EDITORIAL ADVISORY BOARD

CURRENT DIAGNOSIS 7

Edited by REX B. CONN, M.D.

Professor of Pathology and Laboratory Medicine,
Emory University School of Medicine
Director, Clinical Pathology Laboratories,
Emory University Hospital, Atlanta, Georgia

W.B. SAUNDERS COMPANY
Philadelphia London Toronto Mexico City Rio de Janeiro Sydney Tokyo

W. B. Saunders Company: West Washington Square
Philadelphia, PA 19105

1 St. Anne's Road
Eastbourne, East Sussex BN21 3UN, England

1 Goldthorne Avenue
Toronto, Ontario M8Z 5T9, Canada

Apartado 26370—Cedro 512
Mexico 4, D.F., Mexico

Rua Coronel Cabrita, 8
Sao Cristovao Caixa Postal 21176
Rio de Janeiro, Brazil

9 Waltham Street
Artarmon, N.S.W. 2064, Australia

Ichibancho, Central Bldg., 22-1 Ichibancho
Chiyoda-Ku, Tokyo 102, Japan

Current diagnosis. 1966–
Philadelphia, W. B. Saunders Co.

v. ill. 28 cm.

Biennial.
Editors: 1966– H. F. Conn, R. J. Clohecy, and R. B. Conn.

1. Diagnosis. I. Conn, Howard Franklin, 1908–1982 ed. II. Clohecy, Robert J., ed. III. Conn, Rex B., ed.
[DNLM: W1 CU788CX]

RC71.A13 616.075 66-15617 MARC-S

Library of Congress [8308]

Listed here is the latest translated edition of this book together with the language of the translation and the publisher.

Spanish (*1966-67 Edition*) - Editorial Labor, Barcelona, Spain

Italian (*1971 Edition*) - Editrice Universo, No. 1, Via G.B Morgagni, Rome, Italy

Greek (*1974 Edition*) - Anglo-Hellenic Agency, Athens, Greece

Japanese (*1974 Edition*) - Hirokawa Publishing Company, Tokyo

Current Diagnosis—7

ISBN 0-7216-2713-7 Made in the United States of America. Press of W. B. Saunders Company. Library of Congress catalog card number 66-15617.

Last digit is the print number: 9 8 7 6 5 4 3 2

Contributors

Pasquale Accardo, M.D. Associate Professor of Pediatrics and Adolescent Medicine, St. Louis University School of Medicine. Director, Knights of Columbus Developmental Center, Cardinal Glennon Memorial Hospital for Children, St. Louis, Missouri.
Failure to Thrive

Robert E. Albertini, M.D. Clinical Professor of Medicine, Pennsylvania State University, College of Medicine. Hershey, Pennsylvania. Director, Department of Thoracic Medicine, Geisinger Medical Center, Danville, Pennsylvania.
Chest Pain

Samuel S. Ambrose, M.D. Professor of Surgery/Urology, Emory University School of Medicine. Chief of Urology, Emory University Hospital. Active Staff, Egleston Hospital for Children and Grady Memorial Hospital, Atlanta, Georgia.
Carcinoma of the Kidney

David M. Asher, M.D. Medical Officer, National Institute of Neurological and Communicative Disorders and Stroke, National Institutes of Health. Instructor in Pediatrics and Oncology, Johns Hopkins University School of Medicine. Adjunct Physician, Johns Hopkins University Hospital, Baltimore, Maryland.
Viral Encephalitis and Encephalopathy

Barbara A. Baker, M.D. Endocrinologist, Diabetologist, Springer Clinic. Staff, St. Francis Hospital, Tulsa, Oklahoma.
Empty Sella Syndrome

Marwan Balaa, M.D. Fellow, Division of Digestive Diseases, Department of Medicine, University of North Carolina, Chapel Hill, North Carolina.
Functional Disorders of the Gastrointestinal Tract

James A. Bartley, Ph.D. M.D. Assistant Professor of Pediatrics, University of Iowa College of Medicine. Clinical Director, Regional Genetic Consultation Service, Division of Medical Genetics, Department of Pediatrics, University of Iowa Hospitals and Clinics, Iowa City, Iowa.
Teratogenic Agents

James W. Bass, M.P.H., M.D. Professor of Pediatrics, Uniformed Services University of the Health Sciences (Tripler Army Medical Center Medical Center affiliate). Clinical Professor of Pediatrics, University of Hawaii, School of Medicine. Chairman, Department of Pediatrics, Tripler Army Medical Center, Honolulu, Hawaii.
Whooping Cough

Frank J. Baumeister, Jr., M.D. Clinical Associate Professor of Medicine, University of Oregon Health Sciences Center. Director, Endoscopy Unit, Good Samaritan Hospital and Medical Center, Portland, Oregon.
Peptic Ulcer

Robert W. Beart, Jr., M.D. Assistant Professor, Mayo Medical School; Head, Section of Colon and Rectal Surgery; Consultant in Surgery, Mayo Clinic. Staff Surgeon, Methodist Hospital, St. Mary's Hospital, and Mayo Clinic, Rochester, Minnesota.
Intestinal Obstruction

Theodore V. Benderev, M.D. Instuctor in Urology, Department of Urology, Northwestern University School of Medicine, Chicago, Illinois.
Carcinoma of the Prostate

William Berenberg, M.D. Professor of Pediatrics, Harvard Medical School. Senior Associate, Children's Hospital, Boston, Massachusetts.
Varicella (Chickenpox)

C. Warren Bierman, M.D. Clinical Professor of Pediatrics, University of Washington School of Medicine. Head, Division of Allergy, Children's Orthopedic Hospital and Medical Center, Seattle, Washington.
Asthma in Childhood

Fred E. Boehmke, M.D. Clinical Instructor in Surgery, State University of New York at Buffalo. Attending Staff, Buffalo General Hospital, Sisters Hospital of Buffalo, and St. Francis Hospital, Buffalo, New York.
Anorectal and Perianal Disorders

Timothy Patrick Bohan, Ph.D, M.D. Fellow, Division of Pediatric Neurology, Department of Pediatrics, Duke University Medical Center, Durham, North Carolina.
Reye's Syndrome

Herbert L. Bonkovsky, M.D. Professor of Medicine and Director of the Hepatology Laboratory, Dartmouth Medical School. Attending Physician, Mary Hitchcock Memorial Hospital, Hanover, New Hampshire. Chief, Division of Digestive Diseases, Veterans Administration Medical Center, White River Junction, Vermont.
The Porphyrias

Harisios Boudoulas, M.D. Professor of Internal Medicine, Ohio State University. Director, Division of Cardiology, Ohio State University Hospitals, Columbus, Ohio.
Syncope

Jerry E. Bouquot, D.D.S., M.S.D. Chairman and Professor, Department of Oral Pathology, West Virginia University School of Dentistry. Professor, Department of Pathology, West Virginia University School of Medicine. Professor, Departments of Oral Surgery and Hospital Dentistry, West Virginia University School of Dentistry, Morgantown, West Virginia. Director, Oral Pathology Clinical Consultation Service, West Virginia University School of Dentistry. Consultant, Pittsburgh Children's Hospital, Pittsburgh, Pennsylvania. Consultant, Veterans Administration Hospitals in Clarksburg, Martinsburg, and Beckley, West Virginia.
Neoplastic and Non-neoplastic Lesions of the Oral Mucosa

William H. Boyce, M.D. Professor of Urology, Department of Surgery, The Bowman Gray School of Medicine. Staff, The North Carolina Baptist Hospital, Winston-Salem, North Carolina.
Obstructive Nephropathy

Jonathan C. Boyd, M.D. Fellow in Urology, The Bowman Gray School of Medicine. Staff, The North Carolina Baptist Hospital, Winston-Salem, North Carolina.
Obstructive Nephropathy

Philip A. Bromberg, M.D. Professor of Medicine and Director, Division of Pulmonary Diseases, University of North

Carolina School of Medicine. Attending Physician, North Carolina Memorial Hospital, Chapel Hill, North Carolina.
Atelectasis

Audrey K. Brown, M.D. Professor and Vice Chairman, Department of Pediatrics, State University of New York, Downstate Medical Center. Attending Pediatrician and Director, Pediatric Hematology/Oncology, State University Hospital and Kings County Hospital Center, Brooklyn, New York.
Neonatal Jaundice

Paul Brown, M.D. Medical Director, Laboratory of Central Nervous System Studies, National Institute of Neurological and Communicative Disorders and Stroke, National Institutes of Health, Bethesda, Maryland.
Acute Viral Encephalitis

Leonard H. Brubaker, M.D. Professor of Medicine, Medical College of Georgia. Attending Physician, Talmadge Hospital. Consultant, Veterans Administration Hospital, Augusta, Georgia.
Neutropenia and Agranulocytosis

J. Bruni, M.D. Assistant Professor of Medicine, University of Toronto. Staff Neurologist, Wellesley Hospital, Toronto, Ontario, Canada.
Epilepsy and Other Convulsive Disorders

John A. Bryan, M.D. Assistant Professor, Department of Pathology and Laboratory Medicine, Emory University School of Medicine. Director, Clinical Virology Laboratory. Assistant Director, Clinical Microbiology Laboratory, Emory University Hospital, Atlanta, Georgia.
Laboratory Diagnosis of Viral Infections

Russell K. Brynes, M.D. Associate Professor of Pathology and Laboratory Medicine, Emory University School of Medicine. Staff, Emory University Hospital, Atlanta, Georgia.
Acquired Immunodeficiency Syndrome (AIDS)

Herbert J. Buchsbaum, M.D. Professor of Obstetrics and Gynecology University of Pittsburgh School of Medicine Director of Gynecologic Oncology, McGee Women's Hospital Pittsburgh, Pennsylvania.
Benign and Malignant Uterine Corpus Tumors

David C. Budson, M.D. Staff, Clinical Pulmonary Medicine and Internal Medicine, Kaiser-Permanente Medical Center, Vallejo, California
Atelectasis

Brian P. Buggy, M.D. Assistant Professor of Medicine, Medical College of Wisconsin. Consultant in Infectious Diseases, St. Luke's Hospital, Milwaukee, Wisconsin.
Brucellosis

F.N. Burt, M.D. Staff, Providence Hospital, Southfield, Michigan; Sinai Hospital, Detroit, Michigan.
Peripheral Venous Disease

Blake Cady, M.D. Associate Professor of Surgery, Harvard Medical School. Coordinator of Surgical Oncology, Harvard Surgical Service, New England Deaconess Hospital, Boston, Massachusetts.
Evaluation of Breast Masses and Symptoms

Andrei Calin, M.D., M.R.C.P. Consultant Rheumatologist, Royal National Hospital for Rheumatic Disease, Bath, England.
Reiter's Syndrome

Carlos C. Campbell, M.D., M.P.H. Chief, Malaria Branch, Division of Genetic Diseases, Center for Infectious Diseases, Centers for Disease Control, Atlanta, Georgia.
Malaria

D. Erskine Carmichael, M.D. Clinical Associate Professor of Obstetrics and Gynecology, University of Alabama Medical Center. Attending Obstetrician and Gynecologist, St. Vincent's Hospital, Birmingham, Alabama.
Endometriosis

Richard L. Carpenter, M.D. Chief Resident, Department of Otolaryngology, Washington University. Staff, Barnes Hospital, Jewish Hospital of St. Louis, John Cochran Veterans Hospital, Children's Hospital of St. Louis, and County Hospital of St. Louis, St. Louis, Missouri.
Tumors of the Larynx and Pharynx

James T. Cassidy, M.D. Professor of Medicine and Pediatrics, University of Michigan Medical School, Ann Arbor, Michigan.
Pain in the Extremities and Back

William T. Cave, Jr., M.D. Associate Professor of Medicine and Oncology, University of Rochester School of Medicine. Head, Endocrine Unit, St. Mary's Hospital. Senior Associate Physician, Strong Memorial Hospital, Rochester, New York.
Thyroiditis

Samuel Charache, M.D. Professor of Medicine and Pathology (Laboratory Medicine), Johns Hopkins University School of Medicine. Active Staff, Laboratory Medicine. Director, Hematology Division, Department of Laboratory Medicine, Baltimore, Maryland.
Hemoglobinopathies

Carol Cheney, M.D. Scripps Clinic and Research Foundation, La Jolla, California.
Cystic Fibrosis

Michael Cherington, M.D. Associate Clinical Professor of Neurology, University of Colorado Medical School, Denver, Colorado.
Botulism

Rod Cherrie, M.D. Adjunct Assistant Professor, Department of Surgery/Division of Urology, UCLA School of Medicine, Los Angeles, California.
Intrascrotal Masses and Tumors

John F. J. Clark, M.D. Professor of Obstetrics and Gynecology, Howard University College of Medicine. Obstetrician–Gynecologist, Howard University Hospital, Washington, D.C.
Rubella

C. G. Clough, M.B., M.R.C.P. Senior Registrar in Neurology, Queen Elizabeth Hospital, Birmingham, England.
Migraine and Its Variants

Lewis Cogen, M.D. Attending Rheumatologist, Maine Medical Center, Portland, Maine.
Bursitis and Tendinitis

Herbert J. Cohen, M.D. Professor of Pediatrics and Rehabilitation Medicine, Albert Einstein College of Medicine. Director, Children's Evaluation and Rehabilitation Center, and Director, Rose F. Kennedy Center, University Affiliated Facility, Bronx, New York.
Mental Retardation

Robert W. Colman, M.D. Professor of Internal Medicine and Thrombosis, Temple University School of Medicine. Chairman, Thrombus Research Center; Section Head, Hematology/Oncology; Attending Hematologist, Temple University Hospital, Philadelphia, Pennsylvania.
Hemorrhagic Disease Due to Disseminated Intravascular Coagulation and Fibrinolysis; Hemorrhagic Diseases Due to Circulating Anticoagulants

Marcel E. Conrad, M.D. Professor of Medicine, University of South Alabama. Attending Hematologist and Oncol-

ogist, University of South Alabama, Mobile, Alabama.
Acute Leukemia

Avram M. Cooperman, M.D., Professor of Surgery, New York Medical College, Valhalla, New York. Director of Surgery, St. Clare's Hospital, New York, New York.
Diseases of the Gallbladder and Biliary Tract; Acute and Chronic Pancreatitis; Pancreatic Cysts and Neoplasms.

Austin J. Corbett, M.D. Clinical Associate, Department of Medicine, Division of Rheumatology, University of Iowa Hospitals and Clinics. Attending Rheumatologist, University of Iowa Hospitals and Clinics, Iowa City, Iowa.
Periarteritis Nodosa

Gibbons G. Cornwell, III, M.D. Professor of Medicine, Dartmouth Medical School. Chief, Section of Hematology and Oncology, Dartmouth-Hitchcock Medical Center, Hanover, New Hampshire.
Multiple Myeloma and Other Plasma Cell Disorders

Joseph N. Corriere, Jr., M.D. Professor and Director, Division of Urology, The University of Texas Medical School. Chief, Urology Services, The Hermann Hospital, Texas Medical Center. Consultant, Shriners Hospital for Crippled Children, Texas Medical Center. Academic Staff, St. Joseph Hospital, Houston, Texas.
Prostatitis and Urethritis

Stanley W. Coulthard, M.D. Professor, Chief, Section of Otorhinolaryngology, University of Arizona Health Sciences Center. Consultant, Attending Physician, Surgery, Veterans Administration Hospital; Kino Community Hospital; Tucson Medical Center; and El Dorado Hospital. Consultant, Surgery, Northwest Hospital, Tucson, Arizona.
Disorders of the Paranasal Sinuses

Jacques Couvreur, M.D. Professeur Agrege Associe Faculté Saint Antoine; Staff Hopital Trousseau, Paris, France.
Toxoplasmosis

Elizabeth A. Cowden, M.D., M.R.C.P. Assistant Professor of Medicine, University of Manitoba, Faculty of Medicine. Head, Section of Endocrinology and Metabolism, St. Boniface General Hospital, Winnepeg, Manitoba, Canada.
Hyperprolactinemia

Yvonne E. Cummings, M.D. Associate Professor of Medicine, Division of Nephrology, University of Southern Florida College of Medicine. Attending Nephrologist, Tampa General Hospital, Tampa, Florida.
Glomerulonephritis

Maria Da Costa, M.D. Associate Professor of Medicine, State University of New York, Downstate Medical Center, Brooklyn, New York.
Pernicious Anemia and Other Megaloblastic Anemias

David S. Dahl, M.D. Professor and Chairman, Department of Neurology, Milwaukee Clinical Campus of the University of Wisconsin School of Medicine. Head, Section of Neurology, Department of Medicine, Mt. Sinai Medical Center, Milwaukee, Wisconsin.
The Comatose Patient

John K. Davidson, M.D., Ph.D. Professor of Medicine; Director, Diabetes Unit, Emory University School of Medicine. Attending Diabetologist, Grady Memorial Hospital and Emory University Hospital, Atlanta, Georgia.
Hypoglycemia; Diabetes Mellitus

Scott F. Davies, M.D. Assistant Professor of Medicine, University of Minnesota. Director, Pulmonary Medicine, Department of Internal Medicine, Hennepin County Medical Center, Minneapolis, Minnesota.
Systemic Mycotic Diseases

Harry L. Davis, M.D. Professor of Medicine; Chief, Division of Pulmonary Medicine, University of Tennessee Center for the Health Sciences. Medical Director, Pulmonary Laboratory and Department of Respiratory Therapy, St. Joseph Hospital. Consulting Staff, Baptist Memorial Hospital and St. Francis Hospital, Memphis, Tennessee.
Chronic Cough

Jean B. de Kernion, M.D. Professor of Surgery/Urology, UCLA School of Medicine. Director for Clinical Programs, Jonsson Cancer Center, Los Angeles, California.
Intrascrotal Masses and Tumors

Ludo De Keyser, M.D. Fellow in Endocrinology, UCLA Hospital, Los Angeles, California.
Hypothyroidism

Frederick W. Derks, M.D. Assistant Professor of Internal Medicine, Section of Infectious Diseases, Louisiana State University School of Medicine. Senior Staff Physician in Internal Medicine, Charity Hospital of Louisiana, New Orleans, Louisiana.
Rickettsial Diseases

Georges Desmonts, M.D. Chief, Laboratoire de Sérologie Néonatale et de Recherche sur la Toxoplasmose, Institut de Puériculture de Paris, Paris, France.
Toxoplasmosis

Vincent T. De Vita, Jr., M.D. Professor of Medicine, The George Washington University School of Medicine. Clinical Director, National Cancer Institute, Clinical Centers of the National Institutes of Health, Bethesda, Maryland
Malignant Lymphomas

Frank B. Diamond, Jr., M.D. Clinical Assistant Professor, University of South Florida College of Medicine, Department of Pediatrics. Staff, Morton Plant Hospital, C.L.W. Mease Hospital, Dunedin Medical Center Hospital, Largo, Florida; All Children's Hospital, St. Petersburg, Florida.
Delayed Sexual Maturation and Sexual Precocity

Hugh C. Dillon, Jr., M.D. Professor of Pediatrics and Microbiology, University of Alabama, School of Medicine. Physician, University Hospital, The Children's Hospital of Alabama, Birmingham, Alabama.
Acute Pharyngitis

Salvatore Di Mauro, M.D. Professor of Neurology, College of Physicians and Surgeons, Columbia University. Staff, Columbia Presbyterian Hospital, New York, New York.
Myoglobinuria and Myopathy of Storage Disease

John H. Dirckx, M.D. Medical Director, University of Dayton Student Health Center, Dayton, Ohio.
Infectious Mononucleosis

Kenneth W. Dumars, M.D. Professor of Pediatrics and Obstetrics; Chief, Division of Developmental Disabilities and Clinical Genetics, University of California, College of Medicine, Irvine, California. Staff, University of California at Irvine Medical Center and Children's Hospital of Orange County, Orange, California.
Approach to Genetic Disease; Recognizable Congenital Syndrome Due to Single-Gene Abnormalities

Nancy L. Dunn, M.D. Assistant Professor of Pediatrics, Medical College of Virginia/Virginia Commonwealth University, Children's Medical Center. Consultant, Pediatric Hematologist, St. Mary's Hospital, Richmond, Virginia.
Leukocytosis and Leukemoid Reactions

Herbert L. Du Pont, M.D. Professor and Director, Program in Infectious Diseases and Clinical Microbiology, University of Texas Medical School. Staff Physician, Hermann Hospital, Houston, Texas.
Viral Diarrhea

James R. Eckman, M.D. Associate Professor of Medicine, Emory University School of Medicine. Staff, Grady Memorial Hospital, Atlanta, Georgia.
Anemias Due to Decreased Erythrocyte Production

John H. Edmonds, Jr., M.D. Professor of Medicine and Cardiology, Bowman Gray School of Medicine of Wake Forest University. Director of Heart Station, North Carolina Baptist Hospital/Bowman Gray Medical Center, Winston-Salem, North Carolina.
Pericarditis

James W. Edmondson, M.D. Professor of Medicine, School of Medicine, Indiana University Medical Center. Staff Physician, Indiana University Hospitals. Attending Physician, Veterans Hospital and Wishard Memorial Hospital, Indianapolis, Indiana.
Hypoparathyroidism

John E. Edwards, Jr., M.D. Associate Professor of Medicine, UCLA School of Medicine, Los Angeles, California. Chief, Division of Infectious Diseases, Department of Medicine, Harbor/UCLA Medical Center, Torrance, California.
Opportunistic Mycoses

George E. Ehrlich, M.D. Adjunct Professor of Clinical Medicine, New York University School of Medicine, New York, New York. Vice President, CIBA-GEIGY Corporation, Pharmaceuticals Division, Summit, N.J.
Osteoarthritis

Edward R. Eichner, M.D. Professor of Medicine, University of Oklahoma School of Medicine. Chief of Hematology–Oncology, University of Oklahoma Health Sciences Center. Attending Physician, Oklahoma Memorial Hospital and Oklahoma City Veterans Administration Hospital, Oklahoma City, Oklahoma.
The Sideroblastic Anemias

Esther Eisenberg, M.D. Assistant Professor, Department of Obstetrics and Gynecology, University of Pennsylvania School of Medicine. Clinical Assistant Obstetrician–Gynecologist, Pennsylvania Hospital, Philadelphia, Pennsylvania.
Functional Menstrual Disorders

F. Henry Ellis, Jr., M.D., Ph.D. Clinical Professor of Surgery, Harvard Medical School. Chief of Staff, Section of Thoracic and Cardiovascular Surgery, Lahey Clinic Medical Center, Burlington Massachusetts; Division of Thoracic and Cardiovascular Surgery, New England Deaconess Hospital, Boston, Massachusetts.
Diaphragmatic Hernias

Peter A. Emerson, M.D., F.R.C.P., F.A.C.P. Dean, Westminster Medical School, University of London. Consultant Physician, Westminster Hospital, London, England.
Disorders of the Pleura

Celia J. Emery, B.Sc., Ph.D. Scientific Officer, Royal Hallamshire Hospital, Sheffield, England.
Influenza

Richard W. Emmons, M.D., Ph.D. Chief, Viral and Rickettsial Disease Laboratory, State of California Department of Health Services, Berkeley, California.
Rabies

David N. F. Fairbanks, M.D. Clinical Professor of Otolaryngology, George Washington University School of Medicine. Active Staff, Sibley Memorial Hospital, Washington, D.C.
Otitis Media, Otitis Externa

Z. Myron Falchuk, M.D. Associate Professor of Medicine, Harvard Medical School. Associate Physician, New England Deaconess Hospital and Brigham Women's Hospital. Investigator, Center for Blood Research, Boston, Massachusetts.
Gluten-Sensitive Enteropathy

Robert J. Fass, M.D. Professor, Departments of Medicine and Medical Microbiology and Immunology, The Ohio State University College of Medicine. Attending Physician, The Ohio State University Hospitals, Columbus, Ohio.
Tetanus

Robert Fekety, M.D. Chief, Division of Infectious Diseases; Professor of Internal Medicine, University of Michigan Medical Center, Ann Arbor, Michigan.
Brucellosis

Jerome M. Feldman, M.D. Associate Professor of Medicine, Duke University. Chief, Endocrinology Section, Durham Veterans Administration Medical Center, Durham, North Carolina.
Pheochromocytoma

Yehudi M. Felman, M.D. Clinical Professor in Dermatology and Lecturer in Preventive Medicine and Community Health, State University of New York–Downstate Medical Center, Brooklyn, New York. Lecturer in Public Health, Columbia University, New York, New York. Consultant, Dermatology, Maimonides Hospital and Community Hospital. Attending Physician in Dermatology, Kings County Hospital, Downstate University Hospital, Flatbush General Hospital, Kings Highway Hospital, and Baptist Medical Center, Brooklyn, New York.
Gonococcal Infection

William A. Ferrante, M.D. Head, Department of Internal Medicine, Section on Gastroenterology, Ochsner Clinic and Alton Ochsner Foundation Hospital. Senior Visiting Physician, Charity Hospital of Louisiana, New Orleans, Louisiana.
Gastrointestinal Hemorrhage

Peter H. Forsham, M.D., M.A. Professor of Medicine and Pediatrics, University of California at San Francisco. Senior Physician, University of California Hospitals, San Francisco, California.
Cushing's Syndrome

John W. Francfort, M.D. Transplantation Research Fellow; Assistant Instructor in Surgery, University of Pennsylvania School of Medicine; Hospital of the University of Pennsylvania, Philadelphia, Pennsylvania.
Acute Appendicitis

Donald Fraser, M.D., Ph.D. Professor, Departments of Paediatrics and Physiology, Faculty of Medicine, University of Toronto, Research Institute, The Hospital for Sick Children. Senior Staff Physician, The Hospital for Sick Children, Toronto, Canada.
Rickets and Osteomalacia

S. Douglas Frasier, M.D. Professor of Pediatrics and Physiology/Biophysics, University of Southern California School of Medicine. Chief, Division of Pediatric Endocrinology, Los Angeles County/USC Medical Center, Los Angeles, California
Short Stature

Eugene P. Frenkel, M.D. Professor of Internal Medicine and Radiology, University of Texas Health Science Center, Southwestern Medical School. Chief of Hematology/Oncology, Parkland Memorial Hospital, Dallas, Texas.
Acquired Hemolytic Anemia

Stanford B. Friedman, M.D. Professor of Pediatrics; Head, Division of Behavioral Pediatrics, University of Maryland School of Medicine, Baltimore, Maryland.
Behavioral Problems in Children and Adolescents

Henry G. Friesen, M.D. Professor and Head, Department

of Physiology; Professor, Department of Medicine, Faculty of Medicine, The University of Manitoba. Staff, Health Sciences Centre, Endocrinology and Metabolism, Winnipeg, Manitoba, Canada.
Hyperprolactinemia

J. Timothy Fulenwider, M.D. Assistant Professor of Surgery, Emory University School of Medicine; Emory University Hospital; Grady Memorial Hospital; and Henrietta Egleston Hospital for Children. Assistant Chief of Surgery, Atlanta Veterans Administration Medical Center, Atlanta, Georgia.
Evaluation of Abdominal Pain in Adults

Daniel E. Furst, M.D. Associate Professor, Department of Medicine, Division of Rheumatology; Attending Rheumatologist, University of Iowa Hospitals and Clinics, Iowa City, Iowa.
Periarteritis Nodosa

Wesley Furste, M.D. Clinical Professor of Surgery, Ohio State University School of Medicine. Chairman, Department of Surgery, Mount Carmel Medical Center, Columbus, Ohio.
Tetanus

D. Grant Gall, M.D., F.R.C.P.(C.) Professor of Pediatrics and Internal Medicine, University of Calgary. Head, Division of Pediatric Gastroenterology and Nutrition; Director, Alberta Children's Hospital, Calgary, Alberta, Canada.
Chronic Diarrhea and Malabsorption

Robert A. Garrett, M.D. Professor of Urology (Pediatrics), Indiana University School of Medicine. Active Staff, Riley Hospital for Children, Indiana University Hospitals, Wishard Memorial Hospital, and Veterans Administration Hospital, Indianapolis, Indiana.
Tumors of the Ureter and Urinary Bladder

Pierce Gardner, M.D. Professor of Medicine and Pediatrics, Pritzker School of Medicine, University of Chicago. Director, Infectious Diseases Training Program, University of Chicago Hospital, Chicago, Illinois.
Varicella (Chickenpox)

J. Bernard L. Gee, M.D. Professor of Medicine, Yale University School of Medicine. Attending Physician, Yale-New Haven Hospital, New Haven, Connecticut.
Pneumoconiosis

Richard H. Glew, M.D. Professor of Medicine, Molecular Genetics and Microbiology, University of Massachusetts Medical School. Chief, Infectious Disease Service, The Memorial Hospital, Worcester, Massachusetts.
The Acute Infectious Disease Syndrome

Philip M. Gold, M.D. Associate Professor of Medicine, Loma Linda University School of Medicine. Medical Director, Respiratory Care and Pulmonary Intensive Care Unit, Loma Linda University Medical Center. Consultant, Jerry L. Pettis Memorial Veterans Administration Hospital, Loma Linda, California.
Chronic Obstructive Pulmonary Disease

Paul Gonick, M.D. Professor of Surgery, Urology, Hahnemann University. Attending Urologist, Hahnemann University Hospital, St. Agnes Medical Center, and West Park Hospital, Philadelphia, Pennsylvania.
Dysuria, Pyuria, and Hematuria

David S. Gordon, M.D. Professor of Medicine, Associate Professor of Pathology, Emory University School of Medicine. Attending Physician, Emory University Hospital. Consultant, Emory Clinic, Atlanta, Georgia.
Immunodeficiency

Jack M. Gorman, M.D. Assistant Professor of Clinical Psychiatry, College of Physicians and Surgeons, Columbia University. Director, Biological Studies Unit, New York State Psychiatric Institute. Assistant Attending Psychiatrist, Presbyterian Hospital, New York, New York.
Anxiety Disorders

Mateel S. Graham, M.D. Assistant Professor of Internal Medicine, University of Texas Health Science Center, Southwestern Medical School. Attending Hematologist-Oncologist, Parkland Memorial Hospital, Dallas, Texas.
Acquired Hemolytic Anemia

Sam D. Graham Jr., M.D. Assistant Professor, Emory University School of Medicine. Staff Urologist, Emory Hospital, Grady Memorial Hospital, and Henrietta Egleston Hospital for Children. Chief, Urology, Veterans Administration Medical Center, Atlanta, Georgia.
Carcinoma of the Kidney and Renal Carcinoma

John T. Grayhack, M.D. Herman L. Kretschmer Professor of Urology; Chairman, Department of Urology, Northwestern University Medical School, Chicago, Illinois. Staff, Northwestern Memorial Hospital, Veterans Administration Lakeside Hospital, Children's Memorial Hospital, and Evanston Hospital.
Carcinoma of the Prostate

William B. Greenough, III, M.D., Associate Professor of Medicine and Microbiology, The Johns Hopkins University, Baltimore, Maryland; Director, International Centre for Diarrhoeal Disease Research, Dacca, Bangladesh.
Cholera

Monte A. Greer, M.D. Professor of Medicine; Head, Section of Endocrinology, Oregon Health Sciences University School of Medicine, Portland, Oregon.
Hyperthyroidism

John P. Griffin, M.D. Clinical Professor of Pulmonary Medicine, University of Tennessee Center for Health Sciences. Chief, Pulmonary Disease Section, Veterans Administration Medical Center. Staff Physician, Baptist Memorial Hospital and University of Tennessee Hospital, Memphis, Tennessee.
Lung Abscess

George T. Griffing, M.D. Assistant Professor of Medicine, Boston University School of Medicine. Section of Endocrinology and Metabolism, University Hospital, Boston, Massachusetts.
Primary Aldosteronism

Robert C. Griggs, M.D. Professor of Neurology, Medicine, Pathology, and Pediatrics, University of Rochester School of Medicine and Dentistry. Neurologist, Strong Memorial Hospital, Rochester, New York.
The Periodic Paralyses

Robert L. Hackney, Jr., M.D. Associate Professor of Medicine, Howard University College of Medicine. Attending Staff, Internal Medicine, Pulmonary Division; formerly Chief, Pulmonary Division, Howard University Hospital, Washington, D.C.
Sarcoidosis

D.R.W. Haddock, M.D., F.R.C.P., D.T.M. & H. Senior Lecturer in Tropical Medicine; Honorary Consultant Physician, Liverpool School of Tropical Medicine, Liverpool, England.
Amebiasis

Stephanos J. Hadziyannis, M.D. Professor of Internal Medicine, University of Athens, School of Medicine. Attending Physician and Head of the Liver Research Unit, Second Department of Medicine, Hippokration General Hospital, Athens, Greece.
Echinococcosis

Henry Haimovici, M.D. Clinical Professor Emeritus of Surgery, Albert Einstein College of Medicine. Senior Consultant and Chief Emeritus, Vascular Surgery, Montefiore Hospital and Medical Center, Bronx, New York.
Chronic Arterial Occlusive Disease of the Lower Extremity

W. Kenneth Haisty, Jr., M.D. Assistant Professor of Medicine and Cardiology, Bowman Gray School of Medicine of Wake Forest University. Attending Physician, Director of Clinical Electrophysiology, North Carolina Baptist Hospital–Bowman Gray Medical Center, Winston-Salem, North Carolina.
Pericarditis

Katerina Haka-Ikse, M.D., F.R.C.P.(C.), F.A.A.P. Associate Professor of Pediatrics, School of Medicine, University of Toronto. Senior Staff Physician, Hospital for Sick Children, Toronto, Ontario, Canada.
Delayed Development

Michael J. Halberstam, M.D. Associate Professor, George Washington University Hospital, Washington D.C. Editor, *Modern Medicine.* Member, Institute of Medicine.*
Fatigue

W. Dallas Hall, M.D. Professor of Medicine; Director, Division of Hypertension, Emory University School of Medicine and Grady Memorial Hospital, Atlanta, Georgia.
Chronic Renal Failure

Philip C. Halverson, M.D. Fellow, Division of Allergy/Immunology, University of Iowa Hospitals and Clinics, Iowa City, Iowa.
Hypersensitivity Pneumonitis

Stephen C. Hammill, M.D. Assistant Professor of Medicine, Mayo Medical School. Consultant, Division of Cardiovascular Diseases and Internal Medicine, Mayo Clinic and Mayo Foundation, Rochester, Minnesota.
Cardiac Arrhythmias

Ala B. Hamoudi, M.D. Clinical Professor of Pathology, Ohio State University. Pathologist, Department of Laboratory Medicine, Children's Hospital, Columbus, Ohio.
Histiocytosis X

James W. Hanson, M.D. Professor of Pediatrics, University of Iowa College of Medicine. Chairman, Division of Medical Genetics, Department of Pediatrics, University of Iowa Hospitals and Clinics, Iowa City, Iowa.
Teratogenic Agents

Robert C. Hartmann, M.D. Professor of Medicine, University of South Florida College of Medicine. Consultant, James A. Haley Veterans Administration Hospital. Attending Physician, Tampa General Hospital, Tampa, Florida.
Hereditary Elliptocytosis (Ovalocytosis); Hereditary Spherocytosis; Paroxysmal Nocturnal Hemoglobinuria

Ivan R. Harwood, M.D. Associate Professor, University of California at San Diego, La Jolla, California. Staff, University Hospital Medical Center, and Chief, Pediatric Pulmonary and Cystic Fibrosis Center, San Diego, California.
Cystic Fibrosis

Arthur Haut, M.D. Professor of Medicine, Division of Hematology and Oncology, University of Arkansas College of Medicine, Attending Physician in Medicine, Hematology, and Oncology, University Hospital. Consultant in Hematology and Oncology, Little Rock Veterans Administration Hospitals, Little Rock, Arkansas.
Iron Deficiency Anemia

Javad Hekmatpanah, M.D. Professor of Neurosurgery, University of Chicago. Professor, Section of Neurosurgery, University of Chicago Hospitals and Clinics, Chicago, Illinois.
Brain Abscesses

Jane E. Henney, M.D. Deputy Director, National Cancer Institute, National Institutes of Health, Bethesda, Maryland.
Malignant Lymphomas

Robert E. Hermann, M.D. Clinical Professor of Surgery, Case-Western Reserve University. Chairman, Department of General Surgery, Cleveland Clinic, Cleveland, Ohio.
Pancreatic Cysts and Neoplasms

Karl R. Herwig, M.D. Associate Clinical Professor, Department of Surgery/Urology, School of Medicine, University of California at San Diego. Head, Division of Urology, Green Hospital of Scripps Clinic, La Jolla, California.
Cystic Disorders of the Kidney

Charles E. Hess, M.D. Professor of Internal Medicine, Hematology/Oncology Division, University of Virginia School of Medicine. Staff, University of Virginia Hospital, Charlottesville, Virginia.
Diseases of the Spleen; Lymphadenopathy

Jonathan Hiatt, M.D. Assistant Professor of Surgery, UCLA School of Medicine, Los Angeles, California. Staff, Harbor/UCLA Medical Center, Torrance, California.
Hepatic and Perihepatic Abscess

Chesley Hines, Jr., M.D. Clinical Associate Professor, Department of Medicine, Tulane University School of Medicine. Visiting Staff, Ochsner Foundation Hospital and Charity Hospital of Louisiana, New Orleans, Louisiana.
Gastrointestinal Hemorrhage

Monto Ho, M.D. Professor of Medicine, University of Pittsburgh School of Medicine. Chief, Infectious Diseases, Presbyterian-University Hospital, Pittsburgh, Pennsylvania.
Cytomegalovirus Infections

John E. Hodgkin, M.D. Clinical Professor of Medicine, University of California, Davis, School of Medicine. Medical Director, Center for Health Promotion and Rehabilitation, and Respiratory Care and Pulmonary Rehabilitation, St. Helena Hospital and Health Center, St. Helena, California.
Bronchiectasis

Stephen F. Hodgson, M.D. Assistant Professor, Mayo Medical School, Consultant, Rochester Methodist Hospital and St. Mary's Hospital, Rochester, Minnesota.
Empty Sella Syndrome

Arno R. Hohn, M.D. Professor of Pediatrics (Cardiology), Los Angeles; Director, Division of Cardiology, Children's Hospital of Los Angeles, Los Angeles, California.
Normal Heart Murmurs in Children

David R. Holmes, Jr., M.D. Associate Professor of Medicine, Mayo Medical School. Consultant, Division of Cardiovascular Diseases and Internal Medicine, Mayo Clinic and Mayo Foundation, Rochester, Minnesota.
Cardiac Arrhythmias

G. Richard Holt, M.D. Assistant Dean for Student Affairs; Associate Professor of Otorhinolaryngology and Oral and Maxillofacial Surgery, The University of Texas Health Science Center, San Antonio, Texas.
Masses in the Neck

Mark Holzberg, M.D. Department of Dermatology, Emory University School of Medicine, Atlanta, Georgia.
Invasive and Noninvasive Mycotic Diseases of Skin

Linton C. Hopkins, M.D. Associate Professor of Neurology, Emory University School of Medicine. Staff, Emory Uni-

*Deceased.

versity Hospital and Grady Memorial Hospital, Atlanta, Georgia.
Congenital Myopathies and Mitochondrial Myopathies; Muscular Dystrophies; Endocrine Myopathies; Motor Neuron Diseases

Simon Horenstein, M.D. Professor and Chairman, Department of Neurology, St. Louis University, St. Louis, Missouri.
Metabolic Encephalopathy

Charles A. Horwitz, M.D. Professor of Laboratory Medicine and Pathology, University of Minnesota Medical School. Associate Pathologist, Mt. Sinai Hospital, Minneapolis, Minnesota.
Acute Transfusion Reactions

Peter Howard, D.M.(Oxon), F.R.C.P. Reader in Medicine, University of Sheffield. Consultant Chest Physician, Royal Hallamshire Hospital, Sheffield, England.
Influenza

R. Rodney Howell, M.D. Professor and Chairman, Department of Pediatrics, The University of Texas Medical School at Houston. Chief of Pediatrics, Hermann Hospital, Houston, Texas.
Hereditary Disorders of Carbohydrate Metabolism; Mucopolysaccharidoses

R. L. Huckstep, C.M.G., M.D., F.R.C.S., F.R.A.C.S. Professor, Faculty of Medicine, University of New South Wales, Sydney, Australia. Professor, Faculty of Medicine, Makerere University, Kampala, Uganda.
Typhoid Fever

Clara V. Hussey, M.D. Professor of Pathology, Medical College of Wisconsin. Senior Attending Physician, Milwaukee County Medical Complex, Froedtert Memorial Lutheran Hospital. Consultant, St. Luke's Hospital, Milwaukee, Wisconsin.
Hemophilia and Other Inherited Coagulation Disorders

Harry Iland, F.R.A.C.P., F.R.C.P.A. Research Associate, Division of Hematology-Oncology, Duke University Medical Center, Durham, North Carolina.
Chronic Granulocytic Leukemia; Myelofibrosis/Agnogenic Myeloid Metaplasia and Essential Thrombocythemia; Polycythemia Vera

Robert R. Jacobson, M.D., Ph.D. Chief, Clinical Branch, National Hansen's Disease Center, Carville, Louisiana.
Leprosy

Janine Jason, M.D. Chief, Epidemiologic Studies, Division of Host Factors, Center for Infectious Diseases, Centers for Disease Control. Visiting Faculty, Emory University School of Medicine, Atlanta, Georgia.
Child Abuse or Maltreatment

Joseph E. Johnson, III, M.D. Professor and Chairman, Department of Medicine, Bowman Gray School of Medicine of Wake Forest University. Chief of Medicine, North Carolina Baptist Hospital, Winston-Salem, North Carolina.
Relapsing Fever

K.M. Johnson, M.D. Director, Hazardous Viruses Program, U.S. Army Medical Research Institute of Infectious Diseases, Frederick, Maryland.
Viral Hemorrhagic Fever

Philip C. Johnson, M.D. Clinical Instructor, The University of Texas Health Science Center at Houston. Staff Physician, Hermann Hospital, Houston, Texas.
Viral Diarrhea

Thomas W. Johnson, M.D. Professor and Director, Division of Dermatology, Department of Medicine, Meharry Medical College. Physician, G.W. Hubbard Hospital, Nashville, Tennessee.
Granuloma Inguinale, Lymphogranuloma Venereum

William G. Johnson, M.D. Associate Professor of Clinical Neurology, College of Physicians and Surgeons, Columbia University. Associate Attending Neurologist, Presbyterian Hospital and Neurological Institute, Columbia-Presbyterian Medical Center, New York, New York.
Sphingolipidoses

C. Conrad Johnston, Jr., M.D. Professor of Medicine, Indiana University School of Medicine. Attending Physician, Veterans Administration Medical Center. Staff Physician, Indiana University Hospitals. Program Director, General Clinical Research Center, Indiana University School of Medicine, Indianapolis, Indiana.
Hypoparathyroidism

J. Heinrich Joist, M.D., Ph.D. Professor of Medicine and Pathology, St. Louis University School of Medicine. Director, Division of Hematology/Oncology. Attending Physician, St. Louis University Hospital. Consultant, St. Mary's Health Center, Deaconess Hospital, Cardinal Glennon Memorial Hospital for Children, and John Cochran Veterans Administration Medical Center, St. Louis, Missouri.
Bleeding Due to Vascular and Platelet Disorders

Frederick L. Jones, Jr., M.D. Clinical Professor of Medicine, Pennsylvania State University College of Medicine, Hershey, Pennsylavania. Chairman, Department of Medicine, Geisinger Medical Center, Danville, Pennsylvania.
Chest Pain

Henry E. Jones, M.D. Professor and Chairman, Department of Dermatology, Emory University School of Medicine. Staff, Emory University Hospital, Atlanta, Georgia.
Invasive and Noninvasive Mycotic Diseases of Skin

William E. Josey, M.D. Associate Professor of Gynecology and Obstetrics, Emory University School of Medicine. Attending Obstetrician annd Gynecologist, Emory University and Crawford W. Long Hospitals, Atlanta, Georgia.
Infection and Inflammation of the Female Genital Tract

M. Bashar Kahaleh, M.D. Associate Professor of Medicine, Medical University of South Carolina. Attending Rheumatologist, Medical University of South Carolina, Charleston, South Carolina.
Scleroderma

Emily J. Kahlstrom, M.D. Assistant Professor of Pediatrics, University of Southern California. Director, Respiratory Disease Center, Los Angeles County–University of Southern California Medical Center, Los Angeles, California.
Viral Pneumonia

Robert L. Kaiser, M.D. Visiting Lecturer on Tropical Public Health in the School of Public Health, Harvard University, Boston, Massachusetts. Director, Division of Parasitic Diseases, Centers for Disease Control, Atlanta, Georgia.
Malaria

Ruth K. Kaminer, M.D. Associate Professor of Pediatrics, Albert Einstein College of Medicine. Director, Infant and Preschool Unit, Children's Evaluation and Rehabilitation Center. Attending Pediatrician, Abraham Jacobs Hospital, Bronx, New York.
Mental Retardation

Stuart S. Kassan, M.D. Assistant Clinical Professor of Medicine (Rheumatology), University of Colorado Health Sciences Center. Attending Physician, University Hospital, Lutheran Medical Center and St. Anthony Hospital, Denver, Colorado.
Sjögren's Syndrome

Irvin A. Kaufman, M.D. Assistant Adjunct Professor of Pediatrics, University of California at San Diego, La Jolla, California. Director, Inpatient Services, Children's Hospital and Health Center, San Diego, California.
Genetic Defects of Amino Acid Metabolism and Transport

Arnold F. Kaufmann, D.V.M., M.S. Chief, Bacterial Zoonoses Activity, Division of Bacterial Diseases, Center for Infectious Diseases, Centers for Disease Control, Atlanta, Georgia.
Leptospirosis

John S. Kaufmann, M.D., Ph.D. Associate Professor of Medicine and Pharmacology, Bowman Gray School of Medicine of Wake Forest University. Staff, North Carolina Baptist Hospital, Winston-Salem, North Carolina.
Carcinoid Tumor and Carcinoid Syndrome

Louis L. Keeler, M.D. Clinical Associate Professor of Urology, Thomas Jefferson University, Philadelphia, Pennsylvania. Chief of Urology, Our Lady of Lourdes Medical Center. Attending Urologist, West Jersey Health System.
Acute Infections of the Urinary Tract

A. Paul Kelly, M.D. Professor of Internal Medicine/Dermatology, Charles R. Drew Postgraduate Medical School; Associate Professor of Dermatology, University of California at Los Angeles School of Medicine. Chairman, Division of Dermatology, King/Drew Medical Center, Los Angeles, California.
Syphilis

David F. Keren, M.D. Associate Professor of Pathology and of Microbiology and Immunology; Staff, University Hospital, The University of Michigan, Ann Arbor, Michigan.
Whipple's Disease

Harry L. Keyserling, M.D. Assistant Professor of Pediatrics, Emory University School of Medicine. Attending Physician, Grady Memorial Hospital and Henrietta Egleston Hospital for Children, Atlanta, Georgia.
Herpes Simplex Virus Infections

Robert F. Kibler, M.D. Professor and Chairman, Department of Neurology, Emory University School of Medicine. Staff, Emory University Hospital and Grady Memorial Hospital, Atlanta, Georgia.
Vertigo

Thomas W. Kiernan, M.D. Associate Professor of Medicine, Marshall University School of Medicine. Chief of Staff, Veterans Administration Medical Center, Huntington, West Virginia.
Cirrhosis of the Liver

Paul E. Klotman, M.D. Assistant Professor of Medicine, Department of Medicine, Division of Nephrology, Duke University Medical Center and Durham Veterans Administration Medical Center. Staff Nephrologist, Durham Veterans Administration Medical Center, Durham, North Carolina.
Peripheral Edema

Sang Whay Kooh, Ph.D., M.D. Associate Professor, Departments of Paediatrics and Physiology, Faculty of Medicine, University of Toronto. Associate Professor, Research Institute; Senior Staff Physician, The Hospital for Sick Children, Toronto, Canada.
Rickets and Osteomalacia

Lawrence R. Krakoff, M.D. Professor of Medicine and Chief, Hypertension Division, Mount Sinai School of Medicine. Attending Physician, Mount Sinai Hospital, New York, New York. Consultant, Bronx Veterans Hospital, Bronx, New York.
Hypertension

Roger Kurlan, M.D. Assistant Professor of Neurology, University of Rochester, School of Medicine and Dentistry. Associate Neurologist, Strong Memorial Hospital, Rochester, New York.
The Dementias

Catherine U. Kyong, M.D. Assistant Professor of Pediatrics; Attending Pediatric Specialist, Pediatric Infectious Disease; Medical University of South Carolina, Charleston, South Carolina.
Measles

Paul W. Ladenson, M.D. Assistant Professor of Medicine, Johns Hopkins University School of Medicine. Chief, Thyroid Unit, Johns Hopkins Hospital. Head, Division of Endocrinology and Metabolism, Sinai Hospital, Baltimore, Maryland.
Thyroid Tumors

John C. Laidlaw, M.D., Ph.D. Professor of Medicine, McMaster University Faculty of Health Sciences. Physician, Chedoke-McMaster Hospital, St. Joseph's Hospital, and Hamilton Civic Hospital, Hamilton, Ontario, Canada.
Acute Adrenocortical Insufficiency

John R. Lake, M.D. Associate Professor of Medicine; Fellow, Gastroenterology, University of California at San Francisco. Attending Physician, University of California Medical Center, San Francisco, California.
Jaundice

Peter M. Lamont, M.B., F.R.C.S. Senior Registrar in General Surgery, Sheffield and Chesterfield Hospital with initial tenure at the Royal Hallamshire Hospital, Sheffield, England.
Peritonitis and Intra-abdominal Infection

Richard K. Lange, M.D. Professor of Clinical Medicine, Tulane School of Medicine. Staff, Department of Rheumatology, Ochsner Clinic and Ochsner Foundation Hospital, New Orleans, Louisiana.
Gout

Eric B. Larson, M.D. Associate Professor of Medicine and Adjunct Associate Professor, Health Services, University Hospital, School of Medicine, University of Washington. Attending Physician, University Hospital, Seattle, Washington.
Fever of Unknown Origin

John Laszlo, M.D. Professor of Medicine, Duke University Medical Center. Staff, Division of Hematology-Oncology, Duke University Hospital, Durham, North Carolina.
Chronic Granulocytic Leukemia; Myelofibrosis/Agnogenic Myeloid Metaplasia and Essential Thrombocythemia; Polycythemia Vera

Robert L. Lebowitz, M.D. Associate Professor of Radiology, Harvard Medical School. Director of Uroradiology, The Children's Hospital, Boston, Massachusetts.
Lower Urinary Tract Obstruction in Children

Daniel H. Lederer, M.D. Assistant Professor of Medicine, Brown University Program in Medicine. Director, Pulmonary Disease Division, The Miriam Hospital, Providence, Rhode Island.
Hemoptysis

Garrett Lee, M.D. Director of Research, Western Heart Institute, St. Mary's Hospital and Medical Center, San Francisco, California.
Congestive Heart Failure

E. Carwile Le Roy, M.D. Professor of Medicine; Director, Division of Rheumatology and Immunology, Medical University of South Carolina. Attending Rheumatologist, Med-

ical University of South Carolina, Charleston, South Carolina.
Scleroderma

Robert I. Levy, M.D. Professor of Medicine, College of Physicians and Surgeons, Columbia University. Attending Cardiologist, Presbyterian Hospital, New York, New York.
Disorders of Lipid Transport

Richard P. Lewis, M.D. Professor of Internal Medicine, The Ohio State University. Director, Division of Cardiology, The Ohio State University Hospitals, Columbus, Ohio.
Syncope

Samuel Lifshitz, M.D. Associate Professor, Obstetrics and Gynecology, University of Texas Southwestern Medical School. Attending Physician, Parkland Memorial Hospital, St. Paul Hospital, and Baylor University Medical Center, Dallas, Texas.
Ovarian Tumors; Benign and Malignant Uterine Corpus Tumors

Charles J. Lightdale, M.D. Associate Professor of Clinical Medicine, Cornell University Medical College. Director, Diagnostic Gastrointestinal Unit, Memorial Sloan-Kettering Cancer Center, New York, New York.
Malignant Tumors of the Colon and Rectum

John A. Linfoot, M.D. Clinical Professor of Medicine, University of California, Davis, California. Director, Endocrine-Metabolic Service and The Pituitary Center, Alta Bates Hospital, Berkeley, California. Consultant, Veterans Administration Hospital, Martinez, California.
Acromegaly

Jack M. Lockhart, M.D. Attending Rheumatologist, Gundersen Clinic and La Crosse Lutheran Hospital, La Crosse, Wisconsin.
Ankylosing Spondylitis

Linda Loney, M.D. Instructor in Pediatrics, St. Louis Children's Hospital, St. Louis, Missouri.
Nephrotic Syndrome

Joshua Lynfield, M.B., B.Ch. Professor of Clinical Pediatrics, New York University School of Medicine. Attending Physician, University and Bellevue Hospital Center. Associate Attending Physician, Beth Israel Hospital Center, New York, New York.
Rheumatic Fever

Neil R. Mac Intyre, M.D. Assistant Professor of Medicine, Duke University Medical Center. Medical Director of Respiratory Care Services and Pulmonary Function Laboratory, Duke University Medical Center, Durham, North Carolina.
Sleep-Related Respiratory Dysfunction

James A. Madura, M.D. Professor of Surgery, Indiana University School of Medicine. Attending Staff, Indiana University Medical Center Hospitals, Indianapolis, Indiana.
Small Bowel Tumors

Jonathan M. Mann, M.D., M.P.H. Clinical Associate Professor of Pediatrics, University of New Mexico School of Medicine, Albuquerque, New Mexico. State Epidemiologist, Health Services Division, New Mexico Health and Environmental Department, Santa Fe, New Mexico.
Plague

Donald E. Manning, M.D. Associate Professor of Psychiatry, Emory University. Chief of Psychiatry, Emory University Hospital, Altanta, Georgia.
Personality Disorders; Somatoform and Dissociative Disorders

Luis A. Marco, M.D. Professor of Psychiatry and Human Behavior; Professor of Pharmacology, Jefferson Medical College of Thomas Jefferson University, Philadelphia, Pennsylvania. Associate Chief of Staff for Research and Development, Veterans Administration Medical Center, Coatesville, Pennsylvania.
Schizophrenia

David M. Marcotte, M.D. Bowman Gray School of Medicine, Clinical Professor of Psychiatry; Medical College of Wisconsin, Clinical Professor of Psychiatry, Winston-Salem, North Carolina. Medical Director, ASA Cumberland Hospital, Fayetteville, North Carolina.
Psychosexual Disorders

Philip D. Marsden, M.D. Professor of Tropical Medicine, University of Brasília, Brasília, Brazil.
Leishmaniasis

Susan G. Marshall, M.D. Fellow, Allergy and Immunology, University of Washington School of Medicine, Seattle, Washington.
Asthma in Childhood

Dean T. Mason, M.D. Physician-in-Chief, Western Heart Institute, St. Mary's Hospital and Medical Center, San Francisco, California
Congestive Heart Failure

Elmo F. Masucci, M.D. Associate Professor of Neurology, Georgetown University School of Medicine. Assistant Chief, Neurology Service, Veterans Administration Medical Center, Washington, D. C.
Peripheral Neuropathy

John R. Mathias, M.D. Associate Professor of Medicine, University of Florida College of Medicine and Gainesville Veterans Administration Medical Center. Staff Gastroenterologist and Associate Director, Division of Gastroenterology and Nutrition, Gainesville Veterans Administration Hospital, and Shands Hospital, Gainesville, Florida.
Dysphagia, Esophageal Obstruction, and Esophagitis

Robert L. Mayock, M.D. Professor of Medicine, University of Pennsylvania School of Medicine. Senior Consultant, Pulmonary Disease Section, Department of Medicine, Hospital of the University of Pennsylvania, Philadelphia, Pennsylvania.
Tuberculosis and Diseases Due to Other Mycobacteria

Michael R. McClung, M.D. Associate Professor of Medicine, Oregon Health Sciences University. Chief, Section of Endocrinology, Portland Veterans Administration Medical Center, Portland, Oregon.
Hyperthyroidism

Layton McCurdy, M.D. Director, Department of Psychiatry, Pennsylvania Hospital. Psychiatrist-in-Chief, The Institute of Pennsylvania Hospital. Clinical Professor of Psychiatry, University of Pennsylvania School of Medicine, Philadelphia, Pennsylvania.
Affective Disorders

Willie McDaniel, M.D. Assistant Professor, Radiology, Howard University College of Medicine. Director, Nuclear Medicine, Howard University Hospital, Washington, D.C.
Sarcoidosis

William C. McGarity, M.D. Professor of Surgery, Emory University School of Medicine. Assistant Chief of Surgery, Emory University Hospital, Atlanta, Georgia.
The Evaluation of Acute Abdominal Pain in Adults

Douglas B. McGill, M.D. Professor of Medicine, Mayo Medical School. Attending Gastroenterologist, Mayo Clinic, St. Mary's Hospital, and Methodist Hospital, Rochester, Minnesota.
Intestinal Disaccharidase Deficiency

John E. McGowan, Jr., M.D. Professor of Pathology and Laboratory Medicine; Professor of Medicine (Infectious Diseases); Emory University School of Medicine. Director, Clin-

ical Microbiology, Grady Memorial Hospital, Atlanta, Georgia.
Bacterial Diarrheas

Donald M. McLean, M.D. Professor of Medical Microbiology, University of British Columbia. Consultant in Microbiology, Health Sciences Centre Hospital and Children's Hospital, Vancouver, British Columbia, Canada.
Aseptic Meningitis and Viral Meningitis

Michael E. McLeod, M.D. Professor of Medicine, Duke University School of Medicine; Physician, Duke University Hospital, Durham, North Carolina.
Chronic Abdominal Pain

W. Robert Meadows, M.D. Associate Professor of Medicine, Loyola University, Stritch School of Medicine, Maywood, Illinois; Chief of Graphics, Edward Hines, Jr., Veterans Administration Hospital, Hines, Illinois.
Cardiomyopathy

James C. Melby, M.D. Professor of Medicine and Physiology, Boston University School of Medicine. Head, Section of Endocrinology and Metabolism, University Hospital, Boston, Massachusetts.
Primary Aldosteronism

Nancy L. Meryhew, M.D. Assistant Professor of Medicine, University of Minnesota School of Medicine, Minneapolis, Minnesota.
Rheumatoid Arthritis

Ronald P. Messner, M.D. Professor of Medicine, University of Minnesota School of Medicine, Minneapolis, Minnesota.
Rheumatoid Arthritis

Roger W. Miller, M.D. Physician, St. Mary Corwin Hospital and Parkview Episcopal Hospital, Pueblo, Colorado.
Disorders of the Paranasal Sinuses

Paul F. Milner, M.D. Professor of Pathology and Medicine, Medical College of Georgia. Attending Hematologist, Eugene Talmadge Memorial Hospital, Medical College of Georgia, Augusta, Georgia.
Thalassemia

Robert D. Mitchell, M.D. Professor of Medicine, Loma Linda University School of Medicine. Attending Physician, Loma Linda University Medical Center and Jerry L. Pettis Memorial Veterans Administration Hospital, Loma Linda, California.
Anorexia, Nausea, and Vomiting

K.A. Monsur, M.B., D.C.P., D. Bact. F.R.C. Path. Senior Consultant, International Centre for Diarrhoeal Disease Research, Dacca, Bangladesh.
Cholera

M. Brittain Moore, Jr., M.D. Dermatologist, Watson Clinic. Consulting Staff, Lakeland Regional Medical Center, Lakeland, Florida.
Chancroid

David M. Morens, M.D. Associate Professor, Department of Tropical Medicine and Medical Microbiology, University of Hawaii School of Medicine. Attending Physician, Leahi Hospital, Honolulu, Hawaii.
Coxsackievirus and Echovirus Infections

Kenneth M. Moser, M.D. Professor of Medicine, University of California, San Diego, School of Medicine. Director, Pulmonary and Critical Care Division, University Medical Center, San Diego, California.
Pulmonary Embolism and Infarction

Clifton F. Mountain, M.D. Professor of Surgery; Head, Thoracic Surgery; and Chairman, Thoracic Oncology, The University of Texas System Cancer Center, M.D. Anderson Hospital and Tumor Institute, Houston, Texas.
The Diagnosis of Pulmonary Tumors

Haralampos M. Moutsopoulos, M.D. Professor of Medicine, University of Ioannia School of Medicine. Chairman, Department of Medicine, Hatzikosta General Hospital, Ioannina, Greece.
Sjögren's Syndrome

S. Grant Mulholland, M.D. Professor and Chairman, Department of Urology, Thomas Jefferson University Medical School. Chairman, Department of Urology, Thomas Jefferson University Hospital, Philadelphia, Pennsylvania.
Infections of the Urinary Tract

Patrick J. Mulrow, M.D. Professor of Medicine, Medical College of Ohio, Toledo, Ohio.
Chronic Adrenal Insufficiency

David M. Nagorney, M.D. Assistant Professor and Consultant in Surgery, Mayo Medical School. Staff Surgeon, Rochester Methodist Hospital, St. Mary's Hospital, and Mayo Clinic, Rochester, Minnesota.
Intestinal Obstruction

André J. Nahmias, M.D., M.P.H. Professor of Pediatrics and Pathology; Associate Professor of Community Health, Emory University School of Medicine. Chief, Infectious Disease and Immunology Divisions, Pediatric Services, Grady Memorial Hospital and Henrietta Egleston Hospital for Children, Atlanta, Georgia.
Herpes Simplex Virus Infections

G. David Neal, M.D. Assistant Professor, University of Texas Health Science Center. Staff, University of Texas Medical Center Hospital and Audie Murphy Veterans Administration Hospital, San Antonio, Texas.
Masses in the Neck

Albert D. Newcomer, M.D. Professor of Medicine, Mayo Medical School. Attending Gastroenterologist, Mayo Clinic, St. Mary's Hospital, and Methodist Hospital, Rochester, Minnesota.
Intestinal Disaccharidase Deficiency

William A. Newton, Jr., M.D. Professor of Pathology and Pediatrics, Ohio State University. Chief, Department of Laboratory Medicine, Children's Hospital. Pediatric Hematologist/Oncologist, Formerly Chief, Division of Pediatric Hematology/Oncology, Children's Hospital, Columbus, Ohio.
Histiocytosis X

Ronald Lee Nichols, M.D. Henderson Professor and Vice Chairman, Department of Surgery; Professor of Microbiology and Immunology, Tulane University School of Medicine. Attending Surgeon, Tulane Medical Center Hospital, Charity Hospital of Louisiana, New Orleans, Louisiana.
Gas Gangrene and Similar Anaerobic Soft-Tissue Infections

Linda J. Nims, M.S. Supervisor, General Microbiology, New Mexico State Laboratory, Scientific Laboratory Division, Albuquerque, New Mexico.
Plague

Philip T. Ninan, M.D. Assistant Professor and Director, Anxiety Disorders Research Program, Department of Psychiatry, Emory University School of Medicine. Staff Psychiatrist, Emory University Hospital and Veterans Administration Hospital, Atlanta, Georgia.
Substance Use Disorders

William L. Nyhan, M.D., Ph.D. Professor and Chairman, Department of Pediatrics, University of California at San Diego, La Jolla, California. Staff, University Hospital Medical Center, San Diego, California.
Genetic Defects of Amino Acid Metabolism and Transport

John B. O'Connell, M.D. Assistant Professor of Medicine, Loyola University, Stritch School of Medicine. Attending Cardiologist, Loyola University, Maywood, Illinois.
Cardiomyopathy

Joseph H. Ogura, M.D.* Rindburg Professor and Head, Department of Otolaryngology, Washington University, St. Louis, Missouri.
Tumors

Marcelo R. Olarte, M.D. Assistant Professor in Clinical Neurology, College of Physicians and Surgeons, Columbia University. Assistant Attending Neurologist, New York Neurological Institute, Columbia Presbyterian Medical Center, New York, New York.
Dermatomyositis and Polymyositis

James A. Olive, D.M.D., M.D. Assistant Professor, Medical College of Wisconsin. Senior Attending Physician, Milwaukee County Medical Complex. Director of Blood Bank, Froedtert Memorial Lutheran Hospital, Milwaukee, Wisconsin.
Hemophilia and Other Inherited Coagulation Disorders

E. V. O'Loughlin, M.B., B.S., F.R.A.C.P. Fellow in Pediatric Gastroenterology, University of Calgary; Division of Pediatric Gastroenterology and Nutrition, Alberta Children's Hospital, Calgary, Alberta, Canada.
Chronic Diarrhea and Malabsorption

John M. O'Loughlin, M.D. Clinical Instructor in Medicine, Harvard Medical School. Assistant Clinical Professor, Tufts University School of Medicine. Chairman, Department of Allergy and Dermatology, Lahey Clinic Medical Center. Senior Staff Physician, Lahey Clinic Medical Center, Boston, Massachusetts.
Asthma in Adults

Newton G. Osborne, M.D., Ph.D. Professor of Obstetrics and Gynecology, Howard University College of Medicine. Chief of Gynecology, Howard University Hospital, Washington, D.C.
Rubella

J. T. Parer, M.D., Ph.D. Professor and Director of Obstetrics, University of California at San Francisco. Associate Staff, Cardiovascular Research Institute, San Francisco, California.
Pregnancy

John S. Parks, M.D., Ph.D. Professor of Pediatrics, Emory University School of Medicine. Pediatric Endocrinologist, Henrietta Egleston Hospital for Children and Grady Memorial Hospital, Atlanta, Georgia.
Congenital Adrenal Hyperplasia

George W. Paulson, M.D. Kurtz Professor and Chairman, Department of Neurology, College of Medicine, Ohio State University. Staff, Ohio State University Hospitals, Columbus, Ohio.
Tetanus

Zbigniew Pawlowski, M.D., D.T.M. & H. Professor in Medical Parasitology, Medical Faculty, Poznań, Poland. Senior Medical Officer, Parasitic Diseases Programme, World Health Organization, Geneva, Switzerland.
Trichinosis

J.M.S. Pearce, M.D., F.R.C.P. Consultant Neurologist, Chief, Hull Royal Infirmary, Yorkshire, England. Director, Headache Clinic, Birmingham, England.
Migraine and Its Variants

Gary S. Pearl, M.D., Ph.D. Assistant Professor of Pathology, Emory University School of Medicine. Attending Pathologist, Emory University Hospital, Atlanta, Georgia.
Spinocerebellar Degenerations

John H. Per-Lee, M.D. Associate Professor, Department of Surgery (Otolaryngology), Emory University School of Medicine. Staff, Emory University Hospital, Grady Memorial Hospital, Veterans Administration Hospital, and Henrietta Egleston Hospital, Atlanta, Georgia.
Vertigo

Carl A. Perlino, M.D. Associate Professor of Medicine, Emory University School of Medicine. Hospital Epidemiologist, Grady Memorial Hospital. Consultant Physician in Infectious Diseases, Emory University Clinic, Atlanta, Georgia.
Bacterial Pneumonia

Leonard J. Perloff, M.D. Associate Professor of Surgery, University of Pennsylvania School of Medicine and Hospital of the University of Pennsylvania. Director of Vascular Surgery, Philadelphia Veterans Hospital, Philadelphia, Pennsylvania.
Acute Appendicitis

Robert H. Peter, M.D. Professor of Medicine, Duke University School of Medicine. Attending Cardiologist, Duke University Medical Center, Durham, North Carolina.
Pulmonary Hypertension

C. J. Peters, M.D. Chief, Medical Division, U. S. Army Medical Research Institute of Infectious Diseases, Frederick, Maryland.
Viral Hemorrhagic Fevers

Paul C. Peters, M.D. Professor and Chairman, Division of Urology, The University of Texas Health Science Center. Attending Staff, Parkland Memorial Hospital, Baylor University Medical Center, Presbyterian Hospital, Children's Medical Center, Veterans Administration Hospital, Medical Arts Hospital, and John Peter Smith Hospital of Fort Worth, Dallas, Texas.
Benign Prostatic Hypertrophy

Robert G. Petersdorf, M.D. Vice Chancellor, Health Sciences; Dean, School of Medicine, University of California at San Diego, La Jolla, California.
Fever of Unknown Origin

John A. Phillips, III, M.D. Associate Professor of Pediatrics, Johns Hopkins University School of Medicine. Active Staff, Department of Pediatrics, Johns Hopkins Hospital, Baltimore, Maryland.
Hemoglobinopathies

James R. Philp, M.D. Professor of Medicine, Division of Infectious Disease and Immunology, Bowman Gray School of Medicine, Winston-Salem, North Carolina.
Relapsing Fever

Henry A. Pitt, M.D. Assistant Professor of Surgery and Physician, UCLA Medical Center. Staff, Sepulveda Veterans Administration Medical Center, Los Angeles, California.
Hepatic and Perihepatic Abscess

Jack D. Poland, M.D., M.P.H. Affiliate Professor, Department of Microbiology, Colorado State University. Physician, Center for Infectious Diseases, Centers for Disease Control, Fort Collins, Colorado.
Colorado Tick Fever

Herbert F. Polesky, M.D. Professor of Pathology and Laboratory Medicine, University of Minnesota School of Medicine. Director, Minneapolis War Memorial Blood Bank, Minneapolis, Minnesota.
Acute Transfusion Reactions

Hiram C. Polk, Jr., M.D. Professor and Chairman, Department of Surgery, University of Louisville School of Med-

*Deceased.

icine. Norton-Kosair-Children's Hospital, University Hospital, Veterans Administration Medical Center, Jewish Hospital, Louisville, Kentucky.
Peritonitis and Intra-abdominal Infection

Konstantinos S. Polyzoidis, M.D. Cerebrovascular Research Fellow, Division of Neurosurgery, Emory University School of Medicine, Atlanta, Georgia.
Cerebrovascular Disease

Bertram A. Portin, M.D. Clinical Professor of Surgery, State University of New York at Buffalo. Chief, Colon and Rectal Surgery, Sisters of Charity, Buffalo General Hospital, Erie County Medical Center, and St. Francis Hospital, Buffalo, New York.
Anorectal and Perianal Disorders

Benjamin L. Portnoy, M.D. Consultant, Infectious Diseases, Diagnostic Clinic of Houston, Houston, Texas.
Rat-Bite Fever

Bernard Portnoy, M.D. Professor of Pediatrics and Preventive Medicine, School of Medicine, University of Southern California. Staff, Los Angeles County–USC Medical Center, Los Angeles, California.
Viral Pneumonias

Charles M. Poser, M.D. Lecturer on Neurology, Harvard Medical School. Professor of Neurology, Boston University School of Medicine. Attending Neurologist, Beth Israel Hospital. Staff Neurologist, Veterans Administration Outpatient Clinic, Boston, Massachusetts.
Multiple Sclerosis

Aluizio Prata, M.D. Full Professor of Tropical Medicine, University of Brasília. Hospital Presidente Medici. University of Brasília, Brasília, Brazil.
American Trypanosomiasis

Gregory Prazar, M.D. Staff, Exeter Hospital, Exeter, New Hampshire.
Behavioral Problems in Children and Adolescents

Jean H. Priest, M.D. Professor of Pediatrics, Associate Professor of Pathology, Emory University. Attending Physician, Grady Memorial Hospital, Atlanta, Georgia.
Chromosomal Disorders

Kevin C. Pringle, M.B., Ch.B., F.R.A.C.S. Associate Professor of Surgery, University of Iowa, College of Medicine, and the University of Iowa Hospital and Clinics, Iowa City, Iowa.
The Acute Abdomen in Childhood

Robert E. Pumphrey, M.D. Clinical Professor, George Washington School of Medicine. Senior Attending Physician, Sibley Memorial Hospital, Children's Hospital National Medical Center, and George Washington University Hospital, Washington, D.C.
Otitis Media, Otitis Externa

Eugene A. Quindlen, M.D. Professor of Neurosurgery, University of South Alabama College of Medicine. Chief, Neurosurgical Service, University of South Alabama Medical Center, Mobile, Alabama.
Intracranial Neoplasms

Bruce S. Rabin, M.D. Ph.D. Associate Professor of Pathology, University of Pittsburgh. Director, Division of Clinical Immunopathology, University Health Center of Pittsburgh, Pittsburgh, Pennsylvania.
Diagnostic Problems in Immunosuppressed Patients

Albert Augustus Ramage, M.D. Fellow in Gastroenterology, Medical College of Georgia, Augusta Georgia.
Neoplasms of the Stomach

Raymond V. Randall, M.D. Professor of Medicine, Mayo Medical School. Consultant, Rochester Methodist Hospital and St. Mary's Hospital, Rochester, Minnesota.
Hypopituitarism; Empty Sella Syndrome

Patricia M. Randels, M.D. Clinical Professor of Psychiatry and Human Behavior, Jefferson Medical College of Thomas Jefferson University, Philadelphia, Pennsylvania. Chief, Psychogeriatric Unit, Veterans Administration Medical Center, Coatesville, Pennsylvania.
Schizophrenia

T. K. Sreepada Rao, M.D., F.A.C.P. Associate Professor of Medicine, Downstate Medical Center, State University of New York. Acting Director, Renal Diseases Division, Downstate Medical Center. Medical Director, Hemodialysis Units, Kings County Hospital, Brooklyn, New York.
Acute Renal Failure

Morton I. Rapoport, M.D. Vice Chancellor and Chief Executive Officer, University of Maryland Medical System, Baltimore, Maryland.
Tularemia

Robert R. Recker, M.D. Professor of Medicine, Chief of Endocrinology, Creighton University School of Medicine. Staff, St. Joseph Hospital and Veterans Administration Hospital, Omaha, Nebraska.
Osteoporosis

Helen C. Redman, M.D. Professor of Diagnostic Radiology, University of Texas Health Science Center at Dallas. Staff, Vascular and Interventional Radiology, Parkland Memorial Hospital, Dallas, Texas.
Aneurysms of the Aorta

Peter A. Rice, M.D. Associate Professor of Medicine, Boston University School of Medicine. Associate Physician, Medical Service and Director, Clinical Immunology Laboratory, Boston City Hospital, Boston, Massachusetts.
Acute Bacterial Meningitis

Hal B. Richerson, M.D. Professor, Department of Internal Medicine, University of Iowa School of Medicine. Director, Allergy–Immunology Division, University of Iowa Hospitals, Iowa City, Iowa.
Hypersensitivity Pneumonitis

E. Chester Ridgway, M.D. Associate Professor of Medicine, Harvard Medical School. Chief, Thyroid Unit, Massachusetts General Hospital, Boston, Massachusetts.
Thyroid Tumors

Michael H. Rivner, M.D. Assistant Professor of Neurology, Medical College of Georgia. Director of the Electromyography Laboratory, and Attending Physician, Neurology, Talmadge Memorial Hospital. Attending Neurologist, Veterans Administration Hospital, Augusta, Georgia. Consultant in Neurology, Eisenhower Medical Center, Fort Gordon, Georgia.
Diagnosis in Disorders of Neuromuscular Transmission

James Roberson, M.D. Assistant Professor, Department of Orthopaedics, Emory University. Attending Staff, Emory University Hospital, Grady Memorial Hospital, and Atlanta Veterans Hospital, Atlanta, Georgia.
Septic Arthritis

Stephen H. Robinson, M.D. Professor of Medicine, Harvard Medical School. Chief of Hematology and Clinical Director, Department of Medicine, Beth Israel Hospital, Boston, Massachusetts.
Anemia

Alan M. Robson, M.D. Professor of Pediatrics, Washington University School of Medicine. Director, Division of Pediatric Nephrology, St. Louis Children's Hospital, St. Louis, Missouri.
Nephrotic Syndrome

Charles R. Roe, M.D. Professor of Pediatrics and Chief, Division of Genetics and Metabolism. Department of Pediatrics, Duke University Medical Center, Durham, North Carolina.
Rye's Syndrome

Allen W. Root, M.D. Professor of Pediatrics, Associate Chairman, Department of Pediatrics; Head, Section of Pediatric Endocrinology, University of South Florida, Director, University Teaching Service, All Children's Hospital, St. Petersburg, Florida. Staff, General Hospital, Tampa, Florida.
Delayed Sexual Maturation and Sexual Precocity

Milton D. Rossman, M.D. Assistant Professor of Medicine, University of Pennsylvania School of Medicine. Medical Coordinator, Fiberoptic Bronchoscopy Service; Member, Respiratory Committee; Hospital of the University of Pennsylvania, Philadelphia, Pennsylvania.
Tuberculosis and Diseases Due to Other Mycobacteria

Sheldon P. Rothenberg, M.D. Professor of Medicine, State University of New York, Downstate Medical Center, Brooklyn, New York.
Pernicious Anemia and Other Megaloblastic Anemias

Daniel Rotrosen, M.D. Assistant Professor of Medicine, University of California School of Medicine, Los Angeles, California.
Opportunistic Mycoses

Randall G. Rowland, M.D., Ph.D. Associate Professor of Urology, Indiana University School of Medicine. Attending Physician, Indiana University Hospital. Consultant in Urology, Wishard Memorial Hospital and Indianapolis Veterans Administration Hospital, Indianapolis, Indiana.
Tumors of the Ureter and Urinary Bladder

Robert K. Rude, M.D. Associate Professor of Medicine, University of Southern California School of Medicine. Staff, Los Angeles County/University of Southern California Medical Center and Orthopaedic Hospital, Los Angeles, California.
Primary Hyperparathyroidism

Hussain I. Saba, M.D., Ph.D. Associate Professor, University of South Florida. Attending Staff, Tampa General Hospital and James A. Haley Veterans Hospital. Consulting Staff, University Community Hospital, St. Joseph's Hospital, Town and Country Hospital, and Brandon Community Hospital, Tampa, Florida.
Hereditary Elliptocytosis (Ovalocytosis); Hereditary Spherocytosis; Paroxysmal Nocturnal Hemoglobinuria

Arun Samanta, M.D. Assistant Professor of Medicine, New Jersey School of Medicine, and University of Medicine and Dentistry of New Jersey, Newark, New Jersey. Acting Chief of Digestive Diseases, Veterans Administration Medical Center, East Orange, New Jersey.
Cirrhosis of the Liver

Don M. Samples, M.D. Associate Clinical Professor of Medicine, Tulane University School of Medicine. Senior Staff, Associate Chairman, Department of Medicine, Head, Section on Hematology and Medical Oncology, Ochser Foundation Hospital, New Orleans, Louisiana. Consultant, South Louisiana Medical Center, Houma, Louisiana.
Iron Storage Disease

Charles V. Sanders, M.D. Professor of Medicine and Microbiology, Louisiana State University School of Medicine. Head, Adult Closed Care Unit, Charity Hospital, New Orleans, Louisiana.
Rickettsial Diseases

Donald B. Sanders, M.D. Professor of Medicine, Duke University Medical Center. Director, Electromyography Laboratory, and Attending Neurologist, Duke University Hospital, Durham, North Carolina.
Myasthenia Gravis

George A. Sarosi, M.D. Professor, Division Director of General Medicine, Vice Chairman for Professional Affairs, University of Texas Medical School, Health Science Center, Houston, Texas.
Systemic Mycotic Diseases

John A. Saryan, M.D. Instructor of Pediatrics, Tufts University School of Medicine. Courtesy Staff, Children's Hospital Medical Center, Boston, Massachusetts. Senior Staff Physician, Lahey Clinic Medical Center, Burlington, Massachusetts.
Asthma in Adults

Edward Warren Savage, M.D. Professor, Obstetrics/Gynecology, Charles R. Drew Medical School, Adjunct Associate Professor, University of California at Los Angeles. King/Drew Medical Center, St. Francis Hospital Center, UCLA Hospital and Clinics, Memorial Hospital of Gardena.
Tumors of the Vulva, Vagina, and Cervix

Ernst J. Schaefer, M.D. Associate Professor of Medicine, Tufts University School of Medicine. Staff, Endocrinology Division, New England Medical Center, Boston, Massachusetts.
Disorders of Lipid Transport

William Schaffner, M.D. Professor and Chairman, Department of Preventive Medicine; Professor and Chief, Division of Infectious Diseases, Department of Medicine; Vanderbilt University School of Medicine. Epidemiologist and Attending Physician, Vanderbilt University Hospital, Nashville, Tennessee.
Psittacosis

Bruce F. Scharschmidt, M.D. Associate Professor of Medicine; Attending Physician, University of California at San Francisco, Affiliated Hospitals, San Francisco, California.
Jaundice

Eliot Schechter, M.D. Professor of Medicine, University of Oklahoma Health Sciences Center. Director, Cardiac Catheterization Laboratory, Oklahoma City Veterans Administration Medical Center; Attending Physician, Oklahoma Memorial Hospital, Oklahoma City, Oklahoma.
Ischemic Heart Disease

I. Herbert Scheinberg, M.D. Professor of Medicine, and Head, Division of Genetic Medicine, Albert Einstein College of Medicine. Attending Physician, Bronx Municipal Hospital Center, Bronx, New York.
Hepatolenticular Degeneration (Wilson's Disease)

W. Michael Scheld, M.D. Associate Professor of Internal Medicine and Neurosurgery, University of Virginia School of Medicine. Attending Physician, University of Virginia Affiliated Hospitals, Charlottesville, Virginia.
Infective Endocarditis

Alvin H. Schmaier, M.D. Assistant Professor of Internal Medicine, Thrombosis and Pathology. Attending Hematologist/Oncologist and Director, Temple University Hospital Coagulation Laboratory, Philadelphia, Pennsylvania.
Hemorrhagic Disease Due to Disseminated Intravscular Coagulation and Fibrinolysis; Hemorrhagic Diseases Due to Circulating Anticoagulants

George P. Schmid, M.D. Physician, Bacterial Zoonoses Activity, Division of Bacterial Diseases, Center for Infectious Diseases, Centers for Disease Control, Atlanta, Georgia.
Leptospirosis

Stephen W. Schwarzmann, M.D. Associate Professor of Medicine, Emory University School of Medicine. Chief, In-

fectious Diseases, Emory University Hospital, Atlanta, Georgia.
Bacterial Pneumonia

Harold H. Scudamore, Ph.D., M.D. Clinical Associate Professor of Medicine, University of Wisconsin Medical School, Madison, Wisconsin. Attending Physician, St. Clare Hospital, Monroe, Wisconsin.
Gastritis

John M. Seaman, M.D. Chief, Rheumatology Section, Medical Center, Wright-Patterson Air Force Base, Ohio.
Collagen Diseases

Leonard B. Seeff, M.D. Associate Professor of Medicine, Georgetown University School of Medicine. Chief, Gastroenterology and Hepatology, Veterans Administration Medical Center, Washington, D. C.
Viral Hepatitis and Its Differential Diagnosis

Thomas F. Sellers, Jr., M.D. Professor of Community Health, Emory University School of Medicine. Physician, Grady Memorial Hospital and Emory University Hospital, Atlanta, Georgia.
Diphtheria

John T. Sessions, Jr., M.D. Professor of Medicine, University of North Carolina School of Medicine. Attending Physician, North Carolina Memorial Hospital, Chapel Hill, North Carolina.
Functional Disorders of the Gastrointestinal Tract

Barry Shannon, Ph.D. Clinical Assistant Professor, Departments of Pediatrics and Pathology, Ohio State University. Head, Immunology Section, Department of Laboratory Medicine, Children's Hospital, Columbus, Ohio.
Histiocytosis X

Hiromi Shinya, M.D., Ph.D. Clinical Professor of Surgery, Mount Sinai School of Medicine. Chief, Surgical Endoscopy, Beth Israel Medical Center, New York, New York.
Benign Polyps of the Colon

Dana L. Shires, Jr., M.D. Professor of Medicine; Director, Division of Nephrology, University of South Florida. Director, Kidney Transplant Service, and Attending Nephrologist, Tampa General Hospital, Tampa, Florida.
Glomerulonephritis

Ira Shoulson, M.D. Associate Professor of Neurology and Medicine, University of Rochester School of Medicine and Dentistry. Senior Associate Neurologist, Strong Memorial Hospital, Rochester, New York.
The Dementias

Robert Silber, M.D. Professor of Medicine, New York University School of Medicine. Director, Division of Hematology, University Hospital and Bellvue Hospital. Attending Physician, University Hospital, Bellvue Hospital and Veterans Administration Hospital, New York, New York.
Chronic Lymphocytic Leukemia

Frederick R. Singer, M.D. Professor of Medicine, University of Southern California School of Medicine. Los Angeles County/University of Southern California Medical Center, Orthopaedic Hospital, Los Angeles, California.
Primary Hyperthyroidism

Alice Faye Singleton, M.D., M.P.H. Assistant Professor of Pediatrics at Charles R. Drew Postgraduate Medical School and University of California at Los Angeles. Director, Pediatric Health Services Research, King/Drew Medical Center. Director, Ambulatory Pediatric Division, King/Drew Medical Center, Los Angeles, California.
Syphilis

Michael R. Skeels, Ph.D. Adjunct Faculty, University of New Mexico School of Medicine. Chief, Biological Sciences Bureau, New Mexico Scientific Laboratory Division, Albuquerque, New Mexico. Director, Oregon Public Health Laboratory, Oregon Health Division, Portland, Oregon.
Plague

Ronald Skowsky, M.D. Associate Professor of Medicine, Department of Medicine, California College of Medicine, University of California, Irvine, California. Chief, Endocrinology/Metabolism Section, Veterans Administration Medical Center, Long Beach, California.
Diabetes Insipidus

Richard T. Smith, M.D. Fellow, Baylor College of Medicine, Houston, Texas.
Normal Murmurs in Children

Thomas F. Smith, M.D. Assistant Professor and Chief, Division of Allergy/Immunology, Department of Pediatrics. Instructor, Department of Microbiology and Immunology, Grady Memorial Hospital. Attending Physician, Pediatric Allergy, Immunology, and Pulmonary Diseases, Henrietta Egleston Hospital for Children, and Grady Memorial Hospital, Atlanta, Georgia.
Immunodeficiency

Charles A. Sninsky, M.D. Assistant Professor of Medicine, University of Florida College of Medicine and Gainesville Veterans Administration Medical Center. Staff Gastroenterologist, Shands Hospital and Gainesville Veterans Administration Medical Center, Gainesville, Florida.
Dysphagia, Esophageal Obstruction, and Esophagitis

Robert T. Soper, M.D. Professor of Surgery, University of Iowa, College of Medicine, and the University of Iowa Hospital and Clinics, Iowa City, Iowa.
The Acute Abdomen in Childhood

William G. Speed, III, M.D. Associate Professor of Medicine, The Johns Hopkins University School of Medicine. Active Staff, The Johns Hopkins Hospital, Baltimore, Maryland.
Headache and Facial Pain

Charles H. Spencer, M.D. Assistant Professor of Pediatrics, Louisiana State University School of Medicine. Attending Pediatric Rheumatologist, Charity and Children's Hospitals, New Orleans, Louisiana.
Juvenile Rheumatoid Arthritis

Thomas J. Spira, M.D. Chief, Clinical Immunology Laboratory, Division of Host Factors, Center for Infectious Diseases, Centers for Disease Control. Clinical Assistant Professor of Medicine and Pediatrics (Infectious Diseases), Emory University School of Medicine, Atlanta, Georgia.
Acquired Immunodeficiency Syndrome (AIDS)

Robert L. Stahl, M.D. Teaching Assistant in Medicine, New York University School of Medicine. American Cancer Society Clinical Research Fellow, Senior Fellow in Hematology, New York University Medical Center, New York, New York.
Chronic Lymphocytic Leukemia

Brian D. Steg, M.D. Fellow in Cardiology, Bowman Gray School of Medicine of Wake Forest University, Winston-Salem, North Carolina.
Pericarditis

James C. Steigerwald, M.D. Associate Professor of Medicine, University of Colorado School of Medicine. Staff, Colorado General Hospital, Veterans Administration Hospital, and Denver Hospital, Denver, Colorado.
Systemic Lupus Erythematosus

Herman Steinberg, M.D. Clinical Professor of Medicine, Cornell University College of Medicine. Attending Physician, The New York Hospital, New York, New York.
Chronic Ulcerative Colitis and Crohn's Disease

Irmin Sternlieb, M.D. Professor of Medicine and Associate Director, Liver Research Center, Albert Einstein College of Medicine. Attending Physician, Bronx Municipal Hospital Center, Bronx, New York.
Hepatolenticular Degeneration (Wilson's Disease)

G. Thomas Strickland, M.D., Ph.D., D.C.M.T. Director and Professor, International Program, and Professor of Microbiology, University of Maryland School of Medicine, Baltimore, Maryland. Director, International Center for Medical Research, Lahore, Pakistan.
Parasitic Infection of the Intestinal Tract

John Studd, M.D., M.R.C.O.G. Consultant Obstetrician and Gynecologist, King's College Hospital, London, England.
Menopause

Thomas R. Swift, M.D. Professor and Chairman, Department of Neurology; Program Director, Neurology Residency Training Program, Medical College of Georgia. Attending Neurologist, Eugene Talmadge Memorial Hospital; Consultant, Veterans Administration Hospital, Dwight David Eisenhower Army Medical Center, University Hospital, and Department of Offender Rehabilitation Hospital, Augusta, Georgia.
Diagnosis in Disorders of Neuromuscular Transmission

Francis J. Tedesco, M.D. Professor of Medicine, and Chief, Gastroenterology, Medical College of Georgia, Augusta, Georgia.
Neoplasms of the Stomach

Ronald F. Teitler, M.D. Clinical Instructor in Surgery, State University of New York at Buffalo. Attending Surgeon, Buffalo General Hospital, Sisters Hospital of Buffalo, and St. Francis Hospital, Buffalo, New York.
Anorectal and Perianal Disorders

John M. Tew, Jr., M.D. Professor and Chairman, Department of Neurosurgery, University of Cincinnati Medical Center. Attending Staff, The Christ Hospital, Children's Hospital Medical Center, Deaconess Hospital, Cincinnati General Hospital, and Good Samaritan Hospital, Cincinnati, Ohio. Consulting Staff, Clinton County Memorial Hospital, Wilmington, Ohio; Clermont County Hospital, Batavia, Ohio; Booth Hospital and St. Elizabeth Hospital, Covington, Kentucky; St. Luke Hospital, Ft. Thomas, Kentucky.
Neuralgias of the Trigeminal, Glossopharyngeal, and Facial Nerves

Jeremy H. Thompson, M.D., F.R.C.P.I., F.A.C.P. Professor of Pharmacology, UCLA School of Medicine, Los Angeles, California. Internist and Clinical Pharmacologist, Santa Monica Hospital and St. Johns Hospital, Santa Monica, California.
Drug Reactions

Jesse E. Thompson, Jr., M.D. Assistant Professor of Surgery, UCLA School of Medicine, Los Angeles, California. Olive View Medical Center, Department of Surgery, Van Nuys, California.
Hepatic and Perihepatic Abscess

Suzie C. Tindall, M.D. Assistant Professor of Surgery (Neurosurgery), Emory University School of Medicine. Chief, Neurosurgical Service, Grady Memorial Hospital, Atlanta, Georgia.
Trauma of the Central Nervous System

Harold Tucker, M.D. Assistant Professor of Medicine, The Johns Hopkins University School of Medicine. Attending Gastroenterologist, Greater Baltimore Medical Center, Baltimore City Hospitals, and the Johns Hopkins Hospital, Baltimore, Maryland.
Diverticular Disease of the Colon

J. Blake Tyrrell, M.D. Associate Clinical Profesor of Medicine, University of California at San Francisco. Senior Physician, University of California Hospitals, San Francisco, California.
Cushing's Syndrome

William N. Valentine, M.D. Professor of Medicine, University of Southern California at Los Angeles School of Medicine, Center for the Health Sciences, Los Angeles, California.
Hereditary Anemias Due to Abnormal Red Cell Enzymes

Peter J. Vandermeer, M.D. Chief Resident, Department of Otolarynology; Assistant Clinical Instructor, Washington University Medical School. Chief Resident, Washington University Teaching Hospitals, St. Louis, Missouri.
Tumors of the Larynx and Pharynx

Dennis W. Vane, M.D. Clinical Instructor, Department of Surgery, Ohio State University. Clinical Instructor, Section of Pediatric Surgery Columbus Children's Hospital and Ohio State University Hospitals, Columbus, Ohio.
Small Bowel Tumors

Andre J. Van Herle, M.D. Professor of Medicine, UCLA School of Medicine, Los Angeles, California.
Hypothyroidism

Harry Van Loveren, M.D. Chief Resident, University of Cincinnati Medical Center, Department of Neurosurgery, Cincinnati, Ohio.
Neuralgias of the Trigeminal, Glossopharyngeal, and Facial Nerves

Thomas A. Vargo, M.D. Assistant Professor, Baylor College of Medicine; Chief, Intensive Care Service and Associate in Cardiology, The Lillie Frank Abercrombie Section of Cardiology, Texas Children's Hospital, Houston, Texas.
Congenital Heart Disease

Eric C. Vonderheid, M.D. Associate Professor of Dermatology, Temple University School of Medicine. Attending Dermatologist, Skin and Cancer Hospital, Temple University Hospital, Philadelphia, Pennsylvania.
Mycosis Fungoides and Sézary Syndrome

Robert A. Waugh, M.D. Associate Professor of Medicine, Duke University Medical Center, Durham, North Carolina.
Valvular Heart Disease

Thomas E. Weiss, M.D. Chairman Emeritus, Section on Rheumatology, Ochsner Clinic and Alton Ochsner Medical Foundation. Staff, Ochsner Foundation Hospital, New Orleans, Louisiana.
Gout

B. J. Wilder, M.D. Professor of Neurology, University of Florida College of Medicine. Chief, Neurology Service, Veterans Administration Medical Center, Gainesville, Florida.
Epilepsy and Other Convulsive Disorders

Jeanette Wilkins, M.D. Professor of Pediatrics, University of Southern California School of Medicine. Physician, Specialist, Los Angeles County–University of Southern California Medical Center, Los Angeles, California.
Mumps

Julian C. Williams, M.D., Ph.D. Assistant Professor of Pediatrics, University of Texas Health Science Center at Houston. Pediatrician, Hermann Hospital, Houston, Texas.
Hereditary Disorders of Carbohydrate Metabolism; Mucopolysaccharidoses

Lester F. Williams, Jr., M.D. Professor and Chairman, Division of Surgery, Boston University School of Medicine. Surgeon-in-Chief, University Hospital. Director, Surgical Services, Boston City Hospital, Boston, Massachusetts.
Vascular Disease of the Mesentery

Sidney J. Winawer, M.D. Professor of Clinical Medicine, Cornell University Medical College. Chief, Gastroenterology Service, Department of Medicine, Memorial Sloan-Kettering Cancer Center, New York, New York.
Malignant Tumors of the Colon and Rectum

Terence D. Wingert, M.D. Assistant Professor of Internal Medicine, Medical College of Ohio, Toledo, Ohio.
Chronic Adrenal Insufficiency

Madelaine M. Wohlreich, M.D. Clinical Associate, Department of Psychiatry, University of Pennsylvania School of Medicine. Clinical Assistant Psychiatrist and Staff Psychiatrist, Consult-Liaison Service, Pennsylvania Hospital. Associate Psychiatrist, Institute of Pennsylvania Hospital, Philadelphia, Pennsylvania.
Affective Disorders

Douglas L. Wood, M.D. Assistant Professor of Medicine, Mayo Medical School. Consultant, Division of Cardiovascular Diseases and Internal Medicine, Mayo Clinic and Mayo Foundation, Rochester, Minnesota.
Cardiac Arrhythmias

James H. Wood, M.D. Assistant Professor, Division of Neurosurgery, Emory University School of Medicine. Director, Cerebral Blood Flow Laboratory, Emory University Hospital, Atlanta, Georgia.
Cerebrovascular Disease

Harry T. Wright, Jr., M.D., M.P.H. Professor of Pediatrics, University of Southern California School of Medicine. Head, Division of Infectious Diseases and Virology, Children's Hospital of Los Angeles, Los Angeles, California.
Poliomyelitis

Melvin D. Yahr, M.D. Professor and Chairman, Department of Neurology, Mt. Sinai School of Medicine, City University of New York. Neurologist-in-Chief and Director of Neurology, Mount Sinai Hospital, New York, New York.
Extrapyramidal Disorders

David Yashon, M.D. Professor of Neurosurgery, Ohio State University. Associate Attending Neurosurgeon, St. Anthony's Hospital, Columbus, Ohio.
Expanding Intraspinal Lesions

K. Randall Young, Jr., M.D. Fellow in Pulmonary Medicine, Yale University School of Medicine, New Haven, Connecticut.
Pneumoconioses

Roscoe C. Young, Jr., M.D. Associate Professor of Medicine, Department of Medicine, Division of Pulmonary Diseases, Howard University Hospital, Washington, D.C.
Sarcoidosis

Lawrence Zaslow, M.D. Associate Clinical Professor of Medicine, Tulane University School of Medicine. Visiting Physician, Charity Hospital. Attending Physician, Veterans Administration Hospital, Touro Infirmary, and East and West Jefferson General Hospital, New Orleans, Louisiana.
Hay Fever

Preface

During the four years since publication of the sixth edition of *Current Diagnosis,* there have been impressive developments in the technology used in medical diagnosis: new generations of CT scanners; improved methods of ultrasound imaging, including two-dimensional echocardiography; digital subtraction angiography; and myriad new laboratory tests. However, most new technology merely replaces older technology that has become obsolete; it cannot be substituted for skillful questioning and examination of the patient, nor can it replace clinical judgment. These observations provide the rationale for *Current Diagnosis.* The editorial objective in this edition remains unchanged from that of previous editions: to provide the practicing physician with an up-to-date reference that gathers into one volume the best available information on medical diagnosis. This completely revised and rewritten edition represents more than simply adding the factual information that has accumulated since publication of the last edition; it provides a critical examination of all of the available information, new and old. To accomplish this, new contributors have been selected to present their concepts and to discuss their understanding of current diagnostic practices.

As in previous editions, the first part of the book presents discussions of the differential diagnosis of commonly encountered clinical problems. This is followed by sections covering specific disease entities or clinical conditions. Authors have been requested to provide precise definitions and to discuss presenting signs and symptoms as well as relevant physical findings. Indications for laboratory tests and imaging studies are presented, and characteristic findings are discussed in sufficient detail to permit accurate interpretation. Perhaps equally important, procedures rendered obsolete by new technology are identified, and the hazards of invasive procedures are pointed out. The most important potential errors in following the recommended diagnostic approach are included under the heading "Pitfalls in Diagnosis."

Readers of previous editions of *Current Diagnosis* may notice, in addition to much new material, several new sections. Psychiatry now receives appropriate additional attention in a separate section. Completely new sections on disorders of the immune system, disorders of growth and development, and recognizable congenital syndromes have been added. New articles have been incorporated in the appropriate sections on evaluation of patients with suspected genetic disorders, child abuse, and the acquired immunodeficiency syndrome (AIDS), and the material presented in a number of the sections has been reorganized to enhance the usefulness of the book.

Current Diagnosis is not intended to be a comprehensive textbook of medicine, which must include information on etiology, pathogenesis, and treatment as well as diagnosis. It is intended as a convenient, one-volume source of the best information available to assist the physician in achieving a correct diagnosis as efficiently as possible. Since the book will be used primarily when there is a diagnostic problem, the contributors have been asked to go beyond the "textbook picture" to include information that will be useful in evaluating patients with atypical and perhaps misleading manifestations. The most frequent diagnostic problem is one in which the physician suspects that a patient has a certain condition and in which the most direct and definitive methods for confirming the provisional diagnosis must be found. An article on the specific problem should assist the physician in accomplishing this. Another common situation is one in which the physician must choose between an unknown number of possible diagnoses. To meet this need, we have incorporated numerous cross references and an extensive index that lists the symptoms, signs, and findings mentioned in the book.

To accomplish our ongoing objectives, we have invited more than 300 leading medical authorities, both in the United States and abroad, to summarize their accumulated experience and to present it in a manner most convenient and useful to the practicing physician. Contributors are selected not only because they are familiar with current advances in medical knowledge, but also because they are practicing physicians who apply this information in their daily patient care activities. I am grateful for the cooperation of these busy physicians, and I sincerely acknowledge each author's part in the success of *Current Diagnosis.*

An important group of individuals who played key roles in preparation of this edition are the members of the Board of Editors. Their continuing advice during preparation of the book was invaluable in identifying important omissions, arranging the sequence of articles, and settling the few controversial issues that arose. Four authors, Donald Manning, Linton Hopkins, Jean Priest, and John Bryan also deserve special recognition for their advice on the articles covering psychiatry, disorders of skeletal muscle, genetic disorders, and viral diseases, respectively.

Special thanks go to my editorial assistant, Eileen Jones, for her competent help in organizing the manuscripts, proofs, and correspondence, and to my wife, Vicky, who probably would have preferred the missed family vacations, concerts, and social events, but patiently put up with a recluse husband working on a book.

Although the name of the publishing company is always indicated on the cover, it is individuals who publish books, and I would like to thank the following persons at the W. B. Saunders Company who have been responsible for this edition of *Current Diagnosis*: John J. Hanley, President; Albert E. Meier, Editor in Chief; Lisette Bralow, Associate Medical Editor; Carol Robins Wolf, Copy Editor; Laura Tarves, Production Manager; and William Donnelly, Designer.

It is with deep regret that we acknowledge the death of the senior editor for the first six editions, Howard F. Conn. Howard died April 17, 1982, a time when the initial plans for this edition were being formulated. His contribution to medical publishing was truly unique. In addition to six editions of *Current Diagnosis,* he edited 35 annual editions of *Current Therapy* and, with Robert E. Rakel, two editions of *Family Practice.* Howard will be missed not only by his family, friends, and colleagues, but by an entire generation of American physicians who benefited from his editorial knowledge and skills.

REX B. CONN, M.D.

Contents

Section Three
EAR, NOSE, AND THROAT

Section Four
RESPIRATORY SYSTEM

Section Five
CARDIOVASCULAR SYSTEM

Section Six
BLOOD AND BLOOD-FORMING ORGANS

Section Seven
GASTROINTESTINAL TRACT

Section Eight
METABOLIC DISEASES

Section Nine
ENDOCRINE SYSTEM

Section Ten
NERVOUS SYSTEM AND MUSCLE

Section Eleven
PSYCHIATRY

Section Twelve
SKELETAL SYSTEM

Section Thirteen
GENITOURINARY SYSTEM

Section Nineteen
RECOGNIZABLE CONGENITAL SYNDROMES

Section Twenty
DISEASES OF UNKNOWN CAUSE

Section Twenty-One

Section One

CLINICAL PROBLEMS—DIFFERENTIAL DIAGNOSIS

FEVER OF UNKNOWN ORIGIN

By Eric B. Larson, M.D.
Seattle, Washington

and Robert G. Petersdorf, M.D.
La Jolla, California

Fever is a cardinal manifestation of disease that is encountered commonly in medical practices. Most febrile illnesses are brief, lasting less than 2 weeks. The cause is usually obvious and is most likely a viral or bacterial infection of the respiratory, urinary, or gastrointestinal tract. The fever and accompanying illness typically remit spontaneously or following specific therapy. When fever is prolonged or due to a more serious disease, such as pneumonia, neoplasm, tuberculosis, or abscess, the diagnosis can often be made without difficulty. Occasionally, however, a patient has a febrile illness in which the cause of fever is obscure and escapes recognition despite numerous attempts at determining the correct diagnosis. Patients with persistent unexplained fever are said to have "fever of unknown origin," or FUO.

The label FUO should be reserved for patients who meet fairly rigid criteria for the syndrome:

1. The presence of fever for at least 3 weeks.
2. A documented temperature of at least 38.3°C (101°F) on several occasions.
3. Failure to make the diagnosis after at least 1 week of intensive study.

These criteria eliminate patients with common, short-lived bacterial and viral infections, patients in whom the diagnosis is obvious, and patients with fever caused by the sequential occurrence of unrelated illnesses. The patient with FUO deserves a carefully executed and planned diagnostic approach, which is usually not required for febrile patients who fail to meet these criteria.

DIFFERENTIAL DIAGNOSIS

The differential diagnosis of FUO is long, complex, and imposing. Experience with FUO patients has yielded some general principles that make the diagnostic task easier. First, FUO is not usually caused by rare diseases; rather, most patients have relatively common diseases that present in an atypical fashion. Second, the patient's environment and personal characteristics are important in analyzing the clinical picture; the common causes of FUO in southeast Asia are different from those in the continental United States, and those of adults differ from those of children. Third, the patient frequently presents with a clinical clue, or clues, that when pursued with the differential diagnosis in mind, results in the correct diagnosis. Because a clue may have been overlooked, it is important to go over the patient again and again, repeating the history and physical examination, reviewing the chart and diagnostic studies, thinking about the patient's problem, and discussing it with colleagues.

The differential diagnosis is also simplified by dividing the causes of FUO into five categories: infections, neoplasms, connective tissue diseases, granulomatous diseases, and miscellaneous causes of fever. The frequency distribution of patients in these categories will vary from place to place. Table 1 lists some of the diseases causing FUO in the United States.

Infections

Pyogenic infections in the abdomen are common and easily overlooked in patients with FUO. As causes of FUO, they tend to occur in spaces that produce few localizing signs and symptoms. The clue to a *subphrenic abscess* may be an abnormal finding in the chest, such as a pleural effusion, or pain in the shoulder. *Liver abscess* may present with fever as the only symptom and sign. *Splenic abscesses* are usually associated with bacteremia of unknown source. *Diverticular abscess* occurs in older persons and may be suggested if fever occurs after an enema, or it may present with pneumaturia. Obstructive jaundice and fever should always suggest pyogenic hepatobiliary disease. In any case, attention must *always* be given to the abdomen as a location for cryptic infection causing prolonged, undiagnosed fever.

Although *tuberculosis* is becoming less common among native-born Americans, it is still a common cause of FUO. It is more likely to occur in nonwhites, and when it causes FUO, it is typically extrapulmonary. The tuberculin test may be positive or negative, but a negative PPD with a positive control indicating intact delayed hypersensitivity makes tuberculosis most unlikely. Prolonged infections in compromised hosts should suggest the possibility of *atypical mycobacterial, fungal,* or other opportunistic infections. Because fungal and mycobacterial diseases are common causes of FUO, mycobacterial and fungal cultures of biopsied tissue are usually indicated in patients with FUO.

Table 1. Diseases Responsible for Fever of Unknown Origin (FUO)

- Infections
  - Pyogenic infections
    - Abdominal, upper
      - Subphrenic abscess
      - Hepatic abscess
      - Subhepatic abscess
      - Splenic abscess
      - Cholecystitis, gallbladder empyema
      - Cholangitis
      - Lesser sac abscess
    - Abdominal, lower
      - Diverticular abscess
      - Appendiceal abscess
      - Pelvic abscess
    - Renal infections
    - Osteomyelitis
    - Sinusitis
    - Mycotic aneurysm
    - Wound infection
    - Catheter infection
  - Mycobacterial and granulomatous infections
    - *Mycobacterium tuberculosis*
    - Atypical mycobacterial infection
    - Fungal and higher bacterial infections (candidiasis, histoplasmosis, nocardiosis, actinomycosis)
  - Bacteremias
    - Subacute bacterial endocarditis
    - Brucellosis
    - Gonococcemia
    - Listeriosis
    - Meningococcemia
  - Viral, rickettsial, and chlamydial infections
    - Cytomegalovirus
    - Epstein-Barr virus (infectious mononucleosis)
    - Coxsackie B virus
    - Q fever
    - Psittacosis
  - Parasitic infections
    - Amebiasis
    - Trichinosis
    - Malaria
- Infections *(continued)*
  - Spirochetal infections
    - Syphilis
    - Borrelia recurrentis (relapsing fever)
- Neoplasms
  - Tumors of the reticuloendothelial system
    - Lymphoma, Hodgkin's disease
    - Leukemia
    - Malignant histiocytosis
    - Angioimmunoblastic lymphadenopathy
    - Lymphomatoid granulomatosis
  - Solid tumors
    - Hypernephroma
    - Hepatoma
    - Pancreatic carcinoma
    - Atrial myxoma
    - Other intra-abdominal tumors
  - Metastatic tumors
    - From gastrointestinal tract
    - From lung, kidneys, bone
    - Melanoma
- Collagen diseases
  - Systemic lupus erythematosus
  - Rheumatic fever
  - Still's disease (juvenile rheumatoid arthritis)
  - Giant cell arteritis or polymyalgia rheumatica
  - Polyarteritis nodosa
  - Hypersensitivity vasculitis
- Granulomatous diseases
  - Sarcoidosis
  - Regional enteritis, granulomatous colitis
  - Granulomatous hepatitis
  - Erythema nodosum
- Miscellaneous causes
  - Drug fever
  - Factitious fever
  - Multiple pulmonary emboli
  - Subacute thyroiditis
  - Hematomas, usually associated with cryptic trauma
  - Familial Mediterranean fever
  - Nonspecific pericarditis
  - Whipple's disease
- Undiagnosed FUO

Other common pyogenic infections cause FUO when their presenting signs and symptoms are overlooked or when they are not considered in the differential diagnosis. *Urinary tract infections* can cause prolonged fever when they are associated with *obstruction, abscess* formation, or anatomic abnormalities. *Osteomyelitis* may turn into FUO when back pain is overlooked or ignored. *Sinusitis* causing FUO may cause symptoms that the patient considers unimportant. Finally, a recent surgical scar or intravascular medical device should always be considered a possible source of infection and fever. Prompt detection of *wound* or *catheter infection* may obviate the need for an extensive FUO "workup."

Undiagnosed *subacute bacterial endocarditis* is a rare cause of FUO in these days of frequent and effective blood cultures. However, the diagnosis may be obfuscated in patients who receive antibiotics at the time cultures are taken. For this reason, patients with cardiac murmurs and intravenous drug abusers who are being evaluated for prolonged fever should have blood cultures taken for several days after antibiotics are discontinued, particularly if cultures were not taken before chemotherapy was instituted.

Patients with *infectious mononucleosis* may present with FUO, but the Monospot and heterophile agglutination tests plus the clinical picture should make the diagnosis easy. *Cytomegalovirus* infections also cause prolonged fever, lymphadenopathy, and chemical hepatitis.

Some infections are suggested by epidemiologic clues. *Brucellosis* occurs in animal workers (farmers, veterinarians, slaughterhouse personnel); *psittacosis* in parrot fanciers and pet store operators; *Q-fever* in persons tanning animal hides and in patients with culture-negative endocarditis; *malaria* in travelers to endemic areas; and *borreliosis* in patients with recurrent fever who have stayed in mountain cabins or have camped in tick-infested areas. *Amebiasis* usually causes FUO in persons traveling outside the United States when it is complicated by hepatic abscess or hepatitis.

Neoplasms

Neoplasms of the reticuloendothelial system are more likely to present with fever than are solid tumors. They cause problems in diagnosis when there is no overt evidence of abnormal tissue or when the pathologic diagnosis is uncertain. *Hodgkin's* and *non-Hodgkin's lymphoma* present as FUOs when the disease is confined to the abdomen or the retroperitoneal areas. The usual solution is to find abnormally enlarged or situated areas of lymphoid tissue by imaging techniques and then to obtain that tissue for pathologic study. When acute *leukemia* causes FUO, blast cells are usually not present in the peripheral smear. Anemia, leukopenia, and/or thrombocytopenia are common, and the diagnosis eventually becomes evident on examination of the bone marrow. Patients with a prior diagnosis of lymphoma or leukemia who have fever are usually suffering from an acute infection. Occasionally, obscure fever is the only sign of relapse in a patient who has enjoyed a period of remission from lymphoma.

Hypernephroma and *hepatoma* are solid tumors that are well known to cause prolonged fever. Other solid tumors causing FUO are usually located in the abdomen. Metastatic or local disease of the bone or lung will cause fever but rarely escapes detection. The clinical inaccessibility of parts of the abdomen has been markedly mitigated by ultrasonography, CT scanning, endoscopic retrograde cholangiopancreatography (ERCP), transhepatic cholangiography, and other imaging techniques. *Metastatic cancer* causing FUO is most likely to be present in the liver.

Patients with cancer and FUO frequently have few localizing signs on physical examination, and laboratory data may be nonspecific. Palpable masses, organomegaly, and abnormal liver chemistries are important clues. The diagnosis can be made definitively only by biopsy of lymph nodes, bone marrow, or abnormal masses.

Collagen or Connective Tissue Diseases

Most of the so-called collagen or connective tissue diseases present with fever either as a manifestation of the disease or one of its complications. Widely available and vastly improved diagnostic tests, like the antinuclear antibody test, have made it unusual for an illness like *systemic lupus erythematosus* (SLE) to cause FUO. Nonetheless, it is essential to determine by careful evaluation that infection is not causing fever in patients with SLE, rheumatoid arthritis, scleroderma, dermatomyositis, or other vasculitides. For patients receiving steroids or cytotoxic drugs, who are at even higher risk for infection, this distinction is particularly important.

The collagen diseases for which there are no serologic tests are more difficult to diagnose and seem to be more common causes of FUO. *Still's disease,* or juvenile rheumatoid arthritis, does occur in adults; is characterized by particularly high fevers, rash, intense arthralgias, and myalgias; and tends to be recurrent. *Giant cell arteritis* and *polymyalgia rheumatica* should be considered in older patients with fever and anemia, and *polyarteritis nodosa* tends to occur in men in their 40s and 50s. Giant cell arteritis may be diagnosed by temporal artery biopsy, whereas angiography should precede biopsy in polyarteritis nodosa.

Granulomatous Diseases

Both *sarcoidosis* and *erythema nodosum* commonly present with fever, and an exhaustive evaluation to find an alternative explanation for fever in these patients is usually not necessary. Fever is often the only manifestation of *granulomatous hepatitis.* A history of drug ingestion, especially antibiotics, can often be elicited. Often these patients will benefit from anti-inflammatory therapy, usually corticosteroids, if the fever does not remit spontaneously. Patients eventually diagnosed as having *granulomatous colitis* or *regional enteritis* may have prolonged fever in the absence of gastrointestinal symptoms.

Miscellaneous Causes

Although not reported as a frequent cause of FUO, drug fever should be considered in febrile patients because the treatment is very easy, consisting of removal of the offending agent and, if effective, obviates the need for extensive evaluation. *Factitious fever* should come to mind in febrile young women with a history of psychiatric illness; those closely associated with the health professions; and those with recurrent, unexplained bouts of pyrexia associated with atypical fever patterns. Table 1 lists some other miscellaneous causes of FUO, which should be considered in the differential diagnosis.

DIAGNOSTIC FAILURE

In 5 to 20 percent of patients with FUO, all attempts at diagnosis are futile. Fortunately, the fever usually disappears after several weeks and the patient recovers. In general, these patients look well despite fever, and, aside from a variety of laboratory abnormalities, the examination is noncontributory. The causes of resolved, undiagnosed FUO are generally thought to be hypersensitivity reactions or undiagnosed viral infections. A small group of patients have recurrent or prolonged fever that does not resolve spontaneously. These patients may require suppression of fever with steroids. In most of them, a definitive cause of fever is never established.

DIAGNOSTIC APPROACH

In the face of such a large number of diagnostic possibilities, there is no standard approach to the clinical problem of FUO. Each patient must be evaluated individually with careful history and thorough physical examination, which often bear repeating. Diagnostic procedures should be selected after careful consideration of the features of each case, with particular attention to the epidemiologic setting in which these illnesses occur and to clues, however subtle they may be. All previous diagnostic tests, records, and biopsies should be systematically reviewed. Before embarking on an elaborate workup, the obvious must not be overlooked. First, fever should be carefully documented. Discordant readings suggest manipulation of the thermometer; should such a pattern emerge, the diagnosis of factitious fever should be strongly suspected. If no fever is documented, the diagnostic workup should be postponed and the patient followed for recurrence of fever. Any drugs likely to cause drug fever, especially antibiotics, should be discontinued. Generally, this poses little or no risk to the patient. If the fever resolves, no further workup is necessary.

Laboratory Tests

Given the wide variety and large number of blood tests performed, it is surprising how infrequently they actually provide new information or help make the diagnosis. For this reason, blood tests should not be ordered reflexly but should be tailored to specific, ongoing diagnostic hypotheses. Among blood chemistries, the so-called liver enzymes (alkaline phosphatase, gamma glutamyl transferase, and transaminases) and muscle enzymes (creatine phosphokinase) may suggest disease in those organs causing fever. A complete blood count (CBC) and erythrocyte sedimentation rate (ESR) usually provide only nonspecific information. Anemia, leukopenia, and thrombocytopenia may be clues to preleukemia. A bone marrow biopsy is useful to confirm this diagnosis. Immunologic tests are frequently requested in evaluating FUO patients, but they rarely yield useful diagnostic information, presumably because immunologic diseases have been culled out by these tests before fever became prolonged.

Among the most useful laboratory tests are microbiologic studies. Sequential blood cultures, but no more than four to six, should be incubated both aerobically and anaerobically. Biopsy or surgical specimens should be appropriately stained and cultured for bacteria, acid-fast bacilli (AFB), and fungi. If disseminated tuberculosis or mycosis is suspected, bone marrow or tissue biopsy specimens are frequently the only means for making the diagnosis. Serologic tests for amebiasis or brucellosis are occasionally helpful.

Radiographic Studies and Diagnostic Ultrasound

Although chest x-rays are often considered "routine," they may provide evidence for tuberculosis, lymphoma, carcinoma, or an abnormal diaphragm contour suggesting subphrenic abscess. The intravenous pyelogram, sinus x-rays, spine films, and upper gastrointestinal tract (GI) series are of value if there are other clues suggesting disease in these organ systems.

Ultrasonography has become an important aid to detection of intra-abdominal disease. It is likely to be helpful in detection of subphrenic, subhepatic, splenic, and occasionally hepatic abscess as well as adenopathy and other masses in the abdomen or retroperitoneum. Computed tomography (CT) is extremely helpful in many of the same conditions. Both CT scanning and ultrasonography are especially useful in "opening up" the abdomen. Computed tomography has replaced lymphangiography as the best way to image the retroperitoneum. False-positive and false-negative results, however, are still a problem even with such sensitive techniques as CT scans.

Angiography is rarely needed. However, an occasional patient with polyarteritis nodosa may be diagnosed with aortography and renal angiography. Cardiac ultrasound should not be routine but may suggest the correct diagnosis in cardiac myxoma.

Radioisotope Scans

Among radioisotope scans, the liver-spleen scan is perhaps the most useful, given the frequency with which pathology, especially abscess, is found in those organs. The gallium scan, in our experience, is not sufficiently accurate to be considered a first-line study, primarily because false-positive and false-negative results are very frequent and tend to be extremely misleading. However, an occasional patient with intra-abdominal abscess is diagnosable only with this technique. Lung scans are helpful when pulmonary emboli are suspected. Most patients with prolonged fever owing to osteomyelitis have x-ray changes and do not require a bone scan, but the bone scan is clearly useful in patients with fever, bone pain, and no x-ray changes. New and promising radioisotope imaging techniques appear frequently. Currently, the one in vogue is Indium 111 (^{111}In) leukocyte scanning. Its role in the diagnostic evaluation of FUO remains to be determined.

Examination of Tissue

Histologic examination of tissue is often the quickest, most efficient, and least expensive method of establishing a diagnosis of FUO. The bone marrow biopsy is frequently useful in diagnosing leukemia, lymphoma, tuberculosis, or metastatic disease. It should be considered in all patients with an abnormal CBC. Lymph node biopsy is often diagnostic, provided the node(s) is abnormally located or significantly enlarged. Temporal artery biopsy may be useful in diagnosing giant cell arteritis and should be performed in older persons with unexplained fever, mild headache, generalized aches and pains, and an elevated sedimentation rate. Muscle biopsy should be done in patients with suspected vasculitis or myositis, particularly if the limb is painful. Biopsies of other tissues such as skin, lung, gastrointestinal tract, or bone are useful when there are clues pointing to an abnormality in these organs. Liver biopsy is most useful in granulomatous hepatitis, but it should not be considered a routine procedure in FUO.

Exploratory laparotomy remains an important and direct approach to the diagnosis of FUO, particularly when pyogenic infection of the right upper quadrant or intra-abdominal carcinomatosis is suspected. However, "blind" laparotomy should be discouraged when there are no clinical signs, imaging studies or other data that clearly point to the abdomen as the source of fever. An FUO "work-up" does not include routine exploration of the abdomen, and this practice cannot be condoned.

Therapeutic Trials

In general, therapeutic trials add confusion to an already confusing situation and they should be employed only as a last resort. When they are used, these trials should be as specific as possible and should be aimed at a single disease that might be causing fever.

Nonspecific use of antibiotics in patients with FUO often obfuscates the clinical picture and impedes arriving at the correct diagnosis. These drugs should be used only after careful consideration of the problem and then for the most likely infection, not "several." The undesirable consequences of therapeutic trials, including drug toxicity, superinfection, interference with culture results, and misinterpretation of a coincidental fall in temperature, should be carefully weighed against their potential benefits.

CONCLUSIONS

The excitement of making the correct diagnosis in FUO is enhanced by the knowledge that the patient, once diagnosed correctly, is likely to benefit from therapy. Except for patients with malignancy, most patients with FUO either will be cured or will improve dramatically with specific medical or surgical therapy. Therefore, it is incumbent upon every physician to pursue the diagnosis conscientiously and with vigor. Each patient should be considered a unique intellectual challenge for whom a "shotgun" diagnostic workup is inappropriate. More importantly such a patient is a sick and distressed individual who deserves the most thoughtful and compassionate care of which we physicians are capable.

THE ACUTE INFECTIOUS DISEASE SYNDROME

By Richard H. Glew, M.D.
Worcester, Massachusetts

The patient with an acute infectious disease may present with diverse complaints and physical signs, and it is critically important for the physician to recognize the varied clinical clues that suggest that an infection may be responsible for the patient's illness. Although the most common manifestation of infection is fever, the febrile response may be blunted or absent during an acute infection in many patients such as neonates, the aged, and patients with renal failure or those receiving therapy with corticosteroids, salicylates, or other nonsteroidal anti-inflammatory agents. Moreover, fever commonly occurs in many noninfectious illnesses, including collagen vascular diseases; allergic reactions (to drugs, blood products); neoplastic diseases (especially lymphomas, primary and metastatic tumors of the liver, renal cell carcinoma, and, less often, colon carcinoma); hemorrhage (retroperitoneal, subarachnoid, intra-articular); microcrystalline arthritis (gout, pseudogout); and pulmonary embolism. Nevertheless, it is prudent to consider that fever is due to infection until extensive diagnostic efforts have failed to document an infection. Most infectious diseases do not produce characteristic fever profiles. Classically, patients with malaria exhibit regular febrile cycles, with chills and fevers occurring every third day counting the day of occurrence as the first day (tertian pattern, seen with *Plasmodium vivax, P. ovale,* and *P. falciparum*) or every 72 hours (quartan pattern, seen with *P. malariae*); however, most patients who reside in areas nonendemic for malaria and who acquire infection during travel manifest hectic, unremitting symptoms rather than classic periodicity. A biphasic, camel-backed fever course is commonly noted in patients with leptospirosis or dengue, but these illnesses are relatively uncommon in the United States and are usually seen in patients with a history of animal exposure (leptospirosis) or travel (dengue).

Chills may occur in patients experiencing abrupt, rapid temperature rises, but true bone-shaking, teeth-rattling chills (rigors) are strongly suggestive of an acute bacterial infection (although malaria commonly is associated with repeated, dramatic rigors as well). A single chill is commonly one of the earliest symptoms noted by patients with pneumococcal pneumonia, cellulitis, and erysipelas. Repeated chills in a patient with pneumonia should suggest the likelihood of necrotizing pneumonia involving *Staphylococcus aureus* or gram-negative bacilli such as Klebsiella. Recurrent chills and hectic fevers are common in patients with localized, pyogenic infections (abscesses, cholangitis).

HISTORY

The first priority in the evaluation of a patient suspected of harboring an infectious disease is to determine whether the patient's past history indicates a predisposition to infections that are likely to be fulminant or fatal. This predisposition may be due to (1) the debilitating nature of the underlying disease (e.g., acute leukemia, obstructing lung carcinoma, and chronic renal, cardiac, or pulmonary insufficiency); (2) the severity of the associated infection (e.g., *S. aureus* bacteremia-endocarditis in a hemodialysis patient or parenteral drug abuser, gram-negative bacillary pneumonia or peritonitis in the chronic alcoholic, *Pneumocystis carinii* pneumonia in a patient with lymphoma); or (3) the adverse interaction of host and parasite (e.g., *Streptococcus pneumoniae* bacteremia in asplenic patients, Salmonella infections in patients with hemoglobinopathies). In recent years, severe infections due to opportunistic pathogens (e.g., *P. carinii* pneumonia, intestinal cryptosporidiosis, nontuberculous mycobacterial infection) have been described in patients with the acquired immunodeficiency syndrome (AIDS), which occurs primarily in promiscuous homosexual men but also is seen in parenteral drug abusers and in a few other high-risk groups.

Epidemiology. Are there epidemiologic clues in the patient's history that may suggest specific infectious causes? The patient's geographic and ethnologic roots may reveal exposure to appropriate animals or animal products as a source of brucellosis, bovine tuberculosis, or echinococcosis. Recent exotic travel may have exposed the patient to malaria, dengue, typhoid fever, hepatitis (A, B, or non-A, non-B), amebiasis, giardiasis, yellow fever, or leishmaniasis. However, even within the continental United States there are regional and seasonal variations in the distribution of infections: coccidioidomycosis in the southwestern United States, histoplasmosis largely in the Mississippi and Ohio river valleys, babesiosis and Lyme disease along the northeast coastal regions and adjacent offshore islands, and plague from the Rocky Mountains westward. Despite its name, Rocky Mountain spotted fever is most commonly acquired during the warm months along the mid-Atlantic coast, particularly in the Carolinas. The various arbovirus encephalitides exhibit characteristic distribution as to locale and season (usually summer incidence in temperate areas). Occupational and avocational history may reveal exposure to sporotrichosis (gardeners), anthrax (handlers of raw wool, hides, or bones, especially products originating outside the United States), brucellosis (slaughterhouse workers), tularemia (hunters or trappers of rabbits, squirrels, muskrats, or other rodents), leptospirosis (exposure to rats, cattle, dogs), toxoplasmosis (cat owners, especially if involved in the handling of litter boxes), psittacosis (parrots, pigeons), or salmonellosis (turtles). A history of animal-related trauma may suggest cat-scratch disease (typically via scratches or bites by young cats), *Pasteurella multocida* cellulitis or osteomyelitis (penetrating bite by cat or dog), or rabies (skunks, bats, foxes, dogs, and cats).

Knowledge of any illness in members of the patient's household and community may be important. Many viral syndromes such as influenza and enterovirus infections exhibit seasonal clusterings with notable peaks of incidence in the community. Such viral illnesses as well as infections due to *Mycoplasma pneumoniae* and Group A Streptococcus tend to spread throughout families, often with widely varying manifestations in different family members. One should ask if any member of the household has ever had tuberculosis, or if anyone has recently been ill with hepatitis or dysentery.

In the case of a febrile patient recently hospitalized or otherwise under medical care, additional historical avenues must be explored. Recent anesthesia predisposes patients to pulmonary infections. A history of antecedent dental manipulation may provide a clue to the diagnosis of bacterial endocarditis. Administration of antibiotics may alter a patient's normal endogenous microbial flora, increasing susceptibility to colonization and infection by drug-resistant and often unusual organisms, including gram-negative bacteria and fungi. Corticosteroids produce broad, potent immunosuppression and may predispose the patient to opportunistic infections by a variety of organisms. Moreover, many chronic illnesses are commonly associated with a tendency to develop specific infectious problems: staphylococcal pyarthrosis in patients with rheumatoid arthritis, pneumococcal peritonitis in children with nephrotic syndrome, brain abscess in patients with cyanotic congenital heart disease, gram-negative peritonitis in patients with cirrhosis, and malignant external otitis (with *Pseudomonas aeruginosa*) in patients with diabetes mellitus.

Symptoms. Localization of the infection in a patient may be facilitated by a history of pain (headache, pleurisy, flank pain, joint or bone pain), organ dysfunction (altered consciousness, cough, symptoms of congestive heart failure, dysuria), or organ irritability (diarrhea, urinary frequency). Unfortunately, many systemic, febrile illnesses, including viral infections (influenza, infectious mononucleosis), severe bacterial infections (endocarditis, Salmonella enteric fever), and protozoan infections (malaria) commonly produce spuriously localizing complaints such as headache, low back pain, arthralgias, and abdominal pain.

The temporal sequence of symptoms often provides guidance in determining the alacrity with which medical evaluation should be accomplished. A rapidly fulminant clinical course in a critically ill, febrile patient mandates a rapidly paced diagnostic evaluation and prompt therapeutic intervention, whereas a patient with a protracted, insidious history warrants a more studied, laborious approach. Moreover, the evolution of clinical events and the occurrence of seemingly unrelated symptoms may shed light on the patient's more obvious presenting complaint. For example, a prior history of otitis media or sinusitis may be recalled in the history of a patient subsequently brought to the physician with meningitis or brain abscess; the patient with staphylococcal pneumonia often relates a history of initial recovery from an earlier influenza syndrome, followed by the appearance of a productive cough, chest pain, fever, and chills; and the patient with monoarticular gonococcal pyarthrosis commonly describes recent migratory polyarthralgias and papulopustular skin eruption.

PHYSICAL EXAMINATION

Examination of the skin and mucous membranes may provide a variety of diagnostic clues in the infected patient. A primary infection of the skin (cellulitis, lymphangitis) may be noted. There may be evidence of disseminated infection such as the pustular lesions of staphylococcal or gonococcal septicemia, the petechial rash of Rocky Mountain spotted fever or meningococcemia, the varied rashes of secondary syphilis, the papulovesicular lesions of varicella, and the many dermatologic manifestations (subungual or conjunctival splinter hemorrhages, Osler's nodes, Janeway lesions) of bacterial endocarditis. Cutaneous eruptions may reflect infection on the basis of toxin production (scarlet fever) or immunologic mechanisms (erythema nodosum). Finally, exanthems (often characteristic) may be seen in patients with noninfectious febrile illnesses such as drug reactions, sarcoidosis, juvenile rheumatoid arthritis, and systemic lupus erythematosus. The patient with one of the severe systemic vasculitides may exhibit bilateral, palpable purpuric lesions or necrotic papules over the extremities. The optic fundi should be examined for evidence of endocarditis (Roth spots), disseminated candidiasis (fungal endophthalmitis), or miliary tuberculosis (choroidal tubercles). Enlarged lymph nodes may indicate an infection in the region drained by the nodes or may be a manifestation of systemic disease (infectious mononucleosis, secondary syphilis, miliary tuberculosis, lymphoma). Moreover, there may be prominent regional lymph nodes draining the site of primary cutaneous inoculation with infectious agents that subsequently have produced disseminated infection: tularemia, plague, syphilis, lymphogranuloma venereum, and cat-scratch disease.

Examination of the chest may demonstrate the presence of an effusion of pneumonia; however, in viral and mycoplasma pneumonia, physical findings may be minimal despite the demonstration of extensive pulmonary involvement by chest roentgenogram, and effusions, when present, are small. Auscultation of the heart may disclose a rub typical of pericarditis or murmurs suggestive of endocarditis. Examination of the abdomen may demonstrate diffuse tenderness and guarding suggestive of peritonitis or local findings related to cholecystitis, appendicitis or abscess. Occasionally, impressive abdominal findings (tenderness, diminished bowel sounds) can be seen in patients with extraperitoneal infections such as pyelonephritis or lower lobe pneumonia. Splenomegaly may be due to local disease (splenic abscess or infarction) but more commonly occurs as part of a systemic infection such as bacterial endocarditis, malaria, brucellosis, or typhoid fever as well as in noninfectious conditions such as lymphoma and various collagen vascular diseases. Examination of bones and joints for local tenderness or swelling, effusion, or restricted motion may suggest pyarthrosis, osteomyelitis, or systemic rheumatologic disease such as rheumatoid arthritis, systemic lupus erythematosus, or gout. Rectal and pelvic examination may demonstrate prostatic abscess, perirectal abscess, or pelvic inflammatory disease (including pelvic abscess). Abnormalities found on neurologic examination can suggest meningitis, encephalitis, brain abscess, or cerebral infarction secondary to septic emboli.

LABORATORY FINDINGS

The hematologic hallmarks of pyogenic bacterial infection are neutrophilic leukocytosis, increase in the number of immature granulocytes, and the presence within neutrophils of vacuolization and toxic granulation. However, severe and overwhelming infection due to bacterial septicemia or typhoid fever may be associated with neutropenia, and neutrophilic leukocytosis has been described in patients with several viral infections (influenzal pneumonia) or granulomatous infections such as miliary tuberculosis. Eosinophilia can be seen in patients with trichinosis, drug reactions, and exfoliative skin disorders including scarlet fever. Red blood cell production may be suppressed by a variety of infections, but anemia (usually normochromic and normocytic) is most likely to occur in chronic infections. Hemolysis with acute onset of anemia may be seen in bacteremia due to *Clostridium perfringens.* Although the causative mechanisms are poorly understood, anemia in malaria may be moderately severe and out of proportion to the level of parasitemia.

A chest roentgenogram may reveal evidence of pneumonia, pulmonary infarction, lymphadenopathy, or pericardial or pleural effusion, all of which can be inapparent on physical examination. An abdominal roentgenogram may reveal the presence of genitourinary stones, renal calcification due to tuberculosis, peritonitis, free intraperitoneal air indicative of rupture of a viscus, bowel displacement or spasm secondary to an adjacent abscess, or intraluminal air-fluid levels suggestive of functional or anatomic obstruction.

Examination of the urinary sediment may demonstrate pyuria suggestive of urinary tract infection. Microscopic hematuria is compatible with bacterial endocarditis, collagen vascular disease (systemic lupus erythematosus, polyarteritis nodosa, Wegener's granulomatosis), or renal tuberculosis but may also be seen with bacterial urinary tract infections, particularly cystitis.

Abnormal collections of fluid, including pleural effusions, ascites, joint effusions, and pericardial effusions, should be aspirated diagnostically (and often therapeutically for relief of pain or mechanical compromise) unless the procedure would be technically dangerous or the fluid collection is seemingly unrelated to an obvious focus elsewhere. A lumbar puncture to obtain cerebrospinal fluid must be performed immediately if there is any possibility of meningitis, and should be included in the initial evaluation of the critically ill, febrile patient whose sensorium is difficult to interpret, such as with infants and the demented. It is important to remember that the diagnostic value of such fluids may be reduced after antibiotic therapy has been instituted. All such body fluids should be subjected to cell counts, Gram stain, and determination of sugar and protein concentrations. Special studies may be indicated, including polarizing microscopy of joint fluids for crystals, acid-fast stain of fluids in cases of possible tuberculosis, determination of rheumatoid factor titers, and serologic testing of cerebrospinal fluid (CSF) for syphilis reactivity. In the patient suspected of having pneumonia, sputum should be obtained for Gram stain and culture (as well as for acid-fast stain and culture in the patient with possible pulmonary tuberculosis). In most patients, an adequate specimen can be obtained by expectoration, aided by direct supervision by a physician. If spontaneous efforts are unsuccessful, chest physical therapy plus ultrasonic nebulization under the direction of a respiratory technician often will produce a satisfactory sputum specimen (i.e., containing polymorphonuclear leukocytes and few squamous cells). In the unconscious patient, nasotracheal suctioning may be utilized. Transtracheal aspiration should be employed only in a cooperative, alert patient without bleeding diathesis in whom there is a likelihood of bacterial pneumonia but who is unable to produce expectorated sputum, particularly when unusual pathogens (e.g., gram-negative bacilli or anaerobes) are suspected to be present. Gram or Wright stains of stool specimens may reveal the presence of polymorphonuclear neutrophils, suggestive of inflammatory diarrhea due to Salmonella or Shigella, pseudomembranous colitis, or inflammatory bowel disease.

The clinical microbiology laboratory is of tremendous value, since cultures of various body fluids can confirm the presence of an infectious disease and provide positive identification and indicate susceptibility of the invading organism to various antimicrobial agents. Specimens of blood (at least two samples from separate venipunctures) and urine (well-supervised clean-catch or catheterized specimen) should be routinely obtained. Any purulent drainage, easily aspirated collections of pus, abnormal body fluid collections (joint, pericardial or pleural fluid, ascites), and CSF (when central nervous system infection is suspected) should be cultured routinely for bacteria. Special handling and plating techniques to ensure survival of anaerobic organisms should be utilized when infection due to anaerobes is suspected (intra-abdominal or intrapelvic infections, foul odor, gas in tissues). Similarly, special media should be utilized if disease due to mycobacteria or fungi is suspected, although some fungi, including Candida species and *Cryptococcus neoformans,* are able to grow on routine bacterial media. Although viral diagnostic laboratories are not commonly available and their services are frequently expensive, the isolation of a significant viral pathogen (e.g., cytomegalovirus) may enable the physician to make a definitive diagnosis and avoid further diagnostic evaluation.

Serologic tests are widely available and are often of more value than the virology laboratory in confirming the diagnosis of viral infection as well as infections due to other organisms (*Mycoplasma pneumoniae, Legionella pneumophila,* leptospira, and rickettsiae), which are difficult to isolate from patients. However, since a rising or falling (at least fourfold) serologic titer is more indicative of recent infection than a single positive titer, which may simply indicate prior infection, serologic tests usually provide only retrospective or confirmatory diagnostic information. Nevertheless, on admission, patients with an enigmatic clinical picture should have serum frozen and stored for possible later use in serologic testing. On the other hand, the presence of cryptococcal antigen in cerebrospinal fluid can be detected quickly by immunologic testing and is the most sensitive test available for diagnosing cryptococcal meningitis. Similarly, the presence of the heterophile antibody is indicative of infectious mononucleosis due to the Epstein-Barr virus. Several studies have suggested potential value in the rapid detection of bacterial or fungal antigens by counter-immunoelectrophoresis or chromatographic methods, but the clinical utility of these tests is not yet known.

Skin tests, particularly those of the delayed hypersensitivity type (e.g., tuberculin), may be of diagnostic value. However, a positive skin test simply indicates that exposure to the antigen has occurred in the past and does not signify active infection. Moreover, anergy is commonly seen in patients with lymphoma, sarcoidosis, terminal malignancy, or overwhelming infection such as miliary tuberculosis; it may occur temporarily in patients with viral illnesses such as mumps, measles, and smallpox and may decline temporarily following immunization against these viruses.

Although abnormalities of blood chemistries may reflect nonspecific manifestations of severe infection, they may also indicate primary or predominant involvement of a specific organ. Abnormalities of liver function studies occur in patients with viral hepatitis, cholangitis, leptospirosis, infectious mononucleosis, or liver abscess (bacterial or amebic). Renal function abnormalities may occur in patients with bacterial septicemia and shock, acute pyelonephritis with bilateral papillary necrosis, disseminated candidiasis, leptospirosis, severe falciparum malaria, or fulminant vasculitis.

Infrequently, it may be necessary to obtain biopsy material for histopathologic examination and culture in order to establish a diagnosis. Caseating tubercles in pleura, bone marrow, lymph nodes, or liver are strongly suggestive of tuberculosis but can also be seen in patients with disseminated histoplasmosis and brucellosis, whereas noncaseating tubercles are characteristic of sarcoidosis. Muscle biopsy is often helpful in the diagnosis of trichinosis. Finally, lung biopsy (transbronchial via bronchoscopy or as an open surgical procedure) may be necessary for prompt diagnosis of opportunistic pulmonary infection in the immunocompromised host with fever and pulmonary infiltrates.

CHEST PAIN

By Robert E. Albertini, M.D.
and Frederick L. Jones, Jr., M.D.
Danville, Pennsylvania

Chest pain, although one of the commonest symptoms encountered in clinical practice, often represents a major diagnostic challenge. Its many and varied sources include the skin and its deeper structures, musculoskeletal and neural components of the chest wall, parietal pleura, major bronchi, myocardium, pericardium, other mediastinal structures, cervical spine, and abdominal viscera. Occasionally it is of psychogenic origin.

HISTORY

A carefully taken history is the most important part of the diagnostic process. Attentive listening, supplemented when necessary by specific questions, should elicit the following characteristics of the patient's pain: location, intensity, duration, frequency, radiation, circumstances causing aggravation or relief, associated symptoms, the patient's perceived need for and use of analgesics, and whether or not pain interferes with activities.

EXAMINATION

The examination should begin while taking the history by carefully observing the patient's facial expressions, tone of voice, position, and use of the hands to describe and localize pain. Obviously severe pain, hypotension, marked tachycardia, sweating, painfully restricted breathing, pallor, cyanosis, high fever, and agitation are critical signs. Careful palpation of the bony thorax should be carried out, lightly at first, but then with firm pressure using two fingers in the area where pain is described and also over the costochondral, chondrosternal, and xiphisternal areas and the cervical and dorsal vertebrae. Muscle groups in the area should be firmly compressed or squeezed and the shoulders and dorsal and cervical spines put through their full ranges of motion. Auscultation of the heart and lungs is primarily of value in detecting pneumothorax, pleural or pericardial friction rubs, cardiac murmurs, gallop rhythm, and signs of pleural fluid or pulmonary consolidation. Finally, the abdomen should be examined for signs of subdiaphragmatic inflammatory processes and the extremities for evidence of thrombophlebitis or inequality of the arterial circulation. A tentative diagnosis or at least a narrow differential list should now be possible.

LABORATORY STUDIES

Posteroanterior and lateral chest roentgenograms and usually an electrocardiogram are obtained routinely as part of the initial evaluation. Additional studies may be indicated, but these should be selected as a second step and tailored to the differential diagnosis. They may include radiographic studies of the decubitus thorax, ribs, cervical spine, and dorsal spine; lung scans; bronchoscopy; thoracentesis and pleural biopsy; cardiac exercise studies; echocardiography; aortic and pulmonary angiography; cardiac enzyme determinations; assessment of venous patency in the lower extremities; barium esophagram and esophageal motility studies; and radiographic contrast, ultrasonographic, and endoscopic evaluation of the upper abdominal structures.

THE DECISION PROCESS

The evaluation of chest pain requires a series of decisions. The first is whether or not a disease process that may represent an immediate threat to life is possibly responsible for the pain. Here it is helpful to recall that critical illnesses usually cause acute, often severe, pain and frequently are accompanied by such distressing features as pleurisy, intense dyspnea, cyanosis, tachycardia, sweating, high fever, hypotension, and restlessness. The patient perceives he is ill and usually presents as an emergency. Chest pain unlikely to be of immediate life-threatening etiology has often been recurrent over days or weeks, is unassociated with the physical signs just noted, and does not interfere with daily activities or prompt the patient to take medication. It is usually described with concern but not fright. A list of symptoms and findings that aid in making this distinction is represented in Table 1. There are many gradations between these two predominant presentations. Nonetheless, after a careful evaluation, the correct decision can usually be made rather easily.

The next decision, actually a corollary of the first, concerns the urgency of the evaluation and where it should be carried out. Potentially life-threatening illnesses require immediate assessment where full diagnostic facilities are available, i.e., in an emergency room or inpatient facilities of a hospital. Otherwise, an ambulatory setting is satisfactory, with selected studies being performed in an orderly scheduled manner.

Table 1. Differential Features in Evaluation of Chest Pain

Urgent Hospital-Based Evaluation Advisable	Orderly Ambulatory Evaluation Appropriate
Acute, obviously severe pain	Pain recurrent over weeks to months
Presence of risk factors for or past history of coronary or thromboembolic disease	No interference with activities
Physical findings of	Analgesics not used
Hypotension	Associated with localized chest wall tenderness
Rapid tachycardia	Aggravated by motion of neck or shoulders
Cyanosis	Patient concerned but not alarmed
Profuse sweating	
High fever	
Agitation	
Signs of congestive heart failure	
Signs of deep thrombophlebitis	
Pleural or cardiac friction rub	
Abdominal tenderness or rigidity	
Inequality of arterial circulation	

Eventually, a third decision is necessary as to the precise etiology of the pain or, if this is uncertain, the possible causes that must be further investigated. This determines what kind of further laboratory evaluation—and eventually what kind of treatment—is indicated. Accordingly, it is appropriate to consider individually those disorders that are responsible for chest pain in all but a small fraction of those who present with this compaint.

CHEST WALL PAIN

The most common cause of chest pain in adults is strain of the costochondral or chondosternal joints. Here, a careful history is virtually diagnostic. Discomfort may be sharp and brief or dull and aching. The pain is intermittent and does not seem to require analgesics or suspension of usual activities. The pain is often aggravated by motion of the trunk, especially rolling over in bed. Radiation to the shoulder or arm, but rarely the forearm, is common. A highly important and virtually diagnostic clue appears when patients are asked to show where the pain occurs and they point with one or two fingers to a site on the anterior thorax. Surprisingly, a history of specific stress or direct trauma is rarely obtained. Careful palpation with successive pressure on each of the second through fifth costochondral and chondrosternal joints invariably elicits tenderness at one or more of these sites. *Tietze's syndrome*—tender swelling of a costochondral junction—is quite rare, much overemphasized, and of the same etiology and prognosis as simple ligamentous strain at these joints. Occasionally, the xiphisternal joint may be solely involved (*xiphodynia*).

There are numerous other causes of chest wall pain. *Herpes zoster* presents as burning pain along a thoracic dermatome with the characteristic cutaneous eruption present or eventually appearing. *Mondor's syndrome* is a form of thrombophlebitis involving a subcutaneous vein in the anterior axilla; it is identified by palpating a thick tender cord lateral to the breast. *Gynecomastia,* if it is the cause of chest pain, is readily obvious on physical examination. *Rib fractures* that are due to trauma or coughing are associated with highly tender areas over the ribs in the midaxillary or anterior axillary line. *Intercostal neuritis* often appears in epidemic form and causes a superficial lancinating or electric shock pain along a thoracic dermatome which is aggravated by motion, cough, and sneezing but—unlike pleural pain—not by deep breathing. Finally, a variety of *"rheumatic" causes* related to strains of muscles and their ligamentous attachments to bone and joints may cause pain. Sometimes a specific act of overexertion—e.g., splitting logs or heavy lifting—may be recalled by the patient, but frequently the precise precipitating event is inapparent. Pain of this etiology either is sharp, momentary, and precipitated by motion or is aching and poorly localized. Rest in the position of maximum comfort invariably brings relief.

PULMONARY AND PLEURAL PAIN

The pulmonary parenchyma and the visceral pleura are devoid of pain receptors, whereas the parietal pleura has rich sensory innervation. Consequently, even extensive lung lesions are not painful unless the parietal pleura or chest wall becomes involved by the disease process. Pleural pain (pleurisy) is highly characteristic, being distinguished by its sharp, unilateral, stabbing features and its clear relationship to inspiration and sudden movements of the thorax. Coughing and sneezing may produce intense distress. The patient often seeks relief by lying on the affected side or, when upright, by bending the trunk in that direction. Irritation of the central diaphragmatic pleura causes radiation of pain to the shoulder top. When the peripheral diaphragmatic pleura is involved, pain may be felt solely in the distribution of lower thoracic dermatomes extending as far down as the iliac crest; commonly an acute abdominal illness is the initial impression. A pleural friction rub heard on auscultation is diagnostic, but this finding is not invariably present.

Pleuritic pain can occur in a variety of conditions and ranges in severity from mild to intense. *Acute bacterial pneumonia* and *pulmonary embolism* are the most common causes of acute pleuritis. Pulmonary emboli rarely occur without risk factors being present (see article on this topic). Fever greater than 38.5°C (101.3°F), shaking chills, leukocytosis greater than 15,000/cu mm, purulent sputum, and a predominant organism on Gram stain of the sputum favor the diagnosis of pneumonia. Tachycardia, tachypnea, percussion dullness, bronchial breathing, rales, and a pleural rub are common to both disorders and hence are not helpful as distinguishing features. Pulmonary infiltrates may be present in both, but the absence of an infiltrate makes pneumonia unlikely. Pulmonary ventilation and perfusion scanning is of diagnostic value if the scans show unmatched defects that are clearly of a segmental or lobar nature. Otherwise, pulmonary angiography will be required. Arterial blood gases will determine the severity of hypoxemia, but they are of no benefit in the differential diagnosis.

When pleuritic pain is associated with hemoptysis, *bronchogenic carcinoma* with malignant pleural effusion should be considered; in this instance, fiberoptic bronchoscopy is often diagnostic. The pain of *malignant pleural effusion* is insidious in onset and is usually a constant, boring ache increased by deep breathing. Weight loss, a strong smoking history, or a previous known malignancy (particularly in breast, lung, ovary, or gastrointestinal tract) strongly favors the diagnosis. When pleural fluid is present (best demonstrated on the lateral decubitus view), thoracentesis and pleural biopsy will often lead to the diagnosis. *Malignant mesothelioma* is the only primary malignancy of the pleura. A history of asbestos exposure is apparent in approximately 75 percent of patients with this rare tumor. Open biopsy is usually required for the diagnosis. *Connective tissue diseases* commonly have associated pleural disease at some point in their course. The diagnosis is usually apparent from associated multisystemic abnormalities and the assessment of serologic markers such as rheumatoid factor and antinuclear antibody (ANA).

Pneumothorax may occur spontaneously or as a result of trauma. It should be strongly considered in relatively tall, thin young persons with acute onset of pleuritic pain and dyspnea, as well as in older patients with chronic obstructive lung disease. In anyone who has suffered recent trauma, *hemothorax* or *hemopneumothorax* may be the culprit. Chest roentgenograms are diagnostic in all these conditions.

CARDIAC PAIN

Fear that chest pain is caused by heart disease motivates most persons to seek medical evaluation. A carefully taken history usually excludes or suggests this possibility more effectively than examination or laboratory studies. The pain of *myocardial ischemia* ranges from that of angina pectoris to myocardial infarction. Typically, angina is seen in persons over 35 years of age and is provoked repeatedly by exertion, emotional stress, and heavy meals. It is perceived as requiring rest, which brings relief within a few minutes, and described—often with a fist against the sternum—as pressing, heavy, or squeezing rather than painful. Pain may radiate to the shoulders, arms, inner forearms, neck, and jaws. Coronary insufficiency or myocardial infarction causes similar pain, but it is usually more severe and accompanied by profuse sweating, restlessness, and fear of death. The electrocardiogram may be indicative or suggestive of myocardial infarction, or it may be nondiagnostic. When clinical suspicion remains high, the patient requires hospitalization for cardiac monitoring and serial cardiac enzymes and electrocardiograms.

Chest pain may also occur with valvular or myocardial disease. *Asymmetrical septal hypertrophy* and *aortic valvular insufficiency* may cause angina by decreasing coronary blood flow and creating increased myocardial oxygen demand. The former may be suspected in the presence of a systolic ejection murmur that does not radiate well to the base of the heart and a double-peaked carotid pulse. Echocardiography is diagnostic. The decrescendo diastolic murmur of aortic valvular insufficiency provides the diagnostic clue to this condition. Echocardiography and left heart catheterization confirm the diagnosis and quantitate the degree of insufficiency. Patients with *mitral valve prolapse* may also experience nondescript recurrent pain. Characteristically, a midsystolic click is followed by a late systolic murmur; however, one or both of these findings may be absent. The diagnosis is easily made by echocardiography.

The pain of *pericarditis* may be pleuritic in nature, but it is more commonly described as steady, substernal, aggravated by swallowing, and relieved by bending forward. Pericarditis is frequently characterized by a two- or three-component friction rub, best heard with the patient leaning forward. If large amounts of pericardial fluid are present, heart sounds are diminished and signs of peripheral hypoperfusion may be present. The electrocardiogram frequently shows characteristic changes consisting of nonreciprocal ST segment elevation with subsequent T-wave inversion. When enough fluid is present to cause tamponade, pain usually is a minor symptom and findings related to decreased cardiac output predominate. Echocardiography is the preferred method for assessing pericardial effusion. Open pericardial biopsy is often indicated to establish the exact etiology.

PULMONARY HYPERTENSION

Increased pulmonary arterial pressure may cause pain which mimics that of myocardial ischemia in its substernal location, duration, constricting quality, and relation to exertion. Here, the most common acute process is massive pulmonary embolism. Chronic pulmonary hypertension may be associated with multiple recurrent pulmonary emboli, pulmonary vasculitis, and mitral stenosis.

DISORDERS OF THE MEDIASTINUM

Mediastinal cysts are usually asymptomatic, but a large cyst as well as an aneurysm of the ascending thoracic aorta may cause a deep, constant substernal ache. *Dissecting aneurysm* of the thoracic aorta is associated with excruciating, unremitting anterior chest pain, which may be described as ripping through to the midscapular area or down into the abdomen. The pain is usually accompanied by agitation, profuse sweating, and fear, a clinical presentation suggesting myocardial infarction. Associated findings of a new aortic insufficiency murmur and loss of pulses in the neck, left arm, or both legs in a patient with a history of atherosclerotic disease, hypertension, ankylosing spondylitis, or Marfan's syndrome should alert the clinician to this diagnosis. The plain chest film is often quite suggestive of the diagnosis, but angiography is usually required for confirmation.

Inflammation of the trachea and proximal bronchi, such as occurs in acute tracheobronchitis, causes a deep, aching substernal discomfort that is particularly aggravated by the invariable coughing that accompanies it.

Esophageal or diaphragmatic disorders can easily mimic cardiovascular symptomatology. Severe substernal pain with a burning quality caused by *reflux esophagitis* or *esophageal spasm,* most commonly associated with a *hiatal hernia,* may radiate to the neck or jaws. The pain is commonly relieved by swallowing an antacid or food. Barium swallow, esophageal radionuclide studies, endoscopy, and motility studies help in establishing the diagnosis.

Pain following severe vomiting may be due to *esophageal rupture.* This may cause widening of the mediastinum or development of a left pleural effusion with a low pH and a high amylase content. Endoscopy of the upper gastrointestinal tract is usually diagnostic.

Diaphragmatic rupture may occur spontaneously as a result of a congenital muscle defect or as a result of previous injury, usually of the penetrating type. The history of a previous bullet or knife wound of the thorax should generate suspicion. Herniation of abdominal contents into the chest may be suggested on plain chest films and is confirmed by barium contrast studies.

OTHER SOURCES OF CHEST PAIN

Chest pain may originate outside the thorax from structures in the neck or abdomen. *Cervical radiculopathy,* usually the result of degenerative arthritis or a protruding intervertebral disc, is an uncommon source. *Disorders of the subdiaphragmatic structures* are more frequently seen. These include hiatal hernia, chronic or acute cholecystitis, gastric ulcer, chronic pancreatitis, liver and pancreatic abscesses, infections of the subdiaphragmatic spaces, and the splenic flexure syndrome. In these conditions, abdominal symptoms and signs are also present and tend to predominate. More comprehensive discussions of the diagnosis of these disorders will be found in their appropriate chapters.

PSYCHOGENIC PAIN

Pain of psychogenic origin is usually described as diffuse, constantly present, and aggravated by any effort, however trivial. It is invariably associated with dyspnea, fatigue, and other somatic symptoms. Despite complaining of persistent pain, the patient almost never takes analgesics and does not permit symptoms to interfere with pleasurable activities. Usually the pain is of months to years in duration and has allegedly baffled other physicians. Psychogenic pain is particularly common in emotionally disturbed children and adult women. Again, a careful history is the most important diagnostic tool, but radiologic and laboratory studies are almost inevitably necessary.

CHRONIC COUGH

By Harry L. Davis, M.D.
Memphis, Tennessee

The ability to cough is an important defense mechanism of the respiratory system. Sporadic coughing is a frequent occurrence that often results from an acute respiratory infection or minor exposures to bronchial irritants and usually is of no concern. However, a cough that has become persistent or recurrent should never be considered to be normal but should be regarded as a possible warning that serious disease may be present or developing.

CAUSES OF CHRONIC COUGH

Perhaps the most common cause of a chronic cough is the habitual smoking of tobacco, especially in the form of cigarettes. Unfortunately, this cough is considered to be "normal" by many individuals and seldom is the symptom that causes the patient with early chronic bronchitis or emphysema to seek medical care. Thus, a valuable warning goes unheeded and the patient may receive no advice or therapy until the disease progresses to the stage at which significant shortness of breath becomes a problem. Even the physician may underestimate the ultimate importance of a "cigarette cough." It should be emphasized that chronic exposure to cigarette smoke from smoking parents or other contacts has been shown to increase the incidence of acute respiratory infections and asthma attacks in infants and small children. Therefore, it seems likely that daily exposure to tobacco smoke in the air may be an unrecognized cause of chronic cough in this age group.

A chronic cough should always be investigated and the cause determined, if possible. A logical sequence should be followed in the investigation in order to arrive at a diagnosis as efficiently as possible, sparing the patient the discomfort and expense of procedures that may not be required or are unlikely to yield specific information. Occasional patients may require repeated evaluation before a definite diagnosis can be made.

The possible causes of a chronic cough are numerous. Many of the more commonly encountered etiologies are listed in Table 1.

PHYSIOLOGY OF COUGH

Knowledge of the normal physiology of cough is helpful in understanding its pathogenesis. The sequence in a voluntary cough consists of the following major events: (1) a deep inspiration, followed by closure of the glottis; (2) the development of high pressure within the thoracic cavity by forceful contraction of the muscles of expiration; and (3) sudden opening of the glottis, resulting in a generalized narrowing of the lumen of the tracheobronchial tree and a rush of air through all its ramifications, carrying with it accumulated secretions and inhaled foreign particulate matter.

Cough is initiated by stimulation of receptors in the tracheobronchial tree by inflammation, chemical irritation, or mechanical stimulation such as that caused by inspissated mucus plugs or a foreign body. The cough reflex is mediated through a cough center in the medulla by way of the glossopharyngeal and vagus nerves. Stimulation of the auricular branch of the vagus nerve may initiate cough in some instances.

Certain diseases, such as chronic bronchitis and obstructive emphysema, are associated with severe impairment of the normal clearance mechanisms, which results in a reduction in cough effectiveness. This loss of efficiency greatly increases the frequency and duration of a chronic cough.

Although cough is a protective mechanism that usually occurs as a result of stimulation of the cough receptors within the lungs, it is also under volitional control and may occur in the absence of such stimulation. Many patients are seen who cough as a nervous habit or as a manifestation of anxiety.

DIAGNOSIS

The history and physical examination are perhaps of the greatest importance in the evaluation of chronic cough and will point to the correct diagnosis in the majority of patients, although confirmation by means of specific laboratory procedures may be required. The history and physical examination should not be confined to the respiratory system, since vital clues may be found remote from the lungs. In taking the history, the physician may find it helpful to consider the observations of relatives or associates, since the patient may not be aware of some of the details if the cough has developed insidiously.

History

The major goal of the history taking is the analysis of certain characteristics of the cough in order to narrow the differential diagnosis. Onset and duration, time of day it occurs, type and quantity of sputum production, environmental exposures and personal habits, and associated clinical manifestations are especially important.

Chronic cough is often insidious in onset, and the duration may be difficult to determine. This is especially true in patients with chronic obstructive pulmonary disease (COPD) and chronic infections, but it is also likely to be the case when cough is caused by extrinsic pressure or upper respiratory tract disease. The onset is usually abrupt when cough is caused by pulmonary congestion or multiple embolization, aspiration, or exposure to a bronchial irritant. Cough caused by bronchial obstruction resulting from a neoplasm or foreign body may begin abruptly and may be associated with recurrent or slowly resolving pneumonitis.

The time of day a cough is most troublesome often gives valuable clues to the diagnosis. Early morning productive cough is characteristic of COPD and suppurative lung disease because of the accumulation of

Table 1. Causes of Chronic Cough

Causes
Upper respiratory tract disease
Chronic rhinitis or sinusitis with postnasal drainage*
Chronic pharyngitis
Disease of the larynx
Chronic laryngitis
Polyposis
Cancer*
Elongated uvula
Lower respiratory tract disease
Infections
Mycobacterial infections*
Fungus infections*
Pneumonias*
Laryngotracheobronchial irritation
Tobacco smoking
Occupational exposure
Industrial dusts
Chemical fumes
Atmospheric pollution
Household aerosols
Hot or cold air
Chronic obstructive lung disease*
Bronchial asthma*
Bronchitis and bronchiolitis
Obstructive emphysema
Cystic fibrosis (children and young adults)*
Localized obstruction with atelectasis
Inspissated secretions
Neoplasms*
Foreign body
Eroding broncholith
Aspiration
Gastroesophageal reflux*
Hiatal hernia with regurgitation
Incompetent cardia
Achalasia
Esophageal diverticulum*
Dysphagia due to stroke or other neurologic disease
Suppurative pulmonary disease
Bronchiectasis*
Lung abscess*
Lower respiratory tract disease *(continued)*
Extrinsic pressure on airways
Aortic aneurysm*
Mediastinal tumors
Enlarged lymph nodes
Pleural disease*
Pleuritis with effusion
Empyema
Mesothelioma
Asbestosis
Hypersensitivity pneumonitis*
Bronchopulmonary aspergillosis
Farmer's lung
Air conditioner lung
Bird fancier's lung
Diseases of uncertain etiology
Sarcoidosis*
Fibrosing alveolitis
Histiocytosis X*
Collagen diseases*
Cardiovascular disease
Pulmonary embolic disease
Pulmonary congestion
Left ventricular failure
Mitral stenosis
Pulmonary edema from any cause
Nonrespiratory causes
Subphrenic abscess
Adenomatous thyroid
Stimulation of auricular branch of vagus nerve
Impacted cerumen
Foreign body
Otitis externa and media*
Hair touching tympanic membrane
Stimulation of certain afferent pathways
Psychogenic causes
Chronic anxiety reaction
Psychogenic cough tic (common in children and adolescents)

*See articles on these topics.

pulmonary secretions during the night. Cough caused by extrinsic pressure on the airways may occur throughout the day and night, is usually dry, and often has a brassy quality. Chronic cough occurring primarily during the night may occur as a result of several different types of disease. Pulmonary congestion, caused by left ventricular failure or mitral stenosis, often occurs a few hours after the patient has gone to bed and frequently is associated with paroxysmal nocturnal dyspnea and orthopnea. Aspiration of retained food or gastric contents caused by cardiospasm, esophageal diverticulum, stricture, or the presence of a hiatal hernia may occur primarily when the patient is in the supine position; therefore, cough related to aspiration is usually worse at night. Aspiration caused by dysphagia as the result of a stroke or other neurologic disease may occur at any time during the day but is more likely to occur during eating or drinking. Cough as a manifestation of bronchial asthma may be most severe during the night in patients allergic to feathers or other materials in the bedding. Chronic cough is a commonly unrecognized symptom of asthma in infants and children. Cough occurring during physical exertion primarily may be a manifestation of exercise-induced asthma or incipient pulmonary congestion. Cough may awaken patients with bronchitis or emphysema, who must clear their lungs of secretions before obtaining relief.

Careful analysis of the type and quantity of sputum produced is very important, and the physician should observe a specimen of sputum while taking the history. A persistently dry cough suggests that the cough is produced by a mechanical stimulation, either by extrinsic pressure on the airways or by an intrinsic mass such as a neoplasm, an eroding node, a foreign body, or inspissated plugs of mucus. Cough caused by allergy or by chemical irritation may be dry in early cases. Psychogenic cough is virtually always nonproductive. Production of copious amounts of purulent sputum suggests the presence of bronchiectasis, a draining lung abscess, or severe chronic bronchitis, but it may also be indicative of cystic fibrosis in a child or young adult. The sputum of pulmonary edema is thin and foamy in character and pink-tinged. The sputum of the asthmatic patient is mucoid and tenacious, often containing casts of mucus. Occasionally, patients with an eroding calcified lymph node may expectorate gritty material or small bits of calcified tissue. The presence of blood in the sputum seldom is helpful in arriving at a diagnosis but does serve to emphasize the pathologic nature of the cough and underscores the need for a thorough search for a diagnosis.

The environmental exposures and personal habits of the patient should be carefully explored to investigate the possibility of exposure to occupational or household irritants that may be the cause of a chronic cough. This will include a detailed record of the patient's smoking habits and occupational history as well as a history of travel and of exposure to recognized sources of infection such as caves or the roosting places of birds. Inquiry should be made concerning known exposure to tuberculosis.

Associated clinical manifestations often give the clues that lead to an early diagnosis. The presence of hoarseness indicates disease of the larynx. A history of fever, night sweats, and weight loss suggests the possibility of chronic infection, lymphoma, or collagen disease. Shortness of breath experienced primarily during exertion is indicative of chronic bronchitis or emphysema, whereas acute shortness of breath occurring during the night is more likely to indicate heart failure. Syncope caused by a prolonged paroxysm of coughing is most likely to occur in patients with chronic obstructive lung disease.

Physical Examination

Clues to the cause of a chronic cough may be found in any part of the body; this emphasizes the need for a complete examination. Observation of the patient while taking the history usually will provide an opportunity to study the nature of the cough, including the character of the sputum. The presence of accumulated secretions may be obvious from the cough, even though the patient may be unable to produce a sample of sputum for inspection. The patient's ability to cough effectively should be evaluated, since chronic cough may result from any abnormality that causes the cough to be weak and ineffective. The patient should be observed for other evidence of disease, such as labored respiration, cyanosis, or the presence of skin lesions. Psychogenic cough often has an artificial character and appears to be disproportionate to the objective evidence of abnormality.

The presence of chronic sinus disease or chronic pharyngitis will be discovered by careful examination of the upper respiratory tract. Examination of the ears will reveal the presence of impacted cerumen, large hairs, foreign bodies, or inflammation of the middle ear or external auditory meatus. Examination of the thyroid will detect the presence of large adenomas that may be compressing the trachea. Enlarged nodes in the neck and supraclavicular areas may be a clue to neoplastic disease or granulomatous infection. The presence of neck vein distention may be observed in patients with congestive heart failure or cor pulmonale. The use of the accessory muscles of respiration indicates reduction of vital capacity and points to the presence of serious restrictive or obstructive pulmonary impairment.

Examination of the chest is perhaps the most important diagnostic procedure in the evaluation of chronic cough and will indicate the correct diagnosis in many cases. Examination of the heart may reveal a gallop rhythm, cardiomegaly, and other evidence of heart failure or the murmur of mitral stenosis. Inspection will detect abnormalities of lung expansion, hyperinflation, or paradoxic motion of the lower rib margins (Hoover's sign), which is seen in advanced emphysema. The absence of normal fremitus and breath sounds aids in differentiating fluid or atelectasis from consolidation, which is characterized by increased fremitus and bronchial breathing. Percussion may reveal the hyperresonance of emphysema or the dullness of consolidation, atelectasis, or fluid. Auscultation should be carried out over each segment of both lungs. Reduced breath sounds or prolonged expiration may indicate the presence of emphysema. Coarse rhonchi or coarse moist rales cleared by coughing are characteristic of chronic bronchitis and bronchiectasis. High-pitched generalized wheezing usually signifies the presence of obstructive lung disease with a bronchospastic component such as asthma or chronic asthmatic bronchitis, but it may occasionally be caused by a localized obstructing lesion such as a tumor or foreign body. When localized obstruction is suspected, wheezing at the site of the obstruction may be elicited by comparing the breath sounds over both lungs during repeated forced expirations. Evidence of early COPD may be detected by listening to the chest during a forced expiration. Subclinical asthma often has recurrent cough as an early manifestation and may be discovered by asking the patient to breathe rapidly for a few seconds following which wheezing may be heard. Moist rales heard in the lung bases may be indicative of heart failure. However, rales may be caused by stasis, especially in elderly or bedfast individuals. These rales usually are eliminated by deep breathing. Small areas of pneumonitis may cause no abnormal physical findings during quiet breathing, but rales may be heard during inspiration following an expiratory cough.

The presence of an enlarged tender liver may add support to a diagnosis of congestive heart failure or cor pulmonale. Tenderness over the liver may be the principal clue to a diagnosis of subphrenic or hepatic abscess. Examination of the extremities may reveal cyanosis, clubbing, edema, or evidence of vein disease that may be a source of pulmonary emboli.

A neurologic examination should be performed on all patients with chronic cough in which the cause is obscure. Insidious episodes of aspiration caused by difficulty in swallowing may be present in patients with cerebrovascular disease or neuromuscular disease, such as amyotrophic lateral sclerosis, myasthenia gravis, or chronic impairment from poliomyelitis. Muscular dystrophy may be a cause of chronic cough in young children.

X-ray Examinations

Posteroanterior and lateral chest x-rays should be performed on all patients with chronic cough, since many diseases produce anatomic changes that can be detected by x-ray long before they produce abnormal physical findings. Comparison of current films with those taken previously often is of great value in dating the onset and in establishing the acute or chronic nature of the disease. The physician should inquire about the existence of previous films, and they should be obtained for comparison if possible. Although a definitive diagnosis usually cannot be made from the chest x-ray alone, the roentgenographic abnormality is virtually always helpful in indicating the most appropriate diagnostic measures.

Special x-ray examinations may be indicated in selected cases. Lordotic views of the apices of the lungs may reveal evidence of granulomatous disease, and tomograms are often of value in determining whether or not calcium is present in solitary nodules or if cavitation is present. Fluoroscopy is useful in determining paralysis of the diaphragm or cardiac chamber enlargement. Sinus x-rays should be obtained if chronic sinusitis is suspected. Bronchograms are indicated when bronchial obstruction is suspected distal to the main segmental orifices or when bronchiectasis is suspected that may be localized and amenable to surgical resection. Bronchograms present some hazard to elderly patients and those with advanced impairment of pulmonary function; therefore, bilateral bronchograms should not be performed at one sitting in patients with marginal breathing reserve. Since the emphasis today in the management of bronchiectasis, lung abscess, and tuberculosis is largely medical and surgery is used only very infrequently, bronchography is indicated in only highly selected patients.

Lung scanning and arteriography may aid in the diagnosis of pulmonary embolism and infarction. Lesions of the esophagus and upper gastrointestinal tract usually require studies with radiopaque media, although evidence of such diseases may be present in the routine view of the chest. A tracheoesophageal fistula may be discovered occasionally during an esophagram.

Although the ultimate role of computed tomography (CT) in the evaluation of the chest is still somewhat unsettled, it appears to have definite value in selected cases involving disease in the mediastinum and in the detection of pulmonary metastases when conventional x-rays and tomography are negative or indecisive. Computed tomography has the advantage of being useful in determining the density of lesions and therefore is helpful in determining whether the lesion is a cyst or a solid tumor. Eventually, it may be possible to discriminate between benign and malignant solitary nodules with a high degree of accuracy.

Sputum Examinations

The information that can be obtained from gross inspection of the sputum has been stressed in previous paragraphs. Bacteriologic studies should be conducted for common pyogenic bacteria, tubercle bacilli, and fungi. Cytologic examination of the sputum should be performed if neoplastic disease is a reasonable possibility. Blastomycosis is occasionally diagnosed initially during this cytologic examination. Microscopic examination of the sputum may reveal an increased number of eosinophils and mucus plugs indicative of asthma, phagocytes containing hemosiderin suggestive of chronic pulmonary congestion, or evidence of infestation with parasites.

Careful instruction of the patient to collect a deep cough sputum specimen at the moment of awakening is very important in those patients whose cough appears to be nonproductive. A suitable sputum container must be available at the bedside when the patient awakens. If sputum cannot be obtained by voluntary coughing, sputum induction may be carried out by ultrasonic nebulization or other means of humidification. Gastric washings should be cultured if tuberculosis is suspected and sputum cannot be obtained. Nasotracheal suctioning or transtracheal aspiration, in skilled hands, is a possible approach to obtaining sputum from patients who cannot cooperate.

The presence of blood in the sputum is an indication for bronchoscopy unless a definite diagnosis is made by other means.

Other Clinical Laboratory Examinations

Many of the vast number of clinical laboratory procedures that are available may be helpful in the evaluation of patients with chronic cough. However, only a few of the most important can be discussed here. The presence of polycythemia may suggest chronic hypoxemia, leading to further study with arterial blood gas studies and red blood cell mass and blood volume determinations. The presence of either leukocytosis or leukopenia, although never diagnostic, may aid in the differentiation of infections and may indicate the likelihood that the disease is not infectious. The presence of eosinophilia may be the initial clue that the cough is a manifestation of asthma or a hypersensitivity pneumonitis.

Serologic studies may be helpful in many infections. Complement fixation tests or cold agglutinins may be positive in mycoplasmal infections. Certain fungal infections, such as histoplasmosis, may be diagnosed by rising titers of antibodies. Precipitin tests are helpful in diagnosing hypersensitivity diseases caused by certain thermophilic fungi or molds, such as farmer's lung, bird fancier's disease, or air conditioner lung. Serum protein electrophoresis is invaluable in identifying the infrequent patient with recurrent infections related to agammaglobulinemia.

Evidence in the urine of renal disease combined with abnormal findings in the chest x-ray suggests the possibility of Goodpasture's syndrome, Wegener's granulomatosis, or one of the collagen diseases.

The presence of cystic fibrosis is confirmed in the laboratory by the demonstration of an abnormally high level of chloride in the patient's sweat.

Pulmonary Function Studies

In the evaluation of patients with chronic cough, spirometry and other pulmonary function studies serve primarily to confirm the presence of chronic obstructive lung disease or other impairment that has been suspected from the history, physical examination, and chest x-rays. Response to a bronchodilator may indicate the presence of a bronchospastic component and may lend support to the impression that the patient's cough is an expression of hitherto undiagnosed bronchial asthma. Use of the methacholine challenge test may aid in diagnosing bronchial asthma in those patients who do not have evidence of bronchospasm. In such patients, the need for bronchoscopy may be obviated by the demonstration that their cough is a manifestation of asthma. Since there may be some risk to the patient during a methacholine challenge test, a physician should always be present and appropriate emergency drugs and equipment readily available. Exercise testing may be important in patients suspected of having exercise-induced asthma.

Analysis of flow-volume loops may be helpful in demonstrating obstructing localized lesions of large or upper airways. The presence of such lesions should be confirmed by bronchoscopy and biopsies taken, if indicated.

Diffusing capacity measurements are helpful in differentiating chronic bronchitis or asthma from anatomic emphysema and the evaluation of patients suspected of multiple small pulmonary emboli.

If the patient is being considered for exploratory laparotomy or open lung biopsy, pulmonary function studies will have value in determining the degree of breathing reserve present and whether the patient is a suitable candidate for surgery.

Endoscopy

Patients with intractable chronic cough whose condition remains undiagnosed usually will require bronchoscopy as part of their evaluation, even in the absence of abnormal findings on physical examination or x-ray unless a definite diagnosis such as asthma can be established. The possibility of discovering small lesions that are undetectable by other means makes bronchoscopy a necessary procedure if the examination is to be complete. Other indications for bronchoscopy are (1) evidence of bronchial obstruction on physical examination or chest x-ray, (2) unexplained hemoptysis, (3) the presence of persistent mass lesions near the hilar areas, or (4) pneumonitis that remains unresolved on repeated x-rays. Specimens of secretions for bacteriologic and cytologic study should be obtained during bronchoscopy as well as a biopsy when a lesion is visualized.

Because of the more thorough visualization that is possible, the initial bronchoscopy should virtually always be performed with a flexible fiberoptic instrument unless a foreign body is suspected or the patient is coughing up large amounts of blood. Bronchial biopsy and transbronchial lung biopsy have been very helpful in diagnosing conditions such as sarcoidosis, and bronchial brushing has been of value in identifying the organism responsible for many different types of infections.

Direct laryngoscopy should be performed when hoarseness is present or when disease or paralysis of the vocal cords is suspected. When feasible, a biopsy should be taken of any lesions that are discovered.

Esophagoscopy may be important in certain cases in which disease of the esophagus is suspected but not clearly diagnosed by x-ray. Biopsy specimens and washings for cytology taken during esophagoscopy are especially helpful in the diagnosis of neoplastic disease.

Surgical Procedures

Histologic examination of tissue is frequently necessary before a specific diagnosis can be made, and biopsy procedures should not be delayed if, in the physician's judgment, other measures are not likely to give conclusive information, or the patient's chances of recovery will be compromised by prolonged delay. In those patients with a pleural effusion, thoracentesis and pleural biopsy should be performed prior to resorting to a surgical procedure in most instances. In a high percentage of cases with effusion, these measures ultimately will yield a diagnosis. Supraclavicular or cervical nodes are frequently diagnostic in patients with neoplastic or granulomatous disease of the respiratory tract, although specific diagnosis of chronic infections may depend upon the results of special stains and cultures of the tissue. Mediastinoscopy with biopsy may be of value in patients with enlarged paratracheal or hilar nodes or a mass in the anterior mediastinum. In selected cases, a mediastinotomy incision may be a satisfactory approach for biopsy of a node or other disease in or near the mediastinum.

Lung biopsy is frequently necessary in patients with diffuse infiltrative lesions of the lungs in which a diagnosis cannot be established by other means. Open lung biopsy has the advantage of allowing limited exploration of the chest and is preferred by many physicians. However, in experienced hands, needle lung biopsy is an acceptable technique in selected cases and should be considered in poor-risk patients with accessible lesions and in patients with localized peripheral lesions with evidence of pleural reaction. Needle aspiration of the lesion may be sufficient to make a diagnosis in difficult cases, such as *Pneumocystis carinii* or opportunistic fungal infections.

Bone marrow aspiration or biopsy may reveal evidence of granulomatous infection or neoplastic disease. Skin and muscle biopsy should be obtained when diffuse vasculitis is suspected. Liver biopsy may be helpful in diagnosing disseminated granulomatous infections or sarcoidosis.

Tissue and bone marrow specimens should be studied bacteriologically as well as histologically.

Psychiatric Evaluation

The diagnosis of psychogenic cough should not be made entirely by exclusion but should be supported by evidence of an emotional reaction such as chronic anxiety, which could explain its development. Psychogenic cough tic, or habit cough, is especially common in children and adolescents. Fortunately, most psychogenic cough problems can be diagnosed and managed by an understanding family physician. However, in patients in whom the cough appears to be a manifestation of a neurosis or psychosis and is interfering with the patient's ability to function, more intensive psychiatric investigation is definitely indicated after possible organic causes have been ruled out.

HEMOPTYSIS

By Daniel H. Lederer, M.D.
Providence, Rhode Island

The term *hemoptysis,* defined as expectoration of blood, implies a source of bleeding from anywhere in the respiratory tract below the glottis, including the subglottal larynx, trachea, bronchi, and lung parenchyma. Hemoptysis may occur as blood-streaked sputum or as gross blood. One must differentiate hemoptysis from bleeding arising in the nose, mouth, or pharynx; from upper gastrointestinal tract hemorrhage with hematemesis; and from factitious bleeding. A careful examination of the nose and throat, including indirect laryngoscopy, may identify a bleeding site in those areas. Hematemesis produces blood that is usually dark, has an acid pH, and is mixed with food particles, whereas blood from the respiratory tract is more often bright red and alkaline in pH and on microscopy may show hemosiderin-laden macrophages. On occasion a malingerer may try to simulate hemoptysis by self-inflicted trauma to the mouth or pharynx or by drinking blood and then expectorating it.

Once it is clear that bleeding is from the respiratory tract, the approach to an etiologic diagnosis is based on a consideration of the more likely causes of bleeding. Table 1, although not all-inclusive, lists the more common causes of hemoptysis along with several others that are important to recognize if present. Bronchitis may be either acute or chronic. Bronchiectasis may occur as an isolated entity or as part of the immotile cilia syndrome, in which some patients will also have sinusitis and dextrocardia (Kartagener's syndrome); bronchiectasis is a common finding in patients with cystic fibrosis. Hemoptysis may be a feature of bacterial pneumonias, especially necrotizing pneumonias caused by anaerobes, staphylococci, or gram-negative bacilli. Bleeding may occur from a region of tuberculous pneumonia or from a mycotic aneurysm within a tuberculous cavity. Varicella and influenza pneumonias frequently cause hemoptysis, as can a variety of fungal infections or parasitic diseases such as amebiasis and paragonimiasis. A fungus ball can form in a pre-existing cavity, the usual organism being an Aspergillus species.

Hemoptysis may be the first sign of bronchogenic carcinoma or of bronchial adenoma, which is actually in most cases a low-grade carcinoma that tends to be highly vascular. A pulmonary arteriovenous fistula may occur alone or as part of the syndrome of hereditary hemorrhagic telangiectasia. An aortic aneurysm may cause hemoptysis if there is rupture into a bronchus. Broncholithiasis causes hemoptysis when calcified material from a lymph node or, less often, from

Table 1. Some Causes of Hemoptysis

Inflammatory conditions
Bronchitis*
Bronchiectasis*
Bacterial pneumonias*
Tuberculosis*
Lung abscess
Viral pneumonias
Fungal infections
Parasitic diseases
Fungus ball
Neoplasms
Bronchogenic carcinoma*
Bronchial adenoma
Cardiovascular diseases
Pulmonary embolism with infarction*
Mitral stenosis*
Left ventricular failure*
Pulmonary arteriovenous fistula
Aortic aneurysm
Vasculitides
Goodpasture's syndrome
Wegener's granulomatosis
Trauma
Lung contusion
Penetrating wound
Tracheobronchial tear
Miscellaneous
Broncholithiasis
Foreign body aspiration
Iatrogenic
Coagulopathies

*Commonly encountered.

lung parenchyma erodes into a bronchus. Hemoptysis may occur as a sequela of bronchial or lung biopsy or of intravascular catheterization. Coagulopathies, either as manifestations of specific diseases or secondary to anticoagulant administration, may unmask localized respiratory tract pathology.

HISTORY

In the evaluation of the patient with hemoptysis, certain historical features or symptoms may favor specific diagnoses. A chronic productive cough occurring over years suggests chronic bronchitis or bronchiectasis. The recent onset of cough, purulent sputum, and fever is more likely due to acute bronchitis or pneumonia. Fetid sputum is characteristic of infection by anaerobic bacteria and is often associated with necrotizing pneumonia or lung abscess, the latter often preceded by an episode of depressed consciousness. Patients with a past history of tuberculosis, histoplasmosis, or coccidioidomycosis may have broncholithiasis. The sudden onset of dyspnea and pleuritic chest pain is consistent with pulmonary embolism with infarction, while orthopnea and paroxysmal nocturnal dyspnea are common symptoms of left ventricular failure or mitral stenosis. The patient with a history of weight loss may have bronchogenic carcinoma or tuberculosis. Cigarette smoking predisposes to chronic bronchitis and bronchogenic carcinoma. A history of infertility in a man should raise the question of immotile cilia syndrome. Sinusitis may be associated with bronchiectasis or Wegener's granulomatosis.

Patients who have received cytotoxic drugs or steroids, especially when severely granulocytopenic, are at increased risk for infection by fungi such as Aspergillus species, and those with lymphoma or sarcoidosis who have received steroids are prone to develop cryptococcosis. A patient may have contracted disease during travel to or residence in endemic areas for histoplasmosis, coccidioidomycosis, or paragonimiasis. A history of dysentery raises the possibility of an amebic hepatic abscess with extension into the lung. One must ask the patient specifically about trauma, aspiration of a foreign body, and anticoagulant medications.

PHYSICAL EXAMINATION

As in the history, certain findings may suggest specific diagnoses. For example, small red telangiectases on the skin, lips, and oral or nasal mucosa are characteristic of hereditary hemorrhagic telangiectasia. The typical rash of varicella should be easily recognized. Periodontal disease is often associated with anaerobic infections. There may be ecchymoses or puncture wounds indicating chest trauma. Both pulmonary arteriovenous fistula and pulmonary embolism can at times cause an audible bruit. A localized wheeze may result from an obstructing lesion in a bronchus such as a tumor or foreign body. Clubbing is often seen in bronchiectasis, lung abscess, bronchogenic carcinoma, and arteriovenous fistula; when clubbing is accompanied by tenderness of long bones and arthritis involving the wrists, ankles, or knees (hypertrophic osteoarthropathy), carcinoma is highly likely. Evidence of deep venous thrombosis should raise suspicion of pulmonary embolism. Axillary or supraclavicular lymphadenopathy may yield a diagnosis of carcinoma. Rales and signs of right ventricular failure suggest the presence of left ventricular failure or mitral stenosis, the latter often associated with a loud first heart sound and low-pitched apical diastolic murmur.

LABORATORY PROCEDURES

In all instances of hemoptysis, routine studies should include a complete blood count, prothrombin time, partial thromboplastin time, bleeding time, urinalysis, blood urea nitrogen (BUN), and tuberculin test. In addition, sputum should be examined for cytology and both stained and cultured for acid-fast bacilli and fungi. When an anaerobic infection is suspected, transtracheal aspiration or transbronchoscopic culture with a protected microbiology brush will yield specimens for culture that are not contaminated by oropharyngeal organisms.

When the clinician suspects a specific diagnosis, additional testing will be indicated. Both sputum and stool may show the ova of Paragonimus species. A patient with a fungus ball will usually have detectable serum precipitins to Aspergillus antigens. Electron-microscopy of sperm or respiratory tract mucosa will show abnormalities of ciliary morphology in the immotile cilia syndrome. Pilocarpine iontophoresis and measurement of sweat chloride may help confirm a suspected diagnosis of cystic fibrosis. When amebiasis is being considered, one should examine the stool for cysts and obtain an indirect hemagglutination serology test. Long bone films will show subperiosteal new bone formation in hypertrophic osteoarthropathy. Azotemia associated with hematuria, especially when red cell casts are present, may lead to a diagnosis of Goodpasture's syndrome or Wegener's granulomatosis; in over 90 percent of patients with early Goodpasture's syndrome, circulating antibody to basement membrane can be demonstrated by serum radioimmunoassay or immunofluorescence.

CHEST ROENTGENOGRAM

It is important to review the chest films early in the evaluation of the patient with hemoptysis, since in some cases roentgenographic findings may lead to a decision to initiate respiratory isolation procedures in order to protect other patients and staff. A single cavity or multiple cavities in a region of consolidation may represent an abscess or necrotizing pneumonia. Inhomogeneous consolidation involving posterior portions of one or both upper lobes, often with cavitation, is highly suggestive of tuberculosis. A round opacity in a pre-existing cavity, usually in an upper lobe and often capped by a thin rim of air, is almost always a fungus ball. In bronchiectasis, one may see multiple 1- to 2-cm–diameter cysts, ring shadows, or the parallel "tram lines" caused by peribronchial fibrosis. Lobar or segmental atelectasis may be due to obstruction by a foreign body or tumor. A pleural-based region of consolidation, often with an associated pleural effusion, suggests pulmonary infarction. Left ventricular enlargement, pulmonary vascular engorgement, and signs of interstitial or alveolar pulmonary edema indicate left ventricular failure. The combination of enlargement of the left atrium, right ventricle, and pulmonary vessels, along with basilar nodular densities that may be ossified, is the classical roentgenographic pattern of mitral stenosis. An enlarged aortic shadow may represent an aneurysm. Calcified mediastinal nodes or multiple parenchymal calcifications may be present with broncholithiasis. One may see rib fractures that account for pulmonary laceration; if upper ribs are fractured, the clinician should suspect an associated tracheobronchial tear.

BRONCHOSCOPY

Bronchoscopy is often the most useful procedure in establishing a diagnosis in patients with hemoptysis; if the procedure is done while active bleeding is occurring, the site of bleeding can usually be identified. Because it allows better visualization, the flexible (fiberoptic) bronchoscope is preferable to the rigid bronchoscope except in cases of massive hemoptysis or foreign-body aspiration. Bronchoscopy is especially useful in the diagnosis of bronchogenic carcinoma and bronchial adenoma, and it may provide valuable bacteriologic information, via microbiology brush specimens, in abscess or necrotizing pneumonia. Because of the possibility of neoplasm, virtually all patients with hemoptysis should at some time undergo bronchoscopy.

OTHER DIAGNOSTIC PROCEDURES

Fluoroscopy will often show the pulsatile nature of an arteriovenous fistula. *Tomography* of the mediastinum may show a broncholith penetrating an airway. With the exception of cystic bronchiectasis, in which routine films will show a characteristic pattern, *bronchography* is necessary to make a definitive diagnosis of bronchiectasis but is usually reserved for patients in whom surgery is contemplated; it can produce false-positive results in the presence of atelectasis, which causes shortening and distortion of bronchi, or viral tracheobronchitis, which causes mucosal ulceration.

Radionuclide lung scanning is especially useful when it is normal, thereby ruling out pulmonary embolism, or when it shows one or more segmental perfusion defects with preservation of ventilation, a pattern which, in the proper clinical setting, is considered highly specific for pulmonary embolism, although false-positive results can occur. A radionuclide flow study may demonstrate an arteriovenous fistula. *Pulmonary angiography* can provide a definitive diagnosis of pulmonary embolism or arteriovenous fistula and is especially important in the latter because approximately a third of patients have more than one fistula.

Other tests may be helpful in specific clinical situations. *Bronchial arteriography* may be necessary to localize a site of bleeding, especially when the chest roentgenogram is normal or when parenchymal abnormalities are widespread. *Echocardiography* shows a characteristic pattern in mitral stenosis, and cross-sectional imaging can determine the mitral orifice area. *Lung biopsy* may be necessary to diagnose Wegener's granulomatosis, Goodpasture's syndrome, or occasionally a fungal or parasitic infection; the clinical situation will determine whether the transbronchial approach or an open procedure is preferable.

COURSE AND COMPLICATIONS

The course of patients with hemoptysis depends on the nature of their underlying disease and whether it is correctly diagnosed and treated. It is important to quantitate the amount of bleeding, since massive hemorrhage (at a rate greater than 250 ml per 24 hours) should be considered a medical emergency, because of the risk of asphyxia, and requires close observation by a surgeon because prompt surgical intervention may be necessary. In approximately 10 percent of patients with hemoptysis, no diagnosis is obtained; these patients must be observed over time and re-evaluated periodically.

MASSES IN THE NECK

By G. Richard Holt, M.D.
and G. David Neal, M.D.
San Antonio, Texas

The diagnosis of neck masses is much more sophisticated than when the article on this subject was first written for this text. Recent advances in conventional roentgenologic tomography, radionuclide scintography, and computed tomography (CT) have greatly improved our diagnostic radiologic capabilities. Ultrasound capabilities and fine-needle aspiration have also provided valuable information to the clinician. Additionally, the refinement of the flexible fiberoptic endoscope has provided a means of identifying abnormalities in patients difficult to examine by conventional means. The goals in the diagnosis of a neck mass are to separate the benign from the malignant and the surgical from the nonsurgical. By means of a basic series of diagnostic tests coupled with a precise history and physical examination, the correct diagnosis may be obtained more than 90 per cent of the time. The evaluation of masses in the neck will be outlined in this article, first in general terms and then by specific pathologic conditions.

HISTORY

Much valuable information can be obtained by a historical review. The length of time since onset of the mass is very important, with most benign lesions exhibiting a slow growth pattern and the malignant lesions presenting a faster progression. In the absence of symptoms of infection or inflammation, a rapidly growing mass is more likely to be malignant than one of slower growth. The age of the patient is quite important; a mass in a child is more likely to be benign or inflammatory than in an adult, whereas a unilateral neck mass in a patient over 55 years of age carries an 80 per cent risk of being malignant. Accompanying symptoms such as pain, swelling, fever, or an association with pharyngitis or stomatitis points toward an infectious origin. Malignant tumors do not commonly have pain associated with them until the tumor is large or is infiltrating cranial nerves. Epistaxis, nasal obstruction, and a mass in the neck are the three main presenting symptoms for nasopharyngeal carcinoma and cancer of the nasal cavity.

Eliciting a history of exposure to possible etiologic agents may be helpful; prior exposure to domestic and feral animals might raise suspicion of histoplasmosis, brucellosis, or tularemia. A long history of tobacco and alcohol abuse will suggest a malignant process.

Any additional health-related information can be helpful: is the patient diabetic or immunocompromised; is there a history of hemoptysis, hematuria, or melenic stools? The more comprehensive the medical history, the more likely one is to identify information which may point to a possible etiology.

PHYSICAL EXAMINATION

An orderly head and neck examination should be performed. The presence of a conductive hearing loss on tuning fork examination and the finding of a middle ear effusion on pneumatic otoscopy may raise suspicion of carcinoma or an angiofibroma of the nasopharynx. The entire skin of the head and neck, including the scalp, should be examined for lesions such as basal cell epithelioma, squamous cell carcinoma, and malignant melanoma. Proptosis, decreased visual acuity, or altered visual fields and diplopia indicate involvement of the orbit by a space-occupying mass. Tumors within the nasal cavity and paranasal sinuses may reach relatively large size before causing symptoms. A mass in the nose, fullness in the cheek, and bulging of the palate with loosening of the teeth are late signs of sinus tumors.

Examination of the salivary glands may reveal a diffuse fullness or a well-circumscribed mass. Bimanual palpation of the submandibular and sublingual glands may reveal an otherwise undetectable mass. Many intraoral lesions are very difficult to find unless every area of the mouth and tongue is inspected; the dentures must be removed for an adequate examination. The use of the mirror for examining the nasopharynx, hypopharynx, and larynx provides the best view of these structures. If the patient is difficult to examine, use of the flexible fiberoptic nasopharyngoscope under topical anesthesia has proved valuable in obtaining an initial view of the upper aerodigestive tract.

Palpation of the neck requires the use of both hands. The normal laryngeal crepitus found on movement of the larynx against the vertebral bodies should be elicited; its absence suggests a mass effect in larynx or esophagus. Careful palpation of the carotid vessels may reveal a carotid body tumor or aneurysm. The presence of a thyroid mass in association with a lateral neck mass strongly raises the question of a thyroid neoplasm. Finally, the mass itself is palpated; its firmness, tenderness, size, and mobility are all important parameters and should be recorded. If a primary tumor is located, the neck disease should be classified according to the tumor-node-metastasis (TNM) clinical staging system.

A complete physical examination is obviously indicated in the 5 to 8 per cent of cases in which a neck mass represents metastasis from a lesion below the level of clavicle. Cancer of the breast, stomach, lung, kidney, and reproductive system are all capable of producing metastases to the neck.

LABORATORY DATA

There are a number of laboratory tests that should be performed in the evaluation of a neck mass, which, if positive, can direct the clinician to an expedient diagnosis. The complete blood count with differential may indicate an elevated leukocyte count with a bacterial infection or an elevated atypical lymphocyte count when infectious mononucleosis is present. Hematuria seen on a urinalysis may indicate the possibility of a renal cell tumor. Liver function tests may be abnormal in both viral systemic infections and in widely disseminated neoplastic diseases. If the calcium and inorganic phosphate are abnormal, a parathyroid adenoma should be suspected. Any patient who presents with hoarseness and cough associated with a neck mass should have several sputum specimens evaluated for the presence of bacteria or abnormal cytology and for acid-fast bacteria with acid-fast and fluorochrome stains. Thyroid function studies should be obtained only if the neck mass is low in the neck or if there is an indication of altered metabolism. Other laboratory tests can be ordered as indicated by presentation of the mass and other physical or chemical findings.

RADIOGRAPHY

A number of conventional roentgenograms are helpful in evaluating a neck mass. Lateral and anteroposterior soft-tissue views of the neck may demonstrate a cervical rib (often mistaken for a neck mass when present), calcification within the mass (possible dermoid), or deviation of the air passage. A chest x-ray examination is certainly mandatory to look for evidence of pulmonary infection, masses, or congenital abnormalities (Fig. 1A). Paranasal sinus films are indicated when a neck mass is located in the posterior triangle of the neck or when some aspect of the examination indicates the possibility of an occult sinus tumor. Thyroid and salivary scans using low-dose radionuclides are indicated when the mass is along the lower neck or mandible. If no evidence of a primary tumor is found in the head and neck to account for a suspicious neck mass, further systemic evaluation is indicated, including barium swallow, upper gastrointestinal tract series, barium enema, and intravenous pyelography. If the mass is proved to be malignant on subsequent biopsy, liver, spleen, and bone scans should be performed to identify distant metastases for TNM staging.

Conventional tomography has been helpful in identifying possible lesions in the paranasal sinuses, orbit, palate, larynx, and lung. Although these tomograms are largely being supplanted by computed tomography, they still are useful in identifying bony erosion or widening of a cranial nerve foramen.

The diagnosis of neck masses within the last few years has been greatly aided by the use of computed tomography. These scans can be multiplanar (lateral, axial, coronal), with other views reconstructed by the computer memory as required. With each generation of CT scanners, ability to diagnose smaller lesions with greater accuracy is improved. The CT scan can identify the size and location of the mass as well as its composition and density (Fig. 1B). With intravenous contrast, it can assess vascularity of the mass. It is possible also to identify a deep neck abscess or a branchial cleft cyst using CT scanning. Only a few patients will require a CT scan to assist in diagnosis of a neck mass, but in equivocal or difficult cases it can be very valuable.

Arteriography is employed when there is indication by enhanced CT scanning, Doppler ultrasound, or

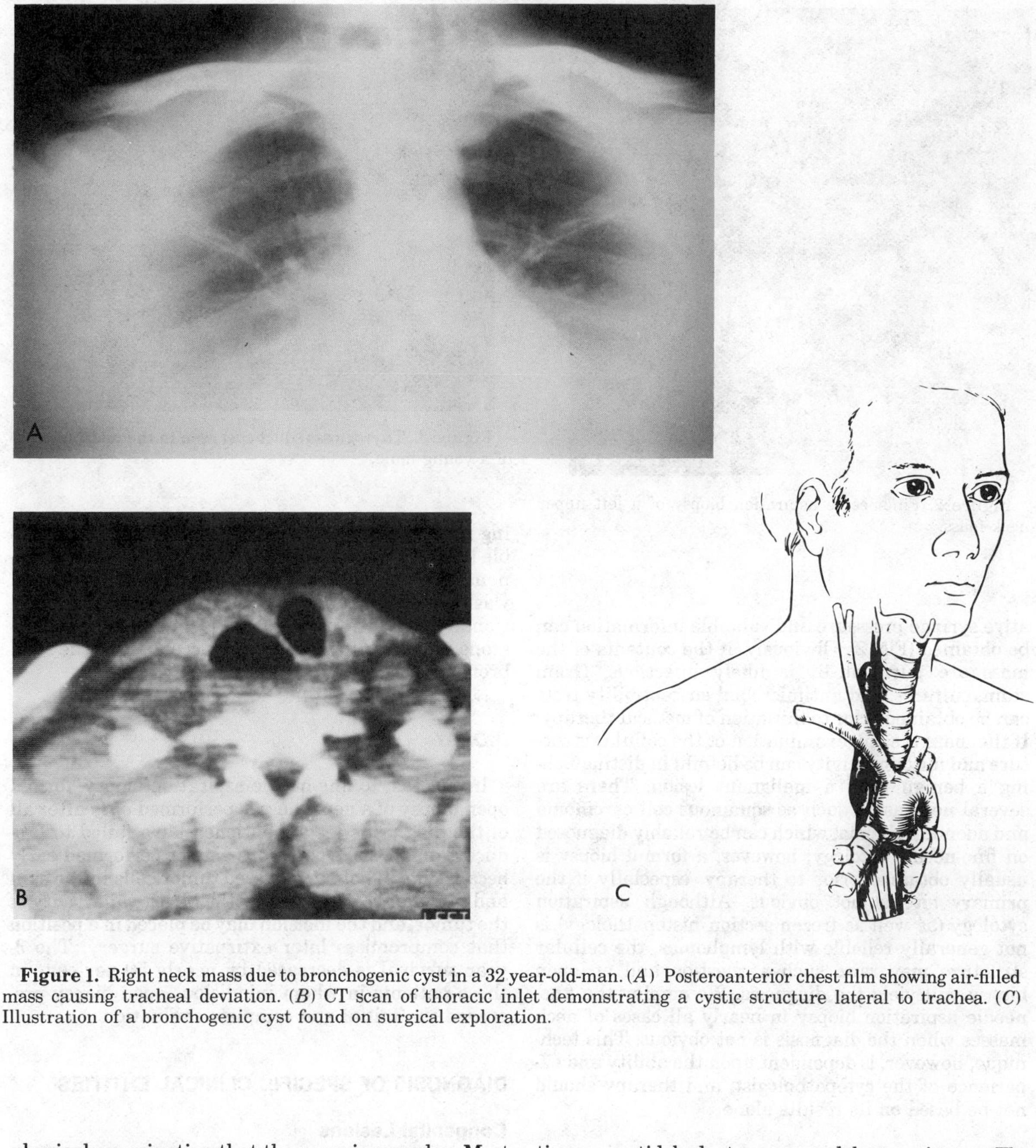

Figure 1. Right neck mass due to bronchogenic cyst in a 32 year-old-man. (*A*) Posteroanterior chest film showing air-filled mass causing tracheal deviation. (*B*) CT scan of thoracic inlet demonstrating a cystic structure lateral to trachea. (*C*) Illustration of a bronchogenic cyst found on surgical exploration.

physical examination that the mass is vascular. Most vascular masses can be diagnosed by the CT scan and confirmed by arteriography. The arteriogram also gives precise information on the feeder vessels to the mass and provides a vehicle for embolotherapy, if indicated.

ULTRASOUND

Ultrasound examination of a neck mass often provides valuable information. Two methods of ultrasound evaluation are commonly employed. The *Doppler ultrasound velocimeter* gives both an audible and metered reading of vascular flow to the mass and can identify arteriovenous fistulae and malformations, carotid body tumors, and hemangiomas. The *A-scan* commonly employed in orbital and thyroid mass diagnosis can also be employed on other neck masses; it can differentiate a solid from a cystic mass and can identify involvement of surrounding tissue such as periosteum or muscle. Ultrasonography is helpful in the evaluation of thyroid masses prior to fine-needle aspiration.

FINE-NEEDLE ASPIRATION CYTOLOGY

As clinicians and cytopathologists have gained more experience in fine-needle aspiration cytology, its clinical reliability has greatly improved. Any neck mass can be aspirated through a fine needle with neg-

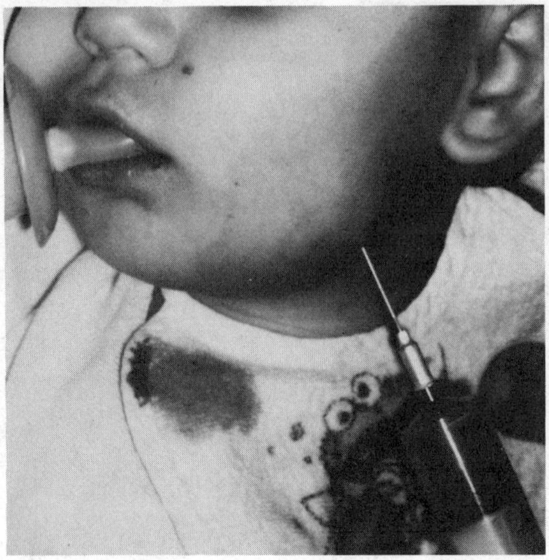

Figure 2. Fine-needle aspiration biopsy of a left upper neck mass.

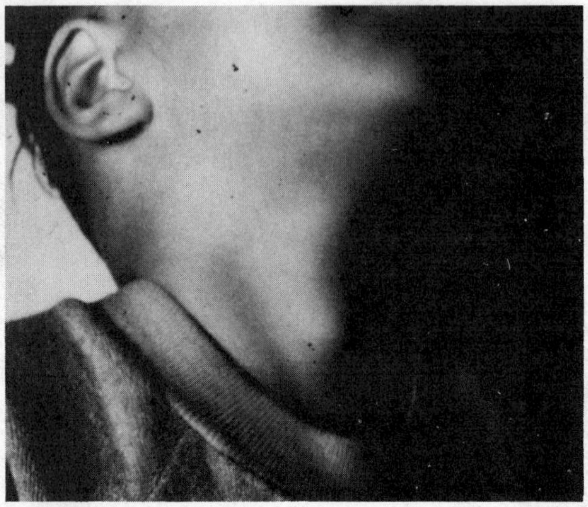

Figure 3. Thyroglossal duct cyst seen in the midline neck of a young male.

ative syringe presssure and valuable information can be obtained (Fig. 2). Obviously, if the contents of the mass are purulent, it is likely infectious; Gram stain, cultures, and antimicrobial susceptibility tests can be obtained prior to initiation of medical therapy. If the mass is solid, examination of the cellular structure and mitotic activity can be helpful in distinguishing a benign from a malignant lesion. There are several neoplasms, such as squamous cell carcinoma and adenocarcinoma, which can be reliably diagnosed on fine-needle cytology; however, a formal biopsy is usually obtained prior to therapy, especially if the primary site is not obvious. Although aspiration cytology (as well as frozen section histopathology) is not generally reliable with lymphomas, the cellular structure may raise such a question and an open biopsy will yield the diagnosis. We employ the fine-needle aspiration biopsy in nearly all cases of neck masses when the diagnosis is not obvious. This technique, however, is dependent upon the ability and experience of the cytopathologist, and therapy should not be based on its results alone.

ENDOSCOPY

Initially in the evaluation, indirect mirror or flexible fiberoptic endoscopy is performed. If there is a lesion in the upper air and food passages exposed to these visualizations, it will usually be seen. However, some lesions are not readily visible or are located in the lower air and food passages and require formal endoscopy for evaluation. Any mass in the neck should be considered metastatic from a head or neck primary tumor until proven otherwise.

Most diagnostic endoscopy is performed under general anesthesia, although local and topical anesthesia may be employed. Nasopharyngoscopy, laryngoscopy, bronchoscopy, and esophagoscopy are performed using rigid endoscopes, headlight, and mirror. Any visible lesions are biopsied and sent for frozen and permanent histopathology. When indicated, bronchial washings for culture and cytology are obtained. Occasionally, the use of the flexible fiberoptic bronchoscope is utilized to view areas inaccessible to the rigid bronchoscope.

BIOPSY

In contrast to fine-needle aspiration biopsy, formal open biopsy of a neck mass is performed *only* after all of the diagnostic tests mentioned have failed to produce a diagnosis. Open biopsy is not performed early because it can potentially seed tumor cells to the skin and lymphatics, it may alter the biological activity of the tumor, and the incision may be placed in a position that compromises later extirpative surgery. The 3-year survival is decreased by nearly 50 per cent in those patients in whom injudicious open biopsy preceeded the initial and complete evaluation.

DIAGNOSIS OF SPECIFIC CLINICAL ENTITIES

Congenital Lesions

Masses in the neck may be remnants of embryologic structures that failed to involute completely. For reasons that are not entirely known, these cysts usually become evident in the second or third decade but have rarely been found in the elderly. Generally, *branchial cleft cysts* will present as a mass 4 to 5 cm near the anterior border of the sternomastoid muscle in the midneck. A history of size fluctuation is common, but these masses never regress completely. *Fistulas* or *sinus tracts* also may persist from the same embryologic origins. If a tract is evident, diagnosis is aided by injection of a radiopaque contrast material in conjunction with a lateral neck radiograph. The *thyroglossal duct cyst* is derived from midline structures and is generally found immediately above the larynx

(Fig. 3). The history is apt to be one of gradually increasing size, and most present between 5 and 20 years of age. The radionuclide thyroid scan should be obtained to diagnose ectopic functioning thyroid tissue. Rarely, all of the functional thyroid tissue will be found in this midline position and its removal without replacement therapy could cause myxedema in adults and growth retardation in children (see article on this topic).

Other congenital lesions that occur in the first year of life are the *hemangioma* and *lymphangioma*. Either can grow rapidly to cause marked deformity or life-threatening airway problems. Because of their tendencies to wax and wane and even resolve spontaneously, they are best followed conservatively as long as possible. Diagnosis can be made by ultrasonography and CT scan. The type of lymphangioma that is called *cystic hygroma* generally presents superficially in the parotid or submandibular region and can be easily transilluminated. It also has a characteristic consistency similar to that of a water-filled sponge that refills slowly after compression. *Teratomas* and *dermoid cysts* are subcutaneous rests of embryologic tissue. They are solid tumors that are evident at birth or soon thereafter. Their presence near the midline makes airway obstruction common, but in other cases they grow slowly. Their embryologic origins are unclear, but they are most frequently found near the region where the fusion of paired structures has occurred. A lateral soft-tissue roentgenogram may demonstrate calcified mesodermal structures.

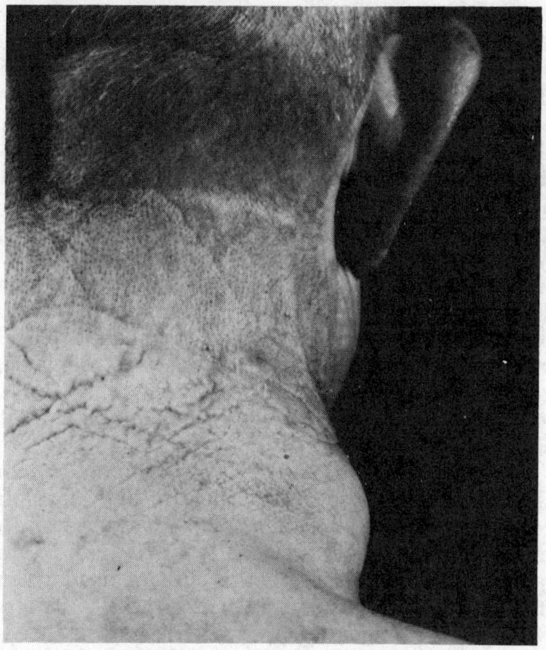

Figure 4. Cervical lymphadenitis resulting from disseminated histoplasmosis in a 52-year-old farm worker.

Infection and Inflammation

Neck masses of *infectious origin* are usually found in lymphatic tissue (Fig. 4), but the salivary glands can also enlarge as a result of viral or bacterial causes. These masses are for the most part tender and may be associated with localized edema or fluctuance. Bacterial lymphadenitis is the most common cause of neck masses in the young and usually responds to antibiotic agents. However, *scrofula* (tuberculous lymphadenitis) will persist until the lymph node is removed. The ingestion of nonpasteurized milk is rare in the United States, but atypical strains of mycobacteria also cause cervical lymphadenitis. The tuberculin skin test is only weakly positive or negative in these individuals, making preoperative diagnosis largely dependent on the history of exposure and acid-fast stains of aspirated material.

Systemic fungal infection will rarely cause enlargement of cervical lymph nodes, but *actinomycosis* is seen as a "woody" induration of the tissues around the mandible simulating a submandibular mass. The presence of sinus tracts and yellowish particulate drainage ("sulfur granules") is characteristic of cervicofacial actinomycosis.

Toxoplasmosis and *cat-scratch disease* are both systemic infections transmitted through cats in which cervical lymph node enlargement may be prominent. Diagnosis in these rests with confirmed immunologic titers and histopathologic findings on fine-needle aspiration cytology or open biopsy. Skin tests for cat-scratch fever are available through certain institutions conducting active investigations.

Neoplastic Disease

Acquired tumors of the head and neck may be benign or malignant; the diversity of structures in the region makes it a site of many histologic types. Metastases to the regional lymph nodes of the neck are particularly common for epithelial malignancies of the scalp, face, ears, nasal, and oral and pharyngeal cavities. The probability of finding a primary tumor is directly related to the diagnostic acumen of the physician. It is important to recognize the patient who is a candidate to develop these malignancies, which are etiologically related to heavy tobacco and alcohol use. The diagnostic evaluation for suspected tumors involves indirect and direct endoscopy, fine-needle aspiration, radiography of suspected areas, and open biopsy only as a last resort.

Benign tumors of the neck are rarely multiple, as in the case of bilateral carotid body tumors. In general, they do not grow rapidly and are not intimately related to the major chains of lymph nodes. CT scans, ultrasonography, and arteriography are usually required to make the diagnosis. *Thyroid tumors,* whether benign or malignant, are best diagnosed with radionuclide scan, ultrasound, and fine-needle aspiration (see article on this topic). In florid hyperthyroid states, it is possible to hear a bruit over the thyroid but this is rare. Carotid body tumors may not have an audible bruit but can be heard on audible Doppler ultrasonography. A tortuous or S-shaped carotid artery can mimic a neck mass, as can an arteriovenous fistula or an aneurysm of the carotid artery.

Salivary gland tumors are best identified by their location under the body of the mandible or near its angle. It is not uncommon for the tumor to appear in the neck and thus present a diagnostic problem. A positive technetium scan will strongly suggest Warthin's tumor of salivary tissue, but it may be positive in other salivary tumors, such as the mixed tumor. Thin-needle aspiration biopsy has come to play a greater role in the diagnosis of salivary masses, but it will always be difficult to be truly confident that the tissue sampled actually came from the palpable mass. Therefore, an open biopsy utilizing a superficial parotidectomy is the definitive approach. A slowly progressive paralysis of the facial nerve strongly suggests a hidden parotid malignancy that can often be identified on CT scan performed in conjunction with sialography.

The *neurofibroma* and *schwannoma* are tumors that arise from the nerve sheath. Neuromas are caused by the proliferation of axons at the site of nerve damage. They are usually single and are frequently painful or dysesthetic. Tumors of neurolemmal origin are frequently multiple, arising in patients with von Recklinghausen's neurofibromatosis. The tumor may arise from any nerve, and the proliferation may be so extensive that local gigantism results. The presence of hyperpigmented café au lait spots confirms the diagnosis and should encourage a search for other lesions such as pheochromocytoma and tumors of the cerebellopontine angle. Malignant degeneration of neurofibromas is not infrequent in neurofibromatosis, making it more important to follow these lesions closely or excise them when possible. Peculiar bony defects in the lateral-posterior skull and a J-shaped sella turcica can also be seen on skull radiography in this disease.

Malignant lymphomas and *Hodgkin's disease* often present with multiple enlarged cervical lymph nodes. Careful examination of the axilla and inguinal regions may reveal the systemic nature of the problem. Needle biopsy will seldom obtain enough tissue for complete diagnosis but will distinguish lymphoma from carcinoma. The consistency of lymphomatous nodes is soft and rubbery, as distinguished from the firmness of squamous carcinoma. It is rare that a lymphoma patient will not have systemic symptoms like malaise, night sweats, fever, or pruritus. Weight loss is a sign that is common to most malignancies, whether primary or metastatic in the neck. Laminograms of the chest, liver scan, and CT scans of the abdomen will help stage the lymphoma after diagnosis in the neck.

Metastases to cervical lymph node chains from tumors of the head and neck such as thyroid, squamous carcinoma, melanoma, and salivary neoplasms are common. Cancer of the oral cavity is easily seen, but is unfortunately sometimes missed (see article on this topic). The symptoms of dysphagia, otalgia, or pain on swallowing acidic juices are typical of oropharyngeal malignancies that cannot be seen without a mirror examination or without the use of a flexible nasopharyngoscope. Small tumors of the vocal fold present early because they cause hoarseness, but lesions of the epiglottis, false vocal cord, or pyriform fossae are much more occult. The nasopharynx has historically been the most common site of origin in patients presenting with neck metastasis from an unknown primary. Computed tomography will often demonstrate a large tumor, and conventional tomography can identify widening of the foramen lacerum, the most common route of intracranial spread. Biopsies of this area are usually obtained presumptively during endoscopy if the appearance is normal because the tumors tend to grow submucosally. As stated previously, patients with significant alcohol or tobacco exposure should undergo examination of these areas under anesthesia before excisional biopsy of the suspicious lymph node.

There is no contraindication to needle aspiration cytology of metastatic nodes, and this can frequently direct the diagnostic search in a more appropriate direction. Lower cervical lymph node chains are subject to metastatic spread from cancer below the clavicle via the thoracic duct. The finding of adenocarcinoma in a cervical lymph node suggests that the gastrointestinal tract, kidneys, breast, and gonads must also be investigated. The finding of squamous carcinoma mandates a thorough search of the upper airway for a primary site utilizing all of the diagnostic entities outlined in this chapter. The prognostic significance of a cervical metastasis from a head and neck malignancy is less ominous than that from a distant adenocarcinoma.

SUMMARY

The diagnosis of masses in the neck should start with a comprehensive history and physical examination, and a careful, considered evaluation of the likely etiologic sites should be undertaken. The indicated radiographic evaluation may include skull and sinus roentgenography, salivary and thyroid scans, conventional tomograms, and computed tomography of the neck. Additional information can be gained by utilizing ultrasonography, fine-needle aspiration cytology, and arteriography. Formal endoscopy with biopsies of any suspicious mucosal lesion should precede an open biopsy of the neck mass. In children, the mass is most likely to be inflammatory or congenital, and the diagnostic evaluation may be limited to skin tests, chest radiography, and needle aspiration of the mass. Definite therapy usually proceeds after the immediate infection has resolved.

THE ACUTE ABDOMEN IN CHILDHOOD

By Robert T. Soper, M.D.
and Kevin C. Pringle, M.B.,Ch.B., F.R.A.C.S.
Iowa City, Iowa

The mechanisms that produce the acute abdomen are virtually identical in all age groups: gastrointestinal obstruction and perforation, peritonitis, massive hemorrhage (gastrointestinal or intraperitoneal), and visceral infarction. Only abdominal wall abnormalities and delivery-related visceral injuries are totally unique to the newborn. However, the disorders that provoke these acute abdominal crises in children are quite different from those in the adult, and furthermore, they are expressed clinically in more variable and obtuse patterns. These variations in cause and clinical manifestations are striking even among children of different ages, fully justifying our subdividing this discussion into at least four age groups: neonatal, infant, preschool, and school.

NEONATAL AGE (First Month of Life)

Protrusions of abdominal viscera through congenital defects in the abdominal wall are problems that are totally unique to the neonatal period. Although embryologically different in origin, both *omphalocele* (herniated viscera covered by a thin, translucent sac) and *gastroschisis* (no sac) present common problems of infection and loss of body temperature and fluids that mandate immediate surgical correction. Inspection suffices for diagnosis postnatally; ultrasound of the gravid uterus allows prenatal diagnosis.

The rare *rupture of solid viscera* (spleen, liver, adrenal) occurring during the trauma of vaginal delivery is also a uniquely neonatal problem. Diagnosis is suspected when a large newborn or one who is the product of a difficult labor develops pallor, abdominal distention, tachycardia, and shock during the first few hours of life. Examination of the gradually distending abdomen reveals shifting dullness and a fluid wave; diagnosis is confirmed by a bloody peritoneal tap.

The other types of neonatal abdominal emergencies tend to present as some mix of repeated vomiting (usually bilious) and abdominal distention. The more proximal the lesion, the earlier the bilious vomiting occurs with less abdominal distention.

Congenital duodenal obstruction is heralded by persistent vomiting, usually bile-stained, in a newborn who is the product of a pregnancy complicated by polyhydramnios. Physical examination reveals a scaphoid abdominal contour. Plain upright radiographs show the classical "double-bubble" air-fluid level of distended stomach and duodenum. Duodenal atresia is the most common cause of complete obstruction; since about 30 per cent of these babies have Down's syndrome, the characteristic facies and single palmar crease and other physical stigmata of this syndrome should be sought. Partial congenital duodenal obstructions are caused by duodenal stenosis or extrinsic obstructions by Ladd's bands (midgut malrotation) or annular pancreas, which are distinguishable best at operation. In addition to the "double-bubble," plain radiographs show driblets of gas in downstream bowel. The threat posed by midgut volvulus to the viability of the midgut mandates a carefully done contrast study of the upper gastrointestinal (GI) tract that forces barium past the duodenum; failure of the barium column to cross to the left of the vertebral column documents malrotation; and a beak-like cutoff to the barium column confirms volvulus. Emergency laparotomy is then undertaken.

Jejunoileal obstructions in the newborn are usually complete and are secondary to in utero vascular insults to the developing fetal intestine. The injury-repair response to the more minor vascular insults generates simple stenosis or an obstructing membrane; at the other extreme, major segments of bowel may infarct and disappear to significantly shorten the intestine. Recurrent bile-stained vomiting is the rule, associated with jaundice in one third and failure to pass meconium per rectum in two thirds. A proximal obstruction is associated with polyhydramnios, and after delivery, inspection reveals a scaphoid abdomen. A tense and shiny distended belly characterizes ileal obstruction, often with visible "laddering" of the obstructed bowel loops. Plain radiographs show air-fluid levels in distended bowel loops of roughly similar size, the number and distribution of which allow an estimate as to the approximate level of the atresia. Barium contrast studies of the colon usually are normal and therefore do not help in diagnosis. Occasionally, intraperitoneal calcification is seen on the plain radiographs, representing calcification of meconium which spilled into the free peritoneal cavity at the time of intestinal ischemia. Rarely, a large accumulation of meconium develops in the peritoneal cavity, known as a giant meconium cyst, owing to a persistence of the bowel perforation until delivery. The meconium cyst tends to displace gas-containing bowel into different areas of the abdominal cavity, depending upon its location. Laparotomy is necessary to distinguish among these entities.

Meconium ileus is an obstruction caused by undigested, inspissated, tenacious meconium impacting in the terminal ileum. It almost always is associated with cystic fibrosis of the pancreas and generalized mucoviscidosis. Diagnosis is suspected with a family history of cystic fibrosis or in a newborn with a distended abdomen which is shiny and tense with visible vascular patterns and who is vomiting green material. Plain radiographs are suggestive of meconium ileus rather than atresia if the distended and obstructed bowel loops vary in size and contain air bubbles entrapped in the tenacious meconium. Diagnosis is confirmed on contrast enema, which shows meconium filling defects in a small colon and meconium tightly impacted in the terminal ileum. In the well-hydrated baby, hypertonic water-soluble contrast material will pull enough water into the terminal ileum to disimpact the inspissated meconium and allow its expulsion per rectum without surgical intervention. However, one third of the babies with meconium ileus have a complication of volvulus or perforation of the obstructed bowel that mandates surgical correction.

Atresia can occur most anywhere in the intra-abdominal colon but is much less common than in the small bowel because of the dual colonic blood supply. Atresia produces a complete colonic obstruction that occasionally can be detected on the plain films if the distended colon loops are distinguishable from obstructed small bowel loops; if not, contrast enema will fill a collapsed colon up to the point of the atresia, beyond which material will not pass. Final confirmation awaits laparotomy.

Neonatal Hirschsprung's disease is characterized by failure to pass meconium during the first 24 hours of life associated with a gradually distending abdomen and bile-stained vomiting. Examination reveals a distended, shiny, and tympanitic abdomen, and rectal examination reveals an empty rectum tightly wrapped around the examining finger. In about half of the babies, the tip of the examining finger will enter the dilated ganglionated bowel, which provokes an explosive gush of gas and liquid per rectum upon withdrawing the finger. Plain radiographs reveal air- and fluid-distended bowel loops, with no rectal gas. Carefully done contrast study of the colon may show a smaller distal aganglionic bowel with dilated bowel at the transition to ganglionated intestine, usually in the rectosigmoidal area. Lateral and oblique views are recommended for better bringing out of the transition zone; only small amounts of barium are used because barium is just as difficult for the baby to expel as stool. Rectal manometry (if available) shows a failure of the internal anal sphincter to relax when the rectal ampulla is distended by a balloon. Further diagnostic confirmation is afforded by a transanal biopsy of the rectum. This can be achieved without anesthesia by suction technique or a small punch biopsy forceps to allow histologic investigation of the submucosal layer for ganglion cells. Rarely, in Hirschsprung's disease the obstructed and distended ganglionated colon perforates, and the baby's condition rapidly worsens with signs of shock, sepsis, and respiratory distress. Plain radiographs confirm free air, mandating laparotomy for final diagnostic confirmation and exteriorization of the perforation.

The *meconium plug syndrome* is a temporary anorectal obstruction secondary to inspissated meconium. Meconium is not passed per rectum during the first 24 hours of life by a baby with a progressively distending abdomen and bile-stained vomiting. Physical examination confirms the distended and tympanitic abdomen, and rectal examination detects thick, tenacious plugs of meconium in the anorectum. Plain radiographs reveal air- and fluid-distended loops of intestine with no rectal gas. Obstruction is relieved explosively when the meconium plug is expelled; this occurs spontaneously or in response to digital rectal examination, therapeutic enemas, or contrast study of the colon. In our experience, about half of the babies with meconium plug syndrome turn out to have no other abnormality; the other half are ultimately found to have either Hirschsprung's disease or cystic fibrosis, so that both of these possibilities are diagnostically explored in babies with the clinical manifestations of the meconium plug syndrome.

Anorectal atresia is suspected in the baby who does not have a normal perineal anus; usually these babies gradually develop abdominal distention with bile-stained vomiting. Physical examination should include critical inspection of the perineum for an ectopic or absent anal opening and for evidence of a rectoperineal fistula or a fistula from the rectum into the vagina (in females) or into the urethra (in males) as manifested by pneumaturia or meconium in the urine. Radiographs are taken in true lateral projections after the baby has been upside down for 3 or 4 minutes with thick barium pasted over the perineal skin. The distance between the perineal marker and the lowest air-distended loop of bowel helps to distinguish between low atresias (the rectum has descended through the levator sling) and the high atresias (the rectum terminates above the levator sling). Injection of contrast material through any available fistula helps define diagnosis; if in doubt, a neonatal colostomy should be established, after which contrast material can be introduced into the downstream bowel to more precisely document the details of the atresia.

Neonatal gastrointestinal perforations have been described in every part of the gastrointestinal tract from stomach to rectosigmoid. Any of the aforementioned obstructing mechanisms can perforate proximal to the obstruction if diagnosis and treatment are delayed or neglected. However, perforations that are not secondary to neglected obstruction do occur. Neonatal gastric perforations occur either spontaneously (when large volumes of air are acutely swallowed) or following forceful passage of a stiff nasogastric tube. Gastric perforation is heralded by acute deterioration of a previously well newborn who rapidly develops signs of shock, associated with a distended, tender tympanitic abdomen. Plain radiographs show large volumes of free air in the peritoneal cavity with a single large fluid level on erect or decubitus views. Final diagnosis is confirmed at laparotomy.

Stress ulcers in the newborn occasionally develop in the latter half of the first week of life and clinically present either with free air (perforation) or massive upper gastrointestinal hemorrhage with shock, hematemesis, and melena occurring simultaneously. Diagnosis of perforated ulcer (usually duodenal, occasionally gastric) is suggested by pneumoperitoneum and a spreading peritonitis, confirmed at laparotomy as a punched-out perforation without a linear quality. The stress ulcer that bleeds in the newborn is diagnosed clinically by the rapid onset of massive upper gastrointestinal hemorrhage, hematemesis, and melena. Upper GI contrast studies usually do not show the punched-out ulcer crater. Because endoscopy at present cannot be carried out in these young patients, diagnosis is based on clinical suspicion alone. Saline lavage of the stomach and blood transfusions suffice to tide the patient over 85 per cent of the time, laparotomy being required in the minority both to confirm diagnosis and to stay the bleeding by suture ligatures to the base of the ulcer.

Neonatal necrotizing enterocolitis usually develops during the first 2 weeks of life in the stressed baby who is born prematurely. The condition is preceded by several hours of refusing feeds or by bile-stained vomiting associated with some abdominal distention. Early plain radiographs show a paralytic ileus pattern and later films reveal pneumatosis intestinalis, usually involving the distal ileum or right colon, these being the most common locations of necrotizing enterocolitis. Untreated patients, or those in which the condition is unusually severe, progress to necrosis of the involved bowel with free air visible on plain radiographs. Gas bubbles within the portal vein are a radiographic sign of advanced disease. Abdominal wall erythema, edema, signs of peritoneal irritation, and the presence of a tender mass are all evidence of advanced disease. Metrizamide contrast study of the colon will show the diagnostic thumbprinting of involved bowel, but the procedure is not recommended at the present time because of the danger of bowel perforation. Nasogastric suction and systemic antibiotics are started when necrotizing enterocolitis is first suspected, and in the majority of patients, these measures halt progression of the disease. Laparotomy confirms the diagnosis when the bowel is perforated or if the disease rapidly progresses clinically or radiographically in the face of adequate treatment. Paracentesis yielding brownish fluid that on Gram stain shows cells and bacteria documents impending perforation and mandates laparotomy.

INFANCY (1 Month to 2 Years of Age)

Hypertrophic pyloric stenosis is the most common surgically amenable disease that produces protracted vomiting in the baby 3 to 6 weeks of age. These babies characteristically do not vomit the first few days or weeks of life, which distinguishes this condition from the truly congenital causes previously discussed. Vomiting is postprandial, is never bile stained, and becomes progressively more frequent and forceful as the days go by. These features allow a historical distinction to be made from *achalasia,* the common gastroesophageal reflux pattern of effortless regurgitation favored by the supine position, which is another common cause for vomiting in this age group. The child with pyloric stenosis passes a reduced number and quantity of stools as the days go by, which is associated with weight loss and dehydration. Physical examination confirms these latter findings. Abdominal inspection reveals characteristic gastric hyperperistaltic waves sweeping from the left rib cage across the epigastrium to just beyond the midline, which can best be triggered by feeding a bottle of glucose water. The physician can then witness the clear vomitus and forceful nature of the vomiting that is triggered by the feeding. Diagnosis is complete if the so-called "olive" mass of the hypertrophied pylorus can be palpated in the epigastrium or right upper abdominal quadrant; this mass is firm, movable, and nontender. Rarely, when the history or age group is atypical or if the examiner fails to palpate the "olive," upper gastrointestinal contrast study will reveal the characteristic "shouldering" imprint of the proximal end of the hypertrophied pyloric muscle in the antrum as well as the elongated "string sign" of barium in the attenuated pyloric channel. Final diagnostic confirmation is achieved at laparotomy after appropriate correction of the dehydration and characteristic hypochloremic, hypokalemic alkalosis.

Intussusception is the most common cause of intestinal obstruction in the baby from 3 to 18 months of age. History reveals the sudden onset of acute and severe abdominal colic lasting 15 to 30 seconds, during which time the baby drops his toy, lies down, draws up his knees, and screams out in pain. When the colic has passed, he will then play or return to previous activity and appear to be perfectly well for 15 to 20 minutes until the next bout of colic develops. Occasionally, the colicky pain lasts for several minutes and the pain-free interval between attacks may vary in duration. The child will often vomit once or twice during the first few attacks of pain. After a few hours have passed, these babies tend to refuse feedings and to appear pale and listless between attacks of colic. About 12 to 18 hours into the illness, altered blood admixed with stool may appear in the diaper. This alarming passage of so-called "currant jelly" stool usually brings the baby in for diagnosis.

Physical examination reveals pallor in a listless, apathetic, and unwell baby, and often the physician has the opportunity to witness a bout of colic to verify the parental history. The baby often sleeps between episodes of colic, allowing careful abdominal palpation to detect a tubular and transversely oriented right upper quadrant abdominal mass that is easily separable from liver edge. In the late or neglected patient, bile-stained vomiting, abdominal distention, and intestinal obstruction develop, the mass now being palpable under the left rib cage with downstream advancement of the intussusception. Early plain abdominal radiographs may show only a nonspecific gas pattern, but often with absence of gas in the right lower quadrant where the cecum usually lies. In the more delayed or neglected case, a typical pattern of small bowel intestinal obstruction may be apparent, and in rare cases free air from a perforation of necrotic bowel might be seen in decubitus and upright radiographs in the baby who presents clinically with evidence of generalized peritoneal irritation. Rectal examination confirms altered blood in the stool.

With the exception of the baby with a confirmed or suspected perforation, all babies with intussusception should have a diagnostic contrast enema, which characteristically shows "hold-up" of the contrast at the lead point of the intussusception with the classical "coiled spring" appearance of small amounts of barium slipping around the leading edge of the intussusception. Attempts at therapeutic hydrostatic reduction under fluoroscopic control are permitted in babies lacking either high-grade small bowel obstruction or radiographic or clinical evidence of perforation. Babies who fail hydrostatic reduction or who are not candidates for attempted reduction should have the diagnosis confirmed at laparotomy.

Incarcerated or strangulated indirect inguinal hernia is the next most common cause of small bowel obstruction in young babies. Irritability, gradually increasing abdominal distention, evidence of abdominal discomfort, and bile-stained vomiting are the hallmarks of the history, lasting several hours and associated with reduction or absence of stool and gas passed per rectum. Physical examination reveals a distended abdomen with hyperactive bowel sounds. Often, only careful inspection of the inguinal area will disclose the characteristic firm mass in the inguinal canal or scrotum that confirms diagnosis. Plain radiographs show dilatation and laddering of the obstructed small bowel loops. Erythema or exquisite tenderness of the mass mandates early laparotomy to confirm diagnosis and reduce the hernia, which may be strangulated. Lack of these signs justifies attempts at nonsurgical reduction.

Regrettably, *child abuse* is not an uncommon cause of the acute abdomen in the child who is too young either to defend himself or to articulate the cause of his distress. Manifestations of injury will vary from ruptured solid organs, with intraperitoneal bleeding and shock, to pancreatitis to rupture of hollow viscera, each with its own separate set of radiographic and clinical findings. One should suspect deliberate injury if a disparate and misleading parental history suggests innocent or minor trauma which produces a disastrous intra-abdominal injury of the aforementioned type. A history of previous episodes of trauma, bruise marks, or skin abrasions and injuries in varying stages of resolution and radiographic evidence of old bone injuries heighten the suspicion of child abuse. Reporting the possibility to the appropriate authorities is mandatory (see article on child abuse).

Recurrent bouts of *partial intestinal obstruction* in infants can be secondary to congenital causes such as intestinal stenosis, annular pancreas, and midgut malrotation. Duodenal stenosis and annular pancreas produce intermittent bile-stained vomiting in a youngster with a scaphoid abdomen. Plain abdominal radiographs may show modest dilatation of the stomach and first part of the duodenum with only small amounts of gas distal to the obstruction. Upper GI contrast studies will show a narrowing of the duodenal lumen, intrinsic in a baby with duodenal stenosis and extrinsic in the baby with annular pancreas. Laparotomy confirms the diagnosis. The baby with midgut malrotation may have intermittent volvulus or duodenal obstruction manifested by bile-stained vomiting, abdominal discomfort, and failure to thrive. Plain radiographs show air- and fluid-distended stomach and duodenum if the main obstruction is extrinsic and in the duodenum because of so-called Ladd's bands, but with intermittent volvulus may reveal a disparate picture which ranges all the way from distended loops of air-filled small bowel to a totally "gasless" abdomen. Whenever this diagnosis is suspected, carefully performed upper GI contrast study will rapidly confirm that the fourth part of the duodenum fails to cross to the left of the midline. The beaklike cutoff characteristic of midgut volvulus may also be seen. Emergency laparotomy confirms the diagnosis. Babies with this clinical picture who evidence shock or signs of peritoneal irritation should have emergency laparotomy without any further study in order to salvage potentially strangulated midgut.

Hirschsprung's disease, which does not produce high-grade neonatal obstruction, is capable of producing a bewildering complex of signs and symptoms during the second and third months of life; thereafter, the condition gradually settles down into a more predictable clinical picture of severe and unrelenting constipation. Early in infancy, failure to thrive, protein-losing enteropathy, intermittent abdominal distention, alternating constipation and diarrhea, and recurrent vomiting can all be seen in patients with congenital aganglionosis. Enterocolitis, the most feared complication of the disease, is common during these first months of infancy and is characterized by acute and sudden worsening in the general condition of an infant in this clinical setting, associated often with failure of gas or stool passage per rectum, worsening abdominal distention, pallor, shock, and bilious vomiting. The clinical deterioration may be devastatingly rapid. Plain radiographs will reveal air- and fluid-distended bowel loops, sometimes with the characteristic appearance of pneumatosis intestinalis or perhaps with free air, indicating a perforation. Rectal examination usually demonstrates an empty rectum wrapped around the examining finger. Very carefully performed contrast enema reveals a narrowed rectum, funneling into dilated bowel at the transition point, often with "thumbprinting" evidence of submucosal edema. Colostomy is justified after appropriate intensive supportive and resuscitative treatment. Passage of a large-bore rectal tube may afford rapid relief of distention.

The older infant who escapes the complication-prone first 3 months of life gradually settles down into a typical constipation picture that resists all of the usual therapeutic measures. These babies are fussy, fail to thrive in a normal fashion nutritionally, and have distended abdomens, which improve only when the bowels are induced to move by enemas or laxatives. Physical examination reveals a softly distended abdomen, often with palpable lumps of stool. Again, rectal examination tends to show a narrowed rectum, perhaps with firm stool at the fingertip. Plain radiographs reveal an enlarged and distended colon, characteristically with no air in the rectum. Contrast enemas are almost always diagnostic, showing narrow distal aganglionic bowel funneling into dilated megaintestine at the point of histologic transition from aganglionic to normal intestine. Rectal manometry and transanal biopsy both confirm the diagnosis.

Symptomatic *Meckel's diverticulum* usually manifests itself by significant lower intestinal bleeding or signs of small bowel obstruction. The second year of life is the most common age for symptoms to develop, although ultimate diagnosis may not be made for several years, depending on the frequency and severity of the symptoms. The bleeding episodes may be associated with abdominal discomfort, but they are not associated with hematemesis or blood retrieved by nasogastric tube. However, the blood is admixed with stool and maroon in color; the blood loss does not characteristically occur rapidly enough to produce shock but usually does reduce the hemoglobin level measurably. Intestinal obstructions that are associated with vitellointestinal remnants can be acute and complete or partial and intermittent. These variables determine the degree and duration of abdominal distention, colic, and bile-stained vomiting as well as the plain abdominal radiographic evidence of small bowel obstruction. A radioactive technetium scan shows abnormal uptake in a Meckel's diverticulum, which contains ectopic gastric mucosa in most cases, although both false-negative and false-positive examinations have been reported. Gastrointestinal contrast studies, both from below and above, are not diagnostically helpful. Usually, diagnosis is confirmed at laparotomy.

PRESCHOOL AGE (2 to 5 Years)

The preschool child is peculiarly free of acute abdominal crises because of a diminishing incidence of the congenital and acquired causes discussed earlier and because appendicitis is still a rarity at this stage. Blunt abdominal trauma in a child of this age is apt to be incurred at play, is more common in boys than in girls, or is secondary to vehicular accidents in which the child is either a pedestrian or a rider. Child abuse diminishes as the child gets old enough to identify the abuser, and the injuries incurred at a younger age by uncertain gait and judgment change into the improved neuromuscular coordination of the preschooler.

Primary peritonitis has become a rare cause of the acute abdomen at any age, particularly since the introduction of antibiotics. Children with the nephrotic syndrome who are being treated with steroids or have an immunologic deficiency are predisposed to develop this peritonitis. *Pneumococcus* is the most common organism isolated. The abdominal pain of primary peritonitis is acute and severe, and it is associated with tachycardia, a high temperature, elevated white blood cell count, and decreased appetite *from the beginning of the illness.* Physical examination reveals a flushed and ill child with generalized abdominal distention and tenderness, both direct and rebound. Abdominal paracentesis yields syrupy mucopurulent fluid that contains gram-positive cocci. A high clinical index of suspicion is essential, and intravenous fluids and penicillin will confirm the diagnosis by the rapid disappearance of the acute abdominal complaints. Laparoscopy or laparotomy to exclude perforated appendicitis is justified when diagnosis is in doubt.

Rarely, an acute abdominal state is produced in a youngster of this age who *ruptures a solid tumor,* such as a Wilms' tumor or neuroblastoma. The history will divulge the often minor episode of trauma to the abdomen, perhaps preceded by subtle signs of abdominal enlargement. Physical examination reveals a slightly tender abdominal mass, usually filling the loin, associated with modest signs of peritoneal irritation. Plain radiographs show bowel loops displaced from the location of the mass. Paracentesis yields a bloody return. Ultrasound is an additional helpful diagnostic study. Laparotomy confirms diagnosis.

Appendicitis is rare under the age of 5, and it is different enough from the same disease in the older child to justify special consideration. Appendicitis is reportable in the newborn, extremely rare under 2 years of age, and quite unusual in the patient who is under 5 years. This rarity, plus the nonspecific nature of its incipient signs and symptoms and the inability of the young to communicate, combine to yield an appalling 80 percent incidence of perforation with generalized peritonitis at the time the patient is first brought in for diagnosis. The triggering mechanism of appendicitis in the very young is the same as it is in the older child: obstruction to the lumen of the appendix. In the very young, the obstruction is more apt to result from submucosal lymphoid hyperplasia of the appendix rather than a fecalith, which is more common in the older child. Another important difference is the rapidity with which the disease progresses from obstruction to perforation in the very young, requiring only a few hours; this in turn is likely due to the tiny appendiceal lumen, abundant lymphoid tissue, vigorous reaction (edema, pus) to infection, and the ineffective mechanisms in the very young to localize inflammation. A thin and short omentum contributes to the last item.

Clinically, appendicitis in the very young child is a short, nonspecific, and acute illness culminating within hours in generalized peritonitis. Fever, flushed face, irritability, and refusal of feedings herald the disease. Copious vomiting ensues, generally bile-stained, with ill-defined evidence of abdominal pain associated with distention, oliguria, dehydration, and sometimes diarrhea. In 12 to 24 hours, a healthy baby becomes acutely and critically ill.

Inspection reveals dehydration in a crying or apathetic baby who is acutely ill with a high temperature (up to 40°C, or 104°F) and tachycardia. Attempts at physical examination are generally resisted, although the severely shocked infant may react in an apathetic and listless manner. The exquisitely tender abdomen is typically distended, tympanitic, silent, and board-like, with little evidence of a mass or other localizing signs. Rectal examination may reveal a boggy and tender cul-de-sac. The critically ill child may show minimal peritoneal signs until normal fluid and electrolyte balance has been restored. The white blood cell count is elevated, but it may be disarmingly normal or even low in the very ill. Urine is scanty, concentrated, and ketotic. Serum electrolyte concentrations are elevated (dehydration), and the blood pH is low.

Vigorous resuscitation with nasogastric suction, intravenous fluids, and broad-spectrum antibiotics is mandatory to lower body temperature and pulse rate, to reverse the signs of dehydration, and to improve renal function. Plain radiographs show a paralytic ileus picture. Safe emergency laparotomy to confirm diagnosis may be undertaken only in the baby who has been properly resuscitated.

SCHOOL AGE (5 to 16 Years)

Study of the acute abdomen in the school-age child and adolescent essentially involves a review of appendicitis and its differential diagnosis as well as abdominal trauma and its evaluation. Appendicitis is without doubt the most common cause for the acute abdomen in older children and adolescents and is the most common justification for emergency laparotomy.

Appendicitis occurs with increasing frequency throughout childhood, peaking in incidence from 12 to 16 years of age, with progressive diminution in both older and younger age groups. Further, the complication rate (perforation and peritonitis) steadily diminishes in the older child as his cooperativeness and ability to render a dependable history improve and as his ability to cope with inflammation becomes more effective.

Appendiceal lumen obstruction initiates the appendicitis cycle, commonly triggered by concretions of stool and undigested food residue known as fecaliths. A history of vague, difficult-to-describe central abdominal pain of 2 or 3 days' duration is typical, associated with anorexia and nausea with occasional vomiting. As the appendiceal inflammation spreads transmurally to involve parietal peritoneum, the pain gradually becomes sharper and better described, localizing to the right lower abdominal quadrant. Appendicitis pain disturbs sleep patterns and alters normal daytime behavior and play. Physical examination reveals a somewhat ill and slightly dehydrated youngster with mild abdominal distention. Bowel sounds are usually hypoactive but present. Palpation reveals maximum tenderness, often with some guarding, localized to the right lower abdominal quadrant. Light fingertip percussion of the abdomen often is a most sensitive way to localize tenderness without provoking exquisite pain and an uncooperative child. Involuntary guarding accompanies localization of pain; voluntary spasm relaxes when the patient's attention is drawn from himself or when he inhales, whereas involuntary guarding remains. Rectal examination is often unremarkable. Unless the child is obviously ill, it is always illuminating to ask the patient to get off the bed and walk. There is a world of difference in how this is accomplished by a well child, when compared with a child with appendicitis.

Plain radiographs of the abdomen either are normal or may show mild evidence of paralytic ileus; a calcified appendolith should be closely looked for. Extension of the right hip often increases pain, as does physical motion. The body temperature is mildly elevated and the white cell count usually is between 10,000 and 15,000 with a modest shift to the left. This clinical picture clearly justifies laparotomy to confirm the diagnosis.

If by chance the appendix lies retrocecally or down in the pelvis adjacent to the sigmoid colon or bladder, the parietal peritoneum-somatic innervation component is absent and the clinical picture remains vague and difficult to define both by history and physical examination. Obliteration of the right psoas shadow on x-ray film suggests a retrocecal appendicitis, in which case the psoas sign should be markedly positive and the lumbar spine might flex to the right side. Dysuria and a few blood cells in the urine suggest a perivesical location of the appendix, and diarrhea and an exquisitely tender cul-de-sac on rectal examination suggest a so-called "pelvic appendicitis." Whereas constipation resulting from paralytic ileus is characteristic of inflammation of a normally located appendix, an inflamed appendix juxtaposed to the sigmoid colon may trigger hyperperistalsis and diarrhea.

Delay in diagnosis allows perforation to occur, with signs of sepsis and paralytic ileus, generalized peritoneal irritation producing a boardlike abdominal rigidity in a silent abdomen. Less commonly, delay is associated with several days of a "flulike" illness, and examination may then detect a moderately tender mass in the right lower abdominal quadrant or cul-de-sac without signs of generalized peritoneal irritation. This so-called "missed appendicitis" with perforation is well tamponaded and walled off into an abscess cavity adjacent to the appendix. Nasogastric suction, parenteral fluids, and antibiotics may produce a rapid enough improvement to delay appendectomy to a later symptom-free interval (see article on appendicitis).

The differential diagnoses of appendicitis in the older child are legion and must include all of the possible inflammatory diseases of the abdomen in childhood. However, gastroenteritis and mesenteric lymphadenitis are the two most common nonsurgical causes that need to be excluded. *Gastroenteritis* usually has more vomiting followed by diarrhea than appendicitis and is commonly associated with a similar illness in classmates or neighborhood children. Temperature and white blood cell count are not as consistently elevated in gastroenteritis as in appendicitis, and abdominal examination shows minimal tenderness and mild distention of a generalized nature with no localizing signs or involuntary guarding. Bowel sounds are often extremely hyperactive but are not obstructive in pitch. Rectal examination confirms the diarrhea, and further observation allows confirmation of diagnosis as the disease runs its course.

Mesenteric adenitis is often preceded by an upper respiratory tract infection, with later vague abdominal discomfort that often begins in the right lower abdominal quadrant and is intermittent. Body temperature is higher with mesenteric adenitis than with appendicitis, but there is no white cell count elevation or shift. Abdominal examination reveals only mild right lower quadrant abdominal tenderness that is not well localized or acute and is not accompanied by involuntary guarding; in the cooperative older child, deep-seated nodules may be palpated in the right lower quadrant, confirming the diagnosis. Observation and re-examination show either no progression or gradual improvement. In the occasional case that is indistinguishable from appendicitis, a carefully done barium enema might exclude the latter by completely filling the appendix without any signs of adjacent inflammation. Laparoscopy helps document a normal appendix, but in children it requires a general anesthetic. Simple observation often allows clear distinction to be made with no other diagnostic maneuver necessary.

Occasionally, acute *transmural granulomatous enterocolitis* (Crohn's disease) of the terminal ileum cannot be distinguished from appendicitis. In a cooperative or sedated patient, one may palpate the tubular, tender mass of an ileitis. A previous history of similar episodes is often helpful, as is occult blood in the stool. A carefully performed barium enema will often clearly distinguish the two, as will laparoscopy. Occasionally, laparotomy is required for diagnosis (see article on Crohn's disease).

Rarely, other acute abdominal conditions produce an acute abdomen that cannot be totally differentiated from appendicitis: right lower lobe pneumococcal pneumonia, acute pyelonephritis, rheumatic fever, lead colic, abdominal epilepsy, sickle cell crisis, and acute cholecystitis. Pelvic inflammatory disease should be considered in older girls. Direct questioning as to any sexual activity must be reserved for a time when the parents have been excluded from the room.

As school-age children grow into adolescence, they are increasingly subject to blunt abdominal trauma, especially boys. These injuries are usually acquired in contact sports, playground activities, falls, and pedestrian or vehicular accidents. This history is extremely important to obtain, but the physician may occasionally be deliberately misled by the apprehensive child who wishes to protect playmates from punishment.

Contusion of the abdominal wall is a simple and common result of abdominal trauma, provoking no underlying visceral injury. However, it may be severe enough to cause abdominal pain, tenderness, and rigidity. Observation and repeated examination often suffice to exclude more serious intra-abdominal injuries, occasionally helped by ultrasound examination, plain radiographs, or paracentesis.

The spleen, liver, and kidney are the three solid organs most commonly injured by blunt abdominal trauma, in decreasing order of frequency. *Rupture of the spleen* in a child occurs relatively easily because it has only a thin capsule and is only partially protected by a very elastic left lower rib cage that is easily deformed by an impacting blow without producing rib fracture. Pain of a ruptured spleen occurs immediately and can be either localized to the left upper abdominal quadrant or spread in a more generalized fashion with free extravasation of blood; 15 per cent of patients will have the pain accentuated by deep inspiration, which radiates the pain to the left shoulder tip (Kehr's sign). Examination of the child with a ruptured spleen reveals left upper abdominal quadrant tenderness and perhaps guarding. The white blood cell count is mildly elevated, and serial hematocrits tend to fall with fluid resuscitation. Plain radiographs may show medial displacement and serration of the greater curvature of the stomach gas shadow and downward displacement of the splenic flexure of the colon. A stable child with suspected splenic trauma can be admitted to hospital and observed while fluid resuscitation is commenced. Abdominal paracentesis yielding a bloody return, ultrasound, computed tomography (CT), liver-spleen scan, and arteriograms all may confirm splenic injury, but usually these measures are not needed. Laparotomy for diagnostic confirmation should be carried out in the patient in shock who is unstable and requires significant blood replacement.

Fortunately, *liver lacerations* are fairly uncommon in children because they are seen with multiple system injuries incurred usually in automobile-associated accidents and are associated with significant mortality. Rapid intra-abdominal blood loss provokes shock and pallor with a distending abdomen. When confirmed by paracentesis, immediate laparotomy is undertaken coincident with aggressive resuscitation.

Contusion or laceration of the kidney in children produces hematuria and flank pain, sometimes with a visible and palpable mass. Urinalysis and pyelography confirm diagnosis, as do ultrasound and CT scan.

Upper abdominal trauma in the younger child, often resulting from an impaling injury, may produce pancreatic injury or intramural duodenal hematoma. *Pancreatic injury* often produces vague upper abdominal discomfort associated with anorexia and occasional vomiting, which often takes 24 to 48 hours to become significant enough to justify a visit to a physician. Abdominal examination reveals epigastric tenderness and perhaps skin contusion. Diagnosis is supported by elevations of the serum and urine amylase and ultrasonic or CT scan detection of an enlarged pancreas, perhaps with peripancreatic collections of fluid.

Intramural hematoma of the duodenum follows a similar impaling injury to the epigastrium, but after an initial few hours of epigastric discomfort, it often is strangely asymptomatic for the 1 or 2 days it takes for the submucosal hematoma to obstruct the lumen. At this time, bile-stained vomiting ensues, which brings the patient in for examination. Physical examination shows only epigastric tenderness with contusion and hematoma marks of injury. Diagnosis is afforded by an upper gastrointestinal contrast study showing the characteristic narrowing, obstruction, and "coiled spring" appearance, usually in the second, third, or fourth part of the duodenum. Diagnosis is confirmed when obstruction disappears after a few days of nasogastric suction and intravenous fluids and nutrition.

EVALUATION OF ACUTE ABDOMINAL PAIN IN ADULTS

By J. Timothy Fulenwider, M.D.
and William C. McGarity, M.D.
Atlanta, Georgia

Acute abdominal pain is one of the most frequently occurring maladies prompting emergency consultation. Although it is true that 40 to 50 per cent of patients examined in the emergency room have nonspecific abdominal pain of indeterminate cause that results in no adverse clinical sequelae, from 5 to 15 per cent of such patients will have natural, spontaneous disorders requiring surgical intervention. Establishing the correct, yet expeditious, clinical diagnosis of acute abdominal pain can be one of the most challenging tasks confronting physicians, despite the recent explosion of sophisticated radiographic and laboratory investigations. The vast majority of episodes of abdominal pain can be explained if the examiner accepts the indispensable role of a complete and orderly history and physical examination and relates data collected to prior knowledge of anatomy, embryology, and physiology. It is improbable that any present or future radiographic or laboratory examination will supersede the importance of mature clinical judgment and experience in managing the patient with acute abdominal pain, although these modalities are useful adjuncts when diagnostic specificity is paramount and the clinical condition permits their use.

The problems facing the examiner of the patient with acute abdominal pain are summarized as follows: (1) What is the most likely diagnosis and pathophysiology? (2) Does the patient require surgical consultation and operative intervention? (3) If an operation is deemed necessary, what is the "safe" interval of resuscitation and investigation? (4) How can judgmental errors be identified, and what price must the patient pay for errors in diagnosis?

Some of the most catastrophic diseases requiring operation may be ushered in by the subtlest of clinical symptoms and signs; however, the most excruciating abdominal pain may have a purely medical explanation yet mimic the "acute surgical abdomen." The term "acute surgical abdomen" used here is medical slang referring to a heterogeneous group of abdominal conditions requiring rapid decision-making and operative intervention. The presence of either localized or generalized peritonitis is implied in this definition, and the early detection of either generally warrants consideration of operation. Intestinal obstruction and acute gastrointestinal bleeding are usually included categorically, since their detection also requires prompt surgical intervention but rarely features peritoneal signs as presenting complaints.

This article is devoted to the early detection of spontaneously occurring, natural diseases of surgical importance. Although the evaluation of blunt and penetrating abdominal trauma is also critically important, the delay in diagnosis of traumatic abdominal conditions is usually much shorter than the delay in recognition of spontaneously occurring disease. Since delay in diagnosis is known to adversely influence the outcome of such natural disorders, this article will focus upon the history, physical examination, pathophysiology, and differential diagnosis of the "acute abdomen" in an effort to sharpen diagnostic acumen of examiners challenged by the patient with acute abdominal pain.

ANATOMY AND PATHOPHYSIOLOGY OF ABDOMINAL PAIN

Pain is the subjective, unpleasant sensation arising from the central nervous system's interpretation of peripherally received noxious stimuli. The expression of similar degrees of pain by different individuals is highly variable and modified by the following psychologic factors: (1) personal interpretation of the consequences of the injury or stimulus, (2) previous experience (conditioning), (3) psychologic stability, (4) personality, and (5) cultural background. Precise quantitation of an individual's pain has defied clinical measurement, yet it is this unpleasant and purely subjective sensation that physicians must correctly interpret and provide relief for. However, the physician must resist the temptation to alleviate this pain promptly with the use of narcotics or other potent analgesic measures because interpretation of this signal of tissue injury may be the only clue to the correct diagnosis. Dulling the patient's sensorium may foil serial abdominal examinations, mask evolving clinical patterns, and delay proper therapy. Compassion should prevail once the correct diagnosis has been established and treatment begun, and appropriate analgesics should be administered.

Abdominal pain may be categorized into three major types: (1) visceral (protopathic) pain, (2) parietal (somatic, epicritic) pain, and (3) referred pain. Each of these types has different sensory characteristics, neural pathways, and clinical significance. An appreciation of evolving abdominal pain patterns and characteristic referral distribution is frequently clinically useful in narrowing the spectrum of differential diagnosis.

Visceral Pain. Because there are no specific nociceptors, free nerve endings in the visceral walls and soft tissues of the abdominal wall provide the "starting blocks" of the abdominal afferent pain pathways. Pain arising from any hollow abdominal viscus is triggered by any maneuver or condition that increases intramural tension. Distention occurring with obstruction or violent contraction such as a gut hypermotility disorder will create discomfort. Distention of the capsules of solid viscera, such as the liver, spleen, and kidney, creates similar abdominal discomfort. The rapidity and magnitude of "stretch" determine the severity of the visceral discomfort, which is characteristically described as dull, aching, poorly localized, often midline, and frequently associated with secondary autonomic reflexes such as sweating, tachycardia, pallor, and nausea.

In general, the abdominal discomfort arising from a viscus is referred topograpically to the abdominal wall dermatome from which the diseased organ also receives innervation. The quality of visceral discomfort is usually described as "cramping, burning, boring, gnawing," with the diffuseness and midline-referral best explained by the overlapping, multisegmental innervation, and paucity of free nerve endings in the visceral walls and capsules when compared with the density of somatic innervation. The anterior abdominal surface referral of pain of visceral origin may be integrated with embryologic development: Visceral pain of foregut origin, e.g., from the biliary tract, liver, stomach, duodenum, pancreas, and spleen, is referred to the epigastrium, whereas visceral pain arising from organs of midgut origin, e.g., the small intestine and colon (to the level of the splenic flexure), is referred to the periumbilical region. Pain arising from viscera of hindgut origin, e.g., left colon, is generally referred to the hypogastrium. This knowledge of embryology and abdominal wall expressions of visceral pain is invaluable in determining the regional origin of the discomfort.

Noxious abdominal stimuli, other than intramural or parenchymal tension, include bacterial and chemical inflammation exemplified by the irritation created by metabolites of bacterial origin; mediators of inflammation such as bradykinin, histamine, serotonin, and prostaglandins; anaerobic metabolites that are due to ischemia; and naturally occurring visceral contents such as hydrochloric acid, bile, blood, and urine. The severity of abdominal pain associated with chemical or bacterial stimuli depends upon the rapidity of exposure, volume, duration of irritant contact, and inherent noxious potential; for example, peritoneal exposure to hydrochloric acid from a perforated peptic ulcer elicits an intense and immediate pain response in contrast to large volumes of blood, which initially creates minimal peritoneal irritation.

Neural transmission circuitry of afferent impulses of visceral pain involves unmyelinated, C fibers which pass through the splanchnic ganglia and sympathetic chain via the splanchnic nerves, entering the dorsal roots of their respective nerve cell bodies via the white rami communicantes. Upon entering the spinal cord, these nerve fibers travel several segments through the tract of Lissauer before terminating with dorsal horn cells. Branches are also sent directly to the posterior horn. The visceral afferents decussate through the anterior commissure and ascend in the lateral spinothalamic tracts, ending in the reticular formation of the medulla, midbrain, or thalamic nuclei. Both cerebral postcentral gyri ultimately receive afferent terminations from both sides of the body, thus accounting for the ability to perceive and interpret peripheral pain following massive destruction of one cerebral hemisphere.

Table 1. Viscera: Their Afferent Innervation and Referral Pain Patterns

Organ	Afferent Innervation	Extra-abdominal Referral Pain Zones
Esophagus	Thoracic sympathetics—unnamed	Neck, anterior and posterior trunk—usually at precise level of disease Less commonly to supraclavicular and medial upper extremity regions
Hepatic suspensory ligaments, Glisson's capsule, central diaphragm, pericardium	Phrenic nerve (C_{3-5})	Supraclavicular regions
Biliary tree, stomach, pancreas, small bowel, peripheral diaphragm	Greater splanchnic nerve, celiac plexus (T_{6-9})	Scapular tip; upper to mid-dorsal midline
Colon, appendix, pelvic viscera	Lesser splanchnic nerve, superior mesenteric plexus (T_{10-11})	Dorsal, lumbosacral region
Sigmoid colon, rectum, renal pelvis and capsule, ureter, testes	Least splanchnic nerve, inferior mesenteric plexus (T_{11}–L_1)	Groin, flank, lumbosacral regions
Bladder, rectosigmoid colon	Hypogastric plexus (S_{2-4})	Sacral region

Parietal Pain. Extension of a visceral inflammatory process to involve the parietal peritoneum stimulates free nerve endings lying in the submesothelial areolar tissue. The pain created is generally more intense and well localized than its visceral counterpart. These somatic nerve impulses travel in C and A-delta (small, myelinated) nerve fibers within peripheral nerves. The dermatomes subtended by afferents responsible for mediating abdominal parietal pain include T_6 through L_1.

Referred Pain. With increasing intensity of the visceral pain, discomfort may be felt in a region remote from the primarily diseased viscus. This referred pain is characteristically well localized, usually superficial, and occasionally associated with cutaneous hyperesthesia. Referred pain is usually concomitantly felt with its abdominal counterpart and intensified by abdominal compression. On very rare occasions, the referred pain may be the solitary clue to the diagnosis of remote abdominal visceral disease. Classically, referred pain is exemplified by pain of gallbladder origin referred to the supraclavicular fossa or right scapular tip, and cardiac pain referred to the cervical, acromial, and mandibular regions or ulnar aspect of the left arm. Subdiaphragmatic inflammation such as created by a subphrenic abscess, perforated ulcer, hepatic abscess, or ruptured spleen may be referred to the ipsilateral supraclavicular fossa. Similarly, pancreatic inflammatory diseases frequently are associated with pain referral to the dorsal spine and posterolateral thorax, whereas the pain of ureteral colic may radiate to the groin, testicle, or medial thigh. Knowledge of the spinal levels of afferent innervation of the viscera and their usual dermotome representation is very helpful in determining the source of abdominal discomfort (Table 1).

Pain impulses from the esophagus are conveyed through unnamed thoracic sympathetic nerves that enter the spinal cord through the dorsal root. Esophageal pain is produced primarily by conditions leading to obstruction, inflammation, penetration, or perforation. The pattern of pain referral of an esophageal disorder generally allows precise localization by the patient in the majority of cases. On rare occasions, a cervical esophageal disorder may refer pain to the epigastrium; however, involvement of the intra-abdominal esophagus virtually never gives rise to cervical pain unless perforation has produced subphrenic peritonitis. Glisson's hepatic capsule, the triangular and coronary ligaments, splenic capsule, central portion of the diaphragm, and pericardium are innervated by the phrenic nerve; thus, the pattern of pain referral corresponds to the third through fifth cervical dermatomes. The peripheral portion of the diaphragm, biliary tree, stomach, pancreas, and small bowel receive afferent impulses via the greater splanchnic nerve, which travels through the celiac plexus with dermatome representation at thoracic segments 6 through 9. The colon, appendix, and pelvic viscera are innervated by the lesser splanchnic nerve with afferents passing through the mesenteric plexus and dermatome segments corresponding to the 10th through 11th thoracic segments. The sigmoid colon, rectum, renal pelvis and capsule, ureter, and testes are innervated by the least splanchnic nerve and are topographically represented by the 11th thoracic through the first lumbar dermatomes. The urinary bladder and rectosigmoid colon send afferents through the hypogastric plexus to the spinal cord from the second through fourth sacral nerve roots. These visceral afferent pathways and typical patterns of pain referral should be committed to memory, since knowledge of these circuits is indispensable in deciding probable sources of the abdominal complaint.

Thus far, emphasis has been upon the distinction of visceral and somatic pain and their significance as well as recognition of primary and referral patterns of abdominal pain. Integration of pertinent historical data with knowledge of such pain patterns produced by specific disease states directs further investigation and facilitates expeditious diagnosis and therapy.

APPROACH TO THE PATIENT WITH ACUTE ABDOMINAL PAIN

Evaluation of the patient with abdominal pain always begins with a detailed, painstaking history and thorough physical examination, since there are few conditions other than exsanguinating hemorrhage that demand immediate surgical intervention. The history and physical examination remain paramount in the diagnosis of abdominal pain, for most decisions regarding operation are made predominantly on the basis of history and physical examination and are rarely influenced solely by other investigations.

The examiner should determine the onset, quality, location, duration, and precipitating events of the acute abdominal pain in addition to those maneuvers, medications, or physiologic events (micturition, defecation) that alleviate or aggravate the discomfort. Relevant symptoms and signs that preceded the acute event may be helpful in differential diagnosis; for instance, the history of several weeks of nocturnal, deep, boring epigastric pain may forecast the catastrophic presentation of a perforated peptic ulcer. A previous history of similar abdominal discomfort, treatment regimens, outcome, and assigned diagnoses is also beneficial. Essential components of the history also include a list of previous operations, family history, medications (especially anti-inflammatory and immunosuppressive agents), and co-existing medical diseases that might influence the presentation of the illness, treatment, or morbidity and mortality if operation is necessary. A complete review of systems, including menstrual history, is an essential ingredient of the complete history.

The history that is collected by an experienced, calm examiner not only provides the essential clues to diagnosis but also serves to establish rapport with the patient, allay anxiety created by the acute illness, and consequently allow a more meaningful physical examination. It is often useful to ask the patient to point to the area of most intense pain. Mapping of the area of pain by the patient's outstretched hand implies poor localization—a feature combined with "dull, aching, cramplike" qualities suggests a visceral origin without parietal peritoneal irritation. Localization of the abdominal pain, such as indicated by the patient's index finger, with intensification by coughing, straining, or jarring of the examination table is suggestive of parietal inflammation, either primary (e.g., spontaneous bacterial peritonitis of cirrhosis) or secondary (e.g., extension of the visceral inflammation to the abdominal wall). The intensity of this latter type of pain frequently overshadows a visceral component; however, both patterns may coexist and blend imperceptibly in the presentation of the acute illness.

The best example of the evolution of these pain patterns is the classical description of acute appendicitis —the initial complaints of dull, periumbilical discomfort are poorly localized and are due to obstruction of the appendiceal lumen. Over the next 12 to 24 hours, the pain migrates to McBurney's point in the right iliac fossa as the appendiceal inflammatory process extends to involve the parietal peritoneum. Subsequently, the pain becomes more intense and well localized, since the inflammation progresses as a result of suppuration.

Another pattern of abdominal pain is that of intermittent, visceral discomfort with a variable-length, crescendo-decrescendo pattern referred to as "colic," which implies obturation of a hollow viscus. Examples include impaction of a calculus in the cystic duct of the gallbladder, intestinal obstruction, or ureteral obstruction. Initially, the abdominal pain is poorly localized, becoming more intense and well localized with extension of the inflammatory process to the parietal peritoneum. With obstruction of any viscus, initially there are no peritoneal signs; therefore, diagnosis delayed until the development of abdominal rigidity is frequently accompanied by gangrenous changes that portend high mortality rates.

Abdominal pain that arises from perforation of a hollow viscus is frequently characterized by an explosive onset of severe somatic pain owing to massive contamination by caustic chemical and bacterial agents contacting a large surface of sensitive parietal peritoneum. Examples include perforation of a peptic ulcer or free perforation of a colon diverticulum. Abdominal pain caused by visceral ischemia characteristically reaches peak intensity within minutes to hours, is initially visceral in nature, and disproportionately severe when compared with the abdominal physical findings.

The classic example of this pain pattern is the superior mesenteric artery embolus which accounts for about 5 per cent of peripheral arterial emboli. With acute occlusion of a chronically stenotic superior mesenteric artery, there is frequently the past history of weight loss, moderate to severe postprandial visceral discomfort, and "food fear" created by the ingestion of meals. Early diagnosis of mesenteric ischemia is essential for survival, but all too frequently the diagnosis is delayed because of failure of the examiner to consider this possibility.

Abdominal conditions associated with inflammatory visceral pathology characteristically demonstrate a slow, graded transition from visceral to somatic abdominal pain as the inflammatory process extends to the parietal peritoneum. Examples of these conditions include Crohn's disease, diverticulitis, and hemorrhage, as intraperitoneal bleeding also represents a common cause of abdominal pain. Conditions associated with intraperitoneal bleeding such as traumatic liver rupture, splenic laceration, or ruptured ectopic pregnancy all are associated with a paucity of early peritoneal signs, since blood is a relatively weak peritoneal irritant. Over the course of several hours, physical signs of peritonitis may become prominent but never of the intensity created by a similar volume of gastric juices.

Frequently, the pattern of pain referral is helpful but rarely of sufficient diagnostic specificity to incriminate one organ system or reliably localize the problem to an abdominal viscera. An example of such diagnostic confusion is the scenario of vague, right upper quadrant colic of several hours' duration referred to the tip of the scapula or interscapular region. Such a classic presentation of acute biliary colic may dupe the unwary examiner who does not consider the differential diagnostic possibilities, which include acute, inferior myocardial infarction, dissecting aortic aneurysm, or acute pulmonary embolus. Therefore, one must not depend solely upon the pattern of pain referral to make a definitive diagnosis.

The physical examination begins as soon as the examiner enters the patient's room. Note should be made of the patient's grimacing or other facial expressions, the affect of the patient toward his discomfort, the patient's seeking postures of comfort, and signs of autonomic stimulation such as sweating, cutaneous pallor, or contraction of the erector pili muscles. The patient with obstruction of a hollow viscus usually writhes incessantly with flexion of the hips and abdomen in search of the elusive position of comfort. Patients with abdominal pain due to severe, generalized parietal peritonitis prefer immobility, shallow breathing, and avoidance of any movement that increases peritoneal tension. A comprehensive physical examination is essential; however, the examiner must gingerly approach the patient with acute abdominal pain. A handshake or gentle stroking of the patient's brow is effective initial physician contact, since it portrays compassion and reassures the patient that the examiner will not inflict unnecessary discomfort. All too frequently, the hasty, brusque examiner elicits voluntary abdominal muscle guarding, which masks intraperitoneal clues and precludes meaningful serial abdominal examinations. The abdominal examination should always begin with inspection for protuberance, asymmetry, discoloration, abnormal venous collaterals, and external hernias.

Following inspection, the examination continues with auscultation of the frequency and pitch of intestinal sounds, bruits, venous hums, and peritoneal friction rubs. Gentle pressure upon the stethoscope during auscultation has proved useful in detecting early involuntary guarding resulting from reflex muscle hypertonicity associated with parietal peritonitis. Since the patient is distracted during abdominal auscultation, a more reliable assessment of abdominal tenderness is obtained that can be compared with the findings of manual palpation. A marked discrepancy in the pain response after these maneuvers (i.e., an exaggerated pain response from manual palpation when compared with that from stethoscope pressure) may disclose the patient's tolerance to pain and even detect the malingering patient.

The earliest indication of parietal peritonitis is involuntary guarding resulting from muscular hypertonicity, which is considered a protective reflex. With early, localized peritonitis only one quadrant of the abdomen may demonstrate involuntary guarding; therefore, a comparison of muscular tonicity in multiple abdominal regions is important. Palpation should begin gently with the fingertips in an area remote from the site of most intense pain. Often simple percussion with the fingertips, causing peritoneal reverberation, will indicate peritonitis. When these findings are detected with light percussion, it is unnecessary to elicit "rebound tenderness"—the pain produced by slow abdominal wall depression with quick release of the examining hand. Both maneuvers, when positive, imply parietal peritonitis; therefore, deep palpation and release only inflict pain without yielding additional diagnostic information. A note of caution is warranted regarding the examiner's interpretation of the patient's response to the quick-release maneuver used to detect rebound tenderness. If the examiner does not explain the maneuver to the patient, quick release of the examiner's hand may startle the patient and the examiner may interpret the response as indicating rebound tenderness. This erroneous interpretation could lead to unnecessary celiotomy because of the implications of the presence of parietal peritonitis.

Following light palpation, deeper examination follows and must include a search for visceromegaly and abdominal masses, noting the mobility, tenderness, dimensions, or obscurity caused by voluntary abdominal wall tension. Voluntary tension of the abdominal wall musculature will mask intra-abdominal masses, whereas true abdominal wall masses will remain unchanged in contour. Gently stroking the skin with the fingertip or tongue depressor may elicit hyperesthesia in the dermatome shared by the diseased intraperitoneal organ. This test is helpful only if positive, for its absence does not preclude the possibility of peritonitis. No abdominal examination is complete without a thorough inspection and palpation of the external genitalia, pelvic structures, and rectum.

Finally, it must be mentioned that the presence of audible peristalsis in no way excludes the diagnosis of peritonitis. Additionally, abdominal silence may be due to either peritonitis of surgical importance or other causes for adynamic ileus, for instance, hypokalemia, hypomagnesemia, or extra-abdominal sepsis.

The decision for and timing of operation are almost invariably made on a clinical basis. A normal laboratory or roentgenologic examination can never confidently exclude the possibility of the acute abdomen. All laboratory investigations should be considered adjunctive to diagnosis and management of the primary disease and comorbid conditions that might influence the outcome of the acute illness. With established peritonitis, time should not be wasted unnecessarily on tests and procedures intended to specify the diagnosis—especially with generalized peritonitis. However, a few basic laboratory tests are essential in patient management. Such tests include a complete blood count, urinalysis with microscopic examination, electrolyte package, amylase, creatinine and blood urea nitrogen (BUN), serum glutamic-oxaloacetic transaminase (AST, SGOT), and bilirubin. A chest x-ray, ECG, and arterial blood gases are helpful in excluding acute thoracic conditions such as pneumonitis, myocardial infarction, and pulmonary embolus, which may mimic the acute abdomen. Other tests such as plain and upright abdominal x-rays, intravenous pyelography, ultrasonography, computerized axial tomography, arteriography, liver-spleen scintigraphy, and barium or water-soluble contrast studies may be selectively utilized if the clinical condition warrants and permits time for these examinations.

There does exist a small subset of patients who, because of age, low intelligence, altered consciousness, or neurologic injuries, will remain impossible to evaluate accurately by history and physical examination alone. In this group, peritoneal lavage through a catheter placed percutaneously in the midline below the umbilicus may provide diagnostic clarification. The method is similar to that originally described for the investigation of blunt abdominal trauma. Basically, 1000 ml of crystalloid (or 10 to 15 ml/kg) is instilled into the peritoneal cavity over a period of 5 to 10 minutes. After dwelling for 10 minutes, the siphoned effluent is examined for red blood cells, white blood cells, bacteria, vegetable fibers, bile, and amylase. Normal peritoneal fluid contains a few red cells, an occasional polymorphonuclear leukocyte, and no organisms or bile. The amylase content is usually less than or equal to that of the plasma. It should be remembered that the abdominal examinations following peritoneal lavage may be influenced by the local tenderness following abdominal puncture or the possible low-grade chemical peritonitis created by lavage solutions.

A basic knowledge of the most frequent abdominal problems leading to emergency operation is helpful in the differential diagnosis of acute abdominal pain. In regional trauma centers, blunt and penetrating abdominal trauma is the most common indication for emergency celiotomy. In regional trauma centers, almost 60 per cent of emergency abdominal operations are performed for abdominal trauma. Excluding traumatic indications, the most frequently occurring natural diseases requiring emergency operation are acute appendicitis and intestinal obstruction—each accounting for approximately one third of emergency operations, with perforated ulcer and acute cholecystitis collectively accounting for approximately 15 per cent of the cases. In almost all reported series, acute appendicitis, intestinal obstruction, perforated gastroduodenal ulcer, and acute cholecystitis—in that order—account for the overwhelming majority of indications for emergency celiotomy. One must note that the single most frequent condition initially misdiagnosed and later requiring emergency operation is acute appendicitis. Other less common indications for surgical intervention include intra-abdominal abscess, acute pancreatitis, and acute colonic diverticulitis.

THE ACUTE ABDOMEN IN PREGNANCY

Acute abdominal pain is a frequent complaint during pregnancy. The majority of these episodes are vague, deep, abdominal colics thought to arise from fetal movement, expansion of the uterus, Braxton-Hicks uterine contractions, or traction upon the broad ligament. Nausea and vomiting are also frequently problematic—especially in the first trimester. The physiologic changes of elevated basal body temperature, tachycardia, leukocytosis, dilutional anemia, and an elevated erythrocyte sedimentation rate are also normal during pregnancy. These frequent nonspecific complaints and laboratory findings may also be the prelude to a number of catastrophic abdominal diseases that may afflict the pregnant patient. Displacement of pelvic viscera by the gravid uterus, the high prevalence of gastrointestinal complaints, and the natural reluctance to carry out radiographic or other invasive diagnostic techniques all compound the diagnostic challenge during examination of the pregnant patient with acute abdominal pain. It is estimated that 1 in 500 pregnancies will be complicated by an acute abdominal condition requiring exploratory celiotomy. Of these explorations, one third will be considered negative with fetal wastage occurring in one fourth of those patients explored.

Acute appendicitis is the most frequent general surgical indication for emergency celiotomy in pregnancy. Approximately 1 in 1200 pregnancies is complicated by this acute disease. The diagnosis is frequently delayed until the development of gangrenous appendicitis because of cephalad and lateral migration of the appendix displaced by the enlarging uterus. This displacement by the gravid uterus and counterclockwise rotation of the appendix causes the appendix to lie superior to the right iliac crest, overlying the right kidney, by the seventh or eighth month of gestation. The omentum is also displaced superiorly and unable to confine the progressive inflammatory process; thus, the gravid uterus forms the medial wall of an evolving appendiceal abscess. It would appear that the incidence of spontaneous abortion is related to the extent of the suppurative process rather than to celiotomy or general anesthesia alone. Early diagnosis and excision of the appendix prior to gangrenous changes should be accompanied by maternal and fetal mortalities that approach zero; however, with the development of intra-abdominal sepsis, spontaneous abortion will occur in approximately a third of pregnancies. Other less common diagnoses of surgical importance during pregnancy include torsion, rupture, or intracystic hemorrhage of ovarian cysts, acute cholecystitis, perforated peptic ulcer, and acute pancreatitis.

The puerperal period is generally uncomplicated and rarely associated with abdominal discomfort. The rarity of complications during this period may dampen diagnostic suspicion while abdominal wall laxity impairs the development of abdominal muscular tension secondary to intraperitoneal inflammation, leading frequently to unimpressive physical findings. The most common complications of surgical importance during this puerperal period are acute appendicitis and acute intestinal obstruction.

THE ACUTE NONSURGICAL ABDOMEN

The acute nonsurgical abdomen refers to a heterogeneous group of metabolic, infectious, allergic, endocrinologic, and hematologic conditions that create abdominal symptoms and signs that mimic those of surgically treatable conditions. No discussion of abdominal pain would be complete without considering this group of disorders best treated without the scalpel. Approximately one fourth of instances of the "acute abdomen" are later found to have a medical explanation for symptoms initially thought to be of surgical importance. Approximately one fifth of these patients undergo celiotomy that is considered unnecessary for cure but is obviously beneficial in establishing the correct diagnosis. The major causes of abdominal pain that mimic the acute abdomen are due to intraluminal, hollow viscus infections or to intraperitoneal infections. Infectious agents usually causal of the gastroenteritides, including Shigella, Salmonella, Coxsackie, and Yersinia, are predominant etiologic agents.

Conditions predisposing to ascites, such as nephrotic syndrome and cirrhosis with portal hypertension, are also important factors in peritonitis of bacterial origin. Although the routes of peritoneal access of the bacteria remain speculative, the existence of primary peritonitis in these diseases is well established. Approximately 5 to 15 per cent of those with ascites secondary to cirrhosis will have spontaneous, primary bacterial peritonitis. The mortality associated with recognized cirrhotic spontaneous peritonitis varies between 70 and 85 per cent in the United States. The majority of these infections are due to aerobic, coliform bacteria, with *Escherichia coli* accounting for approximately 50 per cent of infections. Anaerobic or microaerophilic bacteria are found in approximately 6 per cent of cases, but as many as 50 per cent of these primary infections are polymicrobial. The most commonly found organisms in primary peritonitis associated with nephrosis are the hemolytic streptococci and pneumococci. Other conditions associated with primary bacterial peritonitis include chronic renal failure or any disease state associated with immunosuppression, acute phlegmonous gastritis, and systemic lupus erythematosus. An important dictum is that all ascites, whether the origin is known or unknown, warrants sampling for Gram stain and fungal slide preparation, cultures, white blood cell count and differential, lactate levels, and pH, in addition to the other biochemical studies including protein, lactate dehydrogenase (LDH), amylase levels, and other pertinent studies.

Supradiaphragmatic infections and ischemic or embolic events may also produce severe abdominal pain. Leading the list of such conditions are acute pneumonitis—especially lower lobe involvement, acute myocarditis or myocardial infarction, and acute pericarditis. The importance of the routine chest x-ray films and ECG cannot be overemphasized; yet the physician must maintain a high index of suspicion because of the unacceptably high morbidity and mortality associated with general anesthesia and abdominal operations concomitant with these acute thoracic conditions.

The collagen vascular diseases are associated with multiple systemic clinical syndromes, and abdominal pain is a frequent complaint of patients with these diseases. Systemic lupus erythematosus, scleroderma, dermatomyositis, and polyarteritis nodosa are all associated with degenerative, fibrosing, and inflammatory changes in small arteries in virtually every organ

Table 2. Medical and Extra-abdominal Conditions That May Mimic the Acute Abdomen

Cardiopulmonary	**Metabolic-Hematologic**
Myocardial infarction	Diabetic ketoacidosis
Congestive heart failure	Uremia
Myocarditis	Addisonian crisis
Pericarditis	Hyperthyroidism
Pulmonary embolus	Hyperparathyroidism
Acute pneumonitis	Hyperlipidemia
Acute pleuritis	Sickle cell, other hemolytic crises
Empyema	Acute intermittent porphyria
Pneumothorax	Leukemias
Dissecting aortic aneurysm	Dysproteinemias, cryoglobulinemia
	Hemochromatosis
Drugs—Poisons	Henoch-Schönlein purpura
Lead, arsenic, mercury poisoning	
Ergot alkaloid poisoning	**Collagen-Vascular**
Drug, sedative withdrawal	Systemic lupus erythematosus
Cholinomimetic overdose	Polyarteritis nodosa
Methyl alcohol poisoning	Dermatomyositis, polymyositis
Anticoagulant complications	Rheumatoid arthritis
Vinca alkaloids	Scleroderma
Anticholinergic toxicity	Acute rheumatic fever
Neurologic	**Other**
Compression radiculopathy	Black widow spider envenomation
Acute myelitis, arachnoiditis	Familial Mediterranean fever
Tabes dorsalis	Malaria
Causalgia	Hereditary angioneurotic edema
Herpes zoster	Abdominal epilepsy
	Rectus sheath hematoma
Genitourinary	Bornholm disease
Ureteral colic	Clicking rib syndrome
Acute pyelonephritis	Fractured ribs
Acute prostatitis	
Seminal vesiculitis	

system. Many patients require chronic steroid or other immunosuppressive medications to suppress their symptoms because of the vasculitis associated with these diseases. These anti-inflammatory agents may mask the development of abdominal symptoms and signs of acute disease, leading to a delay in diagnosis and consequently high morbidity and mortality rates. Physicians must be warned of the hazard of relying on steroid therapy alone in the treatment of acute abdominal pain, since the deposition of circulating immune complexes may lead to focal visceral ischemia, necrosis, and perforation—the physical findings being masked by steroids. Diagnostic peritoneal lavage may be of benefit in diagnosis of conditions of surgical importance in these patients.

There are many other metabolic, endocrinologic, and hematologic conditions associated with acute abdominal pain that simulate the acute abdomen of surgical importance. A list of such diseases is included in Table 2; however, a discussion of each disease state is beyond the scope of this chapter. One can readily understand the complexity of these pseudosurgical conditions—particularly when the leisure in decision making and work-up is inherently short. Nonetheless, there are certain historical physical clues that should heighten suspicion of a medical condition accounting for the acute abdominal pain. Important historical features include unusual food or foreign body ingestion, accompanying dermatitis, arthralgias or arthritis-associated urologic symptoms, changes in urine color, or previous steroid or immunosuppressive treatment. Physical findings that might suggest a medical basis for abdominal pain include bizarre mental changes with motor deficits or sensory disturbances such as vibratory or joint position abnormalities. The Argyll-Robertson pupil, lipemia retinalis, unexplained lymphadenopathy, pleural or pericardial friction rubs, splenomegaly, vaginal or urethral purulent discharges, skin eruptions or purpura, or arthropathies are also significant.

Only a complete awareness of the existence of these multiple medical causes for acute abdominal pain will lead to their consideration in the individual case. Despite the most comprehensive examination performed by an astute, experienced clinician, many episodes of acute abdominal pain will require diagnostic celiotomy; however, one must realize that in the absence of preoperative objective findings, the yield from diagnostic celiotomy will be low.

SUMMARY

The diagnosis of acute abdominal pain can be one of the most challenging tasks for the clinician despite the availability and the sophistication of currently available diagnostic techniques. No test to date has superseded the importance of a compulsory history and physical examination in determining the propriety of operation or the safety of observation with serial examinations. Accordingly, the authors have focused upon the history and physical examination, as these are the foundations of the diagnosis of acute abdominal pain.

GASTROINTESTINAL HEMORRHAGE

By Chesley Hines, Jr., M.D.
and William A. Ferrante, M.D.
New Orleans, Louisiana

Gastrointestinal hemorrhage can be one of the most urgent medical problems when it is massive and one of the most frustrating of problems when the bleeding is occult.

For diagnostic purposes, it is helpful to divide gastrointestinal hemorrhage into two areas: bleeding above the ligament of Treitz (upper gastrointestinal bleeding) and bleeding below this site (lower gastrointestinal bleeding).

BLEEDING ABOVE THE LIGAMENT OF TREITZ

Bleeding from a site above the ligament of Treitz is characterized by hematemesis and melena. The vomited blood may be red if it is coming from the esophagus or is high in the stomach, while blood originating in the distal stomach or duodenum often has the appearance of "coffee grounds," resulting from the action of stomach acid on the blood. Blood passed via the rectum is usually tarry black and sticky; however, on occasion, when the hemorrhage is massive, the blood may be maroon or even red.

Etiology

Following are the most common sources of bleeding above the ligament of Treitz:

1. Ulcerations in the stomach or duodenum.
2. Acute erosive gastritis.
3. Esophageal varices.
4. Hiatal hernia.
5. Esophagitis.
6. Esophageal tears.
7. The Mallory-Weiss syndrome (a linear tear at the cardioesophageal junction).
8. Carcinoma and lymphoma of the stomach.

Less common causes of upper gastrointestinal bleeding are as follows:

1. Carcinoma of the esophagus.
2. Esophageal ulceration.
3. Benign tumors of the stomach.
4. Benign and malignant tumors of the duodenum.
5. Hereditary telangiectasia (Osler-Weber-Rendu syndrome).
6. Uremia
7. Pseudoxanthoma elasticum.
8. Hemobilia.

Historical Information

A tentative diagnosis of the site of bleeding can often be made from the history alone. Bleeding from a duodenal or benign gastric ulcer may be massive or occult. There may or may not have been typical symptoms of peptic ulcer disease preceding the hemorrhage. Ulcerating gastric carcinomas usually bleed slowly, or they may not bleed at all. Gastric lymphomas commonly bleed, but rarely massively. Abdominal pain of a steady nature is often present in both gastric carcinoma and lymphoma. Gastritis, especially that induced by aspirin, phenylbutazone, or indomethacin, may cause massive bleeding. The combination of alcohol ingestion at night followed by aspirin the following morning produces a particularly bloody gastric mucosa. Esophageal varices usually produce sudden eruption by mouth of red or partially clotted blood. The bleeding from varices usually continues steadily until the patient's blood volume has been significantly depleted. A history of alcoholism or previous hepatitis may lead to the suspicion of varices. Blood produced from the Mallory-Weiss syndrome is usually red and is preceded by at least one episode of retching. Esophagitis occurring alone or above a hiatal hernia may cause bleeding, but the bleeding is usually a slow ooze. Minor bleeding from the gastric mucosa in the hiatal hernia may occur also. The typical symptoms of pyrosis and water brash will point to the diagnosis of these conditions.

Physical Findings

A rectal examination is the most important part of the physical examination of a person with a history of gastrointestinal hemorrhage, especially if the hemorrhage has not been observed by the examiner. The material on the examining glove will usually be black if the bleeding is coming from the upper part of the gut.

The skin may be pale and clammy if the patient has bled massively. These skin findings are usually accompanied by a rapid pulse and a falling blood pressure. Spider angiomas may be observed if the patient has cirrhosis. Dilated superficial veins of the abdominal wall may be seen in portal hypertension. The characteristic chamois-colored plaques of pseudoxanthoma elasticum may be noticed in skin folds, and the angioid streaks in the retina may confirm this diagnosis.

Splenomegaly is often a good indicator of portal hypertension, and esophageal varices should then be suspected. The liver may be enlarged in nutritional cirrhosis but may be very small in postnecrotic cirrhosis. Both types of cirrhosis create portal hypertension. Even when portal hypertension and varices are present, bleeding may still be due to a gastric or duodenal ulcer or gastritis.

Diagnostic Procedures

The hemoglobin and hematocrit levels obviously must be obtained in a patient with gastrointestinal hemorrhage. The presence of blood in the stool should be confirmed by laboratory analysis.

Probably the single most important diagnostic procedure in the evaluation of a patient with upper gastrointestinal tract hemorrhage is the insertion of a nasogastric tube. This is especially important in the patient with melena who has not vomited blood. Blood in the gastric aspiration usually indicates that the bleeding has occurred above the ligament of Treitz. The absence of blood in the aspirate virtually excludes bleeding from the esophagus or stomach; however, it does not exclude bleeding from the duodenum. If blood is present in the stomach, the nasogastric tube should be left in place, and chilled saline lavage should be performed at frequent intervals. This not only provides an assessment of the rapidity of bleeding but often seems to slow or stop the bleeding, apparently by cooling the gastric mucosa.

Endoscopy should be performed prior to barium studies in a patient in whom active bleeding is suspected. In the patient with occult bleeding, a barium study of the upper gastrointestinal tract should first be obtained. Endoscopy is then indicated.

If the site of occult upper gastrointestinal tract hemorrhage escapes discovery by these techniques, it may be located by using a recently developed nuclear medicine scanning technique involving radioactive technetium-labeled sulfur colloid or technetium labeled red blood cells.

Arteriography of the celiac and superior mesenteric arteries may be useful when these diagnostic procedures have failed to reveal a bleeding site or when bleeding has occurred repeatedly with no site found.

BLEEDING BELOW THE LIGAMENT OF TREITZ

If the site of bleeding is below the ligament of Treitz, blood passed via the rectum may be maroon, magenta, or red, depending upon the proximity to the anus and how rapidly the blood has traversed the bowel. Hematemesis is a rare occurrence.

Etiology

Gastrointestinal hemorrhage from a site distal to the duodenum is most commonly caused by the following conditions:

1. Hemorrhoids.
2. Diverticulosis coli.
3. Angiodysplasias.
4. Chronic ulcerative colitis.
5. Crohn's disease of the ileum or colon.
6. Carcinoma of the colon (especially the ascending colon and cecum).
7. Ulceration of gastric mucosa in Meckel's diverticulum.

Less common causes follow:

1. Benign and malignant tumors of the small bowel.
2. Amebiasis.
3. Infections with Shigella and Salmonella.
4. Vasculitis.

Historical Information

The patient with hemorrhoidal bleeding has probably bled intermittently from hemorrhoids for many years. The bleeding is usually red. The blood may cover the stool, drip into the toilet bowl, or be so minor that it only stains the toilet tissue.

Bleeding from diverticulosis is arterial, tends to be acute, and most of the time is quite severe.

Angiodysplasias may bleed both acutely and massively, but they also have the potential for bleeding intermittently and occultly. Bleeding angiodysplasias of the arterial venous malformation type are usually in the right colon. However, other types of angiodysplasia, such as hemangiomas or telangiectasia, may be found in any area of the intestine, particularly in young individuals. In patients with angiodysplasias, recurrent hemorrhages are common, occurring at a rate of 85 per cent, whereas in diverticular disease the chance of recurrent bleeding after conservative control is 25 per cent after the first bleeding episode and 50 per cent after the second.

Carcinoma of the distal colon may lead to the passage of bright red blood in or around the stool, whereas carcinoma of the right side of the colon usually causes occult bleeding.

Bleeding via the rectum is a prominent feature of ulcerative colitis. The clinical presentation of amebiasis may be very similar. In Crohn's disease, bleeding is usually occult or does not occur at all in the early stages; but when bleeding does occur, it may be massive. The other symptoms of inflammatory bowel disease, such as diarrhea, abdominal cramps, fever, and weight loss, may be present also.

Ischemia of the bowel is usually due to a low flow state of the small terminal arterioles and commonly follows major surgery or a serious illness. A major embolus to a large vessel may occur in a patient following a myocardial infarction or in a patient with a cardiac arrhythmia or valvular heart disease. Abdominal pain is usually a prominent complaint in bowel ischemia.

Salmonella and Shigella infections are usually accompanied by fever and systemic symptoms of infection.

The passage of red or maroon stool in a child should cause one to suspect bleeding from a Meckel's diverticulum. The episodes of bleeding are usually characterized by intermittent, infrequent bouts of gross, but not massive, lower gastrointestinal bleeding.

Physical Findings

The physical examination may or may not be helpful. As in bleeding from above the ligament of Treitz, the rectal examination is the most important part of the physical examination in a person with lower gastrointestinal tract bleeding. The color of the blood on the glove may give an approximate idea of the source of the blood. External hemorrhoids may be seen immediately to be the source of bleeding. Palpation of the abdomen may reveal a mass in a patient with carcinoma of the colon. A generalized tender abdomen may be present in inflammatory bowel disease and bowel ischemia. There may be abdominal distention if a toxic megacolon is impending. The abdomen may also be tender in infections with Shigella and Salmonella, especially in the right lower quadrant.

Diagnostic Procedures

Figures 1 and 2 are schematograms for diagnostic approaches to acute and chronic lower gastrointestinal bleeding.

Proctosigmoidoscopy is the most useful diagnostic procedure. Bleeding from internal hemorrhoids, carcinoma of the rectum, distal colonic polyps, and di-

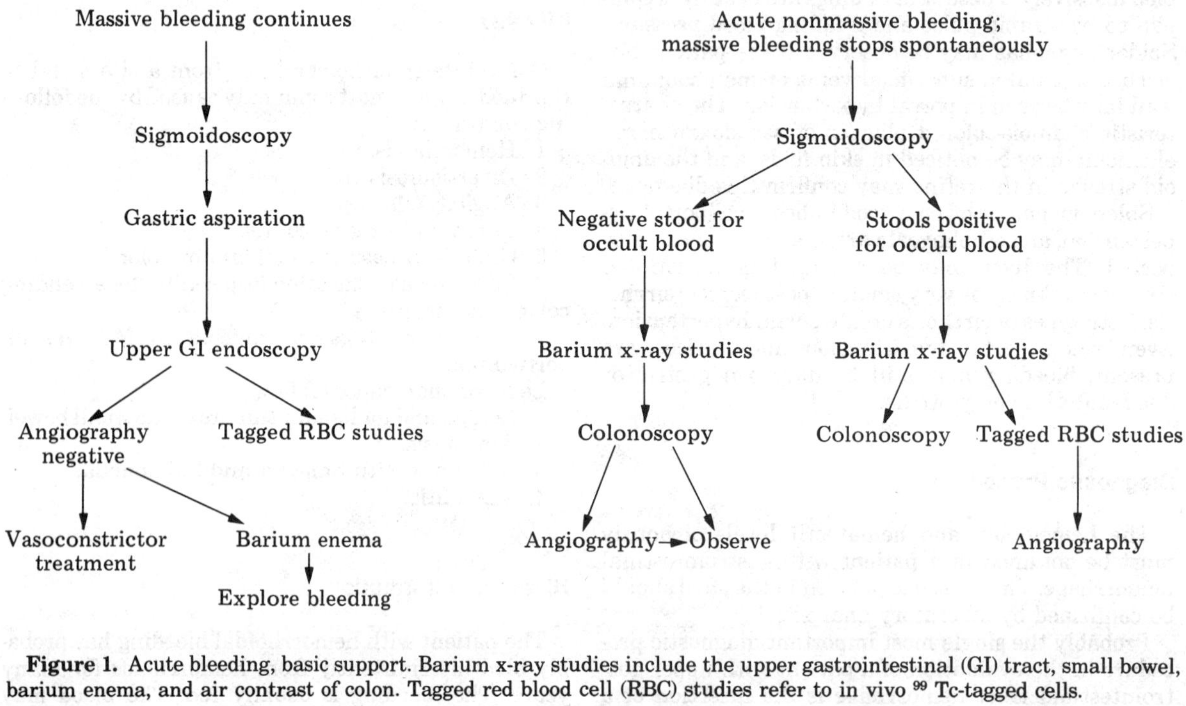

Figure 1. Acute bleeding, basic support. Barium x-ray studies include the upper gastrointestinal (GI) tract, small bowel, barium enema, and air contrast of colon. Tagged red blood cell (RBC) studies refer to in vivo [99] Tc-tagged cells.

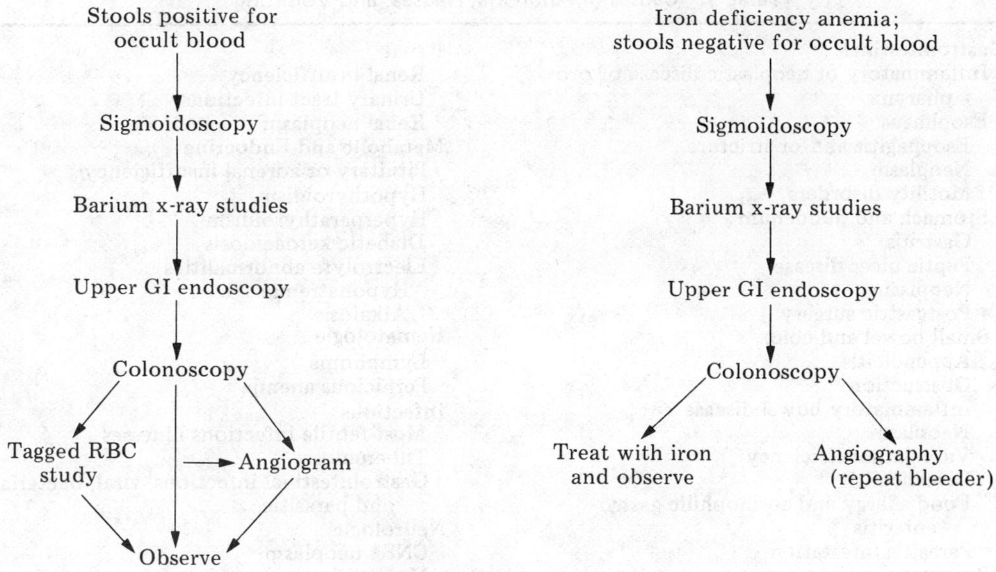

Figure 2. Chronic blood loss.

verticula can be seen with this examination. Mucosal abnormalities seen may lead to the diagnosis of ulcerative colitis, Crohn's disease of the anus or rectum, ischemic colitis, bacterial infection, or amebiasis. Even if the bleeding site is not found within the range of the sigmoidoscope, the procedure serves importantly to narrow down the area of bleeding in question.

A barium study of the colon may demonstrate a carcinoma of the colon, diverticulosis, the characteristic "thumbprinting" of bowel ischemia, or the mucosal changes of chronic ulcerative colitis and Crohn's disease of the colon and terminal ileum. Small bowel tumors may or may not be demonstrated by a barium study; however, polyps in the small bowel usually can be seen. A Meckel's diverticulum is almost never demonstrated by barium x-rays; however, a Meckel's scan using technetium pertechnetate can be diagnostic.

Arteriography of the superior and inferior mesenteric arteries may reveal the site of bleeding if the rate of bleeding is 0.5 ml per minute or greater. This test may be indicated as the first choice after proctosigmoidoscopy, especially in massive bleeding. We have also found it useful in those patients who have bled on several occasions and in whom no site has been found by other means. Arteriography may reveal an arteriovenous fistula that could not be seen with barium studies. Occlusion of the large or small vessels supplying the bowel may be demonstrated in ischemia of the bowel.

Colonoscopy is often useful in locating the site of occult lower gastrointestinal bleeding; it is not useful in massive hemorrhage.

A recent nuclear medicine technique utilizing radioactive ^{99m}Tc-tagged cells may be useful in discovering the cause of lower gastrointestinal bleeding as well as upper gastrointestinal hemorrhage.

ANOREXIA, NAUSEA, AND VOMITING

By Robert D. Mitchell, M.D.
Loma Linda, California

Anorexia is a loss or lack of appetite for food. It may be temporary or intermittent and is a very general symptom. By itself, it is not a good subject for differential diagnosis because of its presence with many illnesses. It may be caused by or associated with a wide variety of emotional and physical disease conditions, from depression to widespread malignant disease. When persistently present with other more specific symptoms, it becomes very significant. When it is the presenting complaint, a careful history, system review, and physical examination must be done to look for additional clues to guide further investigation. When persistent, it usually results in weight loss and other findings of protein-calorie deficiency.

There are centers in the hypothalamus that are concerned with appetite. Electrical stimulation of the lateral hypothalamic center in the experimental animal will cause an increase in intake of food. Stimulation of the medial hypothalamic area called the "satiety center" stops the intake of food. In the human, this process appears more complex, being influenced by the senses and by the cerebral cortex.

Anorexia is present in many gastrointestinal diseases, but it is not limited to diseases of that system. Anorexia may be a prominent symptom with malignancies, with acute and chronic infections, with metabolic and electrolyte disturbances, with emotional depression, as well as with anorexia nervosa. Many

Table 1. Causes of Anorexia, Nausea, and Vomiting

- **Gastrointestinal**
  - Inflammatory or neoplastic disease of oropharynx
  - Esophagus
    - Esophagitis and/or stricture
    - Neoplasm
    - Motility disorders
  - Stomach and duodenum
    - Gastritis
    - Peptic ulcer disease
    - Neoplasm
    - Postgastric surgery
  - Small bowel and colon
    - Appendicitis
    - Obstruction
    - Inflammatory bowel disease
    - Neoplasm
    - Vascular insufficiency
    - Diverticulitis
    - Food allergy and eosinophilic gastroenteritis
    - Parasitic infestation
  - Pancreas
    - Pancreatitis, acute and chronic
    - Neoplasm
  - Liver and gallbladder
    - Hepatitis
    - Alcoholic liver disease
    - Neoplasm, primary or secondary
    - Congestive hepatomegaly
    - Hepatic abscess
    - Cholecystitis, cholelithiasis, cholangitis
    - Biliary obstruction, intra- or extrahepatic
  - Peritoneum and mesentery
    - Peritonitis
    - Mesenteritis
    - Neoplasm, primary or metastatic
    - Retroperitoneal malignancies
- **Cardiovascular**
  - Congestive heart failure
  - Pericarditis
  - Myocardial infarction
- **Pulmonary**
  - Pulmonary insufficiency
  - Neoplasm
  - Pulmonary infections
- **Renal**
  - Renal insufficiency
  - Urinary tract infections
  - Renal neoplasm
- **Metabolic and Endocrine**
  - Pituitary or adrenal insufficiency
  - Hypothyroidism
  - Hyperparathyroidism
  - Diabetic ketoacidosis
  - Electrolyte abnormalities
    - Hyponatremia
    - Alkalosis
- **Hematologic**
  - Lymphoma
  - Pernicious anemia
- **Infectious**
  - Most febrile infectious illnesses
  - Tuberculosis
  - Gastrointestinal infections, viral, bacterial and parasitic
- **Neurologic**
  - CNS* neoplasm
  - Meningitis
  - Brain abscess
  - Degenerative and vascular CNS diseases
  - Migraine
  - Labyrinthine disturbance
  - Tabes
- **Psychiatric and Psychogenic**
  - Psychogenic vomiting
  - Depression
  - Schizophrenia
  - Anorexia nervosa
  - Acute psychoses
  - Neuroses
- **Miscellaneous**
  - Alcoholism
  - Drugs
    - Digitalis
    - Appetite suppressant drugs
    - Narcotic drugs
    - Side effect of many drugs
  - Withdrawal from addicting drugs
  - Vomiting of pregnancy
  - Collagen vascular disease

*CNS = Central nervous system.

medications produce anorexia as a possible or even frequent side effect.

Anorexia nervosa is a condition usually occurring in young women, and it is variously considered to be a result of depression, a psychologic alteration, or a dysfunction of the hypothalamic appetite-satiety centers. Although it is well documented that many measurable endocrine abnormalities can be present, they may be the result rather than the cause of anorexia nervosa.

Depression may be the etiology of anorexia; however, before this is accepted as the diagnosis, the patient should have a thorough evaluation to rule out a hidden malignancy or infection that may be the cause of the depression. Table 1 lists some of the possible etiologies of anorexia, nausea, and vomiting.

Nausea is the sensation that warns of impending vomiting. Subjectively it may be quite variable, but objectively it may be associated with increased salivation and decreased gastric motility; it may also be associated with profuse sweating, pallor, bradycardia, hypotension, and other autonomic effects, depending on the severity of the sensation. Nausea may precede an episode of vomiting, or it may persist for a considerable period without vomiting actually occurring. Vomiting is usually preceded by nausea, but it also can occur with little or no feeling of nausea associated with the episode. Nausea, as with anorexia, may be a manifestation of a wide range of both gastrointestinal and nongastrointestinal diseases. Other associated symptoms and findings help to determine the cause.

Vomiting is the forceful expulsion of gastric contents. Retching is the forceful effort of vomiting with-

Table 2. Differential Features of Some Common Causes of Vomiting*

	Onset, Duration, and Character	Character of Vomitus	Associated Findings	Key Lab Data
Gastrointestinal Disorders				
Pyloric obstruction	Long time after meals; often nocturnal; projectile in infants	Retained food from previous meals	Ulcer history; succussion splash	Large volume aspirate; hypochloremic, hypokalemic alkalosis
Gastric cancer	Gradual onset; initially after heavy meals; free periods	Normal gastric contents, bile, blood or "coffee grounds"	Belching, early satiety; anemia; lymphadenopathy	X-ray and/or endoscopy
Alcoholic gastritis	Begins during or shortly after alcohol binge, lasts hours or days	Much mucus and bile; may be fresh blood	Signs of present and past alcohol abuse	Early endoscopy (usually unnecessary)
Intestinal obstruction	Sudden onset; persists till obstruction relieved	First food, then bile, then fecal-smelling material	Colicky pain, constipation, diffuse tenderness, increased bowel sounds, visible peristalsis	X-ray
Biliary colic	Sudden onset	Normal contents	Pain in RUQ† radiating to back and shoulder; chills; cholangitis; jaundice	X-ray
Pancreatitis	Sudden	Normal contents	History of alcohol or biliary disease; severe pain; shock	Elevated amylase; peritoneal aspirate
Central Nervous System Disorders				
Brain tumor	Sudden or gradual onset; no nausea	Normal contents	Headache; fits; neurologic signs	CT scan
Brain abscess	Same as for tumor	Normal contents	Headache; fever; ear problems; history of trauma	CT scan
Meniere's	Sudden onset	Normal contents	Tinnitus and hearing loss	Caloric tests and audiometry
Migraine	Gradual onset	Normal contents	Unilateral headache; sensory abnormalities	Relieved by parenteral ergotamine
Digitalis intoxication	Sudden onset	Normal contents	Cardiac findings; diarrhea	ECG abnormal
Systemic Disorders				
Diabetic acidosis	Gradual; increasing	Normal contents	Lassitude; polyuria, polydipsia; epigastric pain; acetone smell, Kussmaul breathing	Blood glucose, ketones high, and acidosis present
Uremia	Frequent and recurrent often before breakfast	Normal contents; blood terminally	Kussmaul breathing; lassitude; nocturia	Elevated BUN and creatinine

*Reprinted from Douglas, A. P.: Anorexia, nausea, and vomiting. In Conn, H. F., and Conn, R. B. (eds.): *Current Diagnosis*, 6th ed. Philadelphia, W. B. Saunders Company, 1980.

†RUQ = Right upper quadrant.

out loss of significant amounts of gastric contents, and when persistent, it is often described as "dry heaves." It may precede vomiting or continue after emptying of the stomach. Regurgitation occurs with little or no effort as though the stomach or esophagus were just "running over" and often is associated with a weak or ineffective lower esophageal sphincter.

Vomiting occurs by contraction of the pylorus and antrum, relaxation of the fundus, and probably the lower esophageal sphincter, while the abdominal muscles and diaphragm contract forcing contents out of the compressed stomach into the relaxed esophagus and through the mouth. This occurs after inspiration with suspension of respiration and closure of the glottis and elevation of the soft palate to prevent aspiration of vomitus. Reverse peristalsis, postulated by some, has not been shown to occur. The whole series of events is coordinated through a vomiting center in the medulla. This vomiting center receives stimuli via afferent fibers from viscera or from a chemoreceptor trigger zone located in the floor of the fourth ventricle, which is sensitive to certain chemicals and to other stimuli.

Nausea and vomiting may occur as a result of acute emotional stress, following an episode of syncope, or associated with severe pain or headache. It may result from medication either by central effect (digitalis, emetine, apomorphine) or effect on gastric mucosa (some antibiotics, antirheumatic drugs in some individuals). Other visceral stimuli such as myocardial infarction, abdominal inflammation, or mesenteric vascular occlusion result in nausea and vomiting. Distention of the stomach, duodenum, small bowel, biliary tree, and colon also regularly provide stimuli for nausea and vomiting.

The characteristics of the vomiting may be of help in diagnosis. Morning vomiting is seen with pregnancy. The alcoholic often vomits in the morning on arising, coughing, or brushing the teeth. The patient with partial gastric resection also may vomit before breakfast or sometimes soon after eating. Patients with labyrinthitis or Meniere's disease may vomit with motion of the head, and patients with migraine vomit at time of the severe headache. Emotional or psychogenic vomiting usually occurs in close relationship to eating, while pyloric obstruction results in vomiting hours after eating, usually in late afternoon or evening. Projectile vomiting is usually associated with brain tumors. The presence of blood in the first vomitus indicates an upper gastrointestinal cause. Blood present in subsequent vomitus the same day may be a result of esophageal laceration caused by the vomiting (Mallory-Weiss syndrome).

If gastric outlet obstruction is suspected, the presence of hydrochloric acid (HCl) suggests ulcer, whereas the absence of acid is more consistent with carcinoma. Presence of bile indicates duodenogastric reflux. Bile is usually present in prolonged vomiting unless pyloric obstruction is also present. Fecal odor of vomitus indicates bacterial overgrowth consistent with intestinal obstruction or the infrequent gastrocolic fistula. Additional differential features of some common causes of vomiting are listed in Table 2.

Anorexia, nausea, and vomiting are symptoms or manifestations of a more basic disease process. Their relative importance depends on such factors from the history as duration, frequency, persistence, presence of blood, weight loss, pain, fever, jaundice, diarrhea, and previous health history. This, with the appropriate physical examination and basic laboratory studies, will usually give the physician enough information to point to one of the body systems as outlined in Table 1. If there is still insufficient direction, one should proceed with barium x-rays of the gastrointestinal tract. More definitive studies are usually suggested by the additional positive or negative findings and a further consideration of the list of possibilities.

CHRONIC ABDOMINAL PAIN

By Michael E. McLeod, M.D.
Durham, North Carolina

Chronic abdominal pain can be defined as pain that is constant, as occurring daily over weeks to years, or as reoccurring attacks with pain-free intervals.

The history of the pain is most important and will help the physician decide whether any laboratory, x-ray, or other abnormalities observed are related to the patient's pain history. For example, hyperamylasemia may be due to macroamylasemia which occurs in 1 per cent of the population and is therefore unrelated to the pain history. Similarly, gallstones may be asymptomatic.

Severity of the pain will vary, depending on the intensity of the stimulus and type of pathologic process. Perception of the pain will be modified by the patient's cultural background, previous experience with pain, interpretation of its possible meaning, secondary gain, and distracting elements in the immediate environment. Depression and anxiety also lower the pain threshold. Presence of central nervous system damage may also modify perception and characterization of pain. Medication may modify the intensity (e.g., analgesics) or the pathologic process producing the pain (e.g., steroids and antibiotics).

Functional pain will represent a significant proportion of patients with chronic abdominal pain and can be defined as pain in the presence of normal physical, laboratory, and x-ray examinations and unrelated to any physiological variables such as eating, defecation, physical movement, and so on. Of course, the hysterical patient, the pain-prone personality, and the depressed patient may also develop structural disease independent of the psychophysiologic problems. Functional abdominal pain is real and is probably related in many instances to increased motility or altered perception of normal motility. These patients require physiologic interpretation of this diagnosis, and surgery should not be performed for unrelated x-ray or laboratory abnormalities. Secondary autonomic effects such as tachycardia, nausea, pallor, sweating, or hyperventilation can be seen as concomitants of functional pain as well as physical causes of abdominal pain.

The medical history must be comprehensive and must include consideration of systemic diseases, such as lupus serositis, that produce abnormalities in the abdominal area. Systemic symptoms such as weight loss, fever, and night sweats, as well as findings such as anemia, elevated sedimentation rate (ESR), and hypoalbuminemia, will help in assessing the potential seriousness of the pain. A history of other chronic pain syndromes such as intractable headaches or diffuse myalgias increases the likelihood that the abdominal pain may be functional. Similarly, patients with previous multiple operations without findings of well-established pathology and brief periods of pain relief followed by the same pain or a new pain syndrome have a high likelihood of functional abdominal pain.

Assessment of the patient's performance level in terms of energy, sleep pattern, appetite, and weight will also help in assessing the impact of the abdominal pain on general health and well-being.

APPROACH TO THE PATIENT

There are four categories of abdominal pain: visceral pain, parietal pain, referred pain, and pain of indeterminate origin.

Visceral Pain

Visceral pain arises from afferent nerves innervating the peritoneum overlying the retroperitoneum, mesentery, bowel, and gallbladder. The pain develops secondary to stretching of muscular tubes or to muscular activity, i.e., spasm or stretching secondary to inflammation and edema. Muscular tube pain is usually described as cramping. It may occur in waves, as with small bowel pain, lasting 30 to 45 seconds with intervals free of pain, or it may be a steady pain as seen in biliary colic and less commonly in renal colic. Muscular tube pain results in the patient pacing the floor and in inability to find a comfortable position. Palpation of the area produces little or no effect. Visceral pain, because of bilateral splanchnic nerve innervation and a paucity of nerve endings, is poorly localized and frequently described by the patient as midline in location and diffuse. Whereas muscular tube pain may start and stop abruptly, lasting minutes, hours, or days, pain related to inflammation usually develops over days because the pathophysiologic events involved in the inflammatory process require time to evolve. Expanding masses such as pancreatic tumor, pancreatic pseudocyst, or aortic aneurysm will produce pain by stretching the visceral peritoneum and may also involve branches of the posterior cerebrospinal nerves thus producing back pain.

Parietal Pain

Parietal peritoneum is innervated by branches of the cerebrospinal axis; as a result, parietal pain is more accurately localized. Inflammation and, less commonly, stretching of the parietal peritoneum produce pain. This pain usually develops when organs coming in contact with overlying parietal peritoneum are involved in an inflammatory process as in cholecystitis, appendicitis, ileitis, or diverticulitis, or in generalized peritonitis such as that following perforated ulcer. The pain is aggravated by factors that stretch the parietal peritoneum (i.e., coughing, jarring movements, or palpation), and the patient resists being moved. Voluntary muscle guarding is often present, and the patient may manifest involuntary contractions and rigidity of the abdominal wall muscles. Rebound pain is related to inflammation of the parietal peritoneum. Voluntary flexion of the abdominal wall will decrease the intensity of parietal pain, whereas this will increase the intensity of pain arising from structures within the abdominal wall (i.e., rectus sheath hematoma or incisional hernia).

Referred Pain

Referred pain is perceived in areas remote from the origin of the pathology. Biliary colic may be felt in the right infrascapular area, and ureteral pain in the testicle and anterior thigh. Leaking aortic aneurysm, a retroperitoneal structure, may produce similar radiation of pain into the testicle and thigh because of irritation of the third and fourth lumbar nerve roots. Conversely, pleural pain, especially from the diaphragmatic pleura, may be felt in the upper abdomen. Abdominal pain may also arise from diabetic neuropathy or, rarely, to nerve root compression due to a herniated thoracic disc or extradural metastatic lesion. These pains will frequently manifest a radicular pattern and will be associated with decreased sensory perception.

Pain of Indeterminate Origin

Finally, there are instances of abdominal pain in which the exact mechanism is less clearly understood. Sickle cell crisis, lead colic, acute intermittent porphyria, and hyperlipidemia are examples. Hyperlipidemia may also be an etiologic factor in pancreatitis.

HISTORY

In order to identify the organ producing the pain and the pathophysiologic process involved, changes in the pain over time, response to physiologic variables, and associated changes in organic function must be determined. Constant epigastric pain radiating through to the back, accompanied by changing liver function studies, has a different meaning if the history reveals that preceding the constant pain there was daily periodic epigastric pain relieved by food. A duodenal ulcer penetrating into the area of the common bile duct would then be a logical diagnosis. The location of the pain and its radiation will also help determine the organ system of origin. This is discussed next. Changes in body position may also alter pain. The fetal position may reduce pain of pancreatic origin or that due to small bowel ischemia. The supine position may induce more esophageal reflux and aggravate esophagitis. Changing character of the pain may also help determine separate pathologic processes in the same organ. A patient with gallstones may experience recurrent attacks of colic lasting 15 to 45 minutes, later experiencing an episode of cholecystitis with fever and tenderness lasting 2 to 5 days.

Physiologic factors that aggravate or alleviate pain also help indicate the organ system involved. Ingestion of food tends to help or, less commonly, aggravate peptic pain. Food frequently precipitates pain emanating from the small intestine, whether because of partial small bowel obstruction or mesenteric angina. Food frequently aggravates existing pancreatic pain. Relief of lower abdominal discomfort with passage of gas or defecation is compatible with colon discomfort, although it does not identify the cause—which might be obstructing colon carcinoma, irritable bowel, or aerophagia. The time of day at which pain occurs may be important, particularly in relationship to peptic pain that is rhythmic, is worse on an empty stomach, and frequently awakens the patient between 12 and 2 A.M.

Depression can be associated with functional abdominal pain. The patient is frequently awakened between 3 and 5 A.M. with abdominal pain, at times associated with other intestinal symptoms such as nausea or diarrhea. Lower abdominal pelvic pressure awakening the patient in the early morning hours may also be a depressive equivalent. In contrast, biliary colic and the pain of cholecystitis occur randomly, unrelated to food or time of day, for example. Constant pain gradually increasing in intensity suggests either an expanding mass, such as tumor, abscess, cyst, or aneurysm, or a complication of tubular pain with fistulization (i.e., ileitis, diverticulitis, or penetrating ulcer). Functional pain may also be constant, but these patients will usually manifest normal laboratory data and x-ray results and in general will not report physiologic variables changing their pain. Functional pain is frequently described as having multiple characteristics such as throb, burn, ache, or sting occurring at different times, and the pain will frequently migrate to different areas of the abdomen. These patients frequently manifest other chronic pain syndromes and have a disproportionate alteration in their performance level with excessive fatigue and altered sleep in the absence of objective abnormalities.

Small and large bowel are uncommon sources of chronic pain unless there has been transmural extension of the disease process (i.e., Crohn's disease, diverticulitis). Otherwise, constant pain from the small or large bowel would point to impending strangulation. Other tubular pains, such as biliary or ureteral, will depend on the rate of obstruction and may be absent if obstruction is gradual (i.e., carcinoma of the pancreas) or severe (in the case of a stone).

PHYSICAL EXAMINATION

Physical examination must be comprehensive, looking for remote pathology that might relate to the abdominal pain. A left supraclavicular node from pancreatic or gastric cancer, clubbing with small bowel Crohn's disease, and pleural effusion secondary to a subdiaphragmatic process will be helpful clues. Inspection of the abdomen may reveal distention related to bowel loops, ascites, or organomegaly. Asymmetry of the abdomen with respect to distention and firmness should be noted. Massive enlargement of the liver to the iliac crest secondary to fat or tumor can be misinterpreted as a firm rectus muscle. Gentle palpation of the abdominal wall may reveal defects in scars with herniation of bowel or metastatic tumor around the umbilicus. A rectus sheath hematoma may be detected or a soft spleen tip that might be missed by deeper palpation. The response of the pain to palpation both with the abdominal wall relaxed and voluntarily flexed should be evaluated. The colon can frequently be felt in the left lower quadrant as a tubular structure and the cecum palpated in the right lower quadrant as a soft rounded mass. Less commonly, the transverse colon can be felt in the asthenic individual. However, the colon should not be hard or fixed and there should be little or no discomfort associated with palpation. Crohn's disease of the ileum may present with a thickened palpable loop of small bowel. The right kidney can normally be palpated. A palpable gallbladder is usually related to common bile duct obstruction often secondary to tumor.

The effect of respiratory movement on a palpable mass in the upper abdomen should be observed. If the mass is retroperitoneal, such as pancreas, lymph node, or aorta, it will not move, whereas liver, spleen, colon, gastric masses, or tumor deposits in the omentum will tend to move with inspiration. If pain is radicular, notation of areas of anesthesia should be carried out looking for nerve root lesions. An electromyogram may be helpful. In the case of lower abdominal pain, a careful pelvic exam should be carried out to evaluate tubes, ovaries, and uterus. Careful examination of the back for costovertebral angle or paravertebral muscle tenderness may help point to a renal, hepatic, retroperitoneal, or paraspinus process.

DIAGNOSTIC STUDIES

Laboratory, x-ray, and endoscopic studies will provide objective findings that should be interpreted carefully with respect to the patient's history before assuming that abnormalities are related to the patient's complaint. In the instances of recurring attacks, observations ideally should be made during the attacks. Common bile duct stone or recurrent pancreatitis may produce serial changes in liver enzymes or amylase, respectively, coinciding with the attacks. Flat plate films and upright films of the abdomen may reveal air-fluid levels, sentinel loops, and obliterated psoas shadows compatible with obstruction, local ileus, or edema. Serial changes in the white blood cell count and sedimentation rate also provide objective data during the attack. In addition, anemia, hypoalbuminemia, and positive stool guaiac will provide supportive data for a structural cause for the patient's pain. In the case of suspected pancreatitis, a serum calcium determination should be made after the attack has subsided, since a transient decrease in calcium during the attack might mask hypercalcemia as an etiologic factor in pancreatitis. If biliary colic or recurrent pancreatitis is suspected, examination of the bile for cholesterol crystals should be carried out. Small stones 1 mm or less in size are associated with cholesterol crystals in a high percentage of patients. These small stones may be missed by ultrasound and oral cholecystography. Administration of gallbladder dye may produce a transient increase in serum bilirubin, creating the false impression of a common bile duct event; it has also been reported to produce false elevations in serum and urine amylase. Hyperlipidemia, particularly phenotypes I and V, should be evaluated because significant elevations in triglycerides have been associated with recurrent attacks of abdominal pain, many of which are related to pancreatitis. Hyperlipidemia can also cause inhibition of serum amylase activity, and urine amylase should be evaluated with measurement of amylase clearance and hourly amylase excretion. Other laboratory studies may include erythrocyte basophilic stippling for lead toxicity, sickle cell preparation, haptoglobin concentration for hemolytic crisis, fluorescent antinuclear antibody (FANA) test for lupus serositis, porphobilinogen for acute intermittent porphyria, Venereal Disease Research Laboratory (VDRL) for tabes dorsalis, and C-1-esterase in patients with recurrent small bowel pain. Familial Mediterranean fever will produce an elevated sedimentation rate, and laparoscopy may demonstrate evidence of peritonitis. Urinalysis may reveal protein; red blood cells with the passage of stones, crystals, clots, sloughed tumor, or papillae; or chyluria in the presence of lymphatic obstruction.

In rare instances, patients may have paroxysmal attacks of abdominal pain associated with alterations in consciousness and abnormalities on encephalograph (EEG). Although seizures arising from the limbic brain are rare, if suspected a sleep EEG with nasopharyngeal leads can be obtained. The majority of patients with suspected seizure disorders and abdominal pain prove to be hysterical, but a few well-documented cases with abnormal EEGs have demonstrated excellent response to phenytoin.

Radiologic evaluation should begin with a KUB film of the abdomen. The plain film may reveal calcification of the pancreas or milk of calcium bile; the latter may look like a functioning gallbladder. Barium in the upper tract may mask pancreatic calcification. Calcification in the wall of an aneurysm or thorotrast in the liver, spleen, or lymph nodes may be a clue to expanding aneurysm or complicating angiosarcoma. Air-fluid levels and the sentinel loop of an ileus have been mentioned. A chest x-ray may reveal pleural effusion, and laboratory examination of the fluid (e.g., amylase cytology and cultures) may have important implications regarding a subdiaphragmatic process. Proctoscopy and barium enema exam should be done if the patient is suspected to have colonic pain. A laxative preparation should be avoided if partial small or large bowel obstruction is suspected. Colonoscopy is rarely helpful in patients with pain except where there are equivocal x-ray findings which need evaluation with visual observation and biopsy. Ultrasound or pelvic computed tomography (CT) may be helpful if a mass in the lower abdominal area is suspected. An ovarian carcinoma involving the bowel serosa may create bowel pain and may be easily missed on bowel x-ray. It should be emphasized, however, that the finding of an ovarian cyst or uterine fibroid should not be assumed to relate to the patient's lower abdominal pain.

If gastroduodenal disease is suspected, upper gastrointestinal (GI) x-ray, especially with the newer air-contrast techniques, provides excellent detail. The barium study is more sensitive in demonstrating extrinsic mass effects and abnormalities in motility. However, endoscopic examination provides a better assessment of esophageal symptoms, particularly mucosal inflammation, and will demonstrate subtle mucosal disease in the stomach frequently missed by x-ray. However, endoscopic findings of superficial gastritis or erosion should not be considered a cause of the patient's chronic pain syndrome. The small bowel can be evaluated with a standard upper GI series and small bowel follow-through; but if partial obstruction is suspected, a primary tube or small bowel enema should be carried out.

The hepatobiliary area and pancreas can be evaluated by ultrasound providing information on gallstones, size of intrahepatic ducts, metastatic lesions, and presence of pancreatic cysts or tumors. The intravenous cholangiogram, because of its low sensitivity and specificity and relatively high complication rate, should not be used in evaluating the common bile duct unless bowel anatomy precludes endoscopic retrograde cholangiography and pancreatography (ERCP) and primary transhepatic cholangiography is unsuccessful. The ^{99m}Tc cholescintigraphy (HIDA) scan can help diagnose acute cholecystitis by demonstrating the isotope in the common bile duct with failure to fill the gallbladder.

If solid organs such as liver, spleen, kidney, or lymph nodes are suspected as the cause of pain, ultrasound, abdominal CT, and ERCP would be the methods of choice, depending on the organ. The asthenic patient without tissue planes separated by fat is best evaluated with ultrasound, whereas the patient with obesity or with bowel gas is better evaluated by abdominal CT. When available, ERCP is considered to be the most sensitive method to evaluate pancreatic anatomy. Angiography has been less useful since the development of ultrasound and abdominal CT. However, ischemic disease of the small bowel can be diagnosed only by demonstration of 60 per cent narrowing of the combined cross section of the celiac, superior mesenteric, and inferior mesenteric arteries along with evidence for collateral circulation. Occasionally, a vascular tumor such as carcinoid may be seen on angiography and may be missed by contrast studies of the bowel. Laparoscopy and exploratory laparotomy are rarely helpful if the history, laboratory, and x-ray studies are not able to focus on a specific area of potential pathology. However, on occasion tuberculous peritonitis, familial Mediterranean fever, or Fitzhugh-Curtis syndrome secondary to gonococcal perihepatitis may be diagnosed in this way.

It is important to emphasize that disease processes change over time, and repeated x-rays and laboratory studies may show changes at a later date. In addition, different techniques such as the air-contrast upper GI or barium enema may reveal abnormalities that single-contrast methods have missed. The primary tube or small bowel enema exam may also show findings missed on the conventional small bowel follow-through exam.

ORGAN SYSTEM PAIN

The *esophagus* is included in this discussion of abdominal pain because pain in the lower substernal and subxiphoid area may arise from the distal esophagus. Pain in the esophagus is well localized to the area of pathology except in approximately 10 per cent of patients who will have pain referred to the suprasternal notch from distal esophageal pathology. Pain is generally of two kinds: (1) the burning type, related to mucosal ulceration or inflammation, or (2) the pressure or squeezing type, usually related to motility disturbances. The pain may radiate through to the back and may be aggravated by the act of swallowing and by factors that induce reflux such as the supine position, bending, or large meals. Aspiration, dysphagia, and weight loss may be associated with pain in this organ.

Pain arising from the *stomach and duodenum* is usually felt in the epigastric region to the right of the midline in the case of the duodenum and in the lower chest and left epigastrium in the case of gastric ulcers in the body and cardia. Pain arising from these structures usually is related in some way to meals, either with relief or with accentuation of pain. The quality of the pain may vary from classic "burning" or "gnawing" to an ache or a cramp. Ulcer pain is rhythmic unless there has been penetration or obstruction by the ulcer. Transmural tumor involvement will also produce constant pain and may be felt in the back if there has been posterior penetration. Symptoms associated with gastroduodenal disease may include early satiety, retentive vomiting, bleeding, succussion splash after prolonged fasting, anorexia, or weight loss.

Solid organs including *liver, spleen, and kidney* will not generate pain unless the capsule is stretched or inflamed. Pain in these instances will generally be well localized to the area of the organ and will be aggravated by movements such as deep breathing or turning in bed and by direct palpation or compression.

Biliary pain secondary to stone will present as a muscular tube pain with brief intense random attacks of steady epigastric or right upper quadrant and occasionally right subscapular pain lasting 15 to 60 minutes. The second pattern of pain relates to inflammation of the gallbladder. This pain will last from 2 to 5 days and can be aggravated by movement, breathing, and so on. Fatty food intolerance, postprandial bloating, and pain precipitated by cholecystokinin injections relate better to functional bowel syndrome than to gallbladder disease. Biliary colic is associated with normal laboratory findings unless the stone is in the common bile duct. Then chills, fever, and rapid changes in liver enzymes and amylase may occur within hours. Cholecystitis is associated more predictably with fever and elevation in the white blood cell count. Shaking chills in this setting is a late complication occurring 4 to 6 days into the illness and is more indicative of impending empyema.

Pancreatic pain may be midepigastric or right or left upper quadrant, but it is felt more often in the midline. An expanding mass—a tumor, a pseudocyst, or an inflammatory process—produces the pain. Involvement of the parietal peritoneum is infrequent in inflammation of the pancreas, and rigidity and rebound are uncommon. Pain coming from the pancreas will usually last days to months, depending on the nature of the process; it is uncommon for such pain to occur as brief attacks of less than 12 hours. Pancreatic pain is frequently aggravated by eating and can be reduced when the patient assumes the fetal position. Associated symptoms, including diarrhea, steatorrhea, jaundice, diabetes, or duodenal obstruction, may occur with benign or malignant disease of the pancreas. A palpable mass in the epigastrium unaffected by breathing may be noted. The gallbladder may also be palpable secondary to common bile duct obstruction and the spleen as a result of splenic vein thrombosis secondary to contiguous inflammation or tumor.

Small bowel pain is usually tubular in character, waxing and waning and lasting 15 to 45 seconds with pain-free intervals, until late in the evolution of the attack, when the pain may become constant because of increasing distention of the bowel loops. Vomiting may provide temporary relief of the pain. In fixed low-grade obstruction (e.g., as in Crohn's disease), food may precipitate the cramping type of pain. If the pathologic process is inflammatory and transmural, it may involve parietal peritoneum and may create localized peritoneal pain as well as tubular pain. Hence, a flare-up of Crohn's disease may manifest as both local tenderness and cramping pain of partial obstruction. Small bowel ischemia pain will occur with food ingestion and usually is related to volume of food; in these instances, patients frequently develop a fear of eating and show weight loss.

The *descending colon and the sigmoid colon* tend to elicit pain in the hypogastrium. This pain is described as cramping, but it tends to be more sustained and can be relieved by defecation or passage of gas. However, the transmural inflammatory process of Crohn's disease or diverticulitis may produce parietal peritoneal pain and local tenderness. The right colon is said to refer pain to the periumbilical area. The hepatic and splenic flexures of the colon produce pain in the respective quadrants, lower chest, and subscapular area; at times the pain will be referred to the shoulder. These pain patterns, when associated with changing bowel habits and relief with flatus or defecation, help point to the colon as the source of pain and the need for a barium enema examination.

The *ovaries, fallopian tubes, uterus, and rectum* may create pain in the suprapubic area or sacral area and may be associated with rectal pressure and urgency.

Renal and ureteral pain can be related to the renal capsule and renal pelvis with a localized aching type of pain in the costovertebral angle (CVA) area with pain on palpation or compression. Ureteral obstruction tends to produce pain in the lower quadrants and referred pain in the testes and anterior thighs.

Retroperitoneal structures, including the aorta, iliac arteries, and lymph nodes, may elicit back pain or poorly localized anterior pain with radiation into the thigh and testes with involvements of L_3 and L_4 nerve roots.

Neuropathic pain should be considered if the pain follows a radicular pattern and is associated with a sensory loss over the area of the pain. A thoracic disc (rare), extradural tumor metastasis, diabetic neuropathy, or tabes dorsalis should be considered.

CONCLUSION

One of the most common errors made in the diagnosis and treatment of abdominal pain is the assumption that findings on physical examination, x-ray, or laboratory testing relate to the patient's history of pain.

Hiatus hernia, nephroptosis, gallstones, peptic deformities, and ovarian cysts may be erroneously blamed as the cause of pain syndromes. Adhesions are also frequently stated to be a cause of pain when all studies are negative. Unless there are objective changes in bowel anatomy on plain films and barium x-rays and unless the pain is compatible with partial obstruction, adhesions should not be used as an explanation for chronic and recurrent pain syndromes. In those instances when surgery has been carried out for adhesions without objective findings, it is not uncommon for patients to have their pain resolve for 2 to 6 months and then return or reoccur in a different location. The temporary relief is presumably related to the placebo effect of surgery rather than correction of a pathological abnormality. Accordingly, the results of any therapeutic trial should be interpreted with caution in view of the approximately 35 per cent response rate to placebo in most treatment studies in which a placebo has been used.

NEONATAL JAUNDICE

By Audrey K. Brown, M.D.
Brooklyn, New York

DEFINITION

In the first week of life, almost every newborn infant has a plasma bilirubin concentration that is higher than that seen at any time later in life in normal children or adults. Jaundice can be visually appreciated in the neonate when the plasma bilirubin reaches approximately 5 mg/dl. More than 50 per cent of infants will become jaundiced during the first week of life. Because the condition is so common, the term *physiologic jaundice* has been used to describe this phenomenon.

There is still some usefulness for this term when we approach the question of differential diagnosis of neonatal jaundice. By using this term, we recognize a degree and extent, as well as a time of appearance and disappearance, of both jaundice and bilirubinemia that do not connote pathology or require either investigation or treatment. If we define the limits of physiologic jaundice, we can then use the term *neonatal hyperbilirubinemia* to encompass the degree of bilirubinema that exceeds these limits, whether in degree or extent.

Table 1. Hyperbilirubinemia: Criteria for Investigation of Neonatal Jaundice

Criteria
Jaundice appearing within the first 24 hours of life
A rate of increase in serum bilirubin concentration greater than 5 mg/dl/24 hr on any day
Serum bilirubin level $\geq$ 10 mg/dl at any time
Persistence of jaundice or serum bilirubin $>$ 3 mg/dl beyond 1 week of age
Any direct-reacting (conjugated) bilirubin $\geq$ 1.5 mg/dl

LIMITS OF PHYSIOLOGIC JAUNDICE

In full-term infants, the limits of jaundice and bilirubinemia attributable to factors related to developmental physiology are easier to recognize than in very immature, preterm infants. Nevertheless, the limits of this phenomenon outlined in Table 1 are useful in all but the most immature infants.

As can be seen, jaundice visible within the first 24 hours of life is never to be excused as physiologic; it should always serve as a signal of an abnormal process. The most likely cause is increased red blood cell destruction with attendant formation of excess bilirubin. This early appearance of jaundice is abnormal because it represents a rate of rise in plasma bilirubin of more than 5 mg/dl within 24 hours, since, as indicated previously, icterus is not apparent in the neonate at lower bilirubin concentrations. Further, a rate of rise in plasma bilirubin concentration of this degree, i.e., 5 mg/dl/24 hours, is abnormal on any day and usually indicates increased bilirubin production rather than poor clearance alone.

In full-term infants, physiologic jaundice becomes apparent between the second and third day of life, peaks between the third and fourth day, and disappears before the end of the first week of life. It is important to record both bilirubin levels and the appearance of jaundice in relation to the infant's age in *hours* in order to be certain that the course of jaundice is within acceptable limits or is clearly signaling abnormality.

In preterm infants the plasma bilirubin concentration peaks later and may not begin to clear until the sixth or seventh day of life. This is because of delay in a development of the capacity to metabolize bilirubin rather than to excessive formation of bilirubin, and the ultimate level of bilirubin in the plasma of these infants is, on the average, higher than that seen in term infants and the peak occurs later. The daily rate of rise in plasma bilirubin concentration remains less than 5 mg/dl/24 hours but continues for a longer period than in term infants. The more immature infants can be expected to develop the capacity to clear bilirubin later than those who are mature. However, it should be noted that even preterm infants are not usually jaundiced in the second week of life, indicating that, in general, the phenomenon of birth speeds up the development of mechanisms for bilirubin conjugation and clearance.

In both term and preterm infants, the presence of direct-reacting (conjugated) bilirubin in the plasma is evidence of an abnormality and should never be excused as physiologic. It is an indication of an obstruction in the route of clearance of conjugated bilirubin from the hepatic cell or biliary system.

One of the most difficult criteria to set as a limit of physiologic jaundice is a maximum plasma bilirubin concentration. More than 90 per cent of term infants have peak plasma bilirubin concentrations less than 7 mg/dl in the course of neonatal jaundice, and the mean peak bilirubin is about 5 mg/dl. Since less than 10 per cent of normal full-term infants will have bilirubin levels in excess of 10 mg/dl and because one mode of therapy for hyperbilirubinemia, namely phototherapy, is not very effective at bilirubin concentrations in excess of 10 mg/dl, we arbitrarily select this level as the limit of physiologic bilirubinema. In practice this represents a minimal level of bilirubin that should be investigated so that some underlying cause will not be overlooked. It is not an automatic signal for therapy, and certainly no therapy should be instituted for jaundice without first attempting to define its cause.

These limits of physiologic jaundice should serve to help recognize two distinct types of pathology, one related to the underlying cause and the other related to the concentration of bilirubin itself.

HYPERBILIRUBINEMIA

We use the term "hyperbilirubinemia" to identify abnormal patterns of jaundice as well as exaggerated degrees of bilirubinemia, so that only one word is needed to identify the overall problem of jaundice in the newborn. This is not to be overlooked or excused as a *physiologic* phenomenon. Infants whose pattern of neonatal hyperbilirubinemia and jaundice differs from these expected features may have an underlying disorder such as hemolysis, infection, or deranged hepatic function. Jaundice often serves as the most obvious herald of such pathology and should be considered by the physician as a signal alerting him to unrecognized and possibly treatable disorders. In such cases the underlying disorder, rather than the degree of hyperbilirubinemia itself, may require specific therapy.

The second type of pathology to which one is alerted when these limits are exceeded is, of course, related to the abnormal concentration of bilirubin that is potentially toxic to the brain of the newborn human infant. This relates chiefly to three situations: (1) the early rapid rise in plasma bilirubin associated with hemolysis; (2) prolonged hyperbilirubinemia in infants with disorders that disturb the development of the capacity of the liver to conjugate and clear bilirubin such as infection, inborn errors of metabolism, or respiratory distress; and (3) continued excessive red cell destruction from hemolysis, enclosed hemorrhage, or polycythemia.

The third type of pathology is the little-understood phenomenon of kernicterus with very low levels of plasma bilirubin, which is found at post-mortem in as many as 6 to 10 per cent of very small, sick, acidotic, preterm infants.

DIFFERENTIAL DIAGNOSIS OF NEONATAL HYPERBILIRUBINEMIA

Recognition of deviations from the pattern of physiologic jaundice serves as the prime step in differential diagnosis of neonatal jaundice. Other considerations unique to the interpretation of neonatal bilirubin values appear in Table 2. Emphasis must again be placed on the consideration of the infant's age in relation to the concentration of plasma bilirubin during the neonatal period. A given concentration of bilirubin (for example, 10 mg/dl) has a vastly different connotation at 1 hour of life than at 72 hours of life and still another meaning at 10 days of age. At 1 hour of life, or even within the first 24 hours of life, such a level is almost certainly due to hemolysis or some other form of increased red cell degradation, but at 72 hours of life it may simply be the expression of delayed development of the capacity to conjugate bilirubin. At 10 days of age, it would have to be due to an abnormal process, either affecting hepatic function alone or occurring in combination with hemolysis.

Table 2. Features of Fetal Bilirubin Metabolism

Bilirubin formation
Slightly increased production from red blood cell destruction
Enzymatic conversion of heme to biliverdin to bilirubin
Transport-unconjugated bilirubin
Low albumin level with diminished bilirubin binding per gram of albumin
Transported across placenta for maternal clearance
Hepatic metabolism
Limited uptake of unconjugated pigment
Development of ligands during gestation
Limited development of formation of UDPGA*
Limited conjugation of bilirubin to bilirubin diglucuronide
Excretion
Some limitation of excretion of bilirubin diglucuronide from hepatic cell
Some deconjugation of bilirubin diglucuronide in intestine by β-glucuronidase
↑ Intestinal reabsorption of unconjugated bilirubin; ↑ enterohepatic shunt
Limited amount of bilirubin in meconium

*UDPGA = Uridine diphosphoglucuronic acid.

Such considerations compel the physician to accurately record the age at which a sample is taken for determination of bilirubin. For at least the first 4 days of life, the age should be recorded in hours rather than in days.

It is also extremely useful to plot each bilirubin value graphically in relation to the infant's age so that the rate of increase or decrease can be appreciated. All too often, physicians miss the significance of the bilirubin value because they consider the process static rather than dynamic and try to interpret a bilirubin value at the time it is reported, rather than considering the age at which it was drawn. Further, no laboratory determination can be considered in a vacuum, least of all in the neonatal period when adaptive developmental processes can change rapidly.

Fundamental to differential diagnosis of neonatal jaundice is consideration of the infant's gestational age as well as postnatal age, since immaturity changes the interpretation of delayed clearance of bilirubin and also alters the potential risk of bilirubin encephalopathy.

Another feature unique to the differential diagnosis of neonatal jaundice is the necessity of taking into consideration prenatal and natal factors that may be contributory. Maternal diet, disease, or drugs can influence the infant's bilirubin metabolism, some by promoting hemolysis (drugs); others by predisposing to prematurity (disease, socioeconomic status); and others, such as maternal diabetes, through combined effects (i.e., immaturity and polycythemia), which can exaggerate neonatal hyperbilirubinemia. In the breast-fed infant in particular, maternal factors may have a continued influence on the pattern of jaundice in the infant.

CAUSES OF NEONATAL HYPERBILIRUBINEMIA

Major causes of hyperbilirubinemia in the neonate are listed in Table 3. All of these conditions should be considered as superimposed upon a basic predisposition of the neonate to accumulate bilirubin because of the tenuous balance already existing between production of bilirubin and the developing capacity for its clearance in the immediate neonatal period. We will discuss some of these causes in relation to the diverse mechanisms that can accentuate the tendency of the neonate to accumulate bilirubin.

Prematurity: Persistence of Fetal Bilirubin Metabolism

The clearance of bilirubin during fetal life is not dependent upon its conjugation and excretion into the intestine; clearance is accomplished by means of the placenta to the maternal circulation. Conjugation of bilirubin by the fetus is not only unnecessary, it could actually interfere with clearance during intrauterine life, since only bilirubin in the unconjugated form crosses the placenta and there is no fetal excretion. On the other hand, if the fetal pattern of bilirubin persists into postnatal life, unconjugated bilirubin accumulates in the infant. It is the persistence of some of the features of the fetal pattern of bilirubin metabolism that accounts for the basic propensity of the newborn to accumulate the pigment in the unconjugated form. The principal features of prenatal bilirubin metabolism are outlined in Table 2. Although the persistence of any of these features in the neonate will contribute to the degree to which bilirubin may accumulate, the major determinant is the degree to which the capacity to conjugate bilirubin has developed.

It is also evident that the earlier a preterm infant is born, the more fetal-like are the metabolic pathways. It is no surprise that the capacity to clear bilirubin takes longer in such infants and the degree of bilirubinemia is more exaggerated than in term infants. The persistence of some features of fetal bilirubin metabolism of premature infants is a major cause of hyperbilirubinemia; more than 60 per cent of infants weighing less than 2000 gm at birth have peak bilirubin levels greater than 10 mg/dl during the first week of life and more than 40 per cent of such infants have levels greater than 15 mg/dl.

Table 3. Causes of Unconjugated Neonatal Hyperbilirubinemia

- Physiologic jaundice
- Hemolytic diseases
  - Hemolytic disease of the newborn, resulting from isoantibodies
    - Rh, ABO, and minor blood group incompatibilities
    - Maternal autoimmune hemolytic anemia
  - Hemolytic disease of the newborn, resulting from inherited intracorpuscular defects
    - Hereditary spherocytosis
    - Enzyme deficiencies (e.g., G-6-PD,* pyruvate kinase, etc.)
  - Drugs and chemicals
    - Vitamin K_3
    - Naphthalene
    - Novobiocin
- Neonatal sepsis
  - Bacterial sepsis
  - Viral infections
    - Cytomegalic inclusion disease
    - Congenital rubella
    - Disseminated Herpes simplex
  - Congenital toxoplasmosis
  - Congenital syphilis
- Resorption of large hematomas
- Metabolic disorders
  - Galactosemia
  - Crigler-Najjar syndrome
  - Breast milk jaundice
  - Transient familial neonatal hyperbilirubinemia
  - Maternal diabetes

*G-6-PD = Glucose-6-phosphate dehydrogenase.

Maternal Diabetes

Infants of diabetic mothers frequently exhibit an exaggerated degree of neonatal unconjugated hyperbilirubinemia. Since these infants may have associated problems such as immaturity, hypoglycemia, polycythemia, and/or respiratory distress with hypoxia, a specific metabolic factor has not been defined. In general, the pattern of jaundice seen in these infants is that of delayed development of the capacity to conjugate bilirubin. Peak serum bilirubin levels are both higher and later in the first week of life than those of infants of comparable weight from nondiabetic mothers.

Drugs and Environment

Many factors, including drugs and environmental agents, can influence the development of the bilirubin conjugating system; some serve as inducing agents, others as inhibitors or competitors. When attempting to diagnose the nature of hyperbilirubinemia, every effort should be made to identify such agents. Investigation of an epidemic of hyperbilirubinemia occurring in two hospitals led to the discovery that use of a phenolic disinfectant detergent used to clean bassinets and mattresses was associated with the condition.

Breastfeeding and Breast Milk

Although controlled studies of the influence of breastfeeding on the development of hyperbilirubinemia have not uniformly shown an association, it is generally agreed that breast-fed infants often have exaggerated neonatal bilirubinemia. This has been ascribed in part to limited caloric intake and may invoke the same response as seen in starvation. In some infants, however, a different factor related to the breast milk rather than to the feeding pattern appears to be responsible. A small percentage of breast-fed infants have a progressive hyperbilirubinemia from about the fourth day of life that may peak at 10 or 15 days with serum bilirubin levels of 10 to 30 mg/dl. If breastfeeding is continued, elevated bilirubin levels may persist and normal levels of less than 2 mg/dl may not be reached until the infant is 3 to 12 weeks of age. The most useful diagnostic test is interruption of breastfeeding. This will be followed by a prompt decline in the serum bilirubin level within 48 hours. If nursing is resumed, there is often an associated rise in the level of serum bilirubin to about 3 mg/dl but the previous degrees of hyperbilirubinemia are not seen subsequently.

Intestinal Obstruction

High intestinal obstruction, such as pyloric stenosis, is often associated with indirect-reacting hyperbilirubinemia. Although diminished glucuronyl transferase has been reported in children with pyloric stenosis, the common denominator that explains the association may be related to prolonged intestinal transit time. This allows greater opportunity for reabsorption of bilirubin and augmentation of the enterohepatic shunting or recycling of bilirubin. A similar factor may in part explain the jaundice seen in situations characterized by poor intestinal motility and evacuation such as in delayed feeding and cretinism.

Hemolytic Disease Resulting from Isoimmunization

ABO System. Twenty per cent of newborn infants are ABO heterospecific with their mothers; they are type A or B and the mother type O. About one third to one half of these infants will show serologic evidence of erythroblastosis, but fewer than 10 per cent will have hyperbilirubinemia. Hydrops fetalis has not been described in this type of erythroblastosis. Intrauterine diagnosis is not necessary and should not be attempted.

Anemia is usually moderate, and the peripheral blood smear characteristically displays spherocytes and polychromasia. The reticulocyte count is usually increased above 5 per cent, which is the upper limit of normal during the first few days of life. Definitive diagnosis is made by demonstrating antibody in the infant's blood to his own cell type. This may be done by demonstrating either a positive direct or indirect Coombs' test. Antibody may also be identified by eluting it from the infant's red blood cells. These tests should be performed, since the finding of heterospecific blood types between mother and child is not sufficient evidence that there has been transplacental passage of IgG anti-A or anti-B antibody or that there is hemolytic disease of the newborn.

Early jaundice (icterus precox) was the first clue to the existence of this entity and remains the major sign for its recognition in the nursery. Bilirubin concentrations of 10 mg/dl are often seen within the first 24 hours of life. If the bilirubin is accumulating this rapidly from hemolysis, it may not be controlled by phototherapy alone and exchange transfusion may be necessary to remove both the sensitized cells and the bilirubin. Further, even if jaundice and hemolysis appear to be moderate in the first week of life, red cell destruction will continue in the presence of antibody and infants should be carefully followed to detect anemia, which may develop later.

The Rh System. On the red blood cell, there are in the Rh system—or, more precisely, the CDE system—six genetically determined antigens grouped in three sets: Cc, Dd, and Ee. It is the presence of the D antigen that determines whether an individual is called Rh positive. The antigens are inherited in two sets of three, one set contributed by each parent. For example an infant might inherit the set CDe from an Rh-positive father and cde as the set from the mother. The infant would have the Rh genotype CDe/cde, and because he had the D antigen, he would be Rh positive. If the mother were genotype cde/cde and had no D antigen she would be Rh negative, would recognize red blood cells from such an infant or fetus as bearing a foreign antigen, and could mount an antibody response. These antibodies, as IgG antibodies, could cross the placenta and destroy fetal D-positive cells. It is important to remember that a mother can form antibodies to any of these antigens that she does not possess. This includes c or e as well as C, D, or E. For example, a mother homozygous for C can form antibodies to c.

Unlike A and B antigens—which are ubiquitous in nature—the Rh antigens are found only in the red cell membrane; their presence is essential for the normal function of that membrane. This difference in the distribution of these antigens is responsible for many of the clinical differences in the two types of hemolytic disease of the newborn. These differences include the fact that ABO incompatibility can occur in the first pregnancy, since sensitization to A and B can occur without exposure to red cells.

Further, the naturally occurring anti-A and anti-B antibodies are mainly IgM and do not cross the placenta. About 50 per cent of group O women with group A or B fetuses make some IgG antibodies to A or B that can cross the placenta; however, only some of that antibody attaches to the red cell, since A and B antigens are present in other tissues. This probably accounts for both the lack of significant hemolysis in utero as well as the relatively milder hemolytic process after birth in infants with ABO hemolytic disease.

In contrast to ABO incompatibility, it is essential to determine prenatally whether an Rh-negative mother has antibodies to the red cells of her fetus, and, indeed, if an antibody titer is found, amniocentesis must be done to determine whether the fetus is affected. Amniotic fluid spectrophotometric examination can be used to predict with great accuracy (95 per cent) the degree to which the fetus is affected. An objective comparison of deviation from linearity of the absorbance spectrum at 450 nm, the "delta O.D. at 450 nm," correlates with the bilirubin concentration in the amniotic fluid. This accumulates as a result of intrauterine hemolysis and thus accurately reflects the severity of the disease in the fetus.

These procedures are carried out to determine whether the fetus is destined to die in utero; the procedures are monitored closely in sensitized women so that if fetal death is likely, preparation can be made for either intrauterine transfusion or early delivery, depending on other considerations, chiefly gestational age and the state of pulmonary development.

Although accurate assessment of fetal hemolysis and anemia is possible, it is not possible to predict antenatally whether an infant with Rh hemolytic disease will have severe hyperbilirubinemia and kernicterus. It has been observed that infants who have hemolyzed a great deal before birth may actually have relatively mild degrees of hyperbilirubinemia, since the pigment from the cells destroyed during fetal life is, of course, cleared by the mother. On the other hand, severely anemic infants, when jaundiced at or shortly after birth, can have evidence of obstructive jaundice, and the direct-reacting fraction of bilirubin in the plasma may be elevated along with the indirect-reacting component.

It is important when taking a history in cases of Rh hemolytic disease to determine whether problems in any previous pregnancies were related to antenatal events such as stillbirth or to postnatal events such as hyperbilirubinemia, exchange transfusion, or kernicterus. Such postnatal events relate to the infant's ability to clear bilirubin and are not predictive of the next infant's potential for intrauterine death. On the other hand, a history of previous stillbirth from hemolytic disease usually indicates that the next affected fetus will also be severely affected in utero at about the same time or slightly earlier. It should be noted, however, that women who have had no stillbirths or severely affected fetuses do not have to anticipate progression in the expression of hemolytic disease with each successive pregnancy as was once thought.

Early jaundice and a rapidly rising bilirubin level must be considered as signs of hemolytic disease in the newborn until it proves not to be. The direct Coombs' test is positive in any hemolytic disease caused by isoimmunization. In ABO hemolytic disease it may not be demonstrable in all cases, particularly if the diagnosis is not sought until after the first few days of life. The indirect Coombs' test and/or elution of antibody may be necessary.

If the Coombs' test is positive, the ABO and Rh types of the mother and infant must be determined and the mother's blood screened for antibodies. The performance of a Coombs' test should be routine on all cord blood samples. Cord blood bilirubin levels above 2.8 mg/dl are abnormal and usually indicate a hemolytic process.

The neonatal expression of Rh hemolytic disease varies widely. Some infants have severe anemia and hydrops during fetal life. Others who are born with only moderate anemia may become profoundly jaundiced and may develop bilirubin encephalopathy. Some infants have such a mild course in the first few days of life that it might go unrecognized until the mild but prolonged course of hemolysis leads to appreciable anemia after a few weeks. Hemolysis can continue as long as the antibody persists in the infant; this can be identified by the Coombs' test.

Cord blood hemoglobin values of less than 14 gm/dl are indicative of anemia; when the hemoglobin is in the range of 11 gm/dl in infants with hemolytic disease, it is worthwhile to perform an exchange transfusion to stop the process by removing the sensitized cells. Infants with cord hemoglobin values in the range of 9 gm/dl may have signs of impending heart failure, and a packed cell exchange transfusion may be required. The volume of such an exchange should be about 100 ml in a term infant. It should be emphasized that serial hemoglobin and bilirubin values should be obtained in order to follow the course of the disease, avoid severe anemia, and prevent kernicterus. When sequential hemoglobin values are compared, it should be remembered that in the neonate, capillary values are about 2 gm/dl higher than venous values. It is desirable to obtain blood samples from consistent sites.

Reticulocytosis is seen in infants with hemolytic disease and can range from above 10 per cent to more than 50 per cent. Although a few normoblasts can be seen in the peripheral blood of normal infants on the first day of life, circulating erythroblasts are the hallmark of severe hemolysis. They may also be seen in the peripheral blood of infants who have had severe chronic blood loss in utero, usually due to chronic fetomaternal blood loss. The latter can be identified by examination of the maternal blood for the presence of fetal cells by the Betke-Kleihauer technique of acid elution. In contrast to infants with hemolysis, infants whose anemia is due to blood loss do not usually develop hyperbilirubinemia.

Non-immune Hemolytic Diseases

There are many types of hemolytic processes that manifest in the newborn infant, and all can mimic the features of erythroblastosis except the Coombs' test. Inborn errors of red cell metabolism can be expressed as hemolytic disorders in the immediate neonatal period and can be specifically diagnosed with appropriate assessment of altered red cell morphology or enzymes or both.

Hereditary spherocytosis frequently is initially expressed as hyperbilirubinemia. Spherocytes can be identified in the peripheral blood of the infant and often in a parent. It is particularly useful to examine the blood from both parents when a hereditary hemolytic disorder is considered as the probable cause of jaundice.

Many black infants with glucose-6-phosphate dehydrogenase (G-6-PD) deficiency will develop some hemolysis and hyperbilirubinemia in the neonatal period under the oxidative challenge of infections or drugs. Although normal newborn infants have normal or increased red cell glucose-6-phosphate dehydrogenase, 10 to 14 per cent of black male infants and 2 per cent of black female infants are deficient in this enzyme. Preterm infants with this enzymatic defect frequently develop hyperbilirubinemia, and there is some evidence that a similar phenomenon is found in term infants as well. Oxidative agents, such as drugs, which trigger hemolysis may enter the fetus from the mother or may be acquired by infants during breast feeding. One of the common trigger events for sudden hemolysis and jaundice in these infants is infection. Kernicterus occurs if the hyperbilirubinemia reaches toxic levels. Some red blood cells appear as blister cells or as distorted and fragmented red cells during the course of hemolysis. Spontaneous Heinz bodies can be seen in red cells on blood smears stained with methylene blue. Since this disorder is a sex-linked recessive, it is useful to determine red cell G-6-PD in the mother's blood; the reticulocytosis in the infant may interfere with interpretation of the infant's enzyme value.

Other Causes of Increased Bilirubin Production

Hemorrhage. Intracranial and other forms of enclosed hemorrhage contribute significantly to increased bilirubin production. One gram of hemoglobin degrades to 34 mg of bilirubin, and, in infants with limited capacity to conjugate bilirubin and with very limited plasma volume, serum bilirubin concentration can increase as rapidly as in some cases of overt hemolytic disease. Anemia can develop and reticulocytosis can be seen within 48 hours, so that the differential diagnosis with hemolytic disease may seem difficult. The use of ultrasonography has greatly facilitated the diagnosis of intracranial, particularly intraventricular, hemorrhage, which appears to occur in about 40 per cent of preterm infants weighing less than 1250 gm at birth. This finding probably accounts for some of the extreme variability in the extent of the hyperbilirubinemia of the premature infant.

Sepsis and Jaundice. Neonatal jaundice can be an important clue to the presence of infection in the newborn infant. The infections may be bacterial, viral, spirochetal, or protozoal. The infection might be one that was acquired in utero, such as cytomegalovirus or toxoplasmosis. In such cases, one commonly finds abnormal liver chemistries and an elevated direct reacting as well as total bilirubin.

An elevated direct-reacting fraction of bilirubin is always abnormal even if it is only 2 or 3 mg/dl. The commonest cause of such elevation is infection; sepsis and pyelonephritis are frequently found. Urinalysis as well as cultures of blood and urine should be performed. *Escherichia coli* is often the offending agent.

The presence of direct-reacting (conjugated) bilirubin in the blood of infants is indicative of obstruction to the secretion of bilirubin diglucuronide from the hepatic cell, of inability to secrete bile in general (intrahepatic cholestasis), or of impairment of flow through the major bile ducts as in extrahepatic biliary atresia or with a choledochal cyst. In infants it is commonly a sign of liver cell injury. In infections such as cytomegalic inclusion disease, histologic sections of the liver often reveal intracellular as well as intracanalicular accumulation of bile pigment. In any form of obstructive jaundice, both indirect- and direct-reacting bilirubin are found in the blood.

A major differential diagnosis to be made in this combined type of hyperbilirubinemia is, of course, between hepatitis and biliary atresia. It is most important to determine whether the obstruction is partial or complete. Accurate assessment of the presence of significant amounts of urobilinogen in the urine and bilirubin in the stool is helpful, as is the determination of excretion of rose bengal. PIPIDA (a ^{99m}Tc-labeled derivative of iminodiacetic acid) scans are often but not always helpful in defining atresia of the bile ducts. The ultimate diagnostic test when complete obstruction is present is limited exploration and biopsy. Definition of extrahepatic biliary atresia should be made before the infant is 6 weeks of age, since cirrhosis develops rapidly and renders useless certain surgical procedures, such as the Kasai operation, that might be performed to promote the clearance of bile.

Metabolic causes of combined indirect as well as direct-reacting hyperbilirubinemia include alpha$_1$-antitrypsin deficiency and galactosemia as well as other inborn errors of metabolism that lead to hepatic derangement and which can be excluded by specific enzymatic and other appropriate laboratory tests.

JAUNDICE

By John R. Lake, M.D.
and Bruce F. Scharschmidt, M.D.*
San Francisco, California

Jaundice may be defined as a condition in which the sclerae, mucous membranes, skin, and urine become abnormally yellow as a result of an increased concentration of bilirubin in the blood. To be detected clinically, the bilirubin concentration must usually exceed 3 mg/dl. This "threshold" depends upon whether the bilirubin level is rising or falling, since it requires time for the bilirubin to accumulate in tissues. In patients with darkly pigmented skin, icterus may be most easily detected in the mucous membranes, tympanic membranes, or sclerae.

Jaundice can result from a variety of causes ranging from life-threatening hemolytic or hepatic disorders to innocuous impairment of hepatic bilirubin transport. Its differential diagnosis is, therefore, a most interesting and challenging clinical problem. The most important task of the clinician is to identify disorders, such as biliary obstruction, for which specific therapy is required. In order to better understand the differential diagnosis of jaundice, it is helpful to briefly review normal bilirubin metabolism.

NORMAL BILIRUBIN METABOLISM

Bilirubin is produced from the catabolism of heme (Fig. 1). Daily bilirubin production averages approximately 4 mg/kg, of which about 70 per cent results

*Supported in part by NIH Grant AM-26270 and a grant from the Giannini Foundation.

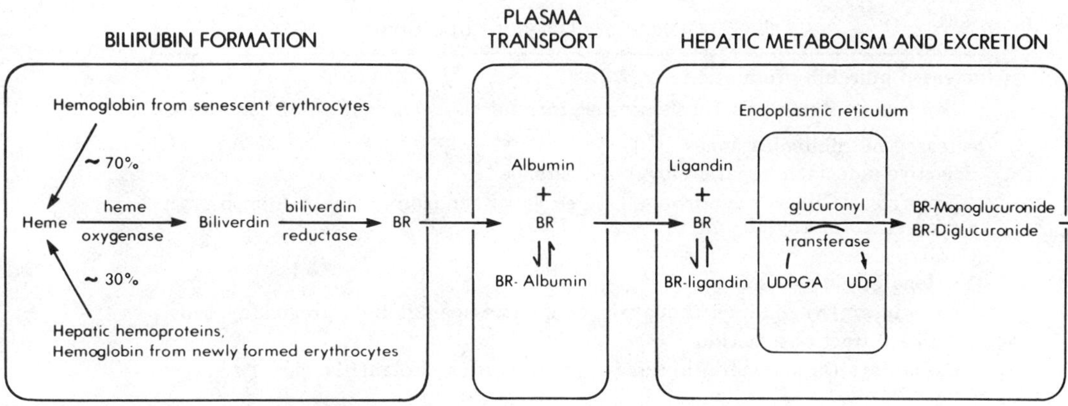

Figure 1. Overview of normal bilirubin (BR) metabolism.

from the catabolism of heme released from senescent erythrocytes. Most of the remaining 30 per cent of bilirubin production results from the breakdown of nonhemoglobin hemoproteins primarily present in the liver, such as cytochrome P-450. A small fraction of daily bilirubin production is the result of premature destruction of newly formed erythrocytes, a process termed "ineffective erythropoiesis."

Heme is first converted to biliverdin by the microsomal enzyme heme oxygenase. Hemoglobin heme is converted to biliverdin primarily in mononuclear phagocytic cells in the spleen, liver, and bone marrow. Biliverdin is then converted very rapidly to unconjugated bilirubin by the cytosolic enzyme biliverdin reductase. Unconjugated bilirubin circulates in plasma tightly bound to albumin. Hepatic uptake of unconjugated bilirubin shows characteristics of carrier-mediated transport, including saturability and competition by other organic anions. Once in hepatocytes, bilirubin binds to cytosolic proteins such as ligandin, thereby decreasing the amount of bilirubin available for reflux back into plasma. Water-insoluble unconjugated bilirubin is conjugated in the hepatocyte by joining glucuronic acid, and occasionally other sugars, in ester linkage to one or both propionic acid groups, thereby converting bilirubin to a water-soluble molecule. Formation of the mono- and diglucuronide is catalyzed by the microsomal enzyme UDP-glucuronyltransferase. Conjugated bilirubin is then transported across the canalicular membrane into the bile. Approximately 80 per cent of the bilirubin excreted into bile is of the diglucuronide form. Most of the remaining 20 per cent is present as the monoglucuronide, with unconjugated bilirubin normally present in bile in trace amounts only. Bilirubin moves from the bile to the terminal ileum and colon, where it is deconjugated and subsequently converted by bacterial enzymes to colorless compounds called urobilinogens. About 20 per cent of urobilinogen is reabsorbed, and 90 per cent of the reabsorbed fraction is re-excreted in the bile with the remainder excreted in the urine.

MEASUREMENT OF BILIRUBIN IN SERUM

Normal serum bilirubin concentration in adults is less than 1.0 mg/dl. Bilirubin is conventionally measured in the serum by a diazo reaction, in which bilirubin couples with a reagent, such as diazotized sulfanilic acid, to form a colored product that is quantitated spectrophotometrically. Conjugated bilirubin tends to react "directly" in this assay, that is, without the addition of an "accelerator" such as alcohol or urea. Total bilirubin is obtained by performing the assay in the presence of an "accelerator," which facilitates the reaction of unconjugated bilirubin with the diazo reagent. The indirect fraction is calculated by subtracting the direct fraction from the total bilirubin concentration.

The conventional diazo reaction is relatively nonspecific, and the direct- and indirect-reacting fractions are relatively inaccurate measures of conjugated and unconjugated bilirubin, respectively. Newer, more specific techniques have shown that essentially all of the plasma bilirubin in healthy adults is unconjugated. The conventional diazo technique also tends to yield higher values for the total bilirubin when compared with more specific techniques. This is particularly true for patients with hepatocellular disease. This is probably due to the detection of bilirubin covalently bound to albumin which accumulates in hepatobiliary disease and is not measured by the newer techniques. A chromatographic assay that permits quantitation of this pigment fraction covalently bound to serum albumin has been described. For practical purposes, however, the diazo technique is quite satisfactory and rarely creates a great deal of confusion.

DIFFERENTIAL DIAGNOSIS OF JAUNDICE

The differential diagnosis of jaundice (Table 1) can be divided into two major pathophysiologic categories: bilirubin overproduction and decreased bilirubin clearance.

Bilirubin Overproduction

Bilirubin overproduction is most commonly caused by hemolysis. Certain rules of thumb are occasionally useful in assessing the role of hemolysis as a cause of hyperbilirubinemia. First, chronic steady-state hemolysis cannot by itself account for a sustained

Table 1. Differential Diagnosis of Jaundice

Increased bilirubin production
Examples: Hemolysis, ineffective erythropoiesis, reabsorption of hematomas
Decreased bilirubin clearance
Selective defects in hepatic bilirubin clearance
Examples: Gilbert's syndrome, Crigler-Najjar syndrome, Dubin-Johnson syndrome, Rotor's syndrome
Cholestasis
1. Hepatocellular disease
Examples: Drug-induced hepatitis, congestive heart failure, pregnancy, sepsis
2. Biliary tract obstruction
Examples: Choledocholithiasis, tumor, sclerosing cholangitis, chronic pancreatitis

bilirubin concentration greater than 4 to 5 mg/dl. Concentrations consistently above this level usually indicate the additional presence of hepatic dysfunction. In contrast, acute hemolysis can result in a bilirubin production rate that transiently exceeds the excretory capacity of even a normal liver and may cause striking bilirubin elevation and occasionally conjugated hyperbilirubinemia. Ineffective erythropoiesis may also be increased in certain disease states and can cause hyperbilirubinemia. Examples of this include megaloblastic anemia from either B_{12} or folic acid deficiency, iron deficiency anemia, sideroblastic anemia, thalassemia minor, polycythemia vera, aplasia, and lead poisoning. One other cause of bilirubin overproduction is the resorption of large hematomas.

Selective Defects in Hepatic Bilirubin Metabolism or Transport

Hyperbilirubinemia and jaundice may also result from decreased hepatic bilirubin clearance owing to a hereditary defect in either the hepatic metabolism or transport of bilirubin. These syndromes are outlined in Table 2.

Gilbert's syndrome, once considered a rarity, has been shown by several population surveys to have a prevalence of 5 to 7 per cent in Caucasian populations of the United States and Western Europe. Gilbert's syndrome results from a decreased hepatic clearance of unconjugated bilirubin, but the precise mechanism for this remains unclear. Serum bilirubin concentration in these patients may rise two- to threefold with fasting, with dehydration, or following the administration of nicotinic acid. Bilirubin concentrations decrease following the administration of phenobarbital because of the induction of UDP-glucuronyltransferase. Gilbert's syndrome may present as mild scleral icterus in the second or third decade of life. More commonly, though, the bilirubin elevation is insufficient to produce clinical jaundice and patients with Gilbert's syndrome present with unconjugated hyperbilirubinemia identified on routine multiphasic biochemical screening. Although a wide variety of symptoms have been associated with the disorder, they are very nonspecific and are probably not attributable to Gilbert's syndrome itself.

Many view the diagnosis of Gilbert's syndrome as one of exclusion. In reality, an extensive exclusionary work-up is seldom indicated and the diagnosis can usually be established by the repeated demonstration of normal liver function tests in an asymptomatic individual with a mild elevation in the serum concentration of unconjugated bilirubin. Although liver biopsy permits structural liver disease to be ruled out and is employed in a few special centers to demonstrate a reduced activity of UDP-glucuronyltransferase, most authorities do not recommend liver biopsies for the routine work-up of Gilbert's syndrome because of the small associated risk. Extensive biliary visualization procedures are also unnecessary. Normal fasting and postprandial concentrations of bile acids have been shown to be helpful in excluding liver disease. Although overt hemolysis needs to be ruled out, it has been shown that up to half of patients with Gilbert's syndrome may have mild decreases in red blood cell survival by ^{51}Cr-labeling techniques. The major reason to establish the diagnosis of Gilbert's syndrome is to reassure the patient and to avoid unnecessary surgical procedures (e.g., cholecystectomy, splenectomy).

Crigler-Najjar syndrome (congenital nonhemolytic jaundice) is an uncommon cause of unconjugated neonatal hyperbilirubinemia caused by the absence of glucuronyltransferase activity (Type I) or markedly reduced glucuronyltransferase activity (Type II). The majority of patients with the Type I Crigler-Najjar syndrome develop kernicterus and die in the neonatal period. Patients with the Type II Crigler-Najjar syndrome and occasional survivors with the Type I syndrome may reach adulthood. These patients have bilirubin concentrations of 5 to 40 mg/dl, all of which is unconjugated (Table 2). Liver function is otherwise normal, and the patients with the Type II syndrome are usually asymptomatic. A diagnostic trial of phenobarbital should produce a drop in the bilirubin level in patients with Type II Crigler-Najjar syndrome, but not Type I. Other causes of neonatal jaundice resulting from impaired bilirubin conjugation are discussed in the preceding article.

Hereditary transport defects (Dubin-Johnson syndrome, Rotor's syndrome) resulting in conjugated hyperbilirubinemia are more easily confused with hepatobiliary disease (Table 2). These rare syndromes are characterized by mild jaundice and serum bilirubin levels between 1 and 5 mg/dl, mostly conjugated.

Table 2. Hereditary Defects in Bilirubin Transport

	Gilbert's Syndrome	Crigler-Najjar Syndrome (Congenital Nonhemolytic Jaundice) Type I	Type II	Dubin-Johnson Syndrome	Rotor's Syndrome
Incidence	≤ 7% of population	Rare	Uncommon	Rare, up to 1:1300 in Iranian Jews	Rare
Identified defects in bilirubin metabolism	(1) Decreased hepatic uptake (2) Decreased glucuronyl transferase activity	Absent glucuronyl transferase activity	Markedly decreased or absent glucuronyl transferase activity	Impaired bilirubin excretion	Impaired bilirubin excretion
Plasma bilirubin concentration (mg/dl)	Total: ≤ 3 in absence of hemolysis or fasting Conjugated: ≤ 0.1 by new assays	Total: 17–50 (usually > 20) Conjugated: 0	Total: 6–45 (usually < 20) Conjugated: 0	Total: 1–25 (usually < 7) Conjugated: averages 60% of total	Total: 1–20 (usually < 7) Conjugated: averages 60% of total
Inheritance	Autosomal dominant (?)	Autosomal recessive	? Autosomal dominant with variable penetrance	Autosomal recessive	Autosomal recessive
Physical findings	Occasional scleral icterus	Jaundice, findings of kernicterus in infants; seizures, myoclonus athetosis, incoordination, retardation in young adults	Jaundice, findings of kernicterus only rarely present	Jaundice, occasional hepatomegaly	Jaundice
Plasma BSP disappearance rate	Decreased in some patients (45 min retention ≤ 15%)	Normal	Normal	Slow initial disappearance in some patients (45 min retention ≤ 20%); frequent secondary rise at 90–120 min)	Markedly slow initial disappearance (45 min retention 30–50%), no secondary rise
Diagnosis	Clinical and laboratory findings; measurement of serum bile acids if available; liver biopsy not routinely necessary	Clinical and laboratory findings; no reduction in plasma bilirubin concentration by phenobarbital	Clinical and laboratory findings; partial reduction in plasma bilirubin concentration by phenobarbital	Clinical and laboratory findings including BSP disappearance and urinary coproporphyrins; liver biopsy shows coarse dark pigment in centrolobular cells	Clinical and laboratory findings including BSP disappearance and urinary coproporphyrins; liver biopsy shows no dark pigment
Treatment	Phenobarbital rarely indicated	No generally effective, practical, and safe treatment available	Phenobarbital if indicated	No specific treatment available; avoid estrogens	No specific treatment available
Prognosis	Normal	Usually death in infancy; rarely, later onset of neurologic damage	Usually normal; kernicterus occurs only rarely	Probably good	Probably good

Liver function tests are normal with the exception of an increased retention of bromosulfophthalein. The two syndromes may be distinguished by the presence of black pigment in the liver in Dubin-Johnson syndrome, by differences in urinary coproporphyrin excretion, and by differences in plasma bromosulfophthalein disappearance.

Cholestasis

The other etiologies of jaundice all reflect the presence of cholestasis, that is, impaired bile formation and/or bile flow resulting from extrahepatic biliary tract obstruction or hepatic parenchymal disease. Even in cholestasis, however, increased bilirubin production may be an important contributing factor (e.g., hemolysis complicating viral hepatitis or ineffective erythropoiesis caused by folate deficiency complicating alcoholic hepatitis).

Cholestasis can be subdivided into intrahepatic and extrahepatic causes. Intrahepatic causes include conditions in which the hepatocyte is unable to excrete bile even though the major ducts are patent. Included are both acute and chronic viral hepatitis of any etiology, most commonly the B and non-A non-B viruses, but occasionally the Epstein-Barr virus or cytomegalovirus. Drugs or toxins are a common cause of intrahepatic cholestasis, with alcohol, phenothiazines, and estrogens most commonly incriminated. Other causes of intrahepatic cholestasis include primary biliary cirrhosis, congestive heart failure, sepsis, pregnancy, infiltrative diseases of the liver, and liver disease in infancy. A total listing of causes of intrahepatic cholestasis is beyond the scope of this article. The other major cause of cholestasis is extrahepatic biliary obstruction, most commonly due to a neoplasm or gallstone. This topic is discussed in the article on diseases of the gallbladder and biliary tract.

APPROACH TO THE PATIENT WITH JAUNDICE

Most conditions causing jaundice can be diagnosed or at least suspected based on the clinical history, physical examination, and routine laboratory tests. A practical approach to the patient with jaundice is outlined in Figure 2. Although such an algorithm is useful as an illustration of a systematic approach, it is important to emphasize that no algorithm is applicable to all patients. Under some clinical circumstances, it may be appropriate to skip certain steps or move in directions not indicated by the algorithm. Certain such selected situations will be illustrated by example in the discussion to follow.

Clinical Evaluation

There are aspects of the patient's history that may aid in the differential diagnosis of jaundice. The presence of itching should alert one to the presence of cholestasis. Although the identity of the "pruritogen(s)" is controversial, bile salts in the skin are the most likely candidates. A history of dark urine implies the presence of increased levels of bilirubin conjugates in the serum and represents a clue to the presence of cholestasis, Rotor's syndrome, or Dubin-Johnson syndrome. The presence of clay-col-

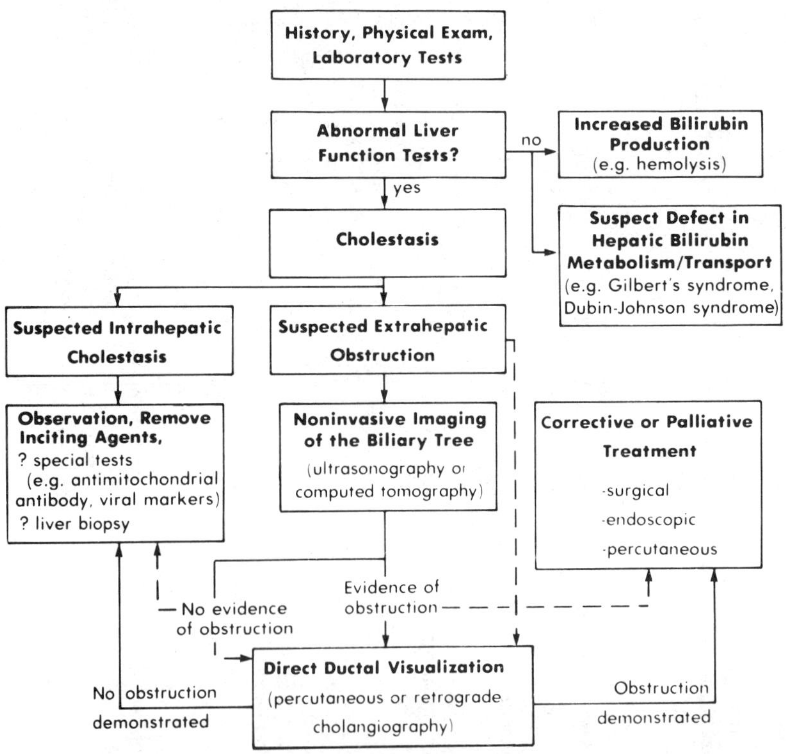

Figure 2. Outline of a clinical approach to the patient with jaundice.

ored (acholic) stool implies severe cholestasis. Although initially thought to result from diminished fecal bilirubin and urobilinogen excretion, this is probably not correct, since patients with the Type I Crigler-Najjar syndrome excrete minimal bilirubin into bile but have normal colored feces. The presence of abdominal pain should alert one to a diagnosis of biliary disease.

The physical examination may also be of assistance in the differential diagnosis of jaundice. Estimates of the degree of hyperbilirubinemia may be obtained from the physical examination. As mentioned previously, a bilirubin level of 3 mg/dl or greater is usually required for the detection of scleral icterus. Mucous membrane or cutaneous icterus generally requires higher concentrations. The presence of occult blood in the stool may represent a clue to a periampullary neoplasm or hemobilia. Cholestasis also may produce markedly elevated cholesterol levels that may result in cutaneous xanthomas.

Laboratory Tests

Often the most assistance in evaluating the cause of jaundice comes from laboratory studies. A basic work-up of a patient with jaundice requires a complete blood count (CBC), reticulocyte count in selected cases, and liver function tests including measurement of serum bilirubin concentration and serum transaminase and alkaline phosphatase activities. If liver function tests are normal, one should think of either hemolysis, ineffective erythropoiesis, or a selective defect in hepatic bilirubin transport such as Gilbert's syndrome.

A CBC, reticulocyte count, and examination of the peripheral blood smear will usually indicate the presence of hemolysis or a condition associated with increased ineffective erythropoiesis. Lactate dehydrogenase activities (particularly isoenzyme 1), decreased serum haptoglobin concentration, or the presence of urinary hemosiderin may also assist in the diagnosis of hemolysis. If the patient is anemic and the reticulocyte count is inappropriately low, this should suggest ineffective erythropoiesis.

If the CBC, reticulocyte count, and liver function tests are normal, Gilbert's syndrome should be considered. The increase in serum bilirubin concentration that accompanies Gilbert's syndrome and disorders associated with hemolysis or ineffective erythropoiesis is characteristically unconjugated, particularly if the new assays, alluded to earlier, are employed. In contrast, the hyperbilirubinemia that accompanies the Dubin-Johnson and Rotor's syndromes is partially or predominantly conjugated (Table 2).

If liver function tests are abnormal, the jaundice is very likely a manifestation of cholestasis. Cholestasis is characteristically accompanied by increased activities of gamma glutamyltransferase, 5'-nucleotidase, leucine aminopeptidase, and alkaline phosphatase in serum. Alkaline phosphatase has been most intensively studied and can be measured in most clinical laboratories. Unlike the case with bilirubin or bile acids, an elevated alkaline phosphatase activity in serum does not reflect diminished biliary excretion but, rather, increased synthesis and, possibly, increased release of this enzyme into the circulation. This same mechanism may be operational for the other enzymes, such as 5'-nucleotidase or leucine aminopeptidase, which are also located on the plasma membrane. Although increased activity of these enzymes is characteristic of cholestasis, elevations do occur in other situations. Alkaline phosphatase activity may be increased in certain bone disorders and in pregnancy. Gamma glutamyltransferase (GGT) activity may be increased by numerous enzyme-inducing drugs, as well as alcohol, in the absence of a hepatic disorder. It is not found in bone, and a normal value therefore suggests that an elevated alkaline phosphatase activity is of bony origin. Leucine aminopeptidase is also present in virtually all tissues, but elevated serum levels are seen only in hepatobiliary disease, particularly biliary obstruction, and pregnancy. Again, this enzyme is used primarily in evaluating the significance of an elevated alkaline phosphatase activity. Other laboratory abnormalities that may accompany cholestasis include elevated concentrations of cholesterol and lipoprotein X in serum. The elevation in serum bilirubin concentration that accompanies cholestasis is due largely to an increase in the conjugated fraction.

With either parenchymal liver disease or biliary obstruction, the normally efficient hepatic clearance of bile acids from portal venous blood is impaired. Indeed, elevated serum bile acids are a more sensitive indicator of cholestasis than is hyperbilirubinemia. Although a normal bile acid level is helpful in excluding a cholestatic disorder and may aid in making a diagnosis of Gilbert's syndrome, elevated values are nonspecific and are not useful in the differential diagnosis of cholestatic jaundice. Measurement of serum bile acid levels is presently not available in most laboratories.

APPROACH TO THE PATIENT WITH JAUNDICE DUE TO CHOLESTASIS

Clinical and Laboratory Evaluation

In practice, jaundice is usually a manifestation of cholestasis and the differential diagnosis of cholestasis is the most common and perhaps most important distinction faced by the clinician. It is particularly critical that the patient with biliary obstruction be identified so that appropriate treatment may be instituted.

Clinical clues to the presence of extrahepatic obstruction are outlined in Table 3. The value of the patient history, physical examination, and routine laboratory tests in the differential diagnosis of jaundice has been reaffirmed by a recent prospective study in which over 90 per cent of cases of proven obstructive jaundice were correctly suspected on the basis of clinical evaluation alone. Laboratory tests of particular value in the differential diagnosis of cholestasis include serologic tests for hepatitis B virus infection (see the article on Viral Hepatitis), antimitochondrial antibodies (positive in 85 per cent or more of patients with primary biliary cirrhosis sometime during the

Table 3. Clinical Clues to Extrahepatic Obstruction

History
1. Abdominal pain suggestive of biliary or pancreatic disease
2. Previous biliary surgery
3. Prolonged or intermittent cholestasis
4. Absence of exposure to potential hepatotoxins (e.g., drugs), and absence of hepatitis exposure and hepatitis-like symptoms

Physical examination
1. Palpable gallbladder or abdominal mass
2. High fever suggestive of cholangitis
3. Occult blood in stool
4. Absence of stigmata of chronic liver disease
5. Abdominal tenderness

Laboratory studies
1. Disproportionate elevation of bilirubin, alkaline phosphatase
2. Elevated amylase
3. Complete normalization of a prolonged prothrombin time following vitamin K administration
4. Negative serologic markers for viral hepatitis, chronic active hepatitis, primary biliary cirrhosis

course of the disease), and serum amylase activity (often elevated with pancreatic or biliary tract disease).

Techniques for Imaging the Biliary Tree

If extrahepatic obstruction is suspected on the basis of clinical grounds, further evaluation to determine the site and nature of the obstruction is warranted (Fig. 2). A reasonable next step is the use of a noninvasive study such as *ultrasonography* or *computed tomography* to determine whether the intra- and/or extrahepatic biliary system is dilated, implying mechanical obstruction. Because of its lesser expense and the lack of radiation exposure, ultrasonography is preferred to computed tomography (CT) as a first procedure. Ultrasonography and computed tomography will demonstrate ductal dilatation in 85 per cent or more of patients with jaundice due to biliary obstruction. Both techniques may also yield additional information such as the presence of stones in the gallbladder or the presence of a pancreatic mass.

False-negative examinations have resulted from errors in interpretation and have also been reported in patients with sclerosing cholangitis. False-negative results may also occur in the presence of cirrhosis, presumably because of poor distensibility of the hepatic parenchyma. Gallstones, which commonly produce only partial or intermittent biliary obstruction, may also fail to cause ductal dilatation, and both techniques frequently fail to detect stones in the common duct. If dilated bile ducts are detected, it is generally appropriate to further define the location and perhaps nature of the obstruction with direct cholangiography, either by endoscopic retrograde cholangiography or by percutaneous transhepatic cholangiography. Because false-negative ultrasonographic or CT studies do occur, direct cholangiography is also appropriate even if one or both of these studies are negative if the clinical suspicion of biliary obstruction is high. Indeed, in certain selected situations such as the evaluation of recurrent symptoms suggestive of biliary disease in a patient who has previously undergone cholecystectomy, direct ductal visualization may be appropriate as a first procedure. For a detailed description of retrograde and percutaneous cholangiography, along with their specific indications and risks, the reader is referred to the article "Diseases of the Gallbladder and Biliary Tract."

Other Tests

A wide variety of other tests, discussed next, are sometimes employed in the work-up of the jaundiced patient. However, because these tests lack sensitivity and specificity, they are not routinely indicated but may be helpful under certain circumstances.

Technetium-99m sulfur-colloid scans are useful primarily in the detection of intrahepatic mass lesions, which occasionally may produce striking cholestasis when strategically located. Overall, the diagnostic yield of a liver scan in the work-up of jaundice is low when compared with that of computed tomography or ultrasonography.

Anecdotal reports have suggested that *hepatobiliary scintigraphy* with technetium-99m dimethyl acetanilide imminodiacetic acid (HIDA) may be useful in the evaluation of jaundice. HIDA is taken up by hepatocytes and excreted into bile in detectable amounts even in patients with moderately severe cholestasis and hyperbilirubinemia. The detection of HIDA in the bile ducts but not in the gallbladder is a generally reliable indicator of cystic duct obstruction in the previously healthy patient, but false-positive and false-negative results occur frequently in alcoholic patients or in those receiving parenteral nutrition. Some prospective studies have indicated that the utility of HIDA scanning in the differential diagnosis of cholestasis is limited. Moreover, radionuclide scans are unable to provide the same sort of resolution available with direct cholangiography and complete failure of the extrahepatic ducts to visualize is of no help in distinguishing intra- from extrahepatic cholestasis.

Intravenous cholangiography, although generally

Table 4. Causes of Cholestasis That Can Mimic Extrahepatic Obstruction

Viral hepatitis	Primary biliary cirrhosis
Alcoholic hepatitis	Postoperative cholestasis
Benign recurrent cholestasis	Parenteral nutrition
Pregnancy	Hodgkin's disease
Sepsis	Drugs (e.g., estrogens, phenothiazines, rifampin)
Infiltrative liver disease (e.g., amyloidosis, sarcoidosis)	Inherited disorders (e.g., arteriohepatic dysplasia)
Hepatic neoplasia	Sickle cell disease
Hepatic abscess	

classified as noninvasive, is associated with a 4 to 10 per cent incidence of adverse reactions, including a 1 per cent incidence of serious hypersensitivity reactions. Moreover, the test is unreliable. Even in patients with a serum bilirubin concentration < 3 mg/dl, duct opacification is not adequate to permit a definitive reading in up to 45 per cent of cases and no ductal visualization is generally achieved with bilirubin concentrations exceeding 3 mg/dl. Thus, intravenous cholangiography has no role in the routine evaluation of jaundice. *Oral cholecystography* is also of no value in the work-up of the jaundiced patient. It will generally not visualize the gallbladder when the serum bilirubin concentration exceeds 3 mg/dl and provides no direct information about the ductal system.

Despite anecdotal reports suggesting that *liver biopsy* in patients with biliary obstruction might be associated with an inordinate risk of complications such as peritonitis, larger series suggest that the risk of liver biopsy is not greatly increased as long as the prothrombin time (< 3 seconds prolonged) and platelet count (> 80,000 per cu mm) are acceptable. Nonetheless, liver biopsy is not indicated in the routine work-up of jaundice because (1) histologic findings diagnostic of obstruction are often absent in patients with proven obstruction and (2) even if histologic changes suggestive of a diagnosis of biliary obstruction are present, the biopsy generally provides no information regarding the location or nature of the obstruction. The principal role of a liver biopsy in the jaundiced patient is in the differential diagnosis of difficult or confusing cases of intrahepatic cholestasis.

Hepatic Disorders that May Mimic Obstruction

In most cases, the distinction between intra- and extrahepatic causes of cholestasis can be readily made on the basis of a thorough clinical evaluation. However, it is important for the clinician to be aware of certain hepatic disorders that may sometimes present with very prominent cholestasis suggestive of extrahepatic obstruction. Examples are listed in Table 4. Even these entities can usually be correctly suspected on the basis of clinical evaluation. The most important causes of intrahepatic cholestasis to identify are obviously those that are potentially treatable or reversible on withdrawal of the offending agent. In some instances (e.g., alcoholic hepatitis, amyloidosis) liver biopsy may permit a specific diagnosis. However, in most instances (e.g., cholestatic hepatitis, drug- or estrogen-induced cholestasis, benign recurrent cholestasis, cholestasis related to sepsis) liver biopsy typically demonstrates only cholestasis with variable hepatocellular necrosis, findings which by themselves do not permit a specific diagnosis.

It is also worth emphasizing that biliary and hepatocellular disease often coexist. For example, the incidence of gallstones is known to be increased in cirrhotics, and in one study 39 per cent of patients with primary biliary cirrhosis were found to have gallbladder stones. Thus, known hepatocellular disease should not dissuade one from pursuing possible biliary disease suspected on clinical grounds.

SUMMARY

The differential diagnosis of jaundice remains one of the most interesting and challenging problems encountered in clinical practice. The correct diagnosis is generally apparent on clinical evaluation, and the work-up of the patient with cholestasis and suspected obstruction has been greatly facilitated by the advent of new techniques for visualizing the biliary system. The challenge to the clinician is to minimize the time, expense and patient risk necessary to establish a diagnosis and institute treatment.

THE COMATOSE PATIENT

By David S. Dahl, M.D.
Milwaukee, Wisconsin

Coma is synonymous with brain failure. This can be brief, such as a simple syncope, or it can be prolonged. If the episode is brief, before neuronal failure has a chance to become irreversible, the patient potentially can have a total recovery. The length of coma, however, is of extreme importance: seconds to minutes of coma caused by certain conditions such as hypoxia can produce irreversible brain damage and even brain death. Therefore, diagnosis must be made quickly and accurately. In many circumstances, the need to treat is so great that some supportive therapeutic measures must be instituted from the beginning and must proceed concomitant with the diagnostic investigations. A thorough and systematic approach is mandatory.

Often no history is available, but even shreds of history from rescue squad members, bystanders, or information from Med-Alert bracelets and wallet contents are most important and can help focus the inquiry. In general, the physical examination supplies the earliest objective data. There are certain elements of the neurologic examination that are particularly useful in evaluating a comatose patient. Fortunately, these procedures can be done rather quickly.

NEUROLOGIC EXAMINATION

The neurologic examination of the unconscious patient concentrates on five specific areas of assessment. The evaluation should be done before the traditional aspects of the examination (e.g., funduscopic exam, deep tendon reflexes, plantar responses) are performed but after the usual vital signs are observed. These areas are as follows.

Level of Consciousness. The comatose patient appears to be asleep. Frequently the patient can be aroused to some degree by verbal stimulus or shaking. If this does not arouse the patient, the examiner should quickly administer a painful but harmless stimulus. Sometimes the patient does not arouse at all but may exhibit a stereotyped motor response. (See discussion under the topic of motor responses to be discussed.)

Respiratory Pattern. The respiratory pattern varies with specific processes. With bilateral diencephalic dysfunction, Cheyne-Stokes respirations, a pattern of cyclic alternating apnea and hyperventilation waxing and waning in a smooth crescendo-decrescendo fashion, can be observed. This pattern can be seen in the waking state. With damage to the upper brain stem, central neurogenic hyperventilation can occur. This consists of sustained, rapid, and fairly deep hyperpnea. Other breathing patterns, such as ataxia or apneusis, are of grave prognostic implication. Hypoventilation is often seen with toximetabolic coma and is easily missed.

Spontaneous and Provoked Ocular Movements. In the absence of focal lesions, the eyes are conjugate or slightly divergent and are frequently roving. Conjugate deviation of the eyes toward the side implies a supranuclear process. A destructive anterior hemispheral lesion will show conjugate eye deviation toward the side of the lesion and away from the hemiparetic side, a destructive pontine lesion away from the lesion and toward the paretic side. Downward and binasal eye deviation indicates a pretectal or thalamic lesion but can also be seen in some encephalopathies.

Dysconjugate gaze implies an infranuclear lesion. A number of rare and bizarre eye movements, such as ocular bobbing or nystagmoid jerking of a single eye, indicate brain stem dysfunction.

Ocular motility can be tested in two ways: by the oculocephalic reflex (doll's eye maneuver), or the oculovestibular reflex (ice water calorics). The oculocephalic reflex should not be performed unless a fractured neck can be ruled out. The examiner elicits the oculocephalic reflex by quickly rotating the head from side to side. This procedure provides no useful data when the patient is awake. If consciousness is lost but the brainstem is intact, the eyes will move conjugately in a direction opposite that of the head movement. If the brainstem is damaged, this response will be attenuated or even absent so that the eyes do not move in relation to the head.

The oculovestibular reflex need be done only if a broken neck cannot be ruled out or if the oculocephalic response is uncertain or negative. This reflex is elicited by positioning the head 30° above the horizontal and then injecting a stream of ice water into the external auditory canal to chill the petrous bone. The external auditory canal should be visualized before the test to ascertain that the tympanic membrane is intact. In a conscious or psychogenically unresponsive patient, nystagmus toward the opposite side will occur. In a comatose patient with an intact brain stem, the eyes will slowly and conjugately deviate toward the stimulated ear. If the brain stem is damaged, the eyes will not move or they may show a dysconjugate response.

Pupillary Responses. The technique requires that a very bright light stimulus be used and that it be directed as best as possible in the line of the visual axis. Darkening the surroundings may help accentuate the reaction. Sometimes a hand lens should be used in examining the pupils for minimal movements. Metabolic diseases usually produce small but reactive pupils. Anticholinergic agents and anoxia lead to bilaterally wide and fixed pupils. A herniated medial temporal lobe (uncus) results in an ipsilateral fixed and dilated pupil because of compression of the third cranial nerve. Midposition but bilaterally fixed pupils can be seen in midbrain compression from above but can also be seen with glutethimide intoxication. Pinpoint pupils with minimal light reactivity can be seen in lesions of the pons but can also be seen with opiate overdose.

Motor Responses. Much information can be obtained from using nociceptive but harmless stimulation and observing the response. The blink response is a variant of the corneal reflex. It can be elicited by touching the eyelashes lightly. Perception is through the trigeminal nerve, tegmental pathways in the lower half of the pons, and motor output via the seventh nerve. If the blink response is equivocal or unobtainable, the true corneal reflex should be elicited with observation of eyelid tone and also the presence or absence of Bell's phenomenon (reflex upward deviation of the eyes in response to forced closure of the eyelids). Presence of the latter indicates normal function of the brain stem between the nuclei of the third nerve and the seventh nerve.

A traditional sensory examination cannot be performed, but some assessment of the sensory system can be determined. A lack of response could be due to loss of sensation, loss of efferent responses, or a coma so deep that there is no central processing.

Painful stimuli should be administered to the distal portions of all four extremities as well as both sides of the head. Pressure on the base of the nails by the edge of the examiner's own fingernail is appropriate technique. The face can be stimulated by squeezing the supraorbital nerve at the uppermost margin of each orbit.

In light coma, the motor responses may be purposeful withdrawal or a defensive response such as trying to push the stimulus away. A facial grimace should also be observed.

At a deeper level of coma, a decorticate response can be seen; the arms adduct, the elbows and the wrists flex, and the lower limbs extend and inwardly rotate. The head and upper back may extend somewhat.

At yet deeper levels of coma, a decerebrate posture may be seen; the arms are in extension with hyperpronatation of the forearms and more intense leg extension and back and neck hyperextension. At even deeper levels of coma, no response may be seen. Asymmetrical responses are also of great importance and imply structural neurologic damage.

The Glasgow Responsiveness Scale provides a reasonable quantitation of consciousness and calls attention to precoma states such as lethargy. This scale measures eye opening, motor response, and verbal response to stimulation. The scoring range is from 3 in the deepest coma to a maximum of 15 in a fully conscious patient. Eye opening is worth 4 points if done spontaneously, 3 if in response to speech, 2 if in response to pain, and 1 if no response. The best motor response is recorded as 6 if the patient obeys commands, 5 if he responds to annoying stimulation, 4 if there is withdrawal of a limb from stimulation, 3 if there is decorticate posturing, 2 if there is decerebrate posturing, and 1 if there is no response. Asymmetrical responses are also noteworthy. Verbal responses are scored as 5 points if the patient is oriented, 4 if able to converse but in a confused fashion, 3 if conversation is inappropriate, 2 if speech is incomprehensible, and 1 if there is no verbal response. The scale values are easily recorded and are more specific than using such terms as "obtunded" or "stuporous." The Maryland Coma Scale is a newer alternative that includes other eye findings and avoids the confusion of quantifying untestable observations.

Obviously some parts of the neurologic examination such as assessment of cerebellar function cannot be done. The deep tendon reflexes provide surprisingly little useful information. It is extremely important, however, to examine the ocular fundi; papilledema reflects increased intracranial pressure, preretinal hemorrhage suggests subarachnoid bleeding, and emboli may be seen at retinal arteriole branching points.

INITIAL ASSESSMENT AND EMERGENCY MANAGEMENT

With these requisite observations in mind, it is appropriate to consider the overall conduct of the approach to the comatose patient. The physician must be ready to institute elements of emergency management whenever necessary during the assessment phase. A brief review of these principles is in order.

As the diagnostic process begins, the patient's unclothed body should be closely inspected, especially for signs of trauma, skin discoloration, needle tracks, or unusual odors at the same time that vital signs are being measured. Airway assessment and assurance of oxygenation are of prime importance in this phase. The patient may need to have endotracheal intubation. Blood pressure, pulse, cardiac rate, and rhythm must be checked quickly. Access to the circulation should be established and necessary blood samples drawn at this time. (This is discussed further under the topic of emergency laboratory evaluation later in this article.) After specimens are drawn, an intravenous line should be attached. Fifty to 100 mg of thiamine should be injected next, before glucose is given, to avoid provoking Wernicke's syndrome. Then, 25 grams of glucose (50 ml of 50 per cent solution) should be given through the intravenous line; this will prevent hypoglycemic brain damage and will not injure a person who is not hypoglycemic. If seizures are occurring, it is appropriate to begin treatment at this time (see article on the epilepsies and other convulsive disorders). Body temperature should be ascertained and attempts made to normalize a deviant temperature.

Before lumbar puncture is performed on a comatose patient, thorough funduscopy and computed tomographic (CT) scanning should be performed. This will also permit assessment of intracranial pressure. In an infant, palpation of the fontanelle can provide a quick estimate of intracranial pressure. Increased intracranial pressure should be suspected if there is progressive deterioration with repeated assessments. Treatment may have to be instituted early by means of hyperventilation and osmotic agents.

If overdosage of drugs, alcohol, narcotics, tranquilizers, hallucinogens, or other substance is suspected, one must be prepared to intervene with appropriate antidotes if available.

A crucial observation is to determine that the cervical spine is not fractured. In cases of trauma, especially head injuries, the neck must be assumed to be broken until proved otherwise by x-ray examination; any movement of the patient should be carried out with the neck held in slight extension and traction, maintaining its relationship with the thoracic spine. When it is determined that the neck is intact, the patient must be examined for nuchal rigidity.

Where a team is available, it is helpful for one physician to take responsibility for assessment and another one to institute early therapeutic interventions. Various monitors and repeat assessments of vital signs by nursing personnel are also mandatory. Arterial blood gases should be drawn to assess acid-base balance.

If meningoencephalitis is strongly suspected, even the time to do a CT scan may be critical and it should be bypassed in order to obtain cerebrospinal fluid for microbiologic study and chemical analysis.

EARLY DIAGNOSTIC CONSIDERATIONS

As the early information is developing from the available history, the general physical examination, and the specific neurologic profile discussed earlier, the physician should be formulating a diagnostic impression. As with other neurologic problems, it is helpful to first consider an anatomic diagnosis (where is the lesion or dysfunction?) and then seek to make an etiologic-pathologic diagnosis (what is the actual process?). As noted before, coma represents brain failure, which can be divided into two large categories:

Table 1. Major Features of Coma Types

Etiology	Respirations	Pupils
Supratentorial lesion		
Cerebral hemispheral disease	Normal, sighing, or Cheyne-Stokes patterns	Normal or small, reactive
Uncal herniation	Normal or sighing early, central neurogenic hyperventilation seen late	Ipsilateral dilatation early
Diencephalic	Normal, sighing or Cheyne-Stokes patterns	Small and reactive
Subtentorial lesions		
Midbrain (can be damaged also from rostrocaudal progression of supratentorial lesions)	Cheyne-Stokes or central neurogenic hyperventilation	Midposition, irregular fixed
Pontine	Shallow, rapid or slow and irregular (ataxic)	Midposition and fixed (pressure from above), or pinpoint and sluggish (local processes)
Diffuse intracranial and toximetabolic processes	Varies with causes, especially acid-base balance; frequently hypoventilation	Small, equal, reactive, usually pinpoint with opiates. Dilated and fixed with glutethimide intoxication
Psychogenic unresponsiveness	Normal	Reactive

1. Primary brain failure from an event within the cranial cavity.
2. Secondary brain failure from extracranial or nonanatomic process.

It is helpful to subdivide these processes further into:

1. Supratentorial masses or destruction.
2. Subtentorial masses or destruction.
3. Diffuse intracranial processes.
4. Toximetabolic coma.
5. Psychogenic unresponsiveness (Table 1).

(Note that diffuse intracranial processes and toximetabolic coma look alike clinically.)

After the problem is narrowed down to this point, it is time to be concerned about actual etiologic agents or pathologic processes (Table 2).

EMERGENCY LABORATORY EVALUATION

Computed tomography has revolutionized the approach to diagnosis of structural brain diseases. If a supratentorial lesion is suspected, a CT scan should be performed as soon as the patient is reasonably stable. If a CT scan is not available, carotid angiography or a radionuclide brain scan should be done. Skull films waste time and should not be done unless palpation of the scalp and skull suggests a depressed skull fracture. The CT scan is invaluable in demonstrating bleeding, mass lesions, midline shifts, and edema. However, early and relatively small infarcts are often missed with the initial CT scan.

Blood specimens obtained initially should be sent for measurement of glucose, electrolytes, creatinine, or urea, and possibly osmolality. Arterial blood gases should be obtained as well. Additional specimens can be drawn as indicated for measurement of sedative and toxic drugs, liver function tests, coagulation studies, endocrinologic tests, and serologic or cultural tests for infectious agents. The urine should be analyzed for sedative and toxic drugs in addition to routine studies.

The electroencephalogram (EEG) is a physiologic test that is very useful for assessing coma. However, it is rarely used in emergent situations. The EEG may show diffuse slowing that is roughly proportionate to the level of consciousness. The EEG may also show focal abnormalities (masses, seizure foci). The EEG is normal, all things being equal, in patients with psychogenic unresponsiveness.

SOME SPECIFIC CAUSES OF COMA

Epidural Hematoma. An epidural hematoma may develop when a skull fracture line crosses the groove of the middle meningeal artery. Blood under arterial pressure rapidly collects between the dura and the skull, compressing the brain from the side. If the patient has been rendered unconscious from the precipitating trauma, consciousness may briefly return only to decline again as the expanding mass of blood presses inexorably upon the brain. This lucid interval has been described in a fair number of such patients. As consciousness declines, a dilated pupil appears ipsilateral to the hemorrhage and contralateral to the hemiparesis. On occasion the brain stem is moved so far across the midline that it impinges on the edge of the tentorium, thus damaging contralateral corticospinal fibers that will cross over to the ipsilateral side below this secondary lesion. This con-

Table 1. Major Features of Coma Types (Continued)

Eye Movement	Motor Responses	Miscellaneous
Tonic conjugate deviation toward side of destructive lesion or away from irritative focus	Hypotonia on side opposite lesion, paresis or paratonia seen in semicoma	Abnormal reflexes on side opposite the lesion Progression of lesion shows rostral to caudal dysfunction
Loss of movement of ipsilateral eye to oculocephalic or oculovestibular maneuvers, seen late. Third nerve palsy in repose (eye down and out)	Contralateral paratonia and paresis or diminished contralateral movements to noxious stimuli. Asymmetrical decorticate or decerebrate responses (late)	
Roving eye movements, normal oculocephalic and oculovestibular responses	Paratonias, paresis early, decorticate responses	
Impaired oculocephalic and oculovestibular responses; eyes may be dysconjugate	Decerebrate responses to stimulation	Upward eye movements limited when there is upward transtentorial herniation
Eyes immobile; if local process, may show deviation toward more paralyzed side	Decerebrate responses; legs may flex to local stimulation	
Roving in repose. Normal reflex responses, but reduced or absent when coma is very deep	Any response or none, depending on severity, but mostly symmetrical; mixed loss and preservation of function at same level	Slow evolution of coma with preceding organomental behavior, headache, stupor, asterixis, myoclonus, or seizures
Intact blink reflex, lids close actively, oculocephalic response unpredictable, nystagmus seen with oculovestibular testing	Normal tone, withdrawal, or no response	No pathologic reflexes present

sequence is referred to as a false localizing sign and demonstrates the importance of being able to analyze the total pattern of findings. Death may result unless the pressure is quickly relieved by surgical intervention.

Trauma to the head should always be highly suspected in alcoholics, those with serious mental illness, those with convulsive disorders, and combative patients.

Cerebellar Hemorrhage. This entity accounts for about 12 percent of parenchymal intracranial hemorrhages. If the diagnosis can be made promptly, many patients can be treated successfully by posterior fossa decompression. If there is any history available, typically there is a story for occipital headache, nausea and vomiting, dizziness, unsteadiness, and dysarthria. However, some cases evolve so quickly that the patient has little time to express these complaints. Those that present with coma show irregular respirations, pinpoint pupils, absent oculovestibular responses, and quadriplegia. A CT scan provides considerable information. If the patient is not yet comatose, emergent surgery can produce excellent results. Since subtentorial lesions can expand upward through the tentorium and downward through the foramen magnum, decompression from above the tentorium or a lumbar puncture may actually worsen the herniation.

Anoxic Encephalopathy. This entity is a good example of toximetabolic brain disorder caused by a number of circumstances that reduce oxygen delivery to brain cells. If the process is prolonged, secondary brain failure can evolve into a primary brain failure, that of cortical laminar necrosis. This process can occur quickly. Total ischemic anoxia lasting longer than 4 minutes will cause irreversible damage. This outcome can occur even more rapidly if there is superimposed pre-existing cerebral vascular disease, or conversely can be delayed in rare instances where hypothermia provides some protective effect such as drowning in cold water, especially with children.

Psychogenic Unresponsiveness. A number of serious mental disorders, such as the dissociative state in a person of hysterical temperament or the catatonic stupor of schizophrenia, can render an individual seemingly unresponsive. Table 1 demonstrates the findings that show that the person is physiologically awake. An amytal interview can be both diagnostic and briefly therapeutic; however, such individuals are often seriously mentally ill and should be evaluated by a psychiatrist.

PITFALLS IN THE DIAGNOSIS OF COMA

It is easy to assume that all observations made in the heat of rapid assessment are acute and new. Nonetheless, there are circumstances where pre-existing disease such as an old stroke or neurologic complications of diabetes can lead to some confusion in assessment (Table 3). This is especially important to consider when the assessment suggests brain death.

BRAIN DEATH

This occurs when irreversible brain damage is so extensive that there is no potential for recovery and no maintenance of the body's internal homeostasis. Mechanical means may preserve breathing and circulation for a time under these circumstances. Our modern medical technology is no better illustrated than by our ability to keep an essentially brainless body "living" for extended periods with respirators, cardiovascular drugs, antibiotics, and so on. However, this is a prolonged and essentially futile exercise that is expensive both financially as well as emotionally for family and medical staff. Therefore, the concept of brain death and what to do about it has evolved.

In a government document published in 1981,* these issues are discussed and one particular recommendation is made. The Uniform Determination of Death proposal says the following:

> An individual who has sustained either (1) irreversible cessation of circulatory and respiratory functions, or (2) irreversible cessation of all functions of the entire brain, including the brain stem, is dead. A determination of death must be made in accordance with accepted medical standards.

Table 2. Causes (Etiology or Pathology) of Coma

Supratentorial brain disease (mass lesions pressing on brain or intraparenchymal masses or destruction)
Neoplasm (usually subacute evolution), subdural hematoma or empyema, epidural hematoma, intracerebral hematoma (traumatic or spontaneous, hypertensive or secondary to vascular malformation), infarct (thrombotic), abscesses, and brain edema accompanying all of the above. The increasing volume of these lesions indirectly causes brain stem dysfunction.

Subtentorial brain disease
Brain stem or cerebellar infarcts, hemorrhages or neoplasms, subdural and extradural hematomas, abscesses, granulomas, neoplasms (coma late), and central pontine myelinolysis.

Diffuse cerebral disorders
Anoxic-ischemic encephalopathy (partially or totally irreversible brain disease from prolonged ischemia or hypoxia), meningitis, encephalitis, vasculitis, subarachnoid hemorrhage (ruptured vascular malformation or trauma), concussion (brief), status epilepticus, and postictal states (usually brief). Also primary neuronal or glial disorders (e.g., progressive multifocal leukoencephalopathy.)

Toximetabolic processes
Hypoxia, cofactor deficiency (e.g., thiamine); systemic diseases (diabetes, sepsis); organ failures (e.g., liver, kidney); imbalance of water, electrolytes, hormones, and acid-base environment; disordered temperature regulation; and exogenous poisons including drugs.

Psychogenic unresponsiveness
Conversion reaction, catatonic stupor, and malingering.

*_Defining Death: Medical, Legal and Ethical Issues in the Determination of Death._ President's Commission for the Study of Ethical Problems in Medicine and Behavioral Research. Library of Congress, July 1981.

Table 3. Pitfalls in the Diagnosis of Coma

Findings	Possible Causes
Pupils fixed	Anticholinergic drugs Pre-existing disease
No oculovestibular reflexes	Anticholinergic drugs Ototoxic drugs
No respiration	Posthyperventilation apnea Neuromuscular blocking agents
No motor activity	Neuromuscular blockers "Locked in" state Sedative drugs
Isoelectric EEG	Sedative drugs Anoxia Hypothermia Encephalitis

It is hoped that all states will adopt this standard Uniform Determination of Death proposal; so far only a minority of states have their own brain death statutes. The statute is of considerable importance to transplant programs that require the donation of healthy organs and to families, since the support of a living corpse is very expensive financially and emotionally.

The question then is: What are "acceptable" medical standards?

Table 4 delineates the criteria for the diagnosis of brain death. These are slightly modified criteria from the Cornell Affiliation Hospitals, New York.

One should point out that the EEG does not replace all of the rest of these criteria. The EEG can be considered optional except when there are potential legal implications or when plans are made to salvage organs for transplant.

Most patients on artifical respirators have a Pa_{O_2} and a Pa_{CO_2} below normal levels, indicating little respiratory drive from the increased plasma CO_2. Therefore, as a final determining event, the patient is respired with 100 per cent oxygen for 10 or 20 minutes, then the respirator is disconnected. Oxygen is delivered through a catheter to the trachea at the rate of about 6 liters per minute. Apneic oxygenation for 10 minutes thus allows the Pa_{CO_2} to rise without danger of hypoxia and assures that the respiratory threshold is exceeded. If no breath is taken during this period of time, all further resucitation can be discontinued. In some transplant programs, the respirations and circulation may need to be artificially maintained until the tissues to be transplanted have been removed.

ETHICAL AND LEGAL CONSIDERATIONS

From a legal standpoint, death of the brain has been more or less explicitly accepted as indicating death of the entire individual. Unfortunately, most states have not enacted brain death statutes. Nonetheless, if the above guidelines are followed, there can be little cause

Table 4. Criteria for Diagnosis for Brain Death*

Nature and duration of coma
Known structural disease or irreversible systemic cause
Drug intoxication or hypothermia ruled out
Six hours' observation
Absence of cerebral function
No behavioral or reflex response to noxious stimuli above foramen magnum level
Isoelectric electroencephalogram, minimum of 30 minutes at 5–10 μV/mm.
Absence of brain stem function
Fixed pupils
No oculovestibular responses to 50 ml ice water calorics
Systemic circulation may be intact
Purely spinal reflexes may be maintained
Apneic during oxygenation for 10 minutes

*Modified from the Cornell Affiliation Hospitals, New York. Published by Plum, F., and Posner, J. B.: *The Diagnosis of Stupor and Coma*, 3rd ed. Philadelphia, F. A. Davis Co., 1980.

for legal action. It is absolutely necessary, however, that the physician and family be in close communication as well as agreement. If there is no agreement, the physician must pursue educational efforts with the family. Anecdotal reports abound of people awakening from prolonged coma. The brain-dead individual often gives the appearance of life: the moving chest, the pulsing vessels, the bodily warmth sometimes making it difficult for the family to accept the situation. Appropriate consultation and recommendation for input from a spiritual advisor may be helpful, and the nursing staff can be invaluable in promoting good communication about this decision. It is recommended in transplant cases that two other physicians with no stake in the transplant should be involved in the brain death opinion. This situation always calls for the greatest tact and relational skills of the sensitive physician.

HEADACHE AND FACIAL PAIN

By William G. Speed, III, M.D.
Baltimore, Maryland

The differential diagnosis of headache may be simple or complex. To begin with, one should have a concept of the classification of headache. A reasonable and workable classification is presented in Table 1.

The differential diagnosis depends on the characteristics and pattern of the headache. Establishing the pattern of a headache requires a thorough and detailed history and, at the very least, a modified physical examination with emphasis on the head, neck, and neurologic system. Obtaining a proper headache history is a time-consuming but essential process, since without a clear concept of the total headache pattern, the correct diagnosis cannot be made (Table 2). If one obtains the history data (as outlined in Table 2) in a careful and comprehensive way, a clear pattern of headaches should emerge.

TYPES OF HEADACHE

Migraine

In this disorder there is an inherited profound instability of cranial vascular regulation. In all forms of migraine, there are a *vasoconstriction* phase and a *vasodilatation* phase. When intracranial vasoconstriction is of sufficient degree to produce ischemia, and therefore neurologic symptoms, the attack is called *classic migraine.* The symptoms produced depend on the areas of ischemia. The following symptoms may occur: scintillations, scotomata, homonymous hemianopsia, diffuse blurring of vision, amaurosis fugax, dysarthria, dysphasia, loss of depth perception, confusion, total global amnesia, impaired thought processes, hemiparesis, hemiplegia, hemianesthesia, paresthesia, impairment of consciousness, unconsciousness, vertigo, and ataxia.

The vasodilatation phase is associated with sterile inflammation of the vessel wall, and this combination produces the pain of migraine. As a rule, the vasoconstriction phase precedes the vasodilatation phase, but the two phases may not be sharply separated; hence neurologic symptoms and headache may coexist. When there is no demonstrable neurologic manifestation, the headache is called *common migraine.*

Normally migraine is a recurrent disorder, usually occurring one to three times a month; however, the frequency may vary from one to two attacks a year to three or four or more per week and sometimes on a daily basis. The duration of the attack may range from hours to a few days or more, and the intensity of the pain may vary from mild and annoying to severe and totally incapacitating. The vessels involved in pain

Table 1. Headache Classification

Vascular	Muscle contraction
Migraine	Episodic or chronic
Classic	Myofascial pain dysfunction syndrome (sometimes called temporomandibular joint (TMJ) syndrome)
Common	Cervical degenerative arthritis/discogenic disease
Hemiplegic	Post-traumatic (some)
Ophthalmoplegic	
Basilar artery	Traction and inflammation
Cluster	Tumor, hematoma, aneurysm, cranial arteritis, intracranial infections, diseases of EENT,* cranial neuralgias
Episodic	
Chronic	
Toxic or metabolic	
Hyperpyrexia	
Hypoxia	
Carbon monoxide	
Nitrates	
Tension (some)	
Post-traumatic (many)	
Hypertension	

*EENT = Eye, ear, nose, and throat.

Table 2. Headache History

Types (Is more than one type present?)	Emotional history
Onset	Tension, nervousness, or anxiety symptoms
Frequency	Depression, including history of crying spells and suicidal thoughts
Duration	Fatigue
Location	Sleep patterns
Range of severity	Marital adjustments
Neurologic symptoms and their time-sequential relationship to headache	Perfectionism
Other associated symptoms or signs, e.g., nausea, vomiting, lacrimation, rhinorrhea, ptosis, pupillary change	Chronic worrying
Family history	
Emotional status	

are the external carotid artery, the internal carotid artery, and the basilar artery systems. Essentially, any area of the head and face may be involved alone or in any combination, but most often migraine involves the temporofronto-ocular areas. The headaches are frequently unilateral and may shift sides during an attack. Many patients have bilateral attacks of migraine interspersed with their unilateral headaches, and there are some patients whose headaches are only bilateral. The pains are likely to be pounding and throbbing, but the absence of these characteristics does not exclude the diagnosis of migraine. Nausea and/or vomiting are common accompaniments.

The headache attacks may be precipitated or aggravated by exposure to various odors such as gasoline, diesel fuel, exhaust fumes, paint, perfume, and tobacco smoke, as well as a low barometric pressure, and by the ingestion of certain foods such as aged cheese, alcohol, avocados, bacon, bananas, pods of broad beans, canned figs, chicken livers, chocolate, citrus fruits, coffee (including decaffeinated coffee), fermented sausage, pickled herring, hot dogs, nuts, onions, tea, and yogurt.

Although the vascular instability of migraine is extremely vulnerable to emotional stress, tension, anxiety, apprehension, worry, anger, hostility, and depression, it is not a primary psychological disorder. It is incorrect to classify these headaches as being due to tension or "nerves."

There are subsets of migraine that should be recognized in the differential diagnosis of headaches, since these varieties may simulate life-threatening disease.

Hemiplegic Migraine. This variety is thought to be due to a prolonged ischemic aura involving the cerebral cortex and producing hemiplegia. The hemiplegia is usually followed by unilateral headache; that is, it may precede the headache as an aura or it may accompany the headache and in rare instances may outlast the headache. It is more likely to be seen in infants or very young children, but it does occur in adults. Hemiplegic migraine is recognized by its repetitive character and sequential relationship to headache.

Basilar Artery Migraine. This variety results from prolonged profound ischemia of the vertebrobasilar artery system, which produces vertigo, dysarthria, diplopia, ataxia, and sometimes impairment of thought or loss of consciousness. The headache usually follows these symptoms and is likely to be occipital in location. It is more likely to occur in youngsters.

Ophthalmoplegic Migraine. This variety is thought to occur from compression of the third, fourth, and sometimes sixth cranial nerves in the cavernous sinus by a dilated and edematous carotid artery associated with the nasal dilatation of migraine. There is diplopia, impairment of eye movement, and a unilateral fixed dilated pupil occurring during the headache phase. The headache is likely to be experienced behind or over the eye on the same side as the ophthalmoplegia. In patients who have repeated attacks, it is usual for the paralysis to be transient in the beginning but later to persist for a few days to many months; in rare instances, certain palsies may become permanent.

The presentation of these varieties of migraine is called *complicated migraine* and may be confused at times with stroke, tumor, or aneurysm. The diagnosis may be suspected by history of previous episodes usually occurring in childhood and associated with a strong family history of migraine. (Further discussion of migraine can be found in the article on migraine and its variants.)

Cluster Headache

This is a male-dominated vascular headache disorder that can appear at any age, but most occur between 20 and 40 years of age. Its pattern and characteristics are so distinct that the diagnosis should be readily apparent.

This type of headache usually occurs in "clusters" that continue for weeks or months. When a cluster continues without remission for a period of 6 to 12 months, it is considered *chronic.*

There are short attacks of pain (15 to 120 minutes), one to three attacks per 24-hour period—frequently nocturnal and always unilateral—and the same side persists during a cluster. Pain involves the eye, temple, cheek, jaw, and teeth, and at times the pain may extend to the occipital area. The intensity of the pain is almost always severe and excruciating and is described as boring, burning, gnawing, pounding, and throbbing. Frequently associated with cluster headache are homolateral rhinorrhea, nasal congestion, lacrimation, and reddened eye. There may be homolateral miosis and ptosis, which are usually transient but at times become permanent. Nausea is uncommon and vomiting is rare. The attacks may be precipitated by drinking alcohol or by lying down to take a nap. It is not uncommon for attacks to occur nocturnally, usually a couple of hours after going to sleep. Patients with migraine tend to seek a dark and quiet room and do not want to be disturbed, whereas patients with cluster headache tend to pace and want to get out of bed when an attack occurs. A patient presenting with a typical cluster headache pattern does not need any laboratory or radiologic procedures to establish the diagnosis.

Toxic or Metabolic Headache

A diffuse, nondescript, usually throbbing headache may be seen as the result of vasodilatation secondary to a toxic or metabolic process such as very high fevers or hypoxic states as in respiratory distress syndromes or anemia. These conditions should not present any diagnostic difficulty, since the underlying problem is usually apparent.

A more subtle variety of toxic vascular headache is seen in mild degrees of carbon monoxide poisoning. As an example, an individual driving to and from work with the windows closed in an automobile with a defective muffler may experience nondescript, diffuse, mild, throbbing, aching headache. The key factors here are the nondescript nature of the headache and the subtle relationships to the times of day, such as pain occurring shortly after arriving at work or shortly after coming home at night. These headaches are rather rare, and a high index of suspicion is needed for the physician to think about such possibilities. A carbon monoxide blood level will establish the diagnosis.

Sometimes the use of nitrates in individuals who have coronary insufficiency may produce a significant degree of vascular headache. More subtly, a diffuse, usually low-grade headache or aggravation of an existing migraine process may be seen in hypertensive individuals who are being treated with reserpine. Reserpine depletes serotonin, which in turn results in vasodilatation and hence may aggravate an existing migraine.

Hypertensive Headache

These are dull, diffuse, aching, throbbing headaches that may be generalized, unilateral, or occipital. Most often they are worse in the early hours of the day, usually beginning after midnight, sometimes wakening the patient from sound sleep, but more commonly present on awakening and then diminishing in intensity after the person arises and becomes active. There are no characteristics of these headaches that permit a specific diagnosis of this disorder. Hypertensive headache is suspected only when the blood pressure is elevated—and it need not be markedly elevated—and when a therapeutic trial of an antihypertensive agent (other than reserpine) will prove the diagnosis. This headache will promptly disappear with appropriate control of the hypertension. If the headache persists despite appropriate blood pressure control, a more complete evaluation is indicated and probably should include an enhanced computed tomographic (CT) scan of the head.

Muscle Contraction Headache

There are episodic and chronic varieties of this disorder. As in the previous headaches described, the pattern of these headaches either establishes the diagnosis or indicates a high probability of its presence.

The episodic variety is common and may involve the temporofrontal, vertex, or occipitocervical region, separately or in any combination. The patient describes tight pressure, squeezing, or aching; the episodes are usually triggered by fatigue, an acute family crisis, or peaking of stressful workloads. This variety does not present a problem to the patient or the physician, since it invariably subsides with the removal of the stressful trigger.

Table 3. Secondary Chronic Muscle Contraction Headaches

This disorder may be secondary to the following:

- Disturbances of the eye (inflammation, muscle imbalance)
- Nasal or paranasal inflammation
- Temporomandibular joint dysfunction
- Disorders of the neck (degenerative arthritis, ankylosing spondylitis, and discogenic disease)
- Inflammation secondary to systemic disorders, such as viral infections
- Trauma, including nerve entrapment
- High cervical or posterior fossa tumor (slow-growing astrocytoma or meningioma)
- Vascular headaches

One chronic variety of this disorder is constant and unremitting and may be present for weeks, months, years, or decades without any significant periods of freedom. The areas involved are the same as those in the episodic variety, and the characteristics of the pains are similar; in addition, however, these patients may complain of soreness, tight headbands, weight-like sensations, and a feeling like that of a tight skullcap. The diagnosis in patients who present with these symptoms is somewhat more difficult because there are a number of underlying conditions that produce this pattern of headache (Table 3).

When the physician is confronted by a chronic unremitting headache of this type, it is imperative that the aforementioned conditions be excluded at the beginning of the diagnostic process. For the most part, this does not create a significant problem. For example, systemic disorders such as viral infection or inflammation of the eyes and nasal and paranasal structures are usually readily apparent. Temporomandibular joint (TMJ) dysfunction can be suspected by tenderness on palpation of the joint or by a clicking sound in this joint, which is easily discernible with a stethoscope. One should be cautious about this diagnosis, however, because a primary disturbance in the TMJ is seldom at the basis of chronic muscle contraction; therefore, the term *myofascial pain dysfunction syndrome* is a more appropriate one to use. If, on examining the neck, one obtains excellent mobility without evidence of muscle tightness or restriction of movement, the more diffuse chronic headache is unlikely to be due to cervical arthritis or discogenic disease, regardless of what x-ray films show. High cervical or posterior fossa tumors are difficult to exclude because they may give no neurologic signs until they have been present for long periods.

For the most part, chronic muscle contraction headaches are related to none of the disorders described in Table 3 but are associated with tension, anxiety, depression, repressed hostility or anger, unresolved dependency needs, or psychosexual conflicts. Even though the diagnosis may be apparent from the pattern just described, an enhanced CT scan of the head should be done if the headache is not readily controlled on appropriate management programs.

Chronic Post-traumatic Headache

Almost anyone who injures his head will have pain and tenderness at the site of impact for hours or several days and then will become free of symptoms. The chronic variety represents those headaches that have persisted for more than 2 months following an injury.

Chronic headache resulting from trauma may mimic almost any type of chronic recurring headache. It may be constant or intermittent and may involve any areas of the head—e.g., it may be frontal, temporal, vertex, occipital, alone or in any combination; it may be unilateral, bilateral, or generalized; and patients may exhibit more than one type of headache concurrently. Pains are described variously as aching, pressing, squeezing, expanding, burning, stabbing, throbbing, pounding, feeling like a band around the head, or resembling an ache located deep inside the head. If vascular mechanisms are involved, they may be aggravated by bending over, coughing, straining, being exposed to loud noises and bright lights, and jarring the head.

The mechanisms involved are as follows:

1. *Muscle contraction.* This is the most frequent cause of chronic post-traumatic headache. It is clinically indistinguishable from the chronic muscle contraction headache unrelated to trauma (detailed previously).

2. *Vasodilatation.* Pulsating, pounding, and throbbing are common in some post-traumatic headaches. Diagnosis of the vascular nature of the headache is established not only by the throbbing pulsatile character of the pain but also by the fact that these headaches may respond to the use of ergotamine tartrate. Although many of these are nonmigrainous vascular headaches, both classical and common migraine can be precipitated by head injury as well as by an aggravation of an already existing migraine disorder. Trauma may precipitate the first attack of migraine in the susceptible individual, may increase the frequency and/or severity of pre-existing migraine, and occasionally may produce features compatible with chronic migraine. The diagnosis ultimately depends on proper interpretation of the pattern of the headache.

3. *Combined muscle contraction and vasodilatation.* This combination is quite common when both muscle contraction factors and vasodilatation are occurring simultaneously. The term *mixed-type headache* describes this entity.

4. *Scar formation.* If the soft tissues of the head are injured, an area of localized tenderness may result, apparently based on the entrapment of sensory nerve endings as a result of locally damaged tissue or the entrapment in a scar. The latter results from traumatic myositis, fibrositis, or periostitis. These headaches are felt for the most part around the site of the injury, and the pain may be intermittent or continuous. The involved site is always strikingly tender to finger pressure, making the diagnosis easy.

5. *Vascular dilatation, muscle contraction, and scar formation.* These processes may occur simultaneously in the same patient.

6. *Injuries to neck structures.* Injuries to the superficial and deep structures of the neck involving muscle, ligaments, discs, bones, or nerve roots can produce cervical pain that may be referred to the head. The popular term "whiplash injury" describes the sudden hyperextension of the neck followed by hyperflexion, usually as a result of a rear-end collision. Most patients, shortly after such an accident, complain of diffuse muscle soreness followed by neck and head pain. The head pain component may be limited to the occipital area, or it may spread to involve the vertex and the temporofrontal and retrobulbar areas as well. This is usually a dull pressure, squeezing pain, at times with a throbbing component. Neck pain is usually considerably aggravated by any attempt to move the neck. The head and neck pain of the chronic variety may last for many months or longer. Exacerbation of pre-existing arthritis or discogenic disease may occur. In some cases, the occipital neurovascular bundle (made up of the occipital nerve, artery, and veins) at the level of or near the occipital ridge may be traumatized at the time of the original injury, or it may be traumatized secondarily as a result of prolonged muscle contraction or chronic vascular dilatation. The resultant headache is called *occipital neuralgia.* The diagnosis is rather easily established by the presence of considerable localized pain and tenderness brought out by thumb pressure over the occipital ridge where the occipital neurovascular bundle crosses (approximately 2 inches lateral to the occipital cervical juncture).

The history and physical examination will usually establish the diagnosis of chronic post-traumatic headache with reasonable certainty. However, because of the potential medicolegal problems surrounding most headache injuries, certain x-rays, such as a cervical spine film and an enhanced CT scan of the head, may be indicated.

Cranial Arteritis

This is a disorder of the older age group. Essentially all patients with this disorder are over the age of 50, and most are over the age of 60. When a headache begins for the first time in someone over the age of 50 or when a change in the characteristics of a previous recurring headache occurs, cranial arteritis should be high on one's list of suspected disorders. It affects both sexes, women somewhat more than men, is characterized by painful inflammation of the cranial artery, and is associated with general systemic signs and symptoms such as malaise, weight loss, fever, sweating, and weakness. At times the symptoms are subtle, and the patients' complaints have been mistaken for depression. The sedimentation rate is usually quite elevated, and there is a mild to moderate elevation of the leukocyte count.

The headache is nonspecific but is most likely to be diffuse or generalized. There is often aching, throbbing, or burning, and the pain varies from moderate to severe in intensity. The scalp is frequently tender to touch, particularly along the course of the cranial arteries. Pulsation of the arteries may be present or absent. Intermittent claudication of the jaws sometimes occurs.

Since there is a significant potential for blindness to occur in this disorder as a result of optic nerve ischemia secondary to ophthalmic arteritis, it is imperative that the diagnosis of cranial arteritis be made promptly. There should be a high order of suspicion from the symptoms just described, and the prompt use of prednisone, 60 mg a day, or its equivalent should be instituted. If the diagnosis is correct, prompt resolution of the headache and its symptoms will occur within 24 to 72 hours—one of the most dramatic symptom responses seen in any medical disorder. If the response does not occur within 72 hours, the diagnosis should be reassessed.

Once the diagnosis is presumably confirmed by the response to prednisone, a biopsy of an involved artery should be obtained. A delay of several days for the therapeutic trial with prednisone does not alter the pathologic findings. A negative biopsy result does not exclude the diagnosis—the arterial lesions may "skip"; hence a generous segment of artery should be removed and a diligent search should be made by a pathologist for the changes characteristic of cranial arteritis.

Brain Tumors

Headache associated with brain tumors may be mild to severe, and in a number of cases there may be no headache at all. Headache is more likely to occur with rapidly expanding tumors producing traction on pain-sensitive structures in the head. Headache may be a prominent finding with increased intracranial pressure. One should be suspicious of a brain tumor in an individual previously free of headache who develops the insidious onset of headache with a relentless progression of the intensity and duration. The presence of neurologic abnormality intensifies the suspicion of a tumor.

Although there are no outstanding characteristics of the headache produced by a brain tumor, patients describe a deep, aching, steady, dull pain usually not rhythmic and seldom throbbing. These headaches may be intermittent or continuous and may be relieved by simple analgesics or ice compresses. Such headaches rarely interfere with sleep, may be aggravated by coughing or straining, and are likely to be somewhat worse in the morning than later in the day. Vomiting occurs with displacement or compression of the medulla and sometimes is projectile, since it may be unaccompanied by nausea. Headaches, when occipital or suboccipital, may be associated with stiffness or aching of the muscles in the neck and tilting of the head toward the side of the tumor. A CT scan of the head, particularly with enhancement, should be carried out in any patient in whom there is suspicion of a brain tumor. Small posterior fossa tumors are likely to be missed in the absence of enhancement. (Intracranial neoplasms are discussed in a later article.)

Aneurysm

Aneurysms that do not bleed or produce neurologic signs do not produce headache. Expressed another way, an asymptomatic aneurysm is asymptomatic.

Hematoma

Hematomas may cause headache. If a patient is conscious following a head injury, headache may be a prominent early sign of epidural hematoma because the pain-sensitive vascular structures in the dura separate from their attachment to the skull. As the size of the hematoma progresses, the patient may become restless and combative before lapsing into unconsciousness. The headache, therefore, is only one of the progressive steps in the signs and symptoms of an epidural hematoma and does not create a problem in diagnosis.

Subdural hematomas are commonly accompanied by headache that has no specific characteristics of its own. Over time there is usually a progression of signs of brain compression, but these may be as nonspecific as apathy, inappropriate behavior, and confusion. Presentation of such a group of symptoms would certainly indicate the need for a CT scan of the head.

Cranial Neuralgia

Tic douloureux is an episodic, recurrent, unilateral facial pain syndrome. It most often begins after the age of 50 and is seen more often in women than in men. It involves predominantly the second division of the cranial nerve, less frequently the first and third divisions. The pains may involve any part of the face, but they never occur below the ramus of the jaw or behind the ear. The pain is characterized by extremely high-intensity jabs lasting less than 20 to 30 seconds, followed at times by a period of relief lasting a few seconds to a minute, again followed by another jab of pain. Repeated episodes may occur for minutes to as much as an hour. A cardinal sign is the presence of trigger zones (areas of increased sensitivity on the face, particularly about the nares and mouth), which set off the attack when they are stimulated often by trivial sensations. These patients tend to avoid touching and washing the face, shaving, biting, or chewing. An episode may even be triggered by talking or by exposure to very light drafts.

Glossopharyngeal neuralgia is a similar phenomenon, but the symptoms are related to the distribution of the glossopharyngeal nerve. The same sort of pain felt in tic douloureux may be experienced in the pharynx, the tonsils, and the ear and may be precipitated by swallowing, yawning, or eating. Syncope may occur during an attack of glossopharyngeal neuralgia, presumably secondary to asystole resulting from stimulation of the vagus system as well.

Table 4. Conditions Associated with Facial Pain

Post-herpetic neuralgia	Angina pectoris
Anesthesia dolorosa	
Lethal midline granuloma	Myocardial infarction
Multiple sclerosis	Raeder's paratrigeminal syndrome
Lesion of cerebellopontine angle	
Intra- or extraspinal abnormalities C_{1-3}	Glaucoma, iritis, retrobulbar neuritis
Central pain from brain stem	TMJ* syndrome (myofascial pain dysfunction syndrome)
Central pain from thalamic area	
Tic douloureux	Migraine
Apical petrositis (Gradenigo's syndrome)	Cluster
Inflammation or malignancy of sinuses	Atypical facial neuralgia
Inflammation of teeth or gums	Occipital neuralgia
Fifth nerve compression	Cranial arteritis
Impaction of nasal septum	Tolosa-Hunt syndrome
Carotidynia	Conversion reaction
Post-traumatic syndrome	Depressive equivalents

*TMJ = Temporomandibular joint.

Pain relief is often dramatic with anticonvulsant therapy such as carbamazepine (Tegretol), 200 mg two or three times daily. In some patients if symptoms persist, phenytoin (Dilantin) may be added. If there is no response to these medical therapies, surgical intervention is indicated. (These neuralgias are discussed in a later article.)

Sinusitis

Acute sinusitis almost invariably produces head or facial pain, depending on the sinuses involved. A diagnosis is relatively easily made, usually by history and evidence of nasal or paranasal infection. Chronic or long-standing recurrent head or facial pain is seldom if ever related to underlying inflammation of the sinuses. (Disorders of the sinuses are discussed in a later article.)

Atypical Facial Neuralgia

This is a category of facial pain that is poorly understood. It represents those facial pains that do not result from migraine, cluster headache, cranial neuralgias, dental, nasal, or paranasal infection. The clinical picture is usually one of persisting, unrelenting, deep-seated, aching pain in the face that is not limited to areas supplied by a single cranial or cervical nerve; also, there are no trigger zones. The pain may be unilateral or bilateral and is frequently associated with mood changes such as depression, anxiety, or hysterical features. Although this type of facial pain is usually chronic, it may be episodic. Some pains are due to vascular dilatation, some to muscle contraction, and some to undoubtedly psychogenic factors. It is a difficult diagnosis to make and is primarily one of exclusion. It is important to recognize the presence of this type of facial pain, since it is unrelieved by such procedures as the cutting of nerves; alcohol injections; operations on the teeth, mastoid process, nasal structures, and sinuses; cocainization of the sphenopalatine ganglion; resection of superior cervical sympathetic ganglion; evulsion of the supra- or infraorbital nerve; and subtotal section of the sensory root of the fifth cranial nerve.

There are a number of conditions to be considered in the presence of facial pain, not all of which can be discussed in detail here. A list is contained in Table 4. The diagnosis depends on recognition of the underlying disorder.

SUMMARY

Comments made at the beginning of this section should be re-emphasized. The differential diagnosis of head and facial pain depends on understanding the diversified patterns produced by a variety of headaches and learning the technique of history taking so that appropriate data are obtained.

SYNCOPE

By Harisios Boudoulas, M.D.
and Richard P. Lewis, M.D.
Columbus, Ohio

DEFINITION

Syncope is defined as a temporary loss of consciousness that is due to a reversible disturbance of cerebral function. Presyncope and near syncope are less well defined entities but probably represent lesser degrees of the same disorder. The loss of consciousness in syncope and the altered consciousness in presyncope reflect an impairment in cerebral cellular metabolism usually resulting from a generalized or localized reduction of cerebral blood flow or an inadequate concentration of metabolic substrate necessary for brain function. Complete interruption of cerebral perfusion for 2 to 3 seconds results in a feeling of faintness, often described as "dizziness" or "giddiness"; if prolonged to 10 seconds, loss of consciousness results.

Clinically, syncope must be differentiated from a wide variety of complaints often referred to as "spells." These episodes may signify anything from transient and sudden weakness to a clouding or loss of consciousness, acute episodes of vertigo, a complete loss of consciousness, and even sudden death. No cardiovascular symptom alarms the patient more and no disorder of the circulation demands more careful diagnostic appraisal than the complaint of a sudden or transient loss in consciousness.

Syncope and presyncope can be conveniently classified into three major categories: (1) vasodepressor, (2) cardiovascular, and (3) noncardiovascular syncope (Table 1). As an initial approach to the diagnosis in the

Table 1. Classification of Syncope

- Vasodepressor
- Cardiovascular
  - Cardiac
    - Obstructive
    - Arrhythmic
  - Vascular
    - Orthostatic
    - Cerebrovascular
    - Reflex
- Noncardiovascular

patient complaining of sudden loss of consciousness, it is essential to attempt to distinguish the underlying cause in terms of the three basic mechanisms: vasodepressor, cardiovascular, and noncardiovascular syncope. This differentiation is accomplished in the majority of patients through careful attention to the basic clinical examination, history, physical examination, electrocardiogram (ECG), and chest x-ray (Fig. 1). The following discussion of the diagnostic evaluation of the patient with syncope presents this pattern of diagnostic consideration.

VASODEPRESSOR SYNCOPE

Approximately 15 to 25 per cent of young individuals experience one or more episodes of vasodepressor syncope (common faint). Syncope that is of a vasodepressor origin is rare in otherwise normal individuals after 35 years of age.

Clinically, vasodepressor syncope is characterized by a fall in arterial pressure with or without bradycardia; is associated with impairment or loss of consciousness and loss of motor tone; and is accompanied by variable expressions of autonomic overactivity, as evidenced by pallor, sweating, nausea, and mydriasis. After recovering consciousness, the patient is noted to have persistence of pallor, sweating, and nausea, associated with a tendency for recurrence of syncope if the upright posture is resumed prematurely.

The common faint may occur as a response to sudden emotional stress, or it may occur in a setting of real, threatened, or fantasied injury. The reaction is not infrequently brought on by venipuncture or the sight of blood and is also observed after a sudden painful experience such as that occurring during surgical manipulation or following severe tissue injury. It is particularly likely to occur in certain environmental settings such as in a hot and crowded room, especially if the individual is fatigued, hungry, or ill or has recently experienced blood loss. The common faint is usually encountered when the patient is in an upright or sitting posture, rarely occurring while the patient is recumbent. The primary circulatory disorder in vasodepressor syncope is a marked fall in peripheral vascular resistance, which is the essential factor responsible for the fall in arterial pressure and the diminished perfusion pressure to the brain.

Vasodepressor syncope is not uncommon in patients with cardiovascular disease. Syncope of this type may be observed in patients with aortic stenosis, with various forms of congenital heart disease, and with primary pulmonary hypertension.

The history is of essential interest in the diagnostic workup of the patient with sudden loss of consciousness resulting from vasodepressor syncope. Indeed, knowledge of the premonitory symptoms, the associated environmental circumstances, and the postsyncopal findings often leads to the proper diagnosis. Of importance in the evaluation of the patient with an episode of vasodepressor syncope is the consideration as to whether it is an isolated event or one that is symptomatic of underlying cardiovascular disease. The finding of a completely normal clinical examination is helpful in this differentiation, particularly in the younger patient. In the older patient, however, there is often sufficient question as to an underlying cardiovascular disorder to dictate a more complete evaluation, including noninvasive and invasive tests as outlined in the following sections.

CARDIOVASCULAR SYNCOPE

If a fainting episode is not found to be typical for vasodepressor syncope, it must be explained by one or more of a wide variety of other causes. Cardiovascular syncope may be cardiac or vascular in origin. In cardiac syncope and in most cases of vascular syncope, global cerebral ischemia is present.

Cardiac Syncope

Either severe obstruction to cardiac output or disturbances of cardiac rhythm can produce cardiac syncope (Table 2). Obstructive cardiac lesions and arrhythmias frequently coexist, and indeed one abnormality may accentuate the other. The diagnosis of lesions producing mechanical obstruction to flow can usually be made by a careful history and physical examination. The recognition of arrhythmias is more difficult because of their transient nature.

Obstructive Cardiac Syncope

Obstruction to cardiac output may result from pathologic lesions or structural abnormalities of the left or right side of the heart. On the left side it is most

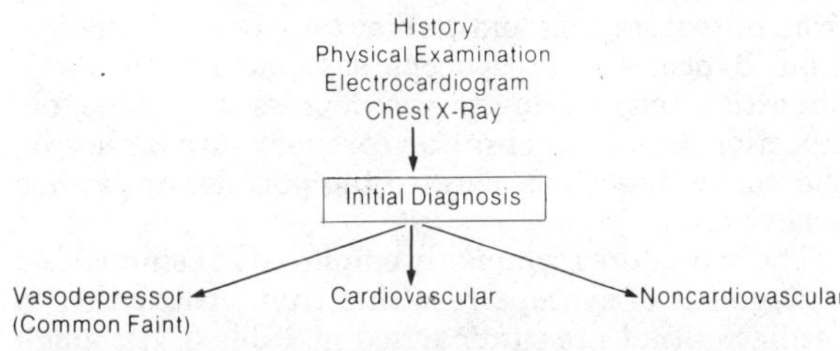

Figure 1. Basic schema for diagnostic evaluation of syncope. The differentiation in vasodepressor, cardiovascular, and noncardiovascular syncope is accomplished in the majority of patients with the history, physical examination, chest x-ray, and electrocardiogram. (Reproduced with permission from Boudoulas H., et al.: The clinical diagnosis of syncope. In Harvey, W. P., et al. (eds.): *Current Problems in Cardiology.* Copyright © 1982 by Year Book Medical Publishers, Inc., Chicago.)

Table 2. Cardiac Syncope

Obstructive	Arrhythmic
Left heart	*Bradycardia*
Aortic stenosis	Sinus bradycardia or sinoatrial exit block
Hypertrophic cardiomyopathy	Reflex bradycardia
Prosthetic valve malfunction	Atrioventricular block
Myxoma	Pacemaker malfunction
Mitral stenosis	*Tachycardia*
Cardiac tamponade	Ventricular tachycardia
Aortic dissection	Supraventricular tachycardia
Right heart	Frequent premature ventricular beats (PVBs)
Eisenmenger's syndrome	Pacemaker malfunction
Tetralogy of Fallot	
Primary pulmonary hypertension	
Pulmonary embolism	
Pulmonary stenosis	

likely the result of aortic stenosis, hypertrophic cardiomyopathy, prosthetic valve malfunction, or left atrial myxoma.

The most common causes of syncope with obstruction to right ventricular output are Eisenmenger's syndrome (left-to-right shunt with pulmonary hypertension), tetralogy of Fallot, primary pulmonary hypertension, pulmonary embolism, and pulmonary stenosis.

Syncope, particularly with exertion, is a major symptom of aortic stenosis (effort syncope). Syncope associated with effort (often immediately after exertion) is also observed in patients with hypertrophic cardiomyopathy, pulmonic stenosis, tetralogy of Fallot, and primary pulmonary hypertension. If an adult woman with no cardiac murmur has experienced effort-related syncope, primary pulmonary hypertension should be suspected.

A left atrial myxoma or a malfunctioning prosthetic valve may obstruct left ventricular filling, leading to a marked and sudden lowering of cardiac output and syncope. The obstruction to left ventricular inflow in atrial myxoma may be posturally induced. Mitral stenosis and cardiac tamponade may also produce cardiac syncope, particularly if tachycardia or other arrhythmias supervene. However, syncope resulting from mitral stenosis and cardiac tamponade is uncommon. Syncope or presyncope associated with aortic dissection may be due to vasodepressor syncope, obstruction to the cerebral or coronary circulation by the aortic dissection, cardiac tamponade, or cardiac arrhythmia.

The procedures commonly employed in establishing a diagnosis of syncope resulting from obstruction to cardiac output are summarized in Table 3. Although the history and physical examination usually suggest the diagnosis, complete noninvasive evaluation is often necessary to establish the severity of the underlying disease. The routine electrocardiogram is of diagnostic importance in indicating the presence of atrial or ventricular hypertrophy and associated disorders of conduction and rhythm. The chest roentgenogram may reveal telltale dense calcification at the aortic or mitral valve areas. Image intensification fluoroscopy may detect such valvular calcification when this finding is absent on the chest roentgenogram. The chest roentgenogram often reveals additional data concerning the state of the central and peripheral pulmonary circulation, lending clues to the diagnosis of left- and right-sided obstructive disease at either the cardiac or pulmonary vascular level. The first suggestion of congenital heart disease is often made by the chest film. Image intensification cinefluoroscopy is of special usefulness when prosthetic valve dysfunction is under consideration.

In the modern era, the echocardiogram has become critical to the diagnosis of obstructive cardiac disease and is of great value in establishing a diagnosis of aortic stenosis, hypertrophic cardiomyopathy, mitral stenosis, left atrial myxoma, aortic dissection, or pericardial effusion (which may be associated with tamponade) as a cause of syncope. The echocardiogram is also useful in the detection of prosthetic valve dysfunction and in the diagnosis of congenital heart disease as causes of syncope. Radionuclide angiography adds to the diagnosis in certain cases with congenital heart disease. Graphic recordings of the pulse and heart sounds, including the determination of the systolic time intervals, add to the diagnosis and to the evaluation of the severity of several entities associated with recurrent syncope. Thus, the finding of a prolonged left ventricular ejection time is consistent with hemodynamically significant aortic valvular stenosis or hypertrophic cardiomyopathy. Arterial blood gases and combined ventilatory and perfusion nuclear lung scanning may be highly informative in the diagnosis of pulmonary embolism. If noninvasive tests remain inconclusive, cardiac catheterization and cinecardiography may be required to establish the diagnosis.

Arrhythmic Cardiac Syncope

Either extreme of ventricular rate (bradycardia or tachycardia) can depress cardiac output to a point of critical hypotension and syncope. Arrhythmias are a common cause of syncope and must be considered in all cases in which an obvious mechanism is not evident. The most common arrhythmias producing syncope or presyncope are profound sinus bradycardia or sinoatrial exit block, high-grade atrioventricular block, ventricular tachycardia, supraventricular

Table 3. Cardiac Syncope—Diagnostic Evaluation

Obstructive	Arrhythmic
Image intensification fluoroscopy	Ambulatory monitoring
Echocardiography (M-mode and 2–D)	Exercise testing
Graphic methods and systolic time intervals	Electrophysiologic studies
Radioisotopic methods (radionuclide angiography, pulmonary ventilation-perfusion scan)	
Catheterization-angiography	

tachycardia, frequent premature ventricular beats, and pacemaker malfunction (Table 2).

Many patients with cardiac conduction and/or rhythm disturbances leading to syncope are not aware of their arrhythmias. The occurrence of syncope with cardiac arrhythmias often depends on the magnitude of concurrent hemodynamic disturbances. Thus, patients with normal cardiac function can tolerate the changes in heart rate and rhythm that accompany most cardiac arrhythmias. If there is obstruction to cardiac output or severe myocardial failure, a rapid change in heart rate and rhythm may be associated with a sudden and profound reduction in cardiac output. The appearance of symptoms during cardiac arrhythmias may also be related to the patient's posture, level of wakefulness, arterial pressure, and blood volume at the time of the rhythm disorder. Thus, patients with recurrent arrhythmias may not experience presyncope or syncope with every episode of the arrhythmia.

A most challenging diagnostic dilemma faces the physician who suspects arrhythmic syncope. Such patients often have evidence of underlying cardiovascular disease, and a definite linkage between the presence of an arrhythmia and the occurrence of syncope is often difficult to establish. Methods used to study arrhythmias include the routine electrocardiogram, exercise testing, ambulatory electrocardiographic monitoring, and electrophysiologic studies (Table 3). Because of the transient nature of most arrhythmias, the routine electrocardiogram is of limited value. The electrocardiogram, however, is useful in identifying patients with electrophysiologic abnormalities that may predispose to syncope, such as the presence of a remote or recent myocardial infarction, the Wolff-Parkinson-White syndrome, or the occurrence of a prolonged QT interval. Although identification of second- and third-degree atrioventricular block on the electrocardiogram is very useful, the presence of bundle branch block is not a reliable predictor of syncope.

Cardiac arrhythmias may be provoked by exercise in the patient with episodic rhythm disorders. Clinical and physiologic studies support the use of this approach as a means of uncovering suspected arrhythmias. It should be noted, however, that there is a better chance, statistically, for detecting transient arrhythmias on prolonged ambulatory monitoring than with exercise. Although long-term observation of cardiac rhythm can be accomplished in a hospital monitoring unit, experience has shown that ambulatory monitoring is more efficacious when the patient is allowed to perform ordinary daily activities.

With patients in whom ambulatory monitoring and an exercise challenge fail to reveal an arrhythmic basis for syncope, electrophysiologic studies employing intracardiac recordings should be used. These studies make it possible to localize abnormalities to various sites, such as the sinus node, atrium, atrioventricular node, His bundle, and Purkinje system; pacemaker automaticity can also be assessed. With patients in whom supraventricular or ventricular tachycardia is suspected as the cause of syncope, the arrhythmia may be provoked by the introduction of premature atrial or ventricular impulses at the time

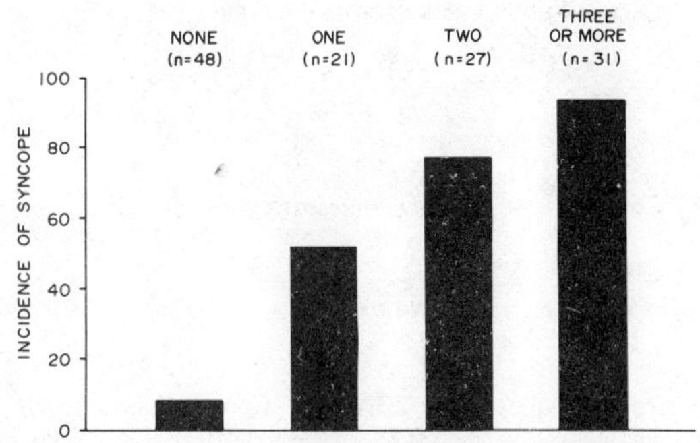

Figure 2. Relationship between the number of electrophysiologic abnormalities and syncope. The frequency of syncope is plotted against the electrophysiologic abnormalities, which include sinoatrial recovery time, sinoatrial conduction time, atrial-to-His interval, His-to-ventricular depolarization interval, or atrioventricular block at slow rates during atrial pacing. (From Boudoulas H., et al.: Electrophysiologic risk factors of syncope. J. Electrocardiol. 11:339, 1978. Used by permission.)

the intracardiac electrophysiologic recordings are made. This approach may define the mechanism of the tachycardia as well.

In regard to electrophysiologic studies, patients who have syncope on the basis of transient sinoatrial dysfunction or an atrioventricular conduction defect usually have two or more electrophysiologic abnormalities (Fig. 2). The likelihood of syncope increases as the number of electrophysiologic abnormalities increases. Syncope is unlikely to be caused by sinoatrial dysfunction or atrioventricular conduction defects if these abnormalities are not detected during electrophysiologic studies. In our experience, in patients with no obvious cause of syncope or presyncope during the routine clinical examination and in whom arrhythmia is strongly suspected, the arrhythmic cause of the symptoms has been detected by ambulatory monitoring in approximately 50 per cent of cases, by electrophysiologic studies in 60 to 70 per

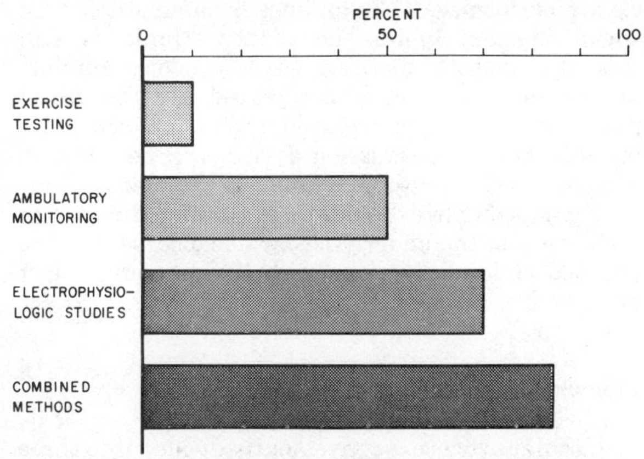

Figure 3. Detection of arrhythmia in patients with no obvious cause of syncope. The sensitivity of each method alone and in combination in defining arrhythmias as a cause of syncope. (Reproduced with permission from Boudoulas H., et al.: The clinical diagnosis of syncope. In Harvey, W. P., et al. (eds.): *Current Problems in Cardiology.* Copyright © 1982 by Year Book Medical Publishers, Inc., Chicago.)

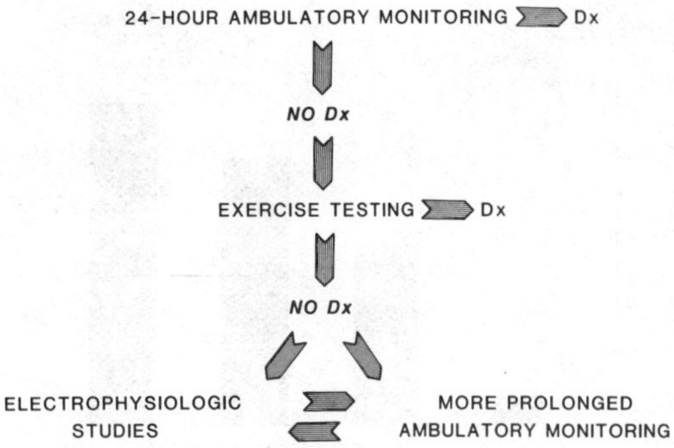

Figure 4. Diagnostic approach for evaluating a patient suspected of having arrhythmic syncope. Dx = Diagnosis.

cent and with exercise testing in 10 per cent. The use of all of these methods in combination has detected the cause of syncope in 80 to 85 per cent of patients (Fig. 3).

Our diagnostic approach in evaluating the patient suspected of having arrhythmic syncope follows the algorithm summarized in Figure 4. Initially 24-hour ambulatory monitoring is performed. If the patient experiences syncope or presyncope during monitoring and if a cardiac arrhythmia is observed simultaneously, it is clear that the syncope is caused by the arrhythmia. If the patient experiences syncope during 24-hour monitoring and no concurrent arrhythmia is detected on a technically adequate recording, arrhythmia can probably be ruled out as a cause of the syncope. If no syncope occurs during a 24-hour monitoring period and if a significant arrhythmia is found (e.g., ventricular tachycardia and/or atrioventricular block), it remains most probable that the patient's symptoms are related to the arrhythmia; that is, the arrhythmia recorded on ambulatory monitoring may not be of sufficient duration or severity to overwhelm circulatory adaptation. If no arrhythmia is found after an adequate trial of ambulatory monitoring, an exercise stress test is next performed. If exercise testing discloses no arrhythmia, electrophysiologic studies are performed. If the findings from all studies are within normal limits and if arrhythmia is still strongly suspected as the cause of syncope, ambulatory monitoring should be repeated and the use of patient-activated electrocardiographic recordings using telephonic transmission devices can be tried. In patients with syncope secondary to cardiac arrhythmia, complete diagnostic evaluation directed at the nature of the underlying cardiac disease must be pursued assiduously along with the maneuvers just described.

Vascular Syncope

Vascular syncope is conveniently divided into three major categories: (1) orthostatic, (2) cerebrovascular, and (3) reflex syncope (Table 4.)

Table 4. Vascular Syncope

Orthostatic syncope (orthostatic hypotension)
Cerebrovascular
Reflex
Vasovagal
Carotid sinus hypersensitivity
Cough
Postmicturition
Glossopharyngeal neuralgia

Orthostatic Syncope (Orthostatic Hypotension)

When a normal individual assumes the upright posture, the attendant gravitational stresses on the circulation are compensated by several mechanisms, such as reflex arteriolar and venous constriction, acceleration of heart rate, and mechanical factors—including the venous valvular system, compression of the leg muscles, and decreased intrathoracic pressure. The increased autonomic activity during upright posture is reflected in an increase in plasma catecholamine levels.

Chronic orthostatic hypotension is a disorder in which the autonomic factors compensating for the upright posture are inadequate or absent. Assumption of the upright posture in such patients is associated with a prompt fall in arterial pressure. Hypotension is progressive over a period of seconds to minutes, depending on the degree of loss in the adaptive reflex responses, until perfusion pressure to the brain becomes inadequate to sustain consciousness. When the recumbent posture is resumed, there is rapid return toward normal in arterial pressure and consciousness is regained. The failure of reflex hemodynamic adaptation in the upright posture in chronic orthostatic hypotension is a reflection of an overall deficiency in autonomic function.

Orthostatic hypotension with syncope is observed in a variety of clinical situations (Table 5), including

Table 5. Orthostatic Syncope—Common Causes*

Volume depletion or venous pooling
Prolonged bed rest
Prolonged standing
Pregnancy
Dehydration
Excessive diuresis
Bleeding
Varicose veins
Adrenal insufficiency
Pharmacologic agents
Antihypertensives
Diuretics
Nitrates
Arterial vasodilators
Calcium channel blocking agents
L-dopa
Phenothiazines
Other tranquilizers
Neurogenic hypotension
Neuropathy
Spinal cord disease
Surgical sympathectomy
Prolonged exposure to zero gravity
Idiopathic hypotension

*With permission from Boudoulas, H., et al: The clinical diagnosis of syncope. In Harvey, W. P., et al. (eds.): *Current Problems in Cardiology.* Copyright © 1982 by Year Book Medical Publishers, Inc., Chicago.

physiologic disturbances, such as prolonged bed rest, prolonged standing, or pregnancy; conditions associated with blood volume depletion or venous pooling, such as dehydration, excessive diuresis, hemorrhage, adrenal insufficiency, and varicose veins; and complicating side effects of pharmacologic agents, such as antihypertensives, diuretics, nitrates, and arterial vasodilators, including calcium channel blocking agents, levodopa (L-dopa), phenothiazines, or other tranquilizers. Orthostatic hypotension is also common in the presence of faulty reflex control of arterial pressure, such as that occurring in patients with spinal cord disease and neuropathies involving the autonomic nervous system (neurogenic hypotension)—i.e., tabes dorsalis, syringomyelia, diabetic neuropathy, subacute combined sclerosis, peripheral neuritis, alcoholic neuropathy, Wernicke's syndrome, porphyria, amyloidosis, and spinal cord transsection. A similar picture is seen following surgical sympathectomy, with pharmacologic blockade of the autonomic ganglia, and in drug-induced suppression of sympathetic nerve activity. Hypotension after prolonged exposure to zero gravity in astronauts may be related to transient loss of reflex control of arterial pressure.

There is, in addition, an idiopathic form of chronic orthostatic hypotension in which no etiologic factor has been elucidated. Such idiopathic orthostatic hypotension has been described in association with progressive neurologic abnormalities, including rigidity and tremor, ataxia, and upper and lower motor neuron abnormalities. This usually sporadic association of autonomic and peripheral neurologic abnormalities has been reported to have a familial association.

Orthostatic syncope is best diagnosed on the basis of history and physical examination. In our experience, the most common reason for missing the diagnosis of orthostatic syncope is the failure to adhere to the fundamental step of measuring the blood pressure with the patient in the supine and upright postures.

Table 6. Cerebrovascular Syncope

Common types
Atherosclerotic
Thrombotic
Embolic
External mechanical compression
Other (pulseless disease)
Common sources of cerebral emboli
Atherosclerotic plaque
Endocarditis (infective, noninfective)
Calcific valves
Prosthetic valves
Mitral valve prolapse
Intracardiac thrombus or tumor

Cerebrovascular Syncope

The common causes for syncope or presyncope in cerebrovascular disease are summarized in Table 6. Reduction of cerebral blood flow by atherosclerotic obstruction, thrombus, or embolism can result in a variety of syndromes, ranging from a transient ischemic attack to a cerebrovascular accident. Altered consciousness is a prominent feature of cerebrovascular disease when the carotid vertebrobasilar arterial system is involved. In some patients, the symptoms are due to arterial embolism arising from an atherosclerotic plaque or thrombus in the arteries supplying the brain. Cerebral emboli may originate from the cardiac chambers or valves as well. Patients with the mitral valve prolapse syndrome and those with intracardiac thrombus or tumor, in particular, are subject to such embolic episodes.

The internal carotid and the vertebral arteries may be mechanically compressed during certain movements of the head or neck. This is especially common when severe osteoarthritis, vertebral arterial occlusive disease, or both are present. These attacks may follow turning of the head or hyperextension of the neck, and the episodes may mimic carotid sinus syncope.

The specific symptoms of a transient ischemic attack are, of course, determined by the area of brain that is most depleted of its blood supply. The presence of transient focal neurologic symptoms and the findings of a carotid bruit or a localized diminution in the amplitude of the carotid arterial pulse will suggest the diagnosis.

With extensive occlusive involvement of the origins of the brachiocephalic vessels, such as that occurring in patients with pulseless disease (aortic arch syndrome, Takayasu's arteritis), syncope and presyncope occur with a high degree of frequency. With lesser degrees of cerebral vascular inflow occlusion, transient lowering of arterial pressure, such as that occurring immediately following the assumption of the upright posture, may be followed by vague symptoms that suggest impaired or marginal cerebral blood flow.

Impairment or loss of consciousness associated with upper extremity exercise has been described and characterized as the *subclavian steal syndrome.* This syndrome is caused by major occlusive disease of the proximal subclavian artery. With the decrease in vascular resistance accompanying upper extremity exercise, blood flow is shunted via the circle of Willis retrograde from the vertebral artery to the distal subclavian artery on the affected side. The consequent loss of blood flow to the cerebral circulation induces symptoms of cerebral ischemia. This syndrome is diagnosed by the findings of diminished brachial arterial pressure on the affected side, a bruit that is maximal over the supraclavicular area, and the induction of symptoms by exercise of the involved extremity.

The diagnostic procedures employed in the evaluation of the patient with suspected cerebrovascular syncope are summarized in Table 7. Evaluation of the

Table 7. Cerebrovascular Syncope—Diagnostic Evaluation

Ophthalmodynamometry
Doppler flow studies
Cervical spine, skull x-ray
Echocardiography (2–D)
Computed tomography
Electroencephalography
Cerebral angiography
Digital subtraction angiography

cerebral circulation is of paramount importance in the diagnosis of syncope resulting from cerebrovascular disease. Initially, noninvasive methods are performed. In select patients, additional studies such as electroencephalography and computed tomography (CT) may be indicated to better define functional and anatomic abnormalities that may underlie syncope of cerebrovascular origin. With patients in whom cerebral emboli are suspected, two-dimensional (2-D) echocardiography may be necessary to rule out an intracardiac source for such events. If noninvasive procedures prove inconclusive, cerebral angiography may be indicated to establish the severity of the disease and to identify whether surgical intervention is indicated. Digital subtraction angiography is a promising new diagnostic modality that will probably prove to be of great diagnostic value in patients with suspected cerebrovascular syncope.

Reflex Syncope

Under the classification of reflex syncope, primary consideration will be given to five clinical entities: (1) vasovagal syncope, (2) carotid sinus syncope, (3) cough syncope, (4) postmicturition syncope, and (5) glossopharyngeal neuralgia.

Vasovagal Syncope. Reflex suppression of atrial pacemaker activity or of atrioventricular conduction by the vagus plays a key role in several forms of syncope. In rare instances, syncope may occur in individuals without evidence of heart disease as a result of reflex cardiac asystole. The term "vasovagal syncope" is applied to such syncope in which the entire reflex arc is located within the vagal system. Syncope associated with distention of an esophageal diverticulum and pathologic lesions in the larynx and mediastinum has been explained on this basis. A similar mechanism for cardiac standstill arising from vagal reflex activity has been attributed to syncope following distention of the viscera, fainting associated with irritation of the pleura or peritoneum, the cardiac asystole associated with esophagoscopy or bronchoscopy, and the syncope associated with cardiospasm. Syncope that occurs early in the course of acute inferior myocardial infarction is usually vasovagal in origin; sinus node ischemia, acute left ventricular dysfunction, and decreased peripheral vascular resistance may also play a role in syncope associated with inferior infarction. Recurrent syncope of this type is often relieved or prevented by administration of anticholinergic agents (e.g., atropine sulfate) in adequate dosage.

Carotid Sinus Syncope. Massage or compression of the carotid sinus in normal persons is often attended by transient slowing of the heart rate and mild hypotension. In patients with carotid sinus syndrome, stimulation of the carotid sinus by pressure or massage can produce syncope of three kinds:

1. The cardioinhibitory type, manifested by profound bradycardia, sinus standstill, or atrioventricular block and prevented by atropine.
2. The vasodepressor type, manifested by a profound hypotensive response without bradycardia and blocked by epinephrine but not by atropine.
3. A central type, without bradycardia or hypotension, that is not influenced by atropine or epinephrine and is best classified as a form of *noncardiovascular syncope.*

Carotid sinus syncope is observed most commonly in elderly patients, many of whom have diffuse atherosclerosis or other organic heart disease. Such carotid hypersensitivity is observed far less frequently in patients of similar age without heart disease. These considerations have led to the impression that it is the associated cardiac disease and not age per se that predisposes to the problem of carotid sinus hyperirritability and syncope in the aged.

Carotid sinus syncope has been observed in patients with disease localized to the carotid sinus area, such as neoplasm and inflammatory masses in the neck. In patients with a hyperirritable carotid sinus reflex, symptoms of lightheadedness and impaired consciousness may be initiated by relatively minor stimulation of the carotid sinus and by head motion, shaving, or a tight collar.

Cough Syncope. In this kind of syncope (also called "tussive syncope"), loss of consciousness occurs following a paroxysm of vigorous coughing. This syndrome is particularly frequent among robust individuals with chronic bronchitis and a "hacking cough." Several factors may be implicated in the mechanism of cough syncope, including a sharp decrease in cardiac output, peripheral vasodilatation or bradycardia by reflex mechanisms, a marked increase in cerebrospinal fluid pressure, an increase in cerebral vascular resistance induced by the hypocapnia of coughing, and a "concussive" effect caused by the sudden rise in intracranial pressure.

Postmicturition Syncope. Micturition syncope—or, more properly, postmicturition syncope—is often seen in adult men with nocturia. During or immediately following voiding, there is a sudden loss of consciousness, often without premonitory symptoms. Many such persons give the history of drinking large quantities of alcoholic beverages before retiring. It has been suggested by some investigators that the loss of consciousness in these circumstances is related to a sudden reflex decrease in peripheral vascular resistance stimulated by the precipitous fall in intra-abdominal volume. Others have considered the loss of consciousness to be related to typical vasodepressor syncope accentuated by such factors as the Valsalva maneuver and the peripheral vasodilation associated with sleeping in a warm bed and recent alcohol consumption.

Glossopharyngeal Neuralgia. An unusual form of reflex syncope is that associated with glossopharyngeal neuralgia. The patient experiences a sudden loss of consciousness—the result of profound bradycardia and arterial hypotension—at the height of a paroxysm of pain.

With regard to reflex syncope, careful attention to the patient's history is critical to the diagnosis. The

Table 8. Combined Causes of Syncope

Arrhythmia
Volume depletion
Decreased peripheral resistance
Obstruction to cardiac output
Obstruction to cerebral flow

Table 9. Conditions Associated with Noncardiovascular Syncope

Hypoxia
Hypoglycemia
Hyperventilation
Convulsive disorders
Vertigo
Hysterical syncope
Syncopal migraine

circumstances in which the episode occurs and its recurrence when the procedure is repeated establish the diagnosis.

Combined Causes of Syncope

In many instances, particularly in the older age groups, several factors are responsible for syncope. Although each factor may be unable to produce syncope alone, a combination of precipitating factors depletes cerebral blood flow sufficiently to induce loss of consciousness (Table 8). Thus, the occurrence of a transient arrhythmia in a volume-depleted patient with obstructive cardiac disease who experiences sudden lowering of peripheral resistance following exercise may be associated with an episode of syncope. Each of these changes in circulatory dynamics alone may be unassociated with symptoms.

NONCARDIOVASCULAR SYNCOPE

The differential diagnosis of syncope and presyncope often includes a group of disorders wherein suddenly impaired consciousness is not primarily related to alterations in cardiac output, cardiac rhythm, or arterial pressure. These forms of syncope that we refer to as syncope of noncardiovascular (or noncirculatory) origin may be caused by primary disorders of cerebral function, profound alterations in cerebral metabolism, or psychologically induced behavioral mechanisms (Table 9).

Hypoxia

Fainting that results from hypoxia may be related primarily to the lack of oxygen or to an episode of vasodepressor syncope initiated during a period of oxygen lack. With cardiovascular disease, pulmonary insufficiency, and anemia, symptoms of hypoxia occur at lesser degrees of oxygen deprivation. The environmental setting in which impaired consciousness that is caused by hypoxia occurs usually leaves little difficulty in differentiating it from other forms of syncope.

Hypoglycemia

Severe hypoglycemia is associated with weakness, sweating, a sensation of hunger, confusion, and altered consciousness. The symptoms are unrelated to posture and usually respond promptly to food ingestion or intravenous glucose administration. Impaired consciousness in hypoglycemia is usually associated with sinus tachycardia and is rarely accompanied by hypotension.

Hyperventilation

In normal persons, anxiety is regularly accompanied by varying degrees of hyperventilation. In the hyperventilation syndrome, anxiety is associated with an inordinate degree of hyperventilation. The symptoms of hypocapnia dominate the clinical picture under these circumstances and may actually replace the anxiety as the major discomfort.

Early during the episode, the patient complains of smothering, a tightness in the chest, and a feeling of suffocation. Later, there appears confusion, a sense of unreality, bewilderment, and, in time, a feeling of panic. Associated with these symptoms may be numbness and paresthesia of the extremities and circumoral areas. The symptoms persist in the supine, sitting, or recumbent posture. The symptoms abate after the patient's anxiety is allayed and the hyperventilation ceases.

One may aid the resolution of symptoms of hypocapnia by having the patient rebreathe in a paper or plastic bag. It is notable that although consciousness is impaired, actual loss of consciousness usually does not occur. The heart rate during hyperventilation is frequently rapid, and although arterial pressure may decrease slightly, there is no profound hypotension.

Convulsive Disorder

The differentiation of the various forms of syncope of circulatory origin from the transitory loss of consciousness that occurs during a generalized convulsive seizure is often made on the basis of history alone. One form of epilepsy, i.e., the akinetic form of petit mal, does offer particular difficulty in differentiation. The finding of an abnormal electroencephalogram suggesting cerebral arrhythmia between episodes of unconsciousness is most helpful in this differentiation.

Vertigo

Though recurrent episodes of vertigo may first be described by the patient as a loss or impairment of consciousness, careful attention to the history will often reveal the nature of this symptom. In true vertigo there is a keen sense of movement, either of the environment or of the patient. Falling may be abrupt; it is due not to weakness of postural muscles but to loss of balance. Nausea, pallor, and cold perspiration may suggest vasodepressor syncope, but the lack of true loss or impairment of consciousness, the increased distress with head movement, and the associated nystagmoid movements of the eyes, together with the finding of a normal arterial pressure and pulse, will help differentiate the syndrome.

Hysterical Syncope

Hysterical syncope is of particular importance because it may mimic altered consciousness of an organic origin. Hysterical episodes occur most frequently in young adults, often with severe emotional illness and in the presence of an audience. The patient slumps gently, even gracefully, to the floor or in a convenient chair, typically without injury or awkwardness. The episode is of varying duration and may last for as long as an hour or more. Although the patient is unresponsive to verbal stimulation, there is often evidence that consciousness is not lost and there are no abnormalities in pulse, arterial pressure, or skin color.

Syncopal Migraine

Symptoms suggesting syncope are rarely if ever encountered in ordinary types of migraine. In rare instances in which the basal arterial system is involved (as opposed to the more usually affected carotid system), the premonitory aura of migraine terminates in a period of unconsciousness of several minutes' duration. When the patient awakens, there is severe headache, typically in the occipital area. The period of unconsciousness is associated with no apparent circulatory change.

It has been our experience that noncardiovascular syncope is diagnosed most effectively on the basis of a careful history. All too often, the patient with noncardiovascular syncope is subjected to extensive and costly laboratory testing without the benefit of a complete clinical examination.

SUMMARY

In this review we have attempted to include all the conditions known to produce or mimic syncope. In clinical practice, many of these are rare. In our experience the following are the most common causes of syncope: vasodepressor syncope (common faint), rhythm disturbances, orthostatic hypotension, and aortic stenosis. However, a combination of mechanisms leading to syncope may well be the most common etiology, and by its very nature, the most difficult to diagnose.

FATIGUE

By Michael J. Halberstam, M.D.*
Washington, D.C.

If you would like to know the epidemiology, differential diagnosis, and prognosis of fatigue as the presenting symptom in office practice, don't bother checking the standard medical literature. I have, and it's worthless. There is no more telling indictment of academic medicine and its separation from the real world of patient care than the articles listed under "Fatigue" in *Index Medicus.* Therein are listed for each year a host of articles on muscle physiology ("Aldolase activity during fatigue in isolated muscles of frog, *Rana hexadactyla*") and on clinical psychology ("Effect of fatigue and alcohol on observer perception"), but next to nothing on fatigue in clinical practice. During the years 1966 to 1978 not a single article appeared with any actual data on the outcome of tired patients. This article attempts to remedy this lack.

Fatigue is one of the most common presenting symptoms in a clinician's office. Variants of "I just don't seem to have any energy," "I'm tired all the time," and "I don't seem to be able to get out of bed" are extremely common as the spontaneously expressed chief complaint. Furthermore, many patients who present with symptoms ostensibly related to another system ("I think I have the flu") quickly sort themselves into the category of fatigue. (The "flu" turns out to be of 6 months' duration and characterized not by cough or fever, but by loss of energy.)

In an attempt to quantify the picture of fatigue in the office practice of internal medicine, I kept a running score sheet of new patients over a 2-month period. In addition, I asked two internist colleagues of mine, with separate practices and with different patient populations, to keep track of patients presenting with fatigue. They (and others) were asked to recall cases in which unexplained fatigue was eventually linked to organic disease.

From this study (which is continuing), certain facts emerged that should come as no surprise to the primary care physician, but that should be helpful in formulating a systematic approach to fatigue.

AN APPROACH TO DIAGNOSIS

1. In office practice, fatigue as the sole or major presenting symptom is overwhelmingly due to psychologic disarray, usually depression.
2. The history will indicate the correct diagnosis in over 90 per cent of the patients.
3. When the history is equivocal, the basic laboratory tests will establish the diagnosis in all but a handful of the remaining patients.
4. Despite the massive predominance of psychologic factors as the cause of primary fatigue, occasional cases are caused by unsuspected organic illness. Some of the more common of these rarities are discussed below.

Primary Causes. The clinician's empiric observation that most primary fatigue is caused by depression was borne out in my office study. Of 38 patients presenting with fatigue and its variants, only one had organic disease. My practice is an urban one, canted toward young-to-middle-aged patients, about 60:40 white and black, and predominantly middle class with a smaller proportion of blue-collar workers. There are no active farmers, ranchers, or factory workers in the patient population. The practices of my two col-

*Deceased.

leagues vary somewhat from mine in patient age and social background, but not in occupation. While figures are not available from their practices, their observations support the notion that depression is by far the commonest cause of fatigue. Simple overwork as a cause of fatigue is rare in my experience—most people enjoy hard work and recognize the physiologic fatigue that accompanies it. It is the man who is underworked and bored who is more likely to bring his fatigue to a doctor's attention.

Importance of the History. The history usually makes the diagnosis. When "lack of energy" is the chief complaint, when it has been present over a month, when it is unaccompanied by weight loss, documented fever (not "I feel like I've got a low-grade temperature"), when there has been no persistent localized pain, when there has been no other dramatic change in the systems review, psychologic factors are almost surely the cause. Look for a recent loss or separation in the patient's life.

It is crucial in history-taking to make sure that you and the patient are talking about the same thing. In particular, the patient should be questioned specifically about whether "tiredness" means generalized fatigue or localized muscle aching. The other crucial distinction is between fatigue and shortness of breath. Of course, some patients with severe cardiorespiratory disease complain primarily of "breathlessness." This is often the equivalent of dyspnea at rest. Genuine fatigue of over a month's duration without any other evidence of systemic illness is rarely caused by organic disease. There are, however, instances in which the history can keep one pointed in the direction of somatic illness. These will be discussed.

Role of Laboratory Testing. While the history may strongly suggest depression and while the physical examination may be, and usually is, unrevealing, the patient presenting with persistent fatigue deserves an appropriate laboratory work-up. Anemia, hypocalcemia, hypokalemia, uremia, and hypothyroidism in their earlier or less severe forms may all be apparent on laboratory tests and not on physical examination. I have seen experienced clinicians examine a patient with a hematocrit of 30 ml/dl and fail to detect any physical evidence of anemia. I've done so myself, particularly with Blacks and Orientals. Renal failure can creep up insidiously with no localizing signs or symptoms until a creatinine of 3.0 is detected on a "routine" scan. Significant adult-onset diabetes (not merely a 2-hour after-meal glucose of 160, but 300 or 350) can present without polyuria, polydipsia, or weight loss. Besides a urinalysis, a chest x-ray can be unexpectedly helpful. Hodgkin's disease, sarcoid, and malignancies may all shout their presence from a chest x-ray in the total absence of any pulmonary symptoms.

These tests—complete blood count with sedimentation rate, sequential multiple analysis (SMA), electrolytes, urine, x-ray—are the basic minimum in laboratory testing for chronic, global fatigue. The cost-cutters and Medicare, indeed, may even quibble about the morality of doing electrolyte testing on a 24-year-old woman who has been tired for 2 years. They are correct in believing that it is unlikely that the test will be abnormal, but you are correct in ordering it. Anyone who has been tired for 2 years deserves a work-up for what is unlikely as well as for what is likely.

Further laboratory testing depends on the case, and particularly on the physician's intuition about whether the basic cause is somatic or psychologic (for the purposes of this discussion I will accept a total separation of the two, acknowledging that they are inseparable). Physician intuition is nothing mystical but rather a computer-like summation of past personal experience, the medical literature, and clues provided by the patient.

When the Cause Is Organic. Time after time I have seen interns and residents label patients as "crocks" because the patients did not arrive displaying gross manifestations of their disease. After all, hospitalized patients usually *do* present far-advanced evidence of illness or they would be treated or diagnosed on the outside. Confronted with a patient complaining of persistent fatigue (or persistent pain or persistent dizzy spells) and with no other abnormalities, the house officer and the inexperienced practitioner is likely to offer up a psychologic etiology and go on to "sicker" patients. There is no more grievous error. As foolish as it is to persist in laboratory testing on a patient with endogenous depression, it is worse to miss the only curable case of Addison's disease you are ever going to see. There are ways to minimize this risk.

Neurosis and depression rarely strike suddenly in middle age. Most of the time, but not always, there is a long history of hypochondriasis or of mild depression, the kind that brings 27-year-old lawyers into your office when they haven't been able to find the right sort of mate or the proper kind of job. But when a 45-year-old woman walks into your office complaining of recent onset of fatigue and has no past history and no present evidence of depression, watch out! Do not make the House Officer's Mistake—do not diagnose psychologic disease just because there is no immediate evidence of somatic disease. Depression is *not* a diagnosis of exclusion. In addition to fatigue, there are other confirmatory physical sensations that accompany it, and, most convincingly, the patient usually has psychologic evidence of depression. The depressed patient who presents to a family practitioner or internist (as opposed to a psychiatrist) may not immediately announce, "I'm depressed," but will on questioning say "My job is just a job—I don't enjoy it any more" or "I don't know . . . it seems that my wife and I hardly talk any more."

The fatigued patient who steadfastly denies any problem besides fatigue and whose lifestyle data support this statistically deserves an extra-hard search for organic illness. (Be suspicious of the recently separated parent who says he or she feels "just great except I can't get out of bed in the morning.") If the blood tests were all normal 4 weeks ago and the patient still feels bad, repeat the tests. If everything is normal and the only symptom is a mild queasiness in the abdomen, don't forget about the early abdominal nodes in lymphoma. Thyroiditis can have absolutely no specific signs and symptoms; the only early clue may be an elevated sedimentation rate. If all the initial laboratory work is normal except for a white blood cell count of 6900 per cu mm with 85 per cent polys, it is not all normal. Something is going on. Find a toehold somewhere from which you can advance the diagnostic work-up. That vacation trip may have provided your patient with a low-grade infestation of Giardia and the intestinal symptoms may have long since been masked by a slight, generalized, persistent malaise. The elevated mean corpuscular volume (MCV) may be the only evidence that your patient has been less than candid in giving you his drinking history. Remember that rheumatoid arthritis and, indeed, most of the autoimmune diseases can have as their harbinger only a sudden, profound fatigue. Look for abnormalities of the globulins and don't be afraid to order a fluorescent antinuclear antibody test (FANA) in the absence of flagrant lupus. It is axiomatic that any medicine the patient is taking may be causing fatigue; "elimination pharmacology" is a logical first step.

In my own experience and that of my colleagues, infectious disease is rare today as the cause of primary fatigue, although low-grade Salmonella infections can sometimes be overlooked, particularly in the elderly. The major disease seen today that presents as fatigue and fatigue alone is malignancy, particularly lymphoma. Here is an example in which the low-grade fever so typical of hypochondria ("My temperature got up to 99.2, but that's high for me. I usually run 97") may in fact be another early manifestation of tumor. Not every patient with persistent fatigue should or can have every laboratory test, and certainly few need to be hospitalized for a diagnostic work-up. Yet, if the clinical context suggests organic disease, if there is no positive evidence of depression, and if the clinician's suspicions remain strong enough, all the technology of modern medicine may be brought to bear on the problem. The third-party payers and the house officers may grumble, but the physician's job is to make the diagnosis in the hard cases as well as the easy ones. If one remembers that every disease must have its first symptoms and that the first symptom may be very vague and very mild, fewer large mistakes will be made. Symptoms are the early warning signal of disease. They will almost always appear before the physical examination becomes abnormal and often before laboratory results are out of line. A convincing history for organic disease is as significant as a hematocrit of 32, and needs to be studied just as thoughtfully.

PAIN IN THE EXTREMITIES AND BACK

By James T. Cassidy, M.D.
Ann Arbor, Michigan

HISTORY

Since pain is subjective, a sensation of discomfort, it is crucial that the physician determine precisely what a patient means by a complaint of pain and its exact location. In general, the history is indispensable for categorizing the origin of the patient's complaint, be it musculoskeletal, vascular, or neural. The physical examination aids the diagnostician in being more precise, or it may suggest a disorder that otherwise might have been overlooked. Laboratory studies are helpful in delineating the systemic extent of a disorder or, if uniformly negative, in corroborating a diagnosis of nonorganic pain.

The pain described by the patient should be placed in the context of other problems that have been experienced and of the past medical history. The occurrence of constitutional symptoms, such as fatigue, malaise, or weight loss, raises the suspicion of systemic disease. Fever and chills are characteristic of an acute illness. A recent history of trauma suggests a variety of possibilities of direct injury to a structure that results in pain. A past history of other disease, particularly malignancy, or of familial disorders, such as diabetes mellitus, may be important in explaining the recent onset of pain in a patient. In this regard, a family history of ankylosing spondylitis, psoriasis, or inflammatory bowel disease may point directly to a likely cause of arthritis or back pain.

The manner in which a patient describes pain is often revealing of cause. Bizarre descriptions are suggestive of psychologic disorders. Organic pain is usually well localized by the patient and follows a classic distribution for each disease. Pain that is everywhere or nonanatomic in its distribution or radiation is often more easily attributed to psychologic disturbance than to identifiable organic causes.

Neurogenic pain is often described as burning, or shooting; a paresthetic component is common. Vascular pain is often acute in onset, severe, and throbbing. It may be exacerbated or relieved by rest, depending upon its etiology. Pain arising from lesions of bone may be of any degree of severity and may be particularly difficult for a patient to describe. Bone pain is often worse at night or may be exacerbated by lying down. Muscular and joint pain is often described as aching and is frequently associated with stiffness. It is generally well localized to the site of the problem.

TYPES OF PAIN

Pain will be considered in three categories: that which is referred, that which arises from local causes, and that which reflects systemic disease.

Referred Pain

Pain may be well localized, but the site of localization may not correspond to the area of the primary lesion. The two predominant sources of referred pain are the thoracic and abdominal cavities. Pain referred to the left pectoral area, the shoulder, and the distribution of the ulnar nerve in the upper extremity may have its origin in the cardiovascular system and may represent ischemic heart disease or aortic aneurysm, or it may arise in the mediastinum and surrounding thoracic cage. Anginal pain is described characteristically as substernal crushing discomfort brought on by exertion and relieved by rest. It radiates often to the shoulder and the ulnar distribution in the arm. The deltoid area is often spared in this type of referred pain.

Pain referred from the abdominal cavity is related often to diaphragmatic irritation. When it involves the right shoulder, it may represent subphrenic abscess or hepatic disease. Acute cholelithiasis causes right shoulder pain that radiates also to the inferior border of the right scapula. Left shoulder and arm pain may represent an injured spleen, hemoperitoneum, pancreatitis, or gastric disease. A hiatus hernia can duplicate the pain of angina pectoris but is also associated with complaints of peptic distress.

Pain referred to the lower extremities from intra-abdominal disease is much less frequent. However, the pain of appendicitis may radiate along the iliopsoas muscle into the thigh. Abdominal aneurysm, nephrolithiasis, and diseases of the rectum, uterus, bladder, and prostate may be the origin of referred pain to the hip, groin, or knee. Occasionally, dysmenorrhea is associated with radiation of pain to the lower extremity.

Local Causes of Pain

Intrinsic. Any form of *superficial trauma* to an extremity, such as a contusion or burn, will result in inflammation and pain. Pain in an extremity that results from local causes is usually felt at the site of the injury. However, disease of the hip may be perceived by the patient as pain in the knee, and disease in the knee may cause pain in the foot. Therefore, a careful, systematic history related to contiguous joint structures should always be taken.

Superficial disorders of the skin and soft tissue are usually readily apparent. Contact dermatitis, eczema, cellulitis, paronychia, and infections such as maduromycosis and erysipelas may be encountered. *Idiopathic, nonsuppurative panniculitis* may be limited to the extremities. *Adiposis dolorosa* is a curious disorder in which subcutaneous lipomas are painful. Acute pain from *plantar warts* or from a *hard corn* over a metatarsal head should be differentiated from pain arising from disorders such as a neuroma. *Calluses and bunions* may be painful over points of contact in the feet.

Forms of *acute trauma to the skin* such as chilblain, frostbite, immersion foot, and trench foot are accompanied by the pain of ischemia and nerve involvement and may progress to gangrene. In the child these may lead eventually to maldevelopment of the extremity and bones. Pain arising from regional lymph nodes involved by tumor or infection is localized to the area of the nodes and is accompanied by tenderness or fluctuance.

Sprains, fractures, and dislocations are usually self-evident. Fractures of the os calcis, the navicular bone, or the metatarsal bones (march or fatigue fractures) may cause pain on walking, and their subtle roentgenographic signs can be easily overlooked during the immediate post-traumatic period. Periosteal hematomas following an injury may be responsible for many weeks of gradually subsiding pain and tenderness over the affected area. Certain traumatic causes of pain may be forgotten by the patient. An acromioclavicular separation or rotator cuff tear may present as a diagnostic problem of pain in the shoulder on movement. This type of pain may be referred to the mid–upper arm. In the knee, a torn semilunar cartilage or ruptured collateral ligament may masquerade as a monarthritis.

Fibrositis is a disorder of the superficial tissues that causes stiffness, aching, and ease of fatigue. Painful subcutaneous or fascial nodules can occasionally accompany this disease. Some of these nodules may represent herniation of fat through fascial orifices. *Nonarticular rheumatism* is an allied disorder that does not respond generally to salicylates and is made worse by sudden changes in temperature or by air conditioning. A *Dupuytren contracture* is characterized by progressive fibrosis of the soft tissue of the palm and flexor side of the fingers.

A *localized myositis* may be an unusual accompaniment of a rheumatic disease. *Tenosynovitis* is a more frequent inflammatory manifestation of a connective tissue disease or may result from repeated trauma in certain occupations such as typing or piano playing. Sudden *tendon rupture* may occur in the clinical setting of a tenosynovitis or from nodule formation within the tendons in rheumatoid arthritis. Acute localized pain and disability may accompany rupture of major tendons such as the biceps, the Achilles, or the plantaris after prolonged or forceful exertion. Localized tenosynovitis may be one of the causes of painful heel pads and plantar spurs. *Calcific tendinitis* may occur as a dystrophic disorder or be part of the pseudogout syndrome. Ligaments may also undergo calcification. *Pellegrini-Stieda disease* is an example of calcification in the medial collateral ligament of the knee. *Metatarsalgia* may be part of generalized osteoarthritis, or it may result from localized weakening of the supporting tissues of the feet. Pain in this disorder often radiates up the anterior surface of the foot and shin. Flexible flat feet are not associated with pain; symptoms occur only when the feet are rigid.

Other afflictions of the musculoskeletal system are somewhat less well defined. The *restless leg syndrome* may occur alone, it may be related to psychologic stress, or it may be accompanied by nocturnal leg cramps of metabolic or atherosclerotic origin. *Growing pains of childhood* appear to be associated with overuse of muscles. They are to be distinguished from the leg discomfort of rheumatic fever that is associated with tenosynovitis and is most prominent behind the knee in the hamstring tendons. *Writer's cramp* is a response to long periods of use of fine muscles. In contrast, prolonged immobilization of an extremity may be followed by use or causalgic pain.

Some of the most acutely painful disorders are associated with diseases of blood vessels or nerves. Pain that extends along an extremity and crosses over joints and muscle groups or is confined only to the distal part may be related to a vascular or neurologic lesion. *Ischemia* resulting from arterial thrombosis or embolism has a sudden onset. It is quite often described as throbbing or is noted to be synchronous with the pulse. Ischemia may also cause paroxysms of severe neuritic pain. Occasionally the pain is tardy in appearance and then gradually increases with the passage of time. It may be accompanied by marked pallor in the affected part and other evidence of generalized arterial disease, such as atherosclerosis, or of valvular heart disease in the case of embolism. The pain is distal to the site of the lesion, and objective evidence of arterial disease at the initiating locus may be lacking. Relief of symptoms with dependency of the extremities suggests arterial ischemia.

Intermittent claudication is characterized by cramping pain in the muscles of the lower extremities brought on by exercise. There is latency of onset, and the pain subsides after a short rest. *Atherosclerosis of the iliac vessels* cause pain not only in the legs but also in the hips and buttocks. This pain is brought on by walking and is relieved by rest. It is not related to bending and lifting. Diseases such as *thromboangiitis obliterans* should be thought of in a young man who is a smoker and, in an older man, *arteriosclerosis obliterans* should be considered. These diseases are bilateral in most cases but may start unilaterally. Each may, in turn, be associated with trophic changes or gangrene of the digits. Certain other symptom complexes are related to arteriosclerotic disease. In the *Leriche syndrome,* ischemic pain is localized to the buttocks, thigh, and calf, and it is associated with impotence in the male. *Shin splints* are a unique type of ischemic pain in the anterior tibial compartments accompanied occasionally by actual muscle necrosis. They are brought on by extreme overactivity and are most common in the young and untrained runners.

Aneurysms of peripheral vessels are not common but may be seen in certain locations such as the popliteal space. They are often traumatic in origin. *Raynaud disease or phenomenon* occurs most frequently in the upper extremities and is caused by disturbances of sympathetic tone or generalized vascular diseases, as in scleroderma. Each acute episode is precipitated by cold or emotional conflict. The fingers undergo a series of color changes associated with initial numbness and later with frank pain that is usually mild but can be intense. *Acrocyanosis,* although it has many of the same characteristics, is more chronic and often not associated with an important element of discomfort.

Thrombophlebitis causes pain and tenderness at the site of venous inflammation, with relief following elevation of the extremity. Pain or resistance to movement in milder cases may be elicited in a calf muscle by dorsiflexion of the foot. The pain of venous thrombosis is usually mild to moderate and is seldom severe. It is constant in character and is made worse by activity or standing. *Postphlebitic syndromes* of chronic venous obstruction may follow repeated episodes of disease and are characterized by aching, edema, and tiredness in the legs after long periods of dependency. Recurrent, superficial thrombophlebitis may be associated with occult malignancy. Deep varicosities or superficial venules may rupture in otherwise normal individuals and cause sudden stinging pain at the site of extravasation. Painful *disorders of the lymphatics* are less common and occur predominantly with infections. Lymphangitis may result in symptoms of inflammation and, if chronic, cause elephantiasis of the extremity.

The association of pain in the extremities or back with *neuropathy* is worthy of emphasis. Pain, numbness, or dysesthesia in the innervation of a superficial nerve results from localized pressure in the entrapment syndromes. Symptoms of pain and tenderness of the involved nerve trunk are often present proximal to the point of entrapment, a situation that may cause confusion if not appreciated. The most common example is the *carpal tunnel syndrome* in the upper extremity. The patient experiences pain, numbness, tingling, and paresthesia in the distribution of the median nerve that are often worse at night. These symptoms may be referred to the elbow in *acroparesthesia* or the *pronator syndrome.* The carpal tunnel syndrome may be caused by a fracture of the wrist or repeated trauma, or it may be associated with systemic diseases such as multiple myeloma, rheumatoid arthritis, hypothyroidism, diabetes, or cirrhosis of the liver. It may also occur transiently in pregnancy. *Meralgia paresthetica,* pain and hypesthesia in the anterolateral aspect of the thigh, is the result of entrapment of the lateral femoral cutaneous nerve as it passes through the attachment of the inguinal ligament.

Pressure on a nerve by a tumor may cause paresthesia and loss of sensation or excruciating pain that is often described as burning or stabbing. Objective documentation of muscular weakness and atrophy will follow the innervation pattern of the affected nerve. *Neurofibroma* or *hereditary neurofibromatosis* may result in a variety of syndromes, depending on the area of involvement. Plantar digital neuroma or the Morton toe may mimic metatarsalgia or vascular disease of the foot. The patient should be able to pinpoint the source of pain between the toes.

Sudeck atrophy is a post-traumatic osteoporosis that follows nerve injuries. *Causalgia* is a type of severe pain that may be related to post-traumatic vasomotor disturbances, or it may be secondary to coronary artery disease. The resting pain of the *shoulder-hand syndrome* is a dramatic example of this type of disorder and is unresponsive to the usual analgesic or anti-inflammatory measures. The most frequent involvement in the lower extremities is in the sciatic distribution. Other types of post-traumatic disorders are usually not accompanied by pain in their chronic stages. A *Volkmann contracture* is the classic situation in the upper extremity.

Localized joint pain is an important cause of a painful extremity. Characteristically the pain of joint disease will be exacerbated by movement of the specific joint. *Monarthritis* may be present at one phase in the development of a systemic disease such as rheumatoid arthritis, or it may be related to a traumatic or congenital abnormality. Some of the anomalies of the hip joint are illustrative of congenital or acquired disorders that result in localized joint pain. These are *coxa vara, slipped capital femoral epiphysis,* and *protrusio acetabuli.* Each occurs at a characteristic age and is accompanied initially by pain, weakness, or stiffness of the leg and a limp and later by restriction of movement. Hip disease is associated with pain localized to the anterior or medial thigh and does not cause isolated pain in the buttock.

Osteonecrosis with or without trauma may play a

role in coxa plana and the various forms of *osteochondritis dissecans.* The latter affects most commonly the knee, ankle, hip, elbow, and shoulder. Symptoms result from the loose body present within the joint and include pain, weakness, catching, or locking. *Fibrous dysplasia of bone* may lead to an abnormal shape or configuration of an extremity or may be symptomatic with repeated stress. *Hereditary multiple exostoses* are not usually a cause of pain but may be if the disorder results in abnormal forces upon muscle attachments or in secondary osteoarthritis.

Acute momentary pain over a joint, brought on by stress, may result from *rupture of the synovial membrane.* Inflammatory disease invariably precedes such an occurrence. Ectasia may result, and dissection into contiguous facial planes may cause swelling and discomfort. A *Baker cyst* starts in the popliteal space and dissects into the calf. Similar disorders occur in the antecubital fossa or at the shoulder. Localized forms of synovial disease such as a *ganglion* are often tender on direct pressure or stress or in the extreme ranges of joint movement.

Bursitis may be related to trauma or to systemic diseases such as gout or rheumatoid arthritis. Pain is caused by any movement of the extremity and radiates distally. Redness and warmth of the overlying tissues are usually present along with extreme tenderness. The most common bursae that are affected are the subacromial, olecranon, prepatellar, and posterior calcaneal. Subacute symptoms are associated more commonly with the superficial trochanteric, ileopectineal, and ischiogluteal bursae. Bursitis may be difficult to distinguish on history from the periarthritis that often accompanies it. In periarthritis there is subacute inflammation of the surrounding tissues, ligaments, and muscles. The shoulder is the most common site of involvement. Onset is often insidious, and pain is associated intially with the extreme ranges of motion, particularly abduction and elevation. Aching occurs at night, and there is persistent morning stiffness. More advanced disease results in continuous aching and diffuse tenderness.

Bone pain is usually well localized to an area of the back or extremity but may be referred to a contiguous joint if the cause of the pain involves the end of a long bone. Pain arising from bone is often described by the patient as throbbing. There is usually nocturnal aggravation, and the pain is accentuated by pressure over the area of involvement. Discomfort may result from periosteal hemorrhage, as in scurvy, hemophilia, or trauma, or it may be associated with periostitis secondary to tumor and infection. The pain of *Paget's disease* is related in part to structural changes of the bone and in part to inflammation. At first the pain may come on only with use of a lower extremity. *Osteosarcoma* may arise in areas of pagetic bone or may occur as a solitary lesion. Pain in osteosarcoma is localized to the site of the lesion and has the characteristics of bone pain. Spontaneous fractures occur in areas of neoplastic involvement. *Osteomyelitis* may arise as an acute hematogenous disease in the long bones of children or may be secondary to trauma. A *solitary bone cyst* may mimic a tumor and be symptomatic through a fracture or deformity. *Idiopathic migratory osteoporosis* is an unusual bone disease of unknown cause that produces acute pain in and around a joint.

Extrinsic. Extremity pain, numbness, paresthesia, and weakness may arise from pressure on a nerve or vessel before they enter the extremity. A *cervical rib* may result in pain in the upper limb from radicular compression of the brachial plexus and subclavian vessels. Ulceration and gangrene may develop if vascular obstruction is severe.

A *ruptured intervertebral disc* may occur in either the cervical or lumbar spine. Prodromal symptoms include pain and stiffness in the neck with eventual radiation into the arm or pain in the back on movement with subsequent sciatica. Distal pain may be of two types: a deep, vague referred pain, and pain of brief duration from pressure of a herniated nucleus pulposus on nerve roots that is superficial, sharp, shooting, and associated with numbness and paresthesias.

Pain along the base of the neck radiating to both shoulders may indicate a lesion affecting the C_{3-4} nerve roots of the cervical spine. Circumferential pain in the chest or abdomen is generally associated with a lesion of the thoracic spine and pain that extends down the leg from the buttocks is related to a lower lesion. The symptom complex of sciatica is the most common and results in pain or paresthesia of the lower extremity. Symptoms are exaggerated by coughing or sneezing. If the sacral segments are involved, the pain is in the calf, and the Achilles reflex is decreased or absent. If the lumbar nerve roots are involved, the pain is localized to the quadriceps muscle. Pain in the distribution of the sciatic nerve may be caused by tumors of the spinal canal. This pain often occurs at night or during rest and will be relieved by activity. Sciatic pain may also be related to the neuritis or neuropathy of metabolic diseases such as diabetes mellitus. Pressure on the cervical cord by a herniated nucleus pulposus or tumor may also produce pain in both lower extremities that tends to be deep and aching but may be burning.

Pain in the extremities may arise secondary to *structural abnormalities of the lower lumbosacral spine.* Asymmetry of the posterior articulating facets, sacralization of the fifth lumbar vertebra, or spondylolysis may be asymptomatic or may cause pain in the back and buttocks and radiating pain into the legs. Such a disorder may be difficult to distinguish from that related to disc disease. *Syringomyelia, hematomyelia,* and *central cord tumors* are rare causes of distal pain. *Tumors of the cauda equina* are associated with pain, paresthesia, and motor disturbances of the lower extremities. A similar disorder may be one of the complications of *ankylosing spondylitis. Hypertrophic pachymeningitis,* a *fracture dislocation of a vertebral body,* or a *calcified ligamentum flavum* may cause pain or paralysis, depending upon the area of the cord that is involved. *Infection of a vertebra or intervertebral disc* results in similar acute complaints accompanied by fever and other constitutional symptoms.

Certain *hernias,* such as those occurring in the obturator or femoral canals, result in pain radiating into the lower extremity. Pressure in the sciatic notch or the pyriformis syndrome may mimic the symptoms of degenerative joint disease.

Pain Associated with Systemic Disease

Systemic disease is a common cause of extremity pain. A symmetric distribution should suggest systemic disease, whereas trauma would be more characteristically associated with pain that is asymmetric. *Polyarteritis* causes cramps characteristic of ischemia, aching of inflamed muscle, or neuropathy with paresthesia from involvement of the vasa nervorum. A clinical triad in the middle-aged male with polyarteritis consists of hypertension, abdominal pain, and paresthesia of the lower extremities.

The patient with *polymyalgia rheumatica* is usually elderly, and the pain is characterized as a moderately severe aching in the trunk and girdle musculature. It seldom, if ever, involves only the distal extremities and is not a cause of weakness. The site of the discomfort tends to be slowly migrating. Polymyalgia rheumatica may be associated with a giant cell arteritis and lead to ischemia of the ophthalmic artery. Headache, scalp tenderness, and claudication are suggestive of the latter disorder. The erythrocyte sedimentation rate (ESR) is markedly elevated in these conditions.

Osteonecrosis occurs in alcoholism or steroid therapy or may be associated with vasculitis. If it involves the femoral head, the patient will have pain early in the course of the disease along the inner aspect of the thigh on weight bearing. Intense pain of acute onset associated with cyanosis may be the first symptom of embolism in an extremity. *Caisson disease,* although it involves predominantly the viscera and central nervous system (CNS), may also be accompanied by plantar neuralgia. Specific types of *poisoning,* such as ergotism, may cause digital ischemia. *Bacterial endocarditis* may be accompanied by arthralgia or, less commonly, arthritis and is often associated with peripheral evidence of embolization.

Pulmonary or pleural disease, particularly when apical, results in pain in the extremities that is either referred or related to direct involvement of a nerve or vessel. The *Pancoast tumor* causes arm pain by compression or invasion of the brachial plexus. Other evidence of malignancy is often present. An unusual and sometimes dramatic cause of extremity pain is *hypertrophic pulmonary osteoarthropathy* secondary to bronchogenic tumor or metastatic pulmonary disease, chronic suppuration, or endocrine abnormalities. Quite often, the bone pain in osteoarthropathy is so severe that the patient will not move the extremities or allow anyone to touch them. Periosteal tenderness along the shafts of the bone is characteristic. Clubbing of the digits is sometimes present in this disorder, or it may arise from other causes such as congenital heart disease. It is usually asymptomatic in the latter condition.

Back pain may be caused by *penetrating peptic ulcers, pancreatic lesions,* or *renal disease.* The site of the pain is often localized in an area specific for the disease, generally does not radiate, is not made worse by motion of the back, and is almost always accompanied by other suggestive manifestations of the disorder. Specific kidney pain is felt in the flank or costovertebral angle, whereas pancreatic or peptic ulcer disease is localized to the midback. *Esophageal disorders* may be felt in the midthoracic area by the patient. *Disease of the prostate or uterus* can cause low back pain. Any type of metastatic disease to the spine or multiple myeloma will result in bone pain, quite often made worse by lying down. *Aneurysms of the aorta* may cause a boring excruciating pain in the back and distal symptoms and signs of vascular insufficiency.

Renal disease seldom causes extremity pain per se. An exception is uremia, in which pain is often of muscular or neurogenic origin and may be accompanied by tetany. The various other causes of tetany with tingling, numbness, or stiffness in the extremities need to be considered in the differential diagnosis. Hypocalcemia from malabsorption or hypoparathyroidism is frequently implicated.

There are other endocrine and metabolic abnormalities that may be responsible for extremity pain. Neuropathy or ischemia leading to gangrene is seen in advanced diabetes mellitus. The first sign of a metabolic bone disease such as *osteitis fibrosa cystica* may be pain on weight bearing in the lower extremities. Metabolic bone pain is often localized to the back from progressive compression fractures of the vertebral bodies. *Acromegaly* may cause pain in muscles, bones, or joints, and it leads to accelerated osteoarthritis. This disorder and *hypothyroidism* may be accompanied by generalized aching as an early symptom. Less frequently, patients with *hyperthyroidism* may have similar complaints. *Primary adrenal insufficiency,* or Addison disease, also causes pain, aching, and stiffness in the muscles. The *steroid-withdrawal syndrome* is a type of pseudorheumatism that is accompanied by similar complaints of pain and stiffness and often by systemic features such as fever.

Any disorder involving the sensory areas of the central nervous system may result in dysesthesia or pain. The patient may not be able to localize the pain precisely with a CNS lesion. *Cerebral tumor, vascular accident,* or *multiple sclerosis* should be considered. The patient may also be aware of other unpleasant sensations and yet have difficulty defining them precisely. Extremity pain may be part of the aura of *epilepsy* or *migraine. Phantom limb* is a curious disorder in which the patient feels extremity pain after amputation as if the extremity were still present. In some cases this type of pain is associated with a traumatic neuroma in the stump. *Tabes dorsalis* may cause lancinating pain in the legs. There may also be insensibility to pain in syphilis, as in Charcot arthropathy. Patients with *Parkinson's disease* often complain of stiffness and awkwardness more than actual pain and discomfort. *Transverse myelitis, amyotrophic lateral sclerosis,* and *progressive muscular atrophy* are accompanied by extremity pain that corresponds to the level of involvement of the cord.

Peripheral neuropathy is generally bilateral when associated with systemic disease. The irritative sensory phenomena begin in a stocking-or-glove distribution and then spread proximally. Symptoms may be mild, consisting of numbness or tingling, or they may be severe with constant burning pain. They may also be interpreted by the patient as muscle tenderness. Toxic polyneuropathy is related occasionally to alcoholism or to heavy metal intoxication. *Pink disease,* or acrodynia, is seen in infants and is associated with discoloration of the hands and feet, gastrointestinal complaints, pain in the joints and digits, and muscular weakness.

Porphyria and other rare genetically determined disorders, such as *Refsum's disease,* are accompanied by severe forms of neuropathy. Paralysis and abnormal porphyrin excretion in the former disease and ataxia in the latter should alert the clinician to these possibilities.

Acute infectious polyneuritis or radiculitis may be associated with a variety of organisms. In herpes zoster, intense, superficial pain in a dermatome distribution precedes the onset of vesiculation. It may mimic angina if in the distribution of C_8 to T_1 on the left. Paralysis or sensory dysfunction is seen after trauma to a nerve. *Axillary paralysis,* or the *Saturday night syndrome,* is a classic example of this type of disorder. *Hysteria* or *hyperventilation* should be considered in any seemingly neurogenic disorder of the extremities that is not otherwise explained. The latter is characterized by tingling in the hands and face associated with sighing respirations and anxiety. It may represent a psychoneurotic manifestation, or be the first sign of a serious occult disorder such as coronary artery disease.

Myalgias are commonly seen in association with connective tissue diseases, with acute viral infections, or after exercise. Painful cramping of muscles may occur with metabolic or electrolyte disturbances such as *hypokalemia, hypocalcemia, hypomagnesemia,* and *hyponatremia.* A rare cause of progressive rigidity of muscles with episodes of severe, sustained muscle spasm is the *stiff-man syndrome.*

Cramping in the muscles may be an early symptom of *muscular dystrophy, dystrophica myotonia, myotonia congenita, paroxysmal myoglobinuria, rhabdomyolysis,* and the *McArdle syndrome* or another hereditary enzyme deficiency in muscle. Night cramps in the calves may be idiopathic or the result of overactivity, or they may be related to metabolic disturbances such as hyponatremia or imbalances in calcium or magnesium. *Polymyositis* and *dermatomyositis* are inflammatory diseases of muscle that may be associated in the adult with underlying malignancy. The aching pain, tenderness, and weakness in these syndromes affect primarily the proximal musculature of the extremities and the girdle areas.

Nutritional deficiencies such as beriberi, pellagra, pyridoxine deficiency, and pernicious anemia may cause neurogenic pain in the extremities. The extremity pain associated with scurvy is caused by subperiosteal hemorrhages. Microfractures of bone may be symptomatic in osteomalacia. An excess of vitamin A may also cause extremity pain.

Systemic infections may result in pain of varying severity in the extremities. *Dengue fever* and *coccidioidomycosis* are characterized by extreme degrees of musculoskeletal pain in some patients; dengue fever is often referred to as "break-bone fever" and coccidioidomycosis as "valley rheumatism." Painful periosteal nodules or abscesses may be seen in *typhoid fever. Influenza* causes a well-known syndrome of muscular pain and stiffness. Acute muscular pain precedes the onset of paralysis in *poliomyelitis. Diphtheria* causes a toxic neuritis and paralysis. *Granulomatous reactions* of known or unknown cause, such as those of tuberculosis, syphilis, leprosy, and sarcoid, may be symptomatic when they involve muscles or nerves of the extremities. The subcutaneous nodules of *erythema nodosum* are painful and tender and may occur alone or in association with an acute arthritis, often located predominantly in the ankle. The acute muscular pain and tenderness of *trichinosis* is often preceded by a history of gastrointestinal distress and is accompanied by constitutional and systemic symptoms. *Toxoplasmosis* is a parasitic infestation that causes an acute vasculitis and muscular pain.

Certain *hematologic disorders* are associated with pain in the extremities. The crisis of sickle cell anemia is characterized by microinfarctions in bone and muscle. Leukemia in the child may be accompanied by an acute arthritis or periarthritis that arises from increased pressure within the metaphyses of the bones. The subperiosteal hemorrhages of hemophilia may resemble those seen in scurvy. Repeated episodes of intra-articular hemorrhages and pain are also characteristic of this disease.

Neoplasms may be associated with a neuropathy that is incidental or the primary cause of the patient's debility. Bronchogenic carcinoma, carcinoma of the breast, leukemia, and lymphoma are among the most frequent disorders that elicit a reactive neuropathy. Metastatic disease may appear as a solitary, painful nodule in an extremity or joint before the primary tumor is suspected.

The many forms of polyarthritis are beyond brief description. The course of joint involvement, if this can be discerned from the medical history or periodic observation of the patient, may be of inestimable diagnostic value. *Rheumatoid arthritis* may involve one or more joints and vary from asymptomatic swelling or effusion to incapacitating joint pain. It is accompanied by gelling and stiffness of muscles and joints in the morning. *Osteoarthritis,* on the contrary, may be secondary to trauma in a single joint or may occur as a primary generalized disease. Pain upon use and stiffness late in the day in the weight-bearing joints are characteristic symptoms. The patient will often feel relatively well after a short rest or in the morning. *Ankylosing spondylitis* is primarily an inflammatory disease of the spine but may also be accompanied by peripheral disease of the large or girdle joints. *Psoriatic arthritis* and *lipoid dermatoarthritis (multicentric reticulohistiocytosis)* are associated with characteristic skin lesions. The *Reiter syndrome* is diagnosed by recognizing a complex of urethritis, conjunctivitis, keratodermia, and arthritis. It may involve any peripheral joint or the spine and is associated particularly with heel pain that may be accompanied by inflammatory periosteal calcaneal spurs. *Ulcerative colitis, regional enteritis,* and *Whipple disease* may be accompanied by a peripheral arthritis or spondylitis.

There are a variety of other diseases that involve connective tissues. *Systemic lupus erythematosus* (SLE) is accompanied by inflammatory disease of joints and periarticular tissues that may be indistinguishable from the clinical presentation of rheumatoid arthritis. The arthritis and fasciitis of SLE are characteristically transient, and the severity of pain experienced by the patient may be out of proportion to the degree of objective change. A sensory neuropathy that can be severe and intractable to treatment may accompany this disorder. The musculoskeletal symptoms of polyarteritis and polymyositis have already been mentioned. *Scleroderma* is not associated with a prominent arthritis but is characterized by acrosclerosis and the Raynaud phenomenon. *Acute rheumatic fever, gout,* and *infectious arthritis* account for the most extreme degrees of joint inflammation and pain.

The initial swelling and pain in patients with *polychondritis* are localized to the cartilage of a joint, ear, or bridge of the nose. Certain disorders are characterized by a periodicity of symptoms. One of these is *familial Mediterranean fever,* with its characteristic bouts of acute synovitis and abdominal or thoracic pain. *Amyloidosis* is one of the miscellaneous group of disorders of unknown cause that results in musculoskeletal symptoms. On occasion it may mimic rheumatoid arthritis.

Other types of arthritis are associated with known biochemical or endocrine abnormalities. *Ochronosis* causes degenerative arthritis of the peripheral joints and spine with periodic acute inflammation. *Xanthoma tuberosum* and certain of the *hyperlipoproteinemias* are accompanied by a mild tendinitis or arthritis. Intermittent claudication may also occur in these disorders. *Gout* is perhaps the best known of the metabolic abnormalities associated with joint disease. The first attack is often in the large toe; any joint may be involved in its subsequent course. *Gouty arthritis* is acute and self-limited initially, and the pain may be extreme. The patient may be unwilling to move the affected joint or to even allow bed covers to lie on it. Chondrocalcinosis may be asymptomatic or may be associated with pseudogout. The latter mimics gout closely in clinical presentation except for the joints involved and a relative lack of response to traditional medical therapy or colchicine. The serum urate is normal in pseudogout.

The arthritis of *serum sickness* or *drug hypersensitivity* may not be acutely painful, and the extremity may be only swollen. Constitutional symptoms such as fever are usually present. A burning sensation and pruritus are characteristic of angioneurotic edema. The other exudative syndromes of *erythema multiforme,* such as the *Stevens-Johnson syndrome* and *Behçet disease,* may be accompanied by an acute synovitis. *Henoch-Schönlein purpura* presents as arthritis, abdominal pain, and nonthrombocytopenic purpura.

Certain inherited or congenital disorders involve connective tissues and are associated with hydrarthrosis. Recurrent joint effusions and fractures of the long bones are seen in *osteogenesis imperfecta.* Superficial ulcers on the lower extremities that may be quite difficult to heal are characteristic of certain forms of the *Ehlers-Danlos syndrome.* The various diseases associated with *abnormalities of glycosaminoglycans* are accompanied by joint enlargement and generalized muscular stiffness. The Hurler and Morquio syndromes are examples. *Spondyloepiphyseal dysplasia* is often associated with progressive musculoskeletal stiffness, as in the Morquio syndrome, but the child's intelligence is not affected.

PHYSICAL EXAMINATION

Careful physical examination is of major importance in the evaluation of pain. The following comments deal mainly with examination of the extremities and back, although it is assumed that a complete examination has been performed in order to detect the many systemic diseases and other disorders that produce referred pain. The history will usually have suggested certain diagnostic possibilities, and the physical examination can be directed accordingly. It is helpful in evaluation of physical findings to compare symmetric areas of the paired upper and lower extremities. Each extremity is evaluated carefully, system by system, starting with the skin and proceeding on to the peripheral vessels, neuromuscular system, and bones and joints. Examination of the back is also based on inspection, palpation, testing of range of motion, and observation of the walk.

Skin

The great majority of primary skin disorders, including those resulting from physical injury and infection, can be diagnosed readily on the basis of the history and physical examination. In addition, many systemic diseases produce cutaneous manifestations. Erythema nodosum, for instance, with its characteristic crops of tender erythematous nodules in the pretibial regions, may be associated with a variety of diseases, including bacterial, viral, and fungal infections; drug reactions; sarcoidosis; and systemic lupus erythematosus. The syndrome of erythema nodosum, arthritis, and bilateral hilar adenopathy occurs commonly with sarcoidosis. Erythema marginatum, an evanescent, erythematous, macular, or papular eruption affecting the trunk and proximal extremities, with central clearing as the outer border of the lesion advances, is characteristic of rheumatic fever. The lesions of the characteristic rash of juvenile rheumatoid arthritis are evanescent, salmon pink in color, and macular, varying from 2 to 6 mm in diameter. They may become confluent, and the larger lesions generally exhibit central clearing with a zone of pallor around the periphery of each lesion. This rash is usually not pruritic.

The hyperkeratotic skin lesions of keratodermia blennorrhagica, occurring on the palms and soles and occasionally on the trunk or extremities, are associated with the Reiter syndrome. Lesions of the mucous membranes, especially superficial circinate ulcerations of the glans penis (balanitis circinata), also occur frequently in this disorder. The classic butterfly rash of SLE, often associated with sunlight sensitivity, is readily recognized, but less classic cutaneous involvement is more frequent. The lesions may be purpuric or urticarial. Small erythematous lesions of the finger tips, especially around the nail folds, are also characteristic. Alopecia is common. Dermatomyositis may be associated with skin lesions similar to those observed in lupus. Heliotrope discoloration of the upper eyelids is characteristic and is accompanied in the acute phase by periorbital edema.

Symmetric violaceous, atrophic lesions over the dorsum of the small finger joints may provide diagnostic aid. The skin may be quite edematous in early scleroderma; as the disease progresses, the skin becomes indurated, fibrotic, and atrophic and is bound firmly to underlying structures. Contractures result in decreased joint motion or deformity and ulcerations may occur at the finger tips.

Nodular lesions within or beneath the skin should be sought, since they may be of considerable diagnostic value. The subcutaneous nodules of rheumatoid arthritis occur frequently on the extensor surfaces of the elbows and forearms and over other bony prominences and pressure points. They constitute the most nearly specific histopathologic lesion of the disease. Rheumatic fever nodules tend to be smaller and more transient. They may occur over bony surfaces but are also frequently found in tendons. Neither of these types of nodules is tender or painful. Tophaceous deposits of monosodium urate monohydrate, diagnostic of gout, are as common in the extremities as in the helix of the ear. Palpebral xanthelasmas, eruptive xanthomas, and xanthomatous deposits in skin or tendon occur frequently in the hyperlipoproteinemias. Although not often symptomatic themselves, they may suggest a predilection to severe artherosclerotic disease. In addition, patients with type II hyperlipoproteinemia often have a migratory polyarthritis with features somewhat similar to those of rheumatic fever, whereas patients with types III to V have hyperuricemia and develop clinical gout. Calcific deposits in skin and subcutaneous tissue occur in scleroderma and dermatomyositis. The multiple tumors of neurofibromatosis are often visible or palpable along the course of a peripheral nerve. Although usually painless, they may become symptomatic if sufficiently large or strategically located so as to cause pressure on contiguous structures or if they undergo malignant change. Lipomas are generally asymptomatic, but in an uncommon condition, adiposis dolorosa, painful subcutaneous nodules occur, sometimes in association with systemic symptoms, peripheral neuropathy, or endocrine adenomas.

The nails should be carefully examined, especially for evidence of clubbing. Clubbing that is accompanied by periostitis and new bone formation at the ends of the long bones in association with an arthritis that may mimic rheumatoid arthritis may reflect the presence of a pulmonary neoplasm as in hypertrophic osteoarthropathy. Splinter hemorrhages beneath the nails are seen in bacterial endocarditis and may be associated with clubbing, myalgias, arthralgias or arthritis, and osteomyelitis. Similar lesions may be seen in trichinosis and polyarteritis. Paroxysmal episodes of extreme pain may be precipitated by pressure over a glomus tumor, which occurs as a small, reddish-gray lesion beneath the nails or as a subcutaneous nodule elsewhere on the distal extremities.

Peripheral Vessels

The most helpful physical finding in obliterative arteriosclerosis is a decrease in or an absence of arterial pulsations. The peripheral arteries should be carefully inspected and palpated. The arterial walls may exhibit thickening, tortuosity, beading, or calcification. Early arterial insufficiency results in loss of hair on the dorsum of the great toe or entire foot. The nails appear thickened, opaque, and ridged longitudinally. The skin may feel cold and appears dry, shiny, smooth, thin, or inelastic. The digits may display pallor and distal areas of necrosis or ulceration. Livedo reticularis may be a cutaneous manifestation of the vasculitic syndromes.

The effect of position on blood supply should be carefully evaluated if obliterative arterial disease is suspected. Generally an involved extremity will display pallor on elevation and rubor or cyanosis on dependency. When a healthy extremity is moved from an elevated to a dependent position, normal skin color returns within 5 to 10 seconds and the superficial veins refill within 10 to 15 seconds. These changes are greatly delayed in the presence of arterial obstruction. If the site of obstruction is distal, normal arterial pulses may be found at the wrist or ankle. Compression tests may be useful in this situation in the hand. The examiner first occludes the radial artery while the patient makes a tight fist to force blood from the hand; the patient then opens the fist while the examiner maintains pressure over the radial artery. Failure of the hand to regain normal color within 3 seconds signifies occlusion of the ulnar artery or the ulnar side of the palmar arterial arch. The radial side of the arch is then evaluated by repeating the maneuver while the ulnar artery is compressed.

Thromboangiitis obliterans, or Buerger's disease, is much less common than arteriosclerosis obliterans, produces similar manifestations of arterial insufficiency, and is classically associated with a migratory superficial thrombophlebitis. The arteries lack the rigidity and beading of arteriosclerosis, and calcification is usually absent or minimal on x-ray examination. Arterial pulses are absent distal to the sudden obstruction of blood supply to an extremity from peripheral embolism. Pallor and often blotchy cyanosis are present. The limb is cold, and there is a decrease in or loss of sensation and inability to move it.

Arteriovenous fistulae in the extremities are most often the result of some penetrating injury that is likely to be evident on inspection. Local pulsatile swelling and increased warmth are present. A bruit, usually accompanied by a palpable thrill, may be heard over the fistula.

Major veins in the upper and lower extremities should be inspected and palpated for evidence of dilation, tortuosity, thickening, or tenderness. It is important that leg veins be examined while the patient is standing to avoid missing varicosities. Varicose veins appear prominent, tortuous, and increased in caliber. Edema is usually present if the patient has been ambulatory. Thrombophlebitis of the superficial veins produces tenderness of the involved segment. The overlying skin is red, swollen, and tender. The vein becomes palpable as a firm, cordlike structure as the thrombus organizes. Thrombophlebitis of the deep veins produces tenderness along the course of the involved segment, especially in the calf region, where pain is accentuated by dorsiflexion of the foot. Tenderness should also be sought in the plantar veins and along the course of the femoral vein in the thigh. Measurement of the circumference of the extremities at corresponding levels is helpful diagnostically.

If venous valves have been destroyed in the process of organization and recanalization of a thrombus, the flow of blood in the upright position may be reversed from the deep to the superficial veins and a chronic, postphlebitic syndrome may result. Changes of stasis dermatitis appear about the ankle, including brownish discoloration, redness, thickening, scaling, superficial oozing, and eventually ulceration.

The lymphatic vessels that accompany veins are not normally visible. A red streak along the course of the lymphatics leading from an area of infection, with enlarged, tender regional lymph nodes, is indicative of acute lymphangitis. Chronic lymphatic obstruction produces elephantiasis with persistent severe swelling and induration of one or both lower extremities. It may result from malignancy affecting the inguinal lymph nodes or from filariasis, or it may occur in a familial form.

Neuromuscular System

Pain in the extremities or back may result from disorders of the peripheral nerves or central pain pathways. Physical examination should always include evaluation of the sensory and motor systems and reflex status. Neurologic examination may be brief in routine and obviously non-neurologic conditions but should be thorough and comprehensive when indicated. Superficial pain sensation should be tested with a pin in both proximal and distal sites, looking for differences on the two sides of the body. The demonstration of a sensory level is helpful in localizing a spinal cord lesion. Any area of relative or absolute anesthesia should be outlined as accurately as possible by testing outward from the area of abnormality to determine whether it is in the distribution of a nerve root or peripheral nerve. Vibratory sensation, tested with a 128-cycle tuning fork over the lateral malleoli and wrist, is affected generally before motion and position sense.

Muscles should be inspected and palpated for any differences in size, atrophy or hypertrophy, symmetry of position or contour, abnormality of consistency, or abnormal movements. Fasciculations or fine tremors of muscle fibers are indicative of lower motor neuron disease, whereas grosser involuntary movements are suggestive of extrapyramidal involvement. If tremor is present, one should determine whether it is most prominent at rest and relieved by voluntary movement, as the resting tremor of Parkinson's disease, or if it is accentuated by voluntary movement, as the intention tremor of multiple sclerosis. The former condition is associated with rigidity, an increase in muscle tone that results in cogwheeling on passive motion of the part. Spasticity or an increase in muscle tone is seen in upper motor neuron disease and flaccidity or a decrease in lower neuron disease. Myotonia, increased irritability, and delayed relaxation of muscle can be tested by observing the response to percussion of affected muscles, especially in the forearm or thenar areas. Muscle strength should be evaluated in both proximal and distal regions and compared bilaterally. The biceps, triceps, brachioradialis, patellar, and Achilles reflexes should be tested routinely. Hypoactive or absent reflexes are found in many diseases and result from abnormalities in any part of the reflex arc. A pathologic increase in reflexes usually associated with clonus, however, is indicative of upper motor neuron disease. Similarly, the presence of a positive Babinski response is a definitive sign of pyramidal tract disease.

Involvement of a single peripheral nerve or mononeuropathy may be the result of direct trauma or pressure and traction on a nerve with interruption of blood supply as the result of some occupational injury or abnormal position. The entrapment syndromes represent an important cause of peripheral mononeuropathy in both the upper and lower extremities. The commonest of these is the carpal tunnel syndrome, which has already been described. Symptoms of this disorder are aggravated by tapping over the nerve on the palmar aspect of the wrist (Tinel sign). Motor signs include weakness and atrophy of the thenar muscles. Other entrapment syndromes involve the ulnar, sciatic, obturator, peroneal, and posterior tibial nerves.

Peripheral neuropathy or polyneuropathy may result from numerous systemic disorders, and differentiation from the primary myopathies is important if the predominant manifestations are motor. In neuropathy, weakness usually appears first and is more severe distally, whereas polymyositis affects the proximal muscles predominantly. Tendon reflexes tend to be decreased or lost early in neuropathy and late, or not at all, in myopathy. Fasciculation, if present, is an indication of destruction of the anterior horn cells. Sensory involvement does not occur with myopathy. In neuropathy it appears early and is prominent distally in a stocking-or-glove pattern. Tactile, vibratory, and position senses show variable loss, again, distally more than proximally.

Polymyositis is an inflammatory myopathy in which muscle weakness and atrophy are most severe proximally in the shoulder and hip muscles. Contractions may develop. When associated with cutaneous involvement, especially about the eyelids and articular surfaces, the disorder is termed dermatomyositis. Trichinosis may produce a similar degree of severe muscle tenderness. The myopathies associated with thyrotoxicosis and adrenal corticosteroids are more apt to be characterized by atrophy and weakness than by tenderness. The hereditary muscular dystrophies are an important cause of weakness and atrophy of the trunk and proximal limb muscles but are seldom a cause of pain. Pseudohypertrophy, in which enlargement of muscle groups with weakness is seen, may be prominent in early cases of some of these disorders.

Examination of the back should be initiated by inspection of contour, range of motion, and walk. Palpation and percussion for discrete areas of pain or tenderness are next performed. Degenerative disc disease commonly involves the lower lumbar spine and is a frequent cause of low back pain with radiation into the buttocks and lower extremities. Neurologic signs include a sensory loss in the foot or leg, weakness of the dorsiflexors of the foot or of the calf muscles, and loss of the Achilles or patellar reflexes. Localization of the pain and other signs may be help in identifying the nerve root(s) involved. Compression of the corticospinal tracts may result in upper motor neuron signs at lower levels, including weakness, hyperactive tendon reflexes with clonus, and extensor plantar responses. Symptoms arising from cervical cord disease are not aggravated by coughing or sneezing, nor are they relieved by rest or immobilization; pain arising from herniation of a lumbar disc is made worse by stretching the nerve root by sharp dorsiflexion of the foot (Spurling's sign), and a positive straight leg–raising test is present (Lasègue's sign).

Pain, often associated with discoloration and swelling of the upper extremity, may result from a number of conditions producing compression in the thoracic outlet. These syndromes are designated according to the causative mechanism, i.e., scalenus anticus, cervical rib, costoclavicular, or hyperabduction syndrome. The Adson maneuver is helpful in detecting compression in the interscalene triangle in the first and second of these syndromes: The patient inhales and holds a deep breath; hyperextends the neck; and then turns the head toward the side being examined, then in the opposite direction, while the examiner notes any decrease in the volume of the radial pulse. The costoclavicular syndrome is produced by pressure on the subclavian artery and vein in the space between the clavicle and first rib. The test for this involves having the patient draw the shoulders downward and backward (the exaggerated military position) and observing whether the radial pulse is obliterated and whether the patient's symptoms reproduced. The hyperabduction syndrome results from compression of the subclavian vessels or brachial plexus in the supraclavicular triangle or at the point at which these structures pass beneath the pectoralis minor tendon. It produces symptoms in persons who sleep with their arms over their heads or whose occupations involve working in this position. It is tested for by having the patient abduct and elevate the arm above the head while the examiner notes any dampening or obliteration of the radial pulse or reproduction of the typical symptoms.

Bones and Joints

In approaching the problem of joint pain, it is critical to determine whether there are associated objective findings. In some diseases, as in early gout, there may be a convincing history of arthritis, although there may be no findings if the patient is examined in the interval between attacks. Joint pain, often associated with myalgias, in the persistent absence of positive findings suggests some variety of the fibrositis syndrome or psychogenic rheumatism. Hypothyroidism may produce a similar picture. Diffuse joint and muscle discomfort without objective findings is also characteristic of polymyalgia rheumatica, an entity that is assuming increasing importance because of its association with temporal arteritis and sudden blindness.

If objective joint findings are present, it is important to differentiate between inflammatory and noninflammatory signs. The former suggest rheumatoid arthritis and related disorders, whereas the latter indicate a degenerative or post-traumatic disorder. Joint swelling, which is probably the commonest sign, is usually apparent on inspection and palpation but may be difficult to detect when minimal in degree. Normal joints may appear to be swollen in the presence of atrophy of surrounding muscles. Swelling may be the result of effusion, thickening of the periarticular soft tissues, or hypertrophy of cartilage or bone. The latter type of swelling is characteristic of degenerative joint disease and in the hands is located characteristically in the distal and proximal interphalangeal and first carpometacarpal joints. Inflammatory signs and synovial cyst formation may be present early but are not generally prominent and tend to subside after several years.

In rheumatoid arthritis and other inflammatory joint diseases, the overlying skin may be red and warm. The joints are usually tender to palpation and painful on motion. The swelling is fusiform, diffuse, and symmetric. The location of involved joints may provide diagnostic aid. Rheumatoid arthritis in the hand, for example, tends to affect the proximal and metacarpophalangeal joints and to spare the distal joints. An acute arthritis involving the great toe is likely to be gout, whereas a similar attack in a knee may represent gout but is more apt to be pseudogout. A number of other diagnostic possibilities, including specific infectious arthritis, need to be considered. Migratory polyarthritis affecting the large joints is characteristic of rheumatic fever. More persistent involvement of relatively few large joints is seen in ankylosing spondylitis and the Reiter syndrome. These diseases are frequently the cause of persistent pain and tenderness in the plantar aspect of the heel. Painful swelling of the sternomanubrial joint is most suggestive of ankylosing spondylitis. Distal interphalangeal involvement, often lending a sausage-like appearance to the affected finger or toe, is suggestive of psoriatic arthritis or the Reiter syndrome.

The possibility that "joint" pain may originate from periarticular structures, such as ligaments, bursae, or bones, needs to be considered. Effort should be made to localize symptoms and physical findings as accurately as possible and to relate them to specific anatomic structures. Shoulder pain is often the result of calcific tendinitis and bursitis rather than arthritis; tenderness is sharply localized to the subacromial area at which point the supraspinatus and other tendons insert into the greater trochanter of the humerus. Pain is usually aggravated by abduction and rotation of the shoulder, whereas arthritis produces pain on motion in all directions. Persistent *periarthritis* may result in adhesive capsulitis with progressive loss of motion until the familiar frozen shoulder results. *Bicipital tenosynovitis* produces pain and tenderness in the bicipital groove and over the long head of the biceps tendon. Pain is accentuated by maneuvers requiring contraction of the biceps muscle. Shoulder pain associated with inability to initiate or maintain abduction is often the result of tendon rupture or of tears in the musculotendinous cuff of the glenohumeral capsule. In the shoulder-hand syndrome, a form of reflex sympathetic dystrophy, pain and limitation of motion in the shoulder with dusky cyanosis, edema, and causalgic pain in the hand are present. Later, atrophy of the skin and subcutaneous tissues, contractures of the digital and palmar fascia, and patchy osteoporosis on x-ray examination may develop.

The olecranon bursa at the tip of the elbow is a frequent site of trauma and involvement in rheumatoid arthritis and gout. Swelling is often severe and accompanied by marked tenderness and erythema and increased warmth of the overlying skin. Tenderness sharply localized to the medial or lateral epicondyles of the humerus reflects the presence of epicondylitis in tennis elbow. *De Quervain disease,* a stenosing tenosynovitis of the long abductor and short extensor tendons of the thumb, is characterized by tenderness over the radial styloid process and is made worse by having the patient grasp the thumb by the forefingers and deviate the wrist ulnarly. The familiar ganglion, a cystic swelling of the tendon sheaths on the dorsum of the wrist, is usually associated with mild or no discomfort, but it may be painful. In the hip region, pain and tenderness over the greater trochanter may result from trochanteric tendinitis or bursitis. Hip pain from any cause is often referred to the knee. A normal physical examination in a patient complaining of knee pain should include careful examination for hip disease.

Internal derangements of the knee may produce sharply localized tenderness. Tenderness medially or laterally in the joint space between femur and tibia suggests a torn or damaged meniscus, whereas tenderness extending more proximally over the medial or lateral femoral condyles suggests involvement of the collateral ligaments. Further delineation of the area of involvement can be made by abducting and adducting the leg with the patient supine and the lower thigh anchored by the examiner's hand. Abduction decreases pressure on the medial meniscus and increases pressure on the lateral meniscus, while relaxing the lateral collateral ligament and increasing tension on the medial collateral ligament. Thus, if this maneuver increases pain laterally, it points to the lateral meniscus as the site; if it produces pain medially, the medial collateral ligament is incriminated. With adduction, the situation is reversed; production of pain medially suggests a lesion of the medial meniscus, and lateral pain suggests a disorder of the lateral collateral ligament. Painful locking of the knee may result from a loose body in the joint or a movable fragment attached to a meniscus or other internal structure. Lateral instability of the knee may be demonstrable with stretching or tearing of the collateral ligaments. Forward and backward instability with the knee flexed at 90° indicates an abnormality of a cruciate ligament. Forward instability indicates anterior cruciate ligament involvement and posterior instability, a disorder of the posterior cruciate ligament. The prepatellar bursa may be inflamed in *housemaid's knee.* In addition to trauma and the major rheumatic diseases, infection should be considered a possible cause.

Bone tenderness is determined by firm pressure over the bony structures. It may reflect the presence of fracture, periostitis, osteomyelitis, neoplasm, or metabolic bone diseases. Periostitis may result from infection of underlying bone, subperiosteal hemorrhage, or hypertrophic osteoarthropathy. Bony enlargement and deformity may be apparent in Paget's disease.

LABORATORY EXAMINATIONS

Acute Phase Reactants. Elevation of the acute phase reactants is an indication of an acute infectious or inflammatory response. The most commonly employed examination is the Westergren ESR. The speed of sedimenting of a column of red blood cells is directly related to the concentration of certain proteins of the blood such as fibrinogen and the degree of anemia. An elevated ESR is an index of pyogenic or inflammatory activity and a normal ESR is associated with noninflammatory or degenerative conditions. Other acute phase reactants include C-reactive protein and the serum immunoglobulins. These may serve as confirmatory tests for a questionable change in the ESR. If all are within the normal range, it is unlikely that the patient has an inflammatory disease.

Specific Antibody Assays. A number of specific assays are useful in an evaluation for extremity or back pain and are often positive in infectious, rheumatic, or other autoimmune conditions. The most generally employed are the latex agglutination test for rheumatoid factors, an antinuclear antibody test, and the lupus erythematosus (LE) cell preparation. Abnormalities in these examinations are associated with specific inflammatory diseases such as rheumatoid arthritis and SLE. The presence of rheumatoid factors and antinuclear antibodies may also be a phenomenon of the acute phase response or aging. A more specific test for SLE is assay for anti–double-stranded DNA antibodies. Other tests for antibodies related to infectious diseases may be ordered when indicated. An antistreptolysin O titer or a Streptozyme test is useful when considering rheumatic fever as a diagnosis.

Although components of the complement sequence may respond as acute phase reactants and may be elevated in inflammatory diseases, they are quite often depressed to below normal values in disorders characterized by immune complex formation and *in vivo* fixation of complement. Specific depression of complement components is also seen in certain hereditary deficiencies of the proteins of the complement pathway. Circulating immune complexes may also be detected by determining cryoglobulins or specific immune complex determinations, such as Clq-binding or Raji cell assay.

Blood Chemistry. Assay for serum calcium, phosphate, and alkaline phosphatase activity is useful in differentiating certain lesions of bone. Elevations of other enzymes such as serum glutamic oxaloacetic transaminase (SGOT), creatine kinase, and aldolase are characteristic of disease of skeletal muscle. Although not specific for inflammatory muscle disease, the sequential course of the serum concentrations of these enzymes may be helpful in diagnosis of the less classic and more subtle examples of these myopathies.

Synovial Fluid Examination. The presence of excess fluid in a joint may reflect inflammation, trauma, hemorrhage, or infection, and, when the diagnosis is uncertain, is an indication for aspiration and synovial fluid examination. The fluid should be characterized for gross appearance, cell and differential count, and mucin clot, and a search with a polarizing microscope should be made for crystals. In infectious arthritis, specific bacteria may be identified by Gram stain and culture.

Radiologic Examinations. X-ray examination of the back or joints is invaluable in the diagnosis of arthritis of these structures. Most, if not all, of the rheumatic diseases have specific radiologic appearances. In addition, x-ray examination may point to the presence of a tumor, infection, or fracture. Newer methods of visualization involving bone scans, computed tomography (CT), and nuclear magnetic resonance imaging will greatly aid in differentiating the causes of extremity or back pain. Contrast studies such as arthrography can also be used to delineate disruption of the internal joint structures. Myelography is generally indicated if surgery is considered for a ruptured intervertebral disc or if there is reason to suspect an intraspinal tumor.

Electromyography and Nerve Conduction Studies. These tests are useful in providing evidence for objective muscular or neurologic lesions. Delay in nerve conduction is characteristic of the entrapment syndromes. Many inflammatory, atrophic, and degenerative muscle diseases have characteristic electromyographic findings.

Histocompatibility Testing. Medicine is on the threshold of defining immunogenetic relationships among many of the diseases that result in pain in the extremities and back. Although the presence of HLA-B27 lymphocyte antigen is characteristic of ankylosing spondylitis, this is not a useful diagnostic test in a single patient. These genetic tests will, however, be rewarding in delineation of epidemiologic and family studies.

Biopsy. Pathologic examination of a tissue or bone specimen may be definitive for making a diagnosis. Clinically, muscle biopsy is often the most useful in providing specific histopathologic classification of myopathy or vasculitis. In selected cases, biopsy of a bone, nodule, or synovial tissue may be indicated.

DYSURIA, PYURIA, AND HEMATURIA

By Paul Gonick, M.D.
Philadelphia, Pennsylvania

DYSURIA

Any degree of discomfort or pain while urinating is considered dysuria. Dysuria is usually associated with frequency and is a nonspecific symptom indicating an inflammatory condition of the lower ureter, bladder, urethra, or prostate, or of an adjacent organ (ileum, appendix, sigmoid colon, fallopian tube, or vagina). Dysuria without pyuria or hematuria may be due to turbulent urine flow secondary to a urethral stricture, stenosis, or diverticulum. Occasionally, no cause can be determined (urethral syndrome).

PYURIA

Pyuria is recognized as the presence of more than five white blood cells per high-powered microscope field (WBC/HPF) in centrifuged urine for men and children and more than 10 WBC/HPF for women. A positive leukocyte esterase dipstick is also considered significant pyuria. The exact cell count per milliliter of urine will vary depending upon urine osmolality, pH, age of sample, degree of inflammation, and method of centrifugation. An inflammatory lesion in or near the urinary tract will result in pyuria. General disease processes that cause pyuria are listed in Table 1. Infection is the most common cause and can be confirmed by obtaining a urine culture.

The diagnostic approach for determining the reason for the patient's pyuria is to first localize the site of inflammation and then determine into which of the six general categories the history, examination, and laboratory findings best fit.

Urine analysis can furnish leads for further investigation. Pyuria with proteinuria (usually with tubular casts) suggests renal disease. Bacteria seen in the uncentrifuged urine and confirmed by significant growth upon culture indicate infection. One must consider tuberculosis or a fungal infection with pyuria in an acid urine without bacterial growth on routine culture media. The urine sediment may show the typical crystalline structure of compounds that form urinary calculi (calcium oxalate, calcium phosphate, uric acid, and cystine). The urine may be separated into first, second, and post-prostate massage samples to differentiate urethritis from cystitis, pyelonephritis, and prostatitis. When collecting a urine sample, care must be taken to prevent contamination with vaginal secretions especially in obese women.

Further investigation of the urinary system can be performed with excretory urography, sonography,

Table 1. Causes of Pyuria

Infection
Kidney, ureter, bladder, urethra, prostate, seminal vesicles
Adjacent organs—ileum, colon, appendix, fallopian tubes, cervix, vagina
Anatomic abnormalities
Strictures, diverticula, foreign bodies, urinary obstruction
Metabolic abnormalities
Calculi, crystalluria
Trauma
Immune diseases
Glomerulitis, focal and diffuse interstitial nephritis, transplant rejection
Malignancies

Table 2. Causes of Hematuria

- Mechanical obstructions
  - Calculi
  - Strictures, bands, vessels
  - Prostatic enlargement
  - Renal cysts
- Infections and Inflammation
  - Bacteria—enteric or tubercular
  - Fungus, virus, parasites
  - Sterile inflammation (interstitial cystitis)
  - Verumontanitis, urethritis, prostatitis
  - Inflammation of adjacent organs
- Neoplasms—benign and malignant
  - Primary urinary system
    - Kidney
    - Ureter
    - Bladder
    - Prostate
    - Urethra
  - Metastatic
  - Local invasion (e.g., from cervix, colon)
  - Endometriosis
- Trauma
  - Acute—blunt or penetrating
  - Chronic—jogging, bicycling, boxing
  - Severe exercise
  - Foreign bodies and catheters
- Immunologic
  - Glomerulopathies
- Congenital anomalies
  - Urinary system
  - Vascular system
    - A–V fistula
    - Varices
- Hematologic
  - Coagulopathies
  - Anticoagulant states
  - Hemoglobinophathies
    - Sickle cell trait or disease
    - Mediterranean anemia
- Vascular
  - Infarcts—venous or arterial
  - Emboli
  - Hypertension
  - Vasculitis
- False
  - Vaginal, penile, or scrotal bleeding
  - Pigmenturia
    - Porphyria
    - Hemoglobinuria
    - Myoglobinuria
    - Food (beets)
    - Drugs

computed tomography (CT), nuclear scanning, and cystoscopy. Excellent investigative means of examining the urinary organs are available, and they invariably lead to identification of the cause of pyuria.

HEMATURIA

Hematuria is considered to be the presence of three or more red blood cells in a high-power microscope field from a centrifuged urine sample or a positive Hematest. As a general rule, it does not matter whether hematuria is gross or microscopic; the diagnostic considerations are the same.*

The general disease processes considered are listed in Table 2. The initial diagnostic approach requires a detailed history, physical examination, urine analysis, complete blood count, prothrombin time, partial thromboplastin time, and serum creatinine.

History. If pain was present at the onset of hematuria, was it dull or acute and colicky (resulting from a stone or blood clot causing obstruction)? Was the blood noticed only at the beginning or end of the urinary stream (bleeding from bladder neck or prostate) or throughout (kidney or bladder lesions)? Dysuria along with hematuria may indicate an infection or lower ureteral calculus. Fever usually means there is an infection or a renal malignancy.

A family history of renal disease may indicate sickle cell trait or disease (usually in a black patient) or hereditary nephropathy (e.g., Alport's syndrome), or it may be happenstance. Query is made about previous operations and illnesses (iatrogenic obstruction, adjacent organ malignancy or inflammation), fad diets urinary calculi, vitamin deficiency), exercise habits, smoking habits, use of "recreational" drugs, use of medications, and allergies.

Physical examination includes observation of the skin for bruises, petechia, and telangiectasia; a funduscopic examination for hemorrhages or exudates from hypertension or emboli; palpation and auscultation of the heart for rhythm, murmurs, or rubs; palpation and auscultation of the abdomen for masses, bruits, bowel sounds, tender areas, or a distended bladder; palpation and inspection of the genitalia for a bleeding site at the urethral meatus, cervix, vagina, or labia; and palpation in the rectum for masses, prostate size and consistency, presence of blood, and color of feces.

Laboratory Investigation. The initial blood work should make evident most hematologic bleeding disorders. The urine analysis is helpful in diagnosing the immunologic diseases (significant proteinuria or casts in the sediment), infections (bacteria), inflammatory disease (pus or white cell casts or positive leukocyte esterase on dipstick), or calculi (identifiable crystals).

If the diagnosis is still indefinite, imaging techniques such as intravenous urography, ultrasonography, computer-assisted tomography, nuclear imaging, cystoscopy (still the best method of identifying bladder pathology), retrograde pyelography, antegrade percutaneous urography, aortography, and venography may be utilized to locate and determine the cause of the hematuria.

*According to Stamey, asymptomatic microscopic hematuria caused by a glomerular lesion may be diagnosed by finding typical distorted, misshapen, or thick-walled red corpuscles. (Stamey, T.F.: Office examination of urinary sediment in the diagnosis of urinary tract disease. American Urologic Association meeting April 21, 1983.) If this report is confirmed, many patients with microscopic hematuria can be spared the risks, discomfort, and expense of urinary tract "imaging" to rule out other lesions.

PERIPHERAL EDEMA

By Paul E. Klotman, M.D.
Durham, North Carolina

Peripheral edema is an important clinical sign indicating an alteration in Starling forces, either systemically or locally. It is a clue to underlying diseases that may require treatment. Only rarely does the edema itself actually need therapeutic attention. The physical characteristics of the edema, its severity, and distribution all give important clinical information concerning its etiology.

QUANTITATING EDEMA

Most normal people have trace edema. The best method for assessing the presence of edema is to compress the skin firmly against the tibia for 5 to 10 seconds using the thumb. By quickly lifting the thumb and then passing the index finger over the compressed area, one can feel an indentation. If a slight indentation is palpable, the patient has "trace edema." Trace edema reflects normal interstitial fluid volume and is one of the clinical signs suggesting an adequate extracellular volume. Any degree of edema greater than trace palpable edema reflects an alteration of Starling forces and some degree of pathophysiology. The quantitation of edema as one plus or four plus is imprecise and descriptive. For this reason, these indices are only useful to the individual observer who is following a particular patient. There are better methods of quantitating total body sodium and water, particularly body weight, so that qualitative indices are rarely useful. The descriptions *no edema, trace palpable edema,* or *massive edema* convey the appropriate images, and if one wants to quantitate the edema, it is better to simply measure the degree of indentation in millimeters.

DISTRIBUTION OF EDEMA

Gravitational forces enhance edema formation by increasing vascular hydrostatic pressure and opposing lymphatic flow from the periphery. Therefore, peripheral edema appears initially, or is most severe, in dependent portions of the body. In an ambulatory patient, the lower extremities are the most likely site for edema formation. When a patient is bedridden, presacral edema may predominate. Asymmetric edema suggests local alterations in Starling forces, whereas bilaterally symmetric edema suggests a systemic etiology.

Generalized edema is usually detected as bilateral lower extremity edema, but it can be so massive that it involves all extremities, the trunk, and the face. Massive generalized edema is referred to as *anasarca.* Occasionally, the earliest presentation of generalized edema is in a single extremity owing to the presence of previous trauma, venous insufficiency, or impaired lymphatic drainage. Thus, the distinction between bilateral and unilateral edema can be arbitrary and misleading. However, bilateral edema is a useful sign of a more generalized phenomenon and unilateral edema is more indicative of local disease. Causes of generalized edema and localized edema are summarized in Table 1.

GENERALIZED EDEMA

Systemic changes in Starling forces produce generalized edema. Thus, increases in hydrostatic pressure or capillary permeability and reductions in plasma oncotic pressure or lymphatic drainage would promote edema formation. Diseases that produce generalized edema are common and are usually easily diagnosed by history, physical, and laboratory examination. Therapy should be aimed at the underlying condition and not at the peripheral edema.

Cardiovascular Diseases

Congestive Heart Failure

Both "high-output" and "low-output" congestive heart failure (see article on this topic) produce enhanced renal sodium retention and peripheral edema, particularly in the setting of cardiac decompensation. In congestive heart failure, a combination of reduced renal blood flow, increased hydrostatic pressure, and reduced interstitial lymphatic drainage may all contribute to the generation of peripheral edema.

A history of cardiac failure should be relatively easy to elicit. Patients will complain of orthopnea, paroxysmal nocturnal dyspnea, or dyspnea on exertion. Physical examination should reveal signs of compromised cardiac function, including an enlarged heart, an S_3 or summation gallop, and jugular venous distention. Laboratory data may contribute to the diagnosis by revealing a blood urea nitrogen (BUN) to creatinine ratio greater than 10, suggesting prerenal azotemia. Urinalysis may be remarkable for an increase in osmolality and specific gravity and a decrease in urinary sodium concentration, suggesting a reduction in renal blood flow. Chest x-ray may reveal an increased heart size, and an electrocardiogram may demonstrate evidence of ischemic heart disease. Peripheral edema will resolve if the underlying hemodynamic disturbance can be improved.

Right Ventricular Heart Failure

Right ventricular failure may complicate a posterior or inferior myocardial infarction. Peripheral edema accumulates rapidly as a result of the rise in right ventricular end-diastolic pressure, which increases the venous hydrostatic pressure and reduces lymphatic drainage from the interstitium. Systemic cardiac output falls, and renal sodium retention occurs. Severe jugular venous distention is present, and there may be evidence of tricuspid regurgitation manifested by a large jugular venous CV wave, a pulsatile liver, and ascites. The diagnosis is made by the combination of clinical findings and typical pressure rela-

Table 1. Causes of Generalized and Localized Edema

Generalized Edema	Localized Edema
Cardiovascular Diseases Congestive heart failure Right ventricular failure Pulmonary hypertension Pericardial disease Vena caval obstruction Arteriovenous fistulae	*Vascular Diseases* Venous diseases Venous insufficiency with varicosities Deep venous thrombophlebitis Vascular anomalies
Renal Diseases Acute renal failure Chronic renal insufficiency Nephrotic syndrome	*Localized Lymphedema* Primary lymphedema Congenital lymphedema Lymphedema praecox Lymphedema tarda Secondary lymphedema—obstruction Malignancy Granulomatous disease Filariasis Radiation-induced Postsurgical Synovitis
Liver Diseases Hepatitis Cirrhosis Chronic biliary obstruction Hepatic venous congestion	
Generalized Lymphedema	
Altered Systemic Capillary Permeability Diabetes Angioedema Sepsis	*Recurrent Lymphangitis*
	Local Changes in Capillary Permeability Ischemia Cellulitis Local trauma, surgery or burns Vasculitis
Hypoproteinemic States Nephrotic syndrome Liver disease Protein-calorie malnutrition	*Autonomic Dysfunction* Cerebrovascular accident Reflex sympathetic dystrophy
Drug-Associated Drugs with mineralocorticoid effects Sympatholytic drugs Vasodilators Nonsteroidal anti-inflammatory agents	*Synovitis-Associated* Local inflammation Ruptured Baker's cyst Lymphatic obstruction
Idiopathic Cyclic Edema	
Edema of Pregnancy	

tionships found by right heart catheterization. Colloid and crystalloid infusions are usually required to maintain an adequate cardiac output. Although this sodium load markedly exacerbates the accumulation of peripheral edema, therapy should be directed toward the maintenance of an adequate cardiac output.

Pulmonary Hypertension

Generalized peripheral edema frequently accompanies pulmonary hypertension (see article on this topic). As pulmonary resistance increases, patients may experience vague chest pain or dyspnea on exertion. Physical examination reveals evidence of increased venous pressure with jugular venous distention. Cardiac examination may reveal a right-sided S_4 gallop, an accentuated pulmonic closure sound, and, with severe pulmonary hypertension, paradoxical splitting of the second heart sound. Tricuspid insufficiency commonly occurs. A chest x-ray may provide evidence of pulmonary hypertension manifested by right ventricular hypertrophy, large pulmonary arteries, and attenuation of the small pulmonary vascular branches. When there is coexistent left ventricular failure, left-sided chamber enlargement and cephalization of the pulmonary vasculature will also be present. If left ventricular failure is severe enough, radiographic evidence of pulmonary edema may be present. A chest x-ray may also provide clues to the underlying etiology, (e.g., chronic obstructive lung disease, interstitial fibrosis). The electrocardiogram may reveal right ventricular hypertrophy or a right bundle branch block pattern.

A ventilation perfusion lung scan may be useful in detecting recurrent pulmonary emboli. More often the scan is useful in indicating suspicious areas of ventilation and perfusion mismatch where a limited pulmonary angiogram may be performed (assuming pulmonary pressures do not exclude a limited vascular procedure).

Right heart catheterization will document the pulmonary pressures. Since an attempt at treatment of the peripheral edema may well exacerbate the low cardiac output, an attempt at therapy should be undertaken only in patients who are symptomatic from their massive edema.

Pericardial Disease

Jugular venous distention, ascites, and peripheral edema may be the only physical findings of chronic constrictive pericarditis (see article on this topic). The edema accumulates as venous hydrostatic pressure increases and as lymphatic drainage from the periphery decreases. When patients are symptomatic, it is usually due to the low cardiac output state typical of chronic constrictive pericarditis. Patients may complain of exertional fatigue and dyspnea or vague substernal chest pain. Most often, the onset of disease is insidious and the progression sufficiently slow to obscure the diagnosis. A pericardial friction rub, or "pericardial knock," may be audible. Neck veins are distended, and a prominent Y descent should be apparent. The electrocardiogram can be useful, frequently demonstrating reduced QRS voltage. The chest x-ray may indicate a normal or small heart size.

Calcification of the pericardium may be present. An echocardiogram can confirm the presence of a thickened pericardial membrane and small ventricular dimensions. Right heart catheterization should demonstrate "equalization of pressures" in such a way that pulmonary, right ventricular, and right atrial end-diastolic pressures are roughly equivalent. Laboratory examination can reveal a decrease in plasma albumin if there is sufficient liver disease from chronic hepatic congestion. Unless symptomatic, peripheral edema should be ignored and therapy should be directed toward relief of the constriction. In this setting, diuretics should be avoided, since they may further lower the cardiac output by reducing venous filling pressure.

Vena Caval Obstruction

Vena caval obstruction in the thorax or abdomen can produce bilateral extremity edema and, depending upon the level of obstruction, may be associated with ascites formation. Both the increase in venous hydrostatic pressure and the reduction in lymphatic drainage contribute to the formation of peripheral edema.

Superior vena caval obstruction occurs most often as a complication of lung cancer with direct mediastinal invasion. Extrinsic compression of the superior vena cava produces edema of the face and upper extremities and is associated with dilated and tortuous superficial veins visible along the anterior superior chest wall, neck, and face. Chest x-ray may reveal the underlying lung cancer, but mediastinal tomograms or chest CT scan may be required to better delineate mediastinal structures.

Inferior vena caval obstruction produces bilateral lower extremity edema often associated with ascites. Usually, obstruction is extrinsic and results from compression by a malignancy. Lymphomas, prostatic carcinoma in men, and genital carcinoma in women are the most common causes of malignant obstruction of the inferior vena cava. Renal cell carcinoma occurs in both men and women but is much less common. Obstruction can also occur from the intrinsic propagation of a clot into the inferior vena cava from a renal vein or iliac vein thrombus.

Finally, hypercoagulable states may present with vena caval obstruction. Abdominal x-rays rarely yield a diagnosis. Ultrasound or CT scan of the abdomen may reveal soft-tissue masses. However, a venogram or contrast CT will likely yield more definitive information, particularly with regard to the level and degree of obstruction.

Arteriovenous Fistulae

Arteriovenous fistulae promote renal sodium retention, presumably as a result of the lowering of peripheral vascular resistance. Chronically, fistulae may produce cardiac decompensation and the combination of renal sodium retention and increased hydrostatic pressure may produce significant peripheral edema.

Renal Diseases

Renal diseases are associated with peripheral edema for at least two reasons. Both acute and chronic forms of renal failure impair sodium excretion, and this may produce a net positive sodium balance. Second, renal losses of albumin in the nephrotic syndrome can be great enough to lower plasma oncotic pressure and promote fluid movement from the intravascular to the interstitial space.

Acute Renal Failure

In most forms of acute renal failure (see article on this topic), renal blood flow, glomerular filtration rate, and renal excretion of sodium are impaired significantly. The patient's history will reflect the underlying etiology of the acute renal failure. It may be consistent with a systemic vasculitis, toxin exposure, recurrent urinary tract infections, bladder outlet obstruction, or stones. In acute glomerulonephritis, edema formation is frequently greater than that observed in other forms of acute and chronic renal failure, despite equivalent levels of renal function. The pattern of edema is also different, with more frequent involvement of the hands and face, particularly in a periorbital distribution.

In all forms of acute renal failure, the laboratory examination is particularly important and may suggest the diagnosis. Blood urea nitrogen and plasma creatinine concentrations are elevated. Urinalysis may reveal significant proteinuria, hematuria, pyuria, tubular elements, cellular casts, or crystalluria. Therapy of acute renal failure should include the careful balancing of sodium intake with sodium output. The edema of some patients may respond to loop diuretics, but in others dialysis may be required to manage sodium and water excess.

Chronic Renal Insufficiency

Patients with chronic renal failure (see article on this topic) lose the ability to concentrate urine and conserve sodium maximally. The diurnal variation of urine output is lost, and many patients complain of nocturia and polyuria. The presence or absence of edema reflects the net balance between sodium intake and output. The diagnosis of chronic renal insufficiency is easily made by laboratory examination, revealing an elevated BUN and plasma creatinine and reduced creatinine clearance. Urinalysis may reveal mild to moderate degrees of proteinuria or hematuria, but elements suggesting acute disease are absent. Nephrotomograms usually reveal small kidneys. Therapy of edema should be directed toward sodium balance by reducing sodium intake and promoting sodium excretion with loop diuretics.

The Nephrotic Syndrome

The nephrotic syndrome (see article on this topic) is defined as the urinary excretion of 3.5 grams or more of protein per day, hypoalbuminemia, hypercholesterolemia, and peripheral edema. The proteinuria reflects changes in glomerular capillary permeability. A patient's presenting complaint is often mild to severe peripheral edema. The nephrotic syndrome may be associated with a glomerulopathy, neoplastic disease, or collagen vascular disease, or it may be caused by exposure to toxins or to a variety of medications. There are also inherited forms of renal disease with associated nephrotic syndrome. Physical examination reveals soft, generalized, pitting edema. The other symptoms and signs are consistent with the underlying disease process. Laboratory examination reveals an abnormally low plasma albumin and elevated cholesterol concentration. Blood urea nitrogen and plasma creatinine concentrations may be normal or elevated. Urinalysis is remarkable for heavy proteinuria. A 24-hour urine collection will reveal a daily protein excretion of 3.5 grams or more.

Most patients with nephrotic-range proteinuria, normal kidney size, and normal renal function should undergo a renal biopsy. In general, the edema of the nephrotic syndrome can be treated successfully with bed rest, sodium restriction, and diuretics. Corticosteroids are appropriate for the treatment of certain underlying glomerular diseases (nil lesion or idiopathic membranous glomerulonephritis) and are used in hopes of preserving renal function. They are rarely needed for the treatment of proteinuria and edema, although occasionally patients with nephrotic syndrome are refractory to diuresis by any modality short of hospitalization or the administration of corticosteroids.

Liver Disease

A variety of liver diseases are associated with ascites and peripheral edema. Acute and chronic hepatitis, cirrhosis, and chronic biliary obstruction are particularly potent stimulators of sodium retention by the kidney. The stimulus to sodium retention is unknown, but increased circulating aldosterone levels, a reduction in "effective plasma volume," and changes in intrarenal prostaglandins may all be important. In addition, impaired hepatic synthesis of albumin and a marked reduction in peripheral lymphatic drainage contribute to the altered Starling forces that allow peripheral edema to accumulate. Hepatic venous outflow obstruction appears to be more important to the development of edema and ascites than does portal hypertension.

With an acute hepatitis, patients may provide a history of jaundice, weight loss, nausea, vomiting, abdominal pain, pruritus, and an enlarged tender liver. With chronic liver disease, patients may present with the stigmata of cirrhosis: spider angiomata, gynocomastia, small testes, and splenomegaly. With biliary disease, abdominal pain may be a more prominent feature of their illness. Laboratory examination of the plasma may reveal elevated transaminase, alkaline phosphatase, and bilirubin concentrations. Plasma albumin concentration may be reduced, depending upon the nutritional status of the patient and the rate of hepatic albumin synthesis. This reduction in plasma oncotic pressure may further exacerbate peripheral edema formation.

Idiopathic Cyclic Edema

Periodic and recurrent edema may occur in women prior to the onset of menopause. Typically, patients are obese and many have a family history of diabetes. The edema is generalized and symmetric, occurring at the end of the day in dependent parts of the body. Patients may also complain of swelling of the hands, feet, breasts, and back. Episodes of edema are unrelated to the menstrual cycle. The etiology of this phenomenon is unknown, and other diseases that may lead to peripheral edema formation should be excluded. Treatment should be limited to patients who are symptomatic from their edema.

The Edema of Pregnancy

The majority of women experience lower extremity edema during pregnancy. There are a variety of factors that predispose the pregnant patient to peripheral edema, including intense sodium retention with expansion of the extracellular space, an increase in aldosterone secretion, a reduction in peripheral resistance with an increase in venous capacitance, a reduction in plasma oncotic pressure, and an increase in venous hydrostatic pressure due to mechanical pressure from the gravid uterus. This edema is usually confined to the lower extremities but on occasion may be more generally distributed. Patients usually respond to the simple maneuvers of elevating the legs and assuming the lateral recumbent position while sleeping. Mild sodium restriction may be helpful, but diuretics should not be used during pregnancy.

Generalized Lymphedema

Obstruction to lymphatic outflow may produce either local or more generalized edema. Initially, the physical characteristics of lymphedema are similar to those of edema from other causes. However, chronic lymphedema becomes firm and resistant to pitting.

When bilateral lymphedema occurs after the age of 40, it is usually secondary to obstruction of the lymphatics in the abdomen or thorax. The most common cause of lymphatic obstruction in this age group is a malignancy, usually a lymphoma or carcinoma of the prostate in men or carcinoma of the genital tract in women. Virtually any malignancy, however, can produce lymphatic obstruction. Physical examination may reveal lymphadenopathy, and occasionally soft-tissue masses may be detected in the abdomen. In men, examination of the prostate may demonstrate a mass and an elevated serum acid phosphatase may support the diagnosis of prostatic carcinoma. In women, a pelvic exam may yield evidence of a genital carcinoma. Biopsy is required for a definitive diagnosis. Lymphangiography, ultrasound, or a CT scan of the pelvis and abdomen may demonstrate the obstructing tumors.

Altered Systemic Capillary Permeability

Any disease process that increases peripheral capillary permeability will allow the movement of proteins into the interstitial space and produce generalized peripheral edema.

Diabetes

Diabetes alters the basement membranes of capillaries, possibly as a result of glycosylation of basement membrane proteins. Peripheral edema may develop coincident with the onset of diffuse microangiopathy. Associated cardiac and renal disease may exacerbate sodium retention and enhance edema formation. The patient will have other physical manifestations of diabetes and demonstrate impaired glucose tolerance.

Angioedema

Angioedema is due to altered peripheral capillary permeability in response to histamine release. This is usually a local phenomenon, but some forms of angioedema may produce edema in a more generalized distribution. For example, the cold-induced urticaria-angioedema syndrome usually is a generalized phenomenon occurring after cold exposure. There are both hereditary and acquired forms of this disease. In response to a reduction in skin temperature, patients experience a pruritic urticarial eruption that may be diffuse and that may coalesce to produce generalized angioedema. The hereditary form is transmitted as an autosomal dominant gene, and a family history may suggest the diagnosis. In the acquired forms, which are the most common, the etiology remains obscure. Occasionally, this condition has been associated with cryoglobulinemia.

Septic Shock

Septic shock has also been associated with the diffuse "capillary leak syndrome" resulting from an increase in capillary permeability. Most commonly, this occurs with gram-negative sepsis. It is frequently associated with adult respiratory distress syndrome and probably shares similar capillary pathophysiology. Patients are usually quite ill and are frequently intubated on a medical intensive care unit. Peripheral edema in this condition may be exacerbated by positive pressure ventilation, which both increases venous hydrostatic pressure and reduces lymphatic flow to the thorax. Therapy should be aimed at treating the sepsis, and edema control is rarely a consideration.

Hypoproteinemic States

Any disease that reduces plasma oncotic pressure will tend to promote the production of peripheral edema. The role of reduced plasma oncotic pressure in the formation of the edema associated with nephrotic syndrome and with liver disease has been discussed previously.

Several other diseases may also lead to a reduction in plasma albumin and produce peripheral edema by similar mechanisms. For example, patients with *protein-calorie malnutrition* may have a sufficiently low plasma oncotic pressure to produce both ascites and peripheral edema. In children with kwashiorkor, edema may be localized to the lower extremities, but in severe cases the edema may be more generalized. In adults, a reduction in serum albumin may occur as a result of protein-calorie malnutrition due to anorexia, nausea, and vomiting, as well as impaired hepatic synthesis of albumin. Physical examination will frequently yield evidence of both dehydration and chronic malnutrition. Patients appear cachectic with significant loss of muscle mass and temporal wasting. In adults, protein-calorie malnutrition may occur in the setting of chronic alcoholism, malignant disease, malabsorption, protein-wasting enteropathy, or primary psychological disorders associated with impaired intake, such as anorexia nervosa. The physical examination may provide evidence of an underlying malignancy with hepatic metastases.

In *chronic alcoholism,* the stigmata of chronic liver disease are usually present. In contrast, *anorectic patients* are generally young and most often female and the diagnosis will be obvious by history. Serum protein will generally be lower than 6 gm/dl, and serum albumin falls below 2.8 gm/dl. The BUN:creatinine ratio may also be reduced from its normal value of 10:1 to less than 6:1. Other associated *nutritional deficiencies* and *anemia* are commonly associated with chronic alcoholism.

Drug-Related Edema

A variety of medications produce generalized edema. These drugs can be categorized into roughly four groups by their mechanisms of action. Drugs that promote renal sodium retention because of their mineralocorticoid-like effect include estrogen or progesterone-containing compounds (birth control pills) and corticosteroids. Second, many antihypertensive agents promote renal sodium retention, including the sympatholytic agents alpha methyl dopa, clonidine, guanethidine, and prazosin. Third, vasodilators such as hydralazine HCl, diazoxide, minoxidil, and nitrates are particularly potent in their sodium-retaining properties. Finally, nonsteroidal anti-inflammatory agents reduce sodium excretion in humans and may lead to the generation of peripheral edema.

LOCALIZED EDEMA

Localized edema, like generalized edema, occurs as a result of altered Starling forces. Local changes in hydrostatic pressure, capillary permeability, or lymphatic drainage are the most likely contributors to edema generation in a single extremity. Because of its localization, the underlying etiology of the edema is usually easily diagnosed. As in generalized edema, therapy should be directed to the underlying condition and not to the edema itself.

Venous Diseases

Venous Insufficiency

Venous insufficiency as a result of multiple varicosities produces an asymmetric pattern of edema that may involve one or both legs. Venous insufficiency may complicate deep venous thrombophlebitis, obesity, portal hypertension, or vena caval obstruction. When edema is due to varicosities, it frequently resolves with leg elevation at night and is exacerbated after prolonged upright posture. With chronic venous insufficiency, there may be an increase in pigmentation of the skin of the lower extremities, particularly in the pretibial region. Posterior tibialis and dorsalis pedis pulses are normal. The diagnosis is made by history and physical examination.

Deep Venous Thrombophlebitis

Deep venous thrombophlebitis is one of the most common causes of unilateral lower extremity edema. Edema occurs as a result of venous obstruction and local inflammation with changes in vascular permeability. Most often, thrombophlebitis occurs in previously diseased vessels, particularly when there is venous outflow obstruction in the pelvis or abdomen or from extrinsic compression by a ruptured Baker's cyst. Patients may give a history of previous trauma to the extremity or previous abdominal or pelvic surgery.

The pain of deep venous thrombophlebitis is acute in onset and frequently occurs after prolonged immobilization. The patient may be febrile, and the extremity is enlarged, erythematous, and warm. The opposite extremity should be used to compare size. Precise measurement of the circumference of the calf at a fixed point below the tibial plateau can be a useful parameter to follow. The extremity is usually tender and a venous "cord" may be palpable. Forceful dorsiflexion of the foot frequently produces pain in the calf (Homans' sign).

Another useful sign in distinguishing the pain of thrombophlebitis from other causes is to compress the calf against the tibia between the thumb and fingers. With deep vein thrombophlebitis, this maneuver will produce more pain than will compression of the muscles of the calf between the thumb and fingers without pressing against the tibia.

When deep venous thrombophlebitis is suspected, the diagnosis should be confirmed by venography or a Doppler flow study of the deep venous system. If a patient has recurrent episodes of deep venous thrombophlebitis without an obvious anatomic abnormality, other possible etiologies should be entertained. For example, tumors, compression by local lymph nodes, congenital venous bands, or localized joint disease may all contribute to the recurrence of thrombophlebitis.

Vascular Anomalies

Arteriovenous (AV) fistulae can produce edema localized to a single extremity. In dialysis patients, the creation of an AV fistula is frequently accompanied by temporary edema of the extremity. An increase in venous hydrostatic pressure and postsurgical disruption of lymphatic drainage probably contribute to this phenomenon. Some authors have postulated that an associated reflex autonomic dystrophy occurs after the creation of a fistula. In general, this is a self-limited process and eventually resolves.

Arteriovenous fistulae may also occur spontaneously or as a result of trauma. In the presence of a chronic fistula, the extremity is usually swollen and edematous and may be larger than the opposite limb. A thrill can be palpated, and a bruit is frequently audible in the involved extremity. An arteriogram will demonstrate the vascular anomaly.

Localized Lymphedema

Localized lymphedema can occur in any extremity, although lower extremities are much more commonly involved than upper extremities.

Primary Lymphedema

Primary lymphedema is a disease characterized by defective lymphatic drainage from an extremity. This disease may be inherited, or it may occur sporadically. Primary lymphedema may be congenital, or it may develop between the ages of 10 and 35 (lymphedema praecox) or after the age of 40 (lymphedema tarda). Of the inherited forms, lymphedema praecox is by far the most common. It is painless in onset, occurs most frequently in women, and usually begins insidiously with dorsal foot edema. This dorsal "hump" occurs typically at the onset of lymphedema.

The diagnosis can be established by family history, age of onset, and lymphangiography. The lymphangiogram will reveal hypoplasia in the vast majority of cases (approximately 80 per cent), hyperplasia and tortuosity in 5 to 10 per cent, and gross dilatation of the lymphatics in the remaining 5 to 10 per cent. Lymph node biopsy of the involved limb may reveal nodular fibrosis. Primary lymphedema is usually unilateral, but bilateral involvement may occur in as many as 20 per cent of cases.

Secondary Lymphedema

Secondary lymphedema occurs as a result of obstruction or recurrent infection and inflammation. Unless the thoracic or abdominal lymphatics are involved, the edema is usually localized to a single extremity. Obstruction of the lymphatics can occur following surgery or localized radiation therapy. Intralymphatic obstruction results from invasion by carcinoma, lymphoma, or granulomatous diseases including sarcoidosis, tuberculosis, lymphogranuloma venereum, and syphilis. In tropical climates, filariasis with the nematodes *Wuchereria bancrofti* and *Brugia malayi* is common and can produce massive lymphatic obstruction and subsequent elephantiasis. On occasion, synovitis, particularly when complicated by a ruptured Baker's cyst, can produce localized extrinsic lymphatic obstruction.

Local inflammation with lymphatic obstruction is most often confused with deep venous thrombophlebitis. A venogram may be useful in excluding venous disease. Appropriate cultures and serologies can help in the diagnosis of granulomatous diseases. When lymphedema occurs as a result of obstruction from tumor or granuloma, the patient may give a history consistent with a systemic illness and physical examination may reveal localized or diffuse lymphadenopathy. Following local radiation, overlying skin may demonstrate atrophic changes. Lymphedema complicating synovitis should be obvious by physical examination. Lymphangiography, CT scan, or ultrasound can usually define the anatomic causes of obstructions when present.

Lymphangitis

Lymphangitis may accompany cellulitis or lymphatic obstruction. Its onset is usually heralded by spiking fever with chills and the appearance of a systemic illness. An examination of the extremity reveals reddened lymphatic channels that appear as streaks from an area of central inflammation. Local lymphadenopathy is frequently present. Cellulitis and lymphangitis are also commonly confused with deep venous thrombophlebitis. Because of the obvious differences in treatment, these entities are important to distinguish. Again, a venogram is frequently required to demonstrate a lack of deep venous involvement.

Local Changes in Capillary Permeability

Ischemic Injury

Ischemic injury to a limb will increase capillary basement membrane permeability and produce local edema. Common causes of ischemic injury include trauma, surgery, atherosclerotic disease (particularly in diabetics), systemic emboli, vasculitis, and severe infections. History and physical examination should provide clues to the underlying etiology. Occasionally, occult mitral valvular stenosis will present with a systemic embolus that lodges in a peripheral artery. An echocardiogram can help evaluate mitral valve thickening, valve motion, and the presence or absence of valvular vegetations. Fungal endocarditis in drug abusers has, on occasion, presented with an ischemic extremity following the embolization of a large fungal vegetation.

Local Infection

Local infections such as cellulitis or lymphangitis will produce edema of the surrounding tissue. The area involved will be erythematous and warm. There may be evidence of previous trauma or a central area of vascular insufficiency. The intradermal injection of sterile saline using a 25-gauge needle followed by aspiration may yield identifiable organisms by Gram stain and culture. Blood cultures should be obtained as well. Cellulitis is most commonly due to either streptococcal or staphylococcal infections, but in diabetics, mixed aerobic and anaerobic infections are more common.

Autonomic Dysfunction

Several poorly understood syndromes associated with autonomic dysfunction may cause edema localized to an extremity. Edema may occur following a cerebrovascular accident or in association with one of the reflex sympathetic dystrophies. For example, the shoulder-hand syndrome may complicate an acute illness, typically a myocardial infarction or stroke, or it may follow trauma to the upper extremity. The acute onset of shoulder pain coincides with the onset of edema of the extremity (usually the hand). Alterations in autonomic tone affect both intravascular hydrostatic pressure and lymphatic drainage and may be responsible for the edema formation. Patients may experience intense pain, hyperesthesias, and marked vasomotor changes with vasodilatation, alternately followed by vasoconstriction in the extremity. Other autonomic changes occur in the limb as well. Therapy should be directed at the acute illness rather than at the edema.

DISORDERS MIMICKING PERIPHERAL EDEMA

Several disorders are characterized by swollen legs but without true pitting edema. For example, obese patients may have enlarged legs as a result of fat deposition but without edema. Lipedema is an unusual syndrome of severe, painful swelling of both legs, associated with obesity and rapid weight gain, that does not improve with rest or leg elevation. The legs are exquisitely tender to palpation. The skin is thickened and woody in appearance. However, the lymphatic drainage and venous drainage of the leg are normal.

Tumors may also cause swelling of the legs without edema. Benign tumors include cavernous venous hemangiomas, fibromyxomas, and lipomas. The most common malignant tumors that produce an enlarged leg without edema are the various sarcomas.

Myxedema is a unique form of "edema" that accompanies hypothyroidism and that can also be seen in a small percentage of patients with Graves' disease. Pretibial thickening of the skin that is nonpitting and that represents the subcutaneous deposition of mucopolysaccharides is present. Patients will have the signs and symptoms of thyroid disease, and a laboratory evaluation of thyroid function will confirm the diagnosis.

Other rare causes of an enlarged limb without edema include rupture of a gastrocnemius muscle and deep fungal infections.

SUMMARY

The presence of edema is common and represents an important clinical sign. Although the differential diagnosis of edema is extensive, a systematic approach to the patient can be based upon the distribution of edema. Since edema formation represents an alteration in the balance of Starling forces, the underlying disease processes can be evaluated in a simple and straightforward manner. One should not be satisfied with a diagnosis of "edema"; rather, the discovery of edema should prompt a search for its cause. Therapy should be guided by the underlying disease, and treatment of the edema should be reserved for those patients who are symptomatic. Only rarely does edema represent an actual threat to the patient's health, and in those few instances an attempt at therapy is appropriate.

ANEMIA

By Stephen H. Robinson, M.D.
Boston, Massachusetts

Very often an anemic patient may fail to have any significant symptoms or signs and the anemia is detected on the basis of routine blood counts. A logical laboratory evaluation based on two primary measurements, the red blood cell indices and the reticulocyte count, complemented by examination of the peripheral blood smear, will ordinarily lead to an understanding of the general nature of the anemia, which then can be confirmed by specific laboratory tests such as measurements of the serum iron and total iron-binding capacity (TIBC) and the serum concentrations of vitamin B_{12} and folic acid, or tests for different types of hemolytic anemia. Nevertheless, it remains important to inquire about pertinent symptoms and to investigate the patient for physical signs that may have discriminatory value in ascertaining the nature and cause of the anemia.

SYMPTOMS

As already mentioned, many patients have no symptoms even when the anemia is of moderate severity. This is presumably because the decrease in hemoglobin concentration has occurred over a relatively long period of time, permitting physiologic adaptation by the patient. A more precipitous decrease in hemoglobin concentration (and usually in intravascular blood volume as well)—e.g., with active gastrointestinal bleeding—may be accompanied by profound pallor, weakness, and indeed circulatory collapse.

Patients with more chronic forms of anemia may of course complain of fatigue and a decrease in exercise tolerance. They are sometimes noted to look pale by friends or family members, although pallor is a rather subjective criterion for anemia. It is not uncommon for older patients with anemia to present with cardiac symptoms such as angina or congestive heart failure. Myocardial oxygenation becomes impaired when the hematocrit falls below a level of about 30 per cent, often precipitating anginal pain in patients with preexisting coronary disease. Congestive heart failure is a fairly common mode of presentation in elderly patients with chronic anemia (e.g., pernicious anemia), in which the anemia leads to a high output state that finally exceeds the cardiac capacity.

In interviewing the patient with anemia, it is always worthwhile to ask several questions that may shed light on the cause of the problem. First, one should inquire about any history of gastrointestinal bleeding, since acute or chronic blood loss may lead to anemia with virtually any type of red blood cell indices. It is also useful to determine whether there is any past or family history of jaundice because this would suggest the possibility of congenital hemolytic disease. A history of the early development of gallstones in the patient or family members would also suggest the possibility of hemolytic anemia. Finally, one should inquire about pica, since a craving for ice, starch, or clay occurs in some patients with iron deficiency anemia.

PHYSICAL SIGNS

There are several physical signs that the physician should look for in the investigation of an anemic patient. The physician may try to gauge the presence or the severity of anemia by the degree of pallor of the conjunctiva, mucous membranes, or nail beds, but the laboratory determinations of course become the final arbiters of anemia. Severe anemia may sometimes be associated with mild fever and flame-shaped retinal hemorrhages. The presence of jaundice, which in the presence of anemia may impart a "lemon yellow" color to the patient's complexion, would suggest the presence of hemolysis or ineffective erythropoiesis (the destruction of early red cell precursors in the bone marrow).

A shiny, depapillated, red tongue (glossitis) is occasionally found in patients with severe iron deficiency or megaloblastic anemia. Indeed, patients with these disorders sometimes complain of a sore tongue. Glossitis is often accompanied by cheilosis (cracking and

Table 1. Blood Cell Values in a Normal Population

	Men	Women
White cell count, × $10^3/\mu l$ blood	7.25 (3.9–10.6)	7.28 (3.5–11.0)
Red cell count, × $10^6/\mu l$ blood	5.11 (4.4–5.9)	4.51 (3.8–5.2)
Hemoglobin, gm/dl blood	15.5 (13.7–17.7)	13.7 (11.7–15.7)
Volume packed RBC, ml/dl blood	46.0 (39.8–52.2)	40.9 (34.9–46.9)
Mean corpuscular volume, μm^3/red cell	90.1 (80.5–99.7)	90.4 (80.8–100.0)
Mean corpuscular hemoglobin, pg/red cell	30.2 (26.6–33.8)	30.2 (26.4–34.0)
Mean corpuscular hemoglobin concentration, gm/dl RBC	33.9 (31.5–36.3)	33.6 (31.4–35.8)
Platelet count, × $10^3/\mu l$ blood	248 (148–348)	248 (148–348)

*The range given is the mean ± 2 standard deviations. Adapted from Williams, W.T., et al.: *Hematology*, 3rd ed., New York, McGraw-Hill, 1983.

fissuring about the corners of the mouth), but both of these signs are rather nonspecific and may be found in a variety of states of nutritional deficiency. Koilonychia, i.e., concavity or "spooning" of the nails, is quite specific for iron deficiency anemia but is found only rarely and usually occurs with chronic, severe iron deficiency.

Lymphadenopathy would suggest the presence of an infectious or neoplastic process affecting the lymphoid organs, which might account for an accompanying anemia. Splenomegaly may be found in association with a large variety of hematologic problems, including different types of hemolysis, lymphoproliferative and myeloproliferative diseases, and certain infectious illnesses. It may occasionally be seen in deficiency states such as iron deficiency or pernicious anemia.

Nutritional anemias may be associated with peripheral neuropathies. Upper motor neuron defects, in particular when associated with loss of posterior column sensory modalities (such as position sense and especially vibration sense) in a patient with a macrocytic anemia, would strongly suggest that one is dealing with vitamin B_{12} deficiency. Under these circumstances, rapid diagnosis and therapy are indicated, because this "subacute combined systems disease" of vitamin B_{12} deficiency may be largely irreversible.

LABORATORY EVALUATION

Definition of the type of anemia usually rests on the laboratory findings. Table 1 presents normal basic hematologic values for men and women. There is some debate as to which index of anemia is the most useful. The packed cell volume, or hematocrit, when measured by centrifugation, is one of the most accurate measurements in clinical medicine. However, most clinical laboratories now utilize electronic counters and the hematocrit is measured as the product of the red blood cell count and mean corpuscular volume (MCV). The hemoglobin concentration is probably the most functional measurement of whether or not a patient is anemic. Indeed, in a mild hypochromic anemia such as that due to early iron deficiency, one may have a more or less normal hematocrit but a subnormal hemoglobin concentration because of the poor hemoglobinization of the packed erythrocytes. When measured electronically, the red blood cell count is quite an accurate measurement but is not commonly used to assess the degree of anemia.

If the laboratory values indicate that the patient is anemic, one should repeat the determinations to ensure that the values are correct and were not performed on another patient. Once having determined that the patient is indeed anemic and having searched for all possible clues in the history and physical examination, one would proceed to use the laboratory in a logical and cost-effective way in order to ascertain the type of anemia, after which more specific tests can be used to make a precise hematologic diagnosis. A general approach to the evaluation of the anemic patient is outlined in Table 2, and the following discussion is based on this approach.

The anemic patient should of course have a white blood cell and differential cell count as well as an estimate of platelet number to determine whether anemia is the sole hematologic problem or whether it is accompanied by abnormalities of the white cells and/or platelets as in the various forms of acute and chronic leukemia, aplastic anemia, or myelophthisic disorders. Focusing specifically on the red cell problem, we ask two major questions: What is the morphologic classification of the anemia, and is the anemia due to decreased red blood cell production or to increased red blood cell loss?

Morphologic Classification. If the red blood cells are microcytic and hypochromic, the anemia is due to

Table 2. Major Steps in the Diagnostic Evaluation of Anemia

1. Check white blood cell and differential count, platelet count
   Is anemia part of a more general hematologic problem (e.g., acute or chronic leukemia, aplastic anemia)?
2. Measure red cell indices; corroborate by blood smear (to look for heterogeneous population)
   Microcytic, hypochromic red blood cells
   - Iron deficiency
   - Chronic disease (infection, inflammation, malignancy)
   - Thalassemia
   - Sideroblastic anemia

   Macrocytic red blood cells
   - Reticulocytosis
   - Nonmegaloblastic
     - Liver disease
     - Hypothyroidism
     - Some instances of "aregenerative" anemias (e.g., aplastic anemia, acquired pure red cell aplasia)
     - Primary acquired sideroblastic anemia
   - Megaloblastic
     - Vitamin B_{12} or folic acid deficiency
     - Other causes

   Normochromic, normocytic red blood cells
   - Acute hemorrhage or hemolysis
   - Some cases of aregenerative anemia (aplastic anemia, acquired pure red cell aplasia)
   - Marrow replacement (leukemia, fibrosis, tumor)
   - "Secondary anemias"
     - Chronic disease
     - Renal insufficiency
     - Endocrine insufficiency (hypopituitarism, hypoadrenalism, hypogonadism)
3. Examine peripheral blood smear
   White blood cell and platelet number and morphology
   Red cell morphology
   - Size and shape
   - Different red cell populations
   - Polychromatophilia
   - Specific clues to diagnosis (e.g., spherocytes, red blood cell fragments)
4. Measure reticulocyte count
   Increased—marrow response to blood loss (hemorrhage or hemolysis); occasionally early release due to myelofibrosis, tumor invasion of marrow, or extramedullary hematopoiesis

   Decreased—inability of the marrow to respond to anemia (if sufficient time has elapsed for a reticulocyte response to occur)
5. Check several stool samples for occult blood
6. Bone marrow aspiration and biopsy
   Indicated when the etiology of the anemia remains unclear, to search for neoplastic disease involving the marrow, and to ascertain iron stores

a defect in hemoglobin synthesis. If the anemia is macrocytic and there is evidence of megaloblastic change, there is a disorder of DNA synthesis and cell division as in vitamin B_{12} or folic acid deficiency. If the red blood cells are normochromic and normocytic, multiple possibilities exist, as will be described.

Morphologic classification of the anemia is accomplished using the red blood cell indices—the MCV, mean corpuscular hemoglobin (MCH), and mean corpuscular hemoglobin concentration (MCHC)—which are now measured routinely and with great precision by the modern electronic counters that are used in most clinical hematology laboratories. Indeed, electronic measurement of the MCV can detect mild degrees of microcytosis or macrocytosis that cannot be appreciated by microscopic examination of the peripheral blood smear. Nevertheless, it is imperative that the peripheral blood smear be inspected microscopically in all instances of anemia. Electronic counters provide only the average value for the red cell size and hemoglobin content and therefore fail to discriminate the presence of more than a single red cell population, as might be found in a patient with acquired sideroblastic anemia. Moreover, characteristic and sometimes diagnostic changes in the size and shape of the red blood cell can be appreciated only through the microscope. For example, the presence of spherocytes in large numbers suggests that one is dealing with either congenital spherocytosis or immunohemolytic anemia. Moreover, abnormalities in white blood cell or platelet morphology may lead the physician to conclude that the anemia is part of a more global hematologic process, such as one of the forms of leukemia.

Production/Loss Classification. Is the anemia due to decreased red blood cell production or increased red cell loss? This is the second major question that one should ask when evaluating a patient with anemia. It is most simply answered by measuring the reticulocyte count in the peripheral blood, although it is sometimes necessary to examine the bone marrow for the degree of erythroid activity as well. A decreased or even a normal reticulocyte count in the presence of substantial anemia indicates that the bone marrow is not capable of a normal erythroid response and that the anemia is due at least in part to impaired bone marrow function. It must be kept in mind, however, that it takes a few days for a reticulocyte response to be generated in response to acute anemia and thus it may be necessary to wait 3 to 5 days to ensure that the marrow has had adequate time to respond to a recent anemic stress.

There are two general pathophysiologic causes of decreased red blood cell production by the bone marrow. When reticulocytopenia is accompanied by a decreased number of erythroid precursors in the bone marrow, one is dealing with erythroid hypoplasia. Occasionally, however, the decreased reticulocyte count in the peripheral blood is accompanied by an increased number of erythroid precursor cells in the marrow, a constellation of findings indicative of ineffective erythropoiesis. Ineffective erythropoiesis is observed in disorders such as megaloblastic anemia, thalassemia, and sideroblastic anemia; in these conditions, the abundant red blood cell precursors in the bone marrow are destroyed prematurely before they can mature into effective circulating reticulocytes.

When anemia is accompanied by an increase in the number of reticulocytes, the bone marrow is probably responding adequately and the anemia is doubtless due to an increased loss of red blood cells from the circulation. Most commonly, this is due to hemorrhage, underlining the importance of examining the patient for bleeding, particularly from the gastrointestinal tract. If there is no evidence of hemorrhage, the reticulocytosis is probably in response to hemolysis, i.e., an increased rate of red blood cell destruction. Hemolysis is associated not only with reticulocytosis but usually also with an increase in the serum concentrations of unconjugated bilirubin and lactate dehydrogenase (LDH), a decreased serum haptoglobin level, and often, but not always, characteristic changes in the morphology of the red blood cells on the peripheral smear.

Occasionally, one may see a mild factitious reticulocytosis that is not due to an effective bone marrow response to anemia but instead is the result of premature release of reticulocytes from an abnormal bone marrow compartment, e.g., a bone marrow that is compromised by the invasion of tumor cells or fibrous tissue or bone marrow proliferation that is taking place in extramedullary sites such as the liver or spleen. In these instances, however, the reticulocytosis is usually accompanied by characteristic changes in the peripheral blood including the presence of immature granulocytic forms, nucleated erythroid cells and abnormal red cell shapes, particularly teardrop-shaped erythrocytes.

TYPES OF ANEMIA

Let us now review briefly the major classes of anemia based on assessment of red cell size and hemoglobin content combined with the use of the reticulocyte count.

Microcytic, Hypochromic Anemias. If the red blood cell indices and peripheral smear indicate that the red blood cells are microcytic and hypochromic, one is doubtless dealing with one of four types of anemia, all of which are associated with characteristic changes in iron metabolism. Thus, identification of a microcytic and / or hypochromic anemia calls for measurement of the serum iron concentration and TIBC. It is frequently also important to determine whether iron stores are present in the bone marrow. This can be ascertained by direct marrow examination or, alternatively, by measurement of the serum ferritin concentration. Like bone marrow iron stores, serum ferritin concentrations are low with iron deficiency anemia and normal or high in the three other causes of microcytic hypochromic anemia.

Iron deficiency anemia is by far the most common cause of microcytic hypochromic anemia or, indeed, of anemia in general. (See article on this topic.) In this condition the serum iron is low, the TIBC high, bone marrow iron stores are depleted, and serum ferritin concentrations are low.

In the *anemia of chronic disease,* there is a defect in the reutilization of iron released from senescent red blood cells, leading to a low serum iron associated with normal or increased bone marrow iron stores and serum ferritin concentration. Characteristically, the TIBC is low. This abnormality in iron reutilization gives rise to hypochromia (and, less commonly, microcytosis) in only somewhat fewer than half of all patients with anemia due to chronic infection, inflammatory states, or malignant disease.

The *thalassemias* are reviewed in detail in a later article. Briefly, these are a group of hereditary disorders of hemoglobin synthesis that occur primarily in Mediterranean and Asiatic people. In the heterozygous or minor form of thalassemia, the patient may be only minimally anemic but the red blood cell indices nevertheless show marked microcytosis and the peripheral blood smear may reveal prominent red cell abnormalities including microcytes, target cells, and other unusual red cell forms. The thalassemias, particularly the severe homozygous forms of the disease, are usually associated with iron-loading, and the serum iron is typically high, often almost saturating a normal or somewhat subnormal TIBC.

Increased iron stores and an elevated serum iron are also characteristic of the group of disorders known as the *sideroblastic anemias.* The diagnostic feature of this group of disorders is the presence of ringed sideroblasts, i.e., red cell precursors with a ring of iron granules surrounding the nucleus, found on Prussian blue stain of the bone marrow aspirate. Sideroblastic anemia may be found in a number of settings. (See later article on this topic.) In its most common form, primary acquired sideroblastic anemia, there is often a dimorphic red cell population in which hypochromic cells are accompanied by macrocytic erythrocytes;

thus, the red cell indices may show a mild macrocytic anemia and the hypochromia may not be evident unless one examines the peripheral blood smear.

Macrocytic Anemias. Mild degrees of macrocytosis (with the MCV usually less than 105) may be found with *reticulocytosis,* since immature reticulocytes leave the bone marrow prematurely in response to anemia. This should be evident in the form of polychromatophilia (large gray erthrocytes) on inspection of the peripheral blood smear and can be further documented by doing a reticulocyte count.

Inspection of the peripheral blood smear should also reveal whether a macrocytic anemia is associated with megaloblastic changes. In well-developed instances of *megaloblastic anemia* (see later article), the MCV will usually be very high, in excess of 110 and sometimes as high as 120 to 130. However, milder or earlier cases may be associated with only minor degrees of macrocytosis. In megaloblastic anemias, there is often a heterogeneous array of red cell shapes and sizes, including a population of oval macrocytes on the peripheral smear. There is almost invariably hypersegmentation of the neutrophils, i.e., forms containing six or more discrete lobes. Finally, megaloblastic anemias are usually associated with leukopenia and thrombocytopenia as well as anemia. Confirmation of the fact that the patient has a megaloblastic process can be obtained by examining a bone marrow aspirate for characteristic morphologic abnormalities.

Macrocytosis, usually of moderate degree, may also be seen in the absence of reticulocytosis or megaloblastic change. In these instances, the peripheral blood smear usually shows round rather than oval macrocytes and the MCV is characteristically less than 110. Perhaps the most common cause of nonmegaloblastic macrocytic anemia is the *anemia of liver disease.* Occasionally one may see this kind of macrocytosis in anemia associated with *hypothyroidism,* although several different forms of anemia have been associated with the latter disorder. As mentioned, many patients with *primary acquired sideroblastic anemia* have moderate macrocytosis in addition to a population of hypochromic erythrocytes. Finally, many patients with "aregenerative" anemias (e.g., aplastic anemia, acquired pure red cell aplasia, or the anemia seen after the administration of marrow suppressive drugs) may be mildly to moderately macrocytic. In these instances and in the sideroblastic anemias, the macrocytes appear to represent erythroid cells released prematurely from a bone marrow containing relatively few normal erythroid precursor cells that are responding to large amounts of erythropoietin. Paradoxically, the reticulocyte count in these patients is usually not increased.

Normochromic, Normocytic Anemias. When the red cell indices reveal a normochromic normocytic anemia, the physician confronts a broad array of diagnostic possibilities. Indeed, the same type of anemia may present with different red cell indices in different patients so that the same disorder is sometimes listed in more than one morphologic category (Table 2).

In the case of *acute hemorrhage or hemolysis,* before substantial reticulocytosis ensues, the red cells will be of normal size and will show a normal hemoglobin content unless previous hemorrhage has produced some iron deficiency. Reticulocytosis will then lead to the presence of polychromatophils on the peripheral smear and usually mildly macrocytic red cell indices. Although some patients with *aregenerative anemias* (such as aplastic anemia or pure red cell aplasia) have macrocytic cells, others have normochromic normocytic erythrocytes. The *anemia of chronic disease,* usually implying chronic infection, inflammatory disease or malignancy, is hypochromic only about 40 per cent of the time and only rarely is substantially microcytic and hypochromic; even though the characteristic defect in iron reutilization is generally present, the red cells in these patients are most commonly normochromic and normocytic. The anemia that accompanies *marrow replacement* by leukemia, fibrosis, or tumor is usually also normochromic and normocytic, as are the anemias that accompany *renal or endocrine insufficiency.*

Thus, particularly when anemia is normochromic and normocytic, one must rely on the reticulocyte count to help determine whether the anemia is due to decreased red blood cell production or to increased red blood cell loss, always keeping in mind the fact that increased loss will engender a reticulocyte response only after several days. Measurement of the serum iron and TIBC may help to implicate a chronic disorder. In other instances, a bone marrow aspiration and biopsy may be necessary to determine whether abnormal cells are present in the marrow compartment.

COMMENTS ON LABORATORY TESTS

Peripheral Blood Smears. As indicated earlier, microscopic examination of a well-prepared and stained peripheral blood smear is essential in the evaluation of all anemic patients. This will allow the physician to examine the white cells and platelets for abnormalities in either number or morphology and the red cells for polychromatophilia, characteristic changes in size and shape, and the presence of different red cell populations that might not be reflected by the red blood cell indices. Moreover, only by examining the peripheral smear will one be able to detect specific morphologic abnormalities of the red blood cell such as spherocytes, red blood cell fragments, teardrop deformity, or other abnormalities that may point to a specific hematologic diagnosis.

Reticulocyte Count. We have already referred to the importance of doing a reticulocyte count in virtually all anemic patients in order to determine whether the cause of the anemia is decreased red blood cell production in the bone marrow or increased loss (hemorrhage or hemolysis) from the peripheral blood. We have also indicated the occasional instances in which a mild reticulocytosis is due to early release of these cells from a bone marrow that is compromised by tumor or fibrosis or from red blood cell production in extramedullary locations.

The reticulocyte count is expressed as the percentage of the total red blood cells that contain RNA, as determined by staining with a dye such as new methylene blue. However, this does not take into account the fact that the patient may be severely anemic with a marked reduction in the red cell count. A so-called "absolute" reticulocyte count may be calculated by multiplying percentage of reticulocytes by the total red blood cell count. This value then has to be corrected for the early release of reticulocytes that occurs with the response of the bone marrow to erythropoietin in anemic states. Because these bone marrow reticulocytes now persist in the peripheral blood for 2 or 3 days rather than the 1 day during which normal reticulocytes lose their RNA, the absolute reticulocyte count must be divided by a factor of 2 or 3 in the presence of marked reticulocytosis and polychromatophilia. Correcting the reticulocyte percentage for the total red blood cell count and for the premature entry of marrow reticulocytes into the peripheral blood yields a "reticulocyte index," which serves as a reliable estimate of effective new red blood cell production by the bone marrow.

Testing Stool Samples for Occult Blood. Testing several stool samples over a prolonged period of time is important in any patient in whom the cause of anemia is unclear. It is an essential procedure in male or postmenopausal female patients with iron deficiency anemia. Gastrointestinal bleeding is a very common cause of anemia and may of course represent an early sign of malignancy in the gastrointestinal tract. It should be emphasized that the bleeding may be intermittent and several negative stool samples do not eliminate the possibility that the patient has bled in the past and may bleed again in the future.

Blood loss can produce anemia with virtually any kind of red cell indices. Acute loss of blood before there is a reticulocyte response produces a normochromic normocytic picture. When a reticulocyte response occurs, the indices may show mild macrocytosis. With chronic bleeding, iron deficiency may ensue and produce a microcytic hypochromic anemia. With both acute and chronic blood loss, reticulocytosis and iron deficiency may coexist and, depending upon the severity of the two processes, the red cell indices might fall in any category; however, examination of the peripheral blood smear should show both polychromatophilia and a microcytic hypochromic population of red blood cells.

Bone Marrow Examination. This is not required in all or even most patients with anemia, since the diagnosis can often be made on the basis of the red cell indices, peripheral blood smear, reticulocyte count, and the more specific tests (e.g., serum iron and TIBC, serum bilirubin and haptoglobin concentrations, serum vitamin B_{12} and folic acid levels) that these call into play. When the cause of anemia remains obscure, however, the bone marrow may reveal the presence of neoplastic diseases, dysplastic changes consistent with a "preleukemic" disorder, or other abnormalities best discernible by marrow examination. Moreover, the iron stain will indicate whether or not the patient is iron deficient if this issue remains in doubt on the basis of the serum iron and TIBC. In addition, one may find ringed sideroblasts when individual red blood cell precursors stained for iron are examined under high magnification, yielding a diagnosis of sideroblastic anemia. Unless a bone marrow aspiration is being performed primarily to assess iron stores, a trephine biopsy is usually also indicated, since this is the most sensitive means of discerning the presence of neoplastic cells in the marrow compartment.

LYMPHADENOPATHY

By Charles E. Hess, M.D.
Charlottesville, Virginia

INTRODUCTION

From a diagnostic standpoint, lymphadenopathy presents one of the most challenging problems in all of clinical medicine. Not only are enlarged lymph nodes frequently missed on physical examination, more importantly, a systematic approach is often not followed when these patients are evaluated. Too often a lymph node biopsy is either performed unnecessarily or not done when clearly indicated to establish a diagnosis.

DIAGNOSTIC APPROACH

The major decision in most cases is whether or not to perform a lymph node biopsy to rule out a malignant neoplastic process. If the lymphadenopathy is localized and is secondary to inflammation in the area drained by the enlarged lymph node or nodes, or if generalized and secondary to a well-defined systemic illness (e.g., viral infection, systemic lupus erythematosus), a lymph node biopsy is generally not indicated. When making this decision, there are several factors that are very helpful; these include: (1) age of the patient, (2) clinical history, (3) physical examination, (4) anatomic location and extent of the lymphadenopathy, and (5) proper selection of laboratory investigations that may establish a diagnosis without the need for lymph node biopsy.

Age of Patient. Hypertrophy of lymph nodes and other lymphoid tissue (e.g., adenoids, tonsils) is often a normal physiologic process in infants and children. In addition, the occurrence and extent of lymphadenopathy in response to a variety of stimuli such as viral and bacterial infections and vaccinations are much greater in infants and children than in adults. This age difference is of such importance to warrant an almost totally different diagnostic approach to patients before and after puberty. In children with either localized or generalized lymphadenopathy, an infectious cause usually is easy to demonstrate and lymph node biopsy is not indicated. Other than treatment of the underlying infection when indicated, follow-up to document resolution of the lymphadenopathy is all that is needed.

The strikingly enlarged lymph nodes that are seen in infectious mononucleosis in young adults should not be biopsied if the clinical history, physical findings, and, more importantly, the serologic studies are consistent with that diagnosis. Not only is lymph node biopsy unnecessary to make a diganosis, but histiopathologic interpretation of these lymph nodes presents a very difficult differential diagnostic problem, particularly when attempting to distinguish the changes from those found in non-Hodgkin's lymphomas, Waldenström's macroglobulinemia, and lymphocyte-predominant Hodgkin's disease. Other reactive processes (e.g., postvaccinal lymphadenitis, syphilis, toxoplasmosis, drug-induced lymphadenopathy) present similar problems with histiopathologic interpretation. Because of these problems, most hematopathologists will demand the results of a careful history and physical examination and a serologic test for syphilis, toxoplasmosis, and heterophile antibody before rendering a final interpretation in such cases.

Clinical History. A careful clinical history is invaluable in the evaluation of the patient with lymphadenopathy and frequently leads one to a correct diagnosis without the need for lymph node biopsy. The mode of onset and the duration of the lymphadenopathy are very important factors. In addition, specific inquiries regarding drugs, allergies, animal exposure, and occupation should be made. Tender, painful lymph nodes that appear and progress over a period of a few days or weeks are often secondary to an inflammatory process in the area drained by the lymph nodes. The diagnosis in such patients may be obvious, as in a patient with unilateral cervical lymphadenopathy secondary to dental infection, or it may be very difficult, as in a patient with cat-scratch fever with lymphadenopathy involving the epitrochlear, axillary, and supraclavicular areas if a history of exposure to cats is not obtained.

Enlarged nontender lymph nodes in the epitrochlear, axillary, femoral, and inguinal areas are often seen in patients with certain occupations in which recurrent and usually minor injury to the extremities occurs. Generalized and usually asymptomatic lymphadenopathy also is found in patients with such chronic dermatologic disorders as eczema. The lymphadenopathy that occurs as a part of the hypersensitivity reaction to anticonvulsant drugs presents a particularly difficult clinical and histiopathologic diagnostic problem; the atypical hyperplasia in these lymph nodes may be very difficult and at times impossible to distinguish from Hodgkin's disease. If the lymphadenopathy does not regress after the drug is stopped, a repeat biopsy is recommended.

Physical Examination. The physical examination is equally important. One should become very familiar with the normal anatomy of the lymphatic system. In general, a lymph node that is larger than 1 cm in diameter should be considered enlarged. When palpating for enlarged lymph nodes, the physician must "take off the boxing gloves." Lymph nodes that are only minimally enlarged or fixed to underlying tissue may not be appreciated if one does not use a "gentle" approach; enlarged supraclavicular and axillary nodes are missed most frequently (a Valsalva maneuver may aid in detecting supraclavicular lymphadenopathy).

The size, shape, and consistency of lymph nodes are also very important when deciding whether to do lymph node biopsy or which lymph node to biopsy. Lymph nodes that are enlarged but flat, smooth, and relatively soft are usually normal or show only hyperplasia if biopsied. When the enlarged lymph node is irregular and has a rubbery or hard consistency, biopsy usually reveals involvement by a malignant neoplastic process, such as lymphoma or carcinoma, or by sarcoidosis.

Enlarged, tender lymph nodes are usually secondary to infection, either primary in the lymph node or in the area drained by the lymph node. One must keep in mind, however, that patients with lymphoma, particularly with Hodgkin's disease, may occasionally present with tender, painful lymphadenopathy. If the enlarged lymph node is fluctuant and is not secondary to an obvious distal site of infection, a needle aspiration for special stains and culture will often give a diagnosis and thus avoid the need for biopsy; a diagnosis of tuberculous lymphadenitis can often be made by aspiration alone. In lymphadenitis secondary to bacterial infection, the lymph node may become very large and fluctuant, particularly in children, and require incision and drainage as part of the treatment.

A careful examination for the presence of splenomegaly or hepatomegaly, or both, should be performed in all patients with lymphadenopathy. The presence of splenomegaly usually indicates a systemic process (e.g., infectious mononucleosis, chronic lymphocytic leukemia, lymphoma) and will often direct attention to investigative studies other than lymph node biopsy that will lead to the diagnosis.

Anatomic Location and Extent of Lymphadenopathy. When lymphadenopathy is confined to one lymph node region or when it involves two or more regions that are contiguous with each other, a thorough knowledge of disorders that are known to affect lymph nodes and other structures in that particular area is invaluable. An effort should be made to eliminate inflammatory disease before performing a diagnostic lymph node biopsy. Unilateral lymphadenopathy in the neck or in an extremity is often due to infection of structures drained by those lymph nodes (inguinal lymphadenopathy secondary to an infected wound of that extremity, an enlarged submental node secondary to tooth abscess).

There are situations in which an infectious cause, although highly suspected, cannot be established; in such instances, only treatment of the infection when indicated and close follow-up to document resolution of the lymphadenopathy are required. In cat-scratch fever, the distribution of the lymphadenopathy (unilateral involvement of the epitrochlear, axillary, and supraclavicular lymph nodes) and the clinical course, if associated with a history of a cat scratch or just contact with a cat, constitute a good example of such a disorder. A similar clinical picture may be seen in rat-bite fever, bubonic plague, sporotrichosis, anthrax, or rickettsial disease or with any infective agent for which the portal of entry is the skin.

There are several nonmalignant disorders that show a predilection for certain lymph node regions; these include rubella, oculoglandular syndrome, sinus histiocytosis with massive lymphadenopathy, syphilis, sarcoidosis, pneumoconiosis, angiofollicular mediastinal lymph node hyperplasia, lymphogranuloma venereum, and acute mesenteric lymphadenitis. In *rubella,* enlarged posterior auricular—and, less commonly, suboccipital and posterior cervical—lymph nodes are very characteristic and in certain instances a diagnostic finding. *Oculoglandular syndrome* involves anterior auricular lymphadenopathy associated with a variety of inflammatory lesions of the eyelids and conjunctivae (e.g., rubella, trachoma, cat-scratch fever).

Sinus histiocytosis with massive lymphadenopathy is a benign disorder of unknown cause that occurs in children and young adults and is characterized by painless massive cervical lymphadenopathy, usually bilateral; fever; neutrophilia; and an elevated erythrocyte sedimentation rate (ESR). The lymphadenopathy progresses slowly over a period of a few weeks to several months and regresses after 6 months to several years. Histiopathologically, there is marked histiocytic infiltration in the sinuses of the lymph node; a biopsy is necessary to rule out a malignant neoplastic process.

The bilateral epitrochlear lymphadenopathy of *syphilis* has long been considered of diagnostic importance in secondary syphilis but is more commonly due to recurrent injury to the hands in people who do manual labor; lymph node biopsy generally is not indicated. Bilateral hilar lymphadenopathy in an asymptomatic patient or in association with erythema nodosum is so characteristic of *sarcoidosis* that a diagnosis usually can be made without biopsy confirmation. Close follow-up for several months is mandatory, however, to document resolution. In *pneumoconiosis,* the parenchymal lung involvement is frequently accompanied by bilateral hilar lymphadenopathy. *Angiofollicular mediastinal lymph node hyperplasia (Castleman's disease)* is a disorder characterized by the presence of either a large solitary mediastinal mass or intra-abdominal involvement. Biopsy reveals an atypical hyperplasia, with either an interfollicular plasma cell infiltration or a hyaline-vascular pattern. The disorder is usually self-limiting, but a biopsy for documentation and close follow-up is necessary.

In *lymphogranuloma venereum,* unilateral inguinal lymph node enlargement is a characteristic finding. *Acute mesenteric lymphadenitis* is characterized by recurrent abdominal pain in children and young adults and often mimics acute appendicitis.

Lymphadenopathy that is confined to certain lymph node regions also has diagnostic importance in the evaluation of a patient for a suspected malignant neoplasm. Isolated supraclavicular lymphadenopathy is frequently due to either metastases from an intrathoracic or intra-abdominal malignant neoplasm or malignant lymphoma. Generally, isolated left supraclavicular lymphadenopathy is seen more with intra-abdominal malignant neoplasms, whereas isolated right supraclavicular lymph node involvement is seen more often with intrathoracic malignant lesions. Even in the absence of palpable lymphadenopathy, a scalene node or "fat-pad" biopsy may be very helpful in the evaluation of intrathoracic lesions.

Intra-abdominal or retroperitoneal lymphadenopathy, particularly if gross enough to be felt on physical examination of the abdomen, is usually due to a malignant process. Abdominal exploration and biopsy should be performed if necessary to establish a diagnosis. If a malignant lymphoma is found, a staging procedure (splenectomy, bone marrow biopsy, and multiple liver biopsies) may be indicated, particularly in cases of Hodgkin's disease, and should be performed at the same time. Patients with moderate to marked enlargement of retroperitoneal lymph nodes often present with backache. If the back pain is associated with other findings (e.g., fever, weight loss, night sweats), a thorough search should be made for retroperitoneal lymphadenopathy. The bipedal lymphangiogram and, more recently, sonography and computed tomography of the abdomen and pelvis have aided greatly in the diagnosis of intra-abdominal lymphadenopathy. If these tests are normal, intra-abdominal lymphadenopathy essentially is eliminated. Isolated mesenteric lymphadenopathy may escape detection by all of these techniques, and require abdominal exploration to document.

Generalized lymphadenopathy, defined as involvement of two or more noncontiguous lymph node regions, occurs in a variety of disorders. Not only is lymph node biopsy unnecessary in many instances, but if performed, it usually reveals only nonspecific histiopathologic change. Disorders frequently associated with generalized lymphadenopathy include viral infections, toxoplasmosis, dermatopathic lymphadenopathy, connective tissue disorders, chronic lymphocytic leukemia, malignant lymphomas, and sarcoidosis.

In *viral infections,* generalized lymphadenopathy occurs much more frequently in children and young adults than in older adults. In most of these infections the diagnosis can be made from the clincal course of the illness (e.g., rubella, rubeola). The diagnosis of infectious mononucleosis usually requires examination of a peripheral blood smear for presence of atypical lymphocytes and a serologic test for heterophil antibody. Diagnosis can be very difficult if the clinical findings suggest infectious mononucleosis and the test for heterophil antibody is negative. There are several viral infections that can produce this "seronegative infectious mononucleosis-like illness" (e.g., cytomegalovirus, viral hepatitis, adenovirus, influenza). A lymph node biopsy is not helpful except to rule out a malignant neoplastic process.

The acquired form of *toxoplasmosis* frequently presents with generalized lymphadenopathy. The clinical course may mimic infectious mononucleosis (approximately 10 per cent of seronegative infectious mononucleosis is due to toxoplasmosis). The diagnosis is established by demonstrating a rise and fall in antibody titer to the protozoan *Toxoplasma gondii* using the toxoplasmosis dye test; the titers may not start to rise for 3 weeks after onset of illness. A high titer that does not change with time may occasionally be found in lymphomas. A lymph node biopsy is usually performed in most patients because of the long course of the illness and the prominence of the lymphadenopathy, especially in the cervical area. Although the histiopathologic findings are not pathognomonic (hyperplasia and aggregation of histiocytes in and around germinal centers), they are characteristic and should lead to other studies to establish the diagnosis. The cysts or organisms of *T. gondii* are rarely seen in the sections.

Dermatopathic lymphadenopathy is seen most often with exfoliative dermatitis and mycosis fungoides. Lymph node biopsy is frequently necessary in patients with mycosis fungoides to evaluate for systemic spread of this lymphoma. Of the *connective tissue disorders,* generalized lymphadenopathy is most often seen in active rheumatoid arthritis and systemic lupus erythematosus. Unless an associated malignant neoplastic process is suspected, a lymph node biopsy is not indicated.

A cardinal feature of *chronic lymphocytic leukemia* is generalized lymphadenopathy. A lymph node biopsy is not indicated, since the peripheral blood and bone marrow findings are diagnostic. With *malignant lymphomas,* generalized lymphadenopathy is much more common in non-Hodgkin's lymphomas, particularly in the more differentiated lymphocytic types. A lymph node biopsy and interpretation, preferably by a hematopathologist, is necessary for diagnosis.

Although generalized lymphadenopathy is one of the most characteristic clinical findings in *sarcoidosis,* a lymph node biopsy is indicated in most patients to confirm the diagnosis. Because of the increased incidence of nonspecific granulomatous reactions in lymph nodes and other organs in Hodgkin's disease, multiple lymph node biopsies may be indicated to eliminate Hodgkin's disease if the clinical course is atypical for sarcoidosis.

Other disorders such as bacterial infections (brucellosis, secondary syphilis, leptospirosis), hypersensitivity drug reactions (anticonvulsant drugs), and hyperthyroidism may occasionally be associated with generalized lymphadenopathy.

Laboratory Investigation. A thorough knowledge of which laboratory studies to obtain on the basis of the clinical features of a particular patient is mandatory in order to arrive at a diagnosis promptly and avoid unnecessary lymph node biopsies. Most of these studies, and the clinical situations in which they should be performed, have been mentioned in this article. Generally, before a lymph node is biopsied, a white blood cell count and a careful inspection of a peripheral blood smear should be done. The selection of other studies before making a decision to do a lymph node biopsy must be individualized (e.g., a bone marrow biopsy and aspiration is preferred to lymph node biopsy if leukemia is suspected).

LYMPH NODE BIOPSY PROCEDURE

Once a decision is made to perform a lymph node biopsy, there are certain guidelines that must be followed in order to obtain the information necessary to make a diagnosis. The selection of which lymph node to biopsy is critical. Because of the chronic changes (such as scarring) that are frequently present in lymph nodes in the inguinal region, biopsy in this area should be avoided if possible. In general, the largest lymph node in the area selected for biopsy should be removed. All too often, smaller nodes are removed that show only reactive changes secondary to a malignant neoplastic process in a larger, adjacent lymph node; this is particularly true in Hodgkin's disease. Multiple lymph node biopsies are indicated in some patients to rule out a malignant neoplastic process. These repeat biopsies may be indicated during the initial work-up or on follow-up if the lymphadenopathy progresses.

Proper handling and processing of the lymph node also is very important. The specimen should be placed in formalin as soon as possible and fixed for 24 hours. Because of the slow penetration of the formalin, larger lymph nodes should be sectioned into smaller pieces prior to being placed in the formalin. If a frozen section is desired, only a portion of the lymph node should be submitted for this study, the rest being processed as just discussed. If lymph node imprints are obtained, the lymph node should be sectioned one or more times prior to being placed in formalin. Several "touch" preparations and smears should be made for Wright stain and other special stains (e.g., periodic acid-Schiff [PAS], nonspecific esterase) as indicated. These preparations are helpful in the subclassification of non-Hodgkin's lymphomas.

Other studies that are helpful in the differential diagnosis of malignant neoplastic disorders, but unfortunately are available only in certain centers at the present time, include electron microscopy and immunologic studies (e.g., immunofluorescent stains, lymphocyte typing). Lymph node cultures are not indicated routinely but are important studies to obtain if the clinical manifestations suggest an infectious process or if the lymph node reveals necrosis when sectioned.

APPROACH TO GENETIC DISEASE

By Kenneth W. Dumars, M.D.
Irvine, California

The subjects of disease and/or malformations due to genetic mechanisms have not received major emphasis in medical education, for even today approximately 25 per cent of medical schools offer no formal course in medical genetics. It is this author's bias that many physicians regard inherited disease with a degree of finality not characteristic of their perception of a severe infection or even a neoplastic disorder; after all, they might ask, whoever considered altering one's genetic material? The approach that "you shouldn't tamper with Mother Nature" is under challenge. For now, the science of genetics is focusing on how to prevent disease by turning a gene on or off, for example, the sickle cell gene. Genetics is on the threshold of identifying persons at risk for degenerative disease such as cancer, or replacing missing enzymes that are responsible for inborn errors of metabolism, such as phenylketonuria or mucopolysaccharidosis. Parents who are normal in appearance and in function but are at risk for delivering a genet-

Table 1. Mendelian Disorders*

Mode of Inheritance	Verschuer 1958†	1966 (1st ed.)	1968 (2nd ed.)	1971 (3rd ed.)	1975 (4th ed.)	1978 (5th ed.)	1983 (6th ed.)
Autosomal Dominant	285	269 (+568)‡	344 (+449)	415 (+528)	583 (+635)	736 (+753)	934 (+893)
Autosomal Recessive	89	237 (+294)	280 (+349)	365 (+418)	466 (+481)	521 (+596)	588 (+710)
X-linked	39	68 (+51)	68 (+55)	86 (+64)	93 (+78)	107 (+98)	115 (+128)
Total	412	574 (+913)	692 (+853)	866 (+1,010)	1,142 (+1,194)	1,364 (+1,447)	1,637 (+1,731)
Grand Total	412	1,487	1,545	1,876	2,336	2,811	3,368

* Adapted from McKusick, V.A.: *Mendelian Inheritance in Man: Catalogs of Autosomal Dominant, Autosomal Recessive and X-Linked Phenotypes*, 6th ed. Baltimore, Johns Hopkins University Press, 1983.

† *Lehrbuch der Humangenetik.* Munich: Urban and Schwartzenberg, 1958.

‡ Numbers in parentheses refer to unasterisked entries; the other numbers refer to asterisked entries, which are considered to represent confirmed loci.

ically handicapped child can be identified. Genetic technology is rapidly expanding the number of mutant genes which can be detected in the *heterozygous* or carrier state prior to conception and in the *homozygous* conceptus.

This article will briefly describe and include:

1. The frequency of genetic disorders.
2. A genetic work-up.
3. Genetic mechanisms of disease transmission.
4. Signs and symptoms that should trigger a physician's suspicion that a disease is genetic in origin.
5. A glossary of genetic terms.

FREQUENCY OF GENETIC DISEASE

Information on the frequency of genetic disease in society is necessary for a number of reasons. It is essential for our understanding of chronic illness that is caused by genetic mechanisms. It is a starting point for our assessment of the burden within the societal gene pool. And finally, population surveillance allows monitoring the manifestations of mutant genes that may be affected by the environment, specifically chemical mutagens and the proliferation of nuclear energy and exposure to radiation.

A number of population studies estimate that 9.4 of each 100 liveborn infants will suffer from a genetic disease during their lifetime. Precise data regarding the frequency of genetic disorders are difficult to obtain because of late onset of many genetic diseases, lack of knowledge regarding precise mode of inheritance, and failure of ascertainment because of incomplete or inaccurate vital records. McKusick's catalogs* of mendelian disorders will enhance accurate statistics. Over the past 25 years, there has been an almost tenfold increase in the number of mendelian disorders recognized (Table 1). There is no absolute increase in the incidence of genetic disease, for many disorders formerly regarded as "congenital malformations" or "mental retardation of unknown origin" are now recognized as specific entities resulting from mendelian or chromosomal, or multifactorial, inheritance.

Current data indicate that 22 per 10,000 liveborn infants will suffer from a mendelian disorder; 20 per 10,000 from chromosomal anomalies causing detectable defects:† 428 per 10,000 from congenital malformations; and 473 per 10,000 from other multifactorial malformations. The majority of children affected by genetic disease(s) will be recognized within the first year of life; however, it is estimated that of the 9.4 per 100 live-born infants affected, 12 per cent of these (120 per 10,000 live-born infants) will suffer from a genetic disorder that will not be manifest until after age 20.

Additional data indicate that 40 to 50 per cent of all spontaneous abortions are due to chromosome anomalies. An indication of the societal economic burden is revealed by studies of hospital admissions; approximately 30 per cent of admissions to children's hospitals are for the management of genetic disease.

GENETIC WORK-UP

As with any medical evaluation, following a routine is advisable. A genetic work-up is time-consuming and requires the following:

1. A family pedigree.
2. Complete medical evaluation of the proband and oftentimes other members of the family.
3. Appropriate laboratory, radiologic, histopathologic, and electrodiagnostic procedures.
4. Treatment plan to include informing the proband/family, specific therapies, and/or supportive care.

Family Pedigree. Constructing a family pedigree, using universally accepted symbols, is the first and most important step in a genetic work-up (Fig. 1). Initially, it is useful to review the clinical aspects of the disease in question. Preface the drawing of a family

*McKusick, V. A.: *Mendelian Inheritance in Man: Catalogs of Autosomal Dominant, Autosomal Recessive and X-Linked Phenotypes,* 6th ed. Baltimore and London, Johns Hopkins University Press, 1983. This contribution is a necessity on every medical geneticist's bookshelf. An invaluable compendium providing excellent references.

†The greater frequency (given in a later article) 0.5 per cent applies to all chromosome abnormalities, including balanced translocations—which do not produce abnormalities in the carrier.

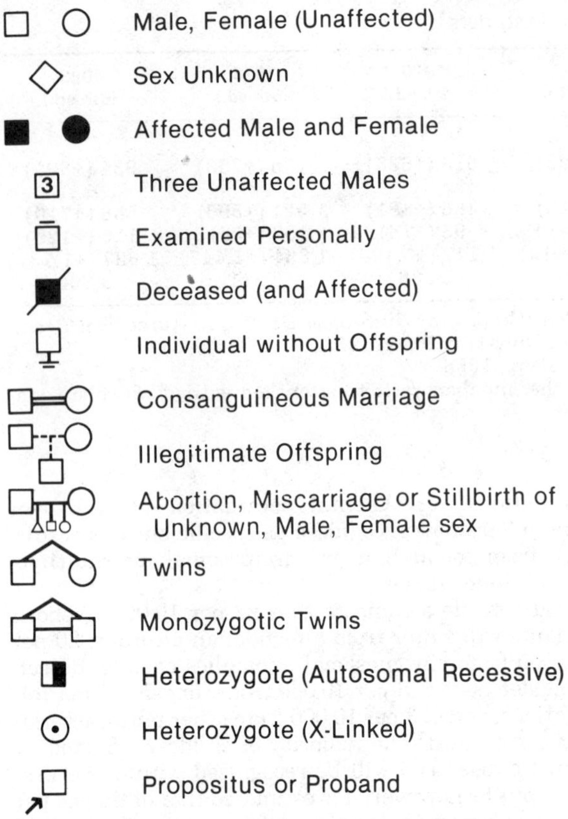

Figure 1. Symbols to be used in compiling pedigree.

pedigree with an explanation as to information needed and allow the consultand to observe drawing. In addition to information about the familial occurrence of the disease under consideration, it is advisable to inquire about additional genetic conditions such as malformations, mental retardation, neurologic disorders (especially late-onset diseases), history of infertility, spontaneous abortion, stillbirths, and newborn deaths. It is also informative to obtain a history of multifactorial degenerative disorders such as cancer, diabetes, and neurologic and mental disorders, including affective disorders, schizophrenia, and premature senility.

Begin the pedigree with the consultand, proceed to his/her sibs, to the parents, then laterally to the parents' sibs and offspring, and then to the previous generation(s). In general, it is difficult and often unreliable to extend a family pedigree beyond three generations unless representatives of a previous generation(s) are present.

An accurate diagnosis is imperative; for example, "mental retardation" is not an accurate diagnosis. Mental retardation can be the result of different genetic mechanisms, such as Down's syndrome (chromosomal), X-linked mental retardation, or microcephaly (mendelian); or the disorder may not be genetic at all but associated with the neuropathology of prematurity or an intrauterine infection.

Most cancers are not genetic in origin; however, there are certain cancers that clearly can be transmitted in a mendelian fashion, such as medullary carcinoma of the thyroid or cancer of the breast or bowel. "Cancer families" do exist wherein a variety of malignant tumors cluster within a family. Patients with a number of genetic disorders are at risk for cancer, such as leukemia in Down's syndrome and in the chromosome breakage syndromes.

Additional practical suggestions are as follows:

1. Obtain a release of information from the consultand in order to contact other family members.
2. Note the date on which pedigree was obtained.
3. Enter the year of birth, not the age of individuals.
4. Record maiden names of women.
5. Obtain addresses of relevant family members.
6. Obtain the cause of death(s).
7. Inquire specifically regarding infant deaths, stillbirths, and abortions. Repeated stillbirths and/or spontaneous abortions may be the result of a familial chromosome translocation.
8. Ask whether the mother and father are blood-related. Consanguinity may be the clue that suggests autosomal recessive disease. Similar last names in previous generations may be a clue to relatedness.
9. Mistaken paternity or illegitimacy can be puzzling and should be gently elicited.
10. Despite the fact that a disorder seems to be dominant or X-linked recessive, obtain information from both sides of the family; such data may be revealing.

However, a number of obstacles may present themselves:

1. Even with examination of the patient/proband, a specific diagnosis may not be possible. In our genetic clinic, we are unable to determine the exact diagnosis in 50 per cent of the patients referred.
2. The affected individual may have died when modern diagnostic techniques were not available or when no autopsy was conducted.
3. The diagnosis may have been in error.

Medical Evaluation of the Proband and Other Family Members. After completing the pedigree and medical history, a complete general medical, frequently a neurologic, or, in the case of a child, more often a developmental examination must be completed on the proband. When examining patients with malformations, and particularly if suspicious of a syndrome, the physician should quantitate dysmorphic features. Anthropometric tables are available* and provide norms for facial features, linear growth, secondary sex characteristics, hair patterns, and dermatoglyphics. These can be used to aid in establishing

*Bergsma, D. (ed.): *Birth Defects Compendium,* 2nd ed. New York, Alan R. Liss, Inc., 1979. (A catalogue providing good clinical description of developmental and genetic disorders; however, it is not a "genetics textbook.")

Goodman, R. M., and Gorlin, R. J.: *Atlas of the Face in Genetic Disorders,* 2nd ed. St. Louis, C.V. Mosby Co., 1977. (An excellent text providing brief descriptions and photographs accurately depicting those facial features characteristic of many genetic disorders.)

Smith, D.: *Recognizable Patterns of Human Malformations.* Philadelphia, W.B. Saunders Company, 1976. (In addition to brief descriptions of common congenital and genetic disorders, a diagnostic approach and norms for anthropometric data are provided.)

Table 2. Signs and Symptoms of Genetic Disease

Signs and Symptoms of Genetic Disease	Chromosome Karyotype	Specific Enzyme	Hormone	Blood and Urine Amino Acid Chromatography	Organic Acids	Gene Probe	Blood and Rh Type	Sweat Chloride	Coagulation Studies	Immunoglobulin, Complement and Leukocyte Function	Biopsy R = Rectal S = Specific Tissue	Electrodiagnostics	Hemoglobin Electrophoresis
A. Manifestations at birth or shortly thereafter													
1. Malformations	X												
2. Deformations	X												
3. Ambiguous genitalia	X	X	X										
4. Hypo- or hypertonia	X	X		X	X								
5. Seizures or coma		X		X	X	X							
6. Metabolic acidosis		X			X	X							
7. Hyperammonemia		X		X	X	X							
8. Bleeding									X				
9. Hyperbilirubinemia		X					X						
10. Meconium ileus								X					
11. Abnormal screen for inborn errors		X		X									
12. Anemia													X
B. Initial manifestations after newborn period													
1. Mental retardation	X	X		X	X								
2. Hypo- or hypertonia	X	X		X	X	X						X	
3. Neurologic deterioration		X		X	X	X					R	X	
4. Growth failure	X		X										
5. Disproportionate growth		X											
6. Visceromegaly		X				X						X	
7. Recurrent infections						X				X			
8. Anemia													X
9. Chronic renal disease		X											
10. Liver dysfunction		X					X						
11. Bleeding or hemarthrosis									X				
12. Malignancy	X										S		
C. Initial manifestations adolescent and adult years													
1. Selected malignancies	X										S		
2. Failure sex maturation	X		X										
3. Infertility	X												
4. Repeated SABs*	X												
5. Neurologic deterioration		X		X							R and S	X	
6. Selected anemias													X

*SABs = Spontaneous abortions.

normality or quantitate variation from the norm. Examination of old family photographs may aid in the diagnostic process. Perhaps a single odd facial feature or growth discrepancy may be found as a familial or a racial feature. The clinical features of a genetic disorder may change over the period of growth (aging). Examination of old photos may reveal clinical features more easily visible in earlier years. Examination of relevant family members may reveal microsymptoms of the genetic disease in question or identify familial facial features or growth abnormalities. It is necessary to document relevant diagnoses in family members using previously completed studies.

Laboratory, Radiologic, Histopathologic, and Electrodiagnostic Procedures. There are a large number of genetic disorders, many with confirmatory laboratory tests (Table 2). This means the physician must be aware of the specific disorder and the specific tests available. With certain exceptions, a chromosome karyotype is not useful in the study of mendelian disorders. Likewise, amino acid chromatography or enzyme determinations are not generally useful in the diagnosis of a chromosomal disorder.

Additional specific testing that will be increasingly available is the development of disease-specific probes and gene linkage. The availability of DNA probes for specific genes may allow detection of individuals who are homozygous or heterozygous for a mutant allele at that gene locus. This would occur in the following way.

A mutant gene may be associated with base changes in the nucleotide sequence in noncoding regions close to the site of the mutation. These base changes may lead to changes in reactivity of the DNA with restriction endonuclease enzymes (i.e., enzymes that cut DNA). It is possible, then, to identify individuals who carry the mutant gene allele because they show a different pattern of DNA fragments on electrophoresis compared with persons with the normal allele. This association of restriction endonucleic polymorphism with a mutant gene has been used in the prenatal diagnosis of sickle cell disease and phenylketonuria (PKU). Of course, it is essential when these analyses are carried out that samples from parents and, if possible, siblings be analyzed.

In certain rare instances, it has been demonstrated that the base substitution in the coding region of DNA, which leads to gene mutation, also leads to a change in reactivity of the DNA with a specific restriction endonuclease. The base substitution leading to the sickle mutation results in altered reactivity with the restriction enzyme Dde I; this alteration allows direct detection of the presence of the mutant allele.

An additional diagnostic methodology will employ gene linkage. Though a probe may not be available for a specific disorder, identification of gene loci linked to the locus for a specific disease can be carried out; thus identification of the associated or linked genes will aid in the establishment of a diagnosis. This has been effectively employed in diagnosis of myotonic dystrophy using secretor locus.

Treatment Plan. Treatment of genetic disorders is outside the scope of this text. Nonetheless, a variety of surgical, medical, dietary, and replacement modalities are used to treat selected genetic disorders. It is also apparent there are many genetic disorders for which there is no specific treatment. This fact makes it imperative that adequate time be made available to the proband, consultand, or family in order to completely describe the disease process, the risks of occurrence or recurrence, and those supportive measures and agencies available to aid the affected. This requires time outside of the ordinary 5- to 10- minute office visit. Harper's *Practical Genetic Counseling** is an excellent source for the general physician.

GENETIC MECHANISMS OF DISEASE TRANSMISSION

The phenotype consists of a person's physical and behavioral characteristics, some of which are primarily determined by the environment, some by genetic endowment (genotype). Traits or characteristics of an individual—normal or abnormal (disease)—are the result of gene-environment interaction. Those disorders that are clearly genetic in origin, such as PKU or Down's syndrome, are altered by the environment, in the former by diet and in the latter by developmental therapy. Disorders that are clearly environmental, such as pneumococcal pneumonia or beta streptococcal infections, are influenced by our immune system, which is clearly under genetic control.

Genetic disorders can be transmitted by:

1. Chromosomal inheritance.
2. Mendelian inheritance.
3. Multifactorial inheritance.

Chromosomal Inheritance

Disorders that are caused by one too many or one too few chromosomes (aneuploidy) are described by Dr. Priest in Section 19 and will not be repeated. However, familial chromosome abnormalities due to reciprocal and to robertsonian translocations can mimic mendelian inheritance (pseudomendelism).

Reciprocal Translocation. In this situation, there occurs in a parental gamete an exchange of fragments between two or more chromosomes. In the balanced state, the individual's phenotype is normal; there are still 46 chromosomes, but the chromosomal structure is altered. Upon meiosis, the affected parent may contribute a haploid complement that is unbalanced and that may result in an abnormal infant.

Figure 2 demonstrates a 1-month-old infant with features commonly found with Brachmann-de Lange syndrome and, in this instance, associated with a chromosome abnormality: one chromosome No. 2 appeared too long and had a duplicated piece of chromosome No. 3 attached. The father had a similar abnormality in one No. 2, but in addition had one abnormally short chromosome No. 3 (Fig. 3). Prior to conception of the father, breaks occurred in chromosomes Nos. 2 and 3; upon union, the fragments from the long arms of these chromosomes exchanged sites (Fig. 4). Thus, the father had a balanced translocation: He had the correct amount of chromosomal material, but it was rearranged. Family studies revealed that the father had given the balanced translocation to one daughter and two normal chromosomes to a second daughter. The father and carrier daughter both appeared normal; however, their offspring might receive the unbalanced, the balanced, or the normal chromosome sets.

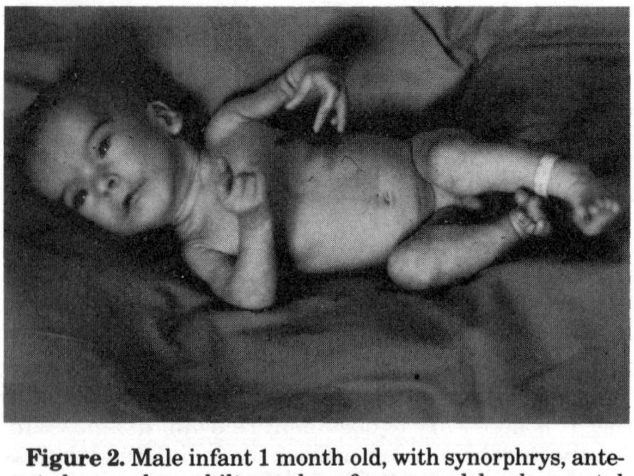

Figure 2. Male infant 1 month old, with synorphrys, anteverted nares, long philtrum, long fingers, and developmental delay.

*Harper, P.S.: *Practical Genetic Counseling.* Baltimore, University Park Press, 1981. (An excellent, slim text providing accurate information in a brief, readable, and sometimes witty fashion often found in British publications. The author is now a Welshman.)

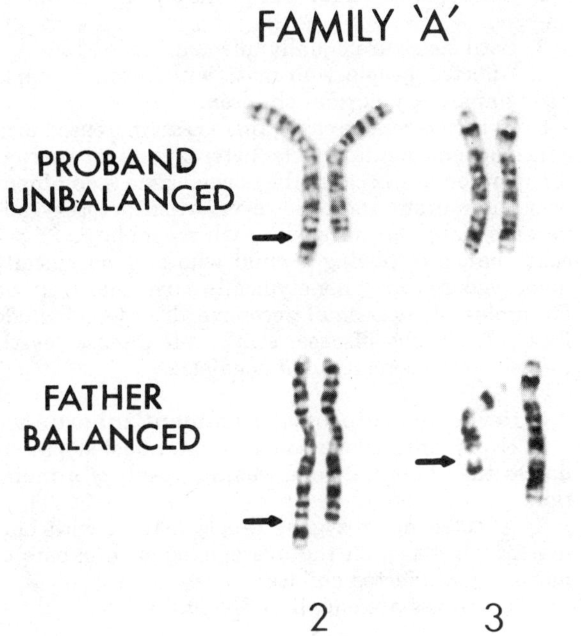

Figure 3. Balanced reciprocal translocation with exchange of fragments between distal long arms of chromosomes Nos. 2 and 3 (*bottom*). Normal chromosomes are on the right. Arrows indicate the rearrangement. In the affected baby (top), one chromosome 2 (left) is abnormal with an extra piece of no. 3 attached. Both No. 3 chromosomes are normal; thus an unbalanced translocation is present.

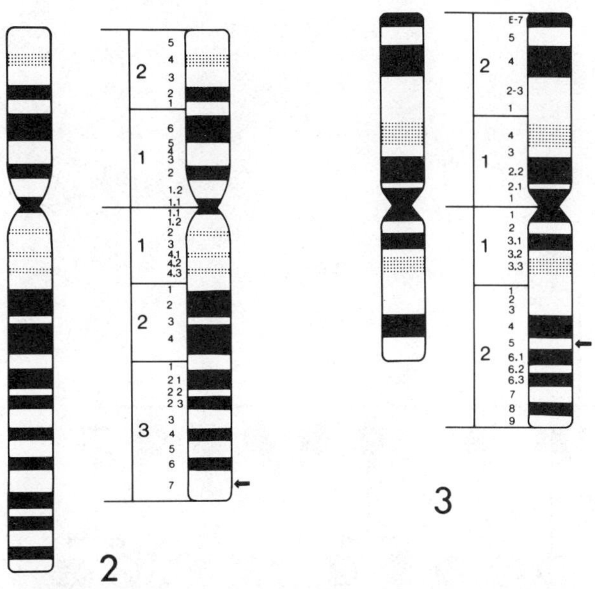

Figure 4. Idiogram demonstrating break points on chromosomes Nos. 2 and 3 (arrows). Normal chromosomes are on the right.

Robertsonian Translocation or Centric Fusion. In this situation, two chromosomes literally fuse. In the balanced state, the individual's phenotype is normal but only 45 chromosomes are present. Meiosis may result in an unbalanced gamete with the occurrence of an abnormal conceptus. Robertsonian translocations affect primarily those acrocentric chromosomes responsible for Down's syndrome (trisomy 21) or Patau's syndrome (trisomy 13). Figure 5 reveals the union of an ova containing an abnormal recombinant chromosome plus the normal 21, with the normal sperm haploid complement. The child, though having a normal number of chromosomes, has an abnormal chromosomal mass containing an extra 21, thus suffering from Down's syndrome.

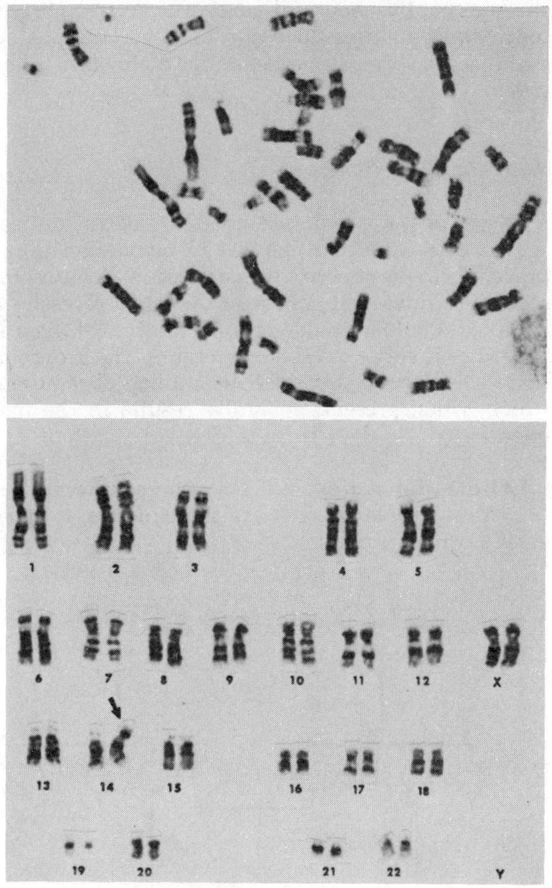

Figure 5. Representation of the chromosomes found in a single-cell nucleus from a child with Down's syndrome (*top*). Karyotype demonstrating three No. 21 chromosomes (*bottom*). The third No. 21 chromosome has joined with a No. 14 chromosome and is termed a robertsonian translocation.

Translocations can be de novo so that the only future children in the family at an increased risk are those conceived by this de novo affected proband. The risk of recurrence in the reciprocal or robertsonian balanced translocation carrier varies, depending upon whether the mother or the father is carrier of the balanced state. If the father is a carrier, the risks are small, 3 to 5 per cent, because he produces both normal and abnormal sperm. Normal sperm has a selective advantage over the abnormal. The mother has but a single ovum, and in that situation the recurrence risk is closer to 20 per cent. Affected families frequently have a history of repeated spontaneous abortion because of the decreased viability of a chromosomally abnormal conceptus. These chromosome abnormalities do occur in a vertical fashion within a family and thus can mimic mendelian inheritance.

Mendelian Inheritance

There are approximately 3000 known diseases proved or suspected to be due to mendelian inheritance. These diseases are transmitted in an autosomal recessive, autosomal dominant, X-linked recessive or X-linked dominant mode of inheritance. Y-linked inheritance is very rare, if it ever occurs. The Y chromosome represents the sex-determining chromosome which, when present, generally results in the male phenotype.

Criteria for Autosomal Recessive Inheritance

1. Most people affected are the children of apparently normal parents.

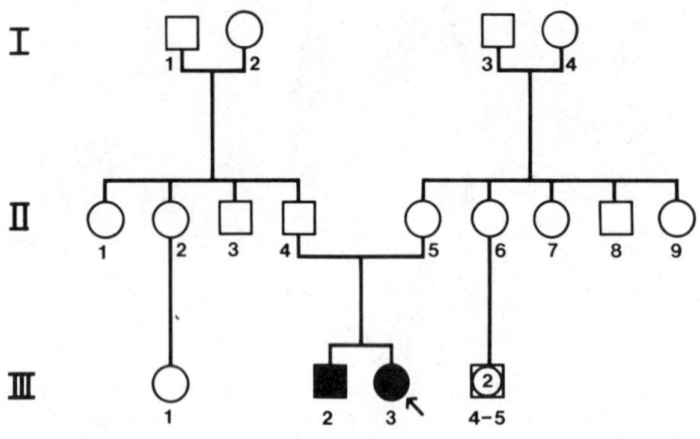

Figure 6. Pedigree of a family who have two children with phenylketonuria (PKU). Note a "horizontal" inheritance, the abnormality appearing only in a sibship.

2. Often, more than one child in a sibship is affected.
3. Both sexes are equally affected.
4. Affected people who mate with normal people have apparently normal children.
5. In rare recessive cases, there is an increased incidence of consanguinity. The heterozygote (or carrier) is asymptomatic because the normal gene is dominant over the mutant gene. However, when heterozygous parents mate, they face with each pregnancy a 25 per cent chance of having a child who is genotypically homozygous, thus phenotypically abnormal (Fig. 6). Examples of autosomal recessive disorders include PKU, Tay-Sachs disease, sickle cell disease, cystic fibrosis, microcephaly, and achalasia.

Criteria for Autosomal Dominant Inheritance

1. Every affected person has one affected parent unless the abnormal gene was the result of a mutation.
2. Affected heterozygous people mating with normal people have, on the average, equal numbers of normal and affected children.
3. The sexes are equally affected.

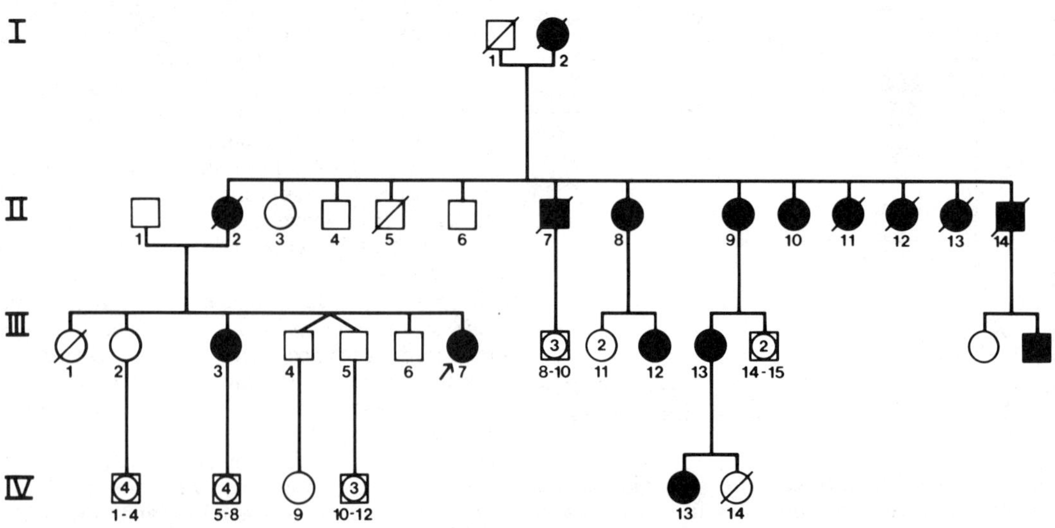

Figure 7. Pedigree of a family demonstrating vertical inheritance found in an autosomal dominant disorder, Huntington's disease. Individuals represented by II_5 and III_1 committed suicide, a frequent occurrence in families affected with this devastating disorder.

4. Normal family members do not transmit the abnormality to their children (Fig. 7). In this situation, the abnormal gene is dominant over the normal gene. Many of the autosomal dominant disorders present with structural malformations that are not as disabling as the more globally involved autosomal and X-linked recessive disorders. Autosomal dominant disorders are frequently associated with a high rate of mutation, and a disease may seem to skip a generation because of incomplete penetrance or lack of expression of the disease.

Criteria for X-linked Recessive Inheritance

1. Affected fathers do not transmit the mutant gene to their sons but do transmit it to all their daughters, who are then heterozygous (carriers).
2. Heterozygous mothers transmit the genes to half their sons, who are enzyme-deficient, and to half their daughters, who are then heterozygous.
3. Homozygous mothers transmit the gene to all their sons, who are then enzyme-deficient. Commonly occurring X-linked recessive disorders include X-linked mental retardation, Duchenne type muscular dystrophy, and hemophilia (factor VIII deficiency) (Fig. 8). X-linked recessive disorders occur almost exclusively in the male offspring; however, one can occasionally see these disorders in females owing to the occurrence of XO female and to lyonization. In order to maintain genetic equilibrium, one of the X chromosomes in the female is randomly inactivated and can be seen in somatic cells as a Barr body or X chromatin body. If the X chromosome carrying the mutant gene for muscle dystrophy is inactivated, these cells will not express the disease; however, should the X chromosome carrying the normal gene be inactivated, these cells can express muscle dystrophy, albeit a milder variety of the disease (lyonization).

Criteria for X-linked Dominant Inheritance

1. Affected males transmit the trait to all their daughters and to none of their sons.
2. Transmission by females follows the same pattern as autosomal dominant inheritance.
3. In rare X-linked dominant disorders, affected females are twice as numerous as affected males. In this case, the father with X-linked disease transmits the disorder only to his daughters, whereas the heterozygous mother passes the trait on to 50 per cent of her offspring, and the homozygote to 100 per cent of hers regardless of sex (Fig. 9). The pedigree is very similar to autosomal dominant disease, but is distinguished by the fact there is no male-to-male transmission and the number of females affected exceeds that of males affected.

Multifactorial Inheritance

Multifactorial inheritance is responsible for such traits as height, skin color, blood pressure, and intelligence. This mode of inheritance is also responsible for the transmission of a large variety of structural malformations such as spina bifida cystica (SBC) with myelomeningocele, cleft lip/cleft palate, and club foot. The term "multifactorial" implies an interrelationship between the environment and the genome, and this interrelationship is clearly established in twin studies. Let us assume that Q syndrome is purely a genetic disorder. Given that assumption, when Q syndrome occurs in twins with the same genome (monozygotic or MZ), both twins will always have the same syndrome. But if Q syndrome occurs in twins who do not have the same genome (dizygotic or DZ), concordance for Q syndrome would be no more common than in siblings. If Q syndrome were purely envi-

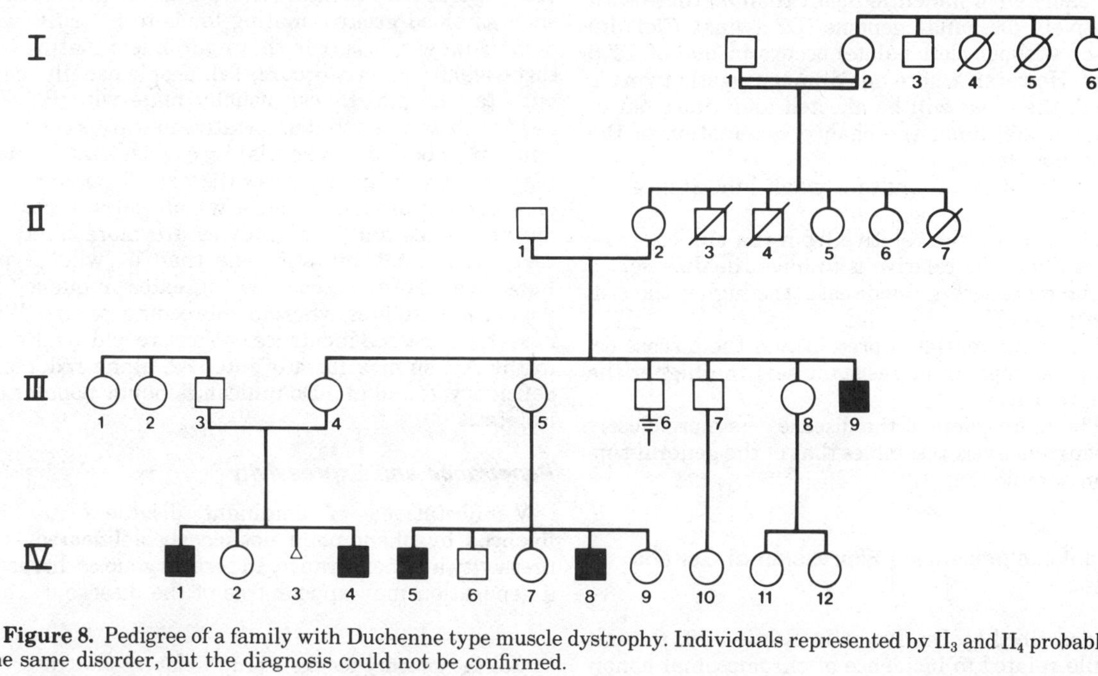

Figure 8. Pedigree of a family with Duchenne type muscle dystrophy. Individuals represented by II_3 and II_4 probably had the same disorder, but the diagnosis could not be confirmed.

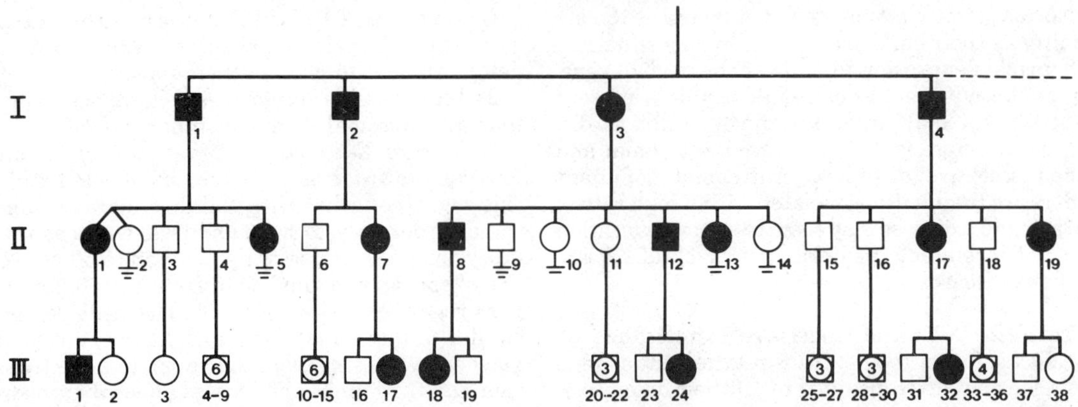

Figure 9. A partial pedigree from a family with familial hypophosphatemia (Vitamin D–resistant rickets). The pattern is similar to autosomal dominant inheritance but differs in that there is no male-to-male transmission and all daughters of affected males are also affected. (Adapted from McKusick, V. A.: *Mendelian Inheritance in Man*, 6th ed. Baltimore and London. Johns Hopkins University Press, 1983.)

ronmental, the incidence of Q syndrome would be very similar in MZ and DZ twins.

Disorders of multifactorial inheritance are not primarily genetic or environmental in origin; they are a product of this interaction. The cleft lip/cleft palate shows this interaction. Concordance in MZ twins is much greater than in DZ twins. This implies that even though the genome is identical as in MZ twins, the effect of a teratogen upon that genome may vary. However, the more similar the genome, the more likely it is that the end result (in this instance cleft lip/cleft palate) will be the same. The effects of a teratogen upon persons with a relatively dissimilar genome (DZ twins) will be less reproducible. These empirical observations imply that genetic forces have a powerful influence over the ultimate results of an environmental insult. Persons with an identical genome (MZ twins) react in a more predictable fashion to the same environmental insult than do those with a relatively dissimilar genome (DZ twins). Cleft lip (with or without cleft palate) occurs in one of 1200 infants. However, where one of monozygotic twins is affected, the other will be affected four times out of ten, about 400 times the chance expectation of the general population.

Characteristics of multifactorial inheritance include the following:

1. The further the relative from the clinical case, the less likely the relative is to have the disease.
2. The more severe the disease, the higher the risk to relatives.
3. If sex differential is present and the disease occurs in the opposite or resistant sex, the higher the risk to relatives.
4. The more common the disease, the more closely the recurrence risk resembles that of the general population sample (Fig. 10).

Mechanisms Influencing Expression of Genetic Disease

As described by Dr. Priest in Section 19, the one variable related to incidence of chromosomal abnormalities is maternal age. Penrose first described the maternal age relationship to Down's syndrome. Perhaps nondisjunction occurs with equal frequency in the male, but because of the numbers of sperm produced and the selective advantage of the normal sperm, a strong paternal age dependency cannot be demonstrated.

The frequency of recessive disorders is influenced by a number of phenomena. All of us carry a number of recessive mutant genes; however, because of the rarity of specific recessive disorders and a predominance of random mating (panmixis), the frequency of recessive disorders is minimized. Hardy and Weinberg* first quantitated a genetic equilibrium based upon random mating: any one genotype at a specific locus has a purely random probability of occurrence dependent upon the gene frequency within the general population. For many traits, i.e., biologic markers such as blood groups, mating tends to be truly random. However, it is true that nonrandom mating (assortative) frequently occurs. Tall people usually mate with tall people, Blacks usually mate with Blacks, Jews with Jews, so that assortative mating is common and can be positive. A special type of assortative mating, consanguinity, increases the risks for occurrence of a genetic disease because we all carry recessive mutant genes and our relatives are more likely to carry that same mutant gene than a "wild" type. Recessive disorders occur with greater frequency in population isolates wherein inbreeding occurs. Witness the increased incidence of Von Creveld syndrome in the Amish or a form of intersex, alpha reductase deficiency, found in a Dominican Republic population isolate.

Penetrance and Expressivity

Manifestations of dominant disorders are influenced by phenomena not clearly delineated—expressivity and penetrance. In certain genetic diseases, a generation may appear free of the disease so that

*See the glossary for the Hardy-Weinberg law.

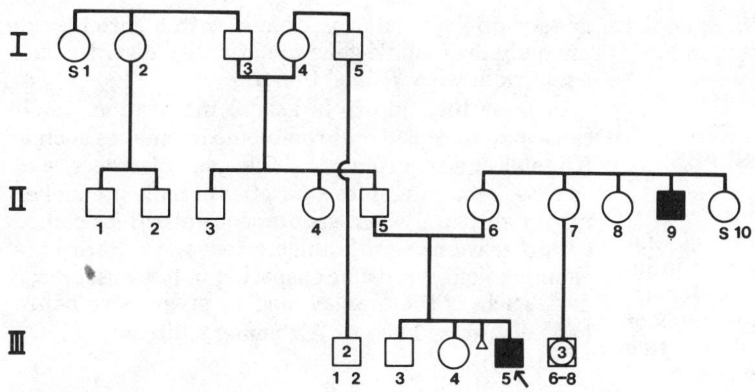

Figure 10. Pedigree of a family with neural tube malformation, a multifactorial disorder. Note spontaneous abortion immediately prior to proband, a frequent occurrence.

contrary to the definition of dominant transmission, an affected child may be born to nonaffected parents. This phenomenon may occur as a result of variable expression of the disease or variable penetrance. Genetic disorders, as with other diseases affecting mankind, can present with varying degrees of severity; a dominant disorder may be present with a degree of subtlety so as to be almost invisible or overlooked in a parent.

For example, tuberous sclerosis may present in a child with seizures, mental retardation, ash leaf spots, and adenoma sebaceum, a truly devastating disease. However, the parent may appear perfectly normal and have no symptoms, but with a brain computed tomographic (CT) scan evidence of one or more intracranial tuberi may be found.

Some dominant disorders may produce no abnormality in the parent (nonpenetrant), yet offspring can be affected. Postaxial polydactyly may be nonpenetrant in the parent, yet the child may be born with polydactyly.

Penetrance and expressivity occurring in genetic disease can be illustrated by comparison with beta hemolytic streptococcal infections. An individual may be a carrier of the beta hemolytic streptococcus, yet the organism may produce no disease in that individual (nonpenetrant). In others carrying the organism symptoms can occur, ranging from a mild pharyngitis with few systemic effects to an acute illness with severe systemic effects (variable expression).

New Mutations

An additional mechanism responsible for the occurrence of a dominant disorder in a child with normal parents is a point mutation. In this situation, there is a preconceptual change in the genotype of the egg or sperm, and when union with a normal gamete takes place, disease occurs in the offspring.

Unlike the situation with variable expression and penetrance, we have a greater understanding of the molecular phenomenon occurring with mutation, even though we may not be able to totally explain the cause of the molecular abnormality. It is presumed that ionizing radiation is responsible for most, though not all, mutations. Mutations occur with increasing frequency in the older male, perhaps a result of wear and tear produced by a lifetime of exposure to ambient ionizing radiation. It is estimated that a point mutation occurs in 10^6 gametes.

Mutations, though a mechanism for evolutionary change, are predominantly undesirable and produce deleterious traits. Mutations also explain the constancy of certain genetic disorders in the population. Certain genetic diseases are of a severity such that reproduction (fitness) is markedly reduced. For example, the reproductive fitness of a patient with Duchenne muscular dystrophy or tuberous sclerosis is low. Yet the disease does not diminish in frequency but remains constant over the passage of time. This means that new cases or new mutations are constantly occurring. Thus, the lower the reproductive fitness of an individual with a dominant genetic disease, the higher the frequency of mutation, whereas the closer to normal the reproductive fitness, the lower the incidence of mutation. For example, Huntington's disease, with its late onset, seldom interferes with reproduction, and it is apparent that spontaneous mutations seldom if ever occur.

Heterogeneity: Several Genes, One Effect

Our perception of individual genetic disorders has changed over the recent past and will continue to change. Disorders that were perceived to be a single entity have been subdivided into a number of disorders with similar characteristics (phenotypes) but clearly different genotypes (splitting). Deafness is a case in point, for parents with phenotypic autosomal recessive deafness upon mating may have all normal-hearing infants, thus demonstrating a "non-allelism of recessives." At one time, PKU was perceived to be due to a deficiency of a single liver-specific enzyme, phenylalanine hydroxylase. We now know the identical phenotype can be caused by a defect in biopterin synthesis, which is not totally corrected by diet. These phenomena are not unique to the realm of genetics because not too many years ago, dropsy, arthritis, and jaundice were thought by many to be single entities.

Pleiotropy: One Gene, Several Effects

Separate and distinct clinical entities may be caused by the same genetic abnormality (lumping). For example, steroid sulfatase deficiency may cause two separate clinical entities. During reproductive age, there may occur delayed onset of labor with an increased frequency of stillbirths. However, steroid sulfatase deficiency in postnatal life produces an X-linked icthyosis. A gene or gene pair may, and often does, affect multiple organ systems. For example, the eyes, heart, and skeletal systems are affected in Marfan's syndrome.

SIGNS AND SYMPTOMS OF GENETIC DISEASE

Although the gene or chromosome abnormality is present at and before birth, manifestations of that abnormal genotype may not appear until later in infancy, in childhood, or even in adult years. Genetic etiology must be considered when there are signs or symptoms present, as listed in Table 2. This listing does not imply that all seizures in infancy or that all anemias or cancer in adult years are genetic. Nonetheless, a portion of the disorders producing these symptoms are genetic in origin and, therefore this etiology should be considered.

Malformations in the neonate, though always congenital, are not always genetic. Approximately 15 per cent of malformations occurring in the neonate are of a genetic origin. Deformation is less often genetic in origin, but it occurs because of an unusual fetal position often associated with abnormalities of the maternal uterus. Any time one detects biochemical abnormalities such as hyperammonemia, metabolic acidosis, or hyperbilirubinemia, a genetic etiology must be considered. The occurrence of seizures, hypotonicity, or hypertonicity suggests a genetic and often progressive neurologic disorder.

There are numerous initial manifestations occurring after the newborn period that suggest genetic etiology. Changes in growth—failure to thrive or disproportion in size—as well as visceromegaly, particularly if associated with neurologic or mental deterioration, are often genetic. The occurrence of a malignancy in a child must raise the possibility of genetic etiology, be it associated with a chromosome anomaly or a single-gene abnormality disorder such as aniridia with Wilms' tumor.

In later life, failure of sexual maturation should cause one to consider chromosome anomalies such as Klinefelter's syndrome or single-gene disorders, such as those occurring in the varieties of male pseudohermaphroditism. Repeat spontaneous abortions can occur in a woman with undetected cystic fibrosis. A genetic etiology must be suspected in late-onset disorders, such as the ataxias, and in progressive neurologic disorders, such as Alzheimer's disease.

SUMMARY

During the routine evaluation of patients, the physician needs to be aware of the family pedigree. The importance of accurate physical assessment cannot be overemphasized, including anthropometric measurements in the infant and assessment of the developmental milestones, along with documentation of minor physical abnormalities. Only by maintaining a degree of suspicion will the physician detect genetic disorders and thus institute early treatment and accurate family counseling. Additional information is available to the physician.*

*Thompson, J.S., and Thompson, M.W.: *Genetics in Medicine,* 3rd edition. Philadelphia, W.B. Saunders Company, 1980. (An excellent overview of human genetics.)

Vogel, F., and Motulsky, A.G.: *Human Genetics: Problems and Approaches.* New York, Springer-Verlag, 1979. (A comprehensive and rather ponderous text, but recommended for those who wish to pursue in depth the fascinating arena of human genetics.)

Glossary of Genetic Terms

A priori probability: The probability calculated on theoretical grounds prior to experimental verification of the theory.

Acentric: Indicating a chromosome (or chromatid) that lacks a centromere.

Acrocentric: Indicating a centromere that is placed almost terminally so that its chromosome has one long arm and one very short arm.

Aggregation, familial: An increased number of cases in one family or in a geographic area. This does not permit any inference about the mode of inheritance; however, such a term is more likely correlated with autosomal recessive inheritance and the founder effect.

Alleles (Allelomorphs): Alternative forms of a gene found at the same locus on homologous chromosomes and segregating at meiosis, one given to an individual from each parent.

Anaphase: That phase of mitosis or meiosis following metaphase and preceding telophase during which the two longitudinal halves of the replicated chromosomes are migrating to opposite poles of the cell.

Aneuploidy: A condition in which there is an abnormal number of individual chromosomes, not in a multiple of the number for basic set—for example, monosomic: containing only one representative of a specific pair of chromosomes; trisomic: containing three representatives of a specific pair of chromosomes.

Ascertainment: The finding or selection of families for inclusion in a genetic study.

Assortive mating: Mating of individuals who are more similar phenotypically than if mating were random.

Autosome: Any chromosome that is not a sex chromosome; there are 22 pairs of autosomes in humans.

Barr body: The sex chromatin as seen in somatic cells of the female; named for the discoverer of sexual dimorphism in somatic cells, Dr. Murray Barr. See *Sex chromatin.*

Basis defect: A homogeneous defect of a structural or chemical nature that forms the basis of the multiple symptoms of a hereditary disease.

Carrier: An individual who carries a single recessive gene, either autosomal or X-linked, that is, a heterozygote.

Centromere: A localized, nonstaining region of the chromosome that attaches to a spindle fiber and controls chromosome migration at anaphase.

Chromatin: A nucleoprotein substance in cell nuclei that stains with basic dyes. Upon condensation during early prophase it becomes the chromosome.

Chromosome: Basophilic organelle formed by condensation of the chromatin at the time of cell division, the number and morphology being relatively constant within members of the same species.

Chromosome map: Relative location of genes on a given chromosome.

Clone: A group of cells derived by mitotic divisions from a single ancestral cell.

Codominance: State in which each gene produces its characteristic effect in the heterozygote, as in the AB blood genotype, which produces both A and B antigens.

Concordant: Indicating the possession of a certain trait in both members of a twin pair.

Congenital: Relating to a character present at or dating from birth, either of genetic or of environmental origin.

Consanguinity: Mating between relatives.

Consultand: The person, in a genetic counseling situation, whose genotype is being evaluated; often the parents of an affected child.

Coupling: Linkage phase in which two dominant alleles are on one chromosome and the two corresponding recessives on the homologous chromosome. Antonym: *repulsion.*

Crossing over: Exchange of parts of homologous chromosomes resulting in chromosomes with new genetic combinations.

Deletion: Loss of a segment of a chromosome; in a diploid cell only one representative of the segment being present.

Dermatoglyphics: Study of the patterns of the ridged skin involving the palms, fingers, soles, and toes.

Dicentric: Presence of two centromeres in one chromosome.

Diploidy: Presence in a cell of a chromosome set containing twice the haploid gametic number.

Discordant: Indicating the presence of a trait in one member of a pair of twins and not the other.

Dizygotic twins: Two-egg twins for which the genetic relationship is the same as that for full sibs.

DNA (deoxyribonucleic acid): Nucleic acid of the chromosomes in which genetic information is coded.

Dominant: A trait that is expressed phenotypically in both the heterozygous and the homozygous condition.

Euchromatin: Regular staining material of most of the chromosome. See *Heterochromatin.*

Euploidy: Presence in a cell of an exact whole-number multiple of the gametic (haploid) chromosome number.

Expressivity: Degree of quality of the phenotypic expression of a gene or group of genes.

Familial: Describing a condition which is more often present in two or more members of a family group than would be expected on a null hypothesis.

Fitness: Relative number of progeny left by an individual.

Forme fruste: Minimal manifestations of a disorder.

Fragment (of a chromosome): A product of chromosome breakage that may or may not have a centromere. Also used to describe minute supernumerary chromosomes of undetermined origin.

Gamete: Mature germ cell with normally a haploid chromosome number.

Gene: Portion of a chromosome that performs as a unit of heredity.

Gene frequency: Proportion of gametes in a population that carries a particular allele.

Genetic code: Base triplets of DNA and RNA that carry the genetic information specifying the selection of particular amino acids.

Genetic marker: A readily recognizable gene which can be used in family and population studies.

Genome: A haploid set of chromosomes and the corresponding set of genes.

Genotype: Genetic composition of an individual inherited from the parents, sometimes referring to the sum of genes of an individual or just alleles at a given locus.

Haploidy: Presence of a single set of chromosomes, that is, the number present in normal gametes; there are 23 in humans.

Hardy-Weinberg law: If two alleles (D and d) occur in a randomly mating population with the frequency of p and q, respectively, where $p + q = 1$, the expected proportions of the three genotypes are DD = p^2, Dd = 2pq, and dd = q^2. These remain constant from one generation to the next. Mutation, selection, migration, and genetic drift can disturb the Hardy-Weinberg equilibrium.

Hemizygote: A gene located on the nonhomologous portion of the X chromosome in the male is in the hemizygous state since it lacks its partner gene or allele.

Heterochromatin: A part of the chromosome material that stains differently from the rest of the chromatin, especially in some stages of the division cycle.

Heterogeneity: The commonly observed phenomenon of identical phenotypes caused by different genes. Frequently mild variations can be detected by refined methods. Heterogeneity of genetic disease is a corollary of the axiom that the phenotype is not a necessary indication of the genotype.

Heterozygote: A genotype with two different alleles at a locus.

Holandric: Indicating transmission from father to son, such as traits inherited through genes in the Y chromosome.

Homozygote: A genotype with two identical alleles at a locus.

Inborn error of metabolism: A defect which is determined at a particular gene locus and which results in block or diversion of a metabolic pathway.

Inversion: A chromosomal segment that has been turned 180 degrees. It is pericentric when the centromere is included in the inverted segment, paracentric when it is not.

Isochromosome: A chromosome with two identical halves joined to a common centromere.

Karyotype: Orderly arrangement, by size and morphology, of the chromosomes from one cell; by extension also used to mean the chromosomal complement of a cell line or an individual.

Lethal gene: A gene which is incompatible with survival either in heterozygotes or in homozygotes.

Linkage: Occurrence on the same chromosome of two or more loci.

Locus (loci): Point (or points) location on homologous chromosomes where alleles will appear.

Malformation: A primary structural defect resulting from a localized error of morphogenesis, for example, cleft lip, which is distinguished from *deformation*—an alteration in shape and/or structure of a previously normally formed part, such as torticollis.

Meiosis: Two specialized cellular divisions, producing the germ cells containing a haploid genome.

Messenger RNA (mRNA): A nucleic acid of high molecular weight that carries genetic information from the gene to the ribosome.

Metacentric: Indicating a centromere in a position such that a chromosome has two arms of approximately equal length.

Metaphase: That phase of mitosis or meiosis following prophase and preceding anaphase when the chromosomes, having been replicated, are aligned at the equatorial plane of the cell.

Mitosis: Process of replication of somatic cells. See also *Anaphase, Metaphase, Prophase,* and *Telophase.*

Monosomy: Absence from a somatic cell of one chromosome of a homologous pair.

Monozygotic twins: One-egg twins, which therefore have identical genotypes.

Mosaic: An individual composed of two or more cell lines, recognizably different in karyotype, that were derived from one zygote.

Multifactorial: Pertaining to a phenotype which has arisen through interaction of many causes, genetic and environmental.

Multiple alleles: More than two gene forms at one locus.

Mutant: An altered gene or an individual showing the phenotypic effects of such a gene.

Mutation: A change of a gene from one allelic form to another; sometimes used more broadly to include chromosomal aberrations.

Mutation rate: The rate at which mutations occur at a given locus; expressed as mutations per gamete per locus per generation.

Nondisjunction: Failure of chromatids or chromosomes to separate and migrate to opposite poles at mitosis or meiosis, resulting in unequal distribution of homologous chromosomes to daughter cells at cell division.

Penetrance: Frequency with which a particular genotype shows a recognizable phenotype.

Phenotype: Observed trait for an individual.

Pleiotropy: Multiple phenotypic effects of a single locus.

Polygenic: inheritance of a trait involving a number of genes without a major environmental component. See *Multifactorial.*

Polymorphism: Simultaneous occurrence of two or more different genotypes in the population, whose ratio is kept in equilibrium by means of selection.

Polyploidy: Any euploid number of chromosomes except haploid (N) and diploid (2N); for example triploidy (3N), tetraploidy (4N).

Population genetics: Study of the genetic characteristics and forces of change for a group of individuals.

Proband: Starting case from which a genetic investigation is undertaken.

Prophase: First phases of mitosis or meiosis during which the chromosomes become visible, the nuclear membrane disappears, and, the centriole having divided, the two parts migrate to opposite poles of the cell.

Recessive: A trait expressed only when the genotype is homozygous.

Recombination: Formation of new combinations of genes at meiosis.

Repulsion: Linkage phase in a double heterozygote in which the two dominant alleles are on opposite chromosomes.

Ribosome: Cytoplasmic particle concerned with protein synthesis.

Ring chromosome: Chromosome with the two ends fused to form a continuous circle.

RNA (ribonucleic acid): A nucleic acid formed upon a DNA template and taking part in the synthesis of polypeptides.

Satellite: Small terminal portion of some chromosomes separated from the remainder of the chromosome by a secondary constriction.

Sex chromatin: A deeply staining, characteristically shaped nuclear body formed by the condensation of an X chromosome and seen in a high proportion of cells from normal females.

Sex chromosome: The X or Y chromosome.

Sex influenced: A trait which is not sex-linked in its pattern of inheritance but is expressed differently (either in degree or in frequency) in males and females.

Sex-limited: Indicating appearance of a trait in only one sex.

Sex-linked: Indicating location on the X or Y chromosome; usually used more specifically to refer to genes on the X; also used for traits caused by such genes. See *X-linked, Y-linked.*

Sib, sibling: Brother or sister.

Telophase: That phase of mitosis or meiosis during which chromosomes have reached opposite poles of the cell and are being incorporated into new nuclei and during which cytoplasmic cleavage is completed.

Translocation: Interchange of material between two nonhomologous chromosomes. A mutual exchange, each chromosome both losing and gaining a segment, is called reciprocal translocation.

Trisomy: Presence in an otherwise diploid cell of one extra complete chromosome, in this instance three homologues being present. When only part of an extra chromosome is present, this is termed partial trisomy.

X-linked: Indicating location of genes on the X chromosome or traits determined by such genes.

Y-linked: Indicating location on the Y chromosome or traits determined by such genes.

Zygote: The fertilized egg cell from which the new individual develops.

CHILD ABUSE OR MALTREATMENT

By Janine Jason, M.D.
Atlanta, Georgia

DEFINITION

Definitions of child abuse or maltreatment have broadened over the past 20 years and now, in most states, include purposefully inflicted physical injury, sexual or emotional maltreatment, and neglect of any individual younger than 18 years of age. The abuse often, but not necessarily, is perpetrated by the child's caretaker(s). Physicians are required by law to report any case of suspected child abuse to the appropriate local state agency, generally a protective services agency. A high index of suspicion is needed for this diagnosis to be made accurately. The following information will provide diagnostic clues for the clinician, who must be constantly alert to the possibility of child abuse.

PRESENTING SIGNS AND SYMPTOMS

Physical Abuse

History is an important key to diagnosing physical abuse. Purposeful injury should be suspected when the history of the traumatic event is vague, is improbable, or does not fit the injury observed, as well as when there has been a delay in seeking medical care. The person bringing the child for medical care is often not the one described as present at the time of injury. The adult seeking care for the child may appear indifferent to or, alternatively, overly anxious about the injury. If this individual is the parent, he or she may openly admit to occasionally hitting the child with a closed fist or an object, to kicking or burning the child, or to throwing things at the child. These acts of violence are usually explained as being forms of discipline. When questioned, the parent may describe himself or herself as isolated or lacking assistance with child care.

The child should also be interviewed. This should be done privately and in a nonthreatening fashion. He or she should not be pressured into contradicting the parent's story, but responses differing from the parent's should be calmly recorded by the examiner.

Physical examination is highly suggestive of child abuse when any of the findings in Table 1 are present without a clear and probable explanation. Observation of the parent's responses during the examination can be extremely useful in supporting a diagnosis of physical abuse (Table 2).

Laboratory examination should include a hematocrit if blood loss appears possible. Radiologic evaluation should include skull films if a skull fracture is suspected, and a skeletal survey to look for old fractures, metaphyseal or epiphyseal injury, or subperiosteal hemorrhage. Ideally, all lesions and bruises should be photographed in case documentation is needed in court.

Differential diagnoses include accidental injury. Although the following diagnoses are uncommon, they also should be considered: leukemia or a bleeding disorder as a cause of bruising, and osteomyelitis, periostitis, or osteogenesis imperfecta as a cause of bone lesions not associated with other signs of trauma or maltreatment.

Table 1. Findings Suggestive of Physical Child Abuse

Nonresponsive affect
Soft-tissue bruises
Multiple bruises
Bruises in different stages of healing
Bruises that occur before a child can walk
Shaped bruises (e.g., the outline of a hand, cord, gag, or rope)
Burns in areas which the child could not reach on his or her own body
Shaped burns (e.g., the outline of a cigarette tip, iron, or heating grate)
Buttock burns
Any head trauma
Cephalohematoma
Sternal, scapular, or skull fracture
Transverse or spiral fractures
Joint dislocation
Abdominal trauma
Comatose state of unknown cause

Table 2. Parental Behavior to Observe During Examination

Attitude toward child
Eye contact with child
Response to crying
Ability to comfort
Ability to support child
Need for child's support
Mode of disciplining child

Sexual Abuse

Sexual abuse can be broadly defined as the instigation, by coercion or force, of active or passive participation by a child or adolescent in any nonpeer sexual activity. The child will usually present in one of three fashions: (1) a history of possible or confirmed assault; (2) genital, urethral, or anal injuries, lesions, or discharge; or (3) nonsexual behavioral changes or problems.

As with physical abuse, a carefully taken history is the key to a diagnosis of sexual abuse. As in a case of suspected physical abuse, the child may appear guilt-ridden. The young child may seem sexually precocious or provocative for his or her age; however, this apparent sexual precocity is the result, not the cause, of sexual assault. Alternatively, the child may be extremely apprehensive or even hysterical about the physical or genital examination. Any child presenting with penile, scrotal, or vaginal injuries or with a sexually transmitted disease (STD) should be suspected of having been abused unless peer sexual activity is acknowledged. Because multiple physical examinations should be avoided, it is important to plan all necessary tests before the examination. If examination by a specialist appears necessary, it should be conducted, if at all possible, by one specified individual to minimize the emotional trauma associated with repeated examinations. As with physical abuse, photographic documentation of injuries may be indicated.

Laboratory evaluation is outlined in Table 3. Immediate treatment of physical injury or of STD is indicated when these are present. However, prophylactic STD treatment, before diagnosis, is not indicated unless there is evidence that the assailant was infected.

Emotional Abuse and Neglect

These forms of child maltreatment are poorly defined, difficult to diagnose in a short-term clinical set-

Table 3. Laboratory Procedure For Evaluating Sexual Abuse*

Laboratory management of children with genital symptoms or a history of sexual assault
Mandatory immediate tests
1. Gram stain of any discharge for intracellular gram-negative diplococci
2. *Neisseria gonorrhoeae* cultures from cervix/vagina, urethra, anus, and throat, as indicated by history; confirm positive cultures with sugar utilization test
3. Syphilis serology
4. Pregnancy test in postmenarcheal girls
5. Wet preparation of trichomonads
6. Test for presence of semen, if history is positive for recent assault
Recommended immediate tests (if available)
1. *Chlamydia trachomatis* cultures
2. *Ureaplasma urealyticum* cultures
Follow-up tests
1. *N. gonorrhoeae* cultures
2. Syphilis serology
3. *C. trachomatis* cultures (if available)
4. *U. urealyticum* cultures (if available)
5. *Herpes simplex* virus cultures, if suspicious lesion appears
6. Repeat pregnancy test, if appropriate
Mandatory follow-up tests
1. Test of cure 3–7 days after treatment of proved *N. gonorrhoeae* infection
2. Repeat syphilis serology if another STD† confirmed
3. Follow-up culture of any previously cultured pathogen
Laboratory management of children with suspected sexual abuse because of behavioral symptoms
Complete history and physical should include vaginal/cervical and anal cultures in girls or penile and anal cultures in boys for *Neisseria gonorrhoeae*
Consider other nontraumatic tests for STD
1. Syphilis serology
2. Wet preparation for trichomonads
3. Others as appropriate and available
Consider pregnancy test

*Adapted from Kramer, D.G., and Jason, J.: Sexually abused children and sexually transmitted diseases. Rev. Inf. Dis., 4:S883, 1982.

†STD = Sexually transmitted disease.

ting, and, by any definition, even more prevalent problems than physical or sexual abuse. Furthermore, physical and sexual abuse, when they occur, tend to do so in combination with emotional abuse and/or neglect. This category of abuse will rarely appear as the presenting problem but rather may be an underlying cause of, or a finding unrelated to, the presenting complaint. This type of abuse should be considered a possibility when the parent-child interaction appears to be poor (Table 2) or when the child is having behavioral problems, appears to receive inadequate care, or is not thriving nutritionally or developmentally.

Despite diagnostic difficulties, it is important not to overlook these diagnoses for two reasons. First, at least three subcategories—i.e., failure to thrive, malnutrition, and failure to receive needed medical care —are best handled in a medical setting and, if left untreated, can have long-term medical complications. Second, protective services agencies are generally understaffed and thus unable to provide adequate long-term follow-up for these problems. Places that provide ongoing medical care are often better equipped, trained, and staffed to manage these patients.

As with other forms of abuse, the history is an important clue in making a diagnosis. It should deal in depth with family history; developmental milestones; previous medical care; dietary habits; social network; participation and achievement in school; interactions with peers, siblings, and parents; and episodes of criminal behavior, drug abuse, or alcohol abuse. Particular note should be made of the parent's knowledge of the child and his or her general concern for the child's well-being. It is especially important to note the parent's interaction with the child during the taking of the history and physical exam (Table 2).

On examination, note the child's general state of care and hygiene; attitude toward self, parent, and examiner; and developmental status. He or she should be examined carefully for signs of recent or past abuse. Height and weight should be compared with the norms for the age and sex-matched population. Ideally, past measurements should be obtained for comparisons over time. All children below the third percentile for height and/or weight should be investigated further. For infants and young children, this may require in-hospital evaluation. Laboratory evaluation should include hematocrit, serum lead level, and, if the child's growth is retarded, endocrinologic assessment and radiographic appraisal of bone age. (See the section on disorders of growth and development.)

COURSE AND THERAPY OF CHILD ABUSE

Child abuse rarely occurs as a single event. The immediate goals of therapy should thus be both the treatment of acute damage and the prevention of further harm. Treatment is inadequate unless it assures long-term management, including the psychological and social rehabilitation of the child and family and the prevention of further family dysfunction.

Three points merit emphasis. First, the physician should not be reluctant to report suspected child abuse. Protection of the child should be of paramount importance, and a physician cannot be sued if a suspected diagnosis of child abuse proves to be in error. Second, when the physician's approach is sympathetic, the doctor-patient (parent) relationship can generally be maintained. Finally, if a diagnosis of abuse is suspected, evaluation and therapy are best handled by a multidisciplinary team, including physicians, psychiatrists, psychologists, child development specialists, social workers, protective services' legal counsel, and trained lay personnel.

Section Two

INFECTIOUS DISEASES

BACTERIAL DIARRHEAS

By John E. McGowan, M.D.
Atlanta, Georgia

DEFINITION

Diarrhea (increase in fluidity, frequency, or volume of bowel movements) may be due to any of several bacterial organisms. The most common causes in the United States are Salmonella species (both *typhi* and nontyphoid strains), Shigella species, Campylobacter species, and certain strains of *Escherichia coli.* In special situations, one must also consider *Clostridium difficile, Yersinia enterocolitica, Vibrio parahemolyticus, Bacillus cereus, Staphylococcus aureus,* Clostridium species, and *Vibrio cholerae* (both 01 and non-01 strains). Cases associated with *Salmonella typhi* are discussed elsewhere in this book, as are cases due to viruses or parasites.

The term "bacterial dysentery" has been employed as a synonym, but this is less often used today because it is interpreted by some as referring to diarrhea cases with certain clinical or laboratory characteristics suggesting inflammation, and others consider the phrase to be a synonym for shigellosis.

CLINICAL PICTURE

The most important aspect of establishing a diagnosis is to differentiate diarrhea cases with bacterial etiology from those due to nonbacterial causes (e.g., viruses, parasites) and from those due to noninfectious conditions (e.g., inflammatory bowel disease, chemical diarrhea). This often is difficult to do because there are no findings that invariably distinguish one group from the other. For example, the concurrent presence of fever or lower abdominal pain with diarrhea makes bacterial etiology more likely, but fever or abdominal pain also can be present with amebiasis, granulomatous colitis, ulcerative colitis, or a number of other entities. Thus, one must evaluate the presence or absence of several different factors to decide whether bacterial etiology is likely.

Factors relating to the patient's symptoms, other historical points, and physical examination that may affect the decision-making process are listed in Table 1. This table reveals useful clues, but no single item or group of points can establish a bacterial etiology for diarrhea with absolute certainty.

Since pathognomonic signs or symptoms are not available, it is useful to synthesize the information in Table 1 and decide which of the following forms of illness is best fit by a given patient. Because different groups of bacteria are more likely to cause each of these syndromes, such classification aids in choosing further diagnostic studies. Although there is considerable overlap among the groups, two main forms can be distinguished:

1. Watery diarrhea, without blood or mucus prominent in the gross appearance of the stool. Systemic symptoms (e.g., fever history, headache, malaise) are rare. Nausea and/or vomiting are common. Abdominal pain is less prominent than for the second syndrome (to be described); when present, it often is localized to the periumbilical area. Profuse stool production often is matched by gaseous distention and flatulence as prominent parts of the picture.

This pattern is most often due to nonbacterial pathogens; when bacteria are the cause, they are more likely to be toxigenic *E. coli, S. aureus, B. cereus,* Clostridia, or Vibrios. Nontyphoidal salmonellosis must be considered as well.

2. Initial watery diarrhea, if present at all, followed by cramps, tenesmus, and frequent but scanty (relatively small-volume) stools containing mucus and/or blood. Pain often is localized to the lower abdomen or rectum. Nausea and/or vomiting usually is mild or absent. Fever is usual, and may be rather high; other constitutional symptoms (e.g., headache) are also frequent.

This picture often arises from bacterial infection, and usually is due to more invasive pathogens: Shigella species, Campylobacter species, certain *E. coli, Y. enterocolitica,* or *V. parahemolyticus.* However, in less severe infections, most of these bacterial agents also can cause a watery diarrheal illness similar to the first syndrome described earlier. Salmonella in particular can be associated with either of the two forms or (more likely) with combinations of the two.

LABORATORY PROCEDURES

The clinical features must be considered before specifying the laboratory tests to be performed. In mild cases of watery diarrheal disease in an otherwise healthy individual, one may at times presume that the disease will be self-limited. Laboratory testing may be optional in this situation. For most other cases, at least some of the following tests routinely will be utilized.

Table 1. Clinical Features Aiding Diagnosis of Bacterial Diarrhea

History of current illness

1. *Acute onset?* An acute onset makes infectious etiology more likely, although inflammatory bowel disease (e.g., granulomatous colitis) also may begin abruptly.
2. *Fever noted?* Fever makes inflammatory disease more likely; it enhances possibility of bacterial or parasitic cause (but inflammatory bowel disease and other conditions possible, too). In the afebrile patient, bacterial etiology still possible but is less likely.
3. *Tenesmus present?* Same significance as fever.
4. *Stools bloody and/or mucoid?* Presence of blood or mucus emphasizes bacterial organisms as likely cause, although other causes (e.g., anal fissure) still possible.
5. *Stool frequency and volume?* Scanty, frequent stools increase chances for bacterial etiology.

Other historical points

1. *Antibiotic therapy?* Recent administration of antimicrobials increases likelihood of *Clostridium difficile*. Some antibiotics may cause diarrhea as a direct chemical effect.
2. *Other drugs?* Antimetabolites and some other drugs can produce diarrhea. Laxative abuse often is overlooked as cause unless patient is specifically asked about this.
3. *Unusual diet?* Herbal teas, other "health foods," increased fiber in diet, and so on, may produce diarrhea.
4. *Other cases known?* Occurrence in outbreak fashion can indicate possible cause.
   a. Day care center source—suspect Shigella, Campylobacter (but rotavirus or Giardia also described in this setting).
   b. Food- or waterborne source can be vehicle for many different bacteria; incubation period between ingestion and symptoms can help identify responsible agent.
   c. Secondary cases occurring in family members more characteristic of Shigella and Salmonella than of other bacterial agents common in the United States.
5. *Recent travel?* Travel history to certain areas emphasizes possibility of certain bacteria.
6. *Male homosexual?* If so, this emphasizes likelihood of Shigella, Campylobacter (but giardiasis, amebiasis, gonococcal or chlamydial proctitis and/or anal fissure also present with increased frequency in this group).

Physical examination

1. *Pain location?* Pain localized to lower abdomen or rectum enhances likelihood of bacterial disease.
2. *Anal fissure?* Presence may explain illness, but possibility of concurrent bacterial cause still requires evaluation.
3. *Splenomegaly or adenopathy?* See article on typhoid.
4. *Rectal exam?* Rectal prolapse suggests shigellosis or other bacterial cause. Fecal impaction may explain illness.
5. *Seizures?* In children, presence of associated seizures increases suspicion of bacteria as cause.
6. *Skin rash?* Rose spots of typhoid, erythema nodosum of yersiniosis can help guide further studies.
7. *Arthritis or myositis?* Presence suggests possibility of Yersinia, Salmonella, early "limb pain" of Campylobacter.

Evaluation of Stool

Gross Examination. Presence of blood and/or mucus should be investigated. Malabsorption produces frothy, foul-smelling, greasy stools that suggest the presence of Giardia or post-rotavirus lactose intolerance.

Fecal Leukocytes. Microscopic examination of the stool for white blood cells can be helpful in differentiating among the several bacterial causes. A small amount of stool (use mucus instead, if present) is placed on a microscope slide, a drop of methylene blue and saline is added, the solution is mixed, and a coverslip is placed over the solution. The slide is examined using the "high dry" objective of the microscope. If numerous white blood cells are seen, shigellosis, salmonellosis, Campylobacter, and Yersinia are the most likely bacterial cause. However, noninfectious etiologies like ulcerative colitis or other inflammatory bowel diseases can also produce this picture. Absence of polys does not exclude these pathogens, and a number of other bacteria (e.g., *C. difficile*) may or may not have a white cell response noted, depending on how severe a focal response is produced in an individual case.

Stool Culture. Most laboratories routinely culture only for Salmonella, Shigella, and Campylobacter; a specific request is required before culture is performed for other bacterial pathogens mentioned in this article. Few clinical laboratories are equipped to identify the presence of invasive or toxigenic *E. coli* or *Clostridium perfringens.* Thus, one must be familiar with the limits of testing provided by an individual laboratory and make special test requests when the data in Table 1 suggest these to be of value.

Routine stool culture for bacteria requires fresh stool specimens, since a number of organisms (especially Shigella) are inhibited by other stool flora and by the lowering of pH that occurs with time after stools are passed. If a delay of more than 2 hours is anticipated, the specimen should be placed in a transport medium (e.g., Cary-Blair). Refrigeration is discouraged, since low temperatures result in a decrease of stool pH. Although one specimen is often adequate, submission of two or three specimens collected at spaced intervals over 2 or 3 days increases the likely yield.

The routine culture of stool for bacterial pathogens includes inoculation of selective and differential agar media; using these, most Salmonella, Shigella, and Campylobacter organisms can be recovered within 24 to 48 hours. Some organisms are present in very low numbers in stool. For example, Salmonella and Shigella ordinarily are present in large numbers in stool only during the first 3 to 5 days of diarrheal disease. Later, an enrichment process may be necessary to detect their presence in stool; this likely will delay the organism identification by 1 to 2 days.

If alerted by the patient's physician, many hospital laboratories can test for Yersinia and Vibrio organisms (special media and incubation temperatures are needed). These identifications also may require more time than the routine culture studies.

Toxin Assay. Many laboratories now can test for the toxin produced by *C. difficile.* This usually requires a special request to the laboratory, in the appropriate clinical circumstances.

Blood Cultures

If an invasive organism such as Salmonella is suspected, or if an invasive bacterial infection is suspected from the clinical features of the illness (e.g., high fever), blood cultures should be obtained. At least two cultures at separate times, drawn with separate venipunctures, give a satisfactory chance of recovering the organism.

Other Diagnostic Tests

For cases in which bacterial etiology is suspected but not easily confirmed, proctosigmoidoscopy may be useful. Not only can a bacterial cause be established, but nonbacterial agents (especially parasitic) and noninfectious etiologies (such as villous adenoma, inflammatory bowel disease) can also be recognized. The technique is especially useful in detecting plaques of pseudomembranous colitis (direct visual inspection) and in obtaining samples from colonic mucosa that provide the best yield for confirmation of *E. histolytica* infection.

POTENTIAL ERRORS AND PITFALLS IN DIAGNOSIS

As noted in the discussion on clinical features, there are no pathognomonic signs, symptoms, or laboratory features confirming or denying bacterial etiology for diarrheal illness. The diagnosis depends on synthesis of several clinical and epidemiologic factors, combined with selective laboratory testing.

Most clinical laboratories will not routinely culture stool specimens for all possible bacterial pathogens. Instead, routine stool culture usually is performed for Salmonella, Shigella, and Campylobacter, and the laboratory depends upon the patient's physician to make a special request for additional studies if other pathogens seem likely. Some bacterial agents of diarrheal disease cannot readily be confirmed in the usual clinical laboratory even if special request is made. In addition, one must keep in mind that diarrheal disease associated with *C. difficile* is identified by toxin assay rather than by stool culture.

CHOLERA

By K. A. Monsur, M.B., D.C.P., D. Bact.
Dacca, Bangladesh
and W. B. Greenough, III, M.D.
Baltimore, Maryland

DEFINITION

Cholera, also called "Asiatic cholera," is an acute diarrheal disease caused by *Vibrio cholerae,* which is present in large numbers in the stool of the patient, especially in the acute stages of the disease. An exotoxin is produced by the vibrios, which causes loss of solutes and water at a rapid rate that may exceed one liter per hour. There is no structural damage to the gut epithelium, and the natural course of illness rarely exceeds 5 days. There is no phase of tissue invasion or bacteremia, and all effects are topical on the intestinal mucosa.

A variety of terms, such as "cholera gravis," "choleraic diarrhea," and "cholera asiatica," have been used to describe the different clinical forms of the disease. These terms have no value except to emphasize the geographic extent or severity of the disease. Because a similar clinical condition can be caused by other agents, the diagnosis of cholera cannot be confirmed unless *V. cholerae* is isolated from the stool. The disease occurs only in humans, and it is generally believed that humans are the only reservoir of infection. Several studies indicate that the organism may sometimes persist in a suitable aquatic environment for a long time, and it may occasionally be possible for the infection to originate from the environment without coming directly from humans.

ETIOLOGY

Traditionally it was believed that only the classical biotype of *V. cholerae* caused cholera. The pandemics of the 1960s proved beyond a doubt that the El Tor biotype can also cause the identical disease in a global epidemic form. Both the classical and El Tor biotypes possess a common O antigen, and either organism will be agglutinated by antiserum against other *V. cholerae* possessing this group antigen. All organisms with this antigen are designated as *V. cholerae* 01. For each of the classical and El Tor biotypes of *V. cholerae* 01,

Table 1. Average Plasma and Stool Values in Cholera Patients and of Commonly Used Rehydration Fluids

	Plasma			Cholera Stool		Rehydration Fluids				
		Cholera				Intravenous				
	Normal	*Adult*	*Child*	*Adult*	*Child*	*DTS**	*Ringer's Lactate*	*5:4:1†*	*½ Darrow's with 25% Glucose‡*	*Oral ORS§*
Concentrations (mEq/L)										
Na^+	140	141	138	135	105	118	131	134	61	90
K^+	4.5	4.5	4.0	15	25	13	4	13	17.5	20
Cl^-	103	107	110	100	90	83	111	99	52	80
HCO_3^-	25	9	12	45	30	48	29	48	26	30
Glucose¶	90	180	165	—	—	50	—	—	250	111

* DTS = Diarrhea treatment solution.
† 5:4:1 = 5 gm NaCl, 4 gm $NaHCO_3$, and 1 gm KCl per liter; also known as Dhaka solution. In this solution the bicarbonate can be replaced by acetate for a more stable solution.
‡ This solution is widely used for the treatment of diarrhea but because of its low sodium content has not been tried for cholera.
§ ORS = Oral rehydration salts. Each packet contains NaCl—3.5 gm, $NaHCO_3$—2.5 gm, KCl—1.5 gm, and glucose—20 gm. To be dissolved in 1 liter of water for drinking.
¶ Plasma glucose in mg/dl; intravenous solution in gm/liter.

there are two serotypes, Ogawa and Inaba. Rarely an intermediate serotype Hikojima is found that shares both Ogawa and Inaba antigens. All these serotypes produce toxin, can cause similar clinical diseases, and can occur in epidemic or sporadic modes.

The definition of *V. cholerae* now includes all those non-01 strains of vibrios that are similar biochemically and are related on the basis of DNA homology to *V. cholerae* 01. Such non-01 strains are commonly referred to as nonagglutinating vibrios (NAGs) or noncholera vibrios (NCVs). Some of them produce toxins and may occasionally cause sporadic cases of cholera-like diarrhea or even limited epidemic outbreaks. Under this new definition, many of these NAGs, which previously would have been considered quite different, are now classified as *V. cholerae.*

PATHOGENESIS

Infection is always acquired by mouth. Parenteral infection is not known. After being swallowed, the organisms must survive the acidity of the stomach. This is why the challenging dose either has to be high or has to be protected by a food vehicle. After leaving the stomach, the organisms remain localized in the intestine, multiply there, attach to the lining epithelium, and excrete a toxin—but they never invade the body. The toxin is also not absorbed into the blood or body fluids. The disease is, therefore, strictly an intoxication of gut epithelium.

The toxin has two components—A and B. Component B, which is larger and antigenic, is made up of five identical subunits that attach to a specific GM_1 ganglioside in the epithelial cell wall. The toxin moiety A then enters the cells, where it locks the enzyme adenylate cyclase in its fully activated state. This causes an increase in cyclic AMP in the cell, blocks normal absorption of sodium, and initiates full secretion of chloride ions with consequent increased outpouring of water and small solute molecules. This effect lasts at least 24 hours and possibly for the functional life span of the gut epithelial cell, which is almost 72 hours. This explains why, once the diarrhea starts, even complete sterilization of the intestine with antibiotics will not stop diarrhea in less than 24 hours. There is no structural damage to the epithelial cells. An alternate glucose and amino acid–dependent pathway for absorption of sodium ions remains unaffected, permitting oral rehydration therapy (ORT), which is now being extensively used in many countries (Table 1).

EPIDEMIOLOGY

A variable proportion of those who become infected develop clinical symptoms. Asymptomatic carriers have no manifestation of illness and are detectable only by laboratory isolation of *V. cholerae* from stool or retrospectively by detection of a rise in circulating antibody against an antigenic component of the organism. The incubation period varies from 24 hours to about 5 days, with an average of about 1 to 2 days, and seems to vary inversely with the number of organisms ingested. Among those who develop symptoms, the severity varies from a mild intestinal upset to severe watery diarrhea, leading to collapse, shock, and—if untreated—death, which may occur in less than 24 hours.

The case-to-infection ratio for classical biotype has been reported as 1:3. For the El Tor biotype, this can be as high as 1:25 or even 1:100. In Bangladesh, El Tor has also been found to have a 1:4 case-to-infection ratio.

Cholera is primarily a disease of persons living under unhygienic conditions. Physicians and nurses, who care for patients without special isolation precautions, rarely contract the disease, suggesting that with simple hygiene, such as hand washing, transmission is uncommon, even when there is direct contact.

Infected persons usually excrete the organisms for less than 1 week. Chronic carriers have been documented for the El Tor biotype but are extremely uncommon. When this occurs, it is due to infection of the gallbladder, which probably occurs retrograde via the bile duct and not through blood.

CLINICAL PICTURE

Typically, cholera, in its most severe form, is a dramatic illness and has a terrifying effect on the community. The disease starts as an acute diarrhea, usually without abdominal pain. Vomiting may appear early. The diarrhea rapidly increases in severity, and the volume of stool may be as high as 15 to 20 liters in 24 hours. In early stages, rates of 2 liters per hour have been seen. The stool is initially bile-stained but gradually becomes white with a slight "fishy" odor and contains flakes of mucus—commonly described as "rice watery." The patient becomes rapidly dehydrated and goes into vascular collapse, and the skin becomes cold, clammy, and wrinkled. If the skin is pinched, skin folds persist. Eyes are sunken and the facies drawn and anxious looking. Severe muscle cramps and extreme thirst ensue. In severe cholera, if the patient is left untreated, the fluid deficit rapidly reaches 10 to 12 per cent of the body weight. A normal adult can die as early as 3 to 4 hours after onset, although this is the exception.

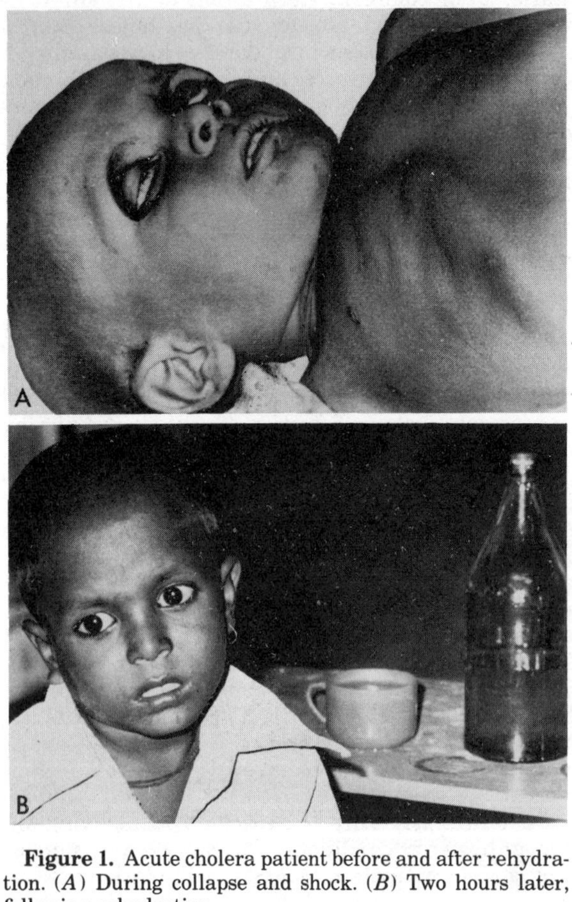

Figure 1. Acute cholera patient before and after rehydration. (*A*) During collapse and shock. (*B*) Two hours later, following rehydration.

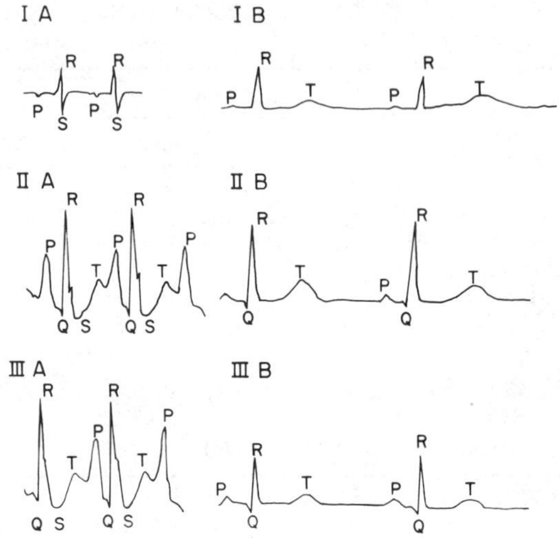

Figure 2. Electrocardiographic changes in cholera. (*A*) Leads I, II, and III during shock. (*B*) Leads I, II, and III during convalescence.

As dehydration increases, the blood pressure falls and radial pulse volume becomes diminished, thready, or even imperceptible, but femoral and carotid pulses are clearly palpable until a later stage. Intense thirst develops, and there are severe muscular cramps. The urine volume decreases and mouth and eyes become dry, but sweating may persist. Oral and axillary temperatures fall below normal, but rectal temperature may be slightly elevated, especially in children. Respiration rate increases. Metabolic acidosis produces significant pooling of blood in the lungs and is a major cause of pulmonary edema if the patient is rehydrated without correction of the base deficit. Deep Kussmaul type respiration associated with uncorrected base deficit may develop within 24 hours after start of treatment if this deficit is allowed to persist. Recovery is usually prompt with full replacement of fluid and electrolytes (Fig. 1). If untreated, the patient remains cyanotic and stuporous. If shock is long-standing, renal failure can occur.

Untreated, the illness lasts from 24 hours to about 7 days, and the mortality is about 50 per cent. In untreated patients, electrocardiographic changes include right axis deviation, relative or absolute, peaked P waves, and tall tented T waves. These abnormalities disappear with rehydration (Fig. 2). Cardiac arrhythmias are occasionally noted, particularly if improper replacement solutions are used.

LABORATORY FINDINGS

As a result of the loss of water and small solute molecules, the plasma specific gravity and protein concentrations increase in proportion to the losses. The leukocyte count also increases as a part of these phenomena. Since anemia is common in many patients before onset of the disease, the rise of hematocrit with dehydration may be masked by preceding anemia. If shock is allowed to persist, all associated changes characteristic of the body's response to this emergency can be measured.

Fecal osmolality increases above normal but does not exceed the plasma values. Fecal sodium concentration approaches that of plasma at high output rates. Stool potassium and bicarbonate concentrations exceed those of plasma.

Plasma proteins and formed elements of the blood are absent in stool or present in traces. The main protein found in cholera stool is IgA secretory immune globulin probably derived directly from gut-lining immunocytes. The loss of bicarbonate leads to a drop in plasma bicarbonate level and in arterial pH.

Plasma potassium may initially be normal or slightly elevated even when potassium depletion is severe because of acidosis. However, correction of base deficit results in rapid transfer of potassium into the cells, producing significant hypokalemia unless simultaneous replacement is given. Serum sodium and chloride are normal (see Table 1 for plasma and stool values). Total serum osmolality is normal or slightly elevated. Other blood solutes are normal. Serum SGOT (AST) and alkaline phosphatase are normal or slightly elevated. Serum glucose is usually slightly elevated as with other solutes but may fall to hypoglycemic levels during therapy, especially in children, if glucose is not provided.

COMPLICATIONS

In untreated patients, renal failure leading to uremia and death may occur. In those dying of uremia, autopsy findings of acute tubular necrosis secondary to prolonged hypotension exist. This can be prevented by simple volume deficit replacement promptly and completely and by keeping pace with further losses to prevent recurrence of shock.

Acute pulmonary edema is now a rare complication, occurring only if rehydration is not accompanied by simultaneous correction of acidosis. Sudden death from cardiac arrhythmia due to hypokalemia can occur if adequate replacement of potassium during correction of metabolic acidosis is not attended to. Paralytic ileus is seen in children during treatment and is attributed to inadequate replacement of potassium.

Children with cholera may occasionally develop altered consciousness or even seizures after initiation of rehydration therapy. In some patients this is associated with hypoglycemia; in others it is due to cerebral edema when inappropriate solutions have been used, but in some the cause is unknown. Seizures not associated with hypoglycemia are frequently followed by stupor or coma, which are poor prognostic signs.

Cholera occurring in the third trimester of pregnancy is associated with high risk of fetal mortality and precipitate labor, independent of the degree of vascular collapse experienced.

DIAGNOSIS

General Considerations. An identical clinical condition can be caused by a number of other enteric pathogens among which enterotoxigenic *E. coli* is the most important. The diagnosis of cholera must, therefore, be confirmed by the isolation of *V. cholerae* from stool and cannot be made from the clinical picture alone. However, for the purpose of management a working diagnosis of cholera is justified on the basis of the clinical picture, and if rates of fluid loss exceeding one half liter per hour are sustained after admission, the diagnosis is more likely. When caused by other agents, the resulting physiologic and metabolic abnormalities (and, consequently, treatment and management) are the same. Thus, treatment is not dependent on a precise microbiologic diagnosis and should begin immediately at the start of diarrhea with oral rehydration therapy (ORT).*

In the early stages of the acute disease, *V. cholerae* is present in the stool in very large numbers, and since the organism grows easily on most noninhibitory culture media such as MacConkey's or E.M.B. agar routinely used for isolation of enteric pathogens, laboratory diagnosis in acute disease should normally present very little problem. *V. cholerae*, which ferments sucrose and produces indol, will not agglutinate with any of the Salmonella-Shigella antisera routinely used for diagnosis of enteric pathogens and would ordinarily be discarded as a nonpathogen by many laboratories unless cholera is considered. During a bacteriologic examination, the most common cause for missing the diagnosis is failure to consider the possibility of *V. cholerae* as the cause of the disease. This commonly occurs with the first few cases in the early stages of an outbreak, especially when the disease strikes an area where cholera was previously unknown.

Bacteriologic Diagnosis. In acute cholera, the organisms are present in the stool in large numbers and an experienced observer will be able to make a presumptive bacteriologic diagnosis by observing the characteristic motility of the organism in the watery stool. This can be done even in the field using a battery operated, pocket-sized, dark-field microscope. The identity of the organism can be further confirmed if the motility stops when monospecific (Ogawa or Inaba) antiserum against *V. cholerae* (without preservative) is added to the stool preparation. This presumptive diagnosis, though sometimes helpful, must never be taken as final and should always be confirmed by growing the organism from the stool. Fluorescent microscopy using fluorescein-labeled antibody, if available, can also provide direct, accurate diagnosis from stool. In acute disease the organisms will grow in large numbers if the stool is inoculated on a selective medium for cholera such as thiosulfate citrate bile salt sucrose agar (TCBS) or taurocholate tellurite gelatin agar (TTGA). On TCBS the organism gives fairly large, slightly flat, smooth yellow colonies,

*Composition of oral rehydration salts (ORS): NaCl—3.5 gm; $NaHCO_3$—2.5 gm; KCl—1.5 gm; glucose—20 gm for 1 liter of water.

and on TTGA the colonies are gray with a black center and have a slightly milky halo around each. A slide agglutination test can be carried out directly from growth on TTGA but is not always satisfactory from growth on TCBS. Growth from TCBS should preferably be subcultured on an agar slant or a Kligler iron agar before doing slide agglutination.

In the milder cases, in the later stages of the disease, during convalescence and in carriers, the organism may be present in stool in only small numbers and special selective media are necessary to isolate the vibrio in the presence of other competing organisms. The most commonly used selective plating media are TCBS and TTGA. Before plating, the inoculum may be enriched for *V. cholerae* by passing it through an enrichment medium such as alkaline bile peptone broth. Alkaline bile peptone broth with added tellurite can also be used as a good transport medium. For transportation from the field, when nothing else is available, even ordinary blotting paper soaked in stool can be wrapped with several layers of polythene and sealed in a polythene envelope. For safety it should be put in a second envelope and sent to the laboratory for isolation of *V. cholerae.* This will enable a positive isolation in most cases.

Serology. There is a rise of vibriocidal, agglutinating, and antitoxic antibody titers after an attack of cholera. But since the disease is of short duration, serologic reactions have not been found to be very useful for diagnosis in individual patients. A rise of vibriocidal antibody titer at the community level may be taken as evidence of a recent outbreak of cholera.

TYPHOID FEVER

By R. L. Huckstep, C.M.G., M.D., F.R.C.S., F.R.A.C.S.
Sydney, Australia

INTRODUCTION

Typhoid fever in the mid-1980s is still endemic in many of the developing countries of the world, and epidemics also occur in North America, Europe, and other economically rich countries, usually where a carrier has infected a static water supply, ice cream, or some other food. In March 1973, for instance, 65 confirmed cases were reported near Miami, Florida, from contaminated well water.

Two large epidemics of typhoid fever occurred in the 1960s in Zermatt in Switzerland and in Aberdeen, and many other epidemics have been reported from Europe and North America since then. They have caused consternation, as the United States, Switzerland, and Britain have supposedly high standards of education and hygiene and pure water supplies. The World Health Organization in 1979 reported a total of 373,522 cases of typhoid fever. There were no fewer than 266,204 from India, 22,935 from Indonesia, and 24,939 from Bangladesh. The United States had 449 reported cases, England and Wales 221, Spain 2466, and Italy 4257. There were also many thousands of new cases from other parts of the world. When it is realized that only a fraction of all new cases of typhoid are diagnosed or reported, and that for each new case there are many asymptomatic carriers, it will be apparent that the problem is a huge one. It will remain so until a protective vaccine is developed that is considerably better than the present typhoid, paratyphoid A, and paratyphoid B (TAB) vaccine, which gives relatively incomplete protection.

Over 20 cases in the Aberdeen epidemic alone occurred among people who had had previous TAB vaccine inoculation. This indicates even more the importance of maintenance of high standards of hygiene as the first line of defense and reinforces the statement about the relative lack of value of TAB vaccine. The drug that is still the first choice in treatment (chloramphenicol) is potentially dangerous, while the disease still has an appreciative mortality, even when treated adequately and well. The asymptomatic carrier is difficult both to trace and to treat, and an epidemic such as the one in Aberdeen, with well over 400 confirmed cases, is bound to leave both known and unknown carriers in its wake.

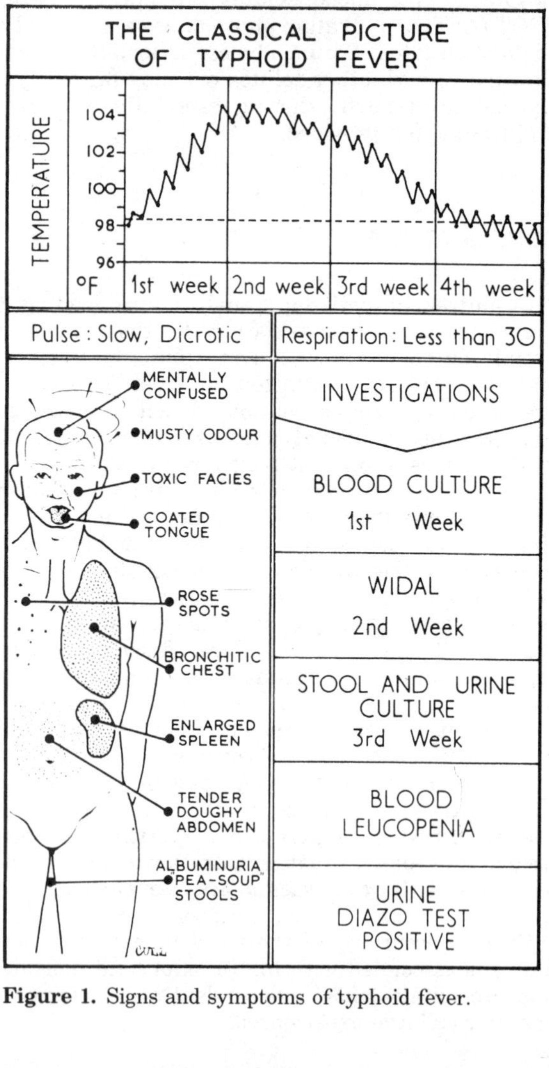

Figure 1. Signs and symptoms of typhoid fever.

The diagnostic criteria given in this article are based on a series of over 1300 typhoid cases that I treated in East Africa from 1954 to 1972. Nine hundred and seventy-five of these patients were documented, and much of the material in this article is the result of investigation of these cases, most of which has been already reported in the monograph entitled "Typhoid Fever and Other Salmonella Infections."

CLINICAL DIAGNOSIS

During an epidemic the problem of diagnosis is simplified (Fig. 1). Many isolated cases of typhoid, however, still occur each year, as mentioned earlier, in the United States, Britain, and Europe, and these cases may be misdiagnosed, especially if mild or asymptomatic.

Typhoid fever and the paratyphoid fevers may present identical diagnostic problems, and the clinical and laboratory pictures are similar in most respects.

The severity of an attack of typhoid depends not only on the dosage and virulence of the particular organism but also on the resistance of the patient and the stage of disease at the time treatment is started. Epidemics undoubtedly vary, and those occurring in the developing countries of the world tend to be more severe, possibly because of the combination of more virulent strains of organisms, larger doses of bacteria, late diagnosis and treatment, and low resistance of patients.

SYMPTOMS

The symptoms of typhoid fever (Fig. 2) may be quite variable and range from a completely asymptomatic patient, only diagnosed on routine stool culture, to a patient with extremely virulent and rapid onset of a disease very much like a severe Salmonella gastroenteritis.

A good clinical history is essential, and this may be difficult to obtain if the patient is mentally dull or confused. Delirium and mental confusion are particularly likely to occur in patients who are seen relatively late in this disease.

The incubation period is usually from 10 to 14 days, but it may vary from 7 to 21 days, and sometimes is even less than 7 days. In the Aberdeen outbreak the first two students to be affected became ill after an incubation period of only 5 days. In the case of the paratyphoid fevers the incubation period is shorter than in typhoid.

A history of exposure to a likely infected source is important, as in the case of a recent trip to a country with endemic typhoid such as Spain, Italy, or Mexico. Infected water, milk, and ice cream are still the most important worldwide sources of infection despite the epidemics in Britain caused by contaminated meat from South America.

The insidious onset helps to differentiate typhoid from influenza, gastroenteritis, acute bronchitis, malaria, and bacillary dysentery. In children the onset tends to be much more sudden, and the diagnosis is therefore more difficult. Massive infection in adults may also cause an acute onset similar to that seen in influenza or gastroenteritis.

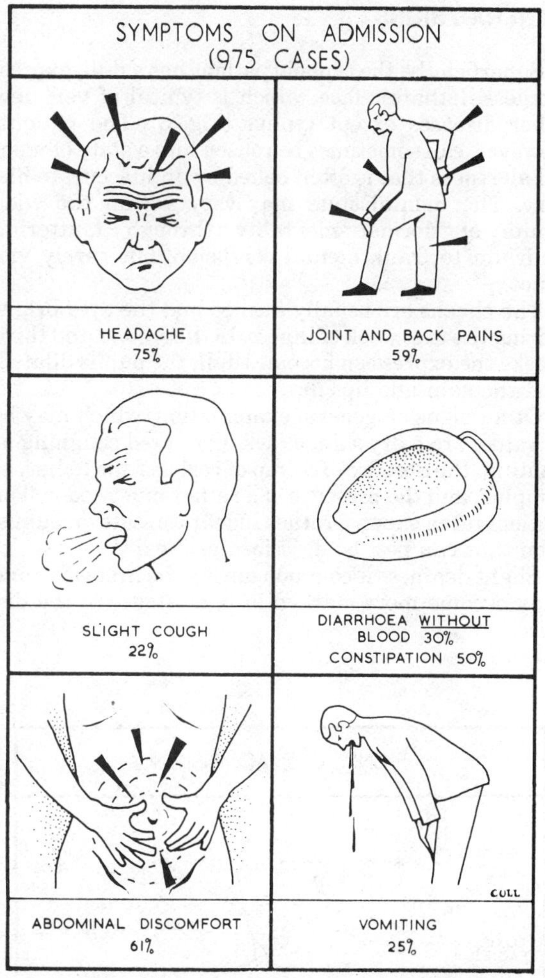

Figure 2. Some of the varied symptoms of typhoid fever seen on admission.

General malaise, anorexia, and lassitude early in the disease are almost invariable symptoms, and they tend to be longer-lasting than in many other conditions. Headache is common, usually occurring within the first 2 days, and is generally dull and continuous rather than acute.

Vague abdominal discomfort is an early symptom and very common. Vomiting tends to be mild and not sustained. Constipation occurs more frequently than diarrhea, but if diarrhea does occur, it is nearly always without blood, a useful point of differentiation from bacillary dysentery. Diarrhea plus vomiting is rare in typhoid but common in gastroenteritis.

Mild joint pains and backache are common, but the joints are *not* swollen except following the rare complication, typhoid arthritis, in which case the pain is not usually severe. A dry cough is common but tends to be slight unless a complication has supervened. Epistaxis sometimes occurs and varies from epidemic to epidemic.

GENERAL SIGNS

Superficially, the typhoid patient has a dull, expressionless, lethargic face, which is typical of very few other diseases except typhus (Fig. 3). The patient, however, can sometimes be roused into a state of mental alertness that is often belied by an inaccurate history. The mental state may vary within the wide limits of normal mentality through muttering delirium to frank mental confusion, but rarely violence.

The cheeks are usually flushed and the eyes bright during the first week of illness. In the second and third weeks the expression becomes dull, the pupils dilated, and the skin and lips dry.

Other signs on general examination, which may be of value, are a dry skin, a lack of marked coughing or sputum, the absence of a crop of vesicles due to herpes simplex, and the presence of a rather musty odor. The patient often shows a rather indefinite state on admission that can best be described as "toxic."

Slight deafness is common during the first week and may become more marked in later stages of the disease.

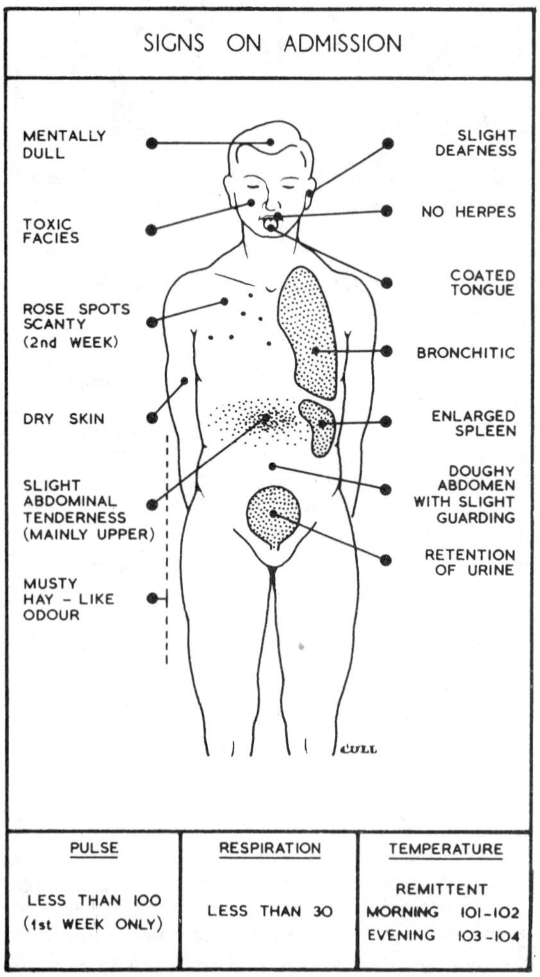

Figure 3. Admission signs. The so-called "toxic facies" is typical of few other diseases.

Rose spots usually occur between the seventh and tenth day of illness. Each spot lasts for 3 to 4 days and then disappears completely. The spots may continue to appear for another 1 to 2 weeks. The spots are rose-colored, slightly raised, and fade on pressure. They occur mainly on the abdomen and chest and occasionally on the back, upper arms, and thighs. The spots usually number less than 12 in typhoid but are more numerous in the paratyphoids. Their presence and number bear no relation to the severity of the attack. They *can* be seen on black skin, despite teaching to the contrary, and a drop of oil will make them easier to see.

SPECIFIC SIGNS

1. Pyrexia. Fever varies greatly in typhoid, and the classic temperature pattern may be present only in the untreated and uncomplicated cases. The classic chart in the untreated case shows a stepladder rise during the first week with an evening rise of about 2°F (1.1°C) and a morning fall of about 1°F (0.55°C). Toward the end of the first week the temperature usually reaches about 104°F (40°C), and during the second week the evening temperature is about 103 to 104°F (39.4 and 40°C) with a morning temperature of about 101 to 102°F (38.3 to 38.8°C).

The pyrexia in the third week in an uncomplicated case begins to fall in much the same way as it rose, i.e., a fall of 2°F (1.1°C) in the morning with a rise of 1°F (0.55°C) in the evening. There are many other temperature patterns, and this may lead to difficulty, especially if the patient is seen late or a complication has set in. A sudden rise at an early stage of the disease may be due to a complication such as typhoid lobar pneumonia, and a sudden fall may be seen in the later stages of the disease or after a complication such as sudden intestinal hemorrhage or perforation. A low pyrexia may occur in mild cases or occasionally in older patients. In the paratyphoid fevers the pyrexia tends to be lower than in typhoid. A rise in pyrexia in convalescence may be due to a relapse or a complication.

The temperature after treatment with chloramphenicol usually shows a drop to normal in about 4 days, but there is a latent period during the first 2 days when very little alteration is noted.

Thus it can be seen that the temperature pattern in typhoid may be deceptive. In the typical uncomplicated case, however, it can be a very useful clinical sign, especially when correlated with other diagnostic criteria.

2. Respiratory System. In the majority of cases the respiration rate is from 20 to 30 breaths per minute. It is rare to find a rate of over 30 breaths per minute in adults, which is a useful differential diagnostic sign from lobar pneumonia.

A bronchitic chest is a common finding, and 56 per cent of my patients presented with this. This finding may vary from a few rhonchi to a frank acute bronchitis. It may be of considerable diagnostic value, especially when correlated with the typical abdominal findings of typhoid fever, and together these constitute the two most valuable diagnostic signs.

3. Cardiovascular System. The pulse rate is classically described as a bradycardia. A better description, however, is that the pulse rate is relatively slow compared with the temperature during the first week of illness and it seldom exceeds 100 beats per minute. It also tends to be dicrotic. In children and in severe cases the pulse rate may be much more rapid, even during the first week of illness.

4. Gastrointestinal System. The tongue may be dry and coated on admission. In severe cases it may be covered by a brown fur on the dorsum with a marked diminution of saliva, especially during the second and third weeks in an untreated patient.

The abdominal signs of most value are a combination of slight upper abdominal tenderness in the liver and splenic regions, while a tender palpable spleen may be a valuable positive finding in countries where hypersplenism is uncommon. There is often slight guarding and generalized tumidity of the abdomen similar to the "doughiness" of tuberculous peritonitis, and moderate abdominal distention is common in the second and third weeks of illness.

5. Central Nervous System. There is often some mental dullness in typhoid, although this may not be present in mild cases of paratyphoid.

Meningism may be seen at an early stage of the disease, sometimes mimicking a true meningitis. There may be neck retraction, photophobia, and severe headache, which gradually regresses as the ordinary signs of typhoid develop. Meningism is particularly common in children.

6. Skeletal System. The patient may complain of joint, muscular, and back pains on admission. Clinical examination, however, is usually negative.

7. Genitourinary System. Apart from retention of urine, which may occur in the early stages, there are no early signs attributable to the genitourinary system.

INVESTIGATIONS

1. Simple Ward Tests. The stool in typhoid should always be inspected. The "pea soup" stool of the classic papers on typhoid fever is less frequent now that purgatives are not given in typhoid, but it should always be looked for.

Blood in the stool early in the illness indicates a diagnosis of bacillary dysentery rather than typhoid fever.

Albuminuria is an extremely common finding in typhoid but is of little diagnostic value.

2. Simple Laboratory Tests. The blood slide for malarial parasites should be examined in all cases in which the possibility of malaria exists.

The white blood cell count is a useful test in typhoid, and a low count with a relative lymphocytosis is commonly seen. The converse is much truer, and a white blood cell count of over 10,000 per cu mm with a leukocytosis is very much against a diagnosis of enteric fever, except in children.

The stool specimens examined for ova and entameba may be useful in differentiating schistosomiasis and amebiasis from the more chronic forms of typhoid in endemic areas.

3. Diazo Test of Urine. The froth of the urine of typhoid patients turns red when mixed with diazo reagents. This test can be performed quickly in the ward and is very useful, especially during an epidemic. Eighty to 90 per cent of the typhoid patients in the author's series who were tested gave a positive reaction at some stage of their illness, while only 5.7 per cent of control patients gave a positive reaction. The reaction is particularly likely to be positive in a pyrexial patient between 5 and 14 days after the onset of the illness. Laboratory details of the test have been described elsewhere.

The diazo reaction is particularly useful when the blood has been sterilized by chloramphenicol or the Widal reaction invalidated by previous TAB vaccine inoculations. It has definite limitations but is a quick screening test in countries where typhoid is widespread and particularly where laboratory facilities are scarce.

4. Culture of the Typhoid Bacillus. Culture of the typhoid bacillus is the only sure method of making the diagnosis of typhoid fever.

A blood culture may be positive at any stage of the clinical illness, particularly during the first week. Chloramphenicol usually sterilizes the blood within 2 hours, and it is therefore important to take a blood sample before chloramphenicol is started.

Blood clot culture, however, has been shown to be positive more often than whole blood culture, and it may remain positive several days after the administration of chloramphenicol.

Stool culture is not positive as often as blood culture. It is, however, a valuable diagnostic test, and several stool specimens should always be cultured. Contrary to the usual teaching, it is often positive before the third week of illness and may be positive at any stage of the disease.

Urine culture is not positive as often as stool culture, and then only after the second week of illness. Culture of pus from abscesses and postmortem culture will occasionally yield a positive result when other results have been negative.

5. Agglutination Tests. The diagnostic value of the Widal reaction has been diminished by the widespread use of TAB vaccination. In an unimmunized patient it does not become positive until after 7 to 10 days of illness.

In an endemic area, or in patients who have had previous TAB vaccine inoculations, the H antibody level can be raised by many nonspecific illness and therefore yields little specific data. The O antigen agglutination is of much more value, and an O antigen agglutination of 1:200 in a patient with a rising titer and a pyrexia clinically resembling typhoid is very suggestive of typhoid but is not diagnostic. In patients in nonendemic areas who have not had previous TAB vaccine, the Widal reaction is of much greater value.

DIFFERENTIAL DIAGNOSIS

Typhoid fever may be confused with a large number of diseases. In the United States and Britain the diagnosis is particularly liable to be missed in isolated cases, while in the tropics many conditions may resemble typhoid fever.

1. Paratyphoids A, B, and C. The laboratory is usually required as the final authority. The paratyphoids tend to run a milder course with profuse rose spots. Geographic distribution sometimes simplifies the matter; the paratyphoids are rare in East Africa, but paratyphoid B is not uncommon in Britain.

2. Salmonella Infection and Gastroenteritis. Salmonellae, the dysentery group, and staphylococci may occasionally cause an invasive illness that resembles typhoid fever with bacteremia. Usually, however, the gastrointestinal symptoms are more acute than the general manifestations and the pyrexia much lower and of shorter duration.

3. Other Diseases in Differential Diagnosis. There are many other conditions that may mimic typhoid fever. A careful history and examination, with the aid of the laboratory when necessary, will often resolve the difficulty.

Malaria may be mistaken for typhoid in countries where both are endemic, but a history of previous attack, the more rapid onset, the shivering and sweating, the high early pyrexia, the relative infrequency of abdominal symptoms and signs, and a positive blood slide all point to a diagnosis of malaria.

Influenza may also be confused with typhoid, but it is usually of much more rapid onset, with high temperature, severe sore throat, cough, and the absence of a palpable spleen and rose spots.

Bacillary dysentery seldom causes much difficulty in diagnosis. The onset is usually acute, with severe bloody diarrhea, although in mild cases the blood may be absent. Diarrhea with blood is rare in early typhoid. The signs and symptoms in dysentery are usually abdominal and remain so, the mental state and chest being clear.

Typhus and other rickettsial infections are important to consider in the differential diagnosis, as both typhus and typhoid can cause a febrile illness with delirium, chest signs, and abdominal discomfort. In typhus, however, the onset is acute and the temperature high at an early stage. Shivering attacks are common at the onset, and prostration is rapid. The rash is quite different (brownish-red in color and much more profuse) and does not fade on pressure as does the rose spot in typhoid. There is a leukocytosis, and the Weil-Felix test becomes significantly positive at about the tenth day.

In economically poor countries pulmonary tuberculosis and atypical abdominal tuberculosis are probably the most difficult diseases to differentiate from typhoid fever. The pyrexia and vague symptoms and signs may be very similar, and an x-ray of the chest or laboratory confirmation of typhoid may be the only sure method of diagnosis.

Brucellosis may cause difficulty, but the onset tends to be more insidious, the patient is alert, and a painful joint is frequently present. Trypanosomiasis in endemic areas should also be considered in the differential diagnosis.

The other diseases that enter the diagnostic field are too numerous to mention individually. Suffice it to say that there are few conditions that cannot mimic, or be mimicked by, typhoid fever.

TYPHOID AS A COMPLICATION

Typhoid itself may first present as a complication such as typhoid pneumonia, meningitis, orchitis, nephritis, or abscess (Fig. 4). An acute abdominal emergency may prove to be a perforated ileum in an otherwise unsuspected case of typhoid fever.

COMPLICATIONS

There are many complications in typhoid fever, and it may sometimes be difficult to differentiate between a complication and the natural course in so variable a disease. Complications are often associated with the gross toxemia and prostration of the disease and are especially common if nursing care is inadequate.

1. General Complications. The general complications include typhoid abscesses, boils, bedsores, otitis media, Zenker's degeneration of muscle, severe mental confusion, deafness, severe dehydration, and tonsillitis.

The importance of typhoid abscesses is that they are often missed, as they tend to be deep in the buttocks.

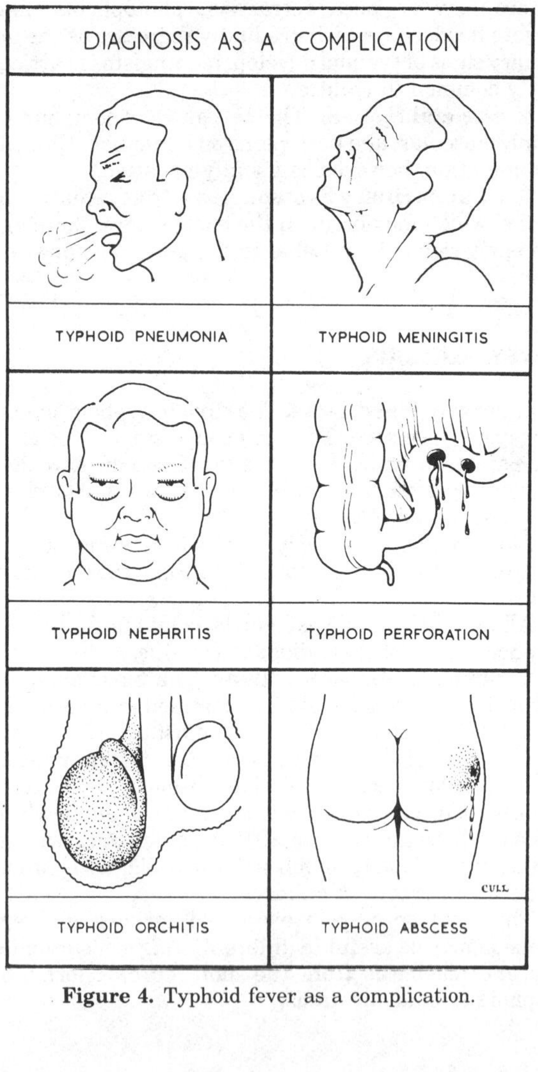

Figure 4. Typhoid fever as a complication.

They may, however, be superficial and present exactly like boils.

Zenker's degeneration of muscle is rare, but it may affect other muscles besides the classic site of rectus abdominis.

Mild deafness is common, but severe inner ear deafness is rare. Other complications are mainly due to intercurrent infection or difficulties of nursing in a debilitated patient.

2. Medical Complications. The medical complications include acute bronchitis and frank typhoid lobar pneumonia, toxic myocarditis, venous thromboses, hemolytic anemia, acute typhoid nephritis, typhoid meningitis, and peripheral neuritis.

Acute bronchitis is so common that it should be considered a manifestation of the disease itself rather than as a complication. Typhoid lobar pneumonia presents with the typical symptoms and signs of lobar pneumonia except that "rusty" sputum is uncommon and the white blood cell count low; it responds well to chloramphenicol.

Myocarditis is extremely common, particularly in the very toxic patient. The cardiac muscle is affected, even in convalescence, and this is shown by a rapid deterioration of the cardiovascular system in a relapse or after administration of a general anesthetic.

Typhoid meningitis, which is rare, must not be confused with meningism, which is common. Mild hemolytic anemia is fairly common in the very toxic typhoid patient. A marked degree is rare, and the mortality rate is high.

Febrile albuminuria is common, but a true acute typhoid nephritis is rare. Peripheral neuritis and "tender toes" should be treated with large doses of vitamin B complex, which should also be given in typhoid fever as a prophylactic measure.

3. Major Surgical Complications. The major surgical complications of typhoid fever may include parotitis, intestinal perforation and hemorrhage, acute cholecystitis, paralytic ileus, orchitis, pyelitis, cystitis, retention of urine, empyema, arthritis, and osteomyelitis.

Intestinal perforation may be associated with peritonitis. This is one of the most serious complications of typhoid and rarely occurs before the third week of illness. Diagnosis may be difficult, and many of the usual symptoms are masked by the general toxic state of the patient and by local adhesions around the leakage. In many cases, especially in the very sick, the first indication of perforation may be the presence of free fluid, either generalized or localized, with deterioration of condition of the patient, absent bowel sounds, and vomiting. Sometimes the classic signs of perforation will occur, but deterioration in the general condition is always rapid.

Intestinal hemorrhage may be a very serious complication of typhoid fever; it usually occurs from 14 to 21 days after the onset of the illness and is often "silent." The patient may bleed small amounts from several areas, or there may be a massive silent hemorrhage, and the first evidence may be a shocked patient with very pale conjuctivae.

Typhoid cholecystitis, like cholecystitis due to other organisms, occurs more frequently in women than in men. Diagnosis may be difficult because of the upper abdominal tenderness that is often present in typhoid fever.

Paralytic ileus may be secondary to a perforation or primary to a severe toxemia. Intestinal obstruction may be due to a localized abscess or adhesions.

Typhoid orchitis usually occurs in convalescence, while acute pyelitis is more common than is generally recognized. Typhoid arthritis and osteomyelitis are uncommon, and a true typhoid spine is rare and a late complication. Infection of bones due to other salmonellae, however, such as *Salmonella typhimurium,* is common, especially in sickle cell anemia.

CONCOMITANT DISEASES

In tropical countries concomitant diseases such as bacillary dysentery, malaria, amebiasis, and worm infestations are common. They should always be borne in mind, as they may confuse the diagnosis.

TYPHOID FEVER IN CHILDREN

The incubation period in children tends to be shorter and the onset more acute than in adults, and in some cases the disease simulates a gastroenteritis due to other causes. The child often, but by no means invariably, has a less severe attack than the adult, with pyrexia settling earlier. Complications tend to be less common, but when they do occur they usually progress more rapidly. Dehydration and mineral loss may be particularly severe.

TYPHOID FEVER IN PRIMITIVE CONDITIONS

Despite the publicity given to outbreaks in the United States, Britain, and Europe, the problems associated with them are trivial compared with the rest of the world. Most cases occur in countries in which hygiene is poor, equipment and trained medical and nursing staff are in extremely short supply, and transportation to hospitals is sometimes nonexistent.

Diagnosis must be made mainly on clinical findings plus simple tests such as a low blood cell count and the diazo test for urine. Confirmation is obtained from a single specimen of clotted blood that can be used for both culture and the Widal reaction, while a culture of feces in glycerol will allow for delay in transport of the specimen. Finally, in doubtful cases, a therapeutic test with chloroquine for malaria, penicillin for pneumonia, and sulfaguanidine for bacillary dysentery may be unscientific but is essentially practical.

THE CARRIER

The screening of all patients, suspects, and contacts is essential in countries in which adequate medical facilities exist. Three, and preferably six, negative stool and urine cultures and a negative Vi antigen test of blood should be the minimum requirements before a proved case of typhoid is discharged from hospital.

THE PARATYPHOID FEVERS

The paratyphoid fevers A, B, and C resemble typhoid fever and usually, but not always, run a milder course. *Salmonella paratyphi,* however, requires a medium in which to multiply, and meat pies, synthetic cream, and milk are the usual vehicles for this. Paratyphoid fever resembles other nonspecific salmonella infections in this respect, and paratyphoid B may occasionally also have an onset similar to Salmonella gastroenteritis. Despite this, paratyphoid fever is primarily an invasive type of disease like typhoid fever.

Paratyphoid A, however, is less likely to cause complications than typhoid fever but is more likely to relapse. Paratyphoid B, which is common in Europe, is milder than typhoid but is more likely to result in carriers and to cause jaundice, thromboses, and suppurative lesions. Paratyphoid C differs clinically from typhoid fever and the other paratyphoids by causing more septicemic manifestations such as arthritis, cholecystitis, and abscesses, with little in the way of gastrointestinal lesions.

CONCLUSIONS

The enteric fevers, and particularly typhoid fever, are still very much a worldwide problem, and many hundreds of thousands, if not millions, of new cases occur each year throughout the world. It will be many years before the hygiene of the world is improved and the incidence of the disease drastically diminished.

In the future, it will be not only the practitioner in the hygienically backward country who will have to contend with the disease but his colleagues in the so-called developed countries as well. As air travel increases, so will actual cases in visitors and vacationers returning from abroad and also epidemics caused by unknown carriers. Other sources of infection, such as preserved foods from abroad, will also undoubtedly continue to be a source of infection, as it will obviously be impossible to examine every can of meat or improve world standards of hygiene overnight. Sooner or later the practitioner will fall into the diagnostic trap that the sporadic unsuspected case presents, unless he constantly bears in mind the many guises of this "international" disease.

ACKNOWLEDGMENTS

I am indebted to the Managing Director of Churchill Livingstone for permission to reproduce Figures 1–4 from my monograph, "Typhoid Fever and Other Salmonella Infections," 1962.

BRUCELLOSIS

By Brian P. Buggy, M.D.
and Robert Fekety, M.D.
Ann Arbor, Michigan

SYNONYMS

In 1887, Brucellae were first isolated from the spleens of British soldiers dying on the island of Malta from a disease then called Malta fever. This disorder has also been known as undulant fever or Mediterranean fever, and is frequently called Bang's disease or "infectious abortion" by farmers and veterinarians.

DEFINITION

Brucellosis is an infectious disease transmitted to humans by animals or animal products containing bacteria of the genus *Brucella.* Brucellae are aerobic, non–spore-forming, gram-negative rods that do not ferment carbohydrates or form a capsule in vivo.

Human disease is caused primarily by four species of brucellae: *B. abortus, B. suis, B. melitensis,* and *B. canis. B. abortus* is isolated from cattle and is the sole etiologic agent in 35 per cent of human disease. *B. suis* is most commonly isolated from swine (domestic and feral) and causes approximately 17 per cent of human brucellosis in the United States. Swine had been the source of the majority of human infections until 1974, but the incidence has declined. Exposure to both cattle and swine accounts for another 30 per cent of cases. *B. melitensis* is found in sheep and goats and, although an unusual cause of brucellosis in the United States, is the most common cause worldwide. *B. canis* (usually derived from dogs) is a rarely documented agent of human disease. *B. ovis* from rams and *B. neotomae* from the desert wood rat are potential sources of brucellosis but have never been documented to cause human disease. Brucellae have also been isolated from deer, caribou, horses, mice, cats, and chickens, but their role as reservoirs of the organism has not been established.

Brucellae can persist within phagocytic and lymphoid cells, and adequate cellular immunity is required to resist or contain infection. Apparently healthy animals can shed brucellae in their milk for years. The organisms are killed by pasteurization but may persist for several weeks in unpasteurized dairy products, such as cheese and butter.

Epidemiologic data reveal that 170 cases of brucellosis in humans were reported to the Centers for Disease Control in 1981. This continues an almost uninterrupted decline since 1947 in the number of reported human cases, although the frequency has been relatively constant since 1978. Most (80 per cent) represent newly acquired infections, 10 per cent are relapsing or chronic, and in the remaining 10 per cent the patient's prior status could not be ascertained. Iowa, Virginia, Texas, and California account for one half of all cases.

Brucellosis is acquired as a result of contact with infected animals (living or recently slaughtered), their products of conception, their dairy products (raw milk or unpasteurized cheese and butter), and, rarely, laboratory exposures or accidental injection of the strain intended for cattle vaccination ("Strain 19 disease"), which almost always occurs in veterinarians. The majority of human infections occur in slaughterhouse and packing plant workers, livestock producers, meat inspectors, and veterinarians. The age and sex distribution of disease mirrors these occupations, with 80 per cent occuring in men between the ages of 20 and 60 years. Organisms gain entry through broken skin, via the conjunctivae, or by ingestion. Recent epidemiologic data have also strongly supported a role for the aerosol inhalation of organisms, especially in abattoir and laboratory workers.

PRESENTING SIGNS AND SYMPTOMS

There are no pathognomonic signs or symptoms of brucellosis, but fever is the most common presenting complaint. The average incubation period is 1 to 3 weeks. Asymptomatic infection is at least ten times as frequent as symptomatic infection. The onset of symptoms is equally divided between acute and subacute presentations. Fever occurs in almost all patients with acute brucellosis and less often in chronic disease. The majority of patients also experience weakness, malaise, shaking chills, profuse sweats, anorexia, and weight loss averaging 15 to 20 pounds in the first 2 to 3 weeks. Approximately one fourth of patients also describe arthralgia of the large joints (true arthritis is rare), myalgias, cough, back pain, and headache. Constipation, diarrhea, nausea, retro-orbital pain, tinnitus, insomnia, and impotence are also seen. Infection with *B. abortus* is usually milder than that with *B. suis* or *B. melitensis.*

B. canis also causes a relatively milder disease process that is almost always self-limited. This organism was first described in 1966 in kennel-bred beagles, but it also exists in domestic and wild dog populations as well as in raccoons, foxes, and coyotes. From 1967 to 1977, 18 cases in humans were reported. In 13 patients the diagnosis was made by blood (12) or abscess (1) culture, and in five by serology. Pet dogs were the source in eight cases, eight were related to occupational exposure (six laboratory accidents), and the source was unknown in the remaining two.

PHYSICAL EXAMINATION

Apart from fever and weight loss, there are few objective physical findings in acute brucellosis. Diffuse lymphadenopathy and splenomegaly are present in approximately one third of patients, reflecting lymphoreticular localization of this initially bacteremic disease. Hepatomegaly is present in only 10 per cent. A variety of skin manifestations have been reported in 5 to 10 per cent of patients. Brucellosis is one of the diseases that can produce petechiae on the palms and soles. Small papular lesions on the trunk, erythematous patches over the bridge of the nose (similar to those seen with systemic lupus erythematosus), and erythema nodosum-like nodules on the legs (both shin and calf) have also been reported. With chronic disease, physical findings are either absent or reflect localization of the disease process.

COURSE AND COMPLICATIONS

If acute disease is diagnosed within 1 month of onset and appropriately treated, almost all patients will be cured. Less than 5 per cent will suffer a relapse in some form. Untreated brucellosis resolves in the vast majority of instances over 3 to 6 months, but most chronic disease and localized complications evolve from these untreated patients. Since brucellosis is initially a bacteremic disease, subsequent problems can occur literally anywhere in the body. Most common sites of metastatic infection include the spine, joints, kidney, spleen, epididymis, lung, liver, and heart. Although rare, the most lethal form of the disease is endocarditis. Thus, chronic brucellosis can present as osteomyelitis (usually vertebral), suppurative arthritis, epididymitis, orchitis, nephritis, cystitis, optic neuritis, encephalitis, meningitis, soft-tissue abscess, lung abscess, endocarditis, myocarditis, and with the skin lesions already mentioned.

LABORATORY FINDINGS

The white blood cell count is usually normal and occasionally depressed. A relative lymphocytosis is often seen. Pancytopenia is uncommon and usually occurs in long-standing disease. Liver function tests and erythrocyte sedimentation rate are nonspecifically increased in acute disease. Aerosol inhalation may produce a miliary pattern on chest x-ray, and long-standing disease may show calcifications in the spleen.

In acute untreated disease, 50 to 75 per cent of blood cultures will be positive. However, for optimal detection, the laboratory must be informed of the possibility of brucellosis and must be asked to incubate the cultures for 3 to 4 weeks. Three to four separate pairs of blood cultures are sufficient. In relapsing or chronic disease, blood cultures are almost never positive. Cultures of other tissues are occasionally rewarding, most often from the bone marrow, liver, spleen, and lymph nodes. Again, if brucellae are being specifically sought, the laboratory must be notified to assist in identification and to be aware of this biohazard. The addition of erythritol to culture media and a CO_2-enriched atmosphere will facilitate growth.

Culture of blood, tissue, or abscess material is the best diagnostic test for brucellosis. However, except for blood cultures in acute disease, the yield on cultures is generally low and bacteriologic confirmation of the disease occurs in no more than 20 per cent of patients. There are six species of *Brucella* and 16 biotypes (three of *B. melitensis,* nine of *B. abortus,* four of *B. suis*), and these are differentiated by dye inhibition tests, bacteriophage lysis, urease activity, production of hydrogen sulfide, and requirement for carbon dioxide.

Diagnosis is most often made serologically, since cultural confirmation is uncommon. The tube-agglutination test, introduced in 1936, has remained the standard serologic test in the United States. A standard suspension of heat-killed bacilli is used, which is agglutinated by a group antiserum against *B. melitensis, B. abortus,* and *B. suis. B. canis* requires a separate reagent, and titers against this organism must be specifically requested. A fourfold increase in antibody titer is significant for diagnosis at any time, and a minimal or stable titer of 1:160 or greater is suggestive of recent infection. Chronic infections typically are either negative or have titers of 1:80 or less. Almost all (97 per cent) recently infected individuals will be seropositive within 3 weeks after disease onset. The current tube-agglutination test measures both IgG and IgM antibodies. IgM is reflective of recent infection, can be determined after 2-mercaptoethanol treatment of serum, and typically disappears within 3 months of infection, leaving a monovalent IgG as the long-standing antibody. The limitations of the tube-agglutination test include a prozone phenomenon, which means that agglutination may not occur unless the serum is diluted several hundredfold (this is due to the presence of blocking antibodies). False elevations in antibody titer resulting from the use of the brucellin skin test (no longer available) and false elevations due to recent infection with or immunization against tularemia or cholera also occur. *Campyl obacter fetus* and *Yersinia enterocolitica* can also induce agglutinins that react in this test. Admission titers of patients acutely infected with brucellae average 1:1280, with a range of 1:640 to 1:5120. Successful treatment will result in a slow fall in titers to 1:80 after one year. A negative titer (with no prozone phenomenon) at any time of the illness essentially excludes naturally occurring brucellosis.

PITFALLS IN DIAGNOSIS

The diagnosis of brucellosis is relatively easy to make in a person who is in contact with animals or animal products and has an acute illness with fever, sweats, myalgias, and arthralgias. Cultural (blood) or serologic evidence is likely to be present. The clinical presentation of acute brucellosis, however, can be easily mimicked by influenza, infectious mononucleosis, toxoplasmosis, viral hepatitis, thyrotoxicosis, systemic lupus erythematosus, adult rheumatic fever, tuberculosis, leptospirosis, and typhoid fever. Diagnosis becomes much more difficult in the patient with a chronic process manifested by malaise and weight loss, especially in someone with past or continued exposure to the organism. Tuberculosis, sarcoidosis, Hodgkin's disease, non-Hodgkin's lymphomas, and metastatic carcinoma are the likely masqueraders in the chronic setting. Since serology is less likely to be helpful in chronic disease, the importance of biopsy and culture of any suspicious lesion cannot be overemphasized. Therapeutic trials with tetracyclines or trimethoprim-sulfamethoxazole are usually not helpful and are not recommended.

TULAREMIA

By Morton I. Rapoport, M.D.
Baltimore, Maryland

DEFINITION

Tularemia is an acute bacterial infection with remarkable similarity to plague. It is caused by the gram-negative coccobacillus *Francisella tularensis.* This disease is encountered worldwide and is epizootic and enzootic in numerous species of animals. Recent reports have emphasized domestic cats as an important reservoir of human infection. In addition, a variety of acarina and insects, including ticks and deer flies, have been established as vectors in the transmission of the disease.

The clinical course of this disease is dependent on the route of infection. While tularemia can be divided into five basic clinical patterns, frequent overlap can hinder definitive categorization. Variant forms of the disease include ulceroglandular, oculoglandular, enteric or typhoidal, and pulmonary. Most human infections are of the ulceroglandular type, although primary and secondary pulmonary infections are frequently encountered.

The infection may be transmitted by arthropod vector or animal bite, by handling of infected animal tissues, or by exposure to infected aerosols. Diagnosis is frequently suspected by historic exposure; however, only serologic and cultural findings are confirmatory.

CLINICAL COURSE

The various forms of infection, while occasionally overlapping, are distinctly different and generally reflect the route of inoculation. The two major types of infection, pulmonary and ulceroglandular, are both associated with prominent lymphatic involvement.

Ulceroglandular Tularemia. Direct inoculation of the organism is associated with ulceroglandular infection. Patients with this illness become clinically ill within 1 week of contact. The classic lesion begins as a small erythematous papule that rapidly progresses to ulceration. Within 1 to 2 days, regional lymph nodes are noted to enlarge and become painful. In many patients systemic influenza-like symptoms, including chills and fever, headache, and toxicity, become manifest. Occasionally, the inoculation site and the regional lymphatic involvement go unrecognized and constitutional and pulmonary symptoms predominate. These latter infections may be mistaken for primary pulmonary infections. In the more typical patients with ulceroglandular tularemia, the lymph nodes are the most prominent sites of involvement. Over a period of several weeks, tender nodes become fluctuant and may progress to suppuration and frank drainage. Microscopic examination of the lymph nodes shows large numbers of organisms in association with granulomatous lesions and abscesses remarkably similar to tuberculous infection.

A mortality rate of 3 to 7 per cent has been reported in ulceroglandular infection.

Pulmonary Tularemia. Primary pulmonary infection or pneumonia due to *Francisella tularensis* is almost invariably associated with inhalation of the organism, although the circumstance of exposure may vary widely. Hunters and trappers may be exposed to aerosols during the process of skinning and dressing game, farm workers can be exposed during threshing of grain that has been contaminated by rodent feces, and laboratory workers likewise can be exposed in the process of diagnostic or cultural handling of the organism. It should be noted that the organism is exceedingly infectious and inhaled counts of as few as 10 organisms may be associated with disease.

The incubation period varies between 2 and 4 days and tends to reflect the intensity of the aerosol. Illness is abrupt in onset with constitutional symptoms becoming most prominent. Initial symptoms including headache, chills, high fever, and malaise with nonproductive cough are recognized. With delayed diagnosis or therapy the illness proceeds to a more virulent form characterized by bloody sputum, prostration, and refractory hypoxemia. In as many as 50 per cent of patients, physical findings may be absent and therefore not reflective of the fulminance of the disease.

More reliable diagnostic findings include a radiologic picture that shows diffuse bronchopneumonic or lobar infiltrate. In addition, pleural effusion and hilar or mediastinal adenopathy may be associated with parenchymal involvement.

Rarely, as just noted, secondary pulmonary involvement may be encountered in patients with advanced ulceroglandular disease. These patients may present with severe toxicity in association with advanced roentgenologic evidence of parenchymal and mediastinal disease.

Untreated or delayed treatment of pulmonary infection is associated with a mortality rate considerably higher than that encountered with ulceroglandular disease, possibly as high as 30 per cent.

Oculoglandular Tularemia. Considerably less common is the infection caused by direct inoculation of the organism into the mucous membranes of the eye. Diagnosis is frequently delayed because of the relatively nonspecific complaints and findings. Symptoms of severe pain, lacrimation, and photophobia may be encountered. Physical findings include formation of yellowish-white granulomatous lesions on the palpebral conjunctiva. In addition, conjunctival suffusion, chemosis, or conjunctival edema is also present. Characteristically, regional lymph nodes, particularly preauricular and cervical, may be enlarged and tender. Delayed recognition may result in corneal perforation or optic atrophy.

Typhoidal Tularemia. Much less common is the enteric or typhoidal form of tularemia associated with infection by the oral route. The organism has been isolated from mud and water, and water-borne infection has been documented.

Chills and high fever in association with nausea, vomiting, diarrhea, and severe abdominal pain may suggest a diagnosis of typhoid fever. Similarity to typhoid may extend to development of ulcerative lesions in the gastrointestinal tract as well. Complications including significant gastrointestinal hemorrhage and perforation may also be encountered. The mortality rate approximates that experienced with pulmonary tularemia.

LABORATORY DIAGNOSIS

Leukocyte counts and acute phase reactants are of little diagnostic value in that they may be normal or slightly increased. Using selected media, isolation of the organism from ulcers, secretions, blood, and biopsy specimens serves to establish the diagnosis given. The organism is easily propagated on glucose cystine blood agar (GCBA). Extreme care in the handling of this organism is required because of its remarkable propensity for producing laboratory infection. Similarly, laboratory animal inoculation is discouraged, owing to the frequency of laboratory-acquired disease.

Surprisingly, serologic diagnosis may be extremely useful even in the early diagnostic process. Indeed, significant increases in agglutinating antibodies may be detected within the first 10 to 14 days of clinical illness.

As with most serologic studies, diagnosis is established most effectively using paired or sequential sera in an effort to document titer increases. In tularemia, the importance of sequential sera is also underscored by virtue of the characteristic persistence of antibodies for many years. Cross-reactivity of serum obtained from patients with brucellosis has also been reported, although comparative studies will reflect higher titers using the homologous antigen.

A diagnostic intradermal skin test using a purified killed suspension of *F. tularensis* as described by Foshay is highly specific. Positive reactions are encountered after one week of illness and reactivity persists for many years. The reaction is analogous to the tuberculin reaction in that inoculation intradermally is followed by an erythematous indurated papule within 48 hours in patients with positive reaction.

PITFALLS IN DIAGNOSIS

Ulceroglandular tularemia must be distinguished from the myriad conditions that are associated with cutaneous ulceration and draining lymphadenopathy. These include plague, cat-scratch fever, rat-bite fever, anthrax, lymphogranuloma venereum, and sporotrichosis and other cutaneous fungal infections, including histoplasmosis and coccidioidomycosis. While historic and epidemiologic information may exclude most diagnostic possibilities, serolgic and cultural data are particularly relevant to the array of conditions that mimic ulceroglandular tularemia.

Pulmonary tularemia must be distinguished from a variety of pulmonary infections not readily diagnosed by bacteriologic smears. These include primary fungal infections, mycoplasma infection, Legionnaires' disease, rickettsial infections (specifically, Q fever), and an acute viral infection, particularly influenza.

PLAGUE

By Jonathan M. Mann, M.D., M.P.H.
Santa Fe, New Mexico
Linda J. Nims, M.S.
and Michael R. Skeels, Ph.D.
Albuquerque, New Mexico

SYNONYMS

Infection with *Yersinia pestis* is properly called plague. Common synonyms include bubonic plague (which actually refers to a particular clinical form of the disease), the "Black Death" (reference to the second great plague pandemic of the 14th century), or pest.

DEFINITION

Plague is a zoonosis, a disease of rodents that can be spread to humans. Animal populations infected with plague can be divided into three groups: maintenance hosts, amplification hosts, and incidental hosts. Maintenance hosts are rodents less likely to die from plague, thereby providing a constant reservoir for the disease. In the United States, this group includes mice, pack rats, and wood rats. The amplification hosts are rodents much more susceptible to fatal plague infection, so that epizootics generally follow the introduction of *Y. pestis* into these animal populations. The amplification hosts of plague in the United States include ground squirrels, rock squirrels, and prairie dogs. Incidental hosts are animals that may acquire disease yet play little known role in plague ecology, such as lagomorphs (rabbits) and carnivores (dogs, cats, coyotes, bobcats). Plague infection can be transmitted to humans from any of these groups of animals.

Plague can be transmitted from infected animals to humans either by fleas or by direct contact. Fleas ingesting blood meals from plague-infected animals may become vectors for disease spread. Flea-borne spread is the most common route of plague acquisition in the United States (approximately 85 per cent of cases) and tends to occur in the warmer months of the year (May through September). The second route of transmission involves the handling (usually skinning) of plague-infected animals, with exposure to *Y. pestis* in animal blood and body fluids. The direct contact route accounts for about 15 per cent of cases in the United States that typically occur in the late fall, winter, or early spring. The incubation period of plague is 2 to 6 days.

In addition, humans infected with *Y. pestis* can develop a pneumonia as a result of hematogenous spread of the organism (e.g., pneumonic plague, to be discussed). In some cases, persons with plague pneumonia cough viable plague bacilli into the air and these bacteria-laden droplets can be inhaled by and infect close contacts. The potential for person-to-person spread of plague pneumonia is extremely important. Primary plague pneumonia (plague acquired directly from another person) is a highly virulent and frequently fatal disease with a brief incubation period (1 to 4 days).

Historically, plague pandemics have affected large areas of the world. Foci of animal plague currently exist in Africa, Asia, South America, and North America, and more than 1000 cases of human plague are reported each year to the World Health Organization. Plague was apparently introduced into the United States at the end of the 19th and beginning of the 20th century on ships traveling from plague-enzootic areas of the world. In the early part of this century, plague was primarily a problem among rodents in and immediately around port areas of the Western and Gulf Coasts. Following changes in ship sanitation practices and campaigns to eradicate port rodents (rats), plague disappeared from the Gulf Coast. However, in the American West, plague spread to peridomestic rodents near port city foci and then into the sylvatic (wild) rodent populations. Animal plague has since been documented in 15 states west of the 100th meridian. From 1950 to 1982, human plague cases occurred in ten Western states (Arizona, California, Colorado, Idaho, Nevada, New Mexico, Oregon, Texas, Utah, Wyoming). In the United States, an average of 11 cases of human plague have been reported each year from 1970 to 1979, with a 14 per cent case-fatality ratio. Groups at particular risk of plague infection include residents of rural areas of the American West, hunters, trappers, and veterinarians.

PRESENTING SIGNS AND SYMPTOMS

Plague infection exists in three major clinical forms: bubonic, primary septicemic, and primary pneumonic. These major forms can be complicated by metastatic infections of the meninges or lungs. In addition, less common clinical forms of plague include pharyngeal, cutaneous, and endophthalmic plague.

Bubonic Plague. Bubonic plague is characterized by an exquisitely painful lymphadenitis (the bubo). The onset of illness is usually rapid, with fever, malaise, and appearance of the bubo. Buboes are usually unilateral and are most often inguinal/femoral in location, but may be axillary, cervical, or epitrochlear. Buboes are extremely tender and often exhibit overlying erythema and perinodal edema. The constellation of acute onset of fever, malaise, and exquisitely painful lymphadenitis is characteristic of bubonic plague.

Primary Septicemic Plague. Primary septicemic disease is plague infection in the absence of a detectable bubo. Primary septicemic plague is clinically indistinguishable from other causes of community-acquired bacterial sepsis and is characterized by the acute onset of fever, malaise, or prostration that progresses rapidly if appropriate antibiotics are not administered.

Primary Pneumonic Plague. As mentioned, a patient with plague pneumonia can spread *Y. pestis* to close contacts. The early symptoms of primary pneumonic plague include acute onset of fever and malaise or prostration. A cough may be initially absent, but coughing, including production of bloody sputum, follows within hours to 1 day after onset. Other than the severity and rapid progression of disease, no features reliably distinguish plague pneumonia from other bacterial pneumonias.

COMPLICATIONS OF PLAGUE INFECTION

In some patients with bubonic or primary septicemic disease, the most readily identifiable feature is a metastatic focus of plague infection such as meningitis or secondary pneumonia. Plague meningitis presents with signs and symptoms typical of bacterial meningitis; plague pneumonia has already been described. In addition to these specific infectious complications, plague patients may experience diverse problems associated with sepsis, including shock, disseminated intravascular coagulation, and adult respiratory distress syndrome.

COURSE OF PLAGUE INFECTION

Unless treated with appropriate antibiotics, plague is rapidly progressive and death may occur within 3 to 6 days after onset. Metastatic spread of disease can complicate either bubonic or primary septicemic plague, especially when treatment is delayed. Plague infection does not respond immediately to antibiotic therapy. An increase in well-being should be anticipated within 1 to 2 days after initiation of appropriate antibiotics; however, fever lysis may not occur for 5 to 7 days and the bubo may actually continue to enlarge (although becoming less tender and with reduced inflammation) during the first several days. For most patients, plague is an acute illness resulting in a 1- to 2-week hospitalization followed by complete recovery with no sequelae.

PHYSICAL EXAMINATION

The physical findings depend upon the clinical form of plague. Bubonic plague, which accounts for approximately 85 per cent of all plague cases, is characterized by the bubo. Early in the illness, the bubo may be quite small and firm, yet is exquisitely tender. As the illness progresses, the bubo enlarges and becomes more fluctuant, with overlying erythema and perinodal edema. Physical findings in primary septicemic plague are nonspecific and relate to sepsis and its manifestations. Meningeal plague and plague pneumonia exhibit typical physical findings of acute bacterial meningitis and pneumonia.

DIAGNOSTIC PROCEDURES

Laboratory Procedures. Rapid laboratory diagnosis of plague is essential, given the importance of this diagnosis for personal (prompt initiation of effective antibiotics) and public health (allay concerns, prevent person-to-person spread of pneumonic plague). The peripheral leukocyte count can provide nonspecific support for a diagnosis of plague; in most cases, either a leukocytosis, a left shift in the differential count, or both are present. However, specific early diagnosis requires microscopic examination and culture of clinical specimens, most commonly bubo aspirate or blood and occasionally cerebrospinal fluid, sputum, or other material.

Bubo aspirates are obtained using a large (25- to 50-ml) syringe and a 19- to 20-gauge needle. Following skin preparation, the bubo should be entered and suction applied. Even if no aspirate is visible following this procedure, try to express fluid from within the needle and also submit the needle and syringe for culture. In addition, when no visible aspirate is obtained with this method, repeat by first injecting a small volume of nonbacteriostatic saline into the bubo and then withdrawing the fluid. Care must be taken to avoid aerosolization during bubo aspiration and specimen preparation. Several blood cultures should also be obtained from all patients prior to instituting antimicrobial therapy. It is important to notify the laboratory promptly about specimens from suspected plague cases. In addition, suspected plague specimens should always be handled in a Class II Type A Biological Safety Cabinet.

Direct Immunofluorescence and Stained Smears. A rapid diagnosis of human plague may be made by direct immunofluorescent (IF—usually called fluorescent antibody, or FA testing) examination of bubo aspirate, cerebrospinal fluid, sputum, bacterial isolates, or other material. About 90 per cent of bubo aspirates from cases of plague will be positive by this test, which is performed at the Centers for Disease Control, Atlanta, Georgia, and certain state health laboratories. A negative IF on a clinical specimen does not rule out the diagnosis of plague.

Gram stains of bubo aspirates, sputum, or cerebrospinal fluid from plague patients will reveal gram-negative rods. These organisms are more visible and usually appear "safety pin-like"—bipolar with a clear center—with a Wayson, Wright, or Giemsa stain. On smears from a liquid blood culture medium, the bacilli appear in chains rather than as single cells.

Culture and Identification of *Y. pestis*. In culture, *Y. pestis* grows well on blood agar, producing pinpoint (< 1 mm) colonies after 24 hours' incubation at 35°C. These colonies are seen more easily if low magnification (10X) is used. By 3 days, isolated colonies will be 1 to 2 mm in diameter. With magnification, they have a characteristic "beaten copper" appearance, shiny but with many shallow indentations on the surface. Positive cultures will usually show colonies at 48 hours, but negative plates should be incubated 1 week before discarding.

Y. pestis does not grow well in the presence of other microorganisms. If it is not the predominant bacterium in a mixed infection, animal inoculation may be necessary to obtain a pure culture. A saline suspension of the specimen is inoculated subcutaneously into mice. If the specimen is heavily contaminated, the surface of the skin is scratched with a needle and the specimen is rubbed into the broken skin. The mice are examined daily, and a direct IF exam is made on the liver and spleen at death. Mice surviving 3 weeks are killed, and a direct IF is performed. Cultures are inoculated from those specimens which are IF-positive.

Once isolated, the identity of *Y. pestis* is confirmed by a direct IF test, a bacteriophage test, and biochemical reactions. A specific phage isolated from *Y. pestis* will cause lysis of the organism at 25°C. The key biochemical reactions are shown in Table 1. Note that although *Y. pestis* does not ferment lactose or sucrose, its slow growth may require 48 hours on triple sugar iron (TSI) agar to reach the typical K/A (alkaline/acid) reaction of a glucose fermenter. Either conventional media or a rapid identification system such as API or Micro ID may be used for biochemical tests.

Because plague and tularemia may have similar clinical presentations, specimens from suspected plague cases should also be cultured for *Francisella tularensis* by inoculating chocolate agar and Thayer-Martin agar.

Radiologic Evaluation. A chest roentgenogram is mandatory for all patients with suspected or confirmed plague in order to rule out plague pneumonia. Roentgenograms in patients with plague pneumonia may demonstrate rapidly progressive alveolar pulmonary infiltrates, nodular densities, hilar adenopathy, and pleural effusions. In some cases x-ray findings are not specific for plague pneumonia but may reflect shock, adult respiratory distress syndrome, or disseminated intravascular coagulation.

Serology. A retrospective diagnosis of plague may be established serologically by the use of the indirect hemagglutination test. Paired specimens should be obtained at the onset of illness and 3 weeks later. A fourfold or greater increase in titer is considered evidence of recent infection. A single convalescent titer of $\geq 1{:}10$ is considered positive in a patient with no history of previous infection or immunization. Tularemia should also be considered and an agglutination test for *F. tularensis* antibodies performed simultaneously.

Animal Specimens. Human plague is usually acquired zoonotically; therefore, we often examine animals (using the IF test) as a component of public health plague surveillance and control. From rodents and lagomorphs, the spleen and liver are tested. If the animal has decomposed greatly, bone marrow from a long bone may be used. In the infected cats we have examined, *Y. pestis* is most frequently found in abscess material. Dogs that roam in plague-enzootic areas can be monitored for antibodies to *Y. pestis*.

Other Diagnostic Procedures. Plague is one of the few diseases commonly encountered in the United States in which a bacteremia of sufficient magnitude to permit visualization of *Y. pestis* organisms in the peripheral blood smear may occur. However, this finding is usually limited to severe cases and may not appear until late in the course of illness. Therefore, while careful examination of the peripheral blood smear may be useful, it should not be considered a highly sensitive or routine method for plague diagnosis.

POTENTIAL ERRORS AND PITFALLS IN DIAGNOSIS

Plague is an uncommon disease, even in endemic areas of the American West. Typical bubonic plague, while not difficult to recognize in retrospect, may be initially unsuspected in favor of more common causes of acute lymphadenitis such as staphylococcal or streptococcal disease. In addition, signs and symptoms of tularemia may closely mimic plague infection. Primary septicemic illness can be considered only if a high level of suspicion for plague infection is entertained. The essential problem in plague diagnosis is consideration of a rare disease. This problem is compounded in areas of the country that do not experience endemic plague, for travelers can easily acquire plague in the West and return to their homes during the incubation period of disease. Suspected plague cases should be reported immediately to the health department; consultation and assistance are available from state health departments and the Centers for Disease Control.

Table 1. Reactions of *Yersinia pestis*

Test	Reaction	Test	Reaction
Fermentation of			
Glucose	Acid	H_2S (TSI*)	–
Lactose	–	Indol	–
Mannitol	Acid	Methyl red	+
Sucrose	–	Voges-Proskauer	–
Maltose	Acid	Lysine decarboxylase	–
Xylose	Acid	Arginine dihydrolase	–
Rhamnose	–	Ornithine decarboxylase	–
Oxidase	–	Esculine hydrolysis	+
Motility	–	Coagulase	+
Urease	–	Growth on MacConkey Agar	Poor
Citrate (Simmons)	–		

*TSI = Triple sugar iron.

WHOOPING COUGH

By James W. Bass, M.D.
Oahu, Hawaii

SYNONYMS

Pertussis, chin cough, tosferira (Spanish), Keuchhusten (German), coqueluche (French), and pertoss (Italian).

DEFINITION

Whooping cough is an infection of the respiratory passages characterized by prolonged and protracted episodes of cough, usually ending in an inspiratory whoop. Greater than 95 per cent of cases are caused by *Bordetella pertussis* and less than 5 per cent by *B. parapertussis,* with *B. bronchiseptica* an even rarer cause of the disease. Recent studies have also etiologically implicated certain adenoviruses alone or in concert with *B. pertussis* organisms. Whooping cough is highly contagious with attack rates from 80 to 100 per cent in susceptible household contacts. The disease confers a fairly high degree of lasting immunity. Immunization produces relative protection, most field trials showing 70 to 80 per cent reduction in attack rate in vaccinees. This lasts only 2 to 3 years with declining protection thereafter and little or no evidence of protection after 12 years. Although the incidence of the disease has declined dramatically over the past few decades, a small number of cases have still been reported annually throughout the United States. The case fatality rate is now less than 1 per cent in this country; however, this disease is still a serious threat to young infants under 6 months of age. Most deaths occur in the 2- to 3-month-old age group. Whooping cough is still a major cause of sickness and death in developing countries throughout the world where broad-scaled immunization against the disease has not been achieved.

PRESENTING SIGNS AND SYMPTOMS

After an incubation period of 10 days (range, 5 to 16) the disease presents as a simple cold with nasal stuffiness, clear mucosal discharge, and a cough. This is referred to as the "catarrhal" stage and usually lasts 6 to 7 days. It may on some occasions persist up to 2 weeks, whereas in others it may be so mild as to even go unrecognized.

COURSE

The cough of the catarrhal stage worsens, and the subsequent clinical course of the disease varies depending upon age. Violent paroxysms of cough occur, numbering from only several to numerous bouts daily. This "paroxysmal" stage of the disease lasts from 1 to 3 weeks, but usually averages about 2 weeks in duration. In infants under 6 months these severe paroxysms of cough are usually so exhausting as to leave the infant limp, cyanotic, and apneic; death may occur if resuscitation measures are not immediately instituted. The characteristic whoop is seldom heard in these small, weak infants. In older, stronger infants and preschool children, the cough is usually followed by the classic inspiratory whoop which most often leads to the diagnosis. School-age children and young adults may simply have severe paroxysmal coughing bouts without a whoop. The "convalescent" stage of whooping cough consists of a persistent occasional cough for an additional 3 to 4 weeks, the whole illness then lasting a total of several weeks. *Formes frustes* of whooping cough do occur, with the entire illness so modified as to resemble only a mild cold with an occasional cough.

PHYSICAL EXAMINATION

Pertussis organisms are not invasive beyond the ciliary border of the tracheobronchial mucosa, so that fever does not occur unless complications develop. Thick tenacious nasal and tracheobronchial secretions cause nasal obstruction and sometimes choking episodes if aspiration occurs. These, along with frequent bouts of severe paroxysmal cough, often produce numerous facial petechiae, primarily around the eyelids and cheeks and on the neck. Conjunctival and scleral hemorrhages may be extensive. Epistaxis is common. When the disease is severe, there may be puffy edema of the face, most pronounced in the periorbital tissues. Laceration of the frenulum of the tongue may develop as a consequence of repeated protrusions of the tongue against the lower incisors with cough paroxysms. Scattered, coarse wet rales and rhonchi are commonly heard; fine moist rales are not heard unless pneumonia complicates the disease. Vomiting occurs frequently at the termination of severe cough paroxysms. In small infants, this may lead to dehydration and metabolic alkalosis with tetany. Weight loss and malnutrition may develop if the course is protracted.

COMPLICATIONS

High fever seldom occurs unless complications ensue. Atelectasis, bronchopneumonia, and otitis media are the most frequent complications. Convulsions may occur in small infants, with severe and persistent paroxysmal bouts of cough complicated by cyanosis and apnea. They may occur at any time during the course of illness but are more commonly seen in the earlier paroxysmal stage. A transient hemiplegia (Todd's paralysis) may follow these seizures when they are severe. Convulsions followed by lethargy progressing to coma are an ominous sign; should recovery occur, prominent neurologic residua are often seen.

LABORATORY FINDINGS

The white blood cell count with differential smear is a most helpful diagnostic aid. An absolute lymphocytosis is usually observed, with the total white cell count often above 20,000 cells per cu mm and the differential smear showing greater than 60 to 70 per cent small mature lymphocytes. Lymphocytic leukemoid reactions with counts varying from 50,000 to 125,000 per cu mm are most often seen in association with severe complications. In younger infants, particularly those under 6 months of age, the characteristic lymphocytosis of whooping cough is frequently absent. The erythrocyte sedimentation rate is normal or, more frequently, low. Should it become elevated, a secondary complication should be suspected. The chest x-ray may show hilar peribronchial infiltrates, producing the "shaggy heart" appearance characteristic of whooping cough. Lobar atelectasis, particularly involving the right upper lobe, as well as a patchy segmental atelectasis occurs commonly. Fluffy alveolar infiltrates diagnostic of secondary bacterial pneumonia develop in about 10 per cent of children with the disease.

Most large medical centers and state laboratories can now quickly confirm the presence of *B. pertussis* organisms by the use of fluorescent antibody staining. Smears are made from posterior nasopharyngeal swabs of patients suspected of having the disease, and these can be tested by skilled technicians in a few minutes. Fluorescent antibody staining is more sensitive than culture and often remains positive even after effective antibiotic administration has cleared the patient of viable organisms. Best results in the culturing of *B. pertussis* organisms are achieved utilizing calcium alginate nasopharyngeal swabs smeared directly onto fresh Bordet-Gengou medium containing 20 per cent sheep's blood. Characteristic, small pinpoint metallic-like colonies with a mercurial sheen are first noted after 72 hours or more incubation at 37°C. Swabs taken from the oropharynx and cough plate specimens yield less reliable results. The nasopharyngeal smear for fluorescent antibody (FA) studies and culture is usually positive within the first 1 to 2 weeks of illness. Organisms disappear thereafter, and these tests are seldom positive after 3 to 4 weeks.

PITFALLS IN DIAGNOSIS

The most common pitfall in the diagnosis of whooping cough is the frequent absence of the whoop in infants under 6 months of age and in the older child and adult, causing the clinician to fail to suspect the diagnosis. Another is the misconception that immunization confers protection against the disease. Vaccine protection is relative and declines considerably with time, so that prior immunization does not preclude the diagnosis of whooping cough in a patient otherwise suspected of having the disease.

DIPHTHERIA

By Thomas F. Sellers, Jr., M.D.
Atlanta, Georgia

Diphtheria is an acute bacterial infection, usually involving the upper respiratory tract, characterized by the formation of a thick "grayish-white" eschar, or pseudomembrane. The name is derived from the Greek word "diphthera" meaning "leather" and refers to the leathery appearance of the pseudomembrane.

The causative organism, *Corynebacterium diphtheriae,* is not invasive. It produces its local and systemic effects by the production of a potent exotoxin which causes local necrosis, and, when it is absorbed into the circulation, myocardial and peripheral nerve damage.

CLINICAL COURSE

After the incubation period of 1 to 7 days, the disease usually begins as a small exudate on the tonsils or elsewhere in the pharynx, but it may be located almost anywhere in the upper respiratory tract, including anterior and posterior nares, or larynx. On occasion, the infection may occur in the skin, eye, ear, or vagina, alone or in combination with a respiratory site.

The initial infection may not be associated with any symptoms at first, but as it spreads to involve adjacent structures, local soreness and swelling will develop. Sore throat is an almost universal symptom but may not be as painful as other common throat infections. Nonspecific symptoms of nausea, vomiting, and headache may occur.

At first the exudate can be removed easily; however, as toxin-induced tissue necrosis begins, the typical pseudomembrane forms and spreads. With progression of the disease, the pseudomembrane may spread and coalesce to cover tonsils, pharynx, uvula, or palate. As the necrotic process involves deeper structures, the pseudomembrane becomes densely adherent so that it cannot be easily removed, and where it is disturbed, it may bleed. This characteristic of the exudate is an important diagnostic clue. The membrane is whitish at first, becoming grayer and darker, depending upon the amount of underlying hemorrhage which occurs. Local lymph nodes may become enlarged and tender. Fever is usually low-grade. There may be slight leukocytosis, but white blood cell (WBC) counts rarely exceed 15,000/cu mm. Indeed, fever above 38°C and WBC counts over 10,000 are signs of poor prognosis in diphtheria or indicators that another disease may be present, such as streptococcal infection. The frequent indolent and apparently benign beginning of diphtheria is particularly treacherous, misleading the clinician as to the cause of the disease and the dangerous course it may follow.

With further local spread of the disease, considerable local swelling of tissues and lymph nodes may ensue, causing the so-called "bull neck" appearance due to enlargement of the tissues of the submandibular area and anterior neck. At times the edema of the neck may become extensive, brawny, warm, and tender, obscuring the underlying structures, including enlarged lymph nodes, which may become evident only after the edema has subsided. Neck swelling is not a constant feature, however.

Although the upper respiratory tract is the site of diphtheria infection in most patients, infections do occur elsewhere, particularly in the skin. These present as a variety of lesions, resembling at times common impetigo, ecthyma, or leg ulcers produced by chronic venous insufficiency. The lesions tend to have a dirty, irregular eschar and show little evidence of local tenderness, redness, or swelling. Such lesions are more frequently encountered in tropical areas, but they have characterized epidemics of mixed pharyngeal and cutaneous diphtheria which have occurred in temperate climates. Although serious late toxin-mediated complications may follow cutaneous diphtheria, the morality rate is low compared with the pharyngeal forms.

The course of untreated diphtheria is highly variable. The infection may remain well localized and contained, or it may spread with alarming rapidity. Some cases are so fulminating that the patient is desperately ill within a few hours of apparent onset. The variable courses diphtheria may take are probably due to differences in toxin production by the organism and to differences in immunity of the host.

COMPLICATIONS

The complications of diphtheria follow two different paths: one, the consequence of respiratory obstruction by the pseudomembrane; the other, the result of effects of diphtheria exotoxin absorbed into the circulation.

If the pseudomembrane extends downward to involve the lower respiratory tract, obstruction to the flow of air may occur. With involvement of the larynx and trachea, dyspnea becomes increasingly evident. Severe coughing and stridor may occur with great rapidity, requiring immediate intubation or tracheostomy. Because of the adherent nature of the pseudomembrane, little sputum is produced until later, when the membrane separates. In severe cases, the membrane may actually form a cast of the trachea and upper bronchi. The larger surface area involved increases the absorption of the endotoxin, adding to the danger of this form of the disease.

The effect of the exotoxin on the heart represents the second great danger of diphtheria resulting in either myocarditis, conduction disturbances, or both. Myocarditis usually begins sometime in the first or second weeks of illness. Rhythm disturbances usually occur in the second week or later. Mild electrocardiographic changes such as mild ST segment or T wave abnormalities may be seen in as many as 50 per cent of cases, but significant myocardiopathy is uncommon —perhaps 5 to 10 per cent.

In patients with myocardiopathy, the heart sounds may become muffled and the pulse rapid and weak. The patient exhibits profound weakness and lethargy. As congestive heart failure develops, the patient becomes progressively more dyspneic, pale, and sweaty. Severe epigastric and right upper quadrant pain may result from acute congestion of the liver. An S_3 gallop is commonly heard. Electrocardiograms may show varying degrees of conduction disturbances, including bundle branch or complete heart block and ectopic beats. Sudden death may ensue from arrhythmia, or the patient may expire in cardiogenic shock or intractable congestive heart failure. The prognosis for recovery in such patients remains poor despite remarkable advances in the treatment of acute myocardial disease generally. Case-fatality rates for all forms of diphtheria in the United States have declined from about 15 per cent to 1 per cent over the past decade (1973–1983). This change is mainly due to improved immunization status and increased numbers of the milder cutaneous form of diphtheria being reported. The contribution of highly technical intensive care for cases of diphtheria is probably small. If the patient does recover, the arrhythmias and other cardiac manifestations regress slowly and usually completely, although accounts of residual myocardial fibrosis have been made.

Cranial nerve and peripheral nerve palsies may also occur in the second week or later. Most common is paralysis of the soft palate, resulting in a tendency to regurgitate liquids and food when the patient attempts to swallow, and in a nasal quality to the patient's speech. Involvement of other cranial nerves—chiefly III, VI, and VII—may also occur, causing impairment of eye movements and focusing. Weakness of extremities, foot drop, and loss of deep tendon reflexes may also occur. Very rarely, paralysis of muscles of respiration may cause severe, even fatal, respiratory failure. Recovery of impaired peripheral nerve function is gradual but usually complete.

CARRIERS

Individuals may become asymptomatic carriers of *C. diphtheriae* even when adequately immunized, and contacts of diphtheria cases should be examined and cultured. Sometimes lesions may be found of which the individual is unaware, especially in the anterior nares, a location which apparently rarely leads to significant disease itself but may be an important source of spread to others.

DIAGNOSIS

Diagnosis is of unusual importance in the management of diphtheria. Much weight must be placed on making an early clinical diagnosis because prompt administration of antitoxin is crucial to successful treatment. Since antitoxin itself carries a considerable risk of morbidity, rarely even mortality, the diagnosis of diphtheria must be reasonably accurate as well.

The first step is the clinical suspicion that is aroused by the pharyngeal exudate, noting its appearance, location, and tendency to spread. Examination of a direct smear of the pharyngeal exudate is of doubtful usefulness. Few persons have had sufficient experience to recognize the diphtheria organism when mixed with other throat bacteria. Many organisms such as saprophytic diphtheroids may be difficult to distinguish from pathogenic *C. diphtheriae,* and the inability to see typical bacterial forms does not exclude diphtheria as a diagnosis. It is necessary, therefore, to make a decision based on the clinical features of the disease whether to begin treatment with antitoxin. An immunization history may be useful. If the patient has good evidence of having completed a prescribed course of diphtheria toxoid immunization, usually in the form of diphtheria-pertussis-tetanus (DPT) vaccine injections in childhood, the risk is greatly reduced that the disease is diphtheria or that serious complications will ensue if it is diphtheria. In such cases, it may be appropriate to await the results of cultures and rely on antibiotics. For nonimmune individuals or those whose immune status is partial or unknown, however, one cannot rely upon antibiotics to prevent the complications due to diphtheria toxin. Waiting to learn the results of bacterial culture before administering diphtheria antitoxin may be regretted.

The classical Schick test has no application in the diagnosis of diphtheria. It measures susceptibility to diphtheria toxin (lack of antitoxin), but its results come too late to be of much usefulness.

CULTURES

Using cotton or potassium alginate swabs, cultures should be obtained both from the throat and nasopharynx as well as from any other suspected sites such as skin lesions and immediately placed on appropriate media. Ideally three media are used: Loeffler's or Pai media, tellurite agar, and blood agar plates. If the throat swab must be sent some distance, it should be placed in a silica gel packet before transport. After 2 to 4 hours incubation at 37°C, a smear from the Leoffler's medium may be stained with methylene blue (Loeffler's) and examined for the typical *C. diphtheriae* morphology. The organisms are pleomorphic, club-shaped rods that tend to lie in "V" or "L" shaped arrangements. Small clumps of such organisms give the so-called "Chinese letters" appearance. The presence of intracellular, purple "metachromatic" granules may impart a beaded appearance to the bacillus. Such characteristics, while not conclusive, may help establish a tentative diagnosis of diphtheria.

After 24 hours incubation, the appearance of typical colonies on the Loeffler's or tellurite medium confirmed by methylene blue stain smears will permit the laboratory to make a presumptive diagnosis and to proceed with further testing to determine whether the organism produces toxin, the ultimate criterion for identification of pathogenic *C. diphtheriae.*

Several tests are used to determine toxicity: guinea pig inoculation, tissue culture testing, and modified Ouchterlony technique. The latter is most commonly used. Since confirmation of toxin production may take several days, this information is rarely of use to the clinician who must decide whether to treat or not, based on the initial findings as emphasized earlier. A confirmed isolation of toxigenic *C. diphtheriae,* however, is of great importance epidemiologically because the first clinical case may indicate the presence of more disease in family and community contacts.

Bacteriologically, *C. diphtheriae* organisms may be classified into three types: *gravis, mitis,* and *intermedius.* Although more severe disease and epidemics have been said to be associated with the *gravis* and *mitis* types, such distinctions are of little value in the diagnosis and treatment of the disease.

Theoretically, the concept of using fluorescent antibody stains to identify *C. diphtheriae* directly on fresh throat swab material is very attractive, but it has not proved to be sufficiently practical for routine use.

PITFALLS IN DIAGNOSIS

There are several pitfalls in the diagnosis and differential diagnosis of diphtheria. The disease has become quite uncommon in the areas of the world where diphtheria toxoid immunizations have been well carried out. Many physicians may have never seen a case, and when faced with a patient with pharyngitis may tend to think of streptococcal or infectious mononucleosis etiology first and of diphtheria not at all. Even if diphtheria is considered, the need to treat likely cases promptly with antitoxin without waiting for bacteriologic confirmation is a concept of which many physicians are unaware.

Diphtheria may simulate common conditions. Hemolytic streptococci and many viruses are frequent causes of acute pharyngitis which must be differentiated.

Streptococcal pharyngitis or tonsillitis tends to show more diffuse redness and more local soreness. The exudate tends to be localized to the tonsils, and, being purulent and not necrotic, it is not deeply fixed. Fever is usually higher, and there is a greater tendency to leukocytosis than in diphtheria.

The marked anterior cervical soft-tissue swelling of diphtheria may simulate peritonsillar abscess but must not be incised, since there is no purulent matter to be drained and the procedure may increase the absorption of diphtheria toxin.

Infectious mononucleosis may present with an extensive exudate, but fever and pharyngeal soreness are usually more pronounced. Enlargement of lymph nodes elsewhere than the anterior neck and splenomegaly are other physical clues. Agranulocytosis and leukemia may also cause a severe pharyngeal inflammation but the cause will be easily revealed by a differential WBC count. Viral causes of pharyngitis other than infectious mononucleosis rarely produce an exudate, despite at times considerable fever and constitutional reaction.

Occasionally, diphtheria may invade the larynx initially and cause symptoms that resemble croup or the even more severe acute obstructive laryngitis. In such suspected cases, laryngoscopic examination is indicated.

Cutaneous diphtheritic ulcers may resemble impetigo or chronic infected wounds such as leg ulcers due to chronic venous insufficiency. Cultures are necessary to differentiate.

Diphtheria has become a rare disease in many parts

of the world but remains a problem where immunization against the disease does not reach most of the population. It is ironic that the diagnosis is most likely to be missed with tragic consequences in those areas where prevention has been most successful because physicians may not be alert to the possibility of diphtheria, its diagnosis and treatment.

GAS GANGRENE AND SIMILAR ANAEROBIC SOFT-TISSUE INFECTIONS

By Ronald Lee Nichols, M.D.
New Orleans, Louisiana

Postoperative infectious complications continue to be the most frequent cause of morbidity and mortality in the surgical patient. The most frequently encountered infections are relatively easy to diagnose and involve the surgical wound, the intra-abdominal cavity, or the urinary or respiratory tracts. Rapidly spreading soft-tissue infections caused by anaerobic endogenous bacteria are rare but often catastrophic because of the confusion produced by the clinical presentation which frequently leads to delay in initiating appropriate therapy. Many of these infections clinically simulate clostridial myonecrosis, the most dreaded and severe form of anaerobic soft-tissue infection (Table 1).

GAS GANGRENE (CLOSTRIDIAL MYONECROSIS)

General Principles

Among the most serious surgical infections are those caused by anaerobic clostridia. Gas gangrene, produced by *Clostridium perfringens,* is a destructive process of the muscle associated with local crepitance and extreme systemic signs of toxemia. An antecedent event such as trauma, gunshot wound, frostbite, or intestinal surgery exposes muscle and subcutaneous tissues to these ubiquitous organisms. In the proper environment of tissue necrosis, low oxygen tension, and adequate concentrations of amino acids and calcium, the clostridial spores introduced from the external environment or the gastrointestinal tract germinate with production of the potent alpha toxin.

Bacteriology

Clostridia are gram-positive, spore-forming, obligate anaerobes that are widely present in soil contaminated with animal excreta. In humans, their normal residence is the gastrointestinal and the female genital tracts, although these organisms can be isolated occasionally from the surface of the skin and from the mouth. At present, there are over 60 recognized species of clostridia, in addition to many isolates that do not fit the accepted taxonomy.

The most important of the histotoxic species involved in gas gangrene is *C. perfringens.* This organism is relatively aerotolerant and exhibits "stormy fermentation" in milk. It is the fastest growing clostridial species, with a generation time of 8 minutes under ideal conditions. *C. perfringens* produces alpha toxin, which is a phospholipase C (lecithinase) that splits lecithin into phosphoryl choline and diglyceride. Its activity can be inhibited by specific antitoxin. The alpha toxin has been associated with gas gangrene; it is known to be hemolytic, to destroy platelets, and to cause widespread capillary damage.

Myonecrosis is caused by *C. perfringens* in 80 per cent of patients. The remaining causative agents are *C. novyi, C. septicum,* and *C. bifermentans.* Other species that have on occasion been involved are *C. histolyticum, C. sporogenes, C. fallax,* and *C. tertium,* but the proof of their etiologic role is rather tenuous. The wounds themselves frequently are contaminated with other aerobic and anaerobic bacteria, especially when the abdominal wall is primarily involved.

Pathogenesis

The pathophysiology of gas gangrene is necrosis of muscle owing to a compromised blood supply, either through direct injury or underlying vascular disease, in association with contamination by potential pathogens. The conditions for elaborating of the toxin are a low tissue oxidation-reduction potential, anoxia, and local necrosis. These conditions are fulfilled in traumatic wounds associated with sepsis.

The history of gas gangrene has been intimately tied to warfare, since traumatic wounds, gross contamination, and delay in surgical management are characteristic of battlefield conditions. We have come to recognize that this disease also occurs in peacetime, although the epidemiology is somewhat different. The current experience in metropolitan centers is that 60 per cent of cases are related to trauma—one half are caused by automobile accidents; and the remainder are crush injuries, industrial accidents, or gunshot wounds acquired in our urban combat zones. Other cases of gas gangrene occur postoperatively following colon resections, ruptured appendix, perirectal infection, perforated bowel, and biliary tract or gastroduodenal surgery. A small group of cases of gas gangrene can be traced to vascular insufficiency, usually in diabetics who develop disease in the stump following amputation. Overall, the experience in peacetime is that two thirds of gas gangrene cases occur in the extremities and one third in the abdominal wall.

Clinical Features

The *incubation period* of gas gangrene is usually 8 hours to 2 days, with an average of 36 hours, following the initiating event, which is either trauma or a surgi-

Table 1. Differential Diagnosis of Anaerobic Soft-Tissue Infections

Characteristic	Clostridial Myonecrosis (Gas Gangrene)	Clostridial Cellulitis	Anaerobic Streptococcal Myositis	Synergistic Necrotizing Cellulitis	Necrotizing Fasciitis
Systemic toxicity	Extreme	Absent–mild	Moderate	Moderate–severe	Moderate–severe
Wound pain	Severe	Mild	Occurs late	Moderate–severe	Mild
Tissue induration	Absent	Absent	Absent	Absent	Present–hard
Gas	Present–late	Present	Present	Variable	Variable
Appearance of skin	Tense, white, or gangrenous with bullae	Variable	Red, swollen	Swollen, red, or gangrenous	Brawny; pale red or gangrenous
Muscle death	Always–extensive	None	Rare—localized	Rare—focal	Rare—localized
Gross characteristic of exudate	Thin, serous; may be sweetish or putrid	Putrid, brown	Seropurulent, sour	Purulent, putrid	Variable
Gram stain of exudate	Few neutrophils, gram-positive rods	Abundant neutrophils, gram-positive rods	Many neutrophils, gram-positive cocci	Variable neutrophils, mixed organisms	Many neutrophils, variable, sometimes mixed organisms
Etiology	Clostridia	Clostridia	Anaerobic streptococci (± aerobic streptococci, staphylococci)	Mixed aerobic–anaerobic streptococci, Bacteroides, and coliforms	Aerobic and anaerobic streptococci and staphylococci; occasionally Bacteroides
Surgical therapy	Extensive removal of all infected muscle	Excision of involved superficial tissue	Debridement of involved necrotic tissue	Debridement of involved necrotic tissue	Excision of involved fascia and other necrotic tissue
Antibiotic therapy	Penicillin	Penicillin	Penicillin	Aerobic-anaerobic coverage	Aerobic-anaerobic coverage

cal procedure. There is a sudden onset of *pain* in the wound, increasing in severity and extending somewhat beyond the original borders over the next several hours. The skin initially becomes edematous and tense. It changes in color from an initial pale appearance to a magenta hue, often accompanied by large, hemorrhagic bullae. A thin, watery discharge appears early in the course. It may have an unpleasant, foul-sweet odor and on microscopic examination there are abundant gram-positive rods with a remarkable *paucity of inflammatory cells.* The patient initially has a tachycardia that cannot be explained by the height of fever or circulatory changes. Subsequently, a high fever (38 to 40°C), shock, and renal failure ensue.

The *appearance of the involved muscle* is characteristic in gas gangrene, being quite unlike any other soft-tissue infection. It must be viewed by direct surgical exposure since many of the changes are not apparent when inspected through the edges of a traumatic wound. Initially, the muscle is pale and edematous, appearing as a piece of steak which has been seared over a charcoal fire. The muscle, however, does not contract when cut with a scalpel, and further dissection usually reveals beefy red, nonviable muscle tissue. As the disease progresses, the muscle becomes frankly gangrenous, black and extremely friable, but by this time the patient is near death. It is important to establish the diagnosis of myonecrosis as early as possible in order to resect all devitalized, necrotic tissue.

The *mental status* of a patient with gas gangrene is an extraordinary feature of the disease process. Despite profound hypotension, renal failure, and advancing crepitance, these patients may be remarkable alert, showing extreme sensitivity to their surroundings. They feel their impending doom, and a sense of terror can be read in their furtive gaze. This intense mental awareness is mercifully suspended just prior to death, when the patient lapses into toxic delirium and eventually into coma.

Diagnosis

The *sine qua non* for diagnosis of gas gangrene is *direct visualization of the muscle* to determine the characteristic appearance of the disease. In patients in whom the infection is limited to the skin and subcutaneous tissue at operation (clostridial cellulitis), debridement is easier and prognosis much improved. The clinical features, as described above, should arouse suspicion early in the course, so that the disease can be recognized and surgically managed with haste. Gas in the wound and surrounding tissue is a relatively late finding; by the time crepitance is appreciated, the patient may be beyond hope of survival. X-ray of the affected site reveals gas in the tissues with dissection along the fascial planes, but, again, this tends to be a late finding. A great help is obtained by examining a gram-stained slide of the wound discharge for the presence of clostridia and absence of inflammatory cells. Needle aspiration of the active margin of the skin infection is helpful when wound discharge is not present. Approximately 15 per cent of blood cultures are positive, but this finding occurs late in the course of the infection.

Complications

The mortality in gas gangrene is 40 to 60 per cent. It is highest in infections involving the abdominal wall and lowest in those affecting a single extremity. Among the signs that prognosticate a poor outcome are *leukopenia, low platelet count, intravascular hemolysis,* and severe *liver* or renal impairment.

Hypotension is an early sign of gas gangrene and can lead to *renal failure* and *irreversible shock.* Release of alpha toxin into the bloodstream can cause severe *hemolysis,* with hemoglobinemia, hemoglobinuria, and renal cortical necrosis. This diagnosis is established by measuring free hemoglobin in the urine and plasma and by examining the peripheral blood smear for the characteristic red blood cells with crinkled, shaggy edges. Such hemolysis is more common in uterine gas gangrene, although it is occasionally seen in infections involving the limbs if there is extensive muscle involvement.

OTHER ANAEROBIC SOFT-TISSUE INFECTIONS

There are several spreading infections other than clostridial myositis or cellulitis that involve the soft tissues. As in the case of the clostridial infections, the keystone to successful treatment is rapid early diagnosis.

Anaerobic Streptococcal Myositis

This infection is a more indolent process than aerobic streptococcal infections. It is caused by various species of anaerobic streptococci (peptostreptococci). Involvement of the muscle and fascial planes usually follows trauma or a surgical procedure. There may be *severe* local pain. The overlying skin appears as a gangrenous wound which emits a foul, watery brown discharge. Bleb formation is common, and crepitus may be apparent in the surrounding tissue. Gas formation can be extensive, with tracking into the adjacent healthy tissues. On inspection of the muscle, there is redness and edema with some local destruction. However, there is no myonecrosis and the muscle contracts when cut with the scalpel. Although there usually is generalized toxicity and fever, the patient is not as ill as a person with gas gangrene.

Diagnosis

The initial approach to a crepitant skin infection is obtaining a sample of exudate for Gram stain and opening the wound for inspection of muscle and soft tissue. The major distinctions between the diseases caused by anaerobic streptococci and clostridia (Table 1) are as follows:

1. Systemic effects are less prominent with the streptococcal form. This infection does not cause hypotension and renal failure, as does clostridial disease.

2. On inspection, the involved muscle remains viable in streptococcal disease, although there may be inflammatory reaction and edema. True myonecrosis is not found.

3. The anaerobic streptococcal form can produce considerable gas, which occurs early in the course,

whereas clostridial infections tend to have less gas, and it is usually a late development.

4. The discharge from the wound in streptococcal myositis is a thin, brown fluid which shows Gram-positive cocci and numerous neutrophils. By contrast, the discharge in gas gangrene shows gram-positive rods but no neutrophils.

Synergistic Necrotizing Cellulitis

This is a highly lethal polymicrobial infection which produces extensive necrosis of the skin and soft tissues with progressive undermining along fascial planes. The process may be rather indolent at first, presenting after 7 to 10 days of mild symptoms. Patients are often afebrile or have only low-grade fever, lacking systemic toxicity in the early stages of the infection. The initial lesion in the skin is a small area of necrosis or a reddish-brown bleb with extreme local tenderness. However, the superficial appearance belies the widespread destruction of the deeper tissues. By direct inspection through skin incisions there is extensive gangrene of the superficial tissues and fat with gelatinous necrosis of fascia and muscle. The discharge is brown, rather thin, and watery, with a foul odor; such exudate has been labeled *"dishwater pus."* Gram stain reveals a *mixed flora* with abundant polymorphonuclear leukocytes. Gas can be palpated in the tissues in 25 per cent of patients.

The most common site of involvement is the *perineum,* seen in one half of patients. The major predisposing causes are *perirectal abscess* and *ischiorectal abscess;* these conditions track to the deeper structures of the pelvis, leading to a severe form of the disease. A more superficial form involves the buttocks without extension to deeper muscles.

Approximately 40 per cent of patients have involvement of the thigh and leg. Some infections arise in the adductor compartment of the thigh, often extending from an infected amputation stump, or accompany diabetic gangrene. Lesions in the lower leg usually are associated with vascular disease or diabetic foot ulcers. The remaining 10 per cent of cases occur in the upper extremities or in the neck, most frequently in patients with vascular disease or diabetes.

Predisposing Conditions. Seventy-five per cent of patients have diabetes mellitus, which may be relatively mild and discovered at the time of admission. However, some patients present with ketoacidosis. Cardiovascular and renal disease are seen in 50 per cent of patients. Obesity is common, being found in over half of patients.

Bacteriology. This is a mixed aerobic-anaerobic infection, consisting of organisms that have their origin in the intestinal tract. Of the aerobes, coliforms are most common, such as *Escherichia coli,* Klebsiella, and Proteus. The anaerobes include Bacteroides, Peptostreptococcus, Peptococcus, Clostridium, and Fusobacterium. Approximately a third of patients have positive blood cultures, usually growing a coliform, Bacteroides or Peptostreptococcus.

Differential Diagnosis. Several infections of the skin can be mistaken for synergistic necrotizing cellulitis:

1. *Gas gangrene.* This clostridial infection is more dramatic in presentation, often associated with renal failure, high fever, and severe toxicity. The most striking feature in gas gangrene is myonecrosis, in which the muscle initially has a pale, white appearance followed by a mushy red color, eventually leading to black gangrene. The overlying skin is extensively involved with blebs and hemorrhagic necrosis. Abundant gas is found in the subcutaneous tissues. Gram stain of the exudate from gas gangrene shows few polymorphonuclear leukocytes and an abundance of large, gram-positive rods.

2. *Progressive synergistic bacterial gangrene (Meleney's gangrene).* This is an indolent process, involving the skin and subcutaneous tissues without extensive tracking into deeper structures. Gram stain of the outer zones reveals gram-positive cocci.

3. *Necrotizing fasciitis.* Although systemic toxicity may be severe, the necrotizing component is confined to the fascial planes, with relative sparing of the superficial layers of the skin and surrounding muscles. There is relatively little exudate, and the pathogen on Gram stain or culture is often a single organism, such as *Staphylococcus aureus,* Group A Streptococcus, Peptostreptococcus, or Bacteroides.

4. *Fournier's gangrene.* This is a variant of synergistic gangrene which involves the scrotum and penis, presenting with an explosive onset. It occurs in relatively healthy men, usually 25 to 50 years of age, although rare cases have been reported in the neonate and in the elderly. One half of patients have no preceding infection; the remaining individuals have one of the following conditions:

a. Ischiorectal abscess.
b. Perianal fistula.
c. Erysipelas of the perineum.
d. Bowel disease (rectal carcinoma, diverticulitis).
e. Scrotal trauma.
f. Prior urogenital surgery.
g. Urogenital infections, especially those involving the periurethral glands.

In recent times, this disease has been observed in alcoholics who develop pressure sores of the scrotum and perineum by sitting in the same position in a drunken stupor. There is also an association with diabetes mellitus. Dissection of pancreatic juice through the retroperitoneum has, on rare occasion, presented as scrotal gangrene.

The route of infection is thought to be via Buck's fascia, spreading alone the planes of dartos fascia of the scrotum and penis. The infection may then extend to Colles' fascia of the perineum and even to Scarpa's fascia of the abdominal wall. At the outset this tends to be superficial gangrene, limited to the skin and subcutaneous tissue and extending to the base of the penis. The testes and spermatic cord usually are spared. There may be extension to the perineum and the anterior abdominal wall through the fascial planes.

Necrotizing Fasciitis

This is a relatively rare infection involving subcutaneous tissues with extensive undermining and

Table 2. Signs of Necrotizing Fasciitis

Clinical Feature	Number of Patients Affected (%)
Cellulitis	90
Edema	80
Skin discoloration or gangrene	70
Anesthesia of involved skin	Frequent*

*True incidence unknown.

tracking along fascial planes. Although originally associated with "hemolytic streptococci" (Group A *Streptococcus pyogenes*), it is apparent that the disease can be caused by other microorganisms, including anaerobic streptococci, *Staphylococcus aureus,* Bacteroides, and a mixed anaerobic-aerobic flora.

Clinical Features

Extension from a skin lesion is seen in 80 per cent of patients. The lesion often is trivial, such as a minor abrasion, insect bite, injection site (in the case of heroin addicts), or abscess (perirectal most frequent). Rare cases have been reported in women with Bartholin's gland abcess, from which the infection has spread to fascial planes of the perineum and thigh. The remaining 20 per cent of patients have no visible skin lesion.

The initial presentation is that of that of cellulitis which advances rather slowly. Over the next 2 to 4 days, however, there is systemic toxicity with high temperatures. The patient is disoriented and lethargic. The local site shows the features listed in Table 2.

The most distinguishing clinical feature is the *wooden-hard* feel of the subcutaneous tissues. In cellulitis or erysipelas the subcutaneous tissues can be palpated and are yielding. However, in fasciitis the underlying tissues are firm, and the fascial planes and muscle groups cannot be discerned by palpation. It is often possible to observe a broad erythematous track in the skin, along the route of the fascial plane as the infection advances cephalad in an extremity. If there is an open wound, probing the edges with a blunt instrument permits ready dissection of the superficial fascial planes well beyond the wound margins. There is remarkably little pain associated with this procedure.

Bacteriology

Monomicrobial Form. Pathogens in this group are Group A beta hemolytic *Streptococcus pyogenes, Staphylococcus aureus,* and anaerobic streptococci (Peptostreptococcus). Staphylococci and hemolytic streptococci occur in about equal frequency, and approximately one third of patients will have both pathogens simultaneously. Most patients acquire their infection outside the hospital. The majority of these infections present in the extremities, approximately two thirds in the lower extremity.

There is often an underlying cause such as *diabetes, arteriosclerotic vascular disease,* or *venous insufficiency with edema.* In some instances a chronic vascular ulcer changes into a more acute process. The mortality in this group is high, approaching 50 per cent in patients with severe vascular disease.

Polymicrobial Form. An array of anaerobic and aerobic organisms can be cultured from the involved fascial plane, from 1 to 15 bacteria, with an average of five pathogens in each wound. The most common organisms, found in various combinations, are listed in Table 3.

The polymicrobial infections are associated with four clinical settings:

1. Surgical procedures, especially bowel resections, and penetrating trauma can be complicated by cellulitis leading to superficial fascial dissections.

2. The infection can involve the buttocks and perineum and may have been preceded by a decubitus ulcer, minor trauma, or perirectal abscess. As a result of the proximity of the anus, contamination by fecal bacteria is universally present.

3. In heroin addicts, the upper extremities are frequently involved at the site of injection. Because the needles and "works" are contaminated, unusual organisms such as Citrobacter and Pseudomonas can be isolated in association with the anaerobes listed above.

4. The lesion can spread from a Bartholin's abscess or a minor vulvovaginal infection. Some infections have been associated with pudendal block anesthesia during delivery. While mixed infections are usually noted in this setting, there may be a single pathogen, particularly anaerobic Streptococcus.

Diagnosis

It may not be possible to diagnose fasciitis upon first seeing the patient. Overlying cellulitis is a frequent accompaniment. That the process involves the deeper fascial planes is suggested by the following features:

1. Failure to respond to initial antibiotic therapy. Cellulitis usually improves, with lowering of fever and reduction in local signs, within 24 to 48 hours. Fasciitis is a more stubborn infection which shows little improvement in the initial few days.

2. Hard *"wooden feel"* of the subcutaneous tissue, extending beyond the area of apparent skin involvement.

3. Systemic toxicity, often with altered mental status.

Another diagnostic consideration initially is *erysipelas.* However, this condition has raised, sharply defined borders that are bright red and often associated with streaking lymphatics in a caudad direction. The overlying skin usually is tender. Most importantly, the red border advances rapidly so that a mark made with a pen at the edge will demonstrate

Table 3. Organisms Commonly Present in Polymicrobial Necrotizing Fasciitis

Anaerobes	Aerobes
Bacteroides	*Escherichia coli*
Peptococcus	Klebsiella
Peptostreptococcus	Citrobacter
Clostridium	Pseudomonas

progression within 1 to 2 hours. Necrotizing fasciitis, on the other hand, moves more slowly, does not have a discrete border, and is not particularly tender; indeed, it may be anesthetic.

The most important diagnostic feature of necrotizing fasciitis is the appearance of the fascial planes. Upon direct inspection, the fascia is swollen and dull gray in appearance, with stringy areas of necrosis. A thin, brownish exudate oozes from the wound. Even upon deep dissection, there is no true pus. Extensive undermining of surrounding tissues is present, and the fascial planes can be dissected with a gloved finger or a blunt instrument.

A Gram stain of the exudate demonstrates the pathogens and provides an early clue to therapy. Gram-positive cocci in chains suggest streptococcal disease (either group A or anaerobic); large, gram-positive cocci in clumps suggest *Staphylococcus aureus* or Peptococcus. A mixed flora would suggest polymicrobial infection.

Cultures are best obtained from the deep tissues. If the infection has developed from a contaminated skin wound such as a vascular ulcer, the bacteriology of the superficial wound is not necessarily indicative of the deep tissue infection. An array of coliforms, staphylococci, and various streptococci can be isolated from the ulcer, but the fascia may have a pure culture of a single organism such as anaerobic streptococci or *Staphylococcus aureus.* Direct needle aspiration of the advancing edge has been advocated as a means of obtaining material for culture, but this technique is nearly always unproductive. A definitive bacteriologic diagnosis can only be established by culturing the fascia at operation or by positive blood culture.

CONCLUSIONS

This group of severe, spreading, life-threatening infections challenges all surgeons to the limit. Successful therapy depends on a rapid diagnosis; appropriate, specific antibiotic therapy; and, most importantly, aggressive surgical excision and debridement. The presumptive diagnosis must be made on the basis of clinical presentation and Gram stain studies of the wound exudate. Definitive culture and sensitivity results, which often require several days, should be used to modify, if necessary, empiric antibiotic therapy.

RHEUMATIC FEVER

By Joshua Lynfield, M.B., B.Ch.
New York, New York

Rheumatic fever is a complication of a group A beta-hemolytic streptococcal pharyngitis. The use of antibiotics to treat streptococcal infections has resulted in a marked decrease in incidence of rheumatic fever. Antibiotic prophylaxis, maintained after a first attack, effectively prevents recurrences.

Host factors are important in determining who acquires acute rheumatic fever. Recent serologic studies showed that 60 per cent of children with rheumatic fever but only 14 per cent of controls were positive for the 883 alloantigen carried on the D locus of the HLA complex.

The first attack of rheumatic fever usually occurs between the ages of 5 and 15 years. Children are more likely to present with carditis than adults. Recurrences are usually seen within 5 years. Recurrent attacks of rheumatic fever mimic the initial attack—e.g., an individual with polyarthritis without carditis in the initial attack will be unlikely to develop carditis in a recurrent attack.

One to 4 weeks after streptococcal pharyngitis, rheumatic fever manifests itself by the appearance of acute migratory polyarthritis, carditis, subcutaneous nodules, erythema marginatum, and (later) chorea, either singly or in combination. Because none of these alone is pathognomonic of this disease, Jones devised criteria for diagnosis, which have been modified by the American Heart Association (*Circulation,* 32:664, 1965). These are listed in Table 1. In order to make the diagnosis, at least two major or one major and two minor criteria should be present. The major manifestations include polyarthritis, carditis, subcutaneous nodules, erythema marginatum, and chorea. Erythema marginatum should probably be changed to a minor manifestation because it does not carry the same weight as the other major criteria. The minor manifestations include fever, arthralgia, previous rheumatic fever or rheumatic heart disease, and laboratory manifestations of activity, such as an elevated erythrocyte sedimentation rate or C-reactive protein and prolongation of the PR interval on the electrocardiogram. Evidence of a preceding streptococcal infection greatly strengthens the diagnosis; absence of such evidence throws doubt on the diagnosis except in cases of chorea or long-standing carditis.

The diagnosis is easiest to make at the beginning of an attack, when the physician can evaluate the acute manifestations by direct observation. Later, after the joint manifestations subside, diagnosis becomes more difficult, since more reliance must be placed on the history. It may be impossible to determine whether the patient had myalgia, arthralgia, or arthritis; to evaluate a transient heart murmur which has disappeared; or to distinguish chorea from nervous tics or erythema marginatum from other rashes by history.

The onset of rheumatic fever is variable. Sometimes it appears with dramatic suddenness, ushered in by fever and polyarthritis. Its onset may be more insidious, with low-grade fever and arthralgia. It may even be subclinical, detected later by the appearance of a characteristic murmur, such as that of mitral stenosis. Fever is usually present except in chorea, and is usually low-grade or moderate. Sore throat, epistaxis, abdominal pain, and vomiting may be presenting symptoms. Occasionally, right lower quadrant pain associated with rheumatic fever may simulate appendicitis.

JOINT MANIFESTATIONS

Migratory polyarthritis is the most frequent major manifestation of acute rheumatic fever. The inflammation starts in one joint, then subsides and moves to

Table 1. Revised Jones Criteria

Major Manifestations	Minor Manifestations
Carditis	Clinical
Polyarthritis	Previous rheumatic fever or rheumatic heart disease
Chorea	Arthralgia
Erythema marginatum	Fever
Subcutaneous nodules	Laboratory
	Acute phase reactions, erythrocyte sedimentation rate, C-reactive protein, leukocytosis
	Prolonged P–R interval

Plus

Supporting evidence of preceding streptococcal infection (increased ASO or other streptococcal antibodies, positive throat culture for group A Streptococcus, recent scarlet fever)

involve another or several other joints over a period of several days. Individual joint involvement lasts from 1 to 5 days; all joint symptoms usually subside within 2 to 4 weeks. Most commonly, large joints are involved, usually the knees and ankles. However, the hips, elbows, shoulders, and wrists may also be involved. Uncommonly, the small joints of the hands and feet are involved; exceptionally, the spine or temporomandibular joints, which are far more frequently involved in rheumatoid arthritis, are involved. Occasionally, arthritis is not migratory and only involves a single joint, particularly if treatment has been started early. It may be advisable to withhold anti-inflammatory treatment until the diagnosis is definite.

A clear-cut distinction must be made between arthritis, a major manifestation, and arthralgia, a minor manifestation. Arthritis is characterized by pain, limitation of motion, swelling, warmth, redness, and tenderness of the affected joints. The pain may be very severe especially if the slightest movement, active or passive, is attempted. In fact, a characteristic feature of rheumatic arthritis is the extreme tenderness of the joint. A child may be seen to flinch in anticipation of pain when seeing the examiner's hand approach the inflamed joint. Redness may be mild and limited to a small area over the joint. When arthritis is severe, fluid may be present in the joint. The fluid in such cases is turbid, contains leukocytes, and is sterile on bacteriologic culture.

Arthralgia can be distinguished from arthritis by the absence of swelling, warmth, redness, tenderness, and significant limitation of motion of the joint. Arthralgia should not be lightly dismissed, as it may be a clue to the presence of carditis, particularly in a child with a history of low-grade fever and lassitude. Myalgia may be confused with arthralgia.

The arthritis and arthralgia of rheumatic fever respond dramatically to aspirin therapy. If joint symptoms persist or recur while on adequate salicylate therapy, and particularly if the spine and small joints are involved, rheumatoid arthritis should be considered. Rheumatic fever, unlike rheumatoid arthritis, does not result in permanent joint deformities. Polyarthritis may also occur in systemic lupus erythematosus, periarteritis nodosa, anaphylactoid purpura, and serum sickness. If arthritis involves only a single joint, septic arthritis should be promptly ruled out by performing a joint aspiration. Gonococcal infection can produce mono- or polyarthritis. Osteomyelitis, leukemic joint involvement, and the arthralgia of sickle cell anemia have been mistakenly diagnosed as rheumatic fever. Transient synovitis of the hip following a streptococcal pharyngitis should be distinguished from rheumatic fever.

CARDITIS

Carditis is the most serious manifestation of rheumatic fever. It may result in congestive heart failure or even death during the acute phase of the disease. The late manifestations of rheumatic heart disease are valvular deformities, especially of the mitral and aortic valves.

The diagnosis of carditis depends upon the recognition of a new significant heart murmur. In recurrent attacks when a murmur is already present, development of cardiac enlargement, pericarditis, or congestive heart failure is acceptable for diagnosis even in the absence of a new heart murmur. Tachycardia is usually present and excessive for the degree of fever.

The commonest murmur, that of mitral insufficiency, is recognized by the presence of a Grade II to IV/VI blowing, high-pitched pansystolic murmur maximal at the apex and transmitted toward the axilla. A soft murmur may be intensified by listening with the patient turned into the left lateral position. Even if the murmur is less than Grade II/VI in intensity, it is significant if it is blowing in character and maximal at the apex. The murmur of mitral insufficiency in acute rheumatic carditis does not increase when the patient stands, which differentiates it from the murmur of mitral valve prolapse, which is unmasked or intensified by assuming the standing position.

In patients with mitral insufficiency, a low-pitched mid-diastolic murmur (the Carey-Coombs) may be heard at the apex following the third heart sound. This murmur should be differentiated from the diastolic murmur of mitral stenosis, which has a presystolic accentuation and is not preceded by a third heart sound.

The murmur of aortic insufficiency appears much less frequently as a manifestation of carditis than the murmur of mitral insufficiency. It is usually associated with mitral insufficiency but may appear alone.

It is a soft, high-pitched, blowing, early diastolic murmur along the left sternal border, best heard during held expiration with the patient sitting up and leaning forward or supine. Often the patient with aortic insufficiency has a systolic ejection murmur along the left sternal border, which should lead to a careful search for the aortic diastolic murmur that is less obvious. If aortic insufficiency is present as an isolated finding, great care must be taken to rule out bacterial endocarditis as the cause of the murmur.

An innocent murmur may lead to the misdiagnosis of carditis, especially if it appears for the first time during an attack of rheumatic fever, precipitated by tachycardia, fever, and anemia. The two most common types of innocent murmur are the diffuse vibratory, low-pitched, groaning or somewhat musical, short systolic murmur best heard over the precordium, and the systolic ejection murmur, which is best heard along the left sternal border and is usually maximal over the pulmonary area. In cases of doubt about the significance of a systolic murmur, the new technique of Doppler ultrasound may be of help. Another method of clarifying the diagnosis in the patient with questionable carditis is the use of Neo-Synephrine, 0.09 mg/kg, given subcutaneously. In the patient with a significant murmur, auscultation or phonocardiography at the height of the pressor response demonstrates that the murmur becomes more clearly pansystolic and louder and an early aortic diastolic murmur may be unmasked. In the patient with an innocent murmur, the test is negative.

The electrocardiogram in rheumatic fever may show prolongation of the PR interval, which is not necessarily a sign of carditis. In the absence of carditis, it is used as a minor criterion for the diagnosis of rheumatic fever.

CHOREA

Chorea may be the sole manifestation of acute rheumatic fever and may occur up to 6 months following a streptococcal pharyngitis. Chorea may occur following an attack of polyarthritis and/or carditis while signs of carditis are still present but almost never concurrently with polyarthritis. It may begin months after all signs of polyarthritis and/or carditis have disappeared, when all laboratory findings have returned to normal.

Chorea is usually seen between the ages of 5 and 15 and is more common in females. In adults, it occurs mainly during pregnancy.

This central nervous system disorder is characterized by emotional instability, purposeless movements, and muscular weakness. It is a self-limiting disease, lasting an average of 3 months but sometimes persisting for as long as a year. During the initial stage of chorea, the child may be restless and irritable, is apt to drop things, and displays a grimace. As the disease progresses, the involuntary movements become more frequent and more extensive, involving most muscle groups, especially those of the upper extremities, feet, legs, tongue, and face. The movements are abrupt and jerky, and muscular force is diminished. The severity varies from mild involuntary movements to violent continual activity, totally incapacitating the patient.

During sleep the movements disappear. The contrast between the sleeping and waking state is remarkable. The same person who a few moments before was sleeping quietly on waking goes out of control in a frenzy of purposeless activity. Coordinated activities such as speech, eating, and writing are affected. The child may be unable to walk, talk, sit up, or feed himself. Physical signs include the "milking grip"—a waxing and waning of power on gripping the examiner's hand, and the development of flexion and extension movements of the wrists when the arms are held above the head. Chorea may be unilateral. There is no sensory loss. A tic or habit spasm may be confused with chorea; the movements of a tic are repetitive and unassociated with muscular weakness.

ERYTHEMA MARGINATUM

Erythema marginatum is a rare manifestation of rheumatic fever. These asymptomatic skin lesions usually involve the trunk, especially the abdomen, occasionally appearing on the limbs and sparing the face. They are flat or slightly raised and are annular or arcuate; they have sharp, erythematous margins that blanch on pressure and pale centers. They may coalesce to form serpiginous patterns. The lesions are transient, disappearing or changing during the course of a single day. They may subsequently reappear in the same area, with a tendency to intermittent recurrences over a period of weeks or months.

SUBCUTANEOUS NODULES

Subcutaneous nodules are rare but may be seen in the patient with carditis as a late manifestation. The nodules are usually located over bony prominences, especially the elbows, knuckles, knees, and ankles. They may also occur over the scalp and spine. They are not erythematous. The nodules are firm and nontender, freely movable, not fixed to overlying skin or underlying bone, and tend to persist for weeks. Their diagnostic value is limited because they appear late, when the diagnosis is already obvious.

LABORATORY TESTS

Laboratory tests important in the diagnosis of acute rheumatic fever are concerned with the documentation of a recent streptococcal infection and the degree of inflammatory activity.

Throat cultures are not of great value because a significant number of normal individuals carry streptococci in their throats. The best evidence of a recent streptococcal infection consists of a rising antibody titer. Antibody titers rise within 1 week of infection, reaching their peak in 3 to 5 weeks. After 2 months, titers may be declining or low. The most widely used antibody test is the antistreptolysin O titer (ASO), which is elevated (333 Todd units or above) in 75 per cent of patients with acute rheumatic fever. Where the results are inconclusive, other antistreptococcal tests such as the antihyaluronidase or antiDNAase B can be performed and at least one will be positive in 90 per cent of patients with acute rheumatic fever. The Streptozyme slide test screens for multiple antibodies to streptococcal products and may provide evidence of a recent streptococcal infection when the ASO is negative. Inability to document a recent streptococcal infection casts serious doubt on the diagnosis of rheumatic fever.

Evidence of acute inflammatory activity such as an elevated erythrocyte sedimentation rate and C-reactive protein should be demonstrable. The blood count may show a moderate polymorphonuclear leukocytosis and a mild normochromic anemia.

Laboratory data should always be evaluated in conjunction with the clinical findings and the modified Jones criteria, so that undue emphasis is not placed on a minor manifestation, e.g., arthralgia, because of an elevated ASO, C-reactive protein, and sedimentation rate.

Many other diseases share some symptoms and signs with rheumatic fever, and additional laboratory tests as well as careful clinical evaluation may be necessary to establish the correct diagnosis.

GONOCOCCAL INFECTION

By Yehudi M. Felman, M.D.
Brooklyn, New York

Neisseria gonorrhoeae, the causative organism of gonorrhea, primarily infects the human anogenital tract and oropharynx. The production of symptoms depends on both host factors and the strain of *N. gonorrhoeae* involved. The presence of these symptoms, in turn, influences patient promptness in seeking treatment, which subsequently affects the size of the infected pool. While it is generally believed that males experience profound symptoms and women manifest few, this may relate to the nature of health facilities surveyed and the types of complaints with which patients present. For example, sexually transmitted disease clinics generally draw symptomatic males and their asymptomatic contacts, who are often brought to treatment as a result of epidemiologic investigation known as contact tracing. Hospital emergency rooms attract the symptomatic female patient, with pelvic inflammatory disease (PID) the most frequent diagnosis. Often the male contacts of women with gonococcal PID have *asymptomatic* urethral gonorrhea.

SYMPTOMS

The probability that an uninfected male will acquire gonorrhea from an infected female is roughly 20 per cent per exposure. The risk of an uninfected female acquiring the disease from an infected male is 40 per cent per exposure. A symptomatic infection may manifest itself 3 to 5 days after the patient has sexual contact with an infected individual.

In men, gonococcal urethritis is generally characterized by dysuria and a purulent urethral discharge. The quality of the discharge is not particularly diagnostic. A scanty, watery discharge may be produced by *Neisseria gonorrhoeae,* just as a thick, yellow discharge may have a nongonococcal etiology. Laboratory tests, and not clinical appearance, are essential for accurate diagnosis. Although 50 to 75 per cent of infected females have asymptomatic infections, this means that a good number of women have symptomatic infection. Female patients with symptomatic endocervical gonorrhea may experience lower abdominal pain, vaginal discharge, and, occasionally, abnormal uterine bleeding. Because these symptoms are not pathognomonic for gonorrhea and since other organisms may obscure the diagnosis of coexisting gonococcal infection, specific testing is imperative.

Symptomatic rectal gonorrhea in females and in male homosexuals is characterized by rectal pain, pain on defecation, change in bowel habits, or the presence of pus, blood, or mucus in the stool. Infection at the rectal site occurs primarily in patients who practice anal receptive intercourse but can result secondary to cervical infection by anorectal contamination with gonococci-laden exudate. Because symptoms of anorectal infection can be nonspecific, the clinician must have a high index of suspicion among patients presenting with anorectal complaints, particularly trauma due to anal intercourse, fissures, hemorrhoids, condylomata, and inflammation resulting from substances used as lubricants. Anorectal gonorrhea occurs in about 50 per cent of homosexual men with gonococcal infections.

Symptoms of oropharyngeal gonorrhea may range from acute exudative pharyngitis to febrile tonsilitis. A normal-appearing throat is quite usual, however. The infection is transmitted primarily by fellatio, though cunnilingus can be a mode of transmission. As patients are reluctant to volunteer that they engage in oral-genital contact, it is best to assume such activity in sexually active patients and wise to perform the appropriate diagnostic test to determine whether a gonococcal infection is present, particularly when another body site is infected.

COMPLICATIONS

Local complications of acute gonococcal urethritis include prostatitis, epididymitis, inguinal lymphadenopathy, and urethral stricture. Since symptomatic men seek treatment promptly and effective therapy is available, complications of gonorrhea have declined over the years. The increase in asymptomatic infections may offset this trend. Ten per cent of men who acquire urethral gonorrhea have onset of symptoms delayed until as much as 2 weeks following exposure. In another 3 per cent, symptoms fail to develop until 6 months following exposure. It is unclear what long-term effects asymptomatic individuals will experience by harboring gonococci for extended periods.

Pelvic inflammatory disease is the leading complication of gonorrhea among women. Of gonococcal and nongonococcal etiologies, infection ascends from the cervix to the fallopian tubes, usually during menstruation. Symptoms include lower abdominal pain, fever, and elevated white blood cell count. The diagnosis of PID is made by bimanual pelvic examination when adnexal tenderness is noted upon palpation. Yellowish endocervical discharge, uterine tenderness, and cervical motion tenderness may all be present but not specific for PID. Pelvic inflammatory disease is a major contributor to sterility and is responsible for ectopic pregnancies and chronic pelvic pain. Owing to the serious consequences of the infection, PID should be considered in the differential diagnosis of all sexually active women who present with surgical abdomens. Treatment should be initiated immediately and sex contacts should be examined for asymptomatic infection.

Disseminated gonococcal infection (DGI) is the most common infectious cause of acute arthritis in the United States. The arthritis-dermatitis syndrome begins with an initial bacteremic stage characterized by fever, chills, tenosynovitis, polyarthralgias, positive blood cultures, and pustulovesicular skin lesions. The skin lesions are the hallmark of the condition, appearing in roughly 50 to 65 per cent of patients. They are found predominantly on the distal portions of extremities. Early lesions progress from papule to pustule within 24 hours, then evolve into a vesicle or bulla. A second type of lesion may appear as a hemorrhagic bulla with a surrounding erythematous area. Focal petechiae over the digits or medial aspects of the ankles are another possible dermatologic manifestation.

The second phase of DGI, the septic joint phase, is characterized by monoarticular arthritis and synovial fluid that yields *N. gonorrhoeae* on culture. Skin lesions are absent or in the process of resolution, and blood cultures are often negative.

Patients with DGI are generally asymptomatic with respect to the primary site of infection, and cultures should be taken from all potentially infected sites. Pharyngeal infections do have a role in the genesis of DGI, and therefore an oral culture should be performed on all patients with DGI.

Gonococcal conjunctivitis occurs in adults when fingers freshly contaminated with exudate accidentally reach the eyes. The disease presents as a purulent conjunctivitis with profuse discharge and is more often than not unilateral. Adult gonococcal conjunctivitis is often associated with infection at another site in the same patient. When conjunctivitis and urethritis simultaneously occur, it is important to consider the diagnosis of Reiter's syndrome. (See article on this topic.)

EXAMINATION

In examining a male for asymptomatic urethral gonorrhea, a careful physical examination is required to reveal a small amount of discharge unnoticed by the patient himself. If no discharge is obtained by urethral stripping, introduction of a calcium alginate swab should be effected to obtain a specimen.

Endocervical specimens should be obtained by using a speculum that has not been lubricated, since surgical jelly will inhibit the growth of gonococci on culture.

Anoscopy is useful in the diagnosis of anorectal gonorrhea. A sample of mucus or pus for culture can be obtained with a bacteriologic loop, paddle, or calcium alginate swab.

LABORATORY PROCEDURES

Determining gonococcal infection is accomplished by identifying the organism with one of several diagnostic tools. The Gram-stained smear is by far the most commonly used method. It requires a minimum of equipment and is fast, cheap, and simple enough for an office-based practice. Positivity of the Gram smear is over 90 per cent in symptomatic males and about 50 per cent in symptomatic females.

To prepare a Gram-stained smear, place a sample of exudate on a clean glass slide by rolling the swab on the slide so that microscopic morphology will not be distorted. The smear should be allowed to air dry and fixed with heat prior to staining by passing the slide quickly through the flame of a Bunsen or alcohol wick burner several times in succession. After fixing, the slide is placed in a crystal violet solution, the primary stain, for 60 seconds and washed with tap water. Iodine solution is then applied for 1 minute and the slide is once again washed in water. The third step is to decolorize with 95 per cent ethanol for 5 to 10 seconds. In the last step, the counterstain safranin is used. After 60 seconds, the slide can be rinsed and examined under the microscope. Positive smears reveal gram-negative diplococci (pink-stained from safranin uptake) that are within polymorphonuclear leukocytes. For urethral specimens, positive smears are diagnostic and treatment should be initiated. Positive cervical and anal smears likewise warrant immediate treatment of patients. A confirmatory culture is always necessary to rule out penicillinase-producing *Neisseria gonorrhoeae* (PPNG) strains.

Selective culture media such as Martin-Thayer medium or New York City medium, which inhibit the growth of organisms other than *N. gonorrhoeae* and *N. meningitidis,* should be chosen to increase the yield of gonococci. Inoculated plates should be placed in a carbon dioxide–rich atmosphere for incubation. An oxidase-positive reaction occurs with the use of an indicator, which turns deep purple in the presence of Neisseria. Gram-stained smears of colonies should be done to confirm the morphology. In the absence of an office incubator, commercial growth-transport systems are available to maintain specimens until they reach a laboratory.

Blood cultures and synovial fluid cultures should be taken from patients with disseminated gonococcal infections.

POTENTIAL ERRORS AND PITFALLS IN DIAGNOSIS

Failure to take an adequate sexual history can lead to serious errors in diagnosis. For example, a urethral smear from a patient seeking treatment for gonorrhea will do nothing to detect the infection in the patient who primarily engages in anal-receptive intercourse. Patients require diagnostic tests on parts of the body they use in sexual activity; when these sites are asymptomatic, they should be cultured.

The gonococcus is not the only Neisseria to colonize the anogenital and oropharyngeal canals. In oral infections, sugar fermentation tests are required to determine the species of diplococci present, as *N. meningitidis* is a frequent oral colonizer. *N. meningitidis* is also frequently a colonizer of the anal canal in homosexual males, making the sugar fermentation test useful.

Penicillinase-producing *N. gonorrhoeae* strains have been found with increasing frequency in the United States, associated with travel to the Far East, and have been seen in patrons of local prostitutes. These strains should be suspected for all cases of treatment failure in which symptoms do not abate and in which there is neither indication of re-exposure or misadministration of medications. Commercially available indicators to test isolates for penicillin sensitivity should be incorporated in all culture tests for gonorrhea.

CHANCROID

By M. Brittain Moore, Jr., M.D.
Lakeland, Florida

SYNONYMS

Soft chancre, ulcus molle, Ducrey's disease (infection).

DEFINITION AND PRESENTING SIGNS AND SYMPTOMS

Chancroid, the most common of the minor venereal diseases, produces, after a short incubation period, painful, tender, multiple superficial ulcerations in the anogenital region, associated with inflammatory regional lymphadenopathy. It is caused by the gram-negative Streptobacillus *Hemophilus ducreyi,* a fastidious organism only in regard to its growth requirements on artificial media.

CLINICAL COURSE AND PHYSICAL FINDINGS

One to three days after exposure, an exquisitely tender, small, painful, ragged ulceration appears (following an evanescent papule or pustule), most commonly just proximal to the glans penis, at the site of first entry of the Ducrey bacillus. By autoinoculation, multiple lesions often develop on skin and mucous membrane in direct apposition to the primary lesion(s). The ulcerations grow rapidly with undermining and coalescence and may encircle the penis at the coronal sulcus. Tender regional lymphadenopathy occurs within a week and is bilateral in up to 50 per cent of cases. Unilocular fluctuation develops several days later. Despite the severity of the local inflammatory disease, constitutional symptoms (low-grade fever, malaise) are rare.

Immunity does not develop well, and reinfection is common. Reported cases are 20 to 50 times as frequent in males as in females, but it has been shown that women may harbor the organism as part of their vaginal flora for prolonged periods without symptoms.

COMPLICATIONS

If the condition is untreated or if treatment is delayed, foul-smelling, phagedenic ulcerations and chronically draining, suppurative regional lymphadenopathy develop. Phimosis or paraphimosis is common, and urethral fistulae may develop when intraurethral lesions are present.

LABORATORY AIDS

With great difficulty, *Hemophilus ducreyi* can be grown on blood agar at 37 C (98.5 F) from material taken from beneath the undermined edges of ulcers. New selective media, especially supplemented heart infusion agar with vancomycin, have increased dramatically our ability to rapidly isolate and identify the organism. Smears from ulcers or lymph node aspirates stained with Gram or Wright stain may be helpful *if* the short gram-negative Streptobacillus can be found. Usually, it cannot, and these studies are time-consuming and disappointing. A much more helpful direct immunofluorescent staining procedure has been developed and should be used where available.

Years ago an intradermal skin test (Igo-Reenstierna) was used. Generally, it did not become positive before the third week of infection, thus limiting its usefulness in the fast-moving venereology practice of today in which acute conditions are treated immediately. The material for this skin test is not presently available commercially.

There is no serologic test for chancroid.

PITFALLS IN DIAGNOSIS (DIFFERENTIAL DIAGNOSIS)

The differential diagnosis includes granuloma inguinale, lymphogranuloma venereum, syphilis, and anogenital herpes simplex infection.

Granuloma inguinale is excluded by absence of pain and regional lymphadenopathy as well as by its diagnostic findings on biopsy. Lymphogranuloma venereum is excluded by absence of genital lesions at the time of presentation and by the character of the suppurative lymphadenopathy (unilocular in chancroid, multilocular in lymphogranuloma venereum).

Primary syphilis with multiple chancres can be ruled out by negative darkfield examination of *painful, nonindurated,* "dirty" chancroid lesions associated with *tender* lymphadenopathy as contrasted with indurated, nontender syphilitic chancres accompanied by rubbery, discrete, nontender satellite buboes. The serologic tests for syphilis detecting reagin (e.g., Venereal Disease Research Laboratory [VDRL], and rapid plasma reagin [RPR]) are reactive in only about 50 per cent of those with primary syphilis on first examination but will become reactive soon (and always within 1 month after appearance of primary lesion) if no antitreponemal therapy is administered.

Chancroid is most often confused with secondarily infected anogenital herpes simplex infection in which prompt erosion of the grouped vesicles occurred before the patient or examining physician saw them, or with primary herpes *without* secondary infection. After syphilis is excluded, a therapeutic test with tetracycline is reasonable. Before syphilis is excluded, sulfonamide therapy can be given without interfering with the diagnosis of syphilis.

Failure to recognize syphilis with multiple chancres is the most serious pitfall in the diagnosis of chancroid, and there is little reason for this to happen. Overdiagnosis of herpes infection as chancroid is of little consequence.

Incision and drainage of an abscessed lymph node for material for culture and sensitivity determinations should not be done, for chronic draining sinus tracts may persist despite adequate treatment. Material should be aspirated only through a needle inserted through normal adjacent skin (preferably above the node).

Chancroid is almost never seen in a circumcised male and, for all practical purposes, rarely occurs in anyone with good hygiene. As our standard of living has improved, the incidence of chancroid has decreased and the relative frequency of its most common differential diagnostic problem, genital herpes simplex infection, has increased.

GRANULOMA INGUINALE

By Thomas W. Johnson, M.D.
Nashville, Tennessee

SYNONYMS

Granuloma venereum, Donovanosis, ulcerating granuloma of the pudenda, granulomatosis, infective granuloma, sclerosing granuloma, granuloma contagiosa, chronic venereal sores.

DEFINITION

Granuloma inguinale is a chronic ulcerogranulomatous disease caused by the microbacillus *Donovania granulomatis,* also referred to as the Donovan body. Although the disease is worldwide in its distribution, it is more common in tropical and subtropical areas. The frequency of cases of this disease is low. Primary manifestations of the disease involve the genitalia in a majority of patients, and the disease is generally considered to be one of low contagiousness.

PRESENTING SIGNS AND SYMPTOMS

The incubation period of granuloma inguinale may vary from 8 days to 4 months with an average of 14 to 50 days. The majority of patients are in the age group from 20 to 45 years, although the disease has been reported in infants and children. The incidence is greater in males than in females.

The initial lesion is a solitary, plane, flat-topped papule or subcutaneous nodule of the skin or mucous membranes and occurs on the external genitalia in over 90 per cent of the patients. Extragenital lesions, when present, usually represent sites of autoinoculation from primary lesions of the genitalia and most commonly involve the lips, oral cavity, face, neck, upper trunk, posterior aspects of the hands, and the digits. Direct orogenital contact may also account for the presence of extragenital lesions. Pain is not a prominent symptom of the primary lesion, which breaks down within a few days of its initial occurrence to yield a shallow, well-demarcated ulcer with a rolled edge and a vivid, pink base of granulation tissue. Extension of the lesion may occur by contiguity through advancement of the border of granulation tissue or by autoinoculation in satellite or more distant locations with eventual coalescence of lesions. The lesions may undergo spontaneous arrest or continue to spread slowly, especially in warm, moist intertriginous areas. Eventually, untreated or inadequately treated lesions progress to marked atrophic, depigmented scarring. The intervention of secondary infection complicates the course of the lesions and increases the possibility of systemic complications and debility.

CLINICAL COURSE

With the exception of the primary lesion, which rapidly sloughs to form a shallow, well-demarcated ulcer, the course of granuloma inguinale is characterized by a slow, progressive spread of granulomatous tissue. Spontaneous arrest of the spread can occur, or the lesions may continue a destructive course for many years. Superinfection of the lesions may occur with fusospirochetal organisms with resultant acceleration and accentuation of the destructive process. Lymph node involvement, although not characteristic of granuloma inguinale, can occur with the formation of indurated swellings or fluctuant abscesses (pseudobuboes) that eventually rupture and add to the ulcerative process. Hematogenous dissemination of the organisms is rare.

PHYSICAL EXAMINATION

The initial lesion tends to occur on the external genitalia of the male and on the labia, clitoris, and fourchette in the female. Characteristically, the lesion is a solitary, plane papule or subcutaneous nodule that breaks down in a few days to form a shallow, well-demarcated ulcer with a pink, velvety base and rolled edges of granulation tissue. A serosanguineous exudate is present. Four clinical types of granulation tissue are seen: (1) Nodular—pink to beefy red, well-defined, exuberant granulation tissue. (2) Ulcerovegetative—the most frequently observed type. Extension occurs by contiguity or by the formation of satellite papules and nodules that eventually ulcerate and coalesce with the parent lesion. Serpiginous borders are characteristic, and the formation of deep scars may occur. (3) Hypertrophic—formation of large, granulomatous lesions. (4) Cicatricial—rapidly forming areas of fibrosis are interspersed among areas of ulcerations. Secondary keloid formation may occur as well as hypopigmentation and depigmentation.

COMMON COMPLICATIONS

The most common complication of granuloma inguinale is superinfection with fusospirochetal organisms. A rapidly spreading, destructive ulceration covered by a foul-smelling exudate results. Interference of the lymphatic drainage from extensive genitoinguinal scarring may result in pseudoelephantiasis of the external genitalia, particularly in females. In males, penile destruction and deformities may occur. Cicatricial narrowing of the urethra, vagina, and anus may also occur. Squamous cell carcinomas of the penis, vulva, and cervix may develop, particularly in those instances in which the disease has a protracted course.

LABORATORY FINDINGS

Slide Preparations. It is essential that the clinical diagnosis of granuloma inguinale be confirmed by demonstration of the causative organisms, the Donovan bodies, in smear preparations. This is best done by obtaining a small specimen from the granulation tissue at the border of an ulcer, crushing the specimen between two clean glass slides, and then smearing the specimen on the slides by rubbing the slides together as they are separated. Smears can also be made from a punch biopsy by smearing the undersurface of the specimen on a slide prior to placing the specimen into a fixative solution. Slides should be air dried and then stained by Gram, Giemsa, Wright, or pinacyanole stain. Giemsa stain is preferred. Donovan bodies are rod-shaped microorganisms that can usually be demonstrated in the large mononuclear cells found in the granulation tissue. They occur individually or in clusters, have a bipolar appearance owing to the concentration of chromatin material found at both ends, and may contain a well-developed capsule. Morphologically and antigenically (based on capsular antigens) they closely resemble Klebsiella sp. By Gram stain, the organisms are gram-negative; by Giemsa stain, the organisms are red. Wright-stained organisms are bluish to deep purple surrounded by a pink capsule; with pinacyanole stain, they are blue-black with a pink capsule. Material aspirated from pseudobuboes can also be used for staining purposes.

Biopsy. Because of the possibility of squamous cell carcinoma occurring at the site of lesions of granuloma inguinale, a biopsy is recommended. As stated previously, the biopsy specimen is suitable for the preparation of a smear prior to essential fixation for histopathologic processing. The histopathology reveals an absence of the epidermis in the center of the lesion with acanthosis at the border of proportions sufficient for it to be called pseudocarcinomatous hyperplasia. A dense infiltrate is present in the dermis, composed predominantly of histiocytes and plasma cells. Scattered throughout this infiltrate are a small number of lymphoid cells. Donovan bodies are present within a variable number of histiocytes. Donovan bodies are best demonstrated by Giemsa or silver stain.

Culture. Culture is generally not a useful, practical means of isolating the organisms because of the need for special enriched medium under strict cultural conditions.

PITFALLS IN DIAGNOSIS

In spite of the apparent decreasing incidence of granuloma inguinale, the disease must be considered a diagnostic possibility in the presence of chronic ulcerogranulomatous processes. This is particularly significant if the lesions involve the genital, genitoinguinal, or perineal areas. Syphilis, chancroids, and lymphogranuloma venereum, in particular, must be considered on a differential basis as well as tuberculosis (ulcerative type), streptococcal and phagedenic ulcers, and squamous cell carcinoma. Clinical impressions must be confirmed by laboratory identification of the causative organisms.

LYMPHOGRANULOMA VENEREUM

By Thomas W. Johnson, M.D.
Nashville, Tennessee

SYNONYMS

Lymphopathia venereum, lymphogranuloma inguinale, Durand-Nicholas-Favre disease, climatic bubo, tropical bubo, lymphogranulomatosis inguinalis, poradenitis.

DEFINITION

Lymphogranuloma venereum is an infectious disease that primarily involves the lymphatic system. The causative agent belongs to the genus Chlamydia and is known as *Miyagawanella lymphogranulomatosis.* The organisms are morphologically indistinguishable from other microorganisms in this group (also called PLT [psittacosis-lymphogranuloma-trachoma],

Miyagawanella, and Bedsonia). They range from 0.2 to 1 μm in diameter, and are obligate intracellular parasites that contain both DNA and RNA.

The disease is worldwide in its distribution, although there is a marked concentration of cases in tropical and subtropical areas. In the United States, the majority of cases are reported from the southeastern states. Transmission of the infection occurs almost exclusively venereally, although the occurrence of cases in laboratory workers and medical personnel tends to implicate other routes of infection. Cases are reported more frequently in the male than in the female, suggesting the possibility that subclinical infection is more prevalent in the female than in the male.

PRESENTING SIGNS AND SYMPTOMS

The incubation period of lymphogranuloma venereum may vary from 5 to 21 days. The primary lesion is frequently painless and inconspicuous and tends to heal rapidly. In many instances its presence is not noticed by males, and rarely is noticed by females. The lesion usually occurs on the genitalia and consists of a solitary papule, solitary vesicle, or small cluster of vesicles that may rupture, leaving a nonindurated, shallow erosion of 2 to 3 mm in diameter with an erythematous halo.

From 7 to 30 days after the appearance of the primary lesion, regional lymphadenopathy occurs as a result of lymphatic and hematogenous dissemination of the organisms from the site of initial entry. The enlarged nodes are initially firm, tender, and discrete. As the condition progresses, the nodes tend to become matted together, considerably enlarged, and adherent to the surrounding tissue. Frequently, they are bisected by a depression formed by the inelastic Poupart ligament, forming an upper and a lower portion. When this occurs, it is quite characteristic of lymphogranuloma venereum. Multilocular abscesses may form with eventual rupture onto the skin, forming multiple fistulous openings through which a seropurulent exudate may drain. Healing may occur slowly with the formation of puckered, retracted scars.

In the male, the primary lesion occurs most frequently on the glans penis, on the prepuce, and in or near the urethral meatus. In most instances, lymphadenopathy is unilateral, but it may be bilateral.

In the female, the primary lesion usually occurs intravaginally, perivaginally, in or around the urethra, or on the cervix. Lymphadenopathy then involves the nodes found in the perirectal, rectosigmoidal, anorectal, sacral, and hypogastric chains. Signs and symptoms of the disease will occur late in the course of the infection.

In those instances in which primary infection occurs within the anal or rectal canals, initial symptoms may include a mucopurulosanguineous discharge from the rectum, obstipation, tenesmus, and pain.

Systemic signs and symptoms of the disease may include chills, fever, sweating, headache, weight loss, arthralgias, myalgias, and polyarthritis. Hepatosplenomegaly may occur. Urticarial, scarlatiniform, erythema multiforme-like, and papulopustular eruptions may occur.

COURSE

Evidence would suggest that in many instances infections with lymphogranuloma venereum may not progress beyond the occurrence of the primary lesion. This evidence is based upon the presence of complement-fixing antibodies for lymphogranuloma venereum in persons with no documented evidence of recent or remote presence of overt disease. Progression of the disease results from early dissemination from the initial site of entry by way of the lymphatic and blood systems, with subsequent disease manifestations restricted mainly to the lymphatic drainage of the site of initial invasion. Although the primary lesion tends to heal without scarring, the later stages of the disease may progress to scar formation with all the related consequences. Scarring sequelae are most marked in females, in whom any of the following could occur: (1) cicatricial stenosis of the urethra and vagina, (2) rectal strictures and fibrosis of the rectal wall, (3) perirectal and perianal abscess, (4) vaginovesical and vaginorectal fistulas, (5) elephantiasis of the genitalia, or (6) fibrous growth around the anus. The homosexual male may develop the rectal and anal complications.

Extragenital primary lesions are rare but can occur on the lip, tongue, and finger. Regional lymphadenitis may occur and may result in Parinaud's syndrome. Sclerokeratitis, uveitis, and iridocyclitis may also occur.

PHYSICAL EXAMINATION

The primary lesion of lymphogranuloma venereum is essentially asymptomatic and inconspicuous and regresses rapidly. Usually it is not a prominent feature as a sign of the disease. When noted, however, it initially occurs as a small papule, vesicle, or cluster of vesicles that rupture to leave a small, shallow erosion with a halo of erythema. The lesion may be located on the glans, on the prepuce, or within the urethral meatus in the male and on the vulva, urethra, vaginal vault, or cervix in females. When genitorectal contact occurs, the lesion may occur in the perianal or anal areas.

Prominent as a feature of the disease are the findings related to the lymph nodes. When the lymphatic drainage of the primary lesion dictates, the inguinal nodes, either unilaterally or bilaterally, are involved. Early nodes are enlarged, matted, and adherent to the overlying skin, which may become discolored. Discoloration may vary from a violaceous to a dusky hue, depending upon the basic pigmentation of the individual. Longitudinal cleavage of the enlarged, matted nodes by the inelastic Poupart ligament is characteristic of lymphogranuloma venereum. In some patients spontaneous resolution may occur at this stage, although in the majority of patients the enlarged node will develop multilocular abscesses with subsequent rupture and drainage of a seropurulent exudate from fistulous tracts. Subsequent healing by scar tissue formation results in a puckered cicatrix.

In the female, vulvar enlargement, ulceration, and subsequent scarring may occur. There may be progressive ulcerations of the labia, urethra, and vagina with eventual cicatricial stenosis of the urethra and vagina. Proctocolitis and anorectal strictures may occur. Such strictures are also seen in homosexual males and may be detected on rectal examination.

Systemic findings include chills, fever, sweating, headache, weight loss, arthralgias, myalgias, polyarthritis, hepatosplenomegaly, and skin eruptions such as urticarial, scarlatiniform, erythema-like, and papulopustular eruptions. Generalized lymphadenopathy may also be present.

COMMON COMPLICATIONS

Pneumonitis, meningitis, meningoencephalitis, and cystitis can occur as complications of infections by the causative agent of lymphogranuloma venereum. Other complications may be seen in spite of adequate treatment of the disease. Strictures, which are the complication of greatest consequence, occur more frequently in females than in males. Strictures of the colon usually occur within 10 cm of the anal orifice and frequently within 5 cm. Ulcerative colitis–like syndromes with potential intestinal obstruction and/or perforation of the rectum and rectosigmoid areas may occur. Strictures of the urethra in females, along with fistulas and fenestrations of the clitoris and labia minora, may also occur. There may be elephantiasis of the genitalia secondary to lymphatic and lymph node scarring. Recotovaginal fistulas are seen in females, and pararectal abscesses and sinuses are seen in females and homosexual males. Squamous cell carcinomas of the penis, vulva, bladder, anus, and rectum are frequently associated with lymphogranuloma venereum.

LABORATORY FINDINGS

Peripheral Blood. Peripheral blood changes are nonspecific with positive findings relating to systemic signs only.

The Frei Test. This is an intradermal test that detects a state of hypersensitivity to the causative agent of lymphogranuloma venereum. The antigen, known commercially as Lygranum C.F., is derived from the infected yolk sacs of chick embryos, and normal yolk sac material is utilized as a control.

The test is performed by injecting 0.1 ml of the antigen intradermally into the flexural surface of the forearm and 0.1 ml of the control material into a similar area of the opposite forearm. A positive test is reflected by the occurrence of an area of focal induration at least 5 mm or greater in diameter within 48 to 96 hours after injection with a control area of focal induration 5 mm or less in diameter. The severity of the skin test reaction, which can progress to the point of ulceration, does not correlate with the severity of the infection. The skin test becomes positive 12 to 40 days after the onset of adenitis and usually remains positive for life. In approximately 20 per cent of cases, false-positive reactions may occur. A test that is negative in the early stages of the disease should be repeated at a later date; once the test is positive, repeated tests will not alter the degree of the response.

Complement Fixation Tests. A positive complement fixation test may precede a positive intradermal skin test (Frei test). The test utilizes an antigen specific for the chlamydial group of microorganisms, prepared from infected yolk sacs of chick embryos or infected mouse lung suspensions or extracts, which gives a complement fixation reaction when mixed with serum from patients infected with lymphogranuloma venereum. A titer of 1:40 or more is significant; typically, early in the disease, a titer of up to 1:160 will occur. Later higher titers (e.g., 1:640) may occur, and an increase in titer (fourfold or greater) in two successive tests is considered diagnostic. Cross-reactions occur in patients who have been infected with or have recovered from psittacosis, ornithosis, cat-scratch disease, and viral pneumonia, inasmuch as a species-specific antigen for lymphogranuloma venereum, although possible through specific extraction procedures of infected yolk sac material, is not stable enough for routine use.

The sensitivity of the complement fixation test for lymphogranuloma venereum renders it a more significant and useful test than the Frei Test.

Viral Cultural Techniques. Inoculation of either the yolk sacs of chick embryos or brains of mice with blood, purulent exudate, excised lymph nodes, or cerebrospinal fluid can result in isolation of the causative organism. These techniques are not done routinely in most laboratories, however.

PITFALLS IN DIAGNOSIS

Lymphogranuloma venereum must be differentiated from other sexually transmitted diseases such as herpes simplex, syphilis, chancroids, and granuloma inguinale. It must also be differentiated from such diseases as actinomycosis, tuberculosis, tularemia, plague, lymphomas, ulcerative colitis, and carcinoma.

The disease must be considered in a differential diagnosis when presenting signs and symptoms would tend to dictate. All positive confirmatory tests must be carefully interpreted, and negative tests should be repeated at appropriate intervals.

PSITTACOSIS

By William Schaffner, M.D.
Nashville, Tennessee

SYNONYMS

Parrot fever, ornithosis.

DEFINITION AND EPIDEMIOLOGY

Psittacosis is a systemic infection caused by *Chlamydia psittaci.* This obligate intracellular agent, formerly thought to be a virus, now is considered a specialized bacterium.

First discovered in parrots, psittacosis is a zoonotic infection of many avian species including canaries, pigeons, and turkeys. Psittacosis in humans results from exposure to aerosols from contaminated bird droppings, feathers, or infected tissues. Infected birds may be asymptomatic or may have an illness characterized by poor feeding, greenish diarrhea, lethargy, and ruffled feathers. Over 100 cases of human disease are reported annually to the Centers for Disease Control; the majority are associated with exposure to pet birds. Almost 20 per cent of cases, however, do not demonstrate a history of direct bird exposure. Exposure to the psittacosis agent may be indirect; cases have occurred following brief presence in a room which previously had contained an infected bird. The occupational or recreational activities of pet store and zoo employees, veterinarians, and pigeon fanciers place them at risk for psittacosis. Outbreaks of the disease have occurred among workers in poultry processing plants. Infection has not been acquired by handling or eating dressed poultry or game birds. Human-to-human transmission is very rare.

PRESENTING SYMPTOMS AND SIGNS

The onset of psittacosis resembles that of other pneumonic infections and can vary considerably. After an incubation interval of 1 to 2 weeks, the disease often begins abruptly with chills and high fever, but onset also may occur slowly with gradually worsening fever and malaise. Severe headache is common. Systemic symptoms include anorexia, myalgias, abdominal pain, nausea, and vomiting.

A dry, hacking and persistent cough may appear at the onset or only after several days of illness. Small amounts of mucoid, blood-streaked sputum may be produced. A few patients have epistaxis. The respiratory rate is elevated; severe infections are accompanied by dyspnea and cyanosis.

Chest examination usually reveals only rales, but psittacosis also can produce the signs of lobar consolidation. Pleural and pleuropericardial friction rubs are heard occasionally. The pulse may be slow relative to the height of the fever (pulse-temperature dissociation). This finding also has been recognized in some patients with typhoid fever, brucellosis, Legionnaires' disease and other intracellular bacterial infections. Hepatomegaly and splenomegaly (in 10 to 70 per cent of patients) have been noted. Indeed, when splenomegaly is present in a patient with an obscure pneumonitis, the diagnosis of psittacosis should be considered strongly. A fleeting macular pale erythematous rash (Horder's spots) is sometimes noted.

RADIOLOGIC EVALUATION

Chest x-ray films often reveal more extensive pulmonary infiltrates than would have been expected from the physical examination. The usual findings are patchy interstitial infiltrates in both lung fields, most prominently in the basilar segments. Involvement of only one lung and dense lobar consolidation also are seen, however. It is important to note that lobar consolidation does not "rule out" the diagnosis of psittacosis.

COURSE

Without specific antibiotic therapy, psittacosis may cause a grave illness with extensive pulmonary involvement, hypoxia, disorientation, and meningismus. Although the response to therapy may be prompt, a desultory response is quite common. Thus, the administration of tetracycline cannot be used as a "therapeutic trial," nor should fever persisting after 3 or 4 days be interpreted as a therapeutic failure. Because relapses may occur, treatment should be prolonged.

COMPLICATIONS

Extrapulmonary manifestations are rare except in fatal cases. These include pericarditis, myocarditis, encephalitis, and granulomatous hepatitis. A few patients with endocarditis have been described. In these patients, repeated blood cultures were negative; but *C. psittaci* was demonstrated in involved heart valves obtained at surgery or autopsy.

LABORATORY PROCEDURES

Routine laboratory studies do not assist in the diagnosis. The white blood cell count ranges from mild leukopenia to modest leukocytosis. The urinalysis may show slight proteinuria. The serum glutamic oxaloacetic transaminase (SGOT, AST), glutamic pyruvic transaminase (SGPT, ALT), and alkaline phosphatase often are modestly elevated. The bilirubin level is almost always within normal limits. The electrocardiogram usually is normal, but in the more severely ill it may show evidence of myocarditis or pericarditis. The Gram stain of sputum reveals only alveolar macrophages, a few polymorphonuclear leukocytes, and a scant mixed bacterial flora.

The diagnosis of psittacosis usually is made by a fourfold rise in complement-fixing (CF) antibodies in acute and convalescent serum specimens. This test usually is not performed in hospital laboratories; specimens must be sent to state or other reference facilities. Also, antibiotic treatment often delays the appearance of antibodies for 6 to 8 weeks. A final late-convalescent serum specimen should be obtained during follow-up visits after the patient has been discharged from the hospital. Thus, serologic confirmation of the diagnosis may not be available during the patient's hospitalization for acute illness. Some patients with Legionnaires' disease have increases in psittacosis CF titers and represent the only major limitation of the test's specificity.

Because attempts to isolate the agent expose technologists to the hazard of laboratory-acquired infection, this procedure has no place in routine practice.

PITFALLS IN DIAGNOSIS

Since psittacosis presents as an influenza-like illness with varying clinical manifestations, the diagnosis may not be considered. A history of contact with birds often is the sole diagnostic clue. The diagnosis may first be entertained when a patient with pneumonia without an obvious bacterial cause does not respond to penicillin ("penicillin-resistant pneumonia"). If present, splenomegaly should suggest the possibility of psittacosis. Illnesses that produce a similar clinical presentation include Legionnaires' disease, influenza, mycoplasma pneumonia, brucellosis, and tularemia, among others. If the history suggests psittacosis, tetracycline therapy should be administered and serum specimens obtained for later serologic testing. All cases should be reported promptly to local public health authorities.

TUBERCULOSIS AND DISEASES DUE TO OTHER MYCOBACTERIA

By Milton D. Rossman, M.D.
and Robert L. Mayock, M.D.
Philadelphia, Pennsylvania

TUBERCULOSIS

Synonyms

Consumption, galloping consumption, phthisis.

Definition

Tuberculosis is a chronic infectious disease caused by the organism *Mycobacterium tuberculosis* or, more rarely, *Mycobacterium bovis.* Although greater than 80 per cent of patients will have pulmonary involvement, any organ system can be involved.

Presenting Symptoms and Signs

Pulmonary tuberculosis frequently develops without any striking clinical evidence of disease. However, since the disease has a wide spectrum of manifestations, ranging from skin test positivity with negative x-rays to far advanced pulmonary tuberculosis, a variety of clinical presentations also may occur. Ordinarily, until the disease is moderately or far advanced, as shown by changes on the chest roentgenogram, symptoms are minimal and often attributable to other causes, such as excessive smoking, hard work, pregnancy, or other debilitating conditions.

Symptoms. Symptoms may be divided into two categories: constitutional and pulmonary. The constitutional symptom most frequently seen is one of fever, low-grade at the onset but becoming quite marked if and when the disease progresses. Characteristically, the fever develops in the late afternoon and may not be accompanied by marked symptoms. With defervescence, usually during sleep, sweating occurs—the classic "night sweats." Other signs of toxemia, such as malaise, irritability, weakness, unusual fatigue, headache, and weight loss may be present. With development of caseation necrosis and concomitant liquefaction of the caseation, the patient will usually notice cough and sputum often associated with mild hemoptysis. Chest pain may be either diffuse on the involved side or localized and pleuritic. Shortness of breath usually indicates extensive disease with widespread involvement of the lung parenchyma or some form of tracheobronchial obstruction and therefore usually occurs late in the course of the disease.

Signs. Physical examination of the chest is ordinarily of minimal help early in the disease. At this stage, the principal finding over areas of infiltration is fine rales detected on deep inspiration followed by full expiration and a hard, terminal cough—so-called "post-tussive rales." This is found particularly in the apices of the lungs, where reactivation disease has its onset in a large majority of patients. As the disease progresses, more extensive findings are present, corresponding to the areas of involvement and the type of pathology. Allergic manifestations may occur, usually developing during the primary infection at the time of onset of the immune response to tuberculosis. These include erythema nodosum and phlyctenular conjunctivitis. Erythema induratum—involvement of the lower leg and foot with redness, swelling, and necrosis—probably represents a combination of local subcutaneous bacterial infection with an allergic response; it should not be confused with erythema nodosum, considered to be due to circulating immune complexes with resultant localized vascular damage. Initially, erythema nodosum occurs in the dependent portion of the body and, if the reaction is severe, may be followed by more disseminated lesions.

Course

Tuberculosis is transmitted from one individual to another by the airborne route. An individual who has sputum that is positive for *M. tuberculosis* will nebulize live tubercle bacilli into the air. Only those droplets that remain suspended in the air (5 microns or less) are small enough to penetrate to the air spaces of the lungs (the site of the initial lesion in tuberculosis). On rare occasions, direct cutaneous inoculation of *M. tuberculosis* can occur (prosector's warts).

As just indicated the lung is the major portal of entry in the majority of patients with tuberculosis. The first contact with the organism results in few or no clinical symptoms or signs. The tubercle bacillus usually sets up a localized infection in the periphery of the lung, where it has been deposited by inhalation. Body defenses appear to have little effect on the organism until the time of development of tuberculin hypersensitivity (4 to 6 weeks). At this time, mild fever and malaise will develop, and occasionally the other hypersensitivity manifestations (as described) are noted.

In the majority of patients, no additional evidence of tuberculosis will develop and the process will be contained by the local and systemic defenses. Since the primary pulmonary focus is usually subpleural, rupture into the pleural space may result in the development of a tuberculous pleurisy with effusion. This is usually accompanied by the classic but nonspecific symptoms of pleurisy. Local spread to the hilar lymph nodes is a common occurrence and from there via the bloodstream to other areas of the body. It is this hematogenous dissemination of the organisms that results in the pulmonary and extrapulmonary foci that are responsible for the major clinical manifestations of tuberculosis. Radiographically, spread is manifested by enlargement of the lymph nodes with later calcification, both of the lymph nodes and the parenchymal lesion. This is the classic "Ghon complex" and is suggestive not only of an old tuberculous infection but also of other granulomatous diseases, such as histoplasmosis. Progressive (reactivation) tuberculosis usually develops after a period of dormancy and arises from the sites of hematogenous dissemination (e.g., pulmonary, pleural, lymph node, bone, renal, and meningeal).

Untreated, tuberculosis will result in symptomatic disease in 10 per cent of individuals within 2 years of the initial infection. Between 10 and 20 per cent of the remaining individuals will become symptomatic from tuberculosis at some time during their lives. Although most individuals are infected with tuberculosis during childhood, over 80 per cent of newly diagnosed cases of tuberculosis occur between the ages of 45 and 65. Thus the first infection with tuberculosis frequently is clinically insignificant and unrecognized. In the majority of patients, the disease stays dormant either indefinitely or for many years, and when a breakdown occurs, it may be secondary to a decrease in body immunity.

Common Complications

Pleural effusion is a relatively uncommon manifestation, particularly of primary tuberculosis, occurring in 3 per cent of clinical cases. Tuberculous pleural effusions are almost always due to rupture of subpleural foci of tuberculosis that may not be evident radiologically. The effusions in tuberculosis are unilateral and mild to moderate in extent. The presence of bilateral effusions in tuberculosis usually means a miliary spread. The natural course of a tuberculous pleural effusion is to resorb gradually; it often disappears completely or causes minimal changes, which can be seen on the chest radiograph.

Miliary tuberculosis is a term used to describe a fatal (if untreated) form of tuberculosis. In this form of the disease, the host is unable to contain the spread of the organisms after hematogenous dissemination. The hematogenous dissemination occurs normally in the course of the primary infection or occasionally when a focus of reactivation tuberculosis ruptures into a blood vessel. Only when the host cannot contain these disseminated lesions does miliary tuberculosis develop. This syndrome may present as either an acute febrile illness (with fever, headache, and prostration) or as a chronic subtle illness (with fever, weight loss, and weakness). The diagnosis will usually be suspected because of disseminated small nodules (about the size of millet seeds, i.e., 1 to 3 mm) on the chest radiograph. Diagnosis can be confirmed by sputum smear and culture in 70 per cent of cases, although transbronchial biopsy, bone marrow aspirate, or liver biopsy will frequently be needed to confirm that a granulomatous process with acid-fast bacilli is present.

Prior to chemotherapy, *meningitis* had been invariably fatal. If the condition is not recognized and treated early, significant neurologic deficits still frequently occur. Although most cases of tuberculous meningitis are thought to occur within a year after the primary infection, over half of the cases that are seen today occur in adults. As in miliary tuberculosis, this complication may develop either abruptly or slowly. A subependymal tubercule, a tuberculoma, or a parameningeal focus will rupture into the subarachnoid space, and the tubercle bacilli will spread throughout the cerebrospinal fluid. Examination of the spinal fluid will frequently reveal 50 to 200 cells per cu mm with a lymphocytosis. The cerebrospinal fluid (CSF) protein is elevated and the glucose is depressed. Although acid-fast bacilli will be seen only 25 per cent of the time, in over 75 per cent of patients tubercle bacilli can be cultured from the fluid.

Renal tuberculosis is frequently an asymptomatic illness until there is very advanced disease. Because of the greater blood supply to the renal cortex, hematogenous dissemination of tubercle bacilli will be to the renal cortex. When the infection descends into the medulla, spread throughout the genitourinary tract frequently occurs. Sterile pyuria may be the only sign of renal tuberculosis. Confirmation of the diagnosis by urine culture is absolutely essential since saprophytic acid-fast bacilli are frequently found in the urine.

Pott's disease is the name applied to tuberculosis of the spine. The focus of tuberculosis usually involves the anterior portion of a vertebral body near an intervertebral disc. The presence of collapse with anterior wedging of the vertebral bodies and a surrounding inflammatory reaction should always raise the suspicion of tuberculosis. Needle-aspiration biopsy or open biopsy is necessary to confirm the diagnosis.

Unusual Complications of Pulmonary Tuberculosis

Rarely, *empyema* caused by tuberculosis may result from a primary infection with an associated tuberculous pleural effusion. However, the latter usually clears, and empyema is more common later in disease associated with debility and loss of resistance to infection. It is usually a part of a progressive, extensive parenchymal infection with caseation and cavitation, the presumed sources for pleural contamination.

Although a relatively uncommon complication of tuberculous infection, the development of a *pneumothorax* requires prompt attention. One postulated theory of etiology is rupture of a cavity that connects the tracheobronchial tree with the pleural space, creating a bronchopleural fistula. In this instance, contamination of the pleural space with caseous material results in spread of the infection to the pleura which, because of the tendency to produce pleural fibrosis with expansion failure, should be corrected immediately. A second possible mechanism is the development of a submucosal bronchiolar lesion with air trapping in an acinus or subsegment that causes the development of a bleb. Rupture of this bleb allows air to enter the pleural space, often without tuberculous infection of the pleura. However, both occurrences should be treated with rapid expansion of the lung by tube suction to avoid the possibility of further infection and fibrosis of the pleura with entrapment of the lung. A *bronchopleural fistula* may persist after these episodes of pneumothorax and, especially if untreated, often results in major problems as a result of the tuberculous infection's becoming complicated by secondary invaders ("mixed" empyema).

Minor endobronchial disease is a common occurrence in tuberculosis but usually involves the distal bronchi. Resected lung specimens frequently show either ulceration or stenosis of the draining bronchioles or bronchi. *Bronchial stenosis* of significance may occur in the major bronchi but is rare. At times it results from involvement of the central lymph nodes draining into the lobar bronchi with caseation, ulceration, and fibrosis. Since fibrosis caused by tuberculosis tends to contract and aggravate the stenosis, resection of the involved lung segment may be required after chemotherapy has resolved the active inflammatory reaction.

The same endobronchial processes may result in *bronchiectasis* owing to destruction of the bronchial wall. This is usually distal and frequently occurs in the upper lobes. "Dry" bronchiectasis (without sputum) often is the result of prior pulmonary tuberculosis and may manifest itself chiefly as low-grade hemoptysis.

After treatment of extensive tuberculosis, the patient may be left with open, healed cavities as well as areas of bronchiectasis. Colonization of these areas can occur with a variety of infectious agents. Usual ororespiratory flora may produce the syndrome of "wet" bronchiectasis, i.e., with sputum production. Other mycobacteria may be recovered during the development of inactivity, and at one time they were considered to be a sign of healing. The presence of other pathogenic mycobacteria brings up the possibility of a dual infection, especially when found early in the disease.

The presence of Aspergillus species is common in badly damaged lung areas, especially those that are cavitary. In England, up to 34 per cent of clinically healed tuberculosis patients who have residual cavities develop positive precipitins to Aspergillus species and up to 17 per cent have demonstrable cavitary "balls," presumed to be aspergillomas or "fungus balls." This may be due in part to the increased incidence of Aspergillus noted in the United Kingdom, both in the environment and as an infective agent. (See the article on Opportunistic Mycoses.)

Massive hemorrhage is a dramatic event, frequently terminal, occurring in advanced cases of tuberculosis. Mild hemoptysis itself is very common in acute infection and not infrequently calls attention of an otherwise unconcerned patient to the presence of serious disease. Rupture of a mycotic aneurysm of a branch of the pulmonary artery (Rasmussen aneurysm) has been well publicized as a cause of death; an aspergilloma may be associated with severe and fatal hemorrhage. However, less well defined major hemorrhages may also occur.

Resection of the involved area has been the most widely used method of control; unhappily, many patients die before this can be accomplished and often (as in the case of aspergillomas) the areas are multiple, thus not lending themselves to excisional therapy. The extensive disease found in these patients often mitigates against surgery, since functional lung tissue necessary for survival must often be removed along with the diseased area.

During the acute infectious phase of the disease, two interesting complications have been reported: the *syndrome of inappropriate antidiuretic hormone excretion (SIADH), and a reset osmostat.* Both manifest themselves by an abnormally low sodium value. However, the former is associated with all of the clinical and renal abnormalities associated with SIADH. A reset osmostat is characterized by decreased serum osmolality without clinical symptoms and the obligatory renal salt wasting found in SIADH. Both conditions disappear with control of the infection but should be differentiated from each other, since SIADH requires that metabolic controls usually be employed.

Laboratory Procedures

Routine laboratory examinations are rarely helpful in establishing or suggesting the diagnosis. A mild normochromic normocytic anemia may be present in chronic tuberculosis. The white blood cell count is often normal, and counts over 20,000 per cu mm would suggest another infectious process; however, a leukemoid reaction may occasionally occur in miliary tuberculosis but does not occur in tuberculosis confined to the chest. Although a "left shift" in the differential white blood cell count can occur in advanced disease, these changes are neither specific nor useful.

Other nonspecific tests that may be elevated in active tuberculosis include the sedimentation rate, alpha-2 globulins, and gamma globulins. The finding of pyuria without bacteria by Gram stain is suggestive of renal involvement. Liver enzymes (transaminases and alkaline phosphatase) may occasionally be elevated prior to treatment. However, this is usually due to concomitant liver disease secondary to other problems such as alcoholism rather than to tuberculous involvement. Since the drugs used in the therapy of tuberculosis are often associated with hepatotoxicity, it is important to quantitate any hepatic abnormalities prior to treatment. On rare occasions, the serum sodium may be depressed as a result of the inappropriate secretion of ADH (already described). This occurs only in advanced pulmonary tuberculosis.

Tuberculin Skin Testing

All tuberculin that is currently available for skin testing is prepared from a protein precipitate of a filtrate of a heat-killed culture of *M. tuberculosis* (purified protein derivative—PPD). A positive delayed hypersensitivity reaction (48-hour reaction) to tuberculin is a useful marker of the occurrence of a prior primary infection. When the reaction is strongly positive—greater than 10 mm induration to 5 toxic units (TU) of PPD given by intradermal injection (Mantoux)—the test is considered to be diagnostic of a prior primary infection. A positive multipuncture skin test (Tine, Mono-Vacc, Heaf, or Aplitest) should always be checked with an intradermal skin test. False-positive reactions occur primarily for two causes. First, sensitization to another Mycobacterium species could have occurred. These reactions are generally small (between 5 and 10 mm of induration) although occasionally they may be large. Purified protein derivatives prepared from different Mycobacterium species cannot be used to differentiate the species that sensitized an individual. Second, vaccination with bacille Calmette Guérin (BCG) can cause severe reactions to PPD. However, when more than 2 years have elapsed since the vaccination, a large reaction to PPD should be considered diagnostic of at least a primary infection with tuberculosis, if not actual disease.

False-negative reactions to PPD are more of a problem than false-positive reactions. Faulty technique may be the most common cause of a false-negative reaction. In all situations in which tuberculosis is suspected and in which a negative PPD is observed, the test should be repeated. A state of immunosuppression may be the cause of a false-negative PPD. This could be induced by a disease state (viral infection, cancer, collagen vascular disease, sarcoidosis, or malnutrition) or by therapeutic intervention. Testing with multiple agents ("anergy panel") is the best means to document a state of immunosuppression. (See article on Diagnostic Problems in Immunosuppressed Patients.) On rare occasions, specific immunosuppression to tuberculin may occur.

Chest Radiography

The chest radiograph is the single most useful study for suggesting the diagnosis of tuberculosis. The appearance of the radiograph differs in primary and reactivation tuberculosis.

Primary Tuberculosis. In contrast to reactivation tuberculosis, which usually involves the superior and dorsal segments, parenchymal involvement in primary tuberculosis can involve any segment of the lung. In the primary infection, there is only a slight predilection for the upper lobes; in addition, anterior as well as posterior segments can be involved. The air-space consolidation appears as a homogeneous density with ill-defined borders, and cavitation is rare except in malnourished or other immunocompromised patients. Miliary involvement at the onset is seen in less than 3 per cent of cases, most commonly in children under 2 to 3 years of age.

Hilar or paratracheal lymph node enlargement is a characteristic finding in primary tuberculosis. In 15 per cent of patients, bilateral hilar adenopathy may be present. More commonly the adenopathy is unilateral. Unilateral hilar adenopathy or unilateral hilar and paratracheal adenopathy are equally common. Massive hilar adenopathy may herald a complicated course.

Atelectasis with an obstructive pneumonia may result from bronchial compression by inflamed lymph nodes or from a caseous lymph node that ruptures into a bronchus with resultant atelectasis and tuberculous pneumonia. Obstructive "emphysema," or a localized hyperinflated segment, at times precedes atelectasis. The segments most frequently involved are the anterior segment of the right upper lobe or the medial segment of the right middle lobe. Right-sided collapse is twice as common as left-sided collapse. Residual bronchiectatic changes may persist after the obstruction has cleared.

An isolated pleural effusion of mild to moderate degree may be the only manifestation of primary tuberculosis. However, the most common radiographic appearance of primary tuberculosis is a normal radiograph.

Reactivation Tuberculosis. Although reactivation tuberculosis may involve any lung segment, the characteristic appearance and distribution usually suggest the disease. In 95 per cent of localized pulmonary tuberculosis, the lesions will be present in the apical or posterior segment of the upper lobes or the superior segment of the lower lobes. The anterior segment of the upper lobe is almost never the only manifest area of involvement. A radiologist may attempt to describe the activity of a lesion based on its radiographic appearance, but the documentation of activity is best left to bacteriologic and clinical evaluation. Too often a lesion described as inactive or stable by radiograph will progress to symptomatic tuberculosis.

The typical parenchymal pattern of reactivation tuberculosis is of an air-space consolidation in a patchy or confluent nature. Frequently there are increased linear densities to the ipsilateral hilum. Cavitation is not uncommon, but lymph node enlargement is rarely seen. As the lesions become more chronic, they become more sharply circumscribed and irregular in contour. Fibrosis will lead to volume loss in the involved lung. The combination of patchy pneumonitis, fibrosis, and calcification is always suggestive of chronic granulomatous disease, usually tuberculosis.

The cavities that develop in tuberculosis are characterized by a moderately thick wall, a smooth inner surface, and the lack of an air-fluid level. Cavitation will frequently be associated with endobronchial spread of disease. Radiographically, this will appear as multiple, small acinar shadows.

Bacteriologic Examination

A firm diagnosis of tuberculosis requires bacteriologic confirmation. It is important to remember that a positive acid-fast smear is not specific for *M. tuber-*

culosis. Other mycobacteria, both saprophytes and potential pathogens, can be acid-fast. Thus, culture of *M. tuberculosis* is the only absolute way of confirming the diagnosis.

Freshly expectorated sputum is the best sample to stain and culture for *M. tuberculosis*. Twenty-four hour sputum samples are frequently overgrown with mouth flora and are much less useful. If the patient is not spontaneously producing sputum, an induced sputum is the next best specimen for study. This can be obtained by having the patient breathe an aerosol of isotonic or hypertonic saline for 5 to 15 minutes. If the patient cannot cooperate to give a spontaneous sputum sample, a gastric aspirate to obtain swallowed sputum may be useful. This must be obtained in the morning before the patient arises or eats.

In the majority of patients, this procedure will be successful in obtaining positive material for culture. Smears of gastric contents for acid-fast bacilli are of limited value because of the presence of ingested nontuberculous acid-fast bacilli. With a few patients, one may have to resort to bronchoscopy. Because the local anesthetics used during fiberoptic bronchoscopy may be lethal to *M. tuberculosis*, specimens for culture should be obtained using a minimal amount of anesthesia. However, irritation of the bronchial tree during the fiberoptic bronchoscopy procedure will frequently leave the patient with a productive cough. Thus collection of the postbronchoscopy sputum can be another valuable source of diagnostic material. In the absence of a positive sputum smear and before initiating therapy, biopsies and cultures should be attempted of any sites that appear to be involved.

In 1980, only 71 per cent of the cases of tuberculosis reported to the Centers for Disease Control had the diagnosis confirmed by positive culture. In an additional 10 per cent of the cases, only the smear was positive. In 20 per cent of reported cases, both the smears and the cultures were negative. Thus, in a significant number of cases, the diagnosis of tuberculosis had been made in the absence of bacteriologic confirmation. In these cases, the diagnosis was made by a combination of a positive skin test, compatible chest radiograph, biopsy material containing granulomas, and a therapeutic trial.

Therapeutic Trials

Since confirmation of tuberculosis by culture requires 4 to 6 weeks, most patients are started on therapy prior to confirmation of the diagnosis. When the diagnosis is not confirmed by culture of *M. tuberculosis,* the response of the patient to the therapeutic trial may be important in deciding whether or not the patient has had active tuberculosis. This most commonly occurs in an asymptomatic middle-aged individual with apical scarring and a positive skin test to PPD. Clearing of the chest radiograph in response to therapy would be evidence for active tuberculosis and an indication for a full therapeutic course. Failure of the radiograph to change after 6 to 8 weeks would be evidence of old or inactive tuberculosis, and the patient would be a candidate for prophylactic therapy. Similarly, clearing of an undiagnosed exudative pleural effusion in a patient with a positive PPD would be considered as evidence of active tuberculosis.

Potential Errors and Pitfalls in Diagnosis

Since tuberculosis today is a disease most frequently present in older individuals, the major differential diagnosis is usually between tuberculosis and carcinoma of the lung. An important concept to remember is that carcinoma may cause a focus of tuberculosis to spread; thus tuberculosis and carcinoma of the lung may be present simultaneously. In patients with simultaneous presentation of carcinoma and tuberculosis, the diagnosis of tuberculosis frequently is made first and the diagnosis of carcinoma is delayed for several months. Thus if the radiograph and the clinical situation suggest carcinoma but the sputum contains acid-fast bacilli, further procedures to diagnose carcinoma may still be indicated. Isolated involvement of the anterior segment of the upper lobe, isolated involvement of the lower lobe, or the presence of irregular cavities would suggest carcinoma, and further diagnostic work-up may be indicated despite acid-fast bacilli in the sputum smear.

Any type of infectious or granulomatous disease may be radiologically identical to tuberculosis. Three broad categories must be distinguished: fungi (histoplasmosis, coccidioidomycosis, and blastomycosis); bacteria (*Pseudomonas pseudomoniae*); and other mycobacteria (mainly *M. kansasii* and *M. intracellulare*). Culture of the organism from the patient's sputum is the best way to differentiate these diseases, although serum antibody titers to fungi are also valuable.

Common bacterial pneumonias are usually easily differentiated from tuberculosis. The localized alveolar infiltrate on the chest radiograph and the prompt response to antibiotic therapy usually differentiate bacterial pneumonia from tuberculosis. When in doubt, a bacterial pneumonia should be treated first and tuberculosis therapy withheld until adequate sputums have been obtained and the response to antibiotics determined. Lung abscesses can usually be differentiated from tuberculous cavities by (1) the prominent air fluid level, (2) the more common lower lobe distribution, and (3) the clinical situation (i.e., association with seizures, alcoholism, dental caries, and so on).

DISEASES CAUSED BY OTHER MYCOBACTERIA

Definition

Diseases caused by nontuberculous mycobacteria should always be referred to by the specific organism that is causing the disease and the site of involvement (e.g., pulmonary disease due to *M. kansasii*).

Presenting Symptoms and Signs

The presenting symptoms and signs of the infections caused by nontuberculous mycobacteria can be identical to those of tuberculosis. Although any organ can be infected, the pulmonary, lymph node, soft-tissue, and skeletal systems are the ones most frequently affected. Disseminated involvement can also occur (Table 1).

Pulmonary symptoms are indicative of a chronic inflammatory process. Cough, night sweats, low-grade fever, and weight loss will usually be present for several months. These mycobacterial infections will often occur in already damaged lungs. Thus the disease will occur commonly in middle-aged white men with a history of chronic bronchitis, emphysema, prior tuberculosis, bronchiectasis, chronic aspiration, pneumoconiosis, or cancer. Because many of the nontuberculous mycobacteria can be found in the soil, a geographic localization of these cases can be found. *M. kansasii* is frequently reported from Texas, Chicago, Kansas City, England and Wales, whereas *M. intracellulare* is most frequent in the southeastern United States, Western Australia, and Japan. However, pulmonary disease caused by both of these mycobacteria can be found almost anywhere. A history of contact with other patients with nontuberculous mycobacterial disease is not helpful, since person-to-person transmission of these diseases has not been documented.

Cervical lymphadenitis, or "scrofula," is most common in children younger than 10 years old. Commonly, only a single node is involved, but occasionally multiple nodes are involved. As much as 75 per cent of all granulomatous cervical adenitis may be due to nontuberculous mycobacteria, particularly *M. scrofulaceum*. Although the nodes are initially small, firm, and painless, they may become fluctuant and rupture. Sinus formation with prolonged drainage is not uncommon.

Superficial skin disease is most commonly caused by direct inoculation. Swimming pool granuloma is usually caused by *M. marinum* at sites of local abrasions. The lesions begin as papules and progress over 2 to 3 weeks to shallow ulceration and scab formation. *M. fortuitum* infections are usually caused by trauma or surgical wounds.

Disseminated disease can occur in an immunosuppressed host. Childhood immune deficiencies, hematologic malignancies, immunosuppressive therapy, or corticosteroids have been associated with disseminated mycobacterial infections. Of particular interest is the recent description of disseminated *M. intracellulare* infection in patients with acquired immune deficiency syndrome (AIDS). This illness has been described in homosexuals, hemophiliacs, Haitians, and heroin abusers. Disseminated nontuberculous mycobacterial infection is just one of many unusual conditions acquired by patients with AIDS. (See Section 15 for an article on AIDS.)

Laboratory Procedures

Routine laboratory tests are of little use in the diagnosis of nontuberculous mycobacteria. Skin testing with proteins prepared from cultures of mycobacteria were thought at one time to be useful in identifying a particular species. However, it is now known that PPDs made from various mycobacteria cannot be used to diagnose specific mycobacterial infections. In particular, neither the size of the PPD reaction nor the type of PPD utilized can be interpreted to identify a species of mycobacteria that is infecting an individual.

Specialized laboratories are usually necessary to correctly identify specific mycobacteria. The Runyon classification of mycobacteria based on growth rate and pigment production (Table 2) can be used only as a rough guide for specific mycobacterial identification. A total of 14 different tests may be necessary to correctly identify all the various species of mycobacteria.

Because the nontuberculous mycobacteria can colonize the skin, bronchial tree, or urine, one must be very careful in interpreting a positive culture to indicate infection. In addition, since nontuberculous mycobacteria have been cultured from water samples, false-positive cultures can occur. Thus multiple positive cultures are necessary to confirm the diagnosis. In particular, at least three consecutive positive sputum cultures containing at least 100 colonies per cul-

Table 1. Nontuberculous Mycobacterial Disease of Man*

Disease	Common Species	Unusual Species
Pulmonary disease	*M. avium/intracellulare* *M. kansasii*	*M. xenopi* *M. szulgai* *M. simiae* *M. scrofulaceum* *M. fortuitum*
Lymphadenitis in children	*M. scrofulaceum* *M. avium/intracellulare*	*M. kansasii* *M. fortuitum*
Swimming pool granuloma	*M. marinum*	
Local abscess	*M. fortuitum*	
Skeletal	*M. kansasii* *M. avium/intracellulare*	*M. fortuitum* *M. marinum*
Disseminated	*M. avium/intracellulare* *M. kansasii*	*M. fortuitum* *M. scrofulaceum*

*Case reports of disease caused by nontuberculous mycobacteria other than those listed above are in the literature.

Table 2. Classification of Nontuberculous Mycobacteria

Group	Skin Test	Growth Rate (Days)	Pigment	Niacin
Photochromogens (pigment is light-dependent)				
M. kansasii	PPD-Y	7–21	Yellow	–
M. marinum				
Scotochromogens (pigment is not light-dependent)	PPD-G	7–21	Yellow-orange	–
M. scrofulaceum				
Nonchromogens (no pigment)				
M. intracellulare	PPD-B	7–21	Buff	–
M avium	PPD-A	7–21	Buff	–
Rapid growers				
M. fortuitum	PPD-F	3–7	None	–

ture should be found before one attributes a pulmonary infiltrate to a nontuberculous mycobacteria. Positive cultures from tissue samples that are normally sterile are usually considered diagnostic of a mycobacterial infection. However, one must be aware that the water used in the culture media can be contaminated with mycobacteria. Thus the contaminated water, rather than the tissue sample, may be responsible for the positive culture. For these reasons, it is always preferable to have multiple positive cultures of nontuberculous mycobacteria.

LEPROSY

By Robert R. Jacobson, M.D., Ph.D.
Carville, Louisiana

Leprosy (Hansen's disease) is a chronic infectious disease caused by *Mycobacterium leprae.* It primarily involves the skin, peripheral nerves, eyes, and mucous membranes, although in the more advanced forms bacilli may be found nearly anywhere in the body outside the central nervous system.

There are four types of leprosy. The earliest in all cases is referred to as *indeterminate.* This may self-heal or progress to one of the three common clinical types, depending on the extent of the defect in the patient's cell-mediated immune response toward *M. leprae.* In those with the most intact response, the disease is kept localized and develops into *tuberculoid leprosy,* often referred to as TT disease under the Ridley-Jopling classification. In those with the poorest response, the disease disseminates, developing into *lepromatous leprosy* (LL). Between these two extremes is the broad borderline (*dimorphous*) portion of the leprosy spectrum, often subdivided into borderline-tuberculoid (BT), mid-borderline (BB), and borderline-lepromatous (BL).

There are more than 12 million cases worldwide and over 4000 in the United States. Most cases in the United States are detected among aliens, with only about 15 per cent of all new cases during the last decade being found in native-born residents.

CLINICAL COURSE

The diagnosis of leprosy should be considered in any patient with skin lesions and sensory loss. The disease usually begins with cutaneous and neural manifestations (sensory and/or motor), and a history of repeated injuries as a result of loss of sensation, particularly in the extremities, may be noted.

Indeterminate disease commonly presents as a hypopigmented, sometimes erythematous, macule on the face, extremities, or buttocks in which diminished sensation may be detected. It is usually singular, although occasionally more than one lesion may be found. As noted above, if not detected and treated, this form of leprosy is self-healing or it progresses to one of the other forms.

Tuberculoid disease usually presents as a single, large macular lesion which in the classic case is hypopigmented, scaly, and anesthetic with a raised, well-defined margin. Less commonly, the lesions are purely macular or plaquelike. Only peripheral nerves in the vicinity of the lesions are likely to be involved, as evidenced by enlargement, tenderness, and/or diminished function. Usually the disease is stable, although occasionally it may downgrade immunologically to the borderline type.

Lepromatous disease is usually generalized at the time of diagnosis, although occasional cases are detected very early and may have relatively localized disease. It most commonly presents as a papular and nodular eruption. It may also begin as faint erythematous macules with vague margins that tend to increase in number, enlarge, and coalesce, or it may present as diffuse disease with no distinct lesions, except perhaps for a slight generalized erythema. There may be partial (lateral portion) or complete loss of eyebrows and eyelashes, diminished body hair, and enlargement of the earlobes. Although seldom seen today, very advanced cases sometimes have such extensive facial infiltration that a corrugated appearance, the so-called "leonine" facies, develops. Infiltration of the upper respiratory tract occurs and may lead to varying degrees of nasal stuffiness, epistaxis, and hoarseness. Advanced cases occasionally have a perforated nasal septum and, less commonly, collapse of the nose. In the eyes, tiny lepromatous papules involving the conjunctiva, sclera, and episclera with beading of the corneal nerves may occur, together with loss of corneal sensation and diminished tearing. Sensory loss in lepromatous cases is usually present at the time of diagnosis. It commonly begins on the dorsal portions of the distal extremities and may progress to more extensive loss of sensation on the hands and feet as well as extending proximally. Very advanced, long-standing cases sometimes have almost total body sensory loss, but this is rarely seen at the time of diagnosis. Many different peripheral nerves may be involved, including the great auricular, ulnar, radial cutaneous, median, peroneal, sural, and facial. Motor loss at the time of diagnosis is less common than with borderline cases but may develop in the course of chronically active disease and/or reactive episodes.

The presentation of borderline leprosy varies considerably from the tuberculoidlike lesions that may be seen in BT cases to the lepromatouslike lesions of BL disease. Between these two extremes an endless variety of skin changes may occur. Borderline-tuberculoid (BT) lesions tend to be large and annular, macular, or plaque-like, with diminished sensation in many of them. Midborderline (BB) lesions may be similar occasionally with satellite lesions nearby, but they are generally smaller and the sensory loss may occur within the lesions or in the lepromatous pattern. Borderline-lepromatous (BL) lesions are usually small and similar to lepromatous with sensory loss in the lepromatous pattern. Since the disease tends to downgrade immunologically without treatment, it might have started as BT but may be essentially BL at diagnosis, producing a variety of skin lesions and a mixed tuberculoid-lepromatous pattern of sensory loss. Nerve involvement tends to be extensive in all borderline cases, and motor loss is often present at the time of diagnosis.

Leprosy-related reactions are more common after treatment has begun, but they may occur beforehand and thus be a presenting symptom. A Type 1 or reversal reaction will typically present with fever, neuritis, edema, and erythema of pre-existing lesions, which may progress to ulceration, new lesions, adenopathy, and a high white blood cell count. Type 2 reactions (erythema nodosum leprosum, or ENL) usually present with erythematous, frequently painful nodules; these may be few and develop sporadically or may appear quickly in large numbers and are nearly always accompanied by fever. Less commonly, the lesions are erythema multiforme–like, pustular, hemorrhagic, or ulcerating. Neuritis, arthralgias, leukocytosis, iridocyclitis, lymphadenitis, pretibial periostitis, orchitis, and nephritis may also occur.

Neuritis may be manifested by enlargement of the nerve, pain, tenderness, paresthesias, and sensory or motor loss. The most common sites of motor involvement are (1) the ulnar and median nerves, producing a partial or complete claw hand deformity with flattening of the hypothenar eminence and thenar webspace and wasting of the interosseous muscles; (2) the common peroneal nerve, leading to a footdrop; and (3) the posterior tibial nerve, resulting in clawed toes. Less commonly, facial nerve paralysis may be seen and rarely the radial nerve (wrist drop) is involved, but only in patients who have ulnar and median nerve paralysis.

Testicular atrophy is sometimes seen in a newly diagnosed case, although it is more common with long-standing disease. Gynecomastia is also occasionally present.

PHYSICAL EXAMINATION

This should include careful inspection of the skin to determine the extent of involvement and type of lesions; a sensory examination; motor strength testing in the face, hands, and feet; palpation of peripheral nerves; and examination of the eyes. The typical skin lesions encountered have been described previously, but nodules, papules, plaques, and/or macules are seen.

Sensory loss may include the modalities light touch, pain, and temperature. Testing for these sensations is done with a cotton wisp or weighted hairs, pinprick, and two test tubes filled with cold and hot liquids, respectively. At least, typical lesions and the extremities should be tested for sensory loss. The ability to sweat is also lost in insensitive areas, which may appear dry and scaly, particularly in a dry climate.

The face should be inspected for seventh nerve paralysis and the hands for evidence of ulnar and median nerve involvement, such as muscle wasting and inability to extend the fingers fully. The feet should be checked for muscle wasting, inability to extend the toes, and footdrop. The ulnar nerve at the elbow, the median and superficial radial cutaneous at the wrist, the great auricular in the lateral neck crossing the sternomastoid muscle, the common peroneal in the popliteal fossa passing down around the neck of the fibula, and the sural behind the lateral malleolus should all be gently palpated bilaterally for enlargement and tenderness.

Examination of the eyes should include checking for loss of eyebrows and eyelashes, lagophthalmos, decreased corneal sensation, decreased tearing, pupillary shape and response to light, and any evidence of iridocyclitis such as circumcorneal hyperemia. The nose is examined for a septal perforation, and the hands and feet should be inspected for injuries.

DIAGNOSIS

Diagnosis in a patient suspected of having leprosy on the basis of the history and physical examination is confirmed by skin scrapings and biopsy. Nerve conduction velocities and a lepromin test also provide useful information in some patients. Routine laboratory studies will provide relatively little assistance. *M. leprae* may be detected in the buffy coat of a spun-down blood specimen from a patient with advanced disease, but this test is seldom done. The erythrocyte sedimentation rate is usually elevated and false-positive serologies are occasionally seen, but any other abnormalities would generally be related to complications such as a leukocytosis in a patient having a reaction.

Skin scrapings are taken by pinching the skin to diminish blood flow, wiping the area with an alcohol sponge, and making a small slit about 5 mm long and 4 mm deep with a sterile razor blade or scalpel. Any blood is wiped away, the slit is gently scraped, and the material transferred to a microscopic slide to form a moderately thick smear in a circular area about 5 to 6 mm in diameter. The slide is fixed in 10 per cent formalin for 15 minutes and rinsed in tap water. Staining for acid-fast bacilli is then done by the Fite-Faraco method. The morphologic index (MI) and bacteriologic index (BI) are then determined. The MI is the percentage of bacilli that appear normal insofar as the size, shape, and uniformity of staining are concerned. This value usually ranges from 0 to 5 per cent at various sites in a newly diagnosed case and correlates to some extent with viability, since when the MI falls to zero (0) at all sites on treatment, bacilli isolated from that patient will no longer routinely grow in the mouse footpad system. The BI is a semilogarithmic scale used to quantify the number of bacilli seen. It ranges from 0 to 6+, as shown in Table 1. Typically the BI will be 0 on skin scrapings and 0 to 1+ on biopsy in an indeterminate or tuberculoid case. The BI on both skin scrapings and biopsy will normally range from 0 to 2+ in BT, 2 to 4+ in BB, 3 to 5+ in BL, and 4 to 6+ in LL patients.

A biopsy may be taken from any representative lesion. It is, however, generally better to perform a biopsy on the more active margin in a tuberculoid or similar BT lesion, being careful to take the specimen from entirely within the lesion and not to include normal skin. Biopsies from patients with no distinct lesions may be taken from any site where bacilli were found on skin scrapings, normally choosing the area with the highest BI. When no lesions are present and skin scrapings are negative but the diagnosis is suspected on the basis of sensory loss, a biopsy can be done from the insensitive area or a nerve biopsy can be considered. Some sections from the biopsy are stained with hematoxylin-eosin for evaluation of the histopathology and others with a Fite-Faraco stain for acid-fast bacilli. The MI and BI are determined by the latter stain just as on skin scrapings. Indeterminate lesions histologically appear as a chronic nonspecific dermatitis. The infiltrate will be seen around nerves, and the bacilli are most likely to be found in dermal nerves. Tuberculoid disease is characterized by epithelioid cell granulomas containing occasional giant cells and surrounded by lymphocytes. The infiltrate may extend up to the dermis, and nerves may be invaded and destroyed to the point of being unidentifiable. It is usually difficult to find bacilli, but they are most likely to be located in nerves. Lepromatous disease is characterized by an extensive infiltrate of foamy histiocytes separated from the epidermis by a clear zone. The infiltrate is present around nerves but may not invade them except in advanced cases. Numerous bacilli will be found within the histiocytes and in nerves, particularly in the Schwann cells. The infiltrate in borderline cases is tuberculoidlike in BT disease with lymphocytes, epithelioid and giant cells, and very few bacilli. As the disease moves toward BL, the infiltrate becomes mostly macrophages and a clear zone becomes prominent, bacilli increase in numbers, and nerve involvement becomes mainly perineural rather than intraneural. Lymphocytes are plentiful until the LL end of the spectrum is approached, at which time they nearly disappear.

Table 1. The Bacteriologic Index (BI)

BI	
0	No bacilli in 100 OIF*
1+	1–10 Bacilli per 100 OIF
2+	1–10 Bacilli per 10 OIF
3+	1–10 Bacilli per OIF
4+	10–100 Bacilli per OIF
5+	100–1000 Bacilli per OIF
6+	Over 1000 Bacilli per OIF

*OIF = Oil immersion fields.

Peripheral nerves may show evidence of diminished function on nerve conduction studies prior to clinical evidence of involvement being noted. Thus this test is sometimes useful in difficult cases and when a neuritis is present to accurately evaluate subtle changes in function.

The lepromin test is a useful measure of an individual's ability to generate a cell-mediated immune response to *M. leprae,* but it is not a diagnostic test and is not readily available in the United States. It has some value in indeterminate cases, since patients with a negative response may require more prolonged treatment than those who are positive. It is also helpful in evaluating contacts because patients with a positive response are generally considered nonsusceptible. It is a heat-killed suspension of *M. leprae* given like a tuberculin test (0.1 ml injected intradermally). The tuberculin-like Fernandez response is read at 48 hours and the Mitsuda response at 21 days. A nodule of 3 mm or more at 21 days, often going on to ulceration, is considered positive. The test is positive in TT and BT cases, negative in BL and LL cases, and sometimes positive or negative in BB or indeterminate cases.

DIFFERENTIAL DIAGNOSIS

Leprosy will seldom be confused with other diseases if the patient is carefully evaluated. Various skin conditions likely to be confused with it usually do not have sensory loss and other evidence of neural involvement. Cutaneous sarcoid has occasionally been misdiagnosed as leprosy, but acid-fast bacilli will not be found and biopsies will not show involvement of dermal nerves. Other mycobacterial skin infections are sometimes misdiagnosed as leprosy; however, these are cultivatable (whereas *M. leprae* is not), and neural involvement is not present. A variety of other dermatologic conditions have been referred to the National Hansen's Disease Center at Carville, misdiagnosed as leprosy over the years, including necrobiosis lipoidica diabeticorum, lymphomatoid granulomatosis, and cutaneous leishmaniasis. Occasionally, leprosy presents coexistent with another disease and the negative (for leprosy) findings in such a patient—if only the nonleprosy lesions are biopsied or scraped—may be misleading. Furthermore, hypopigmented macules or other lesions may be misdiagnosed as leprosy on contact examinations unless sensory testing, skin scrapings, and/or biopsies are also done to confirm the diagnosis.

CONTACT EXAMINATIONS

The diagnosis of leprosy obligates the physician to perform contact examinations on the other members of the household. Basically, the approach would be similar to that already outlined. The findings may be more subtle, however, so that detection of the disease and confirmation of the diagnosis may be somewhat more difficult. Usually the contacts are asked about any sensory loss or "numbness." The physician follows this with a brief inspection of the skin in good light, looking for any lesions suspect of leprosy. Second, the hands and feet are inspected for any evidence of motor loss or muscle atrophy or for findings that might indicate sensory loss, such as a plantar ulcer. Commonly involved peripheral nerves are palpated for evidence of enlargement and/or tenderness, and the head is examined for loss of eyebrows, perforation of the nasal septum, or enlarged earlobes. A brief sensory exam utilizing a cotton wisp and/or pinprick may be done by checking any suspect skin lesions and the distal extremities. If any findings suggest a diagnosis of leprosy, skin scrapings and a biopsy are indicated. With some experience, the entire examination takes very little time. It should be repeated every 6 to 12 months for at least 5 years for household contacts, and in this way any cases among this group will be detected early, usually before any significant nerve damage occurs.

LABORATORY DIAGNOSIS OF VIRAL INFECTIONS

By John A. Bryan, M.D.
Atlanta, Georgia

Viruses are living microorganisms that range in size from 50 to 300 nanometers (nm) and multiply only inside living cells of susceptible hosts. Presently, some 400 to 500 viruses are known to infect humans. Viruses cause a significant proportion of the morbidity and mortality attributable to the common infectious diseases found throughout the world. Many viral infections occur in epidemic form; some have the potential for nosocomial spread; and others result in persistent, latent infection and/or transformation of human cells.

Traditionally, methods for viral diagnosis consisted primarily of isolation/identification of viral agents using cell culture systems, embryonated hens' eggs, or animals (e.g., guinea pigs and adult or suckling mice); alternatively, or in conjunction with isolation/identification procedures, serologic techniques were utilized to demonstrate a significant (fourfold) rise in specific antibody titer in "paired" (acute and convalescent) sera collected approximately 2 to 4 weeks apart.

Historically, these approaches were of limited usefulness clinically because of limited availability and the time required—3 to 4 weeks for completion of testing and submission of results. Presently, however, the situation is vastly different. Modern equipment, advances in isolation/identification techniques, and improvements in procedures for collection of specimens have considerably shortened the time required for viral diagnosis. With current isolation methods, many viruses produce a cytopathic effect (CPE) in cell culture within 5 to 6 days, and some (e.g., herpes simplex virus [HSV]) will produce CPE in 1 to 2 days. Furthermore, new rapid techniques for viral identification have further shortened the time required for diagnosis to less than 24 hours. Using these new developments, it is now possible for even a small microbiology laboratory possessing only minimal equipment and space to specifically diagnose many viral diseases within a clinically useful period of time.

The present general applicability and capability for rapid viral diagnosis are associated with direct benefits to both patients and hospital staff and indirect benefits to the community (Table 1). Important among these are the institution of specific antiviral therapy or prophylaxis for some viral diseases, the avoidance of antibiotics in primary viral respiratory infections, and the reduction in health care costs derived from earlier hospital discharge.

COLLECTION AND TRANSPORT OF SPECIMENS

All specimens submitted to the laboratory for viral studies should be accompanied by the information

Table 1. Benefits of Viral Diagnosis

Institution of specific prophylaxis or therapy
Avoidance of unnecessary laboratory tests, antimicrobial therapy, and prolongation of hospital stay
Clarification of prognosis
Recognition and control of viral disease(s) in hospital and community
Early warning of virus disease with epidemic potential
Active and passive immunization of persons at risk
Prevention and control of nosocomial viral infection
Isolation of patients
Special measures to control hospital spread
Identification of the role of viruses in diverse clinical syndromes
Identification of new viruses of clinical importance
Education and training of physicians and health care workers
Accumulation of data for research in viral diseases

Table 2. Information to Accompany Specimens

Full name of patient and clinician
Address of hospital or clinic
Age of patient
Sex of patient
Clinical diagnosis/viral agents(s) suspected
Main clinical and laboratory findings
Date of initial symptom onset
Brief summary of illness course, including antibiotic treatment
Pertinent epidemiologic information (e.g., similar illness in family or community, travel/exposure/immunization history, occupation)
Type of specimen(s)
Date(s) and time(s) collected

listed in Table 2. Selection of the proper specimen(s) to collect is critical for accurate viral diagnosis and should be determined by the nature of the illness (e.g., respiratory, gastrointestinal), and the particular viral agent(s) suspected (Table 3). Prior consultation between the clinician and the laboratory can facilitate this process and save valuable time. Since the amount of virus in a patient is usually at a maximum during or very shortly after the appearance of initial symptoms and declines rapidly thereafter, any specimen for virus isolation must be collected as soon as possible following onset of disease. Specimens for viral isolation can be taken at postmortem examination, since this permits direct access to affected organs (Table 4). However, the specimens must be collected aseptically and within a few hours after death.

Procedures for collection and transport of specimens are outlined in Table 5. Generally, specimens should be immediately placed at 4°C (wet ice or cold packs)—not frozen (−5°C)—and promptly transported to the laboratory and processed as soon as possible. For transportation and/or storage requiring up to 5 days, hold the specimen(s) at 4°C; if a longer time is anticipated before processing, hold the specimen(s) at −70°C. Repeated freeze-thawing of specimen(s) should be avoided, since a drop in the viral titer may result; if freezing and thawing are necessary, it is best to freeze at −70°C and thaw at 25°C. Commonly used media for transport include modified Stuarts or Hanks and Leibovitz-Emory. Several commercial swab transport media systems are available. Specimens taken at postmortem examination for viral isolation must not be placed in fixatives.

BASIC METHODS FOR LABORATORY DIAGNOSIS

The three basic approaches to the laboratory diagnosis of viral infections are (1) direct examination of clinical materials for virus or viral antigens, (2) isolation/identification of viruses from clinical specimens, and (3) serologic diagnosis. These are outlined in Table 6.

Direct Examination

Direct examination of clinical specimens permits the most rapid recognition and identification of viral agents. Direct methods include electron microscopy (EM), cytopathology (CP), fluorescent antibody (FA) techniques, and solid-phase immunoassays (SPIA). Electron microscopy and cytopathology permit direct ultrastructural visualization of viral particles or identification of nuclear/cytoplasmic inclusions and other cellular alteration by light microscopy. With FA and SPIA, the specimen is incubated with an antibody that is specific for the virus (viral antigen) to be identified and examined for the presence of specific fluorescence (FA), radioactivity, or color change (SPIA).

Electron Microscopy

Electron microscopy is most applicable for investigation of viral infections in which the concentration of virus in the clinical specimen is at least 10^6 to 10^7 particles per milliliter. The specimen must also be free of background debris to permit detection and definitive identification of virus morphology. Many types of specimens can be examined, including feces, serum, urine, vesicle fluid, brain tissue, or other tissues such as warts. Direct EM (DEM) is useful for the rapid diagnosis of viral gastroenteritis syndromes (rotaviruses, parvoviruses, adenoviruses, coronaviruses, astroviruses, and caliciviruses), vesicular lesions (HSV, varicella zoster virus [VZV], and vaccinia-variola viruses), congenital cytomegalovirus (CMV) infection, hepatitis A virus (HAV) infection, papillomatous lesions (molluscum contagiosum), and warts (papillomaviruses).

Following appropriate preparation (i.e., dilution—suspension, mincing, homogenization, centrifugation, clarification), clinical specimens are placed on copper grids (Formvar-carbon-coated, 400 mesh are commonly used), negatively stained with 2 to 4 per cent phosphotungstic acid, and examined directly for the presence of viruses. Enhancement techniques can be used to increase the sensitivity of EM when examining clinical specimens with virus titers lower than 10^6 particles per milliliter. Pseudoreplica and agar gel diffusion can be used to concentrate and purify clinical specimens and are useful procedures for identifying rotaviruses in feces and CMV in urine. Immune EM (IEM) provides a means for direct observation of the interaction of virus with homologous antibody. This technique is useful for the specific identification of small particles difficult to visualize by DEM and viral agents that cannot be isolated using conventional methods. Immune EM has permitted identification of the agents of acute nonbacterial gastroenteritis (astroviruses, caliciviruses, and parvoviruses), and HAV.

Cytopathology

Cytopathology is useful in identifying many common viral infections that produce characteristic cytopathic effects in cytologic preparations or tissue sections. Certain types of cytopathologic change are quite specific, and some are even diagnostic for specific viral infections. The cytopathologic effects of infections with many common viral agents are listed in Table 7. Specimens from vesicular skin and mucosal lesions may be obtained by scraping the edge of the "unroofed" lesion with a sterile swab or scalpel blade

Table 3. Choice of Specimens for Diagnosis

Disease and Common Etiologic Viral Agents	Clinical Specimens for Viral Isolation/Identification*	Other†
Respiratory		
Adenoviruses, enteroviruses, HSV, influenza viruses, parainfluenza viruses, mumps virus, RSV	Throat swab; nasopharyngeal aspirate, wash, swab (influenza, RSV); urine (mumps)	Paired sera
Meningitis-Encephalitis		
Arboviruses, enteroviruses, HSV, mumps virus, rabies virus	Throat swab; stool/rectal swab; CSF; blood (arbovirus); urine (mumps); brain biopsy (HSV)	Paired sera; corneal impression smear and/or skin biopsy for immunofluorescence assay (rabies)
Myocarditis-Pericarditis		
Group B coxsackieviruses, influenza viruses, CMV, mumps virus	Throat swab; stool/rectal swab; urine (CMV, mumps); pericardium, pericardial fluid	Paired sera
Exanthems-Enanthems		
Adenoviruses, enteroviruses, rubella virus, HSV, VZV, vaccinia virus	Throat swab; stool/rectal swab; urine (rubella virus); vesicle fluid or swab (HSV, VZV, coxsackievirus, vaccinia)	Paired sera; smear of lesion scraping for cytopathology and immunofluorescence
Eye		
Adenoviruses, HSV, enteroviruses	Throat swab; conjunctival swab/scraping; corneal scrapings	Paired sera; smear of scrapings for cytopathology and immunofluorescence
Gastrointestinal		
Adenoviruses, rotaviruses, parvoviruses (Norwalk-like agents)	Stool/rectal swab	Paired sera; rotaviruses and parvoviruses cannot be cultivated in conventional cell cultures; must use direct EM, immune EM, or other immunological methods for detection
Other		
Infectious mononucleosis (EBV, CMV) Viral hepatitis (HAV, HBV, NANBV)	Throat swab (CMV); urine (CMV); leukocytes (CMV) not routinely attempted	Paired sera; demonstration of respective serologic markers associated with HAV or HBV infection. NANBV infection is a diagnosis of exclusion at present

*Cell culture; direct methods such as electron microscopy (EM), fluorescent antibody (FA), and enzyme-linked immunosorbent assay (ELISA).

†Serologic tests for all adenoviral and enteroviral serotypes are not generally available; virus isolation and specific serologic identification are preferred.

Abbreviations: HSV = Herpes simplex virus; RSV = respiratory syncytial virus; CMV = cytomegalovirus; VZV = varicella zoster virus; EBV = Epstein-Barr virus; HAV = hepatitis type A virus; HBV = hepatitis type B virus; CSF = cerebrospinal fluid; NANBV = hepatitis non-A, non-B viruses.

and fixing the prepared slide in 95 per cent ethanol, Zenker's solution, or Bouin's solution. Specimens for diagnosis of respiratory infections include cells in sputum and bronchial washings and brushings. Cerebrospinal fluid, effusions, and urine can also be processed and the cells from these fluids stained and examined for specific viral-induced changes.

Fluorescent Antibody Techniques

Fluorescent antibody methodology relies on the fact that fluorescent compounds such as fluorescein isothiocyanate (FITC) can be coupled with antibody molecules at locations that do not affect the immunologic specificity of the antibody. The FITC-labeled antibody molecule can bind specifically to the homologous viral antigen, and the reaction can be visualized microscopically using ultraviolet light. Fluorescent antibody techniques are reliable for the diagnosis of numerous viral infections, including those caused by respiratory syncytial virus (RSV), influenza viruses, parainfluenza viruses, adenoviruses, mumps virus, rubeola virus, rubella virus, rabies virus, HSV, VZV, CMV, vaccinia virus, and some arenaviruses, arboviruses, and enteroviruses. Fluorescent antibody techniques can be used for the detection of viral antigens in clinical specimens and in cell cultures inoculated with clinical materials or for detection and quantitation of serum antibodies following viral infection (vide infra). When used in conjunction with virus isolation, FA tests will often be positive prior to detection of CPE in tissue culture (often 1 or 2 days postinoculation).

The two basic FA methods are the direct and the indirect techniques. With direct staining, the FITC-labeled viral immunoglobulin binds directly to the homologous viral antigen in the clinical specimen. With indirect staining, the viral immunoglobulin, which binds to its homologous viral antigen, is not FITC-labeled; rather, an FITC-labeled antispecies immunoglobulin is employed to detect the specific viral antigen-antibody complex. Indirect testing is more

Table 4. Postmortem Specimens of Choice for Viral Diagnosis

Syndrome	Specimens
Respiratory	Lung, tracheal swab, blood
Central nervous system	Brain, spinal cord, cerebrospinal fluid, feces, blood
Cardiovascular	Myocardium, pericardium, pericardial fluid, feces, blood
Undiagnosed febrile illness	Brain, liver, lung, pleural fluid, spleen, kidney, blood, feces, skin lesions, pharyngeal swab, peritoneal fluid
Hepatitis	Liver, feces, blood

sensitive; however, the direct test has several advantages over the indirect tests, including greater specificity, a cleaner background (less nonspecific fluorescence), and fewer manipulations and reagents. The direct method permits detection of viral antigens only, whereas the indirect method can be used for detection of either viral antibody or antigen. Conjugated reagents are commercially available for direct FA detection of the following viruses: HSV 1 and 2 (monovalent or bivalent); influenza A and B; parainfluenza 1, 2, 3; mumps; RSV; CMV; VZV; Epstein-Barr virus [EBV]; rubella; rubeola; and adenovirus. Reagents for indirect FA staining are commercially available for HSV 1 and 2 viruses, CMV, VZV, EBV, and RSV.

Specimens that can be used for FA diagnosis include frozen sections of tissue, impression smears, lesion scrapings, resuspended cells from centrifuged sediment, and occasionally, if ample material can be recovered, specimens in viral transport media (see Tables 3, 4, and 5). After preparation, the slides are air-dried completely and fixed in acetone at 4°C for 10 minutes. Slides to be stored for long periods of time must be kept at -70°C.

Staining by the direct method consists of two stages. In stage one, acetone-fixed cells are covered with FITC-conjugated viral immunoglobulin (conjugate) and then incubated in a moist chamber. In stage two, the excess conjugate is rinsed away and the slides are examined with a fluorescent microscope. The viral antigens will exhibit yellow-green fluorescence.

The indirect method of staining consists of three stages. In stage one, acetone-fixed cell preparations are incubated with unlabeled antiviral immunoglobulin. In stage two, the specimens are rinsed of excess immunoglobulin and again incubated, this time with FITC-labeled antispecies immunoglobulin, which will specifically detect the unlabeled antiviral immunoglobulin. In stage three, the excess conjugate is rinsed away and the slides are examined for the presence of the same yellow-green fluorescence. The indirect staining method has the advantage of requiring only one conjugate (FITC-labeled antispecies immunoglobulin) for detecting a number of antigen-antibody reactions.

Conjugates for both direct and indirect staining are titrated at dilutions of 1:5, 1:10, 1:20, and 1:40 in 0.01M phosphate-buffered saline to determine optimum working conditions. The optimal staining dilution of a conjugate is one that results in 3 to 4+ specific fluorescence of infected cells, no fluorescence in controls, no more than 1+ fluorescence with heterologous viruses, and no fluorescence in noninfected control cells.

Strict criteria must be used in interpreting FA results. Nuclear and/or cytoplasmic staining is seen with influenza viruses, rubeola virus, adenoviruses, CMV, VZV, and HSV; cytoplasmic staining alone occurs with RS, parainfluenza, vaccinia, rabies, rubella, and mumps viruses. False-positive fluorescence can be encountered with leukocytes, mucus, and yeasts; leukocytes have immunoglobulin Fc receptors that nonspecifically bind conjugates. False-negative tests can occur when viral antigens or antibodies are present in low titer. Virus laboratories should use conventional virus isolation and serologic tests to confirm FA test results until such time as technical proficiency has been achieved and the accuracy and reliability of FA testing adequately demonstrated.

Solid-Phase Immunoassays

Solid-phase immunoassay detects viral antigens or antibodies by using as an indicator either a radioactive label (radioimmunoassay—RIA) or the action of an enzyme attached to a substrate (enzyme-linked immunosorbent assay—ELISA). Although three different methods of antigen detection (competitive, direct, and indirect) are in use, the indirect method is currently the most popular. This method involves addition of the clinical specimen to a mixture containing a capture antibody attached to a solid phase. Unbound antigen is washed away, and an unlabeled detector antibody is added and unbound antibody washed away. Finally, a labeled antispecies indicator antibody is added that is measured visually or spectrophotometrically (ELISA) or in a radioactive counter (RIA). The indirect method is highly sensitive because of amplified binding, but it also suffers from nonspecific reactions owing to binding of nonspecific antibodies. Specimens most appropriate for detection of viral antigens by ELISA are serum, urine, sputum, and nasopharyngeal secretions.

Serum may be tested directly, but other specimens must be processed (e.g., dilution, centrifugation, clarification) prior to testing. The SPIA procedures have been developed for the detection of HAV and hepatitis type B virus (HBV), rotaviruses, adenoviruses, HSV, RSV, influenza A, CMV, and group A coxsackieviruses. Commercial kits (ELISA) are currently available for identification of HAV, HBV, HSV, and rotaviruses. The ELISA techniques appear to be supplanting RIA procedures as methods of choice for the rapid diagnosis of many viral diseases. The ELISA tests are stable and superior to RIA procedures in that no radioactive reagents or expensive isotope counters are required. Furthermore, with ELISA techniques, one can use the light or electron microscope and a permanent specimen record is available. Results can be either quantitative or qualitative. However, ELISA methods require multiple wash procedures and some substrates have been shown to be carcinogenic. In ad-

Table 5. Procedures for Collection and Transport of Specimens for Viral Studies

Specimen	Collection	Transport
Throat	Swab posterior pharynx	Swab in transport media*
Nasopharynx	Insert flexible wire swab into nasopharynx, rotate and remove	Swab in transport media*
Nasal wash	Tilt patient's head back (approx. 70°): insert rubber bulb syringe (1 oz tapered with 3–5 ml PBS) until nostril occluded); squeeze and aspirate	Sterile screw-capped container
Sputum	Deep cough specimen	Sterile screw-capped container
Fecal swab	Insert swab 3–5 cm into rectum	Swab in transport media*
Stool	Collect 4–6 gm of a fresh stool specimen	Sterile screw-capped container
Urine	Clean-voided first morning urine; 2–3 specimens on successive days	Sterile screw-capped container (10–20 ml)
Dermal /genital lesions	Aspirate vesicle fluid from fresh lesions; rupture vesicle, scrape surface (margins) to obtain fluid and cells from base of lesion	Tuberculin syringe with 26-gauge needle; swab in transport media;* clean glass slide in 95% ethanol (cytology)
Cerebrospinal fluid or other body fluids	Qualified personnel should collect fluid under sterile conditions	Sterile screw-capped container (1–2 ml)
Eye		
Conjunctiva	Press swab firmly against inflamed areas	Swab in transport media*
Corneal lesions	Corneal scrapings collected by qualified personnel	Extract in transport media (fluid)*
Tissue	Take specimen from area directly adjacent to affected tissue	Sterile screw-capped container with transport media (fluid)*
Blood		
Culture	Collect early during acute phase of illness†	Heparinized sterile tube (5 ml)
Serology	Two or more serum specimens at least 2 to 3 weeks apart	Sterile tube (5 ml)

*Transport media: modified Stuarts, modified Hanks, and Leibovitz-Emory; other commercially available viral transport media or systems.

†Attempts to isolate viruses from blood are usually fruitless because of the extremely brief period of viremia with most viral infections.

Abbreviations: PBS = Phosphate-buffered saline.

dition, many tissues have endogenous peroxidases (particularly red blood cells); therefore, steps to inactivate these endogenous enzymes must be incorporated in ELISA systems that utilize peroxidase.

Isolation/Identification of Viruses from Clinical Specimens

Virus isolation takes more time than rapid methods for viral diagnosis but offers some advantages. It is a more sensitive technique, since it provides for host system amplification of small amounts of virus in clinical specimens. A broad array of viral agents can be detected and concentrated in a preparation that is free of the background debris usually present in clinical specimens. Host systems for isolation/identification of viruses from clinical specimens include cell cultures, embryonated hens' eggs, and laboratory animals. Most diagnostic virology laboratories that perform virus isolation utilize cell lines; specimens requiring inoculation into hens' eggs or laboratory animals are usually sent to state or federal or other specialized virology laboratories. The relative efficacy of isolation of many common viral pathogens is shown in Table 8.

Cell Cultures

Cell lines are of three types: primary, diploid, and heteroploid. Primary cultures are those started from cells, tissues, or organs taken directly from the organism. When a cell culture is subcultured for the first time, it becomes a cell line. Primary cell lines (secondary cell cultures) have been subcultured only a few times and usually retain the appearance and virus sensitivity of the primary cell culture. Diploid cell lines are those in which at least 75 per cent of the cells have the same karyotype as the original species and the cells can survive for approximately 50 passages. In heteroploid cell lines, less than 75 per cent of the cells have the same karyotype as the original species; heteroploid lines that have demonstrated the potential to be subcultured indefinitely in vitro (at least 70 times) are termed *continuous* lines (also *established* or *immortal* lines).

The availability of cell cultures and media from commercial sources has made diagnostic virology fea-

Table 6. Basic Methods for Laboratory Diagnosis of Viral Infections

Direct examination of clinical materials for virus or viral antigens
Electron microscopy
Cytopathology
Fluorescent antibody techniques
Solid-phase immunoassays
Isolation/identification of viruses from clinical specimens
Cell culture systems
Embryonated hens' eggs
Animals
Serologic diagnosis (conventional methods)
Neutralization
Hemagglutination-inhibition
Complement fixation
Fluorescent antibody
Passive hemagglutination

sible for many clinical microbiology laboratories. Cell cultures are commonly used to isolate a wide variety of human viruses (Table 9). Primary monkey kidney (rhesus, or cynomolgus, occasionally African green) is often used for primary cell lines. These are versatile cells that support the growth of many myxoviruses, enteroviruses, and adenoviruses. Most monkey cell lines, however, are contaminated with simian viruses; this requires the addition of specific antisera to inactivate these agents. Diploid cell lines are usually of human origin. Many commercial varieties are available. Diploid cells are inexpensive and susceptible to a broad range of viruses including VZV, HSV, adenoviruses, and enteroviruses; diploid cell lines are best for isolation of CMV. Continuous or "established" cell lines are derived from malignant tumors (HEp-2, HeLa) and quite readily support the growth of adenoviruses and HSV; continuous lines are especially good for isolation of RSV.

Table 7. Cytopathology of Common Viral Infections

Cellular Change	Agents
Inclusions	
Intranuclear	Adenoviruses HSV VZV
Intracytoplasmic	Parainfluenza viruses RSV Rabies virus Vaccinia virus
Both	Rubeola virus CMV
None	Influenza viruses Mumps virus Rubella virus
Multinucleation ("giant" cells)	HSV VZV Rubeola virus RSV Parainfluenza viruses
Enlargement	CMV HSV Adenoviruses

Abbreviations: HSV = Herpes simplex virus; VZV = varicella zoster virus; RSV = respiratory syncytial virus; CMV = cytomegalovirus.

Table 8. Relative Efficacy of Isolation of Some Human Viral Pathogens

Viruses commonly and easily isolated by routine cell culture techniques
Adenoviruses
Group B coxsackieviruses
Echoviruses
HSV
Influenza viruses
Polioviruses
Vaccinia virus
Viruses more difficult to isolate by virtue of viral instability or requirement of special conditions
Measles virus
Mumps virus
Parainfluenzaviruses
Rhinoviruses
Rubella virus
Viruses best isolated in animal systems
Arboviruses
Group A coxsackieviruses (most)
Lymphocytic choriomeningitis virus
Rabies virus
Viruses isolated only by specialized laboratories
EBV
HAV
HBV
Rotavirus
Parvovirus and Norwalk-like agents

Abbreviations: HSV = Herpes simplex virus; EBV = Epstein-Barr virus; HAV = hepatitis type A virus; HBV = hepatitis type B virus.

Clinical specimens are processed and inoculated into one or more appropriate cell cultures and observed daily for 2 to 3 weeks for the presence of CPE. Most viruses produce a CPE in cell culture; moreover, the type of CPE (e.g., ballooning, grapelike clustering of cells, syncytia formation), the length of time required for CPE to develop, and the cell cultures in which the characteristic CPE occurs are all important elements in the tentative identification of the isolated virus. Most viruses will produce CPE in 5 to 6 days, and many show CPE in only 1 or 2 days. Herpes simplex virus produces CPE very rapidly; 50 per cent of isolates show CPE in 24 to 48 hours and 90 per cent show CPE by 3 to 4 days. Fluorescent antibody testing of cell culture fluids at 24 hours can be used as an adjunct to shorten the time required for virus isolation results. Viral antigen presence can often be demonstrated by FA in scattered, loose cells in the supernatant prior to appearance of CPE. Specific viral identification following isolation can be made using FA or ELISA methods or by viral neutralization with specific antisera.

Embryonated Hens' Eggs

Inoculation of hens' eggs is useful for isolation of certain viral and other infectious agents and for production of some vaccines. Influenza viruses grow well in the amnionic cavity of hens' eggs; amplification of viral titers is achieved because the embryo swallows

Table 9. Cell Cultures for Viral Isolation

Virus	Primary	Diploid	Heteroploid*
Adenoviruses		•	•
Group B coxsackieviruses	•	•	
Echoviruses	•	•	
Polioviruses	•	•	
Influenza viruses	•		
Parainfluenza viruses	•		
RSV			•
HSV		•	•
VZV		•	
CMV		•	
Rubeola virus	•		
Rubella virus	•	•	

*Lines with demonstrated potential to be subcultured indefinitely in vitro.

Abbreviations; RSV = Respiratory syncytial virus; HSV = herpes simplex virus; VZV = varicella zoster virus; CMV = cytomegalovirus.

and inhales the amnionic fluid, thereby increasing the number of infected cells. Yolk sac inoculation is also helpful in the isolation and identification of rickettsiae and chlamydia, which can cause infections closely mimicking those of many viral agents.

Laboratory Animals

Inoculation of laboratory animals has been employed for the identification of the arboviruses, group A coxsackieviruses, and rabies—agents that do not grow readily in cell lines or eggs.

Serologic Diagnosis

The basis for the serologic diagnosis of virus infection is the demonstration of seroconversion or a significant increase in circulating homologous viral antibody over the course of illness. Paired sera are obtained 14 or more days apart and tested in parallel. A fourfold or greater rise in the titer of homologous antibody is consistent with a recent infection. Unfortunately, the converse (a fourfold antibody decrease) cannot be viewed with the same significance as a fourfold rise.

Conventional Methods

Conventional serologic methods include neutralization, hemagglutination-inhibition (HI), complement fixation, and fluorescent antibody and passive hemagglutination tests. Neutralization tests are markedly specific and are utilized for identifying virus subtypes, antigenically different strains, and immunotypes. Neutralization tests are more sensitive than conventional in vitro tests for detecting antibody of long duration. However, neutralizing antibody appears early and persists, necessitating collection of serum early in the course of illness in order to demonstrate a significant rise in titer. Neutralization tests have several disadvantages, which include the need for expensive living host systems, the requirement of longer time (usually 7 to 10 days), and the fact that some viruses (HSV, arboviruses) are difficult to neutralize.

Hemagglutination-inhibition tests measure antibody directed against viruses that agglutinate red blood cells of certain species; the antibody binds to the hemagglutinin site on the virus and thus blocks the reaction. The advantages of HI testing include no requirement of living host systems and the rapid achievement of results (in hours) compared with neutralization tests. The HI tests are widely used in serodiagnosis and screening for previous rubella and influenza infection. These tests do have some disadvantages: Not all viruses hemagglutinate, nonspecific binding substances in sera may give false-positive results, test sensitivity is markedly dependent on viral antigen concentration, and some viruses cause hemagglutination only over a narrow range of pH.

The complement fixation (CF) test is widely used for serologic diagnosis, even though CF tests are less sensitive than neutralization and HI tests. The CF antibodies disappear rapidly, compared with HI and neutralizing antibody; therefore, CF tests are not recommended for determination of immune status of individuals or populations (serosurveys). Viral CF antibody (usually of IgG-specificity) appears later in the course of infection than neutralization or HI antibodies which appear early and are usually of IgM-specificity. Complement fixation testing often permits demonstration of a fourfold or greater rise in antibody titer, whereas neutralizing and HI antibodies often are stable in paired sera. However, CF tests are not good for the diagnosis of all viral infections because some viral agents fail to stimulate a CF antibody response following infection; also other groups of viruses (enteroviruses, rhinoviruses) commonly exhibit within-group heterotypic antibody responses that preclude demonstration of a significant antibody rise following infection.

For antibody detection by FA procedures, the somewhat more cumbersome indirect FA (IFA) method must be used. Therefore, IFA serology is usually reserved for occasions in which other sensitive and specific in vitro tests for antibody are not available (lymphocytic choriomeningitis virus [LCM] and EBV infection) or when other tests yield equivocal results. The sensitivity and specificity of IFA are equivalent to those of neutralization and HI antibody testing. False-positive results occur with some viruses (especially CMV) that induce formation of nonviral cytoplasmic IgG receptors, which bind conjugate in infected cells and produce nonspecific fluorescence.

Passive hemagglutination (PHA) testing is based on the fact that red blood cells "sensitized" with tannic acid, glutaraldehyde, or chromic chloride adsorb viral antigens onto their surfaces and can be used in PHA tests to demonstrate viral antibody in sera. In contrast to direct hemagglutination, agglutination in the PHA test is mediated by antibody. The PHA tests are not readily used, since concentrated and purified virus is essential to avoid competition from nonviral host proteins. Furthermore, antigen-coated red blood cells are unstable and must be prepared frequently. Passive hemagglutination testing is used to assay for antibody to viruses that do not hemagglutinate directly and for which neutralization tests are cumbersome or insensitive. The PHA tests are approximately a thousand times more sensitive than complement fixation tests for detecting antibody to the hepatitis B surface anti-

Table 10. Serologic Diagnosis of Viral Hepatitis

			Interpretation
Hepatitis A			
anti-HAV (IgM)	*anti-HAV**		
+	–		Acute (recent) infection (within previous 6 mos.)
–	+		Remote infection (6–12 mos. ago or longer)
Hepatitis B			
HBsAg	*anti-HBc*	*anti-HBs*	
+	+	–	Active infection (acute or chronic)†
–	+	–	Active infection (most likely acute)†,‡
–	+	+	Resolved recent infection (mos.–years)
–	–	+	Resolved remote infection (years)
Hepatitis NANB			
Persistently negative markers indicative of *acute* HAV or HBV infection in patient with clinical/laboratory evidence of acute viral hepatitis (must exclude drugs, toxins, alcohol, ischemia, CMV, EBV, etc.)			Presumptive acute NANB viral hepatitis

* Combined IgM and IgG specificity.
† Clinical correlation, clinical and laboratory follow-up are essential for specific diagnosis.
‡ The vast majority of chronic HBV infections are characterized by presence in serum of both HBsAg and anti-HBc.
Abbreviations: HAV = Hepatitis type A virus; anti-HAV = hepatitis A antibody; HBV = hepatitis type B virus; HBsAg = hepatitis B surface antigen; anti-HBc = hepatitis B core antibody; anti-HBs = hepatitis B surface antibody; NANB = non-A, non-B; CMV = cytomegalovirus; EBV = Epstein-Barr virus.

gen (anti-HBs) and are used primarily as a means of titering anti-HBs in individual sera and immunoglobulin pools.

General Considerations

As a general rule, 2 to 5 ml of serum should be obtained as early as possible on patients evaluated for a viral work-up. Then, if viral isolation or direct methods yield negative or equivocal results, a convalescent serum can be obtained and the paired sera examined for titers of antibody to the suspect viral agent(s). This approach falls short when infection is due to a viral agent belonging to a large group of closely related viruses, such as the echoviruses or adenoviruses, because of major heterotypic cross reactions among the subgroup antigens. In addition, false-positive or false-negative serologic results can occasionally occur. Specifically, false-positive CMV or HSV antibody increases may be observed in patients with other viral or mycoplasma infections (presumably due to "stress activation") and false-negative results are sometimes encountered with infections in infants (especially with respiratory viruses, CMV, and rubella) and immunocompromised patients.

Although paired sera are preferred for viral diagnosis, in certain circumstances single serum specimens can also be useful for this purpose. Single sera can be of value in demonstrating presence of viral antibody of IgM-specificity within the first few weeks after infection. This is particularly applicable for diagnosis of VZV, EBV, CMV, rubella virus, and coxasackievirus infections. Establishing the presence of IgM-specific antibody to HAV (anti-HAV[IgM]) is now the procedure of choice for diagnosis of this disease (Table 10). It must be borne in mind, however, that even IgM-specific antibody determinations are not always diagnostic. There may be an increase in IgM-specific antibodies with reactivation or reinfection; this is especially common with VZV, CMV, HSV, and EBV agents. Furthermore, high IgM titers may persist for prolonged periods (6 months or more) following CMV or rubella virus infections and heterotypic antibody responses have been observed during CMV and EBV infections. Moreover, false-positive tests for IgM antibody have been regularly encountered in patients whose serum also contains rheumatoid factor.

Immunoglobulin G specific antibody levels in single sera can be of value in determining the immune status of individuals at high risk for rubella, mumps, VZV, and other viral infections. When there is sufficient accumulated experience regarding the expected antibody responses during infection and the early convalescent period, the magnitude of an antibody titer may permit a presumptive diagnosis of a recent infection. Specifically, HI antibody titers of $\geq$ 1:160 to Western equine encephalitis (WEE) or St. Louis encephalitis (SLE) viruses and CF antibody titers of $\geq$1:128 to influenza B virus are distinctly unusual except in association with recent infection. Nevertheless, in the final analysis, it must be emphasized that individual antibody titers are subject to great variation and titers in single serum specimens must be interpreted with caution.

Serologic panels can be of value for viral diagnosis for situations in which the clinical syndrome is established (e.g., meningitis, encephalitis, pneumonia, exanthems) but any of several viral agents could be responsible for the infection. A central nervous system (CNS) panel would include testing paired sera with antigens specific for HSV, mumps virus, WEE.

SLE, and Eastern equine encephalitis (EEE), and California encephalitis viruses (and perhaps LCM and selected enteroviruses). A respiratory viral antigen panel might include influenza A and B; RSV; parainfluenza, 1, 2, and 3; adenoviruses (and perhaps mycoplasma and chlamydia). Similar panels could be prepared for other clinical syndromes of presumed viral etiology (see Table 11).

Special Considerations

Serologic diagnosis is less expensive than viral isolation, and currently a wide variety of reagents are available from numerous commercial sources. However, there are special considerations that apply to the serologic diagnosis of viral diseases. The first is that serology as a primary means of diagnosis requires paired sera collected at least 10 to 14 days apart, thereby making the diagnosis retrospective and usually of less clinical value.

Another consideration is that the type of antibody test to be employed must be tailored to the specific syndrome and viral agent(s) suspected. For example, too many serotypes exist among the enteroviruses (echoviruses and coxsackieviruses) to attempt specific serologic diagnosis initially; the only sensible approach is to first isolate and specifically identify the viral agent and then confirm the infection by demonstrating a significant antibody response. Then, for some viruses, particularly EBV and HBV, testing for antibodies directed against different antigenic components aids diagnostic specificity. During primary EBV infection, antibody (combined IgM and IgG specificity) to the viral capsid antigen (VCA) appears early; IgM-anti-VCA persists for a maximum of 2 to 3 months following infection, while anti-VCA (IgG) persists for life. Antibody to the Epstein-Barr nuclear antigen (EBNA) appears late (2 to 6 months after onset) and persists for life (Table 12). These EBV-specific serodiagnostic tests are required for Paul-Bunnell-Davidsohn heterophile-antibody-negative cases of infectious mononucleosis (IM) or IM-like illnesses to differentiate those caused by EBV from those due to infection with CMV, other viral agents, and *Toxoplasma gondii.*

Table 11. Serologic Panels for Viral Diagnosis

Syndrome	Suggested Composition of Viral Antigen Panel
Central nervous system	HSV 1 and 2 mumps virus WEE, EEE viruses SLE, CE viruses
Respiratory	Influenza A and B viruses RSV parainfluenza viruses adenoviruses
Exanthem-Enantham	rubeola virus rubella virus enteroviruses* HSV 1 and 2† VZV†
Myocarditis-pericarditis	Group B coxsackievirus, types 1–5 Influenza A and B viruses

*Best diagnosed by virus isolation.
†If rash is vesicular.
Abbreviations: HSV = Herpes simplex virus; WEE = Western equine encephalitis; EEE = Eastern equine encephalitis; SLE = St. Louis encephalitis; CE = California encephalitis; RSV = respiratory syncytial virus; VZV = varicella zoster virus.

Table 12. Serodiagnosis of Epstein-Barr Virus Infection

Antibody	Recent Infection	Remote Infection
anti-VCA* IgM	+	–
IgG	+	+
anti-EA†	+	–
anti-EBNA‡	–	+

*VCA = Viral capsid antigen; anti-VCA (IgM) persists for 2–3 months after infection, anti-VCA (IgG) persists for life.
†EA = Early antigen; anti-EA persists for 3–4 months after infection.
‡EBNA = Epstein-Barr nuclear antigen; anti-EBNA appears approximately 6 months after infection and persists for life.

Infection with HBV can be classified as acute (recent), chronic (active), or remote (recovery) by employing a combination of tests for the presence of HBsAg, anti-HBc and anti-HBs (Table 10). The diagnosis of non-A, non-B viral hepatitis infection can be inferred by combining tests for HAV and HBV and excluding the presence of serologic markers of acute infection with these agents (Table 10).

Finally, serologic diagnosis is useful for situations in which viral isolation is difficult to achieve because of a very abbreviated period of viral excretion (e.g., infection with the arboviruses and some respiratory viruses).

INFLUENZA

By Celia J. Emery, B.Sc., Ph.D.
and Peter Howard, D.M. (Oxon), F.R.C.P.
Sheffield, England

Influenza is an acute pyrexial illness that affects mainly the bronchial tree with systemic manifestations. There are three types of viruses: A, B, and C. Types A and B are indistinguishable clinically. The C types are frequently found but rarely cause respiratory symptoms or other illness.

STRUCTURE OF THE VIRUS

The virus has a type-specific genome, made of ribonucleic acid (RNA), which is covered with a protein envelope. Polypeptide surface antigens project through the envelope. A soluble S antigen is common to all A types, and a different S antigen is characteristic of all B types. The two most important surface antigens are undoubtedly the hemagglutinin and the neuraminidase. These are called H and N, respectively. They describe the antigenic characteristics of the virus, but in contrast to most other types of virus they are subject to change. This characteristic confers a remarkable infectivity. Previous population immunity becomes obsolete, giving rise to quite extraordinary worldwide illness before immunity is reestablished. A small change in surface antigens is defined as a *drift,* a major change as a *shift.* Shifts in Type A viruses have been responsible for pandemics typified by the 1918/1919 Spanish flu and the 1957 Asian flu. Changes in Type B viruses are slower, and the infectivity of the virus is rather less. This gives the host immunity a better chance of establishing itself.

In the past 50 years, epidemiologic studies have described pandemics occurring approximately every 11 years or so. All have proved to be due to Type A viruses. Since 1933 the two main antigens, hemagglutinin and neuraminidase, have been numbered. Hence the 1933 epidemic has been labeled H_0N_1, the 1947 epidemic, H_1N_1. This gave way to H_2N_2 in 1957, leading to H_3N_2 in 1968. There has not been a major pandemic throughout the world for some years. Virologists are awaiting with some trepidation the next major shift. The importance of immunity was demonstrated in the 1977 epidemic, which was curiously due to the re-emergence of H_1N_1 virus seen during the years 1947 to 1956. Persons who had contracted the disease earlier were immune during its later resurgence. This was an important clinical observation, since it demonstrates that if an effective vaccine could be found, long-lasting immunity may be effective in controlling disease. Pandemics are characterized by attack rates of 25 to 50 per cent and by high morbidity. Mortality certified as due to influenza rises sharply; at the same time, there is an increased mortality in the elderly or in those chronically ill with chest or heart disease from complications. Lesser epidemics at more frequent intervals have been associated with drift of surface antigens, Type B viruses, or both.

CLINICAL FEATURES

Typical influenza begins with fever, headache, and muscle pains. The incubation period is short, from 1 to 5 days, and the onset of clinical symptoms abrupt. Fever is associated after a few hours with progressive prostration, anorexia, and severe weakness. Shivering is common but only at the onset. The respiratory symptoms commence with sore throat, stuffy or runny nose, hoarseness of the voice, and after 1 to 2 days substernal soreness. Coincident with the substernal soreness an irritating nonproductive cough appears. The voice may be lost temporarily.

On examination the patient looks flushed and later perspiring; the eyelids are swollen, and the conjunctivae are injected. Mucous membranes of the throat and nasal passages are injected, and there is a watery discharge from the nose. There is usually a tachycardia, but blood pressure is normally maintained. Moist sounds may be heard at the bases of both lungs, and there may be rhonchi. Tenderness of muscles to pressure is often a feature. Meningism is sometimes detected, but there are usually no other specific neurologic signs.

This description pertains to a major illness lasting up to 10 days, but most attacks are less severe, particularly when influenza B is the organism. All degrees of severity have been recorded. In mild cases, slight fever lasting 24 hours or less and transient upper respiratory tract symptoms are the only manifestation, in which case influenza is not suspected and the diagnosis is confused with other common cold viruses. Even in major epidemics, the severity of symptoms may vary among members of the same family.

In mild cases, in adults or children, the illness may be over in 3 to 4 days. In the more severe cases, fever and prostration may last 1 to 2 weeks, to be followed by a period of several weeks' return to normal health. During this latter period, an irritating cough (occasionally productive of white or mucopurulent sputum), fatigue, and mental depression are common.

COMPLICATIONS

In the normally healthy person, influenza is rarely fatal. Respiratory complications, however, are of great importance to the elderly, the debilitated, and those with chronic obstructive airway disease. The virus causes an intense inflammation of bronchial and tracheal mucosa with denudation, leaving the submucosa exposed and bleeding. The most common complications are therefore laryngitis, tracheitis, bronchitis and bronchiolitis, and pneumonia. Secondary invading organisms are the principal cause of these complications. All the usual pathogens may be involved, such as Pneumococcus (*Streptococcus pneumoniae*) and *Haemophilus influenzae,* but the most important and the rarest is *Staphylococcus aureus.* The complications with these organisms occur in high-risk patients after either Type A or B infections, giving rise to a secondary swinging fever and radiologic signs of pneumonia, lung abscess, or empyema. Great care must be exercised in protecting these patients by prompt recognition and treatment of complications with appropriate antibiotics.

Other complications, such as myocarditis, encephalitis, or psychotic episodes, are uncommon.

DIAGNOSIS

The specific diagnosis of influenzal infections is technically complicated and can be only summarized here. Isolation and identification of the virus by growth in various culture media and serologic confirmation of infection by rising titers of antibodies are the two major tests used.

To isolate the virus, nasal washings or throat swabs are taken and the material is inoculated into monkey kidney tissue culture or amniotic fluid of fertilized chicken eggs. The samples usually have to be mixed with antibiotics in the culture media to avoid contamination with bacteria. Once harvested, the virus is identified by hemagglutination of fowl erythrocytes. A complement fixation test for the S soluble antigen will differentiate between A and B types but not between the different A subtypes. The A influenza surface antigens are typed using specific antisera.

The second method detects a rise of antibodies in convalescent serum to the hemagglutinin and neuraminidase surface antigens using the hemagglutinin/neuraminidase inhibition (HI, NI) tests. A fourfold rise of antibodies from the first day of illness over a period of 3 weeks is considered diagnostic. The tests are lengthy to perform because inhibitors in serum have to be removed. Two new somewhat simpler tests are under evaluation. The serial radial diffusion technique tests for both hemagglutinin and neuraminidase antigens, and the serial radial hemolysis procedure tests for the hemagglutinin antigen. Correlations between these two new tests and the standard methods of measuring antibodies are still required. Serial radial hemolysis, which takes only 24 hours, correlates well with the HI test and looks promising. Because of the high morbidity and mortality from complications in susceptible groups, a quick, easy diagnostic test for influenza that will distinguish it from a multitude of other virus infections is needed.

ANTIVIRAL AGENTS

Few specific antiviral agents are active against the influenza viruses. Amantadine and rimantadine have proved to be of only mild potency.

Studies on a possible interferon effective against influenza virus have so far proved disappointing, but better preparations are expected to be tested shortly. Thus the treatment of influenza remains largely symptomatic with appropriate antibiotics for the various infective complications.

IMMUNIZATION

There are two major types of vaccine, *killed* and *attenuated live.*

Killed vaccines are usually polyvalent, containing formaldehyde-treated virus embodying the same strains as those of the most recent epidemics. Resulting immunity lasts from 1 to 2 years but is less effective in the second year. Drifting of the antigens reduces the protection, which is best against homologous virus.

The second type of vaccine uses a live attenuated virus. An active virus with required antigens is mixed with a previously attenuated virus, and the two inoculated together produce progeny that show less virulence but that are still capable of infecting to induce a useful antibody response. Live attenuated vaccine is inoculated nasally, and by so doing, it is hoped to confer mucosal membrane immunity at the site of virus entrance as well as a systemic antibody response. A great deal of work has gone into live attenuated vaccines in recent years. Despite this, it is fair to say at the present time that a wholly satisfactory live attenuated vaccine has not been produced. As the virulence falls, the immunity conferred also falls.

THE FUTURE

Influenza remains one of the few pandemic viruses without effective control. Killed vaccines are recommended, but on account of the shift and drift of the surface antigens an effective vaccine is rarely available against new pandemic viruses. Attenuated live vaccines, which offer theoretical advantages of less reactogenicity but good immunity, have not yet proved satisfactory.

There are risks of epidemic spread unless genetic stability of the viruses can be assured. Work has started to produce a specific vaccine using gene-engineered bacteria in attempts to induce stability. There is always the risk of a virulent virus re-emerging and causing serious pandemics of the sort witnessed in 1957 and 1968. At present there is an uneasy truce between current viruses and the community.

INFECTIOUS MONONUCLEOSIS

By John H. Dirckx, M.D.
Dayton, Ohio

Infectious mononucleosis (IM) is an acute communicable disease caused by the Epstein-Barr virus (EBV) and characterized by fever, lymph node enlargement, lymphocytosis, and a distinctive antibody response. The disease occurs most commonly between the ages of 15 and 25. Transmission is usually salivary, by direct oral contact or sharing of food or eating utensils; rarely is it acquired by transfusion of blood or fresh plasma. The incubation period is 30 to 50 days. Spontaneous recovery after 3 to 4 weeks is the rule, with lifelong immunity to further attacks. Live virus may continue to be shed in the saliva for months or years after recovery.

CLINICAL FEATURES

Symptoms. Onset may be abrupt or insidious. In virtually all cases there is some fever, accompanied by enlargement of lymph nodes of which the patient may be unaware. The presenting and most conspicuous symptom is usually severe pharyngitis, but throat symptoms are absent in 10 to 20 per cent of patients. Most patients complain of both weakness (lack of energy) and lethargy (an urge to sleep 12 to more hours a day).

Chills, headache, myalgia, anorexia, and nocturnal restlessness may occur as in any febrile illness. Gastrointestinal and respiratory symptoms are not usual. About half of patients have painless edema of the eyelids. Less than 10 per cent have jaundice, and less than 5 per cent have morbilliform or urticarial rashes. Ampicillin will induce a maculopapular trunk rash, after a latent period of 5 to 10 days, in almost anyone who takes it during the acute phase of IM. Some patients notice a sense of fullness in the left upper quadrant of the abdomen, especially after eating, because of splenomegaly. Severe abdominal pain is uncommon and suggests splenic rupture.

Physical Findings. Erythema and edema of the pharynx may be extreme. Most patients with pharyngitis have a shaggy, ivory to greenish-gray exudate over the tonsils. In about half, a sprinkling of fine red petechiae can be seen around the junction of the hard and soft palate. Any lymph nodes may be swollen, but those of the posterior cervical chains are usually most prominent. The nodes of IM are large, firm, discrete, and nontender. Tender anterior cervical nodes are a nonspecific finding in pharyngitis.

The spleen is enlarged and somewhat tender in a third to half of patients. Repeated or vigorous palpation of the spleen is unwise because it may cause rupture. Hepatomegaly is not commonly seen even in the presence of jaundice, but the liver may be tender to fist percussion.

Course. Fever and sore throat usually reach their peak by the second week. Spontaneous recovery by the third or fourth week is usual. Lingering weakness and lethargy are seldom seen in patients who have not been subjected to prolonged bed rest. In children the clinical picture is often very mild. In older adults, lymph node enlargement may be less conspicuous but the febrile period tends to be longer (3 to 4 weeks).

Complications, which are rare, include airway obstruction (which is due to pharyngeal edema), tonsillar hemorrhage, rupture of the spleen after minor trauma, hemolytic anemia, thrombocytopenia, severe hepatic dysfunction, and various neurologic disturbances, including Guillain-Barré syndrome.

LABORATORY STUDIES

Hematology. The hematologic changes of IM usually appear during the first week of illness, are well established by the second or third week, and seldom last more than 6 weeks. The hallmark of IM is the appearance in the peripheral blood of many atypical lymphocytes, or Downey cells—large mononuclear cells with irregularly staining cytoplasm and bizarre, highly variable nuclei. Atypical lymphocytes are T lymphocytes mobilized against B lymphocytes infected with EBV.

Lymphocytosis is both relative (50 per cent mononuclear cells in a blood film) and absolute (4500 lymphocytes per cu mm). In addition, at least 10 per cent of white blood cells (WBC) are atypical lymphocytes. The total WBC count is usually between 10,000 and 20,000 per cu mm but may remain in the normal range even when lymphocytosis is fully developed.

Serology. Infectious mononucleosis elicits formation of two unrelated types of antibody. The heterophile antibody, which appears during the acute phase in about 90 per cent of patients, was for several decades an essential diagnostic criterion for the disease. Although indirect immunofluorescence studies for specific viral antibodies now provide more accurate identification of EBV infection and are indispensable in research, heterophile antibody remains the most widely used serologic indicator of IM.

Heterophile antibodies are IgM globulins that agglutinate sheep red blood cells (RBC), as demonstrated by the Paul-Bunnell test. In the Davidsohn modification of this test, heterophile antibodies other than those of IM are removed from the serum by absorption with guinea pig kidney. After such absorption, a heterophile titer of 1:56 is presumptive, but not certain, evidence of IM.

Heterophile antibody appears during the first week of illness in about 70 per cent of patients and by the third week in 85 to 90 per cent. Seldom can this antibody be detected more than 3 months after recovery. A false-positive heterophile has been reported in rheumatoid arthritis, Hodgkin's disease, and tularemia. It is also believed to occur at times as an anamnestic response to fever, months or years after recovery from IM. The heterophile remains negative in 5 to 10 per cent of patients. Children are somewhat less likely than adolescents and adults to form heterophile antibody in IM.

Qualitative slide tests have largely supplanted the heterophile titer in clinical practice because of the ease and rapidity with which they can be done. Since these tests use horse RBC instead of, or along with, sheep RBC and may not include a guinea pig kidney absorption step, they respond to a different spectrum of heterophile antibodies. They are nonetheless highly reliable. False-positive slide tests have been reported in hepatitis, rubella, cytomegalovirus (CMV) and adenovirus infection, leukemia, and pancreatic carcinoma. Heterophile antibody as detected by agglutination of horse RBC may persist for as long as 18 months after recovery from IM.

Antibodies to components of the EBV are formed in every case of IM. Tests for these antibodies are more specific than the heterophile titer or slide tests, but they are more expensive and their availability is still limited. Early in the course of IM—indeed, usually before the onset of symptoms—an IgM antibody to the viral capsid antigen (VCA) appears in the serum. It rises rapidly, reaches peak levels by the second week of illness, and disappears after about 6 months. This is a highly specific indicator of recent or active IM, but unless serum is taken very early in the acute phase, it is nearly impossible to demonstrate a fourfold rise in anti-VCA.

IgG antibodies to VCA are also formed. About 90 per cent of patients show these antibodies during the first week of illness, and all show them by the third week. Since IgG antibody to VCA persists throughout life, its detection does not prove recent or active IM. It does, however, indicate either present or past infection and immunity to future attacks.

Antibody to EBV nuclear antigen appears 3 to 4 weeks after onset of illness and persists throughout life. Its absence, coupled with presence of antibodies to VCA, indicates active infection with EBV. Testing for antinuclear antibody is not widely available.

Other Diagnostic Studies. Tests of liver function are typically abnormal. The bilirubin may exceed 6 mg/dl, and liver enzymes, particularly alkaline phosphatase, may rise to very high levels for a few days. Significant or permanent impairment of liver function is, however, quite rare. Hemolytic anemia or thrombocytopenia may be detected, but these are seldom of clinical significance. About one third of patients with IM have false-positive complement fixation tests for antibody to CMV. False-positive serologic tests for syphilis and anergy to tuberculin have also been reported. Throat cultures have detected beta-hemolytic streptococci in one third of patients in some series, but in my experience the incidence of streptococcal infection is much lower. Electrocardiographic changes compatible with myocarditis are frequently seen but are probably not significant. A chest x-ray may show large hilar nodes.

CRITERIA FOR DIAGNOSIS

Infectious mononucleosis has an undeserved reputation as a protean disease because its initial presentations vary, the clinical picture sometimes evolving slowly over a period of days. When IM is accurately defined, virtually all cases will be found to fit the pattern. Because no one sign is pathognomonic, three independent diagnostic indicators are needed for a firm diagnosis:

1. *Clinical*: Fever and posterior cervical lymph node enlargement.
2. *Hematologic*: 4500 lymphocytes/cu mm, and 10 per cent atypical lymphocytes.
3. *Serologic*: Positive slide test for IM, *or* heterophile titer of 1:56 or greater after guinea pig kidney absorption, *or* rising titer of anti-VCA, *or* positive anti-VCA with negative antinuclear antibody.

A WBC and differential and a slide test for IM should be obtained in all patients suspected of having the disease. If laboratory tests are negative or inconclusive during the first week of illness, they should be repeated in 4 to 7 days. A tube of serum drawn at the first visit should be stored in case specific antibody studies are needed later.

If lymphocytosis has not appeared by the third week of illness, the diagnosis of IM can be excluded. When hematologic criteria are met but the slide test remains negative, a heterophile titer should be done. If this is also negative, the patient with a typical clinical picture can be regarded as having heterophile-negative IM.

If doubt persists as to the diagnosis—especially if leukemia, lymphoma, or a severe form of hepatitis is under consideration—specific antibody studies should be done for EBV, CMV, and toxoplasmosis. Certainly these studies should precede lymph node biopsy or marrow aspiration.

DIFFERENTIAL DIAGNOSIS

Since specific therapy for IM is not available and the disease nearly always resolves without complications or sequelae, establishing a firm diagnosis of IM may be less important than ruling out more serious diseases. Many acute viral infections cause fever and lymphadenitis, but IM alone causes both atypical lymphocytosis of more than 10 per cent and a positive heterophile agglutination or IM slide test. The enlarged nodes of rubella are entirely different from those of IM: smaller, fewer in number, tender, and located at or above the hairline posteriorly.

Severe pharyngitis may suggest streptococcal infection, Vincent's angina, or diphtheria. Jaundice and abnormal liver function tests are common to a wide range of hepatic diseases. Eyelid edema is seen in trichinosis and nephritis. In each case, appropriate laboratory tests should supply differentiating clues.

Atypical lymphocytes may be seen in other viral infections (rubella, measles, hepatitis A and B, herpes simplex), in Hodgkin's disease, in sarcoidosis, and occasionally in normal persons. In these conditions, the atypical lymphocytes rarely exceed 10 per cent of all WBC and they tend to be smaller and more constant in morphology than those of IM. Atypical lymphocytes may exceed 10 per cent in CMV infection and toxoplasmosis. Both of these diseases also cause fever, splenomegaly, and disturbances of liver function, but pharyngitis is not common in either and tests for heterophile and EBV antibodies are negative. It should be remembered that one third of patients with IM have positive serologic tests for CMV and that false-positive slide tests for IM have been reported in CMV.

RUBELLA

By Newton G. Osborne, M.D., Ph.D.
and John F. J. Clark, M.D.
Washington, D.C.

SYNONYMS

German measles, 3-day measles, red measles, rubeola notha, röteln, rosalia idiopathica.

DEFINITION

Rubella is a disease caused by a member of the alphavirus group of the Togaviridae. The virus spreads by aerosol dissemination, enters the upper respiratory tract, and multiplies there. From the nasopharynx and the oropharynx, it disseminates to the cervical, suboccipital, and postauricular lymph nodes and gains entrance to the bloodstream. Infection with rubella virus may cause an acute illness, the severity of which is greatly influenced by age. If acquired antenatally, rubella may have severe effects on organogenesis and somatic development.

PRESENTING SIGNS AND SYMPTOMS

Rubella is a disease that may be acquired postnatally or antenatally. When acquired postnatally, the site of implantation is the mucosa of the upper respiratory tract. Primary multiplication occurs in the respiratory epithelium and local lymph nodes, to be followed by viremia and virus shedding from the throat. In children, malaise and fever are usually mild or absent. A rash may be the first sign of the disease.

A prodrome is seen primarily in adolescents and adults and consists of malaise, myalgia, headache, and tender, swollen suboccipital, postauricular, and posterior cervical lymph nodes, which often precede the rash by up to a week. The nodal enlargement may persist for 2 weeks following the rash. The rash begins as small pink macules appearing over the face and behind the ears and spreading to the neck, trunk, and extremities. The individual areas are elevated, giving the skin a sandpaper texture. Some patients may exhibit discrete macular areas on the soft palate.

The course of uncomplicated rubella is short, with the rash vanishing usually by the third day and the patient feeling well by then.

When rubella occurs during pregnancy, the fetus may escape infection completely, it may be infected subclinically with no apparent pathologic consequences, or there may be damage to single or multiple organs and tissues. Transmission to the fetus can occur whether or not the maternal infection is symptomatic. Intrauterine infection occurs in the course of maternal viremia. Once the fetus becomes infected, the virus persists in the fetal tissues throughout gestation and into postnatal life. Viral replication in fetal tissues interferes with cellular multiplication and retards organogenesis. Spontaneous abortion or gross structural defects may result. The degree of fetal damage is related to the gestational age at the initial time of infection. Teratogenesis occurs when infection involves the conceptus prior to the 60th day after nidation. The most serious fetal effects are observed when maternal infection is acquired during the first month of pregnancy. The incidence of congenital anomalies declines sharply after the first trimester, and the defects are less pronounced when the infection is acquired after 16 weeks of gestation. Rubella acquired during the second half of pregnancy may still produce active postnatal disease, including pneumonitis and encephalitis. Fetal damage may be so subtle that mental retardation, deafness, and vestibular dysfunction may not be detected before the child enters school.

The spectrum of abnormalities that can occur with the congenital rubella syndrome is wide (Table 1). The most common abnormalities are cataracts, cardiac anomalies, and deafness. Approximately 20 per cent of infants born to mothers infected during the first 3 months of gestation will have signs of congenital rubella. However, infants with minimal or no apparent involvement at birth may subsequently develop signs of congenital disease that most commonly involve auditory, ocular, and central nervous system anomalies.

Rubella infection during the first 8 weeks of pregnancy produces cardiac defects, cataracts, and glaucoma in the offspring. Hearing loss can occur with infection up to 16 weeks. Although multiple handicaps can occur in children afflicted with intrauterine rubella, the problems most commonly reported are auditory and visual impairment, congenital heart disease, small stature, and a variety of less common afflictions such as cerebral palsy and diabetes mellitus.

Table 1. Abnormalities Associated with Congenital Rubella

Common abnormalities	Less frequent abnormalities *(continued)*
Cataracts	Meningoencephalitis
Growth retardation	Micrognathia
Deafness	Microphthalmia
Cardiovascular lesions	Jaundice
Hepatosplenomegaly	
Less frequent abnormalities	**Rare abnormalities**
Thrombocytopenic purpura	Microcephaly
	Brain calcification
Interstitial pneumonitis	Glaucoma
Central nervous system defects	Hepatitis
	Immune defects
Psychomotor retardation	Diabetes

COURSE

Rubella is a disease of short duration when acquired postnatally. Virus is shed from the pharynx of infected persons from approximately 7 days before to 5 days after onset of the rash. Droplet dissemination is maximum at the time of the rash. The rash may last 2 to 4 days. Systemic symptoms can occur in the absence of a rash. The patient may also be totally asymptomatic.

COMPLICATIONS

Complications associated with rubella are not common. The most frequent is arthralgia, chiefly in young women, and even less commonly, arthritis. Joint symptoms are usually self-limited and clear spontaneously within a week, but in severe cases they may persist for several weeks. Myalgia, tenosynovitis, and peripheral neuritis may accompany arthritis. Thrombocytopenic purpura, gingivitis, and encephalitis have been described, but they are extremely rare. Recovery from these conditions is usually complete. Progressive rubella panencephalitis has been reported to be associated with dementia, which can occur years after the disease.

PHYSICAL EXAMINATION

The presence of a fine, discrete, red rash that started as small macules over the face and behind the ears and spread to the neck, trunk, and extremities is characteristic. The presence of postauricular and posterior cervical nodes is probably the most common feature. Thus, the history of a prodrome with the presence of a characteristic rash of 2 to 3 days' duration and the presence of swollen suboccipital, postauricular and/or posterior cervical nodes are presumptive signs of rubella but are not definitively diagnostic.

LABORATORY PROCEDURES

The definitive diagnosis of rubella is confirmed by the laboratory. It is possible to identify individuals with an active infection, susceptible individuals, immune individuals, and individuals who have had a recent infection. All of these categories are of epidemiologic importance. The hemagglutination inhibition (HAI) test is the most useful. The rubella virus agglutinates the erythrocytes of various animals, and the HAI test depends on the ability of the rubella antibody to prevent this agglutination. Immune persons have antibody titers ranging from 1:16 to 1:512.

A high titer does not necessarily indicate a recent infection. Roughly 6 per cent of immune individuals will have an antibody titer of 1:512. The HAI test does not identify individuals whose titers have markedly decreased although they had been previously infected or vaccinated. Nonspecific lipoprotein inhibitors can produce an apparent titer of 1:8.

A pregnant woman exposed to rubella should be tested for immunity within 7 days of exposure. Any antibody present in the maternal serum is indicative of immunity at this time. Since antibody first appears at the time of rash, the susceptible patient should be scheduled to return 5 days after the presumed incubation period (or 14 to 21 days after the first visit).

The original serum sample obtained during the first visit should be divided into two equal units and labeled. One sample is submitted for serologic testing, and the second sample is frozen to be submitted for paired testing when the second sample is collected at the second visit. Because of the variability of rubella titer, a valid serologic diagnosis requires an eightfold increase in titer between the pre- and postconvalescent specimens, titered in duplicate and under identical test circumstances. Pregnant women suspected of having rubella should be scheduled to be seen at the gynecology clinic, never at the obstetrical clinic. If the repeat titer is negative, the pregnant patient should be monitored through the 14th week of gestation, when fetal organogenesis is complete.

The demonstration of IgM-specific antibody indicates a recent primary infection. The HAI antibody titers of 1:32 or less are not likely to represent a recent infection. If the titer is greater than 1:128, it is prudent to obtain a sample for determination of the presence of IgM (rubella within 3 to 7 weeks) and for complement fixing (CF) antibodies specific for rubella (infection within the last 4 to 6 months). IgG and IgA antibodies can be detected subsequent to IgM.

Virus isolation by tissue culture techniques is possible, but the procedure is too lengthy and complicated to be useful in pregnancy when rapid diagnosis is essential.

The probability of overt congenital rubella is greater than 50 per cent when maternal infection occurs during the first month. It is about 25 per cent in the second month, 10 per cent in the third month, and 1 to 2 per cent in the fourth month. The demonstration of an elevated cord IgM level by radial immunodiffusion is evidence of intrauterine infection, even if no clinical signs of congenital rubella are evident at birth. Cord HAI or IgG may represent passive maternal antibody transfer. Isolation of the virus in the immediate neonatal period is definitive evidence of intrauterine involvement. The virus may be isolated from the throat, urine, or spinal fluid of the child. Viral replication persists in spite of humoral antibody production during intrauterine life and may continue in the postnatal period.

A latex agglutination cord assay kit called the Rubascan has been developed. It can be performed at room temperature, and the results are read in 10 minutes. The Rubascan is sensitive and accurate. It compares favorably with HAI and enzyme-linked immunosorbent assay (ELISA) tests, but it cannot be used for detection of rubella-specific IgM antibody.

PITFALLS IN DIAGNOSIS

Extreme care must be exercised in the interpretation of antibody levels. If there is incomplete removal of nonspecific inhibitors of hemagglutination or incomplete absorption of agglutinins from sera, erroneous HAI titers may be reported. This is the reason for running paired sera titered in at least duplicate under identical laboratory circumstances. The HAI test requires the removal of nonspecific lipoprotein inhibitors that may mask the detection of rubella antibody. For the serologic diagnosis of rubella, an eightfold rise in titer must be established between two specimens run simultaneously and in duplicate under identical circumstances.

The absence of overt stigmata at birth does not exclude the possibility of congenital disease. A small percentage of infected infants may appear to be normal by all gross parameters and develop ultimately clinical signs such as retinopathy, deafness, microcephaly, or motor retardation, which bare the underlying diagnosis. The absence of cord IgM does not rule out the diagnosis. The titers of mother and infant IgG may be similar as a result of the presence of passively transferred maternal IgG. In this case, serum from both mother and infant should be tested again after 3 to 6 months. The mother's titer will be essentially unchanged, but the infant's titer should have declined unless there is rubella infection, in which case it will have remained elevated or even increased. An exception occurs when there are abnormalities in the infant's humoral immunity, which happens rarely in congenital rubella, but such children usually have other stigmata of rubella.

RUBELLA IMMUNIZATION

Since January 1979, the RA 27/3 strain of live rubella vaccine has been used in the United States. This vaccine is highly immunogenic and is the only one infective by the intranasal route. A reinfection rate, usually inapparent, may occur in 9 per cent of vaccinated individuals. The importance of reinfection depends on whether it is associated with viremia and therefore a hazard to the fetus if it occurs in a pregnant woman. The RA 27/3 vaccine may induce transient arthralgia or arthritis, especially in adults but rarely in children.

The small amounts of vaccine-virus shed from the pharynx of vaccinees has not proved to be communicable. Thus, susceptible children whose mothers are pregnant should be immunized to prevent infection with the wild virus in the children. Although there are no reports of congenital rubella as a result of inadvertent immunization of susceptible pregnant women, pregnancy is still an absolute contraindication to vaccination with rubella virus vaccine. Immunization during the postpartum period is not a contraindication for breast-feeding.

Women who have no detectable rubella antibody are susceptible. In a small percentage (less than 10 per cent) of naturally immune women who had rubella during childhood, low levels of antibody may go undetected. These immune women usually fail to respond to inoculation of live attenuated rubella vaccine. After the second inoculation, such women may be considered immune. There is no need to repeat the immunization.

MEASLES
(Rubeola)

By C. U. Kyong, M.D.
Charleston, South Carolina

SYNONYMS

Rubeola, red measles.

DEFINITION

Measles is an acute, highly contagious, generalized viral infection caused by paramyxovirus, characterized by fever, coryza, conjunctivitis, cough, and a specific exanthem (Koplik's spots), followed by a confluent maculopapular (morbilliform) rash. The rash begins on the face and neck and spreads downward to involve the entire body. The illness reaches its climax between the second and third day of eruption followed by rapid subsidence of fever, coryza, and conjunctivitis. The incubation period is 8 to 12 days. Measles is a self-limited disease. Treatment is mainly supportive.

PRESENTING SIGNS AND SYMPTOMS

Fever. The temperature generally climbs in a stepwise pattern until the fifth or sixth day of illness. Occasionally, the temperature curve may be biphasic. At times, the temperature may reach its peak by the end of the first day and remain elevated for the remaining prodromal and early rash period. In uncomplicated measles, the temperature falls rapidly between the second and third day after onset of the rash.

Coryza. The coryza of measles is indistinguishable from that of a severe common cold. It clears rapidly after the patient becomes afebrile.

Conjunctivitis. Conjunctival injection may occur in the early prodromal period. Subsequently, extensive conjunctival inflammation, an increase in lacrimation, and photophobia develop. The conjunctivitis disappears shortly after the fever subsides.

Cough. The cough is caused by the inflammatory reaction in the respiratory tract. Five to 10 days after the rash has covered the body, the cough subsides.

Koplik's Spots. Such spots are pathognomonic and occur 2 days prior to appearance of the rash. These lesions were described by Koplik in 1896 as "small irregular spots of bright red color, in the center of each red spot is seen a minute bluish-white speck." There may at first be only two, three, or six such spots on the buccal mucosa. These lesions can be so small and delicately colored that only a strong direct light source will bring out the characteristic red halo and bluish-white center.

Rash. The rash begins as an erythematous maculopapular eruption and generally develops 3 to 4 days after the onset of illness. It appears first on the face and neck and then progresses caudally. The rash tends to be confluent and begins to fade by the third day. Areas first to develop a rash will be the first to undergo fading.

Other Manifestations. Generalized lymphadenopathy is noted in moderate to severe illness. Anorexia and malaise are usually present in the febrile period. In infants, diarrhea may occur.

FORMS OF MEASLES

Hemorrhagic Measles (Black Measles)

This rare, severe, often fatal type of measles may occur in immunocompromised hosts. The illness begins with high fever, followed by convulsions, delirium, respiratory distress, and extensive confluent hemorrhagic eruption. Disseminated intravascular coagulation may be severe and uncontrollable.

Modified Measles

"Modified measles" is defined as measles virus infection made milder by the presence of antibodies. This type of measles commonly develops in children who have been passively immunized with immune serum globulin after exposure to the disease or in infants whose transplacental passive immunity has only partially waned. The prodromal period is short (1 or 2 days). The patient may have either no fever or a low-grade one. The coryza, cough, and conjunctivitis are minimal. Koplik's spots may not be present. The rash is generally mild and sparse.

Atypical Measles

"Atypical measles" refers to an unusual clinical pattern of measles virus infection that occurs predominantly in adolescents and young adults who have previously received inactivated measles vaccine. The illness is characterized by 2 to 3 days' prodrome of high fever, cough, headache, myalgia, and abdominal pain, followed by the development of an unusual rash that is most pronounced peripherally. The rash is usually maculopapular, but it may be urticarial, vesicular, or petechial. Pulmonary involvement (focal infiltration, hilar adenopathy, pleural effusion) and transient hepatitis also are common features of atypical measles.

PHYSICAL FINDINGS

The development of a generalized maculopapular rash preceded by a 3- to 4- day period of fever, cough, coryza, and conjunctivitis associated with pathognomonic Koplik's spots should enable one to diagnose measles.

COMPLICATIONS

Bacterial otitis media is one of the most common complications of measles. Pneumonia may result from (1) an extension of the viral infection, (2) a superimposed bacterial infection, or (3) a combination of both. Acute encephalitis is the most serious complication, which occurs in only about 0.1 per cent of those with measles. It occurs most commonly between the second and sixth days of the rash. The course may be mild and brief (60 per cent), or it may progress rapidly and result in death (15 per cent). Between these two extremes exist many variations. Many children suffer permanent brain damage.

Subacute sclerosing panencephalitis (SSPE) is a rare, ultimately fatal disease caused by persistent measles virus infection. The onset of SSPE occurs many months or years after the initial infection. The illness is characterized by insidious and progressive behavioral and intellectual deterioration associated with awkwardness, stumbling, and falling. Seizures, mental deterioration, and death occur in the late stage of the disease. (See the article on Subacute and Chronic Viral Encephalitis and Encephalopathy).

Other complications include transient depression of cell-mediated immunity, bacterial cervical adenitis, bronchitis, laryngotracheitis, subclinical hepatitis, mesenteric adenitis, appendicitis, and purpura.

LABORATORY FINDINGS

Leukopenia and lymphopenia are frequently seen but hematological findings are non-specific.

Isolation of the virus is difficult. The techniques most commonly used to confirm measles serologically are hemagglutination inhibition (HI) and complement fixation (CF) tests. A fourfold or greater increase in antibody titer confirms measles. An additional serodiagnostic test, the staphylococcal protein A (SPA) absorption test, has recently been developed to measure measles-specific IgM antibody.

PITFALLS IN DIAGNOSIS

An intensified immunization program with live attenuated measles vaccine has been effective in causing a progressive decline in the incidence of measles in the United States. Measles virus infection is now often sporadic, occurring in older children or adults without known exposure. Therefore, it can present considerable difficulty in diagnosis. The early problem-oriented differential diagnosis prior to appearance of the rash is likely to be febrile bronchitis and nonpurulent conjunctivitis. In patients with atypical measles, because of its unusual forms of rash, the diagnosis may be mistaken for Kawasaki disease, Rocky Mountain spotted fever, streptococcal infection, mycoplasma pneumonia, enteric virus infection, meningococcemia, infectious mononucleosis syndrome, leptospirosis, toxic shock syndrome, or psittacosis. Proper recognition of this syndrome will prevent unnecessary diagnostic procedures.

VARICELLA (Chickenpox)

By Pierce Gardner, M.D.
Chicago, Illinois
and William Berenberg, M.D.
Boston, Massachusetts

DEFINITION

Varicella is a highly contagious disease of childhood, caused by a large DNA virus and characterized by (1) a well-defined incubation period, and (2) a vesicular rash that typically occurs in successive crops and is most marked on the trunk. In healthy children, the disease is usually mild with clinical symptoms limited to the skin; but in immunosuppressed children and adults, life-threatening illness caused by deep visceral involvement is not uncommon. After a primary infection, varicella virus generally persists in a latent form in dorsal root sensory ganglia. In response to various stresses, the virus may reactivate to produce herpes zoster (shingles), a painful vesicular eruption in a dermatomal pattern most commonly seen in adults. Lifelong immunity to exogenous varicella infection usually follows the primary infection. Patients with either chickenpox or herpes zoster represent a source of infection to susceptible persons.

PRESENTING SIGNS AND SYMPTOMS

The classic presentation of varicella is that of a young child (highest incidence between 2 and 8 years of age) with a history of exposure to chickenpox 10 to 21 days previously (usually, 14 to 16 days), who has mild prodromal symptoms of malaise and low-grade fever, followed within 12 to 36 hours by a centripetal (maximally truncal) rash. Early recognition of varicella is of greatest importance in the hospital setting, where exposed immunosuppressed children with no previous history of varicella should be identified and treated with zoster immune globulin (ZIG) or plasma in order to prevent or modify the clinical course of varicella. Since the benefit of passive immunization of exposed contacts is greatest during the period immediately after exposure, early recognition of the index case is important for optimal management. Recipients of zoster immune globulin or plasma who do develop modified varicella often have a prolonged incubation period (up to 42 days) and prolonged clinical course (with prolonged viral shedding).

PHYSICAL EXAMINATION AND COURSE

Typically, the rash begins with erythematous macules that rapidly progress to papules, which vesiculate to form the classic "dewdrop on a rose petal." Itching is a common and sometimes intense early symptom. In contrast to vaccinia and variola, the lesions are located in the superficial layers of epidermis and have thin, easily ruptured walls. The vesicular lesions are often elliptical, rarely exceeding 3 to 4 mm in diameter. Drying results in central depression (umbilication) of vesicles, followed by crusting. Characteristically, successive crops of vesicles appear for 3 or 4 days after the first rash, so that in a given area lesions may be seen in all stages of development from macules to vesicles to lesions that are becoming encrusted. Only rarely do new lesions appear after the seventh day of rash except in immunocompromised hosts. Lesions may involve any mucous membrane, most commonly the mouth, conjunctiva, or genital area, producing local irritation and pain. Local lesions may account for the occasional complaints of abdominal pain, dysuria, and cough. The evolution of the lesions from vesicles to crusting is variable but is usually complete within 7 to 10 days. Once crusted, the lesions are probably no longer contagious. Temporary depigmentation is common, but generalized scarring is rare in the absence of secondary bacterial infection. Systemic symptoms and fever are generally mild. The presence of high fever or significant toxicity should lead the physician to suspect one or more of the complications listed below.

Rarely, a hemorrhagic form of varicella has been noted, marked by high fever and hemorrhage into vesicles and other areas. This often fatal syndrome appears to be related to intravascular coagulation of clotting factors and platelets and has been noted predominantly in children with impaired host defenses (i.e., leukemia).

COMPLICATIONS

Secondary Bacterial Infection. Skin lesions often become superinfected by staphylococci or streptococci. Impetigo and cellulitis are the most common infections and may in severe cases result in generalized sepsis or metastatic infections (especially septic arthritis). Poststreptococcal sequelae, including glomerulonephritis or rarely acute rheumatic fever, may occur.

Pneumonia. Chest infiltrates can be detected roentgenographically in as many as 16 per cent of patients with varicella. Respiratory symptoms are usually mild or absent. Clinically, significant pneumonia has been detected most frequently in adults and immunosuppressed patients. Symptoms of cough and tachypnea typically begin several days after the rash appears. In certain patients, severe hemorrhagic pneumonitis with marked impairment of respiratory function may cause life-threatening illness. This complication is important to recognize, as preliminary studies suggest that antiviral agent adenine arabinoside (Ara A) or acyclovir may be of therapeutic benefit.

Varicella pneumonia also may be complicated by bacterial superinfections, most commonly with *Staphylococcus aureus.* The bilateral nodular densities characteristic of varicella pneumonia may subsequently calcify and appear indefinitely on chest x-rays.

Dissemination to Other Viscera. Involvement of the liver and other viscera is rare except in the immunosuppressed patient. Fever, right upper quadrant pain, toxicity, and elevated hepatocellular enzymes are the hallmarks of hepatic involvement by varicella. Widespread visceral dissemination is associated with high mortality. Neonates who contract varicella are also at increased risk of visceral involvement. The risk is greatest for infants developing the rash at age 5 to 11 days or born of mothers with onset of varicella within 4 days of delivery. Early recognition of disseminated varicella is important because prompt therapy with antiviral drugs may be beneficial.

Central Nervous System Complications. Varicella has now supplanted measles as the most commonly identified cause of fatal encephalitis in the pediatric age group. Encephalitis, which occurs approximately once per 3000 cases, usually represents a postinfectious encephalitis in which hypersensitivity mechanisms are thought to be important in the pathophysiology. Characteristically, the symptoms of headache, altered sensorium, meningeal irritation, and secondary fever begin 3 to 7 days after the appearance of the rash. Cerebrospinal fluid pleocytosis (predominantly lymphocytes) and protein elevation are common. Although many patients recover completely, death occurred in approximately 10 per cent, as reported to the Centers for Disease Control. Residual neurologic deficit is not uncommon.

Other neurologic complications of varicella include cerebellar ataxia, transverse myelitis, polyneuritis, and aseptic meningitis. Recovery from these complications is usually complete. Lumbar punctures performed on children with varicella often show mild pleocytosis (lymphocytes) in the absence of neurologic signs or symptoms.

Coagulation Complications. Thrombocytopenic purpura or disseminated intravascular coagulation with hemorrhage into vital organs may occur in unusual cases.

Rare Complications. Varicella infection of the cornea may threaten vision. Lesions in the larynx may produce edema with airway obstruction requiring tracheostomy. On occasion, varicella, as well as a number of other infectious agents, has been associated with Reye's syndrome (acute fatty degeneration of the liver together with "toxic" encephalopathy, often with hypoglycemia), or myocarditis.

LABORATORY FINDINGS

Laboratory tests are seldom necessary to secure the diagnosis of varicella. However, if doubt exists, the following tests are useful:

1. Examination of scrapings of the vesicle base (stained with Wright or Giemsa stain) usually will reveal multinucleated giant cells, often with inclusions. These cells may also be seen in herpes simplex but not in other diseases associated with vesicles.
2. Acute and convalescent sera taken 14 days apart may be expected to show an elevation of complement-fixing and neutralizing antibodies.
3. Demonstration of virus can be achieved by isolation in human tissue culture or by direct electron microscopy of scrapings from the base of a lesion.

Differential white blood cell count and urinalysis are seldom of diagnostic importance.

PITFALLS IN DIAGNOSIS

The characteristic epidemiology and clinical appearance usually serve to distinguish varicella from other diseases associated with vesicles. Early lesions may be confused with insect bites, dermatitis herpetiformis, eczema vaccinatum, eczema herpeticum, smallpox, or rickettsialpox. Later lesions may be confused with pemphigus or bullous impetigo. With the exception of infections caused by herpes simplex, none of these diseases is associated with multinucleated giant cells in scrapings of the vesicle base, and microscopic demonstration of these giant cells by Giemsa or Wright stained smears (see above) is a most useful rapid diagnostic test. Hemorrhagic chickenpox may mimic meningococcemia, but epidemiologic and other clinical features provide a basis for differentiation.

MUMPS

By Jeanette Wilkins, M.D.
Los Angeles, California

SYNONYM

Epidemic parotitis.

DEFINITION AND EPIDEMIOLOGY

Mumps is an acute communicable disease of viral etiology with worldwide distribution. The infectious agent is an RNA virus belonging to the Paramyxovirus group. Mumpsvirus infections occur year-around with peak incidence in late winter and spring. Its seasonal pattern has remained unchanged since the introduction of the Jeryl Lynn strain mumps virus vaccine into the United States in December 1967.

Some infants may be susceptible to mumps at birth; the remainder become susceptible following the loss of passively acquired immunity of maternal origin usually by or shortly after 6 months of age. Epidemics occur at 2- to 3-year intervals. As a result of the highly infectious nature of the mumpsvirus and ease of intrafamilial spread, infection is often acquired at an early age. Attack rates of 70 per cent have occurred among susceptibles following the introduction of mumps into a household. In our experience, 19 per cent of infants and children between 1 and 2 years of age had serologic evidence of prior mumps infection before the availability of a means for active immunization. Peak age for the acquisition of mumps is stated to be 4 to 6 years, and by 15 years of age greater than 90 per cent of many populations may have experienced infection with this virus. Deliberate exposure through active immunization with the live, attenuated vaccine virus has the potential for eliminating clinical disease in most vaccine recipients. There is no sex predilection for infection with mumpsvirus, although complications have been more common in males.

PRESENTING SIGNS AND SYMPTOMS

Following the inoculation of respiratory epithelium by infectious viral particles that are present in the salivary and respiratory secretions of diseased individuals, a nonimmune person may develop clinical or subclinical infection following an incubation period of 17 to 21 days. Incubation periods as short as 8 days and as long as 35 days have been reported. Inoculation may result from droplet nuclei or by direct contact.

Early signs of infection are nonspecific for mumpsvirus and include malaise and fever. Some patients may have, in addition, a headache and/or anorexia. It is important to appreciate that the mumpsvirus, during the incubation period, may disseminate by way of the bloodstream to all tissues of the body. The ability of the virus to propagate in distant tissues or target organs away from the portal of entry is manifested following the immunologic attack by the host's T cells on virus-infected cells within these organs. Therefore, the severity of disease in each infected organ will be due to summation of viral toxicity to cells and to the intensity of the local cell-mediated immune response. Approximately 30 per cent of all individuals infected with mumpsvirus will remain asymptomatic and infection will be recognized only through the utilization of cultural and serologic techniques.

The common localization of mumpsvirus in the exocrine glands around the portal of entry has led to the belief that mumps is parotitis with or without submaxillary or submandibular gland involvement. Signs or symptoms of selective localization in organs or tissues away from the portal of entry have been termed complications. However, since the histopathology produced in all organs is similar, the clinical signs and symptoms point to those particular organs or glands of the body in which the virus has most successfully replicated.

Exocrine Glands

Parotid Glands. The most common organs showing disease with mumpsvirus are the parotid glands. Disease is manifested by bilateral or unilateral enlargement of these glands. Their sudden increase in size within their restrictive capsules leads to painful swelling. Swollen glands are visually recognizable and palpable in their location at the angles of the jaw. The ear lobe may be pushed out and upward. Erythema and induration are notably absent. The orifice of Stensen's duct is often reddened in the presence of gland involvement. Findings similar to that noted in the parotid glands are also seen with primary infection of the submandibular and submaxillary glands and the orifices of Wharton's ducts. Pain may be intensified by the ingestion of foods containing substances that increase parotid and/or salivary gland secretions or act as irritants when eliminated from the body by this route.

The period of communicability coincides with the period of virus excretion from the parotid and/or salivary glands, i.e., 7 days before onset to approximately 3 days after the onset of gland enlargement. As a rule, an individual is considered noninfectious when the glands have returned to their normal size; this occurs in most by around 8 days after the onset of enlargement.

An inconstant finding with parotid and in particular with salivary gland enlargement is pitting edema over the sternum and the anterior and anterolateral chest wall. Obstruction to the lymphatics draining the area is the proposed mechanism. Occurring in approximately 6 per cent of cases, it usually appears 5 to 8 days after the onset of disease and persists for up to 5 days.

Testes. Localization of mumpsvirus in the testes is not uncommon, and clinical disease may occur in 18 to 36 per cent of males over 15 years of age. In contrast, an incidence of 0.4 per cent is reported in prepubertal males. Orchitis may develop without parotitis but is most commonly observed as parotitis is beginning to subside. The restrictive tunica albuginea promotes painful enlargement. Unilateral disease is more common. Isolated epididymitis may occur infrequently; it is more likely to be associated with orchitis. Hydrocele and/or scrotal edema may be concurrent findings. With intense enlargement of the testis, there may be some reduction in size because of atrophy. However, sterility as a complication of mumps is uncommon.

Ovaries. The ovaries of postpubertal females are also vulnerable to the localization of mumpsvirus. Pain and edema in the areas of the ovaries and the right and left lower quadrants point to their being infected. Oophoritis in the female is seen clinically less often than orchitis in males.

Pancreas. Although the pancreas may be a frequent site for mumpsvirus localization, pancreatitis is rarely diagnosed. Epigastric pain, vomiting, nausea, and pain on deep palpation over the area of the pancreas will be signs and symptoms for this gland's infection. With intense involvement the pancreas may be palpable in individuals with a scaphoid abdomen.

The temporal association of the onset of diabetes following mumps points to a role for mumpsvirus in the initiation of this disease. Infection of the beta cells of this gland is inferred.

Pancreatitis in patients with cystic fibrosis can be devastating. Death has resulted from mumps in this population.

Breasts. Breasts are rare targets for mumpsvirus localization. Mastitis is diagnosed by the painful, nonerythematous swelling of one or both breasts. Either sex is vulnerable to mumpsvirus mastitis. Like all of the other distant organs or glands involved, breast infection can occur in the presence or absence of parotitis and may appear before, during, or after the onset of parotid swelling.

Central Nervous System

Brain and Meninges. Fever in association with headache and vomiting with or without nuchal rigidity are signs and symptoms of mumpsvirus localization in the meninges. Mumpsvirus is considered the leading cause of aseptic meningitis, a usually benign, self-limited disease with no sequelae. In the absence of parotid swelling, unequivocal diagnosis requires isolation of the virus from the cerebrospinal fluid (CSF). Meningitis is the most common CNS infection with mumpsvirus infection.

A CNS examination from patients with meningitis shows pleocytosis with a predominance of lymphocytes. White blood cell counts <500 per cu mm are found in the majority of cases; cell counts up to 2500 per cu mm have been reported. The protein concentration is minimally elevated, although concentrations >100 mg/dl have been present. Most patients, if indicated, will require a single lumbar puncture. Symptoms and signs often abate subsequent to the spinal tap, and the spinal tap may be considered therapeutic. Peculiar to mumps meningitis has been hypoglycorrhachia. Glucose concentrations in the CSF <20 mg/dl are rare. It should be appreciated that abnormal CSF parameters may persist for a prolonged period of time after all other signs and symptoms of mumpsvirus infection have resolved, usually by 1 and at most 2 weeks after onset. The persistence of cells and especially increased protein concentration in the CSF of some patients have not correlated clinically with late sequelae.

Seizures, coma, and personality changes are indications of an underlying encephalitis. It is estimated that for every one million cases of natural or wild mumpsvirus infection, 2600 cases of encephalitis may occur. Although recovery from encephalitis may be complete a 1.4 per cent mortality rate has been realized.

Ependymal cells are selectively vulnerable to infection with mumpsvirus. The resultant ependymitis may be followed by obstruction of the aqueduct of Sylvius after ependymal cell dropout and scarring. Hydrocephalus has occurred as early as 3 months to as late as 4 years after postnatally acquired mumpsvirus infection. It is conceivable that those patients with persistently elevated CSF protein following aseptic meningitis might have a mild degree of transient or permanent obstruction to the flow of CSF from an occult ependymitis.

Transverse myelitis and polyradiculitis are rarely seen with mumps infection.

Cranial Nerves. Of the 12 cranial nerves, the eighth is the most commonly associated with mumps infection. Although the vestibular portion may be affected, the auditory branch is associated with the greatest morbidity. An abrupt hearing loss may occur that is most often unilateral. Twenty per cent of the cases have bilateral involvement. The sensorineural deafness may be permanent or associated with varying degrees of recovery. Deafness may occur coincident to or closely following parotid gland enlargement.

Facial nerve palsy and/or paralysis have also been associated with mumpsvirus infection. Likewise, the optic nerve, when diseased, may present clinically as optic neuritis or papillitis. Optic atrophy may be a sequela of mumpsvirus involvement of this cranial nerve.

Miscellaneous Organ Localization

Attesting to the generalized spread of this virus throughout the body have been the isolated reports of the following disease states: (1) thyroiditis, (2) myocarditis, (3) pericarditis, (4) arthritis, (5) dacryoadenitis, (6) conjunctivitis, (7) scleritis, (8) uveitis, (9) keratitis, (10) hepatitis, and (11) nephritis.

Although rarely diagnosed clinically, infection of the kidney probably occurs in most, if not all, individuals with mumps. The virus *in vitro* and presumably *in vivo* replicates effectively in renal tissue. Viruria has been detected up to 13 days after the onset of parotitis. Fatal nephritis has been noted rarely. It has been postulated that if specific and sensitive testing of renal function were employed, some degree of compromise would be demonstrated in most individuals with uncomplicated mumpsvirus infection.

DIAGNOSTIC TESTS

The confirmation of a clinical diagnosis of mumps requires the cultivation of the virus or the demonstration of a significant rise in mumps-specific antibody in the serum of an infected individual. Mumps skin tests have been unreliable, and none is available commercially as an indicator of immune status.

Few laboratories with the capability of carrying out techniques for mumpsvirus isolation are readily available to the practicing physician. However, mumpsvirus can be successfully isolated from the saliva and urine as long as 8 and 14 days, respectively, after the onset of clinical disease. For optimum chances for recovery of the virus special handling, storage and transport of specimens is necessary and instructions should be obtained from the contracted laboratory prior to their being obtained. In addition to the above, mumpsvirus has been isolated from CSF, blood, breast milk, and infected tissues. State or local health departments can offer helpful information regarding viral isolation.

Serologic techniques have been the most widely used methods for the evaluation of patients with mumps. The ideal test should be technically simple, specific, and relatively inexpensive. The following tests have been developed to detect antibody to the mumpsvirus:

1. Complement fixation (CF) test.
2. Hemagglutination inhibition (HI) test.
3. Virus neutralization tests (Nt), which include the plaque reduction technique.
4. Immunofluorescence (IF) test.
5. Radioimmunoassay (RIA).
6. Enzyme-linked immunosorbent assay (ELISA).

Until recently, the CF and HI tests have been the most often utilized. However, the CF and HI tests lack specificity for mumpsvirus, since cross-reacting antibodies to parainfluenzae viruses are also detected, if present, in the patient's serum. In addition, nonspecific inhibitors, which are difficult to remove from the serum, may prevent the detection of low levels of antibody with the HI test. Unfortunately, the most sensitive Nt tests are more costly and technically more difficult to perform. The ELISA and IF tests are now available for introduction into clinical laboratories.

During infection with mumpsvirus, antibodies are

Table 1. Differential Diagnosis of Parotid Swelling*

I. Infectious
   - Viral: mumps, parainfluenza types 1 and 3, coxsackievirus A, echovirus, lymphocytic choriomeningitis, influenza A
   - Bacterial: Acute suppurative parotitis (staphylococcal, pneumococcal, occasionally gram-negative bacilli), recurrent parotitis (primarily *Streptococcus viridans*), typical and atypical mycobacterial parotitis
   - Other: trichinosis, actinomycosis

II. Obstructive
   - Sialolithiasis
   - Papillary trauma (including ill-fitting dentures)
   - Foreign body in Stensen's duct
   - Parotid-masseter hypertrophy-malocclusion syndrome
   - Chronic sialectasis
   - Tumor of duct

III. Tumors or cysts
   - Benign and malignant parenchymal tumors
   - Hemangiomas
   - Lymphangiomas
   - Cysts, congenital and acquired

IV. Drugs
   - Iodides ("pyelography mumps")
   - Isoproterenol
   - Phenylbutazone, oxyphenylbutazone
   - Bromide poisoning
   - Chronic heavy-metal poisoning (lead, mercury)
   - Thiocyanate
   - Thiouracil
   - Phenothiazines

V. Metabolic
   - Malnutrition (protein deficiency?)
   - Rapid refeeding after malnutrition
   - Obesity
   - Diabetes mellitus, overt and latent
   - Alcoholism (malnutrition?)
   - Gouty parotitis
   - Uremic parotitis

VI. Miscellaneous
   - Sarcoidosis (uveoparotid fever)
   - Mikulicz's disease—Sjögren's syndrome—benign lymphoepithelial lesion
   - Waldenström's macroglobulinemia
   - Systemic lupus erythematosus
   - Fatty atrophy
   - Menopausal hypertrophy
   - Excessive starch ingestion
   - Cystic fibrosis
   - Fibrous parotitis
   - Pneumo-parotitis (glass blowers, trumpet players)
   - "Anesthesia" mumps

VII. Conditions resembling parotitis
   - Intraparotid, anterior cervical, lymphadenitis
   - Lymphoma
   - Dental abscess
   - Severe otitis externa
   - Caffey's disease (infantile cortical hyperostosis)
   - Cervicofacial actinomycosis
   - Masseter hypertrophy (bruxism, excessive gum-chewing)
   - Branchial cleft cysts
   - Prominent transverse process of atlas

*Reprinted from Marcy, M.: Mumps. In Conn, H.F., and Conn, R.B.: *Current Diagnosis*, 6th ed. Philadelphia, W.B. Saunders Company, 1980.

induced against the S (soluble, internal ribonucleoprotein core) and the V (viral outer envelope) antigens. The S antibodies usually appear within the first week of illness, and the V antibodies appear 1 or 2 weeks later. Thus in the convalescent stage, both antibodies will be demonstrable at their highest levels. With the passage of time, levels to both antibodies decrease, the S antibodies at a faster rate than the V antibodies. The HI test measures antibody to the V antigen, whereas the CF, RIA, Nt, IF, and ELISA measure antibody to both the S and V antigens. Serum should be obtained as soon as possible after the onset of symptoms (acute serum) and 3 to 4 weeks later (convalescent serum). A fourfold or greater rise in titer in the convalescent serum is suggestive of recent mumpsvirus infection.

The peripheral white cell count can be depressed, normal, or elevated with mumpsvirus infection. Leukopenia with an absolute lymphocytosis is frequently seen with "atypical lymphocytes" or virocytes present. Leukemoid reactions with white blood cell counts up to 60,000 per cu mm have been noted. Plasmocytosis in the peripheral blood may also be a feature of mumps infection.

Serum amylase will be elevated with parotid and/or pancreatic involvement in mumps. Elevation may be seen in the absence of parotid gland enlargement. Increased levels of amylase in the urine may persist after serum levels have returned to normal. The differentiation of isoamylases of pancreatic or parotid gland origin requires sophisticated techniques and is impractical. Most have turned to the determination of serum lipase levels to evaluate patients for associated pancreatitis.

The urinalysis should be normal in patients with mumps. The finding of microscopic hematuria, proteinuria, and especially red cell casts should point to the presence of nephritis.

DIFFERENTIAL DIAGNOSIS

It is expected that the widespread use of mumps vaccine will reduce the prevalence of wild virus. With the reduction in clinical disease those conditions, other than mumps, that have been characterized by parotid swelling will become more apparent (Table 1).

COLORADO TICK FEVER

By Jack D. Poland, M.D.
Fort Collins, Colorado

SYNONYMS

None in common usage; for a frequently used misnomer, see Pitfalls in Diagnosis.

DEFINITION

Colorado tick fever is an acute febrile disease caused by a virus transmitted to humans by the adult stage of the Rocky Mountain wood tick (*Dermacentor andersoni*). This arbovirus is maintained in nature by transmission between the immature stages (larvae and nymphs) of the wood tick and small rodents. The adult tick typically feeds on larger mammals, including humans when they encroach on the tick's habitat.

Known human exposure is thus limited to the distribution of this tick vector—principally mountainous regions of Colorado, Wyoming, Montana, Idaho, Oregon, Washington, South Dakota (the Black Hills region), California, Nevada, and Utah. The four-corners area of Arizona and New Mexico and the southwestern border of Canada are marginal to the habitat for this tick, and only a few human exposures have been traced to these areas.

In the past decade, between 100 and 300 cases have been reported annually from Colorado and from 0 to 50 from the other western states. Detection and reporting of large numbers of cases from Colorado and its adjacent states reflects a combination of high clinical awareness, a high incidence of transmission to humans in the Rocky Mountains, and readily available state or federal laboratories capable of testing for CTF infection.

PRESENTING SIGNS AND SYMPTOMS

From 3 to 6 days after tick exposure, the patient experiences an abrupt onset of fever, myalgia, headache, malaise, lethargy, retro-orbital pain, and photophobia. Stiff neck, abdominal pain, or lower back pain are often reported, but these may reflect the severity of the myalgia. Less frequent complaints include sore throat, nausea, vomiting, diarrhea, or a transient truncal rash. An attached tick is reported in about half of confirmed cases; ticks are found on clothing or other personal items in 30 to 40 per cent; 10 to 15 per cent of patients report finding no ticks. Two examples of infection have been documented in persons who had not traveled to CTF-tick infested areas: an elderly Colorado woman who laundered clothes for college students, and a 6-year-old boy whose father had returned from a Colorado mountain fishing trip 3 days prior to onset of the child's illness.

COURSE

Acute symptoms last for 5 to 10 days. Only half of confirmed patients have the biphasic fever and illness pattern considered typical, in which an acute illness with fever of 101°–103°F for 2 or 3 days is followed by a 2-day remission, then recrudescence, often with higher fever and more severe morbidity; rarely, a third relapse is reported. About two thirds of adults and one third of children have a prolonged period of malaise lasting 3 or more weeks. About 20 per cent of patients are hospitalized, children more frequently than adults.

COMPLICATIONS

No complication is common. Only two fatalities are known. Both were children, ages 4 and 9, and both had bleeding diatheses. Other syndromes that have rarely developed in association with CTF infections include encephalitis with full recovery, pericarditis, epididymo-orchitis, and atypical pneumonia. The latter two complications developed during the early convalescent period (9 to 10 days after onset of illness).

Insufficient data exist on CTF during pregnancy to suggest whether or not adverse fetal effects might result. Follow-up of eight women in the past decade who had CTF at various stages of gestation has shown no adverse effects on either the pregnancy or the offspring. One of these women delivered an infant with multiple anomalies that were not considered to have been related to the mother's CTF infection. In a 1950 report, a pregnant woman spontaneously aborted 2 weeks after she had acquired acute CTF.

PHYSICAL FINDINGS

The typical patient has no physical findings of diagnostic significance. Intensity of the symptoms, specifically myalgia, headache, retro-orbital pain, fever, and dehydration, often results in such severe morbidity that the possibility of a more serious infection, such as Rocky Mountain spotted fever (RMSF) (see article on Rickettsial Diseases), is difficult to dismiss. The brief appearance of a rash, though often truncal in distribution, may further confound the clinical picture and precipitate precautionary antibiotic therapy for RMSF.

LABORATORY FINDINGS

Leukopenia, with white blood cell (WBC) counts below 3000/cu mm to as low as 700/cu mm, develops in most CTF patients and thus strongly supports the clinical and epidemiologic suspicion of this diagnosis. Of considerable importance, however, is the observation that WBC counts are often in the high normal range for the first 2 days of illness, necessitating sequential counts to demonstrate WBC depression. Thrombocytopenia also occurs in virtually all CTF patients; again, sequential platelet counts are often required to demonstrate this. Platelet counts are preferred over an appraisal of the peripheral smear for "adequacy" of platelets. Platelet counts of from 20,000 to 95,000 per cu mm are common. Other evidence of coagulopathy (elevated fibrin split products, increased prothrombin time, overt bleeding tendency, or petechiae) is rarely reported.

In 1981, leukopenia was reported in only 34 per cent of suspected CTF patients who were negative, compared with 90 per cent of confirmed CTF patients. Also the leukopenia of the CTF-negative patients was not as profound, with most falling between 3500 and 4500 per cu mm. Depressed platelet counts are also frequently reported in CTF-negative patients, but, as with leukopenia, this depression is not as profound, most of the lower counts in CTF-negative patients exceeding 150,000 per cu mm.

In the few bone marrow studies done, maturation arrest of all three circulating blood cell precursor series is evident and undoubtedly is instrumental in the marked depression of circulating leukocytes and platelets. It is of interest, however, that anemia is not a feature of CTF infection.

The tropism of CTF virus for bone marrow results in infection of all circulating blood cell precursors. The virus remains sequestered in circulating red blood cells for the life of the cell, long after clinical recovery. This poses a risk of transmission to recipients of blood transfusions donated by persons either incubating CTF or recently recovering from CTF. Confirmation of CTF infection can be accomplished by obtaining an acute phase blood sample and sending (at ambient temperature) both the clot and the serum in separate tubes to a state Health Department laboratory. Clinical and epidemiologic information, *especially the date of onset of illness,* is essential for appropriate processing of these diagnostic samples. The virus is present in high titer in the serum for the first 5 days of illness and in the red blood cell fraction for 10 to 14 days. The virus is readily isolated by inoculating these specimens into suckling mice. The CTF virus can also be demonstrated in the infected red blood cells by direct fluorescent antibody examination.

Confirmation can also be accomplished by testing paired sera if the convalescent serum is obtained at least 3 weeks after onset for the neutralizing (N) antibody test or at least 4 weeks after onset if the complement fixation (CF) test is used. Detectable N antibody is slow to develop, probably because of antibody binding caused by prolonged viremia. With properly spaced sera, the N antibody test rarely fails to confirm a CTF infection, but false-negative CF tests occur in 20 to 25 per cent of patients even when the convalescent phase serum is obtained at 4 weeks. Detectable indirect fluorescent antibody (IFA) develops concurrently with N antibody (often by the 14th day), but the IFA titer is usually higher ($\geq$ 1:40) in contrast to low (1:10 or 1:20) N titers in early convalescent sera. In later convalescent sera, N antibody titers are equal to or higher than indirect fluorescent antibody (IFA) titers.

OTHER DIAGNOSTIC PROCEDURES

The marked thrombocytopenia without clinical evidence of a bleeding disorder may stimulate additional studies of coagulation pathways. At present these studies are of no recognized diagnostic importance. There is also no known pathophysiologic significance of the transiently elevated serum glutamic oxaloacetic transaminase (SGOT, AST) or alkaline phosphatase levels occasionally noted.

POTENTIAL ERRORS AND PITFALLS IN DIAGNOSIS

The initial symptom complex of CTF is indistinguishable from RMSF, a rickettsial disease that is most prevalent in the eastern United States but that may be transmitted in the western states by the same tick vector that transmits the CTF virus. Rocky Mountain spotted fever is uncommon in the western states, with from 0 to 5 cases reported annually in Colorado. Suspected CTF patients should be instructed to watch for the typical RMSF rash and to report it promptly to the physician. Other summer diseases that are clinically similar to CTF include relapsing fever (borreliosis) (see related article), tularemia (see related article), and enterovirus infections, especially the coxsackie B viruses (see related article), which often produce severe myalgia. A biphasic illness is not unique to CTF, as it is also reported in a high proportion of CTF-negative patients. In 1981, we documented a coxsackie A viremia in a child with suspected CTF and a biphasic illness.

That CTF patients, particularly children, must be examined for persistently attached ticks was illustrated by an incident (1981) in which a child developed an ascending paralysis concurrent with laboratory-confirmed CTF. Removal of two engorged ticks, discovered during hospitalization, resulted in rapid neurologic recovery.

Appropriate laboratory testing is sometimes impeded by a failure of clinicians to discriminate between the two tick-borne diseases (CTF and RMSF) when specimens are submitted with a request that they be tested for "tick fever," a *misnomer* signifying neither agent specifically. Appropriate tests are likely to be applied in these situations only if sufficient clinical and epidemiologic information is supplied to implicate the suspected etiologic agent.

HERPES SIMPLEX VIRUS INFECTIONS

By Harry L. Keyserling, M.D.
and Andre J. Nahmias, M.D.
Atlanta, Georgia

Infections with herpes simplex viruses (HSV) are very common. The clinical spectrum is broad, varying from a completely asymptomatic infection to severe and fatal disease. There are two serotypes:

1. Type 1 (HSV-1), which generally *but not always* causes infections above the waist.
2. Type 2 (HSV-2), the agent responsible for most *but not all* infections below the waist (Table 1).

The serotype cannot be determined by clinical manifestations but may often be suspected by the method of transmission and the age of the patient. Thus, sexually transmitted genital infections are almost always HSV-2; with cunnilingus or fellatio, the genital infection is most often HSV-1. After the neonatal period, when most infections are HSV-2, infections in children and adolescents (unless they are sexually abused) are almost always HSV-1. Common areas of infection include the mouth, eyes, genital sites, and skin. The infection tends to be more severe locally in immunocompromised hosts and can disseminate to visceral organs, particularly in neonates or in severely malnourished children. Immunopathologic disease occurs occasionally in the form of erythema multiforme or Stevens-Johnson syndrome associated with orolabial or genital herpes.

Transmission requires close contact between infected and uninfected mucosal or skin surfaces. Although autoinoculation from one site to another can occur occasionally, there is no evidence in humans that the virus can be acquired from inanimate objects such as toilet seats.

Serologic surveys indicate that the prevalence of HSV-1 and/or HSV-2 antibodies depends on the age, socioeconomic status, and sexual patterns of populations studied. Thus, the prevalence of HSV-1 antibodies is higher in low socioeconomic than in higher socioeconomic groups; the prevalence of HSV-2 antibodies is low in children and nuns and high in prostitutes.

A primary infection occurs when an individual is initially infected with either HSV-1 *or* HSV-2. Prior to the infection the patient is seronegative, and following the infection antibodies can be detected. Many primary infections are mild and are often not clinically evident to either patient or physician—because the lesions are not present, they are not characteristic, or they occur in internal areas such as the cervix or urethra. The incubation period for a primary infection is 3 to 15 days.

The virus also establishes a latent infection in sensory and/or autonomic neurosystem ganglia. Recurrent infections, clinically manifest or asymptomatic, occur intermittently and at varying frequencies in different individuals. Mechanisms responsible for the maintenance of the latent state and stimuli that induce recurrences are poorly understood. Virus may be recovered from many anatomic sites (saliva, tears, vaginal secretions) when no clinically manifest signs or symptoms are noted.

Precipitating events that are associated with recurrences include fever, physical trauma, ultraviolet light (sunshine), and intensive suppression of cell-mediated immunity. Some individuals report that emotional stress often precedes a recurrence.

Clinical manifestations of herpetic disease depend on the individual's age, immune competence, and herpes antibody status. Prior infection with one herpes virus type does not prevent exogenous reinfection at the same or different anatomic site with another type, although clinical symptoms will generally be milder. Exogenous reinfection with the homologous type can also occur occasionally.

OROLABIAL INFECTION

Primary oral infection (herpes stomatitis, herpes pharyngitis) usually occurs during childhood but may also be acquired by orogenital contact later in life. The spectrum of infection is variable, ranging from asymptomatic seroconversion to numerous oral lesions requiring hospitalization for parenteral rehydration. If symptoms occur, the patient usually complains of a sore mouth or sore throat and pain with swallowing. Ulcerative lesions of the tongue, gingiva, palate, or buccal mucosa may be noted. Fever and cervical adenopathy can be present. Constitutional symptoms

Table 1. Body Sites That Can Be Involved by Herpes Simplex Virus*

Commonly Involved Sites	Infrequently Involved Sites
Oral cavity[1AS†,‡,§]	Larynx[3A], trachea[3A], lungs[3A],
Lips[1B]	Esophagus[3A], stomach[3A], intestines[3A],
	Pancreas[3A], liver[3A], spleen[3A]
Penis[2B], *vulva*[2B], vagina[2BS], cervix[2BS]	Urethra[2BS], prostate[2BS], seminal vesicle[2BS], anus[2B], bladder[2CS], kidneys[3A], adrenals[3A]
Eyes—*Cornea*[1B], conjunctiva[1AS]	Lens[2A], choroid[2A], retina[2A]
Skin—*Above the waist*[1B]	Heart[3A], bone marrow[3A]
—*Below the waist*[2B]	
—*Hands*[3B]	
Sensory ganglia—Trigeminal[1S]	Brain[1A], meninges[2A], spinal cord[3A]
—Sacral[2S]	
Sympathetic or parasympathetic ganglia[X]	
Salivary and lacrimal glands[X]	
Peripheral blood[X]	
Lymph nodes[X]	
Placenta and cord[X]	

* Modified from Shore, S., and Nahmias, A.: Immunology of herpes simplex viruses. In Nahmias, A., and O'Reilly, R. (eds.): *Immunology of Human Infection: Part II. Viruses and Parasites: Immunodiagnosis and Prevention of Infectious Diseases.* New York, Plenum Press, 1982.

† The herpes simplex virus (HSV) type most usually found:
1 = HSV–1; 2 = HSV–2; 3 = About equal frequency or dependent on type of host (e.g., newborn).

‡ Clinical form most usually seen:
A = Primary; B = Recrudescent; C = About equal frequency; S = Frequently subclinical; X = Information too incomplete regarding frequency of involvement, HSV type or clinical form.

§Italics = Those sites in which the diagnosis has heretofore most commonly been made clinically (and often erroneously).

of malaise, myalgia, headache, and fatigue are common. Rarely the infection may extend to involve the esophagus, larynx, or trachea. The primary infection resolves in 1 to 3 weeks. Chickenpox may cause oral lesions similar to herpes simplex but can usually be differentiated by the generalized skin eruptions. Certain enteroviruses induce ulcerative lesions that are indistinguishable from herpes simplex on clinical examination. Irradiation, malnutrition, Stevens-Johnson syndrome, and the mucositis associated with immunosuppression therapy can also cause oral ulcers that may resemble those of primary herpes simplex.

Asymptomatic shedding of virus in saliva is common (2 to 5 per cent of adults). Febrile illness of nonherpetic etiology will often trigger herpetic recurrences that may cause difficulty interpreting positive throat cultures for herpes. For instance, isolation of the virus from the throat of an adult with encephalitis is no proof of the herpetic etiology of the central nervous system (CNS) disease.

Recurrent labial herpes (fever blisters, cold sores) are often preceded by 12 to 48 hours of prodrome symptoms: burning, itching, numbness, tingling, paresthesias. Precipitating events include fever, ultraviolet light (sunlight exposure), and physical trauma. Stress and menstruation have also been associated with recurrences. The patient presents with single vesicles or groups of vesicles at the vermillion border of the lips; the vesicles then form ulcers that crust and heal without scarring. Pain associated with recurrent lesions is generally mild. Viral shedding is brief (average 3 days), and complete healing usually occurs after a week.

Aphthous stomatitis (canker sores) is very often confused with recurrent herpes simplex, since both diseases recur and are precipitated often by similar stimuli. The major distinguishing factor is that recurrent herpes rarely causes intraoral lesions.

GENITAL INFECTION

Genital herpes is usually transmitted during sexual intercourse; either genital-genital, oral-genital, or anal-genital. Autoinoculation from an extragenital site, such as the mouth to the genital region, may occur and has been well documented in children. Primary genital infection is less common than primary oral infection and is more common in the higher socioeconomic populations, since lower socioeconomic individuals are more usually infected with oral HSV-1 prior to the onset of sexual activity. In the United States, HSV-2 is generally recovered from 90 per cent of initial cases of genital herpes; however, in some other countries with perhaps different sexual patterns, over half the genital isolates may be type 1. It appears that recurrent genital infections are less common with HSV-1 than with HSV-2 and that the reverse may be true regarding oral infections.

Primary or first episodes of nonprimary (antibody present before infection) herpes are usually more severe than recurrent infections. The ratio of asymptomatic infections to cases of clinically manifest disease is unknown, although shedding of virus in cervicovaginal secretions is not infrequent (up to 3 per cent of random samples) in women with a prior history of genital herpes. The spectrum of disease in women includes cervicitis, vaginitis, urethritis, vulvar lesions, and rarely progression of infection to intrapelvic organs. Disease in males may involve the penis, scrotum, urethra, or perineum; proctitis has been reported in homosexuals. Asymptomatic urethral shedding in males has also been demonstrated. Ascending herpes cystitis (ulcerative lesions of the bladder) is uncommon. Systemic symptoms, including fever, myalgias, headaches, and fatigue, are common findings in primary infections. Approximately 10 per cent of patients will demonstrate evidence of meningitis (stiff neck, photophobia, emesis, mononuclear cerebrospinal fluid [CSF] pleocytosis). The meningitis does not progress to encephalitis, is self-limited, infrequently recurs, and is rarely accompanied by neurologic sequelae.

Local manifestations include bilateral vesicular ulcerative lesions of the skin and mucous membranes that are often painful and pruritic. Vaginal discharge in women, rectal discharge in homosexual men with proctitis, dysuria, and tender inguinal adenopathy may occur. The lesions progress from vesicles to ulcers, then pustulate, forming crusts. Local symptoms gradually increase for the first week, then resolve during the second week of disease. Skin lesions heal without scarring by the third week. Virus can be recovered from the cervix in over 90 per cent of women with primary vulvar infections and about 40 per cent of those with nonprimary first vulvar infections. Mean duration of viral shedding from external genital lesions is 10 days. Autoinoculation to extragenital sites (mouth, hands, eyes, skin) and secondary bacterial or yeast infection may occur.

Recurrent episodes are experienced by at least 75 per cent of individuals with clinically manifest genital herpes. Skin and mucous membrane lesions are the most common symptoms. Dysuria can occur in females but is infrequent in males. More than half of patients exhibit a prodrome consisting of pain, burning, itching, paresthesias, or frank neuralgia within 1 to 2 days of the onset of lesions. Mean viral shedding from the vesicular or ulcerative lesions is 4 days and complete healing averages 10 days. Occasionally, the prodrome is not followed by a clinically apparent outbreak, although viral shedding may occur. Systemic symptoms are uncommon in recurrent disease, and the degree and duration of pain is less. The cervix is concomitantly involved with recurrent vulvar lesions in approximately 15 per cent of cases. It should be emphasized that recurrent cervical herpes is often not accompanied by external lesions.

There are numerous infectious and noninfectious diseases that have clinical manifestations similar to genital herpes. Ulcerative sexually transmitted infections include syphilis, chancroid, lymphogranuloma venereum, and granuloma inguinale. Ulcerative lesions in syphilis are painless in contrast to herpetic ulcers. Chancroid and herpes have clinical features that are similar, but chancroid is uncommon in the United States except in local outbreaks. Superficial bacterial pyoderma in the genital area may be confused with the crusting pustules of a resolving herpes outbreak. Vesicular skin lesions of the rare case of herpes zoster in the sacral or inguinal dermatomes would be clinically indistinguishable from herpes simplex. Noninfectious ulcerative diseases that may be similar to herpes include trauma related to sexual intercourse, contact dermatitis, inflammatory bowel disease, Stevens-Johnson syndrome, and Behçet's syndrome. Multiple small vesicular lesions that coalesce are characteristic of herpes simplex (with the exception of zoster). The recurrent nature of herpes simplex is helpful in the differential diagnosis. Also helpful is the fact that HSV is the only agent associated with prodromal symptoms which occur in over 50 per cent of patients with recurrent disease.

SKIN INFECTIONS

The skin of any body site may be infected with HSV-1 or HSV-2. If the integumentary barrier is compromised (e.g., in burn victims or in patients with eczema), disease is more severe and can occasionally disseminate to visceral organs. Trauma to the skin allows a portal of entry for the virus. Examples include herpes of thumb-sucking tots and herpes gladiatorium, which occurs with contact sports such as wrestling or rugby. In primary infections, fever, lymphangitis, and regional lymphadenopathy may occur. Dermatologic lesions are vesicular and heal without scarring unless secondary infections are present. Herpetic whitlow is an occupational hazard for medical personnel, dentists, and respiratory therapists. Surgical incision and drainage of skin infections are contraindicated. Recurrence of skin lesions almost always occurs at the same location and is often accompanied by a prodrome. Cutaneous herpetic infections are often misdiagnosed as bacterial pyodermas, contact dermatitis, or herpes zoster.

OCULAR INFECTIONS

In the United States, ocular herpes is the leading cause of corneal blindness that is due to an infectious agent. Primary infection results in an acute follicular keratoconjunctivitis or, less commonly, pseudomembranous conjunctivitis. Conjunctival injection, irritation, pain, photophobia, and mucoid discharge are present. Bacteria, chlamydia, or other viruses may cause similar manifestations, but the discharge is usually purulent in bacterial conjunctivitis. Adenoviral conjunctivitis is often confused with herpes conjunctivitis, since both agents commonly cause preauricular adenopathy. Slit-lamp examination strongly supports the diagnosis of herpes if watery vesiculations of the lids are present. Fluorescein staining will assist in demonstrating the corneal ulcerations.

Recurrent ocular disease is usually manifest as corneal involvement and less commonly as conjunctivitis alone. Symptoms include flaring, photophobia, and irritation. Although dendritic ulcers are almost pathognomonic, there are many infectious and noninfectious corneal conditions that may sometimes confuse the diagnosis, particularly in cases presenting late.

Disciform keratitis is the most common complication of ocular infection and is thought to be caused by delayed hypersensitivity to HSV antigens. Disc-shaped stromal edema is noted, and white corneal precipitates may be noted. Interstitial keratitis, immune ring, and limbal vasculitis are uncommon manifestations of herpetic infection thought to be mediated by immune complex hypersensitivity reactions. In severe cases, corneal perforation occurs.

CENTRAL NERVOUS SYSTEM INFECTIONS

Herpes encephalitis in patients over 6 weeks of age occurs in 1 in 100,000 to 1 in 500,000 individuals per year and is almost always due to HSV-1 ($\geq$ 98 per cent). The CNS infection may occur as a primary infection, as a recurrent infection, or possibly as a reinfection with a new HSV strain. Disease occurs in all age groups and in both sexes. Because mortality is 70 per cent without treatment, early diagnosis is essential for the initiation of appropriate antiviral therapy. Brain biopsy is currently the only method for a definitive diagnosis of HSV encephalitis, both in regard to specific therapy for the virus and for any other treatable cause of the syndrome. There are numerous infectious agents associated with encephalitis, and treatment is available for bacterial (abscess, parameningeal infection), mycobacterial, and fungal pathogens. Of the many viruses that cause encephalitis, HSV is the only viral agent shown in controlled studies to respond to specific therapy (vidarabine). Epidemiologic information (travel, tuberculin exposure, animal exposure) is important but unfortunately is often not helpful in distinguishing herpes from other causes of encephalitis. However, an encephalitis occurring in the winter or spring is more likely to be herpetic than in the summer or fall, when enteroviruses and arboviruses are common.

Findings compatible with herpes encephalitis include acute febrile encephalopathy, headache, seizures, autonomic dysfunction, CSF pleocytosis (predominantly mononuclear cells), and elevated CSF protein. Greater than 90 per cent of patients have at least one focal neurologic sign such as hemiparesis, cranial nerve deficits, visual field loss, dysphasia, ataxia, or focal seizures. Most herpetic infections are located in the temporal lobe and clinical, electroencephalogram (EEG), or radiologic focalization to that area is most suggestive of a herpetic etiology, requiring a brain biopsy.

Neuroradiographic diagnostic techniques are helpful, if positive, and can guide the neurosurgeon to the appropriate biopsy site. Computed tomographic (CT) and brain scans are normal approximately half the time when the patient is first evaluated but usually are positive at a later time. The EEG shows localization in 80 per cent of cases. The CSF analysis may show a mononuclear pleocytosis (in 95 per cent of cases), increased red blood cells (85 per cent), and elevated protein (80 per cent).

Prior history of skin herpes, orolabial herpetic lesions, or isolation of herpes from saliva is not helpful, since many nonherpetic causes of encephalitis will trigger a recurrence of herpes. This does not apply to neonates because isolation of virus from any anatomic site in a neonate with evidence of encephalitis would be diagnostic for herpes encephalitis. Viral isolation from CSF in adults is low (about 4 per cent) and is higher in neonates (25 to 40 per cent).

Examination of brain biopsy material will often suggest a herpetic infection by histologic demonstration of inflammation with associated intranuclear inclusions. Unfortunately, there are often false-positive and false-negative pathologic results when compared with isolation of virus from the brain specimen. Similarly, it may not be possible to demonstrate the virus by electron microscopy or its antigens by immunologic methods. Another problem less commonly encountered is the possibility of a falsely negative brain biopsy virus culture. This may occur by sampling error (e.g., surgical procedure on left temporal lobe when infection was present in the right temporal lobe) or culture of edematous material rather than an infected portion. Therefore, a negative brain biopsy result does not absolutely rule out herpes encephalitis.

Many attempts have been made to diagnose herpes encephalitis without a brain biopsy. Neither a fourfold rise in titer nor antibody tests in the serum definitively separate brain biopsy–positive and –negative individuals. Cerebrospinal fluid antibody titers and ratios of serum/CSF antibodies are helpful only retrospectively, since the serologic changes are generally not noted in the first 2 weeks of disease. Moreover, these assays have a sensitivity of only 80 per cent and specificity of 80 per cent. Several investigators are evaluating techniques to detect HSV antigens in CSF samples. The sensitivity of these assays, particularly in the early phase of the disease, is about 50 per cent and approximately 10 percent are falsely positive. Efforts are currently being directed to improving such tests to enable an early specific diagnosis to be made for optimal therapy.

NEONATAL INFECTION

Most neonates acquire their infections from exposure to the mother's infected genital tract near the time of delivery. Transplacental infection is rare. Postnatal infection from maternal nongenital sites, nosocomial transmission in nurseries, and from exposure to infected family members occur uncommonly. Estimates of incidence rates in the United States vary from 1 in 3000 to 1 in 15,000 live births. About one half of infants will be born prematurely. Only 30 per cent of women will have clinical evidence of genital herpes at the time of delivery. Infants are predisposed to severe disease during the first month of life. Prior to the use of antivirals, mortality was 60 per cent, with less than 25 per cent of infants being normal after follow-up. Neurologic and ocular sequelae are common. Pregnant women with genital herpes or histories of genital herpes in their male partners should be monitored for active infection in the third trimester to decrease the risk of infection to the newborn. Cesarean delivery is recommended if infection near the time of delivery is detected.

Neonatal infections can be classified into disseminated and localized forms. Disseminated disease involves infection of multiple organs including liver, adrenals, lungs, kidneys, heart, skin, and brain. Infants may present with temperature instability, irritability, lethargy, poor feeding, jaundice, seizures, respiratory distress, hepatosplenomegaly, petechial rash, shock, or disseminated intravascular coagulation. Bacterial, fungal, or enteroviral sepsis has a similar clinical presentation. In addition, other neonatal entities such as intraventricular hemorrhage, necrotizing enterocolitis, congenital metabolic defects, and congenital heart disease have features in common with advanced herpetic infections. Localized disease may affect the brain (meningoencephalitis), or it may be limited to the eye (conjunctivitis, keratitis), mouth (oral ulcers), or skin (vesicles). Progression of mouth, eye, or skin disease to involvement of the brain or visceral organs occurs in about 75 per cent of infected infants. Skin vesicles must be differentiated from other dermatologic entities that cause vesiculopustular lesions in the neonatal period.

INFECTION IN THE IMMUNOCOMPROMISED HOST

Transplant patients (renal, heart, liver, bone marrow) and individuals on immunosuppressive regimens for neoplastic disease are predisposed to unusual or severe localized infections with herpes simplex. Severe malnutrition, extensive burns, and generalized eczema of the skin occasionally result in disseminated disease. Most primary congenital immunologic defects (except Wiskott-Aldrich syndrome) and the acquired immune deficiency syndrome (AIDS) are not associated with life-threatening HSV infections.

Mucosal and skin infections tend to become deep and necrotic. Extension of the disease to the esophagus, trachea, and lungs may occur. When invasive disease occurs, the liver is the organ most frequently involved. Pneumonia and visceral dissemination to other organs, such as the adrenals and kidneys, is similar to the spectrum of disease that occurs in neonates. It should be noted that brain involvement does not appear to occur any more often in the immunocompromised host than in a normal host.

LABORATORY DIAGNOSTIC TECHNIQUES

Isolation of herpes simplex virus in the virology laboratory is still the best method for documenting infection. Serologic tests have little usefulness in clinical diagnosis to date. For viral isolation, skin, oral, eye, genital, and rectal specimens are obtained by swabbing the area of involvement and transferring the material into viral transport media. Body fluids (urine, CSF) or biopsy specimens (lung, liver, brain) should be collected in sterile containers. Special media, such as the Leibovitz-Emory media, are available for storage and transport at room temperature. Most other transport media should be kept at 4°C or frozen at –70°C. Storage at temperatures of –20°C will result in rapid inactivation of the virus. Aliquots of the samples can be inoculated into many types of tissue culture cell lines that will support viral replication. Growth is rapid, and most positive specimens will be detected between 1 and 4 days after inoculation.

Several methods, including immunofluorescence and peroxidase techniques, are available for typing the virus as HSV-1 or HSV-2. Restriction endonuclease analysis of viral DNA is a powerful tool for identifying strains that are epidemiologically related. Laboratories are also developing methods that provide antiviral susceptibility tests for HSV, now that more than one antiviral may be effective and that drug resistance is becoming recognized.

Rapid detection of virus is possible by cytologic techniques using Papanicolaou (Pap), Wright, or Giemsa stains. Smears or scrapings show multinucleated giant cells. The Papanicolaou stain is preferred because it also reveals the intranuclear inclusions characteristic of herpetic infection (including varicella zoster). The Pap smear has a sensitivity of 75 to 80 per cent when interpreted by an experienced cytologist. Electron microscopy by the pseudoreplica method frequently shows positive results when vesicular fluid or tissue specimens are examined. Herpesviruses cannot be differentiated by regular electron microscopy and require specific immune electron microscopic tests for specific diagnoses of HSV. Immunologic methods, such as immunofluorescence, immunoperoxidase, radioimmunoassay (RIA), or enzyme-linked immunosorbent assay (ELISA) are most useful at present to confirm HSV in tissue cultures inoculated with suspect samples. The value of these methods for direct demonstration of viral antigens in clinical specimens is not yet well established and awaits systematic comparative studies with the virus isolation method.

PITFALLS IN DIAGNOSIS

Because of the increasing interest with HSV infections in recent years, it is important to elucidate what we believe to be pitfalls in diagnosis at the various levels—epidemiologic, clinical, and laboratory. The last factor is a cause of particular concern because physicians sometimes accept the accuracy of new laboratory tests before having the opportunity for adequate clinical evaluation. The premature or inappropriate use of such tests may lead to incorrect decisions regarding therapy or to psychological trauma as a result of an erroneous diagnosis. Now that possible preventive and therapeutic approaches have become available, or as these are being experimentally ascertained, correct diagnosis has also become even more important.

Epidemiologic Considerations

Herpes simplex virus as a cause of disease in a newborn is suspected more readily if the mother and/or father had genital herpes, particularly if laboratory-confirmed, or if the mother had orogenital sexual relations with a man with labial herpes close to the time of delivery. It should be stressed, however, that as the incidence of genital herpes is rising (about 5 to 10 per cent of pregnant women may give a positive history of genital herpes), and since up to 50 per cent of individuals may have orolabial herpes, one should be cautious when interpreting the epidemiologic information.

Clinical Considerations

As noted earlier and as shown in Table 1, some herpetic diseases tend to be diagnosed clinically. We believe that *no* individual should be diagnosed as having genital herpes without some laboratory confirmation because that patient's life will often be traumatized psychologically thereafter. It is also important that no child, or the parents, be told that he has genital herpes without laboratory confirmation; when genital herpes is diagnosed, one should not assume that the infection was acquired sexually. Autoinoculation from mouth to genitals is common in children, and the virus should be typed; if type 1, autoinoculation would be the most likely source and the onus of sexual abuse would be diffused.

Ocular herpes may be overdiagnosed and overtreated with topical antivirals resulting in toxic effects on the eye. Unfortunately, an effective combined regimen with antivirals/debridement makes corneal cultures unavailable when trying to establish effectiveness of antivirals. In recalcitrant cases isolation of virus for susceptibility testing may be helpful.

As noted earlier, outside the newborn age group, brain biopsy is currently necessary for diagnosing herpes encephalitis prior to antiviral therapy. A history of associated findings of mucocutaneous herpes is often a red herring and is not useful in a child or adult. A significant isolate will be needed even more for susceptibility tests if the resistance of HSV to some antivirals continues to increase. In the case of a newborn, the presence of an associated herpetic lesion (skin, mouth, eyes) is sufficient and does not require a brain biopsy. Also, in the immunocompromised host, laboratory diagnosis is mandatory prior to antiviral therapy.

Laboratory Considerations

Viral Identification. As mentioned, viral isolation is the current preferred method of diagnosis. It is important for the physician to become familiar with the optimal methods for obtaining and transporting specimens. Cultures should be obtained early in the course of illness, since the period of active viral shedding is short (1 to 5 days) in recurrent oral and genital herpes. There are kits that provide cell culture and immunologic tests for detecting virus for laboratories without tissue culture facilities. Reliability of such commercial tests, as well as local expertise in interpretation of positive or negative results, is greatly dependent on quality control, both by the company and local laboratory. Caution is therefore necessary when using such kits.

More rapid direct tests for identification of herpes are also prone to many problems regarding sensitivity and specificity. Physicians should be cautious when interpreting results obtained with such assays that may be used to label someone as having genital herpes.

There is a need for rapid diagnosis for early treatment in neonates and compromised hosts. One may therefore accept a lesser degree of specificity, balancing false-positive results with possible improved outcome from early therapy. Conventional virologic isolates would still be required for confirmation. There is a very great need for rapid diagnosis of genital herpes close to delivery for possible cesarean sections. The development of newer assays and methodologies, such as monoclonal antibodies, will hopefully provide such rapid tests in the not too distant future.

Serologic Tests. There are large numbers of serologic tests currently available to measure antibodies to HSV. A few laboratories are also able to differentiate HSV-type antibodies and antibodies to specific viral proteins. Unfortunately, most laboratories are using a complement fixation test that is usually grossly insensitive in comparison to such assays as ELISA. Pitfalls in interpretation are many (Table 2), and the old maxim regarding the significance of a fourfold rise in antibody titer is full of problems in cases of HSV. Occasionally patients or their sexual contacts wish to know if they have antibodies to HSV-2. Most such type-specific antibody tests have at least a 10 per cent false-positive and 10 per cent false-negative rate. At present, the use of such assays may cause more problems than are prevented or resolved. However, current work to make such tests more specific should provide methods to detect asymptomatic genital herpes that develops or that is reactivated during pregnancy.

Table 2. Serologic Methods for Detection of Herpes Simplex Virus Antibodies, Type-Specific Antibodies, and Serum Class Antibodies*

Method	Total Antibodies	Type-Specific Antibodies	Serum Class Antibodies (IgG, IgA, IgM)
Complement fixation (CF)	+	+	–
Neutralization (various tests)	+	+	–
Passive hemagglutination (PHA)	+	Inhibition PHA	–
Immunofluorescence (IF)	+	+	+
Radioimmunoassay (RIA)	+	+	+
Enzyme-linked immunosorbent assay (ELISA)	+	+	+
Complement-dependent antibody cytotoxicity (CDAC)	+	–	–
Antibody-dependent cell cytotoxicity (ADCC)	+	–	–

*Adapted from Nahmias, A.J.: The laboratory diagnosis of herpes simplex virus infection: Prospects and problems. Diagnostic Horizons 1:1, 1977.

COXSACKIEVIRUS AND ECHOVIRUS INFECTIONS

By David M. Morens, M.D.
Honolulu, Hawaii

NOMENCLATURE AND TAXONOMY

The coxsackieviruses are named after the city in New York where they were first isolated in 1948. The term *echovirus* is derived from an acronym for *e*nteric *c*ytopathic *h*uman *o*rphan, reflecting skepticism about their association with disease that briefly followed their discovery in 1951. Both are members of the Picornavirus family (which includes aphthoviruses, caliciviruses, enteroviruses, and rhinoviruses) and the Enterovirus genus, which is composed of the following four subgroups: polioviruses, coxsackieviruses, echoviruses, and "enterovirus types."

The original basis for classification of the first three of these subgroups was type of, or absence of, pathology in suckling mice. However, since subsequent experience with biochemical, physical, and tissue culture characterization of different viruses revealed the artificiality of reliance upon mouse pathology, it was decided in 1969 to retain the names of the 67 viruses already designated as polio-, coxsackie-, or echoviruses and to call newly discovered viruses "enterovirus" to be followed by a chronological number; e.g., for the first virus discovered after the change in terminology, "enterovirus 68." Enterovirus types 68 through 72 have been identified thus far. There are 29 coxsackieviruses and 31 echoviruses. The echoviruses are numbered from 1 to 34, except echovirus types 8, 10, and 28, which were deleted when shown to belong to different virus groups or when shown to be not unique. The coxsackieviruses are further divided into coxsackie A viruses (23 types designated coxsackie A1 through A24, A23 having been deleted) and the coxsackie B viruses (six types designated B1 through B6). There is no group-specific antigen that can be detected in serologic tests.

EPIDEMIOLOGY

The epidemiology of enteroviruses is nearly as confusing as the nomenclature. There are 60 coxsackie- and echoviruses, each one of which may cause a variety of disease syndromes. Most viruses have been associated with some of these syndromes (e.g., aseptic meningitis) but not with others (e.g., carditis). For all types except those associated with acute hemorrhagic conjunctivitis (AHC), there is a high rate of subclinical infection. Since virtually all of the enteroviruses can produce a spectrum of distinct disease syndromes, it is not surprising that almost all enterovirus syndromes can be caused by a number of different types. However, it is not important that the physician appreciate the complexity of this overlapping syndrome scheme. The nonpolio enteroviruses can be thought of as homogeneous for the purpose of clinical diagnosis. The physician must be familiar with the clinical and epidemiologic picture in his or her locality, but determination of the viral etiology is left to the virology laboratory in situations in which attempts at isolation (with or without identification of the specific type) seem warranted.

Transmission is by both the fecal-oral and respiratory routes. Foodborne and waterborne transmission are uncommon. Nosocomial transmission, particularly within nurseries, has been documented. Persons of all ages are affected, but children are more likely to be symptomatically infected than adults. Males are more likely to be symptomatically infected than females, the male : female ratio, dependent upon the specific type, being as high as 8 : 1 for some syndromes.

Although type-specific circulating antibody usually presumed to be associated with lifelong immunity appears 1 to 2 weeks after infection, reinfections with the same type have been documented. And, since many enteroviruses may cause a particular syndrome, it is possible for an individual to have an identical illness (e.g., aseptic meningitis, hand-foot-and-mouth disease) more than once. Though the incubation period for most coxsackie- and echovirus infections varies from a day or two to several weeks, for most acute syndromes it is in the range of 3 to 5 days.

Coxsackie- and echoviruses are worldwide in distribution. In temperate climates they circulate only in the summer, beginning in May or June in the northern hemisphere and disappearing by October, with peak activity in the July-August-September period. In the tropics enteroviruses may circulate year-round. In a particular geographic area such as a city or county, seasonal enterovirus activity is variable and seemingly mercurial. For example, five or ten enterovirus types may cocirculate during the summer months of one year, only a few of which are associated with recognized outbreaks. The next year, a few of the same viruses return, others disappear, and still others appear on the scene for the first time. Sometimes virus types associated with specific syndromes (e.g., aseptic meningitis) are associated with different syndromes (e.g., febrile exanthem) in other communities or at other times in the same community, or they may be associated with no recognizable syndrome. Furthermore, many enterovirus syndromes are frustratingly nonspecific, simulating a host of infectious and noninfectious diseases.

Because of these confusing aspects of enteroviruses, it is important to be aware of enterovirus activity *in one's own community.* It cannot be emphasized strongly enough that the crucial keys to diagnosis of coxsackie- and echovirus infections are:

1. Knowledge of the seasonal pattern of occurrence in the area.
2. Familiarity with enterovirus activity within the community.

I remember a large inner-city hospital where every spring senior housestaff would delight interns and medical students by successfully predicting influxes to the clinic of children with aseptic meningitis in late June. While such precision may only be possible in facilities serving large stable population centers, physicians practicing in medium and large sized communities may be rewarded by:

1. Developing a high index of suspicion as the enterovirus season (characteristic of the area) approaches.
2. Looking for an increase in sentinel syndromes that are possibly associated with enteroviruses (e.g., aseptic meningitis) or that are fairly distinctive (e.g., herpangina).
3. Checking periodically with the county or state health department laboratory or a university-based laboratory to learn which viruses are being isolated in the community.

A provisional diagnosis of infection with an enterovirus can be made by consideration of the epidemiologic characteristics of enterovirus activity in the community, history of present illness, and physical examination (to be discussed next). Helpful questions to ask in the history taking include those about a common-source outbreak and whether the patient has been exposed to a person with the same illness (e.g., pleurodynia) or to a person with some other illness possibly caused by the same enterovirus, within the expected incubation period.

LABORATORY DIAGNOSIS

Routine laboratory tests, including the white blood cell (WBC) count, WBC differential, and erythrocyte sedimentation rate, are not helpful in the diagnosis of coxsackie- and echovirus disease, except to the extent that they may rule out other conditions considered in the differential diagnosis. In adults the WBC count is normal or low normal. In children it may be elevated, a nonspecific finding associated with a number of infectious and noninfectious stresses.

With the exception of AHC, which will be discussed in more detail later in this article, the single most important element in confirmation of infection with all of the enteroviruses is a stool culture. During the course of illness, virus is almost always present in the stool and may persist for weeks. Throat and nasopharyngeal swabs are also likely to be positive early in those enterovirus syndromes associated with respiratory symptoms. Many enteroviruses can be recovered from the cerebrospinal fluid (CSF) if the sample is either inoculated immediately or frozen immediately for subsequent testing. Isolation from blood and tissue is variable. Isolation from unruptured vesicles should be attempted with a 27-gauge needle or, less ideally, by swabbing the base of a freshly ruptured vesicle.

Stool samples are two to three times as likely as rectal swabs to yield an enterovirus. Proper technique specifies placing a fresh 4- to 8-gm stool sample in a glass jar and taking it directly to the virology laboratory for emulsification, centrifugation, and inoculation. In the absence of a virus isolation or a very high index of suspicion of a specific enterovirus type, serodiagnosis is impractical. Obtaining acute and convalescent serum specimens is *not* a high priority when enterovirus disease is suspected but may be helpful in excluding other illnesses.

NONSPECIFIC FEBRILE ILLNESS

Nearly all enteroviruses produce febrile illnesses that are regarded as nonspecific because they are not associated with exanthem, enanthem, or neurologic or visceral involvement. Most such illnesses are either influenzalike or are associated with minor upper respiratory tract symptoms such as pharyngitis. They are commonly seen in preschool children and are virtually impossible to diagnose with certainty on a clinical basis alone. Such illnesses are likely to be seen as part of an outbreak of an enterovirus type associated with different syndromes, particularly febrile exanthematous disease and/or aseptic meningitis. In this case, an index of suspicion of an enterovirus etiology is raised, since most other viruses that cause influenzalike illnesses either are not prevalent in the summer (e.g., influenza) or do not cause such a variety of symptoms (e.g., adenoviruses).

EXANTHEM WITH FEVER

Perhaps the most common of the recognizable enterovirus syndromes is that of fever and rash. Most of the echo- and coxsackie B viruses can cause pink maculopapular rashes that are nonspecific and similar in appearance to each other (Fig. 1). Rashes are common in children but much less so in adults. Exanthem is usually accompanied by or preceded by fever of several days' duration, but other signs and symptoms are absent. The rash is usually concentrated on the trunk, especially when associated with defervescence. Echovirus type 9 has been noted to appear first on the face and evolve in a pattern mimicking measles. Echovirus type 16 has been associated with

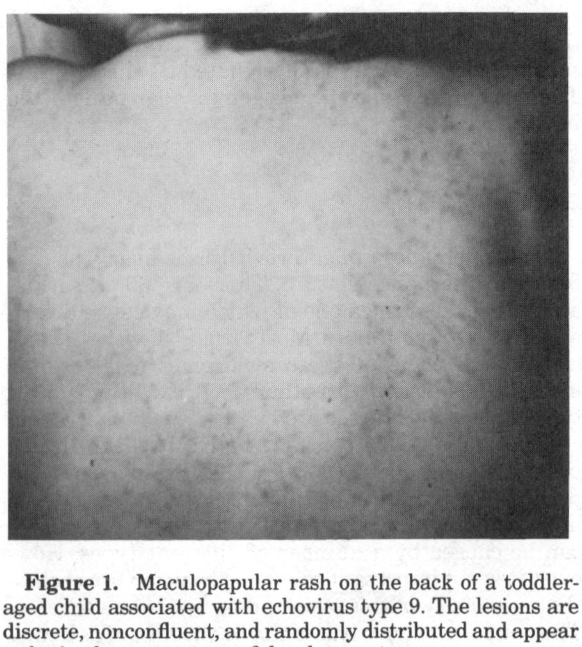

Figure 1. Maculopapular rash on the back of a toddler-aged child associated with echovirus type 9. The lesions are discrete, nonconfluent, and randomly distributed and appear to be in the same stage of development.

"Boston exanthem disease," a supposedly distinctive syndrome of fever and florid morbilliform or rubelliform rash appearing at the time of, or shortly after, defervescence, and the variable presence of herpangina-like ulcers.

Although the exanthem associated with echo- or coxsackievirus B disease varies greatly, a typical clinical picture is that of simultaneous appearance of hundreds of discrete or grouped pink, salmon-colored, or red truncal macules or low papules 2 to 8 mm in diameter. The lesions blanch upon pressure with a glass slide and may appear to wax and wane over the few days of their presence. Papules are often surrounded by a halo of faint blanching. Pruritus is uncommon. The exanthem is rarely impressive. There is typically a high proportion of affected persons with fever in whom the rash is either absent or not recognized. Petechial, urticarial, and other unusual exanthems have occasionally been reported.

The differential diagnosis often includes measles, rubella, and atypical measles, all of which can be excluded by history of vaccination and careful examination. Kawasaki disease has such a characteristic evolution that it is not a source of diagnostic confusion. Roseola infantum is a specific disease or syndrome that may be difficult to exclude unless viral isolation is made. Arbovirus infections (e.g., dengue) can sometimes be ruled out on the basis of geographic distribution of the vectors.

Coxsackie A viruses may also be associated with pink maculopapular rashes but are more noteworthy for their ability to cause vesicular rashes. The best known and most distinctive of these syndromes is *hand-foot-and-mouth disease* (not to be confused with foot-and-mouth disease of cattle, which is caused by an aphthovirus). Hand-foot-and-mouth disease is classically associated with coxsackievirus A16 but may also be caused by coxsackievirus A5 and others. Children 1 to 5 years old are at greatest risk. The condition usually begins with a mild febrile or nonspecific afebrile illness accompanied by the appearance of multiple discrete red macules of about 4 mm on the palms, soles, ventral surfaces of the fingers and toes, and buttocks (Fig. 2). Sometimes the lesions do not progress beyond this stage. More typically, they vesiculate, becoming white or gray flaccid vesicles containing infectious viruses that represent a source of contagion when they break down. When present, lesions on the buttocks all but confirm the diagnosis of hand-foot-and-mouth disease.

The differential diagnosis includes varicella, the lesions of which are more central in distribution, and disseminated herpes simplex disease. A neonate with such vesicular lesions must be presumed to have herpesvirus disease until proven otherwise; vesicular enterovirus disease is uncommon in newborns. The enanthem of hand-foot-and-mouth disease is similar to that of herpangina (to be discussed), an unsurprising fact when it is considered that some of the same viruses are associated with both diseases. Hand-foot-and-mouth disease may appear in incomplete forms. Many enteroviruses, especially the coxsackie A viruses, may cause vesicular exanthems in other than the characteristic pattern of hand-foot-and-mouth disease.

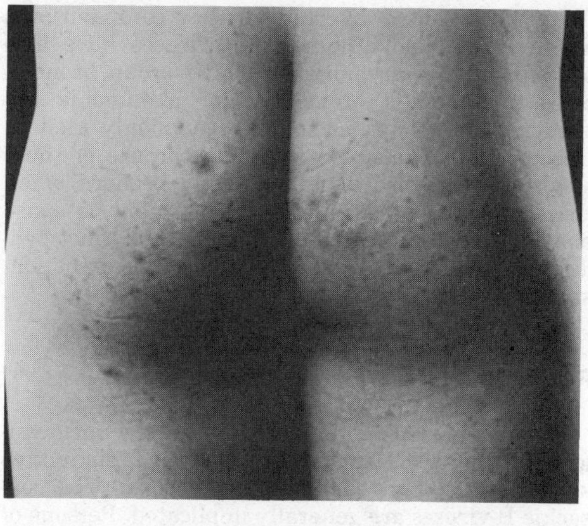

Figure 2. Exanthem of hand-foot-and-mouth disease. The papules are distributed over the buttocks. On the upper left buttock, one of the papules is beginning to vesiculate.

ENTEROVIRUS ENANTHEMS

Two distinct syndromes of enanthem have been associated with enteroviruses: herpangina and lymphonodular pharyngitis. Herpangina, derived from the same Greek root (meaning "to creep") as that of the unrelated herpesviruses), has been linked to numerous coxsackie A viruses and is most commonly seen in grade school and preschool children. Following onset of fever, sore throat, anorexia, and constitutional symptoms, there appear 2-mm red or burgundy-colored macules on the soft palate or fauces. The lesions rapidly vesiculate to become small white vesicles or, when broken down, shallow ulcers with intensely red bases. Some children may refuse to eat or drink because of the discomfort associated with swallowing. The lesions are usually in the posterior oral cavity, in contrast to primary herpetic gingivostomatitis and aphthous stomatitis, conditions included in the differential diagnosis.

Lymphonodular pharyngitis has rarely been observed since first described in the medical literature. It has been associated only with coxsackievirus A10. Pharyngitis is associated with the simultaneous appearance of discrete papules (not nodules) of infiltrating lymphocytes surrounded by a red halo at the base. These papules have white or yellow crowns that neither vesiculate nor ulcerate.

RESPIRATORY ILLNESS

In individual patients the coxsackie- and echoviruses have been associated with a variety of conditions of the upper and lower respiratory tract, most notably upper respiratory infections (URIs). There is nothing characteristic of URIs caused by enteroviruses. They may be clinically indistinguishable from those caused by rhinoviruses, coronaviruses, adenoviruses, and others. Enteroviruses have also been linked to pharyngitis, laryngitis, croup, bronchiolitis, pneumonitis, bronchitis, and pneumonia. Although such conditions may be commonly seen in infected individuals, community outbreaks of these syndromes are not usual, probably because when there is sufficient circulation of an agent to cause enough recognizable cases, other more distinct syndromes appear and overshadow the occurrence of nonspecific respiratory tract syndromes.

PLEURODYNIA

Pleurodynia (epidemic pleurodynia, epidemic myalgia, Bornholm disease) is an impressive, distinctive syndrome usually seen in epidemic form. The coxsackie B viruses are generally implicated. Persons of all ages may be affected, especially grade school children. The acute onset is characterized by fever, constitutional symptoms, and sharp pleuritic chest pain, which is often worse in adults. In children, pleuritic pain may be referred to the abdomen. In adults and most children, the pain is piercing, bilateral, and localized to the area of the lower rib cage. The intercostal muscles may be sore. Patients may avoid exertion in an effort to prevent the pain of deep inspiration. Similarly, patients may "force" frequent shallow coughs rather than cough deeply. Some patients spontaneously increase their respiratory rate while decreasing volume, attempting to avoid deep inspiration, which may be painful. It is not unusual for adult men to fear they are having a myocardial infarction. Older boys and men have been noted to develop unilateral orchitis in association with pleurodynia (to be discussed). The chest roentgenogram is typically normal, but the diagnosis is usually easy to make on clinical-epidemiologic grounds.

ASEPTIC MENINGITIS

Outbreaks of aseptic meningitis, which occur every summer in many developed countries, indicate widespread community transmission of one or more coxsackie- or echoviruses, reinforcing the importance of looking for other syndromes caused by the same viruses. Outbreaks of aseptic meningitis may also be seen in camps, schools, or sports teams. Enterovirus infections are among the most common causes of meningitis in the summer, causing both sporadic and epidemic cases. School-age children appear to be at greatest risk, although all ages may be affected, including infants. In older children or adults, onset of nausea, vomiting, irritability, and meningeal signs follows 2 to 3 days of prodromal illness, which is often nonspecific in nature. Infants may not have meningeal signs but may be irritable, may be disinterested in feeding, or may appear distressed. In severe infant infections, floppiness, hypotonia, pallor, and grunting respirations may appear. There is controversy over the degree to which enteroviral meningitis/encephalitis in infancy causes mental retardation. Especially with cases of aseptic meningitis caused by echoviruses, rash may be present (see Exanthem with Fever, already discussed).

Once the diagnosis is suspected on clinical-epidemiologic grounds, it can be confirmed by lumbar puncture, which usually reveals clear and colorless CSF, normal glucose, normal or slightly elevated protein, and moderate pleocytosis of mononuclear cells. Neutrophils may prevail early in the course of illness, but there is a rapid shift to mononuclear predominance. Many coxsackie- and echoviruses can be cultured from the CSF (to be discussed). It is more important to first rule out bacterial or partially treated bacterial meningitis, as well as mycobacterial, fungal, protozoal, and parasitic meningitis when these enter into the differential diagnosis. Also included in the differential diagnosis are other causes of viral meningitis. It is particularly important to consider arboviruses, since they are prevalent during the same season, may be associated with rash, and may appear clinically similar.

ENCEPHALITIS

There is much epidemiologic and clinical overlap between encephalitis and aseptic meningitis caused by coxsackie- and echoviruses. There is a tendency for enteroviral aseptic meningitis to be diagnosed in children and encephalitis in adults. Oftentimes patients will have evidence of both, e.g., meningeal signs, photophobia, mental dullness, somnolence, or clouded sensorium, confusion, or delirium. However, enterovirus encephalitis is normally not as severe as that associated with other viruses. There is rarely clinical evidence pointing to an enterovirus infection. The differential diagnosis includes herpes simplex encephalitis, for which treatment is available. Other neurologic abnormalities, including ataxia, are occasionally seen.

PARALYSIS

Many coxsackie- and echoviruses have been associated with paralytic disease similar to poliomyelitis. In fact, these other enteroviruses were first discovered by investigation of cases of paralysis thought to be due to polioviruses. History of completed trivalent poliovirus vaccination helps to rule out the diagnosis of poliomyelitis and suggests other enteroviruses. Cases are invariably sporadic. Onset and initial progression of disease mimics that of poliomyelitis: A prodrome of fever and constitutional symptoms lasting a day or two is followed by sudden onset of flaccid paralysis of one or more limbs over a period of 1 to 2 days. Bulbar involvement is rare, and the prognosis is considerably better than that of poliomyelitis, with complete recovery in most cases.

MYOCARDITIS AND PERICARDITIS

Enteroviral carditis is almost exclusively caused by coxsackie B viruses. There is a predominance of males at all ages, including infancy. (Infantile enteroviral carditis, which may be associated with multisystem disease, is discussed separately.) There is a predilection for myocarditis to occur in healthy young men. It is a rare complication of enterovirus infection seen sporadically in large community outbreaks in which other disease syndromes predominate.

Myocarditis is variable in onset. There may be 1 to 2 weeks of respiratory or other prodrome. Patients may present with fever, anxiety, radiating or nonradiating precordial pain, irregular cardiac rhythms, and signs and symptoms of congestive heart failure, including tachypnea, dyspnea, and orthopnea. The electrocardiogram (ECG) may indicate ischemia or even infarction. Reported findings include ST-T wave abnormalities, Q-T abnormalities, conduction defects such as partial or complete bundle branch block, ectopic atrial/ventricular beats, atrial flutter, fibrillation, and others. Creatine kinase (CK), lactate dehydrogenase (LD), and transaminases (SGOT, AST; SGPT, ALT), may all be elevated. The disease course is often prolonged, lasting weeks or even months. In some cases there is rapid deterioration and death as a result of infarction, arrhythmia, or failure.

Pericarditis (acute benign pericarditis) is caused by the same coxsackie B viruses that cause myocarditis. It is more commonly a disease of adults than of children, presenting with acute onset of fever and tachycardia. Diagnosis is usually made on the basis of clinical findings, including examination and ECG. Diagnosis may be made during evaluation of other symptoms, especially those of the respiratory tract, including pleurodynia and pleural effusion. Small pericardial effusions may occur. Spontaneous resolution is expected.

NEONATAL ENTEROVIRUS DISEASE

Infants are most susceptible to serious complications of enteroviral disease, particularly during the neonatal period. There is a spectrum of disease severity, ranging from inapparent infection, to illness with or without rash, to a fulminant course culminating in death. Most dramatic is a syndrome of severe neonatal disease, sometimes referred to colloquially as "viral sepsis." This condition usually appears on the second to twelfth days of life. Onset is often abrupt with irritability, refusal of feeding, and in some cases rash. The temperature may be normal, elevated, or decreased and is a poor indicator of infection in the neonatal period. Many organ systems may be involved, and thus a variety of signs and symptoms are possible. But given the infant's limited behavioral and physiologic repertoire, localizing signs may not be apparent despite the presence of meningitis, carditis, or other involvement. Myocarditis is likely to manifest as tachycardia, respiratory distress, weak cry, cyanosis, mottling, and organomegaly. Tachypnea and grunting respirations may supervene. Cerebrospinal fluid pleocytosis is typical. Signs of meningeal and cerebral involvement may overlap. Hepatitis and jaundice usually indicate multisystem involvement and a poor prognosis. The physician must not wait for localizing signs to appear. Signs of infectious and noninfectious diseases in neonates are rarely specific, and all such neonates must be hospitalized for a complete work-up.

Since it is usually impossible to rule out bacterial disease immediately, most neonates are started on antibiotic therapy after a lumbar puncture is done and appropriate bacterial cultures obtained. Although diagnosis of severe neonatal enterovirus disease can be made only by the virology laboratory, the physician may have a high index of suspicion if it is summer, if there is community enteroviral illness, particularly with coxsackie B viruses, and if there is history of illness in the mother or other family member. Occasionally, nosocomial outbreaks of enterovirus disease are seen, but these should not occur if there is adequate infection control.

In severe neonatal disease, the prognosis is poor. For neonates with mild illness, particularly those *not* caused by coxsackie B viruses, and for older infants, the prognosis is much better, with complete recovery to be expected.

CONJUNCTIVITIS

Mild conjunctivitis has occasionally been associated with several of the coxsackie- and echoviruses. Involvement may be unilateral or bilateral, is nonspecific, and resolves in a matter of days.

Acute hemorrhagic conjunctivitis is one of the most unique and recognizable of all the enterovirus syndromes. It appeared first in West Africa in the late 1960s, became pandemic in the 1970s, and first caused epidemics in the Western Hemisphere in 1981, when a major outbreak occurred in southern Florida, with smaller outbreaks elsewhere in the United States and Canada. An epidemic occurred in American Samoa the same year, and numerous imported cases from Oceania and South America were noted. Some of the same factors that make AHC such an unusual enterovirus syndrome are also those that make it of extreme importance to public health: high population susceptibility, extreme contagion, short incubation period, rapidity of spread, and presumed amenability to public health intervention, in which the physician may play a key role.

Acute hemorrhagic conjunctivitis occurs in epidemics and is typically associated with high attack rates. All age groups are affected, adults to a greater degree than in many other enterovirus syndromes. Once a household index case occurs, there may be rapid, complete intrafamily transmission. Intraschool transmission is to be expected unless school exclusion policies are instituted. There is more likely to be spread of AHC in crowded urban areas of low socioeconomic status and imperfect hygiene. Transmission is thought to occur by direct contact with infectious eye secretions either by means of the hands or by such fomites as towels and washcloths or bed linen. Transmission within the physician's office may be mediated by improperly cleaned instruments (e.g., tonometers). Nosocomial transmission can also occur.

The incubation period is shorter than for any other enterovirus, averaging about 24 hours, often as little as 12 hours. Onset is sudden, to the point of being precipitous. Patients may think they have suffered an acute foreign body injury. Most patients report profound irritation, foreign body sensation, pain, burning, redness, and swelling of the lids and periorbital soft tissues. Symptoms either begin bilaterally or rapidly become so. Subconjunctival hemorrhage is seen in greater than 95 per cent of patients, although some hemorrhages may be pinpoint in size. In other cases, there is dramatic crimson subconjunctival hemorrhage. Patients are remarkably free of extraocular signs and symptoms. There is rarely fever, coryza, or other evidence of contiguous spread. Severity becomes maximal within a day or so, then slowly resolves over 7 to 10 days.

Diagnosis during an epidemic need only be clinical. Almost all outbreaks have been associated with enterovirus type 70 (one of the newly discovered viruses not designated as either a coxsackie- or an echovirus). Others have been associated with a variant of coxsackievirus A24. Because enterovirus type 70, in particular, is difficult to culture in the laboratory, the clinical diagnosis is of major importance. When necessary, culture can be attempted from scrapings of fresh conjunctival cells. Cultures from tears are less desirable, and those of stool are of little value.

Complications include keratitis, which is rarely clinically significant. Although of no benefit, steroids do not cause rapid deterioration as they may with ocular herpes simplex infections. During the 1981 epidemic in Miami, Florida, there were a number of cases of secondary gonococcal and Proteus ophthalmitis resulting from the home remedy of instilling urine into the eyes. Certain epidemics of enterovirus type 70 have been associated with poliomyelitislike paralysis. This is thought to be a rare complication, on the order of less than 1 in 10,000 cases of conjunctivitis.

MISCELLANEOUS SYNDROMES

Epidemic *gastroenteritis* is not caused by enteroviruses. Some patients with enterovirus infection, especially children, may have nausea, vomiting, or diarrhea, typically as part of another enterovirus syndrome. Cases of diarrhea or vomiting seen in office pediatrics, likewise, are not normally caused by enteroviruses.

Hepatitis is only rarely caused by the well-characterized enteroviruses, except as part of multisystem disease in neonates. *Hepatitis A,* caused by the newly designated enterovirus type 72, is discussed in another article.

Acute enteroviral *pancreatitis* associated with the coxsackie B viruses occurs in persons of all ages. *Juvenile diabetes mellitus* has been linked epidemiologically, and occasionally by isolation, to various viruses, most notably coxsackievirus B4. However, the association is unproved. *Reye's syndrome* has also been linked to various enteroviruses by virtue of their isolation from affected patients. Such isolations are probably coincidental.

Other syndromes linked rarely or questionably to enteroviruses include sudden infant death syndrome (SIDS), glomerulonephritis, hemorrhagic and nonhemorrhagic cystitis, hemolytic-uremic syndrome, acute arthritis, orchitis, myositis, rhabdomyolysis, poly- and dermatomyositis, and lymphadenitis.

COXSACKIEVIRUS AND ECHOVIRUS INFECTIONS IN THE IMMUNOCOMPROMISED HOST

Persons with congenital or acquired immunodeficiency and those receiving steroids, immunosuppressive chemotherapy, and extensive radiation may be at increased risk of a serious outcome when infected with an enterovirus. Although relatively little is known about the typical course of enterovirus disease in such patients, persistent infections, including persistent CNS infections, have been noted, as have cases of polymyositislike and dermatomyositislike illnesses.

CYTOMEGALOVIRUS INFECTIONS

By Monto Ho, M.D.
Pittsburgh, Pennsylvania

The cytomegalovirus (CMV) of man has been found to cause an increasing number of different diseases in patients of all ages, whereas previously it had been thought exclusively to be the cause of a rare but fatal congenital syndrome. These include congenital cytomegalic inclusion disease (CID), spontaneous CMV mononucleosis (heterophile-negative mononucleosis), post-transfusion (CMV) mononucleosis, CMV infection in the immunosuppressed, and disseminated CMV infection. Involvement of specific organ systems may be called CMV pneumonitis, CMV retinitis, CMV hepatitis, and so on. Proper diagnosis requires familiarity with these disease syndromes and confirmation by appropriate laboratory examinations.

The one important characteristic of the biology of this virus—as well as all the other viruses of the herpesvirus group (herpes simplex types I and II, varicella zoster, and Epstein-Barr viruses—EBV)—is that they infect large segments of the population during early life without causing apparent disease. Hence, disease is an unusual manifestation of infection and one should always try to elicit host factors that may dispose the patient to disease.

CONGENITAL AND PERINATAL INFECTIONS

Congenital CID is the most severe form of congenital infection, which occurs in about 10 per cent of all infants who are infected in utero. In its florid form, the neonate is smaller than normal at birth and presents with jaundice, hepatosplenomegaly, a petechial rash, and involvement of multiple organs and systems. Microcephaly, motor disability, chorioretinitis, and cerebral calcifications may be seen. Congenital anomalies or defective development may occur in the central nervous system, but otherwise, unlike in the rubella syndrome, they are unusual. Immediately at birth or shortly thereafter, there may be lethargy, respiratory distress, convulsive seizures, and hemorrhagic phenomena associated with thrombocytopenia. The child may die shortly after birth. Survival may be complicated by microcephaly, mental retardation, and motor disability. Less severe infections may present only one or a few of the manifestations listed. It may be difficult to distinguish CID from other congenital or perinatal infections, particularly toxoplasmosis. Demonstration of the virus in urine, blood, or other tissues is essential for diagnosis.

Most congenitally infected infants are apparently normal at birth, but some may develop symptoms later in life. Failure to thrive and pneumonitis resulting from CMV may occur within a few months, and evidence of hepatitis may arise years later. Irreversible liver disease is unusual. More insidious and irreversible are neurologic sequelae that may not be detected until school age. The most important are unilateral or bilateral neural hearing loss and mild mental retardation characterized by low or borderline I.Q.

Neonates may also be infected by the mother perinatally, i.e., during birth or by outside sources shortly after birth. The most important cause of serious postnatal infection is transmission of CMV to neonates by exchange transfusion with blood containing CMV. Symptomatic disease and death may result. Otherwise most perinatal infections are usually asymptomatic. Some authors believe that the transmission of CMV by blood to neonates may be prevented by the use of blood from seronegative donors.

INFECTIONS IN THE NORMAL SUBJECT: CMV MONONUCLEOSIS

Symptomatic CMV infection may occur in normal children and adults. Cytomegalovirus mononucleosis in adults may be clinically indistinguishable from EBV or heterophile-positive mononucleosis. Not all heterophile-negative mononucleosis is caused by CMV. Other causes are EBV and toxoplasmosis.

Cytomegalovirus mononucleosis has the following distinguishing features. It occurs later in life than EBV mononucleosis, usually at age 25 to 35. It is not associated with severe pharyngitis or lymphadenopathy. The clinical hallmarks are prolonged fever, lymphocytosis or lymphopenia with atypical lymphocytes, and hepatitis. The latter may be asymptomatic except for mild elevations of serum SGOT (AST) and SGPT (ALT) levels. Jaundice and marked hepatomegaly are uncommon. The liver biopsy may show noncaseating granulomas, indistinguishable from those of tuberculosis or sarcoid. Other less common manifestations are skin rashes, which may be associated with ampicillin administration; pneumonitis; conjunctivitis; myocarditis; thrombocytopenia; hemolytic anemia; aseptic meningitis; encephalitis; and chorioretinitis. The Guillain-Barré syndrome is thought to be a sequela to some CMV infections. The course of most CMV infections is benign, and recovery is usually complete.

The history should include an attempt to identify a source of infection, although "spontaneous" cases are not unusual. Multiple transfusions of blood or leukocytes, particularly over 10 units, are an important source of infection. Cytomegalovirus mononucleosis can occur after any major surgical procedure if associated with multiple transfusions. It has been described in patients after surgery for trauma, abdominal operations, open heart surgery, or organ transplantation. It is an important cause of postoperative fever of unknown origin.

Another source of infection is related to the sexual habits of the patient. Cytomegalovirus infection is probably transmitted by intimate oral contact, heterosexual intercourse, and male homosexual intercourse, particularly of the passive genital-anal type. The acquired immunodeficiency syndrome (AIDS), particularly common in male homosexuals, may be associated with CMV infection. It is not clear which part of the syndrome, if any, is due to CMV. It may be involved in producing the inanition, fever, leukopenia, reversed T helper lymphocyte over T suppressor lymphocyte ratio, immunosuppression, or Kaposi's sarcoma. It is also not clear whether these patients with AIDS have primary, repeated, or reactivated infections. Reactivated infections are dormant, latent infections in the host that become active. In AIDS, CMV and pneumocystis may act synergistically to cause *interstitial pneumonia* (discussed next; see also the article on AIDS).

INFECTIONS IN THE IMMUNOSUPPRESSED

Cytomegalovirus infection occurs in practically all patients approximately 2 to 3 months after major organ transplantation. Most cases represent latent infections that have been activated by iatrogenic immunosuppressive measures. Primary or *de novo* infections may be transmitted by the grafted organ, such as the kidney or heart. In most patients, the infection is asymptomatic. Cytomegalovirus infection is also common in patients on cytotoxic chemotherapy or in those receiving any cytotoxic immunosuppressant such as azathioprine, cyclophosphamide, and methotrexate. Cyclosporine also predisposes to CMV infection.

Symptomatic disease is more common after primary infections and in patients who are more severely immunosuppressed. Hence, the proportion of symptomatic patients may vary from 10 to 60 per cent of all those infected. The clinical picture may be the same as that described for CMV mononucleosis. In the more severely affected, CMV infection may not be associated with any atypical lymphocytes and lymphopenia rather than lymphocytosis is more common. Fever and mild hepatitis are almost invariable features. Complications are more common and more severe. Pneumonitis, retinitis, ulcerations in the gastrointestinal tract that may produce bleeding, or disseminated disease may occur. In the marrow transplant recipient, CMV pneumonitis is a particularly serious problem, often associated with a graft-versus-host reaction and death.

Cytomegalovirus pneumonitis is more likely to show an *interstitial* than an *alveolar* pattern. Nodules and even cavities demonstrable by x-ray may occur. Respiratory complaints are usually of less than 2 weeks' duration. Fever, nonproductive cough, and dyspnea with hypoxia may be present. Hypoxia is a poor prognostic sign. The clinical picture may be difficult to distinguish from bacterial, fungal, and particularly pneumocystis pneumonia. Indeed, in many cases of CMV pneumonitis in this group of patients, one or more of these agents may be present together with CMV. In the marrow transplant recipient, the pulmonary manifestations of a graft-versus-host reaction may also obscure the picture. Isolation of the virus from lung tissue is necessary for definite diagnosis.

Cytomegalovirus retinitis may be asymptomatic and discovered only by funduscopic examination. Or the patient may complain of blurred vision, decreased visual acuity, or scotomata in one or both eyes. The course is frequently progressive and irreversible. Most cases have occurred in transplant patients, often beyond the first 3 months after surgery. There are in the fundi white, granular necrotic patches that may be superimposed on flame-shaped intraretinal hemorrhages. Vascular sheathing may be a poor prognostic sign. The lesions begin in the periphery of the retina but may eventually involve central vision. Remissions and relapses are common. Diagnosis is usually circumstantial, i.e., a compatible funduscopic picture and laboratory evidence of systemic infection elsewhere.

LABORATORY DIAGNOSIS

Disease due to CMV cannot be diagnosed without laboratory aid. The simplest and quickest laboratory test is demonstration of the virus in urine, blood buffy coat, or throat. This is done by culturing the virus in human fibroblast cell cultures. Results may be available in 5 days, but usually 1 or 2 weeks are required, depending on the amount of virus in the sample. Congenital infection is diagnosed by demonstration of viruria immediately after birth. This may be done by inoculation of cell cultures or by electron microscopy, which is less time consuming. Virus cultured 1 month or more after birth may represent postnatally acquired infection. The presence of virus in the urine, blood, or throat in an adult with a clinical picture consistent with CMV mononucleosis is usually sufficient for diagnosis. Asymptomatic carriers among normal subjects may confuse the picture, but such carriers are rare after childhood. Some male homosexuals, immunosuppressed patients, or pregnant women may have asymptomatic viruria. Culture of the virus has been found to be more sensitive than anatomic diagnosis, whether in the lung or other tissue, and it is also more sensitive than looking for inclusion-bearing cells in urine.

The presence of serum IgM antibodies against CMV demonstrable by immunofluorescence is an indication of acute, active, or persistent infection. It is, however, neither entirely sensitive nor specific. False-positive tests may occur in the presence of rheumatoid factor. IgM antibodies may persist for varying lengths of time after infection. In adults, IgM antibodies may occur after a primary initial infection or after a reactivated infection in immunosuppressed patients.

Demonstration of a rise in IgG antibodies by an immunofluorescent or complement fixation test is reliable evidence of an active infection. The problem is that demonstration of a rise requires examination of a late convalescent serum and the results may be too late to be clinically relevant. A single titer of IgG antibodies is usually worthless, since most adults are seropositive. Even a high titer does not necessarily mean active infection because quantitation of titers is poorly standardized in diagnostic laboratories. Antibody rises are demonstrable in practically all types of postnatal CMV infections and occur even in immunosuppressed patients, since most immunosuppressive drugs do not prevent antibody synthesis. However, severe infections in such patients may occur without an antibody rise. The absence of a response is prognostic of a poor outcome.

Antibody responses also occur in transplacental and perinatal infections. The presence of specific IgM antibodies against CMV in cord blood is useful in the diagnosis of transplacental infections, but the presence of IgM antibodies is not as specific or sensitive as virus isolation. Antibody rises in neonates may also be obscured by passively transferred maternal antibody. Hence, serologic diagnosis in the first months of life may be difficult. If the mother is seronegative, the presence of antibody in a neonate may indicate a postnatal infection, particularly if a rise in titer can be shown.

The distinction between a primary *de novo* infection and a reactivated latent infection in patients who show a serologic rise requires examination of a serum sample before infection. This may not always be available. Primary infections occur in initially seronegative subjects.

VIRAL DIARRHEA

By Philip C. Johnson, M.D.
and Herbert L. DuPont, M.D.
Houston, Texas

In the last 10 years, viral agents have been recognized as a major cause of acute gastroenteritis worldwide. Rotaviruses are the most important agents in wintertime diarrhea of infants and children under the age of 3 years, and they may account for as much as 10 per cent of travelers' diarrhea. Norwalk agent and other Norwalk-like agents have been associated with waterborne, foodborne, and person to person–transmitted outbreaks in all ages. Other viral agents, including coronavirus, minireovirus, adenovirus and calicivirus, have been associated with gastroenteritis based on finding the viral particles in feces using electron microscopy. Their overall importance remains to be determined.

ROTAVIRUS

Rotavirus is a double-stranded RNA virus, approximately 70 nm in diameter, with an outer capsule morphologically resembling a wheel with radiating capsomeres for spokes. Initially referred to as orbivirus, duovirus, and a reovirus-like agent, it is now known as a distinct genus in the family Reoviridiae.

Rotaviruses have been identified in a wide range of mammalian species. The Nebraska calf diarrhea virus (NCDV) strain has been designated the reference strain because it is related immunologically to human rotavirus and, in contrast to the human agent, is easily propagated on tissue culture.

Viral diarrhea caused by rotavirus is most common in children 6 months to 2 years of age. It occurs during the winter months in temperate zones and with predominance during the rainy season in the tropics. Adult contacts of ill children usually have asymptomatic infections, but overt illness in adults has been described. The role of breastfeeding in protecting infants from the disease has been strongly suggested but is not yet proven. From animal studies and intestinal biopsies in children, the sites of infection of rotavirus are the duodenum and the proximal small bowel. Diarrhea is presumably caused by the loss of the absorptive ability of the small intestine secondary to observed inflammatory cell infiltration of the lamina propia with alteration of the mucosa, shortening of the villi, and hyperplasia of the intestinal crypts. Loss of brush border disaccharidases occurs, but there is no change in adenyl cyclase activity.

After an incubation period of 2 to 4 days, vomiting and watery diarrhea occur in afflicted children. Occasionally, vomiting is the only clinical symptom. Fever occurs in over 50 per cent of patients. The illness lasts 5 to 7 days with diarrhea generally persisting longer than vomiting when both are present. Viral shedding in the feces is greatest on the third and fourth day of the illness and continues throughout the symptomatic period. Fecal-oral spread accounts for further infections among close family members.

Since the small bowel is affected and the inflammatory lesion is limited, fecal leukocyte determination is negative when stools are examined microscopically employing a methylene blue stain. Diagnosis can be established by several methods, including counterimmunoelectrophoresis, radioimmunoassay, fluorescent virus precipitin testing, and electron microscopy. Enzyme-linked immunosorbent assay (ELISA) methods, including a commercially available kit (Rotazyme), are clinically the most useful because of their simplicity, convenience, and high sensitivity. A similar ELISA method has more recently been developed for the diagnosis of enteric adenovirus.

There are a multiple but limited number of rotavirus strains that are pathogenic for man. High serum antibody titers to one rotavirus type may not be protective against infection with like or different types. For this reason, and from adult volunteer studies in which jejunal IgA levels were measured, it is speculated that secretory type-specific IgA antibody in the small intestine may be the best protection against rotavirus infection. Efforts at developing an effective oral vaccine against rotavirus are presently under way.

NORWALK AND OTHER NORWALK-LIKE AGENTS

Although Norwalk agent was the first well-characterized viral particle shown to be commonly associated with diarrhea, less is known about the epidemiology and biologic properties of this agent than for those of rotavirus. The Norwalk agent is a small, round, nonenveloped particle, 27 nm in diameter, isolated originally from an outbreak of gastroenteritis in elementary school children in Norwalk, Ohio. Antigenetically dissimilar particles, 26 to 27 nm in diameter, were later found in outbreaks in several areas, including Hawaii; Montgomery County, Maryland; and Snow Mountain, Colorado, in the United States and Dichling and Cockle in England. These agents are described as Norwalk-like, although it is unknown whether their genome is composed of RNA or DNA.

In contrast to rotavirus, the Norwalk agent and other Norwalk-like agents cause isolated outbreaks of gastroenteritis. The Norwalk agent is the best studied. It was shown to have been involved in 42 per cent of 74 outbreaks of acute nonbacterial gastroenteritis investigated by the Centers for Disease Control from 1976 to 1980. These studies relied on a radioimmunoassay of paired sera that measured antibody to the Norwalk agent. Most of the reported outbreaks of Norwalk illness were waterborne where water supplies and swimming pools became contaminated. Chlorination may not have prevented the outbreaks. Foodborne outbreaks have been related to raw oysters and salads. The outbreaks have occurred year-round in both children and adults.

Disease in animals caused by these agents has not been described, but in volunteer studies with Norwalk and Hawaii agent, the virus was shown to infect the proximal small bowel, leading to pathologic changes similar to those seen with rotavirus infection. Brush border enzymes are decreased, but levels of adenyl cyclase remain unchanged. Diarrhea is probably caused by malabsorption and vomiting by virus-induced reduction in gastric emptying.

The incubation period in outbreaks and in volunteer studies is 1 to 2 days. Symptoms range from vomiting with or without diarrhea, usually in children, to diarrhea alone in adults. Low-grade fever, abdominal cramps, malaise, and headache may also be present. Symptoms last for 1 or 2 days. Although the primary mode of spread is fecal-oral, respiratory spread may occur.

The diagnosis of Norwalk illness should be suspected whenever there is an outbreak of gastroenteritis in a relatively closed population such as a school, church camp, or even a community-wide epidemic.

Fecal leukocyte determination is negative. The diagnosis can be made from paired sera using Norwalk agent RIA or by immunoelectronmicroscopy of fecal filtrates. These tests are available only in a few research centers. Cell culture of the Norwalk-like agents so far has been unsuccessful and an ELISA method is unavailable.

Local jejunal IgA production may be important in acquiring immunity to Norwalk illness, but this remains to be proved. In volunteer studies, experimental infection resulted in resistance to reinfection for at least 14 weeks. Infection with Norwalk agent is protective against infection with the Montgomery County agent and vice versa, but does not protect against infection with the Hawaii agent. Further understanding of these agents awaits their classification and propagation.

VIRAL HEMORRHAGIC FEVERS

By K. M. Johnson, M.D.
and C. J. Peters, M.D.*
Frederick, Maryland

At least 15 membrane-bound RNA viruses are known to cause the syndrome of acute hemorrhagic fever. All but one are exotic to North America; therefore, the critical step in recognizing them is to take a detailed travel history from any patient returning from abroad who presents with fever of unknown origin or with fever and bleeding manifestations. As a practical guide, these diseases, their geographic and ecologic localization, and their estimated incubation periods are given in Table 1. Except for hemorrhagic fever (HF) with renal syndrome, a travel history for the 3 weeks prior to onset will account for possible acquisition of all of these diseases.

SYNONYMS

With the isolation and characterization of specific etiologic agents, former synonyms for these syndromes have largely disappeared. An exception is hemorrhagic fever with renal syndrome (HFRS), which has been described in many countries and languages. Terms for this condition still in common use are hemorrhagic nephrosonephritis, epidemic hemorrhagic fever, Korean hemorrhagic fever, and nephropathia epidemica.

PRESENTING SIGNS AND SYMPTOMS

Many of the viral hemorrhagic fevers (VHF) present in a similar rather nonspecific manner, and thus initial clinical manifestations are usually not helpful in making a specific diagnosis. Significant or pronounced departures from this general picture will be given in individual disease descriptions. Acute onset of fever, headache, and severe, usually generalized myalgia are the rule. A flushed face, neck, and upper trunk and conjunctivitis are common features that indicate early vascular involvement; nausea, vomiting, and/or diarrhea may be present.

THERAPEUTIC TESTS

There are no specific therapeutic tests for any of the forms of VHF; moreover, therapy itself is almost completely supportive and centers on management of fluid and electrolyte balance, prevention and treatment of shock, treatment of coagulation disorders, and therapy for secondary bacterial infection. An exception is Argentine hemorrhagic fever (AHF) (and presumably Bolivian hemorrhagic fever—BHF), in which administration of convalescent human plasma has been shown to dramatically reduce mortality.

In most instances of VHF, conventional management of shock is indicated, with the understanding that (1) hypovolemia from vascular leakage is a common phenomenon but is the overriding consideration only in dengue hemorrhagic fever (DHF) and severe cases of HFRS, and (2) myocardial and other circulatory defects impose important limitations on vigorous fluid administration.

Hemorrhage per se is rarely life-threatening, and blood transfusion is not usually required. The exception is Congo-Crimean hemorrhagic fever (CCHF). Thrombocytopenia is usual in patients with an overt bleeding diathesis. Limited data on coagulation factors fail to establish specific defects, and available evidence suggests that disseminated intravascular coagulation (DIC) is not a fundamental mechanism in many VHF but may be important in Marburg-Ebola (M-E) HF and possibly in CCHF. In these diseases, heparinization may be cautiously undertaken; replacement therapy has never been evaluated but would be reasonable for patients pursuing an unfavorable course.

POTENTIAL ERRORS AND PITFALLS IN DIAGNOSIS

The differential diagnosis of viral hemorrhagic fevers presents two distinct problems. One is distinguishing among possible VHF agents in patients who have visited areas where more than one such agent is endemic. Tropical Africa, where at least five distinct agents are present (Table 1), is the continent of greatest concern. Agents related to the virus causing HFRS may be found throughout the world, adding this possibility to individual geographic candidates. The second problem centers in distinguishing among other causes of syndromes similar to viral hemorrhagic fever that might be found anywhere in the world. These include malaria (a given patient might have malaria and VHF), typhus, spotted fever group rickettsiae, leptospirosis (Weil's disease), typhoid or paratyphoid fever, meningococcemia, acute leukemia, idiopathic thrombocytopenia, viral hepatitis, and a variety of conditions in which the unusual patient exhibits acute signs of damage to the hepatic and/or vascular-coagulation systems. We have been asked repeatedly to perform viral studies on material from patients living in the United States who developed severe illnesses clinically resembling VHF but have never incriminated any of the known agents.

INDIVIDUAL VIRAL HEMORRHAGIC FEVERS

Yellow Fever (YF)

Definition. A mosquitoborne disease presently limited to tropical and rural portions of Africa and South America.

*The views of the authors do not purport to reflect the positions of the Department of the Army or the Department of Defense.

Table 1. Parameters of Viral Hemorrhagic Fevers (VHF) Pertinent to Travel Histories of Febrile Patients Who Are Possibly Infected

Disease	Geographic Region	Ecology	Incubation Period (days)
Yellow fever (YF)	Tropical South America and Africa	Sylvan; forests and savannahs	3–6
Dengue HF (DHF)	Tropical SE Asia, Pacific Islands, Cuba	Urban; young children most affected	2–5
Argentine HF (AHF)	Argentina; parts of Buenos Aires, Cordoba, Santa Fe Provinces	Rural agricultural corn harvest; mostly males	7–14
Bolivian HF (BHF)	Foci in eastern Beni Province, Bolivia	Rural but house associated; both sexes affected equally	7–14
Lassa fever (LF)	West Africa, Senegal to Nigeria	Rural but house associated; hospital transmission occurs	5–16
Marburg-Ebola HF (M-E)	Central and East Africa; wider on continent (?)	Rural; primary transmission unknown; person-person important	7–16
Congo-Crimean HF (CCHF)	Southern USSR to Pakistan, SW China, Middle East, much of Africa	Rural; close association with large domestic animals	2–7
Kyasanur Forest disease (KFD)	Western India, focal	Rural; man-modified forests	3–8
Omsk HF (OHF)	NW Siberia	Rural agriculture, winter muskrat associated cases	3–8
Hemorrhagic fever renal syndrome (HFRS)	Asia, Europe, Scandinavia world-wide (?)	Rural; urban (Rattus); laboratory rats	10–40

Abbreviations: HF = Hemorrhagic fever.

Presenting Signs and Symptoms. Relative bradycardia, vomiting frequent.

Course. Highly variable. Many patients experience no progression of disease; they have mild elevations of hepatic enzyme levels, and they convalesce rapidly. Others pursue one of two courses: fulminating toxemia with gastrointestinal hemorrhage, shock and death; or progressive hepatic damage without shock, which leads to clinical jaundice and, after resolution of fever, to serious but reversible renal tubular failure.

Physical Examination. Flushed face, bradycardia, anxious, "toxic" appearance. Evidence for capillary leak syndrome; petechiae; gum bleeding; other hemorrhages from membranes. Epigastric tenderness *without* organomegaly. Usually no pulmonary signs, narrowed pulse pressure, jaundice by fifth day of illness.

Laboratory Procedures. Lymphopenia followed by lymphocytosis, thrombocytopenia, prothrombin and partial thromboplastin time prolongation, fibrin split products. The SGOT (AST) to $>$ 2000 U/liter; the SGPT (ALT) lower; bilirubin, direct and indirect, to 20 mg/dl; albuminuria to 5 gm/liter or greater; BUN $>$ 100 mg/dl late.

Diagnostic Procedures. Virus isolation from blood, first 5 days; specific IgM antibodies, day 6 onward.

Pitfalls in Diagnosis. Individual cases of yellow fever originating in Africa might be confused with Lassa fever (LF), Marburg (MBG), or Ebola (EBO) hemorrhagic fever, Rift Valley fever (RVF), or CCHF. Occurrence of jaundice is common only in YF and RVF.

Dengue Hemorrhagic Fever

Definition. A mosquitoborne disease affecting mainly children in the urban tropics of southeast Asia and, more recently, Cuba.

Presenting Signs and Symptoms. Fever, nausea, vomiting. Depending on severity and duration of illness, there may be dehydration, narrow pulse pressure, petechiae, or coffee-ground vomitus.

Physical Examination. Petechiae on face, axillae, upper chest. Slight hepatomegaly. Skin may be dry and hot, or in shock it may be very damp, cool, and mottled brownish. Edema of face and hands may be present.

Course. A shock crisis due to severe capillary leak syndrome 3 to 5 days after onset of illness represents the major clinical challenge. It usually occurs abruptly and lasts no more than one day. Convalescence is rapid.

Laboratory Procedures. Relative lymphocytosis with normal or elevated white blood cell (WBC) count is common. Hemoconcentration (hematocrit to 50 or greater) and hypoalbuminemia (total protein $<$ 6.5 gm/dl) occur prior to onset of shock, and there is thrombocytopenia ($<$100,000 per cu mm) and albuminuria (1 to 5 gm/liter). Complement is activated through the classical pathway, and C_3 split products circulate during the shock crisis. There may be mild

Table 2. Some Significant Differences in Clinical Course of Arenaviral Hemorrhagic Fever Seen in New World (AHF–BHF) and Old World (LF) Infections

	Onset	Fever Duration	Hepatitis	Neurologic Signs	Bleeding	Shock	Other Findings
AHF–BHF	Insidious	5–10	Very mild	Major*	Very common	Common	Moderate renal impairment
LF	Insidious	7–20	Variable, often major	Minor†	Unusual (15%)	Not common	Many; eighth nerve deafness, pericarditis, pleural, other effusions

*Encephalopathy; may be severe but no direct virus invasion.
†Meningitis; uncommon but there is virus invasion of brain.
Abbreviations: AHF–BFH = Argentine and Bolivian hemorrhagic fever; LF = Lassa fever.

elevations of SGOT, but there is never jaundice; the rapid convalescence indicates that little damage to hepatic parenchyma occurs.

Diagnostic Procedures. When first seen, most patients have very high dengue virus antibodies and they may have specific IgM antibodies. Virus isolation is very difficult, probably because most patients are experiencing at least second-degree dengue infection.

Pitfalls in Diagnosis. The major pitfall is meningococcemia. Another is believing that a patient returning from endemic areas has DHF on the basis of fever plus a positive tourniquet test. Dengue hemorrhagic fever is almost never seen among travelers, but *dengue fever* is.

Arenaviral Disease

Definition. Three rodent-borne diseases are caused by distinct members of the arenavirus family. These are Argentine hemorrhagic fever (AHF), caused by Junin virus; Bolivian hemorrhagic fever (BHF), which is due to Machupo virus infection; and Lassa fever (LF), attributed to Lassa virus. Epidemiology is determined by the behavior of the individual and of specific rodents, which are chronically infected and transmit the viruses by shedding them into the environment in urine. All three are rural infections. Rodents transmitting BHF and LF come into contact with the population most often in or near human dwellings, whereas Junin virus is acquired in the extensive corn cultivars of Argentina.

Presenting Signs and Symptoms. Insidious onset. Severe myalgia often with low back or substernal accentuation. Conjunctivitis, strong facial and upper trunk blush.

Physical Examination. Few specific findings; organomegaly rare. Pneumonitis, pleural effusion, pericardial effusion with friction rub may be seen with LF. Pharyngitis initially emphasized in LF descriptions is neither a constant feature nor a specific enough feature to be of diagnostic value. Also eighth nerve deafness, unilateral or bilateral, occurs in about 5 per cent of LF patients.

Clinical Course. Very similar for AHF or BHF; distinct for LF (Table 2). Six to 10 days after symptoms begin, the former pursues either a course marked by shock and hemorrhage or a central nervous form beginning with intention tremors, dysarthria, and inability to swallow, proceeding to generalized clonic and tonic convulsions and death. Cerebrospinal fluids (CSF), however, are normal. Mixtures of these two forms may be seen. Convalescence usually takes several weeks.

Lassa fever is a more protracted disease. Fever may continue for 2 to 3 weeks. There is much greater damage to hepatic parenchyma and lungs; heart and kidneys may be affected. A maculopapular rash may be present during the first week. Many patients do experience a hypovolemic, mildly hemorrhagic shock crisis, but many more do not. Convalescence is also slow in LF.

Common Complications. All three diseases are immunosuppressive, and secondary bacterial infections, particularly of the lungs, are both common and life-threatening.

Laboratory Procedures. See Table 3 for a differential summary.

Diagnostic Procedures. Virus isolation from blood is the only practical measure for AHF and BHF; in the latter, a majority of specimens are negative and daily samples are thus important. Antibodies are not detectable until the patient is well into convalescence. Most Lassa patients develop specific IgM antibodies during acute illness, and 30 to 40 per cent show positive results on admission. Viremia is common, and severely ill patients have antigenemia detectable by enzyme immunoassay.

Potential Errors and Pitfalls. Hemorrhagic forms of AHF and BHF should present little diagnostic problem if careful attention is paid to geographic travel history. Neurologic forms, however, may be confused with a variety of other acute conditions, principally viral encephalitis. Cerebrospinal fluid findings should sort this problem.

Lassa fever, in contrast, may be confused with other West African hemorrhagic fevers such as nonicteric cases of YF and RVF. Lassa fever is such a protean disease that it may be attributed to many other agents. Malaria, typhoid fever, tuberculosis, and acute urinary tract infection are four of the favorites named by West African physicians. Fever, plus a history of residence or travel in rural West Africa, should raise suspicion of this disease.

Table 3. Clinical Pathologic Findings in Argentine-Bolivian Hemorrhagic Fever and in Lassa Fever

	Leukopenia	Platelets↓	Hemo-concentration	Coagulation Factors	Urine Protein	CPK GOT	Bilirubin	CSF
AHF–BHF	Pronounced (< 2000)	Reduced (< 100,000)	Significant (Hct > 48)	Mild changes; DIC very rare	Abnormal (1–5 gm)	Normal to slight elevations		Normal
LF	Unusual; normal count usually	Low normal (> 100,000)	Significant in less than 20% (Hct > 45)	Not sufficiently studied	Abnormal (1–5 gm)	Greatly elevated (> 2000 CPK > GOT)	Slight increase	WBC; increased protein; virus present

Abbreviations: AHF–BHF = Argentine and Bolivian hemorrhagic fever; LF = Lassa fever; Hct = hematocrit; CPK = creatine phosphokinase; GOT = glutamic oxaloacetic transaminase; CSF = cerebrospinal fluid; WBC = white blood cell; DIC = disseminated intravascular coagulation.

Rift Valley Fever

Definition. This is a mosquitoborne, contact, or aerosol-transmitted disease of domestic livestock and humans in sub-Saharan Africa. A major epizootic-epidemic occurred in highly susceptible animal and human populations in Egypt, 1977–78.

Presenting Signs and Symptoms. Typically nonspecific.

Clinical Course. Typically, the patient has highest temperature (to 40°C) and feels worst on the first day of illness. All signs and symptoms usually subside within 2 to 4 days.

Physical Examination. Unremarkable. Conjunctival injection may be present.

Complications. Three principal complications have been recognized. Although definitive data are lacking, it is believed that none of these occurs in more than 1 per cent of infections. The most severe is hemorrhagic diathesis with severe hepatic injury. This syndrome—marked by major clotting defects, probable DIC, and jaundice—emerges during the febrile period and has a poor prognosis.

Two other complications occur several days after the patient has become afebrile. One is acute retinitis, which has been shown to be the product of a sclerosing vasculitis. Depending on the area of the retina involved, there may be significant unilateral or bilateral loss of vision, which may be temporary (edema) or permanent (infarction and scarring). The other late manifestation is acute encephalitis with confusion, meningismus, paresis, and convulsions. There is cerebrospinal fluid pleocytosis, protein elevation, and extremely high antiviral antibody level but no detectable virus. Death may ensue, or there is variable slow recovery, often with significant mental and motor residua.

Laboratory Procedures. In uncomplicated cases, leukocytes are usually normal or there is acute lymphopenia. Hemorrhagic cases show evidence of major acute hepatic injury: elevated transaminases, bilirubin, and alkaline phosphatase; thrombocytopenia, increased prothrombin time, and other coagulation defects are also present. Retinitis patients apparently have no abnormal clinical pathology, and encephalitis patients display only CSF abnormalities. More than a single complication has not been observed in a given patient.

Diagnosis. Most patients experience high viremia for 2 to 4 days, permitting ready isolation of RVF virus or detection of antigenemia by enzyme immunoassay (EIA). Retinitis and encephalitis patients have serologic evidence of recent RVF infection (rising antibody titers or presence of serum IgM by IFA or EIA).

Pitfalls and Errors in Diagnosis. Other potential causes of HF in Africa are brought to mind. The hemorrhagic form might also be confused with delta-hepatitis B virus infection. Leptospirosis and herpes encephalitis in the neurologic disease form may be confusing. Interestingly, there is no serious arbovirus encephalitis described from Africa. Untreated cerebral falciparum malaria is a critical diagnostic differential.

Marburg and Ebola Fevers (Green Monkey Disease)

Definition. These are clinically indistinguishable viral diseases with unknown natural reservoir and transmission to man. Cases with high mortality have been recognized in Central, East, and South Africa and on one occasion in Germany and Yugoslavia, where transmission was traced to infected monkeys imported from Uganda. These diseases have a significant rate of transmission from patients to providers of medical care.

Presenting Signs and Symptoms. Usually nonspecific; dry cough prominent in a minority of patients.

Physical Examination. Most patients exhibit few signs or symptoms of diagnostic value. Bradycardia is common, as is a flushed, agitated "toxic" appearance. A characteristic maculopapular rash occurs during the course of Marburg disease and in some patients during the course of Ebola HF.

Clinical Course. Illness is marked by an inexorable progression of pathologic damage to multiple organs. Chemical hepatitis, usually without jaundice, is pronounced. Petechiae and mucous membrane hemorrhages appear. Protracted vomiting and intense epigastric pain have been accompanied by hyperamylasemia, although reduced renal clearance complicates interpretation. Finally, at the end of about 1 week, hypovolemic shock, accompanied by purpura and uncontrollable bleeding from venipuncture sites, occurs and is usually followed by death. Mortality from Marburg infection averages 30 per cent and, in three separate Ebola fever outbreaks, ranged from 55 to 90 per cent!

Laboratory Findings. Leukocyte counts are normal or sometimes depressed throughout illness, but thrombocytopenia is almost always present by the third day of disease. Coagulation parameters have been measured in only a few patients, but fibrin split products have been found late in the course of disease, strongly suggesting that DIC is at least a terminal event.

Liver transaminase elevations to 1000 to 2000 U/liter are common, but bilirubin levels are normal or only slightly elevated. Amylase levels may be elevated but are rarely above 800 U/liter. The urine may contain 1 gm/liter of albumin or more, accompanied by tubular casts and microscopic hematuria. Urea nitrogen may be increased as well but rarely rises to 100 mg/dl.

Diagnostic Procedures. Most patients are highly viremic throughout the course of illness, and isolation of the agent from blood is a simple if hazardous procedure. Virus-specific antibodies rarely appear until after the acute crisis is weathered.

Pitfalls and Errors in Diagnosis. These are mainly the other forms of HF of Africa, but prominent abdominal pain and diarrhea may lead to erroneous diagnosis of acute gastroenteritis. Travel history should help. Unless the patient has visited West Africa, Lassa fever is unlikely. A yellow fever outbreak would likely be known either to the patient or to national public health authorities. Other diseases leading to confusion are similar to those discussed for Rift Valley Fever.

Congo-Crimean Hemorrhagic Fever

Definition. Congo-Crimean hemorrhagic fever is a tickborne disease, occasionally transmitted by aerosols or fomites. It occurs in rural areas of southern portions of the Soviet Union, neighboring China, Pakistan, the Middle East, and Africa. Major foci of infection with annual occurrence of cases are best documented in the Soviet Union. About one in six human infections is clinically apparent, and the mortality is about 20 per cent.

Presenting Signs and Symptoms. After a 1-week incubation period, abrupt onset of fever and other nonspecific signs occur, including vomiting and diarrhea.

Physical Examination. Bradycardia and conjunctival suffusion are common. Hepatomegaly occurs in about half of cases, splenomegaly rarely.

Clinical Course. Bleeding manifestations appear about day 4 of illness and usually progress. Fine petechiae appear and often develop into frank *purpura hemorrhagica,* particularly over pressure points. The nose, the gums, the vagina, and especially the gastrointestinal tract are the main sites of hemorrhage, which at times may be life-threatening per se, a condition observed otherwise only in occasional VHF patients. Secondary bacterial pneumonia is common. A fatal outcome, generally between 8 to 12 days after onset, is heralded by either neurologic signs, such as stiff neck and coma, or by hypovolemic shock coincident with lysis of fever. Convalescence is protracted, and occasional patients suffer from chronic peripheral neuritis.

Laboratory Procedures. Panleukopenia and thrombocytopenia are nearly universal and may be severe (< 2000 WBC and 50,000 platelets). Transaminases are usually elevated and may exceed 2000 U/liter; in rare cases, there is bilirubin elevation sufficient to produce mild clinical jaundice. Renal function is generally preserved until shock occurs, but generous amounts of albumin are present along with microscopic hematuria. Coagulation parameters have not been measured, except for prothrombin time, which is increased. Although not proven, DIC may occur late in the course of severe illness.

Diagnostic Procedures. Isolation of virus from blood of patients during the initial 4 days of symptoms is the only proven method for specific diagnosis. Survivors do not produce detectable antibodies for 1 to 2 weeks after fever abates.

Pitfalls and Errors in Diagnosis. These are largely as outlined for RVF. In addition, one should exercise caution in relying on urban-versus-rural epidemiology of this disease. Important vector ticks of CCHF parasitize domestic animals that may be quartered or brought to market in the heart of large cities; these ticks are long-lived and may crawl considerable distances in search of a host.

Kyasanur Forest Disease (KFD) and Omsk Hemorrhagic Fever (OHF)

Definition. These are clinically similar syndromes caused by closely related tickborne flaviviruses. They occur in circumscribed areas of western India and western Siberia, respectively. Hemorrhagic manifestations of infection are generally mild, and both agents have high infectivity-to-disease ratios.

Presenting Signs and Symptoms. No specific findings.

Physical Examination. Signs of bronchopneumonia are frequently noted after the third day of illness. There is no organomegaly.

Clinical Course. Patients appear toxic, are uncomfortable, and frequently develop evidence for patchy pulmonary infiltrates about the fourth day of illness coincident with the appearance of a few petechiae, mucous membrane bleeding, and mild albuminuria. Shock ensues 1 to 3 days later in a minority of patients. Kyasanur Forest disease is sometimes marked by encephalitic signs, meningismus, and findings suggesting viral invasion of the brain. Convalescence, as for most other forms of viral HF, is protracted but usually is completed without residua.

Laboratory Findings. Leukopenia is almost invariable, but thrombocytopenia is marked only in the face of severe hemorrhagic diathesis. Radiologic examination confirms the physical findings indicating the development of scattered foci of bronchopneumonia. There is minimal or no evidence for hepatic or renal damage. Coagulation defects, if any, have not been studied in either disease.

Diagnosis. Each virus can be recovered from blood of patients during the early days of illness and frequently from brain tissue at autopsy. No recent work has been done to determine whether specific antibodies or antigen can be detected in clinically ill patients.

Pitfalls and Errors in Diagnosis. These diseases might be readily confused with other causes of acute bronchopneumonia, especially viral or chlamydial, or with tickborne encephalitis caused by antigenically related viruses. For both political and ecologic reasons, it is highly unlikely that either disease will be seen in western Europe or the Americas.

Hemorrhagic Fever with Renal Syndrome

Synonyms. Because the etiologic agent(s) of this syndrome has been discovered so recently and because its geographic and linguistic distribution is so wide, this—of all forms of viral HF—is the one with a phalanx of synonyms.

The principal terms are Korean hemorrhagic fever, epidemic hemorrhagic fever (China, Japan), hemorrhagic nephrosonephritis (Soviet Union), nephropathia epidemica (Scandinavia), and muroid viral nephropathy, the latter a recent proposal to collect all of the disease forms now known to be caused by Hantaan virus (Korean prototype) and related agents.

Definition. Hemorrhagic fever with renal syndrome is a variable clinical entity most characterized by an acute renal tubular lesion, which is caused by a group of antigenically related rodentborne viruses. Chronic infection of rodents with urinary virus excretion and aerosol transmission to humans is the central epidemiologic mechanism. Incubation periods longer than 40 days have been documented, although the mode is thought to be 2 to 3 weeks. Human infection takes place in at least three distinct settings:

1. Rural agricultural or other activities in which contact is made with urine of infected small rodents, usually one or very few species.
2. Urban areas in which rats (Rattus) are chronically infected and play a similar role. This biologic pattern has led to the discovery that similar viruses are found in virtually every major city in the world where sought. This includes the United States.
3. Infection of laboratory workers in medical research centers where rat colonies have somehow become infected.

Presenting Signs and Symptoms. Disease severity and hemorrhagic manifestations are clearly greater in eastern Asia than elsewhere. The description presented here is based on the Asian form of HFRS. The disease presents with high fever, severe myalgia, and prominent facial flush. Conjunctival and palatine injection is common.

Physical Examination. In addition to the usual signs of VHF, patients often exhibit marked lumbar pain accentuated by percussion of the costovertebral angle.

Clinical Course. In severe cases, this represents one of the most remarkable sequences in acute viral disease. The toxic febrile period lasts about 1 week and is marked by the appearance of petechiae on the upper trunk, slight mucous membrane bleeding, progressive proteinuria (which can be massive), a rising hematocrit, and finally, as temperature falls, intractable shock. Surviving patients then enter a severe oliguric phase lasting 7 to 10 days, which may require prompt dialysis to treat uremia, hyperkalemia, or volume overload. From this point, survivors, now reduced further in numbers, must endure 1 to 2 weeks of major diuresis with all its fluid and electrolyte disturbances, together with a clinically fragile vascular system that tends to collapse or override into hypertension whenever balance is lost. Convalescence requires weeks to months but is always complete. Long-term sequelae, in particular impaired renal function, have not been documented.

Laboratory Procedures. As may be surmised from the preceding description, there are many abnormalities, some of which can be spectacular. Early in the disease, blood leukocytes are usually normal. Proteinuria, which may progress to more than 5 gm/liter, together with isosthenuria, is a cardinal feature of this syndrome. Leukocytosis may appear toward the end of the febrile period, and values as high as 50,000/cu mm have been recorded. Protein leakage from the circulation may be so severe as to produce hematocrit values as high as 70 per cent. Coagulation defects have not been well defined. There is little or no chemical evidence for hepatitis.

During the oliguric phase, there is progressive elevation of urea nitrogen, often to concentrations higher than 200 mg/dl. Associated acidotic changes occur, and hyperkalemia may reach clinically significant levels. In diuresis the reverse conditions obtain. Salt loss is major, and hypokalemia is an ever-present danger. Urinary concentrating capacity may require weeks or even months to be fully restored.

Diagnosis. It is extremely difficult to recover virus from any source in acutely ill patients. Fortunately, the vast majority already have specific IgM antibodies when first seen medically. Both phenomena are thought to be related to the variable but relatively long incubation period for this disease.

Pitfalls and Errors in Diagnosis. The full-blown syndrome is readily recognized if suspected. The related Scandinavian disease (nephropathia epidemica) is characterized by fever, abdominal pain, and mild to moderate renal tubular dysfunction, but not hemorrhage or mortality. With the discovery of worldwide infection of Rattus and other rodents by related viruses, this diagnosis should be considered in any patient with fever, proteinuria, and isosthenuria.

The important conditions that might be confused with this syndrome include acute lupus erythematosus, mild or recovering acute tubular necrosis due to toxins or unknown agents, the nephrotic syndrome, and intercurrent infections in a patient with chronic renal failure.

NOSOCOMIAL INFECTION

In addition to their normal patterns of zoonotic transmission to humans, several of the viruses causing hemorrhagic fever have spread directly from person to person, frequently to medical personnel, and under circumstances in which aerosols were possibly or definitely the vehicle of spread. These include Lassa, Marburg, Ebola, Congo-Crimean, and possibly RVF viruses. As such, these agents are regarded as extremely hazardous, requiring maximum biologic containment (P-4) for safe laboratory manipulation. There is, of course, a related need to provide the best isolation of patients and protection of medical personnel available. Therefore, the suspicion of any of these infections in a given patient represents a significant medical emergency. Immediate consultation can be provided by the Centers for Disease Control, Special Pathogens Branch, Atlanta, Ga. (404-329-3308) or the U.S. Army Medical Research Institute for Infectious Diseases, Frederick, Md. (301-663-2227). Diagnostic assistance and advice regarding the management of nosocomial risks also is available.

RICKETTSIAL DISEASES

By Frederick W. Derks, M.D.
and Charles V. Sanders, M.D.
New Orleans, Louisiana

The signs and symptoms of the rickettsial diseases, particularly in the initial phase, are common to many acute infectious diseases. Because differential clinical diagnosis is difficult and specialized laboratory diagnostic procedures are not always readily available, the physician must be aware of the different possibilities and devise a strategy, sometimes empirically based on probability, for the diagnosis of a rickettsialike disease. The clinician must consider all epidemiologic, clinical, and laboratory information that is available.

In general, the rickettsioses are transmitted by arthropod vectors, although Q fever is usually acquired from domestic animals. Since the basic lesion caused by rickettsiae is a vasculitis, a variety of organ systems and clinical presentations may be involved. However, the symptom complex of fever, headache, and rash, even though not always present, should alert the clinician to the possibility of a rickettsial disease. The single most important factor in reducing mortality and speeding convalescence is prompt diagnosis and adequate antirickettsial therapy.

ROCKY MOUNTAIN SPOTTED FEVER

Synonyms

Spotted fever, tick typhus, fiebre manchada, fiebre petequial, febre maculosa, São Paulo typhus.

Definition

Rocky Mountain spotted fever is an acute infectious disease caused by a rickettsial agent, *Rickettsia rickettsii.* It is transmitted to humans by several species of infected ticks and is characterized by fever, skin rash, myalgias, intense headache, and prostration.

Epidemiology

The disease is named from its initial recognition in the mountainous areas of Montana and Idaho. This is currently a misnomer, since in the United States the disease is now much more prevalent along the Atlantic seaboard and in the southeastern states. The range of the disease is limited to North and South America. Rocky Mountain spotted fever is a zoonosis transmitted to humans by several species of ticks. Approximately 80 per cent of patients give a history of tick bite or tick exposure. Aerosol transmission may occur among laboratory personnel involved in rickettsial research.

Clinical Features

Following an incubation period that ranges from 2 days to 2 weeks, averaging 7 days, there is frequently an abrupt onset of severe headache, chills, fever higher than 102°F, generalized myalgias (especially involving the back and legs), malaise, anorexia, and prostration. Other symptomatology may include nausea, vomiting, photophobia, arthralgias, and upper abdominal pain.

The characteristic rash usually appears on about the fourth day (range—2 to 6 days) of illness. It begins as an erythematous macular eruption involving wrists, palms, ankles, soles, and forearms. It rapidly becomes maculopapular and spreads to involve the proximal extremities, trunk and face. In another 3 to 4 days, the lesions become petechial, and in severe cases may coalesce into areas of ecchymoses. Occasionally, the rash may not appear until later in the illness, and rarely the rash may be absent. This increases the difficulty of making the diagnosis. Patients with more severe disease may show profound alterations in the neurologic, cardiovascular, hematologic, and metabolic status. Neurologic abnormalities are often a prominent feature of the illness. Nuchal rigidity, stupor, delirium, coma, and grand mal seizures may occur in addition to severe headaches. A nonproductive cough and localized pneumonitis may be present. Mild to moderate hepatic and splenic enlargement occurs frequently, but jaundice is uncommon.

Laboratory Findings

About half of all patients with Rocky Mountain spotted fever exhibit some degree of thrombocytopenia. This is probably due to margination of platelets at sites of vasculitis. In fulminant cases, diffuse intravascular coagulation gives rise to consumptive coagulopathy characterized by depletion of circulating clotting factors and severe hemorrhagic diathesis. The diffuse vascular damage in Rocky Mountain spotted fever may lead to anemia, hypoproteinemia, hypovolemia, and edema. In severe infections, there may be enough loss of circulating blood volume so that hypotension, azotemia, oliguria, and circulatory collapse occur. Hyponatremia is frequently found in seriously ill patients and is thought to be secondary to inappropriate secretion of antidiuretic hormone. Lumbar puncture may be normal or may show mild pleocytosis and an increase in protein content, but the cerebrospinal fluid glucose concentration remains normal.

Diagnosis

The diagnostic serologic tests that are available usually do not become positive until late in the course of the disease. Two types of serologic tests are generally available. The Weil-Felix agglutination is based on cross-antigenicity between rickettsiae and Proteus OX-2 and OX-19. Proteus OX-K agglutinins are not useful in the diagnosis of Rocky Mountain spotted fever. The complement fixation test uses purified rickettsial antigens. A fourfold or greater rise in serum antibody titers between the acute and convalescent samples in either the agglutination or complement fixation test is diagnostic. Other serologic tests, such as immunofluorescent antibody procedures and microagglutination, are not readily available. Attempts at isolation of the organism by inoculation of tissue cultures is a lengthy procedure and may be hazardous to laboratory personnel.

Promising new approaches to earlier laboratory diagnosis include the immunofluorescence technique on biopsies of skin lesions and the monocyte culture technique. However, in most instances, the disease must be suspected and therapy instituted on clinical grounds. Thus, Rocky Mountain spotted fever should be suspected in patients visiting or living in endemic areas who become ill during the warmer months with an illness characterized by fever, maculopapular or petechial rash, and headache. The diagnosis is extremely likely with a history of tick bite or tick exposure, but the absence of such history does not exclude the diagnosis.

The differential diagnosis includes a variety of febrile rash illnesses. The disease is frequently misdiagnosed as measles, although Koplik spots are absent and measles usually does not occur during the summer months. The petechial rash and neurologic abnormalities may suggest a diagnosis of acute meningococcemia. Other diseases that must be differentiated include the other rickettsioses, typhoid fever, infectious mononucleosis, and the viral exanthemas.

OTHER RICKETTSIAL SPOTTED FEVERS

These are the Eastern Hemisphere tickborne rickettsioses.

Definition

There are three diseases caused by different members of the spotted fever group of rickettsiae that occur in distinct geographic areas of the Eastern Hemisphere: fièvre boutonneuse, Asian tickborne typhus, and Queensland tick typhus (Table 1).

Epidemiology

Each of these diseases is a zoonosis, transmitted to humans by the bite of one or more species of hard-shelled ticks. They tend to occur in distinct geographic areas, as indicated by the name of the disease.

Clinical Features

These three tickborne rickettsioses resemble one another closely. Following the incubation period of approximately 5 to 7 days, the disease is manifested by fever, malaise, myalgia, headache, and conjunctivitis. The primary lesion, present in most cases at the onset of fever, is a small ulcer 2 to 5 mm in diameter with a black center and a red areola. There is usually regional lymphadenopathy. A generalized erythematous maculopapular rash appears on about the fourth day of illness and involves most of the body, including the palms and soles and quite often the face. The rash may become hemorrhagic in severe infections.

The disease usually resolves during the second week. The prognosis is good except in the elderly and debilitated. Sequelae and complications are rare. Thus, these diseases have a short incubation period (5 to 7 days average), a primary lesion (eschar), fever lasting for a few days to 2 weeks, and a maculopapular rash that appears 3 to 5 days after onset of illness.

Laboratory Findings

There are no characteristic changes in the white blood cell count. Transitory proteinuria and hematuria may occur. Nonspecific electrocardiographic changes, a reversal of the albumin/globulin (A/G) ratio in serum, and abnormal liver function tests have been reported. The erythrocyte sedimentation rate (ESR) is usually slightly elevated.

Diagnosis

The clinical diagnosis is based on the presence of the primary lesion, the geographic location, regional lymphadenitis, fever, and the maculopapular rash in a patient who has been exposed to ticks in an endemic area. The definitive diagnosis can be made only in the laboratory. Laboratory findings of greatest importance are those from serologic tests with Weil-Felix and rickettsial antigens. Agglutinins against Proteus OX-2 and OX-19 develop by or during the second week, and complement-fixing antibodies appear shortly thereafter. Microimmunofluorescence will also distinguish these organisms. Differential diagnosis includes meningococcal infections, measles and other viral exanthems, and other rickettsial infections, particularly the typhus fevers.

Table 1. Diseases Caused by Eastern Hemisphere Rickettsial Spotted Fever Group

Disease	Synonyms	Etiology
Fièvre boutonneuse	African tick typhus Kenya tick typhus South African tick bite fever Indian tick typhus	*Rickettsia conorii*
Asian tickborne typhus	North Asian tickborne rickettsiosis	*Rickettsia siberica*
Queensland tick typhus		*Rickettsia australis*

Q FEVER

Synonyms

Query fever, la maladie de Derrick et Burnet.

Definition

Q fever is a rickettsial disease characterized by sudden onset with influenza-like symptoms of fever, chills, sweating, and headache. In fewer than half the patients, an associated pneumonitis may develop. The etiologic agent is *Coxiella burnetti.*

Epidemiology

Q fever is primarily a disease of men rather than women because of occupational exposure. It occurs worldwide and is seen mainly in workers exposed to farm animals, in slaughterhouse workers, and in veterinary personnel. The actual incidence of this disease in humans is unknown, since most infections are undiagnosed. The disease is a zoonosis, but the infection is acquired by humans from inhalation rather than by contact with an arthropod vector.

Clinical Features

After an incubation period of 10 days to 4 weeks, there is a sudden onset of high fever, severe headache, arthralgias, myalgia, and severe malaise. Anorexia, nausea, diarrhea or constipation, and cough are all frequent symptoms. Hyperemia of the posterior pharynx, relative bradycardia, pulmonary involvement, and hepatomegaly are frequently found on physical examination. The rash seen in other rickettsial disease does not occur in Q fever. Myocarditis, pericarditis, endocarditis, encephalitis, pleural effusion, thrombophlebitis, orchitis, parotitis, pancreatitis, nephritis, and thyroiditis may all be associated with Q fever. Prolonged convalescence, lasting up to several months, is the rule even in uncomplicated cases.

Laboratory Findings

X-ray evidence of infiltrates in the lung may be found, and biochemical abnormalities of liver function occur in up to two thirds of patients. With endocarditis, vegetations (frequently large) may be detected on the heart valves. Cerebrospinal fluid findings may be those of aseptic meningitis.

Diagnosis

A diagnosis of Q fever must be considered in a patient with a severe febrile illness of uncertain etiology, especially if accompanied by severe headache, and a history of exposure to livestock or byproducts.

Serologic studies confirm the diagnosis. A fourfold or greater rise in the complement fixation test is diagnostic. This is the most widely used diagnostic study. Agglutination tests may give an earlier diagnosis, since agglutinins rise about a week earlier than complement-fixing antibody. Both the microagglutination and the radioisotope precipitation techniques have been used. The Weil-Felix reaction is not helpful because it is negative in Q fever. The differential diagnosis includes influenza, viral hepatitis, atypical pneumonias, brucellosis, infectious mononucleosis, leptospirosis, toxoplasmosis, cytomegalovirus infection, and typhoid fever.

MURINE TYPHUS

Synonyms

Endemic typhus, fleaborne typhus.

Definition

Murine typhus is an acute febrile disease transmitted to humans by the rat flea. The etiologic agent is *Rickettsia mooseri* (*R. typhi*). The reservoir of this zoonosis is rats and mice, and man is an accidental victim.

Epidemiology

Murine typhus is a zoonosis maintained in a cycle involving rats (and certain other small mammals) with fleas and rat lice as vectors. It is transmitted to humans by contamination of broken skin with infective feces of the vector or by inhalation of dried infective feces. It is not communicable from human to human. Murine typhus is worldwide in distribution, and seasonal incidence of human infection seems to correlate with periods of abundance of vector fleas. In the United States, this occurs in the summer months. Since rats tend to associate with buildings containing food, such as warehouses and grain elevators, the disease is often associated with particular places and occupations.

Clinical Features

Murine typhus is clinically similar to epidemic typhus, except that it is a milder disease. The incubation period ranges from 6 to 14 days and is followed by the onset of fever, headache, myalgia, arthralgia, and rash. The macular or maculopapular rash usually appears on the trunk on the fifth or sixth day after onset of fever and spreads to the upper extremities. Conjunctivitis may occur. The maculopapular rash may be replaced later in the disease by poorly delineated roseolae. Fever lasts approximately 9 to 14 days and terminates by lysis. Myocardial, renal, hepatic, and central nervous system involvement is infrequent. Mortality in untreated patients is approximately 2 per cent, but recovery is usually rapid and without sequelae. Occasionally, if untreated, murine typhus may be severe and debilitating or require 2 to 3 months for convalescence.

Laboratory Findings

The white blood cell count remains normal. The ESR and serum protein concentration are increased. Azotemia is rare.

Diagnosis

The diagnosis of murine typhus may be suspected in a patient with sustained fever, headache, generalized myalgias, rash, and other clinical features, particularly if the person has been exposed to an area where rats are numerous. Cross-reactive antibodies to Proteus OX-19 (Weil-Felix reaction) develop. Serologic methods of choice for diagnosis of murine typhus are the complement fixation test and microagglutination reaction.

Murine typhus can be differentiated from epidemic typhus by the mouse-toxin neutralization test and the microagglutination reaction but not by the complement fixation test. Both a macro- and a microimmunofluorescence test are available for the detection of antibodies in murine typhus. The organism can be isolated by inoculation of the patient's blood into the peritoneal cavity of guinea pigs or white rats. Definitive diagnosis can only be made by isolation of the agent or specific serologic changes.

EPIDEMIC TYPHUS

Synonyms

Louseborne typhus, European typhus, classic typhus, historic typhus, camp fever, war fever, ship fever, jail fever, typhus exanthématique, tifus exantemático, tifus tabardillo, Fleckfieber, and dermotypho.

Definition

Epidemic typhus is an acute infectious disease whose etiologic agent, *R. prowazekii,* is transmitted from human to human by the human body louse. Clinically, it is characterized by sudden onset, a macular rash, sustained high fever of approximately 2 weeks' duration, and an altered mental state.

Epidemiology

The infection involves man and the human body louse. The organism is not transmitted by the louse bite, but louse feces or crushed infective lice contaminates breaks in the skin or bite sites. The disease may also be acquired by inhalation of infective louse feces. Presently, the highest prevalence of epidemic typhus is in the developing countries of Africa and, to a lesser degree, of Latin America and Asia. Although not currently reported from the United States, the potential for this disease remains because of the presence of the louse vector and the number of immigrants susceptible to development of Brill-Zinsser disease (recrudescent form of epidemic typhus).

Clinical Features

The incubation period is from 5 to 23 days, averaging about 11 days. A prodrome of vague malaise and headache commonly occurs. This is followed by the abrupt onset of fever, severe headache, chills, backache, myalgia, and weakness. Constipation is usually present, but nausea, vomiting, and diarrhea are rare. Conjunctivitis, orbital pain, photophobia, and flushing of the face and neck occur frequently. Nonproductive cough is a feature in about two thirds of the cases.

A rash appears between the fourth and ninth day, erupting first on the lateral chest and axillary folds, then spreading to the abdomen and involving the entire body (except the face, palms, and soles) over the next 1 to 2 days. Early, the rash consists of small macular or maculopapular lesions that blanch on pressure. Later, the rash does not blanch; it becomes purpuric and forms groups that do not become confluent. After approximately 10 to 12 days, the rash becomes brownish in color and desquamation occurs during convalescence.

There is also progressive central nervous system involvement that occasionally leads to coma. Splenomegaly, renal insufficiency, cough and tachypnea, tachycardia, hypotension, myocarditis, and gangrene of appendages may occur in severe cases.

Pneumonia is an important complication. Bronchopneumonia developing during the first week is usually rickettsial in origin. During the third or fourth week of disease, about 10 per cent of patients develop secondary bacterial pneumonia. Other common bacterial complications, particularly in untreated patients, are purulent tonsillitis, pharyngitis, otitis media, and parotitis.

Laboratory Findings

During the first week of illness, the white blood cell count is low or normal and only slightly elevated later on. Significant leukocytosis is usually the result of secondary bacterial infection. Anemia, azotemia, and reversal of the serum albumin/globulin (A/G) ratio may occur. Pleocytosis and increased protein may be found in the cerebrospinal fluid. Nonspecific ST- and T-wave changes may be seen on the electrocardiogram, and the chest x-ray may reveal pulmonary infiltrates.

Diagnosis

The clinical diagnosis should be suspected based on the typical rash, headache, high unremitting fever, and signs of central nervous system involvement, particularly during an epidemic or in areas with high incidence of epidemic typhus. Serologic confirmation is most frequently accomplished by the complement fixation test. The microagglutination test and an indirect microimmunofluorescence test are also available for serologic confirmation of the diagnosis. The Weil-Felix Proteus OX-19 reaction is fairly nonspecific. Differential diagnosis of epidemic typhus includes relapsing fever, malaria, measles, yellow fever, and other rickettsioses.

BRILL-ZINSSER DISEASE

Synonyms

Sporadic typhus, recrudescent typhus.

Definition

Brill-Zinsser disease is a recrudescence of epidemic typhus that occurs months to years after the primary attack. The etiologic agent is *R. prowazekii.*

Epidemiology

This disease, which may appear anywhere from a few months to 50 years after the primary infection, is caused by organisms persisting in tissues since the initial attack of epidemic typhus. The factors that precipitate Brill-Zinsser disease are not known. Cases of this disease are important because they represent a potential reservoir for epidemic typhus when louse infestation is present.

Clinical Features

The clinical features are similar to those of classic epidemic typhus but are milder. Fever is usually lower and of shorter duration, rickettsemia is shorter, the rash is less apparent and often absent, complications are infrequent, and fatalities are rare.

Laboratory Findings

Brill-Zinsser disease may have laboratory findings similar to those previously described in epidemic typhus. However, the laboratory abnormalities that do occur are usually much milder than those seen with primary typhus.

Diagnosis

A clinical diagnosis of Brill-Zinsser disease is difficult and depends on a careful history. The Proteus OX-19 Weil-Felix reaction is positive in less than 20 per cent of patients with Brill-Zinsser disease. The complement fixation test is the most frequently used serologic study, but only the indirect microimmunofluorescence test differentiates Brill-Zinsser disease from primary epidemic typhus.

RICKETTSIALPOX

Definition

Rickettsialpox is a miteborne febrile disease distinguished by a primary cutaneous escharlike lesion and a papulovesicular rash. The disease is caused by *R. akari* and is transmitted to humans by the bite of the mouse mite.

Epidemiology

Rickettsialpox is a zoonosis that involves house mice and mouse mites. Man acquires the disease from the bite of this mite. The number of cases of this disease has decreased markedly over the past several years. It is not clear whether the decrease is due to effective control measures or underreporting.

Clinical Features

The incubation period ranges from about 10 to 21 days. This is followed by the sudden onset of fever, chills, malaise, headache, photophobia, and anorexia. Approximately 90 per cent of patients develop an initial lesion (the eschar) at the site of the mite bite about a week prior to the onset of fever. A maculopapular nonpruritic rash begins, usually within the first to fourth day of the fever. The rash involves the trunk, extremities, and mucous membranes, but involvement of the palms and soles is rare. There may be only a few scattered lesions or a generalized eruption. After 2 or 3 days, these maculopapular lesions evolve into a vesiculopapular rash. The vesicles form a crust that falls off, leaving pigmented areas but no scars. The disease resolves spontaneously, and without sequelae, in about 10 to 14 days.

Laboratory Findings

During the acute phase of the disease, there is frequently a leukopenia in the range of 2500 to 5000 cells per cu mm. Lymphocytes tend to predominate, and sometimes large vacuolated mononuclear cells are also present. Heterophil antibody is absent.

Diagnosis

In many cases, the clinical features of the disease are distinctive enough that a presumptive diagnosis can be made. Specific laboratory diagnosis is based on isolation of the organism by inoculation of embryonated eggs or mice and the complement fixation study. The complement fixation reaction cross-reacts with the other members of the spotted fever group of rickettsial diseases. However, the Weil-Felix reaction is negative in rickettsialpox and thus helps to differentiate rickettsialpox from the other spotted fever group of diseases.

Clinically, the disease must be differentiated from varicella, other spotted fever rickettsial infections, murine typhus, infectious mononucleosis, and typhoid fever.

SCRUB TYPHUS

Synonyms

Tsutsugamushi disease, chiggerborne rickettsiosis, miteborne typhus, rural typhus, Japanese river fever, flood fever, Mossman fever.

Definition

Scrub typhus is an acute febrile illness characterized by a primary cutaneous lesion or eschar and a rash. It is caused by *R. tsutsugamushi* and is transmitted to humans by certain larval mites called chiggers.

Epidemiology

This disease is a zoonosis of rats and other small mammals, with man becoming infected as an accidental dead-end host. Scrub typhus is acquired from the bite of an infected larval trombiculid mite (chigger). The classic epidemiologic feature of scrub typhus is its highly focal nature, with outbreaks traceable to common exposure sites. Scrub typhus is distributed throughout eastern and southern Asia and the islands of the western and southern Pacific. In the United States, endemic infection is unknown but a number of cases, imported during the incubation period after infection in an endemic area, have been recognized.

Clinical Features

Following the incubation period, which ranges from 6 to 19 days, the disease has an abrupt onset, with the initial symptom of severe frontal and occipital headache followed within a few hours by high fever and shaking chills. In approximately 60 to 70 per cent of primary infections, a pathognomonic primary lesion, or eschar, develops at the site of chigger feeding. Regional lymph nodes become enlarged and tender. Conjunctival injection, ocular pain, malaise, myalgia, anorexia, apathy, and cough are common features of this disease. The pulse remains relatively slow, and interstitial pneumonitis is common.

Between the third and ninth day, a maculopapular rash appears in 40 to 60 per cent of patients. The rash usually begins first on the trunk and then spreads to the extremities, but it may involve all parts of the body, including the palms and soles. At about the same time, generalized lymphadenopathy, splenic enlargement, and sometimes hepatomegaly occur. During the second week of illness, signs of myocarditis, meningoencephalitis, and nephritis may appear. Without treatment, patients usually defervesce by lysis after approximately 2 weeks of the illness. Convalescence is prolonged, but significant residua are unusual.

Laboratory Findings

Early in the course of the disease, leukopenia, ranging from 1000 to 5000 white blood cells per cu mm, frequently occurs. Later, this resolves to normal or only slightly depressed white blood cell counts. Late in the disease, the count may be somewhat elevated. Occasionally, disseminated intravascular coagulation may develop. Total serum proteins are usually normal or low, but the A/G ratio is frequently reversed. The electrocardiogram may show extrasystoles, variable T-wave changes, shifts in the electrical axis, and variable degrees of atrioventricular (AV) block. Lumbar puncture may reveal elevated cerebrospinal fluid pressure, minimal pleocytosis with mononuclear cell predominance, and elevated protein concentration. Albuminuria is common, azotemia may occur, and serum transaminase levels may be elevated. The serum chloride concentration is often low.

Diagnosis

With no eschar or rash, infectious mononucleosis, dengue and other arboviral infections, leptospirosis, typhoid fever, malaria, and other rickettsial infections should be considered in the differential diagnosis. The possibility of scrub typhus should be strongly considered in the patient with a typhuslike illness, a history of possible exposure in an endemic area, and an eschar associated with regional lymphadenitis.

Laboratory diagnosis is achieved by isolation of rickettsiae by inoculation of embryonated eggs or mice and by demonstration of specific antibody in convalescent serum. The indirect fluorescent antibody test is the current serologic method of choice. The complement fixation test is less specific, and the Weil-Felix test with Proteus OX-K is useful but is not positive in all cases.

TRENCH FEVER

Synonyms

Quintan fever, 5-day fever, shinbone fever, Volhynia fever.

Definition

Trench fever is a louseborne febrile disease characterized by headache and severe muscle, joint, and bone pain. The causative agent is *Rochalimaea quintana,* a rickettsialike organism. It is differentiated from rickettsiae by its ability to grow on artificial media and in the lumen of the louse gut.

Epidemiology

The disease is transmitted to humans through infected louse feces. Infection of humans occurs following inoculation of contaminated feces into abraded skin or conjunctivae. This disease was a major problem during both World Wars, and it continues to occur in parts of North Africa, Mexico, Eastern Europe, and Asia. Since the agent may continue to be isolated from asymptomatic individuals years after their initial infection, humans are considered the principal long-term reservoir of the disease.

Clinical Features

After an incubation period of 9 to 30 days, there is the onset of severe headache, the gradual or abrupt beginning of fever, dizziness, profuse sweating, extreme weakness, and muscle and bone pain, especially in the tibial area. Mild sore throat, neck pain simulating meningitis, and abdominal pain often mimicking appendicitis frequently occur. In 70 to 80 per cent of patients, an erythematous macular or papular rash occurs, often localized on the anterior chest and abdomen, and lasts for only a few days. Splenomegaly and frequently hepatomegaly are also present.

The disease may follow several forms. One form consists of recurrent febrile episodes with intervening afebrile periods of approximately 5 days. Other patterns include a single 3- to 4-day fever, continuous fever for several months, and relapsing fever at irregular intervals for many months. The disease remits even without specific therapy. Convalescence is occasionally protracted, and organisms may circulate in the blood for long periods of time in asymptomatic convalescent patients. Relapses after a year or more of good health have also been described.

Laboratory Findings

Mild to moderate leukocytosis may occur during the acute phase of the disease.

Diagnosis

During epidemics of trench fever, typical cases can be diagnosed on clinical grounds alone. A history of contact with lice during the appropriate incubation period is helpful. The organism can now be cultured on specially prepared media, and specific antibody can be detected by several serologic procedures including complement fixation, passive hemagglutination, and enzyme immunoassay. The differential diagnosis of trench fever includes typhus, dengue, malaria, typhoid fever, influenza, leptospirosis, and relapsing fever.

SYSTEMIC MYCOTIC DISEASES

By George A. Sarosi, M.D.
and Scott F. Davies, M.D.
Minneapolis, Minnesota

The number of fungi that cause invasive disease in humans is quite small. Fungal diseases ordinarily caused by inhalation include diseases caused by the dimorphic pathogenic fungi—histoplasmosis, coccidioidomycosis, and blastomycosis—as well as cryptococcosis, which is caused by the yeast *Cryptococcus neoformans.* Diseases caused by ubiquitous fungi that can colonize mucosal surfaces but invade only under special circumstances include aspergillosis and mucormycosis, caused by opportunistic molds, and candidosis, caused by opportunistic yeast. The wide number of essentially avirulent fungi (including Rhodotorula, Hansenula, Geotrichum, Penicillium, and others) that rarely cause invasive illness in profoundly immunosuppressed individuals are not discussed. Sporotrichosis and maduromycosis are deep mycotic infections ordinarily initiated by inoculation of organisms into subcutaneous tissues and are discussed elsewhere.

Actinomycosis and nocardiosis are caused by higher bacteria rather than by fungi. They are discussed here because of their long historical association with fungal diseases and because their clinical manifestations very closely resemble those of fungal illnesses.

HISTOPLASMOSIS

Histoplasmosis refers to infection by the pathogenic fungus *Histoplasma capsulatum.* This soil fungus is endemic throughout the east central United States, especially along the Mississippi and Ohio river valleys. Heavy concentrations of the fungus are found in excrement of chickens, pigeons, starlings, and bats. Infection is acquired when the mycelium is disturbed and the fungal spores are aerosolized and inhaled.

Clinical Features

Primary Pulmonary Histoplasmosis. Primary pulmonary histoplasmosis may have few or no symptoms. Chest roentgenograms, even in asymptomatic patients, may show patchy areas of pneumonitis and prominent ipsilateral hilar adenopathy. Pleural effusions are uncommon. Patients who are ill become symptomatic between 10 and 14 days after exposure. They have an influenzalike illness with fever, chills, myalgias, and nonproductive cough.

Patients who have been exposed to a large infecting inoculum may present with diffuse nodular infiltrates throughout both lung fields. Such patients are usually quite ill, but most recover uneventfully. A few progress rapidly to respiratory failure and have all the features of the adult respiratory distress syndrome.

The chest roentgenogram may return to normal or may have residual abnormalities. The initial patchy infiltrates may become denser and smaller, forming one or more pulmonary nodules. Central necrosis may result in a dense core of calcium (a "target" lesion). Infrequently, alternate periods of activity and healing may result in characteristic concentric rings of calcium. Lymph node calcification, alone or with a pulmonary nodule, is common. Finally, small "buckshot" calcifications may be scattered over both lung fields, a pattern characteristic of heavy primary exposure and uneventful recovery.

Several uncommon local complications may occur. Extensive fibrosis in the mediastinum can cause vascular compression and may result in superior vena caval syndrome. Inflammatory masses adjacent to the esophagus may cause dysphagia. Calcified nodes may erode into a bronchus and cause hemoptysis and bronchial obstruction with distal infection or volume loss. Pericarditis may also occur.

Chronic Cavitary Histoplasmosis. Upper lobe cavitary histoplasmosis closely resembles reinfection tuberculosis in roentgenographic appearance and in symptomatology. The mechanism of infection, unlike tuberculosis, is primary infection in a patient with abnormal lungs, typically a male middle-aged smoker with some centrilobular emphysema. Acute pulmonary histoplasmosis in such patients usually resolves as it does in patients with normal lungs. However, infected air spaces may persist in a few cases and progress to a destructive fibrocavitary pneumonia. Unilateral or bilateral upper lobe involvement is characteristic, but cavitary disease may occur in other parts of the lung. Most patients have chronic cough and constitutional symptoms, including weight loss, poor appetite, malaise, night sweats, and sometimes low-grade fever.

Disseminated Histoplasmosis. This term refers to progressive extrapulmonary infection. Disseminated histoplasmosis can occur as an overwhelming postprimary spread (most often in young children) with little tendency to granuloma formation despite the presence of massive numbers of organisms in all reticuloendothelial tissues. High fever, diffuse lymphadenopathy, hepatosplenomegaly, and pancytopenia are clinical features. Death may occur within weeks. Among nonimmunocompromised adults, dissemination is most common in the elderly, who often have a smoldering subacute illness many months in duration. Fever is modest. Weight loss, skin and mucous membrane lesions, and well-formed granulomas on biopsy are common features. Disseminated histoplasmosis also occurs as an opportunistic infection in immunosuppressed patients. The illness may resemble the acute infantile or the more chronic adult form of the illness.

Fewer than half of patients with disseminated histoplasmosis have cough, dyspnea, or other pulmonary symptoms. The chest roentgenogram may have a localized infiltrate, but it may also be normal or may reveal a diffuse interstitial pattern, especially in immunosuppressed patients. The clinical picture is variable and often nonspecific; fever is the only universal finding.

Progressive extrapulmonary histoplasmosis is sometimes localized. Examples include central nervous system histoplasmoma, histoplasma meningitis, and isolated gastrointestinal histoplasmosis, which usually involves the terminal ileum.

Diagnostic Tests

Morphology. Histopathologic specimens that reveal macrophages crowded with small (2 to 4 microns) yeast are diagnostic of histoplasmosis. The intracellular organisms can be seen on routine hematoxylin and eosin–stained sections. When there are well-formed noncaseating granulomas, there may be very few organisms. These are extracellular and are seen only in sections that have been silver-stained. The organism may be seen in lung biopsies or mediastinal lymph node biopsies in primary histoplasmosis and in biopsies of bone marrow, liver, or skin and mucous membrane lesions in disseminated histoplasmosis. Biopsies are seldom necessary in primary histoplasmosis but are occasionally done to exclude other more serious diagnoses such as lymphoma or carcinoma. Biopsies are often done in disseminated histoplasmosis and are the best way to quickly prove this diagnosis in a severely ill patient with a febrile systemic illness.

Culture. The organism can be cultured from the sputum occasionally in primary histoplasmosis and quite regularly in chronic cavitary histoplasmosis, although it is almost never identified in potassium hydroxide (KOH) preparations of sputum. Bone marrow aspirate and fragments of liver biopsied by needle are frequently culture-positive in disseminated histoplasmosis. Blood cultures may be positive; although the organisms grow on routine media, they grow more slowly than bacteria. The laboratory must be told that fungi are suspected so that the cultures can be held for a longer time. The problem with fungal cultures is that identification may take several weeks. This is too long for many patients severely ill with disseminated disease. Diagnosis and treatment must be rapid, and histopathology is crucial.

Skin Testing. Intradermal skin testing is performed with histoplasmin. It is a reliable antigen; induration of 5 mm or more at 48 hours indicates that the patient has had histoplasmosis at some time in his or her life. Unfortunately, the test is of little use as a diagnostic test for two reasons. Histoplasmosis is extremely common, and perhaps 40 million persons throughout the endemic area have a positive skin test. Thus, a positive test does not identify an acute illness as histoplasmosis. In addition, about 50 per cent of persons with disseminated disease have a negative skin test. Thus, a negative skin test cannot rule out histoplasmosis in a seriously ill patient. Skin testing should be considered an epidemiologic tool and should not be relied on for diagnosis.

Serologic Diagnosis. Complement-fixing antibodies to mycelial and yeast antigens can be detected 4 to 6 weeks after exposure (at least 2 to 4 weeks after onset of fever). The titers usually decrease gradually over 3 to 12 months but occasionally remain positive at a high dilution for years. Nonetheless, titers against the yeast antigen of 1:16 or greater in a patient with an appropriate history suggest histoplasmosis. However, the majority of patients with primary histoplasmosis will be well before the complement fixation titers become positive, an obvious limitation in diagnosis of an acute illness. Because complement fixation titers are negative in about 50 per cent of immunosuppressed patients with disseminated histoplasmosis, a negative test cannot exclude the diagnosis. However, a high titer is very helpful in pointing to histoplasmosis as a possible cause of an obscure febrile illness.

Immunodiffusion testing for precipitating antibodies to H and M antigens is specific for histoplasmosis. Immunodiffusion becomes positive later than complement fixation following primary infection, and it is less sensitive. It offers no advantage as a screening test other than rapidity and ease of performance.

Radioimmunoassay and enzyme-linked immunosorbent assays (ELISA) offer promise of more sensitive screening tests but are not yet routinely available, nor are they well validated clinically in terms of sensitivity and specificity.

COCCIDIOIDOMYCOSIS

Coccidioidomycosis refers to infection by the pathogenic fungus *Coccidioides immitis.* This fungus is endemic in desert soil in the southwest United States (particularly southern Arizona and New Mexico and the San Joaquin Valley in California) and in adjacent areas of northern Mexico. The infecting arthrospores are spread over long distances by the wind. Exposure to the fungus (as judged by a positive skin test) is nearly universal in highly endemic areas.

Clinical Features

Primary Pulmonary Coccidioidomycosis. Sixty per cent of patients with primary pulmonary coccidioidomycosis have minimal or no symptoms. The other 40 per cent have a febrile illness that resembles influenza and lasts 1 to 3 weeks. Patients have nonproductive cough, myalgias, arthralgias, headache, and fatigue. Pleuritic pain is common early. Dyspnea is unusual in uncomplicated cases. The chest roentgenogram may show a localized alveolar infiltrate or a single nodular density. Ipsilateral hilar adenopathy is not uncommon.

Ninety-five per cent of all patients recover without sequelae. Five per cent have residual abnormalities on x-ray, most commonly thin-walled cavities. Only one or two patients in a thousand will develop disseminated disease. Dissemination occurs most commonly among black and Philippino men (probably as a result of exposure to a large inoculum of spores in dusty outdoor jobs) and in diabetics and pregnant women.

Hypersensitivity manifestations of cell-mediated immunity—such as erythema nodosum, erythema multiforme, arthralgias, and arthritis—occur in up to 20 per cent of cases, a higher incidence than in other deep mycotic infections. They are favorable prognostic indicators. In endemic areas, "desert rheumatism" and "the bumps" are recognized clinical syndromes.

Sterile inflammatory pleural effusions occur in 5 to 10 per cent of cases. Pain may be severe. Of patients with effusions, 50 per cent have erythema nodosum or erythema multiforme, suggesting that the effusions may be manifestations of hypersensitivity.

A persistent thin-walled cavity or a nodule is the most frequent residuum. An occasional patient may develop a chronic fibrocavitary pulmonary process resembling tuberculosis, without distant spread.

Disseminated Coccidioidomycosis. Persistent or recurrent fever may mark the onset of disseminated disease. The illness may be fulminant with rapid development of meningitis, together with multiple bone and skin lesions. Other patients may have a postprimary miliary spread and present with diffuse infiltrates and respiratory failure. Clinically recognizable defects in cell-mediated immunity are common in these patients with rapidly progressing severe illness; many patients have been taking high doses of prednisone for other illness.

For most patients, the onset of dissemination is more insidious. It usually follows primary infection by a few weeks to a few months, but it may occur much later. In many instances, the primary infection was asymptomatic and thus cannot be accurately dated.

Coccidioidal meningitis is the most frequent manifestation of extrapulmonary disease. A granulomatous process at the base of the brain obstructs the flow of cerebrospinal fluid and entraps cranial nerves. Headache may be the only symptom; the level of consciousness is frequently depressed. High fever and a stiff neck are not common. Examination of cerebrospinal fluid reveals a moderate, predominantly mononuclear leukocytosis, often with less than 500 cells per cu mm.

Skeletal disease occurs in 10 to 20 per cent of patients with extrapulmonary coccidioidomycosis. Single or multiple nonreactive lytic lesions occur in long bones, spine, or skull.

Skin lesions usually occur in those with widespread dissemination but may also be the only evidence of dissemination. Individual lesions are verrucous in nature and may mimic basal cell carcinoma.

Diagnostic Tests

Morphology. The pathognomonic feature in tissue sections is a giant spherule ranging in size up to 100 microns and filled with numerous (up to 100,000) small round endospores. The spherule may be identified in hematoxylin and eosin–stained sections and more easily in silver-stained sections. Identification of spherules in KOH-treated specimens of sputum, body fluids, or pus is also diagnostic. The inflammatory reaction seen in tissue is a mixture of granulomatous and pyogenic elements.

Culture. The organism can be cultured on Sabouraud's agar or blood agar. The fungus grows in the laboratory, as in nature, as a mycelium. Arthrospores on the mycelium are extremely infectious. Moreover, similar arthrospores exist on saphrophytic fungi so that cultures are not diagnostic until they have been passed into mice where the spherule characteristic of the tissue phase of growth can develop. Because of these difficulties and because cultures are seldom positive in coccidioidal meningitis—where they would be most useful—cultural identification is not clinically important. Reliance on direct demonstration of organisms, on skin testing, and on serologic testing is adequate for management of most patients.

Skin Testing. Skin tests are usually performed with coccidioidin. The tests are positive in 83 per cent of patients with inactive pulmonary disease, in 67 per cent of patients with active pulmonary disease, in 62 per cent of patients with unifocal dissemination, and in only 38 per cent of patients with widespread dissemination. Attempts to increase sensitivity by using an antigen derived from the tissue phase of growth (spherulin) have not improved the clinical utility of skin testing. Reactivity to either antigen means the patient has at one time had coccidioidomycosis. However, positive skin tests do not mean there is active disease and negative skin tests never exclude the diagnosis.

Serologic Diagnosis. The mycelial phase antigen, coccidioidin, is most useful in detecting humoral antibody response. Serum IgM precipitins can be demonstrated by tube precipitation or by latex agglutination. Precipitins are first detected 1 to 3 weeks after onset of symptoms of primary pulmonary infection in perhaps 75 per cent of cases and generally disappear within 4 months. Latex agglutination is a slightly more sensitive test, but there is a false-positive rate of 6 to 10 per cent.

Serum IgG antibodies that fix complement occur later, mainly in patients with symptomatic primary infections. By 3 months after the initial onset of symptoms, nearly 90 per cent of patients have such antibodies. High titers of complement-fixing antibodies are the hallmark of disseminated disease. Ninety-five per cent of patients without disseminated disease will have titers below 1:32, and 99 per cent will have titers below 1:64. Conversely, 61 per cent of patients with dissemination will have titers of at least 1:32 and 41 per cent, of at least 1:64. These figures refer to results from Dr. Charles Smith's original reference laboratory. The height of a titer will vary somewhat from laboratory to laboratory, and it is important to be familiar with the results from the specific laboratory reporting the test when assessing the significance of a given titer. In general, the titer of complement-fixing antibodies parallels the course of the disease. Rising titers are a poor sign, and falling titers indicate improvement. The exception to the picture described is meningeal disease, in which case serum titers resemble nondisseminated disease unless other foci of dissemination are also present.

Complement-fixing antibodies can be demonstrated in the cerebrospinal fluid of 70 per cent of patients with meningeal disease at the time of initial evaluation and in virtually all patients as the disease progresses. Complement-fixing antibodies cannot be demonstrated in unconcentrated cerebrospinal fluid in the presence of disease outside the central nervous system accompanied by high serum titers. Therefore, a positive complement fixation test on cerebrospinal fluid is diagnostic of meningeal coccidioidomycosis. An exception to this rule may occur when there are epidural abscesses or osteomyelitic lesions abutting the dura.

Counterimmunoelectrophoresis is an easier and more rapid test than is complement fixation and appears to have about the same sensitivity and specificity.

BLASTOMYCOSIS

Blastomycosis refers to infection by the pathogenic fungus *Blastomyces dermatitidis.* This fungus is endemic in the southeastern and south-central United States. Although it is undoubtedly a soil fungus, there have been very few isolations from nature. The endemic area has been mapped out on the basis of individual case reporting. Disease is acquired by inhalation and is most common among those with outdoor jobs and interests. Most cases occur in middle-age men.

Clinical Features

Acute Pulmonary Blastomycosis. This infection may or may not be symptomatic. Patchy areas of alveolar infiltrate usually involve one or both lower lobes. Hilar enlargement may occur, but pleural involvement and cavitation are uncommon. If present, symptoms suggest bacterial pneumonia and include high fever, productive cough, and pleuritic chest pain. Symptoms usually resolve within 2 weeks but roentgenographic abnormalities often persist for months.

Progressive primary infection with continued suppuration and eventual cavitation occurs infrequently. In rare instances, patients have miliary spread of organisms throughout the body, presenting with diffuse bilateral infiltrates and the clinical picture of the adult respiratory distress syndrome.

Chronic Pulmonary Blastomycosis with or without Involvement of Distant Sites. Most clinical cases of blastomycosis present as chronic pulmonary blastomycosis. Patients give no antecedent history of an acute pneumonic illness but have chronic respiratory symptoms of weeks to months in duration. Chronic cough, low-grade fever, night sweats, and weight loss are common complaints. The chest roentgenogram may reveal a single large mass, often perihilar, and may strongly suggest the diagnosis of bronchogenic carcinoma. A more common roentgenographic finding is fibronodular infiltrates with cavitation, which mimics tuberculosis. A rare roentgenographic presentation is a single large cavity, resembling an anaerobic lung abscess.

Involvement of distant sites is common. Two thirds of the patients have skin involvement; one third, bone involvement; and one fifth, genitourinary tract involvement. The occurrence of infection at these sites, in conjunction with a chronic pulmonary infection, not only suggests blastomycosis as a diagnosis but also often provides an easily accessible source of diagnostic material.

Isolated Involvement of Distant Sites. Isolated involvement of skin, bone, or genitourinary tract may occur without past history or present evidence of respiratory infection. Such cases represent progression of disease at sites seeded during asymptomatic primary infection.

Characteristic skin lesions are raised, warty, crusted lesions with irregular borders that occur most commonly on the face and the upper extremities. They mimic basal cell carcinoma but can be distinguished by small microabscesses at the periphery of the lesions.

Bone is the second most common distant site. The spine is involved most frequently, followed by ribs, skull, and long bones. Spine involvement mimics tuberculosis with involvement of two adjacent vertebrae and destruction of the intervening disc space. Lesions may be osteolytic or osteoblastic.

Unlike tuberculosis, blastomycosis seldom involves the kidney or ureter. The prostate, epididymis, and testes may be involved. The usual presentation is a scrotal or prostatic mass or bladder outlet obstruction. Hematuria and/or sterile pyuria are common.

Diagnostic Tests

Morphology. Biopsy specimens of infected tissue reveal an 8- to 20-micron yeast with characteristic wide-necked single budding. The organism is difficult to see in hematoxylin and eosin–stained sections but is readily apparent when the periodic acid-Schiff (PAS) stain or a silver stain is used. The inflammatory reaction consists of a mixed granulomatous and pyogenic response.

The organism can also be identified in sputum, in aspirates of skin lesions, or in prostatic secretions after KOH digestion. The sensitivity of direct smears is not known, but the specificity is virtually 100 per cent when the single budding yeast with broad neck of attachment is identified. Direct diagnosis is also often possible by careful examination of sputum samples prepared for cytologic evaluation with the Papanicolaou stain.

Culture. Biologic material should be cultured on selective media for fungi, including Sabouraud's agar. Some plates should be prepared without cycloheximide and incubated at 25°C. The organism grows slowly, and the plates must be sealed to prevent drying. The colony formation is variable, and the microscopic morphology of the mycelium is not diagnostic. For positive identification, the mycelial form must be converted to the characteristic yeast form by subculture at 37°C. Culture diagnosis often takes 3 weeks or more from the time the specimen is submitted.

Skin Testing. Skin test preparations to date have not been sensitive or specific. Many false-positive results have occurred in patients who had had histoplasmosis, an illness much more common and coendemic over a very large area. There is no commercial skin test antigen available at present.

Serologic Diagnosis. Serologic tests for blastomycosis are not as useful as in the other major mycotic illnesses. The complement fixation test with blastomycin as the antigen was not reliable. Most patients with blastomycosis had a negative test, and most patients with a positive test had histoplasmosis rather than blastomycosis. More recently, an immunodiffusion test using a water-soluble cell wall extract (antigen A) has been reported positive in 80 per cent of cases of blastomycosis. A complement fixation assay using this antigen has also been developed, and work is in progress on an enzyme-linked immunosorbent assay. These recent developments are promising, but the vast majority of all cases of blastomycosis are presently diagnosed by demonstration of characteristic yeast in tissue biopsies and other biologic materials or by culture of the fungus from the same.

CRYPTOCOCCOSIS

Cryptococcosis refers to infection by the encapsulated yeast *Cryptococcus neoformans.* The primary pulmonary infection rarely produces a clinical illness, and most patients present with a subacute or chronic meningitis. The organism is distributed worldwide, in both urban and rural environments, and often grows in pigeon droppings. Half of all patients have an underlying condition that predisposes them to infection such as hematologic malignancy or treatment with immunosuppressive drugs.

Clinical Features

Primary Pulmonary Cryptococcosis. Patients usually have no symptoms. If present, fever is modest. The chest roentgenogram may show a localized lower lobe infiltrate, without associated hilar adenopathy. Infiltrates usually resolve completely without nodules or cavitation. Pulmonary cryptococcosis generally requires treatment only in immunosuppressed patients and then only because the risk of subsequent meningitis is so high.

Central Nervous System Cryptococcosis. Eighty per cent of diagnosed cases involve the central nervous system without evidence of previous or concurrent respiratory infection. Headaches gradually increase in frequency and severity, and there may be mild fever and signs of meningeal irritation. There are usually high-protein and reduced glucose concentrations in the cerebrospinal fluid and a lymphocytic pleocytosis, usually with less than 200 cells per cu mm.

Patients may uncommonly present with a single focus of infection in the brain that acts as a mass lesion. Such patients may have evidence of increased intracranial pressure (nausea, vomiting, change in level of consciousness) and focal neurologic signs.

Disseminated Cryptococcosis. Rapid hematogenous spread to many organs occurs only in immunosuppressed patients. High fever is common. Diffuse infiltrates are present, and there may be respiratory failure. Liver and bone marrow are often involved. Meningitis is usually, but not always, present.

Cryptococcosis can involve the skull, vertebrae, or long bones, even in the absence of severe systemic illness. Bone involvement is much less frequent than in coccidioidomycosis or blastomycosis. Roentgenograms show a destructive focus, without periosteal reaction.

Diagnostic Tests

Morphology. The organism is a single budding yeast with a narrow-necked bud and averages 8 to 12 microns in diameter. The characteristic feature is a carbohydrate capsule of variable thickness. The organisms can be seen well on silver-stained sections, but they cannot be positively distinguished from other yeast unless an unstained halo can be seen surrounding the organisms. Direct demonstration of the capsule by a mucicarmine stain secures the diagnosis. Sections of infected tissues generally show very little inflammatory response.

The presence of the capsule also permits rapid microscopic identification of organisms in cerebrospinal fluid mixed with India ink. Large halos around the organisms are easily seen. This test is positive in about 50 per cent of patients with cryptococcal meningitis and is completely specific for the diagnosis.

Culture. The organism grows readily and quickly at 37°C on most media. The colonies are very mucoid, and microscopic confirmation of the capsule is sufficient for diagnosis. Occasionally, the capsule is lost or markedly reduced in culture, and biochemical tests or mouse inoculation will be necessary for identification.

Cultures of spinal fluid are positive in 80 to 90 per cent of patients with cryptococcal meningitis. Blood cultures are often positive in severe disseminated illness. Positive culture of cryptococcus from cerebrospinal fluid, blood, urine, or aspirates of bone or skin lesions always means cryptococcosis. Interpretation of sputum cultures is more difficult because *Cryptococcus neoformans* (and other related strains of cryptococcus) sometimes colonizes the respiratory tract.

Skin Testing. No commercial skin test is available. The skin test is not likely to prove a valuable diagnostic tool because many normal persons demonstrate delayed hypersensitivity to the organism and immunosuppressed patients may not, even when infected.

Serologic Diagnosis. In cryptococcosis, direct measurement of fungal antigen is important. Capsular material in cerebrospinal fluid and in serum can be detected by a sensitive latex-fixation method. This test is positive in about 95 per cent of patients with meningitis and is more sensitive than culture. False-positive tests for cryptococcal antigen occur in the presence of high titer rheumatoid factor. This is usually not a problem in cerebrospinal fluid and can be minimized in serum by running concurrent controls for rheumatoid factor and by preheating the serum to 100°C, which destroys the rheumatoid factor but not the heat-stable cryptococcal antigen.

Determination of cryptococcal antigen is prognostic as well as diagnostic. Initial high levels in the cerebrospinal fluid or failure of the titer to come down after treatment portend treatment failure or early relapse.

Anticryptococcal antibody can be measured by a variety of techniques including complement fixation. However, many patients with cryptococcal meningitis have negative titers. This test has little value, especially compared with the cryptococcal antigen test.

ASPERGILLOSIS

Aspergillosis refers to infection by any of the numerous members of the genus Aspergillus. These fungi are among the most common life forms on earth. Although these organisms have very low pathogenicity for humans, they may readily colonize mucosal surfaces. They cannot invade unless local or systemic immune defenses are altered. Most infections are caused by *Aspergillus fumigatus.* Other potentially pathogenic species include *A. niger, A. flavus, A. clavatus,* and *A. nidulans.*

Invasive aspergillosis occurs almost exclusively in severely immunocompromised patients and is most common in neutropenic leukemics undergoing intensive chemotherapy. Widespread tissue necrosis occurs initially in the lung, where there may be multiple wedge-shaped areas of pneumonia. The fungus grows in blood vessels, causing thrombosis and infarction of lung; new cavities may form as necrotic material is expectorated. The first symptoms are usually those of an acute pneumonia with cough, fever, dyspnea, and pleuritic pain. The chest roentgenogram usually shows rapidly developing infiltrates that may be wedge-shaped or that may quickly cavitate. Some patients, however, have fever, pleuritic pain, and cough even before the chest roentgenogram becomes abnormal. Such a presentation is suggestive of aspergillosis in the appropriate host, i.e., a febrile neutropenic leukemic. Multiple metastatic abscesses may develop in the brain, liver, heart, and skin.

Infections with Aspergillus are also discussed under the topic Opportunistic Mycoses.

MUCORMYCOSIS

Mucormycosis, also called phycomycosis or zygomycosis, refers to infection by members of several genera of soil fungi including Mucor, Rhizopus, and Absidia. These organisms are ubiquitous in nature and cannot invade a normal host. They can invade the nose, sinuses, and other facial structures of ketoacidotic diabetics, the lungs of leukemics or transplant recipients, and the necrotic skin of burn victims. Infection is angiocentric, and there is extensive tissue necrosis.

Rhinocerebral mucormycosis is the most fulminant invasive fungal disease. Infection begins in the nose; there is a dark bloody discharge from both nostrils. Necrosis of the nasal septum and turbinates is followed by rapid spread to the paranasal sinuses. Ulceration and necrosis of the palate, periorbital cellulitis, and direct invasion of the orbit, eye, and brain soon follow. Major arterial thrombosis contributes to tissue destruction, and cavernous sinus thrombosis is common. Progression of illness can be observed hour by hour, and most patients die in less than a week.

Pulmonary mucormycosis and cutaneous mucormycosis are other forms of infection with these organisms. Mucormycosis is also discussed under the topic Opportunistic Mycoses.

CANDIDOSIS

Candidosis refers to infection by any species of the genus Candida. These organisms are part of the normal stool flora and also may inhabit the mouth, pharynx, and sometimes the trachea and bronchi. They do not invade unless local or systemic defenses are altered. Candidosis is usually caused by *Candida albicans.* Other potentially pathogenic species include *C. parapsilosis, C. tropicalis. C. stellatoidea, C. guilliermondi, C. krusei,* and others. Any species may cause any of the clinical forms of candidosis.

Locally invasive candidal organisms in the mouth, esophagus, bladder, or bowel may seed organisms into the bloodstream. Plastic intravenous catheters, especially when used for hyperalimentation, permit direct seeding. The transient fungemia that occurs would be of no consequence in a normal host. However, the same patients, with overgrowth of Candida on mucosal surfaces and long-term intravenous lines, often have serious underlying illnesses that are being treated with antibiotics, corticosteroids, and antineoplastic chemotherapy. In these patients, hematogenous spread of Candida may cause microabscesses in multiple organs. Patients have fever and chills and may develop renal failure. Nodular skin lesions and endophthalmitis may be clues to the diagnosis. About half of all patients with this form of candidosis have lymphoma or leukemia as their underlying illness. Mortality is high.

Many patients with this septicemic form of candidosis have multiple cerebral microabscesses. Other patients may develop meningitis. Candidal involvement of the central nervous system must be considered in any high-risk host with neurologic signs.

Candidal endocarditis occurs among drug addicts, on damaged valves of patients with previous subacute bacterial endocarditis, and as an early postoperative infection after valve replacement. Vegetations are large and embolize to major arteries. Patients with the septicemic form of candidosis usually develop cardiac microabscesses rather than endocarditis.

Isolated candidal peritonitis may complicate peritoneal dialysis, or it may occur in the setting of spontaneous bacterial peritonitis that is under treatment with antibacterial drugs. A polymicrobial peritonitis with Candida as well as multiple species of bacteria suggests bowel perforation. If the treatment is surgery together with antibacterial therapy but the candidal infection is ignored, the patient may develop invasive candidosis.

Candida infections are also discussed under the topic Opportunistic Mycoses.

ACTINOMYCOSIS

Actinomycosis is a chronic suppurative infection caused by *Actinomyces israelii,* an anaerobic bacterium that is part of the normal flora of the mouth. It can directly invade structures around the mouth and pharynx or can be aspirated into the lung. Hematogenous spread may occur with seeding of distant sites.

Clinical Features

Cervicofacial Actinomycosis. Disease begins in the mouth or oropharynx. Usually, there is a break in the normal protective barrier, for example, around a carious tooth. Infection extends to adjacent bone and burrows through soft tissues, producing multiple abscesses with interconnecting fistulas and sinus tracts draining to the surface. Pus expressed from the sinus tracts usually contains "sulphur granules," the matted hyphal masses that are characteristic of actinomycosis. Surprisingly, there is little pain.

Pulmonary Actinomycosis. This is a chronic, fibrosing and abscess-forming infection that frequently resembles tuberculosis. Direct involvement of the pleural space and adjacent ribs is common, and there may be sinus tracts draining to the surface. Symptoms include fever and cough productive of purulent sputum. Later there may be anemia and weight loss.

Abdominal Actinomycosis. Abdominal disease commonly presents as a fistula draining to the abdominal wall. Access to the peritoneal cavity may occur by hematogenous spread from the mouth or by direct penetration of bowel mucosa, either from within by a fishbone or other sharp object or from without by a penetrating wound. A diseased appendix may be the source of abdominal actinomycosis.

Pelvic Actinomycosis. There have been reports of chronic endometrial infection by Actinomyces species. Most frequently, these are related to intrauterine devices used for contraception. The infection may spread to the fallopian tubes.

Diagnostic Tests

Morphology. The bacterium is a gram-positive rod that grows in thin hyphalike strands. The width of the strands is an order of magnitude less than true fungal hyphae (less than 1 micron, as contrasted to 10 to 20 microns). Tangled masses of organisms form macroscopic specks (1 to 2 mm in size) known as sulfur granules, which are characteristic of this infection.

The inflammatory response is mainly pyogenic. There are multiple abscesses separated by bands of fibrosis and interconnected by fistulous tracts. A granulomatous response is seen at the periphery of the lesion.

Identification of sulfur granules in pus from a draining sinus is diagnostic. Demonstration of characteristic organisms on a Gram stain is diagnostic of actinomycosis if the organism is seen in specimens other than oral secretions, tooth scrapings, or expectorated sputum.

Culture. Direct anaerobic cultures of pus or surgical biopsy specimens are frequently positive. The organism is somewhat difficult to grow and requires strict anaerobic conditions. Small white mycelial colonies appear in 2 to 5 days.

Skin Testing. Skin tests are not used for diagnosis.

Serologic Diagnosis. Serologic tests are not used for diagnosis.

NOCARDIOSIS

Nocardiosis is an acute suppurative bacterial infection caused by *Nocardia asteroides,* an aerobic bacterium. Primary infection is in the lung, but there may be hematogenous spread to other organs, most commonly the brain. Nocardia is not part of the normal oral flora; rather, it is a soil organism. Infection is acquired by inhalation.

Clinical Features

Pulmonary Nocardiosis. This is a rapidly progressive necrotizing pneumonia. Patients have fever, chills, and sweats and may have pleuritic pain. The chest roentgenogram shows one or several large rounded infiltrates, often with central cavitation. Nonproductive cough becomes productive of mucopurulent sputum after cavities are formed. Most infections occur in immunosuppressed patients with underlying illnesses requiring treatment with corticosteroids and/or cytotoxic agents. Brain lesions present as a mass with focal neurologic findings. In appropriate patients, a cavitary lung infiltrate in association with new focal neurologic deficits should suggest nocardiosis. Other metastatic abscesses may occur in the subcutaneous tissues, where they are more accessible to aspiration for obtaining diagnostic material.

Diagnostic Tests

Morphology. The organism can be recognized in sputum or in pus from metastatic abscesses as a gram-positive filamentous rod. As in actinomycosis, the hyphalike threads are much thinner (less than 1 micron) than true fungal hyphae. Nocardia can be differentiated from Actinomyces because it is acid-fast in a modified Ziehl-Neelsen stain. Because it is only weakly acid-fast, the 3 per cent hydrochloric acid used in the acid alcohol step must be replaced with 0.5 per cent solution of aqueous sulfuric acid or the organism will be decolorized. The inflammatory response in tissue is pyogenic and is not distinctive from other necrotizing pneumonias.

Culture. Culture of sputum or of bronchial washings and brushings frequently yields the organism. Nocardia is not a contaminant from the mouth, and culture isolates are always significant. Nocardia is not difficult to grow and can be recovered in 3 to 10 days on fungal media, tuberculosis media, or blood agar.

Skin Testing. Skin tests are not used for diagnosis.

Serologic Diagnosis. Serologic tests are not used for diagnosis.

OPPORTUNISTIC MYCOSES

By Daniel Rotrosen, M.D.
and John E. Edwards, Jr., M.D.
Torrance, California

CANDIDIASIS

Candidiasis is a localized or disseminated opportunistic infection with protean manifestations. Candida organisms are small (4 to 6 microns), thin-walled, ovoid cells that reproduce by budding. Yeast forms, pseudohyphae and hyphae can be seen in clinical specimens. *Candida albicans* can be identified presumptively by germ tube formation in serum or by chlamydospore formation on cornmeal agar. Identification of non-*albicans* species depends on carbohydrate assimilation and fermentation reactions. Candida organisms are found mainly in human and animal sources; when found in soil, hospital environments, and food, contamination from humans or animals is probable. The organisms are normal commensals of man and are found throughout the gastrointestinal tract, on damaged and macerated skin, in the female genital tract, and in the urine of patients with indwelling catheters. Most human infections are due to *C. albicans,* although non-*albicans* species are emerging as frequent pathogens both in the immunocompromised host (particularly *C. tropicalis*) and among intravenous drug addicts.

Predisposing Factors

A number of naturally occurring and iatrogenic factors are known to increase susceptibility to Candida infection. T cell dysfunction (in chronic mucocutaneous candidiasis) and diabetes mellitus predispose to superficial but not disseminated disease. Damage to skin and mucosal surfaces leaves these sites vulnerable to Candida invasion. Iatrogenic factors associated with disseminated candidiasis include use of broad-spectrum antibiotics, immunosuppressive and cytotoxic therapy, intravenous hyperalimentation, use of plastic catheters, and gastrointestinal surgery.

Clinical Features

The clinical manifestations of candidiasis are diverse and depend upon both localization of infection and underlying host disorders.

Mucocutaneous and Gastrointestinal Infections

Thrush. This common form of oral candidiasis is characterized by a creamy-white curdlike pseudomembrane on the tongue, soft palate, and buccal mucosa. The distribution may be either confluent or patchy; the pseudomembrane is composed of desquamated epithelial cells, leukocytes, bacteria, Candida organisms, keratin, and food debris. On scraping, the underlying mucosa is raw, erythematous, and painful. Patients may complain of sore throat, especially on swallowing. Thrush may occur in any age group but is particularly common in neonates, patients with the acquired immunodeficiency syndrome, and those undergoing cancer chemotherapy. Additionally, it has been associated with the use of steroid inhalers in the treatment of asthma. In older children, chronic thrush is usually indicative of chronic mucocutaneous candidiasis.

Candida Esophagitis. Esophageal involvement typically occurs in the setting of hematopoietic or lymphatic malignancy. The lower two thirds of the esophagus characteristically is involved; approximately half of patients with esophageal candidiasis do not have signs of oral thrush. Patients may be nearly asymptomatic but usually complain of painful swallowing, often associated with a feeling of obstruction and substernal chest pain. In profoundly immunocompromised hosts, dissemination theoretically could occur from an esophageal focus. Massive hemorrhage and perforation of the esophagus are infrequent.

Gastrointestinal Candidiasis. In patients with malignancy, candidiasis may involve any segment of the gastrointestinal (GI) tract. Lesions may be either single or multiple and consist of mucosal ulcerations with Candida found deep in the ulcer bed.

Candida Vaginitis. Involvement of the female genital tract usually occurs in the setting of diabetes mellitus, antibiotic therapy, and pregnancy. However, recurrent Candida vaginitis is also seen in the absence of these factors. Symptoms include intense vulvar pruritus, usually accompanied by a thick curdlike discharge. The vagina and labia are typically erythematous; extension to the urethra and perineum may occur.

Cutaneous Candidiasis. Cutaneous involvement is common when skin is traumatized or macerated, or when skin surfaces are in close proximity, providing a warm, moist environment. Manifestations include intertrigo, diaper rash, pruritus ani, folliculitis, balanitis, paronychia, and onychomycosis. Certain cutaneous lesions may be an important clue to the diagnosis of hematogenously disseminated candidiasis. The lesions are characteristically maculonodular or maculopapular but may be pustular, hemorrhagic, or erythematous, or they may mimic ecthyma gangrenosum. Nodular subcutaneous lesions with little or no overlying cutaneous findings have been described.

Chronic Mucocutaneous Candidiasis (CMC). This is a syndrome of Candida infection involving the skin, mucous membranes, nails, and scalp in association with diminished T cell in vitro response to Candida antigens, frequent cutaneous anergy, and polyendocrinopathy, which is seen in approximately 50 per cent of patients. Most forms of CMC begin in infancy or childhood; if untreated, they run a protracted and persistent course. Mucocutaneous involvement may be either minimal or severely disfiguring, as in Candida granuloma. The endocrine dysfunction tends to postdate the cutaneous manifestations, often after an interval of several years. Hypoparathyroidism and Addison's disease are the most common findings; hypothyroidism and diabetes mellitus also occur.

Deep Organ Involvement

Deep organ involvement usually occurs in the course of widely disseminated disease. Virtually any organ can be infected by the hematogenous route. Most patients have fever and signs of sepsis; certain features listed as follows are suggestive of specific organ involvement.

Ocular Candidiasis. Following trauma or eye surgery, Candida can infect virtually any eye structure. Depending on the extent of involvement, patients may complain of eye pain or visual deficit. Once endophthalmitis occurs, the incidence of permanent intraocular damage and blindness is high. Hematogenous Candida endophthalmitis has been increasingly recognized as a sign of systemic infection as well as a localized complication of transient candidemia. Fundal lesions are often demonstrated easily by direct or indirect ophthalmoscopy. They are gray to white and chorioretinal in origin and rapidly extend to involve the vitreous. In profoundly granulocytopenic patients, lesions may not be detected despite active chorioretinal infection, presumably because a cohesive inflammatory mass does not form, owing tc a lack of cellular exudate. Symptoms include eye pain, loss of visual acuity, and floating scotomata.

Central Nervous System (CNS) Candidiasis. Candida meningitis usually occurs in the setting of disseminated infection or as a neurosurgical complication, particularly following placement of a ventricular shunt. Signs of meningeal irritation are usually present. In disseminated candidiasis, the brain parenchyma is frequently involved with diffuse microabscess formation resulting in lethargy, obtundation, or localizing neurologic signs.

Cardiac Candidiasis. Candida myocarditis is a frequent autopsy finding in patients who die with disseminated candidiasis. Clues to the diagnosis are profound hypotension, severe congestive heart failure (CHF), and ECG changes suggestive of cardiac involvement. Multiple small abscesses are scattered throughout the myocardium.

Candida endocarditis arises as complications of narcotic abuse and prosthetic valve implantation. The clinical features resemble those of bacterial endocarditis; however, arterial emboli to large vessels are a prominent feature. Most cases of Candida prosthetic valve endocarditis occur within 2 months of valve implantation; infection may also occur late (years after surgery).

Urinary Tract Candidiasis. Candida cystitis is most often a complication of prolonged bladder catheterization or diabetes mellitus. Symptoms may be absent, or they may mimic bacterial cystitis. Candida cystitis often resolves spontaneously, although candiduria may persist for prolonged periods. Upper tract involvement may develop by the ascending route or by hematogenous spread to the kidney, resulting in renal abscess or diffuse pyelonephritis. Fungus ball formation in the renal pelvis or ureter may result in partial or complete urinary tract obstruction.

Skeletal Candidiasis. Candida osteomyelitis and Candida arthritis most often arise as complications of candidemia. Localization to the spine and intervertebral disc space is common. Symptoms may be minimal and, following transient candidemia, may be delayed for weeks or months.

Pulmonary Candidiosis. Candida pneumonia is uncommon and occurs predominantly in the severely immunocompromised host. Pulmonary infection may develop following aspiration or by hematogenous spread to the lung. Chest x-ray findings are nonspecific; isolation of Candida from sputum must be interpreted in proper perspective. Definitive diagnosis requires biopsy evidence of parenchymal lung invasion.

Syndrome of Disseminated Candidiasis and Candidemia. In the setting of severe host debility, dissemination of Candida to multiple organs is common. Kidney, brain, myocardium, and eye are most often involved; organs less frequently involved include skin, muscle, lungs, gastrointestinal tract, and endocrine glands. Symptoms are usually nonspecific; diligent and repetitive examination for signs of dissemination is indicated.

Great care should be taken not to dismiss a positive blood culture for Candida as harmless and spontaneously resolving. Most patients with candidemia will require therapy.

Laboratory Findings

Mucocutaneous Infection

Scrapings from involved areas should be examined by Gram stain or 10 per cent potassium hydroxide (KOH) mount; typical blastospores, hyphae, and pseudohyphae should be readily found.

In patients with Candida esophagitis, barium swallow may show characteristic mucosal irregularities as well as shoulder defects, diverticulae, fistulae, and esophageal dilation. Similar findings may be seen in Herpes esophagitis. Definitive diagnosis is made by endoscopy with biopsy.

Deep Organ Involvement and Disseminated Candidiasis

Routine blood studies and x-rays may suggest involvement of a particular organ but are not helpful in specific diagnosis. Definitive diagnosis of deep organ involvement is based on biopsy demonstration of the organism invading tissue with confirmation by culture. In general, a presumptive diagnosis of disseminated candidiasis is made on clinical grounds. In the proper clinical setting, biopsy and isolation of Candida from skin lesions, muscle, bone, synovial fluids, or cerebrospinal fluid (CSF) may confirm the diagnosis.

Although Candida grows well in vented blood cultures, fungemia is detected in only about 50 per cent of patients with disseminated candidiasis. Reports suggest that lysis/centrifugation culture systems may slightly increase the yield of blood cultures. Several serologic techniques for antibody are available; their usefulness is limited by frequent false-negative titers in immunocompromised patients and occasional false-positive titers in patients with intestinal or mucosal colonization. In a clinical setting compatible with disseminated candidiasis, Candida precipitins in high titer or seroconversion is evidence in support of the diagnosis, but this finding must be interpreted cautiously. Techniques to identify circulating Candida antigens and metabolites are currently under investigation.

Pitfalls in Diagnosis

Comprehensive and repetitive clinical evaluation is of critical importance in establishing the diagnosis of disseminated candidiasis. Common pitfalls are exclusion of disseminated candidiasis or Candida endocarditis because of negative blood cultures and attributing a positive culture to a "skin" or "laboratory" contaminant. Clinicians occasionally disregard non-*albicans* blood or tissue isolates based on the misconception that they are nonpathogens. It may be extremely dangerous to assume that a positive blood culture for Candida represents "benign" candidemia. Repetitive clinical and laboratory evaluation should be pursued to exclude the presence of disseminated disease. The evaluation should consist of serial examinations including ophthalmoscopy, repeat cultures, and x-ray studies and scans as indicated. Diagnosis and treatment should not be based solely on isolation of Candida from superficial sites such as sputum or wounds. Over-reliance on Candida serologies can result in serious error because of the limited sensitivity and specificity of available tests.

ASPERGILLOSIS

Members of the genus Aspergillus can produce varied clinical syndromes in the normal and immunosuppressed host. Disease manifestations result from local or widespread tissue invasion, colonization of preformed cavities, and antigenic stimulation.

Aspergillus species are exceptionally ubiquitous in nature and can be found in foods, growing in soil, in vegetation, and in airborne dust. Disease is usually acquired by inhalation of airborne spores, although numerous case reports suggest that skin of operative sites may be the primary focus of infection. Hospital renovation and construction have been associated with an increased frequency of disease in immunocompromised patients.

Aspergillus fumigatus is responsible for the majority of cases; *A. flavus, A. niger,* and other species are less commonly implicated. Speciation is based on colonial morphology and microscopic examination of the spores and fruiting bodies. Aspergillus hyphae in tissues are 2 to 4 microns wide, even in diameter, usually septate, and dichotomously branched. A distinguishing feature of Aspergillus infection is its propensity to invade blood vessels and to cause subsequent thrombosis and infarction.

Invasive Aspergillosis

Clinical Features

Most cases of invasive aspergillosis occur in the setting of severe immunocompromise resulting from the management of hematopoietic and lymphoreticular malignancies and organ transplantation. Corticosteroids, cytotoxic agents, and broad-spectrum antibiotics have been administered in the majority of cases, though a causative role for the latter has been questioned. Less often, invasive aspergillosis has been noted as a complication of cardiac surgery, collagen vascular disorders, and chronic granulomatous disease of childhood. There is no apparent age or sex predilection. Clinical features will be described according to sites of involvement.

Pulmonary Aspergillosis. The lung is the organ most frequently involved in invasive aspergillosis; in most series, over 90 per cent of patients have pulmonary involvement manifesting as necrotizing bronchopneumonia, infarction, solitary or multiple abscesses, microabscess formation, or lobar consolidation. Usual findings include unremitting fever associated with pulmonary infiltrates, nonproductive cough, dyspnea, and tachypnea. Symptoms usually progress despite antibiotic therapy or recur after an initial response. Invasion of pulmonary vessels with occlusion and thrombosis may result in pulmonary infarction and hemorrhage in up to one third of patients. The clinical course in these patients is notable for the sudden occurrence of dyspnea, pleuritic chest pain (often accompanied by a pleural rub), tachycardia, gallop rhythm, and cough with occasional hemoptysis.

Extrapulmonary Dissemination. Among immunocompromised patients with invasive pulmonary aspergillosis, widespread dissemination occurs in 25 to 50 per cent. Sites frequently involved are the gastrointestinal tract, CNS, heart, kidney, liver, thyroid, and skin. Dissemination from a nonpulmonary focus is rare. Infection may occur at any level of the GI tract; ulcerative esophagitis is the most common lesion. Biopsy demonstrates invasion by fungal hyphae at the ulcer base. Ulcers are generally deeper than those seen in Candida esophagitis, particularly when vascular invasion and infarction have occurred. In the latter situation, extension of the lesion to the serosal surface is not uncommon and fatal perforation and hemorrhage may occur. Similar lesions may occur throughout the GI tract. The exact role of steroid and cytotoxic therapy in the pathogenesis of these lesions is unclear. With severe oropharyngeal or esophageal involvement, patients may complain of painful swallowing. In patients with intestinal perforation and massive hemorrhage, symptoms may be masked by concomitant steroid administration.

Central nervous system involvement may occur by direct extension from the paranasal sinuses and orbit or by hematogenous dissemination. Solitary or multiple abscesses may develop, accompanied by vascular invasion, thrombosis, and infarction. Diffuse meningeal and spinal cord infection are rare. The clinical features are variable and nonspecific; common findings are depression, lethargy, confusion, obtundation, seizures, coma, and focal neurological deficits. Central nervous system involvement may be rapidly progressive and result in death in a matter of days. Alternatively, it may persist for weeks or months.

Renal and hepatic abscesses with areas of infarction are common and, in most cases, clinically silent. With extensive liver involvement, right upper quadrant tenderness may be present.

Cardiac infection may arise hematogenously, by direct extension from the lung, or as a complication of cardiac surgery. In the latter case, Aspergillus prosthetic valve endocarditis often presents with major arterial emboli superimposed on typical features of infective endocarditis. In the immunosuppressed patient with disseminated aspergillosis, myocardial abscesses, myocarditis, pericarditis, coronary thrombosis, and nonvegetative endocardial plaques may be found. Vegetative valvular endocarditis is extremely rare. The clinical picture is nonspecific. Signs of congestive failure may be prominent. Pericarditis is rarely symptomatic.

Cutaneous manifestations may develop by means of hematogenous dissemination or as a primary focus of infection in traumatized areas. Necrotizing plaques, subcutaneous granulomas, abscesses, and maculopapular lesions have been described.

Laboratory Findings

Routine blood studies may reflect specific organ involvement or underlying disorders, but they are not helpful in the definitive etiologic diagnosis. The roentgenographic features are variable in invasive pulmonary aspergillosis. Chest x-ray may be normal in up to one third of the patients who are studied acutely at the onset of respiratory symptoms.

The earliest findings are solitary or multiple nodules that may rapidly progress to extensive consolidation, patchy bronchopneumonia, cavitation, or wedge-shaped, pleural-based lesions. Arterial oxygen tension is usually well preserved despite extensive radiographic involvement. Sputum cultures rarely yield Aspergillus, and when positive, can be considered only presumptive evidence of invasive disease. Definitive diagnosis requires biopsy proof of parenchymal lung invasion with confirmation by culture. The organism is readily seen with periodic acid–Schiff (PAS) and methenamine silver stains but may be poorly visualized with hematoxylin-eosin.

Isolation of *A. flavus* from nasal surveillance cultures has been correlated with invasive pulmonary and disseminated disease. However, the cost-effectiveness of surveillance cultures and their overall utility in early diagnosis has been questioned. Even with widely disseminated disease, Aspergillus species only occasionally can be isolated from blood, bone marrow, urine, or CSF. Blood cultures are positive in less than 10 per cent of well-documented cases of Aspergillus endocarditis. Definitive diagnosis of disseminated disease requires documentation by biopsy and culture.

Serologic tests have been of limited utility in the diagnosis of invasive aspergillosis. Conversion of serum precipitin titer (as determined by counterimmunoelectrophoresis [CIE], enzyme-linked immunosorbent assay [ELISA], or passive hemagglutination) is correlated with invasive disease, but the interpretation of single titers and the incidence of false-negative titers remain problematic. Techniques to detect circulating Aspergillus antigens are under investigation.

Pitfalls in Diagnosis

Recent studies have demonstrated an improved prognosis with early diagnosis and therapy in invasive aspergillosis. Unfortunately, antemortem diagnosis remains unusual. Failure to consider the diagnosis or to pursue it aggressively is a major pitfall. Culture results and serologies, if available, must be interpreted in proper perspective.

Aspergilloma

Clinical Features

Patients with a variety of chronic lung disorders may develop aspergillomas occupying pre-existing cavities, cysts, and ectatic airways. The fungus ball is a mass of aspergillus mycelia growing in airway secretions, or in some cases, in devitalized lung tissue. The fungus ball may be attached to the cavity wall, but invasion of the wall and surrounding parenchyma is unusual. Underlying diseases include tuberculosis, histoplasmosis, sarcoidosis, chronic bronchitis, and bronchiectasis. The symptoms and prognosis are generally related to the underlying condition. Hemoptysis is frequent and may be massive.

Laboratory Findings

The roentgenographic features are characteristic but not pathognomonic. Localization is typically to the apical segments of the upper lobes; the aspergilloma appears as a rounded intracavitary density usually surrounded by an air crescent; calcification of the fungus ball may occur. Lesions may resolve spontaneously. Sputum cultures and bronchial washings yield Aspergillus species in the majority of cases. Precipitin reactions are nearly invariably positive when aspergilloma is seen on chest x-ray.

Allergic Bronchopulmonary Aspergillosis

Clinical Features

Allergic bronchopulmonary aspergillosis (ABPA) is characterized by bronchospasm, pulmonary infiltrates, central bronchiectasis, and evidence of hypersensitivity to Aspergillus antigens. Patients typically present with wheezing, dyspnea, and cough that may be productive. Expectoration of mucus plugs occurs in up to 50 per cent of cases. Minimal hemoptysis, fever, and pleuritic chest pain may be present. The bronchospastic component of ABPA is thought to be a Type I (IgE-mediated) hypersensitivity reaction. Chronic sequelae, possibly mediated through a Type III (immune complex–mediated) hypersensitivity reaction, include pulmonary fibrosis, bronchiectasis, and restrictive lung disease.

Laboratory Findings

A number of immunologic findings are associated with ABPA. Peripheral eosinophil counts and total IgE levels are elevated and correlate well with disease activity. Immediate skin reactivity to Aspergillus antigens may be present; however, it also is found in asthmatics without other evidence of ABPA, in patients with aspergilloma and with other chronic lung diseases, and in normal controls. Serum precipitins to Aspergillus antigens by CIE or double gel immunodiffusion are detected in most patients with ABPA. False-positive results may occur in the aforementioned conditions. Chest roentgenograms show acute patchy infiltrates with an upper lobe predilection. Bronchography may show saccular proximal bronchiectasis and has been used to confirm the diagnosis of ABPA in patients with a compatible syndrome and laboratory features. Aspergillus species can be isolated from sputum in approximately two thirds of cases.

Chronic Necrotizing Pulmonary Aspergillosis

Clinical Features

Chronic necrotizing pulmonary aspergillosis (CNPA) is an indolent, cavitating pulmonary process caused by invasion of lung parenchyma by Aspergillus. The disease typically occurs in middle-aged patients with a background of chronic lung disease. Predisposing pulmonary disorders include inactive mycobacterial disease, chronic obstructive pulmonary disease (COPD), pneumoconiosis, and prior radiation therapy in the area of involvement. Mild systemic immunocompromise (resulting from diabetes mellitus, connective tissue disorders and low-dose corticosteroid therapy) has been implicated as a potential factor in pathogenesis. Frequent complaints are fever, weight loss, cough, and sputum production. Symptoms may be present months to several years prior to diagnosis and the long-term course is uncertain. The outcome is usually favorable with amphotericin B or combined medical-surgical therapy.

Laboratory Findings

Diagnosis can be difficult because the clinical findings mimic infection due to anaerobic bacteria, mycobacteria, and other fungi. The chest roentgenogram shows infiltrative and cavitary disease with a predilection for the upper lobes. Cavity formation may be complicated by development of a mycetoma. Serum precipitins against Aspergillus are usually present. Definitive diagnosis requires demonstration of parenchymal lung invasion with confirmation by culture.

MUCORMYCOSIS

Mucormycosis refers to opportunistic infection caused by members of the family Mucoraceae; these include the genera Rhizopus, Absidia, and Mucor. Mucoraceae are ubiquitous saprophytes found in nature in decaying vegetation, in soil, and as laboratory contaminants. The majority of human infections occur by inhalation of fungal spores or by direct invasion of nasal mucosa, sinuses, skin, and gastrointestinal tract. The fungal hyphae show a predilection for blood vessel invasion, which results in thrombosis, hemorrhagic infarction, and extension across tissue planes. Hyphae are irregularly wide (6 to 50 microns) and nonseptate with right angle branching; they are seen well with PAS and methenamine silver stains but may be missed with hematoxylin-eosin. Clinical manifestations and histopathology are identical in disease due to Rhizopus, Absidia, and Mucor. Speciation is determined in vitro, based on differences in morphology and physiology.

Rhinocerebral Mucormycosis

Clinical Features

Rhinocerebral mucormycosis generally occurs in the setting of poorly controlled diabetes mellitus; both clinical and experimental evidence implicates acidosis (and not hyperglycemia) as the primary factor predisposing to rhinocerebral infection. Other predisposing conditions include uremia, infant diarrhea with acidosis, and hematologic malignancy. Rarely, rhinocerebral mucormycosis may be the initial manifestation of diabetes mellitus.

Infection begins in the nasal cavity or palate and extends to the paranasal sinuses, ethmoids, and retro-orbital region and into the brain. The disease may be fulminant and progress to death within a few days, or it may become indolent. Early symptoms include headache, lethargy, proptosis, and visual loss. The latter finding, due to retinal artery occlusion, is helpful in distinguishing rhinocerebral mucormycosis from pyogenic cavernous sinus thrombosis, in which visual impairment is mild and occurs late if at all. As orbital involvement progresses, paralysis of the second, third, fourth, and sixth cranial nerves results in ptosis, pupillary dilatation, and ophthalmoplegia. The trigeminal and facial nerves are frequently involved; thrombosis of the cavernous sinus and internal carotid artery with contralateral hemiplegia may occur. Meningismus is unusual, even with extensive CNS involvement. Black necrotic lesions on the palate or nasal mucosa and drainage of black pus from the eye are diagnostic clues, but similar lesions may occur with infection due to *Pseudomonas aeruginosa* and Aspergillus species.

Laboratory Findings

Routine blood studies reflect the severity of underlying disorders. Radiologic studies are useful in demonstrating extent of disease. Findings include clouding of the sinuses and evidence of bone destruction. Angiography may show aneurysms, luminal narrowing due to thrombosis, or occlusion of the internal carotid and ophthalmic arteries. Computed tomography (CT) may demonstrate retro-orbital involvement. Common CT findings include thickening of the medial rectus muscle, opacification of the orbital apex, and enlargement of the optic nerve. Orbital venography may reveal obstructive changes within the orbit and cavernous sinus. Examination of CSF usually shows slightly increased fluid pressure, moderate pleocytosis with approximately 50 per cent polymorphonuclear cells, and slight protein elevation; hypoglycorrhachia is uncommon and culture is negative. Definitive diagnosis requires biopsy demonstration of characteristic broad, nonseptate hyphae invading tissue. Blood cultures are rarely positive; cultures of biopsy and autopsy specimens are frequently negative.

Pulmonary Mucormycosis

Clinical Features

Seventy-five per cent of cases of pulmonary mucormycosis occur in patients with leukemia, lymphoma, or profound neutropenia. The remainder are seen associated with diabetes, renal failure, or burns;—rarely in otherwise healthy individuals. The characteristic lesion is thrombosis of pulmonary vesels with infarction. Hemorrhagic bronchopneumonia is common, as well as concomitant infection due to bacteria, viruses, and other fungi. Fever, cough, and dyspnea usually occur. Hemoptysis and pleuritic pain are uncommon.

Laboratory Findings

Roentgenographic findings are variable and include patchy infiltrates, consolidation, cavitation, and, rarely, pleural effusion and fungus ball formation. There is no lobar predilection. Radiographs typically show rapid progression, but chronic pulmonary lesions have been reported. Mucor is rarely isolated from sputum or blood. Diagnosis requires biopsy proof of pulmonary parenchymal invasion.

Disseminated Mucormycosis

Disseminated mucormycosis occurs in the same setting as pulmonary mucormycosis, and in most patients dissemination is thought to arise from a primary focus in the lung. Widespread infection is characterized by vessel invasion with thrombosis and ischemic necrosis of surrounding tissues. Organs commonly involved include spleen, kidney, heart, gastrointestinal tract, liver, pancreas, and brain. Concomitant bacterial, viral, and fungal infection is frequent and antemortem diagnosis is unusual. Mucor is rarely isolated from body fluids and secretions.

Gastrointestinal Mucormycosis

Gastrointestinal mucormycosis occurs infrequently in the temperate zone. It is more often seen in tropical and subtropical countries associated with kwashiorkor. Other predisposing conditions include amebic colitis, typhoid, pellagra, gastric ulcers, and corticosteroid treatment. The stomach is most frequently involved, followed by the colon. Both invasion and colonization of gastric ulcers can be seen; in the latter instance, prognosis is favorable. Complications include intestinal perforation, hemorrhage, and obstruction. Widespread dissemination from a primary gastrointestinal site may occur. Diagnosis is based on biopsy evidence of tissue invasion.

Miscellaneous Mucor Infections

Several forms of cutaneous mucormycosis have been described. Primary cutaneous lesions have occurred in diabetics and burn patients; use of Elastoplast bandages has been associated with the development of cutaneous mucor under the application site of the bandage. Wound infections and infection at injection sites are described. Dissemination from cutaneous sites may occur. Conversely, cutaneous lesions resembling ecthyma gangrenosum may develop in severely immunocompromised patients.

Mucor endocarditis has occurred de novo and complicating implantation of prosthetic valves. The clinical features resemble other forms of fungal endocarditis with bulky vegetations and emboli to major vessels.

Pitfalls in Diagnosis

An aggressive approach is warranted when mucormycosis is suspected on clinical grounds. The major pitfall in diagnosis is failure to consider mucormycosis and proceeding promptly to histopathologic examination of suspicious lesions. Negative fungal cultures should not dissuade the clinician when mucormycosis is suspected. There are no serologic tests currently useful in the diagnosis of mucormycosis. Blood cultures are nearly always negative.

MISCELLANEOUS OPPORTUNISTIC MYCOSES

A variety of disseminated mycoses are seen infrequently but are increasing in importance. *Candida glabrata* (formerly *Torulopsis glabrata*) causes urinary tract and systemic infections with clinical features similar to other Candida infections. *Petriellidium boydii* (formerly *Allescheria boydii*) is the most common cause of Madura foot in the southeastern United States. The infection is characterized by granulomatous induration and brawny edema of the foot with formation of draining sinus tracts. *P. boydii* has been increasingly recognized as a pathogen in the immunocompromised host. Widely disseminated disease and a variety of focal *P. boydii* infections are described. These have included endocarditis, myocarditis, bone and soft-tissue infection, sinusitis, endophthalmitis, pneumonia, and intracavitary mycetoma. Proper identification is important, since the organism is usually, but not always, resistant to amphotericin B. Imidazoles appear promising in petriellidiosis.

In the severely compromised host, disseminated infection may be due to a variety of relatively "nonpathogenic" fungi. Case reports describe widespread involvement with saccharomyces, rhodotorula, geotrichum, drechslera, penicillium, and curvularia; dissemination may occur in sporotrichosis, chromomycosis, trichopytosis, and trichosporosis. Diagnosis of these unusual infections requires biopsy evidence of tissue invasion with confirmation by culture. Serologic tests are not available in these unusual mycoses.

The endemic mycoses (coccidioidomycosis, histoplasmosis, blastomycosis, and paracoccidioidomycosis) and cryptococcosis may present in the normal or immunocompromised host. These infections are discussed in other chapters.

INVASIVE AND NONINVASIVE MYCOTIC DISEASES OF SKIN

By Mark Holzberg, M.D.
and Henry E. Jones, M.D.
Atlanta, Georgia

This article is restricted to the discussion of fungal diseases of cutaneous origin. Since many species of fungi elicit a variety of well-defined clinical syndromes, each cutaneous syndrome is discussed separately in consideration of the extent or pathologic depth of cutaneous involvement (Table 1).

PITYRIASIS VERSICOLOR

Synonyms

Tinea versicolor, dermatomycosis furfuracea, chromophytosis, tinea flava, liver spots.

Diagnostic Criteria

1. Chronic, mild infection of the upper stratum corneum characterized by discrete and confluent furfuraceous, discolored, mildly scaly macules affecting principally the upper chest, back, and upper extremities caused by *Pityrosporum orbiculare* (*P. ovale*).

2. Round, budding yeasts and short, infrequently branched hyphae found by direct examination of a potassium hydroxide (KOH) preparation of epidermal skin scrapings.

Table 1. Noninvasive and Invasive Fungal Skin Disease in Relation to Pathologic Extent of Involvement

Disease	Integument						
	Glabrous Skin	*Palms and Soles*	*Hair*	*Nails*	*Mucosa*	*Subcutaneous Invasion*	*Opportunistic Hematogenous Dissemination*
Pityriasis versicolor	+	–	–	–	–	–	–
Dermatophytosis	+	+	+	+	–	–	–
Candidiasis	+	+	–	+	+	–	+
Chromoblastomycosis	+	+	–	–	–	+	–
Maduromycosis	+	+	–	–	–	Bone	–
Mucormycosis	+	+	–	–	+	Arteries	+
Sporotrichosis	+	+	–	–	+	Lymphatics	+

Epidemiology

Pityrosporum orbiculare (*P. ovale*) is a part of the normal human flora and is especially dense in the scalp and upper trunk. However, special circumstances lead either to fungal overgrowth or to a decrease in squamous cell turnover and disease ensues. One such special circumstance is an environmental condition in which a rise in temperature and humidity leads to perspiration and maceration. Disease is more clinically evident and very prevalent in the tropics and subtropics. Other predisposing factors include malnutrition, excess plasma cortisol levels, seborrheic dermatitis, pregnancy, oral contraceptives, and possibly genetic predisposition. Although pityriasis versicolor may be found in all races, ages, and both sexes, the patient is most often a postpubertal white male. The disease is rare in the elderly.

Disease occurs when the saprophytic yeast form changes to the pathogenic mycelial form. It is the mycelial form that is responsible for melanocyte changes and corresponding pigmentary changes. Epidermis isolated from hyperpigmented lesions reveals large melanosomes; hypopigmented areas reveal small melanosomes. Evidence that lipid-derived dicarboxylic acid elaborated by the organism is associated with both a tyrosinase inhibitor effect and a melanosome cytotoxic effect is gaining acceptance as the mechanism responsible for achromic lesions.

Clinical Manifestations

Pityriasis versicolor is essentially extracorporal and outside the domain of host response. This superficial infection is usually brought to the patient's attention for cosmetic reasons. It presents as numerous small hypopigmented to darker-brown furfuraceous macules that soon form a fine scale and become concrescent (Fig. 1). Clinically apparent areas are usually limited to the upper chest, back, and arms. Infection may spread to involve areas as low as the popliteal fossae or as high as the scalp. The patient usually becomes aware of infection after sun exposure when affected areas fail to tan normally and become hypopigmented or, occasionally, hyperpigmented. There is sometimes an inflammatory response, and some patients report mild itching. Papular lesions are occasionally seen perifollicularly. In more long-standing disease, both hypopigmented and hyperpigmented areas—representing younger and older lesions, respectively—may coexist on the same patient. A clinical variant called *pityriasis versicolor alba* or *achromia parasitica* is found in the tropics in dark-skinned infants. The primary features of this variant are the usual diaper-area distribution and marked depigmentation.

Complications rarely occur. If the organism invades the hair follicle or sebaceous glands in large numbers, an inflammatory folliculitis may occur, most commonly in young adults.

Laboratory Procedures

Direct examination of epidermal scales from affected areas by a KOH preparation is essential for diagnosis. Involved scales are placed on a glass slide to which 10 to 20 per cent KOH is added. The slide is gently heated to optically clarify the specimen and then is studied microscopically with reduced substage lighting. Examination reveals pathognomonic, 4-micron, thick-walled, spherical, budding yeasts with short, infrequently branched, septate mycelium. Parker Quick Ink can be added to the KOH solution to stain hyphae for easier identification. This procedure confirms the diagnosis, and culture is not necessary.

Potential Errors and Pitfalls in Diagnosis

Several epidermal scrapings with careful inspection may be required for diagnosis. Only one microscopic field with characteristic fungi is necessary to confirm one's suspicion. Partially treated infection or application of ointments may interfere with obtaining a positive KOH preparation. The presence of scale should differentiate pityriasis versicolor from pigmentary disorders such as vitiligo. Pityriasis versicolor is usually less inflammatory and possesses a finer scale than pityriasis rosea, erythrasma, seborrheic dermatitis, tinea corporis, secondary syphilis, and pinta.

DERMATOPHYTOSIS

Epidemiology

A closely related keratophilic group of fungi gives rise to a variety of clinical syndromes, all grouped

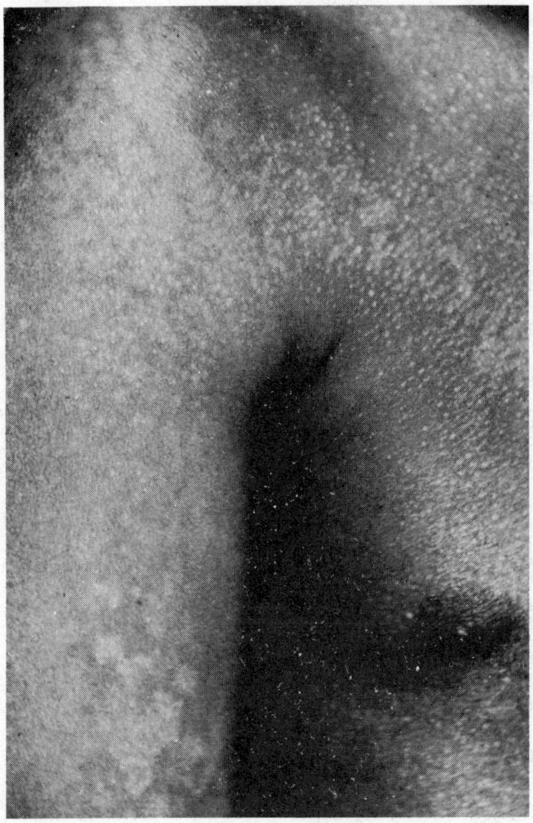

Figure 1. Pityriasis versicolor of the upper chest and arms.

under the term *dermatophytosis*. Dermatophytic fungi are restricted to the cornified layers of the skin, hair, and nails, with the severity of disease correlating with the species of dermatophyte present and the vigor of the host immune response. With dermatophytes leading essentially an extracorporal existence, skin damage and the resulting signs and symptoms actually occur as a host response to fungi or their metabolic products. The closely related dermatophytes are classified into three imperfect genera: Trichophyton, Microsporum, and Epidermophyton. These keratolytic fungi are similar in taxonomy, nutritional keratin requirements, metabolism, and antigenicity.

Each of these dermatophytes has evolved a certain equilibrium with a specific host. In order to survive on the epidermis of these hosts, dermatophytes had to evolve mechanisms by which they could evoke the least host inflammatory response possible so that infection could be maintained. In this natural evolution from soil saprophytes (geophilic fungi) to keratin-invading organisms, specific dermatophytes sought an equilibrium with a specific host. Zoophilic fungi are more at equilibrium with animal hosts, as are anthropophilic fungi with humans. There are even further degrees of equilibrium within anthropophilic fungi: *Microsporum audouinii* evokes the least host response in European children, as does *M. ferrugineum* in Asians and *Trichophyton concentricum* in Pacific islanders. In each of these respective hosts, it is unclear whether the least proteolytic enzymes, diffusible irritants, and toxins are elaborated or whether the respective host evokes a lesser host immune response to this special species. However, when a dermatophyte inhabits a nonpreferred host, as does the zoophilic *M. canis* when infecting humans, the unknown but requisite event(s) occurs that leads to a vigorous inflammatory reaction. Epidermal shedding is increased, a clinically intense reaction is apparent, and the dermatophyte is shed from the host's colonized skin. Dermatophytes are therefore classified according to preferred hosts for diagnostic, epidemiologic, and pathogenic purposes (Table 2).

In the United States, the dermatophytoses are second in prevalence only to diseases of the sebaceous glands (acne) among all skin conditions. Over 90 per cent of all males have had at least one transient dermatophyte infection by middle age. This high prevalence is due to certain common predisposing factors. Maceration, as caused by either climate (humid subtropics) or anatomic site (toe webs), is responsible for an increase in colonization. Maceration, plus a heavy fungal bombardment, helps to make tinea pedis a common condition in dormitories and locker rooms. Close contact favors spread, as found in family-centered tinea capitis. Any condition impairing cellular-mediated immunity (CMI) results in chronic, minimally inflamed infections. Atopy—typically allergic rhinitis and bronchial asthma and not atopic dermatitis—appears to be related to an increased incidence of extensive, noninflammatory infection and a decreased likelihood of spontaneous regression. In addition to person-to-person transmission, fomites play an important role. *Trichophyton mentagrophytes* is commonly isolated from locker room floors, *M. audouinii* may be found in hair brushes and on the backs of theater seats, and *Epidermophyton floccosum* is readily recovered from towels and underclothing.

Clinical Manifestations

In all types of dermatophytosis, with the possible exception of white-spot tinea unguium, infection begins with an inoculum that grows by downward mycelial invasion into the dead layers of the integument. Restriction of downward movement may be due to the depletion of essential nutrients (perhaps iron) or active resistance by host mechanisms. Lateral

Table 2. Dermatophytic Species* and Their Preferred Hosts

Geophilic	Zoophilic	Anthropophilic
M. gypseum	*M. canis*	*E. floccosum*
M. fulvum	*T. mentagrophytes* var. *mentagrophytes*	*M. audouinii*
	T. verrucosum	*M. ferrugineum*
		T. rubrum
		T. tonsurans
		T. mentagrophytes var. *interdigitale*
		T. schoenleinii
		T. concentricum

*Abbreviations refer to Trichophyton, Microsporum, and Epidermophyton.

spread of the mycelium may continue unless the inflammatory process causes shedding of the colonized skin. Hair follicles act as fungal reservoirs. Variations in this schema relate to the host, the dermatophyte species, and the anatomic site. The initial course is silent and subclinical for approximately 1 to 5 weeks when the second period of infection occurs: the visible, symptomatic, host-parasite interaction phase. In this period, CMI to dermatophyte antigen is expressed, causing an inflammatory reaction, particularly at the advancing centrifugal "ringworm" border. Inflammation can be expressed as erythema, vesicles, or pustules. Exposure to host defense mechanisms leads, in most cases, to a resolution phase (shedding) when clinical signs disappear. If CMI does not occur, a chronic, intermittent, or continuous infection ensues. Thus, two basic types of syndromes are found: an acute inflammatory infection, and a chronic noninflammatory infection.

Since dermatophyte species are so closely related, they all may elicit clinically well-defined syndromes based on anatomic location, more so than genus or species. Each syndrome is designated by the word "tinea," followed by the word for the related anatomic location, e.g., tinea capitis. Each clinical syndrome forms a distinct entity and will be discussed individually.

Laboratory Procedures

Material may be collected on the same glass slide as that used for direct examination, and subsequently a portion can be transferred to culture. Skin scrapings and white-spot tinea unguium scrapings are accomplished with the use of a sterile blunt scalpel blade held at a right angle to the skin surface. Samples yield best results if taken from the active border of the lesion. Broken, fluorescent, lusterless hairs should be plucked and examined microscopically.

To prepare a slide specimen, 10 to 20 per cent KOH is added to optically clarify the specimen. Mild pressure is applied with a coverslip to create a thin layer, and the mixture is heated gently, without boiling. After cooling and "ripening," the specimen is ready for observation. Material selected for direct examination of onychomycosis should come from the soft subungual debris in invasive subungual onychomycosis and from superficial scrapings in superficial, white-spot onychomycosis. For direct examination of nail material, a drop of 3:2 20 per cent KOH to pure DMSO is added to the material on a glass slide for clarification. Recognition of hyphae and spores in a background of artifacts requires experience and skill.

Cultures should be taken of suspicious lesions on standard Sabouraud's agar or Dermatophyte Test Media, even if they are KOH-negative. Because of the large variety of causative agents in onychomycosis, culture identification is imperative in order to look for all etiologic agents by both Sabouraud's universal media and selective media.

Some forms of tinea capitis fluoresce with 360 nm ultraviolet (UV) light. A Wood's lamp should be used in a darkened room. Because of the changing etiology of tinea capitis and an increase in nonfluorescent types, cultures are necessary in ringworm of the scalp.

Tinea Capitis

Synonyms

Ringworm of the scalp and hair, tinea tonsurans, herpes tonsurans.

Diagnostic Criteria

1. Fungal invasion of the hair shaft characterized by lesions varying from subclinical, noninflamed, and minimally scaly to ulcerating, scarring, alopecious, and inflammatory infections affecting the scalp, eyebrows, and eyelashes caused principally by *T. tonsurans, M. audouinii,* and *M. canis.*
2. Fungal hyphae and spores by direct examination of a KOH preparation of affected hairs and epidermal scrapings.
3. Culture is necessary for diagnosis.
4. Fluorescence of affected areas may be confirmatory in certain ectothrix infections, mainly *M. canis.*

Clinical Manifestations

The presentation of tinea capitis is related to the type of hair invasion and the degree of host response. Hair invasion is characterized as either endothrix (mycelial invasion with fragmentation into spores within the hair shaft) or ectothrix (mycelial invasion with fragmentation into spores external to the hair shaft). In general, anthropophilic infections have the least inflammatory response; geophilic and zoophilic infections have the most. Because of these factors, several clinical syndromes can be recognized:

Gray-Patch Ringworm. *Microsporum audouinii,* in Europe and less commonly in the United States today, and *M. ferrugineum,* in Asia, produce an anthropophilic, small-spored, ectothrix hair infection. It usually begins in prepubertal boys as a mild hair infection that is mildly erythematous, papular, and scaly. These papules soon scale, producing a pale plaque with grayish, brittle, lusterless hair that may break off above the scalp. Centrifugal spread in a ringworm distribution reveals numerous broken hairs within the patch. Regression is usually spontaneous, often occurring at puberty. A Wood's lamp detects a brilliant green fluorescence in occult lesions and reveals the true extent of manifested gray-patch ringworm.

Black-Dot Ringworm. Principally *T. tonsurans,* in Eurasia and very commonly today in the Americas ($\geq$ 95 per cent of all tinea capitis in the U.S.A.), and less commonly *T. violaceum,* in southern Europe and the Far East, produce an anthropophilic, large-spored, endothrix hair infection. Black-dot ringworm presents as a minimally inflammatory, minimally scaly, diffuse, patchy baldness. Hairs break at the follicular orifice, giving the characteristic "black-dot" appearance. Infection is frequently chronic, continuing into adulthood. Inflammatory, kerion-type infections may also be seen. Endothrix infections do not fluoresce.

Mildly Inflammatory Ringworm. *Microsporum canis,* responsible for approximately 5 per cent of scalp infections in the United States, produces a zoophilic, small-spored, ectothrix infection. Tinea capitis

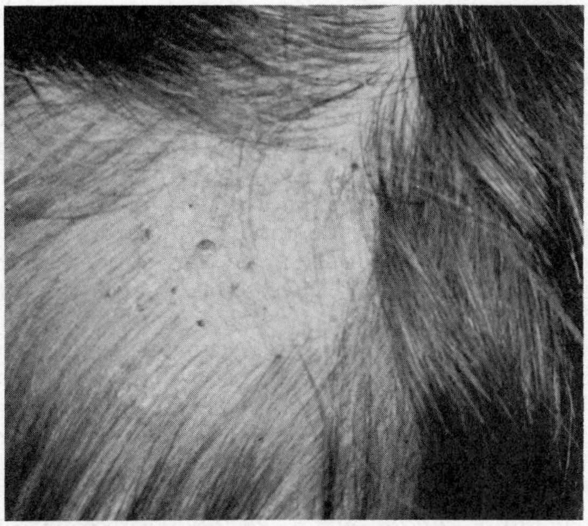

Figure 2. Mild inflammatory tinea capitis, resulting from *Trichophyton tonsurans.*

syndromes should be considered as a spectrum with overlap, and *M. canis* illustrates this point best. *Trichophyton tonsurans* can produce a similar picture. Infection is usually mildly inflammatory, producing an area of hair loss (Fig. 2). Less commonly, a gray-patch syndrome occurs. Infection may progress to kerion, keloid, and severe inflammation. A Wood's lamp usually reveals a green fluorescence.

Kerion. *Trichophyton mentagrophytes* and *T. verrucosum,* both ubiquitous dermatophytes, produce a zoophilic, large-spored, ectothrix infection. An intense inflammatory reaction usually found in rural areas and acquired by cattle, kerion is characterized by a suppurative, pustular folliculitis with thick crusting, matting of surrounding hairs, and frequent lymphadenopathy. Bacterial superinfection may occur, sinus tracts may form, and in rare instances mycetoma-like grains are visible. This process resolves in scarring and permanent, patchy alopecia. No fluorescence is found with a Wood's lamp.

Favus. *Trichophyton schoenleinii*—in Europe, the Middle East, the near East, and rarely in the United States—produces an anthropophilic infection. Favus usually presents in children as discrete, cup-shaped crusts called scutula, which develop perifollicularly and become a confluent mass of yellow crusting. Removal of the crust creates an oozing, erythematous surface. Glabrous skin and nails can also be affected. Favus rarely involutes, leaving scarring and permanent alopecia.

Tinea capitis can be complicated by a dermatophytid ("id") reaction, although less commonly than when associated with tinea pedis. Grouped vesicles or an eczematoid reaction occur at a distal site in response to the primary scalp infection. These lesions, which are devoid of organisms, spontaneously clear with cure of the primary infection.

Potential Errors and Pitfalls in Diagnosis

Tinea capitis may be confused with other diseases causing an inflammatory, patchy alopecia. Seborrheic dermatitis and psoriasis usually involve more scale with unbroken hair of normal integrity. Other diseases important in the differential diagnosis include lupus erythematosus, alopecia areata, impetigo, and secondary syphilis.

Tinea Corporis

Synonyms

Tinea circinata, tinea glabrosa, ringworm of the body.

Diagnostic Criteria

1. Infection of the stratum corneum and villous hair follicles characterized by lesions varying from simple scaling to erythematous and vesicular lesions to deep granulomata affecting glabrous skin caused by allergic and foreign body reaction to the dermatophytes.
2. Fungal hyphae and spores by direct examination of a KOH preparation of epidermal scrapings or material plucked or scraped from an involved follicle.
3. Culture is necessary because of the small number of fungi present and the resulting large numbers of falsely negative KOH tests.

Clinical Manifestations

In contrast to tinea capitis, dermatophytes causing tinea corporis are basically ubiquitous with no predilection for geographic location. A variant of tinea corporis may be found in the beard area. This condition is commonly known as tinea barbae. In fact, the name tinea corporis is applied to all glabrous skin infections, even if the infection is on the arm, leg, or dorsum of the hand or foot. Three basic lesions are recognized in tinea corporis, and each entity will be discussed separately.

Noninflammatory Lesions. *Trichophyton rubrum, E. floccosum, T. tonsurans,* or *M. canis* causes a subclinical, centrifugal, spreading infection that manifests itself clinically when host defense comes into play. At that time, the lesion appears as an erythematous, raised, swollen, annular, discrete ring with a scaly, relatively cleared center (Fig. 3). With exposure to a heavy inoculum, several discrete lesions may develop and become confluent, leading to polycyclic "ringworm" borders, or they may become psoriasiform or plaquelike. *Trichophyton rubrum* has the greatest tendency for extreme chronicity.

Inflammatory Lesions. *Trichophyton mentagrophytes, T. verrucosum,* and occasionally almost any of the other dermatophytes cause annular-appearing lesions as just described, with the exception that there is now a central area of vesicles and crusts that resolves, leaving a central postinflammatory hyperpigmentation. Inflammatory lesions are often small in size but may be multiple.

Tinea Imbricata. *Trichophyton concentricum,* in the Pacific Islands and in South and Central America, begins as an area of scaling that soon spreads centrifugally. In the area of central clearing, a new focus begins, leading to the appearance of repetitive, inwardly directed, scaly, concentric rings covering most of the

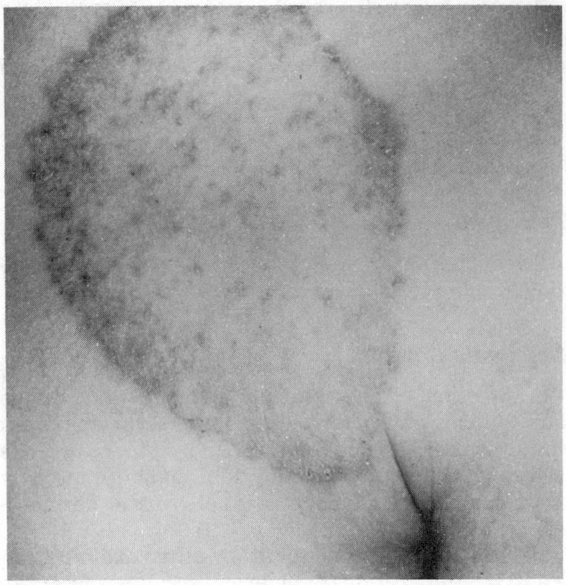

Figure 3. Centrifugally spreading tinea corporis, leaving a relatively cleared center.

body. Susceptibility to this cosmetically disfiguring, but sometimes culturally accepted, form of tinea corporis is thought to be inherited as an autosomal dominant gene, with the first contact being spread from mother to infant. Pruritus, at times intense, can lead to secondary lichenification.

Potential Errors and Pitfalls in Diagnosis

Clinically distinct lesions should actually be thought of on a continuum because atypicalities in these lesions are common. Tinea corporis can be confused with psoriasis, pityriasis rosea, erythema annulare, numular eczema, lichen planus, contact dermatitis, pityriasis versicolor, granuloma annulare, and annular secondary syphilis and other scaly lesions. Distribution is important in distinction from these diseases. Any scaly body rash should be scraped for possible KOH positivity.

Tinea Cruris

Synonyms

Jock itch, gym itch, dhobie itch, eczema marginatum, ringworm of the groin.

Diagnostic Criteria

1. Infection of the stratum corneum characterized by discrete, raised, erythematous margins with a central thin, dry, epidermal scaling affecting principally the groin, perineum, and perianal regions, most commonly in men, caused by *E. floccosum, T. rubrum,* and *T. mentagrophytes.*
2. Fungal hyphae and spores by direct examination of a KOH preparation of epidermal scrapings.
3. Culture is necessary because of the large numbers of falsely negative KOH tests.

Clinical Manifestations

Infection with *T. rubrum* in the United States and *E. floccosum* more commonly in Europe presents as erythematous, arciform plaques with sharply raised borders, at times vesicular, beginning on the thigh area that is in contact with the scrotum. Both the penis and the scrotum are usually symptomatically spared. Lesions are commonly bilateral, usually spreading downward farther on the left than on the right as a result of the lower scrotal sac on that side. The lesion spreads serpiginously owing to varying rates of spread. An incomplete central clearing gives the appearance of a brown to red, mildly scaly, marginated plaque. Pruritus and erythema are more common in acute infection, becoming more lichenified and plaquelike in more chronic lesions. *Epidermophyton floccosum* infections have a tendency to remain localized, but *T. rubrum* and *T. mentagrophytes* may disseminate to other cutaneous areas.

Fungal elements present in skin scales are recovered in such intimate surroundings as showers, locker room floors, clothing, and rugs. When spores enter occlusive areas, as in the thigh area, colonization is more likely. Individuals with diabetes, neurodermatitis, and obesity (macerating conditions) or those living in hot humid areas are at greater risk of developing tinea cruris.

Potential Errors and Pitfalls in Diagnosis

Candida infection is often confused with tinea cruris. However, infection with *Candida albicans* frequently produces weeping areas with a less distinct, raised margin and satellite pustular lesions, often occurring in diabetics and in women with vaginal candidiasis. Seborrheic dermatitis is more often symmetric and psoriasis more scaly and plaquelike. Other important considerations are contact dermatitis, erythrasma, lichen planus chronicus, intertrigo, and bacterial infections.

Tinea Pedis

Synonyms

Athlete's foot, ringworm of the foot.

Diagnostic Criteria

1. Infection of the stratum corneum characterized by lesions varying from mild, chronic, scaly patches to acute, exfoliative pustules and bullae affecting principally the feet and toes caused more commonly by *T. rubrum, T. mentagrophytes,* and *E. floccosum* and less commonly by *T. violaceum.*
2. Fungal hyphae by the direct examination of a KOH preparation of epidermal scrapings.
3. Multiple cultures are necessary because of frequent obscuring bacterial overgrowth.

Clinical Manifestations

Tinea pedis is among the most common infectious diseases of the world. However, it is unknown why only certain people are susceptible. It is said that tinea pedis is the penalty of civilization and the wearing of shoes. Occlusion leads to macerating conditions favoring both overgrowth of the dermatophyte and destruction of the stratum corneum. This condition is greater between the fourth and fifth toes. Infection is most often acquired as a teenager, the incidence of infection increasing with age. However, repetitive exposure, as occurs in locker rooms and common bathing facilities, leads to infection earlier in life. Respiratory atopics appear to be more prone to chronic, papulosquamous, hyperkeratotic infection, especially with *T. rubrum*. Three representative clinical types of foot (and hand) infection are actually on a continuum and will be discussed.

Chronic Intertriginous (Interdigital). *Trichophyton rubrum, T. mentagrophytes,* and *E. floccosum* are each capable of causing a chronic peeling of dead, white, macerated epidermis. Skin fissures and raw, erythematous, weeping epidermis are found beneath. Usually, beginning in the web spaces, a foul odor becomes apparent and pruritus is especially intensified with warm weather and bacterial overgrowth.

Chronic Papulosquamous Hyperkeratosis (Moccasin Tinea Pedis). *Trichophyton rubrum* and *T. mentagrophytes* cause thick, red plaques covered by thin, silvery scales that, if extensive enough, involve the whole foot to cause a "moccasin foot" (Fig. 4). This is a chronic, persistent condition that may persist for years or decades, despite therapy.

Dermatophytic infection of the palmar aspect of the hand (tinea manuum) appears identical to this hyperkeratotic variety, except in a different anatomic location. Tinea manuum may occur alone, but it is usually found on one hand associated with tinea pedis of both feet ("one hand-two feet" syndrome).

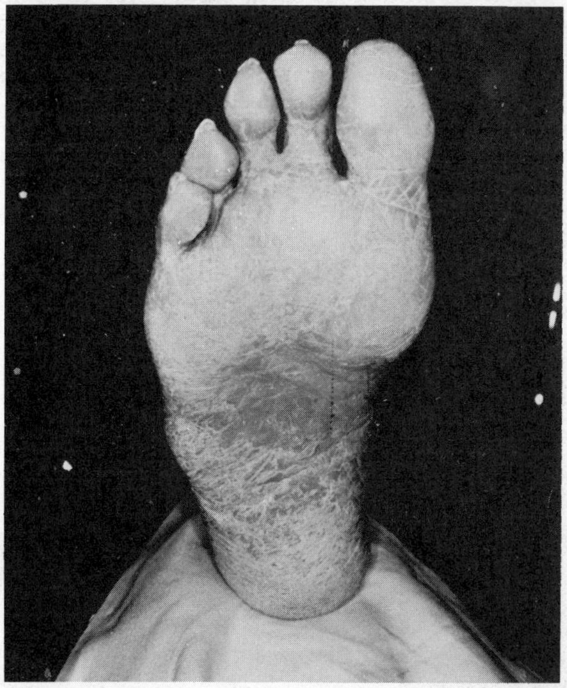

Figure 4. "Moccasin foot" hyperkeratotic tinea pedis, caused by *Trichophyton rubrum.*

Vesiculobullous. *Trichophyton mentagrophytes* and, less commonly, *T. rubrum* cause vesicles, pustules, and occasionally bullae, usually in the intertriginous areas but soon spreading to the dorsum of the foot, and, less commonly, to the anterior surface. Dermatophytes can be recovered from the top of the roofs of these vesicles. Rupture occurs, leaving dry, ragged, denuded areas. Resolution usually occurs spontaneously, but symptoms may recur, especially in warm weather.

Potential Errors and Pitfalls in Diagnosis

Because bacterial overgrowth may cloud the picture of interdigital tinea pedis, several cultures may be needed to confirm a suspected case. Many conditions may clinically mimic tinea pedis: bacterial infection, contact dermatitis, pustular psoriasis, Reiter's syndrome, secondary syphilis, erythrasma, idiopathic hyperkeratosis, acrodermatitis perstans, dermatitis repens, erysipelas, pyodermas, candidiasis, arsenical keratosis, fixed-drug eruption, mycetoma, and pityriasis rubra pilaris. Culture and clinical suspicion are most helpful in differentiation.

Onychomycosis

Synonyms

Tinea unguium, ringworm of the nail.

Diagnostic Criteria

1. Invasion of the nail plate characterized by lesions varying from patches or pits on the nail plate to an invasive, subungual infection caused by dermatophytes (principally *T. rubrum* and *T. mentagrophytes*), Candida sp., and other fungi: *Scopulariopsis brevicaulis, Hendersonela tortuloidea, Scytalidium hyalinum, Fusarium oxysporium,* Cephalosporium sp., and Aspergillus sp.
2. Fungal hyphae and spores by direct examination of a KOH/DMSO (dimethyl sulfoxide) preparation of nail scrapings.
3. Culture examining both dermatophyte and nondermatophyte possibilities is imperative.

Epidemiology

Onychomycosis refers to fungal invasion of the nail unit. At present a wide variety of fungi, represented by dermatophytes, Candida sp., and many other fungi, are found as etiologic agents of onychomycosis (Table 3). It is imperative from a therapeutic standpoint to detect the causative fungus responsible.

Clinical Manifestations

Two distinct clinical types are commonly encountered:

Invasive Subungual Dermatophytosis. A mild paronychia usually precedes invasion of the lateral or

Table 3. Etiologic Agents in Onychomycosis

Clinical Type	Dermatophytes	Candida	Other Fungi*
Fingernail subungual onychomycosis	+++	±	±
Toenail subungual onychomycosis	+++	+	+++
Finger or toenail superficial white-spot onychomycosis	+++	−	−

* *Scopulariopsis brevicaulis, Hendersonela tortuloidea, Scytalidium hyalinum, Fusarium oxysporium,* Cephalosporium sp., and Aspergillus sp.

distal nail edge by the dermatophyte. A yellowish nail plate spot enlarges, leaving the nail plate brittle and thickened (Fig. 5). Irritation by the fungus causes abnormal, soft, friable keratin production and accumulation, lifting the nail plate and often causing cracking. The nail plate darkens in color. The plate may appear separated from the underlying nail bed as in onycholysis, but this is actually due to the dermatophyte separating the plate into lamellae. Dermatophyte infection may lead to total nail plate destruction, but the nail matrix is never entered. A more widespread form of invasive subungual onychomycosis with involvement of the total thickness of the nail plate occurs in chronic mucocutaneous candidiasis patients.

Superficial White-Spot Onychomycosis. This clinical type of onychomycosis occurs exclusively in toenails and produces little symptomatology. It appears as a discrete, irregularly bordered, powdery, white, superficial nail plate infection, being either single or multiple in number.

Potential Errors and Pitfalls in Diagnosis

Invasive dermatophytosis of the nail can be confused with other discoloring, thickened nail plate abnormalities: onychogryphosis, onychophagia, neoplasms, psoriasis, and viral and bacterial infections. Congenital diseases (nonmycotic leukonychia, pachonychia congenita) can cause abnormalities that mimic superficial white-spot tinea unguium. Mees' lines, contact irritants, trauma, and onychomycosis may also produce similar white areas in the nail plate.

Since only the dermatophytes are sensitive to griseofulvin and ketoconazole, it is imperative to document the causative agent so as not to inappropriately subject the patient to one of the oral antifungal agents.

CANDIDIASIS

Synonyms

Candidosis, moniliasis, thrush, dermatocandidiasis, mycotic vulvovaginitis, muguet.

Diagnostic Criteria

1. Primary or secondary infection of the skin and mucous membranes characterized by lesions varying from an inflammatory irritation to acute and chronic suppuration to granulomatous reaction affecting the skin, nails, mouth, throat, and vagina caused principally by *C. albicans.*
2. Yeast or mycelium found on Gram stain or KOH preparation of mucosal secretions or cutaneous scrapings.
3. Culture is necessary for diagnosis, using fresh and possibly multiple specimens.

Epidemiology

Several species of Candida, particularly *Candida albicans,* are a group of dimorphic, saprophytic yeasts that constitute normal flora of the alimentary tract and mucocutaneous regions. They exist in two forms: (1) the *commensal* state, consisting of the approximately 7-micron oval yeast, and (2) the *pathogenic* state, consisting of a mycelial phase. Candida species

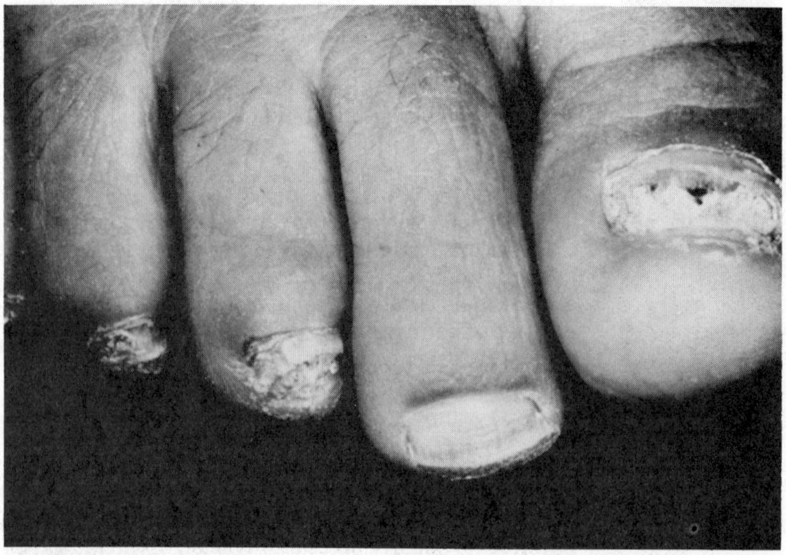

Figure 5. Invasive subungual onychomycosis producing a thickened, brittle nail plate of the toes.

are normally present in the mouths and intestines of healthy adults and in the vagina and perianal areas of many normal females. This carriage rate increases to 25 per cent for women who are pregnant or are taking oral contraceptives. Perianal colonization in babies may occur, followed by diaper rash.

Although the normal adult has a high innate ability to reject infection, the very young and the elderly are more susceptible. Factors that predispose to opportunistic Candida species are basically of two types: exogenous and endogenous. Macerating conditions, such as those encountered in the inframammary folds, perianal skin, and intertriginous areas, are an example of an exogenous factor. Moisture may play a role in a lessened integrity of the stratum corneum and its ability to act as a defensive host barrier. The entire cutaneous barrier may be breached with indwelling catheters, dentures, surgical procedures, injections, and thermal burns. There are many endogenous risk factors leading to an opportunistic, invasive disease state. Before a resident flora is established in infancy, infection may be prominent, often clearing without therapy as the infant ages. Antibiotics, leading to a change in the normal flora, may increase the number of Candida organisms in the same way. Physiologic changes, such as pregnancy and steroid and endocrine imbalances (particularly diabetes mellitus), are endogenous predisposing factors. Finally, general debility and immune system compromise, such as T cell defects and iron deficiency–dependent immune defects in chronic mucocutaneous candidiasis (CMCC), predispose to candidiasis. It appears that *C. albicans*, which is part of the normal human flora, can reverse its morphology from the saprophytic yeast phase to a pathogenic mycelial phase under these predisposing conditions.

Clinical Manifestations

Candidiasis presents differently at different sites and is also involved in allergic conditions. Because of the multiplicity of clinical presentations, discussion will follow the site of infection.

Cutaneous Involvement. Intertriginous candidiasis, common in any glabrous, occlusive skin fold, is the most common cutaneous candidal infection occurring either in patients with occlusive, macerated, flexural areas (obesity) or in patients with metabolic conditions that predispose them to an increase in fungal colonization (diabetes, chronic alcoholism). Erythema and exudation of a "scalded" appearance begin in an occluded area but soon spread to form a scalloped border with punctate surrounding satellite vesicle or pustular lesions (Fig. 6). Characteristic subcorneal pustules form and occasionally break, leaving exposed, eroded, ragged, raw surfaces.

A common condition identical to adult infection occurs in the perineum in infants, especially when chronically damp diapers are changed infrequently. Bluish-brown nodules and granulomas, representative of host response to the candidal infection, represent a rarer clinical variant of this disease.

Candida Paronychia. A combination of trauma and frequent immersion in water, commonly occurring in housewives, bartenders, and chefs, predisposes these individuals to paronychial colonization with Candida species. Erythema and induration of the nail folds and loss of the cuticle are due primarily to Candida infection, but other bacterial species are often present. Commonly, invasion results in a thick, grooved, brown discolored nail.

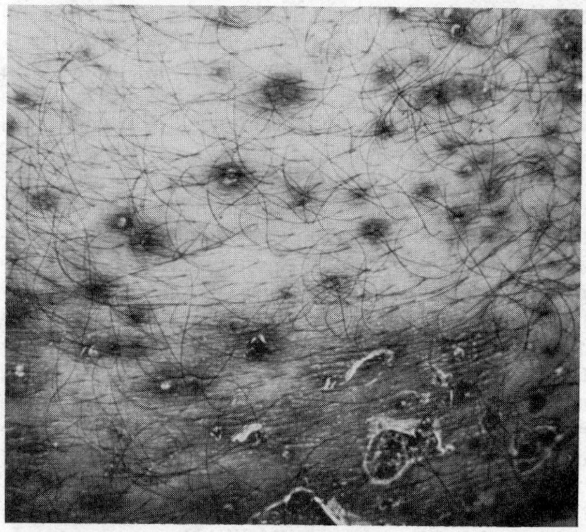

Figure 6. Cutaneous candidiasis of the intertriginous groin with characteristic surrounding satellite lesions. (Courtesy of Marilynne McKay, M.D.)

Mucocutaneous Involvement. There are three distinct common forms of mucocutaneous Candida infection.

The first form, *oral candidiasis,* is a master of disguise in the mouth. Oral thrush is the most common. Thrush consists of discrete to confluent, creamy, "curdlike" pseudomembranes attached to a red, oozing, epithelial base, most commonly on the tongue, gums, and buccal or palantine mucosa. Thrush is most common in infancy when the baby's mouth has a low pH similar to the maternal gravid carrier promoting Candida growth. A black hairy tongue is a prominent feature of acute atrophic oral candidiasis. Although the etiology is not clear, characteristic hypertrophy of the papillae occurs, usually following antibiotic therapy. Median rhomboid glossitis, a loss of the papillae in a diamond-shaped area on the dorsum of the tongue, may become more chronic in other areas of the mouth, resembling leukoplakia. Erosive, erythematous, painful, chronic, atrophic candidiasis results from poor dentition, poorly fitting dentures, or in association with orthodontic appliances. Steroids and antibiotics may lead to a chronic oropharyngeal candidiasis. A true candidal angular chelitis characterized by pain and cracked, fissured sores at the angles of the mouth presents with surrounding primary satellite lesions.

Genital and *perineal candidiasis* is a second form of mucocutaneous infection. Vulvovaginal thrush appears as a creamy, "curdlike," foul-smelling vaginal discharge and as patches of gray pseudomembranes on a red vaginal mucosa. Pruritus and soreness are associated symptoms. Patients are usually sexually active individuals. Pregnancy, antibiotic therapy, and diabetes mellitus are all thought to be predisposing conditions. Candidal balanitis, especially in the sexual partner of a patient with vulvovaginitis (conjugal candidiasis), occurs on the glans penis most commonly in uncircumcised males. White pustules and vesicles with surrounding erythema may lead to erosions and soreness in this condition.

The third form, *chronic mucocutaneous candidiasis,* is actually a group of syndromes caused principally by lymphocyte and endocrine system defects and is characterized by persistent Candida infection of areas prone to incidental candidiasis. This infection usually first presents in children or young adults and may be only one of several opportunistic pathogens infecting the child. Glabrous skin is often involved, and lesions may be granulomatous. Lesions can go on to be more extensive and present as verrucous in quality. The mouth, esophagus, vocal cords, and paronychxis can be involved, leading to severe scarring. Pyogenic infections, vitiligo, alopecia areata, and dermatophytosis are associated findings in CMCC patients.

Laboratory Procedures

Scrapings from cutaneous and mucocutaneous surfaces can be examined directly with 10 to 20 per cent KOH (as described for dermatophyte infections) or with Gram stain. Culture of a moist mucosal or skin site is not helpful in a suspected case of candidiasis because of the high normal carriage rate. A positive culture does not necessarily prove the presence of infection. However, a characteristic KOH preparation demonstrating the pathogenic mycelial phase does confirm a suspected case of candidiasis. If specimens are not fresh, a disproportionate mycelial growth may occur, clouding the significance of the microscopic picture.

Potential Errors and Pitfalls in Diagnosis

Candida can appear in virtually every location of the body. It is, therefore, important that all suspicious lesions be examined by both smear and culture. Oral thrush may be confused with leukoplakia, lichen planus, or tertiary syphilis. Scrapings and culture will differentiate Candida intertrigo from dermatophytosis, bacterial intertrigo, seborrheic dermatitis, flexural psoriasis, and familial benign pemphigus. Probably the most confusing differential diagnosis involves genital and perineal candidiasis. Trichomonas and other bacteria can also produce a vulvovaginitis. Psoriasis, lichen sclerosis, and contact dermatitis can affect the vulva, producing similar clinical pictures. Candidal balanitis must be differentiated from herpes simplex virus infections, lichen planus, bacterial infections, and psoriasis.

CHROMOBLASTOMYCOSIS

Synonyms

Chromomycosis, verrucous dermatitis, phaeosporotrichosis, cladosporiosis, dermatitide verrucosa chromoparasitaria, infections by dematiacious fungi.

Diagnostic Criteria

1. Chronic infection of the skin and subcutaneous tissue characterized most commonly by slow-growing, verrucoid, cutaneous nodules resembling the florets of cauliflower and affecting principally the lower legs and feet at the site of inoculation of the causative fungus: principally, *Fonsecaea pedrosoi, F. compacta, Phialophora verrucosa,* and *Cladosporium carrionii* and, less frequently, *Cladophialophora ajelloi* and *Rhinocladiella aquaspersa.*

2. Brownish, spherical bodies (medlar bodies, "copper pennies") seen microscopically on direct examination by the addition of a drop of KOH/DMSO to a slide on which a black dot isolated from the surface of the lesion has been placed.

3. Culture is necessary for identification of the organism.

Epidemiology

Dematiacious fungi are soil-inhabiting and thrive on decaying vegetation and rotting wood. Inoculation of the fungus via skin puncture leads to infection. In rural communities, male agricultural workers who do not wear shoes are most often exposed to the causative organisms. Infection is commonly found in the Americas, southern Europe, Africa, and Australia.

Clinical Manifestations

Because there is a high natural resistance to infection, only under repeated exposure or trauma does infection ensue. If infection does occur, a foreign-body granuloma with abscess formation develops. The mycelium, spores, and sclerotic fungal cells appear pigmented.

Infection takes the form of several basic clinical lesions. Chromoblastomycosis is the form of fungal infection most frequently encountered. Trauma on exposed areas implants the fungus cutaneously and subcutaneously to produce localized, slow-growing, cauliflower-like, verrucoid nodules and flat, annular plaques with an active border and atrophic centers (Fig. 7).

Traumatized lesions are violaceous in color, have a friable, smooth, less keratinized surface, and may bleed profusely. Black dots on the surface of these lesions are mixtures of inflammatory remains (e.g., hemosiderin) and the organism. Black dots can be used for the direct microscopic visualization of the organism. Lesions are usually painless; however, if secondary infection occurs, pain and pruritus may ensue. Other rarer forms of this disease are represented by subcutaneous or intramuscular cysts (phaeohypomycotic cyst) and benign colonization (phaeomycotic cutaneous colonization).

Laboratory Procedures

The most successful method for direct examination as an aid in diagnosis involves visualizing a surface "black dot" with KOH/DMSO for sclerotic, round, "medlar body" cells. Also seen are transitional hy-

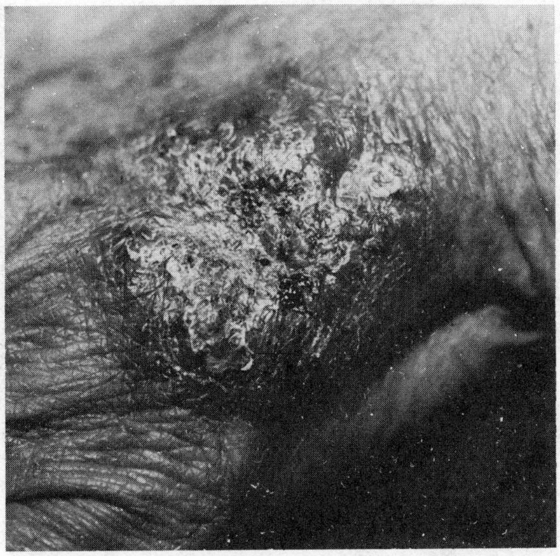

Figure 7. Chromoblastomycosis of the hand; early changes.

phae. Culture is necessary for identification of the organism and utilizes a combination of physiologic and morphologic properties.

Potential Errors and Pitfalls in Diagnosis

Blastomycosis resembles chromoblastomycosis closely, but usually the former is more pustular, having more sharply raised borders. Yaws, lupus vulgaris, lupus erythematosus, leprosy, leishmaniasis, tertiary syphilis, and other fungal diseases should be carefully considered in the differential diagnosis.

MADUROMYCOSIS

Synonyms

Madura foot, mycetoma.

Diagnostic Criteria

1. Localized, chronic infection of the skin, subcutaneous tissues, and bone characterized by suppurating abscesses, draining sinuses, granulomata, and the presence of colored grains affecting principally the feet and hands caused by a diverse group of fungi (Table 4).
2. Triad of tumefaction, draining sinus, and grains.
3. Broad, branching, septate filaments found by direct examination of a KOH preparation or Gram stain of crushed, colored granules.
4. Culture from a deep biopsy sample is necessary.

Epidemiology

Eumycetes, such as Madurella and Cephalosporium, are common inhabitants of soil and decaying vegetation commonly in the tropics and subtropics and, less frequently, in North America. These fungi usually gain entrance to the body after minor penetrating injuries. Maduromycosis is especially common in Sudan and Mexico, where barefoot adult male rural laborers are subjected to repeated environmental exposure and poor nutritional and hygienic conditions. Although incubation periods range from one to several months, the disease is not disabling until several years after the initial injury.

Table 4. Species Associated with Mycetoma and Characteristic Grain Color

Species	Grain
Phialophora jeanselmei	White to yellow
Madurella grisea	Black
Madurella mycetomatis	Brown to black
Leptosphaeria senegalensis	Black
Pyrenochaeta romeroi	Black
Monosporium apiospermum	White to yellow
Neostudina rosatii	Yellow to brown
Cephalosporium falciforme	White to yellow
Cephalosporium recifei	White to yellow

Clinical Manifestations

Inoculation via a minor injury leads to the formation of a granulomatous, painless nodule that softens and discharges a serous to purulent material through sinus tracts. Surrounding induration is responsible for the characteristic convex plantar surface found on examination of infected feet. The infection is locally invasive, extending to the subcutaneous tissue and rarely to bone and ligaments. Secondary surrounding nodules form, giving the area an irregularly lumpy appearance. The total clinical picture is one of swollen areas on the extremities draining pus and containing characteristic colored granules.

As is true with other invasive fungal infections, there is a high degree of natural immunity in the normal host to the invasive pathogen. If infection occurs, it develops slowly with varying periods of quiescence and activity. Disease is generally localized. Resolution may occur with massive fibrosis, giving the area a hard, tumorlike appearance.

Laboratory Procedures

Laboratory examination of colored granules in the mycetomatous discharge not only confirms the diagnosis of maduromycosis but also differentiates actinomycetes from eumycetes. Granule color varies with the causative organism (Table 4). It is necessary, however, to submit several specimens for culture for both diagnosis and pharmacologic sensitivities. X-ray examination of bones may be important to confirm clinical suspicion of osteomyelitis.

Potential Errors and Pitfalls in Diagnosis

Tumefaction, draining sinuses, and grains can also be found in bacterial infections. This condition is termed *botryomycosis.* Actinomycosis, yaws, elephantiasis, cellulitis, and osteomyelitis can also be confused with mycetoma. Eumycotic infection caused by

Sporothrix and Coccidioides species should also be considered in the differential diagnosis.

MUCORMYCOSIS

Synonyms

Phycomycosis, hyphomycosis, zygomycosis.

Diagnostic Criteria

1. Acute and rapidly developing infection of cutaneous and subcutaneous tissues also affecting other organ systems of debilitated patients characterized by lesions varying from plaques and pustules to ulcerations, abscesses and painful nodules affecting principally the rhino-facio-cranio area, lungs, gastrointestinal tract, and skin with a predilection for arterial vessels caused by several genera of the order Mucorales.
2. Thick-walled, nonseptate hyphae with right-angle branching found on direct examination of a KOH preparation of material from skin scrapings, discharge, or biopsy.
3. Culture is necessary for diagnosis.

Epidemiology

Mucormycosis is caused by several species of the genera Rhizopus, Rhizomucor, Mucor, and Absidia, all of the order Mucorales. These fungi are ubiquitous, existing on decaying vegetation and organic material, but they grow especially well at acid pH, high glucose concentrations, and a temperature above 37°C. Therefore, diabetic ketoacidosis in particular is associated with this infection. In addition, patients with leukemia or lymphoma, acidotic patients, chemotherapy and immunosuppressed patients, burn patients, malnourished children, and renal failure patients are predisposed to mucormycosis.

Clinical Manifestations

Fungi that cause mucormycosis are truly opportunistic. It takes certain predisposing conditions to penetrate a highly innate immunity to these essentially avirulent organisms. Once disease occurs, it is acute and fulminant, especially in the diabetic in whom the disease may take on a rapidly fatal course. The two most important characteristics of infection, no matter where it occurs, are these:

1. These fungi have a predilection for the arterial system, commonly causing emboli and resultant tissue necrosis.
2. Black, necrotic pus is produced.

Several clinical syndromes are encountered, regardless of the etiologic agent.

Rhinocerebral Mucormycosis. Caused principally by the Rhizopus species, this has been the most common form seen in the United States and usually occurs with underlying diabetic ketoacidosis. Infection usually begins with spore inhalation, leading to colonization in the upper turbinates or palate. Cellulitis and a black necrotic discharge develop following an episode of poorly controlled diabetes mellitus. Patients initially complain of headache, lethargy, and visual loss. Orbital cellulitis carries a poorer prognosis with central nervous system invasion retro-orbitally or through the ethmoids. Arterial blood vessel invasion is a common complication, leading to cavernous sinus thrombosis and internal carotid artery thrombosis. Disease rapidly terminates in death after approximately 10 days, carrying an overall mortality of 80 to 90 per cent.

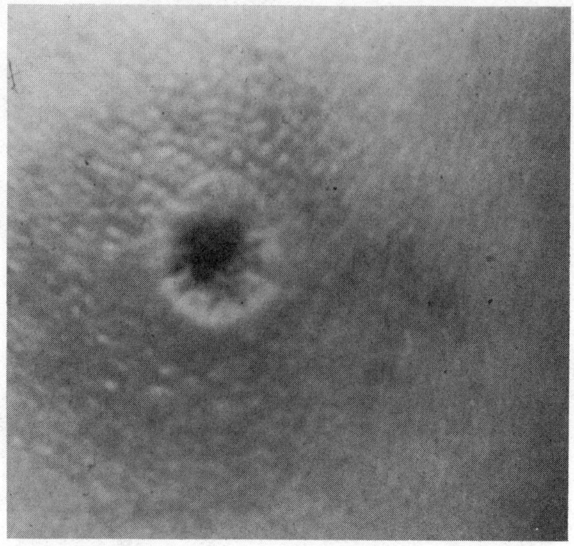

Figure 8. Primary cutaneous aspergillosis of the arm, which closely mimics primary cutaneous mucormycosis. (Courtesy of Steve Estes, M.D.)

Cutaneous Lesions. Rapidly fatal disease can occur in burn patients, diabetics, and, more commonly today, in immunocompromised and immunosuppressed patients. Two forms of cutaneous lesions can be found:

1. Breaks in the skin barrier may lead to primary lesions characterized by plaques, pustules, abscesses, and ulcerations (Fig. 8).
2. Disseminated lesions from hematogenous spread, beginning as painful ecchymotic nodules, may result in necrosis, ulceration, and eschar formation.

The development of mucormycosis in immunosuppressed, hospitalized patients has been associated with the application of certain types of bandage dressings.

Pulmonary and Abdominal Mucormycosis. Severe infection in these sites has become increasingly common in oncology patients, compromised because of therapy.

Laboratory Procedures

Direct examination by KOH preparation may lead to few fungal elements, especially in black pus or discharge specimens. Repeated KOH examinations are necessary. Histopathologic demonstration of the organism plus recovery on culture is critical to diagnosis. Culture on standard laboratory media is easily accomplished and necessary. Laboratory values may be of some assistance: a high fasting blood glucose, low serum carbon dioxide, and a white blood cell (WBC) count of 10,000 to 30,000 per cu mm are common.

Potential Errors and Pitfalls in Diagnosis

Rhinocerebral mucormycosis may be confused with pyogenic cavernous sinus thrombosis, which is not associated with early retinal artery occlusion and early visual loss. Radiographically, this form of mucormycosis may resemble epidermoid carcinoma.

SPOROTRICHOSIS

Synonyms

None.

Diagnostic Criteria

1. Chronic infection of cutaneous or subcutaneous tissues characterized by nodular lesions which suppurate, ulcerate, and drain—usually along a lymphatic distribution—affecting principally the skin with secondary spread from subcutaneous lesions to articular surfaces, bone, and muscle caused by *Sporothrix schenckii.*
2. Culture is the definitive procedure for diagnosis.
3. Serum sample for serologic diagnosis may be helpful.

Epidemiology

Sporothrix schenckii is often found in temperate and tropical zones. It is the most common invasive fungus in Mexico and is prominent in the mining areas of South Africa. In these areas, this fungus may colonize the individual having high natural resistance, or it may exist on decaying vegetation, sphagnum moss, or timber; however, it does not gain entrance unless some minor trauma occurs, e.g., inoculation with a splinter or thorn. Adult males most commonly present with sporotrichosis because of occupation and exposure.

Clinical Manifestations

This opportunistic organism creates a granulomatous necrotic reaction in one of three different clinical presentations.

Lymphocutaneous Sporotrichosis. After traumatic inoculation of spores subcutaneously, a small, hard, nonfixed, nontender nodule forms; this nodule may ulcerate, forming a chancre. If untreated, the organism spreads via the lymphatics to produce similar buboes along a lymphatic drainage pattern (Fig. 9). This is the most common form of sporotrichosis. An ulcer on a distal extremity, with a chain of similar lesions and local or regional lymphadenopathy extending proximally up the extremity, is almost pathognomonic. If untreated, the infection may become chronic, although some cases have healed spontaneously.

Fixed Cutaneous Sporotrichosis. In these patients, disease is restricted to the primary site of inoculation and may become hypertrophic or verrucous. This course leads to recurrent periods of activity, followed by quiescent periods. This form may occur where *S. schenckii* is highly endemic and where the population can be shown to be sensitized to the organism by a sporotrichin test.

Extracutaneous and Disseminated Sporotrichosis. These rarer forms of primary sporotrichosis are found in the bone, periosteum, synovium, eye, sinuses, meninges, and, not uncommonly, lungs.

Laboratory Procedures

Serology and culture play a prominent role in diagnosis. The yeast cell agglutination test and latex particle agglutination test are very sensitive indicators of sporotrichosis. Samples of discharges and aspirates are easily cultured on almost any media. However, since so few organisms are present in tissue and dis-

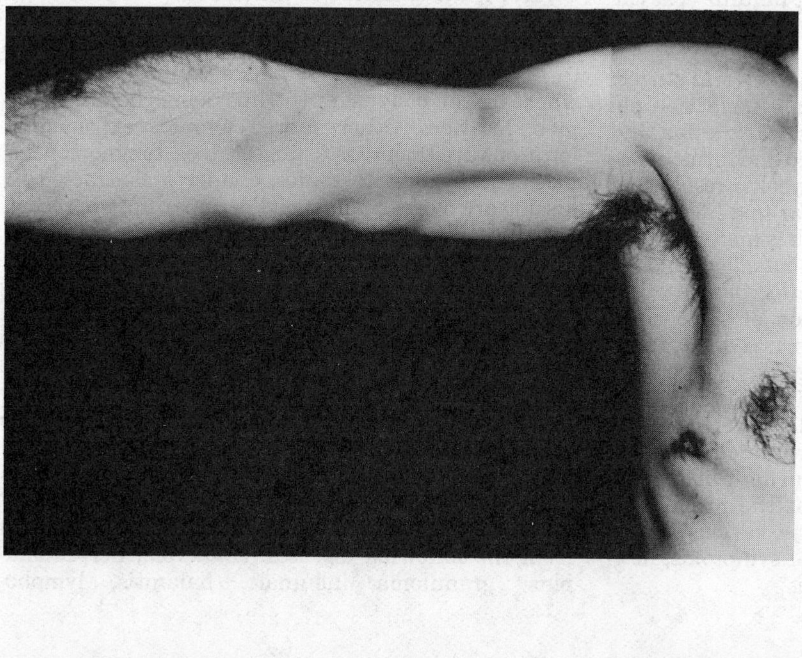

Figure 9. Ulcerating nodules of lymphocutaneous sporotrichosis following a lymphatic drainage pattern. (Courtesy of Steve Estes, M.D.)

charge fluid, both KOH preparation and histopathology may be fruitless.

Potential Errors and Pitfalls in Diagnosis

There are many diseases, especially infectious in etiology, that may mimic sporotrichosis. Nocardia, actinomycoses, and mycobacterial infections lead the list. Lesions of a granulomatous nature are especially confusing.

SYPHILIS

By A. Paul Kelly, M.D.
and Alice Faye Singleton, M.D., M.P.H.
Los Angeles, California

SYNONYMS

Lues venerea, pox, morbus gallicus, "the French disease," "bad blood," "hair cut," "old Joe," and "sif."

DEFINITION

Syphilis is an infectious disease caused by the spirochete *Treponema pallidum.* It is usually transmitted from person to person by intimate contact, but it may be acquired prenatally and by blood transfusion. The disease is characterized by the florid primary and secondary types, which resolve and enter into a period of latency that may progress into a tertiary stage.

PRESENTING SIGNS AND SYMPTOMS AND COURSE

Since all stages of syphilis may mimic other medical problems it is often called the "great imitator"; as Sir William Osler said, "He who knows syphilis, knows medicine."

Syphilis in an adult passes through several stages: inoculation during sexual contact, an incubation period of approximately 3 weeks; a *primary* lesion and silent systemic dissemination for 1 to 2 months; a *secondary* stage of approximately 6 weeks; resolution; and a latent stage lasting from 1 year to a lifetime or progressing to a *tertiary* stage, which is manifested by central nervous system, cardiovascular, and granulomatous lesions. *Congenital syphilis,* on the other hand, results from the transmission of spirochetes from an infected mother to the fetus. It is divided into early and late stages and stigmata.

Primary Syphilis. The initial lesion of primary syphilis is the chancre, which usually develops at the site of treponemal inoculation after an incubation period of 9 to 90 (average 21) days. During this incubation period, spirochetes multiply at the inoculation site, in regional lymph nodes, and in various organs throughout the body. Constitutional symptoms, however, are absent in primary syphilis.

Since syphilis is usually transmitted by sexual contact, most chancres appear on the genitals. They begin as papules that ulcerate. The typical ulcer (chancre) has a smooth, well-defined, raised border with a hard and finely granular base. Sometimes, owing to secondary infection, the ulcer may be covered with a yellowish crust or have a necrotic base. Chancres are usually solitary but may be multiple. They vary in size from a few millimeters to 1 to 2 cm in diameter, and although most are annular, they may assume any morphologic appearance. Typically, they are painless, although extragenital and secondarily infected lesions are often painful.

The neighboring lymph nodes usually become enlarged, hard, nonsuppurative, and nontender ("satellite bubo") within a week after the chancre appears. The nodes have a rubbery consistency, are discrete, and are not adherent to the skin or underlying tissues; there is no overlying erythema or skin change. Initially, the adenopathy associated with genital chancres is unilateral but subsequently becomes bilateral. Approximately one third of the patients with primary syphilis have no adenopathy. In addition, lymphadenopathy is not usually detectable in patients with cervical or rectal chancres.

In males most chancres appear on the penis, especially on the prepuce, coronal sulcus, frenulum, or glans. In infected females the most common sites are the labia majora, labia minora, and the fourchette. Fourchette chancres are often multiple and coalescent. Common, but often missed because they are not looked for, are chancres of the male urethra, which may be accompanied by mucoid discharge. In females, urethral and cervical lesions often go unnoticed.

In homosexual men, the sites most frequently involved with chancres are the anus and rectum. Here, such lesions often present with itching, discharge, painful defecation, constipation, or occasional bleeding. Although chancres are classically considered to be painless, those of the rectum are often quite painful. In male homosexuals, the extragenital site most frequently involved with primary lesions is the oral cavity. In lesbians, however, syphilis of the oral cavity is rare, while chancres of the lips may be seen more often than those of the oral cavity itself.

Foreplay and various sexual practices may give rise to extragenital chancres, which can be found anywhere on the body, with the lips being the most common location. Other more common extragenital locations are the breasts, fingers, toes, tongue, tonsils, face, and eyelids. In males, chancres contracted by kissing are more common on the upper lip, whereas in females they usually appear on the lower lip.

Since the primary lesions of syphilis are often asymptomatic, they may go unrecognized and untreated. Without treatment they usually heal within 3 to 6 weeks, leaving a thin atrophic scar.

Syphilis secondary to blood transfusion or puncture wounds is often devoid of a chancre in the primary stage and usually presents with signs and symptoms of the secondary stage. This appearance of secondary lesions without a primary chancre is called "syphilis d'emblée."

Clinically, primary syphilis should be differentiated from the following diseases: chancroid, herpes simplex, granuloma inguinale, balanitis, lymphogranuloma venereum, carcinoma, trauma, and fixed drug eruption.

Secondary Syphilis. In untreated individuals the secondary stage of syphilis occurs 2 to 12 (average 3) weeks after the appearance of the chancre or within 6 months (average 2) after exposure. A resolving primary chancre may still be present when secondary lesions appear. Secondary syphilis is the most contagious stage of early syphilis, because there are usually many contagious lesions in contradistinction to a single lesion of primary syphilis.

Patients with early secondary syphilis often have influenza-like symptoms: fever, headache, sore throat, malaise, anorexia, and generalized arthralgia. Generalized painless lymphadenopathy, as well as spleen and liver enlargement, may also occur.

Skin lesions are usually the hallmark of secondary syphilis. They may be macular, papular, follicular, papulosquamous, or pustular. Any of these types may occur singly or, more commonly, in combination. Vesiculobullous lesions do not occur in adults but may be seen in congenital syphilis. Except for follicular skin lesions, eruptions are usually nonpruritic. Initially, they are usually generalized and symmetrical, often becoming localized. Untreated lesions of secondary syphilis may last from weeks to months.

Macular lesions of secondary syphilis are copper-colored in light-skinned persons and of a deep brown hue in persons with dark skin, in whom they often go unrecognized. These lesions tend to be discrete and oval, following the lines of cleavage, especially on the trunk. The face is usually spared.

Papular lesions are the most common and characteristic skin manifestation of secondary syphilis. They may arise in macular lesions or independently. Their color varies according to the skin color of the patient: reddish-brown (salmon) on light skin and brown to gray on dark skin. Papular lesions are usually diffuse and symmetrical, with the most characteristic location being on the palms and soles. Macular and papulosquamous lesions also appear on the palms and soles. Here, because of the induration of the lesions and the thickness of the epidermis, they often appear flat or slightly elevated. Discrete, hyperkeratotic, centrally pitted papules (syphilis cornée) may appear on the palms and soles. Occasionally, a large papule may be surrounded by smaller satellite papules, producing a configuration called corymbiform (corymbose) syphilis. Split eroded papules at the corners of the mouth are also diagnostic of syphilis.

Grouped papules may coalesce to form annular ("nickel and dime") lesions, which are most commonly seen on the midface. Contrary to popular belief, they are seen in whites as well as in blacks. Lesions of condyloma lata are whitish moist papules and plaques that occur in moist intertriginous areas, especially the anogenital region. Lesions may vary from few to many in number. Clinically they are similar to lesions of condyloma acuminata. Papulosquamous lesions are common and must be differentiated from psoriasis, pityriasis rosea, and drug eruption.

Pustular lesions are usually the last to appear in secondary syphilis. They may resemble impetigo, acne, or chickenpox. A rare form, characterized by necrosis and ulceration with systemic symptoms, is called "lues maligna" or "malignant syphilis."

The skin lesions of secondary syphilis usually heal without scarring in 2 to 10 weeks, regardless of whether or not the patient is treated.

Mucous membrane lesions may occur alone or with any of the cutaneous lesions just discussed. They are usually 1- to 2-cm grayish-white erosions that may be surrounded by a dull erythematous margin (mucous patch). The lips, oral mucosa, tongue, pharynx, and larynx are most often involved. When the larynx is involved, a sore throat or hoarseness, or both, may occur. Mucous membrane lesions are highly infectious and usually last for several weeks, but they may be present for only a few days.

Alopecia is a common manifestation of secondary syphilis. It may present either as a diffuse thinning of the scalp hair or as patchy hair loss, giving the characteristic "moth-eaten alopecia." The scalp lesion resembles alopecia areata, whereas when the eyebrows are involved, the hair of the lateral portion is lost, resembling changes seen in leprosy and hypothyroidism. The hair loss is temporary and nonscarring regardless of whether or not the patient receives treatment.

Since secondary syphilis is a systemic disease, signs and symptoms often originate from organs other than the skin. These may appear in any time relationship to the skin lesions. Most patients disregard constitutional symptoms but with thorough questioning often admit to headache, sore throat, low-grade fever, malaise, arthralgias, and anorexia. Generalized lymphadenopathy usually precedes the skin lesions, with the cervical, epitrochlear, popliteal, and suboccipital nodes being characteristically involved. As in primary syphilis, the nodes are nontender, discrete, and rubbery in consistency. Concomitant spleen and (less commonly) liver enlargement may be present. Ophthalmic lesions may consist of iritis, uveitis (decreased vision, eye pain, photophobia, tearing) and corneal opacities. Nephropathy, probably secondary to immune complex deposition, may cause proteinuria and edema. Anorexia, nausea, vomiting, and epigastric pain secondary to ulcerations or strictures, or both, may be present. Syphilitic myositis characterized by aching muscles and progressive proximal muscle weakness, without muscle wasting, may occur. Severe aching pains of the long bones (osteocopic pain) are sometimes present; however, this is more common in congenital syphilis. Bone destruction, especially of the frontal bone, tibia, and clavicle, has been reported. Headaches may indicate acute syphilitic meningitis. Additional (although uncommon) central nervous system findings are transverse myelitis, nerve deafness, papilledema, and thromboses of the cerebral or spinal arteries. Other often neglected findings are transient electrocardiographic abnormalities, which clear with adequate treatment.

Latent Syphilis. Even without treatment the signs and symptoms of secondary syphilis clear in 2 to 8 weeks. Latent syphilis then supervenes. Latent syphilis is that stage in which, although there are no clinical signs and symptoms of the disease, serologic tests for syphilis are reactive. Latency is divided into two periods: early and late. There is disagreement as to the duration of early latency. Some experts use 2 years from the onset, others use 4. Regardless, in early latency approximately one half of the patients may have one or more relapses of mucocutaneous secondary syphilis, especially during the first year of infection. Therefore, early latency, along with the primary and secondary stages, is considered to be part of infectious syphilis. As the time of latency increases, the infectiousness decreases. At the end of this stage approximately two thirds of patients will enter the late latent phase and the other third will enter the tertiary stage.

Late latent syphilis of more than 4 years' duration is not communicable, except in pregnant women who, if not treated, may transmit syphilis to the fetus. Also, if the spinal fluid examination is negative at 4 years, it will probably remain so for the lifetime of the patient, unless he or she is reinfected. Approximately one half of late latent patients do not develop tertiary syphilis and become seronegative.

Tertiary Syphilis. Tertiary syphilis may involve any organ system, but cutaneous, bone, cardiovascular, and central nervous system lesions predominate, developing 5 to 20 years after the primary stage (although a small percentage of cases occur earlier or later).

Gummatous lesions may develop in any organ system, but the skin, liver, and bone are the most common sites. These lesions are usually benign, but lethal cases have been reported secondary to heart or brain involvement. Cutaneous gummas often begin as erythematous or "flesh"-colored, painless nodules that enlarge slowly and are often arranged in a polycyclic fashion. Sometimes these nodules ulcerate, forming noduloulcerative lesions. The nodular lesions heal without residua, but ulcerative lesions usually heal with atrophic scars and hyperpigmentation. Some lesions start as deep subcutaneous indurations with an overlying dusky-red appearance of the skin or mucous membrane. They rapidly break down and form punched-out ulcers with an arciform border.

These lesions tend to be quite destructive, often causing damage to the underlying bone and cartilage with resulting perforation of the hard palate or nasal septum. Serologic tests for syphilis are always positive in patients with active gummata, but spirochetes are not demonstrable in the lesions. This fact has led many syphilologists to postulate that gummas result from a hypersensitivity reaction rather than from direct tissue invasion by the spirochetes. Gummas are not infectious.

Neurosyphilis. Neurosyphilis develops in approximately 10 per cent of patients with untreated syphilis. It is more frequent in males than in females and is seen more frequently in whites than in blacks. Although invasion of the central nervous system occurs during early stages of syphilis, symptoms usually do not appear for at least 2 years after the initial infection. Neurosyphilis occurs in two forms: meningovascular and parenchymatous, but the classic clinical presentation of each type is usually not observed because routine antibiotic treatment of nontreponemal disease alters the pattern of disease.

In asymptomatic neurosyphilis there is no clinical evidence of disease, the patient having been identified because of positive routine serologic tests. Spinal fluid examination usually reveals an increased leukocyte count (5 or more per cu mm), a total protein concentration of over 40 mg/dl, and a positive serologic test for syphilis (STS). In tabes dorsalis the spinal fluid examination is normal in approximately 20 per cent of the patients.

Meningovascular syphilis (syphilitic meningitis) may be acute or chronic. Acute involvement (within the first 2 years of infection) is manifested by symptoms of headache, fever, stiff neck, and a positive Kernig's sign. It is rare, occurs usually in males, and may clear with or without treatment.

The clinical manifestations of chronic meningovascular syphilis vary according to which blood vessels or areas of the central nervous system are involved. Vessel involvement may cause psychosis, dizziness, mental confusion, aphasia, and hemiplegia. Extraocular muscle and facial palsies result from chronic meningitis of the base of the brain. Vertex involvement results in headache, seizures, increased intracranial pressure, nausea, and vomiting. Optic neuritis or optic atrophy or both may result from syphilitic inflammation of the optic nerve. Other cerebral manifestations may include irregularity and inequality of the pupils with a normal reaction to accommodation but a sluggish reaction to light (Argyll Robertson pupil) and inequality of deep tendon reflexes.

Degeneration of the ganglion cells and axons may result in parenchymatous neurosyphilis. There may be frontal lobe involvement (general paresis) or involvement of the posterior columns and posterior roots of the spinal cord (tabes dorsalis). The midbrain and sympathetic nervous system may also be involved in tabes.

Initially, paresis is often associated with subtle nonspecific symptoms such as headache, insomnia, poor concentration, and behavioral changes before overt mental changes are noted; some patients, however, may have seizures that are diagnosed as epilepsy and other patients may have small strokes that are usually diagnosed as a cerebrovascular accident. The full-blown mental symptoms consist of varied psychoses such as mania, euphoria, dementia, depression, and schizophrenia. Neurologically, the symptoms may be varied, but slurring of speech and pupillary irregularities are common.

The classic symptoms of tabes dorsalis are ataxia, lightning pains, paresthesias, visceral crises, bladder disturbances, impotence, and diplopia. Ataxia is manifested by loss of position sense (high stepping-slapping gait), especially in the dark. Lightning pains occur most commonly in the legs. They start suddenly, are severe and intermittent, and may last for minutes or days. Abdominal pain with visceral crises may be so severe that patients undergo surgery. The classic Argyll Robertson pupil or optic atrophy or both may be present. Loss or impairment of pain sensation may lead to trophic joint changes (Charcot's joints), the knee being the most common joint affected. Loss of deep pain sensation may lead to chronic indolent ulcers on the soles or toes (mal perforant).

The signs and symptoms of paresis and tabes dorsalis may coexist in the same patient (taboparesis).

Cardiovascular Syphilis. Cardiovascular involvement may occur as early as 5 years after primary infection but is seldom detected before 10 years and may not be discovered for 30 years after primary involvement. There are no early electrocardiographic changes. Approximately 10 per cent of untreated syphilitics will develop cardiac disease, males being more frequently affected than females.

The basic lesion of cardiovascular syphilis is aortitis, which has been reported only in acquired syphilis. In aortitis the elastic tissue of the media and the intima is destroyed and is replaced by rigid fibrous tissues, producing saccular aneurysms that may be filled with organized blood clots. The ostia may become narrowed, leading to myocardial ischemia and (rarely) death.

Involvement of the aortic valve rings and cusps may produce incompetence, resulting in regurgitation of the blood in the left ventricle. A diastolic murmur is produced that is best heard in Erb's area with the patient sitting and leaning forward in forced expiration. The pulse rises and falls quickly (Corrigan's, collapsing or water-hammer pulse).

Large aortic aneurysms may exert pressure and cause problems with the trachea, bronchi, lungs, vagal nerve, diaphragm, recurrent laryngeal nerve, and vertebrae.

Congenital Syphilis. *Treponema pallidum* will not pass through the placenta until after weeks 16 to 20, apparently because the Langhans' cell layer of the placenta, which completely atrophies by week 16, prevents its passage. As a result, congenital syphilis dates from after the fourth or fifth month of gestation. If a mother is adequately treated before this time, the product of gestation will have no evidence of syphilis.

Congenital syphilis is classified as early (up to 2 years, wherein the lesions are infectious); late (2 years and later, with primarily noninfectious lesions); and stigmata (permanent changes resulting from the disease in either stage).

Early Congenital Syphilis. The disease in the newborn is extremely variable in severity of onset. Local skin findings may erupt in an infant who appears to be quite well. Other infants may present with snuffles (coryza) and mucosal fissures or patches, rashes, and periostitis and osteochondritis; a disseminated maculopapular rash, particularly prominent on the palmar and plantar surfaces, associated with mucous membrane lesions; or a classic picture of snuffles and rhagades, with hepatosplenomegaly and a generalized rash. Other clinical presentations include those of an isolated anemia, thrombocytopenia, leukocytosis, jaundice, lymphadenopathy, fever, and failure to thrive. What is most difficult for the practitioner is that an infant may be entirely well, with negative serology, only to subsequently develop the full-blown disease.

Vesiculobullous lesions ("syphilitic pemphigus") are the earliest skin manifestations of congenital syphilis, often being present at birth. This is the only time of life when syphilis will be associated with a vesicle or bulla. On physical examination, the infant often has grouped vesiculobullous lesions, symmetrically distributed, particularly on the palms and soles. These lesions may also be present at the anorectal junction, periorally and, on rare occasions, may be generalized. The rash may be scant or diffuse, with fluid contents that are serous or seropurulent. Darkfield examination reveals that the contents are loaded with *T. pallidum,* thus being highly infectious. The lesions usually progress to superficial crusted erosions. During this phase, the child may often appear to be gravely ill.

Superficial desquamation, particularly of the palms and soles, is a quite frequent finding. It may, indeed, be the only dermatologic manifestation of congenital syphilis.

Later in onset are macular, papular, maculopapular, and papulosquamous eruptions, which constitute the typical syphilide. The palms and soles may be so intensely involved that they appear to be diffusely inflamed. Cutaneous lesions also appear on the face, chin, buttocks, genitals, and diaper area (presenting as a persistent diaper rash). In moist intertriginous areas, these may progress to become condylomata lata. The eruption may be scant or diffuse in quantity, and of a reddish color. Some experts attribute the development of rhagades (linear circumoral scars) to the secondary bacterial infection of the eruption around the mouth.

Other cutaneous manifestations include circinate lesions, raised plaques, café au lait–like patches, and shallow ulcers.

Mucous patches identical to those of acquired secondary syphilis develop, particularly on the palate, at the commissures of the mouth, and at various mucosal sites of the mouth, nose, anus, and genitals. They begin as maculopapular lesions, developing a central fissure with ulceration, becoming covered with a grayish membrane. The patient usually has accompanying systemic symptoms, including fever and malaise.

Mucous patches in the nose give rise to "snuffles," the signs and symptoms of which are coryza and rhinitis, which do not respond to decongestants and topical medications, and produce symptoms of obstruction. The amount of discharge may be profuse or slight, but the discharge is highly infectious, as demonstrated by a plethora of spirochetes on darkfield examination. It is serosanguineous, mucoid, purulent, or mucopurulent. Eventually, it excoriates the upper lip. By interfering with the development of the nasal bones, the infection in the nose gives rise to syphilitic facies, including the saddle nose (flat nasal bridge), small maxilla, and high-arched palate. The development of rhagades has also been attributed to this manifestation of syphilis.

Bony involvement has been given many names (Parrot's periostitis, osteomyelitis, periostitis, metaphysitis, osteochondritis). It consists of a panosteomyelitis, with most prominent effects on the growth plate of the metaphysis. Bone destruction and bone production are characteristic of this disease. The long bones and skull bones are involved most often, although involvement of the scapulae and ribs has been reported. Symptoms range from none (positive x-ray only) to pseudoparalysis, resulting from pain on motion. One may also find pyarthrosis, crepitation, and dislocation of joints. Pathologic fractures, usually in the metaphysis, have been reported in the diaphysis as well. Untreated bony lesions may resolve without residua or may progress into the bony lesions of late congenital syphilis.

Central nervous system involvement in early congenital syphilis may be the initial manifestation of a florid syphilitic infection. Although symptoms or signs (e.g., bulging fontanel, seizures, nuchal rigidity, increasing head circumference) may be present, it is asymptomatic in half of the patients. There are several forms that the central nervous system disease may take: acute meningovascular syphilis, which has severe sequelae including mental retardation and low-grade hydrocephalus; acute syphilitic meningitis with seizures; and meningoencephalitis.

Visceral involvement includes hepatosplenomegaly, lymphadenopathy, nephrotic syndrome, acute nephritis, and severe hepatitis, among others. Eye lesions include iritis and chorioretinitis. Edema may develop, resulting from hypoproteinemia, the major cause of which is thought to be malnutrition rather than the renal loss of protein. Orchitis, pneumonia, fever, failure to thrive, gastrointestinal disturbances, hemorrhage, and restlessness have also been reported. Death attributed to pulmonary hemorrhage, bacterial infection, or severe hepatitis may occur.

Late Congenital Syphilis. Untreated early congenital syphilis is the origin of late congenital syphilis. Sixty per cent of cases of late congenital syphilis remain latent, however, being diagnosed only by a routine serologic test. Among the 40 per cent that become clinically evident, the spectrum of disease differs widely from that of acquired late syphilis, aside from the fact that cardiovascular syphilis rarely if ever occurs in congenital syphilitics. Except for rhagades and gummas, lesions of the skin are not present. Bone and joint lesions include Clutton's joints and gummatous periostitis. Clutton's joints (chronic syphilitic hydrarthrosis) are characterized by symmetrical painless swellings of knees more often than of elbows or other joints. These lesions present primarily in pubertal or adolescent males. Joint tap produces no *T. pallidum,* but 10,000 to 45,000 white blood cells, primarily lymphocytes, are found. X-ray reveals no bony changes. It is thought that Clutton's joints represent a hypersensitivity reaction to the *T. pallidum.* Treatment with penicillin is ineffectual. Joint tap is followed by a reaccumulation of fluid until the disease burns itself out.

Gummatous periostitis, as in the bony lesions of early congenital syphilis, may be bone-producing or bone-destroying. Bone-producing lesions are found in the tibias (leading to the development of saber shins), phalanges, and skull. Lesions of the scapulae, clavicles, and shoulder girdle have been reported. Sternoclavicular swelling (Higouménakis' sign) has also been described. Bone-destroying lesions occur primarily in the palate, producing palatal perforation. They also occur in the bony ridge of the nose. In contrast to the lesions of early congenital syphilis, wherein the defects in the nose and face result from the *prevention of development* of bones, in late congenital syphilis they result from actual *destruction* of bone. The age of onset is 4 to 20 years.

Visceral lesions include gummas of the liver and other organs.

Central nervous system lesions that are asymptomatic are present in one third of untreated patients lacking other clinical manifestations. A positive spinal tap is the only manifestation of disease in these patients. Symptomatic neurosyphilis occurs in one fourth of untreated congenital syphilitics over the age of 6 years. It consists of parenchymal disease (juvenile tabes dorsalis, juvenile paresis), meningovascular syphilis, and eighth nerve deafness. The last finding, limited to the auditory portion of the nerve, occurs in 25 to 38 per cent of late congenital syphilitics. It may occur in isolation, leading to rapidly progressive deafness. It is characterized by the sudden onset, at age 8 to 10 years, of bilateral, symmetrical, sensorineural deafness. No vestibular signs are present. This finding is often associated with interstitial keratitis or Hutchinson's incisors (an affliction of the permanent incisors, usually the upper central pair but involving other teeth at times) or both.

The most common lesion of late congenital syphilis is interstitial keratitis. Although it usually presents at the same age as does palatal perforation, it may present at any time. Like Clutton's joints, this lesion is thought to result from a hypersensitivity reaction to the *T. pallidum.* The patient presents with acute photophobia, pain, and lacrimation in one or both eyes. Even if the affliction begins unilaterally, however, it eventually—after weeks or years—involves the other eye. The condition leads to progressive corneal opacity and blindness. Treatment with penicillin alone will not be effective. Other ocular lesions include chorioretinitis, vascular occlusion, and optic atrophy. The combination of eighth nerve deafness, Hutchinson's incisors, and interstitial keratitis is called Hutchinson's triad.

Stigmata. By definition, the stigmata of congenital syphilis are the scars and defects that remain as permanent evidence of congenital syphilis. They usually result from the more severe lesions. Stigmata of early congenital syphilis include old chorioretinitis (resulting from active chorioretinitis); frontal bossing (from osteomyelitis of the skull); syphilitic facies (maxillary underdevelopment, high arched palate, saddle nose, resulting from the mucous patches in the nose); rhagades (either from snuffles that excoriate the skin around the mouth, aggravated by grimacing or smiling, or from secondary bacterial infection of moist lesions around the mouth); and pupillary changes from iritis. Hutchinson's incisors and Moon's (mulberry) molars also arise from this stage and may be seen on x-ray prior to eruption.

The stigmata of late congenital syphilis include old chorioretinitis (also arising from active disease), frontoparietal bossing (from sclerotic osteoperiostitis), and saber shins (from the waxing and waning of sclerotic periostitis).

LABORATORY FINDINGS

The clinical diagnosis of syphilis should be confirmed by laboratory tests that demonstrate the presence of spirochetes in the lesions, classic histopathologic findings on biopsy, and/or antibodies in the serum or spinal fluid. Syphilis antibodies are of two main types: those to the organism itself and those secondary to the interaction of the spirochete with the tissue (reagin).

Darkfield Examination

This is the direct visualization of spirochetes in the lesions of primary and secondary syphilis. Darkfield examination of late secondary or tertiary lesions is usually negative. To perform a successful darkfield examination:

1. Abrade the lesion with gauze so as to produce a serous exudate with little or no bleeding.
2. Squeeze the lesion between your gloved thumb and forefinger.
3. Wipe away the first few drops in order to get more spirochetes from the depth of the lesion.
4. Touch the exudate with a glass slide (from the vagina and cervix collect the serum with a capillary pipette).
5. Place a coverslip on the drop of serum, and in order to prevent drying and death of the spirochetes, seal the coverslip with petrolatum.

Oral and genital mucous membrane lesions often have other spirochetes that are confused with *T. pallidum.* Darkfield examination in these patients is best done by injecting 0.5 to 1 ml of sterile saline solution into an enlarged regional lymph node, using the needle tip to macerate the tissue, aspirating the material and examining it for spirochetes. If the patient has used topical antiseptics or if the lesion is secondarily infected, the spirochete may be temporarily destroyed in the surface serum. In these cases, advise the patient to compress the lesions with saline solution 20 to 30 minutes three or four times a day and return in 24 hours for darkfield examination.

Serology

The humoral antibodies produced in syphilis are measured by treponemal and nontreponemal tests. The nontreponemal tests are further divided into flocculation (Venereal Disease Research Laboratory [VDRL] test, Hinton, Kahn, Kline) and complement-fixation (Wassermann, Kolmer) types.

Nontreponemal Tests. There are more than a hundred different nontreponemal tests for syphilis. The most commonly used flocculation tests are the VDRL test and a modification developed for rapid screening, the rapid plasma reagin (RPR) test. The Kolmer is the most commonly used complement-fixation test. The VDRL may be positive in 10 to 25 per cent of the patients having a chancre of 1 week's duration, increased to 50 per cent positivity by the end of the second week of the chancre, and usually reaching 75 per cent positivity in primary syphilis. The reactivity increases to 100 per cent in secondary syphilis but decreases thereafter. A negative test in suspected patients should be repeated at least two times. False-positive tests may be secondary to acute viral infections, bacterial infections, other spirochetal diseases, malaria, leprosy, collagen vascular disease, recent vaccination, chronic intravenous narcotic use, pregnancy, and old age.

An advantage of the VDRL is its quantitativeness. Serum is diluted serially and the test repeated at each dilution until it is no longer reactive. The last dilution producing a positive result is the titer; e.g., a titer of 1:32 means that the serum was reactive at 1:32 (seven-tube dilution) but negative (nonreactive) at 1:64. In active disease the titer usually increases on subsequent testing. If the patient is not treated in late syphilis, the titer remains the same; with treatment, however, it decreases. The VDRL becomes nonreactive with treatment within a year in almost 100 per cent of those with primary syphilis; in 95 per cent of those treated in the secondary stage, it becomes nonreactive within 18 months. Occasionally with nontreponemal tests, the excess production of antibody (especially in the secondary stage of syphilis) results in the prozone phenomenon. Undiluted serum will give a weakly reactive, atypical, or, on rare occasions, nonreactive reading, whereas testing at higher dilutions will give reactive test results.

Treponemal Tests. Treponemal tests are more specific but are more expensive and more difficult to perform. They become positive earlier in primary syphilis and remain positive for indefinite periods of time after treatment. The highest percentage of positive tests is found in secondary syphilis.

One of the most specific tests is the *Treponema pallidum* immobilization (TPI) test, which is a complement-fixation test using live treponema. Owing to the slow development of antibodies, the TPI test becomes reactive later in primary syphilis than do the nontreponemal tests. The test is difficult to perform and is done only at the Centers for Disease Control (CDC) in Atlanta, Georgia, and a few research laboratories. This test should be used only if one suspects syphilis in a patient with any condition that may cause other tests to be falsely positive.

The most widely used treponemal test is the fluorescent treponemal antibody-absorption (FTA-ABS) test. It is quite specific and sensitive, but intravenous narcotic addiction, hypergammaglobulinemia, systemic lupus erythematosus, pregnancy, and rheumatoid arthritis with a high titer rheumatoid factor may cause a false-positive reaction. The FTA-ABS test becomes positive in primary syphilis at approximately the time that the chancre appears and remains positive longer in treated and in late untreated syphilis than any of the treponemal or nontreponemal tests.

Other Tests. Because it is more economical than the FTA-ABS, the microhemagglutination assay for *T. pallidum* (MHA-TP) is replacing the former test in many centers. It is more specific and more sensitive in all stages beyond primary syphilis than the nontreponemal tests. The MHA-TP becomes positive in primary syphilis later than the VDRL and FTA-ABS tests and remains positive longer.

Laboratory Tests in Congenital Syphilis

If the mother is treated late in pregnancy, even if the results for the baby are negative at birth—serologically and clinically—the physician should follow the baby's serology and clinical picture, since these may change. The most difficult diagnosis to make is on the infant whose VDRL titer is the same as the mother's. In this case, one should do the long bone x-rays as soon as possible, since these may be positive early; one should also send a blood specimen for quantitative IgM, which may indicate an intrauterine infection of some kind if the level is over 20 mg per dl. All newborns with suspected or definite congenital syphilis should have a spinal fluid examination. A FTA-ABS-IgM should also be done. If it is positive, it is helpful, although in 10 per cent of cases it may be positive because of anti-IgM produced by the infant in response to other antigens, including maternal IgG, which is passively transferred to the fetus. The major drawback to this test, however, is that it will fail to detect the condition in up to 35 per cent of patients having delayed-onset disease!

Any moist lesion may be examined under darkfield, although this examination may not distinguish between pathogenic and nonpathogenic spirochetes. Other useful tests include a complete blood count with a differential cell count, and cell morphology.

When in doubt, the best regimen is to treat the patient for neurosyphilis. Those physicians who prefer to wait for definitive evidence of the disease may follow the VDRL and clinical picture. If the antibody is passively transmitted to the fetus, the VDRL will decline promptly and become negative by 3 months of age. An increase in titer or the failure of the titer to decline is suggestive of active disease. It is essential to follow the titer until it becomes completely nonreactive because occasionally there will be an initial decrease followed by progressive increases. In late congenital syphilis, it is common for the VDRL titers to vary from measurement to measurement.

Histopathology

The fundamental pathologic changes in syphilis are swelling and proliferation of the endothelial cells and a perivascular infiltrate that is composed of lymphocytes and numerous plasma cells. In tertiary syphilis, one finds these changes in addition to a granulomatous infiltrate of epithelioid and giant cells. Caseation necrosis is often present in the center. Although plasma cells are the hallmark of syphilitic tissue, there are few to none in some biopsy specimens. Spirochetes are difficult to demonstrate except in condyloma lata. If present, they can be demonstrated with silver stains such as the Warthin-Starry of Levaditi's stain. They are more common in the epidermis than the dermis and will not be present if antibiotic therapy has been given prior to biopsy.

DIFFERENTIAL DIAGNOSIS

Primary Syphilis. A genital chancre must be differentiated from chancroid, herpes simplex, granuloma inguinale, erosive balanitis, trauma, and carcinoma. Primary cervical chancres must be differentiated from carcinoma. Extragenital chancres, according to their sites, must be differentiated from various diseases: oral lesions due to tuberculosis, Behçet's disease, herpes simplex, and carcinoma; nipple lesions due to Paget's disease; tonsillar lesions secondary to infectious mononucleosis, agranulocytosis, and acute tonsillitis; finger chancres from paronychiae, sarcomas, carcinomas, felons, or herpetic whitlow; and anal or rectal lesions from cancer, thrombosed hemorrhoids, or Bowen's disease.

Secondary Syphilis. This may mimic any cutaneous disease, and any cutaneous disease may coexist with syphilis. Macular and papular lesions must be differentiated from pityriasis rosea, lichen planus, urticaria pigmentosa, drug eruption, leprosy, sarcoid, infectious mononucleosis, measles, and erythema multiforme. Papulosquamous lesions may resemble psoriasis, pityriasis rosea, seborrheic dermatitis, and tinea. Syphilitic alopecia resembles alopecia areata. Granuloma annulare, sarcoid, and tinea corporis must be differentiated from the annular lesions of secondary syphilis. Hemorrhoids, condyloma acuminata, Behçet's disease, and pemphigus vegetans may resemble condyloma lata. Cutaneous lesions of congenital syphilis must be differentiated from atopic eczema, from diseases causing hepatomegaly and splenomegaly, and from diseases causing lymphadenopathy.

Tertiary skin lesions may resemble any granulomatous disease, especially tuberculosis, leprosy, sarcoidosis, and deep mycoses.

Diagnostic Guidelines. Any patient treated for gonorrhea should have a serologic test for syphilis 6 to 12 weeks later. Darkfield examination of a chancre or an enlarged lymph node is indicated in any patient suspected of having primary syphilis. If the darkfield examination cannot be performed, serum should be drawn for a nontreponemal test. If the test is negative but suspicion remains high, an FTA-ABS should be performed.

Both treponemal and nontreponemal serologic tests are reactive in almost 100 per cent of patients with secondary syphilis. If, however, a false-positive reaction is suspected, a darkfield examination should be performed on all suspected lesions or on a lymph node aspirate.

In late syphilis nontreponemal tests may become negative; therefore, the FTA-ABS or other treponemal tests must be ordered. These patients should all have spinal fluid examinations.

RELAPSING FEVER

By James R. Philp, M.D.
and Joseph E. Johnson, III, M.D.
Winston-Salem, North Carolina

SYNONYMS

Tick fever, fowl nest fever, vagabond fever, bilious typhoid, febris recurrens, spirillum fever.

DEFINITION

Relapsing fever is a systemic infection caused by several spirochetes of the genus Borrelia, resulting in acute febrile episodes alternating with afebrile periods of at least 1 week's duration.

EPIDEMIOLOGY

There are many species of Borrelia that cause the syndrome of relapsing fever. *Borrelia recurrentis,* because it is spread by the human body louse (*Pediculus humanis*) and because man is the only host, has the potential for worldwide distribution. It is currently confined to the Sudan and Ethiopia because of the prevalence of poverty and overcrowding. It may also be encountered in travelers returning from these areas. All other Borrelia species are spread by the bite of soft ticks (Ornithodoros), e.g., *B. duttoni* by *Ornithodoros moubata* in Central and South Africa; *B. turicatae* by *O. turicata* in the southern plains of the United States and Mexico; and *B. hermsii* by *O. hermsi* in the western mountain areas of the United States. However, the wide distribution of tick vectors outside these areas is indicated by a case report from Ohio in 1978. In the tick, the organisms invade all tissues resulting in transovarial spread to the progeny. Ticks can remain infective for years and survive in relation to rodents and other small animals which also act as intermediate hosts for Borrelia species. In consequence, two recent outbreaks have been traced to sleeping in cabins containing rodents' nests and infective ticks.

CAUSATIVE AGENT

Borrelia are slender (10 to 20 X 0.3 micron), loosely coiled (5 to 7 microns), gram-negative, motile spirochetes. The spirochetes undergo repeated antigenic changes, which account for the cyclical recurrences of spirochetemia and fever. Defervescence of fever is by crisis and correlates with the appearance of IgM antibodies to the new antigenic phase. *Borrelia recurrentis, B. turicatae,* and *B. hermsii* have recently been cultured in artificial media. This should facilitate further study and better define the antimicrobial sensitivity spectrum of this group of organisms.

PRESENTING SIGNS AND SYMPTOMS

Following an incubation period of 5 to 11 days, the disease is characterized by the sudden onset of high fever (39 to 41°C) accompanied by rigors, arthralgia, myalgia, and headaches. A macular rash that may become generalized or petechial is often seen.

As a rule, the illness produced by *B. recurrentis* and *B. duttoni* is more severe than that due to the other species. Sequential relapses are similar to the initial episode but are usually less severe with progressively longer intervals between them. Usually there are no more than four relapses in louseborne disease, but as many as ten have been observed in untreated tickborne disease. Between febrile episodes the spirochetes are harbored in the marrow, liver, spleen, and central nervous system. This distribution of organisms along with antigen-antibody interactions and resulting spirochetal lysis and endotoxemia can account for many of the clinical features mentioned. Other findings and complications include hepatosplenomegaly, jaundice, hepatic failure, splenic rupture, coagulopathy, epistaxis, pneumonic involvement, meningitis with pleocytosis, brain hemorrhage, and cardiac dysrhythmias. Rapid resolution of fever by crisis is accompanied by profuse sweating. Hypotension and hypothermia can also occur during the crisis.

DIAGNOSIS

A good travel history is the prerequisite for logical diagnosis and will lead to examination of a *wet* blood film for the presence of motile spirochetes, preferably by darkfield microscopy. Because Borrelia is the only human bloodborne spirochete to stain with aniline dyes, a Wright or Giemsa stain of a thick blood film may also reveal the organisms. For this reason, it is not unusual for a fortuitous diagnosis to be made from a Wright stain of peripheral blood prepared for other purposes. In the acute febrile phase, circulating spirochetes may be found in 70 per cent of cases. An increased yield of positives may be had by examination of buffy coat preparations.

Inoculation of blood into mice is the most sensitive test during the afebrile period. The Weil-Felix test is nonspecific and is of supportive value only. The white blood cell count is unhelpful, since it may be normal, high, or low. In view of the likelihood of such nonspecific clinical findings, the differential diagnosis in the United States should include Colorado tick fever. Rocky Mountain spotted fever, Q fever, leptospirosis, and meningococcal disease. In other geographic settings, malaria, dengue, and Kala-Azar should also be considered.

PITFALLS IN DIAGNOSIS

In view of the nonspecific clinical picture, the main problem is failure to consider the possibility of borreliosis in individuals with an appropriate geographic history.

RAT-BITE FEVER

By Benjamin L. Portnoy, M.D.
Houston, Texas

SYNONYMS

Haverhill fever, sodoku.

DEFINITION

An acute febrile illness following a rat bite may be caused by either *Streptobacillus moniliformis* or *Spirillum minus.* Rat-bite fever is a disease of persons frequently exposed to rats, such as laboratory technicians, inhabitants of impoverished areas, or farmers. The streptobacillary form has also occurred in epidemics from ingestion of contaminated milk or other foods (Haverhill fever).

PRESENTING SIGNS AND SYMPTOMS

Both microorganisms produce a febrile illness with nonspecific symptoms, such as headache, malaise, and nausea. In the streptobacillary form, the rat-bite wound is usually healed at the time of onset of fever, 1 to 7 days following the bite. As the disease progresses, most patients develop a faint macular or papular erythematous eruption that begins on the palms and soles and spreads centrally. Arthralgias are a common complaint.

The spirillary form of rat-bite fever (sodoku) is not very common in the United States. With the onset of fever, over 7 days after the bite, the original wound will become inflamed, and lymphangitis and lymphadenopathy will appear. The rash is limited to extremities and arthritis is rare.

COMMON COMPLICATIONS

Bacterial endocarditis is a complication described in both types of rat-bite fever. *Streptobacillus moniliformis* may produce abscesses and septic joints accompanied by prolonged fever. An L-form of this organism will also lead to prolonged fever unresponsive to the routine treatment with penicillin. For L-forms, tetracycline or streptomycin must be substituted.

LABORATORY FINDINGS

Streptobacillus moniliformis is an aerobic gram-negative highly pleomorphic bacillus. It can be cultured from blood or joint fluid. Culture requires addition of calf serum or ascites fluid to the media, but if enough blood is inoculated into routine blood culture media, there appear to be sufficient nutrients to support growth. Blood or chocolate agar cultures will not cause *S. moniliformis* to grow. Growth appears as a sediment on top of the blood layer in the aerobic blood culture media and as fluffy balls on the blood layer of the anaerobic bottle. The organism gets its name from the odd appearance of older cultures. As the culture ages, the short rods elongate, develop yeastlike medial swellings, and eventually form chains of filaments.

Spirillum minus is a spiral organism with a polar flagellum. It has not been reliably cultured on artificial media, although other Spirillum species have been reported to grow in anaerobic glucose broth containing thioglycollate. Peritoneal inoculation of blood into mice or guinea pigs will yield large numbers of organisms in 5 to 15 days from blood or peritoneal fluid. Darkfield microscopy or Wright-stained smears are used to identify *S. minus.*

No serologic or fluorescent antibody test is clinically available to aid in the diagnosis of either form of rat-bite fever.

PITFALLS IN DIAGNOSIS

The streptobacillary form of rat-bite fever appears strikingly similar to Rocky Mountain spotted fever. The rash, severity of malaise, degree of fever, and headache may be identical in the two illnesses. Since other rodents besides rats and mice may carry *S. moniliformis,* campers who suffer animal bites in spotted fever endemic areas may present a confusing epidemiologic history. A response to penicillin would rule out the rickettsial illness.

LEPTOSPIROSIS

By George P. Schmid, M.D.
and Arnold F. Kaufmann, D.V.M.
Atlanta, Georgia

SYNONYMS

Weil's disease, hemorrhagic jaundice, autumnal fever, Fort Bragg fever, mud fever, swineherd's disease, European swamp fever, pea-picker's disease, seven-day fever, canefield fever, and canicola fever.

DEFINITION

Leptospirosis is an acute infectious disease caused by numerous serovars (serotypes) of the spirochete *Leptospira interrogans.* Although the array of signs and symptoms varies widely among patients, the illness is broadly subdivided into anicteric and icteric syndromes. Either syndrome can be caused by any of the more than 180 *L. interrogans* serovars that are currently recognized.

Leptospirosis has a worldwide distribution. Cases tend to occur individually or in small clusters, with large outbreaks being rare. Leptospirosis infections can occur throughout the year, but are most common in the summer.

Leptospirosis is a zoonosis, with a wide range of domestic and wild animals serving as reservoir hosts. Human infection primarily results from direct and indirect exposure to the urine of infected animals. Indirect exposure, such as swimming in contaminated streams or working in rodent-infested wet environments, is more commonly implicated than direct exposure. Other modes of infection, such as animal bites, handling infected animal tissues, and ingestion of contaminated food and water, are far less important. Person-to-person transmission is extremely rare.

PRESENTING SIGNS AND SYMPTOMS

Between 2 and 20 days following penetration of the organism through mucous membranes or abrasions, illness usually begins abruptly with fever, chills and rigors, intense headache, myalgia, nausea, and vomiting. Muscle pain, often quite marked, is most notable in the calf and lumbar areas, although abdominal myalgia may simulate intra-abdominal disorders and cervical myalgia may simulate meningismus. Conjunctival injection, pharyngitis, hepatomegaly, and a variety of skin rashes may occur in the first several days of illness.

COURSE

The course of illness following onset depends upon which of two clinical syndromes develops—anicteric leptospirosis (90 per cent of cases) or icteric leptospirosis (10 per cent of cases). These clinical syndromes are best understood by a description of the unique pathophysiology of leptospirosis.

Leptospirosis is a biphasic disease with a septicemic and an immune stage. Illness begins with the septicemic stage, which lasts for 4 to 7 days. During this stage, leptospires disseminate widely throughout the body and may be found in the blood, cerebrospinal fluid (CSF), kidneys, and other organs. Direct damage to the various organs by the leptospires is the basis of the initial illness. Following the appearance of antibody, the initial symptoms subside as the leptospires disappear from all organs except the aqueous humor and kidneys. Following this quiescent period, which lasts 1 to 3 days, the immune stage of illness begins and clinical illness in this stage is believed to occur on the basis of the patient's immune response to the leptospires. The biphasic nature of the illness is not always apparent, particularly in icteric leptospirosis.

In both syndromes, the initial signs and symptoms last for approximately 4 to 7 days. During this time, fever, chills and rigors, headache, and myalgia are prominent symptoms. About 50 per cent or fewer patients will also have pharyngitis, cough, nausea or vomiting, abdominal pain, or diarrhea. Skin rashes of varying types may occur. Headache is characteristically intense, and occasionally disturbances in mental status occur. Myalgia most commonly affects the calf, thigh, lumbar, and cervical muscles. Distinct clinical improvement marks the end of the septicemic stage.

In anicteric leptospirosis, the immune stage is generally of lesser duration and severity than the septicemic stage and its most important features are meningitis and leptospiruria. Fever may not be prominent. The severity of meningitis varies, but it usually only lasts a few days and is clinically similar to aseptic meningitis. Not uncommonly, the septicemic phase of illness is very mild and patients initially present with signs and symptoms of meningitis. Conversely, not all patients with anicteric leptospirosis will develop a clinically recognizable immune stage.

Other symptoms may develop during the immune stage. Nonmeningitic neurologic manifestations, including encephalitis, nerve palsies, and myelitis may occur and last for weeks or months. Uveitis typically appears late in the immune stage, even months after the onset of disease.

Unlike the relatively mild illness experienced by persons with anicteric leptospirosis, icteric leptospirosis may be quite severe and results in death in up to 10 per cent of cases. The hallmarks of icteric leptospirosis—jaundice and azotemia—begin in the latter part of the septicemic stage and tend to obscure the biphasic nature of the disease. Jaundice may be quite marked and is a general guide to the severity of disease. Reflecting the lack of significant hepatocellular damage, however, jaundice is not accompanied by signs or symptoms of hepatic encephalopathy. Impairment of renal function, on the other hand, is common and reflected by varying degrees of azotemia and oliguria. In addition, cardiovascular involvement, often with hypovolemia or myocarditis, may be manifested by hypotension and shock. Reflecting the hemorrhagic diathesis of icteric leptospirosis, frank bleeding into the gastrointestinal tract or lungs may occur.

The prognosis in nonicteric disease is excellent, with complete recovery ensuing as the immune stage ends. In icteric disease, death may occur secondary to renal failure, cardiovascular collapse, and hemorrhage; mortality is highest in older persons.

COMMON COMPLICATIONS

Complications occur primarily in patients with icteric disease. Dialysis may be required until adequate renal function returns. Cardiac failure and arrhythmia may require close medical monitoring. Frank hemorrhage may occur into the gastrointestinal tract, leading to hypotension, or into the lungs, causing a hemorrhagic pneumonitis. Acalculous cholecystitis may occur, necessitating operative intervention.

PHYSICAL EXAMINATION

Physical findings are few and nonspecific. Conjunctival suffusion, often in association with photophobia, occurs in about 33 per cent of patients during the septicemic phase of disease. An erythematous pharynx, sometimes with exudate, has been noted in up to 25 per cent of patients. Hepatomegaly occurs commonly in icteric disease and in about 15 per cent of nonicteric patients; splenomegaly has been reported variably. Muscle tenderness helps differentiate leptospirosis from other causes of jaundice. Meningismus is generally not apparent during the septicemic stage of disease despite the presence of intense headache but is often apparent during the immune stage. Skin rashes, usually truncal, are quite variable, although pretibial rashes are characteristic of infection with several serovars.

LABORATORY DIAGNOSIS

General Laboratory Test Findings. Clinical laboratory test results tend to occur in certain patterns, but exceptions are common. In general, test results are most abnormal in icteric patients.

A persistently increased erythrocyte sedimentation rate is the most consistent hematologic finding. In anicteric patients, the total white blood cell (WBC) count is normal to slightly elevated, with relative neutrophilia being common. In icteric patients, leukocytosis with a left shift is usual and may be marked in severe cases. Slight thrombocytopenia and moderate anemia occur in icteric patients with bleeding diathesis.

Serum biochemical abnormalities tend to be inconsistent and not very striking in anicteric patients. The majority, however, do have minimal-to-moderate increases in either their alanine aminotransferase (SGPT, ALT), aspartate aminotransferase (SGOT, AST), alkaline phosphatase (ALP), or lactate dehydrogenase (LD) levels. Less than 50 per cent have elevated blood urea nitrogen (BUN) or creatinine levels.

Icteric patients have increased total serum bilirubin levels, usually less than 20 mg/dl but occasionally reaching 60 to 80 mg/dl. The direct reacting fraction usually predominates because the jaundice is usually due to nonobstructive intrahepatic biliary stasis. Levels of SGPT, SGOT, ALP, and LD are typically elevated, usually two to three times normal and infrequently to the higher ranges typical of acute viral hepatitis. Most icteric patients have elevated BUN (usually less than 100 mg/dl) and creatinine levels (usually 2 to 8 mg/dl). Creatine kinase (MM isoenzyme) levels are commonly elevated in acute leptospirosis due to the skeletal muscle involvement, another potentially useful finding in differentiating leptospirosis from acute viral hepatitis.

Examination of the CSF commonly reveals pleocytosis even in the absence of nuchal rigidity. The total WBC count is usually less than 500 per cu mm. Mononuclear cells usually predominate, but neutrophils may predominate in early illness. In association with pleocytosis, the CSF protein concentration is usually increased (up to 300 mg/dl) but the glucose concentration tends to be normal.

Urinalysis findings are normal to slightly abnormal in anicteric patients, with proteinuria (>2+), pyuria (>5 white blood cells/high power field), or microscopic hematuria (>2 erythrocytes/high power field) being present in less than 33 per cent of patients. In icteric patients, common findings are proteinuria, pyuria, cylinduria, microscopic-to-gross hematuria, bilirubinuria, and urobilinogenuria.

Specific Diagnostic Tests. Specific laboratory confirmation of leptospirosis is a slow process, requiring a minimum of 1 week to a month or more. Because therapy is beneficial only when initiated within 5 days of clinical onset, the ability to make a clinical diagnosis in the absence of specific diagnostic findings is important.

Serologic tests are the most commonly used approach to confirmation. Paired serum specimens, with an interval of 14 to 21 days between specimen collection, are essential for accurate interpretation of test results. A third serum specimen may be necessary because up to 10 per cent of patients fail to develop antibodies within 30 days of clinical onset.

In the United States, the three most common serologic procedures are the macroscopic (slide) agglutination, the microscopic agglutination, and the indirect hemagglutination tests. The slide and indirect hemagglutination tests are screening procedures, the former using a suspension of killed leptospires and the latter using genus-specific antigen coated on sheep red blood cells to detect agglutinating antibody. Although both procedures may detect antibody in the course of illness earlier than the microscopic agglutination test, they are more prone to false-positive reactions. The microscopic agglutination test is the most reliable procedure and entails the testing of serum against a battery of live leptospiral serovars. A fourfold or greater change in agglutinating antibody titer is considered significant. Because a given antigenic grouping may be present in different serovars, a patient's serum commonly agglutinates multiple serovars. Although useful in supporting a clinical diagnosis of leptospirosis, serologic test results do not reliably indicate the identity of the infecting serovar.

Leptospires are slow-growing organisms, and their presence in cultures cannot be detected for days to several weeks after inoculation. Isolation from blood and CSF is generally possible only during the first 10 days of illness. After this period, urine is the optimal culture specimen. Leptospiruria begins in the second week of illness and may persist for 30 days or more. In fatal cases, liver, kidney, and brain are the preferred tissues for culture. Because special culture media and techniques are used, good coordination with the laboratory in specimen collection and processing is essential.

Direct examination of blood, urine, and CSF using a darkfield microscope may reveal leptospires. This approach, however, is an insensitive diagnostic technique, and artifacts such as filamentous extrusions from blood cells are frequently misidentified as leptospires. Leptospires can be demonstrated in tissue sections by silver impregnation techniques suitable for spirochetes such as the Dieterle stain. They cannot be demonstrated with routine bacterial stains.

PITFALLS IN DIAGNOSIS

Because leptospirosis is an uncommon illness, physicians often fail to consider it in the differential diagnosis of patients with meningitis, jaundice, or nonspecific febrile illnesses. Suspicion of the illness together with a history of exposure to potential sources of infection, constitutes the most valuable clue to the diagnosis of leptospirosis.

AMEBIASIS

By D. R. W. Haddock, M.D., F.R.C.P.
Liverpool, England

DEFINITION

Amebiasis has been defined as the condition of harboring *Entamoeba histolytica* with or without clinical manifestations. Most gastrointestinal infections with *E. histolytica* are asymptomatic, the amebae living as commensals in the lumen of, or on the mucosal surface of, the colon. In a minority of patients the organism becomes invasive, causing colonic lesions by means of its proteolytic, cytolytic enzymes; occasionally it spreads by direct extension or by the bloodstream to the liver, pleura, lungs, and, rarely, to the pericardium and brain.

What causes "invasiveness" is not clear. Host immune deficiency, especially virulent strains of amebae, and colonic bacterial infections have all been postulated as factors. *Entamoeba histolytica* is identified by its morphologic characters. Sargeaunt and colleagues have identified 18 isoenzyme types and believe that only two of these show "invasiveness." In Mexico, Biagi found that of 1000 patients with amebiasis, 200 showed evidence of invasive disease and one, hepatic amebiasis. Although 5 per cent of residents in temperate climates pass amebic cysts, invasive amebiasis is very rare. Infection is much more common in the tropics, where 20 per cent of the population may be cyst passers. Male homosexuals in temperate climates have a relatively high incidence of amebiasis.

CLASSIFICATION

Amebiasis is sometimes classified in the following way:

1. *Asymptomatic*—intestinal cyst passers.
2. *Symptomatic intestinal.*
   a. Dysentery.
   b. Nondysenteric colitis.
   c. Ameboma.
3. *Extraintestinal.*
   a. Hepatic: Amebic liver abscess (ALA). (The concept of diffuse amebic hepatitis is not generally accepted.)
   b. Involvement of other organs with or without hepatic involvement.

INTESTINAL AMEBIASIS

Presenting Symptoms

Most people harboring amebae in their gut are asymptomatic. Abdominal symptoms should not be attributed to amebiasis if only cysts are found in the stools. Some cyst passers give a history of previous recurrent diarrheal disease, and about 20 per cent have positive amebic serology suggesting previous invasive disease.

The characteristic history of invasive intestinal amebiasis is of intermittent or chronic diarrhea with the passage of two to six loose stools a day often containing blood and mucus. Lower abdominal cramps are common; constitutional signs such as fever and wasting are usually absent. In very chronic disease, there will be anemia and weight loss. On examination there may be tenderness over the cecum and iliac colon. This type of disease may persist intermittently for months or even years.

In a few patients the onset is abrupt, with severe diarrhea, tenesmus and fever—the illness resembles bacillary dysentery of moderate severity. Rarely, invasive disease is fulminant with severe diarrhea; heavy colonic bleeding; high fever; shock; and a tender, distended abdomen. There is considerable likelihood of colonic perforation and peritonitis; the prognosis is poor—the illness resembling toxic dilatation of the colon in ulcerative colitis. A fulminant course may occur in association with pregnancy or corticosteroid therapy.

Complications

These include peritonitis, pericolic abscess, appendicitis, severe rectal bleeding, colonic stricture (rarely), and extension to the perianal skin. An ameboma is a chronic granuloma around the colon that may lead to obstruction or intussusception. It can mimic carcinoma, appendix abscess, or diverticulitis. A condition of postdysenteric colitis may persist for months after parasite elimination.

There is a tendency to overdiagnose amebiasis in the tropics. On clinical grounds, it is impossible to differentiate amebiasis from other diseases producing a similar picture; therefore, positive parasitologic diagnosis is of prime importance.

AMEBIC LIVER ABSCESS

Presenting Symptoms

The usual presentation is with pain in the liver area. The pain is dragging or pleuritic in nature. There may be right shoulder tip pain due to diaphragmatic involvement. Constitutional symptoms with swinging fever, anorexia, weakness, and wasting are commonly present. A dry cough due to pleural irritation may be found.

If untreated, the abscess extends to and can penetrate the diaphragm, causing pleural effusion and lung involvement. It may burst through the skin, causing cutaneous amebic ulceration; it may reach the pericardium, causing pericarditis; or it may cause peritonitis. Jaundice occurs in 5 to 10 per cent of patients and is usually not deep. Bloodstream spread may occur to lungs or brain.

On examination, the liver is usually enlarged and tender and there is intercostal tenderness over the right lower thorax. Respiratory signs sometimes present include dullness to percussion, diminished breath sounds, and auscultatory crackles over the right base of the lungs. Some patients present with fever of uncertain origin.

Complications

Some complications of ALA are as follows:

1. Pleural effusion, either a sterile reactive one or one infected with amebae.
2. Amebic lung abscess.
3. Pericarditis.
4. Peritonitis.
5. Rupture externally and cutaneous amebiasis.

Other sites occasionally infected include cervix, vagina, penis, bladder, and spleen. Early diagnosis of ALA is vital because it is an eminently treatable condition and, if neglected, is often fatal.

LABORATORY PROCEDURES

Intestinal Amebiasis

The questions to be answered are these:

1. Can the parasite be found in the stools?
2. If so, are only cysts present?
3. Is there evidence of invasive intestinal amebiasis as shown by motile trophozoites containing red blood cells?
4. Is there evidence of extraintestinal amebiasis?

Diagnosis depends upon parasite identification by an experienced microscopist.

Trophozoite Detection. The presence of progressively motile trophozoites of *E. histolytica* containing red blood cells in the stools confirms invasive intestinal amebiasis. The trophozoites are 10 to 40 microns in diameter, having a granular endoplasm and a clear ectoplasm. They contain erythrocytes and are actively motile across the slide. When stained with iron hematoxylin, the nuclei show a small central karyosome and a layer of fine chromatin granules around the nuclear membrane (Fig. 1).

Stools should be examined warm within 15 minutes of passage; otherwise, the trophozoites round up, become immotile, and are difficult to identify with certainty. If rapid examination is impracticable, stools may be preserved in polyvinyl alcohol and stained specimens examined. Iron hematoxylin or Wheatley's trichrome stain can be used to identify specific morphology.

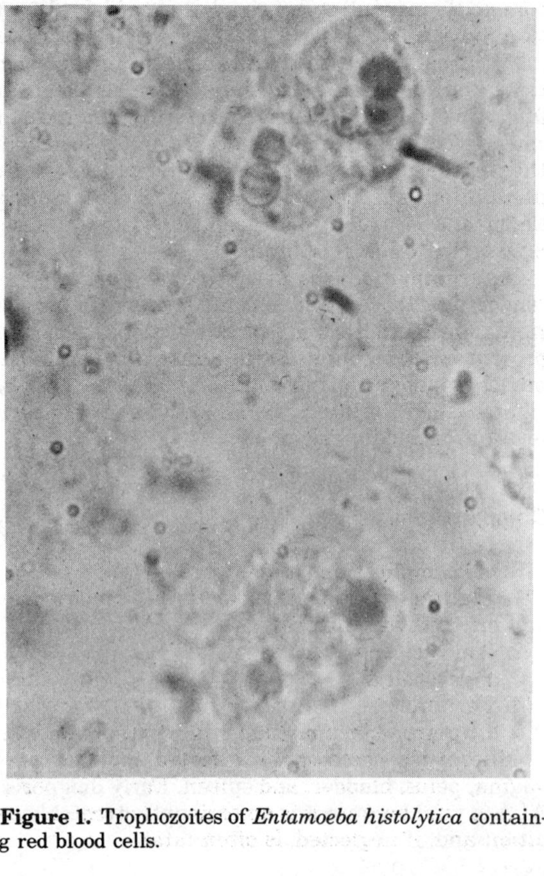

Figure 1. Trophozoites of *Entamoeba histolytica* containing red blood cells.

It is desirable to examine a specimen taken from a portion of stool that contains blood and mucus. Several examinations may be necessary at various intervals. Scrapings or pipette aspirations from lesions on the bowel wall taken at sigmoidoscopy are sometimes positive when ordinary stool examination results are negative. Specimens should be examined before treatment because certain drugs may prevent diagnosis (see Pitfalls of Diagnosis).

Detection of Cysts of *E. histolytica*. Because cyst excretion is intermittent, three daily negative stool specimens are necessary to exclude the diagnosis with 85 per cent certainty (six negatives are said to give 95 per cent certainty). The cysts are spherical or slightly ovoid, grayish in color, have a definite cyst wall, and are 10 to 17 microns in diameter. Rod-shaped chromidial bars may be seen in the unstained cyst. When stained with 1 per cent potassium iodide saturated with iodine crystals, one to four nuclei with the morphologic characteristics described are present. Nonpathogenic cysts are under 10 microns in diameter (*Endolimax nana, Entamoeba hartmanni*) or contain more than four nuclei with appearances different from *E. histolytica* and are often over 17 microns in diameter (*Entamoeba coli*). Cultural methods can be employed using special media.

As previously emphasized, persons passing cysts only cannot be diagnosed as having invasive amebiasis, but such persons are infective. Occasionally both cysts and pathogenic trophozoites are found in the same stool specimen.

Extraintestinal Amebiasis

Identification of E. histolytica in pus from a liver abscess is often difficult or impossible. In ALA, aspiration should be performed only for therapeutic purposes and only if the abscess is very large, if it seems likely to rupture, or if it is not responding to treatment. Amebic pus is characteristically brownish-red in color and contains degenerate liver cells. Examining the last few drops of pus or examining the aspirate after incubation with streptokinase may facilitate the finding of trophozoites (cysts are never present in tissues). Aspirated pus should be cultured for bacteria. Parasites are frequently absent from the stools in extraintestinal amebiasis.

Serologic methods are useful in hepatic amebiasis; the results are positive in about 95 per cent of cases using fluorescent antibody tests (FAT), enzyme-linked immunosorbent assay (ELISA), or hemagglutination techniques. Thus, negative test results make hepatic amebiasis extremely unlikely. Positive results may signify present or past infection. Serologic tests are usually positive in invasive intestinal amebiasis but are of less assistance in diagnosis.

Trophozoites may be found in scrapings or biopsies from cutaneous or genital amebiasis.

RADIOLOGIC EVALUATION

Barium enema is of little help in the positive diagnosis of amebiasis but assists in the exclusion of other conditions that may coexist, such as carcinoma of the colon. In ALA, x-ray of the chest often shows a raised right hemidiaphragm that is immobile on fluoroscopy (Fig. 2). Pleural effusion and lung involvement may also be demonstrated. Ultrasound scanning and isotope scanning of the liver are useful in detection and localization of abscess cavities.

OTHER DIAGNOSTIC PROCEDURES

Sigmoidoscopy. This procedure will often show ulceration in the rectum and sigmoid colon. Amebic lesions are shallow ulcers up to 2 cm in diameter with raised and undermined edges. The ulcers are covered with yellowish exudate, and the intervening mucosa is normal. Aspirates from ulcers should be examined rapidly for trophozoites. Sigmoidoscopy is necessary only if trophozoites cannot be found in the stools or if other pathology is suspected. The procedure is inadvisable in severe disease because there is a definite danger of perforation. A normal sigmoidoscopy using a rigid sigmoidoscope does not exclude invasive intestinal amebiasis, since sometimes lesions are confined to the cecum.

Aspiration of Liver Abscesses. Aspiration is used for therapeutic purposes and rarely solely for diagnosis. Aspiration is conducted under local anesthesia after premedication. The site of aspiration is preferably over the site of an abscess localized by ultrasound; failing this, the site of pointing or maximal tenderness is used. If there is no clearly indicated site, the eighth intercostal space in the anterior axillary line is used, with the needle directed toward the vertebral column and *no deeper* than 9 cm in an adult. A wide-bore bone marrow needle with a trocar is inserted, the latter being removed at intervals and suction applied. If pus is encountered, it is aspirated to dryness. If no pus is found, the aspiration may be repeated once only. The pus is examined microscopically and cultured.

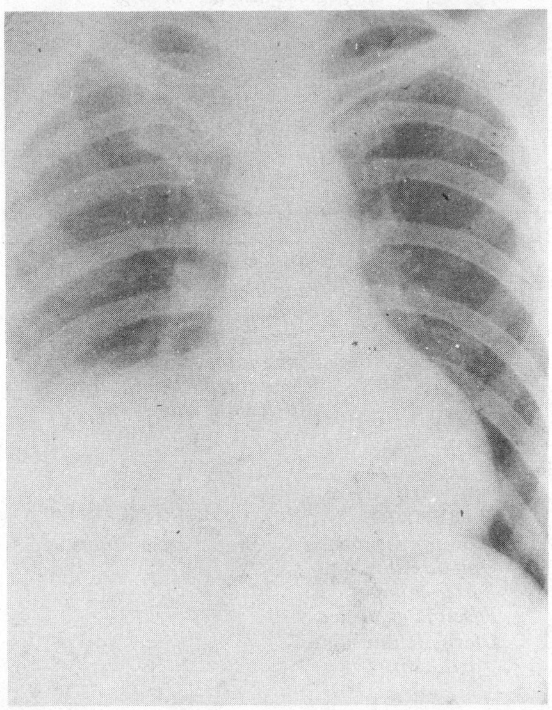

Figure 2. Chest x-ray in amebic liver abscess showing marked elevation of the right hemidiaphragm.

Therapeutic Tests. Therapeutic trials should not be necessary in intestinal amebiasis if skilled parasitologic help is available. The specific diagnosis of ALA may be difficult, particularly when serology and liver scanning are not available. In this event, therapeutic trial with metronidazole is often justifiable. Metronidazole is reasonably specific (although it does act on anaerobic bacteria which can cause liver abscesses), and its toxicity is low. The diagnosis of ameboma is sometimes problematic, but a trial of metronidazole and tetracycline with careful monitoring of progress may be helpful. If improvement is not clear-cut, laparotomy is necessary.

POTENTIAL ERRORS AND PITFALLS IN DIAGNOSIS

It is important not to miss the diagnosis of amebiasis because therapy is very successful and often lifesaving. Disasters due to fulminant invasive amebiasis may occur when steroids are given to patients who are harboring *E. histolytica* in the presence of colitis or other conditions. However, there is a tendency to attribute all chronic diarrhea in the tropics to amebiasis; in fact, tropical malabsorption, giardiasis, and schistosomiasis are other common causes. Amebiasis is common and may coexist with other lesions such as carcinoma of the colon; thus, careful follow-up after therapy is important. The diagnosis of ameboma is sometimes possible only after excision of the mass. The possibility of hepatic amebiasis should be considered in lesions at the base of the right lung, particularly if the liver is palpable.

Inexperienced laboratory workers may misidentify macrophages in the stool as *E. histolytica.* Vital staining with cresyl blue may clarify morphology. Some factors can interfere with detection of *E. histolytica* in the stools, including prior administration of amebicidal drugs, tetracyclines, sulfonamides, laxatives, bismuth and kaolin compounds, barium sulfate used in radiologic studies, and enemas. Stool examination should precede therapy and radiology.

PARASITIC INFECTIONS OF THE INTESTINAL TRACT

By G. Thomas Strickland, M.D., Ph.D., D.C.M.T.
Baltimore, Maryland, and Lahore, Pakistan

Innumerable parasites are capable of infecting the human gastrointestinal tract (Table 1). Some are protozoa; others are helminths. Some are pathogenic; others cause no symptoms. Some are common causes of infection (with hundreds of millions of people parasitized); others are extremely rare. Intestinal parasitic infections are diagnosed by observing the parasite or its ova in the stool. However, useful diagnostic information can be obtained by other techniques.

SIGNS AND SYMPTOMS

Symptoms and signs of illness do not necessarily follow all gastrointestinal parasitic infections.

Asymptomatic. Symptoms have not been associated with some protozoal infections (Table 1). For instance, *Entamoeba hartmanni* cysts and trophozoites are identical in appearance to *Entamoeba histolytica* except that they are smaller. *Entamoeba hartmanni* has not been associated with human disease. The majority of *E. histolytica* infections are asymptomatic cyst passers. *Giardia lamblia* was formerly considered nonpathogenic; it almost always causes minimal or no symptoms in those who have developed immunity.

With one exception, intestinal helminths often cause asymptomatic infections. Patients found to have *Capillaria philippinensis* ova in their stools either had been symptomatic or developed symptoms later. This parasite, unlike all other helminths except *Strongyloides*, multiplies in the gut. Even many patients with schistosomiasis are asymptomatic.

Abdominal Pain. Except for the nonpathogenic protozoa and usually for pinworm (*Enterobius vermicularis*) infection, all of the parasites in Table 1 have been associated with abdominal pain. The most characteristic symptom complex includes anorexia, nausea, and intermittent abdominal distention and cramps, flatulence, and loose stools. Sometimes the patient also has weight loss. This is the most common symptom complex for amebiasis (*E. histolytica* infection) and the only one described for *Entamoeba polecki* and *Dientamoeba fragilis* infections. These symptoms occur during the intestinal invasive stage of intestinal sporozoa infections and during initial egg laying in schistosomal infections. It is the most common presentation for symptomatic patients with ascariasis, hookworm, strongyloidiasis, and trichuriasis.

Table 1. Some Important Intestinal Parasites

Protozoa

Frequently Pathogenic	*Potentially Pathogenic*	*Nonpathogenic*
Ameba		
Entamoeba histolytica	*Entamoeba polecki*	*Entamoeba hartmanni*
		Entamoeba coli
		Iodoamoeba butschlii
		Endolimax nana
Flagellates		
Giardia lamblia	*Dientamoeba fragilis*	*Chilomastix mesnili*
		Trichomonas hominis
Ciliate		
Balantidium coli		
Sporozoa		
	Isospora belli	
	Sarcocystis spp.	
	Cryptosporidium spp.	
	Blastocystis hominis	

Helminths

Nematodes	Cestodes
Ascaris lumbricoides	*Taenia saginata*
Enterobius vermicularis	*Taenia solium*
Necator americanus and *Ancylostoma duodenale*	*Diphyllobothrium latum*
Strongyloides stercoralis	*Hymenolepis nana*
Trichuris trichiura	*Hymenolepis diminuta*
Capillaria philippinensis	*Dipylidium caninum*
Trichostrongylus spp.	

Trematodes

SCHISTOSOMES	INTESTINAL FLUKES	LIVER FLUKES	LUNG FLUKES
Schistosoma mansoni	*Fasciolopsis buski*	*Clonorchis sinensis*	*Paragonimus* spp.*
Schistosoma japonicum and *Schistosoma mekongi*	*Heterophyes heterophyes*	*Opisthorchis* spp.	
*Schistosoma haematobium**	*Metagonimus yokogawai*	*Fasciola hepatica*	
Schistosoma intercalatum	*Echinostoma* spp.	*Fasciola gigantica*	
	Gastrodiscoides spp.	*Dicrocoelium dendriticum*	

* Adult parasites usually occur outside the gut; however, ova may be seen in the stool.

Fecal Mucus and Blood. The passage of mucus and blood in the stool, with or without diarrhea, is a frequent complaint of patients with schistosomiasis, particularly *Schistosoma mansoni* infection. This is more likely to occur in patients with heavy infections and intestinal polyposis and is caused by the passage of ova through the gut wall. Similarly, patients with intestinal amebiasis, hookworm, heavy whipworm (*Trichuris trichiura*) and pseudohookworm (*Trichostrongylus* spp.) infections can pass blood and mucus from the rectum.

Dysentery. Classical dysentery with bloody diarrhea occurs in infections with the two protozoa which have the potential to invade the large bowel mucosa causing ulcerations, *E. histolytica,* and *Balantidium coli.*

Malabsorption. Some parasites which infect the small intestine, i.e., *G. lamblia, Isospora belli, Sarcocystis* spp., *Cryptosporidium* spp., *Strongyloides stercoralis,* and *C. philippinensis*, can cause a chronic malabsorption. Giardiasis, the most common of these, is often characterized by epigastric discomfort and distention, flatulence, intermittent nausea, lassitude, and foul-smelling, loose or watery stools. Weight loss is usual.

Ascending Cholangitis. The liver flukes live in the biliary passages and may cause biliary obstruction and secondary pyogenic cholangitis, with single or multiple liver abscesses. The patient typically has anorexia, fever, chills, an enlarged tender liver, and eosinophilia and may become jaundiced. Occasionally, an aberrant ascaris can obstruct a biliary duct, causing the same symptoms and signs. Ascarids can also cause pancreatitis when they obstruct the pancreatic duct.

Intestinal Obstruction. When ascarids become "coiled up" in the gut, they can cause intestinal obstruction with nausea, vomiting, abdominal pain, and distention. Sometimes an ascaris or pinworm obstructs the appendix, leading to an acute attack of appendicitis.

Ground Itch. A pruritic, erythematous, papulovesicular rash may occur at the sites of penetration of hookworm and schistosome larvae. In the case of the former, this is usually on the feet, the site of contact with contaminated soil. In the case of schistosomiasis, it is associated with exposure to water containing cercariae of human or nonhuman schistosomes; this is called "swimmer's itch."

Larval Pneumonitis. Some intestinal parasites (i.e., *Ascaris lumbricoides,* hookworm, *S. stercoralis, Schistosoma* spp.) have a larval stage that migrates through the lungs. The resulting brief pneumonitis can produce cough, fever, shortness of breath, eosinophilia, and occasionally asthma.

Anemia. Blood loss from heavy schistosome, hookworm (and even *Trichuris*) infections can lead to excessive depletion of iron and proteins. Patients with iron deficiency anemia complain of malaise, weakness, easy fatiguability, and dyspnea on exertion. They are pale, have a tachycardia at rest, may have abdominal distention and in more severe illness (as described in hookworm disease) have congestive heart failure. Geophagy has been associated with severe hookworm disease.

Anal Pruritus. Persons with pinworm infections (enterobiasis) frequently have perianal itching and pain, particularly at night. Gravid female worms crawl out of the anus to deposit eggs on the perineum. Occasionally the parasite may deposit its eggs in the vulvovaginal area, causing an unpleasant pruritus.

EXPOSURE HISTORY

Travel. Intestinal parasitic infections are far more common in the tropics and less developed subtropical countries than they are in the United States. Furthermore, the majority are transmitted by fecal-oral contamination, usually in food and water. Therefore it is important to always take a travel history from your patient. Those most likely to have intestinal parasitic infections include immigrants, travelers to, and residents and students from, less developed countries.

The extent of potential exposure is also important. A missionary who has lived in a rural mission in Zaire is much more likely to have ascaris and hookworm infections than a tourist who took a package tour of China. Until recently, the association of giardiasis and a tour of Leningrad was very strong. Several of the parasites are very focal in their distribution. For instance, intestinal capillariasis has only been described in northern Luzon in the Philippines and (a very few cases) in Thailand.

Unusual Exposure. To become infected with schistosomiasis, the individual must have been exposed to fresh water containing the specific snail intermittent host from which the infectious cercarial stage of the parasite comes. *Entamoeba polecki* is a natural parasite of monkeys; *Cryptosporidium* of cattle; *B. coli* of pigs. Humans infected with these parasites have almost always had exposure to monkeys, cattle (calves), and pigs, respectively. Tapeworms are transmitted by the ingestion of raw or rare beef (*Taenia saginata*), pork (*Taenia solium*) or fresh-water fish (*Diphyllobothrium latum*). The ingestion of raw fresh-water fish (usually in the orient) also can cause infections with *C. philippinensis* or the liver flukes (i.e., *Clonorchis sinensis* and *Opisthorchis* spp.). Another liver fluke, *Fasciola hepatica,* the sheep liver fluke, is an accidental parasite of man in sheep- and cattle-raising areas of the world that are damp.

Unusual Hosts. Promiscuous male homosexuals are more frequently infected with many agents that have a fecal-oral transmission cycle (e.g., *E. histolytica, G. lamblia*). Common parasitic infections of the small bowel (e.g., giardiasis, strongyloidiasis, isosporiasis, cryptosporidiasis) have been reported with increased frequency in patients with acquired immunodeficiency syndrome (AIDS), hypogammaglobulinemias and other immunodeficiency states. Immunologic control appears to be an important factor in these infections.

STOOL EXAMINATION

Examination of the feces and intestinal contents is the method of diagnosing intestinal parasitic diseases. No technique is uniformly successful for detecting parasites in a single stool examination. Since cysts, and to a lesser extent ova and larvae, tend to be excreted intermittently, three or more serial specimens must be examined before an individual can be considered free of infection. This is particularly the case in strongyloidiasis, giardiasis, and amebiasis.

Visual Inspection of Stool. The presence of blood and mucus suggests that a parasite infection may be present. Adult ascarids, pinworms, and tapeworm proglottids are sometimes visualized in the stool.

Direct Smears. Simple emulsions of feces can be prepared in water, saline, or 1 per cent eosin (stains debris but not protozoa) or iodine (stains parasites and background a similar brown color). The entire area under the cover slip should be examined systematically with low magnification (100 X). (See standard tropical medicine and parasitology texts for details.) The high-dry objective (400 X) is used to study those objects that appear to be parasites. A micronmeter is an essential element of the microscope, since size is important for identification.

Motile trophozoites and helminth larvae can be recognized in fresh saline smears, whereas iodine stain is invaluable for identifying amebic and flagellate cysts, since it stains their nuclei and glycogen masses.

Merthiolate-Iodine-Formalin (MIF) Stain and Fixative. The MIF technique enables staining of protozoa cysts and trophozoites while acting as a preservative of these parasites as well as helminth eggs and larvae. With rapid placement in MIF solution, labile organisms (e.g., *D. fragilis* and flagellates) retain their characteristic morphology.

Polyvinyl Alcohol (PVA) Fixative. This is satisfactory for the detection of protozoal cysts and is particularly good for preserving amebic trophozoites. It is the preferred preservative for later preparation of stained slides.

Concentration Techniques. These methods (e.g., zinc sulfate centrifugal flotation and formalin-ether sedimentation) are used to concentrate helminth larvae and eggs and protozoan cysts. However, they are not satisfactory for detecting trophozoites.

Quantitative Egg Counts. Several methods (e.g., Stoll's dilution method, Beaver's direct smear technique, the Kato thick smear technique) are used for evaluation of infections with hookworms, *Ascaris, Trichuris* and *Schistosoma* parasites in which the pathophysiology is related to the intensity of infection.

Staining of Protozoa in Fecal Smears. Among the methods used to stain protozoa are Heidenhain's iron-hematoxylin, phosphotungstic acid-hematoxylin, and trichrome. These stains make it easier to visualize the protozoa and their morphology.

Interpretation of Fecal Smears. It requires some experience to properly identify intestinal parasites in fecal smears. Knowing the size and shape is helpful in identifying protozoa in direct saline smears (Fig. 1). Nematode eggs have a characteristic shape and size (Fig. 2). The larvae of *S. stercoralis* and hookworm may be difficult to differentiate. Trematode eggs range from very small to large (Fig. 3). It is difficult to differentiate ova of *Opisthorchis* spp. from *Clonorchis sinensis* (now considered to be an *Opisthorchis*) and either from ova of *Heterophyes heterophyes* or *Metagonimus yokogawai.* Human cestode infections can be identified by characteristic differences in the mature proglottids or by their ova (Fig. 4). The ova of *T. saginata* and *T. solium* are indistinguishable.

SCOTCH TAPE TEST

The ova of *E. vermicularis* are infrequently seen in the stool. Instead, diagnosis is made by observing the adult worms or finding eggs about the anus. For this purpose the tape slide technique is useful. Transparent adhesive tape is placed over the end of a tongue depressor with the sticky side out. The gummed surface is pressed against several areas of the perianal region, and the tape is then attached to a microscopic slide, sticky side down. The test should be taken in the morning before the patient bathes or defecates. It may be done at home by a parent and should be carried out on two or three mornings, after which the slides are brought to the physician or laboratory for examination. The diagnosis is made by observation of typical embryonated eggs that are flattened on one side.

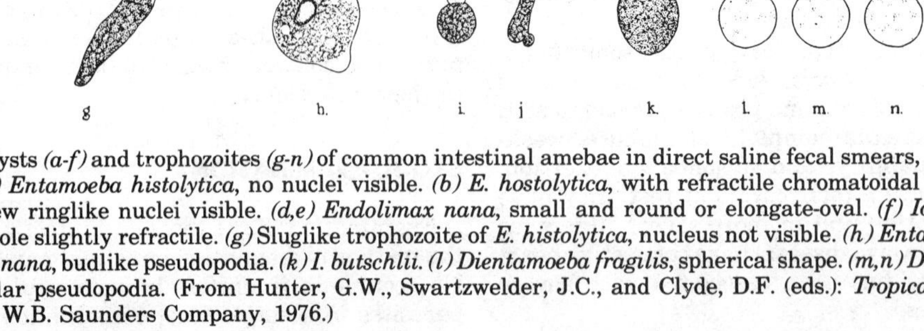

Figure 1. Cysts *(a-f)* and trophozoites *(g-n)* of common intestinal amebae in direct saline fecal smears, fresh, unpreserved, unstained. *(a) Entamoeba histolytica,* no nuclei visible. *(b) E. hostolytica,* with refractile chromatoidal bar. *(c) Entamoeba coli,* with a few ringlike nuclei visible. *(d,e) Endolimax nana,* small and round or elongate-oval. *(f) Iodamoeba butschlii,* glycogen vacuole slightly refractile. *(g)* Sluglike trophozoite of *E. histolytica,* nucleus not visible. *(h) Entamoeba coli,* nucleus visible. *(i,j) E. nana,* budlike pseudopodia. *(k) I. butschlii. (l) Dientamoeba fragilis,* spherical shape. *(m,n) D. fragilis,* triangular and rectangular pseudopodia. (From Hunter, G.W., Swartzwelder, J.C., and Clyde, D.F. (eds.): *Tropical Medicine,* 5th ed. Philadelphia, W.B. Saunders Company, 1976.)

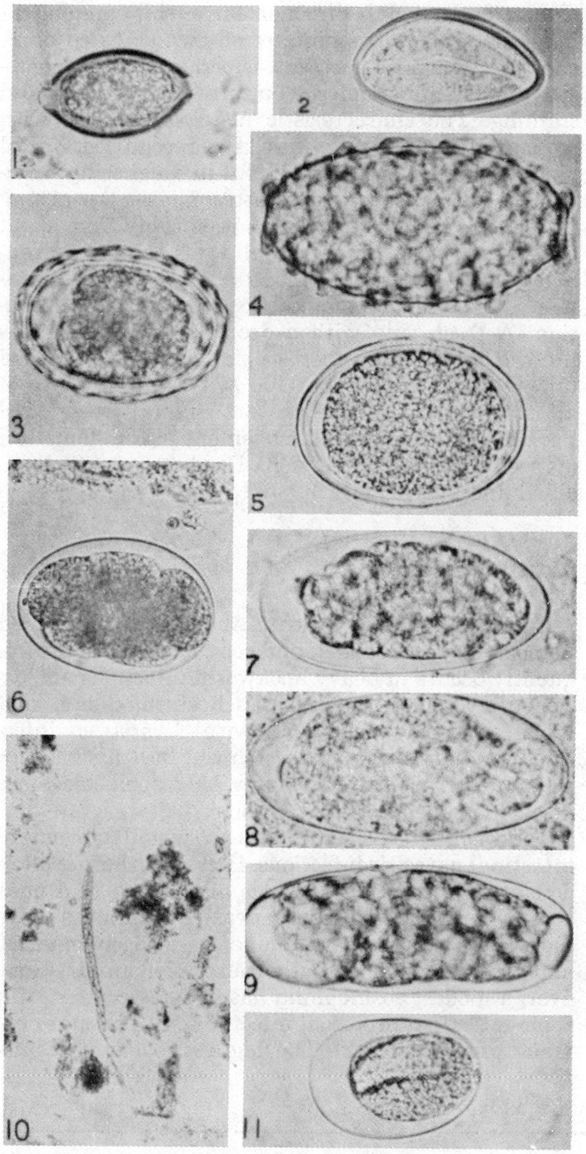

Figure 2. Some common nematode eggs. *(1)* Whipworm, *Trichuris trichiura.* *(2)* Pinworm, *Enterobius vermicularis.* *(3)* Large roundworm, *Ascaris lumbricoides,* fertilized egg. *(4) A. lumbricoides,* unfertilized egg. *(5) Ascaris,* decorticated egg. *(6)* Hookworm egg. *(7)* Immature egg, *Trichostrongylus orientalis.* *(8)* Embryonated egg, *T. orientalis.* *(9)* Egg of *Meloidogne javanica,* a plant nematode sometimes found in stools. *(10)* Rhabditiform larva, *Strongyloides stercoralis,* the stage usually found in the stool. *(11)* Egg of *S. stercoralis,* rarely seen in the stool. All figures 500 X except *(10)* 75 X. (From Hunter, G.W., Swartzwelder, T.C., and Clyde, D.F. (eds.): *Tropical Medicine,* 5th ed. Philadelphia, W.B. Saunders Company, 1976.)

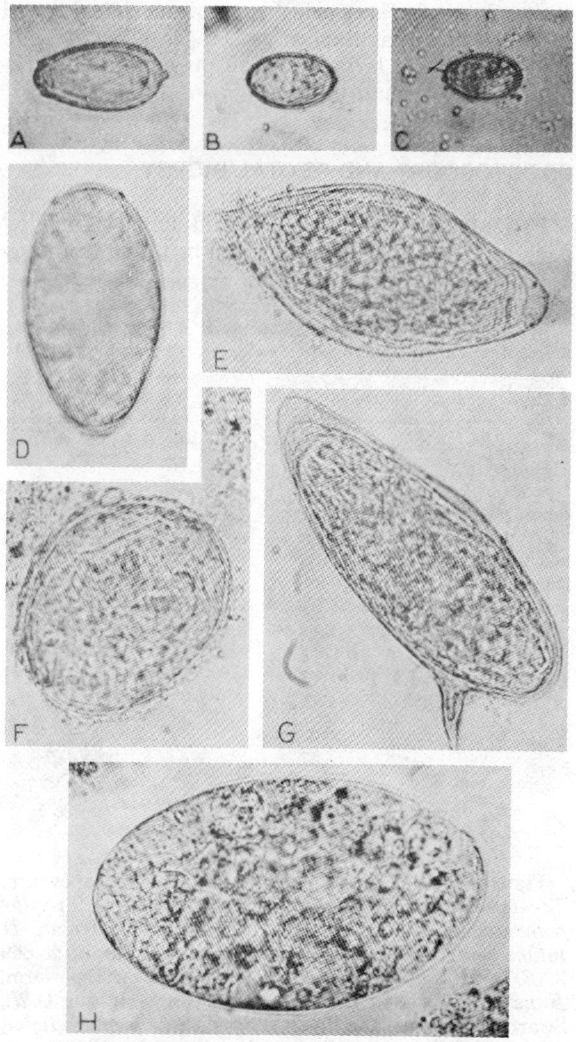

Figure 3. Some trematode eggs. *(A)* Chinese liver fluke, *Clonorchis sinensis.* *(B) Heterophyes heterophyes.* *(C) Metagonimus yokogawai.* *(D)* Lung fluke, *Paragonimus westermani.* *(E)* Vesical blood fluke, *Schistosoma haematobium.* *(F)* Oriental blood fluke, *S. japonicum.* *(G)* Manson's blood fluke, *S. mansoni.* *(H)* Large intestinal fluke, *Fasciolopsis buski.* All figures 500 X except *A,* which is 830 X. (From Hunter, G.W., Swartzwelder, T.C., and Clyde, D.F. (eds.): *Tropical Medicine,* 5th ed. Philadelphia, W.B. Saunders Company, 1976.)

EXAMINATION OF SMALL INTESTINAL FLUID

In the case of some parasites that normally live in the small intestine or biliary ducts (i.e., *G. lamblia, I. belli, Sarcocystis* spp., *Cryptosporidium* spp., *S. stercoralis, C. philippinensis, C. sinensis, Opisthorchis* spp., *Fasciola hepatica*), the ova or larvae may be more easily found in duodenal juice than in the stool. This can be easily performed by intubation and aspiration or by using the simple string capsule method (Entero-Test, Hedeco, Mountain View, Cal.). A direct smear is observed microscopically for parasites and ova. Protozal trophozoites, particularly *G. lamblia,* have been observed attached to the mucosa and in the crypts of small bowel biopsy specimens. An impression smear of the biopsy should be made on a microscopic slide, stained with Giemsa, and examined for trophozoites. The mucus clinging to the biopsy tube may also show parasite larvae as well as trophozoites on direct examination.

The biopsy sample itself may show parasites in the tissues or on the surface. This is particularly true in strongyloidiasis, isosporiasis, cryptosporidiasis, and capillariasis. In capillariasis, all stages of the parasite (i.e., adults, egg, larvae) can be present in the submucosa of the small intestine.

PROCTOSCOPY AND RECTAL BIOPSY

Patients with dysentery should have sigmoidoscopy, at which time scrapings can be taken from any ulcerations noted. A direct smear of this sample will likely detect any trophozoites of *E. histolytica* or *B. coli* which might be present. Ulcerations can be biopsied and examined microscopically after fixation and staining. The characteristic histologic lesions with trophozoites at the margins can be recognized. Rectal biopsy is also sometimes helpful in diagnosing schistosomiasis mansoni and schistosomiasis japonicum. Three or four snips are taken, preferably from small erythematous patches with yellowish centers (or randomly if no lesions are visualized). Part of the specimen is fixed and later undergoes histologic examination. A fresh snip with a drop or two of saline is pressed between two microscopic slides and examined under low magnification (100 X) for the presence of schistosome ova. Viable ova are generally clear and have a slight undulating movement in the flame cell (as seen under oil immersion). Dead ova are often calcified and appear dark.

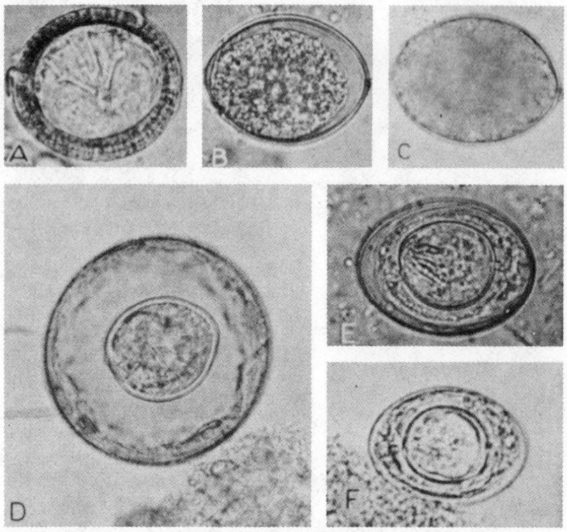

Figure 4. Some cestode eggs. *(A)* Human tapeworm, *Taenia* sp., 750 X. *(B)* Broad tapeworm of man, *Diphyllobothrium latum,* 500 X. *(C)* Broad tapeworm of man, *D. latum,* 500 X. *(D)* Rat tapeworm, *Hymenolepis diminuta,* 650 X. *(E)* Dwarf tapeworm, *H. nana,* 750 X. *(F)* Dwarf tapeworm, *H. nana,* 750 X. Note polar filaments. (From Hunter, G.W., Swartzwelder, T.C., and Clyde, D.F. (eds.): *Tropical Medicine,* 5th ed. Philadelphia, W.B. Saunders Company, 1976.)

BLOOD TESTS

Complete Blood Count. Anemia with reduced hemoglobin, hematocrit, and red blood cell count frequently occurs in heavy hookworm infections and occasionally in trichuriasis, trichostrongyliasis, and schistosomiasis (particularly with *S. mansoni* infections). *D. latum* competes with the host for vitamin B_{12} and in rare instances may be responsible for a pernicious anemia–like syndrome.

Total white blood cell counts are usually normal in intestinal parasitic infections. However, there is often a relative and absolute eosinophila (Table 2). A good rule of thumb is that tissue-invasive helminths cause more eosinophilia than luminal-dwelling helminths, and protozoa do not usually cause eosinophilia. However, a modest eosinophilia has been associated with some intestinal protozoal infections with no other obvious cause (Table 2). The highest levels of eosino-

Table 2. Eosinophilia and Intestinal Parasitic Infections

None or Minimal (<5%)	Inconsistent and Modest (5–10%)	Consistent and Considerable (> 10%)
Protozoa		
Entamoeba histolytica	*Entamoeba polecki*	
Giardia lamblia	*Dientamoeba fragilis*	
Balantidium coli	*Isospora belli*	
Nonpathogens		
Nematodes		
Enterobius vermicularis	*Ascaris lumbricoides*	*Strongyloides stercoralis*
	Hookworm	Tissue migrating larvae (pulmonary symptoms)
	Trichuris trichiura	*Trichostrongylus* spp.
	Capillaria philippinensis	
Trematodes		
	Schistosoma spp.	Hepatic flukes
	Intestinal flukes	Tissue migrating schistosomules and intestinal flukes
Cestodes		
Taenia spp.		
Diphyllobothrium latum		
Hymenolepis spp.		

philia occur when larvae are migrating through the lungs; this is often associated with pulmonary symptoms.

Blood Chemistries. Rarely are other blood tests useful for diagnostic purposes. The liver function test most likely to be abnormal in patients with schistosomiasis mansoni or japonicum or liver fluke infection is the alkaline phosphatase.

Serology. Serum gammaglobulin levels (primarily IgG) are elevated in patients with trematode (best data are available regarding Manson's schistosomiasis) infections and IgE elevations have been documented with most invasive helminth infections.

Diagnostic serologic tests are available at the U.S. Centers for Disease Control in Atlanta, Georgia, for amebiasis, fascioliasis, giardiasis, schistosomiasis, and strongyloidiasis. Serology for schistosomiasis can be helpful in chronic cases and in very early (before eggs are excreted) or light (eggs difficult to find) infections.

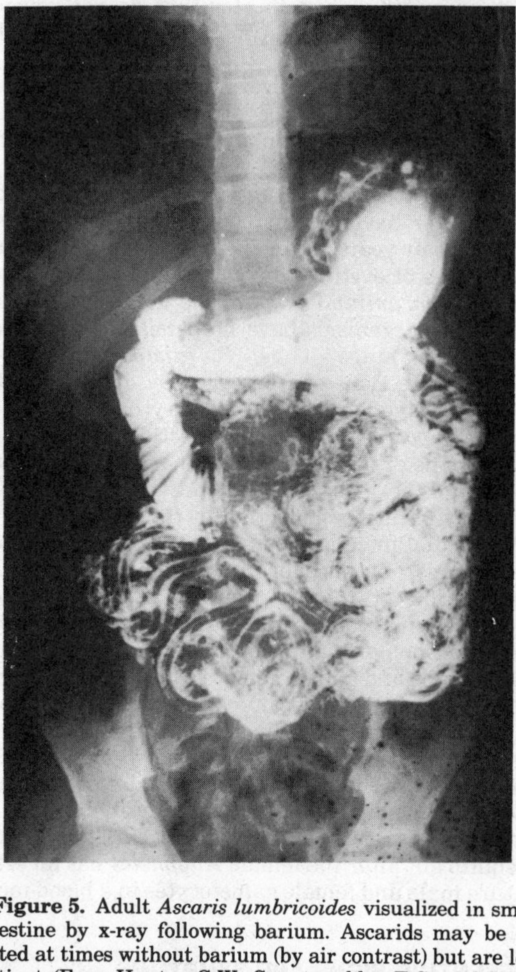

Figure 5. Adult *Ascaris lumbricoides* visualized in small intestine by x-ray following barium. Ascarids may be detected at times without barium (by air contrast) but are less distinct. (From Hunter, G.W., Swartzwelder, T.C., and Clyde, D.F. (eds.): *Tropical Medicine,* 5th ed. Philadelphia, W.B. Saunders Company, 1976.)

The value of serology for the other intestinal parasitic infections (excluding amebiasis) is still questionable.

RADIOLOGIC FINDINGS

Upper Gastrointestinal Series. A small bowel follow-through examination will often show duodenal and jejunal dilation with mucosal edema, pooling of fluid in loops of bowel, and lymphoid nodularity in patients with severe abnormalities due to infections involving the small intestine (i.e., giardiasis, isosporiasis, cryptosporidiosis, strongyloidiasis, capillariasis). Ascaris worms appear on x-ray films as linear tissue densities and a bolus of worms as a tangled thick cord. The worm may be a negative shadow (Fig. 5) in a barium-filled loop of bowel or may ingest the barium itself, revealing a linear opacity about 1 mm wide after the barium column has passed down the gastrointestinal tract. Tapeworms may also be visualized.

Barium Enema. Abnormalities are seldom seen in amebiasis or balantidiasis, with the exception of the rare ameboma, which can be mistaken for carcinoma of the colon. Intestinal polyposis can be occasionally detected in patients with heavy infections with *S. mansoni.* It can be extensive and usually involves the descending colon and rectum.

Hepatobiliary Studies. X-rays of the abdomen can demonstrate hepatosplenomegaly in patients with schistosomiasis and liver fluke infections. Contrast studies of the biliary tract can show radiolucent densities (representing liver flukes and ascarids) in the bile ducts. They also can show abscesses and other abnormalities associated with the biliary obstruction caused by these parasites.

OTHER STUDIES

Newer technologic developments have led to several noninvasive methods that can detect the presence and severity of parasitic infections in the gastrointestinal tract. For instance, liver scans, computed tomographic scans, and sonography can demonstrate and define the extent of abscesses in the liver or the presence of flukes. Sonography can be used to clearly define the extent of Symmers' pipe-stem fibrosis, which is present in many patients with Manson's schistosomiasis.

CONCLUSION

Despite many recent technologic developments in diagnosis, it is still essential to carefully examine the patient's stool to diagnose parasitic infections of the intestinal tract. This procedure is simple and inexpensive and causes no discomfort or danger to the patient.

MALARIA

By Carlos C. Campbell, M.D.
and Robert L. Kaiser, M.D.
Atlanta, Georgia

DEFINITION

Malaria is a disease produced in humans by infection with protozoal parasites of the genus *Plasmodium*. The parasite has a complex life cycle involving a sexual reproductive cycle in female *Anopheles* mosquitoes and asexual replication in human hepatocytes and erythrocytes. Human disease results from erythrocyte infection with one of four species of *Plasmodium: P. falciparum, P. vivax, P. ovale,* and *P. malariae.* Depending upon the infecting species and the prior malaria experience, the human disease spectrum can range from mildly symptomatic to catastrophic and rapidly fatal.

SYNONYMS

The symptoms of malaria were first recognized and described by the ancient Greeks, and during the ensuing millennia, many descriptive terms for the disease were coined. Since the discovery of the causative protozoan in the 19th century, these synonyms for malaria are no longer of other than historic interest. Among the four human malaria species, descriptive terms have evolved for particular fever periodicity because of biologic variations in the duration of the asexual maturation in the erythrocyte, and these terms are still in general use. *Plasmodium vivax* cycles approximately every 46 hours and is termed "benign tertian" (in that the fever recurs every third day). The erythrocytic cycle of *P. falciparum* requires approximately 48 hours to complete and the illness may be severe; hence, it has been referred to as "malignant tertian" malaria. The erythrocytic cycle of *P. malariae* requires approximately 72 hours, a pattern referred to as "quartan" malaria. These descriptive terms, while having a biologic basis, generally have limited diagnostic use; this is because such synchrony of the fever pattern with any of the human malarias may never be present or may dissipate as the infection progresses past the initial waves of erythrocyte invasion, particularly with *P. falciparum* and *P. vivax.*

PARASITE LIFE CYCLE

To understand the bases for the recommendations for malaria diagnoses, it is essential to understand the life cycle of the malaria parasite. Malaria in humans is normally transmitted by the bite of a female *Anopheles* mosquito that is infected with *P. falciparum, P. malariae, P. ovale,* or *P. vivax.* As the mosquito feeds from the human bloodstream, it releases malaria sporozoites, which rapidly enter liver cells (exoerythrocytic stage). After the parasite matures, the liver cell ruptures and releases thousands of merozoites. These invade red blood cells (RBCs), starting the erythrocytic stage of an infection. Within the RBCs the parasites mature, become schizonts, and divide again into merozoites. Finally, the infected RBCs rupture and merozoites repeat the cycle by invading other RBCs. The release of merozoites from erythrocytes initiates the chills and fever of a typical malaria paroxysm. The time required for maturation of the primary exoerythrocytic parasites and initial invasion of the RBCs (the prepatent period) is 7 to 11 days for *P. falciparum, P. vivax,* and *P. ovale;* for *P. malariae* the prepatent period is considerably longer (16 to 28 days).

Sporozoite infections with *P. falciparum* and *P. malariae* mature synchronously in the hepatocyte, and following rupture of the primary tissue schizonts, no parasites remain in the liver parenchyma. In primary infections with *P. vivax* and *P. ovale,* only a proportion of the intrahepatocytic parasites undergo immediate development, leading to infection of RBCs. Those parasites in hepatocytes that do not develop immediately are termed *hypnozoites.* Subsets of the parasite develop following intervals of dormancy of several months or even several years (relapses). Each wave of tissue schizont development can initiate a new cycle of RBC infection and a clinical malaria attack.

Relapses occur when *P. vivax* or *P. ovale* parasites mature after having remained dormant in the liver for months or years, enter the blood, and initiate another series of erythrocytic cycles. Infections caused by *P. falciparum* and *P. malariae* do not relapse because these organisms have no persistent liver (exoerythrocytic) stage. Thus, *P. falciparum* and *P. malariae* infections can be cured by drugs that are active only against the parasite's erythrocytic stages. With *P. vivax* and *P. ovale* infections, therapy directed at the erythrocytic stages may eliminate parasites from the blood but will not prevent relapses caused by parasites persisting in the liver.

Plasmodial infections can be transmitted from person to person by transfer of infected RBCs. Natural transmission of the infection by *Anopheles* mosquitoes requires that sexual parasitic stages (gametocytes) develop during the course of the RBC infection. Mature male and female gametocytes of *P. falciparum* initially appear in the peripheral circulation approximately 7 to 10 days following the onset of parasitemia. For the other three human malaria species, gametocytes appear in the first week of parasitemia. Gametocytes do not replicate in the human host, and they do not produce disease. Fertilization occurs only in the mosquito gut after the female *Anopheles* has ingested mature male and female gametocytes in a blood meal.

PRESENTING SIGNS AND SYMPTOMS

The incubation period (interval from inoculation to onset of malarial symptoms) varies in the nonimmune individual, depending on the species of *Plasmodium.* The exoerythrocytic or hepatic schizogeny produces no tissue reaction or illness. Generally, the incubation period corresponds closely to the prepatent period, since the nonimmune host is extremely sensitive to even very low levels of erythrocyte infection. In *P. falciparum, P. vivax,* and *P. ovale,* the mean incubation period is 10 to 14 days, and rarely longer than 30 days. The incubation period for *P. malariae* may be as long as 30 to 45 days because of its slower exoerythrocytic maturation.

The onset of a malaria attack can resemble an influenzalike illness; fever may persist for several days, accompanied by headache, arthralgias, and malaise. Temperature elevation is the only consistent presenting sign; temperatures in excess of 105°F (41°C) are not uncommon. The classic malaria paroxysm of chills, shivering, high fever, and sweating may not occur. In infants the presenting signs of malaria can be subtle and quite variable and may be characterized by poor appetite, restlessness, and lethargy.

Since the early symptoms and signs of malaria may be quite protean, any patient with a compatible exposure history and febrile illness should be evaluated for the possibility of malaria. Furthermore, with the increasingly widespread prevalence of drug resistance in *P. falciparum,* not even the most credible history of malaria chemoprophylaxis or prior drug therapy should preclude the clinical suspicion of malaria. Failure of prophylaxis, particularly with drugs such as chloroquine and pyrimethamine, is an increasing problem, with the recent development of chloroquine resistance in Africa and its continued spread in Asia and South America. Furthermore, physicians must be aware of the possibility of malaria in patients who have been treated recently for *P. falciparum* and experience a renewal of fever or other symptoms suggestive of malaria.

Persons who have experienced previous malaria infections may have a degree of acquired immunity. That immunity will not prevent subsequent malaria infections, but it may increase host tolerance for low-density infections and limit the maximal parasite density in the blood. Consequently, the incubation period may be prolonged and an appreciable proportion of parasitemias in semi-immune persons may be asymptomatic.

In nonimmune individuals, the course of infections with *P. vivax* and *P. ovale* is marked by periodic paroxysms of fever, initially on a regular basis. After three to four such paroxysms, fever may be continual with daily or every-other-day elevations. The predilection for these species to develop in younger RBCs places a general biologic ceiling on the maximal percentage of RBCs that will be affected. Rarely does the percentage parasitemia (see Laboratory Procedures later in article) exceed 2 per cent of RBCs infected (80,000 per cu mm). Consequently, severe illness, with hemolysis and renal or cerebral compromise, occurs rarely.

Plasmodium malariae infections evolve more slowly because of the 3-day erythrocytic cycle, the relatively small number of daughter merozoites per schizont (average 8 versus 16 for *P. falciparum*), and the propensity for development in more mature RBCs. Peak parasitemias rarely exceed 1 per cent (40,000 per cu mm) RBCs infected. In untreated infections a degree of immunity develops, resulting in a blunting of the paroxysms and in prolonged periods of asymptomatic, low-density parasitemia.

Malignant tertian malaria, caused by *P. falciparum,* can result in fatal illness. These parasites can invade and develop in all circulating erythrocytes, leading to a rapid, exponential increase in parasite density. The risk of complications, including death, is related directly to the percentage of infected RBCs.

PHYSICAL EXAMINATION

The physical examination in the early stages of malaria may be normal, or it may reveal only very nonspecific findings. During the acute paroxysm, a true shaking chill, which is uncontrollable and very dramatic, may be relatively specific for malaria. Similarly, the profuse sweating that occurs at the conclusion of the paroxysm is quite dramatic.

Splenomegaly is a highly variable physical sign. In the acute attack, the spleen tip may be palpated and tender. Generally, greater degrees of splenic enlargement result only following chronic parasitemias in individuals with acquired immunity. Flare-ups of *Herpes labialis,* while not pathognomonic, are a frequent occurrence during an acute malaria attack.

More specific physical examination findings are present, particularly in *P. falciparum* infections, when complications develop.

COMPLICATIONS

Although infections with *P. vivax, P. ovale,* and *P. malariae* are generally not life-threatening, *P. falciparum* infections, if not promptly diagnosed and appropriately treated, can produce severe illness and death. The recognized risk factors that predispose to complications are high parasite density in RBCs, pregnancy, and nonimmune status with respect to prior or recent malarial infections.

In the nonimmune patient, malaria parasite density (percentage RBCs parasitized) increases exponentially during the initial 7 to 10 days of parasitemia. The risk of complications increases appreciably once the percentage parasitemia exceeds 5 to 10 per cent of RBCs infected. Several pathophysiologic processes have been hypothesized to underlie these complications. Infected RBCs attach to capillary endothelial cells as the parasites develop to the schizont stage. This adherence produces "capillary sludging," resulting in vascular occlusion, anoxia, and tissue damage. The RBCs are hemolyzed in the course of the maturation of the malaria parasite, and the degree of hemolysis may exceed that expected on the basis of the parasite density. Researchers have speculated that some degree of RBC destruction is immune-mediated, resulting in complement-mediated hemolysis. As a result, the oxygen-carrying capacity is greatly diminished, and excess free hemoglobin is released, which may compromise renal function.

The most catastrophic complication of *P. falciparum* results from central nervous system impairment. Clinically, cerebral malaria may present as disorientation, stupor, or frank psychosis, or as coma and decerebrate posturing. Recent studies have suggested that cerebral edema is not the principal process underlying the neurologic complications. Generalized seizures are a frequent component of the presenting illness. Not infrequently, however, focal neurologic signs may be observed in patients with *P. falciparum* and no other detectable neurologic disease.

Red blood cell hemolysis results in massive liberation of hemoglobin, leading to hemoglobinuria. Prior to the current era of synthetic antimalarials, this condition was termed "blackwater fever," a condition associated with intermittent quinine therapy or prophylaxis. Hemoglobinemia and hemoglobinuria result from excess hemolysis because of physical, immune, or drug-mediated RBC lysis. Acute renal failure develops frequently during the course of complicated *P. falciparum* infections. Hemoglobinuria may be associated with renal failure. In addition, impaired glomerular perfusion secondary to dehydration and capillary sludging contribute to azotemia.

Thrombocytopenia commonly occurs during infections with any of the human malarias but is most severe with *P. falciparum*. Hypersplenism leading to sequestration of platelets in the spleen develops during the acute attack and is rapidly reversed during recovery following therapy. Excessive bleeding rarely occurs in this condition, even though platelet counts in the range of 20,000 to 50,000 per cu mm occur. Less frequently, thrombocytopenia develops, accompanied by prolongation of the prothrombin time and fibrinolysis, the triad of disseminated intravascular coagulopathy.

During the acute attack, or not infrequently during the recovery phase of a severe *P. falciparum* parasitemia, severe pulmonary failure may develop. The onset may be precipitous, and hypoxemia requiring ventilator support may occur. The syndrome is distinct from pulmonary edema in that congestive heart failure does not occur, the condition is not highly responsive to diuresis, and the chest radiograph demonstrates diffuse alveolar changes. Many researchers have commented on the similarity of this condition to "shock lung" syndrome.

Plasmodium malariae infections that persist chronically, generally with a low, asymptomatic parasitemia, may produce the nephrotic syndrome. Immune complexes are deposited in the basement membrane of the glomeruli, as detected by immunofluorescence. This nephrotic syndrome occurs most typically in children in areas of Africa where *P. malariae* is endemic.

LABORATORY PROCEDURES

Confirmation of infection by *Plasmodium* depends on finding the parasites in the peripheral blood smear. Furthermore, an accurate species determination and quantification of parasite density in the blood depends upon meticulous examination of the smear and is the basis for appropriate therapy and an initial estimate of the risk of complications, including death. When the possibility of a malarial infection exists, prompt and accurate blood film examination is mandatory. Blood smears should be obtained when the diagnosis is considered and should be repeated every 6 to 12 hours until the diagnosis is confirmed or excluded. Collection of blood smears at the time of acute symptoms does not necessarily enhance the sensitivity of the examination. In fact, during the fever-chill paroxysm the majority of parasites tend to be young trophozoites, the stage at which species differentiation is most difficult.

As noted previously, nonimmune individuals may develop malaria at even subpatent parasite densities. Consequently, the examination of thick blood smears is mandatory in order to enhance the sensitivity of the procedure. Thin blood smears should be collected at the same time so that detailed RBC and parasite morphology can be assessed.

Blood smears should be made on glass slides that are free of grease and particulate matter, both of which can confound diagnosis, particularly on thick blood smear. Both the thick and thin blood smears should be obtained from free-flowing blood from a finger stick. Blood smears prepared from anticoagulated blood may fail to stain properly and may show distortions of both RBC and parasite morphology. To prepare the thick smear, apply three 1- to 2-mm drops of blood to the slide in a triangle approximately 1 cm apart. Using the corner of a second clean slide, gently swirl the three drops into a confluent circle 1 to 2 cm in diameter. The blood thickness should be sufficient to just obscure newsprint through the glass. Thick smears should be allowed to dry thoroughly at ambient temperature and protected from dust and insects. Thin blood smears are obtained in the standard manner as for complete blood count and white blood cell (WBC) differential counts.

The thick blood smear should be stained without fixation because preservation of RBC morphology is not desired and dehemoglobinization must occur to permit accurate examination for *Plasmodium* parasites. The thin blood smear is fixed by quick dipping in absolute methanol and air dryed.

Giemsa polychromatic stain is preferred for malaria blood smears. Commercially available Giemsa stain should be strained through filter paper immediately before use to remove precipitated stain, which can result in basophilic particles on smears. For optimal staining, Giemsa reagent should be prepared at 2 per cent concentration at a pH 7.0 to 7.2. To ensure optimal stain results, slides should be stained for 30 to 45 minutes.

A systematic approach to the examination of blood smears will produce the optimal sensitivity and specificity in diagnosis. To determine whether *Plasmodium* parasites are present, the thick blood smear is examined. Considerable experience is required to accurately examine thick blood smears, principally because of the potential presence of confusing, nonparasite objects, including platelets, RBC debris, and stain artifacts. Plasmodial parasites will consist of eosin-staining chromatin and basophilic cytoplasm. Plasmodial pigment will be present in older rings, yet may not be observed in *P. falciparum* infections, in which generally only young trophozoites circulate in peripheral blood.

As a general rule, a minimum of 200 high-powered (500 to 1000X oil immersion magnification) fields are examined before declaring a thick blood film negative for parasites. If only thin blood films are available, 5 to 10 times as many fields must be examined to produce a comparable degree of sensitivity.

In the thick film, the density of parasites can provide a clue to determining the species. Infections with *P. vivax, P. ovale,* and *P. malariae* rarely exceed a parasite density of 1 per cent of RBCs infected, which translates to approximately six to eight asexual parasites per each WBC in the thick smear. Parasitemias in excess of 3 to 5 per cent RBCs infected (25 asexual parasites per WBC) will generally indicate a *P. falciparum* infection. Similarly, if many trophozoites or schizonts are detected in the thick film, it is unlikely that the infecting species is *P. falciparum,* since development of blood stages of *P. falciparum* occurs in the deep vascular circulation.

Precise identification of *Plasmodium* species generally requires examining the thin blood film, where the morphology of infected RBCs and the parasites can be assessed. Many of the distinguishing morphologic characteristics (Table 1) are found to a varying degree in all four species (e.g., RBC distortions in shape or size occur more typically in *P. vivax* or *P. ovale,* but not exclusively). In addition, some are dependent on the quality of staining (e.g., Schüffner's eosinophilic stippling in RBCs infected with *P. vivax* and *P. ovale* may not be present with suboptimal Giemsa staining).

Calculation of parasite density in the blood is important, in that with *P. falciparum* infections the density roughly predicts the likelihood of complications. In addition, serial determination of parasite density permits an assessment of the rapidity and efficacy of the therapeutic response following drug administration. Counting the number of RBCs that contain an asexual parasite(s) in a standard number of RBCs (e.g., 100 for high densities or 1000 in lower-density infections) provides a rapid and reliable quantification of the density of infection. Gametocytes are not included in the count, since they neither replicate nor produce disease in humans.

With *P. falciparum* infections, blood smears should be obtained routinely for 2 to 3 days following therapy or until asexual parasites are no longer detected. Asexual parasites may be found in the blood for 36 to 72 hours following initiation of therapy. If asexual parasites persist until day 7, investigations are indicated to determine whether therapy was actually taken or whether parasite drug resistance is present. Gametocytes of *P. falciparum* can persist for many days following adequate therapy for asexual parasites, and the presence of gametocytes does not imply therapeutic failure.

SEROLOGY

Several serologic test methodologies have been developed for malaria, but only the indirect fluorescent antibody (IFA) is currently available for all human species. The malaria IFA test is available in a very limited number of laboratories, however, because blood-stage parasites are required for each *Plasmodium* species and specialized skills are necessary for test interpretation.

A primary serologic response to *Plasmodium* parasitemia is detectable between days 7 to 10 following patency. The malaria IFA response attains a peak titer at 3 to 4 weeks following initial patency. The maximal titer attained depends on the duration and density of parasitemia; when the parasitemia is of very low density or is treated within the initial 3 to 4 days following patency, the IFA response may be quite low and of short duration. More typically, the IFA serologic response persists for 18 to 24 months following a more prolonged infection.

Interpretation of the IFA serology depends to a great extent on the antigens used for testing. In some laboratories, nonhuman primate malarias are employed because of their ready availability. Titers with these antigens are lower than with the homologous (infecting) species, and obviously no conclusion about the infecting species is possible. Results of IFA serology, when the four human species are available for testing, generally demonstrate a degree of cross reaction among species, yet the species with the highest titer is generally the infecting species.

Malaria IFA serology is neither sufficiently sensitive nor specific to serve as the primary or sole diagnostic test. Serology is of greatest assistance in determining whether a purportedly nonimmune individual has had parasitemia when the individual has had a classic malarial illness and a conclusive blood slide examination has not been possible. Epidemiologically, IFA serology has proved to be a valuable screening test to identify blood donors who have been responsible for transfusion malaria.

Table 1. Distinguishing Morphologic Characteristics of Human *Plasmodium* Species in the Thin Blood Smear

Characteristic	*P. falciparum*	*P. vivax*	*P. ovale*	*P. malariae*
Enlargement of infected erythrocytes	No	Yes	Yes	No
Fimbriated or oval shape of infected erythrocytes	Rare	Rare	Frequent	Rare
Avg. maximum parasite density (% RBCs infected)	No limit	1%	0.5%	0.5%
Schüffner's dots in infected erythrocytes	No	Yes	Yes	No
Number of hours in erythrocytic cycle	48	46	50	72
Multiple infections in erythrocytes	Frequent	Rare	Very rare	Very rare
All stages of parasites in peripheral blood	Rare	Yes	Yes	Yes
Double chromatin dots on parasites	Frequent	Rare	No	No
Sausage-shaped gametocytes	Yes	No	No	No
Number of merozoites per mature schizont	8–20	12–24	6–12	6–12

BLOOD CHEMISTRIES AND COMPLETE BLOOD COUNT

Except for the blood smear examination, no single test or group of routine laboratory results will confirm the diagnosis of malaria. There are, however, several general abnormal test results observed during a malaria attack. Depending on the duration and density of the parasitemia, some degree of anemia will result due to hemolysis. Free hemoglobin in the plasma causes the packed RBC volume (hematocrit) to be lowered generally to a greater extent than the hemoglobin value. The WBC remains normal, or a mild leukopenia is noted. The differential WBC is unchanged, except that eosinophils may be absent during the acute parasitemia. Thrombocytopenia, with platelet counts as low as 20,000 to 50,000 per cu mm, are frequently noted in *P. falciparum* and *P. vivax* infections; this depression of the platelet count may occur with normal fibrinogen levels or the absence of evidence for disseminated intravascular coagulopathy.

Tests for liver function may be mildly abnormal, particularly in complicated *P. falciparum* infections. Elevations in lactate dehydrogenase (LD) levels generally result from RBC hemolysis. To the extent that renal failure occurs in *P. falciparum* infections, resulting either from diminished intravascular volume and renal perfusion or from direct damage to glomeruli, the blood urea nitrogen and creatinine will be elevated.

TOXOPLASMOSIS

By Georges Desmonts, M.D.
and Jacques Couvreur, M.D.
Paris, France

THE ORGANISM

Toxoplasma gondii is a coccidian, the life cycle of which involves the cat and its prey animals. Schizogony and gametogony take place in the small intestine of the cat and end in formation of *oocysts,* which are shed in the feces and which survive and remain potentially infectious for months or even years in soil. This is a source of infection for rodents, birds, and domestic animals. In their tissues, toxoplasma are able to multiply intracellularly; this form of the organism is termed *endozoite* or *tachyzoite.* The organisms then encyst in tissue cells. *Cysts* persist as viable parasites throughout the life of their host, mainly in brain, heart, and skeletal muscle. Cats that hunt or that are fed raw meat become infected, and the cycle is renewed.

Humans are a "dead end" in the life cycle. Infection in humans is frequent because of the numerous sources of the parasite and because of our susceptibility to the different forms of *T. gondii* (Fig. 1). After local invasion, usually via the gut, the organisms spread throughout the body, reaching every organ via lymphatics and the bloodstream, and multiply intracellularly.

Termination of this acute initial stage of infection depends on the development of both cell-mediated and humoral immunity. As a consequence, toxoplasma infection reaches a latent or chronic stage at which encysted parasites persist in the host tissues. The tissue cysts provoke little or no inflammatory response as long as the cyst wall is not disrupted.

Clinical disease, when present, may be observed in the early acute stage of infection or in the chronic stage as well. This is summarized in Table 1.

The prevalence of toxoplasma antibodies among most human populations is high; in most areas of the world, a significant proportion and even the majority of the population have been infected by the parasite. However, it is important to recognize that while toxoplasma infection is widespread, disease due to this infection is relatively uncommon.

LABORATORY DIAGNOSIS

The laboratory methods used for the diagnosis of toxoplasma infection and of the various stages of the infection will be described before we show how the parasitologic and serologic data may be interpreted by the obstetrician, the internist, the pediatrician and the ophthalmologist.

Parasitologic Diagnosis. The organisms present in tissue cells are not easily accessible for examination except at autopsy. When toxoplasmosis is clinically suspected, it is sometimes possible to identify the parasite by inoculation of appropriate tissue specimens or body fluids into laboratory mice. This is shown in Table 2.

The results of the parasitologic examination should be considered in relationship to the clinical manifestations and/or the pathologic findings.

In this connection, one should remember that the presence of organisms is proof of toxoplasma infection, but not necessarily of disease. For example, isolation of toxoplasma from blood or cerebrospinal fluid indicates the presence of endozoites and, therefore, of active and probably acute infection. In contrast, isolation of toxoplasma from muscles after enzymatic digestion is possible in a patient who had a subclinical infection years earlier and whose death was related not to toxoplasma but to another disease. Even cysts in sections of brain or heart have sometimes been an incidental finding.

Serologic Diagnosis. Immunologic methods are the main tools for the diagnosis of toxoplasma infection. The major methods in use are for demonstration of antibodies in serum and body fluids; the intradermal test is not routinely used at the present time.

The principle of the most common serologic tests, the antibody classes involved, and the significance of the different reactions are shown in Table 3. These tests can be considered as falling into two groups:

1. In the first group, the whole unbroken organisms are used as an antigen. Thus, these methods mainly demonstrate antibodies specific for the antigens of the

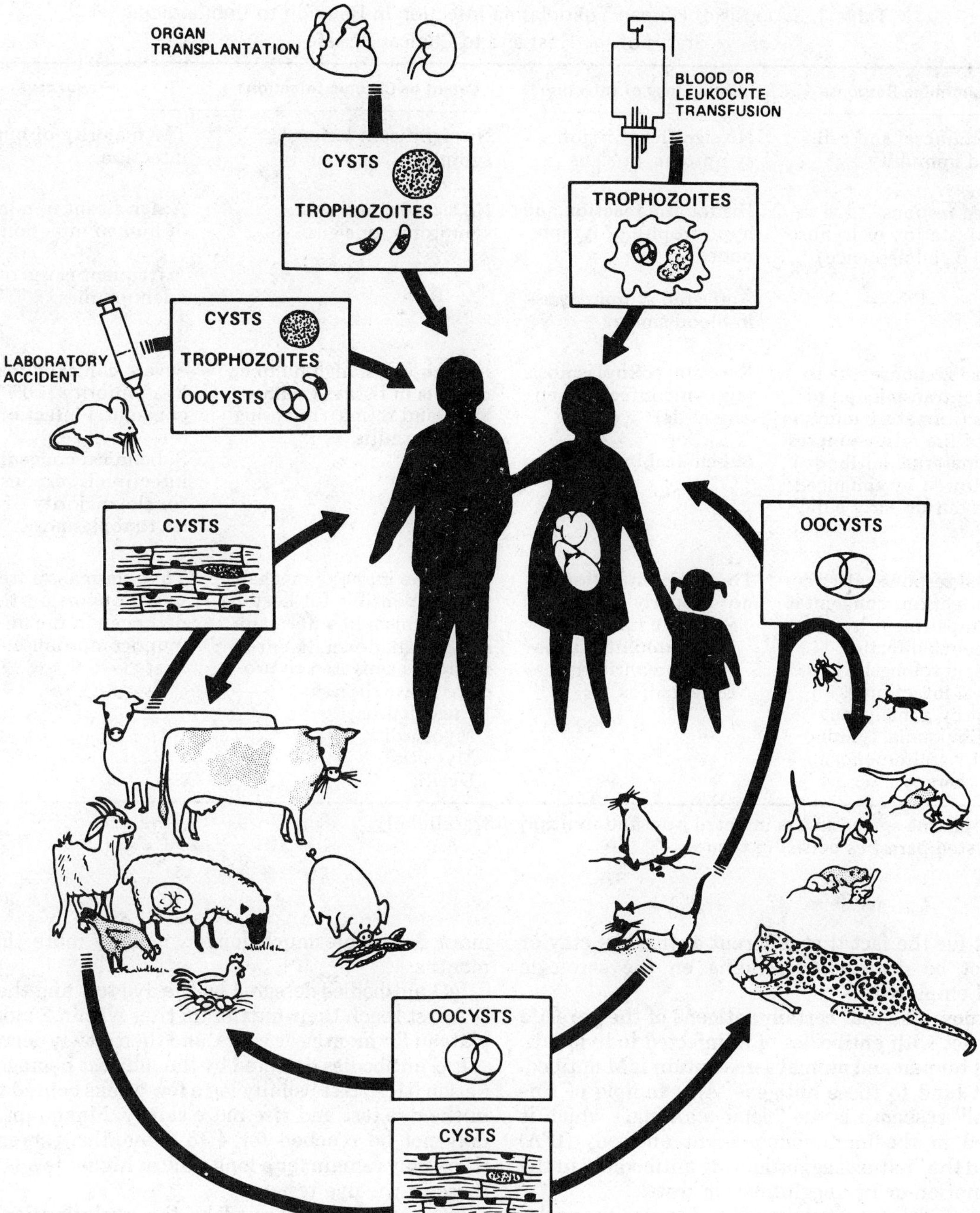

Figure 1. Life cycle of *Toxoplasma gondii.* (From Remington, J.S., and McLeod, R.: Toxoplasmosis. In Braude, A.I. (ed.): *International Textbook of Medicine,* Vol. II, *Medical Microbiology and Infectious Disease.* Philadelphia, W.B. Saunders Company, 1981.)

parasite membrane. These methods are the most widely used and are presently the only ones for which significance is well established.

2. The second group uses an antigenic extract from lysed parasites (a mixture of many different antigens that originate from the cytoplasm and cell membrane). As a consequence, the results of these tests—complement fixation, hemagglutination, latex agglutination, and enzyme-linked immunosorbent assay (ELISA) tests as examples—may differ considerably from one laboratory to another, depending on the way the antigen extract is prepared.

Antibody Response in Toxoplasma Infection. The antigenic structure of toxoplasma is complex. Membrane antigens and cytoplasmic antigens, which are liberated when the organisms are lysed, are involved in the immune response.

Antibodies formed in response to these different antigens differ in their specificity and also in their class and subclass of immunoglobulins. These differences

Table 1. Synopsis of Human Toxoplasma Infection in Relation to Immunologic Status of the Host and to Clinical Disease

Host Immune Response	Acute Stage of Infection*	Latent or Chronic Infection†	Frequency
Normal humoral and cell-mediated immunity	No significant lesion, symptoms, or signs	No significant lesion, symptoms, or signs	The majority of human infections
Enhanced response (due to heavy infestation or to host factors, i.e., adolescence)	Histiocytic reaction and hypertrophy of lymph nodes Activated lymphocytes in blood smears	No significant lesion, symptoms, or signs	A significant minority of human infection A frequent cause of adenopathies
Abnormal response due to congenital transmission of parasites (immature immune system of the fetus; suppression by maternal antibody) later followed by enhanced response during early childhood	Neonatal toxoplasmosis (systemic infection, encephalitis) or Subclinical infection	In both cases, high number of cysts in tissues (mainly brain and retina); relapsing chorioretinitis	Severe clinical disease in a minority (10%) of congenital infections Subclinical congenital infection is responsible for the majority of ocular toxoplasmosis
Abnormal response after acquired infection: congenital defect, impairment by a simultaneous infection (measles, cytomegalovirus, other viral infections), impairment by a malignant disease (leukemia, lymphoma), or by an immunosuppressive therapy	The initial infection is not properly contained: Systemic infection (pneumonitis, hepatitis, nephritis); Encephalitis	When the immune mechanisms responsible for keeping the organism in a dormant state break down, latent infection is activated to produce active disease: Encephalitis Myocarditis Myositis Uveitis	Toxoplasma is a frequent opportunistic pathogen in the immunocompromised host

*Toxoplasma spread in the infected host and multiply intracellularly.
†Encysted parasites persist in tissues.

account for the fact that different antibodies may or may not be detected, depending on the serologic method employed.

We know also that certain antigens of the parasite cross react with antibodies of uninfected individuals. Normal human and animal sera contain IgM antibodies that bind to these antigens. An example of this "normal" response is the "polar staining," which is observed in the immunofluorescent antibody (IFA) test, and the "natural agglutinating antibodies" in the agglutination or hemagglutination test.

In Figure 2 we have attempted to describe the evolution of the IgM and IgG response, as observed with the help of the most currently employed serologic tests: the dye test, the IgM and IgG IFA test, and the hemagglutination test.

Specific toxoplasma antibodies appear within a few weeks after acquisition of infection. The IgM IFA antibodies and dye test antibodies appear first. The IgM antibodies, as detected by the IgM IFA test, usually reach maximum titer within 4 weeks and then decrease to become undetectable after 4 months. Individual variation is considerable: the IgM IFA test may turn negative earlier than 4 weeks, or it may remain positive (usually at a low titer) for months or even years in a minority of patients (less than 5 per cent).

When detected by the immunosorbent assay (ISA), or the double-sandwich ELISA, IgM antibodies remain detectable much longer, usually more than 6 months.

IgG antibodies detected by the dye test and the IgG IFA test reach their maximum titer within 2 months, plateau for months or years, and then slowly decrease.

IgG antibodies detected by the indirect hemagglutination (IHA) test usually lag a few weeks behind those in the dye test and rise more slowly. Maximum titer may not be reached for 4 to 6 months; thereafter, titers may remain for a long time at higher levels than those in the dye test.

IgG antibodies detected by the agglutination test (AG) in the presence of 2-mercaptoethanol (2-ME) usually parallel those in the dye test but frequently rise for a longer time and also persist at high levels for months and years following initial infection.

This prolonged persistence of antibodies, for years and probably for the entire life of the host, is related to the persistence of the parasites in the tissues and to the immunogenic stimulus due to this persistence.

The World Health Organization (WHO) has recommended that titers in toxoplasma antibody tests be expressed in international units (IU) per ml of serum. For this purpose, an international standard reference serum has been prepared by pooling sera taken from patients with an established diagnosis of toxoplasmic lymphadenopathy. This reference serum has a high titer of IgG antibody, which has been defined as 1000

Table 2. Parasitologic Diagnosis

Methods	Indication	Specimen Examined	Comments
Isolation procedures (inoculation into mice)	Toxoplasmic lymphadenopathy	Lymph node biopsy (ground node or needle biopsy)	Must be performed in a laboratory that has experience in this field (animals free of spontaneous toxoplasma infection)
	Neonatal toxoplasmosis	Placenta (after enzymatic digestion)	Infection is preferably proved by both parasitologic and serologic evidence in primary inoculated animals
	Active infection in immunocompromised patient	Blood (e.g., cord blood)	A definitive result may take as long as 6 weeks
		Cerebrospinal fluid	
		Muscle or brain biopsy	
	Autopsy	Brain, heart, muscles (after enzymatic digestion)	
Microscopic examination of specimen	Active infection in immunocompromised patient	Infrequent findings: Lymph nodes, Bone marrow, Cerebrospinal fluid, Brain biopsy, Muscle biopsy	*Endozoites* very difficult to see and identify; crescentic in shape on dry films, nearly spherical in sections; a definite identification based on morphology alone is not possible (immunofluorescence or peroxidase technique is helpful)
	Autopsy	Brain: Smears from tissues taken at periphery of necrotic lesions; In sections, examine normal tissue in vicinity of lesions, for presence of cysts	*Cysts* more easily recognizable; spherical in brain, conforming to the shape of muscle fibers, in heart and skeletal muscles. Microscopic findings should, if possible, be confirmed by isolation of organism

IU per ml. Because the dilution titer (i.e., the reciprocal of the last positive dilution of this serum) by the different techniques used in different laboratories may vary from less than 1:1000 to more than 1:20000, the usefulness of reporting positive results in IU by comparison with this standard serum is obvious.

Serologic Diagnosis of the Presence and Stage of Infection. Except for passively transferred antibodies, the presence of a positive titer in the tests for IgG antibodies establishes the diagnosis of toxoplasma infection. Since titers may remain elevated for years, a single titer, even if very high, does not define whether the infection is acute or chronic.

Tests for IgM antibodies are of considerable help: Absence of IgM most often excludes the diagnosis of acute infection at that time and in the recent past; their presence *suggests* but *does not prove* a recent infection.

To diagnose acute toxoplasmosis, it is necessary to demonstrate a rising titer in serial specimens. This is discussed in Table 4.

Comparison of Serologic Test Results Obtained in Body Fluids with Different Concentrations of Ig. The serologic titer observed in a fluid depends on the number of toxoplasma specific molecules of Ig present in the fluid. Two factors must be considered in this regard:

1. The amount of Ig present in the fluid (e.g., which may be measured by immunodiffusion).

2. The proportion of specific antitoxoplasma antibody molecules among the total pool of Ig molecules. This proportion has been termed "the immune load of IgG," which may be estimated by computing the ratio of antibody units per milligram of IgG. This computation is necessary when considering the significance of a titer in sera with a low immunoglobulin level (infants) or a high level (hypergammaglobulinemic patients) or when one desires to compare titers in body fluids with different levels of immunoglobulins (serum, cerebrospinal fluid, aqueous humor).

A high-immune load (e.g., 100 to 1000 IU of toxoplasma antibodies per milligram of IgG) means that among the cells actually involved in synthesis of the Ig present in the fluid being examined, a high proportion has been stimulated by toxoplasma antigen. A low-immune load (e.g., 1 to 30 IU per mg of IgG) means that this proportion is low.

DIAGNOSTIC PROBLEMS IN GYNECOLOGY AND OBSTETRICS

Acute infection, even subclinical, occurring in a pregnant woman is often transmitted to the offspring and may be responsible for fetal damage.

Chronic infection has repeatedly been suggested as a possible cause of sporadic abortion. The question is still controversial, and the occurrence of abortion associated with latent toxoplasma infection must be exceedingly uncommon. As a rule, in fact, a latent infection may be considered as evidence of immunity and of protection against the risk of giving birth to a congenitally infected child.

In France and in some other countries, serologic screening of women is routinely performed for the prevention of congenital toxoplasmosis; as a consequence of this screening, the obstetrician is faced with three problems:

1. Interpretation of the results of a serologic test performed in a patient who is not yet but who intends to become pregnant (Table 5).

Table 3. Serologic Tests for Toxoplasma Antibodies

Method	Antigen	Principle of Method	Class of Antibody Detected and Comments
Dye test (DT)	Living parasites	Living parasites are lysed and killed by complement when antibody complexes are present on the cell membrane	Identical with neutralizing antibodies Principally IgG Reference test; unfortunately, requires use of living parasites
Immunofluorescent antibody test (IFA)	Dried smears of fixed parasites	Antibody complexes when present on parasite membrane are stained by anti-Ig–labeled serum	May be used to detect Ig as a whole, or IgG, or IgM, depending on specificity of labeled reagent Total IG test is the "standard IFA test" and probably the most widely used for detection of toxoplasma antibodies. Results are usually in good agreement with DT. Sometimes nonspecific staining impedes differentiation between negative and weakly positive sera Specific IgM test: Some false-positive results due to rheumatoid factor (sera should be tested after absorption of RF). Also false-negative results due to competitive inhibition by IgG antibodies
Agglutination test (AG)	Parasites fixed with formalin	Pattern of sedimentation in microtest wells is different, depending on presence of antibody complexes on membrane (carpet) or absence of antibody (button)	Very sensitive to IgM antibody: decrease in titer following 2 mercaptoethanol (2-ME) treatment of serum is suggestive of presence of IgM antibodies Nonspecific reactions are observed due to binding of "natural" IgM antibody on surface of parasites Specific and very sensitive for IgG antibodies if a 2-ME buffer is used as a diluent in test. In these conditions, titers closely parallel those of DT
Immunosorbent assay (IgM ISA)	Parasites fixed with formalin (Particles coated with toxoplasma antigen)	A sample of patient IgM is bound in wells of microtiter plates, prepared with anti-IgM serum Pattern of sedimentation is different if specific IgM present in sample (carpet) or absent (button)	Specific and sensitive method for detection of IgM antibody: No false-positive results with RF No inhibition by IgG antibodies
Complement fixation test (CFT)	Antigens prepared from lysed parasites	Hemolytic complement is adsorbed on antigen-antibody complex and disappears from fluid	Results differ markedly, depending on antigen extract used (membrane or cytoplasma) Now becoming obsolete
Indirect hemagglutination test (IHA)	–	Red blood cells coated with toxoplasma antigen agglutinate in presence of antibody	Widely used Titers may lag several weeks or more behind those in DT and IFA Certain antigen preparations may reveal a double-peak response; the first related to IgM, the second related to IgG Decrease in titer, when serum is treated with 2-ME, is suggestive of an IgM peak Nonspecific reaction may sometimes occur
Enzyme-linked immunosorbent assay (ELISA)	–	Antigen-antibody complexes adsorbed on plastic are detected by an enzyme labeled anti-Ig serum	Will probably be widely used, but needs a more precise knowledge of the parasite antigens May detect total Ig or IgG Detection of IgM is possibly impeded by inhibition (false-negative) and by rheumatoid factor (false-positive)
Double-sandwich (DS) ELISA Reverse ELISA	–	Capture of a sample of patient IgM (see ISA) Demonstration of specific antibody in sample by enzyme-linked assay	Specific and sensitive for IgM antibody; no inhibition by IgG antibody; no false-positive result in presence of rheumatoid factor

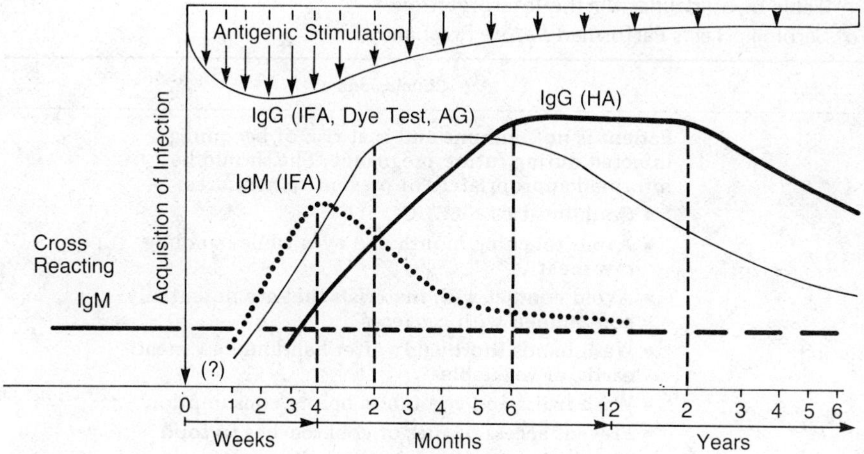

Figure 2. Antibody response to acute toxoplasma infection. IgM antibodies detected by the IgM IFA test are represented by the dotted line; IgG antibodies detected by the IFA, dye test, and direct agglutination test (AG) are shown by the thin solid line; IgG antibodies detected by the hemagglutination test (HA) are shown by the thick solid line. (Modified from the Symposium Bio Merieux, Lyon, France, November 1982.)

Table 4. Practical Guidelines for Serologic Diagnosis of Presence and Stage of Toxoplasma Infection

Tests for IgM Antibodies (*IgM IFA or Preferably ISA or DS ELISA)*	Tests for IgG Antibodies (Paired Samples)*: *Dye Test or IgG IFA Test*	Tests for IgG Antibodies (Paired Samples)*: *Agglutination or Hemagglutination Test (After Treatment of Sera with 2-ME)*	Conclusion (Immunocompetent Host)
(A) Negative	Negative		Uninfected patient First days following acquisition of toxoplasma infection
(B) Positive	Rising titer	Rising titer‡	Acute infection
(C) Positive	High† and stable titer	Rising titer	End of acute stage: infection probably acquired 1 to 6 months before
(D) Positive	High stable titer		Infection acquired months ago (more than 2 months) and probably no longer in acute stage May be locally active (subacute stage)
(E) Negative	High stable titer		Chronic or latent infection, acquired many months or a few years ago Recent infection possible but unlikely
(F) Negative	Low† stable titer		Chronic or latent infection, acquired years ago
(G) Positive	Low stable titer		Chronic infection with persistence of specific IgM (?) Nonspecific IgM reaction (?)
(H) Negative	Rising titers		Relapse during chronic infection (?) Reinfection (?) Acute infection possible but unlikely
(I) Positive	Stable negative		Nonspecific reaction (?) Toxoplasma infection unlikely

* To detect a rise or to assess a stable titer:
Samples of sera should be collected at an interval of 3 weeks apart as a minimum.
Paired sera should be examined in the same laboratory and in the same series of tests.
A specific method for IgG antibodies should be used and not solely a method measuring both IgG and IgM, since a rise in IgG titer might remain unnoticed if occurring together with a decrease in IgM titer.
Tests should be performed with *twofold* dilutions so that a *fourfold* (two tubes) rise can be detected and considered significant.

† A "high" titer is about 1000 IU/ml (range 400 to 12000 IU); a "low" titer is below 300 IU/ml (2 to 200 IU).

‡ The rise in titer may be suppressed if patient has been treated early.

Abbreviations: ISA = Immunosorbent assay; DS ELISA = double-sandwich enzyme-linked immunosorbent assay; IFA = immunofluorescent antibody; ME = mercaptoethanol.

Table 5. Guidelines for the Interpretation of Serologic Tests Performed *Before* Pregnancy

Serologic Results*	Conclusions
Negative (A, I)	Patient is not immune and is at risk of becoming infected during future pregnancy. She should be informed appropriately of preventive measures: • Cook meat to > 66° C • Avoid touching mouth and eyes while handling raw meat • Avoid contact with materials that are potentially contamined with cat feces • Wash hands thoroughly after handling raw meat, earth, or vegetables • Wash fruits and vegetables before consumption • Prevent access of flies or cockroaches to food • Wear gloves when working in the garden • Avoid cat scratches
Chronic infection (D, E, F, G)	Immune patient No risk of congenital toxoplasmosis in future pregnancies
Acute infection (B, C)	No risk or very low risk of congenital toxoplasmosis; nevertheless, pregnancy best postponed for a few months (e.g., 6 months)

*Letters refer to cases described in Table 4.

2. Interpretation of serologic tests in a pregnant woman (Table 6).

3. When an acute infection has been diagnosed in a pregnant woman, estimation of the fetal risk and approach to a prenatal diagnosis of fetal toxoplasmosis (Table 7).

PROBLEMS IN INTERNAL MEDICINE

Toxoplasma infection is very common. Its presence and its stage are relatively easy to determine through the help of appropriate serologic tests (Table 4); but clinical manifestations, when present, may be protean and the problem is to establish the role of toxoplasma in the presenting clinical disease.

The different possible relationships between this infection and the disease are summarized in Table 8; types 2 and 4 will be discussed as current diagnostic problems.

Toxoplasmic Lymphadenopathy

In most cases, in the adolescent and adult, toxoplasmic lymphadenopathy runs an afebrile course with few or no symptoms that suggest an infectious disease (Table 9). The most important differential diagnosis in these cases is malignancy (lymphoma, Hodgkin's disease). It relies on proper interpretation of serologic test results and on the microscopic examination of lymph node biopsies.

Adenopathies are associated with the acute stage of toxoplasma infection. As a consequence, a toxoplasmic origin of adenopathy is practically ruled out if serologic results are those of a chronic infection (Table 4, part F). Diagnosis is easily established if the first sample of serum has been drawn early enough; serologic findings correspond to cases B and C in Table 4. It sometimes happens that the first sample of serum proves negative or positive only for IgM antibody. If so, presence of IgG antibodies in the second sample is diagnostic. Because toxoplasmosis is a frequent cause of adenopathy, it is a good rule to routinely perform a serologic test at the first consultation of a patient with adenopathy, the etiology of which is not obvious.

The diagnosis is not as easily established when the first sample of serum has been drawn too late and the antibody titer is high but stable. In these circumstances, the presence of IgM antibodies is highly suggestive (Table 4, case D); if IgM antibodies are not present (case E, or even H), the diagnosis of toxoplasmic lymphadenopathy should be questioned unless there are characteristic findings on lymph node biopsy.

In summary, two pitfalls are commonly encountered in cases of toxoplasmic lymphadenopathy: misdiagnosis and overdiagnosis.

1. Misdiagnosis is frequent when this infection is not well recognized. Physicians and pathologists frequently do not consider it, and many patients are considered initially to have lymphogranuloma or lymphoma. This has significant and sometimes dangerous therapeutic consequences.

2. There are also instances of overdiagnosis. This occurs when physicians are very aware of the frequency of toxoplasma infection as a cause of enlarged lymph nodes, and they too readily accept a single high titer of antibodies as signifying the diagnosis.

In infants and young children, asymptomatic lymphadenopathy is also frequently associated with toxoplasma infection, but the disease sometimes occurs as an acute, febrile illness lasting for some weeks. Toxoplasma infection is a significant cause of "glandular

Table 6. Guidelines for the Interpretation of Serologic Tests Performed *During* Pregnancy

Serologic Results*	Conclusions
Negative (A, I)	See Table 5. Should be tested again during pregnancy; ideally every 6 weeks, if economically possible
Latent infection (E, F, G)	Immune patient. No risk of congenital toxoplasmosis (except perhaps for a very low risk if case (E) is discovered during the last months of pregnancy in a patient who was not examined earlier)
Acute or recent infection (B, C, D)	See Table 7
Reinfection or relapsing chronic infection (acute infection unlikely) (H)	Probably no risk or very low risk; e.g., chronic ocular toxoplasmosis often relapses during pregnancy. Delivery of child with congenital infection has not been observed in these conditions

*Letters refer to cases described in Table 4.

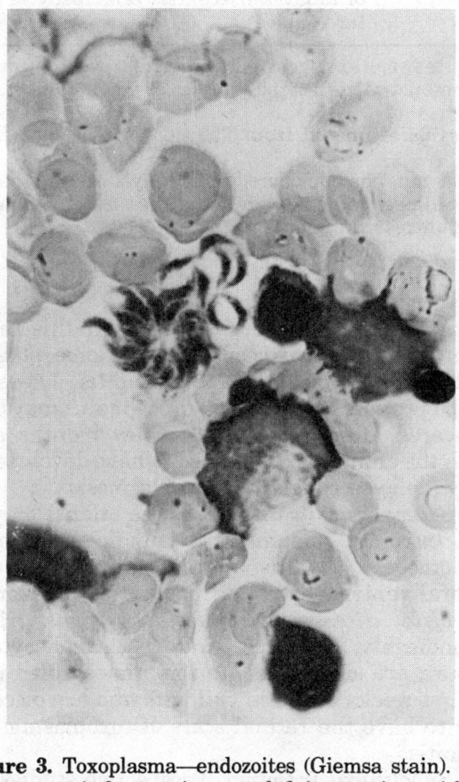

Figure 3. Toxoplasma—endozoites (Giemsa stain). Bone marrow smear is from an immunodeficient patient with systemic toxoplasmosis. (Courtesy of J.P. Barbet.)

fever" in children. Fever is seldom high, but it may be of long duration; adenopathy is generalized (possibly mesenteric as the initial location, causing abdominal pain); pharyngitis is usually absent or discrete, and there is moderate or no splenomegaly. Reactive atypical lymphocytes are present in blood smears but are not as numerous as they are in infectious mononucleosis. Serologic diagnosis is easy (case B, Table 4). There is no cross reaction with heterophil antibodies.

Severe Forms of Acquired Toxoplasmosis

These are mainly observed in patients whose immune response is defective (resulting from a congenital defect or an underlying disease) or impaired (by another infection or by immunosuppressive therapy). More than one cause of impairment is often associated in the same patient, for instance:

1. A depressed cell-mediated immunity due to Hodgkin's disease together with immunosuppressive therapy (cortisone); or
2. Cytomegalovirus infection and immunosuppressive therapy in a patient with an organ transplant.

Impairment of both humoral and cell-mediated immune response may be responsible for the more virulent course of infection and for the severity of disease. If immune defect or immune suppression existed prior to the acquisition of toxoplasma infection, the initial infection may not be contained. This may result in acute progressive systemic infection with fever, lymphadenopathy, rash, pneumonitis, encephalitis, myocarditis, or even hepatitis and nephritis.

Lymph node biopsy shows foci of necrosis with little or no surrounding inflammatory reaction. Toxoplasma endozoites are numerous and easily seen in smears of lymph node tissues. They can also be found in smears of bone marrow (Fig. 3).

These cases are extremely rare. In most patients the disease runs a subacute course, and after a few weeks (or even months) cardiac and neurologic signs become predominant. Myocarditis and encephalitis are the most frequent clinical manifestations of severe toxoplasmosis in an immunodeficient patient.

Encephalitis may also be the result of a relapse when immunosuppressive therapy is initiated in a patient who had acquired toxoplasma infection months or years earlier.

Toxoplasmic encephalitis has a subtle onset and is difficult to recognize. Multiple and highly variable features of central nervous system involvement may

Table 7. Acute Infection During Pregnancy: Practical Guidelines for an Estimation of Fetal Risk*

Time of Acquisition of Maternal Infection	Transmission to Offspring (Risk of Congenital Infection)	If Infection Transmitted†		Comments
		Risk of Abortion or Fetal Death	*Risk of Congenital Disease*	
Shortly before time of conception	Very low risk (below 1%)(?)	Probably high (over 90%)(?)	Probably low (< 10%)(?)	Therapeutic abortions performed in 57 such cases; attempt at isolation of toxoplasma from products of abortion was negative in every case
First trimester of pregnancy	Low risk (about 10%)	High (45%) (?)	High (45%) (?)	Therapeutic abortions performed in 112 such cases; 12 positive isolations of parasites from product of abortion
Second trimester of pregnancy	Frequent (10 to 50%)	Low (< 10%)	High (10 to 25%)	Possible prenatal diagnosis of: Fetal damage by echography (ascites; enlargement of cerebral ventricles) Fetal infection by amniocentesis and sampling of fetal blood (presence of IgM or positive isolation following inoculation into mice is diagnostic)
Third trimester of pregnancy	Very frequent (50 to 100%)	No	Low; severe systemic congenital toxoplasmosis possible in a minority of cases (1%) (?)	If possible, on delivery, placenta should be preserved for inoculation into mice Delayed onset of disease is common weeks or months after birth, principally in premature babies

*The risk to the fetus is related to the time at which maternal acute infection occurred. This time is well defined when seroconversion from negative to positive serologic tests has been demonstrated in serial samples or when clinical signs of infection (lymphadenopathy) are present.

The approximate time of acquisition of infection may sometimes be estimated from Table 4 (B, C, D, and E) if the *first* serologic test performed during pregnancy is positive.

The risk of transmission to the offspring and that of fetal damage must be considered separately since fetal infection may be subclinical in the majority (90% ?) of neonates. The percentages indicated are from the authors' experience; they are not established from statistically controlled studies among untreated patients.

† Estimated as a percentage of infected offspring.

be observed: generalized encephalopathy without localizing signs, or encephalitis with meningeal involvement (cerebrospinal fluid is clear with a moderate increase in cells and a high protein content). Space-occupying masses or multiple mass lesions are not infrequent, suggesting tumor or brain abscess that leads to biopsy and (or) additional surgical intervention. Multiple brain abscesses are one of the most common manifestations of toxoplasmosis in patients with the acquired immunodeficiency syndrome.

Table 10 gives a synopsis of the problems related to severe toxoplasma infection.

PROBLEMS IN PEDIATRICS

What has been termed the classical case—an infant with hydrocephalus, palsies, psychomotor retardation, microphthalmia, chorioretinitis, and intracranial calcifications—has never been the most frequent form of the congenital disease. Such a case might be prevented nowadays through the help of systematic examination of pregnant women and earlier diagnosis of infection in the newborn infant.

Clinical Patterns

One may schematically describe different patterns of congenital infection in the following way:

1. *Neurologic disease of the infant.* In this form the infant may have hydrocephalus or microcephaly, microphthalmia, and/or retinochoroiditis. These signs may be present at birth, or hydrocephalus may be first discovered after a period of a few months during which the child was considered to have developed normally (delayed congenital toxoplasmosis).

2. *Severe systemic disease.* These infants may have rash, purpura, pneumonitis, jaundice, and hepatosplenomegaly. Uveitis and/or enlargement of the cerebral ventricles may or may not be present.

3. *Mild disease, with isolated signs.* Hepatosplenomegaly, jaundice, and/or thrombocytopenic purpura are signs that are sometimes noted during the first weeks of life in children who are discovered later to have the retinal scars of toxoplasmic chorioretinitis.

4. *Subclinical infection.* Prospective studies of acquired toxoplasma infection in pregnant women have revealed that signs or symptoms of congenital disease are present only in a minority of the infected infants (Table 11). In most cases, congenital infection is subclinical.

Figure 4 demonstrates the pathogenesis of congenital toxoplasma infection or disease in relation to the time of maternal acquisition of the infection and to the early or delayed transfer of parasites to the fetus.

Table 12 summarizes the clinical diagnostic problems of congenital toxoplasmosis.

Table 8. Possible Relationship Between Clinical Disease and Toxoplasma Infection

Relationship	Examples
Incidental	Incidence of *acute infection* is between 0.5 and 10% of the non-immune population, per year Prevalence of *chronic* (latent) infection varies from 10% to more than 90% in most adult population Hence, the frequency of coincidence between evidence of toxoplasma infection and unrelated diseases
Specific cause-effect relationship; the observed disease is directly and solely related to virulence of parasite, to inflammatory response, and to specific immune response of host	Toxoplasmic lymphadenopathy Congenital toxoplasmosis Ocular toxoplasmosis
Nonspecific cause-effect relationship; toxoplasma infection has induced a disease or syndrome that might also have been provoked by other infectious agents.	Due to location of inflammation; e.g., around aqueduct of Sylvius (hydrocephalus), or in area related with endocrine functions (precocious puberty, myxedema, diabetus insipidus) Due to the induction of an immunologically mediated syndrome; e.g., thrombocytopenic purpura, disseminated intravascular coagulation, hemolytic anemia, nephrotic syndrome, polymyositis
Opportunistic relationship; pathogenicity of toxoplasma has been enhanced by an immune deficiency	Systemic toxoplasmosis and pneumonitis; when acute toxoplasma infection occurs together with an immunosuppressive infection or in immunodeficient patient Encephalitis, uveitis, myocarditis, myositis; when a chronic infection is reactivated by immunosuppressive therapy

Table 9. Main Features of Toxoplasmic Lymphadenopathy

Feature	Comment
Age of patients	Every age
Symptoms	Nodes may be spontaneously painful when they appear and tender on palpation when recently developed
Aspect	No redness of skin
Size	Moderately enlarged; size of a bean, hazelnut, or almond, seldom more than a walnut
Consistence	Firm but not hard, smooth and uniform, well defined, without edema of overlying skin, not adhering to skin or underlying tissues, never evolving toward suppuration
Location	Possible in every area; the most characteristic and by far the most frequent are: — Posterior cervical, suboccipital, subauricular, submental — Supraclavicular, axillary, pectoral, epitrochlear rather frequent — Seldom inguinal
Number	Most often localized: a single or a few lymph nodes in one area Sometimes generalized: swelling of nodes appearing in another area, after a few days or weeks
Symptoms possibly associated	Asthenia (may be prolonged), headache, myalgia, low fever (in children principally). General condition usually unaffected
Duration	Often long; weeks, months, even a year or longer Clinical evolution benign with spontaneous involution of enlarged nodes.
Leukocytes	Neutropenia, activated lymphocytes, sometimes eosinophilia
Histologic picture	Often characteristic: groups of epithelioid cells scattered along the node; immature sinus histiocytosis and follicular hyperplasia with phagocytosis of nuclear debris Inflammatory infiltrate may sometimes extend into perinodal tissues Sometimes not characteristic: "inflammatory reaction" Sometimes misleading; this picture may be misinterpreted as an early stage of tuberculosis, as sarcoidosis, or as an initial lymphogranuloma or lymphoma

Table 10. Synopsis of Problems Related to Severe Toxoplasmosis

Circumstances	Clinical Disease	Diagnostic Problems	Comments
Patient known to have a deficient immune system (e.g., combined deficiency with agammaglobulinemia)	Subacute progressive toxoplasmosis, with pneumonitis, myocarditis, and encephalitis	Serologic tests remain negative (or passively positive due to injection of gammaglobulins); importance of parasitologic examination	Care should be taken to avoid infection in this patient (see *Table 5* on instructions to pregnant women)
Patient not known to be immunodeficient	Toxoplasmosis has been diagnosed, the course of which is unusually severe (e.g., prolonged high fever, relapsing lymphadenopathy, progressive uveitis, signs of cardiac or central nervous system involvement)	Antibody response may be enhanced with high, persisting titers of both IgM and IgG	Patient immunocompetence should be checked in order to detect a previously unknown immunologic imbalance (e.g., defect in cell-mediated immunity) Patient should be examined for an associated infection, or an underlying malignancy
Patient to receive immunosuppressive therapy (e.g., treatment of malignant disease or transplantation)	Depending on drugs used, treatment may have little effect on immunity to toxoplasma or may interfere not only with development of immunity but also with maintenance of well-established immunity In patient with chronic infection, local relapses may result in progressive uveitis, myocarditis, and mostly encephalitis	A sample of serum should be obtained before treatment and examined to determine either absence or presence and stage of toxoplasma infection; sample should be kept frozen for later comparisons; antibody response to relapse or chronic infection may be very weak	Infection should be avoided in this patient (see *Table 5*) Transfusions are a potential risk, mainly leukocyte transfusion (parasitemia has been demonstrated in asymptomatic patients with chronic myelocytic leukemia)

Table 11. Prospective Study of Infants Born to Women Who Acquired Toxoplasma Infection During Pregnancy: Signs and Symptoms in 108 Infants with Proven Congenital Infection*

Finding	No. Examined	No. Positive	(%)
Prematurity			
Birth weight below 2500 gm	108	4	(3.7)
Birth weight of 2500 to 3000 gm		7	(6.5)
Dysmaturity (intrauterine growth retardation)	108	3	(2.7)
Postmaturity	108	9	(8.3)
Icterus	107	12	(11.2)
Hepatosplenomegaly	108	5	(4.6)
Thrombocytopenic purpura	108	2	(1.8)
Abnormal blood count (anemia, eosinophilia)	105	5	(4.8)
Microcephaly	108	9	(8.3)
Hydrocephaly	108	4	(3.7)
Hypotonia	108	7	(6.5)
Convulsions	108	5	(4.6)
Psychomotor retardation	108	5	(4.6)
Intracranial calcifications on x-ray	103	16	(15.5)
Abnormal EEG	95	8	(8.4)
Abnormal CSF			
Pleocytosis	94	32	(34.0)
Increased protein level		32	(34.0)
Microphthalmia	108	4	(3.7)
Strabismus	108	9	(8.3)
Chorioretinitis			
Unilateral	108	21	(19.4)
Bilateral		6	(5.5)

*Data from cases discussed by Szusterkac, M., Faculté de Médecine, Sainte-Antoine, Paris, 1980; table adapted from Remington, J.S., and Desmonts, G: Toxoplasmosis. In Remington, J.S., and Klein, J.O. (eds.): *Infectious Diseases of the Fetus and Newborn Infant.* Philadelphia, W.B. Saunders Company, 1983, p. 193.

Abbreviations: EEG = Electroencephalogram; CSF = cerebrospinal fluid.

Diagnosis of Infection in the Infant

Definitive establishment of the diagnosis of toxoplasma infection, whether overt or subclinical, depends on demonstration of toxoplasma and/or a specific immune response (antibody production) in the infant. Isolation of parasites should be attempted whenever possible, since the antibody response of a congenitally infected baby may be very weak or delayed.

During the first weeks and months of life, the antibody response may be strikingly different from one patient to another. In some patients, the response may be completely suppressed with no evidence of synthesis of IgM or IgG antibody; the antibodies present in the child's serum seem to be solely of maternal origin. In other newborns, a definite and strong antibody response may be observed, parallel to that which is observed following an acquired infection in the adult, and includes both IgM and IgG antibodies. In most patients, however, the antibody response is weak, delayed, or incomplete; some infants synthesize IgM antibodies, others do not. In addition, synthesis of IgG antibodies may sometimes be present without any evi-

Table 12. Congenital Toxoplasmosis: Circumstances of Diagnosis and Guidelines for Interpretation of the Serologic Test Results of the Mother

Circumstances	Clinical Diagnostic Problem	Maternal Serologic Results and Provisional Conclusions
Diseased infant: Signs suggesting congenital toxoplasmosis are present	Differential diagnosis from neonatal disease due to *Cytomegalovirus*, bacterial sepsis, rubella, syphilis, herpes simplex; also from hemolytic disease of the newborn and hydrops fetalis	Congenital toxoplasmosis* is: D, C, B = probable E = possible A, F, G, I = unlikely
Asymptomatic child: Mother is known to have acquired toxoplasma infection when pregnant	Differential diagnosis between no infection and subclinical infection: if infection present, recognition of potential disease:† fundus, CSF examination, x-rays, echotomography and CT scan of skull	If maternal infection was present before pregnancy or acquired early during pregnancy, congenital infection would not be subclinical; infant is probably *not* infected, if clinically normal‡ If maternal infection was acquired late, subclinical infection is often present in infant‡

* Refer to Table 4.
† Refer to Table 11.
‡ Refer to Table 7.
Abbreviations: CSF = Cerebrospinal fluid; CT = computed tomography.

Table 13. Biologic Diagnosis of Congenital Toxoplasma Infection in the Infant

Age of Infant*	Examination Preformed	Comments
1st days of life	Placenta, blood: inoculation into mice	*cf.* Table 2
	Serologic test for IgM antibody	IgM—ISA double-sandwich ELISA are positive in 70% of cases of congenital infection IgM IFA is positive in only 25%
	Comparison between immune load of maternal and cord serum	Difference is significant if the immune load in cord serum is four times that of maternal serum
15 days	Test for IgM in infant's serum	Positive in cord blood turning negative in serum obtained later suggests possibility of placental leak Negative in cord blood may turn positive when transmission occurred shortly before delivery
1, 2, 4, 6, 8 months	Compare immune load of the recent sample with that of previous samples	An increasing or stable immune load proves synthesis of toxoplasma antibody by the infant A decreasing immune load suggests absence of synthesis due either to absence of infection or to reduction of antigenic stimulus following effective treatment: Surveillance of the immune load is useful for following treatment

*When examination should be performed.
Abbreviations: ISA = Immunosorbent assay; ELISA = enzyme-linked immunosorbent assay; IFA = immunofluorescent antibody.

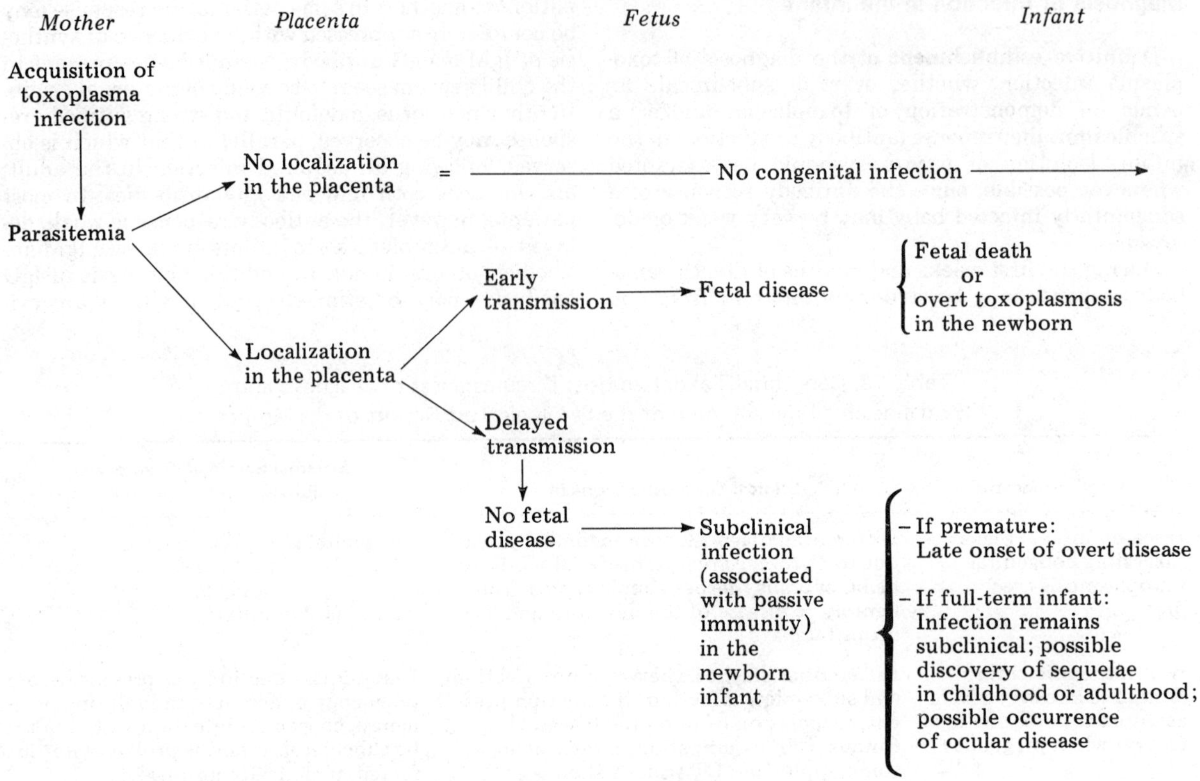

Figure 4. Pathogenesis of congenital infection with Toxoplasma.

dence of synthesis of IgM antibodies. The antibody response is also labile and is easily suppressed when treatment of the child is continued.

It should be noted that strong production of antibody or absence of any specific antibody synthesis may be observed in infants with subclinical infection as well as in those with severe clinical congenital disease.

When specific IgG antibody synthesis is weak, antibody production is difficult to assess as long as passive antibodies of maternal origin are present. As a consequence, in the absence of IgM antibodies a definitive serologic diagnosis of congenital toxoplasma infection may be delayed for several months (sometimes for as long as 6 to 10 months). This is especially true in treated children in whom development of a specific antibody response may sometimes be very slow, weak, and delayed.

Table 13 gives a synopsis of the methods we use to establish the diagnosis in the infant. Some other methods that might also be useful are antigen-specific lymphocyte transformation, attempts at demonstra-

Table 14. Indications for Examination of Aqueous Humor in the Presence of Eye Lesions Suggesting Toxoplasmosis

Age When Observed	Serologic Results*	Conclusion	Indication for Aqueous Humor Examination
Any age	A	Toxoplasmosis excluded	No
Infant	D or E, in mother and child	Congenital toxoplasmosis	No
Child	B, C, D	Probably acquired toxoplasmosis	No
Adolescent	H	Probably toxoplasmosis (congenital or acquired)	No: if antibody titer is high in serum, results of aqueous humor examination will usually be insignificant
	E	Possible, but not proved toxoplasmosis	
Adult	F	Possible toxoplasmosis	Yes

*Letters refer to cases described in Table 4.

tion of antigen in body fluids, and analytic study of antibody complexes. They will not be discussed here because study of their significance is still in progress.

PROBLEMS IN OPHTHALMOLOGY

Toxoplasma infection is one of the most common causes of chorioretinitis and posterior uveitis. Features of the ophthalmoscopic examination are well known and will not be described here. Nevertheless, it should be noted that while some aspects are highly characteristic (the pigmented and necrotic scars), others are not (principally recent edematous lesions). *The diagnosis of ocular toxoplasmosis should never rely solely on the ophthalmoscopic examination.*

The clinical history of patients with ocular toxoplasmosis suggests that the first retinal lesion sometimes occurs during the subacute state, i.e., weeks or a few months after acquisition of the infection. More often, the clinical history suggests that the lesions occurred later, during the chronic stage of the infection, either in patients in whom retinal colonization by the parasite had been subclinical or most commonly in those patients in whom previously unrecognized retinal involvement is proved by the presence of old retinal scars.

Ocular disease is seldom a consequence of postnatally acquired infection; it is most often the result of congenital infection. From available data, it is possible to give a gross estimate of the respective incidence of eye lesions which is probably below 1:1000 of cases of acquired infection, while probably more than 50 per cent of congenital infections result in eye disease, even if subclinical at birth. There is some evidence that early treatment of the infant with congenital infection decreases the incidence of eye disease during childhood and adolescence.

The cause of the inflammation associated with recurrence is still controversial: delayed hypersensitivity reaction to toxoplasma antigens (cyst rupture), parasites resuming their proliferation or, more likely, both. Whatever the mechanism, recurrence is related to the persistence of cysts or of dormant endozoites persisting in tissue cells, years after colonization of the retina.

A major diagnostic problem occurs in the patient who is examined in the chronic stage of infection. Most of the time, such an individual has an antibody titer that is low and not different from antibody titers commonly observed in the normal population. Thus, serologic results do not allow for more than a "presumptive" diagnosis of "possible" toxoplasmic uveitis. Therapeutic trials have not been satisfying because the lesions may get better without treatment. Thus, the result is difficult to evaluate.

Because of this problem, procedures which allow for a definite diagnosis are most valuable. One such method is serologic examination of the aqueous humor obtained by paracentesis of the anterior chamber of the eye. The indications for this are discussed in Table 14 and the results in Table 15.

Table 15. Results of Aqueous Humor Examination

Serum *Immune Load*	Aqueous Humor *Serologic Titer*	 *Immune Load*	Conclusion
Low (1 to 30 IU/mg IgG)	Negative	0	Toxoplasmosis cannot be excluded; negative serologic test in aqueous humor is possible in scarred inactive ocular toxoplasmosis or if puncture is performed too early after a relapse
	Positive	Less than or equal to serum	Toxoplasmosis unlikely; uveitis probably of other origin
		Twice that of serum	Possible toxoplasmosis: threshold significant result
	Positive	More than four times and sometimes 10 or 100 times that of serum	*Ocular toxoplasmosis* (clinical relapse of chronic toxoplasma infection) Low level of total IgG in aqueous is usually associated with self-limited lesions High IgG level associated with important inflammatory reaction and possibly with severe progressive uveitis
High (> 100 IU/mg IgG)	Positive	Usually not significantly different from serum	Ocular toxoplasmosis possible but not proven

AMERICAN TRYPANOSOMIASIS

By Aluizio Prata, M.D.
Brasília, Brazil

SYNONYMS

Chagas' disease, chagasic cardiomyopathy, endemic megaesophagus.

DEFINITION

Chagas' disease occurs as an acute or chronic condition. It is found only in the Western Hemisphere, resulting from infection with *Trypanosoma cruzi;* is usually transmitted by the feces of reduviid bugs of the subfamily Triatominae; and is related to heart, esophagus, and large intestine involvement. Frequently infection is not associated with disease.

TRANSMISSION

Endemic Chagas' disease is a result of socioeconomic status of the population. The reduviid bugs settle in houses with poor hygienic conditions and transmit *T. cruzi* at night when taking a blood meal. The trypanosomes penetrate through skin abrasions or normal mucosa. Transmission can also occur by blood transfusion, congenitally, or by laboratory accident.

PRESENTING CLINICAL MANIFESTATIONS

Chagas' disease must be considered as presenting two phases: acute and chronic.

The *acute phase* occurs about 4 to 12 days after the inoculation of *T. cruzi* in the host by the bug, or 20 to 40 days if transmitted by blood transfusion. It is seen mainly in infants and children, and the following points are important in diagnosis: signs related to the portal of entry of the parasite, manifestations of a generalized infection, and signs of cardiac and central nervous system involvement.

When the portal of entry is the eye, there is unilateral palpebral edema of purplish color, with conjunctival hyperemia and satellite adenopathy. If the penetration of the parasite is cutaneous, the lesion resembles a furuncle. In other cases the portal of entry cannot be seen. The principal systemic clinical manifestations are fever, tachycardia, lymphadenopathy, splenomegaly, and edema. The fever, commonly around 38°C, is higher in the afternoon and is frequently associated with asthenia, anorexia, nervousness, and headache. Tachycardia disproportionate to the height of the fever is a common finding. Slight lymphadenopathy and splenomegaly are frequent. Edema not related to cardiac failure may appear. The clinical manifestations of cardiac involvement are those of an acute myocarditis, frequently accompanied by a pericardial effusion. The heart sounds may be muffled, and gallop rhythm may be present. Some patients develop biventricular failure. Meningoencephalitis is a less frequent finding and appears in infections during the first years of life.

It must be emphasized that in the acute phase there is extreme variation in the frequency in intensity of the clinical manifestations. In the majority of cases, this phase of the disease is not recognized, either because it is misdiagnosed or because the diagnostic signs are not apparent.

Congenital Chagas' disease can be asymptomatic or associated with jaundice, hepatosplenomegaly, cutaneous hemorrhage, and neurologic signs in premature newborns.

The *chronic phase* includes a period of clinical latency in which patients are asymptomatic. In some patients the physical examination may detect a wide and fixed splitting of the second heart sound, usually related to the presence of a complete right bundle branch block. The clinical manifestations may be due to cardiomyopathy, involvement of the digestive tract, and neuronal destruction. The clinical manifestations of chronic Chagas' disease show differences in presenting patterns in different endemic areas.

In the symptomatology of cardiomyopathy, it is possible to distinguish two types: Arrhythmias predominate in one, and manifestations of myocardial failure predominate in the other. The main symptom of patients with arrhythmia is palpitation, accompanied by dizziness and episodes of loss of consciousness in the more severe cases. The manifestations of myocardial failure, when present, are mild to moderate in degree. In chronic Chagas' myocarditis, heart failure is usually biventricular in type, with predominant signs of right ventriclar failure. Symptoms of left ventricular failure do not attain the degree of severity observed in other cardiomyopathies in which there is predominantly involvement of the left ventricle. Thus, patients with cardiac decompensation due to Chagas' heart disease never present with attacks of acute pulmonary edema and orthopnea is not common. Dyspnea on exertion is of moderate degree and not progressive. Crises of paroxysmal nocturnal dyspnea are infrequent. Ascites and palpitation not related to effort are common symptoms in patients with severe heart failure. Thromboembolic phenomena in the pulmonary or systemic circulations occur frequently.

Physical examination reflects the severity of myocardial damage. Patients with advanced cardiac insufficiency present with a small volume pulse, sometimes alternating in character, and a small pulse pressure. Examination of the heart usually reveals cardiomegaly, decreased intensity of the first heart sound, a loud pulmonic component of the second sound, third and fourth heart sounds, and murmurs.

The main symptoms of esophageal involvement are dysphagia and retrosternal pain. As the disease progresses to megaesophagus, regurgitation, sensation of retrosternal fullness, heartburn, eructations, cough, hiccup, and bilateral parotid gland enlargement may also occur. Patients with megacolon present meteorism and occasionally fecaloma.

Neuronal destruction is usual in Chagas' disease, and it is not always recognized by symptoms. One clinical sign of involvement of the spinal cord is abolition of the deep tendon reflexes, especially the Achilles tendon reflex.

COURSE

The manifestations of the acute phase subside within 2 to 4 months in more than 90 per cent of cases. In other cases, the patients die with acute myocarditis or meningoencephalitis. The acute phase is usually followed by a long period of clinical latency. It has been classified as the indeterminate form of Chagas' disease. Many individuals remain symptom-free. The time of appearance of chronic manifestations ranges from 10 to 30 years. In the initial stage of cardiopathy, there may be no symptoms in spite of the presence of electrocardiographic evidence of heart disease. Usually cardiac insufficiency is heralded by dyspnea on exertion and edema of the legs; more than half of the these patients are in the 20- to 40-year age group. The time of survival after onset of cardiac insufficiency ranges from 1 month to 10 years, the majority of deaths occurring within a period of 7 months to 2 years. Many patients with Chagas' disease die suddenly.

COMMON COMPLICATIONS

Episodes of thromboembolism occur frequently. In a small number of patients, they can be the initial manifestation of the disease. Chest pain and cough with hemoptysis occur in association with pulmonary embolism and infarction. Embolism to the lungs may produce acute cor pulmonale and occasionally lung abscess.

In advanced megaesophagus, regurgitated material may produce aspiration pneumonia. Esophagitis is more frequent after surgical dilatation of the cardia. The difficulty in swallowing can result in cachexia. Megacolon can be complicated by sigmoid torsion or fecaloma.

LABORATORY PROCEDURES

In acute Chagas' disease, demonstration of circulating forms of *T. cruzi* is essential for definitive diagnosis even in the inapparent clinical form. This is accomplished by the direct examination of a drop of blood between a slide and coverslip, a stained thick film, the leukocyte buffy coat, or the supernatant from clotted blood. Although it is sometimes difficult to find the parasites in stained films, often the diagnosis is made during a routine white blood cell count. *Trypanosoma cruzi* can be demonstrated by hemoculture or xenodiagnosis with nymphs of triatomid bugs reared in the laboratory. Serologic tests usually become positive a few days after symptoms appear. The reactions most used in Chagas' disease are immunofluorescence, complement fixation, hemagglutination, and enzyme-linked immunosorbent assay (ELISA). Cross reaction is possible with leishmaniasis and *Trypanosoma rangeli* infections. An absolute lymphocytosis is present in nearly all patients. The Paul-Bunnell test is frequently positive and there is an increase in plasma gamma globulins.

In the chronic phase of Chagas' disease, the parasite can be demonstrated by xenodiagnosis and hemoculture if repeated. The same serologic tests as those used in acute Chagas' disease are done. When positive, they do not indicate morbidity but only infection with *T. cruzi.*

RADIOLOGIC EVALUATION

In the acute phase, radiologic studies demonstrate a transitory and variable degree of generalized enlargement of the heart chambers. In the chronic phase, the heart size of patients with mild myocarditis is normal. As the disease progresses, cardiomegaly appears, initially of the left ventricle but later affecting all four heart chambers. There is diminished pulsation on fluoroscopy. Signs of a pleural effusion occur in about a quarter of fatal cases. Rarely there are signs of severe pulmonary congestion. Triangular radiodense areas are associated with pulmonary infarcts. The diagnosis of megaesophagus and megacolon are confirmed by radiological examination.

ELECTROCARDIOGRAPHY

In the acute phase the electrocardiographic changes most frequently seen are sinus tachycardia, a low-voltage QRS complex, a prolonged P-R interval, primary ST-T wave alterations, and a prolonged Q-T interval. Cardiac involvement is detected most frequently when serial observations are made.

In the chronic phase, the most common electrocardiographic changes are due to disturbance in the formation and conduction of the electrical impulse within the heart and in the repolarization of the myocardial ventricular fibers. Ventricular premature beats are very common, and they get worse with the evolution of the disease. They become numerous and multifocal and give origin to runs of ventricular tachycardia, and they are generally associated with electrocardiographic signs of a ventricular conduction disturbance. Complete right bundle branch block is one of most representative disturbances of chronic cardiomyopathy. The association with a left anterior hemiblock suggests a more severe form of heart disease. Atrioventricular blocks, especially first degree A-V block, commonly occur. In many asymptomatic patients the electrocardiographic changes constitute the most important evidence of cardiac involvement.

DIFFERENTIAL DIAGNOSIS

In the differential diagnosis of acute Chagas' disease, one has to consider infectious mononucleosis, toxoplasmosis, acute schistosomiasis, acute glomerulonephritis, endocarditis, tuberculosis, brucellosis, salmonellosis, leukemia, and certain collagen diseases.

It is possible to confuse chronic Chagas' disease with rheumatic heart disease, ischemic heart disease, idiopathic cardiomegaly, alcoholic cardiomyopathy, peripartal heart disease, and endomyocardial fibrosis.

SPECIAL CONSIDERATIONS

The diagnosis of Chagas' disease lies in the analysis of multiple factors: epidemiologic, clinical, parasitologic, serologic, electrocardiographic, and radiologic.

One should think of acute Chagas' disease when a patient, even without sign of a portal of entry, edema, cardiomegaly, or electrocardiographic changes, presents with prolonged fever, tachycardia, slight generalized lymphadenopathy, slight splenomegaly, and lymphocytosis, especially if the patient is a child.

When unexplained fever with lymphocytosis occurs after blood transfusion, the possibility of post-transfusional Chagas' disease must be considered.

Congenital Chagas' disease is a possibility in premature newborns with hepatosplenomegaly, cutaneous hemorrhage, and neurologic signs even if the mother appears healthy.

The diagnosis of chronic Chagas' disease must be considered in patients with one or more of the following findings: clinical symptoms of arrhythmias (dizziness, palpitations and loss of consciousness), cardiac failure with predominance of right-sided failure, congestion, episodes of thromboembolism, cardiomegaly, and suggestive electrocardiographic alterations (complete right bundle branch block, especially if accompanied by left anterior hemiblock and severe ventricular premature beats, complete A-V block), evidence of megaesophagus, or megacolon.

PITFALLS IN DIAGNOSIS

In acute Chagas' disease the specific and diagnostic finding is the presence of *T. cruzi* in the peripheral blood by direct examination or by examination of a thick smear. The parasitemia becomes scanty with evolution of the infection, and the parasites may not be detected.

Serology is the best method for diagnosis in chronic Chagas' disease. A negative serologic test, especially if only a single test is done (and it is important which laboratory does it), does not exclude the diagnosis. Also, demonstrating that a patient is infected with *T. cruzi* does not signify necessarily that the individual has clinical symptoms of Chagas' disease.

LEISHMANIASIS

By Philip D. Marsden, M.D.
Brasília, Brazil

Leishmaniasis has an impressive geographic distribution in the tropics and subtropics, being found in every large land mass with the exception of Australia and New Guinea. Recently it has been suggested that 400,000 new human visceral infections occur a year and that 10 million people are infected. Certainly an underestimate, more cases than this probably occur in South America alone.

Although leishmania show only minor morphologic differences among species in their amastigote or promastigote phase, with biologic, biochemical and immunologic techniques, definite consistent differences can be demonstrated. Over a dozen different techniques exist for such taxonomic identification, and preferences are changing as new techniques are developed. At the moment DNA hybridization to species and monoclonal antibodies to subspecies seem most appropriate, but many aspects of this active research field are still in debate. Since the clinician will rarely have access to these techniques, Table 1 should be valuable in showing the distribution of the main species and subspecies coupled with the type of disease they cause. Unfortunately, more than one species is often present in an area. If conditions exist for the clinician to arrange identification of the parasite, this should be done, because it is in the patient's interest to know. The type of infecting parasite is not the only determinant of disease expression; the host response is probably more important, but unfortunately immunologists have yet to give us sensitive techniques that can be used clinically to understand this aspect. There are rare records of *Leishmania mexicana* species recovered from the nasal mucosa and bone marrow and of *Leishmania tropica* causing visceral disease.

Autochthonous leishmaniasis in Texas has been reported, but American physicians are seeing increasing numbers of cases of cutaneous disease from abroad. Many years ago a series of cases of oriental sore were reported from Philadelphia in Jews who had visited Israel. Since only *L. tropica* exists in Israel, the diagnosis of what species of parasite was responsible for these infections was possible by implication, but in a patient with a skin sore coming from Brazil, *L. mexicana amazonensis, Leishmania braziliensis guyanensis,* and *Leishmania braziliensis braziliensis* may all produce a similar skin lesion. Does it matter? Very much so, because we have good evidence that *L. braziliensis braziliensis* will need three times the normal standard course of pentavalent antimonial (Pentostam) recommended by the Centers for Disease Control (CDC). Pentavalent antimonials (Pentostam or Glucantime) are the preferred initial treatment for all forms of leishmaniasis and are only available from CDC. The diagnosis of leishmaniasis will be discussed in order of frequency of the clinical presentation, namely skin lesions, visceral leishmaniasis (hepatosplenomegaly, anemia, and fever), and mucosal disease (granuloma of the nose, mouth, and upper respiratory passages).

SKIN LEISHMANIASIS

After an infected sandfly bite, the species causing cutaneous leishmaniasis multiply in macrophages in the amastigote form, promoting a skin granuloma of epithelioid cells heavily infiltrated with lymphocytes. Ulceration depends on the degree of necrosis, edema, and vasculitis in the lesion. Closed lesions are common in Old World skin leishmaniasis and members of

Table 1. Speciation of Human Leishmania and Their Principal Geographic Distribution

Name of Parasite	Type of Disease	Geographic Distribution
Leishmania tropica minor	Skin sore	Urban disease in Middle East
Leishmania tropica major	Skin sore	Rural disease in Middle East, southern Russia
Leishmania aethiopica	Skin sore (DCL)†	Ethiopia, Kenya
Leishmania mexicana mexicana	Skin sore	Mexico, other parts of Central America and northern South America above the Andes
Leishmania mexicana amazonensis	Skin sore (DCL)	All countries southeast of the Andean range
Leishmania braziliensis braziliensis	Skin sore mucosal disease	Countries with territory below‡ Amazon river and southeast of the Andean range
Leishmania braziliensis panamensis	Skin sore	Panama, other Central American countries
Leishmania braziliensis guyanensis	Skin sore	Countries with territory north of Amazon river southeast of the Andean range
Leishmania peruana	Skin sore	Peru west of the Andes
*Leishmania donovani**	Visceral disease (Kala azar)	India, Burma, Afghanistan, China, Kenya, Sudan, countries surrounding the Mediterranean sea, Brazil, Venezuela

* Some authorities have subspeciated *L. donovani* (India), *L. d. chinensis* (China), *L. d. archiboldi* (East Africa), *L. d. infantum* (Mediterranean), *L. d. chagasi* (South America); taxonomic work is still in progress to decide the validity of this speciation.

† DCL = Diffuse cutaneous leishmaniasis; also recorded from Dominican Republic, the parasite being unclassified to date. Also a suggestion that in Venezuela another parasite, *L. mexicana pifanoi* may be responsible.

‡ Recent evidence suggests extension of *L. braziliensis braziliensis* as far as Central America. No proof as yet that *L. b. guyanensis* and *L. b. panamensis* are associated with mucosal disease.

the Mexicana complex. The Braziliensis complex is more prone to ulceration. *Leishmania braziliensis braziliensis* causes much necrosis, and large ulcers can be produced in a few weeks. *Leishmania braziliensis guyanensis* is said to be more frequently associated with lymphatic spread, mimicking sporotrichosis, which is common in many endemic areas. Often the ulcer has an infiltrated raised border. It is common in endemic areas particularly in rural dwelling males. The presentations of skin leishmaniasis are so varied that for any skin granuloma this diagnosis must be considered. The histopathology is suggestive but not specific unless leishmanial amastigotes with clearly visualized nuclei and kinetoplasts are seen.

Parasite Detection

Skin biopsies are best taken from the active border of the lesion. The biopsy site should be cleaned with alcohol swabs, and the best method is to take a 5-mm punch. The inferior surface of the biopsy is blotted on filter paper to remove blood, and this surface is then firmly applied to a clean glass slide to make a series of impression smears. The slide is air-dried, fixed in alcohol, and labeled. A Giemsa stain is used, and the slide is scanned for amastigotes. Success in identifying characteristic amastigotes is dependent on time spent at the microscope. The number of parasites in the specimen is related to the age of the lesion (since the host's immune mechanism destroys many) and the species, being most scanty in *L. braziliensis braziliensis.*

The biopsy should then be triturated in sterile saline and inoculated into several tubes of 3N Difco agar medium, held at 26°C, and examined regularly every week for a month. Triturated material can also be inoculated subcutaneously into the nose and feet of a hamster. Mexicana-type parasites grow well in both media, but *braziliensis* type show poor growth and may visceralize. Another biopsy sample should be put in fixative for histology. Pathologists exhibit differing degrees of imagination in their ability to see scanty amastigotes, but in a heavily parasitized lesion they are easily seen.

Immunodiagnosis

Since particularly in infections with *L. braziliensis braziliensis* parasites may be difficult to find, these indirect means are of value in diagnosis. Sometimes a diagnosis is based on a suggestive clinical picture, compatible histology, and a positive skin test without the organism being found.

Leishmanin Skin Test

This is the most reliable skin test in parasitic disease, with more than 90 per cent correlation with active or healed skin leishmaniasis in the New World. One-tenth ml of an antigen of $> 1 \times 10^6$ killed promastigotes (the species does not matter) are injected intradermally in the volar surface of the forearm. An area of induration of > 5 mm after 48 hours is read as positive. Such an antigen should become available in the United States. It has been widely used in South America since 1926, when Montenegro described the test.

Serology

Promastigotes or amastigotes can be used as the slide antigen for an indirect immunofluorescent antibody (IFA) test. There is still some debate as to which antigen is most sensitive, and, if possible, the homologous species to that dominant in the area should be used. Although significant titers can be detected in the majority of patients with active disease in an area of *L. braziliensis braziliensis,* enzyme-linked immunosorbent assay (ELISA) revealed more circulating antibodies. Inasmuch as the IFA cross reacts with sera from patients with *Leishmania donovani* and *Trypanosoma cruzi* infection, interpretation may be difficult in areas where such infections are prevalent. These antibodies are of interest because in some patients they disappear rapidly after treatment and in consequence have been used as a criterion of cure. Since we believe that sometimes live leishmania persist in patients with clinically healed lesions, the value of detecting such antibodies could be important and is the subject of current research.

Special Forms of Skin Leishmaniasis

So protean are the clinical presentations of skin leishmaniasis that it can resemble a boil, a skin cancer, secondary yaws, a deep mycosis, or a varicose ulcer. If the diagnostic plan explained earlier is followed, the correct diagnosis will be made. However, there are three forms of cutaneous leishmaniasis requiring special mention because of their unusual presentations. The first two represent extremes of the spectrum of skin leishmaniasis, so-called polar forms. Both are rare. The concept of the spectrum is not much used in clinical practice since the great majority of patients have histology in the middle of the range.

1. *Diffuse cutaneous leishmaniasis.* This is mentioned in Table 1. It is associated with a depression of cell-mediated immunity and therefore a negative Montenegro test and virtual absence of lymphocytes on skin histology; macrophages are packed with amastigotes. Leishmania are easy to detect and isolate. Clinically, multiple-nodular lesions are present; these progress slowly and never ulcerate. Diffuse cutaneous leishmaniasis closely resembles lepromatous leprosy, and many patients have been discovered in leprosaria.

2. *Tuberculoid leishmaniasis (lupoid leishmaniasis, leishmaniasis recidivans).* This is the other polar form with strong cell-mediated immunity, granuloma formation on biopsy, very scanty parasites, and a strongly positive skin test. Why it does not heal is unknown, but lesions last for years, with central scarring and an active border. This form closely resembles skin tuberculosis.

3. *Post–kala azar dermal leishmaniasis.* This provides a link to the next section. Twenty per cent of Indian and 2 per cent of African patients develop macules, papules, or nodules containing leishmania 1 to 2 years after treatment of their visceral leishmaniasis. Parasites are in higher density in nodular lesions, but hypopigmented macules may be the only sign.

VISCERAL LEISHMANIASIS (KALA AZAR)

This is the rarest of the three great endemic parasitic diseases of warm climates producing hepatosplenomegaly. Consequently the other two, namely malaria and schistosomiasis, always enter in the differential diagnosis. A widespread epidemic of kala azar occurred recently in Bihar.

Patients present with an intermittent fever, anemia, and splenomegaly, often associated with hepatomegaly. Night sweats are common and epistaxis may be the presenting sign. Kala azar affects mainly children, but in India and Africa adult infections are common. Hematologic investigation reveals anemia, leukopenia, and thrombocytopenia. IgG globulins are often elevated to an extraordinary degree (3 to 10 gm per liter), a situation seen only in the paraproteinemias. Hepatosplenic schistosomiasis with salmonella septicemia (an established association) can closely mimic these clinical and laboratory findings. There are differences in the behavior of *L. donovani* in man in different parts of the world. For example, the African and Mediterranean kala forms are much less sensitive to pentavalent antimonial therapy than the types causing disease in India, Brazil, or China. The marked epidemiologic differences (animal reservoirs, sandfly vectors) have resulted in the subspeciation mentioned in the table.

Parasite Detection

Detection is best done by examining bone marrow aspirates. Smears should be Giemsa stained and carefully searched for the characteristic amastigotes. Cultures of 3N Difco medium should be inoculated and read as previously described. The great majority of infections will be diagnosed in this way, although occasionally parasites are detected in liver or gland biopsy sections. The parasite load in established kala azar is heavy. In experienced hands, splenic aspiration is a safe, sensitive procedure. Fatalities occur because prothrombin and bleeding times are abnormal, too big a needle is used, or the physician fails to learn the technique.

Immunodiagnosis

The IFA and ELISA detectable antibodies are present in the circulation, but it is rarely necessary to estimate them in individual patients because the parasite can usually be found.

Differential Diagnosis

The following diseases may be confused with visceral leishmaniasis: lymphoma, leukemia, schistosomiasis, malaria (particularly the tropical splenomegaly syndrome), deposition disorders (Gaucher's disease, amyloidosis, hemochromatosis), brucellosis, typhoid, septicemia, systemic tuberculosis, histoplasmosis, and cirrhosis of the liver with portal hypertension.

MUCOSAL LEISHMANIASIS

Although this is the rarest of the three clinical forms of leishmaniasis, it is not only the most mutilating but also the most difficult to treat. *Leishmania braziliensis braziliensis* is the known causative organism. The position regarding the capacity of *L. brazili-*

ensis guyanensis and *L. braziliensis panamensis* to cause such disease is not known. Rarely, cases are reported outside the Americas. More than 50 cases have been reported from the Sudan, but the nature of the leishmanial species is not clear.

Leishmania braziliensis braziliensis must metastasize frequently via the lymphatic system and bloodstream, and circulating amastigotes settle in the nasal area, which has a rich plexus of porous capillaries. For unknown reasons, weeks, months, or even up to 30 years after the active skin lesion develops, granuloma also appears in the nose. Our difficulty in cultivating this species has made it impossible to study this sequence of metastasis. The first diagnostic step when mucosal leishmaniasis is suspected is to examine the patient's skin in a good light for the characteristic scar of the past skin lesion. Over 90 per cent of patients will have a detectable scar. In the others, the skin infection was probably sufficiently superficial not to leave a mark. The scar is often centimeters in width in *L. braziliensis braziliensis* infections, slightly depressed, and hypopigmented. It resembles a healed burn or mother yaw, both of which can be excluded by history.

The most common mucosal lesion occurs on the nasal septum. Being thin, the septum is cooled by inhaled air, a possible factor favorable to leishmanial growth. The lesion appears initially as a small friable granuloma accessible to biopsy. If untreated, the lesion often grows, the septum perforates, and a varying degree of nasal cartilage destruction occurs. The nose tip dips and broadens, the so-called "tapir nose." In some patients, complaints of obstruction, epistaxis, and tissue being blown from the nose indicate that the lesion is deep in the nose and difficult to access for biopsy.

In about 25 per cent of patients, the granuloma spreads out of the nose to involve the mouth, pharynx, and larynx. The prognosis is much worse in this group with drug therapy, and consequently a careful examination of all these structures in good lighting conditions is necessary. Leishmaniasis of only the palate or a lone laryngeal lesion occur. Involvement of the larynx is indicated by the degree of dysphonia. Dysphagia can also be a symptom. On laryngoscopy under anesthesia, granuloma can sometimes be seen extending down the trachea. Suffocation is a consequence of airway obstruction, and the patient's anterior cervical triangle may be marked by tracheostomy scars.

Organism Isolation

This is difficult, partly because of the inaccessibility of some lesions, but also the numbers of amastigotes in tissues usually are scanty. Impression smears, cultures, and hamster inoculation should be done.

Immunodiagnosis

Both the Montenegro test and tests for circulating antibody are usually strongly positive. A negative skin test may be associated with secondary malnutrition due to difficulty in eating. It is a bad prognostic sign, even with vigorous treatment. The most important differential diagnosis in South America is from *Paracoccidiodes braziliensis* infection which, especially in the mouth, can closely mimic leishmaniasis. On histology, the fungus can usually be seen and always cultured on Sabauraud's medium. A quick diagnostic maneuver, if the patient is in hospital, is to take an anteroposterior chest x-ray, since mucosal blastomycosis is usually associated with lung disease. Other entities that mimic mucosal leishmaniasis are tertiary treponematosis syndromes, particularly gangosa of yaws, leprosy, histoplasmosis, buccal carcinoma, and idiopathic midline granuloma. Leishmanial granuloma of the glans penis or female pudenda is usually a direct inoculation site by a female phlebotomine and not related to metastatic spread. There is one case of sexual transmission to the cervix on record, and other forms of contact transmission are rarely seen.

ECHINOCOCCOSIS

By Stephanos J. Hadziyannis, M.D.
Athens, Greece

DEFINITION AND SYNONYMS

Echinococcosis is a parasitic disease caused by infection with the larval form of tapeworms (cestodes) of the genus *Taenia echinococcus,* phylum *Platyhelminthes,* order *Cyclophyllidea,* family *Taeniidae.* It is characterized by the development of cysts in various organs predominantly in the liver and lung. It is one of the most important zoonoses, has a worldwide distribution, and is a serious human health problem in some areas of the world, particularly in sheep-rearing countries.

Echinococcus means sea urchin (echinus) and grain (coccus); i.e., it is a composite term used to designate both the thorny appearance and the very small size of the tapeworm, particularly of its scolices (heads), which are contained in the cysts.

Echinococcosis is also referred to as *hydatid disease* or *hydatidosis,* from the Greek word meaning watery, a term emphasizing the clear, watery appearance of the fluid content of the cysts (hydatid cysts or simply hydatids), which form in humans and other intermediate hosts.

There are several species and possibly subspecies of the genus *Taenia echinococcus.* The most common and worldwide one causing human disease is *Echinococcus granulosus* or *cysticus.* Another relatively rarer species, *E. multilocularis* or *alveolaris,* can also affect humans, causing a malignant-like disease, mainly of the liver. This is usually described under the terms of alveolar echinococcosis, alveolar hydatid disease, or alveolar hydatidosis, alveolosis, and alveococcosis.

This article deals primarily with echinococcosis caused by the common species *E. granulosus.* When necessary, echinococcosis due to *E. multilocularis* is also briefly discussed, being specifically designated with the adjective *alveolar.* Two other species, *E. oligarthrus* and *E. vogeli,* have also been reported to affect humans. However, the number of described cases is very small and further information will be needed to define the diagnostic features of these diseases.

LIFE CYCLE OF THE PARASITE AND PATHOLOGY

All species of echinococcus are maintained in nature by a cycle of transmission between an intermediate and a definitive host. The cycles of the various species differ only in the species of the hosts involved. The modes of transmission to humans are identical.

Definitive hosts are several carnivorous and omnivorous animals, the usual one for *E. granulosus* being the dog and for *E. multilocularis* the red fox. The mature worms live in the small intestine of the definitive host. In dogs the life span of *T. echinococcus* is 3 to 6 months.

Echinococci are the smallest of all tapeworms (1.5 to 9 mm) and consist of a head (scolex), a neck, and usually three segments (proglottides), the last one being gravid and containing many eggs. The various species and subspecies of *T. echinococcus* can be differentiated morphologically.

Eggs pass in the feces of the definitive host. They contaminate grass and farmland and are ingested by intermediate host animals. Humans can be infected easily, both by handling dogs or by eating contaminated vegetables.

The most frequent intermediate hosts for *E. granulosus* are sheep, cattle, pigs, and occasionally a human, and for *E. multilocularis,* various rodents, especially field mice, and very occasionally a human. With a related species of *E. oligarthrus,* the cat is the definitive host and the small rodent is an intermediate one.

The eggs of Echinococcus have an outer chitinous shell and an inner spherical larva (oncosphere) with six hooklets. They are resistant to temperature and to various physical and chemical agents and may remain viable for as long as 2 or 3 months at –16 to –18°C. Eggs are swallowed by the intermediate host, and the chitinous shell is digested in the duodenum. Embryos are liberated, penetrate the intestinal wall, and are carried by the portal bloodstream until trapped in a small capillary. The first capillary filter is the liver, where about 65 to 70 per cent of the larvae are arrested, and the next most common is the lung (20 per cent). About 10 per cent of the larvae gain access to the systemic circulation, so that almost any organ and tissue of the body can be affected (e.g., the spleen, brain, bone, kidneys).

The parasite develops in the intermediate host into a bladder-like cyst, which grows at a rate of approximately 1 cm per year. The growing hydatid cyst becomes isolated from adjacent tissues by a connective tissue membrane that represents a host defense mechanism. Calcification of this membrane is not exceptional. Inside this outer wall develops a semipermeable laminated cuticle and an inner germinal layer consisting of nucleated epithelium which gives rise to brood capsules. In these capsules, scolices develop which are released into the fluid of the cysts and fall to the bottom by gravity. This is referred to as hydatid sand, and it may contain as many as 400,000 scolices per milliliter. Daughter and granddaughter cysts may develop in the germinal layer, and some cysts may thus become huge (50 cm or more).

In the case of alveolar cysts, these are minute ones containing a jelly-like substance. They have a very thin laminated membrane, are not surrounded by connective tissue, and grow by exogenous budding, forming conglomerates of small vesicles (alveolosis) which penetrate the surrounding tissues. They can metastasize via the circulation, and their growth is considered to be malignant.

Carnivorous and omnivorous definitive hosts eat infected carcasses and offal of intermediate hosts; scolices contained in the cysts are liberated in the duodenum and adhere to the small intestine where they develop into adult worms. The eggs are excreted in the feces and are ingested by intermediate hosts, and the whole cycle starts again.

GEOGRAPHIC DISTRIBUTION

Echinococcosis caused by *E. granulosus* is particularly frequent in Balkan and Mediterranean countries (Greece, southern Italy, Sardinia, the Iberian Peninsula, and Algeria); in the Middle and Far East (India, Turkey, Iraq, Iran, Israel, Lebanon, and Syria); in some South American countries (Argentina, Uruguay, and Chile); and in Africa, mainly in the north, east, and south, with Ethiopia, Sudan, and Kenya representing areas of extremely high incidence. In the past, echinococcosis was also endemic in Cyprus, New Zealand, and Australia but has been eradicated. Echinococcosis is very rare in the United States, where it is encountered mainly in immigrants.

On the other hand, human disease due to *E. multilocularis* is encountered only in the Northern Hemisphere. Alaska, Canada, some areas of Switzerland, Austria, some parts of Germany, and the Soviet Union, including Siberia, are the main regions where it remains endemic.

PRESENTING SYMPTOMS AND SIGNS

Clinical symptoms of echinococcosis do not usually develop until the hydatid cyst has attained a considerable size. Symptoms may be delayed for a period of 20 years or more after the initial infection. Thus, though most infections occur in childhood, the average age of a patient at presentation is about 35 years. As many as 20 per cent of *E. granulosus* cysts of the liver and about 50 per cent of the lung may never cause symptoms. Silent cysts are not an uncommon autopsy finding in endemic areas.

Symptoms and signs are not characteristic. They depend entirely on the organs involved, on the size of the cysts, on the mechanical effects on affected organs and adjacent tissues, and on the development of complications.

Liver. About 70 per cent of the cysts are located in the liver and 90 per cent of these, in the right lobe. Liver hydatidosis is usually manifested after the cyst has attained a size of 10 or even 20 cm. About 50 per cent of the liver cysts are discovered incidentally in patients hospitalized for other reasons. The most frequent presentation is with an enlarged liver or with a slowly growing liver mass, either painless or accompanied by right upper abdominal pain (50 per cent) and discomfort. Patients with liver cysts may occasionally present with symptoms and signs caused by pressure on the biliary tract (obstructive jaundice), on the portal vein (portal hypertension), or on the hepatic veins (Budd-Chiari syndrome). Not rarely, liver echinococcosis may first present with symptoms and signs of the complications discussed later, particularly rupture in the biliary tract (15 to 25 per cent), or with allergic manifestations.

Lung. Patients usually present with cough and chest pain that is not severe and is frequently reported as discomfort or feeling of weight in the chest. Hemoptysis is not rare and may be induced by coughing. Many patients (50 per cent) are completely asymptomatic, whereas others first present with clinical features of some complication, like cyst rupture and infection.

Brain. Hydatidosis may present with symptoms and signs of increased intracranial pressure, convulsions, and sometimes focal neurologic signs. The patients are younger than those with cysts of other organs.

Cardiac. Cysts may be silent or may present with arrhythmias or with pericardial symptoms caused by rupture into the pericardium.

Kidney. Echinococcosis may cause pain, hematuria or altered renal function.

Bone. Echinococcosis often presents as a relatively painless cystic mass or as a pathologic fracture. Soft-tissue cysts also present as painless masses.

Alveolar. In alveolar echinococcosis, 90 per cent of the cysts are located in the liver. Hepatic manifestations are therefore predominant. Usual initial symptoms include vague right upper abdominal pain, epigastric discomfort, anorexia, and weight loss. Jaundice is frequently included among the initial manifestations, in contrast to *E. granulosus,* in which case jaundice is usually related to rupture of a cyst in the biliary tract. The liver is enlarged and sensitive, and its surface is often nodular. Clinical features of pulmonary and brain metastases may also be present.

COURSE

Hydatid cysts increase in size progressively. The rate of their growth is generally slow (1 cm/year) though extremely variable, depending upon the resistance of the involved tissue. With increasing size, complications develop and may cause the death of the patient. However, rupture of a cyst with evacuation of its content (e.g., into intestine or bronchi), may also lead to spontaneous healing. In the natural course of untreated cysts, calcification and death of the parasite are also included; however, calcification should not necessarily be regarded as synonymous with death of the echinococcus.

The course of alveolar echinococcosis is characterized by progressive deterioration, and untreated disease frequently (75 per cent) runs a fatal course in a mean period of 5 years from presentation. The initial manifestations aggravate progressively, and development of massive hepatomegaly, shortness of breath, ascites, and even neurologic signs due to brain metastases is frequently encountered.

COMMON COMPLICATIONS

Complications of echinococcosis due to *E. granulosis* are rupture, infection, and allergic reactions (Table 1).

Rupture. This is the most frequent complication, being either spontaneous following high intracystic pressure and pressure necrosis, or induced by manipulations and trauma. Rupture is a dangerous complication and is usually associated with dissemination, infection, and allergic reactions having a potentially fatal outcome; however, it may occasionally lead to spontaneous healing of the disease.

Liver cysts are usually located in the right lobe (90 per cent) either superficially or deeply. According to their location, rupture can occur:

1. Into the biliary tract (15 per cent) producing pain, obstructive jaundice, and cholangitis with chills and fever.
2. Into the peritoneal cavity, causing generalized infestation and a usually catastrophic syndrome with anaphylaxis and peritonitis.
3. Through the diaphragm (3.5 per cent) into the pleural space, causing pleurisy and empyema containing bile followed by bronchopleural fistula and expectoration of hydatid sand; into the lung and bronchi, causing hepatobronchial fistula; or, rarely, into the pericardium.
4. With perforation; cysts projecting from the liver surface may be in contact with other abdominal organs and can perforate them, e.g., duodenum, colon, right renal pelvis, vena cava, or even the abdominal wall.

Table 1. Major Complications of Echinococcosis

Rupture of liver cyst
Peritoneal cavity
Biliary tract (obstructive jaundice, cholangitis)
Pleural space, lung, bronchi, pericardium (through diaphragm)
Stomach, duodenum, colon, and other sites
Infection
Liver or lung abscess
Subphrenic abscess
Pleural effusion and empyema
Peritonitis
Cholangitis
Septicemia
Allergic reactions
Urticaria and other rashes with pruritus
Fever and eosinophilia
Wheezing
Anaphylactic shock

Rupture of lung cysts may cause pneumonia, anaphylactic shock, pleural invasion, or simply evacuation of the cyst contents through the bronchus by coughing up a salty-tasting clear fluid and pieces of membranes. A coexisting biliary communication may produce biliptysis.

Infection. This complication usually occurs in ruptured cysts, especially of the liver, with invading organisms being introduced through the biliary system. Active infection of the cyst results in death of the scolices, and the condition then presents as liver abscess. A suppurative process in the liver may extend to the subphrenic space, causing a subphrenic abscess, or to the peritoneal cavity, causing peritonitis.

Allergic Reactions. These are relatively common (10 to 25 per cent). With slow leakage of cyst fluid, urticaria, and other allergic manifestations may occur, whereas with cyst rupture or with needle puncture, severe anaphylactic shock may develop. Urticaria, fever, wheezing, abdominal pain, and delirium may accompany such a reaction, which can be fatal.

PHYSICAL EXAMINATION

In the absence of complications and with small cysts, physical findings are usually completely negative. Most patients remain in good health, this being true even for those with cysts that are quite large. Liver cysts of large size deeply located in the organ are accompanied only by hepatomegaly, whereas inferior and high anterior cysts are palpable as rounded, smooth, sometimes tender masses. Cysts in other organs and in soft tissues are also felt as slowly growing, smooth, cystic tumors, but if calcified they may become quite hard.

A characteristic physical sign over a cyst is a vibration or tremor produced by ballottement, known as the "hydatid thrill." But this is very rarely elicited and should not be depended upon for diagnosis.

Physical examination may be negative for cysts but positive for signs indicative of some of the described complications; such findings, particularly in areas in which echinococcosis is endemic, are of considerable diagnostic value.

LABORATORY PROCEDURES

Several laboratory tests aid in diagnosis:

Eosinophil Count. A count above 5 per cent is present in half the cases and above 7 per cent in about one quarter. Eosinophil counts are even higher (up to 20 and 25 per cent) in the presence of ruptured cysts. *Leukocytosis* accompanies an infected cyst.

Liver Function Tests. These are of little value in the diagnosis of uncomplicated hepatic disease, but increased serum bilirubin, alkaline phosphatase, and gamma-glutamyl-transferase (GGT) are found if cysts rupture into the biliary tract or on the rare occasions when pressure is produced on large ducts. Abnormal liver tests are found mostly in alveolar echinococcosis.

Casoni Test. The standardized intradermal Casoni test has been widely used for years, being considered a sensitive diagnostic procedure. Its use is now limited and it may soon be abandoned partly because of a shortage of suitable antigenic material and partly because of the availability of superior tests. The test should be performed with 0.2 ml of sterile hydatid fluid. Characteristic is the development of a wheal within 15 min. The Casoni test results should always be compared with those from a control injection. Results are positive in about 75 per cent of cases, but false-positive reactions may occur in as many as 18 per cent of normal controls.

Immunoserologic Tests. Several are used, aiming at the demonstration of serum antibodies against specific echinococcal antigens. These are the complement fixation test (CFT, or Weinberg test), the indirect hemagglutination (IHA), latex agglutination (LAT), bentonite flocculation (BFT), immunofluorescence (IF), radioimmunoassay (RIA), enzyme-linked immunosorbent assay (ELISA or EIA), immunodiffusion (ID), counterelectrophoresis (CEP) in agarose or cellulose acetate, and immunoelectrophoresis (IE). The results are influenced not only by the sensitivity of each technique but also by the composition of the antigenic material used; by cross reactivities between other serum antibodies and the antigens in the tests; and, of course, by various other factors influencing the titer, class, and specificity of antibodies produced by the host. As a result, none of them is 100 per cent sensitive and entirely specific. In practice it is advisable to use a highly sensitive, easy-to-perform test like IHA, EIA, or LAT and to subject the positive reactions to specificity control by IE or CEP in cellulose acetate, looking for the diagnostic antibodies against the echinococcus-specific arc 5 antigen.

Microscopic Examination. The finding of suspicious material in sputum, gastric juice, bile, or urine in cases of ruptured cysts may be helpful in detecting scolices and parts of membranes. In the case of suspected liver echinococcosis, needle liver biopsy and needle aspiration are contraindicated.

RADIOLOGIC EVALUATION

A plain film of the abdomen may give important information, showing calcified cysts, a calcified rim, or irregular calcifications. Diaphragmatic distortion, an opaque line around the cyst, intrahepatic gas bubbles, and the "water lily sign" (caused by membranes and vesicles floating on the surface of fluid in a cyst) may be detected by radiologic examination in liver echinococcosis.

Cholangiograms are also of value, mainly to check the patency of the biliary system.

Lung hydatids typically appear radiologically as oval opacities or as a cavity with a fluid level. The water lily sign may be positive. In complicated cases, pleural effusion or hydropneumothorax may be detected.

Angiography, once very useful for the differential diagnosis of cysts from tumors and for demonstrating their location, number, and size, has been replaced by computed tomography (CT) and by ultrasonography.

OTHER DIAGNOSTIC PROCEDURES

Radioisotope Scanning. Liver scans are of great value in demonstrating hepatic cysts of size over 3 cm. The cysts appear as cold areas and cannot be differentiated with confidence from tumors.

Ultrasonography. This technique has been found to be extremely helpful in detecting cysts in various organs and is the method of choice in differentiating cystic from solid lesions. It may also help in differentiating between unilocular and multilocular cysts. However, it is not applicable in the diagnosis of lung and other cysts and may also give some false-positive results in neoplastic lesions with central necrosis and cavitation, particularly in hepatocellular carcinoma. Distinguishing hydatid from simple cysts may also be difficult.

Computed Tomography. This is the imaging technique of choice in the diagnosis of echinococcosis. It shows clearly and precisely the presence, number, and size of hepatic, pulmonary, kidney, brain, and other cysts. Computed tomography can easily differentiate echinococcosis from solid tumors and even from abscesses (Fig. 1). However, differentiation from simple cysts is not always possible.

POTENTIAL ERRORS AND PITFALLS IN DIAGNOSIS

The diagnosis of echinococcosis is seldom mistaken in an endemic area, particularly when a cystic swelling is detected and radiography shows compatible findings. Immunologic and other laboratory procedures usually confirm the diagnosis. However, the clinical picture may be extremely puzzling and misleading, particularly in complicated disease, with uncommon localizations of the cysts, and mostly in alveolar echinococcosis, which resembles malignant disease. In such cases, the appropriate confirmatory immunologic tests, which are also positive in *E. alveolaris,* are not ordered and diagnostic errors both by internists and surgeons are quite common. The high degree of suspicion required for diagnosis is practically achieved only in endemic areas. Even so, laboratory procedures may be misleading, giving rise to diagnostic errors. Thus, in patients with calcified or dead cysts, serologic test results may be falsely negative because of low or negative titers of serum antibodies. Confusing serologic results due to nonspecific reactions may also be obtained in patients with other hepatic disorders.

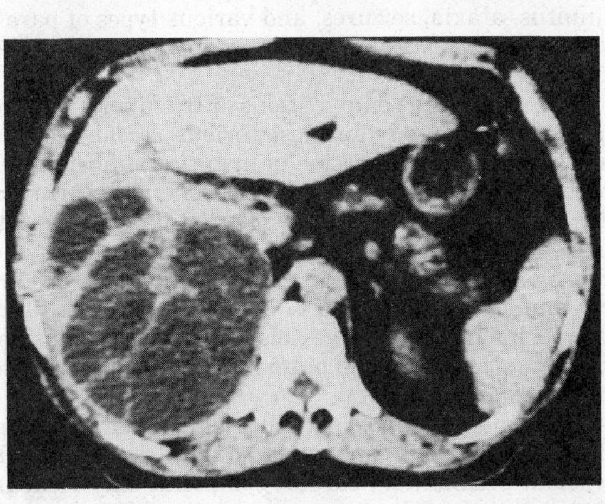

Figure 1. CT scan of the liver showing hydatid disease of the right lobe with multiple daughter cysts and calcification. (Courtesy of Dr. K. Strigaris.)

Lung cysts frequently give negative results in immunologic tests, and radiological appearances may be confused with those of solid tumors.

Intrahepatic calcifications may be due to other causes such as hemangiomas or old bacterial abscesses. They can also be confused with calcifications of adjacent structures such as adrenals, kidney, diaphragm, and costal cartilages, leading to unnecessary or wrong operations.

Errors and pitfalls in diagnosis have been significantly reduced with the use of CT and ultrasonography, but even so multilocular cysts and alveolar disease may still be confused with some neoplastic and other lesions; moreover, a clear-cut distinction between hydatid and simple cysts is not always possible.

TRICHINOSIS

By Zbigniew S. Pawlowski, M.D.
Poznań, Poland

SYNONYMS

Trichinellosis, trichiniasis.

DEFINITION

The term trichinosis implies both the infection with *Trichinella spiralis* and the disease caused by *T. spiralis.*

Trichinella spiralis is a nematode parasitizing the intestinal tract and muscle tissue of humans and many domesticated and wild mammals. The disease in its acute stage is characterized by hypersensitivity reactions, acute myositis, and metabolic disorders. Circulatory, neurologic, and pulmonary complications are not uncommon and may be fatal.

Trichinosis tends to occur in epidemics caused by the same infected meat; however, isolated cases in which the diagnosis may be more difficult are occasionally reported. Trichinosis is now not so common in the United States as it was 30 to 50 years ago, but as many as 206 cases were reported in 1981.

BIOLOGIC BACKGROUND

Trichinosis is acquired by ingestion of *T. spiralis* larvae encysted in meat. Adult worms, which develop in the small intestine, start to produce newborn *T. spiralis* larvae as early as the fifth day after consumption of infected meat. The larvae are carried in the bloodstream to different tissues and organs but develop further only in the muscle tissue. Adult worms may survive in the human intestine for about 2 months, but most of the larvae are produced in the first few weeks. The muscle larvae may live for many years, but usually they die off gradually and become calcified or absorbed.

There are some definite intraspecies variants of *T. spiralis*. An African strain, *T. spiralis v. nelsoni*, causes a relatively mild trichinellosis in humans, whereas an Arctic strain, *T. spiralis v. nativa*, is more likely to cause serious disease.

SYMPTOMS AND SIGNS

Trichinosis is characterized by a remarkable variety of symptoms and signs, which occur in a sequence reflecting the successive pathologic processes.

The abdominal syndrome, consisting of abdominal pain and diarrhea, may be the first to appear as a result of trichinous enteritis. It may also occur or recur between the third and fifth weeks of disease, probably because of a delayed hypersensitivity reaction.

The general trichinous syndrome consists of fever, followed by myalgia and malaise. The pathomechanism of the fever remains unclear; some toxins or immunologic phenomena are suspected to activate endogenous pyrogens. Myalgia is related to acute myositis; there is some spontaneous muscle pain, but intensity normally increases greatly with movement. Immobilization of untreated patients may lead to fixed contractures in the later stage of disease.

The allergic vasculitis, present early in moderate and severe trichinosis, manifests itself in the leakage of fluid from the vascular to the interstitial compartment, best visible as periorbital edema, and in hemorrhages. The latter may occur in many organs, but can be seen most easily in the conjunctiva and as splinter hemorrhages of fingernail beds.

Metabolic disorders such as hypoalbuminemia, hypokalemia, and hypoglycemia are usually related to the intensity of infection and do not occur before the third week of trichinosis. Hypoalbuminemia is clinically expressed by hydrostatic edema and effusions in the peritoneal and pleural cavities. Signs of hypokalemia may best be seen in electrocardiographic (ECG) tracings in the later stages of disease.

COURSE OF TRICHINOSIS

The clinical course of trichinosis usually varies considerably in the individuals involved, even in some epidemic outbreaks. The incubation period of acute trichinosis (fever, myalgia, periorbital edema, eosinophilia) is between 5 and 51 days. Usually it is shorter in severe cases.

Trichinosis may be asymptomatic, or it may have one of these clinical courses.

1. In *asymptomatic* cases, history of exposure and serologic tests (if performed 4 to 8 weeks after ingestion of infected meat) may be the only positive findings; eosinophilia may be transient.
2. In *abortive* cases, eosinophilia is usually present in addition to a few transient signs (some fever and/or myalgia for 1 to 2 days).
3. *Mild* cases usually show a complex of signs (fever, myalgia, periorbital edema) mildly expressed. Fever in patients not treated with steroids is below 38°C and lasts for less than a week.
4. In *moderate* cases, the full complex of signs is well expressed with fever over 38°C for up to 2 weeks and hypoalbuminemia below 3 gm/dl in untreated cases. Complications are still rare and/or transient, and recovery occurs within 5 to 7 weeks.
5. In *severe* cases, the full complex of signs is intensively expressed. Fever above 39°C may be present for more than 2 weeks, hypoalbuminemia may be below 2.5 gm/dl and eosinophilia may be absent. Circulatory, neurologic, and/or pulmonary complications are common. Recovery is slow and takes at least 7 weeks.

COMMON COMPLICATIONS

The diagnosis may be difficult in the later stages of trichinosis, at which time complications appear that dominate the clinical picture. The complications are mainly due to the ectopic migration of *T. spiralis* larvae and/or inflammatory or hypersensitive reactions of the host. Sometimes the complications are secondary, for example, to metabolic disorders.

The orbital manifestations such as periorbital edema or conjunctival hemorrhages are sometimes the first signs suggesting trichinosis. Later on, pain in the eyeball, disturbed vision, photophobia, and blurring may occur.

The neurologic manifestations appear early on or later; they may be of a diffuse or a focal character. Symptoms and signs of meningitis and encephalitis, such as strong headache, insomnia, delirium, and apathy, are usually early and diffuse. Focal manifestations such as hemianopsia, aphasia, anisocordia, tinnitus, ataxia, seizures, and various types of paralysis and paresis usually develop during or after the third week of disease.

Cardiovascular complications of trichinosis are the most frequent and the most serious. Focal necrosis and/or cellular infiltration of myocardial fibers later becomes more diffuse, causing an eosinophilic myocarditis that may eventually evolve into an interstitial myocarditis. The myocardial changes are only one cause of circulatory complications; the others are arrhythmias, adrenal gland insufficiency, and functional changes of blood vessels. Extreme hypotension, thrombosis, emboli, and pulmonary complications are not uncommon.

The major causes of death in trichinosis are myocarditis, encephalitis, and pneumonitis. Sudden death without premonitory cardiac symptoms may occur in the first week of the disease but is more likely to occur later on as a result of pulmonary embolism or paroxysmal tachycardia.

PHYSICAL EXAMINATION

In trichinosis, physical examination is of somewhat limited diagnostic importance. One may suspect trichinosis only by finding symptoms and signs that are not pathognomonic, by having a history of exposure to infected meat, and by finding very high eosinophilia. Trichinosis may be confirmed by the observation of a characteristic clinical course, by a positive reaction to corticosteroid and/or mebendazole treatment, and by positive serologic tests. However, the definitive diagnosis of trichinosis can be based only on finding the parasite.

Fever, myalgia, and malaise are common in many other diseases. However, muscle symptoms and signs have some characteristic features:

1. Pain is referred to the muscles most frequently used (masseters, tongue, extraocular and respiratory muscles, neck, and flexor muscles of the extremities).
2. Because pain increases greatly with movement, patients usually keep their elbows, hips, and knee joints flexed and do not like to change their position.
3. The muscles of the extremities are tender to palpation and painful with induced movement or deeper pressure.
4. Flexor contractions may induce tetanic rigidity.

Far more characteristic, but by no means universal, symptoms of trichinosis include periorbital edema and conjunctival or fingernail hemorrhages.

LABORATORY PROCEDURES

Eosinophilia, leukocytosis, increased activity of some enzymes, and positive specific serologic tests are of much help in the diagnosis of trichinosis.

Eosinophilia is one of the earliest, most common and characteristic findings in human trichinosis. Eosinophilia occurs during the second week after ingestion of infected meat, remains high for several weeks, and gradually declines; it can be diminished by corticosteroid therapy. It is usually well pronounced (1000 to 3000 per cu mm) and protracted for many weeks; only in aborted infections it may be slight (500 cells per cu mm) and transient. In very severe trichinosis, eosinophilia may be as high as 89 per cent or may fall sharply; this is a poor prognostic sign.

Leukocytosis is usually less consistent, less evident, and less persisting than eosinophilia. The count is usually around 15,000 per cu mm, but it may be as high as 50,000 per cu mm.

The leakage of some enzymes from muscle fibers into the serum results in an increase in serum levels of creatine phosphokinase (CPK), aldolase (ALD), and lactate dehydrogenase (LDH) in the second week of disease. Less common and less pronounced is the increase of aminotransferases (AST and ALT).

A high serum creatine level and creatinuria are usually present in intensive trichinosis.

Serologic tests become positive in the third or fourth week of infection. The most sensitive tests are passive hemagglutination (PA) and enzyme-linked immunosorbent assay (ELISA); indirect immunofluorescence (IF) is less sensitive. Flocculation or agglutination techniques with bentonite, latex, or cholesterol are highly specific but have a low sensitivity; the same is true for counterelectrophoresis and double diffusion tests. With the exception of the IF test, which becomes negative after a year, the other tests usually remain positive for a few years. In practice it is good to use two different tests at the same time and to repeat the serologic examination after 10 to 14 days in order to observe a positive conversion or an increase in their titers, which would suggest a recent infection.

PARASITOLOGIC DIAGNOSIS

A definite diagnosis of trichinosis by finding the parasite is important in a sporadic case or in an index case in an epidemic outbreak. Attempts to find adult *T. spiralis* worms in the duodenal content or in the feces are impractical. Finding adult worms in small intestinal mucosa scrapings during postmortem examination has been reported. A few newborn *T. spiralis* larvae can be isolated by filtration of several milliliters of blood through filters with 3-micron pores.

Finding the older larval stages of *T. spiralis* requires biopsy of muscle tissue. Muscle biopsy not only confirms the presence (or absence) of trichinosis but also gives an idea of the intensity of infection and enables identification of the *T. spiralis* strain (by a cross-fertilization test with known strains). The character and intensity of some pathologic changes found in the biopsied muscle tissue may also be helpful for a better understanding of the clinical picture and for decisions concerning specific therapy.

The preferred superficial skeletal muscles for biopsy are the deltoideus of the shoulder or the gastrocnemius of the leg. The muscle sample (0.5 to 1.0 gm) is usually divided into a smaller part (¼) for fixation and subsequent histopathologic examination, and a larger part (¾) for parasitologic examinations. This consists of trichinoscopy (microscopical examination of tiny cuts of muscle compressed between two glass slides) followed by digestion. The same muscle tissue samples used as for trichinoscopy can be digested in 1 per cent pepsin and 1 per cent hydrochloric acid solution at 38°C. After a few hours, the excysted larvae can be collected from the washed sediment. The digestion technique is not practicable for nonencysted *T. spiralis* larvae, i.e., younger than 16 days. After trichinoscopy, a small sample with *T. spiralis* encysted larvae may be fed to mice in order to keep the strain for further investigations.

POTENTIAL ERRORS AND PITFALLS IN DIAGNOSIS

Human trichinosis frequently remains undiagnosed or is incorrectly diagnosed, especially in sporadic or index cases, because of the diversity and wide variation in symptoms and signs during different periods of the disease.

In the incubation period of trichinosis, food intoxication and nonspecific gastroenterocolitis are commonly misdiagnosed. The acute general trichinosis syndrome (fever, myalgia, malaise) is similar to several viral infections as well as to typhoid fever, leptospirosis, rheumatic fever, and septicemia.

The syndrome of allergic vasculitis may be confused with dermatomyositis, periarteritis nodosa, angioneurotic edema, serum sickness, and drug allergy. Neurologic, pulmonary, or cardiac complications may sometimes overshadow other signs and symptoms of trichinosis.

In some severe cases, the lack of eosinophilia or a positive serologic test for typhoid may be misleading.

Trichinosis is most likely to occur in patients living in the well-known endemic areas, but it should also be considered in tourists or hunters visiting exotic states or countries (e.g., Alaska, Hawaii, Egypt, Kenya, Tanzania, Thailand).

Section Three

EARS, NOSE, AND THROAT

OTITIS EXTERNA

By David N. F. Fairbanks. M.D.
Washington, D.C.

DEFINITION AND SYNONYMS

Otitis externa is an inflammatory process of the skin of the external ear canal. The term is inclusive of several differing pathologic entities as noted in the following outline:

1. Acute otitis externa ("swimmer's ear").
2. Otomycosis ("fungus ear," "jungle ear").
3. Seborrheic otitis externa.
4. Allergic otitis externa.

SIGNS, SYMPTOMS, AND PHYSICAL FINDINGS

Acute otitis externa is characterized by severe pain and tenderness in the ear, with a scanty greenish-gray discharge that obstructs the ear canal and impairs hearing. It usually occurs the evening or day after the patient has been swimming or after some other event that allowed water into the ear canal, such as hair washing, showering, or washing the ear with water for removal of ear wax.

The characteristic physical finding is tenderness to pressure on the tragal cartilage. Similar pain is elicited when the ear is pulled. The skin of the ear canal is red and swollen and usually is too tender to allow the examiner to insert the ear speculum. For this reason, and also because of purulent secretions mixed with ear wax, the tympanic membrane is often not seen.

Otomycosis, by contrast, creates little pain, with more of a sensation of itching and blockage of the ear with a fluid that sloshes back and forth. The ear canal contains a whitish secretion the texture of cottage cheese, with surface patches of black, which, on magnified inspection, prove to be fuzzy spores. There is little swelling of the ear canal skin or tenderness of the ear or tragus.

Seborrheic otitis externa is characterized by chronic itching of the ears and a reddened scaly ear canal skin with overproduction of scaly ear wax. It may be the only site of seborrheic dermatitis in the patient, but more often other sites are also affected, such as the scalp. Patients with this condition are prone to develop acute otitis externa easily when water is allowed into their ear canals.

Allergic otitis externa is a reaction to ear drops that have been used to soften ear wax or to treat infection. The history is suggestive. The patient exhibits pain, tenderness, reddening, swelling, and blistering of the ear canal and nearby skin. Another type of allergic reaction occurs against fungal infections of skin elsewhere on the body. It causes itching and scaliness similar to seborrheic otitis externa.

COMPLICATIONS

Necrotizing (malignant) otitis externa involving the ear and scalp and extending intracranially is a rare complication of acute otitis externa. It occurs in elderly, diabetic, or debilitated patients with compromised host defenses.

LABORATORY FINDINGS

Culture studies of secretions in acute otitis externa yield *Pseudomonas aeruginosa* in most instances. Occasionally *Staphylococcus aureus* or *Proteus* will be present. Otomycosis yields *Aspergillus niger.*

PITFALLS IN DIAGNOSIS

Otitis externa is frequently misdiagnosed as acute otitis media because of the pain and otorrhea. Tenderness of the tragus is the distinguishing diagnostic sign because pressure on the cartilage stretches the ear canal skin, creating pain in external canal infections but not in otitis media. Furthermore, the tympanic membrane, when visible, is seen as normal in most external ear infections. Postauricular swelling due to cellulitis and postauricular lymphadenopathy in advanced otitis externa may mimic some signs of acute coalescent mastoiditis, and the mastoid x-rays may even show haziness owing to inflamed overlying skin. However, otitis externa runs a rapid course with pain and swelling appearing in a few days. Mastoiditis, on the other hand, takes 10 to 14 days to develop after the initial onset of acute suppurative otitis media.

Folliculitis or furunculosis of the ear canal skin may mimic acute otitis externa, but the inflammatory lesion is more localized and generally does not extend deeply into the ear canal.

Herpes zoster can affect the ear canal. It also affects the seventh and eighth cranial nerves, creating facial paralysis, neural hearing loss, and vertigo. The ear canal, the ear, and nearby facial skin exhibit painful vesicular eruptions.

OTITIS MEDIA

By David N. F. Fairbanks, M.D.
and Robert E. Pumphrey, M.D.
Washington, D.C.

DEFINITION

Otitis media is an inflammatory process of the middle ear, the anatomic area that includes the tympanic membrane, the ossicles, the mastoid and tympanic air spaces with their mucous membrane linings, and the eustachian tube. The term is inclusive of several differing pathologic entities, as noted in the following outline:

1. Acute otitis media: bacterial or viral infection of the middle ear.
   a. Acute suppurative otitis media.
   b. Acute coalescent mastoiditis.
   c. Acute necrotizing otitis media.
   d. Bullous myringitis.
2. Persistent otis media with effusion: retention of secretions in the middle ear.
   a. Unresolved acute otitis media.
   b. Allergic otitis media.
   c. Baro-otitis.
   d. Congenital-mechanical eustachian tube dysfunction.
3. Chronic otitis media–tympanomastoiditis.
   a. With perforation.
   b. With cholesteatoma.
   c. Tuberculous.

SIGNS, SYMPTOMS, AND PHYSICAL FINDINGS

Acute otitis media is characterized by pain and a stuffy or blocked sensation in the ear. In the first few hours of the disease, the inflammation affects the mucosa of the middle ear space and the eustachian tube, yet the tympanic membrane is deceptively normal: The normal tympanic membrane is somewhat translucent and has the color, thickness, and tensile strength of waxed paper. Minute blood vessels can be seen coursing around the periphery of the membrane and down the long process ("handle") of the malleus bone where it is attached to the membrane. Acute otitis media is first detectable when these vessels become engorged, but the examiner may not detect this change as abnormal unless he or she compares the painful ear with the one on the opposite side.

Within 24 hours the entire tympanic membrane becomes erythematous and overvascularized, and in the ensuing days the membrane loses its concave appearance and bulges because of the accumulation of inflammatory secretions in the middle ear space. The light reflex on the membrane is often (but not always) lost when the membrane bulges. Pus in the middle ear adds a yellow hue to the reddened membrane.

If untreated, the inflammation will lead to such pressure and weakening of the membrane that spontaneous perforation occurs, releasing yellow secretions into the ear canal. The perforation is usually pinhole-sized and is not seen by the examiner if secretions obscure the view. The secretions are usually pulsatile, which reflects the state of vascular engorgement of the membranes.

In acute necrotizing otitis media, the vascular supply of the tympanic membrane is infarcted and the central portions of the membrane become necrotic and virtually disappear, which results in a large horseshoe-shaped perforation. This is seen in children with high fever and concurrent infections such as scarlet fever or measles.

Bullous myringitis appears as blister-like lesions on the surface of the tympanic membrane. They resemble the labial lesions of herpes simplex. Usually they contain only serous clear fluid, but they may become hemorrhagic and look like blood blisters. This type of infection is extraordinarily painful.

Acute coalescent mastoiditis is an extension of acute suppurative otitis media into the mastoid air spaces and bone. It follows the acute episode by about 10 to 14 days and is characterized by a recurrence of pain and ear discharge. Tenderness and swelling behind the ear and a bulging displacement of the ear forward and away from the head are ominous signs.

Persistent otitis media with effusion is a prevalent disease in children and it is occasionally seen in adults as a sequel to acute otitis media with incomplete recovery of eustachian tube function. Any event that compromises the function of the tube will lead to such a condition. Notable examples are allergies of the upper airways, infections of the adenoids and nasopharynx, and the cleft palate deformity. Barotitis, barotrauma, and tympanic squeeze are terms describing malfunction of the eustachian tube during rapid changes in air pressure such as those encountered in airplane travel and scuba diving, especially when the patient has a respiratory infection.

Most adults find the stuffy, blocked sensation in the ear caused by otitis media with effusion distressing enough to seek medical attention. However, many children do not, and the disease is discovered on routine physical examinations or on school screening tests for hearing. Tuning fork tests show better hearing by bone than by air, but not always. Changes in the appearance of the tympanic membrane are subtle and easily overlooked. They include any of the following:

1. Air-fluid levels (bubbles) behind the membrane.
2. Retraction of the membrane with rotation of the malleus handle posterior-superiorly.
3. Discoloration of the membrane due to color in the fluid behind it, usually an amber or "old dishwater" color, but sometimes blue or black from hemorrhage.
4. Increased vascularity and thickening of the membrane with loss of its translucency.
5. Decreased mobility of the membrane to changes in air pressure. This is demonstrated by the application of alternating positive and negative air pressure against the drum, utilizing the pneumatic otoscope. Decreased mobility suggests fluid in the middle ear space. Absent mobility suggests a perforation.

Chronic otitis media is characterized by hearing loss from damage to the tympanic membrane and ossicles, and by recurring drainage from the ear. The tympanic membrane appears thickened with calcific white patches in some patients; in others there are thin atrophic areas, and perforations of various sizes and shapes may be present. Contamination of the middle ear occurs through the perforation whenever the patient allows water to enter the ear, such as when swimming or showering, and this is followed by drainage of yellow-brown or gray pus through the perforation. During such an active infection, the middle ear mucosa (visible through the perforation) is reddened and edematous. When no active infection is present, there are no visible secretions, and through the "dry" perforation the middle ear mucosa is seen as a transparent glistening covering over the white bone.

A "perforation" in the superior part of the membrane may actually be a retraction pocket where skin from the tympanic membrane is inverted into the mastoid air cells. If it becomes large and deep, it will retain the keratin that epidermal cells shed and an epidermal inclusion cyst will develop in the mastoid. This condition is known as cholesteatoma and is today's most common form of mastoiditis. On examination the perforation appears to be filled with cheesy seborrheic debris and, when infected, with foul-smelling discharge.

Tuberculous otitis begins with multiple small perforations that subsequently coalesce into a larger one, and painless drainage with hearing loss ensues.

COMMON COMPLICATIONS

All varieties of otitis media produce a conductive hearing loss. Mastoiditis is the notable complication of otitis media. From the mastoid the infection can extend into the labyrinth (labyrinthitis), intracranially (subdural empyema, brain abscess, meningitis), into the facial or abducens nerves (seventh or sixth nerve paralysis), or into the deep tissue planes of the neck (Bezold's abscess).

LABORATORY FINDINGS

Audiometry reveals the presence and severity of conductive hearing loss characteristic of otitis media. It is unnecessary in acute otitis unless the diagnosis is in question; in otitis media with effusion it aids considerably in confirming the diagnosis. Fluid in the middle ear creates mild losses from 5 to 40 decibels. Patients with small perforations due to chronic otitis media may exhibit no hearing loss; those with larger perforations show mild losses in the range of 20 to 40 decibels. A hearing loss of 40 to 60 decibels suggests destruction of the ossicular chain. Tympanometry (impedance audiometry) showing impaired mobility of the middle ear structures suggests effusion. Exaggerated mobility suggests disruption of the ossicular chain, and failure to obtain an airtight seal suggests a perforation.

Cultures taken from middle ear secretions in acute suppurative otitis media reveal *Streptococcus pneumoniae* and *Hemophilus influenzae* as the predominant pathogens, accounting for 70 per cent of cases (in about equal proportions). *Streptococcus pyogenes* is an occasional pathogen. *Branhamella catarrhalis* is more common and is actually pathogenic. Bullous myringitis may be caused by any of the foregoing, or by the *Mycoplasma pneumoniae* organism. Nasopharyngeal cultures correlate with middle ear cultures in only 50 per cent of instances.

Chronic otitis media pathogens are those of external origin that commonly contaminate open wounds: *Pseudomonas aeruginosa, Bacteroides fragilis, Staphylococcus aureus,* and *Proteus.*

Mastoid x-rays are helpful only when mastoiditis is suspected, and such films are easily overinterpreted since even acute suppurative otitis media produces clouding of the mastoid air cells. However, when the bony partitions between such cells are eroded, the condition is termed coalescent mastoiditis, which is a surgical emergency. Chronic otitis media produces a sclerotic, constricted mastoid air system that has little clinical significance.

PITFALLS IN DIAGNOSIS

Otitis media is probably overdiagnosed as a cause of fever in children. Young children when screaming and restrained often demonstrate a flushed, erythematous appearance not only of the face but the eardrum as well. The appearance is indistinguishable from that of early acute otitis media. The child should therefore be examined when he is quietly sitting in his mother's lap.

Otitis media must be distinguished from otitis externa, since the disease processes and treatments are entirely different.

Earache does not necessarily signal ear infection. Indeed, the ear is the target of referred pain from almost any structure in the head and neck. Ear pain that is transitory, waxing and waning without treatment, is almost certainly a "referred" otalgia. Following is a list of anatomic sites that refer pain to the ear:

1. Temporomandibular joint: dysfunction due to malocclusion, teeth grinding, or faulty chewing patterns.
2. Teeth: caries, abscess, or "cutting" teeth in children.
3. Tonsils: inflammation or tumor, especially ear pain after tonsillectomy.
4. Adenoids and nasopharynx: inflammation or tumor.
5. Sinuses: inflammation or tumor.
6. Salivary glands: inflammation or tumor.
7. Base of tongue: inflammation or tumor.
8. Larynx or hypopharynx: inflammation or tumor.

Any patient with earache, normal-appearing tympanic membrane, and normal hearing deserves a thorough examination of these structures.

DISORDERS OF THE PARANASAL SINUSES

By Stanley W. Coulthard, M.D.
and Roger W. Miller, M.D.
Tucson, Arizona

The nose and paranasal sinuses are considered together from the diagnostic perspective because of the overlap of clinical symptoms and signs. The sinuses are lined by respiratory epithelium and are named after the bones in which they develop. The sinuses and nasal chambers are closely associated with the orbits, base of the skull, oropharynx, and pterygomaxillary spaces. Disorders of congenital, neoplastic, traumatic, and infectious etiologies may present by disturbing the contiguous structures. Diagnosis in each case must identify all of the contributing factors, estimate the stage of disease progression, and anticipate the clinical course and possible complications.

AIDS TO DIAGNOSIS

A thorough history and physical examination to evaluate airway obstruction, pain, and nasal discharge are sufficient for good diagnosis in most clinical cases. The physical must include a complete head and neck direct and indirect examination.

Nasal airway obstruction is not indicative of allergy alone. Fixed nasal obstruction in early childhood would suggest lesser degrees of choanal atresia overlooked in infancy or of severe adenoid hypertrophy. Anterior rhinoscopy after topical decongestion and nasopharyngeal examination confirm the diagnosis. Variable nasal obstruction is associated with nasal septal deformities as well as allergic diatheses. Contributing factors are dependent congestion during sleep, cyclical vasomotor changes, and rebound congestion from rhinitis medicamentosa acquired in self-treatment of the symptoms of obstruction. Onset at middle age may indicate the contribution of flaccid alar tissues with inspiratory nasal collapse or the pharmacologic effects from drugs such as reserpine and prazosin. More distal causes of respiratory compromise such as acquired sleep apnea and primary pulmonary and cardiac diseases may be mistakenly attributed to coexistent nasal abnormalities. Progressive nasal obstruction at any age is a harbinger of neoplasia in the nose, nasopharynx, or sinuses and necessitates a complete evaluation. Granulomatous and infiltrative diseases such as tuberculosis, Wegener's granulomatosis, midline granuloma, mucormycosis, sarcoid, and others must also be considered in such cases.

Pain in sinus disorders is localized over the involved sinuses, except in sphenoid sinus disease, in which case pain may be retro-orbital or referred to the vertex or occiput. It is aching in quality, and its course is related to the underlying disease process. When pain is the predominant or sole symptom, a broader perspective is required. Consideration should be given to common tension and vascular headaches, to neuritic causes with lancinating features and dysesthesias, to pain of occult dental disease, and to temporomandibular joint disease with its many manifestations.

Postnasal drainage of itself is normal; awareness of its presence usually indicates a pharyngeal disorder or nasal abnormality rather than sinus pathology. The character of the discharge, other than that noted on arising, should be assessed for truly purulent features or the presence of blood. Complete nasal and nasopharyngeal examinations are essential in this evaluation.

Current diagnostic adjuncts will be discussed in a following section. Culture of nasal secretions poorly reflects sinus flora in acute infections. Contrast sinography is of historical interest only, and ultrasound has no established place in the diagnostic armamentarium.

PRESENTING SIGNS AND SYMPTOMS

Sinusitis

Sinusitis arises in the setting of obstruction and contamination from viral infection, trauma, allergy, neoplasia, or dental disease. Pain becomes intense when obstruction of the sinus ostium occurs or a dental focus is present, and purulent drainage may diminish or be absent at such times. Dependency or straining typically exacerbates the pain in this instance and toxicity, spread to neighboring sinuses, and complicating orbital or facial cellulitis or central extension are more likely to occur. Unilateral sinusitis especially must occasion concern for a dental or neoplastic basis and requires follow-up until complete resolution is achieved or until the cause is clearly established. In children, a nasal foreign body is the most likely cause.

Chronic sinus infection occurs when specific local causes, such as allergy, nasal polyps, tumors, septal deformities, foreign bodies, or dental foci, are not discovered or managed; when irreversible damage has already occurred to the respiratory membranes; and when cystic fibrosis or local or systemic immune deficiency disorders are present. The history is that of repeated recurrence or relapse with aching discomfort, purulent drainage, and nasal obstruction.

Allergy

Allergy classically presents as episodic seasonal or perennial sneezing, congestion, itching, and rhinorrhea. The patient may or may not be aware of the responsible inhaled or ingested allergens. In cases of perennial allergy, dust, molds, and danders are often responsible. The patient may experience symptoms on retiring or arising in cases of house-dust allergy. Cat dander is a frequent cause of symptoms, although pet owners are reluctant to accept this possibility. Often, the relevance of a cause in the home is convincing only when remission of symptoms is apparent during a vacation or other trip away from the home.

A significant number of allergy patients do not have florid symptoms. They may have symptoms of other sequelae or accompaniments, such as recurrent rhinosinusitis, bronchitis, asthma, or nocturnal cough, or they may have had prior nasal surgery such as polypectomy. In small children, unless there are significant symptoms and an appreciable response to a plain antihistamine, chronic rhinosinusitis and/or adenoid hypertrophy should be suspected.

Neoplasms

Neoplasms of the paranasal sinuses usually present with symptoms of progressive nasal obstruction and changes in nasal secretions. Unsuccessful treatment of infections or obstruction at any age necessitates exclusion of a neoplasm.

Maxillary sinus neoplasms ultimately penetrate the bony confines and produce a mass in the cheek or buccal sulcus; displace teeth or dentures to cause malocclusion; invade the orbital floor, causing hypesthesia, diplopia, and epiphora; or invade posteriorly into the masticator muscles, causing trismus.

Ethmoid and frontal sinus neoplasms may present as a bulge at the medial or superior-medial orbital margins, respectively. Epiphora due to lacrimal obstruction and downward or outward protrusion of the globe may develop. Later, extraocular muscle infiltration may result in diplopia.

Sphenoid and nasopharyngeal neoplasms are often late in manifesting themselves and may in fact present with metastatic nodes below the mastoid tip. Postnasal obstruction and symptomatic drainage, eustachian tube obstruction with middle ear effusion, and, later, pain and optic nerve and extraocular dysfunction are common.

COURSE

Acute sinusitis usually resolves over a 7- to 10-day period, depending on mucosal resolution and re-established aeration of the involved sinus. Chronic sinusitis will respond to a variable degree only when an underlying remediable medical or surgical cause is identified and appropriately treated. Allergy will respond variably, depending on long-term therapy appropriate to the individual case. Neoplastic diseases follow fairly known and predictable courses, depending on the histologic type; and outcome depends on the stage of the disease at the time of correct diagnosis.

PHYSICAL EXAMINATION

The nose is examined with a nasal speculum and head mirror, noting anatomic asymmetries of the septum and turbinates; mucosal color and engorgement; and the amount, nature, and location of secretions. A vasoconstrictor such as ½ per cent Neosynephrine on cotton pledgets is then placed in the nose and the patient is examined for local tenderness over the sinuses, for soft-tissue and orbital involvement, for evidence of eustachian obstruction and middle ear effusion, and for signs of primary or secondary dental abnormalities. Nasopharyngeal mirror examination, including the posterior choanae, is then performed for possible mass lesions and to pinpoint the source of abnormal secretions. The nasal pledgets are removed, and the nasal cavities can then be adequately examined as far as the adenoid pad.

Infections

Nasal membranes are inflamed in acute infections, and purulent secretions may be seen only after suitable decongestion. A middle meatus origin indicates frontal, maxillary, or anterior ethmoid sinus infection. Posterior ethmoid and sphenoid drainage appears posteriorly from above the middle turbinate. When the sinus is draining, tenderness over the sinus is usually absent or mild. When obstruction is complete and the infection is confined, drainage may be scant and tenderness to palpation and percussion exquisite. Dental examination may reveal percussion tenderness of the teeth, oro-antral fistulae, or a periapical phlegmon contributing to and sometimes masquerading as a sinusitis.

Chronic sinus infection produces less severe but more protracted discomfort. Purulent secretions are seen on adequate examination, but the membranes of the nose generally lack the intense inflammation seen in the acute episode and may, in fact, have an atrophic appearance.

Allergies

Nasal membranes are congested in nasal allergy. Although a bluish or pale color is often described, no single appearance is reliably characteristic. Secretions are clear in the absence of supervening infection and plentiful if seen during an acute diathesis. After decongestion, polyps may be visualized in the middle meati or involving the middle turbinates. Nasopharyngoscopy will sometimes reveal striking swelling of the inferior turbinates.

Neoplasms

Neoplasms must be predicated on the above-mentioned setting of slowly progressive obstruction, unilateral purulent drainage, and late development of pain because of their generally nondescript appearance on rhinoscopy. Except for those arising on the anterior septum, most neoplasms are not circumscribed but rather appear as a diffuse fullness, the major expansion of the process occurring submucosally. Most present fairly posteriorly in the nasal passage and may displace the septum to the contralateral side, causing bilateral obstruction later.

In infants and young children, rhabdomyosarcoma, teratoma, dermoids, and meningoceles are to be suspected. Males from childhood on are to be suspected of having a juvenile angiofibroma, especially if epistaxis has occurred. Obviously, biopsy is contraindicated until full radiographic assessment is completed. Squamous carcinoma, inverting papilloma, melanoma, adenocarcinoma, and minor salivary gland tumors are seen in adults. Soft-tissue neoplasms, lymphomas, plasmacytomas, and neurogenous tumors are less commonly encountered. Pain is not common and, if overlooked early, neoplasms will go on to present as deformities of craniofacial structures as previously discussed.

COMPLICATIONS

Acute infections may extend beyond the bony confines of the sinus to cause cellulitis and closed space abscesses in the face and masticator regions. They may penetrate the orbit to cause cellulitis, abscess, or orbital apex syndrome and may cause osteomyelitis of the facial or cranial skeleton; or they may extend centrally by direct or vascular diploic channels to cause meningitis, cerebritis, or intracranial abscesses. Hematogenous spread may occur with septicemia or cavernous sinus thrombosis. Except in the immunologically compromised patient, these complications arise in the setting of complete sinus obstruction. Therefore, when severe pain and toxicity, localized edema and mass effects, or mentation changes occur in acute sinusitis, immediate surgical consultation is indicated in addition to any considered antibiotic therapy.

Mucoceles are cystic expansions due to sinus obstruction of long duration. They may present as slowly developing expansions externally or internally. Reactivation of infection may lead to the complications just mentioned.

The complications of allergies are those of sinus obstruction and secondary infection and of expansion and pressure deformity. The same is true of neoplasms in addition to the prognosis of the disease entity proper.

DIAGNOSTIC TESTS

Sinus x-rays conventionally include the upright Waters, Caldwell, submental-vertex, and lateral views. Often ordered by routine, plain films add little or nothing to management determinations in the majority of patients with acute sinusitis. Mucosal thickening may be present as a residual of a long-resolved sinus infection, from acute or chronic sinusitis, as a residual of prior surgical intervention, from barotrauma, or due to allergic rhinosinusitis. Air-fluid levels reveal only that an exudate is present and clearing mechanisms are impaired—features usually quite evident from clinical evaluation. Opacification only reflects obstruction of the sinus ostium. Rather than obtaining sinus films routinely, a better course might be to elect a trial of medical therapy for the ordinary case, to perform antral irrigation which is both diagnostic and therapeutic in severe cases, and to reserve x-rays for the atypical or unresponsive situations.

When neoplasms, mucoceles, or other destructive processes are suspected, the most efficient course is to obtain specialty examination followed by a possible computed tomographic (CT) scan because of the decided superiority of this modality in differentiating fluid from soft tissue, in detailing bone destruction and displacement, and in providing better definition of the disease relationship to vital structures. Tomography, more informative by far than plain films, is being increasingly replaced by the CT scan.

Biopsy of truly suspicious lesions should not be undertaken in the primary care setting. Full specialized examination and radiographic evaluation based on that assessment should be completed first. Inadequate biopsy may give a misleading diagnosis, and bleeding requiring nasal packing will interfere with further examination and contaminate tissues unnecessarily prior to definitive treatment.

PITFALLS IN DIAGNOSIS

Common pitfalls are the acceptance of the patient's frequent self-conceived diagnosis instead of a careful elucidation of all symptom particulars, incomplete physical examinations, failure to identify contributing factors, the treatment of symptoms and signs in and of themselves, and an undue reliance on radiographic interpretation for diagnosis.

NEOPLASTIC AND NON-NEOPLASTIC LESIONS OF THE ORAL MUCOSA

By Jerry E. Bouquot, D.D.S., M.S.D.
Morgantown, West Virginia

The oral mucosa is as adept in its reflection of systemic disease as it is varied in its production of local disease that may or may not eventually extend beyond the mouth. Although a few systemic diseases with potential presenting signs on the oral mucosa are discussed in this article, emphasis has been placed on the presentation of mucosal lesions somewhat unique to, or commonly seen within, the oral cavity. Many, and occasionally all, of the diagnostic criteria of such entities are based upon close visual and tactile inspection, with special consideration of the intraoral site and the age of the patient. Relatively few sophisticated laboratory aids are required for the final diagnosis of oral complaints.

Lesions of the oral mucosa typically fall into one of the following broad categories: *white plaques or macules; red or pigmented lesions; soft-tissue masses; ulcers;* or *vesicles or bullae.* It has long been established that the diagnosis of such lesions is much more dependent on an understanding of their potential clinical presentations than on a knowledge of their various etiologies. The entities following, therefore, are listed and discussed in groups according to their most common presenting features in an attempt to aid the clinician in arriving at a rapid definitive or differential diagnosis. A quick-reference diagnosis chart is offered in Table 1, with special indication of the potential for malignant transformation for each lesion discussed.

WHITE LESIONS (SLOUGHING)

Candidiasis

Synonyms. Moniliasis, thrush, acute pseudomembranous candidiasis, candidosis, superficial monilial stomatitis.

Candidiasis is an acute or chronic superficial infection of oral or other mucous membranes by the dimorphic yeastlike fungus, *Candida albicans*. *Candida albicans* can be cultivated from most healthy individuals, and only under conditions of altered host resistance is its virulence enhanced enough to produce local, regional, or systemic manifestations of disease.

Candidiasis is found most frequently at either extremity of the age spectrum, presenting usually as curd-like, white plaques that can be scraped off to leave a raw, painful, bleeding surface. Mild cases demonstrate fine whitish papule-like deposits on an erythematous base, while severe cases showing invasion of deeper tissues are characterized by a more tenacious pseudomembrane and/or ulceration. Neonatal oral candidiasis, derived from maternal vaginal fungi, usually becomes evident on the fifth to sixth postpartum day. Adult infections are typically promoted by dry mouth, aging, poor denture hygiene, antibiotic therapy, diabetes mellitus, pregnancy, cunnilingus, and lowered body resistance due to such conditions as malabsorption, primary immune deficiencies, systemic malignancy, corticosteroid therapy, uremia, and various chronic nonfungal infections. An inherited syndrome of candidiasis—Addison's disease—and hypoparathyroidism has been described. The presence of candidal conjunctivitis and paronychial involvement of the nails of the hands is not necessarily indicative of systemic involvement, since direct spread of the fungus may be facilitated by hand-to-mouth and subsequent hand-to-eye contact.

In most otherwise healthy individuals, oral candidiasis is a self-limiting disease that may produce intermittent or continuous burning sensations, tenderness, and/or pain for years if left untreated with topical nystatin. The curd-like pseudomembranes may not always be prominent but can be replaced by a symptomatic erythema or a nonsloughing white plaque. Oral candidiasis in a debilitated patient tends to become deep-seated and to spread to the gastrointestinal and respiratory tracts, necessitating systemic therapy with amphotericin B or ketoconazole.

The most sensitive diagnostic procedure for oral candidiasis is the microscopic identification of pseudohyphae and spores via a suspension in 10 per cent potassium hydroxide; such a preparation will seldom be positive in normal individuals. The organism is cultured on Sabouraud's agar, but a positive culture must be viewed with suspicion because this microorganism can be cultured from a large percentage of healthy mouths. Tissue sections from biopsy may show pseudohyphae or spores when processed with a fungal stain such as MacManus periodic acid–Schiff (PAS), but such sections more often than not will be completely and frustratingly negative. An effective, albeit slow, diagnostic technique is a 4- to 8-week course of Mycostatin vaginal tablets (100,000 units dissolved in the mouth four times a day) or oral suspension (less effective) for those patients with strictly oral manifestations and no underlying systemic process.

Materia Alba

Synonyms. Plaque, food debris.

Materia alba is surprisingly often mistaken for the previously mentioned oral candidiasis because it presents as single or multiple curd-like white plaques on oral membranes. In reality, it is simply a mixture of food debris and bacteria and is understandably most frequent in persons with poor oral hygiene. Unlike candidiasis, materia alba leaves a nontender, nonerythematous mucosal base after being removed with a tongue blade or with gauze.

Aspirin Burn

Synonyms. Chemical burn, contact burn.

The most frequent chemical burn in the mouth is caused by direct application of an aspirin tablet to an aching tooth. Other cases may result, however, from inadvertent application of caustic medications to the mucosa by the dentist or physician. The clinical appearance of such lesions depends on the severity of tissue damage. Mild cases will produce a tender erythema, whereas more severe burns necrose and coagulate the surface of the tissue to produce a diffuse white plaque that can be scraped off to leave a painful, bleeding, erythematous surface.

Unless treated with a protective paste (Orabase), warm salt-water rinses, and a bland diet, these lesions may subject a person to 3 or 4 weeks of oral pain before healing (usually without scarring). Occasionally they become secondarily infected. With palliative therapy, most cases resolve within 7 to 12 days. Esophogeal strictures may result if enough caustic was swallowed, but this is seldom the case except with small children who swallow household cleaners.

Secondary Syphilis

Synonym. Mucous patch.

Mucous patches are smooth-surfaced white plaques with a glistening, opalescent character; they may or may not scrape off easily and are usually painless. The lesions are single or few in number, usually presenting on the tongue, lips, or soft palate 6 to 10 weeks after initial infection. Hoarseness, dysphagia, fever, swollen tonsils, and maculopapulary skin rash are other easily identifiable features that may be present. All moist lesions of secondary syphilis are extremely contagious. Intraoral lesions of secondary syphilis persist for 1 to 3 weeks, after which they resolve without scar formation.

Table 1. Differential Diagnosis and Prognosis for Oral Mucosal Lesions

Appearance of Mucosal Lesion	Differential Diagnoses	Potential for Malignant Transformation
Sloughing White Lesions	Oral candidiasis	–
	Materia alba	–
	Aspirin/chemical burn	–
	Mucous patch (secondary syphilis)	–
Keratotic, Nonsloughing White Lesions	Leukoplakia	+++
	Nicotine palatinus	–
	Tobacco (snuff) pouch	+
	Leukoedema	–
	White sponge nevus	–
	Chronic cheek bite	–
	Lichen planus	+
	Lupus erythematosus	+
	Fordyce granules	–
	White hairy tongue	–
	Geographic tongue	–
Brown-Black Pigmentation	Physiologic pigmentation	–
	Oral melanotic macule	+
	Amalgam tattoo	–
	Peutz-Jeghers syndrome	–
	Black hairy tongue	–
	Malignant melanoma	++++*
Red Lesions	Median rhomboid glossitis	–
	Lingual varicosities	–
	Papillary hyperplasia (palate)	–
	Angular cheilitis	–
	Denture sore mouth	–
	Xerostomia (dry mouth)	–
	Erythroplakia	+++
	Infectious mononucleosis	–
Mucosal Ulcers	Squamous cell carcinoma	++++*
	Traumatic ulcer	–
	Aphthous ulcer	–
	Major aphthous stomatitis	–
	Chancre (primary syphilis)	–
	Gumma (tertiary syphilis)	–
	Behçet's syndrome	–
	Neutropenia	–
	Agranulocytosis	–
	Necrotizing ulcerative gingivostomatitis	–
Blisters and Blister-like Lesions	Mucocele (and ranula)	–
	Epidermoid cyst	–
	Herpes simplex	–
	Herpangina	–
	Hand-foot-mouth disease	–
	Erythema multiforme	–
	Pemphigus vulgaris	–
	Benign mucous membrane pemphigoid (BMMP)	–
	Bullous lichen planus	+
Soft-Tissue Masses	Pyogenic granuloma	–
	Peripheral giant cell granuloma	–
	Irritation fibroma	–
	Epulis fissuratum	–
	Papilloma	–
	Phenytoin gingival hyperplasia	–
	Verrucous carcinoma	++++*
	Squamous cell carcinoma	++++*

*This lesion is already a malignancy.

A smear examined with dark-field microscopy will demonstrate motile spirochetes. (For suggested approaches to the laboratory diagnosis of this disease, the reader is referred to the article on syphilis.)

WHITE LESIONS (NONSLOUGHING)

Leukoplakia

Synonyms. Benign hyperkeratosis, oral callus, linea alba, white patch, keratosis, smoker's keratosis.

Leukoplakia is a rather common oral lesion in the United States, being seen in approximately 4 per cent of adult mouths. It typically appears as a chronic, nontender, smooth-surfaced, nonindurated white plaque of variable thickness; thin lesions appear gray and somewhat translucent. The clinical appearance is derived from a simple excess of the keratin layers of the mucosa; however, a variable amount of dysplasia may be seen within the deeper cell layers of the epithelium. The name "leukoplakia" in the dental profession is used in a strictly clinical sense to refer to a keratotic white patch that cannot be scraped off and cannot be given another more specific name. This usage differs somewhat from the medical profession's lexicon which defines "leukoplakia" as absolutely demonstrating microscopic dysplasia of the affected epithelium. The latter definition works well for vaginal and uterine cervix leukoplakias, but the presence of teeth in the mouth and the chronic mechanical trauma inherent in the process of mastication often leads to simple callus formations that are clinically indistinguishable from the so-called "premalignant" leukoplakias. Since these nonpremalignant, callus-type leukoplakias constitute about 50 per cent of all leukoplakias, it seems most practical to discontinue the microscopic dysplasia implication of the term and use the more simple clinically oriented definition.

Oral leukoplakia, especially the premalignant variants, is seldom seen in persons younger than 35 years of age. The typical leukoplakia patient is a male, 50 years or older, who smokes heavily and has been aware of his leukoplakia for at least 2 years prior to professional diagnosis. Usual sites include the buccal and commissural mucosae, but lesions of the oral floor and ventral tongue are much more worrisome because they carry a considerably higher rate of malignant transformation. The keratotic lesion of the hard palate that is called "smoker's palate," or nicotine palatinus, is not considered to transform often into malignancy.

Biopsy of affected tissues is essential and may have to be repeated numerous times during subsequent follow-up visits for those lesions too large for complete initial removal. Staining affected tissues with a metachromatic dye prior to biopsy may be helpful, in that such dyes seem to selectively stain for dysplastic epithelium (inflammatory *or* neoplastic). Oral smears are discouraged in leukoplakia lesions because the thickened keratin layer does not allow the clinician to scrape down to the deeper epithelial cells, i.e., those cells most likely to be dysplastic. Serologic testing for syphilis should be performed in patients with keratotic lesions of the dorsum of the tongue, since this is quite an unusual site for leukoplakia except in tertiary syphilis ("syphilitic glossitis").

Nicotine Palatinus

Synonyms. Nicotine stomatitis, smoker's palate, nicotinic palatal leukokeratosis.

Heavy tobacco smokers, especially pipe and cigar smokers, will usually develop a slight, diffuse grayish-white appearance to the hard palate. With time, this appearance often alters to that of a thick, fissured, painless, white patch involving the entire hard palate. Small red depressions with elevated white keratotic halos are an almost constant feature of the more severe cases of nicotine palatinus, representing the inflamed ductal orifices of the numerous mucous glands of the palate. If a patient is a denture wearer, the lesions will be confined to mucosa not covered by the denture base. Patients are predominantly middle-aged or elderly males who may present with keratotic white plaques elsewhere in the mouth or throat.

With cessation of the smoking habit, nicotine palatinus will diminish rapidly and many lesions will completely disappear within 4 to 8 weeks. This entity is, in fact, a form of smoker's leukoplakia and was for that reason once thought to be premalignant; however, it must be strongly emphasized that this is no longer considered to be the case: Nicotine palatinus is *not* now considered to be a precursor to oral malignancy. Diagnosis and prognosis depend on the anatomic site. Smoker's keratoses elsewhere in a patient's mouth *are* considered premalignant.

Smears are useless in diagnosing this entity. Biopsy will demonstrate nonspecific hyperkeratosis with minimal dysplasia, but nicotine palatinus is so characteristic clinically that microscopic evaluation is usually not necessary.

Tobacco Pouch

Synonyms. Snuff pouch, snuff keratosis, snuff dipper's lesion.

Chronic tobacco or snuff chewers will often develop a well-circumscribed white or grayish-white, opalescent, fissured plaque of the vestibular mucosa of the area in which they habitually place their tobacco or snuff. This lesion often has a soft velvety feel, and further palpation of tobacco chewers' cheeks will usually reveal a distinct "pouch" caused by the chronic stretching of the cheek muscles in the area. No erythema, ulceration, or pain is associated with this lesion, and it usually takes at least 5 to 10 years to become manifest. Tobacco pouches may gradually show a thick, white, leathery surface, but most remain unchanged for decades. Although it is rare for a malignancy to develop from such lesions, when this does occur, the cancer produced is most likely to be a verrucous carcinoma which is a unique form of low-grade epithelioma that may locally enlarge for years without metastasis. Biopsy will show hyperkeratosis and/or intracellular edema of superficial epithelial layers; however, the characteristic clinical appearance combined with a history of tobacco or snuff chewing usually precludes the necessity of microscopic evaluation. Biopsy is definitely indicated for any ulceration or tumefaction, as these may show early malignancy.

Leukoedema

This condition most often presents as a filmy opalescence or a whitish-gray wrinkling of the entire cheek mucosa bilaterally. It shows a racial predilection for blacks, is not associated with smoking or chronic irritation, and is usually manifest during young adulthood. There is no ulceration, erythema or pain associated with it. Once manifest, this "variation of normal anatomy" remains constant throughout life. There is no malignant potential.

Smears are of no value. Biopsy will show characteristic hyperkeratosis and/or intracellular edema of superficial epithelial layers, but microscopic evaluation is usually not necessary because of the characteristic clinical appearance. White sponge nevus and chronic cheek bite must be included in a differential diagnosis.

White Sponge Nevus

Synonyms. Cannon's disease, congenital leukokeratosis, familial white folded dysplasia of mucous membranes, oral epithelial nevus.

This inherited disorder results from defective tonofibrils and typically presents as white or opalescent grayish-white, corrugated plaques of the buccal, gingival, oral floor, or lingual mucosae. The lesions may be congenital or appear as late as puberty and may occasionally be found on mucosa of the esophagus, vulva, vagina, anus, rectum, and nose. The condition persists unchanged throughout life. There is no malignant potential. Buccal smears show paranuclear and perinuclear condensation of cytoplasm. Biopsy demonstrates marked spongiosis of the epithelium and is rather characteristic, although similar to the epithelium of leukoedema and chronic cheek bite.

Many of the following entities are not discussed in this article, but all present oral lesions similar to white sponge nevus and should therefore be ruled out before a final diagnosis is made: hereditary benign intraepithelial dyskeratosis (Witkop's disease), leukoedema, pachyonychia congenita, dyskeratosis congenita, Darier's disease, and chronic cheek bite.

Chronic Cheek Bite

Synonyms. Cheek and lip biting, marsicatio buccarum, chronic lip bite.

Nervous individuals will occasionally develop a habit of sucking and "chewing" on their lips and cheeks, resulting in a macerated hyperkeratosis that is a white, often corrugated plaque with erythematous patches representing erosions or areas where the patient has peeled off the keratin layer of the epithelium. This condition is especially frequent in college and professional students, but it may be seen at any age. The lesion is often bilateral, and occasionally small hematomas may be seen. This lesion will become more severe during times of increased stress and will otherwise persist as long as the habit persists. It has absolutely no tendency to develop into cancer. The lesion will disappear if the patient abandons the habit. Smears are not helpful, and biopsy will show nonspecific spongiosis and hyperkeratosis; neither technique is recommended, therefore, except to rule out dysplasia in the epithelium. Leukoedema and white sponge nevus must be included in a differential diagnosis of this entity.

Lichen Planus

Synonyms. Lichen ruber planus, erosive lichen planus, bullous lichen planus.

Lichen planus is a rather common skin disorder of probable autoimmune etiology. Up to 40 per cent of lichen planus patients manifest oral mucosal lesions, and many patients present with *only* oral lesions.

A variety of keratotic white patterns may occur on the oral mucosa of patients with lichen planus: reticular, annular, and/or plaque-like lesions are most often seen on the buccal mucosa. Occasional patients will also demonstrate erythematous areas of erosion, ulceration, atrophy, or blister formation. The typical patient is a middle-aged female who is "nervous," and although the cheeks are the most likely site, any oral membrane may be affected. A metallic taste or a burning sensation may accompany the oral lesions; the ulcers and bullae, when present, are painful. Skin lesions, when present, are small bluish-silver, flat-topped plaques or nodules that tend to coalesce and/or scale. Fine grayish lines (Wickham's striae) may be present on the surface of skin lesions, and pruritus may be prominent. The genital mucosa may also be affected.

Oral lesions may follow or precede skin lesions of lichen planus, or they may be the only lesions to ever develop. Once present, the lesions may last for months or years. The erosive or bullous forms, especially, tend to last a lifetime. If the disease does disappear in time, the patient should be informed that recurrences are common. Squamous cell carcinoma has occasionally developed in a pre-existing lichen planus, especially of the erosive or bullous type.

The clinical manifestations of this disease are often so specific that no further testing need be performed. If such is not the case, however, biopsy of the oral keratotic areas will provide a definitive microscopic diagnosis demonstrating a band-like lymphocytic infiltrate of the lamina propria, hydropic degeneration of the basal cell layer, and hyperkeratosis. Oral lesions of lupus erythematosus often mimic lichen planus.

Lupus Erythematosus

Lupus erythematosus, a so-called collagen disease "of unknown etiology," is a multisystem disorder that may be systemwide or that may affect only a few tissues. Rather characteristic oral lesions may be the first presenting signs or symptoms. (For a detailed discussion of extraoral aspects of this disease, refer to the article on systemic lupus erythematosus.)

Systemic and discoid lupus erythematosus present oral manifestations that are quite similar, although oral involvement is much more common with the systemic type. Oral lesions may present as erythematous papules, plaques, or ulcerations covered by a nonspecific white membrane, but more typically they present as rounded, well-circumscribed, slightly elevated white plaques (with a reticular or radial appearance) on an erythematous base. Centrally located areas of atrophy or ulceration are occasionally seen. Such oral lesions are usually painless and found most frequently on the lips, buccal mucosa, and palate. Palatal petechiae and gingival hemorrhage may be later signs of lupus erythematosus in the mouth. Patients treated with chloroquine or hydroxychloraquine may show a diffuse brown-black pigmentation of palatal mucosa that is of no clinical consequence.

White oral lesions may last for years; ulcerative and atrophic oral lesions heal in weeks or months with a tendency toward scar formation. There may be an increased tendency for individuals with discoid lupus erythematosus to develop squamous cell carcinoma within lip scars.

Biopsy of an intraoral white lesion of lupus erythematosus may be definitively diagnostic of the disease, but this is often not the case, especially with the systemic variant. Characteristic microscopic findings would include liquefactive degeneration of basal cells; atrophy and mild hyperparakeratosis of the epithelium; and a marked cellular infiltrate of lymphocytes and plasma cells beneath the epithelium, in addition to vasculitis and fibrinoid degeneration of perivascular and subpapillary connective tissue. The fibrinoid degeneration and a thickened basement membrane stain positively with the PAS stain. Deposits of immunoglobulins and complement have been demonstrated in the basement membrane of oral lesions as areas of granular fluorescence. IgM and complement are most frequently found, IgG less frequently, and IgA rarely.

Fordyce Granules

Synonym. Fordyce's disease.

Heterotopic, usually nonfunctioning, sebaceous glands are seen in about 80 per cent of the population as numerous, small, yellowish-white papules or superficial granules of the buccal mucosa, labial mucosa, and retromolar pad area. They are typically bilateral and asymptomatic and occasionally present a cauliflower-like appearance from coalescence of many glands (called sebaceous adenomas by some authorities). Rarely, patients will complain of altered taste, presumably secondary to sebum extrusion.

Fordyce granules increase in number until puberty or shortly thereafter, with no change after body growth stops. Because clusters of these glands may appear as nodular white plaques, they are occasionally mistaken by the patient or physician as carcinoma, but they are, in fact, completely benign and have no tendency to undergo malignant transformation. Most cases are so characteristic clinically that no further testing is necessary; however, biopsy showing normal sebaceous glands, with or without ductal attachment to the overlying mucosal epithelium, will provide a definitive diagnosis.

Hairy Tongue

Synonyms. White hairy tongue, black hairy tongue, yellow hairy tongue.

Hairy tongue is a harmless elongation of the filiform papillae of the tongue to such lengths that they resemble hair. The condition is thought to be provoked by irritation from poor oral hygiene, antibiotic therapy, habitual use of oxidizing agents in oral preparations, and systemic disease debilitation. Chromogenic bacteria, food debris, tobacco, coffee, radiotherapy, and various coloring agents in medications and candies alter the normal white hairy tongue to a yellow, brown, or black appearance.

Numerous long, thin, white discolored hair-like papillae are found on the dorsum of the tongue, especially toward the posterior aspect. Pain is not usually a feature, unless secondary infection by *C. albicans* occurs, but the hairs may be long enough to produce a gagging problem and alteration of taste may be present. The condition is self-limiting and is remedied by treating the underlying systemic problem, eliminating the causative medicaments, and/or brushing the tongue daily.

This entity is usually so characteristic clinically that further testing is unnecessary; however, biopsy or scrapings will reveal hyperkeratinized elongated papillae and bacterial or fungal aggregates.

Geographic Tongue

Synonyms. Benign migratory glossitis, glossitis areata migrans, wandering rash.

This rather common disorder has an unknown etiology and typically presents as irregularily shaped red patches and white patterns resembling a map on the dorsum and lateral surfaces of the tongue. The erythematous patches represent areas of desquamated filiform papillae and are usually surrounded by a small white rim of sloughed keratocytes and necrotic debris. The pattern of the lesions continuously changes and the "map" noticed initially may be completely altered within a week's time. The condition is unusual in children and is usually asymptomatic unless secondarily involved with *C. albicans* or a limited bacterial infection. Similar changing lesions have recently been reported on vestibular mucosae.

The changing patterns of geographic tongue may persist for years with no detrimental effect. Spontaneous remissions and recurrences may be observed. Although the tongue involved in such a disorder can look quite unusual, there is no tendency for malignant transformation. Biopsy will reveal a microscopic appearance similar to psoriasis, but such a procedure is hardly ever indicated because the lesion is readily diagnosed clinically.

BROWN-BLACK PIGMENTED LESIONS

Physiologic Pigmentation

Synonyms. Racial pigmentation, negroid pigmentation, melanoplakia.

Dark-complexioned people, especially blacks, frequently have single or multiple nonblanching brown macules of various configurations and sizes on their oral mucosa. Such pigmented macules are most frequently found on the gingivae; the buccal and palatal and labial mucosa are sites of lesser predilection.

The lesions are present from childhood and should not change size in an adult; there is no malignant transformation potential.

Biopsy will show melanin pigment within the basal cell layer of the epithelium, but this technique is usually not required because the clinical appearance is so often diagnostic.

Oral Melanotic Macule

Synonyms. Ephelis, freckle, lentigo, oral melanosis.

Single, nonblanching, brown macules on the oral mucosa of whites are extremely rare phenomena that can affect any site and become manifest in middle-aged and older persons. They are usually painless, less than 1 cm in greatest diameter, well circumscribed, of the same consistency as normal mucosa, and of fairly recent onset.

Oral melanotic macules seem to reach their full maturity rapidly and then remain unchanged indefinitely. The major dilemma for the clinician lies in the fact that developing malignant melanomas are clinically similar or even indistinguishable from this benign macule. Therefore, excisional biopsy of all doubtful lesions is strongly recommended and is essential for all lesions larger than 1 cm in greatest diameter.

Biopsy will show melanin pigment within the basal cell layer of the epithelium as well as within histiocytes of the lamina propria.

Amalgam Tattoo

Synonym. Amalgam pigmentation.

Abrasion of oral membranes during tooth preparation will allow dental amalgam particles to be entrapped within the soft tissues, producing a smooth, irregularly outlined brown-black, nonblanching macule. Patients are often completely unaware of the initiating traumatic episode. The majority of amalgam tattoos will demonstrate radiopaque particles on radiographs. Graphite, dirt, asphalt, and so on may produce a similar lesion if traumatically introduced to oral soft tissues. The pigmented area remains unchanged after its initial appearance; the particles will not work their way to the surface, as with many other entrapped foreign bodies. The major complication is the occasional inability to differentiate between this entity and early malignant melanoma.

Radiographs may detect the metal particles producing this lesion, otherwise a biopsy is required to microscopically reveal them. These particles are birefringent and seldom show evidence of a surrounding inflammatory reaction. The particles are usually not found within histiocytes but rather are seen to be deposited along reticulum fibers.

Peutz-Jeghers Syndrome

Synonyms. Familial polyposis, intestinal polyposis II, periorofacial lentigines, visceral polyposis.

Peutz-Jeghers syndrome is an inherited disorder with two main features: mucocutaneous melanotic pigmentation and benign intestinal polyposis.

All patients with this syndrome present with numerous small brown-black or blue-gray pigmented macules of the lips, and 90 per cent have buccal mucosa macules; however, any oral membrane may be involved. About half of the patients will have similar pigmented macules on the skin around the facial orifices. The pigmentation usually appears in infancy, which is usually a decade or more before the hamartomatous polyps appear in the intestines. Rarely, the pigment is present without polyps.

The skin pigmentation tends to fade somewhat after puberty, but this is not true for the intraoral macules. The oral lesions do not transform into malignancy. Intussusception, colic pain, and melena may result from the intestinal polyps; a few cases of malignant transformation of these benign polyps have been reported.

Biopsy of the skin or oral macules will show melanin pigmentation of the basal cell layer, but this technique is usually not necessary because the clinical appearance is so characteristic. Examination of the gastrointestinal tract by proctoscopic and roentgenographic means is recommended. The following disorders may also present with multiple pigmented macules of the oral mucosa and should be ruled out before a final diagnosis is made: Addison's disease, Albright syndrome, drug ingestion (chloroquine), argyria, secondary syphilis, malignant melanoma, multiple melanotic macules (freckles), and physiologic pigmentation.

Malignant Melanoma

Primary melanomas of oral mucosa are relatively rare, appearing as painless, raised, soft, brown-black lesions that may or may not be ulcerated or hemorrhagic. They tend to arise de novo, but they may arise from a pre-existing nevus or oral melanotic macule. Palatal and maxillary alveolar mucosae are definite sites of predilection for oral melanomas, accounting for approximately 80 per cent of all such neoplasms. The location of pigmented oral lesions, therefore, is of prime diagnostic importance.

This tumor occurs most often in men and usually in the older population, with the greatest prevalence being seen in the sixth decade. Oral melanomas are unusual in that they seldom present as the superficial spreading variant but rather as the nodular, invasive form. This, plus a strong tendency toward early and widespread metastasis, helps to account for the tragically low (5 per cent) 5-year survival rate for this disease.

Early excisional biopsy is suggested for any pigmented oral lesion that meets one of the following criteria: elevated above the mucosal surface; larger than 1 cm in greatest dimension; unexplained etiology; and a duration of less than 1 year. A differential diagnosis that includes oral melanoma should also include oral melanotic macule, amalgam tattoo, nevus, chloroquine pigmentation, and mucosal discoloration secondary to Addison's disease.

RED MUCOSAL LESIONS

Median Rhomboid Glossitis

Synonym. Cherry patch tongue.

This anomaly typically presents as a painless, smooth, or nodular red area (0.5 to 2.5 cm) in the posterior midline of the tongue. The red appearance is caused by the loss or lack of normal lingual papillae in the area. Because this entity is seldom reported in children, current speculation implicates *C. albicans* as a causative agent, but many authorities still consider this to be a simple developmental phenomenon in which the tuberculum impar remains attached to the tongue surface rather than becoming embedded in the body of the tongue. Rarely, the surface may be white and keratinized or may be painful. These lesions generally persist for years or a lifetime after diagnosis.

Treatment with nystatin will reduce any tenderness but will not diminish the erythematous patch appreciably. While usually unnecessary, a biopsy of the area will provide an accurate diagnosis, showing pseudoepitheliomatous hyperplasia of an inflamed and degenerate epithelium. One should be concerned about doing a biopsy of this area of the tongue, however, because it is also the most common site for a lingual thyroid.

Lingual Varicosities

Synonyms. Caviar tongue, phlebectasia linguae.

Oral varicosities, or distended veins, are a very common occurrence in older individuals and typically present as superficial, painless, bluish blebs, or tortuous vessels on the ventral surface of the tongue. These lesions blanch on palpation, are usually bilateral, are occasionally seen on the lip mucosa, and occasionally are grouped so densely as to mimic a hematoma or hemangioma. Phleboliths may be palpated or radiographically visualized. Lingual varicosities slowly increase with age, but the rate is such that problems rarely develop, even in persons with numerous phleboliths. No laboratory aids are needed for diagnosis.

Papillary Hyperplasia of the Palate

Synonyms. Palatal papillomatosis, inflammatory papillary hyperplasia.

This is an inflammatory tissue response to chronic infection, probably by *C. albicans,* beneath a full or partial denture.

Papillary hyperplasia is invariably confined to the palate and conforms to the patient's denture-bearing areas. Typical lesions consist of multiple red, edematous nodules, each of which is about 1 to 2 mm in diameter. The nodules often crowd together so as to appear clinically alarming. Tenderness and hemorrhage are occasional features, as are occasional white keratosis and/or fibrosis of long-standing lesions. About 10 per cent of denture wearers have papillary hyperplasia of their palates, especially those who do not remove their dentures at night, but occasionally a case will be seen in a patient who does not wear dentures.

The condition persists indefinitely and may become more fibrous, but a dramatic return to normal is often seen in those patients who are willing to forgo their dentures for 4 to 8 weeks. Although this lesion can appear clinically aggressive, it has no tendency toward malignant transformation, a concept that is contrary to the implications in the older literature.

Although this entity is usually so clinically distinctive that it precludes further testing, biopsy will show a characteristic microscopic appearance of multiple inflammatory, edematous polyps with pseudoepitheliomatous change.

Angular Cheilitis

Synonyms. Angular cheilosis, perlèche.

This entity consists of erosions and fissures of the labial commissures secondary to *C. albicans* infection, poor denture construction, vitamin B-complex deficiency, and other factors.

As a person ages, a skin fold tends to develop at the corners of the mouth (commissure area), which is constantly moistened by saliva, and the area eventually may become eroded, cracked, or macerated. Tenderness and a burning sensation are common complaints. This is generally a chronic or recurrent condition that will not improve unless the initiating factor is removed.

Smears for *C. albicans* identification can be used diagnostically, as can the use of a topical Mycostatin cream. Vitamin therapy and/or denture reconstruction may also be used in a "diagnostic" fashion: If the cheilitis disappears with therapy, the clinician can assume that the proper etiology has been determined.

Denture Sore Mouth

Synonyms. Denture-related candidiasis, denture stomatitis, chronic atrophic oral candidiasis.

Denture sore mouth is an inflammatory atrophy of palatal mucosa secondary to trauma and Candida overgrowth beneath a poorly fitting denture, especially one left in overnight during sleep. Approximately 20 per cent of all cases are produced by a mixed bacterial infection.

The mucosa beneath the upper denture is fiery red and slightly edematous with possible petechiae and/or a burning sensation. The patient will have had the denture for some time and may also show evidence of other infection by *C. albicans,* i.e., papillary hyperplasia of the palate, smooth and red tongue, angular cheilitis, and generalized burning sensation of all oral membranes. Rarely, the white curd-like manifestation of candida will be present. Without treatment with nystatin antibiotics, tissue conditioners and improved denture hygiene, this inflammatory process will remain indefinitely.

Smears for *C. albicans* identification may be tried but are less successful than with acute pseudomembranous candidiasis.

Xerostomia

Synonym. Dry mouth.

Xerostomia is not a disease but a nonspecific clinical condition of decreased salivation leading to minimal washing and lubrication effect for the oral tissues. A wide variety of underlying systemic conditions may produce xerostomia, including numerous drugs, sialadenitis, Sjögren's syndrome, Mikulicz's disease, Heerfordt's syndrome, hereditary ectodermal dysplasia, head and neck radiotherapy, diabetes mellitus, anemias, vitamin A deficiency, and simple aging.

Xerostomia patients often complain of soreness, burning, and pain of the oral membranes, which appear very atrophic and erythematous. The tongue often demonstrates a marked loss of papillae in addition to erythema and burning. Increased caries susceptibility, intolerance to dentures, and speech or mastication difficulties are common features. Secondary infection by *C. albicans* may produce angular cheilitis and more intense pain.

Unless the underlying causative factors are corrected, xerostomia will remain a problem indefinitely and the patient will be forced to use artificial saliva. The diagnosis of this condition is clinical; however, methods are available to accurately assess salivary flow in patients.

Erythroplakia

Synonyms. Red patch, carcinoma in situ, erythroplasia of Queyrat.

Traditionally, "white patches," or leukoplakias, have been considered to be the most worrisome oral mucosal lesions relative to their potential for malignant transformation. More recently, however, it would appear that the "red patches," or erythroplakias, have a far greater chance of developing into a carcinoma. These small, velvety, painless, well-defined red macules usually show epithelial dysplasia or carcinoma in situ at their first biopsy.

Erythroplakia patients are usually older than 50 years of age and are usually male. The oral floor, ventral surface of the tongue, and buccal mucosae are most often involved. Erythroplakia may be admixed with a leukoplakia lesion, in which case "speckled leukoplakia" is the preferred term.

Chronic, painless, erythematous plaques of the oral mucosa are unusual enough to warrant excisional biopsy and microscopic examination of all such lesions. Staining the living tissues with a metachromatic dye may reveal previously undetected foci of dysplastic epithelium.

Infectious Mononucleosis

Synonyms. Glandular fever, kissing disease.

Infectious mononucleosis is a febrile condition affecting the lymphorecticuloendothelial system and the blood and is probably caused by the Epstein-Barr and other viruses. (For a discussion of extraoral involvement see the article on this disease elsewhere in the book.)

Oral lesions of infectious mononucleosis may be the first indication of the disease; these include palatal petechiae, sore throat, tender and hemorrhagic gingivae, tonsillitis, ulceration of oral and pharyngeal membranes, and/or generalized oral tenderness and redness. Cervical nodes are usually enlarged and tender.

Oral and pharyngeal involvement usually resolves within 5 to 14 days of onset. Since palatal petechiae are an early and very characteristic sign of this disease process, the clinician should be aware of the fact that several other conditions will produce a similar phenomenon, e.g., measles, hemophilia, leukemia, severe cough, purpuras, fellatio trauma, hereditary hemorrhagic telangiectasia, and Fabry's disease.

ORAL ULCERS

Squamous Cell Carcinoma

Synonyms. Squamous epithelioma, oral cancer.

Oral cancers, 90 per cent of which are squamous cell carcinomas of the mucous membranes, comprise approximately 5 per cent of all human malignancies and are diagnosed in about 12 persons per 100,000 of the population each year in the United States. Paradoxically, oral cancer—from a body cavity that is readily accessible for inspection and biopsy—has a poor prognosis: a 20 to 30 per cent 5-year survival rate. This paradox is tragically emphasized by the fact that 5-year survival for early and small (less than 1.5 cm in greatest dimension) mouth cancers is better than 60 per cent, and in certain locations better than 80 per cent! Early detection is of far more prognostic importance than the quality or type of treatment provided an oral carcinoma patient.

The typical patient with oral malignancy is older than 55 years; the disease is seldom seen before 40 years of age. Two thirds of these patients are males, although the sex differential becomes less striking for lesions in the more posterior aspects of the mouth and oropharynx. Few etiologic factors are significant: Tobacco and alcohol abuse seem to be the only important contributors to this disease, as well as sunlight for lesions of the lower lip. Some authorities consider chronic mechanical trauma and poor oral hygiene to be of etiologic significance, but this theory has recently become less popular.

The lateral posterior border of the tongue, the oral floor, and the lower lip vermilion comprise the sites for more than 75 per cent of all oral malignancies. Carcinomas in the mouth are seldom painful unless secondarily infected; typically, they have been present for at least 18 months prior to definitive diagnosis. These cancers have several clinical forms: (1) an indurated ulcer with rolled borders and a necrotic base; (2) a hemorrhagic, semifirm, sessile outgrowth with ulceration or white keratinization of the surface; and (3) a deeply infiltrating or scirrhous lesion that is firm upon palpation but has relatively few surface manifestations. Carcinoma of a sun-damaged lower lip often appears as a small chronic or recurrent scaling ulcer in the area where the patient holds a cigarette or pipe. Positive ipsilateral cervical nodes are seen in 40 per cent of all oral cancer patients at the time of diagnosis, and this greatly diminishes the prognosis for those persons.

Incisional biopsy is the diagnostic tool for this disease and should be considered essential for *all* unexplained, painless oral ulcerations that do not heal within 2 to 3 weeks. It should be remembered that squamous cell carcinoma could be hidden within a long-standing lesion of oral leukoplakia or erythroplakia. A final reminder: Persons with a history of a previously treated oral malignancy carry a 9 to 20 per cent chance of developing a *second* primary oral cancer and must, therefore, be followed carefully.

Traumatic Ulcer

Synonym. Denture sore spots.

This very common oral ulcerative lesion may be induced by mechanical, chemical, or thermal trauma and presents as a quite painful ulcer or crater with a clear or usually white pseudomembrane base and a red inflammatory halo of the surrounding mucosa. The size of the ulcer varies according to the severity of the trauma and there may be multiple lesions present at one time. Denture sore spots appear 1 to 7 days after placement of a new prosthesis and may be nothing more than a painful area of erythema. Ulcers on the vermilion border of the lips usually have a crusted surface because of the absence of saliva. Cervical lymphadenitis is common.

Most traumatic ulcers heal uneventfully within 7 to 10 days, but ulcers in areas that are continually receiving trauma may take 3 to 5 weeks or more to heal. Oral ulcers of longer duration should undergo biopsy, especially if nonpainful. These lesions will show a nonspecific inflammatory reaction under the microscope.

Numerous systemic diseases may lead to ulceration of oral membranes secondary to very mild trauma, and such ulcers often take an extended period of time to heal. Such diseases include diabetes mellitus, chronic and cyclic neutropenia, agranulocytosis, leukemia, and immunodeficiency states. Oral ulcers in such diseases may, in fact, be the first evidence of the disease.

Aphthous Ulcers

Synonyms. Canker sores, aphthous stomatitis, recurrent aphthous stomatitis, minor aphthous ulceration.

This is a common, self-limiting but recurring ulcerative condition of oral mucosa of unknown etiology. A host of theoretical causation factors, including trauma, psychological stress, bacteria, autoimmunity, endocrine dysfunction, and allergy, have been postulated.

Patients are often aware of a burning sensation in the affected mucosa during the prodromal stage; the mucosa becomes focally erythematous, then necrotic. Lesions are usually single or few in number and tend to recur with or without identifiable irritating factors. The typical lesion is a round to oval, very painful ulceration between 3 and 10 mm in diameter with a grayish-white fibrinous base and a red inflammatory halo around the periphery. These lesions are especially prominent on the lip, cheek, and tongue mucosae and occasionally reach 2 to 2.5 cm in diameter.

Young adults seem to be most often affected, but in truth, no individual of any age is immune to these frustrating lesions. The ulcers heal without scarring in 10 to 14 days; recurrences may continue indefinitely at 1 to 12 episodes annually. Severe involvement may produce lymphadenitis, fever, and/or malaise, and the pain may make eating quite difficult.

Culturing scrapings from an aphthous ulcer will prove nonproductive because of contamination by large numbers of bacteria normal to the oral environment. Biopsy will show only nonspecific ulceration.

Major Aphthous Stomatitis

Synonyms. Sutton's disease, periadenitis mucosa necrotica recurrens, Mikulicz's aphthae, recurrent scarring aphthae.

The individual oral ulcers in this nonhereditary condition of unknown etiology are similar to routine aphthous ulcers, except that they may be larger, deeper, and more numerous, and they tend to heal with scar formation. Remissions are short, and it is not unusual for a new ulceration to appear before a previous one has healed. Onset of these painful ulcers can take place at any age but is more common around puberty. Occasional involvement of laryngeal or genital mucosae has been noted.

A leukocyte and differential count will rule out agranulocytosis and neutropenia; biopsied tissue shows nonspecific ulceration, and therefore the procedure is not recommended.

Syphilitic Chancre and Gumma

Synonym. Lues, primary and tertiary syphilis.

The oral chancre of primary syphilis develops at the inoculation site 12 to 40 days after sexual contact. The lesion is a painless, round to oval, clean-based, indurated ulcer that usually begins as a nodule; if located on the lip, the lesion often has a crusted surface. Painless swelling of regional lymph nodes is common, and occasionally multiple chancres are seen. The oral chancre is an extremely contagious lesion.

The tertiary lesions of oral syphilis involvement consist of indurated and keratotic syphilitic glossitis, or painless gummatous infiltration of either the palate or tongue and occasional other oral sites. The gummas necrose to form sharply outlined, punched-out ulcers that may have a granular appearance to their bases; they are usually single lesions and are not considered contagious.

Oral chancres heal without scarring within 2 to 4 weeks. Oral gummas heal with occasional scarring after several months; palatal gummas may perforate the bony palate before healing occurs. Syphilitic glossitis is considered to carry a malignant transformation rate of 25 to 30 per cent.

Biopsy should be performed on oral gummas in order to rule out squamous cell carcinoma, tuberculosis, histoplasmosis, blastomycosis, lethal midline granuloma, Wegener's granulomatosis, sarcoidosis, necrotizing sialometaplasia, and other chronic ulcerative/nodular disease entities.

(For a more detailed discussion of syphilis, see the article on this topic in Section 2.)

Behçet's Syndrome

Synonyms. Behçet's disease, cutaneomucouveal syndrome, recurrent genito-oral aphthosis and uveitis with hypopyon.

Behçet's syndrome is made up of the triad of aphthous stomatitis, genital ulcerations, and recurrent uveitis with hypopyon. Its etiology is unknown. Not all components of the syndrome are present at any given time.

The oral ulcers of Behçet's syndrome resemble typical aphthous ulcers with a painful white pseudomembrane ulcer base surrounded by an erythematous halo. They are often the initial sign of the disease, which typically affects young adults, especially males. These ulcers extend into the pharynx or esophagus, resulting in dysphagia. This syndrome is characterized by a tendency to recur, often several times annually. Joint, cutaneous, neurologic, and gastrointestinal complications are not uncommon. There are no diagnostic laboratory aids available yet for this disease.

Cyclic Neutropenia

Cyclic neutropenia is a possibly inherited defect of early hematopoietic stem cells that manifests as periodic decreases of neutrophilic leukocytes in the peripheral blood. Clinical disease appears and regresses spontaneously according to the altering leukocyte count. Cyclic neutropenia presents orally as multiple shallow ulcerations (with or without erythematous rimming) and severe ulcerative gingivitis that leads to alveolar bone loss or premature periodontitis. The gingivitis and ulceration typically recur every 3 to 4 weeks and persist for 5 to 8 days before healing; these recurrences correspond to depressions in the leukocyte count, and healing occurs as these counts return to normal. Mild fever, malaise, otitis media, headache, joint pain, and sore throat are often present during neutropenic episodes.

The disease lasts throughout life, although spontaneous improvement in adulthood has been reported occasionally. Early loss of dentition from periodontitis is common. Hematologic examinations may have to be repeated weekly until a depression or complete absence of neutrophils is noted in peripheral blood. Biopsy of oral ulcers shows them to be agranulocytic, but this is not necessarily diagnostic.

Agranulocytosis

Synonyms. Malignant neutropenia, agranulocytic angina.

Agranulocytosis is an acute disease characterized by marked leukopenia. This condition most often occurs as a cytotoxic sensitivity response to a wide variety of drugs. The lowered resistance to infections seen in agranulocytosis leads to typical ulcerative lesions of the gingiva and buccal or palatal mucosae. The lesions are well defined with a gray-brown to yellow-green base and are without an erythematous rim. The patient complains particularly of sore throat and dysphagia, and regional lymph nodes may be enlarged. Gingival ulceration and necrosis are commonly seen. Oral lesions of this disease tend to worsen continually as long as the leukopenia persists untreated. Periodontal involvement may lead to loosening of teeth and sequestration of alveolar bone. Secondary infection may lead to a fatal outcome.

The hemogram shows a marked decrease or complete absence of mature granulocytes. (The reader is referred to the article on Neutropenia and Agranulocytosis for more detail.)

Necrotizing Ulcerative Gingivostomatitis

Synonyms. Vincent's disease, trench mouth, fusospirochetal infection, acute necrotizing ulceromembranous gingivitis.

Necrotizing ulcerative gingivostomatitis is an acute or subacute gingival inflammation of young adults probably caused by a combination of vibrios, hemolytic streptococci, certain viruses, and poor oral hygiene.

This disease, with its marked predilection for males in their early twenties, is characterized by tender, swollen, red gingival papillae that rapidly undergo painful ulceration, producing almost pathognomonic punched-out erosions of these papillae. The free gingiva becomes covered with a gray pseudomembrane while pain, tenderness, and bleeding cause great difficulty in eating. Halitosis (fetor ex ore) and excessive salivation are marked, as is regional lymphadenitis. Low-grade fever, headache, and malaise are common. The condition may spread to the pharynx or other oral sites if the patient's resistance is low.

With treatment the condition subsides within 48 hours; without treatment it can continue on for months or lead to septicemia, cancrum oris (noma), or death in debilitated patients. Spontaneous remission and healing also may occur in 1 to 3 weeks. Recurrences are common.

The diagnosis is made clinically, but peripheral blood will show a mild leukocytosis with a relative lymphomonocytosis. Microscopic demonstration of fusobacteria or spirella is of no value because these organisms may normally be found in the mouth.

VESICLES AND BULLAE

Mucocele

Synonyms. Mucus retention phenomenon, mucus retention cyst, ranula.

A mucocele is a subepithelial pooling of mucus resulting from the traumatic rupture of a salivary gland duct. Occasionally, obstruction of such a duct results in distention and subsequent epithelial-lined cyst formation without the escape of mucus into connective tissues. When the large ducts of the sublingual or submandibular glands are involved, *ranula* is the term used for the resultant oral floor lesion.

A mucocele usually appears suddenly on the lower lip mucosa as a soft, fluctuant, transparent or blue "blister" of 2 to 10 mm in diameter. The lesions are occasionally tender, occasionally multiple, and have a characteristic history of disappearing after rupture only to reappear several hours to several weeks later. The ranulas of the oral floor are large, often displacing an entire side of the floor; they tend to be more painful than their smaller counterparts on the lips, and they are often associated with pain and enlargement during or after meals.

Recurrences are common unless the causative salivary gland is removed surgically. Occasionally, a small mucocele will transform into a pyogenic granuloma and subsequently sclerose into an irritation fibroma.

Biopsy will demonstrate pools of mucus within a fibrovascular connective tissue with mild sialadenitis of adjacent salivary glands.

Epidermoid Cyst

Synonyms. Epidermal cyst, dermoid cyst, epidermoid inclusion cyst.

Epidermoid or dermoid cysts of the mouth are usually located in the floor and are typically sessile or somewhat pedunculated, yellow-white, painless nodules 2 to 8 mm in diameter. The thinness of the overlying mucosa often imparts a semitransparent, cystic appearance to these lesions reminiscent of pustules. Although young adults most frequently present with these cysts, no age is exempt.

Most epidermoid cysts of the mouth remain small and innocuous indefinitely. Occasional deep-seated lesions of the oral floor will reach the size of an egg and may interfere with speech and swallowing.

Biopsy will show a keratin-filled cyst lined by mature stratified squamous epithelium with or without skin appendages. The clinical differential diagnosis for such a lesion should also include lymphoepithelial cyst and lipoma.

Herpes Simplex, Primary and Secondary

Synonyms. Acute herpetic gingivostomatitis, herpetic stomatitis, recurrent herpes simplex, herpes labialis, fever blisters, cold sores.

This is an acute vesicular infection by the herpes simplex ectodermotropic virus. This virus belongs in the common group with that of herpes zoster, chickenpox and probably cytomegalic inclusion virus. *Herpesvirus hominis type 1* produces oral and paraoral lesions and is pantropic in affected newborn infants, and *Herpesvirus hominis type 2* produces genital disease (herpes genitalis). The primary attack, or herpetic gingivostomatitis, usually occurs in early life, although clinical disease is seldom severe enough to be called to the attention of a parent or physician. Regardless of whether the primary infection is clinical or subclinical, recurrent (secondary) herpetic lesions develop later in many persons; it has been estimated that up to 90 per cent of the adult population are carriers of the virus.

Primary infection with *Herpesvirus hominis type 1* occurs between 1 and 5 years of age and is characterized by multiple vesicular eruptions of the gingival, labial, and buccal mucosae that rupture rapidly, leaving painful, raw, yellow-white, pseudomembranous erosions with red inflammatory halos. There is considerable gingival swelling, halitosis, and increased salivation, with frequent yellow crusting of the vermilion border of the lips. Systemic involvement includes high fever, irritability, dehydration, malaise, headache, dysphagia, and regional lymphadenitis.

Recurrent herpes simplex (herpes labialis) almost invariably presents as multiple and coalescing clear vesicles at the vermilion border of the lips. These painful vesicles rapidly rupture, becoming covered with a yellow-brown crust; for 1 or 2 days prior to their formation, the patient is often aware of a tingling or burning sensation in the area. Recurrences generally are quite self-limiting and occur at the same sites; rarely, intraoral recurrent herpes is noted on the gingiva or hard palate. Regional lymphadenitis and fever are absent in recurrent disease.

A variety of stimuli may precipitate recurrent herpes simplex, including fever, respiratory infection, sunlight, nonspecific gastroenteritis, food allergy, menstruation, and mechanical trauma.

Primary and secondary herpes simplex lesions both heal spontaneously without scarring within 10 to 14 days. Recurrence of the primary form is extremely rare, and when occurring in older patients, should lead to a suspicion of leukemia or an immunodeficient condition.

Complications of infection by herpes simplex virus are numerous and varied. Herpetic meningocephalitis or generalized herpes simplex of the newborn infant, characterized by central nervous system and visceral involvement, commonly is fatal. Eczema herpeticum (Kaposi's varicelliform eruption) is a herpetic infection of a primary eczema, is most often seen in infants and young children, and may terminate fatally. Herpetic conjunctivitis may produce edema and hyperemia of the palpebral conjunctiva, keratitis, corneal ulceration, and vesicles of the eyelids. Inoculation herpes simplex is a primary form of the infection that is most often seen on the fingers of dentists, physicians, and dental hygienists who have examined patients with clinical disease.

Late in the course of a primary herpes simplex infection, the antiherpes antibody titer is elevated; this is noted earlier in secondary infections. Paul's test, inoculation of an affected patient's saliva onto a rabbit cornea, will produce typical dendritic keratitis within 24 to 48 hours. A biopsy of an intact vesicle or a smear of a ruptured lesion demonstrates characteristic cells with ballooning degeneration, multinucleation, or the presence of eosinophilic intranuclear inclusions (Lipschütz bodies), but such cells can also be seen in herpes zoster and varicella vesicles.

Herpangina

Synonyms. Aphthous pharyngitis, coxsackievirus group A infection.

Herpangina, produced by Group A and B coxsackie viruses, is limited to the soft palate and oropharynx in children; extension anteriorly is rare. After a 2- to 9-day incubation period, the disease presents with rapid onset of sore throat, fever, malaise, headache, muscle ache, and cervical lymphadenitis. The clinical findings in the mouth and pharynx significantly aid diagnosis, presenting as fewer than a dozen small reddish vesicles of the soft palate, uvula and fauces, usually painful, symmetric, and rapidly ruptured.

The disease usually resolves in 2 to 6 days; rarely, acute parotitis, meningitis, or hemolytic anemia may result.

Herpangina is usually distinctive enough to be diagnosed clinically; however, serologic tests for virus-neutralizing and complement-fixing antibodies may be performed. The virus can be isolated from hamsters or mice after inoculation of scrapings from the ruptured vesicles.

Hand-foot-and-mouth disease, herpes zoster, and recurrent intraoral herpes simplex must be included in a differential diagnosis of this entity.

Hand-Foot-and-Mouth Disease

Synonym. Aphthous fever.

This acute, contagious infection, caused by several coxsackieviruses, almost invariably occurs in children and presents lesions with a pathognomonic distribution: oral cavity, hands, and feet. The virus has an estimated incubation period of 2 to 6 days; a subfebrile stage and mild malaise are common. The oral lesions are located primarily on the lips and buccal mucosa, sparing the posterior mouth and oropharynx. Initial lesions are red papules, 2 to 10 mm in diameter, which become gray-white vesicles within 1 or 2 days; total numbers of mucosal and skin vesicles range from 20 to 100, with only five to ten in the mouth. After the vesicles rupture, painful ulcers with white or gray pseudomembranous bases remain. Regional lymphadenitis is rare. Spontaneous healing of all lesions occurs within 1 to 2 weeks.

This disease is usually diagnosed clinically; however, complement fixation and inoculation of guinea pigs or suckling mice may be used for isolation and diagnosis of the virus. Smears from ruptured vesicles may demonstrate intracytoplasmic eosinophilic inclusion bodies.

Erythema Multiforme

Synonyms. Erythema multiforme exudativum, Stevens-Johnson syndrome, ectodermosis erosiva pluriorificialis.

Erythema multiforme is a dermatologic disorder that is probably a hypersensitivity reaction and is often, but not invariably, precipitated by allergens such as antibiotics and viruses, especially the herpes simplex virus. Infection or initial drug intake might precede erythema multiforme by 1 to 3 weeks.

This disease usually manifests in young adults, and a variety of skin and mucosal lesions are found, often on a single individual. Upper respiratory tract infection, fever, malaise, and arthralgia may be early features. Typical oral lesions consist of erosions and bullae that rapidly burst to leave large, painful ulcerations with white pseudomembranous bases. Although any oral membrane may be affected, the lips are almost constantly affected, often producing a thick hemorrhagic crusting. Skin lesions may be bullae, solid macules, or target-like macules (pathognomonic, if present); occasionally oral lesions are seen without skin manifestations. Severe involvement of skin, oral mucosa, conjunctival mucosa, and genital mucosa, with a tendency toward leukopenia, is known as the Stevens-Johnson syndrome.

This disease runs its course in 2 to 5 weeks, and recurrences are uncommon. Once recurrence does occur, however, the patient may suffer periodic bouts for a decade or more. Rarely, a fulminating course, complicated by secondary infection, may lead to a fatal outcome.

The diagnosis is made on the basis of clinical information. A microscopic examination of a bullous lesion will generally show the bulla to be subepithelial, thereby ruling out pemphigus vulgaris, but biopsy findings are otherwise nonspecific. A differential diagnosis for this disease should include chemical burns, pemphigus vulgaris, and benign mucous membrane pemphigoid. Immunofluorescence of fresh or frozen tissue will rule out the latter two entities.

Pemphigus Vulgaris

Pemphigus vulgaris is an autoimmune dermatologic disorder of middle-aged and older individuals, especially those of Semitic extraction.

Oral lesions are invariably present during the course of the disease and often precede the development of skin lesions by several years. The typical oral and skin lesions are bullae of varying sizes that rupture rapidly to leave painful ulcers with gray-white pseudomembranous bases. These bullae tend to arise from clinically normal skin or mucosa and, in fact, may be produced on normal surfaces by lateral pressure or friction (Nikolsky's sign). Eye and genital mucosae tend to be spared in the early stages of this disease, as opposed to erythema multiforme or benign mucous membrane pemphigoid.

The disease becomes more severe at varying rates, with or without spontaneous remissions and exacerbations. Long-term systemic steroid therapy usually controls the disease; if left untreated, it progresses to death, resulting from dehydration, septicemia, or cachexia toxicity.

Biopsy of skin or oral bullae will reveal intraepithelial blister formation immediately above the basal cell layer. Smears of intraoral bullae may demonstrate detached acantholytic epithelial cells with characteristically enlarged, hyperchromatic nuclei (Tzanck cells). Antibodies against the epithelial cells of the skin or oral mucosa can be found in vivo in the intercellular cement regions or circulating in the blood. Direct or indirect immunofluorescent procedures will demonstrate binding of IgG and complement to the cell membranes of the spinous epithelial layer.

Benign Mucous Membrane Pemphigoid (BMMP)

Synonyms. Pemphigoid, mucous membrane pemphigoid, cicatricial pemphigoid.

This chronic, nonfatal autoimmune disorder of middle-aged and elderly individuals resembles bullous pemphigoid, except that its lesions have a strong predilection for mucous membranes.

The condition is characterized by bullous lesions of the oral, conjunctival, and genital mucous membranes. The oral bullae are usually few in number and may last for 1 or 2 days before rupturing to leave slightly tender ulcerations with white or gray pseudomembranous bases. Erythema of the oral mucosa is a constant feature, often persisting for several weeks after the ulcers have healed. The eye erythema and bullous formation is found on both bulbar and palpebral conjunctivae and, unlike the oral lesions, tends to heal with scarring (symblepharon or synechiae formation). Occasionally, skin, pharyngeal, laryngeal, esophageal, nasal, and anal lesions are noted. Oral lesions usually precede those of the conjunctiva or genitalia.

This disease follows a protracted course characterized by periods of exacerbation and remission. Individual oral lesions heal without scarring within 2 to 4 weeks, but repeated conjunctival involvement may lead to corneal cloudings, loss of cilia, and cicatricial fibrous bands. The major complication of this disease is entropion with blindness in about 30 per cent of patients with uncontrolled lesions.

Biopsy reveals subepithelial bullous formation, which is nonspecific but does rule out pemphigus vulgaris. Antibasement membrane antibodies in serum can be detected, and direct immunofluorescence demonstrates that immunoglobulins and complement are bound to the epithelial basement membrane.

SOFT-TISSUE MASSES

Pyogenic Granuloma

Synonyms. Granuloma pyogenicum, proud flesh, pregnancy tumor, hormonal tumor, epulis granulomatosum (if developing in tooth socket).

Pyogenic granuloma is a common type of inflammatory hyperplasia in the mouth or on the skin; it is essentially exuberant overgrowth of granulation tissue in response to local trauma or infection. These growths are especially common in a tooth socket after recent extraction and in the later stages of pregnancy, at which time they may be multiple and associated with prominent gingivitis. Puberty and birth control medications may produce lesions similar to those seen in pregnancy.

The lesions typically present as soft, painless, ulcerated, easily bleeding polypoid masses with broad bases. They usually are quite vascular in appearance, but the necrotic surface areas are often covered by a white, sloughing, pseudomembrane that resembles pus, hence the "pyogenic" terminology. Pus, however, is seldom a feature of this lesion. Pyogenic granulomas may occur at any age, being especially prone to occur in young adults and in females.

These lesions often have an alarmingly rapid onset, may become 2 cm or more in diameter, and commonly recur after conservative surgical removal, but they have no malignant potential. Pyogenic granulomas of pregnancy (pregnancy tumors) are especially known for their dramatic diminution in size postpartum. More typically, pyogenic granulomas tend to fibrose with time, eventuating in typical irritation fibromas.

Biopsy will be diagnostic, showing marked neocapillary proliferation, edema, and inflammatory cells of both the acute and chronic type.

Peripheral Giant Cell Granuloma

Synonyms. Peripheral giant cell reparative granuloma, peripheral giant cell tumor, giant cell epulis, epulis granulomatosum (if developing in a tooth socket).

Peripheral giant cell granulomas are common inflammatory hyperplasias of the periodontal ligament and by definition, therefore, must arise on the gingival tissues or from a tooth socket. The exact etiology of this entity is unknown but appears to be local trauma or infection.

These lesions are typically deep red, easily bleeding, painless, often ulcerated, and usually nodular polyps or broad-based masses on the gingiva of middle-aged individuals, especially females. Unlike pyogenic granulomas, they do not tend to be multiple, are not more common in pregnancy, and occasionally become 4 to 5 cm in diameter, but clinical resemblance to pyogenic granulomas is otherwise remarkable. Peripheral giant cell granulomas may form palpable and radiographically visible bone deep in their bulk. Occasionally a peripheral lesion is contiguous with its intraosseous counterpart, the central giant cell granuloma.

After a rapid onset, these lesions become quiescent and may eventually diminish in size and fibrose into a typical irritation fibroma. Because of the deep periodontal origin of peripheral giant cell granulomas, they have an even greater tendency than pyogenic granulomas to recur, but malignant transformation has not been reported.

Biopsy will be diagnostic, showing numerous multinucleated giant cells scattered throughout a cellular connective tissue stroma. Large, multiple, or actively recurring lesions should lead the clinician to check the patient's serum calcium, phosphorus, and alkaline phosphatase levels, as peripheral giant cell granulomas are clinically and microscopically indistinguishable from the "brown tumors" of hyperparathyroidism.

Irritation Fibroma

Synonyms. Inflammatory fibrous hyperplasia, traumatic fibroma, fibrous epulis, fibroepithelial polyp.

Irritation fibromas are very common inflammatory hyperplasias of fibrous connective tissue which form in response to acute or chronic mechanical trauma or infection. Several oral lesions gradually fibrose and transform into irritation fibromas (e.g., mucoceles, pyogenic granulomas, and peripheral giant cell granulomas), but more commonly the lesions are firm and fibrous from their early stages.

Irritation fibromas are typically firm, nonhemorrhagic, nontender polypoid masses of the buccal, labial, or other mucosal surfaces. They are usually smooth-surfaced and of normal coloration, but they may be lobulated and may be white from keratinization of the surface. Although they occasionally reach 3 to 4 cm in diameter, the great majority are less than 1 cm in diameter.

These lesions grow slowly, and growth stops as they mature. There is no malignant potential, and recurrence after conservative surgical removal is uncommon.

Biopsy will be diagnostic, showing dense collagenic connective tissue covered by a normal mucosal epithelium.

Epulis Fissuratum

Synonyms. Denture injury tumor, inflammatory fibrous hyperplasia, denture hyperplasia.

This common oral lesion is an inflammatory hyperplasia of fibrous connective tissues resulting from the chronic inflammation or mechanical irritation caused by ill-fitting dentures.

Epulides fissurata are typically elongated, firm, nonhemorrhagic, nontender folds of tissue located along the edge of a loose-fitting denture; several redundant folds may be present. While they are usually of normal coloration, acute trauma or superimposed inflammation may produce an erythematous and ulcerated surface. Similar folds of fibrous tissue occur on the crest of an alveolus that has undergone marked bone resorption. Occasionally, leaf-shaped epulides occur under the denture base, and these may produce a bony concavity in the palate as a result of pressure atrophy of palatal bone.

Epulides fissurata develop slowly and have a limited growth potential. After maturation the lesions remain indefinitely, and even after surgical removal they tend to recur unless the offending denture is corrected or replaced. These lesions may look alarming clinically, but they are not considered to be premalignant.

The clinical appearance of denture hyperplasia is usually diagnostic, but biopsy will show characteristic fibrous and collagenic hyperplasia.

Papilloma

Synonym. Squamous papilloma.

The papilloma is a relatively common, benign neoplastic proliferation of mucosal epithelium that is similar clinically and microscopically to the common wart (verruca vulgaris) of the skin. It may be initiated by a virus, as are warts, but such a virus has not yet been isolated.

The papilloma is typically a single soft, nonhemorrhagic, nontender, papillomatous or cauliflower-like growth on a stalk. Typically small and white (keratinized surface), they may reach several centimeters in size and may be normal or red in color with a pebbled, rather than papillary surface. This lesion is most frequently seen on the tongue and soft palate of a middle-aged or older individual; it is occasionally multiple and can be seen in children. After initial slow growth, papillomas remain unchanged indefinitely. Unlike papillomas from the larynx and nasal sinus, oral papillomas do not tend to transform into squamous cell carcinoma.

Biopsy is diagnostic, demonstrating numerous finger-like projections with connective tissue cores running to the stalk of the lesion. White lesions show hyperkeratosis of the covering epithelium.

Phenytoin Gingival Hyperplasia

Synonyms. Dilantin gingivitis, Dilantin gingival fibromatosis, diphenylhydantoin hyperplasia, phenytoin gingivitis.

Phenytoin gingival hyperplasia is a fibrous hyperplasia of the gingivae arising as a side effect of diphenylhydantoin used in the control of epileptic convulsions and other neurologic disorders.

Phenytoin intake often results in a firm, nonhemorrhagic, nontender, fibrous enlargement of all gingival tissues, occasionally to the point of completely covering the teeth with fibrous tissue. Unless secondarily inflamed, phenytoin gingivae are of normal coloration.

This fibrous gingival overgrowth continues slowly while the patient is taking the drug, and recurrence after surgical removal is common. The severity of the condition is usually related to the patient's oral hygiene and the duration of therapy; gingival hyperplasia may be avoided in patients with excellent oral hygiene.

History and clinical appearance offer the best diagnostic potential, but biopsy will demonstrate a uniform, avascular proliferation of collagenic connective tissues.

Verrucous Carcinoma

Synonyms. Snuff dippers' cancer, Ackerman tumor, oral florid papillomatosis.

Verrucous carcinoma is a very low-grade form of squamous cell carcinoma that is seen almost exclusively in the oral cavity and larynx. It is the malignancy most likely to develop in the area where tobacco or snuff chewers keep their "quid" (i.e., in a "tobacco pouch") and accounts for no more than 5 per cent of all oral malignancies.

This lesion has a distinctive clinical appearance, being found usually in the mandibular buccal sulcus and presenting as a large, painless, papillary mass that is typically white but may appear pink or red on its surface. The tumor is neither as firm to palpation as the other forms of squamous cell carcinoma nor as prone toward surface ulceration or hemorrhage. Such malignancies often demonstrate considerable lateral spread but are remarkable in their lack of deep invasion, even after several years. Underlying muscle and bone can be progressively destroyed in this disease, however, and such destruction must therefore be evaluated prior to the initiation of treatment.

The average age of patients with verrucous carcinoma is about 65 years, with many more being found in men than in women, except in those areas where snuff dipping is more popular with women. A period of at least 20 years of tobacco chewing or snuff dipping is required for the development of this particular malignancy, and the usual verrucous carcinoma has a duration of several years prior to definitive diagnosis. Prognosis is quite good: at least 80 per cent of affected patients survive for 5 years after surgical removal.

Although verrucous carcinoma has a rather well-defined clinical appearance, incisional or excisional biopsy is required for proper diagnosis. The clinician must be sure to remove a large enough tissue wedge to ensure that the pathologist can determine the general morphology of the lesion, since the individual cells are almost always so well differentiated that they appear benign. Microscopically, this tumor presents a pattern of multiple projecting folds of squamous epithelium with a marked acanthosis, ballooning rete pegs, deep parakeratin-lined clefts, and the appearance of "pushing" into adjacent tissue. Smears are virtually useless in the diagnosis of this cancer.

ACUTE PHARYNGITIS

By Hugh C. Dillon, Jr., M.D.
Birmingham, Alabama

SYNONYMS

Tonsillitis, tonsillopharyngitis, septic sore throat; or simply, sore throat.

DEFINITION

The syndrome of acute pharyngitis as discussed in this article includes those respiratory tract infections in which the primary manifestations are related to inflammation of the pharyngeal mucosal and lymphoid tissues. Although sore throat may accompany many forms of upper respiratory tract infection as well as noninfectious illness, the term "acute pharyngitis" is generally used in describing a well-localized infection in which acute sore throat is the predominant manifestation.

ETIOLOGIC AGENTS

No attempt is made here to list all infectious agents known to be associated with acute pharyngitis. Group A beta hemolytic streptococci are the principal bacteria that cause the syndrome. Group C and G streptococci may cause a similar acute illness, and less often group B streptococci may produce sore throat. *Neisseria gonorrhoeae* and *Corynebacterium diphtheriae* also produce acute exudative pharyngitis. Classical diphtheria is no longer common in well-developed countries; gonococcal pharyngitis has become more common. Many viral agents can produce sore throat. Acute pharyngitis is associated with several serotypes of adenovirus; coxsackievirus, influenza virus, herpes simplex virus, and parainfluenza viruses are others of importance. Adenoviruses are more likely to produce an acute pharyngitis resembling streptococcal pharyngitis, but coxsackievirus infections often produce vesicular eruptions in the throat or mucous membranes of the mouth. The syndrome of infectious mononucleosis is associated with a number of agents, including Epstein-Barr (EB) virus, toxoplasma, or cytomegalovirus.

PRESENTING SIGNS AND SYMPTOMS

The signs and symptoms associated with acute pharyngitis caused by various infectious agents may be quite similar. Clinical features alone cannot be relied upon for establishing the etiology. It is useful to intially consider features typical of streptococcal pharyngitis as an example of an acute pharyngitis in which the diagnosis can be established by relatively simple means, the throat culture.

Streptococcal pharyngitis is most common in school-aged children and adolescents and tends to follow seasonal patterns with late fall and late winter–early spring peaks in incidence. Seasonal patterns and age distribution are therefore of some value in predicting risk of streptococcal disease. Signs and symptoms of typical streptococcal pharyngitis, especially in children beyond 4 years of age, include an abrupt onset of painful sore throat, fever, chills or chilly sensations, headache, and occasionally stomachache. Acute abdominal pain is especially common when streptococcal pharyngitis is accompanied by scarlet fever. In more severe acute streptococcal pharyngitis, dysphagia may be pronounced and the child may drool or continually expectorate rather than swallow secretions. Anterior cervical lymph nodes are tender and often lead to referred pain to the ear on the affected side. Physical findings reveal a fiery red throat, edematous lymphoid tissues, exudate on mucosal surfaces, and in severe infections, including patients with scarlet fever, petechial lesions on the palate and uvula. A marked enanthem is characteristic of scarlet fever.

These features make streptococcal infection a likely diagnosis, and development of the fine erythematous papular rash of scarlet fever is a pathognomic sign. However, throat cultures should be done to confirm a streptococcal diagnosis even in the presence of scarlet rash. Obviously, not all cases of streptococcal pharyngitis are considered typical or severe, and the clinical spectrum of disease varies from mild or even subclinical illness to the more severe form. In the author's experience, the combination of an abrupt onset of illness in which exudative pharyngitis and tender cervical lymph nodes are evident has provided the best clinical clues for predicting streptococcal etiology.

Adenoviral infection in the young preschool child may resemble streptococcal pharyngitis in the older child. Adenoviral infections are more likely to be associated with additional nonspecific findings including cough, which is not a common feature of streptococcal pharyngitis. Coxsackie viral infections usually differ seasonally from streptococcal or adenoviral infections and include a variety of clinical expressions: oropharyngitis with buccal mucosal lesions as well as exanthems. These infections may also be accompanied by gastrointestinal complaints. Patients with influenza often have sore throat with localized erythema, but additional clinical manifestations and progression of the illness soon make it apparent that this illness differs from the acute pharyngitis of streptococcal or adenoviral infection. Myalgia is a common complaint in sore throat caused by influenza virus.

Gonococcal pharyngitis should be suspected in sexually active adolescents or young adults who present with an acute exudative pharyngitis if the throat culture is negative for streptococcus. A history of oral-genital contact may be elicited and, if so, is supportive of the likelihood of gonococcal pharyngitis.

Patients with infectious mononucleosis may present initially with clinical features much like those in children with streptococcal pharyngitis. The throat culture is commonly negative, however, unless the patient happens to be a coincidental carrier of streptococcus. Less often, one may encounter a patient with active streptococcal pharyngitis and the syndrome of infectious mononucleosis. Although the acute features of infectious mononucleosis and streptococcal pharyngitis are similar, the former disease tends to be somewhat less abrupt in onset, but clinical manifestations tend to persist considerably longer. Generalized systemic signs and symptoms, along with malaise, progressive weakness, anorexia, and occasionally mild depressive illness, may occur in patients with infectious mononucleosis.

COURSE OF INFECTION

The clinical course of an acute pharyngitis varies in relation to a number of factors. These include initial clinical severity of illness, etiologic agent, host-age range, therapy, and presence or absence of complications. Patients with streptococcal pharyngitis are usually promptly treated, but even untreated patients may have a self-limited infection that improves considerably within 3 or 4 days. Infants and young children with certain viral infections, including adenoviral disease, may be ill somewhat longer, and, as the illness progresses, may develop more systemic complaints. As noted previously, the course of infectious mononucleosis is quite variable but may include a protracted illness extending for weeks.

COMMON COMPLICATIONS

Complications of acute pharyngitis are also related to a number of features, including etiologic agent and therapy in particular. Any viral infections associated with acute upper respiratory tract involvement, including those in which acute pharyngitis is the principal manifestation, may be complicated by suppurative infections including otitis media and acute sinusitis. (See the articles on these topics.) It is also important to recognize that certain viral agents, such as adenovirus, that produce the pharyngitis syndrome may also produce lower respiratory tract infection, including pneumonia. Lower respiratory tract infection, therefore, does not necessarily reflect a suppurative complication but may be an extension of the initial infection.

Complications associated with streptococcal infection are of particular interest. Suppurative complications, though less frequent in this antibiotic era, are still of some concern. These include otitis media, sinusitis, and peritonsillar or retropharyngeal abscess. Nonsuppurative complications of streptococcal pharyngitis have attracted considerable attention over the years, in particular acute rheumatic fever. Acute rheumatic fever may be a complication of untreated or improperly treated acute streptococcal pharyngitis in which the offending organism persists for a number of days or weeks. (See the article on rheumatic fever.) Acute glomerulonephritis may be a complication of either streptococcal pharyngitis or streptococcal skin infection. (See the article on glomerulonephritis.) Appropriate treatment (penicillin) of acute streptococcal pharyngitis to eradicate the offending organism will prevent acute rheumatic fever. There is less evidence that treatment of either throat or skin infection uniformly prevents the development of acute glomerulonephritis. However, only limited types of group A streptococci are known to cause nephritis, and unless such "nephritogenic" types are present, the risk of nephritis is essentially nil.

PHYSICAL EXAMINATION

Physical findings in acute streptococcal and other forms of pharyngitis have been mentioned previously. The physical examination in patients with streptococcal pharyngitis usually fails to reveal abnormalities other than those directly related to the acute throat infection and associated cervical lymphadenitis. An obvious exception is scarlet fever, in which the typical rash of this disease appears. It is often most marked in the covered areas and on flexor surfaces of the arms. After several days the rash of scarlet fever begins to peel, resulting in a branny desquamation, often associated with considerable pruritus. Should complications such as sinusitis, otitis media or peritonsillar abscess occur, physical findings will reflect these various conditions. Patients with streptococcal infection may also have acute urticaria, and care should be taken to distinguish this from urticaria secondary to antibiotic hypersensitivity reaction.

LABORATORY FINDINGS

The simplest and most direct laboratory approach to the patient with acute pharyngitis is the throat culture. This documents or excludes the presence of group A beta hemolytic streptococci. Positive throat cultures in patients with acute manifestations are sufficient reason to make an etiologic diagnosis of streptococcal disease; negative throat cultures are sufficient to exclude the diagnosis of streptococcal disease. In general, patients with acute streptococcal illness have larger numbers of beta hemolytic streptococci present in the throat than do healthy children who are carriers. Occasionally a patient may have large numbers of streptococcus present in throat culture during coincidental, nonstreptococcal respiratory tract infection. Since one cannot exclude a contributing role for the streptococcus, such patients are treated for streptococcal disease.

Throat cultures can be easily done, even in office practice, provided appropriate materials and good techniques are employed. Cultures may be grown aerobically or under partial CO_2; overnight growth for 18 to 24 hours at 37°C is sufficient. It is important to estimate the quantity of organisms present and document that beta hemolytic streptococci are group A, since the latter group is responsible for streptococcal complications. A simple laboratory test, the bacitracin disc test (done on the primary blood agar plate), demonstrates inhibition of growth of group A streptococci in the presence of low concentrations of bacitracin; non–group A strains such as B, C, and G are not inhibited.

Many clinicians believe that a peripheral white blood cell count is of benefit in evaluating the patient with acute pharyngitis. A leukocytosis with left shift is more likely to occur in streptococcal, rather than nonstreptococcal, pharyngitis, but some patients with clinical and bacterial evidence of streptococcal disease may have an equivocal finding or a normal blood count. Peripheral blood smears are useful when infectious mononucleosis is suspected; one should look for the characteristic atypical lymphocytes. The sedimentation rate and C-reactive protein may be elevated or positive more often in patients with streptococcal infection than those with non-streptococcal disease; however, neither of these tests is specific.

In infectious mononucleosis a Mono Spot Test and heterophile antibody titers are of value; the latter should be done on acute and convalescent sera to confirm the diagnosis. Certain antibody tests are of value for demonstrating an immune response to group A streptococcal infection but are of little or no value in the acute illness. Antibody titers are best interpreted when acute and convalescent titers are done. Since the latter are not usually available in uncomplicated cases, streptococcal antibody titers find their most important use in evaluating patients with suspected streptococcal complications such as rheumatic fever or nephritis, or in the occasional patient with recurrent sore throat and persistent positive streptococcal cultures in whom the question—infection versus carriage—arises. A number of streptococcal antibody tests are available, the most commonly used being anti-streptolysin O and anti-DNAse B. The former is a classical antibody test for patients with pharyngitis and streptococcal complications of sore throat, while the latter is of use in both respiratory and skin infections caused by group A streptococcus.

THERAPEUTIC TESTS

There are no useful therapeutic tests for aiding the clinician in the differential diagnosis of acute pharyngitis. Indeed, one should avoid the temptation to interpret a clinical response in the patient given one or two doses of antibiotic because of the variability of the clinical course of most forms of acute pharyngitis including streptococcal disease.

POTENTIAL AREAS OF PITFALLS IN DIAGNOSIS

The first and most important consideration in evaluating the patient with acute pharyngitis is to take an appropriate history and perform a careful physical examination to document the nature of the illness. These observations, in addition to an understanding of the epidemiologic features of common respiratory tract infectious agents, are of great value in the initial evaluation. The appropriate use of throat culture, as indicated, should distinguish streptococcal from nonstreptococcal disease. It is important to perform this simple procedure properly: The common pitfalls in streptococcal bacteriology are an inadequate throat swab, inadequate or poor quality of culture media, or an inexperienced person attempting to interpret the throat culture results. When gonococcal pharyngitis is suspected, it is important that appropriate culture media and cultural conditions be employed for the recovery of the organism, which is more fastidious than the streptococcus and requires different media and cultural conditions. (See article on Gonococcal Infections.)

Much has been written about the difficulty in distinguishing streptococcal infection from carriage. The majority of acutely ill patients with pharyngitis and a positive streptococcal throat culture do not pose a clinical problem in diagnosis or management. Patients who become "problems" because of recurrent symptoms, repeat positive cultures, or both may require additional or sequential evaluation, including careful assessment of clinical features at the time throat cultures are done, estimates of numbers of streptococci present in each culture, and determination of the pattern of streptococcal antibody response. It is important not to *overestimate* the problem of distinguishing carriage from infection. A patient who remains asymptomatic and who harbors small to moderate numbers of streptococci in the throat over time without manifesting significant antibody change is very unlikely to be at risk for streptococcal complications. In particular, one should not subject an asymptomatic child to repeated courses of penicillin in an effort to eradicate small numbers of beta hemolytic streptococci.

TUMORS OF THE LARYNX AND PHARYNX

By Joseph H. Ogura, M.D.*
Richard L. Carpenter, M.D.
and Peter J. Vandermeer, M.D.
St. Louis, Missouri

Tumors of the pharynx and larynx are relatively uncommon and frequently present with minimal early symptoms. This often results in a lack of clinical suspicion and a delay in diagnosis and, therefore, treatment. A thorough approach to patients with complaints relating to the pharynx and larynx is important. This involves a complete history, physical examination, and appropriate diagnostic evaluation.

The pharynx is the musculomembranous sac, divided into the nasopharynx, oropharynx, and the hypopharynx. The nasopharynx extends from the posterior choanae to the level of the soft palate. The oropharynx extends from the soft palate to the level of the hyoid bone; the anterior margin is the anterior tonsillar pillar. The hypopharynx extends from the hyoid bone to the lower border of the cricoid cartilage. The larynx extends from the epiglottis, aryepiglottic

*Deceased.

folds, and arytenoids to the inferior margin of the cricoid. The lining of this sac consists primarily of squamous mucosa with scattered glandular elements. Waldeyer's ring is a circular band of lymphoid tissue that includes the lingual and pharyngeal tonsils, adenoids, and other smaller aggregates of lymphoid tissue.

Tumors in this region are varied and classified as congenital, neoplastic, and inflammatory.

CONGENITAL LESIONS

Congenital lesions of the pharynx and larynx include thyroglossal duct cysts, mucosal cysts, laryngoceles, diverticuli, and hemangiomas. Thyroglossal duct cysts or incompletely descended thyroid glands may present in the pharynx as midline masses of the base of tongue or anteriorly in the neck. Small mucosal retention cysts appear frequently in the tonsils, vallecula, or epiglottis. Unless they enlarge greatly or cause symptoms of a foreign-body sensation or obstruction, they may be left alone.

Within the larynx, cysts of the laryngeal ventricle may be either fluid-filled mucoceles or air-filled laryngoceles. These may cause significant voice change or airway obstruction. They may extend from the interior of the larynx out into the neck.

Pharyngoesophageal or Zenker's diverticuli present with dysphagia, odynophagia, and regurgitation of food, and this is often complicated by aspiration pneumonia. While thought to be congenital lesions, they are usually seen in middle-aged patients.

Hemangiomas may present throughout the pharynx and larynx. A common site is the palate, but they also present in the subglottic region and may cause severe respiratory obstruction. They may be associated with cutaneous hemangiomas.

Vertebral osteophytes may present as firm, immobile posterior pharyngeal masses causing symptoms of dysphagia.

NEOPLASTIC LESIONS

Benign tumors in this region are relatively rare when compared with malignancies. In order of decreasing frequency they include papillomas, chondromas, neurofibromas, leiomyomas, angiofibromas, myomas, and chemodectomas. In many patients the diagnosis is obvious on examination.

Papillomas may occur as single or multiple warty growths. A chondroma will present most often as a smooth mass arising from the cricoid or thyroid cartilage. Neurofibromas present throughout the larynx and pharynx and are most commonly associated with von Recklinghausen's disease. Leiomyomas present as smooth rounded submucosal masses in the larynx and pharynx. Angiofibromas are highly vascular tumors occurring almost exclusively in the nasopharynx of adolescent males. Myomas usually present as red excrescent masses in the arytenoid regions. Chemodectomas present as cystic masses in the ventricle or false vocal cord region.

Of malignant neoplasms, approximately 95 per cent are squamous cell carcinomas of the mucous membranes. They are strongly associated with tobacco use. Metastasis to regional cervical lymphatics is common.

Prognosis depends on the stage of tumor at diagnosis, the presence of metastatic spread, and the region involved (Fig. 1). In general, laryngeal cancer has a good prognosis with high cure rates. The best cure rates are for glottic carcinoma (Fig. 2). Supraglottic and transglottic tumors are still highly curable lesions, as are tonsillar and base of tongue tumors (Fig. 3). Piriform recess and posterior pharynx carcinomas have a dismal percentage of cures in spite of maximal therapy.

INFLAMMATORY LESIONS

Inflammatory processes, including bacterial, viral, and granulomatous disease, often present as pharyngeal and laryngeal masses. The masses may enlarge in response to inflammation and may suppurate to form abscesses. With asymmetric enlargement in what is otherwise thought to be an inflammatory condition, lymphomas should be suspected.

HISTORY

Patients with tumors of the pharynx and larynx are often symptomatic for several months prior to evaluation. Symptoms are often vague, nonspecific, and varied. They include a foreign-body sensation in the throat, dysphagia, odynophagia, hoarseness, stridor,

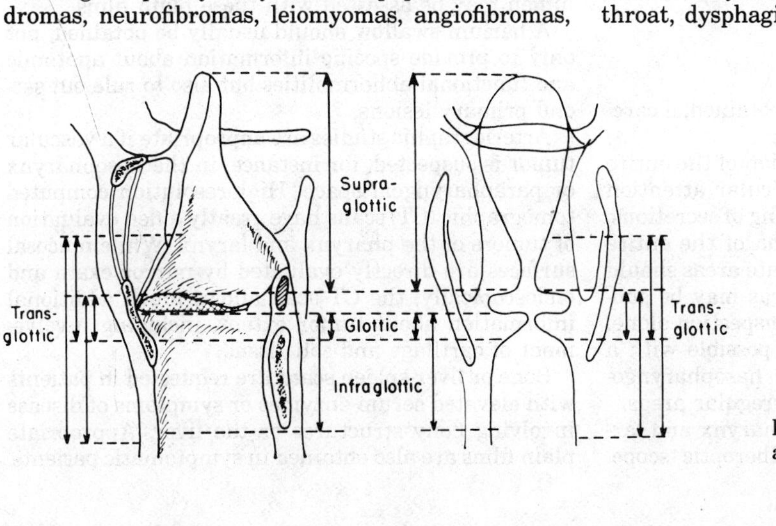

Figure 1. Primary site classification for laryngeal tumors. *Left,* lateral view; *right,* anterior view.

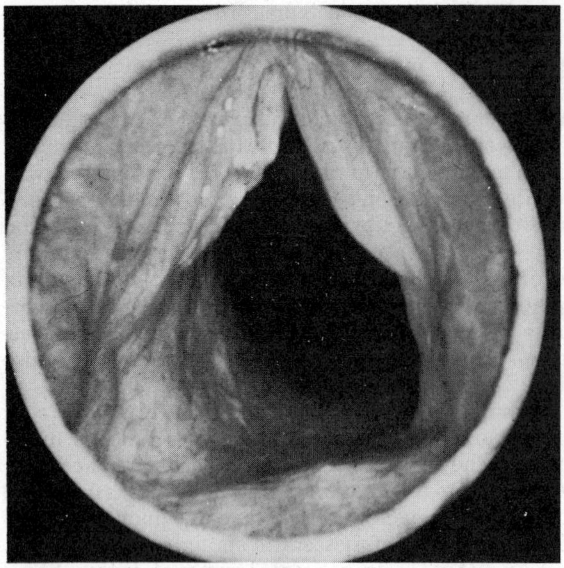

Figure 2. A squamous cell carcinoma of the true vocal cord as seen endoscopically.

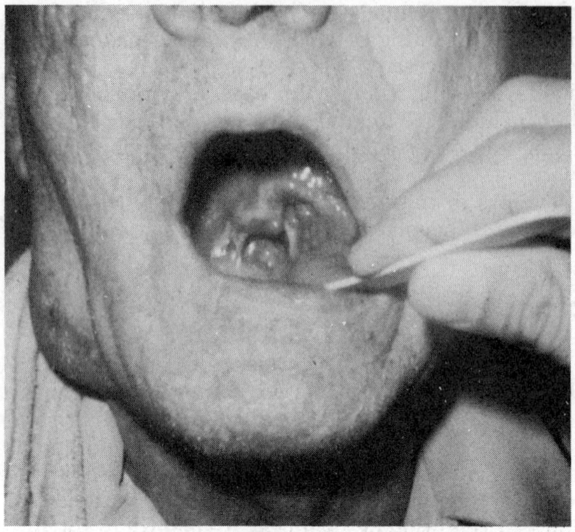

Figure 3. Large squamous cell carcinoma of the tonsil with associated neck metastases in an elderly man.

otalgia, hemoptysis, cough, or weight loss. Occasionally a tumor may be asymptomatic and therefore discovered only on routine examination.

A patient with any of these symptoms should be questioned as to their duration and severity. A review of associated illness, other tumors, tobacco and alcohol use, prior radiation treatments, trauma to the head and neck, and family history of similar tumors should also be done.

Tumors of the nasopharynx are often initially asymptomatic but may cause nasal stuffiness, epistaxis, or a unilateral serous otitis media. For this reason, all adults with a unilateral serous otitis media should have examination of the nasopharynx.

Oropharyngeal and hypopharyngeal tumors are often associated with pain, dysphagia, weight loss, a foreign-body sensation, localized bleeding, or referred otalgia. Tumors in the parapharyngeal space may present as masses in the tonsillar fossa. Tumors of the larynx typically present very early with hoarseness and much later with stridor.

PHYSICAL EXAMINATION

After a thorough history has been obtained, a careful physical examination is indicated.

Using a bright light source, inspection of the entire oropharynx is performed, with particular attention directed to swelling, asymmetry, pooling of secretions, or bleeding or friable areas. Palpation of the entire floor of mouth, tongue, tonsil, and palate areas should be done because tumors in these areas may be submucosal and not readily detected by inspection alone. Visualization of the nasopharynx is possible with a nasopharyngeal mirror or fiberoptic nasopharyngoscope. Note is taken of bleeding or irregular areas.

Indirect visualization of the hypopharynx and larynx is possible with a mirror or fiberoptic scope. Masses or granular areas of the vallecula, epiglottis, piriform sinuses, and laryngeal interior are often obvious to the trained observer. Vocal cord paralysis is often a finding with more advanced laryngeal carcinomas. It is important to be aware that up to 10 per cent of carcinomas in these areas have synchronous second primary cancers and that as many as 20 per cent of these patients will have an unassociated second primary lesion within 5 years. Therefore, a complete evaluation of the upper aerodigestive tract is mandatory.

Physical examination is not complete without palpation of node-bearing areas of the head and neck, since these areas are commonly involved by regional metastasis.

RADIOGRAPHIC EVALUATION

Soft-tissue and airway films may demonstrate a nasopharyngeal mass or an air-fluid level in a diverticulum or laryngocele. Glottic and subglottic lesions may be obvious, and the caliber of the laryngeal lumen may be assessed with these plain films.

A barium swallow should usually be obtained, not only to provide specific information about anatomic and functional abnormalities but also to rule out second primary lesions.

Arteriographic studies are appropriate if a vascular tumor is suspected, for instance, in the nasopharynx or parapharyngeal space. High-resolution computed tomographic (CT) scans have greatly aided evaluation of tumors of the pharynx and larynx. While mucosal surfaces are directly evaluated by mirror exam and endoscopically, the CT scan allows much additional information about tumor extent, including involvement of cartilage and soft tissue.

Bone or liver-spleen scans are requested in patients with elevated serum enzymes or symptoms of disease involving bony structures or the liver. Appropriate plain films are also obtained in symptomatic patients.

ENDOSCOPY

After a complete history, a physical examination, and a radiographic work-up are completed, direct endoscopy should be performed. Laryngoscopy, nasopharyngoscopy, and esophagoscopy should be performed by an experienced endoscopist or head and neck surgeon. Biopsy and mapping of lesions are performed at this time. In addition, if preoperative radio therapy or chemotherapy is planned, the margins of the tumor are tattooed. Secondary lesions are searched for. In patients for whom nutrition has been a problem, early nutritional consultation and evaluation with hyperalimentation (enteral or intravenous) are helpful in avoiding complications of surgery.

CONCLUSION

Though tumors of the pharynx and larynx often present with vague symptomology, they are often malignant. Treatment that will succeed in conserving function and in curing the patient depends upon early recognition of such tumors. All patients with symptoms referrable to the pharynx and larynx should have prompt, thorough, and expert evaluation.

Section Four

RESPIRATORY SYSTEM

THE DIAGNOSIS OF PULMONARY TUMORS

By Clifton F. Mountain, M.D.*
Houston, Texas

The great majority of tumors originating in the lungs are primary lung cancers. Tubercular and fungal granulomas and hamartomas are the most common benign lesions. Since there are few absolute criteria of benignity of masses occurring in the lungs, the diagnostic procedures obviously overlap.

LUNG CANCER

Synonyms. Lung cancer, bronchogenic carcinoma, bronchial carcinoma, carcinoma of the lung, bronchiogenic carcinoma, bronchial adenoma, bronchiolar carcinoma. The term *bronchogenic carcinoma* is in general use as a synonym for lung cancer. This is somewhat misleading because it implies a bronchial origin for all lung carcinomas, which may not be true. Carcinomas account for over 90 per cent of malignant lung tumors. Carcinoids (bronchial adenoma) comprise 5 to 10 per cent. Variants of the carcinoid type, called *cylindromas* or *adenoid cystic carcinoma,* occur less frequently; and mucoepidermoid carcinoma, which can occur in young children as well as in elderly persons, is rare.

Definition. Primary cancer of the lung refers to those malignant tumors arising within the lung, for the most part from the epithelium of the tracheobronchial tree. The incidence of the major histologic types may vary according to geographic location, to the type of population surveyed, or even to the sophistication of the available pathology service. For example, Table 1 shows the frequency of each cell type diagnosed at our institution (The University of Texas M.D. Anderson Hospital) during a recent 4-year period. Owing to the nature of the specialized cancer center, fewer "early" resectable patients are seen and the higher proportion of adenocarcinoma and small cell patients reflects the preponderance of "late" stage patients referred for investigational treatment programs. Further, a highly specialized pathology team, including an electron microscopist, is involved in the classification process.

*Supported by DCT-NCI Contracts NO1-CM-77149 and NCI-CM-07417.

Squamous Cell Carcinoma

Historically, squamous cell carcinoma has been the most prevalent cell type. It is most commonly linked with cigarette smoking, although an increased incidence of adenocarcinoma and small cell carcinoma is also reported among smokers.

Squamous cell carcinoma arises in the basal cells of the bronchial epithelium; it is usually centrally located in the segmental or larger bronchi. Squamous cell carcinoma is the only cell type with a recognized phase of dysplasia and carcinoma in situ distinct from invasive carcinoma.

Precarcinoma and preclinical and clinical phases are demonstrated.

Precarcinoma. The precarcinoma phase may last for several years, during which time dysplastic nuclear changes in the cells in the sputum are observed. Careful follow-up at short intervals is indicated for such patients with dysplastic cells in the sputum, as they are at high risk for developing squamous cell carcinoma.

Preclinical Phase. In this phase of development, malignant squamous cells are found in the sputum and the source of the tumor is not seen on chest x-rays. These tumors can usually be localized by meticulous fiberoptic examination of the tracheobronchial tree, preceded by careful examination of the upper airway to rule out a nasopharyngeal or laryngeal primary.

Clinical Phase. This phase begins when the tumor can be visualized on the chest film or has caused bronchial obstruction resulting in atelectasis and pneumonia. These signs and symptoms are usually indicative of more advanced disease; however, many patients first seen in the clinical phase still have disease that is amenable to complete resection. The best outcome, overall, is usually achieved for patients with squamous cell carcinoma.

Adenocarcinoma

Adenocarcinoma arises from the epithelium of much smaller bronchi than those in which squamous cell carcinoma occurs. Thus it is primarily a peripheral tumor and is the most frequent type of tumor found in this location. A strong association has been noted between scarring of the lungs and the development of adenocarcinoma; however, there is evidence that adenocarcinoma produces typical central foci of scarring due to vascular involvement.

Adenocarcinoma is the most common type of lung tumor diagnosed in women. Its incidence is reportedly increasing, and this is apparently a real increase, not

Table 1. Frequency of Lung Cancer by Cell Type*

Cell Type	Per Cent
Squamous cell carcinoma	32.3
Adenocarcinoma	38.5
Large cell, undifferentiated	3.2
Small cell, undifferentiated	22.3
Other	3.7

* Data from The University of Texas, M.D. Anderson Hospital and Tumor Institute, Houston, 1975–1978.

related to the increased incidence of lung cancer in women or to refinements in histologic classification.

The outcome for patients with adenocarcinoma is, overall, poorer than that achieved for the squamous cell group. Patients with stage I disease have as good or better survival rates following resection as squamous cell patients, but any further progression of stage forewarns of much poorer prognosis, even in patients whose disease is technically resectable. Adenocarcinoma, although slower to progress, exhibits a metastatic pattern similar to that of small cell carcinoma, with a predilection for central nervous system metastases. It differs from small cell carcinoma in that the brain is often a single site of metastasis in the absence of widespread dissemination. The histologic and radiographic distinction between primary lung cancer and pulmonary metastasis may be difficult in patients known to have adenocarcinoma elsewhere and who have a peripheral nodule seen on chest x-ray.

Bronchioloalveolar carcinoma (bronchoalveolar, bronchiolar, alveolar cell) is a subtype of adenocarcinoma arising in the terminal bronchioalveolar area. It grows on the walls of the distal air spaces and disseminates through the airways. Bronchioloalveolar carcinoma is associated with scarring, as are other peripheral tumors, but the etiology of this tumor is unknown. In our own work, we have not shown a significant survival advantage for this cell type over that of adenocarcinoma in resected patients with stage I disease. However, it is a biologically favorable tumor, in that it tends to remain confined to the lungs even when extensive local growth and spread is observed.

Large Cell Carcinoma

Large cell undifferentiated tumors are characterized by a lack of differentiating features seen in the other cell types. In the presence of a significant amount of intracellular mucin, these tumors are usually classified as adenocarcinoma. Some large cell carcinomas, called *giant cell carcinomas,* exhibit large numbers of multinucleate cells and some having a clear cytoplasm, are called *clear cell carcinoma.* The giant cell type, which is uncommon, usually follows a fulminant course. Large cell tumors tend to be bulky and more peripheral than squamous cell tumors. Their biologic behavior and response to therapy is generally similar to that of adenocarcinoma; however, they may have less propensity for distant metastasis.

Small Cell Carcinoma

There are differing theories regarding the origin of small cell carcinoma; however, it is generally regarded as a form of bronchogenic carcinoma arising from bronchial epithelium which has, in some cases, biochemical and ultrastructural properties similar to those seen in tumors of the APUD system (tumors that cause secondary clinical effects by secreting polypeptide hormones). These tumors tend to occur in a central location, but they may be located peripherally.

Small cell carcinoma is characterized by very rapid growth and early dissemination outside of the chest. It is not uncommon for a small cell carcinoma, even when it presents as a small peripheral lesion, to have metastasized widely to the mediastinum or to distant organs at the time of diagnosis. There is no preclinical phase, and patients usually come to clinical attention because of symptoms caused by rapidly spreading disease, or in some cases, ectopic hormone production.

Small cell carcinomas are classified in three subtypes: (1) oat cell, one of the most distinctive lung cancers histologically; (2) intermediate cell; and (3) combined, usually with squamous cell carcinoma. In this latter case, small cell remains the primary classification. It has been proposed that these subtypes have an influence on prognosis; however, this has not been definitively determined.

There appears to be an increasing incidence of small cell carcinoma among women, greater than that observed in men. In recent years, significant progress in prolongation of median survival time has been made in the treatment of patients with this disease through the use of polychemotherapy and combined modality programs.

Bronchial Carcinoid

Bronchial carcinoids, or adenomas, are uncommon tumors, accounting for less than 10 per cent of all lung tumors. They do, however, represent a larger proportion of all tumors excised. These tumors are slow-growing but frequently are locally invasive and occasionally metastasize. They grow as polypoid masses that bulge into the bronchial lumen, but mucosal ulceration is infrequent. This intraluminal growth produces clinical symptoms such as cough, hemoptysis, bronchiectasis, emphysema, and atelectasis.

The older term, "bronchial adenoma," has been replaced with the designation "bronchial carcinoid," since 90 per cent of these tumors are of the carcinoid type. Bronchial carcinoids belong to the APUD class of tumors, and electron microscopy reveals the neurosecretory granules characteristic of such tumors. They may produce one or more of a number of biologically active substances, such as 5-hydroxytryptamine (serotonin) or adrenocorticotropic hormone (ACTH); however, a classic carcinoid syndrome or Cushing's syndrome is rarely seen. Most bronchial carcinoids do not have secretory activity, and although they do metastasize to intrapulmonary lymph nodes, to the liver, and elsewhere, a relatively benign course over a long period of time is characteristic.

Complete surgical removal usually provides a very good outcome.

Variants classified according to histologic pattern as cylindroma, adenoid cystic carcinoma, and mucoepidermoid carcinoma (which is rarely seen) are derived from submucosal bronchial glands and resemble tumors of salivary gland origin. The cylindromatous type is more likely to metastasize than the carcinoid pattern.

BENIGN LUNG TUMORS

Benign Mesenchymal Tumors

Benign lung tumors are rare. The hamartoma is the most common type. It is slow-growing and usually appears on chest x-rays as a "coin" lesion in asymptomatic individuals. A small proportion may be endobronchial, but most are found in the periphery of the lung. This tumor is composed mainly of mature hyaline cartilage; however, the recent report of Bateson, who reviewed the pathology in 305 cases, showed 41 per cent of these tumors to contain adipose tissue. It has been suggested that a preoperative diagnosis of hamartoma can be made by computed tomography (CT) density measurements in those patients with solitary pulmonary nodules containing mixed fat and soft-tissue densities. This may be particularly helpful when the characteristic calcific pattern is absent. Malignant change in these tumors is extraordinarily rare, but some may increase in size and become symptomatic. If there is no excessive risk to thoracotomy, the tumors are usually removed.

The incidence of lipomas, fibromas, neuromas, and leiomyomas in the lung is very low, and most of these tumors are not clinically significant. Generally, they are removed for diagnosis and to prevent continuing growth and subsequent possible airway obstruction. The bronchial chondroma is a very uncommon tumor that arises from bronchial rings and thus is inseparable from the wall of the bronchus.

Granuloma

The term "granuloma" is used to designate chronic inflammatory lesions that occur in the form of a mass resembling a tumor. Such masses of granulation tissue develop in response to certain chronic infections, the most common being tuberculosis (tuberculoma), histoplasmosis, and coccidioidomycosis. Any organism, however, that can incite a granulomatous reaction is capable of producing a mass, and such lesions are clinically relevant in the differential diagnosis of lung neoplasms. The incidence of infective granulomas may be related to the geographic distribution of endemic fungal areas. Noninfectious granulomas, small pulmonary nodules, or larger masses are produced by some diseases such as sarcoidosis, silicosis, and coal worker's pneumonconiosis. Wegener's granulomatosis and rheumatoid nodules are less common. Necrobiotic lung nodules are a rare manifestation in rheumatoid arthritis; however, they can present a diagnostic problem if they precede the arthritis or the detection of circulating rheumatoid factor. In those cases of undiagnosed lung opacities, a search for rheumatoid factor and personal or family history of rheumatoid disease is worthwhile.

Freundlich has categorized benign masses radiologically into those with smooth and those with irregular borders, as shown in Table 2. He notes that benign solitary masses with grossly irregular, but usually not finely serrated, borders, almost always are inflammatory and granulomatous. Granulomas usually are calcified in a laminated or speckled fashion, and many cavitate. As a result of the past infection, any of the granulomas may have scars and satellite lesions around the mass.

Other Benign Lesions

There are a number of rare benign neoplasms and non-neoplastic disorders of uncertain histogenesis, such as so-called sclerosing hemangioma, benign clear cell tumor, and inflammatory pseudotumor. So-called sclerosing hemangioma and benign clear cell tumors appear on x-ray as circumscribed, noncalcified, noncavitating peripheral masses. As the name implies, so-called sclerosing hemangioma is characterized by marked proliferation of small blood vessels, usually focal within the tumor. It has a specific histologic appearance, and when it is removed the diagnosis is readily apparent. Benign clear cell tumors are rare and have the distinguishing histologic feature of abundant intracytoplasmic glycogen, which is not present in other tumors.

The inflammatory pseudotumor (plasma cell granuloma, pseudotumors, histiocytoma, xanthoma, solitary mast cell tumors, pseudoneoplastic pneumonitis) is a non-neoplastic pulmonary mass made up of a variety of different types of cells. Inflammatory pseudotumor is uncommon but is found in disproportionate numbers in younger patients. In children younger than 16 years old, it is the most common, isolated, primary tumor-like lesion. Roentgenographically, it appears as a solitary solid nodule with smooth borders located in the lung parenchyma. About half of the patients with this tumor have symptoms related to the lungs, such as cough, hemoptysis, shortness of breath, and pain. The etiology is unknown, and the lesion is not associated with systemic disease or other abnormalities. Surgical removal is usually necessary to establish the diagnosis and the prognosis is usually excellent.

PRESENTING SIGNS AND SYMPTOMS

Unfortunately, bronchogenic carcinoma is a great mimic of less serious diseases in the chest. Indeed, it has no specific symptoms unique unto itself. It can masquerade as any benign respiratory ailment and is generally asymptomatic in its earliest stages, such as in the precarcinoma phase of squamous cell carcinoma, previously described, in which 6 or 8 years may be required before the tumor becomes roentgenographically visible.

Table 2. Benign Masses*

Solitary with Smooth Borders	Solitary with Irregular Borders	Multiple with Smooth Borders	Multiple with Irregular Borders
Granulomas (tuberculous, fungal†)	Nocardiosis†	Fungal granulomas†	Wegener's granulomatosis†
Hamartoma (adenoma)	Actinomycosis†	Septic emboli†	Nocardiosis†
A–V malformation	Wegener's granulomatosis†	Rheumatoid nodules†	Primary lymphoma
Hematoma	Chronic pneumonitis	Echinococcosis†	Fungal granulomas†
Bronchogenic cyst	Rounded atelectasis	A–V malformations	Sarcoid granulomas†
			Conglomerate silicosis
			Fibrotic masses of coal worker's pneumoconiosis
			Chronic pneumonitis

*Reproduced with permission from Freundlich, I.M.: *Pulmonary Masses, Cysts, and Cavities: A Radiologic Approach*. Copyright © 1981 by Year Book Medical Publishers, Inc., Chicago.
†Cavitation common.

The likelihood of the presence of lung cancer in a given patient will be based on the integration of information regarding the disease itself with a carefully detailed history of the patient's lifestyle, smoking history, alcohol intake, workplace, familial disease record, and record of past illnesses. The relationship between lung cancer and smoking is based on the excess of lung cancer deaths among smokers and the observation that less than 10 per cent of patients with this disease are nonsmokers. Older age groups are those predominantly affected, and the male:female ratio is 3:1. Higher incidence rates are reported for urban compared to rural areas. A number of occupational exposures, such as asbestos workers and those exposed to arsenic, chromium, nickel, and ionizing radiation in various types of mining, particularly uranium, have been identified. The number of persons exposed to these industrial hazards is limited, but they all apparently present a more serious problem combined with smoking. A genetic component is recognized in lung cancer, as well as in other malignancies. There are inadequate data, however, to demonstrate an hereditary etiology. It is of interest that a relationship between deficient dietary vitamin A intake and lung cancer has been reported recently.

Symptom Pattern

A pattern of symptomatology that creates a high index of suspicion for lung cancer includes (1) chronic cough, (2) change in pulmonary habit, (3) hemoptysis, (4) wheezing in the absence of a history of asthma, (5) recurrent episodes of pneumonia, (6) fever and weakness, (7) weight loss, and (8) chest pain. Symptoms of more advanced disease include (1) hoarseness, (2) exertional dyspnea (with bronchial obstruction), (3) obvious supraclavicular lymph nodes, (4) shoulder and arm pain (associated with brachial plexus involvement by apical tumor, (5) dysphagia, and (6) Horner's syndrome.

More than half the people who develop lung cancer have had bronchitis for years, and very often the symptom bringing the patient to seek clinical attention is a worsening of the "smoker's cough." In regard to this symptom pattern, which is common to heavy cigarette smokers, the paradox must be acknowledged that the majority of smokers do not develop lung cancer and some persons who never smoke do develop the disease. Nevertheless, bronchial carcinoma is the most common cancer in the Western world, and it is essential to exclude its presence in any patient in whom the chest disease is symptomatic.

Extrathoracic Manifestations of Lung Cancer

About 10 per cent of lung cancer patients will present with primary or coexisting extrapulmonary manifestations of their disease. Indeed, the earliest symptoms and signs may be systemic in nature. Extrapulmonary manifestations can, in themselves, be life-threatening, and they frequently complicate the clinical picture. An increased awareness of the systemic effects of lung cancer has been evident in recent years (Table 3). The most commonly encountered extrathoracic manifestation of bronchogenic carcinoma is that of clubbing of the nails, which occurs in 8 to 12 per cent of patients and most frequently is associated with squamous cell carcinoma. Gynecomastia is almost as common and frequently accompanies hypertrophic pulmonary osteoarthropathy. Polyarthritis and migratory thrombophlebitis are less commonly observed, but they are more apt to be presenting symptoms that take the patient to the physician.

The presence of unusual hormonal syndromes in patients with lung cancer has been observed for many years, but the development of contemporary methods of bioassay and immunoassay has been necessary to understand the mechanism of their production. Sensitive tests for these substances have been developed and applied in the search for a specific marker for "early" lung cancer, even if the clinical syndrome is not present. The relationship of cell type to ectopic hormone production is shown in Table 4. Two new markers, serum neuron-specific enolase and bombesin have been reported to characterize small cell lung cancer.

History

A very common history is that of a patient over 50 years of age with a long history of heavy cigarette

Table 3. Extrathoracic Nonmetastatic Manifestations of Lung Cancer*

Skeletal	**Vascular**
Clubbing	Thrombophlebitis
Hypertrophic pulmonary osteoarthropathy	Nonbacterial endocarditis
Dermatologic	**Endocrine**
Acanthosis nigricans	ACTH, ADH, MSH
Erythema gyratum repens	Calcitonin
Pigmentation	Parathormone
Renal	Growth hormone
Nephrotic syndrome	Gonadotropin
Neurologic	Prolactin
Leukoencephalopathy	Gastric inhibitory peptide
Cerebellar degeneration	Vasoactive intestinal peptide
Polymyositis	**Systemic**
Myasthenia-like syndrome	Weakness
Hematologic	Weight loss
Anemia	Anorexia
Leukemoid reaction	Taste disturbance

*Reproduced with permission from Margolese, R.G., et al.: Recent advances in management of lung cancer. In MacLean, L.D., et al. (eds.): *Advances in Surgery*, vol. 15. Copyright © 1981 by Year Book Medical Publishers, Inc., Chicago.

Abbreviations: ACTH = Adrenocorticotropic hormone; MSH = melanocyte-stimulating hormone; ADH = antidiuretic hormone.

smoking and a change in pulmonary habit. The patient has a chronic cough that initially was dry and hacking but subsequently became productive of mucus. The patient has frequent bouts of pneumonia and may be aware of wheezing. With the passage of time, if unattended, the sputum will become tinged with blood, and some degree of exertional dyspnea will be present. Persistent fever and a general malaise will accompany a persistent pneumonitis that is not responsive to appropriate antibiotics. The patient will frequently complain of thoracic discomfort or deep-seated pain.

If the lesion is peripheral and invasive of the chest wall, the factor of pain will become the most important item in the patient's history. Particularly with lesions of the left main bronchus, dysphagia or dysphonia may be the initial symptom. In the case of tumors located in the extreme apex of the lung (often referred to as superior sulcus or Pancoast's tumor), the patient will almost invariably present with a history of pain about the shoulder and down the arm associated with muscle wasting and possible weakness in the affected extremity. When this "painful apical syndrome" is associated with local destruction of the second or third rib and/or of the corresponding thoracic vertebral bodies accompanying Horner's syndrome, it is known as Pancoast's syndrome. This symptom complex is, of course, related to invasion of the brachial plexus and paralysis of the sympathetic ganglion.

Tumors that arise in a more central location are likely to cause atelectasis, and the symptoms of obstructive pneumonitis with ill-defined chest pain are more commonly encountered. With the progress of such lesions, evidence of mediastinal lymph node involvement or direct mediastinal extension may become evident in the patient's history. A change in the tonal quality of the voice may be noticed by the patient, or, more frequently, by a close member of the family. This indicates involvement of the recurrent laryngeal nerve and is more commonly associated with lesions arising within the left hilar structures. Patients may also present with signs and symptoms of superior vena caval obstruction.

It is not uncommon for a patient to present with signs and symptoms of hematogenous dissemination as the first evidence of pulmonary cancer. Abnormalities related to the central nervous system and bone pain are the most frequent presenting symptoms of distant metastasis. Other sites of distal spread, such as the liver or adrenal glands, may be as common but are usually clinically silent.

Course of the Disease

The observed clinical course of bronchogenic carcinoma is dependent upon (1) functional status of the patient at the time of symptom onset, (2) biologic behavior of the specific cell type, (3) stage of the diseases at the time of diagnosis, (4) type of therapy utilized, and (5) tumor-host relationships. Long-term control of the disease is dependent upon 100 per cent tumor cell eradication by whatever treatment is implemented.

PHYSICAL EXAMINATION

Physical findings associated with lung cancer may be minimal or even absent. Systemic manifestations with pallor and physical evidence of weight loss generally signify advanced disease. Tachycardia and fever may accompany atelectasis and obstructive pneumonitis. In examination of the head and neck, palpation of the supraclavicular and scalene lymph nodes is extremely important to discover metastatic nodes. There is a high correlation between the clinician's judgment with respect to metastatic nodes in this area and positive findings at biopsy. Indirect laryngoscopy should be done if mediastinal involvement of the recurrent laryngeal nerves is suspected. The presence of Horner's syndrome with sinking in of the eyeball, ptosis of the upper eyelid, constriction of the pupil, and narrowing of the palpebral fissures in association with anhidrosis would indicate paralysis of the sympathetic chain which is most commonly associated with a malignant lesion. Examination of the cranial nerves may suggest cerebral metastasis. Neck vein distention, prominence of veins of the anterior chest wall, and symptoms of lightheadedness when bending over all suggest superior vena caval obstruction. Tracheal deviation indicates a mediastinal shift, usually to the side of atelectasis, although it may be displaced in the opposing direction by tumor.

Simple inspection of the thorax and observation of the ventilatory habit is often helpful in the initial evaluation of ventilatory reserve. Localized tenderness suggests a point of chest wall invasion or metastasis to rib. In percussion of the lungs, one can detect

Table 4. Relationship of Cell Type to Ectopic Hormone Production*

	Small Cell		Squamous Cell		Adeno-carcinoma		Large Cell	
	No.	*Per Cent Positive*	*No.*	*Per Cent Positive*	*No.*	*Per Cent Positive*	*No.*	*Per Cent Positive*
ACTH								
Abnormal control pattern or ACTH > 80 pg/ml	190	36	36	0	20	25		
Ectopic ACTH syndrome	202	5	36	0	20	0		
Vasopressin SIADH	264	23	18	0	12	25		
Calcitonin	226	51	137	20	60	33	24	33
Hypercalcemia (no bone metastases)	112	0	60	25	20	0	32	6
Beta-hCG	130	19	62	13	45	24	11	9

*Modified from Bondy, P.K.: The pattern of ectopic hormone production in lung cancer. Yale J. Biol. Med., 54: 181, 1981 (with permission).

Abbreviations: ACTH = Adrenocorticotropic hormone; SIADH = syndrome of inappropriate secretion of antidiuretic hormone; hCG = human chorionic gonadotropin.

the decreased resonance of atelectasis, obstructive pneumonitis, and pleural fluid as well as the hyperresonance of pneumothorax. Paralysis of the diaphragm may be detected by percussing the magnitude of its excursions. In auscultation of the lungs, a rhonchus is indicative of partial occlusion of the tracheobronchial tree.

On examination of the abdomen, if hepatomegaly is present, tumor metastases indicative of far-advanced disease must be ruled out by laboratory examinations.

In examination of the extremities, clubbing of the fingers is a common finding, as indicated previously. It should be remembered, however, that clubbing may be familial or idiopathic. In the presence of lung cancer, such clubbing is frequently associated with hypertrophic pulmonary osteoarthropathy, with joint swelling and subperiosteal growth of bone. Evidence of arthritis and arthropathy should be sought out, not only because of its association with bronchogenic carcinomas but also because it frequently gives a lead to diagnosing benign pulmonary disorders such as rheumatoid lung, sarcoidosis, and tuberculosis. Evidence of peripheral thrombophlebitis should also be sought.

COMPLICATIONS

The most common complication of lung cancer is secondary infection. Atelectasis or obstructive pneumonitis will be present in approximately 60 per cent of all cases. Pleural effusion occurs in approximately 12 per cent of patients at the time of first presentation. Hemoptysis is quite common and may lead to a fatal hemorrhage. Involvement of the mediastinum by direct tumor extension or metastasis to the mediastinal lymph nodes is very common. As a result, phrenic nerve paralysis or paralysis of a recurrent laryngeal nerve is a frequent complication of lung cancer.

Direct extension of tumor into the esophagus with tracheo-esophageal fistulae communicating with the left mainstem bronchus is seen as an unusual complication. Vena caval obstruction is relatively rare (less than 2 per cent) except in small cell carcinomas (10 per cent).

LABORATORY FINDINGS

Radiologic Examination

The standard roentgenographic examination of the chest with posteroanterior and lateral projections is the most useful single examination for the objective detection of intrathoracic disease. Comparison with previous films is invaluable for detecting abnormalities in the early stages of development and for identifying the origin of such abnormalities. The most common radiologic presentations of bronchogenic carcinoma are the presence of a central lesion suggested by the hilar or mediastinal mass or a peripheral nodule or infiltrate.

The Solitary Nodule

A nodular lesion in the lung can result from a number of agents, as described earlier. The classic study of Steele and coworkers in 1964, which documented the results of 887 patients with asymptomatic solitary pulmonary nodules, showed that up to 56 per cent of such lesions may be malignant, depending on the population examined. These authors, confirming what was generally accepted at the time, concluded that most solitary nodules must be resected if malignancy is to be ruled out. The only findings in this report eliminating the possibility of malignancy in the patients studied were roentgenographic evidence of dense or concentric calcification, or the presence of a nodule over a number of years without change in size. The advent of refinements in imaging techniques, needle biopsy and more definitive information about the etiology of lung cancer have influenced this concept.

Theros has shown that calcification, which is best demonstrated by tomography, in peripheral carcinomas is rare. A single fleck of calcium in the center of a nodule, diffuse homogeneous, diffuse stippled, lamellated, or "popcorn" calcification is evidence of a benign process. In many instances, benign lesions have not been shown radiologically to contain calcium but histologic examination has confirmed significant amounts that were undetected. Computed tomography, which has greater density resolution, may show calcium not seen by standard techniques in some of these nodules, thereby eliminating further invasive procedures.

Siegelman and co-workers reported a technique in which very thin CT slices are made through the nodule. The density is estimated by averaging density numbers within the nodule and deriving a representative CT number. These investigators reported a mean CT number of +92 Hounsfield Units (HU) in 45 malignant tumors studied, none of which had more than one CT number greater than 175 HU. A mean CT number greater than 164 HU was documented for 20 of 33 benign tumors. The authors thus conclude that a solitary pulmonary nodule having a mean CT number greater than 164 HU can be presumed to be benign and should be followed radiographically at 6-month intervals. Using this method, 60 per cent of the benign lesions in the Siegelman report were confirmed. If a lesion considered probably malignant or probably benign is not confirmed by CT, needle biopsy is required. In 3 to 15 per cent of cases, needle biopsy will be negative or not diagnostic.

The decision for thoracotomy in patients with undiagnosed lung lesions will depend primarily on the physician's assessment of a number of interrelated facts and findings including the patient's risk profile in regard to age, sex, and carcinogen exposure, operative risk, and all other clinical elements that may pertain, i.e., growth rate of the lesion, if it is known, and the possible consequences of a delay in diagnosis in a given situation. This holds true from the initial presentation through planning and carrying out the diagnostic plan. Radiologically identical masses cannot be given identical interpretations, and the nonradiologic data may be the most important factor in pursuing an appropriate course of action.

Midzone and Central Lesions

The most common appearance for bronchogenic carcinoma is a mass lesion greater than 3 cm in diameter located centrally in a major bronchus. These masses present in the hilar or perihilar areas with an irregular or lobulated contour. Frequently it is not clear whether the hilar enlargement is the primary tumor or lymphadenopathy, or both. X-ray evidence of a segmental or lobar pneumonia generally accompanies partial bronchial obstruction. Distal atelectasis is, therefore, a very common finding. Special views of the chest may prove helpful. The lordotic position is useful in investigating lesions in the apices that are usually obscured by the clavicles and upper ribs on standard chest films. Inspiratory and expiratory films permit an objective assessment of diaphragmatic excursion. The lateral decubitus film is helpful in determining the presence of free interpleural fluid.

Conventional Tomography

Tomographic evaluation of the major airways and their surrounding structures is one of the most useful studies, since it permits demonstration of lesions otherwise obscured by surrounding or overlying structures. Tomograms more clearly demonstrate the peripheral characteristics of lesions and are extremely useful in establishing cavitation and the nature of cavity walls as well as the presence and patterns of calcification, if it is present. The 55° oblique tomogram is useful in patients with central lesions and a normal-appearing or questionable hilus. If no hilar adenopathy is shown on oblique tomograms, it is very unlikely that mediastinal involvement will be found at the time of surgery.

Computed Tomography

The development of CT has provided a new perspective in radiologic evaluation of the chest. Computed tomographic scanning of the lung is useful in the evaluation of noncalcified pulmonary nodules, in detection of metastatic involvement of the chest, in staging for selected patients, and in treatment planning for primary thoracic malignancies. It has some value in differentiating pleural from parenchymal processes and in directing needle biopsies. Most transthoracic needle biopsies are accomplished with fluoroscopic or ultrasound guidance, but in very small processes in difficult locations CT may provide more safety and accuracy. Computed tomography is an excellent method for demonstrating the presence of underlying lung parenchymal abnormalities when loculated pleural effusions or massive pleural effusions obscure underlying pathologic parenchymal processes.

The superiority of this modality for mediastinal imaging results from the unique cross-sectional imaging format. The relationship of a pathologic process to anatomic structures such as direct extension of a primary tumor into the mediastinum or chest wall is readily shown. Computed tomography is indicated in patients with abnormal hila and no definite mediastinal or chest wall involvement on conventional studies. The value of CT in determining calcification not shown by conventional radiographic techniques has been described in the discussion of solitary nodules. Essential information for radiotherapeutic planning is obtained from CT evaluation, since it provides superior information regarding the total extent of involvement and the lung volumes to be treated. This has permitted radiation therapists to more precisely define the area to be treated and to evaluate the results of treatment. We use CT to resolve questionable mediastinal involvement shown by standard radiographs or hilar and mediastinal tomograms and to demonstrate local invasive tumor extent in superior sulcus tumors, in those with involvement of the chest wall, and in those thought to invade vascular structures. We are currently studying, in a prospective investigation, the definitive contributions of CT, and also of nuclear scanning, in our diagnostic and evaluative schema for lung cancer. The cost-effectiveness of these imaging modalities and the effect of the findings on subsequent patient management are two important questions to be resolved. All imaging techniques are limited by the fact that lymph node enlargement does not always signify tumor involvement and nodes involved with tumor are not always enlarged.

Gallium Scanning

Gallium 67 scanning has been recommended by DeMeester and co-workers as a reliable means of assessing involvement of the mediastinum in patients with primary lung cancer and for selecting patients for mediastinoscopy. It is useful if uptake is shown over both the primary tumor and the mediastinum; however, false negatives in one third of all cases have been noted. Adenocarcinomas apparently concentrate gallium least and account for the majority of false-negative reports.

Bronchography

There have been few indications for bronchography since the advent of the fiberoptic bronchoscope. However, in patients with recurrent hemoptysis, when other techniques fail to provide an etiology, bronchography may be used. The cause of persistent or recurrent pneumonia of undetermined etiology also may be evaluated by bronchography. Pulmonary function changes that affect patients following bronchography, such as reduced lung volumes, air flow rates, and diffusing capacity, limit its use.

Pulmonary Angiography

The refinement of noninvasive imaging techniques has limited the indications for pulmonary angiography for staging and the determination of resectability. However, in the marginal patient with a central lesion of the left lung under consideration for surgery, pulmonary angiography may be indicated, since this procedure can provide evaluation of the vascular margin.

Respiratory Cytopathology

It cannot be stressed too strongly that the establishment of an objective and specific diagnosis is essential to the proper management of patients with intrathoracic malignant disease. All findings of the history and physical examination and selective x-ray examinations are essential to the diagnostic and evaluative process, but none of these methods is specific for lung cancer. The success of pulmonary cytology for the detection of lung cancer cells in spontaneous cough and induced sputa, bronchial washings, bronchial brushings, fine-needle aspiration biopsies, and pleural and pericardial effusions is reflected in the high percentage of preoperative positive diagnoses. A definitive diagnosis can be made in 80 to 90 per cent of all patients and specific identification of cell type is possible in the great majority of cases. Careful instruction of the patient in obtaining a series of sputum samples, three consecutive early morning cough specimens, and persistence by the physician in collecting multiple specimens from each patient are important if a high diagnostic yield from sputum examination is to be obtained. Additional specimens are obtained by bronchial washings and brushings at the time of endoscopy, and the rate of false-positive cytologic diagnoses will be in the order of 1 per cent. Almost invariably, the false-positive diagnosis will be made in the presence of acute infection with bronchiectasis or in association with active pulmonary tuberculosis. An occasional false-positive specimen will be found in association with a pulmonary infarct.

The efficacy of cytologic techniques obviously is related to the quality of specimens and their processing; thus, the predominant factor in a false-negative diagnosis is shown to be unsatisfactory specimens. Squamous cell carcinoma and undifferentiated small cell carcinoma in a central tumor site are significantly correlated with positive cytologic diagnoses. Large peripheral adenocarcinoma may be easily detected by sputum samples, but small (less than 3 cm) peripheral lesions are not as readily diagnosed. However, needle aspiration biopsy of these small peripheral tumors has been reported 87 per cent accurate.

Occult Carcinoma

Refinement of sputum cytologic techniques has been responsible for the diagnosis of an increasing number of cases termed "occult" carcinoma of the lung. In these instances of preclinical squamous cell carcinoma, the patient clearly has a positive sputum cytology but all of the roentgenographic studies have been negative. The site of the primary lesion, therefore, is unknown. Meticulous examination of the tracheobronchial tree with bronchial brushings will usually provide localization of malignant cells. A new approach to the diagnosis of preinvasive lesions is fluorescence bronchoscopy, which involves the use of hematoporphyrin derivative (Hpd). This dye is accumulated and retained in malignant tissue and emits a red fluorescence upon excitation by violet light. Preliminary investigations have been reported showing that this technique is able to localize carcinoma in situ or small cancer plaques that are not visible by white-light bronchoscopy. At this time, however, the methodology is still highly investigational and expensive. Hpd has the side effect of making the patient very light-sensitive for 3 weeks or more following its use.

The use of routine sputum cytologic examinations and chest x-rays for screening groups of individuals at high risk for developing lung cancer is under evaluation by the National Cancer Institute Cooperative Early Lung Cancer Group. The high-risk groups include men over 45 years of age who are chronic, excessive cigarette smokers. Three investigational programs have been under way for several years at the Johns Hopkins Hospital, Memorial Cancer Center, and the Mayo Clinic. All three programs show that the screening procedures detect a higher proportion of resectable cases than is found in unscreened controls or in the general population. The screening techniques have not been successful in detecting stage I patients with undifferentiated small cell carcinoma. Seventy to 90 per cent of the patients under surveillance found to have stage I non-small cell lung cancer are projected to achieve long-term survival; but at this time, no significant differences in lung cancer mortality between the screened and the unscreened groups has yet been shown. However, the value of using these techniques for close follow-up of patients at high risk for developing lung cancer has been shown, since stage I non–small cell lung cancer is potentially curable.

I am personally convinced that disease extent at the time of treatment is a proxy of survival and that, over time, the results of early detection will impact on survival in this disease. This belief is also expressed by others, such as Martini, who notes that if the treatment of lung cancer is to be of any value in prolonging survival, it is more effective when the tumor burden is small and the individual is still healthy; this means early detection, early diagnosis, and early treatment.

Needle Biopsy

Fine-needle aspiration biopsy is becoming increasingly acceptable as a nonoperative method of obtaining a histologic diagnosis when other cytologic or histologic sampling such as sputum cytology, brush biopsy, and bronchoscopy with biopsy have not yielded definitive results. Improvements in technology such as the development of thin-walled, narrow-gauge needles, and image intensifiers that permit fluoroscopic localization and biopsy of small lesions, along with improved cytologic evaluation have made this approach a valuable addition to the diagnostic process for chest disease. There are differences of opinion regarding the indications for needle biopsy. I believe that, in general, nonoperative biopsy procedures are not indicated if both definitive diagnosis and treatment can be accomplished by open thoracotomy. However, others suggest that needle biopsy is indicated to make a cytologic or histologic diagnosis on newly discovered parenchymal lung masses that are potentially malignant and operable or inoperable lung lesions that have increased in size or have not been seen on previous chest radiographs, particularly in heavy smokers over 40 years old. There is general agreement on the use of this technique to obtain a diagnosis in patients who are not candidates for surgery and in whom a definitive diagnosis is required for alternative therapeutic planning. Our policy for the decision regarding needle biopsy is the same as that for other diagnostic procedures. It must be based on integration of clinical data with the acknowledged risk of the procedure in a given patient and on the implications of a false-negative diagnosis. We do not feel that a histologic diagnosis is required preoperatively in every patient.

Because a painful apical syndrome and a Pancoast-type syndrome may result from causes other than a carcinoma in the apex of the lung, tissue diagnosis is regarded as essential prior to implementation of either preoperative or definitive Roentgen therapy. In such a clinical situation, this can be achieved by needle biopsy using a posterior approach through the third intercostal space immediately adjacent to the medial aspect of the scapula. Unless the lesion is directly adjacent to the chest wall with obliteration of the pleural space, the procedure is best performed under fluoroscopic control using the biplane image intensifier.

Pneumothorax is the most frequent complication of needle biopsy. Its incidence ranges from 5 to 20 per cent. The frequency and degree of pneumothorax are influenced by age and sex, size and depth of the lesion, the number of punctures, the presence of emphysema and fibrosis, and the experience of the operator. The highest incidence of this complication may be anticipated in patients over 70 years of age owing to the presence of emphysema and fibrosis. Local pulmonary bleeding and hemoptysis occur in some patients; however, this is rarely of a serious nature and is usually spontaneously resolved.

False-negative reports may occur in 5.5 per cent to 15.7 per cent of all cases. The incidence of false-negative diagnosis drops if the "negative" report is based on at least three representative samples from different sites of the tumor.

In patients under investigation for non–small cell lung cancer, the routine use of liver, brain, and bone scans for the detection of metastasis is not worthwhile in the absence of clinical symptoms or laboratory findings indicative of metastatic disease. Routine scans and bone marrow biopsy of the iliac crest are indicated in patients with small cell carcinoma, since widespread metastasis at the time of diagnosis is common.

Pleural Effusion

When a pleural effusion is present, it should be examined for the presence of malignant cells. At the same time, a specimen should invariably be submitted for bacteriologic study. In a patient with suspected lung cancer, the presence of any fluid usually indicates an extremely grave prognosis. This remains true whether or not malignant cells have been observed in the specimen.

ENDOSCOPY

Bronchoscopy

Bronchoscopy plays a dual role in establishing the diagnosis in situations in which other diagnostic techniques have been ineffective and in estimating the extent of disease, thereby aiding the evaluation of resectability. Diagnostic bronchoscopy is indicated in any patient with unexplained pulmonary symptoms or signs and when a radiologic abnormality exists that is not specifically diagnosed.

An evaluative bronchoscopy should be performed whenever the sputum cytology is positive for malignant cells and there is no obvious evidence of disseminated disease. If there is evidence of metastatic disease easily accessible to biopsy, bronchoscopy is obviated. Because of the small but definite risk associated with bronchoscopy, it is best that the procedure be performed in a hospital setting. The most common serious complications are (1) adverse reaction to anesthesia, (2) arrhythmias and possible cardiac arrest, and (3) hemorrhage following biopsy.

Although fiberoptic bronchoscopy is used in more than 95 per cent of the patients being evaluated for primary lung cancer, the rigid scope is not obsolete. The rigid bronchoscope permits direct visualization of the hypopharynx, larynx, trachea, mainstem bronchi, bronchus intermedius, and both lower lobe bronchi with some of the segments of the lower lobes. Direct biopsy within this range of visualization is possible by utilization of right-angle, foreoblique, and retrograde telescopes. The lobar orifices and segmental orifices can be visualized, although they are beyond the range of biopsy. The rigid instrument is used for biopsy of vascular tumors, since excess bleeding can be controlled by packing. Endobronchial resection of tumors or granulation tissue, biopsies of the carina or major spurs, and transbronchial needle aspiration of mediastinal or hilar tumors can be accomplished using the rigid scope. If the diagnosis of malignancy has not been established objectively or if the cell type is unknown, every effort should be made to obtain tissue at bronchoscopy. Frequently this information can be obtained by bronchial washing and aspiration with cytologic examination if the cancer lies beyond the range of biopsy or the range of vision.

Because the diagnosis has been established in most instances by cytologic examination, the role of bronchoscopy becomes increasingly important in evaluating resectability. Evidence of recurrent nerve involvement with paralysis of the vocal cord, invasion of the trachea, broadening and fixation of the carina, or presence of a tumor within 2 cm of the carina all suggest nonresectability. In selected patients with tumors located near the carina that are biologically favorable, sleeve lobectomy with tracheobronchial reconstruction may be feasible.

The Flexible Bronchofiberscope

The introduction of the flexible bronchofiberscope has markedly increased both the visible and biopsiable range of the endoscopic procedure. A transnasal insertion using a nasopharyngeal airway is the most commonly used technique in the United States; however, the use of the endotracheal tube is preferred by some. The instrument can be directed into segmental bronchi of all lobes and into the subsegmental divisions of the fourth and fifth order. In addition, minute flexible nylon brushes can be passed beyond the fifth order divisions toward the periphery of the lung, and these have proved highly successful in yielding cytologic diagnoses.

Bronchial brushings or the technique of curettement under fluoroscopic control also provides a reliable and safe approach to the diagnosis of peripheral tumors. A yield of 85 per cent with the flexible bronchofiberscope compares favorably with an average yield of 30 to 40 per cent by rigid endoscopy. Even with coin lesions less than 2 cm in diameter, the diagnostic yield with the flexible scope is greater than 60 per cent. Fiberoptic bronchoscopy is an exceedingly safe procedure with an incidence of major complications and mortality of less than 1 per cent.

Transbronchial Biopsy

Transbronchial biopsy is a relatively new technique. It is performed with the fiberoptic bronchoscope, which is guided directly or, in most cases, fluoroscopically into the lung segment containing the lesion for biopsy. It is useful in the diagnosis of parenchymal lesions without pleural, mediastinal, or gross airway involvement in which fiberoptic bronchoscopy fails to permit observation of the lesion. It is a safe procedure with various complication rates ranging from 5 to 15 per cent. Pneumothorax is the major complication, and, as in the case in needle biopsy, it is increased in elderly patients with emphysema. It is used primarily in the diagnosis of diffuse lung disease but has been used for the diagnosis of nodular lesions, providing reported diagnostic yields of 66 to 88 per cent in bronchogenic carcinoma.

Esophagoscopy

Esophagoscopy should be performed at the time of bronchoscopy in any patient having difficulty in swallowing. It is also indicated for the evaluation of a bronchoesophageal fistula.

Mediastinoscopy

Between 50 and 70 per cent of lung cancer patients have positive mediastinal lymph nodes at the time of diagnosis. It is obvious, therefore, that objective assessment of mediastinal involvement in lung cancer patients is critical to appropriate management. Both resectability and survival are highly correlated with the presence or absence of mediastinal metastases. Thus, information regarding this element of disease extent is of considerable prognostic value. Ideally, both the diagnosis of bronchogenic carcinoma and the evaluation of tumor extent should be determined without major surgical intervention. Exploratory thoracotomy, especially if it is done when there is nonresectable disease, has a significant morbidity and mortality. Indirect methods of mediastinal evaluation by roentgenographic examination have been discussed earlier.

A number of surgical techniques have been introduced for evaluation of the mediastinum. Of these, *transcervical mediastinoscopy* (Carlens) has achieved the widest acceptance. This procedure permits direct surgical exploration and biopsy of the middle and posterior portions of the superior mediastinum. The procedure is reserved for those patients who have been examined by conventional methods and for whom the results of bronchoscopy and sputum cytology are available. It is particularly useful in patients when questions of diagnosis and resectability remain unsolved.

It is important to appreciate anatomic features as they relate to the extent of the examination. The mediastinoscope lies directly anterior to the trachea and beneath the pretracheal fascia. The lymph nodes of the anterior mediastinum are not accessible because the instrument is posterior to the innominate artery and vein and to the arch of the aorta. Mediastinoscopy permits biopsy and examination of both peritracheal regions, the subcarinal space, and about 2 to 3 cm along each mainstem bronchus. There is a remarkably low index of morbidity and mortality associated with the procedure. There are differences of opinion regarding indications for mediastinoscopy, primarily in the selection of patients for the procedure. We find it useful in all patients with lung cancer who are surgical candidates, except those with peripheral "coin" lesions and a normal-appearing mediastinum, and in patients with true Pancoast's tumors.

In 5 to 9 per cent of patients, mediastinoscopy will give the only objective evidence of carcinoma. Criteria for nonresectability according to this technique are as follows: (1) a diagnosis of undifferentiated small cell carcinoma, (2) involvement of contralateral paratracheal lymph nodes, (3) involvement of ipsilateral paratracheal lymph nodes in the upper half of the intrathoracic trachea, (4) direct invasion of mediastinal structures, and (5) mediastinal lymph node involvement with adenocarcinoma (except for patients that are candidates for investigational adjuvant treatment). In addition, patients with evidence of gross extracapsular spread are not candidates for definitive resection. Mediastinotomy is of particular value in evaluating lesions arising within the left upper lobe. Because of the relationship of these tumors to the aortic arch, they are frequently underevaluated at mediastinoscopy. As described earlier, we are currently evaluating, in a prospective manner, the contribution to the diagnostic and evaluative schema of the various methods of imaging the chest. The information obtained is being correlated with the findings from mediastinoscopy and thoracotomy.

Pleuroscopy

Pleuroscopy is carried out using the fiberoptic bronchoscope or mediastinoscope. With the bronchoscope, the site of incision is usually along the posterior axillary line. The instrument is inserted into the pleural space, which can be explored visually. All of the costal pleural space and much of the mediastinal and diaphragmatic pleural space can be visualized. Fluid, if present, is aspirated, and if lesions are encountered, biopsies are taken. In patients with massive pleural effusion, talc can be placed over the pleural surface in order to produce adhesions.

Pleuroscopy is of value in the work-up of patients with undiagnosed pleural effusion in whom needle aspiration and closed-needle biopsy of the pleura have not yielded a positive diagnosis. It is also indicated when pleural involvement either by direct extension or by metastatic spread is suspected in patients with bronchogenic carcinoma.

ANCILLARY PROCEDURES

It can be shown that clinical judgment is quite valid in assessing the presence of metastases in the scalene and supraclavicular areas. A suspicious palpable lesion in this region, therefore, is a prime indication for direct biopsy. If such nodes are positive on microscopic examination, exploratory thoracotomy is contraindicated. In the absence of palpable nodes in the scalene region, biopsy is not indicated because the diagnostic yield is extremely small and much more can be learned by examination of the mediastinum.

Pulmonary Function Tests

Since most patients with lung cancer have coexisting chronic obstructive lung disease, some measure of the functional integrity of the lung is a prerequisite to surgical intervention. Spirometry, with measures of vital capacity, flow rates, volume, and maximum breathing capacity, along with arterial blood gas analysis, helps to estimate residual function. An analysis of regional function by Xenon 133 radiospirometry provides an excellent method for the assessment of patients in whom the functional status is borderline. A high correlation has been observed between the decrease in regional circulation and survival rate. More than 90 per cent of patients with lung cancer are found to have zonal defects in the tumor-bearing lung, whereas 50 per cent will have significant zonal derangement on the contralateral side. The preoperative assessment of regional pulmonary function is, therefore, of great value for proper patient management.

Exploratory Thoracotomy

If histologic confirmation of malignant disease has not been established in the course of a thorough diagnostic evaluation, exploratory thoracotomy must be considered. Approximately 10 per cent of all cases of bronchogenic carcinoma will require exploratory thoracotomy for objective diagnosis. In the final analysis, resectability in all cases can be definitely determined only at exploratory thoracotomy. In the absence of physiologic contraindications, early exploratory thoracotomy with resection is advocated for solitary pulmonary nodules in which there is no visible calcification or where there is an increase in size on serial x-ray films (particularly if the patient is over 35 years of age).

SEQUENCING OF STUDIES

Many of the studies undertaken in the patient with suspected lung cancer have a dual function. They provide input toward establishing a definitive diagnosis, and they develop information relative to a valid assessment of the extent of disease. Studies should be undertaken in an orderly and logical progression. The clinician should seek the optimum pathway to answer two essential questions:

1. What is the definitive diagnosis?
2. What is the furthest measurable extent of disease?

The diagnostic and evaluative process need proceed only to the point where these answers are provided. The selection of diagnostic tests should be stratified, from those with the least risk and cost to the patient to those which carry substantial morbidity or mortality. Thus, the extremes of definitive diagnosis are the sputum examination at one end of the spectrum and exploratory diagnostic thoracotomy at the other. Frequently, the extent and complexity of evaluation are inversely proportional to the extent of disease. Thus, a patient with a classical history of lung cancer, an appropriate x-ray abnormality on standard chest roentgenogram, and a palpable scalene node should have sputum examinations and lymph node biopsy. This may constitute all of the studies necessary to select proper management. Thus, costly and traumatic intermediate steps such as mediastinoscopy and bronchoscopy may be obviated. In such a case, the physiologic studies can also be simplified as it becomes known that the patient is not operable. Conversely, if a patient meets all of the criteria of operability as one progresses through radiologic evaluations, bronchoscopy, and mediastinoscopy, in-depth functional analysis is usually indicated. Thus, the patient requiring the most intensive study may frequently have the best prognosis.

DIAGNOSTIC PITFALLS

The failure to persistently and vigorously pursue a program of diagnostic evaluation to rule out the presence of malignancy in patients with a suggestive history or with cardinal signs and symptoms of lung cancer is the principal pitfall in the clinical evaluation of chest disease. An individual over 40 years of age with a history of heavy cigarette smoking, chronic cough, deterioration of cough, and expectoration of sputum must be considered to have lung cancer until proven otherwise. Similarly, any patient with a history of hemoptysis that is not related to bleeding in the nasopharynx, the oral pharynx, or gums, must be considered to have a pulmonary malignancy until this diagnosis can be objectively excluded.

Perhaps the most common error of all is to overlook the possibility of lung cancer in a patient with a history of recurrent bouts of pneumonia or with an unresolved pneumonic infiltrate. Furthermore, in a patient with a prior history of pulmonary infectious disease, it must not be assumed that recurrent signs and symptoms of chest disease are etiologically related to the initial diagnosis. The diagnosis of lung cancer must always be considered in the differential diagnosis.

CHRONIC OBSTRUCTIVE PULMONARY DISEASE

By Philip M. Gold, M.D.
Loma Linda, California

The term chronic obstructive pulmonary disease (COPD) is applied to a group of disorders having in common the physiologic abnormality of airflow limitation. The most important of these are asthma, chronic bronchitis, and emphysema. This article will emphasize the diagnosis of chronic bronchitis and emphysema.

SYNONYMS

Chronic obstructive respiratory disease, chronic airflow limitation, chronic airway disease or dysfunction, chronic obstructive airway disease, asthmatic bronchitis, pink puffer, blue bloater.

DEFINITION

Chronic bronchitis is characterized by the excessive production of mucus associated with cough and sputum production. A strict definition requires that the patient have suffered from cough on most days of the week for at least three consecutive months during two consecutive years and that other diseases associated with excessive mucus production have been excluded. *Emphysema* is a disease characterized by an increase in the size of the airspaces distal to the terminal bronchioles associated with destruction of the alveolar walls. It is apparent that the diagnosis of chronic bronchitis is a clinical one made upon the basis of an appropriate history of cough and sputum production, whereas the diagnosis of emphysema rests upon pathologic findings. In some patients one or the other diagnosis predominates; however, in the majority of patients, emphysema and chronic bronchitis coexist and a precise classification is impossible. It is for this reason that the generic term COPD has found utility.

SIGNS AND SYMPTOMS

Cough and sputum production are often the initial symptoms of COPD. A majority of patients are not particularly concerned about these symptoms and minimize their import. For this reason, symptoms of cough and sputum production often do not bring the patient to the physician; however, their presence is uncovered during routine health examinations or evaluation of other problems. Cough is usually most severe in the morning after awakening or in the evening after retiring and may or may not resolve during the daytime hours. Sputum varies in amount and character. Exacerbations associated with infection or increased inflammation result in increased sputum volume. Sputum changes from either clear and watery or white and mucoid to thick and yellow-green or brown in color. Sputum viscosity increases during exacerbations, and patients may complain of the inability to raise sputum easily. Prolonged coughing or inflammation may result in blood streaking or frankly bloody sputum.

Shortness of breath is the symptom for which COPD patients most frequently seek medical attention. The medical history often discloses that the symptom has been insidious in onset. When present, dyspnea should be quantified in terms of the patient's usual activity. In retrospect, many patients recognize having gradually curtailed certain activities because of dyspnea. As their COPD progresses, dyspnea occurs with less strenuous activities. Ultimately patients may complain of dyspnea at rest and may be unable to eat or to talk without severe breathlessness.

Shortness of breath may be aggravated by body position as well as by activity. In far advanced disease, mechanical disadvantage of the diaphragm in the supine position leads to orthopnea. Additional factors that aggravate shortness of breath in COPD include intercurrent infection and exposure to irritating fumes and odors such as cigarette smoke, cooking odors, perfume, and ambient air pollution. Further, many patients find that their symptoms are improved or aggravated by changes in temperature, humidity, or barometric pressure.

In addition to cough and dyspnea, airway narrowing may result in wheezing, which is frequently a presenting symptom of COPD.

Many nonspecific symptoms accompany advanced COPD. Chronic hypoxemia and obliteration of the pulmonary vascular bed may lead to pulmonary hypertension and cor pulmonale. Affected patients present with fatigue, bloating, and edema. At one time such patients were thought to have chronic bronchitis and were referred to as "blue bloaters." A contrasting group of patients with far advanced disease and intense dyspnea complain of anorexia and weight loss. These patients were referred to as "pink puffers" and were thought to have emphysema. It is now believed that the presence of severe, symptomatic obstructive pulmonary disease indicates the presence of emphysema.

During the evaluation of patients with COPD, certain areas of medical history should be reviewed in detail. These include the smoking history, history of childhood respiratory infections, history of allergic disorders, sleep history, occupational history, and family history. All may play a significant role in the pathogenesis of COPD.

PHYSICAL EXAMINATION

Many patients with COPD recognize that they are more comfortable if they breathe slowly through pursed lips and find that they can breathe more efficiently when sitting forward in a chair with their arms supported. This characteristic posture associated with the appearance of chronic distress or apprehension is characteristic of the patient with advanced COPD. Further, such patients will be observed to use the accessory muscles of the neck and shoulder girdle in respiration. Chest configuration in patients with COPD varies from barrel-chested to emaciated. Cyanosis is an unreliable sign of COPD, present only when there is in excess of 5 gm/dl of reduced hemoglobin, a level likely to be present only during episodes of acute respiratory failure.

Chest examination of the patient with COPD often discloses signs of overinflation, including lungs that are hyperresonant to percussion and diaphragms that are low, flat, and immobile. In addition to the characteristic breathing pattern just described, inspection may reveal paradoxical movement of the diaphragm, especially when the patient is in the supine position. Normally during inspiration the diaphragm descends, intra-abdominal pressure increases, and the abdomen moves outward, as does the chest. Owing to respiratory muscle fatigue in severe COPD, the abdominal wall may move inward paradoxically during inspiration. Auscultation of the chest reveals a prolonged expiratory phase. Forced expiration may be timed with a stethoscope placed over the sternum or trachea. Normal individuals should be able to exhale their entire vital capacity within 4 seconds. Inspiratory and/or expiratory wheezing and noisy breathing may be present. In patients with severe pulmonary overinflation, breath sounds are distant or entirely absent. Medium and coarse crackles early in inspiration are frequently heard in patients with chronic bronchitis.

The point of maximal impulse (PMI) is often observed and palpated in the subxyphoid region. Heart tones are diminished or may be heard only in the subxyphoid area. If cor pulmonale develops, cardiac auscultation reveals an accentuated pulmonic second sound and examination discloses a right ventricular heave, distended neck veins, tender hepatomegaly, and peripheral edema. Patients with severe airway obstruction often develop wide swings of pleural pressure with respiration, and this may result in a significant pulsus paradoxus.

Advanced COPD may result in anorexia, and many patients eat little because of intolerable breathlessness. In such patients the increased work involved in breathing requires considerable caloric expenditure. For these reasons, many patients with far-advanced COPD are severely emaciated.

COURSE

Cigarette smoking is the major factor in the pathogenesis of COPD. Owing to the generous physiologic reserve of the lungs, pathologic processes begin 20 to 30 years prior to the onset of symptoms. In some patients with chronic bronchitis, symptoms do not progress beyond the stage of cough and mucus hypersecretion. For such patients some have advocated specifying a diagnosis of "simple" chronic bronchitis. These patients have a good prognosis and normal life expectancy. It is believed that those patients with chronic bronchitis who ultimately develop symptoms of cor pulmonale or severe dyspnea and respiratory failure have emphysema in addition to mucus hypersecretion.

Spirometry has served as a useful prognostic tool in following the course of COPD. In particular the forced expiratory volume in 1 second (FEV_1) and its change over time have served as indicators of disease severity. Mild exertional dyspnea may occur when the FEV_1 is less than 2 liters. When the FEV_1 is less than a liter, many patients have dyspnea with moderate to mild exertion.

The rate at which tests of expiratory flow decline over time is significant. For example, in male nonsmokers the FEV_1 falls by approximately 32 ml per year. In patients with COPD, the annual decline in FEV_1 is 56 to 84 ml per year. In those patients in whom the FEV_1 is less than half the predicted value, patient survival is approximately 10 years. When the FEV_1 is less than one third the predicted value, survival is approximately 4 years.

Because pulmonary function tests are more sensitive than clinical findings, abnormal spirometric tests may lead to a diagnosis of COPD before patients are aware of illness. It is believed that cessation of smoking at this point may result in return to or toward normal lung function and life expectancy. Once symptoms of COPD develop, the course of the illness is progressive. Treatment following the onset of symptoms may improve quality of life but does not appear to influence the natural history of the disease. In some patients the clinical course is inexorably downhill; in the majority, however, progress of the disease is characterized by recurrent exacerbations and remissions.

COMMON COMPLICATIONS

The most frequent complication in patients with COPD is the acute exacerbation of a stable or slowly progressive process. This commonly occurs because of a superimposed viral, mycoplasma, or bacterial infection. Most often, the patient will complain of an upper respiratory tract infection that, within a short period, "settles in the chest." Such infection may result in purulent bronchitis with no infiltrates observed on chest x-rays; however, in some cases unequivocal pneumonia develops. In addition to infection, other factors responsible for acute exacerbation include exposure to irritants, including air pollutants; noncompliance with treatment; use of sedative or hypnotic drugs; and concomitant congestive heart failure.

Those patients with COPD who require upper abdominal or thoracic surgery are subject to increased risk of postoperative pulmonary complications including atelectasis, pneumonia, and respiratory failure.

Right ventricular enlargement due to pulmonary hypertension is a complication of severe COPD. The signs and symptoms of cor pulmonale have been described. Whether left ventricular dysfunction occurs solely as a complication of COPD is controversial. The weight of evidence suggests that it does not. Nonetheless, in patients with pre-existing heart disease, cardiac failure may develop, in part, because of severe respiratory dysfunction. Furthermore, patients with unstable COPD are subject to a variety of arrhythmias, and, in particular, frequently suffer from multifocal atrial tachycardia.

Recently it has been recognized that patients with COPD are at risk of developing respiratory sleep disorders with an increase in the number and duration of apneas that occur during sleep.

Fluid and electrolyte problems also complicate COPD. These arise, in part, as a complication of therapy with steroids and diuretics but also occur as a complication of the pulmonary disease itself.

Problems encountered most frequently include hyponatremia due to syndrome of inappropriate antidiuretic hormone secretion (SIADH) and metabolic alkalosis due to hypokalemia and/or hypochloremia. Patients who develop respiratory failure due to hypoventilation demonstrate respiratory acidosis.

Pneumothorax may occur in patients with COPD as a result of rupture of subpleural blebs or bullae. In those patients in whom pulmonary function is already marginal, pneumothorax may lead to respiratory failure.

LABORATORY PROCEDURES

A diagnosis of COPD requires an appropriate index of suspicion, a careful history and physical examination and a minimal number of laboratory tests. Posteroanterior and lateral chest x-rays and spirometry should be done in all patients suspected of COPD. Spirometry should be performed by qualified personnel using standardized equipment and techniques. Patients are asked to perform an expiratory forced vital capacity maneuver and reproducible spirometric tracings are obtained. From these tracings, a variety of spirometric indices can be computed. Those of greatest value include the FEV_1 and the forced expiratory flow rate between 25 and 75 per cent of vital capacity (FEF_{25-75}). The measured values are compared with predicted values based upon the patient's age, sex, and height.

The FEV_1 is the simplest and most frequently reported spirometric value. In the absence of restrictive disease, FEV_1 results in 20 per cent or 1.65 standard deviation (SD) below predicted values indicate airway obstruction and, in the appropriate clinical setting, validate the diagnosis of COPD. Spirometry is often performed before and after a bronchodilator in an effort to assess the reactivity of the airways. Physicians should recognize that lack of a bronchodilator response does not imply that patients will not improve clinically with a comprehensive management program.

In special circumstances, other tests of pulmonary function may be required in the evaluation of patients with COPD. Lung volume measurements by gas dilution or plethysmography may be useful to quantify the degree of pulmonary overinflation. When the distribution of ventilation is severely inhomogeneous, as is often the case in COPD, gas dilution methods will underestimate lung volume measurements. Measurement of the diffusing capacity for carbon monoxide (DLCO) provides information regarding oxygen transfer in the lung, a function, in part, of lung surface area. A significant reduction of the DLCO in COPD patients is thought to indicate the presence of emphysema. When evaluating patients for disability or when trying to distinguish between cardiac and respiratory causes of dyspnea, the physician may find that exercise studies of pulmonary function are required.

Arterial blood gases, although nonspecific, analyze the gas exchange function of the lungs and serve as a baseline against which to measure improvement or deterioration. Blood gas measurements are required to document the necessity for oxygen therapy (Pao_2 less than 60 mm Hg) if such is required. Normal blood gas values at sea level are: Pao_2, 75–110 (age-dependent), $Paco_2$ 35–45, pH 7.35–7.45. An increase in $Paco_2$ indicates alveolar hypoventilation and is associated with a fall in pH (respiratory acidosis). A fall in $Paco_2$ indicates alveolar hyperventilation and is associated with an increase in pH (respiratory alkalosis).

Because patients with obstructive sleep apnea may present with signs and symptoms of cor pulmonale and some patients with COPD have complicating sleep apnea, questions regarding excessive snoring, hypersomnolence, and sleep apnea are an important part of the clinical history in patients with COPD and aid in differential diagnosis. If sleep-disordered breathing is suspected, a formal sleep study in a sleep laboratory should be done. (See the article on Sleep-Related Respiratory Dysfunction.)

A small number of patients with emphysema suffer from an inherited deficiency of the enzyme alpha$_1$-antitrypsin. Such patients generally develop signs and symptoms of emphysema at an early age, and their disease progresses rapidly. The family history is usually positive. When a genetic basis for emphysema is suspected because of clinical history, measurement of the alpha$_1$-antitrypsin level and phenotype are appropriate. Afflicted individuals have extremely low or no detectable levels of the enzyme and are usually of the ZZ phenotype. If alpha$_1$-antitrypsin deficiency is identified, enzymatic screening of family members is appropriate.

RADIOLOGIC EVALUATION

The chest x-ray is neither a sensitive nor a specific tool in the diagnosis of COPD. Nevertheless, certain findings occur with relative frequency. Pulmonary overinflation is a common finding. It is characterized by hyperlucent lung fields; an increase in the retrosternal clear space; widening of the rib spaces; and low, flat diaphragms. Flattening of the diaphragms may be appreciated only on on the lateral view of the chest. The heart often appears small and centrally located unless the patient suffers from concomitant cor pulmonale or cardiac disease. Redistribution of blood flow to the apices is common and often results in an erroneous impression of congestive heart failure. Patients with pulmonary hypertension have prominent central pulmonary arteries and pulmonary vascularity tapers abruptly toward the periphery of the lung. Bronchitic patients often demonstrate thickening of the bronchial walls and an increase in nonspecific linear makings is seen, especially at the lung bases. Some radiologists have referred to these findings as the "dirty chest."

OTHER DIAGNOSTIC PROCEDURES

Electrocardiography is often obtained during the initial evaluation of patients with COPD. Peaked P waves or P pulmonale correlates with pulmonary overinflation. Right axis deviation or right ventricular hypertrophy may be identified in patients with cor pulmonale. The electrocardiogram (ECG) frequently shows low voltage and clockwise rotation.

Sputum examination is often of value in evaluating patients with COPD. During exacerbations, polymorphonuclear leukocytes (PMNs) and eosinophils (EOSs) may be responsible for purulent sputum. The PMNs and EOSs cannot be distinguished on the Gram stain but can be by Wright stain or by microscopic examination of an unstained "wet" mount of sputum. The PMNs suggest an infectious or inflammatory basis for exacerbation; the EOSs suggest aggravation of an allergic process. Many chest specialists believe that persistent sputum eosinophilia indicates inadequate bronchodilator or steroid therapy. Gram stain and culture of sputum during exacerbation may play a role in appropriate antimicrobial selection.

POTENTIAL ERRORS AND PITFALLS

Asthma is a disease that is characterized by increased reactivity of the trachea and bronchi and that changes spontaneously or in response to therapy. Occasionally patients with asthma are incorrectly labeled as bronchitics or emphysematous, and it is not uncommon that patients with chronic bronchitis or emphysema are incorrectly diagnosed as having asthma. Often the problem is a semantic one having to do with imprecise usage and the unique terminology used to describe COPD in one geographic area, as opposed to that in another.

A more significant error is the incorrect diagnosis of COPD in patients whose primary problem is cardiac dysfunction. Careful physical examination concentrating on the presence of an S_3 or S_4 heart sound, weight gain, edema, and comparison of heart size and lung vasculature on sequential x-rays may aid in the differential diagnosis. Since similar risk factors coexist in both heart and lung disease, occasionally congestive heart failure is incorrectly interpreted as an exacerbation of COPD and vice versa. When the diagnosis cannot be resolved on the basis of clinical or radiographic findings or an empiric trial of therapy, Swan-Ganz catheterization is required.

Since cough and sputum production may indicate the presence of bronchogenic carcinoma and since risk factors for COPD and lung cancer overlap, physicians must be alert to the possibility of lung cancer in patients with known COPD. Hemoptysis, a change in the character of cough, or unexplained weight loss should be thoroughly evaluated.

The presence of COPD may complicate the diagnosis of pulmonary embolism. The symptom of breathlessness is common to both disorders and may lead to incorrect diagnosis. Further the presence of severe COPD is invariably associated with abnormal ventilation and perfusion scans, which are usually considered indeterminate with regard to ruling in or ruling out pulmonary embolism. For this reason, when the diagnosis of pulmonary embolism is seriously considered in patients with COPD, pulmonary angiography is required for clinical decision making.

SUMMARY

Chronic bronchitis and emphysema are common illnesses with major economic impact, morbidity, and mortality. Diagnosis is frequently made after a prolonged asymptomatic period at a time when, with current management techniques, the natural history of the disease cannot be influenced in a significant way. The diagnosis can be made readily with an appropriate clinical history and simple pulmonary function tests. Furthermore, the diagnosis can be made prior to the onset of symptoms with readily available, noninvasive spirometric tests. Such testing is appropriate in chronic cigarette smokers and other adults at risk of developing COPD.

BRONCHIECTASIS

By John E. Hodgkin, M.D.
St. Helena, California

DEFINITION

Bronchiectasis is defined as irreversible dilatation of one or more bronchi (those larger than 2 mm in diameter) as a result of destruction of the muscular and elastic components of the bronchial wall. This dilatation of bronchi may be local or generalized. Although clinical manifestations or the plain chest x-ray may lead one to suspect the presence of bronchiectasis, bronchography is generally necessary to make the diagnosis because the disorder is defined in morphologic terms.

INCIDENCE

Bronchiectasis used to be a relatively common disorder, but its incidence has decreased markedly in the last few years. This marked reduction in incidence is directly related to the advent of antimicrobial therapy. In addition, the use of vaccines to prevent such diseases as measles, pertussis, and influenza have markedly reduced the prevalence of childhood disorders which are commonly followed by a secondary bacterial respiratory infection.

The precise incidence of bronchiectasis in the population today is unknown. Several decades ago, the presence of bronchiectasis was quite obvious since the majority of patients with this disorder died at a relatively early age as a result of the disorder or its complications. However, today, while bronchiectasis may coexist with other respiratory disorders such as chronic bronchitis and pulmonary emphysema, it uncommonly is a direct cause of death and patients with this disorder live to a considerably older age than was the case several decades ago.

CLASSIFICATION

In 1950, Lynne Reid described the pathologic-roentgenographic correlation of bronchiectasis. This disorder was classified into three groups: *cylindrical bronchiectasis, varicose bronchiectasis,* and *saccular (cystic) bronchiectasis.*

Cylindrical Bronchiectasis (Fig. 1). The diameter of the bronchi is only slightly increased and their lumens end squarely and abruptly as a result of thick, purulent material plugging the smaller distal bronchi and bronchioles. In Dr. Reid's study, the number of branches of the bronchial tree from the main bronchus to the periphery (normally 17 to 20) was considered to be normal in this type of bronchiectasis.

Varicose Bronchiectasis (Fig. 2). Dilatation is greater than in the cylindrical type, and the margins of the bronchi are irregular, resembling varicose veins. The number of patent bronchial subdivisions is markedly reduced (e.g., 4 to 8).

Saccular Bronchiectasis (Fig. 3). The number of bronchial subdivisions is also markedly reduced. As the name suggests, the bronchi have the appearance of sacs or cysts which often have air fluid levels.

Although these classifications may be useful from a roentgenographic standpoint, they are of little practical significance, since there is no specific relationship among the various classifications and the causative factors. The different forms, in fact, may be seen within the same lung.

Bronchographic differentiation between chronic bronchitis and mild cylindrical bronchiectasis may be difficult because slight cylindrical dilatation of bronchi may be seen with chronic bronchitis. Reversible bronchitis (pseudobronchiectasis) may be seen in patients with segmental or lobar atelectasis following pneumonia (Fig. 4). Ulcerations of the bronchial mucosa following viral infections may appear as irregular dilatation on a bronchogram. Re-expansion of an atelectatic area of lung results in a reversal of the shortening and broadening of bronchi. Since it may take several months for bronchographic appearance of airways to return to normal following pneumonia, it is best to wait 4 to 6 months following an episode of pneumonia before performing bronchograms if one is attempting to assess for the presence of bronchiectasis.

PATHOGENESIS

In the pre-antimicrobial and pre-vaccine era, necrotizing respiratory infections were the most com-

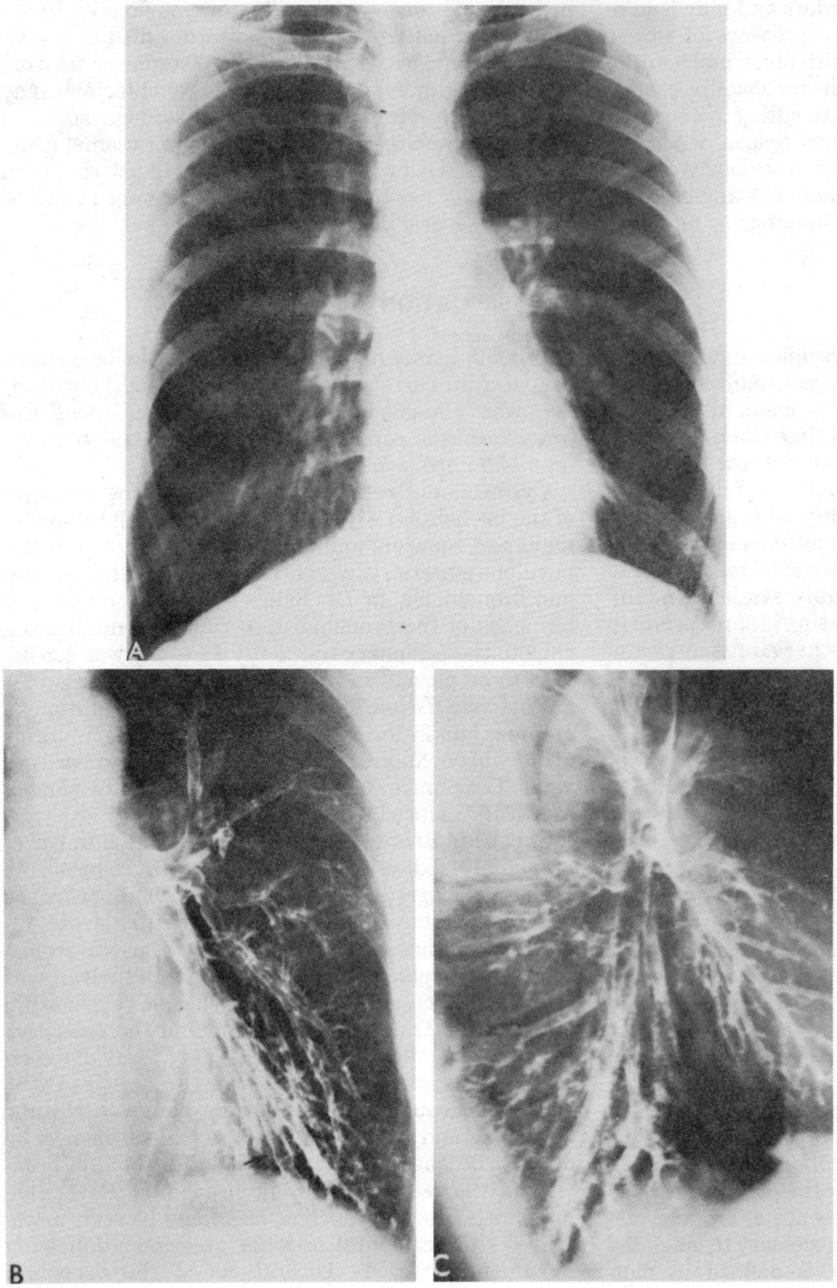

Figure 1. Cylindrical bronchiectasis. *(A)* A posteroanterior roentgenogram demonstrates a slight elevation of the left hemidiaphragm, chiefly in its posterior portion (see *C*). The linear markings in the basal segments are more prominent than normal and have lost their sharp definition. Elsewhere, the lungs appear normal. A left bronchogram in posteroanterior *(B)* and lateral *(C)* projection reveals uniform dilatation of all basal bronchi of the left lower lobe; prominent transverse striations are present in the lateral basal bronchus (arrow). All bronchiectatic segments end abruptly, and there is little or no peripheral filling. The remainder of the bronchial tree is normal. In lateral projection, note the crowding of the bronchiectatic segments and the elevation of the posterior portion of the hemidiaphragm, both findings indicating moderate loss of volume. Cinefluorographic studies revealed normal bronchial dynamics. This 31-year-old man had a history of productive cough dating from an attack of whooping cough and bronchopneumonia as a child. Pulmonary function studies were normal. (Reprinted by permission from Fraser, R.G., and Pare, J.A.P. (eds.): *Diagnosis of Diseases of the Chest,* volume III, 2nd ed. Philadelphia, W.B. Saunders Company, 1979.)

mon cause of bronchiectasis. One could usually get a history of severe pneumonia, either as a primary infection or as a complication of measles, pertussis, or influenza. The severe inflammation led to damage to the elastic and muscular components of the bronchial walls.

Since the advent of antimicrobial therapy, an increasing percentage of cases are associated with other structural abnormalities, deficiencies or diseases. These may be divided into two categories which can affect structure: (1) congenital and hereditary disorders and (2) acquired disorders.

Congenital disorders, such as bronchogenic cysts, cul-de-sacs, and bronchomalacia, may lead to infection in the involved airways and subsequent bronchiectasis. *Kartagener's syndrome,* which has a high familial incidence, is characterized by situs inversus, sinusitis, and bronchiectasis. Recent studies have shown that patients with this syndrome have a structural abnormality of the microtubular system of the cilia. Electron microscopy of spermatozoa and of nasal and bronchial mucosa demonstrates a lack of dynein arms or other structural abnormalities of the microtubules of the cilia. Patients with these ciliary abnormalities are included in a new group of genetically determined disorders called the *immotile-cilia syndrome.* Kartagener's syndrome is but one variety of this new group of disorders that make one prone to stasis of secretions, infection, and subsequent bronchiectasis.

Cystic fibrosis, inherited as a mendelian recessive

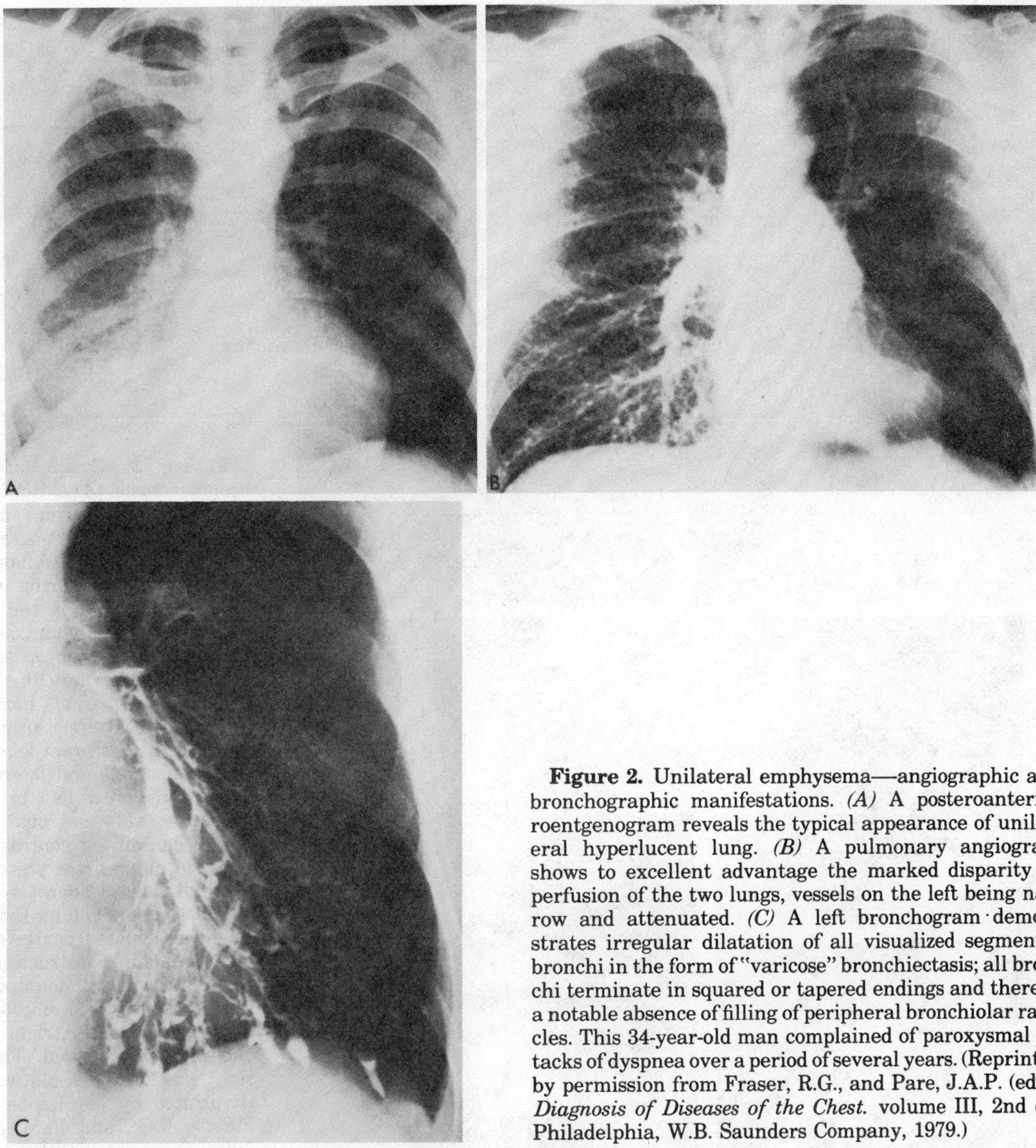

Figure 2. Unilateral emphysema—angiographic and bronchographic manifestations. *(A)* A posteroanterior roentgenogram reveals the typical appearance of unilateral hyperlucent lung. *(B)* A pulmonary angiogram shows to excellent advantage the marked disparity in perfusion of the two lungs, vessels on the left being narrow and attenuated. *(C)* A left bronchogram demonstrates irregular dilatation of all visualized segmental bronchi in the form of "varicose" bronchiectasis; all bronchi terminate in squared or tapered endings and there is a notable absence of filling of peripheral bronchiolar radicles. This 34-year-old man complained of paroxysmal attacks of dyspnea over a period of several years. (Reprinted by permission from Fraser, R.G., and Pare, J.A.P. (eds.): *Diagnosis of Diseases of the Chest.* volume III, 2nd ed. Philadelphia, W.B. Saunders Company, 1979.)

disorder, affects exocrine gland function throughout the body. Secretion of thick, tenacious mucus in the lungs leads to airway obstruction, infection, and bronchiectasis. To date, no defect in cellular or humoral immunity or structural defect in cilia has been identified to account for this disorder. Cystic fibrosis is characterized by sodium and chloride concentrations in sweat greater than 60 mEq/liter in children and 80 mEq/liter in adults. (See the article on this topic.)

The *yellow nail syndrome* is characterized by lymphedema, pleural effusion, bronchiectasis, and yellow nails. The syndrome results from hypoplasia and atresia of the lymphatic system. Bronchial cartilage deficiency, as seen in the *Williams-Campbell syndrome,* also leads to bronchiectasis. Congenital or hereditary deficiencies in the immune mechanism may predispose the patient to recurrent respiratory infections and bronchiectasis. These would include a deficiency of gamma globulin, defect in cell-mediated immunity, and deficiency in phagocytic function, e.g., chronic granulomatous disease of childhood or Chédiak-Higashi disease.

Acquired disorders that predispose to bronchiectasis include mucoid impaction, as seen with pulmonary aspergillosis; bronchial obstruction by neoplasms or aspirated foreign bodies; and bronchostenosis associated with tuberculosis. Bronchiectasis has been demonstrated in conjunction with *unilateral hyperlucent lung (Swyer-James or Macleod's syndrome)* (Fig. 2), and with *alpha$_1$-antitrypsin deficiency.* Bronchiectasis may also follow the aspiration of corrosive chemicals, particularly hydrocarbons such as kerosene. The repeated aspiration of gastric fluid into the lungs, e.g., with hiatus hernia or other esophageal disorders may also lead to bronchiectasis.

It is now generally agreed that bronchial obstruction does not lead to bronchiectasis simply because of the mechanical obstruction but by causing impaired clearance, stasis of secretions, and secondary bacterial infection. Some patients with severe bronchial asthma and associated stasis of thick secretions may

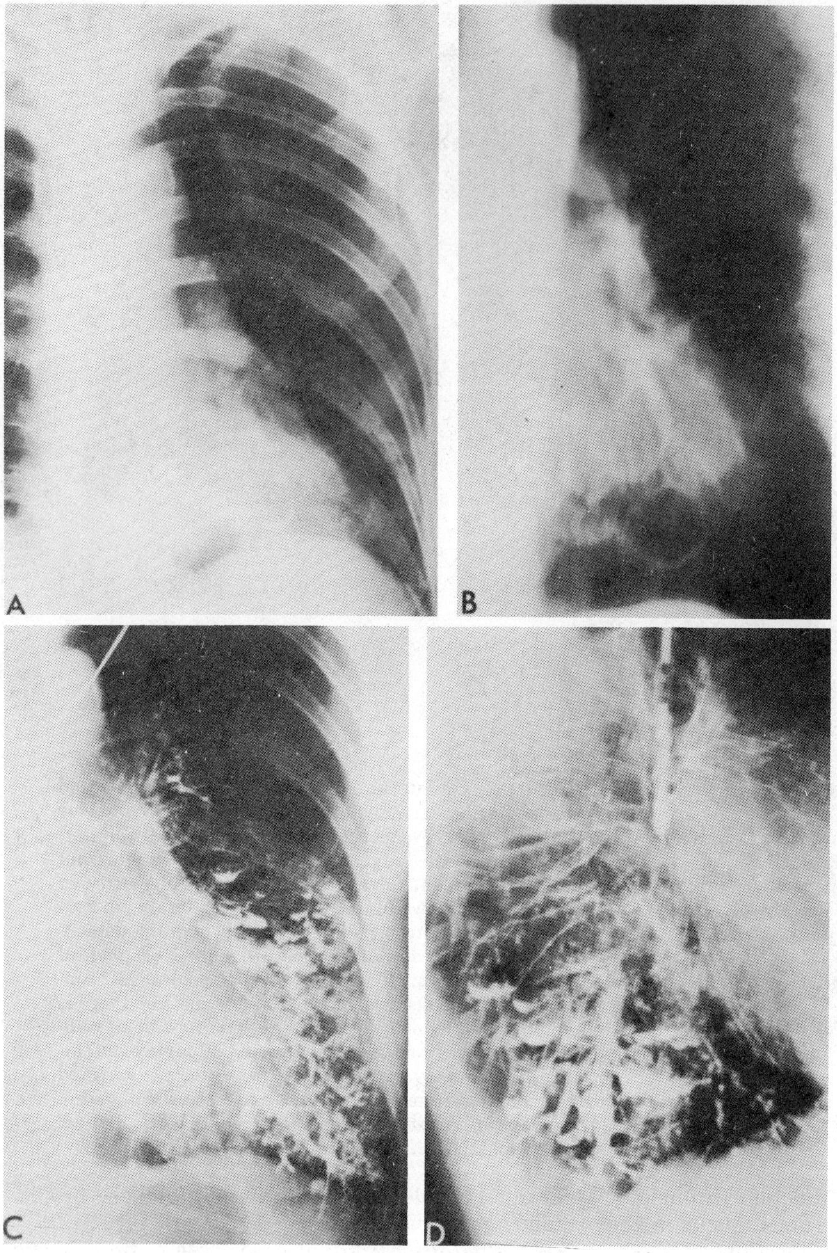

Figure 3. Cystic (saccular bronchiectasis. *(A)* A view of the left hemithorax from a posteroanterior roentgenogram reveals two or three well-defined cystic spaces measuring almost 3 cm in diameter in the lower portion of the left lung, seen to better advantage on an anteroposterior tomogram *(B)*; several patchy shadows of increased density are scattered throughout much of the left lower lobe. Posteroanterior *(C)* and lateral *(D)* projections of a left bronchogram reveal numerous cystic spaces containing contrast material in many areas presenting as fluid levels. There is somewhat less loss of volume than one might anticipate from the extensive bronchial destruction, an observation that undoubtedly reflects the presence of considerable emphysema. A right bronchogram was normal. The patient was a 46-year-old woman. (Reprinted by permission from Fraser, R.G., and Pare, J.A.P. (eds.): *Diagnosis of Diseases of the Chest*, volume III, 2nd ed. Philadelphia, W. B. Saunders Company, 1979.)

end up with generalized bronchiectasis. It is now believed that bronchiectasis does not spread from one area of the lung to another but instead generally represents a systemic disturbance that predisposes the entire lung to bronchiectasis.

DIAGNOSIS

Clinical Findings

The classic clinical presentation of bronchiectasis includes cough, sputum production, intermittent episodes of hemoptysis, and recurrent respiratory infections. Dyspnea is also common with generalized disease. The signs and symptoms vary greatly, and are dependent on such things as the severity, extent, and location of the bronchiectasis. For example, in upper lobe bronchiectasis there may be little or no sputum production on a chronic basis, leading to the term *dry bronchiectasis.*

The typical history of onset of symptoms during infancy or early childhood, in association with frequent respiratory infections through childhood and adolescence, and the production of copious quantities of foul-smelling sputum is now uncommon. Because of antibiotics and vaccines, the onset of bronchiectasis at an early age is becoming infrequent. Although chronic bronchitis is also characterized by a chronic productive cough, occasional hemoptysis, and recur-

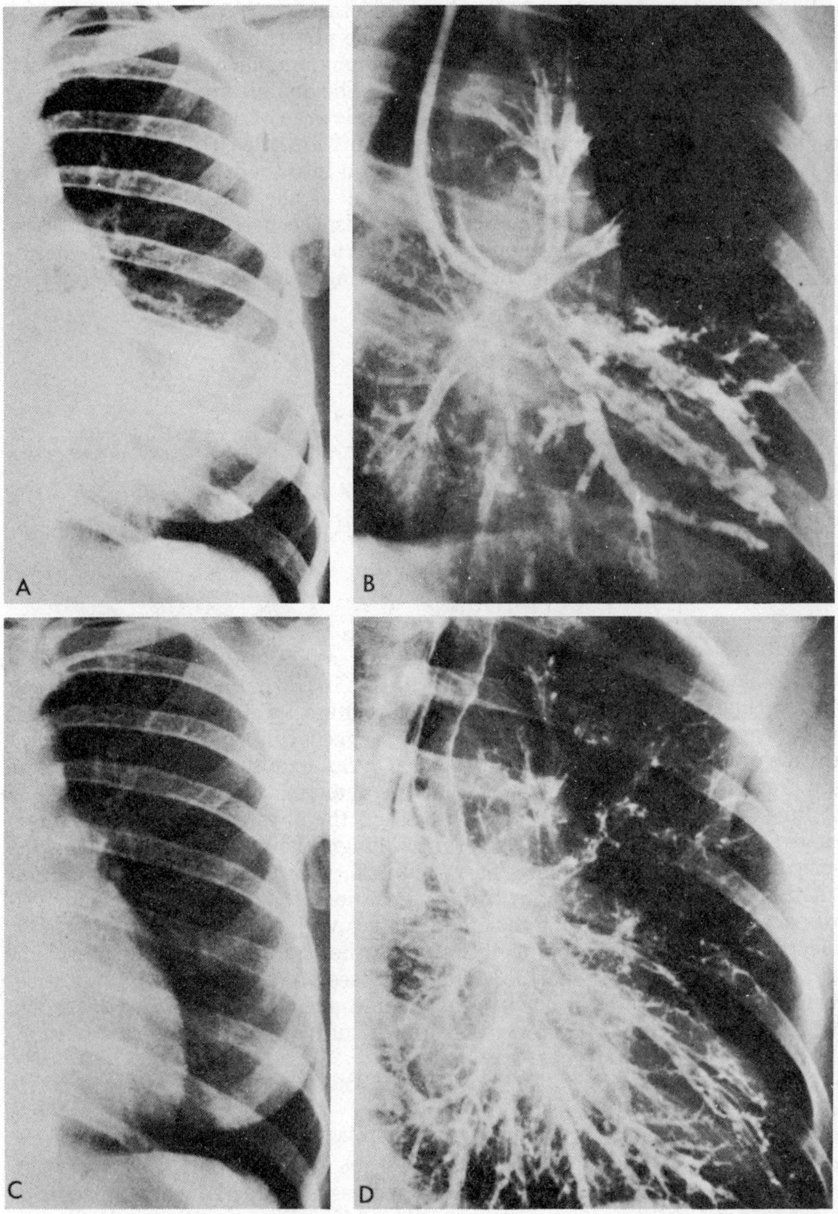

Figure 4. Reversible bronchiectasis. A 26-year-old woman was admitted to the hospital for the first time with an acute pneumonia of the lingula *(A)*. During each day of her convalescence, she coughed up a cup of greenish, purulent sputum, and because of this symptom she was referred for bronchography 3 weeks after the onset of the acute pneumonia. The bronchogram *(B)* revealed moderate cylindrical and varicose bronchiectasis of both segments of the lingula. Subsequent treatment was supportive only, and her symptoms gradually diminished. One year after the acute pneumonia, a posteroanterior view of the left hemithorax (C) reveals a normal appearance of the left lung. Bronchography performed at this time *(D)* shows a normal bronchial tree; the lingular segments show none of the deformity observed a year previously. (Reprinted by permission from Fraser, R.G., and Pare, J.A.P. (eds.): *Diagnosis of Diseases of the Chest,* volume III, 2nd ed. Philadelphia, W. B. Saunders Company, 1979.)

rent infections, the production of large quantities of yellow-green sputum, and a history of recurrent pneumonias in a local region of the lung would be suggestive of bronchiectasis.

Streaks of blood in the sputum occur commonly with bronchiectasis, and an episode of frank hemoptysis is not uncommon. Rarely, life-threatening hemoptysis may occur from erosion into a bronchial artery. Relatively uncommon manifestations include clubbing of the fingers, metastatic abscesses, e.g., brain abscesses, lung abscesses, and amyloidosis. With severe generalized bronchiectasis, cor pulmonale and respiratory failure may develop.

The major physical finding is that of rales in the area of the bronchiectasis. If generalized disease is present, or if localized bronchiectasis is associated with chronic bronchitis, rales are commonly heard over both lung fields.

Laboratory Findings

The complete blood count (CBC) is generally normal; however, leukocytosis signifying infection and anemia reflecting chronic infection may be present. Urine analysis is normal except for those rare cases in which proteinuria resulting from amyloidosis occurs. The sputum may be loaded with polymorphonuclear leukocytes and bacteria when infection is present. Gram stain and culture of the sputum may help determine the responsible organism during episodes of bacterial infection. The electrocardiogram may show evidence of cor pulmonale in patients with severe generalized bronchiectasis.

Pulmonary function studies vary with the extent and severity of disease. Patients with localized disease may suffer little or no functional impairment; however, ventilation/perfusion mismatching would be demonstrated in the involved area by such techniques as radionuclide lung scans. In patients with generalized bronchiectasis, a pattern of obstructive airway disease would be observed, e.g., reduction in flow rates (and perhaps in the forced vital capacity as a result of air trapping), and an increased residual volume: total lung capacity ratio. The total lung capacity, when the patient is stable, would generally be within normal limits; however, it may be reduced if the bronchiectasis is associated with significant segmental or lobar atelectasis. The arterial oxygen tension (Pa_{O_2}) may be reduced and the alveolar-arterial PO_2 difference increased as a result of mismatching of ventilation and perfusion.

Patients with recurrent episodes of respiratory infection should have an immunologic work-up to detect diseases resulting from immunodeficiency. Sweat electrolyte studies are essential to detect the presence of cystic fibrosis. Electron microscopy studies of spermatozoa and bronchial or nasal mucosa are necessary to diagnose the *immotile-cilia syndrome.*

Roentgenographic Findings

The plain chest x-ray reveals changes suggestive of bronchiectasis in most patients with this disorder. Typical changes on the plain roentgenogram include an increase in size and loss of definition of lung markings in the involved area of lung, a crowding of lung markings (associated with loss of lung volume), the presence of cystic or saccular shadows sometimes containing air fluid levels, and in severe disease the presence of a "honeycomb" pattern. Although the plain x-ray may strongly suggest the presence of bronchiectasis, bronchograms are mandatory to establish the diagnosis unequivocally.

Bronchography is usually performed under topical anesthesia by instilling radiopaque liquid iodine compounds through a catheter in the tracheobronchial tree. The location of the catheter, and thus area of lung being studied, is determined under fluoroscopy. The insufflation of powder, i.e., tantalum, into the airways has been investigated as an alternative to the instillation of liquid; however, it has not found widespread acceptance. Bronchography should not be performed during an exacerbation of the disease, and in fact should only be performed after secretions have been cleared from the lungs as much as possible. Vigorous clapping and postural drainage prior to bronchography can help improve airway patency. As a general rule, it is best to only study one lung at a time to avoid respiratory difficulty in patients with generalized disease.

Since in most patients the management of the bronchiectasis is similar to that for chronic bronchitis, bronchograms should not be done routinely simply to demonstrate the presence of bronchiectasis. It should be reserved for those patients with recurrent episodes of pneumonia in whom localized bronchiectasis is suspected or in those patients with recurrent severe hemoptysis. In both of these situations, bronchography would be justifiable since surgical resection would be under consideration. Bronchography can document the sites of bronchiectasis so that more effective postural drainage can be prescribed.

Flexible bronchoscopy may be useful in the patient with bronchiectasis. The flexible bronchoscope may be used to select a specific area of lung to be studied and then radiopaque liquid instilled through a catheter that has been inserted into the tracheobronchial tree through the channel of the flexible bronchoscope. Bronchoscopy may also be useful in clearing thick, tenacious secretions from the lung as well as in identifying the site of bleeding in a patient with hemoptysis.

LUNG ABSCESS

By John P. Griffin, M.D.
Memphis, Tennessee

DEFINITION

Abscess of the lung refers to the roentgenographic detection of cavitation in the pulmonary parenchyma, with a contained air-fluid level. There are only nonspecific findings to suggest this syndrome in most clinical settings until x-ray examination of the chest is performed. Having detected the presence of single or multiple "abscesses," the physician initiates an interesting differential diagnosis including pulmonary disorders of congenital, vascular, degenerative, and suppurative or granulomatous infectious etiology. Although some illnesses will remain undiagnosed after appropriate studies, the majority of "primary" or "idiopathic" lung abscesses are now recognized as consequences of aspiration and as being due to anaerobic bacterial infection, usually with multiple microorganisms.

SIGNS AND SYMPTOMS

Primary lung abscess is suspected when an acute or subacute, usually febrile, illness with a solitary air-fluid–containing infiltrate on x-ray, follows an episode of aspiration. Therefore, patients with a known convulsive disorder, with a history of recent general anesthesia, and with comatose states associated with the abuse of alcohol or drugs, most often develop this disease. Even greater likelihood of lung abscess is present if additional history is obtained of poor dental hygiene, upper respiratory tract infection, or of potential foreign body aspiration such as a fractured tooth or food material (e.g., meat chunks or peanuts). The anaerobic bacterial species implicated in the tissue necrosis and suppuration are those resident in the oropharynx and periodontal areas and often considered commensal flora, although they are present in greater numbers when pyorrhea is evident. Complaints of foul breath, sore throat, purulent postnasal discharge, and painful teeth or antral "fullness" might be helpful. Although high fever and toxicity are sometimes present, it is often impressive how little systemic response might be present in a patient with liquefaction of lung tissue. Respiratory symptoms often include cough, pleuritic chest pain, or hemoptysis, but major dyspnea and wheeze are unusual. Sputum is usually scant at onset but increases in purulency and volume with progression of the illness, finally becoming copious and foul-smelling. There is a stepwise reversal of these sputum characteristics with successful treatment. Physical examination is nonspecific, with occasional signs of localized consolidation or of complicating empyema but rarely with evidence of major cavitation such as cavernous breathing. Signs and symptoms sometimes may be almost nonexistent, or they may be those suggestive of another etiology such as pneumonia, lung cancer, pulmonary infarction, or granulomatous infection.

DIAGNOSIS

The diagnosis of idiopathic lung abscess should be approached by exclusion. Skin testing with purified protein derivative intermediate strength and sputum smears for acid-fast bacilli are indicated to detect tuberculosis. Sputum smears and culture plus appropriate serologic testing are helpful in detecting pulmonary mycoses, such as histoplasmosis, blastomycosis, coccidioidomycosis, cryptococcosis, and sporotrichosis in its primary pulmonary form. Since Aspergillus species are found as normal respiratory flora, histologic study would be necessary to establish this infection; the crescentic radiolucency with a central mass effect consistent with aspergilloma ("fungus ball") might be detected. Necrotizing pneumonia with aerobic organisms, e.g., Klebsiella, Proteus, and Pseudomonas species, and less often staphylococci and selected serotypes of pneumococci, are best identified by Gram-stained smear and culture of lower respiratory secretions, of blood and of pleural fluid. "Skinny" needle percutaneous aspiration of lung material with fluoroscopic localization, is being increasingly used because of the good yield of pathogenic organisms and the growing recognition of its safety, despite earlier fear of producing a bronchopleural fistula. Pulmonary infarction with secondary excavation often due to superinfection can be approached by lung scanning or angiography, or with septic infarction by identification of a distal infection from which metastatic spread likely occurred.

In patients who are heavy smokers, it is well to suspect bronchogenic carcinoma in a newly detected abscess lesion. Development of an air-fluid level might be the result of necrosis in large tumors that have outgrown their blood supply or may be due to proximal airway obstruction with poor drainage and distal infection by necrotizing organisms. Cytology may be positive; however, diagnostic bronchofiberscopy is usually necessary to establish the tumor cell type and to interpret the pathogenesis of the abscess, which are important treatment considerations. Infected bronchial cysts or fluid-filled infected bullae in emphysema may appear to be lung abscesses. Bronchography and pulmonary function studies are often ordered in this setting, but the most practical information is obtained from chest x-rays taken prior to the present illness.

Primary or idiopathic lung abscess is therefore the likely diagnosis after the relatively exhaustive workup outlined. Clinical investigation has clearly implicated anaerobic bacterial infection in this disorder. Treatment must be directed against these microorganisms for a successful outcome, but in most patients the infecting agents will not be identified. This is due to the unavailability in most community hospitals of the sophisticated microbiology laboratory necessary to perform modern anaerobic cultural studies, particularly with reference to species identification and their susceptibility to antimicrobial drugs. If special cultures are attempted, it should be realized that sputum is an unsatisfactory specimen because of large concentrations of anaerobic organisms resident in the upper airways. Thoracentesis fluid and blood are acceptable specimens for culture but are usually not helpful. Transthoracic needle aspiration of the lung has been increasingly used for anaerobic studies; opinion is mixed as to the value of transtracheal aspirates for this purpose. Recently, sleeved-catheters have shown promise for bronchoscopic culturing when successfully introduced into the vicinity of the abscess lesion.

Radiologic examination has been emphasized in the identification and attempted localization of the abscess. Traditionally, idiopathic abscess is favored in certain regions of the lung, by position of the patient at the time of aspiration and by the law of gravity. Although increased frequency is seen in the right lung, in the posterior segment of the upper lobes, and in the superior segment of the lower lobes, there are many exceptions in clinical practice. Differential diagnosis of "abscess" includes consideration of the predominance of granulomatous disease in the upper lobes and of pulmonary infarction in the lower lobes. Computed axial tomography (CAT) of the thorax is being increasingly used, but its role in the evaluation of the patient with lung abscess has not been established. Computed tomographic scanning has been reported to be helpful when peripheral lung abscess and empyema are indistinguishable by conventional techniques. Computed tomography may make the distinction by demonstrating lung tissue partially surrounding a peripheral parenchymal consolidation or air bronchograms within it. A smooth interface with the chest wall suggests than an empyema is present (analogous to the extrapleural sign).

COMPLICATIONS

Resolution of lung abscess ordinarily requires drainage via the endobronchial route. Usually this is relatively continuous after identification of the abscess on x-ray, since bronchial communication must be present to manifest the characteristic air-fluid level. In some patients, drainage is delayed and then occurs suddenly, with large volumes of pus not only capable of bronchogenic spread of infection, but in some instances filling the airways and impairing gas exchange in such a way that acute respiratory failure and even death can result. Another dreaded complication, representing a surgical emergency, is development of pulmonary gangrene due to involvement of adjacent vasculature and often signified by continuous and possible life-threatening hemoptysis. Frank empyema is a common complication, suggesting a communication with the pleural space but infrequently resulting in bronchopleural fistula because of the intense inflammatory response and its tendency to reseal any communication. Anaerobic lung abscess is now regarded as a pleuropulmonary syndrome because of the high frequency of initial pleural involvement as a characteristic of this infection. Historically, lung abscess was often complicated by metastatic brain abscess, but this is a rarity in the antibiotic era.

The clinical course of primary lung abscess is ordinarily limited to a 4- to 6-week period. Sometimes the course and initial response to treatment suggest the idiopathic variety, but recurrent or persistent respiratory or systemic symptoms might suggest diagnostic error. Cultural results for TB and fungal etiologies will not be available until late in the illness. Bronchofiberscopy, if not performed earlier, should be obtained at this time to exclude a proximal obstructing neoplasm, or occasionally to identify and, if possible, to remove foreign bodies when no initial history of their aspiration was elicited. Localized bronchiectasis, with subsequent recurrent infection with possible hemoptysis, can result from tissue necrosis during the early course of lung abscess. Cavitary defects in the lung may persist for months to years; however, surgical resection is no longer considered necessary in most instances, since little subsequent illness appears to result from these residual x-ray abnormalities. Finally, recurrence of lung abscess is a definite possibility if predisposing conditions, such as severe dental caries, chronic alcoholism, or a seizure disorder, are not successfully treated.

BACTERIAL PNEUMONIA

By Carl A. Perlino, M.D.
and Stephen W. Schwarzmann, M.D.
Atlanta, Georgia

Pneumonia can be defined simply as inflammation of the parenchyma of the lung, or pneumonitis, due to either infectious or noninfectious causes. Pneumonia from any cause is usually accompanied by nonspecific symptoms and signs referable to the organ system involved, such as cough and dyspnea, and by systemic signs such as fever. Noninfectious causes such as pulmonary emboli with infarction, atelectasis, immunologic diseases such as lupus erythematosus, Goodpasture's syndrome, and farmer's lung are often diagnosed only after infectious etiologies have been excluded and the epidemiology and laboratory evaluation suggest a specific noninfectious cause.

Infectious etiologies of pneumonia are given in Table 1. The examples listed are not all-inclusive but suggest the large number of pathogens that require consideration when a patient presents with pneumonia. Overall, mycoplasma, viruses, and bacteria are the most common causes of infectious pneumonia. Bacterial infections are probably the most common cause of pneumonia in the adult population, whether the infection is community- or hospital-acquired. The ability to diagnose bacterial pneumonia and distinguish between the various possible bacterial etiologies is of obvious importance, since effective, specific antimicrobial therapy can decrease the morbidity and mortality of this disease.

DIFFERENTIATION OF BACTERIAL PNEUMONIA FROM THE "ATYPICAL" PNEUMONIA SYNDROME

The term "atypical" pneumonia was coined in the early decades of the 20th century to describe those patients who presented with a constellation of symptoms and signs distinctly different from those of lobar pneumococcal pneumonia. The etiology of "atypical" pneumonia usually includes nonbacterial agents such as mycoplasma and viruses. Bacterial pneumonia can often be distinguished from "atypical" pneumonia on the basis of the epidemiology of the disease, the symptoms and signs of the infection, and, occasionally, laboratory studies. The epidemiology of the infection is least helpful in distinguishing between bacterial and "atypical" pneumonia, while the symptoms associated with the infection usually will aid the examiner in making the diagnosis. Specific examples follow.

The time of year in which an infection occurs is important only occasionally in distinguishing bacterial from "atypical" pneumonia. Legionella infections occur commonly in the summer months, whereas pneumonia due to influenza or adenovirus occurs during the colder months of the year. However, certain bacterial pneumonias also occur more commonly during the winter, e.g., pneumonia due to pneumococci. Gram-negative bacillary pneumonias and mycoplasma infections occur year-round.

In most cases of bacterial pneumonia, a contact history with an infected individual is not obtained, since these infections are usually secondary to aspiration of

Table 1. Infectious Etiologies of Pneumonia

Viral	**Fungal**
Influenza	Histoplasmosis
Adenovirus	Coccidioidomycosis
Herpes, cytomegalovirus	Aspergillus
Chlamydia	**Bacterial**
	Streptococci
Mycoplasma	Staphylococci
	Enterobacteriaciae
Rickettsia	Pseudomonas
Q Fever	Legionella
	Anaerobic bacteria
Parasitic	Nocardia
Pneumocystis	Neisseria
Ascariasis	**Mycobacterial**

potential pathogens from the mouth and oropharynx, rather than transmission from person to person or from an environmental source. An exception would be epidemic Legionella pneumonia, a bacterial infection secondary to inhalation of infectious organisms from the environment. In contrast to bacterial pneumonias, viral infections due to adenovirus or influenza are usually transmitted from person to person.

The onset of infection, whether acute or subacute, is seldom helpful in distinguishing bacterial from mycoplasma or viral infections. Viral infections of the upper respiratory tract may predispose to bacterial infection and give the impression of a subacute course prior to diagnosis. Occasionally a patient with an upper respiratory tract infection will have a sudden shaking chill, or rigor, followed by symptoms of pneumonia, a sequence of events seen in pneumococcal pneumonia. However, influenza may begin with one chill. Other symptoms such as the presence or absence of fever, the height of fever, the severity of dyspnea, the presence of chills (as distinguished from "chilliness") are nonspecific symptoms and are not often useful in distinguishing bacterial pneumonia from the "atypical" pneumonia syndrome.

One feature that may distinguish between these two syndromes is the type of sputum production associated with cough. The sputum of bacterial pneumonia is most often copious, purulent, and occasionally "rusty" colored, while the sputum of an "atypical" pneumonia is usually scant or, often, absent. Sputum produced by a patient with legionnaires' disease is initially scant, becoming more mucopurulent later in the disease, and is occasionally blood-tinged.

Complaints of chest pain on coughing and inspiration may be elicited from patients with either bacterial pneumonia or the "atypical" pneumonia syndrome. The examiner must be careful to be specific in the questions regarding this symptom. Bacterial pneumonias will often be associated with inflammation of the visceral pleura secondary to alveolar infection, resulting in a true pleuritic pain, pain associated with cough or deep inspiration localized approximate to the area of inflammation and felt in the peripheral aspects of the chest wall. Viral or mycoplasma infection is associated with pain on cough found in the middle, anterior chest and is due to bronchial inflammation.

The most helpful symptoms that distinguish between bacterial pneumonia and the "atypical" pneumonia syndrome are those of headache, myalgia, and arthralgia. These symptoms, and to a lesser extent nausea and vomiting, are more likely to be associated with the latter syndrome and are less commonly found in bacterial pneumonias. The exception to this finding is legionnaires' pneumonia, which may mimic "atypical" pneumonia in that these symptoms are present, while the presence of true pleuritic chest pain suggests the bacterial etiology of this disease.

Unfortunately, the physical signs of pneumonia are less helpful than the symptoms in distinguishing between bacterial and "atypical" pneumonias unless the infection is associated with a true lobar consolidation in the former case or interstitial inflammation in the latter. Lobar consolidation, most often associated with bacterial pneumonias, such as those due to the pneumococcus or *Klebsiella pneumoniae,* is distinguished by findings of local dullness, egophony, vocal and tactile fremitus, rales, and splinting. True interstitial infection, most often associated with viral pneumonia, is remarkable for the lack of abnormal findings found by percussion or auscultation of the chest. Many bacterial pneumonias and mycoplasma infections give rise to a bronchopneumonia with rales associated with the area of infection, but lacking true lobar consolidation, and it is difficult to distinguish between bacterial and "atypical" etiologies in this circumstance.

Using the chest roentgenogram, a distinction can also be made between bacterial pneumonias and the "atypical" pneumonia syndrome in a manner similar to the differences demonstrated by the physical examination. A roentgenographic picture of true lobar consolidation is characteristic of bacterial disease. Interstitial infiltrates are more likely to represent viral infection, whereas bronchopneumonia may be common to either. The presence of a pleural effusion is more likely to indicate bacterial pneumonia.

Other laboratory studies such as measurements of liver enzymes are of little help in differentiating between the two syndromes, since hepatocellular inflammation can occur in either. Finally, the total leukocyte count and differential white blood cell count add only modest information useful in distinguishing between these two syndromes. A leukocyte count of greater than 20,000 per cu mm with immature forms is likely to represent bacterial infection, whereas normal or slightly elevated counts may be seen with either syndrome. Similarly, leukopenia, thought by many to be indicative of viral disease, is occasionally found associated with bacterial pneumonia and sepsis.

Common diagnostic features associated with bacterial pneumonia are found in Table 2.

ESTABLISHING THE ETIOLOGY OF BACTERIAL PNEUMONIA

The causative agent of a case of bacterial pneumonia can be suggested by the clinical setting in which the infection occurs but is established only by specific

Table 2. Features Helpful in the Diagnosis of Bacterial Pneumonias

Epidemiology
- Winter months: Pneumococcus
- Summer months: Legionellosis

Symptoms
- Purulent sputum production
- True pleuritic chest pain
- Lack of systemic symptoms of headache, myalgias, or arthralgias

Signs
- Lobar consolidation

Laboratory
- Lobar consolidation on roentgenogram
- Associated pleural effusion on roentgenogram
- WBC* > 20,000 per cu mm

*WBC = White blood cell count.

laboratory evaluation. Unfortunately, the causative agent may remain unidentified, pointing out the limitations of our current diagnostic ability.

Host factors, such as associated disease, will increase the likelihood of infection with certain pathogens because of alterations in specific host defense mechanisms. Bacterial pneumonia occurring in a young, healthy adult is most likely due to pneumococci. These organisms are commonly found as part of the oropharyngeal flora and are enclosed in a polysaccharide capsule that makes phagocytosis by alveolar macrophages and polymorphonuclear leukocytes difficult. Relatively unrestricted growth of these bacteria thus may occur when they are aspirated and reach the alveolar space. Increasing age of the patient increases the likelihood of pneumococcal infection as well as of legionnaires' disease. Cigarette smoking also increases the risk of infection with either of these two pathogens. Patients with sickle cell disease or abnormalities in immunoglobulin synthesis are likely, in the absence of more severe immune deficits, to be infected with encapsulated organisms, such as the pneumococcus or *Hemophilus influenzae.*

Infection with influenza virus has been associated with secondary bacterial pneumonia due to *Staphylococcus aureus* as well as pneumococci and *H. influenzae.* The patient with obstructive pulmonary disease and chronic bronchitis has chronic lower airway colonization associated with *H. influenzae* and pneumococci, and pulmonary infections with these organisms are common. Pneumonia due to gram-negative bacilli (Klebsiella, *Escherichia coli*) also must be thought of in this patient group. The alcoholic patient is prone to infection with pneumococci and gram-negative bacilli, but the alcoholic patient with significant periodontal infection and a history of loss of consciousness or seizures is likely to have infection due to anaerobic bacteria that may lead to putrid lung abscess or pneumonia. Gram-negative bacteria and staphylococci are common causes of hospital acquired pneumonia, but anaerobes and pneumococci must be considered as well.

Patients with disease resulting in significant immunosuppression, such as leukemia, lymphoma, and organ transplantation, who develop bacterial pneumonia are likely to be infected with gram-negative bacilli and occasionally Nocardia. It becomes apparent that as the patient becomes more immunologically compromised, the etiology of bacterial pneumonia is more often due to less virulent, but more antibiotic-resistant, organisms.

The symptoms and signs associated with infection are not usually of sufficient specificity to aid in the prediction of the bacterial etiology of the disease. Legionnaires' disease and pneumonia due to anaerobic bacteria may be exceptions to this statement. As noted in the previous section, the patient with legionnaires' disease often develops disease during the summer, the symptoms of a minimally productive cough becoming more productive with time. Pleurisy and associated complaints of headache, myalgia, and diarrhea suggest the disease. The patient with anaerobic pulmonary infection may present with a subacute course and complain of foul-smelling, copious sputum, especially when the infection is complicated by necrotizing pneumonia or lung abscess. Apart from this example, the types of sputum produced by a patient with bacterial pneumonia is of little diagnostic significance. Infection with *K. pneumoniae* is often said to produce thick, tenacious sputum, but this finding has uncertain diagnostic significance.

Whereas epidemiologic data and the clinical presentation of infection can suggest a specific bacterium as the cause of pneumonia, bacteriologic diagnosis depends on the demonstration of bacteria in infected body fluids or secretions by Gram stain and culture. Positive cultures from blood or infected fluid (empyema) from patients with pneumonia are considered to be diagnostic of the organisms causing the infection. Thus, if fluid is seen on chest roentgenogram in a patient with fever and pulmonary infiltrates, a specimen of pleural fluid must be obtained by thoracentesis *before* antibiotics are started. In addition to the total cell count, differential, total protein, lactate dehydrogenase (LDH), glucose content, and pH, an aliquot of the fluid is centrifuged and Gram stained while another aliquot is sent for aerobic and anaerobic cultures. Similarly, blood cultures (one or two sets) obtained before antibiotics are started will be positive in 10 to 20 per cent of pneumonia due to pneumococci and occasionally will be positive when the pneumonia is due to gram-negative bacilli.

Cultures of expectorated sputum will grow organisms that may be infecting the lung but will also reflect organisms colonizing the oropharynx, thus giving potentially false-positive data. Furthermore, because of poor collection techniques, the specimen cultured may contain predominantly oropharyngeal secretions, not true sputum, and give useless data. Because of these problems in interpreting the results of sputum cultures in absence of ancillary data, it is mandatory to examine the sputum Gram stain. Microscopic evaluation of the sputum will give data as to the origin of the specimen; e.g., a specimen containing a predominance of squamous epithelial cells obviously originates in the oropharynx or mouth, whereas a specimen containing predominance of neutrophils can be assumed to originate in the infected lung. The predominant organisms seen on Gram stain of expectorated sputum containing primarily neutrophils can be identified according to morphology and staining characteristics and the information used to choose initial therapy. Specifically, the sputum Gram stain is examined to determine whether the predominant flora is gram-positive elliptical cocci (pneumococci or streptococci), gram-positive, round cocci (staphylococci), large gram-negative bacilli (Enterobacteriaciae), or short gram-negative diplococci (Neisseria). In addition to the predominant flora, intracellular organisms (inside neutrophils) should be noted as likely pathogens. Organisms associated with squamous epithelial cells are of little diagnostic significance. The bacteriologist can also use these results to assist in selecting probable pathogens from the culture plate.

Sputum cultures can also give false-negative data in regard to organisms that have rather fastidious growth requirements. This is especially true with pneumococci, which may be identified from cultures of sputum in only 20 to 50 per cent of patients with true pneumococcal pneumonia. Other techniques, such as the quellung reaction or the detection of pneumococcal polysaccharide from sputum by counterimmunoelectrophoresis, can be used to definitively identify pneumococci as the cause of the infection. *Legionella pneumophila* is rarely recovered from cultures of expectorated sputum because of overgrowth by faster-growing bacteria. Direct fluorescent antibody stains of sputum or lung tissue or cultures of normally sterile tissue such as lung may be helpful in the diagnosis of legionnaires' disease. Serology is confirmatory.

Anaerobic lung infections can be suspected when an appropriately performed Gram stain demonstrates a mixture of organisms, gram-negative bacilli, gram-positive cocci, and gram-positive bacilli, i.e., usual mouth flora. Cultures of expectorated sputum are inappropriate for demonstrating anaerobes because of the ubiquitous contamination of specimens passing through the mouth by the anaerobic flora of the area. Techniques for obtaining specimens of sputum that bypass the oropharynx, such as transtracheal aspiration or direct aspiration of infected lung, may be useful in obtaining specimens adequate for culture of anaerobes. These techniques may also prove useful in obtaining specimens for bacteriologic cultures when specimens obtained by expectoration are unavailable. Specimens obtained by nasotracheal suction or by fiberoptic bronchoscopy should be considered equivalent to expectorated sputum for diagnostic accuracy.

VIRAL PNEUMONIA

By Emily J. Kahlstrom, M.D.
and Bernard Portnoy, M.D.
Los Angeles, California

Viruses are responsible for over 95 per cent of acute respiratory disease among all age groups, ranging from the common cold to bronchitis-bronchiolitic syndromes. Viral agents also cause the majority of community-acquired pneumonias characterized by diffuse pulmonary infiltration, an unusual radiographic manifestation of bacterial pneumonia. The prevalent organisms and frequency of disease vary by age group. Pneumonia, representing the most severe manifestation of viral respiratory tract infection, occurs in 1 to 5 per cent of infected individuals. The incidence of total lower respiratory tract disease decreases with age; from 240 per 1000 per year in infants to 134 per 1000 per year in older children. The rate decreases to 34 per 1000 by late adolescence.

The most common agent producing acute lower respiratory tract disease, severe enough for hospitalization, in the infant is respiratory syncytial virus (RSV). It produces a clinical syndrome characterized by rhinorrhea, cough, and low-grade fever followed in 1 to 2 days by rapid respiration, chest retraction, and wheezing. The peak of respiratory distress usually lasts no more than 3 to 4 days, with return of respiratory rate, abnormal blood gases, and radiographic abnormalities to normal within 10 days. Twenty per cent of these infants may have a protracted course with persistent wheezing and hyperinflation of the lungs, persistent evidence of continued airway obstruction as demonstrated by physiologic studies, and persistent abnormalities of gas exchange lasting as long as several months. Approximately 3 per cent of hospitalized infants will require assisted ventilation. Respiratory syncytial virus is responsible for annual midwinter to early spring epidemics and is the major cause of pneumonia in infants under 12 months of age. The reason some infants develop bronchiolitis while others develop pneumonia is unknown. Other agents such as the adenoviruses, parainfluenza viruses, and influenza viruses are causative agents of bronchiolitis and pneumonia in a smaller number of infants.

In the adult, type A influenza is probably the virus most pathogenic for the respiratory tract. Approximately 60 to 75 per cent of patients will be mildly ill or have inapparent infection, 25 per cent will be bedridden, and 5 per cent will have pneumonic involvement. The onset may be minor with upper airway involvement or more abrupt with chilliness, nasal congestion, rhinorrhea, slight pharyngitis, conjunctival irritation, headache, malaise, and aching with or without fever. Those patients with pneumonic involvement will have an intensification of signs and symptoms within the first days, with paroxysmal cough; scant mucoid, mucopurulent or bloody sputum; and tachypnea lasting for a few days to two weeks or longer. Fever may be absent or present to 40°C (104°F) for up to 2 to 5 days. Secondary bacterial invaders, most commonly the pneumococcus and *Staphylococcus aureus* and less often *Hemophilus influenzae* and group A streptococci, will account for the majority of deaths.

The onset of bacterial complications tends to occur late in the illness, with evidence of more sputum production and recurrence of shaking chills and dyspnea. The radiograph is more likely to show segmental, lobar, or focal pneumonia superimposed on the diffuse process of uncomplicated influenzal pneumonia. Unfortunately, the signs and symptoms of secondary infection cannot always be differentiated from the primary process until the bacterial infection is very far advanced. Adenoviruses, especially in military recruits, are also occasional causes of pneumonia in those over 20 years old.

Other viruses that may attack the lung include both measles and varicella. Varicella pneumonia occurs in approximately 10 to 15 per cent of adults and in less than 1 per cent of children, although it has been reported in patients from 4 days of age to 71 years.

DIAGNOSTIC APPROACH

Pneumonia, a microbial disease of the lung, involving alveoli and/or the interstitial supporting structures of the lung, may be caused by rickettsiae, bacteria, fungi, and parasites as well as by the viruses already mentioned. *Mycoplasma pneumoniae* is a particularly important agent, since it causes 40 to 45 per cent of pneumonia cases in epidemic periods unless influenza infection is prevalent in the community. Mycoplasmal pneumonia is a disease of school-aged children and young adults, particularly college students and military personnel. Tuberculosis must always be considered, particularly in recently arrived Hispanic or Asian populations. Clinical, radiographic and laboratory features are the mainstay for a presumptive diagnosis because identification of a specific microbe can be difficult in an individual patient and diagnostic tests may be equivocal.

The clinical presentation of RSV pneumonia in infancy and influenza A pneumonia in the adult is described in the introductory text of this article. Physical signs are variable, depending upon the severity of disease. There may be facial flushing and conjunctivitis. Pharyngeal mucosa may be inflamed with occasional excoriation. Cervical lymph nodes are rarely enlarged or tender. Tachypnea and nasal flaring may be the only obvious signs of pneumonia, since the suppressed breath sounds and rales may be absent initially. Cyanosis will be noted only in the severest cases. True consolidation is not a feature of viral pneumonia. Bronchophony or egophony is an indication of secondary atelectasis or consolidation due to secondary bacterial infection. Febrile convulsions may complicate the course, particularly in infants and children with influenzal viral pneumonia. Gastrointestinal disturbances and altered states of cerebral consciousness are associated with adenoviral infections. Pericarditis, myocarditis, meningoencephalitis, and mesenteric adenitis may occur rarely in patients with viral pneumonia. These represent an integral part of the viral infection rather than a complication of viral pneumonia.

Roentgenographic changes include ill-defined localized structural accentuation of the bronchi and an interstitial reticulonodular pattern. The pattern may involve one or more lobes, usually lower, with the density being greatest at the hilum. Mottled densities of atelectasis and lucent areas of emphysema often are seen. Pleural effusions are uncommon and when present are small. Radiographic changes may persist for weeks or longer.

Laboratory changes include a total white blood cell count that is usually normal; however, both leukopenia and leukocytosis occur. The erythrocyte sedimentation rate may increase slightly. Monocytic cells predominate in the sputum. Bacterial superinfection is uncommon except in influenza and measles.

DIFFERENTIAL DIAGNOSIS

Bacterial complications of viral pneumonia, some pneumonias of bacterial origin, and pneumonias due to mycoplasmosis, coccidioidomycosis, histoplasmosis, Q fever, toxoplasmosis, psittacosis-ornithosis, and tularemia may be clinically indistinguishable from viral pneumonias. These may be identified by epidemiologic features, course of the disease, and identification of their causative agents.

For viral isolation, sputum or nasopharyngeal washings or swabs in veal infusion broth or tissue culture fluid may be sent to the laboratory fresh, or frozen if delayed more than 1 day. A presumptive diagnosis is possible in 5 to 10 days. Ten milliliters of serum drawn early and refrigerated to compare with a convalescent specimen drawn 10 days to 3 weeks later will show a fourfold rise in specific antibody titer. These procedures are not useful for a timely diagnosis to differentiate viral pneumonia from other microbial pneumonias that require prompt therapy.

Bacterial complications of viral pneumonia and primary bacterial pneumonias may be suspected when high fever, leukocytosis with shift to the left, purulent sputum, true pneumonic consolidation, or purulent effusion is present. Roentgenographic findings of dense consolidation, moderate or large effusions, pneumatocoeles, or frank abscess is also characteristic of bacterial pneumonia.

Culture of the nose and throat is not useful in diagnosis, since bacteria capable of producing pneumonia are commonly present in normal individuals. Examination of expectorated sputum is of more diagnostic value. Specimens may be obtained from infants and young children by direct suctioning of sputum at the larynx but are difficult to interpret because of contamination with saliva. A pure culture of certain organisms such as *S. aureus* or *H. influenzae* (which are uncommon nasopharyngeal organisms) provides suggestive evidence of a bacterial etiology, but a specimen that yields mixed flora is useless.

Transtracheal aspiration of sputum from a cannula passed through a needle inserted through the cricothyroid membrane will yield a single organism 75 per cent of the time. This procedure is useful if an anaerobic organism is suspected or if the adult patient cannot cooperate with expectorated sputum samples. Complications make this technique generally unsuitable for the child under 10 years of age. It should be considered only when serious pneumonia is present that has not responded to empiric therapy.

Blood cultures are indicated in patients with serious pneumonia who have temperatures greater than 38.9°C (102°F). Depending on the etiologic agent, bacteremia may be present in 10 to 25 per cent of patients. The absence of fever in the very young infant does not rule out bacteremia.

Direct lung puncture and aspiration are the only direct ways to obtain fluid for bacterial culture. The technique is attended rarely by serious complications such as pulmonary hemorrhage or pneumothorax. This procedure should be reserved for when the patient is seriously ill, when the cause is uncertain, and when the patient has not responded to antibiotic therapy.

Mycoplasmal Pneumonia. This condition may be indistinguishable from viral pneumonia. The diagnosis should be suspect in the child over 5 years, in the adolescent, or in the young adult during a summer or autumn epidemic when influenza has not been documented in the community. Cold agglutination of erythrocytes occurs in 10 per cent of mild attacks, in 50 per cent generally, and in 80 per cent of severe attacks but may occur in other types of nonbacterial pneumonia. Approximately one quarter of cold agglutinin-positive pneumonias are not caused by *M. pneumoniae.* Culture of *M. pneumoniae* on agar or in broth requires a specialized laboratory and 2 weeks to

3 months for specific diagnosis. Similarly, a fourfold rise in specific antibody titer may take several weeks.

Immunofluorescent microscopy of sputum or pleural fluid directly stained with fluorescent antibody is particularly valuable but not readily available in most laboratories. Therefore, diagnosis remains presumptive and choice of initial therapy may be determined by epidemiologic considerations and clinical presentation.

Coccidioidomycosis. This disease (see article on Systemic Mycotic Diseases) must be suspect if the patient has pneumonia in an endemic area or has recently arrived from an endemic area. The clinical presentation may be indistinguishable from viral pneumonia. Endemic areas include the southwestern United States, the western plateau of Mexico, and areas of Central and South America.

The most common roentgenographic changes include parenchymal consolidation, occurring mainly in the lower lobes, which may be homogeneous or mottled, segmental or nonsegmental. Hilar and mediastinal lymph node enlargement may be associated with the pneumonia or may occur alone in contrast to the usual absence in patients with viral pneumonia. Pleural effusion is present in 19 per cent of patients. Tension pneumatocoeles are particularly characteristic of coccidioidomycosis. The coccidioidin skin test, 0.1 ml of a 1:100 dilution (and occasionally a 1:10 dilution) injected intradermally is usually positive 12 to 20 days following clinical illness. The serum precipitin test becomes positive late in the second or early in the third week of illness. Complement-fixing antibodies appear somewhat later, at 4 to 6 weeks into illness.

Sputum showing the characteristic spherules or a positive growth of *Coccidioides immitis* on Sabouraud's medium may be the earliest confirmation of the diagnosis. However, the sputum is not uniformly positive.

Gastric aspirations are not useful.

Histoplasmosis. This condition causes pneumonia in the central and eastern portions of the United States, notably in the Ohio, Mississippi, and St. Lawrence River valleys, but it has also been reported from South and Central America, India, Malaya, and Cyprus. Skin testing, serologies, and sputum cultures are standard diagnostic measures. (See the article on Systemic Mycotic Diseases.)

Q Fever. Q fever is caused by *Coxiella burneti,* a rickettsia-like microbe. The disease is systemic and worldwide and produces a viral-like pneumonia. Cattle, sheep, and goats are carriers. Infection attacks laboratory personnel and persons handling hides, wool, goat hair, and infected meat. Drinking raw milk has been implicated. Diagnosis may be established in special laboratories by isolation of Coxiella from the sputum, blood, urine, or pleural exudates. A greater than 1:32 complement-fixing antibody titer during convalescence confirms the diagnosis. (See the article on Rickettsial Diseases.)

Toxoplasmosis. This is a widespread, generally inapparent infection in humans indicated by antibody in 20 to 80 per cent of various populations. (See the article on toxoplasmosis.) Rarely, systemic disseminated disease occurs, generally in debilitated patients, newborn infants who acquired their infection transplacentally, and in the generally immunosuppressed. Diagnosis is made by the Sabin-Feldman dye test, and rising complement-fixation, hemagglutination, and indirect fluorescent antibody tests.

Psittacosis-Ornithosis Pneumonia. This form of pneumonia should be considered when the patient has had close contact with sick or healthy birds. Pet bird owners and poultry workers are at risk. The organism is a filtrable, intracellular, coccoid parasite closer to rickettsia than viruses. The illness may be indistinguishable from viral pneumonia. *Chlamydia psittaci* may be detected in stained sputum smears or in cultures of sputum, blood, or lung. Fluorescent antibody may aid in early diagnosis. Complement-fixing antibodies appear late. (See the article on psittacosis.)

Tularemic Pneumonia. This disease is caused by *Francisella tularensis,* a gram-negative, nonmotile bacillus. The disease is rare but has been reported from all areas of the United States and Canada. The pulmonary form of tularemia, resulting from inhalation of organisms, is chiefly a problem in laboratory workers but may be suspected in butchers or hunters, especially those handling rabbits or hares. Cultures can be made directly from sputum. Serial agglutination tests permit a positive diagnosis, with the antibody titer rising 8 to 10 days after onset of infection. (See the article on tularemia.)

Differential Diagnosis in Infants. Lower respiratory tract disease (LRD), or pneumonitis, in the infant under 3 months of age has been attributed to viral etiology in over 95 per cent of cases despite the fact that older careful epidemiologic and laboratory work failed to identify a specific agent in over half of infants studied. Recent studies in hospitalized infants between 1 and 3 months of age suggest that single infections occur in 74 per cent of infants whereas mixed infections occur in 26 per cent. The four most common infectious agents isolated include *Chlamydia trachomatis* (25 per cent), *Ureaplasma urealyticum* (21 per cent), cytomegalovirus (20 per cent) and *Pneumocystis carinii* (18 per cent).

The clinical characteristics of pneumonitis associated with *C. trachomatis* have been described most extensively. It is generally a specific syndrome characterized by gradual onset, afebrile course, bilateral radiographic interstitial infiltrates, the presence of preceding or concurrent conjunctivitis in nearly half of the cases, and peripheral eosinophilia in many infants. The untreated course tends to be more protracted than the usual viral pneumonias. Unfortunately, clinical characteristics are not specific enough to differentiate LRD caused by these agents from that caused by RSV and other respiratory viral agents. With chlamydial pneumonia, epithelial scrapings of the tarsal conjunctiva or nasopharynx may reveal intracytoplasmic inclusion bodies. The etiologic agent may be isolated in the laboratory, in tissue culture, and in the yolk sac of embryonated eggs.

Urea urealyticum requires specialized culture methods similar to *M. pneumoniae* or an indirect immunofluorescent method (IFA) for detection of antibody. Neither technique is readily available and must be requested specially. Cytomegalovirus infection may be confirmed by culturing CMV from urine and saliva or by demonstrating a complement-fixing or fluorescent antibody rise.

be diagnosed only by open lung biopsy under general anesthesia. Bronchoalveolar lavage for diagnosis in the older immunosuppressed patient looks promising for diagnosis, but technical difficulties preclude its use in infants and children. Most of these illnesses are self-limited and do not require timely differentiation from viral pneumonia. However, chlamydial pneumonia will resolve more rapidly when treated with erythromycin. Although untreatable, CMV is important to diagnose for isolation and prognostic purposes.

The clinical importance of *P. carinii* infection for the nonimmunosuppressed infant under 3 months of age remains to be determined. However, seriously ill patients, particularly those requiring respiratory support, should be considered for a therapeutic trial with trimethoprim/sulfamethoxazole. Such a trial without biopsy does have a greater risk in the older immunosuppressed patient in whom the infection is often polymicrobial. The immunosuppressed patient should have therapy started on empiric grounds but confirmed as soon as possible by biopsy to confirm the diagnosis and to exclude other treatable agents such as candidiasis and atypical mycobacteria.

HYPERSENSITIVITY PNEUMONITIS

By Philip C. Halverson, M.D.
and Hal B. Richerson, M.D.
Iowa City, Iowa

DEFINITION

Hypersensitivity pneumonitis (extrinsic allergic alveolitis, HSP) is an allergic inflammation of the lung parenchyma secondary to the repeated inhalation of a variety of etiologic agents, including organic dusts and simple chemicals. Histopathology typically reveals a granulomatous interstitial pneumonitis with variable degrees of distal bronchiolitis obliterans. In early stages, granulomata are prominent and fibrosis is mild. In some patients, the disease may progress to end-stage fibrosis.

Farmer's lung, caused by the inhalation of thermophilic actinomycetes in "moldy" hay, is the prototype. Other examples of hypersensitivity pneumonitis developing in a variety of occupational and domestic environments are listed in Table 1. Identification of the source of exposure, which may in some cases challenge the most astute clinician, is essential for a definitive diagnosis and future management.

PRESENTING SIGNS AND SYMPTOMS

The presentation may be acute, subacute, or chronic, depending on frequency, intensity, and duration of inhalational exposure and perhaps on host or other factors determining immunopathogenesis. Both systemic and respiratory symptoms may occur. In the *acute form,* influenza-like symptoms often predominate, consisting of chills, fever, sweating, myalgias, lassitude, headache, and nausea which come on 2 to 9 hours after exposure, peak typically between 6 and 24 hours, and last from hours to days. Respiratory symptoms such as cough and dyspnea are common but not universal. The *subacute form* may appear gradually over several days to weeks, is marked by cough and dyspnea, and may progress to severe dyspnea with cyanosis leading to urgent hospitalization. The *chronic form* has an insidious onset over a period of months with increasing cough and exertional dyspnea. Fatigue and weight loss may be prominent complaints.

Physical examination may be within normal limits or may disclose bibasilar or more generalized crepitant inspiratory rales in any of the forms of presentation. Fever is common after acute exposure. Cyanosis may be seen in severe disease. Clubbing is not expected.

COURSE

Symptoms, signs, and other manifestations of hypersensitivity pneumonitis disappear within days, weeks, or months in most patients if the causative agent is no longer inhaled. Transformation to a chronic fibrotic stage with continued antigen exposure has been documented.

Individualization of environmental control is reasonable. Continued symptomatic febrile episodes indicate a failure of environmental control. If the patient remains asymptomatic in or out of the offending environment, the prognosis is generally good, although even complete removal from the incriminated environment may not prevent progression, depending at least partially on the age of the patient and the period of continued exposure to the antigen with concurrent symptoms.

LABORATORY PROCEDURES

Following acute exposure, a neutrophilia and lymphopenia are common. Mild elevations in erythrocyte sedimentation rate, C-reactive protein, rheumatoid factor, and immunoglobulins of IgG, IgM, or IgA isotypes may be present occasionally, reflecting acute or chronic inflammatory changes. Antinuclear antibodies are not common.

Precipitins. The attempted demonstration of precipitating antibodies against suspected antigens, such as those listed in Table 1, is an important part of the diagnostic work-up. If found, precipitins indicate sufficient exposure to the causative agent to generate an immunologic response. Although at one time considered important in disease pathogenesis, precipitins are currently considered simply as markers of exposure to an antigen source. Precipitins are not demonstrable in all patients, and available antigens are not standardized.

False-negative results may occur because of poor antigens or the wrong choice of antigens. Extraction of antigens from the patient's environment may at

Table 1. Examples of Hypersensitivity Pneumonitis

Disease	Antigen	Source of Antigen
Farmer's lung	Thermophilic actinomycetes, Aspergillus species	Contaminated hay, grain, silage
Bird fancier's, breeder's or handler's lung	Parakeet, pigeon, dove, chicken, turkey proteins	Avian droppings
Humidifier or air-conditioner lung	Thermophilic actinomycetes, *Aureobasidium pullulans*, amebae, other	Contaminated water in humidification aerosols, vaporizers, sprays
Woodworker's lung	Wood dust; Alternaria	Oak, cedar, mahogany dusts; pine and spruce pulp
Sauna taker's lung	*A. pullulans*, other	Contaminated sauna steam
Bagassosis	Thermophilic actinomycetes	Contaminated bagasse (sugar cane)
Malt worker's lung	*Aspergillus fumigatus, Aspergillus clavatus*	Moldy barley
Mushroom worker's lung	Thermophilic actinomycetes, other	Mushroom compost
Sequoiosis	Pullularia, Graphium species	Redwood sawdust
Maple bark stripper's disease	*Cryptostroma corticale*	Maple bark
Cheese worker's lung	*Penicillium casei*	Moldy cheese
Suberosis	Cork dust mold	Cork dust
Pituitary snuff taker's lung	Animal proteins	Heterologous pituitary snuff
Coffee worker's lung	Coffee bean dust	Coffee beans
Miller's lung	*Sitophilus granarius* (wheat weevil)	Infested wheat flour
Bathtub refinisher's lung	Toluene diisocyanate (TDI)	Porcelain surfacing catalyst
Chemical worker's lung	Toluene diisocyanate (TDI), methylene diisocyanate (MDI), phthallic anyhdride, vinyl chloride, other	Polyurethane foam, varnishes, plastics, synthetic rubber manufacturing, meat wrapping and labeling, other

times be helpful. The antibody response in some patients may be too meager to give a precipitin reaction using the traditional Ouchterlony double immunodiffusion technique. More sensitive methods may yield more positive results, but such results may lead to clinical confusion.

False-positive precipitin reactions are quite common with traditional techniques and must be interpreted with careful clinical correlations. For example, in a chart review of all inpatients and outpatients for whom a HSP precipitin battery was ordered at University of Iowa Hospitals during 1982–1983, we found 63 positives (25 per cent) among 252 ordered. Of those patients with positive results, four were diagnosed as having HSP, and three others as having allergic bronchopulmonary aspergillosis or fungus ball. Ten patients had clinical findings compatible with HSP, but they were diagnosed as having idiopathic pulmonary fibrosis, sarcoidosis, or histoplasmosis; in these patients, further follow-up is needed for definitive diagnosis. Forty-six (73 per cent) of the precipitin-positive patients had clinical findings incompatible with or irrelevant to HSP.

In vitro Tests for Cell-Mediated Immunity. The pathogenesis of hypersensitivity pneumonitis most likely involves antigen-specific T cell subsets responsible for delayed hypersensitivity (the so-called T_{DH} cell). No *in vitro* test has been shown to demonstrate T_{DH} effector activity reliably. Until such a test is found, there is no place in the routine diagnostic work-up for measures of cell-mediated immune responses, e.g., antigen- or mitogen-induced blastogenesis or release of lymphokines such as macrophage migration inhibitory factor (MIF).

RADIOLOGIC EVALUATION

The chest x-ray is sometimes normal even in symptomatic patients. The acute phase may be associated with a small, poorly defined, uniform, rather discrete and diffuse nodulation, occasionally symmetrically sparing the apices or bases. A diffuse, soft, stringy, or patchy interstitial infiltrate may also be seen with or without nodulation. In the chronic fibrotic phase, the linear element becomes more distinct and the periphery may be more prominently involved. Honeycombing may eventually develop and nodulation remain. As the condition progresses, loss of volume accentuates these changes. Abnormalities never or rarely seen in hypersensitivity pneumonitis include pleural effusion or thickening, hilar adenopathy, calcification, cavitation, atelactasis, and coin lesions.

PULMONARY FUNCTION TESTING

Pulmonary function studies typically show a restrictive pattern with decreased compliance and impaired gas exchange. Following acute exposure, there is a decrease in forced vital capacity and 1-second forced expiratory volume (FEV_1) with maintenance of flow rates. Changes in small airways may result in an increase in closing volume and in nonuniform ventilation distribution with disturbance in ventilation-perfusion relationships contributing to hypoxemia and impaired diffusing capacity. As the chronic stage develops into progressive fibrosis, changes of airway obstruction may become increasingly prominent.

OTHER DIAGNOSTIC PROCEDURES

Skin Testing. Antigens prepared and used experimentally in patients with hypersensitivity pneumonitis and appropriate controls have been irritating and nondiscriminatory. Skin test antigens are not available. Skin testing is therefore neither appropriate nor practical at this time.

Inhalational Challenge. Inhalation of aerosolized material suspected as causative in individual patients has produced acute changes and substantiated the clinical impression in many reports. Few of these reports have included appropriate controls. No standardized antigens or techniques are available. In one recent study, positive findings most helpful included fever, neutrophilia, lymphopenia, decreased forced vital capacity, and decreased exercise minute ventilation.

In many patients, purposeful exposure to the suspected natural environment may be practical, useful, and preferable to laboratory challenge. Interpretation of results may be difficult and routine use of either method of inhalational challenge is not recommended, especially in patients with forms of the disease other than simple, acute, recurrent, transient attacks.

Bronchoalveolar Lavage. Many centers are using fiberoptic bronchoscopy and bronchoalveolar lavage to aid in diagnostic evaluation of interstitial lung disease. Hypersensitivity pneumonitis and sarcoidosis are typically associated with an increase of lymphocytes, particularly T cells, whereas idiopathic pulmonary fibrosis is characterized by the presence of neutrophils in lavage fluids. Insufficient information is now available to know to what extent this procedure is useful in the routine diagnostic work-up of interstitial lung diseases.

Lung Biopsy. In patients without sufficient clinical criteria to make a definitive diagnosis, lung biopsy may be indicated, especially to rule out other diseases requiring different treatment. Open lung biopsy will usually provide adequate material, whereas transbronchial biopsy may not. Although the histopathology is distinctive, it is not pathognomonic. When the biopsy is taken during the active phase of disease, typical findings include an interstitial alveolar infiltrate consisting of plasma cells, lymphocytes, and occasional eosinophils, usually with accompanying granulomata. Interstitial fibrosis is common but most often mild in earlier stages of the disease. Some degree of bronchiolitis is found in about half the cases, and foreign-body material demonstrable by polarized light is often seen. Vasculitis is not a feature.

Differentiation of HSP from infectious fungus disease requires careful search for fungal elements. Hypersensitivity pneumonitis differs from sarcoidosis in that a variable infiltration of lymphocytes and plasma cells occurs involving the pulmonary parenchyma at sites distant from granulomas, whereas in sarcoidosis such infiltrates are found only in and around the granulomas. Another distinguishing feature is that in sarcoidosis, but not HSP, granulomas are found in perivascular and intramural areas of blood vessels. With these clues, the biopsy, if justified, should greatly help to establish the diagnosis.

THERAPEUTIC TESTS

Removal of the causative agent from the patient's environment, or of the patient from the incriminated inhalant, should be followed by improvement in most cases within days, weeks, or months and will help confirm the diagnosis.

POTENTIAL ERRORS AND PITFALLS IN DIAGNOSIS

The diagnosis of HSP should be initially considered in any patient with a history of recurrent pneumonias or with interstitial lung disease, as well as in those with typical presentations of acute, subacute, or chronic HSP. Recurrent pneumonias also require that immune deficiency syndromes, especially hypoimmunoglobulinemia, be ruled out. (See the article on Immune Deficiency Diseases.)

Idiopathic interstitial fibrosis (cryptogenic fibrosing alveolitis) may resemble HSP clinically; autoimmune phenomena are more common in idiopathic interstitial fibrosis, and bronchopulmonary lavage (above) may be helpful. Histopathology is distinctive except in end-stage lung. Cystic fibrosis should be included in the differential diagnosis. (See the article on this topic.) Eosinophilic pneumonias are usually accompanied by striking eosinophilia and are often associated with bronchial asthma; neither of these features is expected in HSP. Allergic bronchopulmonary aspergillosis is a variant of eosinophilic pneumonia occurring in an extrinsic asthmatic, but is sometimes confused with HSP because of the presence of precipitating antibodies to *Aspergillus fumigatus.* (See the article on Opportunistic Mycoses.) Collagen vascular diseases, granuloma-vasculitis syndromes, and sarcoidosis are usually multisystem diseases, whereas HSP is confined to the lung.

A condition termed *pulmonary mycotoxicosis* (more recently "atypical" farmer's lung) occurs in patients massively exposed to moldy silage and is manifested by fever, chills, and cough within a few hours. Precipitins are not present, suggesting that prior sensitization is not required.

In general, a history of exposure to moldy hay, birds, or other incriminated occupational or environmental inhalants in a patient with clinical and radiologic features consistent with HSP should lead to the demonstration of serum precipitins to the suspected antigen and an established diagnosis, confirmed by avoidance of the agent involved. Occasionally, other diagnostic procedures are required. The diagnosis is often difficult in domestic exposures such as humidification and air conditioning systems. A careful environmental history is essential, and at times the physician must inspect the patient's environment personally.

PNEUMOCONIOSIS

By J. Bernard L. Gee, M.D.
and K. Randall Young, Jr., M.D.
New Haven, Connecticut

The term pneumoconiosis simply means lungs full of dust; it does not necessarily imply a disease, either pathologically or clinically. Thus, there are benign and disease-producing pneumoconioses. However, all dust deposition evokes alveolar macrophage mobilization within the airspaces, a phenomenon most commonly seen in cigarette smokers. Some increased reticulin formation may be detectable, but there is little tissue injury or repair. These benign forms are due to mixed dust, iron (siderosis), tin (stannosis), soot, and coal-dust (in the early stages of coal-worker's pneumoconiosis, CWP).

By contrast, other pneumoconioses are characterized by three general types of reaction.

1. The noncaseating granuloma associated with immune reactions. This will be discussed in relation to beryllium (other hypersensitivity reactions to biologic materials are treated in the article on hypersensitivity pneumonitis).
2. The foreign-body granulomata, in which macrophage ingestion of the particle may occur without a full cellulohumoral immune response, e.g., talc.
3. The more common and disabling fibrosing pneumoconioses that are due to silica, asbestos, and so on.

This classification, though useful, is oversimplified because beryllium and talc can also cause lung fibrosis. Likewise, there is increasing modern evidence that such connective tissue cells as the fibroblast (which makes collagen and other tissue matrix materials such as fibronectin) is subject to humoral regulation by such classical immune system cells as the macrophage and lymphocyte and also by intact granulomata. The particles responsible for these fibrous pneumoconioses are phagocytosed by resident and recruited alveolar macrophages. Even in the absence of classical immunosensitization, these macrophages can be involved in the regulation of fibroblast activity and in the injury process to lung connective tissue. Likewise, the phagocytic activity of these macrophages evokes the release of neutrophil chemoattractants, which both mobilize and activate the latter cell. The activated neutrophil can cause injury to lung cells and matrix by two general mechanisms: *oxidant* (superoxide anion, H_2O_2) and *proteolytic* (collagenase, elastase, and other proteases). These neutrophil determinants are particularly relevant to asbestosis.

The term pneumoconiosis does not usually include neoplasia, asthma, or the predominantly airway mucosal changes of simple nonobstructive bronchitis.

GENERAL APPROACH TO THE DIAGNOSIS OF PNEUMOCONIOSIS

Although there are certain features, notably in chest x-rays, that are highly suggestive of the diagnosis of specific pneumoconioses, the diagnosis eventually rests on the combination of a carefully taken work history and the clinical-radiologic-pulmonary functional constellation. Invasive procedures such as lung biopsies may be useful in some instances but are not generally required. We will indicate these components of the diagnostic approach.

Work History

A painstakingly detailed history is essential and frequently very time-consuming. Ideally, the patient should list all jobs chronologically, including the time spent in those occupations. The job titles and locations of the work place will often suggest diagnoses to the physician, particularly if he or she knows the community. However, specific questions as to specific agents are the next requirement. Is a construction worker using asbestos roofing? Is a boilermaker or a maintenance worker who is also a part-time insulator using or removing old asbestos? If a miner, what does the worker mine? If coal, is it hard or soft coal? Where does the coal miner work? At the coal face (most exposed), i.e., a hard-header? If a rubber products worker, does this person use talc? Does the worker know the grade of talc (i.e., is it "contaminated" with asbestos fibers)? A machinist may be exposed to oils, dusts, coolants, benign metals (stainless steels) or hard metals, the latter occurring in tool repairers. Metals present problems because the worker may not know what is in the alloy, particularly at scrap metal processing plants. Specific inquiries at the workplace are appropriate, but the worker can often bring labels of the materials in use. The precision of the work history depends on the tenacity and knowledge of the physician. A simple question—"Do you work with asbestos?"—may be misleading (the worker used it in a ceiling last week!) or inadequate (maintenance or railroad workers often are not aware if they are using it unless instructed, often by their union).

Industrial hygiene surveys may rarely be required (e.g., beryllium levels), but a visit to the work site by an informed physician can be useful.

Radiology

Conventional chest radiology alone is needed. Aside from recognizing specific patterns and their association with specific pneumoconioses, there is great value in reading these in a standard manner. This standardization has merits in minimizing inter-observer error.

It permits a quantification of disease and correlates with dust contents, at least in CWP and silicosis. It permits consistent epidemiologic studies and medicolegal opinions, notably in regard to workmen's compensation. This classification is based on the size, shape, and profusion of the opacities. It was introduced primarily for the common pneumoconioses (CWP and silica). It is termed the *ILO U/C International Classification.* Although it is not essential for the general physician to pass the formal examination for certification as a qualified reader, some familiarity with it stimulates precision and is important educationally.

Pulmonary Function Tests

Conventional tests are appropriate, and the only point in relation to our subject is the advisability of maintaining permanent records, particularly of any spirometric tracings involved in measures of forced vital capacity (FVC), forced expiratory volume at one second (FEV_1) and even diffusing capacity (DL_{CO}). All spirometric test records should be retained in suspected cases to avoid medicolegal quarrels.

Bronchoalveolar Lavage

This benign procedure of bronchoscopic saline lavage of the airways and alveoli with an examination of cellular and chemical constituents has become increasingly employed in the diagnosis and management of lung disorders. For the pneumoconioses it has limited use. In mineral dust diseases it has no place. In metal diseases it may be useful, as we shall see.

ASBESTOSIS

Definition

Asbestosis is a diffuse fibrosing alveolitis due to inhalation and retention of a number of forms of fibrous silicates, mainly chrysotile, and the amphiboles crocidolite and amosite. The term does not apply to pleural effusions or fibrotic pleural plaques, in spite of the high frequency of the latter following asbestos exposure.

Pathogenesis

The term *fibrosing alveolitis* correctly implies an inflammatory response with progressive fibrosis. The inflammatory response is characterized by macrophage, lymphocyte, and fibroblast proliferation. Lung lavage studies suggest an intra-alveolar neutrophil leukocytosis and free collagenase to be common in established cases. There is a particularly intense cellular and fibrotic reaction in the small and terminal airways. Progressive fibrosis occurs and honeycombing is the ultimate result. Asbestos bodies can be observed; phase contrast and electron microscopy can characterize the fiber number and types.

Clinical Features

Asbestosis presents as cough, progressive dyspnea on exertion and, where severe, breathlessness at rest. Finger clubbing occurs in 10 per cent of cases. End-inspiratory fine rales commonly occur in the disorder. Chest x-rays show initial changes of either ground glass or of fine small opacities. Pleural, interlobar, and pericardial plaques, frequently calcified, in a patient with parenchymal x-ray abnormalities should indicate the diagnosis, particularly where they are bilateral.

The radiologic differential diagnosis of asbestosis is very large and includes all the common diffuse lung diseases. Of these the most important are idiopathic pulmonary fibrosis (cryptogenic fibrosing alveolitis), the fibrosis associated with systemic connective tissue disorders (e.g., rheumatoid arthritis), and the fibrotic end stages of eosinophilic granulomata. The predominance of lower zone distribution and the absence of bullae distinguish asbestosis from fibrotic sarcoidosis. Eosinophilic pneumonitis is more common in women and occurs more frequently peripherally in the upper zones but can be indistinguishable from asbestosis. Low-grade pulmonary edema can trap the unwary, but heart size and Kerley B lines should differentiate.

In the presence of pleural plaques, the differential diagnosis of asbestosis is limited but bilateral tuberculosis is plausible and pleural fibrosis due to sequential pneumothoraces can be a problem occasionally.

Lung Function

The classical features of restrictive disease occur in established cases and include reduction in *all* volumes: vital capacity (VC), FEV_1, functional residual capacity (FRC), residual volume (RV), and total lung capacity (TLC). Reduced DL_{CO} is the rule in these cases. In early disease, VC and FEV_1 may be about 80 per cent predicted (i.e., low normal range), and DL_{CO} can be of help where it is less than 70 per cent predicted. These features are in no way pathognomonic but provide supporting and functionally relevant data.

Pathology Tests

Asbestos bodies in the sputum certainly suggest the diagnosis, but the latter still depends on above features together with an appropriate work history. Lung biopsies are nonspecific. Lavage may show free alveolar space leukocytosis, but this is not essential for the diagnosis. In certain cases, for research purposes autopsy material may be submitted for a transmission electron microscopic mineralogic analysis to define the number and type of fibers.

SILICOSIS

Definition

The disorder is a fibrotic reaction to inhalation and deposition of dust that contains silicon dioxide. This disorder used to be far more prevalent, but improvements in mining techniques and dust control have lessened (but not eradicated) the disorder. The disease takes two forms, acute and chronic silicosis.

Acute Silicosis

The acute form requires either massive exposure (as in tunneling) or some other associated exposure, notably alkali which is mixed with silica to cause abrasive soap powders. The disease has a variable progression rate, but death can occur in a few years. The illness is characterized by fever, cough, progressive dyspnea, weight loss, and an x-ray picture of diffuse perihilar fluffy opacification. The differential diagnosis includes pulmonary edema, Goodpasture's syndrome, hypersensitivity pneumonitis, and alveolar proteinosis. The occupational history is the only clue to the correct diagnosis.

Chronic Silicosis

Pathogenesis

Silica, deposited in the lung, calls for alveolar macrophage mobilization, and these cells phagocytose the particulate silica, which is highly cytotoxic for macrophages. It causes disruption of the membrane around the phagocytic vacuole. This leads to lysosomal enzyme autodigestion of the macrophage cytoplasm and such intracytoplasmic and subcellular organelles as the mitochondrion. Thus, ingestion by and autolysis of macrophages permit silica recycling and impair lung defenses against such organisms as *M. tuberculosis.* Silica also causes macrophages to release fibroblast-stimulating factors, among which is interleukin I. For uncertain reasons, silica produces focal fibronodular lesions as opposed to the diffuse fibrosis seen with asbestos.

Clinical Features

Classical chronic silicosis is a slowly progressive disorder that, in the early and uncomplicated forms, is not directly associated with any symptoms. Many of the symptoms are due to smoking, which causes cough, sputum, and airway obstruction and hence effort dyspnea. The evidence for progression is radiologic. In the complicated form, i.e., progressive massive fibrosis (PMF), serious problems develop, with progressive dyspnea to dyspnea at rest, arterial desaturation, and congestive heart failure. Physical signs are frequently absent until the end stages.

In PMF, associated tuberculosis is a most important risk. Activation may be suggested by hemoptysis, fever, and weight loss. Sputum smears and cultures are essential. All patients with silicosis should be tested with tuberculin, and most authorities recommend long-term antituberculosis chemoprophylaxis. The major diagnostic features, apart from the history, are radiologic. Radiologically, silicosis shares with sarcoidosis a superior symmetric distribution of the disease, which is characteristically nodular. Complicated silicosis is defined radiologically as conglomerate masses greater than 1 cm in diameter. These are characteristically upper- and sometimes midzone lesions. They are associated with linear stranding from the base of the masses to the diaphragm, which often becomes tented. The area around the masses shows hyperlucency and loss of vasculature. Pleural disease is uncommon and, where present, should raise the possibility of mixed exposures (tremolite, other asbestos materials, and silica).

Unlike sarcoidosis, lymph node enlargement is infrequent, but the nodes show a characteristic ring calcification known as "eggshell" calcification. This is very common in silicosis and very rare in sarcoidosis. In the absence of eggshells, symmetrical upper lobe nodulation suggests tuberculosis but the clinical picture and work history should differentiate silicosis from tuberculosis. Care should be taken to consider their coexistence.

Lung Function

Early disease is not associated with functional abnormalities, but some loss of VC, FEV_1, TLC, and lung compliance occur with advancing disease. The complicated forms show clear reductions in the above with low DL_{CO} and arterial desaturation.

Occupations

Mining is the most obvious work activity associated with silicosis. Other occupations include work related to foundries, blast furnaces, potteries, glass making, stone cutting, quarries, abrasives manufacturing, fillers in the paint industry, and boiler scaling.

COAL WORKER'S PNEUMOCONIOSIS

Definition

Simply, CWP is coal dust accumulation in the lung and tissue reaction thereto.

There are, however, some variations in the usage of the term in the United States, the United Kingdom, and Europe. These center on the role ascribed to silica in coal worker's lung disorders. We suggest that:

1. There is clearly an entity, CWP, specifically due to coal dust in the absence of measurable silica in the coal or without excess (i.e., not above that in normal non-coal workers) silica in the autopsied lung:
2. Similar entities occur in graphite workers who are not exposed to coal:
3. There are perhaps some variations in coal worker's lung disease which may be ascribed to silica.
4. Broadly speaking, the prevalence and severity of the lesions bear a direct relation to lung coal dust content and coal rank. (High-rank coal gives off more heat on combustion than does low-rank coal.)
5. Silicosis can also occur in coal workers notably in areas of hard rock.

Pathology

In its simple form, CWP is characterized by the coal macule, which is easily recognized in sectional slices of inflated formalin-fixed autopsy lungs (Gough sections) as a black nodule, sometimes with focal emphysema. Histologically the macule shows pigmented alveolar macrophages with some increased reticulin and collagen.

The macule is situated around the terminal bronchiole. In some instances centroacinar emphysema occurs. In complicated CWP, the lesions are similar to silicotic PMF except that they may contain coal dust.

Clinical Features

In its simplest form, CWP probably has no symptoms and certainly has no physical signs. Cough, sputum, and overt dyspnea are usually due to cigarette smoking, but cough and sputum without overt airway obstruction may be present. However, where present, this may reflect large airway mucosal changes (i.e., industrial bronchitis) rather than CWP per se. In the complicated form, dyspnea occurs and is progressive. Ultimately there is arterial desaturation and heart failure supersedes.

In spite of the initial provisions of the Black Lung Act, there is no evidence that simple CWP is either disabling or shortens life span. From the diagnostic viewpoint, *simple* CWP remains a radiologic diagnosis based on the chest x-ray of a person with an appropriate work history. Clinical, physiologic, and other studies are diagnostically useless.

Lung Function

Although there are certain minor physiologic changes, these are not diagnostic of CWP. The changes are small decreases in FEV_1, increases in RV and FRC and probably increases in peripheral airway resistance. Slight loss in DL_{CO} and slight increases in the dead space: tidal volume ratio may be seen. It should be stressed that 80 per cent of coal workers filing claims under the Black Lung Act have lung function abnormalities that do not even approach usual social security disability criteria.

RADIOLOGY

These were discussed under other sections and are similar to (though the lesions are often smaller and less discrete than) those observed in silicosis. Eggshell calcification is most unusual. Complicated CWP or PMF is defined as any shadow with a diameter greater than 1 cm. Simple CWP lesions progress slowly, and x-rays should be taken at 5-year intervals.

Caplan's syndrome is characterized by peripherally situated lesions varying between 0.5 and 5 cm in diameter. These may calcify, and effusions may also occur. There is a variable temporal relation to the development of rheumatoid arthritis. The disorder occurs in early CWP. The mechanisms are unclear.

MISCELLANEOUS MINERAL DUST PNEUMOCONIOSES

Numerous materials produce nodular, symmetric, usually predominantly upper lobe lesions without symptoms, without major lung function abnormalities, and without reduction in life expectancy. Some pneumoconioses are due to minerals with high radiodensity (barium—baritosis; iron—siderosis; tin—stannosis; antimony; zirconium; and rare earth metals). This group represents the sources of benign pneumoconioses. Diagnosis is obvious from the occupational history.

Other non-benign pneumoconioses result from talc (nodular, diffuse fibrotic, and mixed forms). Pleural plaques may be seen. Birefringent plating and acicular particles together with foreign-body granulomata may be evident pathologically. "Talc" is a vague term, mineralogically speaking. Talc may include silica or tremolite (like asbestos). Kaolin (China clay) may also cause nodular and massive fibrosis.

LUNG DISEASE CAUSED BY HARD METALS

Tungsten carbide is a metal of extreme hardness and resistance to heat and is widely used in manufacturing drills, tools, and armaments. In the process of producing tungsten carbide, tungsten and carbon are mixed and heated to a very high temperature (presintering) and cobalt is added to provide a matrix for tungsten carbide crystals. Other metals such as titanium, tantalum, and nickel may be added, depending on the desired properties of the final product. Paraffin is added to the powdered metal to provide the proper consistency for pressing it into shapes, and the metal is then deparaffinized and heated in a furance (sintering) to form the hard metal. At many points in this process, fine dusts containing both tungsten and cobalt may be generated that can be inhaled by workers in the area. Hard metal lung disease from tungsten (or tungsten carbide pneumoconiosis) can be encountered in workers exposed to any stage of this process. Three general forms of respiratory illness may be found in these workers: asthma, bronchitis, or diffuse interstitial lung disease.

Asthma

Asthma in hard-metal workers shows many features similar to other occupational asthmatic syndromes. Workers experience typical symptoms of wheezing, cough, and dyspnea upon exposure to the work place, with these symptoms abating over the weekend or during other periods away from work. During vacations or other extended work absences, their symptoms may be completely relieved. Pulmonary function testing reveals the characteristic changes of obstructive lung disease-diminished forced expiratory volumes in 1 second (FEV_1) and maximum midexpiratory flow rate (MMEFR), with relatively normal forced vital capacity (FVC). The FEV_1:FVC ratio is below normal. These parameters usually return toward normal when the worker is removed from exposure, although some patients have developed severe persistent asthma. Patients' symptoms and flow rates may improve following bronchodilator administration. The chest radiograph is usually normal.

Considerable evidence suggests that cobalt is the agent responsible for the hypersensitivity reaction in hard-metal worker's asthma, and in some cases challenge tests with cobalt alone have reproduced the obstructive findings.

Bronchitis

Bronchitis, characterized by cough and sputum production without significant airways obstruction, may also be seen in workers involved in tungsten carbide production, or it may be present together with the asthmatic symptoms.

Diffuse Fibrosing Interstitial Lung Disease

This condition has been recognized in hard-metal workers in many countries. The clinical features of this illness resemble those of idiopathic pulmonary fibrosis (IPF). Disease is not usually seen with less than about 10 years of exposure but occasionally may present earlier. Early in the course, there is usually cough with the production of only scanty sputum. This is followed by progressive dyspnea occurring first only with exertion and then at rest. Physical examination reveals tachypnea, rales on auscultation and, in advanced cases, clubbing and evidence of pulmonary hypertension. The chest radiograph demonstrates bilateral nodular and linear densities and cannot readily be distinguished from that seen in IPF. Analysis of arterial blood gases frequently shows hypoxemia with further desaturation following exercise. Pulmonary function tests show primarily a restrictive defect with loss of lung volume (low FVC and total lung capacity). Biopsy specimens of lung tissue characteristically show infiltration of alveolar and interstitial regions with large multinuclear macrophages and desquamation of type II alveolar cells. There may be at times a granulomatous reaction. Later cases reveal extensive fibrosis. Crystals of tungsten carbide may be seen on electron microscopy, and tungsten can be demonstrated by elemental analysis of lung tissue. Although cobalt is considered to be important in the pathogenesis of these lesions, cobalt may not be found in lung tissue because of its high solubility in body fluids and rapid excretion.

A recent report indicates that bronchoalveolar lavage of patients with interstitial disease caused by hard-metal exposures may demonstrate the presence of bizarre multinucleated macrophages, a helpful but nonspecific finding.

Although patients with hard-metal worker's pneumoconiosis may respond to removal from the exposure and administration of corticosteroids, the disease may be progressive, with death resulting from pulmonary hypertension and the resultant cor pulmonale.

LUNG DISEASE CAUSED BY BERYLLIUM

Beryllium is a soft metal with the properties of extremely light weight and high tensile strength, and it has wide application in the space, x-ray, and nuclear fields. Several beryllium salts and alloys are used for the production of electronic devices, nonsparking tools, dental alloys, and engine parts. The metal is chiefly prepared from beryl ore (beryllium aluminum silicate).

In the past, the chief source of occupational beryllium exposure was in the manufacture of fluorescent light bulbs in which beryllium phosphors were used as a coating. With the substitution of less toxic substances as coating materials, the importance of this exposure source has lessened. Presently the major groups at risk for beryllium exposure are those workers involved in the machining, drilling, and welding of the metal and its alloys or those working with beryllium oxide in ceramics industries.

Beryllium may be absorbed through either the lungs or the skin and can give rise to both acute and chronic respiratory illness.

Acute Berylliosis

Inhalation of large concentrations of beryllium *acutely* may cause a syndrome of tracheobronchitis and chemical pneumonitis. Within 72 hours of exposure, the nasal and oral membranes become hyperemic and swollen. The development of tracheitis and bronchitis is characterized by a hacking dry cough often accompanied by substernal pain. There may be ocular irritation, and there is often evidence of an erythematous papular and vesicular rash on exposed areas.

Following large exposures, there may develop a chemical pneumonitis which is occasionally fatal. The patient experiences sudden dyspnea, cough, and chest discomfort. Blood-streaked sputum may be present. Examination reveals cyanosis, tachycardia, tachypnea, and rales on auscultation. The chest radiograph may resemble pulmonary edema with diffuse bilateral infiltrates. Arterial blood gases reveal hypoxemia, which may be profound. The extent of the pulmonary function abnormalities depends upon the severity of the illness, usually demonstrating lowered lung compliance and abnormal diffusing capacity.

Treatment with oxygen and corticosteroids usually leads to a benign course with complete resolution of signs and symptoms within 1 to 4 weeks. Occasional cases will require mechanical ventilation, and fatalities have occurred. It is felt that about 10 per cent of individuals may progress to chronic berylliosis even without further exposure.

Chronic Berylliosis

Chronic berylliosis is a granulomatous disease that may affect many organs throughout the body, including the lungs. Respiratory disease is usually the most prominent manifestation of beryllium-induced illness and may appear as soon as several months following exposure or may not present until 10 to 15 years later.

Berylliosis very closely resembles sarcoidosis in its clinical manifestations. The earliest symptom is dyspnea on exertion, which usually progresses and may become severe. Dry cough is frequently a prominent complaint. There may be constitutional symptoms such as malaise, anorexia, and weight loss. The disease may progress to severe pulmonary fibrosis in advanced cases. Spontaneous pneumothoraces may be seen, and some 20 per cent of patients will exhibit clubbing. Like sarcoidosis, hepatic and splenic involvement occurs not uncommonly.

Physical examination is nonspecific and will reveal rales in the lungs and occasionally hepatomegaly. The skin lesions just described may be evident. In contrast to sarcoidosis, ocular involvement and erythema nodosum are not seen and parotitis is reportedly rare.

The chest radiograph usually demonstrates nodular, granular, or linear parenchymal densities sometimes accompanied by bilateral hilar adenopathy. Advanced cases may show fibrosis and/or cyst formation.

The abnormalities seen on pulmonary function testing are nonspecific and are similar to those seen in IPF, hypersensitivity pneumonitis, sarcoidosis, or other interstitial lung diseases. Mild or early disease is marked by arterial oxygen desaturation more pronounced on exercise. The DL_{CO} is commonly low and may be used to follow cases during therapy. More advanced disease usually manifests a "restrictive" ventilatory defect with low FVC and TLC and preservation of the FEV_1:FVC ratio.

Routine laboratory tests are usually not helpful in differentiating berylliosis from sarcoidosis or other similar illnesses. Hypercalcemia and hyperuricemia may occur in both berylliosis and sarcoidosis. In both berylliosis and sarcoidosis, serum immunoglobulin levels (especially IgG) may be elevated. There has been no agreement among authorities on the utility of serum angiotensin-converting-enzyme (ACE) determinations in distinguishing the two diseases; some investigators have reported similar elevations of ACE levels in both conditions. The Kveim test is usually negative in berylliosis but is also frequently negative in sarcoid, limiting its usefulness.

Histologic examination of lung tissue or lymph nodes reveals noncaseating granulomata in berylliosis, and there may be a variable amount of cellular infiltration of alveolar walls.

The diagnosis of berylliosis rests upon a history of beryllium exposure; characteristic clinical, radiographic, and physiologic findings; and demonstration of the nonspecific histologic features. Elemental analysis of lung tissue obtained by open biopsy for quantitation of beryllium is important. Amounts greater than 0.02 μg beryllium per gram of dried tissue are usually seen in cases of berylliosis, but these levels may also be seen in lungs of individuals exposed to the metal but without clinical evidence of berylliosis.

A hypersensitivity reaction to beryllium is felt to be important in the pathogenesis of this disease, and evidence of this hypersensitivity may be elicited by a number of methods. Patch testing of the skin with a beryllium salt will frequently cause formation of a papular lesion that is granulomatous on biopsy. Cells retrieved from the lung by bronchoalveolar lavage contain a high percentage of lymphocytes, and both these lymphocytes and those from peripheral blood will proliferate and release macrophage migration inhibitory factor (BeMIF) when challenged with beryllium salts. The clinical and diagnostic value of these tests is just beginning to be assessed, and their medicolegal evidentiary standing has not yet been tested in the courts.

LUNG DISEASE CAUSED BY OTHER METALS

Although beryllium and hard metals (tungsten-carbide/cobalt) are the causes of the major metal-related respiratory syndromes, exposure to other metals may also be associated with lung disease or asymptomatic radiographic changes.

Cadmium is extremely corrosion-resistant and is widely used in electroplating. Respiratory exposure may occur in those workers involved in smelting ore during processing of the metal or in individuals firing or welding cadmium-plated metals and alloys.

Within 3 to 4 hours of exposure to cadmium fumes, a syndrome of mucous membrane irritation may develop, presenting with rhinitis, sore throat, cough and chest pain. Some patients may have a more severe illness with myalgia, dyspnea, hemoptysis, fever, cyanosis, and atelectatic rales in the chest. The chest radiograph may resemble pulmonary edema, or there may be only vague mid- and lower-lung zone infiltration. If extremely severe, the syndrome may be fatal, but in survivors all the defects resolve completely. Cadmium exposure may also cause renal tubular dysfunction with resultant proteinuria and occasional aminoaciduria.

There has been considerable debate over whether chronic cadmium exposure causes pulmonary emphysema. Most authorities seem to agree that no definite causal link between the two can be proved.

Aluminum metal and bauxite (aluminum oxide) have been known to cause pulmonary fibrosis and associated spontaneous pneumothorax. Analysis of lung tissue in these cases shows greatly increased aluminum levels.

Inhalation of numerous metals may cause radiographic changes that are often striking, but these metals (in the absence of concomitant exposure to silica) are such elements as do not cause respiratory symptoms. They are listed here: iron (siderosis), tin (stannosis), titanium, barium (baritosis), and antimony. Vanadium, mercury, and manganese have been associated with tracheobronchial irritation and bronchitis.

Finally, a syndrome known as *metal fume fever* sometimes occurs after the inhalation of fumes generated by welding, cutting, and melting metals. It is an influenza-like illness characterized by myalgias, fever, headaches and malaise. The onset is acute and resolution is complete within 1 to 2 days. It may occur more commonly following time away from work and thus has also been termed "Monday morning fever."

ATELECTASIS

By David C. Budson, M.D.
Vallejo, California
and Philip A. Bromberg, M.D.,
Chapel Hill, North Carolina

DEFINITION

Translated literally from its Greek source, atelectasis means "imperfect stretching." The term was originally applied to a lung or a portion of lung that did not fill with air at birth but was later used to denote collapse of a previously expanded portion of lung. Atelectasis has been defined by a number of authors as any state associated with a loss of lung volume. This definition, unfortunately, includes the loss of volume owing to pulmonary fibrosis, for which a category of "cicatrization" or "contraction" atelectasis has even been designated. However, the loss of volume secondary to fibrosis is due to replacement of alveoli with fibrous tissue rather than to the collapse of intact alveoli, and in reality, few clinicians or physiologists think of fibrosis in the lungs as a form of atelectasis. It would seem, therefore, that a better definition of atelectasis would be "the collapse of anatomically intact alveoli associated with a loss of lung volume."

CLASSIFICATION

The most rational classification of atelectasis is based on an understanding of the mechanisms that are responsible for maintaining lung volume and the ways in which these may be altered. On the basis of a discussion of these mechanisms, we will describe three general types of atelectasis: relaxation atelectasis, atelectasis related to altered surfactant, and resorption atelectasis.

Lung Elastic Recoil and Relaxation Atelectasis. The force with which the lungs tend to collapse at a given volume (retractive pressure or elastic recoil) arises from elastic forces in lung tissue as well as surface-related forces at the alveolar-air interface. At functional residual capacity (FRC), the elastic recoil of the lung is balanced by the passive expansile tendency of the chest wall, resulting in a subatmospheric intrapleural pressure. (At lung volumes higher than FRC, active inspiratory muscle contraction is required to balance the increased lung elastic recoil.) Alteration of the resting position of the chest wall or interference with the coupling of the chest wall to the visceral pleural surface, which may occur with thoracoplasty, pneumothorax, or pleural effusion, may allow retraction of the underlying lung. A similar mechanism is responsible for retraction of lung tissue adjacent to a space-occupying lesion in the lung parenchyma (e.g., solid masses, cysts, bullae, or lobar emphysema in infants). This form of atelectasis is referred to as *passive* or *relaxation atelectasis.* Other synonyms include *mantle atelectasis* and *compressive atelectasis,* but the latter term is not entirely accurate since the lung in this situation collapses owing to its own passive recoil rather than to active compression.

Surface Forces and Atelectasis. Surface forces also contribute to the tendency of the lung to retract, and high surface tensions at the alveolar-air interface render alveoli unstable, particularly at low lung volumes and low distending pressures. Alveoli are lined by a phospholipid-containing surface active film, or surfactant, that promotes alveolar stability by its inherent property of lowering surface tension as alveolar surface area decreases. If surfactant activity is reduced by impaired synthesis, destruction, or increased removal, alveoli become unstable and collapse. This form of atelectasis has been variously termed *adhesive, congestive,* and *nonobstructive atelectasis.* It is likely to be spotty or focal but is often diffuse in distribution. Deficiency of lung surfactant due to decreased synthesis is well established in the neonatal respiratory distress syndrome, in which diffuse atelectasis is a prominent feature.

Normal lung expansion is thought to be necessary for continual renewal of surfactant, and conditions associated with decreased transpulmonary pressure (e.g., recumbency, obesity, ascites, and diaphragmatic weakness) may predispose to atelectasis. The resulting alveolar collapse in such cases may be inapparent radiographically, so-called *microatelectasis* or *miliary atelectasis,* or it may result in linear radiographic densities, so-called *discoid* or *plate-like atelectasis.* Altered surfactant has also been implicated in atelectasis associated with pulmonary thromboembolism and a variety of other lung insults.

Airway Obstruction and Resorption Atelectasis. The maintenance of noncollapsed alveolar units depends on the patency of the airways supplying these units. If these airways are blocked, and if there are no other pathways by which air may enter these units, then the remaining air distal to the obstruction is gradually absorbed until collapse occurs. This is usually termed *resorption* or *obstruction atelectasis.*

Airway obstruction may result from intraluminal causes such as a neoplasm, foreign body, blood clot, or mucus plug, or from extrinsic compression by a neoplasm, enlarged lymph nodes, an aortic aneurysm, or an enlarged left atrium. In addition, airway narrowing from bronchoconstriction, secretions, or intramural edema may act in concert with any partial intrinsic or extrinsic obstruction to cause complete obstruction. Although collapse of a lobe or segment may be due to obstruction of its supplying main airway, it may also occur as a result of obstruction of multiple small airways, with the more proximal larger airways remaining widely patent.

Atelectasis is not an inevitable result of bronchial obstruction. Even an obstruction that appears bronchoscopically to be "complete" may allow enough air to pass to avoid atelectasis, although total obstruction may then result from minor additional changes in the airway. An obstructing tumor or foreign body may at times behave as a check-valve, permitting air to enter the obstructed region during inspiration but preventing its egress, leading to the paradoxical situation of hyperinflation of the obstructed region, characteristic of foreign body aspiration in children.

The development of obstructive atelectasis may also be modified by pneumonic consolidation or the accumulation of fluid in the air spaces distal to an obstruction. Infection is a common complication of obstructing neoplasms or foreign bodies, and consolidation developing distal to an obstruction may at least partly counteract the collapse that would usually result from air resorption. In acute obstructive atelectasis, there is often some degree of exudation of fluid in the alveolar spaces that again limits the volume loss. This exudation is a result of the increasingly negative pleural pressure that occurs with collapse and that is transmitted to the interstitial space, pulling fluid from the vascular bed. This accumulation of fluid distal to an obstruction has been referred to as the "drowned lung." If the obstruction persists, excess fluid is gradually absorbed, resulting in further volume loss.

The composition of the inspired gas mixture is important in the development of collapse following bronchial obstruction. Nitrogen is poorly soluble in blood and is slowly absorbed from a closed space. Replacement of nitrogen (which comprises 78 per cent of room air) by high concentrations of oxygen or by highly soluble anesthetic gases (both of which are relatively rapidly absorbed) hastens the collapse that may occur following bronchial obstruction. Also, lung units that are very poorly ventilated but not totally devoid of air may be converted to completely collapsed units if their gas composition is changed to one that may be absorbed at a rate faster than can be replaced by inspired ventilation.

Finally, the development of atelectasis following bronchial obstruction may be modified by the presence of collateral ventilation, i.e., ventilation of alveoli by pathways other than direct airway connections. Diminished collateral ventilation to the right middle lobe, compared with other lobes, is thought to be an important factor in the development of chronic or recurrent atelectasis of this lobe, so-called *middle lobe syndrome*.

CLINICAL FEATURES

The clinical features of atelectasis depend on the volume of lung involved, the acuteness or chronicity of the collapse, the mechanism by which the collapse occurs, and the underlying disease or conditions that predispose the patient to developing atelectasis.

Symptoms and Physical Signs. In all cases, the history and physical examination should be directed toward revealing the underlying disease or conditions responsible for the atelectasis. It is important to seek clues for foreign-body aspiration, bronchial neoplasms, conditions associated with bronchial plugging (e.g., asthma, cystic fibrosis, or pneumonia), conditions associated with decreased diaphragmatic mobility (e.g., neuromuscular diseases, sedation, obesity, and the postoperative period), and conditions associated with nitrogen washout (e.g., administration of anesthetic gases or of high concentrations of oxygen).

In general, dyspnea, tachypnea, and tachycardia are more prominent with collapse that occurs acutely and involves larger volumes of lung than with collapse that evolves gradually, is chronic, or involves only small losses of volumes. In the former circumstance, there is usually an increase in tidal volume and respiratory frequency, leading to increased total minute ventilation and hypocarbia. This ventilatory response results from a vagal reflex induced by the effects of lung deflation on pulmonary stretch receptors, irritant receptors, or both. Stimulation of arterial chemoreceptors may also contribute to the increased ventilation when atelectasis results in significant arterial hypoxemia.

Fever and cough may be present owing to either the underlying condition or to the development of secondary infection. Unproductive cough may also be a result of stimulation of irritant receptors by deflation. Chest pain, usually of a pleuritic nature, is often a prominent feature of pneumonia, pneumothorax, or pleural effusions, but it may also occur with acute obstructive atelectasis secondary to mucus plugging.

The chest examination in resorption atelectasis reveals signs of absent air entry (dullness to percussion, decreased breath sounds, decreased fremitus, and inspiratory lag). If the collapse is extensive enough, there may be tracheal or cardiac deviation toward the atelectatic side, and hemidiaphragmatic elevation and rib space approximation on the atelectatic side, all a result of more negative local pleural pressures. With relaxation atelectasis due to a space-occupying process, there are also decreased breath sounds over the affected region. The percussion note, however, depends on the nature of the space-occupying process—whether it is air or fluid. The mediastinum shifts away from the atelectatic side owing to local pleural pressure becoming less negative. With a large pneumothorax or pleural effusion, the rib spaces may also be widened owing to expansion of the thoracic cage; i.e., part of the volume of fluid in the pleural space is taken up in the expansion (relaxation) of the chest wall. If there is enough mediastinal shift, as in the case of a "tension" pneumothorax, the volume of the contralateral lung may also be seriously compromised.

Arterial Blood Gases. Arterial blood gases reflect the effects of atelectasis on total ventilation and on the distribution of ventilation and perfusion. As previously indicated, decreased arterial P_{CO_2} and a corresponding rise in pH may occur in acute collapse because of an increase in total ventilation. However, respiratory acidosis is more likely in a patient with severe underlying lung disease. Hypercapnia and acidosis are also frequent accompaniments of the neonatal respiratory distress syndrome. This is due to the immature infant's inability to increase total ventilation enough to eliminate the high P_{CO_2} that is present at birth as well as to the presence of multiple alveolar units that maintain ventilation but are poorly perfused (increased dead space).

A widened alveolar-arterial oxygen tension difference is frequently an important feature of atelectasis. Overt hypoxemia usually results from the persistence of pulmonary arterial blood flow to lung units that are completely unventilated, resulting in increased venous admixture of the blood entering the systemic circulation (a right-to-left shunt). Hypoxemia resulting from this mechanism is characterized by its unresponsiveness to the administration of increased concentrations of oxygen, in contrast to hypoxemia resulting from less extreme ventilation-perfusion inequality or from overall alveolar hypoventilation, in which increased inspired oxygen concentrations cause a substantial increase in arterial P_{O_2}.

A number of factors may affect the pulmonary arterial blood flow to atelectatic lung, thereby determining the degree of intrapulmonary shunting and hypoxemia that occurs. Two very important factors are the state of lung inflation and the alveolar oxygen tension. Pulmonary vascular resistance is increased at low lung volumes (particularly below residual volume), owing to passively decreased caliber of the conducting vessels. Alveolar hypoxia is known to cause active local pulmonary arterial vasoconstriction. Both of these mechanisms may act to decrease pulmonary blood flow to atelectatic lung (which is both deflated and hypoxic), thereby limiting the extent of right-to-left shunting and arterial hypoxemia. However, following acute obstructive atelectasis as well as collapse from pneumothorax, there is commonly a prompt fall in arterial P_{O_2}. Usually the degree of hypoxemia is not as great with pneumothorax as with resorption atelectasis, and in the former the P_{O_2} usually reverts toward normal within hours, whereas in the latter situation significant hypoxemia is more likely to persist.

Several factors may contribute to these differences. With resorption atelectasis, the increased negative pleural pressure on the side of the collapse causes the contralateral lung to hyperinflate. If there is enough overinflation of that lung, its capillaries are compressed, thus increasing pulmonary vascular resistance, and limiting the amount of pulmonary blood flow that can be diverted away from the collapsed lung. In addition, some recent experimental work has indicated that the local hypoxic pulmonary vasoconstrictor response may be attenuated by the presence of systemic hypoxemia operating via arterial chemoreceptors. Such an effect might create a self-perpetuating mechanism for hypoxemia. Another consideration is that if infection develops distal to a bronchial obstruction, pneumonic consolidation might maintain pulmonary blood flow to that region.

Also of importance in determining the degree of hypoxemia caused by intrapulmonary shunting are the effects of posture, exercise, and mixed venous oxygen saturation. The distribution of pulmonary blood flow is greatly affected by hydrostatic pressure differences, with the most dependent lung regions receiving the greatest proportion of pulmonary arterial blood. The blood flow to an atelectatic region may therefore increase when that region is placed in a dependent position. Blood flow to an atelectatic lung may also increase with exercise. Finally, in the presence of intrapulmonary shunt of blood through an atelectatic area, the oxygen saturation of the mixed venous blood will affect the degree of desaturation in the systemic arterial blood. For the same degree of shunt, as a fraction of total cardiac output, there will be greater arterial oxygen desaturation if the mixed venous oxygen saturation is low. Conditions that are associated with low mixed venous oxygen saturations, such as anemia, low cardiac output, or increased O_2 consumption, may therefore magnify the degree of arterial hypoxemia resulting from atelectasis.

Hypoxemia is a major feature of the extensive atelectasis characteristic of the neonatal respiratory distress syndrome. The right-to-left shunt in this condition is often quite large (up to two thirds of the cardiac output) and is attributable mainly to perfusion of nonventilated alveoli, although shunts through the foramen ovale or patent ductus arteriosus are also contributory. Surface atelectasis of a more limited nature, such as diffuse microatelectasis or more focal plate-like atelectasis, is characterized by an increased alveolar-arterial oxygen gradient owing to perfusion of nonventilated alveolar units. Atelectasis of this sort may produce no clinical findings other than hypoxemia.

Re-expansion and Complications. Elimination of a bronchial obstruction or removal of a space-occupying process, such as pneumothorax, large pleural effusion, or large emphysematous bulla, often results in re-expansion of a collapsed lung or lobe with relief of symptoms and of hypoxemia. Similarly, one or two full lung inflations can reverse the microatelectasis seen in conditions associated with decreased diaphragmatic movement. Several factors, however, may interfere with expansion of the collapsed region, even when the initiating cause of the collapse is reversed. In a completely airless lung or lobe such as that resulting from resorption atelectasis, considerable pleural negative pressures are required to overcome the surface forces of apposed alveolar walls and bring about their reopening. The critical opening pressure required to expand alveoli in lungs that are atelectatic owing to nonresorptive mechanisms is not as great, because some gas may remain trapped in bubbles within the terminal air-spaces; i.e., the lung or lobe is not as completely airless as in resorption atelectasis. The large opening pressure required to expand lungs or lobes following removal of an offending obstruction may not be attainable by patients with respiratory muscle weakness, and in this circumstance atelectasis may persist despite removal of the obstruction that initiated the atelectasis. It is also possible that surfactant may be altered with long-standing atelectasis, especially if there is complicating infection or if local pulmonary blood flow is markedly decreased, and this may hinder the ability of the lung to re-expand.

Following the obstructive atelectasis, infection and inflammation frequently develop because of impairment of mucociliary clearance and the cough mechanism in the bronchial tree distal to an obstruction. Bronchiectasis, with chronic suppuration and scarring, is a complication of long-standing atelectasis, and may prevent complete re-expansion of the involved portion of lung, leading to chronic respiratory impairment if the volume loss is great enough. In relaxation atelectasis, however, bronchial clearance mechanisms are more likely to be maintained, and secondary infection is not as great a problem as in obstructive atelectasis. However, long-standing pleural effusions or pneumothoraces may result in pleural changes limiting re-expansion of the collapsed lung.

A well-recognized complication of collapse owing to pneumothorax or pleural effusion is the development of unilateral pulmonary edema following the rapid re-expansion of the underlying collapsed lung. The setting in which this may occur is that of a large pneumothorax or hydrothorax that is rapidly removed after having been present for at least several days. The pulmonary edema is usually limited to the side of the re-expanded lung. The development of edema may be preceded by a sensation of chest tightness and coughing during the thoracentesis, following which symptoms of respiratory distress may develop. Typically, such edema resolves spontaneously within a few days. The pathogenesis of re-expansion pulmonary edema is not well understood, but it is clearly noncardiogenic and may be at least partly related to a sudden marked increase in negative intrapleural pressure. This pressure is transmitted to the lung and may alter Starling forces in a way that leads to the transudation of fluid from the microvascular bed.

RADIOLOGIC FEATURES

The definitive diagnosis of atelectasis is made with the posteroanterior and lateral chest roentgenograms. The importance of the lateral projection cannot be overemphasized. In the case of right middle lobe collapse or lingular collapse, it is the lateral view that most clearly demonstrates the triangular densities cast by these collapsed lobes, the findings on the frontal projection being more subtle. The lateral projection is also extremely useful in differentiating complete pulmonary collapse from massive consolidation or massive pleural effusion. In the case of total lung collapse, the contralateral lung becomes hyperinflated and the anterior mediastinum is displaced to the affected side, rotating laterally and posteriorly. This gives the appearance on the lateral projection of increased depth and radiolucency of the retrosternal airspace as well as a general increase in density posteriorly. In the case of massive consolidation or effusion, the x-rays passing through the chest in the lateral projection are absorbed uniformly and no such differences in radiolucency or density are observed.

Resorption (Obstructive) Atelectasis. The basic radiologic principles governing lobar and segmental atelectasis secondary to bronchial obstruction are similar, the differences between them owing only to the volume of lung that is collapsed. Generally, collapse results in a triangular density with its apex directed toward the hilum and its base situated on the pleura. Descriptions of distinctive roentgenographic patterns cast by each individual lobe or segment are beyond the scope of this article but may be found in several excellent references.* The basic radiologic signs common to lobar and segmental collapse will be discussed briefly.

Since atelectasis involves the loss of lung volume, the direct sign of lobar collapse is displacement of interlobar fissures. With lesser degrees of volume loss in segmental collapse, displacement of fissures is usually minimal. Indirect signs of atelectasis include increased radiodensity of the collapsed zone, crowding of bronchovascular markings, and signs that occur because of compensation for the volume loss. These signs include hemidiaphragm elevation, mediastinal and hilar displacement, compensatory overinflation of nonobstructed lung, and approximation of ribs.

Hemidiaphragmatic displacement is a more prominent feature of lower rather than upper lobe atelectasis, and mediastinal shift is generally a more helpful sign in upper lobe collapse, in which tracheal position may be assessed. (The degree of mediastinal shift is always greatest in the region of the major pulmonary collapse.) Compensatory overinflation of the non-collapsed portion of the involved lung is a helpful sign, but since it takes time to develop, it is not helpful immediately following collapse. In contrast, mediastinal and diaphragmatic displacement tends to be greatest acutely and becomes less prominent as atelectasis becomes chronic. Hilar displacement occurs more predictably in upper lobe than in lower lobe collapse and is more marked the longer the atelectasis has been present. Rib approximation may be noted in situations of chronic volume loss but is generally not a reliable compensatory sign in atelectasis.

Two conditions that may sometimes be confused radiologically with lobar collapse are consolidation and encapsulated pleural fluid. In consolidation without collapse, there is no displacement of the interlobar fissures. Encapsulated pleural fluid can be more difficult to distinguish but may be suspected from its rounded contours, the presence of pleural thickening elsewhere in the thorax, and the absence of air bronchograms. Computed axial tomography is very useful in defining these lesions.

The presence or absence of an air bronchogram may be a useful clue in atelectasis. If enough bronchial obstruction occurs to cause air resorption from the parenchyma, it must also cause all air to be absorbed from the bronchial tree. In the situation in which pneumonitis develops distal to such an obstruction and the degree of consolidation prevents significant volume loss, the absence of an air bronchogram may help in identifying the primary process as an obstructing lesion with a secondary infection rather than a simple bacterial pneumonia.

Relaxation (Passive) Atelectasis. A discussion of the radiographic features of pneumothorax and pleural effusion will not be attempted here except to indicate several important features of the collapse associated with these conditions. In the case of a large pneumothorax or pleural effusion, many of the compensatory signs of obstructive atelectasis are reversed. Hence, if there is any shift of mediastinal and hilar structures, it is to the side away from the atelectasis. Similarly, in the case of pneumothorax, the chest springs outward as the underlying lung collapses so that the distance between ribs is widened rather than narrowed. The collapse resulting from pneumothorax produces no increase in radiodensity until approximately 90 per cent of the lung is collapsed. This is due to the presence of air in the pleural space anterior and posterior to the collapsed

*See Felson, B.: *Chest Roentgenology.* Philadelphia, W.B. Saunders Company, 1973; and Fraser, R.G., and Paré, J.A.P.: *Diagnosis of Diseases of the Chest,* 2nd ed., vol. 1. Philadelphia, W.B. Saunders Company, 1977.

lung, as well as to the concomitant decrease in pulmonary blood flow that occurs with pneumothorax. In contrast to the absence of an air bronchogram with resorption atelectasis, an air bronchogram is usually present with relaxation atelectasis. This may provide a useful clue in lung collapse secondary to pneumothorax, in which case the absence of an air bronchogram may be indicative of an otherwise unsuspected endobronchial obstruction.

Surface Atelectasis. As indicated before, this form of atelectasis commonly exists without any radiographic manifestations, the diagnosis of "microatelectasis" being inferred from the presence of mild or moderate hypoxemia in the appropriate clinical setting. Plate-like atelectasis, which has similar pathophysiologic significance, is manifested radiographically by single or multiple linear densities ("Fleischner's lines"),1 to 3 mm in thickness and up to several centimeters in length, always extending to a pleural surface. They are usually located in the lung bases, unilaterally or bilaterally, and are horizontal or slightly oblique in orientation. These areas of atelectasis are usually transient, often appearing or disappearing within a few hours. Despite this, they are important to recognize because of the pathophysiologic significance they have in terms of ventilation-perfusion abnormalities.

The radiographic appearance of the extensive atelectasis seen in the neonatal respiratory distress syndrome (hyaline membrane disease) is that of a diffuse mottling and granularity with prominent air bronchograms.

OTHER ROENTGENOGRAPHIC STUDIES

Oblique projections may permit better visualization of a collapsed segment, depending on which segment is involved. Regular lung tomography and computed axial tomography may help define segmental collapse that is not as apparent on ordinary chest roentgenograms. These techniques may also be valuable in identifying enlarged lymph nodes or tumors that have caused a lobe or segment to collapse. Bronchography may be useful when chronic collapse occurs with a patent lobar or segmental bronchus, in which case peripheral plugging of multiple small airways may be demonstrated.

FIBEROPTIC BRONCHOSCOPY

Fiberoptic bronchoscopy, which allows direct visualization of the tracheal bronchial tree to the level of subsegmental bronchi, is an invaluable aid in identifying various causes of obstructive atelectasis. Endobronchial obstructions such as tumors, foreign bodies, blood clots, or mucus plugs may be identified, or extrinsic bronchial compression may be noted. Material may be aspirated for cultures and cytologic examination, and brushings and biopsies of lesions may also be obtained. In the case of obstructive atelectasis due to mucus plugging or foreign bodies, fiberoptic bronchoscopy may be therapeutic as well as diagnostic.

OTHER LABORATORY TESTS

Pulmonary function tests such as spirometry, lung volumes, and carbon monoxide diffusing capacity are not helpful in the diagnosis of atelectasis per se, but may be quite useful in the diagnosis of such underlying pulmonary diseases as asthma or chronic bronchitis, and in the evaluation of pulmonary functional impairment resulting from chronic atelectasis.

Other laboratory tests such as urinalysis, complete blood count, eosinophil count, blood chemistries, and sputum examination are essential in evaluating the underlying conditions and should be selected on the basis of the clinical setting.

PULMONARY EMBOLISM AND INFARCTION

By Kenneth M. Moser, M.D.
San Diego, California

DEFINITION

Venous thrombi may originate in any of the systemic veins and, less commonly, in the right cardiac chambers. When such thrombi detach, are carried to the pulmonary vasculature, and lodge in the pulmonary arterial vessels, pulmonary embolism has occurred. Occasionally, embolism leads to pulmonary infarction, that is, hemorrhage, collapse and, rarely, actual death of the lung tissue distal to the embolic destruction.

PATHOGENESIS

Since pulmonary embolism is but a complication of venous thrombosis, the pathogenesis of embolism is the pathogenesis of venous thrombosis. The basic factors involved in the genesis of venous thrombosis are stasis, injury to the vascular intima, and thrombogenic alterations in the coagulation system. These alterations are poorly understood, and there are no specific coagulation measurements that reliably predict thrombotic tendency (aside from the rare heritable condition of antithrombin III deficiency). However, stasis or intimal injury or both occur in a number of well-recognized clinical contexts, in which the incidence of venous thrombosis and pulmonary embolism is high. Such situations include the postoperative period, pregnancy and the postpartum state, traumatic injuries (particularly to the pelvis and lower extremities), burns, congestive heart failure, and any cause of prolonged immobility. Obesity and cancer are other known risk factors. A number of studies have disclosed a substantial incidence of venous thrombosis and pulmonary embolism in all of these "high-risk" situations.

NATURAL HISTORY

In approaching the diagnosis of pulmonary embolism, it is important to recognize its natural history. Embolism is a dynamic disorder. After an embolus lodges in the vasculature, it undergoes changes over hours to days. Most frequently, resolution of the embolus occurs due to fibrinolysis. This is a relatively rapid process that in man can result in total dissolution of the embolus over a period of several days. With even minimal dissolution, an embolus may move distally, obstructing a smaller segment of the pulmonary vasculature.

If fibrinolytic resolution proceeds slowly, emboli resolve by the process of organization—fibroblastic ingrowth followed by endothelialization. This "scar" leaves a permanent, though usually quite small, residual in the vessel wall. Rarely, fibrinolysis and organization lead to little resolution, and extensive, chronic obstruction persists.

Additionally, recurrence of emboli may develop from the original thrombotic source; or, in some instances, the embolus itself may grow further in situ by accretion of platelets and fibrinogen.

Thus, the status of the patient with pulmonary embolism may change rather rapidly in terms of symptoms, signs, and the findings on certain laboratory tests.

Another consideration of diagnostic importance is the factors that condition the severity of the cardiopulmonary consequences of embolism. One major one is the *extent* of obstruction per se; i.e., the more vascular bed is occluded, the more severe the impairment of cardiac and pulmonary function. Another is the release of vasoactive and bronchoactive amines (e.g., serotonin) from the platelets that are known to coat emboli. Such a sequence occurs in dogs and may occur in man. Finally, the pre-existing cardiopulmonary status of the patient conditions the consequences. Patients with reduced function may have serious responses to relatively small emboli; otherwise healthy individuals may tolerate rather extensive embolism with minimal symptoms.

Pulmonary infarction is an uncommon consequence of embolism. In individuals without prior cardiopulmonary disease, it occurs in well under 10 per cent; in those with prior disease, it occurs in as high as 40 per cent. This fact is important diagnostically because the clinical and laboratory findings of *infarction* are absent in the majority of patients with *embolism.*

DIAGNOSIS

Conceptually, there are two major categories of approach to the diagnosis of embolism: (1) by detection of the consequences of embolism, and (2) by direct visualization of the emboli.

Consequences. Among the potential consequences are symptoms and physical findings, i.e., the clinical diagnosis of embolism. Unfortunately, the clinical diagnosis is notoriously unreliable. Signs and symptoms of embolism are nonspecific; they are shared with many other cardiopulmonary diseases. Therefore, they suggest—but cannot make—the diagnosis. The most common symptom of embolism is *dyspnea of sudden onset.* In general, the more extensive the occlusion, the more severe the dyspnea. A sense of "impending doom" is commonly reported. Substernal chest discomfort, mimicking that which occurs with coronary occlusion, may be reported, usually with extensive obstruction; syncope may occur. Pleuritic chest pain and hemoptysis are less frequent symptoms because they are manifestations of infarction, which follows embolism in a minority of patients.

Among physical findings, *tachycardia* is the most common. Cardiac examination is frequently otherwise normal; only with embolism of sufficient magnitude to cause significant pulmonary hypertension are such findings as palpable right ventricular "tap" along the left sternal border, a right ventricular S_3, fixed splitting of the second sound, and accentuation of the pulmonary closure sound detected.

The lung fields are usually clear to examination. With infarction, a pleural rub and the physical findings of consolidation and pleural effusion may be present. Clinical evidence of peripheral venous thrombosis is absent in more than 50 per cent of patients with embolism. Fever, usually not exceeding 101.5°F (40.5°C), occurs in a minority of patients, particularly in those with infarction.

Thus, symptoms and signs are often quite modest, particularly when small emboli occur in patients with no pre-existing cardiopulmonary disease. In all patients, the findings are nonspecific. Therefore, definitive diagnosis of embolism depends upon laboratory tests.

The majority of such tests, again, mirror the consequences of embolism and so are variable and nondefinitive. Leukocytosis often occurs but does not assist in diagnosis, although it rarely exceeds 20,000 per cu mm. There are no definitive "blood tests" that confirm or rule out embolism. Serum glutamic oxaloacetic transaminase (SGOT), lactic dehydrogenase (LDH), fibrin degradation products, and other tests proposed have such a high incidence of false-positive and false-negative results that they are useless. The most frequent electrocardiogram pattern shows only tachycardia; occasionally, with extensive obstruction, evidence of acute right atrial and ventricular overload is seen ("S_1, Q_3 pattern," peaked P waves, nonspecific ST-T changes, R axis shift). The chest roentgenogram is notoriously unreliable. Without infarction, one looks for disparities in the size of major pulmonary arteries that *should* be of similar size, or regional hypoperfusion—both are subtle and nondiagnostic findings. With infarction, pulmonary infiltrate(s) or pleural effusion(s) or both may be seen. Despite prior suggestions, there are no shapes or locations of infiltrate that are definitive for infarction, except that all do abut a pleural surface.

Similar nonspecificity characterizes the values of arterial blood gases seen in embolism. It is certainly true that some degree of hypoxemia is common in embolism, and that the more extensive the occlusion, the more frequent and severe the hypoxemia (low Pa_{O_2}). However, it is equally true that (1) a normal Pa_{O_2} (> 80 mm Hg) is seen in a substantial proportion of patients with embolism, and (2) hypoxemia is common in many nonembolic disorders that mimic embolism. Therefore, whereas measurement of the Pa_{O_2} is useful in patient management, it is not a valuable diagnostic tool.

The only laboratory tests affected by embolic consequences that are at all reliable are the perfusion and ventilation lung scans. A perfusion lung scan should be performed in all patients suspected of embolism. The reason for this is that a normal, six-view (posterior, anterior, both laterals, both posterior obliques) well-performed perfusion ($\dot{Q}$) scan excludes the diagnosis of embolism. While a negative $\dot{Q}$ scan in embolism is a theoretical possibility, no angiographically proven embolus with a negative scan (performed immediately before or after) has been reported.

But what if the scan is "positive," that is, shows one or more "defects" indicative of reduced or absent pulmonary blood flow? It is true that many disorders other than embolism can cause such abnormalities in the distribution of pulmonary blood flow. It is becoming evident that the diagnostic specificity of an abnormal perfusion scan is related to the size of the defect(s), their relationship to chest x-ray abnormalities, the coexistence of known cardiopulmonary disease, and the relationship between perfusion defects and the results of a radionuclide ventilation (V) scan. For example, in my view, the discovery of segmental or larger perfusion defects in a patient with no known cardiopulmonary disease is very compelling evidence of pulmonary embolism. Depending on the clinical context, such a finding may suffice as an indicator of embolic disease. However, if these criteria are not satisfied or if the potential risks of heparin therapy are high, additional confirmation is useful.

Such confirmation is worth seeking by performing a ventilation scan in patients with segmental or larger perfusion defects not matched to chest x-ray infiltrates. We have not found the $\dot{V}$ scan useful in patients with subsegmental defects or defects *limited to* areas of radiographic infiltrates. The use of the $\dot{V}$ scan (most commonly done with a radioactive gas such as xenon 127 or xenon 133) is based on the physiologic fact that vascular obstruction (including embolism) produces a zone of the lung in which *perfusion* is absent but *ventilation* remains normal. Thus embolism results in $\dot{V}/\dot{Q}$ "mismatch" (normal $\dot{V}$, absent $\dot{Q}$), whereas parenchymal pulmonary diseases (e.g., emphysema) result in $\dot{V}/\dot{Q}$ "match" (abnormal $\dot{V}$ and abnormal $\dot{Q}$). However, the *technique* of $\dot{V}$ scanning is crucial to proper interpretation. First, with proper doses of radionuclides, a $\dot{V}$ scan can and should be performed immediately after an abnormal $\dot{Q}$ scan is obtained. The prior $\dot{Q}$ scan does not interfere with interpretation of the $\dot{V}$ scan. Second, a "single breath" $\dot{V}$ scan is not satisfactory. The most useful component of the $\dot{V}$ study is the *wash-out* phase. Therefore, the study should be performed by having the patient rebreathe xenon 133 to equilibrium (wash-in), then wash-out. Patients with embolism wash-in and wash-out normally. Patients with parenchymal disease wash-in and, particularly, wash-out slowly or not at all. The $\dot{V}$ study should be done in that view (e.g., posterior) in which the $\dot{Q}$ defect(s) is best seen.

Should a $\dot{Q}$ scan be done in someone with an infiltrate on chest x-ray? Yes, because emboli often (more than 30 per cent) are multiple, and characteristic $\dot{V}/\dot{Q}$ "mismatch" may be seen in other noninfiltrated zones of the lung.

How reliable is the finding of segmental or larger $\dot{Q}$ defects mismatched by $\dot{V}$ scan results in the diagnosis of vascular occlusion? In my judgment, the finding is highly reliable (90% +). One need go further diagnostically only when such a $\dot{V}/\dot{Q}$ result is not obtained or certain therapeutic procedures (such as embolectomy and inferior vena caval ligation) are being contemplated.

Procedures That Visualize Emboli. At present, short of thoracotomy, only one procedure is available by which an embolus can be directly visualized: pulmonary angiography. However, the limitations of this procedure must be weighed against its benefits. First, it is an invasive procedure that is not without some risk. Second, both risk and yield are conditioned by the experience of those performing the angiogram. When angiograms are performed infrequently, the risk is increased, the quality of the study reduced, and the interpretation rendered uncertain. Even pulmonary angiograms of high quality are not "easy" to interpret. Those of poor quality may be impossible to evaluate.

Third, there are only two diagnostic findings by angiogram: the "filling defect," in which the thrombus creates a negative image within the stream of opaque medium, and the "cutoff," in which there is abrupt cessation of the dye stream. Other findings such as absence of capillary filling are nonspecific and nondiagnostic.

One advantage of performing angiography is that the hemodynamic status of the patient also can be determined; that is, pulmonary arterial pressure, cardiac output, and so forth can be measured.

Thus, our indications for angiography are (1) the presence of an experienced angiographic team, and (2) the need for a high degree of diagnostic certitude either because of the equivocal nature of other studies (or lack of access to them) or the contemplation of high risk or high morbidity medical or surgical therapy.

OTHER DIAGNOSTIC CONSIDERATIONS

New techniques are being introduced that may allow visualization of emboli. The two most promising are direct labeling of emboli with gamma-emitting radionuclides (e.g., indium 111–labeled platelets) and fiberoptic angioscopy (transvenous insertion of a fiberoptic device directly into the pulmonary arterial system). The true potential of these techniques awaits elucidation.

Another approach suggested by some is to study the lower extremities for deep venous thrombosis (in lieu of angiography). Whether this is done by contrast venography, impedance phlebography or radiofibrinogen leg scan, the thesis is the same: if there are no venous thrombi present, the diagnosis of embolism is highly unlikely. Unfortunately, this attractive thesis is flawed. In my experience, some 20 per cent of patients with emboli do not have evidence of venous thrombosis in the legs. How can this be, if more than 95 per cent of all emboli arise from leg thrombi? Our presumption is that, in these patients, the entire thrombus detached as an embolus. (In a small additional percentage, the emboli arose from the right cardiac chambers.)

Furthermore, venous thrombi can occur in patients whose cardiopulmonary symptoms are not due to emboli. Thus, although establishing the presence or absence of venous thrombosis certainly is useful in planning the management of patients with embolism, it does not allow exclusion (or inclusion) of the diagnosis of embolism.

Finally, it should be noted that the extent of diagnostic "work-up" in a given patient that needs to be completed before therapy is instituted depends heavily on the potential risk of that therapy in the specific patient. Unless that risk is high (e.g., bleeding due to heparin), therapy usually is initiated before such procedures as scans and angiograms are obtained.

PULMONARY HYPERTENSION

By Robert H. Peter, M.D.
Durham, North Carolina

The lungs receive the total cardiac output, yet the pulmonary vasculature functions as a low-pressure and low-resistance system. The normal mean pulmonary artery pressure is less than 15 mm Hg and the pulmonary vascular resistance is less than 2 units (mm Hg/ml/min). The elastic pulmonary arteries larger than 1 mm in diameter passively distend to accept volume, while the muscular pulmonary arteries between 100 and less than 1000 microns in diameter can dilate and constrict in response to flow, hypoxia, oxygen, and certain drugs. Pulmonary artery vasoconstriction can lead to medial hypertrophy, which presumably enhances more vasoconstriction, with less ability to vasodilate. Progressive pathologic changes of increased elastica, intimal proliferation, and eventually fibrinoid changes with obliteration of the vessels with an "arteritis," thrombosis, and further reduction of pulmonary vessels, creating more severe pulmonary hypertension, can occur. Peculiar plexiform lesions are seen in the small pulmonary arteries of patients with far advanced pulmonary hypertension secondary to schistosomiasis, primary pulmonary hypertension, and Eisenmenger syndrome. Right-sided heart failure and all the complications of low output with congestion to the body below the level of the heart can occur. The cause of pulmonary hypertension should be vigorously sought, since some causes are reversible or at least treatable.

CLASSIFICATION OF PULMONARY HYPERTENSION

Pulmonary hypertension can result from a number of causes, but all are either pre- or postpulmonary capillary in origin (Table 1). Conditions that elevate the pressure in the left atria or pulmonary veins or raise left ventricular end diastolic pressure to abnormal levels can elevate pulmonary pressure. These can be classified as postcapillary in origin and include any illness that causes left ventricular failure or elevations in left atrial pressure. As examples, patients with acute myocardial infarction and left ventricular failure can have a rise in pulmonary artery pressure to a significant degree. Patients with severe mitral stenosis can have high left atrial pressures and at times severely elevated pulmonary pressures exceeding that expected for the rise in left atrial pressure. This is believed to be due to a vasoconstriction in the pulmonary arteriolar bed, an additive precapillary cause for the pulmonary artery pressure rise.

Precapillary causes for pulmonary hypertension can occur when there is obliteration of vessels, as in recurrent pulmonary emboli or pulmonary arteritis. Primary pulmonary hypertension probably begins as a muscular pulmonary artery vasoconstrictive situation and progresses to a severe obliterative artery disease with laminar intimal fibrosis, fibrinoid necrosis, arteritis and plexiform lesions. Infiltrative lung diseases, recurrent infective processes, and other causes of parenchymal lung disease can bring about loss of functioning lung (loss of vessels), or hypoxia-induced pulmonary artery vasoconstriction. There are many diseases of various etiologies that can involve the precapillary pulmonary vascular bed to cause pulmonary hypertension.

SYMPTOMS

Like systemic hypertension, pulmonary hypertension has no symptoms until there is compromise in the cardiac output. The first symptom is often dyspnea on exertion, since the cardiac output is compromised with exercise. Nonspecific symptoms such as weakness and fatigue are common. Patients will often complain of exertional substernal pain that is felt to be due to "right heart angina." A nonspecific dry cough is often present.

As the patient's condition progresses from exertional decrease in cardiac output to resting decrease in cardiac output and right-sided failure, ankle and foot edema, leg edema, and even ascites will often occur, compromising the patient's respirations and ability to ambulate. The patient will often become agitated, profoundly anxious, and depressed. Palpitations late in the illness suggest ventricular arrhythmias. Syncope on effort is also common late in the disease, and sudden death is a frequent terminal event in pulmonary thromboembolism, primary pulmonary hypertension, and Eisenmenger physiology congenital heart disease.

It should be pointed out that patients with postcapillary origin pulmonary hypertension will often have symptoms secondary to lung congestion, since pulmonary venous pressure elevation will lead to pulmonary congestion and a secondary elevation in the pulmonary artery pressure. An example of this type of hypertension would be mitral stenosis with a markedly elevated left atrial pressure and symptoms

Table 1. Pathophysiologic Classification of Pulmonary Hypertension

Precapillary Origin	Postcapillary Origin
Eisenmenger congenital heart disease	Left ventricular failure
Peripheral pulmonary artery stenosis	Mitral valve disease
Extrinsic pulmonary artery compression	Pulmonary veno-occlusive disease
Primary pulmonary hypertension	Cor triatriatum
Pulmonary thromboembolism	Left atrial myxoma or thrombus
Pulmonary schistosomiasis	Extrinsic pulmonary vein compression
Pulmonary arteritis	
Hypoventilation syndrome	
Chronic parenchymal lung disease to include:	
Kyphoscoliosis	
Pulmonary fibrosis	
Bronchiectasis	
Sarcoidosis	
Cystic fibrosis	
Scleroderma	
Pneumoconiosis	
Hypoxic obstructive airway disease	
Infiltrative cancer	

referrable to pulmonary congestion prior to pulmonary hypertension and right heart failure.

PHYSICAL EXAMINATION

The physical examination may be essentially normal in early precapillary origin pulmonary hypertension. There may be little to suggest pulmonary hypertension except for a mild right ventricular lift and/or a loud, palpable pulmonary closure sound. If the patient is a thin female, this could indeed be a normal finding or missed because it is felt to be a normal finding.

On visual examination, the patient with pulmonary hypertension may be cyanotic. This could be due to a low cardiac output and a wide arteriovenous oxygen difference, with the venous blood very dark and the arterial blood normally saturated. Cyanosis could also be from a right to left shunt caused by Eisenmenger physiology or a patent foramen ovale with right to left shunting from a high-pressure right atrium to a normal-pressure left atrium. Clubbing is often present in patients with Eisenmenger physiology who are cyanotic.

Because of noncompliance in the right ventricle, a prominent jugular venous pulse A wave is often seen. If tricuspid insufficiency is present, visible V waves may be noted in the neck veins and, if profound, a pulsatile liver may be seen and felt. A prominent A wave would not be expected in an Eisenmenger shunt, or atrial or ventricular septal defect. With long-standing right ventricular hypertrophy that occurred during childhood growth, a more prominent left rib cage may be noted. On examination, there is often a left parasternal (right ventricular) lift, and a systolic pulmonary artery thrust in the second to third left interspace adjacent to the sternum, indicative of a dilated pulmonary artery. A loud and palpable pulmonary closure sound is noted, and at auscultation right atrial and ventricular gallops can be heard. A pulmonary ejection click is often heard along the left sternal border. Murmurs of tricuspid and pulmonary insufficiency are a late occurrence in pulmonary hypertension. Signs of right-sided failure with leg edema, enlarged liver and, eventually, ascites can occur. There is often a conspicuous absence of a pulmonary flow murmur, particularly in those patients with low cardiac outputs who are far along with their disease.

ELECTROCARDIOGRAM

The electrocardiogram can be helpful in diagnosing right ventricular hypertrophy (RVH), even though the left ventricle so dominates the electrical forces of depolarization that RVH may not be seen. In the absence of pulmonary stenosis, RVH is almost always caused by pulmonary hypertension. The classic findings are (1) right axis deviation, (2) QR deflection in lead V1 or $>$ 6 mm R wave in lead V_1, (3) sum of SI and R III $>$ 10.5 mm, (4) sum of R and S waves in lead V_1 greater than 15 mm, (5) asymmetric ST-T wave depression in leads V_{1-3}, the so-called right ventricular "strain pattern," (6) "P-Pulmonale" P waves of right atrial enlargement as manifest by a tall (3 mm) peaked P wave in lead II, AVF, III, and/or V_1.

There may be subtleties that suggest RVH, such as only one or two of the preceding findings. Patients with severe chronic obstructive emphysematous lung disease may have very low diaphragms and poor R wave progression in leads V_{1-3} as those electrodes are placed above where the heart lies in the chest cavity. The strain pattern, right axis deviation or P-Pulmonale may still be present.

The bifid P wave configuration in leads II, AVF, and III ("P-Mitrale") or a negative terminal P wave deflection in lead V_1 suggests left atrial enlargement and is seen in mitral stenosis. Thus, electrocardiographic criteria for left atrial enlargement and RVH can suggest a more specific diagnosis when pulmonary hypertension is suspected (Fig. 1, *A* and *B*).

CHEST X-RAY

The chest x-ray, utilizing oblique projections, may give valuable information in the diagnosis of pulmonary hypertension. Bulging of the right ventricle against the sternum in the lateral projection and the region of the right ventricular outflow tract in the left anterior oblique projection is seen in right ventricular enlargement (Fig. 2). In the postanterior projection, the cardiac silhouette may be normal in dimension despite RVH. However, the right and particularly the left pulmonary artery segments may be quite prominent. Pronounced pruning in the distal one third of the peripheral lung vessels is seen in far advanced pulmonary hypertension (Fig. 3). Dilated superior pulmonary veins and a double density to the right cardiac border in the posteroanterior projection (suggesting left atrial enlargement) would suggest mitral stenosis is the cause for the other roentgenographic findings of pulmonary hypertension. A large right ventricle and pulmonary trunk in a patient with diffuse fibrocystic lung changes or kyphoscoliosis with obliteration of lung space would suggest that pulmonary hypertension is present.

Widening of the superior cardiac silhouette indicative of superior vena cava and azygos vein engorgement can often be seen in patients with right-sided failure, and is almost always indicative of pulmonary hypertension except in the presence of primary tricuspid regurgitation not due to pulmonary hypertension. Other x-ray findings attributable to right heart failure are enlargement of the liver and spleen, pleural effusions, and a "ground-glass" appearance of ascites on abdominal films.

In pulmonary veno-occlusive disease, the left atrial shadow should be normal, but Kerley B lines and a superior pulmonary venous vascular shift may be present.

ECHOCARDIOGRAM

The two-dimensional and M-mode echocardiogram can be helpful in diagnosing RVH, but is of little value in diseases in which chest or lung configuration makes the quality of the tracing poor (such as in chronic obstructive emphysematous pulmonary disease or kyphoscoliotic lung disease). The echocardiogram can be particularly helpful if the pulmonary valve can be visualized. In normals, there is an atrial systolic wave form (A wave dip) which begins the opening of the pulmonary valve as seen with M-mode (Fig. 4*A*). This is attenuated or absent in pulmonary hypertension (Fig. 4*B*). The right ventricle can be seen to be hypertrophied and/or dilated in pressure and pressure-volume overload. The ventricular septum is flattened

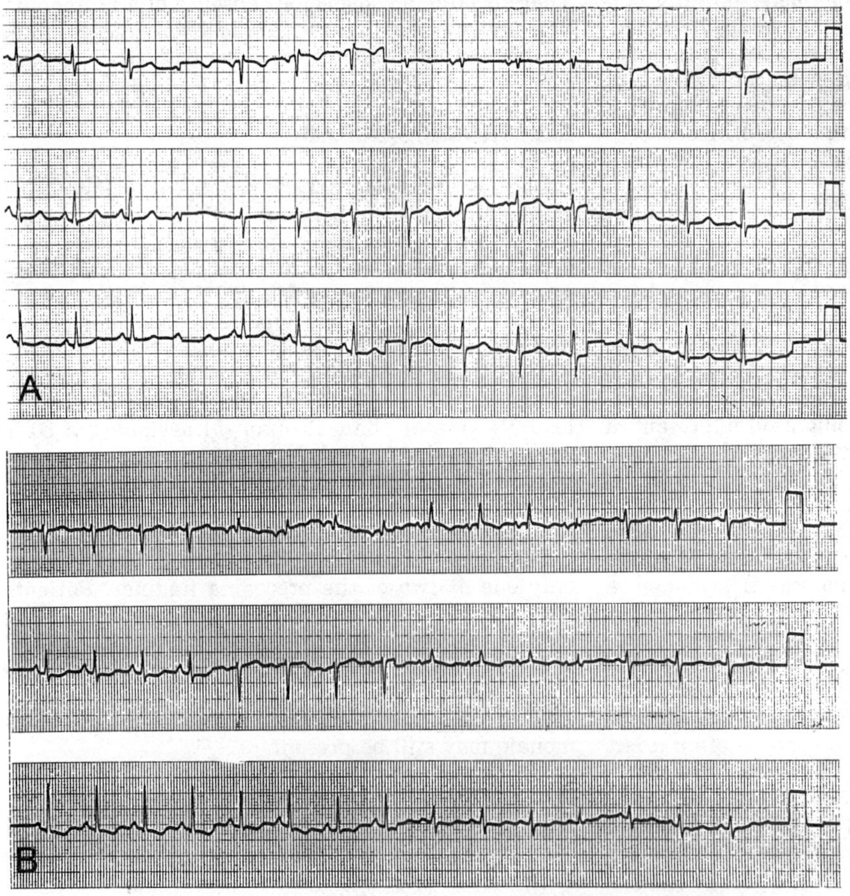

Figure 1. *(A)* An almost normal electrocardiogram in a 23-year-old woman with clinically mild mitral stenosis. The negative terminal P wave in lead V_1 suggests left atrial enlargement. *(B)* Three years later, marked right axis deviation in the frontal plane with a QR deflection in lead V_1 of RVH has occurred. The left atrial enlargement criteria persist, and severe mitral stenosis with pulmonary hypertension was found at cardiac catheterization. Leads are in the following order:
I AVR V_1 V_4
II AVL V_2 V_5
III AVF V_3 V_6

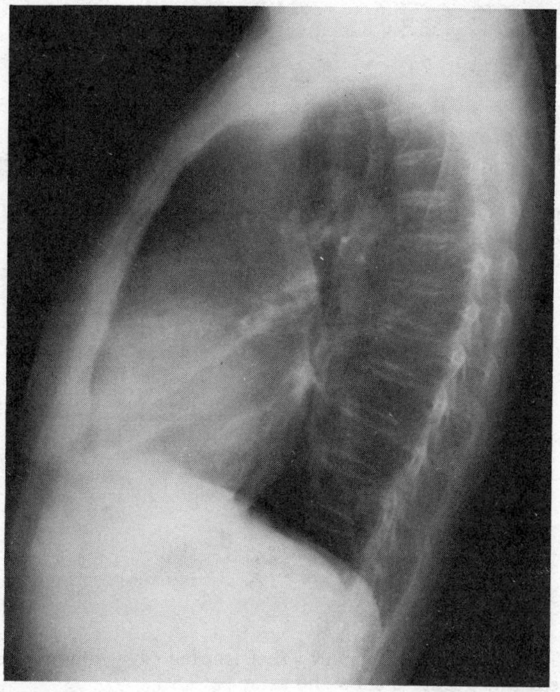

Figure 2. Lateral chest x-ray in a 54-year-old woman with severe chronic mitral insufficiency and pulmonary hypertension. The large right ventricle bulges against the sternum. The left ventricle and atria are also enlarged.

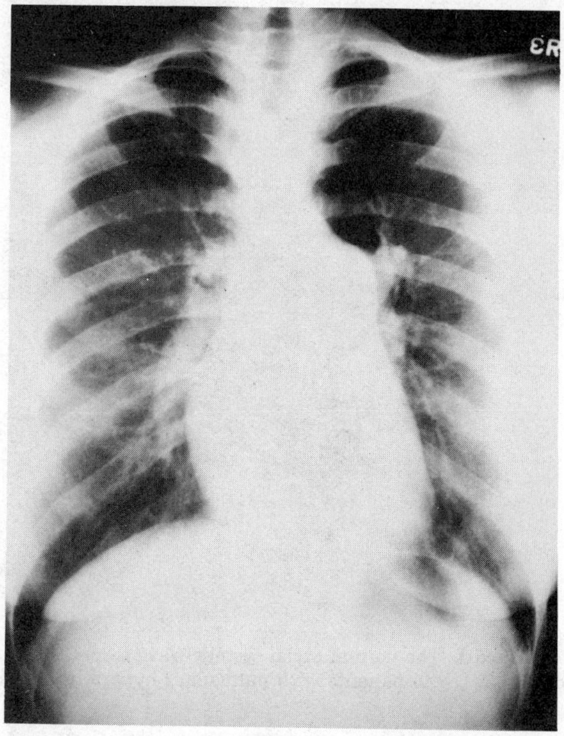

Figure 3. Posteroanterior chest x-ray in an 18-year-old woman with primary pulmonary hypertension. The right and left pulmonary arteries are large, and distal pulmonary artery pruning in the lateral lung fields is present.

("pancake septum") and paradoxic septal motion suggests pulmonary hypertension (Fig. 5). The right ventricular pre-ejection period is prolonged. Contrast echocardiography may show a right to left shunt at the atrial level, suggesting either an Eisenmenger physiology right to left shunt, or an open foramen ovale in a patient with primary pulmonary hypertension. A deformed immobile mitral valve with a large left atrium in the presence of other findings consistent with pulmonary hypertension would indicate mitral stenosis with secondary pulmonary hypertension. Intracardiac tumors (left atrial myxoma), extrinsic compressive masses to the heart, and cor triatriatum may be suggested by echocardiographic findings, particularly with two-dimensional capabilities. Likewise, complex congenital heart defects with pulmonary hypertension (i.e., truncus arteriosus and transposition of the great vessels without pulmonary stenosis) can often be diagnosed.

DOPPLER FLOW STUDIES

The Doppler flow tracings recording flow velocity across the valves to and from the low-pressure right ventricle and high-pressure left ventricle are quite distinct. When pulmonary hypertension occurs, the pulmonary closure to tricuspid opening time interval increases and the pulmonary artery flow velocity profile looks like the aorta velocity pulse. That is, pulmonary artery blood flow acceleration increases and in some patients it can approach that seen in the aorta. If tricuspid regurgitation is present, the Doppler velocity tracing looks like that seen in high-pressure mitral regurgitation instead of the usual tricuspid regurgitation low-velocity jet.

PULMONARY FUNCTION TESTS AND ARTERIAL BLOOD GASES

Pulmonary hypertension secondary to parenchymal lung disease of chronic bronchitis-emphysema is different from that produced by primary pulmonary hypertension or the causes of post-capillary pulmonary hypertension. In patients with primary pulmonary hypertension, there is usually no alveolar hypoventilation (and, therefore, no resultant hypoxemia or hypercapnea), hyperinflation, wheezing, or pulmonary edema. Results of pulmonary function studies should be close to normal. Of course, there can be an abnormal Po_2 if elevated right atrial pressure has opened a foramen ovale with some right to left shunting. The Pco_2 should be normal. In Eisenmenger congenital heart disease, the Pco_2 is normal while the Po_2 is low and not appreciably changed with breathing 100 per cent oxygen.

Hypercapnea and hypoxemia are common in pulmonary hypertension secondary to chronic parenchymal lung disease. Breathing 100 per cent oxygen may not always raise the Po_2 to normal, but arterial saturation should approach 100 per cent. Pulmonary function studies can differentiate obstructive from primarily restrictive lung disease, though often a mixture is seen. Severe kyphoscoliosis and obesity in their

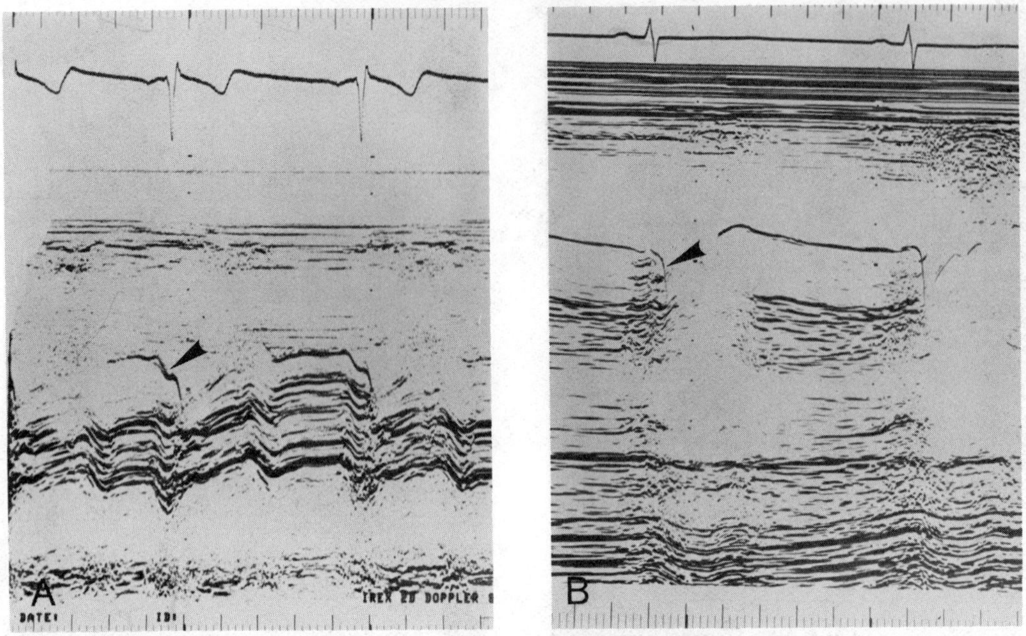

Figure 4. The normal atrial systolic wave form (arrow) at the beginning of pulmonary valve opening *(A)* is diminished or absent *(B)* in patients with pulmonary hypertension. Figure 4*B* and Figure 3 show the same patient.

pure form are examples of restrictive lung disease, whereas pneumoconiosis and chronic bronchitic asthma are examples of obstructive disease.

In postcapillary pulmonary hypertension, the lungs become stiff as pulmonary venous engorgement increases. The vital capacity, maximum midexpiratory flow rate, dynamic compliance, and carbon monoxide flow rate fall as pulmonary hypertension increases, while the airway resistance increases. Relief from the cause for pulmonary venous hypertension can eventually reverse these abnormal pulmonary function studies.

VENTILATION PERFUSION LUNG SCAN AND PULMONARY ARTERIOGRAPHY

A question often raised is whether a patient has chronic pulmonary emboli or primary pulmonary hypertension. The ventilation-perfusion scan ($\dot{V}$-$\dot{Q}$ scan) can often help differentiate between recurrent pulmonary emboli and primary pulmonary hypertension. A low probability scan for pulmonary emboli should obviate the need to do a pulmonary angiogram. The pulmonary angiogram in a patient with severe pulmonary hypertension secondary to chronic pulmo-

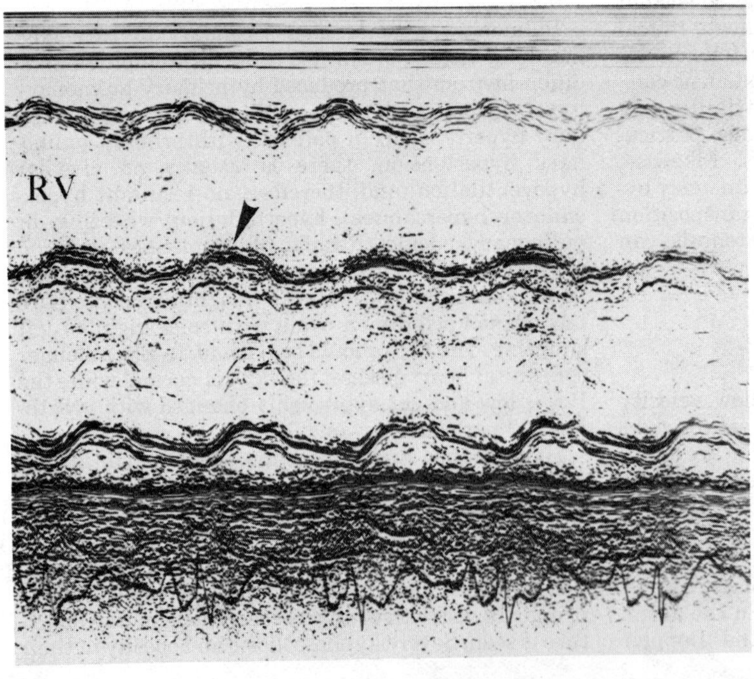

Figure 5. Paradoxic septal motion (arrow) and right ventricle (RV) dilatation in a 23-year-old woman with mitral stenosis and pulmonary hypertension.

nary emboli or with primary pulmonary hypertension has a significant mortality risk and should be done only when other likely causes for pulmonary hypertension are not found. A high probability $\dot{V}$-$\dot{Q}$ scan is also felt by many to be enough probable evidence for recurrent pulmonary emboli to use anticoagulant therapy.

LUNG BIOPSY

Though not without hazard, the lung biopsy can be helpful in differentiating causes of pulmonary hypertension, particularly those inflammatory causes that are reversible or partially reversible. Some feel that the only way to differentiate recurrent pulmonary artery microemboli and pulmonary veno-occlusive disease from primary pulmonary hypertension is by lung biopsy.

CARDIAC CATHETERIZATION AND PULMONARY ANGIOGRAPHY

Cardiac catheterization is the definitive test used to determine the degree of pulmonary hypertension. In precapillary causes of pulmonary hypertension, the left atrial pressure is abnormally elevated. Right and left heart cardiac catheterization with angiography can assess ventricular function, mitral gradients in mitral stenosis, whether left ventricular failure (high left ventricular end-diastolic pressure and no mitral gradient) or congenital heart defects are present. Green dye curves can indicate where the shunt is, and by measuring oxygen consumption and blood saturations from various areas in the cardiopulmonary circuit, pulmonary and systemic blood flows can be calculated. High-pressure and high-flow atrial or ventricular septal defects may still be closed surgically if the pulmonary resistance calculates near normal or less than one half systemic resistance.

In patients with primary pulmonary hypertension, some of the vasodilators (hydralazine and nifedipine) have been shown to lower pulmonary resistance and increase cardiac output. Patients with cor pulmonale secondary to parenchymal lung disease, usually those with chronic bronchitis-emphysema, may also respond to vasodilators with a 20 per cent drop in pulmonary resistance and 20 per cent or more increase in cardiac output. Although patients with precapillary pulmonary hypertension may clinically benefit from vasodilator therapy, deleterious side effects may preclude therapy and should not be tried unless hemodynamic benefit is proved.

DISORDERS OF THE PLEURA

By Peter A. Emerson, M.D.
London, England

DRY PLEURISY

This term is applied to fibrinous pleurisy with fibrinous exudate only. There is pain on inspiration, sneezing, and rib cage movements, and characteristically a pleural rub is heard.

Dry pleurisy is most commonly due to disease in the underlying lung. Any of the conditions causing pleurisy with effusion may present initially as dry pleurisy before the fluid accumulates. When a patient has a persistent dry pleurisy but an apparently normal chest radiograph, several conditions should be particularly considered. Tuberculosis can cause a low-grade dry pleurisy that can persist for months. The tuberculin test will be positive. Rheumatoid disease can be accompanied by dry pleurisy. Sometimes it is the presenting feature of systemic lupus erythematosus. Trauma can cause simple bruising of the parietal pleura with pain and a pleural rub that may persist long after the pain has subsided. A shallow pneumothorax may cause pleural friction as the lung re-expands; this presents as an apparent dry pleurisy. Dry pleurisy may be associated with pleural plaques owing to asbestos exposure in addition to being an initial presentation of a pleural mesothelioma. Radiation and certain cytotoxic drugs such as methotrexate can cause dry pleurisy. Although often diagnosed, viral infections rarely cause dry pleurisy unless there is pneumonia. An exception is epidemic myalgia, but even in this condition a pleural rub is unusual and an effusion rare.

EPIDEMIC MYALGIA (BORNHOLM DISEASE)

As its name suggests, this is primarily an infection of intercostal muscle caused by the coxsackievirus Group B. Pain is severe, as is indicated by one of its eponyms, "the devil's grip"; it is aggravated by all movements of the chest and associated with intercostal tenderness. Pain in the shoulder from involvement of the diaphragm is common. Fever is not always present, and the erythrocyte sedimentation rate (ESR) is normal or only slightly raised. Characteristically, the pain and any fever may subside and recur several times before finally settling.

The diagnosis may be made by virus isolation from throat washings or stools during the acute phase but usually is made by the demonstration, in paired sera, of a rising titer of complement-fixing and neutralizing antibodies to one of the Group B coxsackieviruses.

PLEURAL EFFUSIONS

The cause may be obvious from pre-existing disease or from an easily demonstrated underlying lung lesion, but we are concerned with the presenting problem of fluid in the pleural space without obvious evidence of an underlying lung lesion. Fluid may be in the general pleural space or located between lobes, above the diaphragm, or against the chest wall or mediastinum.

Radiographic Appearances. Fluid causes a dense homogeneous opacity. A moderate-sized effusion in the general pleural space appears as a triangular shadow based on the diaphragm with the apex curving up and out into the axilla. If one thinks of the lung as a balloon being pushed down into the chest half full of water, the reason for the increased radiographic density going up into the axilla is obvious. The upper level of the fluid is in fact always horizontal but is only seen as a horizontal fluid level if there is air as well as fluid in the pleural space (hydropneumothorax).

If radiographs are taken first upright and then in the lateral decubitus position, the fluid, unless encysted, can be observed to collect in the most dependent part of the pleural space and thus can be differentiated from consolidation and other conditions.

Computed Tomography. Computed tomography (CT) scanning is more sensitive than the chest radiograph or conventional tomograph for the detection of pleural nodules or larger tumors, especially when there is a considerable collection of fluid in the pleural space. Fluid can be differentiated from solid tumor by the various densities revealed by the CT numbers and the fact that positioning the patient alters the relative position of the fluid. Air replacement of all or some of the fluid can be used when any doubt remains.

Ultrasound. Ultrasound can be useful in the localization of pleural fluid prior to aspiration. Whereas the plain chest radiograph does not differentiate between pleural thickening and pleural fluid, especially if encysted, ultrasound demonstrates fluid as an echo-free space between the chest wall and the lung-pleura interface. The extent and depth of this space give the precise extent and localization of the pleural fluid.

Diagnostic Pneumoperitoneum. The use of ultrasound now elucidates the problem of infrapulmonary collections of fluid and subdiaphragmatic infections, so pneumoperitoneum is no longer necessary. It can still be useful in demonstrating the small diaphragmatic defects referred to later. The air passes through into the pleura.

Examining the Fluid. The chest radiograph does not indicate whether the fluid is serous fluid, pus, chyle, or blood. This can only be determined by aspirating a small sample of fluid from any significant collection of fluid in the pleural space.

SEROUS EFFUSIONS

Cytologic examination of the fluid is of prime importance. Malignant cells can be identified in about 50 per cent of patients with malignant pleural effusions, but false-positive tests are reported in about 3 per cent of instances, particularly in effusions complicating pulmonary infarction. Polymorphs favor an inflammatory cause other than tuberculosis when the predominant cells are lymphocytes. However, polymorphs are often replaced by lymphocytes in any serous effusion of some weeks' duration. Eosinophilia in the pleural fluid most commonly occurs when there has been some minor extravasation of blood into the pleural space, for instance in pulmonary infarction. Pleural eosinophilia may also accompany peripheral blood eosinophilia as in polyarteritis nodosa and allergic lung disease. Bacteriologic examination by direct smear and culture for tuberculosis and other organisms is essential.

Chemical studies on pleural fluid are not practically helpful except in the diagnosis of effusion complicating acute pancreatitis, when the pleural fluid amylase concentration may be much in excess of that in the serum. The pleural fluid glucose is low in infections and effusions owing to rheumatoid disease. If infection can be excluded, a very low pleural fluid glucose ($<$ 20 mg/dl) is virtually diagnostic of rheumatoid effusion.

Needle biopsy of the pleura using an Abrams or Cope needle (taking several specimens) should be done at the time of initial diagnostic aspiration in all patients with undiagnosed pleurisy with effusion. Adequate biopsies are obtained in about 85 per cent. True-positive results may be expected in about 65 per cent of patients whose effusions are due to tuberculosis and in about 50 per cent of those due to malignancy. A report of nonspecific inflammation does not exclude the more specific diagnoses. In these patients and those in whom a satisfactory biopsy is not obtained, the choice lies between thoracoscopy and pleural biopsy, limited thoracotomy and pleural biopsy, and full thoracotomy. The choice must depend on the circumstances and skills available. Provided that sufficient fluid can be aspirated and replaced with air, thoracoscopy and pleural biopsy will be the method of choice. When this is not possible, one or another form of thoracotomy is necessary.

The conditions listed in Table 1 must be considered when diagnostic aspiration yields straw-colored serous fluid.

PURULENT EFFUSIONS (EMPYEMA)

The following are causes of pus in the pleural space: lung infections such as lung abscess, pneumonia, tuberculosis, and fungal infections; subphrenic abscess; bronchopleural fistula, especially after lung resection; penetrating chest wounds with rupture of the esophagus. Sometimes there is no clinical evidence of a lung infection and the empyema appears to be the primary event—this is more likely to occur in diabetic patients or patients who are immunologically compromised.

Usually the diagnosis is made when an obvious collection of fluid in the pleural space is aspirated and pus is present. Severe and persistent pain suggests the presence of pus as opposed to serous fluid. Sometimes, however, the diagnosis is difficult and delayed. The underlying or preceding cause may not be apparent and the patient has some or all of the following indications: chronic ill health with persistent or intermittent low fever; peripheral blood polymorphonucleocytosis, anemia and raised erythrocyte sedimentation rate (ESR); finger clubbing; and unusual chest radiographic appearances that are difficult to interpret because they represent pockets of pus encysted along the chest wall or mediastinum or between lobes.

The key to the diagnosis is to keep in mind all the alternatives and to do chest aspiration, preferably after localizing any pockets by ultrasound.

CHYLOTHORAX

Chylothorax is an unusual condition that is classically due to rupture of the thoracic duct. The duct may be ruptured by a nonpenetrating injury causing stretching of the thoracic duct over the vertebral bodies, such as landing from a jump, vomiting, and even coughing.

Usually a latent interval occurs after the injury. The duct ruptures and chyle starts to collect under the mediastinal pleura; the subpleural collection of chyle may resemble a tumor. Then a week or month later the pleura gives way and the chyle escapes into the pleural space. The patient becomes short of breath and develops the physical and radiologic signs of chylothorax.

The thoracic duct is more likely to rupture if it is blocked centrally by, for instance, a mediastinal tumor; at other times it may actually be eroded by tumor. Other rare causes of obstruction are filariasis and tuberculosis.

Chylous Reflux. Apart from rupture of the thoracic duct in its mediastinal course, chylothorax may also occur when there is reflux of chyle and distended tributary lymphatics have ruptured, sometimes causing multiple small fistulas that weep chyle. This condition of chylous reflux is not necessarily associated with malignant disease. There may be a developmental blockage of the thoracic duct system.

Diagnosis of Chylothorax. The diagnosis may be suspected from the chest radiograph because the fat content of the collection of chyle makes it less radiopaque than other effusions. Confirmation depends on the aspiration of the chyle.

HEMOTHORAX AND HEMORRHAGIC EFFUSIONS

It is not always easy to distinguish between a blood-stained effusion and a true hemothorax. An originally serous effusion may be complicated by bleeding, especially if the patient is treated with anticoagulants; when primary bleeding occurs into the pleural space, there is always a reactive outpouring of serous fluid that then dilutes the blood. For this reason, it is useful to measure the hemoglobin concentration of the fluid. Even in frank hemothorax, it will seldom be above 50 per cent and as time passes, the concentration falls further. Hemorrhagic effusions may be expected to have a concentration of under 10 per cent.

Causes of Hemothorax. The majority of cases of hemothorax and hemopneumothorax follow penetrating or nonpenetrating injuries to the chest. Spontaneous hemopneumothorax occurs when spontaneous

Table 1. Causes and Characteristics of Serous Fluid in the Pleural Space

Cause	Characteristics
Malignant disease, e.g., mesothelioma; metastatic carcinoma from lung, breast, ovary; also reticuloses and myeloma	Effusions often blood-stained and contain neoplastic cells; pleural needle biopsy positive in about 50 per cent of patients; thoracoscopy and biopsy useful
Tuberculosis, e.g., post-primary tuberculosis in young adults or complicating established disease, usually in older persons	Straw-colored lymphocytic fluid; tubercle bacilli rarely seen on direct smear but grow on culture in about 60 per cent of patients; needle pleural biopsy diagnostic in about 65 per cent; tuberculin test positive
Postpneumonic effusions	Serous fluid with polymorphs initially; untreated may proceed to empyema; causative organisms may be isolated
Effusions secondary to subdiaphragmatic abscess or liver infection—whether amebic or simple abscess	Serous fluid with polymorphs; usually sterile unless an empyema develops; ultrasound diagnostic
Asbestos effusions: benign pleural effusions; may be recurrent and occur unrelated to mesothelioma; usually evidence of parenchymal lung change due to asbestosis	Serous effusion: Cytology pleomorphic but no neoplastic cells and pleural biopsy nonspecific; history of asbestosis raises specter of mesothelioma; CT scan after aspiration clear
Effusions due to acute pancreatitis	Serous fluid with amylase activity in the pleural fluid (500 to 2000 units), higher than in the blood; at autopsy pleura shows fat necrosis
Pulmonary infarction	Straw-colored or blood-stained fluid; sometimes has a raised eosinophil content
Acute rheumatic fever	Pleurisy with or without effusion in 10 per cent of cases
Rheumatoid disease	Serous effusion; pleural fluid glucose much lower than the serum glucose; rheumatoid factor positive as in blood
Systemic lupus erythematosus	A common manifestation; cytology pleomorphic; LE cells seen but more usual to identify antinuclear antibodies and DNA antibodies in blood
Polyartertis nodosa	Serous effusion with high eosinophil content
Radiation pleurisy	Serous effusion usually several weeks after therapy; cytology pleomorphic; no malignant cells
Adverse drug reactions, e.g., intramuscular methotrexate, oral practolol	Drug history is the clue. There may be others!
Lymphatic deficiency	Persistent serous effusions, usually bilateral and larger on one side than on the other, may occur in patients with other developmental lymphatic deficiencies manifested by lymphedema and yellow nails
Massive onset of effusion (usually right-sided) complicating ascites owing to malignant peritoneal involvement, ovarian fibroma (Meigs' syndrome), liver cirrhosis	Due to a small rupture of the tendinous part of the diaphragm; therefore ascitic and pleural fluids have the same characteristics; aspiration of pleural fluid relieves the ascites; communication can be demonstrated by pneumoperitoneum or other methods
Transudates caused by cardiac failure or hypoproteinemia due to nephrotic syndrome, liver cirrhosis, protein-losing enteropathy	Cause usually clinically obvious; clear straw-colored fluid with few cells, low protein, low lactate dehydrogenase activity

pneumothorax is complicated by bleeding from a ruptured adhesion. In the majority of patients who present with blood, but no air, in the pleural space, there has recently been a hemopneumothorax from which the air, but not the blood, has been reabsorbed. Other causes of hemothorax are bleeding from pleural metastases and such rarities as endometriosis of the pleura.

Causes of Hemorrhagic Effusions. These are pleural metastases, pulmonary infarction, and tuberculous effusions (rarely).

PLEURAL FIBROSIS AND CALCIFICATION

Pleural Plaques. Local plaques on the parietal pleura are normally discovered on routine chest radiographs of persons who have been exposed to asbestos dust, either industrially or in the environment. A holly leaf pattern of calcification may develop and plaques are mainly seen on the chest radiograph when they are tangential to the x-ray beam on the lateral chest wall or along the diaphragm. There is almost certainly a relationship between the presence of such plaques and the eventual development of mesothelioma.

More Extensive Pleural Thickening. More extensive fibrosis of the visceral pleura occurs when the parenchyma of the lung is more extensively involved by asbestosis. It also occurs following incompletely resolved pleuropulmonary infections, after hemothorax and thoracotomy, as a result of radiation fibrosis, and rarely as an adverse drug reaction, for example, to intramuscular methotrexate. A particular

Table 2. Examples of Occurrence and Causes of Pneumothorax

In otherwise healthy young adults (usually males 5:1)	Lungs are usually normal apart from localized apical scars with associated bullae.
In patients with chronic lung disease with airflow obstruction	Older patients with chronic bronchitis and emphysema; asthmatics.
After certain invasive diagnostic and therapeutic procedures	Lung, pleural, liver biopsies; anesthetic blocks; operations on cervical fascia; acupuncture.
After trauma	Penetrating and nonpenetrating chest injuries.
Complicating neonatal respiratory distress syndrome	As a complication of IPPV, especially if PEEP used.
Complicating localized lung disorders	Tuberculosis; lung abscess; hydatid disease; metastases from bone sarcoma
As a common complication of rare disease	Tuberous sclerosis; lymphangioleiomyomatosis; eosinophilic granuloma; connective tissue disorders.
Decompression	In divers and air travelers.

Abbreviations: IPPV = Intermittent positive pressure ventilation; PEEP = positive end-expiratory pressure.

apical form of fibrosis occurs in ankylosing spondylitis.

PNEUMOTHORAX

Table 2 shows the various causes of pneumothorax. The onset is usually signaled by the sudden onset of pain in the chest laterally and usually in the shoulder, accompanied by progressive shortness of breath. The pleural leak may seal itself spontaneously (closed pneumothorax); it may remain freely open so that the pleural space freely communicates with the atmosphere (open pneumothorax); or it may act as a one-way valve allowing air into the pleural space when the patient raises the intra-alveolar pressure by coughing or forced expiration. In this case air is never allowed out, so that the intrapleural pressure gets progressively greater (tension pneumothorax). This results in collapse of first the ipsilateral lung; then the mediastinum is displaced and may even collapse the contralateral lung.

The clinical and radiologic signs of pneumothorax are as would be expected and are usually obvious. Difficulties arise, however, when the pneumothorax is a quite shallow one. The classical physical signs will be absent, but if the pneumothorax is on the left, there may be a "pleural click"; this is heard, not just with the stethoscope, but often by the patient and sometimes by other people in the room. It is due to a curious amplification of the heart sounds by the acoustic conditions of the shallow left pneumothorax. It is sometimes mistaken for the mediastinal crunch (Homan's sign) of pneumomediastinum.

When a pneumothorax is suspected but not seen on the routine chest radiograph taken in inspiration, it is essential to take a film in full expiration.

PRIMARY PLEURAL TUMORS

Fibroma of the pleura is uncommon, and there is seldom an effusion unless the tumor becomes malignant. Clubbing is almost invariable, and hypertrophic pulmonary osteoarthropathy may occur.

Diffuse malignant mesothelioma is becoming more common. It is now recognized that the development of a mesothelioma of the pleura or peritoneum is often etiologically related to inhalation of asbestos, particularly crocidolite, up to 40 years previously. Contact with asbestos may have amounted only to living near or walking through the factory or merely cleaning workers' clothing—very much less than is required for the development of pulmonary asbestosis or even pleural plaques. It is also common in certain villages in Turkey where the size of the rock strata crystals are the same as those of asbestos, with obvious implications. The name of one of the villages translated into English is "Pain in the Chest."

The course is often more benign than for other pleural malignancies, and the patient may survive for several years. Pain and shortness of breath result from the pleural involvement, but episodes of pulmonary infarction may occur and give rise to additional contralateral chest pain.

The effusion is usually blood-stained and rapidly recurs after aspiration. Malignant mesothelial cells may be recognized on microscopy of the fluid.

The tumor does not metastasize to distant organs until late, but it is locally invasive, involving the chest wall, extruding through needle tracts or incisions or growing into the mediastinum or through the diaphragm. The tumor may also break through to the skin over areas where x-ray therapy has been given. For these reasons any interference does more harm than good and should be resisted. Patients who are left alone live longest.

SLEEP-RELATED RESPIRATORY DYSFUNCTION

By Neil R. MacIntyre, M.D.
Durham, North Carolina

Recent advances in sleep research have led to an increased awareness that important cardiorespiratory adjustments occur during various stages of sleep and that these can have profound physiologic effects, particularly in patients with underlying cardiorespiratory disease. This article is designed to address the respiratory changes that occur during sleep, relate them to specific sleep-associated respiratory syndromes, and then describe appropriate diagnostic approaches.

NORMAL RESPIRATORY FUNCTION DURING SLEEP

Normal sleep has several well-defined stages that can be classified by electroencephalographic (EEG) criteria. These stages represent discrete levels of central nervous system function during sleep and are often grouped under two general categories:

1. *"Quiet" sleep* is characterized by progressive slowing of the EEG through four separate stages. Quiet sleep is often referred to as non-rapid eye movement sleep (NREM) and is felt to represent the "restorative and reparative" period of sleep,

2. *Rapid eye movement (REM) sleep* is characterized by intensive EEG activity and the rapid eye movements from which this stage derives its name. This phase is felt to represent the "synthetic" period of sleep. During a typical sleep period, normal subjects experience each of these stages in repetitive 90- to 120-minute cycles.

Normal sleep affects respiratory function through both central nervous system (CNS) and direct intrapulmonary effects.

Central Nervous System Effects

Interactions of the CNS–respiratory system (Fig. 1) are coordinated through the respiratory controller in the brainstem. Output from the controller is to the respiratory muscles, and input into the controller is from the reticular activating system (RAS), cerebrum, chemoreceptors, stretch receptors, and irritant receptors. The function of the controller is to:

1. Be the ventilatory "pacemaker."
2. Protect the lungs from aspiration through action of the upper airway muscles.
3. Coordinate the respiratory system to perform communicative and other behavioral activities.

During sleep, all of these CNS–respiratory interactions are affected. As a normal subject progresses through stages 1 to 4 of NREM sleep, there is decreasing RAS and cerebral input into the respiratory controller and a change in the homeostatic "set point" for Po_2 (downward) and Pco_2 (upward). These result in a periodic breathing pattern in the lighter stages of NREM sleep (stages 1 and 2) followed by a regular, but decreased, breathing pattern in the deeper stages of NREM sleep (stages 3 and 4).

During NREM sleep, CNS responsiveness to CO_2 appears reduced but responsiveness to hypoxia, stretch receptors, and irritant receptors are near normal. Upper airway muscle tone and coordination with respiratory movements are also normal. In contrast, the very striking CNS activity that occurs during REM sleep is accompanied by irregular breathing patterns (with apneic periods lasting up to 20 seconds occurring up to four times per sleep hour) and a pronounced decrease in responsiveness to both chemoreceptor (Po_2 and Pco_2) and mechanical receptor (stretch and irritant) input. Additionally, upper airway motor tone is markedly reduced during REM sleep.

Direct Intrapulmonary Effects

A smaller minute ventilation with fewer sighs results in a small amount of atelectasis and ventilation perfusion ($\dot{V}/\dot{Q}$) mismatching during normal sleep. Along with this is a reduction in irritant receptors responsiveness (as noted previously) and a slowing of mucociliary clearance activity. These effects can result in retained secretions and further atelectasis and $\dot{V}/\dot{Q}$ mismatching. Bronchomotor tone fluctuations have also been noted during REM sleep.

ABNORMAL RESPIRATORY FUNCTION DURING SLEEP

Respiratory dysfunction during sleep can be grouped into disorders affecting CNS–respiratory interactions and those affecting the lung directly. Disorders in the former category can be further divided into ventilatory control abnormalities (irregular breathing and sleep apnea syndromes) or airway protection abnormalities (the nocturnal aspiration syndromes) (Fig. 2).

Sleep-Related Ventilation Control Abnormalities

As noted, periodic breathing during stages 1 and 2 NREM sleep and apneic periods during REM sleep can occur in normal subjects. However, there are clearly distinct clinical syndromes characterized by much more frequent and prolonged sleep related apneic periods (usually more than ten per sleep hour and lasting 10 to 100 seconds each). These apneas are categorized as either central (apneas due to a lack of CNS respiratory stimulation) or obstructive (apneas due to occlusion of the upper airways by the tongue or flaccid pharyngeal musculature). Although the obstructive apneas can be a result of specific upper airway anatomic abnormalities (Table 1), most are not. In fact, central and obstructive apneas frequently occur together in the same patient and the concept has developed that each type of apnea is actually a different manifestation of respiratory controller dysfunction—the central apneas reflecting abnormalities in the pacing mechanism, the obstructive apneas reflecting abnormalities in the coordination of the upper airway musculature with respiration.

Sleep apneas may be associated with specific disease processes (Table 1) but often there is no clear etiology. There are, however, certain risk factors associated with the more commonly diagnosed obstructive variety: male sex, increasing obesity (perhaps due to fat infiltrates in the hypopharynx), alcohol or sedative use, and possibly obstructive airway disease. An additional risk factor is a history of snoring. Many authorities, in fact, would argue that this very common sleep

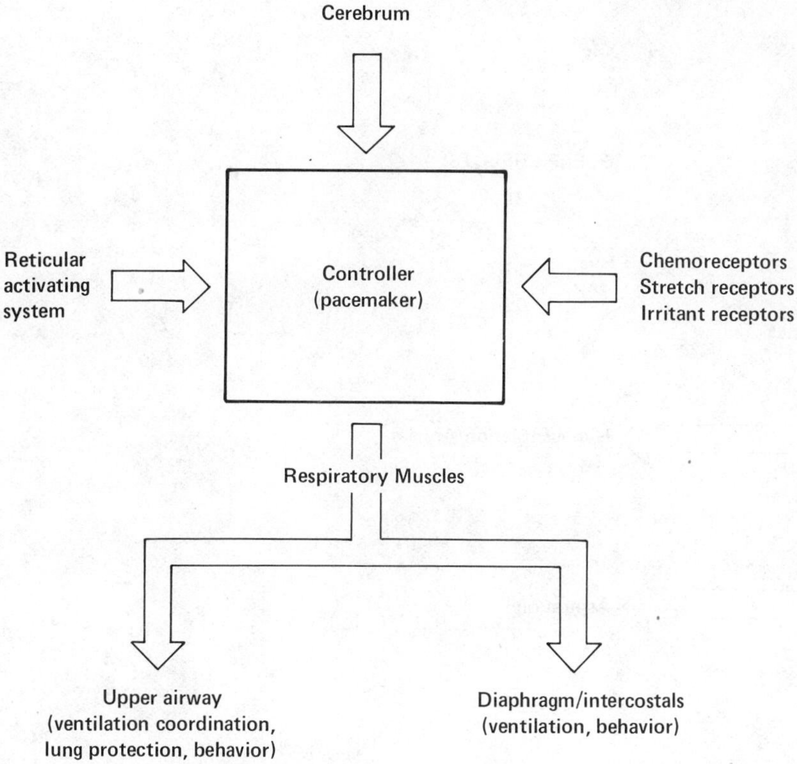

Figure 1. Respiratory interactions of the central nervous system.

phenomenon is, in itself, a mild form of obstructive sleep apnea.

Typical patients with true sleep apnea syndromes experience hundreds of apneas each night. These can occur during all stages of sleep but are particularly severe during REM sleep. During each apneic period, there is progressive hypoxemia and hypercapnea. These result in transient hypertension (both systemic and pulmonary), bradycardia, and often other cardiac arrhythmias. The termination of the apneas are felt to be due to either metabolic changes that develop during the apneic periods or, during REM sleep, a cerebrally initiated event. If the apneas are obstructive in nature, a loud noisy snore often accompanies apnea termination. There is typically either a lightening of sleep or arousal. However, the subject usually quickly resumes sleep and the cycle repeats. Chronic sleep apnea with episodic hypoxemia may result in fixed pulmonary hypertension, cor pulmonale, and polycythemia. Sleep fragmentation and inability to progress to deeper stages of quiet sleep result in the behavioral and personality changes associated with sleep deprivation.

Patients with the syndrome often first present with complaints of daytime somnolence and personality disturbance. Associated symptoms are listed in Table 2. A careful history taken from the patient's bed partner often reveals an awareness of the apneic spells and, in the obstructive variety, loud snoring.

The physical exam may reveal obesity (particularly in the obstructive variety) or one of the specific causes of sleep apnea (Table 1). Other physical signs associated with sleep apneas include systemic hypertension and signs of pulmonary hypertension and cor pulmonale. Routine laboratory findings are nonspecific, but an elevated hemoglobin and radiologic or electrocardiographic evidence for pulmonary hypertension and cor pulmonale may be present.

Table 1. Disorders Associated with Sleep Apnea

Disorder
Central Apnea
Bulbar poliomyelitis, encephalitis
Brain stem infarction
Brain stem neoplasm
Cervical cordotomy
Spinal surgery
Primary (idiopathic) hypoventilation syndrome
Obstructive Apnea
Adenotonsillar hypertrophy
Adenotonsillar lymphoma
Acromegaly
Myxedema
Micrognathia
Temporomandibular joint disease
Goiter
Myotonic dystrophy
Shy-Drager syndrome

The diagnosis of the sleep apnea syndrome is established by measuring respiratory function during sleep. As mentioned, merely observing the patient asleep can often reveal the repeated apneic periods. However, to establish the diagnosis and assess its functional significance, several other parameters must be measured (Table 3). These should include a continuous measurement of arterial oxygen saturation, heart rate, air flow, and ventilatory effort. Optional parameters include EEG and electrooculograms to characterize sleep stages, continuous

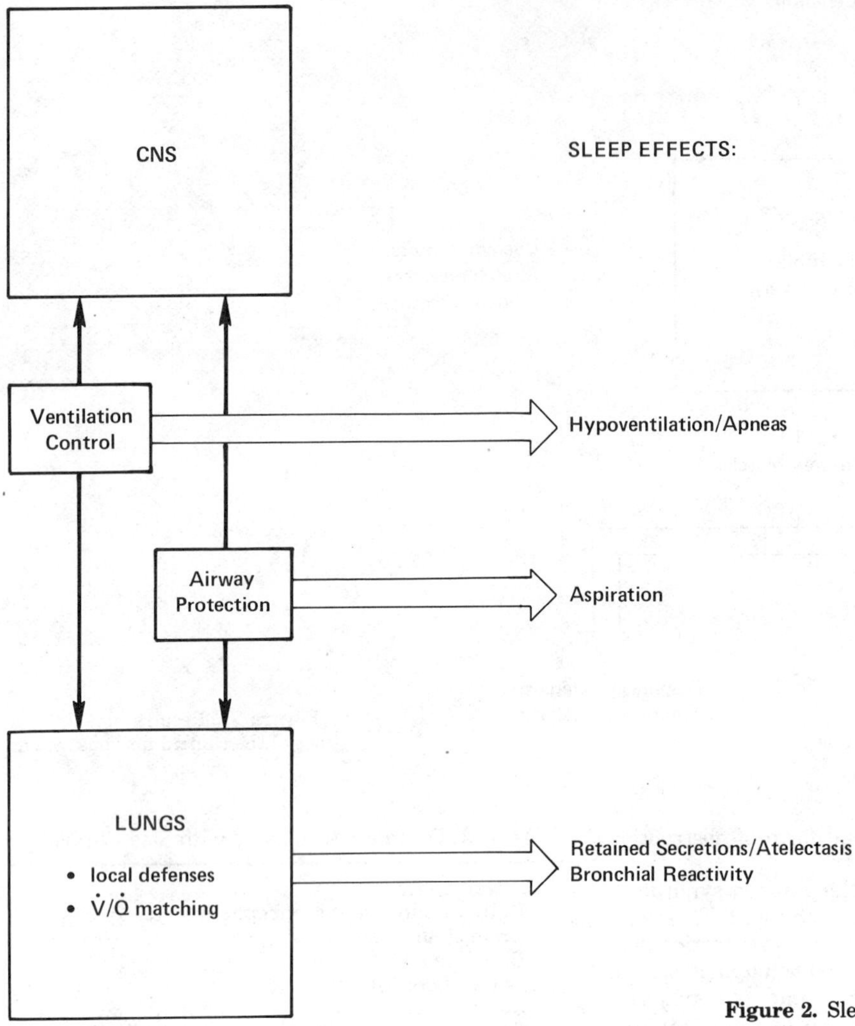

Figure 2. Sleep effects on respiratory function.

pulmonary artery or systemic artery pressure, genioglossus electromyograms to characterize upper airway muscle function, and periodic arterial blood gases to quantitate actual levels of Po_2 and Pco_2. From the above, it is possible to:

1. Document the number and duration of apneas.
2. Quantitate the effects of these apneas on gas exchange and cardiac function.
3. Describe whether the apneas are primarily central in origin (apneas without any ventilatory efforts), obstructive in origin (apneas with ventilatory effort but no air flow), or a combination of both.

Sleep-Related Aspiration Syndromes

It is important to realize that sleep-related impairment of pulmonary defenses in both the upper airway (decrease irritant receptor function and muscle coordination) as well as in the lung itself (decrease cough, mucus clearance) can predispose to aspiration. This can, in turn, result in primary lung disease (e.g., lung abscess or recurrent pneumonias) or worsen underlying chronic lung conditions. The diagnosis should be suspected in patients with these conditions and is often presumptive in patients with chronic lung disease and recurrent infections. Specific diagnostic approaches include careful examination of the upper airway, lung scanning after nasopharyngeal instillation of radioactive tracers to assess direct aspiration, or esophageal pH measurements to assess for gastric reflux. (See the article on Dysphagia, Esophagitis, and Esophageal Obstruction.)

Sleep-Related Direct Lung Abnormalities

As noted above, sleep is associated with a decrease in minute ventilation and a small amount of atelectasis and $\dot{V}/\dot{Q}$ mismatch. While in normal subjects these changes have minimal physiologic effect, in abnormal subjects with underlying lung disease, these changes can have profound effects on oxygen delivery. Moreover, in these abnormal subjects, the decrease in cough and mucociliary clearance associated with sleep may result in excess retained secretions and further worsening of the $\dot{V}/\dot{Q}$ mismatch. Bronchial motor tone fluctuations during REM sleep may also

Table 2. Sleep Apnea Syndromes: Clinical Symptoms

Excessive daytime sleepiness
Nocturnal insomnia
Noisy snoring (obstructive apnea)
Abnormal motor activity during sleep
Intellectual and personality changes
Sexual impotence
Morning headache

result in bronchospastic episodes in sensitive individuals. Complicating all of this is the fact that, as noted, sleep reduces metabolic and mechanical feedback mechanisms (particularly during REM sleep) such that potential compensatory responses are blunted.

Sleep-related hypoxemia should be strongly suspected in any patient with chronic lung disease in whom evidence of pulmonary hypertension, cor pulmonale, or polycythemia exists despite an awake arterial P_{O_2} above 60 mm Hg. Likewise, chronic lung disease patients with nocturnal cardiac arrhythmias, chest pains, or episodes of shortness of breath should be suspected of having episodic sleep-related hypoxemia.

To make this diagnosis, a continuous nocturnal recording of arterial oxygenation (as described) is appropriate. This should be accompanied by a continuous ECG recording to document arrhythmias or other cardiac abnormalities that might be associated with these hypoxemic episodes. Optional parameters would include blood pressure measurements and periodic arterial blood gas sampling during sleep.

Table 3. Continuous, Noninvasive Methods Available for Measuring Cardiorespiratory Function During Sleep

Parameter	Methods
Arterial oxygenation	Oximetry Transcutaneous monitor
Heart rate and rhythm	Electrocardiograms
Ventilatory flow	Oronasal thermistors Oronasal CO_2 concentrations Inductive plethysmograph Mask/Pneumotach
Ventilatory effort	Inductive plethysmograph Esophageal balloon pressure Diaphragmatic/intercostal electromyograms

Section Five
CARDIOVASCULAR SYSTEM

HYPERTENSION

By Lawrence R. Krakoff, M.D.
New York, New York

The past several decades have been a dramatic period of change for recognition of systemic arterial hypertension as a treatable risk factor in prevention of future cardiovascular disease. Efficacy of antihypertensive drug therapy in reduction of morbidity and mortality due to cerebrovascular disease, congestive heart failure, malignant hypertension, and aneurysm is now well accepted. Coronary heart disease has been reduced to a lesser extent by antihypertensive therapy *per se,* yet there is evidence that lowering of arterial pressure, when combined safely with other preventive strategies, may be effective. These trends have led to an emphasis on the treatment of hypertension with corresponding minimalization of diagnostic effort largely because of cost/benefit considerations. However, the recent development of remarkable new technologies for hormone assay, specific blockade of the renin-angiotensin system, and visualization of organs by sonographic and radiographic techniques have provided the tools for improved and safer diagnostic precision in detection of secondary hypertension. In addition, there are promising approaches to the definition of hypertension that may assist in the selection of those more likely to benefit from therapy. The advances in the diagnostic aspects of management of hypertension include emerging methods for assessing future risk and for "staging" the degree of cardiovascular pathology that has already occurred but that has been previously hidden from older techniques. This review will focus on the most useful of the traditional and emerging methods for diagnostic assessment of the hypertensive patient.

DIAGNOSTIC STRATEGY

Emergencies

Management of hypertensive patients may be viewed as a sequence of decisions as depicted in Figure 1. Few patients will require immediate hospitalization for hypertensive emergencies. Malignant hypertension, defined as a rapidly increasing arterial pressure, usually with the diastolic exceeding 130 mm Hg, accompanied by retinal hemorrhages, exudates, and papilledema, and evidence of deteriorating renal and cardiac function with or without encephalopathy, has become an uncommon entity because of effective detection and treatment of hypertension at earlier stages. Appearance of malignant hypertension should raise the question of renal artery stenosis, scleroderma, or occasionally a rapidly progressing nephritis. Unfortunately, malignant hypertension still occurs in a few patients with essential hypertension who have been undetected or untreated because of their isolation from the medical care system.

Sudden increases in arterial pressure that may require emergency medical attention may occur in pheochromocytoma and acute glomerulonephritis. Unanticipated sudden withdrawal of antihypertensive medication (especially related to the central acting antiadrenergic drugs such as clonidine, methyldopa, or guanabenz) may cause abrupt and impressive increases in pressure. Severe hypertension with headache may occur as the result of ingestion of tyramine-containing foods in patients taking monoamine oxidase (MAO) inhibitors (e.g., tranylcypromine).

Hypertensive crises due to catecholamine excess that occur in pheochromocytoma, clonidine withdrawal, or the MAO-inhibitor/tyramine syndrome respond well to adrenergic alpha receptor blockade with phentolamine. Use of this agent has diagnostic significance, but is not entirely specific as some patients with accelerated essential hypertension or with hypertension due to chronic renal disease may also have reduction in pressure when given phentolamine. The $alpha_1$ receptor antagonist, prazosin, may reduce pressure in pheochromocytoma. Its effectiveness in other states of catecholamine excess remains to be established.

The other conditions requiring emergency management of hypertensive patients indicated in Figure 1 are complications of pre-existing hypertension and should be detected and treated with dispatch by conventional methods.

Management of Outpatients

Most patients with hypertension will, after detection, proceed to an evaluation in an office or clinic for management in an ambulatory care setting. The left-hand sequence of Figure 1 indicates this pathway. The

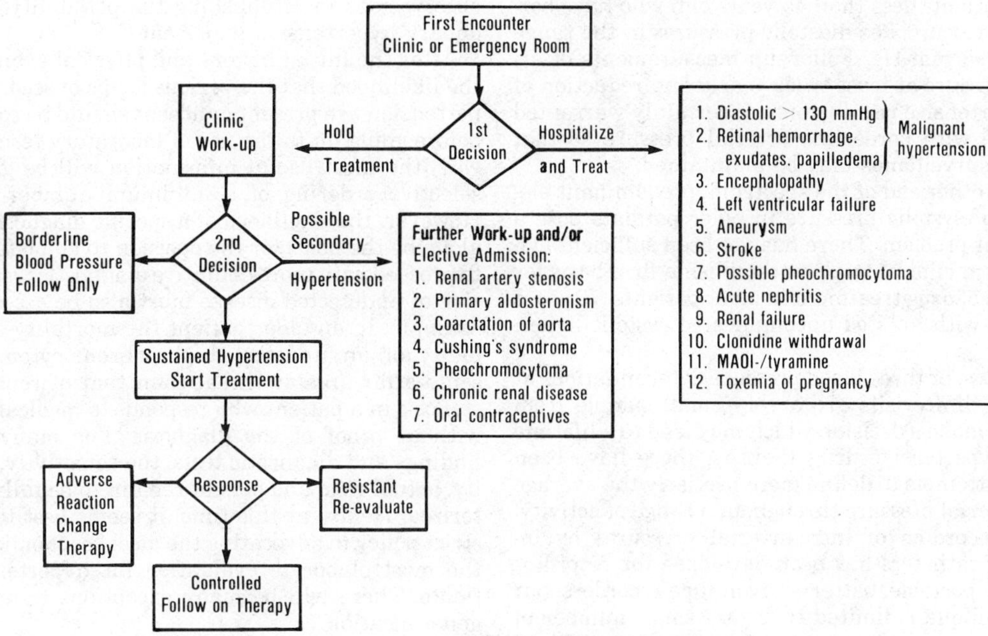

Figure 1. Scheme for diagnosis and management of hypertensive patients.

office or clinic evaluation should efficiently achieve several goals:

1. The level of systemic arterial pressure should be established with sufficient accuracy for a decision that antihypertensive drug therapy is or is not warranted.
2. The likelihood of reversible secondary hypertension should be defined by an appropriate screening assessment.
3. The overall cardiovascular risk status of the patient should be assessed for design of therapy addressed to nonhypertensive risk factors.
4. The presence or absence of existing cardiovascular morbidity will be documented.
5. Pertinent factors in the comprehensive medical evaluation will be detected and likelihood of response to one or more antihypertensive drugs will be elicited. For example, a history of asthma will indicate a contraindication to the use of beta receptor blockers.
6. Some consideration of the mechanisms accounting for elevated blood pressure may be included in the initial evaluation of hypertensive patients prior to institution of drug therapy.

Follow-up evaluations will be made in patients in order to re-evaluate the level of pressure in untreated patients with borderline situations, for assessment of antihypertensive therapy and of other risk factors, and for intervention. Those patients who do not respond to drug therapy in a satisfactory manner but who are deemed to be compliant will require reevaluation for the possibility that underlying potentially reversible secondary hypertension is present. With more effective antihypertensive drug therapy now available, it seems likely that fewer patients will reach the stage at which comprehensive evaluation for secondary hypertension will take place because of failure to respond to medical management as the only indication.

LEVEL OF ARTERIAL PRESSURE

The level of arterial pressure prior to treatment remains the most important single factor in assessing the potential benefit of blood pressure reduction for the individual patient. In the making of this decision, the diastolic pressure has been the basis for therapy in all clinical trials of antihypertensive drug therapy. It has become accepted in the United States to begin treatment in *all* patients with diastolic pressures of 105 mm Hg and above.

For those with lower levels of diastolic pressure on one or more occasions, the indications for starting drug therapy are less clear. The High Blood Pressure Detection and Follow-up Program (HDFP), 1977, intervention study conducted in the United States was based upon a two-step screening process. The *first* stage employed home screening and only those with diastolic pressure ≥ 95 mm Hg were chosen for a second screen in special clinics. At the *second* screen, those with diastolic measurements of 90 or more were entered into the treatment protocol. Of those called hypertensive at the first (home) screen, about one third were normotensive at the second screen. In the Australian clinical trial for treatment of mild hypertension, a diastolic pressure of 95 mm Hg on two occasions in the same clinic was used as the basis for entry into the treatment limb. Reanalysis of the results of this study has led to the suggestion that an average diastolic pressure of less than 95 mm Hg after three separate measurements should not warrant treatment but only continued observation. In no clinical trial of treatment for mild hypertension (diastolic 90 to 104 mm Hg) has there been proof of benefit for those less than 50 years of age upon entry, despite sustained therapy for 5 years. It seems most appropriate, then, to withhold antihypertensive drug therapy for young patients (less than 45 years old) who have borderline pressure, i.e., diastolic pressures in the range of 90 to 95 mm Hg. Follow-up measurements of arterial pressure at least twice yearly and reduction of nonhypertensive risk factors are certainly warranted for those with borderline arterial pressure so that medical surveillance may be maintained.

At the other end of the spectrum, predominant elevations of systolic pressure in older patients pose a persistent problem. There has not been sufficient evidence from clinical trials to establish a firm basis for any form of drug treatment in older patients (70 years or more) with isolated uncomplicated systolic hypertension.

Since two or three blood pressure determinations at office or clinic visits are a very small sample from which to make a decision which may lead to a lifetime of antihypertensive drug therapy, there have been several attempts to define more precisely the average daily arterial pressure throughout a range of activity. Direct recording of intra-arterial pressures by indwelling catheters has been developed for recording on small, portable, battery-driven tape recorders, but this technique is limited to a very small number of subjects engaged in research studies. Home blood pressure recordings may have some merit. Portable devices for automatic indirect blood pressure recording are now being employed in research studies and may become available for clinical use. Preliminary studies indicate that such devices may reveal patterns of increased arterial pressure during job-related activity, for example, compared with home, office, or clinic settings. Such information may be useful for designing appropriate therapy once the correlations between arterial pressure in various settings and long-term cardiovascular morbidity are known. Home blood pressure determinations by knowledgeable patients may be helpful in achieving compliance with therapy and in assessing the effect of recently prescribed drugs. However, not all patients are comfortable in monitoring their own therapy in this fashion. The decision to request this effort from patients is very much an individual one.

SEARCHING FOR SECONDARY HYPERTENSION

Initial Steps

A careful, complete, and pertinent medical history and physical examination remain the foundation for assessment of hypertensive patients with regard to curable or reversible disease. Symptoms that are characteristic of pheochromocytoma should be considered in the history as well as a family history of multiple endocrine neoplasia. Use of oral contraceptive pills or excessive licorice ingestion require careful questioning for detection. There are many other examples that underscore the role of the history. Similarly, the detection on physical examination of an abdominal bruit, the typical appearance of Cushing's syndrome, or the reduced peripheral pulses of coarctation of the aorta indicate the extraordinary specificity of these observations in establishing the possibility that secondary hypertension is present.

After the initial history and physical examination, the likelihood that the various forms of secondary hypertension are present or absent should be considered before going on to the use of laboratory tests. In this way, the most useful information will be gained by selective ordering of a minimum number of tests. However, the likelihood of a specific diagnosis cannot alone be the basis for the decision to go no further or to proceed with more definitive diagnostic testing. The risk of undetected disease must also be assessed. For example, in an older patient the mortality and morbidity of an undetected pheochromocytoma represents a far greater threat than that of renal artery stenosis in a patient who responds to medical therapy without proof of the diagnosis. For many clinical findings and diagnostic tests, the sensitivity, specificity, actual risk, and benefit remain to be fully characterized. Hence, at this time, it seems best to avoid a strict policy in advocating the most "economic" versus the most elaborate evaluation for hypertensive patients. There will be many exceptions to any broad generalization.

Specific Etiologies and Mechanisms

Pheochromocytoma-Catecholamine Excess. These tumors of chromaffin cell origin are most often detected because of a history of symptoms suggesting catecholamine excess or a family history of multiple endocrine neoplasia—Type II. However, the vagueness of many symptoms and the ease with which they may be dismissed as due to anxiety or stress suggests that biochemical screening for pheochromocytoma be done at least once in many patients with hypertension despite the rarity of the disease. The excretion of catecholamine metabolites—the metanephrines or vanillylmandelic acid (VMA) — in carefully timed samples or expressed as micrograms per milligram urine creatinine remains the most reliable initial test in biochemical detection of chromaffin tumors. Unequivocally negative tests from reliable laboratories, when coupled with little or no clinical suggestion, virtually exclude the diagnosis of pheochromocytoma. When the clinical picture is strongly suggestive and/or borderline metanephrine or VMA levels are found, further testing is needed for biochemical definition. In those with a compatible clinical picture and high levels of catecholamine metabolite excretion, diagnostic effort should be shifted to the anatomic localization of the tumor(s).

Measurement of plasma catecholamine concentration may be helpful in establishing the diagnosis of pheochromocytoma. When the tumor is present, marked increases in plasma norepinephrine concentration (usually more than 1000 picogms per milliliter) may be observed. Plasma epinephrine concentration may be increased in pheochromocytoma, but this occurs less often than increased norepinephrine.

Some hypertensive patients with symptoms suggestive of pheochromocytoma have mild elevations of plasma catecholamine concentration that are in a borderline range for the presence of tumor. Administration of clonidine, the alpha receptor agonist, suppresses plasma norepinephrine concentration by 50 per cent or more in essential hypertension but has little suppressive effect in patients with pheochromocytoma.

Pheochromocytomas and other adrenal neoplasms may be detected with the intravenous pyelogram if tumors are large. However, this technique is far too insensitive for many neoplasms. Use of abdominal sonography and computer-assisted tomography (CT scans) have markedly improved the precision of anatomic localization. Recently, an isotopic scanning technique employing ^{131}I benzylguanidine has been developed and appears to be promising for localization of small pheochromocytomas that may be missed by other methods. It has been suggested that this test may be especially useful in detecting the early stage of adrenomedullary hyperplasia that occurs in familial endocrine neoplasia—Type II. The very rare occurrence of pheochromocytomas in the chest may be detected by chest x-ray or plain tomography: The CT scan appears to be the most accurate. (See the article on Pheochromocytoma.)

Mineralocorticoid Excess. Hypertension due to mineralocorticoid excess is nearly always associated with reduced serum potassium, hypokalemia. However, in its most common form, primary aldosteronism, mineralocorticoid hypertension is often asymptomatic and has no characteristic features on physical examination—hence the need for obtaining a serum potassium concentration in all hypertensive patients prior to drug therapy. (See the article on Hyperaldosteronism).

An exception is the occasional association of primary aldosteronism with acromegaly in which the typical physical findings of growth hormone excess are combined with hypertension and hypokalemia. The other characteristic biochemical finding in hypertension due to mineralocorticoid excess is suppression of plasma renin activity as a result of feedback upon renin release by chronic salt retention resulting from prolonged excess steroid secretion. The various causes of mineralocorticoid excess are given in Table 1. The very rare disorders resulting from deficiency of adrenal enzymes in pathways of steroid synthesis are associated with characteristic findings on physical examination, usually early in life. Precocious puberty or virilization with hypertension suggest the 11-OHase deficiency. Absence of secondary sex development and primary amenorrhea indicate the 17-OHase deficiency (see the article on this topic.)

Hypertension, hypokalemia, and suppression of plasma renin activity with *reduction* of aldosterone secretion may result from chronic ingestion of natural licorice, which contains glycerrhyzic acid, a plant mineralocorticoid. A similar form of pseudoaldosteronism may be due to exposure to 9-alpha-fluorocortisol (Florinef) as therapy for orthostatic hypotension. In Europe, pseudoaldosteronism has been reported as a result of the use of nose drops containing potent synthetic mineralocorticoids.

In adult hypertensives with mineralocorticoid excess, the most likely cause will be aldosteronism due

Table 1. Syndromes of Mineralocorticoid Excess

Primary aldosteronism
Idiopathic aldosteronism
Deoxycorticosterone excess
18-Hydroxydeoxycorticosterone excess
17-α-Hydroxylase deficiency
11-β-Hydroxylase deficiency
Cushing's syndrome (some)
Pseudoaldosteronism
Licorice ingestion
9α-fluorocortisol, Florinef
Steroid nose drops

either to a functioning adrenal adenoma (Conn's syndrome) or to bilateral adrenal hypersecretion of the salt-retaining steroid. The former condition is suggested by a greater degree of deviation from normal in reduction of serum potassium (usually less than 3.0 mEq/liter) and in plasma renin activity (often undetectable by radioimmunoassay). Also, in Conn's syndrome, or true primary aldosteronism, plasma aldosterone concentration is elevated to its greatest extent in the morning, falling throughout the day following the pattern of plasma cortisol. In idiopathic or pseudoprimary aldosteronism, plasma aldosterone concentration, although elevated, responds normally with an increase in upright posture following the pattern of plasma renin activity. It has also been reported that cyproheptadine, a serotonin antagonist, selectively reduces plasma aldosterone concentration in idiopathic aldosteronism after suppression of adrenocorticotropic hormone (ACTH) release by dexamethasone.

Adrenal tumors 1.0 cm or larger may be seen on CT scan; about two thirds of aldosterone-secreting adenomas fall in this range. Confirmation of unilateral secretion of aldosterone by adrenal venous catheterization and sampling will be necessary as a presurgical step and is usually combined with retrograde adrenal phlebography (venography), which provides more direct visualization of the tumors. Functioning adrenal adenomas have also been localized through the use of radioisotopic scanning employing ^{131}I-iodocholesterol.

Adrenal neoplasms that secrete large amounts of desoxycorticosterone or other weak adrenal mineralocorticoids will also cause hypertension as a result of mineralocorticoid excess. When cortisol production is also elevated, these patients will have the characteristics of Cushing's syndrome. (See the article on this topic.) The presence of Cushing's syndrome with evidence of massive overproduction of both cortisol and mineralocorticoids suggests an adrenal carcinoma or an oat cell carcinoma of the lung, which is synthesizing huge quantities of ACTH-like peptides.

Hypertension with suppressed or low plasma renin activity and normal serum potassium is quite common, occurring in 20 to 30 per cent of those with essential hypertension (more often in blacks and those 60 years of age and older), and in many with chronic renal disease. These patients often respond well to diuretics, suggesting that salt and water retention play a significant pathogenetic role in raising arterial pressure. However, at present there is little evidence that these forms of low renin hypertension are due to excess production of known mineralocorticoids.

Glucocorticoid Excess. Hypertension due to pure or predominant glucocorticoid excess may occur in Cushing's syndrome of the benign type due to an adrenal adenoma or to dysregulation of pituitary secretion of ACTH. Most often, the cause is the use of pharmacologic doses of synthetic steroids in the course of treatment for a condition requiring these agents. Hypertension in these circumstances is not invariably associated with hypokalemia. Furthermore, plasma renin activity is not suppressed but may be normal or elevated. Like the oral contraceptive pills, glucocorticoids may increase plasma renin substrate (angiotensinogen). When naturally occurring Cushing's syndrome is suspected, consideration of a pituitary, adrenal, or extra-adrenal neoplasm should be made and appropriate radiologic evaluations are necessary; the use of CT scanning is extraordinarily helpful.

Renovascular Hypertension. Stenosis of the main renal arteries or their branches may cause hypertension. Arterial narrowing may be due, in younger patients, to a group of dysplasias of various layers of the arterial wall (the fibromuscular dysplasias). In older patients or those with several risk factors for atherosclerosis, atherosclerotic renal artery stenosis may be present either as a primary cause of hypertension or as a complicating event in the course of pre-existing high blood pressure. Severe atherosclerotic bilateral renal artery obstruction may produce hypertension and accompanying renal insufficiency. Renal artery stenosis may be due to neurofibromatosis in the course of von Recklinghausen's disease, and retroperitoneal tumors, occasionally pheochromocytoma, may compress renal arteries as an additional cause of hypertension.

In younger hypertensive patients with fibromuscular dysplasia of the renal artery, the finding of a subcostal or upper abdominal bruit, often high-pitched and lasting from systole into diastole, is a highly specific sign. Many older patients have systolic abdominal bruits that have little diagnostic significance.

Renovascular hypertension not infrequently first appears with a severe onset, marked elevation in pressure, and advanced retinopathy with hemorrhages and exudates. A rapid increase in pressure in a previously well-controlled mild hypertensive should also suggest the possibility of intercurrent renal artery narrowing. Once suspected, the presence of renovascular hypertension need not be proved unless invasive therapy, surgery, or transluminal balloon angioplasty is contemplated.

Medical management of suspected renovascular hypertension is entirely feasible, now that there are several effective and well-tolerated drugs for management of severe hypertension, including converting enzyme inhibitors, i.e., captopril and enalapril, which block the renin-angiotensin system. Most (about 60 per cent) patients with renovascular hypertension have evidence of increased activity of the renin-angiotensin system when assessed by measurements of plasma renin activity during standardized conditions of sodium intake or after stimulation by furosemide, and by the response to specific inhibition of the renin system. Infusion of saralasin, a peptide antagonist of angiotensin II receptors, significantly reduces arterial pressure in most patients with renovascular hypertension. Administration of captopril also causes significant reduction in pressure in high renin states such as renal artery stenosis. Reduction in blood pressure due to these agents may be observed in high renin essential hypertension, a cause of false-positive interpretations in the search for renovascular hypertension. Similarly, false-negative saralasin tests may occur in patients with bilateral renal artery stenosis or when patients with unilateral stenosis are not sufficiently depleted of sodium before angiotensin blockade. Thus, functional assessment of the renin-angiotensin system may be quite helpful in defining the patient with renovascular hypertension but should not preclude anatomic assessment of the renal vasculature when the diagnosis is to be completely excluded.

In the past, screening for renovascular hypertension has relied upon intravenous contrast urography and radioisotopic renal scanning for detection. These techniques have been successful in many instances, but the relatively high frequency of both false-positive and false-negative tests (10 to 20 per cent), plus the cost of these procedures, has been a continuing problem. Furthermore, the intravenous pyelogram and the renal scan do not provide visualization of the renal arteries but reveal only indirect evidence of reduced renal blood flow in instances of unilateral main renal artery narrowing or subtotal renal infarction. Recent improvement in computerized image enhancement of radiopaque dye during its arterial phase after intravenous injection has been provided by the technique of digital subtraction vascular angiography, or imaging (the DVI). The DVI has been employed for visualization of carotid, renal, and peripheral arteries. Although the DVI is still being improved, images of main renal arteries are quite distinct but resolution of renal artery branches and intrarenal vessels are not of the quality seen by selective renal arteriography. Nonetheless, the DVI appears to be a superior method for out-patient evaluation of patients for renal artery stenosis and may reduce the need for renal arteriography by more specific selection of those with lesions of the main renal arteries.

Our own practice is to combine the DVI with blood samples obtained from the renal veins for measurement of plasma renin activity by employing a femoral vein catheter for both purposes. Patients can be prepared for renal venous sampling, as is usually done, by previous administration of furosemide, or, more recently, captopril. It is highly likely that a patient with no main renal artery lesion detected by the DVI and no lateralization of renin production by renal vein sampling does not have unilateral renal pathology as a cause for correctable hypertension. However, the true incidence of false-negative assessments by this approach remains to be established. On the other hand, detection of main renal artery lesions by the DVI coupled with lateralization of renin production in the case of unilateral stenosis indicates a high likelihood of cure or substantial improvement in the patient's hypertension by balloon angioplasty or vascular surgery.

Retrograde femoral arteriography with injection of dye into the aorta or the renal arteries still has a place in management of patients with renal artery stenosis.

However, the promise of increased diagnostic precision offered by the DVI suggests that arteriography will be limited to use as a presurgical evaluation or will be performed in the course of transluminal angioplasty in order to document the degree of arterial dilatation that has been achieved by the procedure.

Other Forms of High Renin Hypertension. Excess production of renin by one kidney may occur as a result of intrarenal arterial stenosis or obstruction of a small branch with ischemia or segmental infarction. In addition, renal cysts and hydronephrosis may cause unilateral renin secretion. These conditions are usually detected radiographically or by sonography of the kidney. Occasionally, unilateral renin production occurs as a result of small vessel disease, nephrosclerosis, or the collagen-vascular diseases in which there is a greater degree of pathology in one kidney compared with the other. Such conditions are documented by lateralization of renin production by samples taken during bilateral renal vein catheterization when coupled with radiologic proof that there is no other cause for unilateral renin secretion.

Several types of renin-secreting tumors have been described. *Hemangiopericytomas* of the renal cortex are small benign neoplasms that may cause severe hypertension due to secretion of renin with resultant secondary aldosteronism and hypokalemia. These rare tumors are small (less than 2 cm) and require selective renal arteriography for visualization. *Wilms' tumor,* the malignant renal neoplasm of childhood, may secrete large quantities of renin. These may produce abnormal large molecular weight forms of the enzyme that have unusual characteristics on gel filtration resembling stored or precursor forms (pro-renins). Recently, a pancreatic carcinoma has been described which also produced enormous quantities of abnormal forms of renin. Thus, it may be of interest to screen any patient with severe hypertension and a malignancy for a hyperreninemia and to consider that elevations of pro-renin (as measured by acid or trypsin activation) may be present. The biochemical similarity of the renins to other acid proteases suggests that, in theory, these proteins may arise from a variety of malignant cells.

High renin essential hypertension occurs in 10 to 15 per cent of all those with primary or essential hypertension. These patients are often young and may or may not have resting tachycardia. Some have evidence of a hyperadrenergic state as documented by elevated plasma norepinephrine concentration. Plasma renin activity is usually elevated to a mild or moderate degree. There is no radiologic evidence of unilateral renal disease or renal arterial pathology and renal vein renin determinations do not indicate lateralization of renin secretion. These patients often respond remarkably well to small doses of beta receptor–blocking drugs, e.g., propranolol 20 to 40 mg twice daily or atenolol 50 mg once daily.

Most patients with malignant hypertension will have elevated plasma renin activity, especially if they have lost weight and have little evidence of pre-existing renal disease. Renal artery stenosis, acceleration of essential hypertension, scleroderma, and occasionally other collagen-vascular diseases may be the underlying etiologies for malignant hypertension. The role played by activation of the renin-angiotensin system and resultant secondary aldosteronism provides the basis for effective therapy. These patients may respond dramatically to inhibition of the converting enzyme by captopril with excellent control of arterial pressure and correction of hypokalemia. There may be little requirement for additional antihypertensive therapy in some patients, so that the response to captopril serves as a diagnostic as well as a therapeutic intervention.

Coarctation of the Aorta. Congenital coarctation of the aorta is a cause of hypertension early in life that is usually detected on the basis of reduced pulsation in the arteries of the lower extremities. This condition may occur in conjunction with other congenital cardiac defects and is associated with Turner's syndrome or ovarian dysgenesis. On physical examination, excessive pulsation of the supraclavicular arteries may be evident. Plain x-rays of the chest often reveal dilation of the left subclavian artery, a reduced aortic knob, and post-stenotic dilation of the descending thoracic aorta, combined to form the "3" sign. Notching of the ribs is also often observed as a result of collateral circulation from the internal mammary system to the intercostal arteries. Coarctation of the lower thoracic aorta is much less common than the typical narrowing just beyond the site of the ductus arteriosus. Case reports document that acquired aortitis, perhaps a variant of Takayasu's or "pulseless" disease, may involve the suprarenal aorta and cause coarctation.

Confirmation of the diagnosis of coarctation requires visualization of the aorta, usually by arteriography. Use of digital vascular imaging by intravenous injections has yet to be documented but may be useful in some circumstances. Some patients with hypertension due to coarctation of the aorta have evidence of increased activity of the renin-angiotensin system. There may be elevation of plasma renin activity or depressor responses to administration of drugs that block the renin-angiotensin system, i.e., saralasin or captopril.

Oral Contraceptive Hypertension. Women in the child-bearing age group who are hypertensive should be considered for the possibility of oral contraceptive hypertension until this is excluded by history. At one time, oral contraceptive hypertension was considered as one of the more common forms of secondary hypertension in premenopausal women. In recent years, this diagnosis is less often made. It may be that a reduced occurrence of oral contraceptive hypertension is due to a combination of better detection of women with early hypertension prior to use of the birth control pill and to reduced content of synthetic estrogens in more recent formulations. In women suspected of this diagnosis, the oral contraceptive pill should be withdrawn and a period of 6 months allowed for reversal of the hypertension. Plasma renin substrate (angiotensinogen), the precursor of angiotensin I, is elevated in women taking oral contraceptives. However, this measurement does not correlate with the level of pressure. In women who have persistent hypertension long after withdrawal of the pill, one should consider other causes of secondary hypertension or recognize that essential hypertension is present and treat accordingly.

NONHYPERTENSIVE RISK FACTORS

The long-term risk of future cardiovascular disease in hypertensive patients depends not only upon the level of arterial pressure before treatment but also upon the presence or absence of several other factors. In general, for American populations, white women have the lowest incidence of complicating events with or without therapy. In contrast, black men have the worst outcomes as a result of hypertensive cardiovascular disease. White men and black women have morbidity rates which fall between these two extremes.

The well-defined risk factors that have emerged from the Framingham experience have pervasive influences upon outcome in hypertensive as well as normotensive populations. Cigarette smoking, hypercholesterolemia, and diabetes are well documented for their effect. The separate significance of HDL and LDL cholesterol concentrations have recently been shown to have strong prognostic correlation. The separate roles of long-term exercise and weight (as independent factors) remain controversial, yet there is some epidemiologic documentation that the pattern of increased exercise in adult life is a protective one against cardiovascular disease. Thus, the hypertensive patient should be assessed to establish an overall profile of reversible risk factors. Comprehensive therapy will then address all of these for maximal reduction of risk.

STAGING HYPERTENSIVE PATIENTS

Ordinarily, the natural history of untreated hypertensive patients is described as a long silent period when hypertension alone is present then followed by the progressive appearance of arteriosclerotic pathology—stroke, cardiac enlargement and failure, and renal insufficiency. Atherosclerotic manifestations may be interwoven: coronary artery disease and peripheral arterial insufficiency. In the most severely affected patients, malignant hypertension may occur or dissection of the aorta may take place. Early detection of the hypertensive patient implies that therapy begins long before complicating cardiovascular events will have occurred.

Despite the success of large-scale screening programs, many hypertensive patients have detectable abnormalities in cardiac, renal, and occasionally neurologic function when first identified as hypertensive. There is, therefore, the need to survey these systems carefully at the outset, as the presence of abnormality attributable to cardiovascular disease worsens prognosis considerably. Hypertensive patients should have careful assessment of cardiac, neurologic, and renal function. Beyond the detailed medical history and physical examination, simple measures will ordinarily suffice: an electrocardiogram, chest x-ray (at 2-year intervals), multichannel serum chemistries, and a urinalysis. Results of the recently concluded Multiple Risk Factor Intervention Trial (MRFIT) indicate that electrocardiographic abnormalities suggestive of left ventricular hypertrophy or ischemia are important factors in determining the outcome of therapy.

Recent studies document the improved sensitivity of M-mode echocardiography for detection of the early stage of left ventricular hypertrophy in hypertensive patients, compared with the ECG or chest x-ray. Evidence of early hypertrophy is often a basis for more aggressive antihypertensive therapy in those with mild hypertension. However, clinical trials have yet to demonstrate that this approach is correct. At the present time, use of echocardiography for staging in uncomplicated hypertensives cannot be considered routine. Cost-benefit considerations suggest that the ECG remain the preferred technique for detecting cardiac enlargement in most patients.

FOLLOW-UP EVALUATIONS

Hypertension is a chronic disorder and appropriate long-term follow-up is an important part of the management scheme even when reversible forms of secondary hypertension have been treated successfully. Recurrence of hypertension occurs in nearly half of those with primary aldosteronism several years after removal of the tumor. Pheochromocytoma may recur. Renal artery stenosis may also reappear or advance from trivial to significant narrowing. Clearly, those given antihypertensive drug therapy need to be monitored for their blood pressure response and for possible adverse reactions. As of this writing, there is considerable controversy about management of hypokalemia, a common consequence of many diuretic agents. Despite antihypertensive therapy, hypertensive patients remain overly susceptible to intercurrent cardiovascular disease, which should be detected at the earliest possible stage by appropriate measures. Yearly re-evaluations for cardiac function (ECG), neurologic status by examination, and renal function by BUN and/or serum creatinine are warranted. Periodic assessment of nonhypertensive cardiovascular risk factors is appropriate.

ISCHEMIC HEART DISEASE

By Eliot Schechter, M.D.
Oklahoma City, Oklahoma

The coronary circulation supplies oxygen and nutrients to myocardial cells to provide for their needs, which, as a result of the constant activity of the heart, are high and continuous. The coronary circulation receives about 5 per cent of the total cardiac output at rest, and because of the high metabolic demands of the heart, virtually all the available oxygen is extracted from the blood as it circulates through the coronary arteries. As a result, when increased oxygen is required, it must be provided by increased flow because increased extraction can provide only a very limited reserve.

The heart utilizes the major portion of oxygen and nutrients to support contraction and the development of pressure. Oxygen demand, therefore, is proportional to systolic pressure, systolic time, and myocardial contractility. An increase in any of these parameters may cause the demand to exceed the supply even in the face of normal coronary arteries and thus produce signs and symptoms of myocardial ischemia.

Coronary blood flow, on the other hand, is primarily a diastolic event. During diastole the gradient between aortic pressure and intramural myocardial pressure is greatest and the resistance of myocardial vessels is lowest. Supply is thus determined by diastolic time, by the diastolic gradient between the aorta and left ventricle, and by the state of the coronary vascular bed itself. A reduction in any of these may reduce supply enough to induce myocardial ischemia in the face of a normal demand.

The ratio of diastolic supply to systolic demand determines the presence or absence of ischemia. This has been called the *endocardial viability ratio,* since the endocardium is often the first area to show the effects of myocardial ischemia. A decrease in supply or an increase in demand will decrease the endocardial viability ratio and, if sufficiently marked, will result in myocardial ischemia.

Ischemic heart disease may result from conditions such as valvular disease, which increase the demand, or from coronary obstructions, which decrease the supply. Only the latter will be considered in this article.

Myocardial ischemia may make itself manifest in several ways:

1. The symptom of angina pectoris or chest pain.
2. Alterations in the functional state of the myocardium. These may occur electrically, with ischemia producing changes in repolarization on the electrocardiogram (ECG) or the appearance of arrhythmias, or mechanically, with ischemia impairing systolic and/or diastolic function.
3. Injury to myocardial cells with recovery.
4. Necrosis of cells with eventual scarring (myocardial infarction).

Ischemic heart disease may present with various clinical pictures. As in all conditions, there is an asymptomatic or subclinical stage. Patients may suffer from stable or unstable angina. Myocardial infarction with or without complications may occur. Unfortunately, in some patients sudden death is the first symptom. Though it is tempting to consider these stages as progressive, except for the fact that subclinical disease precedes clinical manifestations, this is unfortunately not true. Each stage of the disease poses specific diagnostic problems and will be considered separately.

SUBCLINICAL ISCHEMIC HEART DISEASE

Subclinical ischemic heart disease implies the presence of obstructive lesions in the coronary arteries without symptoms, signs, or objective evidence of myocardial ischemia. Recognition of subclinical disease is important from a preventive standpoint, since interventions or modifications of risk factors may slow or prevent progression of the disease. More importantly, it is vital in selected populations such as the military, aircraft pilots, and interstate truck drivers, in whom a sudden catastrophic presentation of ischemic heart disease would pose a serious threat, not only to these individuals but to others as well. For diagnosing subclinical coronary artery disease, we must depend upon screening tests. These tests must be sensitive; that is, they must pick up nearly all individuals with disease. This requires a tradeoff in that good screening tests are not specific; that is, there are many false-positive results.

The history, by definition, in these patients is negative. Physical examination may reveal other conditions, such as aortic stenosis, that may be associated with myocardial ischemia. These conditions are discussed elsewhere in this book. There are no physical findings of subclinical coronary artery disease, although tendon xanthomata, hypertension, and nicotine-stained fingers may suggest individuals at high risk.

The resting ECG is not a valuable screening test. Electrocardiographic changes, especially in the resting tracing, represent myocardial damage and are rare in asymptomatic individuals. In early disease, supply at rest is usually adequate to meet demand and ischemia does not occur.

The exercise electrocardiogram was believed to hold promise for screening, since it was positive in most patients with ischemic heart disease, but this work was based upon hospitalized patients in whom the incidence of coronary disease was high. In a healthy population where the incidence of disease is low, the incidence of false-positive results has been reported as high as 60 per cent, and, coupled with a 15 per cent false-negative rate, makes the test of little value. This difference in the results of a test may be explained by reviewing Bayes' theorem, which states that the value of a diagnostic test depends not only upon its sensitivity and specificity but on the prevalence of disease in the population studied. Several simple formulas are necessary to define these terms:

$$\text{Sensitivity} = \frac{\text{Number of true positive tests}}{\text{Number of patients with disease}}$$

$$\text{Specificity} = \frac{\text{Number of true-negative tests}}{\text{Number of normals}}$$

$$\begin{array}{l}\text{Predictive accuracy}\\ \text{of a positive test}\end{array} = \frac{\text{Number of true-positive tests}}{\text{All positive tests}}$$

$$\begin{array}{l}\text{Predictive accuracy}\\ \text{of a negative test}\end{array} = \frac{\text{Number of true-negative tests}}{\text{All negative tests}}$$

To apply this to an actual example, consider two populations of 1000 patients being screened for coronary disease. One consists of middle-aged or older men hospitalized for chest pain, a population with a high incidence of coronary disease, arbitrarily set at 90 per cent. The second is a population of young individuals with no symptoms (e.g., military pilots), a population with a low incidence of coronary disease, arbitrarily set at 5 per cent. Let us assume a test has a sensitivity of 85 per cent (15 per cent false-negative results) and a specificity of 90 per cent (10 per cent false-positive tests). We can make the calculations seen in Table 1.

As is obvious, this hypothetical screening test would be of value in the low-risk population for confirming the absence of disease since, with a negative test, one could be 99 per cent certain that the patient was normal. A positive test, however, would carry only a 31 per cent possibility of the disease existing, and thus most patients with a positive test would be normal and would require further study before a diagnosis could be made. Conversely, in a high-risk population a positive test would confirm the presence of disease, whereas a negative test would reduce the possibility of disease only moderately to 40 per cent.

In low-risk populations, the use of a screening test with good sensitivity can exclude disease but does not establish the diagnosis in those with positive tests. Exercise ECG testing has a fair sensitivity, and this has been improved somewhat by utilizing combinations of exercise electrocardiograms with either thallium perfusion scans or radioisotope nuclear ventriculograms. These increase the sensitivity somewhat, but specificity remains a problem.

In summary, in the asymptomatic patient suspected of subclinical coronary disease, the first step in evaluation is an exercise screening test combining electrocardiography with an exercise nuclear ventriculogram (since thallium for the perfusion scan is more expensive and more difficult to obtain). If the screening test is positive, coronary angiography will be required to establish whether or not obstructive coronary disease is present.

STABLE ANGINA PECTORIS

In stable angina pectoris the patient has reproducible symptoms of ischemia with stress. Pathophysiologically this occurs when the coronary reserve is adequate at rest but cannot meet the increased demand of stress with an appropriate increase in blood flow because of the presence of obstructive lesions.

The history is the most valuable part of the examination and, unfortunately, the one in which the art of medicine is more important than the science. There is no substitute for experience and practice.

Table 1. Predictive Values for a Screening Test for Myocardial Ischemia in High-Risk and Low-Risk Populations

	Low Risk	High Risk
Test		
Sensitivity	85%	85%
Specificity	90%	90%
Patients		
Total	1000	1000
No. with disease	50 (5%)	900 (90%)
No. normal	950	100
True-positive	43	765
False-positive	95	10
True-negative	855	90
False-negative	8	135
Predictive value		
Positive test	31%	99%
Negative test	99%	40%

Angina pectoris has four characteristic features that should be sought in taking the history:

1. Its location.
2. Its character.
3. Its relation to stress.
4. Its duration.

Each of these characteristics should be explored individually in obtaining the patient's history.

Anginal pain is more commonly retrosternal than precordial. It may radiate, usually to the left shoulder and upper arm, sometimes to the neck and jaw, and occasionally to the right side of the chest or right shoulder. The pain may occur in the typical retrosternal location with radiation occurring if the precipitating factors are continued or if the attack is unusually severe. Of importance in the history is the fact that location and radiation are constant from attack to attack in a given patient and remain so even with the development of myocardial infarction.

More of a problem for the physician obtaining the history is the character of the symptom. The discomfort (and patients more often perceive angina as a discomfort than as a pain) varies widely from person to person. It is often mild or vague, and when asked about experiencing chest pain, many patients with angina will give a negative reply. If allowed to describe other discomforts, however, significant symptoms are often found. Patients describe angina as a "heavy feeling," a "weight on the chest," a "tight band around the chest," or sometimes just an "uneasy feeling." Helpful in this regard is the so-called "Levine sign." This finding, named after Dr. Samuel Levine, is present when the patient, in attempting to convey what he feels, makes a squeezing motion with the hands in a graphic attempt to convey the sensation.

It is not unusual for patients to consider anginal discomfort to be indigestion, since angina may occur following meals (to be discussed), or for the angina to be overshadowed by other less serious but more painful chest discomforts.

Since myocardial ischemia results from a supply-demand imbalance, and since this is usually precipitated by stress, the relationship of anginal discomfort to stress is, in my mind, one of the helpful diagnostic features. The patient has no symptoms at rest, but with exercise, emotion, a heavy meal, or other factors that increase oxygen demand, the symptom occurs. Although some variation from day to day occurs, the amount of stress required to precipitate angina is remarkably constant. Under controlled conditions it can be shown that the systolic demand (heart rate × systolic blood pressure) at which angina occurs is similar from day to day. With stress, angina gradually builds up as stress is continued. Rarely, patients report that with continued stress the pain subsides, the so-called "walk-through" phenomenon.

Just as stress produces supply-demand imbalance and therefore angina, rest restores the balance and the angina subsides. With cessation of activity, anginal symptoms subside gradually over a period of 2 to 10 minutes. Pain of very brief duration, several seconds to a minute, is seldom angina. Similarly, pain of long duration—over 20 minutes, if due to ischemia—represents infarction or at least unstable angina.

Based upon my assessment of these four characteristics (location, character, relation to stress, and duration), I classify the patient's symptoms as definite angina, probable angina, probably not angina, and definitely not angina. In a large study it has been shown that if, based on a careful history, a cardiologist thought that the patient's pain was definitely angina, there was a 98 per cent incidence of obstructive coronary atherosclerosis. If the cardiologist thought that the pain was definitely not angina, only 2 per cent of the patients had obstructive coronary disease.

Sometimes, in doubtful cases, the response to nitroglycerin can be helpful. Because the use of this drug is so familiar to the public, there is often a strong placebo response and therefore the test must be controlled. The patient is given two bottles, one of nitroglycerin and one of saccharin, labeled "A" and "B," and is instructed to alternate their use, putting a tablet under the tongue each time he suffers an attack of pain. The patient is to keep an accurate (timed with a watch) record of the duration of each attack and which tablet was utilized. Distinct shortening of the attacks with nitroglycerin compared with saccharin favors a diagnosis of angina; an equal response to both suggests either a placebo effect or non-ischemic pain.

Physical examination is of limited value in evaluating a patient with ischemic heart disease. It serves to rule out causes of ischemia other than obstruction of the coronary arteries. The most frequent of these are hypertensive cardiovascular disease, aortic stenosis, and hypertrophic cardiomyopathy with or without subvalvular obstruction. These are discussed elsewhere in this volume and are not further amplified here.

Examination of a patient during an attack of chest pain is more helpful than examination at rest. The appearance of certain physical findings during pain is of much more use than findings that are present continuously. Findings that should be sought include an S_4 or atrial gallop (resulting from the increased atrial contribution to filling of the ischemic ventricle with its reduced compliance), a late systolic mitral regurgitant murmur (due to failure of the ischemic papillary muscle to contract and prevent late systolic regurgitation), and a palpable precordial bulge (resulting from abnormal expansion of the ischemic segment during systole). The response to carotid sinus massage is also helpful. If slowing of the heart rate is obtained, the pain will often disappear promptly, possibly as a result of reduction in demand, since at a slow rate the rate pressure product is lower or due to reflex coronary dilatation as a result of vagal stimulation. The test is performed by massaging the carotid sinus while listening to the heart sounds or feeling the pulse to document the change in rate. Ask about changes in the pain if rate slowing is obtained. In the absence of slowing, the test is of no significance and a negative test does not exclude ischemic pain.

Objective tests are of limited value in a patient with classic angina. The incidence of coronary obstruction in these patients is sufficiently high that a positive test adds little to our diagnostic certainty and a negative test is more than likely a false-negative one.

Noninvasive, objective recordings that may be utilized include electrocardiography and various nuclear studies. A resting electrocardiogram is of limited value but may reveal an old myocardial infarction which would strongly suggest the presence of obstructive coronary disease. An electrocardiogram during pain is more helpful because it may reveal significant ST segment shifts confirming that the pain is due to myocardial ischemia. The presence of ST elevation, especially with either atrioventricular conduction disturbances or ventricular arrhythmias, suggests that the coronary disease is spasm of an epicardial vessel with or without underlying atherosclerotic obstruction.

Because myocardial ischemia is most often present with stress, exercise testing is widely utilized. Myocardial perfusion may be monitored by electrocardiographic recordings. ST segment shifts indicate ischemia, but this test has a sensitivity of about 75 per cent in patients with obstructive coronary disease and may give false-positive results in a significant number of patients who are particularly troublesome diagnostic problems (e.g., young women with atypical pain). (A flat ST segment depression of at least 1 mm, lasting 0.08 second after the J point, is the most widely used criterion for a positive test.) Adding thallium nuclear imaging, which provides pictures of myocardial perfusion during exercise and rest, increases both the sensitivity and specificity but also the expense of the test. Exercise nuclear ventriculography allows evaluation of the ejection fraction and segmental wall motion. This provides evidence of overall myocardial function (rather sensitive but not very specific) as well as segmental wall motion (more specific but less sensitive) as evidence of myocardial ischemia.

I find the greatest diagnostic value of exercise testing for stable chest pain is in patients with an intermediate risk of coronary disease when a positive test strongly favors the diagnosis of angina and a negative test makes its likelihood very low. It is also of value, especially using thallium imaging, for assessing the functional ability of patients with established coronary disease and in assessing the significance of equivocal lesions demonstrated on angiography. For example, a 50 per cent narrowing of a vessel would be a significant lesion if, with exercise, the patient showed ECG changes, a thallium defect, or wall motion abnormalities of the portion of the myocardium supplied by the vessel in question.

Coronary angiography is the cornerstone of diagnosis in patients with ischemic heart disease. In a patient with classic angina in whom the presence of coronary disease is almost certain or in a patient with equivocal findings in whom the diagnosis must be established or excluded with certainty (for example, a pilot), I would proceed directly with angiography. In most symptomatic patients, management is dictated directly by the anatomy. Patients with left main obstruction or with three-vessel coronary artery disease and abnormal (perhaps even with normal) left ventricular function have been shown to have a better survival with surgical than with medical therapy. Symptomatic patients with single-vessel disease may be offered coronary angioplasty, which has a lower morbidity and expense and approximately equal results to coronary artery bypass surgery. Patients may have coronary artery spasm, which can often be demonstrated at catheterization utilizing ergonovine as a provocative test. Such patients should be treated with nitrates and calcium-blocking agents but not beta-blockers. These subgroups of patients comprise two thirds to three fourths of those undergoing angiography (the remainder are patients with two-vessel disease), and thus in most patients the data from catheterization and angiography will dictate management.

The risk of coronary angiography in patients without other complicating problems is very low (mortality of 1 per 5000 to 10,000 angiograms), and the risk: benefit ratio is thus very high. Recent economic studies have shown that proceeding directly with angiography in patients with typical symptoms of ischemia rather than progressing through a series of noninvasive tests is the most cost-effective means of making an accurate diagnosis.

UNSTABLE ANGINA

The syndrome of unstable angina has, in the past, been called pre-infarction angina, intermediate coronary syndrome, impending infarction, and accelerated angina, to name just a few. The term *unstable angina* is preferable, since it more accurately describes the situation—a patient whose course may progress either to infarction or to stable angina.

Several clinical pain patterns comprise the syndrome of unstable angina. An increase in the frequency or severity of pain in patients with previously stable angina and the recent onset (less than 4 weeks) of severe and disabling angina are two of the most common patterns. Of more concern is the development of angina at rest or the presence of prolonged pain, which may be due to either unstable angina or myocardial infarction, since this implies that the supply-demand imbalance is so severe that even resting myocardial oxygen needs cannot be met.

The initial evaluation of a patient with unstable angina involves the exclusion of myocardial infarction, to be discussed. Many patients stabilize after admission to a coronary care unit (CCU), in which case evaluation as discussed under Stable Angina is appropriate. If the patient continues to present an unstable picture after CCU admission, urgent angiography is imperative so that appropriate surgical plans can be made. The risk of angiography in a patient with continuing unstable pain is significantly decreased if intra-aortic balloon counterpulsation is employed prior to angiography.

ACUTE MYOCARDIAL INFARCTION

The final syndrome to be discussed in the spectrum of ischemic heart disease is that of acute myocardial infarction. Here the blood supply to the myocardium has been sufficiently compromised, most often by thrombotic occlusion of a vessel with severe underlying atherosclerosis, so that there is actual necrosis of myocardial tissue. The severe ischemia produces characteristic symptoms, and the death of tissue characteristic electrocardiographic, enzymatic, and scintigraphic changes.

Because of the total interruption of blood supply to the myocardium, the pain of myocardial infarction frequently occurs at rest and lasts hours rather than minutes. Although often more intense, it does not differ significantly in location and character from the patient's usual angina. It may be associated, if cardiac function is significantly impaired, with feelings of anxiety and impending doom, probably due to increased circulating catecholamines, as well as cold, clammy skin due to poor peripheral perfusion. This history of prolonged pain, which is otherwise characteristic of the patient's angina, is the most important early diagnostic clue to myocardial infarction. Confirmation of infarction is most often obtained by electrocardiographic and enzymatic changes. The characteristic electrocardiographic changes early (less than 4 hours after infarction) include elevation of the ST segments and high peaking of the T waves due to ischemia and injury. Subsequently, the T wave progresses from peaked to deeply inverted, and there is a loss of R-wave amplitude or development of Q waves in the electrocardiographic leads recording the area of infarction. The necrotic myocardium releases intracellular enzymes, the earliest and most specific being the MB isoenzyme of creatine kinase (CK or CPK). This can be detected in the blood 6 to 8 hours after infarction and returns to normal 2 to 3 days later. Elevation of the total CK is less specific, since the majority of CK is the MM fraction, which is also released from skeletal muscle. Isoenzyme fraction 1 of lactate dehydrogenase (LD or LDH) is also relatively specific for myocardial damage. LDH appears in the blood approximately 12 hours after infarction and returns to normal in 5 to 7 days. Elevations of these enzymes with the appropriate time course to their rise and fall is diagnostic of myocardial infarction and is especially useful in patients in whom the ECG is not diagnostic because of left bundle branch block, preexisting myocardial infarction, or the location and size of the infarction. It is helpful to order isoenzymes of CK and LDH every 8 hours on the first day of infarction and daily thereafter, since a small infarction may produce a rise and fall within, or very close, to the normal range. A very high enzyme level implies an extensive amount of myocardial necrosis and may be associated with a poor prognosis.

At the present time, nuclear techniques have only limited application in the diagnosis of myocardial infarction. Thallium scintigraphy gives an image of myocardial perfusion. A patient with an occluded vessel will show a resting perfusion defect in the distribution of this vessel. The application of this technique to the diagnosis of acute infarction is limited, since thallium has a short half-life and cannot be kept on hand for use when a patient presents. Further, a resting perfusion defect could represent either a new or old occlusion, thus limiting the diagnostic value of the study.

Radionuclide ventriculography can identify wall motion abnormalities and, inferentially, areas of impaired perfusion. Again these could be new or remote abnormalities. This technique has its greatest application in evaluating ventricular function in patients with myocardial infarction to assist in their management and to assess their prognosis. The most useful diagnostic technique is hot spot imaging with pyrophosphate. Because mitochondria in areas of infarcted tissue bind calcium, an isotope-tagged compound with calcium affinity will localize in areas of infarcted tissue and thus produce a hot spot image of the area of infarction. Technetium 99m pyrophosphate is such an agent. These scans show their greatest positivity 4 to 7 days after myocardial infarction but have limited sensitivity, in part because of the uptake of the isotope by the liver, spleen, and overlying skeletal elements of the chest. The test is especially useful in a patient who presents several days after the presumed infarction when the ECG changes may be stable and cannot be differentiated from an old scar, and the enzymes have already returned to normal. There have been some data suggesting that certain patterns on pyrophosphate scans, particularly a stippled or "donut" appearance, indicate a poorer prognosis than do other patterns.

SUMMARY

The diagnostic approach to patients with ischemic heart disease depends upon the clinical syndrome: asymptomatic, symptomatic (either typical or atypical, stable or unstable), or acute myocardial infarction. A skillfully obtained history is most important. The therapeutic approach to symptomatic patients with ischemic heart disease depends upon demonstration of the anatomy at angiography. Patients with left main or three-vessel disease are best treated by surgery, patients with single-vessel disease may be offered coronary angioplasty, and patients with normal coronary arteries but coronary spasm should be treated with nitrates and calcium entry blocking agents but not with beta-blockers. Catheterization and angiography constitute a mainstay of diagnosis. Present noninvasive tests offer some assistance in selecting patients for angiography, since those with normal exercise performance seldom have multivessel disease, while those who are severely limited usually do, and in evaluating the extent of myocardial dysfunction. Ultimately, however, the diagnosis most often depends on demonstration of the coronary anatomy, and angiography must be at least considered in the work-up of every patient.

CONGESTIVE HEART FAILURE

By Dean T. Mason, M.D.
and Garrett Lee, M.D.
San Francisco, California

In the past two decades, improved understanding of the hemodynamic and mechanical mechanisms of cardiac contraction has provided precise definition of the heart failure state. *Heart failure* is the abnormal condition in which disturbed cardiac performance is primarily responsible for the inability of the heart to pump blood at a rate commensurate with systemic metabolic requirements at rest and during activity. Heart failure is considered to be *compensated* when cardiac output is maintained at a normal level by reserve systems principally inherent in the ventricle, often with congestive features and other signs and symptoms attending the operation of these adaptive processes. *Decompensated* congestive heart failure (CHF) evolves with chronic low cardiac output despite maximal activity of cardiocirculatory protective mechanisms.

This article initially considers the regulation of cardiac performance in clinical CHF, then delineates the bedside approach and important noninvasive and invasive techniques available to the physician for assessment of the nature and degree of cardiac dysfunction as well as for determination of the specific heart diseases causing CHF.

PATHOPHYSIOLOGIC MECHANISMS

Fundamental Causes of CHF

Recent findings obtained from experimental and clinical studies on the control of force and velocity of ventricular contraction have clarified that the function of the intact heart is governed by intimate integration of four principal determinants that regulate stroke volume and cardiac output:

1. *Preload* (ventricular end-diastolic volume).
2. *Contractility* (variable force of ventricular contraction independent of loading).
3. *Afterload* (intraventricular systolic tension during ejection).
4. *Heart rate.*

The first two determinants are fundamental intrinsic mechanisms inherent in the contractile machinery of the myocardium, whereas the last two are largely under extrinsic autonomic modulation. The terms *cardiac function* and *ventricular performance* are used in the general sense to refer to the combined action of these determinants of cardiac output and not necessarily to the single determinant, contractility itself. The disturbed mechanisms operative in all types of clinical heart disease can be evaluated and accurately characterized within the framework of isolated or composite disorders of these four major determinants of cardiac performance. The development of improved techniques and concepts for the assessment of cardiac function in patients by both hemodynamic methods and myocardial mechanics has provided the means for differential analyses of the nature and degree of the roles of each of these fundamental determinants and their interrelations with cardiac compensatory mechanisms governing stroke output in CHF.

Underlying Causes of CHF

Clinical heart disease can be broadly classified on a pathophysiologic basis according to three general forms of cardiac functional abnormalities:

1. *Primary contractility disturbance,* as in idiopathic or ischemic myocardial disease.

2. *Diastolic mechanical inhibition* of cardiac performance (ventricular underloading) in which ventricular hypertrophy does not develop, as in restricted ventricular filling in mitral stenosis or pericardial tamponade.

3. *Systolic mechanical overloading* of the ventricle characterized by excessive pressure loading, as in aortic stenosis or essential hypertension, or increased volume loading, as in mitral or aortic regurgitation. In systolic ventricular overloading and in primary inotropic disorders, CHF occurs when there is substantial depression of contractility; decompensation ensues when the impairment of contractile state becomes particularly severe.

Precipitating Causes of CHF

In CHF that is unresponsive to standard medical therapy, in addition to the systematic evaluation of the nature and degree of heart disease, careful consideration of the possibility of noncardiac conditions simulating or perpetuating cardiac dysfunction is essential. The common abnormalities that mimic heart disease include pulmonary embolism, other bronchopulmonary disorders, thyrotoxicosis, pheochromocytoma, adrenal tumors and insufficiency, metastatic carcinoma, various forms of anemia, and hepatic and renal diseases.

Several conditions may contribute to the persistence of the CHF state in any type of heart disease: hyperthyroidism, hypothyroidism, anemias, atrial fibrillation and other tachyarrhythmias, heart block, pulmonary embolism, bacterial endocarditis, pulmonary and urinary tract infections, hepatic and renal diseases, hypertension, ingestion of large quantities of alcohol, obesity, excessive physical activity, increased salt and water intake, electrolyte disturbances, abnormalities of acid-base balance, and excessive use of opiates.

Finally, complications of cardiovascular drug therapy may perpetuate or worsen pump function, such as cardiac depression due to large doses of antiarrhythmic agents, relatively low blood volume because of too vigorous diuretic therapy, and rhythm and conduction disturbances induced by digitalis toxicity.

Cardiac Compensatory Mechanisms

When systolic hemodynamic overloading or a primary defect in contractility is imposed on the heart, there are three principal compensatory mechanisms available to it that provide a limited amount of ventricular reserve for the direct support of cardiac function and its fundamental goal of maintaining a normal level of cardiac output:

1. The *Frank-Starling principle.*
2. Ventricular hypertrophy.
3. The sympathetic nervous system.

Deleterious symptoms necessarily accompany the operation of these compensatory mechanisms in their primary role of sustaining stroke volume, and these symptoms restrict the extent to which the adaptive systems can be used.

Ventricular Dilation. The Frank-Starling preload mechanism of ventricular dilation is immediately utilized to aid the ventricle in maintenance of cardiac output in the presence of an excessive systolic hemodynamic (particularly volume) overload or primary inotropic disturbance. The increased end-diastolic volume permits more forceful contraction, and the greater ventricular size allows ejection of a larger stroke volume with less shortening of the circumferential fibers. On the other hand, the effectiveness and reserve capacity of the Frank-Starling system are encroached on when the contractile state is diminished, since its ascending limb becomes less steep and flattened with its apex decreased in amplitude so that the reduced maximal stroke volume possible must be delivered at an abnormally high level of end-diastolic pressure. Thus, the failing ventricle has a lowered and depressed function curve and exhibits decreased systolic response to preload increments. Furthermore, operation of the Frank-Starling preload mechanism by the ventricles for maintaining cardiac output is obligatorily associated with pulmonary and systemic congestion, and increased myocardial systolic tension; thereby the price for use of this reserve system is dyspnea and peripheral edema, along with increased cardiac oxygen needs.

Ventricular Hypertrophy. An increase in the number of contractile units by development of ventricular hypertrophy provides a relatively quickly responsive second compensatory system in support of cardiac output in systolic mechanical (particularly pressure) overloading and in contractile state impairment. Thus, protein synthesis is stimulated by excessive intramyocardial tension, which appears to serve as the mechanical-biochemical transducer or coupling mechanism responsible for accelerated production of ventricular mass. Since extensive ventricular hypertrophy results in relative myocardial ischemia, due to cardiac oxygen demands in excess of delivery capacity of even the normal coronary circulation, angina pectoris may attend marked use of the reserve mechanism of hypertrophy.

In addition to the increase in oxygen requirements because of greater muscle mass, myocardial oxygen utilization is also enhanced by the Frank-Starling and adrenergic adaptive mechanisms. Thus, at a given ventricular mass, *myocardial oxygen consumption* is principally determined directly by three hemodynamic-related variables:

1. Intramyocardial systolic tension (governed by systolic pressure and cardiac size).
2. Heart rate.
3. Contractile state.

Ventricular dilation and increased sympathetic activity raise the first two of these factors above normal levels in CHF.

Sympathetic Nervous System Activity. Besides ventricular dilation and hypertrophy reserves, the dysfunctioning heart has immediately available some inotropic support provided by adrenergic activity. Thus, the ventricles are richly innervated by sympathetic fibers in which increased impulse traffic, through release of its endogenous neurotransmitter, norepinephrine, and consequent myocardial beta receptor stimulation, is capable of improving contractility and increasing frequency of contraction. There is abundant evidence that sympathetic activity is augmented in CHF. Paradoxically, however, norepinephrine is reduced in the hypertrophied myocardium because of its defective synthesis, and the dysfunctioning ventricle is largely deprived of this rapidly responsive compensatory mechanism. On the other hand, adrenergic support is partially restored to the failing heart as the result of increased circulating norepinephrine because of its increased synthesis in the peripheral vasculature and adrenal medulla. The symptoms accompanying utilization of sympathetic assistance include tachycardia, tachyarrhythmias, and those due to redistribution of peripheral blood flow such as excessive sweating, cool skin, and oliguria.

Extracardiac Compensatory Mechanisms

It is clear that a state of systemic arteriolar and venous constriction is characteristic of human CHF. This vasoconstriction compensates for the reduced performance of the heart in support of central and peripheral circulatory function.

Arteries. The increase in total systemic vascular resistance provides a peripheral circulatory mechanism by which arterial pressure is maintained in the face of a low cardiac output. This arteriolar constriction in CHF is produced mainly by increased sympathetic nervous activity and by a stiffness component in the arteriolar wall. In contrast to the failing myocardium, there are increased labile stores of norepinephrine in the arteriolar beds of skeletal muscle in patients with CHF. The altered mechanical properties of the arterioles in CHF result from increased sodium and water content in the vessel itself and are responsible for the decreased systemic arteriolar dilator capacity in CHF patients.

With failure of the heart as a pump, there is decrease in blood flow to most regions of the body. However, since the uniform reduction of flow to all areas might result in critical decline of tissue oxygen tension in some organs, in severe CHF this reduction of flow is not uniform and redistribution of flow occurs.

In advanced CHF, blood flow to the renal and cutaneous circulations is reduced disproportionately more than to other areas. At the same time, coronary blood flow remains normal at all stages of CHF in the absence of coronary arterial disease and blood flow to skeletal muscle and brain tends to be preserved except with marked CHF. Thus, adrenergic-mediated vasoconstriction occurs in the kidneys and skin and thereby blood is diverted to the heart, brain, and skeletal muscle, which have high metabolic requirements relative to flow. As a consequence of these regional adjustments in heart failure, there is deterioration of renal function and impairment of the dissipation of heat generated by the metabolic processes within the body. This is the mechanism that may underlie the heat intolerance and body temperature elevations experienced by some CHF patients.

Veins. The overall systemic venous capacitance bed is relatively indistensible in CHF and thereby affords another peripheral circulatory mechanism for the aid of the failing heart. Thus, the adrenergic-induced increase of venous tone is accompanied by a shift of blood in the systemic venous reservoir toward the central circulation, which augments venous return to the heart and assists in utilization of the Frank-Starling mechanism to maintain cardiac output by elevating ventricular diastolic filling. In addition to these alterations in venous tone at rest in CHF, during exercise there is an excessive rise in venous tone and central venous pressure mediated by increased sympathetic nervous activity and thereby enhanced return of blood to the impaired ventricle.

Kidneys. By their influence on total blood volume through action on salt and water balance, renal mechanisms contribute actively to the altered hemodynamics comprising the heart failure state. Thus, with reduced renal blood flow, which may occur prior to reduction of cardiac output due to increased adrenergic activity and redistribution of total blood flow, the kidneys retain sodium and water, which increases the intravascular volume, thereby enhancing ventricular filling and use of the Frank-Starling mechanism for control of cardiac output.

The detection and quantification of occult impairment of sodium excretion in patients with heart disease constitutes the basis of the *oral sodium tolerance test.* Early in CHF, blood flow to the kidney is reduced to a greater extent than reduction of glomerular filtration rate; thereby the filtration fraction is increased and the reabsorption of sodium rises in the proximal convoluted tubules. It is speculated that this increased reabsorption of sodium in CHF is the result, in part, of insufficiency of an undefined hormonal substance that normally causes proximal renal tubular sodium rejection. In addition, with more advanced CHF, the renin-angiotensin-aldosterone system is activated, and inappropriate increased secretion of antidiuretic hormone occurs as well, thus leading to enhanced sodium and water reabsorption in the distal tubules. Unlike normal subjects who exhibit diuresis with adrenergic blockade, in persons with CHF any tendency for an antiadrenergic effect to enhance sodium excretion is overcome by worsening of the depressed cardiocirculatory status, which produces further retention of sodium and water.

Functional Classification of Clinical CHF

The primary objective of the compensatory mechanisms in clinical CHF is to maintain basal cardiac output at a normal level. Therefore, initial CHF symptoms are related to unfavorable side effects necessarily resulting from the action of these mechanisms in performance of their role. Late CHF symptoms are due to low cardiac output, which is the last hemodynamic variable to become abnormal when myocardial function is reduced.

From these observations, the clinical manifestations of advancing CHF develop initially (Class II functional classification of the New York Heart Association) with dyspnea on exertion (early use of the Frank-Starling mechanism), fatigue with more than ordinary activity (reduced response of cardiac output with exercise due to diminished cardiac contractility), exertional angina pectoris (ventricular hypertrophy with consequent increased myocardial oxygen demands), and excessive tachycardia and sweating with exercise (augmented sympathetic discharge). In the next phase, as the condition worsens (Class III), dyspnea, fatigue, angina, tachycardia, and sweating occur with ordinary activity (further depression of contractility with increased use of compensatory mechanisms). These result finally in deterioration (Class IV) with weakness, cachexia, mental confusion, oliguria, and hypotension in addition to the other symptoms at rest (due to reduced basal cardiac output and poor organ perfusion despite maximal use of compensatory mechanisms).

There may be considerable overlap between the relations of altered hemodynamics and clinical features. Thus, when diuretic treatment reduces congestive symptoms and concurrently reduces availability of the Frank-Starling mechanism, a Class III patient may be converted to Class II symptoms with reduced cardiac output at rest. Furthermore, these patient functional classes comprise a continuum rather than discrete categories. In Class II (congestion with moderate activity) and Class III (congestion with mild activity), heart failure is compensated (normal basal cardiac output), and in Class IV (congestion at rest) decompensation (low basal cardiac output) occurs. It is evident from this consideration of the correlation of clinical signs and symptoms with pathophysiologic mechanisms that the traditional clinical classification of CHF is principally based on deleterious expressions of the activity of compensatory mechanisms and not directly on the evaluation of this condition's fundamental hemodynamic variable (cardiac output), the maintenance of which is responsible for CHF symptomatology.

CLINICAL FEATURES

The clinical manifestations of heart failure vary considerably and are dependent upon a number of factors such as the specific etiology of heart disease, the actual cardiac chambers disturbed by the disease process, the degree and rate of development of cardiac dysfunction, and the precipitating causes of CHF.

Symptoms

Pulmonary Congestion. The cardinal symptom complex related to left heart failure (that of shortness-of-breath, due to pulmonary congestion) may occur with increasing severity: exertional dyspnea, orthopnea, paroxysmal nocturnal dyspnea, rest dyspnea, and acute pulmonary edema. Progressive degrees of pulmonary capillary and venous distention produce *exertional dyspnea, orthopnea* (supine dyspnea), and *rest dyspnea* as engorged vessels encroach upon small airspaces and cause lung stiffness, restricted ventilation, decreased vital capacity and tidal volume, peripheral airway trapping with increased dead space, and ventilation-perfusion alterations with consequent widened alveolar-arterial oxygen difference and hypoxemia. Further, bronchial congestion leads to the dyspnea equivalent of *cough,* which may become productive when mucus secretion is stimulated. The presence of pulmonary interstitial edema induces attacks of *paroxysmal nocturnal dyspnea,* and bronchospasm resulting from extravascular swelling of bronchial mucosa causes episodes of *cardiac asthma.* Alveolar edema with transudation and expectoration of blood-tinged sputum underlies *acute pulmonary edema,* while rupture of distended bronchial capillaries can result in hemoptysis.

Lowered Cardiac Output. Impaired cardiac output response to physical activity brings about *easy fatigability,* and diminished resting stroke output results in *cerebral symptoms* and even syncope. Sympathetic-induced redistribution of regional blood flow away from the kidneys during physical activity subsequently leads to the diurnal pattern of *nocturia* with resting recumbency relatively early in CHF, whereas oliguria occurs with renal failure and is a late finding in CHF when basal cardiac output is markedly depressed.

Systemic Congestion. The principal symptoms of right heart failure relate to congestion of the liver and gastrointestinal tract. These include right upper quadrant discomfort, anorexia, nausea, and constipation.

Physical Signs

Depressed Cardiac Contractility. Early impairment of ventricular contractility is usually accompanied by a low-frequency *early diastolic gallop (S_3)* audible with the stethoscope bell placed lightly over the apex of the appropriate ventricle. *Presystolic atrial gallop (S_4)* may also be heard with ventricular dysfunction; this finding does not necessarily denote ventricular decompensation but rather represents decreased diastolic compliance of the corresponding ventricle. In sinus tachycardia, third and fourth heart sounds usually merge during diastole to produce a *summation gallop.* Third heart sounds may be heard in normal adolescents and young adults, and fourth heart sounds are often heard in apparently normal older individuals. Since the rate of left ventricular pressure rise is diminished during isovolumic systole with depressed contractility, there is *first heart sound decreased intensity* in left ventricular failure. Left ventricular ejection may also be delayed with myocardial failure; thus, *paradoxical second heart sound splitting* may occur (pulmonic component of the second sound precedes aortic component) in which second heart sound splitting widens during expiration, in contrast to normal second heart sound splitting increasing with inspiration.

Pulsus Alternans. With severe left ventricular dysfunction, relatively evenly spaced alterations of strong and weak peripheral pulses may occur with each beat. This phenomenon, known as pulsus alternans, is observed most commonly in aortic stenosis, systemic hypertension, cardiomyopathies, and coronary artery disease. While the precise mechanism leading to the development and perpetuation of pulsus alternans is not firmly established, it is generally regarded that there is alteration of force of ventricular contraction due to variations in contractility, preload, electrical excitability, and refractoriness. In some patients, pulsus alternans may persist for several days, whereas in other individuals it may be initiated by a premature ventricular contraction and last for only a few beats. In general, discrepancy between amplitude of strong and weak beats and duration of the phenomenon are directly related to depression of left ventricular contractile state.

Dicrotic Pulse. Palpable dicrotic carotid pulsation may occur in left ventricular pump failure. Normally, carotid pulse rises rapidly to its peak or anacrotic shoulder coincident with peak carotid blood flow (percussion wave). The subsequent tidal wave descending limb is interrupted by a dicrotic notch (coincident with aortic valve closure). The dicrotic notch is followed by a small upward diastolic wave (normally not palpable). In left ventricular failure with reduced stroke volume and cardiac output, however, the characteristic percussion wave decrease in amplitude and rate of rise result in increased amplitude of dicrotic pulse, which often becomes palpable. Also in left ventricular failure, the carotid pulse ejection period may become shortened because of diminishhed stroke volume and elevated peripheral vascular resistance.

Elevated Sympathetic Tone. Other abnormalities in the systemic arterial tree are caused by increased sympathetic activity of CHF. The resting heart rate is increased with excessive rise in pulse rate after minimal exertion, as well as mild diastolic hypertension with narrow pulse pressure. Increased sympathetic tone also produces venoconstriction, which contributes to increased jugular venous pressure. Increased sympathetic activity with low cardiac output in CHF results in redistribution of peripheral blood flow among the body's organs. Thus, relatively less blood flow is delivered to the cutaneous and renal circulations, causing decreased skin temperature, heat intolerance, and often prerenal azotemia. Distal extremities become cool, increased sweating occurs, and peripheral cyanosis results from increased oxygen extraction with oxygen desaturation in cutaneous veins.

Peripheral Cyanosis. The bluish cutaneous color of cyanosis is best visualized in the oral mucous membranes, tongue and lips, around the mouth, conjunctiva, digital nail beds, fingers, and hands. This abnormal coloration is usually not seen until systemic arterial oxygen saturation becomes less than 85 per cent. Cyanosis is either central or peripheral in origin. Central cyanosis, seen principally in the facial and digital areas, results from intrapulmonary admixture or generalized hypoventilation with diminished ventilation-perfusion and from right-to-left intracardiac shunting in congenital heart diseases. Peripheral cyanosis, limited to the extremities, occurs with marked stasis of blood in CHF with low basal cardiac output, shock states, peripheral arterial or venous obstructive disease, and intense limb vasoconstriction such as cold environment or Raynaud's phenomenon.

Ventricular Hypertrophy. Chronic left ventricular failure ultimately results in progressive left ventricular hypertrophy, which can easily be perceived by precordial palpation. In concentric hypertrophy without dilation, left ventricular hypertrophy produces increased amplitude and duration of the apical pulse with the patient in the left lateral position, often without modification of its location. In hypertrophy with reduced left ventricular compliance, palpation reveals prominent presystolic pulsation caused by left atrial contraction in the presence of diminished ventricular distensibility. With right ventricular hypertrophy, abnormal outward motion along the left sternal border occurs during systole.

Ventricular Dilation. Left ventricular dilation, occurring as a compensatory mechanism to maintain normal resting cardiac output, is appreciated by precordial palpation. With the patient supine, the normal left ventricular impulse occurs during isovolumic systole in the fourth or fifth intercostal space medial to the midclavicular line. An apical impulse lateral to the midclavicular line is indicative of left ventricular dilation. Segmental dyssynergy of the left ventricular anterior wall and apex in coronary heart disease also causes cardiac enlargement with lateral apical pulse sustained in its outward motion during systole. Left ventricular dilation also causes widening of the mitral valve ring and disturbance of papillary muscle function with consequent incompetence of the mitral valve leaflets. Thus, left ventricular dilation itself may lead to some degree of mitral regurgitation which is characterized by an accompanying murmur, commonly pansystolic at the cardiac apex, best heard with the patient in the left lateral decubitus position. Similarly, right ventricular dilation can lead to tricuspid regurgitation with a systolic murmur, often increased in intensity during inspiration, heard best at the left lower sternal border.

Excessive Left Ventricular End-Diastolic Pressure. Left ventricular failure produces an increase in left ventricular end-diastolic pressure and in left atrial pressure, which is transmitted to the pulmonary capillaries via an increase in pulmonary venous pressure. When pulmonary capillary hydrostatic pressure exceeds colloid osmotic pressure, there is fluid transudation into interstitial spaces leading to increased lung extravascular fluid and *pulmonary edema.* Interstitial edema leads to alveolar edema, with pulmonary rales detectable by chest wall auscultation.

Pleural Effusion. Pleural effusions are also common in chronic CHF. It is not well recognized that hydrothorax most often occurs with right heart failure or biventricular failure; increased systemic venous pressure is more important than elevated pulmonary capillary pressure in pleural effusion formation.

Valsalva Maneuver. The engorged pulmonary vasculature in left heart failure produces a characteristically abnormal Valsalva response (forceful expiration against closed glottis). Normally a brief initial rise in systemic arterial pressure (representing sudden blood flow from the pulmonary bed into the left heart) occurs, and arterial pressure then falls (reflecting decreased cardiac output resulting from diminished venous return); this in turn stimulates reflex carotid baroreceptor sympathetic-induced vasoconstriction. With discontinuation of expiration, sudden release of thoracic cavity positive pressure causes a brief additional drop in arterial pressure. Then arterial pressure normally rises immediately above pre-

Valsalva control arterial pressure accompanied by reflex bradycardia. The striking post-Valsalva arterial pressure overshoot is due principally to continued reflex sympathetic vasoconstriction. In contrast, with left ventricular failure the pulmonary reservoir maintains left ventricular filling throughout the maneuver. Consequently, stroke volume ejected from the impaired left ventricle is maintained and systemic blood pressure remains elevated. Since systemic blood pressure does not fall, and thus increased baroreceptor stimulation is absent, forced expiration release results in neither post-Valsalva systemic blood pressure overshoot nor reflex bradycardia.

Excessive Right Ventricular End-Diastolic Pressure. Visual inspection of the jugular veins permits a remarkably accurate estimation of *central venous pressure* and, in turn, right heart failure, since with elevation of right ventricular end-diastolic pressure right atrial pressure rises. Elevated venous pressure is best observed in the right external and internal jugular veins, with the patient's head elevated so that the blood-oscillating column top can easily be noted. With the patient supine, the head of the bed is tilted upward until the jugular veins begin to empty in a pulsating meniscus representing the blood column summit. Central venous pressure is equal in centimeters of water to this meniscus height measured relative to the right atrium, which serves as the column's lowest point or zero level. At the bedside, column height is estimated using the superior sternal angle as reference point, since the right atrium is approximately 5 cm below the sternal angle. With the patient's head elevated approximately 30°, the vertical distance between the sternal angle level to oscillating blood column top is normally less than 3 cm. Thus, this 3 cm plus the 5 cm from the sternal angle to right atrium equals 8 cm of blood, or approximately 11 mm Hg. The central systemic venous pressure is elevated when the vertical distance between the highest point of the visible pulsation of the jugular vein is greater than 3 cm above the sternal angle.

Peripheral Edema. Peripheral edema is generally found in chronic right heart failure as a result of elevated systemic venous pressure and salt and water retention from diminished renal perfusion. Edema formation occurs in the dependent body portions, usually in the pretibial areas, and can be differentiated from lymphedema by characteristic pitting with mild finger pressure. Noncardiac edema, usually more diffuse in location, is caused by chronic renal disease, profound hypoalbuminemia, Cushing's disease, and premenstrual period. In primary hepatic cirrhosis, ascites is proportionally greater than ankle edema. Facial edema rarely occurs in CHF and is most commonly the result of superior vena caval obstruction or strenuous respiratory efforts due to chronic obstructive lung disease.

Abdominal Examination. In right heart failure, elevation of right atrial pressure increases venous pressure throughout the entire systemic venous bed. This leads to engorgement of abdominal organs with *hepatomegaly* and occasionally splenomegaly. These organs are tender with acute congestion. Severe tricuspid regurgitation causes the liver to pulsate during systole. In addition, peripheral edema and *ascites* occur in severe chronic right heart failure. A useful maneuver to elucidate borderline right ventricular failure is the *hepatojugular reflux,* in which pressure applied by the open hand to the right upper quadrant increases venous return to the right heart. Since the failing right ventricle is unable to accept this increased venous return, the maneuver elicits an abnormal rise in jugular venous pulse in addition to accentuating the prominent V wave of tricuspid regurgitation.

Chest Roentgenogram. The frontal chest film serves as a useful screening test for the presence of CHF by virtue of changes in cardiac size and configuration combined with abnormalities of the lung fields. Normally, in the erect position, there is better perfusion of the lung bases than the apices. When left atrial, pulmonary venous, and capillary pressures become elevated, interstitial and perivascular edema develops, particularly in the lung bases where hydrostatic pressure is greatest. The consequent pulmonary vessel compression in the lower lobes causes equalization of vascular size throughout the lung fields with modest increase in pulmonary capillary pressure. *Pulmonary vascular redistribution,* manifested by greater prominence of upper lobe vascularity, takes place with moderate elevation of pulmonary capillary pressure. Marked increase in pulmonary capillary pressure leads to interstitial edema characterized by *septal Kerley's lines* of interlobar interstitial edema, perivascular blunting of peripheral vessels, and subpleural fluid accumulation between the lung and adjacent pleural surface. Severely excessive pulmonary capillary pressure results in alveolar edema and large pleural effusions.

NONINVASIVE TECHNIQUES FOR ASSESSING CARDIAC FUNCTION

Systolic Time Intervals

The simultaneous recording of the ECG, phonocardiogram, and carotid arterial pulsations allows indirect determination of total electromechanical systole ($Q\text{-}S_2$ interval: beginning of QRS complex to the first high-frequency vibration of the second heart sound), left ventricular ejection time (LVET: onset of upstroke to incisural notch on the carotid tracing), and the pre-ejection period (PEP: electromechanical systole minus ejection time). In patients with primary and secondary abnormalities of myocardial contractility, often before the onset of overt CHF, the pre-ejection period usually lengthens while the ejection time shortens. Thus, the ratio of the pre-ejection period to ejection time (PEP:LVET) provides a useful index of cardiac function, permitting relative separation of patients with diminished contractility from normal subjects. In patients with heart disease, the PEP:LVET ratio appears to be sensitive to diminished contractile state in the cardiomyopathies, systemic arterial hypertension, and chronic coronary artery disease.

In valvular heart disease, however, the index is somewhat less accurate owing owing to concomitant chronic pressure and volume overload. Acute myocardial infarction usually results in normal or variable PEP, whereas the LVET is abbreviated. In serial studies in individual patients, PEP is altered by acute changes of preload or afterload alone, in addition to changes in contractility. Digitalis tends to shorten both PEP and LVET. Leg exercise in patients with angina pectoris due to coronary artery disease leads to an increase of LVET, whereas this interval is unchanged with exercise in normal subjects. PEP normally shortens with exercise and remains unchanged in patients with angina. Left intraventricular conduction defects produce lengthening of PEP without alterations of LVET. In the presence of left ventricular conduction disturbances, determination of the isovolumic contraction time as the measure of pre-ejection duration appears to offer potential advantages over PEP, since the isovolumic contraction time is not influenced by variations of QRS depolarization time among different ventricles.

Echocardiography

The ability to image the left ventricle and other heart chambers by ultrasound has led to intense interest in the evaluation of cardiac function by echocardiography. Echocardiographic measurements of left ventricular dimension have been utilized in the evaluation of cardiac performance, as have indices of left ventricular volume, stroke volume, and ejection fraction derived from simple dimensional measurements. The velocity of dimensional shortening has also been calculated from echocardiographic recordings of the left ventricle, as have the thickness and motion patterns of the walls of the left ventricular chamber. In addition, aberrations of valvular motion patterns, such as mitral and pulmonic valve abnormalities in the setting of elevated left ventricular end-diastolic pressure and pulmonary hypertension, have been utilized in the evaluation of cardiac function.

Left Ventricular Size. A measure of left ventricular size, or left ventricular dimension, may be obtained continuously throughout the cardiac cycle by an M-mode echogram through the body of the left ventricle in a plane just below the mitral leaflets. Furthermore, the thickness of both the interventricular septum and posterobasal wall may also be computed at any point of contraction or relaxation. The cube of the echographic left ventricular end-systolic and end-diastolic dimensions provides corresponding left ventricular volumes. Thus, stroke volume may be determined as the difference between end-diastolic and end-systolic volumes, and ejection fraction as stroke volume related to end-diastolic volume.

To obtain the optimal left ventricular minor axis dimension, it is necessary to record an echo that traverses the interventricular septum and left ventricular posterior wall simultaneously, in an area just below the major deflection of the mitral leaflets. Numerous investigators have shown close correlation between echographic left ventricular volumes and those obtained by contrast cineangiography. However, echographic volumes are unreliable in the presence of extreme left ventricular dilation or substantial areas of left ventricular segmental dyssynergy. These discrepancies are exaggerated in systole as compared with diastole.

Two-dimensional echocardiography has made a significant contribution to the evaluation of left ventricular size by ultrasound. Thus, by enabling visualization of the entire ventricular circumference, a two-dimensional echocardiogram avoids the difficulty of analyzing a dimension of the left ventricle through an area that is not representative of the overall size of this chamber. In addition, cross-sectional echocardiography provides visualization of the left ventricle in multiple planes so that biplane estimations of actual left ventricular size may be achieved.

Right Ventricular Size. Estimation of the size of the right ventricle is difficult by M-mode echocardiography owing to the shape of the right ventricle as well as to technical problems of clearly defining the endocardial surface of the right ventricular anterior wall. Thus, the clinical utility of such measurements has not always been of great value. Rather, the size of right ventricular dimension can be compared with that of left ventricular dimension in a semiquantitative fashion; right ventricular size is normally less than half that of the left ventricle.

Two-dimensional echocardiography has an important role in estimation of the size of the right ventricle. Thus, the four-chamber view obtained by positioning the ultrasonic transducer at the point of maximal cardiac impulse has enabled the accurate visualization of right ventricular circumference. Such measurements have been found to correlate well with independent measurements of chamber size obtained by other techniques and have proved of value in distinguishing normal subjects from patients with volume overload of the right-sided cardiac chambers.

Left Ventricular Wall Thickness. The ability of ultrasound to evaluate left ventricular wall thickness provides an important attribute of echocardiography. There is close correlation of left ventricular wall thickness by echography with values obtained at operation, at necropsy, and by left ventricular angiography. Echocardiography accurately predicts the presence of left ventricular hypertrophy in nearly all patients with this abnormality. Thus, left ventricular posterior wall thickness on echogram provides a reliable index of left ventricular hypertrophy and has been utilized in the calculation of left ventricular mass.

Echocardiography also allows quantitative estimation of the width of the interventricular septum. Comparison of left ventricular posterior wall and interventricular septum widths has proved to be of major importance in distinguishing ventricular hypertrophy due to hypertensive cardiovascular disease from that produced by hypertrophic cardiomyopathy; hypertensive disease results in concentric left ventricular hypertrophy, whereas hypertrophic cardiomyopathy presents with asymmetric septal hypertrophy primarily involving the interventricular septum.

Left Ventricular Posterior Wall Motion. Examination of the extent and velocity of circumferential fiber shortening and of the temporal sequence of segmental left ventricular contraction has been utilized in the assessment of ventricular performance in patients with a variety of cardiac disorders. Echocardiography provides a unique noninvasive method for the recording of the velocity and amplitude of left ventricular wall motion, as well as the sequence of contraction and the extent of wall thickening during systole. The contractile characteristics of the portions of the left ventricular wall accessible to ultrasound examination include both the interventricular septum and the left ventricular posterior wall. At the onset of ventricular ejection, the left ventricular posterior wall moves anteriorly toward the ultrasound transducer; anterior motion is rapid at first but then is progressively reduced until termination of systole. During diastole, the left ventricular posterior wall moves posteriorly with greater velocity of motion in early diastole than in late diastole.

Measurements of posterior wall contraction on echography reflect the performance only of that myocardial segment. However, echocardiography is capable of accurately detecting alterations in the contractile pattern of the posterior wall, such as those induced by pharmacologic agents or exercise, and thus provides a sensitive method for assessment of the effects of interventions upon posterior wall motion or for the serial evaluation of cardiac performance in individual patients.

Interventricular Septal Motion. In contrast to the uniform contractile pattern of the posterior wall, the normal motion of the interventricular septum has been found to be heterogeneous. The most superior portion of the interventricular septum, representing the membranous septum, typically exhibits a slight anterior motion during systole. In contrast, the apical portion of the septum characteristically reveals a substantial posterior systolic motion approximating the posterior wall as ejection occurs. The middle portion of the interventricular septum (the segment recorded in the area of the mitral leaflets) represents a transition zone in which septal motion is usually notched or flat, but may be either slightly wholly anterior or posterior. In addition to heterogeneous motion, the echo from the entire interventricular septum displays a prominent notch at the end of ejection and the beginning of diastole.

The echographic contractile pattern of the interventricular septum provides important information regarding the status of cardiac performance. Inappropriate or paradoxical anterior systolic motion of the interventricular septum indicates right ventricular volume overload. It has also become recognized that the contractile pattern of the septum undergoes a characteristic echographic alteration in left bundle branch block; the interventricular septum exhibits a rapid, sharp, posterior peak that occurs within 100 msec of the onset of the QRS complex and is followed by a sustained paradoxical anterior motion. Furthermore, septal dyssynergy (either akinesis or dyskinesis) occurs in primary cardiomyopathies, idiopathic hypertrophic subaortic stenosis, constrictive pericarditis, and the postoperative state after sternotomy. In addition, coronary artery stenosis disturbs the contractile pattern of both the interventricular septum and posterior wall. An important clue to the presence of ischemia is the absence of septal thickening in addition to abnormal motion.

Velocity of Circumferential Fiber Shortening. The velocity of circumferential fiber shortening (V_{CF}), as determined from the left ventricular cineangiogram, has been found to be a useful indicator of left ventricular performance and also estimates left ventricular contractility. V_{CF} can be quantitated with echocardiography as mean V_{CF} by the equation

$$(Dd\text{-}Ds)/(ET \cdot Dd);$$

where Dd is end-diastolic dimension, Ds is end-systolic dimension, and ET is ejection time (measured as the time from onset of QRS on the electrocardiogram to the peak posterior wall contraction, minus 50 msec for isovolumic contraction).

Echographic V_{CF} provides a useful index of ventricular performance, especially in the presence of valvular heart disease or cardiomyopathy. The good correlation of echographic V_{CF} with ventricular function in some patients with segmental wall abnormalities due to coronary disease may be related to the hyperkinesis of the uninvolved myocardium. Preservation of a normal or increased amplitude of contraction of one ventricular wall may be the principal echographic feature that distinguishes coronary patients with CHF from those with congestive cardiomyopathy in whom wall motion is characteristically diffusely depressed. Echographic V_{CF} is affected by alterations in ventricular afterload and, to a lesser extent, ventricular preload. Thus, V_{CF} measured by ultrasound reflects overall cardiac pump performance rather than myocardial contractility specifically.

Nuclear Cardiology

Noninvasive radioisotopic techniques for the instantaneous wide-field imaging of the cardiac blood pool provide determination of global and regional left and right ventricular function, as well as important information regarding cardiac chamber anatomy and intracardiac shunts. Both equilibrium gated and first-pass scintigraphic cardiac blood pool methods can be utilized for these purposes.

Multiple-Gated Equilibrium Blood Pool Scintigraphy. By combining a computer with an Anger-type single crystal scintillation camera and gating device, it is possible to obtain images of the cardiac blood pool during selected segments from the entire cardiac cycle. The resulting scintigraphic information can be used to form a ventricular equilibration activity-versus-time curve. Since the number of counts emitted from the blood pool radiopharmaceutical (^{99m}Tc-labeled autologous red blood cells) is proportional to the blood volume in a given region after background subtraction, the ventricular activity-versus-time curve represents a relative volume-versus-time curve of the left ventricle. From this curve, ejection fraction can be measured by comparing peak-to-valley radioactivity concentrations.

The multiple-gated equilibrium technique has proved to be an accurate method for assessing regional wall motion and left ventricular ejection fraction. It has been particularly valuable for a number of indications in evaluating cardiac function in both acute and chronic coronary artery disease patients.

Since, in the asymptomatic stage, most coronary patients have normal wall motion and normal left ventricular ejection fraction at rest, an important development has been exercise scintigraphy in which left ventricular performance is assessed by multiple-gated equilibrium cardiac blood pool scintigraphy at rest and during bicycle exercise. In normal subjects, ejection fraction rises during exercise and no regional wall motion abnormalities develop. In contrast, in coronary patients, ejection fraction typically falls during exercise or fails to rise and new regional wall motion abnormalities develop.

First-Pass Blood Pool Scintigraphy. In contrast to equilibrium blood pool scintigraphic techniques in which images are taken over a period of minutes, the first-transit scintigraphic cardiac blood pool studies require only a few seconds to perform. These studies may be used for evaluation of ventricular function and, in addition, are well suited for assessment of the pattern of blood flow through the heart. The radiopharmaceutical usually employed is ^{99m}Tc in the simple sodium-pertechnetate form. For data acquisition, the first-pass study involves the collection of scintigraphic data during the initial transit of the radioactive bolus through the chambers of the heart. Multiple-gated images of the first transit can be obtained by temporal summation of counts from corresponding segments of the cardiac cycle obtained over several cycles during the first pass utilizing a multicrystal scintillation camera. Thus, the correct distinction is between first pass and equilibrium studies rather than first-transit and gated studies. Ejection fraction is measured with the first-transit method by monitoring the cyclic oscillations in count rate over the left ventricle during the initial transit of the radioactive bolus.

CARDIAC CATHETERIZATION

In evaluation of the principal determinants of cardiac performance in heart disease, it is possible to measure precisely ventricular preload (end-diastolic pressure, volume, and tension) and afterload (Laplace relation in which systolic tension is directly equated with the product of ventricular systolic pressure and radius). However, it is considerably more difficult to assess accurately contractility (inotropism or contractile state) of the intact human heart. There are two general approaches to evaluation of contractility and function of the heart:

1. Its pump (hemodynamics) performance characteristics.
2. Its muscle (mechanics) performance characteristics.

Hemodynamic Performance

In the traditional approach of pump analysis, the contractile state can be estimated qualitatively by standard hemodynamic variables of ventricular function of *cardiac output* (normal $>$ 2.50 L/min/M^2), stroke volume, systolic ejection rate, and left ventricular *end-diastolic pressure* (normal $<$ 13 mm Hg); and the more complex measurements of left ventricular end-diastolic volume, *ejection fraction* (normal $>$ 0.60)), stroke work, stroke power, and ventricular mass.

Although these hemodynamic variables provide considerable useful information about cardiac function and directional inotropic differences, they are indirect and qualitative indicators of cardiac contractility. The sensitivity of cardiac pump measurements in the evaluation of contractility is increased by determining the hemodynamic response to certain interventions such as exercise and alterations in ventricular loading. Further, inotropic estimation is improved by evaluating hemodynamic responses within the concept of the Frank-Starling principle (ventricular function curve), which relates pump performance characteristics such as cardiac output to left ventricular end-diastolic pressure.

Mechanical Performance

It has become possible to clinically examine contractility in terms of muscle mechanics which describe the force, velocity, and length properties of the ventricular myocardium. In the numerical assessment of contractile state, the mechanical events occurring during both the isovolumic and ejection phases of systole have been characterized. Thus, mechanical measures of inotropic state have been developed along two general lines:

1. *Isovolumic indices* utilizing dp/dt (rate of ventricular pressure rise).
2. *Ejection indices* employing V_{CF} (circumferential fiber shortening rate).

It has been difficult to evaluate the validity and accuracy of these indices of contractility in the intact heart, since there is no standard measure of this property of the myocardium with which they can be compared. Nevertheless, the mechanical indices provide qualitative and quantitative estimation of contractility alterations in single patients in response to interventions and of basal contractile state between different patients.

CARDIAC ARRHYTHMIAS

By Stephen C. Hammill, M.D.
David R. Holmes, Jr., M.D.
and Douglas L. Wood, M.D.
Rochester, Minnesota

Cardiac arrhythmias occur in a wide variety of patients, ranging from the asymptomatic patient with occasional premature atrial complexes to the one with ventricular tachycardia or ventricular fibrillation who dies suddenly. The physician caring for patients with disturbances in cardiac rhythm must evaluate the disturbance correctly because prognosis and therapy are based on the diagnosis. Harm can come to the patient if a rhythm disturbance is diagnosed as being benign when, in reality, the disturbance is potentially life-threatening. In this circumstance, the physician may decide not to treat such a patient and serious consequences can result. Similarly, the patient with a benign cardiac arrhythmia, whose arrhythmia is misdiagnosed and believed to be life-threatening, may suffer undue anxiety and side effects due to the therapy because of improper diagnosis.

This article describes the presenting symptoms and the associated physical findings in patients with disturbance of cardiac rhythm. The various disturbances in rhythm will be defined, and newer diagnostic techniques that can be performed in the physician's office or at the patient's bedside will be described. Finally, several syndromes associated with cardiac arrhythmias will be discussed.

SYMPTOMS ASSOCIATED WITH CARDIAC ARRHYTHMIAS

Obtaining an accurate clinical history from a patient with suspected cardiac arrhythmias is extremely important. Patients can be asymptomatic; or they can have variable symptoms of palpitations, chest pain, dyspnea, diaphoresis, lightheadedness, near-syncope and syncope, and may die suddenly. Because patients may have similar symptoms not associated with disturbances in cardiac rhythm, these symptoms are not pathognomonic of cardiac arrhythmias.

The variable clinical presentation depends on hemodynamic consequences of the arrhythmia, associated clinical problems, and the unique awareness that each patient has of his heart rhythm. In turn, the hemodynamic consequences of the arrhythmia are dependent on:

1. The heart rate during the arrhythmia.
2. The presence or absence of atrioventricular (AV) synchrony.
3. The effect on coronary blood flow.
4. The effect on cerebral blood flow.
5. The duration of the arrhythmia.
6. The effect of reflex responses to the arrhythmia.
7. Associated cardiac or extracardiac abnormalities.

The goal in taking the patient's history is to document the presence or absence of an arrhythmia, establish the relationship between the arrhythmia and the clinical symptoms, identify the type of arrhythmia and its precipitating cause, and establish the presence or absence of associated clinical problems that may affect the arrhythmia.

Palpitations

Palpitations are probably the most common symptom of patients presenting with arrhythmias. Although physicians define palpitations as a change in heart rate, rhythm, or contractility, patients are not bound by such a definition and, more frequently, describe their symptoms as flip-flops, fluttering, or skipping. It is helpful, in this regard, to have the patient illustrate the cadence of his specific complaint by tapping out the rhythm with his hand. Alternatively, the physician may tap out several cadences and have the patient select the appropriate one. This, plus specific questioning in terms of onset and termination of the arrhythmia, the duration, and regularity or irregularity, helps the experienced clinician narrow the etiologic possibilities. Subsequent sections will describe the typical history associated with the various rhythm disturbances.

Lightheadedness, Near-Syncope, and Syncope

A brief disturbance in normal consciousness is a common presenting symptom. When it is an isolated occurrence with an adequate explanation, the physician is seldom consulted. However, if the disturbance recurs, it may become a matter of concern and may require that one weigh such episodes as evidence of an underlying disease and distinguish syncope on the basis of a disturbance in the cardiac rhythm from epilepsy, vertigo, hyperventilation, and many other conditions (Table 1).

The terms "syncope" and "faint" can be used interchangeably and refer to a transient, rapid, or even abrupt disturbance of consciousness associated with an inability to maintain postural tone. This is due to a global compromise in cerebral perfusion. The patient with disturbance in cardiac rhythm may present with a decrease in global perfusion. This results in various degrees of lightheadedness, near-syncope, and syncope.

Syncope due to a cardiac abnormality results from a transiently diminished cardiac output secondary to cardiac arrhythmia (Table 2) or to reduced stroke volume. The major cardiac abnormalities that result in syncope include cardiac arrhythmias, ischemic heart disease, valvular heart disease, and congenital anomalies of the heart. The onset of cardiac syncope is usually more rapid than the onset of other types of fainting; in fact, it may be so sudden that there are no premonitory symptoms. If symptoms occur, they consist of lightheadedness, nausea, blurring of vision, a sense of rapid heart action, or other cardiac distress. Recovery may be equally rapid. In general, the patient is not left with lingering postsyncopal discomfort. A significant proportion of patients with cardiac syncope exhibit anoxic convulsions during the spell. A distinguishing characteristic of cardiac syncope is that it may occur with the patient in either the recum-

Table 1. Major Clinical Types of Syncopal Disorders

Vasodepressor or vasovagal syncope
Orthostatic syncope due to poor postural adjustment (orthostatic hypotension)
Cardiac syncope due to cardiac arrhythmias (see Table 2): ischemic heart disease, valvular heart disease, and congenital heart disease
Syncope due to primary pulmonary hypertension
Carotid sinus syncope:
Cardioinhibitory type
Vasodepressor type
Glossopharyngeal-vagal syncope
Cerebrovascular syncope
Micturition syncope
Pressor-postpressor syncope

Table 2. Disturbances in Cardiac Rhythm Associated with Syncope

Sick Sinus Syndrome
- Sinus arrest
- Sinoatrial conduction block
- Tachycardia-bradycardia syndrome

Supraventricular Tachyarrhythmias
- Atrial fibrillation
- Atrial flutter
- Atrial tachycardia
- Paroxysmal supraventricular tachycardia due to re-entry within the atrioventricular node or a concealed accessory atrioventricular pathway
- Anomalies resulting in enhanced atrioventricular conduction during supraventricular tachycardia
  - Wolff-Parkinson-White syndrome
  - Lown-Ganong-Levine syndrome
  - Enhanced atrioventricular node conduction

Atrioventricular Dissociation
- Type I atrioventricular block (hypervagotonia)
- Type II atrioventricular block (His-Purkinje disease)
- Complete heart block due to:
  - Congenital heart block
  - Drug toxicity (digitalis, verapamil, quinidine, lidocaine, phenytoin)
  - Electrolyte disturbances
  - Valvular heart disease
  - Myocarditis (viral, rheumatic fever, toxoplasmosis, syphilis, mumps, diphtheria)
  - Coronary artery disease
  - Infiltrative cardiomyopathy (amyloidosis, sarcoidosis, hemochromatosis)
  - Collagen vascular disease
  - Cardiac tumors (primary, metastatic)
  - Degenerative diseases (Lenegre's disease, Lev's disease)
  - Neuromuscular diseases (Duchenne's and myotonic dystrophy, Friedreich's ataxia)

Ventricular Tachyarrhythmias
- Ventricular tachycardia
- Ventricular fibrillation
- Prolonged Q-T syndrome
  - Primary (Jervell and Lange-Nielsen syndrome, Romano-Ward syndrome)
  - Secondary (quinidine, procainamide, disopyramide, hypokalemia, hypocalcemia, hypomagnesemia, cerebral contusion, stroke)

bent or the upright position. Syncope due to cardiac arrhythmias occurs with excessively slow or fast heart rates, causing severely reduced cardiac output. Any disturbances in cardiac rhythm may be transitory and are not necessarily found at subsequent examination. Episodes of syncope should be related to changes in position, since orthostatic hypotension can result in near-syncope or syncope and occurs commonly in elderly patients and patients taking cardiovascular medications.

Chest Pain, Dyspnea, and Diaphoresis

Patients with a disturbance in cardiac rhythm, whether it be an excessively fast or slow rate, may present with chest pain, dyspnea, or diaphoresis. These patients may have associated cardiac abnormalities, including impaired left ventricular function or coronary artery disease. With an excessively fast or slow heart rhythm, the cardiac output decreases, resulting in decreased coronary artery and systemic perfusion. This decrease may result in angina secondary to poor coronary perfusion or in diaphoresis due to sympathetic discharge as a response to hypotension. If left ventricular function worsens, left ventricular end-diastolic pressure may increase, resulting in increased pulmonary venous pressure and in dyspnea.

Specific attention must be directed to the clinical setting in which cardiac arrhythmia occurs, the presence of precipitating factors, and associated clinical problems. The presence of reproducible precipitating factors such as exercise, caffeine use, and alcohol intake has important implications in terms of diagnosing the rhythm disturbance. The physician may not find evidence of a rhythm disturbance when the precipitating factor is absent. In order to identify the rhythm disturbance, the physician may need to record the patient's rhythm in the presence of a known precipitating factor.

As previously mentioned, the variable clinical presentation of arrhythmias is dependent, in part, on associated clinical problems. These clinical problems may be responsible for an arrhythmia and may affect the treatment. For example, paroxysmal supraventricular tachycardia or paroxysmal atrial fibrillation occurring in a patient with severe aortic stenosis may require a different evaluation from that of paroxysmal supraventricular tachycardia occurring in a young, otherwise healthy patient whose paroxysmal supraventricular tachycardia is related to emotional upset, anxiety, or excessive caffeine use.

Care must be taken during the evaluation of patients with rhythm disturbances to obtain detailed information concerning associated cardiovascular, central nervous system, pulmonary, and other organ system diseases which may affect not only the presentation of the arrhythmia but also the clinical treatment and outcome.

SUDDEN DEATH

The increasingly widespread use of paramedical personnel trained in cardiopulmonary resuscitation has increased the numbers of patients who survive cardiac arrest. Most such patients die suddenly from ventricular tachycardia or ventricular fibrillation. *Sudden death* is generally defined as death within 24 hours of the onset of symptoms; death within the first hour of the onset of symptoms is termed *instantaneous death.* Instantaneous death is almost always due to ventricular fibrillation, which is either primary or the result of ventricular tachycardia.

PHYSICAL EXAMINATION

Although electrocardiographic recording techniques are critical in the diagnosis of cardiac arrhythmias, information obtained from the physical examination often can allow the diagnosis of a rhythm abnormality to be made when an electrocardiogram alone is insufficient for this purpose. The jugular venous pulse, the arterial pulse, and heart sounds are the most important physical findings in the bedside diagnosis of cardiac arrhythmias. In addition, the physical examination can aid in the diagnosis of diseases associated with the various arrhythmias.

The jugular venous pulse reflects atrial activity. When used in conjunction with the arterial pulse to provide timing, the jugular venous pulse can aid in the diagnosis of atrial ventricular dissociation. So-called *cannon A waves* occur in the jugular venous pulse when the right atrium contracts against the closed tricuspid valve. When a cannon A wave occurs coincident with arterial pulsation during episodes of tachycardia, the rhythm may be either supraventricular tachycardia with a short P-R interval or ventricular tachycardia with 1:1 ventriculoatrial (VA) conduction. During supraventricular tachycardia with 2:1 AV block, cannon A waves may be noted during every other atrial cycle and are coincident with the arterial pulse. In atrial flutter, flutter waves can sometimes be detected in the jugular venous pulse. Cannon A waves in the presence of bradycardia are suggestive of atrioventricular block. During an episode of ventricular tachycardia, the physician may detect a falling blood pressure, the association of angina pain, congestive heart failure, or pulmonary edema.

Other physical findings during ventricular tachycardia depend on the relationship of the atrial rhythm to the ventricular tachycardia. Patients who demonstrate 1:1 retrograde conduction during tachycardia have a regular cannon A wave in the jugular venous pulse with each beat and have a constant intensity of the first heart sound. Patients with ventriculoatrial dissociation and a regular atrial rhythm have intermittent cannon A waves in the jugular pulse, variation in the intensity of the first heart sound, and beat-to-beat variation in the systolic blood pressure. In patients who also have atrial fibrillation, there are no cannon A waves and the first heart sound is constant.

The most useful heart sound in the diagnosis of rhythm abnormalities is the first one. Alterations in the intensity of the first heart sound in patients with regular tachycardia are suggestive of atrioventricular dissociation, either atrioventricular junctional tachycardia or ventricular tachycardia. The intensity of the first heart sound is not a useful sign in the presence of irregular tachycardias because of the alterations of the intensity caused by changes in the length of the cardiac cycle.

The physical examination also should be directed at detecting underlying cardiac abnormalities and systemic diseases that may be the cause of the rhythm disturbance or affect the presentation of the arrhythmia.

DISTURBANCES IN CARDIAC RHYTHM: DISORDERS OF IMPULSE FORMATION

The following paragraphs outline the most common disorders in cardiac rhythm encountered by the physician. Key terms used in the evaluation of cardiac arrhythmias are defined in the glossary at the end of this article.

Sinus Arrest

Sinus arrest results in an absence of activation of the atrium with no discernible P waves visible on the electrocardiogram (Fig. 1). If there is no escape rhythm, syncope may occur.

Sinus Tachycardia

Sinus tachycardia is a rhythm mechanism that is sinus in origin with a rate of more than 100 beats per minute (bpm). Sinus rhythm is the normal rhythm of the heart and occurs when the impulse arises in the sinus node at a normal rate and is conducted through the atria. Sinus rhythm varies significantly, depending on factors that include body temperature, emotion, neurohumoral status, and physical exertion. The sinus rate increases in response to emotional disturbance, physical exertion, and temperature. The maximal rate observed during sinus rhythm occurs with exercise and varies with age. In healthy young persons, the rate may exceed 200 bpm, whereas in elderly persons it seldom exceeds 140 bpm. When sinus tachycardia occurs in the absence of physiologic factors, evaluation should be performed to determine the underlying cause.

Sinus Bradycardia

Sinus bradycardia is a rhythm with sinus mechanism that is slower than 60 bpm. However, a high

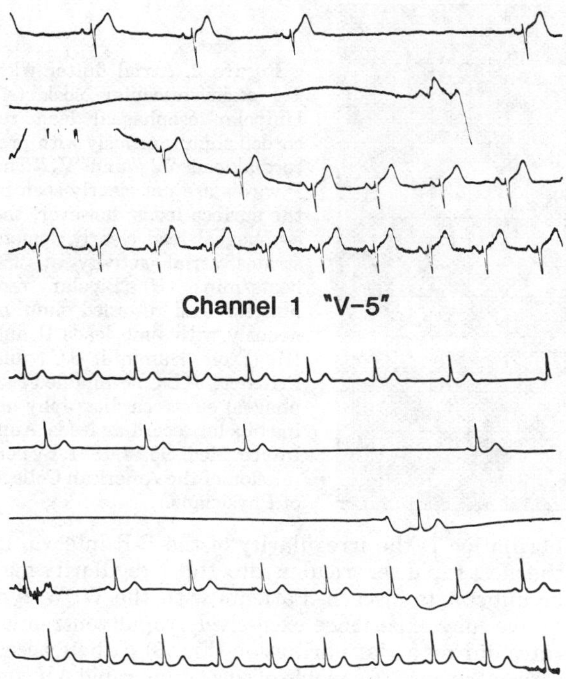

Figure 1. Sinus arrest documented with 24-hour ambulatory monitoring. Channel 2 records "V_1" and demonstrates a sinus bradycardia with a sinus pause followed by sinus arrest. The patient then experiences syncope, resulting in the baseline artifact. Sinus rhythm then resumes. Channel 1 records "V_5" and again demonstrates sinus rhythm with episodes of sinus pause and sinus arrest.

proportion of persons in good physical condition have heart rates between 50 and 60 bpm. A rate of 50 bpm is probably a better cutoff point to differentiate normal sinus rhythm from sinus bradycardia.

Periodic Sinus Arrhythmia

The rate of the normal sinus mechanism is influenced by the sympathetic and parasympathetic nervous systems and exhibits a periodic change that can be synchronized to respiration. This is termed "periodic sinus arrhythmia" and is more pronounced in children and young adults than in older persons. This rhythm disturbance is not pathologic; however, on occasion it may be difficult to distinguish it from an ectopic atrial rhythm or sinoatrial conduction block.

Atrial Premature Complexes

Atrial premature complexes (APCs) are observed commonly in healthy persons. The frequency of APCs increases in persons who have heart disease that results in abnormal atrial musculature or atrial size. In APCs, the P wave has a different shape than during normal sinus rhythm and occurs early in the cardiac cycle. The APCs may be seen very early in the cardiac cycle, at the same time as the T wave; these early P waves are considered to be "buried" in the T waves and can be identified because they deform the T waves. Such APCs may occur too early to be conducted to the ventricle, owing to refractoriness that results from the normal sinus beat, giving the appearance of an atrioventricular conduction block or a sinus pause. However, if the T wave is analyzed, the abnormal P wave can be found, leading to the diagnosis of a nonconducted APC. On occasion, owing to the prematurity in the cardiac cycle of APCs, the resulting QRS complex may be aberrantly conducted. If the abnormal P wave is not observed in the cardiac cycle, the aberrant QRS complex may be misdiagnosed as a premature ventricular complex.

Atrial Flutter

Atrial flutter and atrial fibrillation are among the most frequent causes of supraventricular tachycardias that are encountered clinically. Each is frequently associated with organic heart disease; however, either may be present in patients who have no obvious heart disease. Atrial flutter may be transitory or chronic (Fig. 2). It occurs commonly with acute myocardial infarction and after cardiac surgery in adults and may be seen in children with congenital heart disease. Typical electrocardiographic features of atrial flutter are an atrial rate of 300 bpm with a narrow QRS complex and 2:1 atrioventricular conduction with a ventricular rate of approximately 150 bpm. Atrial activity during atrial flutter causes a specific alteration in the surface electrocardiogram, giving the baseline a very characteristic sawtooth appearance. The atrial rate during atrial flutter ranges from 250 to 300 bpm, although the rate is remarkably close to 300 bpm in most patients, with very little beat-to-beat variation (usually less than 20 msec).

The physiologic characteristics of the AV node require that AV block be present in virtually all cases of atrial flutter. The most common conduction ratio in patients with untreated atrial flutter is 2:1 AV block, which provides the typical ventricular rate of 150 bpm. Higher grades of AV block in patients not treated with digitalis, beta receptor blocking agents, or calcium receptor blocking agents suggest the presence of AV nodal disease or enhanced vagal tone. Drugs that impair AV nodal conduction, specifically digitalis and verapamil, also will cause higher grades of AV block. In some patients, the typical flutter waves may not be evident on the electrocardiogram and, in this circumstance when the diagnosis is in doubt, carotid sinus massage (discussed later) may be a helpful diagnostic maneuver. Carotid sinus massage increases AV block and allows typical flutter waves to be appreciated on the electrocardiogram. In patients with accessory atrioventricular pathways (Wolff-Parkinson-White [WPW] syndrome), impulses may be conducted from the atrium to the ventricle without delay in the AV node during atrial flutter. This rhythm is often poorly tolerated and causes hemodynamic collapse.

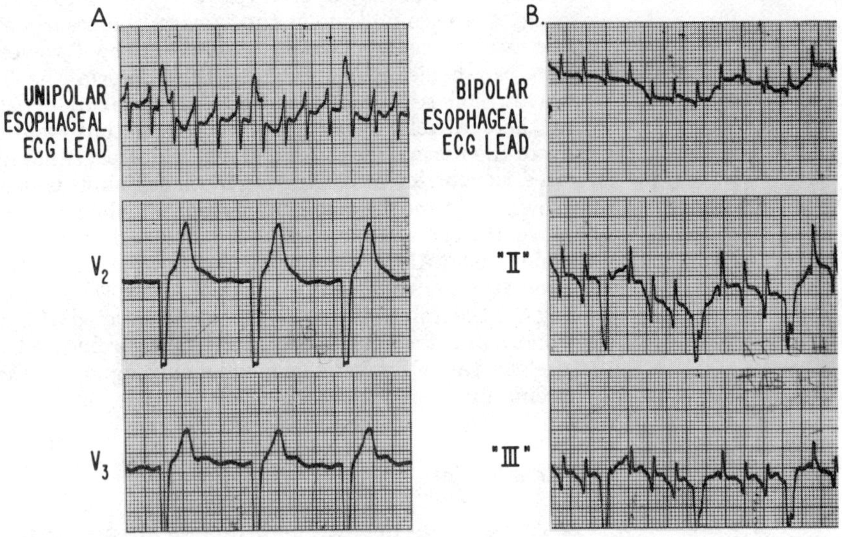

Figure 2. Atrial flutter with 4:1 atrioventricular block. (*A*) Unipolar esophageal lead recorded simultaneously with precordial leads "V_2" and "V_3." The P waves are not clearly seen in the surface leads; however, the esophageal lead clearly demonstrates atrial activity at 280 beats/min. (*B*) Bipolar esophageal lead recorded simultaneously with limb leads II and III. (From Hammill, S.C., and Pritchett, E.L.C.: Simplified esophageal electrocardiography using bipolar recording leads. Ann. Intern. Med., 95:14, 1981. By permission of the American College of Physicians.)

In addition to patients who have accessory AV pathways that result in rapid conduction during atrial flutter, there is a group of patients who demonstrate enhanced AV nodal conduction. These patients may have what represents the end of the spectrum of AV nodal conduction properties, or they may actually have conduction tracts that allow accelerated conduction to occur within the AV node. Whatever the cause, such patients have rapid ventricular responses during atrial flutter and are usually more symptomatic, presenting earlier with paroxysmal atrial flutter.

Atrial Fibrillation

Atrial fibrillation is a common supraventricular arrhythmia and may occur in patients with and without organic heart disease. This rhythm is so common that it coexists with many other arrhythmias and conduction defects. Although the atria are continuously depolarized and therefore not subject to other atrial arrhythmias, a combination of AV junctional arrhythmias and ventricular arrhythmias is common in patients who have atrial fibrillation. Some of these rhythms are related to the treatment of atrial fibrillation with drugs such as digitalis. Perhaps one of the most common associated AV junctional rhythms is that of nonparoxysmal AV junctional tachycardia, which is related to digitalis intoxication.

The initiation of atrial fibrillation is usually by an APC. Although an APC may strike the atrial vulnerable period and cause atrial fibrillation as the initial rhythm, brief periods of rapid atrial tachycardia may actually precede the development of characteristic atrial fibrillation. Typically, the electrocardiogram in atrial fibrillation shows a rapid, irregular tachycardia in which P waves are absent. QRS complexes are generally normal, and the ventricular rate in patients with untreated atrial fibrillation generally ranges between 130 and 200 bpm. The ventricular rate can be accelerated by the coexistence of thyrotoxicosis, fever, catecholamines, catecholamine-like drugs, or conditions that enhance the tone of the sympathetic nervous system. Although a cardinal feature of atrial fibrillation is the irregularity of the R-R interval at the most rapid ventricular rate, this irregularity may be difficult to discern. Patients with the WPW syndrome may experience excessively rapid ventricular rates during atrial fibrillation (Fig. 3) if their accessory pathways are capable of sustaining rapid AV conduction.

Paroxysmal Supraventricular Tachycardia

Also called paroxysmal atrial tachycardia, paroxysmal supraventricular tachycardia (PSVT) is characteristically abrupt in onset and termination and variable in duration. The rate of such rhythms varies between 150 and 230 bpm, with a narrow QRS complex. However, patients may exhibit rate-related aberrant conduction and consequently may have a widened QRS complex during episodes. These tachycardias may last from several minutes to hours or even days, and they may occur in patients with or without identifiable heart disease. Patients with normal hearts generally tolerate the arrhythmia well, except for the symptoms of palpitation or awareness of a rapid heart beat. Patients with coexisting organic heart disease may complain of dyspnea or chest pain or may have symptoms of lightheadedness, near-syncope, or syncope. Very rapid episodes of PSVT may cause severe hemodynamic compromise in patients with associated cardiovascular disease.

The causes of PSVT vary. In approximately 60 per cent of patients, PSVT is due to re-entry within the AV node (Fig. 4); in 30 per cent of patients, PSVT is due to re-entry that utilizes the normal AV conduction system in the antegrade direction and a concealed accessory pathway in the retrograde direction (Fig. 4); and in the remaining 10 per cent of patients, PSVT is due to re-entry within the sinoatrial node or the atrium.

PSVT Due to Re-entry Within an AV Node. The electrocardiogram during PSVT related to AV nodal re-entrant tachycardia shows a regular tachycardia with a rate of 150 to 230 bpm and a narrow QRS complex. Characteristically, the P waves in AV nodal

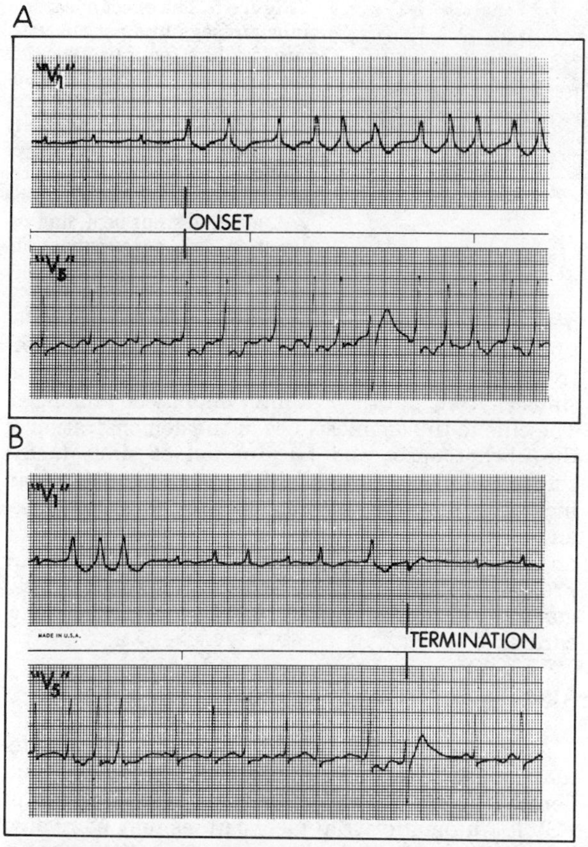

Figure 3. Atrial fibrillation recorded by 24-hour ambulatory monitoring in a patient with the Wolff-Parkinson-White syndrome. (*A*) The onset of the atrial fibrillation is observed in this panel, where precordial leads "V_1" and "V_5" are recorded simultaneously. (*B*) Termination of the atrial fibrillation. The rhythm is irregular with varying degrees of preexcitation and normal atrioventricular node conduction, resulting in fusion beats of different QRS configuration.

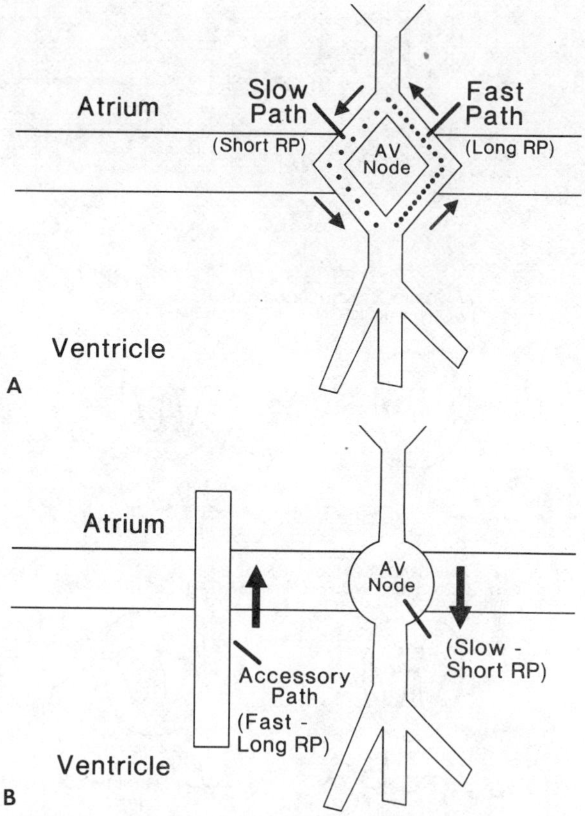

Figure 4. Mechanism of paroxysmal supraventricular tachycardia due to re-entry within the atrioventricular node and utilizing an accessory atrioventricular pathway. *(A)* Panel demonstrates re-entry within the atrioventricular node with antegrade conduction down the slow pathway (short refractory period) and retrograde conduction via the fast pathway (long refractory period). *(B)* Re-entry utilizing an accessory atrioventricular pathway with antegrade conduction down the atrioventricular node (slow pathway, short refractory period) and retrograde conduction via the accessory pathway (fast pathway, long refractoy period). RP = Refractory period.

re-entrant tachycardia occur simultaneously with the QRS complex or shortly thereafter. Long R-P intervals in patients with supraventricular tachycardia are suggestive of PSVT that utilizes a concealed accessory pathway or paroxysmal junctional reciprocating tachycardia. AV nodal re-entrant tachycardia often will abruptly terminate with vagal maneuvers, including the Valsalva maneuver and carotid sinus massage (Fig. 5).

An unusual form of AV nodal re-entrant tachycardia that causes incessant tachycardia is paroxysmal junctional reciprocating tachycardia, and this form behaves differently from AV nodal re-entrant tachycardia, previously described. In this atypical AV nodal re-entrant tachycardia, the tachycardia is persistent and the R-P interval is long. Affected patients generally do not respond well to treatment.

PSVT Due to Re-entry Utilizing a Concealed Accessory Pathway. Supraventricular tachycardia may occur in patients with accessory pathways. Patients with the WPW syndrome may have various rhythms associated with their accessory pathways. The accessory pathway in the WPW syndrome can conduct in either an antegrade or a retrograde direction or both. Conduction in the antegrade direction leads to the common delta wave, which represents a fusion beat of activation proceeding by way of the accessory pathway and the AV node. In patients with PSVT due to a concealed accessory pathway, the pathway is not capable of antegrade conduction, thus resulting in the absence of the delta wave on the electrocardiogram and the designation as a concealed bypass tract (Fig. 6). The diagnosis of a concealed accessory pathway is made at the time of an electrophysiologic study.

The clinical presentation of patients with tachycardia that utilizes a concealed accessory pathway is similar to that of patients with PSVT due to re-entry within the AV node. In patients with a concealed AV pathway, the electrocardiogram shows a rapid regular rate of 150 to 230 bpm and a normal QRS complex during the tachycardia (Fig. 7). The P wave may be abnormal, and the R-P interval is frequently lengthened. Functional bundle-branch block is more likely in patients with supraventricular tachycardia that utilizes a concealed pathway. This rhythm disturbance may be initiated by a change in sinus rate or a

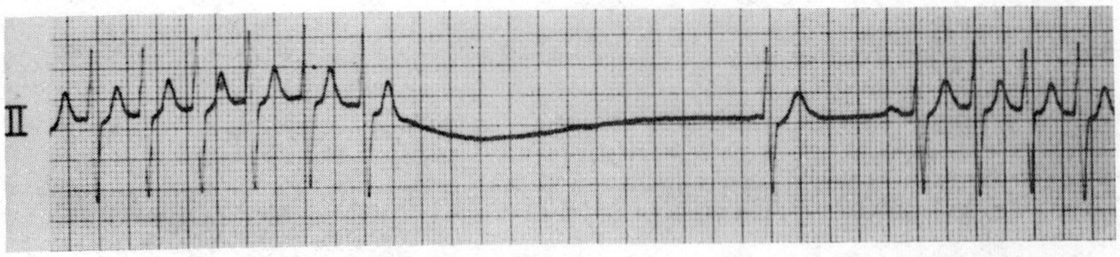

Figure 5. The effect of carotid sinus massage in a patient with paroxysmal supraventricular trachycardia utilizing a concealed accessory atrioventricular pathway. Limb lead II demonstrates a slight slowing of the tachycardia with abrupt termination, followed by an escape beat, a single sinus beat, and resumption of paroxysmal supraventricular tachycardia.

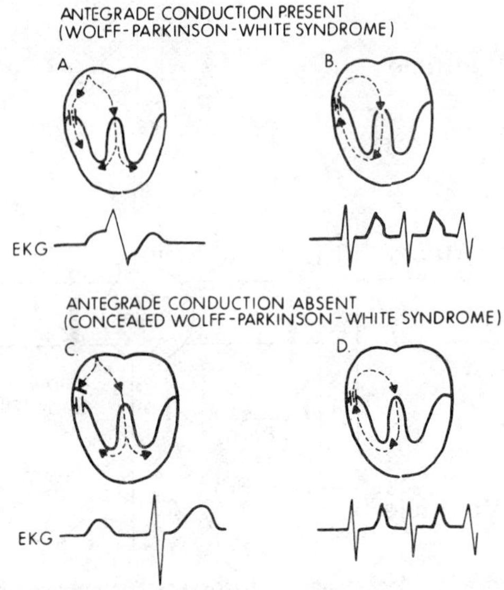

Figure 6. Accessory atrioventricular pathways demonstrating bidirectional and unidirectional conduction. (*A*) Schematic representation of a normal sinus beat in a patient with an accessory pathway capable of bidirectional conduction (the Wolff-Parkinson-White syndrome). Antegrade conduction is present down the accessory pathway, and the ECG complex is a fusion complex formed by activation via the accessory pathway and the normal atrioventricular conduction system. (*B*) Re-entrant tachycardia is demonstrated with antegrade conduction down the atrioventricular node-His Purkinje system and retrograde conduction using the accessory pathway. The QRS complex is narrow because the ventricle is being activated entirely by the normal conduction system. (*C*) There is no antegrade conduction down the accessory pathway (unidirectional conduction or concealed conduction) and the QRS complex after a sinus impulse is normal. (*D*) Re-entrant tachycardia again utilizes the atrioventricular node-His Purkinje system in the antegrade direction and an accessory pathway in the retrograde direction. (From Hammill, S.C., and Pritchett, E.L.C.: Dynamic electrocardiography in the investigation of supraventricular tachycardia and tachycardia associated with the preexcitation syndromes. In Campbell, R., and Murray, A. (eds.): *Dynamic Electrocardiography.* Edinburgh, Churchill Livingstone [in press].)

critically timed atrial or ventricular premature depolarization. Similarly, critically timed APCs and ventricular premature complexes can terminate the tachycardia, since both the atrium and the ventricle are required components of the re-entrant circuit.

PSVT Due to Re-entry Within the Sinoatrial Node. An unusual mechanism of PSVT is due to re-entry within the sinoatrial node. The patient often notices the abrupt onset of a rapid episode of palpitation and similarly the abrupt termination. The electrocardiogram shows a P wave identical to that during sinus rhythm, but the P-R interval may be prolonged. The clue to the diagnosis lies in the demonstration of the abrupt onset and termination of sinus tachycardia, not in association with known factors that can increase sinus rate, such as emotion, fever, exercise, and medications. The tachycardia may be initiated by an atrial premature depolarization or a ventricular premature depolarization, and vagal maneuvers will generally abruptly slow and then terminate the tachycardia.

Atrial Tachycardia

Atrial tachycardia that involves either an automatic mechanism or an intra-atrial re-entry, independent of the sinus node or AV node, is a rare form of PSVT. Automatic atrial tachycardias may be related to the effects of certain drugs (digoxin) or certain disease entities, such as chronic obstructive lung disease with multifocal atrial tachycardia. Intra-atrial re-entry tachycardias are rare in adults and are seen in less than 5 per cent of patients with PSVT. These tachycardias occur most commonly in younger adults and adolescents.

Typically, paroxysmal atrial tachycardia begins suddenly, marked by symptoms of palpitation or rapid heart beat. Spontaneous termination of attacks of paroxysmal atrial tachycardia is less common than observed in other forms of PSVT, other than paroxysmal junctional reciprocating tachycardia. Paroxysmal atrial tachycardia differs from PSVT in that it is relatively insensitive to vagal maneuvers, although AV nodal block may be produced.

During episodes of paroxysmal atrial tachycardia, the heart rate generally ranges from 140 to 200 bpm. The P wave configuration is different from that noted in sinus rhythm, depending on the location of the re-entrant or automatic focus, and the P-R interval is also variable. Generally, a long P-R interval indicates an origin at some distance from the AV node and a short P-R interval indicates an origin near the AV node.

Multifocal Atrial Tachycardia

Multifocal atrial tachycardia is diagnosed when there are frequent APCs with P waves exhibiting three or more distinct shapes, a heart rate greater than 100 bpm, and a variable P-P interval. The rhythm most often occurs in patients with decompensated chronic obstructive lung disease. Generally, the

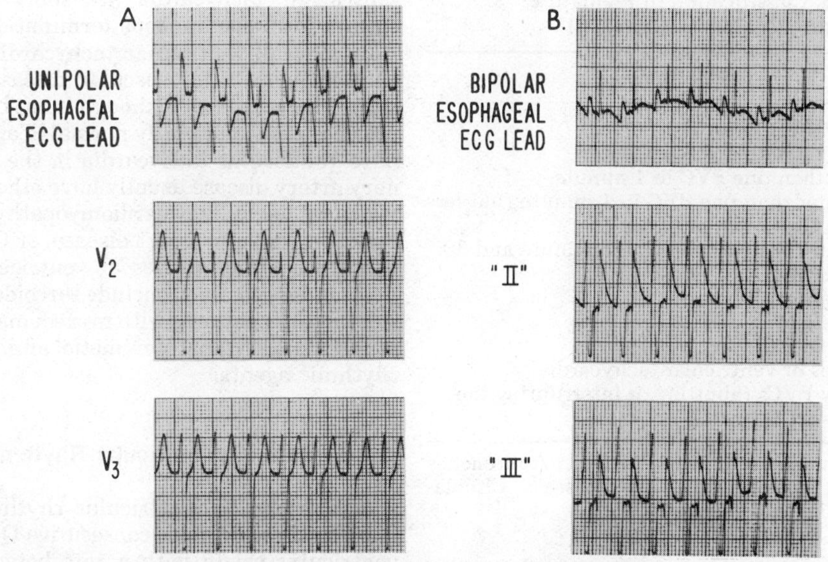

Figure 7. Paroxysmal supraventricular tachycardia utilizing a concealed atrioventricular accessory pathway. (*A*) Unipolar esophageal lead recorded simultaneously with precordial leads V_2 and V_3. The rate of the tachycardia is 170 beats per minute, and atrial activation can be observed to follow ventricular activation by approximately 160 ms. *(B)* Bipolar esophageal lead recorded simultaneously with limbs II and III. The bipolar esophageal lead records distinct atrial depolarizations that are approximately three times the magnitude of the ventricular depolarization. This patient had an accessory pathway located in the left lateral atrioventricular groove at the time of electrophysiologic study. (From Hammill, S.C., and Pritchett, E.L.C.: Simplified esophageal electrocardiography using bipolar recording leads. Ann. Intern. Med., 95:14, 1981. By permission of the American College of Physicians.)

arterial blood gases and serum electrolyte levels are abnormal and the patient is being treated with catecholamines and theophylline medications. This form of tachycardia is highly resistant to treatment with antiarrhythmic agents, and the use of digoxin may result in digitalis toxicity.

Premature Ventricular Complexes

Premature ventricular complexes (PVCs) have the following electrocardiographic features: no premature P wave precedes the QRS complex; the QRS complex is premature, wide, and often bizarre in appearance; and the S-T segment and T wave are opposite in direction to the QRS complex. There are two broad classifications: simple and complex.

Simple PVCs exhibit the following characteristics:

1. They occur beyond the T wave of the preceding QRS complex.
2. Their shape is uniform.
3. They occur in an isolated fashion and do not present as pairs or triplets.
4. They generally exhibit constant coupling intervals to the preceding QRS complex.

The simple type of PVC is frequent in the general population, occuring in 35 to 60 per cent of healthy young adults during 24-hour ambulatory monitoring. As persons increase in age, the frequency of such PVCs increases such that approximately 70 per cent of patients between the age of 40 and 60 years have simple PVCs, and these simple PVCs are seen in most persons older than 60 years of age. Persons with simple PVCs who do not have cardiac disease do not require treatment. However, the physician must not overlook the fact that sudden death occurs in persons who were previously believed to be healthy and normal. Therefore, when examining a patient who has simple PVCs, the physician must evaluate for the presence of associated cardiac or electrolyte abnormalities before assuring the patient that the rhythm disturbance is benign.

Complex PVCs occur in pairs, triplets, or more prolonged runs of ventricular tachycardia; occur during the vulnerable period of the cardiac cycle (R-on-T phenomenon); and have more than one configuration. A relationship exists between the complexity of PVCs and the risk of developing ventricular tachycardia and fibrillation in patients with cardiac disease. Patients who have complex ventricular ectopy in the apparent absence of cardiac disease only rarely experience life-threatening ventricular arrhythmias.

Lown and Wolf have proposed criteria that attempt to correlate the complexity of ventricular arrhythmias with the risk of sudden death (Table 3). This grading scale has received some criticism, specifically with regard to the high level of severity given to the R-on-T phenomenon; however, the grading system does provide a useful framework within which to evaluate PVCs and to decide which patients require therapy.

Ventricular Tachycardia

Ventricular tachycardia is due to abnormal impulses originating from areas of the specialized conduction system or ventricular myocardium which are distal to the bundle of His and is defined as three or more ectopic ventricular complexes with a rate of 100 to 250 bpm (Fig. 8). The ability of patients to tolerate an episode of ventricular tachycardia generally de-

Table 3. Classification of Premature Ventricular Complexes (PVC)*

Grade	PVC Complexity
0	No PVCs
1	Less than 30 PVCs per hour
1a	Less than one PVC in 1 minute
1b	Greater than one PVC in 1 minute (but less than 30 PVCs per hour)
2	Greater than one PVC in 1 minute and 30 per hour
3	Multiform PVCs
4	Repetitive PVCs
4a	Couplets
4b	Salvos or ventricular tachycardia
5	Early PVCs (abutting or interrupting the T wave)

*Modified from Lown, B., and Wolf, M.: Approaches to sudden death from coronary heart disease. Circulation, 44:130, 1971.

pends on the rate of the tachycardia and the state of the cardiovascular system. In patients with poor myocardial function and a rapid tachycardia, there is often hemodynamic deterioration, resulting in diminished coronary artery perfusion and ventricular fibrillation. In contrast, patients with well-preserved myocardial function may tolerate ventricular tachycardia for a prolonged period. Ventricular tachycardia is often referred to as being *sustained* or *nonsustained*. Sustained ventricular tachycardia refers to an episode that is prolonged, lasting at least 30 seconds, and generally requires termination by antiarrhythmic drugs, anti-tachycardiac pacing techniques, or electrocardioversion. Nonsustained runs of ventricular tachycardia are short (three beats or longer), with spontaneous termination.

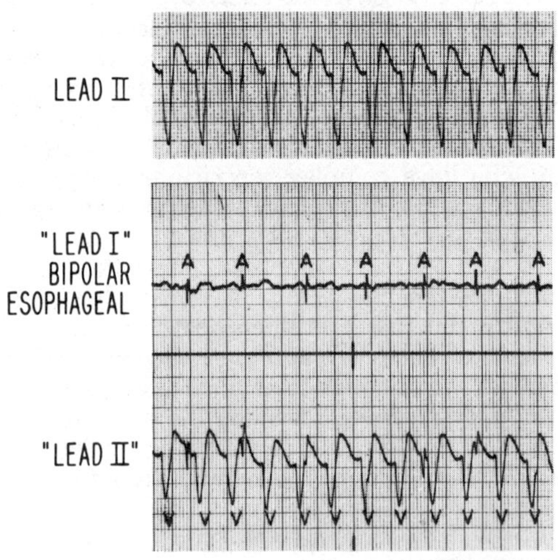

Figure 8. Ventricular tachycardia. Limb lead II demonstrates a QRS complex 120 ms wide and a ventricular rate of 160 beats per minute. "Lead I" records a bipolar esophageal lead simultaneously with limb "lead II." Atrioventricular dissociation is present, confirming that this rhythm is ventricular tachycardia. A = Atrial depolarization; V = ventricular depolarization.

In general, ventricular tachycardia is observed in patients with cardiovascular disease (usually coronary artery disease), although it has been described in patients with apparently normal hearts. Patients who have ventricular tachycardia in the absence of coronary artery disease usually have other cardiac abnormalities, including cardiomyopathy, mitral valve prolapse, valvular heart disease, or Q-T interval prolongation. Other causes of ventricular tachycardia that are less common include sarcoidosis, initiation of treatment in patients with myxedema, and such drugs as digitalis, sympathomimetic amines, and antiarrhythmic agents.

Accelerated Idioventricular Rhythm

Accelerated idioventricular rhythm (AIVR) is defined as three or more consecutive QRS complexes of ventricular origin with a rate between 50 and 100 bpm. Since the rate in AIVR is reasonably slow, the atrial rhythm is often easy to identify. Sinus rhythm with atrial ventricular dissociation is often present, and the sinus and ventricular rates are often similar enough that sinus capture with fusion beats can be observed. As the sinus rate increases, either during sinus arrhythmia or after slight exercise or the administration of atropine, fusion QRS complexes will be observed, followed by the reinstitution of sinus rhythm. The rhythm is generally easy to diagnose because of the rate, the obvious AV dissociation, and the presence of fusion beats. This rhythm is most often observed during acute myocardial infarction, occurring in about 15 per cent of patients.

Ventricular Parasystole

Ventricular parasystole is an automatic ventricular rhythm that is independent of the dominant sinus rhythm. The two cardinal features for the diagnosis of this ventricular rhythm disturbance are a varying coupling interval of the PVCs to the sinus beat and a common denominator for interectopic intervals. In general, the rate of the parasystolic focus is considerably slower than the sinus rate, and the key factor that permits parallel independent activity of a ventricular focus and the sinus focus is entrance block, protecting the ventricular focus. Entrance block allows the parasystolic focus to maintain its rhythm without being depolarized by the dominant sinus rhythm.

Ventricular Flutter and Ventricular Fibrillation

Ventricular flutter is rarely noted in patients because this rhythm is not stable and tends to convert to either sinus rhythm or ventricular fibrillation. The rhythm almost always results in severe, symptomatic hemodynamic impairment. Ventricular fibrillation is the most catastrophic cardiac arrhythmia and is likely to occur with myocardial ischemia, infarction, electrolyte disturbance, hypothermia, electrocution, and drug toxicity. Cardiac output ceases during ventricular fibrillation, resulting in a patient who is pulseless, with loss of consciousness and often convulsions. If this rhythm is not converted to a hemodynamically effective one within 3 to 4 minutes, the patient will most often die. The rate of ventricular flutter is 300 bpm or more, with the usual rates being 240 to 300 bpm. The flutter waves are large sinusoidal or zig-zag waves, and QRS complexes cannot be clearly distinguished from ST-T waves. Ventricular fibrillation is defined as the absence of QRS complex and T waves and the presence of low-amplitude baseline undulations on the electrocardiogram.

DISTURBANCES IN CARDIAC RHYTHM: DISORDERS IN IMPULSE CONDUCTION

Sinoatrial Block

Sinoatrial block occurs when an impulse that is generated in the sinus node fails to activate the atrium. This impulse may be delayed within the sinus node or blocked before the atrium is activated. Sinoatrial block can occur in first-, second-, or third-degree conduction delay, as described for AV block. First-degree sinoatrial block cannot be identified on the surface electrocardiogram, whereas second-degree sinoatrial block is the most common form diagnosed electrocardiographically. Sinoatrial block is identified when the patient shows no beat on the electrocardiogram where the R-R interval, encompassed by the dropped beat, is exactly twice the normal R-R interval and no P wave can be observed.

Atrioventricular Block

Atrioventricular block is usually classified as first-, second-, or third-degree. *First-degree* AV block presents as prolongation of the P-R interval, with the site of the conduction delay generally being in the AV node. On occasion, first-degree AV block can be due to conduction delay distal to the bundle of His.

Second-degree AV block is of two types.

Type I. Type I presents with characteristic Wenckebach periodicity and occurs within the AV node. It has the following characteristics:

1. The P-R interval is prolonged with each successive cycle until a P wave fails to be conducted to the ventricles, resulting in a long R-R interval.
2. The longest R-R interval is less than twice the shortest R-R interval.
3. The first P-R interval after the blocked P wave is always the shortest one.
4. In subsequent cycles, the P-R interval lengthens progressively, and this increase is characteristically greatest in the cycle after the blocked P wave.
5. After the second cycle, the increment in the P-R interval becomes smaller and smaller, accounting for the progressive shortening of the R-R interval after the longest R-R interval.

Type II. Type II second-degree block in the AV node is due to block that occurs below the AV node in the His-Purkinje system. This type of block is recognized by the sudden failure of a P wave to be conducted to the ventricles. Type II AV block occurs without any previous lengthening of the P-R interval and often occurs in patients with bundle-branch disease. When AV conduction with a 2:1 conduction ratio is present, it is not possible to be certain about the site of AV block. However, if the QRS complex is normal, the block is most likely a type I AV block and located in the AV node. If the QRS duration is prolonged, either type I or type II block is likely.

In *third-degree* AV block, the atria are under control by one rhythm, whether it be sinus rhythm, atrial fibrillation, or atrial flutter, and the ventricles are under control by a second rhythm (Fig. 9). Atrioventricular dissociation exists with a ventricular escape rate of between 35 and 55 bpm. The R-R intervals are almost always regular, the site of block is usually below the AV node, and the atrial rate is faster than the ventricular rate.

The clinical features associated with AV block are variable and depend on the degree of block. First-degree AV block causes no symptoms, and only rarely does type I second-degree AV block result in symptoms. This type of block often accompanies a transient problem, such as acute rheumatic fever, acute inferior myocardial infarction, or digitalis intoxication. Rarely, type I AV block can progress to third-degree AV block. Type II AV block is usually associated with progression of disease in the His-Purkinje system (bundle-branch block), and this condition is likely to progress to complete heart block. Such patients often have symptoms of near-syncope or syncope. Finally, third-degree AV block is likely to be symptomatic because of the slow ventricular rate. Such patients experience lightheadedness, near-syncope, and syncope.

DIAGNOSTIC METHODS USED TO AID IN IDENTIFICATION OF CARDIAC ARRHYTHMIAS

The crucial information needed by the physician who is attempting to diagnose the mechanism of a cardiac arrhythmia is an electrocardiographic recording performed during the episode of symptoms. This recording can then document whether a rhythm disturbance is the cause of the symptoms and can aid in diagnosing the mechanism of the arrhythmia. The 12-lead electrocardiogram and long rhythm strips are important when attempting to diagnose a rhythm disturbance; however, such rhythm strips are recorded only rarely in a patient with a history suggestive of a rhythm disturbance. During the initial evaluation of such a patient, it should be determined whether the patient has ever had an electrocardiogram recorded during a symptomatic arrhythmia. Obtaining such electrocardiographic documentation may obviate the need for further testing and can facilitate the selection of the proper treatment regimen.

Several methods are available for recording an electrocardiogram during the rhythm disturbance. These methods include transtelephonic electrocardiographic monitoring, 24-hour ambulatory monitoring, and the treadmill exercise test.

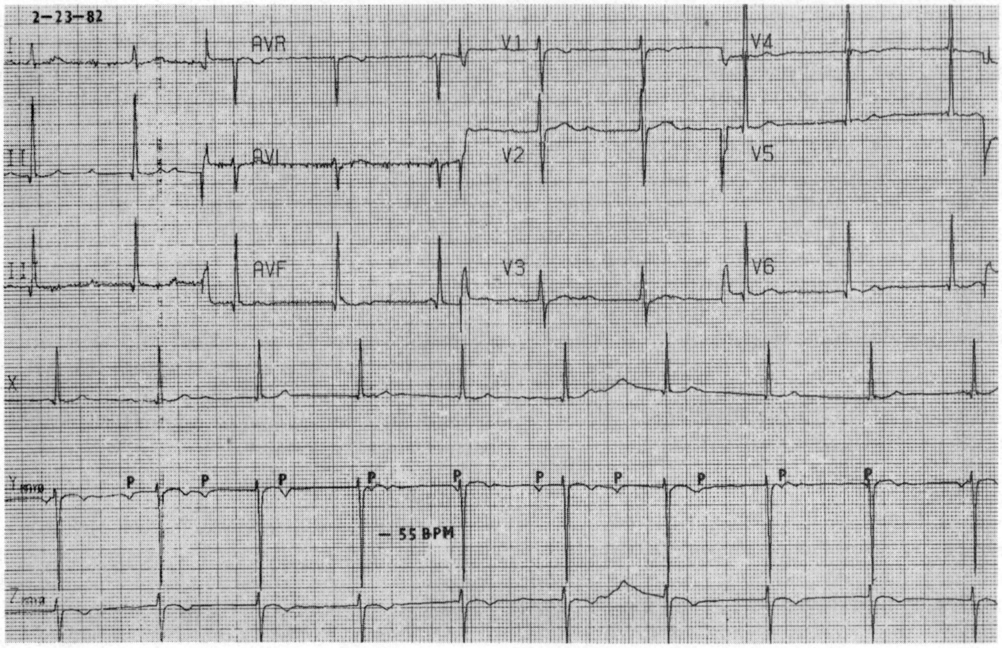

Figure 9. Complete heart block. Twelve-lead ECG with a ventricular rate of 55 beats per minute and a QRS complex of normal configuration. Atrial activity (*P*) is regular and unrelated to ventricular activity.

Transtelephonic Electrocardiographic Monitoring

Because of the intermittent nature of arrhythmias, there has been considerable interest in the development of event recorders that can be used for long-term monitoring. Several commercial systems are available, including transmitters for patients with pacemakers. With the onset of symptoms, the patient attaches the system, using wrist, axillary, or precordial electrodes, and then transmits the electrocardiogram over the telephone. The most important advantage of this system is that the electrocardiogram can be recorded during a patient's symptoms (Figs. 10 and 11). Often the telephone transmission of an electrocardiogram during symptoms provides more information than does conventional 24-hour ambulatory monitoring. Of interest, approximately one fourth of patients who transmit during a typical spell have a normal electrocardiogram. This finding is of great help in counseling such patients.

The technique does have limitations; some systems are cumbersome and involve either wrist or axillary electrodes, which may be difficult to use. The patient must be able to detect the arrhythmia and then have time to transmit it. This requires access to a receiving center and telephone. If the patient rapidly suffers serious hemodynamic consequences such as near-syncope and syncope soon after the onset of the arrhythmia, the transtelephonic monitoring system is obviously not helpful. The system may not be beneficial in patients whose spells are of very short duration.

A monitoring system with a memory loop that can be activated by the patient and then transmitted to a receiving center, at the patient's convenience, has been introduced. These and other advances should increase the role that transtelephonic monitoring has in the evaluation of arrhythmias. Such a system is important because the rhythm is recorded during a patient's symptoms. The patient then feels confident that the physician has identified the mechanism of the rhythm disturbance while symptoms are being experienced and not just a rhythm disturbance that may be detected by electrocardiographic recording but unrelated to the symptoms.

24-Hour Ambulatory Monitoring

Development of a portable device for the long-term recording of electrocardiograms has greatly facilitated evaluation of paroxysmal rhythm disturbances. Since its original description by Holter, the technique has assumed increasing importance. At present, major indications for ambulatory monitoring include:

1. Documentation of symptomatic and asymptomatic rhythm disturbances.
2. Documentation of the cardiac rhythm during symptoms that could be related to a cardiac origin (e.g., fainting spells).
3. Documentation of the effect of treatment regimens on rhythm disturbances.
4. Evaluation of pacemaker function.
5. Evaluation of the risk of subsequent events in patient subgroups (e.g., postmyocardial infarction).

Present systems use multiple channels that aid in differentiating artifact and QRS and P waves. In addition, combined blood pressure and ambulatory monitoring systems are available that can provide hemodynamic information on the effect of arrhythmias and also elucidate whether fainting spells are related to arrhythmias or to hypotension alone.

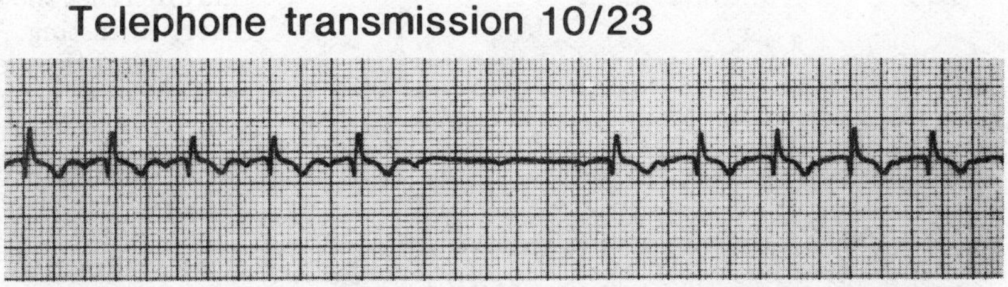

Figure 10. Atrioventricular conduction block recorded by transtelephonic monitoring. In the center of the rhythm strip, two P waves are not followed by QRS complexes.

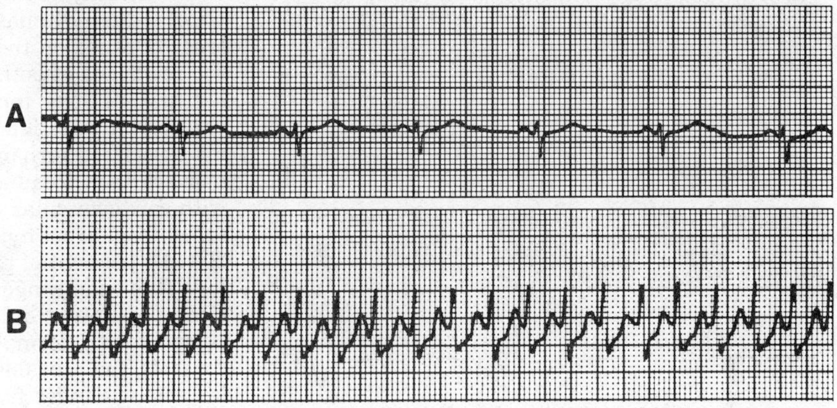

Figure 11. Paroxysmal supraventricular tachycardia recorded by transtelephonic monitoring. (*A*) Panel demonstrates a baseline recording with the patient in sinus rhythm. (*B*) Panel demonstrates PSVT recorded during an episode of symptomatic palpitations.

In applying the technique of 24-hour ambulatory monitoring in patients with rhythm disturbances, three major factors are important to remember: the intermittent nature of symptoms and rhythm disturbances; the spontaneous variability of rhythm disturbances; and the wide range of normal findings.

Because of the intermittent nature of patients' symptoms, diagnostic ambulatory monitoring cannot be obtained in all patients. This makes estimation of the sensitivity of the technique difficult. Approximately 25 per cent of patients who have histories consistent with cardiogenic syncope have symptoms during the initial 24 hours of ambulatory monitoring. If the recording time is extended beyond 24 hours, the detection of additional significant arrhythmias will be increased. Obviously, patient selection influences the outcome of these studies significantly, and in patients with remote and infrequent spells, this technique may not be helpful.

The reproducibility of the findings of ambulatory monitoring has stimulated considerable interest. There is significant variability in arrhythmias from day to day and hour to hour. This variability is seen in both simple and complex ventricular ectopy, and the variability can be circumvented by increasing the duration of monitoring from 24 to 48 hours.

It is important to consider the range of normal findings on ambulatory monitoring because many patients with arrhythmias are asymptomatic. In a patient undergoing evaluation of cardiogenic syncope, the finding of sinus node arrest (Fig. 1) at the time of syncope during a 24-hour monitoring period makes the clinical decision easy. When the same patient has only evidence of simple ventricular ectopy and syncope does not occur during the study, the decision is considerably more difficult. Ambulatory monitoring in patients who are without apparent heart disease has documented a relatively wide range of arrhythmias. The range of heart rate in healthy young males may range from 37 to 180 bpm during waking hours and from 33 to 115 bpm during sleeping hours. During sleeping periods, approximately one fourth of normal persons have heart rates of less than 40 bpm and sinus pauses of greater than 1.75 seconds. Transient second-degree AV block has been documented in 2 to 6 per cent of trained athletes and young, otherwise healthy males and females. These arrhythmias often occur during sleep and appear to be vagally mediated. Both APCs and PVCs are frequently found in healthy individuals, although the absolute number in any specific person is low. The frequency of such arrhythmias increases with age.

The 24-hour ambulatory monitoring technique has been used in patients with episodic dizziness, lightheadedness, syncope, and palpitations in an attempt to correlate symptoms with the electrocardiogram. The results of ambulatory monitoring in these patients are variable, depending in part on the selection of patients for evaluation, the specific complaint, and the frequency of the episodes. In 50 to 60 per cent of patients with syncope, palpitations, or lightheadedness, significant arrhythmias will be documented that could account for their symptoms (Figs. 1 and 12). It is important to note that symptoms such as dizziness and palpitations may not correlate with arrthythmias and conversely that patients with major cardiac arrhythmias may in fact be asymptomatic. Physicians should be aware that artifact recorded by ambulatory monitors may mimic significant arrhythmias (Fig. 13).

Exercise Testing

Exercise testing is frequently used in the detection of arrhythmias. Major indications include:

1. Exercise-induced palpitations or exercise-induced symptoms consistent with a primary rhythm disturbance.

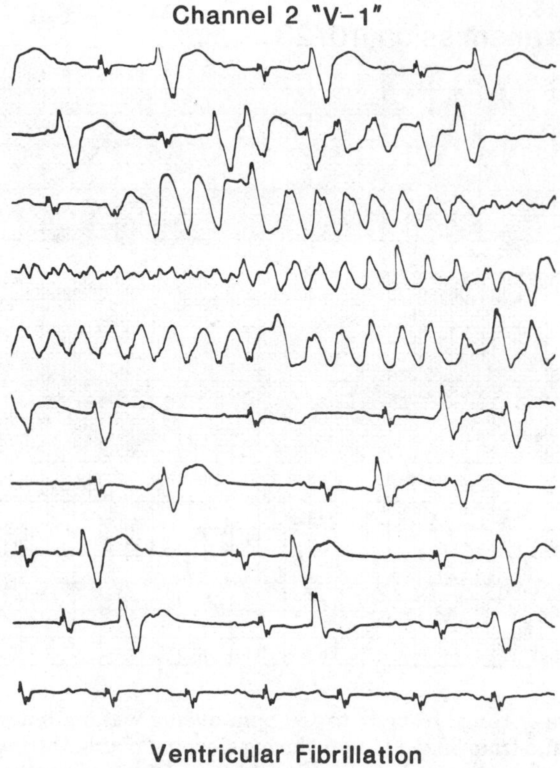

Figure 12. Ventricular arrhythmia recorded during 24-hour ambulatory monitoring. Channel 2 records "V_1" and demonstrates a bigeminal rhythm with episodes of a rapid tachycardia of irregular configuration. The rate of the tachycardia is initially 300 beats per minute and is presumably ventricular flutter. The tachycardia then degenerates into a brief run of a ventricular rhythm compatible with fibrillation, followed again by ventricular flutter, and finally conversion back to sinus rhythm with frequent premature ventricular complexes.

2. Evaluation of the effect of exercise on supraventricular and ventricular ectopy documented during 12-lead electrocardiography or during 24-hour ambulatory monitoring.

3. Detection and classification of ventricular ectopy in specific patient groups, including those with coronary artery disease, hypertrophic obstructive cardiomyopathy, and mitral valve prolapse.

With the use of this technique, several important aspects must be considered:

1. The recording system and exercise protocol used.
2. The type, frequency, and significance of arrhythmias detected during exercise testing in normal and abnormal patients.
3. The spontaneous variability and reproducibility of exercise-induced arrhythmia.

Technical aspects of the recording system have an important role in the detection and evaluation of exercise-induced arrhythmias. The capability of monitoring multiple leads can provide significant information that is of particular importance in distinguishing aberration from ventricular ectopy. In addition, some authors have found that continuous monitoring or real-time playback review of analog tape recordings may increase the yield of arrhythmia detection during exercise testing. The amount of exercise performed also affects the yield of arrhythmias. The incidence of arrhythmias increases during maximal or near-maximal exercise testing.

Exercise-induced arrhythmias are frequent both in normal controls and in patients with cardiac disease. Supraventricular arrhythmias (Fig. 14) with sinus node dysfunction, atrial ectopy, and short paroxysms of atrial tachycardia, as well as a wide range of ventricular arrhythmias (Fig. 15), are seen. The prevalence depends on the population studied; in general, the incidence of both supraventricular and ventricular arrhythmias increases with increasing patient age. Asymptomatic supraventricular arrhythmias are not associated with increased mortality and morbidity and are seen frequently in normals and in patients with cardiovascular disease.

Ventricular arrhythmias have been documented in 20 to 60 per cent of patients undergoing exercise testing. This wide range relates to differences in the patient population studied and the protocol used. In patients with normal coronary arteries or in normal controls, the prevalence of exercise-induced ventricular ectopy ranges from 10 to 15 per cent. This contrasts to that in exercise testing in patients with established coronary artery disease, in whom as many as 60 per cent may have ventricular ectopy. In patients with coronary artery disease, increased ventricular ectopy is often associated with more extensive coronary artery disease, left ventricular dysfunction, and exercise-induced ischemia with S-T depression.

Ventricular tachycardia or ventricular fibrillation is uncommon during treadmill exercise testing. Both rhythms occur in less than 1 per cent of patients and may occur either during the exercise test or the recovery period. Ventricular tachycardia is usually of short duration, but occasionally it is sustained. Such rhythm disturbances may be present in patients without obvious heart disease, but they are generally seen in patients with coronary artery disease. A frequent indication for exercise testing is for the evaluation of ventricular ectopy documented during 12-lead electrocardiography or ambulatory monitoring. Unfortunately, the suppression of resting ventricular ectopy by exercise does not reliably indicate the absence of significant coronary artery disease.

Exercise testing also has been used in other patient groups, such as patients with hypertrophic cardiomyopathy and mitral valve prolapse, in an attempt to document arrhythmias and identify patients at risk for sudden death. In patients with hypertrophic cardiomyopathy, both supraventricular and ventricular arrhythmias are common during exercise. Approximately 50 per cent of selected patients with hypertrophic cardiomyopathy undergoing exercise testing develop supraventricular arrhythmias, with 25 per cent having complex ventricular ectopy. Similarly, as many as 75 per cent of patients with mitral valve prolapse have both documented symptomatic and asymptomatic ventricular and supraventricular arrhythmias.

Exercise testing has been used in patients with conduction defects, such as sinus node dysfunction and AV block, to determine the response to exercise. It

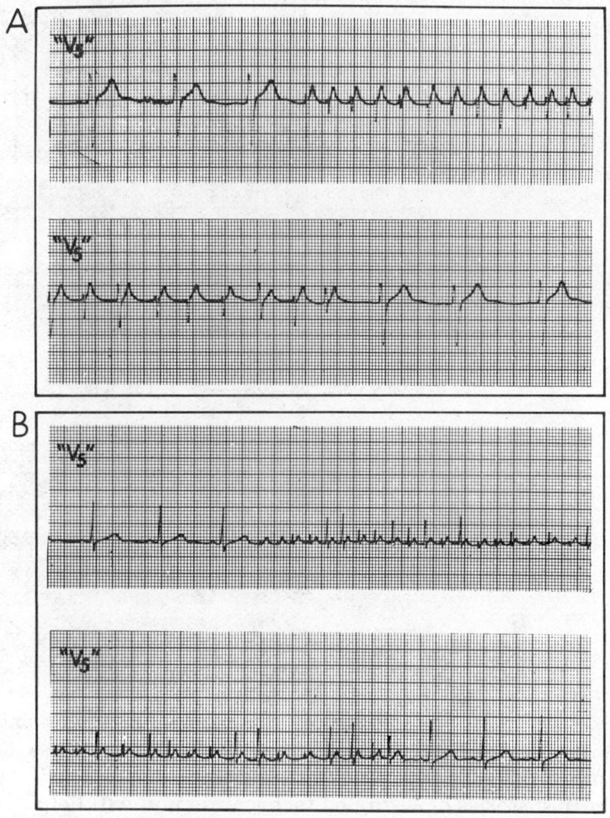

Figure 13. Artifact recorded during 24-hour ambulatory monitoring. (*A* and *B*) Data are shown from two patients with artifact recorded during 24-hour monitoring. Surface lead "V_5" records a rapid rhythm with a narrow QRS configuration in both patients. This rhythm abnormality was artifact due to battery failure and intermittent slowing of the tape, resulting in a compressed rhythm.

may be possible to identify the level of AV block using exercise testing. Block occurring at the level of the AV node and related to increased vagal tone improves during exercise, whereas block occurring in the His-Purkinje system usually is not affected by exercise.

Spontaneous variability and the reproducibility of exercise-induced arrhythmias are important factors in the evaluation of patients using exercise testing. Reproducibility of exercise testing performed on subsequent days or several years apart has not been evaluated fully; however, there is a suggestion that exercise testing is not reproducible when comparing the events found during one episode of exercise with those found during a second episode.

Ambulatory Monitoring versus Treadmill Exercise Testing

Ambulatory monitoring and the treadmill exercise test have specific strengths and potential weaknesses. The former gives a higher yield of ventricular and atrial arrhythmias. However, treadmill exercise testing in some patients will provoke arrhythmias not seen during ambulatory monitoring. In addition, important information on exercise tolerance, blood pressure response to exercise, and S-T segment changes is also available with exercise testing. The pathophysiology of arrhythmias provoked by exercise, of course, may be different from that seen with ordinary activity. If a patient who is suspected of having cardiac arrhythmia relates his symptoms to exertion, he should undergo exercise treadmill testing in an attempt to reproduce the clinical situation that is associated with the rhythm disturbance.

Ambulatory Monitoring versus Transtelephonic Event Recording

Limited information is available for comparing ambulatory monitoring with telephone transmitter event recorders. Patients who have very infrequent symptoms may benefit from the use of a transtelephonic monitoring device. The patient who has well-defined episodes of palpitations lasting several minutes and occurring irregularly is an ideal candidate for use of the transtelephonic monitoring system. In contrast, the patient who has frequent brief episodes of symptoms suggestive of cardiac arrhythmia will benefit from 24-hour ambulatory monitoring.

Electrophysiologic Testing

In the evaluation of arrhythmias, the techniques previously described may fail to provide diagnostic information, may not be appropriate, or may not be applicable. In these clinical settings, invasive electrophysiologic testing is often used. The correct diagnosis in patients with episodic arrhythmias may be difficult unless the episode occurs during monitoring or exercise testing or can be documented with a transtelephonic monitoring system. In these patients, electrophysiologic testing is valuable in documenting the anatomic and physiologic substrates for arrhythmias. The electrophysiologic test can reproduce su-

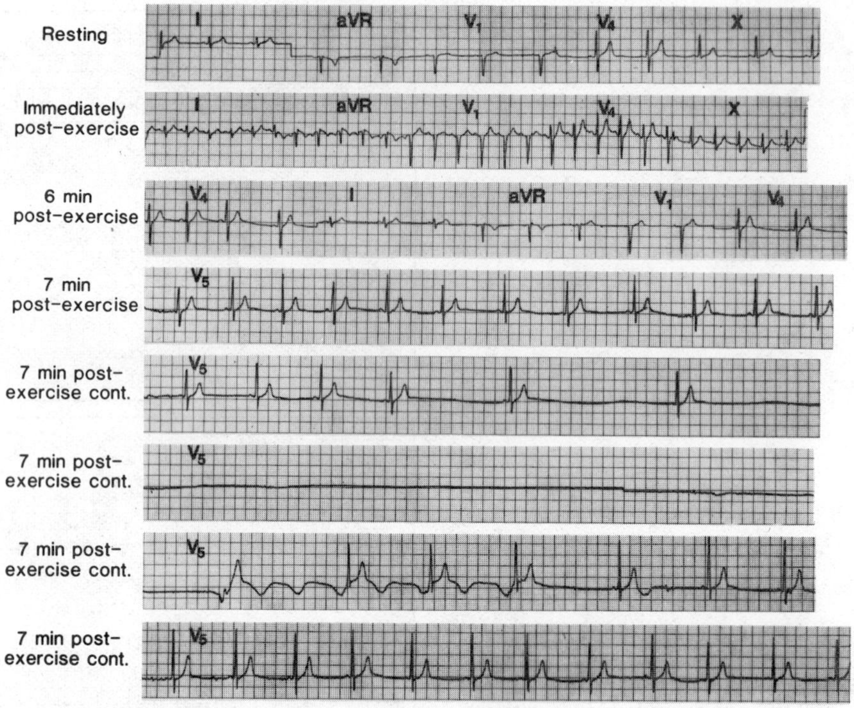

Figure 14. Sinus pause followed by sinus arrest after exercise stress testing.

praventricular or ventricular arrhythmias in patients with histories of sustained tachycardia and will help to identify the specific mechanism and cause of presumed tachycardias.

Patients who survive a cardiac arrest pose major clinical problems, particularly if the arrest was not related to acute myocardial infarction. In these patients, the risk of recurrence is substantial and the reliance on noninvasive ambulatory monitoring or exercise testing to detect the underlying arrhythmia may not be helpful or clinically advisable. Electrophysiologic testing has been used with increasing frequency to reproduce and document the clinical arrhythmia and to determine the most appropriate means of therapy. This method is generally reserved for patients who have symptoms that are suggestive of a disturbance in cardiac rhythm and in whom noninvasive testing has not identified the cause or for patients who are suspected of having life-threatening arrhythmias. Electrophysiologic testing should be performed by physicians experienced with the technique.

DIAGNOSTIC TECHNIQUES USEFUL IN PATIENTS PRESENTING WITH TACHYCARDIA

When confronted with a patient who is in the midst of a cardiac arrhythmia, the physician must diagnose the mechanism of the rhythm disturbance. The patient who has hemodynamic compromise during the rhythm disturbance may require cardioversion, either chemically or electrically, before the rhythm disturbance can be diagnosed with certainty. In the patient who presents with a rhythm disturbance that is hemodynamically stable, evaluation in addition to routine electrocardiography and extended rhythm strip may need to be performed. Such evaluation includes recording atrial activity from the esophagus and right atrium and the use of carotid sinus massage and drugs that alter AV conduction. These techniques establish the relationship of the atrium and ventricle during the episode of tachycardia, thus allowing for proper identification of the mechanism of the tachycardia.

Carotid Sinus Massage

Physiologic maneuvers used in association with an electrocardiographic recording during an episode of tachycardia can be helpful in the diagnosis of the mechanism of the arrhythmia. Such maneuvers are most commonly performed during episodes of supraventricular tachycardia in order to identify more clearly the atrial and the ventricular activity.

The most common physiologic maneuver utilized is carotid sinus massage (Fig. 5). External pressure applied to the area of the carotid body at the bifurcation of the external and internal carotid arteries (below the mandibular angle) with a gentle massaging motion will stimulate the baroreceptors of the carotid sinus, which in turn will increase vagal tone significantly. Increased vagal tone influences the AV node and causes increased AV block and may allow recognition of P waves that previously were not apparent. Therefore, the most important application of carotid sinus massage is to assist the analysis of a rapid, regular tachycardia when P waves are not easily seen. In patients with wide QRS complex tachycardias and

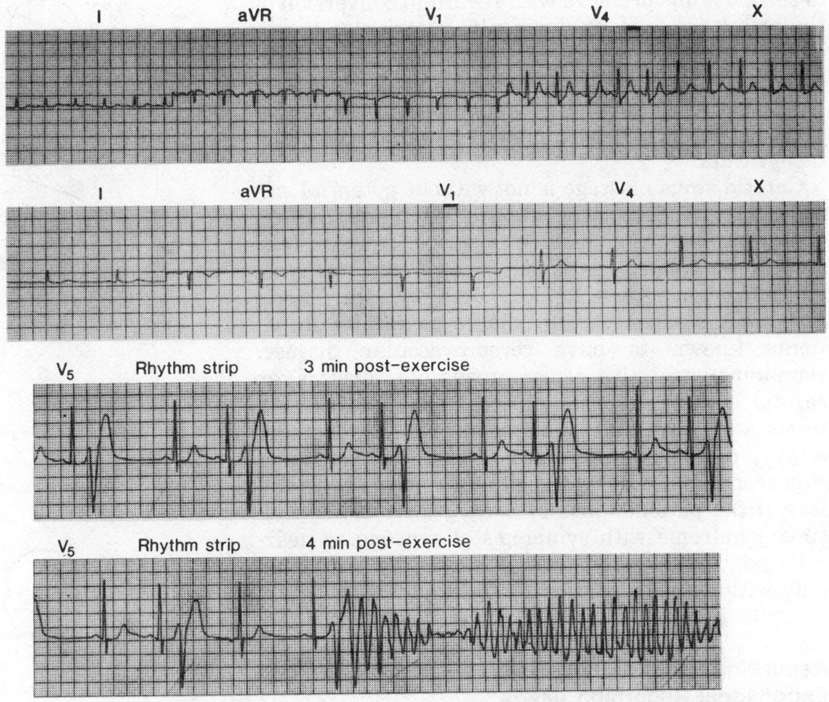

Figure 15. Premature ventricular complexes and ventricular fibrillation occurring 3 minutes after exercise stress testing.

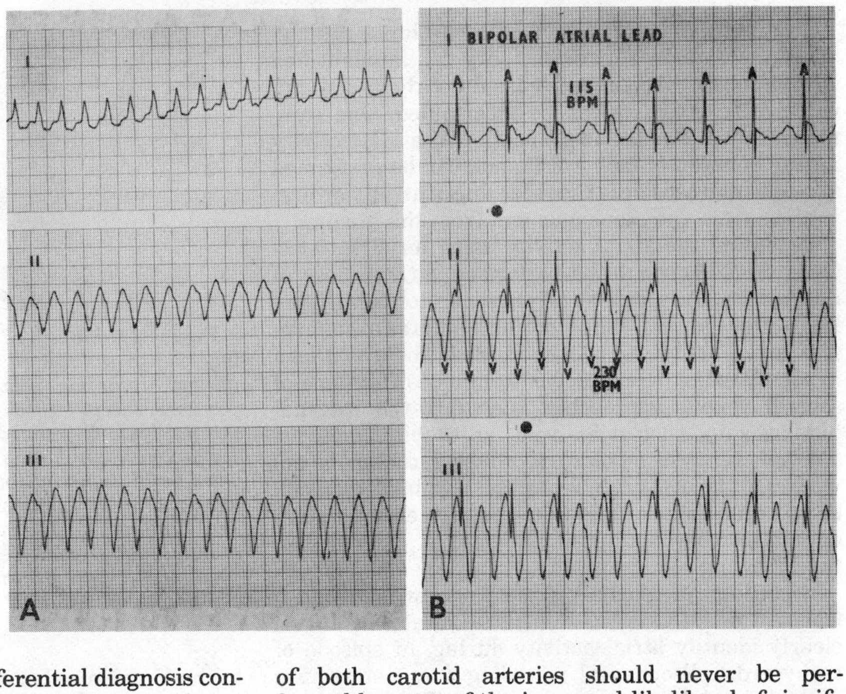

Figure 16. Ventricular tachycardia. (*A*) Panel demonstrates tachycardia with a rate of 270 beats per minute and a QRS width of 160 ms. (*B*) Panel records a bipolar lead in the right atrium on channel 1 with limb leads II and III. Atrial activity (*A*) with a rate of 115 beats per minute is observed using the bipolar atrial lead. The ventricular rate (V) is 230 beats per minute. Ventriculoatrial conduction is present with 2:1 ventriculoatrial block.

poorly defined P waves, the differential diagnosis concerns sinus tachycardia, PSVT, atrial flutter, and ventricular tachycardia.

Carotid sinus massage must be performed carefully. The patient should be placed in a supine position, the neck being allowed to relax. The head is then turned away from the right carotid artery for massage of the right carotid artery. If no response is elicited after 10 to 20 seconds of very light massage, more firm pressure is exerted. In any instance, firm massage should not continue for more than 5 seconds. If no response is obtained on one side, contralateral carotid sinus massage may be performed. Simultaneous massage of both carotid arteries should never be performed because of the increased likelihood of significant adverse effects.

The general response of sinus tachycardia to carotid sinus massage is a gradual slowing before the premassage rate is resumed. Characteristically, PSVT due to re-entry within the AV node or to utilization of an accessory pathway demonstrates an all-or-none response to carotid sinus massage, either terminating abruptly or changing little if at all. In atrial flutter, the degree of AV block is increased with carotid sinus massage, which allows better visualization of flutter waves. Ventricular tachycardia responds only rarely to carotid sinus pressure with regard to conversion of the tachycardia. More commonly, ventricular tachycardia associated with 1:1 retrograde activation of the atria may demonstrate increased ventriculoatrial block and allow for better identification of AV dissociation, establishing the diagnosis of ventricular tachycardia.

Carotid sinus massage is not without potential significant risks, especially in elderly patients. Significant complications include syncope, convulsions, stroke, prolonged asystole, ventricular tachyarrhythmias, or adverse hemodynamic reflexes. Therefore, carotid sinus massage should be avoided in patients known to have cerebrovascular disease, symptoms suggestive of cerebrovascular disease, or carotid artery bruits on physical examination. Patients who have sick sinus syndrome may demonstrate a prolonged sinus arrest after the conversion of supraventricular tachycardia to sinus rhythm. Therefore, if the patient's history is suggestive of the sick sinus syndrome with symptoms of syncope or near-syncope, carotid sinus massage should be performed only with extreme caution, if at all.

Recording Atrial Activity Using Atrial and Esophageal Recording Leads

The mechanism of a cardiac arrhythmia is diagnosed more easily if atrial activity can be identified with certainty and the relationship of the atrial and ventricular activities can be ascertained. One technique that allows the identification of atrial activity during episodes of tachycardia and can be performed at a patient's bedside is the recording of atrial depolarizations from the esophagus and from the atrium.

Recording the atrial activity using an atrial electrode (Fig. 16) should be performed with the use of fluoroscopy. This allows the physician to identify the location of the tip of the recording lead so as to confirm that atrial activity is being recorded. The atrial lead is passed using percutaneous techniques from one of several venous approaches, including the internal jugular vein, subclavian vein, antecubital vein, or femoral vein. A bipolar recording catheter is advanced to the atrium, where atrial depolarization can be recorded using either special equipment or a standard electrocardiographic machine, as described in the following paragraphs.

Recording an esophageal electrogram has been a frequent solution to the difficulties of attempting to clearly identify atrial activity during an episode of tachycardia. Esophageal recording does not require sophisticated fluoroscopy equipment. The usual technique for esophageal electrocardiography in the bedside diagnosis of arrhythmias involves connecting a unipolar recording lead positioned in the esophagus to the V_1 terminal of a standard electrocardiographic machine (Fig. 17). This technique improves discrimination of the P wave compared with that in standard surface electrocardiographic leads, but it requires patience, experience, and skill. The P wave obtained with a unipolar recording lead is generally smaller than the associated QRS complex and may be difficult to identify during rapid ventricular rhythms (Fig. 18).

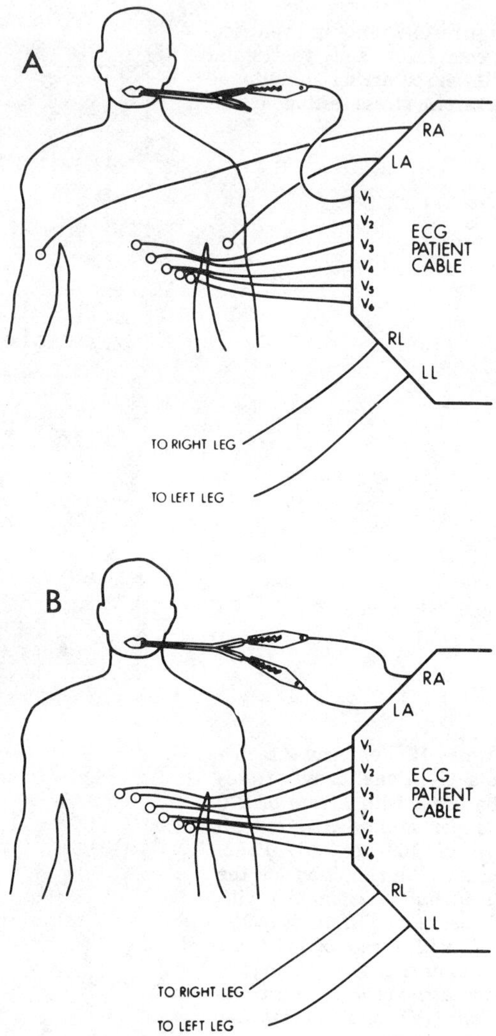

Figure 17. Method of connecting the esophageal recording lead to a standard ECG machine. (*A*) Unipolar esophageal recording with all ECG leads in their usual positions, except for lead "V_1," which is attached to the esophageal lead. (*B*) Panel demonstrates the method of recording a bipolar esophageal lead. Again, all leads are in their usual positions, except for the right and left arm leads, which are attached to the esophageal lead. (From Hammill, S.C., and Pritchett, E.L.C.: Simplified esophageal electrocardiography using bipolar recording leads. Ann. Intern. Med., 95:14, 1981. By permission of the American College of Physicians.)

Instead of using a unipolar recording lead attached to the V_1 terminal of a standard electrocardiographic machine, we favor recording the esophageal electrogram using a bipolar recording lead (Fig. 17). Bipolar recordings are made by placing the right-leg, left-leg, and precordial terminals of the patient's cable in their usual positions. The right-arm and left-arm terminals are each connected to one electrode of the bipolar recording lead in the esophagus (or right atrium if a transvenous electrode is used) with an alligator clip.

The electrocardiographic machine must be capable of recording three channels simultaneously. The channel selector is positioned in the 1-2-3 mode. Channel 1 records a bipolar electrogram from the esophagus, and channels 2 and 3 record bipolar electrographic signals between the esophagus and the left leg. The lead in the esophagus is then positioned to show maximal amplitude of the P wave.

Two recording electrodes that are ideal for recording atrial activity from the esophagus are an endocardial lead, originally designed for permanent pacing (Fig. 19) (Medtronic, model 6904, Minneapolis), and a swallowed bipolar pill electrode described by Arzbaecher (Fig. 20). Both electrodes are flexible and thin and are not associated with significant gagging and esophageal discomfort—problems previously associated with larger esophageal recording leads.

The leads are passed through the nares until they reach the back of the pharynx. The patient then swallows water, and the lead is slowly advanced to the esophagus. The bipolar recording allows for large distinct P waves to be recorded on channel 1 of the electrocardiographic machine. The amplitude of the P wave in channel 1 is three to four times larger than that of the associated QRS complex when comparison is made with the old style of unipolar recording, in which the P wave is of lower amplitude than the QRS complex (Figs. 2, 7, and 18).

The esophageal electrogram is valuable in patients who have supraventricular tachycardia of unclear etiology because the lead helps to differentiate atrial flutter from PSVT. The lead is advantageous in identifying atrial activity in patients who have tachycardia with a wide QRS complex, in which the differential diagnosis includes atrial flutter and PSVT with aberrant conduction and ventricular tachycardia.

Using the proximal lumen of a Swan-Ganz catheter as a salt-bridge to record atrial activity has been advocated by others; however, we have not found this technique to be reliable (Fig. 21).

SUPRAVENTRICULAR TACHYCARDIA WITH ABERRANCY VERSUS VENTRICULAR TACHYCARDIA

It is very important and often difficult to differentiate ventricular tachycardia from supraventricular tachycardia with aberrancy (Figs. 8, 16, and 22). A patient who presents with a tachycardia that has a wide QRS complex and hemodynamic deterioration should have electrical cardioversion performed immediately. However, if the patient is tolerating the episode of tachycardia, the physician should make all attempts at diagnosing the cause of the tachycardia before terminating it. The most useful technique is to obtain a 12-lead electrocardiogram with a long rhythm strip and then perform carotid massage in an attempt to more easily identify P waves if they are not readily apparent. If atrial activity remains obscure, atrial activity should be recorded using a bipolar recording lead from the esophagus or atrium.

Despite the most careful scrutiny of a surface electrocardiogram, it is often difficult to determine the origin of a tachycardia. Electrophysiologic investigation has helped to determine the relative importance of the following in differentiating supraventricular from ventricular tachycardia by use of the surface electrocardiogram: rate and regularity of the tachycardia, relationship of the ventricular and atrial activity during tachycardia, width of the QRS complex, shape of the QRS complex, and fusion beats during tachycardia (Table 4).

Tachycardia Rate

The ventricular rate during tachycardia does not help to distinguish supraventricular tachycardia with aberrancy from ventricular tachycardia. The most common ventricular rates range from 170 to 200 bpm for supraventricular tachycardia and from 130 to 170 bpm for ventricular tachycardia. However, rates less than 120 and more than 200 bpm are found with both types of tachycardia. In both the supraventricular and the ventricular types, the tachycardia is generally regular. Occasionally, in ventricular tachycardia, there is a variation of 10 to 50 msec between two ventricular complexes. Changes of more than 20 msec in regularity can be observed in 20 per cent of patients with ventricular tachycardia and in less than 10 per cent of patients with supraventricular tachycardia.

Atrioventricular Relationship

Recording the atrial activity by use of an esophageal or atrial recording lead helps to evaluate the relationship of atrial and ventricular activities if atrial activity cannot be identified on the electrocardiogram. The presence of AV dissociation has long been used as a clue in identifying ventricular tachycardia. It has been well established that patients with ventricular tachycardia can have a 1:1 AV relationship. Such patients have retrograde VA conduction.

In general, VA conduction is often intact during ventricular tachycardia, with 30 per cent of patients demonstrating 1:1 VA conduction, 20 per cent demonstrating incomplete VA block, and the remaining 50 per cent having no VA conduction. As the ventricular rate increases during ventricular tachycardia, the frequency of VA conduction block also increases, such that less than 10 per cent of patients with a ventricular rate exceeding 200 bpm will demonstrate 1:1 VA conduction.

In patients with ventricular tachycardia who have a 1:1 atrial and ventricular relationship due to retrograde VA conduction, the P waves will proceed from the low to the high portion of the atrium, with an axis of −90°. Such P waves occur shortly after the completion of the QRS complex and are similar to P waves associated with PSVT due to re-entry within the AV node and PSVT dependent on an accessory AV pathway that is present near the atrial septum.

During an episode of tachycardia with a wide QRS complex, the tachycardia is most likely ventricular in origin if P waves are seen that are normal in shape and independent of the ventricular rhythm. If no P waves are seen, or if there is 1:1 AV relationship, the tachycardia can be either supraventricular or ventricular.

Finally, if 2:1 VA conduction is observed, the diagnosis is ventricular tachycardia because this relationship is only rarely produced by a rhythm other than ventricular tachycardia. On occasion, carotid sinus massage can help dissociate atrial activity from ven-

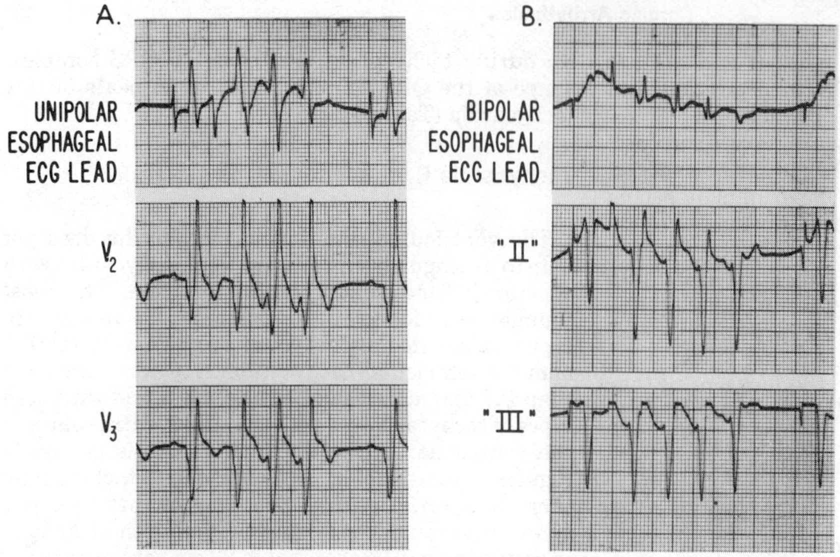

Figure 18. Contrasting atrial premature complexes recorded using a unipolar esophageal lead with a bipolar esophageal lead. (*A*) Panel demonstrates a unipolar esophageal lead recorded simultaneously with surface leads "V_2" and "V_3." Atrial premature complexes are present; however, the atrial depolarization is difficult to discern from ventricular depolarization in the unipolar esophageal lead recording. (*B*) Atrial premature complexes are again present; however, the bipolar esophageal lead clearly demonstrates atrial depolarization without interference from QRS depolarization.

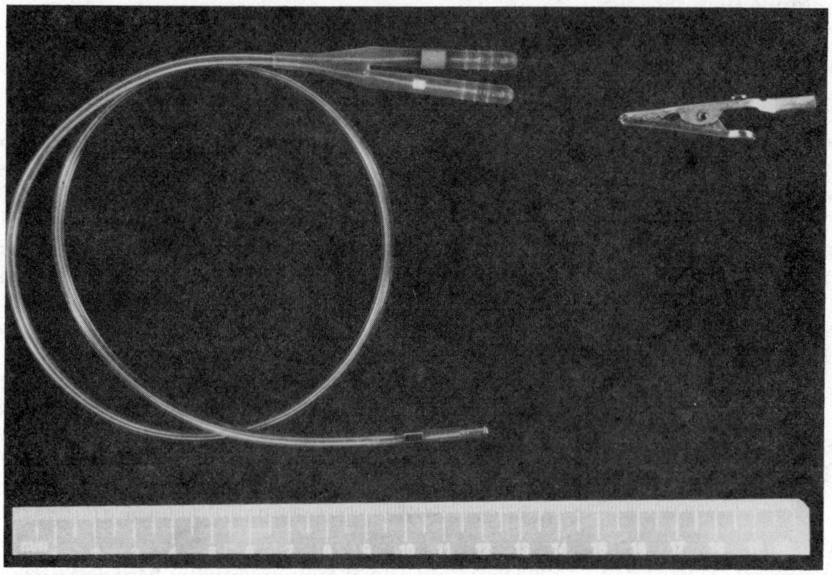

Figure 19. Typical endocardial permanent pacing lead used for recording a bipolar electrogram from the esophagus.

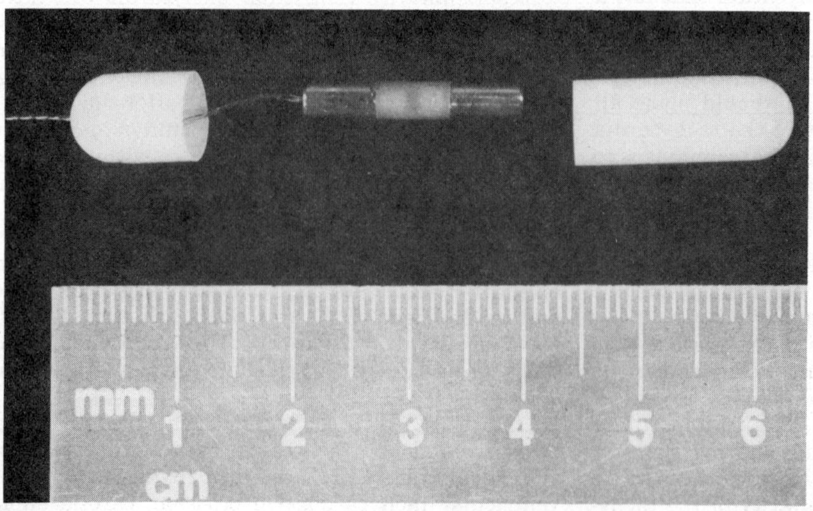

Figure 20. Pill electrode used for recording a bipolar electrogram from the esophagus.

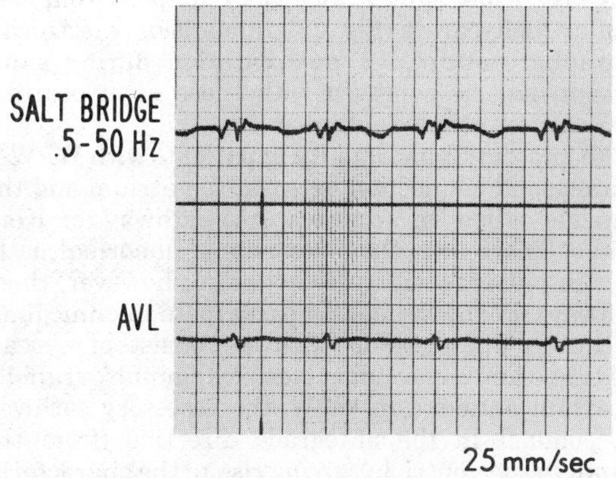

Figure 21. Recording an atrial electrogram using the proximal lumen of a Swan-Ganz catheter as a salt-bridge. The salt-bridge is filtered at 0.5 to 50 Hz, and atrial activity can be observed as it is recorded simultaneously with surface lead AVL. However, the atrial activity is difficult to separate from ventricular activity, and during a rapid ventricular rhythm, this technique may not provide adequate information.

tricular activity during ventricular tachycardia and establish the diagnosis.

QRS Width and Configuration

The width of the QRS complex during tachycardia can help identify whether it is supraventricular or ventricular in origin. In general, when a tachycardia exhibits a QRS duration longer than 140 msec (if the baseline QRS is normal), it is ventricular tachycardia. However, ventricular tachycardia also may be present with QRS complexes of less than 140 msec and occasionally of less than 100 msec. If ventricular tachycardia originates near the origin of the His bundle, the QRS configuration will be narrow. This occurs because the ventricles are depolarized simultaneously from a focus that originates in the intraventricular septum. It is generally believed that ventricular tachycardia in which there is a right bundle-branch block pattern originates in the left ventricle, and a ventricular tachycardia with a left bundle-branch block pattern originates in the right ventricle. However, recent observations have demonstrated that nearly 100 per cent of patients with right bundle-branch block patterns will have the tachycardia originating from the left ventricle and more than 80 per cent of patients with a left bundle-branch block pattern also will have the tachycardia originating in the left ventricle. Approximately 15 per cent of patients with left bundle-branch block configuration during ventricular tachycardia will have the tachycardia originating in the right ventricle, and, in general, these patients do not have associated coronary artery disease.

Fusion Beats

Fusion beats appear in approximately 12 per cent of patients with ventricular tachycardia and are important findings in differentiating supraventricular from ventricular tachycardia. The fusion beat combines the morphologic features of the supraventricular complex and the complex formed by the ventricular tachycardia. The presence of fusion beats on the surface electrocardiogram during tachycardia generally is suggestive of a ventricular origin.

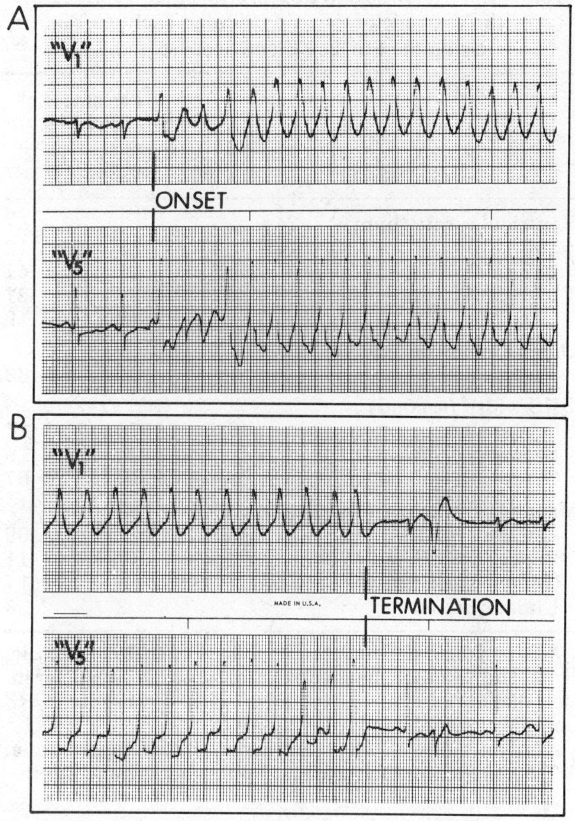

Figure 22. Tachycardia with a wide QRS complex recorded during 24-hour ambulatory monitoring. (*A*) Surface leads "V_1" and "V_5" are recorded simultaneously and demonstrate the onset of tachycardia. The tachycardia has a QRS width of 120 ms and is regular, and the rate is 200 beats per minute. (*B*) Termination of tachycardia. The mechanism of this tachycardia was determined to be antidromic re-entrant tachycardia, using an accessory atrioventricular pathway for conduction in the antegrade direction and the atrioventricular node for conduction in the retrograde direction in a patient with the Wolff-Parkinson-White syndrome and an accessory pathway located in the left lateral atrioventricular groove.

The H-V Interval

The relationship of the His bundle depolarization to the onset of the QRS complex (H-V interval) is important in establishing the origin of a tachycardia; however, this information can be obtained only during electrophysiologic testing. If the mechanism of a tachycardia remains obscure despite recording atrial activity using an esophageal or atrial recording lead, it may be necessary to perform intracardiac recording

Table 4. Differentiating Supraventricular Tachycardia with Aberrancy from Ventricular Tachycardia Using the Surface Electrocardiogram*

	Percentage of Patients	
	SVT	*VT*
Ventricular rate (bpm)		
100–130	1	13
130–170	27	47
170–200	60	21
> 200	12	19
One-to-one atrial and ventricular relationship	100	33
QRS width (second)		
0.12 or less	76	14
Between 0.12 and 0.14	24	19
Greater than 0.14	0	67
Mean QRS axis (frontal plane)		
−30° or less	7	69
Between −30° and +90°	47	11
Greater than +90°	43	17
Undetermined	3	3

*Data from Wellens, H.J.J., Bär, F.W.H.M., and Lie, K.I.: The value of the electrocardiogram in the differential diagnosis of a tachycardia with a widened QRS complex. Am. J. Med., 64:27, 1978.

Abbreviations: SVT = Supraventricular tachycardia; VT = ventricular tachycardia; bpm = beats per minute.

and programmed stimulation. This technique should be performed by physicians trained in this procedure.

The following observations are more commonly made during ventricular tachycardia when attempting to differentiate this rhythm from supraventricular tachycardia with aberrancy: atrial ventricular dissociation; superior QRS axis; QRS width exceeding 0.14 second; monophasic or biphasic QRS complexes in V_1 resembling those in right bundle-branch block; Q-R or Q-S in V_6 resembling those in left bundle-branch block; and fusion complexes.

SYNDROMES ASSOCIATED WITH DISORDERS IN CARDIAC RHYTHM

Wolff-Parkinson-White Syndrome

Ventricular pre-excitation exists when any part of the ventricular myocardium is activated by an impulse originating in the atrium earlier than would be expected if the impulse reached the ventricle by way of the normal specialized conducting tissues. The most common pre-excitation syndrome is the WPW syndrome. The clinical significance of WPW is due to the increased incidence of arrhythmias associated with pre-excitation. In addition, the electrocardiographic pattern observed in patients with pre-excitation often gives rise to bizarre electrocardiographic tracings during tachycardia, which can be a source of tremendous diagnostic difficulty in attempting to diagnose atrial flutter or PSVT with conduction down the accessory pathway, resulting in a wide QRS complex from ventricular tachycardia (Fig. 22). In addition, electrocardiographic patterns of pre-excitation during sinus rhythm may be confused with those of myocardial infarction or other conditions.

The anatomic abnormality in patients with WPW is an abnormal connection between the atrium and the ventricle called an accessory AV pathway, or Kent bundle. There are other locations of abnormal pathways in patients with pre-excitation; however, these pathways do not frequently participate in clinical arrhythmias. The accessory pathway consists of myocardial tissue and can conduct electrical impulses rapidly in certain patients. In WPW, the accessory pathway can conduct in the antegrade direction (from the atrium to the ventricle), giving rise to the characteristic findings on the electrocardiogram. Activation of the ventricle results from a fusion via the normal conducting AV node and the accessory pathway. This results in abbreviation of the P-R interval (classically less than 0.1 second) and an abnormal QRS complex due to eccentric depolarization of the ventricles by the accessory pathway. The eccentric ventricular depolarization with fusion results in a delta wave and a QRS duration greater than or equal to 0.12 second.

It is important to note that not all patients with WPW have a short P-R interval. If there is prolonged conduction within the atrium and the accessory pathway is remote from the AV node, the P-R interval may approach normal.

The incidence of the electrocardiographic pattern of pre-excitation described as WPW has been reported to vary from 0.1 to 3.0 per 1000 and shows no age predilection. Atrioventricular accessory pathways that are involved in tachycardias and are capable of antegrade conduction have been associated with certain heart disease, specifically Ebstein's anomaly of the tricuspid valve, in which as many as 10 per cent of patients so affected will have pre-excitation, usually involving a pathway located in the right ventricular free wall. There is an association reported between left-sided bypass tracts and mitral valve prolapse. In most patients with WPW, however, no disease is present, even though pre-excitation is found.

Many patients with accessory pathways manifest arrhythmias, the most common of which is PSVT, which uses the normal AV node and His-Purkinje system as the antegrade limb of the re-entrant circuit and the accessory pathway as the retrograde limb of the re-entrant circuit. This type of tachycardia is termed *orthodromic.* Initiation of a typical attack of tachycardia results when a premature beat blocks the accessory pathway and then conducts with a physiologic delay down the normal conduction tissue of the AV node, which results in a QRS complex without pre-excitation. The wave of excitability then spreads throughout the ventricle and reaches the accessory pathway, which can sustain conduction so that it occurs in the retrograde direction across the pathway, allowing re-excitation of the atrium. As a result, a re-entrant circuit has been established and tachycardia is initiated.

A less common type of re-entrant tachycardia in patients with accessory pathways is referred to as *antidromic reciprocating tachycardia.* In this circumstance, the accessory pathway functions as the antegrade limb of the re-entrant circuit and the retrograde limb is made up of the AV node. This type of tachycardia occurs in approximately 5 per cent of patients with PSVT associated with WPW. Since the impulse travels from the atrium to the ventricle down the AV bypass tract, the electrocardiogram during tachycardia reveals a P wave just preceding the pre-excited ventricular complex and a wide QRS complex, which may be confused with ventricular tachycardia (Fig. 22). The electrocardiogram during sinus rhythm demonstrates the typical WPW characteristics of a short P-R interval and a delta wave.

Patients with WPW are susceptible to the development of very rapid ventricular rates during atrial fibrillation or atrial flutter. During atrial fibrillation the QRS complex will be wide, owing to ventricular pre-excitation. However, conduction down the AV node will occasionally result in a normal QRS complex or fusion complexes (Fig. 3). The ventricular rate and the configuration of the QRS complex depend on the refractory periods of the AV node and the accessory pathway. Patients with an accessory pathway can experience ventricular rates as fast as 350 bpm during atrial fibrillation or atrial flutter, which may deteriorate to ventricular fibrillation and cause sudden death. Such patients should be evaluated further with electrophysiologic testing.

Mitral Valve Prolapse

In general, mitral valve prolapse is considered a benign condition; however, a low but significant incidence of sudden death does occur. In most patients, the cause of the sudden death appears to be secondary to ventricular arrhythmia. During 24-hour ambulatory monitoring, patients with mitral valve prolapse have a higher incidence of ventricular arrhythmias than otherwise normal patients. These patients also exhibit an increased incidence of supraventricular arrhythmias, including APCs, atrial fibrillation, atrial flutter, and PSVT. They also have a higher incidence of left-sided accessory pathways that may conduct in the antegrade direction (WPW syndrome) or only in the retrograde direction (concealed accessory pathway).

The most significant rhythm abnormalities in patients with mitral valve prolapse are the ventricular arrhythmias, and these range from isolated PVCs to frequent multiform PVCs and ventricular tachycardia. The overall incidence of sudden death is not known, although a review of several series of patients with mitral valve prolapse noted a 1.4 per cent incidence. These groups were probably biased because of symptoms and obvious cardiac signs; however, the condition of mitral valve prolapse may be a relatively important cause of sudden death in patients who are otherwise young and healthy.

Patients with mitral valve prolapse and suspected ventricular arrhythmias should be evaluated with 24-hour ambulatory monitoring. This technique may identify potentially life-threatening arrhythmias; however, because such monitoring is merely a sample in time, arrhythmias may not occur during that time. If necessary, 24-hour ambulatory monitoring can be continued until arrhythmias are recorded. If a patient's episode of palpitation lasts long enough to allow the use of a telephone transmitter, this technique can be very helpful in identifying the cause of a patient's symptoms.

Some patients with mitral valve prolapse may have serious arrhythmias during exercise stress testing. This is an appropriate initial examination to perform in an attempt to induce the arrhythmias in patients who have symptoms suggestive of tachycardia. A normal exercise stress test does not exclude the possibility of sudden death at a later date, and the significance of ventricular ectopy, in the absence of ventricular tachycardia induced at the time of exercise, is not known. Patients with documented ventricular arrhythmias or episodes of syncope may benefit from electrophysiologic testing.

Patients with mitral valve prolapse have abnormalities of their electrocardiograms. Approximately 80 per cent of patients who have mitral valve prolapse and die suddenly demonstrate S-T segment and T wave changes on their electrocardiograms. Unfortunately, these changes are not specific. Q-T interval prolongation is present in approximately 25 per cent of patients with mitral valve prolapse who die suddenly. Little is known about the incidence of Q-T prolongation or S-T segment and T wave changes in patients with mitral valve prolapse who have no symptoms suggesting tachycardia. In general, such changes on the electrocardiogram in patients with mitral valve prolapse should raise the suspicion of significant ventricular arrhythmias, and these patients should be evaluated further with 24-hour ambulatory monitoring and exercise stress testing.

Sick Sinus Syndrome

Sinus node dysfunction is an important syndrome resulting in disturbances in cardiac rhythm. The sick sinus syndrome is a general term used to describe disorders of sinus node function that result in a failure of the sinus node impulse to activate the atrium (sinoatrial conduction block) or a failure of the sinus node to adequately perform its pacemaking function (sinus pause or sinus arrest) (Fig. 1). A major subset of the sick sinus syndrome is the tachycardia-bradycardia syndrome, which is characterized by episodes of supraventricular tachycardia and sinus bradycardia. At the termination of supraventricular tachycardia, there is often prolonged delay before sinus rhythm returns. Patients may experience syncope during this transition phase from paroxysmal tachycardia to sinus rhythm. Generally, sinus node dysfunction is found in association with abnormalities of the subsidiary pacemakers in the AV node and the His-Purkinje system such that they do not maintain an adequate cardiac rhythm during the absence of sinus node activity. Supraventricular arrhythmias associated with the tachycardia-bradycardia syndrome include atrial fibrillation, atrial flutter, and atrial tachycardia.

Symptoms in patients with the sick sinus syndrome may be intermittent and are often difficult to correlate with findings on the electrocardiogram. In identifying episodes of tachycardia and bradycardia that the patient is unaware of, 24-hour ambulatory monitoring may be helpful. Symptoms include syncope, dizziness, and palpitation, and cerebrovascular accidents due to thromboembolism are observed in the tachycardia-bradycardia syndrome. The increased risk of cerebral embolization is presumably due to alterations in the atrial rhythm.

Patients may present with sinus arrest, sinus pauses, or significant sinus bradycardia of 25 to 40 bpm. On occasion, atrial standstill may be observed; this is most commonly associated with cardiomyopathies and infiltrative diseases of the heart. Obviously, for significant sinus bradycardia or sinus pauses to occur, there must be malfunction of subsidiary pacemakers in the region of the AV junction and specialized conduction system.

Atrial fibrillation may occur in patients with sick sinus syndrome as a result of the atrial enlargement and fibrosis that has been the initial cause of the sinus node dysfunction. Such patients will have severely prolonged sinus node recovery after attempted electrocardioversion of their atrial fibrillation. If it is suspected that patients with atrial fibrillation have underlying sick sinus syndrome, they should undergo cardioversion with caution, if at all. One clue that may help the physician identify patients with sinus node dysfunction as the cause of their atrial fibrillation is that such patients may have coexistent AV node dysfunction and a slow ventricular rate during atrial fibrillation.

Hypertrophic Cardiomyopathy

Patients with hypertrophic cardiomyopathy are known to have an increased incidence of sudden death when compared with otherwise normal patients. Approximately 70 per cent of patients who die suddenly are younger than 30 years of age, with 50 per cent of patients having no functional limitations and 15 per cent of patients performing sedentary or minimal physical activity at the time of sudden death. Most of these patients probably die from ventricular arrhythmias. Of patients with hypertrophic cardiomyopathy who have symptoms suggestive of arrhythmias, 80 per cent will demonstrate PVCs, 50 per cent will have grade II ectopic activity, and 15 per cent will have short runs of ventricular tachycardia. It is difficult to delineate clinical variables that identify a subgroup of patients with hypertrophic cardiomyopathy who are at an increased risk for sudden death. However, two variables that may be helpful are a predilection for sudden premature death in families with known hypertrophic cardiomyopathy and the presence of asymptomatic ventricular tachycardia on 24-hour ambulatory monitoring.

Congenital Heart Disease

Recent advances in surgical techniques and improved postoperative care have increased the survival of patients undergoing correction of congenital heart defects. These patients are now approaching adulthood, and the long-term sequelae of these repairs are assuming more importance to the cardiologist. Patients may present with arrhythmias that existed before surgery, including atrial fibrillation, atrial tachycardia, and PSVT.

Generally, surgery does not eliminate these arrhythmias. Patients with congenital heart surgery also experience atrial ventricular block, including complete heart block, as a complication of their operations. Ventricular arrhythmias are the most significant arrhythmias of patients who have had congenital heart surgery. Data on the incidence of ventricular tachycardia in this group of patients are scarce, but information is becoming available with regard to certain subsets of patients, including those with repair of tetralogy of Fallot. The long-term electrophysiologic consequences of repair of tetralogy of Fallot include atrial ventricular conduction defects, intraventricular conduction defects, ventricular arrhythmias, and sudden death. Electrophysiologic study of a few such patients has suggested that one cause of sustained ventricular tachycardia after repair of tetralogy of Fallot is re-entry at the site of the previous operation in the right ventricular outflow tract. The development of significant ventricular arrhythmias in patients who have had total correction of tetralogy of Fallot is uncommon, and it remains unclear why certain patients will experience ventricular tachycardia. Patients with repair of tetralogy of Fallot who present with frequent and severe ventricular arrhythmias or documented recurrent ventricular tachycardia should undergo electrophysiologic testing to characterize the rhythm disturbance and determine the most appropriate therapeutic approach.

Congenital Heart Block

Congenital complete heart block implies that the atrium and the ventricles beat independently (complete AV dissociation). Congenital heart block can be diagnosed when a young patient has a slow pulse and AV block is seen on his electrocardiogram and there is no evidence of an infectious process that may have resulted in AV block during childhood. The incidence of congenital heart block is approximately 0.4 per cent, and it is generally detected during the perinatal period. In approximately 10 per cent of patients, the diagnosis will not be made until they are older.

Congenital heart block can be diagnosed on the surface electrocardiogram. The P waves and QRS complexes are unassociated, and the atrial rate is usually faster than the ventricular rate. The AV block is generally located in the region of the AV node in patients who have a normal QRS complex and a ventricular rate of 60 bpm or more. In contrast, in patients who have a slow ventricular escape rhythm and a wide QRS complex, the block is usually within or distal to the bundle of His. Unfortunately, there is overlap with regard to the level of AV block and the findings on the surface electrocardiogram. Intracardiac recordings can establish the level of block.

Twenty-four-hour ambulatory monitoring may be helpful in evaluation of the patient with congenital heart block. This allows the physician to evaluate the heart rate during various levels of activity and determine if bradycardia is persistent. It also allows for identification of ventricular arrhythmias that may be precipitated with exercise.

Patients with congenital heart block also should be evaluated using exercise testing. This allows the physician to evaluate the response of the escape focus to exercise. In general, patients who can increase their heart rates the most during exercise have block in the region of the AV node. Usually, such patients can lead relatively normal lives without the need for a permanent pacemaker. Exercise stress testing also can determine whether ventricular arrhythmias can be precipitated with exercise. Patients with congenital heart block will have an increased incidence of significant ventricular arrhythmias as they become older. The increased incidence of ventricular arrhythmias during exercise may place the patient at a higher risk for sudden death, and such patients may respond favorably to implantation of a permanent pacemaker. This question is currently under evaluation. After diagnosing congenital heart block, the physician should further evaluate the patient using 24-hour ambulatory monitoring and exercise stress testing. If a persistent bradycardia is present that does not respond well to exercise or if there are ventricular arrhythmias, the patient should be considered for an electrophysiologic study and the implantation of a permanent dual-chamber physiologic pacing system.

Aortic Valve Replacement

Sudden death is a complication of aortic valve disease even after successful aortic valve replacement has been performed and the hemodynamic burden imposed by aortic regurgitation and aortic stenosis has been improved. Sudden death occurs in a small percentage of patients after aortic valve replacement and is most likely a consequence of ventricular arrhythmias. More than 90 per cent of patients with aortic valve replacement will demonstrate significant ventricular arrhythmias, including multiform PVCs in 90 per cent, bigeminy in 60 per cent, couplets in 60 per cent, and ventricular tachycardia in 35 per cent.

After aortic valve replacement, most patients have significant ventricular arrhythmias, and the relationship of these ventricular arrhythmias to the occurrence of sudden death has to be inferred. Patients with aortic valve replacement exhibiting ventricular tachycardia by 24-hour ambulatory monitoring should be further evaluated for antiarrhythmic therapy. Patients who have symptoms of near-syncope or syncope suggestive of prolonged episodes of tachycardia should be evaluated by 24-hour ambulatory monitoring and exercise stress testing and considered for electrophysiologic investigation.

Aggravation of Ventricular Arrhythmias by Antiarrhythmic Drugs

The use of ambulatory monitoring and exercise stress testing has enabled the physician to identify patients with significant ventricular arrhythmias who are at risk for sudden death. Once the patient with complex PVCs is identified, treatment is instituted in an attempt to suppress the ventricular arrhythmia by the use of antiarrhythmic drugs. Frequently drug therapy fails to control the arrhythmia despite achieving "therapeutic" blood levels. Each antiarrhythmic drug has the potential of making the ventricular rhythm disturbance worse in an individual patient. This constitutes a significant threat to the patient being treated for ventricular arrhythmias and undoubtedly has accounted for iatrogenic fatalities, which could have been prevented had the physician been aware of this adverse reaction. Quinidine was the first drug to be associated with a paradoxical increase in ventricular tachycardia and ventricular fibrillation.

Less well appreciated is the potential for other antiarrhythmic drugs to worsen ventricular arrhythmias. The aggravation of arrhythmias also has been noted with lidocaine, procainamide, disopyramide, propranolol, metoprolol, aprindine, mexiletine, tocainide, amiodarone, and pindolol. The worsening of ventricular arrhythmias occurs with plasma drug concentrations in the therapeutic range; the incidence is between 6 and 16 per cent.

The physician who is caring for patients with significant ventricular arrhythmias should realize the potential that each antiarrhythmic drug has for worsening the ventricular arrhythmia. The physician must assess not only whether the antiarrhythmic drug is effective and has not resulted in toxicity but also whether the drug has not resulted in a paradoxical increase in the frequency of the ventricular arrhythmias.

Arrhythmogenic Right Ventricular Dysplasia

In 1972, Uhl described a group of patients with right ventricular dysplasia in whom the right ventricle was paper-thin, with apposition of the endocardium to the epicardium. Since this initial description, patients have been identified who have right ventricular dysplasia with right ventricular musculature that is partially or totally absent and replaced by fibrous and fatty tissue.

This abnormality is confined to the right ventricle, and if the dysplasia is extensive, there will be roentgenographic evidence of cardiomegaly and congestive heart failure in early childhood. However, such patients may survive to adulthood and have asymptomatic cardiomegaly. The dysplasia can be limited to certain portions of the right ventricle, with minimal impairment in cardiac function. Such patients may present with ventricular tachycardia of right ventricular origin. They have the following characteristics:

1. The male-to-female ratio is 2.7:1 with a mean age, by the time of hospitalization, of 39 years.
2. All the patients have ventricular tachycardia of left bundle-branch block configuration.
3. All patients have inverted T waves over the right precordial leads on a surface electrocardiogram.
4. The heart generally demonstrates cardiomegaly with abnormal pulmonary vasculature.

5. Right ventricular angiography or two-dimensional echocardiography will demonstrate contraction abnormalities of the right ventricle.

The diagnosis should be considered in patients who have ventricular tachycardia of unknown cause, especially if the tachycardia has a left bundle-branch configuration on the surface electrocardiogram.

Liquid Protein Diets

The protein supplement fast is recognized as an effective means of weight reduction; however, patients taking the liquid protein diet have an increased incidence of sudden death. Electrocardiograms performed on such patients often demonstrate a prolongation of the Q-T interval and decreased QRS voltage. Unfortunately, studies designed to evaluate the liquid protein diet in a prospective fashion have found no abnormalities on the 12-lead electrocardiogram in patients who subsequently develop significant ventricular arrhythmias.

The mechanism of sudden death in patients taking low-protein diets remains unclear. Deficiencies of protein, electrolytes, trace elements, and micronutrients (such as essential fatty acids) may have a role in the development of significant ventricular arrhythmias. This type of diet program is not recommended, and patients on such diets should undergo 24-hour ambulatory monitoring and should be warned of the increased incidence of ventricular arrhythmias and sudden death. Routine chemical determinations and metabolic balance studies have failed to identify patients at risk for cardiac complications; therefore, the physician and patient can have a false sense of security if only serum electrolytes are monitored.

Torsades de Pointes

Dessertenne described a rare ventricular arrhythmia in 1966, which he termed *torsades de pointes* (Fig. 23). This arrhythmia may be misclassified as ventricular tachycardia or ventricular fibrillation; however, it is a distinct rhythm disturbance. Torsades de pointes can be distinguished from ventricular fibrillation by its unusual response to conventional treatment; antiarrhythmic drugs that prolong the Q-T interval may aggravate the frequency and duration of episodes of torsades de pointes. Such drugs include quinidine, procainamide, and disopyramide.

The electrocardiographic pattern in torsades de pointes is distinct, with episodes of alternating electrical polarity such that the peaks of the QRS complexes appear to twist around an isoelectric line. The alternating cycles may be seen to move in and out during episodes of rapid tachycardia with uniform configuration and polarity.

The rhythm disturbance generally terminates spontaneously; however, a fatal outcome is possible. The rhythm has been reported to occur at all ages and often without evidence of associated heart disease. The rate of the tachycardia varies between 160 and 280 bpm and is usually initiated by a PVC occurring late in diastole. Torsades de pointes virtually always occurs in the setting of prolongation of the Q-T interval, and a prominent U wave is frequently present. Our present state of knowledge with regard to this rhythm disturbance suggests that torsades de pointes should not be diagnosed solely from the morphologic appearance of the tachycardia and that there also should be supportive evidence of associated delay in myocardial repolarization (Q-T interval prolongation).

The relationship among conventional ventricular tachycardia, torsades de pointes, and ventricular fibrillation remains unclear. Torsades de pointes appears to be a rhythm disturbance that is transitional between ventricular tachycardia and ventricular fibrillation. Any disturbance that results in Q-T prolongation can cause torsades de pointes. Such disturbances are listed in Table 5. This rhythm disturbance is associated with syncope in patients with the syndrome of congenital Q-T prolongation both without (Romano-Ward) and with (Jervell and Lange-Nielsen) deafness. The rhythm also occurs frequently in the setting of pronounced bradycardia or complete heart block, possibly due to a variation in sympathetic tone of the cardiac nerves and the consequent aggravation of the dispersion of repolarization that is already present at slow heart rates. In patients who have syncope after being started on quinidine therapy, torsades de pointes is the most likely cause. The incidence of Q-R prolongation with therapeutic quinidine levels is between 0.5 and 8.8 per cent. Other causes of torsades de pointes include the use of procainamide, disopyramide, organophosphorus insecticide poisoning, phenothiazines, liquid protein diets, and possibly tricyclic antidepressants after overdosage. Hypokalemia is an important cause of torsades de pointes, and there have been case reports of hypomagnesemia in association with torsades de pointes. Although Q-T prolongation occurs with myocarditis, myocardial infarction, and variant angina, torsades de pointes is rare in these settings.

Unless recognized, torsades de pointes secondary to antiarrhythmic medications will be made worse if antiarrhythmic treatment is increased. The proper therapy is to discontinue the offending antiarrhythmic agent in such patients and restart a new antiarrhythmic agent that does not result in Q-T prolongation but does suppress the initial ventricular arrhythmia.

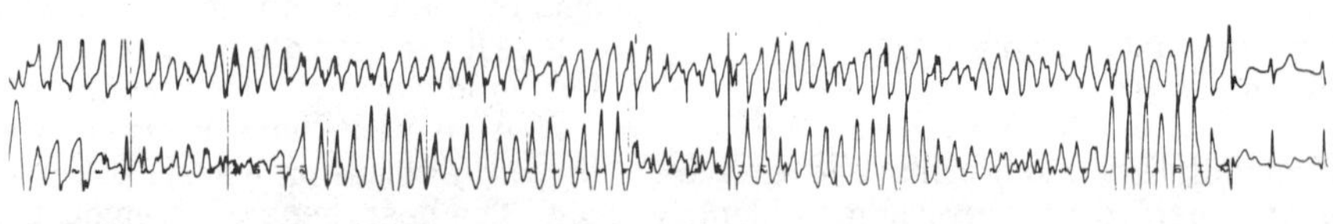

Figure 23. A rhythm strip recording an episode of torsades de pointes in a patient with congenital Q-T prolongation.

Table 5. Conditions Associated with Torsades de Pointes

Electrolyte Abnormality
- Hypokalemia
- Hypomagnesemia (rare)
- Hypocalcemia (rare)

Drug-Related
- Antiarrhythmic agents (quinidine, procainamide, disopyramide, amiodarone, lidocaine, aprindine)
- Psychotropic agents (phenothiazines, tricyclic antidepressants)
- Organophosphate poisoning

Liquid Protein Diets

Cardiac Disease
- Ischemia
- Myocarditis
- Bradycardia (sinus node disease, atrioventricular block with a slow escape rhythm)

Central Nervous System Disease
- Intracranial trauma
- Subarachnoid hemorrhage
- Pneumoencephalography

Congenital Syndromes
- Romano-Ward
- Jervell and Lange-Nielsen

Lown-Ganong-Levine Syndrome

The Lown-Ganong-Levine syndrome (LGL) is diagnosed in patients with paroxysmal tachycardia whose electrocardiograms demonstrate a P-R interval of less than 0.1 second and a normal QRS complex. Arrhythmias associated with the LGL syndrome include atrial fibrillation, atrial flutter, PSVT due to re-entry within the AV node, re-entry within the atrium, or re-entry utilizing a concealed accessory pathway, ectopic atrial tachycardia, and ventricular tachycardia. Patients with this syndrome demonstrate enhanced conduction and shortened refractoriness of the AV node which presumably allows supraventricular tachycardias to cause a more rapid ventricular rate. These patients are thus more likely to be symptomatic than patients with normal AV nodal conduction.

Carotid Sinus Hypersensitivity

The recognition that the carotid sinus reflex has not only physiologic but also clinical implications is as old as the discovery of the reflex itself. Numerous accounts have appeared in the medical literature of syncope and even convulsions in response to mechanical manipulation of the carotid sinus in man. Persons so affected were believed to have a hyperactive carotid sinus reflex. As a logical extension of this observation, the sinus reflex was studied as a possible cause of spontaneously occurring syncope and a relationship was shown to exist in some patients. Spontaneously occurring carotid sinus symptoms with or without syncope are referred to as the carotid sinus syndrome.

The term *hyperactive carotid sinus reflex* applies when digital stimulation of the carotid sinus results in pronounced slowing of cardiac rate or in cardiac asystole accompanied by a decrease in systemic blood pressure. In some patients, only the blood pressure decreases while cardiac rhythm remains unaffected. In general, cardiac asystole of 3 seconds or more and a decrease in systolic blood pressure of 50 mm Hg or more are clearly abnormal responses to carotid sinus massage. A slowing of heart rate by 30 to 40 per cent, cardiac asystole lasting 2 seconds, and a decrease in blood pressure of 30 mm Hg constitute a borderline response.

The incidence of a hyperactive carotid sinus reflex is extremely low during the first three decades of life, but it increases steadily thereafter. Males are affected twice as often as females; the reflex may be evoked more easily from the right than from the left sinus, and it may be present bilaterally. This reflex may be present in elderly persons and not be responsible for episodes of syncope. Such persons may have syncope on the basis of another disturbance in cardiac rhythm, which will be overlooked if the evaluation is stopped after carotid sinus hypersensitivity is identified.

While the hyperactive carotid sinus reflex has limited clinical significance and does not give rise to spontaneous symptoms, the *carotid sinus syndrome* (also called spontaneous carotid sinus syncope) is clinically significant, with symptoms occurring spontaneously. Most patients exhibiting abnormal sinus sensitivity on manual testing do not suffer spontaneous carotid sinus syncope. Conversely, patients with spontaneous sinus syncope usually do have a hyperactive reflex. The two may be closely related, differing perhaps only in matters of severity. By definition, the diagnosis of spontaneous carotid sinus syndrome can be established if spontaneously occurring symptoms of dizziness, blurring of vision, faintness, or fainting can be reproduced by stimulation of one or both carotid sinuses, provided carotid blood flow is preserved during the test.

The spontaneous syndrome has been divided into the cardioinhibitory type (with bradycardia or asystole with or without systemic hypotension) and the vasodepressor type (not associated with a cardiac slowing but only a decrease in blood pressure). This division is nearly always made on the basis of the patient's response to the sinus stimulation test, since one is rarely able to study the patient during one of these spontaneous attacks.

In most patients suffering from spontaneous carotid sinus syncope, no obvious cause for the spells can be identified. Causes of carotid sinus syncope include forced head turning while backing up an automobile, hyperextension of the neck, and working overhead. Other local trigger factors include pressure of constricting neckwear, stretching of the skin over the neck when shaving, and carrying heavy shoulder loads. Pathologic changes adjacent to the carotid sinus, such as thyroid tumors, carotid body tumor, and inflammatory and malignant lymph nodes, are other extravascular conditions that may precipitate the spontaneous syndrome.

Repetitive Monomorphic ("Benign") Ventricular Tachycardia

Gallavaridin was the first physician to suggest there may be a benign form of ventricular tachycardia. He described a ventricular arrhythmia characterized by single and double PVCs and brief episodes of ventricular tachycardia. The bursts of tachycardia were usually three to ten complexes long, and all ectopic QRS complexes exhibited a uniform configuration. The intervening sinus complexes were normal, and the ventricular arrhythmia occurred alternating with normal sinus complexes. This tachycardia has subsequently been called benign ventricular tachycardia, type II paroxysmal ventricular tachycardia, and repetitive paroxysmal ventricular tachycardia.

The arrhythmia is usually associated with a good prognosis; however, sudden death has been reported. The arrhythmia occurs in younger patients who do not demonstrate significant heart disease and may persist for years, although spontaneous resolution has been reported. Occasionally, patients will experience congestive heart failure during the incessant ventricular tachycardia.

Patients with this form of ventricular tachycardia have the following clinical characteristics:

1. The mean age is approximately 35 years.
2. In general, a long history of arrhythmia is present before evaluation.
3. Only rarely is there a history of syncope, and most patients are either asymptomatic or complain only of palpitations.
4. Most patients have no evidence of underlying heart disease, although an occasional patient may present with mitral valve prolapse.
5. Episodes of tachycardia tend to occur in clusters as demonstrated by 24-hour ambulatory monitoring.

Patients with this syndrome who were followed up for 8 years since the arrhythmia was first recognized showed no episodes of sudden death or progression of symptoms. It was reported that the ventricular tachycardia resolved spontaneously in approximately 30 per cent of patients when evaluated 4 years after the initial evaluation. In this group of patients, the incidence of mortality secondary to ventricular arrhythmia is low, and antiarrhythmic drug therapy is generally used only for the relief of symptomatic palpitations.

SUMMARY

The diagnosis of cardiac arrhythmias remains challenging. New techniques have facilitated the identification of symptomatic and asymptomatic rhythm disturbances. However, the physician must identify not only the mechanism of an arrhythmia but also the presence of associated cardiac and extracardiac abnormalities that affect the clinical presentation of the arrhythmia. Thus, the appropriate treatment of patients with a rhythm disturbance is based on accurate diagnosis and evaluation by the physician.

Glossary of Cardiology Terms

Aberrant conduction: The result of conduction that does not proceed normally through the atrioventricular conduction system. Aberrant conduction can be a consequence of left or right bundle-branch block, left anterior or posterior fascicular block, or ventricular pre-excitation due to an accessory atrioventricular pathway.

Antegrade conduction: Conduction that proceeds from the atrium to the ventricle. The conduction can be over the normal atrioventricular conduction system or an accessory atrioventricular pathway.

Atrioventricular association: The normal sequential activation of the atria and ventricles by a single impulse.

Atrioventricular dissociation: Activation of the atrium and ventricles by independent impulses.

Automatic rhythm: Automatic rhythms can occur throughout the heart and result when cells undergo spontaneous diastolic (phase IV) depolarization, reaching threshold at a rate that is faster than the rate of the normal sinus rhythm.

Concealed conduction: The effect of incomplete penetration of an impulse that can result in the following unexpected findings on an electrocardiogram: (1) a spontaneous pacemaker that demonstrates pauses; (2) failure of an impulse to propagate normally, resulting in high-grade block; and (3) prolongation of conduction, resulting in first-degree conduction block.

Conduction intervals:

P-R interval: The time from the onset of the P wave to the onset of the QRS complex.

H-V interval: The time from the onset of depolarization of the His bundle to the onset of ventricular activity (usually recorded by an endocardial electrode).

V-A interval: The time from the onset of ventricular activity to the onset of atrial activity. This measurement is usually obtained using intracardiac recordings or recordings of atrial activity from the esophagus.

R-P interval: The time from the onset of ventricular activity to the onset of atrial activity as manifested by the P wave. This interval is present when there is retrograde conduction from the ventricle to the atrium.

Q-T interval: The time from the onset of the Q wave to the termination of the T wave.

P-P interval: The time between two consecutive P waves.

R-R interval: The time between two consecutive QRS complexes.

Escape complex: Any complex that occurs later than the time of the next expected complex.

Nonparoxysmal: An arrhythmia that is present most of the time and neither starts nor terminates abruptly.

Normal atrioventricular conduction system: Also referred to as the *specialized conduction system.* Comprised of the atrioventricular node, His bundle, and Purkinje fibers.

Paroxysmal: An arrhythmia that is present intermittently and has an abrupt onset and an abrupt termination.

Premature complex: Any complex that occurs earlier than the next expected normal complex.

Re-entrant rhythm: Also referred to as a reciprocating rhythm, this rhythm abnormality can occur in any location within the heart. A re-entrant circuit is made up of two functionally distinct pathways that join proximally and distally to create a closed conduction circuit. A critically timed impulse will encounter this circuit at a time when one of the limbs is refractory to conduction and the other limb is able to maintain conduction (unidirectional block). The conduction proceeds slowly down the unblocked pathway, thus allowing the previously blocked pathway time to recover its ability to conduct the impulse. As the impulse reaches the distal end of the second pathway, it returns to the proximal common pathway, thus completing the re-entrant circuit. If a single re-entrant beat is produced, this is known as a *re-entrant echo,* or *reciprocating beat.* If the electrical impulse continues to move around the re-entrant circuit, a re-entrant tachycardia develops. Re-entry may involve a *micro*circuit that includes small areas within the heart, such as the atrioventricular node or areas of ventricle associated with myocardial infarction, or a *macro*circuit that involves larger areas of the heart, including the atria, ventricles, or His-Purkinje system.

Refractory Periods:

Relative: Prolongation of conduction of a premature impulse marking the end of the full recovery period.

Functional: The shortest interval that can be obtained between two consecutively conducted impulses.

Effective: The longest interval between two impulses that fails to be conducted through the tissue.

Retrograde conduction: Conduction that proceeds from the ventricle to the atrium. The conduction can be over the normal atrioventricular conduction system or an accessory atrioventricular pathway.

Supraventricular: Impulses that originate proximal to or within the His bundle.

Ventricular: Impulses that originate distal to the His bundle.

VALVULAR HEART DISEASE

By Robert A. Waugh, M.D.
Durham, North Carolina

Even though the incidence of rheumatic fever in the United States is declining, rheumatic valvular heart disease remains with us. In addition, other congenital and acquired valvular diseases are being recognized with increasing frequency due, in part, to the emergence of new technologies such as echocardiography. Finally, the increasing age of the United States population has allowed emergence of a variety of acquired degenerative valvular diseases.

This section deals primarily with valvular heart disease in the adult but touches briefly on other heart diseases as they relate to the clinical presentation, physical examination, and differential diagnosis. Since patients frequently present without a "label," the history and physical examination will be dealt with in a topical format (rather than a disease format) followed by a more detailed discussion of the clinical course and complications, differential diagnosis, and laboratory evaluation of various specific valvular entities. The salient historical and physical findings grouped according to type of valvular heart disease are also summarized in Tables 1 through 8.

HISTORY

Symptomatic Mechanisms

Patients with valvular heart disease may present in a variety of modes ranging from the asymptomatic state to full-blown heart failure. Asymptomatic patients are more likely to have either mild valvular disease (e.g., the usual patient with mitral valve prolapse) or volume overload problems such as aortic and mitral valve regurgitation. Symptoms typically arise, however, when the dysfunction is severe enough to cause problems with electrical function (arrhythmias), mechanical function (heart failure), and/or myocardial perfusion (chest pain). On occasion, the defect may alter the hemodynamics sufficiently (in the absence of heart failure) that the patient can perceive the alteration as, for example, in symptomatic neck vein pulsations due to tricuspid regurgitation or the large stroke volume of aortic regurgitation. In some instances, symptoms may arise when intracardiac clots or vegetations embolize and cause pain and/or significant target organ dysfunction. Although there is a general correlation between symptoms and severity, this is not invariable as, for example, when atrial fibrillation and/or systemic embolization supervene in relatively mild mitral valve disease. Finally, although the symptomatic manifestations arising from various perturbations in cardiac function can

Table 1. History and Symptoms in Aortic and Mitral Valve Disease

	Murmur	Arrhythmia	Heart Failure	Chest Pain
Aortic stenosis (AS)	If congenital, noted from early age by numerous examiners; in older patient, noted more recently and may have been labeled innocent	Unusual in youth/early adulthood; with increasing age, PVCs and atrial fibrillation are more frequent	Exertional syncope a common initial complaint in the younger patient; exertional dyspnea and CHF, more common early sign in the older patient	Exertional angina a common initial symptom in younger patient; angina frequent at some time in the course, regardless of age
Chronic aortic regurgitation (AR)	Rarely noted in childhood unless in association with rheumatic fever; long asymptomatic interval before symptoms develop	PVCs common, producing "hard beats" or "chest thumping," most noticeable lying on left side	Left-sided CHF common; syncope less common than in AS	Angina more common in luetic AR because of associated coronary ostial stenosis; nocturnal angina may occur with sleep-related drop in heart rate and blood pressure
Acute AR	Acute illness may be initial presentation; prior murmur not uncommon	Arrhythmias uncommon unless superimposed on chronic valve disease	Precipitous onset with marked pulmonary congestion; hypotension common	Unusual unless embolic coronary disease or pericarditis develops
Mitral stenosis (MS)	Frequently missed even after onset of symptoms	PACs and paroxysmal atrial flutter/fibrillation common	Exertional dyspnea and nonproductive cough prominent early symptoms; hemoptysis occurs relatively early; pulmonary edema with stress such as exercise, pregnancy, and atrial fibrillation	With pulmonary hypertension and right ventricular hypertrophy, anginal syndrome common
Chronic mitral regurgitation (MR)	Noted early, sometimes from the episode of rheumatic fever; with isolated MR, well tolerated for long periods	Atrial ectopy and fibrillation even more common than with MS	CHF reflects progressive left ventricular dysfunction and/or arrhythmia and is usually gradual in onset; fatigue prominent	Rarely part of clinical picture unless CAD a concomitant feature
Mitral valve prolapse (MVP)	Variable from childhood to old age	Controversial, may reflect study of selected populations; possibly increased incidence of long Q-T interval; palpitations commonly due to sinus tachycardia	Occurs with significant MR (a minority of patients); most are asymptomatic; when dyspnea and fatigue occur, usually noncardiac etiology	Most patients do not have chest pain; in symptomatic patients, pain usually distinctly nonanginal; classic angina may occur with normal coronaries but atherosclerosis and MVP may coexist
Acute MR	May be presenting manifestation or superimposed on prior mitral murmur	Sinus rhythm is usual	Acute, fulminant	May occur with endocarditis due to coronary embolization or pericarditis

Abbreviations: CHF = Congestive heart failure; CAD = coronary artery disease; PVC = premature ventricular contractions; PAC = premature atrial contractions.

accurately identify the underlying mechanism (e.g., palpitations due to an arrhythmia), a particular symptom per se is not diagnostic of underlying valvular heart disease. (See Tables 1 and 2.)

Rheumatic Fever

Rheumatic fever produces symptoms that may or may not be associated with acute valvular dysfunction (in particular, mitral and aortic regurgitation) and/or chronic valvular dysfunction (principally mitral stenosis with or without concomitant mitral regurgitation and aortic regurgitation with or without concomitant aortic stenosis). With acute rheumatic fever, the valvular dysfunction is typically not severe and symptoms are overwhelmingly those of arthritis, carditis (if myocardial involvement causes heart failure), and/or chorea as well as more nonspecific complaints such as fever, malaise, and fatigue. In patients with a prior history of rheumatic fever, one should always see if it is possible, in retrospect, to substantiate the diagnosis. Commonly, further questioning reveals that a murmur was heard in the past as a part of a physical examination or during a febrile illness and that the patient was told that he or she "has had" or "must have had rheumatic fever in the past." From that moment on, the patient will respond affirmatively to queries concerning prior rheumatic fever. If there have been no major Jones' criteria (arthritis, chorea, subcutaneous nodules, erythema marginatum, or carditis—the last three particularly difficult to diagnosis in retrospect), one should seriously question the diagnosis of rheumatic fever. Finally, acute rheumatic fever may be subclinical or unrecognized, and approximately 50 per cent of patients with proven rheumatic mitral stenosis have no convincing history of rheumatic fever.

Heart Murmur

Patients should always be queried about the prior detection of a heart murmur including when it was first heard, how consistently it was observed over time, and the reactions of the examining physician and/or the parents. A murmur heard at birth or early

Table 2. History and Symptoms in Pulmonic and Tricuspid Valve Disease

	Murmur	Arrhythmia	Heart Failure	Chest Pain
Pulmonic stenosis (PS)	If congenital, noted from early age by numerous examiners	Unusual	Right-sided CHF may occur, rarely in infancy or childhood and more commonly in the fourth to sixth decades; if mild to moderate, usually stable and well tolerated	May occur with severe RVH
Low-pressure pulmonic regurgitation (PR)	Usually in youth or young adulthood; common after repair of PS	Unusual	When congenital, if high fetal pulmonary vascular resistance weathered, usually no CHF (but combination of PDA and PR may be poorly tolerated); acquired increases in pulmonary pressure in adult (e.g., myocardial infarction) may worsen degree and cause right-sided CHF	No
High-pressure PR	Detected during evaluation of left-sided heart disease or causes of pulmonary hypertension; commonly mistaken for AR	When present, due to primary process (e.g., pulmonary embolism); may cause syncope	Right-sided CHF common but primarily due to pulmonary hypertension, the cause of PR exertional syncope when severe; low output fatigue a prominent complaint	Anginal syndrome with severe pulmonary hypertension and RVH
Tricuspid stenosis (TS)	Often missed in setting of left-sided VHD	High incidence of atrial fibrillation, particularly when associated with rheumatic mitral disease	With associated left-sided VHD, disproportionate right-sided CHF may be a clue to presence of TS	No
Low-pressure tricuspid regurgitation (TR)	If mild, frequently missed or misinterpreted; if more severe, usually detected in setting of primary cause (e.g., endocarditis)	With Ebstein's anomaly, frequent A–V junctional reentry due to right-sided accessory pathway	Occasionally causes right-sided CHF, but with normal pulmonary artery pressure, well tolerated for long periods	With endocarditis, pulmonary infarction may occur
High-pressure TR	Often missed or misinterpreted in setting of other murmurs or other nonvalvular heart disease	If combined with mitral valve disease, atrial fibrillation common and occasionally causes syncope because of associated pulmonary hypertension	Right-sided CHF with abdominal visceral congestion; left-sided CHF symptoms may diminish with the advent of TR	Frequent, if due to pulmonary hypertension

Abbreviations: VHD = Valvular heart disease; CHF = congestive heart failure; RVH = right ventricular hypertrophy; AR = aortic regurgitation; PDA = patent ductus arteriosus; A–V = atrioventricular.

in follow-up is suggestive of aortic or pulmonary stenosis. A significant murmur first detected later in childhood (e.g., preschool physical examination) is likely to be secondary to a left to right shunt such as atrial septal defect, ventricular septal defect, or patent ductus arteriosus because these murmurs become manifest only after the fetal pulmonary vascular resistance drops, allowing the shunt to occur. An *innocent murmur* classically is present in youth or young adulthood, is variable from one examination to the next, and is accompanied by the advice that it will be outgrown; physical activity is not restricted. Significant murmurs, on the other hand, are associated with advice to restrict activity, regular follow-up, the denial of life insurance, or rejection from military service.

Arrhythmias

Symptoms from arrhythmias are quite common and not necessarily indicative of underlying valvular heart disease. They may arise from isolated premature beats, sustained tachyarrhythmias, and significant bradyarrhythmias. When such arrhythmias occur with significant valvular heart disease, they are likely to be sensed by the patient because of the underlying hemodynamic abnormalities.

Palpitations. Palpitations, defined as an awareness of one's own heartbeat, most commonly reflect isolated premature beats felt by the patient as "flip-flop" or "skip" sensations. With aortic regurgitation, the post-premature beat has an even larger stroke volume that may be appreciated as a "thump" or "hard beat." On occasion, shaking of the bed in association with this post-premature beat's augmented stroke volume may be noticed, a "bedside ballistocardiogram." With premature atrial beats, underlying mitral valve disease should be considered. Unfortunately, since premature atrial and ventricular beats may present with the same symptomatic manifestations and are common in valve disease of all varieties, isolated palpitations are not particularly helpful in differentiating the type of valve disease. This is particularly true in respect to *mitral valve prolapse;* that is, several clinical investigators have reported an increased incidence of a variety of arrhythmias, but more recent studies have shown that the incidence of arrhythmias in patients with palpitations is independent of associated mitral valve prolapse. In contrast asymptomatic subjects, both with and without mitral valve prolapse, show no difference in the incidence of arrhythmias. It may be that the reported association is more a matter of selection in the population studied, but further research is needed to clarify this point.

Sudden rapid and irregular palpitations are highly suggestive of generalized atrial re-entry (atrial fibrillation), and underlying mitral valve disease is common. When such generalized atrial re-entry is slower and regular (atrial flutter), it may be difficult, by history, to differentiate from atrioventricular (A-V) junctional re-entry (so-called "PAT"), an arrhythmia not necessarily indicative of underlying valvular heart disease. With atrial flutter-fibrillation, disproportionate dyspnea should suggest underlying heart disease. Indeed, well-compensated patients with mitral stenosis (e.g., Class I or early Class II) may develop pulmonary edema when atrial fibrillation supervenes because abbreviated diastole during the arrhythmia causes a disproportionate rise in left atrial and pulmonary venous pressure.

Alterations in Consciousness. Although it is unusual for presyncope/syncope to occur with supraventricular tachycardias (in the absence of Wolff-Parkinson-White accessory conduction), an occasional patient with severe mitral stenosis or any severe valvular disease with concomitant left ventricular dysfunction may experience syncope during atrial fibrillation with a rapid ventricular response. Bradycardias, the classic arrhythmia for presyncope/syncope, occur with left-sided valvular heart disease when calcification of the mitral annulus and/or aortic valve extends into the proximal interventricular septum, erodes the conduction system, and causes heart block. Syncope in aortic valve disease may occur secondary to an arrhythmia, but the more usual cause is the inability to augment *forward cardiac output*—a type of acute heart failure.

Chronic Myocardial Dysfunction

Chronic Left Heart Failure. When symptoms of left heart failure (dyspnea, orthopnea, paroxysmal nocturnal dyspnea, and nocturia) occur with a positive history of rheumatic fever or heart murmur or with a negative history of other causes of heart failure (such as coronary artery disease, hypertension, and alcohol ingestion), the possibility of valve disease should always be considered. A long asymptomatic interval between the first detection of a heart murmur and the onset of left heart failure suggests a left-sided regurgitant lesion; a shorter asymptomatic interval is more characteristic of a left-sided stenotic lesion. In the younger patient with aortic stenosis, left heart failure is less common than syncope or chest pain initially; in the older patient, left heart failure is a common initial symptom.

Chronic Right Heart Failure. Isolated right-sided failure with peripheral edema and symptoms of abdominal visceral congestion (nausea, vomiting, and abdominal pain) may be due to tricuspid stenosis or tricuspid regurgitation with concomitant pulmonary hypertension. In the absence of pulmonary hypertension, tricuspid and pulmonary regurgitation are well tolerated as long as right ventricular function remains well compensated. Even relatively severe congenital pulmonary valve stenosis may be tolerated well into middle age. Peripheral edema as an initial manifestation of left-sided valvular heart disease is unusual and typically occurs only after a period of symptomatic left heart failure. Thus, when cardiac edema occurs in isolation, it may be due to right-sided valvular heart disease, particularly with tricuspid stenosis or concomitant pulmonary hypertension; however, when cardiac edema precedes the symptoms of left heart failure or when the two develop relatively simultaneously, one should think of other causes such as cardiomyopathy.

Fatigue. Fatigue is a notoriously nonspecific complaint and most frequently represents depression, but patients with valvular heart disease and inadequate forward cardiac output characteristically experience severe fatigue. One helpful point in differentiating fatigue from these causes is that after a night's rest, patients with heart disease wake up feeling well, only to become more fatigued as the day progresses; in contrast, patients with depression typically find that their fatigue improves as the day goes on. Not infrequently, fatigue and peripheral edema gradually replace left-sided congestive symptoms, reflecting progressive left ventricular dysfunction, poor cardiac output, tricuspid regurgitation, and curtailment of activity levels.

Cough. A nonproductive cough, particularly with recumbency, may indicate pulmonary venous congestion secondary to left heart failure and is frequent in patients with mitral stenosis.

Acute Myocardial Dysfunction

Presyncope/Syncope. Acute left heart failure (defined as the inability to appropriately augment cardiac output) is one mechanism for syncope in patients with severe aortic stenosis, as with severe obstruction to blood flow there may be an inability to augment stroke volume in response to stresses such as exercise and, in concert with venous and arteriolar vasodilatation, resultant hypotension, and syncope. This mechanism, and particularly the inability to augment forward output, may also explain syncope in patients with other blood flow–obstructing lesions such as severe mitral stenosis with pulmonary hypertension. In each instance, a relationship to exertion is typical. As previously mentioned, presyncope/syncope may also be secondary to an arrhythmia, and this differential diagnosis needs to be kept in mind.

Congestive Symptoms. Occasionally, the combination of a tachyarrhythmia and mild valve disease may cause acute decompensation, as in the instance of mitral stenosis and atrial fibrillation. Acute left heart failure in the setting of chest trauma or a febrile illness is suggestive of leaflet disruption secondary to either traumatic avulsion or endocarditis.

Chest Pain Syndromes

Anginal Chest Pain. The combination of angina and a heart murmur should always suggest aortic outflow tract obstruction, although it by no means helps to localize the site (supravalvular, valvular, and subvalvular) and an occasional patient with pure aortic regurgitation may also present with angina. There is also nothing about the anginal syndrome per se that helps to differentiate isolated aortic valve disease from that occurring in combination with coronary artery disease. Approximately 10 to 15 per cent of patients with mitral stenosis (particularly with pulmonary hypertension) may develop angina in the absence of coronary artery disease, presumably from ischemia of the hypertrophied right ventricle. Chest pain from embolism to the coronaries has also been reported.

Atypical Chest Pain. Mitral valve prolapse patients, particularly early in their course, have a chest pain syndrome that is usually highly atypical for angina (nonexertional, nonsubsternal, lasts for hours to days, and is unrelieved by nitroglycerin) and is more suggestive of anxiety. With time and continued interaction with the health care system, the pain syndrome may evolve to classic angina. In one series of young women presenting with chest pain, however, the chest pain could not be related to the presence or absence of prolapse. It seems likely that much of the reported association between chest pain and prolapse stems from the highly selected nature of the mitral valve prolapse population studied but, as in the instance of arrhythmias, further research is needed to clarify this issue.

Chest Wall Tenderness. Patients with a variety of imagined or real heart disease, including valvular heart disease, frequently complain of chest wall discomfort (particularly in the left inframammary area) that is more likely to occur in the left lateral decubitus position. The pathophysiology of this complaint is unknown, but it is not infrequently related to an appreciation of the heartbeat when lying on the left side and is more likely with left ventricular enlargement.

Altered Hemodynamics

Hemoptysis. Hemoptysis may occur in patients with mitral valve disease and particularly mitral stenosis. When it is due to rupture of endobronchial veins, hemoptysis is characterized by the expectoration of gross blood (as opposed to the blood-streaked sputum typical of bronchitis or the pink sputum of pulmonary edema). Such hemoptysis is usually not life-threatening and does not reflect severity, since it typically occurs early in the course of pulmonary venous hypertension.

Neck Pain. Neck pain pulsating in synchrony with the heart beat due to stretching of the carotid sheath occurs rarely in patients with severe aortic regurgitation.

Pulsations of the Neck and Body. Patients with aortic regurgitation may be aware of neck pulsations secondary to bounding carotid pulses or head pounding, and, in some patients, shaking of the bed causes the patient to seek help for tremor or seizures. Neck pulsations may rarely be a manifestation of giant A waves caused by tricuspid stenosis or, more likely, right ventricular hypertrophy with decreased right ventricular compliance (as, for example, in pulmonary hypertension). Most commonly, symptomatic neck vein pulsations are due to the C-V or "S" waves of tricuspid regurgitation. These venous wave forms are classically noted in men while they are shaving.

Miscellaneous Symptoms

Peripheral Embolization. The heart is a classic source of emboli with the symptomatic manifestations a function of their origin (right versus left side), character, size, and distribution. Emboli may lodge (1) in the lungs or coronary arteries, producing infarction and chest pain syndromes; (2) in the brain, producing strokes; (3) in the abdominal viscera, producing pain and/or altered function (e.g., painful splenic infarction, hematuria and/or renal insufficiency, ischemic bowel necrosis); or (4) in other peripheral vasculature (and most commonly the lower extremities) producing acute and/or chronic arterial insufficiency. Emboli are particularly likely with endocarditis and with mitral valve disease in association with either chronic or recurrent atrial fibrillation.

PHYSICAL EXAMINATION

As mentioned, patients do not usually present with a valvular "label." This section presents a sequential analysis of the physical examination. The "five-finger" approach popularized by Harvey is used to discuss the patient's general appearance, venous pulse, arterial pulse, precordial pulses, and auscultation, including how each relates to the differential diagnosis of underlying valvular heart disease. (See Tables 3 through 8.)

General Appearance

A marfanoid habitus should always suggest the possibility of aortic regurgitation and/or mitral regurgitation secondary to mitral valve prolapse. Other than this particular appearance, sex or body habitus is not helpful in diagnosing mitral valve prolapse because skeletal muscle deformities (straight back, pectus excavatum, scoliosis) are common in the absence of prolapse, and, although more common in the female, prolapse is not at all uncommon in men. Valvular pulmonic stenosis is the most common cardiac anomaly associated with Turner's syndrome.

Venous Pulse

The venous pulse may be altered by arrhythmias, by primary tricuspid valve disease, and by left-sided heart disease that produces pulmonary hypertension, decreased right ventricular compliance, and/or regurgitation in the tricuspid valve. Analysis of the venous pulse includes evaluating central venous pressure, respiratory variation, and morphology. (See Tables 3 and 4.)

Estimated Central Venous Pressure

The estimated mean central venous pressure in mild mitral and aortic valve disease is normal (7 to 8 cm of water or less), but when the valve disease is severe enough to cause left heart failure pulmonary hypertension ensues, causing right ventricular hypertrophy and, eventually, right ventricular failure with

Table 3. Pulses in Aortic and Mitral Valve Disease

	Venous Pulse	Arterial Pulse/Blood Pressure	Precordial Pulse
Aortic stenosis (AS)	Normal until late in disease then elevated CVP and giant A wave; rarely, giant A wave occurs early	Small, narrow pulse pressure with thrill/shudder particularly over left carotid; in older patient, pulse pressure and upstroke may seem normal; transmitted bruits common, loudest over left carotid	Apex nondisplaced, enlarged and sustained with palpable atrial gallop common; if associated AR or CHF, then laterally displaced; in patients under age 50, an S_4 correlates with severe gradient
Chronic aortic regurgitation (AR)	Same as AS	Large pulse with wide pulse pressure and brisk upstroke; if severe, bisferious; diastolic BP less than 60 mm Hg common.	Apex enlarged, laterally displaced and hyperdynamic with palpable S_3 common; with CHF or concomitant AS, may be sustained
Acute AR	Usually normal; increased CVP a late and ominous finding	Brisk upstroke but amplitude and pulse pressure may not be particularly widened; diastolic BP may not be significantly lower	Sustained, nondisplaced with palpable S_3 common; diastolic thrill at LSE may be present
Mitral stenosis (MS)	Elevated CVP with C-V wave common; if NSR, giant A wave; with atrial fibrillation, dominant Y descent	Normal unless severe, then small pulse	1. Systolic impulse at upper LSE due to dilated pulmonary artery 2. Sustained systolic impulse at LLSE with palpable S_4 due to RVH common; with advent of TR, palpable S_3 may also occur
Chronic mitral regurgitation (MR)	Normal until late in disease course or until atrial fibrillation supervenes, then dominant Y descent	Brisk upstroke if moderate to severe with well-maintained left ventricular function	1. Apex enlarged, sustained; if more than moderate MR, inferolaterally displaced with palpable S_3 common 2. If severe, late systolic impulse at LLSE due to right ventricle being thrust anteriorly by systolic expansion of posteriorly located left atrium and pulmonary veins
MR secondary to mitral valve prolapse (MVP) and mitral apparatus dysfunction	Normal	Normal	Apex usually normal; with MVP, a minority show midsystolic retraction; if severe, apex sustained and inferolaterally displaced with palpable S_3; apical systolic thrill common
Acute MR	Giant A wave common	Brisk upstroke with normal pulse pressure; rarely dicrotic	Apex normally located but enlarged and sustained; palpable S_4 and/or S_3 common and with sinus tachycardia, summation gallop frequent

Abbreviations: BP = Blood pressure; RVH = right ventricular hypertrophy; LSE = left sternal edge; CVP = central venous pressure; LLSE = lower left sternal edge; CHF = congestive heart failure; NSR = normal sinus rhythm; S_3 = ventricular gallop; S_4 = atrial gallop.

a progressive rise in the central venous pressure. With mitral stenosis (compared with the other left-sided valvular lesions), such changes occur earlier in the disease course and result in systemic venous hypertension with or without associated changes in the venous pulse morphology (to be discussed). With more advanced aortic valve disease (usually in association with left ventricular dysfunction), subtle elevations of the central venous pressure are frequent, particularly in the absence of diuretic therapy. Even with severe mitral regurgitation, the central venous pressure is usually normal until late in the disease course because the dilated, compliant left atrium forms a low-pressure reservoir that protects the pulmonary veins from the effects of mitral regurgitation. In mitral regurgitation, it is far more likely that the morphology of the venous pulse will become abnormal secondary to an atrial arrhythmia. In even relatively severe valvular pulmonic stenosis, the central venous pressure is typically normal although a giant A wave may make estimation of the "mean" central venous pressure difficult. Similarly, with isolated, low-pressure tricuspid regurgitation of mild degree, the estimated central venous pressure is typically normal. When more severe, the prominent C-V or "S" wave may make visual integration of the venous pulse and estimation of the mean central venous pressure difficult. With tricuspid regurgitation and pulmonary hypertension, marked elevations of the central venous pressure are common.

Regardless of the type of valvular heart disease, in an untreated patient with right heart failure an elevated central venous pressure is the rule.

Respiratory Variation

In all valvular heart disease, there is a normal inspiratory drop in venous pressure. Kussmaul's sign (an inspiratory rise in venous pressure) has been reported with severe right heart failure regardless of the etiology (including valvular heart disease), but most commonly this is a "pseudo"-Kussmaul's sign; during expiration the venous structures are full and phasic pulsations minimal or inapparent, but with inspiration the venous pressure falls normally, allowing the low-pressure venous wave forms to become apparent. If one has not discerned the elevation in venous pressure, this inspiratory appearance of the phasic venous wave forms leads to the mistaken conclusion that the venous pressure is rising with inspira-

Table 4. Pulses in Pulmonic and Tricuspid Valve Disease

	Venous Pulse	Arterial Pulse/Blood Pressure	Precordial Pulse
Pulmonic stenosis (PS)	Normal CVP unless severe; giant A wave usual	Typically normal unless severe, then may be small	If more than mild, sustained systolic impulse at LLSE due to RVH; palpable S_4 also common; systolic thrill middle to upper LSE (particularly post-exercise)
Low-pressure pulmonary regurgitation (PR)	Normal	Normal	If more than mild: 1. Systolic impulse at ULSE due to dilated pulmonary artery 2. Hyperdynamic systolic impulse at LLSE due to volume overloaded right ventricle
High-pressure PR	Elevated CVP and giant A wave common due to associated right ventricular hypertrophy and failure	Normal unless severe, then may be small	Systolic impulse at ULSE due to dilated pulmonary artery; sustained systolic impulse at LLSE commonly with palpable S_4; both impulses are secondary manifestations of pulmonary hypertension and RVH
Tricuspid stenosis (TS)	Increased CVP; if NSR, giant A wave; with atrial fibrillation, Y descent is abbreviated	Abnormal as function of any associated left-sided rheumatic valve disease	If isolated, no RV or pulmonary artery impulse; otherwise abnormal as function of associated left-sided rheumatic valve disease
Low-pressure tricuspid regurgitation (TR)	C-V waves if more than mild; estimation of mean CVP may be difficult due to systolic filling of neck veins	Usually normal	If moderate to severe, hyperdynamic systolic impulse at LLSE with palpable S_3
High-pressure TR	Elevated CVP with C-V waves usual; atrial fibrillation common and may make detection of C-V wave difficult	Usually normal unless severe pulmonary vascular disease, then may be small	Systolic impulse at ULSE due to dilated pulmonary artery; sustained systolic impulse at LLSE with palpable atrial gallop due to RVH from pulmonary hypertension; if severe, palpable ventricular gallop may occur

Abbreviations: RVH = Right ventricular hypertrophy; ULSE = upper left sternal edge; LLSE = lower left sternal edge; CVP = central venous pressure; NSR = normal sinus rhythm; S_3 = ventricular gallop; S_4 = atrial gallop.

tion. Thus, an inspiratory rise in the venous pressure should suggest the presence of constrictive pericarditis.

Venous Pulse Morphology—Normal Sinus Rhythm

With left-sided valvular disease, the venous pulse morphology becomes abnormal secondarily when pulmonary venous and arterial hypertension eventuate and cause abnormal right ventricular compliance and/or function. As mentioned, such changes are likely earlier in the course of mitral stenosis where, in addition to an elevated central venous pressure, there are giant A waves reflecting augmented right atrial systole in response to decreased right ventricular compliance. Such changes characteristically occur much later in the course of mitral regurgitation and aortic valve disease, usually with the advent of left ventricular dysfunction, failure, and resulting pulmonary hypertension. Giant A waves, on the other hand, are an early feature of tricuspid stenosis and of pulmonary valve stenosis, particularly if of more than mild degree. Primary (or low-pressure) tricuspid regurgitation, if more than mild, and tricuspid regurgitation in association with pulmonary hypertension produce easily discernible C-V waves with a large Y descent in early diastole (Fig. 1).

Venous Pulse Morphology—Arrhythmias

Any of the arrhythmias may produce alterations in the venous pulse morphology, but this discussion will be limited to the alterations in venous pulse morphology secondary to atrial fibrillation, an arrhythmia frequently secondary to mitral valve disease. With atrial fibrillation there is a loss of coordinated atrial systole and, therefore, of the A wave. There is also a loss of coordinated atrial relaxation and, therefore, X descent. To the examiner's eye, this produces a dominant Y descent (Fig. 2). Since the same changes may occur with mild to moderate tricuspid regurgitation in the setting of atrial fibrillation, it may be very difficult to differentiate isolated atrial fibrillation from atrial fibrillation with associated tricuspid regurgitation. With more severe tricuspid regurgitation, however, the typical systolic C-V wave (that is frequently palpable) occurs along with pulsation of the earlobes and/or liver, findings rarely seen with atrial fibrillation alone even with an elevated venous pressure.

Arterial Pulse and Blood Pressure

The blood pressure should be measured in both arms, noting the pulse pressure and the diastolic level. The arterial pulses should be examined for presence or absence, symmetry, volume (or amplitude), and morphology (upstroke and systolic/diastolic contour). For timing and evaluation of morphology, the carotid artery is most convenient and likely to provide useful information. Occasionally alterations in wave form such as a bisferiens or dicrotic pulse (to be discussed) may be more prominent in a peripheral artery. The normal arterial pulse is easily palpable and is appreciated as a single brief tap by the examining

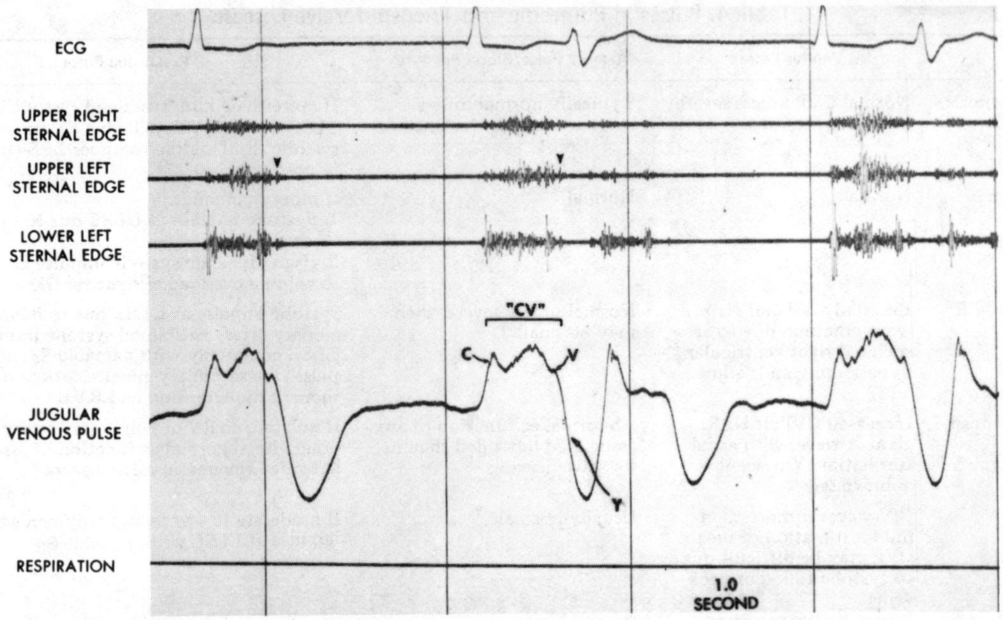

Figure 1. This jugular venous pulse tracing, from a 59-year-old man with atrial fibrillation and moderately severe rheumatic aortic and mitral valve disease, shows a "C-V" wave of tricuspid regurgitation caused by right ventricular dilatation from pulmonary hypertension and not intrinsic rheumatic tricuspid valve disease. Note also the absence of an A wave and the dominant Y descent. The holosystolic murmur at the lower left sternal edge is tricuspid regurgitation. An opening snap (small arrowhead) is well recorded at the upper left sternal edge, a common finding in rheumatic mitral valve disease.

finger. As with the jugular venous pulse, there is the potential for each of the various parts of the arterial pulse to become altered by underlying valvular disease.

Blood Pressure and Pulse Volume

With mild valve disease, the arterial pulse and blood pressure are typically normal. A small arterial pulse and narrow pulse pressure may occur with severe obstruction to blood flow and/or a reduced forward output (as, for example, in severe mitral stenosis) and are particularly likely with severe aortic stenosis. (Note, however, that in the older patient with significant aortic stenosis, a normal blood pressure and pulse volume may occur.)

Normal pulses are usual with mitral and right-sided valve disease as long as cardiac output is well maintained. Aortic regurgitation, if more than mild, produces a large pulse (wide pulse pressure) and a low diastolic pressure. If severe, a diastolic blood pressure of less than 60 mm Hg is typical. (Note that with acute severe aortic regurgitation, the diastolic pressure may be misleadingly high.) These pulses are frequently described as bounding, collapsing, or "water hammer" in character. They are reflected peripherally as capillary pulses, and over the femoral arteries as pistol shot sounds and "to and fro" bruits.

Arterial Pulse Morphology—Upstroke

Obstruction to blood flow and/or a poor cardiac output at any valvular level may produce a small pulse volume, but aortic stenosis stands alone in producing a slow-rising pulse (the classic parvus et tardus—small and late pulse) which when present indicates significant fixed left ventricular outflow tract obstruction. (Remember that supravalvular and subvalvular membranous aortic stenosis may produce similar abnormalities in the arterial pulse.) A brisk arterial upstroke with a normal pulse volume occurs with severe mitral regurgitation and well-compensated left ventricular function, presumably owing to rapid left ventricular contraction. In aortic regurgitation, a brisk upstroke is usually due to the increased stroke volume and peripheral arteriolar vasodilation (the latter due to unknown factors).

Arterial Pulse Morphology—Contour

Most valve disease, including mild aortic regurgitation, produces an arterial pulse that has a single systolic peak. With moderate to severe chronic aortic regurgitation (with or without associated aortic stenosis), however, accentuation of the initial percussion wave and the subsequent reflected tidal wave produces a bifid or bisferious pulse (Fig. 3). Acute severe aortic regurgitation may, on occasion, not demonstrate these changes. This bifid systolic pulse (with two peaks of about equal height) needs to be differentiated from the bifid spike-and-dome arterial pulse of hypertrophic obstructive cardiomyopathy (with a more rounded, less prominent second peak) and from the bifid or dicrotic arterial pulse that is usually secondary to congestive cardiomyopathy but may occur with severe mitral regurgitation and a reduced forward output. A dicrotic arterial pulse is usually easier to detect, compared with a bisferious pulse, since the second peak is diastolic and therefore more widely separated from the first peak.

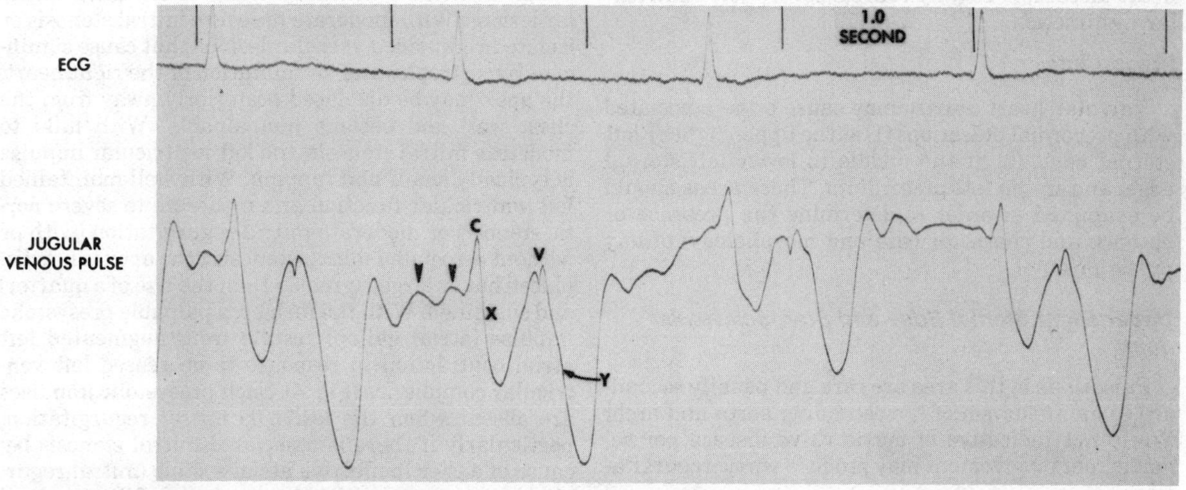

Figure 2. This tracing, from a 37-year-old woman with mitral regurgitation, shows the effects of atrial fibrillation on the jugular venous pulse in the absence of tricuspid regurgitation. Note the dominant Y descent and the small fibrillation waves (arrowheads). There is no A wave but a small X descent remains because of the caudal movement of the entire heart with ventricular systole. C=C wave: V=V wave.

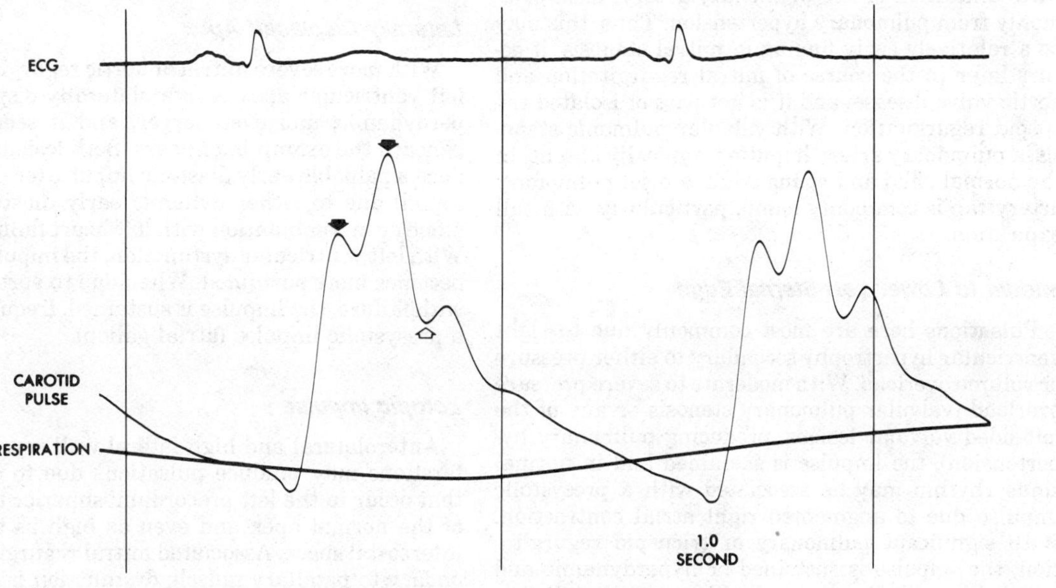

Figure 3. This carotid pulse tracing, from a 40-year-old man with moderately severe aortic stenosis and regurgitation, shows a bifid or bisferious contour. Note the two systolic peaks (closed arrowheads). The end of systole occurs at the dicrotic notch (open arrowhead) and is followed by a small dicrotic wave.

Arterial Thrills/Bruits

A systolic thrill over the carotid pulse is the palpable equivalent of a bruit and reflects turbulent blood flow from either intrinsic carotid vascular disease or transmission from the left ventricular outflow tract. Thrills or bruits secondary to aortic valve disease are associated with a precordial systolic thrill and murmur that is typically maximal at the upper right sternal edge. Carotid bruits, on the other hand, become louder as one inches up the neck, are not as harsh, and may be associated with a pulse that is diminished to palpation. Thrills impart a buzzing or vibratory sensation to the examining finger but when particularly coarse, may be appreciated as a "shudder." Carotid thrills and bruits occur with significant aortic stenosis but may be seen with pure aortic regurgitation as well. Thrills and bruits from aortic valve disease radiate best to the left carotid because of the more direct route of transmission. Supravalvular aortic stenosis, on the other hand, may transmit the stenotic jet best to the right carotid.

Miscellaneous Changes in the Arterial Pulse

Pulsus alternans reflects underlying left ventricular dysfunction and is not a predictive sign of underlying valvular disease, although it may be easier to detect with aortic regurgitation because of the larger arterial pulse. Similarly, pulsus paradoxus is not predictive of underlying valve disease and occurs due to a variety of mechanisms. When present with valvular heart disease, it usually reflects severe left ventricular dysfunction.

Precordium

Valvular heart disease may cause or be associated with precordial pulsations (1) at the upper right or left sternal edge, (2) at the middle to lower left sternal edge, and in the left precordium. These areas should be examined in order to determine the presence or absence and character (size and morphology) of any pulsations.

Upper Right Sternal Edge and Sternoclavicular Joint

Pulsations in this area are rare and usually secondary to an aneurysm of the ascending aorta and arch. While not indicative of aortic valve disease per se, aortic root involvement may produce aortic regurgitation.

Upper Left Sternal Edge

An impulse at the second left intercostal space indicates dilatation of the pulmonary artery, most commonly from pulmonary hypertension. Thus, this may be a relatively early finding in mitral stenosis; it occurs later in the course of mitral regurgitation and aortic valve disease; and it is not part of isolated tricuspid regurgitation. With valvular pulmonic stenosis, a pulmonary artery impulse is typically absent. In the normal child and young adult, a brief pulmonary artery tap is commonly found, particularly with full expiration.

Middle to Lower Left Sternal Edge

Pulsations here are most commonly due to right ventricular hypertrophy secondary to either pressure or volume overload. With moderate to severe pressure overload (valvular pulmonary stenosis or any of the left-sided valvular lesions, producing pulmonary hypertension), the impulse is sustained and in normal sinus rhythm may be associated with a presystolic impulse due to augmented right atrial contraction. With significant pulmonary or tricuspid regurgitation, the impulse is sustained or hyperdynamic and may be associated with a palpable early diastolic impulse (i.e., a right ventricular third heart sound). With severe mitral regurgitation, a palpable right ventricular impulse may occur in the absence of pulmonary hypertension due to systolic expansion of the posteriorly located left atrium and pulmonary veins that in turn thrusts the heart anteriorly and causes a late systolic impulse. The combination of an enlarged, laterally displaced left ventricular impulse (to be discussed) and this late parasternal systolic impulse produces a characteristic seesaw rocking motion to the precordium. Once again, in the normal child or young adult, a brief right ventricular tap may be felt along the lower left sternal edge, particularly with full expiration.

Nondisplaced Apex

A normal apical impulse (within 10 to 12 cm to the left of the midsternal line, fourth or fifth intercostal space) is the rule with mild right- or left-sided valvular lesions. With moderate to severe mitral stenosis or isolated right-sided valvular lesions that cause significant hypertrophy and/or dilatation of the right heart, the apex may be displaced posteriorly away from the chest wall and become nonpalpable. With mild to moderate mitral stenosis, the left ventricular impulse is typically small and tapping. With well-maintained left ventricular function and moderate to severe aortic stenosis or moderate mitral regurgitation (with or without associated mitral stenosis), the apex is nondisplaced but enlarged (greater than the size of a quarter) and sustained. With the former, a palpable presystolic impulse (atrial gallop) results from augmented left atrial contraction in response to decreased left ventricular compliance (Fig. 4). Such presystolic impulses are absent when the lesion is mitral regurgitation, particularly if there is associated mitral stenosis because of either ineffective atrial systole (mitral regurgitation) or restricted left ventricular filling (mitral stenosis). With acute severe mitral or aortic regurgitation, the apex is initially normally located but enlarged and sustained with palpable gallops common.

Laterally Displaced Apex

With more severe mitral or aortic regurgitation, the left ventricular apex is inferolaterally displaced, hyperdynamic, and even larger, and it seems to roll beneath the examining fingers. Both lesions may produce a palpable early diastolic impulse (or third heart sound) due to either dynamic early diastolic filling alone or in combination with left heart failure (Fig. 5). With left ventricular dysfunction, the impulse usually becomes more sustained. When due to aortic stenosis with failure, the impulse is sustained, frequently with a presystolic impulse (atrial gallop).

Ectopic Impulse

Anterolateral and high lateral wall myocardial infarctions may produce pulsations due to dyskinesia that occur in the left precordium superior to the area of the normal apex and even as high as the second intercostal space. Associated mitral regurgitation secondary to papillary muscle dysfunction is common.

Precordial Thrills/Palpable Heart Sounds

Thrills may identify significant valvular disease and should be characterized as to their location and timing. Aortic stenosis produces a thrill at the upper right sternal edge and in the suprasternal notch. Valvular pulmonic stenosis causes a systolic thrill at the upper left sternal edge and in the suprasternal notch as well. In both instances, the thrill may be brought out or accentuated by exercise or by having the patient sit up, lean forward, and breathe out fully. An apical systolic thrill is most commonly due to mitral regurgitation secondary to mitral apparatus dysfunction (e.g., ruptured chordae, mitral valve prolapse) although in an occasional older patient with an increased anteroposterior diameter and kyphosis, the thrill of aortic stenosis may be best appreciated at the lower left sternal edge or apex. Conversely, in an occa-

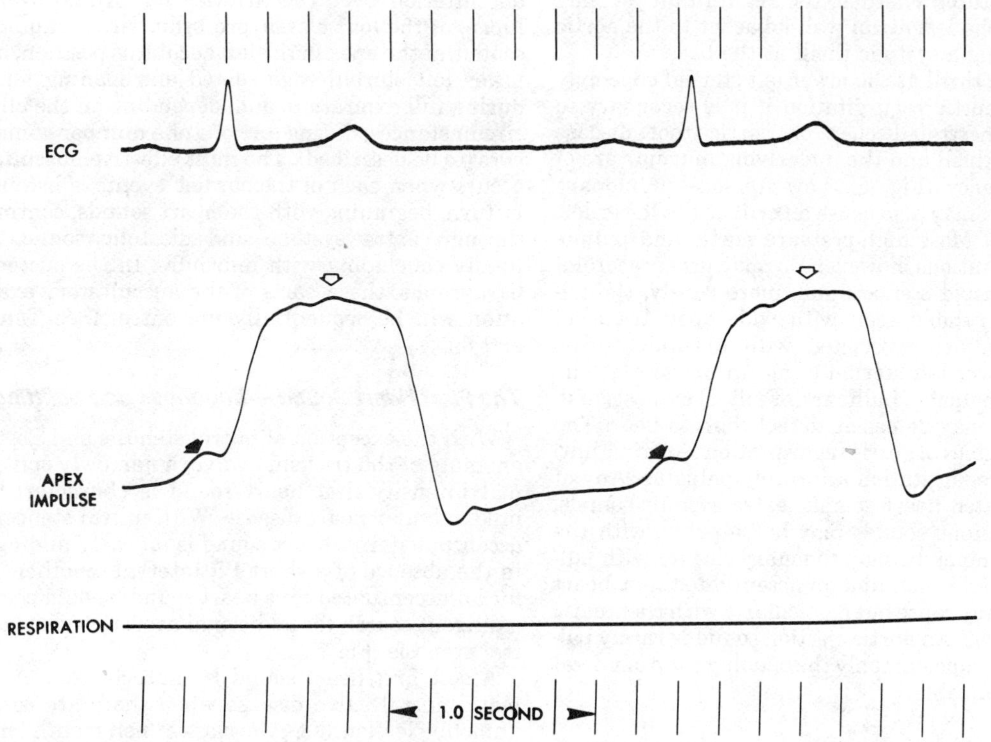

Figure 4. This nondisplaced apex impulse, recorded from a 46-year-old woman with moderately severe aortic stenosis, shows an A wave (closed arrowheads) that was palpable and a sustained systolic contour (open arrowheads).

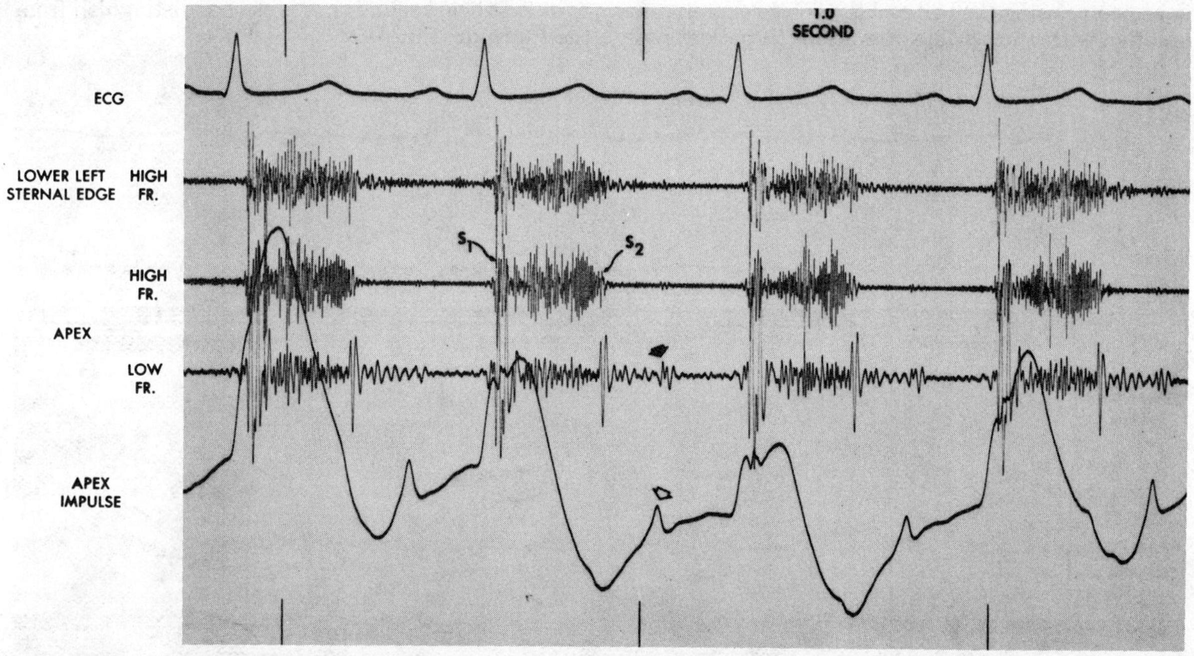

Figure 5. This apex impulse, from a 62-year-old man with severe chronic mitral regurgitation, was recorded 14 cm to the left of the midsternal line in the sixth intercostal space. There is both a palpable (open arrowhead) and audible (closed arrowhead) third heart sound. Note that the apex impulse has no A wave and that there is no fourth heart sound on the apex phonocardiogram. This patient's mitral regurgitation was due to mitral valve prolapse, explaining the well-preserved first heart sound (S_1), the late systolic accentuation of the murmur, and its radiation to the lower left sternal edge.

sional patient with mitral regurgitation due to prolapse or ruptured chordae, the regurgitant jet may impinge on the left atrial wall adjacent to the aortic root producing a systolic thrill at the base.

A diastolic thrill at the lower left sternal edge may accompany aortic regurgitation if it is secondary to either a fenestrated cusp or aortic root disease wherein the thrill and the underlying murmur are of lower frequency (Fig. 6). Low-pressure pulmonary regurgitation may also cause a thrill at the lower left sternal edge. Most high-pressure aortic and pulmonary regurgitations, however, do not cause precordial thrills. Tricuspid stenosis and, more rarely, the tricuspid flow rumble seen with wide open tricuspid regurgitation are associated with diastolic thrills along the lower left sternal edge. An apical diastolic thrill is the palpable hallmark of mitral stenosis and, on occasion, may be easier to feel than to hear. The diastolic rumbles of aortic regurgitation (Austin Flint) and mitral regurgitation are rarely palpable. Any of the accentuated heart sounds, extra systolic sounds, or extra diastolic sounds may be palpable, with the two most common being pulmonary closure with pulmonary hypertension and an accentuated first heart sound from any cause but particularly with rheumatic mitral stenosis. An aortic ejection sound is rarely palpable, but not uncommonly the opening snap of mitral stenosis is palpable.

Auscultation

As with the other parts of the evaluation of the patient with suspected valvular disease, systematic auscultation is also key. Auscultation should proceed in sequence using the bell and the diaphragm in combination with appropriate alterations in patient position. A minimal cardiovascular examination includes auscultation over the arteries for bruits, over the lungs, at the four classic precordial areas supine and seated, at the apex in the left decubitus position, at the lower left sternal edge seated and leaning forward during full expiration, and, depending on the clinical circumstances, during any one of a number of maneuvers (to be described). The most effective auscultation occurs when each of the cardiac events is listened to in turn, beginning with the heart sounds, continuing through extra systolic and diastolic sounds, and finally concluding with murmurs. In the succeeding paragraphs, these parts of the auscultatory examination will be sequentially presented. (See Tables 5 and 6.)

The First Heart Sound—Loudness and Splitting

With the exception of mitral stenosis and Ebstein's anomaly of the tricuspid valve, a narrowly split, normal intensity first heart sound is characteristic of mild valvular heart disease. With mitral stenosis, an accentuated first heart sound is an early finding and in the absence of a short PR interval (another cause for an accentuated first heart sound) should occasion a diligent search for additional acoustic events of mitral stenosis (Fig 7).

A soft first heart sound is characteristic of rheumatic mitral valve disease when there are calcified immobile leaflets (e.g., the classic "fish mouth" mitral valve) and no effective coaptation causing little or no deceleration of blood flow. With mitral regurgitation, it is frequently difficult to characterize the intensity of the first heart sound because it is masked by the holosystolic murmur. With holosystolic mitral regurgitation due to mitral valve prolapse, there is a prominent first heart sound that is easy to distinguish from the murmur (Fig. 5).

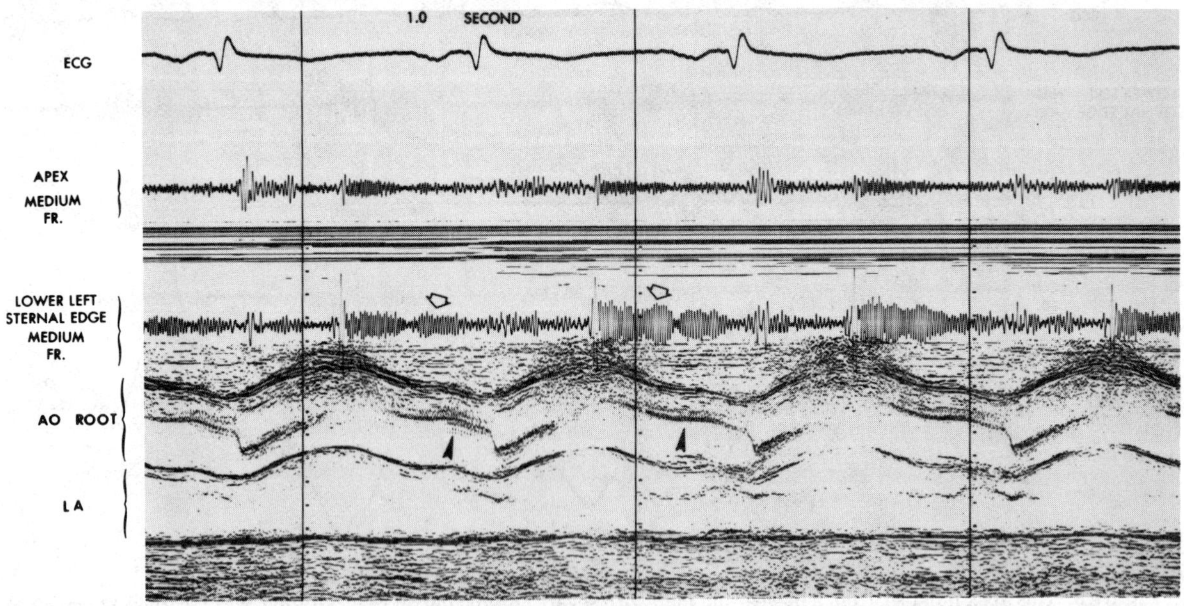

Figure 6. This simultaneous echophonocardiogram, from a 58-year-old man with endocarditis who developed aortic regurgitation because of a fenestrated cusp, shows a medium-frequency, vibratory (or musical) murmur maximal at the lower left sternal edge (open arrowheads). Note that the aortic valve also vibrates in diastole (closed arrowheads). This diastolic murmur was also easily palpable. AO root = aortic root; LA = left atrium.

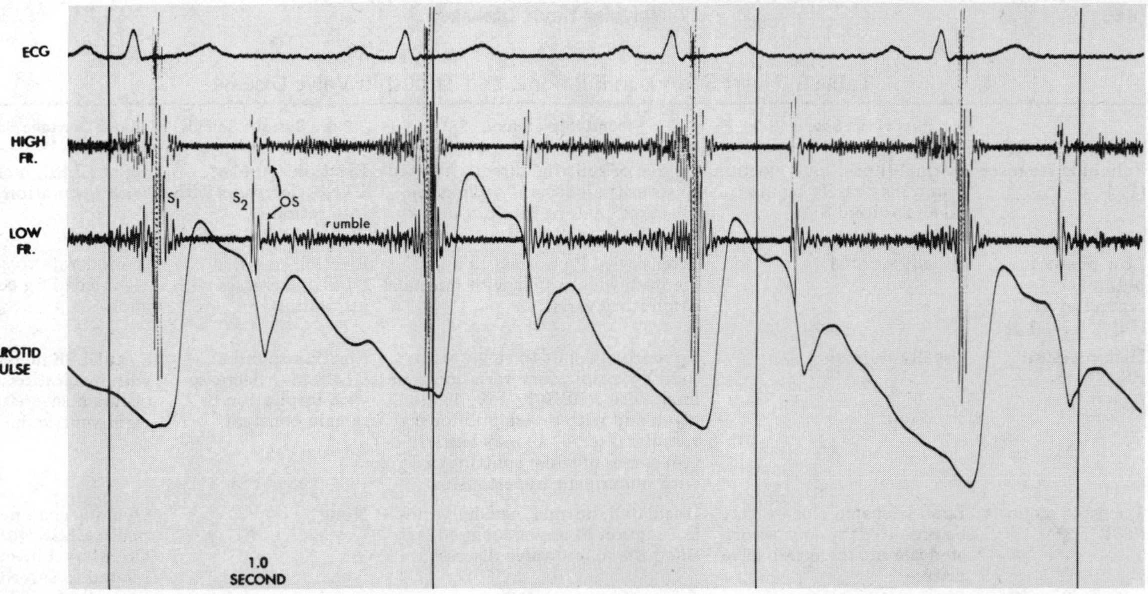

Figure 7. This phonocardiogram, from a 36-year-old woman with moderately severe mitral stenosis, shows the classic bedside features of rheumatic mitral stenosis with a markedly accentuated first heart sound (S_1), an opening snap (OS), and a long holodiastolic murmur (rumble) that demonstrates presystolic accentuation. In this patient, the first and second heart sounds, the opening snap, and the diastolic rumble were all palpable as well.

Table 5. Heart Sounds in Aortic and Mitral Valve Disease

	First Heart Sound (S_1)	Second Heart Sound (S_2)	Extra Systolic Sounds	Extra Diastolic Sounds
Aortic stenosis (AS)	Normal unless heart failure, then diminished	If congenital, A_2 usually well preserved; if severe, paradoxic splitting occurs; with progressive calcification and immobility, A_2 softens	Ejection sound at URSE and apex common if preserved leaflet mobility	Apical S_4 common and in a young patient predicts severe gradient; but in older patient, S_4 common because of associated disease and not predictive of severity
Chronic aortic regurgitation (AR)	Same as AS	If severe, soft aortic component of S_2	Ejection sound at URSE and apex common with bicuspid leaflet but also occurs in other aortic valve disease as well as in aortic root disease	Apical S_3 common in severe disease even without failure
Acute AR	Soft to absent due to presystolic mitral valve closure	Soft to absent A_2; P_2 may be accentuated	None unless pre-existent aortic valve disease—then ejection sound	Apical S_3 common
Mitral stenosis (MS)	Loud, snapping, and frequently palpable	With pulmonary hypertension, P_2 loud and S_2 single or narrowly split with little or no respiratory variation	Ejection sound at ULSE due to pulmonary hypertension	Apical opening snap 30–120 msec after S_2 with A_2–OS interval inversely proportional to severity; left-sided gallops rare
Chronic mitral regurgitation (MR)	Soft and obscured by murmur unless due to MVP	If severe, widely split; P_2 normal intensity until late in disease, then accentuated	None	S_3 common if severe; S_4 rare
MR secondary to mitral valve prolapse (MVP) and mitral apparatus dysfunction	Normal to increased; if MVP, even with significant MR may be loud	Normal unless severe MR, then widely split	Nonejection apical middle to late systolic click(s) with MVP	Mitral valve opening sound may occur with MVP; S_3 with severe MR and/or LV failure
Acute MR	Normal, but frequently obscured by murmur	Widely split with loud P_2	None	S_3 and S_4 common

Abbreviations: URSE = Upper right sternal edge; ULSE = upper left sternal edge; A_2 = aortic component of second heart second; P_2 = pulmonic component of second heart sound; S_3 = verntricular gallop; S_4 = atrial gallop; LV = left ventricular; TR = tricuspid regurgitation; OS = opening snap.

Table 6. Heart Sounds in Pulmonic and Tricuspid Valve Disease

	First Heart Sound (S_1)	Second Heart Sound (S_2)	Extra Systolic Sounds	Extra Diastolic Sounds
Pulmonic stenosis (PS)	Normal (note: loud ejection sound may rarely be mistaken for loud S_1)	Degree of splitting directly related to severity; if severe, A_2 may be obscured by long murmur and P_2 becomes very soft	Ejection sound at ULSE; decreases with inspiration	S_4 at LLSE, increases with inspiration
Low-pressure pulmonary regurgitation (PR)	Usually normal	Intensity of P_2 normal to augmented; widely split with normal respiratory variation	Ejection sound at ULSE: decreases with inspiration	If moderate to severe, right-sided S_3 common
High-pressure PR	Usually normal	S_2 narrowly split to single with loud P_2; respiratory variation minimal; with RBBB, P_2 may be delayed and with severe pulmonary vascular disease, A_2 may be early—two causes of wider splitting of S_2 with pulmonary hypertension	Ejection sound at ULSE may decrease with inspiration or remain constant	S_4 at LLSE increasing with inspiration; S_3 occurs if severe or right ventricular failure
Tricuspid stenosis (TS)	Loud tricuspid closure may be obscured by any associated rheumatic mitral valve disease	If isolated, normal; usually varies as function of any associated left-sided rheumatic valve disease	None	Opening snap maximal at LLSE with S_2–OS interval inversely related to severity; typically found with mitral opening snap as well
Low-pressure tricuspid regurgitation (TR)	With Ebstein's anomaly, widely split with loud tricuspid component (sail sound); otherwise normal to obscured by murmur	With Ebstein's anomaly, widely split with soft, late P_2; with isolated TR, P_2 is rarely early enough to cause paradoxic splitting	Usually none unless nonejection click(s) with tricuspid prolapse; sail cound of Ebstein's anomaly may be mistaken for nonejection click	If more than mild, S_3 at LLSE, increasing with inspiration
High-pressure TR	Normal to diminished loudness; may be obscured by murmur	Narrowly split or single with loud P_2 and little or no respiratory variation (same as for high-pressure PR)	Ejection sound at ULSE; may be fixed or vary with respiration	If more than mild or right heart failure, S_3 at LLSE that increases with inspiration

Abbreviations: ULSE = Upper left sternal edge; LLSE = lower left sternal edge; RBBB = right bundle branch block; A_2 = aortic component of second heart sound; P_2 = pulmonic component of second heart sound; S_4 = atrial gallop; S_3 = ventricular gallop.

Aortic valve disease with associated left ventricular dysfunction may also cause reduced acceleration and deceleration of blood in association with mitral valve coaptation and, therefore, a softer first heart sound. With acute severe aortic regurgitation, there is preclosure of the mitral valve and a soft to absent first heart sound, but chronic aortic regurgitation with a long PR interval can also cause a soft first heart sound. Severe mitral stenosis may cause delayed mitral valve closure due to high left atrial pressure, usually with a single first heart sound but occasionally with reversed splitting.

Ebstein's anomaly of the tricuspid valve in the absence of an accessory pathway causes wide splitting of the first heart sound (60 to 120 msec typically) with an accentuated, delayed tricuspid closure sound—the "sail sound." As with right bundle branch block, this wide splitting is due to a right-sided conduction delay that may be lost when there is an associated right-sided accessory pathway.

The Second Heart Sound—Loudness and Splitting

Normal respiratory splitting is the rule with mild right- or left-sided valvular heart disease. The widest degrees of splitting occur with valvular pulmonic stenosis, with a linear correlation between right ventricular systolic pressure and the degree of splitting. With severe valvular pulmonic stenosis, the pulmonary component also softens dramatically. Narrow splitting of the second sound with little or no respiratory variation, or a single, loud second sound due to an accentuated pulmonary component, is characteristic of pulmonary hypertension and is a relative early finding in mitral stenosis but occurs much later in mitral regurgitation and aortic valve disease. When pulmonary hypertension is due to acute severe or chronic mitral regurgitation, persistent wide splitting with a loud pulmonary component occurs because of shortened left ventricular ejection time and early aortic valve closure.

Paradoxical splitting of the second heart sound (in the absence of left bundle branch block) is typical of severe aortic stenosis and is easiest to appreciate in the younger patient who retains at least some aortic valve mobility. In the older patient with calcific aortic stenosis, the intensity of the aortic component characteristically softens, making the appreciation of paradoxical splitting difficult. Rarely, with severe tricuspid regurgitation, pulmonary closure may occur early and may precede aortic valve closure, producing paradoxical splitting.

Extra Systolic Sounds—Ejection Sounds

Ejection sounds occur either in association with dilatation of a great vessel or with an abnormal semilunar valve. Left-sided ejection sounds may occur with significant hypertension, but they are most likely to occur with aortic valve disease and in particular congenital aortic valve disease (Fig. 8). Other causes of aortic valve ejection sounds include rheumatic, luetic, and calcific aortic valve disease. Aortic ejection sounds follow the mitral component of the first heart sound by 50 to 70 ms, are best appreciated at the upper right sternal edge and over the left ventricular apex, and show little or no respiratory variation.

Right-sided ejection sounds occur due to pulmonary hypertension or congenital pulmonary valve disease (either stenosis or regurgitation), are loudest at the upper left sternal edge and soften with inspiration. The latter occurs because inspiration augments filling of a noncompliant right ventricle and causes doming or opening of the valve so that at the onset of systole, there is less abrupt deceleration of blood flow (Fig. 9). Respiratory variation is most likely with pulmonary

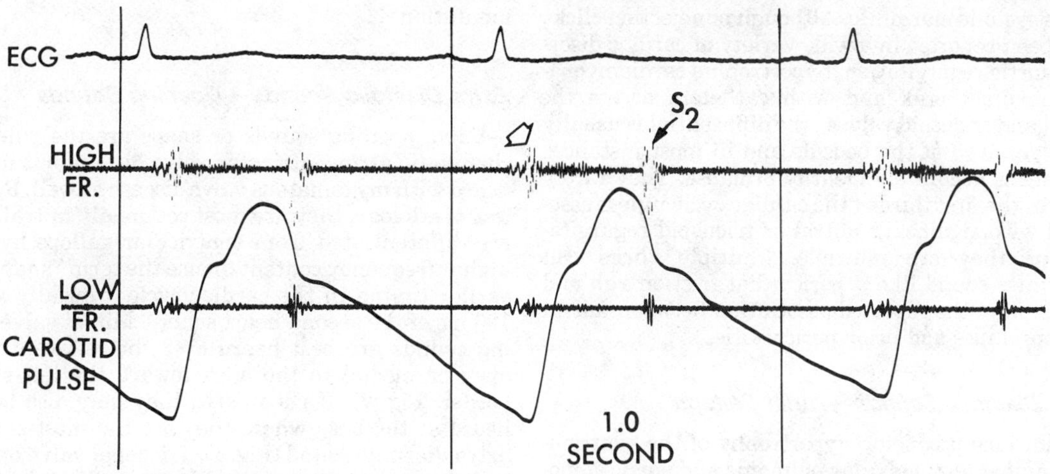

Figure 8. This phonocardiogram, from a 38-year-old man with a bicuspid aortic valve and mild aortic stenosis, shows an aortic ejection sound (open arrowhead) best recorded on the high-frequency tracing at the upper right sternal edge. This ejection sound was also well recorded at the apex. S_2 = Second heart sound.

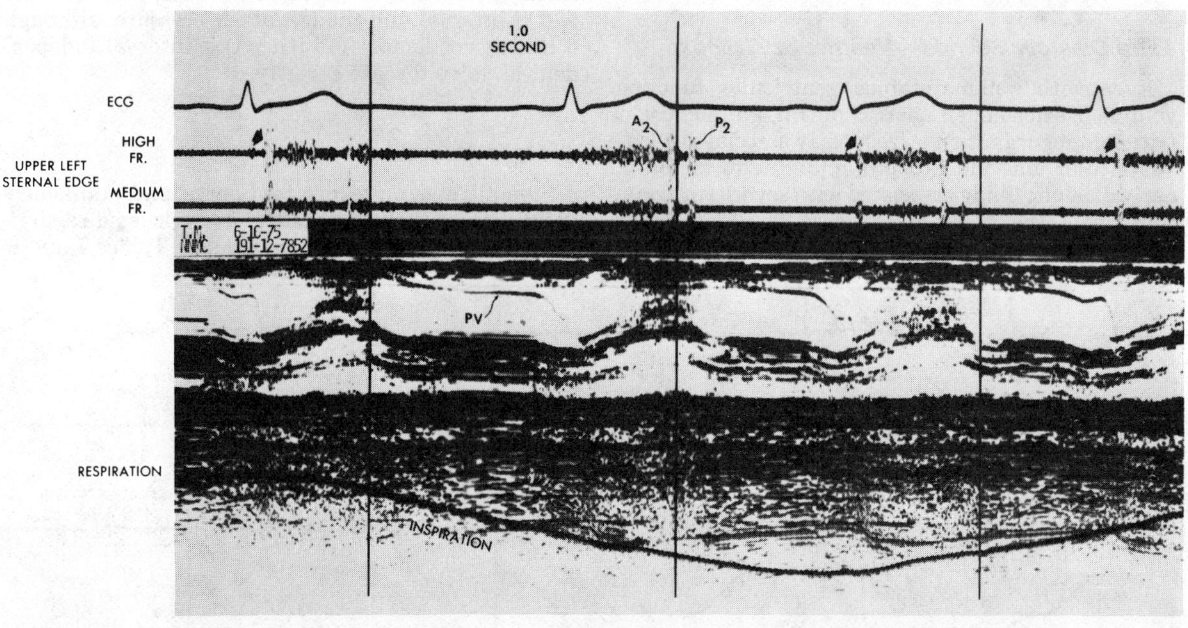

Figure 9. This simultaneous echophonocardiogram is from a 16-year-old male with mild to moderate valvular pulmonic stenosis. Note that during expiration a loud ejection sound (arrowheads) is seen. During inspiration the ejection sound virtually disappears (second complex) coincident with inspiration-induced right ventricular filling, causing presystolic opening of the pulmonary valve (PV). During expiration, the valve is fully closed at the onset of ventricular systole resulting in greater deceleration and a louder ejection sound. Note also the degree of splitting (A_2, P_2) of the second heart sound, the well-preserved pulmonic component (P_2), and the midsystolic murmur, all features of mild to moderate pulmonary valve stenosis.

valve disease but may also occur with pulmonary hypertension.

Extra Systolic Sounds—Nonejection Clicks

Nonejection clicks are the acoustic hallmark of mitral and/or tricuspid valve prolapse. They occur in middle to late systole, are usually well localized to the apex or lower left sternal edge (Fig. 10), and may or may not be associated with a murmur (see the discussion of systolic murmurs). Although nonejection clicks have been reported in a wide variety of cardiac disorders (aortic regurgitation, hypertrophic cardiomyopathy, pneumothorax and with catheters across the mitral and tricuspid valves), the differential is usually easily resolved at the bedside and in most instances such clicks accurately identify prolapse. They rarely occur in the first third of the cardiac cycle unless associated with significant mitral or tricuspid regurgitation or they are multiple. Multiple clicks can sometimes sound like a pericardial friction rub and may explain the reported association between mitral valve prolapse and prior pericarditis.

Extra Diastolic Sounds—Atrial Gallops

Conditions producing hypertrophy of the ventricular chamber (e.g., valvular pulmonic and aortic stenosis), because of the resulting decrease in compliance, are frequently associated with low-frequency gallop sounds due to augmented atrial systole. A right-sided versus a left-sided atrial gallop may be differentiated by where it is best heard (lower left sternal edge versus the apex, respectively) and by the inspiratory augmentation of the former.

Extra Diastolic Sounds—Ventricular Gallops

Even with well-maintained ventricular function, volume overload due to aortic, mitral, pulmonary, or tricuspid regurgitation is frequently associated with a ventricular diastolic gallop (Fig. 5) due to torrential early diastolic filling associated with severe regurgitation (from the great vessel with semilunar valve regurgitation and from the atria with atrioventricular valve regurgitation). It is noteworthy that even mild tricuspid or mitral stenosis is usually sufficient to prevent the generation of the third heart sound associated with tricuspid or mitral regurgitation, respectively. At the bedside, differentiating the explosive onset of the diastolic rumble from a third heart sound may be difficult unless there is a palpable gallop. As in the case of atrial gallops, right-sided ventricular filling sounds are differentiated by their location (lower left sternal edge) and inspiratory augmentation.

Extra Diastolic Sounds—Opening Sounds

Valve opening sounds or snaps are the rule with rheumatic atrioventricular valve disease but may be heard with myxomatous valve disease as well. Regardless of etiology, they are most commonly mitral. They are differentiated from ventricular gallops by their higher frequency content (hence the term "snap") and earlier timing in the cardiac cycle (typically within 120 ms of the second heart sound). Mitral valve opening sounds are best heard over the left ventricular apex or medial to the apex toward the left sternal border (Fig. 7). If rheumatic, they may also be well heard at the base where they are the most common extra diastolic sound (Fig. 1). Tricuspid valve opening sounds are best appreciated at the lower left sternal edge and, in an occasional patient with both mitral and tricuspid valve disease, two snaps may be appreciated in this area. Rheumatic mitral valve opening snaps may be more difficult to hear when there is concomitant aortic valve disease and become softer with progressive immobility of the valve. When rheumatic, there is an inverse relationship between the A_2-OS interval and the left atrial pressure, although a number of factors influence this interval independent of valve disease severity.

Systolic Murmurs

Stenotic and/or regurgitant aortic and pulmonary valve disease, as well as mitral and tricuspid regurgitation, causes systolic murmurs. (See Tables 7 and 8.)

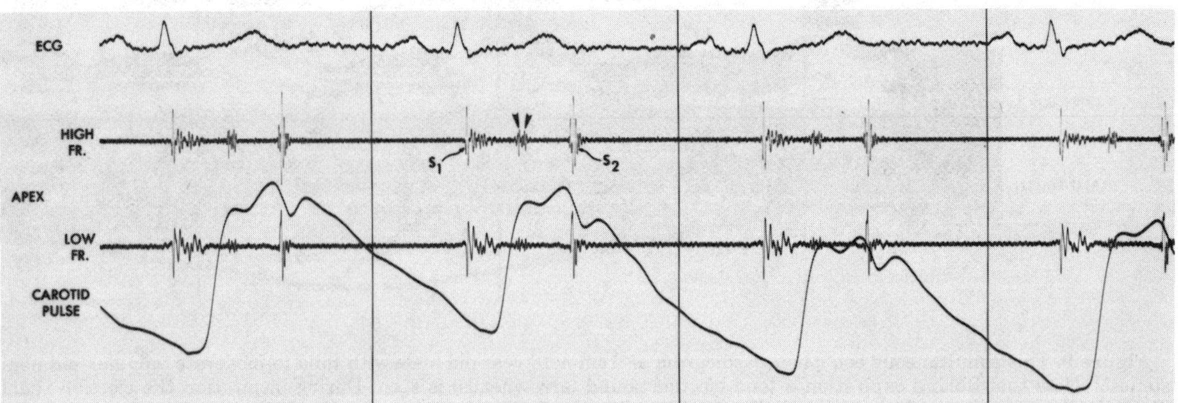

Figure 10. This apex phonocardiogram, from a 29-year-old woman with mitral valve prolapse, shows two narrowly spaced midsystolic clicks (arrowheads). S_1 = First heart sound; S_2 = second heart sound.

Table 7. Murmurs in Aortic and Mitral Valve Disease

	Murmurs	Response to Interventions
Aortic stenosis (AS)	Medium-frequency (harsh) systolic diamond-shaped murmur beginning after S_1 or with ejection sound and ending before S_2; maximal at URSE and radiates well to neck and apex; in absence of failure or concomitant AR, length and time of peaking, correlates well with severity; at apex, murmur commonly has higher frequency and more musical character	Increase after a PVC, after amyl nitrite, and with isotonic exercise; variable response to squatting; decreases during Valsalva strain
Chronic aortic regurgitation (AR)	1. High-frequency diastolic decrescendo murmur beginning with S_2 and frequently extending to S_1 of next beat; maximal at base and LLSE seated with expiration 2. Medium-frequency systolic, diamond-shaped murmur beginning with ejection sound and ending before S_2; maximal at URSE and apex and due to flow or concomitant AS; may be late peaking and radiate to neck even without associated AS 3. Low-frequency (rumbling) mid-diastolic to presystolic apical murmur (Austin Flint), if moderate to severe AR 4. With left ventricular dilatation, apical blowing holosystolic murmur radiating to left axilla due to mitral regurgitation from apparatus dysfunction	Diastolic murmur increases with squatting, isometric exercise; decreases post–amyl nitrite and with Valsalva strain; Austin Flint murmur decreases with amyl nitrite
Acute AR	1. Harsh to musical diastolic decrescendo murmur beginning with or after S_2 and if severe, ending in mid-diastole due to equilibration of left ventricular and aortic root pressures; maximal at base and at LLSE seated and leaning forward 2. Medium-frequency systolic diamond-shaped murmur beginning after S_1 and ending before S_2; maximal at base and radiates to neck and apex; due to increased flow across diseased aortic valve 3. If severe, apical Austin Flint rumble (see chronic AR)	Diastolic murmur response same as with chronic AR
Mitral stenosis (MS)	1. Low-frequency (rumbling) decrescendo diastolic murmur with length proportional to severity; in NSR, presystolic accentuation usual but may occur as well in atrial fibrillation during runs of rapid conduction: maximal at apex 2. With pulmonary hypertension, secondary murmurs of PR and TR are common	Increases with amyl nitrite and isotonic exercise
Chronic mitral regurgitation (MR)	1. High-frequency holosytolic plateau-shaped murmur: maximal at apex and radiating to left axilla 2. If severe MR, low-frequency mid-diastolic murmur, maximal at apex	Systolic murmur decreases with Valsalva strain and amyl nitrite; increases with isometric exercise and squatting; unchanged following a PVC
MR secondary to mitral valve prolapse (MVP) and mitral apparatus dysfunction	1. High-frequency systolic crescendo murmur beginning in midsystole and extending to S_2; maximal at apex but may radiate to base, LSE; if harsh or musical (whooping), is frequently palpable; with progression, becomes holosystolic and frequently retains late systolic accentuation 2. If severe, rumbling, mid-diastolic apical flow murmur (see chronic MR)	Late systolic murmur louder and later with squatting; longer with amyl nitrite, usually not louder unless whoop- or honk-induced; earlier and occasionally louder with standing; longer and usually not louder during Valsalva strain
Acute MR	1. Medium- to high-frequency decrescendo systolic murmur beginning with S_1 and ending before S_2; maximal at apex but may radiate to LSE or base and simulate aortic obstruction 2. Rumbling mid-diastolic apical flow murmur common	Same as chronic MR

Abbreviations: URSE = Upper right sternal edge; LLSE = lower left sternal edge; LSE = left sternal edge; PVC = premature ventricular contraction; S_1 = first heart sound; S_2 = second heart sound; NSR = normal sinus rhythm; PR = pulmonary regurgitation; TR = tricuspid regurgitation.

Outflow tract murmurs are harsh (or medium frequency), begin after the first heart sound, end before semilunar valve closure of the great vessel and outflow tract from which they arise, and are crescendo-decrescendo or diamond-shaped (Figs. 6, 8, and 9). In the absence of significant associated aortic or pulmonary regurgitation and with well-maintained ventricular function, murmur duration and time of peaking bear a direct relationship to severity. When there is semilunar valve regurgitation (particularly with aortic valve disease), the systolic murmur may be loud, long, and late-peaking, with little or no associated stenosis.

Aortic stenosis murmurs are best heard at the upper right sternal edge and radiate prominently to the carotids, particularly on the left. Such murmurs are also well heard at the apex, where they are higher-frequency (the so-called Gallavardin effect), leading to the mistaken conclusion that there is concomitant mitral regurgitation. Pulmonary valve murmurs are characteristically best heard at the upper left sternal edge and radiate to the left infraclavicular area. With severe pulmonary valve stenosis, the murmur may extend beyond and obscure the aortic component of the second heart sound.

Mitral and tricuspid regurgitation also produce systolic murmurs that, as a rule, are easily differentiated from outflow tract murmurs. The murmur of mitral regurgitation is classically holosystolic, blowing (or high-frequency) in character and maximal at the apex, and radiates to the left axilla. In mitral regurgitation due to apparatus dysfunction (e.g. left ventricular dilatation, mitral valve prolapse), the murmur may begin in middle to late systole but typically extends to the second heart sound with a crescendo character (Fig. 11). Although mitral apparatus dysfunc-

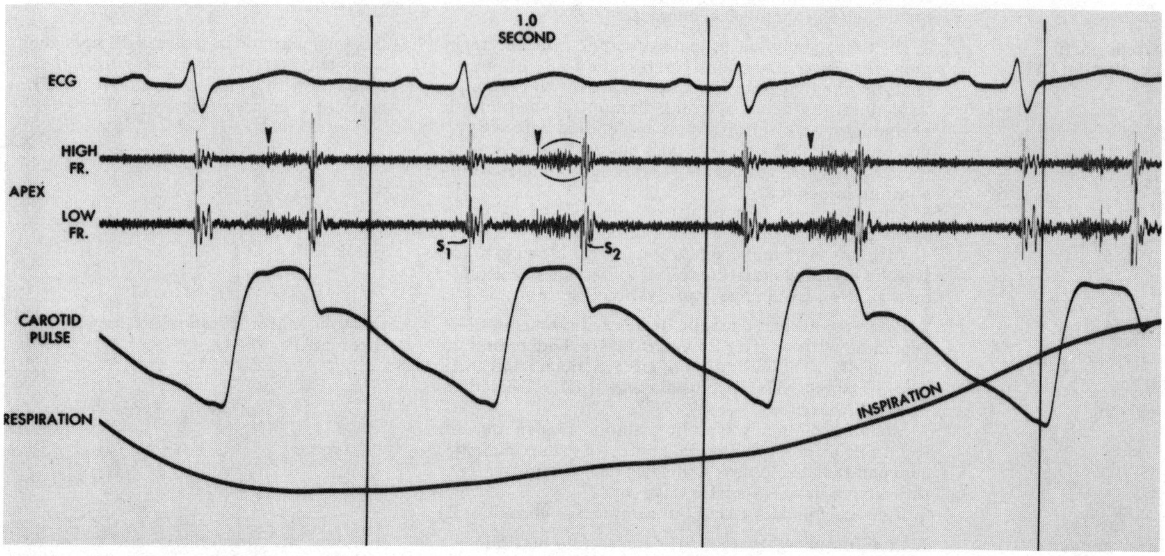

Figure 11. This apex phonocardiogram, from a 46-year-old woman with mitral valve prolapse, shows a midsystolic click (arrowheads) and a late systolic murmur (bracket) that begins roughly with the click and extends to the second heart sound (S_2). The last complex may show a late systolic click as well. S_1 = First heart sound.

Table 8. Murmurs in Pulmonic and Tricuspid Valve Disease

	Murmurs	Response to Interventions
Pulmonic stenosis (PS)	Medium-frequency (harsh) systolic diamond-shaped murmur, beginning after ejection sound with length and time of peaking directly related to severity; may extend to or through A_2	Increases with amyl nitrite inhalation and exercise and decreases during Valsalva strain
Low-pressure pulmonary regurgitation (PR)	1. Low- (rumbling) to medium-frequency early to mid-diastolic murmur, beginning after P_2 and ending well before S_1: maximal at middle to upper LSE 2. Medium-frequency early- to mid-systolic diamond-shaped murmur, beginning after S_1 and ending well before S_2: maximal at ULSE and due to flow into dilated pulmonary artery	Variable response to amyl nitrite; if mild, may increase; no response to squatting; increases with inspiration
High-pressure PR	1. High-frequency diastolic decrescendo murmur beginning with S_2 and usually ending well before S_1 of next cycle: maximal at middle to lower LSE 2. Medium-frequency early- to mid-systolic diamond-shaped murmur ending well before S_2: maximal at ULSE and due to flow into dilated pulmonary artery	Variable response to amyl nitrite depending upon pulomnary vascular reactivity; typically does not change greatly; no response to squatting; may increase with inspiration
Tricuspid stenosis (TS)	Low- (rumbling) to medium-frequency murmur, beginning after opening snap with duration directly related to severity: If NSR, presystolic accentuation: maximal at LLSE	Increases with amyl nitrite inhalation, exercise, and inspiration
Low-pressure tricuspid regurgitation (TR)	1. Medium- to low-frequency holosystolic murmur: may be plateau-shaped or decrescendo: maximal at middle to lower LSE 2. If moderate to severe, mid-diastolic, low-frequency (rumbling) murmur: may begin with S_3 and is maximal at LLSE	Increases with amyl nitrite inhalation; variable response to squatting; both murmurs may augment with isotonic exercise and inspiration
High-pressure TR	1. High-frequency (blowing) holosystolic plateau-shaped murmur: maximal at LLSE. 2. If moderate to severe, mid-diastolic low-frequency (rumbling) murmur: may begin with S_3 and is maximal at LLSE	Usually increases with amyl nitrite, inspiration, and isotonic exercise; no change with squatting

Abbreviations: S_1 = First heart sound; S_2 = second heart sound; S_3 = ventricular gallop; A_2 = aortic component of second heart sound; P_2 = pulmonic component of second heart sound; LSE = left sternal edge; ULSE = upper left sternal edge; LLSE = lower left sternal edge; NSR = normal sinus rhythm.

tion murmurs may be high-frequency in character, they commonly have a more harsh, mixed frequency content, or they may even be musical, producing the classical precordial "honk" or "whoop." These murmurs may also demonstrate a great deal of variability in their frequency content, either on a beat-to-beat basis or in response to various interventions, and when they are musical or harsh are typically palpable as well. Their pattern of radiation may also be quite distinctive, in that depending on the direction of the regurgitant jet into the left atrium, they may radiate preferentially to the left sternal edge or base (Fig. 5).

Diastolic Murmurs

Diastolic murmurs may arise from regurgitation of either semilunar valve, from stenosis of either atrioventricular valve, from diastolic flow across a regurgitant atrioventricular valve in the absence of stenosis, or when there is severe aortic regurgitation (the Austin Flint murmur).

Mitral stenosis produces a diastolic rumbling (low-frequency) murmur that is well localized to the apex and may be heard only in the left lateral decubitus position after an intervention (see the discussion of bedside maneuvers following). With sinus rhythm and mild stenosis, the murmur may be confined to presystole, but with more severe mitral stenosis the murmur begins shortly after the opening snap, decrescendos toward the middle of diastole, and then demonstrates presystolic accentuation (Fig. 7). The length of the murmur is normally directly related to the severity of the stenosis, but with tachyarrhythmias even mild mitral stenosis produces a "holodiastolic" rumble. With atrial fibrillation, the presystolic accentuation is lost, particularly during long R-R intervals. With runs of rapid conduction, however, and with retained leaflet pliability, presystolic accentuation of the murmur may remain. This is because with rapid conduction the shortened diastole causes a rise in left atrial pressure that imparts greater kinetic energy to the column of blood flowing into the ventricle in early diastole after mitral valve opening. With ventricular systole, left ventricular pressure rises and begins to close the mitral valve, which with continuing antegrade flow and a decreasing mitral valve orifice size causes presystolic accentuation of the rumble.

Tricuspid stenosis is best appreciated as a low- to mid-frequency diastolic murmur along the lower left sternal border that increases with inspiration. Diastolic rumbles also occur with severe mitral or tricuspid regurgitation in the absence of stenosis due to torrential blood flow back across the valve in early to mid-diastole.

Aortic regurgitation produces a blowing (high-frequency) diastolic decrescendo murmur that begins with S_2 and may extend to the first heart sound of the next cycle. This murmur may be heard at the upper right sternal edge but is usually best heard at the lower left sternal edge with the patient seated and leaning forward during full expiration. When aortic regurgitation is due to a fenestrated cusp, the diastolic murmur may have a musical or vibratory character (Fig. 6). With acute severe aortic regurgitation, the murmur may be misleadingly short as aortic root and left ventricular pressures equilibrate in mid-diastole. With acute aortic regurgitation, regardless of chronicity, an apical mid-diastolic rumble (the Austin Flint murmur) may occur due to premature mitral valve closure analogous to the previously cited mechanism for presystolic accentuation of the rumble with atrial fibrillation.

Pulmonary regurgitation resulting from pulmonary hypertension also produces a high-frequency diastolic decrescendo murmur that is maximal along the left sternal edge. Low-pressure pulmonary valve regurgitation produces a distinctive mid-diastolic low-frequency (rumbling) murmur that is maximal at the lower left sternal edge. This murmur may be very difficult to differentiate from tricuspid stenosis. All of these right-sided murmurs may augment with inspiration.

The Response of Murmurs to Bedside Maneuvers

During the continued strain phase of a *Valsalva maneuver,* virtually all murmurs, with the exception of those due to hypertrophic cardiomyopathy and mitral valve prolapse, diminish. The former may dramatically augment, whereas the latter typically does not become much louder (unless a "whoop" is induced) but begins earlier in the cardiac cycle. Following release of a Valsalva maneuver, blood pressure increases and the clicks and/or murmur of prolapse are louder and/or later (Fig. 12).

Amyl nitrite inhalation is helpful in differentiating aortic outflow tract murmurs from mitral regurgitation, wherein the former augment and the latter soften. Amyl nitrite inhalation is also helpful in differentiating an Austin Flint murmur of aortic regurgitation from mitral stenosis. The fall in afterload lessens aortic regurgitation and therefore the Austin Flint murmur, while mitral stenosis is accentuated because of the tachycardia and the increase in cardiac output. The response of the murmur following a *premature ventricular contraction* is helpful in differentiating systolic outflow tract murmurs from mitral regurgitation, wherein the former augment and the latter are unchanged. *Squatting* primarily produces an increase in afterload and accentuates aortic regurgitation and mitral regurgitation, whereas aortic valvular stenosis may either increase or decrease.

COURSE, COMPLICATIONS, DIFFERENTIAL DIAGNOSIS, AND LABORATORY EVALUATION

Aortic Stenosis

Course/Complications

Patients with aortic stenosis secondary to commissural fusion or a unicommissural valve may present at a young age with syncope, chest pain, or, more rarely, congestive heart failure. Younger patients with calcification of a bicuspid leaflet may present with the

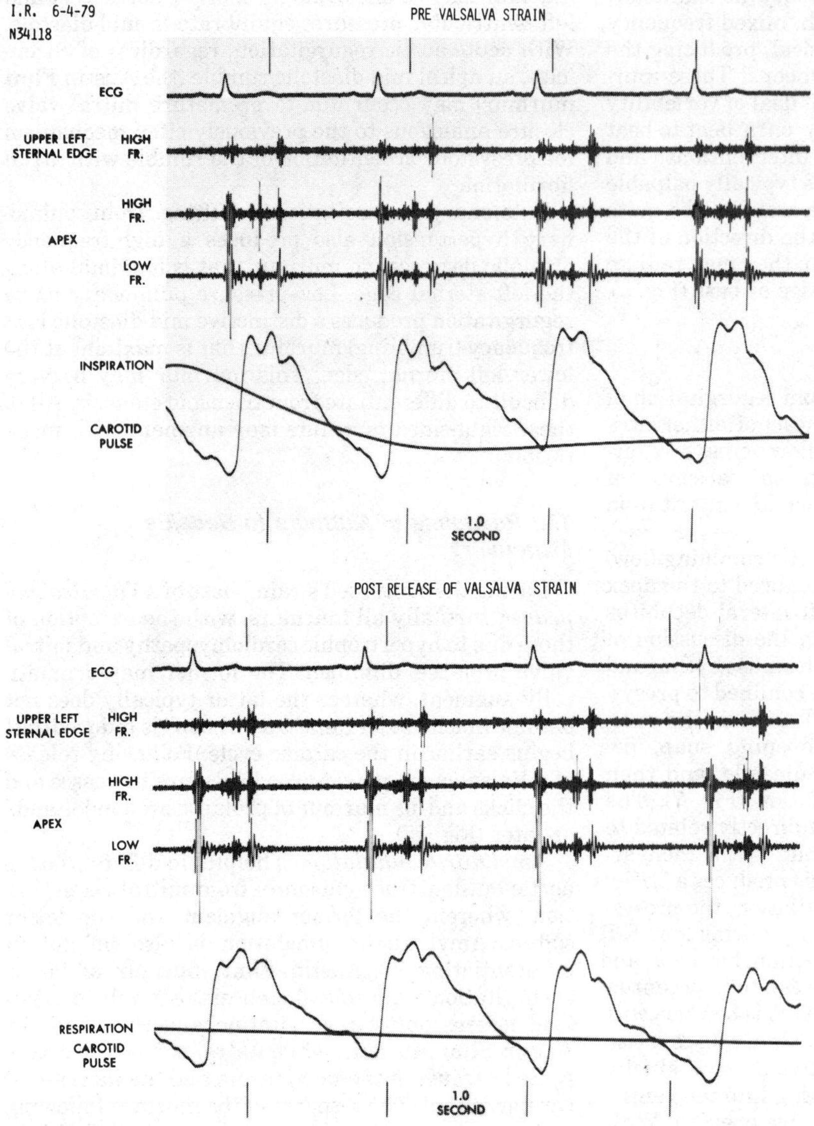

Figure 12. Baseline apex phonocardiogram (top panel) from a 63-year-old man with mitral valve prolapse who had two loud midsystolic clicks with a mid- to late systolic murmur. Following release of a Valsalva strain (bottom panel), there was an increase in blood pressure with the clicks becoming louder and later in systole. There was also mild accentuation of the late systolic murmur.

same symptoms. The older the patient, the more common is congestive heart failure as the presenting complaint. Once heart failure, syncope, or angina occurs, the average life expectancy is between 1½ to 5 years, with heart failure carrying the most dire prognosis. Emboli occur when there is associated endocarditis, a common complication. Sudden death, usually in association with exertion, is more common in children but can occur at any age.

Differential Diagnosis

The differential diagnosis includes subvalvular membranous stenosis, supravalvular stenosis, hypertrophic obstructive cardiomyopathy, aortic sclerosis and, rarely, fungal endocarditis. With supravalvular stenosis, the murmur radiates prominently to the right side of the neck, whereas in subvalvular aortic stenosis the murmur is loudest along the lower left sternal edge and radiation to the neck is not prominent. Hypertrophic obstructive cardiomyopathy has a distinctly different carotid contour and apex impulse (classically triple due to a large A wave and bifid systolic contour) and response to the Valsalva maneuver. With an aortic sclerosis murmur, the differential becomes difficult when hypertension and/or coronary artery disease have altered left ventricular function and/or produced symptoms. When the murmur occurs with a normal second heart sound, a normal apex impulse, no diastolic murmur or ejection sound, and normal simple laboratory tests, the diagnosis of aortic sclerosis is reasonable, with the realization that it may be a harbinger of subsequent stenosis. Fungal endocarditis occurs in a typical clinical setting, and there is usually associated regurgitation.

Laboratory Evaluation

The ECG in significant aortic stenosis shows left ventricular hypertrophy. In the younger patient, this may be manifested by voltage alone without concomitant ST-T wave changes. Sinus rhythm is the rule, although 15 to 20 per cent of patients over the age of 65 develop atrial fibrillation.

The chest x-ray shows concentric left ventricular hypertrophy, and the plain film may show a calcified aortic valve. In the older patient, calcification is invariable on fluoroscopy and its absence should lead to serious reconsideration of the diagnosis. In the younger patient, the aortic root may show poststenotic dilatation with a normal arch and descending aorta, but in the older patient this is unusual and the aorta shows changes compatible with the patient's age.

Echocardiography typically shows a heavily calcified, immobile aortic valve (Figs. 13 and 14). Indeed, in an adult, if one or more leaflets move normally, aortic stenosis is virtually excluded. In the young patient with commissural fusion, however, normal leaflet mobility may occur despite a marked gradient.

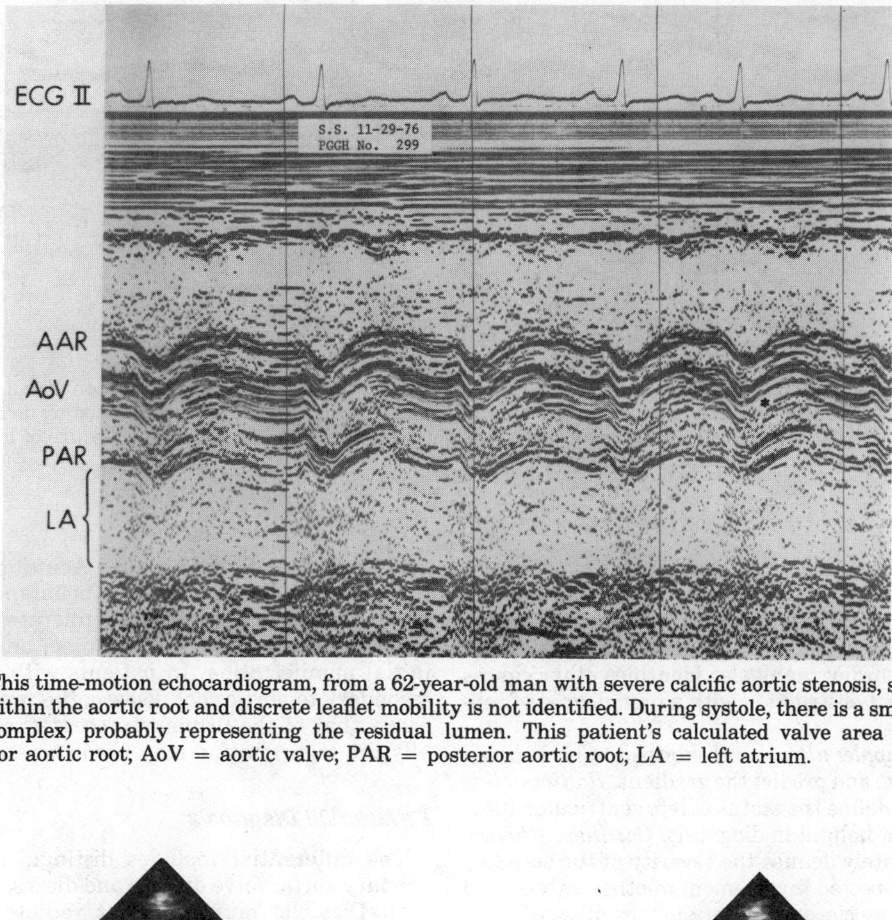

Figure 13. This time-motion echocardiogram, from a 62-year-old man with severe calcific aortic stenosis, shows multiple linear echoes within the aortic root and discrete leaflet mobility is not identified. During systole, there is a small clear space (asterisk-last complex) probably representing the residual lumen. This patient's calculated valve area was 0.65 cm². AAR = Anterior aortic root; AoV = aortic valve; PAR = posterior aortic root; LA = left atrium.

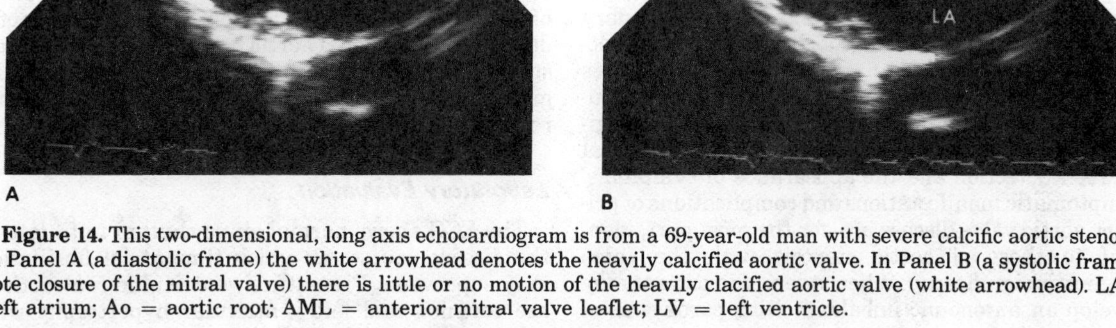

Figure 14. This two-dimensional, long axis echocardiogram is from a 69-year-old man with severe calcific aortic stenosis. In Panel A (a diastolic frame) the white arrowhead denotes the heavily calcified aortic valve. In Panel B (a systolic frame—note closure of the mitral valve) there is little or no motion of the heavily clacified aortic valve (white arrowhead). LA = Left atrium; Ao = aortic root; AML = anterior mitral valve leaflet; LV = left ventricle.

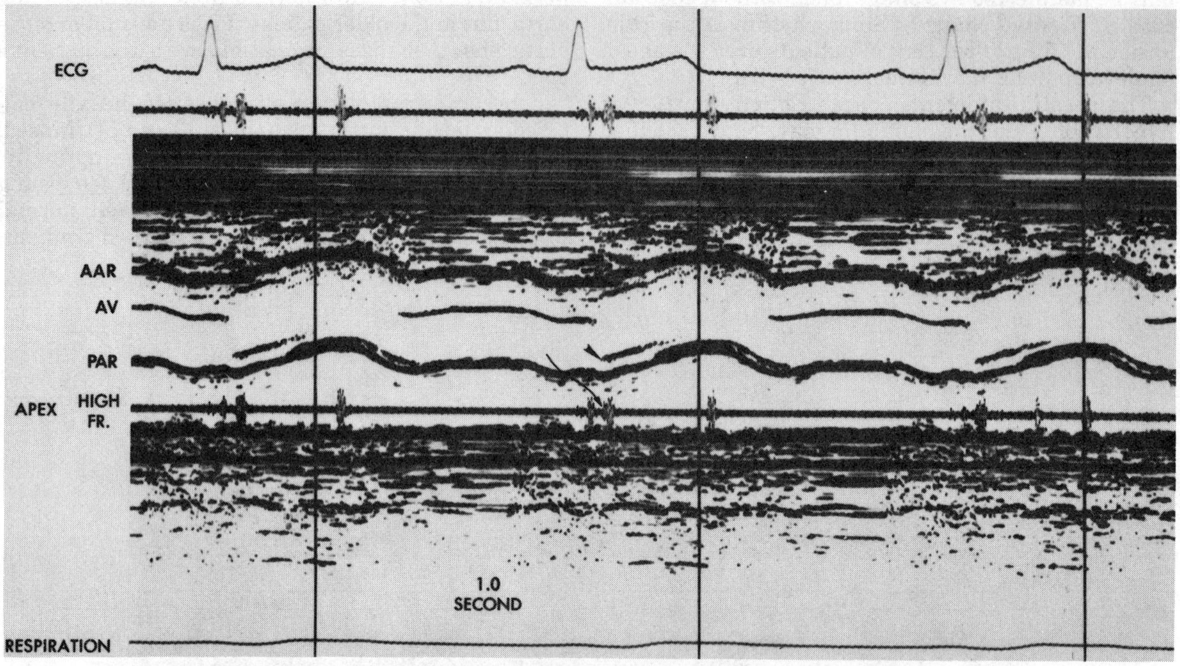

Figure 15. This echophonocardiogram, from a 29-year-old man with an isolated aortic ejection sound secondary to a bicuspid valve, shows that the onset of the ejection sound (curved arrow) coincides with peak opening (arrowhead) of the aortic valve (AV). Note also that the aortic valve echo is slightly eccentric, one characteristic feature of bicuspid leaflets. AAR = Anterior aortic root; PAR = posterior aortic root.

In the younger patient, a bicuspid leaflet may be seen (Fig. 15), but with a severely calcified aortic valve the echo is not particularly helpful in differentiating between calcification of a bicuspid versus a tricuspid leaflet. Echocardiography also identifies other causes of outflow tract obstruction with a high degree of reliability.

Finally, *Doppler ultrasound* shows promise in being able to localize and predict the gradient. *Radionuclide imaging* can define the status of left ventricular function but is not helpful in diagnosis. *Cardiac catheterization* accurately defines the severity of the stenosis, reveals unsuspected involvement of other valves, and defines any associated coronary artery disease.

Aortic Regurgitation

Course/Complications

Aortic regurgitation is multifactorial in etiology, ranging from primary valve disease (rheumatic, congenital, traumatic, and infective) to those secondary to disease of the aortic root (e.g., hypertension, dissection, syphilis, ankylosing spondylitis) or structures supporting leaflet insertions (membranous ventricular septal defect). Patients with chronic aortic regurgitation may enjoy a long asymptomatic interval between detection and the appearance of symptoms. Symptomatic manifestations and complications of primary aortic valve disease are, for the most part, identical to those of aortic stenosis with the same prognostic significance. When severe, the patient may develop an autonomic imbalance with paroxysms of tachycardia and diaphoresis. Acute severe aortic regurgitation due to traumatic, spontaneous, or infective leaflet disruption is poorly tolerated and may supervene at any time in the course, or it may be an initial manifestation. In patients with regurgitation secondary to aortic root disease, the prognosis is generally that of the primary process, though occasionally the regurgitation may predominate.

Differential Diagnosis

The differential includes distinguishing between primary aortic valve disease and diseases of the aortic root. Diastolic murmurs that radiate prominently along the right sternal edge are a clue to root disease, although frequently the murmur radiates prominently along the lower left sternal edge regardless of etiology. With an associated long systolic "flow" murmur, this "to and fro" murmur needs to be distinguished from causes of a continuous murmur, such as coronary arteriovenous (A-V) fistula or ruptured sinus of Valsalva aneurysm, and from a ventricular septal defect with associated aortic regurgitation. High-pressure pulmonary regurgitation may minic aortic regurgitation, but the other typical findings of aortic regurgitation are absent.

Laboratory Evaluation

The ECG shows normal sinus rhythm until late in the disease course, at which time atrial fibrillation may supervene. Premature ventricular contractions are common and left ventricular hypertrophy with strain is prominent (Fig. 16). With acute regurgitation, the ECG is typically normal.

The chest x-ray shows left ventricular enlargement with displacement of the apex inferolaterally. With pure aortic regurgitation, calcification of the aortic valve is minimal. Dilatation of the aortic root, arch, and descending aorta is present (Fig. 17). Signs of pulmonary venous congestion are minimal until late in the disease course. With acute aortic regurgitation, the heart size may be normal or only minimally increased with marked pulmonary venous congestion.

Echocardiography accurately characterizes the aortic root dimension and morphology and mobility of the aortic valve. It can also detect subclinical rheumatic mitral valve involvement and thereby identify a rheumatic etiology for the aortic regurgitation. Echocardiography can also detect aortic vegetations and, with severe acute regurgitation, presystolic closure of the mitral valve, an ominous prognostic sign (Fig. 18). High-frequency diastolic flutter of the mitral valve (sensitivity approximately 85 per cent) and ventricular septum also identify aortic regurgitation (Fig. 19).

Doppler ultrasound shows promise as a sensitive technique for detecting high-frequency diastolic turbulence in the left ventricular outflow tract. Radionuclide imaging is not particularly helpful in diagnosis, but does show promise in evaluating left ventricular function and in therapeutic decision making. Cardiac catheterization with aortic root angiography confirms the diagnosis, provides a gross estimation of severity, defines the status of left ventricular function, and detects concomitant lesions.

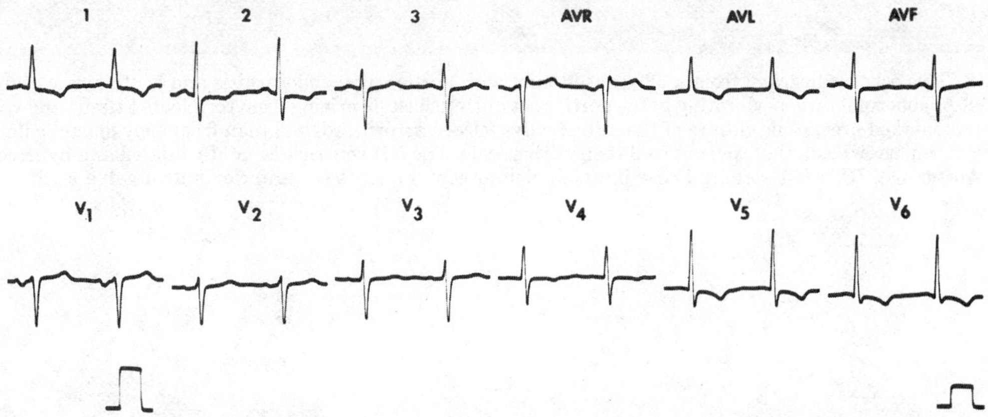

Figure 16. This electrocardiogram, from a 42-year-old man with severe aortic regurgitation, shows ST-T wave changes in leads I, II, AVL and V_5–V_6, left atrial enlargement (note the diphasic P wave with a prominent negative component in V_1), and increased voltage (note that leads V_2–V_6 are half standard). These changes are typical of left ventricular hypertrophy with "strain."

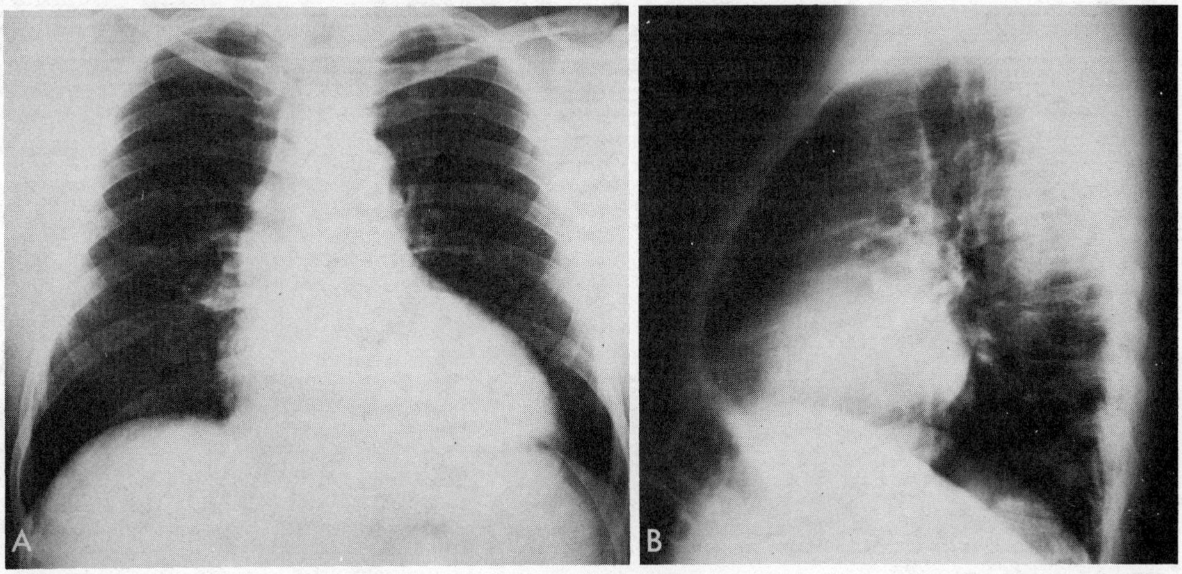

Figure 17. These x-rays are from a 39-year-old man with severe aortic regurgitation. The posteroanterior view (*A*) shows cardiomegaly with a left ventricular contour and dilatation of the aortic root, arch, and descending aorta. The lateral view (*B*) confirms left ventricular enlargement. Pulmonary vasculature is normal.

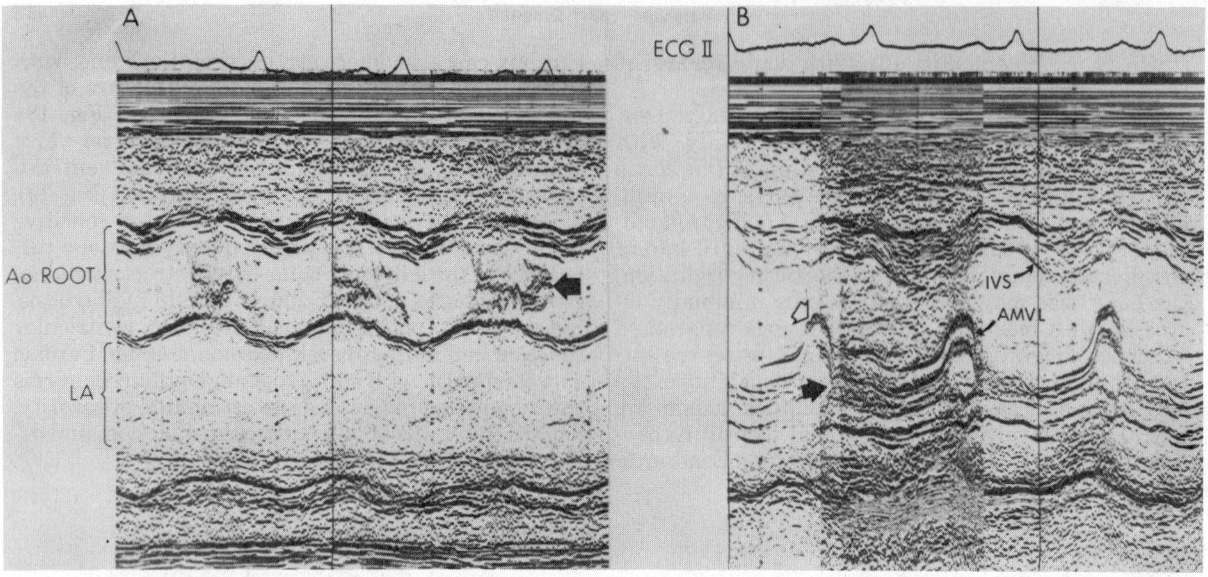

Figure 18. This echocardiogram, from a 38-year-old man with aortic valve endocarditis and acute aortic regurgitation, shows (Panel A) abnormal targets vibrating in the aortic root during diastole arising from torn leaflet tissue and vegetations. Panel B shows marked presystolic closure of the mitral valve (closed arrowhead) and high-frequency diastolic flutter of the mitral valve (open arrowhead) that was not well seen at this scale. The left ventricle is mildly dilated and hypercontractile. Ao Root = Aortic root; LA = left atrium; IVS = interventricular septum; AMVL = anterior mitral valve leaflet.

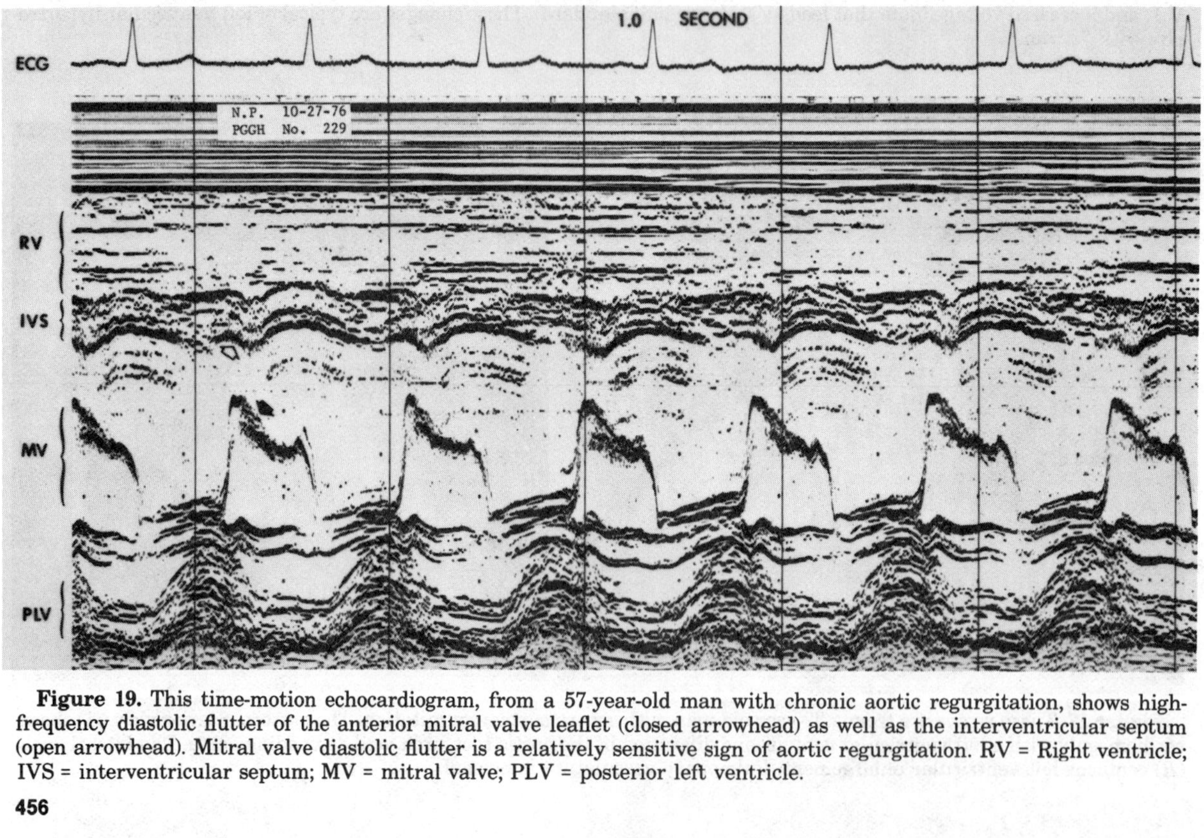

Figure 19. This time-motion echocardiogram, from a 57-year-old man with chronic aortic regurgitation, shows high-frequency diastolic flutter of the anterior mitral valve leaflet (closed arrowhead) as well as the interventricular septum (open arrowhead). Mitral valve diastolic flutter is a relatively sensitive sign of aortic regurgitation. RV = Right ventricle; IVS = interventricular septum; MV = mitral valve; PLV = posterior left ventricle.

Mitral Stenosis

Course/Complications

Mitral stenosis is most commonly rheumatic and is rarely congenital or due to leaflet infiltration with mucopolysaccharides. There is usually a long latent period between the initial attack of rheumatic fever and the subsequent appearance of symptoms. Dyspnea on exertion and palpitations are common early in the course. Hemodynamic stresses such as pregnancy are usually poorly tolerated, with peak symptoms occurring during the last part of the second trimester. Atrial fibrillation occurs in over 50 per cent of patients and accounts for further symptomatic deterioration. Pulmonary emboli occur and add to the degree of pulmonary hypertension. Systemic embolization occurs at any time and is more frequent when atrial fibrillation is present.

Differential Diagnosis

The differential diagnosis includes left atrial tumors (and classically left atrial myxoma), ball valve thrombi (most frequently in association with mitral stenosis) and a rare congenital lesion—cor triatriatum—in which stenosis proximal to the mitral valve occurs. Atrial septal defect may mimic mitral stenosis when there is atrial fibrillation, a diastolic tricuspid flow rumble, a right ventricular impulse, and wide splitting of the second heart sound (with the delayed pulmonary component being mistaken for an opening snap).

Laboratory Evaluation

The ECG shows left atrial enlargement in sinus rhythm, but "coarse" atrial fibrillation is frequent. With progression, increasing right ventricular hypertrophy occurs (Fig. 20).

The chest x-ray may show mitral valve calcification, and left atrial enlargement is invariable. With progression, pulmonary venous congestion, Kerley B lines, enlargement of the pulmonary artery and right ventricular hypertrophy occur (Fig. 21). The left ventricle and aorta are usually normal.

Echocardiography can accurately measure left atrial size and identify mitral valve thickening, a reduced diastolic slope (indicative of a reduced rate of ventricular diastolic filling), a small A wave, and a paradoxic posterior leaflet (Fig. 22). When all four of these valve changes are present, the predictive accuracy for rheumatic mitral valve disease is assured, although none of the findings accurately predicts severity. Two-dimensional echocardiography shows central "tethering," can accurately measure the mitral valve orifice (Fig. 23), and identifies enlargement of the pulmonary artery and the right side of the heart typical of more severe mitral stenosis.

Doppler ultrasound can accurately locate and quantitate the severity of the gradient (Fig 24). Cardiac catheterization with angiography documents the pressure gradient across the mitral valve, and, in concert with measurement of cardiac output, allows calculation of mitral valve orifice area (typically 1.5 cm^2 or less in surgical stenosis). Associated mitral regurgitation and other valvular lesions can be detected and the status of pulmonary vascular resistance measured.

Mitral Regurgitation

Course/Complications

Mitral regurgitation may result from primary valvular disease (rheumatic mitral valve disease, mitral valve prolapse, annular calcification, ruptured chordae, endocarditis) or, secondarily, from processes that interfere with normal coaptation (e.g., papillary muscle dysfunction secondary to left ventricular aneurysm). The prognosis is generally a function of severity and the underlying etiology. Rheumatic mitral regurgitation usually has at least some associated mitral stenosis that imposes an additional burden and earlier complications. Mitral valve prolapse with mild to moderate regurgitation generally remains stable unless ruptured chordae or endocarditis supervenes.

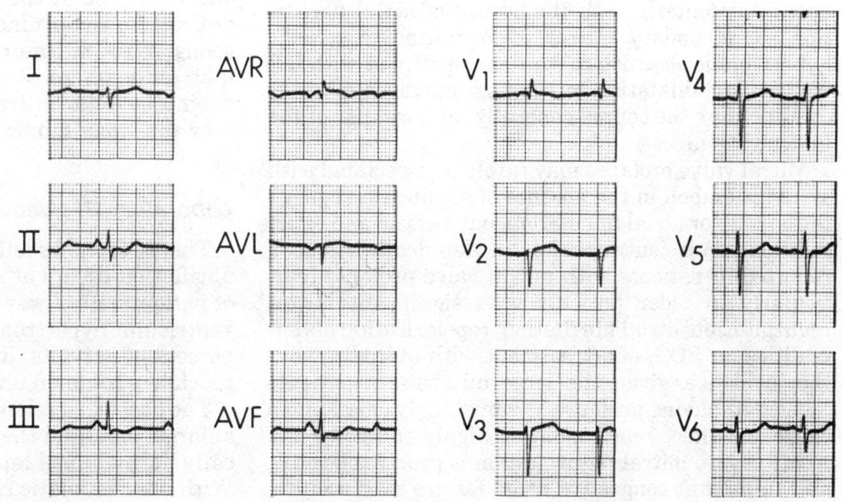

Figure 20. This electrocardiogram, from a 37-year-old woman with severe mitral stenosis who had remained in normal sinus rhythm, shows right axis deviation, a QR complex in lead V_1, and an R/S ratio less than 1 in lead V_6, all features of severe right ventricular hypertrophy.

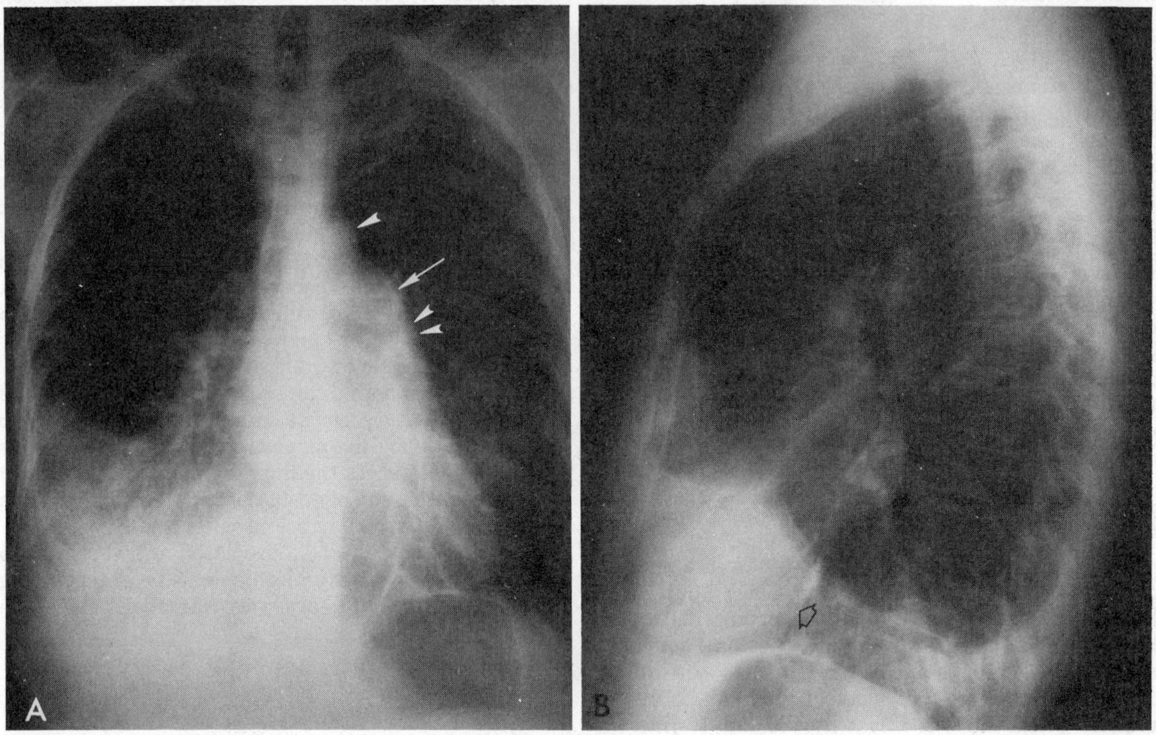

Figure 21. These x-rays reveal severe mitral stenosis in a 36-year-old woman. The posteroanterior view (*A*) shows a normal aortic knob (single arrowhead), with a dilated pulmonary artery (single arrow), and left atrial appendage (double arrowheads). There is also left atrial enlargement and a right pleural effusion. Kerley-B lines also are noted in the right lung above the effusion. The lateral view (*B*) confirms left atrial enlargement (closed arrowheads), a normal left ventricle (open arrowhead), and right ventricular enlargement.

Chronic isolated mitral regurgitation is well tolerated because the dilated left atrium acts as a low-pressure reservoir and the pulmonary venous pressure remains normal or minimally elevated until late in the disease course. With the advent of abnormal left ventricular function and/or atrial fibrillation, congestive symptoms with fatigue and palpitations occur. Atrial fibrillation is even more common than in mitral stenosis, and systemic emboli, though less common than in mitral stenosis, are frequent particularly with the advent of atrial fibrillation. In secondary mitral regurgitation (e.g., with hypertrophic obstructive cardiomyopathy or with left ventricular dilatation producing mitral apparatus dysfunction), the course generally mirrors that of the underlying process.

Mitral valve prolapse may rarely be associated with systemic emboli in the absence of significant regurgitation and/or atrial fibrillation, but a cause-and-effect relationship is controversial. Sudden death has been reported in patients with mitral valve prolapse (particularly in older patients with significant mitral regurgitation, atrial fibrillation, repolarization abnormalities on ECG, and treatment with quinidine) but the incidence, given the large numbers of patients labeled as having prolapse, is vanishingly small and a cause-and-effect relationship is highly controversial. Acute severe mitral regurgitation is poorly tolerated, and fulminant congestive heart failure may occur.

Differential Diagnosis

The differential diagnosis includes tricuspid regurgitation (particularly when the right ventricle is dilated and the murmur is prominent over the left precordium), ventricular septal defect, left atrial tumors, hypertrophic obstructive cardiomyopathy, and aortic sclerosis when the murmur radiates prominently to the apex. Aortic sclerotic murmurs at the apex are nonholosystolic, but with a soft first and second heart sound the length of the murmur may be difficult to determine. Careful attention to the response of the murmur to respiration, where it is maximal, and where it radiates usually provides the diagnosis. Acute mitral regurgitation produces a murmur that may mimic aortic or pulmonary stenosis.

Laboratory Evaluation

The ECG shows left atrial enlargement, and atrial fibrillation occurs at some point in up to 85 per cent of patients. ST-T wave changes are common, and left ventricular hypertrophy is seen in approximately fifty percent of patients. Right ventricular hypertrophy is much less common unless there is associated stenosis.

The chest x-ray shows left ventricular and left atrial enlargement, and the pulmonary vasculature is typically normal until late in the disease course (Fig. 25). With nonrheumatic mitral regurgitation, the leaflets

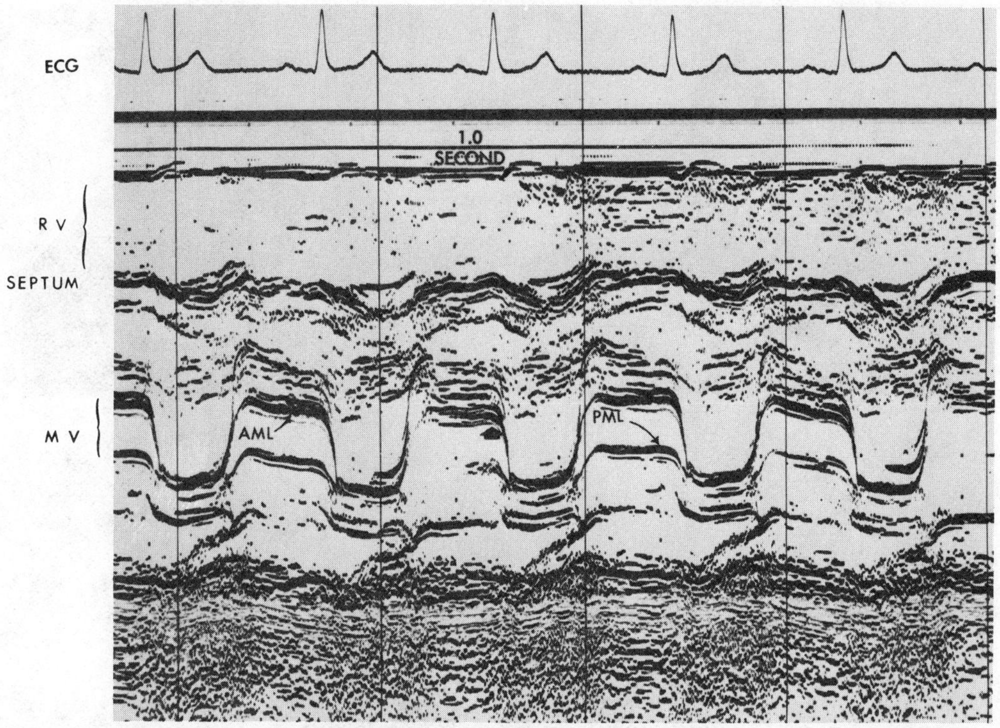

Figure 22. This time-motion echocardiogram, from a 41-year-old woman with rheumatic mitral stenosis, shows thickened anterior (AML) and posterior (PML) mitral leaflets, a reduced diastolic slope, a diminutive A wave, and paradoxic diastolic posterior leaflet movement. RV = Right ventricle; MV = mitral valve.

are typically not calcified, but calcification of the mitral valve annulus along with aneurysmal dilatation of the left atrium may be seen on the lateral plain film and/or fluoroscopy. With long-standing disease, the left atrial wall may be calcified as well.

Echocardiography can accurately define the etiology in rheumatic mitral regurgitation, and even with little or no associated stenosis the changes cited previously for mitral stenosis are seen. Mitral valve prolapse (Fig. 26), mitral valve vegetations with or without leaflet disruption (Fig. 27), and calcification of the mitral valve annulus are also etiologic findings. With severe mitral regurgitation, systolic expansion of a large left atrium occurs and the left ventricle is dilated and hyperdynamic.

Doppler ultrasound detects high-frequency turbulence in the left atrium with a gross relationship between the extent of turbulence and severity. Radionuclide angiography can detect left atrial enlargement and define left ventricular function but is not particularly helpful in diagnosis. Cardiac catheterization with left ventricular angiography confirms the diagnosis, provides an assessment of left ventricular function, assesses the pulmonary vascular resistance, and is able to identify associated abnormalities.

Pulmonary Stenosis

Course/Complications

When it is rheumatic, pulmonary stenosis is invariably associated with severe mitral, tricuspid, and usually aortic involvement, and the clinical course is overwhelmingly that of the associated valvular heart disease. It occurs frequently in malignant carcinoid but is rarely prognostically important. When it is congenital (the most common cause) and of mild to moderate severity, the stenosis is typically stable and normal longevity is common. When severe, right ventricular dilatation and failure cause tricuspid regurgitation and right heart failure that may be intractable, and survival beyond the sixth decade is uncommon. Angina and exertional syncope may occur, but sudden death is rare. Endocarditis occurs but is unusual. Not infrequently, there may be hypertrophy of the muscular right ventricular outflow tract and the course may be complicated by superimposed subvalvular stenosis.

Differential Diagnosis

The differential diagnosis includes an innocent murmur, any condition producing pulmonary flow murmurs such as atrial septal defect, muscular subvalvular pulmonic stenosis, and a high membranous intraventricular septal defect.

Laboratory Evaluation

When stenosis is mild, the ECG is usually normal. When moderate to severe, right ventricular hypertrophy is usual.

On chest x-ray, pulmonary vascularity is usually normal. When severe, pulmonary blood flow may be decreased with more blood flow to the left lung be-

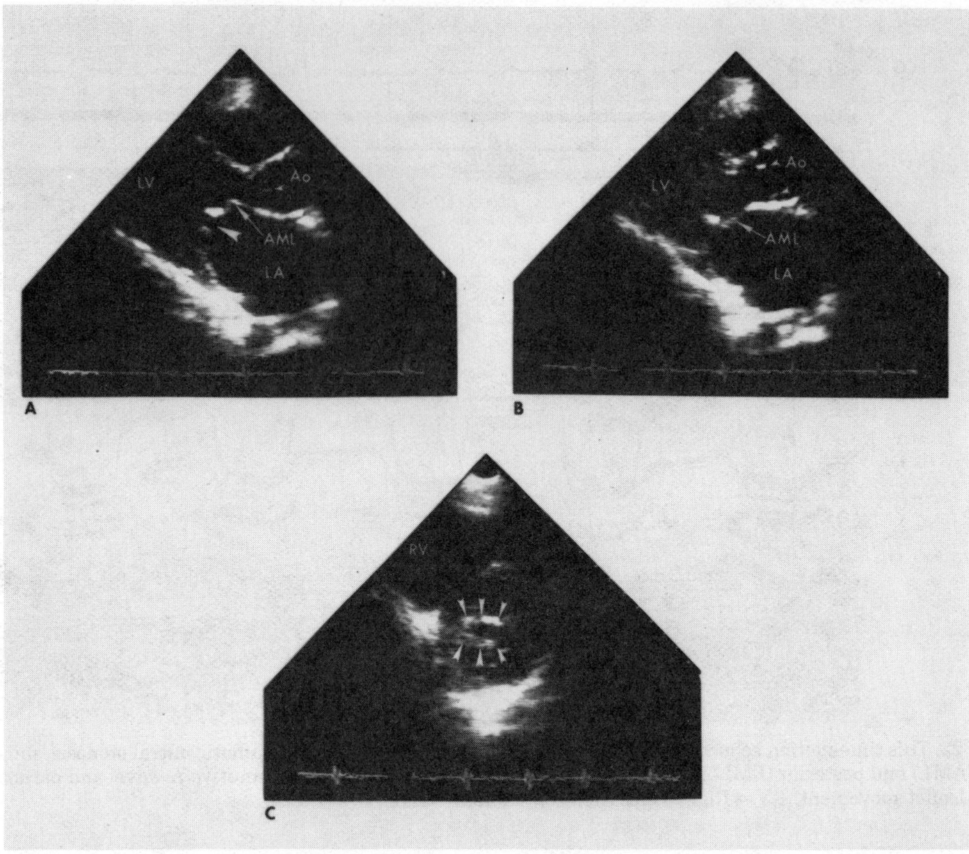

Figure 23. This two-dimensional echocardiogram is from a 43-year-old woman with rheumatic mitral stenosis. Panel A (longitudinal axis-diastolic frame) shows central tethering of the mitral leaflet tips with bowing of the anterior leaflet (AML) into the left ventricular outflow tract. The large white arrowhead denotes the mitral valve orifice, and the small white arrowhead denotes the closed aortic valve within the aortic root (Ao). The left atrium (LA) is moderately enlarged. Panel B (longitudinal axis-systolic frame) shows opening of the aortic valve (small arrowheads) and closure of the mitral valve—note the disappearance of the orifice and bowing of the anterior mitral leaflet (AML) toward the left atrium (LA). In Panel C (cross section-diastolic frame), the white arrowheads outline the thickened anterior and posterior leaflets. The central darker area is the mitral valve orifice, which can be accurately planimetered with a close correlation to that found at catheterization and/or surgery.

cause of preferential streaming. The pulmonary artery shows prominent poststenotic dilatation even with milder degrees of stenosis (Fig. 28); with moderate to severe lesions, right ventricular enlargement is present.

The echocardiogram shows hypertrophy of the free right ventricular wall and septum. The pulmonary valve may demonstrate a large A wave and, with inspiration, doming to the "open" position (Fig. 9).

Doppler ultrasound can localize the site of turbulence and shows promise in quantitating the severity as long as right ventricular function is well maintained. Radionuclide imaging may show abnormalities of right ventricular function but is not helpful in diagnosis. With cardiac catheterization, the site and severity of the stenosis can be identified. Angiography of the right ventricular outflow tract may show thickening of the leaflets with a domed configuration in systole and poststenotic dilatation of the pulmonary artery.

Pulmonary Regurgitation

Clinical Course/Complications

The course of pulmonary regurgitation may be subdivided according to whether it is due to pulmonary hypertension or due to primary valvular disease with normal pulmonary artery pressures. With high-pressure pulmonary regurgitation the clinical course mirrors that of the underlying cause, with right heart failure and concomitant tricuspid regurgitation, exertional syncope, and anginal chest pain common. Sudden death is rare. Low-pressure pulmonary regurgitation secondary to idiopathic dilatation of the pulmonary artery, congenital valvular regurgitation, and leaflet disruption secondary to surgery, trauma or, rarely, endocarditis is well tolerated as long as well-maintained right ventricular function and normal pulmonary vascular resistance prevail. Symptoms, when they appear, are those of right heart failure.

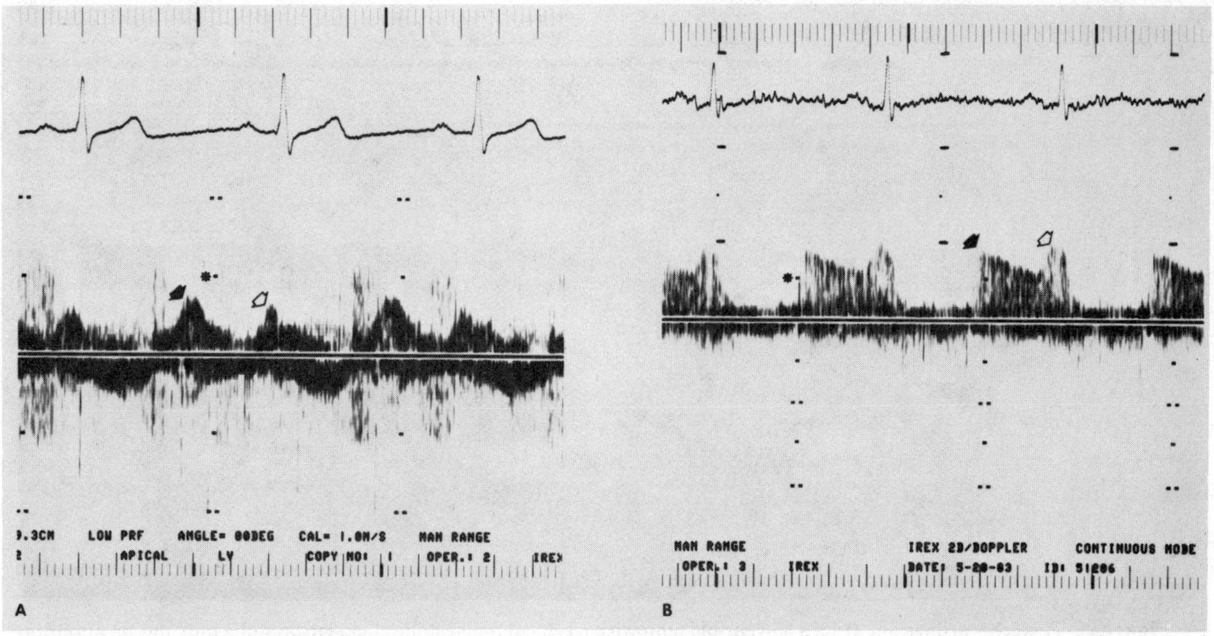

Figure 24. These Doppler tracings are from a normal patient (Panel A) and a patient with moderately severe mitral stenosis (Panel B). Note that both panels show increased turbulence in early diastole following opening of the mitral valve (closed arrowheads) and presystolic turbulence corresponding to atrial systole (open arrowheads). The asterisk on each panel denotes a calibration signal of 1 meter per second. The normal patient (Panel A) shows no significant turbulence during the entire diastole cycle. The mitral stenosis patient (Panel B), however, shows abnormal diastolic turbulence approaching 2 meters per second in early diastole and exceeding this in presystole. Note also that the turbulence fails to diminish rapidly in mid-diastole, another correlate of mitral stenosis wherein a continuing pressure gradient from left atrium to left ventricle causes turbulent blood flow throughout diastole.

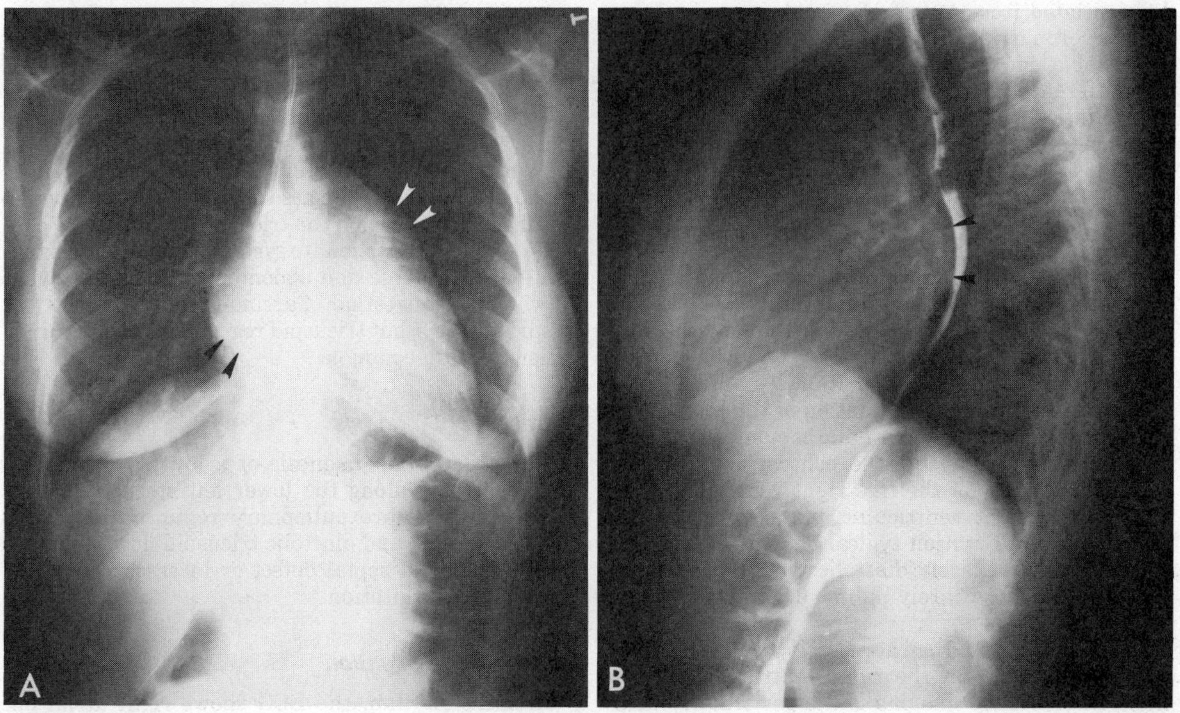

Figure 25. These chest x-rays are from a 21-year-old woman with isolated mitral regurgitation. The posteroanterior view (*A*) shows marked enlargement of the left atrial appendage (white arrowheads) and normal pulmonary vasculature. The lateral view (*B*) shows the enlarged left atrium indenting the barium filled esophagus (black arrowheads). Note the absence of right ventricular enlargement.

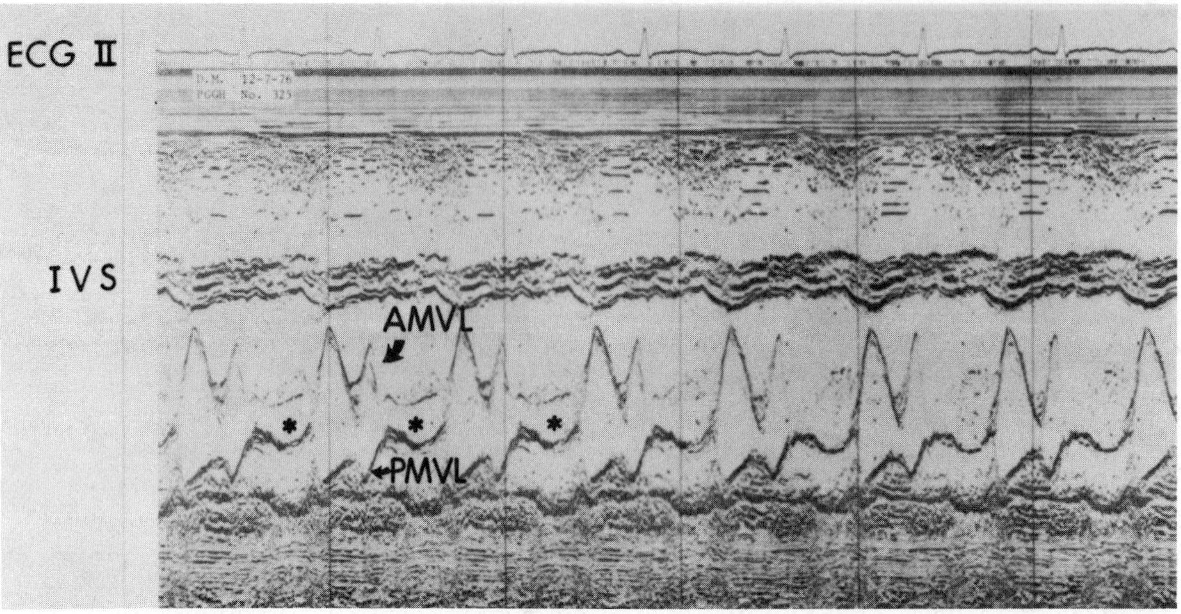

Figure 26. This echocardiogram, from a 35-year-old man with a typical midsystolic click–late systolic murmur on auscultation, shows midsystolic posterior bowing of the leaflets (asterisks) typical of mitral valve prolapse. IVS = Interventricular septum; AMVL = anterior mitral valve leaflet; PMVL = posterior mitral valve leaflet.

Differential Diagnosis

The differential diagnosis of high-pressure pulmonary regurgitation is principally that of aortic regurgitation. If a concomitant systolic pulmonary murmur is prominent, this "to and fro" murmur must be differentiated from causes of a continuous murmur such as coronary arteriovenous fistula, ruptured sinus of Valsalva aneurysm, and patent ductus arteriosus. The differential diagnosis of low-pressure pulmonary regurgitation includes tricuspid stenosis, right atrial myxoma, and atrial septal defect.

Laboratory Evaluation

With high-pressure pulmonary regurgitation, the ECG shows right ventricular hypertrophy and frequently mirrors the underlying condition as, for example, in mitral stenosis. With low-pressure pulmonary regurgitation, the ECG may be normal and frequently shows an r' or R' in V_1.

The chest x-ray shows dilatation of the pulmonary artery and right ventricular enlargement. Depending on severity and etiology, the echocardiogram may show hypertrophy of the free right ventricular wall and septum, right ventricular dilatation and paradoxic septal wall motion typical of right ventricular volume overload. Rarely, diastolic tricuspid valve flutter and even more rarely pulmonary valve diastolic flutter may be seen.

Doppler ultrasound can accurately localize the diastolic turbulent jet in the right ventricular outflow tract. Radionuclide imaging is not particularly helpful in diagnosis. Cardiac catheterization provides supportive evidence when there is equilibration of the pulmonary and right ventricular pressures during middle to late diastole. Angiography shows the dilated right heart and pulmonary artery. A pulmonary angiogram may provide supportive evidence if there is more pulmonary regurgitation than can be accounted for by the catheter being across the pulmonary valve.

Tricuspid Stenosis

Clinical Course/Complications

With rare exceptions, tricuspid stenosis is rheumatic and occurs with associated rheumatic mitral and aortic disease. The clinical course is usually overshadowed by that of the associated left-sided valvular lesions but on occasion the tricuspid stenosis may contribute to disproportionate systemic venous hypertension with anasarca and abdominal discomfort owing to visceral congestion. Carcinoid may produce tricuspid stenosis, but tricuspid regurgitation or a mixed lesion is more common.

Differential Diagnosis

The differential diagnosis of a low-frequency diastolic murmur along the lower left sternal edge includes low-pressure pulmonary regurgitation, right atrial myxoma, and diastolic tricuspid flow murmurs due to an atrial septal defect or in association with tricuspid regurgitation.

Laboratory Evaluation

In sinus rhythm, the ECG shows right atrial enlargement and, with associated mitral valve disease, left atrial enlargement as well. Atrial fibrillation is common. Most frequently, the ECG reflects the associated mitral valve and/or aortic valve disease.

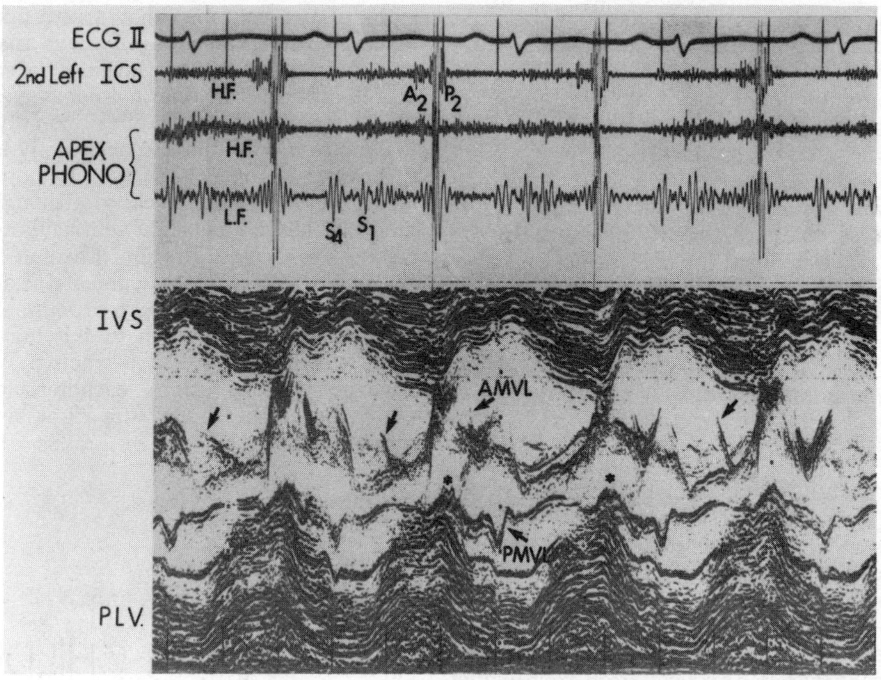

Figure 27. This simultaneous echophonocardiogram, from 47-year-old man with bacterial endocarditis of the mitral valve and acute mitral regurgitation, shows wide splitting of the second heart sound (A_2, P_2) with a markedly accentuated pulmonic component (P_2) and a loud apical fourth heart sound (S_4). The echo shows variable targets (arrowheads) in systole, coarse diastolic vibration of the anterior mitral valve leaflet (AMVL), and an abnormal posterior mitral valve leaflet (PMVL) within the mitral valve orifice (asterisk) in diastole. These are all typical features of mitral valve endocarditis with torn chordae and/or flail leaflet.

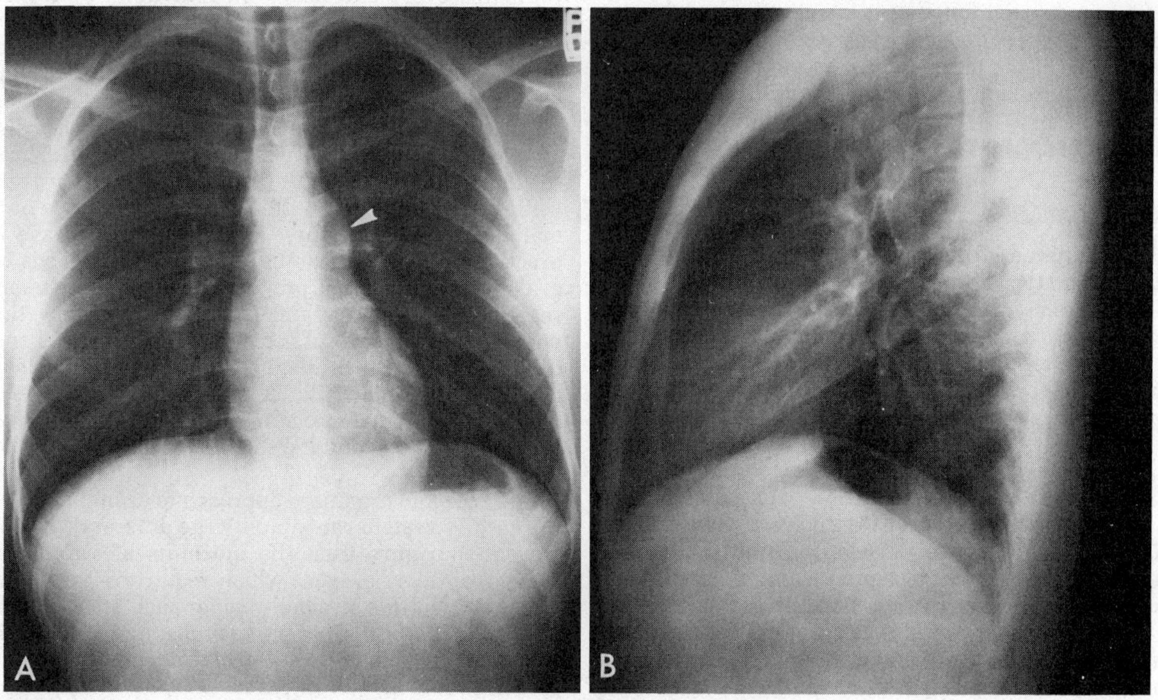

Figure 28. These chest x-rays are from a 16-year-old man with moderate pulmonary valve stenosis. The posteroanterior view (*A*) shows a prominent pulmonary artery (white arrowhead) due to post-stenotic dilatation. The remainder of the cardiovascular silhouette and pulmonary vasculature is normal. On the lateral view (*B*), there is little or no right ventricular hypertrophy.

When tricuspid stenosis is severe and isolated, the chest x-ray shows marked enlargement of the right atrium with normal pulmonary vasculature and little or no enlargement of the right ventricle.

Echocardiography defines right atrial size and abnormal tricuspid valve motion analogous to that seen with rheumatic mitral stenosis.

Doppler ultrasound can accurately localize and predict the site and gradient. Radionuclide angiography has little role. Cardiac catheterization defines the site and severity of the stenosis, the presence of any associated tricuspid regurgitation and the extent and severity of involvement of the mitral and aortic valves.

Tricuspid Regurgitation

Clinical Course/Complications

Tricuspid regurgitation is frequently present in patients with significant heart disease, but it is infrequently recognized. It may be due to primary valve disease from prior surgery, infection, trauma, prolapse, rheumatic scarring, or malignant carcinoid. It occurs with pacing catheters across the tricuspid valve, and removal of an old wire may occasionally cause significant tricuspid regurgitation from leaflet avulsion. Syncope is uncommon and suggests right atrial tumor, particularly if positional. The most common cause of tricuspid regurgitation, however, is secondary to right heart failure with right ventricular dilatation and tricuspid valve apparatus dysfunction. The clinical course mirrors that of the underlying cause, and when tricuspid regurgitation occurs with normal pulmonary pressures and well-maintained right ventricular function, it is well tolerated for long periods. With pulmonary hypertension, the symptoms are those of the primary process in addition to right heart failure and fatigue. Atrial fibrillation is common and, with right heart failure, pulmonary emboli may occur.

Differential Diagnosis

The differential diagnosis includes mitral regurgitation with atypical radiation of the murmur, ventricular septal defect, subvalvular right ventricular outflow tract obstruction, and right atrial myxoma. Careful attention to the neck veins and to the character and behavior of the murmur with respiration usually confirms the diagnosis.

Laboratory Evaluation

In sinus rhythm, the ECG shows right atrial enlargement. When secondary to right ventricular dilatation, the electrocardigraphic features are those of the primary process. Atrial fibrillation is common.

The chest x-ray with isolated tricuspid regurgitation shows right atrial and right ventricular enlargement. When secondary to right ventricular dilatation, the chest x-ray reflects the underlying primary process.

Echocardiography documents right atrial and right ventricular dilatation and may show paradoxic septal wall motion. The rapid injection of saline into a peripheral arm vein may show free reflux of microcavitations into an inferior vena cava that, in addition, may be dilated and pulsatile. The echocardiogram also identifies a rheumatic etiology, vegetations, right atrial myxoma, and Ebstein's anomaly.

Doppler ultrasound can accurately localize systolic turbulence in the right atrium. Radionuclide imaging is not helpful diagnostically, although it can document right atrial and right ventricular dilatation typical of severe regurgitation. Cardiac catheterization shows elevations in the right atrial and ventricular end diastolic pressure and a prominent systolic wave in the right atrium such that it may resemble the right ventricular pressure tracing. With secondary tricuspid regurgitation, catheterization identifies the cause of the underlying right ventricular dilatation.

NORMAL HEART MURMURS IN CHILDREN

By Richard T. Smith, M.D.
and Arno R. Hohn, M.D.
Charleston, South Carolina

The discovery of a heart murmur in an otherwise healthy child is a frequent dilemma confronting the primary health care provider. Certain investigators have estimated that as many as 80 per cent of children have a heart murmur at some point in their life. This contrasts with the incidence of congenital heart disease, which is around 8 cases per 1000 children. Thus, the importance of murmur triage is obvious. However, while much has been written and said about the normal heart murmur, these discussions may leave a practicing physician confused about the methods of evaluation and lack of practical guidelines for referral. Specific diagnosis and terminology used by the physician are important because of the emotional and behavioral impact the diagnosis of heart murmur has on the family and child. A sense of security in the diagnosis of normal murmur on the part of the physician is very important and should be communicated to the family.

The use of an organized approach to examination of the cardiac system can simplify the differentiation of normal murmurs from the murmurs of significant structural heart disease, which require referral and treatment. In this section, we offer such an approach to enable the primary care provider to arrive confidently at the diagnosis of normal murmur. This approach should also allow the identification of patients having structural heart disease who require referral to a cardiac center for further evaluation, treatment and/or subacute bacterial endocarditis (SBE) prophylaxis.

TERMINOLOGY

An extremely wide variety of descriptive terms has been applied to heart murmurs. In one classic chapter on "innocent" murmurs, 74 synonyms for the normal murmur were listed. Many of the terms persist in the literature and in the minds of physicians today. A frequently misused term is "functional" when it is applied to the normal heart murmur not suspected to be the result of pathology. However, the term *functional murmur* actually refers to the heart murmur of anemia, fever, or other high-output states. The term *innocent murmur* also is frequently used but implies inherent abnormality to the anxious parent. The American Heart Association now advocates the description *normal murmur* to apply to the murmurs so frequently noted in childhood that are not associated with structural abnormalities. This characterization has the obvious benefit of describing in no uncertain terms the realities of this finding.

MURMUR EVALUATION

Once the murmur is discovered and the child's history again examined for suggestions of cardiac pathology, a thorough examination of the cardiovascular system should follow (Fig. 1). It must be kept in mind that there are many similarities between normal systolic murmurs and those produced by a wide variety of heart defects; therefore, *all murmurs should be evaluated in light of the company they keep.*

The cardiac examination begins with observation. The heart, which has neither volume overload, as would be the case for many shunt lesions, nor pressure overload, as would be the case for stenotic lesions, should be reflected in a quiet precordium to the eye and to the touch. The presence of a thrill, marked heaves or lifts, and/or hyperdynamic precordial activity should suggest pathology. The initial observation should also include a careful search for cyanosis and clubbing. Observation and palpation are followed by auscultation. Each auscultatory area should be examined in sequence (Fig. 2). The back and axilla should also be examined. Important aspects of the murmur to consider are its position in the cardiac cycle, its intensity, point of maximal intensity, and its quality.

The first and second heart sounds are then considered. In pediatrics, the second heart sound is of great diagnostic importance and should be carefully evaluated in the second left intercostal space (the pulmonic area). Its two components (aortic closure, the first component, and pulmonic closure, the second component) should be identified, and their intensities should be equal. Respiratory variation should also occur with a widening of the separation between the two components during inspiration. Normality of the second heart sound with splitting of its components is important evidence against physiologically significant heart disease. Finally, all cardiac examinations should include evaluation of pulses in the upper and lower extremities, ruling out any discrepancy in intensity and/or timing of the pulses, as well as determination of blood pressure in the four extremities.

At this point in the evaluation, if any concern remains that the heart murmur reflects congenital or acquired heart disease, it is then appropriate to obtain a chest x-ray and an electrocardiogram. Abnormali-

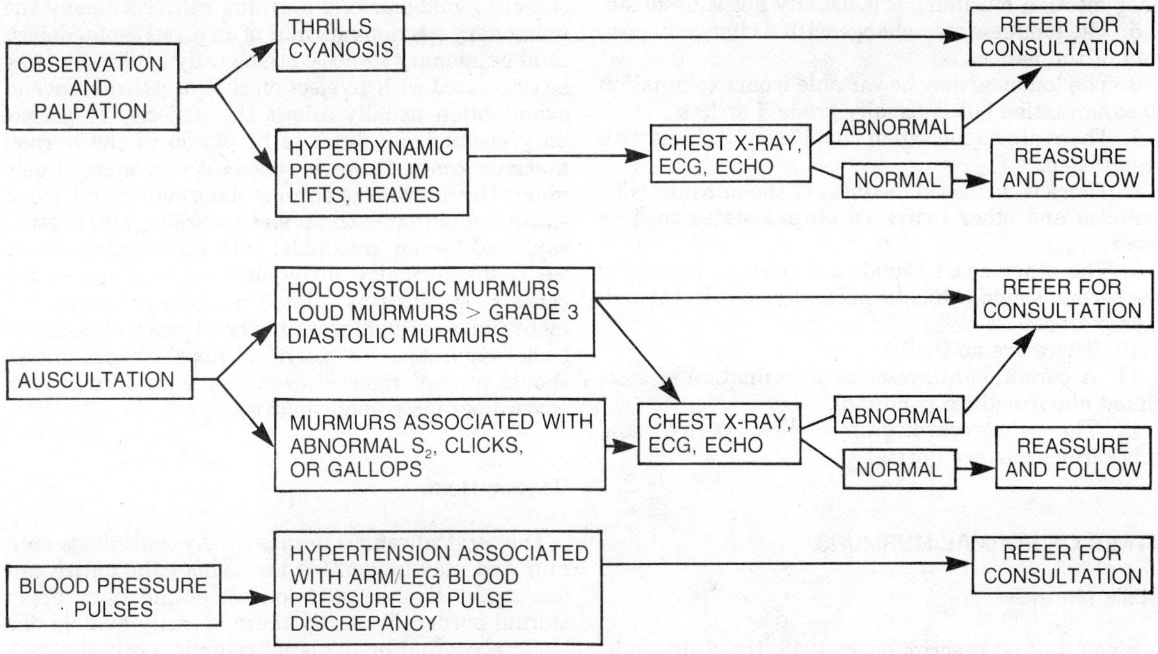

Figure 1. Clinical evaluation of a child with a heart murmur. This idealized flow chart is an outline for management of the heart murmur based on the physical examination. This chart does not cover all situations, and management should, of course, be individualized according to the overall situation. *Hypertension* refers to systolic or diastolic blood pressure outside the 95th percentile, as defined by the Task Force on Blood Pressure Control in Children (Pediatrics, 59 [Suppl]: 797, 1977).

ties suggested by either of these two studies should prompt referral. It should be remembered, however, that apparent normality by examination, x-ray, and electrocardiogram does not rule out a heart defect. During the last few years development, refinement, and proliferation of the two-dimensional (2-D) echocardiogram has led to its currently revered status as a noninvasive tool in the evaluation of the cardiovascular system. More recently, this tool has begun to become available to the practicing physician and may aid in the detection of minor abnormalities such as bicuspid aortic valve or mitral valve prolapse. When indicated and available, the 2-D echocardiogram can be used in addition to the electrocardiogram and chest x-ray to offer even more definitive evidence for normality in the equivocal situation.

CHARACTERISTICS OF A NORMAL HEART MURMUR

The most common types of normal murmurs and their associations have a number of readily identified characteristics that in most cases allow them to be recognized by auscultation (and physical examination) alone. These characteristics are as follows:

1. They are systolic in timing.
2. The duration is usually short and early in systole (generally not beyond the first two thirds of systole), allowing a murmur-free systolic period to be identified prior to the second heart sound.
3. They are loudest usually along the left sternal border, in either the second or third left intercostal space *or* in the fourth or fifth intercostal space medial to the apex.
4. Although transmission does occur (as in pulmonary ejection murmur), it is usually not widespread.
5. The loudness may change with a change in position of the patient.
6. The loudness may be variable from examination to examination but is usually grade 3 or less.
7. There are no consistent changes in loudness with respiration.
8. There is increased loudness of the murmur with exercise and other increased output states such as fever.
9. The other heart sounds are normal, especially the second sound, which is normally split in the pulmonic area.
10. There are no thrills.
11. A careful cardiovascular examination of associated abnormalities is normal.
12. The electrocardiogram, chest x-ray, and echocardiogram are normal.

TYPES OF NORMAL MURMURS

Still's Murmur

Since its first description in 1918, the Still's murmur has been described by a vast number of terms, including "twanging string," honking, groaning, and many others. The adjectives now used most frequently to describe this murmur are vibratory or musical. Located at the fourth or fifth left intercostal space (Fig. 3), it occurs in early to mid-systole, allowing a murmur-free interval to be noted before the second sound; is louder in the supine position; and does not radiate. It is a low-pitched murmur with a frequency measured by phonocardiography of 70 to 160 cycles per second (Table 1). The origin of the Still's murmur remains unknown.

Careful evaluation of the timing and quality will allow the Still's murmur to be distinguished from the holosystolic murmurs of a ventricular septal defect (long or pansystolic and harsh) and mitral insufficiency (late or pansystolic and blowing). Location, quality, and absence of a click will allow its differentiation from the murmurs of bicuspid valves and aortic and pulmonary stenosis. When the rest of the previously listed characteristics of the normal murmur are noted, the diagnosis of Still's *normal* murmur may be made with confidence.

Pulmonary Ejection Murmur

The pulmonic ejection murmur has been demonstrated to be produced by normal turbulent flow at the pulmonary valve. The murmur is somewhat harsher and higher in pitch (90 to 130 cycles per second) than the Still's murmur. Also similar to the Still's murmur, it is louder in the supine position. Unlike the Still's murmur, the specific characteristics of the pulmonary ejection murmur do not usually aid in the differentiation from pulmonary ejection murmurs produced by congenital heart disease. This fact again emphasizes the importance of judging this murmur by the company it keeps, i.e., the findings which accompany it. For example, a wide fixed splitting of S_2 and often a rumbling mid-diastolic murmur will accompany the pulmonary ejection murmur of an atrial septal defect. Mild pulmonary stenosis is generally louder and may be associated with an ejection click or a thrill. Careful examination usually allows the majority of pulmonary ejection murmurs to be placed in the normal murmur group. However, a subset may more closely mimic the murmur of cardiac abnormality and necessitate evaluation with an electrocardiogram, chest x-ray, and, when available, 2-D echocardiogram to verify the normalcy of the murmur. Findings on the chest x-ray, such as dilated pulmonary artery segment, mild cardiomegaly in the absence of straight-back syndrome, or more obvious abnormalities, should prompt referral even in the absence of electrocardiographic abnormalities.

Venous Hum

The cervical venous hum is a truly continuous murmur and may be audible throughout the entire cardiac cycle. It is usually loudest at the right upper sternal border. Typically there is easily audible diastolic accentuation. This murmur is easily differentiated from the pathologic continuous murmurs, such as those of the patent ductus arteriosus (PDA) or arteriovenous (A-V) fistula by its diminution or disappearance in the supine position or with light stetho-

Table 1. Characteristics of Normal Childhood Murmurs

	Still's	Pulmonic Ejection	Venous Hum	Supraclavicular Bruit	Cardiorespiratory
Timing	Early to mid systolic	Early to mid systolic	*Continuous* with diastolic accentuation	Systolic	Late systolic
Duration	Short	Short	Continuous	Short	Last half of systole
Location	4th or 5th left intercostal space	2nd or 3rd left intercostal space	Infraclavicular usually on right	Supraclavicular fossa, usually on right	Border of heart and lung
Transmission	Usually none	Occasionally to lung fields	Upper chest and lower neck	To the carotids	None
Loudness	Grade 3 or less	Grade 3 or less	Grade 3 or less	Variable	Variable
Effect of Respiration	None	None	No change	None	Disappears with expiration
Effect of Exercise	May increase	Increases	May increase	May increase	Variable
Effect of Posture	Louder when supine	Louder when supine	Disappears when supine, changes with head rotation	None	Variable
Phonocardiogram	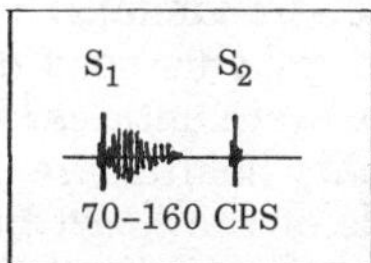 S_1 S_2 70–160 CPS	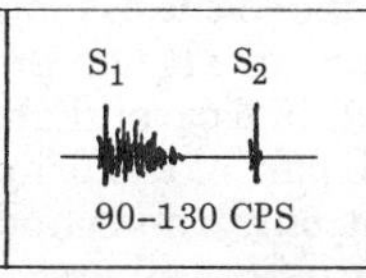 S_1 S_2 90–130 CPS	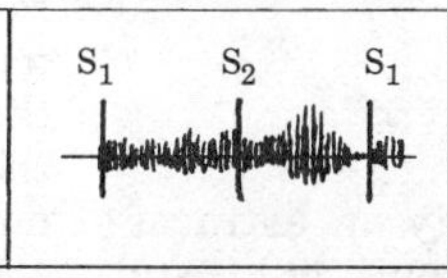 S_1 S_2 S_1	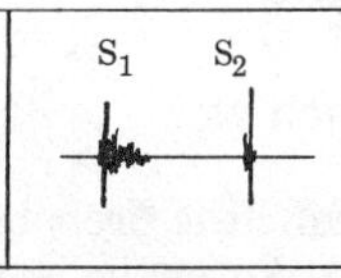 S_1 S_2	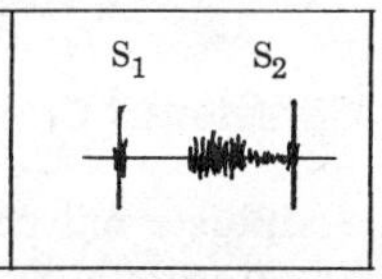 S_1 S_2

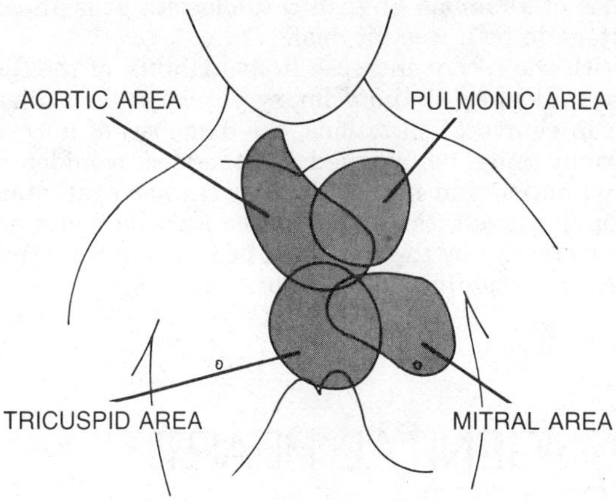

Figure 2. Normal auscultatory areas.

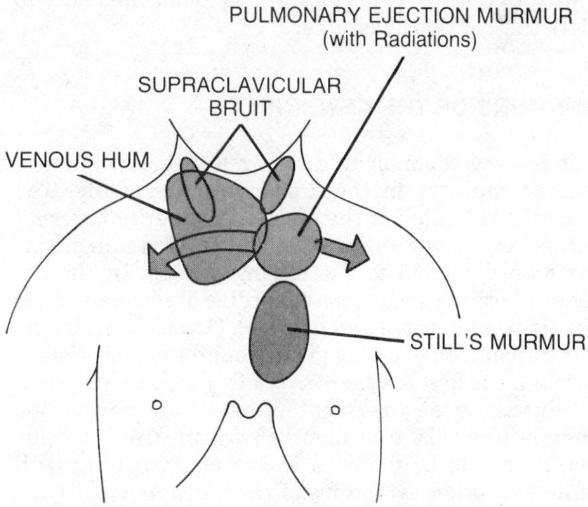

Figure 3. Locations of common murmurs in childhood.

scope pressure over the jugular vein of origin. Changing of the position of the head also frequently affects the intensity of this murmur. The venous hum is very common, with frequency estimates ranging from 30 to 80 per cent in preschool and school-aged children. The simple maneuvers just mentioned will readily differentiate this common murmur from other continuous murmurs and eliminate the need for referral.

OTHER NORMAL MURMURS AND SOUNDS

The Supraclavicular Arterial Bruit

This murmur is generally heard over the clavicles, most frequently on the right side. Accentuation with exercise may occur, but the murmur is not usually affected by posture. When this murmur is suspected, the examiner may occlude the subclavian artery by compression of the first rib, causing the murmur to disappear.

The Cardiorespiratory Murmur

This unusual normal murmur is thought to be of extracardiac origin, produced by the impact of the heart on the lung. This fact is reflected in its location at the heart-lung margin. Its timing and loudness are usually quite variable and are affected by respiration. Logically, expiration usually causes the murmur to disappear.

Characteristics of the normal murmurs described under the previous five subheadings are summarized in Table 1.

The Cephalic Bruit

The cephalic bruit is very commonly noted during childhood. It is usually heard over the occipital or parietal regions of the skull. The murmur may be either systolic or continuous and is usually quite soft. In the absence of other abnormalities, this murmur is without clinical significance in childhood. When noted after the teen-age years, the presence of intracranial pathology must be considered.

The Xiphisternal Crunch

The xiphisternal crunch is probably an extracardiac sound usually heard over the seventh left costal cartilage where the xiphoid and sternum articulate. This sound is not a murmur and is mentioned only to alert the cautious examiner.

MURMURS OF THE NEWBORN

It is very common to discover a soft, low-pitched, systolic murmur in the first few hours of life. The murmur is located at the middle to upper left sternal border and may radiate to the lungs. This murmur is commonly related to the closing ductus. In the absence of other suggestions of cardiac abnormalities, it should be only noted and followed. Occasionally a similar murmur may be noted and found to be persistent through the first few months of life, reaching its greatest intensity at the point of maximal physiologic anemia (6 weeks to 3 months). Again, this murmur needs only to be followed in the absence of growth failure or other symptoms of cardiac abnormality.

MANAGEMENT OF THE NORMAL MURMUR

The optimal management of normal murmurs is readily divided into broad age-group categories. For example, murmurs discovered early in life which fulfill the clinical criteria of the normal murmur require only confident reassurance and routine reevaluation during the health maintenance visits. Those murmurs that persist into school age or are discovered for the first time at that point, especially when associated with parental anxiety, should be evaluated by electrocardiogram, chest x-ray, and an echocardiogram (if indicated and available). If these tests are normal, confident reassurance is again the appropriate course of action. If the murmur continues to be noted into the teen-age years and is again surrounded by anxiety and/or the desire to participate in team sports, a pediatric cardiac consultation may be expedient. Of course, anxiety on the part of either the family or the physician may dictate referral at any time.

Once the child has been labeled as normal, he or she should, of course, be treated accordingly and allowed full activity without limitation. This point of view is supported by a large number of studies that have concentrated on children carrying the diagnosis of normal murmur. These studies evaluated children for any evidence of associated increase in morbidity and mortality; however, none was found. Insurance carriers seem now to be uniform in their acceptance of these statistics, and insurability is unchanged by the presence of a normal murmur.

CONCLUSION

Although traditionally much confusion has surrounded the diagnosis and management of heart murmurs in all age groups, this need not be so. We feel that in a careful and systematic cardiac evaluation on the part of the primary health care provider, in which not only the sounds of the heart but its physiologic status as well are considered, the differentiation of the normal murmur from one requiring referral is readily possible and simple. When a question of a murmur's presence is raised, it may be helpful to consider the advice of a famous English cardiologist: "It is an advantage to be a wee bit deaf."

With the recent increase in availability of the 2-D echocardiogram to the primary physician for utilization in equivocal situations, the diagnosis of normal murmur may be reached with added confidence. Those patients in need of further cardiac evaluation through consultation can then be identified and appropriate care by the combined health care team provided in virtually all situations.

CONGENITAL HEART DISEASE

By Thomas A. Vargo, M.D.
Houston, Texas

In the first year of life, congenital malformations are the second leading cause of death, with congenital heart disease (CHD) accounting for one third of these deaths. For the practitioner to have an impact on

CHD, he or she must be able to diagnose heart disease in the neonate. For many physicians, it is difficult to do this. The two main reasons are (1) the unfamiliar manifestations of heart disease in an infant and (2) the problems in performing a physical examination on an infant's cardiovascular system. This article emphasizes the manifestations of heart disease in infants and will attempt to show that while it may be difficult to diagnose individual heart defects, it is relatively easy to diagnose abnormalities in cardiovascular function in infants and children.

CONGENITAL HEART DISEASE IN THE NEWBORN

Cyanosis

The differential diagnosis of cyanosis in an infant can be a dilemma for the practitioner. Cyanosis in the newborn is usually due to cardiac disease, pulmonary disease, or brain dysfunction. In general, these three can be differentiated by the breathing pattern. Infants with cyanosis due to cardiac disease can have either normal respirations or rapid, shallow respirations (tachypnea). Those with cyanosis from pulmonary disease have deep, grunting respirations (hyperpnea). Infants whose cyanosis is due to brain dysfunction have depressed respirations (hypoventilation or apnea).

Newborns with cyanosis due to cerebral depression of respiration have retention of carbon dioxide, hypoxemia, and lethargy; these infants show immediate improvement in the cyanosis when they are stimulated to breathe. When this is performed, the elevated carbon dioxide and depressed oxygen levels both rapidly return to normal.

The main cardiac defects that cause life-threatening cyanosis in the newborn are:

1. Transposition of the great arteries.
2. Forms of pulmonary atresia in which the only blood supply to the lungs is via a ductus arteriosus (ductus-dependent lesions).
3. The obstructed form of total anomalous pulmonary venous return.

Clinically, it can be difficult to distinguish infants who have cyanosis due to heart disease from those who have lung disease. Table 1 lists clinical and laboratory findings that favor heart disease or lung disease in newborns.

Table 1. Differential Diagnosis of Neonatal Heart Disease and Lung Disease

Favors Heart Disease
Tachypnea
"Peaceful" cyanosis (cyanosis without respiratory distress)
Normal $PaCO_2$
PaO_2 less than 150 mm Hg while breathing 100% O_2
Gross ECG abnormality
Echocardiogram abnormality
Cardiomegaly
Favors Lung Disease
Hyperpneic, grunting respirations
Cyanosis with respiratory distress
Elevated $PaCO_2$
PaO_2 greater than 150 mm Hg while breathing 100% O_2
Prematurity
Birth trauma and asphyxia
Fetal distress or meconium staining

Compared with children and adults, newborns have polycythemia. Frequently, infants with hemoglobin levels above 20 gm/dl will appear to be cyanotic because of their plethoric appearance. These infants have normal arterial oxygenation, and they appear entirely healthy except for their plethora. Sometimes arterial blood gas determination may be necessary to distinguish a normal newborn with plethora from an infant with a cyanotic form of CHD.

Congestive Heart Failure

Congestive heart failure (CHF) occurs in approximately 25 per cent of all cases of CHD, and over 90 per cent who develop CHF do so in the first year of life, usually early in infancy. Heart failure developing within 3 hours after birth is usually due to:

1. Hypoplastic left heart syndrome.
2. A large shunt through a peripheral arteriovenous (A-V) malformation.
3. A cardiomyopathy due to birth asphyxia.

Although most congenital cardiac lesions can cause CHF in the first month of life, the main defects are:

1. Transposition of the great arteries.
2. Interrupted aortic arch.
3. Coarctation of the aorta.
4. Complex cardiac abnormalities.

There are many children with CHD who have large intracardiac defects at birth, but who do not develop CHF until approximately 1 month of age. This is because pulmonary vascular resistance is elevated at birth, and thus, there is minimal, if any, intracardiac shunting. As pulmonary vascular resistance diminishes during the first month of life, left-to-right intracardiac shunting then develops, and the gradual increase in pulmonary blood flow eventually becomes large enough to cause CHF.

Hereditary Diseases

Whenever an infant is born with noncardiac congenital malformations, there is an increased possibility of a cardiac malformation being present. Also, many genetic disorders have an increased incidence of CHD; the most notable examples are Noonan's syndrome, Turner's syndrome, Down's syndrome, Marfan's syndrome, and the Holt-Oram syndrome. There are many other chromosomal and genetic disorders that are associated with and that cause CHD. Rather than listing all of the possibilities, the author recommends that whenever a practitioner examines an infant who appears to have a genetic syndrome or multiple congenital anomalies, the patient also be evaluated for the possibility of CHD.

CONGENITAL HEART DISEASE IN CHILDREN

If a baby is born with CHD and has no cardiovascular symptoms during infancy, the child will most likely remain asymptomatic or have relatively minimal cardiac symptomatology during childhood. The development or worsening of cardiac symptoms in older children and adults with CHD is usually not due directly to the defect itself but is usually due to a complication or sequelae of the cardiac lesion. There are five main reasons for the development of cardiovascular symptoms in older children, adolescents and adults:

1. Ventricular contractility diminishes, such as from a large left-to-right shunt eventually causing poor ventricular function.
2. Pulmonary vascular disease develops and the patient begins shunting right-to-left with resulting cyanosis.
3. An arrhythmia develops.
4. Cardiac surgery is performed, and a complication occurs.
5. A "catastrophic event" may occur. Cerebral vascular accidents, brain abscesses, bacterial endocarditis, and hypercyanotic spells are the most common catastrophic events that occur in children with CHD and most frequently occur in children who have cyanotic forms of CHD.

LABORATORY EVALUATION OF CONGENITAL HEART DISEASE

By history and physical examination, the practitioner should be able to diagnose an abnormality of cardiovascular function in the infant and child with CHD. Laboratory tests provide important additional diagnostic clues. With electrocardiography and roentgenography, most practitioners are able to diagnose most cases of CHD and frequently will be able to diagnose the specific lesion. With echocardiography and cardiac catheterization, an exact anatomic diagnosis can be made.

Electrocardiogram

Electrocardiograms (ECGs) are relatively nonspecific in diagnosing individual congenital heart lesions; however, they are of much value in determining the amount of atrial enlargement and ventricular hypertrophy. Right atrial enlargement is diagnosed if the P wave is taller than 2½ to 3 mm (by standardization, 10 mm = 1 millivolt). Left atrial enlargement is diagnosed if the duration of the P wave is greater than 0.09 to 0.10 seconds, especially if the P wave has a biphasic ("M") shape.

Right ventricular hypertrophy is fairly accurately diagnosed by ECG. If a qR pattern is present in lead V_1, right ventricular hypertrophy is almost certainly present. A positive T wave in lead V_1 in the child, and in infants older than 1 week of age, is a sign of right ventricular hypertrophy. Right axis deviation is another sign of right ventricular hypertrophy. On the other hand, left axis deviation is not a sign of left ventricular hypertrophy in childhood. Left ventricular hypertrophy is usually present if there is T wave inversion in lead V_6. Left ventricular hypertrophy usually can be diagnosed if the left precordial R wave voltage is abnormally increased. Table 2 lists the normal R wave voltages at various ages. If the R wave in lead V_1 is greater than normal, right ventricular hypertrophy can be diagnosed. Similarly, if the R wave in V_6 is greater than normal, left ventricular hypertrophy can be diagnosed.

Chest Roentgenography

The majority of patients with CHD have an abnormal chest x-ray, and the specific type of CHD is occasionally diagnosed accurately from the configuration of the cardiac silhouette.

It is important to examine the x-ray film thoroughly before evaluating the heart and lungs. Situs inversus, sometimes with dextrocardia, may be present and the practitioner must determine whether the heart and stomach are on the left or right side. Thoracic vertebral anomalies, especially hemivertebrae, are commonly associated with CHD.

Pneumonia is stated to be more frequent in CHD. However, pneumonia is probably overdiagnosed in CHD. Many cases of so-called pneumonia are really cases of children who have unexplained fever and who happen to have increased pulmonary vascular markings that are misdiagnosed as pneumonia.

The peripheral pulmonary vascular markings are an important diagnostic aspect of a chest x-ray film. Diminished pulmonary vascular markings almost always signify right-to-left shunting with decreased pulmonary blood flow. Increased pulmonary vascular markings usually mean increased flow from a left-to-right shunt, though they may be due to pulmonary edema from left heart failure or pulmonary venous obstruction. The Eisenmenger syndrome (intracardiac right-to-left shunting because of elevated pulmonary vascular resistance) shows large central pulmonary arteries, but the peripheral pulmonary vessels are diminished in size and have an x-ray pattern similar to "a tree in winter."

Enlargement of the lymph channels is usually due to pulmonary venous obstruction or massive pulmonary blood flow. Engorgement of the lymph channels is seen on the chest x-ray film as small linear densities called Kerley B lines. These lines lie horizontally along the outer parts of the lower lateral lung fields and are about 2 mm wide and 1 to 2 cm long.

Table 2. Maximal Normal R Wave Values

Age	Lead V_1 (in mm)*	Lead V_6 (in mm)*
0–1 month	25	21
2–12 months	20	20
1–8 years	18	24
9–11 years	16	24
12–16 years	16	22
>16 years	14	21

*10 mm = 1.0 mV.

Dilatation of the heart will be noticed on the chest x-ray. In CHD, the main cause of dilatation of the heart is left-to-right shunting with volume overload of the specific cardiac chambers that have the excessive recirculation of blood. Other causes of ventricular dilatation in CHD include myocardial muscle failure and regurgitation through a cardiac valve.

Enlargement of the right atrium is usually seen as a convex dilatation extending along the entire right cardiac silhouette from the diaphragm to the superior vena cava. Enlargement of the left atrium is usually diagnosed by a circular density in the middle of the cardiac silhouette, along with the left bronchus being displaced superiorly. Left ventricular enlargement displaces the cardiac apex downward, while right ventricular enlargement displaces the cardiac apex upward. In CHD, the ventricular anatomy may be so abnormally altered that it may be impossible to definitely state which ventricular chamber is enlarged.

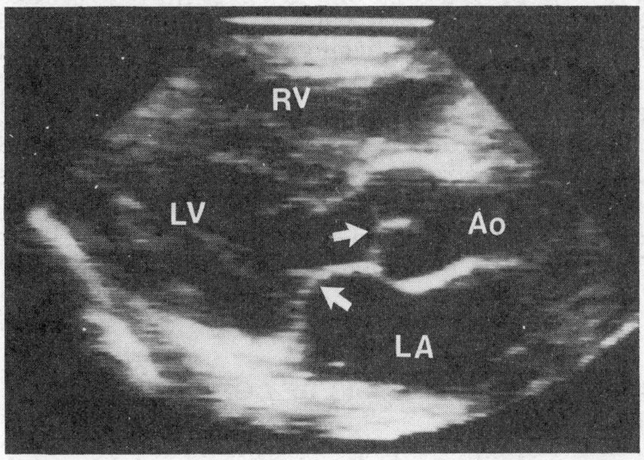

Figure 1. Long axis two-dimensional (2-D) echocardiogram from a normal heart. Two-dimensional echocardiograms show a pie-shaped thin slice of the heart. Cardiac chambers and vascular lumens show up as black areas, while cardiac structures (e.g., valves, septa, vascular walls) show up as white areas. By taking multiple echocardiographic views, an echocardiographer can spatially reconstruct a three-dimensional image of the heart and then usually accurately determine what type of cardiac lesion is present. For example, if a ventricular septal defect were present, the ventricular septum would contain a black area which would communicate with both the left ventricle and the right ventricle; if this were an echocardiogram of hypoplastic left heart syndrome, the left atrium, left ventricle, aorta, mitral valve, and aortic valve would all be markedly diminutive compared with the size of the right ventricle, right atrium, and tricuspid valve. The text describes the 2-D echocardiographic findings for individual congenital heart lesions. RV = Right ventricle; LA = left atrium; LV = left ventricle; Ao = aorta. Arrows point to mitral and aortic valves.

Echocardiography

Echocardiography has become one of the most valuable tools in the diagnosis of CHD. The recent improvement in echocardiographic diagnoses has been dramatic. Echocardiography has eliminated the need for catheterization in many cases of CHD.

M-mode echocardiography was first used routinely approximately 10 years ago. Because the equipment for M-mode echocardiography is relatively inexpensive and has been used by most pediatric cardiologists, it will continue to be utilized for a few years more. However, it is now being surpassed by two-dimensional (2-D) echocardiography, which is much superior in diagnosing specific congenital cardiac defects.

Photographic pictures of 2-D echocardiograms, as shown in Figures 1 and 2, do not do justice to the importance of this entity in the diagnosis of the CHD. Two-dimensional echocardiography must be seen "in motion" to appreciate its value. Every cardiac lesion listed in this article can be diagnosed by 2-D echocardiography. By combining various echocardiographic views, one can reconstruct a three-dimensional image of the heart. Additionally, views obtained from the suprasternal notch and subxiphoid area usually will delineate all of the major blood vessels entering and exiting the heart.

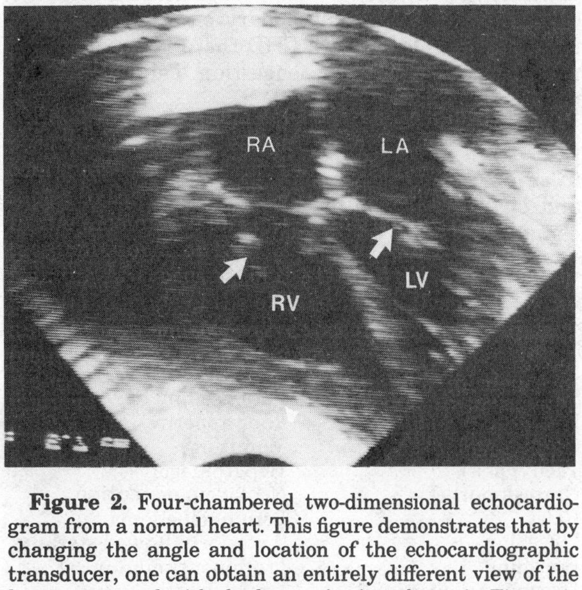

Figure 2. Four-chambered two-dimensional echocardiogram from a normal heart. This figure demonstrates that by changing the angle and location of the echocardiographic transducer, one can obtain an entirely different view of the heart compared with the long axis view shown in Figure 1. RV = Right ventricle; LV = left ventricle; LA = left atrium; RA = right atrium. Arrows point to tricuspid and mitral valves.

Cardiac Catheterization

At the present time, cardiac catheterization (which in this article, by definition, will also include angiography) is the usual means of diagnosing most congenital heart lesions. As experience in echocardiographic diagnosis improves, it is predicted that relatively few cardiac catheterizations will be performed in children with CHD. The author recognizes that throughout this article there are many statements about the value of echocardiography versus cardiac catheterization in the diagnosis of CHD. These comments reflect the author's personal prejudice for echocardiography. It should be re-emphasized that in most pediatric cardiology centers, cardiac catheterization is the usual and preferred way to diagnose most congenital heart lesions. The resolution of angiographic pictures of the heart is much superior to echocardiographic views. A thorough cardiac catheterization study will frequently demonstrate anatomic details that cannot be visualized by echocardiography. Cardiac catheterization is also necessary for determining the magnitude of intracardiac shunts and for obtaining intracardiac blood pressures.

FUNCTIONAL DIAGNOSIS OF CONGENITAL HEART DISEASE

Before discussing individual congenital heart lesions, we will review some general principles of diagnosis in CHD. The author believes it is more important for the practitioner to make a diagnosis of cardiac dysfunction than a specific anatomic diagnosis. It is essentially impossible for the practitioner to know all the clinical features of every CHD. However, it is easy to diagnose an abnormality of cardiovascular function in the infant, child, and adolescent. Abnormalities of cardiovascular function can be divided into three categories: congestive heart failure, low cardiac output, and arterial hypoxemia.

Congestive Heart Failure (CHF)

Congestion (retention of fluids) is the major manifestation of heart failure in infancy. In CHD, CHF is usually due to a structural abnormality, such as a large ventricular septal defect with left-to-right shunting, rather than any intrinsic impairment of myocardial function. Congestive heart failure can occur from decreased myocardial contractility in CHD, but this is less common and usually occurs later in childhood or adulthood. While congestion can involve only the systemic or pulmonary circulation, in the majority of children with CHD there is usually both pulmonary and systemic congestion. Table 3 lists the major manifestations of CHF.

Pulmonary congestion can range from mild interstitial edema with minimal respiratory manifestations to severe pulmonary edema with blood-tinged froth and cyanosis, the latter being due to poor gas exchange.

Table 3. Congestive Heart Failure (CHF)

Minimal respiratory manifestations*	Exercise intolerance*
Severe pulmonary edema	Growth failure
Blood-tinged froth	Poor feeding
Cyanosis	Poor appetite
Tachypnea†	Vomiting
Nurses poorly†	Hepatomegaly†
Rales	Neck vein distention
Wheezing	Peripheral edema
Coughing	Anteriorly bowed sternum
Dyspnea on exertion*	Prominent pulmonary vascularity

*The most common manifestations in the child and adolescent with CHF.

†The most common findings in the infant with CHF.

In the infant, tachypnea is a major sign of pulmonary congestion, commonly with respiratory rates of 60 to 130 per minute. The elevation of the respiratory rate is directly proportional to the amount of pulmonary congestion. The tachypnea is frequently not noted by the parents because the infant's respirations are shallow. However, the parents will usually note that the infant nurses poorly. This is mainly due to the rapid respiratory rate, which does not allow the infant time to stop breathing and suck. In infants, rales may not be heard in CHF because the respiratory excursions are shallow; this can be true even when significant pulmonary congestion is present. While crying or breathing deeply, the rales may become audible.

Wheezing and coughing occur with pulmonary congestion but are not present in all cases, and "cardiac asthma" is not common in children. The older child with pulmonary congestion usually has dyspnea on exertion, though sometimes this is mild and is apparent only if the child's activity is carefully compared with that of peers. The growth failure that occurs is due to the increased respiratory rate that causes both poor feeding, as mentioned, and an increased metabolic rate, which is also present in children with CHD. Furthermore, systemic venous congestion with engorgement of the liver and portal venous system can cause nausea and vomiting.

Hepatomegaly is the most common sign of systemic venous congestion. Neck vein distention is present in children with systemic congestion, but it is not easily recognized in infants because of their relatively short, thick necks. Peripheral edema in children is first noted in the face, especially periorbitally, rather than in the extremities. The chest will have an anteriorly bowed sternum with a bell-shaped configuration owing to decreased lung compliance. With pulmonary congestion, chest x-ray films invariably show increased pulmonary vascularity.

Decreased Cardiac Output

Low cardiac output may be due to:

1. A large intracardiac left-to-right shunt in which the majority of the cardiac output recirculates through the lungs, resulting in an inadequate flow of blood to the systemic circulation.
2. Mechanical restriction of blood flow, such as from a stenotic aortic valve.
3. Poor ventricular contractility.

Table 4 lists the major manifestations of decreased cardiac output.

Tachycardia and vasoconstriction of the skin are the earliest signs of acutely decreased cardiac output. Vasoconstriction of the skin is manifested by paleness, decreased skin temperature, and poor capillary filling. A narrow pulse pressure with diminished pulse volume is a sign of markedly decreased cardiac output; in these cases, pulsus alternans and pulsus paradoxus may occur. Sweating is due to stimulation of the sweat glands by the autonomic nervous system. Oliguria is an early manifestation of decreased cardiac output but is usually not recognized unless the urine output is measured.

Generalized fatigue, lack of stamina, dyspnea on exertion, and pulmonary edema occur in older chil-

Table 4. Decreased Cardiac Output

Tachycardia†
Vasoconstriction of the skin†
Narrow pulse pressure
Pulsus alternans
Pulsus paradoxus
Sweating†
Oliguria
Generalized fatigue
Lack of stamina*
Dyspnea on exertion*
Pulmonary edema
Gallop rhythms
Decreased intensity of the first heart sound
Syncope

*The most common manifestations in the child and adolescent with congestive heart failure.

†The most common manifestations in the infant with congestive heart failure.

dren whose cardiac output is inadequate—these manifestations also occur in children who have pulmonary congestion. In CHF, the symptoms are due to excessive circulation of blood through the lungs or obstruction to pulmonary venous drainage. In cases with a decreased cardiac output due to poor cardiac muscular contractility, pulmonary congestion and edema may occur from elevated left ventricular diastolic pressures. Gallop rhythms are usually found in patients with decreased cardiac output. Poor ventricular cardiac contractility causes a decreased intensity of the first heart sound. Syncope occasionally occurs from a low cardiac output but is relatively rare in children.

Arterial Hypoxemia

Cyanosis is not visible until there is approximately 3 gm/dl of unsaturated hemoglobin, which corresponds with an arterial oxygen saturation of approximately 80 per cent. The ability to recognize clinically arterial oxygen desaturation depends upon: the degree of hypoxemia, the amount of desaturated hemoglobin, and the experience of the observer. We have noticed many intensely cyanotic patients who were not recognized to be cyanotic by either their parents or personal physician. Cyanosis is best seen in the palms, soles, nail beds, and mucous membranes.

Cyanosis in CHD is usually due to intracardiac right-to-left shunting, though occasionally to pulmonary edema. Patients with pulmonary edema usually have marked improvement in their arterial oxygen saturation and color when high concentrations of oxygen are administered. In those with intracardiac shunting of venous blood, administration of oxygen changes the arterial oxygen saturation minimally.

Infants and children with cyanosis due to pulmonary edema have tachypnea and the other signs of pulmonary congestion mentioned earlier. Those with cyanosis due to intracardiac shunting have normal respirations at rest. With exercise, the intracardiac right-to-left shunting increases and the cyanosis worsens; dyspnea on exertion, limited exercise tolerance, and hyperpnea develop during activity. Some children who have minimal right-to-left shunting will have normal coloration at rest but will become cyanotic with exercise.

Paroxysms of hypoxia most commonly occur in tetralogy of Fallot (ToF) and are therefore frequently called "tet" spells, though those spells can occur in any lesion in which there is right-to-left shunting with pulmonary stenosis or pulmonary atresia. These spells tend to occur in children who are younger than 2 years of age, and most frequently occur shortly after the child has awakened from sleep. During these spells, the child suddenly develops paroxysms of hyperpnea and hypercyanosis. If the spell is severe, acidemia, convulsions, brain damage, and death can occur.

Older children with ToF and those who have similar heart defects typically squat following exercise. Squatting decreases right-to-left shunting and increases pulmonary blood flow. Newborns with severe cyanosis do the equivalent of squatting by sleeping in a knee-chest position as soon as they can do so, usually by 3 to 5 months of age.

Clubbing, another well-known sign of arterial hypoxemia, does not occur before 3 months of age, even in cases of severe cyanosis. Clubbing is first detected as a fullness at the base of the thumb nail.

Heart Murmurs

Murmurs are overemphasized as the primary means of diagnosing CHD. Less than one fourth of all infants with CHD who have an easily heard murmur by 2 years of age will have a murmur heard in the first week of life. Typically, the two most serious types of newborn cardiac defects—transposition of the great arteries and hypoplastic left heart syndrome—have no murmur at all. Thus, if we rely upon a murmur to diagnose CHD, we will miss many serious cases of CHD. However, in essentially all cases of CHD, significant changes in cardiovascular function will be present; and if the practitioner is concerned about making a functional diagnosis, most cases of CHD will be diagnosed whether or not a murmur is present.

SPECIFIC CONGENITAL CARDIAC LESIONS

I have arbitrarily divided CHD into an acyanotic and a cyanotic group (Table 5). Many children with so-called acyanotic lesions actually have cyanosis, such as those who have right-to-left shunting secondary to obstructive pulmonary vascular disease, or those who are cyanotic due to pulmonary edema.

On the other hand, some children with cyanotic lesions are not visibly cyanotic because the right-to-left shunting is not that great. I have seen patients with every one of the lesions listed in the cyanotic group who were not clinically cyanotic.

Atrial Septal Defect (ASD)

Defects may occur anywhere in the atrial septum. The most common defect is the ostium secundum ASD. The next most common ASD is a defect in the

Table 5. Congenital Heart Disease

Acyanotic
Left-to-right shunts
Atrial septal defects
Ventricular septal defects
Endocardial cushion defects
Patent ductus arteriosus
Obstruction to blood flow
Pulmonic valvular stenosis
Aortic valvular stenosis
Coarctation of the aorta
Cyanotic
Primarily right-to-left shunts
Tetralogy of Fallot
Tricuspid atresia
Complex lesions with pulmonic stenosis or atresia
Primarily bidirectional shunts
d-Transposition of the great arteries
Hypoplastic left heart syndrome (aortic valve atresia)
Total anomalous pulmonary venous return
Truncus arteriosus
Complex lesions without pulmonic stenosis or atresia

septum primum, which is a form of endocardial cushion defect and is discussed in that section.

Clinical Features. Atrial septal defects are twice as common in females as in males. Patients with the Holt-Oram syndrome have a high incidence of ASD. The two most common findings in this syndrome are an ASD and a "digitalized" thumb (a thumb that has three phalanges and looks like a finger). Symptoms are usually minimal, if present at all, in children with ASDs. Congestive heart failure is rare in patients with ASDs and usually occurs only if the patient has an associated lesion. During childhood, dyspnea on exertion and decreased stamina are the most common symptoms; frequently, however, the symptoms are mild and they may not be recognized.

The main murmur present in an ASD is a grade II-III/VI short midsystolic ejection murmur heard in the pulmonic area. This murmur sounds similar to an innocent pulmonary ejection murmur. A widely split second heart sound is the classic finding in an ASD, with the two components of the second heart sound usually split more than 0.04 seconds during both inspiration and expiration. Patients with smaller shunts from an ASD or those with pulmonary hypertension usually do not have this constant and wide splitting of the second heart sound. The most diagnostic physical finding of an ASD is a third heart sound gallop or low-pitched early to midsystolic murmur heard over the tricuspid area with the intensity of the gallop or murmur increased during inspiration. This is a difficult "sound" to hear, and for most practitioners it is not heard except in the most prominent cases.

Chest X-ray. The chest x-ray film usually reveals moderate cardiomegaly with increased pulmonary vascular markings, with prominence of the right atrium and pulmonary artery segment. As with all left-to-right shunts, the enlargement of the pulmonary vascular markings and the size of the heart is proportionate to the amount of shunting.

Electrocardiogram. The ECG invariably has an rsR' pattern in the right precordial leads. This pattern is a type of mild right ventricular hypertrophy due to dilatation of the right ventricle and morphologically resembles an incomplete right bundle branch block. The height of the r and R' waves in lead V_1 usually exceeds the normal values listed in Table 2.

Echocardiogram. M-mode echocardiography reveals a dilated right ventricle. In the typical case, paradoxical septal motion is noted with the ventricular septum moving abnormally toward the right ventricle during systole rather than toward the left ventricle.

Two-dimensional echocardiography will pinpoint the exact location of the ASD and will demonstrate how well the right ventricle contracts. If 2-D echocardiography shows that all of the pulmonary veins enter normally and that the rest of the cardiovascular structures are normal, many cardiologists will send such patients to surgery without cardiac catheterization.

Cardiac Catheterization. A left-to-right shunt at the atrial level with slight elevation of right ventricular systolic pressure and a mild systolic pressure gradient across the pulmonic valve will be demonstrated. Angiograms by injection in the left atrium will demonstrate the defect in the atrial septum.

Complications and Diagnostic Pitfalls. A small percentage of patients with ASD develop pulmonary hypertension as teen-agers or adults. The section on ventricular septal defects discusses the clinical diagnosis of pulmonary hypertension. Mitral valve prolapse is more common in patients with ASDs. Prolapse is diagnosed by hearing a late to midsystolic click in the apical area; the click is frequently followed by a plateau-shaped systolic murmur. Atrial arrhythmias occasionally occur in patients who have ASDs. Some patients with long-standing dilatation of the right ventricle from the left-to-right atrial shunting develop right ventricular dysfunction, which causes systemic venous congestion. Right ventricular dysfunction is rarely present in the child.

The main differential diagnosis in patients with ASDs is some form of partial anomalous pulmonary venous return, in which one or more pulmonary veins drain into the right atrium. Clinically, partial anomalous pulmonary venous return is identical to ASD. If operation is contemplated and cardiac catheterization is not performed, one should ascertain by 2-D echocardiography that all the pulmonary veins do enter into the left atrium.

Ventricular Septal Defect (VSD)

The clinical signs of VSD were first described by Roger, and now a small VSD is known as a "maladie de Roger." Eisenmenger later described a cyanotic patient who had a large VSD. We now use the name "Eisenmenger" to mean pulmonary hypertension due to obstructive pulmonary vascular disease with right-to-left shunting. The tissue surrounding VSDs frequently continues to grow after birth, and approximately 50 per cent of VSDs will spontaneously close in the first few years of life.

Clinical Features. Congestive heart failure is common in the child who has a VSD, though usually it does not develop until the infant is about 1 month of age. At birth, pulmonary vascular resistance is elevated and equal to systemic vascular resistance, so that there is minimal flow across the VSD early in infancy. As pulmonary resistance decreases during the first 2 months of life, left-to-right shunting increases. Thus, CHF, if it is going to develop, usually does so within 1½ to 2 months of age.

The classic finding in a VSD, besides the signs of CHF, is the systolic murmur. The murmur of a VSD is usually not heard during the first few days of life because of the minimal flow across the VSD during that time. Usually the murmur is first heard at the initial routine follow-up newborn physical examination. The murmur of a VSD is loudest at the left lower sternal border. These murmurs are plateau-shaped, begin with the first heart sound, and are usually holosystolic (except for some small VSDs which have ejection murmurs instead). In small VSDs, the murmur is high-pitched; in larger-sized VSDs, the murmur is harsher and more medium-pitched. When the left-to-right shunt is equal to the cardiac output, a third heart sound or low-pitched mid-diastolic apical murmur is present.

Those patients with a VSD who have mild obstructive pulmonary vascular disease have minimal symptoms. Those who have severe pulmonary vascular obstruction have arterial hypoxemia due to right-to-left shunting. When pulmonary artery pressure is equal to systemic pressure, the second heart sound is loud and single.

Chest X-ray. Chest x-ray films reveal cardiomegaly, usually with enlargement of the left atrium being most obvious. Pulmonary vascular markings and cardiac size are proportionate to the magnitude of the left-to-right shunt. Patients with Eisenmenger's syndrome have normal sized hearts along with very large central pulmonary arteries but diminished peripheral pulmonary vascularity.

Electrocardiogram. The ECG in patients with a small VSD is normal or shows mild left ventricular hypertrophy. With a moderate-sized VSD, the ECG usually shows left ventricular hypertrophy. With large VSDs, the ECG will show biventricular hypertrophy or right ventricular hypertrophy if the pulmonary vascular resistance is elevated.

Echocardiogram. M-mode echocardiography reveals dilatation of the left atrium and left ventricle in those who have left-to-right shunting. Usually, the left atrial diameter will be at least 1.3 times that of the aortic diameter if there is significant left-to-right shunting (this is known as an increased LA/Ao ratio). M-mode echocardiography is relatively imprecise in locating VSDs.

On the other hand, 2-D echocardiography usually shows the exact location and size of the VSD. At the present time, the resolution of 2-D echocardiography will show VSDs as small as 2 mm in diameter. Two-dimensional echocardiography will show if tissue is growing into the defect and will suggest whether or not the VSD may be in the process of spontaneously closing.

Cardiac Catheterization. Cardiac catheterization is performed in the patient with a VSD primarily for measuring the magnitude of the shunt and for determining the pulmonary artery pressures and resistance. Cardiac catheterization will delineate the exact area and size of the VSD and also will determine whether associated cardiac anomalies are present.

Complications and Diagnostic Pitfalls. The main complication of a VSD is the development of the Eisenmenger syndrome. Because of the possibility of developing irreversible pulmonary hypertension, I recommend that all infants who are thought to have a VSD with significant left-to-right shunting or pulmonary hypertension have cardiac catheterization performed at 3 to 6 months of age.

The clinical manifestations of a patient developing increased pulmonary vascular resistance include:

1. Diminishing symptoms of CHF.
2. Increasing intensity of the second heart sound.
3. Diminishing of the intensity of the murmur.
4. Decreasing heart size and vascular markings on x-ray.
5. Decreasing left atrial and left ventricular dimensions by echocardiography.

Unfortunately, the clinical manifestations of Eisenmenger's syndrome may not be evident until after the patient has developed irreversible pulmonary hypertension.

Endocardial Cushion Defect (ECD)

Endocardial cushion defects are also known as *atrioventricular canals* because of the large defect in the contiguous portions of the atrial and ventricular septa. In the complete form of ECD, a VSD is present. In the incomplete form, the ventricular septum is intact; this form of ECD is also known as an ostium primum ASD because of the large ASD in the septum primum portion of the atrial septum. Dysplasia of the mitral and tricuspid valves occurs, and mitral valve insufficiency is invariably present.

Clinical Features. There is a high incidence of ECDs in Down's syndrome. Patients with ECDs, like those with VSDs, do not have murmurs or CHF at birth, but by 1 month of age both are common. Children with ECDs, especially those with the complete form, develop marked CHF.

The most consistent finding in ECD is a systolic mitral valve insufficiency murmur, which is a holosystolic, plateau-shaped, medium- to high-pitched murmur heard maximally at the apical area with radiation to the left axilla. In the complete form of ECD, a systolic murmur of a VSD is present and is heard maximally at the left lower sternal border. In the incomplete form of ECD, the physical findings are similar to those of an ostium secundum ASD with a widely split second heart sound, a tricuspid diastolic gallop or murmur, and a pulmonic systolic ejection murmur. A mitral diastolic murmur or third heart sound gallop is present in almost every patient with an ECD. In those who have most of their left-to-right shunting at the atrial level, the diastolic murmur or gallop is louder in the tricuspid area than in the mitral area.

Chest X-ray. Chest x-ray films show striking cardiomegaly and prominent pulmonary vascularity, especially in the complete form. Right atrial enlargement is usually very noticeable.

Electrocardiogram. Left axis deviation of the QRS complex is almost always present in ECDs. Incomplete forms of ECDs usually have a QRS axis of −30 to −60°. The complete forms usually have a QRS axis of −60 to −90°. Right ventricular hypertrophy with an rsR' pattern in lead V_1, similar to what is found in ostium secundum ASD, is present in most cases of incomplete ECD. Patients with the complete form usually have biventricular hypertrophy on their ECG, similar to patients with VSD. If pulmonary vascular resistance is elevated, right ventricular hypertrophy (RVH) will be present.

Echocardiogram. M-mode echocardiography usually shows an abnormal mitral valve with the valve appearing to cross the ventricular septum during diastole. Although the mitral valve does not actually cross the septum, the mitral and tricuspid valves reflect the echoes in such a way that it appears as if it does. This finding is pathognomonic of an ECD. Frequently the VSD will be seen in the complete form. In the incomplete form of ECD, paradoxical ventricular septal motion is commonly noted.

Two-dimensional echocardiography will reveal the large defect present in all cases of ECD and will almost always distinguish between the incomplete and the complete forms. In the complete form, the ASD and VSD appear as one large defect with the mitral and tricuspid valves appearing to be located in the middle of the combined defect. Frequently these two valves unite into a common atrioventricular valve with no attachments to the ventricular septum; this abnormality can usually be demonstrated by echocardiography.

Cardiac Catheterization. At this time, catheterization should be performed on all patients with ECD both for determining the pulmonary vascular resistance and for confirmation of the diagnosis. Left ventricular angiocardiograms show distortion of the left ventricle resulting from the abnormal mitral valve. Frequently the angiocardiogram resembles a swan or goose, with the left ventricle being the body and the aorta the neck (also known as a gooseneck or swan neck deformity).

Complications and Diagnostic Pitfalls. It is believed that patients with ECDs develop irreversible pulmonary hypertension earlier than patients with an isolated VSD. This is thought to be especially true in the child who has Down's syndrome.

Because of the high incidence of ECDs in Down's syndrome and because newborns with an ECD may be asymptomatic and may not have murmurs, we recommend routinely performing an ECG, and an echocardiogram if available, as part of the initial newborn physical examination in all infants with Down's syndrome.

Clinically, the main differential diagnosis of the incomplete form of ECD is an ostium secundum ASD. The complete form of ECD is most commonly clinically confused with VSD. The ECG and echocardiogram will clarify whether or not an ECD is present.

Patent Ductus Arteriosus (PDA)

The normal ductus arteriosus functionally closes at 10 to 15 hours of age and is anatomically closed by 2 to 3 weeks of age. Persistence of the PDA is common in the premature infant.

Clinical Features. Most premature infants with a PDA have the respiratory distress syndrome or hyaline membrane disease. Full-term infants and children with a PDA have CHF, as listed in Table 3. The symptoms of CHF are in proportion to the amount of left-to-right shunting. Patients with large left-to-right shunts have striking CHF, while those with small PDAs and minimal shunting frequently are asymptomatic.

Murmurs of a PDA are usually continuous and have a "machinery" quality to them. "Machinery" refers to a continuous murmur which has a change in pitch and intensity during diastole. "Continuous" means that the murmur begins in systole and continues into diastole. The murmur of a small PDA begins after the first heart sound, peaks at the second heart sound, and fades away by the last third of diastole. The murmur of a moderate-sized PDA is louder, lasts longer, and is harsher. The murmur of a large PDA may or may not continue into diastole.

If pulmonary hypertension or lung disease is present, the murmur of a PDA may be absent. Bounding pulses are present in all cases of PDA with left-to-right shunting. The larger the shunt, the more prominent the pulses.

Chest X-ray. Chest x-ray films show cardiomegaly and increased pulmonary vascular markings, both proportionate to the degree of shunting. In most cases, enlargement of the left atrium and left ventricle predominates. Though enlargement of the ascending aorta is supposedly common in a PDA, the author has not found this sign to be helpful.

Electrocardiogram. The ECG in most patients with PDAs shows left ventricular hypertrophy. Those with a minute amount of left-to-right shunting have normal ECGs. In patients with pulmonary hypertension, biventricular hypertrophy is present. In patients with Eisenmenger's syndrome, right ventricular hypertrophy is present.

Echocardiogram. M-mode echocardiography shows enlargement of the left atrium, the left ventricle, and the aorta in PDA. The left atrium enlarges more than the aorta, and this causes an increased LA/Ao ratio ($>$ 1.3/1).

Two-dimensional echocardiography shows enlargement of the left atrium and left ventricle. Suprasternal notch 2-D echocardiography will show the ductus arteriosus in most patients. Two-dimensional echocardiography is especially valuable in diagnosing persistence of a PDA in premature infants because in these patients the murmurs are frequently not continuous or may not be present if the lung disease is severe.

Cardiac Catheterization. Catheterization is usually not necessary for diagnosing a PDA. If the PDA is not accurately located by 2-D echocardiography, we recommend cardiac catheterization prior to surgical closure.

Complications and Diagnostic Pitfalls. Lesions having murmurs that mimic PDA include:

1. Aortic stenosis with aortic valve insufficiency.
2. A functional venous hum.
3. Some types of vascular rings.

4. Arteriovenous malformations of the brachiocephalic vessels.
5. Pulmonary arteriovenous malformations.
6. Truncus arteriosus.

Pulmonic Valvular Stenosis (PS)

Children who have PS usually have fusion of the three pulmonic valve commissures. The severity of stenosis corresponds to the amount of fusion.

Clinical Features. The majority of children with PS are asymptomatic. Those with moderate and severe forms occasionally have dyspnea on exertion or exercise intolerance. Some infants with very severe narrowing of the pulmonic valve have cyanosis attributable to right-to-left shunting at the atrial level.

Patients with PS have a grade II-V/VI ejection murmur heard maximally at the left upper sternal border with radiation to the anterior neck, axillae, and back. In mild cases, the murmur peaks before midsystole. In moderate and severe cases, the murmur peaks later in systole. The stenosis is proportional to the duration of the systolic murmur, with mild cases having short murmurs and severe cases having long murmurs. Pulmonic ejection clicks are frequently heard in mild and moderate cases and occasionally heard in severe cases of PS.

Chest X-ray. Chest x-rays in PS are generally normal except for enlargement of the main pulmonary artery due to poststenotic dilatation. The pulmonary vascular markings are normal in PS, except in the newborn with the most severe form who has right-to-left atrial shunting. These babies have diminished pulmonary markings secondary to the decreased pulmonary blood flow.

Electrocardiogram. In PS the right ventricular systolic pressure correlates well with the height of the R wave in the precordial leads. The systolic pressure (in mm Hg) is approximately five times the height (in mm) of the R wave in lead V_4R. The R wave in lead V_1 can be used for this estimation if the S wave is absent in lead V_1.

Echocardiogram. M-mode and 2-D echocardiography are of minimal usefulness in PS. The amount of right ventricular hypertrophy can be measured by echocardiography, but this is not accurate. The main reason for performing echocardiograms in PS is to ascertain that no other cardiac abnormalities are present.

Cardiac Catheterization. This procedure is required to determine if the stenosis is severe enough to recommend operation. A thickened, poorly mobile pulmonic valve is usually well visualized when a right ventricular angiocardiogram is performed. Cardiac catheterization is also necessary in PS to make sure that the patient does not have an associated muscular subvalvular stenosis or supravalvular pulmonary branch stenosis.

Complications and Diagnostic Pitfalls. The murmurs and findings of supra- and subvalvular pulmonic stenosis are similar to PS. In subvalvular pulmonic stenosis, the murmur is heard along the left sternal border at a lower level than in PS and does not have an ejection click. In pulmonary branch stenosis the murmurs are transmitted to the axillae and back more loudly than in PS. Pulmonary branch stenosis and PS are common in Williams' syndrome, in Noonan's syndrome, and in babies who were born of mothers who had rubella during pregnancy.

Infants with severe PS who are cyanotic are prone to sudden death and should be considered surgical emergencies.

Aortic Valvular Stenosis (AS)

The most common form of AS is due to a bicuspid aortic valve. A mildly deformed bicuspid aortic valve is a very common congenital cardiac defect, with many cases not being recognized until adulthood; some cases are probably never detected. Markedly dysplastic aortic valves with rudimentary cusps are usually seen only in infants; this form is known as "critical AS."

Clinical Features. Infants who have critical AS usually have CHF with pulmonary edema and low cardiac output. The majority of children with less severe forms of AS are asymptomatic, though occasionally some have fatigue, dyspnea on exertion, syncope, and chest pain. In AS there is a low-pitched, harsh, grade II-V/VI ejection murmur that is heard maximally at the right upper sternal border with radiation both to the apical area and to the neck. Patients who have AS should always be examined for an early diastolic high-pitched decrescendo murmur of aortic insufficiency because the aortic valve may be both stenotic and insufficient. Apical ejection clicks are frequently present in AS. Diminished pulse volume with a narrow pulse pressure is usually present only in severe cases of AS.

Chest X-ray. The chest x-ray film in AS is often normal. Sometimes a dilated ascending aorta will be noted. Pulmonary venous congestion will be seen in infants who have severe AS. The heart size is usually normal in AS, even in those who have exceedingly hypertrophied left ventricles.

Electrocardiogram. The ECG shows left ventricular hypertrophy in all but the mildest cases of AS. The correlation of the severity of the stenosis with the ECG is not as high as in PS. ST segment depression and T wave inversion, which are signs of left ventricular hypertrophy with ventricular strain, suggest that the AS is severe.

Echocardiogram. M-mode echocardiography is best used in AS for determining the amount of left ventricular hypertrophy. In general, the thicker the left ventricular muscle, the more severe the stenosis. M-mode echocardiograms will show an eccentric aortic valve if the valve is bicuspid. M-mode echocardiography is good for recognizing subaortic narrowing but is not as valuable in detecting supravalvular aortic stenosis.

Two-dimensional echocardiograms will show the abnormal aortic valve and how dysplastic it is. It will also show whether or not subvalvular aortic stenosis is present. This procedure will demonstrate narrowing of the ascending aorta if supravalvular aortic stenosis is present. Both 2-D and M-mode echocardiograms will usually differentiate discrete fibrous subvalvular narrowing from hyperdynamic muscular subvalvular narrowing, such as idiopathic hypertrophic subaortic stenosis.

Cardiac Catheterization. This procedure should be done in all patients with AS, except for those in whom one is convinced that the narrowing is mild. The primary reason for cardiac catheterization is to determine the gradient across the aortic valve and to visualize the exact location of the aortic stenosis (i.e., subvalvular, valvular, or supravalvular).

Complications and Diagnostic Pitfalls. Valvular aortic stenosis must be differentiated from supra- and subvalvular forms of aortic stenosis. Patients with supravalvular aortic stenosis usually have a higher blood pressure in the right arm than in the left arm because of streamlining of blood flow. Supravalvular aortic stenosis is frequently present in patients who have Williams' syndrome.

Sudden death may occur in children with AS and is more common in those who have a strain pattern on their ECG.

Coarctation of the Aorta (CoA)

Many authors classify CoA into an infantile and adult type, with the former known as *preductal* CoA and the latter as *postductal* CoA. However, most now doubt that this classification is valid; instead it is believed that in almost all cases the CoA is immediately adjacent to the ductus arteriosus or ligamentum arteriosum.

Clinical Features. CoA is the most common cause of CHF from 7 to 30 days of age. Beyond the newborn period, symptoms from CoA are rare in childhood.

The usual murmur heard in patients with CoA is a grade II/VI aortic ejection murmur that is due to a bicuspid aortic valve. Approximately 80 per cent of patients with CoA have a congenitally bicuspid aortic valve. The most consistent finding in CoA is diminished lower extremity pulses compared with upper extremity pulses. If the CoA is severe, the pulses will be absent in the lower extremities. If the CoA is mild, the lower extremity pulses may be only slightly decreased in intensity. In CoA during childhood, collateral blood vessels are usually not palpable around the thorax and ejection murmurs are usually not audible over the back. Systemic hypertension in the upper part of the body is common in CoA and is even present in some infants.

Chest X-ray. Chest X-ray films in CoA usually reveal a normal heart size and normal pulmonary vascular markings, though infants with heart failure from CoA have cardiomegaly and increased pulmonary vascular markings. In older children, teen-agers, and adults with CoA, one can frequently determine the exact site of the CoA by locating a constricted area in the upper portion of the descending thoracic aorta. Rib notching is seen in 75 per cent of adults with CoA but is rarely seen before age 1 and is not commonly seen in children until age 5.

Electrocardiogram. In infants with CoA, the ECG invariably shows right ventricular hypertrophy. This may be due to one of the associated cardiac anomalies commonly found with CoA, namely mitral stenosis, hypoplasia of the left ventricle, and subaortic stenosis. In older children with CoA, the ECG is normal in over half of the cases; in most of the others, mild left ventricular hypertrophy is present.

Echocardiogram. M-mode echocardiography is of little value in the diagnosis of CoA, though it will usually determine whether associated cardiac anomalies are present. On the other hand, suprasternal notch 2-D echocardiography can localize the coarctation segment and show how constricted it is.

Cardiac Catheterization. Though many surgeons perform surgery for CoA on older children without catheterization, we recommend that catheterization be performed prior to surgery to determine the exact location and severity of the CoA. Preoperative catheterizations will also determine whether associated cardiac defects are present.

Complications and Diagnostic Pitfalls. The main "problem" in CoA is forgetting to palpate the femoral pulses in all cases of hypertension. The author has seen two teen-agers who were being treated for essential hypertension whose hypertension was actually due to undiagnosed coarctation of the aorta. Cerebral bleeding episodes, common in adults, rarely occur in children. Though hypertension occurs in many children with CoA, the complications of hypertension are rarely noted in childhood.

CoA is common in Turner's syndrome.

Tetralogy of Fallot (ToF)

While ToF is thought to consist of four abnormalities, basically there are two. One is a VSD. The other is underdevelopment of the right ventricular outflow tract with subpulmonic stenosis, pulmonic valvular stenosis, and hypoplasia of the pulmonary arteries. In some cases of ToF, there is complete absence of the main pulmonary artery, this variant is also known as pseudotruncus arteriosus or pulmonary atresia with VSD.

Clinical Features. Classically, patients with ToF are cyanotic. However, many newborns with ToF are not cyanotic until a few months of life. This is because there is continued growth of muscular and fibrotic subpulmonic tissue after birth, so that ToF is, in essence, a progressive lesion during infancy.

Squatting following exercise, cyanosis, clubbing, and paroxysmal hypoxic episodes are common in ToF. These have been discussed in the section on arterial hypoxemia.

The murmur of ToF is due to subvalvular pulmonic stenosis; it is heard maximally at the left upper and midsternal border and is of ejection quality. Patients with pseudotruncus arteriosus do not have systolic murmurs; they usually have continuous murmurs from the ductus arteriosus or other collateral blood vessels which, by necessity, must supply all of the pulmonary blood flow. The second heart sound in ToF is single; it is diminished in intensity over the pulmonic area but is loud over the remainder of the precordium. An ejection click is frequently present.

Chest X-ray. Chest x-ray films typically reveal a boot-shaped heart (coeur en sabot). Usually the typical boot-shaped heart is seen only in children who are cyanotic. The concave area of the "boot" occurs at the left upper to midcardiac silhouette and is primarily due to the underdevelopment of the right ventricular outflow tract. A right-sided aortic arch is present in 25 per cent of patients with ToF. Pulmonary vascular markings are diminished except for those newborns who have relatively mild pulmonic stenosis at birth.

Electrocardiogram. Except in some newborn infants, the ECG shows right ventricular hypertrophy. Usually lead V_1 has an abnormally tall R wave with a positive T wave.

Echocardiogram. Both M-mode and 2-D echocardiograms are diagnostic in ToF and show a large aorta that overrides both the left and right ventricular cavities with the VSD noted to be directly beneath the aortic valve. Echocardiography will also frequently reveal the hypoplasia of the main pulmonary artery and its branches.

Cardiac Catheterization. Prior to performing surgery in ToF, cardiac catheterization is necessary. Usually the intracardiac anatomy is well defined by echocardiography; however, cardiac catheterization must be performed to delineate the exact size of the pulmonary arteries. Whether or not corrective surgery can be performed in ToF is determined primarily by the size of the pulmonary arteries.

Complications and Diagnostic Pitfalls. Paroxysms of hypoxia ("tet spells") are the most serious common complication of ToF. (See the section on arterial hypoxemia in this article.)

Tricuspid Atresia (TA)

In TA, there is an atretic dimple where the tricuspid valve should be. There are many forms of TA; however, most cases have a small VSD, a hypoplastic right ventricle, and diminished pulmonary blood flow.

Clinical Features. The majority of patients with TA are cyanotic. Occasionally, those who have increased pulmonary blood flow or those who also have transposition of the great arteries are not cyanotic. Children with TA do not always have a murmur. However, because most have a small VSD, a murmur is usually heard and is similar to the murmur of a small VSD, i.e., a medium-pitched plateau-shaped systolic murmur heard maximally at the left lower sternal border. If the pulmonary blood flow is by way of a PDA rather than a VSD, the patient will have a continuous murmur in the left upper anterior chest. Because of elevated right atrial pressures, hepatomegaly is frequently present.

Chest X-ray. Chest x-ray films in TA show diminished pulmonary vascularity and a rounded contour to the left cardiac silhouette. Right atrial enlargement is frequently noted also. Variants which have increased pulmonary blood flow have increased pulmonary vascular markings.

Electrocardiogram. In most cases of TA, the ECG has left axis deviation and left ventricular hypertrophy. Right atrial enlargement is also frequently present.

Echocardiogram. On M-mode echocardiography, no tricuspid valve can be visualized and the right ventricle appears hypoplastic. The cardiovascular abnormalities present in TA are usually well defined with 2-D echocardiography.

Cardiac Catheterization. Because there are many forms of TA and many complex lesions that are similar to TA, cardiac catheterization should be performed in all patients with TA to determine the exact intracardiac anatomy.

Complications and Diagnostic Pitfalls. Teenagers and young adults with TA frequently develop left ventricular myocardial failure. Many of these patients die in their twenties and thirties because of the significantly diminished left ventricular contractility that occurs at this time.

d-Transposition of the Great Arteries (d-TGA)

Transposition of the great arteries means that the aorta originates from the right ventricle and the pulmonary artery from the left ventricle. In dextro-transposition of the great arteries (d-TGA), the aortic valve is anterior to the pulmonic valve and *is usually located to the right of* the pulmonic valve. This is known as d-TGA to distinguish it from certain complex forms of CHD in which there is levo-transposition of the great arteries (l-TGA); in the latter, the aortic valve *is usually located to the left of* the pulmonic valve. d-TGA is the only lesion in which the pulmonary and systemic circulations are parallel with each other, as shown in Figure 3.

Clinical Features. Patients with d-TGA are usually markedly cyanotic. Most have CHF also. Because of increased pulmonary blood flow, children with d-TGA do not squat, except for those infrequent cases that have an associated large VSD and significant PS. Systolic murmurs are usually not present in d-TGA unless the patient has a VSD or PS. Frequently apical diastolic murmurs or gallops are present. The second heart sound in d-TGA is loud and single.

Chest X-ray. The chest x-ray film in d-TGA frequently shows an "egg on a string." The "string" is due to a narrow upper mediastinum. The "egg" is due to right ventricular hypertrophy and dilatation forming the narrow end of the egg and to right atrial enlargement forming the larger end of the egg. In infants only 50 per cent have this x-ray finding. Pulmonary vascular markings are usually markedly increased in d-TGA, except for those patients who have associated PS.

Electrocardiogram. The ECG invariably shows RVH in d-TGA. Biventricular hypertrophy and left ventricular hypertrophy are found only in those few cases in which the right ventricle is congenitally hypoplastic.

Echocardiogram. It is difficult to diagnose d-TGA by M-mode echocardiography, though if the aortic valve is noted to be to the right of and anterior to the pulmonic valve, one can suspect d-TGA. M-mode echocardiographic determination of d-TGA frequently requires measuring systolic time intervals to distinguish the pulmonic from the aortic valve, and this can be inaccurate.

With 2-D echocardiography, one can easily diagnose d-TGA by demonstrating that the aorta rises from the right ventricle and that the pulmonary artery rises from the left ventricle.

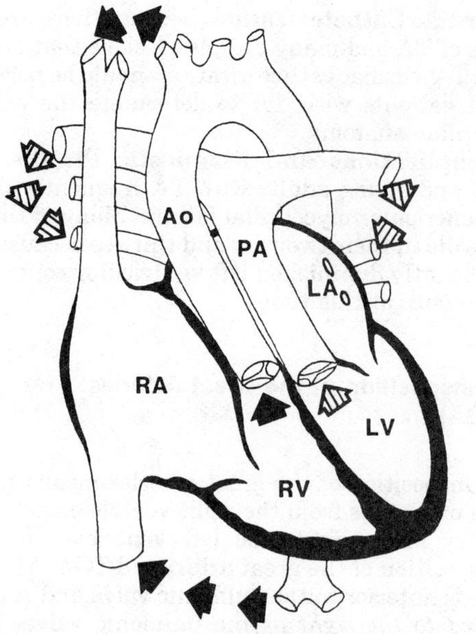

Figure 3. Diagrammatic representation of dextro-transposition of the great arteries (d-TGA). The dark arrows represent nonsaturated systemic venous blood, and the striped arrows the fully saturated pulmonary venous blood. In d-TGA, the nonsaturated blood primarily returns to the systemic circulation resulting in marked arterial hypoxemia. Similarly, the majority of the fully saturated pulmonary venous blood returns to the pulmonary circulation.

Actually, this diagram represents a situation incompatible with life, since there is no mixing of the two circulations. However, it does emphasize three concepts: (1) there must be a communication between the pulmonary and systemic circulations for infants with d-TGA to survive (e.g., atrial septic defect (ASD) or patent ductus arteriosus (PDA)). (2) No matter how great pulmonary blood flow is, the patient will remain cyanotic because systemic blood preferentially reenters the aorta. (3) The systemic and pulmonary circulations are "parallel" to each other, and, therefore, the flow in one circulation may be much greater than in the other. In d-TGA, pulmonary blood flow is usually abnormally increased, which is why patients with d-TGA usually have congestive heart failure (CHF). PA = Pulmonary artery; RV = right ventricle; LA = left atrium; LV = left ventricle; Ao = aorta; RA = right atrium.

Cardiac Catheterization. In all newborns with d-TGA, cardiac catheterization is indicated, partially to confirm the diagnosis, but primarily to perform balloon atrial septostomy at the time of catheterization. In d-TGA, ventricular angiograms will demonstrate conclusively that the aorta arises from the right ventricle and that the pulmonary artery arises from the left ventricle.

Complications and Diagnostic Pitfalls. Those patients who have d-TGA who do not have an ASD, but who instead have mixing by way of a VSD or PDA, usually have marked CHF and pulmonary hypertension. Children with d-TGA, especially those who also have a VSD or PDA, are more likely to develop irreversible pulmonary vascular disease than children with other forms of CHD.

Babies with d-TGA frequently die in the latter half of the first week of life, at which time the ductus arteriosus and/or foramen ovale closes. Early diagnosis of d-TGA is mandatory so that creation of an ASD by balloon atrial septostomy can be performed.

Hypoplastic Left Heart Syndrome (Aortic Valve Atresia)

Most physicians use the terms "hypoplastic left heart syndrome" and "aortic valve atresia" interchangeably. Since aortic valve atresia (AVA) more correctly describes this lesion, this is the term that will be used in this section. In AVA, there is an exceedingly hypoplastic left ventricle with atresia of both the mitral and aortic valves so that the only systemic blood flow is by way of retrograde flow from the pulmonary artery to the ductus arteriosus and then to the aorta.

Clinical Features. Aortic valve atresia is the most common congenital heart lesion causing CHF, low cardiac output, and death in the first week of life. Newborns with AVA usually have both shock and marked pulmonary congestion. Systolic murmurs are usually not present in infants with AVA. Peripheral arterial pulses are diminished significantly in AVA. The second heart sound is loud and single.

Chest X-ray. Pulmonary blood flow is always increased in AVA because right ventricular blood preferentially flows to the pulmonary circulation rather than across the ductus arteriosus to the systemic circulation. Thus, chest x-ray films in AVA reveal significant cardiomegaly and increased pulmonary vascular markings.

Electrocardiogram. The ECG shows marked right ventricular hypertrophy. This is primarily because the left ventricle is very diminutive but also because the right ventricle is markedly enlarged.

Echocardiography. A skilled echocardiographer can diagnose AVA by both M-mode and 2-D echocardiography. With either type of echocardiogram, the extreme hypoplasia of the mitral valve, left ventricle, aortic valve, and ascending aorta is easily visualized.

Cardiac Catheterization. Aortic valve atresia can be diagnosed by injecting radiopaque contrast material through an umbilical artery catheter positioned in the descending aorta near the ductus arteriosus; an anteroposterior chest x-ray film taken approximately one-half second after the injection will reveal the markedly hypoplastic ascending aorta with filling of the coronary arteries from that injection. In the few instances when the diagnosis is uncertain, a complete cardiac catheterization is necessary.

Complications and Diagnostic Pitfalls. Aortic valve atresia is almost always incompatible with life, and the majority of babies with this condition die in the first week of life. Because of the hopeless nature of AVA, it is my belief that most pediatric cardiologists, *at this time,* should inform the parents of the poor prognosis and not continue further medical therapy. However, it is mandatory to determine absolutely that the patient has AVA. New surgical procedures, though still somewhat in the experimental stage, may prove successful in AVA; by the time this text is published, newer operations may negate my statement about not pursuing therapy in these infants.

Total Anomalous Pulmonary Venous Return (TAPVR)

In TAPVR, the pulmonary venous blood always enters the right atrium, usually via an anomalous venous channel, before entering the left atrium. There are three types of TAPVR: supracardiac, intracardiac, and infracardiac. This condition also consists of an obstructed and nonobstructed form, depending upon whether or not there is anatomic obstruction to pulmonary venous emptying.

The most common form of TAPVR is the *supracardiac* type in which the pulmonary veins enter into a common venous structure behind the heart; this structure then drains into an anomalous vein, which empties into the innominate vein and then into the right atrium. In most cases of supracardiac TAPVR, pulmonary blood flow is unobstructed.

In the *intracardiac* type of TAPVR, the pulmonary veins enter into some cardiac structure, usually the coronary sinus. In almost all these cases, pulmonary blood flow is unobstructed.

In *infracardiac* TAPVR, the pulmonary veins drain into an anomalous channel that penetrates the diaphragm and then enters either the portal venous system or the inferior vena cava. Almost all cases of infracardiac TAPVR are obstructed.

Clinical Features. Most cases of unobstructed TAPVR are minimally cyanotic, whereas those who have the obstructed type of TAPVR are markedly cyanotic. Patients with TAPVR invariably have CHF, those with the obstructed form usually have marked pulmonary edema. Newborns with infracardiac TAPVR have striking hepatomegaly because the pulmonary venous blood flows through the liver via the portal venous system. These infants frequently are jaundiced.

Loud systolic murmurs are not common in TAPVR. Those with the nonobstructive type have grade II-III/VI pulmonic ejection murmurs and tricuspid diastolic murmurs similar to what is heard in patients with ASDs. Murmurs are usually not present in obstructed forms of TAPVR. The second heart sound is usually loud and frequently is single.

Chest X-ray. The chest x-ray film in the nonobstructive type of TAPVR shows cardiomegaly, a large main pulmonary artery, and increased pulmonary vascular markings. Newborn infants with the obstructed form of TAPVR have normal- to small-sized hearts and a fine reticular pattern of their lungs.

Electrocardiogram. The ECG in TAPVR invariably shows right ventricular hypertrophy.

Echocardiogram. M-mode echocardiography is of little value in the diagnosis of TAPVR because it is difficult to visualize the pulmonary veins with M-mode echocardiograms. On the other hand, 2-D echocardiography can determine the location and drainage of the pulmonary veins in both those with TAPVR and those with normal hearts. However, diagnosing TAPVR by 2-D echocardiography requires a skilled echocardiographer, high-quality ultrasonic equipment, and a quiet, cooperative patient.

Cardiac Catheterization. This procedure should be performed in all newborns suspected of having TAPVR. Catheterization will accurately depict the type of TAPVR that is present. The pressure measurements obtained will determine whether pulmonary venous drainage is obstructed.

Complications and Diagnostic Pitfalls. Obstructed forms of TAPVR usually require emergency surgery for survival. The main differential diagnosis of a newborn with a normal heart size and a reticular pulmonary pattern is hyaline membrane disease or some other primary lung disorder versus the obstructed form of TAPVR. These can usually be distinguished from each other by inserting an umbilical venous catheter into the right atrium. Patients with hyaline membrane disease have lower oxygen saturations in the right atrium than in a systemic artery; the opposite is true in TAPVR.

Truncus Arteriosus

In truncus arteriosus, the pulmonary artery and aorta arise from a short common arterial trunk that originates from both the left and right ventricles. In truncus arteriosus, there is only an "aortic valve," more properly called a *truncal valve.*

Clinical Features. Though truncus arteriosus is classified as a cyanotic lesion, most patients are not cyanotic or are only minimally cyanotic. Because excessive pulmonary circulation occurs in most cases, the predominant symptoms are those of CHF. Occasionally, infants with truncus arteriosus also have insufficiency of their truncal valve. Usually these babies have severe CHF.

Continuous murmurs are commonly heard throughout the chest. Infants with truncal valve insufficiency have a high-pitched early diastolic decrescendo murmur at the left midsternal border. A systolic ejection click is frequently present. An apical diastolic murmur or gallop is usually present. The second heart sound is usually single, though many patients with truncus arteriosus do have a split second sound. Bounding pulses are present in most cases. Patients who have elevated pulmonary vascular resistance with decreased pulmonary blood flow are cyanotic, may not have bounding pulses, and frequently do not have murmurs.

Chest X-ray. The chest x-ray film in truncus arteriosus reveals cardiomegaly, with left atrial enlargement usually well visualized. Pulmonary vascular markings are increased if pulmonary blood flow is increased. A right aortic arch occurs in one third of patients with truncus arteriosus.

Electrocardiogram. The ECG in truncus arteriosus usually shows left ventricular hypertrophy or biventricular hypertrophy. If pulmonary vascular resistance is markedly elevated, right ventricular hypertrophy will be present.

Echocardiogram. In truncus arteriosus, echocardiograms show a common large truncal valve and short arterial trunk overriding both ventricles. With M-mode echocardiography, it is sometimes difficult to distinguish truncus arteriosus from ToF because the pulmonary artery cannot be seen in many cases of ToF. However, with 2-D echocardiography, the pulmonary artery and pulmonic valve are easily visualized so that one can usually differentiate truncus arteriosus from ToF.

Cardiac Catheterization. Because there are many lesions other than ToF which may be misdiagnosed as truncus arteriosus, even with 2-D echocardiography, cardiac catheterization should be performed. The injection of contrast material into the ascending aorta will usually demonstrate both the aorta and the pulmonary artery arising from the common truncus arteriosus.

Complications and Diagnostic Pitfalls. Lesions that are misdiagnosed as truncus arteriosus include ToF, pseudotruncus arteriosus, PDA, and VSD.

Complex Congenital Heart Defects

There are many other types of CHD, such as absence of the pulmonic valve, Ebstein's anomaly, pulmonary atresia with intact ventricular septum and l-TGA. There are also multiple combinations and permutations of all the lesions described in this article.

Patients with complex heart defects can present with any type of abnormal cardiac finding. A child with a complex defect may be intensely cyanotic if pulmonary blood flow is restricted because of severe pulmonic stenosis, pulmonary atresia, Eisenmenger's syndrome, or any cause of obstruction to pulmonary blood flow such as mitral stenosis. Conversely, if pulmonary blood flow is not obstructed, a patient with a similar lesion may instead have marked pulmonary edema. Thus, patients with complex cardiac defects will have manifestations of CHF, decreased cardiac output, or arterial hypoxemia, depending upon their intracardiac anatomy and hemodynamics.

A child who has a complex cardiac defect may have congenital absence of the spleen (asplenia). Children with asplenia and CHD have severe cardiac anomalies and frequently have situs inversus. If asplenia is present, Howell-Jolly bodies will usually be seen on routine blood smears. Since children with asplenia can die of sepsis within a few hours of the onset of their illness, the practitioner must always check for the presence of a spleen in any child who has complex CHD, situs inversus, and Howell-Jolly bodies.

INFECTIVE ENDOCARDITIS

By W. Michael Scheld, M.D.
Charlottesville, Virginia

SYNONYMS

Subacute bacterial endocarditis, acute bacterial endocarditis, infectious endocarditis.

DEFINITION

Infective endocarditis is an infection of the endocardium, most commonly along the line of closure of the valve leaflets. Other intracardiac (e.g., mural endocardium, septal defects) or extracardiac loci (e.g., arteriovenous or arterioarterial shunts, coarctation of the aorta) may also be involved and lead to a similar clinical syndrome. The pathogenesis, diagnosis, and principles of therapy are similar for all these intravascular infections.

Based on the usual progression of the untreated disease, endocarditis was classified historically into "acute" ("malignant") or "subacute" ("lente") forms. The acute form was characterized by a fulminant course with systemic toxicity, death in days to weeks, and association with pyogenic cocci (e.g., *Staphylococcus aureus,* pneumococci, gonococci, and group A beta-hemolytic streptococci). In contrast, the subacute form was characterized by an indolent presentation with nonspecific symptoms, death in weeks to months, and association with viridans streptococci. This classification is less useful today, since it is recognized that both syndromes may be caused by the same organisms (e.g., enterococci), may lead to identical complications, and are often caused by nonbacterial pathogens. Thus, classification based on the specific etiologic agent, with appropriate implications for therapy, is now preferred.

The disease is not rare and accounts for 0.15 to 5.4 patients per 1000 admissions in United States hospitals. A male sex predominance (1.7 : 1) is found consistently, and infective endocarditis now affects an older patient population, with 54 per cent of cases between 31 and 60 years of age.

The demographic features of infective endocarditis have undergone striking changes in the antibiotic era. With the decline in acute rheumatic fever, rheumatic heart disease is now the underlying structural defect in 37 to 76 per cent of cases. Other types of heart disease have assumed greater importance as the underlying substrate for the development of infective endocarditis. These include congenital heart disease (especially bicuspid aortic valves in elderly males, patent ductus arteriosus, ventricular septal defect), degenerative cardiac lesions in the elderly (e.g., calcified mitral annulus, arteriosclerotic cardiovascular disease), asymmetric septal hypertrophy, and the mitral valve prolapse syndrome.

Two other forms of infective endocarditis have been recognized with increasing frequency: endocarditis in intravenous drug abusers, and prosthetic valve endocarditis. It is now apparent that many cases are acquired nosocomially in seriously ill hospitalized patients subject to intravascular access procedures, including hemodynamic monitoring and hyperalimentation. Although approximately 90 per cent of cases of infective endocarditis are still caused by streptococci or staphylococci, recent trends have emphasized the wide variety of etiologic agents responsible, including gram-negative aerobic bacilli, fastidious gram-negative organisms (e.g., *Hemophilus* or *Cardiobacterium sp.*), diphtheroids, rickettsiae, chlamydia, and fungi (e.g., *Candida* or *Aspergillus sp.*).

PRESENTING SIGNS AND SYMPTOMS

The presenting manifestations of endocarditis are so protean that these patients may present to physicians in virtually any specialty of medicine. Many of the initial complaints are nonspecific. Fever is an important finding and may peak at night (or twice daily in gonococcal endocarditis). Fever may be absent in the elderly and in patients on antimicrobial therapy or when the disease is complicated by renal failure or severe congestive heart failure.

An organic heart murmur is present in over 90 per cent of patients with endocarditis, especially when the disease is of long duration. A new or changing murmur is helpful diagnostically but occurs in only about 10 per cent of cases. A new regurgitant murmur signifies functional valve disturbance by large vegetations or valve (or chordae) rupture and suggests that surgical intervention may be necessary.

Other nonspecific complaints are present in over 50 per cent of the cases, including chills, sweats, weakness, malaise, anorexia, weight loss, cough, and dyspnea. Cough and hemoptysis due to pulmonary emboli (and/or infarction) are the presenting features in the majority of drug addicts with endocarditis affecting the tricuspid valve. Musculoskeletal symptoms may be prominent and cause the patient to present to the rheumatologist or orthopedic surgeon. Musculoskeletal symptoms are the initial complaint in 27 per cent of endocarditis patients. These include back pain, myalgia, arthralgia, and mono- or oligoarticular arthritis. Neurologic findings are useful diagnostically and may be an ominous feature; they are found in approximately 40 per cent of cases. A stroke, secondary to embolic infarction or hemorrhage, was a common finding in the preantibiotic era and this complication now occurs in approximately 20 per cent of cases, especially with mitral valve involvement. Other neurologic findings at presentation (or developing during the disease course) include alterations in mental status (e.g., delirium, coma), blindness, paralysis, altered sensation, or psychiatric manifestations.

Most cases of endocarditis now present with an indolent course developing over weeks to months. When an inciting event (e.g., dental extraction) can be identified, the time interval from the procedure to the first symptoms of endocarditis is less than 2 weeks in 85 per cent of cases. Some patients with endocarditis present with a fulminant course, evolving in hours to days. It is important to emphasize that staphylococcal endocarditis with fulminant onset and petechiae or purpura may be confused with acute meningococcemia, Rocky Mountain spotted fever, or overwhelming sepsis in the splenectomized patient.

COURSE

In the preantibiotic era, untreated infective endocarditis was almost uniformly fatal, with survival in only 1 to 2 per cent of cases. Uncontrolled infection was the usual cause of death. Today, the outcome is dependent on the underlying condition of the host, the pathogen, and appropriate antibiotic selection. With appropriate treatment, the patient's clinical condition improves gradually with reduction of fever to normal by 1 week, depending on the infecting organism. Despite achieving sterile blood cultures after 2 to 6 days on appropriate antibiotics, sterilization of the vegetations with avoidance of relapse requires prolonged antimicrobial therapy, usually 2 to 4 weeks for penicillin-sensitive streptococcal endocarditis and 4 to 6 weeks for enterococcal or staphylococcal endocarditis.

Despite the introduction of new antibiotics, the mortality rate of infective endocarditis is still 30 to 35 per cent, unchanged from the early 1950s. Medical therapy alone is almost uniformly unsuccessful in prosthetic valve or fungal endocarditis, and surgical intervention with valve replacement is mandatory for cure. Congestive heart failure is the major cause (47 to 55 per cent) of death in infective endocarditis today; some of these deaths are preventable by more aggressive surgical management. Other major causes of death are cerebral emboli (30 per cent of deaths), mycotic aneurysm rupture, and renal failure.

PHYSICAL EXAMINATION

Intermittent or remittent low-grade fever (38.3 to 38.8°C; 101 to 102°F) with nightly elevations is present in more than 90 per cent of cases of infective endocarditis. High fever ($\geq$ 39.5°C) is unusual and suggests an acute staphylococcal etiology. Fever may be absent in the elderly and if renal failure or congestive heart failure develops.

The cardiac examination will reveal an organic heart murmur in more than 90 per cent of patients with endocarditis and reflects the underlying valvular pathology and/or changes induced by the endocarditis process itself. Aortic and mitral murmurs are most common and may be associated with findings of congestive heart failure (e.g., rales, third heart sound). A changing murmur has been emphasized as of diagnostic importance but occurs in only 5 to 10 per cent of cases. These changing murmurs may reflect acute valvular destruction (especially with *S. aureus* endocarditis) or other factors (e.g., anemia) developing during the disease course. Tricuspid regurgitation may be present with right-sided endocarditis in drug addicts and may be accompanied by distended neck veins, a positive hepatojugular reflux, and hepatomegaly. Regurgitant murmurs in patients with prosthetic valve endocarditis usually reflect paraprosthetic leaks secondary to valve dehiscence.

Examination of the lungs may reveal the findings of congestive heart failure, especially with aortic valve involvement. Signs of consolidation or pleural involvement (e.g., effusion, friction rub) may be present due to pulmonary emboli or infarction in intravenous drug abusers with tricuspid valve endocarditis.

Splenomegaly occurs in 25 to 60 per cent of endocarditis patients and is most common with prolonged duration ($\geq$ 6 weeks) of disease. Splenic infarction or abscess due to emboli may result in pain and tenderness in the left upper quadrant, a splenic friction rub, or a left pleural effusion. Abdominal, flank, or back findings are highly variable, however, and reflect the potential for embolic infarction, hemorrhage, or abscess formation in virtually any organ or blood vessel.

Major cerebral emboli may result in aphasia, hemiplegia, sensory losses, ataxia, cranial nerve deficits, homonymous hemianopsia, or other focal neurologic signs. Cerebritis (especially with staphylococcal endocarditis), meningitis, abscess, or hemorrhage from rupture of a mycotic aneurysm may result in alterations in sensorium, confusion, delirium, coma, or meningeal signs. Funduscopic examination may reveal Roth's spots (oval, pale lesions surrounded by hemorrhage, usually near the disc) in 5 per cent of cases, retinal artery emboli, flame hemorrhages, or panophthalmitis with extension into the vitreous. None of these findings is specific for endocarditis.

The cutaneous manifestations of endocarditis, although relatively unusual findings at the present time, may be useful diagnostically. A livedo reticularis rash may be the only cutaneous sign seen in a few patients with endocarditis. Petechiae or purpura develops in 20 to 40 per cent of endocarditis cases and are found on the conjunctivae, buccal mucosa, palate, or distal extremities. Petechiae are red or purple, do not blanch on pressure, and may fade or become brown within several days. These lesions are due to capillary hemorrhage. *Osler's nodes* are firm, painful, raised, red-purple lesions 2 to 10 mm in the pads of the fingers or toes. These lesions typically appear and resolve within several days. The pathogenesis of Osler's nodes is controversial; in acute staphylococcal endocarditis they are of embolic origin, but the microscopic appearance in subacute streptococcal cases suggests a vasculitic process. *Janeway's lesions* are flat, macular, red or hemorrhagic painless areas usually found on the palms or soles. These lesions are embolic in origin with subcutaneous abscess formation and strongly suggest *S. aureus* as the etiologic agent. *Splinter hemorrhages* are linear pigmented streaks beneath the nail beds. Although commonly due to trauma, splinter hemorrhages are more suggestive of endocarditis if present in the proximal nail bed and are bright red, reflecting fresh hemorrhage. Clubbing of the digits, rarely seen in endocarditis patients today, reflects either long-standing disease or congenital heart disease as the underlying cardiac substrate leading to endocarditis as a complication.

This discussion has emphasized the presenting symptoms and signs of infective endocarditis. Many of these may develop after hospital admission, even in patients receiving appropriate therapy. The importance of daily examinations—especially cardiac, skin, and funduscopic—during hospitalization of patients with presumed endocarditis with incomplete evidence at admission cannot be overstressed.

COMMON COMPLICATIONS

The complications of infective endocarditis may be classified as intracardiac or extracardiac. Congestive heart failure is the most common complication and cause of morbidity and mortality in this disease. Heart failure may result from valvular insufficiency or obstruction due to the vegetation or perforation, or loss of supporting valvular structures. The abrupt onset of heart failure with aortic insufficiency and premature closure of the mitral valve requires urgent surgical intervention. Other intracardiac complications include myocardial infarction (embolic, thrombotic); myocardial or valve ring abscess with consequent arrhythmias, heart block, or valvular insufficiency; mycotic aneurysm of coronary arteries; sinus of Valsalva aneurysm; and rarely pericarditis, seen most commonly with staphylococcal or pneumococcal endocarditis.

The extracardiac complications of endocarditis may be divided between embolic or vasculitic origins. Emboli may be bland (noninfectious) or suppurative, may result in infarction with or without abscess formation, and may affect virtually any organ. The most common sites of embolic involvement are brain, lung (with right-sided endocarditis), spleen, skin, joints, and the peripheral arterial circulation. Large peripheral emboli are suggestive of a fungal etiology. Emboli to the vasa vasorum may result in the development of mycotic aneurysms in any blood vessel. Rupture of a cerebral mycotic aneurysm with subarachnoid and/or intracerebral hemorrhage is usually fatal.

In endocarditis of long duration, a hypocomplementemic vasculitis may ensue secondary to immune complex deposition. The most important manifestation of this process in endocarditis is renal failure with an active urinary sediment, but the vasculitis may also involve skin (with palpable purpura at times simulating thrombotic thrombocytopenic purpura), central nervous system, joints (with effusion), abdominal organs, and the myocardium.

As a result of the long treatment courses required for endocarditis, complications of antimicrobial therapy are encountered frequently. Superinfections with resistant bacteria or yeasts are common and treatment of bacterial endocarditis may be supplanted by the development of fungal endocarditis (usually *C. albicans*). Adverse reactions due to the beta-lactam antibiotic employed may include skin rash or other hypersensitivity phenomena, drug fever, interstitial nephritis, hemolytic anemia, diarrhea (with pseudomembranous colitis), and leukopenia. Nephrotoxicity and ototoxicity due to the aminoglycoside component of the usual treatment regimens are common and may be accentuated by the coadministration of vancomycin or a cephalosporin.

LABORATORY PROCEDURES

The most important laboratory procedure for the diagnosis of endocarditis is the blood culture. The bacteremia (or fungemia) of infective endocarditis is usually low-grade ($\leq$ 100 organisms per ml of blood), continuous, and persistent. Hence, if any blood culture is positive, all are usually positive. Three sets of properly timed blood cultures are usually sufficient for diagnosis. Persistently negative blood cultures are found in 5 to 10 per cent of endocarditis cases and are usually due to prior antimicrobial therapy or presence of fastidious microorganisms requiring special culture procedures (e.g., anaerobes, diphtheroids, *Hemophilus* sp., *Brucella* sp., fungi, or vitamin B_6—requiring streptococci). Blood cultures are rarely positive in fungal endocarditis except when of candidal etiology (approximately 50 per cent positive). The diagnosis of fungal endocarditis is often suggested after special stains and culture of large emboli removed surgically from peripheral blood vessels.

Various nonspecific hematologic abnormalities are documented commonly in infective endocarditis and include normocytic, normochromic anemia of chronic disease, usually with a hematocrit greater than 30 per cent (acute hemolytic anemia is seen rarely); a mild leukocytosis with a left shift (often with more than 15,000 cells per cu mm in acute suppurative endocarditis due to pyogenic cocci); thrombocytopenia secondary to destruction within an enlarged spleen or disseminated intravascular coagulation (unusual); and an elevated erythrocyte sedimentation rate. These manifestations resolve gradually with successful therapy.

Abnormalities of the urinary sediment are common in infective endocarditis and include proteinuria with microscopic hematuria (up to 60 per cent of patients); gross hematuria (rare); red blood cell or white blood cell casts; and significant bacteriuria, especially in enterococcal or staphylococcal disease. These manifestations may result from embolic renal infarction or abscess, focal glomerulitis, or immune complex–mediated glomerulonephritis. The latter lesion may result in renal failure (approximately 5 to 10 per cent of endocarditis cases overall), especially in patients with prolonged duration of the disease; the lesion resolves with successful therapy.

Because of the neurologic findings, the cerebrospinal fluid (CSF) is often examined in endocarditis patients. The CSF is usually sterile, but frank meningitis may be present with pneumococcal (and rarely, streptococcal) endocarditis. A polymorphonuclear leukocytosis, elevated protein, and decreased glucose in sterile CSF are typical findings in staphylococcal "cerebritis."

Serologic abnormalities are common in infective endocarditis but are usually not diagnostic. These include positive rheumatoid factor in 50 per cent of cases more than 6 weeks in duration; positive antinuclear factor (about 10 per cent of cases); false-positive serologic test for syphilis; hypocomplementemia in cases with immune complex–mediated glomerulonephritis; cryoglobulinemia in nearly 100 per cent of cases, usually without clinical manifestations; macroglobulinemia; hypergammaglobulinemia; and circulating immune complexes detected by the Raji cell assay. Antibodies to teichoic acid in *S. aureus* cell walls in a titer of greater than 1:4 by immunodiffusion are diagnostic of serious disease due to this organism, including endocarditis, osteomyelitis, or metastatic abscess formation. All of these serologic abnormalities should resolve with successful therapy; a rise in titer or reappearance may signify uncontrolled infection or relapse.

RADIOLOGICAL EVALUATION

The chest radiograph is rarely useful in the diagnosis of endocarditis. Right heart involvement with pulmonary emboli may cause scattered peripheral pulmonary infiltrates, pleural effusions, cavity formation, or pneumatoceles in acute staphylococcal infection. The plain chest radiograph may reveal findings of congestive heart failure or the underlying cardiac lesion (e.g., calcified mitral annulus).

When rupture of a mycotic aneurysm is suspected on clinical grounds, arteriography is indicated for precise localization prior to surgical intervention. An aortic root dye injection is done commonly in complicated cases prior to surgery to delineate the altered anatomy (e.g., valve ring or myocardial abscess, sinus of Valsalva aneurysm) accurately.

Various radionuclide scanning procedures are helpful occasionally. A brain scan or computed tomography may demonstrate cerebritis or brain abscess; abdominal abscesses may be revealed by liver-spleen scan or an abdominal ultrasound examination. Detection of intracardiac vegetations by gallium scan, ^{99m}technetium-labeled antistaphylococcal antibody, or ^{111}indium platelet deposition are promising techniques but are still experimental. "Pseudorelapses" with recurrent bacteremia may occur as a result of metastatic abscesses or osteomyelitis, especially in *S. aureus* infections. These metastatic deposits are occasionally detected by gallium scans.

OTHER DIAGNOSTIC PROCEDURES

Two-dimensional echocardiography is a very useful procedure in the diagnosis and therapy of infective endocarditis. This procedure may localize vegetations larger than 2 mm, estimate myocardial contractility and ejection fraction, detect significant valvular insufficiency before congestive heart failure supervenes, document premature closure of the mitral valve with severe aortic regurgitation, and gauge the therapeutic response. Some authors believe that echocardiographic demonstrable vegetations are a poor prognostic sign and serve as an indication for surgery; others disagree. Nevertheless, an enlarging vegetation on repeat echocardiographic examination during treatment, along with other clinical parameters, may indicate that early surgical intervention is necessary.

THERAPEUTIC TESTS

Routine disc sensitivities of antibiotics for the infecting organism are not adequate alone to determine the therapy of infective endocarditis. Quantitative determinations of the minimum inhibitory and minimum bactericidal concentrations (MIC, MBC) of candidate antibiotics against the patient's isolate by broth-dilution or other standard methods are mandatory in all cases to allow proper drug selection. Assays of antibiotic combinations for "synergism" are very helpful in enterococcal endocarditis or when an unusual organism (e.g., gram-negative bacilli or coccobacilli, diphtheroids) are isolated. Serum bactericidal titers should be measured to assure adequacy of therapy. The "peak" serum bactericidal titer, drawn 30 minutes after conclusion of intravenous infusion, should be maintained at a dilution of 1:8 or greater if possible. When aminoglycosides are employed in therapy, peak and trough serum levels of these compounds should be measured to minimize toxicity and to permit rational dosage alterations.

PITFALLS IN DIAGNOSIS

The most common error in the diagnosis of infective endocarditis is failure to consider and pursue this diagnosis. As noted, the manifestations of endocarditis are extremely protean; this disease must be considered in febrile patients with a poorly defined infectious focus (even in the absence of a significant heart murmur), especially in individuals who appear to have a multisystem disease. This diagnosis should be entertained in any patient with structural valvular disease who develops congestive heart failure or clinical deterioration, even if afebrile. An unexplained cerebrovascular event in a young individual or development of fever in an intravenous drug abuser should also suggest endocarditis, and prompt collection of blood cultures is necessary.

Although some authorities suggest that *S. aureus* bacteremia in patients with a removable intravascular focus of infection (e.g., intravenous catheters, shunts) may be treated with short courses of antibiotics for 10 to 14 days, this practice will not eradicate a coexistent endocarditis, which is commonly present in this setting. Unless endocarditis can be excluded with reasonable certainty, long-term therapy should be administered. Finally, endocarditis must be considered in any prosthetic valve recipient who develops fever, increasing hemolysis, or valvular dysfunction of any type.

CARDIOMYOPATHY

By W. Robert Meadows, M.D.
and John B. O'Connell, M.D.
Maywood, Illinois

SYNONYMS

The term cardiomyopathy has largely replaced such others as idiopathic cardiomegaly, myocardosis, and myocardiopathy—in the latter instance, probably because of greater ease in pronunciation. The term primary myocardial disease continues to be used but must be limited to idiopathic cardiomyopathy or some intrinsic disease of the myocardium not present in other organs. In recent years the separation of cardiomyopathies into congestive (or dilated), hypertrophic, and restrictive/obliterative has allowed for a greater precision of terminology by focusing on the most important characteristic of each of these different types.

DEFINITION

Cardiomyopathy is heart muscle disease that arises without relation to gross congenital malformations or the pressure or volume overload secondary to pulmonary or systemic hypertension, valvular disease, systemic arteriovenous fistula, or the left-to-right shunts of congenital heart disease.

The *congestive-dilated type* is most commonly idiopathic, but it is frequently associated with alcoholism and occasionally is peripartal in onset. Although necropsies and endocardial biopsies in the established case of the disease show only fibrosis and other nonspecific findings, some instances of acute myocarditis may evolve into this condition. Possibly viral in origin, the process may then persist as an autoimmune phenomenon. The congestive-dilated type, being the most common, will receive the most extensive discussion here. An etiologic classification is presented in Table 1; many of the entities listed in the table are rarely encountered.

Hypertrophic cardiomyopathy is characterized by small ventricular chambers and by an increase in muscle mass. The hypertrophy usually involves the septum to a greater extent than the remaining myocardium, but the concept of this disease also embraces *concentric* hypertrophy. Left ventricular outflow tract obstruction may or may not be present, or it may be induced by maneuvers or drugs that decrease the size of the left ventricular cavity. Left ventricular stiffness resulting from the hypertrophy gives rise to impairment of diastolic filling, and the resultant increase in pressure transmitted to the pulmonary veins is probably responsible for the dyspnea these patients experience. Chest pain, frequently indistinguishable from angina pectoris, occurs and may be the result of inadequate oxygenation of the increased myocardial mass by coronary arteries of normal caliber or the subendocardial ischemia resulting from impaired diastolic relaxation. Syncope and dizziness are other important symptoms. But there may be no symptoms, and the condition may be discovered on the echocardiogram of an asymptomatic relative of a patient with known disease.

Physical findings include a systolic murmur whose intensity may decrease on squatting and increase on standing (maneuvers altering the left ventricular dimensions and thus the outflow tract obstruction). The murmur is heard at the left lower sternal border and the apex and is not transmitted to the carotids. The pulse is bifid, and the apical thrust may be double, because of a presystolic component, or triple, the third component occurring with the bulge resulting from the outflow tract obstruction. This type of cardiomyopathy may be associated with lentiginosis, Friedreich's ataxia, and possibly pheochromocytoma and neurofibromatosis.

Also infrequently seen is the restrictive type. This is most frequently due to amyloid infiltration of the myocardium or endomyocardial fibrosis with or without eosinophilia, but it is also seen in some cases of hemochromatosis, sarcoidosis, or myocardial fibrosis of any etiology. Systolic function may be maintained in the presence of impairment of diastolic filling, in

Table 1. Etiologic Classification of Cardiomyopathies

Idiopathic
Infective (Inflammatory)
- Viral
  - Enteroviruses (Coxsackie, ECHO, polio)
  - Arbovirus (dengue)
  - Herpesviruses (varicella, cytomegalovirus)
  - Paramyxoviruses (mumps)
  - Orthomyxoviruses (influenza)
  - Poxviruses (variola and vaccinia)
- Rickettsial (Rocky Mountain spotted fever, typhus, Q fever)
- Bacterial (*Corynebacterium diphtheriae*)
- Fungal (*Cryptococcus neoformans, Candida albicans*)
- Protozoal (*Toxoplasma gondii, Trypanosoma cruzi*)
- Metazoal (*Schistosoma mansoni, Trichinella spiralis*)
- *Mycoplasma pneumoniae*

Endocrine
- Hyperthyroidism and hypothyroidism
- Pheochromocytoma
- Acromegaly

Nutritional and Other Deficiencies
- Beri-beri
- Kwashiorkor
- Hypophosphatemia
- Hypokalemia
- Selenium deficiency

Metabolic and Storage Diseases
- Diabetes mellitus
- Hemochromatosis
  - Idiopathic
  - Acquired (multiple transfusions, excessive iron intake)
- Glycogen storage disease
- Glycolipid deposition (Fabry's disease)
- Mucopolysaccharidosis (Gargoylism)
- Glycosyl ceramide deposition (Gaucher's disease)
- Gangliosidosis (Tay-Sachs disease)

Connective Tissue Disorders
- Systemic lupus erythematosus
- Polyarteritis nodosa
- Rheumatoid arthritis
- Progressive systemic sclerosis
- Polymyositis-dermatomyositis

Infiltrative
- Amyloidosis
- Sarcoidosis
- Neoplastic

Drugs, Toxins, Hypersensitivity
- Chronic alcoholism
- Anthracyclines
- Cobalt
- Methylsergide
- Lithium
- Tricyclic antidepressants
- Emetine
- Arsenic
- Solvent abuse (Trichloroethylene)
- Sulfonamides
- Methyldopa
- Penicillin
- Irradiation

Muscular Dystrophies and Neuromuscular Disorders
- Progressive muscular dystrophies
  - Pseudohypertrophic (Duchenne's), limb-girdle, and facioscapulohumeral types
- Myotonic muscular dystrophy
- Friedreich's ataxia

Miscellaneous Unclassified
- Ischemia
- Peripartal
- Endomyocardial fibrosis

contrast to dilated cardiomyopathy, in which systolic function is impaired.

PRESENTING SYMPTOMS AND SIGNS OF CONGESTIVE-DILATED CARDIOMYOPATHY

The onset of symptoms of congestive failure may be insidious or abrupt. Usually left heart failure appears first and is followed later by signs of right heart failure. Very occasionally, failure manifestations are right-sided only. It is not unusual for the patient to state that he has had a "cold" some weeks before the appearance of more definite symptoms of left heart failure. Although the patient may have had an upper respiratory tract infection, it is equally possible that the initial symptoms of left heart failure have been interpreted as a "cold" by the patient. Paroxysmal nocturnal dyspnea and orthopnea are prominent symptoms, sometimes occurring before the patient is aware of exertional dyspnea. A nonproductive cough occurring or worsening at night is a further complaint. The patient may state that he is unable to sleep in bed and must sit up in a chair all night in order to breathe.

Pulmonary crepitations may or may not be present at this stage, and the chest x-ray may show surprisingly clear lung fields. Sinus tachycardia, particularly in the younger patients, is usually present, but atrial fibrillation occurs in a minority. A gallop rhythm is a characteristic finding. While tachycardia persists, it may not be possible to decide whether the gallop sound is in early diastole or is presystolic. In fact, as the rate slows with treatment, one may be able to hear both an S_3 and an S_4, and it then can be assumed that the earlier finding was a summation gallop. The eventual appearance of a systolic murmur may be due to papillary muscle dysfunction and/or dilation of the mitral annulus. The latter, however, is usually only mild. The lack of an increase in intensity of the murmur in the beat following a premature beat is evidence that it is mitral or tricuspid in origin and not aortic. If atrial fibrillation is present, changing cycle lengths will again have no effect on the intensity of the murmur. Murmurs often disappear with treatment, and this is probably secondary to the decrease in ventricular dilatation.

The apical impulse may not be well localized, and there may be precordial hyperactivity reminiscent of the right ventricular volume overload of atrial septal defect. This apparently is due to the abutment of the dilated heart against the chest wall. In other instances, a well-localized apical thrust displaced to the left is palpated. A presystolic impulse, particularly in the left lateral position, is commonly felt. This may occur even when the concomitant S_4 is too low-pitched to be heard. Jugular venous pulsations with the patient at 45 degrees or more should be sought. These can be seen best by allowing an interplay of shadows across the neck.

In a minority of patients the blood pressure will exceed 140/90 when first seen, and the question of a hypertensive etiology will arise. This can be best resolved if there is sufficient documentation of blood pressure readings in the past. Hypertension, either the result of or the cause of congestive failure, tends to fall with bed rest and diuretics. If it recurs in the post-hospital convalescence while the patient is out of failure, it obviously is most likely not the result of failure. The "high pressure stasis" of congestive failure was noted long ago by Sahli (1901), and we know no more today why this occurs in some patients and not in others than physicans of his day. Moreover, in an occasional patient no consensus will be reached as to whether it is cause or effect even at autopsy.

When sought for, pulsus alternans will frequently be detected at some time during the course of the disease. Since this phenomenon is best demonstrated by lowering the left ventricular filling pressure, it may first appear during convalescence. Topical nitroglycerin seems to bring this finding out probably by the mechanism described. Patients should be sitting or standing while being examined for this sign.

A dicrotic pulse is a common accompaniment of this disease. If not palpated (at the brachial artery), it may be demonstrated by direct pressure recording especially if distal occlusive pressure is applied. It is related to the low stroke output as well as the distensible, compliant arterial system found in younger subjects.

COURSE

The course is variable and unpredictable. Some patients have a rapidly downhill course, others linger on for years with recurrent bouts of failure. In some, especially those with a peripartal onset, further episodes of failure do not occur, and recovery by clinical criteria is complete. Similarly, those patients with an alcoholic history will often have a prolonged remission and probable cure if they stop drinking. During remissions the heart size as shown on x-ray is likely to decrease sometimes to normal, only to enlarge again with the onset of another episode of failure. This observation has been called the "accordion heart." Each exacerbation tends to become longer and each remission shorter until finally the patient dies of congestive failure.

A minority of patients will complain of chest pain during the course of their illness. Although usually atypical for such, in some this will be indistinguishable from angina pectoris. Others will have epigastric pain which appears to be related in some unknown way to the left heart failure but may possibly be secondary to acute distention of the liver.

Atrial and ventricular arrhythmias are common, and a significant number of patients will develop atrial fibrillation. Life-threatening ventricular arrhythmias are not usually a problem but may dominate the clinical picture in a small minority. Death is sudden in about 30 per cent.

COMPLICATIONS

Systemic and pulmonary emboli occur in about 20 per cent of cases and arise from the mural thrombi commonly found in the ventricles and atrial appendages at autopsy. Peripheral venous thrombosis, as in any type of congestive failure, is the most likely source of pulmonary emboli. Emboli may occur very early in the course of the disease, and, when systemic, may rarely so dominate the clinical picture as to divert the attention of the physician away from the heart to some other organ.

CHEST X-RAY

The cardiac silhouette at the time of onset of symptoms may show little or no enlargement, but with well-established symptoms and signs cardiomegaly without selective chamber enlargement will be present. The aortic knob will be conspicuously small for the size of the cardiac shadow. Congestive changes in the lung fields may or may not be prominent.

ELECTROCARDIOGRAPHY

The electrocardiogram (ECG) is almost always abnormal. Left ventricular hypertrophy and left bundle branch block are the most frequent findings. Left bundle branch block occurs more frequently in dilated cardiomyopathy than it does in atherosclerotic heart disease. Deep T wave inversion, in some patients suggestive of subendocardial ischemia, may revert to normal in those patients who recover from their disease. Q waves suggestive of myocardial infarction occasionally are seen. In amyloidosis, low voltage and a small or absent R in V_{1-3} are characteristic findings. Myocardial sarcoidosis occasionally gives rise to Q waves as a reflection of fibrosis and granulomatous infiltration.

ECHOCARDIOGRAPHY

Echocardiography reflects the characteristic features of dilated cardiomyopathy, of which atrial and ventricular dilatation and poor wall motion are the most prominent. The mitral echoes are in a midposition from the septum and posterior wall in a chamber with both increased diastolic and systolic dimensions. The distance of the anterior leaflet to the septum at its maximal early diastolic opening (E point-septal separation) is increased. The separation of the anterior and posterior leaflets during diastole is decreased, as is the rate of opening of the anterior leaflet. Both are reflections of the decreased flow through the valve. The normally smooth line reflecting systolic anterior leaflet closure is interrupted by a notch (the B point) just prior to ventricular contraction. This is a sign of poor left ventricular function and often an elevated left ventricular end diastolic pressure. The posterior wall measurement provides evidence for the presence or absence of left ventricular hypertrophy. Two-dimensional echocardiography has the added ability of demonstrating segmental wall motion abnormalities that may be present occasionally in cardiomyopathy but that are more suggestive of coronary disease. Mural thrombi may also be picked up by this method.

Restrictive cardiomyopathies are characterized by thickening of the interventricular septum and the posterior and right ventricular walls. The E-F slope of the anterior leaflet of the mitral valve may be decreased, a reflection of the increased stiffness of the left ventricle. The diastolic dimension of the left ventricular cavity is normal or reduced, and the motion and systolic thickening of the septum and frequently the posterior wall are decreased, as is the systolic-diastolic change in dimension. The atria may be enlarged secondary to the decreased diastolic compliance of the ventricles. Two-dimensional echocardiography of amyloid cardiomyopathy further reveals striking "granular sparkling" appearance of the echoes reflected from the amyloid in the ventricular myocardium. In addition, it demonstrates in some instances thickening of the interatrial septum, papillary muscles, and valves.

RADIOISOTOPIC IMAGING

Radionuclide ventriculography is a noninvasive tool that supplements the echocardiogram providing the clinician with an estimate of ventricular size, a reproducible ejection fraction, and a qualitative assessment of segmental wall motion of the left ventricle. At first it seemed that this would be an ideal diagnostic tool to separate instances of ischemic cardiomyopathy with segmental wall motion abnormalities from other types of congestive-dilated cardiomyopathies with uniform decrease in wall motion. However, segmental wall motion abnormalities are now recognized as occurring with nonischemic cardiomyopathy. Also of some value is the wall motion of the anterobasal segment. This is reduced in congestive-dilated cardiomyopathy and frequently normal in the ischemic variety. The addition of supine bicycle exercise to radionuclide angiography may improve diagnostic accuracy. Some individuals with non-ischemic cardiomyopathy will have an increase in the ejection fraction with exercise, but others (without coronary disease) will have a decrease, as in those with coronary disease. Thus, radionuclide ventriculography has limited usefulness in the differentiation of these two types of congestive-dilated cardiomyopathy except when a definite aneurysm is found.

The same is true for ^{201}thallium imaging during exercise. Here again, both types may show one or more perfusion defects. These are most frequently reversible in nonischemic disease, but fixed defects are also found. However, these fixed defects are likely to exceed 40 per cent of the outer left ventricular perimeter in ischemic cardiomyopathy and to be less than that in nonischemic disease. Also, reverse redistribution perfusion defects, in which the perfusion abnormality first appears or gets much worse on reimaging 3 to 4 hours later, may be a phenomenon limited to some cases of ischemic disease. The cause of perfusion defects in cardiomyopathy is not known. In some instances, fixed defects may be due to myocardial fibrosis or the granulomata of sarcoid.

Radionuclide ventriculography finds its greatest usefulness in the serial determination of ejection fractions in the follow-up of potentially reversible cardiomyopathy (e.g., alcoholic and peripartal) and in those undergoing specific therapy, as well as confirming clinical impressions in the general management of these cases.

SPECIFIC CARDIOMYOPATHIES

Special mention is made of cardiac amyloidosis, sarcoidosis, hemochromatosis, and inflammatory cardiomyopathy. Cardiac amyloidosis is a disease of the older age group, being uncommon below the age of 45. The clinical picture may be that of biventricular congestive failure or, if the restrictive defect dominates, may more closely resemble constrictive pericarditis. Differentiation from the latter is important so as to avoid a thoracotomy in anticipation of a pericardiectomy. Chest pain may resemble angina pectoris. The restrictive aspects will be picked up by echocardiography and radionuclide ventricular angiography. ^{99m}Technetium pyrophosphate imaging of the myocardium shows dense diffuse uptake in patients with cardiac amyloidosis. The sensitivities and specificities of this test are unknown. However, it appears to be a promising screening test for the detection of myocardial amyloid. Biopsy of various tissues, of which the rectal wall has been the most useful, will make the diagnosis. However, it is even better to do endomyocardial biopsy, since occasionally amyloidosis is limited to the heart. Various arrhythmias and conduction defects are common, particularly in the presence of digitalis. Congestive failure is relentless, and death usually occurs 1 to 2 years after the onset of symptoms.

Cardiac sarcoidosis may present as congestive cardiomyopathy in the apparent absence of sarcoid elsewhere. It is likely to be considered idiopathic under these circumstances. ^{201}Thallium perfusion imaging of the myocardium in patients with sarcoidosis consistently shows irreversible perfusion defects that cannot be discriminated from ischemic or idiopathic cardiomyopathic heart disease. Endomyocardial biopsy may or may not demonstrate sarcoid. The granulomas have a predilection for the cephalad portion of the ventricular septum, and complete heart block occurs in a significant minority of cases. Ventricular arrhythmias occur, the clinical course is typically short, and death is frequently sudden. It is not unusual for these cases to develop a ventricular aneurysm.

Although commonly associated, congestive failure due to hemochromatosis can occur in the absence of diabetes, pigmentation of the skin, and hepatomegaly. Cardiac involvement is most likely to occur in the younger patient, liver disease in the older patient. In early stages, a restrictive pattern may be noted on echocardiography, but later a dilated cardiomyopathy is likely to develop. Atrial arrhythmias are common, atrioventricular block and left ventricular arrhythmias less so. The clinical course is short. Repeated phlebotomies may favorably alter the somber prognosis. When the diagnosis is suspected, serum iron, iron-binding capacity, and ferritin values should be obtained. All will be elevated. Endomyocardial biopsy may make the diagnosis. In the absence of facilities for the latter, liver biopsy will be the most useful test. These patients are frequently HLA-B8 positive.

Persistent inflammation following viral infection has been purported to cause the clinical syndrome of congestive-dilated cardiomyopathy, but until recently only indirect lines of evidence supported these claims. These included high titers of enteroviral antibodies in cardiomyopathic patients and the increased incidence of congestive-dilated cardiomyopathy on follow-up of patients who recovered from acute viral myocarditis. With the advent of safe techniques of endomyocardial biopsy, this diagnosis can now be confirmed during life and immunosuppressive treatment may be initiated for this reversible lesion. The incidence of unsuspected myocarditis in patients with congestive-dilated cardiomyopathy has been reported as high as 25 per cent. Inflammation-avid isotopic screening with ^{67}gallium imaging may be used to select a subset of congestive-dilated cardiomyopathic patients who are likely to have inflammation on biopsy. Although elevated serum creatine phosphokinase, acute phase reactants, and audible pericardial friction rubs are common during acute viral myocarditis, these abnormalities do not occur with this chronic, more indolent phase of the disease. A defect in lymphocyte suppressor cell function may be detected in the laboratory but will not separate patients with active inflammation from those whose inflammatory process has "burned-out." In some centers, therefore, ^{67}gallium scanning and endomyocardial biopsy are part of the routine diagnostic evaluation in patients with congestive-dilated cardiomyopathy.

PITFALLS IN DIAGNOSIS

Ischemic cardiomyopathy can be confused with other types of dilated cardiomyopathy. Both may or may not have chest pain; both may or may not have pathologic Q waves on ECG. On therapeutic grounds it would not be profitable to attempt to distinguish between them if it were not for the possibility of a ventricular aneurysm or highly obstructive left main coronary artery disease causing the congestive failure. Both are indications for surgery. Usually a ventricular aneurysm is recognized by characteristic ECG findings, chest x-ray, echocardiography, or radionuclide ventriculography. An exercise stress test suggests left main coronary artery disease, but the ST segment depression is not always marked. It would appear, then, that the greatest assurance that one is not dealing with one of these conditions can be had by left ventricular and coronary angiography as soon as possible after the onset of congestive failure.

Mitral valve disease is suggested by the apical systolic murmur that is frequently present. Likewise, the summation gallop may be confused with the diastolic rumble of mitral stenosis. With treatment early in the clinical course of the disease, the heart rate is likely to slow down to normal and the heart size frequently decreases. Under these circumstances, the summation gallop becomes an S_3 and an S_4 and the systolic murmur decreases in intensity or disappears. This sequence of events does not occur with intrinsic valvular disease. Echocardiography is especially useful in ruling out calcification or thickening of the valve, mitral valve prolapse, and ruptured chordae tendineae. Radionuclide ventriculography also assists in the differentiation, since most cases of dilated cardiomyopathy will have ejection fractions below 25 per cent whereas mitral regurgitation due to intrinsic valve disease will have ejection fractions above 40 per cent.

Aortic stenosis with severe failure is frequently misinterpreted as dilated cardiomyopathy. The cardiac enlargement and subdued murmur secondary to the low cardiac output are the misleading features. It is important to have an index of suspicion for this possibility because some of these patients are salvageable with skilled surgery. Echocardiography or the finding of calcium in the aortic valve on fluoroscopy will be confirmatory, making it obvious that cardiac catheterization for a precise diagnosis is imperative.

A large pericardial effusion, especially if symptomatic because of tamponade, may be confused with dilated cardiomyopathy. Echocardiography readily demonstrates the epicardial-pericardial separation that is present.

PERICARDITIS

By John H. Edmonds, Jr., M.D.
Brian D. Steg, M.D.
and W. Kenneth Haisty, Jr., M.D.
Winston-Salem, North Carolina

Pericarditis is an inflammation of the visceral and parietal pericardium, the enveloping membranes of the heart. Inflammatory reactions may be fibrinous, serofibrinous, hemorrhagic, or purulent. The clinical course may be acute or chronic, and pericarditis may result from a specific infection or some other disease or condition (Table 1). Acute idiopathic pericarditis occurs most frequently and is usually uncomplicated, but relapses may occur. The clinical incidence is lower than the necropsy incidence, since some cases have few symptoms and are undiagnosed. In addition to signs of acute inflammation, pericardial effusion may develop with or without cardiac compression (tamponade), and a few cases may proceed to chronic pericardial constriction.

Table 1. Important Etiologies of Pericarditis

Acute idiopathic (benign, nonspecific)
Infections (viral, bacterial, tuberculous, associated with bacterial endocarditis, fungal, parasitic, rickettsial)
Neoplasms (metastatic and primary)
Trauma
Metabolic disorders (uremia, myxedema, hypoalbuminemia)
Connective tissue diseases (rheumatic fever, rheumatoid arthritis, lupus erythematosus, scleroderma)
Diseases of the heart and adjoining structures (acute myocardial infarction, Dressler's syndrome, postpericardiotomy syndrome, dissecting aortic aneurysm, esophageal diseases, pulmonary diseases)
Drug reactions (anticoagulants, procainamide, hydralazine)
Miscellaneous (cardiac surgery, radiation, pacemaker lead perforation, cardiac catheterization)

SYMPTOMS

Sharp chest pain is the primary symptom of acute pericarditis and is almost always increased by inspiration. Location is usually substernal but may include the supraclavicular area, shoulder, or back. The pain may be mild, moderate, or severe, lasting several days, or it may last longer without therapy. Characteristically, the pain is lessened by sitting up and may be increased with coughing or swallowing. Anxiety and a sensation of dyspnea may occur with the increased pain on inspiration. However, true dyspnea does not occur without effusion and some degree of cardiac compression. Other general symptoms may occur related either to the inflammatory process or associated disease.

SIGNS

A three-component pericardial friction rub is pathognomonic of acute pericarditis, but it may be evanescent and overlooked without repeated auscultation in different positions. It has a grating or scratchy quality, may wax and wane, and is heard best with the diaphragm of the stethoscope. The rub is usually loudest at the left mid-to-lower sternal border but may be heard over the entire precordium. Showing slight respiratory variation, the rub may be distinguished from murmurs by its superficial and scratchy quality and by three distinct components that coincide with ventricular systole, ventricular diastole, and atrial systole. Patients with atrial fibrillation show only a two-component rub, since the atrial component is missing. If the pleura is involved, a pleuropericardial rub may be heard. Other physical signs related to associated diseases occur.

DIAGNOSTIC TESTS

The electrocardiogram (ECG) is the most helpful laboratory test and characteristically evolves in a four-stage pattern. Stage 1 shows concave ST segment elevation in most leads except AVR, and sometimes V_1, without reciprocal changes. PR segments may be depressed, mainly in limb leads. The ST segments return to the baseline during stage 2. Stage 3 shows T wave inversion resembling diffuse myocardial ischemia. Stage 4 shows a return to normal. The electrocardiogram may be atypical in some cases, depending on the time of recording. Also, normal variant electrocardiograms showing "early repolarization" may occasionally be confused with stage 1 changes. The leukocyte count and erythrocyte sedimentation rate may be normal or slightly increased. Cardiac enzymes are negative. Chest x-ray and echocardiogram are normal unless pericardial effusion or an associated cardiac disorder is present.

DIFFERENTIAL DIAGNOSIS

Major differential diagnoses include acute myocardial infarction and pleuritis. Less commonly, acute pulmonary embolism and dissecting aortic aneurysm may present diagnostic problems. Usually careful evaluation plus cardiac enzymes, chest x-ray, arterial blood gases, pulmonary scan, and echocardiogram will establish the diagnosis.

PERICARDIAL EFFUSION AND TAMPONADE

Pericardial effusion may occur with any of the etiologies listed in Table 1. Small effusions may result in few if any symptoms. Large effusions, or those that accumulate rapidly, may produce symptoms and life-threatening cardiac compression (tamponade).

Symptoms, Pathophysiology, and Etiologies

The patient may be asymptomatic or may have symptoms related to the associated disease or to pressure on adjacent structures, i.e., precordial discomfort, tachypnea, dyspnea, or cough. Cardiac compression, or tamponade, occurs when the effusion accumulates rapidly enough to interfere with ventricular filling. When pericardial pressure approaches or is equal to right atrial pressure, ventricular filling is decreased, leading to a decreased cardiac output, a fall in blood pressure, and eventually shock. Important causes of cardiac tamponade are breast carcinoma, lung carcinoma, uremia, chronic dialysis, trauma, cardiac rupture, dissecting aortic aneurysm, and rarely (during cardiac catheterization or with a pacemaker lead) perforation.

Signs

Pericardial effusion due to inflammation is usually associated with a rub, while effusion due to other causes may not cause a rub. With small to moderate effusions, neck venous pulsations, heart sounds, heart rate, and percussion of cardiac dullness are all normal. With large effusions, neck veins are distended, heart rate is increased, heart sounds are decreased, and cardiac dullness is increased. An increase in central venous pressure is the initial result of cardiac compression and can be recognized by examination of the neck veins in most patients. Rarely, Kussmaul's sign, an inspiratory increase in venous pressure, may be present. Pulsus paradoxus, an inspiratory drop in the blood pressure greater than 10 mm Hg, can be detected by careful sphygmomanometry. Intra-arterial pressure monitoring, when feasible, is more accurate and suitable for repeated determinations. Thus, patients with cardiac compression have distended neck veins, increased heart rate, muffled heart sounds, a drop in blood pressure, and a paradoxical pulse. Third heart sounds are almost never present.

Diagnostic Tests

The ECG shows low-voltage, nonspecific ST and T changes, and low-grade sinus tachycardia. If tamponade develops, the QRS, T, and P waves may show direction changes on alternate beats, i.e., electrical alternans. Chest x-ray may show a globular-shaped cardiac silhouette enlargement with clear lung fields. A minimum of 250 ml of pericardial fluid is required to produce the chest x-ray changes.

Echocardiography is a safe, easy, sensitive test that can readily demonstrate the presence of pericardial fluid even when only 25 to 50 ml are present. The pericardial sac is a potential space that may fill with echo-free fluid. The fluid causes echocardiographic separation between the mobile left ventricular wall and the immobile posterior pericardium as well as between the anterior right ventricular wall and the chest wall. Both M-mode and two-dimensional (2D) echocardiography are excellent techniques, but 2D is more accurate and is particularly useful with loculated effusions. Excessive cardiac movement, "the swinging heart," can be observed on 2D echo with large effusions. When paradoxical pulse is present, the interventricular septum may be seen to move into the left ventricle during inspiration, thus reducing left ventricular dimensions and associated cardiac output.

On occasion, radioisotopic scans may aid in detecting pericardial effusions.

Aspiration of pericardial fluid may be necessary for fluid analysis or relief of tamponade. This procedure has risk and should be done only by experienced personnel in the operating room, coronary care unit, or catheterization laboratory. Careful monitoring of the exploring needle by ECG or echo is necessary. Opinions still differ as to whether needle approach or surgical approach is better. Surgical approaches are safe and offer the additional advantage of obtaining tissue biopsies. The procedure of choice will vary with individuals and institutions.

Course

The type of associated disease determines the course. Pericarditis due to inflammation can resolve with proper diagnosis and treatment. Patients with neoplasms, uremia, and other serious disorders have poorer prognoses and require careful, frequent evaluations.

CHRONIC CONSTRICTIVE PERICARDITIS

An uncommon sequel to acute pericarditis is fibrosis, calcification, and thickening of pericardial layers producing chronic constriction. This may follow any type of acute pericarditis, usually developing slowly over a period of years. Often the primary cause is unknown with no antecedent history, making diagnosis difficult. Likely causes are specific infections, trauma, connective tissue diseases and radiation therapy.

Symptoms

Dyspnea, abdominal swelling, and edema are the most frequent symptoms. Less common symptoms are fatigue, cough, and orthopnea.

Signs

Elevated venous pressure is present in all cases and can be suspected by careful evaluation of the neck veins, which shows the elevated pressure, a rapid Y descent, and perhaps an increase in the venous pulse during inspiration. Hepatomegaly is present in the majority of cases, with ascites and peripheral edema almost as common. Pleural effusion, a small paradoxical arterial pulse, and pericardial knock are noted less frequently. The pericardial knock is a high-frequency diastolic sound occurring 0.06 to 0.10 seconds after the aortic component of the second heart sound and is thought to be due to the sudden cessation of rapid ventricular filling. Friction rubs are rare.

Diagnostic Tests

The ECG usually shows low-voltage and nonspecific ST-T changes. Atrial fibrillation is present in 25 per cent of patients. Intra-atrial conduction defects are common. Ventricular hypertrophy and bundle branch blocks suggest other diagnoses.

On chest x-ray the heart size may be small, normal, or slightly increased. Pericardial calcification encircles the heart in 50 per cent of patients. Pleural effusions are common, but pulmonary congestion is uncommon. Cardiac fluoroscopy may show decreased cardiac pulsations and pericardial calcifications.

The diagnosis usually can be confirmed by cardiac catheterization. The right atrial pressure is always elevated exceeding 9 mm Hg with deep X and Y descents occuring in the right atrial pressure pulse. Systolic pressure in the right ventricle is normal or slightly elevated. Right ventricle and left ventricle end-diastolic pressures, pulmonary artery diastolic pressure, and mean right atrial and left atrial pressures all tend to be equal. The square root sign is present in the right ventricle and left ventricle pressure pulses in most cases. A fluid volume challenge has been reported to help distinguish myocardial disease from occult constrictive pericardial disease.

Echocardiography is helpful in excluding other diagnoses. There is no specific pattern in constrictive pericarditis, although abnormal ventricular septal motion and pericardial thickening have been observed in some patients.

Differential Diagnosis

Restrictive cardiomyopathy, hepatic cirrhosis, cor pulmonale, occult left heart disease, and tricuspid valvular disease may be confused with constrictive pericarditis. A computed tomographic (CT) scan may help distinguish constrictive pericarditis from restrictive cardiomyopathy. Difficult diagnostic problems can usually be resolved with cardiac catheterization. Rarely, surgical exploration may be necessary.

Here are some diagnostic pointers:

1. Characteristic chest pain, friction rub, and ECG changes will establish the diagnosis of acute pericarditis in most cases.
2. The normal variant ECG showing "early repolarization" may be confused with stage 1 ECG changes.
3. Pericardial effusion is readily recognized by echocardiography.
4. Any patient with pericardial effusion should be monitored carefully for possible development of cardiac tamponade.
5. Constrictive pericarditis should be considered in all patients with chronically increased jugular venous pressure.

ANEURYSMS OF THE AORTA

By Helen C. Redman, M.D.
Dallas, Texas

Aneurysms are a life-threatening form of cardiovascular disease. As the population enjoys a longer life, the number of atherosclerotic aneurysms increases. Mycotic, traumatic, and dissecting aneurysms with their rather high morbidity and mortality continue to occur, and there is no reason to anticipate a decline in their inciting events. Full diagnostic evaluation of any aneurysm will help to ensure proper surgical or medical management. The diagnostic approach for all types of aneurysms has undergone significant change in the last decade. New techniques with low morbidity such as ultrasound and computed tomography have been developed. Digital angiography has become a useful approach.

DEFINITION

An aneurysm is defined as a focal dilatation of an artery or vein. This definition is somewhat misleading, since aneurysms are often fusiform and not discrete, and dissecting aneurysms may not dilate the aorta beyond its original dimensions. *True aneurysms* involve the entire vascular wall, and at least one of these layers must be intact. Atherosclerosis is the most frequent cause of true aneurysms, though acute or chronic infection or degenerative vascular disease such as cystic medial necrosis can also cause true aneurysms. *False* or *pseudoaneurysms* have a wall of perivascular, vascular, or adventitial tissue and are usually traumatic in origin. Deceleration injury to the thoracic aorta can produce a false aneurysm just distal to the left subclavian artery where a traumatic laceration frequently occurs. *Dissecting aneurysms,* the third major category, are caused by a tear in the intima, allowing blood to dissect into the medial layer of the aortic wall. Dissections may be focal but are more often extensive. Dissecting aneurysms usually occur in patients with long-standing hypertension or medial cystic necrosis. Trauma is another cause of dissection, which may present in an unusual fashion, since the dissection can be isolated to a small part of the aorta and can originate anywhere.

Aneurysms of all types can be found throughout the thoracic and lumbar aorta. The most common occurrence is development of an atherosclerotic aneurysm of the abdominal aorta between the origin of the renal arteries and the aortic bifurcation. Nearly three quarters of all aortic aneurysms occur in this location. Abdominal aneurysms involving the origins of the celiac, superior mesenteric, or renal arteries do occur but are uncommon. Similarly, aneurysms extending both above and below the diaphragm are rare. More frequently, a widened thoracolumbar aorta is part of a diffuse atherosclerotic ectasia of the entire vascular bed. Purely thoracic aneurysms are the second most common group of atherosclerotic aneurysms, accounting for about one quarter of aortic aneurysms. These occur throughout the thoracic aorta but are most commonly seen near the arch.

Dissecting aneurysms should be considered separately from other aneurysms because their appearance, symptomatology, usual causes, diagnosis, and therapy are all specific to dissection. Dissecting aneurysms are generally classified by point of origin and extent. Though there are several classifications in the literature, the one proposed by DeBakey in 1965 has found the greatest acceptance. In his scheme, Type I dissection starts at the aortic root and extends across the aortic arch into the descending aorta. It may extend into the iliac arteries. Type I is a common form of dissection. Type II is limited to the ascending aorta and, except in Marfan's syndrome, is uncommon. Type III begins in the descending thoracic aorta just beyond the origin of the left subclavian artery and extends distally. It may also involve the iliac arteries. In addition to these three types, trauma may cause a focal dissection anywhere along the aorta. Nontraumatic dissections occasionally will originate at a point quite distal to the left subclavian artery.

PRESENTING SIGNS AND SYMPTOMS

Atherosclerotic aneurysms are generally asymptomatic and are therefore incidental findings until they become large enough to press on a vital structure causing pain, nerve dysfunction, or obstruction or until they are leaking. The location of the aneurysm will determine the type of symptoms that occur. Pain, especially acute pain, is an alarming development, since it raises the question of rapid expansion, leakage, or impending rupture. Thoracic aneurysms produce a deep ache or pain in the upper back that may have a insidious or abrupt onset. Leaking abdominal aneurysms cause either abdominal pain or lower back pain, which is generally severe. Though aneurysms may rupture without warning, more often they leak before frank rupture occurs. Attention to early symptoms may permit successful reparative surgery to take place. Surgery is much more difficult when the patient is hypotensive and bleeding massively.

Mycotic aneurysms usually occur in patients with a known septicemia. Intravenous drug abusers, for example, develop these lesions. Mycotic aneurysms are fast-growing and have a significant potential for rupture. The septic course of the patient will often obscure symptoms of a developing mycotic aneurysm.

Dissecting aneurysms also present with pain that is often described as searing or tearing. The pain usually radiates to the back and may change as the dissection progresses. Symptoms may also be caused by occlusion of branch vessels or hemorrhage into the pleural space or retroperitoneum.

COURSE AND COMMON COMPLICATIONS

If untreated, virtually all aneurysms will progress to rupture with exsanguination. The time course is highly variable and unpredictable. Mycotic aneurysms tend to progress rapidly and can rupture within days of their onset. Dissecting aneurysms may decompress by developing enough re-entry sites to stop progression spontaneously, but more often they increase in length and size, eventually either rupturing or occluding the branch arteries. Atherosclerotic aneurysms develop much more slowly and may remain unchanged for months or years. The more fusiform atherosclerotic aneurysm can present as a dilated aorta for years before it can legitimately be called an aneurysm. Likelihood of rupture is related to size and probably also to rapidity of enlargement. Aneurysms over 10 cm in diameter are at extremely high risk of rupture, whereas those over 7 cm are at significant risk. Definable saccular aneurysms greater than 4 or 5 cm in diameter generally should be evaluated for potential surgical repair.

DIAGNOSIS

Most aneurysms are discovered during evaluation for other reasons. Thoracic aneurysms are seen on routine chest films, or a pulsatile mass may be felt in the abdomen during a physical examination. Confirmation of the initial diagnostic idea can be reached in several ways. Added studies may be needed if surgical intervention is considered. The clinican should be versed in current diagnostic modalities in order to reach a diagnosis in the most efficient, economical, and noninvasive fashion possible. Since dissecting aneurysms are different from other aneurysms in presentation and diagnosis, they will be discussed separately.

Plain Films

A thoracic aneurysm will look like a mass that is adjacent to some portion of the thoracic aorta on standard chest films (Fig. 1). If a series of films is available, it may be possible to determine whether the lesion has a vascular origin. More often, routine films cannot determine whether a mass is adjacent to or arising from the aorta. Oblique views or tomography may give added information but, as a rule, additional procedures will be needed. In the abdomen, plain films are often of use in determining the presence of an aneurysm when it has calcification in its wall. Although a routine anteroposterior film may demonstrate the calcified mass, more often a left posterior oblique film and a lateral film will be needed. Care must be taken to avoid confusing a calcified superior mesenteric artery with a wall of an aneurysm. When a leaking or rapidly enlarging aneurysm is the clinical concern, an abdominal film may be adequate to answer the question, since it will show a midline mass. However, more specific information will be desirable in most situations and the clinician must choose among several diagnostic modalities.

Ultrasound

Ultrasound is a simple, noninvasive procedure that can be tolerated by virtually all patients. It is limited by the lack of transmission of ultrasound through bone and air. Therefore evaluation of thoracic aneurysms can rarely be accomplished by ultrasound. In the abdomen, however, ultrasound is quite successful (Fig. 2). Both static and real-time ultrasound can be used to identify the aneurysm, obtain accurate measurements of the lumen and amount of clot, and determine relationship of the aneurysm to the aortic bifurcation and to the origins of the celiac and superior mesenteric arteries. Growth of an aneurysm can be easily followed, and leakage is seen as a para-aortic increase in soft tissue. These factors make ultrasound an ideal modality for the evaluation of abdominal aneurysms. It will be unsuccessful only in patients with massive amounts of bowel gas and in some patients with marked obesity.

Computed Tomography

Computed tomography (Fig. 3) can evaluate the aorta in its entirety. Accurate measurements can be made of the aortic size, and repeat examinations can easily be performed. If the computed tomography is done without intravenous contrast material, there is no morbidity. In most patients, however, contrast material will be needed at least during the first examination to evaluate luminal size or to demonstrate that a

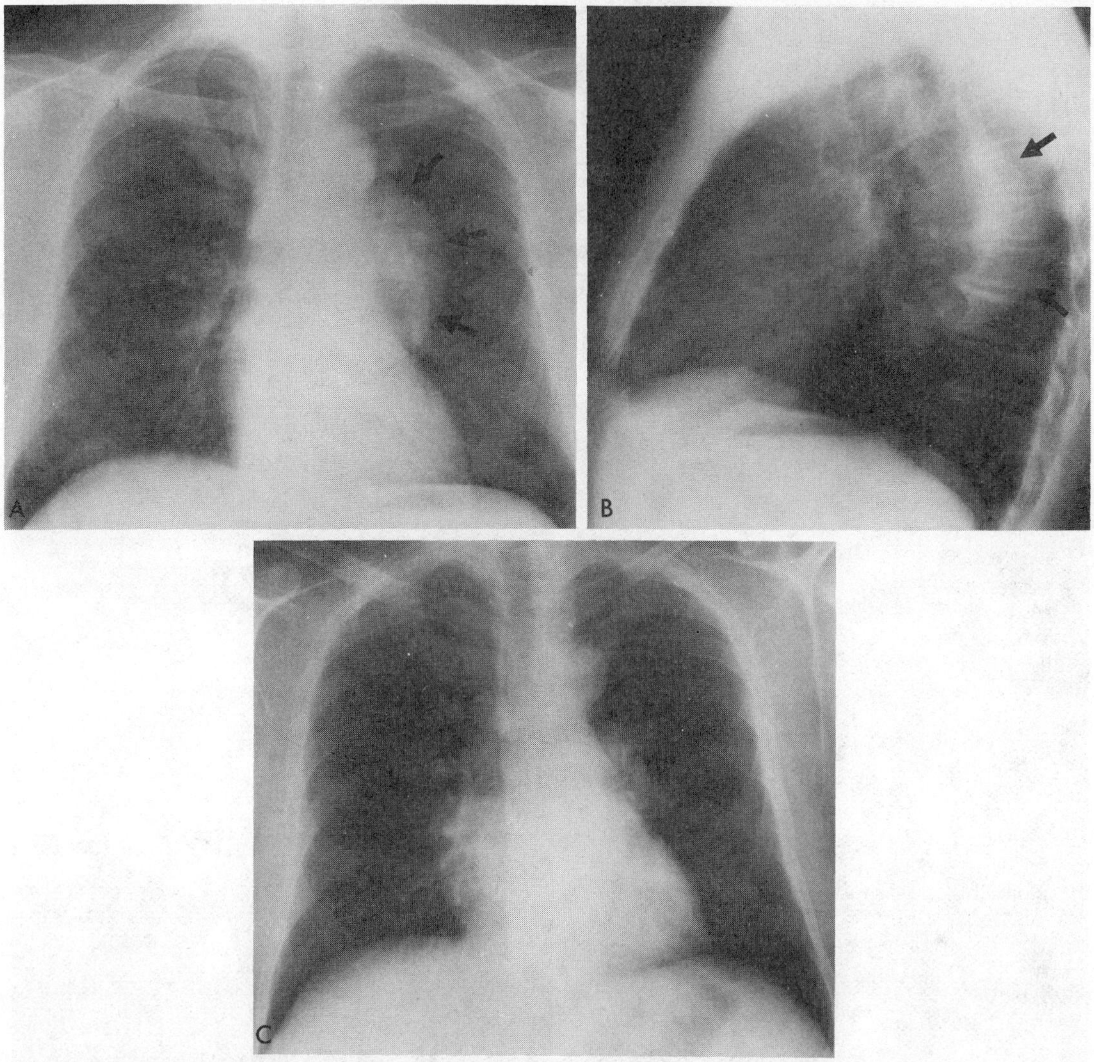

Figure 1. Chest films. (*A*) Posteroanterior view of the chest in a 60-year-old man reveals a mass (arrows) obscuring the left hilum. The aortic knob is well seen, but the descending aorta can not be identified. (*B*) Lateral view of the chest taken at the same time demonstrates that the aorta is elongated. There is a focal aneurysm (arrows) of the descending aorta distal to the origin of the left subclavian artery. (*C*) Posteroanterior chest film on the same patient taken 3 years earlier demonstrated only mild elongation of the thoracic aorta. The left hilum was seen.

para-aortic mass is indeed an aneurysm. Follow-up studies may not require contrast material. Cardiac pulsation limits resolution in the thorax, but generally not enough to impede diagnosis of an aortic aneurysm. A completely clotted aneurysm may appear as a para-aortic mass. Calcification in the wall of such a mass should suggest the correct diagnosis. As a rule, however, computed tomography will accurately identify aneurysms.

Computed tomography does require that the patient be able to lie flat and suspend respiration for a few seconds. It may also require 200 ml or more of 60 per cent contrast material. In the face of dehydration, diabetes, or depressed renal function, this may be a significant drawback. If angiography is also needed urgently, the total volume of contrast material may be unacceptable. When angiography is contemplated, the clinician and radiologist should carefully consider how the computed tomogram is performed and if it is needed.

Angiography

Injection of contrast material into the aorta is considered by many to be the final answer to the diagnosis of aortic aneurysms. This can no longer be considered an accurate statement, though angiography has a major place in the evaluation of aneurysms.

Historically, aortography was accomplished by large intravenous injections of contrast material. Filming time was related to the circulation time. Development of percutaneous angiographic techniques made arterial injection near the aneurysm the procedure of choice. Though introduction of an arterial

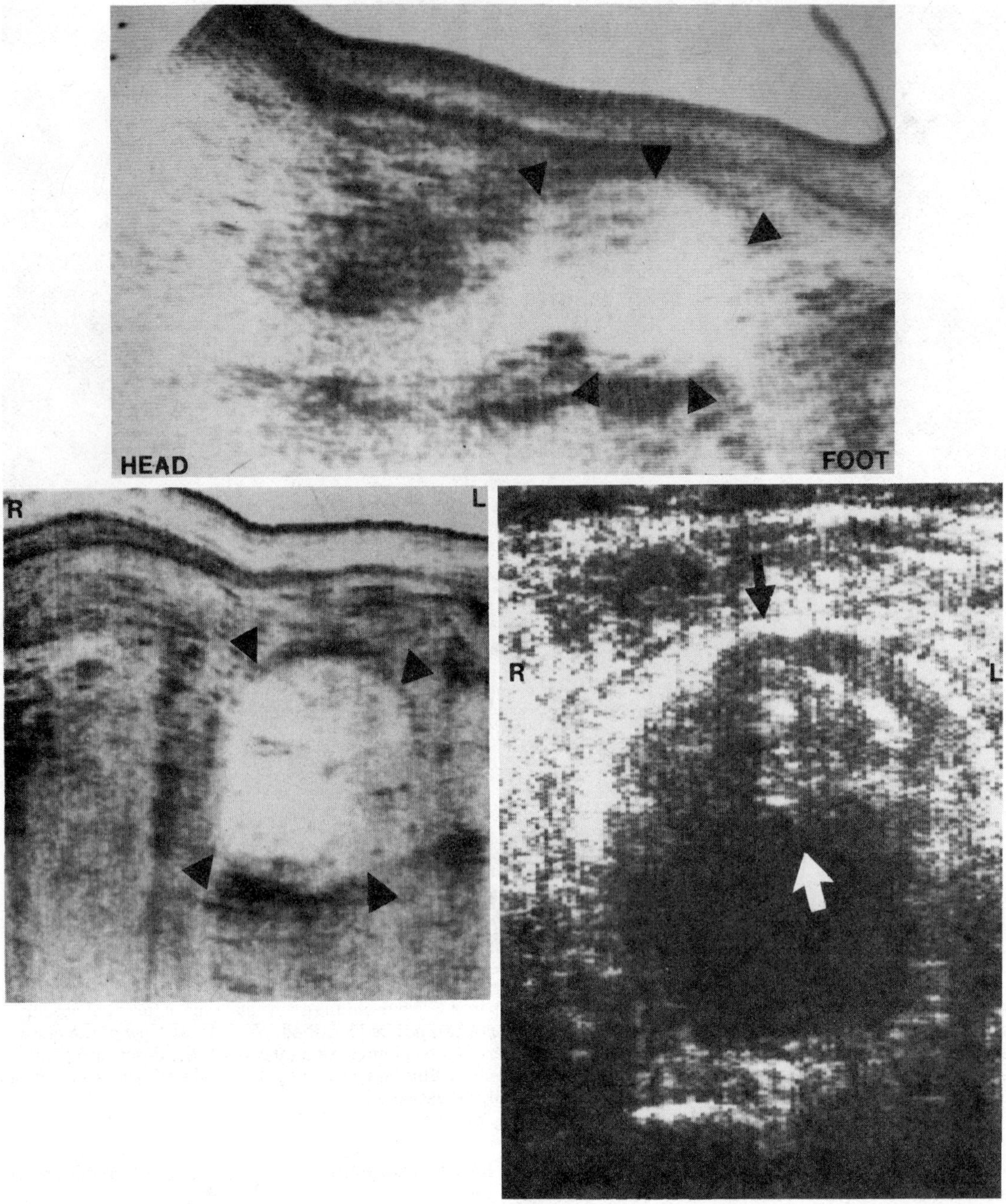

Figure 2. The use of ultrasound in evaluating abdominal aneurysm. (*A*) Parasagittal scan about 2 cm to the left of midline demonstrates the aorta expanding into a focal aneurysm (arrowheads) that measures 8 cm in anteroposterior dimension. There is a clot in the anterior aspect of the aneurysm. (*B*) Transverse scan through the aneurysm (arrowheads.) Transverse dimension is about 7 cm at this level. Clot is seen mostly on the left of the aneurysm. (*C*) Real-time ultrasound, freeze frame of transversal section. Real time ultrasound demonstrates lumen (black arrow) and clot (white arrow) to better advantage, although a single freeze-frame image is less pleasing to the eye. Ultrasound will also demonstrate leakage, when present, around the aneurysm.

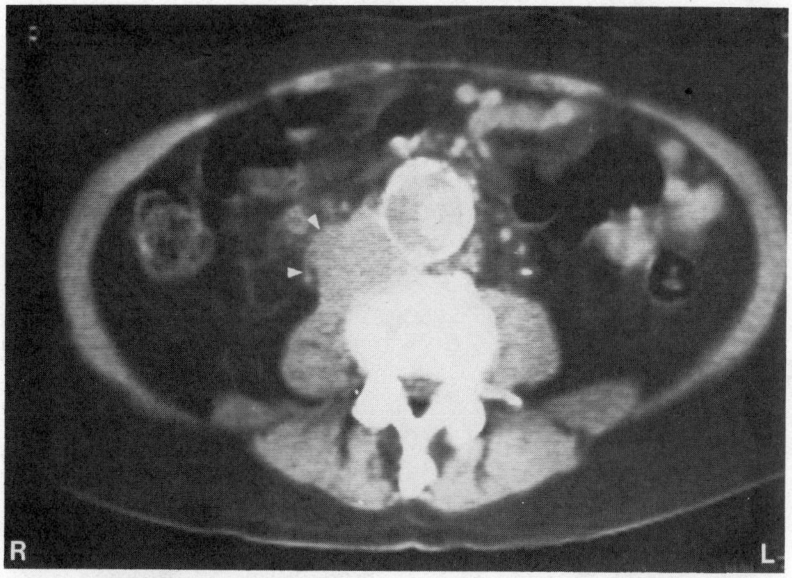

Figure 3. CT scan of the abdomen at about L_3 in a 69-year-old man with metastatic prostatic carcinoma and an abdominal aortic aneurysm. The mass (arrowheads) immediately to the right of the aorta is adenopathy engulfing the inferior vena cava. The aorta itself is enlarged and has a densely calcified wall. Computer measurement of the diameter of the aneurysm was 3.5 cm. This section was obtained within seconds of an intravenous bolus injection of 50 ml of 60 per cent contrast medium. The lumen of the aorta is opacified. It is oval in configuration and lies in the left lateral aspect of the aorta. The crescentic material to its right is clot.

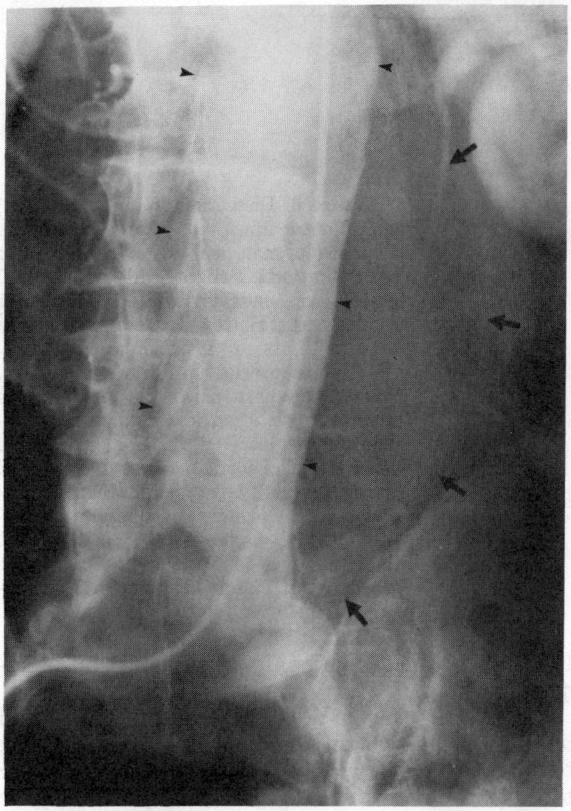

Figure 4. Abdominal aortogram in a 74-year-old man with an enlarging abdominal aneurysm. The catheter has been placed at the level of T_{12}, and injection of contrast material has been made. The opacified aortic lumen (arrowheads) is only mildly dilated and certainly could not be called an aneurysm. The arrows point to a curvilinear calcification that is in the aortic wall. At surgery, the outer dimension of the aneurysm was about 7 cm and there was a very thick laminated clot. If the calcification were missed or not present, it would be easy to conclude that no aneurysm existed angiographically.

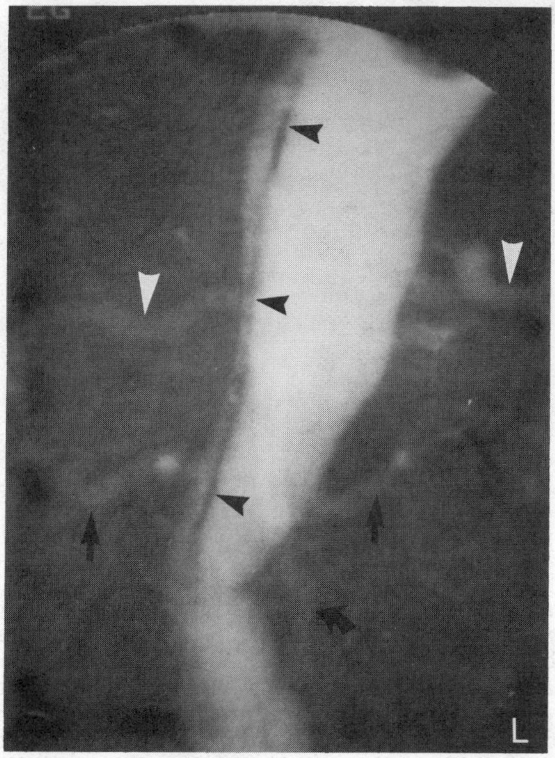

Figure 5. Single frame from an intravenous digital subtraction angiogram with fluid centered in the abdomen reveals an intimal flap (arrowheads) located primarily to the right of the aorta. The renal (arrows) and superior mesenteric (curved arrow) arteries are filled, as are branches of the celiac axis (arrowhead). The right renal artery arises from the false channel, whereas the remainder of the arteries arise from the true lumen. The distal end of the dissection is not clearly seen and may extend distal to the field of view. (Courtesy of Diana Guthaner, M.D., Stanford Medical Center.)

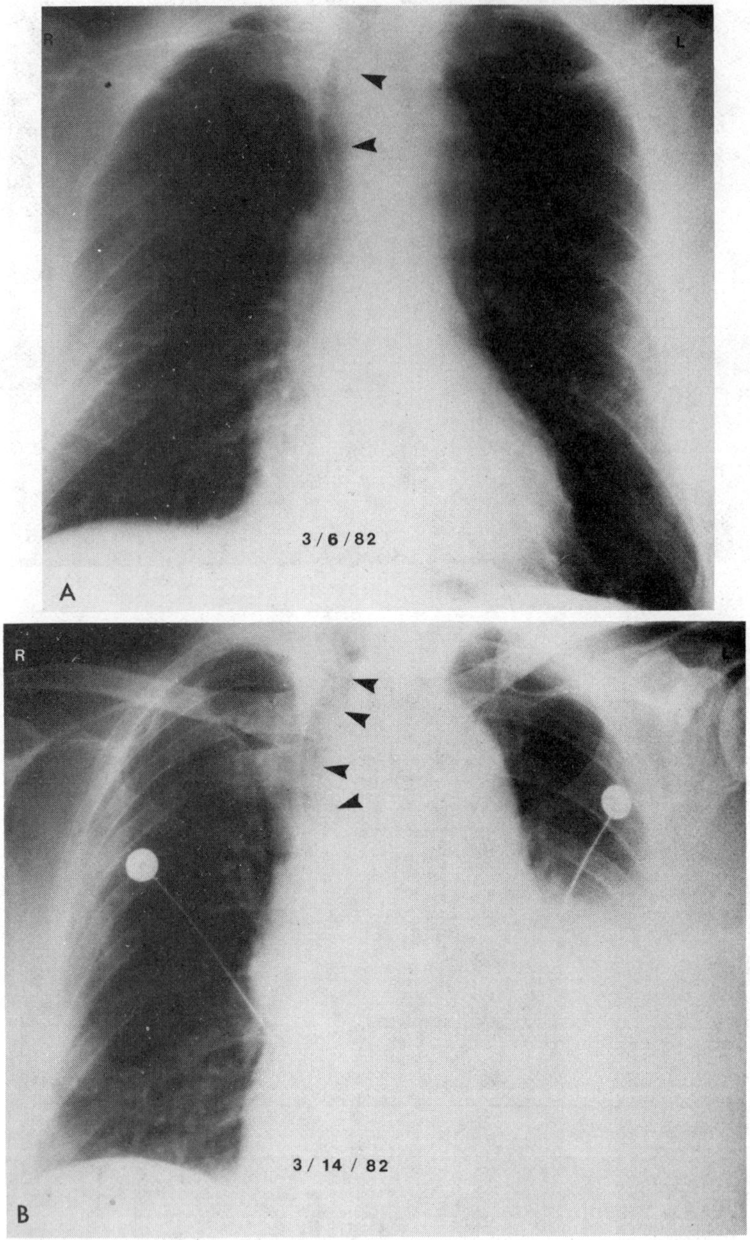

Figure 6. Dissection on chest films. (*A*) Initial chest film taken in a hypertensive 57-year-old man who was having chest pain. The aorta is slightly dilated. The trachea (arrowheads) is deviated to the right by the aorta. However, the film is within normal limits for a patient of this age. (*B*) Posteroanterior chest film 8 days later, when the chest pain was much more severe, shows a marked change. The trachea (arrowheads) is further deviated to the right. The aortic arch is widened, and there is a large left pleural effusion. This rapid change is strongly suggestive of dissection. The diagnosis of Type III aortic dissection was confirmed by angiography. (Courtesy of Diana Guthaner, M.D., Stanford Medical Center.)

catheter carries some morbidity, this type of study was the best method available for studying aneurysms for about 20 years. Limitations were primarily in determination of amount of clot present (Fig. 4). More recently, with the development of digital subtraction angiography, arterial catheterization can often be avoided. The study is performed through a centrally placed venous catheter and therefore can be done on an outpatient basis when appropriate.

Digital subtraction angiography relies on computer manipulation of a faint image, and technical advances are still occurring rapidly. At the present time, digital techniques are seriously hindered by motion, including peristalsis and breathing. The field of view is rather small often requiring several injections to evaluate a lesion of any size. In some patients, a digital subtraction study using a small arterial injection may be more diagnostic than using the intravenous route. In still others, conventional angiography will be required.

The need for each or all of these studies will depend on the clinical problem. Many surgeons are unwilling to operate on the basis of computed tomographic or ultrasonic data alone. Mycotic aneurysms may be multiple, and angiography is the best survey modality. On the other hand, ultrasound can very adequately follow the progression of an infrarenal saccular aneurysm. Therefore, the choice of diagnostic modality will depend on the acuity of the problem and the overall plan for its management.

DISSECTING ANEURYSMS

Dissecting aneurysms initially present with pain or hemorrhage or both. As a rule, immediate medical or surgical therapy will be undertaken when the diagnosis is established. Choice of therapy will depend in part on a detailed evaluation of the extent of the dissection. For this initial evaluation, angiography is the most suitable modality, since it will not only demonstrate the extent of the dissection but will also demonstrate any occluded branch arteries. The method can be either conventional arterial catheter angiography or digital subtraction angiography (Fig 5). Intravenous digital angiography is less likely to have serious complications, but the need to study the aorta from its root to the end of the dissection may require more contrast material than can be safely given in a short period of time. Arterial catheterization can be safely performed in the presence of a dissection and may be the better approach in a given patient.

For clinical situations in which the diagnosis is less apparent or when a dissection is being followed, other diagnostic modalities have a place. The chest film may show marked widening of the aorta (Fig. 6) and development of pleural fluid. Displacement of calcification in the aortic wall used to be considered useful in making the plain film diagnosis of dissection, but this finding can be simulated by calcification in a clot and therefore be misleading. Ultrasound of the aortic root or abdominal aorta may show the false channel and intimal flap. Aortic insufficiency may also be seen. Computed tomography (Fig. 7) with contrast material will show both channels very well and is probably the modality of choice for following medical therapy.

CONCLUSION

It is not reasonable to make hard and fast rules for the diagnostic approach to aneurysms, since the approach should vary with the clinical situation at hand. It is important therefore for the clinician to be aware of the modalities which are available so that the proper sequence of procedures may be chosen for each patient.

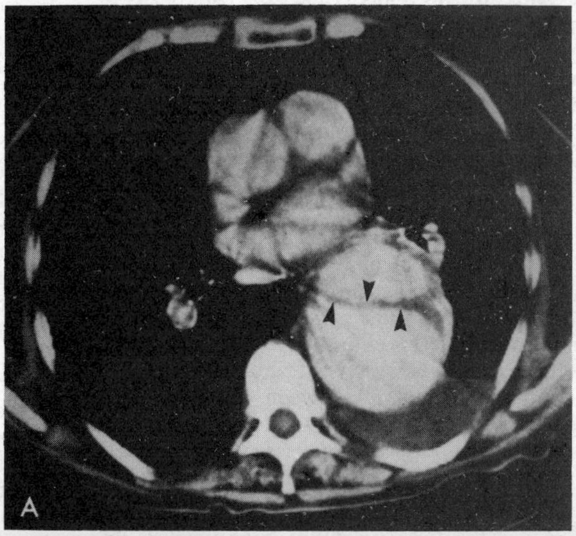

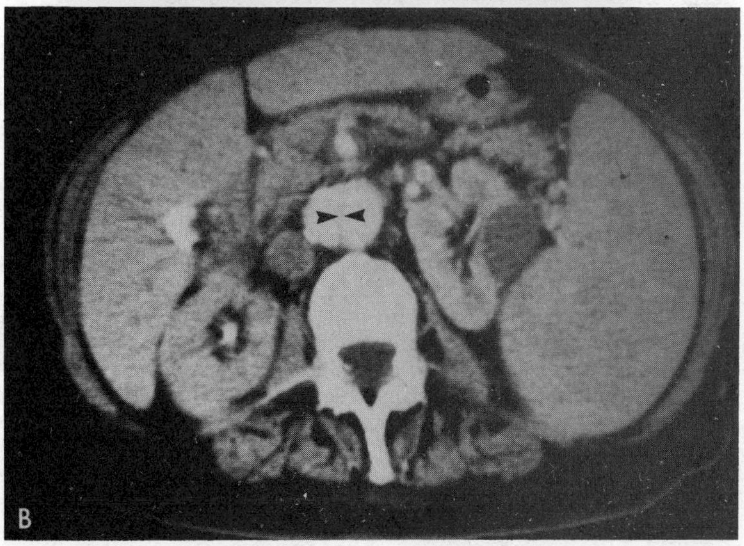

Figure 7. Dissection on computed tomography. (*A*) CT section taken in midthorax reveals marked dilatation of the descending aorta. Contrast medium has been injected and an intimal flap (arrowheads) separating the true and false lumens is outlined. Patient was known to have a dissection and was being followed with CT studies. Development of a left pleural effusion prompted this study. (*B*) CT section through upper abdomen reveals that the dissection extends into the abdominal aorta. The intimal flap (arrowheads) is now nearly vertical in orientation. There is a left renal cyst and the spleen is enlarged. (Courtesy of Diana Guthaner, M.D., Stanford Medical Center.)

CHRONIC ARTERIAL OCCLUSIVE DISEASE OF THE LOWER EXTREMITY

By Henry Haimovici, M.D.
New York, New York

Atherosclerosis is the most common cause of chronic arterial disease of the lower extremities, in contrast to thromboangiitis obliterans (Buerger's disease), which is by far a much rarer entity.

THROMBOANGIITIS OBLITERANS (TAO)

Until about 1950 this entity was diagnosed fairly often. Thereafter its incidence decreased dramatically. Based on Mayo Clinic data (1963), an eightfold decline in its rate over the past 25 years has been estimated. The reason for this decline is rather obscure. The age at clinical onset of the disease is known to be between 20 and 35 years. Ninety per cent of cases occur in men and only 10 per cent in women.

TAO involves the lower extremities more commonly and usually more severely than it does the upper. It begins in medium-sized or small arteries. The lesions are distinctly segmental and follow an episodic course. Larger arteries (popliteal, femoral, or brachial) may also be affected if the disease is severe and progressive. In the major arteries (aorta, iliac) the distinctive lesions of TAO have never been reported.

Migrating thrombophlebitis, in contrast to atherosclerosis, is often the presenting feature in many patients and is considered to be a specific component of TAO. The course of TAO is characterized by periods of remission and relapse directly attributable to cigarette smoking. Relationship between recurrence of the disease and its progression with resumption of tobacco smoking is quite striking. Arteriography may reveal features considered specific of TAO, of which the most significant is the smooth outline of the arterial tree, in constrast to intimal irregularities so characteristic of atheromatous lesions. While these arteriographic signs may be important in the differential diagnosis, they are not pathognomonic. Noninvasive methods for evaluating the hemodynamics in TAO are important and are described later in this article in the discussion on atherosclerosis.

The vascular lesions of TAO are those of an inflammatory process. Their histopathology has been, and still is, the subject of much controversy. This may be partially due to the relatively wide spectrum of lesions, ranging from the acute stage to the healed thrombus. Absence of both intimal atheromatous plaques and medial calcification is an important negative finding necessary to rule out atherosclerosis. A definitive diagnosis may sometimes require a biopsy of an occluded vessel or examination of specimens obtained at amputation or at autopsy.

In brief, TAO is a rare entity but distinct from arteriosclerosis (ASO). It begins at an earlier age than does ASO. Thrombophlebitis may precede the appearance of calf claudication and the upper extremities are often involved. Ulcerations and gangrenous changes of toes and fingers are due to involvement of the small arteries and are the source of severe to excruciating pain. Complete abstinence from tobacco smoking and local management of lesions may limit tissue loss. Lumbar or thoracic sympathectomy or reconstructive surgery may be indicated in selected patients. Otherwise, staged amputations are the alternative.

ATHEROSCLEROSIS

The pathogenesis of atherosclerosis, despite recent progress, is not entirely elucidated. In its simplest definition, atherosclerosis, a degenerative process, is characterized by lipid deposition in the tissue layer that lines the arteries and by focal fibromuscular proliferation.

Structural Features

The atherosclerotic process may be divided into three major stages.

1. The *asymptomatic* stage is represented early by fatty streaks and later by fibrous plaques. The *fatty streaks* appear soon after birth. Lipids are found in the intima, some of it being in macrophages, as foam cells or intimal smooth muscle cells. *Fibrous* plaques appear later on, increasing slowly between the second and fourth decades.

2. The *potentially symptomatic* stage is characterized by lesions in which secondary changes such as calcification, hemorrhage, and ulceration occur.

3. In the *symptomatic* stage, due to complicated lesions, the changes just described result in marked occlusion of the vessel. The chronologic relationship between these three stages is still uncertain. However, a great deal of evidence indicates that this process begins in childhood and does not become apparent until middle or late age. At an advanced stage, the endothelial lining is disrupted, leading to a thrombotic occlusion at the site of the atheromatous plaque.

Atherogenic Mechanisms

The most important of the atherogenic risk factors are metabolic, chemical, physical, biological, and mechanical. Of these, the origin of lipids and their role in atherogenesis have received the greatest attention from biologists and clinicians alike. It is well known that arterial lesions cannot generally be produced experimentally without an increased intake of cholesterol and fat. In the past 20 years, biochemical studies of blood lipoproteins in humans have become a matter of considerable interest.

There are four main types of lipoproteins, which are classified according to their size and density:

1. Chylomicrons.
2. Very low density lipoproteins (VLDL).
3. Low-density lipoproteins (LDL).
4. High-density lipoproteins (HDL).

Of these four types, it is currently accepted that LDL may play the most important role in atherogenesis. It is generally accepted that most lipids enter the arterial wall in a lipoprotein vehicle by crossing the endothelial barrier. The major components of the lipid composition of the atheromatous lesions derive from the circulating cholesterol and other lipids, particularly in the form of LDL. Clinically, the determination of HDL seems to be an important index of the risk factors concerned with cholesterol. An increased HDL is indicative of a negative risk factor for coronary atherosclerosis as well as for peripheral. This lipoprotein fraction has been found to be consistently higher in animal species resistant to atherosclerosis. The reason for the protective effect of HDL in humans is not known.

Other factors important in atherogenesis are arterial hypertension and diabetes mellitus, the latter representing a most serious prognostic feature.

Distribution of Atherosclerotic Lesions

The atherosclerotic process usually involves somatic and visceral arteries in various degrees. Knowledge of the relative incidence of distribution of arterial lesions is largely lacking. Most studies have focused attention either on the peripheral arterial tree or individual visceral arteries. In general, it is recognized that the pathologic features of atherosclerosis are quite variable from individual to individual and from one arterial segment to another. As a result, the patterns emerging from the innumerable combination of lesions are varied and complex. However, in terms of location and extent of the atherosclerotic process, in the lower extremity it is possible to identify a certain number of regional patterns that lend themselves into an overall classification of three major groups: aortoiliac, femoropopliteal, and tibioperoneal-pedal.

Aortoiliac Arteriosclerotic Occlusive Disease. The atherosclerotic process of the aortoiliac segment may begin at the bifurcation or most frequently in one or both common iliac arteries. The development of these lesions is slow, insidious, and progressive. From a clinical pathologic standpoint it may be emphasized that this syndrome ("Leriche's syndrome") may go through two distinct phases—stenotic and occlusive. The reported incidence of these two phases varies with published statistical studies. The degree of stenosis and occlusion of the infrarenal abdominal aorta and that of the iliac arteries is also variable. The variability of these anatomical features is translated into a great number of patterns that in turn determine the clinical manifestations, prognosis, and management. The degree of ischemia is further complicated by the often associated atherosclerotic stenosis or occlusion of the femoral-popliteal or tibioperoneal vessels.

Collateral circulation in aortoiliac occlusive disease varies according to whether the lesions are confined to this segment or are combined with lesions below the inguinal ligament.

The intermittent claudication in this group is characterized by pain affecting primarily the thigh or back musculature. In combined lesions the dominant pain is mostly in the calf and much less above. Some degree of atrophy of the lower extremities is present, which may be symmetrical or asymmetrical, depending on the degree of arterial involvement. Femoral pulses may be diminished in stenotic arterial lesions but are absent in complete and extensive occlusions. Audible bruits may be heard over the distal iliac or femoral vessels.

Evaluation of these lesions, in addition to the physical examination, is achieved by the noninvasive Doppler methods, as mentioned later. If surgery is contemplated, translumbar or transfemoral aortography and arteriography are essential.

Indications for arterial reconstruction depend on the severity of the intermittent claudication or the nonhealing of ulcers or gangrenous changes of the toes. Although aortoiliac occlusive disease confined to this segment may go on for years before serious ischemic manifestations occur, in the combined patterns with distal occlusive disease the process is progressive and usually requires reconstruction, mostly of the proximal arterial tree, for adequate revascularization of the lower extremities.

Femoral-Popliteal Arteriosclerotic Occlusive Disease. The occlusive process of the femoral-popliteal segment is the commonest lesion of the lower extremity, especially in patients over 60. It has been estimated that, of the 73,000 reconstructions of major arteries performed in the United States every year, more than 20,000 (over 27 per cent of the total) involved the femoral-popliteal segment. These statistical data reflect both the high incidence of these lesions and the widespread use of surgical procedures for their reconstruction.

The extent and location of the lesions in the femoral-popliteal segment are extremely variable. Initial lesions are characterized by mild to severe stenosis. One of the most common locations is at the junction between Hunter's canal and the initial segment of the popliteal. Another frequent location is in the distal popliteal or below the origin of the anterior tibial. A complete occlusion of the superficial femoral artery may occur from Hunter's canal up to the bifurcation of the common femoral. The incidence of isolated lesions of the femoral-popliteal segment is much smaller than that of those combined with the proximal or distal arterial tree.

Clinical manifestations consist of intermittent claudication of variable degrees, rest pain without or with ulcers or gangrene of the toes or foot when the occlusive process is quite widespread and when it affects also the distal vessels (see later discussion).

Tibioperoneal Occlusive Disease. Occlusion of leg arteries alone occurs in over 25 per cent of the patients. Combined occlusions of leg arteries with other arterial segments occur in all the other arterial locations. Comparison of the incidence of various patterns in nondiabetic and diabetic groups shows that the atherosclerotic process is more discrete in the nondiabetic and more diffuse in the diabetic group. Involvement of a single artery of the leg is noted more often in nondiabetic than in diabetic patients. Conversely, occlusion of two or all three leg arteries occurs in about two thirds of the diabetic and only in about one third of the nondiabetic patients. This is of considerable importance when considering revascularization of the leg and foot in the presence of limb-threatening, severe ischemia.

Collateral pathways compensating for the different patterns of occlusion are provided by pre-existing major branches of the femoral, popliteal, and leg arteries. Their efficiency depends on the extent of the occlusive process of the major branches as well as of the involvement of the profunda femoris, which is the major collateral of the thigh and leg. The alternate collateral pathways for the salvage of the foot are provided by the dorsalis pedis and plantar arteries through the pedal anastomotic networks. The main arterial arch of the foot is completed in a dorsoplantar direction. The existence of these dorsal and plantar arterial arches providing the metatarsal arteries will determine whether any proximal reconstruction of the arterial tree would be successful enough to salvage the foot and prevent the need for amputations.

Clinical Manifestations

The clinical manifestations of chronic arterial insufficiency, as just stated, vary with the location and extent of the vascular lesions. They are divided into three major groups of increasing severity: intermittent claudication, rest pain, and ischemic ulcers and gangrene.

Intermittent claudication, indicating inadequate blood supply to contracting leg and foot muscles, varies in intensity according to the degree of arterial involvement. Mild to moderate intermittent claudication is generally not considered an indication for reconstructive surgery. By contrast, marked intermittent claudication, greatly restricting the patient's walking ability often to the point of disability, is a major indication. This is especially true if this symptom is a serious handicap in the lifestyle of a younger person. However, an older inactive person whose livelihood is not threatened by this type of claudication is not to be considered a candidate for reconstruction, especially if systemic manifestations of arteriosclerosis are present.

The degree of intermittent claudication is largely related to the extent and progression of the arterial disease. In the course of the evolution of the arteriosclerotic process, a superimposed acute segmental occlusion may occur, with a corresponding sudden aggravation of the claudication. In such instances, arterial reconstruction may assume a more urgent indication than in the chronic stage.

Rest pain is a well-known clinical indication of advanced arterial insufficiency and is due to a fall in the blood flow when the limb is in the supine position. Clinically, rest pain involves the toes and the adjacent metatarsal area and occurs mostly at night. The patient awakes and hangs the involved limb over the side of the bed to relieve pain. If further dependency of the limb is necessary to improve the capillary flow, the patient walks about the room before he can return to sleep. In a further advanced stage, rest pain may become continuous and be present not only during the night but also during waking hours. Associated signs of end-stage ischemia often present are a cold, anesthetic or a cold, edematous, and discolored foot.

Ischemic ulcerative and gangrenous lesions, to be amenable to reconstructive arterial surgery, should be localized either in the toes or the heel or a combination thereof. In these patients, use of antibiotics and avoidance of any trauma will usually limit the lesions to a small area. However, spreading gangrene may occur if local infection is not controlled, especially in diabetic patients, if a venous thrombosis is superimposed and if cardiac failure is present.

In attempting to establish any therapy, it is important to take into account:

1. The type of onset.
2. The age of the patient.
3. The pattern of occlusive arterial disease.
4. The presence of diabetes.

The mode of onset may be insidious, sudden without prior claudication or sudden with prior claudication and a combination of associated trauma, venous occlusion, arterial embolism, and vasospastic conditions. As to age, the majority of patients fall within the sixth, seventh, and eighth decades and over 80 per cent are males. It is noteworthy that the relative age incidence in nondiabetic and diabetic patients varies inversely with the advance in decades. In a study of vascular lesions in these two groups of patients by me and my colleagues, there were slightly more than 50 per cent under the age of 60 in the nondiabetic group, whereas only 33 per cent were found in the diabetic group. Conversely, after the age of 60 the incidence in the diabetic group was 67 per cent and 48.6 per cent in the nondiabetic group.

Diabetic foot lesions deserve a special mention. They are frequently associated with, and sometimes dominated by, two other important clinical manifestations: diabetic neuropathy and local infection. The association, in varying degrees, lends to the lesions a truly characteristic clinical picture, often referred to as the "diabetic foot." Because of their quasi-specificity, these lesions justify a separate description. The clinical manifestations may be classified under the following four headings:

1. Arteriosclerosis obliterans.
2. Peripheral neuropathy.
3. Infection.
4. Combined lesions.

In treating a diabetic, one has to take into account the possibility of the three major factors in order not to overlook any of them.

Clinical Evaluation of Arterial Insufficiency

Prior to undertaking noninvasive instrumental or arteriographic assessment of the arterial insufficiency, its clinical evaluation is the most important part of the physical examination. The *color* of the leg, especially of the foot and toes, in the supine and dependent, as well as elevated, positions, may provide a clue as to the severity of the arterial ischemia at the capillary level. The *temperature* of the skin, examined under basal conditions, may provide an indication of the degree and the location of the arterial impairment, especially if there is a difference between the two sides. Unilateral foot coolness or coldness carries a significant sign of ischemia. It is interesting to note that in an occlusion of the distal superficial femoral or proximal popliteal, *the knee* on the affected side is much warmer than on the contralateral side. This finding, which I call "hyperemic knee sign," indicates an increased collateral circulation around the knee provided by the genicular system and branches of the profunda femoris. The difference between the two knee temperatures may range from 2° to 5°F.

Systematic *palpation* of all the pulses from the abdominal aorta down to the pedal ones should provide a first indication about the degree and location of the arterial occlusion. *Auscultation* along the arteries from the abdominal aorta down to the popliteal may indicate the presence of marked stenosis when a systolic bruit is audible. *Oscillometry,* when other noninvasive methods for evaluation are not available, will provide semiquantitative information concerning the amplitude of the pulsations and should be carried out at several levels of the extremity on both sides. Today, the *Doppler ultrasonic* blood velocity determination is commonly used and is an important means for comparative flow assessment and for localizing the lesions. A permanent record of these blood velocities and blood wave determinations should be kept for future reference. Usually these noninvasive methods are carried out by experienced technicians in especially equipped vascular laboratories. Thus, the interpretation of the graphic flow patterns, analysis of segmental pressure measurements, and interpretation of postexercise ankle blood pressure obtained with this method may aid greatly in the evaluation of the arterial insufficiency and help in deciding the type of treatment to be applied.

Clinical Assessment of General Condition

A routine systematic evaluation of all the vital organs is essential, especially if patients are considered for arterial surgery: electrocardiogram (ECG); cerebral symptomatology; the renal function, especially in diabetic patients; a chest film; blood pressure determinations over a period of several days; and a complete lipid profile.

Arteriographic Evaluation

If surgery is contemplated, a comprehensive assessment of the arterial lesions of the lower extremity is mandatory and should include the entire arterial tree from the terminal abdominal aorta to the pedal vessels. This method is essential to provide information not only about the lesions of the femoral and popliteal arteries but also about the state of the aorta and iliac arteries (inflow tract) as well as about the tibial and pedal vessels (outflow tract). This can be achieved by serial aortoarteriography, performed under general anesthesia and consisting of a percutaneous puncture of both common femoral arteries and using Teflon catheters. Bilateral arteriography should be carried out routinely since in the majority of instances the arteriosclerotic process involves both lower extremities. Interpretation of arteriographic findings is usually not difficult, especially in centers in which angioradiology is a specialized section of the x-ray department. Patients with symptomatic arterial insufficiency rarely display arterial lesions of a monosegmental type and the lesions are most often multiple and complex.

The complete occlusion of a segment is easily interpretable, but intimal lesions encroaching upon the lumen are often difficult to assess in terms of their hemodynamic significance. The degree of stenosis assigned to an atheromatous lesion radiologically visible may be often misleading. Operative findings are usually more severe than the arteriographic outline would indicate. The nature of the lesions may range from a soft atheromatous to a hard fibrous or calcified plaque. The extent of the latter is rarely detectable from the angiographic image. Because of possibility of misinterpretation of these observations, it is essential to obtain an adequate opacification of the angiographic outline of the entire vascular tree.

Diagnosis of the nature and degree of chronic arterial insufficiency of the lower extremity can be achieved by clinical, noninvasive, and arteriographic evaluations. Classification of the lower extremity arterial insufficiency is I, intermittent claudication ranging from mild to severe; II, rest pain; and III, ulcers or gangrene.

Conservative management is indicated in most cases, except in those patients in whom conservative measures fail to relieve rest pain or heal minor ulcers or limited gangrene of toes. Reconstructive surgery is then indicated.

PERIPHERAL VENOUS DISEASE

By F. N. Burt, M.D.
Southfield, Michigan

Classification of venous diseases is difficult because it is common for the type and severity of the signs and symptoms to be more reflective of individual patient variations than of the extent of the primary pathology.

Clinically important disorders of the veins of the legs are characterized by the presence of intravascular thrombosis or valvular incompetence. These conditions may coexist and may even be causally related. Congenital abnormalities may also contribute to the development of venous disease, particularly in superficial venous insufficiency.

The syndromes of peripheral venous lesions are determined by their anatomic location.

LOWER EXTREMITY

Venous disease of the leg must be included in the differential diagnosis of all patients presenting with any one of four types of clinical syndromes:

1. Acute pain and swelling of the leg(s).
2. Chronic edema of the legs in conjunction with stasis pain, pigmentation, cellulitis, or ulceration.
3. Prominent superficial veins (varicose veins).
4. Patients at high risk for thromboembolic disease, presenting themselves for screening.

THROMBOPHLEBITIS

Thrombophlebitis is the generic name for all conditions having intraluminal thrombus in veins. The name is somewhat misleading, however, because the inflammatory component (phlebitis) is not a direct determinant of the severity of the disease. This inflammation, however, is responsible for many of the signs and symptoms upon which the diagnosis is based.

Recent information regarding the etiology of thrombophlebitis has added little to the observations of Virchow when he described his "triad" of etiologic factors:

1. Slowed venous blood flow.
2. Damage to the vein intimal surface.
3. "Hypercoagulable" states.

Etiologic considerations have little impact on the diagnosis of thrombophlebitis.

Clinical presentations of thrombophlebitis can be described in terms of four characteristics. Cases must be alike in all four characteristics before they can be considered similar. The characteristics are:

1. Vein system (superficial or deep).
2. Most proximal location (below knee, above knee, pelvis).
3. Evidence of propagation.
4. Evidence of embolization.

Superficial Thrombophlebitis

The diagnosis of superficial thrombophlebitis is straightforward. Patients' complaints are those of localized pain and swelling in the leg. The patient may volunteer the relationship of the symptoms to a previously noted varicose vein.

Physical examination shows variable degrees of erythema and tenderness along the course of a superficial vein. The presence of palpable thrombus within the vein completes the pathognomonic syndrome.

It is characteristic for findings of subfascial, popliteal, or femoral tenderness or fullness to be absent.

Vascular laboratory evaluation is indicated to rule out the possibility of subclinical extension of thrombus into the deep venous system. (See the discussion on deep thrombophlebitis later in this article.)

The course is usually self-limited, but patients should be continuously monitored for evidence of clot propagation toward the saphenofemoral junction, the occurrence of which should prompt anticoagulation or saphenous vein ligation and excision.

The differential diagnosis of superficial thrombophlebitis is limited to cellulitis, which is easily distinguished because of its involvement of skin remote from veins and by the absence of palpable thrombus. Cellulitis is typically associated with fever and leukocytosis.

Uncomplicated superficial thrombophlebitis is important only because of the patient discomfort which it causes.

The presence of subfascial, popliteal, or femoral tenderness or palpable thrombus should prompt evaluation of the patient for the presence of concurrent deep vein thrombosis (DVT) (see the discussion of deep thrombophlebitis).

Deep Thrombophlebitis

Deep thrombophlebitis is clinically important because of two distinct sequelae.

The risk of pulmonary embolus is higher the further up the leg the thrombus extends and is variously reported as occurring in 20 to 50 per cent of patients with iliac vein involvement. The morbidity and mortality produced by pulmonary embolus are considerable, particularly in the elderly and debilitated.

The processes of clot propagation, fixation to the vein wall, fibrosis, and recanalization destroy the valves in the involved vein, producing obligatory venous hypertension, the so-called "postphlebitic" syndrome. This condition extracts marked morbidity in a slowly progressive course that may become apparent only many years after the phlebitic episode. (See the section on chronic venous insufficiency later in this article.)

Patients who have had thromboembolic disease of any type have a higher than normal risk of recurrent deep thrombophlebitis and should be carefully observed and kept away from medications and activities that might further increase their risk.

For these reasons, the diagnosis of deep thrombophlebitis has an importance extending far beyond the control of the patient's presenting symptoms. An accurate and objective diagnosis must be made if serious sequelae are to be avoided.

The diagnosis of DVT (Fig. 1) is more difficult than generally appreciated. Accuracy in predicting the presence of deep thrombophlebitis on the basis of history and physical findings is only 50 per cent even in experienced hands. It is for this reason that the vascular laboratory has played an expanded role in the diagnostic process in recent years.

Objective Tests in the Diagnosis of Deep Vein Thrombosis

Venography. Contrast venography is considered to be the definitive test for the presence of deep thrombophlebitis. It has several drawbacks, however. There is considerable expense associated with venography, and the test is uncomfortable for patients, so that many are unwilling to undergo follow-up procedures. The contrast medium has been reported to cause thrombophlebitis in as many as 15 per cent of patients undergoing venography. The venous anatomy may be so distorted in patients with severe postphlebitic changes that a new thrombus may not be identifiable. Most physicians are reluctant to perform venography during pregnancy.

Doppler Venous Flow Study. A Doppler blood flow velocity detector, in experienced hands, can detect alterations in venous hemodynamics associated with DVT. The test is time-consuming and, in addition, is generally considered to be inadequate for establishing an objective diagnosis when used alone. Specificity and sensitivity are around 75 per cent.

Limb Plethysmography. A thrombus large enough to obstruct main venous channels in the leg produces measurable abnormalities in limb size under conditions of maximum venous outflow. Various means of measuring these subtle changes in the circumference of limb segments are in use for the diagnosis of venous thrombosis. Techniques based on electrical impedance of the limb, changes in resistance of strain gauges wrapped around the limb, and pressure changes in transducers applied to the surface of the limb segment all give similar results. The tests are easily performed. They are about 85 per cent sensitive in detecting venous abnormalities but may be only 75 per cent specific for acute active venous thrombosis.

Phleborheography. This is an air plethysmographic method for the detection of deep vein thrombi. Its testing technique assesses venous flow under nearly normal conditions with a filled venous system rather than measuring venous outflow. The test can often distinguish acute DVT from chronic venous disease. It has sensitivity and specificity in the 92 per cent range. The errors occur primarily in patients with thrombi confined to the calf.

^{125}I Fibrinogen Scan. Given intravenously, a bolus of fibrinogen will attach itself to an actively forming thrombus. Serial counting of radioactivity in the legs after the administration of ^{125}I tagged fibrinogen can localize thrombi. The test is very sensitive to small soleal clots, which are missed by other techniques. It can only sense actively expanding thrombi. The reliability of fibrinogen scanning is less in the pelvis, and false-positive results are common from injury, effusions, and other similar causes. The test is widely used in Europe for clinical diagnosis, but reports from the United States suggest that some of the positive results are not indicative of clinically significant disease. The method is used widely for screening postoperative patients. A similar technique using tagged streptokinase has been described.

Isotope Venography. Technetium injected into a foot vein allows a gamma camera image of the veins to be developed. The technique has been reported to be

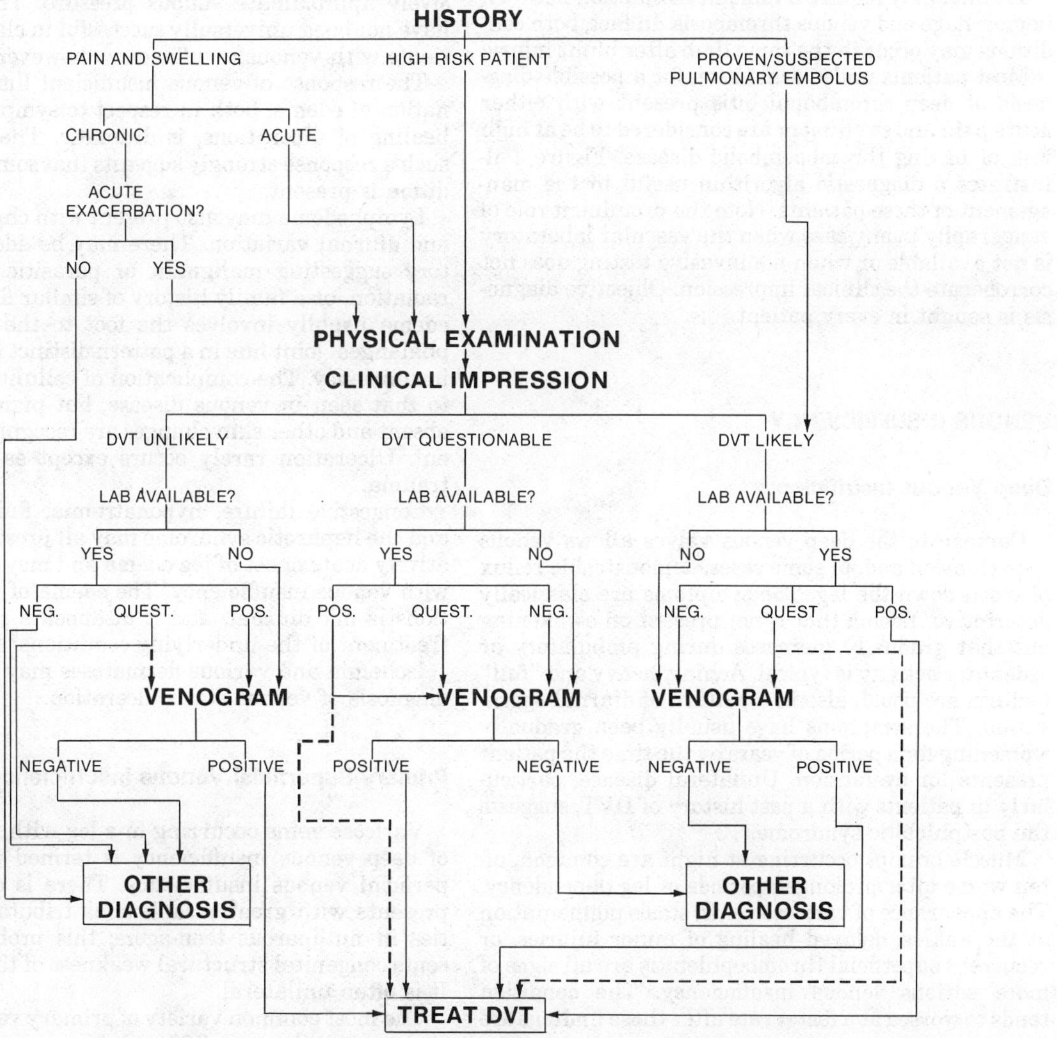

Figure 1. Procedures for diagnosing deep vein thrombosis (DVT).

accurate, but it is not widely used. It shares some of the disadvantages of contrast venography without giving as definitive a result.

Coagulation Studies. Numerous efforts to measure by-products of thrombosis or thrombolysis as means of detecting active thrombophlebitis have been undertaken. The results have not been encouraging to date. It remains possible that differential measurement of such products between both legs may be helpful.

Differential Diagnosis of Deep Vein Thrombosis

The differential diagnosis of DVT includes many other conditions, both common and rare.

Spontaneous rupture of the plantaris or other muscle usually occurs during exercise with a sensation of "being shot." Ecchymosis rapidly develops in most cases. Recognition of this usually clear-cut syndrome is important, as heparinization may cause significant hemorrhage if instituted in the face of acute muscular injury.

Hemorrhage into a soft-tissue tumor has produced a clinical picture identical to the classic description of DVT.

Trauma may require a difficult distinction between hemorrhage and venous thrombosis. In fact, both conditions may occur in the same limb after blunt injury.

Most patients under evaluation for a possible diagnosis of deep thrombophlebitis present with either acute pain and swelling or are considered to be at high risk of having thromboembolic disease. Figure 1 illustrates a diagnostic algorithm useful in the management of these patients. Note the prominent role of venography in any case when the vascular laboratory is not available or when noninvasive testing does not corroborate the clinical impression. Objective diagnosis is sought in every patient.

VENOUS INSUFFICIENCY

Deep Venous Insufficiency

Damage to the deep venous valves allows venous hypertension and, in some cases, demonstrable reflux of blood down the leg. The symptoms are classically descriptive. Edema that is not present on awakening but that gradually increases during ambulatory or sedentary activity is typical. Aching, heavy and "full" feelings are usual, also in a pattern of diurnal aggravation. The symptoms have usually been gradually worsening for a period of years by the time the patient presents for evaluation. Unilateral disease, particularly in patients with a past history of DVT, suggests the postphlebitic syndrome.

Muscle cramps occurring at night are common, often worse after prolonged periods of leg dependency. The appearance of varicose veins, stasis pigmentation at the ankles, delayed healing of minor injuries, or recurrent superficial thrombophlebitis are all signs of more serious venous insufficiency. The condition tends to worsen at a faster rate after these findings are present.

Signs of severe and chronic damage to the legs include ulceration, cellulitis, and fibrotic contraction of the pigmented skin. These are signs of a leg in need of rapid medical attention, often requiring hospitalization.

The diagnosis of chronic venous insufficiency is made on clinical grounds. A possible role of the vascular laboratory is beginning to evolve.

Doppler flow evaluation can reliably identify valvular incompetence if the vein can be localized. The phleborheograph shows changes in respiratory waves and the foot-emptying curves, which suggest venous insufficiency, but they are not specific.

Descending venography, in which contrast medium is injected in the iliac veins and pictures are taken to record the downward cascading of the contrast in response to gravity, provides an impressive and semiquantitative method of study of these patients. This method is considered a requirement before undertaking surgical reconstruction of the incompetent venous system because it localizes incompetent valves.

Direct measurement of ambulatory venous pressures has been shown to quantitatively assess incompetence. Recent investigations have suggested that photo or strain gauge plethysmography can noninvasively approximate venous pressure. These studies have not been universally successful in classifying patients with venous insufficiency, however.

The response of venous insufficient limbs to elimination of edema, both in respect to symptoms and to healing of ulcerations, is dramatic. The absence of such a response strongly suggests that some other condition is present.

Lymphedema may also present with chronic edema and diurnal variation. There may be additional history suggesting malignant or parasitic disease, irradiation, or a family history of similar findings. The edema usually involves the foot to the metacarpophalangeal joint line in a pattern distinct from venous insufficiency. The complication of cellulitis is similar to that seen in venous disease, but pigmentation is absent and other skin changes are recognizably different. Ulceration rarely occurs except as a result of trauma.

Congestive failure, hyponatremia, fluid overload, and the nephrotic syndrome may all present with relatively acute onset of leg edema and may be confused with venous insufficiency. The edema of these conditions is not diurnal, and it disappears rapidly with treatment of the underlying conditions.

Ischemia and various dermatoses may confuse the diagnosis of venous stasis ulceration.

Primary Superficial Venous Insufficiency

Varicose veins occurring in a leg with no stigmata of deep venous insufficiency is termed primary superficial venous insufficiency. There is a form that presents with greater saphenous tributary varicosities in nulliparous teen-agers; this probably represents congenital structural weakness of the vein wall. It is often unilateral.

The most common variety of primary varicose veins occurs after the age of 25 and, in women, after pregnancies. The condition is usually asymptomatic at first. Patients may later develop pain limited to the prominent veins themselves.

Other patients develop a syndrome of discomfort, edema, and even ulceration similar to that described in deep vein insufficiency. There is some difference of opinion as to whether such symptoms ever occur in the absence of some degree of deep venous incompetence.

Secondary Superficial Venous Insufficiency

The most common form of varicose veins is that in which progressive and recurrent superficial varicosities are associated with deep venous insufficiency. Patients have the symptoms of the underlying deep vein incompetence. Direct symptoms from the varicose veins themselves are rare. The significant portion of this condition is the deep vein abnormality, and it must be diagnosed and evaluated independently of the varicose veins. (See the preceding section on deep venous insufficiency.)

UPPER EXTREMITY VENOUS DISEASES

Superficial phlebitis of the arm is usually chemical in origin, following intravenous drug administration in a medical setting. It is almost entirely a self-limiting and nonthreatening condition. Embolization is not thought to occur from this condition. Drug addicts may have superficial phlebitis on a septic basis with the attendant signs of sepsis.

Axillary vein thrombosis is usually a dramatic clinical event, presenting with edema, venous collateral distention, and blue discoloration of the arm and deltoid area. Onset is usually over a period of less than 24 hours, and may follow strenuous exercise by the patient (effort thrombosis). Diagnosis is by venography. Noninvasive testing has not been well standardized for arm thromboses. Doppler studies can be misleading because of the potentially large collateral around the shoulder. Pulmonary embolization has been documented from axillary thrombosis but is considered to be rare.

Section Six

BLOOD AND BLOOD-FORMING ORGANS

ANEMIAS DUE TO DECREASED ERYTHROCYTE PRODUCTION

By James R. Eckman, M.D.
Atlanta, Georgia

SYNONYMS

Hypoproliferative anemia, normochromic normocytic anemia, aregenerative anemia.

DEFINITION

Hypoproliferative anemias result from an absolute reduction in the production of erythrocytes, usually caused by a quantitative reduction in the numbers of red blood cell precursors in the bone marrow. Relative hypoproliferation is seen when there is an inadequate response of the bone marrow to demands for increased production of erythrocytes. The cardinal laboratory manifestations are a reduction of the hemoglobin and hematocrit with a low reticulocyte count. Most of these anemias present with normal mean corpuscular volume and mean corpuscular hemoglobin concentration; that is, they are normochromic normocytic.

A useful diagnostic classification is based on whether the anemia occurs as an isolated phenomenon or with associated alterations in white blood cell and platelet numbers. This diagnostic classification is outlined in Table 1. Such a classification does not address the pathophysiologic etiologies, which are frequently complex, but does assist in effective definition of the diagnostic possibilities. Because as all of these disorders have a component of decreased erythrocyte production, quantitative and qualitative evaluation red cell precursors by bone marrow examination is frequently useful in the diagnostic approach.

ISOLATED DECREASE IN ERYTHROCYTE PRODUCTION

Anemia is usually the only significant hematologic abnormality in these disorders. The leukocyte and platelet counts are generally within the range of normal.

Anemia of Chronic Inflammation

Synonyms

Anemia of infection, anemia of chronic diseases, anemia with inflammatory block, simple chronic anemia.

Definition

The anemia of chronic inflammation occurs in association with long-standing infection, malignancies, and rheumatoid diseases. The anemia results from a modest reduction in red cell survival without compensatory increase in erythrocyte production and from defective reutilization of iron. The usual recycling of iron, which is released by catabolism of hemoglobin from senescent red cells, is blocked so that iron accumulates in the reticuloendothelial system and is not available for production of hemoglobin in new erythrocytes. The exact etiology of this disorder is unclear. This is the most common anemia encountered in a hospital-based practice and is second only to iron deficiency as a cause of anemia in the population as a whole.

Symptoms, Signs, and Course

The anemia of chronic inflammation is mild and usually asymptomatic. The patient may manifest symptoms of the underlying chronic infection, malignancy, or rheumatologic disorder. Physical findings are related to the nature of the chronic disease. This anemia will improve with control of the chronic illness. Without effective treatment of the underlying disease, the reduction in hemoglobin will persist but usually not cause significant morbidity.

Laboratory Findings

The reduction of hemoglobin is mild with values ranging from 9 to 12 gm/dl. The mean corpuscular volume (MCV) and mean corpuscular hemoglobin concentration (MCHC) are usually normal. The red cells appear normocytic and normochromic on blood smear. In about one third of patients, the MCV is reduced and the red cells appear mildly microcytic and hypochromic. The corrected reticulocyte count is less than 2 per cent. The white blood cell and platelet counts are normal unless affected by the underlying disease. Elevations in white cell counts are seen with chronic infections, and elevations in platelet counts may be seen with abscesses, tuberculosis, and malignancies.

Table 1. Anemias Due to Decreased Erythrocyte Production: Diagnostic Classification

Isolated Decrease in Red Blood Cell Production
Anemia of chronic inflammation
Anemia of renal insufficiency
Pure red cell aplasia
Secondary to endocrine deficiency
Decreased Red Blood Cell Production with Alterations in Leukocyte and Platelet Production
Aplastic anemia
Leukemias
Myelophthistic anemias

Classic iron studies reveal reduction in serum iron, in total iron-binding capacity, and in transferrin saturation. The serum ferritin is usually elevated or normal. The bone marrow is normocellular with slight elevation in the myeloid:erythroid ratio. "Prussian blue" stains for iron show a characteristic pattern of increased storage iron and decreased or absent sideroblasts and siderocytes. The percentage of erythroid precursors staining for iron is generally less than 5 per cent.

Errors and Pitfalls in Diagnosis

The coexistence of iron deficiency and the anemia of chronic inflammation is not uncommon and presents difficult diagnostic problems. Routine iron studies become unreliable for the detection of iron deficiency in the presence of chronic inflammation. Values for serum iron and transferrin saturation completely overlap in these two disorders. The elevation in total iron-binding capacity, which is diagnostic of iron deficiency, may be suppressed with chronic inflammation. The serum ferritin is very useful in this setting. A serum ferritin of less than 12 ng/dl is diagnostic of iron depletion. In the absence of hepatocellular damage or certain malignancies such as Hodgkin's disease, a value of greater than 100 ng/dl effectively excludes iron depletion. Values between 12 and 100 ng/dl require bone marrow evaluation to establish iron status. This distinction is important because the anemia of chronic inflammation is unresponsive to iron therapy, and the presence of iron deficiency suggests increased blood loss, which is frequently a symptom of gastrointestinal and genitourinary pathology.

Anemia of Renal Insufficiency

Definition

Chronic renal insufficiency is associated with reduction in hemoglobin concentration, which in general parallels the severity of the loss of kidney function. The pathophysiology of the anemia of chronic renal disease is complex. Marrow production of erythrocytes is decreased secondary to a less than appropriate increase in erythropoietin levels for the degree of anemia. This results from loss of hormone production by the diseased kidney. There is also a less than appropriate response of erythroid precursors to stimulation by erythropoietin. Increased loss of erythrocytes occurs secondary to a reduced survival and through increased bleeding. Volume overload may further reduce hemoglobin concentration independent of reductions in red cell mass by increasing the plasma volume. Anemia usually occurs when the creatinine clearance is below 50 ml per minute per 1.73 sq m and progresses in parallel to the loss of renal function until the hemoglobin concentration is in the range of 5 to 7 gm/dl.

Symptoms, Signs and Course

The anemia of renal insufficiency is usually well tolerated because tissue oxygen delivery is maintained by a right shift of the oxygen dissociation curve. Symptoms of weakness, fatigue, dyspnea, and anorexia are usually related to the uremia. Pallor occurs secondary to the anemia. Edema, hypertension, and signs of heart failure are caused by fluid overload from the renal failure. The anemia becomes more severe as the renal function deteriorates but frequently results in little added disability. Improvement in renal function and dialysis may moderate the severity of the anemia.

Laboratory Findings

The anemia is normochromic and normocytic with a corrected reticulocyte count of less than 2 per cent. Peripheral smear may show burr cells and target cells with severe renal failure. Iron studies and folate and vitamin B_{12} levels are normal in uncomplicated cases. The bone marrow is usually normocellular with some degree of erythroid hypoplasia. Iron stores and sideroblasts are normal.

Other laboratory abnormalities help support this diagnosis. The blood urea nitrogen and creatinine levels are elevated. With moderate or severe anemia, the serum phosphate level is usually elevated, the calcium level is depressed, and a metabolic acidosis is present secondary to the renal failure.

Errors and Pitfalls in Diagnosis

Deficiency of iron and folic acid occurs in higher frequency in patients with renal failure. Iron deficiency occurs because of increased blood loss from bleeding and dialysis. Folic acid deficiency may occur because of poor dietary intake and increased loss with dialysis. The serum ferritin is very useful in determining iron status, and serum and red cell folate levels are reliable in untransfused patients with renal insufficiency.

Pure Red Cell Aplasia

Synonyms

Aplastic crisis with hemolytic anemia; erythroid hypoplasia, red cell aplasia, erythroblastopenia in adults; Joseph-Diamond-Blackfan syndrome in children.

Definition

These anemias are caused by a relatively isolated decrease in production of erythrocytes secondary to a reduction in the number of erythroid precursors in the bone marrow. Acute forms usually are seen in individuals with chronic hemolytic anemias following infection or administration of certain drugs. Chronic forms have an onset in early childhood or may be acquired later in life. The childhood form (Joseph-Diamond-Blackfan syndrome) usually has an onset within the first two years of life and may have a genetic basis. The acquired form may have an onset at any age and is associated with thymoma in about one half of reported cases. Responsiveness to steroids, coincident diseases, and laboratory findings suggest an immune etiology for many of the cases.

Symptoms, Signs and Course

The anemia in these disorders is usually severe, causing symptoms of weakness, fatigue, and dyspnea with exertion. Patients with the acute form frequently, but not invariably, have a past history of chronic hemolytic anemia and a history of an antecedent viral syndrome. Adults with the chronic form occasionally have myasthenia gravis, rheumatologic diseases, or thyroid disease. Physical examination reveals pallor in most patients. There may be physical findings related to the chronic hemolytic state in those with acute red cell aplasia. Those with the chronic form may have evidence of iron overload, hepatic dysfunction, and congestive splenomegaly.

Acute red cell aplasia is usually self-limited and responds to support by red cell transfusion. The chronic forms have variable courses. Thymectomy in adults with thymoma may induce a remission. Steroids, immunosuppression, or antithymocyte globulin may induce remissions in children and adults. Patients that do not respond to treatment require chronic transfusion, which induces iron overload resulting in endocrine, hepatic, and cardiac failure.

Laboratory Findings

Severe anemia with reticulocytopenia is the rule. The anemia is usually normochromic and normocytic. In the majority of patients, the white cell and platelet counts are normal. Serum iron and transferrin saturation are elevated. The bone marrow is normocellular with normal numbers of myeloid precursors and megakaryocytes. Erythroid precursors are severely reduced in number or absent.

Adult patients with the chronic form may have autoantibodies to red cells, heterophile antibodies, antinuclear antibodies, and false-positive tests for syphilis.

Radiologic Evaluation

In adults, chest x-ray may show an anterior mediastinal mass with a coexistent thymoma. Computerized tomography of the chest should probably be performed when plane films are negative to exclude small thymomas.

Errors and Pitfalls in Diagnosis

Acute red cell aplasia may be the first manifestation of folic acid deficiency in individuals with chronic hemolytic anemia. Megaloblastic changes are usually evident in the myeloid and erythroid precursors, but serum and red cell folic acid levels should probably be routinely determined. The first manifestation of spontaneous or drug-induced aplastic anemia may be red cell aplasia. Drugs capable of inducing aplastic anemia should be discontinued, and a bone marrow should be repeated if there is a fall in the white blood cell or platelet count over time.

Anemia Secondary to Endocrine Deficiencies

Definition

Hypothyroidism, androgen deficiency, and adrenal insufficiency are associated with mild anemias. The anemia of hypothyroidism probably results from decreased erythropoietin production due to decreased metabolic demands for oxygen. Androgen deficiency in males results in anemia, as androgens both increase erythropoietin production by the kidney and increase the effect of erythropoietin on the bone marrow. Adrenocortical hormones increase erythrocyte production through unknown mechanisms. Pituitary insufficiency results in decreases of thyroid, adrenal, and gonadal hormones; causing a moderately severe anemia.

Symptoms, Signs and Course

In general, the symptoms and physical findings are related to the underlying hormonal deficiency and not the anemia. The hemoglobin level increases with correction of the hormonal deficiency by replacement therapy.

Laboratory Findings

The anemia is usually normocytic and normochromic with a reduced reticulocyte count. The MCV may be elevated in hypothyroidism. The white cell count and platelet count are normal; however, adrenal insufficiency may be accompanied by an absolute neutropenia and eosinophilia with a relative lymphocytosis. Iron studies and vitamin B_{12} and folate levels are normal in uncomplicated cases. The bone marrow is normocellular to slightly hypocellular with mild to moderate erythroid hypoplasia.

The laboratory findings of the primary endocrine deficiency predominate. These are outlined in the appropriate articles on endocrine deficiencies.

Errors and Pitfalls in Diagnosis

The most common error is to attribute the weakness and fatigue to the anemia and to not consider the presence of an endocrine abnormality. This is particularly true in hypothyroidism. The anemia of adrenal insufficiency may be masked by a concomitant reduction in plasma volume, becoming apparent only after fluid replacement.

Pernicious anemia occurs with higher frequency in individuals with immune-mediated hypothyroidism and adrenal insufficiency. It is important to look for megaloblastic changes in the smears and bone marrows of individuals with these disorders. Determination of vitamin B_{12} levels should be done in hypothyroid patients with macrocytosis.

DECREASED ERYTHROCYTE PRODUCTION WITH ALTERATIONS IN LEUKOCYTE AND PLATELET PRODUCTION

The diagnostic considerations are altered when there is concomitant reduction or elevation of the white cell count, platelet count, or both. Bone marrow destruction, failure, or replacement all cause anemia with reductions in white cell or platelet counts. The anemia in this setting is also normochromic and normocytic, and the reticulocyte count is low. Bone marrow examination with bone marrow biopsy is almost always indicated when an anemia is accompanied by significant alteration of leukocyte and platelet counts.

Aplastic Anemia

Definition

Aplastic anemia is characterized by pancytopenia with severe reduction in the numbers of erythrocytic precursors, granulocytic precursors, and megakaryocytes in the bone marrow. The etiology of this reduction appears to be damage to the pleuripotent stem cell compartment by radiation, drugs, viruses, or immunologic mechanisms. In about one half of cases, the underlying mechanism is not identified. Administration of sufficient ionizing radiation to the bone marrow results in aplasia. A large number of chemicals and drugs have been associated with aplastic anemia. Benzene, chloramphenicol, nonsteroidal anti-inflammatory drugs, gold salts, and antineoplastic agents are those most commonly implicated. Viral hepatitis may cause severe marrow aplasia. There is growing evidence that a number of cases may result from cellular or antibody-mediated immune suppression of stem cell proliferation.

Symptoms, Signs and Course

Patients may present with weakness and fatigue secondary to the anemia, fever, and infection from the neutropenia and with bleeding from thrombocytopenia. Physical findings include pallor, petechiae, ecchymoses, retinal hemorrhages, and gum bleeding. Fever is usually present only with secondary infections. Because the spleen is almost never palpable, the presence of splenomegaly should suggest other causes of marrow failure.

The outlook for patients with severe aplastic anemia is not good, with a median survival of about 6 months. Death usually is caused by bleeding or infection. With less severe reduction in white cell and platelet counts, the prognosis is improved; however, iron overload is a problem when chronic transfusion is required. Spontaneous remissions do occur, especially when marrow toxic agents are withdrawn. Bone marrow transplantation in children and young adults greatly improves the outlook in severe aplastic anemia. Antithymocyte globulin shows promise for older patients and for those without a bone marrow donor.

Laboratory Findings

The anemia is normochromic and normocytic with severe reticulocytopenia. White cell and platelet counts are also markedly reduced. Lymphocytes predominate on the peripheral smear. Bone marrow aspiration reveals absence of erythrocytic precursors, granulocytic precursors, and megakaryocytes. There may be relative or absolute increases in plasma cells, lymphocytes, and tissue mast cells. Trephine marrow biopsy is mandatory for establishing this diagnosis because similar aspirates may occasionally be seen when the bone marrow is infiltrated by tumor or fibrosis. The biopsy in aplastic anemia confirms the absence of marrow elements showing only fat and small islands of lymphocytes, plasma cells, and occasional marrow elements.

Serum iron levels and transferrin saturation are increased. Serum B_{12} levels are occasionally low for unknown reasons. Iron kinetic studies show very low plasma iron turnover and marrow iron incorporation with increased uptake in the liver and spleen.

Errors and Pitfalls in Diagnosis

The most common error in the diagnosis of aplasia is reliance upon the marrow aspirate alone. The aspirate may appear severely hypocellular in situations of marrow replacement. In addition, there may be an appearance of immaturity in the remaining marrow elements, leading to the diagnosis of leukemia. Such a mistake could have devastating consequences if therapy for leukemia is initiated.

Leukemia and Myeloproliferative Syndromes

Definition

Anemia is a very frequent occurrence in patients that present with leukemia or other myeloproliferative disorders. Chronic myelogenous and lymphocytic leukemias usually present with increased white cell counts and normal or increased platelet counts. Acute leukemias present with elevated or reduced white cell counts and thrombocytopenia. Myeloproliferative syndromes often present with anemia and may have high, low, or normal white blood cell and platelet counts.

Symptoms, Signs, and Course

These disorders present with weakness, fatigue, bleeding, and infection. Pallor is frequent. Splenomegaly, hepatomegaly, lymphadenopathy, petechiae, and ecchymoses may be present. The anemia usually improves with control of the leukemic process. The ultimate prognosis depends on the natural history of the underlying disorder and effectiveness of treatment. Marrow failure with bleeding and infection is the most common cause of death.

Laboratory Findings

The anemia is normochromic and normocytic with a low reticulocyte count. Peripheral smear usually shows immature white blood cells and nucleated red blood cells. Bone marrow aspiration may be difficult (dry tap) and usually shows a hypercellular marrow with increases in immature cells. Erythroid precursors and megakaryocytes are reduced in number. Bone marrow biopsy is very hypercellular with predominance of the leukemic cells.

Other laboratory abnormalities include increases in lactate dehydrogenase and uric acid levels. Iron levels and transferrin saturation are increased. Serum and red cell folate may be low.

Errors and Pitfalls in Diagnosis

Acute leukemias presenting with pancytopenia may be mistaken for aplastic anemia or myelophthistic anemia. Bone marrow aspiration and biopsy will usually result in a correct diagnosis.

Myelophthistic Anemia

Definition

Myelophthistic anemias result from replacement of the bone marrow by malignancy, fibrosis, or granulomas. Malignant processes that frequently involve the marrow include lymphomas, myeloma, lung cancer, breast cancer, prostate cancer, and renal cell tumors. Myelofibrosis can be seen as a primary bone marrow disease or secondary to malignancy or autoimmune diseases. The most common granulomatous disease involving the marrow is tuberculosis; however, sarcoidosis and fungal diseases can also occasionally cause marrow replacement.

Symptoms, Signs and Course

These disorders usually all present with weight loss, weakness, and fatigue. Bone pain or tenderness is frequently present. Fever may be present as a symptom of the underlying illness or as the result of coexistent infection. Physical examination reveals pallor. Petechiae or ecchymoses may be present when the platelet count is reduced. Splenomegaly is the rule. Hepatomegaly and lymphadenopathy may also occur.

The myelophthistic anemia will improve if treatment of the underlying condition is effective. The prognosis is very guarded if effective treatment is lacking.

Laboratory Findings

The anemia is usually normochromic and normocytic. The white cell and platelet counts are generally depressed but may be elevated in malignancy or tuberculosis. The peripheral smear is characteristic, showing nucleated red cells and early white cells (leukoerythroblastotic reaction). Teardrop-shaped red cells, schistocytes, and rouleau may be present. Bone marrow aspiration and biopsy should always be obtained when these findings are seen on a peripheral smear.

Bone marrow aspiration may be difficult and misleading. The aspirate may be normal or hypocellular because the infiltration is often patchy. Trephine biopsy usually reveals the nature of the infiltrating progress. Special stains and cultures should be obtained when granulomas are present. Reticulum stains may be required to demonstrate myelofibrosis.

Radiologic Evaluation

Plain x-rays may show lytic or blastic lesions in cases with solid tumors, lymphomas, and myeloma. Radionuclide bone scans can also be positive in this setting. Myelosclerosis may be demonstrated radiologically in cases of advanced myelofibrosis.

Errors and Pitfalls in Diagnosis

Severe megaloblastic anemias can present with pancytopenia and cause a leukoerythroblastic reaction with teardrop-shaped red cells and schistocytes. The evaluation of MCV and megaloblastic changes in the marrow allow easy differentiation. In megaloblastic anemias, vitamin B_{12} or folate levels will be low.

Occasionally the marrow involvement is patchy and the marrow infiltration is missed on original biopsy. The presence of a leukoerythroblastotic reaction strongly suggests marrow invasion, and repeat biopsy should be obtained if originally negative.

PERNICIOUS ANEMIA AND OTHER MEGALOBLASTIC ANEMIAS

By Maria da Costa, M.D.
and Sheldon P. Rothenberg, M.D.
Brooklyn, N.Y.

The first description of a patient with pernicious anemia is ascribed to Thomas Addison of Guy's Hospital in London. In 1855 in his famous manuscript, *On the Constitutional and Local Effects of Diseases of the Suprarenal Capsules,* he included a rather incidental description of a particular type of anemia. He called this "idiopathic anemia" and suggested that it was due to "some form of fatty degeneration." His description did not include the microscopic examination of the blood, the characteristic signs and symptoms of jaundice and glossitis, or the neurologic abnormalities associated with pernicious anemia. The observation by microscopists between 1875 and 1890 emphasized the diagnostic importance of "giant" red blood cells or "macrocytes" and the large nucleated red cells with dispersed nuclear chromatin or "megaloblasts" in these fatal idiopathic anemias. By the turn of the century, the microscopic appearance of the blood, together with the symptoms and physical signs noted by bedside clinicians, led to the recognition of a distinct pathologic condition appropriately called "pernicious anemia." It slowly became evident that pernicious anemia was not uniformly fatal and spontaneous remissions did occur. Indeed the term "progressive pernicious anemia" was first used in 1872 in Zurich by Anton Bierman, who stated that this "anemia was found among poor people, especially women about 30 years of age who were pregnant." It appears, therefore, that Addison and Bierman each described patients with megaloblastic anemia, the former most likely due to vitamin B_{12} deficiency and the latter to folate deficiency.

Since these early descriptions of megaloblastic anemia, a wealth of information has accumulated about the etiology, biochemistry, physiology, and morphology of these disorders. As a result, it has become very simple to identify and successfully treat most patients with this disease. Nevertheless, despite this knowledge, and the newer techniques of diagnosis available, such as electronic sizing of cells, radioisotopic absorption tests, and radioassays of serum vitamin B_{12} and folate, problems in the diagnosis and management of megaloblastic anemias in clinical practice are not infrequently encountered. This article outlines the salient features in the investigation and diagnosis of these disorders and comments on some of the changes in the evaluation of these patients because of the newer laboratory techniques available.

DEFINITION

The megaloblastic anemias are due to disordered deoxyribonucleic acid (DNA) synthesis in the hematopoietic cells of the bone marrow. This impairment of DNA maturation slows cell replication, results in the characteristic nuclear-cytoplasmic asynchrony manifested by the relatively larger nucleus containing lacy chromatin in replicating cells, and leads to macrocytosis of erythrocytes and hypersegmentation of polymorphonuclear granulocytes. These hematologic manifestations of megaloblastic anemia are similar, irrespective of the etiology.

SYNONYMS

The terms pernicious anemia, macrocytic anemia, and megaloblastic anemia are sometimes used interchangeably, but they are not always synonymous. Megaloblastic anemias have multiple causes. Pernicious anemia is a specific entity in which vitamin B_{12} deficiency resulting in a megaloblastic anemia is due to lack of gastric intrinsic factor as a result of atrophic gastritis and loss of parietal cells. In clinical practice the most common cause of the naturally occurring megaloblastic anemias are vitamin B_{12} or folate deficiency. The use of chemotherapeutic cytotoxic agents that inhibit DNA synthesis may also induce megaloblastic hematopoiesis.

DIAGNOSIS OF MEGALOBLASTIC HEMATOPOIESIS

The widespread use of automated electronic blood counters which provide an accurate measurement of the mean corpuscular volume (MCV) of the red blood cells has resulted in a significant improvement in the recognition and diagnosis of megaloblastic anemia. Since macrocytosis is one of the earliest changes noted in the blood count and may occur well before anemia or clinical symptoms are manifested, these instruments have made possible the very early recognition of megaloblastic anemia. The general availability of the MCV has also led to the recognition that macrocytosis can occur with other disorders associated with normoblastic hematopoiesis, and the frequency with which this occurs makes a bone marrow examination necessary to exclude megaloblastosis.

The normal MCV in adults is 83 to 96 femtoliters (fl) with a mean of 88 fl. With some electronic counters, the normal range can extend to 101 fl. The MCV of a newborn infant has a range of 96 to 112 fl, with a mean of 104 fl for the first few months of life. The MCV is a very constant parameter, with only minor variation of 1 to 3 fl in a properly calibrated instrument, and persistent increases in the MCV above normal require investigation.

The causes of macrocytosis are shown in Table 1. Macrocytosis without megaloblastic hematopoiesis is usually mild, the MCV seldom exceeding 110 fl, and is not accompanied by a corresponding increase in the mean corpuscular hemoglobin (MCH).

The diagnosis of megaloblastic hematopoiesis is made by examination of the peripheral blood and bone marrow. The abnormalities of the peripheral blood frequently appear early, before the anemia, and

Table 1. Causes of Macrocytosis

Physiologic
Newborns
Macrocytosis with Megaloblastic Maturation
Vitamin B_{12} deficiency
Folate deficiency
Chemotherapeutic agents that interfere with DNA synthesis (e.g., antimetabolites, alkylating agents)
Congenital enzyme deficiencies (e.g., Orotic aciduria, Lesch-Nyhan syndrome)
Macrocytosis with Normoblastic Hematopoiesis
Reticulocytosis due to hemolysis or in response to hemorrhage
Excess alcohol intake without folate deficiency
Liver disease
Aplastic and hypoplastic anemias including pure red cell aplasia
Sideroblastic anemia
Hypothyroidism
Preleukemic syndromes with refractory anemia
Myeloid metaplasia (this may be secondary to associated folate deficiency)
Fictitious Increase in the Mean Corpuscular Volume
Cold agglutinins with a high thermal amplitude
Blood left at room temperature (causes swelling of the red cells)
Marked leukocytosis in the presence of anemia

become more marked as the severity of the anemia increases. The MCV and MCH are increased, but the mean corpuscular hemoglobin concentration (MCHC) is normal. The earliest morphologic changes are multilobed granulocytes and a nearly uniform macrocytosis, which tend to be oval in shape. This macrovalocytosis later becomes more prominent and is accompanied by a marked anisocytosis, poikilocytois, and fragmentation of the red cells as the anemia progresses. Howell-Jolly bodies, nuclear fragments, and basophilic stippling are commonly present in the red cells when anemia is marked, and nucleated red cells with typical megaloblastic morphology may also appear in the peripheral blood. The reticulocyte count is low because of the bone marrow dyspoiesis.

The leukocyte count is within the normal range in early or mild megaloblastosis. However, hypersegmentation of the neutrophils may be a very early finding, appearing before anemia, and serves to distinguish megaloblastic hematopoiesis from normoblastic macrocytosis. Hypersegmentation is defined as the presence of five lobes in greater than 5 per cent of the neutrophils, or the presence of one or more granulocytes with six or more lobes. Giant neutrophils or macropolycytes may also be present. As the anemia progresses, the number of leukocytes and platelets decreases, the thrombocytopenia in particular being indicative of serious hematopoietic failure.

Bone marrow morphology provides definitive evidence of megaloblastic hematopoiesis and is necessary in all patients except those who have classic findings in the peripheral blood and low concentrations of vitamin B_{12} or folate in the serum. Like the peripheral blood, morphologic changes in the bone marrow parallel the degree of severity of the anemia. The bone marrow is characteristically hypercellular with an increase of all cell lines, but most predominantly in the erythroid series. There is typical megaloblast morphology, and there is failure of the marrow precursors to mature properly, resulting in intramedullary destruction or ineffective hematopoiesis. This results in peripheral pancytopenia. The megaloblastic cells are characteristically large and show "asynchronous" nuclear-cytoplasmic maturation. The nuclei of the erythroid precursors are large and immature with a fine lacy chromatin, while hemoglobinization of the cytoplasm proceeds normally. In mild cases, or if iron deficiency is also present, these megaloblastic changes may be detected only in the late erythroblasts or in only a small proportion of the erythroblasts, but when the anemia is severe, these changes are recognizable at all stages of development. Megaloblastic features are also present in the granulocyte precursors, particularly in the metamyelocytes and myelocytes. The metamyelocytes are large with huge horseshoe-like nuclei. Occasionally, these cells may be present before megaloblastic changes in the erythroblasts are obvious. Megakaryocytes may be increased or decreased, and morphologic changes, multilobulated nuclei containing finely dispersed chromatin, are seen only when the anemia is relatively severe.

The changes in the blood and bone marrow are identical in vitamin B_{12} and in folate deficiency, and examination of the peripheral smear and bone marrow cannot distinguish between the two.

OTHER LABORATORY FINDINGS

Intramedullary hemolysis may elevate the unconjugated bilirubin in the serum to 1.5 to 3 mg/dl, and the serum haptoglobin is low or absent. There is also an increase in urobilinogen in the urine and stool as a consequence of this hemolytic process. Serum lactate dehydrogenase (LD) isoenzymes 1 and 2 are also elevated because of intramedullary destruction of early erythroid precursors; this increase occurs in 90 per cent of patients, sometimes reaching levels of 5000 to 10,000 U/liter. Plasma triglycerides and cholesterol, total and esterified, are often decreased in megaloblastic anemia and return to normal with treatment. Hypogammaglobulinemia has been observed in some patients.

The diagnosis of a megaloblastic anemia is only the first step in the evaluation of the patient. An investigation of the underlying disorder causing the megaloblastic hematopoiesis is essential for proper management and treatment of the patient.

PRESENTING SIGNS AND SYMPTOMS

A careful history and physical examination will often provide evidence of the underlying disorder. Though the hematologic manifestations are virtually indistinguishable in all megaloblastic anemias, there may be unique clinical features that indicate the underlying etiology.

A history of dietary habits, such as excess alcohol consumption or strict vegetarian diet, abnormal bowel function, gastric or other abdominal surgery, and travel to areas where sprue is endemic will provide important clues to the diagnosis.

The presenting symptoms are usually nonspecifically referable to the anemia, and include fatigue, lassitude, palpitation and dyspnea on exertion, and angina. The severity of such symptoms is usually proportional to the anemia and the age of the patient. Deficiency of vitamin B_{12} develops more slowly than folate deficiency, and there may be a remarkable lack of symptoms even with severe anemia because hemodynamic compensatory mechanisms have sufficient time to fully develop.

Gastrointestinal symptoms are common in megaloblastic anemia. Soreness and ulceration of the tongue and buccal mucosa may occur with deficiency of either vitamin, although it is more common with vitamin B_{12} deficiency. Diarrhea and weight loss are also frequent complaints, more so in folate than vitamin B_{12} deficiency. Central nervous system symptoms such as loss of memory, irritability, dementia, and disordered motor function are more specific for vitamin B_{12} deficiency. With more advanced disease, neurologic damage, spastic paraplegia, severe ataxia, loss of sphincter control, and rarely optic atrophy occur with vitamin B_{12} deficiency. Although such neurologic defects usually become manifest when the megaloblastic anemia is obvious, occasionally the hematologic abnormalities may be minimal. This is more common with vitamin B_{12} deficiency in strict vegetarians or in patients who also have a high folate diet or who receive folate supplements.

FINDINGS ON PHYSICAL EXAMINATION

Physical findings depend on the degree of anemia and the associated disorder causing the megaloblastosis. Mild conjunctival icterus and lemon-yellow tint to the skin are typical. The tongue is smooth with atrophic papillae, or there may be glossitis with an inflamed beefy appearance. Occasionally, particularly when anemia is very severe, the spleen may be slightly enlarged as a result of extramedullary hematopoiesis. However, if the spleen is moderately or markedly enlarged, other etiologies must be excluded. Lymphadenopathy and hepatomegaly are not features of megaloblastic anemia per se. Severe anemia may be associated with retinal hemorrhages, and edema with congestive cardiac failure may be present. Bleeding manifestations may appear if there is severe thrombocytopenia, and infections may occur if the neutropenia is marked.

The neurologic defects which are specific for vitamin B_{12} deficiency are the findings of subacute combined degeneration of the spinal cord, i.e., posterior and lateral column pathology. This results in impaired position and vibratory senses, motor weakness with spasticity, hyperreflexia, and pathologic plantar reflexes. There may also be the findings of peripheral neuropathy with impairment of pain and temperature sensation in the glove-or-stocking distribution, but these findings are less specific for vitamin B_{12} deficiency.

The neurologic defects associated with folate deficiency have been less clearly defined. Prolonged drug-induced folate deficiency has been reported to be associated with neuropsychiatric disorders, and in recent years several cases of mental retardation have been ascribed to specific inborn errors of folate metabolism.

Other physical findings depend on associated diseases. These are more likely to be found in patients with folate deficiency, which is usually secondary to another disorder such as malabsorption, alcoholism, or malnutrition.

COURSE

The megaloblastic anemias are among the most satisfying disorders to diagnose and treat since they respond completely to supplementation with the deficient vitamin. Because of early recognition and treatment, one now seldom sees the natural course of these disorders. The anemia will respond completely to administration of the deficient vitamin unless iron deficiency or an underlying medical disorder is also present that suppresses bone marrow function. The severe neurologic disorder that occurs with vitamin B_{12} deficiency may not improve, or—if it does—the response is very slow. If the neurologic symptoms are of recent onset and mild, they can revert completely to normal.

COMMON COMPLICATIONS

The most dreaded complication of the gastric atrophy in pernicious anemia is the development of gastric carcinoma. This occurs in 1 to 3 per cent of patients even after they have been treated with vitamin B_{12}. Several autoimmune disorders that are not complications of the megaloblastic anemia are often associated with pernicious anemia. These are endocrinopathies such as myxedema, thyrotoxicosis, Addison's disease, hypoparathyroidism, and ovarian failure. Mucocutaneous candidiasis, alopecia areata, and vitiligo have also been ascribed to autoimmune disorders associated with pernicious anemia. Acquired hypogammaglobulinemia or an isolated IgA deficiency may also occur in association with pernicious anemia, and such immunodeficiency may lead to infestation with *Giardia lamblia* and bacterial overgrowth, which per se can result in vitamin B_{12} malabsorption.

Iron deficiency has been reported to exist in about 10 per cent of patients with megaloblastic anemia and, though this is not a complication, it may result in an incomplete response to treatment with vitamin B_{12} or folate.

EVALUATION OF A PATIENT WITH MEGALOBLASTIC ANEMIA

After the diagnosis of a megaloblastic anemia has been established from the hematologic and laboratory findings, it is necessary to document the precise vitamin deficiency. Measurements of serum vitamin B_{12} and serum and red cell folate levels are the simplest and most useful laboratory tests and in general provide an accurate diagnosis.

A low serum vitamin B_{12} for all practical purposes indicates deficiency of this vitamin. Newer methods of vitamin B_{12} measurement employing saturation analysis have caused confusion in the interpretation of results because the lower limit of normal varies with the technique. By the microbiologic assay, serum values below 200 pg/ml (200 ng/liter) indicate vitamin B_{12} deficiency, but with some of the radioassay methods serum vitamin B_{12} levels of 200 to 300 pg/ml (200 to 300 ng/liter) may be obtained in deficient patients. Radioassay methods that measure "true" vitamin B_{12} more closely approximate the microbiologic assay, but false low levels have also been observed.

A low serum vitamin B_{12} may be observed in pregnant patients, some patients with a paraprotein in the serum, in 10 per cent of patients with primary folate deficiency, and occasionally in normal subjects in the absence of B_{12} deficiency. Antibiotics and other drugs that inhibit bacterial growth can give falsely low vitamin B_{12} levels with the microbiologic assay. A true normal vitamin B_{12} in the presence of tissue deficiency may be obtained in a patient with a myeloproliferative disorder who has high transcobalamin I serum B_{12}-binding protein. Children with congenital transcobalamin II (TCII) deficiency have normal serum vitamin B_{12} but have a megaloblastic anemia because of the inability of the hematopoietic cells to take up vitamin B_{12}.

The serum folate level (normal, 3.5 to 20 ng/ml) is a less reliable test for folate deficiency. Serum folate levels become reduced quite rapidly after decreased dietary intake, with alcohol consumption, or during a severe illness, even though tissue stores are normal, so that a low serum folate suggests a negative folate balance but not necessarily folate deficiency. A low red cell folate level (< 150 ng/ml) is more indicative of folate deficiency except in vitamin B_{12} deficiency, in which there is impaired retention of folate in the red cells. In vitamin B_{12} deficiency, however, the serum folate is usually normal or high, whereas it is very low if the megaloblastic anemia is due to folate deficiency. Because of these variations it is necessary to measure both vitamins to make a correct diagnosis. Interpretation of the serum levels of these vitamins is shown in Table 2.

If the diagnosis of vitamin B_{12} deficiency is established, the cause must be determined. In over 75 per cent of patients, this is due to pernicious anemia, and it is necessary to show that there is a lack of intrinsic factor. The latter always is associated with histamine or pentagastrin-fast achlorhydria. The diagnosis of pernicious anemia must be precisely documented because if it exists the patient will require parenteral vitamin B_{12} for the rest of his or her life in order to avoid relapse of the anemia and possible neurologic damage.

The presence of circulating antibodies to intrinsic factor is quite specific for pernicious anemia and is found in 50 to 60 per cent of these patients, particularly when the disease occurs at a young age (e.g., below 50 years). Thus, the presence of megaloblastic anemia, low serum vitamin B_{12} level, and intrinsic factor antibodies in the serum can be taken as definitive evidence for the diagnosis of pernicious anemia. On singular occasions, intrinsic factor antibodies are found in autoimmune endocrinopathies, in some patients with atrophic gastritis without clinical evidence of vitamin B_{12} deficiency, and in some relatives of patients with pernicious anemia. Such subjects must be followed carefully for the development of vitamin B_{12} deficiency. Antibodies to gastric parietal cells are present in the serum of about 85 per cent of patients with pernicious anemia; however, these are not specific for this diagnosis, since they are also present in patients with atrophic gastritis in the absence of pernicious anemia.

If intrinsic factor antibodies are lacking in the serum of a patient with vitamin B_{12} deficiency, a series of absorption tests are available. The most commonly used is the Schilling test, in which urinary excretion of radioactive vitamin B_{12} is measured following oral administration. If the urinary excretion is less than 7 per cent of the dose in 24 to 48 hours, malabsorption of vitamin B_{12} is likely. In pernicious anemia, excretion is usually less than 2 per cent. The second part of the test is done 4 to 5 days later, when intrinsic factor is given with the oral tracer dose of vitamin B_{12}. If urinary excretion becomes normal, the vitamin B_{12} deficiency is ascribed to lack of intrinsic factor. This is diagnostic of pernicious anemia. If there is no improvement in vitamin B_{12} absorption with intrinsic factor, it indicates intestinal malabsorption of the vitamin (Table 3). One note of caution must be applied to this interpretation if the Schilling test is done soon after the diagnosis of megaloblastic anemia is made and before the patient has been adequately treated with vitamin B_{12}. In a high proportion of patients with megaloblastic anemia, there may be impairment of vitamin B_{12} absorption through the ileal mucosa because of morphologic changes in the mucosal cells. Absorption of the vitamin, even with intrinsic factor, therefore, may be impaired. We recommend that the Schilling test be deferred for 2 to 4 weeks after the patient has been treated with vitamin B_{12}.

In patients with renal insufficiency or in patients in whom urine collections are unreliable, absorption of radioactive vitamin B_{12} may be determined by measurement of plasma radioactivity 8 to 10 hours after administration of the test dose.

Chronic pancreatitis may affect the Schilling test and suggest malabsorption of vitamin B_{12} even though gastric secretion of intrinsic factor and ileal absorption are normal. The cause is a failure to digest a vitamin B_{12}-binding protein (R-protein) in the intestinal fluid because of lack of pancreatic trypsin. As a consequence, this binder, which has no intrinsic factor activity, sequesters the radioactive vitamin B_{12} used in the Schilling test and prevents its absorption. Actually, clinical vitamin B_{12} deficiency is uncommon in chronic pancreatitis if the dietary supply is adequate because there is then sufficient vitamin to saturate both intrinsic factor and other vitamin B_{12}-binding proteins in the intestinal succus.

If it is not possible to do a Schilling test, the concentration of intrinsic factor may be measured directly in the gastric juice 15 minutes after maximal stimulation with pentagastrin. Absence of secretion of hydrochloric acid 45 minutes after pentagastrin is administered is further evidence for the diagnosis of pernicious anemia. If pernicious anemia is excluded by these studies, other causes of vitamin B_{12} deficiency will have to be sought (Table 3). The most likely cause is malabsorption secondary to disease of the ileum, and evaluation requires appropriate x-ray studies of the small intestine for evidence of anatomic abnormalities or mucosal changes suggestive of sprue. Other studies for malabsorption, including xylose absorption and stool fat content, may be necessary. If there is evidence of a blind loop syndrome, the patient

Table 2. Serum Vitamin B_{12} and Serum and Red Blood Cell Folate Levels in Deficiency States

Deficiency	Serum Vitamin B_{12}	Serum Folate	Red Blood Cell Folate
Vitamin B_{12}	Low	Normal or high	Normal or low
Folic acid	Normal (low in about 10%)	Low	Low
Vitamin B_{12} + Folic acid	Low	Low	Low

Table 3. Causes of Vitamin B_{12} Deficiency

Nutritional
- Strict vegetarians and infants of such mothers

Lack of Intrinsic Factor
- Pernicious anemia—adult type with atrophic gastritis
- Congenital lack of intrinsic factor secretion with normal acid and pepsin secretion
- Total or partial gastrectomy
- Diffuse gastric mucosal damage due to ingestion of corrosives or infiltrative disease of the stomach
- Secretion of functionally abnormal intrinsic factor

Ileal Malabsorption of Vitamin B_{12}
- Tropical sprue
- Ileal resection or bypass surgery
- Ileal diseases such as Crohn's disease, tuberculosis, and lymphoma
- Congenital selective malabsorption of vitamin B_{12} with proteinuria (Imerslund-Gräsbeck syndrome)

Anatomic Abnormalities of the Small Intestine with Bacterial Overgrowth
- Blind loops following gastrointestinal surgery
- Duodenal or jejunal fistulae

Fish Tapeworm (*Diphyllobothrium latum*) Infestation

Congenital Transcobalamin II Deficiency

Drugs
- Neomycin, colchicine, paraminosalicylic acid

may be treated with antibiotics for a few weeks and the first part of the Schilling test repeated (without intrinsic factor). It should now be normal. If intestinal disease is established by these studies, a peroral intestinal mucosal biopsy will be helpful in establishing the nature of the pathology.

In rare instances vitamin B_{12} deficiency will be secondary to TCII deficiency. This usually occurs in early infancy, but some adolescents with this disorder have been described. In these patients, serum vitamin B_{12} is normal but there is impaired intestinal absorption of the vitamin. The diagnosis is established by measuring TCII in the serum.

The etiology of folate deficiency (Table 4) is usually obvious from the history and physical examination. If there is no evidence of malnutrition, alcoholism, or increased requirements for folate, intestinal malabsorption must be ruled out. Absorption tests for folate are not generally available, but evidence of intestinal malabsorption from the xylose absorption test, increased stool fat, and X-rays of the small intestine is usually sufficient for the diagnosis. Peroral intestinal mucosal biopsy may be required to establish the specific pathology.

THERAPEUTIC TESTS

If assays for serum vitamin B_{12} and folate are not readily available, a therapeutic trial with a physiologic dose of the missing vitamin can differentiate folate from vitamin B_{12} deficiency. If vitamin B_{12} deficiency is initially suspected from the history and physical examination, 1 to 2 μg of the vitamin is given parenterally daily and the reticulocyte count is obtained 5 to 8 days later. Reticulocytosis confirms the diagnosis of vitamin B_{12} deficiency. If there is no response, 100 μg of folic acid should be given by injection daily. A reticulocytosis 5 to 8 days later confirms deficiency of this vitamin. This dose of folic acid will not produce a response in vitamin B_{12} deficient patients. In patients who have a history of alcohol abuse, it is not advisable to try folic acid initially because reticulocytosis may occur spontaneously during the first week of hospitalization as a consequence of a good diet or withdrawal of alcohol.

PITFALLS IN DIAGNOSIS

The most common pitfall in the recognition of megaloblastic anemia is failure to identify macrocytosis when it is not the predominant component of the red cell abnormality. That is, if 30 per cent of the red cell population had an MCV of 110 fl and 70 per cent had an MCV of 85 fl, the measured MCV would be 92 fl and would appear to be normal. A similar result would be obtained if there were a dimorphic anemia (i.e., concomitant iron deficiency or thalassemia minor) or if there were an excess population of fragmented red cells. This pitfall can be avoided by careful examination of the peripheral blood smear.

If iron deficiency is also present, erythropoiesis may not appear megaloblastic, but an experienced observer can recognize the giant metamyelocytes of megaloblastic hematopoiesis.

Alcohol excess can result in macrocytosis in the absence of folate deficiency. In this instance, serum folate may be low because alcohol impairs the enterohepatic circulation of folate and a red cell folate measurement is the only simple test to determine whether the patient is folate-deficient.

Patients with chronic pancreatitis may have an abnormal Schilling test for the reason discussed previously. This does not necessarily mean that there is a

Table 4. Causes of Folate Deficiency

Nutritional
- Inadequate intake

Excess Alcohol Ingestion with Nutritional Deficiency of Folate

Malabsorption
- Tropical sprue
- Gluten-induced enteropathy (celiac disease)
- Congenital folate malabsorption
- Crohn's disease (with involvement of proximal small intestine)

Increased Requirements
- Pregnancy
- Infancy
- Chronic hemolytic anemia
- Chronic dialysis
- Increased cell turnover (e.g., myelofibrosis with myeloid metaplasia, psoriasis)

Drugs
- Anticonvulsants—phenytoin, barbiturates
- Oral contraceptives (?)

Inborn Errors of Folate Metabolism
- Methylene tetrahydrofolate reductase deficiency
- Dihydrofolate reductase deficiency (?)

risk of developing vitamin B_{12} deficiency unless dietary intake of the vitamin is low. In such patients the level of serum vitamin B_{12} is more important than the results of the Schilling test to determine a deficiency state.

Finally, interpretation of a serum vitamin B_{12} level should be based on normal values established for the specific assay method used. False low values have been observed when the commercial kit measuring "true B_{12}" has been used. It is, therefore, necessary to correlate the serum vitamin B_{12} measurement with the clinical disorder that prompted this determination.

IRON DEFICIENCY ANEMIA

By Arthur Haut, M.D.
Little Rock, Arkansas

SYNONYMS

Iron lack anemia; anemia of chronic blood loss.

A widely held misconception incorrectly equates *hypochromic microcytic anemia* with *iron deficiency anemia.* That is incorrect because hypochromic microcytic anemia may also result from conditions other than iron deficiency.

DEFINITION

Anemia in which lack of iron per se is the limiting factor in erythropoiesis is correctly termed iron deficiency anemia. When iron deficiency anemia is present, all body iron stores (reserves) are absent and there is insufficient iron to support normal erythropoiesis. It is to be differentiated from *iron depletion,* in which iron stores are less than normal and anemia is absent or, if present, is due to some cause other than lack of iron per se; from *latent iron deficiency,* in which iron stores are fully exhausted but there is sufficient iron to support a normal concentration of hemoglobin in the circulation; and from *iron-deficient erythropoiesis,* a general term referring to less than optimal delivery of iron to the erythron, resulting in hypochromic microcytic erythrocytes. The last situation may occur in some chronic inflammatory diseases and malignancy in the presence of adequate or even increased iron reserves, as well as in actual iron deficiency.

CLASSIFICATION

Iron deficiency anemia may be the most common cause of anemia in the world and is among the leading causes of anemia in the United States. It may be the result of any of a number of conditions that cause a negative iron balance due to excessive loss of iron from the body. Generally this is because of pathologic blood loss, which is often occult. It also results, rarely, from hemosiderinuria, which follows intravascular hemolysis; this may occur with prosthetic heart valves, paroxysmal hemoglobinurias, and other circumstances. Alternatively, insufficient iron in the diet, especially during the phases of rapid growth in infancy and adolescence, and sometimes inadequate absorption of dietary iron, are the responsible mechanisms.

Pulmonary hemosiderosis and the exceedingly rare condition, *congenital atransferrinemia,* are exceptions to the general rule. In these diseases, total body iron stores are normal but they are not available for erythropoiesis because of their sequestration in pulmonary macrophages in the first case, and in marrow macrophages and hepatocytes, for lack of the transport protein, in the second case. The hematologic manifestations in these conditions, nevertheless, are the same as in other causes of iron deficiency anemia.

There are three aspects to the diagnosis of iron deficiency anemia:

1. Recognition of the circumstances in which its presence must be suspected.
2. Definitive tests for establishing or disproving the suspected diagnosis.
3. Recognition and diagnosis of the pathologic state that caused the iron deficiency anemia.

Symptoms and signs (to be discussed) provide the clues that lead to suspicion of iron deficiency anemia. When present, the physician should seek confirmation by ordering the tests listed in Table 1. When positive, the test results establish the diagnosis of iron deficiency anemia. However, the task is not completed until the underlying cause is also diagnosed and treated. Failure to do so might result in recurrence of the anemia or even more serious consequences if, for example, a still curable carcinoma of the colon that had caused occult blood loss were negligently overlooked.

PRESENTING SYMPTOMS AND SIGNS

In the healthy adult male, about 1 mg of iron is lost each day. The same amount is absorbed from a diet that provides about 15 mg of iron, as estimated to be in the average American diet. Unless an additional 0.5 to 1 mg of iron is absorbed daily by the menstruating female and about 2.5 mg daily is absorbed daily during pregnancy and lactation to compensate for the additional loss of iron in those circumstances, iron reserves will be lost and anemia will eventually occur.

For convenience of recall, the symptoms of iron deficiency anemia may be grouped as those (1) common to anemia of any cause, (2) associated with iron deficiency in particular, (3) related to excessive blood/iron loss, and (4) reflecting inadequate diet or absorption of iron.

Symptoms Common to All Anemias

Weakness, fatigue, lassitude, exertional dyspnea, pallid complexion, and tachycardia are common in anemic patients, but these need not occur. Their pres-

Table 1. Results of Differentiating Tests in Iron Deficiency and Simulating Anemias

No.	Test*	Units	Common Test Results: Normal	Iron Deficiency	Thalassemia Heterozygote	Chronic Disease
1	Hemoglobin concentration	gm/dl	Female > 12 Male > 14	4–11	10.5–12.5	7.0–12.0
2	MCV	fl	83–96	70–80	65–77	77–90
3	MCHC	gm/dl rbc	32–36	25–32	29–33	28–34
4	Serum ferritin	μg/l	Female > 20 Male > 30	1–10 1–10	Female > 35 Male > 69	40–100 70–100
5	Plasma iron	μg/dl	65–175	2–40	40–140	25–125
6	TIBC	μg/dl	250–400	275–425	225–425	150–375
7	Transferrin saturation	%	20–50	2–15	20–50	12–60
8	Marrow iron, (Prussian blue stain)	(Visual)	Normal	0–trace	Normal	Normal or increased
9	Marrow sideroblasts	%	17–50	0–8	> 10	6–30
10	Hb A_2	%	2.4–3.0	1.8–2.8	3.0–5.5	2.4–3.0
11	FEP	μg/dl	30–90	200–500	30–90	90–200

*The first four tests usually suffice to identify iron deficiency anemia; 5, 6, and 7 are alternatives to 4; less often, 8, 9, and 11 are required. Test 10 differentiates beta thalassemia heterozygotes from iron deficiency anemia. Tests 7 and 11 are used in population surveys for iron deficiency anemia. The combination of 2 and 10 surveys for beta-thalassemia.

Abbreviations: Hb = Hemoglobin; MCV = mean corpuscular volume; MCHC, mean corpuscular hemoglobin concentration; TIBC = total serum iron-binding capacity; FEP = free erythrocyte protoporphyrin; fl = femtoliters.

ence is not specific for either anemia or iron deficiency. They are least evident when anemia is of gradual onset and progression. They are most prominent when there is the recent or rapid development of anemia.

Symptoms Related to Iron Deficiency Per Se

Dysphagia, especially when accompanied by an esophageal web, brittle finger nails with a spoon-like concave shape (koilonychia), angular stomatitis, and ozena suggest iron deficiency. These, too, are nonspecific.

Symptoms Related to Loss of Blood or Iron

If the history reveals that menorrhagia, metrorrhagia, hematochezia, melena, hematuria, the coffee-colored urine of hemoglobinuria, chronic hemoptysis, epistaxis, or therapeutic, diagnostic, or voluntary phlebotomies (blood donations) have occurred, the setting is ripe for iron deficiency. The underlying conditions are listed in Table 2.

Pregnancy causes an average net loss of about 700 mg of iron (2.5 mg per day). In the absence of dietary supplementation, multiple pregnancies and lactation should be considered as symptomatic evidence suggesting iron deficiency in the anemic woman.

The existence of menorrhagia is notoriously difficult to recognize, even among women patients who are considered to be medically sophisticated. Any of the following should be considered to be provisional evidence of menorrhagia: menstruation for more than seven days; the passage of clots, especially after the first day or of more than about 1 cm in size; the simultaneous use of two or more menstrual pads, or of both pads and tampons; the use of "super" pads or "super" tampons for more than 3 days; or, possibly, the use of more than four pads or tampons daily for more than 1 day.

Occult blood loss is, by definition, not evident from the history. However, it should be suspected if there are symptoms consistent with peptic ulcer, gastritis, or hiatal hernia. The daily ingestion of aspirin or the habitual use of alcohol is associated with gastritis and occult blood loss; hence, such a history implies the possibility of iron deficiency as the cause of anemia. Progressive constipation, intermittent diarrhea, or other major change in bowel habits may be symptomatic of neoplasm or inflammatory disease of the bowel accompanied by occult blood loss.

Symptoms Suggesting Deficient Supply or Absorption of Iron

About 6 mg of iron is estimated to be present with each 1000 kcal of the diet in the United States; less iron is present in the diet in some other countries. Food fadism, which may especially occur in the teenage patient and in the obese, may impair the quantity of iron in the diet. Economic constraints, anorexia, and sociologic and cultural factors also affect the diet and the amount of iron in it. Pica, i.e., the ingestion

Table 2. Predecessors of Iron Deficiency Anemia: Conditions That Most Often Explain Pathologic Blood Loss

Gastrointestinal Tract
Hiatal hernia
Gastritis due to aspirin or alcohol
Gastric ulcer—benign or malignant
Duodenal ulcer, peptic
Leiomyoma—stomach or intestine
Meckel's diverticulum
Hookworm infestation
Regional enteritis, Crohn's disease
Celiac syndrome
Carcinoma of colon or rectum
Polyps of colon or rectum
Diverticulosis coli
Ulcerative colitis or proctitis
Bleeding hemorrhoids
Hereditary hemorrhagic telangiectasia
Genital Tract
Dysfunctional uterine bleeding
Submucosal uterine fibroids
Grand multiparity
Postpartum hemorrhage
Urinary Tract
Chronic hemorrhagic cystitis
Carcinoma of the urinary bladder
Carcinoma of the kidney
Hemoglobinuria and hemosiderinuria
Due to chronic hemolytic anemia with intravascular hemolysis
Paroxysmal nocturnal hemoglobinuria
Paroxysmal cold hemoglobinuria
Cold hemagglutinin disease
Traumatic hemolysis
Prosthetic heart valves
Abnormal natural heart valves (very rarely)
March hemoglobinuria
Respiratory Tract
Recurrent epistaxis
Pulmonary hemosiderosis
Goodpasture's syndrome
Phlebotomy
Therapeutic
Diagnostic, especially with prolonged hospitalization
Volunteer or paid blood donor
Surreptitious

of nonfood substances such as certain clays (geophagia), laundry starch (amylophagia), and ice (pagophagia), suggests the possibility of iron deficiency anemia. Dependence upon milk, which is poor in iron content, as in the diet of infants without food or iron supplements, causes iron deficiency.

Steatorrhea, dumping syndrome, a history of gastric or intestinal resection, and geophagia are historical points that may indicate malabsorption as a cause for iron deficiency anemia.

PHYSICAL SIGNS

Pallor is most common. The sclerae are stark white. Occasionally, atrophy of the lingual papillae may be seen. If koilonychia is found, iron deficiency anemia is strongly suggested. The spleen is rarely enlarged; when it is palpable, it extends only 1 or 2 cm below the left costal margin. The discovery of hemorrhoids or a polyp or mass on rectal examination or by sigmoidoscopy or of uterine myomata on pelvic examination are important clues. The telltale lesions of hereditary hemorrhagic telangiectasia may be found on the vermilion border of the lips or on the tongue, nasal septum, or fingertips, indicating the presence of that rare familial disorder that gives rise to recurrent gross or occult blood loss and then iron deficiency anemia. However important as these symptoms and physical signs may be as a guide, none of them is definitive evidence that iron deficiency anemia is present; they serve only to raise the possibility of that diagnosis. The ultimate conclusion must come from certain laboratory tests (discussed later).

COMMON COMPLICATIONS

The major complications are either cardiovascular or the consequence of failure to diagnose and treat the disease that caused the iron deficiency anemia. Examples of the former relate to the severity of the anemia and include angina pectoris, tachyarrhythmias, and congestive heart failure. Examples of the latter are metastatic carcinoma of the stomach, colon, or kidney; or acute hemorrhage or perforation from a duodenal ulcer. Retinal hemorrhages, papilledema, increased intracranial pressure, and esophageal web are rare complications of iron deficiency anemia.

LABORATORY FINDINGS

Hematologic Tests

Accurate diagnosis of iron deficiency anemia requires positive results on the laboratory tests listed in Table 1. The greater the number of concordant test results, the more likely the diagnosis is correct. Anemia must be present; that is, the hemoglobin concentration in the blood is less than 14.0 gm/dl in the adult male and less than 12.5 gm/dl in the adult female. A value above these limits may nevertheless represent a reduction from the particular patient's prior value within the "range of normal." Hence, in a patient, as distinguished from the presumed healthy subject in surveys of hematologic values, the occurrence of symptoms and signs warrants consideration of anemia when the values are in the lower portion of the "normal range," rather than rejection of that possibility because of strict adherence to any specified cutoff point. In children, the normal hemoglobin concentration is related to age. Less than 11 gm/dl is abnormal, whereas higher values may be subnormal at certain ages of infancy and adolescence.

Given the finding of anemia, then, the following classically signifies iron deficiency anemia:

1. A hypochromic microcytic anemia, as indicated by examination of the Wright-stained blood film and subnormal red blood cell indices, i.e., mean corpuscular volume (MCV) less than 82 femtoliters (fl), mean corpuscular hemoglobin concentration (MCHC) less than 32 gm of hemoglobin per dl of packed red cells.

2. Low serum ferritin.
3. Hypoferremia with an increased total serum iron-binding capacity (TIBC), and less than 16 per cent transferrin saturation.

Any two of the foregoing, in a patient with anemia, confirms the diagnosis; however, discordant, equivocal or conflicting results of these tests require that additional studies be done.

In the development of iron deficiency anemia, the first abnormality is the loss of storage iron; hence, low serum ferritin and absence of marrow iron will occur before anemia develops and before a change in serum iron (SI), TIBC, red cell morphology, or free erythrocyte protoporphyrin (FEP) is found. Examination of the bone marrow usually is not necessary. Furthermore, it is expensive and uncomfortable for the patient, and often even proposing the study is a source of needless apprehension. Bone marrow aspiration, without a biopsy, is indicated when the foregoing tests do not resolve the status of iron stores. If iron is found in any more than trace amounts, the diagnosis of iron deficiency anemia may be excluded. Absence of iron is significant only if an abundance of marrow particles are on the preparation. Lack of adequate marrow particles on the stained thin films prepared from the aspirate or in the sections of clots of the aspirate that were fixed in formalin or Zenker's solution invalidates the test. Either another aspirate or a biopsy is then warranted.

In iron deficiency anemia, the marrow is hypercellular, exhibits erythroid hyperplasia, poor hemoglobinization of the erythroblasts, a low myeloid-to-erythroid ratio, and, most importantly, absent iron stores when evaluated by Perl's reaction (the "Prussian blue" stain) or by examination of wet mounts of unstained, fresh particles. Absence of iron in the bone marrow is a necessary finding in all cases, but the absence of iron, taken alone, does not prove that a particular anemia is due to the lack of iron. That is because iron depletion is common, especially in women, and may be coexistent with an anemia caused by another problem.

Sideroblasts are normoblasts that contain fine ferritin granules, demonstrated as blue dots by Perl's reaction. Sideroblasts are infrequently found in iron deficiency anemia (average of about 2.5 per cent of all normoblasts), whereas in most other kinds of anemia, sideroblasts number 16 per cent or more of the normoblasts. Sideroblastic anemia exhibits both hypochromic and normochromic red cells on the blood film. However, the serum ferritin and serum iron (SI) are not low, and the discovery of large numbers of sideroblasts in the marrow, especially those with a ring of ferritin granules around the nucleus, readily distinguishes this condition from iron deficiency anemia.

An increase in the amount of FEP is characteristic of iron deficiency but is not specific for it. Chronic inflammatory diseases and malignancy have a moderate increase in FEP, whereas lead poisoning results in the highest values of all. Only 20 microliters of blood are required, making this test especially useful in infants and children. The ration of FEB to heme or hemoglobin in the red blood cell is thought to be a more useful index of iron deficiency than the FEP alone.

Many patients display some, but not all, of the various laboratory findings. No single test should be considered the *sine qua non* of the diagnosis of iron deficiency anemia. Rather, the concurrence of findings lends weight to the correctness of the diagnosis. When the anemia is of slight degree or of recent onset, the MCV and MCHC, or both, may be normal. In that circumstance, when symptoms or signs suggest iron deficiency anemia, additional tests are required. The serum ferritin, reflecting body iron stores, would be low (Table 3). The serum ferritin is now preferred over the SI and TIBC because the ferritin values are more constant from day to day, diurnal variation is absent, and there is less frequent interference from other disease states. Other tests useful for the diagnosis of iron deficiency anemia and in differentiating it from anemias that mimic it are given in Table 1.

Still other tests have been described but rarely need to be employed. The enteric absorption and urinary excretion of orally administered radioactive cobalt have been found to be increased in iron deficiency anemia, but such information is rarely clinically useful. The rapid clearance (t ½ of 10 to 20 minutes) of tracer amounts of transferrin-bound radioactive iron from the plasma is characteristic of the physiology of iron deficiency and contrasts with the normal subject (t ½ of 60 to 120 minutes); however, the test is not necessary for ordinary clinical purposes. The urinary excretion of an iron chelate complex after the parenteral administration of deferoxamine or diethylenetriaminepentaacetic acid (DTPA) is less than normal in persons with iron deficiency, whereas in patients with anemias of other causes it would be normal or greater than normal. However, this test is not usually employed because of overlap among groups and because of difficulty conducting it.

Other Biochemical Findings

The normal minor human hemoglobin component, designated hemoglobin A_2, is either slightly reduced or unchanged in iron deficiency anemia. By contrast, in patients heterozygous for beta thalassemia, in whom hypochromic microcytic red cells resemble those of iron deficiency, the hemoglobin A_2 fraction is about twice normal. Column chromatography provides a better measurement of hemoglobin A_2 than the more commonly employed electrophoresis on cellulose acetate because the latter measures the sum of the hemoglobin A_2 and the independently variable enzyme carbonic anhydrase. When both iron deficiency and beta thalassemia coexist, the increase in A_2 may not be found until the iron deficiency is cured. In that circumstance, persistence of microcytosis long after the anemia is improved is the clue to the additional problem.

Urinalysis

Routine urine analysis is normal unless there is hematuria or hemoglobinuria as a sign of the condition that caused the iron deficiency anemia.

Table 3. Laboratory Findings at Stages in The Development of Iron Deficiency Anemia

Stage	Anemia	MCV	MCHC	FER	SI	TIBC	MAR	FEP
Iron depletion	No	N	N	Low	N	N	Low	N
Latent iron deficiency	No	N	N	Abs	N/L	N/H	Abs	N/H
Early iron deficiency anemia	Hb 11+	N/L	N/L	Abs	Low	High	Abs	High
Advanced iron deficiency anemia	Hb 5–10	L	L	Abs	Low	High	Abs	High
Iron deficient erythropoiesis	Any	N/L	N/L	N/H	N/L	N/L	N/H	N/H

Abbreviations: N = Normal; H = high; L = low; Abs = absent; Hb = hemoglobin; / = or; MCV = mean corpuscular volume; MCHC = mean corpuscular hemoglobin concentration; FER = serum ferritin; SI = serum iron; TIBC = total iron-binding capacity; MAR = marrow iron; FEP = free erythrocyte protoporphyrin.

Hemosiderinuria is detected by Perl's reaction on the urine sediment. It is found when iron deficiency is the result of intravascular hemolysis (paroxysmal nocturnal hemoglobinuria, Marchiafava-Micheli syndrome, paroxysmal cold hemoglobinuria, microangiopathic hemolytic anemia, march hemoglobinuria, or turbulence about a prosthetic or, rarely, an abnormal natural heart valve).

THERAPEUTIC TESTS

The ultimate proof of the diagnosis of iron deficiency anemia lies in the complete recovery of the patient and restoration to normal of the laboratory test results that were attributed to this disease when 0.3 gm of ferrous sulfate is taken by mouth once to three times daily. The reticulocyte count should rise from less than 1 per cent to a peak of from 4 to 15 per cent (commonly about 5 to 8 per cent) in about a week. The hemoglobin concentration should rise to normal values in 4 to 8 weeks, regardless of the magnitude of the anemia at the outset, if iron deficiency is the sole cause of the anemia.

However, a therapeutic test should not be used to make the diagnosis of iron deficiency anemia because an increase in the hemoglobin concentration or hematocrit coincident with the administration of iron does not prove a cause-and-effect relationship. For example, improvement in a transient hemolytic anemia, such as that associated with administration of a drug to a patient with erythrocytic glucose-6-phosphate dehydrogenase deficiency, would have occurred whether or not iron was being given. The false inference of iron deficiency anemia would then lead to unwarranted search for pathologic blood loss and failure to protect the patient from subsequent administration of the offending drug.

In particular, one should not administer a combination "hematinic" preparation as a therapeutic test for iron deficiency. The inclusion of folic acid and vitamin B_{12} in such mixtures deprives the physician of the opportunity to confirm the diagnosis by the response to a single agent or to discover by the patient's failure to respond that either the diagnosis was incorrect or a complicating condition is present. Furthermore, a response might be due to the folic acid content and not the iron in such a mixture if the diagnosis were in error. A misdiagnosis or incomplete diagnosis can prove to be costly and detrimental to the patient and, ultimately, to the physician as well.

PITFALLS IN DIAGNOSIS

The serum iron should not be measured or interpreted without simultaneous determination of the TIBC. If the SI is low and the TIBC is not measured, the result may be misleading. The SI may be low in inflammatory diseases and malignancy. In the latter situations, had the TIBC been measured it would have been seen to be low and transferrin saturation would have been found to be normal or elevated rather than low, as in iron deficiency anemia.

Hypochromic microcytic red cells and red cell indices should not be assumed to be due to iron deficiency without additional supporting tests. Patients heterozygous for thalassemia are probably the ones most commonly misdiagnosed as having iron deficiency anemia. In these patients, the hypochromia appears greater on the blood film than that suggested by the MCHC because the leptocytes of thalassemia are thinner than normal red cells and thus appear disproportionately pale. Thalassemia, rather than iron deficiency, should be suspected if the MCV is quite low, 65 to 75 fl, even though the hemoglobin concentration in the blood may be greater than 10 gm/dl. Also, splenomegaly, many target cells on the blood film, severe anemia, or "iron deficiency anemia resistant to treatment with iron" may be found in the patient or family members. In these situations, the serum ferritin and, if necessary, bone marrow iron stores should differentiate thalassemia from iron deficiency because in the former condition iron stores are normal or elevated owing to diversion of iron from the circulating pool of red cells to the reserve pool in the reticuloendothelial system.

Administration of iron by the oral route is not beneficial in anemia not due to iron deficiency and is sometimes harmful. Parenteral administration of iron should be reserved for proven iron deficiency where orally administered iron is not tolerated (for example, in ulcerative colitis and Crohn's disease). Parenteral iron should never be used as a diagnostic test. In patients without iron deficiency anemia, the excess iron cannot be excreted and it can lead to hemosiderosis.

The most common pitfall is to consider the diagnosis to be complete in a patient with iron deficiency before the mechanism for the development of iron deficiency has been discovered. Unless there is incontrovertible proof of grossly inadequate iron intake or of malabsorption, one must look for the source of pathologic blood loss. In the American male adult, a presumption of inadequate dietary iron is almost always wrong.

Even in children with iron-deficient diets and in adults after gastrectomy, pathologic blood loss has often been shown to be a contributing factor to iron deficiency anemia.

THE SIDEROBLASTIC ANEMIAS

By Edward R. Eichner, M.D.
Oklahoma City, Oklahoma

SYNONYMS

Refractory sideroblastic anemia, iron-loading anemia, pyridoxine-responsive anemia, sideroachrestic anemia, chronic refractory anemia with sideroblastic bone marrow.

DEFINITION AND CLASSIFICATION

The sideroblastic anemias comprise a diverse group of disorders having the following features in common:

1. A variable population of hypochromic microcytic red blood cells.
2. Elevated serum iron and elevated saturation of total iron-binding capacity.
3. Ineffective erythropoiesis.
4. Bone marrow findings of erythroid hyperplasia and numerous pathognomonic ringed sideroblasts, i.e., erythroblasts with a ring of Prussian blue–positive iron granules around the nucleus.

The hypochromic red cells reflect impaired heme biosynthesis; the hyperferremia reflects ineffective erythropoiesis (ferrokinetic studies show an increased plasma iron turnover and erythroid iron turnover but a subnormal incorporation of iron into adult red cells); and the ringed sideroblasts reflect the deposition, because of impaired heme formation, of nonheme iron in mitochondria.

Ringed sideroblasts, which are pathologic, must be differentiated from normal marrow sideroblasts. In normal persons, 20 to 80 per cent of the nucleated erythroid cells are sideroblasts, which contain one to six tiny granules of nonheme, ferritin iron. These Prussian blue–positive granules, containing iron beyond that needed for normal heme formation, do not form a ring around the nucleus because they are too few and because they are in the cytoplasm, not in the mitochondria.

Inasmuch as the sideroblastic anemias are heterogeneous, several different classifications have been put forward. Some have divided sideroblastic anemias into primary (either hereditary or acquired), secondary, and pyridoxine-responsive forms. Because some of the hereditary forms are variably pyridoxine-responsive and most of the acquired forms do not show much response to pyridoxine, the classification shown in Table 1 groups sideroblastic anemias into hereditary and acquired forms and the acquired forms are grouped according to presumed common pathophysiology.

Hereditary Types

The *hereditary* sideroblastic anemias are a heterogeneous group with variable response to pyridoxine. More than a hundred cases of congenital, apparently hereditary, sideroblastic anemia have been reported. In the majority (a sex-linked pyridoxine-responsive type), affected males are usually diagnosed in youth, but occasionally not until adulthood. The female carriers (heterozygotes) usually have little or no anemia but have some hypochromic red cells and occasionally a high serum iron. Female heterozygotes tend to have a dimorphic smear, and isolation in such heterozygotes of two red cell populations differing in red cell antigens and in porphyrin content supports the concept of two clones of red cells. Presumably, affected males inherit the X chromosome that codes for a defective delta-aminolevulinic acid synthetase, the rate-controlling mitochondrial enzyme that governs the first step of heme synthesis. In about 20 per cent of patients, large pharmacologic doses of pyridoxine (the coenzyme for delta-aminolevulinic acid synthetase) normalize the hemoglobin—but do not completely correct the peripheral smear or bone marrow—presumably by mass action saturation of the defective apoenzyme with coenzyme. Other patients experience some improvement with pyridoxine therapy, but in about one half the kindreds reported there was no meaningful response. The patients who respond are not nutritionally deficient in pyridoxine; they do not respond to physiologic doses. Recently, four female children with severe sideroblastic anemia without a familial occurrence have been described; one had extensive evaluation which showed a single enzymatic defect—diminished activity of delta-aminolevulinic acid synthetase. Presumably, such patients are homozygotes for an autosomal or X-linked gene.

Table 1. Classification of Sideroblastic Anemias

Hereditary (Variably Pyridoxine-Responsive)
- Sex-linked
- Autosomal recessive

Acquired
- Idiopathic refractory
- Drugs or toxins (reversible), alcohol, chloramphenicol, lead (?), isoniazid (INH), pyrazinamide, cycloserine, azathioprine
- Associated with acute myelocytic leukemia, preleukemia, DiGuglielmo's syndrome, multiple myeloma, aplastic anemia, myelofibrosis, Hodgkin's disease, or other hematologic malignancy
- Complicating other diseases
  - Plausible link—severe malabsorption, certain hemolytic anemias, erythropoietic porphyria, porphyria cutanea tarda
  - Possibly coincidental—rheumatoid arthritis, polyarteritis, systemic lupus erythematosus, thyroid disease, carcinoma

Acquired Types

Sideroblastic anemias that are *acquired* are far more common than those that are hereditary. Of these, the most common is *idiopathic refractory* type, which usually occurs in older adults of both sexes and also gives evidence of being a clonal disease, perhaps from a stem cell mutation. The dimorphic smear suggests two clones of red cells, and the population of smaller, hypochromic cells has elevated protoporphyrin content, decreased iron incorporation, and decreased survival, compared with the population of normal red cells. More recent evidence that idiopathic acquired sideroblastic anemia is a clonal disorder has come from the use of X-linked glucose-6-phosphate dehydrogenase (G-6-PD) isoenzymes as cell markers. In a woman with acquired sideroblastic anemia who was heterozygous for the G-6-PD isoenzymes, analysis of peripheral blood cells showed that the erythrocytes, granulocytes, platelets, macrophages, and B and T lymphocytes all contained the same single G-6-PD isoenzyme and thus came from the same clone. This study also documented the existence of a pluripotent stem cell capable of differentiating into both myeloid and lymphoid progeny. In some ways, the clonal nature of idiopathic acquired sideroblastic anemia resembles that of chronic myelocytic leukemia. In both diseases, acute leukemia evolves (although much less commonly in sideroblastic anemia) which can be either myeloblastic or lymphoblastic. In both diseases, if therapy of the acute leukemia brings about a remission, the bone marrow nonetheless contains a residual defect: the Philadelphia chromosome in chronic myelocytic leukemia and the ring sideroblasts in idiopathic sideroblastic anemia.

Drugs or toxins can cause reversible sideroblastic anemia. Alcohol is probably the most common cause of reversible ring sideroblastic anemia. Up to 30 per cent of skid row alcoholics hospitalized because of complications of alcoholism have folate-deficient megaloblastic anemia with numerous ring sideroblasts, but sideroblastic anemia is uncommon in alcoholics still functioning in the community. Ring sideroblastic changes, along with megaloblastic changes, have been induced in volunteers ingesting alcohol under controlled conditions.

The mechanism by which alcohol induces ring sideroblasts is still being debated. Initially, it was thought that red cell levels of pyridoxal phosphate were subnormal because alcohol inhibited pyridoxine kinase or because acetaldehyde, a metabolite of alcohol, enhanced degradation of pyridoxal phosphate. Recent work suggests that erythrocyte pyridoxine kinase activity is normal in alcoholics and that there is no major intracellular deficiency of pyridoxal phosphate. Furthermore, the effect of alcohol on delta-aminolevulinic acid synthetase is controversial. High concentrations of alcohol inhibit rabbit reticulocyte heme synthesis at the level of delta-aminolevulinic acid synthetase, but a recent study of the activity of bone marrow delta-aminolevulinic acid synthetase in alcoholics with sideroblastic anemia versus normals and patients with idiopathic, acquired sideroblastic anemia showed that patients with idiopathic sideroblastic anemia had diminished activity, as expected, but alcoholics with ring sideroblasts had increased activity, suggesting that the enzymatic or metabolic block from alcohol should be sought at a more distal site in the heme biosynthetic pathway. In this light, it has been shown that erythrocyte activity of aminolevulinic acid dehydrase is decreased in acutely intoxicated patients. On the other hand, one could make the case that alcohol could produce ring sideroblasts without inhibiting the heme biosynthetic pathway. Perhaps the main mechanisms by which alcohol produces ring sideroblasts are (1) direct, toxic, structural damage to mitochondria and (2) rapid cycling of iron because of the ineffective erythropoiesis of the folate deficiency megaloblastic anemia that usually accompanies the ring sideroblastic defect of alcoholism. It may be that the damaged mitochondria cannot handle the incoming iron properly and ring sideroblasts result.

Lead is said to cause ring sideroblasts by inhibiting the heme synthetic pathway at several loci, primarily at aminolevulinic acid dehydrase, but also at delta-aminolevulinic acid synthetase and at heme synthetase. However, the evidence for ring sideroblasts in lead poisoning in humans is remarkably sparse, and lead poisoning perhaps should be dropped from the list of causes of ring sideroblastic anemia in man. Chloramphenicol causes ring sideroblasts primarily by inhibiting mitochondrial protein synthesis and causing ultrastructural damage to mitochondria. Azathioprine has caused anemia with macrocytosis and ring sideroblasts in renal transplant patients and when used for immunosuppressive therapy for autoimmune hemolytic anemia.

The three antituberculosis drugs listed in Table 1 have all caused ring sideroblastic anemia. The main offender, with 25 cases reported, has been isoniazid (INH), which combines with pyridoxal to form a hydrazone that inhibits pyridoxal kinase. The number of reported cases of sideroblastic anemia in patients receiving INH is very small in relation to the widespread use of this drug. Thus, perhaps certain individuals are genetically or nutritionally predisposed to developing ring sideroblastic anemia from INH. In this light, it has recently been shown that the mean erythrocyte pyridoxine kinase activity in American blacks is approximately 50 per cent lower than in American whites. There have been a few reports of ring sideroblastic anemia from pyrazinamide (mechanism unknown) and from cycloserine, which inactivates pyridoxal by binding with it and which also directly inhibits pyridoxine kinase.

Acquired sideroblastic anemia occurs in association with a wide variety of serious and malignant diseases of the bone marrow. This association, along with the aforementioned evidence for clonality of the anemia, suggests that some sideroblastic anemias arise as a mutation of a multipotent marrow stem cell. This concept is further strengthened by the demonstration of chromosomal abnormalities, such as an extra C chromosome, in some patients with sideroblastic anemia, and by certain "leukemia-like" abnormalities when stem cells from sideroblastic marrows are grown in vitro in culture. In one case, three women with idiopathic acquired sideroblastic anemia, each with a structurally abnormal X chromosome (involving band Xq13), developed acute myelomonocytic leukemia. However, each had a very short (months) history of sideroblastic anemia, so the chromosomal defect here may actually have been that of the leukemia, which presumably was incipient at the diagnosis of the sideroblastic anemia. Recent publications have also called attention to the occasional "evolution" of idiopathic sideroblastic anemia into either acute or chronic myelofibrosis; to the unusual occurrence of an antibody-mediated acquired sideroblastic anemia in a child with erythroid hypoplasia who had a response to cytotoxic therapy; and to the appearance of a sideroblastic anemia as a harbinger of acute leukemia in patients treated with cytotoxic agents (and usually radiation therapy also) for Hodgkin's disease, multiple myeloma, or small cell lung cancer.

Ring sideroblastic anemia has complicated diverse diseases. In some instances, a causative association seems plausible. Examples include a patient with severe malabsorption from adult celiac disease treated with folic acid and massive doses of iron, but not with pyridoxine; patients with mechanical hemolytic anemia treated with massive parenteral doses of iron, and a few patients with certain types of porphyria, such as erythropoietic porphyria, in which heme synthetase is deficient, and porphyria cutanea tarda, in which red cell uroporphyrinogen decarboxylase is deficient. In other instances, the relationship may be coincidental. Sporadic cases of sideroblastic anemia associated with rheumatoid arthritis, polyarteritis, systemic lupus erythematosus, thyroid disease, carcinoma, lymphoma, and infectious mononucleosis have been reported, but the mechanisms responsible for the sideroblastic anemia and the relationship, if any, to the associated diseases remain uncertain.

Idiopathic acquired sideroblastic anemia is associated with a variable degree of tissue iron overload, which, in its most severe degree, is indistinguishable from that of hereditary hemochromatosis, even in patients who have received no blood transfusions. Because the frequency of heterozygotes for hereditary hemochromatosis is now thought to be as high as 10 per cent in the general population, most of the patients with sideroblastic anemia and major tissue iron overload may be heterozygotes for hemochromatosis. In fact, in a 1980 Utah study, five of seven men with idiopathic sideroblastic anemia had the HLA-A3 alloantigen, a frequency that matches the frequency of the same alloantigen in hereditary hemochromatosis. This suggests that patients who acquire sideroblastic anemia and also are heterozygous for hereditary hemochromatosis have a major risk of tissue iron overload because of the increased absorption of dietary iron superimposed on the rapid iron recycling of sideroblastic anemia. Of course, most heterozygotes for hereditary hemochromatosis do not acquire sideroblastic anemia; thus it is apparent a second factor is required for the development of this anemia.

PRESENTING SIGNS AND SYMPTOMS

The mode of presentation of the sideroblastic anemia is influenced by the age of the patient and by the type and duration of sideroblastic anemia involved. The sex-linked type occurs mainly in boys and young men who present with pallor but few or no symptoms; the anemia is usually mild to moderate in degree. In up to 50 per cent of these patients, tissue iron-loading occurs slowly, so that in time some patients develop the clinical picture of hemochromatosis. Female heterozygotes usually have little or no anemia, and therefore no symptoms.

Older patients (most are over 50) with idiopathic acquired sideroblastic anemia usually have moderately severe anemia and present with fatigue, but some present with angina, congestive heart failure, or cerebral dysfunction. Nonspecific symptoms of the anemia include easy fatigability, weakness, general lassitude, dyspnea on exertion, headache, and nausea. The symptoms may develop insidiously and be present for years before the patient sees a doctor. Splenomegaly, usually mild but occasionally considerable, occurs in about half of these patients, and hepatomegaly also occurs, although the degree of tissue iron-loading is only mild to moderate in most patients.

In the sideroblastic anemias from drugs or toxins, the clinical picture is usually dominated by the effects of the drug or toxin, or by the associated disease. The typical patient with alcoholic ring sideroblasts is a derelict who has concomitant folate deficiency, malnutrition, and liver disease. With antituberculosis drugs, the anemia develops insidiously after 1 to 10 months on the drug; the patient can present with severe anemia and symptoms therefrom.

When the sideroblastic anemia is associated with another disease, the features of the other disease usually predominate. An exception is the ring sideroblastic anemia that serves as a harbinger of late leukemia in multiple myeloma and in patients in remission from Hodgkin's disease. One study in 1973 showed that 4 of 75 patients with myeloma developed sideroblastic anemia, and within 6 months all 4 developed acute myelomonoblastic leukemia. Late leukemia, which occurs in at least 2 per cent of patients with myeloma, is probably related to the mutagenic effects of melphalan or other alkylating agents, although it may be an unmasking of a hitherto unrecognized aspect of the natural history of myeloma because of the prolonged survival induced by chemotherapy. Late leukemia occurs in up to 5 per cent of patients with Hodgkin's disease, and recently a few such cases of leukemia have been presaged by the appearance of sideroblastic anemia a few months earlier.

PHYSICAL EXAMINATION FINDINGS

Physical findings vary with the type of sideroblastic anemia, the age of the patient, and the severity and duration of the anemia. There may be no findings, there may be only pallor, or there may be tachypnea, hyperpnea, venous distension, hemic murmurs, gallops, rales, edema, and other signs of congestive heart failure. Hepatosplenomegaly is variable. Eventual hemochromatosis, especially in the hereditary forms, can cause hyperpigmentation of the skin, some jaundice, and even testicular atrophy.

LABORATORY FINDINGS

Peripheral Blood

In the hereditary, sex-linked variety, virtually the entire red cell population may be hypochromic and microcytic, with marked variation in size and shape, so that it closely resembles comparably severe iron deficiency or thalassemia. The mean corpuscular volume (MCV) is usually substantially decreased. Female heterozygotes have a dimorphic population, one normal and one hypochromic, microcytic. Patients with idiopathic acquired sideroblastic anemia also have a dimorphic smear, suggesting the emergence of an abnormal clone. One population of red cells is normal to macrocytic (presumably macrocytic because of elevated levels of erythropoietin), while the other, abnormal population (clone) is distinctly hypochromic, microcytic. Although there is great variability, the abnormal clone usually predominates, but the cells of the normal clone are so large the MCV is usually elevated, often in the range of 100 to 115 femtoliters (fl).

Depending upon the severity of anemia, nucleated red cells may be seen. Basophilic stippling (especially in the hypochromic cells) is common, and one usually sees a few siderocytes. Leukocytes and platelets are usually normal, although some patients with idiopathic sideroblastic anemia have moderate to marked thrombocytosis. Hypersegmentation of the polymorphonuclear leukocytes is not seen in these patients. Because of the ineffective erythropoiesis, reticulocytes, which appear as polychromatic cells on Wright stain, are not as frequent as marrow erythroid activity would predict.

In alcoholics, while there are a few hypochromic microcytes, there is not really a dimorphic population, as the macrocytosis of concomitant folate deficiency usually predominates and is associated with hypersegmentation of the polymorphonuclear leukocytes. Likewise, in the sideroblastic anemia from antituberculosis drugs the smear is generally hypochromic and microcytic, not dimorphic.

In sideroblastic anemia associated with acute myelomonoblastic leukemia, a few myeloblasts or monoblasts may be seen in the smear along with other young myeloid forms, and thrombocytopenia. During the preleukemic phase, one may see abnormal neutrophils with stunted granule formation and hyposegmentation, the pseudo-Pelger-Hüet anomaly.

The degree of anemia is variable. Older patients with the idiopathic form usually have hemoglobin concentrations from 7 to 10 gm/dl, whereas young boys with the sex-linked form range from almost normal to as low as 5 gm/dl, and patients taking antituberculosis drugs can present with a level as low as 4 gm/dl. The alcoholics usually have severe anemia with marked megaloblastic features, but if the bone marrow aspiration is not obtained for a week or so in the hospital, the megaloblastic changes can have disappeared while the residual sideroblastic changes are still visible.

Bone Marrow

The bone marrow is hypercellular with marked erythroid hyperplasia. Except in alcoholics, the erythroid series, although often "macronormoblastic" probably because of a high level of erythropoietin drive, is not megaloblastic. In the preleukemic or leukemic forms of acquired ring sideroblastic anemia, the red cell series may be megaloblastoid or may show the multinuclearity (two, four, or even eight nuclei in one erythroblast) characteristic of erythroleukemia. Granulocytic precursors are normal in numbers and maturation, except in preleukemic or leukemic patients who show increased numbers of myeloblasts or promyelocytes and in patients with folate deficiency who show giant myelocytes and metamyelocytes. Megakaryocytes are usually normal, although an occasional patient with idiopathic refractory sideroblastic anemia may have marked thrombocytosis and marked proliferation of megakaryocytes.

The pathognomonic hallmark is the ringed sideroblast best seen on Prussian blue–stained films of aspirated marrow. Characteristically, a dense ring of 10 to 20 coarse blue granules, mainly iron-laden mitochondria, is seen around the nucleus in 40 to 80 or more per cent of the erythroblasts. By electron microscopy, these cells contain massive amounts of nonheme iron as ferruginous micelles within the interstices of the inner cristae of the mitochondria, often producing distortions of the inner membrane of the mitochondria. Iron deposits in the reticuloendothelial cells are often massively increased. In thalassemia major, certain hemolytic anemias, in pernicious anemia, and in some cases of folate deficiency, the erythroblasts, because of high serum iron levels, have increased numbers of small ferritin granules distributed randomly in the cytoplasm. These are not in mitochondria, and these abnormal sideroblasts, which have no pathophysiologic significance, should not be mistaken for ring sideroblasts. When there is doubt as to the location of the iron granules, electron microscopy can resolve the issue.

ADDITIONAL LABORATORY FINDINGS

All sideroblastic anemias characteristically have high-normal or elevated serum iron levels and an increased per cent saturation of the total iron-binding capacity. In some patients with excessive body iron, the serum iron is very high and transferrin is completely saturated. Serum ferritin levels increase in proportion to the progressive expansion of the body iron load.

The erythrocyte protoporphyrin concentration is subnormal (or normal) in the sex-linked, pyridoxine-responsive type, reflecting deficient formation of the precursor delta-aminolevulinic acid. In most of the other types, erythrocyte protoporphyrin level is increased, ranging from 40 to as high as 500 μg/dl, suggesting an accompanying functional deficiency of heme synthetase, either primary, or secondary to mitochondrial iron loading. Most authorities believe the primary abnormality in idiopathic acquired sideroblastic anemia, as in the hereditary forms, is a defective delta-aminolevulinic acid synthetase enzyme, but a minority view still holds that the primary defect is in mitochondrial iron handling with the enzymatic defect secondary. In lead poisoning and erythropoietic porphyria, and in the clone of hypochromic, microcytic cells in preleukemic acquired sideroblastic anemia, protoporphyrin level may be strikingly elevated (over 1500 μg/dl) compared with the normal range of 10 to 35 μg/dl.

Hemoglobin electrophoresis and hemoglobin F and A_2 levels are normal. In up to two thirds of patients with idiopathic refractory sideroblastic anemia, serum and red cell folate levels are low or subnormal and leukocyte alkaline phosphatase values are low. Chromium-labeled (^{51}Cr) red cell survival is usually only slightly shortened, although the survival of the abnormal clone is markedly shortened. Ferrokinetic studies reveal the aforementioned pattern of ineffective erythropoiesis, resulting from destruction of developing red cells within the marrow. Bilirubinemia is usually mild. Tests of hepatic and renal function are normal unless affected by associated disease. Patients with alcoholic ring sideroblasts have subnormal serum levels of pyridoxal phosphate, along with laboratory evidence of folate deficiency, but their red cell content of pyridoxal phosphate may be normal.

BIOCHEMICAL FINDINGS

These have already been adequately covered. The exact pathogenesis of most types of sideroblastic anemia remains unproved, but there are increasing reports of a primary defect in the formation of delta-aminolevulinic acid, presumably because of an abnormality in delta-aminolevulinic acid synthetase, the rate-limiting enzyme of heme synthesis, in both the hereditary and idiopathic acquired forms of sideroblastic anemia. Although the response to pyridoxine in idiopathic sideroblastic anemia is usually disappointing, there are a few reports of partial response to the active form of the coenzyme, pyridoxal phosphate. These reports, however, seem to be a distinct minority, and it seems likely that pyridoxal phosphate will find little or no therapeutic role. As already mentioned, alcoholics with ring sideroblasts have increased, rather than decreased, activity of delta-aminolevulinic acid synthetase. With such diverse causes of ring sideroblasts as heredity, alcohol, chloramphenicol, and antibody-mediated, not to mention idiopathic, it is increasingly obvious that diverse biochemical lesions can cause identical ring sideroblasts.

THERAPEUTIC TESTS

There is no reliable therapeutic test for ring sideroblastic anemia. The diagnosis is made by demonstrating the ring sideroblasts by marrow iron stain.

Perhaps 20 per cent of patients with hereditary sideroblastic anemia will correct their anemia with pharmacologic (50 to 200 mg per day) doses of pyridoxine. Their marrow and peripheral blood will still show subtle abnormalities. If the pyridoxine is discontinued, a full relapse will occur within 2 months. The remaining 80 per cent of patients with hereditary sideroblastic anemia show little or no response to pyridoxine.

Most American investigators agree that most patients with idiopathic acquired sideroblastic anemia show little response to either folic acid or pyridoxine (or pyridoxal phosphate), alone or together. Some British investigators report partial responses to folic acid and/or pyridoxine in apparently similar patients.

Alcoholics respond promptly to withdrawal of alcohol and institution of a nutritious diet. Patients with sideroblastic anemia from antituberculous drugs improve when the drugs are halted or when pyridoxine is given along with the drugs.

COURSE AND COMPLICATIONS

There are two subsets of patients with hereditary sideroblastic anemia. The smaller group are the boys (and rarely girls) who are severely anemic in their first decade and who require frequent transfusions. They follow a course much like that of thalassemia major, with death in childhood. The larger group have a milder anemia, usually first diagnosed in adolescence or early adulthood. They require few or no transfusions and follow a chronic course often progressively complicated by signs of tissue iron overload and, finally, the clinical picture of hemochromatosis. The present and future use of chelating agents by continuous subcutaneous infusion may greatly improve the long-term outlook of such patients by preventing or ameliorating iron overload. Splenectomy is contraindicated in hereditary sideroblastic anemia; it does not improve the anemia, and it may be followed by marked thrombocytosis with lethal thromboembolism. Bone marrow transplantation has not yet been tried in sideroblastic anemia.

Adults with idiopathic acquired sideroblastic anemia can also be divided into two groups. Those with mild, stable anemia not requiring transfusion usually follow a mild, nonprogressive course lasting from 5 to more than 15 years, with most deaths from causes unrelated to the sideroblastic anemia. The prognosis is worse in the other group, those requiring transfusions. These patients tend to die earlier of complications of the anemia; some have a transformation into acute myelomonoblastic leukemia. Although there is no way to predict with certainty whether an individual patient will develop leukemia, there are reports that patients with thrombocytosis (from 500,000 per cu mm to 3 million per cu mm) are less likely to develop leukemia than those with normal or low platelet counts, and that patients with acquired hemoglobin H (beta chain tetramers, also seen in erythroleukemia) are more likely to develop acute leukemia than those lacking this "preleukemic marker" on routine hemoglobin electrophoresis. However, a few patients with marked thrombocytosis have nonetheless developed leukemia. The risk of leukemic transformation in idiopathic sideroblastic anemia is about 10 per cent in the largest analyses (27 out of 268 cases in a recent review), although in smaller series, up to 25 per cent have developed leukemia.

As mentioned, there are no features, not even chromosomal analysis, which enable one to predict who will develop leukemia. In a large analysis, patients who died of acute leukemia tended to have more severe anemia, lower reticulocyte counts, and lower platelet counts. In another analysis, however, none of these routine hematologic measurements served as a predictor of leukemic transformation, although those who developed leukemia tended to have a lesser degree of hyperferremia. Leukemic transformation seems not to occur in hereditary sideroblastic anemia.

PITFALLS IN DIAGNOSIS

The major pitfall in the diagnosis of ring sideroblastic anemia is the failure to think of it and thus the failure to look carefully at an iron stain of an aspirated bone marrow film. The most common misdiagnosis is probably iron deficiency anemia. Oral iron therapy of sideroblastic anemia is, of course, contraindicated because it may augment the tissue iron overload and will not improve the anemia. Sometimes the dimorphic smear is initially confused with iron plus folate or vitamin B_{12} deficiency. The serum iron values should easily separate iron deficiency anemia, with a subnormal serum iron level and a per cent saturation of total iron-binding capacity usually under 15 per cent, from sideroblastic anemia, with a high-normal or elevated serum iron level and a per cent saturation usually well over 70 per cent. Serum ferritin, subnormal in iron deficiency and elevated in ring sideroblastic anemia, should also help in the differential diagnosis. The definitive test is the bone marrow iron stain, which shows absent iron stores and markedly decreased to absent sideroblasts in iron deficiency but shows the pathognomonic ring sideroblasts and increased iron stores in sideroblastic anemia.

Thalassemia major or intermedia presents more difficulty in differential diagnosis because this autosomal recessive anemia shares the hypochromic red cells, the elevated serum iron, the increased marrow iron stores, the tissue iron overload, and even an increase in marrow sideroblasts, although there are few or no actual ring sideroblasts. Other helpful differentiating tests are the frequent Mediterranean ancestry, the equal sex incidence, and the elevation in hemoglobin A_2 or F in thalassemia.

Hypoplastic or *aplastic anemia,* despite the associated high serum iron level, should not be confused with sideroblastic anemia. The red cells in a hypoplastic anemia should look fairly normal, not hypochromic, and the bone marrow will be hypoplastic, not hypercellular with erythroid hyperplasia, as with ring sideroblastic anemia. Marrows in hypoplastic or aplastic anemias do not generally have ring sideroblasts. There are a few instances in which sideroblastic anemia has followed recovery from aplastic anemia.

Primary sideroblastic anemia may be temporarily masked by blood loss. If an elderly patient with idiopathic sideroblastic anemia has major gastrointestinal bleeding, for example, marrow iron may be depleted, serum iron may fall, and ring sideroblasts may disappear. The underlying sideroblastic anemia may nevertheless be suspected because of the dimorphic peripheral smear and a few residual siderocytes which can be confirmed by doing a Prussian blue stain on the peripheral smear. When iron is repleted in such a patient, the ring sideroblastic anemia will again become fully manifest.

HEMOGLOBINOPATHIES

By Samuel Charache, M.D.
and John A. Phillips, III, M.D.
Baltimore, Maryland

Although hemoglobinopathies are defined as clinical disorders produced by abnormal hemoglobins, most abnormal hemoglobins do not cause clinical manifestations and hence are not "hemoglobinopathies." Although they are curiosities to the practicing physician and are not discussed in this article, some of those benign molecules have provided valuable insights into protein structure, anthropology, and evolution. One basic principle used to relegate new hemoglobins to the museum case rather than the medical student's text is this: If a peculiar blood disorder is found in a carrier of an abnormal hemoglobin, all other members of the family who have the hemoglobin should have the clinical disorder and those lacking one should lack the other. The following discussion is based on that principle and touches on sickling, hemolytic anemia, polycythemia and thalassemia-like hemoglobinopathies. Thalassemia syndromes are covered in the next article, and more information is available in other texts. Because of its increasing importance, *prenatal diagnosis* is also included in this article.

SICKLE CELL DISEASE

Nomenclature

Sickle cell disease is a convenient catch-all for the clinical disorders produced by hemoglobin (Hb) S. The term includes primarily sickle cell anemia, sickle thalassemia, and Hb S-C disease, but it also includes unusual combinations such as S-O_{Arab}, S-E, S-$D_{Los Angeles}$, and so on. Sickle cell disease does *not* include sickle cell trait, which is not considered a hemoglobinopathy by the foregoing definition.

Apparently diverse disorders are grouped together because they share two basic processes—vascular occlusion and hemolysis—which are produced by the sickling of red blood cells. The severity and frequency of those two processes depend upon the likelihood that red cells will sickle in vivo at physiologic PO_2 levels whereas Hb SS, S-O, and S-D cells sickle readily, SC cells sickle less readily and S-E and AS* cells do not sickle at all.

Although an in vitro model of sickling may not be completely representative of what happens in vivo, it is convenient to think of the sickling process as being caused by polymerization of deoxygenated hemoglobin molecules into a semisolid gel. Polymerization

*By convention, the hemoglobin in highest concentration is listed first: "AS cells" are sickle trait cells, and the red cells from patients with Hb SC disease could be described as "SC" or "CS," since the proportion of the two hemoglobins is 1:1.

is an extremely concentration-dependent process and can be strongly affected by small changes in mean corpuscular hemoglobin concentration (MCHC). Deoxygenation is, of course, dependent on temperature, pH, and the intrinsic oxygen affinity of the red cells. The deoxyhemoglobin concentration at which a solution gels depends upon the types of hemoglobins present and the proportion of each in the mixture. For mixtures similar to those found in red cells of patients with sickle cell anemia, sickle/Hb C disease, sickle/β^+ thalassemia,* sickle/HPFH,† or sickle trait, the order of gelling concentrations is SS < SC = S thal < S/HPFH < AS. The lower the gelling concentration, the less deoxygenation required, the higher the PO_2 at which sickling occurs, and the more severe the clinical illness. With reflection, it becomes clear that an AS patient with severe cyanotic heart disease could mimic an SS patient, and an SC patient with fever and acidosis could exhibit all the problems usually seen in SS disease.

The importance of MCHC should be stressed, since the naturally low values seen in patients with S/β° thalassemia (or sickle cell anemia coexisting with alpha (α) thalassemia) may account for their relatively mild course when compared with that of patients with sickle cell anemia (whose red cells contain the same hemoglobins, but in higher concentration). Additionally, several modes of experimental therapy (induced hyponatremia, phlebotomy, and the drug cetiedil) all aim at lowering the MCHC.

Fetal hemoglobin (Hb F) should also be emphasized, again because of current therapeutic efforts to increase its production. Hemoglobin F acts as if it does not enter into polymers of Hb S, and red cells containing it sickle less readily than cells containing Hb S alone. Concentrations of Hb F as measured in hemolysates are misleading, for this hemoglobin is found only in some cells ("F cells"). The number of F cells, and perhaps the amount of Hb F per F cell, is determined genetically; in populations in which high numbers of F cells are prevalent, sickle cell anemia tends to be a relatively mild disease.

Sickle Cell Crises

Sickling of red cells produces the two primary manifestations of sickle cell disease, hemolytic anemia and vasco-occlusive events—severity, frequency, and clinical importance depending by and large upon how readily the cells sickle. Since it is not at all clear how hemolytic anemia is produced (membrane loss, cation leaks, fragmentation, and phagocytosis all play some role), it will not be discussed further, although its significance is obvious. Hemolysis is responsible for one type of sickle cell crisis, the "aplastic crisis," in which red cell production ceases abruptly, often following an infection. Similar aplastic episodes occur in other hemolytic anemias and are self-limited, but transfusion may be necessary if the duration of aplasia is unusually long or if the patient's rate of hemolysis is unusually rapid.

Vaso-occlusive events produce the painful crisis of sickle cell disease, which is really infarction or ischemia produced by inflexible sickled cells. The damage may be done by a few cells plugging a small vessel or by a large tangle of cells plugging a larger one. In some instances, vaso-occlusion may be produced by intimal lesions that are themselves due to occluded vasa vasora; or fragments of infarcted bone marrow may break loose and act as emboli. In general, one can say that vaso-occlusion occurs when local conditions (e.g., in bone marrow, spleen, or liver) permit cells to sickle—but in truth, we have no idea why crises occur one day and not the next. It has been suggested that endothelial "stickiness," cell-to-cell interaction produced by fibrinogen, and vasoconstriction play a role in determining the onset of crises, but none of these explanations "works every time."

Two types of crises seen in young children are special types of vaso-occlusive episode. The *hand-foot syndrome,* often symmetric painful swelling of the dorsum and digits of the hand or foot, is probably due to bone infarction; similar lesions can occur in the pretibial area of older patients. *Sequestration crises* are a cause of sudden death in young children. They are produced by stagnation of a major proportion of the blood in abdominal viscera, which in turn can produce very severe anemia, hypotension, and shock. In young children, prompt transfusion is the only effective maneuver. Some pediatricians would consider splenectomy mandatory if the child survives, since such episodes can recur. Milder, and much less frightening, instances of acute splenic engorgement can occur in young adults with persistent splenomegaly. Although the hemoglobin can fall sharply, transfusion may not be necessary.

Acute Complications

Sickle cell lung, or the *acute chest syndrome,* may be a life-threatening event because the associated secondary hypoxemia can be expected to produce severe sickling in all organs. In children, the lung infiltrates and fever must be considered to be due to infection (often with encapsulated bacteria such as *Streptococcus pneumoniae* or *Hemophilus* sp.). In adults, pulmonary infarction is probably more common; if antibiotics are used empirically and the patient improves, it can be difficult to stop the drug despite negative blood and sputum cultures. Great attention must be paid to the arterial PO_2, and vigorous measures should be taken to maintain arterial PO_2 levels above 75 mm Hg.

Infection with encapsulated bacteria is a problem in children, perhaps because they have not yet developed antibodies, because their alternate pathways of complement activation are faulty, and/or because their spleens do not function normally owing to engorgement or infarction. Demonstration of "pits" (actually intraerythrocytic vesicles) by use of Nomarski optics

*In β^+ thalassemia, some Hb A is produced; in β° thalassemia, none is. The Sβ^+ thalassemia patient has SA red cells; the Sβ° thalassemia patient's cells are the same as those of a patient with sickle cell anemia and can be called SS or SF, depending on how much fetal hemoglobin is present.

†Hereditary persistence of fetal hemoglobin.

or phase microscopy is a useful screening test for splenic hypofunction in such children. Prophylactic antibiotics and pneumococcal vaccine have helped, but great caution and a high index of suspicion with a febrile child are the most important therapeutic suggestions one can offer. Salmonella infections (especially osteomyelitis) occur in patients of all ages and may be due to the combination of chronic hemolysis and abundant areas of tissue necrosis.

Strokes occur in patients of all ages, but subarachnoid hemorrhage is probably more common in adults. As noted, lesions of the vasa vasora may account for some large vessel disease. Chronic transfusion therapy is usually advised in children but can be much harder to maintain in adults. Residual paresis and seizures are not infrequent sequels in patients who survive.

The *right upper quadrant syndrome* is usually due to cholecystitis or liver infarction, although *sickle cell lung* can also cause abdominal pain. Gallstones are easy enough to demonstrate, but the question usually concerns their role in the acute illness. Opinions differ (and sometimes strongly!), but we prefer to leave the stones alone unless a history consistent with gallbladder dysfunction can be obtained.

Chronic Complications

As patients grow older, summated small acute lesions tend to produce larger chronic ones, especially in bone and kidney. Treatment of these lesions is no different from care given to patients without sickle cell disease—hip replacement, dialysis, and renal transplantation should all be considered. Many of these patients have had previous transfusions and they tend to be antibody-formers; patients with severe anemia due to renal failure or those with hip necrosis who need surgery may have their treatment thwarted by inability to cross-match blood. Gout and liver disease occur with increased frequency in older patients —the former due to rapid nucleic acid turnover and the latter usually due to a form of cirrhosis following infarctions, not hemochromatosis.

Ankle ulcers, while never a problem in diagnosis, are a frustrating problem for physician and patient. We urge house officers not to culture the lesions, for they always seem to contain antibiotic-resistant staphylococci or *Pseudomonas aeruginosa.* When hospitalized, sicklers with ankle ulcers should be kept away from patients with altered antibacterial defenses and all personnel must adhere to strict hand-washing rules.

HEMOLYTIC ANEMIA

Hemolysis is seen with other hemoglobins as well as with Hb S. The largest group comprises the unstable hemoglobins, whereas hemoglobins C and $D_{Los\ Angeles}$ are different.

Unstable Hemoglobins

The "unstable hemoglobins" are unstable in vitro; in only a few situations have they actually been shown to denature in vivo and be removed from red cells. Methods used to demonstrate instability include heat, incubation with isopropanol (or other almost-nonpolar solvents), and shaking. A variety of molecular lesions produces instability. In general, an amino acid substitution interferes with some sort of stabilizing interaction such as alpha helix formation, interchain bonding, or heme-globin bonding. The methods used to demonstrate instability will cause Hb A to denature too, but the unstable hemoglobins precipitate faster.

Pathogenesis of hemolysis may be due to the altered physical properties of cells containing globs of denatured hemoglobin. The precipitates make the cell stiff, and the cell tends to get torn apart as it struggles to slide through narrow spots in the microcirculation. The precipitates stick to cell membranes and may directly alter their properties or cause membrane lipid oxidation because the process of hemoglobin denaturation in vivo often is associated with liberation of "active oxygen" (e.g., superoxide, peroxide, hydroxyl radicals, singlet oxygen). Oxidized membranes may be stiff or leaky, and the final path of destruction may be similar to that in sickle cell disease.

Unstable hemoglobins may denature spontaneously in vivo as a result of all sorts of "physiologic" stresses (such as the active oxygen generated by phagocytosis) —but denaturation is easily demonstrated if the patient ingests an oxidant drug. Such drugs are the same as those that are a problem in glucose-6-phosphate dehydrogenase (G-6-PD) deficiency and reduced glutathione plays a protective role in both types of hemolysis. Interesting clinical interactions between patient and environment have been described with hemoglobin Zurich and probably exist with other abnormal hemoglobins. High fever can precipitate hemolysis (as high temperature does in the lab), and carbon monoxide from cigarette smoking can protect against hemoglobin denaturation (as it does in various laboratory procedures).

Hemoglobins C and D Diseases

Homozygous Hb C disease is a mild hemolytic anemia in which the blood contains large numbers of microspherocytes. The hemoglobin can be shown to be relatively insoluble under near-physiologic conditions, and the cells can be shown to become stiff when somewhat dehydrated (presumably because the cells shrink and solubility of intracellular hemoglobin is exceeded). Microspherocytes probably form during the life span of the cells as membrane is lost when stiff cells go through narrow conduits. Once enough membrane is lost to form a recognizable microspherocyte, the cell's days are numbered and it is then subject to osmotic as well as mechanical stress.

Homozygous hemoglobin $D_{Los\ Angeles}$ "disease" produced mild hemolytic anemia in one patient, although it did not in several others. The cause of hemolysis was completely unknown. Homozygous abnormal hemoglobins, other than Hb S, C, D, and E (to be discussed), are quite rare, and none has been reported to produce clinical illness. In several instances, the carrier state has been reported in conjunction with α or β° thalassemia; some of those patients are anemic, but the pathogenesis of hemolysis may well involve globin chain imbalance due to the coexistent thalassemia gene (see the article on Thalassemia).

POLYCYTHEMIA, ANEMIA, AND CYANOSIS

Increased oxygen affinity of an abnormal hemoglobin can cause polycythemia as a result of decreased oxygen "unloading" at the tissue level with compensatory increases in erythropoietin production. High-affinity hemoglobins need not have abnormal electrophoretic mobility, and the diagnosis can be made only from measurements of blood or hemolysate oxygen binding. Low-affinity hemoglobins can produce mild anemia or cyanosis, depending upon just how low their affinity is. High-affinity hemoglobins are rare, but they should be considered after the first steps in differential diagnosis of polycythemia. On the other hand, hemoglobins with significantly decreased oxygen affinity are so rare as to not be considered until the last "far out" stages of the diagnostic process. High- and low-affinity hemoglobins, as with many curiosities in medicine, have probably supported many more investigators than they have made patients sick.

THALASSEMIA-LIKE HEMOGLOBINS

Some abnormal hemoglobins are "thalassemia-like" and are produced in such small quantities that the normal globin allele cannot compensate for their low concentration. Hemoglobins like Constant Spring involve production of an elongated globin chain, while Hb Quong-Sze may involve faulty dimer formation in the early phases of globin synthesis.

Much more common are the hemoglobins Lepore and E. The first are hemoglobins produced by crossing over between the δ chain gene (of hemoglobin A_2) and the β chain gene. Whatever it is that diminishes the production of the normal δ chain probably also diminishes the production of Hb Lepore. It should be suspected whenever a hemoglobin with the electrophoretic mobility of Hb S on cellulose acetate at pH 8.6 does not sickle, constitutes only about 15 per cent of the hemolysate, and is associated with microcytosis.

Hemoglobin E is being found in increasing frequency in the United States as a result of immigration of southeast Asians. Carriers have small cells, homozygotes have smaller cells, and genetic compounds with β thalassemia have a condition similar to Cooley's anemia (β thalassemia major). Hemoglobin E is somewhat unstable, but a more important cause of microcytosis may be decreased production of hemoglobin resulting from decreased mRNA. Hemoglobin E moves like Hb C on cellulose acetate electrophoresis but moves like (or nearly like) Hb A on agar.

DIAGNOSIS

The presence of a hemoglobinopathy is usually suggested by the clinical history, a story of similar disease in other members of the family, and abnormal laboratory findings. The latter include anemia (or polycythemia), reticulocytosis or polychromasia, anisocytosis, target cells, poikilocytosis, bilirubinemia, or dark urine (which may not be due to the presence of bilirubin). In an ideal situation, all pertinent information would be provided to the laboratory along with a tube of blood, and those who knew the tests best could decide which were indicated. The following scheme is offered as a second-best plan but one which does have practical advantages.

Cellulose acetate electrophoresis at pH 8.6 is the best all-around screening test, although it will not detect some unstable hemoglobins and some with altered O_2 affinity. Isoelectric focusing yields somewhat better data, but it is too complex a procedure for most routine laboratories. Normal samples, present on every run, delineate the mobility of hemoglobins A and A_2. Hemoglobin S, if present, runs half-way between them, Hb C and E run like A_2, and Hb F runs between A and S.

If the sample shows a sickle trait pattern (AS), a solubility or sickle cell preparation will confirm or reject that diagnosis. If rejected, or if *any other* abnormal pattern is found, the next step is agar electrophoresis at pH 6. This peculiar medium (note, it is *agar,* not agarose) contains a polysaccharide that binds to some, but not all, abnormal hemoglobins and alters the mobility one might expect on the basis of charge alone. As a rule of thumb, it separates Hb A from S, C and F, but nothing else. Because of this behavior, it also distinguishes Hb C from C_{Harlem}, Hb S from G or D, Hb E from C, and so on. Tables of mobility on this medium are available. It should never be ordered as a primary test, and results should always be discussed with an expert.

In many situations, accurate diagnosis is impossible without a family study. Mothers and fathers are best, and children next (since they may have different fathers). A few siblings sometimes provide lucky information, but large numbers of siblings can be very helpful. It can be difficult to get blood from families; interested medical students sometimes overcome great odds in this area.

That's about as far as one can go with routine hemoglobin electrophoresis. Globin chain electrophoresis is available in some laboratories, and it sometimes further refines the diagnosis for abnormal samples. Duplication of the Hb A_2 bands ($\alpha_2{}^A\delta_2$ and $\alpha_2{}^X\alpha_2$) suggests the presence of an α chain variant. Increased fetal hemoglobin, while abnormal, is usually a reflection of some other hematologic disorder.

Decreased amounts of Hb A_2 can sometimes be recognized; they usually reflect iron deficiency. Decreased amounts of Hb S or C (compared with results in other carriers of these hemoglobins) suggest iron deficiency or α-thalassemia, or transfusion with normal blood of a carrier. Very low amounts (3 to 5 percent) of these hemoglobins suggest transfusion of a normal person with Hb AS or AC blood. With practice, increased amounts of Hb Alc (see the article on Diabetes Mellitus) can be recognized—permitting a rare diagnostic coup from the hematology laboratory (i.e., unsuspected diabetes mellitus). Even rarer is a correct "pick-up" of hyperthyroidism, because the carbonic anhydrase band (seen after protein staining) is decreased. The presence of a laboratory computer system, which permits a surreptitious look at data from the chemistry laboratory, can save embarrassment if one seeks to make such startling diagnoses.

Screening of newborns for sickle cell anemia is popular in some areas, but it runs the hazard that technique can outstrip judgment. The goal of such screening is to pick up very young patients and get them into the medical care system very early. It is not clear whether such maneuvers really do prevent death or disability from overwhelming infection or sequestration crises, but it is very clear that if the information is presented to a mother without counseling or without guidance as to how and where the baby can get medical care, harm may be done. On a somewhat different tack, testing the blood is a futile exercise if there is no way to reach the mother because she has been discharged before test results are available. Techniques used for newborn screening vary—some laboratories prefer electrophoresis and others chromatography—but the problem is in counseling, not separation of hemoglobins.

Prenatal Diagnosis

Hemoglobin Synthesis. Prior to 1978, studies of hemoglobin synthesis by fetal red cells were the method of choice for prenatal diagnosis of hemoglobinopathies; they remain the most commonly used procedure for prenatal diagnosis of thalassemia. The techniques necessary to obtain these prenatal samples (fetoscopy and placental aspiration) caused three problems. First, fetoscopy and placental aspiration are technically difficult and are done in relatively few centers. Second, adequate samples are not obtained on the first attempt in about 10 per cent of the fetoscopies and 30 per cent of placental aspirations. Third, fetal losses attributable to the fetoscopy procedure are at least 3.5 per cent.

Once obtained, fetal red cells are incubated with appropriate labeled substrates so that the newly synthesized globin chains are radiolabeled. The α-, β-, and gamma-(γ)globin peaks are separated by chromatography, and the relative amounts of each are quantitated by scintillation counting. Hemoglobinopathies affecting β-globin are detected because the normal β^A-globin peak is replaced by a new peak, and thalassemia syndromes are recognized through imbalance of α and β chain synthesis.

The great majority of the over 1800 fetuses studied by synthetic methods were at risk for β thalassemia; Hb SS, SC, and SO_{Arab} disease constituted less than 10 per cent of cases studied. The error rates reported for these large numbers of cases range from 0.9 to 1.5 per cent.

Amniocyte DNA Analysis. DNA analysis is now routinely used in the prenatal diagnosis of hemoglobinopathies. The primary advantage is that fetal amniotic fluid cells (amniocytes) can be used as a source of DNA. They are obtained reliably by amniocentesis, which does not require the special equipment needed for fetoscopy and is routinely done in many centers. Furthermore, the risk of fetal loss attributable to amniocentesis (less than 0.5 per cent) is relatively low compared with the 3.5 per cent risk associated with fetoscopy.

Blood samples from family members and amniotic fluid samples can be obtained locally and sent to distant laboratories for DNA analysis. Sufficient DNA for analysis can be easily isolated from leukocytes in 10 ml of blood. Enough DNA can often be obtained from 15 ml of amniotic fluid, but these cells can be cultured to provide more DNA if needed. The DNA is digested with a restriction endonuclease such as *Eco*RI or *Mst* II. Since these endonucleases cleave DNA at sites where specific recognition sequences occur, they yield fragments of reproducible size. These DNA pieces are separated by electrophoresis and are then transferred to nitrocellulose membranes. Following hybridization of the bound DNA fragments with a radiolabeled copy of the β- (or other) globin gene sequences, the fragments containing portions of these respective genes appear as bands after autoradiography.

The β^S-gene is easily detected because the sickle mutation alters an *Mst* II recognition site. Since the normal cleavage of DNA does not occur, an abnormally long fragment results which is easily detected. The O_{Arab} and $D_{Los\ Angeles}$ mutations remove an *Eco*RI recognition site so that these genes can be identified by their presence in abnormally large DNA fragments. The Lepore genes also yield abnormal fragments. Certain β° thalassemia genes are smaller because of partial deletions, and in most cases of α thalassemia the α globin genes are completed deleted. Other β variants (Hb C, E, and nondeleted β thalassemia genes) can be detected in most cases by linkage analysis.

DNA analysis has become the method of choice for prenatal diagnosis of many hemoglobinopathies. The error rate is quite low, but in certain cases problems may include:

1. Gross contamination of amniotic fluid with maternal blood.
2. A requirement for family study prior to amniocentesis when linkage analysis is being used.
3. The possibility of nonpaternity with consequent errors in diagnosis when linkage methods are used.
4. The necessity of a 2- to 4- week wait for the analysis.

If the mutation can be directly detected (Hb S, O_{Arab}, $D_{Los\ Angeles}$, some β°, and most α-thalassemias), or if sufficient samples from family members are available to enable linkage analysis studies (most β-thalassemias), prenatal diagnosis by amniocentesis is the method of choice and fetoscopy with its higher risk can be avoided.

THALASSEMIA

By Paul F. Milner, M.D.
Augusta, Georgia

In 1925 Dr. Thomas B. Cooley of Detroit described five cases of a severe childhood anemia with a very poor prognosis. He noted the peculiar mongoloid appearance caused by enlargement of the cranial and facial bones, gross hepatosplenomegaly, and large numbers of nucleated red cells and reticulocytes in the peripheral blood. Cooley distinguished this disease from leukemia, from congenital syphilis, and from other severe anemias of infancy, which had hitherto been grouped together under the name of von Jacsch's anemia. Further reports of "Cooley's anemia" appeared over the ensuing years in the medical literature of America and Europe, and it became apparent that families from Mediterranean countries chiefly were affected by it. It was for this reason that Whipple and Bradford in 1932 coined the term *thalassemia* from the Greek word for sea ($\theta\alpha\lambda\alpha\sigma\sigma\alpha$). In 1936 a Greek clinician, Dr. J. Caminopetros, suggested that the disease was genetically determined. Cooley's anemia is what we now know as homozygous beta (β) thalassemia.

Descriptions of the heterozygous state, or β thalassemia trait, had appeared in the Italian literature back in 1925; microcytosis and hypochromia had been noted, together with increased resistance of the red cells to osmotic lysis, which distinguished it from hereditary spherocytosis. The names of three Italian clinicians, Rietti, Greppi and Micheli, became associated with the condition now called *thalassemia minor.* Not until 1940, however, when Dr. Wintrobe described the typical red cell abnormalities in 40 members of three Italian families living in Baltimore, did the relationship of malattia di Rietti-Greppi-Micheli to Cooley's anemia, and the genetic basis of the disease, become established. Some of these cases were milder, surviving into adult life, and were known clinically as *thalassemia intermedia.* Gradually it became clear that thalassemia is found worldwide; it is very common in some populations, particularly those of the Mediterranean basin and southeast Asia; and it is due to several different but interacting genetic defects of hemoglobin synthesis.

THE GENETIC BASIS OF THE THALASSEMIAS

In order to understand the thalassemias, it is necessary to understand the genetic control of hemoglobin (Hb) synthesis. Hemoglobin is made up of two different types of polypeptide chains: α (alpha) chains, which have 141 linked amino acids, and non-α chains, which have 146 linked amino acids. Alpha chains are common to all three hemoglobin types, but Hb A has β chains, fetal hemoglobin (Hb F) has gamma (γ) chains, and Hb A_2 has delta (δ) chains. The genes controlling α chain synthesis are located in DNA on chromosome 16; genes controlling γ, δ, and β chain synthesis are grouped fairly closely together on the short arm of chromosome 11.

β Thalassemia

When a genetic defect in the DNA controlling β chain synthesis occurs, normal Hb A cannot be formed or it is formed in only very small amounts; this is called β thalassemia. In the heterozygous form, the normal chromosome compensates to a large extent and the hematologic features consist mainly of hypochromia and microcytosis without overt anemia. It is now known that many different defects in the γ-δ-β-gene cluster controlling globin synthesis can produce thalassemia. In subjects with homozygous β thalassemia, the severe defect in β globin synthesis is associated with increased γ globin synthesis and hence an increased proportion of Hb F. In the few red cells that enter the peripheral blood, and in primitive red cell precursors in the marrow, the excess of uncombined α chains is responsible for red cell destruction and gross marrow hyperplasia. Organomegaly results from an attempt to compensate for the ineffective erythropoiesis and severe anemia. Because at birth Hb F is the main respiratory pigment, the symptoms of β thalassemia major are not usually noticed until the child is about 6 months old, at which time the failure of Hb A synthesis, which normally almost completely replaces that of Hb F, becomes apparent.

$\delta\beta$ Thalassemia

Called *F thalassemia* because of the high level of Hb F in heterozygotes, this type of thalassemia is usually caused by a deletion of DNA from chromosome 11, removing all the δ and β gene sequences. The homozygous form is rare, and the affected individuals have 100 per cent of their hemoglobin as Hb F. Compensation is much more efficient than in β thalassemia, and the hematologic and clinical features are therefore milder.

Hb Lepore

This thalassemic gene is the result of a mixup of δ and β gene sequences caused by a mutation that has deleted a segment of DNA between the two genes and joined them into one. The resulting globin chain synthesized makes a hemoglobin with an abnormal electrophoretic mobility, Hb Lepore, which migrates in the position of Hb S. The defect also greatly depresses synthesis of this abnormal chain, resulting in thalassemia trait in heterozygotes and a condition in homozygotes that is clinically indistinguishable from Cooley's anemia. Homozygotes, of course, have no Hb A or Hb A_2 but only Hb Lepore and increased amounts of Hb F. Since the gene is an allele of the β globin gene, double heterozygotes for Hb Lepore and β thalassemia genes occur and genotypic diagnosis may depend on family studies and research techniques.

Hereditary Persistence of Fetal Hemoglobin (HPFH)

This results from deletion of DNA sequences very similar to that causing $\delta\beta$ thalassemia, but for reasons that are not yet clear, γ-chain synthesis is able to compensate almost completely and homozygotes, which are very rare, have 100 per cent Hb F but are not anemic. Although not strictly a thalassemia gene, HPFH is an allele occurring in populations that harbor thalassemic genes and so may interact with them. Double heterozygotes for HPFH and any of the other β or $\delta\beta$ thalassemia genes usually have a clinical picture of thalassemia intermedia and a high proportion, or 100 per cent, Hb F. Family studies and research techniques are necessary to establish the exact genotype.

α Thalassemia

Unlike β globin synthesis, which is controlled by a single gene on chromosome 11, α globin synthesis is controlled by two genes close together on chromosome 16. Deletion, mutation, or defective transcription of DNA sequences in one or both of these genes underlies the syndromes known as the α thalassemias. Although the numerous defects described are complex, the conditions they give rise to are fairly easily recognized. Because α chains are common to all types of hemoglobin, including fetal hemoglobin, α thalassemias give rise to changes that can be detected at birth. Failure of α chain synthesis results in excess γ chains; these combine with each other to form a nonfunctioning pigment called *Hb Bart's,* which, at alkaline or neutral pH, has an electrophoretic migration faster than Hb A. Excess β chains also combine with each other and produce a pigment, with an even faster electrophoretic mobility, called Hb H.

Several allelic genetic defects have been described and are listed in Table 1; different defects tend to be found in different populations. For instance, total deletion of both α chain DNA sequences, referred to as *α thalassemia 1,* is most frequently found in Chinese and southeast Asian peoples of Thailand, Malaysia, Indonesia, and Indochina. For this reason, the homozygous condition is exceptionally rare outside these communities. It causes a stillborn, hydropic fetus in which Hb Bart's, some Hb H, and embryonic hemoglobins are the only pigments present. The heterozygotes have about 3 to 8 per cent Hb Bart's at birth and in later life have markedly microcytic and hypochromic red cells without anemia.

In the allele called *α thalassemia 2,* only one gene is deleted. This is most common in certain black populations, particularly in the western hemisphere and west Africa. Homozygotes have 4 to 5 per cent Hb

Table 1. Genetic Defects That Cause Alpha Thalassemia

α globin genes	Genotype	Phenotype
— α—α — — α—α —	Normal	Normal
— α—α — — ○—○ —	α thal 1 carrier	α thalassemia trait
— α—α — — α—○ —	α thal 2 carrier	"Silent" trait
— α—○ — — α—○ —	α thal 2 homozygote	α thalassemia trait
— α—○ — — ○—○ —	α thal 1/α thal 2 carrier	Hb H disease
— ○—○ — — ○—○ —	α thal 1 homozygote	Hb Bart's hydrops fetalis
— α—α ^{cs}— — α—α —	Hb Constant Spring carrier	"Silent" trait
— α—α ^{cs}— — α—α ^{cs}—	Hb Constant Spring homozygote	α thalassemia trait + Hb CS
— α—α ^{cs}— — α—○ —	Hb CS/α thal 2	α thalassemia trait + Hb CS
— α—α ^{cs}— — ○—○ —	Hb CS/α thal 1	Hb H disease + Hb CS
— ○—α *— — α—α —	Mid East α thal carrier	α thalassemia trait
— ○—α *— — ○—α —	Mid East α thal/α thal 2	Hb H disease
— α—α *— — ○—○ —	Israeli α thal/α thal 1	Hb H disease
—(α—α)*— — α—α —	Shiite α thal carrier	α thalassemia trait
—(α—α)*— —(α—α)*—	Shiite α thal homozygote	Hb H disease

○ = Deleted α chain gene; α^{cs} = Hb Constant Spring α chain gene; α* = intact but defective α chain gene.

Bart's at birth and hematologic features of α thalassemia trait in later life. Heterozygotes, however, are barely distinguishable from the normal, although some have 2 to 3 per cent Hb Bart's at birth.

The third allele is like α thalassemia 2 in its result but, in this type, one of the α genes has a mutation that causes translation of some DNA sequences beyond the termination of the normal gene, resulting in the formation of an aberrant α chain, 172 amino acids long, which forms a very small amount of an abnormal hemoglobin called *Hb Constant Spring.* Homozygotes for this allele have the stigmata of α thalassemia trait with about 5 per cent Constant Spring, but heterozygotes have barely a trace of this hemoglobin, which migrates behind the Hb A_2 band and is easily missed on electrophoresis.

Clinical thalassemia intermedia of mild degree occurs in double heterozygotes for α thalassemia 1 and α thalassemia 2, or α thalassemia 1 and Hb Constant Spring. In such individuals, moderate anemia and splenomegaly are associated with 10 to 15 per cent of Hb H on electrophoresis. The condition is called Hb H disease. In the Middle East and the Mediterranean it now appears that Hb H disease and α thalassemia trait are largely due to α thalassemia alleles with defective rather than absent DNA sequences, or to interaction between such genes and α thalassemia 1 or 2.

THALASSEMIA MAJOR

Synonyms. Cooley's anemia, Mediterranean anemia, homozygous β thalassemia.

Definition. Thalassemia major is a severe anemia that presents in infancy or early childhood and is caused by inheritance of "defective" β thalassemic genes from both parents.

Clinical Features and Course

Symptoms, which include failure to thrive, pallor, irritability, and diarrhea, usually begin between 5 to 6 months of age but may not be apparent until the child is over 1 year old. The spleen and liver become enlarged, and typical facies develop with frontal bossing, prominent cheek bones, and protruding upper jaw, giving a mongoloid appearance. Osteopenia due to marrow expansion causes typical x-ray appearances in the long bones, and pathologic fractures may occur. The skull x-ray may show the typical "hair-on-end" appearance. Physical growth and development are usually delayed, and in untransfused or inadequately transfused patients, menarche and secondary sexual characteristics may be absent.

Complications

Iron absorption is increased in thalassemia major, and blood transfusions increase the iron load; this leads to hemosiderosis, which may lead to cirrhosis and diabetes mellitus. Ultimately, cardiac siderosis causes arrhythmias and cardiac failure. Intercurrent infections, exacerbated by the profound anemia, are a common cause of death. In some cases, hypersplenism, accompanied by leukopenia and thrombocytopenia, may complicate the course and reduces the effectiveness of blood transfusions.

Laboratory Findings

There is severe anemia with hemoglobin concentration of 4 to 5 gm/dl, and a peripheral blood smear that shows gross poikilocytosis, anisocytosis with many microcytes, polychromasia, basophilic stippling, and many poorly hemoglobinized normoblasts. There is often a left shift in the granulocyte series with occasional myelocytes. With hypersplenism there is leukopenia and thrombocytopenia. Concurrent folate deficiency may complicate the picture by adding megaloblastic features to the striking erythroid hyperplasia of the bone marrow. Special marrow preparations, after supravital staining with methyl violet, may show stained inclusions in the cytoplasm of the normoblasts, which consist of denatured free α chains. The reticulocyte count may be only slightly increased; however, indirect serum bilirubin is elevated, and there is a greatly increased catabolism of heme, resulting in abnormal pigmenturia. The serum lactate dehydrogenase (LD) is elevated, as is the alkaline phosphatase, and there may also be elevations of aspartate transaminase (SGOT). Hemoglobin electrophoresis shows predominantly Hb F. The proportion of Hb A_2 may be normal or increased, and there may or may not be some Hb A, depending on the genotype and whether blood transfusions were given prior to diagnosis.

Pitfalls in Diagnosis

The organomegaly, profound anemia, and presence of nucleated red cells, white cell precursors, and possibly thrombocytopenia, may all suggest a leukemic or neoplastic process at first examination. But the low mean corpuscular hemoglobin (MCH) and mean corpuscular volume (MCV) together with the empty appearance of the red cells should suggest the diagnosis. Hb electrophoresis results will confirm it. The patient's parents and family should be examined and blood studies obtained (see the article on hemoglobinopathies). Typical features of thalassemia trait will be found in the red cells of the parents and possibly some siblings. Further tests to establish the type of β thalassemia are best left to laboratory research experts, who can become involved as necessary.

Hb BART'S HYDROPS FETALIS

Synonyms. Homozygous α° thalassemia, homozygous α thalassemia 1.

Definition. A hydropic infant, often stillborn or dying within the hour, whose blood contains Hb Bart's, embryonic hemoglobins and some Hb H, but no normal hemoglobins.

Clinical Findings

The infant is usually delivered prematurely and has a low birth weight despite the edema. There is a high incidence of toxemia of pregnancy in the mothers of these babies. The infant exhibits severe hydrops fetalis with gross pallor and edema. There is marked enlargement of the liver and spleen, but particularly the liver, which fills the distended abdomen.

Laboratory Findings

The blood picture shows severe thalassemic features with a Hb level between 4 and 10 gm/dl. There are numerous nucleated red cells and a variable degree of reticulocytosis. Hemoglobin electrophoresis demonstrates that almost all the hemoglobin is Hb Bart's, which migrates anodally to Hb A; both Hb A and Hb F are missing. There are usually several minor, fast-moving bands consisting of embryonic components and Hb H.

Pitfalls in Diagnosis

The main differential diagnosis is hydrops resulting from Rh or other blood group maternal/fetal incompatibility. Hepatomegaly is usually much less pronounced in Rh isosensitization, and abnormal hemoglobins are not found.

THALASSEMIA INTERMEDIA

Definition. A thalassemic disorder of mild to moderate severity, nor requiring blood transfusion, which may be caused by a variety of β and/or α thalassemic genes.

Clinical Features and Course

Because the anemia is, by definition, only mild to moderate in degree, patients with this syndrome may not present until late childhood or early adult life, or even later. The Hb level is usually between 7 and 10 gm/dl, and splenomegaly, which may be slight or marked, is a constant feature. There may be complaints of lassitude, but frequently the condition is only detected during routine examination for an unrelated intercurrent illness that exacerbated the thalassemia.

Complications

Iron overload with eventual hemosiderosis is a common complication of this type of thalassemia, even in the absence of blood transfusions, and may lead to hepatic and pancreatic dysfunction in later years. Therapeutic iron intake over several years will increase this tendency. Extramedullary erythropoiesis may expand and press on vital organs such as the spinal cord (producing paraplegia), or on the brain (producing symptoms similar to those of meningioma). The spleen may become grossly enlarged, and splenic rupture becomes a hazard.

Laboratory Diagnosis

The mild to moderate anemia, low MCV and MCH, and bizarre red cell morphology are the main clues to the diagnosis. The genetic basis of the disease may be complex. If it is due to β thalassemia genes, Hb F will be increased; this will be seen on Hb electrophoresis, which might also show an abnormal hemoglobin such as Hb E (common in southeast Asians). If Hb H disease is suspected, the electrophoresis strip should be inspected for the minor, fast-moving hemoglobin band of Hb H. Hemoglobin H inclusions can be found in the red cells in the reticulocyte preparation. Hemoglobin Lepore, which migrates in the position of Hb S, can be distinguished from Hb S by a solubility test that will rule out Hb S thalassemia. Further diagnosis as to the type of thalassemia is best left to experts, who will want to study other family members if available.

Pitfalls in Diagnosis

It is important to appreciate that an acquired disorder, such as iron deficiency, may complicate the basic thalassemic defect, further reducing the hemoglobin level. Other causes of ineffective erythropoiesis may have to be excluded by careful physical and laboratory examination. As in all these syndromes, examination of available family members may be most helpful in establishing the basic inherited hemoglobin disorder.

THALASSEMIA TRAIT

Synonyms. Thalassemia minor. Heterozygous β thalassemia. The condition can also be caused by heterozygous α thalassemia 1 or homozygous α thalassemia 2 (Table 1).

Definition. A patient with a microcytic hypochromic red cell morphology, unresponsive to iron therapy, which may or may not be accompanied by mild anemia.

Clinical Features and Course

A few patients may complain of lassitude and tiredness, but there are no clinical findings other than the red cell abnormalities, which are usually first detected unexpectedly during a routine investigation. Anemia may develop during pregnancy and may be unresponsive to iron.

Laboratory Findings

The hemoglobin is usually above 10 gm/dl and the MCV may be as low as 65 femtoliters (fl) or only in the upper 70s. The MCH is appropriately lowered, and frequently this is associated with an increased red cell count. These features should at once alert the physician to suspect thalassemia rather than iron deficiency. Electronic blood cell counters now provide an estimate of the coefficient of variation of red cell size (RDW). This is normal in thalassemia trait because of the minimal anisocytosis, but it is always increased in iron deficiency. Serum iron and transferrin saturation may be helpful if normal, but the ferritin level is more reliable and it should be normal or increased in thalassemia. Hemoglobin electrophoresis may show an increased Hb A_2 band in β thalassemia trait and a band of Hb F in $\delta\beta$ thalassemia trait. The Hb A_2 should be quantified by one of the available microcolumn chromatography techniques. A value greater than 3.5 per cent confirms β thalassemia trait. In α thalassemia trait, rare cells containing Hb H inclusions may be found in suitably stained reticulocyte preparations.

Pitfalls in Diagnosis

The condition is frequently treated as iron deficiency because of inadequate investigation. This may lead to hemosiderosis if continued for many years, as has happened in reported instances. However, iron deficiency may coexist with β thalassemia trait, and in these circumstances the Hb A_2 value, normal initially, may become raised only when the iron deficiency is corrected. In sideroblastic anemia, the smear shows a dimorphic red cell morphology and the RDW is increased, but the condition may have to be carefully excluded in a middle-aged to elderly patient. Because thalassemia is a genetic condition, its features are permanent, and if the condition is suspected, careful follow-up will generally reveal this. Exclusion of acquired disorders is not usually difficult.

HEREDITARY ANEMIAS DUE TO ABNORMAL RED CELL ENZYMES

By William N. Valentine, M.D.
Los Angeles, California

The human erythrocyte, lacking a nucleus, mitochondria, or the capacity to synthesize new protein, is deprived of many metabolic options and hence is peculiarly susceptible to genetically determined abnormalities in its enzymatic machinery. An expanding number of hereditary anemias due to defective red blood cell enzymes are now recognized. Most are hemolytic in type; a few rare syndromes are associated with megaloblastic anemia. The most common hemolytic syndrome is that secondary to defective glucose-6-phosphate dehydrogenase (G-6-PD); the second most common is that associated with severe deficiency of pyruvate kinase (PK) activity. In the last analysis a firm diagnosis rests on the definition of the responsible defective enzyme, and depends upon analytical procedures which, in some instances, are available only in certain research settings. However, screening tests for G-6-PD and PK deficiency are now available in many clinical laboratories.

For the individual practitioner, diagnosis depends upon demonstration of a hemolytic syndrome, exclusion as far as possible of alternative causes of hemolysis, suspicion or documentation of a hereditary etiology, and, often, consultation with a hematologist.

HEMOLYTIC SYNDROMES

From a clinical point of view, suspicion is directed toward a hemolytic syndrome by historical or laboratory evidence of anemia, unexplained jaundice, splenomegaly, and early onset of cholelithiasis. A hereditary etiology is suspect if jaundice and/or anemia is chronic or lifelong and if there is a history of similar syndromes, splenomegaly, or splenectomy in family members. In addition, ethnic background may direct suspicion toward certain hereditary hemolytic disorders.

The nonspecific laboratory hallmarks of chronic hemolysis are greater than normal polychromasia on the Wright-stained blood film, ongoing reticulocytosis unexplained by acute blood loss, and often an elevated indirect-reacting serum bilirubin. Pure hemolysis per se is *never* accompanied by increase in the direct-reacting serum bilirubin or by bile in the urine. However, the latter may be present when hemolytic anemia is complicated by conditions such as transfusion-transmitted hepatitis or cholelithiasis with biliary obstruction due to pigment stones. The importance of documenting and following the reticulocyte count cannot be overstated, but for reasons not clear this simple test is often neglected.

Once clinical and laboratory findings indicative of hemolysis are evident, narrowing the diagnostic possibilities requires exclusion of various causes of chronic hemolysis. Evaluation of the stained blood film by a competent morphologist is a diagnostic must. A negative Coombs' test does not entirely exclude, but renders unlikely, autoimmune hemolytic anemia due to warm agglutinins. With rare exceptions, hemolytic episodes with hemoglobinuria due to cold agglutinins occur only when the latter are present in high titer. Hereditary spherocytosis is characterized by the presence of spherocytes and a positive osmotic fragility test. The latter is rendered more sensitive in mild cases by sterile incubation of blood for 24 hours prior to performing test. Sickle cell disease and other hemoglobinopathies may require special tests including hemoglobin electrophoresis. If the diagnosis is obscure, hematologic consultation is often necessary to provide sophisticated evaluation of morphologic clues and recommendation of diagnostic procedures indicated in the less commonly encountered hemolytic syndromes with or without hemoglobinuria.

G-6-PD DEFICIENCY AND RELATED ENZYMOPATHIES

Defective G-6-PD as a cause of hemolytic anemia in man is the first described, most common, and best known red cell enzymopathy. It affects more than 100 million people. It is X chromosome-linked. Males have full expression of the disorder; females most commonly have less severe manifestations and have two populations of cells, one G-6-PD deficient and the other entirely normal. However, clinical manifestations in females range from those comparable to the male to total absence. In the latter end of the spectrum, deficiency may be undetectable by even the most sophisticated tests and may be recognized only if a male offspring has the disorder. G-6-PD deficiency is not a single disorder, but instead is a large family of syndromes varying widely in clinical manifestations and severity and having in common a mutant gene at the G-6-PD locus. Over 150 separate mutant genes are now documented.

The most commonly recognized diagnostic manifestations are in reality those characterizing the common G-6-PD variant (Type A⁻) which has an incidence of roughly 10 per cent in the black population of North America. G-6-PD deficiency was first defined and the most intensive early studies were conducted in the United States. As a result, the most commonly recognized clinical features of the emerging syndrome were those of the most common variant investigated. The A⁻ mutant gives rise to a clinical syndrome of relatively mild severity. Hemolysis, if present, is episodic and related to certain medications, chemicals, or severe infection. Medications producing oxidative stress result in partial denaturation of hemoglobin and intravascular hemolysis with hemoglobinuria and/or hemosiderinuria. Among drug and chemical agents incriminated with a high degree of certainty as hemolytic in the G-6-PD deficient patient are the following: acetanilid; methylene blue; nitrofurantoin (Furadantin); the antimalarials pamaquine, pentaquine, and primaquine; sulfanilamide; sulfapyridine; sulfacetanide; sulfmethoxazole; toluidine blue; and trinitrotoluene (TNT). Some lists of agents purported to cause hemolysis in deficient subjects include drugs erroneously implicated or whose effects are inadequately documented.

Within 24 hours of ingesting hemolysis-producing medications, patients with this variety of mutant enzyme characteristically experience malaise, often fever, red urine, anemia, and jaundice, all of which begin subsiding after about 8 or 10 days. Only the older red cells are destroyed; the remaining younger cells possess considerable G-6-PD activity, and during or shortly after a hemolytic episode the screening test may be falsely negative.

Patients with G-6-PD deficiency of the A⁻ type can eat fava beans with impunity. However, it should be emphasized that with other variants the clinical manifestations and diagnostic features may be quite different, and in some instances considerably more severe. Some variants found in Mediterranean areas where G-6-PD deficiency is common are associated with severe hemolysis if fava beans are ingested. Moreover, in the more severe syndromes, hemolysis may be constant rather than episodic.

In these patients clinical features are those of a lifelong nonspherocytic hemolytic anemia with splenomegaly. While the individual practitioner may rely on the screening test and the index of suspicion to seek consultative assistance, specially oriented laboratories may not only assay G-6-PD activity by conventional means but may also characterize variants in sophisticated terms of enzyme kinetics, stability, behavior toward cofactors and inhibitors, and in other ways.

G-6-PD is one constituent of a metabolic pathway known as the hexosemonophosphate shunt, which is responsible for protecting hemoglobin against oxidative denaturation. It is therefore closely linked functionally with red cell enzymes responsible for the synthesis of glutathione (the most important and abundant reducing agent in the erythrocyte), with glutathione peroxidase (the enzyme detoxifying harmful peroxides by catalyzing their destruction with reduced glutathione as a cofactor), and with glutathione reductase (the enzyme maintaining glutathione in its reduced state). Hemolytic syndromes associated with nearly complete lack of red cell glutathione due to deficiency of either of the two enzymes responsible for its synthesis are documented, but they are quite rare. In one of these, hemolysis is also associated with cerebellar ataxia; in the other, only hemolysis is present. Even rarer is severe deficiency of glutathione reductase, which in a single patient was associated with favism. These rare causes of hemolysis that are due to enzymopathy currently can be defined only in research laboratories.

PYRUVATE KINASE DEFICIENCY AND RELATED ENZYMOPATHIES

Deficiency of pyruvate kinase (PK) is second only to that of G-6-PD as a cause of hemolytic anemia due to defective enzymes. It can serve as a prototype for other nonspherocytic hemolytic anemias due to defects in enzymes catalyzing the conversion of glucose to lactate—the major energy-generating mechanism available to the anucleate red cell. Deficiency of PK has now been documented throughout most areas of the world.

The diagnostic features are those of lifelong nonspherocytic hemolytic anemia of variable severity associated with splenomegaly, often acholuric jaundice, and frequently with cholelithiasis at an early age. Exchange transfusion may or may not be required for neonatal hyperbilirubinemia. Transfusion requirements may exist from birth, may be absent, or may be present only during periods of stress, such as during infections or in association with surgery. Splenectomized patients continue to have severe hemolysis but may derive very partial benefit from the procedure, which is reserved for those with ongoing transfusion requirements. Hemoglobin is often in the range of 9 to 10 gm/dl, but anemia may range from mild to life-threatening. Although a screening test is available, it should be cautioned that if leukocytes are not removed the test may be falsely negative and that the test fails to detect a number of variants with kinetic abnormalities. Again, the mutant gene products responsible for hemolysis are very pleomorphic, and PK deficiency, like that of G-6-PD, is a family of disorders. Clinical manifestations are linked to hemolysis. Red cell 2,3-diphosphoglycerate (2,3-DPG) levels tend to be very high in PK deficiency, whereas adenosine triphosphate (ATP) tends to be low, although it is sometimes within the normal range. The special characteristics of a given PK variant may be documented by methods not generally available in clinical laboratories.

Other enzymes of the glycolytic pathway, when severely defective, are also associated with hemolytic anemia similar to that seen in PK deficiency. These include the following enzymes: hexokinase (HK), glucose-phosphate isomerase (GPI), phosphofructokinase (PFK), aldolase (ALD), triosephosphate isomerase (TPI), and phosphoglycerate kinase (PGK). All are transmitted as autosomal recessive disorders except PGK deficiency, which, like that of G-6-PD, is X chromosome-linked. Hence a suggestive diagnostic feature sometimes present is the finding of multiple cases in siblings, rather than in parent and child. In X chromosome-linked PGK deficiency, however, children of affected mothers may be normal or affected; PGK-deficient males transmit a defective gene to all of their daughters but to none of their sons. Hexokinase, GPI, and one type of PFK deficiency manifest only as hemolytic anemia. Another form of PFK deficiency exhibits only mild hemolysis but is accompanied by a severe myopathy that dominates the clinical picture. Deficiency of TPI is a severe multisystemic disease. Hemolytic anemia is substantial, but much more ominous is the severe, progressive neurologic dysfunction usually terminating in death during childhood. Deficiency of PGK in males also is associated with neurologic and behavioral abnormalities as well as hemolysis. Severe deficiency of lactate dehydrogenase (LDH) is recognized but does not result in hemolysis or other clinical manifestations. Near total lack of 2,3-DPG, due to a defect in the enzyme responsible for its formation, is also documented. It is not associated with hemolysis, but with mild, clinically asymptomatic erythrocytosis.

Hereditary hemolytic anemia also occurs with certain rare enzymopathies of nucleotide metabolism. Grossly deficient activity of adenylate kinase, the enzyme catalysing the interconversion of adenosine monophosphate (AMP), adenosine diphosphate, (ADP), and ATP, is associated with nonspherocytic hemolytic anemia resembling that of PK deficiency. Clinical and hematologic manifestations require the inheritance of defective genes from each of the two parents. A similar inheritance pattern is seen in severe deficiency of the enzyme pyrimidine 5'nucleotidase, which serves to rid the maturing reticulocyte of pyrimidine products of RNA breakdown. A clinical laboratory clue in affected subjects is a profound, strikingly abnormal increase in cells with basophilic stippling on the Wright-stained blood film. A lead-induced, acquired deficiency of the same enzyme is associated with similar findings and hemolysis in severe lead intoxication. Finally, a rare, dominantly transmitted hemolytic syndrome accompanies an inherited enormous increase (40- to 100-fold), rather than a deficiency, in the activity of the red cell enzyme adenosine deaminase.

Certain rare, inherited enzymopathies are manifested by macrocytic anemia with megaloblastic marrow and findings similar to those seen in pernicious anemia and severe folate deficiency. These include two rare disorders of pyrimidine metabolism associated with oroticaciduria, and diagnosis requires assistance of specialized laboratories. The rarer enzymopathies in general often require special diagnostic assistance even for the practicing hematologist.

HEREDITARY SPHEROCYTOSIS

By Hussain I. Saba, M.D., Ph.D.
and Robert C. Hartmann, M.D.
Tampa, Florida

SYNONYMS

Hereditary hemolytic anemia, familial acholuric jaundice, congenital hemolytic anemia, chronic familial jaundice.

With the greater specificity and clarity provided by the term hereditary spherocytosis, the synonyms are now largely of historical interest.

DEFINITION

Put briefly, hereditary spherocytosis (HS) is an autosomal dominant, chronic hemolytic anemia caused by an unknown erythrocyte membrane defect that in its full expression manifests anemia, intermittent jaundice, and splenomegaly clinically; spherocytic red blood cells (RBC) on blood smear; and in vitro increased osmotic fragility and autohemolysis of such cells. Invariably, splenectomy leads to clinical cure such that in any seeming splenectomy failure, the diagnosis must be seriously questioned or discarded. Hereditary spherocytosis is the first described and most common heritable hemolytic disorder in Northern Europeans with an incidence of about 1 in 5000. It probably occurs in all ethnic groups including blacks, among whom it was formerly thought to be rare.

Inheritance. As expected from autosomal dominant inheritance, the sibling ratio is about 0.5. However, in about 10 to 20 per cent of HS patients, both parents are said to show no demonstrable abnormalities. The degree to which this is due to new mutations or to formes frustes is not known, but one exhaustive family study showed 50 per cent of patients with diagnosed cases of HS to have a mild, compensated hemolytic process and 15 per cent to "appear healthy." Thus, a negative family history by hearsay is inconclusive. Thorough personal historical interview, physical examination, and laboratory studies are necessary. In other families the clinical penetrance of HS may be more striking. Nonetheless, the highly varied clinical picture must be kept in mind in the ensuing discussion, which largely revolves around classic or full-blown clinical manifestations. Recently spherocytic anemia, so severe that it required maintenance transfusions and splenectomy by age 7 months, was described in two sisters with clinically and hematologically normal parents. Spectrin, the most abundant protein of the membrane skeleton of the red cell, was less than 50 per cent of normal in the affected siblings and the inheritance presumed autosomal recessive.

Erythrocyte Defect. The precise nature of the intrinsic membrane defect in the HS red cell remains elusive, but it is manifested by:

1. Decreased ratio of surface area to volume of the RBC.
2. Impaired cellular deformability, causing increased trapping of red cells in the splenic pulp.
3. Enhanced fragmentation during incubation in vitro and during splenic entrapment.

Some studies have identified deficiencies in the quantity or function of spectrin in some HS kindreds. It seems likely that the clinical heterogeneity of HS will become more fully explained as such studies are pursued further. The increased Na^+ leak (flux) accompanied by compensatory increased glycolysis and cation pumping is an accepted feature of the membrane defect but is thought not to be importantly involved in hemolysis since it is not correlated with HS red cell life span.

Regardless of the basic defect of the HS red cell, its shortened survival appears to result from splenic trapping, presumably associated with increased cell rigidity and enhanced by exposure to the deleterious splenic environment of low pH, low glucose concentration, and low O_2 tension. Each passage through the splenic pulp may result in loss of membrane lipid and protein with decrease in surface-to-volume ratio and further increase in rigidity; this becomes a vicious cycle until the cell disintegrates within the spleen and the fragments are then removed by macrophages.

PRESENTING SIGNS AND SYMPTOMS AND PHYSICAL EXAMINATION

The presenting features relate principally to anemia, jaundice, hemolytic crisis, splenomegaly, and the development of gallstones. The greater the severity of HS, the more striking are these features and generally the earlier the detection in life. Thus, severe HS may be manifest in the neonate or in infancy and presumably very mild HS only in old age. Nonetheless, in most cases anemia is first detected in childhood or early adult life. Frequently, jaundice is minimal but can increase in severity with fatigue, exposure to cold, emotional stress, and pregnancy. Even the clinically jaundiced patient with HS is commonly described as "more yellow than sick." However, once significant clinical jaundice sets in, it usually does not clear completely until after splenectomy. Cholelithiasis, hemolytic crisis, and aplastic crisis may also be presenting manifestations and will be discussed under Common Complications.

The spleen is clinically enlarged in about 80 per cent of patients, in the adult usually weighing 800 to 1500 gm. The liver in uncomplicated HS is not significantly enlarged and at the most felt 1 or several cm below the right costal margin. Significant hepatomegaly suggests a complication.

Hereditary spherocytosis is probably a more common cause of neonatal jaundice than generally appreciated. When diligently sought, a history of neonatal jaundice can be obtained from almost one half of the adults with HS. An unusually early or exaggerated form of "physiologic jaundice" of the newborn suggests the possibility. The differential diagnostic problem is compounded by the ordinary "physiologic jaundice" as well as by fetal-maternal ABO incompatibility and sepsis, both of which can be accompanied by jaundice and spherocytosis. Some patients with neonatal HS have received exchange transfusions, and kernicterus has been reported in a few. In others, neonatal manifestation of HS has been a prelude to a severe course, forcing the issue of splenectomy in infancy. On the other hand, the degree of hemolysis in neonatal HS does not necessarily have predictive value as to the future severity of the disease. The various stressful circumstances of the neonatal period may bring out exaggerated hemolysis at that time, only to have the disorder settle down into a milder course later. At birth, pyknocytosis rather than spherocytosis may be present only to be replaced by the latter after a few months.

There are some complications of HS formerly considered prominent but now only rarely noted clinically, probably a phenomenon secondary to better detection of the disorder in its milder forms. These include chronic ankle ulcers, tower skull, and other roentgen findings that are similar to those of sickle cell anemia and thalassemia, albeit usually milder, and that may clear only after splenectomy. Extramedullary erythropoiesis may occasionally lead to paravertebral masses (heterotopia) visible on chest x-ray as well as masses in the renal pelvis.

More than 20 different congenital abnormalities have been described in isolated cases of HS (e.g., of eyes, nose, palate, and digits), but the frequency may be no greater than in the population at large. We have recently seen a large HS kindred with linkage between angioid streaks of the retina and HS. Formerly, retardation of growth and development was prominently mentioned in HS. Nowadays, the threat of future potential retardation is not considered in itself an important factor in the decision for splenectomy in childhood.

COURSE

HS may be manifested or detected at any time from birth to old age. The disorder may remain clinically silent for prolonged periods. Patients most frequently come to medical attention for evaluation of anemia or unexplained jaundice (often attributed to hepatitis), during evaluation of cholelithiasis, or as part of a family study for HS. Mild HS itself is quite compatible with a normal life expectancy. However, the threat of severe and even fatal aplastic crisis and cholelithiasis remains. To obviate this, splenectomy is favored usually *after* the age of 7 if HS is well documented and the spleen is palpable, even if anemia and jaundice are mild. Surgery is usually less upsetting to school and employment records if performed during childhood. Once the spleen is removed (and the gallbladder, if cholelithiasis is present), the patient should have a normal life expectancy free of the complications of HS. However, pediatricians have recently become even more sanguine regarding splenectomy in (early) childhood in any disorder in view of the danger of overwhelming post-splenectomy infections (about 2.5 per cent) which are frequently fatal (about 50 percent).

COMMON COMPLICATIONS

Cholelithiasis. This complication is seen in 43 to 85 per cent of HS patients over the age of 10 but has been detected in children as young as age 3. Multiple pigmented stones, predominantly calcium bilirubinate and hence radiopaque, are usually present. Once cholelithiasis is detected in HS, splenectomy and cholecystectomy are indicated sooner or later. Preoperative work-up should include cholecystogram (and, if necessary, ultrasound visualization of the gallbladder) so that at the time of splenectomy, the patient's condition permitting, cholecystectomy can also be carried out. Preoperative diagnostic gallbladder studies are thus important to guide the surgical planning as well as in the occasional patient to detect "gallstone sand" at times difficult to ascertain solely by palpation of the gallbladder at operation. A particularly serious problem is the blockage of the entire extrahepatic biliary drainage system with thick, tenacious tar-like bile precipitate difficult to remove at surgery and sometimes causing death. All of this serves to emphasize the potentially serious nature of cholelithiasis in HS. Thus, a patient may have a lifelong relatively mild course with HS only to die in older age of the complications of serious cholelithiasis.

Aplastic Crisis. The aplastic crisis of hemolytic disorders was actually first described in HS. Temporary arrest of hematopoiesis occurs with or following infections and occasionally other stress. This leads to marked decrease in marrow normoblasts and peripheral blood reticulocytes. Since red cell survival may be no more than 10 to 20 days, there follows a rapid fall in blood hemoglobin concentration. Obviously multiple family members sharing the same hemolytic disorder may be similarly affected by exposure to the common offending agent (e.g., infection).

Hemolytic Crisis. From time to time the jaundice may deepen and the anemia may increase, often accompanied by abdominal pain, vomiting, tachycardia, and fever. This so-called "crise de déglobulization" has been described less often than the aplastic crisis in recent years. This hemolytic crisis may develop in association with infection thought possibly to occur with secondary splenic hyperplasia and increased sequestration.

Folate Deficiency. "Relative" folate deficiency (owing to increased demands of folate for the accelerated erythropoiesis) in patients with chronic hemolytic disease can be exaggerated, especially by dietary deficiency, intestinal malabsorption, drugs that interfere with folate absorption (e.g., oral contraceptives and certain anticonvulsants), pregnancy, liver disease, or alcoholism. Decrease in reticulocytosis, increased anemia, marrow megaloblastosis, and lastly, response to folate provide the diagnostic features.

Propensity to Infection. Whether there is truly an increased incidence of infections in children with severe HS is a moot question. However, infections can exacerbate the anemia, either by aplastic crisis or by splenic sequestration. Furthermore, it is clear that splenectomy during the first years of life carries a high risk of infection, particularly virulent and overwhelming pneumococcal sepsis and meningitis.

LABORATORY FINDINGS

In common with other hemolytic disorders HS manifests anemia, reticulocytosis, polychromatophilia, occasionally circulating nucleated red cells, marrow erythroid hyperplasia, normal to increased marrow iron, increased unconjugated bilirubin, and absent serum haptoglobin. Hemoglobin concentrations of 9 to 12 gm/dl are commonly seen but during a crisis may fall to 3 to 4 gm/dl. Persistent hemoglobin values less than 8 grams per dl are rare. Reticulocytosis is commonly at 5 to 20 per cent but may be as high as 90 per cent or during aplastic crisis as low as 2 per cent.

Slightly to moderately increased unconjugated serum bilirubin and increased fecal and, less often, urinary urobilinogen reflect the increased erythrocyte destruction and hemoglobin catabolism. Even in the occasional striking increase in serum bilirubin owing to hemolytic crisis, values greater than 6 to 8 mg/dl are suspect for other causes being involved as well, e.g., biliary obstruction or liver disease. The same is true if the conjugated bilirubin increases to greater than 25 to 30 per cent of the total bilirubin. Despite the increase in serum bilirubin, bile pigments and bile salts are absent from the urine in uncomplicated HS, hence the historical designation "acholuric jaundice." Although the red cell destruction is extravascular and hemoglobinemia and hemoglobinuria are not observed, unbound plasma haptoglobin is reduced or absent. Slight leukocytosis and thrombocytosis may also be present.

Examination of the peripheral blood smear usually provides the first specific clue, namely, the presence of a population of small, *densely* staining red cells lacking the normal central pallor. In moderate to severe cases, these microspherocytes are usually present in large proportion and readily detected. If only a few microspherocytes are present, they may often be more readily noted on scanning with the high, dry objective than with the use of oil immersion. The presence of varying proportions of these small spherocytes on the one hand and large reticulocytes and other young red cells on the other hand (as in any overt hemolytic anemia) leads to variable expression of RBC indices. Thus, the mean corpuscular volume (MCV) may be low, normal, or high. The mean corpuscular hemoglobin (MCH) is usually normal. However, as a consequence of the loss of membrane relative to cell volume, the mean corpuscular hemoglobin concentration (MCHC) is usually increased (commonly to 37 to 39 per cent) in the presence of a high proportion of microspherocytes, a finding shared by few other disorders. Thus, anisocytosis may be marked, but poikilocytosis is not usually significant even though a few fragmented forms may be seen. The polychromatophilia reflects the presence of reticulocytes. The presence of spherocytes in other disorders is discussed under Pitfalls in Diagnosis.

DIAGNOSTIC LABORATORY TESTS

The diagnosis of HS requires that it be kept in mind as a possibility and that other causes of chronic hemolysis be excluded. With proper testing the direct Coombs' test is negative as is also the indirect Coombs' test (unless there has been previous transfusion sensitization). The presence of microspherocytes on the peripheral blood smear is obviously the starting point in diagnosis.

Osmotic Fragility. The red cells in HS hemolyze more readily than normal RBCs upon exposure to hypotonic solutions of buffered NaCl (increased osmotic fragility). The saline concentration at which hemolysis begins usually ranges from 0.51 to 0.72 gm/dl but may be as high as 0.85 gm/dl with hemolysis often complete at hypotonic NaCl concentrations at which hemolysis of normal cells just begins. The plotted osmotic fragility curve of HS cells is typically similar in shape to that obtained with normal cells but shifted to higher NaCl concentrations. However, there may be "tails" or "humps" on the curve, owing at the high end of NaCl concentrations to very fragile HS red cells.

"Incubated" Osmotic Fragility. In suspected mild cases exhibiting few spherocytes on blood smear or if the standard test on fresh blood is negative, it is essential to test the osmotic fragility of red cells *incubated* under sterile conditions at 37 C for 24 hours (heparinized or defibrinated blood). It is important to run a control on incubated normal blood since incubation per se increases osmotic fragility. However, the osmotic fragility of HS red cells increases even more strikingly. The use of the "incubated" osmotic fragility test in family studies may be particularly helpful. Patients with only the incubated test positive apparently respond just as well to splenectomy. In neonatal manifestation of HS, incubation of the blood may be required to demonstrate the increased osmotic fragility.

The increase in osmotic fragility in HS does not correlate well with the degree of anemia but does with the degree of spherocytosis. Not unexpectedly, the osmotic fragility may be only minimally abnormal during an aplastic crisis or when iron deficiency complicates HS. Testing has been simplified by the availability of a commercial kit.

Response to Splenectomy. Response to splenectomy with disappearance of anemia, hyperbilirubinemia, and reticulocytosis soon after the operation constitutes a gratifying diagnostic-therapeutic test. Spherocytosis and increased osmotic fragility persist with even more pronounced increments in osmotic fragility of incubated red cells owing to the more prolonged survival in the circulation of cells having potential for such changes upon incubation. It is not an uncommon event for the patient to deny easy fatigability before splenectomy, only to note a most gratifying and unexpected increased sense of well-being and strength after splenectomy. After splenectomy the leukocyte count may be elevated (at times 20,000 to 30,000 per cu mm) for variable and even prolonged periods. This should be ascertained and the patient informed so that in the event of another illness, especially with abdominal pain, the leukocytosis is properly interpreted. Some elevation of the platelet count may also persist for years.

Autohemolysis. Although not always mandatory for diagnosis, the increased spontaneous hemolysis (10 to 50 per cent) of HS blood after incubation under sterile conditions at 37 C for 48 hours is a useful test, especially if in addition it is corrected to normal or near normal (< 4 per cent) by the prior addition of glucose. These findings are characteristic of HS but not completely specific. Autohemolysis may also be increased in autoimmune hemolytic anemias and in hereditary hemolytic anemias owing to enzymatic defects. In the former, the addition of glucose is not usually protective, and in the latter, the response to glucose is variable. Cases have been reported with negative osmotic fragility tests on fresh and "incubated" blood but with spherocytes on smear, positive autohemolysis test for HS and response to splenectomy.

DIAGNOSTIC CLINICAL INVESTIGATIONS

Erythrocyte Survival and Organ Sequestration. Determination of RBC survival with labeled erythrocytes is rarely required for clinical decisions. Enhanced accumulation of radioactivity occurs in the spleen because of its selective trapping of HS RBC.

Family Studies. Strong confirmatory evidence for HS can be provided by the demonstration of clinical and laboratory findings similar to those of the patient in a familial pattern consonant with an autosomal dominant mode of inheritance. As mentioned previously, because of clinical mildness of HS in some family members, a negative family history may be reliable only if personal historical interview and examination and detailed laboratory testing are carried out.

PITFALLS IN DIAGNOSIS

No single test is absolutely diagnostic for HS. The disorder may occasionally be confused with a case of acquired autoimmune hemolytic anemia that is atypical because the conventional direct Coombs' test is negative. Spherocytosis and increased osmotic fragility may be seen in other hereditary or acquired hemolytic disorders. Therefore, appropriate studies to exclude the presence of abnormal hemoglobins, RBC enzymatic defects, RBC antibodies and toxins, and other diseases should be obtained. The spherocytosis and increased osmotic fragility are usually more striking or persistent or both in full-blown clinical HS than in the other disorders. Compared with other disorders with spherocytes, in HS the spherocytes are usually greater numerically, are more uniform in size and shape, and are not accompanied by appreciable numbers of other poikilocytes.

Furthermore, increased autohemolysis in other disorders is not usually corrected by the prior addition of glucose. In contrast to other disorders in which spherocytes are seen, the MCHC in HS is usually greater than 35 per cent. Finally, in extremely difficult cases, splenectomy, unless contraindicated on other grounds, may assist in resolving the issue.

HEREDITARY ELLIPTOCYTOSIS (OVALOCYTOSIS)

By Hussain I. Saba, M.D., Ph.D.
and Robert C. Hartmann, M.D.
Tampa, Florida

DEFINITION

Hereditary elliptocytosis (HE) (or ovalocytosis), when accompanied by overt clinical hemolysis, is similar to hereditary spherocytosis in its clinical manifestations, associated complications, laboratory findings, and clinical cure with splenectomy. Thus, in the *hemolytic* group of HE there is clear-cut anemia, jaundice, and splenomegaly. However, the overtly *hemolytic* group probably comprises only a small proportion of cases of HE (10 to 15 per cent), and the large essentially *asymptomatic* group is difficult to define with precision. The results of recent sophisticated studies suggest a variety of red blood cell (RBC) membrane anomalies indicating a number of subgroups of HE. However, to date the clinical significance of these studies is not fully defined.

The only practical diagnostic feature in the asymptomatic group may be the presence of a morphologic anomaly (i.e., elliptocytosis) on the blood smear. "Ovoid" red blood cells can be seen in a spectrum of shapes from "mildly oval" in up to 15 per cent of red cells in normal blood smears to more exaggerated oval forms in a variety of blood disorders (e.g., macro-ovalocytes in megaloblastic anemias) and finally a mixture of oval and rod-shaped forms comprising 25 to 90 per cent of red cells which is diagnostic for HE. Thus, discrimination must be made as to type and percentage of oval cells.

Although hereditary elliptocytosis is said to be less common than hereditary spherocytosis, significantly increased numbers of elliptical cells have been reported in as many as 4 in 10,000 persons, an incidence similar to that of hereditary spherocytosis. There is no sex predilection, and HE is widespread throughout the world.

Inheritance. As with hereditary spherocytosis, the disorder is autosomal dominant. Linkage of the gene for HE with Rh blood type has been demonstrated in some families with mild or *asymptomatic* HE but not in those with the overtly *hemolytic* form. Although only 10 to 15 per cent have overt hemolysis, data are conflicting regarding the uniformity of hemolytic manifestations within families, in part perhaps because clear-cut differentiation between compensated hemolytic disease and complete freedom from hemolysis has not always been made. Nonetheless, in one family 57 per cent of the members showed signs of hemolysis at one time or another. Thus, the disease within a given family can have a relatively homogeneous expression. During the course of the disease the differentiation between asymptomatic and hemolytic groups may prove to be too arbitrary. It is likely that under certain stresses some of the asymptomatic group may show overt clinical hemolysis.

Erythrocyte Defect. Elliptocytes are characterized by an axial ratio (width-to-length) less than 0.78 (normal about 1.0). Nucleated RBC precursors and reticulocytes are round, not ovoid. Membrane cholesterol appears to be concentrated or polarized to the sites of greatest convexity, and on electron microscopy the hemoglobin appears similarly aggregated in a bipolar arrangement. The red cell glycolytic enzymes are normal as is the hemoglobin type, except in a few sporadic, probably coincidental cases. Upon in vitro incubation HE red cells show an abnormally rapid decline in adenosine triphosphate (ATP) and 2,3-diphosphoglycerate (2,3-DPG) with increased Na^+ efflux. However, neither the degree of these biochemical abnormalities nor the percentage of elliptocytes correlates with the degree of hemolysis in the HE patient. The hereditary elliptocyte appears to share many features with the hereditary spherocyte: abnormal cell shape, selective destruction in the spleen, and probably a somewhat similar membrane permeability defect. However, the specific abnormalities that differentiate the hemolytic forms of of HE from the asymptomatic forms remain to be determined. Recent studies point to abnormalities in the protein (band 4.1) linking spectrin to actin in the RBC membrane skeleton as likely determinants of elliptocytosis in some kindreds.

SYMPTOMS, SIGNS, AND PHYSICAL EXAMINATION

The clinical picture is similar to that of hereditary spherocytosis but is even more variable in its expression, consonant with the extremely large proportion of asymptomatic individuals. Thus, commonly mild elliptocytosis may be an incidental finding in an asymptomatic, nonanemic subject. In symptomatic patients neonatal jaundice, intermittent icterus, anemia, splenomegaly, and aplastic crisis may occur, the last especially in the course of intercurrent disease. There is also, as in hereditary spherocytosis, an increased incidence of cholelithiasis, especially early in life, which may be the lead to medical attention and diagnosis. Occasionally, skeletal deformities are seen as in hereditary spherocytosis. The tip of the spleen may be palpable in patients with definite hemolysis.

COMMON COMPLICATIONS

These are identical to those of hereditary spherocytosis in patients with hemolysis. As in hereditary spherocytosis, it is the complications that are particularly to be feared.

LABORATORY FINDINGS

There may be no laboratory findings except for the presence of elliptical cells on the blood smear. Upon closer scrutiny, a large proportion of supposedly *asymptomatic* patients may show laboratory manifestations of mild, largely compensated hemolysis with hemoglobin concentration of 12 gm/dl or more, reticulocytosis up to 4 per cent, and chromium-labeled (^{51}Cr) RBC survival normal or only slightly reduced.

Ten to 15 per cent of patients (hemolytic group) have a more severe hemolysis with hemoglobin concentrations of 9 to 10 gm/dl, reticulocytosis up to 20 per cent, and decreased red cell T ½ survival, reported as low as 5 days. Some spherocytes and fragmented cells may also be seen on peripheral blood smears. Other laboratory findings of hemolysis with reference to increased hemoglobin catabolism, marrow erythroid hyperplasia, and reduced or absent unbound haptoglobin are present and as cited in the article on hereditary spherocytosis. Although the anemia has been described as normochromic and normocytic, the mean corpuscular volume (MCV) and mean corpuscular hemoglobin (MCH) can be low (50 to 76 cu microns and 18 to 28 pg, respectively). Usually the mean corpuscular hemoglobin concentration (MCHC) is normal. There are no clear-cut differences in RBC morphology between those with overt hemolysis and those with no readily apparent hemolysis.

There is mixed opinion regarding the results of the osmotic fragility and autohemolysis tests in HE, perhaps arising from failure to separate consistently the results in the overtly hemolytic groups from those in the asymptomatic group. A major opinion is that the osmotic fragility tests (on both fresh and incubated cells) and the autohemolysis test are negative when there is no evidence of overt hemolysis, but that all three are positive when active hemolysis is present. Another opinion is that the osmotic fragility test on fresh RBC is normal but that on *incubated* cells, as well as the autohemolysis test, is positive. The abnormal autohemolysis test is supposedly corrected by the prior addition of glucose. In any event, it seems obvious that more work is necessary to clarify the situation.

DIAGNOSTIC LABORATORY AND CLINICAL FINDINGS

Since there are no other pathognomonic findings, the diagnosis revolves around the finding of a significant proportion of appropriate types of oval cells, that is, 25 to 90 per cent of ovalocytes, including rod-shaped forms. To eliminate artifactual effects one should see the oval forms diffusely throughout the smear and not in small collections with the axes all pointing in one direction. Unlike sickle cells, the elliptocytes do not change their shape in sealed fresh preparations. Average dimensions are 8.1 microns long and 5.3 microns wide, but the former may be as large as 12.2 microns and the latter as small as 1.6 microns. The disorder must be differentiated from other causes of mild-to-moderate elliptocytosis, such as thalassemia, sickle cell anemia, iron deficiency, myelofibrosis, macro-ovalocytosis (e.g., as in megaloblastic anemias), and certain red cell enzymopathies. The greater number of elliptocytes in HE, their more uniform size and shape, and the rarity of other poikilocytes in HE stand in sharp contrast to findings in other disorders associated with the presence of ovoid RBC. The number of elliptical forms in a newborn with HE gradually increases until the child is 3 to 4 months of age. Hemolysis and hyperbilirubinemia requiring exchange transfusions have been observed in the newborn, at which time the morphologic picture more closely resembles pyknocytosis rather than elliptocytosis.

Further diagnostic help may be obtained from demonstration of findings in family members in a manner consonant with autosomal dominant mode of inheritance. Response to splenectomy with persistence of the morphologic abnormality in those with the hemolytic form of the disease serves to confirm the diagnosis.

PITFALLS IN DIAGNOSIS

Little confusion exists regarding the patient with a high percentage of elliptocytes on peripheral blood smear, frank hemolysis, splenomegaly, and response to splenectomy. As discussed earlier, the disorder must be differentiated from other causes of mild to moderate elliptocytosis. Appropriate tests should be obtained to exclude red cell enzymopathies, hemoglobin abnormalities, thalassemia, iron deficiency, myelofibrosis, and megaloblastic anemias not only as the primary diagnosis but even as a distinct and separate feature sometimes complicating a case of HE.

PAROXYSMAL NOCTURNAL HEMOGLOBINURIA

By Robert C. Hartmann, M.D.
and Hussain I. Saba, M.D., Ph.D.
Tampa, Florida

SYNONYMS

Strübing-Marchiafava-Micheli syndrome, chronic hemolytic anemia with perpetual hemosiderinuria. The acronym PNH is in common usage.

DEFINITION

Paroxysmal nocturnal hemoglobinuria (PNH), the "great hematologic impostor," has attracted the attention of hematologists far out of proportion to its uncommon occurrence. For many reasons PNH has been considered a rather exotic "clue disorder." For example, it is the only *acquired* hemolytic anemia strictly caused by an intrinsic defect in the red blood cell (RBC). Furthermore, it is the prototype of *intravascular* hemolysis versus the more common type of hemolysis confined to the retiuloendothelial system. Thus, it readily permits the study of the long-term damaging effects of *intravascular* hemolysis on organ function that probably occurs largely from a remarkable chronic thrombotic state. Whatever its basic membrane defect, the crux of the disorder is that the *PNH erythrocyte possesses an exquisite sensitivity to the hemolytic action of complement* in the absence of detectable red cell antibody. This phenomenon is the fundamental basis for the diagnostic tests and presumably the initiating cause for most of the clinical picture.

Incidence. The condition is clearly not as extremely rare as formerly thought (i.e., two per 10^6). Some 85 cases of PNH have been seen at the Royal Postgraduate Medical School in London. Similarly large series have been reported from Asia. The increasing recognition may be due to:

1. Greater awareness and availability of sensitive diagnostic tests.
2. Increasing incidence of aplastic anemia.
3. More prolonged survival in aplastic anemia allowing time for some patients to progress to PNH.

In half of the patients, onset is between the ages of 20 and 50 years. Not rarely it is seen between 10 and 20 years of age, but its onset is exceptional below age 10 and after age 70. The sex ratio is approximately equal. Family studies including those on identical twins have been negative.

Erythrocyte Defect. The membrane defect leading to the exquisite sensitivity to complement hemolysis remains unknown. Deficiency of RBC membrane acetylcholinesterase (AChE) activity is the most consistent biochemical anomaly detected. It may be extremely severe (e.g., 0 to 20 per cent of normal), and some deficient activity is present in all but those with the mildest hemolysis. However, the function of this enzyme in normal red blood cells remains unknown. Furthermore, it is clear from extended studies that the deficiency of AChE activity is not the direct cause of the hemolysis, although the AChE deficiency serves as an excellent marker for that proportion of red cells susceptible to complement hemolysis. There is evidence that combinations of three populations of red cells may circulate in the PNH patient based on sensitivity to complement: Type I with (near-) normal sensitivity; Type II with 3 to 5 times normal; and Type III with 15 to 25 times normal. These findings taken in conjunction with the observed interrelationships between PNH and spontaneous or drug-induced aplastic anemia, acute leukemia, and myelofibrosis have led to the *clonal theory* of PNH. Accordingly, PNH is thought to arise from a clone of precursor cells in the setting of marrow damage.

Electron microscopy has revealed a patchy and pitted RBC surface and abnormal electron-dense material. Attempts to implicate abnormal membrane lipid composition or sensitivity to peroxidation have not met with consistent results. Recently the search has been directed more toward a membrane protein defect. Very recent studies suggest that the susceptibility of PNH RBC to hemolysis in acidified serum relates to a deficiency of a specific membrane protein with complement regulatory activity (decay-accelerating factor [DAF]).

Granulocytes are often reduced in numbers, their phagocytic activity for certain organisms may be reduced, they are more susceptible to complement lysis, and they have reduced alkaline phosphatase activity. Platelets may be reduced in number but usually have a normal life span. They are more sensitive to antibody-induced complement-dependent lysis. Therefore, PNH should be considered a disorder of hematopoiesis rather than just of erythropoiesis.

CLINICAL FEATURES: PRESENTATION, SYMPTOMS, AND SIGNS

The symptoms and signs of PNH are so highly varied that it is impossible to present any typical clinical picture. It is in the main determined by varying combinations, degrees and changing patterns of hemolysis, bone marrow hypoplasia, thrombosis, and infection. At one end of the spectrum exist cases of severe anemia and hemolysis and complicating thromboses and infections; at the other end are quiescent, or "burned-out," cases with little or no anemia or gross hemoglobinuria. These variations exist both between patients and in the same patient at different times. Even in seemingly mild cases, sudden, disastrous complications can occur that require expeditious diagnosis and emergency treatment.

Delay in Diagnosis. Paroxysmal noctural hemoglobinuria has seldom been diagnosed at the start of the patient's illness. Five to 10 years' delay in diagnosis is by no means rare. It is when features other than severe hemolysis dominate the picture that delay in diagnosis may be prolonged.

Hemolysis. Twenty-five to 50 per cent of PNH patients have gross hemoglobinuria at the onset of the disorder, and eventually 80 to 90 per cent develop this manifestation. Typically it is nocturnal with progressive clearing during the day. It may occur in repetitive nocturnal cycles lasting 1 to 14 days (commonly 3 to 5 days). Such attacks occur with extreme variability, ranging from multiple times in a single month to but a few isolated episodes during the entire course of the disease. When carefully studied, it is discovered that the onset is after some 6 to 8 hours of sleep, and hence first noticed in the morning urine. Reversal of day-night sleep patterns proves that the hemoglobinuria is related to sleep. Many elegant studies (including diurnal patterns of pH, cortisol, complement and Mg^{++}) have failed to explain the nocturnal (or sleep) association.

There are, however, many exceptions. With severe episodes, notably those with recognized inciting factors, gross hemoglobinuria may be constant day and night. Inciting factors include infections, exposure to cold, drug and serum reactions, whole blood transfusions, surgery, iron therapy, severe exercise, and possibly certain foods. The common denominators probably include activation of complement and induction of systemic acidosis.

The chronic intravascular hemolysis is manifested by increased plasma hemoglobin, methemalbuminemia, hemoglobinuria, and hemosiderinuria. Clinical jaundice and unconjugated hyperbilirubinemia probably result largely from the catabolism of methemalbumin. *Perpetual hemosiderinuria* is the common denominator for all PNH patients with any degree of disease activity.

Other presentations include those of an ill-defined chronic hemolytic process without gross hemoglobinuria. Such may remain undiagnosed for years until an episode of gross hemoglobinuria provides the clue.

"Aplastic Anemia–PNH" Syndrome. As many as one fourth of PNH patients carry an initial diagnosis of aplastic anemia. When the "aplastic anemia" picture dominates the course, the acid and sucrose hemolysis tests may give relatively weak results and appear largely of secondary interest. Such cases behave clinically more like aplastic anemia.

Physical Findings. As in any hemolytic anemia, pallor and jaundice occur to varying degrees. Clinically detectable splenomegaly is unusual but may occur during episodes of gross hemoglobinuria. However, liver-spleen scans rather consistently reveal some degree of splenic enlargement. The liver may or may not be palpably enlarged. When the clinical picture is dominated by an "aplastic anemia" phase, the physical findings are frequently those associated with hemorrhage and infection.

COMPLICATIONS

The separation of complications from usual clinical manifestations is rather arbitrary, since complications so frequently characterize much of the clinical course.

Infections. Formerly, infections were considered the principal cause of death in PNH, but this is no longer true with the advent of better management of infections in general. Neutropenia and impaired phagocytosis have been cited as factors leading to a propensity to infection. The major consideration is that infection is likely to set off severe hemolysis with gross hemoglobinuria.

Iron Deficiency. Because of the heavy urinary loss of iron in the form of hemoglobin and hemosiderin, iron deficiency develops sooner or later in most cases of PNH. The body distribution of iron is unusual with heavy renal siderosis, but other tissues are usually deficient in iron. Hypochromia may be difficult to appreciate because of macrocytosis owing to a young RBC population. Depression of serum iron may be masked by the ongoing hemolysis and the use of transfusions. Bone marrow examination is usually necessary to detect the iron deficiency. No extensive experience with serum ferritin determinations has been documented. In most PNH patients treatment with oral or parenteral iron precipitates gross hemoglobinuria sooner or later. Indeed, such has been cited as unmasking the diagnosis. Specific replacement treatment of the iron deficiency is thus not only hazardous but probably not highly essential, since iron stores are used at high priority for erythropoiesis.

Transfusion Reactions. Eventually, repeated transfusions of *whole blood* usually provoke episodes of gross hemoglobinuria that may provide the initial tip toward diagnosis. When studied, such patients usually have leukoagglutinins, but these are clearly not the cause of all hemolytic transfusion reactions in PNH. Recently the time-honored concept that whole blood transfusions provoke gross hemoglobinuria has been challenged.

Drug and Serum Reactions. Whether the alleged increased incidence of reactions is unique to PNH or simply what might be expected in a group of chronically ill patients with greater than usual exposure to such agents has not been clarified. In any event, such reactions are apt to induce serious episodes of gross hemoglobinuria, and great care should be exercised with the use of such agents.

Hemorrhage. Despite the relatively high frequency of thrombocytopenia in PNH, thrombosis rather than hemorrhage occurs. Spontaneous hemorrhage is probably more common in those with a predominantly "aplastic anemia" picture.

Association with Other Blood Dyscrasias. The intimate association of PNH with aplastic anemia has already been discussed. In a small number of cases there has been an association with myelosclerosis and myeloid metaplasia. In some the clinical picture of myeloid metaplasia predominated, with the presence of ancillary laboratory features of PNH. In several the presenting picture of myeloid metaplasia was subsequently supplanted by rather typical PNH.

There are now over 20 cases of PNH reported to have terminated in leukemia, usually the acute nonlymphoid type. One patient went the route of successive development of chloramphenicol-induced aplastic anemia, PNH, and acute leukemia. Chromosomal studies have been widely quoted as normal in PNH, and this appears true for cultured lymphocytes from peripheral blood. However, when the *marrow* has been studied, a significant proportion have had varied but important chromosomal abnormalities, suggesting the possibility of slow evolution of a preleukemic state.

Thrombotic Diathesis. Nowadays thrombosis is probably the most common cause of death in PNH. Major, large vein thrombosis has long been recognized, particularly peripheral vein thrombosis, pulmonary infarction, and cerebral and portal vein thrombosis. Only recently has the concept been extended to an undercurrent of chronic, smoldering low-grade thrombosis occurring in small veins and in the microcirculation and leading in some instances to eventual organ damage. The latter probably results in headaches, leg cramps, peculiar skin lesions, abdominal pain, gastrointestinal ulceration, progressive renal damage, and bone changes. Thrombosis is usually venous, but a few cases have been arterial. Autopsy studies reveal that virtually all venous sites have been involved.

The osseous and renal changes in particular simulate those of sickle cell anemia, albeit milder. It had been considered remarkable that renal damage did not occur in PNH despite the severe renal siderosis. There is no solid evidence that renal siderosis per se is significantly harmful. However, when carefully studied, many patients demonstrate varying degrees of microscopic hematuria and proteinuria (distinct from gross hemoglobinuria), fixed hyposthenuria, abnormal tubular function, declining creatinine clearance, and eventually hypertension. Radiologically, there are enlarged kidneys, cortical infarcts and thinning, and papillary necrosis, and in some patients eventual kidney shrinkage, all confirmed by autopsy.

Abdominal Pain. Abdominal pain in PNH can present a particularly difficult diagnostic problem between peptic ulceration; cholelithiasis; and mesenteric, portal, or hepatic venous thrombosis. There is an increased incidence of peptic ulceration in PNH. Cholelithiasis owing to pigmented gallstones occurs. Abdominal pain in PNH should be considered secondary to intra-abdominal thrombosis unless proved otherwise. Repeated attacks of mesenteric venous thrombosis are common in some patients and difficult to define and treat but in most instances clear eventually without sequelae.

Hepatic Venous Thrombosis. Probably the most dread, highly fatal complication of PNH is progressive, diffuse hepatic venous thrombosis (HVT) (Budd-Chiari syndrome) involving not only major venous branches but secondary and tertiary radicles as well. The clinical-laboratory picture of fulminant cases has only recently been crystallized. Diagnosis is suggested by a clinical complex of abdominal pain, low-grade fever, (further) increase in liver size, occasionally liver tenderness, and when the condition is advanced, ascites. Certain laboratory results support the diagnosis of HVT:

1. Further elevation of serum lactate dehydrogenase (LD) and serum glutamic oxaloacetic transaminase (SGOT) (AST) (above baseline elevations due to chronic hemolysis alone).
2. Elevated serum glutamic pyruvic transaminase (SGPT) (ALT).
3. Increased *conjugated* bilirubin (above 25 per cent of total even when the total is relatively low).
4. An elevated titer of fibrin split products.

Abnormal liver scans provide the most useful and least invasive procedure for the diagnosis of HVT and show hepatic and splenic enlargement, unequal distribution of colloid in the various lobes of the liver, rapid changes in pattern and extrahepatic uptake. These changes also occur in advanced cirrhosis and must therefore be interpreted in the proper setting. In HVT there may additionally be a centrally located region of increased radionuclide uptake representing a hypertrophied caudate lobe which is spared by a separate venous drainage into the inferior vena cava. This finding is not observed in typical cirrhosis. Abdominal computed tomographic (CT) scans and inferior vena cavagram may also demonstrate the enlarged caudate lobe.

The rapidly progressing and highly fatal nature of *fulminant* HVT in PNH makes prompt diagnosis and institution of therapy mandatory. Given the typical clinical and biochemical findings plus an abnormal liver scan, heparin should be started immediately. If then deemed necessary, appropriate angiographic studies (e.g., hepatic venogram) can be carried out later. However, with increasing awareness of the clinical, laboratory, and liver scan patterns, angiographic studies, although of interest, should rarely be necessary for the diagnosis. Liver biopsies are generally to be condemned since they rarely show a diagnostic lesion because of the spotty involvement even with *open* liver biopsies, which additionally carry a heavy risk in the face of the severe liver damage. Even needle biopsies carry the disadvantage of delaying the prompt institution of heparin therapy. Exploratory laparotomy for unexplained abdominal pain in PNH in ignorance of the possibility of hepatic venous or other thrombosis is clearly unwarranted. Although there have been but several well-documented cases with survival and return of adequate liver function, earlier diagnosis and treatment may bring better success. At least one early, subclinical case of HVT has been detected by liver scan survey and confirmed by hepatic venogram and is currently on maintenance coumadin therapy.

Pathogenesis of Thrombosis. There have been a legion of studies attempting to interrelate blood coagulation, platelets, and the complement system with respect to thrombosis in PNH. The results have been inconclusive if not conflicting, and to make a long story short, no cohesive, confirmed mechanism has yet been established. One theory relates thrombosis more specifically to a primary qualitative platelet abnormality in PNH.

COURSE

From the foregoing it is apparent that the course of PNH is so highly varied as to defy any simple categorization. Prognosis varies from several years to many decades, with a very few "burned-out" or seemingly spontaneously cured cases. Yet disastrous and even fatal complications can strike at any time. The frequent delays in diagnosis can play havoc with the patient's physical, mental, and financial well-being. Prognosis probably depends ultimately on the size of the patient's complement-sensitive RBC population, the degree of marrow aplasia, and the occurrence of serious thrombotic episodes.

LABORATORY FINDINGS

Although the degree of anemia varies widely, in most cases the hematocrit is less than 30 per cent. There are no distinct erythrocyte abnormalities on blood smears. The RBC indices and blood smear morphology reflect a mixture of macrocytes and polychromatophilia (paralleling the elevated reticulocyte count) and hypochromia owing to iron deficiency. The reticulocyte count ranges widely (e.g., 1 to 40 per cent) but commonly is 5 to 20 per cent.

The leukocyte count is low either regularly or at some time during the disorder in about 50 per cent of patients. It may be less than 1500 per cu mm and then is principally associated with neutropenia. The leukocyte alkaline phosphatase activity is low or even zero but in the "aplastic group" may be normal. Platelet counts are less than 150,000 per cu mm in about two thirds of patients and less than 40,000 per cu mm in one fourth. Although pancytopenia has been cited as characteristic of PNH it is by no means constant from patient to patient nor within the same patient from time to time, and any combination of cytopenias can be seen. Marrow cellularity ranges from extreme hypoplasia to marked erythroid hyperplasia. Marrow iron is usually markedly reduced or absent.

The urine shows periodic gross hemoglobinuria and, in many but not all cases, occult hemoglobinuria in the intervening chronic steady state. In any event, some degree of perpetual hemosiderinuria is a sine qua non for the diagnosis. In active PNH the urine hemosiderin test gives a remarkably strong reaction with marked bluish-black discoloration of the Prussian blue reagents as well as the renal tubular cells in the urinary sediment—a finding strongly suggestive of PNH. Microscopic hematuria and fixed hyposthenuria are hallmarks of chronic renal damage owing to thrombosis. Urinary concentration tests should, however, be carried out with great care in view of the marked thrombotic tendency.

Serum chemistries typically reveal elevated unconjugated bilirubin, LD, and SGOT (AST) activities, as seen with hemolysis from many causes. The additional changes owing to HVT have been discussed earlier in this article. One problem with serum chemistries in PNH is that clotted blood readily hemolyzes in vitro, giving inaccurate values. It is suggested that *heparinized plasma* be used for the usual serum chemistry determinations if hemolysis is marked.

Supported by the Southwestern Medical Foundation—Kinsler Williamson Brown Fund, NIH Grant CA18132 from the National Cancer Institute and the Meadows Foundation.

The following tests are normal in uncomplicated PNH: Coombs' test, osmotic fragility test on fresh RBCs, serum antibodies and immunoglobulins, hemoglobin electrophoresis, and glycolytic as well as membrane enzymes (except for acetylcholinesterase). A few patients have had elevated hemoglobin F.

DIAGNOSTIC LABORATORY TESTS

The specific tests for PNH depend upon the demonstration of complement-sensitive erythrocytes in the absence of RBC antibody.

Sucrose Hemolysis or "Sugar Water" Test. This test depends upon the activation of complement by low ionic strength media. One volume of blood anticoagulated with citrate or oxalate (but not with ethylenediamine tetra-acetic acid [EDTA] or heparin) is mixed with nine volumes of freshly prepared sugar water (1 volume of dry sugar diluted to ten volumes with *distilled water,* not saline). The mixture is incubated at 37°C or room temperature for 30 minutes, centrifuged, and the supernatant inspected for evidence of gross hemolysis. The screening test is made more specific by utilizing saline-washed patient cells and fresh ABO-compatible serum suspended in isotonic buffered sucrose solution and similarly tested.

Acid Hemolysis Test of Ham. This test depends upon the activation of complement by acidification of serum. One part of a 50 per cent suspension of saline-washed patient RBC is added to nine parts of normal ABO-compatible serum after its pH has been reduced by the addition of a small volume of dilute HCl (e.g., 0.2 N HCl). Hemolysis is evaluated after 30 minutes incubation at 37°C.

The sucrose and acid hemolysis tests are the two most useful ones. The sucrose hemolysis test has the advantage of simplicity, not requiring special reagents and temperature and pH control, and is more sensitive. The acid hemolysis test is somewhat more specific. In the sucrose hemolysis test values of <5 per cent hemolysis may occasionally be obtained with non-PNH cells; 5 to 10 per cent hemolysis is considered borderline; and >10 per cent hemolysis definitely positive. Similar considerations hold for the acid hemolysis test. In both tests appropriate controls (which should yield no hemolysis) include the use of complement-inactivated heated serum (56°C for 30 minutes) and testing the patient's (acidified) serum against normal red cells.

Recent studies suggest that when the acid hemolysis test yields a borderline result, advantage may be taken of the PNH RBC's exquisite sensitivity to standard commercial preparations of endotoxin. Pre-incubation of PNH red cells with pyrogen-free saline solutions containing very small concentrations of endotoxin may markedly enhance their subsequent acid hemolysis.

Other diagnostic tests include the thrombin test of Crosby, the "heat test" of Hegglin-Maier, the inulin lysis screening test, and the antibody-induced lysis test. None of these possesses the combination of specificity and simplicity of the sucrose and acid hemolysis tests, but several may be useful in research.

PITFALLS IN DIAGNOSIS

A high index of suspicion is paramount. Since PNH is the "great hematologic impostor," its diagnosis must always be considered in any patient with the following signs: unexplained hemolytic process, hemoglobinuria (especially cola beverage–colored urine on arising with clearing during the day), unexplained hemoglobinuric transfusion reactions, any combination of blood cytopenias, unexplained iron deficiency, precipitation of gross hemoglobinuria with iron therapy, recurrent bouts of abdominal pain, venous thrombosis, and, for that matter, any unexplained anemia. Patients with the condition may be referred by the urologist or nephrologist, particularly when pallor, weakness, and dark urine initially suggest glomerulonephritis or when gross "hematuria" actually turns out to be hemoglobinuria. A strongly positive test for hemosiderinuria is compelling evidence for PNH.

The diagnosis is made by the use of tests for the detection of complement-sensitive erythrocytes. Although these tests are simple in design and concept, false results may be obtained if they are not carefully performed with appropriate controls or if the serum used lacks adequate complement for any reason. An increase in acid hemolysis with 60 per cent of normal sera, but not in sucrose hemolysis, occurs in one variant (HEMPAS) of the rare disorder, hereditary dyserythropoietic anemia.

ACQUIRED HEMOLYTIC ANEMIA

By Mateel S. Graham, M.D.
and Eugene P. Frenkel, M.D.
Dallas, Texas

DEFINITION

The normal red blood cell survives for approximately 120 days, but red cell abnormalities or injury may result in a shortened survival. Increased red cell production by the marrow can compensate when the red cell destruction is only modest (i.e., chromium-labeled (^{51}Cr) red cell survival of greater than 18 days); this is termed a "compensated hemolytic state." If the bone marrow is unable to increase production or if red cell destruction is great, *hemolytic anemia* is seen. This is defined as an anemia resulting from increased red blood cell destruction.

Hemolytic anemias may be congenital or acquired. Congenital hemolytic anemias result from defects intrinsic to the red cell: these defects may involve the cell membrane, hemoglobin, or enzymes responsible for normal erythrocyte metabolism and function. Acquired hemolytic anemias are caused by altered or pathophysiologic mechanisms extrinsic to the erythrocyte, that is, processes affecting inherently normal red blood cells. In the approach to the diagnosis of an acquired hemolytic anemia, a stepwise characterization is possible. Thus, the pathophysiologic mechanisms completely outside the cell include increased sequestration of red cells (e.g., congestive splenomegaly) or the presence of circulating antibodies directed against the red cell (e.g., warm or cold antibodies [autoimmunohemolytic anemia] or alloantibodies [isoimmunization]). The red cell may be directly injured by external trauma to the membrane (e.g., red cell fragmentation syndromes due to external trauma [march hemoglobinuria], turbulent flow around calcific or prosthetic heart valves, or disseminated intravascular coagulation), or internal injury by parasitic infestation (e.g., malaria, bartonellosis). Acquired metabolic abnormalities may result in injury to the membrane (e.g., hypophosphatemia resulting in a rigid membrane, Heinz body formation, copper sulfate intoxication), or produce enzymatic dysfunction (e.g., 5′ nucleotidase deficiency with lead intoxication, pyruvate kinase deficiency with alcoholic hepatitis) with resultant hemolysis. Finally, a rare form of an acquired defect is that of a clonal proliferation of red cells with undue sensitivity to complement-induced lysis (paroxysmal nocturnal hemoglobinuria).

Supported by the Southwestern Medical Foundation—Kinsler Williamson Brown Fund, NIH Grant CA18132 from the National Cancer Institute and the Meadows Foundation.

CLASSIFICATION

By defining the predominant site of red cell destruction, aspects of the clinical expression are described. Thus, when the hemolysis is primarily intravascular, hemoglobinemia and hemoglobinuria are common; and when it is extravascular, reticuloendothelial sequestration occurs.

The pathophysiologic classification presented in Table 1 can be used for the differential diagnostic characterization of acquired hemolytic anemias.

PRESENTING SIGNS AND SYMPTOMS

These depend on the rapidity with which the anemia develops, the degree of anemia, and the underlying cause. In addition, if most of the hemolysis is intravascular, the patient will have hemoglobinuria with passage of dark, cola beverage–colored urine.

Patients with chronic disease states (e.g., renal failure) and those in whom the anemia develops over a prolonged period of time may tolerate moderately severe anemia without symptoms. Patients with an acute hemolytic episode and rapid-onset anemia will present with weakness, shortness of breath, tachycardia, and pallor; in addition, jaundice may be present. In rare patients with severe intravascular hemolysis and shock, renal failure may occur.

The primary underlying disease (e.g., infection or malignancy) may present with symptoms that overshadow those related to hemolytic anemia. In some hemolytic processes, signs and symptoms suggest the true nature of the clinical lesion. For example, in cold agglutinin disease there may be intolerance to cold, Raynaud's phenomenon, and passage of dark urine with exposure to cold. In paroxysmal nocturnal hemoglobinuria there may be recurrent episodes of abdominal pain and thrombotic episodes, in addition to dark urine in the morning. In patients with thrombotic thrombocytopenic purpura, coma or changing neuro-

Table 1. Classification of Acquired Hemolytic Anemia

Extracorpuscular Defect*
1. Hypersplenism or congestive splenomegaly (degree of hemolysis correlates with spleen size)
2. Immune hemolytic anemias
   A. Isoimmune (hemolytic transfusion reactions, erythroblastosis fetalis)
   B. Autoimmune
      1) Autoimmune "warm" antibody types (identified by positive direct antiglobulin [Coombs'] test, IgG, at 37° C)
         a. Idiopathic (chronic cold agglutinin disease)
         b. Secondary (to lymphoproliferative disorders, collagen vascular diseases, infections, drugs; less commonly other neoplastic disorders, sarcoid, malaria)
      2) Autoimmune "cold" antibody types (identified by the presence of cold agglutinins with increasing titer as the temperature is lowered. Positive direct Coombs' with anti-complement sera).
         a. Idiopathic (chronic cold agglutinin disease)
         b. Secondary (post-infections, especially *Mycoplasma pneumoniae*, infectious mononucleosis, other viral infections; lymphoproliferative disorders; rarely, other malignancies)
         c. Paroxysmal cold hemoglobinuria (syphilis, viral infections)
3. Hemolysis associated with red cell fragmentation
   A. Microangiopathic hemolytic anemia (disseminated intravascular coagulation, thrombotic thrombocytopenic purpura, hemolytic uremic syndromes, malignant hypertension, vasculitis, carcinomatosis)
   B. Infections (*Clostridium welchii*, malaria)
   C. Trauma (march hemoglobinuria, prosthetic cardiac valves, calcific aortic stenosis, burns, chemicals)

Extracorpuscular and Intracorpuscular Defects
1. Metabolic abnormalities (hypophosphatemia, uremia, liver disease)
2. Copper (sulfate) intoxication

Intracorpuscular Defects
1. Acquired enzymatic abnormalities (5′ nucleotidase deficiency secondary to lead intoxication)
2. Paroxysmal nocturnal hemoglobinuria
3. Nutritional deficiencies (vitamin B_{12}, folate)

*The majority of acquired hemolytic anemias are due to extracorpuscular defects.

logic signs are seen on presentation. In disseminated intravascular coagulation, clotting abnormalities are more severe than the hemolysis. In idiopathic warm-reacting autoimmune hemolytic anemia, there are generally no signs and symptoms other than those related to the anemia and the rapidity of its onset.

LABORATORY INVESTIGATIONS

These can be divided into two broad categories: those tests that identify the patient with a shortened red cell survival, and those that help identify and confirm the cause. There will, of course, be overlap. Routine laboratory tests usually demonstrate the presence of a hemolytic state.

Complete Blood Count

Anemia to a variable degree will be present. (In patients with minimally shortened red cell survival or with bone marrow compensation, anemia may be minimal.) The mean corpuscular volume (MCV) is normal. Since reticulocytes (polychromatophilic young cells) are large, the MCV may appear elevated; the value can be corrected by subtracting the reticulocyte count from the recorded MCV to provide the true MCV. In chronic intravascular hemolysis (as with prosthetic heart valves), chronic hemoglobinuria results in a loss of iron and a hypochromic microcytic anemia may be seen.

Examination of the Peripheral Smear

This is a critical aspect of the initial evaluation, since it may show evidence of red cell membrane injury and even suggest the cause. Increased polychromasia is evidence of increased red cell production and reflects the reticulocyte count. Red cells may show abnormal sizes (anisocytosis) and shapes (poikilocytosis) with evidence of membrane injury. In autoimmune hemolytic anemia, spherocytosis may be prominent. In microangiopathic states, in addition to microspherocytes, there will be fragmentation of red cells (e.g., helmet cells and schistocytes) and nucleated red cells. In cold-reacting autoimmune hemolytic anemia, there often is clumping and grouping of red cells to form a lake-like pattern.

The white blood cells and platelets may provide important information. Thus, white cells and platelets are often elevated in hemolysis, as evidence of increased marrow turnover. In Evans' syndrome (combined autoimmune hemolytic anemia and idiopathic thrombocytopenic purpura), the platelet count is decreased and large platelets are seen. In microangiopathic states and in disseminated intravascular coagulation, the platelet count is also decreased. In hypersplenism, red cells will be normochromic and normocytic and frequently there is a true pancytopenia (i.e., decreased white cells and platelets). In paroxysmal nocturnal hemoglobinuria, the unusual combination of hypochromic (because of iron loss) red cells with increased polychromasia (red cell repair) suggests a mechanism for chronic intravascular hemolysis.

Reticulocyte Count

An elevated reticulocyte count is evidence of increased production of red cells by the marrow. Normally, the reticulocyte count is 0.5 to 1.5 per cent. In hemolytic anemia, it may be elevated to 10 or 20 per cent. The reticulocyte count should be corrected for the patient's hematocrit:

$$\text{Corrected reticulocyte count} = \frac{\%\ \text{reticulocytes} \times \text{hematocrit}}{45}$$

where the number 45 represents a mean average normal hematocrit.

The reticulocyte index is obtained by dividing the corrected reticulocyte count by 2. A reticulocyte index of 3 or greater indicates increased marrow production of red cells and suggests the existence of hemolytic anemia with repair.

Tests Indicating Red Cell Destruction

Indirect bilirubin is elevated. Its level depends on the total pigment pool (which may be small in severely anemic patients with low hemoglobins) and adequacy of liver function. Hemolysis generally does not produce high values unless there is liver dysfunction. Since indirect bilirubin is protein-bound, the urine is negative for bile.

Fecal urobilinogen is increased in the presence of hemolysis. Again, the degree of increase depends upon the net pigment mass, liver function, and the absence of agents (i.e., antibiotics) in the gastrointestinal tract interfering with normal pigment metabolism.

Urine urobilinogen is increased in hemolysis and the elevation depends on the increased pigment load presented to the gut. It is less reliable, but more readily obtained, than fecal urobilinogen.

Values of *lactate dehydrogenase (LD)* are elevated in patients with intravascular hemolysis because red cells contain substantial amounts of LD.

SPECIAL STUDIES

Plasma Hemoglobin, Urine Hemoglobin, Urine Hemosiderin

Elevated levels are seen in patients with intravascular hemolysis but usually not in those with predominant extravascular hemolysis. Evidence of pink- to mahogany-discolored plasma is a good indication of free hemoglobin. This can be documented by a plasma hemoglobin determination. Free hemoglobin in the serum binds to haptoglobin which is then removed by the reticuloendothelial system, resulting in a depression of the haptoglobin levels. Plasma hemoglobin in excess of the capacity of haptoglobin binding is filtered by the glomerulus, resulting in hemoglobinuria. Hemosiderin-laden tubular cells can be chemically identified by staining the urinary sediment with Prussian blue. Hemosiderinuria may persist for a week after hemoglobinemia clears. Intravascular hemolysis with hemoglobinemia, hemoglobinuria, and hemosiderinuria is most commonly associated with red cell fragmentation, infectious intraerythrocytic causes, and paroxysmal hemoglobinuria (nocturnal or cold).

Serum Haptoglobin Level

Serum haptoglobins are alpha-glycoproteins that have the property of combining with hemoglobin. The normal range is approximately 30 to 200 mg/dl. When hemoglobin destruction exceeds two to three times the normal rate, the serum haptoglobin level will be reduced. Although the level of serum haptoglobin is a reasonable indicator of hemolysis, the values vary considerably: They are decreased in severe hepatocellular disease and elevated in acute or chronic inflammatory disease and in steroid administration.

Red Cell Survival

The survival of radiolabeled (^{51}Cr) red cells provides documentation of a shortened cell survival or hemolysis. The survival can be expressed in relationship to normal red cell life span or alternatively as the "half-life" (T ½) or time in days required for 50 per cent of the radioactive red cells to disappear. The normal half-life is 27 to 32 days. After the radiolabeled cells are administered, gamma emission surface counting over the liver and spleen can identify the selective sites of red cell destruction. Thus, in warm-reacting autoimmune hemolytic anemia, the spleen is the major site of red cell sequestration; in cold-reacting autoimmune hemolytic anemia, red cell destruction is primarily recognized in the liver reticuloendothelial cells.

Bone Marrow

Increased erythroid activity in the bone marrow (the normal erythroid:granulocyte [E:G] ratio of 1:3 may be reversed) is seen as a response to bleeding or hemolysis. This is the marrow attempt at repair, and increased production is reflected in the peripheral blood by the elevated reticulocyte count. With continued high rates of production, relative folate deficiency may develop with resultant megaloblastosis. If marrow injury occurs, increased productivity may not be possible, resulting in a so-called aplastic crisis.

Immunologic Tests

The Coombs' (or antiglobulin) test is the diagnostic criterion of antibody-mediated hemolytic anemia. The majority of the autoimmune hemolytic anemias are caused by warm-reacting antibodies of the IgG class—IgG_1 and IgG_3, predominantly. These antibodies are "incomplete" and do not cause agglutination in vitro unless an anti-human globulin serum (Coombs' serum) is added. The majority of these are anti-Rh antibodies; this can be demonstrated by failure to react with Rh null cells. Cold-reacting antibodies (cold agglutinins or cold hemolysins) are generally of the IgM class, are "complete," and do cause direct agglutination in vitro. They bind to the red cells in the cold and elute as the blood is warmed. They cause hemolysis by the activation of complement. These antibodies are directed against the I (I-i)antigen of the red cell, and the anti-complement Coombs' is positive.

Donath and Landsteiner Test

In paroxysmal cold hemoglobinuria, a rare disorder, the Donath and Landsteiner test will demonstrate binding of the antibody to the red cell in the cold and destruction of the cell when the blood is warmed. This antibody, although cold-reacting, is of the IgG class, directed against the P antigen on the red cell. The hemolysis, often severe, is mediated via complement activation.

Sucrose Hemolysis Test

This is a useful screening test for paroxysmal nocturnal hemoglobinuria, the diagnosis of which is based on the demonstration of complement-sensitive red cells. The sucrose hemolysis test may be positive in a variety of other hematologic disorders including megaloblastic anemias and autoimmune hemolytic anemia.

Ham Test

This acidified serum lysis test is done to establish a definite diagnosis of paroxysmal nocturnal hemoglobinuria. It is almost never positive in other diseases and almost always positive in PNH.

PITFALLS IN DIAGNOSIS

A common pitfall is to misinterpret a peripheral reticulocytosis and associated marrow proliferative response to a recent (occult) bleed as a hemolytic anemia. These are manifestations of marrow "repair" and do not establish a diagnosis. A second error is to consider any hemolytic episode in the adult as an acquired lesion. Both congenital spherocytic and nonspherocytic anemias may be identified for the first time in adult life. Similarly, "oxidative hemolysis" resulting from congenital deficiency of glucose-6-phosphate dehydrogenase may be recognized for the first time in adult life, as an episode is precipitated by drugs, infection, or metabolic lesions.

The patient with a hemolytic anemia may present after the acute process, and hemoglobinuria may not be present. A careful history as to precipitating causes (infection, cold, drugs), symptoms (dark urine, jaundice, back pain), and then an evaluation of the blood smear, reticulocyte count, and follow-up of the patient's course may provide clues to the correct diagnosis.

Finally, in some autoimmune hemolytic anemias, the Coombs' test may not be positive. The clinical pattern of the disease in such circumstances is the best parameter for diagnosis.

It should be emphasized that the pathophysiologic mechanism for the hemolytic anemia should be sought in all cases to help in developing a structured and specific treatment program.

NEUTROPENIA AND AGRANULOCYTOSIS

By Leonard H. Brubaker, M.D.
Augusta, Georgia

SYNONYMS

Granulocytopenia.

DEFINITION

While population studies indicate considerable variation in absolute neutrophil counts (total white blood cell count times fraction of neutrophils in the differential count), neutropenia is customarily defined as a neutrophil count less than 1500 per cu mm. Lower values than this, however, have been observed in asymptomatic and apparently healthy black Americans (especially males), black Africans, and Yemenite Jews.

Agranulocytosis usually refers to the sudden onset of severe neutropenia. Patients taking anticancer or immunosuppressive drugs who develop neutropenia as an expected drug side effect are not considered to have agranulocytosis. The term refers to an idiosyncratic response to a nonmyelosuppressive drug or chemical.

Neutrophil counts below 1000 per cu mm are associated with an increased risk of bacterial infections if the neutropenia is caused by lack of marrow production. If the neutrophil count goes below 500, the risk of fatal infection is much more serious. However, if neutropenia is due to abnormalities of pooling or increased destruction, such a risk is not necessarily present. For the most part, neutropenia is a secondary manifestation of a number of different diseases rather than a primary process.

PATHOPHYSIOLOGIC CAUSES OF NEUTROPENIA

The pathophysiologic causes of neutropenia can be divided into the following categories:

1. Decreased marrow production.
2. Ineffective marrow production.
3. Decreased survival in circulation.
4. Abnormal pooling within the circulation.

Mixed pathophysiologies are sometimes found.

Careful examination of the bone marrow provides considerable insight into the pathophysiologic mechanism of neutropenia, if one bears in mind certain errors of random marrow sampling. For example, the cellularity of the marrow may vary from site to site. In older patients the posterior iliac crest may be markedly hypocellular or even aplastic, whereas the sternal marrow will show the normal cellularity of approximately 30 to 50 per cent cells and the rest fat. Previous radiation of a given bone marrow site may cause this area to be hypocellular while the rest of the marrow may be hypercellular.

There are also potential errors associated with the category of ineffective marrow production. This condition may be properly deduced when the marrow shows megaloblastic changes in the neutrophilic precursors. However, some causes of ineffective marrow production do not produce megaloblastic changes. In these situations the marrow is full of neutrophil precursors in contrast to the circulating blood neutropenia.

Such myeloid hyperplasia can be confused with the appearance of the marrow when the pathophysiologic problem is decreased peripheral blood survival rather than ineffective production. One subtle difference between these two is that in ineffective production the marrow usually has a large number of mature polymorphonuclear neutrophils (polys), whereas in decreased peripheral survival the number of myelocytes, metamyelocytes, and band forms may be normal but there may be a marked decrease in the number of mature polys.

A common cause of abnormal pooling is splenomegaly, regardless of its cause. Splenic pooling or sequestration alone can produce neutropenia in some patients whose spleens are palpable at the umbilical level or below. The degree of splenic pooling is roughly proportional to the spleen size, the same as it is for platelets. Acute neutropenia due to abnormal pooling of neutrophils within the lungs can be produced in clinical situations in which there is a sudden activation of serum complement. Complement-mediated neutrophil pooling occurs during:

1. Hemodialysis and nylon-wool leukopheresis procedures as a trivial problem.
2. Acute antigen-antibody reactions.
3. Endotoxemia.
4. Massive bacterial infections.
5. Shock.

In situations 2 through 5 the complement activation may be massive, and the neutrophil pooling and breakdown in the lung may cause pulmonary edema and other injury.

CAUSES OF NEUTROPENIA GROUPED BY PATHOPHYSIOLOGY

Neutropenia from Drug Damage. Most anticancer or immunosuppressive drugs regularly produce neutropenia from transient depression of committed, actively cycling marrow stem cells. Some drugs in certain individuals may produce unexpectedly prolonged neutropenia. Busulfan, for example, can produce marrow aplasia lasting many months or years. Patients treated sequentially both by radiation of marrow-containing bones and cytotoxic drugs also may have prolonged neutropenia owing to marrow aplasia. Several drugs, chemicals, and other agents may also produce marrow aplasia as an occasional, unpredictable side effect. Examples of these are chloramphenicol, phenylbutazone, benzene, and hepatitis virus. These reactions may lead to pancytopenia or to isolated neutropenia owing to selected suppression of marrow neutrophil precursors (agranulocytosis).

Another form of agranulocytosis due to drugs appears to be related to an immunologic reaction, exemplified by aminopyrine. Following a period of sensitization, the patient has abrupt onset of chills, fever, and collapse caused by the peripheral destruction of circulating neutrophils. These patients can recover quickly when the drug is withdrawn. They evince identical symptoms and develop neutropenia abruptly upon re-exposure to the drug. Immunologic mechanisms may also be responsible for destruction of marrow neutrophil precursors. The drugs most commonly associated with agranulocytosis include phenothiazines, sulfonamides, antithyroid medications, anticonvulsants, and some rarely used analgesics. There is a long list of other drugs reported to be rare causes of agranulocytosis. Every patient who develops neutropenia abruptly should be considered to have a drug-induced or chemically induced neutropenia, and all nonvital drugs should be discontinued.

Other Forms of Neutropenia Due to Decreased Marrow Production

Marrow Stem Cell Defects. A number of congenital syndromes have been described in which neutropenia is produced by lack of marrow neutrophil precursors. If this situation is present at birth the infant usually rapidly dies of infection. Sometimes this type of defect is characterized by a cyclic neutropenia, a condition in which fever, ulcerations of the mouth, skin, anus, or genitals, and extreme neutropenia recur for about 4 to 5 days out of each approximately 21-day cycle. At other times this situation is accompanied by a wide variety of other congenital defects, such as dysglobulinemia or agammaglobulinemia.

Replacement of Bone Marrow. Invasion of the bone marrow by tumors from the lung, breast, or other sites may produce neutropenia, pancytopenia, or some other combinations of cytopenias. The tumor involvement is often nonuniform, one iliac crest being involved and not the other, or the spine being involved and not the iliac crest. A positive bone scan will sometimes indicate the areas of involvement, but often the bone marrow is completely replaced by tumor while the bone scan in the area is negative. Plasma cell myeloma particularly causes that result. Agnogenic myeloid metaplasia may produce neutropenia but the opposite is usually true, since the enlarged spleen in this disease may produce greatly increased numbers of abnormal neutrophils.

Neutropenia Caused by Ineffective Marrow Production. Patients with megaloblastic anemia due to vitamin B_{12} or folic acid deficiency frequently are both thrombocytopenic and neutropenic. The morphologic changes in the marrow are readily apparent, including giant myelocytes, metamyelocytes, and bands and hypersegmented neutrophils in the marrow and circulating blood. The megaloblastic changes in the neutrophils may persist for many days following the vitamin B_{12}- or folate-induced reversion of the red cell changes to normal. Recognition of the persistence of giant bands and hypersegmented neutrophils within the marrow can lead to a diagnosis of pernicious anemia even when the red cell abnormalities have been eliminated by factors in hospital diet or blood transfusions.

Ineffective Marrow Neutrophil Production without Prominent Morphologic Changes. A diverse and vaguely defined group of patients with neutropenia, either isolated or in conjunction with other cytopenias, are considered to have "preleukemia." Several authors prefer the term "myelodysplasia," since only a minority of such patients, including those with refractory megaloblastic and sideroblastic anemias, will develop leukemia. The marrows of these patients are hypercellular and splenomegaly is rarely present. The percentage of blast forms on the marrow smear is slightly to moderately increased. If there are 5 to 20 per cent marrow blasts, the condition is called "refractory" anemia (or neutropenia) with excess of blasts. Sometimes subtle morphologic abnormalities are present, such as a reduced number of primary or secondary granules, or larger than normal primary granules. Hyposegmentation or hypersegmentation of the nucleus may be present.

Neutropenia Due to Decreased Neutrophil Survival. Unequivocal antineutrophil antibodies in association with decreased neutrophil survival in neutropenia have only recently been demonstrated. The passive transfer of maternal antineutrophil antibodies may cause temporary neonatal neutropenia. Acquired antineutrophil antibodies can occur at any age. Several reliable tests for antineutrophil antibodies have now been described.

Occasionally patients with slight or moderate splenomegaly from other causes have severe neutropenia. Several investigators have been able to demonstrate shortened neutrophil survival in these patients.

Neutropenia Due to Abnormal Neutrophil Pooling. Most patients with splenomegaly have sequestration of one or more cellular components of blood in the spleen. However, in the myeloproliferative disorders, extramedullary and medullary hematopoiesis may be balanced against the sequestration owing to splenic enlargement per se. Isotope dilution methods have been used to measure abnormal pooling, but these are no longer available or are unproved. The magnitude of pooling is proportional to spleen size. Splenomegaly and neutrophil pooling are major parts of the pathophysiology of Felty's syndrome (neutropenia, rheumatoid arthritis, and splenomegaly) as well as congestive splenomegaly in association with cirrhosis or other causes. The lung can also be a site of abnormal pooling in patients who have massive complement activation. Examples have been listed previously.

Neutropenia Due to Mixed Pathophysiology. Here, Felty's syndrome is a good example. These patients have been found to have varying degrees of all four of the major pathophysiologic mechanisms.

CLINICAL SYNDROMES INCLUDING NEUTROPENIA

Benign Idiopathic Neutropenia. This is probably a mixture of several disorders that apparently include a variety of pathophysiologic causes. Some patients have a non–sex-linked dominant familial pattern, whereas others have acquired isolated neutropenia. The spleen is usually of normal size. Despite profound neutropenia, there is little risk of infection. Pathophysiologic studies have shown some patients to have shortened neutrophil survival while others have bone marrow production defects.

Felty's Syndrome. A small percentage ($<$ 5 per cent) of patients with rheumatoid arthritis develop neutropenia, which can be moderate to severe. Most of these patients also have splenomegaly, as Felty originally described, but characteristic features may be found in patients who have a normal-sized spleen. The pathophysiology of the neutropenia in these patients is different from one patient to another. Many of them have increased destruction and/or pooling of neutrophils in the enlarged spleen, as shown by pathophysiologic studies and also suggested by the dramatic resolution of neutropenia following splenectomy in many patients. But many patients have decreased marrow production of neutrophils as a partial or total cause of the neutropenia. This presumably is the reason why some patients do not respond to splenectomy but may even be harmed by the procedure. Such patients may die of overwhelming infections in the postoperative period. The marrow failure may be caused by an immunologic reaction: A few patients have been shown by *in vitro* studies to have suppressor T lymphocyte-mediated suppression of marrow neutrophil precursors. One of these patients responded to the administration of prednisone; another responded to splenectomy, which eliminated the suppressor cell activity. Thus, splenectomy could have beneficial effects in addition to the removal of a major site of neutrophil pooling and/or destruction. Unfortunately, there is no good way of predicting in advance which patients with Felty's syndrome may be helped or harmed by splenectomy.

Several investigators have found that patients with Felty's syndrome may have large quantities of IgG on the cell surface, but it is not at all clear whether this represents antibodies directed against neutrophil antigens. Since patients with Felty's syndrome usually have large amounts of intermediate-sized (9 to 15S) immune complexes in circulation, the normal function of neutrophils would cause them to adhere to and phagocytize these complexes due to their activation of serum complement. Indeed, these immune complexes have been demonstrated inside the neutrophils as well as on the surface. It is likely that such stuffing of neutrophils with the immune complexes may interfere with their flexibility, reducing their ability both to get out of the marrow (this pathophysiologic variant has been described) and to get through the spleen. This stuffing may also reduce neutrophil function in other ways, contributing to the well-known tendency for patients with Felty's syndrome to have severe or fatal infections. There is an extraordinarily voluminous literature on the numerous and variable pathophysiologic abnormalities in Felty's syndrome and no agreement on the indications for splenectomy.

Diagnosis of Felty's syndrome is usually simple, since the classic triad is usually present. Diagnostic problems may arise in patients who do not have prominent arthritis. Usually such patients have a high titer of circulating rheumatoid factor of one type or another.

Because of the controversy regarding diagnostic indications for splenectomy in Felty's syndrome, it is hazardous to make suggestions regarding this. Nevertheless, it is our experience that the spleen size and bone marrow picture are helpful in this regard. Patients whose spleens are very large (i.e., more than 5 cm below the costal margin during quiet breathing) are more likely to benefit from splenectomy in our experience. If the bone marrow were hypoplastic with very few neutrophilic precursors and the spleen were only slightly enlarged, we would suggest a diagnosis of decreased marrow neutrophil production. In the latter situation, marrow stimulation with lithium carbonate or treatment with prednisone may be more rational.

Autoimmune Neutropenia. Several syndromes have recently been described in this category. Infants may have an isoimmune neonatal neutropenia caused by maternal antibodies against their neutrophil antigens crossing the placenta. This resolves in 5 to 12 weeks and is not usually associated with severe infections. Should such an infection occur, plasma exchange to eliminate the maternal antibody would be indicated. In contrast, other infants are born without neutropenia but develop this during the first few months of life. These have an autoimmune neutropenia that can be demonstrated in the patient's serum by several methods including neutrophil agglutination, opsonization of test cells, immunofluorescence, and cytotoxicity. These infants have diarrhea and fever from various infections. They have been treated successfully by usual methods for autoimmune diseases.

Adults have been described having severe neutropenia, splenomegaly, and infections related to neoplastic proliferations of Tγ lymphocytes, but the exact description of the Tγ lymphocytes has varied from paper to paper ("helper," "killer," "suppressor"). Antineutrophil antibodies were usually found when they were sought. The nature of the lymphoproliferative disorder has not been clarified, but usually lymphocytosis has been present. A diagnosis of chronic lymphocytic leukemia was sometimes made. Hepatic lymphocytic infiltration, especially in the sinusoids, was often present. The patients almost never had lymphadenopathy.

A severely neutropenic patient with Hodgkin's disease was shown to have serum antineutrophil antibody activity. His neutropenia resolved with prednisone therapy. Perhaps this case was related to the lymphoproliferative syndrome described in the previous paragraph, since there are well known T lymphocyte functional abnormalities in Hodgkin's disease. Autoimmune neutropenia, shown by presence of serum antineutrophil antibodies, has been found also in patients with autoimmune hemolytic anemia, immune thrombocytopenic purpura, collagen vascular diseases, and angioimmunoblastic lymphadenopathy.

Since reliable tests for antineutrophil antibodies have been developed only recently and there are an increasing number of case reports of patients with these syndromes, it is likely that they are far more common than previously appreciated. The virtue of appreciating that neutrophil antibodies are present is that the neutrophil count and predisposition to infection of many such patients can be improved by corticosteroid therapy.

Neutropenia in the Alcoholic. Evidently, this is also a mixture of pathophysiologic abnormalities. Alcohol-related neutropenia, in most cases, is caused by decreased or ineffective marrow neutrophil production. Patients with cirrhosis may in addition have a shortened neutrophil survival and pooling within an enlarged spleen. Since alcohol reduces neutrophil stickiness, a combination of neutropenia and depressed neutrophil function may help account for the frequent severe infections in alcoholics. Folate deficiency and other aspects of malnutrition may also play a role in the neutropenia and infection problem in alcoholics.

Lazy Leukocyte Syndrome. This rare congenital syndrome illustrates that neutropenia can be produced by abnormal neutrophil function. The neutrophils of patients with the syndrome respond poorly to chemotactic factors. The bone marrow appears normally cellular and is without morphologic abnormalities. The neutropenia is caused by the apparent difficulty of marrow neutrophils getting into circulation owing to their lack of response to chemotactic and other factors associated with marrow neutrophil release. Thus, this disorder appears to be a type of ineffective neutrophil production.

Pancreatic Insufficiency with Neutropenia (Shwachman's Syndrome). This is a congenital disorder with exocrine pancreatic insufficiency, neutropenia, dwarfism, and occasionally metaphyseal dysostoses. These patients have frequent infections and may die in infancy or childhood. The bone marrow is hyperplastic. Some patients have had a serum factor that is cytotoxic for neutrophils. This disorder may be differentiated from fibrocystic disease by the lack of chronic pulmonary disease.

Neutropenia with Hypoglobulinemia. This is a congenital disorder of which approximately half the cases are familial. The bone marrow demonstrates abundant early neutrophil forms with little maturation beyond the myelocyte stage. Since these children have two defects in their host resistance to infection, bacterial infections are frequent and severe. At times during bacterial infections, neutrophilia may be noted rather than neutropenia. The pathophysiology of this disorder is obscure.

Cyclic Neutropenia. This disorder, which occurs in both adults and children and is sometimes familial, is characterized by periods of profound neutropenia, accompanied by mouth, skin or anogenital ulcerations, fever, and prostration, lasting for several days. Between episodes the neutrophil count recovers toward normal and the fever, ulcers, and other symptoms disappear. The period from cycle to cycle typically is approximately 3 weeks; this has theoretical importance, since it is approximately twice the time it takes for a neutrophil to mature from its earliest marrow precursor. This means that the disorder is a periodic failure of the marrow, lasting until the profound neutropenia stimulates the marrow to produce more neutrophils. Cyclic neutropenia may be an exaggeration of a normal cycling pattern that usually is well damped by the presence of a large reserve pool of mature marrow neutrophils. Why the ulcers, fever, and symptoms occur is not understood, but ulcers are common in other neutropenic disorders. Recognition of the periodicity is important in making the diagnosis because infection is rarely present and antibiotics do not help. Sometimes the condition goes away spontaneously. A similar disease in grey collie dogs has been cured by bone marrow transplantation.

PRESENTING SIGNS AND SYMPTOMS

Patients with agranulocytosis commonly present with a sore throat, chills, fever, weakness, and shortness of breath. Dyspnea and hypoxia without signs of congestive heart failure usually mean that pneumonia is present even if the chest roentgenogram is negative. The patient may have painful areas in the skin and mouth that may or may not be ulcerated. In contrast, many patients with chronic neutropenia have no symptoms and are discovered accidentally by routine blood counts.

COURSE

Acute agranulocytosis due to drug or chemical toxicity generally has a good prognosis and a short period of disability if the patient's infections can be controlled with antibiotics and the offending drug or chemical removed so that recovery can occur. The benign clinical course of most patients who are treated with anticancer marrow suppressive drugs demonstrates that transient neutropenia, even if severe, may not be associated with infections. Severe neutropenia (neutrophil count below 500 per cu mm), if present for several days, creates an increasing risk of infection. If infection occurs, the patient can die in shock in as short a time as 1 or 2 hours. The patients may recover uneventfully if antibiotics are given promptly and the neutrophil count returns to a normal level.

The course and outcome of chronic neutropenia due to other causes is dependent upon the nature of the associated disease and the pathophysiologic mechanism for the neutropenia.

PHYSICAL FINDINGS

The most specific physical findings concern the evidence of bacterial infections without signs of pus formation. As examples, skin infections may appear to be cellulitis, pneumonia may occur without early radiographic infiltrates, and urinary infections may not be associated with pyuria. Patients may develop multiple areas of cellulitis over the skin from which organisms may be cultured even though no pus is present. Patients who have *Pseudomonas aeruginosa* infections may develop a cellulitis with a central necrotic area (ecthyma gangrenosum). Such findings are characteristic of *Pseudomonas* infections in the setting of neutropenia, but rarely may be seen with *Staphylococcus* infections. Buccal and throat ulcerations are very common.

Other physical findings depend on the underlying associated disorder. For example, patients with physical evidence of rheumatoid arthritis who have splenomegaly probably will also have neutropenia (Felty's syndrome). Patients with enlarged spleens, as previously mentioned, have a strong tendency to pool neutrophils within the spleen and develop neutropenia if they do not have a myeloproliferative disease. The cause of splenomegaly may be elucidated by finding evidence of cirrhosis such as spider angiomas, palmar erythema, gynecomastia, testicular atrophy, and parotid enlargement, suggesting cirrhosis with alcoholism. The physician should be particularly sensitive to evidence of decreased vibration and joint position sense, a smooth tongue, and other signs suggestive of pernicious anemia. A skin rash may be found in some patients with hypersensitivity reactions to drugs. Free hemoglobin in the urine may suggest the presence of paroxysmal nocturnal hemoglobinuria, a rare condition that occasionally is associated with neutropenia.

LABORATORY STUDIES

Peripheral Blood. A number of clues regarding the underlying disorder may be found in the peripheral blood film. Hypersegmented polys and oval macrocytes may suggest that ineffective marrow production (megaloblastosis) is present. Patients who have shortened neutrophil survival with no marrow production problems are likely to have increased numbers of bands in proportion to the number of polys. Metamyelocytes may also be found occasionally in this setting, but the presence of large numbers of metamyelocytes, myelocytes, and more immature forms—especially with nucleated or teardrop red cells—suggests that the patient has myelofibrosis or tumor in the marrow. Many patients with neutropenia have an increased number of monocytes; this condition does not seem to be associated with an increased risk of infection. The presence of increased numbers of monocytes may also indicate that the bone marrow is beginning to recover from prior suppression. Patients with cyclic neutropenia may have an increased number of monocytes during the extremely neutropenic phase. These effects are probably due to the fact that it takes less time to mature from a promyelocyte to a monocyte than from a promyelocyte to a poly. The presence of neutropenia, other cytopenias, and a few circulating blast forms may indicate that the patient has acute leukemia.

Bone Marrow. As mentioned previously, a careful examination of the bone marrow is the most important means of detecting the pathophysiologic and occasionally the etiologic cause of the neutropenia. Lack of marrow neutrophil production may be immediately obvious. The so-called "maturation-arrest" picture can be misleading, however. Some patients' cells do not mature beyond the promyelocyte or early myelocyte stage, and these would appear to be examples of a true maturation arrest. However, neutropenic patients will be frequently found to have abundant neutrophil precursors except for the mature polys. These patients usually have shortened neutrophil survival or abnormal pooling in circulation or both, and the deficiency of polys reflects the premature extraction of these cells from the marrow in conjunction with their peripheral disappearance. On the other hand, the contrast between peripheral neutropenia and abundant polys in the marrow suggests a marrow releasing defect (ineffective marrow production).

Bone marrow biopsy from the iliac crest, the greater trochanter of the femur, or the posterior spine of a vertebra is most important for evaluation of the overall and neutrophilic cellularity. Tumor infiltrations of the marrow are most readily diagnosed by this technique. Large marrow biopsies may disclose variations in cellularity from place to place within the bone marrow and help avoid sampling error.

Other Diagnostic Procedures. Measurement of neutrophil survival with diisopropylfluorophosphate ($DF^{32}P$)-labeled neutrophils has been done in research centers in the past. This drug is no longer available in the United States. Radioactive chromium (^{51}Cr) has been proposed as a substitute, but this chemical labels monocytes and lymphocytes to a greater degree than neutrophils, making its effectiveness in neutropenic patients questionable. A procedure has been described (the "coil test") in which a neutropenic patient is phlebotomized of approximately 400 ml of blood with heparin anticoagulation. The blood is then placed in a hemodialysis coil for 15 minutes, which activates some of the complement in this blood. The activated blood is then returned to the patient. The procedure produces a 5-minute neutropenia followed by an overshoot neutrophilia. The magnitude of neutrophilia is a measure of marrow neutrophil reserves, while the rate of fall-off from the peak neutrophil count to the original baseline value is a measure of the neutrophil survival. The disadvantages of the procedure include the inability to measure neutrophil survival if the bone marrow does not put out enough cells to cause the overshoot neutrophilia and the lack of availability of the test except in a few centers. However, this test can be valuable in discovering the pathophysiologic cause of chronic neutropenia, especially in patients with Felty's syndrome and other patients who present the problem of distinguishing between ineffective neutrophil production and shortened neutrophil life span (previously mentioned as one of the major problems in interpretation of the bone marrow).

References have been made in several published articles to attempts to correlate levels of serum lysozyme and vitamin B_{12}-binding proteins with the neutrophil pathophysiology in neutropenic patients. The experience of most workers is that these tests are not helpful.

Fortunately, many patients have a transient neutropenia and do not require a pathophysiologic workup. In other patients a careful examination of bone marrow gives sufficient evidence of the underlying pathophysiologic abnormality so that no further special tests are needed. Patients in whom more specialized tests are needed are those with Felty's syndrome, chronic idiopathic neutropenia, and patients with splenomegaly who are taking bone marrow suppressive drugs, a relatively common circumstance in patients with renal transplants or lymphomas involving the spleen and marrow.

Antineutrophil antibodies can be determined by several techniques. Frozen serum may be sent to investigators at several locations within the United States for this type of test.

Intravenous injection of small amounts of epinephrine with serial counts of the circulating white cells has been proposed as a procedure for measuring the marginated neutrophil pool. However, this test has not been adequately correlated with the isotope dilution method of determining the marginated neutrophil pool, and some investigators do not consider it reliable. It is rarely used because of this lack of substantiation.

Other tests that may be useful in the diagnosis of the underlying disorder associated with the neutropenia include serum B_{12}, folate, protein electrophoresis, rheumatoid factor, hepatitis-associated antigens, liver-spleen scans, and tests for neutrophil function. A list of diagnostic tests needed for neutropenic patients depends upon the suspected underlying disorders.

LEUKOCYTOSIS AND LEUKEMOID REACTIONS

By Nancy L. Dunn, M.D.
Richmond, Virginia

DEFINITIONS

Leukocytosis may be defined as an increase in the absolute number of circulating leukocytes or white blood cells. The usual upper limit of normal for the total leukocyte count is 10,000 per cu mm, although it may normally be somewhat higher during early childhood. The term leukocytosis is broad and offers no specific clues as to the predominant cell type involved or the degree of cell maturity. The terms *granulocytosis* and *neutrophilia* are often used interchangeably, but the former more correctly refers to increased peripheral blood concentrations of any of the granule-containing white blood cells, including neutrophils, eosinophils, basophils, or monocytes. To be most precise, the terms *neutrophilia, eosinophilia, basophilia, monocytosis,* or *lymphocytosis* should be used to imply increases in the absolute numbers of the individual circulating white cell types.

The term *leukemoid reaction* is used to connote a reactive outpouring of leukocytes which includes immature forms. Often, the total white cell count is in excess of 50,000 per cu mm. This situation may closely resemble leukemia and must be carefully distinguished from it. Once again, one should specify which white blood cell line is involved by referring to neutrophilic leukemoid reactions, eosinophilic leukemoid reactions, and so on.

All of the leukopathic states mentioned may be further subdivided into acute and chronic reactions.

PATHOGENESIS

Leukocyte kinetic studies utilizing radioactive labels have added much to our understanding of the pathophysiology of neutrophilic granulocytosis and leukemoid reactions. Much less is known concerning situations involving other white cell lines, but the mechanisms may well be similar.

Acute granulocytosis is generally caused by a sudden, single stimulus that may be physical or emotional, or it may be caused by a wide variety of drugs, hormones, or toxic agents. In these situations, there is a rapid egress of leukocytes from the marginated peripheral blood pool and/or the bone marrow storage pool. The neutrophil is the main cell type that increases in the majority of these reactions, but certain specific stimuli may preferentially cause an increase of another white cell line. These acute reactions generally last only a few hours.

When the stimulus for the granulocytosis persists, a more chronic reaction, with a somewhat different pathogenesis, develops. The mechanisms involved in these situations may include increased granulocytic proliferation in the marrow with resultant myeloid hyperplasia and delivery of more immature cells to the circulation (i.e., a "left shift"), prolonged granulocyte survival, continued depletion of the marrow storage pools, or a combination of any of these. It is speculated that negative feedback loops regulate the rate of granulopoiesis via some as yet unknown humoral or cellular factors. In these chronic reactions, even more so than in the acute ones, the predominant cell type is dependent on the underlying stimulus.

ETIOLOGIES

Neutrophilic granulocytosis (usually defined as an absolute neutrophil count greater than 8000 per cu mm) may result from a wide variety of causes. Physical or emotional stimuli such as cold, heat, exercise, fear, or panic reactions may elevate the neutrophil count, as may certain pharmacologic agents such as epinephrine, heparin, endotoxin, histamine, corticosteroids, or heavy metals. Infectious etiologies may include bacterial, mycotic, spirochetal, viral, rickettsial, or parasitic disease. Prolonged infection is in many cases also associated with a monocytic and sometimes an eosinophilic reaction. Immature neutrophilic forms may be seen in the more severe infections, such as with disseminated tuberculosis. Neutrophilia is also seen in inflammatory conditions. Neutrophilic leukemoid reactions have long been noted to occur in association with both lymphoproliferative neoplasms and carcinomas, particularly of gastric, bronchogenic, or pancreatic origin. Other causes of leukemoid reactions include metabolic disorders such as thyroid storm, hepatic necrosis, diabetic ketoacidosis, gout, eclampsia, and azotemia. Neutrophilia may also accompany various hematologic disorders such as chronic hemolytic anemias, hemorrhage, transfusion reactions, infectious mononucleosis, postsplenectomy, and myeloproliferative diseases.

Eosinophilic granulocytosis (absolute eosinophil count > 450 per cu mm) may also have a wide variety of etiologies, although most can be categorized as parasitic infections, allergic phenomena, or dermatologic conditions. On a worldwide basis, parasitic infection is probably the most common cause of an increased eosinophil count. It is not the presence of the parasites themselves that elicits the eosinophilia, but rather the tissue granulomatous reaction that occurs when the parasites attach to mucosal surfaces or invade body tissues. Therefore, eosinophilia is more common in helminthic than in protozoal infections, and more common in the more invasive of the helminths. Visceral larva migrans, caused by *Toxocara canis* and *cati,* common dog and cat roundworms (Ascaris), is the most common parasitic cause of eosinophilia in children. Almost all affected children have at least 50 per cent eosinophils, and differential counts of 80 to 90 per cent eosinophils with total white cell counts of 100,000 per cu mm are not uncommon. Most chronic allergic disorders are associated with a mild, persistent eosinophilia. More marked degrees of eosinophilia may be seen in drug reactions and many dermatologic disorders. The eosinophilic leukemoid reactions seen in a group of disorders termed idiopathic hypereosinophilic syndromes may be difficult to distinguish from eosinophilic leukemia. Other causes of eosinophilia include gastrointestinal disorders, malignancies such as Hodgkin's disease, and immune deficiency diseases.

Basophils are the least numerous of the circulating granulocytes, and therefore obtaining an accurate absolute basophil count is difficult unless a direct counting histochemical technique is utilized. Basophilia is common in myeloproliferative disorders, especially chronic myelocytic leukemia (see the article on this topic). Increasing numbers of basophils may actually herald a blast crisis. Basophilia may also be seen in ulcerative colitis, myxedema, and various allergic disorders.

Monocytosis is generally defined as an absolute monocyte count exceeding 750 per cu mm in children or 500 per cu mm in adults. In approximately one half of patients with monocytosis there is an associated underlying hematologic disorder such as leukemia, lymphoma, myeloproliferative syndrome, or neutropenia. Other causes include collagen vascular diseases, nonhematologic forms of malignancy, infections such as tuberculosis or subacute bacterial endocarditis, and chronic inflammatory bowel disease.

Lymphocytosis may occur on either a relative basis (when neutrophil counts are depressed), or on an absolute basis (defined as an absolute lymphocyte count > 9000 per cu mm in infants, > 7200 per cu mm in older children, and > 4000 per cu mm in adults). When evaluating a patient with lymphocytosis, particular attention must be paid not only to the numbers and percentages of lymphocytes but also to their morphologic features, since this may provide important etiologic clues. A relative lymphocytosis is normally seen in early childhood between 4 months and 4 years of age. Marked absolute lymphocytosis can be seen in certain acute infections such as pertussis, infectious mononucleosis, and acute infectious lymphocytosis. Acute infections with moderate relative lymphocytosis include the common childhood exanthems and other viral illnesses, brucellosis, and typhoid and paratyphoid fevers. Chronic infections, drug and allergic reactions, leukemia, thyrotoxicosis, and Addison's disease may also be associated with lymphocytosis.

CLINICAL PRESENTATION

The clinical presentation of patients with leukocytosis or leukemoid reactions may be as varied as the underlying diseases causing these hematologic aberrations. A careful, detailed history and inquiry into the presenting symptoms may provide valuable clues as to the most likely diagnostic possibilities. Similarly, a thorough physical examination, looking in particular for signs of infection or underlying malignant disorders, is also likely to provide important diagnostic clues.

LABORATORY EVALUATION

The laboratory evaluation of these patients should be individually tailored based on the examiner's perception of what the underlying problem may be.

Certainly, every patient should have a complete blood count, including red cell indices, and platelet and reticulocyte counts to determine whether any other hematopoietic cell lines are involved. Examination of a peripheral blood smear is essential, not only to obtain a differential count but also to assess the degree of maturity and/or atypia of the leukocytes; to look for additional signs of infection such as the presence of toxic granulation or Döhle bodies in the leukocytes; and to assess red cell morphology.

Examination of a bone marrow aspirate/biopsy is necessary when malignancy is suspected or cannot be ruled out. Bone marrow smears may also be of diagnostic aid in the work-up of granulomatous or myelophthisic disorders. The marrow itself may be cultured in addition to more routine culture sources in the search for infectious etiologies.

One of the more difficult differential diagnoses to make is distinguishing chronic myelocytic leukemia (CML) from a neutrophilic leukemoid reaction. The peripheral blood and bone marrow may be quite similar in appearance. Two other laboratory modalities may be extremely helpful in this situation. Chronic myelocytic leukemia is characterized by a very low leukocyte alkaline phosphatase (LAP) score and the very frequent (85 per cent) presence of the Philadelphia (Ph^1) chromosome.

In patients with eosinophilia, laboratory evaluation should focus on the search for parasitic infestation or allergic disorders. The presence of immature eosinophilic forms and normoblastemia on peripheral blood smear would point toward a diagnosis of eosinophilic leukemia.

The most important diseases to consider in the patient with basophilia are the myeloproliferative disorders, especially CML. Therefore, these patients would require a bone marrow examination, LAP score, and a karyotype.

When monocytosis is present, the work-up should focus on a search for an underlying hematologic disorder, subacute bacterial endocarditis, or a tuberculous or a chronic inflammatory disorder.

Similarly, the laboratory evaluation of a patient with lymphocytosis will mirror the differential diagnosis of this hematologic manifestation. Some refinement in this laboratory work-up can be achieved by noting the degree of lymphocytosis and the morphologic features of the lymphocytes on the peripheral smear. Extreme degrees of lymphocytosis with essentially normal morphology are seen in pertussis and infectious lymphocytosis. The appearance of greater than 10 to 15 per cent "atypical" lymphocytes is suggestive of a viral infection, such as infectious mononucleosis. A specific diagnosis can often be made with appropriate serologic studies. A predominance of lymphoblasts is usually seen in acute lymphoblastic leukemia, while chronic lymphocytic leukemia is generally characterized by more mature-appearing forms. Bone marrow aspirates, cytochemical stains, and immunologic cell surface marker analysis are important diagnostic laboratory tools in these latter entities.

PITFALLS IN DIAGNOSIS

When evaluating a child with leukocytosis, one must keep in mind age-related normal differences both in the total leukocyte count and in the absolute numbers of the various white blood cell lines. In addition, some episodes of leukocytosis appear to be benign and self-limited. This observation should be remembered when evaluating a well-appearing patient. Close follow-up with serial repeat blood counts may obviate the need for an extensive, costly, and emotionally trying workup.

One final potential pitfall in the diagnosis of these disorders is the prevalent tendency to equate a leukemoid reaction with a diagnosis of leukemia. These two disorders are not synonymous, and patients presenting with the former should have a thorough diagnostic work-up in order to rule out other causes of leukemoid reactions.

ACUTE LEUKEMIA

By Marcel E. Conrad, M.D.
Mobile, Alabama

Human leukemia has been classified with reference to the usual duration of survival and the suspected cell of origin. Thus, the leukemia may be either acute or chronic and either lymphocytic or myelogenous (nonlymphocytic). Paradoxically, newer advances in treatment have made survival in many patients with acute lymphoblastic leukemia and an increasing number of patients with acute myeloblastic leukemia exceed that of the chronic forms of leukemia. Establishing the appropriate diagnostic category for each patient is important because the choice of therapeutic drugs is different for each type of leukemia. The chronic leukemias can usually be distinguished rapidly by morphologic examination of the blood and bone marrow. Most patients have excessive numbers of either mature lymphocytes or maturing granulocytes in their peripheral blood. However, chronic myelogenous leukemia may initially present with blastic transformation and resemble either acute myelogenous or acute lymphoblastic leukemia, and the diagnosis cannot be established without demonstrating the presence of the Philadelphia chromosome (Ph^1). The use of morphologic means alone to distinguish acute lymphoblastic leukemias from acute myelogenous leukemias will result in a significant percentage of incorrect diagnoses. Special histochemical stains are helpful, and newer immunologic techniques promise to permit unequivocal distinction in the near future.

PRELEUKEMIA

Acute leukemia may be preceded by hematologic abnormalities for months or years before a definitive diagnosis can be established. It usually progresses to acute myeloblastic leukemia, but there are occasional reports of acute lymphoblastic leukemia. Preleukemia occurs mostly in older males and is usually manifested by a mild to moderate macrocytic anemia with or without granulocytopenia or thrombocytopenia. The anemia is unresponsive to therapy with vitamin B_{12} or folic acid and may require periodic transfusion. The peripheral smear may show hypogranular neutrophils, ovalocytes, pseudo-Pelger-Huët anomaly, large platelets, and nucleated red blood cells. Hepatomegaly and lymphadenopathy are uncommon, but the splenic tip is palpable in about a third of patients. The bone marrow is usually hypercellular with megaloblastoid features. Ringed sideroblasts may be observed. Chromosomal abnormalities are observed in specimens from about half of preleukemic patients.

ACUTE LEUKEMIA

While there are significant differences in the prevalence of presenting symptoms, signs, and laboratory findings in groups of patients with acute myelogenous versus lymphoblastic leukemia, there are few that are helpful in determining the type of acute leukemia in an individual patient. Although 90 per cent of patients with acute leukemia are under 10 years of age and only 10 per cent of patients over 50 years of age have acute lymphoblastic leukemia, age alone is an unreliable criterion in arriving at the specific diagnosis.

The majority of patients with acute leukemia complain of fatigue or malaise at the time of diagnosis. Fever with or without infection is present in 75 per cent of patients. Bleeding, purpura, weight loss, and bone pain are present in many patients when they are first seen. Exquisite tenderness on pressure over the lower sternum is a useful sign in patients with suspected acute leukemia and is seen in two thirds of them. Moderate but not massive hepatomegaly, splenomegaly, and lymphadenopathy are commonplace in the acute leukemias. The presence of massive lymphadenopathy or multiple large lymph nodes in several anatomic locations is more common in lymphoblastic leukemia. Similarly, a mediastinal mass is rare in acute myelogenous leukemia but is observed in many children with acute lymphoblastic leukemia showing T cell markers.

Most patients with acute leukemia are anemic and thrombocytopenic. The white blood cell count may be normal, decreased, or increased. Blasts are usually seen in the peripheral blood but occasionally are difficult to find in patients with leukopenia. The bone marrow is usually hyperplastic and always shows an increased number of blasts plus progranulocytes. Caution should be exercised in establishing a diagnosis of leukemia in patients with a normocellular or hypocellular marrow because of an increased number of immature cells; this can be observed during recovery from aplasia, agranulocytosis or an aregenerative crisis.

A skilled morphologist can distinguish between acute lymphoblastic and myeloblastic leukemia in 80 to 90 per cent of specimens by light microscopy. Auer rods or Phi bodies can be demonstrated in specimens from half the patients with acute myeloblastic leukemia and are diagnostic of myeloid leukemia. In most patients with acute myeloblastic leukemia, some differentiation toward one of the myeloid cell lines can be detected. The presence of agranular neutrophils, Pelger-Huët anomaly, and megaloblastosis strongly suggests a myeloid leukemia. In erythroleukemia, promyelocytic leukemia, certain of the monocytic leukemias, and those rare instances in which basophilic or eosinophilic differentiation is obvious, morphologic observations permit the diagnosis of myeloid leukemia. Similarly, the morphologic appearance of the cytoplasm and nuclear chromatin permits the experienced morphologist to identify the majority of specimens with classical lymphoid differentiation features. Special stains have been developed to help in more difficult specimens. Sudan black and peroxidase stains detect the presence of lysosomes of granulocytes, and positivity suggests a myeloid leukemia. Specimens that show block positivity in the cytoplasm with periodic acid-Schiff (PAS) stain but no reaction to peroxidase, Sudan black or esterase stains are more likely to be from patients with acute lymphoblastic leukemia.

Table 1. Comparison of Acute Myeloblastic Leukemia and Acute Lymphoblastic Leukemia

	Acute Myeloblastic Leukemia	Acute Lymphoblastic Leukemia
Morphologic features	Auer rods Phi bodies Peroxidase-positive, azurophilic, eosinophilic, or basophilic granules Folded nuclear configuration Megaloblastic erythroblasts Abnormal platelets Low leukocyte alkaline phosphatase score Pseudo-Pelger-Huët anomaly Sudan black–positive	Irregularly clumped nuclear chromatin Clefted nuclei Peroxidase-negative azurophilic granules PAS-positive in block pattern
Surface markers	Detection of anti-AML antigen	E rosette-positive, anti T-Ab-positive Ab against ALL (CALLA) B1 antigen with monoclonal Ab_2 Positive for TdT
Cell growth in semisolid media	Abnormal or poor growth of CFU-C and BFU-E	Normal CFU-C and BFU-E colonies
Cytogenetics	Hypodiploidy	No unique karyotype
Therapy	Response to therapy with anthracyclines and cytosine arabinoside	Response to therapy with prednisone and vincristine

Abbreviations: AML = Acute myeloblastic leukemia; ALL = acute lymphoblastic leukemia; PAS = periodic acid–Schiff stain; TdT = terminal deoxynucleotidyl transferase; BFU-E and CFU-C = erythropoietic progenitor cells.

The enzyme terminal deoxynucleotidyl transferase (TdT) has been used to differentiate the acute leukemias. This enzyme in cells is present in 90 per cent of specimens from patients with acute lymphoblastic leukemia, a third of patients with blastic crisis of chronic myelogenous leukemia, and only 5 per cent of patients with acute myeloblastic leukemia. TdT may be used in combination with immunologic surface markers to permit differentiation of the majority of acute leukemias. During recent years, antibodies have been raised against specific cell surface markers that permit identification of the various categories of both acute myeloblastic and lymphoblastic leukemia. Once they become generally available, the diagnosis of each type of leukemia will probably be standardized. Table 1 compares the characteristics of these two types of leukemia.

ACUTE LYMPHOBLASTIC LEUKEMIA

Acute lymphoblastic leukemia is primarily a disease of childhood with a peak incidence in the first decade of life. The specific diagnosis is established by morphologic and immunologic observations. Therapy provides a confirmation of the diagnosis because it is highly responsive to drugs such as prednisone, vincristine, and asparginase, which are not highly cytotoxic for normal marrow cells and will have little beneficial effect in the treatment of acute myeloblastic leukemia. Indeed, prednisone by itself can accelerate acute myeloblastic leukemia by mobilizing myeloblasts from the marginal pool to produce hyperleukocytosis and cerebral hemorrhage, whereas it is lympholytic in the lymphocytic disorders.

There is developing evidence that acute lymphoblastic leukemia is not a single disease with uniform characteristics; rather there are subclasses that can be distinguished on the basis of the surface markers found on the lymphoblasts. Generally, this divides the patients into those with T or B lymphoblasts, or those with no surface markers (null cell leukemia). The latter appears to be most common and have a better prognosis. Patients with T cell leukemia are more likely to have a mediastinal mass and significant lymphadenopathy. Table 2 shows the French-American-British (FAB) classification of ALL.

ACUTE MYELOBLASTIC LEUKEMIA

The incidence of this disease is increased in humans who have been exposed to radiation, drugs producing aplastic anemia, alkylating agents, and benzene. Acute myeloblastic leukemia may be seen in patients

Table 2. Acute Lymphoblastic Leukemia (French-American-British Classification)

Type	Morphologic Characteristics	Immunologic Characteristics
L1	Small blasts with scanty cytoplasm	T, or non-B non-T (null)
L2	Large cells with variable amounts of cytoplasm	T, or non-B non-T (null)
L3	Large cells with stippled nuclear chromatin and prominent cytoplasmic vacuolation	B

Table 3. Acute Myeloblastic Leukemia (French-American-British Classification)

Type	Morphologic Characteristic Features
Myeloblastic leukemia without maturation (M1)	No or few azure granules and/or Auer rods
Myeloblastic leukemia with maturation (M2)	Maturation at or beyond promyelocyte stage
Hypergranular promyelocytic leukemia (M3)	Abnormal promyelocytes with folded nuclei and numerous Auer rods and azure granules
Myelomonocytic leukemia (M4)	Granulocytic and monocytic differentiation; abnormal monocytes exceed 20% of leukemic marrow cells
Monocytic leukemia (M5)	Monoblasts and promonocytes exceed 80% of leukemic marrow cells
Erythroleukemia (M6)	Abnormal red cell precursors exceed 50% of marrow cells

of all ages, but its incidence increases over the age of 50 years. Symptoms are usually related to the pancytopenia. Hepatosplenomegaly and lymphadenopathy are often present at the time of diagnosis but rarely are prominent features. The peripheral white blood cell count at presentation may be increased, decreased, or normal. However, when the number of blasts in the peripheral blood is excessive (> 100,000 blasts per cu mm), cerebral hemorrhage due to leukostasis is commonplace. This may be the initial manifestation of the disease and can be worsened by the administration of corticosteroids if they are employed without the simultaneous administration of cytotoxic drugs.

A number of subtypes of acute myeloblastic leukemia have been recognized. Their prevalence varies somewhat in different studies because a mixed picture is found in many patients. They have been designated M1 through M6 in the FAB Classification (Table 3). The myeloblastic variant (M1 and M2) includes more than half the patients in most studies. Approximately one third of this group are undifferentiated (M1), and included are patients who are difficult to distinguish from ALL on morphologic grounds alone. Other variants are discussed as follows.

Acute Promyelocytic Leukemia (M3). The predominant cell in the peripheral blood and bone marrow is the promyelocyte. The granules in the cytoplasm may be normal in appearance or abnormally large and oval. A specific chromosomal abnormality with translocation of a portion of chromosome 17 to 15 (15q+, 17q−) has been reported in about two thirds of patients. Disseminated intravascular coagulation is frequently present at the time of diagnosis. Hemorrhage is a prominent feature, and therapy with heparin, fresh frozen plasma and platelet transfusions is often required shortly after diagnosis.

Myelomonocytic Leukemia (M4) and Monocytic Leukemia (M5). The blasts in the blood usually appear more monocytic than those in the marrow. Cytoplasm is more abundant than in the myeloblastic variety and the nuclei of the cells are often folded. Granules may be present in the cytoplasm. The monoblasts usually stain intensely with nonspecific esterase, which is inhibited by fluoride. Intramedullary destruction of leukemic cells is common in these variants, producing increased quantities of muramidase in the blood and urine. Gingival hypertrophy and skin infiltration are more common clinical manifestations than in other forms of leukemia.

Erythroleukemia (M6). The blood and bone marrow may contain erythroid precursors at all stages of maturation and they usually show megaloblastic features, binucleation, nuclear fragmentation, and vacuolated cytoplasm. The clinical course of illness and response to therapy is similar to M1 and M2 variants.

Leukemic Reticuloendotheliosis (Hairy Cell Leukemia). This is a relatively uncommon disorder that is usually initially manifested by splenomegaly and pancytopenia. The peripheral smear shows lymphoid cells with a sky-blue cytoplasm and a nucleus resembling that in a mature lymphocyte. Fine hair-like projections are observed on the surface of the cell. Immunologically these cells may have characteristics of either T cells, B cells, monocyte-macrophages, or a combination of these. A unique feature of these cells is the presence of cytoplasmic acid phosphatase, which is resistant to inhibition by tartaric acid unlike acid phosphatase in normal lymphocytes. Bone marrow is difficult to obtain by aspiration (dry tap). Bone marrow biopsy specimens show increased reticulin fibers with or without frank myelofibrosis. The bone marrow is infiltrated with moderately large cells containing an abundant cytoplasm. Recognition of the disorder is important because it is more responsive to splenectomy than therapy with either corticosteroids or cytotoxic drugs.

POLYCYTHEMIA VERA

By Harry Iland, F.R.A.C.P., F.R.C.P.A.
and John Laszlo, M.D.
Durham, North Carolina

SYNONYMS

Polycythemia rubra vera, primary polycythemia, erythremia, splenomegalic polycythemia, Vaquez-Osler disease. The "spent" phase of the disease is also known as burned-out polycythemia or postpolycythemic myeloid metaplasia.

DEFINITIONS

Polycythemia vera (PV) is one of a group of myeloproliferative disorders (MPD) that are all primary abnormalities of the pluripotent bone marrow stem cell. These disorders are characterized by hyperplasia of the hemopoietic elements (erythrocytic, granulocytic, and megakaryocytic) together with varying degrees of extramedullary hemopoiesis (myeloid metaplasia) occurring predominantly, but not exclusively, in the spleen and reactive fibroblastic proliferation in the marrow. Specific clinicopathologic entities within the MPD are recognized when one cell line is involved to a greater extent than the others.

In the case of PV, there is hyperplasia of all marrow elements; however, the most notable abnormality from a clinical standpoint involves erythroid precursors with expansion of the total red blood cell mass. In the early stages of the disease, extramedullary hemopoiesis (EMH) is usually mild and marrow fibrosis is minimal or absent. A spent phase gradually supervenes in approximately 15 to 20 per cent of cases, characterized by a leukoerythroblastic reaction and teardrop poikilocytosis in the peripheral blood, progressive myelofibrosis (with or without osteosclerosis) and EMH, with increasingly ineffective hemopoiesis leading to anemia. This phase is difficult to distinguish from agnogenic myeloid metaplasia, which arises de novo (see the next article).

PRESENTING SYMPTOMS AND SIGNS

The clinical features, although largely nonspecific, are nevertheless directly attributable to the pathophysiologic processes present in PV. The onset is frequently insidious, and in some patients the disease may be detected as a result of the chance finding of an increased hematocrit (Hct) in an asymptomatic patient. Other patients, however, may present with one of the many complications to be discussed. More than three quarters of the patients are aged 45 to 75 years, with a median of approximately 60 years. The sex distribution shows a slight preponderance of males.

Increased proliferative activity of the bone marrow may be associated with a hypermetabolic state manifested by fatigue, weakness, fever, sweating (especially night sweats), and weight loss. A consequence of the accelerated turnover of hemopoietic cells is increased uric acid production, resulting in hyperuricemia and hyperuricosuria, with clinical acute gout in 5 to 10 per cent of patients. The levels of serum uric acid tend to be higher than those in primary gout.

Expansion of the red cell mass is accompanied by hyperviscosity. This in turn reduces blood flow in both the large vessels and the microcirculation, and largely negates the effect of the increased oxygen-carrying capacity associated with the expanded red cell mass. Sludging of blood flow in small vessels may be further aggravated by thrombocytosis and leukocytosis. The physiologic impact depends not only on the degree of hyperviscosity but also on other factors such as the ability of the blood vessels to accommodate the flow by increasing their diameter. Circulatory disturbances frequently involve the central nervous system, resulting in headache, dizziness, visual disturbances (blurred vision, diplopia, scotomata) and tinnitus. Similar effects in the peripheral and visceral circulation cause erythromelalgia (painful, red extremities), paresthesias and burning sensations, myocardial ischemia (angina, infarction), mesenteric ischemia, intermittent claudication, and thromboembolic phenomena.

Thrombocytosis is commonly present, and platelet function abnormalities have been described. These act together with the hyperviscosity and are in part responsible for the frequent occurrence of both thrombosis and hemorrhage seen in PV. Although epistaxis, cutaneous bleeding, and oral bleeding are the commonest manifestations of the hemorrhagic diathesis, serious and life-threatening hemorrhage may also occur; this is usually related to gastrointestinal bleeding from a peptic ulcer, or it may be associated with surgery or trauma.

Splenomegaly may cause gastrointestinal symptoms of early satiety, abdominal fullness, and left upper quadrant pain. The increased incidence of peptic ulcer seen in PV may be related to increased histamine production by granulocytes (especially basophils). Disturbances in histamine metabolism also appear to be responsible for the pruritus (occurring particularly after a warm bath or shower) experienced by almost half the patients, as well as the less frequent urticaria.

In PV the most significant finding on physical examination is splenomegaly, which is present in about 70 per cent of patients at initial presentation. The etiology of the splenic enlargement is multifactorial and includes EMH, proliferation of the splenic reticulum, and pooling of red cells. Hepatomegaly is less common, but the mechanisms involved are analogous to those in the spleen. Other findings are hypertension, plethoric facies with congestion of the conjunctivae and nasopharyngeal mucosa, retinal venous distention, and peripheral vasodilatation. These features result from the increased blood volume, which in turn is due to the expanded red cell mass and, in

Supported in part by Public Health Service Grant CA-10728 from the National Cancer Institute, Department of Health and Human Services. Dr. Iland is the recipient of a New South Wales (Australia) State Cancer Council Fellowship and Travel Grant-in-Aid.

some patients, to an increased plasma volume. Peripheral cyanosis is occasionally present and can be ascribed to desaturation of hemoglobin (Hb) in red cells subject to stasis.

COMPLICATIONS AND PROGNOSIS

Modern therapeutic regimens involving vigorous management of erythroid production by phlebotomy and/or myelosuppression have resulted in significant increases in median survival, from 18 months to more than 10 years. The major complications limiting survival include thrombosis, hemorrhage, second malignancy (both leukemic and nonleukemic), and postpolycythemic myeloid metaplasia (PPMM). The relative frequencies of these complications are determined to some extent by the therapeutic approach adopted.

Thrombotic phenomena such as cerebrovascular accidents, myocardial infarctions, mesenteric ischemia, peripheral arterial occlusions, and venous thromboembolism constitute the leading causes of morbidity and mortality in PV, particularly among patients treated by phlebotomy alone. The Polycythemia Vera Study Group (PVSG), an international cooperative group dedicated to the study of PV, has demonstrated that the addition of large doses of platelet anti-aggregating agents (aspirin and dipyridamole) to treatment by phlebotomy does not reduce the risk of thrombosis and is associated with an increased incidence of hemorrhage. Thus myelosuppression, which controls the platelet abnormalities as well as the hyperviscosity, is often an essential part of the management of this aspect of PV.

Surgery poses a serious threat to the polycythemic patient because of the great risk of thrombohemorrhagic phenomena. It is essential that the disease be adequately controlled with myelosuppressive therapy before surgical intervention, especially if splenectomy is contemplated (e.g., during the spent phase) in order to prevent extreme thrombocytosis and the catastrophic consequences that may follow. Since up to 90 per cent of the platelet mass is pooled in a grossly enlarged spleen, splenectomy may result in a precipitous rise in the platelet count complicated by massive thrombosis or hemorrhage even in a patient without prior thrombocytosis.

In contrast, second malignancies appear to occur more commonly in myelosuppressed patients; in a randomized study of chlorambucil, ^{32}P, and phlebotomy conducted by the PVSG, a statistically significant excess of acute leukemia in patients treated with chlorambucil became evident after 3 years of therapy. Postpolycythemic acute leukemia is associated with an extremely poor prognosis. Like the blastic transformation of chronic granulocytic leukemia (CGL), complete remission is achieved much less commonly and survival is correspondingly shorter than in adult acute leukemia arising de novo.

Postpolycythemic myeloid metaplasia occurs in a significant proportion of patients. The median duration from diagnosis of PV to the onset of PPMM is approximately 10 years, although it has been suggested that virtually all patients will develop this complication if they survive long enough. Retrospective studies have suggested that ionizing radiation may be a significant factor in the development of PPMM, but there has been no prospective confirmation of this.

A diminishing requirement for phlebotomy or myelosuppression may be the earliest evidence of PPMM. As the process progresses, symptoms of anemia, angina, and cardiac decompensation occur most frequently. The etiology of the anemia is multifactorial and includes ineffective erythropoiesis related to myelofibrosis and EMH, dilutional anemia associated with increasing splenomegaly, and in some patients iron deficiency secondary to gastrointestinal blood loss.

Progressive splenomegaly is an important feature of this phase of the disease, and the patient may present with an "acute abdomen" due to splenic infarction. The other symptoms of splenic enlargement listed earlier also become more prominent. Marked thrombocytosis or thrombocytopenia may develop, exacerbating the bleeding tendency. It is not clear whether platelet function abnormalities are more significant in this phase of the disease than at presentation.

Other features of PPMM include leukoerythroblastosis (circulating myeloid and erythroid precursors), progressive leukocytosis or leukocytopenia, red cell morphologic abnormalities (especially teardrop poikilocytosis), and increasing hepatomegaly. Portal hypertension and ascites are also being increasingly recognized. Shunting of a significant proportion of the cardiac output through the splenic and portal veins as a result of marked splenomegaly, with or without portal or hepatic venous obstruction, is thought to be the basis of this disabling complication. Clearly the shunting of blood acts in concert with the anemia and myocardial ischemia and can precipitate or exacerbate congestive cardiac failure.

Venesection of patients with PV to normal levels of Hb is commonly accompanied by iron deficiency. It is not clear whether the iron deficiency produces significant symptoms in the absence of anemia, though it is a further argument in support of myelosuppression in the long-term management of PV. Symptoms that have been attributed to the iron deficiency include lassitude, irritability, headache, anorexia, glossitis, angular stomatitis, and dysphagia. If these become too troublesome, consideration must be given to the addition of myelosuppressive agents so that iron replacement therapy can be safely administered without precipitating overt polycythemia.

DIFFERENTIAL DIAGNOSIS

Table 1 lists the differential diagnosis of erythrocytosis. Although certain laboratory techniques are helpful in establishing a diagnosis of PV, it is essential that the clinician be aware of the other conditions that are associated with an elevated Hct or Hb. Many of these conditions can be excluded by clinical history and physical examination, whereas others require definitive laboratory investigation.

Table 1. Classification of Erythrocytosis

Polycythemia Vera
Secondary Polycythemia
- Physiologically appropriate increase in erythropoietin
  - High altitude
  - Intrathoracic shunt (right to left)
    - Cyanotic congenital heart disease
    - Cirrhosis
    - Hereditary hemorrhagic telangiectasia
    - Other pulmonary arterio-venous malformations
  - Chronic respiratory disease
  - Alveolar hypoventilation (obesity/somnolence syndrome, Pickwickian syndrome)
  - Defective oxygen transport
    - Smoking (carbon monoxide)
    - High oxygen affinity hemoglobinopathy
    - Congenital reduction in red cell 2,3-DPG
  - Defective oxidative metabolism (cobalt therapy)
- Physiologically inappropriate increase in erythropoietin
  - Renal disorders
    - Renal artery stenosis
    - Renal transplant rejection
    - Cysts
    - Hydronephrosis
    - Renal tumors
  - Endocrine disorders
    - Pheochromocytoma
    - Conn's syndrome
    - Cushing's syndrome
    - Androgen-secreting ovarian tumors
  - Other tumors
    - Uterine fibroids
    - Cerebellar hemangioblastoma
    - Hepatoma
- Hereditary autonomous overproduction of erythropoietin

Relative Polycythemia
- Stress polycythemia (pseudopolycythemia, Gaisböck's syndrome)
- Dehydration

Polycythemia vera complicated by iron deficiency secondary to blood loss must also be distinguished from related MPDs such as essential thrombocythemia (ET). This requires a trial of iron therapy to determine whether the red cell mass or Hb rises to polycythemic levels following correction of the iron deficiency.

DIAGNOSTIC PROCEDURES

Suspicion of PV may be aroused by the presence of the clinical features described above. Additionally, the finding of either an elevated Hct (> 54 per cent in males, > 47 per cent in menstruating females) or Hb (> 18 gm/dl in males, > 16 gm/dl in females), or even a normal Hct or Hb associated with evidence of iron deficiency (hypochromia, microcytosis, and polychromasia) should prompt the physician to consider the possibility of PV. When attempting to determine the cause of erythrocytosis, the clinician will find it helpful to direct the investigations at three questions.

1. *Is the erythrocytosis absolute or relative?* The first step is to measure total red blood cell mass, utilizing the patient's chromium-labeled (^{51}Cr) red cells (normally < 36 ml/kg in males and < 32 ml/kg in females). This procedure should be combined with direct measurement of the plasma volume using ^{125}I-labeled albumin. In this way it is possible to exclude relative polycythemia (stress polycythemia, pseudopolycythemia, Gaisböck's syndrome), which is characterized by either a normal red cell mass and reduced plasma volume or a high-normal red cell mass and low-normal plasma volume. This is an important distinction, since stress polycythemia is probably the most common cause of a chronically elevated Hct and treatment with myelosuppression is inappropriate.

2. *Is there any evidence in favor of polycythemia vera?* If an elevated red cell mass is confirmed, a distinction must then be made between polycythemia vera and the many causes of secondary polycythemia. The blood count is often helpful since many features of MPD may be present, although none is diagnostic of PV per se. They include leukocytosis (> 12,000 per cu mm but usually < 25,000 per cu mm) due predominantly to neutrophilia with or without basophilia, eosinophilia, and occasional circulating myeloid precursors; and thrombocytosis (> 400,000 per cu mm and occasionally > 1,000,000 per cu mm) with or without morphologically abnormal forms. Red cell morphology is usually normal unless iron deficiency is present. The latter is characterized by microcytosis (mean corpuscular volume [MCV] < 80 femtoliters [fl]); hypochromia (mean corpuscular hemoglobin concentration [MCHC] <32 gm/dl); and polychromasia (reticulocytosis > 80,000 per cu mm). The erythrocyte sedimentation rate (ESR) is characteristically low in PV (< 1 mm/hr Westergren), although a high Hct from any cause may have a similarly low ESR. Once the spent phase develops, red cell morphology becomes progressively more abnormal (anisopoikilocytosis with prominent teardrop forms) together with features of leukoerythroblastosis (increasing myeloid immaturity in the peripheral blood and circulating normoblasts). At this stage, the total white cell and platelet counts may rise further or fall to abnormally low levels.

A bone marrow aspirate and biopsy are essential to demonstrate marrow cellularity, iron stores, and the presence or absence of reticulin and fibrosis. Significant hypercellularity (≥ 60 per cent of the cross-sectional area of the biopsy) is present in more than 90 per cent of patients with PV, and one of the most important clues is that in this disorder the marrow shows panhyperplasia (increased erythroid, myeloid, and megakaryocytic cells) in contrast to secondary polycythemia in which hyperplasia is usually limited to the erythroid series. The vast majority of PV patients will have deficient marrow reserves of iron (demonstrated with a Prussian blue stain) even though morphologic or biochemical iron deficiency may not be present. However, none of these marrow findings is diagnostic of PV; an almost identical picture may be found in other MPD, particularly ET. As PPMM develops, serial bone marrow biopsies may show increasing deposition of reticulin (silver stain) and collagen fibrosis (trichrome stain).

In patients without palpable splenomegaly, an estimate of splenic size may be obtained by plain radiography of the upper abdomen and left upper quadrant (with the patient in the recumbent position). Ingestion of a carbonated drink just prior to this procedure improves delineation of the splenic outline. A more precise quantitation of splenic size can be obtained with a ^{99m}Tc liver-spleen scan; this can also provide information about hepatic uptake, which is relevant to the question of whether cirrhosis and hepatoma are causes of secondary polycythemia.

The leukocyte (neutrophil) alkaline phosphatase (LAP or NAP) score is elevated (> 100) in the majority of patients with PV, but it is usually normal in secondary polycythemia (in the absence of infection, inflammation, or hormonal therapy). It is essential to perform this test concurrently with a normal control sample to ensure accurate interpretation.

The serum vitamin B_{12} level, and the unbound B_{12} binding capacity ($UB_{12}BC$) are frequently elevated in myeloproliferative disorders (including PV) because of elevated serum levels of transcobalamins I and III in these conditions. Other laboratory abnormalities in PV patients include hyperuricemia (> 7 mg/dl in 55 per cent) and hyperbilirubinemia (> 1 mg/dl in one third). Hyperhistaminemia is particularly helpful in distinguishing primary from secondary polycythemia, levels > 0.1 μg/ml being present in over 90 per cent of patients with PV. Serum muramidase (lysozyme) levels are also elevated in PV.

A wide variety of platelet function abnormalities has been reported in PV and other MPD, but no single test is diagnostic of PV. Of the many procedures available, spontaneous platelet aggregation in vitro may be helpful in identifying those patients at greater risk of thrombosis. Coagulation tests generally do not contribute to a diagnosis.

The most common cytogenetic abnormality in PV is aneuploidy, which is present in approximately one quarter of previously untreated cases, and the incidence of other abnormalities increases in patients treated with myelosuppressive therapy. Partial trisomy of the long arm of chromosome 1, monosomy 7, and trisomy 9 are the most commonly occurring nonrandom abnormalities in PV, although they also occur in other MPD.

3. *Can secondary causes of erythrocytosis be excluded?* In addition to tests specifically directed at establishing a diagnosis of PV, a number of other investigations may be required to exclude some forms of secondary polycythemia. Estimation of the arterial oxygen saturation is important to exclude secondary polycythemia due to arterial hypoxemia. The arterial saturation should be ≥ 92 per cent in PV; levels below 88 per cent are strongly suggestive of polycythemia due to hypoxemia. Adequate exclusion of the somnolence syndrome may require sleep studies of arterial blood gases and oxygen saturation. Rapid sequence intravenous pyelography is a crucial screening test because of the vast array of renal disorders that can cause secondary polycythemia. Abdominal computed axial tomography is also helpful in visualizing the retroperitoneal area, particularly with regard to adrenal masses.

Hemoglobinopathies associated with increased oxygen affinity (see the article on Hemoglobinopathies) are detectable with starch-gel or agar-gel electrophoresis in at least 50 per cent of cases. If electrophoresis is normal, however, identification requires construction of an oxygen dissociation curve for both whole blood and hemolysate. If both show a reduction in the partial pressure at which Hb is 50 per cent oxygenated (P_{50}), i.e., an increased affinity of Hb for oxygen, a mutant Hb is responsible. However, if only the whole blood P_{50} is reduced, the increased oxygen affinity is probably due to a reduction in red cell 2,3-diphosphoglycerate (2,3-DPG).

A chest x-ray may be helpful in identifying large pulmonary arteriovenous malformations, and the level of carboxy-Hb can be measured in heavy smokers to help determine the contribution of their smoking to the erythrocytosis. The latter is a particularly common problem that must be addressed in the differential diagnosis of PV in smokers. Carboxy-Hb normally constitutes < 1.5 per cent of total Hb; in erythrocytosis caused by smoking, the proportion of carboxy-Hb is usually greater than 6 per cent.

Finally, erythropoietin assays in plasma and urine are helpful in distinguishing PV from secondary polycythemia when no cause for the latter can be found. In PV, erythropoietin levels are usually either decreased or absent, whereas in secondary polycythemia they are increased. Further confirmation is now available in specialized centers using techniques for culture of committed erythropoietic progenitor cells (BFU-E and CFU-E). Whereas these cells normally show a requirement for erythropoietin (to enable proliferation and differentiation), in PV there appear to be two populations, one behaving normally, the other exhibiting autonomous growth char-

Table 2. PVSG Criteria for Polycythemia Vera (PV)

Category A	Category B
1. Increased red blood cell mass Male ⩾ 36 ml/kg Female ⩾ 32 ml/kg	1. Thrombocytosis Platelets > 400,000/cu mm
2. Normal arterial O_2 saturation S_aO_2 ⩾ 92%	2. Leukocytosis White blood cells > 12,000/cu mm
3. Splenomegaly	3. Elevated LAP score > 100 (No fever or infection)
	4. Elevated serum vitamin B_{12} B_{12} > 900 pg/ml or $UB_{12}BC$ > 2,200 pg/ml

Patients are regarded as having PV if either of the following combinations is present:

A1 + A2 + A3

or

A1 + A2 + any two parameters from category B

Abbreviations: LAP = Leukocyte alkaline phosphatase; $UB_{12}BC$ = unbound B_{12} binding capacity; PVSG = Polycythemia Vera Study Group.

acteristics in the absence of erythropoietin. The latter population represents the abnormal clone responsible for the myeloproliferative disorder.

PVSG CRITERIA FOR POLYCYTHEMIA VERA

As can be seen from the preceding section, no single test is readily available to unequivocally establish a diagnosis of PV. The PVSG has therefore proposed a set of criteria to provide maximal exclusion of causes of erythrocytosis other than PV. These criteria are grouped in two categories according to their relative significance (Table 2). The criteria were established in 1968 and have stood the test of time with respect to sensitivity and specificity in the diagnosis of PV.

MYELOFIBROSIS/ AGNOGENIC MYELOID METAPLASIA AND ESSENTIAL THROMBOCYTHEMIA

By Harry Iland, F.R.A.C.P., F.R.C.P.A.
and John Laszlo, M.D.
Durham, North Carolina

MYELOFIBROSIS/AGNOGENIC MYELOID METAPLASIA

Synonyms

Myelofibrosis with myeloid metaplasia, myelosclerosis, osteosclerosis, aleukemic myelosis, chronic erythroblastosis.

Definitions

Myelofibrosis (MF) and agnogenic myeloid metaplasia (AMM) refer to a group of conditions that fall within the spectrum of myeloproliferative disorders (MPD). They are characterized by varying degrees of intramedullary fibrosis and extramedullary hemopoiesis (myeloid metaplasia), together with the findings of a leukoerythroblastic reaction and teardrop poikilocytosis in the peripheral blood. The terms myelofibrosis and agnogenic myeloid metaplasia each emphasize only one pathophysiologic process, yet the majority of patients have evidence of both marrow fibrosis and extramedullary hemopoiesis (EMH). In this discussion, therefore, we will refer to myelofibrosis and agnogenic myeloid metaplasia as a single entity (MF/AMM), and we will also include those patients with marked EMH and minimal fibrosis, to whom the terms "unclassifiable" or "undifferentiated" MPD are sometimes applied. It is not yet clear whether or not the minority of patients who exhibit only fibrosis or only EMH have a course and prognosis different from the more typical cases. Questions such as this are being addressed by the Polycythemia Vera Study Group (PVSG) as part of an ongoing study of various aspects of the MPD.

Like the other chronic myeloproliferative diseases (polycythemia vera, chronic granulocytic leukemia, essential thrombocythemia), the pathophysiology of MF/AMM is based on disordered biology of the pluripotent bone marrow stem cell. Contrary to earlier views, cytogenetic and isoenzyme techniques have shown that the bone marrow fibroblasts are not derived from the abnormal clone of hemopoietic cells, thus establishing the reactive nature of the fibrosis.

The etiology of MF/AMM is unknown in the majority of patients. However, ionizing radiation and toxins (such as benzene) have been implicated in the genesis of some cases. A virtually identical syndrome occurs in up to 20 per cent of patients with polycythemia vera (PV) during the spent phase (postpolycythemic myeloid metaplasia) and in a small number of patients with essential thrombocythemia (ET). Myelofibrosis may be present initially in some patients with chronic granulocytic leukemia (CGL), and a myelofibrotic phase may precede the development of blast crisis in others.

A rapidly progressive and fatal form of marrow fibrosis known as acute myelofibrosis or malignant myelofibrosis has been described. Although there is considerable debate about this entity, in most instances it appears to represent a variant of acute leukemia, the primitive cells frequently having the typical ultrastructural characteristics of megakaryoblasts.

Presenting Symptoms and Signs

Males are affected slightly more commonly than females. The age at diagnosis is 50 to 70 years in the majority of patients, but the age of onset is frequently several years earlier, reflecting the insidious nature of the disease in its early stages. As many as one third of patients are asymptomatic at the time of presentation, the clinician being alerted to the diagnosis only by the chance finding of splenomegaly (the major site of EMH) or of the characteristic abnormalities in the peripheral blood.

The most frequent symptoms are related to anemia (fatigue, weakness, dyspnea); splenic pressure or splenic infarction (early satiety, abdominal fullness, left hypochondrial pain with or without referred shoulder tip pain); a hypermetabolic state (weight

Supported in part by Public Health Service Grant CA-10728 from the National Cancer Institute, Department of Health and Human Services. Dr. Iland is the recipient of a New South Wales (Australia) State Cancer Council Fellowship and Travel Grant-in-Aid.

loss, fever, and night sweats); increased nucleoprotein turnover (urate nephropathy and nephrolithiasis); and accelerated cardiovascular disease (angina, myocardial infarction, congestive cardiac failure). Bleeding occurs in 10 to 20 per cent of patients and is usually mucocutaneous in distribution (epistaxis, petechiae, ecchymoses). Major gastrointestinal bleeding is not uncommon and may arise from peptic ulcers or esophageal varices. Deafness may occur due to otosclerosis. Bone pain is an infrequent initial symptom. Rarely, masses of extramedullary hemopoietic tissue may cause serious complications by virtue of their size and location (e.g., spinal cord compression).

Physical examination reveals splenomegaly in virtually all patients and hepatomegaly in approximately 70 per cent. Splenic size ranges from being just palpable, early in the disease, to massive enlargement extending down to the left iliac fossa and across the midline. Although this is only an estimate, the spleen appears to enlarge by an average of 1 cm per year. Hepatic enlargement is not as dramatic unless the disease is very advanced. Occasionally, marked hepatomegaly follows splenectomy. Other findings include pallor, lymphadenopathy (10 to 20 per cent), petechiae, or ecchymoses. Splenic infarction may be accompanied by a friction rub and a sympathetic pleural effusion. Jaundice and ascites secondary to EMH and portal hypertension may occur, particularly when the latter is complicated by thrombosis of the portal vein, the intrahepatic sinusoids, or the hepatic veins (Budd-Chiari syndrome).

Diagnostic Procedures

A variety of hematologic, biochemical, cytochemical, radiologic, and cytogenetic abnormalities are present, and these can be used to differentiate MF/AMM from other MPD and the various secondary causes of myelofibrosis.

Peripheral Blood. A normochromic anemia is commonly present. This is associated with a mild reticulocytosis (less than 5 per cent) and abnormal red cell morphology (anisopoikilocytosis with prominent "teardrop" forms and circulating nucleated red cells [Fig. 1]). The anemia results from a combination of marrow failure, ineffective erythropoiesis in extramedullary sites, pooling of red cells in the enlarged spleen, mild hemolysis due to hypersplenism, and expansion of the plasma volume associated with splenomegaly (dilutional anemia). Occasionally iron deficiency due to bleeding (hypochromic microcytic anemia), folate deficiency due to the hyperproliferative state (megaloblastic anemia), or severe hemolysis may be contributing factors.

The white blood cell count is elevated in approximately half of the patients at diagnosis but rarely exceeds 50,000 per cu mm. Leukopenia is found in approximately 10 per cent. The differential count reveals mainly mature neutrophilic granulocytes; basophilia and/or eosinophilia may be present. Myeloid precursors are present in the peripheral blood, and together with the circulating erythroblasts they account for the leukoerythroblastic reaction that is present in virtually all patients at diagnosis (Fig. 1).

The platelet count may be low, normal, or high; occasionally counts above 1,000,000 per cu mm are seen. Platelet morphology is often abnormal, with bizarre megathrombocytes and abnormally granulated platelets being present. Circulating megakaryocytic fragments can also be found in the peripheral blood.

Bone Marrow. The bone marrow is often impossible to aspirate, and this produces the "dry tap" of myelofibrosis. Needle biopsy is essential, both to demonstrate fibrosis and to exclude certain other diagnoses.

Several patterns of marrow morphology can be identified in the spectrum of MF/AMM. In some patients marrow biopsy reveals trilineage hyperplasia without collagen fibrosis (trichrome stain), either because the fibrosis is patchily distributed or because the patient has a so-called unclassifiable MPD. There may be some increase in reticulin (silver stain) in these cases. The more usual appearance is of prominent collagen fibrosis with residual foci of hemopoietic tissue, particularly megakaryocytes. Finally, marked hypocellularity may be present, together with intense fibrosis and osteosclerosis (bony trabeculae occupying more than 30 per cent of the marrow cavity). Residual hemopoietic cells consist mainly of clumps of megakaryocytes.

It has not been established whether the natural history of MF/AMM involves progression from panhyperplasia to myelofibrosis and osteosclerosis; however, in view of the fact that these patients tend to deteriorate clinically and hematologically over time, it is likely that progressive histologic changes of this type take place.

Leukocyte Alkaline Phosphatase (LAP). The LAP score is usually normal or high ($>$ 100), although a minority of patients exhibit low levels ($<$ 30).

Cytogenetics. If marrow cannot be aspirated, unstimulated peripheral blood may yield sufficient metaphases for cytogenetic studies. Although karyotypic abnormalities occur frequently, most are nonspecific. The Philadelphia chromosome (Ph^1) does not occur in de novo MF/AMM, and cytogenetic studies have been useful primarily for establishing this important point. However, several nonrandom patterns have been described in MF/AMM and other MPD. These include partial trisomy of the long arm of chromosome 1 (1q), monosomy 7, and trisomy 9. A combination of the first two of these changes may also occur, with translocation of chromosome 7 to the duplicated long arm of chromosome 1; this has been reported only in MF/AMM and postpolycythemic myeloid metaplasia. Banding studies are essential for the precise identification of these abnormalities.

Demonstration of EMH. Fine-needle biopsy of an enlarged spleen or liver will reveal trilineage extramedullary hemopoiesis in MF/AMM, but since the diagnosis can usually be established without this, the risk of hemorrhage associated with the procedure outweighs the benefit in most circumstances. If a tissue biopsy is considered absolutely necessary, laparoscopic biopsy of the liver via a minilaparotomy is recommended because this combines safety with relative simplicity. Preoperative assessment of hemostatic competence is essential, and platelet transfusions should be administered prophylactically.

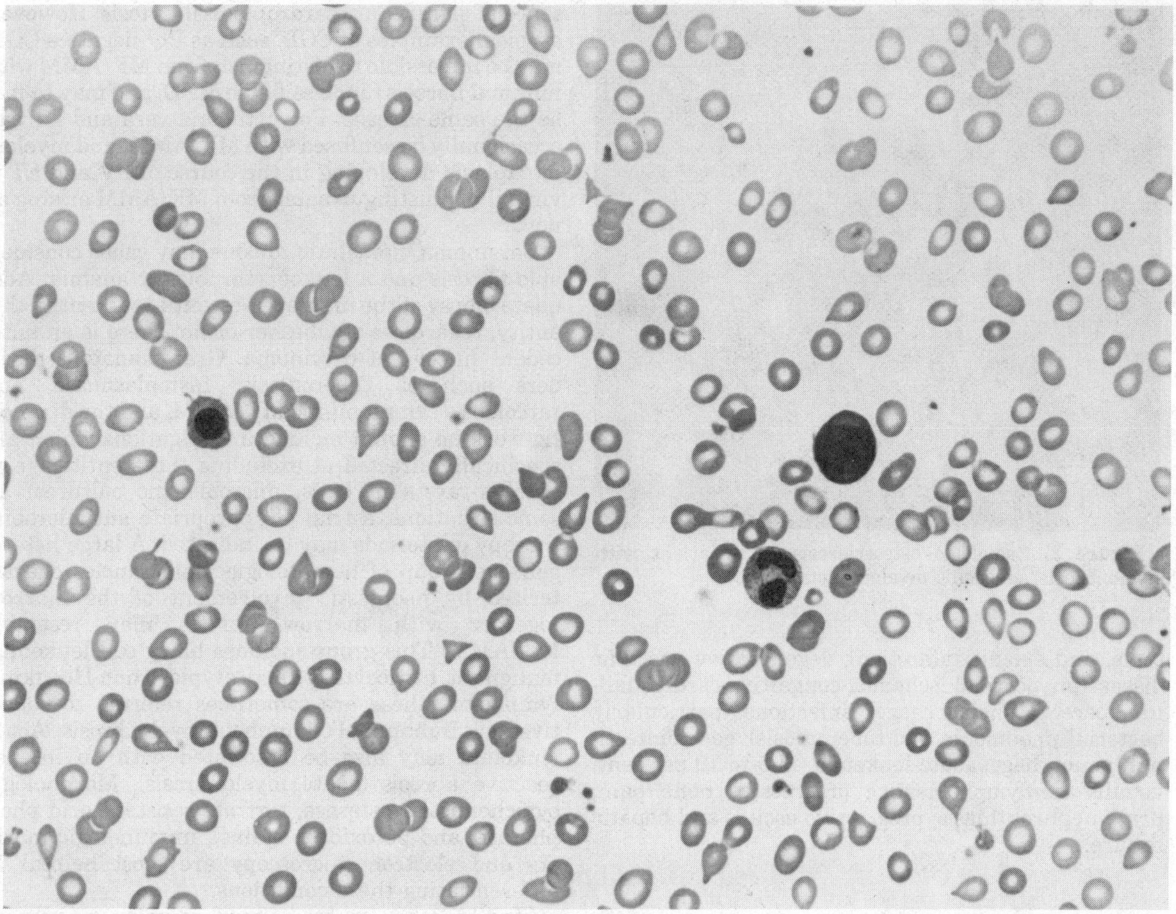

Figure 1. Peripheral blood in myelofibrosis/agnogenic myeloid metaplasia demonstrating a leukoerythroblastic reaction and teardrop poikilocytosis (magnification X400).

Hemostatic Function. A variety of disturbances in platelet function are present in MF/AMM, and these aggravate the hemorrhagic diathesis associated with the quantitative platelet abnormalities. Prolongation of the modified Ivy bleeding time, reduced platelet factor 3 activity, reduced platelet adhesion to glass beads, reduced platelet aggregation (particularly with epinephrine), nucleotide storage pool defects, and reduced lipoxygenase activity have all been described. Occult disseminated intravascular coagulation (DIC) is sometimes demonstrable, with prolongation of the prothrombin time, elevated levels of fibrin degradation products, reduced levels of factors V and VIII, and increased platelet turnover and activation. A diligent search for DIC should be undertaken whenever surgery is contemplated. A normal euglobulin lysis time (> 2 hours) is helpful in differentiating DIC from primary fibrinolysis.

Radiologic Abnormalities. Forty to 50 per cent of patients have demonstrable radiologic osteosclerosis; this is visible in a chest x-ray in most instances. Although various patterns have been described, the most readily recognizable is a diffuse, symmetric increase in bone density involving the axial skeleton (Fig. 2). A chest x-ray is also helpful in excluding secondary causes of marrow fibrosis, such as sarcoidosis and tuberculosis.

Biochemical Findings. Although hyperuricemia and hyperuricosuria are often present, clinical gout is less common. A variety of liver function abnormalities occur, but they are nonspecific and are not useful in establishing the diagnosis or in deciding on management. Serum lactate dehydrogenase (LDH) and histamine levels are usually elevated. Serum vitamin B_{12} levels and unbound B_{12} binding capacity ($UB_{12}BC$) are normal or mildly elevated.

PNH-Like Defect. A defect in the red cells of patients with MF/AMM related to that found in paroxysmal nocturnal hemoglobinuria has been reported by several authors, though it probably is rather uncommon. When it does occur, it may be partly responsible for the severe hemolytic anemia seen in some patients.

Course and Prognosis

Survival in MF/AMM varies considerably; median survival is approximately 5 years from the time of diagnosis. Adverse prognostic factors at the time of presentation include symptoms, significant hepatomegaly, severe anemia, and thrombocytopenia.

The major complications responsible for morbidity and mortality are progressive splenomegaly (with increasing anemia, thrombocytopenia, pressure symp-

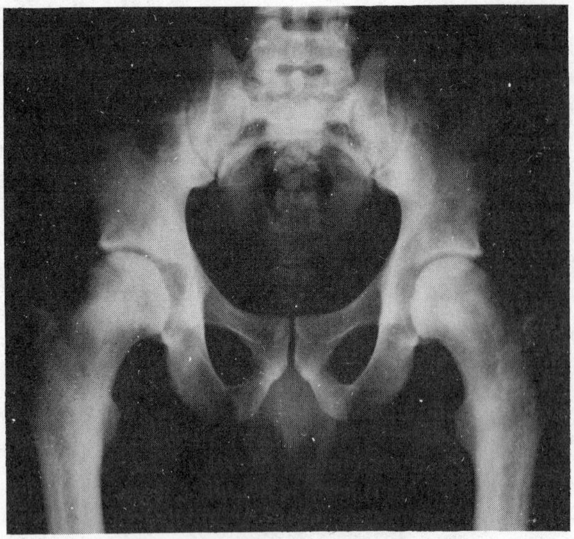

Figure 2. Radiologic osteosclerosis in a patient with myelofibrosis/agnogenic myeloid metaplasia.

toms, and splenic infarction); degenerative vascular disease (myocardial ischemia, congestive cardiac failure, cerebral hemorrhage); infections (particularly bacterial pneumonia and tuberculosis); gastrointestinal hemorrhage; acute leukemia (in 5 to 10 per cent, usually nonlymphoblastic); progressive bone pain; urate nephrolithiasis; progressive ascites and hepatic failure.

Differential Diagnosis

Myelofibrosis/agnogenic myeloid metaplasia must be distinguished from other chronic MPD (Fig. 3) and from other conditions associated with fibrosis of the marrow (Table 1) or prominent splenomegaly. Classic cases of CGL can be recognized by the marked leukocytosis, predominant myeloid hyperplasia in the marrow with little if any fibrosis, presence of the Ph[1] chromosome, low or absent LAP score, and absence of significant teardrop poikilocytosis. However, atypical examples of CGL, such as Ph[1]-negative CGL, may be impossible to distinguish from MF/AMM with minimal fibrosis (unclassifiable MPD) and may in fact be the same disease. Polycythemia vera and ET can occasionally be confused with MF/AMM, and myeloid metaplasia developing in the course of PV and ET is virtually indistinguishable from MF/AMM arising de novo.

Table 1. Differential Diagnosis of Myelofibrosis

Myelofibrosis/Agnogenic Myeloid Metaplasia
Other Chronic Myeloproliferative Disorders
Chronic granulocytic leukemia
Polycythemia vera
Essential thrombocythemia
Overlap myeloproliferative disorders (see Figure 3)
Secondary Causes of Myelofibrosis
Metastatic carcinoma
Granulomatous disorders
Sarcoidosis
Tuberculosis
Histoplasmosis
Hematologic malignancies involving bone marrow
Acute leukemia
Hairy cell leukemia
Malignant histiocytosis
Non-Hodgkin's lymphoma

Carcinoma metastatic to bone may cause considerable fibrosis and a leukoerythroblastic anemia. Adequate biopsy of the marrow is essential to identify this entity, regardless of whether or not there is an antecedent history of carcinoma. Granulomatous disorders such as tuberculosis, histoplasmosis, and sarcoidosis can all mimic MF/AMM, and the diagnostic work-up should include investigations which are specifically directed at excluding these entities (e.g., chest x-ray, skin tests, microbiologic cultures). In some situations, a trial of appropriate antimicrobial therapy or steroids may be indicated. A large heterogeneous group of hematologic malignancies characterized by neoplastic involvement of the marrow together with marrow fibrosis may resemble MF/AMM. This group includes hairy cell leukemia, malignant histiocytosis, and atypical non-Hodgkin's lymphoma; these are sometimes referred to collectively as Duhammel's lymphoid myelofibrosis. Acute leukemia may also be associated with an intense reactive fibrosis (acute myelofibrosis). Morphology, cytochemistry (esterase, tartrate-resistant acid phosphatase, and peroxidase stains), immunologic markers and electron microscopy are most helpful in differentiating these conditions.

Finally, other causes of marked splenomegaly including lipid storage diseases, splenic lymphoma and parasitic infections (malaria and kala-azar) may be confused with MF/AMM. They can be identified by their characteristic morphological appearances in bone marrow, blood or spleen.

ESSENTIAL THROMBOCYTHEMIA

Synonyms

Hemorrhagic thrombocythemia, idiopathic thrombocythemia, primary thrombocythemia, primary thrombocytosis.

Definitions

The last of the chronic myeloproliferative disorders to be recognized was ET. This has proved the most difficult to classify as a discrete entity, since marked thrombocytosis, the characteristic feature of ET, frequently accompanies PV, CGL, and MF/AMM. The major clinical and pathologic manifestations of ET (thromboembolic and hemorrhagic phenomena, splenomegaly, hemopoietic panhyperplasia in the bone marrow), also occur in these other myeloproliferative disorders, particularly PV, making the distinction between these conditions even more difficult. Exclusion of these conditions is necessary before a

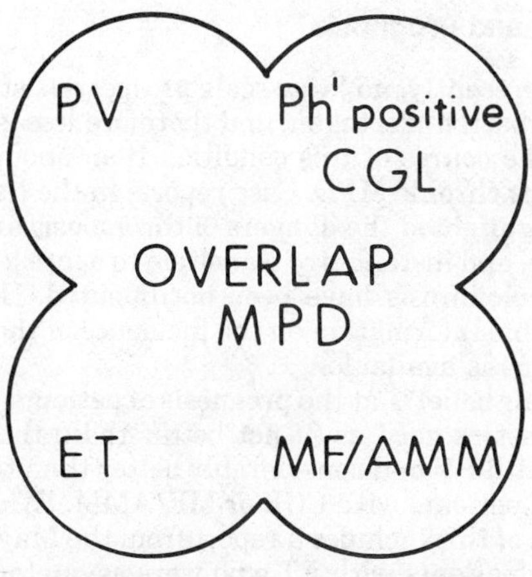

Figure 3. Interrelationship of the chronic myeloproliferative disorders (MPD). This figure schematizes the spectrum of chronic MPD. The peripheral areas represent cases that are distinct enough to constitute well-defined syndromes. The central area represents the "overlap" MPD and includes entities such as Philadelphia chromosome (Ph^1)-negative chronic granulocytic leukemia (CGL); myelofibrosis/agnogenic myeloid metaplasia (MF/AMM) without prominent fibrosis (unclassifiable MPD); Ph^1-positive essential thrombocythemia (ET); fibrotic variants of ET, polycythemia vera (PV), and CGL; and thrombocytotic variants of PV, CGL, and MF/AMM.

diagnosis can be made confidently, and it is in this context that "overlap" MPD pose a major problem (Fig. 3).

Presenting Symptoms and Signs

There is no predilection for either sex. The median age is 60 years, although the advent of automated cell counters has resulted in the recognition of increasing numbers of younger, asymptomatic patients.

Classical descriptions of ET have emphasized the frequent occurrence of major thromboembolic and hemorrhagic phenomena, including thrombosis of the splenic, cerebral, and mesenteric vessels and life-threatening gastrointestinal hemorrhage. Thromboses may develop in either the arterial or venous circulation, especially in the microcirculation; but the expression of symptoms also depends in part on the integrity of the vascular tree. Thus older patients with atherosclerosis, poor collateral circulation, and reduced venous return are more likely to develop vascular complications than are younger patients whose vessels are better able to accommodate changes in blood flow. It is not yet known whether the thrombocytosis per se or the qualitative platelet abnormalities found in ET are primarily responsible for the hemorrhagic diathesis; it is likely that both are contributing factors.

Although the initial clinical presentation may be due to a catastrophic thrombohemorrhagic event, severe complications such as these were notably infrequent in a selected series of prospective studies of ET by the PVSG. The most frequent symptoms were generalized weakness, headache, paresthesias, transient cerebral ischemic attacks (particularly dizziness), and minor bleeding (mainly epistaxis and bruising). Many other manifestations occurred less frequently, including peripheral vascular disease, thrombophlebitis, myocardial ischemia, post-traumatic bleeding (following dental extractions or surgery), gastrointestinal hemorrhage, visual phenomena (amaurosis fugax, dimming or blurring of vision, diplopia), sweating, weight loss, fever, gout, peptic ulcer, left hypochondrial pain, anorexia, and pruritus. The latter occurred much less often in these patients than in patients with PV studied by the PVSG.

Physical examination reveals mild splenomegaly in approximately one third of patients (usually no more than 3 cm below the left costal margin), and minimal hepatomegaly in one sixth. Ecchymoses may be present, but petechiae and purpura are rarely seen.

Diagnostic Procedures

Thrombocytosis is the sine qua non of ET; however, since it is also present in a significant proportion of patients with other chronic MPD, the diagnostic workup for ET necessarily involves a series of investigations directed at excluding these other conditions.

Peripheral Blood. The platelet count is always elevated, usually above 1,000,000 per cu mm, and morphologic abnormalities similar to those found in MF/AMM are frequently present. Similarly, circulating megakaryocytic fragments may be seen.

The hemoglobin (Hb) and hematocrit (Hct) are frequently reduced. In some patients, iron deficiency due to overt or occult blood loss may be responsible, but even when this is excluded, approximately 20 per cent will have a mild degree of anemia (Hb 10 to 12 gm/dl and Hct 31 to 37 per cent). Red cell morphology, in the absence of iron deficiency, shows no characteristic changes. Occasional patients develop evidence of splenic atrophy resulting from splenic infarction; this may be recognized by the presence of Howell-Jolly bodies, siderotic granules, spherocytes, and target cells.

The white blood cell count is elevated (greater than 12,000 per cu mm) in approximately 40 per cent of patients; the elevation is due almost entirely to a neutrophilic leukocytosis. Slight increases in basophils and eosinophils may occur, but the marked elevations seen in CGL are not found. Leukoerythroblastic reactions (circulating myeloid and erythroid precursors) are uncommon and, if present, are not a prominent feature (in contrast to MF/AMM and CGL).

Bone Marrow. Megakaryocytic hyperplasia is always present, and trilineage hyperplasia occurs in 75 per cent of patients. Absence of stainable iron in the bone marrow is also a common finding. Thus the overall appearance is similar to that found in PV, although myeloid and erythroid activity is not as marked, and masses of platelet aggregates are usually seen in the aspirate in ET.

Increased reticulin is present in approximately 25 per cent of patients at diagnosis. The question of whether collagen fibrosis occurs in ET early in the disease is a difficult one; this is an excellent example of the problems created by overlap MPD (Fig. 3). In our experience, patients initially thought to have ET who have any degree of collagen fibrosis at presentation usually have splenomegaly and a leukoerythroblastic reaction as well, and we therefore regard these cases as thrombocytotic variants of MF/AMM rather than as ET. This is more than just a nosologic problem, since the median survival of patients with ET is probably at least twice that of patients with MF/AMM.

Platelet Function. Abnormalities of platelet function similar to those occurring in MF/AMM have been described in the majority of patients with ET. In addition, evidence of platelet hyperaggregability (spontaneous platelet aggregation, circulating platelet aggregates) may be found.

The role of these abnormalities in the genesis of thrombohemorrhagic manifestations is not entirely clear, although several studies have suggested a causal relationship. Tests of platelet function are also very helpful in differentiating ET from reactive thrombocytosis, since the latter condition is not associated with platelet dysfunction.

Cytogenetics. Cytogenetic abnormalities are very uncommon and no patterns specific for ET have been described. However, the Philadelphia chromosome (Ph^1) has on rare occasions been detected in patients with otherwise classical ET, and the PVSG has collected seven such patients in the course of its prospective studies. Interestingly, six of these patients are women. It is not yet known whether these patients will continue to behave as other patients with ET, or whether the hematologic characteristics of CGL (including acute transformation) will evolve.

Cytogenetic analysis also makes it possible to exclude the 5q− syndrome (deletion of the long arm of chromosome 5), which is associated with mild thrombocytosis and megakaryocytic hyperplasia. The other characteristics of this syndrome include macrocytic anemia and hypolobulation of megakaryocytes. This condition appears to represent a variant of the refractory anemias, which are regarded as myelodysplastic syndromes rather than as MPD.

Biochemical Abnormalities. As with the other chronic MPD, increased serum levels of uric acid, LDH, vitamin B_{12}, and $UB_{12}BC$ are occasionally present, though these abnormalities are less frequent and less severe in ET. Pseudohyperkalemia may be found when serum is tested; it is due to excessive release of intracellular potassium from the markedly increased number of platelets during clotting. Simultaneous measurement of plasma and serum potassium will confirm the artifactual nature of the hyperkalemia.

Red Blood Cell Mass and Diagnostic Role of Iron Replacement. Since PV and ET share many clinical and hematologic features, determination of the red cell mass is helpful in differentiating these conditions. The red cell mass is elevated only in PV. If iron deficiency is present, investigation of the red cell mass should be deferred until replacement of iron stores has been achieved with oral iron, since iron deficiency may mask the erythrocytosis of PV.

Leukocyte Alkaline Phosphatase (LAP). The distribution of LAP scores is similar to that seen in MF/AMM.

Course and Prognosis

Until recently, no large-scale prospective studies of ET had been undertaken, and therefore less is known about the course of this condition than about any of the other chronic MPD. Case reports in the literature have highlighted the dangers of thrombosis and hemorrhage, and instances of transition to acute leukemia and myelofibrosis have been documented. However, no reliable information on the incidence of these complications is available.

It is our belief that the prognosis of patients with ET is at least as good as (if not better than) that of patients with PV and considerably better than the prognosis of patients with CGL or MF/AMM. Evidence in support of this includes a report from the Mayo Clinic of eight patients with ET who were asymptomatic at the time of diagnosis and who have remained free of thrombohemorrhagic complications during several years of follow-up despite no attempts at reduction of the platelet count. Furthermore, less than a 5 per cent incidence of transition to acute leukemia or myelofibrosis has been seen in patients studied by the PVSG, who have a median follow-up in excess of 4 years and whose median survival has not yet been reached. (It is probable, however, that any increased incidence of acute leukemia will not become evident until the median follow-up is at least 7 years.)

Although platelet function abnormalities may persist after reduction in the platelet count with myelosuppressive therapy, thrombohemorrhagic phenomena are less likely to occur once the platelet count has been lowered to less than 600,000 per cu mm. For example, the PVSG has shown that when neurologic complications have occurred, 80 per cent did so prior to the institution of myelosuppressive therapy or during subsequent relapses to platelet counts above 600,000 per cu mm. This is the only prognostic variable that has been identified in ET (with the possible exception of platelet function abnormalities).

Splenectomy is thought to be contraindicated because of the extreme thrombocytosis and disastrous thrombohemorrhagic complications that may follow. In fact, surgery of any kind should be undertaken only after thorough evaluation of hemostatic competence and then only if adequate platelet and coagulation factor support is available.

Differential Diagnosis

Essential thrombocythemia must be distinguished from other chronic MPD associated with thrombocytosis, from myelodysplastic syndromes associated with thrombocytosis, and from various conditions in which a reactive thrombocytosis occurs (Table 2).

The MPD which most closely resembles ET is PV, and the importance of iron replacement in excluding masked PV has already been stressed. Chronic granulocytic leukemia is usually easily differentiated from ET by the marked leukocytosis, the Ph^1 chromosome, low or absent LAP activity, marked splenomegaly, and predominant myeloid hyperplasia in the bone marrow. However, overlap cases are being recognized

Table 2. Differential Diagnosis of Thrombocytosis

Essential Thrombocythemia
Other Chronic Myeloproliferative Disorders
Polycythemia vera
Chronic granulocytic leukemia
Myelofibrosis/agnogenic myeloid metaplasia
Overlap myeloproliferative disorders (see Figure 3)
Myelodysplastic Syndromes Associated with Thrombocytosis
5q– syndrome
Idiopathic refractory sideroblastic anemia
Reactive Thrombocytosis
Blood loss and/or iron deficiency
Acute
Chronic
Chronic inflammatory disorders
Rheumatoid arthritis
Inflammatory bowel disease
Polyarteritis nodosa
Infection
Bacterial (e.g., osteomyelitis)
Tuberculosis
Malignancy
Carcinoma
Hodgkin's disease
Splenectomy
Hemolytic anemia

(Ph^1-positive ET), and their relationship to CGL and Ph^1-negative ET is currently under investigation. MF/AMM is distinguished by the presence of marrow fibrosis and prominent extramedullary hemopoiesis.

The 5q– syndrome is distinguished by its characteristic karyotypic abnormality. Another myelodysplastic syndrome that may be associated with thrombocytosis is idiopathic refractory sideroblastic anemia. This is recognized by the dimorphic red cells in the peripheral blood and by the presence of ringed sideroblasts in the marrow when stained for iron (Prussian blue reaction).

Reactive thrombocytosis is a common finding in patients who have a wide variety of clinical conditions (Table 2). In most situations, the underlying process is obvious (e.g., active rheumatoid arthritis, postsplenectomy, acute blood loss), and no investigations specifically directed at the thrombocytosis are indicated. However, iron deficiency due to occult blood loss may cause difficulty in diagnosis, and underlying neoplasms must be excluded whether or not iron deficiency is present. This especially applies to carcinoma involving the gastrointestinal tract, and in particular to carcinoma of the cecum. Bacterial infections and tumors are most likely to be accompanied by thrombocytosis when considerable tissue necrosis and suppuration are present. Hemolytic anemia can be recognized by the marked polychromasia and reticulocytosis in the peripheral blood and the intense erythroid hyperplasia in the marrow; the red cell changes characteristic of the underlying pathophysiologic process may also be obvious (thalassemia, immune hemolytic anemia, Heinz body–positive hemolysis); and if necessary a shortened red cell survival can be demonstrated. A past history of splenectomy for whatever reason may be associated with permanent thrombocytosis. This can coexist with ET, or with other causes of secondary thrombocytosis, and the relative contributions of these conditions to the thrombocytosis can be quite difficult to evaluate.

The following features of reactive thrombocytosis help to distinguish it from ET:

1. Its severity is closely related to the activity of the primary disorder, and it is often self-limited.
2. The platelet count rarely exceeds 1,000,000 per cu mm.
3. Platelet function abnormalities are not present.

CHRONIC GRANULOCYTIC LEUKEMIA

By Harry Iland, F.R.A.C.P., F.R.C.P.A.
and John Laszlo, M.D.
Durham, North Carolina

SYNONYMS

Chronic myeloid, myelocytic, myelogenous or neutrophilic leukemia, splenic leukemia.

DEFINITIONS

Chronic granulocytic leukemia (CGL) is a myeloproliferative disorder (MPD) with the following characteristics noted in the vast majority of patients:

1. Granulocytic hyperplasia in the bone marrow.
2. Granulocytosis in the peripheral blood.
3. Extramedullary hemopoiesis (EMH) in the spleen and liver.
4. Presence of the Philadelphia chromosome (Ph^1) in hemopoietic cells.
5. Reduced activity of leukocyte alkaline phosphatase (LAP).

Following a stable chronic phase of varying duration, virtually all patients with CGL undergo what is loosely termed a *metamorphosis,* or transition to an accelerated phase. Regardless of its clinical or morphologic expression, the accelerated phase of the disease is almost invariably fatal.

The target of the mutagenic event(s) in CGL is the pluripotent bone marrow stem cell, as it is in the other MPD (polycythemia vera, myelofibrosis/agnogenic myeloid metaplasia, and essential thrombocythemia). The result is a neoplastic stem cell that has a proliferative advantage over normal hemopoietic stem cells.

Supported in part by Public Health Service Grant CA-10728 from the National Cancer Institute, Department of Health and Human Services. Dr. Iland is the recipient of a New South Wales (Australia) State Cancer Council Fellowship and Travel Grant-in-Aid.

Evidence is accumulating that this stem cell possesses the potential for differentiation not only along the various myeloid pathways (i.e., granulocytic, monocytic, erythrocytic and megakaryocytic), but also along lymphoid pathways; this is particularly relevant in patients whose metamorphosis involves an acute leukemic transformation.

In most cases of CGL the etiology is unknown, but in some patients a clear association with antecedent ionizing radiation has been seen (e.g., early practitioners of radiology; patients who have had radiation therapy for ankylosing spondylitis; survivors of the atomic bomb blasts at Hiroshima and Nagasaki). The clinical, hematologic, and cytogenetic features of CGL in this subgroup of patients are indistinguishable from those found in patients without a history of exposure to excessive radiation.

CHRONIC PHASE

Symptoms and Signs

Males are affected slightly more than females. The median age is 40 to 45 years, at least 10 years less than for the other chronic MPD. Approximately 10 per cent of patients are Ph^1-negative, and such patients have a somewhat bimodal age distribution with a greater representation in the pediatric age group (juvenile CGL) and in the elderly.

The onset of the disease is insidious, and it is likely that several years elapse between the establishment of a proliferating Ph^1-positive clone of cells and the appearance of symptoms; the diagnosis is rarely made during this asymptomatic phase.

Manifestations of a hypermetabolic state are particularly prominent in CGL, including malaise, lethargy, weight loss, fever, and night sweats. As in other MPD in which there is increased turnover of hemopoietic cells with excessive nucleic acid synthesis and degradation, hyperuricemia and gout may occur. Early satiety, abdominal fullness, and left hypochondrial discomfort or pain are related to the splenic enlargement; anemia causes easy fatiguability and dyspnea. Bleeding manifestations (usually ecchymoses) occur less frequently than in the other chronic MPD and may be due to extreme thrombocytosis (or rarely to thrombocytopenia) with or without associated platelet dysfunction. Bone pain and tenderness, often worse at night, occur in some patients as a result of rapid expansion of the myeloid mass throughout the marrow cavity.

Moderate to marked splenomegaly is almost always present. The spleen may enlarge to the point where it occupies most of the abdominal cavity, producing considerable morbidity from pressure-related symptoms. When splenic infarction occurs, splenic tenderness and a friction rub are demonstrable. Hepatomegaly is often present, but the degree of hepatic enlargement is usually less marked. Occasional patients present with extremely high white blood cell counts (greater than 200,000 per cu mm), resulting in a characteristic clinical syndrome due to leukostasis in small vessels with or without demonstrable hyperviscosity. Such patients may experience mental changes, retinal or cerebral hemorrhages, cutaneous bleeding, cardiopulmonary dysfunction, and peripheral vascular insufficiency.

Patients sometimes present with the clinical and hematologic features of acute leukemia which is found to be Ph^1-positive. Successful remission induction is then followed in some of these patients by the appearance of typical chronic phase CGL, suggesting that metamorphosis from the chronic to the acute phase had already taken place before the initial presentation.

A confusing mode of presentation may be that of a solitary tumor, or chloroma; a paraspinal or other tumor may then easily be mistaken for a sarcoma, particularly when it precedes the blood and marrow manifestations of CGL.

Course and Prognosis

The median survival of patients with CGL is approximately 3.5 years from the time of diagnosis. Although some patients die of intercurrent illnesses or from the complications of therapy, at least 80 per cent will undergo metamorphosis of the disease, which occurs, on the average, about 3 years after diagnosis.

Numerous attempts to identify prognostic variables have been made, but the results are contradictory. Both pretreatment factors and the type of therapy employed appear to influence survival. The pretreatment characteristic with the greatest impact on survival is the Ph^1 status; it is a curious feature that the group of patients who lack the Philadelphia chromosome have a median survival of less than 18 months. Other factors postulated to adversely affect survival include marked splenomegaly or hepatomegaly, male sex, extremes of age, thrombocytosis or thrombocytopenia, anemia, marked basophilia, marked leukocytosis, and prominence of myeloid precursors in the peripheral blood. On the other hand, loss of the Y chromosome has been associated with a better than average prognosis. The type of therapy administered during the chronic phase also affects survival in that untreated patients and those treated only with radiation therapy have shorter survival times than busulfan-treated patients. There is some hope that the use of a less mutagenic chemotherapeutic agent, hydroxyurea, may further prolong survival by delaying the onset of acute leukemic transformations, but randomized controlled studies will be required to establish this point.

Diagnostic Procedures

Clinical, morphologic, cytogenetic and cytochemical changes enable a diagnosis of CGL to be established without difficulty in most instances.

Peripheral Blood. A marked leukocytosis is present (Fig. 1); the diagnosis is rarely made before the white cell count (WCC) exceeds 50,000 per cu mm, and it is above 100,000 per cu mm in about 75 per cent of patients. Maturation of myeloid precursors remains relatively intact in the chronic phase, and thus the leukocyte present in greatest numbers is the seg-

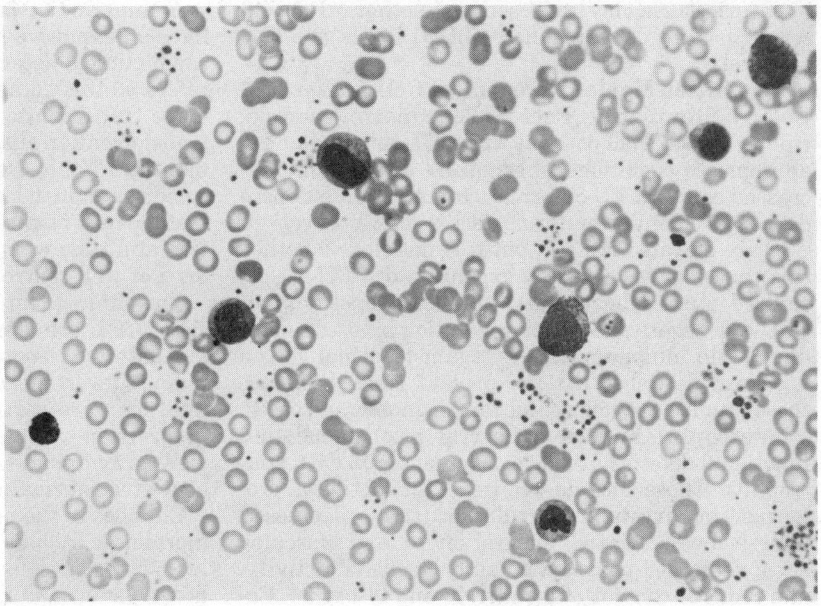

Figure 1. Peripheral blood in chronic granulocytic leukemia demonstrating leukocytosis with numerous myeloid precursors and a basophil (magnification X 400).

mented neutrophil. Although immature myeloid cells (blasts, promyelocytes, myelocytes, and metamyelocytes) are also found in the peripheral blood, the numbers of these cell types are roughly proportional to their degree of differentiation. Spontaneous cycling of the WCC has been noted in a few cases. Increased numbers of basophils and eosinophils are usually present, and the degree of basophilia, particularly, is more marked than in the other chronic MPD. Rare variants of CGL in which eosinophilia or basophilia is the predominant feature are known as chronic eosinophilic or basophilic leukemia, respectively.

Mild anemia (hemoglobin 9 to 12 gm/dl) is usually present in CGL, but the red cells show no diagnostic features. Nucleated red cells may be seen in the peripheral blood, but not to the extent that they are found in myelofibrosis/agnogenic myeloid metaplasia (MF/AMM).

Platelet counts vary from thrombocytopenic levels to marked thrombocytosis; abnormal platelet morphology may be present but is not as prominent as in essential thrombocythemia (ET) or MF/AMM.

Bone Marrow. The peripheral blood findings are usually so typical that examination of bone marrow is often unnecessary. A sternal aspirate or iliac crest biopsy shows marked hypercellularity due almost entirely to granulocytic hyperplasia. Orderly maturation is present, although myelocytes characteristically outnumber metamyelocytes in CGL. Trilineage hyperplasia is much less common than in the other chronic MPD. There may be an increase in the number of megakaryocytes, but they tend to be smaller than those present in ET and polycythemia vera (PV), and prominent erythroid hyperplasia is infrequent, as reflected by the very large myeloid : erythroid ratio. Myelofibrosis is present at diagnosis in less than 5 per cent of patients, and it tends to be associated with more severe anemia.

Cytogenetic Abnormalities. The Ph^1 chromosome arises by translocation of chromosomal material from the long arm of one of the No. 22 chromosomes (22q–). It is present in 80 to 90 per cent of patients with classical CGL; in over 90 per cent of these patients the other chromosome involved in the translocation is the long arm of No. 9 (t[9q34+; 22q11–]). In Ph^1-positive patients, it can be demonstrated in all, or nearly all, unstimulated metaphases obtained from peripheral blood or bone marrow, and it has been identified in the precursors of granulocytes, erythrocytes, platelets, and monocytes. Contrary to earlier views, it is not absolutely specific to CGL. Some overlap is now being observed with other chronic MPD (e.g., Ph^1-positive ET); up to 25 per cent of adult acute lymphoblastic leukemias (ALL) are also Ph^1-positive, although some of these may in fact represent CGL presenting in the form of an acute lymphoblastoid transformation.

Additional cytogenetic abnormalities may be present in the chronic phase before any myelosuppressive therapy; loss of the Y chromosome appears to be associated with a better than average prognosis.

Leukocyte Alkaline Phosphatase. Activity of LAP is reduced or absent in over 90 per cent of patients with Ph^1-positive CGL and is normal (30 to 100) in the remainder. A similar pattern is seen in Ph^1-negative patients, though occasional patients have elevated LAP scores.

Biochemical Abnormalities. Serum levels of vitamin B_{12} and unbound B_{12} binding capacity are markedly elevated in CGL—considerably more so than in other MPD. The increase in the binding capacity of the serum is due largely to the increased amounts of transcobalamin III that are present in CGL granulocytes and released in vitro during clotting. Release of intracellular potassium from the greatly increased number of leukocytes may result in a confusing pseudohyperkalemia. Hyperuricemia and hyperuricosuria may be present as in other MPD, and serum lactate dehydrogenase (LDH) levels are also elevated.

Committed Myeloid Progenitor Cell Assays and Colony Stimulating Factor. Bone marrow and peripheral blood from patients with CGL cultured under appropriate conditions in semisolid agar exhibit increased colony (CFU-c) formation but retain a dependence on colony-stimulating factor (CSF). Levels of CSF are elevated in CGL, but it is not clear whether this causes or is caused by expansion of CFU-c. Specialized studies have shown reduced sensitivity of CFU-c to negative feedback regulation by prostaglandin E, and inhibitory activity against normal CFU-c has been described. At the present time, however, these studies are not useful for diagnostic purposes.

Neutrophil Function. Several biochemical and functional defects have been documented in CGL neutrophils. These include reduced LAP activity, prolonged intravascular circulation time, decreased adhesiveness, delayed emigration to extravascular sites, decreased phagocytic and bactericidal activity, and reduced content of lactoferrin and lysozyme. Except in the case of the LAP score, demonstrating these defects is of more value for the study of the biology of CGL rather than for diagnosis. In spite of these defects, bacterial infections are not a major cause of morbidity and mortality in CGL, and CGL neutrophils function quite effectively when transfused into severely neutropenic individuals.

JUVENILE CGL

Juvenile CGL differs from the adult variety, not only in the age of onset and the absence of the Ph^1 chromosome but in a number of other ways as well. Monocytoid cells are a prominent feature in the peripheral blood and bone marrow; thrombocytopenia and hemorrhage are more common than in adult CGL; the red cells show fetal patterns (e.g., increased fetal hemoglobin); serum and urine muramidase levels are significantly elevated; and CFU-c exhibit mainly monocytic differentiation in vitro. These patients have a poor prognosis and are often unresponsive to busulfan.

METAMORPHOSIS

Several different forms of metamorphosis may occur, though progression from less malignant to more malignant variants is the rule. One form is an *accelerated phase,* in which control of the leukocytosis can only be achieved with increasing doses of previously effective therapy, with a concomitant increase in toxicity. In most cases, this phase rapidly evolves into an *acute leukemic phase,* referred to as *acute,* or *blast, transformation.* The distinction between the accelerated phase and acute transformation depends on the proportion of blasts, since the two forms generally have the same clinical and laboratory features. Acute transformation is defined as greater than 30 per cent blasts in the peripheral blood or bone marrow.

A minority of patients in the chronic phase will have an explosive proliferation of blasts with a more rapid clinical deterioration, and the term *blast crisis* refers to this catastrophic event. Other variants include transition to a *myelofibrotic phase,* with acute transformation usually following in a matter of months. Finally, extramedullary tissues (particularly spleen, lymph nodes, skin, and the central nervous system) may be the initial site of an acute transformation at a time when the marrow still has the appearance of well-controlled chronic phase disease.

The clinical features associated with metamorphosis of CGL are similar to those seen at the time of presentation. Increasing weakness, fatigue, unexplained fever, bleeding, and progressive musculoskeletal pain are particularly common. Recurrence and progression of splenomegaly and hepatomegaly, as well as lymphadenopathy, may herald an incipient acute transformation.

Changes in the peripheral blood that suggest metamorphosis include anemia, increasingly refractory leukocytosis, leukopenia, thrombocytosis, thrombocytopenia, and progressive basophilia. Increasing myeloid immaturity is an ominous sign. Although the LAP score frequently returns to normal during treated chronic phase CGL, further elevation to levels above normal is associated with metamorphosis.

The development of myelofibrosis frequently precedes acute transformation by a few months; the appearance of additional cytogenetic abnormalities suggests clonal evolution, which is thought to be responsible for the transition to acute leukemia. The commonest cytogenetic abnormalities found in this phase of the disease are multiple Ph^1 chromosomes, trisomy 8, and isochromosome or trisomy of the long arm of 17. Finally, changes in the culture characteristics of myeloid progenitors may occur at this stage (e.g., an increasing cluster:colony ratio).

ACUTE PHASE

The survival of patients undergoing metamorphosis varies considerably, depending on the nature of the transition. However, once acute transformation or blast crisis develops, survival is inevitably brief. The major prognostic determinant is the blast cell phenotype. A lymphoblastoid phenotype is demonstrable in 30 per cent of patients on the basis of morphology, terminal deoxynucleotidyl transferase (TdT) positivity, expression of the common-ALL antigen, or presence of intracytoplasmic IgM. Patients with a lymphoblastoid phenotype have a somewhat better prognosis, and TdT positivity is the best prognostic variable. Approximately two thirds of these patients will obtain a complete remission with anti-ALL therapy (vincristine and prednisone). The median survival of such patients, although longer than for those with non-lymphoblastoid transformations, is still significantly shorter than that associated with acute leukemia arising de novo. The karyotype at the time of acute transformation also has some prognostic value. Patients who do not develop additional cytogenetic abnormalities and patients with hypodiploidy have a slightly better prognosis.

DIFFERENTIAL DIAGNOSIS

Chronic granulocytic leukemia must be distinguished from other MPD and from conditions associated with a marked neutrophilic leukocytosis (Table 1). (See the article on Leukocytosis and Leukemoid Reactions.)

Some cases of MF/AMM, ET, and PV have several features in common with CGL, particularly leukocytosis and splenomegaly. The Ph[1] chromosome, the LAP score, and the bone marrow morphology are most helpful in the differentiation of these MPDs, although overlap MPDs occasionally present problems.

Leukemoid reactions (of the myeloid variety) are characterized by a marked neutrophilic leukocytosis, sometimes in excess of 100,000 per cu mm. Myeloid immaturity is not as prominent in most cases, although a differential count closely resembling that seen in CGL is sometimes found. Conditions associated with leukemoid reactions include severe infections (especially tuberculosis), metastatic carcinoma (particularly where bone marrow involvement or considerable necrosis is present), Hodgkin's disease, corticosteroid therapy, hemorrhage and/or hypoxia, severe hemolysis, rebound after marrow depression, and inflammatory disorders (e.g., polyarteritis nodosa). The underlying cause is obvious in many instances, and appropriate therapy will confirm the reactive nature of the leukocytosis. A biopsy will help exclude malignancies involving the bone marrow. The LAP score is usually elevated in leukemoid reactions, and the Ph[1] chromosome is always absent.

An isolated chloroma may pose a major problem in diagnosis unless careful cytologic studies are done to reveal the myeloid nature of the cells. This is an important problem because the location of the tumor may cause serious impairment 3 to 24 months before evaluation shows a clearly leukemic picture.

Table 1. Differential Diagnosis of Chronic Granulocytic Leukemia

Chronic Granulocytic Leukemia
Ph[1]-positive
Ph[1]-negative
Juvenile
Other Myeloproliferative Disorders
Myelofibrosis/agnogenic myeloid metaplasia
Polycythemia vera
Essential thrombocythemia
Overlap myeloproliferative disorders
Leukemoid Reactions
Infection (e.g., tuberculosis)
Malignancy
Carcinoma
Hodgkin's disease
Corticosteroid therapy
Hemorrhage and/or hypoxia
Hemolytic anemia
Rebound after marrow depression
Inflammatory disorders (e.g., polyarteritis nodosa)
Sarcomatous Lesions
Chloroma (granulocytic sarcoma)
True sarcomas

CHRONIC LYMPHOCYTIC LEUKEMIA

By Robert L. Stahl, M.D.
and Robert Silber, M.D.
New York, New York

Chronic lymphocytic leukemia (CLL) is a disease in which monoclonal lymphocytes accumulate in blood, bone marrow, lymph nodes, and sometimes other tissues. It is the most common leukemia in Western society, accounting for 25 per cent of all leukemias. Primarily a disease of the elderly, CLL rarely occurs before the age of 40 years. Ninety per cent of the patients are over the age of 50 years, and the majority are over 60 years at the time of diagnosis. Men are affected twice as often as women. It is a disorder in which survival is highly variable, ranging from less than 1 year to over 10 years. Although the disease is generally responsive to therapy in its early stages, no cure is currently available.

PRESENTING SIGNS AND SYMPTOMS

Over 25 per cent of patients have asymptomatic disease that is discovered on routine physical examination or blood count. The most frequent presenting symptoms are fatigue, malaise, and decreased exercise tolerance. Some patients note enlarged lymph nodes or complain of abdominal discomfort and early satiety due to splenomegaly. Lymphadenopathy is commonly cervical, supraclavicular, or axillary. Inguinal lymphadenopathy is rare. Splenomegaly and/or hepatomegaly develop with disease progression. Unusual areas of involvement include skin, gums, pleura, lung parenchyma, and gastrointestinal or respiratory tract mucosa. Jaundice generally suggests hemolysis, although periportal lymph node enlargement with biliary obstruction can be seen. As the disease progresses, bruising due to thrombocytopenia may occur. Fever when present is almost always secondary to infection.

LABORATORY FINDINGS

The diagnosis of CLL requires the demonstration of sustained lymphocytosis and bone marrow lymphocyte infiltration in the absence of other causes. Normal blood contains 1 to 2000 lymphocytes per cu mm of which 60 to 80 per cent are T cells and 10 to 15 per cent are B cells. In CLL, the absolute lymphocyte count is usually above 15,000 per cu mm. Although both T and B cells are increased in absolute numbers, B cells are preferentially so and account for 40 to 90 per cent of all lymphocytes. Although these cells are mature in appearance and usually indistinguishable from normal lymphocytes, they tend to smudge upon preparation of the blood smear. As the disease progresses, larger forms with nucleoli may be seen. Red blood cell morphology is usually normal. Anemia occurs in 10 to 20 per cent of patients. It is mostly normochromic normocytic. Bone marrow replacement, hypersplenism, or suppressor mechanisms contribute to the anemia. The Coombs' test reveals IgG coating of red blood cells in about 20 per cent of all patients and an immune hemolytic anemia with microspherocytes is seen in 8 per cent. Thrombocytopenia is found in 10 to 20 per cent of cases and is related to bone marrow replacement, hypersplenism, or anti-platelet antibodies. Bone marrow morphology is an indicator of clinical status, with interstitial or nodular lymphocytic infiltration seen in early disease and diffuse infiltration found in advanced stages.

STAGING

On the basis of examination and complete blood count, the patient with CLL can be staged clinically (Table 1). A more recent staging system also considers total lymphoid mass as a factor. Stages 0 and I constitute a favorable prognostic group. Stage III and IV patients have a relatively short survival, whereas prognosis in stage II is intermediate. Generally, disease progression follows a stepwise pattern from earlier to later stages. One exception is patients with lymphocytosis and isolated splenomegaly in the absence of lymphadenopathy; these individuals may have a favorable prognosis.

A number of immunologic alterations are seen in CLL. In 99 per cent of the cases, CLL lymphocytes have surface immunoglobulin and can be classified as B cells. Usually the immunoglobulin is IgM, although IgD or light chains can be seen. In 5 per cent of cases, the same immunoglobulin present on the cell surface is found in the serum and can be detected as a monoclonal protein or M-spike on serum protein electrophoresis. Despite the B cell lymphoproliferation, 50 to 75 per cent of patients are hypo- or agammaglobulinemic, accounting perhaps for the increased frequency of infections, especially pneumonia, seen in these patients. In addition, there is an inverted ratio of helper to suppressor T cells, with the increased number of suppressor cells a probable factor in the hypogammaglobulinemia. The degree of hypogammaglobulinemia increases with advancing stage. Approximately 1 per cent of patients have lymphocytes that form rosettes with sheep red blood cells and are classified as T cell CLL. These patients have massive splenomegaly, marked neutropenia, skin infiltration, modest bone marrow infiltration, and a rapid clinical course.

Table 1. Clinical Staging in CLL

Stage	Definition
0	Lymphocytosis only; peripheral count usually 15,000 per cu mm, marrow population ⩾ 40% Median survival, 150 months
I	Lymphocytosis and lymphadenopathy Median survival, 101 months
II	Lymphocytosis and hepatomegaly or splenomegaly, or both; nodes may or may not be enlarged Median survival, 71 months
III	Lymphocytosis and anemia (hemoglobin < 11 gm/dl); nodes, spleen, or liver may or may not be enlarged Median survival, 19 months
IV	Lymphocytosis and thrombocytopenia (platelets 100,000 per cu mm); anemia or organomegaly may or may not be present Median survival, 19 months

DIAGNOSTIC PITFALLS

Some uncommon disorders can be confused with CLL. Prolymphocytic leukemia is associated with massive splenomegaly and an aggressive clinical course with a median survival of less than 3 years. The malignant cell is large with distinct nucleoli, and white blood cell counts are very high. Hairy cell leukemia is characterized by pancytopenia, modest splenomegaly, difficulty in obtaining bone marrow aspirates, and a variable clinical course. Leukemic cells have fine cytoplasmic projections and give a positive acid phosphatase stain which is tartrate-resistant. "Lymphosarcoma cell" leukemia patients present with marked adenopathy and occasionally massive splenomegaly. The leukemic cells are large with notched nuclei and well-delineated nucleoli, and they have intense surface immunoglobulin, distinct from the weak surface immunoglobulin in CLL. Lymph node biopsy usually reveals nodular poorly differentiated lymphocytic lymphoma. Well differentiated lymphocytic lymphoma with blood involvement is often indistinguishable from CLL. There are two ways to differentiate these entities: CLL lymphocytes form rosettes with mouse erythrocytes, whereas lymphoma cells do not; and CLL lymphocytes do not form caps when exposed to multivalent ligands, whereas lymphoma cells cap normally.

COMPLICATIONS

The most common complications of CLL are bacterial infections, with pneumonia and urinary tract infections occurring most often. Disease progression to an acute leukemia blast crisis, as occurs in chronic myelogenous leukemia, has been reported to occur extremely rarely in CLL. The development of fever, weight loss, rapid lymph node enlargement, and central nervous system symptoms is suggestive of *Richter's syndrome,* which is a very rare transformation to an aggressive lymphoproliferative disorder resembling diffuse histiocytic lymphoma. The incidence of carcinoma in patients with CLL is approximately 9 per cent, as compared with 2 per cent in an age-matched control population, and may be a reflection of the altered immune status in this disorder. Careful monitoring of patients for a new malignancy is therefore in order.

MALIGNANT LYMPHOMAS

By Jane E. Henney, M.D.
and Vincent T. DeVita, Jr., M.D.
Bethesda, Maryland

DEFINITION

The lymphomas are a group of malignant diseases, usually arising in the lymph nodes or in the lymphoid tissues of parenchymal organs such as the gut, lung, or skin, with a characteristic histologic appearance. If untreated, they have a variable but progressive course leading to death.

Malignant lymphomas are generally classified in two groups: Hodgkin's disease in one, and the lymphocytic and histiocytic lymphomas of Rappaport in the other. Each of these groups has been further divided into subcategories. The most common currently used classification of Hodgkin's disease that is readily reproducible and has prognostic relevance was described by Lukes and Butler (Table 1). The other lymphomas until recently were generally described by the Rappaport classification, which has two main subcategories based on lymph node architecture: diffuse and nodular. Lesions with the nodular pattern tend to follow a more indolent course; those with the diffuse pattern, with the exception of those with well-differentiated forms, have a rapid clinical evolution. The nodular and diffuse subtypes are further defined by describing the morphologic features of the cells, such as lymphocytic, histiocytic, and mixtures of the two cell types, the mixed lymphomas.

Classifications based on ultrastructural studies and immunologic techniques delineating T and B cells have recently been proposed by Lukes and Collins and others. A new formulation proposed by an international group of experts who reviewed five major classification systems is compared with the Rappaport System in Table 2.

The term "histiocytic lymphoma" used by Rappaport to designate large histiocytic appearing cells is now known to be a misnomer but is still used by convention. About 80 per cent of all histiocytic and lymphocytic lymphomas are now known to arise from a proliferation of monoclonal B cells, including the lesions in all those patients with nodular forms of the disease. True T cell lymphomas are uncommon and are usually seen in children and adolescents with mediastinal adenopathy and a leukemic blood picture with large convoluted lymphoblasts in the peripheral blood. The only true form of a malignant histiocytic disease is histiocytic medullary reticulosis, although current evidence indicates that the cell of origin in Hodgkin's disease is a histiocyte.

Burkitt's lymphoma is a diffuse lymphoma of the follicular B cells that is primarily observed in African children. In the endemic regions of East Africa and New Guinea, evidence of infection with a herpes-like Epstein-Barr virus has been observed. The child in Africa most commonly presents with extra lymphatic tumor arising from the bone, often the mandible. The American child, on the other hand, presents with disease involving abdominal or pelvic sites, particularly the gastrointestinal tract, and infrequently the jaw is involved. Sites of secondary involvement for the African varieties include frequent spread to the abdominal viscera, ovaries, breast, and meninges and infrequent spread to the bone marrow. Both varieties of disease eventually involve the bone marrow and cerebrospinal fluid in over one third of the patients.

Angioimmunoblastic lymphadenopathy is not considered a histologically malignant disease but rather an extreme form of hypersensitivity reaction. This lymphoma-like systemic disorder most frequently occurs in adults and the clinical features often mimic those observed in the patient with advanced Hodgkin's disease or the other lymphomas. Generalized lymphadenopathy, hepatomegaly, splenomegaly, fever, sweats, and weight loss are often presenting features of this disease. In half of the patients, a generalized pruritic rash may precede the severe constitutional symptoms. In a small number of patients, a history of drug ingestion can be elicited.

Nearly all patients evidence anemia and in 25 per cent it is due to a Coombs' test–positive hemolytic anemia. Leukocytosis and eosinophilia may also be a part of the peripheral blood picture. The majority of patients have a polyclonal hypergammaglobulinemia as well.

When the enlarged lymph nodes are biopsied, alterations can be observed of nodal architecture or complete effacement with a pleomorphic cellular proliferation in which immunoblasts, lymphocytes, and plasma cells predominate. Vascular proliferation and prominent eosinophilic interstitial material are also often seen.

The remainder of the clinical course can vary greatly. Approximately 25 per cent of patients have a long survival, up to 4 years, with or without corticosteroid therapy and never require intensive chemotherapy. Another 25 per cent have a similar survival time but only when intensive chemotherapy is administered. The remaining patients have a rapid downhill course terminating in death regardless of the management approach. Among the terminal events, overwhelming infections, renal failure, and hepatic failure all have been reported.

PRESENTING SIGNS AND SYMPTOMS

Hodgkin's Disease. The young patient (average age 32 in the developed countries) with Hodgkin's disease usually comes to the physician with superficial adenopathy. This lymph node enlargement is usually in the cervical region, but isolated axillary and ingui-

Table 1. Lukes-Butler Histopathologic Classification of Hodgkin's Disease

Lymphocytic predominant
Nodular sclerosis
Mixed cellularity
Lymphocyte-depleted

Table 2. Recommendations of an Expert International Panel on the Formulation* of non-Hodgkin's Lymphoma Compared with the Rappaport Scheme

Panel's Recommendations for Terminology	Rappaport Terminology
Malignant lymphoma Small lymphocytic Consistent with chronic lymphocytic leukemia plasmacytoid	Diffuse well-differentiated lymphocytic
Malignant lymphoma, follicular Predominantly small cleaved cell Diffuse areas Sclerosis	Nodular poorly differentiated lymphocytic
Malignant lymphoma, follicular Mixed, small cleaved and large cell Diffuse areas Sclerosis	Nodular mixed lymphocytic histiocytic
Malignant lymphoma, follicular Predominantly large cell Diffuse areas Sclerosis	Nodular histiocytic
Malignant lymphoma, diffuse Small cleaved cell	Diffuse poorly differentiated lymphocytic
Malignant lymphoma, diffuse Mixed, small and large cell Sclerosis Epitheloid cell component	Diffuse mixed lymphocytic-histiocytic
Malignant lymphoma, diffuse Large cell Cleaved cell Non-cleaved cell Sclerosis	Diffuse histiocytic
Malignant lymphoma Large cell, immunoblastic Plasmacytoid Clear cell Polymorphous Epitheloid cell component	Diffuse histiocytic
Malignant lymphoma Lymphoblastic Convoluted cell Non-convoluted cell	Diffuse lymphoblastic
Malignant lymphoma Small non-cleaved cell Burkitt's Follicular areas	Diffuse undifferentiated

*Modified from the working formulation for clinical usage. Cancer, 49: 2112, 1982.

nal lymph node presentations do occur. This can be either asymptomatic, discrete, or painless, or be associated with symptoms of fever, night sweats, weight loss, and sometimes pruritus. Signs and symptoms not infrequently wax and wane over several months prior to presentation. Fever, night sweats, and weight loss are referred to as "B" symptoms and have been demonstrated to be correlated with more advanced disease and a poor prognosis. Pruritus often accompanies fever but does not have significance when observed as an isolated finding. The disease in young people is often detected by finding mediastinal adenopathy on a routine chest x-ray or a film taken because of a persistent, dry, nonproductive cough. This presentation is most common if the Hodgkin's disease is of the nodular sclerosing variety.

In older patients with Hodgkin's disease, the tumor commonly is associated with fever, night sweats, or both, followed by increasing malaise and weight loss. In some cases, the enlarging lymph nodes are located exclusively in the abdomen. Those patients not having readily apparent lymph node enlargement usually are assigned by the physician a differential diagnosis of fever of undetermined origin. If the diagnosis establishes Hodgkin's disease, the lymphocyte-depleted variety is most frequent. If fever has been among the presenting symptoms in the patient with Hodgkin's disease in either age group, it is usually remittent in nature.

A cyclical fever pattern known as Pel-Ebstein fever has also been observed in the patient with Hodgkin's disease. This temperature pattern is characterized by several days or weeks of fever alternating with afebrile periods. Pain coincident with the consumption of alcohol is uncommon, but when it does occur appears to correlate with heavy eosinophilic infiltration at the sites involved by tumor. Thus this may serve to direct attention to an involved site to biopsy and confirm the diagnosis of Hodgkin's disease. Infrequently, superior vena cava syndrome is the first symptom in a patient with Hodgkin's disease.

Lymphocytic and Histiocytic Lymphomas. Patients with the common nodular poorly differentiated lymphocytic lymphoma (NPDL) present with a more uniform clinical picture than those with the other types. The disease afflicts adults usually over the age of 40. Its occurrence in children is rare, and such a diagnosis should suggest reactive hyperplasia to the physician. The patient with NPDL is commonly asymptomatic at the outset. Painless adenopathy in the cervical, axillary, and inguinal-femoral regions is the common presenting physical finding. Because the lymphocytic lymphoma commonly involves the gastrointestinal tract, large abdominal masses of retroperitoneal or mesenteric lymph nodes that cause acute gastrointestinal problems, including obstruction, hemorrhage, and intussusception, can occur. The symptoms of fever, night sweats, and/or weight loss are less common in patients with lymphocytic and histiocytic lymphomas, and their presence or absence is less related to prognosis.

The lymphadenopathy of the nodular lymphomas may have been present for a long period of time; often, a previous lymph node biopsy may have been interpreted as "atypical" or "hyperplastic." Subsequent review of the initial biopsy and comparison with a second biopsy often reveals that a lymphoma was present from the start. In many patients only one or several enlarged lymph nodes is obvious. Yet when more extensive examination with lymphangiography or other tests is conducted, widespread lymphadenopathy, often symmetric, is easily revealed. The spleen of the patient with NPDL is often enlarged but generally asymptomatic at the onset of the disease. Involvement of the lymphoid tissue in Waldeyer's ring and epitrochlear lymph tissue is a more common clinical problem in patients with NPDL than in Hodgkin's disease. Paravertebral lymphoid masses may result in chylous pleural effusions or ascites or both. It is extremely rare for the central nervous system to become involved, although peripheral nerve compression and epidural tumor masses may develop. Some patients present with a clinical picture of lymphosarcoma cell leukemia, with white blood cell counts as high as 100,000 per cu mm, with evidence of nodular lymphoma in lymph nodes.

In contrast to patients with NPDL, those with the diffuse lymphomas, formerly called *reticulum cell sarcoma,* and diffuse lymphocytic lymphomas often present with localized lymph node enlargement or local extralymphatic manifestation. However, the natural history is more aggressive than in NPDL, with rapid growth of tumor masses. In approximately one fourth of the cases diagnosed, the disease is localized to only one side. The lymph nodes most frequently involved are predominantly located in the neck. Involvement of the gastrointestinal tract, bone, thyroid, testes, brain, and the lymph node tissue of Waldeyer's ring also occurs frequently. The bone marrow is involved initially in less than 10 per cent of the patients and is not commonly involved even late in the course of the disease. Patients with diffuse well-differentiated lymphoma have a natural history that mimics chronic lymphocytic leukemia, except that their disease begins by causing lymph node swelling before involvement of the blood or bone marrow. These patients often present with widespread asymptomatic modestly enlarged lymph nodes.

COURSE

Hodgkin's Disease. The asymptomatic adenopathy of a patient with Hodgkin's disease may wax and wane in size for months prior to diagnosis. Indeed, previous chest x-rays occasionally reveal that evidence of mediastinal widening has been present for several years before the diagnosis. If left untreated slow progression of the disease occurs, commonly by extension to contiguous lymph node areas. Once the hilar lymph nodes have been invaded, the tumor mass usually progresses to involve the pulmonary parenchyma. At some point in the progression of the disease, blood vessel invasion may occur. Involvement of the spleen, an organ that has no afferent lymphatics, occurs frequently in Hodgkin's disease. It suggests that vascular invasion may be a common occurrence, even in patients with apparently localized disease. Later, with further progression of the disease and clear evidence of vascular invasion, the bone marrow, liver, and other viscera are often invaded by tumor. Symptoms, if they had not appeared initially, appear as the volume of tumor increases. Cachexia, complicating infection, and widespread involvement of visceral organs by tumor usually overcome the host and cause death. It should be noted that the development of curative treatments has interrupted this bleak outlook for the vast majority of patients with Hodgkin's disease.

Lymphocytic and Histiocytic Lymphomas. The clinical course of nodular lymphoma is variable. In some, the course is indolent and lymphadenopathy may have been present for years before the diagnosis and may be well tolerated by the patient for 5 years or more after the diagnosis is established. The disease is malignant, however, and although there may be spontaneous regression of lymphadenopathy, clinical progression invariably occurs. In some patients the course of the disease progresses rapidly from the time of diagnosis. These patients may experience difficulties within months of the diagnosis.

When the disease becomes much more aggressive, lymph nodes enlarge rapidly, often in localized sites. Fever, night sweats, and weight loss can occur. If repeat biopsy is performed at the time of progression, the histologic appearance may be observed to have changed from nodular to that of a diffuse lymphoma with effacement of the lymph node. There are many similarities between nodular poorly differentiated lymphoma and the less frequently occurring nodular mixed lymphoma. The latter does differ, however, in overall prognosis, resembling that of those patients with diffuse large cell (histiocytic) lymphoma.

The diffuse lymphomas consist of a number of different types with a variable clinical evolution. The most indolent type is diffuse well-differentiated lymphocytic lymphoma. The clinical course and outcome are nearly the same as in chronic lymphocytic leukemia. When the diffuse small cell type does evolve to a large B cell type, death results from bone marrow failure, that leads to hypogammaglobinemia and subsequent fatal infections. The diffuse poorly differentiated lymphocytic lymphomas and diffuse mixed-cell lymphomas present much like the nodular lymphomas but evolve much more rapidly.

"Histiocytic" lymphoma is highly invasive, and involvement of peripheral nerves, epidural tumors, compression of the vena cava or airways, and destruction of osseous tissue often occur during the course of the disease. The skin, liver, kidneys, lung, and even the brain may be involved. Occasionally, bone marrow invasion results with the appearance of large, undifferentiated cells in the peripheral blood.

HISTOPATHOLOGY

Hodgkin's Disease. The diagnosis and classification of Hodgkin's disease can be made only by biopsy and histopathologic examination of tissue under a light microscope. Aspiration biopsy of lymph nodes never provides enough tissue to adequately subclassify the disease. The Sternberg-Reed cell is the characteristic malignant cell of Hodgkin's disease. If such cells are absent, the diagnosis of Hodgkin's disease should rarely be made. However, the presence of a Sternberg-Reed cell by itself is not diagnostic, since cells simulating Sternberg-Reed cells have been found in patients with mononucleosis and breast cancer. However, if a patient's condition has been previously diagnosed as Hodgkin's disease, the presence of the mononuclear variety of the Sternberg-Reed cell is sufficient to diagnose Hodgkin's disease involving the liver or bone marrow.

Lymphocytic and Histiocytic Lymphomas. The diagnosis of the lymphocytic and histiocytic lymphoma is also made by histopathologic examination of biopsy material usually obtained from lymph nodes. The diagnosis and classification of tissue obtained from other extranodal sites may be more difficult.

PHYSICAL EXAMINATION AND STAGING

Hodgkin's Disease. Accurate staging is vital for planning long-term management (Table 3). The primary physician must take a detailed history, do a through physical examination, and look for any evidence of "B" symptoms. Fever, weight loss of 10 per cent or greater, and soaking night sweats usually mean serious disease. The physician should be cautious to elicit a history of sweats that have taken place before the patient learned of his diagnosis, for soaking night sweats can occur in anxious patients.

The physician should carefully examine every lymph node area of the body. The presence or absence of nodal enlargement should be noted. If enlarged, the size, shape, and consistency of each node should be accurately recorded. The largest lymph nodes in a group should be selected for biopsy. Nodes in areas other than the primary site should be biopsied at the same time, especially if confirmation of spread of disease changes the stage of a patient. An examination of the oropharynx and nasopharynx by indirect laryngoscopy is essential to uncovering Waldeyer ring involvement by lymphoma. Such involvement occurs in less than 1 per cent of patients with Hodgkin's disease but is present in 15 to 33 per cent of patients with non-Hodgkin's lymphoma.

Table 3. Staging Classification for Lymphomas*

Stage	Definition
I	Involvement of a single lymph node region (I) or of a single extralymphatic organ or site (I_E)
II	Involvement of two or more lymph node regions on the same side of the diaphragm (II) or localized involvement of an extralymphatic organ or site and of one or more lymph node regions on the same side of the diaphragm (II_E)
III	Involvement of lymph node regions on both sides of the diaphragm (III), which may also be accompanied by involvement of the spleen (III_S) or by localized involvement of an extralymphatic organ site (III_E) or both (III_{SE})
IV	Diffuse or disseminated involvement of one or more extralymphatic organs or tissues, with or without associated lymph node involvement

The presence of fever, night sweats and/or unexplained loss of 10 per cent or more of body weight in the 6 months preceding admission are denoted by the suffix letter B. The letter A indicates the absence of these symptoms.

Biopsy-documented involvement of Stage IV sites is also denoted by letter suffixes: marrow = M+; lung = L+; liver = H+; pleura = P+; bone = O+; skin and subcutaneous tissue = D+.

*Adopted at the workshop on the staging of Hodgkin's Disease held at Ann Arbor, Michigan, April 1971.

The size of the liver and spleen should be recorded. In Hodgkin's disease, palpable splenomegaly is significant because if this is present, spleen involvement by the disease is likely and thus more generalized disease exists. The technical procedures required for staging patients with Hodgkin's disease under various circumstances are shown in Table 4.

Radiologic examination should include a routine chest film. If positive, whole chest tomography should be performed to identify the extent of mediastinal or hilar adenopathy or evidence of contiguous invasion of the lung from the hilar nodes. Lower extremity lymphangiogram is of paramount importance and should be required unless medically contraindicated. Occasionally, the lymphangiogram will not fill high retroperitoneal lymph nodes. Techniques that can be of use in supplementing lymphangiography are computerized axial tomography and on occasion ultrasound. If a patient is symptomatic with bone pain, separate skeletal survey and a technetium (^{99m}Tc) pyrophosphate bone scan should be performed. The latter is the more sensitive test for identifying bone lesions. Skin, subcutaneous tissue, and breast involvement is more common in patients with advancing systemic disease rather than at initial diagnosis. Bone involvement is also most commonly a sign of advanced disease, but invasion of bone adjacent to massive adenopathy can occur.

Laparotomy should not be considered routine in the staging work-up. Since general treatment strategy may markedly influence the decision to perform a staging laparotomy, the type of treatment to be used by either the radiotherapist or medical oncologist should be considered before a decision is made to operate.

In the United States, the mortality from staging laparotomy in Hodgkin's disease is 1.5 per cent, with a complication rate of approximately 12 per cent. In institutions in which laparotomies are done infrequently, mortality rates up to 6.6 per cent and morbidity rates of more than 25 per cent have been reported. Thus, for some stages of Hodgkin's disease, the operative mortality may exceed the expected death rate at 5 years from the disease!

When performed, the laparotomy should always be complete. The procedure should include at least two needle biopsies of each lobe of the liver, a wedge biopsy of the liver edge, biopsies of suspicious areas, splenectomy, and biopsy of selected lymph nodes in the retroperitoneal area, marked on the lymphangiogram before the operation. Nodes in the porta hepatis should also be biopsied. A postoperative film should confirm that the proper lymph nodes were removed. A wedge biopsy of the iliac bone should also be performed. Lastly, female patients in the reproductive years should have the ovaries moved laterally or centrally to avoid the majority of the radiation ports.

Laparoscopy has now been shown to be a useful alternative approach to laparotomy in staging abdominal disease. The spleen may be the only site involved below the diaphragm. If the spleen does not show evidence of Hodgkin's disease, the liver is almost never involved. Patients having a high risk of liver involvement are those with a positive lymphangiogram result in the region of the para-aortic nodes, those with splenomegaly, or those with poor-risk histology such as lymphocyte-depleted or mixed cellularity types. These patients should have the liver biopsied. This can be done during laparotomy or laparoscopy.

Lymphocytic and Histiocytic Lymphomas. The staging classification developed for Hodgkin's disease is also used in the other lymphomas; the sequence of staging procedures differs, however, because extralymphatic presentations occur more frequently in non-Hodgkin's lymphomas than in Hodgkin's disease.

The histologic patterns of lymphocytic and histiocytic lymphomas correlate with specific disease patterns, response to therapy, and prognosis. Thus the patterns are a valuable aid in determining the staging procedures needed to select the appropriate treatment strategy for a particular patient. Further, since many physicians approach the treatment of Stage III and Stage IV disease in a similar manner, this distinction may be far less relevant in lymphocytic and histiocytic lymphomas than in Hodgkin's disease. Surgical staging clearly should not be considered a routine procedure in patients with lymphocytic and histiocytic lymphomas, since extensive disease can often be identified by simpler diagnostic technique. The major task of staging is to determine whether the patient has limited nodal or extranodal "E" disease, which may be radiocurable (Stage I or II), or disseminated disease, which always requires systemic therapy (Stage III or IV). For patients who, after clinical staging, still appear to have localized disease and are considered eligible for curative radiotherapy, extensive surgical staging evaluation may then be justified. In those whose age or general medical problems limit therapy to local palliation with radiotherapy or systemic treatment with a single drug, few invasive staging procedures are indicated.

Table 4. Staging Work-up of Hodgkin's Disease

1. Adequate surgical biopsy, reviewed by an experienced hematopathologist
2. A detailed history recording the absence or presence of and duration of fever, unexplained sweating and its severity, unexplained pruritus, and unexplained weight loss.
3. A careful and detailed physical examination; special attention to all node-bearing areas, including Waldeyer's ring, and determination of size of liver and spleen
4. Laboratory procedures
   a. Complete blood count, including an erythrocyte sedimentation rate
   b. Serum alkaline phosphatase
   c. Evaluation of renal function
   d. Evaluation of liver function
   e. Bone marrow biopsy if a. or b. is elevated or there is evidence of bone disease by scan or x-ray
5. Radiologic studies
   a. Chest roentgenogram (posteroanterior and lateral) Whole-chest tomography if any abnormality is noted or suspected on the routine chest x-ray
   b. Intravenous pyelogram
   c. Bilateral lower extremity lymphogram Inferior cavography, ultrasonograph, or CT scanning to supplement equivocal lymphographic findings in the high retroperitoneal area
   d. Views of skeletal system to include thoracic and lumbar vertebrae, pelvis, proximal extremities, and any areas of bone tenderness
6. Exploratory laparotomy and splenectomy—only if identification of abdominal disease will change the proposed management plan

LABORATORY FINDINGS

Routine blood counts, erythrocyte sedimentation rate, urinalysis, liver function studies, and renal function studies are all necessary parts of the medical work-up of a patient with lymphoma, but by themselves they do not provide information on the extent of disease or specific organ involvement.

Patients with Hodgkin's disease who do not have symptoms and have disease localized above the diaphragm, with a negative lymphangiogram, do not need the bone marrow examination, since they rarely have bone marrow involvement. In patients with symptoms or the lymphocyte-depleted type, bone marrow involvement is more frequently observed. All other lymphoma patients should routinely have a bone marrow examination. Bone marrow involvement occurs most frequently with diffuse well-differentiated lymphocytic lymphoma and poorly differentiated lymphocytic lymphoma (nodular or diffuse) (50 to 60 per cent) but less frequently with diffuse histiocytic lymphomas (10 per cent). In patients with the diffuse types of lymphoma with bone marrow involvement, cytologic examination of the spinal fluid should be done, since this group of patients are candidates for prophylactic therapy of the central nervous system.

If a bone marrow examination is to be done, a bone marrow biopsy rather than aspiration is required.

Marrow aspiration does not yield results comparable to those obtained by biopsy. This is likely due to the fibrosis and granuloma formation in the marrow of patients with Hodgkin's disease. On smear or section, the myeloid-to-erythroid ratio may be increased and marrow eosinophilia is common; neither finding, however, is diagnostic of marrow involvement. Involvement of the marrow by tumor is demonstrated by finding either classic Sternberg-Reed cells or their mononuclear variant distributed focally or diffusely throughout the bone marrow. Marrow involvement marring the normal marrow architecture is often associated with reticular fibrosis. In a previously diagnosed patient with Hodgkin's disease, intense marrow fibrosis, even in the absence of the characteristic Sternberg-Reed cells, constitutes strong evidence of tumor in the bone marrow. Effective treatment by chemotherapy that results in a remission can lead to total resolution of this type of fibrosis.

Anemia, neutropenia, and thrombocytopenia can occur in either Hodgkin's disease or the other lymphomas and can be, but are not commonly, the consequence of bone marrow involvement. These conditions may also be caused by a variety of other conditions for which a systematic search must be conducted. Among these conditions are hypersplenism, immunologic mechanisms, blood loss secondary to gastrointestinal infiltration and ulceration, or complications of therapy. Patients with Hodgkin's disease frequently demonstrate a moderate normochromic, normocytic anemia associated with low serum iron and low iron-binding capacity but normal or increased iron stores in the bone marrow. This anemia has been shown to be due to both increased destruction and decreased production of red blood cells. In general terms, the anemia correlates with the extent and duration of the disease.

Coombs' positive hemolytic anemia occurs in less than 1 per cent of patients with advanced diffuse or nodular lymphomas and Hodgkin's disease. It is seen with greater frequency in both the diffuse well-differentiated and the diffuse poorly differentiated types of lymphocytic lymphoma. Coombs' negative hemolytic anemia may also be present. Chronic illness resulting in a poor nutritional status and consequent folate deficiency may also contribute to the picture of anemia. Finally, radiotherapy or chemotherapy or both can result in diminished or ineffective erythropoiesis.

A moderate to marked leukemoid reaction is often observed in Hodgkin's disease. This is most common in those patients who are symptomatic. The leukemoid reaction disappears with successful treatment of the underlying Hodgkin's disease and does not indicate involvement of the marrow by tumor.

The leukemic phase of lymphoma is seen most frequently in the lymphocytic lymphomas, usually late in the disease. This type of leukemic invasion of the peripheral blood is rare in other lymphomas such as diffuse histiocytic lymphomas or Hodgkin's disease. In well-differentiated lymphocytic lymphomas, the leukemic cells are usually identical to those seen in chronic lymphocytic leukemia; in the leukemic phase of poorly differentiated lymphocytic lymphoma, they are larger and less mature and often have cleft nuclei, the so-called "buttock" cells. Leukopenia in an untreated patient suggests bone marrow infiltration or hypersplenism. In the patient undergoing therapy, leukopenia is usually due to the therapy. Thrombocytosis occurs occasionally in Hodgkin's disease and even less frequently in the other lymphomas. Frequently following staging splenectomy, the platelet count rises briefly. More often, thrombocytopenia occurs because of bone marrow replacement by lymphoma, hypersplenism, or therapy. Patients with Hodgkin's disease who have pruritus are often found to have a mild elevation of the peripheral eosinophil count.

In about 80 per cent of patients with Hodgkin's disease the erythrocyte sedimentation rate (ESR) is elevated, but less frequently so in lymphocytic and histiocytic lymphomas. The ESR may serve as a useful test to follow disease activity. However, its usefulness is limited by its sensitivity, for it may return to normal when residual disease is obviously still present. It can be a useful test to monitor patients who are in remission to determine the first evidence of recurrence. Caution must be used, however, for extensive radiation therapy may cause the ESR to be elevated for as long as 1 year after treatment without evidence of recurrent tumor. Numerous more complicated and usually more expensive laboratory tests such as C-reactive protein, fibrinogen, serum copper level, and haptoglobin and $alpha_2$ glycoproteins that indicate disease activity have not been shown to be superior to the ESR.

Jaundice may be caused by obstruction of the biliary duct by portal lymph nodes or by infiltration of liver secondary to hematogenous spread. The liver is most frequently involved at diagnosis in the three types of diffuse lymphocytic lymphomas (poorly differentiated, well differentiated, and mixed cell) and less often in histiocytic lymphoma. Splenomegaly or retroperitoneal lymphadenopathy or both can usually be demonstrated. Liver function abnormalities are poor indicators of Hodgkin's involvement of the liver but serve as a useful tool to rule out the presence of other complications or illnesses. In Hodgkin's disease, liver involvement is most commonly seen in patients with mixed cellularity or lymphocytic depletion type who have splenomegaly and symptoms. The differential diagnosis of jaundice must include hemolytic anemia and drug toxicity. Pathologic examination of the liver, spleen, lymph nodes, or bone marrow may show noncaseating granulomas. This sarcoid-like reaction is of no significance and does not indicate involvement of the liver by tumor.

Renal function tests may be abnormal secondary to renal obstruction, hyperuricemia, hypercalcemic nephropathy, or occasionally membranous glomerulopathy owing to immune complex deposition. Rarely, a nephrotic syndrome may result. Generally, other routine blood chemistry tests such as electrolytes, glucose, and blood lipids are normal.

Serum protein abnormalities occur most often in patients with Hodgkin's disease, and less often in the other lymphomas. A polyclonal hypergammaglobulinemia involving $alpha_1$, $alpha_2$, and beta fractions is the most frequent occurrence. This type of elevation is seen in 40 per cent of Hodgkin's disease patients; less frequently in the other lymphomas. Paraproteinemia may occur in lymphocytic lymphomas, especially in diffuse well-differentiated lymphocytic lymphoma, and has occasionally been observed in Hodgkin's disease. Hypogammaglobulinemia may precede the onset of either diffuse well-differentiated or diffuse poorly differentiated lymphocytic lymphoma and occurs eventually in 60 per cent of these patients. This is seen less frequently in advanced Hodgkin's disease. Immunoglobulin levels are usually not decreased in patients with lymphoma. The presence of anergy, or decreased in vitro lymphocyte phytohemagglutinin response, has now been shown to have no influence on prognosis within a given clinical stage when modern therapy is used. Thus routine testing for these findings is unnecessary. This surprising observation indicates that effective antitumor treatment can eradicate disease in patients already immunosuppressed by their disease even when the drugs themselves are immunosuppressive. However, cellular immune function appears to be less affected in lymphocytic and histiocytic lymphoma patients than in Hodgkin's disease.

Radiologic findings such as the demonstration of a mediastinal mass may be the first clue to the diagnosis in an otherwise asymptomatic patient. Nodular infiltrates and pleural effusion secondary to tumor or lymphatic obstruction also occur. If extension of the tumor has led to the pericardium, an effusion and cardiomegaly may be noted on the chest x-ray. Gastrointestinal radiographs may demonstrate any number of abnormalities, including mass lesions, malabsorption pattern, splenomegaly, hepatomegaly, or obliteration of the psoas shadow, especially in patients with lymphocytic or histiocytic lymphoma.

PITFALLS IN DIAGNOSIS

The lymphadenopathy of Hodgkin's disease must be distinguished from adenopathy from other causes. Cervical or axillary adenopathy in young people commonly occurs as a result of infectious diseases with fever. However, headache and pharyngitis that occur in infectious disease usually do not occur in Hodgkin's disease. To be considered in the differential diagnosis are a number of diseases, including infectious mononucleosis, viral disease syndromes, or infection by *Toxoplasma gondii.* Local and lymphatic spread of head and neck cancers should also be included in the differential of older age populations. A good rule of thumb in all patients is that any lymph node 1 cm or larger in diameter that does not show signs of regression after 6 weeks of observation should be biopsied.

A patient presenting with mediastinal and hilar adenopathy may have sarcoidosis or primary tuberculosis. The former is distinguished from Hodgkin's disease in that it is nearly always pan-hilar. Tuberculosis, on the other hand, is unilateral like Hodgkin's disease but almost always has evidence of a resolving pulmonary infection and usually does not cause mediastinal lymph node enlargement. In older patients, one must also include primary tumors of the lung and mediastinum, specifically oat cell and epidermoid carcinomas, in the differential. Reactive mediastinitis and hilar adenopathy owing to histoplasmosis must be considered in patients who live or have traveled in regions where histoplasmosis is endemic. Further, histoplasma mediastinitis can involve the esophagus and should be considered if a history of difficulty in swallowing is obtained and subsequently confirmed by an abnormal esophagram. Occasionally, a biopsy may be necessary to confirm this diagnosis. Hodgkin's disease presenting as "fever of undetermined origin" may remain undiagnosed despite extensive investigations until an exploratory laparotomy is undertaken. Infrequently, patients present with autoimmune hemolytic anemia or idiopathic thrombocytopenia purpura and are found to have Hodgkin's disease only when splenectomy becomes necessary. It is of interest that in some of these cases Hodgkin's disease in the removed spleen has been the only focus of involvement with tumor.

COMPLICATIONS OF HODGKIN'S DISEASE AND LYMPHOCYTIC AND HISTIOCYTIC LYMPHOMA

The complications of lymphoma are many and may be due to progressive enlargement of lymph nodes, involvement of parenchymal organs, and hematologic, metabolic, or immunologic abnormalities.

Progressive lymph node enlargement causes compression or obstruction of surrounding structures such as vascular structures (superior vena cava syndrome), airway, esophagus, the urinary tract, or the gastrointestinal tract. Serious complications may ensue, depending on the site affected.

Direct infiltration of the lymphoma from involved mediastinal lymph nodes into the parenchyma of the lung, pleura, pericardium, and heart may occur. Infiltration from retroperitoneal lymph nodes through lymphatic channels leads to involvement of the gastrointestinal tract and may result in ulceration, perforation, hemorrhage, intussusception, or malabsorption.

Cord compression is the most serious acute neurologic complication caused by growing tumor masses and is usually observed in patients with progressive tumor whose primary treatment has failed. It can be caused by vertebral body involvement with collapse, which is easily seen on x-ray or bone scan, or by invasion of the epidural space from retroperitoneal lymph nodes with compression of the cord or compression of the vascular supply to the cord. Selective electromyelography is a useful way to detect regional denervation, but a myelogram is usually needed to confirm the diagnosis.

Central nervous system involvement may also occur by direct extension of tumor from the mediastinum or retroperitoneum to the spinal canal. Symptoms of cord compression produced in this way occur more often in Hodgkin's disease than with the other lymphomas. This is observed most frequently in those patients who have diffuse histiocytic lymphoma. Cranial nerves and brain may be affected by the lymphomas. Occasionally, lymphomatous meningitis may occur, and lymphoma cells, high protein, and low glucose appear in the spinal fluid. If a patient with diffuse histiocytic lymphoma has bone marrow involvement, a spinal tap is always indicated, since subsequent meningeal involvement occurs with such high frequency that prophylactic intrathecal therapy is recommended.

Bizarre neurologic manifestations occur rarely without demonstrable direct involvement by lymphoma. Progressive multifocal leukoencephalopathy, subacute cerebellar degeneration, myelopathy, and neuropathy have also been described. Occasionally, polymyositis may occur. The differential diagnosis of these central and peripheral nervous system complications includes bacterial and viral meningitis, herpes zoster, and drug toxicity, particularly when drugs such as the vinca alkaloids are used.

The lung may also be involved by direct extension either from mediastinal-hilar lymph nodes or by hematogenous spread. In the lymphocyte-predominant type of Hodgkin's disease and in nodular poorly differentiated lymphocytic lymphoma, the lungs are rarely involved; in contrast, the nodular sclerosis type of Hodgkin's disease frequently involves the lungs. Pleural involvement by lymphoma with malignant effusion may occur with or without lymphoma of the lung. Pneumonia is a frequent complication of treatment and constitutes the major differential diagnosis of lymphoma. Bleomycin, methotrexate, and other drugs used to treat these diseases may cause pulmonary manifestations and their toxicity must be considered in the differential diagnosis of lung disease in patients undergoing treatment.

Skin involvement occurs as part of hematogenous dissemination of the lymphoma. A number of nonspecific skin lesions occur in lymphoma, including excoriations secondary to pruritus, urticaria, erythema multiforme, erythema nodosum, exfoliative dermatitis, and dermatomyositis.

Metabolic abnormalities may occur as a consequence of the lymphoma or therapy. Hyperuricemia is seen most often in patients who have a large volume of tumor. Effective therapy results in a rapid reduction of the tissue mass and may exacerbate the hyperuricemia, leading to a decrease in renal function and infrequently to gouty arthritis. Hydration and administration of allopurinol can prevent these complications. Hypercalcemia occurs in less than 10 per cent of patients, most frequently in diffuse histiocytic lymphoma and Hodgkin's disease of the lymphocyte-depleted and mixed-cellularity types. The hypercalcemia is usually related to destruction of bone by the tumor but may be due to the release of parathyroid-like substance. Hypercalcemia also requires prompt and appropriate therapy.

Infections are common in patients with Hodgkin's disease. Those who have progressive tumor usually die of complications of bone marrow failure, bacterial septicemia, or disseminated fungal infections. Diffuse pulmonary infiltrates may appear in patients who are in remission between cycles of chemotherapy, radiotherapy, or both; infection with the protozoan *Pneumocystis carinii* should be suspected. Patients with Hodgkin's disease are also prone to develop cryptococcosis, either in the form of meningitis or as a primary pulmonary infiltrate with or without meningitis. Herpes zoster occurs in 10 per cent of treated Hodgkin's patients and in 10 per cent of treated patients who have had a splenectomy. Most patients who develop herpes zoster have a few scattered papules outside the involved dermatome; this minimal evidence of spread does not generally warrant systemic treatment.

SUMMARY

Malignant lymphomas can be diagnosed only after biopsy of involved tissue and histopathologic classification. A detailed history, physical examination, supportive laboratory, radiographic, and further biopsy information are useful in documenting the extent of the disease. Following these procedures, the physician is prepared to make appropriate management decisions that can result in long-term disease-free survival for the majority of patients afflicted with these highly treatable tumors.

MULTIPLE MYELOMA AND OTHER PLASMA CELL DISORDERS

By Gibbons G. Cornwell, III, M.D.
Hanover, New Hampshire

MULTIPLE MYELOMA

Synonyms

Plasma cell myeloma, myelomatosis.

Definition

Multiple myeloma may be defined as a neoplastic proliferative disease of plasma cells involving hematopoietic bone marrow throughout the body. The typical presentation of this disease includes bone marrow involvement by immature plasma cells, the presence of a serum and/or urine monoclonal protein produced by the malignant plasma cell clone, evidence of bone marrow failure, and lytic bone lesions. A diagnosis may be difficult in patients with a mild degree of plasmacytosis in the bone marrow and a circulating monoclonal protein of low concentration. For this reason, a number of diagnostic criteria have been established. In general, the diagnosis depends on (1) a bone marrow plasmacytosis of 10 per cent or greater with immature plasma cells present, and/or (2) one or more plasmacytomas. In addition, there must be at least one of the following: (1) a monoclonal IgG or IgA in the serum; (2) a monoclonal kappa or lambda light chain in the urine; or (3) osteolytic lesions on x-ray.

Stage of Disease

Multivariate analyses of disease parameters at diagnosis have permitted classification of patients with multiple myeloma as *good* or *poor* risk or as having *low* (Stage I), *intermediate* (Stage II), or *high* (Stage III) tumor burden (Table 1). In general, patients with renal insufficiency, high levels of monoclonal proteins, severe anemia, and poor performance score have the worst prognosis. Such classifications may determine the rationale for selecting specific therapy in any given patient.

Presenting Signs and Symptoms

The clinical effects of multiple myeloma may be very subtle during early stages of the disease. Patients may present with symptoms of mild anemia only. Anemia associated with back pain or other bone pain should be suggestive of multiple myeloma. The presence of a monoclonal IgG in the serum rarely leads to symptoms of hyperviscosity, although this complication is more common in patients with monoclonal IgA.

Presence of Bence Jones proteinuria (monoclonal free kappa or lambda light chains) increases the risk of renal failure. Patients may rarely present with symptoms of hypercalcemia, but this complication is generally associated with significant bone involvement in patients with prior symptoms of bone pain or pathologic fractures. Because multiple myeloma is usually confined to the bone marrow (although a small number of circulating plasma cells may be found in most patients), generalized organ involvement is not common. The presence of a plasmacytoma, on the other hand, may lead to a wide range of presenting signs and symptoms associated with involvement of the gastrointestinal tract, the spinal cord and nerve roots, or the head and neck.

Course of Disease

Multiple myeloma is usually a slowly progressive disease and, despite the possibility of stabilization with therapy, is rarely cured (less than 5 per cent). Patients eventually die from infection or renal failure, often associated with decreased mobility related to bone disease. Patients with good risk disease (median survival 3 to 4 years) may do very well for extended periods of time on no treatment or conservative therapy. Patients with poor risk disease (median survival 1 to 2 years) generally fail rapidly or show relatively short periods of stable disease irrespective of therapy. Such patients have a course of recurrent infections and complications of bone pain with pathologic fractures, and frequently require blood transfusions as their disease progresses.

Common Complications

Infections. Most patients with a monoclonal serum protein will demonstrate polyclonal hypogammaglobulinemia. This decrease in normal antibody production predisposes patients to gram-positive and

Table 1. Stages of Myeloma

Risk Category (CALGB)	Tumor Burden (Durie and Salmon)*
Good *All of the following:* Hgb ⩾ 8.5 g/dl BUN < 30 mg/dl Performance Score of 0 (Normal) or 1 (Ambulatory) or 2 (< 50% bedridden)	*Low* (Stage I) *All of the following:* Hgb > 10 g/dl Ca^{++} ⩽ 12 mg/dl M protein IgG < 5 gm/dl IgA < 3 gm/dl BJP < 4 gm/day Normal bone structure or solitary plasmacytoma only
Poor *One or more of the following:* Hgb < 8.5 gm/dl BUN ⩾ 30 mg/dl Performance Score of 3 (⩾ 50% bedridden) or 4 (100% bedridden)	*Intermediate* (Stage II) Fitting neither Stage I nor Stage III *High* (Stage III) *One or more of the following:* Hgb < 8.5 gm/dl Ca^{++} > 12 mg/dl M protein IgG > 7 gm/dl IgA > 5 gm/dl BJP > 12 gm/day Advanced lytic bone lesions A = creatinine < 2 mg/dl B = creatinine ⩾ 2 mg/dl

*Durie, B.T.M., and Salmon, S.E.: Cancer, 36:842, 1975.

Abbreviations: BJP = Urinary Bence Jones protein; BUN = blood urea nitrogen; Hgb = hemoglobin; CALGB = Cancer and Leukemia Group B.

gram-negative infections. There is some preliminary indication that patients with certain subtypes of monoclonal antibodies have a greater frequency of infection on the basis of blocked F_c receptors on monocytes and macrophages. To date, it has not been shown that the infection rate can be diminished significantly by prophylactic gammaglobulin or polyvalent pneumococcal vaccine (Pneumovax).

Bone Destruction. Approximately two thirds of patients with myeloma will have lytic bone lesions at diagnosis. These abnormalities are thought to result from the release of an osteoclastic activating factor (OAF) by the malignant clone of plasma cells. For unknown reasons, appropriate compensatory osteoblastic reaction at the site of myelomatous bone lysis is lacking. Consequently, significant repair of lytic bone lesions (as determined by bone x-rays and alkaline phosphatase determinations) occurs in less than 10 per cent of patients. Bone destruction may be stabilized by appropriate therapy, but lytic lesions and osteoporosis may lead to pathologic fractures (including compression of vertebral bodies), particularly in weight-bearing bones. One of the most serious potential complications of tumor growth and bony destruction of the thoracic and lumbar spine is cord and nerve root compression with consequent paraparesis or paraplegia.

Hypercalcemia. This complication occurs as a result of increased bone catabolism and is complicated by dehydration and immobility resulting from pain and weakness.

Renal Insufficiency. Patients with multiple myeloma (especially those with Bence Jones proteinuria) are at risk of renal failure. Light chains are normally reabsorbed and metabolized by renal tubular cells, and it is believed that this process results in renal tubular damage in patients with multiple myeloma. In addition, hypercalcemia, hyperuricemia, and decreased renal perfusion (related to dehydration) may contribute to renal failure.

Hyperviscosity. Although the hyperviscosity syndrome is relatively rare in multiple myeloma, it should be suspected in any patient with confusion or a coagulapathy (with bleeding or thrombosis) of unknown cause. Patients with IgA and IgG_3 are most likely to develop hyperviscosity, presumably on the basis of increased propensity of these proteins to form aggregates. Although most institutions do not measure whole blood viscosity, serum viscosity measurements (normal 1.4 to 1.8) are usually greater than 4.0 in the presence of clinical effects from hyperviscosity.

Laboratory Procedures

Peripheral Blood Counts. A varying degree of anemia (normochromic, normocytic) is common in myeloma as a result of bone marrow failure and, in some patients, shortened red cell survival. As the disease becomes more advanced, pancytopenia is common. The peripheral blood smear will frequently show rouleaux formation resulting from the effects of monoclonal proteins on the surface charge of individual red blood cells.

Bone Marrow. The bone marrow typically shows spotty infiltration, with mature and immature plasma cells, which appears as sheets or nests on biopsy or clot sections. Careful study of individual cells with Wright's or Giemsa stain shows dyssynchrony in maturation of the nucleus and cytoplasm. Immature plasma cells frequently show large nucleoli, often contain cytoplasmic inclusions, and may contain multiple nuclei.

Myeloma Proteins. Ninety-six per cent of patients will show a monoclonal protein in the serum and/or urine. These will be distributed between serum IgG (60 per cent), IgA (20 per cent), IgD (1 per cent) and free urinary light chains only (15 per cent). The ratio of kappa to lambda light chains is 2:1. Eighty per cent of IgGs are subgroup 1 and 93 per cent of the IgAs are subgroup 1.

Miscellaneous. Significant hypercalcemia ($>$ 11.5 mg/dl) occurs in approximately 10 per cent of patients, blood urea nitrogen (BUN) $\geq$ 30 mg/dl in 30 per cent of patients.

X-rays

Lytic bone lesions or compression fractures of vertebral bodies will be present in approximately two thirds of patients, although about 90 per cent of patients will show evidence of osteolysis and/or osteoporosis. Since significant new bone formation does not generally occur in association with the bone lesions, bone scans are usually not helpful. At time of diagnosis, baseline x-rays of the lateral skull, spine, pelvis, and proximal upper long bones are helpful in following the progression of bone lesions.

Potential Errors and Pitfalls in Diagnosis

It is important to distinguish between multiple myeloma and benign monoclonal gammopathy (BMG). The latter disorder occurs in 3 per cent of persons over age 70 and is usually characterized by low levels of circulating monoclonal protein ($<$ 2.0 gm/dl), small numbers of mature-appearing plasma cells in the bone marrow, normal concentrations of polyclonal immunoglobulins, and the absence of lytic bone lesions. Patients with these abnormalities should be followed on a regular basis, since BMG may be associated with systemic illness or, in a small percentage of patients, may evolve into myeloma.

Variants of Multiple Myeloma

Light chain disease is a form of multiple myeloma that is manifest by hypogammaglobulinemia and Bence Jones proteinuria. Solitary or multiple *plasmacytomas* may involve osseous or extraosseous sites. The latter form of plasmacytoma is most likely to involve the head and neck. Patients with these types of tumors should be observed at regular intervals, since a high proportion (especially those with osseous involvement) will eventually develop multiple myeloma.

Plasma cell leukemia is a condition in which plasma cells predominate among circulating leukocytes. Patients generally respond poorly to therapy and have a median survival of approximately 9 months.

MACROGLOBULINEMIA

Primary macroglobulinemia is a variant of diffuse lymphocytic lymphoma or chronic lymphocytic leukemia. By definition, patients have an increased concentration of circulating monoclonal IgM (generally > 2.5 gm/dl) and approximately 25 per cent of patients also have Bence Jones proteinuria. Most patients complain of fatigue, weakness, and bleeding. Anemia occurs as a result of bone marrow failure, hemolysis, and bleeding; thrombocytopenia, neutropenia, and lymphocytosis may also be present. The bone marrow invariably contains increased numbers of small lymphocytes and lymphoplasmacytes. This entity differs from myeloma by the rarity of bone lesions and by greater frequency of lymph node involvement and hyperviscosity. Hyperviscosity represents the greatest threat to the patient, largely by causing thrombotic and bleeding complications.

HEAVY CHAIN DISEASE

Monoclonal fragments of alpha, gamma, and mu heavy chains of immunoglobulins have been described in a small number of patients.

Alpha (α) chain disease usually presents with chronic diarrhea and severe malabsorption. Intestinal biopsies have shown villous atrophy and diffuse lymphoplasmacytic cell infiltration of the mucosa. Lymph nodes, bone marrow, and peripheral blood may contain similar cells. The abnormal protein is secreted by mucosal cells and appears to contain the F_c and hinge regions of the $alpha_1$ heavy chain as well as the J chain. The course of the disease is generally rapidly progressive.

Gamma (γ) chain disease presents with generalized weakness, fever, lymphadenopathy, splenomegaly, and anemia. Bone marrow and other tissues may be infiltrated with plasma cells and lymphocytes, often in association with eosinophils. The circulating monoclonal protein is generally the F_c portion of a γ_1 subclass of IgG. Although the course of disease is variable, rapid progression is usual.

Mu (μ) chain disease is almost always associated with chronic lymphocytic leukemia. It differs from the latter disease, however, in that significant lymphadenopathy is uncommon, plasma cells are usually present and most patients excrete large amounts of kappa light chain in the urine.

PRIMARY AMYLOIDOSIS

Primary amyloidosis is a generalized form of amyloidosis that, although assumed to involve midline organs primarily, is usually widespread at the time of diagnosis. This form of amyloid is associated with a monoclonal immunoglobulin in the serum and/or monoclonal free light chain in the urine in more than 80 per cent of patients. The amyloid fibril protein characteristic of this group of diseases is usually a portion of the N-terminal variable region of lambda or kappa light chain (kappa/lambda = 0.5). In patients with multiple myeloma and amyloidosis (approximately 5 per cent of the latter group), amino acid homology between the amyloid fibril protein and the light chain of the myeloma protein has been present. The presentation at diagnosis depends upon the organ systems most prominently involved. Autonomic neuropathy is common and leads to diarrhea, postural hypotension, and visual difficulties. Direct involvement of the gastrointestinal tract is associated with malabsorption, and cardiac infiltration leads to cardiac enlargement, congestive heart failure, and arrhythmia. Renal involvement is usually limited to the glomeruli and results in nephrosis and edema. A rectal biopsy (including the submucosa) yields a diagnosis in 84 per cent of patients and kidney biopsy in 90 per cent of patients.

MYCOSIS FUNGOIDES AND SÉZARY SYNDROME

By Eric C. Vonderheid, M.D.
Philadelphia, Pennsylvania

SYNONYM

Cutaneous T cell lymphoma.

DEFINITION

Mycosis fungoides and Sézary syndrome are uncommon malignant lymphoproliferative disorders of thymic-derived (T) cells that preferentially infiltrate the skin. The "classical" form of mycosis fungoides (approximately 80 per cent of cases) refers to the sequential evolution of disease with time through three phases of skin involvement, defined imprecisely by the maximal degree of palpable infiltration at lesion sites. The first phase (erythematous, premycotic, or patch phase) evolves into the second phase (infiltrative, mycotic, or plaque phase) and then into the third phase (fungoid or tumor phase) as one or more lesions become raised above the skin surface from accumulation of neoplastic T cells.

The "erythrodermic" form of mycosis fungoides (approximately 15 per cent of cases) refers to the appearance of widespread or generalized erythema that may precede or follow plaque or tumor formation. This clinical presentation interfaces with Sézary syndrome, originally defined as the triad of generalized erythroderma, lymphadenopathy and large atypical mononuclear cells (cellules monstreuses) in the peripheral blood and tissues. Since a small cell variant of Sézary syndrome has been described in recent years, and since leukemic manifestations may occur in patients with extensive plaque or tumor disease, the current definition of Sézary syndrome has become more liberal.

The "tumeurs d'emblée" form of mycosis fungoides (approximately 5 per cent of cases) refers to the appearance of one or more nodules or tumors on otherwise normal skin without the development of antecedent patches or plaques, although these may appear later. This unusual mode of onset is controversial because it is mimicked by other non-Hodgkin's lymphomas involving the skin.

Because of overlapping clinical and cytologic features, mycosis fungoides and Sézary syndrome now are classified under the broader term "cutaneous T cell lymphoma" (CTCL) to emphasize common features of the group. The incidence of CTCL in the United States is one to two new cases per million of population. The disease usually appears after the fifth decade and affects males more often than females by a 2:1 ratio. No racial predilection is known.

PRESENTING SIGNS AND SYMPTOMS

Patients with CTCL (classical mycosis fungoides) usually present with circumscribed erythematous patches or mildly infiltrated plaques, each one tending to differ slightly in appearance from others in terms of size and shape, magnitude of infiltration, color hues or desquamation. Less commonly, patients with CTCL present with multiple erythematous patches that rapidly coalesce into a widespread or generalized erythrodermic state (erythrodermic mycosis fungoides/Sézary syndrome) or rarely present with nodules or tumors (mycosis fungoides "tumeurs d'emblée").

The major symptom that is associated with all forms of CTCL is pruritus, which is quite variable in occurrence and severity. In general, pruritus tends to be more severe in advanced disease and may interfere with normal sleep patterns. Rarely, pruritus may occur in the absence of objective skin infiltration and may be the initial manifestation of disease.

Apart from pruritus, most patients feel quite well even in the presence of advanced disease. Chills, with or without fever, are observed commonly in patients with erythrodermic presentations because of inappropriate loss of heat from the skin. Indeed, absolute hypothermia or concealed fever may be present in this circumstance. Fever may occur in patients with advanced disease and is more often the result of infection than tumor burden.

COURSE

The natural history of CTCL, exclusive of the "tumeurs d'emblée" mode of onset, is highly variable, frequently evolving slowly over many years or even decades. The unpredictable course of early disease presumably reflects poorly understood interactions of factors regulating tumor expansion and host resistance. Clinical and cytogenetic data suggest that the phenomenon of clonal evolution occurs in CTCL, eventually leading to the emergence of subpopulations of cells with increasingly malignant properties.

According to the literature, the median survival of patients with CTCL after histopathologic diagnosis is about 5 years. This figure may be inaccurate, since it is derived from patients who were referred to large treatment centers with relatively severe disease. The prognosis of patients is influenced adversely by extensive or advanced cutaneous involvement, the presence of enlarged superficial lymph nodes, and advanced age (more than 60 years). In one large series, the 5-year survival rate for patients with pretumorous mycosis fungoides involving less than 10 per cent of the skin surface was 90 per cent compared with 70 per cent for patients with more than 10 per cent involvement. The presence of cutaneous tumors and erythroderma resulted in a 5-year survival rate of 40 and 50 per cent respectively. In addition, the frequency of lymph node enlargement parallels the extent of skin involvement and connotes a worse prognosis for any given state of skin involvement, particularly if multiple nodes are present.

These observations reflect the importance that suspected or confirmed extracutaneous disease has on prognosis. Once lymph node involvement is demonstrated histopathologically, the median survival of patients is about 18 months. In late disease, any visceral organ may be involved, most commonly the lungs, spleen and liver, and the median survival probably is between 3 to 6 months. Aggressive therapy with total-skin electron beam radiation or sustained topical chemotherapy with mechlorethamine solutions seems to modify the course of intracutaneous CTCL and may even eradicate (cure) early disease in many instances.

COMMON COMPLICATIONS

Cell-mediated immunity becomes impaired in advanced disease, particularly when extracutaneous involvement is present. In addition, the functional integrity of the skin becomes impaired from extensive infiltration. Thick plaques or tumors frequently ulcerate and become secondarily colonized or infected with bacteria. Episodes of herpes zoster may be severe with widespread dissemination and associated bacterial septicemia. Infections with opportunistic organisms or persistent chronic infection with herpes simplex or Candida may also occur. For these reasons, infection is the most common cause of death of patients with CTCL.

Lymphomatous involvement of internal organs accounts for death in about one third of patients with CTCL. In many instances, the cause of death is difficult to ascertain and is attributed to generalized debility.

PHYSICAL EXAMINATION

The patch phase of "classical" mycosis fungoides is the most difficult to diagnose because significant cellular infiltration at lesions is not a feature. Although any portion of the skin may be involved, lesions frequently appear first on areas normally not exposed to sunlight such as the buttocks, periaxillary areas, or breasts.

Close inspection usually reveals the early lesions of mycosis fungoides to be diverse in size and shape and well demarcated from surrounding normal skin. Several diseased areas may merge together to form a larger patch with a serpiginous outline. In lightly pigmented patients, a subtle variation in erythematous hues from area to area is a characteristic finding (Fig. 1). In darkly pigmented patients, disturbances of melanin pigmentation may be the predominant finding; such patients often present with hypopigmented patches or demonstrate a zone of hypopigmentation surrounding patches (Fig. 2). Likewise, the epidermis may be thin and shiny (varnish-like), mildly scaly, or rarely psoriasiform in appearance. Telangiectasias commonly are present in atrophic areas. Combinations of these changes often produce a variegated appearance to the eruption referred to as *poikiloderma* (Fig. 3).

The early lesions of mycosis fungoides frequently are confused with psoriasis, eczema, tinea, or parapsoriasis. When pruritus is intense, secondary cutaneous changes such as excoriations and lichenification may be present and may make a clinical distinction impossible.

The plaque and tumor phases of "classical" mycosis fungoides are recognized more easily because variably infiltrated lesions occur in association with the patches described. Markedly infiltrated lesions tend to have a more violaceous color than mildly infiltrated ones, thus accentuating the differences in color hues from lesion to lesion. It is not uncommon for some lesions to regress spontaneously without scarring; this phenomenon may produce annular or arcuate patterns which are quite distinctive when present. Alopecia also may occur at lesional sites. Tumors may arise on pre-existing patches or plaques or from otherwise normal skin, and some of these may ulcerate spontaneously.

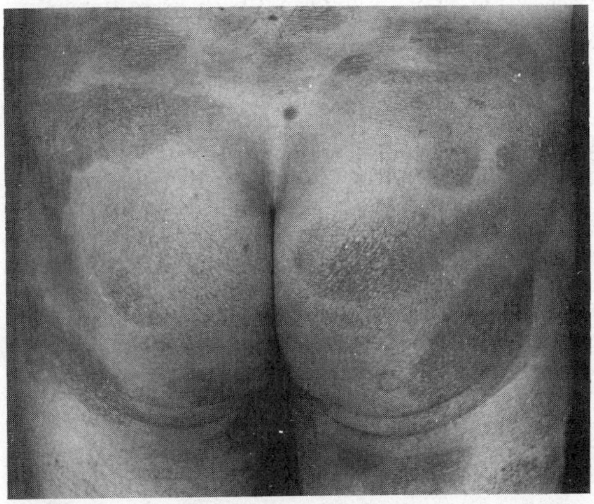

Figure 1. Typical patch-phase mycosis fungoides in a lightly pigmented patient. Note the variation in size, shape, and color hue of lesions.

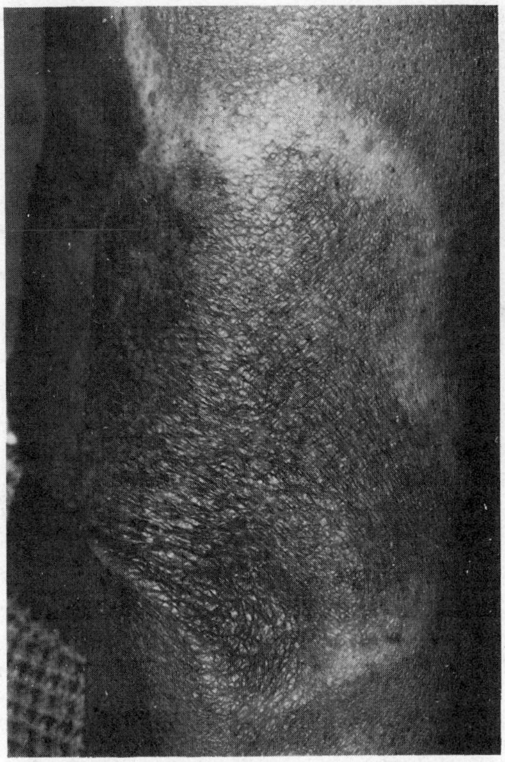

Figure 2. Typical patch-phase mycosis fungoides in a darkly pigmented patient. Note zone of hypopigmentation around the lesion.

Erythrodermic manifestations are usually generalized and may produce marked thickening of the skin of the palms and soles with painful fissuring, nail dystrophy, ectropion formation, and partial or total alopecia. Superimposed plaques or tumors may be present and would suggest the correct diagnosis. The "tumeurs d'emblée" form of CTCL is characterized by one or more nodules, often without alterations in the overlying epidermis.

The general examination usually is unremarkable, even when extensive skin disease is present. The most common finding is palpable lymph nodes that tend to be discrete, firm, and nontender. Peripheral edema may develop in patients with disease on the legs and does not necessarily signify involvement of regional lymph nodes by lymphoma. Spleen or liver enlargement is uncommon except in Sézary syndrome.

LABORATORY PROCEDURES

The diagnosis of CTCL is established most often by skin biopsy. The important histologic features consist of a dermal infiltrate that is located high in the dermis, often abutting against and invading the epidermis. The infiltrate contains an admixture of normal and atypical-appearing lymphocytes, histiocytes, and occasional eosinophils and/or plasma cells. The atypical lymphocytes may have large hyperchromatic nu-

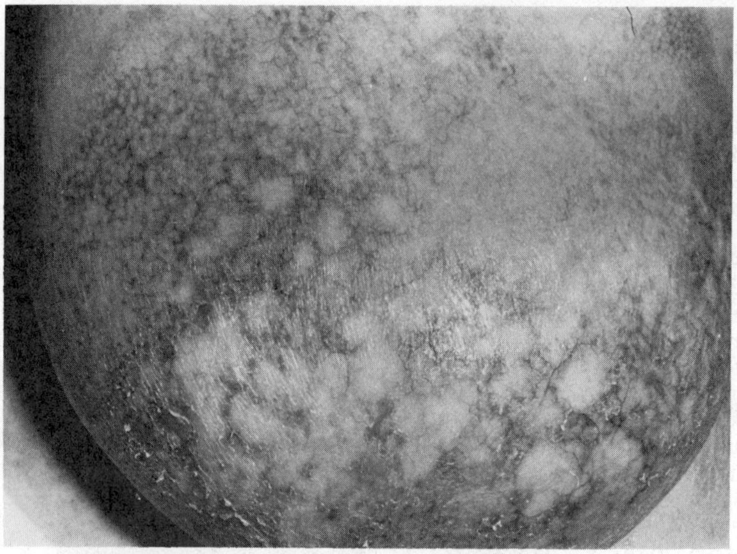

Figure 3. Patch-phase mycosis fungoides presenting as poikiloderma. Such variegated and atrophic changes usually reflect an indolent disease process.

clei (the so-called mycosis cell) or slightly enlarged nuclei with a highly infolded or cerebriform appearance (Lutzner or Sézary cells). The infoldings of cerebriform nuclei are best appreciated on tissue sections cut at 1 micron or by electron microscopy. The presence of clusters of atypical lymphocytes in the epidermis (Pautrier microabscesses) is almost pathognomonic of CTCL. However, on occasion the histopathologic features of CTCL may be closely simulated by benign eczematous dermatoses in which normal activated T-lymphocytes interact with the epidermis.

A lymph node biopsy is indicated on all patients with confirmed or suspected CTCL and palpable lymphadenopathy. The usual histopathologic finding is *dermatopathic lymphadenitis,* which refers to an expansion of the paracortical zones with pale-staining histiocytic cells often containing melanin. Scattered atypical lymphocytes with cerebriform nuclei often are seen, but a pathologic diagnosis of CTCL cannot be made with confidence unless there is marked cellular atypia or effacement of nodal architecture by large numbers of atypical cells. On occasion, diagnostic histopathologic features of CTCL are found in lymph node specimens rather than skin specimens, particularly in patients with erythroderma.

Routine blood studies and urinalysis are normal in most patients with CTCL until the disease is quite advanced. Patients with Sézary syndrome present with a variable leukocytosis with relative lymphocytosis on the complete blood count. Careful examination of blood smears will reveal the cerebriform nuclear morphology characteristic of circulating neoplastic T cells (Sézary cells). In our laboratory, a count of 20 Sézary cells per 100 lymphocytes is considered to be diagnostic of leukemic involvement. Smaller numbers of Sézary-like cells may be found in other forms of CTCL and in benign dermatoses. Electron microscopy, cytochemistry, membrane marker studies, and cytogenetic analysis are useful additional procedures to establish the presence of a neoplastic T cell population in the blood. In addition, the serum IgA or IgE levels may be elevated in CTCL, but this apparently does not have prognostic significance.

RADIOLOGIC EVALUATION

A chest x-ray and computed tomography (CT) of the retroperitoneum are useful noninvasive procedures that may reveal clinically inapparent extracutaneous involvement in patients with advanced CTCL. Bipedal lymphography also may be obtained to evaluate patients for the presence and extent of nodal disease, but it must be remembered that dermatopathic alterations of nodal architecture per se may produce filling defects quite suggestive of lymphoma, particularly in the femoral-inguinal nodes. Therefore a lymph node biopsy always should be performed to assess the significance of abnormal findings on lymphography.

OTHER DIAGNOSTIC PROCEDURES

Liver-spleen and whole-body scintigraphy are not very helpful procedures in detecting occult internal disease, but may be abnormal with gross tumor involvement. At the present time, routine laparotomy for staging purposes does not seem to be advisable.

THERAPEUTIC TESTS

There are no specific therapeutic tests to enhance the diagnosis of CTCL. Physicians must remember that the lesions of CTCL may respond temporarily to treatments used for eczema or psoriasis such as topical or systemic corticosteroids, ultraviolet light, and methotrexate, and this may delay the correct diagnosis.

POTENTIAL ERRORS AND PITFALLS IN DIAGNOSIS

The major potential pitfalls concern difficulty in establishing the diagnosis of CTCL and failure to stage the disease properly once the diagnosis is confirmed.

Early manifestations of CTCL may be quite difficult or impossible to distinguish from benign dermatoses. Adequate tissue sampling (i.e., multiple 3-mm punch biopsies from several representative sites) often enables a histopathologic diagnosis to be made. Physicians also should follow patients closely with suspect presentations such as parapsoriasis and poikiloderma and perform repeat biopsies if there is evidence of the disease worsening. Likewise, biopsies should be taken from patients whose apparent eczema or psoriasis fails to respond to therapy in the expected fashion.

For patients with advanced disease, difficulty may be experienced in distinguishing CTCL from other lymphoproliferative disorders. Tumor-phase mycosis fungoides can be confused with non-Hodgkin's lymphomas involving the skin, and Sézary syndrome can be confused with chronic lymphocytic leukemia. The correct diagnosis will depend on histopathologic features, cellular morphology, cell surface markers, and bone marrow findings.

DISEASES OF THE SPLEEN

By Charles E. Hess, M.D.
Charlottesville, Virginia

The spleen is a unique organ in many aspects. Structurally, the microcirculation with a portion of the blood emptying into the splenic cords (open circulation) is unlike that of any other organ. From a functional standpoint, the exceptional capacity of the spleen for phagocytosis and its active participation in the host immune response result in the spleen's being responsible for many of the clinical and laboratory manifestations of a variety of infectious, malignant, autoimmune, and hereditary disorders. Because the splenic venous drainage is via the portal vein, splenomegaly often is a complication of many primary hepatic disorders that result in portal hypertension. If these and many other structural and functional characteristics of the spleen are not appreciated, a rational approach to the diagnosis of splenic diseases is not possible.

STRUCTURE AND FUNCTION OF THE SPLEEN

The spleen is located in the left upper quadrant of the abdominal cavity, and in healthy adults measures 4 × 8 × 12 cm and weighs less than 200 gm. Anatomically, the spleen is enclosed by a connective tissue capsule with an extensive network of trabeculae that extend into the parenchyma (the white and red pulp). When the spleen is sectioned, the gross appearance is that of a sponge with the pulp tissue occupying the spaces.

The arterial blood supply of the spleen is from the splenic artery, which is a branch of the celiac artery. Upon entering the hilus of the spleen, the artery divides into several trabecular arteries; these in turn give off many branches referred to as central arteries, which enter the white pulp. Many secondary branches of the central arteries penetrate the white pulp and, after further branching, eventually empty into either the reticular meshwork of the marginal zones or the splenic cords (Billroth's cords) of the red pulp. The central artery finally divides into several arterioles called penicilli, which enter into the red pulp. Most of these penicilli empty into the cords (open circulation). Some, however, usually after further branching to become arterial capillaries, empty directly into sinuses (closed circulation). Elements of the blood that travel via the open circulatory route must re-enter the circulation by penetrating the wall of the splenic sinuses, a factor that is very important not only in the normal state but also in the pathogenesis of many disorders affecting the spleen. Venous drainage of the spleen begins in the sinuses, which coalesce to form pulp veins that in turn drain into trabecular veins and finally via the splenic vein into the portal vein.

The white pulp is a loose reticular meshwork that surrounds the central arteries and is composed mostly of lymphocytes and a variable number of plasma cells and macrophages but few red blood cells. The distribution of lymphocytes in the white pulp is similar to that in lymph nodes. There are lymph follicles with germinal centers (Malpighian corpuscles) which are composed of B cells. Surrounding these follicles and also the central arteries (periarterial lymphatic sheaths) are the T cells. A brisk exchange occurs between these lymphocytes and those in the peripheral blood.

There are two major structures in the red pulp, namely the splenic cords and sinuses. The splenic cords are composed of a network of reticular fibers in association with a heterogeneous hematopoietic cell population consisting mostly of lymphocytes, macrophages, red cells, and fewer numbers of granulocytes and platelets. A rich supply of splenic sinuses is located within this meshwork. The reticular fibers that make up the adventitial layer of these sinuses anastamose directly with similar fibers in the cords.

Normal splenic functions in humans include reservoir function; phagocytosis; and lymphocyte proliferation of both T and B cells and antibody formation. The cellular blood elements that normally are sequestered or pooled in the spleen are platelets, lymphocytes, and monocytes. Approximately 30 per cent of the peripheral platelet mass normally is present in the spleen, a factor that probably accounts for the thrombocytosis seen following splenectomy. These pooled platelets are located not only along the endothelial lining of the splenic sinuses but also in the cords, and they slowly exchange with those in the peripheral blood. In the presence of massive splenomegaly, this pool may represent as much as 90 per cent of the peripheral platelet mass and may be the major reason for the thrombocytopenia.

The spleen is rich in lymphocytes and cells of monocyte-macrophage lineage, but what portion of the total body pool of these cells is present in the spleen is not well defined. The lymphocytosis and monocytosis that are commonly seen after splenectomy probably are the result of the removal of the splenic reservoir for these elements.

Although granulocytes and red cells are not sequestered in significant quantities in the normal spleen, in splenomegaly a moderate degree of granulocytopenia and anemia often occur as result of pooling of these cellular elements in the spleen. In some pathologic states associated with splenomegaly, splenic pooling may be the sole mechanism responsible for the anemia, thrombocytopenia, and granulocytopenia present. In such cases, the pooled cells are slowly exchanging with those in the peripheral circulation and usually are not being destroyed or phagocytized at an increased rate.

Phagocytosis by the spleen involves three different processes, namely culling, pitting, and remodeling of cells—mostly red cells. *Culling* refers to phagocytosis and destruction of cells that are defective (e.g., schistocytes, spherocytes) or senescent. Particulate material such as Howell-Jolly bodies and siderotic granules are removed from red cells along with some membrane as red cells squeeze their way through the sinusoidal walls from the cords into the sinuses. The particulate material is then phagocytized by macrophages in the cords. This process is called *pitting*. *Remodeling* refers to the ability of the spleen to trap immature red cells (reticulocytes) until hemoglobinization is completed; during this time some red cell membrane also is lost before a mature biconcave red cell is released.

The spleen's role in the immune response to antigens, especially particulate antigens, has been appreciated for many years. The unique nature of the microcirculation and the ultrastructure of the white and red pulp of the spleen allows for maximum exposure of antigens to the macrophages and lymphocytes to initiate or potentiate an immune response. The splenomegaly commonly seen in association with systemic viral (e.g., infectious mononucleosis), bacterial (e.g., subacute bacterial endocarditis) and protozoal (e.g., malaria) infections is a result of the participation of the spleen in host defense. Although the spleen is not indispensable to the immune response, the rare, but often lethal, post-splenectomy sepsis, usually due to encapsulated organisms such as the pneumococcus, serves as a reminder of the importance of the spleen in host defense under certain circumstances.

DIAGNOSTIC APPROACH

Because most disorders involving the spleen whether of a primary or secondary nature are manifested by splenic enlargement, the diagnostic work-up generally is centered around efforts to determine the etiology of the splenomegaly. If a systematic approach is not followed, many needless laboratory studies are performed, and more importantly, many patients are subjected to unnecessary abdominal exploration and splenectomy. Although some patients, especially children, are said to have "benign splenomegaly" when no underlying etiology is found, this should always be a diagnosis of exclusion and confirmed by long follow-up.

An evaluation of a patient with splenomegaly should always begin with a very careful history and physical examination; this usually leads to performing a few simple and inexpensive laboratory studies that will establish the diagnosis. Infectious causes of splenomegaly are usually seen in children and young adults and in the Western Hemisphere are usually of viral etiology. Infectious mononucleosis is by far the most common offender, particularly in teen-agers and young adults (see the article on this topic). The history, the finding of lymphadenopathy on physical examination, the presence of "atypical lymphocytes" in the peripheral blood, and a positive serology (Monospot test) establish the diagnosis. Other serologic tests (antibody titers to various Epstein-Barr viral antigens) are available, but they are not necessary to confirm the diagnosis in most instances. Because infectious mononucleosis is such a common cause of splenomegaly in young individuals, a Monospot test should be obtained on any patient found to have an enlarged spleen before more invasive procedures are done. It is also important to keep in mind that approximately half of patients with the typical infectious mononucleosis syndrome will have negative serologic studies for the Epstein-Barr virus and that their disease is presumably due to other viruses (e.g., cytomegalovirus). In such cases, careful follow-up is all that is necessary to document resolution of the patient's symptoms and splenomegaly.

Other infectious causes of splenomegaly (e.g., subacute bacterial endocarditis, malaria, typhoid fever, brucellosis) are usually suggested by the history and physical examination and can be confirmed by appropriate blood cultures and serologies. If miliary tuberculosis or a systemic fungal infection is suspected, a bone marrow biopsy for special stains and aspiration for culture will often establish the diagnosis. Liver biopsy is also a very productive procedure in patients suspected of having miliary tuberculosis or other systemic granulomatous disorders. Splenomegaly may be the major clinical manifestation of sarcoidosis, and in most instances the diagnosis can be established by liver biopsy. Occasionally, in an immune-compromised host, splenectomy may be necessary to establish the diagnosis and determine the etiology of suspected fungal (e.g., candidal) abscesses of the spleen. Other infections, particularly those due to protozoal organisms (e.g., leishmaniasis, trypanosomiasis, schistosomiasis) are rarely a consideration in the Western Hemisphere.

Splenomegaly is a common finding in many hematologic disorders, both malignant and nonmalignant. A systematic approach to the examination of the peripheral blood, bone marrow, and lymph nodes is mandatory in order to avoid unnecessary procedures being performed. The differential diagnosis of the leukemias usually can be accomplished from peripheral blood smears or bone marrow biopsy or aspiration specimens with appropriate use of cytochemical, immunologic, and chromosomal analyses. In patients with myelofibrosis and myeloid metaplasia, splenomegaly is a cardinal feature of the disorder (see the article on this topic). Even though the finding of a leukoerythroblastic picture on a peripheral blood smear (teardrop red cells, nucleated red cells, and early myeloid cells) is characteristic, a bone marrow biopsy with special stains to document the presence of the typical bands of fibrosis is necessary for a definitive diagnosis.

In the presence of splenomegaly, a diagnosis of polycythemia vera (see article on this topic) can be confirmed by the findings of an elevated red cell mass ($\geq$ 36 ml/kg in males and $\geq$ 32 ml/kg in females) and an arterial oxygen saturation of $\geq$ 92 per cent. An elevated platelet count, white blood cell count, leukocyte alkaline phosphatase score, and serum vitamin B_{12} level are usually found but are not necessary for diagnosis.

Malignant lymphomas, especially the non-Hodgkin's lymphomas, frequently involve the spleen. Except as a part of a staging laparotomy, splenectomy is rarely necessary to establish a diagnosis. An involved peripheral lymph node usually can be found for biopsy. When an intra-abdominal lymphoma is suspected and in the absence of peripheral lymphadenopathy, the order of procedures should be as follows.

First, bilateral iliac crest bone marrow biopsies and aspirations should be performed. If bone marrow is diagnostic for lymphoma, not only is the diagnosis established, but no further staging is necessary in most instances since by definition the patient has stage IV disease. If the bone marrow is nondiagnostic or equivocal, which is often the case, an abdominal and pelvic computed tomographic (CT) scan should be done, and if positive, an abdominal exploration for diagnosis and staging is recommended. If the scan is normal, a bipedal lymphangiogram should be performed; if positive, proceed with exploration. In patients with Hodgkin's disease, a lymphangiogram may reveal evidence of lymph node involvement in the face of a normal CT scan. In non-Hodgkin's lymphomas, however, the lymphangiogram is rarely abnormal in the presence of a normal abdominal and pelvic CT scan. Primary and isolated lymphomas of the spleen are very rare, so much so that in the face of a normal bone marrow biopsy, normal abdominal and pelvic CT scan, and normal lymphangiogram, other causes of splenomegaly (already discussed and to be discussed) should be ruled out before splenectomy is recommended for diagnostic purposes. The one instance in which a diagnostic splenectomy is indicated occurs when unexplained splenic defects are noted on scan or by ultrasound.

Of the nonmalignant hematologic disorders, the hemolytic anemias, both acquired and congenital, are the most frequent cause for splenomegaly. In each instance, enlargement of the spleen occurs as a result of "work hypertrophy." Hemolysis usually is indicated by an elevated reticulocyte count. If hemolysis is suspected, a reticulocyte count should be performed even though the hematocrit is normal, since some patients will present with a compensated hemolytic process. A thorough family history is important and often points to a possible hereditary form of hemolytic anemia. Careful examination of a peripheral blood smear should be the initial step in the work-up of any patient with hemolytic anemia. If one is not confident in interpreting a blood smear, help should be sought. The morphologic appearance of the red cells often leads one to perform a single test to establish a diagnosis.

In patients with hereditary hemolytic anemias, the characteristic findings include:

1. Microspherocytes in hereditary spherocytosis. Diagnosis may be confirmed by performing osmotic fragility and autohemolysis studies.
2. Target cells, hypochromic microcytes, and basophilic stippling in the thalassemias. Diagnosis is usually established on hemoglobin electrophoresis and by determination of hemoglobin A_2 and F levels.
3. Elliptocytes. If greater than 25 per cent, the diagnosis is usually hereditary elliptocytosis.
4. Stomatocytes. Increased numbers are seen in a variety of hereditary and acquired hemolytic states. In hereditary stomatocytosis they are present in large numbers, and a diagnosis can usually be established by family history together with osmotic fragility and autohemolysis studies.
5. Target cells and hemoglobin C crystals in both homozygous hemoglobin C disease and in hemoglobin SC disease. Hemoglobin electrophoresis will confirm the diagnosis.
6. Extreme microspherocytosis, anisocytosis, and poikilocytosis in hereditary pyropoikilocytosis. Diagnosis is confirmed by demonstrating an increased fragility of the red cells to heat. (These conditions are discussed in various articles.)

Another large group of hereditary hemolytic anemias are those secondary to the various enzymopathies (see the article on hereditary anemias due to abnormal red cell enzymes). These enzyme defects may involve pathways in erythrocyte anaerobic glycolysis, pentose phosphate shunt, glutathione metabolism, or nucleotide metabolism. The peripheral blood findings, although quite variable, are nonspecific (e.g., polychromatophilia, anisocytosis, poikilocytosis, nucleated red cells). Specific enzyme assays usually are not necessary for differential diagnosis. Screening tests such as the pyruvate kinase and G-6-PD screens, the cyanide/ascorbate and autohemolysis tests, will usually point to the pathway involved. Specific enzyme assays are needed to fully define the nature of the defect.

Finally, there are a number of hereditary unstable hemoglobinopathies that are characterized by a Heinz body hemolytic anemia. The peripheral smear, in addition to the usual changes that accompany hemolysis, often demonstrates a severe degree of hypochromia. These unstable hemoglobins usually can be detected by performing either a heat denaturation or isopropanol precipitation test. Hemoglobin electrophoresis may or may not detect the abnormality (see the article on hemoglobinopathies).

The immune hemolytic anemias are, by far, the most frequent acquired hemolytic disorders associated with splenomegaly. Those referred to as autoimmune hemolytic anemia (AIHA) are clinically the most important and may be idiopathic, drug-induced, or secondary to a wide variety of other diseases. A characteristic finding on peripheral smear is autoagglutination of red cells. The differential Coombs' test is an excellent screen but does miss some cases. Various modifications of the test are available and should be used when the situation warrants. Drugs are the most common cause of AIHA and must be considered in every case. In vitro tests can be performed that will establish the association; re-challenge of the patient with a suspected drug should be avoided if possible. Of the many diseases that are associated with an increased incidence of AIHA, the most frequent are the malignant hematopoietic disorders (e.g., lymphomas, leukemias) and the connective tissue diseases (e.g., lupus erythematosus). Others include various infections (e.g., mycoplasma), benign cysts and tumors, and thyroid diseases.

Acquired hemolytic disorders such as paroxysmal nocturnal hemoglobinuria are rare, but they must be kept in mind when working up a patient with hemolytic anemia (see the article on this topic). Splenomegaly also may be seen in patients with chronic iron deficiency anemia and in megaloblastic anemias (e.g., pernicious anemia). Close follow-up is necessary in such cases to ensure that no other underlying disorder has been missed.

Connective tissue diseases such as lupus erythematosus and rheumatoid arthritis frequently are associated with splenomegaly. Felty's syndrome with the characteristic triad of rheumatoid arthritis, splenomegaly, and neutropenia is a frequently overlooked cause of splenomegaly. Patients may be relatively asymptomatic with "burned-out" arthritis. The presence of neutropenia with a variable degree of anemia, a normal platelet count, and positive serologic studies for rheumatoid arthritis establishes the diagnosis.

Congestive causes of splenomegaly present the most difficult diagnostic problems. Intrinsic liver diseases (e.g., cirrhosis) are the most frequent, followed by cardiac dysfunction (e.g., chronic congestive heart failure, constrictive pericarditis), and portal vein or splenic vein obstruction. In most patients with intrinsic liver disease, the history, physical examination, and presence of abnormal liver function studies lead one to obtain a percutaneous liver biopsy, which establishes the diagnosis. Not infrequently, however, patients will present with asymptomatic splenomegaly secondary to hepatic cirrhosis with normal liver function studies. In such patients, the cirrhosis is usually idiopathic.

If there is evidence of portal hypertension (e.g., esophageal varices), a celiac angiogram with venous phase should be performed to rule out portal or splenic vein obstruction prior to liver biopsy. In some patients, the presence or absence of portal hypertension is so critical as to warrant performance of one of several procedures to document. Available procedures include:

1. Wedged hepatic venous pressure.
2. Umbilical vein catheterization.
3. Percutaneous transhepatic portography.
4. Percutaneous transplenic portography.

The choice of technique depends on the expertise available. The wedged hepatic vein technique is most frequently employed, but is often falsely normal in patients with pre-sinusoidal obstruction. Pressures obtained by the transhepatic portal route or by way of umbilical vein catheterization are the most reliable and preferred by the author. Both of these methods, in addition, allow direct dye visualization of the portal venous system. With the availability of such techniques, patients generally should not be subjected to abdominal exploration to evaluate portal hemodynamics or to determine whether intrinsic liver disease is present. Only if the risk of bleeding is high should abdominal exploration be considered as an alternative.

Other rare causes of splenomegaly include the storage disorders (Gaucher's disease), splenic cysts, and hamartomas. Bone marrow and radiographic findings will establish the presence and nature of the storage diseases. Splenic scans are very important to establish the presence of cysts. Splenectomy for diagnostic purpose, as indicated earlier, rarely is necessary if this approach is followed. In some patients the etiology of the splenomegaly will remain unclear. Such patients, in general, should be closely followed. Splenectomy usually reveals only hyperplasia or congestion.

HISTIOCYTOSIS X

By William A. Newton, Jr., M.D.
Ala B. Hamoudi, M.D.
and Barry Shannon, Ph.D.
Columbus, Ohio

SYNONYMS

Eosinophilic granuloma; Hand-Schüller-Christian syndrome, Letterer-Siwe disease.

DEFINITION

In order to discuss the diagnostic aspects of histiocytosis X, it is necessary to make an arbitrary decision about just what is meant when that term is used. This condition is one of many in which proliferation of histiocytes in body tissues is seen, sometimes due to an identifiable cause, but most often not. The resulting clinical manifestations may be similar, even though the pathogenesis may be quite variable.

This article begins by stating that histiocytosis X is an histologically separable entity, readily diagnosed by tissue biopsy. In its simplest form it presents radiologically as a single punched-out area of any bone which histologically has the picture of eosinophilic granuloma. The patient with more extensive involvement has multiple sites of involvement of both bone and soft tissue with the same histologic picture or one that can be easily interpreted as healing or healed eosinophilic granuloma. Diagnostic confusion enters the picture when dealing with the patient with body-wide disease involving skin, lymph nodes, and other organs that have important reticuloendothelial function such as spleen, liver, and bone marrow. Patients who do not show the histologic picture of eosinophilic granuloma in their lesions should not be considered to have histiocytosis X.

HISTOLOGIC DIAGNOSIS

The pathologic picture of eosinophilic granuloma is quite familiar to pathologists and should not be a difficult diagnosis to make in most cases when the process is active and not in a healing phase. It consists of a mixture of several types of cells, but principally of a background of normal-appearing histiocytes mixed with varying numbers of eosinophils and lymphocytes. Often there is a suggestion of a focal reactive process where one sees a central core of degenerating necrotic cells surrounded by sheets of histiocytes mixed with eosinophils. Some lesions show apparent fusion of histiocytes forming multinucleated giant cells. Some show increased fibrosis, probably a healing change.

Another appearance consistent with a healing phase is conversion of the normal-appearing nonvacuolated histiocytes into a lesion in which the histiocytes show marked vacuolization of the cytoplasm. This latter picture had been the basis for an earlier concept that this disease was the result of abnormal storage of cholesterol. If no eosinophils are seen in a biopsy, the diagnosis of histiocytosis X is unlikely. Other types of diffuse histiocytic proliferation do not produce eosinophils, do not show the giant cell change, and rarely show the reactive-like areas of focal necrosis. They may show cellular phagocytosis by the infiltrating histiocytes, usually of red cells, but sometimes both red and white cells. This feature is almost never seen in histiocytosis X. The one important exception to remember in histologic diagnosis of this lesion is that the skin infiltrate almost never shows eosinophils among the histiocytes that characterstically hug the undersurface of the skin epithelium. The most characteristic lesions are to be found in bone, lymph node, and spleen; more rarely in bone marrow and lung; and almost never in the liver.

Nearly all lesions of eosinophilic granuloma show characteristic inclusions in the histiocyte cytoplasm when studied ultrastructurally, namely the Langerhans' granules. Not every cell shows these inclusions, but most lesions show them in 10 to 80 per cent of the histiocytes.

GENETICS

There is no obvious hereditary tendency in patients with histiocytosis X. Greenberger cites one family having identical twins with histiocytosis and several children with concurrent developmental disorders. This suggests a possible genetic factor. Except for its significance in establishing etiology, this type of event is too rare to influence family planning.

CLINICAL SYNDROMES

Isolated single lesions can be seen in either bone or soft tissue, but most frequently in the former. Any bone can be involved, but the skull and flat bones are most common. The nonosseous sites of known incidence are lymph node, skin and perhaps others. When *multifocal,* the sites usually involve bone, lymph node, and skin, and in addition may include gingiva, lung, liver, spleen, brain, and orbit. The most common symptoms at diagnosis include bone pain, lymph node enlargement, skin or gingival involvement, fever, diabetes insipidus, or proptosis. Histiocytosis X is predominantly a disease of children. The younger the age of diagnosis, the more likely that it will be widespread.

DIFFERENTIAL DIAGNOSIS

The histologic diagnosis of isolated primary lesions of histiocytosis X does not present a difficult problem. Occasionally, a reactive process—such as seen in tissue eosinophilia associated with visceral parasitism, with atypical chronic or subacute inflammation, or with Hodgkin's disease where no Reed-Sternberg cells can be demonstrated—can simulate this lesion. Other conditions that can closely mimic the process include Omenn's syndrome, hypereosinophilia, and sometimes chronic granulomatous disease. None of these, however, has the typical acute eosinophilic granuloma histology.

No discussion of differential diagnosis should omit a comment about the patients with widely disseminated disease described by Letterer and Siwe. The patients were mainly infants with hepatosplenomegaly, lymphadenopathy, diffuse cutaneous involvement frequently with pulmonary infiltrates, and with bone marrow involvement associated with lowered peripheral blood elements but not always associated with bone defects. Histologically their lesions showed only histiocytes infiltrating the involved tissues, without the other features of eosinophilic granuloma. Unfortunately, patients with histiocytosis X whose lesions are typically those of eosinophilic granuloma may also have a sufficiently disseminated extent of involvement of the same organ sites to produce the same or similar clinical findings. These groups should be separated by suitable tissue studies, since they are most likely different entities. In fact, the children described by Letterer and Siwe may have had multiple etiologies ranging from graft vs. host disease, intrauterine viral syndromes, immunologic deficiency states, or malignancy of the histiocytic system. The majority of these have a poor prognosis, whereas patients with disseminated eosinophilic granuloma tend to do better.

CLINICAL EVALUATION

The first step in the diagnosis of histiocytosis X is the definitive diagnostic biopsy. If isolated, the organ of principal involvement should be studied, usually bone or lymph node. Since the skin lesion is not fully diagnostic, it should not be the only biopsy site, if at all possible. The next step is to determine the extent of the process. The medical history should include questions concerning skin rashes from birth onward, especially of the scalp and periaural areas. Urinary frequency and volume should be evaluated with respect to possible diabetes insipidus. Bone symptoms may include pain, swelling, and redness at sites of involvement. Dentition development and status should be evaluated. History of possible jaundice or pulmonary insufficiency should be obtained. Symptoms resulting from decreased peripheral blood cells should be asked about, such as purpura, pallor, or fever that might result from neutropenia.

Physical examination should evaluate any skin defects. The rash is frequently a seborrheic dermatitis, but may be less obvious. The distribution of involved skin can be anywhere, but the scalp and ears are frequently the most involved, followed by the diaper area in small children. Occasionally the nails are deformed. The gingiva and dentition should be examined for either loss of teeth, failure of tooth formation, or looseness of teeth associated with mandibular involvement. Peripheral lymph nodes, particularly cervical, may be enlarged, as may be the liver and/or spleen. Pulmonary examination is usually not remarkable, even if the lung radiograph shows involvement. Superimposed pneumonitis, of course, can be present.

RADIOLOGIC STUDIES

Since bone is often involved in histiocytosis X and because any bone can be involved, examination of the entire skeletal system is a must to determine extent of disease. The most accurate method for detection of bone lesions is still routine radiography. The lesions present as punched-out areas of bone lysis without reactive changes at their borders. In contrast to most childhood cancers that involve bone, histiocytosis X lesions are not easily demonstrated by isotopic bone scans. Only about two thirds of lesions demonstrated by x-ray show positive changes by scintiscan. Nonetheless, the two types of examinations are complementary. Bone scans should be done only when radiographs are normal or equivocal.

One of the difficult aspects of studying this disease is interpretation of the stage or degree of activity of the bone lesions. Persistence of radiologic abnormalities may not mean that the process is still active. A lesion may be well along the way to healing and still appear to be an active process. Better tools to evaluate the degree of activity of the disease are needed. Not all patients with punched-out skull lesions have histiocytosis X. One patient presented with a fluctuant midline soft-tissue mass associated with what appeared to be an underlying skull defect; this proved to be a dermoid cyst.

Reports of computed tomographic (CT) studies of histiocytosis X lesions are few, but such studies are said to be more helpful in documenting the soft-tissue mass that frequently accompanies a bone lesion and better differentiates lipomas or dermoid cysts. Sonography may also be helpful in showing the extent of a soft-tissue mass in histiocytosis X lesions.

Lung involvement is not common in patients who have focal bone and soft-tissue sites of involvement. When the disease is more disseminated, it frequently involves the lung. The roentgenographic features are those of nodular or finely reticulonodular infiltrates. Cystic changes are rare; pneumothorax can be seen.

LABORATORY STUDIES

Hematopoietic System

Peripheral blood studies in patients with histiocytosis X may show reduced numbers of circulating blood elements, particularly in children with disseminated disease. Anemia is normochronic, normocytic, frequently with reticulocytosis. Leukopenia and/or neutropenia is usually associated with myeloid hyperplasia of the bone marrow. Similarly, thrombocytopenia, if present, is accompanied by bone marrow megakaryocytic hyperplasia. Despite the fact that the histiocytosis X lesions abound with eosinophils, the peripheral blood rarely shows an increase in this type of cell. Monocytosis of the peripheral blood has been observed, and increased numbers of histiocytes can be seen, particularly in patients with disseminated disease. Rarely do they show phagocytic activity.

Immunologic Aspects

Routine laboratory assays assessing immunocompetence in patients with histiocytosis X fail to identify any consistent abnormalities. Tests including enumeration of T and B lymphocytes in peripheral blood, assessment of the proliferative response of lymphocytes to antigens and mitogens, and quantitation of serum immunoglobulin levels reveal no apparent dysfunction.

Recent evidence supports classifying histiocytosis X as an immunodeficiency disorder. Autoantibodies may be attributable to a suppressor T lymphocyte deficiency. Decreases in suppressor T cells have been observed in numerous autoimmune anomalies including systemic lupus erythematosus and juvenile rheumatoid arthritis. Administration of thymic extract in vivo and treatment of lymphocytes in vitro with the thymic extract apparently reverses the lack of suppressor T lymphocytes, further strengthening the concept that histiocytosis X is an immunoregulatory disorder.

Deficiencies in antibody-dependent, monocyte-mediated cytotoxicity have been reported in patients with histiocytosis X. This is due to an intrinsic defect of the monocyte rather than an inhibitory substance in the serum. Since histiocytosis X is a disorder of the mononuclear phagocyte system, this evidence suggests that persistent functional abnormality may manifest itself in this cell lineage.

More sophisticated methodologies and investigation will provide insight into the immunoregulatory dysfunctions of histiocytosis X and aid the physician in determining the appropriate treatment in dealing with this disease.

Other Laboratory Findings

Initial and serial studies should be done to evaluate functional changes in the liver, lung, and pituitary when clinically suspect. Liver function tests will reflect the presence of chronic liver disease when cirrhosis is significant. Serum bilirubin concentration, serum protein levels, and liver enzyme determinations should be obtained as in any type of liver impairment.

Water deprivation testing may be required to identify mild degrees of partial diabetes insipidus (see the article on this topic). Growth hormone activity should be evaluated in those who show reduced stature.

COURSE

The courses of children with histiocytosis X vary widely, since rarely do any two patients exhibit the same extent of involvement. Those whose disease is limited to a single site, whether in bone or soft tissue, rarely if ever develop a life-threatening problem. Healing is the rule, with or without treatment. When disease is multifocal, it is more often protracted and sometimes fatal. Poor outcome is predicted in patients less than 2 years of age at diagnosis, those with marked splenomegaly, those who have prolonged fever, those with massive nodal involvement, and those with obstructive jaundice. Age seems to be the best indication of outcome, probably because the extent of disease is inversely proportional to age. The infant below a year of age at diagnosis who has multiorgan involvement has the worst prognosis, about 50 per cent survival, while those diagnosed at over 2 years of age have a much better outcome, over 90 per cent survival. The duration of the active phase of the disease is difficult to evaluate, particularly when it involves bone. The usual course lasts months, but it may extend into many years. Since it is not reasonable to do repeated biopsies of involved sites, data to evaluate tissue changes are limited. Several radiographs of a bone lesion may show significant changes long after any symptoms have passed, but structural changes may reflect the healing process rather than disease activity. Eventual loss of all evidence of bone changes is the rule, except for thinning of involved vertebral bodies or bone changes resulting from radiologic damage to developing bone. Other organ systems that may show residual damage with time include the posterior pituitary, liver, and lung. Diabetes insipidus is the most frequent evidence of organ damage in children who survive. This may be associated with growth failure, but not usually. Cirrhosis of severe degree is a principal cause of death, but it may be subclinical in many. Chronic lung changes are very uncommon.

COMPLICATIONS

The most serious acute complications occur in children who have multifocal disease and are receiving therapy for active disease. Infections are common in the severely ill child with widespread lymph node enlargement and hepatosplenomegaly. The responsible organisms are often similar to those detected in children receiving chemotherapy for cancer, for example, *Pneumocystis carinii.* These children may be more susceptible to infection because of a hypersplenic effect of their disease, an underlying immune system inadequacy, immunologic suppression by chemotherapy or radiation, or a combination of these factors. Increased bleeding, particularly epistaxis, is seen frequently in infants who have thrombocytopenia. The chronic complications and sequelae are discussed under course of disease.

HEMOPHILIA AND OTHER INHERITED COAGULATION DISORDERS

By Clara V. Hussey, M.D.
and James A. Olive, D.M.D., M.D.
Milwaukee, Wisconsin

Familial association of excessive bleeding was noted in ancient times. With the development of laboratory tests for evaluating such patients, it was recognized that there were many proteins that interacted to maintain hemostasis.

GENERAL APPROACH TO PATIENTS

The patient with a suspected hemostatic disorder is usually detected during the taking of a history and performance of a physical examination. The history should note any incidence of bleeding or thrombotic symptomatology, duration and frequency of occurrence, and any episodes affecting family members. Bleeding symptoms commonly seen are easy bruising, epistaxis, gum bleeding, prolonged bleeding from cuts, and menorrhagia. Less common are hematoma formation and hemarthrosis. It is important to determine the extent of injury that preceded the bleed and also any medications taken previously as well as during the course of the bleeds. The extent of impairment and the management approach pursued to date should be assessed. The latter, as well as medications taken, are especially important when bleeding occurs during surgery or in the postoperative period.

Family history should include information on the immediate relatives (parents, siblings, children), grandparents, aunts, uncles, and cousins. Drawing a pedigree enables one to determine the inheritance pattern, which can be helpful in establishing a differential diagnosis and in selecting laboratory tests. (See the article in Section 1 on Approach to Genetic Diseases.) In mild bleeding or thrombotic disorders, the family history can be difficult to obtain if the affected family members have not had surgery or injury.

The physical examination should note location and size of ecchymoses. A search for telangiectatic lesions should be made when epistaxis and mucosal bleeding are the presenting symptoms. A patient with hemarthrosis in the acute stage will have a warm to hot swollen joint. After resolution of the hemarthrosis, the joint should be checked for residual limitation of flexion and extension. Table 1 shows the classification of coagulation disorders according to inheritance pattern.

SEX-LINKED RECESSIVE INHERITANCE

The pattern of inheritance in which males are affected and in which the disorder is transmitted by

Table 1. Coagulation Disorders According to Inheritance Pattern

Inheritance Pattern	Disease	Factor	Abnormal Basic Test	Specific Assay
Sex-linked recessive	Hemophilia A	VIII	PTT	VIII:C
	Hemophilia B	IX	PTT	IX
Autosomal dominant	von Willebrand's disease	VIII	PTT, BT	VIII:C VIIIR:Ag VIIIR:RCo
	Dysfibrinogenemia	I	PT, PTT, TT	Fibrinogen
	Antithrombin deficiency	Antithrombin III		Antithrombin III
Autosomal recessive	Afibrinogenemia	I	BT, PT PTT, TT	
	Hypoprothrombinemia	II	PT, PTT	Prothrombin
	Dysprothrombinemia	II	PT, PTT	
	Factor V deficiency	V	PT, PTT	Factor V
	Factor VII deficiency	VII	PT	Factor VII
	Factor X deficiency	X	PT, PTT	Factor X
	Factor XI deficiency	XI	PTT	Factor XI
	Factor XII deficiency	XII (Hageman)	PTT	Factor XII
	Prekallikrein deficiency	Prekallikrein	PTT	Prekallikrein
	No hemostatic defect	HMK	PTT	HMK
	Factor XIII deficiency	XIII (FSF)		Clot solubility
	Antiplasmin deficiency	α_2-Antiplasmin		α_2-Antiplasmin

Abbreviations: HMK = High-molecular-weight kininogen; FSF = fibrin stabilizing factor; BT = bleeding time; TT = thrombin time; PT = prothrombin time; PTT = partial thromboplastin time.

an unaffected (or mildly affected) female is called *sex-linked recessive.* This hereditary pattern is seen in hemophilia A (classic hemophilia or factor VIII deficiency) and in hemophilia B (Christmas disease or factor IX deficiency).

The affected male will have all normal sons, and his daughters will be obligate carriers. The carrier female may have a mild bleeding disorder depending on her circulating level of factor VIII or IX; there is a 50 per cent chance of each son having hemophilia and of each daughter being a carrier.

Hemophilia A (Classical Hemophilia)

Hemophilia A occurs in all degrees of severity ranging from severe to very mild. The disorder is classified as severe if the patient has less than 1 per cent or 0.01 unit/ml of factor VIII : C activity (Table 2) as measured in a one-stage assay using the partial thromboplastin time (PTT).

A patient with *severe hemophilia A* will have spontaneous bleeding after imperceptible trauma and will usually require replacement therapy several times a month. The hemorrhagic complications most commonly seen are hemarthrosis and hematomas. The patient is usually aware that bleeding has occurred before it becomes clinically evident.

Hemarthrosis, bleeding into a joint, is associated with a vague warmth and tingling sensation and/or a sense of mild restlessness or anxiety a few hours before it becomes clinically evident. Initially, there is mild discomfort and slight limitation of motion. If it is untreated, severe pain, joint swelling, and cutaneous warmth, followed by severe limitation of movement, occur. After the bleeding stops, the blood is absorbed over a period of weeks. The blood present in the joint space produces a synovitis that will then predispose the joint to further episodes of bleeding and eventually result in hemophilic arthropathy. The joints most frequently affected are the knees, followed by the elbows, ankles, shoulders, hips, and wrists. Bleeding into other joints is very rare. The first episode of hemarthrosis usually occurs when the child is learning to walk.

Hematomas are another common bleeding manifestation and can be either intramuscular or subcutaneous, or they can be present in other areas such as the neck or tongue or head. Subcutaneous hematomas result from minor trauma and bleeding underneath the skin. This produces a localized warmth and swelling. This type of hematoma is usually of no clinical consequence; however, a hematoma in the neck, tongue, or throat may rapidly obstruct the patient's airway and should be treated immediately. Intramus-

Table 2. Factor VIII Measurements

What has traditionally been called "factor VIII" is now known to be a complex of two distinct molecular entities, the factor VIII procoagulant activity protein and the von Willebrand factor protein. The components of the complex have been characterized by their activity as well as their antigenicity:

VIII:C—the factor VIII procoagulant activity protein which corrects the coagulation abnormality in hemophilia A

VIII:CAg—the antigenic expression of VIII:C

VIIIR:RCo—the von Willebrand factor protein as measured by its ability to promote the agglutination of platelets in the presence of the antibiotic ristocetin

VIIIR:Ag—the antigenic expression of von Willebrand factor

cular hematomas can be small and usually resolve without treatment. Larger intramuscular hematomas may present in a variety of ways; for example, a bleed into the psoas or other muscles in the retroperitoneum may cause pain in the left lower quadrant or pain referred to the groin. Most hematomas in the forearm or in the leg present with swelling, pain, and warmth. If these hematomas are untreated or are inadequately treated, they can undergo fibrinous organization resulting in contractures, pressure on nerves, and muscle wasting. Hemophilic cysts or pseudotumors are another complication of severe factor VIII deficiency. These begin as a hematoma in a muscle or in the subperiosteum that is inadequately treated. As the blood is absorbed and organization starts to occur, the hematoma becomes highly vascular and grows by rebleeding, causing pressure necrosis of the surrounding muscles or bone. The only treatment of the pseudotumors is surgical excision.

Intracranial bleeding in a patient deficient in factor VIII is a medical emergency. This type of bleeding results in death in one out of four hemophiliac patients, half of whom have no history of antecedent trauma.

Moderate hemophilia A is characterized by factor VIII : C activity between 1 and 5 per cent. These patients usually have fewer episodes of spontaneous hemorrhage and require treatment less frequently. Severe hemorrhage will follow any minor trauma and should be promptly treated. These patients must be treated prior to any surgical procedure.

Patients with *mild factor VIII deficiencies* have greater than 5 per cent factor VIII:C activity and usually require therapy only after trauma or for surgery.

The diagnosis of hemophilia A is easy in patients with the severe form. These patients usually present with a family history that shows sex-linked inheritance and hemorrhage that is either spontaneous or related to minor trauma. Laboratory studies show a prolonged PTT, normal bleeding time, low factor VIII : C, and normal factor VIIIR : Ag. The diagnosis of mild hemophilia is more difficult because it must be distinguished from von Willebrand's disease.

Once the diagnosis of hemophilia A has been made and its severity assessed by measurement of factor VIII:C activity, a proper therapeutic regimen must be adopted for each individual patient. This includes a multidisciplinary evaluation of the patient to assess emotional, sociological, and psychological needs in addition to physical needs. A home maintenance program has been instituted in many areas of the United States for individuals with moderate to severe hemophilia. In addition to diagnosis and treatment of patients with hemophilia A, an attempt should be made to diagnose the carrier state and institute appropriate genetic counseling. Frequently, the carrier state can be detected by using the ratio of the VIII : C to VIIIR : Ag levels. In carriers factor VIIIR : Ag levels are usually normal and VIII:C levels are approximately 50 per cent of normal, which would give an approximate 2:1 ratio of VIIIR: Ag to VIII: C (normal ratio 1:1).

The individual who is a hemophilia A carrier or potentially a carrier and who becomes pregnant can have amniocentesis and measurement of factor VIIIC : Ag on a culture of fetal cells. The sex of the child can also be determined. This information can be utilized in deciding whether or not the pregnancy should be terminated to prevent production of a child with classical hemophilia.

Factor VIII Inhibitors

Factor VIII inhibitors arise in 5 to 20 per cent of severe hemophiliacs. Inhibitors rarely occur in patients with moderate or mild disease. Factor VIII inhibitors also arise in a number of individuals without factor VIII deficiency. (See the article on hemorrhagic diseases due to circulating anticoagulants.)

All factor VIII–deficient patients scheduled for elective surgery who have previously received replacement therapy should be screened for a factor VIII inhibitor. Factor VIII inhibitors are time- and temperature-dependent. They can be detected by comparing PTT times performed on a mixture of equal parts of normal and patient plasma prior to and following 2 hours of incubation at 37°C.

Specific inhibitor titers are determined by doing factor VIII:C assays on a series of dilutions of patient plasma in normal plasma after 2 hours incubation at 37°C. The inhibitor levels are reported in units. The most commonly used inhibitor unit in the United States is the Bethesda unit, which is defined as the amount of inhibitor necessary to reduce one unit of factor VIII:C by 50 per cent after incubation at 37°C for 2 hours.

Hemophiliac patients developing an inhibitor can either be low responders, in whom the titer is low and transient, or high responders, who develop a high inhibitor titer that does not disappear. Low responders can be treated with constant infusion of factor VIII concentrates, although an increased quantity is required. The high responder will require other therapeutic modalities such as activated factor IX concentrate.

Hemophilia B (Christmas Disease)

Hemophilia B is a sex-linked recessive disorder similar to hemophilia A. It differs from hemophilia A in that the patient has normal levels of factor VIII:C and decreased levels of functional factor IX. The onset and type of bleeding in hemophilia A and hemophilia B are very similar. The severity of the disorder, as in hemophilia A, is classified as severe if the level of factor IX is less than 1 per cent, as moderate when the level is between 1 and 5 per cent, and as mild if the level is greater than 5 per cent. Symptoms correlate with the severity of the deficiency. The presence and degree of impairment depends on the adequacy of treatment during infancy, childhood, and adult life.

Most individuals who have hemophilia B, while deficient in functional factor IX, have immunologically detectable amounts of factor IX present (CRM^+). Only a small percentage of individuals with hemophilia B are lacking in antigenic factor IX (CRM^-).

The diagnosis of factor IX deficiency depends on a family history of bleeding, a prolonged PPT, and a decreased level of factor IX.

Individuals with factor IX deficiency (CRM^-) have been found who develop inhibitors to the factor IX concentrate.

AUTOSOMAL DOMINANT INHERITANCE

Coagulation disorders occurring in both sexes and in each generation are indicative of autosomal dominant inheritance. This inheritance pattern is seen in von Willebrand's disease, antithrombin deficiency, and dysfibrinogenemia. Mild disorders sometimes require identification of affected family members through laboratory testing in order to confirm the diagnosis.

von Willebrand's Disease

von Willebrand's disease is a congenital disorder commonly diagnosed in adult life. Its expression ranges from very mild to very severe. In severe von Willebrand's disease, the bleeding usually starts to occur in early childhood and tends to become less severe with age. In the mild to moderate forms, the bleeding tendency usually is not recognized until the teens or later and is characterized by mucosal and cutaneous hemorrhages (e.g., epistaxis, bruises, and prolonged bleeding from cuts). Menorrhagia is very frequent, and excessive postpartum bleeding occurs in about a third of patients. Patients may present with excessive bleeding following minor surgery or dental extraction if no replacement therapy is used. In the very severe form, intramuscular hematomas and hemarthroses can occur.

Originally, the most consistent abnormality was prolongation of the bleeding time. That platelet function is altered in von Willebrand's disease is further demonstrated by decreased platelet adhesion to glass beads, and by decreased aggregation with the antibiotic ristocetin (Table 2). Although factor VIII:C levels fluctuate, they are usually in the range of 40 per cent or less. Factor VIIIR:Ag levels are also low and usually are approximately equal to or lower than the factor VIII:C levels.

Currently, the diagnostic criteria for von Willebrand's disease have been expanded and include:

1. A bleeding time that is abnormal at some time.
2. A decreased factor VIII:C level.
3. A decreased factor VIIIR:RCo level in most cases.
4. A quantitative or qualitative abnormality in the factor VIIIR:Ag.

Today, through the use of testing for different components of the factor VIII complex, von Willebrand's disease has been subdivided into two large groups from a genetic point of view. One group, which is very rare, is autosomal recessive. The other group, which is the common form of von Willebrand's disease, is autosomal dominant. The common form of von Willebrand's disease is further divided into at least two types.

von Willebrand's disease is best treated with cryoprecipitate because lyophilized factor VIII concentrate does not contain the large multimeric parts of the factor VIIIR:Ag.

Antithrombin Deficiency

Patients with antithrombin III deficiency present with thrombophlebitis, pulmonary embolism, or mesenteric thrombosis. Since a deficiency of antithrombin requires a specific assay for identification, patients can be selected for study on the basis of a personal or strong familial history of thrombosis. Among patients with this type of history, Bick has given the incidence of antithrombin deficiency as 3 per cent.

The antithrombin assay should be functional rather than immunologic since patients have been reported with normal immunologic levels who have low functional levels. Antithrombin levels of 20 to 70 per cent have been reported with thrombosis. However, some family members with 60 to 70 per cent levels have not developed vascular occlusions throughout their lifetime. Frequently the first thrombotic episode occurs in the teens following trauma, surgery, infections, or use of oral contraceptives. Once the patient has developed a vascular occlusion, recurrences are common. Patients have become asymptomatic while receiving oral anticoagulants or antiaggregating agents such as aspirin. Rare individuals require maintenance on low-dose heparin, especially during pregnancy.

While receiving warfarin, some patients will have an increase in the antithrombin levels. Therefore a normal antithrombin level during warfarin therapy cannot rule out antithrombin deficiency.

Dysfibrinogenemia

Patients with dysfibrinogenemia present with either bleeding or thrombosis. Bleeding, when it occurs, is moderate to severe and involves mucosal areas, or it occurs following trauma or surgery. Patients can also show delayed healing and wound dehiscence. Recurrent thromboembolism is present in many patients with dysfibrinogenemia. These latter patients should be screened for antithrombin deficiency.

The abnormal fibrinogen molecules cause delay in fibrin formation either by slow release of fibrinopeptide A or B or by delay in the polymerization of fibrin. Laboratory tests show low fibrinogen levels when measured as the rate of fibrin formation and a prolonged thrombin time. Frequently there is a prolonged prothrombin time (PT) and partial thromboplastin time (PTT), but usually the bleeding time is normal.

AUTOSOMAL RECESSIVE INHERITANCE

Autosomal recessive inheritance traits can occur in both sexes. The symptomatic patient will be homozygous for the trait, whereas the parents and any unaffected siblings will be heterozygous.

In some instances the heterozygote may be identified by specific laboratory tests. In Table 1 the numerous disorders with this inheritance pattern are listed along with the abnormal basic tests and specific assays by which they can be identified.

Application of specific functional as well as antigenic assays can be used to differentiate those patients having proportional deficiencies of both parameters from those exhibiting a selective deficiency of only the functional aspect.

Afibrinogenemia

Patients with afibrinogenemia may present with umbilical, mucosal, gastrointestinal, or intracranial bleeds. Bleeding occurs in the joints in a small percentage of the patients, but these do not lead to the degenerative joint disease seen in hemophiliacs. The symptomatic patient will have a fibrinogen level too low to produce a fibrin end point in any of the coagulation tests. By salting-out techniques, fibrinogen levels less than 20 mg/dl have been found. Besides a thrombin time (TT), prothrombin time, and partial thromboplastin time of infinity, a prolonged bleeding time (BT) and thrombocytopenia can be seen.

Heterozygotes can be identified by fibrinogen levels of about half normal. In patients with low functional fibrinogen levels, dysfibrinogenemia must be ruled out before the individual can be called a heterozygote.

Prothrombin Deficiency

Prothrombin-deficient patients have a history of bleeding at the time of circumcision, easy bruising, and excessive bleeding with trauma or surgery. Laboratory identification is made by a prolonged prothrombin time and a prolonged partial thromboplastin time with a normal thrombin time and a normal fibrinogen level. The prolonged prothrombin time does not correct with either serum or adsorbed plasma.

Factor V Deficiency

Factor V deficiency is rare, since it has an autosomal recessive inheritance pattern. Depending on the severity of the deficiency, the patient's bleeding may be limited to that during surgery and following major injuries. Laboratory identification can be made by correction of the abnormal prothrombin time with adsorbed plasma and a specific factor V assay.

Factor VII Deficiency

Patients with severe deficiencies (less than 10 per cent) of factor VII have a history of spontaneous intramuscular or intracranial bleeds, epistaxis, and excessive bleeding with trauma, dental extraction, or surgery. Severe menorrhagia occurs frequently. Patients with factor VII levels of 30 per cent or more are usually asymptomatic.

Laboratory identification is made on the basis of a markedly prolonged prothrombin time which corrects by addition of serum, and a normal partial thromboplastin time. A specific factor VII assay can be done for confirmation.

Factor X Deficiency

Depending on the level of factor X activity, patients present with variable bleeding problems, ranging from the severe and life-threatening to that characterized only by excessive bleeding with surgery. Laboratory studies show a prolonged prothrombin time and partial thromboplastin time that correct with the addition of normal serum.

Factors Involved in Initiation of Coagulation and Fibrinolysis

Interaction of factors XII and XI, prekallikrein, and high-molecular-weight kininogen (HMK) results in the activation of the coagulation reactions leading to fibrin formation as well as the conversion of plasminogen to plasmin. In the laboratory, a deficiency of any one of these factors will result in a prolonged partial thromboplastin time and a normal prothrombin time. The partial thromboplastin time will correct with both serum and adsorbed plasma. Prekallikrein and HMK deficiency plasmas show normalization when the activation phase of the partial thromboplastin time is lengthened.

Although patients with factor XI deficiency may have a bleeding disorder, it is mild and usually limited to surgical bleeding. There is, however, no bleeding associated with deficiencies of factor XII, prekallikrein, or HMK. Patients with severe deficiencies of factor XII or prekallikrein have been reported to show increased risk of thromboembolic disorders.

Factor XIII Deficiency

Patients with factor XIII deficiency frequently present with umbilical bleeding. Although spontaneous bleeds occur during childhood, they are not a constant feature. Common problems are slow healing and abnormal scar formation when adequate replacement therapy is not given. Less frequently, patients have epistaxis, gingival bleeds, and musculoskeletal hemorrhage.

Basic laboratory tests are all normal. Since the affected patient is homozygous, factor XIII is virtually absent. The solubility of a clot, formed by recalcification of dilute platelet-rich patient plasma, in 5M urea or 1 per cent monochloracetic acid can be used to identify the patient with this deficiency.

α_2-Antiplasmin Deficiency

Patients who are homozygous for α_2-antiplasmin deficiency have a lifelong history of easy bruising, prolonged bleeding after dental extraction and surgery, and hemarthrosis, but do not experience umbilical bleeding. Since the basic tests are normal, the diagnosis is made with a specific assay of α_2-antiplasmin. The reported cases all show low functional (less than 10 per cent) and low antigenic (less than 1 per cent) levels. There is no consistency in reports of bleeding in heterozygous patients, although their α_2-antiplasmin levels are about half the normal level. Treatment with antifibrinolytic agents such as epsilon-aminocaproic acid (EACA, Amicar) has offered some control of the bleeding disorder in the homozygote.

LABORATORY TESTS

Bleeding Time

The bleeding time is a measure of the time required for blood flow to cease after a standardized cut is made in the skin. Normal values vary with technique used, and therefore the values at each hospital should be obtained from the laboratory.

Factors affecting the bleeding time include vascular constriction, platelets (number and rate of aggregation), and von Willebrand factor deficiency.

Prothrombin Time

The one-stage prothrombin time of Quick detects abnormalities of prothrombin and factors V, VII, and X. Oxalated or citrated plasma is used. In this test, an extract of brain tissue serves as a source of thromboplastin. When thromboplastin is mixed with plasma and calcium chloride, the time for clot formation depends on the limiting factor.

The deficient factor can be replaced, in vitro, using adsorbed rabbit plasma as a source of factor V and fibrinogen and normal aged human serum as a source of factors VII and X. The results of corrections are seen in Table 3.

Partial Thromboplastin Time

Oxalated or citrated plasma is used for the test, and it is important that the plasma be fresh. Equal amounts of plasma and lipid (a substitute for platelets) are mixed and then incubated for 2 to 5 minutes to allow for activation of factor XII and XI in the presence of prekallikrein and HMK. After incubation, calcium chloride is added and the time for fibrin formation measured.

Usually an activating agent such as ellagic acid, celite, or kaolin is incorporated into the test mixture, and the procedure may be referred to as the activated partial thromboplastin time (APTT). Time to fibrin formation is shorter when an activator is used; however, the significance of a prolonged time compared with the control time is the same with or without the activator.

This test, like the coagulation time, will be sensitive to all factors except platelets, factor VII, and factor XIII. There is a definite improvement in the sensitivity of the PTT to the factor deficiencies when compared with the coagulation time. The test is reported to be able to detect deficiencies of 30 per cent or less.

Corrections of the PTT can be performed as shown in Table 4.

Thrombin Time

Adding thrombin to oxalated or citrated plasma will permit measurement of the rate of fibrinogen to fibrin conversion. This reaction is prolonged when heparin and its cofactor (antithrombin) are present.

Delayed polymerization of fibrin occurs when peptides produced from the action of plasmin on fibrinogen or fibrin are present (fibrin split products). Although the delay is proportional to the level of fibrin split products, the thrombin time is sensitive to only some of the peptides obtained from the action of plasmin. Therefore, the thrombin time is not a satisfactory test for determining the total amount of fibrin split products present.

As mentioned earlier, altered fibrinogen, as in the dysfibrinogenemias, affects this test as well as behaving like a fibrinogen deficiency in the partial thromboplastin time and prothrombin time.

Specific Factor Assays

Fibrinogen is assayed either by the rate of fibrin formation or by performing a biuret reaction on a dissolved clot. Specific assays for other coagulation

Table 3. Use of Prothrombin Time to Identify Deficient Factor

Deficiency	Basic PT	PT + Serum	PT + Adsorbed Plasma	PTT
Prothrombin (Factor II)	Abnormal	Abnormal	Abnormal	Abnormal
Factor V	Abnormal	Abnormal	Normal	Abnormal
Factor VII	Abnormal	Normal	Abnormal	Normal
Factor X	Abnormal	Normal	Abnormal	Abnormal

Abbreviations: PT = Prothrombin time; PTT = partial thromboplastin time.

Table 4. Use of Partial Thromboplastin Time to Identify Deficient Procoagulant

Deficient Factor	Basic PTT	PTT + Serum	PTT + Adsorbed Plasma	PT
Factor VIII	Abnormal	Abnormal	Normal	Normal
Factor V	Abnormal	Abnormal	Normal	Abnormal
Factor IX	Abnormal	Normal	Abnormal	Normal
Factor X	Abnormal	Normal	Abnormal	Abnormal
Factors XI and XII PK and HMK	Abnormal	Normal	Normal	Normal
Platelet factor 3	Normal	Normal	Normal	Normal

Abbreviations: PTT = Partial thromboplastin time; PT = prothrombin time; HMK = high-molecular-weight kininogen; PK = prekallikrein.

factors can be done using a mixture of patient plasma with plasma deficient in the factor being measured. Curves are constructed using aliquots of diluted normal plasma with the specific factor-deficient plasma. Factors II, V, VII, and X are measured using the prothrombin time; factors VIII, IX, XI, XII, prekallikrein, and HMK are measured with the partial thromboplastin time.

Antithrombin is measured by its neutralization of thrombin in the presence of heparin. Residual thrombin is measured by action on a synthetic substrate. Similarly, α_2-antiplasmin is measured by neutralization of plasmin, with the residual plasmin measured by its action on a synthetic substrate.

PITFALLS IN DIAGNOSIS

Perhaps the greatest problem lies in obtaining a reliable history. Patients are often impressed by the idea of easy bruising. Epistaxis, especially in children, can be due to "picking the nose." In contrast, however, the patient may accept as normal a symptom such as menorrhagia because other females in the family generally have heavy menstrual bleeding lasting 8 to 10 days.

If the bleeding time is done on a "cold" ear, an erroneous prolongation can be a frequent occurrence. This could be important when the patient is being studied on an outpatient basis.

Every abnormal bleeding time requires a careful check of medication. When possible, having the patient abstain from all medications before doing or repeating the bleeding time is desirable. Medications that have most frequently presented a problem in my experience have been analgesics, anti-inflammatory agents, and tranquilizers.

Since patients with mild hemophilia or mild von Willebrand's disease can have sufficient factor VIII to give normal PTT results, specific factor assays should be done if the bleeding history or family history suggests these disorders.

BLEEDING DUE TO VASCULAR AND PLATELET DISORDERS

By J. Heinrich Joist, M.D., Ph.D.
St. Louis, Missouri

Normal hemostasis, which is the containment of red blood cells (RBC) and other cellular and plasmatic constituents of the circulating blood within the vasculature and the restoration of vascular integrity following vessel wall injury, is dependent on the normal interaction between the vessel wall, platelets, and the blood coagulation/fibrinolytic system. This interaction involves a complex system of tightly integrated and regulated reactions, major parts of which are still incompletely understood. Since this article deals with bleeding disorders due to vascular and platelet disorders, a brief review of the factors and events involved in the initial response of blood to vascular injury, commonly called "primary hemostasis," may be appropriate.

The normal endothelial lining of the vessel wall not only constitutes an effective barrier to prevent escape of the circulating blood constituents but also prevents adherence and activation of platelets and activation of the blood coagulation/fibrinolytic mechanisms. Although certain components of the endothelial surface (such as heparin-like sulfated mucopolysaccharides or glycosaminoglycans) and the ability of the endothelial cells to produce prostaglandin I_2 (prostacyclin) are thought to be important factors, the nature and mechanisms involved in the non-thrombogenicity of the endothelium await full characterization.

When the endothelium is disrupted as a consequence of mechanical, physical, or chemical injury, platelets will swiftly adhere to exposed subendothelial connective tissue structures. This adherence reaction, which appears to be mediated or at least markedly potentiated by plasma factor VIII:von Willebrand factor, involves a change in platelet shape (from disc to sphere), platelet spreading and pseudopod formation. This is followed by the release or selective extrusion of adenosine diphosphate (ADP) and other biologically active substances stored in different platelet granules, and activation of platelet arachidonate metabolism leading to the formation of a number of biologically active intermediates. These include thromboxane A_2, a potent inducer of platelet aggregation and vasoconstriction. Both ADP and thromboxane A_2 may cause platelet aggregation and the formation of the primary hemostatic platelet plug through exposure on the platelet surface of specific binding sites (glycoprotein IIb/IIIa) for fibrinogen, which link the platelets together. In addition, ADP and thromboxane A_2 work synergistically in potentiating the platelet release reaction. In the process of the release reaction, the platelet surface membrane is modified to support high-affinity binding and thus approximation of coagulation zymogens, enzymes, and cofactors (also called platelet factor 3 or procoagulant activity), resulting in the formation of thrombin and fibrin, which stabilizes the hemostatic platelet plug ("secondary hemostasis"). Abnormalities of any of the components of this system—that is, disorders of the vessel wall itself or its supporting structures; a reduction in the mass of circulating platelets; disorders of platelet function; or quantitative or qualitative disorders of zymogens, cofactors, or inhibitors of the coagulation system—may lead to blood extravasation with and sometimes without apparent trauma.

The localization and pattern of bleeding may offer important clues as to the nature of the underlying hemostatic disorder. Thus, petechiae or pinpoint hemorrhages in the skin are more commonly associated with thrombocytopenia or vascular abnormalities, and so-called "spontaneous" (not associated with known trauma) bleeding into joints (hemarthrosis) is extremely rare in patients with hemorrhagic conditions other than disorders of blood coagulation such as classic hemophilia. In contrast, bruises or ecchymoses (bleeding into the skin), hematomata (deep soft-tissue bleeds), and bleeding into the gastrointestinal or urinary tract are common in thrombocytopenia and disorders of platelet function, as well as in abnormalities of blood coagulation and fibrinolysis. Thus, the diagnosis of a bleeding disorder is frequently dependent on careful laboratory evaluation in addition to thorough personal and family history, drug history, and physical examination.

BLEEDING DUE TO VASCULAR DISORDERS

Vascular purpura—bleeding due to abnormalities of the vessel wall—is rare and is usually suspected in patients in whom detailed hemostatic evaluation fails to reveal evidence for abnormalities of platelet number and function or the blood coagulation/fibrinolytic system. The Ivy or the template bleeding time is usually within normal limits. The so-called capillary fragility test (Rumpel Leede test) is frequently abnormal. However, this test not only lacks specificity but appears to be overly sensitive in that it not infrequently gives abnormal results in individuals who have no history of abnormal bleeding. Thus, accurate diagnosis generally depends on careful history, physical examination, examination of biopsy specimens by light and electron microscopy, and immunohistochemical and serologic studies.

Table 1 gives an overview of vascular disorders associated with abnormal bleeding.

Inherited Vascular Disorders

von Willebrand's Disease

Synonyms. vWD, von Willebrand-Jürgens syndrome, vascular hemophilia, angiohemophilia, pseudohemophilia.

Definition. This common familial bleeding disorder has an autosomal dominant mode of inheritance and is characterized by a prolonged bleeding time; low levels in plasma of factor VIII procoagulant activity (VIII: C); factor VIII-related high-molecular-weight antigen (VIIIR: Ag or von Willebrand factor antigen); and factor VIII-ristocetin cofactor activity (VIII : RCo),* which partly reflects factor VIII : von Willebrand factor (VIII : vWF) and promotes interaction of platelets with subendothelial vessel wall structures exposed as a result of vascular injury. Thus, a diminished concentration in plasma of VIII : vWF leads to impaired interaction between platelets and the injured vessel wall (defective platelet adherence)

Table 1. Vascular Disorders Associated with Abnormal Bleeding

- I. **Inherited Disorders**
  - A. von Willebrand's disease
  - B. Hereditary hemorrhagic telangiectasia
  - C. Inherited disorders of connective tissue
    - Ehlers-Danlos syndrome
    - Marfan syndrome
    - Osteogenesis imperfecta
    - Pseudoxanthoma elasticum
- II. **Congenital Disorders**
  - A. Giant cavernous hemangioma
- III. **Acquired Disorders**
  - A. Infections
  - B. Toxins
  - C. Hypersensitivity angiitis
    - Acquired connective tissue disorders
    - Drugs
    - Anaphylactoid purpura
    - Goodpasture's syndrome
    - Erythrocyte autosensitivity
  - D. Degenerative disorders
    - Senile purpura
    - Corticosteroid purpura
    - Scurvy
    - Amyloidosis
    - Diabetes mellitus
    - Acquired angiodysplasia
  - E. Neoplastic diseases
  - F. Purpura without known vascular abnormalities
    - Purpura simplex
    - Mechanical purpura
    - Factitious purpura

*Also abbreviated VIIIR : RCo.

and is thought to be the basis for the prolonged bleeding time. This defect is compounded by the reduction in VIII : C, which leads to impaired thrombin formation and impaired stabilization of the primary hemostatic platelet plug by fibrin. Recent evidence indicates that the antigen expressing VIII : C (VIII : CAg) and the antigen expressing VIII : RCo or VIII : vWF(VIIIR : Ag) are distinct molecular entities that circulate as a complex in plasma, and that normal survival of VIII : CAg (the production of which appears to be under X-chromosomal control in the liver and is normal in vWD) is dependent on normal, autosomally controlled production of VIIIR : Ag, which occurs in endothelial cells throughout the vasculature. Since the primary defect in vWD is impaired production of endothelial cell-derived VIIIR : Ag, the disorder may be considered a vascular one.

von Willebrand's disease appears to be heterogeneous in that, in addition to quantitative reduction in plasma of VIIIR : Ag (vWD type I), variants characterized by the synthesis of qualitatively abnormal VIIIR : Ag multimeric structure (lacking high-molecular-weight multimers) have been reported. These were associated with either decreased (vWD type IIA) or increased (vWD type IIB) platelet aggregation to ristocetin in citrated or heparinized platelet-rich plasma. In addition, there is a rare severe form of vWD that appears to be inherited as an autosomal recessive trait (homozygous or doubly heterozygous form) in which VIII : C is markedly decreased and both VIIIR : Ag and VIII : RCo are virtually absent in plasma as well as in platelets. Finally, a syndrome called pseudo-vWD has been reported. It is characterized by a reduction in VIII : RCo in plasma, a decrease in VIIIR : Ag high-molecular-weight multimers, and mild to moderately severe thrombocytopenia. The primary abnormality in this disorder appears to be an abnormality of platelets that bind VIIIR : Ag more avidly than normal platelets do, leading to a reduction in plasma of VIII : RCo and in high-molecular-weight VIIIR : Ag, as well as thrombocytopenia due presumably to intravascular VIII : RCo-mediated platelet aggregation and accelerated platelet removal from the circulation.

Clinical Features. von Willebrand's disease is probably the most common inherited bleeding disorder after classic hemophilia A. In contrast to classic hemophilia A, the majority of patients with vWD (80 per cent or more) have mild forms of the disease. Thus, estimation of the true prevalence of vWD has been difficult, since patients with mild abnormal bleeding manifestations not infrequently have a normal bleeding time and normal coagulation screening test results, and consequently are not referred for more vigorous and detailed hemostatic evaluation in a specialized laboratory. Females appear to be slightly more frequently affected than males, although this finding could be influenced by the fact that easy bruising in general is more common in females and may lead to increased referral for laboratory evaluation. There is no evidence for racial or ethnic predisposition. Abnormal bleeding manifestations such as easy bruising, frequent epistaxis, and gingival bleeding may occur in childhood, but in many patients the disorder manifests itself in early adolescence or adulthood as bleeding from gums with normal tooth brushing; excessive bleeding after dental extraction, tonsillectomy or other surgical procedures; heavy or prolonged menstrual bleeding (particularly early after menarche); gastrointestinal bleeding; or, less frequently, excessive postpartum bleeding. Petechiae are rarely observed. Spontaneous joint and soft-tissue bleeding is encountered only in rare patients with severe disease. In severely affected patients, excessive bleeding from dental extractions or other surgery may not be controlled without factor VIII replacement in the form of fresh-frozen plasma or cryoprecipitate. In patients with type I vWD, administration of 1-deamino-(8-d-arginine)-vasopressin (DDAVP) may be used as an alternative to replacement therapy because it causes a sufficient increase in VIII : C and VIII : RCo to control excessive bleeding following trauma or prevent abnormal bleeding with elective surgery.

Diagnosis. A prolonged bleeding time in the presence of a normal blood platelet concentration is the hallmark of vWD. However, the bleeding time may fluctuate considerably in the same patient; that is, it may be normal on some and prolonged on other occasions. The activated partial thromboplastin time (APTT) may be slightly to moderately prolonged, but it is frequently normal in patients whose VIII : C levels are greater than 25 per cent of normal. The prothrombin time (PT), thrombin time, and whole blood clot retraction are within normal limits. Factor VIII : C is generally reduced in patients with type I vWD but may be normal in patients with types IIA and IIB vWD. The levels of all other blood coagulation factors are within normal limits. Platelet aggregation in citrated plasma to ADP, epinephrine, arachidonic acid and collagen is normal whereas aggregation to ristocetin may be decreased or absent (types I, IIA, III), increased (type IIB), or normal.

The use of routine screening tests such as bleeding time, platelet count, APTT, and PT, which are available in most clinical diagnostic laboratories, even if coupled with a quantitative assay of VIII : C, is inadequate for establishing or excluding vWD. However, subjection of patients to appropriately detailed and comprehensive laboratory evaluation, which usually means referral to a specialized laboratory with experience and expertise in the diagnosis of bleeding disorders, is associated with a substantial cost and inconvenience to the patient. Thus, the decision whether or not to carry out laboratory evaluation for vWD must be based on a thorough, detailed general medical and bleeding history and family history.

It requires a great deal of judgment on the part of the patient's primary physician as to whether or not the "abnormal" bleeding may indeed be considered abnormal and in some cases whether the patient or the patient's parents are sufficiently concerned about the possibility of a bleeding disorder to warrant full investigation. If the decision is made to carry out laboratory evaluation for vWD, actual referral of the patient to a specialized laboratory is preferable to sending samples of plasma. Under the latter circumstance, the conditions of blood collection and processing and specimen transport may not be adequately controllable and interpretation of test results may be difficult. The patient should be instructed not to take aspirin or other drugs known to interfere with platelet function. Women should avoid estrogen-containing medications for at least one entire cycle, since estrogen administration—as well as pregnancy and liver disease—may raise factors VIII : C and VIII : RCo to normal levels.

Adequate laboratory evaluation for vWD should include the following tests: template bleeding time; blood platelet count; APTT; PT; quantitative estimation of VIII : C, VIIIR : Ag, and VIII : RCo; measurement of platelet aggregation in response to ADP, collagen, arachidonic acid (to exclude a possible, usually aspirin-related, defect of platelet function), and different concentrations of ristocetin; and analysis of VIIIR : Ag multimeric structure (crossed immunoelectrophoresis or agarose gel electrophoresis). The use of this battery of tests should allow either accurate exclusion of vWD or appropriate classification of the disorder (Table 2). There is some evidence that the aspirin tolerance test (template bleeding time before and 2 hours after the ingestion of 300 mg of aspirin) may be useful in the detection of patients with mild vWD. A prolongation of the bleeding time from normal (<8 minutes) to above 15 minutes after aspirin ingestion appears to be highly unusual for normal subjects and strongly suggestive of either vWD or (less commonly) a primary platelet dysfunction. With borderline results, specific tests should be repeated at least once before the diagnosis of vWD is made or ruled out. Accurate classification of vWD has important consequences in regard to the use of appropriate plasma or plasma concentrates in the management of traumatic bleeding or elective surgery. Furthermore, there is recent evidence to suggest that administration of a vasopressin analog (DDAVP) may be effective in controlling or preventing abnormal bleeding in most patients with type I vWD and possibly bleeding with some types of trauma or surgery in type IIA and IIB, whereas this form of treatment or prophylaxis appears to be ineffective in type III vWD patients.

Hereditary Hemorrhagic Telangiectasia

Synonyms. HHT, Osler-Weber-Rendu syndrome.

Definition and Clinical Features. This disorder, which is inherited as an autosomal dominant trait with a high degree of penetrance, is characterized by multiple areas of dilated tortuous capillaries predominantly in the mucous membranes and skin. The abnormal capillaries may reach the size of small venules. They are made up of only a thin layer of endothelium without smooth muscle cell support and may function as arteriovenous shunts that progressively enlarge as the patient ages. The disorder may be due to a focal lack of elastic fibers in the basement membrane. The vascular malformations are commonly close to epithelial surfaces and thus at increased risk of injury.

The vascular malformations are usually small (pinpoint size to 3 mm), slightly elevated, and sharply demarcated red to purple lesions with one or more arms radiating from an eccentric punctum. Because of the preferential localization of the lesions close to epithelial surfaces (lips, tongue, gingiva, nasal mucous membranes, conjunctiva, face, ears, palmar and plantar surfaces, and respiratory, gastrointestinal, and urogenital tracts) bleeding from any of these sites may occur. Lesions in other organs such as liver, spleen, and brain are rare. Epistaxis and gastrointestinal bleeding are by far the most frequent manifestations of the disorder. Iron deficiency anemia is a common complication. The lesions usually develop in childhood and increase in size and number with increasing age. Thus, abnormal bleeding manifestations generally do not occur until adulthood. The disorder seems to affect males and females with equal frequency.

Table 2. Classification of von Willebrand's Disease*

	Type I	Type IIA	Type IIB	Type III
Genetic transmission	Autosomal dominant	Autosomal dominant	Autosomal dominant	Autosomal recessive
Bleeding time	Prolonged	Prolonged	Prolonged	Prolonged
Crossed immuno-electrophoresis	Normal	Abnormal	Abnormal	Variable (mostly abnormal)
VIII:C	Decreased	Decreased or normal	Decreased or normal	Markedly decreased
VIIIR:Ag	Decreased	Decreased or normal	Decreased or normal	Minute amounts or absent
VIII:RCo	Decreased	Markedly decreased	Decreased or normal	Absent
RIPA	Decreased or normal	Absent or decreased	Increased	Absent
Multimeric structure of VIIIR:Ag	Normal in plasma and platelets	Absence of large and intermediate multimers from plasma and platelets	Absence of only larger multimers from plasma, normal in platelets	Variable

Key: VIII:C = Factor VIII procoagulant activity (expressed by VIII:CAg).
VIIIR:Ag = Factor VIII related high-molecular-weight antigen (expresses factor VIII: von Willebrand factor or VIII:vWF).
VIII:RCo = Ristocetin cofactor activity (promotes agglutination of platelets in the presence of the antibiotic ristocetin; expressed by VIIIR:Ag).
RIPA = Ristocetin-induced platelet aggregation in citrated or heparinized platelet-rich plasma.

*Adapted from Zimmerman, T.S., and Ruggeri, Z.M.: Progr. Hemost. Thromb., 6:203, 1982.

Diagnosis. In the presence of the characteristic vascular lesions in the skin or mucous membranes, together with a history of recurrent abnormal bleeding and a family history of abnormal bleeding in both males and females, the diagnosis of HHT is not difficult. The telangiectatic lesions associated with cirrhosis of the liver (spider angiomata) can usually be readily differentiated because of their larger size (0.5 to 2 cm) and the presence of a central bright red, pulsating arteriole. The disease may be difficult to diagnose when the vascular lesions are more discrete or limited to the deep nasopharynx, the gastrointestinal tract, or other internal organs. Endoscopy may be helpful under these circumstances.

Laboratory abnormalities (if present) are usually secondary to the bleeding complications such as acute post-hemorrhagic normocytic, normochromic anemia or microcytic, hypochromic anemia of chronic iron deficiency with or without thrombocytosis. Detailed hemostatic evaluation reveals no abnormalities; in particular, the bleeding time is normal. This is not surprising, since the disorder does not affect the microvasculature in general but is limited to scattered, small, well-defined areas.

Inherited Disorders of Connective Tissue

Several rare disorders of connective tissue due to inborn errors of collagen biosynthesis may be associated with abnormal bleeding.

Ehlers-Danlos Syndrome. This is a rare, heterogeneous connective tissue disorder characterized by abnormal collagen composition in skin, blood vessels, tendons, ligaments, heart valves, and other tissues. Seven different subtypes have been distinguished clinically and genetically. Deficiencies of different enzymes involved in normal collagen biosynthesis have been identified in four of these subtypes. Impaired synthesis of certain species of collagen by fibroblasts apparently leads to changes in the relative distribution of collagen and elastin, and loss of vessel wall connective tissue support. There is evidence to suggest that the abnormal bleeding manifestations associated with this syndrome are due to weakening of the vessel wall with a propensity for rupture, impaired vessel wall retraction after injury, and probably impaired interaction of platelets with the abnormal vessel wall connective tissue.

Patients with Ehlers-Danlos syndrome, particularly the subtype IV (ecchymotic, arterial, or sack type), may exhibit spontaneous bruising, post-traumatic or spontaneous soft-tissue bleeding, gingival bleeding, excessive or prolonged bleeding from tooth extractions, and gastrointestinal bleeding. Hemarthrosis is very rare. The diagnosis is based on recognition of the characteristic features of the disorder such as abnormal looseness of skin and joints, cardiac valve incompetency, and abnormally wide and thin scar tissue. Ultrastructural and biochemical analysis of collagen isolated from a skin biopsy specimen may be helpful in establishing the diagnosis, particularly in patients where the clinical abnormalities are less evident. Although a prolongation of the bleeding time and impaired in vitro platelet aggregation to various stimuli have been reported in a few patients, laboratory evaluation of platelet function and blood coagulation generally reveals no appreciable abnormalities.

Marfan's Syndrome. This syndrome, inherited by an autosomal dominant mode, is characterized by ectopia lentis, unusually long extremities, arachnodactyly, and aortic aneurysm. These abnormalities may be due to a defect in the intermolecular cross-linking of collagen. Mild abnormal bleeding manifestations such as easy bruising may occur. Increased urinary excretion of hydroxyproline has been reported in some patients. Abnormalities of platelet number, in vitro platelet function, or blood coagulation have not been reported. The template bleeding time may be slightly prolonged in some patients.

Osteogenesis Imperfecta. This rare autosomal dominant disorder is characterized by the combination of blue sclera and brittle bones and is thought to be due to a defect in bone matrix formation. Patients usually do not reach adult age. Both abnormal collagen composition and defective collagen cross-linking have been reported. Abnormal bleeding manifestations may include easy bruising, recurrent epistaxis, gastrointestinal tract bleeding, hemoptysis, and, occasionally, intracranial bleeding. Platelet number, platelet function, and blood coagulation are normal.

Pseudoxanthoma Elasticum. Characteristic features of this rare autosomal recessive disorder are the onset in early childhood of easy bruising, petechiae, bleeding from the gastrointestinal and urinary tracts, and the later development (in the second and third decades) of thrombotic occlusion and calcification of arteries leading to peripheral vascular, coronary, and cerebrovascular thromboembolic complications. The basic defect appears to be abnormal formation of elastic fibers in the skin and vascular subendothelium. No abnormalities of platelet number, platelet function, or blood coagulation have been reported.

Congenital Vascular Disorders

Giant Cavernous Hemangioma

Giant cavernous hemangioma (Kasabach-Merritt syndrome) is a rare congenital disorder characterized by variably extensive, frequently multiple, mass lesions involving the skin, soft tissues, and less frequently visceral organs, consisting of tortuous, dilated blood vessels with arteriovenous shunting. Periodic swelling of the lesions, presumably as a result of intermittent obstruction of blood outflow from the hemangioma, is commonly observed. Depending on the size of the lesions, variably extensive hemostatic abnormalities consistent with disseminated intravascular or consumption coagulopathy (DIC) are observed: that is, thrombocytopenia; prolongation of activated partial thromboplastin, prothrombin, and thrombin times; low plasma fibrinogen, factors VIII : C and V; and elevated levels of fibrin/fibrinogen degradation products. Even in the presence of severe DIC due to large hemangiomata, abnormal bleeding usually occurs only in association with accidental trauma or invasive procedures. However, severe and possibly life-threatening bleeding may be encountered with direct accidental trauma to, or surgical incision of, the vascular tumor itself.

Acquired Vascular Disorders

Infections

Infections with a variety of organisms may be associated with abnormal bleeding manifestations. These range from petechiae and small ecchymoses, to generalized bleeding from venipunctures and invasive procedures, to bleeding into the gastrointestinal tract, urinary tract, brain, heart, lungs, and other organs. The pathogenesis of these bleeding complications may be quite varied, ranging from:

1. Direct injury to endothelial cells by the pathogen itself (streptococci, rickettsiae), or one or more of its products (endotoxin).
2. Immune complex–mediated endothelial damage.
3. Thrombocytopenia secondary to direct platelet-pathogen interaction, pathogen-initiated autoimmune platelet antibody formation (predominantly in viral infections), or wide-spread platelet interaction with the damaged vasculature.
4. Endotoxin or immune-mediated vascular injury associated with acute changes in vascular permeability, hypovolemia, and microcirculatory failure as well as activation of platelets and blood coagulation leading to consumption coagulopathy/DIC (*Schwartzmann-Sanarelli syndrome*).

In the vast majority of patients, the bleeding manifestations are mild and clinically inconsequential except that they may offer useful clues as to the particular diagnosis (e.g., scarlet fever, Rocky Mountain spotted fever, septic endocarditis). Generalized bleeding secondary to severe hemostatic failure associated with septicemia may require temporary supportive measures such as replacement therapy with platelet concentrates, fresh-frozen plasma, or cryoprecipitate, in addition to vigorous fluid replacement and antibiotics. Thrombocytopenia may persist for days or even weeks after complete normalization of all other blood hemostatic measurements.

Toxins

Petechiae and ecchymoses have been reported to occur (in the absence of thrombocytopenia or other hemostatic abnormalities) following exposure to drugs (e.g., coumadin, penicillin) or chemicals (e.g., herbicides, insecticides, organic solvents), presumably as a result of direct endothelial injury. The reaction appears to be idiosyncratic, since only certain individuals are affected.

Hypersensitivity Angiitis

Acquired Connective Tissue Disorders. A heterogeneous group of disorders of uncertain etiology, characterized by a variety of autoimmune phenomena, is frequently associated with mild abnormal bleeding manifestations, usually petechiae and ecchymoses with predominant involvement of the lower extremities. This group of disorders includes rheumatoid arthritis, systemic lupus erythematosus, scleroderma, dermatomyositis, Sjögren's syndrome, mixed cryoglobulinemia, hepatitis B, and Wegener's granulomatosis. Skin biopsy of purpuric lesions reveals cuffing of the dermal microcirculation by numerous granulocytes in various stages of viability ranging from normal appearance to complete disintegration ("nuclear dust"). This characteristic pathologic lesion has been named *leukocytoclastic vasculitis* and is the morphologic equivalent of the clinical term "palpable purpura." Bleeding time, blood platelet counts, and results of in vitro platelet function tests and blood coagulation are usually within normal limits. Separation of the various disorders in this group depends on the variable clinical findings; on the demonstration of certain serologic abnormalities (antinuclear antibodies, antibodies to DNA, low levels of serum complement components, cryoglobulin); and on demonstration of various immunoglobulin species, complement, and/or fibrin on the surface or beneath endothelial cells in biopsy specimens from the purpuric lesions.

Drugs. Palpable purpuric skin lesions, in the absence of thrombocytopenia, exhibiting the features of leukocytoclastic vasculitis may be seen in patients exposed to a variety of drugs and other chemicals such as penicillin, iodides, isoniazid, azodyes, aspirin, benzoic acid, chlorothiazides, and oxytetracycline. The appearance of the purpuric skin lesions is usually not associated with any other clinical signs and symptoms.

Anaphylactoid Purpura

Synonyms. Schönlein-Henoch purpura, allergic vascular purpura.

Definition and Clinical Features. This disorder is a form of small vessel vasculitis, principally occurring in children, with a predilection for involvement of skin, intestines, joints, and kidneys. Clinical manifestations include palpable cutaneous purpuric lesions, fever, malaise, headache, arthralgias, abdominal pain, melena, hematuria, and angioedema. Acute glomerulonephritis is a common associated condition. The skin lesions are nonspecific, characterized by the features of leukocytoclastic or necrotizing vasculitis of postcapillary venules. The hallmark of this disorder is the finding of glomerular deposition of IgA in kidney biopsy specimens. This finding and the absence of hypocomplementemia are consistent with the concept that the disorder represents a delayed hypersensitivity type of vasculitis. Drugs and infectious agents (beta-hemolytic streptococci) have been suggested as possible precipitating causes.

When the disorder occurs in children, the onset is usually acute. The purpuric rash occurs early in the course and is usually most marked on the lower extremities but may involve the trunk and upper extremities. Fever, generalized malaise, arthralgia with or without swelling of joints, and abdominal pain may persist for several days. Complete resolution of all signs and symptoms usually occurs within 2 to 3 weeks; however, in some patients, particularly adults, the systemic manifestations may occur in various combinations and at different times. Thus, abdominal pain or arthralgia may precede the appearance of the purpuric skin lesions, and occasionally diagnosis may be difficult when the skin lesions are few and discrete. Although the disorder is usually self-limited with complete resolution of all signs and symptoms within 2 to 3 weeks, in rare cases subacute or chronic glomerulonephritis may develop, leading to renal failure. Other rare complications are convulsions, which are presumably due to cerebral edema, and respiratory failure resulting from edema of the glottis.

Diagnosis. The diagnosis is based on the recognition of the characteristic clinical manifestations already discussed. Whereas histopathologic findings in skin biopsy specimens are nonspecific (varying from leukocytoclastic to necrotizing vasculitis), kidney biopsy may be valuable in establishing the diagnosis (demonstration of glomerular IgA deposition). However, kidney biopsy is generally not indicated in view of the benign, self-limited nature of the disorder. Other laboratory findings are nonspecific. Anemia is absent except in the rare patient with gross gastrointestinal bleeding. However, a positive stool test for occult blood and microhematuria are common, as are mild to moderate albuminuria, and granular and red cell casts. In the acute phase of the disorder, mild to moderate polymorphonuclear leukocytosis may be present. Bleeding time, blood platelet counts, and the results of tests of in vitro platelet function and blood coagulation are typically normal. Some or all of the clinical manifestations of this disorder are shared by certain acquired connective tissue disorders such as systemic lupus erythematosus, rheumatoid arthritis, mixed cryoglobulinemia, hypocomplementemic vasculitis, and the rare vasculitis associated with a malignant tumor. Appropriate studies should be carried out (particularly in adult patients) to exclude these diseases, since they may require specific, aggressive treatment.

Goodpasture's Syndrome. This is a rare disorder characterized clinically by episodic hemoptysis, dyspnea, pulmonary infiltrates, and hematuria. It is thought to be a form of hypersensitivity angiitis due to reaction of autoantibodies with glomerular and alveolar basement membranes and complement-mediated vascular injury. The agents responsible for triggering the abnormal immune response have not been identified. Although occasional cases with spontaneous resolution have been reported, the course in general is progressive: glomerulonephritis with hematuria, proteinuria, and renal failure; episodic dyspnea; pulmonary infiltrates; and hemoptysis varying from microscopic evidence (hemosiderin-laden macrophages in sputum) to occasional death from exsanguination or asphyxia.

The diagnosis is suspected from the clinical manifestations and laboratory findings and is confirmed by the demonstration of antiglomerular basement membrane or pulmonary capillary antibodies in kidney or lung biopsy specimens or of antiglomerular basement membrane antibodies in serum. Bleeding time, blood platelet concentration, and results of coagulation studies are normal.

The disorder must be distinguished clinically from *idiopathic pulmonary hemosiderosis.* This disease, of unknown etiology and pathogenesis, is characterized by chronic, recurrent intrapulmonary blood extravasation leading to pulmonary inflammation and fibrosis, and iron deficiency anemia. There is no evidence of immunologic abnormalities or renal involvement. The chronic hemorrhagic pneumonitis with fibrosis associated with mitral stenosis or other forms of cardiac disease can usually be readily distinguished on the basis of the cardiac manifestations and lack of evidence of glomerulonephritis.

Erythrocyte Autosensitivity

Synonyms. Gardner-Diamond syndrome, autoerythrocyte sensitivity, psychogenic purpura.

Clinical Features. This rare disorder occurs virtually exclusively in middle-aged women with emotional instability or frank personality disorder. It is characterized by the appearance of ecchymoses associated with, and frequently preceded by as long as 24 hours by, pain, heat, and induration of the bruised skin area. There is evidence from serologic and immunohistopathologic studies that the disorder may be a form of immune vasculitis due to sensitization against autologous red blood cell stroma. The skin lesions may vary in size from a few centimeters in diameter to large areas affecting an entire thigh or forearm. Although patients usually deny direct trauma to the painful ecchymotic area, they commonly report a history of preceding trauma or a surgical procedure at a different site. In some patients there is a history of other abnormal bleeding manifestations such as epistaxis, gingival bleeding, gastrointestinal or urinary tract bleeding, or menorrhagia. Additional rare symptoms include episodic abdominal pain, nausea and vomiting, transient visual disturbances, Raynaud's syndrome, syncope, arthralgia, unexplained fever, or transient cerebrovascular ischemic symptoms.

Diagnosis. The diagnosis is suspected on the basis of the patient's general history and the finding of bruises with the unusual feature of marked initial inflammation. The lesions tend to resolve spontaneously within several days to weeks and rarely require more than analgesics for relief of pain. Prompt recognition of the disorder is important to avoid surgical intervention since, particularly in the early phase, the lesions may lack the hemorrhagic component and may be mistaken for cellulitis or a large abscess. The diagnosis of erythrocyte autosensitivity is supported by the appearance of the typical inflammatory-hemorrhagic lesion following intracutaneous injection of 0.1 ml of autologous blood or red blood cell stroma. However, this test may be negative in a third of patients who otherwise fit the diagnostic criteria. Furthermore, positive tests have been reported in some patients with the injection of minute amounts of DNA or a variety of other substances and even saline. Sometimes the lesions can be induced only in an area within the patient's vision or reach. Bleeding time, blood platelet counts, and the results of tests of in vitro platelets, blood coagulation, and fibrinogen are normal.

Degenerative Vascular Disorders

Senile Purpura. This disorder is characterized by sharply demarcated red to purple ecchymotic lesions of variable size that usually occur in areas of the skin that are regularly exposed to sunlight (dorsal surfaces of forearms, hands, legs, face, and neck). They are observed in otherwise healthy older subjects, either spontaneously or with trivial trauma, and frequently leave a residual brownish pigmentation of the skin. The lesions have been attributed to an age-related overall decrease in the number of skin capillaries, atrophy of perivascular connective tissue, a decrease in the collagen content per unit area of skin, and loss of skin and vessel collagen elasticity. The bleeding time is generally normal, but intradermal bleeding may be seen with this test. Blood platelet counts and results of tests of in vitro platelet function and blood coagulation are normal.

Corticosteroid Purpura. Purpuric skin lesions may occur with prolonged administration of corticosteroids or in patients with Cushing's syndrome at the site of striae on the lower extremities. The lesions are thought to be due to changes in connective tissue vascular support similar to those seen in senile purpura.

Scurvy. Severe vitamin C (ascorbic acid) deficiency is associated with a variety of abnormal bleeding manifestations ranging from petechiae, small bruises on the arms and legs, bleeding from swollen gums, epistaxis, and gastrointestinal and urinary tract bleeding, to painful subperiosteal hemorrhages. Bleeding manifestations are thought to be due to defective biosynthesis of collagen in which ascorbic acid functions as an essential cofactor in the conversion of proline to hydroxyproline. Scurvy is common in countries with a high prevalence of malnutrition. All manifestations of scurvy disappear promptly with the administration of Vitamin C.

Amyloidosis. Patients with either primary amyloidosis or amyloidosis associated with paraproteinemia and chronic inflammatory disorders may develop abnormal cutaneous purpuric lesions, usually secondary to trauma, with predilection for the face. Bleeding has been attributed to deposition of amyloid in the skin and blood vessels. Bleeding manifestations may occur in the absence of laboratory hemostatic abnormalities. However, some patients with amyloidosis may develop deficiencies of certain coagulation factors, especially factor X, which may contribute to abnormal bleeding.

Diabetes Mellitus. Recurrent cutaneous purpura may be seen in patients with diabetes mellitus, presumably due to subendothelial small vessel connective tissue alterations similar to those seen in senile and corticosteroid purpura.

Acquired Angiodysplasia. Alterations of capillaries and postcapillary vessels, with arteriovenous malformations similar to those seen in hereditary telangiectasia, may be observed in association with aortic insufficiency, mitral valve prolapse, uremia, and von Willebrand's disease. The lesions are usually multiple and commonly localized in the mucosa of the gastric fundus, the duodenum, and the ascending colon. They may produce recurrent, sometimes life-threatening, bleeding. The pathogenesis of this disorder is not known. When it is associated with von Willebrand's disease or uremia, impaired platelet-subendothelium interaction or uremic thrombocytopathy may contribute to the bleeding manifestations.

Neoplasms

Several rare tumors characterized by neoplastic proliferation of blood vessels are associated with abnormal bleeding. These include Kaposi's sarcoma (a slowly progressive tumor which usually presents with bluish-red to brown macular or nodular lesions in the skin of the lower extremities, but may in later stages involve visceral organs), hemangioendothelioma, hemangiopericytoma, angiosarcoma, angioendothelioma, and proliferating angioendotheliomatosis. Hemostatic abnormalities have not been described, and the bleeding is thought to be due to abnormalities of the endothelial lining of the neoplastic vasculature. Diagnosis is usually suspected on the basis of the clinical presentation and verified by histologic examination.

Purpura without Known Vascular Abnormalities

Purpura Simplex. Easy bruising with petechiae and small ecchymoses on exposed areas of the extremities, occurring with minor trauma or without known trauma, is commonly seen in otherwise healthy women. Bleeding time, blood platelet count, and the results of tests of in vitro platelet function and blood coagulation are normal. Etiology and pathogenesis of this "disorder" are unknown.

Mechanical Purpura (Orthostatic Purpura). Petechiae and small ecchymoses of the lower extremities may occur in healthy subjects after prolonged standing, lifting, or straining. Results of hemostatic tests are normal. The disorder appears to be related to a group of purpuras called progressive pigmented purpura, which includes purpura annularis telangiectodes (Majocchi), progressive pigmentary dermatosis (Schamberg), and pigmented purpuric lichenoid dermatitis (Gougerot-Blum). No structural vascular abnormalities have been identified in this disorder. The cutaneous purpuric lesions may resemble palpable purpura associated with connective tissue disorders or drug hypersensitivity.

Factitious Purpura. On occasion, otherwise healthy-appearing individuals (usually adolescent to middle-aged women) are seen with cutaneous purpura ranging from petechiae to large ecchymoses, as well as deep hematomas predominantly on the extremities. Extensive investigation usually fails to yield evidence for hemostatic abnormalities. The lesions may have an inflammatory component, and thus may be confused with those seen in patients with erythrocyte autosensitization. In such patients, the possibility that the lesions are self-inflicted for the purpose of getting attention from a spouse or lover or as an expression of self-hatred, other emotional disturbances, or a frank personality disorder must be considered. In contrast to patients with psychogenic purpura, evidence for a personality disorder may be more difficult to detect in these subjects, although there appears to be a certain overlap between the two disorders. The finding that the lesions are restricted to areas within reach of the patient's hands may be a clue to the diagnosis. Factitious purpura is not restricted to cutaneous bleeding manifestations, and patients with self-induced hematuria, epistaxis, and gastrointestinal, respiratory, or vaginal bleeding have been reported.

BLEEDING DUE TO PLATELET DISORDERS

When the number of platelets in the circulating blood is markedly reduced or the platelets are functionally impaired, the hemostatic competence of the microvasculature may be impaired. Thus, blood extravasation may occur in response to trauma or even without known trauma, depending on the severity of the thrombocytopenia or platelet dysfunction. The most common bleeding manifestations with such quantitative or qualitative platelet disorders are bleeding into the skin (petechiae, ecchymoses) and mucous membranes (gingival bleeding, gastrointestinal tract bleeding). Paradoxically, abnormal bleeding manifestations may also be observed in patients with markedly increased blood platelet concentrations associated with certain myeloproliferative disorders.

The Thrombocytopenias

Thrombocytopenia is defined as a reduction in the circulating blood platelet concentration below the normal range of 150,000 to 400,000 per cu mm. It is the most common cause of abnormal bleeding. Thrombocytopenia may result from:

1. An inherited or acquired impairment of platelet production.
2. An increased rate of platelet destruction.
3. Abnormal platelet distribution.
4. Dilution.

A classification of the thrombocytopenias based on these pathogenetic considerations is given in Table 3. In some disease states, two or more of these mechanisms may be operative simultaneously.

The general clinical evaluation of a patient with thrombocytopenia should proceed in a sequential fashion and may include the following:

1. Verification of thrombocytopenia, i.e., exclusion of laboratory errors and artifacts (spurious thrombocytopenia) to avoid unnecessary inconvenience, discomfort, anxiety and cost to the patient.
2. Thorough personal history, including history of exposure to drugs and chemicals; family history; and physical examination (petechiae, ecchymoses, lymphadenopathy, hepatomegaly, splenomegaly, rectal examination with stool guaiac test).
3. Complete blood count.
4. Examination of the peripheral blood smear (platelet number, platelet "size," red cell and white cell number and/or morphology).
5. Coagulation screening tests (activated partial thromboplastin time, prothrombin time, fibrinogen, and serum fibrin/fibrinogen degradation products to exclude disseminated intravascular coagulation).
6. Bleeding time. In patients with hyporegenerative thrombocytopenia, the template bleeding time is usually prolonged when the platelet count in blood falls below 100,000 per cu mm, with a linear negative correlation between bleeding time and platelet concentration. In contrast, the bleeding time is commonly normal in patients with even moderately severe thrombocytopenia secondary to increased platelet destruction such as autoimmune thrombocytopenia. This finding appears to be due to the presence in the blood of a high proportion of young, functionally more active platelets in the latter condition. Thus, the test may occasionally be useful in the differentiation between hypo- and hyperregenerative thrombocyto-

Table 3. Classification of Thrombocytopenias

- I. Decreased Platelet Production
  - A. Reduced marrow megakaryocytes
    - 1. Congenital disorders
      - Fanconi's anemia
      - Thrombocytopenia with absent radii
    - 2. Acquired disorders
      - Generalized marrow hypoplasia
        - Radiation
        - Chemicals
        - Drugs
        - Toxins
        - Infections
        - Idiopathic
      - Neoplastic or fibrotic marrow replacement
      - Selective megakaryocytic hypoplasia
      - Drugs, ethanol
      - Infections
      - Autoimmune disorders (systemic lupus erythematosus)
      - Idiopathic
  - B. Normal or increased marrow megakaryocytes
    - 1. Hereditary disorders
      - Wiskott-Aldrich syndrome
      - May-Hegglin anomaly
    - 2. Acquired disorders
      - Vitamin B_{12} or folate deficiency
      - Paroxysmal nocturnal hemoglobinuria
      - Dysmyelopoietic syndromes (erythroleukemia, preleukemia, sideroblastic anemia)
  - C. Disordered regulatory control mechanism
- II. Increased Platelet Destruction
  - A. Immunologic destruction
    - Idiopathic thrombocytopenic purpura
    - Secondary immunologic purpura
      - Systemic lupus erythematosus
      - Evans' syndrome
      - Lymphoproliferative disorders
  - B. Nonimmunologic destruction (consumption)
    - Selective platelet consumption
    - Thrombotic thrombocytopenic purpura
    - Hemolytic uremic syndrome
    - Vasculitis
    - Extracorporeal circulatory assist devices
    - Platelet consumption with disseminated intravascular coagulation
      - Acute infection
      - Disseminated carcinoma
      - Obstetric complications
      - Extensive tissue injury
- III. Abnormal Platelet Distribution
  - A. Increased splenic pooling (splenomegaly)
  - B. Increased vascular pooling (hypothermia)
- IV. Platelet Dilution (Massive Blood Transfusion)

penia in patients in whom bone marrow examination is not possible or inconclusive.

7. Bone marrow aspiration and biopsy to assess the number and morphology of megakaryocytes and to look for the presence of hematologic or nonhematologic neoplasms or fibrosis.

8. Liver-spleen scan, serologic tests for autoimmune disorders (antinuclear antibody, rheumatoid factor, complement, Coombs' test), serum folate, vitamin B_{12}.

9. Tests for platelet antibodies. Qualitative (immunofluorescence) or quantitative (inhibition of complement-mediated RBC lysis, radioimmunoassay immunodiffusion) tests for platelet-associated IgG and antiplatelet antibodies in serum are available in some specialized laboratories. However, the sensitivity of these tests may vary considerably from laboratory to laboratory, and because of low specificity their general usefulness in the evaluation of thrombocytopenia is somewhat limited.

10. Platelet survival studies. Studies of platelet survival using autologous platelets labeled with sodium chromate (^{51}Cr) or indium oxide (^{111}In) are the only definitive means of demonstrating or excluding increased platelet destruction or consumption. Platelet survival and turnover may also be assessed indirectly by a non-isotopic method using measurement of the rate of recovery of platelet prostaglandin production following a single oral dose of aspirin. However, all of these tests are cumbersome, time-consuming, complex, and expensive and thus of limited general clinical usefulness.

Congenital Megakaryocytic Hypoplasia

Neonatal absence or reduction of bone marrow megakaryocytes is associated with Fanconi's anemia and several possibly related disorders characterized by various skeletal anomalies such as bilateral agenesis of the radius or absence of ulna or humerus, cardiac defects, or microcephaly. Fetal injury at 6 to 8 weeks of gestation due to maternal rubella infection and maternal drug exposure (thiazides) have been suggested to be of possible pathogenetic importance. Cutaneous bleeding manifestations are usually present at birth, and early death, frequently due to intracranial bleeding, is common.

Acquired Megakaryocytic Hypoplasia

Generalized Marrow Hypoplasia. Thrombocytopenia is commonly and predictably observed as part of generalized marrow suppression in association with exposure to ionizing radiation or administration of a large variety of chemotherapeutic agents (e.g., alkylating agents, antimetabolites, other cytotoxic drugs). Because of the relatively short half-life of platelets (4 to 5 days), the development of thrombocytopenia is usually rapid, with frequently complete disappearance of megakaryocytes from marrow aspirates or biopsy specimens. Usually, there is prompt recovery within 1 to 3 weeks following cessation of administration of the agents. However, prolonged and occasionally irreversible thrombocytopenia may be seen with some alkylating agents (melphalan, busulfan). Thrombocytopenia as a result of generalized marrow suppression is also observed with exposure to benzene and other toxic chemicals, as an idiosyncratic reaction to certain drugs such as chloramphenicol, as a result of bone marrow injury by infectious agents (hepatitis, infectious mononucleosis), in association with thymoma, and in so-called idiopathic aplastic anemia. In the latter condition, thrombocytopenia and megakaryocytic marrow hypoplasia may precede the development of anemia and granulocytopenia by weeks or months.

Neoplastic or Fibrotic Marrow Replacement. Thrombocytopenia is frequently associated with generalized marrow replacement by neoplastic diseases (leukemia, lymphoma, multiple myeloma, metastatic carcinoma) and myelofibrosis, as well as certain less common disorders such as systemic histiocytosis, Gaucher's disease, and osteopetrosis. In some of these disorders, direct toxic suppression of normal hematopoiesis may be responsible for the cytopenia rather than physical marrow displacement (leukemia, dysmyelopoietic disorders such as sideroblastic anemia, preleukemia, lymphoma, metastatic carcinoma, myeloma).

Selective Megakaryocytic Hypoplasia. Thrombocytopenia without associated reduction in other blood cells may occur as a result of selective toxic suppression of megakaryocyte development by certain drugs such as thiazide diuretics, tolbutamide, and estrogenic hormones. Mild, asymptomatic thrombocytopenia may be observed in up to 2 per cent of patients taking thiazides, indicating that a pharmacologic rather than idiosyncratic mechanism may be involved. Thrombocytopenia may also be seen in infants of mothers taking these drugs. Recovery from thrombocytopenia associated with the use of thiazides may be slow after drug discontinuation. Serologic tests for platelet antibodies have frequently been negative.

Ethanol in large doses has been shown to suppress platelet production in man; this effect may contribute, in addition to nutritional deficiencies, to the thrombocytopenia frequently observed in alcoholic patients.

Selective thrombocytopenia with megakaryocytic hypoplasia has also been observed with certain infections (e.g., hepatitis, infectious mononucleosis) as well as in autoimmune connective tissue disorders, particularly systemic lupus erythematosus. In these disorders, increased pooling of platelets in an enlarged spleen may contribute to the thrombocytopenia.

Hereditary Disorders with Ineffective Thrombocytopoiesis

Moderate to severe thrombocytopenia is one of the characteristic features of the X-chromosomal *Wiskott-Aldrich syndrome* in addition to recurrent infections (due to defects in both cellular and humoral immunity) and eczema. Benign lymphadenopathy is frequently observed. Boys affected with the disorder usually die before the age of 5 from infection, hemorrhage, or a malignant lymphoproliferative disorder. Abnormal bleeding manifestations appear to be due to the combined effects of thrombocytopenia and different forms of platelet dysfunction (storage pool defects, impaired platelet release reaction). Thus the bleeding time is usually longer than expected on the basis of the degree of thrombocytopenia. Platelet size is normal. Since megakaryocyte mass is normal or increased and platelet survival only mildly shortened, the thrombocytopenia appears to be at least in large part due to ineffective thrombocytopoiesis.

The *May-Hegglin anomaly* is a benign autosomal dominant disorder characterized by the presence of well-defined basophilic and pyroninophilic inclusions in granulocytes (similar to Döhle bodies of infection) and abnormally large platelets containing few granules. Mild to moderate thrombocytopenia is present in about one third of affected individuals, but megakaryocytes in the bone marrow are either normal or increased. Patients are usually asymptomatic, but mild abnormal bleeding manifestations may occur. The bleeding time is typically normal but may occasionally be prolonged out of proportion to the degree of thrombocytopenia. In vitro platelet functions are normal.

Acquired Ineffective Thrombocytopoiesis

Thrombocytopenia due to ineffective thrombocytopoiesis is a consistent finding in patients with megaloblastic anemia due to folate or vitamin B_{12} deficiency. Marrow megakaryocyte mass is usually normal or increased, and platelet survival may be moderately shortened. A disproportionate prolongation of the bleeding time, large platelets, and impaired in vitro platelet function may be observed. Similar findings, indicating ineffective thrombocytopoiesis associated with the release into the circulating blood of platelets with abnormal size, morphology, and function, have been described in patients with paroxysmal nocturnal hemoglobinuria and certain forms of dysmyelopoiesis such as erythroleukemia, sideroblastic anemia, and preleukemia.

Disorders of Regulation of Thrombocytopoiesis

Mild to moderate thrombocytopenia secondary to thrombopoietin deficiency or defects in the control by thrombopoietin of platelet production (tidal platelet dysgenesis, cylic thrombocytopenia) is very rarely observed. It is usually not associated with abnormal bleeding manifestations.

Idiopathic Thrombocytopenic Purpura

Synonyms. ITP, autoimmune thrombocytopenic purpura, Werlhof's disease.

Definition. *Acute ITP* is a disorder characterized by sudden onset of thrombocytopenic purpura in otherwise healthy-appearing individuals. Patients may present with extensive petechial hemorrhages, preferentially on the lower extremities and areas exposed to trauma; epistaxis; or gingival, gastrointestinal or genitourinary tract bleeding. Physical examination is otherwise unremarkable; in particular, the spleen is not palpably enlarged. There is usually marked megakaryocytic hyperplasia in the bone marrow with appearance of numerous young basophilic megakaryocytes. The disease occurs predominantly in young children 1 to 3 weeks after a sore throat or cold and is self-limited in over 80 per cent of patients with complete resolution within 2 to 6 weeks without specific treatment. However, acute ITP may present at all ages, and in older children and adults spontaneous resolution is rare; treatment with corticosteroids and/or splenectomy is usually required. Recurrence after recovery is rare.

Chronic ITP occurs predominantly in young and middle-aged adults, with females being affected three or four times as frequently as males. Patients may present with petechiae, easy bruising, and menorrhagia. Physical examination is usually unremarkable, and the spleen is not palpable. Over 90 per cent of adults with chronic ITP fail to undergo spontaneous remission, and the clinical course may be characterized by recurrent remission and relapse.

The autoimmune nature of ITP is suggested by the demonstration of platelet-specific IgG antibodies on platelets and in serum during the acute phase and recurrent exacerbations of thrombocytopenia; by the premature removal of platelets by the spleen (in patients with fulminant disease also in the liver); and by the frequent, though not universal, response (complete or partial) to splenectomy (site of documented platelet destruction as well as antiplatelet antibody synthesis) and immunosuppressive agents such as corticosteroids, azathioprine, and cyclophosphamide. Furthermore, infusion of plasma from patients with acute ITP has been shown to cause thrombocytopenia in normal subjects, and pregnant women with ITP may give birth to infants with thrombocytopenia.

Diagnosis. The diagnosis of ITP is based on the demonstration of:

1. Thrombocytopenia with large platelets (megathrombocytes) on the peripheral blood smear.
2. Normal to increased numbers of mostly immature small megakaryocytes showing low nuclear ploidy, relatively small amounts of basophilic cytoplasm, and little or no evidence of platelet formation.
3. Lack of clinical and laboratory evidence of autoimmune connective tissue disorders.

Demonstration of an increase in platelet-associated IgG or antiplatelet IgG in serum by qualitative or quantitative immunologic assays (available in some specialized laboratories) may be helpful in supporting the diagnosis of ITP. However, these tests have been shown to have relatively low specificity, since positive results may be obtained in patients with a variety of autoimmune disorders as well as in patients with evidence of intravascular platelet destruction (thrombotic thrombocytopenic purpura, hemolytic uremic syndrome, and consumptive coagulopathy or DIC). In severe thrombocytopenia, failure to demonstrate increased amounts of platelet-associated IgG may be used as strong evidence against immune-mediated platelet destruction. Platelet survival studies using isotopic or non-isotopic methods are of limited clinical usefulness in the diagnosis of ITP and have little value in predicting response to specific therapeutic measures such as glucocorticosteroids or splenectomy. A prompt positive response to glucocorticosteroid administration may be used in support of the diagnosis of ITP in patients with a history of drug exposure, since immune-suppressive agents in general do not affect drug-induced immune platelet destruction.

Drug-Induced Immune Thrombocytopenia

Although certain drugs such as thiazide diuretics and tolbutamide may cause thrombocytopenia owing to direct toxic suppression of megakaryocyte production, a much larger number of drugs (including thiazides) have been either documented or strongly suggested to cause thrombocytopenia via immunologic mechanisms. A list of such drugs is given in Table 4.

Clinical Features. The clinical manifestations of drug-induced immune purpura may be indistinguishable from those seen in ITP. Petechiae, ecchymoses, epistaxis, and gingival, gastrointestinal or genitourinary tract bleeding may develop within hours, days, or months of drug administration. Generally, all symptoms and thrombocytopenia clear within 2 to 3 weeks after discontinuation of the offending drug.

Thrombocytopenia may develop as an idiosyncratic reaction via two major mechanisms:

1. Some drugs or their metabolites may act as haptens inducing the formation of antibodies. Interaction of antibody and drug- or drug metabolite-coated platelets in vivo may lead to platelet injury and destruction. This reaction appears to occur only following exposure of the blood to high concentrations of the drug, with subsequent clearance of free drug from the circulation, and high titer of antibody. In vitro platelet agglutination, lysis, and complement fixation may be observed in the presence of drug-coated platelets and drug-free antiserum but not in the presence of either drug or antibody alone. Examples of this type of mechanism may be acetaminophen and penicillin.

2. A drug or drug metabolite may bind to a plasma protein or "carrier" molecule, followed by production of antibodies against the drug/carrier complex (not the drug itself) and formation of drug/carrier/antibody complexes that may attach to platelets nonspecifically ("innocent bystander hypothesis").

Table 4. Drugs That May Produce Thrombocytopenia*

Agents That May Suppress Platelet Production by Selective Suppression of Megakaryocyte Proliferation		
Chlorothiazides	Ethanol	
Estrogenic hormones	Tolbutamide	
Agents That May Provoke Formation of Platelet Antibodies		
Acetazolamide	Diazepam	*p*-Aminosalicylic acid
Allyl isopropylcarbamide (Sedormid) and congeners	Digitoxin	Quinidine
Antazoline	Diphenylhydantoin	Quinine
Carbamazepine	Gold salts	Rifampin
Centulin	Heparin	Sodium valproate
Chlorothiazides	Hydroxychloroquine	Stibophen
Chlorpheniramine	Lidocaine	Sulfamethazine
Chlorpropamide	Methyl-dopa	Sulfathiazole
Desipramine	Novobiocin	Sulfisoxazole
	Organic arsenicals	
Drugs Whose Mechanism of Action May or May Not Be Immunologic		
Acetaminophen	Disulfiram	Phenacetin
Allyl isopropyl barbituric acid	L-Dopa	Phenobarbital
Aminopyrine	Ergot	Phenylbutazone
Amobarbital	Erythromycin	Potassium iodide
Ampicillin	Ethyl-allyl-acetylurea	Prednisone
Aspirin	5-Ethyl-phenylhydantoin	Primidone
Bismuth	Furosemide	Prochlorperazine
Butabarbital	Glymidine	Promethazine
Carbutamide	Heparin	Propylthiouracil
Cephalothin	Heroin	Pyrazinamide
Chloroquine	Hexopropynate	Reserpine
Chlorpheniramine maleate	Iopanoic acid	Sodium salicylate
Chlorpromazine	Isoniazid	Spironolactone
Chlorthalidone	Lincomycin	Streptomycin
Cimetidine	Meperidine	Sulfadiazine
Clonazepam	Meprobamate	Sulfadimetine
Clopamide	Mercurial diuretics	Sulfamerazine
Codeine	Nitrofurantoin	Sulfamethoxazole
Colloidal silver	Nitroglycerin	Sulfamethoxypyridazine
Desimipramine	Organic arsenicals	Tetracycline
Dextroamphetamine sulfate	Oxyphenbutazone	Thiouracil
Diazoxide	Oxytetracycline	Thiourea
Digitalis	Penicillamine	Tolbutamide
Digoxin	Penicillin	Trimethadione
	Pentamidine	

*List does not include all drugs that have been implicated in the causation of thrombocytopenia.

Quinidine, quinine, and Sedormid appear to cause thrombocytopenia via this mechanism. With quinidine/quinine the specific plasma protein carrier molecule may be factor VIIIR:Ag (the high-molecular-weight component of factor VIII that expresses von Willebrand factor activity), since VIIIR:Ag appears to be required for the induction of platelet damage in the presence of antibody and drug in vitro.

Diagnosis. Diagnosis rests on a careful history of recent drug exposure, since the clinical manifestations and blood and bone marrow findings are indistinguishable from those seen in ITP. Patients should be asked to list the medications they have been taking within the last 4 to 6 weeks prior to the onset of hemorrhagic manifestations and also should be specifically questioned in regard to the possible ingestion of some of the known more frequently encountered offenders such as quinidine, quinine (highballs, other beverages), thiazide diuretics, gold, sulfonamides, cimetidine, and Sedormid.

The cutaneous hemorrhagic lesions should be carefully examined. Raised lesions (palpable purpura) should raise suspicion of a possibly drug-induced vasculitis with secondary thrombocytopenia. A number of different tests have been employed for the demonstration of platelet antibodies in serum such as complement fixation, immune injury methods, platelet serotonin release, platelet factor 3 availability, platelet aggregation or agglutination, and inhibition of clot retraction. However, the sensitivity of these assays varies considerably. In general, tests of relatively high sensitivity are quite complex and thus not suitable for the routine clinical laboratory. If drug-induced immune thrombocytopenia is suspected, the prudent course is to discontinue immediately all medications not deemed essential and to replace those that are essential with alternative drugs of different chemical structure. Thrombocytopenia that persists for more than 2 weeks following discontinuation of a suspected offending drug is probably not due to drug-induced immune platelet destruction unless the drug in question is excreted very slowly. The readministration of a suspected drug for the purpose of verifying a causal relationship may be hazardous and cannot be generally recommended.

Post-transfusion Purpura

Severe thrombocytopenia associated with abnormal spontaneous and traumatic bleeding may occur as a rare form of immunologic purpura 5 to 8 days after an otherwise uncomplicated blood transfusion. The disorder has been observed almost exclusively in women with a history of one or more pregnancies. It is almost invariably due to the development of an isoantibody to a platelet antigen, PL^{A1}, which is present in platelets of 98 per cent of the normal population and is absent from the patient's own platelets. The mechanism by which this isoantibody causes destruction of the patient's own platelets, which lack the antibody-inducing antigen, has not been elucidated. Bleeding complications may be severe and thrombocytopenia may persist for up to 8 weeks following a single blood transfusion. The diagnosis should be suspected in patients with sudden onset of purpura shortly after a blood transfusion and verified by demonstration of complement-mediated lysis of normal platelets upon incubation with the patient's serum or plasma and demonstration of specificity of the antibody for the platelet PL^{A1} antigen.

Neonatal Immune Purpura

Immunologic thrombocytopenia in the newborn may be due to passive placental transfer of autoantibodies present in the circulation of a mother with ITP ("congenital ITP"). This disorder may be observed in neonates of mothers with ITP who are in remission following splenectomy but rarely in neonates of mothers with spontaneous or glucocorticosteroid-induced remission.

It may also result from placental transfer of platelet isoantibodies formed in the mother against fetal platelet isoantigens. This isoimmune type of congenital thrombocytopenia thus is similar in mechanism to erythroblastosis fetalis. Immunization to at least four isoantigens has been documented: PL^{A1} (most common), PL^{E2}, $PLGrLy^{B1}$, and $PLGrLy^{C1}$.

Neonatal purpura may occasionally be observed due to passive transfer of maternal autoantibodies induced by drugs or associated with autoimmune disorders (e.g., systemic lupus erythematosus—SLE).

Secondary Immunologic Purpura

Thrombocytopenia may complicate a number of disorders known to be associated with abnormal immunologic responses. In these conditions, the clinical bleeding manifestations are similar to those observed in ITP and the thrombocytopenia appears to result predominantly from accelerated removal of autoantibody-coated platelets by the spleen.

In SLE approximately 10 per cent of patients present with thrombocytopenia, sometimes months or even years before the development of other manifestations of the disease. In SLE, as well as in rheumatoid arthritis, splenomegaly may contribute to the severity of the thrombocytopenia. Tests of antiplatelet antibodies are positive in a high percentage of patients with these disorders.

Autoimmune thrombocytopenia may also be observed in association with autoimmune hemolytic anemia (Evans' syndrome), malignant lymphoproliferative disorders, sarcoidosis, hyperthyroidism, allergic reactions to foods, insect bites, and vaccine administration, as well as in postinfectious states (rubella, infectious mononucleosis, viral hepatitis).

Thrombotic Thrombocytopenic Purpura

Synonyms. TTP, thrombohemolytic purpura, Moschcowitz's disease, microangiopathic hemolytic anemia.

Definition and Clinical Features. This form of purpura is an acute, life-threatening disorder characterized by the clinical spectrum of moderate to severe intravascular hemolysis, thrombocytopenic purpura, fluctuating neurologic signs and symptoms, renal disease, and fever. Although TTP may occur at any age, the peak incidence appears to be in the third decade of life and females appear to be slightly more commonly afflicted than males. Most of the clinical manifestations can be readily explained by the pathologic finding of widespread obstruction of small arterial and capillary vessels in many organs by platelets and fibrin with notable lack of vascular inflammatory cell infiltration.

The anemia appears to be caused by shear fragmentation of red blood cells as they are forced through capillaries (particularly in renal glomeruli) which are partially obstructed by platelets and fibrin. The term *microangiopathic hemolytic anemia* (MAHA) was derived originally from the recognition of the association between hemolytic anemia with red cell fragmentation and small vessel disease in TTP. However, MAHA is currently used to indicate the association of anemia with evidence of red cell fragmentation, seen in a number of conditions characterized by microvascular thrombotic occlusive disease such as hemolytic uremic syndrome, DIC, or connective tissue disorders.

Thrombotic thrombocytopenia purpura has been observed in association with numerous conditions and factors such as infections, vaccination, SLE, Sjögren's syndrome, polyarteritis, drug allergies, pregnancy, and use of estrogen oral contraceptives. Furthermore, reduction of serum complement levels, deposition of immunoglobulins and complement components in vascular lesions, elevated levels of platelet-associated IgG, circulating immune complexes and cytotoxic antibodies to endothelial cells in serum, and lack of a factor in circulating blood that stimulates production of PGI_2 by the vessel wall have been demonstrated in some patients. However, the etiology of the disorder (i.e., the primary cause of the vessel damage which appears to trigger the thrombotic vessel occlusions) is essentially unknown.

Virtually all patients present with fever; moderate to severe anemia; hemorrhagic manifestations; thrombocytopenia; and neurologic manifestations, including headache, mental confusion, hemiparesis, aphasia, ataxia, seizures, sensory changes, and visual disturbances. Renal manifestations, including microhematuria, proteinuria, and elevation of serum urea nitrogen and creatinine, are present in the vast majority of patients. Less common manifestations include respiratory dysfunction, abdominal pain due to pancreatitis or mesenteric vessel occlusion, hepatomegaly, splenomegaly, and chest pain due to myocardial ischemia or infarction.

Diagnosis. One of the most important clues to the diagnosis of TTP is the finding of bizarre red blood cell distortion and fragmentation (schistocytes, helmet cells, teardrop cells) on a peripheral blood smear. Nucleated red blood cells are frequently seen. The reticulocyte count is usually elevated in proportion to the extent of the anemia. Thrombocytopenia is a constant finding and is usually severe with evidence of accelerated release of platelets from the bone marrow (megathrombocytes). Leukocytosis, with or without presence of immature granulocytes, is seen in approximately half of all patients. The bone marrow shows erythroid hyperplasia as well as increased numbers of young megakaryocytes. Careful examination of bone marrow biopsy specimens may show capillaries occluded with hyaline material in a small percentage of patients. The results of coagulation screening tests, plasma fibrinogen concentration, and serum fibrin/fibrinogen degradation products are usually normal. Elevated serum levels of lactate dehydrogenase (LD), hemoglobin, and unconjugated bilirubin; decreased or absent serum haptoglobin; and a positive test for urine hemosiderin are all indicative of intravascular hemolysis. The demonstration of thrombosed small blood vessels in biopsy specimens from gingiva, bone marrow, muscle, or skin may further support the diagnosis of TTP, but this is found in only a third to half of patients.

There is recent evidence that the use of exchange transfusion, plasmapheresis with infusion of 6 to 8 units of normal plasma or plasma infusion alone, together with the administration of high doses of glucocorticosteroids and antiplatelet drugs, may be associated with an overall increase in patient survival of 50 per cent or more. Thus, recognition of the characteristic features of TTP as listed, in particular the combination of anemia with red cell fragmentation and thrombocytopenia, should lead to serious consideration of the possibility of TTP. Vigorous attempts should be made to exclude other conditions known to be associated with MAHA, such as hemolytic uremic syndrome, DIC, connective tissue and other autoimmune disorders, disseminated carcinoma, malignant hypertension, pulmonary hypertension, and eclampsia, as well as several other conditions associated with the red cell fragmentation syndrome such as coarctation of the aorta, valvular heart disease, or prosthetic cardiac valves.

Hemolytic Uremic Syndrome

Synonyms. HUS, Morbus Gasser.

Definition and Clinical Features. Hemolytic uremic syndrome is a rare but serious disorder characterized by acute microangiopathic hemolytic anemia, thrombocytopenia, and rapidly progressive renal failure. It is most commonly observed in infants and young children but may occasionally occur in younger adults. The disorder shares a number of clinical features with and may be pathogenetically related to TTP.

Initial symptoms commonly consist of vomiting and diarrhea followed by acute onset of hemolysis, appearance of dark-red urine, oliguria, anemia, mild jaundice, and bleeding into skin and mucous membranes. Gastrointestinal bleeding may be severe owing to segmental or diffuse intestinal gangrene or colitis. Hepatomegaly is common, but splenomegaly is rare. Neurologic manifestations, including headache, lethargy and drowsiness, transient paresis, and convulsions may be seen, but they are much less common in HUS than in TTP.

Several conditions that seem to predispose to, or be closely associated with, the development of HUS have been described, such as bacterial, rickettsial, or viral infections; vaccinations; autoimmune and immunodeficiency disorders; pregnancy; and use of estrogen oral contraceptives. However, etiology and pathogenesis of the endothelial injury, which in contrast to TTP appears to be more or less restricted to the renal microvasculature, are yet to be elucidated.

The general prognosis of HUS is much more favorable in children (mortality < 5 per cent) than in adults (mortality > 30 per cent, chronic renal failure > 80 per cent) and may have been improved by the recent introduction of exchange transfusions, plasmapheresis, and/or infusion of plasma. Recurrent HUS is occasionally seen.

Diagnosis. The hallmark of and most important clue to the diagnosis of HUS is the association of acute hemolytic anemia with red cell fragmentation, variably severe thrombocytopenia, and rapidly progressive renal failure. The clinical and laboratory features include virtually all of those discussed for TTP. The predominance and greater severity of renal manifestations, and lack of neurologic abnormalities, in the acute phase of the illness tend to favor the diagnosis of HUS over TTP in sporadic cases. Hemostatic abnormalities consistent with DIC are observed in about a fourth of patients in the acute phase of HUS, whereas DIC is distinctly atypical for TTP. Circulating immune complexes have been described in up to half of patients in some epidemic forms of HUS but not at all or much less frequently in others. The differential diagnosis includes many of the conditions associated with red cell fragmentation and renal involvement discussed under TTP.

Vasculitis

Bleeding due to hyperdestructive (consumptive) thrombocytopenia in association with microangiopathic hemolytic anemia may be observed in patients with a number of autoimmune disorders such as SLE, polyarteritis nodosa, and scleroderma as well as in homograft rejection, acute glomerulonephritis, Wegener's granulomatosis, and systemic amyloidosis.

Extracorporeal Circulatory Assist Devices

Mild to moderate thrombocytopenia without DIC, frequently associated with abnormal bleeding, occurs regularly and predictably with the use of cardiopulmonary bypass owing to extensive platelet interaction with the large foreign surfaces of the device, in particular the oxygenator. Thrombocytopenia in this setting is usually complicated by platelet dysfunction (acquired storage pool defect), and the bleeding time is prolonged out of proportion to the degree of reduction in circulating platelets. Recovery from thrombocytopenia and platelet dysfunction generally occurs within 2 to 4 days after bypass, but thrombocytopenia may occasionally persist for 1 week or longer. Variably severe reduction of plasma antithrombin III is commonly observed and may contribute to abnormal bleeding. Similar findings may be observed in patients with defective prosthetic heart valves and during the use of ventricular assist devices.

Platelet Consumption Due to Disseminated Intravascular Coagulation

Thrombocytopenia commonly occurs secondary to intravascular activation of the coagulation system with formation of thrombin; this is perhaps the most potent biologic inducer of the platelet release reaction and platelet aggregation. This condition, which is referred to as DIC, defibrination syndrome, or consumptive coagulopathy, is characterized, in its clinically important form in addition to thrombocytopenia, by a prolongation of the prothrombin time, activated partial thromboplastin time, and thrombin time; reduced levels in plasma of fibrinogen and the labile coagulation factors VIII and V; increased levels of plasma high-molecular-weight fibrinogen complexes; and increased concentrations of fibrin/fibrinogen degradation products in serum.

Thrombocytopenia with DIC is seen in a variety of conditions such as sepsis, disseminated carcinoma, promyelocytic leukemia, abruptio placentae, amniotic fluid embolism, dead fetus syndrome, purpura fulminans, heat stroke, transfusion of incompatible blood, acute fulminant hepatitis or end-stage liver disease, and extensive tissue trauma. Thrombocytopenia secondary to DIC must be distinguished from thrombocytopenia due to decreased platelet production or immune destruction in severely ill patients (intensive care unit!) with prolonged prothrombin time (and possibly prolonged APTT) secondary to vitamin K deficiency.

Abnormal Platelet Distribution Due to Splenomegaly

Mild to moderate thrombocytopenia may occur as a result of abnormal platelet distribution, the principal cause of which is splenomegaly. The spleen, which normally contains approximately one third of the total platelet mass, may increase in size with a variety of acute inflammatory conditions (typhoid fever, infectious mononucleosis), chronic inflammatory conditions (rheumatoid arthritis, malaria), circulatory abnormalities (liver cirrhosis, portal vein thrombosis, chronic cardiac failure), hyperplastic disorders (thalassemia, SLE, myelosclerosis), benign infiltrative diseases (Gaucher's disease, amyloidosis), and malignant infiltrative processes (leukemias, lymphomas).

Hypersplenic thrombocytopenia in many of these disorders is associated with normal or even increased total platelet mass and mild to moderate increases in both platelet production and destruction. The initial recovery of isotopically labeled platelets in the circulating blood is moderately to markedly reduced. In most patients with hypersplenism, thrombocytopenia is associated with anemia and leukopenia. Although the severity of the thrombocytopenia is in general poorly correlated with the size of the spleen, hypersplenic thrombocytopenia is exceedingly rare in the absence of appreciable splenomegaly. Increased platelet pooling in patients with splenomegaly is rarely the sole cause of, but may contribute to, abnormal bleeding manifestations.

Hypothermia

Mild thrombocytopenia occurs predictably with hypothermia (below 25°C), presumably as a result of cold-induced platelet activation and (usually transient) sequestration of activated platelets in the spleen and liver (increased vascular pooling). The disorder is rarely of clinical significance in regard to abnormal bleeding.

Massive Blood Transfusion

Patients with acute massive blood loss frequently develop mild to moderate thrombocytopenia following transfusion of large volumes (> 8 units) of stored blood. Stored blood is usually free of viable platelets, and the recipient's circulating platelets are redistributed in the transfused blood (dilutional thrombocytopenia). Acute massive blood loss itself without blood transfusion is usually not associated with a reduction in blood platelet concentration.

Autonomous Thrombocytosis

Thrombocythemia

Synonyms. Essential thrombocythemia, idiopathic thrombocythemia, hemorrhagic thrombocythemia.

Definition and Clinical Features. Thrombocytosis is defined as a elevation of the circulating blood platelet concentration above the normal upper level of 400,000 per cu mm. It may occur as *reactive thrombocytosis* in association with a number of clinical conditions such as iron deficiency, malignancy, infections and other inflammatory diseases; following splenectomy in patients with ITP or autoimmune hemolytic anemia; as a rebound phenomenon after treatment of vitamin B_{12} or folate deficiency, or withdrawal from alcohol; or in the recovery phase following treatment with certain cytotoxic drugs. The blood platelet concentration in reactive thrombocytosis rarely exceeds 1,000,000 per cu mm and there is no convincing evidence that it is associated with abnormal bleeding.

Thrombocytosis may also occur as an autonomous process that is due to proliferation of an abnormal clone of megakaryocytes and is unresponsive to control mechanisms normally governing platelet production. The disorder, termed *idiopathic or essential thrombocythemia,* predominantly affects middle-aged and older individuals of both sexes and appears to belong to a group of diseases called *myeloproliferative disorders.* It is associated with a high incidence of recurrent bleeding manifestations, particularly epistaxis and gastrointestinal bleeding, as well as thromboembolic complications such as transient ischemic attacks, stroke, myocardial ischemia and infarction, hepatic and mesenteric vein thrombosis, and, in particular, microvascular thrombosis of fingers and toes ("blue finger or blue toe syndrome"). Splenomegaly is found in approximately 80 per cent of patients. The pathogenetic mechanism involved in the development of abnormal bleeding associated with autonomous thrombocytosis, in particular thrombocythemia, is poorly understood. The clinical course is variable but generally benign. In a small percentage of patients, the disorder may terminate in polycythemia vera or acute myeloblastic leukemia.

Diagnosis. At the time of diagnosis, the blood platelet count usually exceeds 1,000,000 per cu mm and may be as high as 14,000,000 per cu mm. The peripheral blood smear shows platelet clumps as well as giant platelets and other bizarre forms. Anemia, if present, is usually due to chronic gastrointestinal blood loss. Mild to moderate granulocytosis with a "shift to the left" as well as slight eosinophilia and basophilia is common. The bone marrow shows marked megakaryocytic hyperplasia, and a mild increase in granulocytic and erythroid precursors may be observed. Leukocyte alkaline phosphatase and serum uric acid and vitamin B_{12} may be elevated. Pseudohyperkalemia due to loss of potassium from the large numbers of platelets during clotting of blood in vitro is not uncommon. The bleeding time may be markedly prolonged or normal and appears to have little or no predictive value in regard to the likelihood of abnormal bleeding or thrombosis. The results of in vitro platelet function tests are highly variable. The most common and perhaps characteristic finding is impaired or absent epinephrine-induced platelet aggregation, apparently due to a deficiency of alpha receptors in platelets produced by the abnormal megakaryocyte clone. Results of blood coagulation screening tests are usually normal.

The differentiation of thrombocythemia from reactive thrombocytosis is usually not difficult in patients with hemorragic or thrombotic complications but may present a challenge in asymptomatic patients with blood platelet counts below or slightly above 1,000,000 per cu mm. In such patients, the demonstration of a prolonged bleeding time and/or defective epinephrine-induced platelet aggregation (in the presence of normal aggregation to ADP, collagen, and arachidonic acid) may support the diagnosis of thrombocythemia.

Thrombocytosis with Other Myeloproliferative Disorders

Autonomous thrombocytosis may be associated with other myeloproliferative disorders such as polycythemia, chronic myelogenous leukemia, and agnogenic myeloid metaplasia (see separate articles on these topics). The clinical hemorrhagic and thrombotic complications are similar to those discussed for thrombocythemia. The bleeding time is frequently prolonged but may be normal. There may be poor correlation between bleeding time and platelet concentration, and the results of in vitro platelet function tests are quite variable.

Disorders of Platelet Function

Abnormal bleeding secondary to platelet dysfunction occurs in a number of different conditions, although it is not as common as that due to thrombocytopenia. It must be considered in any patient with a history of abnormal bleeding and a prolonged bleeding time associated with a normal platelet count and normal blood coagulation test results. However, in some inherited and acquired conditions, platelet dysfunction may be combined with thrombocytopenia. In such patients the prolongation of the bleeding time is characteristically out of proportion to the degree of thrombocytopenia.

In addition to a well-standardized bleeding time procedure, preferably performed on the inside of the upper forearm and with the use of a template device (commercially available), measurement of in vitro platelet aggregation in citrated platelet-rich plasma in response to several different stimuli (ADP, epinephrine, collagen, sodium arachidonate) has become an important tool for confirming and characterizing the platelet functional disorder. This latter test is affected by a number of variables, such as the method of blood collection and preparation of platelet-rich plasma and conditions of storage of this plasma, and requires a substantial amount of technical expertise and experience. Since measurement of in vitro platelet aggregation is sensitive to aspirin and a variety of other medications, it is essential that the patient be advised not to take aspirin for at least 7 days or other medications for at least 24 hours before laboratory evaluation. Disorders of platelet function may be inherited (rare) or acquired (Table 5). Some of the clinically more important or common disorders are discussed next.

Bernard-Soulier Syndrome

Synonyms. BSS, giant platelet syndrome, macrothrombocytopenic thrombocytopathy.

Clinical Features. BSS is a rare familial bleeding disorder, inherited as an autosomal recessive trait, which is characterized by a normal or variably reduced blood platelet concentration, unusually large platelets on peripheral blood smear examination, a variably prolonged bleeding time, and impairment of platelet adherence to subendothelium or foreign surfaces. This defect appears to be due to a selective deficiency (complete or partial) of a single platelet surface membrane glycoprotein, termed GP Ib, thought to be the receptor for factor VIII:von Willebrand factor, which promotes platelet-surface interaction. Bleeding manifestations are highly variable, in terms of both type and severity, even among affected individuals within the same family. Furthermore, there appears to be poor correlation between frequency and severity of bleeding manifestations, bleeding time prolongation, platelet size, or extent of GP Ib deficiency.

Diagnosis. The diagnosis is made by demonstration of absent aggregation of platelets in platelet-rich plasma with ristocetin in the presence of normal aggregation and release in response to ADP, epinephrine, and collagen. In contrast to the finding in von Willebrand's disease, impaired platelet aggregation to ristocetin cannot be corrected by addition of normal plasma or factor VIII : vWF. Bernard-Soulier syndrome must be distinguished from the May-Hegglin anomaly, a disorder also associated with thrombocytopenia and giant platelets. However, in the latter disorder, in vitro platelet function and platelet glycoproteins are normal and patients are usually asymptomatic despite moderate thrombocytopenia.

Another rare disorder associated with thrombocyto-

Table 5. Disorders of Platelet Function

Specific Defect	Hereditary Disorders	Acquired Disorders
Adhesion	Bernard-Soulier syndrome von Willebrand disease	Acquired von Willebrand disease Uremia (?) Drugs (?)
Platelet aggregation	Thrombasthenia Afibrinogenemia	Paraproteinemias Myeloproliferative disorders Drugs (semisynthetic penicillins, dextran) DIC, liver disease, fibrinolytic therapy
Release of granular constituents		
Storage pool deficiency		Cardiopulmonary bypass
Alpha granule	Gray platelet syndrome	Other circulatory assist devices
Dense granule	Hermansky-Pudlak syndrome Chédiak-Higashi syndrome Wiskott-Aldrich syndrome	Immune-mediated release (ITP, collagen vascular disease) Drugs (?) Myeloproliferative disorders DIC syndromes
Primary release mechanism	Cyclo-oxygenase deficiency Thromboxane synthetase deficiency Defect of intracellular Ca^{++} release or Ca^{++} utilization	Drugs (aspirin, other nonsteroidal anti-inflammatory agents Platelet dyspoiesis, e.g., leukemia, myeloproliferative disorders Ethanol (?) Diet (?)
Altered nucleotide metabolism	Glycogen storage disease Fructose-1,6-diphosphate deficiency	
Other mechanisms	Platelet factor 3 deficiency Deficiency of factor Xa receptor	Drugs (?) Diet Viral infections Hypothyroidism

Abbreviations: DIC = Disseminated intravascular coagulation; ITP = idiopathic thrombocytopenic purpura.

penia, variably enlarged platelets, and platelet dysfunction is the so-called *gray platelet syndrome,* in which the platelets are devoid of or deficient in alpha storage granules. Patients with this disorder may have a mild bleeding disorder and impaired platelet aggregation to ADP and other stimuli. Platelets lack the usual granular appearance on peripheral blood smear examination, and electron microscopy reveals a striking deficiency of alpha granules.

Thrombasthenia

Synonyms. Glanzmann's disease, Glanzmann's thrombasthenia.

Clinical Features. Thrombasthenia is a rare autosomal recessive disorder characterized by a markedly prolonged bleeding time; normal platelet number and morphology; and impaired or absent primary platelet aggregation to ADP, epinephrine, arachidonic acid, collagen, and thrombin, and normal to mildly impaired aggregation to ristocetin. The defect in the ability of the platelets to stick to each other in response to all agents except ristocetin is due to the partial or complete deficiency of a glycoprotein complex, termed GP IIb/IIIa, in the platelet plasma membrane. As a consequence of this deficiency, platelets cannot bind fibrinogen, which appears to be the principal protein that facilitates platelet-platelet interaction or platelet cohesion. Platelet adherence to surfaces or subendothelium is normal in this disorder. Glanzmann's thrombasthenia may be a heterogeneous disorder. Thus, a type I associated with GP IIb/IIIa deficiency, absence of detectable platelet fibrinogen, and absent whole blood clot retraction has been distinguished from a type II associated with GP IIb/IIIa deficiency, presence of platelet fibrinogen, and normal to mildly impaired clot retraction.

The extent of abnormal bleeding varies from easy bruising to life-threatening gastrointestinal or intracranial bleeding. Only homozygotes appear to experience bleeding complications, whereas heterozygotes are asymptomatic.

Diagnosis. Diagnosis generally rests on demonstration of a prolonged bleeding time; normal platelet count; impaired or absent primary aggregation to ADP, epinephrine, collagen, and thrombin; and normal to mildly impaired aggregation to ristocetin. Diagnosis can be confirmed by platelet glycoprotein analysis.

Afibrinogenemia

Congenital afibrinogenemia is a rare disorder associated with a wide spectrum of bleeding manifestations ranging from easy bruising and ecchymoses to life-threatening gastrointestinal and intracranial bleeding following head trauma. The bleeding time may be markedly prolonged in some patients with the disorder and normal in others. Platelet aggregation to ADP and epinephrine as well as low concentrations of collagen and thrombin is usually markedly impaired, but it may be normal in response to high concentrations of collagen and thrombin. This latter finding is difficult to explain, since platelets from patients with this disorder contain only traces of fibrinogen.

Inherited Platelet Storage Pool Disorders

Several rare inherited disorders of platelet function have been described in which there is an apparent deficiency of either dense or alpha granules on electron microscopy and absent or reduced release of dense or alpha granule contents in response to collagen or thrombin. Whether these storage pool defects are due to lack of formation of secondary granules or formation of abnormal granules that cannot take up the substances normally stored in these granules has not been determined.

The *Hermansky-Pudlak syndrome* (HPS) is an autosomal recessive disorder characterized by the triad of tyrosinase-positive oculocutaneous albinism; accumulation of ceroid-like material in reticuloendothelial cells of bone marrow and other organ tissues; and a variably severe reduction in platelet-dense granules associated with impaired second phase platelet aggregation to ADP and epinephrine, and impaired platelet aggregation to collagen and thrombin. Approximately half of all patients affected have a mild bleeding disorder. Many of the patients described have been of Puerto Rican origin.

The *Chédiak-Higashi syndrome* (CHS) is also inherited as an autosomal recessive trait in which there is ultrastructural, biochemical, and functional evidence for a dense granule storage pool defect. The disorder is characterized clinically by mild to moderate thrombocytopenia, photophobia, nystagmus, pseudoalbinism, increased susceptibility to infections, hepatosplenomegaly, lymphadenopathy, and early death, due frequently to development of a malignant lymphoproliferative disorder.

The *gray platelet syndrome* (GPS) is a rare disorder characterized by mild thrombocytopenia, mild abnormal bleeding, and the presence of large agranular platelets that appear blue-gray on Wright-stained peripheral blood smears. Whereas dense granules are present in normal numbers, there is virtually complete absence of alpha granules.

Other congenital disorders in which a storage pool defect has been described include the *Wiskott-Aldrich syndrome* and thrombocytopenia with absent radius (TAR).

Inherited Disorders of the Platelet Release Reaction

A few patients have been described whose platelets showed the pattern of normal primary aggregation to ADP and epinephrine followed by rapid deaggregation (lack of second-phase aggregation) and impaired aggregation to collagen (typically seen in patients with platelet-dense granule storage pool disease) but with presence of normal amounts of dense storage granule contents. In some of these patients there was a complete lack of formation of thromboxane A_2 in response to addition of sodium arachidonate (SA) and/or prostaglandin H_2 (PGH_2) consistent with deficiencies of cyclo-oxygenase or thromboxane synthase, respectively. However, in those patients whose platelets responded to PGH_2 but not to SA, the possibility of aspirin-induced inhibition of cyclo-oxygenase could not be definitively excluded. Finally, there is recent evidence for the existence of primary platelet secretion disorders due to a thromboxane A_2 receptor defect and a defect in intracellular platelet Ca^{++} mobilization or utilization. Most of the patients with inherited release abnormalities had only minor abnormal bleeding manifestations or none at all.

Inherited Disorder of Platelet Procoagulant Activity

Several patients have been described with excessive bleeding during menstruation or surgical procedures in whom all tests of blood coagulation, platelet number, and in vivo and in vitro platelet function were normal except for abnormal prothrombin consumption. This was associated with, and thought to be due to, abnormal binding of activated factor X to platelets in response to thrombin. This disorder appears to be exceedingly rare.

Acquired Disorders of Platelet Function

Abnormalities of platelet function occur in a wide variety of acquired clinical conditions. Since they are frequently not associated with abnormal bleeding manifestations, they remain unrecognized. In some conditions, such as the myeloproliferative and myelodysplastic disorders, platelet dysfunction may be secondary to an intrinsic platelet defect, i.e., the formation of structurally and/or biochemically defective platelets by an abnormal clone of megakaryocytes. In other conditions platelet dysfunction may be due to toxic effects of drugs or metabolites (uremia), nonspecific alterations of platelet surfaces (paraproteinemia), or intravascular or extravascular platelet activation (cardiopulmonary bypass). Single or multiple platelet functions may be impaired, and in some conditions the nature and pathogenesis of the platelet functional defect(s) have not been elucidated.

Drug-Induced Platelet Dysfunction Drug-induced platelet dysfunction is among the most common acquired platelet functional disorders. Although many drugs have been shown to cause inhibition of platelet function when added to platelets in vitro, evidence for an effect on the bleeding time or induction of abnormal bleeding following in vivo administration is lacking for most. These agents will not be reviewed here.

Aspirin. Ingestion of a single 300-mg tablet of aspirin by a normal subject will cause predictable suppression of platelet thromboxane A_2 formation, which normally potentiates platelet secretion, particularly at low stimulus concentrations. Absence of second-phase platelet aggregation to ADP and epinephrine, impaired aggregation to collagen, and absent aggregation to sodium arachidonate are the characteristic in vitro findings. These reactions can be observed for up to 7 days after a single dose of aspirin. However, the template bleeding time is found to be prolonged beyond the upper limit of normal (8 minutes) in only 50 per cent of normal subjects following a single dose of aspirin, usually does not exceed 15 minutes, and returns into the normal range within 2 to 4 days. A bleeding time in excess of 15 minutes observed in a subject known to have ingested aspirin recently should raise the suspicion of an underlying hemostatic defect (mild von Willebrand's disease, platelet disorder, coagulation disorder) unmasked by aspirin. It is probably only in such subjects that aspirin or indomethacin may cause abnormal bleeding. Other nonsteroidal anti-inflammatory agents such as sulfinpyrazone, phenylbutazone, sulindac, or ibuprofen have not been shown to cause abnormal bleeding in normal subjects and are in fact used in the management of hemophilic arthritis without apparent increase in the frequency of bleeding episodes in such patients.

Carbenicillin. Carbenicillin, ticarcillin, cephalothin, and several other third-generation semisynthetic penicillins are probably the clinically most important drugs known to cause severe platelet dysfunction associated with abnormal bleeding manifestations. The majority of patients treated with these agents show variably severe prolongation of the bleeding time and impairment of in vitro platelet aggregation to a variety of stimuli. The use of these agents may be of particular concern in regard to the induction or aggravation of a hemostatic defect in patients with renal failure and other pre-existing hemostatic disorders such as anticoagulant therapy, vitamin K deficiency, or thrombocytopenia. The prolonged bleeding time usually returns into the normal range within 24 to 48 hours following discontinuation of the drug. The mechanism by which these agents induce platelet dysfunction appears to be complex but probably involves alteration of agonist receptors on the platelet membrane.

Dextran. Abnormal bleeding may be observed in patients receiving intravenous administration of large volumes of dextran as a plasma expander or for the prevention of venous thromboembolic complications in postsurgical patients. The bleeding time may be prolonged and in vitro platelet aggregation and platelet factor 3 availability may be impaired, presumably as a result of coating of the platelet membrane by the polysaccharide and possibly because of alterations of plasma constituents such as fibrinogen necessary for normal platelet aggregation.

Uremia. Abnormal bleeding is observed in approximately one third of all patients with severe acute or chronic renal failure. Bleeding manifestations commonly include epistaxis, easy bruising, gastrointestinal tract bleeding, and bleeding with venipunctures and other invasive procedures. The platelet count is usually normal, but platelet aggregation in vitro to a variety of stimuli as well as platelet factor 3 availability (prothrombin consumption) is commonly abnormal. The extent of platelet dysfunction in uremia appears to be directly proportional to the degree of renal functional impairment. Partial correction of the bleeding time prolongation and in vitro platelet functional abnormalities may be achieved by peritoneal or hemodialysis. This finding and a number of experimental studies in vitro seem to indicate that the accumulation in plasma of substances toxic to platelets (guanidinosuccinic acid, phenol, and phenolic acids) normally cleared by the kidney is responsible for the impaired platelet function in uremic patients.

Paraproteinemia. Abnormal bleeding occurs commonly in patients with multiple myeloma and Waldenström's macroglobulinemia. Platelet dysfunction, as demonstrated by a prolonged bleeding time as well as impaired platelet aggregation in vitro and abnormal platelet factor 3 availability, is frequently observed in these patients and generally correlates closely with the concentration of the paraprotein in plasma. Platelet dysfunction appears to be more commonly associated with IgA myeloma (compared with IgG myeloma) and IgM paraproteinemia. The mechanisms by which these abnormal immunoglobulins interfere with platelet function are incompletely understood, but accumulation of the paraproteins on the platelet plasma membrane resulting in nonspecific interference with receptor-agonist binding may be largely responsible. Thrombocytopenia, hyperviscosity and interference by the paraprotein with normal fibrin polymerization may contribute to the development of clinical bleeding manifestations.

Myeloproliferative and Myelodysplastic Disorders. Patients with essential or idiopathic thrombocythemia, polycythemia vera, agnogenic myeloid dysplasia or myelofibrosis, and chronic myelogenous leukemia frequently exhibit platelet dysfunction. Various abnormalities, such as giant platelets; abnormal-appearing cytoplasmic granules; abnormal granule centralization in response to platelet stimulation; storage pool defects; defective thromboxane A_2 synthesis; impaired aggregation to ADP, epinephrine, collagen, sodium arachidonate, and thrombin; and abnormal platelet factor 3 availability, have been demonstrated. The bleeding time frequently shows poor correlation with the extent of the platelet functional abnormalities in vitro. Similar abnormalities have been described in patients with other myelodysplastic syndromes such as preleukemia, sideroblastic anemia, refractory anemia, and paroxysmal nocturnal hemoglobinuria, as well as acute leukemia and leukemic reticuloendotheliosis.

Acquired Storage Pool Disorder. Platelet dysfunction associated with a selective depletion of alpha granule contents and alpha granules has been reported in patients undergoing cardiopulmonary bypass operations. The bleeding time is frequently prolonged out of proportion to the extent of thrombocytopenia that occurs commonly in these patients. In vitro studies show impaired second-phase aggregation to ADP and epinephrine and abnormal aggregation to collagen and thrombin. The alpha storage granule defect is thought to be a consequence of platelet activation and release of alpha granule contents triggered by extensive interaction of platelets with the foreign surfaces of the oxygenator and other parts of the extracorporeal circuit of the device. Similar abnormalities may be observed with other circulatory assist devices.

Acquired von Willebrand's Disease. Abnormal bleeding associated with findings characteristic of von Willebrand's disease (type I or IIA) has been reported in a number of patients who lacked a previous personal or family history of a hemorrhagic diathesis. Almost all of these patients had evidence of a malignant lymphoproliferative or autoimmune connective tissue disorder. In some of these patients, all clinical and laboratory abnormalities disappeared following effective treatment of the primary underlying lymphoproliferative disorder. In one patient an IgG antibody that neutralized factor VIII:vWF in vitro but did not affect factor VIII:C was demonstrated. However, in other patients no such inhibitory activity was found in the plasma, and the pathogenesis of the disorder in these cases remains poorly understood.

Liver Disease. Abnormalities of in vitro platelet aggregation to various stimuli have been reported in patients with severe chronic liver disease. However, there is little evidence that platelet dysfunction plays a significant role in the hemorrhagic diathesis associated with liver disease because the bleeding time is usually normal in these patients even in the presence of mild thrombocytopenia.

HEMORRHAGIC DISEASE DUE TO DISSEMINATED INTRAVASCULAR COAGULATION AND FIBRINOLYSIS

By Alvin H. Schmaier, M.D.
and Robert W. Colman, M.D.
Philadelphia, Pennsylvania

SYNONYMS

The term *consumption coagulopathy* describes the utilization of certain coagulation components by the action of thrombin but ignores changes that result from decreased in vivo clearance of activated clotting enzymes and accelerated fibrinolysis. *Defibrination syndrome* is too narrow, describing only the changes in fibrin. *Disseminated intravascular coagulation (DIC)* with its focus on the major pathophysiologic event—accelerated coagulation—is the preferred and widely accepted designation. A better name, not in common parlance, would be *disseminated intravascular coagulation and fibrinolysis,* since primary fibrinolysis is a disease category that has never been rigorously proved to arise in man.

DEFINITION

Disseminated intravascular coagulation is a clinicopathologic condition, not a specific disease state, characterized by an acquired hemorrhagic or thrombotic disorder. It occurs in a wide variety of acute or chronic diseases and is manifest by the simultaneous presence of accelerated systemic coagulation and fibrinolysis. The clinical predominance of bleeding or thrombosis depends on the balance between accelerated fibrinolysis and coagulation. Bleeding states result from the consumption of circulating procoagulants (fibrinogen, prothrombin, and factors V and VIII), the decrease of other zymogens due to activation and in vivo clearance (factors IX, VII, and X), and the presence of circulating fibrin and fibrinogen split products, which in themselves are potent circulating anticoagulants. Thrombotic states arise from activation of the same circulating procoagulants that are not actively cleared from the circulation. The apparent paradox of both bleeding and thrombosis in the same disorder can best be understood by the biochemical products associated with the disorder. If more thrombin than plasmin is present, the disease will manifest as thrombosis; alternatively, if more plasmin is present, bleeding will be the overriding clinical presentation.

PRESENTING SIGNS AND SYMPTOMS

In many instances DIC can be suspected on clinical grounds with a high degree of accuracy; in a few instances it is recognized only because of an increased index of suspicion. In general there are two distinct modes of presentation: acute and chronic.

Acute DIC

In acute DIC, 75 per cent of total patients, the clinical and laboratory features develop rapidly over a few hours to 2 days. The patient is usually critically ill from the precipitating event as well as from DIC. Most inciting etiologies of DIC usually induce a disorder that is acute in nature (Table 1). Rarely, abnormal coagulation tests alone herald the onset of acute DIC. The patient often presents with a multisite bleeding diathesis that can range from oozing to life-threatening hemorrhage. Examination of the skin is of great diagnostic value in these patients with DIC. Patients may show petechiae, purpura, palpable purpura, hemorrhagic bullae, acral cyanosis, gangrene, and wound hematomas.

The recognition that an acquired hemorrhagic diathesis exists is often delayed beyond 2 days in three common situations:

1. The critically ill patient often has multiple catheter insertions, venipuncture sites, and surgical wounds. Oozing of blood can occur at these sites, but the presence of a bleeding diathesis goes unrecognized because the hemorrhage is attributed to the wounds and catheters alone. Similarly, thrombosis of vessels is often attributed solely to the mechanical effects of catheters.
2. When the patient suffers a major hemorrhage from a local site such as a gastrointestinal tract ulcer, other sites of concomitant bleeding, such as a purpura or hematomas, may be overlooked.
3. The occurrence of *acral cyanosis* may be attributed to hypotension or sepsis alone. This combination should be recognized as a clue to acute DIC.

Chronic DIC

In contrast to the acutely ill patient with complicating severe DIC, an individual may have mild or protracted clinical manifestation of consumption coagulopathy or even subclinical disease manifested only by laboratory abnormalities. This form of the disease, occurring 25 per cent of the time, has been termed *subacute* or chronic DIC. Obvious clinical signs of DIC, such as ecchymosis and blood loss, are usually absent in these patients. Although a hemorrhagic presentation secondary to thrombocytopenia and hypofibrinogenemia may occur, many of these patients have symptoms and signs referable to venous thrombosis. The diagnosis is based on clinical suspicion and confirmatory laboratory tests, the most reliable of which are elevations of fibrin split products. Subacute or chronic DIC is associated with a number of etiologies (Table 1), the most common being malignancy. Using malignancy as an example, chronic DIC can take the form of migratory thrombophlebitis, marantic endocarditis with arterial embolization, or microangiopathic hemolytic anemia.

Regardless of its acute or chronic nature, DIC is always a manifestation of an underlying disease or condition. Recognition of the underlying condition may lead to the removal of the cause, the most effective treatment of DIC.

COURSE

The evolution of DIC depends to a great degree on the severity of the condition and on the nature of the

Table 1. Clinical Aspects of Disseminated Intravascular Coagulation (DIC): Etiologic Classification

Inciting Etiologies of Acute DIC	Inciting Etiologies of Chronic DIC
Gram-negative sepsis	Venous thrombosis
Gram-positive sepsis	Neoplasms
Typhoid fever	Retained dead fetus
Acute promyelocytic leukemia	Giant cavernous hemangiomas
Abruptio placentae	Chronic renal disease
Amniotic fluid embolus	Connective tissue disorders
Hypertonic saline abortion	
Trauma	
Snakebite	
Transfusion reactions	
Necrotizing enterocolitis	
Renal homograft rejection	
Purpura fulminans	
Parasites	
Heatstroke	

underlying illness. Mortality associated with acute DIC is high, ranging from 54 to 87 per cent. Mortality is directly related to age, the number of clinical manifestations of DIC, the severity of the laboratory manifestations, and the underlying condition. In some patients, DIC may be acute, but self-limited, particularly as seen with obstetric conditions. In other conditions, such as gram-negative infections, ability to control the DIC may be more difficult than giving specific therapy for the underlying infection. In patients with chronic DIC due to malignancy, the coagulation defect is often ancillary to the inability to treat the underlying condition adequately.

PHYSICAL FINDINGS

The signs reflect the underlying disease. Manifestations of diffuse mucosal bleeding, especially purpura and hematomas, or skin necrosis should alert the physician to the presence of acute DIC. Alternatively, chronic DIC may be suggested by signs associated with the diagnosis of venous thrombosis and pulmonary embolism.

COMMON COMPLICATIONS

Besides the complications arising from the underlying disease, problems arising from DIC relate to hemorrhage, thrombosis, or effects of treatment. Excessive bleeding, in addition to the local effects, frequently results in shock, which in turn may exacerbate the coagulation abnormalities. Thrombi in the glomerular capillaries give rise to renal cortical necrosis; in the adrenals, to the clinical picture of Waterhouse-Friderichsen syndrome; and in the skin, to hemorrhagic necrosis, as seen in purpura fulminans. In the absence of heparin, administration of epsilon-aminocaproic acid, a fibrinolytic inhibitor, may prevent the secondary protective fibrinolysis and thus predispose to disseminated thrombosis.

LABORATORY PROCEDURES

A major difficulty in the diagnosis of patients with DIC has been a lack of accepted criteria. One approach in the laboratory evaluation is to classify available studies according to three categories: screening tests, confirmatory tests, and additional studies. Since the majority of patients with DIC have the acute, severe variety, sequential testing using the screening and confirmatory tests is most helpful. However, in chronic DIC the screening tests are usually slightly abnormal or normal. A high index of suspicion is the best single indication that confirmatory testing should be performed in a patient with a clinical history compatible with chronic DIC.

Screening Tests

Disseminated intravascular thrombosis can be detected by the combination of an abnormal prothrombin time (PT) or activated partial thromboplastin time (APTT), thrombocytopenia, and hypofibrinogenemia. This constellation of findings is usually seen with acute severe DIC. The PT is abnormal ($>$ 15 seconds) in over 90 per cent of patients with DIC. The APTT is also a sensitive screening test for DIC. An abnormal PT and a prolonged APTT combined are most commonly due to DIC in a hospitalized population. Disorders that could lead to similar laboratory findings (vitamin K deficiency, liver disease, and anticoagulants) can usually be excluded on clinical grounds. Moreover, an APTT greater than 100 seconds with an abnormal PT is most commonly due to DIC. The only other clinical state that usually can be associated with these findings is that occurring after heparin administration.

In patients with acute DIC, 70 per cent have clottable fibrinogen levels less than 160 mg/dl. The finding of a normal fibrinogen in a patient suspected of having DIC never excludes the diagnosis, since this protein may have been elevated before the onset of the illness. In a case of suspected DIC, a documented fall in the fibrinogen level from a very high level to one in the normal or low normal range is equally as helpful as one that is absolutely low. On the other hand, a very low clottable fibrinogen is not itself diagnostic of DIC, since end-stage liver disease, L-asparaginase administration, and dysfibrinogenemias can be associated with this finding. The platelet count ($<$ 150,000 per cu mm), like the PT, is abnormal in over 90 per cent of patients with DIC. However, a low platelet count must be shown to be the result of peripheral destruction. A number of the disorders associated with DIC may be associated with thrombocytopenia secondary to bone marrow involvement, resulting in decreased platelet production.

Abnormalities in all four tests establish the diagnosis of DIC in the appropriate clinical situation. However, the rare clinical condition of timber rattlesnake bite can mimic these findings and still not be DIC. The problem in diagnosis in many cases of DIC is that all four of these screening tests may not be abnormal. The finding that only two screening tests are abnormal usually suggests another diagnosis. Thus, confirmatory tests are required to diagnose DIC. Patients with abnormal results for all of the following three tests (PT, fibrinogen, and platelet count) usually have confirmatory evidence for plasmin-induced fibrinolysis. Moreover, in many cases of chronic DIC, only one or none of the screening tests may be abnormal. Thus more specific testing needs to be performed to confirm clinical impressions.

Confirmatory Tests

The most useful test for confirmation of DIC is measurement of fibrin or fibrinogen degradation products (FDP) produced by plasmin digestion. Three tests are available for measuring FDP: Thrombo-Wellco Test, staphylococcal-clumping test, and the tanned red cell hemagglutination inhibition assay. The Thrombo-Wellco Test uses latex particles coated with specific antibody to fibrinogen fragments X, Y, D, and E. It is a rapid, reproducible semiquantitative assay for FDP.

This assay, however, has been noted to give false-positive results in 93 per cent of patients with seropositive rheumatoid factor. The staphylococcal-clumping test, which employs certain strains of coagulase-negative staphylococci that agglutinate FDP, measures mostly fragments X and Y. In most cases of DIC, there is good correlation in findings between the Thrombo-Wellco Test and the staphylococcal-clumping test, although in severe DIC the staphylococcal-clumping assay may be negative because of proteolysis of all X and Y fragments to D and E. The tanned red cell hemagglutination inhibition test, although a technically more difficult and complex assay, is a sensitive and quantitative assay for all forms of FDP. However, the hemagglutination inhibition assay has also been recognized to give false-negative values in in the presence of an anti-D (Rh) antibody. The concentration of FDP by any of these three methods is elevated ($> 5\ \mu g/ml$) in about 95 per cent of patients with DIC. However, it is sometimes difficult to decide what constitutes a significant elevation. In certain conditions, such as liver disease or postoperative states, mild elevations up to 40 $\mu g/ml$ may occur without other clinical or laboratory evidence of DIC. Values greater than 40 $\mu g/ml$ almost always indicate DIC.

Additional Studies

A number of additional studies can be performed to help characterize DIC. Many of these studies are actually more useful in guiding therapy in the management of DIC. These studies, although occasionally useful, generally do not add any more diagnostic information than that given by the screening or confirmatory tests, especially when combined with knowledge of the patient's clinical situation. A helpful maneuver is examination of the peripheral blood smear directly from a finger puncture for evidence of a microangiopathic hemolytic anemia, which produces red cell fragmentation (e.g., helmet cells, schistocytes) and thrombocytopenia. The red cell abnormalities characteristic of a microangiopathic hemolytic anemia may occur in as few as 10 per cent or as high as 50 per cent of patients with DIC; their absence, however, never excludes the diagnosis of DIC. Furthermore, many other disorders, such as march hemoglobinuria, calcific and prosthetic heart valves, malignant hypertension, metastatic carcinoma, thrombotic thrombocytopenic purpura, and hemolytic uremic syndrome, may be accompanied by the same findings on the peripheral blood smear without DIC. In general, if DIC occurs with microangiopathic hemolytic anemia, the findings on the blood smear may suggest the underlying etiology of the DIC rather than determine whether the patient has DIC. For diagnosis, one needs the laboratory evidence provided by the screening and confirmatory tests.

The thrombin time is often used in the diagnosis of DIC. It will be prolonged in the presence of FDP, heparin, or markedly decreased fibrinogen levels and therefore gives no more information than the screening and confirmatory tests. In fact, a fibrinogen level of ≥ 75 mg/dl will usually not prolong the thrombin time. If the DIC is not severe, with a predominant amount of X and Y fragments or fibrin monomer, the degree of FDP inhibition of the thrombin time may be minimal.

Many investigators have reported the utility of specific coagulation factor assays. In an instance of prolonged PT and APTT, the finding of depression of factors II, VII, IX, and X will help distinguish vitamin K deficiency and/or liver disease from DIC. Since thrombin activates factors V and VIII, the finding of low levels of these factors is expected. On the other hand, normal levels of factors V and VIII do not exclude a diagnosis of DIC, since these values may represent decreases from previously elevated values or compensation in a chronic or subacute DIC.

Finally, decreased antithrombin III, protein C, fibronectin, and plasmin levels, and circulating thrombin-antithrombin III and plasmin-alpha$_2$-antiplasmin complexes have been noted in DIC. These studies may be useful in gaining an understanding of the pathogenesis of the disorder or in guiding therapy, but they do not increase diagnostic acumen.

POTENTIAL ERRORS AND PITFALLS IN DIAGNOSIS

Although there is a wide assortment of assays that can be used in the diagnosis of DIC, frequently the patient does not exhibit a classic laboratory picture. There is no substitute for knowledge of the many and complex clinical presentations that characterize DIC. Moreover, since the onset of a coagulopathy is a dynamic situation, serial studies are usually helpful in defining a suspected diagnosis of and as a guide to management in DIC. As indicated previously, a patient with DIC can present in one of two ways: with an acute, severe disorder or with a chronic, indolent one. The laboratory findings supporting these diagnoses are different, reflecting these patterns (Table 2).

In acute, severe DIC the diagnosis is suspected because of clinical evidence of hemorrhage: oozing about venipuncture sites, gum and mucosal bleeding, and positive occult blood in the gastrointestinal tract. The screening laboratory tests will show a prolonged PT and APTT; the latter, usually being more sensitive, is the first to be prolonged. The platelet count usually will be low ($< 100{,}000$ per cu mm), as will clottable fibrinogen (< 150 mg/dl). Platelets, even if not extremely low, exhibit abnormal function by platelet aggregometry owing to the influence of circulating FDP. The patient with severe DIC may have a normal plasma fibrinogen if the concentration prior to the illness was elevated, as seen with sepsis and neoplasia. The confirmatory tests will show that FDPs are elevated to greater than 40 $\mu g/ml$. The thrombin time may or may not be prolonged, depending upon the degree of lowering of fibrinogen and the amount of clot-inhibiting FDP. Factors V and VIII are usually depressed, as are other factors. However, the finding of low factors II, VII, IX, and X alone suggests vitamin K deficiency, whereas liver dysfunction may be associated with deficiencies of the vitamin K-dependent factors, low factor V, and normal factor VIII. Antithrombin III function may also be depressed.

Table 2. Laboratory Variability in Disseminated Intravascular Coagulation (DIC)

Manifestation	Acute, Severe DIC	Chronic DIC
Clinical	Usually hemorrhagic	None or thrombotic
Screening Tests		
PT, APTT	Usually prolonged	Normal
Platelets	Usually decreased	Normal or slightly decreased
Fibrinogen	Usually decreased but may be normal	Usually normal
Confirmatory Tests		
FDP	Strongly positive, usually > 40 μg/ml	Usually positive
Other Assays		
Thrombin time	Normal or abnormal	Usually normal
Factor assays	Decreased factors V, VIII	Normal factors V, VIII
Antithrombin III	May be low	Usually normal

Abbreviations: PT = Prothrombin time; APTT = activated partial thromboplastin time; FDP = fibrinogen degradation products.

In chronic DIC most commonly there are no clinical symptoms of hemorrhage. The diagnosis is suggested by the presence of unexplained thrombosis in a patient suspected or proved to have an underlying malignancy. The incidence of thrombosis is as high as 23 per cent in patients with known malignancy, and thrombosis in a patient with a malignancy makes it well worthwhile to search for the presence of chronic DIC. In chronic DIC (a compensated intravascular coagulation) screening tests reveal a normal PT and APTT, a mildly depressed platelet count, but normal fibrinogen and coagulation factors. The confirmatory tests are positive. The FDP measured by the Thrombo-Wellco Test is usually positive, although instances may occur in which fibrin monomer and X and Y fragment predominate, allowing for a negative Thrombo-Wellco Test but positive staphylococcal-clumping assay. These findings reflect an effective secondary fibrinolytic response that keeps pace with the low-grade intravascular coagulation. Other assays, such as thrombin time and antithrombin III, are usually normal.

HEMORRHAGIC DISEASES DUE TO CIRCULATING ANTICOAGULANTS

By Alvin H. Schmaier, M.D.
and Robert W. Colman, M.D.
Philadelphia, Pennsylvania

SYNONYMS

Circulating anticoagulants is a general term referring to pathologic substances in blood that directly inhibit clotting factors or their reactions. *Acquired anticoagulants, acquired inhibitors,* and *circulating inhibitors* are other broad terms used to describe these substances that interfere with coagulation reactions. *Specific inhibitors* is a term that refers to endogenously arising antibodies that interfere with one coagulation protein by a humoral immune mechanism. *Nonspecific inhibitors* are substances, usually immunoglobulins, that by nonimmune mechanisms (i.e., not through antigen-antibody reactions) interfere with one or more coagulation proteins. This defect is seen in myeloma, a condition in which hyperproteinemic states may interfere with coagulation reactions. *Lupus-like anticoagulant* or *lupus inhibitor* is a term that refers to a unique circulating anticoagulant that appears to be directed toward the reagents in the coagulation factor(s) assay and not to a specific factor or factors. *Circulating antibody* is a term that can be used to describe these anticoagulants, since most, but not all, circulating anticoagulants are antibodies.

DEFINITION

These conditions are acquired disorders, usually caused by circulating substances directed against coagulation proteins or reagents in the coagulation assay. In the vast majority of patients these circulating anticoagulants turn out to be immunoglobulins. However, non-immunoglobulin circulating anticoagulants have been recently recognized. One type of nonimmunoglobulin anticoagulant is the endogenous heparin-like material derived from cells in various hematologic malignancies (myeloma, monocytic leukemia). Regardless of the nature of the anticoagulant, its manifestations result from inhibition of the normal sequence of events leading to the formation of a fibrin clot.

In general, there are two ways in which immunoglobulins in pathologic states can be characterized as circulating anticoagulants:

1. Specific antibodies directed against one coagulation protein.
2. Inhibitors that by non-immune (i.e., not antigen-antibody) interaction alter the interaction of coagulation proteins or the reagents in coagulation protein assays.

The most common examples of a specific antibody are those that arise against factor VIII; the most common example of a circulating inhibitor is the lupus-like anticoagulant.

SPECIFIC ANTIBODIES

Theoretically, an autoantibody can arise against any protein in the coagulation reactions. It has been most commonly reported to occur against factor VIII, but specific inhibitors have also been reported against factor XI, factor IX, factor VII, factor V, von Willebrand's factor, factor XIII (especially after isoniazid administration), and fibrinogen. These latter conditions are relatively uncommon. Antibodies to factor VIII occur in four different circumstances:

1. In patients with congenital factor VIII:C deficiency (hemophilia A).
2. In young women up to 2 years post partum.
3. In patients with immunologic disorders such as systemic lupus erythematosus (SLE).
4. In individuals, usually elderly, who have been previously healthy.

Antibodies to other coagulation proteins have been noted to arise in multiply transfused deficient patients and in patients with underlying immunologic and/or malignant disorders.

Presenting Signs and Symptoms

The signs and symptoms due to an acquired factor VIII antibody relate to the occurrence of spontaneous bleeding, including hemarthroses, in a patient without previous hemorrhagic manifestations. The signs and symptoms may take any form, including hematomas and mucous membrane bleeding. Most commonly, spontaneous factor VIII inhibitors occur in patients with severe hemophilia, the incidence ranging from 8 to 20 per cent in this subpopulation. Postpartum factor VIII inhibitors usually occur within a few months after the birth of the first child or after an interval of 1 year. Factor VIII inhibitors have been noted in patients with rheumatoid arthritis, SLE, penicillin allergy, bronchial asthma, regional enteritis, ulcerative colitis, pemphigus, erythema multiforme, dermatitis herpetiformis, myeloma, and monoclonal gammopathies.

Course of Syndromes Due to Specific Antibodies

The course of the disorder associated with factor VIII antibodies in patients with hemophilia A is variable. Two types of antibodies, characterized as "strong" and "weak," have been reported. In the "strong" variety, titers begin to rise 2 to 3 days following exposure to factor VIII, reaching a maximum within 7 to 21 days. Occasionally, high levels persist even in the absence of re-exposure to factor VIII. "Weak" antibodies may not reappear with re-exposure to factor VIII. The presence of these inhibitors in the hemophilic population may give rise to a severe clinical problem.

Postpartum factor VIII inhibitors, or those in the elderly, also have a variable course; some patients die as a result of the inhibitor, but most of the inhibitors disappear after 12 to 18 months. Inhibitors to von Willebrand factor usually produce a mild bleeding disorder similar to that of von Willebrand's disease.

Laboratory Diagnosis of Specific Inhibitors

Abnormalities on coagulation screening tests will depend on the portion of the hemostatic sequence affected by the inhibitor. They do not make a diagnosis of a specific inhibitor, but point only to the part of the coagulation sequence affected by the inhibitor. Inhibitors to intrinsic coagulation proteins (factors VIII, IX, XI, and XII) will be recognized by a prolonged activated partial thromboplastin time (APTT) but with a normal prothrombin time (PT). Inhibitors to factor VII will produce a normal APTT but a prolonged PT. Inhibitors to factor V—a common pathway protein—will present with prolonged APTT and PT. Inhibitors to von Willebrand's factor will be recognized by a prolonged bleeding time in the presence of a normal PT, APTT, platelet count, and platelet function studies. Inhibitors to fibrinogen rarely produce a prolonged PT and APTT; however, they do cause a prolonged thrombin time and Reptilase time, low fibrinogen when assayed by coagulant activity, and normal fibrinogen by immunologic assay. Since factor XIII is not recognized by routine coagulation screening assays (PT, APTT), a defect in the function of this protein can be recognized only by a specific factor XIII assay.

Identification of a defect in a coagulation protein by screening assays will lead to one of three possibilities to explain the mechanisms responsible for the apparent defect:

1. There may be a true deficiency of the protein.
2. The protein present may be an abnormal molecule that does not function properly.
3. There may be a specific inhibitor or anticoagulant that interferes with the function of the normal protein present.

If an inhibitor is suspected, a simple mixing test consisting of equal volumes of patient plasma and normal plasma used in the PT and APTT may serve to confirm its presence. If a true deficiency exists, mixing equal volumes of normal plasma with patient plasma will correct the abnormal PT and/or APTT. In the presence of a circulating inhibitor, an equal volume mixture will not correct the defect. This screening test for an inhibitor is more sensitive if performed after the mixtures are incubated at 37°C for 1 to 2 hours.

The exact diagnosis of a specific antibody depends upon demonstration of a substance in the patient's plasma that interferes with the specific functional assay for that protein. In order to identify the specific antibody, individual clotting factor assays must be performed by mixing patient and normal plasma in various ratios and comparing the amount of activity observed with that expected. The expected value is calculated from the original activity of the patient's sample and normal plasma performed separately and the ratios of the combined plasmas used in the mixing experiment. In the presence of a specific clotting factor antibody, the observed value will always be less than the expected value. By performing coagulation assays on various ratios of patient plasma to normal plasma, one can titer the level of antibody, that is, determine the level (e.g., 1:10, 1:50) at which the specific inhibitor can no longer be detected. In specific antibody assays, the quantity of reagents in the assay remains constant; only the percentage of patient plasma in the test mixture decreases. For factor VIII antibodies specifically, attempts have been made to "standardize" the measurement and the reporting of specific inhibitors. This standard method expresses potency of the inhibitor in units termed the "Bethesda unit." By definition, one Bethesda unit is the amount of inhibitor present that will inactivate 50 per cent of the factor VIII activity in 2 hours in vitro. However, the designation of an inhibitor unit does not imply that any specific number of factor VIII units infused into the patient will neutralize any specific number of inhibitor units.

Potential Errors and Pitfalls in Diagnosis

Laboratory coagulation abnormalities may be produced artifactually by poor venipuncture technique, high hematocrit (resulting in high citrate and low calcium concentration), and prolonged storage before assay. Evaluation of coagulation samples obtained in glass tubes may also give inaccurate results. Finally, specific antibodies may arise to portions of coagulation proteins that are not involved with the function of that protein. These antigen-antibody complexes may be more rapidly cleared from the circulation, giving a picture of an apparent deficiency. Testing that measures only inhibition of the functional activity of this protein will not recognize this potential situation.

LUPUS-LIKE ANTICOAGULANT

This is a unique coagulation assay inhibitor that was first recognized in patients with SLE. Although it can be seen in 6 to 9 per cent of such patients, the vast majority of individuals with this problem do not have SLE or any similar disorder. The term "lupus anticoagulant" is a misnomer. This anticoagulant, when studied carefully, usually is an immunoglobulin. However, unlike specific coagulation protein inhibitors, these immunoglobulins are not directed against one coagulation protein, but appear to interfere with the phospholipid contained in the reagents of the coagulation assay.

Presenting Signs and Symptoms

The patient with the lupus anticoagulant has no bleeding manifestations and is usually recognized by a prolonged coagulation screening test in the absence of a bleeding history. The recognition of a lupus-like anticoagulant does not necessarily suggest an underlying disorder.

Course

Most patients with lupus anticoagulants will not have abnormal bleeding at the time of surgery. The coexistence of severe thrombocytopenia or hypoprothrombinemia with a lupus anticoagulant, on the other hand, may present a hemorrhagic risk. However, it is unclear whether the risk for hemorrhage in the patient with the lupus anticoagulant is greater than that which might occur in the presence of thrombocytopenia or hypoprothrombinemia alone. Paradoxically, the lupus anticoagulant has been associated with an increased risk for clinical thrombosis.

Laboratory Diagnosis

The hallmark of the lupus anticoagulant is prolongation of all phospholipid-dependent coagulation tests. These include the prothrombin time (PT) and the activated partial thromboplastin time (APTT)—the two main coagulation screening assays. Although historically the lupus anticoagulant was first recognized by a prolonged PT, most observers consider the APTT to be more sensitive. Today the vast majority of patients with lupus-like anticoagulants are recognized first by a prolonged APTT. The sensitivity of the APTT to detect the lupus anticoagulant varies to some extent with the type of reagents used in the APTT.

The specific laboratory diagnosis of the lupus anticoagulant is somewhat difficult. There is no assay that is accepted by all to be specific for this condition. In essence it is a diagnosis of exclusion. Unlike inhibitors directed against specific coagulation proteins, the inhibitor frequently does not exert an increasing effect with increasing incubation times when mixed with normal plasma. One assay that is used to diagnose the lupus-like anticoagulant is called the tissue thromboplastin inhibition (TTI) assay. This test is simply a modified prothrombin time in which the thromboplastin (not the test or control plasma) is diluted and the patient is compared with a normal control. Characteristically, on the TTI, as the clotting time is measured for patient and control sample, the degree of prolongation of the patient sample is greater at the lower thromboplastin concentrations than the control sample, suggesting that the prolongation in the patient sample is more than that which can be ascribed to dilution alone. This test cannot be considered specific for the lupus anticoagulant, since almost any other endogenous or exogenous coagulation abnormality will give an abnormal TTI. Our approach using this test to diagnose lupus anticoagulants is that in the absence of any other coagulation abnormality, an abnormal TTI in an asymptomatic patient suggests the diagnosis.

Potential Errors and Pitfalls in Diagnosis

Since the lupus inhibitor interferes with phospholipid in coagulation assays and because of the marked sensitivity of the APTT to the inhibitor's effect, measurements in one-stage assays for factor XII, prekallikrein, high-molecular-weight (HMW) kininogen, and factors XI, IX, and VIII may be artifactually low. In general, low values obtained on one-stage specific coagulation factor assays do not appear to be due to specific coagulation factor inhibitors. However, occasionally mixing experiments at multiple dilutions do suggest a specific coagulation factor inhibitor. The meaning of this finding is unclear and does suggest that these individuals must be considered to have associated specific factor inhibitors. If appropriate, treatment should be given. The diagnosis of lupus anticoagulant should be made only on the basis of exclusion of specific defects. Although it is the most common cause of an isolated prolonged APTT, diagnostic evaluation of a patient with a prolonged APTT must exclude the presence of mild deficiency of factors XI, IX, and VIII as well as an asymptomatic deficiency of factor XII, prekallikrein, and HMW kininogen before a diagnosis of a lupus-like anticoagulant is made.

ACUTE TRANSFUSION REACTIONS

By Herbert F. Polesky, M.D.
and Charles Horwitz, M.D.
Minneapolis, Minnesota

DEFINITION

Adverse effects occurring during or in the first few hours following a transfusion are defined as *acute reactions*. In various reports, 1 to 7 per cent of recipients develop symptoms that are recognized as acute transfusion reactions. An even larger number of transfused patients may be immunized to white cell or red cell antigens, or they may develop a transfusion-transmitted disease that does not become apparent for weeks to months after the transfusion event. A small group of patients may develop delayed reactions manifested by hemolysis occurring in the first 2 weeks following the transfusion.

SYMPTOMS AND RECOGNITION

The acute complications of transfusion vary from bothersome symptoms to life-threatening emergencies (Table 1). Fortunately, most reactions have little clinical significance; however, in the rare severe reaction, the signs and symptoms are often indistinguishable from those occurring in the benign reactions. Thus, with the exception of hives, any suspicion of a reaction should be considered reason to terminate the transfusion and institute an investigation into the cause. Recognizing that a transfusion patient is having an adverse effect is not always easy. Many of the classic symptoms associated with intravascular hemolysis (e.g., pain and burning at the infusion site, lumbar pain, chest pain, a feeling of oppression, chills) depend on the patient's communicating with personnel in attendance. In many clinical settings in which blood and components are being infused, the patient is unable to provide information about symptoms and one must depend on various signs (e.g., flushing of the face, fever, rapid respiration, hypotension, abnormal bleeding, hemoglobinuria) as indicators of red cell destruction. In some cases the classic signs of a hemolytic transfusion reaction (HTR) are mimicked by changes related to a surgical procedure. Thus in cardiopulmonary bypass, hemoglobinemia and hemoglobinuria are frequently seen even when no blood is used.

Dramatic signs and symptoms of a reaction to other than the red cell component of blood can also occur. Anaphylactic shock occasionally develops after a very small amount of plasma is given to an IgA-deficient patient who has circulating anti-IgA. Chills, fever, nonproductive cough, dyspnea, and pulmonary infiltrates can appear very rapidly when a potent leukoagglutinin is present in the donor's plasma. Similar symptoms can develop when the recipient has antibodies to leukocyte antigens on the donor cells.

In patients receiving granulocyte concentrates, severe pulmonary symptoms, chills, and fever are fairly common. These reactions have been attributed to granulocyte fragments; complement activation; and, in some reports, interaction between white blood cells and amphotericin B. These reactions can be minimized by slow infusion and premedication with di-

Table 1. Acute Complications of Transfusion

Reaction	Relative Frequency (% of Reactions)
Febrile nonhemolytic	50
Urticaria	30
Miscellaneous and undefined	11
Overload	4
Hemolysis	
Delayed	3
Immediate	< 0.1
Dilutional coagulopathy	< 1.0
Potassium toxicity	< 0.01
Citrate toxicity	< 0.01
Air embolism	< 0.01
Anaphylaxis	< 0.01
Septicemia	< 0.01

phenhydramine and/or meperidine. Unless the symptoms are very severe, the infusion is usually not terminated.

Two other dramatic events that occasionally are associated with transfusion are air embolism or infusion of contaminated blood. In the former, signs and symptoms include cyanosis, hypotension, a rapid thready pulse, and syncope; in the latter, fever, shock, and disseminated intravascular coagulation (DIC) usually occur.

Pulmonary edema and cardiac failure can occur if volume overload results from overly vigorous transfusion therapy. Treatment of this complication may require digitalization and venisection to reduce volume. Overload can easily be prevented in most patients by careful attention to the volume infused and by using packed red cells rather than whole blood.

ETIOLOGY

The etiology of most acute transfusion reactions is immunologic. Antibody-antigen reactions leading to complement activation (intravascular hemolysis), release of leukotrienes (bronchospasm and vasoconstriction), or histamine from mast cells (urticaria) underlie most of the symptoms observed clinically. Other complications, such as renal failure, usually are consequences of physiologic changes initiated by the antibody-antigen reaction.

The most serious transfusion reactions are those in which intravascular hemolysis is initiated by infusion of ABO-incompatible blood. These reactions, which often lead to a fatal outcome, usually occur because of errors in properly identifying the tube when drawing a sample for cross-matching or failure to confirm that the unit issued is for the intended recipient. It is because these clerical errors can have such dire consequences that blood banks and transfusion services have rigid identification procedures when drawing patient samples and when starting a transfusion. Reviews of the transfusion-related fatalities reported to the Office of the Biologics of the Food and Drug Administration (as required by CFR 21 section 606.170b) indicate that over 50 per cent were due to ABO incompatibility, most of which occurred because of identification errors. In contrast, patients who receive blood intended for them, and who are considered compatible, based on a type and screen procedure or a crossmatch, almost never develop acute hemolysis.

Adverse effects not related to immunologic events can occur because of hemolysis due to improper storage or administration of blood or because of changes in blood that develop during its storage in the blood bank. Hemolysis can occur if blood is frozen, overheated, or subjected to mechanical trauma or if hypotonic solutions are mixed with the blood. The symptoms are probably related to complement activation and DIC initiated by red cell fragments, since the infusion of stroma-free hemoglobin generally does not cause acute signs or symptoms. Other nonimmunologic effects, such as citrate or potassium toxicity, are rare and occur only when a large volume of blood or plasma is used (massive or exchange transfusion). The rapid infusion of ice cold blood can cause severe pain and muscle cramping and can trigger cardiac arrhythmias.

A febrile reaction to transfusion is probably the most frequently encountered acute adverse effect. This type of reaction often occurs after the infusion has been running from 30 to 60 minutes and is usually caused by antibodies to leukocyte antigens. These antibodies may be directed to HLA antigens found on all white cells and platelets, or they may react with antigens found only on a specific cell type. There is no specific treatment for chills and fever associated with transfusion. As mentioned, these symptoms require stopping the blood. Warming the patient and administering antipyretics is beneficial. Patients with repeated febrile reactions should be tested for leukocyte antibodies. Since in many patients these reactions are related to the dose of infused leukocytes, a trial with leukocyte-poor blood may be indicated. In some multitransfused patients, those with sickle cell disease, thalassemia or paroxysmal nocturnal hemoglobinuria (PNH), routine use of frozen-thawed-deglycerolized red cells is helpful in preventing febrile reactions.

INVESTIGATION

The investigation of a suspected transfusion reaction first must rule in or rule out the presence of acute hemolysis. After the infusion is stopped, a careful check of the unit and a patient ID should be done. This should identify most patients who are receiving ABO-incompatible red cells. If the clinical evaluation suggests that the reaction is allergic, the unit can be restarted after treating the patient with an antihistamine. If the cause of the reaction is not apparent, the next step is to carefully draw a properly labeled blood sample from the patient. This should be sent to the blood bank to be inspected for evidence of hemolysis and for a direct antiglobulin test (DAT). Additional tests may be indicated, depending on clinical findings, review of the clerical work, presence or absence of hemolysis, or a positive DAT.

Further studies may require the use of special techniques to identify weakly reactive antibodies, typing of the patient samples and the units to confirm the presence or absence of specific antigens, and monitoring the patient for biochemical evidence of red cell destruction. If bacterial contamination is suspected, a smear and culture of the unit and remaining blood bag segments can be helpful.

DELAYED HEMOLYTIC TRANSFUSION REACTIONS

Hemolysis related to extravascular destruction of transfused red cells is a much more frequent occurrence than is usually recognized. A very informative study of recipients at the Mayo Clinic identified one delayed hemolytic transfusion reaction (DHTR) per 4000 units transfused. These reactions usually are without clinical symptoms. Recognition depends on suspicion, particularly in patients with unexplained

Table 2. Antibodies Causing Delayed Hemolytic Reactions

Blood Group System	Frequency (% of Reactions)	Usual Specificity
Rh	36	E, c, C
Kidd	30	Jk^a
Duffy	10	Fy^a
Kell	8	K
MNSs	3	M
Multiple	13	

anemia or an episode of hemoglobinuria several days following transfusion. Frequently the possibility of a DHTR is raised when the blood bank obtains a positive antibody screen on a recently transfused patient whose test was nonreactive prior to the previous transfusion. Table 2 shows the antibodies most frequently encountered in extravascular hemolysis. Usually these antibodies are detected at 37°C using antiglobulin techniques. Some may not be detected unless enhancing reagents or enzyme-treated cells are used. Only rarely is a cold-reactive antibody involved in hemolysis, and usually these antibodies will have a wide thermal amplitude. In multitransfused patients, separation of the patient's own cells from the transfused cells by density gradients may be necessary to establish the patient's phenotype. This step is useful in confirming the specificity of the antibody(ies).

There is no specific treatment for a DHTR. It is extremely unusual to observe significant morbidity or mortality following a DHTR. It is important to recognize these reactions and to identify the antibody(ies) involved, since many of these patients will require additional transfusions. Units negative for the antigens to which the patient has antibodies should be selected whenever possible.

Section Seven
GASTROINTESTINAL TRACT

FUNCTIONAL DISORDERS OF THE GASTROINTESTINAL TRACT

By Marwan Balaa, M.D.
and John T. Sessions, Jr., M.D.
Chapel Hill, North Carolina

Functional disorders of the gastrointestinal (GI) tract constitute a group of poorly understood conditions representing a sizable percentage of a specialist's referral patient population and a major cause of morbidity. It is thus not unusual to find increased attention being directed to these disorders in recent times, with a growing number of research projects being developed in an attempt to better characterize them. Table 1 gives a listing of these disorders.

DEFINITION

Disorders of the GI tract can be classified into four groups (Fig. 1):

1. *Structural disorders.* The illness or symptoms in this group are usually referable to an organ in the GI tract that is anatomically distorted at the macroscopic or microscopic level.
2. *Functional disorders.* The symptoms in these disorders are best understood as being secondary to an alteration in the physiologic function of an organ and not associated with any identifiable derangement at the anatomic level.
3. *Psychogenic disorders.* Unlike the first two groups, no anatomic or physiologic derangement can be seen. The symptoms in patients with such a disorder are thought to arise from unconscious mechanisms, whereby mental suffering is expressed through the presence of physical symptoms.
4. *Malingering.* Symptoms are determined by the patient's desire for secondary gain.

The boundaries among the groups are often poorly defined, making it harder for the physician to define the goals of management as well as to define means to reach such a goal.

CHIEF COMPLAINTS

Common to all functional gastrointestinal disorders is a group of nonspecific symptoms including nausea, abdominal pain, abdominal fullness, anorexia, and lassitude, present in varying combinations and proportions. It is not uncommon for these symptoms to be of long-standing duration, with episodes interposed between periods of relative quiescence. Constitutional symptoms, such as fever, chills, unexplained weight loss, jaundice, or change in color of the stool or urine, associated with the patient's complaints should sway one's attention more toward a structural disorder because, by definition, functional disorders are characterized by the absence of such symptoms.

For unclear reasons, patients with functional disorders tend to have symptoms during daytime and rarely if ever are awakened by symptoms at night. If nocturnal symptoms are more often than incidental in a patient's history, one is obliged to rule out some underlying structural disorder.

The final point to be made here relates to stress. Stress is a common denominator in the setting of, or exacerbation of, many diseases belonging to the structural, functional, or psychological group of disorders. The association of symptoms with stress does not make a diagnosis, nor does it characterize the disorder into any of the subgroups.

PHYSICAL EXAMINATION

Patients with functional gastrointestinal disorders have a wide age spectrum, but tend to be crowded on the younger side. The findings on physical examination range from negative to nonspecific and most of the time are related to the abdominal cavity in the form of a poorly localized direct tenderness, typically in the absence of other findings such as masses, bruits, or frank or occult blood in the stools. A more detailed listing of pertinent physical findings will be included in the discussion of particular disorders when applicable.

DISEASE ENTITIES

Esophageal Disorders

Globus

Globus is an abnormal sensation in the throat described as a lump at the level of the cricoid cartilage. The descriptive noun "globus" is historically associated with the adjective "hystericus," but as many writers believe, this is an improper association because the majority of such patients are not hysterical. Female-to-male ratio of such a patient population is 3:1.

Presenting Signs and Symptoms. Aside from the lump sensation, patients are usually asymptomatic and have no history of involuntary weight loss. There is no true dysphagia; some patients report exacerbation, and others have relief of their symptoms with swallowing. Patients often report the relief of symptoms with crying.

Radiologic Evaluation. Upper GI tract barium studies in patients with this disorder more often than not will be normal. Some authors have reported an increased incidence of gastroesophageal reflux. The relation of such a reflux to the globus is not well defined. Osteoarthritic spur formation in the neck area is also described by some authors to be more common in patients with this disorder, but the significance of such a finding and its relation to the patient's symptoms is not well understood.

Other Diagnostic Procedures. No additional tests are necessary to establish this diagnosis. Manometric study of the esophagus, although occasionally showing above-normal pressures in the region of the cricopharynx, does not add to the management and by itself is not diagnostic.

Table 1. Functional Disorders of the Gastrointestinal Tract

Esophagus	**General Gut Involvement**
Globus	Irritable bowel disease
Motor disturbances	Pseudo-obstruction
Stomach	**Biliary Tree**
Gastroparesis	Sphincter of Oddi dyskinesia
Rumination	
Functional vomiting	**Miscellaneous**
Small Bowel	Puritus ani
Lactase deficiency	Dyspepsia
Colon and Rectum	Aerophagia
Constipation	
Functional nonsecretory diarrhea	
Proctalgia fugax	

Motor Disturbances of the Esophagus

This group is discussed in detail in a separate article.

Functional Disorders of the Stomach

Gastroparesis

Gastroparesis is the delay in, or failure of, the stomach to empty its contents. It usually presents as a complication of other diseases, most notably diabetes. Table 2 gives a more complete listing of such underlying disorders.

Presenting Signs and Symptoms. Fullness with vomiting of undigested material several hours postprandially is one of the most frequently observed signs and symptoms. One should also look for manifestations of underlying disease.

Common Complications. Recurrent vomiting with aspiration pneumonia is one of the most common complications. Less frequently, gastric ulcers develop secondary to the long-standing pressure from food particles.

Physical Examination. Findings include a tympanitic left upper quadrant and succussion splash. If the gastric paresis is due to diabetes mellitus, it is quite common that the patient will also have evidence of peripheral neuropathy on physical examination.

Radiologic Evaluation. A simple abdominal film will identify the enlarged, often air-filled, stomach (Magenblase). A barium meal or, better still, a piece of minced meat immersed in barium and swallowed by the patient will show the delay in emptying of the stomach.

Other Diagnostic Procedures. Endoscopic examination of the stomach often helps rule out an ana-

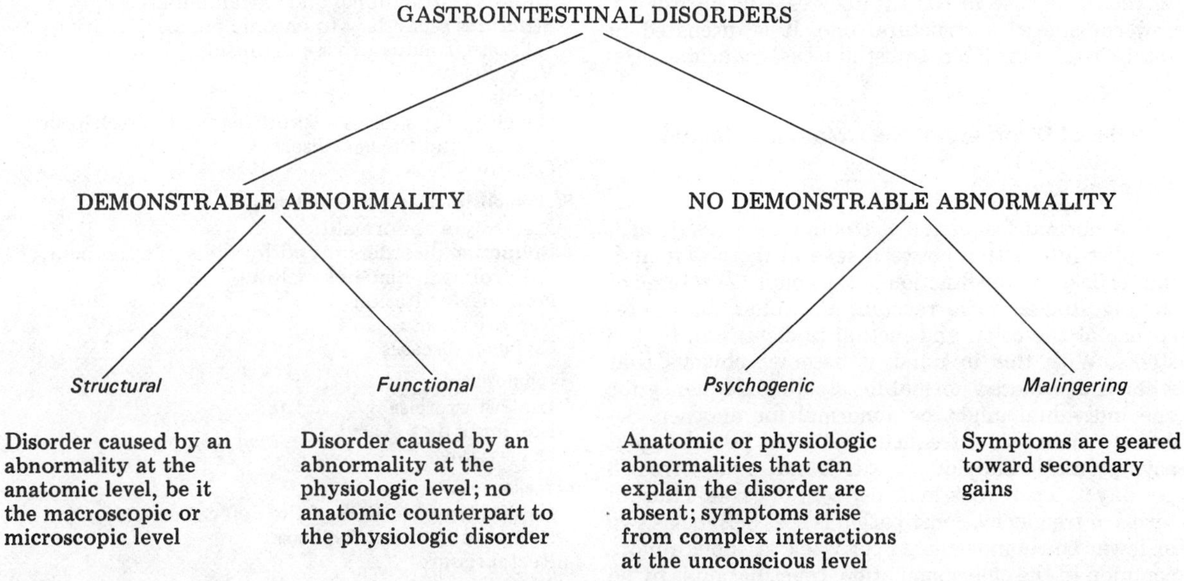

Figure 1. Classification of disorders affecting the gastrointestinal tract.

Table 2. Disorders Having Gastroparesis As A Manifestation

Diabetes
Amyloidosis
Pancreatitis
Superior mesenteric artery syndrome
Annular pancreas
Pyloric hypertrophy
Pyloric channel obstruction
Intestinal pseudo-obstruction

tomic cause of the gastroparesis. Manometric examination of the esophagus can also delineate the extent of the disease, but it does not add much to the knowledge because the majority of patients having both esophageal and gastric motility disturbances will complain of both dysphagia and postprandial fullness.

Rumination

This is often an involuntary act of regurgitation of varying amounts of food into the oral cavity a few minutes postprandially, chewing it again, and then swallowing it.

Presenting Signs and Symptoms. Absence of nausea, pain, dyspepsia, or dysphagia characterizes this act. Patients usually experience rumination under periods of stress and more often than not are brought in by a worrying friend or family member, rather than coming in on their own.

Functional Vomiting

This topic in dealt with in a separate article on Anorexia, Nausea, and Vomiting.

Functional Disorders of the Small Bowel

Until the recent past, lactase deficiency was grouped under functional disorders. However, with the development of cytochemical techniques to show decreased lactase in the enterocytes, this disorder is now considered a structural one. It is discussed in detail in an article on Intestinal Disaccharidase Deficiency.

Functional Disorders of the Colon and Rectum

Constipation

The normal frequency of stooling is a result of a complex interaction between several factors, including (1) basic motor function of the colon, (2) volume of the digested material reaching the colon, and (3) response of the colon and rectum to distention by the stools. With this in mind, it becomes obvious that what is considered normal for stooling frequency for one individual might be abnormal for another. So-called normal stool frequency, studied in a group of asymptomatic individuals, was found to vary from 3 per day to 3 per week in 95 per cent of cases. Thus, in terms of frequency, constipation is best defined as two or fewer bowel movements per week. Although more common in the older population, constipation is by no means limited to one age group. Its severity is often found to increase with advancing age. One of the most important determinants of bowel movements is the so-called gastrocolic reflex. When the stomach is distended, as occurs following a meal, a reflex is set in motion initiating colonic peristaltic waves that propel the colonic contents and culminate in the passage of a stool. A significant number of patients complaining of constipation are found to have a decreased or abolished sensitivity to this reflex. The management of such cases should primarily be directed to retraining the reflex by having the patient attempt to pass a stool following each meal. Other causes of constipation are listed in Table 3.

Presenting Signs and Symptoms. Although a decreased frequency of stooling is often an underlying problem, it rarely constitutes the presenting symptom. The most common presentation is that of a patient complaining of difficulty in passing stools which are often hard and often accompanied by a sense of unsatisfactory defecation. The more severe cases can present with burning pain and even fresh blood coating the stools or being seen on the tissue paper.

Physical Examination. Findings on physical examination are usually related to the increased abdominal pressures needed to move the bowels. These would include internal and external hemorrhoids, rectal prolapse, and perianal tags. Incisional and umbilical hernias are also occasionally found. Anal fissures, caused by the passage of hard stools, are a common cause of dyschezia and a common side effect of constipation. This can further worsen the constipation by suppressing the urge to defecate for fear of the associated pain, thus setting in motion a vicious circle that can be broken only by directing attention to both the fissure and the constipation.

Radiologic Evaluation. Barium enema, though not very helpful in making the diagnosis, should be

Table 3. Structural Causes of Constipation

Obstructive (Obstructive Ileus)
Tumors (intraluminal and extraluminal)
Strictures secondary to chronic mucosal injury by disease, trauma or vascular insults
Volvulus
Hernias
Hirschsprung's disease, short segment Hirschsprung's disease and Chagas' disease
Gallstone ileus
Pseudo-obstructive (Paralytic Ileus)
Electrolyte abnormalities
Endocrine disorders (hypothyroidism, hyperparathyroidism, diabetes mellitus)
Peritoneal irritation
Narcotics
Collagen diseases
Hypomotility
Lack of exercise
Low-bulk diet
Depression
Miscellaneous
Habitual suppression of the defecation urge
Disagreeable toilet facilities
Rectal fissure
Travel

among the first investigative measures taken to help rule out any structural causes for the constipation and identifying a commonly coexistent disease, namely diverticulosis. Other radiologic investigations that have been honored by time include transit time studies with the use of radiopaque markers, both as a pointer to underlying pathology and as a simple means of follow-up for such patients.

Other Diagnostic Procedures. A careful search in the history and physical examination along with logical laboratory and radiologic evaluation can rule out, in a sizable part of the patient population, secondary causes for the constipation. With these ruled out, a therapeutic trial with a high-fiber diet and retraining of the gastrocolic reflex ought to be the next steps in the management.

Other Important Diagnostic Procedures. Other procedures include sigmoidoscopic examination and a rectal manometric study, the latter being performed to rule out any neuromuscular disease of the colon and rectum as an underlying cause for the constipation.

Proctalgia Fugax

This condition in characterized by episodic severe rectal pain caused by spasm of the levator ani and/or the coccygeus muscle. The attacks occur in the absence of any underlying disorder such as fracture of the coccyx, anorectal infection, or chronic prostatitis. It is described as occurring in all age groups with a female preponderance. A common personality trait is the tense, anxious, perfectionist type, described in up to two thirds of patients.

Presenting Signs and Symptoms. Sudden pain in the rectal sphincter area, described as gnawing, grinding, stabbing, or cramping, is characteristic. A typical attack lasts anywhere from a few minutes up to 30 minutes, even awakening the patient from sleep. The attacks tend to occur following bowel action or following various types of sexual activity, and may be associated with priapism in males. Syncope is sometimes the presenting feature occurring with severe attacks.

Physical Examination. It is extremely rare for the patient to present during an acute attack. The few patients examined are described to have a tender, tight band across one or both sides of a lax anal sphincter. Companion findings include varying degrees of autonomic dysfunction; sweating, priapism, or syncope.

Disorders with Generalized Gut Involvement

Irritable Bowel Syndrome

This is the most common of the functional disorders of the gastrointestinal tract. It has no organ predilection, although the colon seems to be a more frequent site of involvement. The underlying pathology is currently viewed as an alteration in the basic electrical rhythm of the bowel which is believed to be the cause of the patient's symptomatology.

Presenting Signs and Symptoms. In patients with this disorder, symptoms do not differ from those outlined in the general discussion. Among the features reported to differentiate between the irritable bowel syndrome and organic disease are loose and/or frequent stools at the onset of pain, relief of the pain by defecation, and abdominal distention. Increase in mucus production, a change in the caliber of the stools, or a sense of incomplete evacuation is also commonly present in patients with irritable bowel syndrome, although not more common than in patients with organic disease.

Radiologic Evaluation. A barium enema is essential in ruling out a colonic lesion that could explain a number of the patient's symptoms, especially when the presentation is in the fourth decade or beyond.

Other Diagnostic Procedures. There is an increased sensitivity to distention of the gastrointestinal tract in patients with the irritable bowel syndrome. Insufflation of the rectum during proctoscopy tends to reproduce the patient's symptoms. Such a finding should not be ignored and, in the absence of findings on physical examination and radiologic evaluation, would strengthen the diagnosis.

Pseudo-obstruction

This disorder is characterized by an abnormal wave progression in the gastrointestinal tract. The site of pathology is not clear. Reports have described this disorder to be associated with malignant neoplasms and with a degeneration of the neuroplexuses.

Presenting Signs and Symptoms. A triad consisting of dysphagia, abdominal distention, and atonic bladder is among the most frequent of presentations.

Diagnostic Procedures. Manometric evaluation of the esophagus, rectal sphincter, and bladder often shows an abnormality in wave progression.

Functional Disorders of the Pancreatic or Biliary Tree

Sphincter of Oddi Dyskinesia

This is a motility disorder of the sphincter of Oddi leading to impedance of the flow of bile, pancreatic juice, or both into the duodenum. Symptoms are thought to arise during contraction of the gallbladder against a hypertonic sphincter of Oddi, leading to dilatation of the extrahepatic biliary tree.

Presenting Signs and Symptoms. The pain reported by patients with this disorder is typical of gallstone attack, occuring postprandially with upper abdominal pain radiating to the subxyphoid area. The majority of patients considered for such a diagnosis have already had surgery on the gallbladder, with postoperative persistence of their symptoms. A small number of patients have had a negative evaluation consisting of a normal ultrasound of the gallbladder, absence of stones on cholangiography, and absence of crystals on microscopic examination of the bile.

Diagnostic Procedures. Sphincter of Oddi dyskinesia is often difficult to differentiate from ampullary stenosis, which most commonly occurs secondary to the passage of stones or surgical trauma. During attacks of pain, elevated levels of serum alkaline phosphatase, amylase, and bilirubin are reported. During cholangiography, a dilated biliary system is often found with a delay in emptying of the common bile duct to more than 45 minutes; this delay is significant only in patients who have had cholecystectomy.

Miscellaneous Disorders

Pruritus Ani

Perianal itching of the functional type occurs without obvious skin lesions, bleeding fissures or hemorrhoids and in the presence of a negative test for pinworms. It is often worsened by periods of anxiety and stress.

Dyspepsia

See the articles on Dysphagia, Esophageal Obstruction, and Esophagitis and on Diaphragmatic Hernias.

Aerophagia

Aerophagia is characterized by an increase in the gas content of the gastrointestinal tract due to an increased swallowing of air. Patients with this disorder are believed to have an increased frequency of dry swallows associated with swallows of bigger volumes of air. The underlying disorder could be excessive salivation, as seen in patients with peptic ulcer disease or in those experiencing anxiety and stress.

Presenting Signs and Symptoms. Increased belching, flatulence and abdominal discomfort related to distention are the presenting symptoms.

Physical Examination. In the stress-related group, findings are typically negative. The interviewer can sometimes observe the patient in the act of swallowing air or can ask the patient to reproduce symptoms by swallowing air.

DYSPHAGIA, ESOPHAGEAL OBSTRUCTION, AND ESOPHAGITIS

By Charles A. Sninsky, M.D.
and John R. Mathias, M.D.
Gainesville, Florida

The function of the esophagus is twofold: first, to transport ingested food from the hypopharynx to the stomach; and second, to prevent the reflux of gastric contents back up into the esophagus. This article addresses three specific areas:

1. Dysphagia for both liquids and solids (motility disorders).
2. Dysphagia for solids (esophageal obstruction).
3. Esophagitis.

Food is transported into the stomach by an organized ring contraction called *peristalsis.* When the act of swallowing is voluntary, the contraction begins in the nasopharynx and traverses the esophagus in an organized fashion (Fig. 1), which is primary peristalsis. Secondary peristalsis occurs in the body of the esophagus and is the result of distention. Both primary and secondary peristalsis are normal events. Contractions that are spontaneous and do not propagate (aperistalsis) are called tertiary contractions. They are always abnormal and are usually associated with chest pain or pain on swallowing (odynophagia), especially when the amplitude is abnormally high.

Dysphagia is the subjective awareness of swallowed contents sticking in the chest or the sensation that they are not moving. Dysphagia for liquids and solids implies that the lack of movement of contents within the esophagus is secondary to an ineffective (low-amplitude) contraction, aperistalsis, or no contraction at all. Dysphagia for solids alone suggests the presence of narrowing of the esophageal lumen, causing partial obstruction. Dysphagia for solids will be discussed under Esophageal Obstruction.

DYSPHAGIA

The lack of effective contractions in the esophagus indicates the presence of a motility disorder. Table 1 lists the more common causes of motor diseases of the esophagus. In general, motor abnormalities are due either to primary muscle disease (myopathy) or to neurologic disease (neuropathy). In addition, these disorders may involve only the upper one third of the esophagus, which is made up of skeletal muscle, or the lower two thirds, which is made up of smooth muscle.

The investigation of esophageal disease consists principally of three specific tests: First, the *barium swallow,* which should include a film record (cine-esophagogram) of swallowing, allows the physician to observe the act of swallowing and is important in diagnosing motility disorders, especially those involving the upper one third of the esophagus. The second test, *esophageal manometry,* allows the actual function of the esophageal muscle to be observed. The standard method at present uses a 6-lumen catheter perfused with water under nitrogen-driven pressure (Arendoffer pump). This low-compliance system allows sensitive and accurate measurements of the upper sphincter, the body of the esophagus, and the lower esophageal sphincter (Fig. 1). If the barium swallow shows no mechanical obstruction, esophageal manometry is essential for all subjects complaining of dysphagia. The third test is *endoscopy,* which allows actual visualization of the anatomy of the esophagus. These three tests are complementary and provide a complete picture of esophageal function.

Muscle Disease

Dermatomyositis (Polymyositis). Polymyositis, an inflammatory disease of skeletal muscle, is of unknown origin and involves the upper one third of the esophagus. (See the article on Dermatomyositis and Polymyositis.) Usually the patient complains of proximal muscular weakness of the upper and lower extremities, which may or may not be associated with

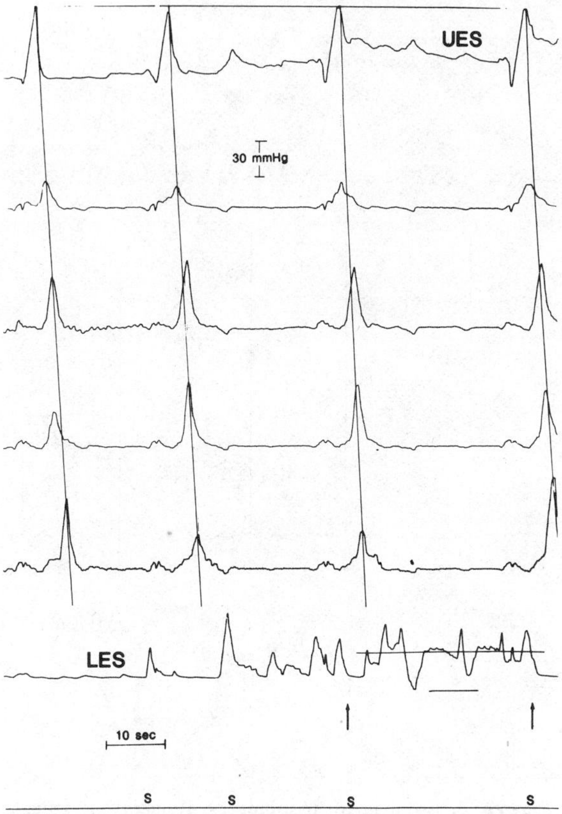

Figure 1. Normal esophageal manometry illustrating the upper esophageal sphincter (UES), normal peristalsis (represented by the slope of the line), and the lower esophageal sphincter (LES). The arrows represent normal relaxation of the LES to intragastric pressure. Swallowing is represented by the symbol (S). A time and pressure constant is also shown.

skin lesions. Muscle tenderness is absent despite the presence of weakness. Skin lesions may consist of spotty or diffuse erythematous or eczematoid lesions, and especially striking, if present is a violet-colored change in skin color over the nose and cheeks of the face. Joint complaints are also common. Dysphagia for liquids and solids may also occur. Usually the dysphagia is localized to the suprasternal notch (space of Burns), although this is not specific. The symptoms of dysphagia for distal esophageal lesions may also be referred to the suprasternal notch. Barium swallow shows impaired function of the upper esophagus, and manometry demonstrates low-amplitude or absent contractions in the upper one third (Fig. 2). Endoscopy reveals normal anatomy. High creatine phosphokinase (CK, CPK) values can confirm the diagnosis. Biopsy of proximal skeletal muscle will show the characteristic histologic lesions. One must keep in mind that polymyositis may precede the diagnosis of certain tumors, especially bronchogenic carcinoma. Elderly patients and those who have lost weight should be suspected of having an occult tumor. Often manometry may give a diagnostic clue, usually showing that the upper third of the esophagus may have weak to absent contractions and then an increase in amplitude as the patient continues to swallow (Eaton-Lambert syndrome).

Muscular Dystrophy (Myotonic Dystrophica). Muscular dystrophy also involves skeletal muscle and occurs predominantly in younger male subjects who have a family history of the disorder. The cause is unknown, but genetic factors are important. Barium swallow may show poor movement of the material in the upper third of the esophagus, and manometry may show that contractions are of low amplitude or are

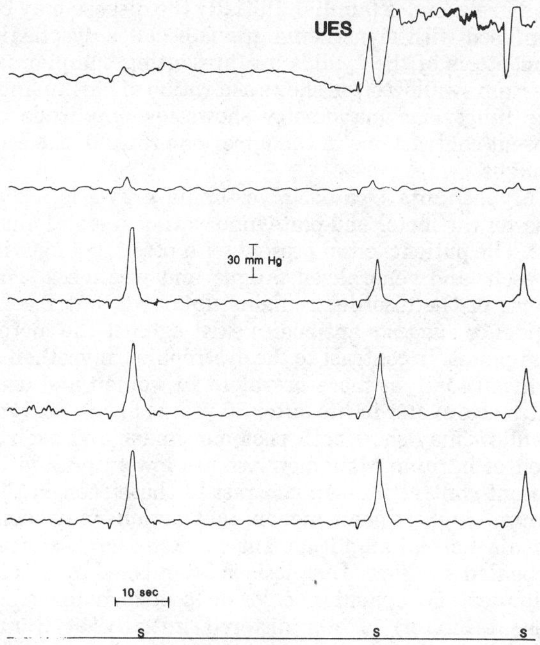

Figure 2. Esophageal manometry illustrating skeletal muscle disease (polymyositis). The upper part of the esophagus has low-amplitude contraction in contrast to contraction of normal amplitude in the lower esophagus. The upper esophageal sphincter (UES) appears normal. Swallowing is represented by the symbol (S). A time and pressure constant is also shown.

Table 1. Motor Disorders of the Esophagus

Lesions in the Upper One Third	**Neurologic Disorders**
Skeletal muscle disease	Achalasia
Polymyositis or dermatomyositis	Diffuse esophageal spasm
Muscular dystrophy	Chagas' disease
Oculopharyngeal dystrophy	**Endocrine Disorders**
Myasthenia gravis	Diabetes mellitus
Neurologic disease	Hypothyroidism
Amyotrophic lateral sclerosis	**Other Disorders**
Multiple sclerosis	Amyloid
Poliomyelitis	Alcoholism
Huntington's chorea	
Diphtheria	
Tetanus	
Lesions in the Lower Two Thirds	
Smooth muscle lesions	
Scleroderma	
Mixed connective tissue disease*	
Lupus erythematosus	
Rheumatoid arthritis	
Scleroderma	

* Involves entire esophagus.

absent. Endoscopy shows normal anatomy. Increased muscle enzyme values (CK or aldolase) and the presence of creatinuria also support the diagnosis. Muscle biopsy findings of single-muscle fiber atrophy with hypertrophy of other fibers are characteristic of muscular dystrophy. (Muscular dystrophy is discussed in a separate article.)

Oculopharyngeal Dystrophy. Oculopharyngeal dystrophy, the cause of which is unknown, is exceedingly rare and is familial. Initially the disease may be confused with myasthenia gravis because dysphagia and ptosis of the eyelids are presenting complaints. Barium swallow often shows aspiration of barium into the lungs, and manometry shows low-amplitude to absent contractions in the upper one third of the esophagus.

Myasthenia Gravis. Myasthenia gravis is a disease of the motor end-plate innervating skeletal muscle. The patients often present with ptosis, changes in speech, and generalized fatigue and weakness. The cause of the disorder remains unknown, but recent evidence suggests antibodies exist against the motor end-plates. In contrast to the dystrophies, myasthenia gravis usually is more prevalent in women and usually occurs later in life (after 30 years of age). Barium swallow may show both poor movement and aspiration of barium. Manometry shows low-amplitude to absent contractions. In contrast to those seen in the Eaton-Lambert phenomenon, contractions may begin with a normal amplitude but quickly decrease after repeated swallows. Diagnosis is established by a Tensilon test: Edrophonium chloride (pseudocholine esterase inhibitor) is administered initially at 2 mg intravenously; if no improvement is observed, an additional 8 mg is given, also intravenously. A positive response is a marked improvement in the patient's muscular strength. The association of thymomas (8 to 10 per cent) with a myasthenia syndrome should be considered. (See the article on Myasthenia Gravis.)

Scleroderma (Progressive Systemic Sclerosis). Scleroderma, a disease involving smooth muscle, begins with small vessel vasculitis and progresses to atrophy of smooth muscle and replacement by fibrosis. The cause remains unknown. Patients may complain of symptoms characteristic of Raynaud's phenomenon and joint symptoms. Skin changes, consisting of tautness of the fingers, hands, and face with ulcerations of the tips of the fingers, may be present. Dysphagia is common in this disorder, and many patients complain principally of heartburn (gastroesophageal reflux disease). Barium swallow examination shows poor to absent contractions in the lower two thirds of the esophagus, and reflux of barium is quite common at the time of fluoroscopy. Manometry discloses aperistaltic contractions of low amplitude in the lower two thirds, but the entire esophagus may be involved. These findings may often be confused with those in achalasia; in scleroderma, however, pressure in the lower esophageal sphincter is usually abnormally lower (< 15 mm Hg) (Fig. 3). In achalasia the lower esophageal sphincter pressure by definition is high (> 35 mm Hg) with incomplete relaxation of the sphincter. In patients with scleroderma, endoscopy may reveal active esophagitis due to reflux disease caused by the low esophageal sphincter pressure and the lack of ability to clear acid because of aperistalsis.

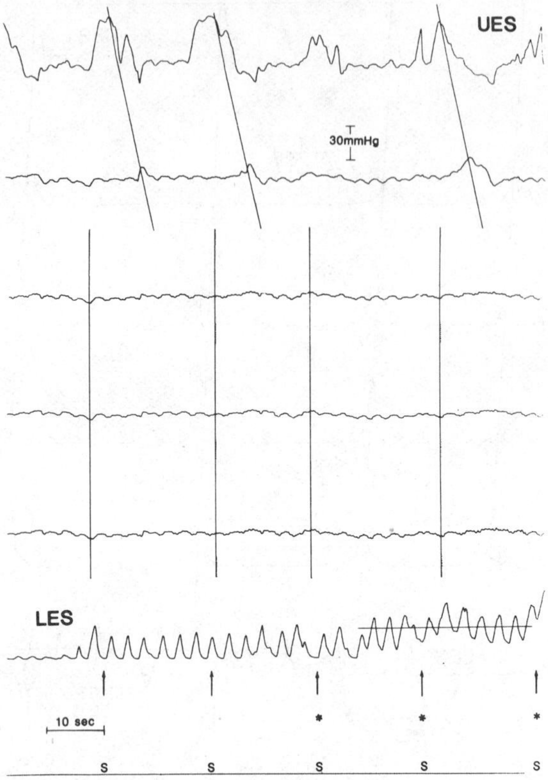

Figure 3. Esophageal manometry illustrating smooth muscle disease of the esophagus (scleroderma). The lower two thirds of the esophagus illustrates aperistalsis (represented by the vertical lines); the upper one third is normal, including the upper esophageal sphincter (UES). The lower esophageal sphincter (LES) is abnormally low, and incomplete relaxation of the sphincter is represented by an asterisk. Swallowing is represented by the symbol (S). A time and pressure constant is also shown.

An antinuclear antibody (ANA) test is often positive in this disorder. In our experience the changes in manometry may precede the development of a positive ANA test by several years.

Aggressive therapy is warranted with the reflux problem in scleroderma because of the altered motility in the body. Chronic untreated esophageal reflux may lead to stricture formation, which would require frequent bougienage. Antireflux surgery should be avoided in this disorder because of the presence of aperistalsis; reflux disease could be converted to iatrogenic achalasia.

Other collagen-vascular disorders, such as systemic lupus erythematosus (SLE), rheumatoid arthritis, or polymyositis, may involve the esophagus. The entire esophagus is usually involved in mixed connective tissue disease, and other vascular markers such as a positive rheumatoid factor, LE cells, or anti-smooth muscle antibodies may be present.

Neurologic Disorders

Table 1 lists the neurologic diseases that affect the esophagus. Two important neurologic diseases that involve the upper one third of the esophagus should be considered.

Multiple sclerosis, a common lesion involving middle-aged adults, may involve the esophagus and result in dysphagia if the lesions affect the innervation to the hypopharynx (ninth nerve) and upper esophagus. *Amyotrophic lateral sclerosis* may involve the esophagus because it is a disease of both the upper and lower neurons. The key to diagnosis is the finding of fasciculations in the extremities. (These two disorders are discussed in separate articles.)

Achalasia

Achalasia involves the lower two thirds of the esophagus and the lower esophageal sphincter. The term literally means "without relaxation." The disease is of unknown etiology and is defined by three specific criteria:

1. Incomplete relaxation of the lower esophageal sphincter.
2. A sphincter pressure that is usually abnormally high (> 35 mm Hg).
3. Aperistalsis of low amplitude (< 35 mm Hg).

Clinically the patient complains of difficulty in swallowing liquids and solids. Often the presence of substernal burning chest pain confuses the entity with reflux disease. Because of the hypertensive lower esophageal sphincter, retention of food and liquid commonly leads to chronic inflammation. Later in the disease process, the esophagus becomes dilated and regurgitation with aspiration may occur. Regurgitation with episodes of coughing and shortness of breath occurs more commonly at night when the subject is lying down. Symptoms of aspiration indicate an emergent condition that warrants immediate therapy. Other symptoms such as associated chest pain suggest the presence of a spasm component (tertiary contractions).

A hypertensive sphincter that fails to relax and tertiary contractions represent a variant of achalasia called *vigorous achalasia.* Weight loss is also common in this disorder. Especially in patients older than 50 years of age, primary achalasia must be distinguished from secondary achalasia. Secondary achalasia is caused by a tumor infiltrating the myenteric plexus and causing manometric changes indistinguishable from those seen in primary achalasia. Similar findings are present in Chagas' disease. Usually these tumors are from spreading adenocarcinomas of the stomach, but they may be from lung, pancreas, lymphoma, or breast. Radiographically the esophagus is usually dilated and shows a retained barium column and an absence of peristalsis. The lower part of the esophagus is shaped like the classic "bird beak," indicative of the hypertensive sphincter. Manometry reveals a lower esophageal sphincter pressure that is abnormally high (> 35 mm Hg) and fails to relax to intragastric pressure on swallowing (Fig. 4). Aperistalsis of low amplitude is present, and in advanced cases contractions are altogether absent. Endoscopy findings are usually normal, but mild to moderate inflammation may be present because of chronic retention of swallowed contents. Resistance is usually encountered at the lower esophageal sphincter, but with gentle pressure a "pop" can be felt as the endoscope enters the stomach. During endoscopy, brushing and biopsy specimens of the lower esophagus must be obtained, especially if any areas appear suspicious.

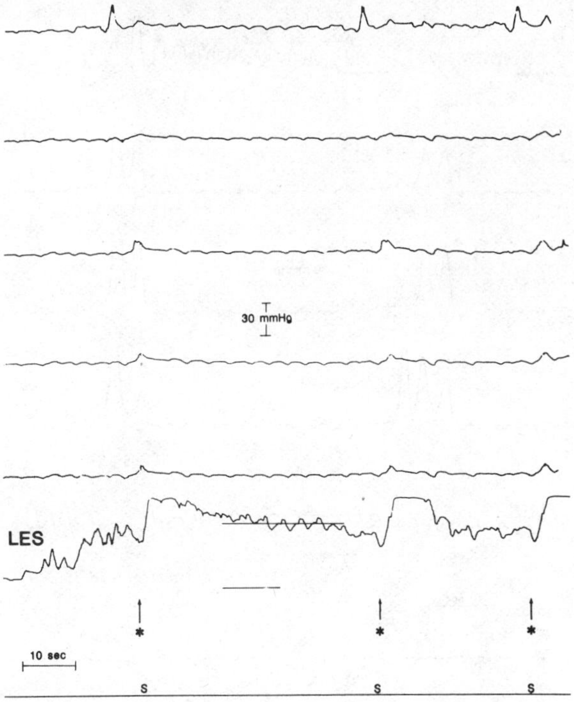

Figure 4. Esophageal manometry illustrating achalasia. The upper third shows normal contractions. Aperistalsis at low amplitude (<35 mm Hg) is shown in the lower esophagus. The lower esophageal sphincter (LES) pressure is abnormally high (>35 mm Hg) and incomplete relaxation at the sphincter is represented by an asterisk. Swallowing is represented by the symbol (S). A time and pressure constant is also shown.

It is important to remember that carcinoma of the esophagus is four to eight times more prevalent in patients with achalasia, which is thought to be secondary to chronic inflammation. Thus achalasia may cause or be caused by carcinoma. Brushings and biopsy will usually not reveal the lesion of secondary achalasia because the lesion is in the myenteric plexus beyond the range of standard biopsy techniques. If carcinoma is suspected as the cause, exploratory thoracotomy may be considered.

Diffuse Esophageal Spasm (Cardiospasm)

Diffuse esophageal spasm consists of a motor disorder of the esophagus in which the patient has chest pain, odynophagia, and dysphagia for liquids and solids. The chest pain may often overshadow the dysphagia; therefore, coronary artery disease is suspected. These subjects often initially undergo cardiac catheterization only to learn that their coronary arteries are normal. Barium swallow usually shows the characteristic "corkscrew" esophagus. Manometry may show several patterns consistent with diffuse esophageal spasm. The classic pattern (Fig. 5) shows spontaneous aperistaltic contractions of abnormally high amplitude (> 75 mm Hg). The lower esophageal sphincter is usually of normal pressure with normal relaxation. If the lower esophageal sphincter pressure is abnormally high with incomplete relaxation and if the body contains tertiary contractions, this pattern is consistent with vigorous achalasia. Other variants

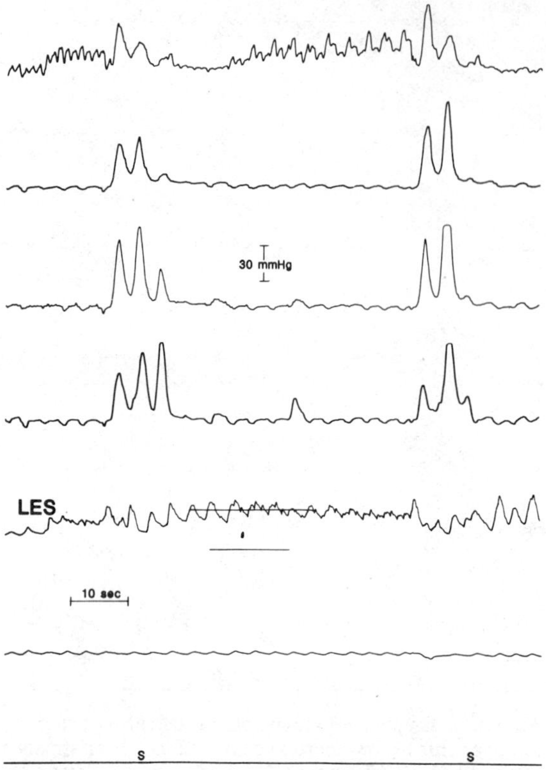

Figure 5. Esophageal manometry illustrating diffuse esophageal spasm characterized by spontaneous and aperistaltic contractions of high amplitude (>75 mm Hg) and a lower esophageal sphincter pressure (LES) of normal amplitude. Swallows are represented by the symbol (S). A time and pressure constant is also shown.

have been described recently, and their importance consists in appropriate recognition. These variants include peristaltic contractions of abnormally long duration (> 25 seconds) or abnormally high amplitude ("nutcracker esophagus") (Fig. 6). Endoscopy findings are usually normal, but tertiary contraction may be seen as one distends the esophagus with air.

Systemic Diseases

Dysphagia for liquids and solids may result from systemic disease states—diabetes mellitus, hypothyroidism, infiltrative disease from amyloid, and alcoholism. These disorders often involve the entire esophagus, and low-amplitude contractions occur with a low esophageal sphincter pressure. Diffuse esophageal spasm may occur as the presenting problem in 5 to 10 per cent of patients with insulin-dependent diabetes.

ESOPHAGEAL OBSTRUCTION

Dysphagia in esophageal obstruction is caused by mechanical narrowing of the lumen, either intrinsically (carcinoma, stricture, web) or extrinsically (mediastinal tumors and vascular anomalies). The initial symptom of dysphagia is difficulty in swallowing solids; with time it progresses to difficulty with both solids and liquids. Unfortunately, dysphagia actually is a late sign of mechanical obstruction, in that the lumen must be reduced by approximately 40 per cent before symptoms occur. A history of dysphagia always indicates the presence of esophageal disease and should always stimulate an extensive diagnostic evaluation.

Esophageal Carcinoma

Two major types of carcinoma involve primarily the esophagus; the most common is *squamous cell carcinoma.* This tumor may involve any part of the esophagus from proximal to distal. In the United States, there appears to be a slightly increased risk to Black men and an association with alcohol ingestion and smoking.

Adenocarcinoma of the esophagus generally either is associated with Barrett's epithelium (to be described), or it arises from the gastric cardia, mimicking a distal esophageal obstruction.

Other predisposing factors leading to esophageal carcinoma include strictures caused by the ingestion of lye, exposure to ionizing radiation, and long-term stasis secondary to untreated achalasia. Clinical associations also exist between esophageal cancer and Plummer-Vinson syndrome and between esophageal

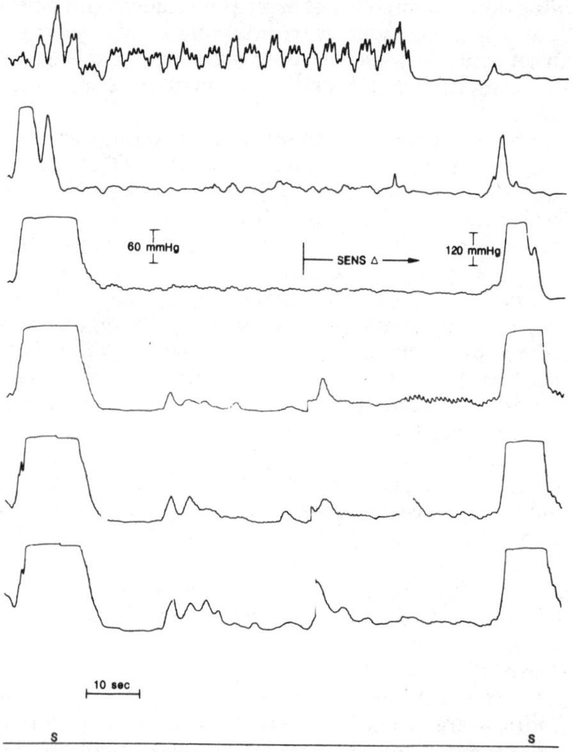

Figure 6. Esophageal manometry illustrating a variant of diffuse esophageal spasm called the "nutcracker" esophagus. Peristaltic contractions of abnormally high amplitude (>75 mm Hg) are illustrated. Swallowing is represented by the symbol (S). A time and pressure constant is also shown.

cancer and tylosis, a rare and genetically transmitted disease characterized by thickened skin of the soles and palms.

Progressive dysphagia and marked weight loss are the most common clinical signs of carcinoma of the esophagus. Substernal pain may also be present and may result from extension of the tumor to the mediastinal space.

Rarely do patients with esophageal cancer have hematemesis, but this can occur in the advanced stages. Massive hematemesis caused by an esophagoaortic fistula has been reported. Other symptoms include hoarseness arising from involvement of the recurrent laryngeal nerve and a tracheal esophageal fistula causing a chronic cough and repeated bouts of aspiration pneumonitis.

The physical examination is usually unremarkable, except for the marked weight loss. In patients with advanced disease, supraclavicular lymphadenopathy or an enlarged liver suggestive of metastatic disease may be palpable.

Because the esophageal lumen must be narrowed by approximately 40 per cent before dysphagia occurs, the disease is at an advanced stage before patients seek medical attention. The barium swallow examination often shows a circumferential lesion of the esophagus with mucosal irregularity. A characteristic ridge or shelf is noted at the superior portion of the tumor. The proximal esophagus is rarely dilated as in achalasia because the lesion progresses so quickly. A suspicious finding on a barium swallow should indicate a need for esophagoscopy, brush cytologic examination, and biopsy of the tumor mass. Brush cytologic findings are more often positive than are those from biopsy specimens. Recently, computed tomography (CT) scanning has been reported to be an excellent method of staging these tumors and assessing their operability.

Strictures, Webs, and Rings

An *esophageal stricture* is a mechanical narrowing that may be benign or malignant. In general, benign strictures are longer than malignant ones and the esophagus is dilated proximal to the stricture. Narrowing of the esophagus may be caused by a reversible process like edema or inflammation or by a process like fibrous tissue narrowing.

An *esophageal web* is a shelf of squamous epithelium that projects into the lumen and generally does not have a lamina propria. If a cricopharyngeal web accompanies iron deficiency anemia, it is referred to as Plummer-Vinson or Patterson-Kelly syndrome.

An *esophageal ring (Schatzki ring),* a projection in the lumen of the distal esophagus, is located at the junction of the esophageal and gastric mucosa. Lined by squamous epithelium on the upper surface and gastric epithelium on the lower surface, this ring consists of smooth muscle and lamina propria.

A range of symptoms may exist with strictures, rings, and webs. Depending on the extent of narrowing, the rings and webs may be found in asymptomatic patients undergoing a barium swallow procedure for other reasons. Symptomatic patients either have chronic intermittent dysphagia for solids or have sudden total esophageal obstruction. The chronic dysphagia may accrue over years, with patients having dysphagia that can be relieved either by regurgitation of the bolus or by "washing" the solid bolus down with liquids. Other patients may have an acute esophageal obstruction with an impacted meat bolus. Total obstruction constitutes a medical emergency. The bolus is usually removed easily during endoscopy, and an evaluation must follow to rule out the process that led to the esophageal obstruction.

A benign stricture of the esophagus usually causes progressive dysphagia from solids to liquids and occurs over months to years. A malignant stricture has an identical progression from solids to liquids, but its development is of a more rapid nature.

Radiographic studies are the primary method of diagnosis. If the lesions are of a minor nature, they may be overlooked by endoscopy, especially with the newer smaller-caliber endoscopes. It is not unusual for an esophageal web to be located by barium swallow, but it is not usually seen by endoscopy because when the instrument is inserted, the web is split. In general, esophageal webs are located in the upper one third on the anterior surface of the esophagus and a cricopharyngeal band is located posteriorly. Lateral and oblique films are necessary to disclose these lesions.

A lower esophageal ring is best seen when the patient performs a Valsalva maneuver to distend the lower esophagus during the barium swallow.

Endoscopy is often both diagnostic and therapeutic and should follow the radiographic procedures to confirm the benign nature of the problem. Cervical strictures may be identified better by rigid esophagoscopy, but this is probably the only indication for this procedure.

Diverticulum

A diverticulum of the esophagus is a sac-like protuberance of one or more layers of the esophageal wall. In contrast to diverticulosis, esophageal diverticula usually involve all three layers and therefore are "real diverticula." In the past, these diverticula have been referred to as "traction" or "pulsion" diverticula, which suggested a possible cause. These terms are no longer used because the etiologies of these lesions are multiple, and "traction" and "pulsion" do not describe the specific process involved.

The most common upper esophageal diverticulum, *Zenker's diverticulum,* occurs immediately above the upper esophageal sphincter. In the past, it has been speculated that Zenker's diverticulum results from motor incoordination at the cricopharyngeal muscle. Recently cine-esophagograms and esophageal manometry have not confirmed this impression. Other forms are mid-esophageal and multiple lower esophageal diverticula and multiple pseudodiverticula.

A single diverticulum may be located above the lower esophageal sphincter; this is referred to as an *epiphrenic diverticulum.*

Small diverticula of the esophagus are generally asymptomatic. The onset and type of symptoms are directly related to the size and location of the diverticulum.

Patients with a Zenker's diverticulum may have a range of symptoms from none at all to transient dysphagia that progresses to regurgitation and pulmonary aspiration. As the sac enlarges, it retains more of the ingested food and may distend to cause an esophageal obstruction. Because of the chronicity of the problem, patients may develop elaborate maneuvers to empty the diverticulum. Other symptoms include a cervical mass or the complaint of halitosis.

Mid- and lower esophageal diverticula tend to be asymptomatic, but on positioning they may cause regurgitation and pulmonary aspiration. It is also important to realize that a patient's symptoms of dysphagia may be caused by the disorder that is causing the diverticulum and not necessarily by the diverticulum itself.

A barium swallow with a cine-esophagogram usually locates the diverticulum. Radiographic studies should always precede endoscopy in patients suspected of having esophageal diverticula to prevent inadvertent perforation of the esophagus. Cine-esophagogram can be coupled with lateral and oblique views of the esophagus to improve the odds of finding this lesion.

Esophageal manometry may be helpful in uncovering a motor disorder that is the cause of the diverticula and in directing the most effective treatment.

Intrinsic Lesions

The most common causes of esophageal obstruction have been discussed, but other less common causes include benign esophageal tumors, cysts, and metastatic lesions. Some of the benign esophageal tumors include lipomas, fibrolipomas, polyps, adenomas, myxofibromas, hemangiomas, lymphangiomas, and papillomas. The most common tumors that metastasize to the esophagus include carcinoma of the breast, melanoma, oat cell carcinoma, and Hodgkin's disease. Occasionally infiltration of the esophagus with leukemia and lymphoma is seen.

The extent and duration of the patient's symptoms are directly related to the size and location of the lesion and to the rapidity with which the obstruction develops. A malignant process, be it primary or metastatic, causes rapid onset of dysphagia that progresses from an inability to swallow solids to an inability to swallow liquids. With a benign tumor there may be a history of progressive dysphagia that spans many months to years. Hoarseness may suggest invasion of the recurrent laryngeal nerve, and a history of hiccups may denote invasion of the diaphragm. The pulmonary complications of repeated regurgitation and aspiration have been discussed previously.

A thorough history and physical exam may suggest the primary site of a tumor that has metastasized to the esophagus. However, small lesions seen in breast carcinoma, melanoma, and oat cell carcinoma may not be obvious and a search for these lesions must necessarily follow.

The diagnosis of intrinsic lesions of the esophagus relies heavily on the history and radiographic studies. Barium swallow frequently identifies the cause of the symptoms, but esophagoscopy is imperative for tissue diagnosis. Biopsies taken at the time of endoscopy frequently clarify the diagnosis. However, submucosal lesions go undiagnosed by this method. The age, medical condition of the patient, severity, and duration of symptoms will direct the evaluation, be it surgical or medical.

Extrinsic Lesions

External compression or displacement of the esophagus may produce esophageal obstruction. Some causes of extrinsic lesions compressing the esophagus include massive left atrial enlargement, mediastinal tumors, cervical osteophytes, arteria lusoria (aberrant right subclavian artery), aortic aneurysms, and other vascular anomalies. Other processes include thyromegaly, cervical lymphadenopathy from benign or malignant causes, and mediastinal fibrosis. As mentioned previously, the symptoms range in severity but dysphagia progressing from an inability to swallow solids to an inability to swallow liquids is common. Partial esophageal obstruction may sometimes be identified only by a careful history while the patient is being evaluated for a primary disorder, such as congestive heart failure secondary to mitral stenosis, thyroiditis, or aortic aneurysm.

In the search for those disorders secondarily affecting the esophagus, other diagnostic tests may be useful, e.g., radiographic studies outlining surrounding esophageal structures. For example, a lateral film of the cervical region will identify prominent cervical osteophytes. CT scanning has been invaluable in disclosing mediastinal, pulmonary, and vascular compression of the esophagus. Angiography may further corroborate the findings of the CT scan.

At esophagoscopy, extrinsic compression of the esophagus is suggested by luminal narrowing with normal overlying mucosa. It is difficult at times to differentiate transmitted pulsation from a true vascular pulsation. In patients with cervical osteophytes, esophagoscopy is a relative contraindication because of trapping of the esophageal wall over the bony prominence, which increases the incidence of perforation.

ESOPHAGITIS

Esophagitis is simply defined as inflammation of the esophagus. Macroscopic changes of the esophageal mucosa at the time of endoscopy include a range of findings from mild erythema to exudate, to erosion, and to frank ulceration. The histologic criteria used by the pathologist to identify esophagitis include a thickened basal layer, constituting more than 15 per cent of the entire epithelial thickness, and elongation of the dermal pegs that reach toward the luminal surface. Biopsy specimens may also show the infiltration of polymorphonuclear leukocytes into the lamina propria. The lowest 2 to 3 cm of the esophagus should be avoided when obtaining suction biopsy specimens because of frequent false-positive results.

Esophagitis may have multiple causes, *gastroesophageal reflux disease* being the most common. Gastroesophageal reflux is secondary to chronic reflux of gastric acid or poor clearing of this acid from the esophagus. Table 2 provides a classification of the multiple causes of esophagitis. It is imperative to recognize that this disease may result from the culmination of a combination of these causes.

Endoscopy will show normal mucosa in 60 per cent of patients with symptoms of gastroesophageal reflux. It is also puzzling to see macroscopic changes of esophagitis in asymptomatic subjects. The most common clinical manifestation of esophagitis is heartburn, usually described as an uncomfortable burning sensation located below the sternum and migrating upward into the neck with a waxing and waning intensity. Heartburn is usually produced by any factor that increases intra-abdominal pressure or decreases lower esophageal sphincter pressure. In certain persons these symptoms can be brought on by excessive bending, tight-fitting clothes, or recumbency. Patients often report that the ingestion of coffee, citrus juices, chocolate, or alcohol precipitates heartburn.

Although some symptoms of esophagitis are characteristic, the chest pain that often accompanies reflux may be indistinguishable from that of other disorders, including myocardial infarction, angina pectoris, or pulmonary embolus. It is imperative for the clinician to differentiate cardiac pain from esophageal pain so that one may appropriately direct the clinical evaluation and subsequent treatment.

Table 2. Causes of Esophagitis

Infections
Moniliasis
Herpes
Tuberculosis
Diphtheria
Scarlet fever
Histoplasmosis
Lactobacillus
Continuous involvement (pharyngitis, tonsillitis, laryngitis)
Syphilitic
Chemical and Physical Agents
Caustic ingesta (lye, ammonia)
Radiation
Acid-peptic reflux
Biliary-pancreatic reflux (alkaline)
Nasogastric indwelling tube
Medication (tetracycline, ascorbic acid)
Stagnation and Trauma
Achalasia
Benign strictures
Malignant strictures (carcinoma, lymphoma)
Trauma
Foreign body
Miscellaneous Causes
Regional enteritis (Crohn's disease)
Sarcoidosis
Pemphigoid
Epidermolysis bullosa
Chemotherapy
Neurogenic (Cushing's disease)
Following burns (Curling)

Besides the classical symptom of heartburn, the other symptoms may be chronic dyspepsia, belching, epigastric fullness, or nausea. Symptoms may also include regurgitation of fluid into the mouth, usually at night or upon bending over. Patients may report that they are awakened by coughing and have either a mouthful of fluid or a pillow wet with gastrointestinal contents. Patients with reflux as the cause of preexisting lung disease or as a significant contributing factor may have markedly improved pulmonary function after appropriate therapy for the esophageal reflux. Another less common symptom of esophageal reflux is "water brash," which refers to the sudden filling of the mouth with a clear, slightly salty fluid probably secreted by the salivary glands.

Odynophagia, painful swallowing, is rarely associated with reflux esophagitis; however, it commonly accompanies infectious esophagitis, specifically candidiasis or herpetic or radiation esophagitis. Therefore, significant odynophagia should alert the clinician to a diagnosis other than reflux esophagitis.

Dysphagia for solids seldom accompanies reflux esophagitis unless it is complicated by a benign stricture or other disorders, including esophageal carcinoma, achalasia, presence of a foreign body, diffuse esophageal spasm, and any factor causing intrinsic or extrinsic compression of the esophagus.

Hematemesis or melena rarely occurs with esophagitis, but may complicate severe forms of the disease. Emergency surgery is almost never, if ever, indicated for this complication.

Although some patients with reflux have a hiatal hernia, not all patients with a hiatal hernia have an incompetent lower esophageal spincter and not all patients with reflux have a hiatal hernia. Hiatal hernia has little, if any, relationship to gastroesophageal reflux. (Hiatal hernia is discussed in a separate article.)

Weight loss is an uncommon feature of reflux esophagitis, but it may be associated with severe erosive disease. Iron deficiency anemia may occur secondary to chronic blood loss, but esophagitis must be confirmed as the cause by appropriate radiographic and endoscopic procedures.

Although accurate diagnosis of esophageal disease can usually be made from the history alone, it is important to confirm a suspicion by one or a combination of diagnostic procedures. From a practical point of view, most patients with minor symptoms typical of gastroesophageal reflux disease do not need an extensive diagnostic evaluation. They often respond to alterations in diet, to antacid therapy 1 and 3 hours after meals, and to avoidance of excessive bending and lifting, recumbency after eating, and tight-fitting clothes. If the patient does not respond to conservative medical therapy or if the history is not characteristic of reflux, a diagnostic evaluation should follow.

Diagnostic Procedures

Although a number of diagnostic studies are available to the clinician, it is important to recognize that the individual tests evaluate specific functions of the esophagus.

The barium swallow examination is useful in determining whether there is a mechanical narrowing of the esophagus or a mucosal abnormality. Unfortunately, the barium swallow is not a very sensitive test. A mucosal abnormality must be moderate to severe before it can be identified by barium swallow, and the changes are not specific for reflux esophagitis. Candida, herpes, and other infectious agents may appear identical to reflux esophagitis on barium swallow examination. The barium swallow is reasonably accurate for evaluating esophageal emptying and can be used to identify spontaneous reflux or in conjunction with provocative maneuvers to induce reflux. However, most radiologists have found that only 15 to 20 per cent of patients who have a good clinical history of esophageal reflux will have spontaneous reflux of barium.

Esophagoscopy by the flexible endoscope is the principal method of visualizing the entire mucosal surface of the esophagus and allowing tissue specimens to be obtained. Small endoscopic biopsy specimens are excellent for ruling out diseases that may mimic reflux esophagitis, but in general they are too small to adequately assess the minor alterations associated with minimal to mild gastroesophageal reflux. A suction biopsy specimen best identifies the specific effects that reflux esophagitis has on the epithelium, but this is seldom warranted.

Current histologic criteria for esophagitis include:

1. Hyperplasia of the basal cell layer of the epithelium.
2. Thinning of the epithelial layer and relative elongation of the papillae (rete pegs).
3. Neutrophils infiltrating the lamina propria.
4. Exudate and erosions of the surface epithelium.

Endoscopy also allows an early tentative diagnosis, depending on the endoscopic characteristics observed, thereby allowing therapy to begin before the disease is histologically confirmed. When appropriate precautions are taken, esophagoscopy is usually well tolerated and complications are rare. Endoscopy is contraindicated in uncooperative patients or those who have unstable medical conditions such as unstable angina or severe chronic obstructive pulmonary disease. Other relative contraindications include prominent cervical osteophytes, which may predispose to esophageal perforation, and the presence of Zenker's diverticulum.

The studies used to evaluate whether or not gastroesophageal reflux occurs are: (1) the pH probe, to measure pH of the distal esophagus; (2) the pH probe that has been expanded to monitor 24-hour pH values; and (3) radioisotope studies. These studies are not routinely available and are almost never required for diagnosis of gastroesophageal reflux, but they may be useful in patients who are refractory to therapy and therefore are referred to tertiary care centers.

The acid perfusion (Bernstein) test can identify whether or not chest pain is caused by esophageal reflux, but the test is rarely necessary when a patient gives a classical description of heartburn. Although it is simple to perform, the test is frequently difficult to interpret. A Bernstein test can give negative results in a patient who has reflux, and its only value is its ability to reproduce the symptoms of patients, providing evidence that the patient's complaints are of esophageal origin.

Esophageal manometry is used to evaluate normal peristalsis of the esophagus and thereby may provide evidence of whether normal clearing mechanisms of the esophagus are present or absent. However, nonspecific motor changes have been associated with esophagitis. Manometry also measures the pressure of the lower esophageal sphincter and is usually less than 5 mm Hg in patients with severe esophageal reflux. This test does not provide evidence that esophageal reflux is occurring, but it does provide objective measurement of the lower esophageal sphincter pressure and quality of esophageal contraction. Most patients with gastroesophageal reflux have lower esophageal sphincter pressures of less than 10 mm Hg.

BARRETT'S ESOPHAGUS

Barrett's esophagus is defined as replacement of the normal squamous epithelium with columnar epithelium. This disorder is thought to be either congenital or acquired, secondary to chronic esophageal reflux. The columnar epithelium may extend variable distances up the esophagus, or it may occur in isolated islands of columnar epithelium. Occasionally, Barrett's epithelium can be grossly identified by endoscopy that reveals salmon-colored mucosa extending above the lower esophageal sphincter, in marked contrast to the glistening white mucosa of squamous epithelium. This impression must be confirmed by histologic specimens that reveal characteristic columnar epithelium. It is imperative that the endoscopist be aware of the location of the normal squamocolumnar junction. Some investigators have suggested that this is a congenital lesion because the fetal esophagus is lined with columnar epithelium and therefore may represent an embryonic disruption in the transition to squamous mucosa. However, recent evidence suggests that it is acquired because it appears more commonly in persons with chronic esophageal reflux. The columnar epithelium may revert to normal squamous mucosa after an antireflux surgical procedure.

Barrett's esophagus frequently ulcerates, usually in the mid-esophagus, and often causes mid-esophageal strictures. Therefore, esophageal carcinoma and Barrett's epithelium are among the most common causes of mid-esophageal ulcer and stricture. Finally, some investigators have reported a 10 per cent incidence of adenocarcinoma in Barrett's epithelium. Treatment of this disorder consists of medical and surgical measures to control esophageal reflux and of yearly endoscopy for early recognition of the tumor.

Symptoms are identical to those of esophageal reflux, but they usually are more severe. Esophageal ulceration, stricture, and bleeding are not uncommon.

The definitive diagnosis of Barrett's esophagus requires the presence of histologically proven columnar epithelium within the esophagus. Multiple biopsy specimens should be carefully obtained during endoscopy with good visualization of the location of the lower esophageal sphincter. Suction biopsy can be aided by manometry to identify the location of the lower esophageal sphincter. Histologically, although the biopsies superficially resemble small bowel epithelium, disaccharidase enzymes are absent and there are no histochemical similarities to either small bowel or gastric epithelium. Others have suggested pertechnetate esophageal scintiscans for the diagnosis, since this epithelium will be labeled by the technetium and can be detected by a gamma camera.

GASTRITIS

By Harold H. Scudamore, M.D., Ph.D.
Monroe, Wisconsin

DEFINITION

Gastritis is a term used to describe inflammation or irritation of the gastric mucosa or infiltration of the stomach wall. Gastritis is actually a spectrum of conditions that may be asymptomatic or that may have a wide variety of symptoms. Gastritis may be classified as acute or chronic, either on the basis of onset and duration of symptoms or on the pathologic analysis of the inflammatory reaction.

The inflammation may be localized to a certain area of the stomach, or it may involve the stomach diffusely. Usually only the mucosa and submucosa are involved, but all layers of the gastric wall may be affected. The gastritis may be graded as mild, moderate, or severe on the basis of histologic examination or endoscopic appearance. Gastritis and duodenitis often occur together, and sometimes esophagitis may be present. Gastritis may also occur in association with peptic ulcer disease or gastric carcinoma.

DIAGNOSTIC METHODS

The most common symptom is epigastric pain that is made worse by eating. In general, the symptoms are not specific but may include any of the following: nausea, vomiting, anorexia, loss of weight, dyspepsia, dysphagia, weakness, hematemesis, melena, or diarrhea. In fact, 30 per cent of upper gastrointestinal hemorrhage is due to erosive or hemorrhagic gastritis. A burning tongue, paresthesias, and neurologic changes may be present with atrophic gastritis and pernicious anemia. A patient with bile reflux gastritis may complain of bitter eructations or bilious vomiting.

In taking the history, the physician should obtain information about the types of medications being used; the amount of alcohol consumed; accidental or intentional swallowing of acids or alkalies; previous operations, especially on the stomach, gallbladder, or bowel; recent radiation or gastric freezing therapy; or known past or present gastrointestinal illnesses.

On physical examination, there is often epigastric tenderness, pallor, or weakness. In some cases there will be glossitis or smooth tongue, neurologic findings of paresthesias or other changes, peripheral lymphadenopathy, or melena noted on rectal exam.

Laboratory procedures may show hypochromic or macrocytic anemia or elevated erythrocyte sedimentation rate (ESR). The serum vitamin B_{12} level would be low and the Schilling test of vitamin B_{12} absorption would be abnormal in atrophic gastritis with pernicious anemia. The bone marrow would usually be megaloblastic. Cultures of blood or gastric contents might be helpful in gastritis due to infections. Gastric analysis and secretory studies are important to check for acid content and bile. It is important to use pentagastrin or Histalog to obtain maximal acid output. From this, the parietal cell mass may be calculated and may be of possible value. Determinations of pepsin, antibodies, enzymes, mucus, and bicarbonate may be helpful in some instances, but they are available only in medical centers. Serum gastrin levels may be of some diagnostic value.

Upper gastrointestinal x-ray studies provide limited help in most cases of gastritis, but may show an increase in mucosal folds in hypertrophic gastritis and a relative decrease in mucosal folds in atrophic gastritis. However, such x-ray studies may show associated conditions of hiatal hernia, gastric or duodenal ulcer, and gastric carcinoma as well as evidence of previous gastric surgery. Upper gastrointestinal x-rays may show evidence of granulomatous, infiltrative, infectious, or corrosive gastritis.

The definitive diagnosis of gastritis is established by gastroscopic examination with visually directed biopsy and possibly brushings for cytology. Sometimes surgical exploration and full-thickness biopsy are needed for diagnosis. When gastritis is strongly suspected, consultation with a gastroenterologist or gastrointestinal endoscopist, and possibly with a gastrointestinal surgeon, is desirable. Gastroscopic inspection has been facilitated by development of flexible fiberoptic gastroscopes. The gastroscopic appearance can be correlated with the histologic analysis by the pathologist, the secretory studies, and the radiographic findings to establish a diagnosis as to type of gastritis, severity of the lesion, and whether acute or chronic.

ETIOLOGIC CLASSIFICATION

Gastritis may be caused by endogenous changes or by exogenous agents or events. It is important to understand etiology and pathogenesis in order to plan diagnostic procedures.

Gastritis of Endogenous Origin

This type of gastritis is often associated with duodenitis and perhaps forms a spectrum encompassing gastroduodenitis, peptic ulcer disease, and gastric cancer. The antrum is usually most severely involved, but the fundus may predominate; or the entire stomach may show changes. The gastritis is produced by an interaction between the destructive forces of hydrochloric acid, pepsin, and possibly regurgitated duodenal contents, bile, and pancreatic enzymes, and the protective action of the mucosal barrier, mucus, bicarbonate, and other factors. Gastrointestinal hormones (e.g., gastrin), genetic factors, immunologic reactions, and emotional conditions may all play a part.

In *bile reflux gastritis* there are additional factors of an incompetent gastroduodenal sphincter, reduced propulsive gastric motility, and/or increased retrograde small intestinal motility. Previous pyloroplasty, gastroenterostomy, Billroth I or II gastroduodenal anastomosis, and vagotomy favor development of this form of gastritis. Bile reflux gastritis also may develop with an intact stomach, especially after cholecystectomy or in the presence of functional gastrointestinal disease.

Atrophic gastritis or *gastric atrophy* represents the advanced stages of chronic superficial gastritis. Intrinsic factor becomes low, and many of these patients develop pernicious anemia. All patients with pernicious anemia have gastric atrophy. Serum vitamin B_{12} levels are often low and the Schilling test is abnormal. Many of these patients have antibodies to parietal cells, suggesting the possibility of an immunologic mechanism. Serum gastrin levels may be high. Atrophic gastritis may be a precancerous lesion; therefore, periodic gastroscopy and biopsy are indicated.

Hypertrophic gastritis is often used to describe gastritis with prominent mucosal folds. In the truest sense, the best example is the uncommon condition of giant rugal folds (Menetrier's disease). It is often associated with a protein-losing gastropathy. A full-thickness biopsy and brush cytology are needed to establish the diagnosis and exclude carcinoma or lymphoma.

Infiltrative gastritis would include lymphoma, pseudolymphoma, and various kinds of polyps.

Eosinophilic gastritis is of unknown cause and may involve all three layers of the stomach wall. It is associated with a peripheral eosinophilia. Food allergy may be a factor. Allergic gastroenteropathy is an example of this type of gastritis.

Gastritis of Exogenous Origin

Many exogenous agents either ingested or directed at the stomach act as irritants to the gastric mucosa to produce gastritis. The many irritants include certain foods or eating habits, hot liquids (e.g., tea), medications, ethyl alcohol, chemicals, infections, inflammatory conditions, irradiation, or freezing.

The most common drug that produces gastritis is acetylsalicylic acid (aspirin). Acetaminophen (e.g., Tylenol) is less irritating but may be associated with gastritis. Indomethacin (Indocin) or other nonsteroidal, anti-inflammatory agents may produce gastritis. Iron or antibiotics may be associated with gastritis. Alcohol is probably the most common cause of both acute and chronic superficial gastritis.

Some chemicals, especially strong acids or alkalies, will produce acute corrosive gastritis. The alkalies also produce a severe esophagitis. Gastritis caused by acid ingestion may go into a chronic stage. Radiation of the stomach to reduce gastric secretion or gastric freezing may produce a gastritis.

PATHOLOGIC TYPES OF GASTRITIS

Acute gastritis is characterized by a polymorphonuclear infiltration of the tunica propria. Necrosis of surface cells and damaged blood vessels may lead to superficial and deep erosions and hemorrhage. The terms "acute gastritis," "acute erosive" or "acute hemorrhagic gastritis," and "acute stress erosions" refer to varying manifestations of the mucosal reaction.

Corrosive gastritis is a severe gastritis with tissue necrosis that may lead to perforation in the acute stage or to scarring and obstruction if it goes into a chronic stage.

Gastritis caused by physical agents such as in irradiation or freezing will produce a superficial gastritis that is self-limited.

Chronic superficial gastritis is characterized by excessive lymphocyte and plasma cell infiltration of the lamina propria. The gastric glands remain normal. *Bile reflux gastritis* is usually this type but will occasionally show erosions or hemorrhage.

Chronic atrophic gastritis and gastric atrophy are diffuse lesions that involve the body and the fundus. There is a loss of gastric glands, a thinning of the mucosa, and a round cell infiltration.

Hypertrophic gastritis shows hypertrophic surface epithelium with normal gastric glands. The extreme form has giant rugae and is known as Menetrier's disease. Other rare types have been described.

Eosinophilic gastritis is characterized by a diffuse infiltration of eosinophils on biopsy.

Granulomatous gastritis includes a variety of lesions involving the gastric wall such as regional enteritis (Crohn's disease), sarcoidosis, and eosinophilic granuloma or infectious granulomas such as those seen in tuberculosis or syphilis.

Infiltrative gastritis due to lymphoma, pseudolymphoma, or various types of polyps may be identified.

In *gastritis due to infections,* viral gastroenteritis is the most common affliction. There is usually both indigestion and diarrhea. Many infectious diseases may be accompanied by an acute gastritis. Phlegmonous gastritis is a rare, serious disease caused by bacterial invasion of the gastric wall, causing a purulent inflammation. If a gas-forming organism (e.g., *Clostridium welchii*) is present, an emphysematous gastritis develops.

CONCLUDING REMARKS

Perhaps the most frequent forms of gastritis are those related to various digestive disorders, usage of medications, and alcohol abuse. Bile reflux gastritis and atrophic gastritis are both fairly common. When symptoms suggest a probable gastritis, a careful history—looking for possible causes—and physical examination are needed. Selected laboratory tests, gastric analysis, and radiologic studies are indicated to help evaluate the condition. The definitive diagnosis of gastritis is established by gastroscopic examination with selective biopsy.

PEPTIC ULCER

By Frank J. Baumeister, Jr., M.D.
Portland, Oregon

Peptic ulcer disease traditionally has been considered to be a single, chronic disease process, the consequence of an imbalance between acid-peptic aggression and intrinsic defense mechanisms of the gastrointestinal mucosa. However, genetic studies, appreciation of the association of peptic ulcer with many different diseases, and observations that a variety of pathogenetic mechanisms may lead to ulceration all suggest that this is a heterogeneous disorder, the end result of which is disruption of vulnerable mucosa adjacent to and exposed to acid and pepsin. Ulceration might then be expected to occur in the distal esophagus, in the stomach, in the proximal duodenum, at or near a surgically constructed gastroenterostomy, or in the ileum adjacent to a Meckel's diverticulum, where the ectopic gastric mucosa lies.

Ulcers may be acute lesions or may represent a chronic process. Acute ulcerations are more often gastric, usually superficial, and frequently multiple. Such lesions may occur under the duress of various kinds of stress or following ingestion of agents known to reduce mucosal resistance to acid-peptic damage. Healing of such lesions will occur once the offending agent is removed or the predisposing condition is corrected. Chronic peptic disease is, however, a lifetime diathesis characterized by recurrences of ulceration, with attendant discomfort and the potential for serious complications of hemorrhage, perforation, and obstruction.

SYMPTOMS AND SIGNS

Pain

An ulcer may exist without any symptoms, and a serious complication may occur as the first indication of its presence. However, abdominal pain is the usual presenting symptom that leads the physician to suspect that an ulcer is lurking. The mechanism producing ulcer pain is incompletely understood, but the classic theory incriminates acid irritation of nerve endings in the ulcer base with resultant local mural muscle spasm. This seems too simplistic, especially in light of recent endoscopic demonstration that typical ulcer distress can persist after an ulcer crater has healed and that pain may disappear even though the crater remains. Ulcer pain, however, can be characteristic and highly suggestive of the diagnosis. It is a visceral pain of foregut origin, and, as such, is located in the midline of the upper abdomen or epigastrium. Variously described as dull, gnawing, burning, or aching, its character is probably less valuable diagnostically than other features. Back radiation to the interscapular region is common. Although this radiation pattern may suggest posterior penetration, duodenal intubation studies with balloon distention have shown that back pain may be produced in most subjects with sufficient distention or in those subjects with low threshold for pain.

Rhythmicity of pain is typical, referring to its occurrence during the day whenever the stomach is empty, and during the night awaking the patient from sleep, with relief promptly following ingestion of food or antacid. It is almost never present in the morning when the patient first arises. The pain will subside or disappear after vomiting, and some patients, in fact, learn to induce emesis for relief of distress.

Periodicity is the term which best describes the characteristic pattern of pain occurring rhythmically and regularly for days or weeks on end, only to disappear spontaneously and to be followed by an asymptomatic period of perhaps several months or longer, after which pain resumes. Thus, *rhythmicity, periodicity,* and *chronicity* are the hallmarks of classic peptic ulcer misery. Unfortunately, this classic presentation is often lacking, and the anamnesis is then less reliable. Experienced clinicians address almost any upper abdominal pain as at least suspicious of peptic ulcer disease and warranting further investigation. The distinction between gastric and duodenal ulcer almost certainly cannot be reliably made on historical grounds alone.

Other Symptoms

Symptoms other than pain occur with ulcer, but are nonspecific and of less diagnostic import. Heartburn and sour regurgitation suggesting esophagitis may in fact occur with peptic ulcer alone. Nausea is uncommon with uncomplicated peptic ulcer, but in a rare instance may be the presenting complaint.

Emesis, too, is not usual, but it may occur, and the genesis of the vomiting is worthy of discussion. That associated with gastric outlet obstruction may occur without significant preceding nausea, infrequently at intervals of 24 to 48 hours, with the emesis containing food ingested many hours prior to vomiting. So-called cyclic vomiting has been considered to be at least suggestive of pyloric channel ulcer, occurring typically approximately 1 hour following a meal, associated with, and subsequently relieving, the attendant epigastric distress. Irritative vomiting occurring immediately after any food or liquid ingestion suggests acute inflammatory antral lesions. These patterns are, however, only suggestive, and cannot be considered diagnostic.

PHYSICAL EXAMINATION

The physical examination is usually unremarkable and offers little in the way of narrowing the search for an ulcer. Epigastric tenderness may or may not be elicited and correlates poorly if at all with the presence or absence of an ulcer crater. Fecal occult blood or melena would certainly lend credence to a suggestive history, but of course could emanate from other sites along the gut.

LABORATORY DETERMINATIONS

Laboratory studies cannot diagnose peptic ulcer disease. Anemia may result from bleeding, but acute hemorrhage is the rule, with iron deficiency from chronic occult blood loss much less common. Polycythemia could indicate polycythemia rubra vera in which the incidence of peptic ulcer is increased. Hypercalcemia may indicate hyperparathyroidism and, therefore, multiple endocrine adenomata with gastrinoma (Zollinger-Ellison syndrome). The serum gastrin level is valuable in this specific instance or once peptic ulcer has been confirmed, but it plays no role in the initial diagnosis of the ulcer itself. Gastric analysis employing pentagastrin or histamine stimulation of gastric secretion need be utilized only rarely. Formerly useful in identifying hypersecretory states or in assessing postoperative anastomotic ulceration, it has been superseded by the now universally available serum gastrin determination.

RADIOGRAPHY

Despite limitations, the conventional barium meal examination remains the most common initial investigation in suspected peptic ulcer disease. Air contrast studies employing ingested carbon dioxide–producing compounds combined with barium are routine in some centers and are thought to yield greater accuracy. Nevertheless, superficial mucosal lesions are often overlooked, and even ulcerations of considerable size can be missed entirely. Proximal gastric ulcers are notorious for escaping detection, sometimes despite a painstaking search with clinical suspicion. The duodenum lends itself better to radiographic scrutiny, and diagnostic accuracy is best in the bulb; however, large craters can hide, and in the presence of deformity the demonstration of a crater is quite difficult. Radiographic demonstration of a duodenal ulcer crater may be diagnostic, but an equivocal or negative study cannot be considered to exclude the diagnosis when suspicion exists. Gastric ulcer or deformity should be further investigated by endoscopy because of the malignant potential of gastric lesions.

ENDOSCOPY

Fiberoptic endoscopy is clearly the most accurate technique for the diagnosis of peptic ulcer. The newer small-caliber instruments are easily inserted and manipulated with minimal discomfort, negligible risk, and remarkable diagnostic yield. Cost is offered as an objection to routine early use of the procedure, but many patients still require endoscopy for precise diagnosis after having undergone a barium meal examination, and one might conversely argue that the availability of a skilled endoscopist obviates the need for radiographic study. Direct endoscopic visualization reveals small, superficial mucosal lesions otherwise undetected. Visually guided forceps biopsy and brushings for cytology allow reliable differentiation of benign from malignant lesions. The bleeding point can be precisely pinpointed in upper gastrointestinal hemorrhage. The postoperative stomach or gastric remnant and gastroenterostomy can be thoroughly examined with accurate differentiation of surgical deformity from inflammation, ulceration, or neoplasm. Only an occasional lesion will be missed by a competent examiner.

COMPLICATIONS

The major complications of peptic ulcer are perforation, hemorrhage, and obstruction. An ulcer may perforate freely into the peritoneal cavity anteriorly or into the lesser peritoneal sac posteriorly or into an adjacent structure, usually the pancreas or the liver. Free perforation presents as a sudden abdominal catastrophe, with excruciating abdominal pain and a rigid, silent abdomen. The patient lies motionless with tachycardia and often hypotension. Free intraperitoneal air, best demonstrated by an upright chest film but also by lateral decubitus or upright abdominal films, can be seen in 75 per cent of cases. A radiographic study utilizing absorbable water-soluble contrast may demonstrate leakage. Endoscopy can be employed if the diagnosis cannot be established by other means. Confined perforation or penetration should be suspected whenever a proven benign ulcer fails to respond symptomatically to appropriate therapy or fails to heal as expected.

Hemorrhage sufficient to produce melena and/or hematemesis occurs in at least 10 per cent of patients with peptic ulcer. Exact identification of the bleeding site and cognition of whether or not there is continued active hemorrhage are critical to charting the best course of management and therapy. This information, of course, is best derived from emergency endoscopy. When vigorous bleeding precludes adequate visualization, gastric lavage via a 34–36 French caliber orogastric tube should be performed, after which endoscopy can usually be successfully accomplished.

Ulcers in the distal stomach or duodenum sometimes obstruct the gastric outlet, usually by acute ulceration with marked edema, and rarely by cicatrix. Typically, emesis is the presenting complaint, but unsuspected obstruction may sometimes be revealed by a barium meal examination or even plain films when a large fluid- and food-filled stomach is demonstrated. It is important to exclude anticholinergic drugs as causative or contributory under such circumstances. Endoscopy is invaluable in clarifying the exact etiology of the blockage. The saline load test is best applied as a predictive assessment after a 48- to 72-hour period of therapy with nasogastric suction and parenteral cimetidine. If 30 minutes after nasogastric instillation of 750 ml of normal saline over 400 ml remains, obstruction persists and surgery may be necessary.

OVERVIEW

Peptic ulcer disease is a common affliction suffered by at least one person in ten sometime during life. Many ulcers are asymptomatic or are only minimally disabling, but as long as an active ulcer crater exists there is a real potential for disaster. Therefore, the diagnosis should be established with certainty. Simultaneously, other, perhaps even more sinister, processes should be excluded as cause for the patient's complaints. A variety of diseases involving the biliary tract, pancreas, and alimentary canal, including both small and large bowel, may masquerade as peptic disease, and the dyspepsia of functional origin may be especially difficult to differentiate from organic illness. A careful history and physical examination may, on occasion, be essentially diagnostic but in another instance may be inconclusive or confusing. The currently available diagnostic armamentarium has been presented, the thorough employment of which should minimize diagnostic errors.

Recurrences are the rule in chronic peptic ulcer disease. Exacerbations of proven duodenal ulcer need only be treated promptly, with further investigations indicated only when the original diagnosis is questioned, complications are suspected, or surgical intervention is considered. The pall of malignant potential, however, hangs over the diagnosis of chronic gastric ulcer and dictates the diagnostic approach. Even though initial endoscopic biopsies and brushings indicate benignancy, serial surveillance is mandatory until there is endoscopic evidence of total healing.

NEOPLASMS OF THE STOMACH

By Albert Augustus Ramage, M.D.
and Francis J. Tedesco, M.D.
Augusta, Georgia

Gastric neoplasms include a variety of tumors arising either from the mucosa (carcinoma or polyps) or from the wall of the stomach (leiomyomas, leiomyosarcomas, and lymphomas). Representing 90 per cent of all gastric neoplasms, gastric carcinoma is clearly the most important of these lesions. Gastric lymphomas follow in frequency representing up to 5 per cent of tumors, with leiomyosarcomas and the benign gastric tumors making up the final 5 per cent. Advances in the ease, availability, and accuracy of double-contrast radiographic examinations and upper gastrointestinal (GI) endoscopy offer some hope—as yet unrealized—of improving the traditionally poor prognosis of these malignancies.

GASTRIC CARCINOMA

The incidence of gastric cancer has declined markedly in the United States over the past 50 years from 28.8 per 100,000 in 1930 to 7 per 100,000 in 1976, and it has fallen from first to fifth as a cause of cancer death in men over the same period. The reasons for this decline are unclear, but similar declines have been seen in several European countries. There is a 2 : 1 male predominance in gastric carcinoma, and the peak age of onset is 55. Achlorhydria, pernicious anemia, gastric polyps larger than 2 cm, and a history of partial gastrectomy are recognized risk factors. The marked geographic and socioeconomic variability in incidence of gastric carcinoma may be related to variable exposure to nitrosamines, though this remains unproved.

Surgical removal remains the only possibility of cure of gastric carcinoma, and the 5-year survival rate for gastric carcinoma has improved little in the past 50 years, remaining at 7 to 9 per cent overall. The only definite improvements in this dismal rate relate to early diagnosis. Up to 11 percent of benign-appearing gastric ulcers may prove to be malignant. This presentation may give the patient a 5-year survival as high as 43 per cent, presumably related to early diagnosis prompted by ulcer symptoms. Likewise, mass screening for gastric lesions in Japan—where there is a high incidence of gastric cancer—has increased the rate of diagnosis of early gastric cancer (i.e., cancer not penetrating the muscularis propria) from 5 to 30 per cent of diagnoses. This subgroup has an 80 to 95 per cent 5-year survival rate.

Symptoms

Symptoms of gastric carcinoma include anorexia, early satiety, nausea, and vomiting. These symptoms arising in patients over age 40 should raise the suspicion of gastric carcinoma. Weight loss, anemia, and obstructive symptoms occur frequently with advanced lesions. The presence of nausea, vomiting, anorexia, and weight loss as well as the simultaneous presence of three or more complaints has proved to be the best predictor of malignancy. Massive bleeding is rare as a presenting complaint. However, many patients have few or no symptoms until the disease is advanced. The vague and nonspecific nature of these symptoms, their insidious presentation, and the relatively high frequency of gastrointestinal complaints in the general population serve to delay the diagnosis of gastric carcinoma. A new concern has been raised that the indiscriminant use of cimetidine may further delay the diagnosis of gastric carcinoma by relieving early symptoms, and the demonstration of partial healing in 70 per cent of ulcers associated with early gastric cancer lends further support to this concern.

Physical Signs

There are no physical signs of gastric carcinoma in its early stage. With extensive local spread or metastasis, pallor, evidence of weight loss, Virchow's node, epigastric mass, pelvic masses, or hepatomegaly may be found. The liver may be palpable even without metastatic disease.

Laboratory Studies

Iron deficiency anemia should prompt an examination of the GI tract unless there is another clear explanation. Megaloblastic anemia may be seen in pernicious anemia—a risk factor for gastric carcinoma. Though massive hematemesis and melena are rare, occult blood is often present in the stool. Gastric pH is helpful only when achlorhydria is demonstrated in the presence of an ulcerating lesion. The presence of gastric acid in no way rules out carcinoma. Elevated alkaline phosphatase suggests hepatic or bony metastases.

At present there is no serum marker of proven utility in the detection of gastric carcinoma or the delineation of high-risk groups. Carcinoembryonic antigen (CEA), alpha-fetoprotein (AFP), and reduced levels of serum pepsinogen I have all been associated with gastric carcinoma, but low predictive accuracy when applied to the general population limits their usefulness. If CEA or AFP levels are initially elevated, they may be helpful in monitoring for recurrence of tumor.

Radiologic Diagnosis

The radiologic examination of the stomach is still the most widely available procedure that can lead to an early diagnosis of gastric carcinoma. The detection of a large exophytic mass is easy by any technique. The challenge in diagnosis remains in the detection of early resectable lesions in ulcers or plaques. The accuracy of single-contrast upper GI series is approximately 80 per cent in the detection of gastric cancers. Double-contrast technique increases detection to 95 per cent, but up to 37 per cent of early gastric carcinomas are read as benign. Signs of malignancy on upper GI series include abnormal mucosal folds, a flat or wavy ulcer base, ulcerations within a mass, or loss of normal distensibility. An ulcer diameter of greater than 21 mm also increases the risk of carcinoma. The radiologic "test of healing" as a test of malignancy is no longer acceptable, since a percentage of malignant ulcers have now been shown to demonstrate at least partial healing on therapy. The detection of a gastric ulcer radiologically is an indication for endoscopy with biopsy and cytologic brushing.

Computed tomographic (CT) scanning is not useful as a screening device for gastric carcinoma, but it is useful in defining local extension or metastasis of carcinoma preoperatively and may obviate operation for staging in some patients who do not need a palliative procedure and who can be shown to have nonresectable disease.

Endoscopy with Biopsy and Cytology

Virtually all lesions such as plaques, ulcers, or masses should be investigated via endoscopy. Direct visualization of tumor is useful, but all studies show significant errors in diagnosis if visualization alone is used. At least seven biopsies should be taken from all sides of the ulcer and from the ulcer base. Recent studies show that this number of biopsies detects greater than 90 per cent of tumors. The addition of directed brush cytology was proven helpful in earlier studies in which biopsy accuracy was lower, but the utility of cytology is now under question. Its usefulness depends on the interest and accuracy of the cytologist performing the study. The high initial accuracy of endoscopy and biopsy has led to diagnosis of 30 per cent of gastric cancer as early gastric cancer in Japan with reduction in the 5-year mortality of the disease.

Endoscopy is clearly superior to radiologic studies in the detection of stomach lesions postoperatively and should be the first-choice technique if there is strong suspicion of gastric carcinoma.

Screening

Routine screening of the general population of the United States for gastric carcinoma is impractical because of a low prevalence of the disease and the high cost of effective screening. In Japan, where the incidence of gastric carcinoma is much higher than in the United States, there was still only 0.15 per cent yield in a mass screening program. Patients who have a history of partial gastric resections have an increased risk of carcinoma beginning about 10 years postoperatively. Pernicious anemia and achlorhydria are recognized as carrying increased risk of gastric carcinoma, though the extent of the increase and whether these conditions warrant screening for carcinoma is a matter of debate. Currently patients with achlorhydria or pernicious anemia have periodic screening examinations, as do patients with a history of partial gastric resections beginning 10 years postoperatively. Family history of gastric carcinoma, intestinal metaplasia, and atrophic gastritis are lesser risk factors and do not warrant screening at present.

LYMPHOMAS

Lymphomas represent less than 5 per cent of gastric neoplasms. They are usually diffuse, non-Hodgkin's lymphomas and may represent part of a disseminated illness or may be primary to the stomach. The stomach and GI tract are frequent locations of extranodal disease. The most common presenting complaint is abdominal pain, simulating the symptoms of ulcer or carcinoma. Lymphoma may also simulate carcinoma both radiologically and endoscopically and may appear as ulcer, polyp, or diffuse infiltration. Only the finding of giant rugal hypertrophy is suggestive of lymphoma. Despite the submucosal origin of the tumor, biopsies may be diagnostic. If endoscopic biopsy fails, surgical biopsy is necessary to document the diagnosis. The differentiation of lymphoma from carcinoma is critical because unlike gastric carcinoma, lymphomas generally respond well to chemotherapy and/or radiation.

LEIOMYOSARCOMA

Leiomyosarcomas are relatively rare malignancies representing approximately 1 per cent of gastric malignancies. The history is similar to that of other malignancies except that hematemesis and melena are more common. On endoscopy or radiographic examination, this appears as an intramural extramucosal mass that may be ulcerative. Brush cytology and biopsy are not likely to penetrate to the actual tumor tissue and are unlikely to yield a diagnosis. The differentiation from gastric carcinoma is important because this tumor has a 50 per cent cure rate with surgery.

BENIGN TUMORS

Only 5 per cent of gastric neoplasms are benign, and gastric polyps and leiomyomas make up most of these.

Ninety-five per cent of gastric polyps are said to occur in achlorhydric persons. Though polyps may rarely cause obstruction or infarction, whether polyps frequently cause any symptoms is unclear. Seventy-five to 85 per cent of gastric polyps are hyperplastic and do not have malignant potential. Only adenomatous polyps are thought to undergo malignant change. Though some series find associated malignancy with 25 to 35 per cent of polyps, this figure seems high. Polyps larger than 2 cm are more likely to be malignant and should be removed. Frequently, removal can be performed endoscopically.

Leiomyomas occur in 16 per cent of autopsies in patients not suspected of having gastric disease. However, clinically significant leiomyomas are rare. Like leiomyosarcomas, they are extramucosal intramural masses. Though they tend to be smaller than leiomyosarcomas, the two can be differentiated only pathologically. Treatment, if required, consists of local resection.

INTESTINAL OBSTRUCTION

By David M. Nagorney, M.D.
and Robert W. Beart, Jr., M.D.
Rochester, Minnesota

Intestinal obstruction is an interruption of the normal transit of gas, liquid, or solid contents through the gastrointestinal tract. Obstruction may result from a discrete mechanical cause or from nonmechanical causes that interrupt the normal propulsive contractions either segmentally or diffusely along the intestinal tract. Regardless of cause, obstruction may be partial or total. The mechanical type may present as a simple obstruction or as a closed-loop obstruction with or without strangulation. Ileus is a nonmechanical type of obstruction in which intestinal motor activity ceases and most frequently occurs after abdominal surgery or after injury to the abdominal cavity. A special clinical syndrome of ileus is *pseudo-obstruction,* in which the signs and symptoms of intestinal obstruction occur without an apparent cause. The specific causes of intestinal obstruction are presented in Table 1.

SIGNS AND SYMPTOMS

The cardinal symptoms of intestinal obstruction are vomiting, abdominal pain, distention, and obstipation. The sequence of presenting symptoms and their severity will depend on the site, degree, and cause of obstruction.

Vomiting

Vomiting is the initial and predominant symptom of foregut obstruction. Vomiting is frequent, often copious, and occasionally projectile. Gastric obstruction results in vomitus of undigested foodstuffs or clear acrid fluid. Bilious vomiting is typical of duodenal or very proximal jejunal obstruction. With progressively distal sites of obstruction, vomiting is less common and is delayed in onset. In fact, vomiting may be absent in distal large bowel obstruction unless marked abdominal distention is present. Feculent vomiting indicates long-standing obstruction of the distal midgut or hindgut with resultant bacterial proliferation within the obstructed lumen. Reflex vomiting may occur acutely with the onset of obstruction.

Pain

Intermittent cramping abdominal pain is the hallmark of midgut obstruction. Pain results from acute distention of bowel between a proximal contracting segment and the distal point of obstruction. The severity of the pain is proportional to the degree and length of the obstructed bowel. The interval between episodes of crampy pain is greater for distal midgut obstruction than for more proximal obstructions, though the interval between cramping episodes is not specific for the site of obstruction. Pain is often absent in patients with foregut obstruction, and discomfort from pressure rather than pain per se is typical of hindgut obstruction. Generally, pain associated with midgut obstruction is periumbilical, and pain with hindgut obstruction is hypogastric. The character of the pain is especially important. Colicky pain with minimal or no discomfort between cramps classically suggests simple obstruction. Change in the pattern of pain, with persistent pain between cramps, or steady, unrelenting pain strongly suggests ischemia.

Abdominal Distention

Abdominal distention reflects both the site and degree of obstruction. Accumulation of gas, liquid, and stool within the obstructed lumen distends the bowel and subsequently the contour of the abdominal wall. Volvulus and acute gastric dilatation may cause an area of localized distention. In general, total obstruction of the distal midgut or hindgut is associated with marked distention. Foregut obstruction causes minimal abdominal distention.

Table 1. Causes of Intestinal Obstruction

I. Mechanical (Dynamic)
  A. Narrowing of lumen, intrinsic lesions
    1. Congenital
      a. Atresia
      b. Stenosis/webs
      c. Imperforate anus, malformations of anus and rectum
      d. Malrotations
      e. Cysts and duplications
      f. Meckel's diverticulum
      g. Vascular rings
    2. Acquired
      a. Inflammatory
        (i) Enteritis
        (ii) Granulomatous disease, specific and nonspecific
        (iii) Diverticulitis
      b. Traumatic (intramural hematoma)
      c. Ischemic—secondary stricture
      d. Neoplastic
        (i) Benign bowel tumor, small or large bowel (leiomyoma)
        (ii) Malignant tumors (adenocarcinoma, melanoma)
  B. Adhesive bands
    1. Congenital (Ladd's)
    2. Traumatic (postoperative)
  C. Hernia
    1. External (inguinal)
    2. Internal
  D. Extraintestinal masses or structures
    1. Abscess
    2. Tumor
    3. Pregnancy
    4. Annular pancreas
    5. Superior mesenteric artery syndrome
    6. Endometriosis
  E. Stomal or anastomotic obstruction
    1. Edema
    2. Stricture
      a. Skin
      b. Fascial
  F. Volvulus

II. Nonmechanical (Adynamic, Paralytic, Functional)
  A. Primary pseudo-obstruction (Ogilvie's syndrome)
  B. Secondary pseudo-obstruction (ileus)
    1. Abdominal causes
      a. Reflex, local causes
        (i) Postoperative
        (ii) Trauma, retroperitoneal hemorrhage
        (iii) Pancreatitis
      b. Infections
        (i) Peritonitis
        (ii) Diaphragmatic inflammation, pneumonia
      c. Ischemia
    2. Extra-abdominal causes
      a. Generalized
        (i) Uremia
        (ii) Sepsis
      b. Neurogenic
        (i) Spinal cord tumors
        (ii) Poliomyelitis
        (iii) Hirschsprung's disease
        (iv) Chagas' disease
        (v) Parkinson's disease
        (vi) Familial autonomic dysfunction
      c. Myogenic
        (i) Myotonic dystrophy
        (ii) Progressive muscular dystrophy
        (iii) Collagen vascular disease (scleroderma)
        (iv) Amyloidosis
        (v) Nontropical sprue
      d. Metabolic
        (i) Endocrine
          (a) Diabetes mellitus
          (b) Hypothyroidism
          (c) Hypoparathyroidism
        (ii) Electrolyte imbalance
          (a) Hypokalemia
          (b) Hypomagnesemia
          (c) Hypocalcemia
      e. Pharmacologic
        (i) Phenothiazines
        (ii) Tricyclic antidepressants
        (iii) Anti-parkinsonian agents
        (iv) Ganglionic blockers
        (v) Cathartic colon (chronic laxative abuse)

Obstipation

Obstipation refers to a complete arrest of the transit of gas, liquid, or stool per anus. It develops late in the course of obstruction because intestinal contents distal to the obstruction will usually be evacuated after total obstruction occurs. Clearly, obstipation is noted earlier in the course of obstruction and more frequently in patients with hindgut rather than midgut obstruction. Alternating diarrhea and constipation may precede obstipation, particularly in patients with partial obstruction initially. In patients with abdominal stomas, it is important to note that an abrupt increase in ostomy output with or without peristomal pain is indicative of partial obstruction.

PHYSICAL EXAMINATION

A thorough physical examination is essential. General inspection will often suggest the severity and acuteness of the obstruction and the patient's nutritional state. Skin turgor and mucous membrane moisture are good indicators of the state of hydration. Tachycardia, narrow pulse pressure, and hypotension reflect either extreme hypovolemia or sepsis. Temperature elevation, when present, is usually low grade unless strangulation or peritonitis is present. Weight loss, jaundice, and lymphadenopathy strongly implicate malignancy as the cause of obstruction. Examination of the chest and heart may reveal a median sternotomy scar, murmurs, or arrhythmias and may suggest an intra-abdominal vascular event secondary to embolism or low cardiac output. Angiography, which has both diagnostic and therapeutic efficacy in this setting, should be performed promptly if this diagnosis is suspected.

Abdominal inspection discloses the degree of distention and the presence of surgical scars or hernias. Skin discoloration or ulceration over abdominal hernias indicates strangulation of the incarcerated viscera. Occasionally visible "peristalsis" of a distended loop of intestine is observed.

Abdominal palpation may reveal only mild or no tenderness over a distended loop in simple obstruction. Marked localized tenderness with guarding is very suggestive of strangulation. Abdominal rigidity and generalized tenderness are associated with perforation and generalized peritonitis. Masses may be due to neoplasms, intussusception, or a closed-loop or strangulated obstructed segment surrounded by omentum. All potential hernia sites must be carefully examined.

Percussion will generally elicit tympany. Localized tympany and distention are commonly seen with volvulus. Auscultation may reveal borborygmi associated with cramping pain. Bowel sounds remain active between the episodic cramps. Infrequent or absent intestinal rushes indicate advanced simple obstruction, strangulation, or generalized peritonitis.

Physical examination is completed by a careful pelvic and rectal examination. Moreover, abdominal stomas must be examined for periostomal hernias or stricture. Finally, re-examination must be performed frequently to determine the course of the obstruction and its treatment.

LABORATORY STUDIES

The major aim of laboratory evaluation in patients with intestinal obstruction is to determine whether significant biochemical or metabolic disturbances are present. Therefore, laboratory studies should be selected to evaluate the overall condition of the patient and to guide treatment. Abnormal findings will be directly related to the degree, duration and site of obstruction, and rapidity of development.

Laboratory studies that are essential for the appropriate management of patients with intestinal obstruction include complete blood count (CBC), measurements of serum sodium, potassium, chloride, amylase, glucose, and creatinine levels, and urinalysis with urine-specific gravity. Additional studies that may provide useful information include determinations of serum phosphate, lactate, alkaline phosphatase, transaminase, bilirubin, protein, and bicarbonate and blood urea nitrogen levels and arterial blood gases.

Obstruction results in an extracellular fluid volume deficit. Because gastrointestinal contents are nearly isotonic, the concentration of extracellular fluid is not changed initially. However, with progressive fluid loss, the hematocrit and hemoglobin concentration increase. A mild leukocytosis (10,000 to 13,000 white blood cells [WBC] per cu mm) may also develop as a result of fluid loss with advanced simple obstruction. A marked leukocytosis (20,000 WBC or greater per cu mm) generally reflects peritonitis from strangulation. Urine-specific gravity and osmolality increase, and urine output decreases. Uncorrected extracellular fluid loss leads to renal insufficiency with an increase in serum creatinine and blood urea nitrogen. Importantly, hourly urine output is the most accurate indicator of volume status. Urine output of 50 ml per hour or greater reflects adequate extracellular volume. Plasma protein concentration will increase transiently with extracellular fluid deficit, but hypoproteinemia is a more important finding and indicates malnutrition.

Alterations in serum electrolytes generally occur late in the course of obstruction. However, significant electrolyte deficits may exist despite "normal" serum concentrations because initial fluid losses are isotonic. Large losses of gastric fluid result in a hypochloremic, hypokalemic metabolic alkalosis. Obstruction distal to a patent ampulla of Vater causes alkaline losses and leads to a metabolic acidosis. Significant volume depletion with cellular hypoperfusion and ischemia or strangulation increases lactic acid production and may result in a profound metabolic acidosis. Importantly, however, lactic acidosis is *not* specific for strangulation. Arterial blood gases are important to assess respiratory mechanics, which may be compromised by abdominal distention.

Elevation of serum amylase may result from pancreatitis or strangulation obstruction. Serum transaminases and bilirubin may be increased with gallstone ileus. Serum phosphate and serum alkaline phosphatase (especially the intestinal fraction) may be markedly elevated with strangulation.

RADIOLOGIC EVALUATION

Plain x-ray examination of the abdomen is the most important diagnostic adjunct. Plain films of the abdomen in supine and upright positions and a posteroanterior chest x-ray should be obtained. If upright films cannot be obtained because of the patient's condition, left lateral decubitus views will suffice.

The patterns of gas and fluid within the bowel are examined initially and may offer some clues to the site and severity of obstruction. Intestinal gas is present normally in the stomach and colon in healthy patients and also in the small intestine in infants. Abdominal films may be normal in patients with foregut obstruction. Gastric outlet obstruction may result in dilatation of the stomach with a large left upper quadrant air-fluid level. Duodenal obstruction may produce an air-fluid level within the proximal duodenum and the stomach, with the so-called "dubble-bubble sign."

The classic stair-step pattern of distended bowel loops with multiple air-fluid levels is typical of midgut obstruction. The presence of valvulae conniventes within centrally located bowel loops and the absence of colonic gas confirm small bowel obstruction. Gas in the biliary tree with these findings in patients without past biliary tract surgery strongly suggests gallstone ileus.

Colonic dilatation confirms hindgut obstruction. Typically, the distended proximal colon is filled with gas and stool. Air-fluid levels are less common in the colon than in the small bowel. Multiple air-fluid levels and colonic distention suggest ileocecal valve incompetence. Hindgut obstruction and a competent ileocecal valve lead to colonic distention only and result in a closed-loop obstruction. Volvulus of the cecum and sigmoid can be recognized by a markedly distended segment of colon. Retrograde contrast studies may reveal a twisting or "bird's beak" deformity at the point of torsion.

Contrast x-ray studies may be useful in defining the site and cause of obstruction in selected patients; however, such studies are not required routinely. Barium is the best agent for examination of the stomach and small bowel because it defines mucosal detail very well and does not become inspissated in the small bowel. Barium and water-soluble contrast are equally effective in confirming the site and cause of large bowel obstruction. A water-soluble medium is preferred, however, when pseudo-obstruction is suspected.

COURSE

The clinical course of patients with intestinal obstruction is extremely variable. Patients with partial obstruction may have recurrent attacks differing in frequency, duration, and intensity. Conversely, patients with a strangulated or closed-loop obstruction often present with fulminant clinical deterioration. Between these extremes are the majority of patients with obstruction who present with a steady progression of signs and symptoms. With obstruction the bowel dilates. Secretions, gas, and debris accumulate within the bowel lumen. The abdomen distends, nausea and vomiting ensue, and bowel movements cease. With strangulation, peritonitis results and generalized sepsis may occur. Continued fluid and electrolyte losses lead to hypovolemia, renal insufficiency, and death unless treatment is initiated.

COMMON COMPLICATIONS

The major complications of intestinal obstruction are fluid and electrolyte loss, acid-base imbalance, and infection. The severity of these complications increases directly with the degree and duration of obstruction.

Fluid loss results from intraluminal sequestration, intramural edema, peritoneal transudation, vomiting, and gastrointestinal suction. Hemoconcentration, hypovolemia, and hypotension result. Oliguria and renal insufficiency follow without rehydration.

Electrolyte loss can be significant. Hypokalemia is the primary abnormality. Obstruction proximal to the ampulla of Vater results in hypokalemic, hypochloremic alkalosis. Metabolic acidosis occurs with loss of upper small bowel fluid which contains both biliary and pancreatic secretions. Acidosis is complicated by increased lactate production from decreased peripheral perfusion or ischemic bowel.

Peritonitis and generalized sepsis are the most feared complications of obstruction. As intestinal fluid accumulates, intraluminal pressure increases, bacteria proliferate, and mucosal ischemia occurs. The intestinal mucosal barrier subsequently becomes incompetent, and bacteremia, endotoxemia, perforation, and peritonitis may follow. Strangulation of an obstructed segment may itself precipitate sepsis or develop as a complication of simple or closed-loop obstruction.

PITFALLS IN DIAGNOSIS

The major diagnostic pitfall of intestinal obstruction is differentiating simple obstruction from strangulating obstruction. Strangulation *cannot* be reliably diagnosed preoperatively. Any suspicion of strangulation in a patient with intestinal obstruction dictates immediate abdominal exploration.

SMALL BOWEL TUMORS

By James A. Madura, M.D.
and Dennis W. Vane, M.D.
Indianapolis, Indiana

In contrast to neoplasms of the stomach and colon, small bowel tumors are relatively uncommon lesions, representing less than 6 per cent of benign and 2 per cent of malignant tumors of the gastrointestinal (GI) tract. These tumors display an amazing variety of histopathologic types, representing the entire gamut of morphologic and embryologic origins. Preoperative and antemortem diagnosis is difficult and rare, given the plethora of vague symptoms often mimicking common GI disorders. Nonetheless, as a group, small bowel tumors are a very interesting collection of lesions, and a high index of suspicion and diligence in investigation are necessary for more accurate preoperative diagnoses and earlier treatment of these perplexing lesions.

PRESENTING SIGNS AND SYMPTOMS

Since the majority of small bowel tumors grow intraluminally or cause extrinsic compression of the lumen, they usually manifest themselves by either intestinal obstruction or hemorrhage. The obstructing lesions can be either partial or total, or they may be the lead point in an intussusception, which in an adult is almost pathognomonic for small bowel tumors. The symptoms most commonly described are pain (usually epigastric or periumbilical), nausea, and vomiting. The intussuscepting lesions usually present with intermittent colicky pain and may be confused with more common problems such as renal or biliary tract disease. In a patient without previous abdominal surgery and with no evidence of hernias, signs and symptoms of small bowel obstruction in the sixth decade of life should cause one to strongly consider the diagnosis of small bowel tumor.

Bleeding lesions may produce any clinical picture from chronic iron deficiency anemia and its attendant symptoms to exsanguinating hemorrhage. In a patient with unexplained iron deficiency anemia who has had negative esophageal, gastric, and colonic examinations, the diagnosis of small bowel neoplasia must be considered.

Lesions in the duodenum, particularly adenocarcinomas, can be readily confused with benign peptic ulcer disease, since they usually present with epigastric pain, nausea, vomiting, and occasionally hematemesis. Onset of painless jaundice is another presenting symptom of tumors in the area of the ampulla of Vater. Lesions lower in the jejunum and ileum tend to be indistinguishable from the more common causes of intestinal obstruction.

In addition, there are a few hereditary diseases which predispose patients to small bowel neoplasia. These diseases include the Peutz-Jeghers syndrome, the association of melanin spots on the oral mucosa, lips, and fingers with multiple hamartomas of the intestinal tract; Gardner's syndrome, the association of soft-tissue tumors, bony exostoses, and intestinal adenomatous polyps; von Recklinghausen's disease, with intestinal neurofibromatosis; and Rendu-Osler-Weber syndrome, in which hemorrhagic telangiectasia involves small bowel mucosa as well as the mucous membranes of eyes, nose and mouth.

Recently, statistical data have confirmed a suspected association of Crohn's disease and subsequent ileal adenocarcinoma as 60 to 320 times more prevalent than in the normal population. Furthermore, the presence of adenocarcinoma in the ileum, a rare location for this histologic tumor, lends even more credence to this association.

Other than producing nonspecific symptoms, small bowel neoplasms are rather clinically quiet lesions until late in the course of their natural history. It has been observed, however, that the majority of symptomatic lesions are malignant, and this is indirectly supported by the larger proportion of benign lesions found incidentally at autopsy. In general, physical examination is rarely helpful in this disease with no particular physical findings; and diagnosis, when made, is by radiologic or endoscopic examination.

TUMOR CHARACTERISTICS

Small bowel tumors are classified into six general categories: adenocarcinoma, carcinoid, lymphomas, sarcomas, metastatic lesions, and benign lesions. Approximately 35 histopathologic varieties have been reported in this group of neoplasms. The adenocarcinomas are the most common and occur most frequently in the duodenum and proximal jejunum, while carcinoids and lymphomas have been found more frequently in the distal small bowel.

The benign tumors include hamartomas, adenomatous polyps, lipomas, leiomyomas, hemangiomas, villous adenomas and fibromas, among others. Among the benign tumors, the leiomyomas and hemangiomas have the greatest tendency to bleed. Villous adenomas are rare lesions, with less than a hundred reported in the world's literature. With the increasing use of endoscopy, however, more of these lesions are being diagnosed. As in the rectal villous adenomas, 25 to 33 per cent are known to be or become malignant. This has great surgical importance, especially for those lesions near or surrounding the ampulla.

Metastatic lesions to the small intestine have been reported most frequently with malignant melanoma, bronchogenic carcinoma, breast carcinoma, choriocarcinoma, and renal cell carcinoma. These lesions are characteristically multiple and occur in the intestinal submucosa.

The carcinoid tumors are perhaps the most intriguing of all the small bowel tumors. (See the article on this topic.) Embryologically they are amine precursor uptake and deamination (APUD) cells, and their incidence of occurrence in the ileum and proximal small bowel is not as high as in the appendix and rectum. The small bowel lesions, however, tend to be multiple, and they metastasize to regional lymph nodes and distant sites more readily. The classic carcinoid syndrome of flushing, diarrhea, bronchoconstriction, and right-sided cardiac valvular disease usually is not seen unless hepatic metastasis has occurred. If any of these symptoms are present, however, urinary determination of 5-hydroxyindoleacetic acid levels may be diagnostic. Some carcinoids have been reported in the duodenal wall; although microscopically indistinguishable from jejunal or ileal lesions, these tumors produce disease complexes similar to those resulting from their embryologic cousins the pancreatic islet cell tumors such as the Zollinger-Ellison syndrome.

The association of small intestinal tumors and Meckel's diverticulum has not been proved to date, but the rarity of these lesions in the general population makes any statistical association circumspect at best.

DIAGNOSTIC TESTS

For tumors beyond the ligament of Trietz, the only accurate preoperative diagnostic examinations are radiologic. In acute obstructions, flat plate and upright abdominal studies may be helpful in determining the level of intestinal involvement, but these studies are not specifically diagnostic of small bowel tumors.

Careful barium studies, on the other hand, have been reported to yield an accurate diagnosis in about 60 per cent of cases. In order to obtain this high level of accuracy, the radiologist must give much time and attention to the so-called fractional small bowel series in which films are taken at frequent intervals as the column of barium progresses caudally. Fluoroscopy during these studies is necessary to "uncoil" the loops of small bowel and to prevent loops of intestine from "hiding" behind one another. Hypotonic duodenography has been very helpful in detection of duodenal lesions. In this technique, the upper gastrointestinal tract is rendered atonic by the use of parenteral propantheline bromide (Pro-Banthine) or glucagon, and air-contrast studies of the duodenum are obtained. Similarly, retrograde small bowel studies have been obtained using the same smooth muscle relaxants to assist in propelling the column of barium from the colon cephalad into the small bowel. In experienced hands, this technique has been reported to demonstrate lesions in a more detailed and accurate fashion. More recently, enteroclysis, an air-contrast antegrade small bowel study, has improved the detection of small lesions significantly. In this technique a nasal tube is passed through the stomach and duodenum into the jejunum, and small amounts of barium and air are given along with Pro-Banthine or glucagon. This gives a remarkably clear air-contrast study of the small bowel, allowing ready examination of the intestinal lumen for lesions.

The common x-ray patterns attributed to small bowel tumors are defective mucosal patterns, narrowing of the intestinal lumen, changes in peristaltic pattern, rigidity of bowel wall (especially in the infiltrative lymphomas), dilatation of bowel proximal to the site of the lesion, and, of course, visible filling defects within the intestinal lumen. Many of these findings may be confused or masked by normal peristalsis or overlapping of loops of gut.

For duodenal lesions, upper gastrointestinal panendoscopy has been shown to be extremely useful. Not only can the lesion be visualized, but endoscopic biopsies can be taken so that the histologic nature of the lesion can be detailed. Up to this point, endoscopic examination of the jejunum and ileum has not been possible from a practical standpoint.

Selective arteriograms of the superior mesenteric artery or celiac axis have been reported to be of some help in locating actively bleeding lesions and in determining anatomic characteristics of the tumors. As yet they have not been reported to be of much use in the diagnosis of small bowel tumors in general. Similarly, computed tomographic (CT) scanning has shown only limited use in the diagnosis of this entity, and then only when the tumors have obtained a significant size.

Etiology of small bowel tumors is unknown, although numerous carcinogenic agents have been used to induce enteric adenocarcinomas in experimental animals.

Treatment of all tumors of the small bowel is surgical excision where technically feasible. This is often not possible because of metastatic invasion of these lesions along blood vessels, which, due to the anatomy of the mesenteric blood supply, frequently makes curative resection impossible. Chemotherapeutic regimens have not shown much benefit in the palliation of these lesions except in the case of lymphoma. Radiation has some palliative benefit in widespread disease for relief of symptoms when resection is not possible. Generally most large series report a 20 to 30 per cent 5-year survival for malignant small bowel tumors.

ACUTE APPENDICITIS

By John W. Francfort, M.D.
and Leonard J. Perloff, M.D.
Philadelphia, Pennsylvania

Although a 15 to 20 per cent incidence of negative findings at laparotomy is high for most pathologic entities, surgeons willingly pay this price for the safe therapy of patients with suspected appendicitis—still a potentially lethal disease—reminding us of the charge to all physicians by Dieulafoy in 1889 that "no one should die of appendicitis." In the United States, over 250,000 appendectomies are performed per year, despite a clearly decreasing incidence of appendicitis since World War II (possibly related to adjunctive antibiotic therapy). It is expected that 7 per cent of the population will develop this disease entity at some time. The mortality for acute appendicitis today is less than 0.1 per cent.

Seventeenth and 18th century Polish and French surgeons described operative drainage of appendiceal abscesses and also suggested, on the basis of autopsy findings, that obstruction of the appendix with fecal matter may lead to inflammation (perityphlitis) and eventual perforation. The term "appendicitis" was first used by Reginald Fitz of Boston in 1886, to call attention to inflammation of the vermiform appendix as the primary lesion and the one to which treatment should be directed, as opposed to the prevalent view of the time that the major pathology was colonic in origin. On April 27, 1887, Sir Frederick Treves of London performed an operation that was deliberately designed to seek and remove an inflamed appendix. His patient was the first to survive such a procedure. Shortly afterward, McBurney's classic description of 11 operative cases appeared.

PATHOGENESIS

Rare in infancy, acute appendicitis has its peak incidence in the teens, at which time the sex distribution is 2:1 in favor of males. At all other ages there is an equal distribution.

Obstruction of the appendiceal lumen can be demonstrated in 75 per cent of specimens resected for acute appendicitis, the most common causes being hyperplasia of the submucosal lymphoid follicles (65 per cent), fecal stasis or a fecalith (30 per cent), foreign bodies (4 per cent), and strictures or tumors (1 per cent). The condition also has been described without obstruction in gastroenteritis (particularly associated with Salmonella, Shigella, Yersinia, and pinworms). Other obstructing entities include postoperative fibrous bands, primary or metastatic appendiceal or cecal tumors, vegetable matter, retained barium, and other parasites. Obstruction of the normal flow of mucosal secretions leads to proliferation of normal intestinal flora, increased intraluminal pressure, infection, and relative ischemia of the appendiceal wall. Obstruction of the lymphatic drainage, venous drainage, and finally arterial flow occurs with continued obstruction. If this goes untreated, eventually gangrene and perforation will occur. Peritonitis, either localized or diffuse, and abscess formation usually signal the presence of a perforated appendix. Periappendiceal abscesses may perforate spontaneously into the bladder, uterus, or vagina, form a fistula to the skin, or provide access to the portal circulation for intestinal bacteria (pylephlebitis), resulting in hepatic abscesses and lethal sepsis.

DIAGNOSIS

Symptomatology

Recent efforts have been made, using a computer-aided univariate discriminant analysis, to provide a more accurate differentiation between patients with acute appendicitis and those with abdominal pain but normal appendices. The results showed that the only features that significantly differed and that suggested appendicitis were sexual (male) predilection, duration of abdominal pain (mean 24 hours), nausea, and anorexia. It was concluded that computer-aided diagnosis was no more effective than unaided clinical diagnosis.

A description of the patient with appendicitis follows.

Abdominal Pain

Over one half of the patients present with a dull, persistent periumbilical ache, which becomes more intense over several hours and eventually localizes in the right lower quadrant. The remaining patients present initially with right lower quadrant pain or continuing diffuse abdominal pain. Although the exact location of the pain appears to depend on the position and length of the appendix, McBurney's explanation of the exact locality of the greatest "sensitiveness" as a point that can be determined by the pressure of one finger 1.5 to 2 inches from the anterior spinous process of the right ilium on a straight line to the umbilicus is one of the classic descriptions in all of medicine.

In approximately two thirds of patients, the appendix lies anterior to or along the medial border of the cecum. Although it lies in the retrocecal position in 30 to 40 per cent of patients, it is fixed to this area only 15 per cent of the time. Its location is retroperitoneal in only 5 to 10 per cent of patients, which results in pain over the iliac crest when the appendix is inflamed. Additional features may include hematuria, urinary urgency, or tenesmus if the appendix lies respectively on the ureter, the bladder, or deep within the pelvis. In the case of situs inversus, left lower quadrant pain is more common. Although perforation of the appendix may lead to temporary relief of the pain as appendiceal intraluminal pressure is relieved, severe symptoms return quite rapidly as peritonitis becomes generalized. Abdominal distention at this point is ominous and signifies peritoneal contamination with gastrointestinal flora.

Nausea and Vomiting

In adults, anorexia and nausea occur in approximately 80 per cent of patients with acute appendicitis. Vomiting, seen somewhat less often, is more common in children, particularly after attempts to eat. Recurrent green or brown vomitus should suggest the possibility of intestinal obstruction. When vomiting occurs before the onset of abdominal pain, diagnoses other than appendicitis should be entertained.

Fever

Although acute appendicitis is usually associated with a low-grade fever (100°F, 37.8°C), many patients are noted to have normal temperatures. Temperatures should always be taken rectally. A temperature above 101.5°F, in combination with shaking chills, suggests appendiceal gangrene or perforation or other entities in the differential diagnosis, such as intestinal infarction, pneumonia, or gastroenteritis.

Obstipation

Obstipation often accompanies the abdominal pain and may prompt the patient to try a cathartic or enema, with little pain relief. Diarrhea, an atypical finding in adults, is not uncommon in children. It is usually mild and may suggest that the inflamed appendix is contiguous with the sigmoid colon or rectum.

Physical Examination

The patient usually lies quietly and appears somewhat anxious and uncomfortable. The pulse rate is usually normal to slightly elevated. Inspection of the abdomen may reveal mild distention, and bowel sounds are normal or slightly decreased. Occasionally, depending on the diffuseness of the peritonitis, bowel sounds will be absent. Very gentle percussion may suggest right lower quadrant dullness. Palpation reveals mild to severe tenderness often associated with a sense of fullness in the right lower quadrant. The tenderness is often most severe at McBurney's point, approximately one third the distance from the iliac spine on a straight line to the umbilicus, and may be associated with rebound. Voluntary guarding is common; however, involuntary guarding or abdominal rigidity suggests peritonitis and perforation. Palpable abdominal masses, although not usually found, suggest perforation with localized abscess formation, or a mass of inflamed omentum and phlegmonous small intestine, or tumor.

Passive extension of the right thigh or flexion against resistance may markedly aggravate the pain (*psoas sign*), suggesting irritation of the right psoas muscle by a posterior appendix. The *obturator sign,* pain elicited by passive internal and external rotation of the flexed hip, suggests that the inflamed appendix is in close contact with obturator internus muscle. Another common finding is *Rovsing's sign,* which is often associated with right lower quadrant rebound tenderness. It is characterized by increased right lower quadrant pain on deep palpation in any other of the abdominal quadrants, particularly the left lower quadrant. Hyperesthesia of the right lower quadrant skin is suggestive of underlying inflammation. Rectal and pelvic examination may reveal cul-de-sac tenderness.

Laboratory Findings

Seventy to 80 per cent of patients with acute appendicitis will have a white blood cell (WBC) count between 10 to 15,000 per cu mm, with a shift to the left. However, no clear correlation exists between the level of the WBC count and the severity of the appendicitis, and, in fact, a normal count may be seen relatively often in the elderly patient. Minimal albuminuria and a few white blood cells may be seen in the urine in 20 per cent of males with acute appendicitis. Greater than 30 red blood cells or 20 white cells per high-power field in a centrifuged specimen of voided urine indicates primary urinary tract pathology.

X-ray Examination

With the exception of an appendiceal fecalith, there are no absolutely reliable radiologic findings in acute appendicitis. Calcified fecaliths, occurring in about 10 per cent of patients, are oval laminated masses identified in the right lower quadrant. Plain films may show a cecal ileus (distended cecum with an air-fluid level) in early stages. Gas in the appendiceal lumen or a mass outside of the cecum may be indicative of a gangrenous or perforated appendix. Late in the course of a complicated appendicitis, there may also be scoliosis to the right, absence of a psoas shadow, and absence of right lower quadrant bowel gas. In patients with positive abdominal findings, some consider barium enema to be contraindicated because of possible perforation of an inflamed appendix; however, it is particularly useful when the abdominal findings are questionable, and recent reports confirm the safety of the study. Significant findings include nonfilling of the appendix (this also occurs in 10 per cent of normals), cecal or terminal ileal spasm, and partial filling of the appendix with a cecal defect suggestive of inflammation or extrinsic compression. Ultrasonography or CT scanning is helpful in eliminating the possibility of tubo-ovarian abscess, ectopic pregnancy, and ruptured ovarian cyst, and laparoscopic examination may be of great help in ruling out these gynecologic conditions.

Differential Diagnosis

The diagnosis of appendicitis is relatively straightforward despite the multiple causes of abdominal pain. In the young patient, one must consider intussusception, gastroenteritis, mesenteric lymphadenitis, inflammatory bowel disease, sickle cell crisis, lead poisoning, and Meckel's diverticulitis. In young women, the list of etiologies also includes pelvic inflammatory disease, twisted ovarian cyst, ectopic pregnancy with rupture, acute pyelonephritis, endometriosis, and *mittelschmerz.* In young men, testicular torsion and epidydimitis must be ruled out. Additional considerations include hepatitis, pancreatitis, ureteral calculus, and, particularly in the older age groups, perforated peptic ulcer, diverticulitis, mesenteric ischemia, ruptured abdominal aortic aneurysm, and colonic carcinoma with or without intestinal obstruction. Finally, for completeness, pneumonia, malaria, diabetic gastroenteropathy, porphyria and the bite of the black widow spider should be remembered.

All of the foregoing conditions have individual characteristics, symptoms, and signs, and many diagnostic tools are available for each one. Four special situations—appendicitis in pregnancy, in infants, in the elderly, and in the immunologically compromised host—will be reviewed separately.

Pregnancy

Although appendicitis complicates only one in every thousand pregnancies, two thirds of the gastrointestinal surgical cases in pregnant women are cases of appendicitis. The rate of occurrence is equal in the three trimesters.

Several diagnostic problems are present. First, although the appendix can be located at McBurney's point in the first trimester, because of uterine enlargement the pain of acute appendicitis can present in the right upper quadrant by the eighth month of the pregnancy, simulating acute cholecystitis. Although nausea and vomiting are quite common, particularly during the early phases of a normal gestation, anorexia and abdominal cramps are suggestive of more severe conditions, such as appendicitis. Mild leukocytosis (11,000 WBCs per cu mm) is common in pregnancy, but acute appendicitis may be unaccompanied by significant temperature elevation possibly related to elevated levels of circulating adrenal steroids. Additional diagnostic considerations are pyelonephritis, twisted ovarian cyst, placental abruption, uterine myomata, and neoplasms.

In cases of perforation of the appendix, fetal loss may be as high as 25 per cent; therefore, early surgical intervention is recommended. Because x-rays are undesirable in the presence of a gravid uterus, laparoscopy may be of use; however, the size of the uterus and the variable position of the appendix prevent uniform success. One helpful physical examination feature is the suggestion that pain of uterine origin may be relieved by change of position, whereas pain from an extrauterine source, such as an acute appendix, will be unrelieved regardless of position.

Children

Because nonspecific abdominal pain is common in children and infants, and because the level of suspicion is lowered by the knowledge that acute appendicitis is rare before 2 years of age, the condition is often discovered only after perforation and peritonitis have supervened. Abdominal pain, fever, vomiting, and anorexia should definitely raise one's suspicion of acute appendicitis. Irritability, flexing of the thighs, and diarrhea are also helpful signs. Because children often cannot give a very good history, two thirds of appendicitis patients in this age group have symptoms for more than 3 days preceding appendectomy. Abdominal distention is one of the more consistent findings. Leukocyte counts are unreliable. A fecalith or an ileus pattern on abdominal x-ray are also suggestive of acute appendicitis.

The Elderly

In older adults the incidence of acute appendicitis is less than 5 per cent. Delay in seeking medical care and the relatively low incidence are probably responsible for the 30 per cent incidence of perforated appendicitis in patients over 60 years of age. The classic symptoms of pain, anorexia, and nausea are less severe, but are present in these patients. Localization to the right lower quadrant appears somewhat later than in younger patients. Physical examination may reveal subnormal temperatures, particularly in the face of an abscess or generalized peritoneal inflammation. As in the child, abdominal distention is relatively common, suggesting mechanical small bowel obstruction. A painless right lower quadrant mass or generalized peritonitis of unknown etiology in the absence of symptoms are not uncommon in these patients.

The Immunologically Compromised Host

Treatment of patients who are immunoincompetent is a regular feature of modern medical and surgical care. Whether the immunologic weakness is related to overwhelming debilitating disease such as carcinoma, malnutrition, uremia, or multiple trauma, or to iatrogenic causes such as cancer chemotherapy or immunosuppression, these patients have a higher incidence of both common and unusual infections. Duodenal ulcer, pancreatitis, and acute colitis comprise 10 to 30 per cent of gastrointestinal complications in immunosuppressed patients. Hepatitis and cecal ulceration are also found with relatively high frequency in these patients. Surprisingly, acute appendicitis is unusual in the immunocompromised host, possibly related to a generalized lymphoid atrophy, particularly in the steroid-treated patient. Nevertheless, because many of the hallmarks of inflammation are lost, gastrointestinal complications in immunosuppressed individuals are associated with a tremendously high morbidity and mortality and should be very high on a differential diagnostic list despite nonspecific features.

CHRONIC DIARRHEA AND MALABSORPTION

By E. V. O'Loughlin, M.D.
and D. Grant Gall, M.D.
Calgary, Alberta, Canada

Chronic diarrhea is a common problem in infancy and childhood. Diarrhea is defined as an excess loss of water and electrolytes in the feces, leading to increased frequency, fluidity, and volume of bowel movements. The following discussion focuses on the mechanisms of diarrhea and an approach to the diagnosis concentrating on the more common pediatric problems. A comprehensive differential diagnosis of chronic diarrhea and malabsorption in infancy and childhood is given in Table 1. Many of these diseases are rare. In general, the majority of infants and young children with chronic diarrhea will be "chronic poopers" in whom no specific disease entity can be identified.

MECHANISMS OF DIARRHEA

In the normal child about 5000 ml of fluid enters the upper small intestine per day; 1000 ml comes from oral ingestion, and the remainder from endogenous secretion. The majority of this fluid is absorbed before reaching the colon. Stool volumes range from 75 to 150 gm/day, of which 65 to 80 per cent is water. Even a small increase in stool volume, as little as 30 to 60 ml, is sufficient to cause the patient to complain of diarrhea.

Three major defects contribute to the production of diarrhea:

1. Osmotic retardation of water absorption.
2. Abnormal water and electrolyte transport.
3. Disorders of transit.

Osmotic

The presence of unabsorbed dietary components in the bowel constitutes an abnormal osmotic load leading to retardation of water absorption. This can result from dietary overloading (e.g., sorbitol-induced diarrhea) or from malabsorption of ingested nutrients, usually carbohydrates. Malabsorbed carbohydrates undergo fermentation by colonic bacteria to organic acids; this further increases the osmotic load. The flux of water into the bowel exceeds absorptive capacity and watery diarrhea results. In osmotic diarrhea the stools are low in sodium, and osmolality exceeds that predicted from the sum of electrolyte concentrations.

Abnormal Water and Electrolyte Transport

Derangement of water and electrolyte transport can be induced by direct mucosal injury or secondary to the effect of intraluminal or circulating factors. The response of the patient depends on the region and extent of intestine involved. Since about 90 per cent of fluid and electrolyte absorption is normally completed by the small intestine, relatively minor abnormalities here may cause diarrhea.

Intraluminal agents that impair water and electrolyte absorption and induce secretion include bacterial enterotoxins (cholera from *Vibrio cholerae* and enterotoxigenic *Escherichia coli*), deconjugated bile salts, and hydroxylated fatty acids. Bacterial deconjugation of bile acids occurs in bacterial overgrowth of the small bowel and when malabsorbed bile salts are acted upon by colonic bacteria. Hydroxy fatty acids are produced from the actions of colonic microflora on unabsorbed dietary fat. Deconjugated bile acids and hydroxy fatty acids are potent secretagogues. Functioning tumors such as carcinoid, pancreatic islet cell tumors, neural crest tumors, and medullary carcinoma of the thyroid secrete humoral agents that stimulate water and electrolyte secretion. With this type of diarrhea, the sum of the electrolyte concentrations in the stool equals osmolality.

Disorders of Transit

Adequate length of small bowel is necessary for digestion and absorption of food. Congenital or acquired short gut may result in inadequate mucosal exposure of intraluminal contents and diminished absorption of nutrients. An intact ileocecal valve is important in controlling intestinal transit and preventing bacterial contamination of the distal small bowel.

Disorders of motility may result in chronic diarrhea and malabsorption. Normal motility is necessary to maintain sterility of the small intestine. Hypomotility allows bacterial overgrowth of the small intestine with resultant absorptive defects. Hypomotility is seen in intestinal pseudo-obstruction, partial anatomic obstruction, and Hirschsprung's disease. Hypermotility can be seen in intestinal infection, laxative abuse, thyrotoxicosis, and functioning tumors.

APPROACH TO DIAGNOSIS

The challenge to the physician is separating those patients in whom chronic diarrhea is a manifestation of underlying intestinal disease from the well chronic pooper. The diagnosis can be established in the majority of patients with a thorough clinical assessment and stool examination.

Clinical Assessment

Initial assessment can reveal whether the child is ill. If so, immediate attention and investigation may be warranted. If not, a "wait-and-see" approach may be far more rewarding than an immediate and costly investigation.

Assessment of appetite, activity, and growth is important. Patients with pancreatic insufficiency frequently have a voracious appetite. The converse is true of patients with celiac disease, who often display anorexia and irritability. Is the patient thriving? If not, a thorough dietary history should be taken. Patients with chronic diarrhea often have frequent manipulation of their diet and severe caloric restriction in an attempt by frustrated parents and physicians to control the stool output, usually without success. Chronological record of dietary milestones may suggest the diagnosis; celiac disease frequently presents within 3 to 6 months of cereal introduction. (See the article on gluten-sensitive enteropathy.)

The consistency, frequency, and type of stool may indicate the presence of underlying disease and may localize pathology to a specific part of the intestinal tract. The presence of blood and mucus usually indicates a colonic problem; steatorrhea and watery diarrhea suggest a problem in the small intestine.

Assessment of general health is important because many gastrointestinal disorders display extraintestinal manifestations. Frequent sinopulmonary infections suggest cystic fibrosis (see related article), primary immune deficiency (see related article), or neutropenia (Shwachman's syndrome). Fever, anemia, arthritis and skin rashes occur in chronic inflammatory bowel disease and in bacterial enteritis. Delay in pubertal development can occur with many chronic diseases, but should alert one to the possibility of Crohn's disease (see the article on Chronic Ulcerative Colitis and Crohn's Disease.

Family history may be helpful. Acute diarrheal disease in other family members suggests an infective agent. Cystic fibrosis, primary monosaccharide intolerance, primary disaccharidase deficiencies and abetalipoproteinemia are inherited. Family history may be positive in celiac disease and in chronic inflammatory bowel disease.

Physical examination includes assessment of growth percentiles, nutritional status, and pubertal development. Plotting of height, weight, and head circumference is mandatory for the assessment of any child with chronic diarrhea. A patient who is growing normally is unlikely to be suffering from significant gastrointestinal disease. Plotting of longitudinal percentiles can give important information about timing and severity of disease and may even suggest the diagnosis. Other indicators of malabsorption and abnormal nutritional status include loss of subcutaneous fat and muscle bulk, peripheral edema (hypoproteinemia), and bruising (vitamin K). Recurrent aphthous ulcers are seen frequently with chronic intestinal disease such as Crohn's disease. Finger clubbing suggests chronic disease and is frequently seen in cystic fibrosis, celiac disease, and Crohn's disease. In performing inspection and digital examination of the rectum, the physician specifically looks for perianal disease, fissures, and fecal impaction; this procedure also affords an opportunity to examine a stool specimen.

Stool Examination

The importance of stool examination is frequently overlooked, but should be considered a routine part of the examination. The presence of numerous white and red cells on microscopy is seen in colonic infection and chronic inflammatory bowel disease but rarely in diarrhea originating in the small bowel. In infants, eosinophils suggest milk protein intolerance. Cysts or trophozoites of *Giardia lamblia* on occasion may be found, but diagnosis, at best, can be made in only 50 per cent of cases by stool examination. Undigested fat is seen as globules of neutral fat that stain orange with Oil Red 0 or Sudan Red. Outside the newborn period, the presence of neutral fat is always abnormal and indicates pancreatic insufficiency. In a child this suggests a diagnosis of cystic fibrosis, or, less likely, Shwachman's syndrome. Care must be taken, since

Table 1. Causes of Chronic Diarrhea and Malabsorption

Bloody Diarrhea	Watery Diarrhea
Infection	Osmotic
Campylobacter	Disaccharidase deficiency
Shigella	Lactase
Salmonella	Sucrase-isomaltase
Yersinia	Glucose-galactose malabsorption
Invasive *Escherichia coli*	Excessive intake, e.g., sorbitol
Cytomegalovirus colitis	Abnormal water and electrolyte transport
Chronic inflammatory bowel disease	Infective
Pseudomembranous colitis	Viral
Milk protein intolerance (infants)	Enterotoxigenic bacteria
Necrotizing enterocolitis	*Giardia lamblia*
Amebiasis	Allergic gastroenteropathy
Hirschsprung's enterocolitis	Cow's milk protein
Diarrhea associated with anal lesions	Soy protein
Steatorrhea	Short gut
Pancreatic insufficiency	Congenital
Cystic fibrosis	Postsurgical
Shwachman's syndrome	Bacterial overgrowth
Malnutrition	Motility disorder
Chronic pancreatitis	Anatomic obstruction
Lipase, colipase deficiency	Laxative abuse
Inadequate bile salt concentration	Immune deficiency disorders
Biliary atresia	Congenital chloride-losing diarrhea
Cirrhosis	Acrodermatitis enteropathica
Cholestatic syndromes	Functioning tumors
Acquired	Pancreatic islet call tumors
Familial	Neural crest tumors
Bacterial overgrowth syndromes	Carcinoid syndrome
Disease or resection of ileum	Medullary carcinoma of thyroid
Inadequate absorptive area	Bile salt malabsorption
Celiac disease	Endocrine disease
Short gut syndrome	Adrenal insufficiency
Cow's milk protein and soy protein intolerance	Diabetes mellitus
Whipple's disease	
Immune deficiency disorders	
Intracellular defect	
Abetalipoproteinemia	
Impaired lymphatic drainage	
Lymphoma	
Intestinal lymphangiectasia	
Constrictive pericarditis	

lubricants and ointments for the buttocks are indistinguishable from neutral fats on microscopy. The presence of meat fibers also indicates pancreatic insufficiency. Excess fatty acids, which are apparent at high power as refractile crystals, suggest a mucosal problem such as celiac disease.

The presence of sugar in the stool can be detected by the use of Clinitest tablets. A small amount of liquid stool is diluted with twice the volume of water, and then 15 drops of this solution together with a Clinitest tablet are placed in a separate tube. The resultant color change is compared with the chart provided. The test needs to be performed immediately to prevent further fermentation of sugars by colonic bacteria. Sucrose is not a reducing substance; if its presence is suspected, it may be necessary to first hydrolyze the sugar with acid before testing. Greater than 250 mg/dl of reducing substances indicates carbohydrate malabsorption. The exception is the breast-fed infant whose stools frequently contain excess lactose in the absence of underlying disease.

Enough information should now be available to the physician to justify a wait-and-see approach or, if the presence of underlying disease is suspected, to guide the subsequent line of investigation.

DIARRHEAL DISORDERS

Chronic Nonspecific Diarrhea

The majority of patients with chronic diarrhea have no identifiable disease and are grouped into the conglomeration known as chronic nonspecific diarrhea. The onset of diarrhea may follow an episode of acute gastroenteritis and is mainly a problem in children younger than 3 years of age. Stools are loose but not watery and may occur four to ten times per day. Despite the frequency of stools, most patients are robust and thriving. The problem is benign and self-limited and is usually of greater concern to the parent than the child. There is no specific therapy. The course, however, may be complicated by multiple dietary manipulations and caloric restriction.

Bloody Diarrhea

Bloody diarrhea usually indicates colonic disease. In infective colitis and chronic inflammatory bowel disease involving the colon, pus cells are readily apparent on microscopy. Diarrhea associated with anal lesions may mimic bloody diarrhea.

Infections

Intestinal infections are usually associated with acute diarrhea but occasionally infections by Campylobacter, Salmonella, and Yersinia and infestation by *Giardia lamblia* can lead to chronic symptoms. *Yersinia enterocolitica* and *Campylobacter jejuni* require special techniques for identification.

Amebic dysentery should be considered in any patient who has traveled to the tropics or who has been in contact with individuals who have. Microscopic identification of trophozoites can be made on fresh stools or rectal mucosal biopsies.

Pseudomembranous colitis should be considered in patients who develop profuse bloody diarrhea following antibiotic treatment. In the majority of cases, proctosigmoidoscopic examination reveals colonic mucosa covered with adherent yellowish white membranes (pseudomembranes). The diagnosis is confirmed by isolation of *Clostridium difficile* and identification of the specific toxin. Both of these procedures require special techniques that are not widely available.

Chronic Inflammatory Bowel Disease

Idiopathic ulcerative colitis and Crohn's disease (see related article) both occur in childhood. In ulcerative colitis, severe bloody diarrhea, abdominal discomfort, urgency to stool, and tenesmus are the usual presenting symptoms. Frequent passage of small stools is the hallmark of rectal inflammation. Patients with Crohn's disease may have a similar presentation, but more commonly complaints of abdominal pain, anorexia, and systemic manifestations including malnutrition, growth failure, and delayed puberty dominate the clinical picture. Chronic inflammatory bowel disease should be suspected in patients with chronic symptoms and negative stool cultures. Diagnosis is based on intestinal radiographic studies, protosigmoidoscopy, and, to a lesser extent, rectal biopsy. Differentiation of ulcerative colitis from Crohn's disease may be difficult. The differential diagnosis rests mainly on distribution of disease. Ulcerative colitis involves only the colon. Diffuse, superficial inflammation of the colonic mucosa nearly always involves the rectum and extends proximally for a variable distance. The entire colon may be involved, but disease in the left colon predominates. On proctosigmoidoscopy, ulcerations are infrequent; the mucosa is red, with loss of vascular pattern, is friable, and bleeds easily.

In contrast, Crohn's disease can involve any area of the gastrointestinal tract, including mouth and anus. Distribution is segmental, and skip lesions are frequent. The majority of the patients (65 per cent) have ileocolonic involvement, 25 per cent small bowel only, and 10 to 15 per cent colonic only. Associated perianal disease is common. In Crohn's disease, the inflammatory process involves all layers of the bowel wall; this explains the frequent occurrence of fistulae and intra-abdominal abscess formation.

Rectal biopsy is not diagnostic, but may aid in the diagnosis. Crypt abscesses and mucosal inflammation are not specific, but suggest ulcerative colitis. Pronounced submucosal inflammation, lymphoid hyperplasia, and granuloma formation strongly support a diagnosis of Crohn's disease.

Protein Intolerance

Chronic diarrhea can be a manifestation of cow and soy protein intolerance. In the very young infant, protein intolerance often presents as colitis. The presence of blood and eosinophils in the diarrheal stool suggests the diagnosis. Improvement of symptoms following withdrawal of the offending protein and exacerbation with rechallenge is diagnostic. Skin testing and specific serum antibodies are not useful aids in the diagnosis.

Steatorrhea

Fat malabsorption results from inadequate pancreatic lipase, insufficient intraluminal bile salts, insufficient absorptive surface, cellular defect, or obstructed lymphatic drainage. When the diagnosis is in doubt, fecal fat excretion as a percentage of fat intake is the only practical technique to determine for certain whether steatorrhea exists.

Cystic Fibrosis

Cystic fibrosis is the most common cause of pancreatic insufficiency in childhood in developed countries. Approximately 90 per cent of patients exhibit pancreatic insufficiency. Most patients present in the first year of life with chronic diarrhea and failure to thrive. Infants frequently have a voracious appetite and may present with severe hypoproteinemia, particularly if fed breast milk or soy protein–based formulae. Patients with milder pancreatic disease may present primarily with pulmonary symptoms.

Diagnosis is suggested by finding meat fibers and neutral fat on stool microscopy and is confirmed by demonstrating sweat chloride or sodium concentrations greater than 60 mEq/liter. Reliability of this simple test depends on the experience of the person doing the test and in obtaining a sufficient quantity of sweat ($>$100 mg). False-positive results can occur in patients with ectodermal dysplasia, glycogen storage disease, and adrenal insufficiency. Falsely low results occasionally occur in patients with hypoproteinemia. If results are equivocal, the test should be repeated.

Celiac Disease (Gluten Enteropathy)

Celiac disease usually presents in the first two years of life, after introduction of cereals into the diet. Irritability, diarrhea, and failure to thrive are common symptoms. Abdominal distention, wasting, and growth failure are usually evident on examination. In general, if a child is thriving, celiac disease is an unlikely diagnosis.

The diagnosis is suggested by the presence of fatty acid crystals on stool microscopy. Diagnosis is based on the characteristic histologic changes of flattened villi and disordered surface epithelium of duodenal mucosa and clinical improvement on gluten withdrawal. The importance of histologic diagnosis cannot be overemphasized, since patients are committed to lifelong dietary restriction of gluten. Skin testing and tests for antigliadin antibodies are unreliable. Tests of mucosal absorptive function such as the D-xylose tolerance test are not diagnostic and do not enable avoidance of small bowel biopsy when celiac disease is suspected.

Shwachman's Syndrome (Pancreatic Exocrine Hypoplasia)

The presence of exocrine pancreatic insufficiency with normal sweat electrolyte levels suggests a diagnosis of Shwachman's syndrome. Pancreatic exocrine insufficiency is associated with bone marrow hypoplasia, short stature, and, less commonly, metaphyseal dysostosis.

Other Conditions

Short gut syndrome, whether congenital or acquired, causes steatorrhea because of inadequate surface area for absorption. Steatorrhea from inadequate intraluminal levels of conjugated bile salts can result from bacterial contamination of the small bowel, disease of the terminal ileum, and severe liver disease. Rarer mucosal defects producing steatorrhea include abetalipoproteinemia and intestinal lymphangiectasia.

Watery Diarrhea

Watery diarrhea usually indicates small bowel disease.

Carbohydrate Malabsorption

In children, chronic watery diarrhea is frequently related to carbohydrate malabsorption from secondary disaccharidase deficiency. This injury is most commonly caused by viral enteritis, but other examples include giardiasis, celiac disease, milk protein intolerance, short gut syndrome, and bacterial overgrowth. In addition, young infants on occasion will develop secondary monosaccharide intolerance after a severe or repeated bouts of viral enteritis.

Primary lactase deficiency is not uncommon in non-Caucasians and usually manifests in later childhood. Other inherited disorders of carbohydrate absorption are rare. Sucrase-isomaltase deficiency presents in infancy after the introduction of sucrose-containing foods. Glucose-galactose malabsorption is a life-threatening disease presenting in the neonatal period.

Younger patients develop explosive watery diarrhea after ingestion of the offending sugar. Bacterial fermentation lowers stool pH and may induce perianal excoriation. Malabsorbed carbohydrate is detected with Clinitest tablets as previously described. Breath hydrogen analysis following oral challenge with a specific sugar is a useful adjunct to diagnosis. Indications for jejunal biopsy are few, but mucosal studies are required to establish the diagnosis of primary sucrase-isomaltase and glucose-galactose malabsorption.

Abnormal Water and Electrolyte Transport

Secretory diarrhea is likely in patients with continued watery diarrhea despite complete bowel rest. Diarrhea is related to decreased absorption, active secretion, or a combination of both. Numerous toxic, humoral, chemical, and mucosal factors have been implicated in secretory diarrheas. While bacterial enterotoxins are a common cause (e.g., *E. coli* enterotoxin in travelers' diarrhea), the disease is usually acute and self-limited. In severe diarrhea that persists with nothing taken by mouth, and stool osmolality is explained by the electrolyte concentrations, consider laxative abuse or humoral factors. Studies are aimed at identifying the specific agent—phenolphthalein in stool water; vasoactive intestinal peptide (VIP), gastrin, or prostaglandins in serum; catecholamines in serum and urine.

SUMMARY OF DIAGNOSTIC APPROACH

Clinical assessment and stool examination in the physician's office will indicate whether the child is ill, and, if so, will point to a likely diagnosis in most. Initial assessment may lead to routine blood tests for anemia and inflammation, stool cultures, examination of stools for parasites, and measurement of sweat electrolytes if cystic fibrosis is a possibility. Serum electrolytes and urea, though frequently performed, are rarely of diagnostic value. Total serum protein and albumin levels provide a rough index of nutritional status and intestinal protein loss. At this point, if the patient is well with normal growth percentiles, further studies are unlikely to be helpful and a wait-and-see approach is justified.

If the patient is ill and initial assessment suggests intestinal disease, admission to the hospital for ongoing investigation may be necessary. Stool collection for assessment of fat absorption, daily volume of stool output, and fecal electrolyte content and osmolality is frequently indicated. Indirect tests of intestinal absorption such as serum carotene measurement and the D-xylose tolerance test have proved to be unreliable. Sugar intolerance can usually be confirmed by examining stools for reducing substances. Oral tolerance tests have been disappointing. Breath hydrogen analysis following oral sugar challenge is a useful test for the patient without obvious carbohydrate malabsorption. It is also useful in patients with suspected bacterial overgrowth.

Radiologic investigation should be restricted to those patients with suspected chronic inflammatory bowel disease or anatomic anomalies. Abnormalities may be seen in other intestinal disorders, but they are usually not diagnostic and expose the patient to needless radiation. The major indication for small bowel biopsy is celiac disease, though intestinal lymphangiectasia, abetalipoproteinemia and Whipple's disease have characteristic histologic features.

Specific investigations can be diagnostic in patients with clinical features suggestive of an unusual disorder. For example, low serum zinc points to a diagnosis of acrodermatitis enteropathica in a patient presenting with failure to thrive, mucocutaneous lesions, and alopecia. Acanthocytic red cells, low cholesterol, and abnormal lipoprotein electrophoresis confirm a diagnosis of abetalipoproteinemia. Differential white cell count and immunoglobulin estimation may lead to a diagnosis of immunodeficiency disease or intestinal lymphangiectasia.

In the majority of patients, severe disease can be excluded or a diagnosis established with thorough clinical assessment, stool examination, and a few simple tests readily performed in the office. In patients who are failing to thrive, caloric restriction should be corrected before intensive investigation, unless evidence strongly suggests underlying disease.

CHRONIC ULCERATIVE COLITIS AND CROHN'S DISEASE

By Herman Steinberg, M.D.
New York, New York

SYNONYMS

Chronic ulcerative colitis (CUC), or nonspecific ulcerative colitis, is often called "proctocolitis." Crohn's disease (CD) is often referred to as Crohn's colitis (proximal colitis, right-sided colitis, transmural colitis, granulomatous colitis), ileocolitis, regional enteritis, terminal ileitis, ileojejunitis, and Crohn's antroduodenitis, depending on the linear distribution of the disease. So-called "idiopathic proctitis" may be either ulcerative colitis limited to the rectum or Crohn's disease, more commonly the former. The terms "inflammatory bowel disease" (IBD) and "idiopathic inflammatory bowel disease" (IIBD) refer to either ulcerative colitis or Crohn's colitis.

DEFINITIONS

Both ulcerative colitis and Crohn's disease are inflammatory conditions of unknown etiology with increased familial incidence, more common in Jews than in non-Jews and in whites than in non-whites, but present in all ethnic groups. The inflammatory process of ulcerative colitis is limited to the mucosa, whereas that of Crohn's disease is transmural with greatest concentration in the submucosa. Neither bacterial nor viral etiology has been established, and it is not known whether the attendant immunologic phenomena, particularly in Crohn's disease, are basic to the pathogenesis or merely epiphenomena. The same uncertainty exists with respect to the emotional disorders that many of these patients suffer. Both diseases tend to develop with an equal sex distribution; the peak incidence of onset is in the second and third decades, but either may occur at any age. Table 1 presents a comparison of features for both diseases.

Ulcerative colitis *always* involves the rectum with or without a variable extent of remaining colon in continuous linear distribution—thus the designation "proctocolitis." The linear extent of the disease may vary from limited rectal disease ("proctitis") to involvement of the rectum and all the remaining colon ("universal ulcerative colitis"). The disease *never* extends into the small intestine, except, rarely, as "backwash ileitis," which is a limited, linear (no more than a few centimeters), insignificant radiologic abnormality.

Ulcerative colitis is distinguished from Crohn's colitis, which may or may not involve the rectum and in which the linear distribution may or may not be segmental—that is, marked by skip areas of uninvolved colon. Distinguishing features of Crohn's colitis include small bowel ("ileocolitis") and occasional gastric and duodenal involvement, as well as a propensity for fistulization. Although Crohn's disease is classified as a granulomatous disease, endoscopic biopsies reveal granulomata less than 10 per cent of the time. Perhaps 10 to 20 per cent of IIBD cannot be categorized with certainty as either ulcerative colitis or Crohn's colitis. Such uncertainty is reflected in the apparent increased incidence of Crohn's colitis in the past two decades; in many centers, Crohn's colitis is as frequent as ulcerative colitis. As indicated above, Crohn's disease may involve any portion of the gastrointestinal (GI) tract, from the stomach to the anus. Esophageal Crohn's disease has been reported as well.

PRESENTING SYMPTOMS AND SIGNS

The symptoms and signs of uncomplicated CUC and CD depend upon the linear distribution of the process (Table 1).

When either disease is limited to the colon, the symptoms and signs are remarkably similar. Activity limited to the rectum may give rise to small-volume bleeding and/or tenesmus. More extensive linear activity causes bloody diarrhea. The accompanying abdominal cramps usually are relieved by defecation, except in fulminant disease. Fever is more common in Crohn's colitis, as are many of the extragastrointestinal manifestations (Table 1). On occasion, the symptoms and signs of the extragastrointestinal manifestations overshadow those of the bowel (see discussion that follows).

Small bowel CD may present with varying degrees of nonbloody diarrhea with or without steatorrhea; abdominal gaseous distress and cramps, unrelieved by defecation if cicatricial (stricture) disease is present; fever; anorexia, nausea and postprandial vomiting, particularly in the presence of luminal narrowing; and, rarely, massive rectal bleeding.

Table 1. Differential Features of Ulcerative Colitis and Crohn's Disease

Feature	Ulcerative Colitis	Crohn's Disease
Anatomic distribution	Continuous linear, always of rectum, with or without varying lengths of colon	Any segment of gastrointestinal tract, often segmental (skip areas)
Granulomata on endoscopic biopsy	No	Rare
(Pseudo)polyps	Yes	Rare
Cobblestoning	No	Yes
Discrete ulcers	No	Yes
Internal fistulas	No	Yes
Perirectal fistulas	Rare	Yes
Palpable abdominal mass	No	Yes
Rectal bleeding	Yes	Yes
"Acute appendicitis"	No	Yes
Fever	Yes	Yes, often out of proportion to gastrointestinal symptoms
Strictures	No	Yes
Free perforation	Yes	Rare
Toxic megacolon	Yes	Rare
Extragastrointestinal manifestations	Yes	Yes, but only with colonic disease
Malnutrition and growth retardation	Rare	Frequent
Carcinoma	Yes	Rare

EXTRAGASTROINTESTINAL MANIFESTATIONS

Arthritis involving the large joints of the lower extremities is episodic, self-limiting, and nondeforming. Ankylosing spondylitis and sacroiliitis may occur.

Cutaneous lesions include erythema nodosum and pyoderma gangrenosum. Oropharyngeal manifestations include aphthous ulcers of the mouth and necrotizing ulcerations of the soft palate.

Ocular manifestations are episcleritis, iritis, and iridocyclitis.

Hepatic and biliary complications include the spectrum of pericholangitis, sclerosing choledochitis or cholangitis, and biliary cirrhosis.

All the extragastrointestinal manifestations are far more common, if not exclusively present, in colonic disease. They are probably immunologically mediated and not primary phenomena with the exception of ankylosing spondylitis and sacroiliitis, which are probably genetic fellow travelers.

COURSE

The linear anatomic distribution of both diseases tends to stabilize permanently early in the course, but it may extend at any time, particularly after surgery in the case of Crohn's disease. Both ulcerative colitis and Crohn's disease are chronic, incurable conditions, except surgically in the case of the former. They usually pursue a cyclic course over the lifetime of the patient, although sustained and seemingly permanent remissions may occur, more commonly in ulcerative colitis. On the other hand, unremittent activity, requiring constant medical supervision, is not unusual. This is particularly true of Crohn's disease patients who develop strictures or enteric fistulae that are not corrected surgically. Periods of exacerbation in either disease may vary greatly in severity, from an ambulatory working status to hospitalization.

There is no medical cure for either disease. So-called spontaneous cures of acute Crohn's disease of the terminal ileum, as seen predominantly in children, probably represent misdiagnosis, perhaps Yersinia ileitis, or some other self-limiting infection. However, proctocolectomy is curative for ulcerative colitis. In a practical sense, the operation is near-curative for Crohn's colitis, since ileostomy recurrences, although not infrequent, are of limited linear extent and rarely lead to a short gut syndrome despite the one to three revisions that may be necessary over a lifetime. Resection of diseased bowel with anastomosis is frequently indicated in Crohn's disease, but the incidence of recurrence in the preanastomotic segment is high (up to 50 to 75 per cent). The patient with Crohn's disease is much more likely to require surgery than the one with ulcerative colitis; more than half the former require operative intervention sometime during the course of their illness.

COMMON COMPLICATIONS

Toxic Megacolon. Far more common in ulcerative colitis than in Crohn's colitis; often preceded by an episode of fulminant colitis and sometimes precipitated by injudicious barium enema examination or excessive use of either spasmogenic antidiarrheal agents or anticholinergic drugs. Suspect it when the patient with colitis manifests one or more of the following: sudden diminution of diarrhea; high fever and tachycardia; and distended, tender abdomen with diminished to absent bowel sounds. Diagnosis is confirmed by flat films of the abdomen revealing 8 cm or greater dilatation of the transverse colon.

Perforation. Far more common in ulcerative colitis than in Crohn's disease; often a consequence of toxic megacolon. Symptoms and signs may be minimized by steroids. Suspect it when there is a sudden appearance of any of the following: increased abdominal pain; loss of bowel sounds and cessation of diarrhea; nausea and vomiting; increased abdominal girth; and hypotension. Diagnosis must be actively pursued in the high-risk hospitalized patient by constant observation. Confirmation of free perforation is by upright and/or decubitus abdominal films, but walled-off perforation is negative for free peritoneal air.

Massive Bleeding. The diagnosis is reasonably obvious in ulcerative colitis, but in small bowel CD or proximal colitis, peptic ulcer disease must be considered, occasionally requiring upper gastrointestinal endoscopy.

Intestinal Obstruction. Rare in ulcerative colitis; common in small bowel CD. When present in ulcerative colitis, rule out carcinoma.

Carcinoma. A complication of long-duration ulcerative colitis of extensive linear distribution. Prophylactic diagnostic measures such as yearly colonoscopy are indicated after 8 to 10 years of universal disease and after 15 to 20 years of left-sided disease. Properly taken multiple biopsies, when expertly interpreted for dysplasia, are helpful in predicting the patient at very high risk for malignant degeneration. The incidence of malignant degeneration in Crohn's disease, although the risk is increased, is far less.

Thromboembolic Disease. A dreaded complication of the seriously ill patient with IIBD. Pulmonary emboli may be the first indication of lower extremity or pelvic phlebitis.

Fistula in Ano and Perirectal Abscess. Far more common in Crohn's disease, particularly if of the multiple tract variety. Abscess in the supralevator space usually lacks a cutaneous tract and presents with high fever and severe perirectal pain.

Internal Fistulas. A complication of Crohn's disease, and never of ulcerative colitis. The most common are ileoileal and ileosigmoid fistulas, which rarely give rise to significant symptoms. Fistulas between the proximal small bowel and the colon, however, may cause severe diarrhea due to bacterial overgrowth of the small intestine.

Choledocholithiasis. A complication of the small bile salt pool consequent upon a diseased or surgically removed distal ileum in Crohn's disease.

Renal Calculi. Oxalate stones due to excessive absorption of dietary oxalate in the patient with small bowel CD and steatorrhea.

Growth Retardation. A dreaded complication of childhood CD, usually in the presence of extensive small bowel disease and/or strictures, but may be seen in colonic disease, either Crohn's or ulcerative colitis. A consequence of poor caloric intake, malabsorption, and/or long-term steroid therapy. Failure of sexual maturation is a feature of the syndrome. The complication of growth retardation should be addressed vigorously prior to epiphyseal closure.

Acute Psychosis. A self-limiting state of severe withdrawal during a period of acute exacerbation of IIBD, usually in a setting of increased steroid dosage.

PHYSICAL FINDINGS

The findings on physical examination will understandably vary with the anatomic distribution, activity, extragastrointestinal manifestations, and complications. Patients with Crohn's disease of the ileocecal region very commonly have right lower quadrant pain and a tender mass. Palpable, bowel-related abdominal masses are not present in ulcerative colitis. A nodular, cobblestone mucosa on rectal examination is diagnostic of Crohn's proctitis. Large, flat, hypertrophied anal skin tags ("elephant ears") are characteristic of Crohn's disease, as is the intractable fistula in ano, although neither finding is diagnostic.

DIAGNOSTIC PROCEDURES

Rigid Tube Sigmoidoscopy. Permits evaluation of the rectum and distal sigmoid with minimal or no clean-out in a sick patient. A distinction between ulcerative colitis, marked by diffuse friability in the absence of discrete ulcers, and Crohn's proctitis, characterized by thickened, nodular mucosa ("cobblestoning") with discrete ulcers often of the aphthous type, can usually be made. In addition, the rigid tube permits an adequate evaluation of the anal canal—fissures and ulcers of the canal are far more common in Crohn's disease. Furthermore, rigid tube examination permits a more satisfactory collection of exudate for microscopic and microbiologic examinations (see below) than does flexible tube examination.

Colonoscopy. Of value particularly in segmental and proximal colitis if the barium enema is negative or equivocal. May have a role in establishing the linear extent of the disease in ulcerative colitis for therapeutic purposes. Hazardous in the acutely ill patient and contraindicated in fulminant disease. A much abused modality in IIBD.

Radiology. The gas pattern of an abdominal flat film may suggest the linear extent of IIBD, particularly in far advanced or fulminant disease, without resorting to contrast study. It is essential for evaluation of suspected perforation and toxic megacolon.

Barium enema usually establishes the linear distribution of pathology, except in low-grade disease, where the contrast study may be negative. It often permits differentiation of ulcerative colitis from Crohn's colitis. The latter is characterized by deep, undermining ulcers on barium silhouette; cobblestoning, long linear ulcers and tiny aphthous ulcers on air-contrast study; and (benign) strictures. Ulcerative colitis is characterized by fine serrations on barium silhouette and multiple (pseudo)polyps; strictures in this disease are malignant until proven otherwise.

As is true of colonoscopy, once the diagnosis has been established, barium enema tends to be an overused procedure in managing patients with IIBD and may be hazardous. It is absolutely contraindicated in very active or fulminant disease. In the face of mild to moderate activity, laxative preparation should be minimized or avoided completely; limiting the diet to fluids for 48 hours, including semi-elemental liquid food supplements, plus a gentle enema, often suffice. The main indication for barium enema in the previously diagnosed patient is to determine possible change in linear distribution or development of malignancy when there has been a clear change in bowel pattern. If the patient is too ill for barium enema, the colon may be studied from above by taking appropriately timed films after ingestion of barium; no cleanout preparation is necessary except for 48 hours of oral fluids as described. Cancer surveillance is best accomplished by colonoscopy rather than contrast study. Water-soluble contrast studies are absolutely contraindicated in patients with inflammatory bowel disease because they may precipitate a fulminant state as a result of both local irritation from the iodide and hyperosmolarity. In addition, the study is often grossly misleading because of osmotic distortion.

Small bowel series is both safe and essential for confirmation of small bowel CD except for the patient with an acute abdomen. Enteric fistulas must be carefully searched for on contrast study. Water-soluble contrast study from above is contraindicated in Crohn's disease, for reasons listed earlier.

PITFALLS IN DIAGNOSIS

Ulcerative colitis and Crohn's disease must be distinguished from "specific" enterocolitides, such as amebiasis, shigellosis, yersinosis, Campylobacter colitis, gonorrheal proctitis, and antibiotic-associated enterocolitis (pseudomembranous enterocolitis), since specific medications are available for these conditions. Furthermore, corticosteroid therapy is hazardous in the specific enterocolitides.

All patients with an initial episode of suspected ulcerative colitis or Crohn's disease should be screened as follows:

1. At least three fresh stools for ova and parasites examined by an experienced parasitology technician or, preferably, examination of endoscopically collected exudate. In extensive linear disease, a serologic test for amebiasis; although a positive test may reflect old, cured infection, a negative result may be helpful in pointing away from amebiasis. Endoscopic biopsy material should be stained (periodic acid–Schiff) for amebae.
2. Stool cultures, properly and promptly plated, for the usual enteric pathogens, as well as Yersinia and Campylobacter.
3. If the linear distribution is limited to the rectum and homosexuality and/or anal intercourse is suspected, rectal exudate is promptly placed on Thayer-Martin medium for gonococcus culture.
4. In a setting of recent antibiotic therapy, as well as in the deteriorating patient with CUC or CD who has been on antibiotics, cytopathic neutralization test for *Clostridium difficile,* if available, or a therapeutic trial of either vancomycin (Vancocin) or metronidazole (Flagyl) is indicated for the possibility of pseudomembranous enterocolitis.
5. A simple smear of rectal exudate or liquid stool diluted with a few drops of saline and stained with methylene blue. The presence of leukocytes serves to *rule out* the secretory diarrheas that often confound the diagnosis of CD.
6. Ischemic bowel disease is a serious differential consideration in the older patient. Despite the observation that most cases of ischemic colitis do not involve the rectum because of hemorrhoidal collaterals, the patient with significant ischemic disease of the lower extremities, as manifested by poor or absent femoral pulses, may develop ischemic proctitis. Under these circumstances, endoscopic appearance cannot be relied on to distinguish ischemic colitis from ulcerative colitis. Characteristic "thumbprinting" of the colon on abdominal flat films is supportive but not diagnostic of the former. Selective mesenteric angiography is helpful in large vessel disease, but is of little use in either small vessel disease or pump failure. In brief, a high index of suspicion of ischemic colitis is warranted in the older individual with a first episode of "ulcerative colitis."
7. Intestinal lymphoma may be limited to the distal ileum, particularly in children. Differentiation from CD is difficult, unless scalloping of the barium silhouette, a radiologic characteristic of lymphoma, is present or unless other features of the illness point to one disease or the other.
8. Intestinal tuberculosis typically involves the ileocecal region without necessarily being accompanied by radiologic evidence of pulmonary tuberculosis. Associated spasm of the supravalvular portion of the cecum (Stirlin's sign) suggests tuberculosis, and colonoscopic biopsy may be helpful. A therapeutic trial of antituberculous therapy is sometimes indicated.

WHIPPLE'S DISEASE

By David F. Keren, M.D.
Ann Arbor, Michigan

DEFINITION

Whipple's disease is a rare systemic disorder that usually has its major manifestations in the gastrointestinal tract. Histologic examination of the gut mucosa discloses the presence of massive numbers of large, foamy, periodic acid–Schiff (PAS)-positive macrophages in the lamina propria. Sometimes the disease is focal and uninvolved villi may be seen. In rare reports, the lamina propria has been uninvolved and the foamy, PAS-positive macrophages are seen only in the submucosa. Regional lymph nodes also contain the foamy PAS-positive macrophages.

The etiology of Whipple's disease is, as yet, unknown. Electron microscopic studies have demonstrated that rod-shaped bacillary bodies measuring approximately 0.25 × 1.5 microns are present within the foamy macrophages and extracellularly in involved tissues. While there has been some debate that several different microorganisms can cause Whipple's disease, this is not the case. The measurements on electron microscopy are relatively constant. Furthermore, an antigenic profile has been described that is also a consistent feature from case to case (Table 1).

The immune system has been thoroughly studied in several patients with Whipple's disease. Most studies agree that there is a decrease in the total number of

Table 1. Reactivity of Bacterial Grouping Antisera with Foamy Macrophage in Whipple's Disease

Antisera to	Case 1	Case 2	Case 3	Control Case
Streptococcus Group A	3*	3	3	0
Streptococcus Group B	3	3	3	0
Streptococcus Group C	1	3	2	0
Streptococcus Group D	1	2	1	0
Streptococcus Group F	0	1	1	0
Streptococcus Group G	4	4	4	0
Shigella A	0	0	0	0
Shigella B	3	3	4	0
Arizona	0	0	0	0
Salmonella polyvalent	0	0	0	0

*Intensity of fluorescence in macrophage graded from 0 to 4+.

T lymphocytes in the peripheral blood of these individuals during active and sometimes inactive Whipple's disease. However, there is much disagreement on whether or not mitogenic responses of the peripheral blood lymphocytes are normal in these individuals. Some reports have found decreased responses to phytohemagglutinin, conconavalin A, and pokeweed mitogen. Other laboratories have refuted these results. It is clear, however, that there is not an overwhelming T or B cell deficiency in these individuals.

Nonetheless, most workers suppose Whipple's disease to be of infectious etiology. Not only are the bacillary bodies always present and always with the same antigenic profile (Table 1) but the disease consistently responds to antibiotic therapy with penicillin, chloramphenicol and sometimes tetracycline.

The lack of an identifiable etiologic agent has been variously attributed to difficulties growing cell wall–defective microorganisms or highly fastidious anaerobic bacteria, which have been suggested as causative agents. The rarity of the disease, together with limited availability of sophisticated microbiologic techniques to perform such cultures, has limited study of the etiologic agent.

PRESENTING SIGNS AND SYMPTOMS

Whipple's disease occurs primarily in previously healthy, middle-aged males. The earliest sign is often a migratory polyarthritis characterized by pain, swelling, tenderness, and warmth over the involved joints. Involvement of serosal surfaces, including pericarditis, pleuritis, and peritonitis, occur, although much less frequently than joint symptoms in patients with Whipple's disease.

Typically, patients do not seek medical attention until they have suffered considerable weight loss due to diarrhea and malabsorption, which often result in a picture of cachexia. Other common presenting features include hyperpigmentation in sun-exposed areas, fever, hypotension, lymphadenopathy, abdominal pain, and central nervous system complaints often referring to personality changes.

The cachexia and extreme weight loss are due to the presence of malabsorption. D-Xylose absorption is frequently decreased as indicated either by inadequate serum levels or poor excretion after a standard oral dose. In addition, fecal fat excretion usually is increased, further confirming the malabsorption. The malabsorption is thought to be due to the physical presence of foamy macrophages with disturbed absorption of nutrients. Also, most of these individuals suffer a protein-losing enteropathy that has been attributed to lymphatic obstruction.

COMPLICATIONS

Many of the complications of Whipple's disease are secondary to the severe malabsorption. These include hypoalbuminemia, anemia, and a prolonged prothrombin time. In addition, patients with Whipple's disease are apt to develop central nervous system symptoms, including personality changes, abnormal reflexes, and impaired vision. These complications relate to involvement of the central nervous system by focal aggregates of the PAS-positive macrophages with focal demyelination. Such central nervous system symptomatology most often occurs when Whipple's disease relapses owing to inadequate treatment. The migratory polyarthritis, which usually involves larger joints, may occur years before the gastrointestinal symptoms become manifest. Articular damage is not found in these cases. Bacillary bodies have been demonstrated to be present in some involved synovial membranes. The hyperpigmentation in Whipple's disease has not been associated with adrenal insufficiency.

DIAGNOSIS

The diagnosis is based upon histologic examination of involved tissues. Most often, this will include a biopsy of the gut mucosa. Usually, biopsies of the small bowel have been the most useful. PAS-positive macrophages can be seen in colonic mucosa of individuals with other disorders. Although the PAS-positive macrophages in the lamina propria of the small bowel are highly suggestive of Whipple's disease, it may be best to perform an antigenic profile in some patients. Recently, patients with the acquired immune deficiency syndrome (AIDS) have been shown to develop gastrointestinal infections with *Mycobacterium avium.* These individuals have the histologic picture of active Whipple's disease with foamy, PAS-positive macrophages stuffing the lamina propria. However, dilated lymphatic channels are not usually seen in these latter patients. An antigenic profile as shown in Table 1 can help distinguish *M. avium*–induced or other non-specific foamy macrophages from those cells involved with Whipple's disease.

LABORATORY FINDINGS

As a result of the malabsorption, several laboratory parameters will be disturbed in these patients. Most patients have a decrease in serum albumin, calcium, and cholesterol, and show an abnormal D-xylose absorption. Hematologic abnormalities include a prolonged prothrombin time, decreased hematocrit and hemoglobin, decreased red blood cell count, and, in some individuals, a striking thrombocytosis with as many as 1,142,000 platelets per cu mm preceding the diagnosis of Whipple's disease. These laboratory abnormalities virtually all resolve with therapy.

ENDOSCOPIC FEATURES

The villi in Whipple's disease are markedly thickened and occasionally club-shaped. The endoscopic corollary of the thickened enlarged villi is a yellow-white granular appearance of the mucosal surface. Occasionally, these thickened villi appear to be yellow-white granules that are lying on top of the mucosa. Interestingly, similar "grains" were described by Whipple in the original case. Study by dissecting microscopy reveals grossly enlarged and distorted villi. Some have likened the appearance of these villi to the pile of a shag rug. By directing endoscopic biopsies to these granular areas, the likelihood of diagnosing Whipple's disease is increased.

LIGHT MICROSCOPIC FEATURES

The lamina propria is usually overstuffed with foamy macrophages, occasional giant cells, and neutrophils. Dilated lymphatic channels and fat droplets further distort the shape of the villi. In many cases, the foamy macrophages can also be found in the submucosa and infiltrating the muscularis propria. The latter feature is important because, rarely, the lamina propria is not involved and the main involvement of Whipple's disease is in the submucosa. Tragically, if the submucosa is not examined in such cases, the diagnosis of Whipple's disease may be missed with fatal results. Foamy macrophages have been found in virtually every organ of the body in one case report or another, emphasizing the systemic nature of Whipple's disease.

THERAPY

Antibiotics are universally successful in treating Whipple's disease. However, it is notable that a wide variety of antibiotics have been used in treating Whipple's disease, such as chloramphenicol, tetracycline, ampicillin, penicillin, and streptomycin, either singly or in various combinations. Early attempts at therapy with adrenocorticotropic hormone (ACTH) and steroids gave only transient symptomatic relief in some cases, but was clearly ineffective in eradicating the infection. Whichever regimen is used, antibiotic treatment of Whipple's disease needs to proceed for a long term because many cases of relapse have been found when therapy was given only for short periods.

PITFALLS IN DIAGNOSIS

Although the histopathologic features of Whipple's disease seem to be pathognomonic, they are not. Foamy macrophages of Whipple's disease merely reflect the fact that the macrophages have engulfed large numbers of microorganisms. Similar foamy macrophages can occur in other infectious processes. Infection with *M. avium* closely resembles Whipple's disease. Since the PAS staining is due to the presence of bacterial glycoprotein, both would be PAS-positive. For specificity, when one is dealing with a possible AIDS patient, acid-fast staining and immunohistologic identification of the antigenic profile shown in Table 1 should be carried out.

When the small bowel biopsy is normal in a patient suspected of having Whipple's disease, the diagnosis has not been excluded. Whipple's disease may be patchy. It is important to direct the endoscopist to biopsy the granular yellow-white areas seen through the endoscope in many cases of Whipple's disease. Whipple's disease may exist in the submucosa and may present primarily with central nervous system manifestation. Characteristic foamy macrophages can be found in some peripheral lymph nodes, and this should be remembered when studying biopsies from individuals suspected of having Whipple's disease. Again, an antigenic pattern profile can help in establishing this diagnosis.

Last, it should be stressed that antigen pattern profiling can be performed on routine formalin-fixed paraffin-embedded tissues. This should allow the pathologist to retrospectively examine tissues involved with foamy macrophages for the presence of Whipple's disease.

GLUTEN-SENSITIVE ENTEROPATHY

By Z. Myron Falchuk, M.D.
Boston, Massachusetts

SYNONYMS

Celiac disease, celiac-sprue disease, non-tropical sprue, gluten-induced enteropathy.

DEFINITION

Gluten-sensitive enteropathy is a disease of the small intestine that results from a unique sensitivity to dietary gluten. The entire small bowel is susceptible to damage characterized by extensive injury to the villus epithelial cells, loss of villus height, and dense inflammation of the lamina propria with infiltration by plasma cells and lymphocytes. The pathologic changes in the small intestine are responsible for the malabsorption and the clinical presentation, since there is interference with normal absorptive capacity. Release of pancreatic and biliary secretions may also be impaired because of deficiencies of pancreozymin-cholecystokinin. The distal small intestine frequently is less abnormal, since gluten is degraded and rendered "harmless" as it travels down the digestive tube. This feature may account in part for some of the clinical vagaries of the disease. The disease is worldwide in distribution, but is rare in Blacks and Orientals.

PATHOGENESIS

The pathogenesis remains elusive, but two general theories exist. One is that deficiency of a peptidase enzyme may give rise to toxic gluten breakdown intermediates; there is little support for this theory. Alternatively, the immune system may give rise to injurious reactions, damaging the surface epithelial cells. Antigluten antibodies as well as sensitized T cells and lymphokine are produced by the intestinal mucosa of patients. These immune products are potentially cytotoxic and have been studied extensively in vitro. Genetic factors are also important since two HLA genes, HLA-B8 and DRW3, are present with markedly increased incidence. A third non-HLA-linked gene is also present in patients.

PRESENTING SIGNS AND SYMPTOMS

The disease typically presents in infancy, after weaning and introduction of cereals into the diet. Wheat, rye, and barley glutens, but probably not oat, are injurious to patients. The peak incidence occurs between the ages of 9 months and 3 years, with a second peak noted in the third decade. Many of the patients who develop the disease later in life have been completely asymptomatic despite evidence that the intestinal lesion is present since weaning. The typical features of the disease are those of the malabsorption syndrome. All nutrients may be malabsorbed. Patients may manifest one or all the features of the syndrome, including diarrhea with foul bulky stools, weight loss, irritability, failure to thrive, tetany, edema, easy bruising, night blindness, bleeding, anemia, osteomalacia, rickets, and iron deficiency. Patients with only a single deficit may be difficult to diagnose. The brush border enzymes are deficient, and lactase deficiency will aggravate the diarrhea. Abdominal pain is rare, but bloating and flatulence are frequent. Neuropathy can occur secondary to vitamin deficiency. Occasionally patients may be constipated.

COURSE

The disease is progressive and can result in death if it remains severe and undiagnosed. Patients have ravenous appetites, compensating for the malabsorbed calories. The start of a gluten-free diet is usually accompanied by a sense of well-being within 48 to 72 hours. The various clinical manifestations may take weeks or months to disappear as the intestinal lesion heals. Restriction of gluten must be complete, since even a small amount of gluten will prevent healing. Once the lesion has healed, some patients will tolerate an occasional indiscretion, while others will have explosive return of symptoms with the smallest amount of gluten.

The disease is sometimes precipitated by gastric surgery and may occur in association with IgA deficiency, juvenile diabetes mellitus, or dermatitis herpetiformis. The latter group of patients has a pruritic skin disease which will show improvement on a gluten-free diet. Their intestinal problem is usually mild.

PHYSICAL EXAMINATION

The physical examination correlates with the degree and severity of malabsorption. In mild cases, it may be normal. Positive findings may include loss of subcutaneous fat, muscle wasting, pedal edema, glossitis and cheilitis, hypotonia, irritability, dry skin, ecchymoses, abdominal distention, and increased bowel sounds. Short stature may be noted, and signs of tetany may be elicited.

COMPLICATIONS

Complications of the disease may be divided between those which are related to the underlying malabsorption, such as bone fractures, hemorrhage, and neuropathy, and those which are incidental to the disease. These include lymphoma and carcinoma of the bowel as well as ulcerative jejunoileitis. The latter may perforate or hemorrhage with dire consequences. In some patients refractory sprue may develop with malabsorption recurring despite a gluten-free diet.

LABORATORY PROCEDURES

The diagnosis is established by a constellation of features. The most important test is small intestine biopsy, which may be obtained with the peroral instrument. The initial biopsy has typical (but nondiagnostic) features of villus flattening, epithelial cell distortion with change from columnar to cuboidal appearance, lamina propria inflammation, and increased crypt mitotic activity. These features disappear with a gluten-free diet, usually within 3 to 6 months, and recur with a short gluten challenge. These three biopsies—before and after a gluten-free diet and after a gluten challenge—must be done to be certain of the diagnosis.

Other laboratory tests include fecal fat measurement. Stool is collected for 3 days while the patient is on a measured fat intake of greater than 70 grams per day. Significant steatorrhea is greater than 7 grams per day. Qualitative assessment of steatorrhea may be made by microscopic examination of stool stained with Sudan III. The D-xylose tolerance test is helpful in distinguishing pancreatic insufficiency with steatorrhea from gluten-sensitive enteropathy. In the former, the D-xylose test is normal; in the latter, it is decreased. Twenty-five grams of xylose are ingested and the urine is collected for the next 5 hours; 4.5 grams of xylose are usually excreted. Since renal disease, gastric atony, ascites, and myxedema may decrease urinary excretion of xylose, a 2-hour blood value should be determined. Normal values are 20 mg/dl or greater. Other tests such as serum cholesterol, carotene, iron, folate, and vitamin B_{12} values are nonspecific and may be abnormal in any malabsorptive disorder.

RADIOLOGIC EVALUATION

The small intestine in patients with malabsorption is generally dilated and filled with fluid. Consequently, one may see these features on the contrast x-ray. Edema will make the folds coarse, and the mucosal pattern will be effaced. The proximal bowel is usually more greatly affected.

OTHER DIAGNOSTIC PROCEDURES

Organ culture of small bowel biopsy in the presence of gluten will duplicate the disease in vitro and may obviate the need for gluten challenge to prove the diagnosis. Human leukocyte antigen (HLA) typing of relatives of patients may identify persons at risk of having clinically undetected disease.

POTENTIAL ERRORS AND PITFALLS IN DIAGNOSIS

The flat intestinal lesion occurs in various other disorders associated with malabsorption syndrome. These include tropical sprue, collagenous sprue, eosinophilic enteritis, agammaglobulinemia, intestinal lymphoma, soy protein allergy, acute viral gastroenteritis, chronic diarrhea of infancy, and giardiasis. Unless the initial diagnosis is confirmed by gluten challenge, a misdiagnosis may result. Lack of response to a gluten-free diet should suggest inadvertent gluten ingestion or a misdiagnosis as the cause. Loss of control in a previously well-controlled patient suggests the onset of a complication such as lymphoma or refractory sprue.

INTESTINAL DISACCHARIDASE DEFICIENCY

By Albert D. Newcomer, M.D.
and Douglas B. McGill, M.D.
Rochester, Minnesota

The disaccharidase enzymes, located in the brush border membrane of the small intestine, hydrolyze di- and oligosaccharides to their component monosaccharides. These include *glucose* and *galactose,* which are actively absorbed, and *fructose,* which is absorbed by facilitated diffusion. Isolated deficiencies of *lactase,* the *sucrase-isomaltase* complex, and *trehalase* may result in intestinal symptoms if sufficient substrate is ingested. Since *maltase* is a composite of several enzymes, clinically significant isolated deficiency of maltase has not been reported.

LACTASE DEFICIENCY

Physiology

Lactose, produced in nature only in the mammary gland of mammals, is hydrolyzed by lactase in the small intestine to glucose and galactose. In contrast to the process with other disaccharides, this hydrolytic step, rather than absorption, is rate-limiting. The crypt cells in the base of the villi contain no lactase, but lactase activity appears as they ascend the villi, with maximum activity in the upper one third to one half of the villus. During the 3- to 4-day life span of the epithelial cells, lactase activity is continually lost and replaced by newly synthesized enzyme. There is also a prominent gradient of enzyme activity along the small intestine with maximum levels achieved in the middle small intestine. A number of intraluminal factors influence activity of lactase. The pH optimum for lactase activity, as well as for the absorption of glucose and galactose, is about 6.0. Thus, hypersecretion of acid inhibits the absorption of lactose. Pancreatic proteolytic enzymes (especially elastase), bile acids, and lysolecithin also influence disaccharidase levels by removing the proteins from the cell membrane and degrading them. Thus, patients with pancreatic exocrine insufficiency have elevated levels of disaccharidases. Another intraluminal factor that apparently lowers disaccharidase activities is the presence of bacteria.

The developmental pattern of lactase activity is genetically programmed. In man, lactase appears in the small intestine toward the end of the first trimester and reaches maximum activity at the time of birth. It remains at this high level through early childhood, but in about 70 per cent of the world's population it declines to a residual level of 5 to 10 per cent, generally before the age of 5 to 6 years but occasionally in the teens and even as late as age 20. A minority of persons maintain high levels of lactase throughout adulthood. This latter group comes primarily from northern and western Europe and includes their overseas descendants.

The "normal" decline in lactase is genetically determined by an autosomal recessive mechanism and is not influenced by dietary lactose. Also, in adults who have either low or persistently high levels of lactase, lactose feeding or deprivation has no effect on the level of lactase activity. In man, there is no evidence that lactase activity is inducible. The rate at which lactase enzyme decreases during early childhood is not known, but in baboons the decline occurs over a number of months. Although definitive studies have not been done, the 5 to 10 per cent residual lactase appears to be identical in structure to the original enzyme present at birth. Almost all other land mammals that have been studied follow this same pattern, with loss of lactase activity following weaning.

Definition

The ultimate definition of lactase deficiency is dependent on the level of mucosal lactase activity and should not be defined in terms of degree of intolerance to lactose. Measurement of lactase activity and determination of the sucrase-lactase ratio of biopsies taken from a standardized location, such as near the ligament of Treitz, provide good separation of subjects into those with low and those with persistently high lactase. In clinical practice, biopsies and assessment of enzyme activity are rarely necessary.

Terminology

The use of various terms for this hereditary delayed-onset loss of lactase activity has caused considerable confusion. Terms such as "lactase deficiency," "hypolactasia," and "hereditary loss of lactase" are preferable because they accurately describe the basic mechanism. "Lactase deficiency" should not be used in the sense of an abnormal state because the aberrant course is actually persistence of lactase activity throughout adulthood. The normal state for man and other land mammals is loss of lactase after weaning. "Alactasia" is inaccurate in that there is 5 to 10 per cent residual enzyme activity. The terms "nondigestion" and "lactose malabsorption" describe the results rather than the primary cause of the condition. These terms are somewhat imprecise, since a number of gastrointestinal states in which lactase activity is normal can be associated with diminished lactose digestion and absorption (e.g., congenital glucose-galactose malabsorption, postgastric surgery, and the short bowel syndrome). The term "lactose intolerance" is frequently used synonymously with the low-lactase state. "Tolerance" and "intolerance" should be used in reference to the symptomatic response of an individual to a defined load of lactose. For example, a lactase-deficient subject may be "tolerant" to one glass of milk and "intolerant" to two glasses. Use of the term "adult lactase deficiency" is confusing, for in most population groups the decline in lactase activity occurs in early childhood. "Milk intolerance" is another imprecise term that is used. A subject with milk intolerance could have any one of several problems, such as low lactase activity, sensitivity to milk protein, malabsorption of glucose-galactose or intolerance to fat.

Geographic Distribution

An intriguing variation in the prevalence of lactase deficiency has been noted in different parts of the world and among various ethnic groups. The prevalence ranges from 1 or 2 per cent among Scandinavians to 99 or 100 per cent among Orientals. With several exceptions, the only populations that maintain lactase are Caucasians living in northern and western Europe and their overseas descendants. The majority of people in almost all other ethnic groups lose lactase activity in childhood. This means that with a high prevalence of lactase deficiency among Blacks, Orientals, Jews, American Indians, and so on, at least 70 per cent of the world's population lose lactase activity in childhood.

How has this peculiar geographic distribution of lactase deficiency arisen? Simoons (1970) observed that groups who have used milk for thousands of years are also those that maintain lactase activity. He postulated that before the introduction of dairying, man followed the same developmental pattern of lactase loss as in other land mammals. With the domestication of animals between 8000 and 4000 B.C., man began using milk in his diet. Simoons proposes that a mutation occurred that resulted in retention of high activity of lactase throughout adulthood. This would provide a selective advantage during periods when food supply was marginal because the person could tolerate more milk as well as digest and absorb more lactose. It has been estimated that if parents with high activity of lactase produced 1 to 3 per cent more children each generation than did parents with lactase deficiency, the current gene distribution could have developed.

Classification

Since lactase does not reach peak activity until birth, the premature infant is born with a relative deficiency of lactase. The clinical significance of *lactase deficiency in prematurity* is questionable, since these infants generally gain weight normally on milk feedings.

Congenital lactase deficiency is extremely rare and is inherited by an autosomal recessive mechanism. In a few patients who have had small intestine biopsies, lactase activity is either undetectable or extremely low, much lower than the 5 to 10 per cent level found in subjects with hereditary delayed-onset lactase deficiency. Studies to date have shown no qualitative differences between the lactase found in adults with persistently high activity and the residual lactase found in subjects with congenital lactase deficiency. In infants with congenital lactase deficiency, diarrhea develops as soon as milk feedings begin and these infants may die from dehydration if the condition is not recognized. The clinical setting is identical to that in congenital glucose-galactose malabsorption; and unless both lactose tolerance and glucose-galactose tolerance tests are done, the correct diagnosis may be missed.

A third type of lactase deficiency is seen in patients with mucosal disease or after removal of a portion of the small intestine. Compared with other disaccharidases, lactase seems to be the most vulnerable to mucosal disease. With damage to the mucosa, as in celiac disease or tropical sprue, lactase is the first to decline and the last to return to normal after treatment. This will directly affect lactose absorption, since hydrolysis is the rate-limiting step. Probably the most common type of *secondary lactase deficiency* occurs in young children with infectious gastroenteritis. Lactase, being the most vulnerable of the various disaccharidases, may remain deficient for several months. An interesting type of secondary lactase deficiency may occur in infants with milk-protein sensitivity and diffuse enteropathy. Another mechanism for insufficient lactase activity is found in patients with a short bowel syndrome. The activity of lactase may be normal on biopsy, but the total amount of enzyme in the entire small intestine may not be sufficient for hydrolysis of a lactose load.

Finally, lactase deficiency may be of the *hereditary delayed-onset variety,* which is the major focus of this article. This type of low-lactase state is inherited by an autosomal recessive mechanism and, of course, the corollary is that persistently high lactase activity is an autosomal dominant trait.

Cause of Symptoms

If the small intestine contains insufficient lactase activity to hydrolyze an ingested load of lactose, the unabsorbed sugar remains in the lumen of the intestine and acts osmotically to retain water. Between 15 and 30 minutes after a lactose load, the person with lactase deficiency may experience symptoms of bloating, cramping, and borborygmi secondary to the osmotic force of lactose within the small intestine. Later, after perhaps 1 to 2 hours, the lactose passes into the colon and is metabolized by bacteria to smaller molecules, such as carbon dioxide, hydrogen, and fatty acids, which further increase the osmotic force and may cause additional bloating and cramping as well as diarrhea and flatus.

Diagnosis

In clinical practice, it is rarely necessary to do a small bowel biopsy and lactase assay in order to diagnose lactase deficiency. In fact, in many instances, either exclusion of milk for a trial period of 1 to 2 weeks or a milk challenge will answer the question of lactase deficiency. If a definite answer is necessary, several screening tests are available.

Lactose Tolerance Test

This test is performed by giving a loading dose of lactose, 2 gm/kg (maximum 50 gm), orally. Serial capillary plasma glucoses are determined over 2 hours (0, 15, 30, 60, 90, and 120 minutes). An increase in the plasma level of glucose of 20 to 25 mg/dl is generally considered the dividing line between a "normal" and a flat curve. Unfortunately, delayed gastric emptying or rapid glucose metabolism can cause a flat curve and thus a false-positive diagnosis of lactase deficiency. On the other hand, the postgastric surgery state with accelerated emptying or diabetes mellitus can cause a normal increase in plasma glucose in patients with lactase deficiency, a false-negative result. Use of venous blood in the lactose tolerance test can result in up to 28 per cent flat curves in subjects without lactase deficiency. By use of capillary blood in the lactose tolerance test, the false-positive flat curves can be largely eliminated, but a significant overlap occurs between 20 and 30 mg/dl. Thus, the lactose tolerance test can be useful if capillary blood is used and a rise in plasma glucose between 20 and 30 mg/dl is considered indeterminate. The symptomatic response to the 50-gm lactose load correlates only roughly with the level of lactase activity. Significant gastrointestinal symptoms will develop in 80 to 100 per cent of lactase-deficient subjects, but about 20 per cent of lactase-sufficient subjects also experience symptoms. If malabsorption of monosaccharides is suspected, a glucose-galactose tolerance test should be done.

Hydrogen Breath Test

Bacteria in the colon are capable of metabolizing unabsorbed nutrients, especially carbohydrates, to hydrogen, which diffuses into the blood and appears in the breath. No mammalian cell has the necessary enzymes to produce hydrogen; thus, any hydrogen that appears in the breath indicates that unabsorbed nutrients have come into contact with large numbers of intestinal bacteria. The number of bacteria in the lumen of the normal small intestine is inadequate to produce measurable amounts of hydrogen in the breath.

The standard way of conducting the hydrogen breath test is to give 50 gm of oral lactose in 250 to 500 ml of water. Breath collections are made at 0 time and at intervals for 4 hours. Breath hydrogen is then measured by means of gas chromatography. The breath can be collected as a single expired sample, which provides results in terms of hydrogen concentration; values of ≥ 20 parts per million (ppm) above the fasting level indicate lactase deficiency.

The hydrogen breath test does not share some of the pitfalls of the lactose tolerance test, in that it does not depend on either the rate of gastric emptying, at least to any great extent, or the rate of glucose metabolism. Instead of measuring the carbohydrate absorbed, as in the lactose tolerance test, the hydrogen breath test depends on the amount of lactose that is malabsorbed, which should be the major focus—since it is the malabsorbed lactose that produces symptoms in lactase deficiency. Subjects undergoing the hydrogen breath test should not smoke before breath collections because tobacco smoke contains hydrogen.

In summary, as a screening test for lactase deficiency, the hydrogen breath test is relatively simple to conduct, noninvasive, and applicable to infants, children, and adults. It appears to be the most accurate screening test available and is superior to the lactose tolerance test and other screening tests.

Fecal pH

The metabolic breakdown products of lactose in the colon include short-chain fatty acids, which may cause a decrease in stool pH. After an oral lactose load, a decrease in pH below 6.0 generally indicates malabsorption of carbohydrate. The test is useful in children, but many false-negative results have been observed in adults. Significant absorption of short-chain fatty acids in the colon probably accounts for these false-negative tests.

Significance

The range of tolerance to lactose is extremely wide among persons with lactase deficiency. Between 80 and 100 per cent of such individuals are intolerant to non-physiologic load of 50 gm of lactose, the amount in one quart of milk. At the other end of the spectrum, milligram amounts of lactose (as in tablets) occasionally have been reported to cause symptoms; however, these anecdotal accounts are poorly substantiated. The critical question is: "What proportion of persons with lactase deficiency are symptomatic after a physiologic load of 12 gm of lactose, equivalent to 1 glass of milk?" Although the literature is controversial on this point, most studies have concluded that the majority of persons with lactase deficiency can drink 1 glass of milk without significant symptoms, especially if the milk is taken with a meal, which would delay gastric emptying of lactose. For reasons that are unclear, children with lactase deficiency tend to be more tolerant of lactose than do adults with lactase deficiency. In subjects with lactase deficiency, the tolerance to lactose increases after ingestion of milk for several weeks.

It is not uncommon for subjects with inherited delayed-onset lactase deficiency to first become symptomatic in adulthood, even though the enzyme loss occurs in childhood. The reason for this delay in symptoms is not known. In some instances, a change in diet, which might include more milk as in pregnancy or in peptic ulcer treatment, brings out symptoms for the first time. Also, patients with lactase deficiency may become symptomatic after gastric surgery, because of accelerated emptying of the stomach. Physicians must be aware that lactase deficiency may be the basis for nonspecific gastrointestinal symptoms, such as abdominal pain, flatulence, borborygmi, bloating, and so forth; but, in fact, most persons with symptomatic lactase deficiency are already aware of intolerance to milk and already have consciously restricted milk to their level of tolerance. There was early hope that lactase deficiency would be a major cause of the irritable bowel syndrome; however, lactase deficiency rarely explains this disorder.

How much nutritional value do persons with lactase deficiency gain from milk? Although much of the lactose in milk is malabsorbed in the small intestine, as much as 85 per cent of the fatty acids produced in the colon by bacterial degradation of lactose is absorbed. The other two major sources of calories in milk, protein and fat, as well as calcium, are for all practical purposes absorbed normally. Postmenopausal women with osteoporosis have an increased prevalence of lactase deficiency which, in part, may relate to long-term diminished calcium intake.

Because of the high prevalence of lactase deficiency among persons in developing countries, the wisdom of providing milk supplements to bolster inadequate diets has been challenged. However, most studies have indicated that the majority of these people, and especially children, appear to tolerate modest amounts of milk when it is distributed throughout the day and given with meals. Nevertheless, the possibility of intolerance must be made known to both the distributors of the milk and the recipients. The Committee on Nutrition of the American Academy of Pediatrics recently concluded that "on the basis of present evidence it would be inappropriate to discourage supplemental milk feeding programs targeted at children on the basis of primary lactose intolerance."

Treatment requires that lactose be restricted to the tolerance level. This does not mean total elimination of lactose from the diet. Lactose-hydrolyzed milk can be produced by incubating milk with a commercial lactase, such as Lact-Aid. Also, fermented milk products, such as cheeses in which lactose has been removed or metabolized, can be used. Based on equivalent protein servings, yogurt has 75 per cent as much lactose as regular milk, cottage cheese 14 per cent and aged cheddar cheese 6 per cent.

SUCRASE-ISOMALTASE DEFICIENCY

Sucrase and isomaltase enzymes are contained in a single complex protein molecule. Sucrase hydrolyzes sucrose to glucose and fructose, and isomaltase hydrolyzes the α-1,6 cross-links of starch. Sucrase-isomaltase deficiency is inherited as an autosomal recessive trait. The onset of symptoms is generally early in life, although several subjects have had the onset during adulthood. The diagnosis can be made by a sucrose tolerance test, performed in the same way as the lactose tolerance test, the hydrogen breath test, and a small intestinal mucosal biopsy with enzyme assay.

TREHALASE DEFICIENCY

Trehalose is a disaccharide found in insects, algae, and mushrooms. Curiously, even though the disaccharide makes up only a tiny fraction of our diets, man has retained a disaccharidase to hydrolyze trehalose. Deficiency of the enzyme trehalase may become manifest as intestinal intolerance to mushrooms.

DIVERTICULAR DISEASE OF THE COLON

By Harold Tucker, M.D.
Baltimore, Maryland

Synonyms

Diverticulosis, diverticula, diverticulosis coli.

Definition

Diverticulosis of the colon refers to the presence of multiple diverticula or outpouchings of the mucosa through the colonic wall. *Diverticular disease* is the term applied to the wide spectrum of clinical conditions associated with colonic diverticulosis. As the pathogenesis and natural history of these various clinical syndromes probably vary, it is important to differentiate these differing expressions of diverticular disease. Asymptomatic diverticulosis is the most common condition and is most often a radiographic or anatomic observation of uncertain clinical significance. Symptomatic diverticular disease may take three forms:

1. An irritable bowel–like syndrome of abdominal pain and altered bowel habits.
2. Diverticulitis, a peridiverticular inflammatory process.
3. Diverticular hemorrhage, massive bleeding from one or more diverticula.

ASYMPTOMATIC DIVERTICULOSIS

The presence of asymptomatic diverticulosis is generally discovered during evaluation of an unrelated problem. It is estimated that four to five times as many cases of asymptomatic diverticulosis remain undetected than are actually diagnosed. The prevalence of diverticulosis increases with increasing age and reaches approximately 50 per cent in patients over 70 years of age. In these asymptomatic patients, physical examination and laboratory studies are unremarkable. Barium enema examination on such patients may demonstrate only a few diverticula, may show multiple diverticula localized to one area (massed diverticulosis), or may show diverticula widespread throughout the entire colon. The natural history of this condition is generally benign, with only about 25 per cent of patients ever experiencing a complication related to their diverticula. Because diverticulosis is very common, pitfalls lie in ascribing other problems to these asymptomatic diverticula.

SYMPTOMATIC DIVERTICULAR DISEASE

Synonyms

Diverticular spasm, painful diverticular disease.

Definition

Symptomatic diverticular disease is a condition characterized by localized abdominal pain associated with diverticulosis, without evidence of any peridiverticular inflammation.

Presenting Signs and Symptoms

The major symptom of this condition is abdominal pain, often associated with altered bowel habits. The abdominal pain is crampy and most often is localized to the left lower quadrant, over the sigmoid colon. During attacks, the patient may also experience constipation or diarrhea. These painful episodes are often fairly discrete and recurrent, but rarely continuous. Bleeding is not a feature of this condition unless it arises from concomitant rectal outlet conditions, such as hemorrhoids or cryptitis. The symptoms are very similar to those of the irritable bowel syndrome. The role of diet and emotions in this disorder is still unclear, but many patients relate an increase in painful episodes following ingestion of certain foods, particularly if fried and fatty, and during periods of increased stress.

The physical examination reveals tenderness over the involved area. A painful, firm cord of sigmoid colon generally can be palpated, but masses are not present. Fever is also notably absent in such cases. The stool is negative for occult blood. Proctoscopic examination is normal, but is often very uncomfortable, particularly if one attempts to reach 25 cm and uses air insufflation.

Course

Symptomatic diverticular disease is generally a chronic recurrent condition marked by painful episodes and symptom-free intervals. The frequency of painful attacks and the duration of symptom-free intervals are highly variable from patient to patient. For the majority of patients, the course is benign without significant morbidity or mortality. Generally, the area of involvement and the mode of presentation during the initial episode remain the same for all future symptomatic attacks, and rarely, if ever, do symptoms emanate from other segments of the colon other than those on the initial presentation. It is unclear whether other complications of diverticular disease, such as diverticulitis or diverticular hemorrhage, occur more commonly in this painful diverticular group than in the asymptomatic group.

There is no evidence that diverticulosis predisposes to colon cancer, although both conditions have been linked to low-fiber diets. Cholelithiasis and a hiatus hernia have been statistically linked with diverticulosis (Saint's triad), although all three conditions are seen with increasing frequency with increasing age of patients and are commonly discovered during evaluation of nonspecific abdominal symptoms.

Laboratory Evaluation

In this painful but noninflammatory condition, the white blood cell count and erythrocyte sedimentation rate (ESR) are normal. The hematocrit is also normal. Stool analysis is negative for occult blood and for enteric pathogens. Abnormalities in any of these laboratory studies should suggest another underlying process.

Radiologic Evaluation

The barium enema examination is the most common method of identifying diverticula. However, except for certain features indicative of diverticulitis (see Diverticulitis, Radiologic Evaluation, in the next section), the radiographic appearance of the colon cannot distinguish the symptomatic patient from the one with symptomatic diverticular disease. There is no correlation between the number or size or extent of the diverticula with the clinical presentation, except to confirm that the painful abdominal area is consistent with the colonic segment containing diverticula. The sigmoid is involved in 90 per cent of cases, accounting for the pain being most frequently encountered in the left lower quadrant. Symptoms may be more persistent and the pain somewhat more diffuse when diverticula occur throughout the entire colon. Evidence of spasm on barium enema examination is a nonspecific finding seen in both asymptomatic and symptomatic groups. Thickening of the muscular wall (myochosis) may be seen in association with the diverticula, but again, this does not correlate with symptoms. The presence of this muscular thickening and shortening in the sigmoid colon in the absence of diverticula has been termed "the prediverticular state."

Besides confirming the presence of diverticula, the barium enema is useful to exclude other causes of abdominal pain. Other conditions with clinical presentations similar to symptomatic diverticular disease include colonic carcinoma, ischemic colitis, and inflammatory bowel disease, particularly Crohn's disease. The radiologic evaluation can help differentiate among these various colonic disorders.

Other Diagnostic Tests

Colonoscopy is also useful in the evaluation of patients with symptomatic diverticular disease, both to diagnose diverticulosis and to exclude other causes for the patient's symptoms. Again, colonoscopy cannot differentiate symptomatic diverticulosis from the asymptomatic condition. Colonoscopy is indicated when the barium enema shows any mucosal abnormality other than the diverticulosis, or when there is less than an optimal study, as often happens when extensive diverticulosis or persistent spasm is encountered.

Proctosigmoidoscopy alone cannot diagnose diverticulosis because the instrument cannot reach far enough proximally to identify the diverticular opening. However, this method is valuable in identifying colonic mucosal disorders that may involve the rectum and rectosigmoid areas, such as ulcerative colitis and neoplastic lesions.

Potential Errors in Diagnosis

The major diagnostic dilemma in this condition is determining that the patient's complaints are in fact related to the diverticulosis and not due to some other underlying disorder with concomitant asymptomatic diverticulosis. This problem is accentuated by the fact that many of the differential diagnostic possibilities occur in the elderly, the same population who have increased prevalence of diverticulosis. In addition, many of these conditions also frequently affect the sigmoid colon, the area most commonly involved with diverticula. Thus, disorders like carcinoma, ischemic colitis, and Crohn's colitis may develop in the setting of pre-existing asymptomatic diverticulosis. Careful attention must therefore be paid to features atypical for symptomatic diverticulosis, such as occult blood loss or even mild hematochezia, weight loss, or an elevated ESR. Total reliance on a barium enema diagnosis of diverticulosis may lead one to overlook other potential problems.

DIVERTICULITIS

Synonyms

Acute diverticular inflammation, left-sided appendicitis.

Definition

Diverticulitis is a complication of diverticulosis resulting from a micro- or macroperforation of a diverticulum with formation of peridiverticular inflammation. This inflammatory reaction may be localized to the pericolic fat with local peritonitis, or the inflammation may be walled off by adjacent structures forming a pericolic abscess. At times, the inflammation may burrow into adjacent organs and form fistulous connections. Free perforation with generalized peritonitis occurs rarely. Diverticulitis usually occurs in the narrow-mouth sigmoid diverticula; only infrequently does it occur in right colonic diverticula. The concept that diverticulitis results from retention of fecal material in an obstructed diverticulum with formation of a retention abscess and mucosal ulcerations has not been substantiated by recent investigations.

Presenting Signs and Symptoms

The major clinical features of diverticulitis are abdominal pain and fever. Pain is most often localized to the left lower quadrant ("left-sided appendicitis") or suprapubic areas. At times, sepsis and its complications, rather than abdominal pain, may be the presenting problem. Nausea, vomiting, and altered bowel function are common associated symptoms. The severity of the clinical symptoms and the mode of presentation depend in large part on the extent of the extradiverticular inflammation.

On physical examination, abdominal tenderness is present, often most impressive over the sigmoid region. Rebound tenderness may also be found as a result of local peritonitis. Occasionally, an abdominal mass is identified, representing either an abscess or an intense inflammatory reaction with adherent loops of bowel. A tender extraluminal mass found on rectal examination should signify the formation of a pelvic abscess. Evidence of some colonic bleeding, either occult blood loss or mild hematochezia, will be found in 25 per cent of patients, but massive hemorrhage is generally not a feature of diverticulitis. Fever is almost always present.

Common Complications

The major complications of diverticulitis are the development of fistulas, abscesses, obstruction, and free perforation.

Fistulas

Fistulous tracks may develop between the colon and any adjacent structures, most commonly forming colovesical, colocutaneous, colovaginal, and coloenteric fistulas. Symptoms suggestive of fistulous formation include the following: *colovesical*—recurrent urinary tract infection, often with multiple organisms, pneumaturia, and even fecaluria; *colocutaneous*—abdominal wall abscesses or cutaneous drainage of purulent fecal material; *colovaginal*—passage of air or stool through the vagina; and *coloenteric*—diarrhea and steatorrhea.

Obstruction

Colonic obstruction may result from luminal compression by the abscess or inflammatory reaction, or the obstruction may be formed by muscular thickening and fibrosis developing with resolution of a single or recurrent episode of diverticulitis. Crampy abdominal pain, distention, and either constipation or diarrhea (leakage around the obstruction) may be the presenting symptoms.

Perforation

Intra-abdominal sepsis may result from the micro- or macroperforation of the diverticulum. Peridiverticular abscess formation is common, but multiple, intra-abdominal abscesses may also occur. Abdominal pain with a tender localized mass is indicative of this complication, but is only infrequently detected on physical examination. Free peritonitis generally presents abruptly with severe diffuse abdominal pain, fever, and diffuse peritoneal findings on examination.

Laboratory Procedures

Laboratory evaluation of patients with diverticulitis almost always reveals a polymorphonuclear leukocytosis with an increase in juvenile forms. The ESR is elevated. Blood cultures may be positive for coliform organisms. The stool may be positive for blood. Sterile pyuria is common secondary to contiguous involvement with the left ureter or bladder.

Radiologic Evaluation

The plain film of the abdomen may be normal or reveal only nonspecific findings. However, careful scrutiny of these films is important to identify extraluminal gas shadows, irregularity and narrowing of the sigmoid colon, or a soft-tissue density compressing the colon. Free air rarely occurs.

Barium enema examination may be very useful in confirming the clinical suspicion; however, as diverticulitis implies perforation, a barium enema has the potential for extending the perforation, for disseminating bacteria into the bloodstream, and for converting a confined process into a more diffuse one. Furthermore, the findings on a barium enema, even when positive, are not entirely specific for diverticulitis. Follow-up examination following resolution of the acute process may be more valuable, in fact, than the initial study in differentiating diverticulitis from other diagnostic considerations. Thus, in cases in which the clinical evidence is very strong in support of the diagnosis of diverticulitis, the barium enema should be deferred until later in the course. However, when there is uncertainty about the diagnosis, a limited study should be performed with primary attention to the sigmoid and left colon and the radiologist be made aware of the concern about diverticulitis.

The features on barium enema that suggest the diagnosis of diverticulitis include:

1. Demonstration of a colonic fistula.
2. Presence of a paracolonic or intramural mass.
3. Extravasation of barium outside a diverticulum.

The finding of diverticulosis with spasm or with the saw-toothed appearance of muscular thickening (myochosis) is not satisfactory radiographic evidence of diverticulitis, since these features may also be seen in symptomatic and asymptomatic diverticular disease.

Although these radiographic features are characteristic of diverticulitis, they may also be seen in other conditions that can coexist with diverticulosis. Crohn's colitis and carcinoma may both cause fistulas and lead to paracolic masses. Therefore, follow-up examination after resolution of the acute inflammatory process is important to document healing of the diverticulitis, disappearance of any paracolic masses, and the presence of normal colonic mucosa. Persistent abnormalities require further investigation.

Other radiographic procedures are also helpful in diagnosing diverticulitis. Computed tomography (CT) and abdominal ultrasonography can identify intra-abdominal abscesses. When positive, these tests can be used to follow the clinical course to complete resolution. An abdominal CT scan is often more helpful in this regard because the ultrasonic patterns may be obscured by bowel gas. Since the sensitivity of this technique in clinical acute diverticulitis is not well defined, a negative scan does not rule out the diagnosis; however, a positive scan for a paracolonic mass can support the diagnosis and avoid the need for an early barium enema. An intravenous pyelogram (IVP) should also be considered prior to any surgical intervention to diagnose left ureteral involvement within the inflammatory mass.

Other Diagnostic Procedures

Endoscopic evaluation of the colon is often needed to exclude other colonic diseases that simulate diverticulitis. Rigid proctoscopy should be performed acutely to identify colitis (i.e., acute infectious or nonspecific ulcerative colitis). This procedure will not confirm diverticulitis, since the area of involvement cannot be reached by the 25-cm rigid sigmoidoscope. Most commonly, marked spasm and narrowing of the lumen will be seen above 15 cm proximal to the anus. The procedure is performed without prior enema administration and without air insufflation.

Endoscopic evaluation of the sigmoid and descending colon by flexible sigmoidoscopy or colonoscopy is relatively contraindicated during acute diverticulitis for fear of extending the colonic perforation. These procedures can be performed after resolution of the acute inflammatory process to exclude other concomitant colonic diseases. This procedure is clearly indicated if the barium enema shows a persistent abnormality. In the acute setting, if the clinical diagnosis remains in doubt despite radiographic studies, a careful, limited endoscopy should be performed while the patient is under close observation.

Potential Errors in Diagnosis

Misdiagnosis of acute diverticulitis can occur in two ways:

1. By overlooking other possible causes for the left lower quadrant pain in a patient with presumed diverticulosis.
2. By overdiagnosis of diverticulitis in a patient with only painful diverticular disease.

Since asymptomatic diverticulosis is common, particularly in the elderly, other colonic disorders often coexist with diverticulosis. As mentioned previously, colonic carcinoma, particularly if perforated, ischemic colitis, and inflammatory bowel disease can readily mimic diverticulitis by producing localized pain, fever, and some bleeding, and can occur in the elderly. Urinary tract infection with pyelonephritis also must be considered as a cause for pain, fever, and an abnormal urinalysis. Gynecologic disorders, such as ovarian cancer, rupture of an ovarian cyst, pelvic inflammatory disease, or an ectopic pregnancy, can mimic the clinical symptoms of diverticulitis. Pancreatitis may also present only with left lower quadrant rather than epigastric pain, since the inflammatory reaction drains into the left colic space. This condition may be difficult to differentiate clinically from diverticulitis without the finding of an abnormal serum amylase. As many of these conditions initially are treated similarly, there is often sufficient time for repeat abdominal examinations, radiographic procedures, and simple observation of the clinical course to differentiate these various conditions.

Another problem is distinguishing inflammatory disease from painful symptomatic diverticular disease. The latter condition may be associated with a mild leukocytosis (less than 12,000 white cells per cu mm), but a marked leukocytosis (greater than 15,000 per cu mm with "shift to the left") and a significant temperature elevation (greater than 100°F orally) are not present. As therapeutic alternatives may vary considerably for these two conditions, particularly in recurrent disease, differentiation should be made as accurately as possible. Objective documentation of inflammation (i.e., fever, marked leukocytosis, elevated erythrocyte sedimentation rate, positive blood cultures, and radiographic evidence of "-itis") rather than subjective impressions relating to the severity of the clinical presentation (abdominal pain and tenderness) should be relied on for the diagnosis of diverticulitis.

DIVERTICULAR BLEEDING

Synonym

Lower GI (gastrointestinal) bleeding.

Definition

Diverticular bleeding results from rupture of a submucosal colonic vessel through the dome or neck of a diverticulum. This hemorrhage into the colonic lumen is generally unassociated with any inflammation of the colonic or diverticular mucosa. Most often, bleeding originates from a right colonic diverticulum in contradistinction to diverticulitis, which most commonly involves a left colon diverticulum.

The frequency of this complication in patients with diverticulosis is uncertain. Previous estimates that 10 to 30 per cent of patients with diverticulosis will bleed are probably gross overestimates, as those figures were derived prior to the use of colonoscopy and angiography to diagnose the source of bleeding. There is no evidence to indicate that pre-existing symptoms of diverticular disease or previous episodes of diverticulitis predispose to diverticular bleeding.

Presenting Signs and Symptoms

The typical presentation is that of an elderly individual having the urge to defecate and suddenly passing blood per rectum. The bleeding is painless, except for some lower abdominal cramps secondary to the purgative effect of intraluminal blood. The severity and rapidity of the bleeding will dictate the clinical presentation. Most commonly, the bleeding is brisk and of sudden onset. The blood passed per rectum may vary in color from bright red to maroon, depending on the activity of the bleed and the rapidity of colonic transit but not on the site of bleeding. The bleeding may be massive, with the patient presenting in shock, or it may be transient and of small volume, resulting in no significant hemodynamic changes. Chronic occult bleeding resulting in iron deficiency anemia is not a feature of diverticular bleeding. Physical findings generally reflect hypovolemia. Orthostatic drop in blood pressure and tachycardia are common findings, but shock is infrequent. Abdominal examination reveals a soft nontender abdomen, free of masses, and with active bowel sounds.

Laboratory Examination

Laboratory tests initially usually reveal only a mild drop in hematocrit, but with continued bleeding, a more profound anemia develops. The anemia reflects an acute blood loss, and evidence by red cell indices or by red cell morphology of iron deficiency anemia should suggest a different diagnosis. Prerenal azotemia may be present.

Course

Bleeding stops spontaneously in about 80 per cent of patients. In the remaining patients, bleeding continues but often in spurts, making diagnostic evaluation difficult. After resolution of the initial episode of hemorrhage, recurrent bleeding occurs in about 25 per cent of patients over a 10-year interval. In patients with two or more episodes of diverticular bleeding, the recurrence rate increases to 50 per cent.

Radiologic Evaluation

A variety of radiologic procedures are available to help diagnose and localize the source of lower GI bleeding. The sequence and timing of these tests depend on the clinical condition of the patient. In a patient with massive hemorrhage, *angiography* may be the initial procedure as it can be both diagnostic and therapeutic; in a patient with persistent but not yet localized bleeding, *radionuclide scanning* can be performed first to localize the bleeding site and to guide further management; and in a patient whose bleeding has stopped, a *barium enema* should be performed to rule out other colonic disorders.

Radionuclide Scanning

Radionuclide scanning for GI bleeding is a relatively new technique that has the following advantages:

1. It is noninvasive.
2. It is more sensitive (i.e., positive at lower bleeding rates) than angiography.
3. It can be performed at the bedside, allowing the critically ill patient to remain in the intensive care unit.

This technique cannot diagnose the etiology of the bleeding; it merely localizes the site of bleeding, i.e., determines whether bleeding is from the right or left colon. This localization can then serve as a useful guide for subsequent angiography or endoscopy.

Two different methods have been used: technetium-sulfur colloid, and technetium-labeled red cells. The former is the conventional radiopharmaceutical used for liver-spleen scans. The material is injected intravenously, and repeated abdominal scans are obtained looking for a collection of the isotope. This technique can detect bleeding at rates as slow as 0.1 ml per minute, but it is limited by a very short half-life within the blood pool. The labeled red cell technique has the advantage of a longer half-life within the blood pool and thus repeated scans can be taken up to 24 hours after injection to detect bleeding. This feature is useful in cases of diverticular hemorrhage, which frequently bleeds intermittently. A negative scan suggests that the bleeding rate is too slow for angiographic detection and in such cases the angiogram can be deferred. Thus, these scans are most useful as screening procedures to define the area (but not the etiology) of bleeding and to predict the success rate of angiography.

Angiography

Angiography should be employed when the patient is still actively bleeding. Minimal bleeding rates of 0.5 to 2.0 ml per minute are needed for successful visualization of a bleeding site by angiography. As bleeding from right-sided diverticula is most common, a superior mesenteric artery angiogram is usually performed first. Extravasation of the dye into a diverticulum and then into the colonic lumen is felt to be diagnostic of a diverticular bleed, but this situation is only occasionally found. Angiography can also identify other potential bleeding sites, such as an arteriovenous malformation (AVM) and vascular tumors.

Barium Enema

The barium enema is a helpful radiographic procedure, but it has significant limitations. This study can confirm the presence of diverticulosis, but it cannot determine the location of the bleeding site, nor can it ever identify an AVM, the other most common cause of massive lower GI bleeding in the elderly. Even when the barium enema shows diverticulosis, other potential bleeding sites (e.g., cancers, polyps, inflammatory bowel disease) can be identified in one third of cases using other techniques (e.g., colonoscopy).

While it is often said that a barium enema can result in the cessation of bleeding, most often such patients have probably already stopped bleeding prior to the barium enema, and the barium can potentially interfere with angiography should rebleeding occur. Thus, a barium enema should be performed only after the patient has been well stabilized and all bleeding has clearly stopped (usually at least 48 hours after the last evidence of active bleeding). An air-contrast barium enema should be utilized in such cases because it is more sensitive in detecting mucosal lesions than a single-contrast study.

Other Techniques

Endoscopic evaluation is an essential component in the diagnosis of diverticular bleeding. Proctoscopy should be performed initially to rule out hemorrhoidal or rectal lesions as causes for the lower GI bleeding. Once bleeding has stopped, colonoscopy should be routinely performed to exclude other potential bleeding sites. Colonoscopy can accurately identify polyps, cancer, ulcerations, and inflammatory or ischemic bowel diseases that may be missed on barium enema. Arteriovenous malformations are now being recognized with increasing frequency because their endoscopic appearance is better appreciated. Emergency colonoscopy has occasionally been utilized to localize the site of bleeding in patients in whom the angiogram is negative. However, this technique is difficult to perform in the actively bleeding patient and good visualization of the mucosa needed to detect an AVM is not always possible.

An upper gastrointestinal source of bleeding must also be excluded. Occasionally patients with duodenal ulcer will present with massive rectal hemorrhage but without hematemesis or reflux of blood into the stomach. This situation can usually be avoided if bile is present in the nasogastric aspirate. Occasionally, upper endoscopy is needed to exclude a gastroduodenal source of bleeding.

Potential Errors in Diagnosis

Errors in diagnosis may arise from incomplete evaluation of rectal bleeding. The diagnosis of diverticular bleeding depends on the exclusion of other conditions rather than on just the positive finding of diverticulosis in a bleeding patient. Judicious use of various diagnostic studies is required, and total reliance on a single test is a potential source of error.

MALIGNANT TUMORS OF THE COLON AND RECTUM

By Charles J. Lightdale, M.D.
and Sidney J. Winawer, M.D.
New York, New York

INCIDENCE

In many areas of the world, particularly in the industrialized West, cancer of the colon and rectum is a common disease. Currently, colorectal cancer develops in approximately 120,000 Americans per year. The disease affects men and women almost equally, with slightly higher rectal cancer incidence in men. In the United States, lung cancer is the most common malignancy in men and breast cancer the most common in women, but colorectal cancer is the single most frequent cancer overall.

ETIOLOGY

Dietary factors may play a major role in the remarkable variation in the incidence of colon cancer in different areas of the world. Japan, for example, although highly industrialized, has a relatively low rate of colorectal cancer, but Japanese migrating to the United States have reached the incidence rate of the general American population within one generation. The incidence of colorectal cancer in Japan, in those who have adopted a more Western type of diet, has also increased. The low-fiber, high-fat diet consumed in more affluent Western countries may alter bowel constituents to produce a carcinogenic environment.

RISK FACTORS

Age

This is the major risk factor in the general population. Both men and women are at low risk until age 40, when the incidence of the disease begins to rise significantly. The risk becomes sharply greater at age 50, and then doubles with each decade, reaching a peak at age 75.

Adenomas

Greater than 90 per cent of primary colorectal cancers are adenocarcinomas, and it is now believed that most, if not all, of these cancers arise from adenomas. These adenomas are commonly identified as polyps in the colon. While the majority of polyps in the colon are not premalignant, the presence of a polyp puts a patient at increased risk for a lifetime. The significance of polyps that are histologically hyperplastic is less clear, but adenomatous polyps have a definite malignant potential, particularly if they have villous features. The larger the size of the polyp, the more likely it is to have villous features. The risk of a polyp's being malignant increases markedly when it becomes greater than 2 cm in diameter. The presence of a polyp indicates a severe abnormality in the underlying mucosa. This basic abnormality seems to be present in a patchy distribution throughout the colon of a patient with an adenomatous polyp. When a single polyp is found, there is a 50 per cent risk of another being present, and there is a continuous risk, estimated at 20 to 30 per cent, for the development of subsequent polyps.

Prior Cancer

A patient who has had one carcinoma of the colon is at risk for additional cancers and adenomas, both immediately and in the future. It is estimated that in 1.5 to 5 per cent of patients with a cancer, a synchronous cancer is present at the time of diagnosis. The risk of a future or metachronous cancer is estimated at 5 to 10 per cent.

Inflammatory Bowel Disease

Ulcerative colitis carries an increased risk for adenocarcinoma of the colon. The risk begins once the disease has been present for 7 years, if the colitis involves the entire colon, and increases with time thereafter. Left-sided disease has a lesser risk, and proctosigmoiditis and proctitis have virtually none. A marker of extreme risk is the presence of severe dysplasia histologically in mucosal biopsies, associated with about a 50 per cent chance of a person's having or developing cancer. Only about 10 to 15 per cent of patients with long-standing ulcerative colitis will have dysplasia. In addition, 10 to 20 per cent of those with ulcerative colitis and cancer will have no evidence of dysplasia.

Patients with Crohn's disease of the colon also have an increased risk for adenocarcinoma, but a much lesser risk than those with ulcerative colitis.

Genetic Factors

Several genetic syndromes have been described that have an increased risk of colon cancer. The most dramatic are associated with the development early in life of multiple colonic adenomas. The best known are called *familial polyposis coli* and *Gardner's syndrome,* which may be variants of the same disease. The colon becomes carpeted by hundreds of small adenomas, usually during adolescence. In Gardner's syndrome there are multiple soft-tissue tumors including desmoids, fibromas, and osteomas, particularly involving the mandible. Polyps of the stomach and small bowel are also seen in both syndromes. These diseases are inherited as autosomal dominants, and affected individuals have close to 100 per cent chance of developing colorectal cancer.

Peutz-Jeghers' syndrome, a genetic disorder associated with hamartomatous polyposis, carries an increased risk for colorectal cancer. Patients with a history of juvenile polyps also have a greater risk, but the risk in these syndromes is considerably less than in familial polyposis coli and Gardner's syndrome.

There are other individuals without polyposis who develop colon cancer and who have a definite family history of colon cancer. In this type of inherited colon cancer, there are usually only a few scattered polyps versus the familial polyposis type. Within this group are two subsets of patients. The first is at risk for colon cancer only. The second is at risk for colon and other cancers, particularly uterine cancer. Cancers of the breast, stomach, pancreas, and skin also occur in these family groups. The risk for both polyps and cancers in these colon cancer families begins in the 20s.

EARLY DIAGNOSIS

The likelihood of recurrent metastatic disease after surgery for colorectal cancer is strongly linked to the stage of the disease at the time of resection. The 5-year survival in all patients is only about 40 per cent. However, if the disease is diagnosed when there is involvement only of the colonic wall (Dukes A and B) and not the lymph nodes (Dukes C) or distant metastases, the 5-year survival is in the range of 70 per cent. The implication is that average survival can probably be improved by greater efforts at early detection. Diagnostic strategy based on an understanding of the natural history of the disease is to evaluate symptoms promptly and to screen high-risk patients who are asymptomatic when the cancer is more likely to be at an early stage. The detection of adenomas in such patients is also important, since their complete removal greatly decreases the probability of cancer developing. The diagnosis and removal of colorectal adenomas thus constitutes a form of secondary cancer prevention.

DIAGNOSTIC METHODS

Fecal Occult Blood Test

This test was reintroduced using guaiac-impregnated filter paper slides in an effort to screen asymptomatic patients for colorectal cancer. The test has been most useful when the patient smears two samples of stool per day onto the slides. A total of six smears over 3 days is obtained with the patient on a high-fiber, meat-free diet. The slides are then tested with a reagent of hydrogen peroxide in denatured alcohol. Several different guaiac-impregnated slides are commercially available.

The nature of the reaction of the guaiac slide test is not well understood. Guaiac, a plant product, is composed of heterogeneous compounds present in varying stages of purity. The positive reaction produced by blood is a result of the pseudo-peroxidase activity of hemoglobin, which interacts with the hydrogen peroxide in the testing reagent. This reaction causes a phenolic oxidation of the guaiac, producing the clear blue color that indicates a positive test.

One problem is that sufficient quantities of blood coming from anywhere in the gastrointestinal tract can lead to a positive test. Even ingested blood can cause a positive reaction, and, therefore, a meat-free diet is recommended. Gastric irritants such as aspirin and alcohol should be avoided during the test period. In addition, anything having peroxidase activity, such as fresh fruit and uncooked vegetables, can produce a positive reaction. Agents that interfere with the oxidation reaction, such as ascorbic acid, may produce a false-negative reaction in the presence of hemoglobin. The high-fiber diet is encouraged to produce a daily stool and to increase the bleeding rate of neoplastic lesions.

Data on results of fecal occult blood testing in the United States are available from two controlled clinical trials. The trials, conducted at the Strang Clinic–Preventive Medicine Institute with the Memorial Sloan-Kettering Cancer Center in New York, and at the University of Minnesota, have involved more than 70,000 patients. Patient compliance with the test has been in the 80 per cent range in the highly motivated participants in the studies. Compliance in the general population or in groups not instructed or educated about the test has been considerably less.

The rate of positive slides in various subgroups of these studies has ranged from 1 to 4 per cent; the false-positive rate has ranged from 0.5 to 3 per cent. Of those patients with a positive test, about half will have an adenoma or a carcinoma on further investigation. The other half will have other benign lesions or no significant abnormalities at all. A crucial finding is that 60 to 80 per cent of the cancers detected by this method are early (Dukes A and B) lesions. This is in contrast to the pathologic stage of symptomatic patients, of whom the majority will have lymph node metastases (Dukes C). These studies are still ongoing, with the goal of determining whether the fecal occult blood test will lead to a mortality reduction from colorectal cancer compared with control patients.

Certainly the fecal occult blood test will not detect all neoplastic lesions that are present. The sensitivity seems to be higher for lesions proximal to the rectosigmoid. False negativity for detection of cancer has been estimated at 10 to 20 per cent and for adenomas, 30 to 70 per cent. A positive test is important and has a role in screening, but other examinations are needed when pursuing a diagnosis of colon cancer.

Sigmoidoscopy

This test is undergoing a major resurgence and reevaluation because of recent improvements in instrumentation. Flexible fiberoptic instruments are replacing the standard rigid 25-cm sigmoidoscope.

A digital rectal examination should precede every sigmoidoscopy. Since it has been estimated that approximately 10 per cent of colorectal cancers can be detected by an examining finger, digital rectal exploration becomes an important part of any physical examination. It should not be omitted without reason.

A sound background of data has accumulated during the past two decades of experience with the rigid 25-cm sigmoidoscope. It is estimated that 50 per cent of colorectal cancers and adenomas can be detected with this instrument. However, the procedure never developed into a popular screening method because it is technically difficult and often markedly uncomfortable, leading to avoidance by patient and physician alike.

When used correctly and rigorously, rigid sigmoidoscopy has been effective. In a study of more than 26,000 asymptomatic patients from the Strang Clinic–Preventive Medicine Institute in New York, 58 cases of rectosigmoid cancer were detected and 88 per cent were early lesions (Dukes A and B). There has been a 90 per cent survival in patients during follow-up for as long as 15 years. Another study showed a mortality reduction for colorectal cancer in a group regularly examined by sigmoidoscope versus a control group. At the University of Minnesota, it was shown over 25 years that rectosigmoid surveillance by sigmoidoscopy, followed by removal of observed polyps, greatly reduced the expected incidence of rectosigmoid cancer. It seems, therefore, that sigmoidoscopy has potential value in screening for cancer as well as in detection and removal of adenomas for interruption of the adenoma-carcinoma sequence. With the lack of utilization of rigid sigmoidoscopy, however, this potential has not been recognized.

Because of the angulation of the rectosigmoid at about 15 cm, most rigid examinations are effective only to about 16 cm before stretching of the sigmoid mesentery produces the cramping pain that frequently requires the termination of insertion. Flexible sigmoidoscopy has been shown in several studies to be much better tolerated, even though the flexible examination may take slightly longer and is more expensive. The knee-chest position is not required. Most examinations are carried out with patients lying on the left side.

There has been a trend in recent decades toward a higher, more rightward distribution of colorectal cancer. In the years 1939 to 1954, a majority of colorectal cancers were found in the rectosigmoid. This is no longer the case, and carrying the usual rigid examination of 16 cm to the easily reached 35 cm with flexible sigmoidoscopy may lead to a significantly higher rate of detection of neoplasms. Recent comparisons of flexible and rigid sigmoidoscopy show an average gain in the diagnosis of cancer and polyps to be greater than 2:1 in favor of the flexible instrument.

The length of the ideal flexible instrument is still controversial. Much of the data generated so far has been obtained by experienced gastroenterologists and colorectal surgeons utilizing instruments measuring 60 to 65 cm. Longer instruments have the advantage of examining more of the colon, and a skilled endoscopist may commonly examine the entire sigmoid colon and some of the descending colon with a 60-cm instrument. It has been estimated that up to two thirds of all colonic neoplasms may be detected using a 60-cm flexible sigmoidoscope.

However, the 60-cm instrument requires considerable training and experience to be used to its full potential. It exposes the patient to increased risks, particularly outside skilled hands, and the longer instruments tend to be more expensive. Shorter flexible instruments with lengths of 30 and 35 cm have proved very easy to master and provide a thorough examination of the rectosigmoid with good tolerance and low risk at reasonable cost. Such instruments may prove to be ideal in the hands of most physicians, with longer instruments used as needed by trained endoscopists.

Barium Enema

This radiologic examination of the colon has undergone a re-evaluation in recent years. There have been improvements in technique with emphasis on better bowel cleansing and double-contrast methodology. High-quality double-contrast radiographs have been effective in demonstrating lesions as small as 0.5 cm. in the colon. Unfortunately, good double-contrast barium enemas are not yet widely available in the United States. When single-column barium enema studies are used, approximately half of the cancers and even more adenomas are missed.

Sigmoidoscopy coupled with double-contrast barium radiography of the colon provides a reasonably thorough and well-tolerated evaluation of the colon in symptomatic patients. For maximum accuracy, double-contrast barium enema is followed by colonoscopy, the two tests providing a synergistically higher diagnostic yield than either alone.

Colonoscopy

The development of the fiberoptic colonoscope and of techniques for the endoscopic examination of the entire colon has produced revolutionary change in the diagnosis of colonic neoplasia during the past decade. With modern instruments, a well-trained endoscopist will reach the cecum more than 90 per cent of the time. Colonic preparation must be thorough, but a variety of methods have proved effective and tolerable. Most commonly, a 48-hour fluid diet is maintained, with an osmotic laxative and tap water enemas prior to the examination. Colonoscopy is usually performed under light sedation using meperidine and diazepam. Skilled examiners maintain patient comfort by avoiding stretching of the mesentery and excessive gas insufflation. The colonic mucosa may be examined in fine detail, and lesions only a few millimeters in size can be biopsied, fulgurated, or excised by cautery snare. Cytologic washings and brushings may also be obtained. The removal of adenomas throughout the colon via colonoscopy theoretically extends secondary cancer prevention from the rectosigmoid to the entire colon. In well-trained hands, colonoscopy is a reasonably safe procedure, with a complication rate of about 0.2 per cent.

A double-contrast barium enema prior to colonoscopy provides the most sensitive combination of examinations for neoplasia. Although the yield of neoplastic lesions is much higher for colonoscopy than it is for barium enema as usually performed, there is false negativity for colonoscopy as well. This false negativity has not been well established for cancers. The potentially difficult diagnostic areas are just proximal to the hepatic and splenic flexures and the medial aspect of the ascending colon, just proximal to the ileocecal valve. In one study comparing colonoscopy with barium enema, colonoscopy had a 6 per cent false-negative rate for adenomas larger than 1.0 cm.

Carcinoembryonic Antigen (CEA)

This glycoprotein was first described in 1965, followed by the development of a radioimmunoassay in 1969 that could detect serum levels in nanogram amounts. Further experiments have shown CEA to be a complex and heterogeneous material that exists on peripheral cell membranes from which it is shed into surrounding body fluids. It is catabolized in the circulation and in the liver and partially excreted in the bile. Commercially available radioimmunoassays have a sensitivity of 0.5 ng/ml, with some interlaboratory variations.

When CEA was first described, it appeared that CEA determinations might constitute a tumor-specific blood test for colon cancer that could enable early diagnosis in asymptomatic patients. This has proved not to be the case. Elevations of CEA have been found in the blood in patients with a variety of malignancies, including gastric, pancreatic, lung, breast, and bladder cancers. In addition, CEA has been identified in the tissues of many normal organs and benign conditions of these organs can produce serum elevations. Elevations of CEA are common in the blood of smokers and in patients with active cirrhosis, pancreatitis, and inflammatory bowel disease.

APPLICATION OF DIAGNOSTIC TESTS

Symptomatic Patients

Cancers of the rectum and colon obstruct, bleed, invade, and perforate. Rectal bleeding is an especially notable symptom suggesting possible colonic malignancy. The character and severity of rectal bleeding do not reliably distinguish benign from malignant disease. For example, hemorrhoidal disease may produce a small amount of blood noted on the toilet tissue, but rectal cancer may cause the same symptom. Profuse bleeding is more likely due to diverticulosis or inflammatory bowel disease, but it may also occur with carcinoma. Melena suggests upper gastrointestinal tract disease, but it can be caused by cecal cancer. Iron deficiency anemia always raises the possibility of an occult colon cancer. A single episode of bleeding may occur as the only symptom of cancer.

Changes in bowel habits with constipation, cramping pain, and narrowed stool caliber may result from diverticulosis as well as cancer involving the left colon. A localized peritoneal abscess may be due to a perforated diverticulum or a cancer. Inflammatory bowel disease or infectious colitis may cause bleeding, tenesmus, urgency, or diarrhea, but colorectal cancer must be a consideration. The most common situation involves symptoms of alternating constipation and diarrhea and abdominal cramps and bloating due to irritable bowel syndrome. In most such patients, a careful history will document long-standing symptoms, which otherwise mimic a partially obstructing cancer of the left colon. Excess discharge of mucus seen in some irritable bowel patients may also represent a highly premalignant villous adenoma. While patients with irritable bowel syndrome do not seem to have a higher incidence of colon cancer, they certainly may still develop this malignancy. A worsening or change in their symptoms requires new evaluation.

Evaluation of symptomatic patients usually begins with a sigmoidoscopy, followed by a barium enema. When a lesion is detected on barium enema, colonoscopy is needed for biopsy. If there is an adenoma found by barium enema, colonoscopy is used to remove it and to examine the entire colon for additional lesions not seen on barium enema. If sigmoidoscopy and barium enema are nondiagnostic or negative, a colonoscopy is also indicated. Again, for the highest diagnostic yield for neoplastic lesions in the colon, a double-contrast barium enema should be performed, followed by total colonoscopy. When used together in this manner, the procedures effectively detect virtually all polypoid lesions.

At times it may be wise to omit an initial barium enema and proceed directly to colonoscopy, for example, in some patients with moderately severe rectal bleeding for whom a delay in diagnosis is unacceptable. An unprepared sigmoidoscopy is prudent when such patients are seen for the first time, however, to diagnose possible inflammatory bowel disease. Active ulcerative colitis may be exacerbated by the usual barium enema or colonoscopy preparations, and these examinations may be deferred until the colitis has been treated and is quiescent. Colonoscopy may also be performed as an initial test to diagnose colon cancer in some patients who cannot tolerate a barium enema. Some elderly patients, for example, are unable to contain the barium even with the use of rectal balloons. Total colonoscopy is easily performed in the great majority of patients without the use of fluoroscopy and is indicated as the first test in all patients where the avoidance of ionizing radiation is a consideration.

The fecal occult blood test is not used in symptomatic patients. Its proper use is in screening asymptomatic individuals. Similarly the CEA test has no role in symptomatic patients because of high false positivity and negativity. It is useful pre- and postoperatively when a diagnosis of colon cancer is made.

Pre- and Postoperative Examination

It is generally desirable to examine the entire colon by colonoscopy whenever a cancer is detected by sigmoidoscopy or barium enema to search for synchronous cancers and adenomas. With small- to moderate-sized adenocarcinomas, colonoscopy can usually be safely done. If considerable manipulation is required, however, as with larger or partially obstructing cancers, an attempt at complete colonoscopy is not advised. In this setting, the colonoscopic examination of the entire remaining colon may be completed 2 to 3 months postoperatively.

Once the colon is cleared of synchronous lesions, periodic endoscopic and radiologic examination of the colon is essential in postoperative follow-up to detect subsequent neoplasms and monitor for recurrence. A repeat air-contrast barium enema and colonoscopy are recommended 1 year after the initial diagnostic examinations. If polyps are encountered, they should be removed endoscopically. The surgical anastomosis should be evaluated, and biopsies and brush cytologic specimens should be taken from any suspicious areas.

Colonoscopy should be performed yearly until the colon is free of adenomas for 2 successive years, and then the examination is recommended at 2- to 3-year intervals. This schedule is based on data indicating that the time for adenomatous tissue to grow from a microscopic lesion to a visible polyp is in the range of 3 years. Performing two successive negative colonoscopies 1 year apart keeps the miss rate of significant lesions to a minimum. Once the colon is cleared, flexible sigmoidoscopy and barium enema are recommended in the interval years between colonoscopies. The National Polyp Study currently in progress will assess whether alterations in this schedule are indicated.

For patients in whom a colon cancer has been diagnosed, it is useful to obtain a preoperative CEA level. An elevated preoperative CEA level seems to place the patient in a higher-risk group for recurrence. If an elevated CEA level does not fall to normal postoperatively, it is likely that there is residual malignant disease. If the CEA level does fall to normal after surgery, it may be followed in a serial manner at 1- to 3-month intervals. Numerous studies have shown that if the CEA level subsequently rises above normal and progresses, there is a high probability of recurrence. This may occur months before the metastasis causes symptoms. The nonspecificity of the test must be taken into account, and many patients will develop recurrence without a rise in CEA. However, a progressive increase in CEA is strong presumptive evidence for recurrent cancer and merits intensive clinical evaluation.

It has not been resolved whether detecting a recurrence on the basis of CEA determinations will lead to prolongation of survival and increased cure rate. When widespread disease cannot be established clinically, exploratory laparotomy in the hope of finding a resectable recurrence has been advocated. Lower levels of increased CEA levels, shorter intervals between increased CEA detection and reoperation, and a slower rate of CEA elevation have been associated with resectability.

Asymptomatic Patients

Screening of asymptomatic people at varying degrees of risk for colon cancer is good medical practice in the United States and in other countries where the overall risk of colon cancer is high. The diagnostic methods recommended vary with the assessment of the degree of risk and can be modified according to available resources, cost, risks, and compliance. Benefits of screening include detecting colon cancer early, diagnosing and removing premalignant adenomas, and identifying high-risk individuals for more intensive surveillance.

Average-Risk Patients

Within the United States, all persons from age 40 to 50 are at risk for colorectal cancers and can be characterized as average-risk patients. Such individuals with no special risk factors should have fecal occult blood testing every year and sigmoidoscopy every 3 to 5 years. The time interval is based on the slow growth of adenomas and on the development of cancer primarily in larger adenomas of at least 1 to 1½ cm in size. The period of this growth and transformation is estimated to take 5 years or more.

A positive fecal occult blood test or the finding of an adenoma on sigmoidoscopy should be followed by prompt evaluation with air-contrast barium enema and colonoscopy.

The measurement of CEA has been studied extensively as a potential serologic screening test for early colorectal cancer. However, in screening average-risk patients, CEA determinations were found to have a false-positive rate of 15 per cent and a false-negative rate of 40 to 60 per cent in nonmetastatic disease. Thus, the test lacks both the specificity and sensitivity to allow for screening. Moreover, patients with elevated CEA levels tend to be those with more advanced cancer. A majority of patients with early stages of disease have a normal concentration of CEA in their blood. Measurements of CEA should not be used as a screening test. The current value of CEA seems to be in the area of surveillance after surgical removal of colon cancer and in assessing the efficacy of treatment of metastatic disease.

Prior Adenomas

Patients with a documented history of removal of colonic adenomas are at increased risk for subsequent adenomas and carcinoma of the colon. Such patients should be evaluated by air-contrast barium enema and colonoscopy. The colonoscopy should subsequently be repeated annually until the colon has been cleared of all adenomas for 2 consecutive years. Based on the slow growth rate of adenomas, it would then be reasonable to re-examine patients at 3-year intervals.

Questions of the time interval between colonoscopic examinations and the role of the barium enema in patients with polyps are currently being addressed by multicenter randomized controlled trials in the United States.

Nonpolyposis Familial Colon Cancer

In these groups, it has been established that cancers develop at a younger age from pre-existing adenomas. These adenomas tend to occur more often on the right side of the colon. Fecal occult blood testing, with a lower sensitivity for adenomas than for carcinomas, is probably of limited value in this group. Similarly, sigmoidoscopy is of less efficacy than in average-risk patients, in whom a majority of adenomas and cancers are within the range of this examination. Therefore, periodic colonoscopy is recommended to determine whether individuals within a suspect family have been affected. The role of barium enema in these patients is questionable, given the lower sensitivity of this test in detecting small lesions and considering the young age of the patients. Once the colon is cleared of all neoplastic lesions by colonoscopy, the surveillance interval can be approximately 3 years. Although the temporal evolution of new adenomas in this group may not be the same as in the average-risk patients, it would seem unreasonable to subject asymptomatic patients to colonoscopy beginning in their 20s and 30s at more frequent intervals.

Polyposis Syndromes

Patients with a family history of familial polyposis or Gardner's syndrome should have a limited flexible sigmoidoscopy to determine whether they are affected; if they are, polyps will always be present in the rectum. Patients should be examined initially during adolescence and then every 6 months to 1 year.

Affected patients are usually treated with subtotal colectomy with anastomosis of the ileum to the rectum. The rectum is subsequently monitored for the development of malignant cells by proctoscopy at approximately 6-month intervals. For patients in whom subtotal colectomy is deferred, e.g., for psychological reasons, the entire colon should be kept under close surveillance using colonoscopy at 6-month to 1-year intervals. Effective cancer control cannot be guaranteed even with such aggressive surveillance, since carcinoma may evolve from any of the hundreds of small adenomas that are usually present. Lavage cytology may be used during the colonoscopy procedure to search for the presence of malignant cells.

Patients with Peutz-Jeghers' syndrome who develop colon polyps usually have multiple polyps present, most commonly above the rectosigmoid. Periodic colonoscopy is indicated in these patients, who should be placed in a program of surveillance similar to that recommended for the nonpolyposis–inherited colon cancer group.

Inflammatory Bowel Disease

In patients with chronic ulcerative colitis involving the entire colon, surveillance using colonoscopy should be started approximately 7 years after the onset of the disease. During colonoscopy, biopsies should be taken systematically throughout the colon for dysplasia and lavage cytology for malignant cells should be obtained. Narrowed or raised areas should be directly biopsied. The timing of examinations, annual versus biannual, has not been firmly established, but the annual examination seems appropriate. Barium enema is not indicated because of its low yield. The carcinomas in ulcerative colitis tend to be flat and infiltrating, rather than polypoid or exophytic, and are difficult to detect by radiography at an early stage.

In patients with only left-sided ulcerative colitis, the risk of developing cancer starts later and surveillance can begin at about 15 years from the onset of disease. Biopsy for dysplasia and lavage cytology is used as in patients with the entire colon involved by ulcerative colitis. Patients with ulcerative colitis involving only the distal descending colon or rectosigmoid carry at least the same risk as the average population and probably slightly more. In some of these patients, the distal disease tends to extend to involve the entire colon. Thus, a surveillance colonoscopy every 2 to 3 years is advocated in this group.

The risk of carcinoma in patients with Crohn's disease involving the colon is greater than the general population but not of the order of magnitude of ulcerative colitis. Dysplasia has been described in Crohn's colitis only rarely. Strictured areas are suspect for carcinoma in both ulcerative colitis and Crohn's, and a barium enema at about 3-year intervals to detect silent strictures is recommended in Crohn's colitis. Strictures in inflammatory bowel disease should be evaluated for malignancy with colonoscopy, biopsy, and brush cytology. The role of surveillance colonoscopy in Crohn's colitis has not been otherwise established. When disease has been present more than 10 years, however, colonoscopy at 2- to 3-year intervals for cancer surveillance would not be unreasonable.

BENIGN POLYPS OF THE COLON

By Hiromi Shinya, M.D.
New York, New York

Benign polyps are the most common lesions of the colon and rectum and are most commonly found in adults over the age of 45 (approximately 10 per cent of this group). Numerous classifications have evolved on the basis of morphologic (gross or histologic) appearances. These polyps may be either pedunculated or sessile. Histologic classifications include hyperplastic (metaplastic), inflammatory, juvenile, hamartomas, and adenomas.

Benign colorectal polyps may be divided into mucosal and submucosal lesions (Table 1). Many are of mucosal origin and non-neoplastic. The hyperplastic (metaplastic) polyp is the most commonly encountered polyp, usually less than 5 mm in diameter. Although benign, the true nature of many of the hyperplastic lesions cannot be determined without total biopsy or removal.

Submucosal polypoid lesions comprise less than 5 per cent of all colonic lesions and include lymphoid polyps (benign lymphomas), lipomas, leiomyomas, carcinoids, granular cell myoblastomas, and endometriomas (rarely a mucosal lesion).

Table 1. Benign Polyps of the Colon

Mucosal Lesions	Submucosal Lesions
Non-neoplastic	Lymphoid polyps
Hyperplastic (metaplastic)	Lipomas
Inflammatory polyps	Leiomyomas
Juvenile polyps	Carcinoids
Hamartomas	Granular cell myoblastomas
Neoplastic	Endometriomas
Tubular adenomas	
Tubulovillous adenomas	
Villous adenomas	

NEOPLASTIC MUCOSAL LESIONS

Adenomas

Definition and Classification

Adenomas are true neoplastic polyps and are considered to be precursors of cancer. Foci of dysplasia and gross cancer are frequently found in the adenomas; adenomas show abnormal cell regeneration; as the size of the adenoma increases, the risk of carcinoma in situ and invasive cancer rises; patients with multiple polyps have a much higher risk of colonic cancer than the general population. The precise time interval over which an adenoma becomes malignant is unknown. The length of time needed for the transformation varies. Data from familial polyposis patients and the occasional so-called malignant polyp observed in situ indicate that an interval of 5 to 7 years is required for the transformation from a benign to a malignant process. We have seen malignant change occur within 2½ years.

We utilize the World Health Organization classification, which divides polyps into three categories: tubular, tubulovillous, and villous adenomas.

Tubular Adenomas. If a polyp contains more than 75 per cent of tubular elements, we classify it as a tubular adenoma. These polyps may be sessile or pedunculated.

Tubulovillous Adenomas. These may also be referred to as villoglandular, or mixed polyps. They are common lesions. Villous and tubular elements are found within these polyps and, by definition, the polyp has more than 25 per cent of tubular and villous components. This polyp is frequently multilobulated and has a variable malignant potential.

Villous Adenomas. These lesions are the least common form of neoplastic polyp. By definition, more than 75 percent of the lesion has villous elements. Villous adenomas are frequently flat and sessile. They may also be pedunculated and may involve a major part of the circumference of the rectum and the colon.

Invasion

Whether colonic adenomas undergo malignant transformation or whether the cancer arises de novo from normal colonic mucosa has been debated. The debate has direct clinical bearing, since laparotomy in the past was required to remove most polyps. Fortunately, colonoscopic polypectomy has made this issue academic, since the removal and analysis of polyps rarely require surgery. Evidence to support the polyp cancer sequence does exist. *Superficial carcinoma* is defined as a lesion in which the carcinomatous cells involve the superficial fibers of the muscularis mucosa but do not invade the muscularis mucosa (intramucosal carcinoma). Although true cancers, these lesions are not malignant in a clinical sense and do not metastasize. The presence of malignant invasive changes in colonic adenomas implies crossing of the muscularis mucosa. Therefore, in invasive carcinoma, malignant cells penetrate through or beneath both layers of the muscularis mucosa. When reporting the histologic appearance of an existing polyp, one must distinguish between superficial and invasive carcinoma because this distinction has important implications regarding management. When cancer cells penetrate the muscularis mucosa, this change must be regarded as *invasive carcinoma.*

Adenomas clearly have the highest potential for malignant change. Using similar criteria to determine malignancy within a polyp, many investigators have found invasive carcinoma within the polyp approximately 5.0 to 6.3 per cent of the time. It is essential that the entire polyp be removed and that adequate tissue sections be made to determine whether the polyp fits the criteria for malignancy. Several observations seem to justify the present theory of the polyp cancer sequence:

1. Foci of dysplasia and frank carcinoma are frequently seen in adenomas, not in normal or hyperplastic mucosa.
2. Unlike normal mucosa, adenomas show abnormal cell regeneration.
3. As polyp size increases, the risk of cancer increases (Table 2).
4. Polyps with severe dysplasia of the epithelium have a very high malignant potential, suggestive of a step-like progression from dysplasia to in situ carcinoma, to microinvasion, to invasion of the muscularis mucosa.
5. Patients with polyps have a higher incidence of carcinoma than the normal population.
6. Many carcinomas show evidence of adjacent benign or adenomatous growths, suggesting origin in the benign tissue, with rapid overgrowth as the carcinoma spreads.
7. Aggressive removal of polyps with stringent follow-up examination can decrease the expected incidence of cancer of the rectum and rectosigmoid.

When a colonic polyp is detected by barium enema or colonoscopy, polypectomy should be performed to ensure that an invasive malignant tumor is not present. Due to the fact that there is strong evidence of a premalignant potential of colonic adenomas, removing benign neoplastic polyps is prophylactic against malignant degeneration. The procedure of choice for removing colorectal polyps has been the technique of snare cautery resection via the colonoscope. Colonoscopic polypectomy can replace the conventional transabdominal approach to most colonic polyps, but it must be done by an experienced colonoscopist. Colonoscopic polypectomy can be performed on an out-patient or in-patient basis, depending upon

Table 2. Size of Adenoma Related to Invasive Carcinoma (Stage IA)*

Size of Adenoma (cm)	Tubular		Tubulovillous		Villous	
	No.	IA (%)	No.	IA (%)	No.	IA (%)
0.5–0.9	1858	6 (0.3)	157	4 (2.5)	42	1 (2.4)
1.0–1.9	2100	75 (3.6)	898	63 (7.0)	260	14 (5.4)
2.0–2.9	499	34 (6.8)	556	60 (10.8)	106	18 (17.0)
3.0+	113	14 (12.4)	206	27 (13.1)	147	21 (14.3)
Total	4570	129 (2.8)	1817	154 (8.5)	555	54 (9.7)

*From Shinya, H.: *Colonoscopy*. New York, Igaku-Shoin, with permission.

the size and nature of the polyps, the patient's general condition, and the operator's preference.

Polyps with Dysplasia or Carcinoma in Situ (Mucosal Carcinoma)

If a pedunculated or a narrow-based sessile polyp has been completely excised endoscopically and shows some evidence of dysplasia or carcinoma in situ, no further resection is required. If a wide-based sessile polyp cannot be excised completely and there is evidence of severe dysplasia or carcinoma in situ, we usually recommend that a segmental bowel resection be performed in the younger patients. For elderly patients or those in poor medical condition, we elect to treat them conservatively and perform colonoscopy at frequent intervals (approximately 1 to 3 months) to determine whether invasive carcinoma is present. Frequent endoscopic resections and coagulations can lead to complete excision of such lesions.

Adenomas with Invasive Carcinoma, Polypoid Carcinoma

Colonoscopic polypectomy is still a relatively new technique. We are currently collecting data to help determine the definitive management of malignant polyps. Most authorities believe that even when a malignant tumor penetrates through the muscularis mucosa, endoscopic polypectomy is sufficient if there is an adequate zone of clearance between the plane of resection and the level of invasion. This is particularly true of pedunculated lesions.

In general, I also agree with this concept. Our experience also militates against recommending abdominal surgery for older patients with malignant polyps. When a malignant lesion extends to or is close to the cauterized tissue, the operator must consider the possibility that all of the malignant tissue has not been excised. Our policy under such circumstances is to recommend colectomy for good-risk patients. In patients with polypoid carcinoma, we are not convinced that endoscopic excision completely fulfills the accepted criteria for adequate cancer surgery and therefore advise surgical intervention for such patients. However, exceptions should be made when there is a long stalk, for the elderly or other poor-risk patients, and for patients who refuse operation. The risk of surgical intervention in elderly patients and those with complicating diseases is carefully weighed against the risk of the possibility of residual carcinoma and lymphatic metastases.

In summary, the absolute indications for colonic resection after the excision of a malignant polyp are:

1. Any residual malignant tumor that is recognized endoscopically.
2. Malignant change that involves the line of resection.
3. Any evidence of lymphatic or vascular involvement in the excised specimen.
4. Carcinoma that is poorly differentiated cytologically (rare).

A relative indication is malignant degeneration close to the line of resection. When no surgical intervention is recommended, colonoscopy offers considerable advantage in permitting the polypectomy sites to be re-examined every few months.

NON-NEOPLASTIC MUCOSAL POLYPS

Juvenile Polyps

Juvenile polyps are hamartomas, not neoplastic polyps. These lesions may appear in adults, although they most often occur in young persons between the ages of 2 and 10. Juvenile polyps are usually found in the rectum and left colon and are rarely seen in the right colon. They are more common in boys than in girls. Since some such lesions bleed, it may be necessary to excise them endoscopically.

Inflammatory Polyps or Pseudopolyps

These are islands of healed mucosa in areas of an ulcerative process of the colon. They are found in ulcerative and granulomatous colitis. They are not premalignant, but they do correlate with the extent and severity of ulcerative activity. When these polyps are symptomatic (bleeding) or arouse suspicion of neoplasm, they should be excised colonoscopically.

Hamartomas

These are defined as an abnormal arrangement of normal tissue. Some have excessive amounts of connective tissue in the lamina propria. At times, the muscularis mucosa proliferates excessively. This type of hamartomatous polyp is seen in Peutz-Jeghers syndrome and is not premalignant. When hamartomatous polyps are less than 1.0 cm in size, there may be difficulty in differentiating them from inflammatory or juvenile polyps. The polyps can be removed endoscopically.

SUBMUCOSAL POLYPOID LESIONS

Lymphoid Polyp (Benign Lymphomas)

Lymphoid polyps are most commonly found in the rectum and rectosigmoid area. They vary in size and are usually not larger than 1.0 cm. These lesions may be mistaken endoscopically for neoplastic or carcinoid polyps. If the lesion is polypoid, particularly when it is located in the rectum up to 10 cm from the anal verge, it may be excised colonoscopically using the snare wire and cautery unit.

Lipomas

Lipomas are the most common benign non-neoplastic, submucosal tumors found in the colon and rectum. They are most frequently located in the colon, usually on the right side. They are uncommon in the rectum. When a lipoma is large, soft, and yellow, the endoscopic diagnosis is easily made. If endoscopic examination reveals the lesion to be a typical lipoma, I believe it should not be excised unless it is less than 1.5 cm in diameter and has a pedicle or a narrow base. A snare wire transection of a lipoma not only may be difficult but also may penetrate the bowel wall. An asymptomatic lesion may be restudied endoscopically on an annual basis or biannually to ensure that it is not growing larger. If symptoms are related to the lesion or if the lipoma is large, firm, and ulcerated, excision is advised, usually by laparotomy.

Leiomyomas

Leiomyomas are smooth-muscle tumors of the colon and rectum. We have removed six such lesions colonoscopically; five were located in the colon and one in the rectum. They were small, ranging in diameter from 0.8 to 1.3 cm, and grossly appeared to be adenomatous lesions. Although these lesions are submucosal or intramural, they can be confused with neoplastic polyps. When these lesions are pedunculated, they may be excised locally by transecting the stalk with the snare wire. If they are sessile and located in the colon, above 10 cm from the anal verge, endoscopic excision is contraindicated.

Carcinoid Tumors

Carcinoids of the colon are most commonly found in the rectum. These lesions grow slowly and have a lower potential for malignancy. They are usually asymptomatic and are incidental findings at colonoscopic examination. The carcinoid syndrome rarely occurs with rectal carcinoids. Endoscopically, carcinoid tumors typically appear as round, tan lesions situated in the submucosa. Usually they are less than 1.0 cm in diameter. Lesions of this size are usually benign. Because of their submucosal location, endoscopic excision is dangerous above the peritoneal reflection. Large lesions, more than 2.0 cm in diameter, are usually invasive and require operative resection. (See the article on Carcinoid Tumors and the Carcinoid Syndrome.)

Granular Cell Myoblastoma

This lesion is a rare submucosal tumor of the gastrointestinal tract and may be found anywhere from the oral cavity to the rectum. Endoscopically, it resembles other submucosal tumors such as carcinoids, lymphomas, and leiomyomas. If the tumor is smaller than 1.0 cm in diameter and is situated in the rectum within the 10-cm level, it may be excised endoscopically for definitive diagnosis. A lesion larger than 2.0 cm in diameter, which would usually be ulcerated, should be excised surgically.

Colonic Endometriosis

Endometriosis involving the colon is not frequently recognized because the diagnosis is difficult. Endometrial implants usually involve the sigmoid colon. Crampy lower abdominal pains, episodic bloody stool, alternating constipation and diarrhea, and small stools are consequences of endometrial implants. Establishing a diagnosis is more difficult, since endometrial tissues are rarely seen in the mucosa of the bowel. A patient with submucosal or mucosal endometrioma and gastrointestinal symptoms usually has deeper involvement of the bowel wall and may require a colotomy to excise the lesion. (See the article on Endometriosis.)

MULTIPLE COLONIC POLYPS (COLONIC POLYPOSIS)

Juvenile Polyposis

Numerous juvenile polyps are found scattered throughout the entire colon. Such cases do not require immediate surgical intervention unless the patient is symptomatic (e.g., growth retardation, anemia). Some physicians believe that the natural history of this entity is that of spontaneous degeneration once the child reaches adolescence. However, others believe that these polyps may change toward the adenomatous types with their attendant risk. This has rarely been reported, and whether these adenomas arise de novo or are a degeneration of juvenile polyps is open to conjecture. We feel that a patient with juvenile polyposis should have the larger lesions excised and examined histologically. If no adenomatous changes are found, these patients can be followed biannually or annually with no need for surgical intervention unless neoplastic changes are demonstrated. Each patient with juvenile polyposis should be individually treated, either endoscopically or surgically, depending upon the family history, age, general condition, and histology.

Peutz-Jeghers Syndrome

In 1921, Peutz described a syndrome of polyposis of the small intestine, associated with pigmented lesions of the skin. In 1949, Jeghers described a polyposis of the intestinal tract with mucocutaneous pigmentation. In 1954, Brewer named this condition Peutz-Jeghers syndrome, which in a classic description consists of mucocutaneous melanotic pigmentation, intestinal polyposis, and a familial history of the disease. The polyps occur throughout the entire gastrointestinal tract but are most commonly seen in the jejunum and ileum, followed in frequency by the colon, rectum, stomach, duodenum, and appendix.

The endoscopic appearance and size of these polyps vary, but they resemble adenomatous polyps. They may be sessile or pedunculated. Histologic examination of the polyps reveals that most are hamartomas (abnormal rearrangement of normal tissue). Treatment of this syndrome is difficult. Because of the diffuse distribution and intermittent growth patterns of the polyp, a definitive prophylactic approach is not possible. Using endoscopy and polypectomy is a relatively conservative approach for polyps that can be reached (i.e., those in the stomach, duodenum, terminal ileum, colon, and rectum). Annual examinations after polypectomy can help keep these areas free of polyps and can reduce the likelihood of complications. However, recurrent intussusception, hemorrhage, or anemia may necessitate surgical intervention after accurate localization.

Familial Polyposis

Familial polyposis is a rare, generalized form of inherited polyposis. The usual feature of this syndrome is the presence of numerous colonic polyps of various sizes. The great danger to the patient is malignant degeneration of the polyps. Usually, from the age of 30, malignant potential is 100 percent. Diagnosis is easily made by barium enema, colonoscopy, or both. All members of the affected patient's family should be examined. Because of the high incidence of cancer of the colon, we recommend subtotal colectomy with ileoproctostomy or a total proctocolectomy. The rectal stump should be examined endoscopically once or twice each year and all remaining polyps should be excised.

Gardner's Syndrome

Gardner's syndrome is an interesting variant of familial polyposis. Here, numerous colonic polyps are seen in association with polyps in the stomach and small bowel. In addition, cutaneous and bony manifestations, such as fibromas, desmoid tumors, sebaceous cysts, osteomas, and other connective tissue tumors, may be present. The colonic polyps, again, are adenomatous and show 100 per cent tendency toward malignant degeneration.

ANORECTAL AND PERIANAL DISORDERS

By Bertram A. Portin, M.D.
Ronald F. Teitler, M.D.
and Fred E. Boehmke, M.D.
Buffalo, New York

An appropriate history, inspection, and palpation are the cornerstones of the physical diagnosis of perianal and anorectal diseases. In order to properly utilize these techniques, it is equally necessary to have a thorough understanding of the anatomy of this region and of the possible pathologic conditions to which this region is subject.

TERMINOLOGY AND ANATOMY

Although anorectal anatomy is constant, the terminology is often variable, confusing, and conflicting. Three general regions are included in the anatomic description. The *perianal area* is limited medially by the anal verge and laterally by an arbitrary distance of 2 to 3 inches. The verge is the external portion of the anal opening. The entire area is covered by skin no different from any other epidermal area. The external sphincters lie subcutaneously surrounding the verge. Lateral to the sphincters are subcutaneous potential spaces that are significant in the development of localized abscesses and fistulas.

The *anal canal* is the terminal portion of the digestive tract. Proximally it begins at the anorectal line. This marks the junction between intestinal mucosa and the squamous epithelium of the anal canal. The first centimeter is a transitional zone similar to that found in other body areas where mucosa meets skin. This transitional zone is the site of the anal crypts and columns, which are important in the development of the common cryptogenic abscess. Distally the anal canal ends at the anal verge.

The third region is the *rectum,* a mucosal tube whose proximal border lies at about the level of the third sacral vertebra. The rectum descends along the hollow of the sacrum for about 10 to 15 cm and ends at the anorectal line. The course of the rectum is in an anterocaudal direction until the last 4 to 5 cm, where there is an approximate 90-degree angulation to a more posterocaudal direction. This angulation is the result of traction by the puborectalis muscle in an anterior direction.

Muscles

The *levator muscles* are a striated series of support slings that extend from the bony pelvis to the region of the lower rectum. The ileococcygeus and pubococcygeus muscles support the lower rectum in a vertical plane, and the puborectalis muscle supports it in a horizontal plane. The puborectalis is responsible for creating and maintaining the anorectal angle. Its integrity is vital for fecal continence.

The *internal sphincter muscle* is a thickening of the most distal portion of the circular smooth muscle layer of the rectum. Its lowest portion actually lies about 1 cm below the anorectal line. Hypertrophy, spasm, and fibrosis of this portion of the internal sphincter is related to the pathogenesis of chronic anal fissure.

The circular rings of skeletal muscle surrounding the anus and anal canal are the *external sphincters.* These muscles are in reality extensions of the levator ani muscles. They are involved with continence and the control of defecation.

Blood Vessels and Lymphatics

The blood supply of the anorectum is important because the most common disease of this region, hemorrhoids, is a vascular condition. The *superior hemorrhoidal veins* drain into the portal system via the inferior mesenteric venous system. Portal cirrhosis may thus be associated with hemorrhoidal disease because of the restricted outflow caused by portal hypertension. Drainage from the middle and inferior hemorrhoidal veins is into the systemic circulation via the internal iliac system. The lymphatic drainage of the anorectum follows the vascular pattern. Perianal and anal canal lymphatics drain to the inguinal lymph nodes. The more proximal lymphatic drainage is cephalad toward the inferior mesenteric and internal iliac nodes.

Innervation

The external sphincters, levators, and sensory portion of the anal canal are supplied by somatic nerves. The autonomic nervous system provides sensation (distention and pressure) of both a stimulatory and inhibitory type through motor innervation of the internal sphincter and the more proximal intrinsic muscles of the rectum. These muscles control propulsion and participate in the defecatory reflex.

PATIENT HISTORY

As is the case with many diseases, a diagnosis can frequently be made by proper history alone. Therefore, knowing what to ask and knowing what the answers indicate is a most important part of the diagnostic process. Bleeding, pain, itching, control problems, stool abnormalities (constipation, diarrhea, foul-smelling stools, frothy stools, acholic stools), and abdominal cramping are the major symptomatology of this region. It is not, however, sufficient to elicit a history of pain. The location, intensity, character, time relationship, relationship to defecation, and relationship to swelling are important factors differentiating the nature of pain. Constipation means different things to many people. Some confuse irregularity with constipation. Others do not appreciate that the diarrhea of fecal impaction is primarily a constipation problem. Therefore, careful questions bordering on tedious attention to minute detail may be rewarding in establishing a diagnosis in a difficult case.

PHYSICAL EXAMINATION

Good illumination, appropriate diagnostic instruments, patient relaxation and comfort, and examiner comfort are the essentials of a good anorectal examination. Either the lateral Sims position or the knee-chest position is satisfactory. In noting pathology, one should remember that the position of examination may vary and that it is important to have a standard reference point. Therefore, one should refer to right and left, posterior and anterior, rather than to positions on the face of a clock.

Inspection

As with any physical examination, inspection is the proper first step. It is well to remember that most patients are apprehensive about rectal examination. Embarrassment, expected discomfort, and fear of the diagnosis all contribute to the apprehension. Patience, gentleness, and conversation may help to allay fear and divert the patient's attention.

The perianal area should be inspected for the various dermatoses. Idiopathic pruritus ani is the most common of these. Differentiation from secondary pruritus, psoriasis, lichen sclerosis, basal cell cancer or Bowen's or Paget's disease may require a trial of nonspecific therapy, hygienic measures, or even biopsy.

Inspection will often provide the diagnosis of para-anal or ischiorectal abscess, external hemorrhoids, thrombotic hemorrhoids, fistula, hidradenitis suppurativa, condylomata acuminata, or fissure. Of course, one should inspect as well the pilonidal area for the telltale intergluteal dimple or sinus. During inspection, valuable information can be gleaned from having the patient bear down. Levator weakness, hemorrhoidal prolapse, or even complete rectal procidentia, cystocele, rectocele, or uterine prolapse may become evident with this maneuver.

Palpation

Tactile examination is done by both palpation of the perianal area and by digital rectal examination. Direct palpation to elicit tender areas can detect such diseases as early deep abscess or coccydynia. Gentle lateral separation of the anus by stretching the buttocks may elicit pain that may provide presumptive evidence of anal canal spasm and an associated anal fissure.

The digital examination, properly done, is a most valuable diagnostic measure. All too often a digital examination is done rapidly and solely for the purpose of ruling out a large rectal cancer. There is far more information to be obtained beyond palpation for a mass lesion. One should develop a habit of circumferential examination beginning and ending at the same point. A well-lubricated finger cot, and the index finger gently inserted with the patient straining, will allow gentle access to the anal canal. The state of the sphincters, both external and internal, and the state of pliability or rigidity of the soft tissues of the anal outlet provide information about sphincter spasm, stricture, and sphincter incompetence. Reassurance and diversion help to relax the patient. Additional questions relative to the patient's history may provide such diversion.

Once the examining finger is inserted, gentle, sequential examination of the rectum and adjacent organs is done. The prostate gland (and sometimes the seminal vesicles), levator muscles, rectovaginal septum, cervix, uterus, cul-de-sac, coccyx, and sacrum all can be evaluated by the examining finger. The diagnosis of internal hemorrhoids cannot be made by digital examination alone. The venous plexus is collapsed by digital pressure, and even large hemorrhoids, therefore, escape detection. Thrombosed hemorrhoids; hypertrophied anal papillae; neoplasms; rectovaginal fistulas; and submucosal, intermuscular, and supralevator abscesses all can be diagnosed by digital examination. If a lesion, such as a deep chronic anal ulcer or fissure, is present, a digital examination is much too painful to pursue without anesthesia. Topical anesthetic ointments generally are of little use. A few milliliters of local anesthesia infiltrated into the painful area will give pain relief and immediate sphincter relaxation, allowing both digital and anoscopic evaluation.

ANOSCOPY

After initial digital examination of the anal canal is done, a well-lubricated anoscope is gently introduced. The pliability and distensibility of the anal sphincter, which have been assessed during digital examination, enable the selection of an instrument of the proper diameter. One should be alert during digital examination to the presence of anal canal pathology that needs to be visualized or that might make the introduction of an instrument too painful for the patient to tolerate. The entire circumference of the anal canal is now visualized through the anoscope. The lining of the canal and lower rectum is examined for changes in the color, consistency, and vascular pattern suggestive of lesions or inflammatory bowel disease. As the anoscope is slowly withdrawn, the internal hemorrhoidal complexes come into view. The patient is asked to strain, and a determination is made of the extent of enlargement and prolapse. Upon further withdrawal of the instrument, the area of the anal crypts and dentate line is examined for lesions in this area. A primary fistulous opening in the base of an anal crypt might be seen, as might hypertrophic anal papillae, anorectal inflammatory disease, or anal canal neoplasm. As the area just distal to the crypt is traversed, anal fissures, if present, can be visualized.

LOWER INTESTINAL ENDOSCOPY

Although the diagnosis of anorectal pathology is the primary concern of this article, subsequent evaluation of the lower intestinal tract in order to rule out additional disease processes is part of a complete colorectal evaluation. Several modalities exist, and the appropriate choice among them must be made, depending upon the experience of the examiner and the clinical situation.

Rigid Sigmoidoscopy

The 25-cm rigid sigmoidoscope provides visual access to the lower rectum and rectosigmoid colon. With the patient either in the knee-chest or the left Sims position, the instrument is gently introduced transanally. This maneuver is accompanied by verbal reassurance from the physician. The sigmoidoscope is passed proximally into the rectum, and, if possible, the rectosigmoid angle is negotiated and further visualization obtained. Introduction of the rigid sigmoidoscope involves careful manipulation in order to reduce discomfort to the patient. The bulk of the examination of the lower colon is accomplished upon gradual withdrawal of the instrument, occasionally aided by the insufflation of small quantities of air. It is not always possible to advance the rigid sigmoidoscope to its full 25 cm. Too vigorous an attempt to do so will cause the patient undue pain and increase the risk of perforation of the bowel. The rigid sigmoidoscope allows an excellent view of the lower rectum and rectal ampulla. Through this instrument, biopsy of pathology and endoscopic polypectomy can be readily performed. The limited diagnostic capability of the rigid sigmoidoscope, however, must be appreciated.

Flexible Sigmoidoscopy

While the diagnostic yield with the rigid sigmoidoscope (cancer, polyps) is approximately 35 per cent, the flexible fiberoptic sigmoidoscope (FFS), 60 cm in length, has increased the diagnostic capability of the examiner to 70 to 80 per cent. Flexible sigmoidoscopy is a slightly more time-consuming examination and requires greater technical expertise. However, when this examination is properly performed, it has been found to have excellent patient acceptance. The visualization of the colonic mucosa is unparalleled. The superior diagnostic yield with this instrument suggests that it ought to be the instrument of choice when sigmoidoscopy is indicated. The FFS can detect lesions in the tortuous sigmoid colon that are unidentifiable on barium enema examination. This ability to achieve an early and accurate diagnosis has allowed more rapid institution of appropriate and effective therapy in a variety of disease conditions. The preoperative confirmation of disease and radiologically suspicious areas of the sigmoid colon can prevent unnecessary surgical procedures.

Flexible sigmoidoscopy is a diagnostic tool. Therapeutic procedures should not be done in an office setting. Were bleeding or perforation to occur, the sequelae might well be extremely hazardous. Such electrosurgical procedures should be performed only in locations where immediate surgical intervention is possible.

Total Colonoscopy

Flexible fiberoptic sigmoidoscopy is never a substitute for total colonoscopy when this latter examination is indicated. Undiagnosed sources of bleeding in the colon require further investigation by total colonoscopy, as does unresolved symptomatology or radiologically suspicious areas beyond the reach of the flexible sigmoidoscope. The electrosurgical removal of polyps, when detected, may be safely accomplished at the time of colonoscopy.

RADIOLOGY

Evaluation of the colon may necessitate barium enema examination in order to rule out undetected pathology beyond the reach of the sigmoidoscope. The choice between standard barium enema examination and an air-contrast enema will depend upon the facilities and skill of the radiologist available and also upon the information required. Specialized studies such as angiography may be indicated in the diagnosis of obscure sources of colonic bleeding. The appropriate combination of endoscopic and radiologic techniques will provide optimal diagnostic certainty.

LABORATORY STUDIES

Hematologic evaluation is occasionally part of a colorectal examination. Determination of the hemoglobin and hematocrit may provide information regarding the extent and duration of colonic bleeding. Liver function tests can provide information as to the presence of intercurrent disease, surgical risk, or the presence of metastatic disease. Carcinoembryonic antigen (CEA) determinations aid in the evaluation and follow-up of cancer of the colon. In the evaluation of patients with anal and perianal condylomata acuminata, serologic studies for syphilis are indicated because the coexistence of these diseases is not uncommon. Recently it has been noted that there is also a coexistence of hepatitis B in patients with condylomata acuminata. Liver function tests and possibly hepatitis B antigen studies should be performed prior to surgical intervention.

In the evaluation of patients with intractable diarrhea, stool and serologic studies for ova and parasites and stool culture for bacterial overgrowth provide information that can lead to the appropriate choice of treatment. Testing of the stool for occult blood can detect the presence of occult neoplasms of the colon. It should be cautioned that in the presence of intercurrent anal canal pathology, false-positive results may occur and treatment of such pathology followed by repetition of the occult blood testing might be considered prior to further extensive work-up. It should be further cautioned that a negative result for stool occult blood does not definitively rule out colon carcinoma or polyps with any degree of certainty when compared with properly combined endoscopic and radiologic evaluation.

PERIANAL AND ANAL CANAL DISEASES

Pruritus Ani

Perianal itching, burning, and irritation are common complaints of the colorectal patient. What begins as a slight tickle, sometimes following a bowel movement, may progress to severe unremitting itching, often worse at night. Scratching and other attempts to alleviate the situation only tend to make the problem worse. Questioning of the patient as to dietary habits may reveal the excessive intake of such substances as spicy foods, beer, tomatoes, chocolate, coffee, tea, or cola drinks. The history might also suggest the presence of pinworms, diabetes mellitus, or allergic reactions to dyes, chemicals, or drugs. On examination, the perianal area is moist and the skin is thickened and exhibits a whitish lichenification. There are corrugated, thickened folds extending radially from the anal verge. Superimposed excoriation from vigorous wiping or scratching may be present and may have caused the patient to observe blood on the toilet paper. Occasional superinfection with fungus may be noted. In the female patient one should note any excessive vaginal discharge.

Bowen's Disease

This condition, manifested by plaque-like thickening and redness of the perianal skin, may mimic pruritus ani. Failure of the condition to respond to antipruritic measures should raise the suspicion of malignancy. Biopsy is then necessary to make the diagnosis of this slow-growing carcinoma in situ. The high association of systemic malignancy with Bowen's disease indicates the necessity for further work-up.

Paget's Disease

Patients with this lesion may present with a complaint of perianal pruritus, which again is unresponsive to antipruritic measures. Examination reveals erythema, eczematoid changes, and either a moist and weeping or dry and scaly lesion of the perianal skin. Paget's disease is neoplastic. Diagnosis is made by biopsy of the lesion.

Squamous Cell Carcinoma of the Anus

The patient with squamous carcinoma of the anus most frequently presents with a complaint of bleeding and pain in the anal region. The assumption that the symptoms are caused by other benign conditions may delay the proper diagnosis. Squamous carcinoma may appear as a hard nodule, grayish in color, in the perianal region or as an indolent anal canal ulceration with raised, rolled, pearly-gray borders. Careful examination and biopsy of suspicious lesions will lead to the appropriate treatment of this malignancy.

Anal Fissure or Ulcer

The patient with an anal fissure presents with a complaint of a tearing or knife-like pain upon defecation. This is frequently accompanied by bright-red rectal bleeding. The pain may persist for hours following a bowel movement. As the disease progresses, the pain becomes severe and unremitting. An anal fissure may be accompanied by either marked constipation or diarrhea. Gentle spreading of the buttocks will reveal the presence of a fissure, most commonly in the posterior midline or sometimes the anterior midline. Often there is an associated external edematous skin tag (sentinel pile). In the presence of marked spasm, digital examination is best done with the aid of local anesthesia in order to avoid causing the patient severe pain. Treatment should be instituted prior to more extensive evaluation. If spasm and pain are not severe, digital examination is done to detect the presence of any additional anal canal pathology. Anoscopy, when possible, will reveal the anal fissure with fibromuscular tissue in its base. Just proximal to the fissure, a hypertrophic anal papilla may be seen. An atypical location of an anal fissure (off the midline) should lead to the suspicion of Crohn's disease, squamous cell carcinoma, or anal canal trauma.

Condylomata Acuminata

Condylomata acuminata (singular—condyloma acuminatum), or venereal warts, appear as raised, tufted, pedunculated collections of pinkish or purplish lesions occurring at the anal verge or within the anal canal. They may be accompanied by excessive moisture, a foul odor, or maceration of the adjacent skin. Itching and pain may also be associated symptoms. Because of the possible sexual transmission of the virus associated with these lesions, an appropriate history should be taken. Also appropriate serologic studies (as mentioned) should be carried out prior to treatment.

Hemorrhoidal Disease

Hemorrhoids are varicose dilatations of the superior and/or inferior hemorrhoidal venous plexuses. Dilatations of the superior hemorrhoidal plexuses are called internal hemorrhoids and originate above the anorectal line. Dilatations of the inferior venous plexuses are called external hemorrhoids and appear at the anal verge, where they are covered by modified anal skin. Increased hydrostatic pressure in the hemorrhoidal veins causes progressive weakening of the fibromuscular attachments of the musculus submucosae ani and results in progressive, saccular, serpiginous dilatation of the venous plexus. This results in prolapse of the venous plexus with its mucosal covering into the distal anal canal with defecation.

Etiologic factors in hemorrhoidal disease include a hereditary propensity, straining at stool, constipation, diarrhea, and pregnancy. A more obscure etiology, such as portal vein hypertension, uncompensated heart failure, pelvic tumors, or carcinoma of the rectum, needs to be ruled out as well. The cardinal symptoms of internal hemorrhoids are bleeding and prolapse. Prolapse may lead to a complaint of the discharge of a foul-smelling, fecally stained, mucoid material from the anal canal, accompanied by secondary perianal irritation. Pain is not a symptom of internal hemorrhoids. If this complaint is present, its cause should be sought elsewhere.

Bleeding from internal hemorrhoids is almost always bright red and ranges from a scant streaking of blood on the stool in the early stages of disease to spontaneous hemorrhage unrelated to defecation in the advanced stages. Indeed this bleeding may reach such significant proportions that a secondary anemia may develop in some individuals.

The prolapse associated with internal hemorrhoids is progressive in nature. Initially patients note that the hemorrhoids spontaneously reduce themselves after defecation. In advanced stages of the disease the prolapse may require manual reduction after a bowel movement. Prolapse may occur spontaneously with exercise and may eventually become constant. In the latter stage of the disease, the patient is exposed to the risk of acute strangulation of the prolapsing hemorrhoids. Upon inspection, one may note the presence of enlarged or possibly thrombosed external hemorrhoids, skin tags at the site of previous external thromboses, and possibly prolapsed internal hemorrhoids as well. Digital examination is usually noncontributory.

The diagnosis of internal hemorrhoids is made during anoscopy. With the anoscope inserted, and with the patient bearing down, one can easily see the bulbous internal hemorrhoids. If the patient continues to strain as the instrument is gently withdrawn, the size of the hemorrhoids and the degree of prolapse may be assessed. Sometimes an actual bleeding site can be identified.

Fistulous Abscess

Fistula in ano is the legacy of an anorectal abscess. In its simplest form, it is a chronic granulating tract connecting two epithelium-lined surfaces: an external opening on the skin, and an internal opening originating in the mucosa of the anal canal usually at the level of an anal crypt.

Cryptogenic abscesses may progress in four directions: downward to form a para-anal abscess, laterally to form an ischiorectal abscess, submucosally to form a submucosal abscess, or proximally to form a high intramuscular or supralevator abscess.

The site of the abscess, its point of origin, and the secondary opening or point of decompression combine to produce a fistulous tract that may be categorized as a low intrasphincteric, trans-sphincteric, or suprasphincteric fistula.

A para-anal abscess presents as a red, tender, ovoid swelling in the para-anal area. This progresses to fluctuance and, if left untreated, eventually leads to skin necrosis and spontaneous decompression of the abscess. Findings from digital examination are usually normal except for some tenderness in the area immediately adjacent to the abscess. The ischiorectal abscess also causes severe pain in the para-anal area. As the disease progresses, a diffuse brawny swelling develops over the ischiorectal fossa and even further out on the buttock. Rectal examination reveals tenderness but rarely extension of the septic process into the rectum, a situation always found in intersphincteric or submucosal abscesses.

In the evaluation of abscesses of the para-anal area, it is important to remember to rule out abscesses arising from other causes such as periprostatic or periurethral glands (which may occur in the male) or Bartholin's gland abscesses (which may occur in the female). It is important also not to confuse post-anal abscesses with pilonidal abscesses, which may occur at the same site.

An anal fistula may occur spontaneously, with no antecedent abscess having been noted by the patient. The patient then presents with a history of discharge and perianal irritation. A fistula is painless, although the patient may develop a secondary pruritus from the continual discharge or episodic pain from small, recurrent, spontaneously draining abscesses. Inspection of the anal region should reveal an external opening or openings at the distal site of the fistula. This secondary opening may be healed over, marked by a raised area of granulation or scar tissue. The skin surrounding this secondary opening may be red and thickened, and irritation from the chronic seepage may be noted. On palpation it may be possible to express pus from the secondary opening of the fistulous tract or to palpate the tract as a thickened cord and trace it back toward its primary opening in the anal canal. Sometimes a fine silver probe can be gently passed along the tract to determine its course back to the anal canal. Digital examination may reveal induration at the site of the primary opening, and on anoscopy the primary opening may be identified either by noting a small amount of purulent material escaping from it or by direct visualization of the opening and passage of a hooked probe into it.

It is important to rule out underlying pathology such as Crohn's disease, colloid carcinoma of the rectum, or lymphogranuloma venereum, all of which may be associated with fistula formation. It is also important to remember that carcinoma may arise from a long-standing fistula.

Crohn's Disease

The most common lesion of Crohn's disease of the anal canal is an atypical fissure. This fissure is distinguished by being a broad-based ulceration that occurs as frequently anteriorly or laterally as it does posteriorly. There may be multiple simultaneous fissures. The skin tags associated with these fissures are edematous, and the ulcers themselves are indolent and undermined and often exude a watery purulent material from their base. The fistulas associated with Crohn's disease are extensive and complicated with undermined edges. They exude purulent material when palpated, and the entire area surrounding them takes on a brawny induration and dusky purplish discoloration. Rectal examination of these patients may show normal findings but in many instances will reveal a secondary stenosis of the anal canal due to the extensive inflammatory changes surrounding it. In many of these instances a biopsy of the ulcer or fistula can be extremely helpful in establishing the differential diagnosis.

ANORECTAL DISEASES

Inflammatory Bowel Disease and Carcinoma

In the evaluation and diagnosis of the patient with anal pathology, the physician must always be alert to the possibility of the simultaneous presence of rectal pathology as well. Thus, in the case of the patient presenting with hemorrhoids and rectal bleeding, it should not necessarily be assumed that the bleeding is coming from the hemorrhoids. A thorough and complete investigation should be done to rule out the possibility of a proctitis or rectal carcinoma that might exist simultaneously.

Inflammatory bowel disease is characterized by a wide range of symptoms ranging from slight looseness of the bowel movements and the passage of blood to severe diarrhea with the passage of liquid fecal material, blood, mucus, and pus. It may also be associated with symptoms of colicky abdominal pain, lethargy, anemia, and pyrexia.

Inspection of the anal area may reveal signs of local complications of the disease such as abscess, fissure, or fistula. Digital examination may reveal the presence of a stenosis or of a granular texture of the mucosa. Sigmoidoscopic examination is of importance, both in defining the extent of the disease above the anal verge and in assessing the severity of the disease by evaluating the degree of granularity and friability of the colonic mucosa and the presence of ulcerations, exudate, or inflammatory polyps. The mucosal biopsy is often a valuable diagnostic aid both for the purpose of confirming the diagnosis and for evaluating the progression or remission of the disease process over a period of time. It also serves an important role in checking for dysplastic changes that may herald the development of carcinoma.

Carcinoma of the rectum is characterized primarily by rectal bleeding associated with a change in bowel habits. Secondary symptoms such as anorexia, weight loss, and rectal or abdominal pain are usually late features of this disease. Digital examination may reveal blood on the finger tip, and palpation of the rectal wall may reveal induration or the raised edge of an ulcerated tumor. Digital examination may reveal also a nodular friable mass extending into the lumen or an annular constricting lesion of the rectum that will not permit the passage of a finger tip through it. In performing the digital examination, it is important to ascertain the location of the tumor, its size, the extent of its invasiveness, and whether or not the lesion is fixed or mobile. Sigmoidoscopic examination permits direct visualization of the lesion and assessment of its size, location, and degree of obstruction. Its microscopic characteristics can be assessed by biopsy. Endoscopy also serves to rule out synchronous lesions and the possibility of adenomatous polyps in adjacent areas of the colon. Barium enema or colonoscopy, performed either preoperatively or postoperatively, is important in ruling out the presence of more proximal synchronous pathology.

Foreign Bodies

Foreign bodies may be divided into two broad categories: those which are ingested and those which are inserted.

Ingested foreign bodies may include fragments of bone, egg shells, seeds, pits, toothpicks, and food materials swallowed either deliberately or inadvertently by the patient. Patients on psychiatric wards have been known to ingest nails, screws, needles, and thermometers.

Inserted foreign bodies include such mundane objects as rectal thermometers and enema tips as well as more unusual objects such as lightbulbs, bottles, vibrators, and the like. The main concern is that these objects, when inserted, will lacerate or necrose the lining of the anal canal or rectum.

Because of embarrassment, history is often sketchy or misleading. Schizophrenic patients also fail to provide adequate history. Diagnosis, therefore, may be accidental following abdominal x-ray films for other disease or following digital or endoscopic examination performed for other reasons.

Removal of foreign objects by the transanal route, and consequent avoidance of laparotomy, should be attempted first. The specific technique of extraction needs to be individualized, depending upon the nature of the object encountered. The mechanics involved often tax the imagination and ingenuity of the physician. Because of the complexity of this problem, removal should be attempted by experienced personnel only.

VASCULAR DISEASE OF THE MESENTERY

By Lester F. Williams, Jr., M.D.
Boston, Massachusetts

SYNONYMS

Mesenteric vascular insufficiency, intestinal infarction, mesenteric infarction, mesenteric venous occlusion, nonocclusive mesenteric ischemia, mesenteric arterial occlusive disease, extensive mesenteric ischemia, segmented mesenteric ischemia, small bowel ischemia, ischemic colitis, chronic intestinal ischemia, or abdominal angina.

DEFINITION

Vascular disease of the mesentery is a spectrum of clinical problems of varying severity and of differing etiologies produced by a primary process that interferes with the blood supply to mesenteric structures. A distinction is made between a vascular process that is the primary event (such as arterial embolism or venous occlusion) and one that is a secondary phenomenon (wherein bowel infarction is the end result of another process such as mechanical small bowel obstruction, which can cause strangulation).

The spectrum is so wide that these clinical problems (with respect to presenting signs and symptoms, course, evaluation, and treatment) are best considered under two separate headings:

1. Extensive mesenteric ischemia.
2. Segmental mesenteric ischemia.

Although there is some overlap within these groups, both with respect to etiology and to area of the bowel involved, most patients' problems fall clearly and easily within one or the other of these headings.

The spectrum of etiologies varies from arterial occlusive phenomena, through venous occlusive phenomena and into hemodynamic or perfusion abnormalities, as seen in nonocclusive mesenteric ischemia. The spectrum of clinical presentation may vary from an acute catastrophic illness manifesting with systemic phenomena and with a localized process within the abdomen, through a bloody diarrheal disease with mild abdominal pain, to asymptomatic or minimally symptomatic obstructive phenomena, as seen in the healing stages of ischemic strictures of the colon. The spectrum of treatment spans observation without intervention until spontaneous healing occurs, through urgent intervention after an aggressive diagnostic approach. The latter may include surgery such as embolectomy, bypass of arterial thrombosis, or resection of the part of the gastrointestinal tract that is involved with venous occlusion. In addition, therapy may be directed toward hemodynamic manipulation of both the patient's systemic and splanchnic circulations.

EXTENSIVE MESENTERIC ISCHEMIA

Presenting Signs and Symptoms

Just as the history of gut ischemia is similar regardless of the cause of ischemia, so the signs and symptoms are similar. The spectrum of clinical presentations is more a reflection of the volume of ischemic damage than of the cause or the location of the ischemia. Gut ischemia is always an acute process, and even patients with chronic intestinal ischemia or abdominal angina show signs and symptoms of recurrent acute attacks. Secondary features, such as weight loss, develop only because the patient, over time, tries to prevent acute episodes. Acute extensive mesenteric ischemia can be suspected on the basis of the history and physical examination. However, a firm diagnosis of its presence and its specific etiology usually requires detailed radiologic study, including arteriography and barium studies, endoscopy, and/or surgical exploration. Analysis using computer techniques for evaluation of relationships between the clinical findings and the specific etiologies for over a hundred cases of mesenteric ischemia has shown that it is not possible to differentiate the patients with occlusion of a major vessel from those with perfusion defects. Furthermore, although the diagnosis can be suspected on clinical grounds, it is frequently not considered.

Pain is the outstanding symptom and is present in almost all cases of intestinal ischemia. In 1500 cases, Jackson noted pain in 98 per cent of the patients ("severe and violent" in 66 per cent). Although some autopsy series note pain in under 50 per cent, in all clinical series there was pain present in over 75 per cent. The pain may be colicky and periumbilical at its onset, but it soon becomes a severe, poorly localized, continuous pain that is not changed by any activity. The pain was insidious in onset and diffuse in location in three of every four patients with perfusion defects. Many associated symptoms have been recorded (vomiting, anorexia, nausea, diarrhea, constipation, melena, and hematemesis), but these are seldom the predominant complaints and they offer little differential information. One of the most characteristic findings with gut ischemia is the lack of significant abdominal abnormalities even when the pain is unbearable. The patient, however, may exhibit evidence of sympathetic activity with restlessness, apprehension, sweating, and hyperactivity, but shock is not present. An early positive physical sign is severe abdominal distention occurring even when peristalsis is present, a finding seen very early in only a few cases (18 per cent) but developing later in most (56 to 80 per cent).

Evidence for gastrointestinal bleeding can also be found in most patients (over 50 per cent), but it is seldom gross except when the colon is involved. With progression of the ischemia, peritonitis becomes manifest (54 to 94 per cent) but is severe in only a few (12 to 38 per cent). A peculiar mottled cyanosis of the abdomen has been observed. When the volume of bowel ischemia is large, dehydration is frequent and severe and shock eventually occurs (in over 60 per cent of poorly treated patients).

The history and/or physical examination may reveal phenomena that could predispose the patient to mesenteric ischemia. Causes of arterial emboli (such as rheumatic valvular disease) or of arterial thrombosis (such as diffuse atherosclerosis) should be noted. Reasons for venous occlusion (such as pancreatic carcinoma, hypercoagulable states) or low flow states (secondary to such conditions as severe congestive failure) should likewise arouse suspicion. Less secure information is provided by observations that seem to rule out common diseases associated with abdominal pain. Patients whose pain is not easily explained by the presence of common diseases should be considered to have mesenteric ischemia if there is the proper setting for arterial or venous occlusion or for a low flow state. Variations in the symptom complex can occur, as in the few patients who manifest abdominal distention, blood loss, or unexplained hypovolemia without prominent pain.

As noted earlier, the diagnosis of acute extensive mesenteric ischemia and identification of its specific cause are seldom possible on the basis of presenting signs and symptoms. Diagnosing the presence of extensive mesenteric ischemia then depends heavily on clinical evaluation.

Course

Hemorrhagic necrosis is the end result for the involved bowel, regardless of the cause of the ischemia. However, the distribution of the lesion along the intestine, the degree of involvement of the wall of the ischemic segment (i.e., full or partial thickness), and the rapidity of the process vary widely with differing etiologies.

With the use of conventional techniques, histologic evidence of change in mucosal cells appears as early as 1 hour after occlusion of the superior mesenteric artery. Several hours are usually required before gross changes are seen. With the electron microscope, some changes can be observed within 10 minutes and extensive changes by 30 minutes. Although damage to the rough and smooth endoplasmic reticulum can be seen within 10 minutes, extensive damage likely associated with significant failure of cellular function is not seen until 30 minutes. By this time, the mitochondria are also affected and their oxygen consumption is decreased by 28 per cent. Interestingly enough, the lysosomal membrane is intact at 30 minutes. Thus, ischemia entails both a metabolic effect and a mechanical effect. The mucosal cells lose their ability to produce mucus, are subject to digestion by intraluminal enzymes, and become permeable to bacteria and other toxic substances. The resultant cellular dysfunction also permits changes in bidirectional flow of fluid and electrolytes as well as luminal loss of plasma. Thus, massive volume loss into the gut lumen develops. The conventional histologic picture following bowel ischemia is one of hemorrhagic necrosis, extensive submucosal edema, some interstitial edema and hemorrhage, and little inflammatory infiltration. A notable exception is the colon, in which inflammatory reaction may be more prominent. The histologic findings are the same, whether the initial process is complete occlusion of a main artery or vein or prolonged severe splanchnic vasoconstriction without any organic occlusion.

Extensive submucosal hemorrhage is manifested clinically as "thumbprints" (a pattern caused by submucosal hemorrhagic edema) on barium studies or hemorrhagic bullae on endoscopic visualization, whereas mucosal destruction is seen as superficial ulceration. One of the hallmarks of ischemic bowel damage is the relatively rapid change in the barium enema or endoscopic picture during the early stages and the very slow change during the later stages. When ischemia is severe enough to involve the muscles of the gut wall, an initial hyperperistalsis is followed by marked distention with disordered mobility. Occasionally, especially in the colon, decreased distensibility is seen. Rarely, full-wall infarction will lead to free perforation or pericolic inflammation.

Healing after an ischemic attack may produce a completely normal bowel or a bowel that is grossly normal but that has histologic abnormalities. Later the ischemic area may contain only hemosiderin-laden macrophages. Some patients develop a stenosis of varying length. Some investigators have found evidence for persistent absorption abnormalities months after an ischemic attack. They suggest that the initial necrosis is followed by rapid regeneration that produces a grossly normal mucosa. This phase is then followed by a much slower one of cellular reorganization into normal functional absorptive tissue.

The rapidity with which the bowel manifests ischemic damage, and thus is associated with changes in physical findings and systemic phenomena (to be described in the section on complications), is related both to the status of collateral circulation before the acute event and to the specific etiologic factor involved. Venous occlusion, which is associated with massive edema of the bowel wall and of the mesentery, manifests severe and very rapid volume depletion phenomena. Arterial emboli, especially if they occur in the absence of diffuse atherosclerosis, are characterized by very acute onset of a distinct episode that progresses over hours. In contrast, nonocclusive mesenteric ischemia—the problem of the low flow state—is most often insidious in onset with progression over days rather than hours. The mildest form of extensive mesenteric ischemia—abdominal angina or chronic mesenteric ischemia—involves only the mucosa, so that there are no abdominal or systemic findings. Because the attack lasts only a few minutes or hours, there is no progression to bowel wall involvement. While an isolated patient may have a specific etiologic diagnosis made on the basis of the signs and symptoms and the early course, experience in all large series has shown great overlap in the clinical picture for each of the etiologic groups. Unfortunately for most patients, this overlap, for both physical findings and laboratory evaluation, continues from the presenting signs and symptoms into the course. Differential observations about specific etiology, and therefore treatment, become manifest only during special radiologic evaluations.

Complications

Complications may be local within the ischemic bowel or within the peritoneal cavity, or systemic with involvement of many organ systems. The clinically relevant changes in mucosal function after an ischemic insult are interference with bidirectional flow of fluid and electrolytes as well as luminal loss of plasma. Thus, there is a massive volume loss into the gut lumen, which becomes manifest from all the signs, symptoms, and consequences of hypovolemia. In addition there may be destruction of the mucosa whereby the gut becomes permeable to bacteria and other toxic substances. These phenomena, which become more obvious when transmural ischemia exists (i.e., in the later stages of any attack or when the process is due to occlusive disease), are manifest from the signs and symptoms of peritonitis. Peritoneal involvement may be localized at first, but it becomes generalized rapidly when extensive amounts of bowel are involved.

The systemic manifestations of mesenteric ischemia are responsible for the descriptions of these entities as catastrophic diseases. The complications are those expected with severe hypovolemia and/or sepsis and primarily involve the cardiovascular, pulmonary, and renal systems. One common manifestation is the metabolic acidosis of poor tissue perfusion. Later in the course of continuing ischemia, all the systemic manifestations of sepsis, with multiorgan failure and its attendant pulmonary, cardiovascular, hepatic, renal, and metabolic consequences, are seen. For many years, specific toxic effects of mesenteric ischemia have fascinated researchers in this field, but the significance of these factors, if they exist, remains in doubt. Death, if it occurs, is due to volume deficits or to the consequences of sepsis. Unfortunately, ischemic gut is capable of perpetuating self-sustaining cycles of volume loss and sepsis even after the original precipitating event has been corrected. Thus, control of volume deficits and of sepsis is as essential as correction of the primary process.

If the process is self-limited, is corrected by proper treatment, or occurs only in a limited segment of bowel, healing may occur without residual defects. Ischemic strictures have been described as a result of ischemic colitis. Some believe absorptive and/or digestive defects can exist when the mucosa has healed to correct ulcerative defects but has not undergone reorganization into normal functional absorptive tissue. The clinical significance of these two healing phenomena is unclear.

Physical Examination

The hallmark of physical examination for a patient with acute extensive mesenteric ischemia is severe abdominal pain when minimal abdominal findings are present. This dichotomy differentiates these lesions from more common conditions such as acute cholecystitis or diverticulitis. Physical findings may support the presence of other features of the acute process such as dehydration, abdominal distention, gastrointestinal (GI) blood loss, or, late in the course, signs of peritonitis. Furthermore, examination may reveal the presence of conditions that would predispose to mesenteric ischemia, such as generalized atherosclerosis, myocardial and/or valvular disease, low flow state, hypercoagulation, or intra-abdominal neoplasms, such as carcinoma of the pancreas.

Laboratory Procedures

Although these patients usually have an elevated white blood cell count with a shift to the left and may have extremely high white cell counts, laboratory evaluation is seldom diagnostic of mesenteric ischemia and never diagnostic of a specific cause for the problem. There may be confirmatory findings for hypovolemia and occasionally of acute blood loss. Over the years many specific tests have been suggested as reasonable screening procedures (e.g., hypoglycemia, base defect, elevated inorganic phosphate, elevated alkaline phosphatase, elevated lactic acid, or changes in intestinal enzymes, mucosal enzymes, creatine kinase and its isoenzymes, lysosomal acid hydrolases). However, none has stood the test of time. Malabsorption has been identified in some patients with abdominal angina, but again it is nonspecific. Persistent metabolic acidosis occurring *after* shock has been corrected suggests mesenteric infarction, but many patients with extensive mesenteric ischemia manifest neither shock nor such a persistent acidosis.

Recent interest in the use of radionuclide studies has shifted from emphasis on direct observations of flow (as mentioned for reactive hyperemia or on the comparison of hot and cold "areas") to wash-out curves for intraperitoneally injected xenon 133. Once again, its specific value remains to be determined.

Radiologic Evaluation

While routine abdominal radiologic studies may suggest the diagnosis of mesenteric infarction because abnormal gas patterns in the bowel wall or liver can be identified, these changes occur so late and so infrequently in adults that they are of limited diagnostic value. In some cases (20 to 25 per cent) such radiologic studies are normal, while in others (40 to 50 per cent) only abdominal distention due to bowel gas can be seen. In the remainder, the abnormal gas pattern may suggest mechanical obstruction of either the small or large bowel. Thus, routine radiologic evaluation provides minimal diagnostic information.

While barium studies may reveal evidence for mesenteric ischemia because of the presence of ulcerations and/or mucosal edema, seen as "thumbprints" in the colon and "pinky" prints in the small bowel, they are seldom necessary for diagnosis of acute extensive mesenteric ischemia. Moreover, the barium would interfere with subsequent angiographic studies, which will be necessary for diagnosis and might be necessary for proper treatment. Thus, most agree that barium studies are contraindicated in these patients.

Angiographic documentation of the specific etiology of mesenteric ischemia is essential for proper therapy and should be obtained preoperatively in all patients. Most agree, then, that all patients with suspected mesenteric ischemia (based upon history, physical findings, laboratory evaluation, and routine radiologic studies) should have an angiogram as soon as the diagnosis is seriously considered. A flush aortogram with both anteroposterior and lateral projections followed when necessary (i.e., when there is no occlusion of the superior mesenteric artery) by selective catheterization of the superior mesenteric artery, occasionally the celiac axis, and/or the inferior mesenteric artery will establish the diagnosis in almost all cases. Easily made diagnoses include acute arterial thrombosis, acute arterial emboli at all levels, and acute venous occlusion. Evaluation of the collateral circulation, particularly on the flush study, may permit decisions about chronic occlusions of the arterial tree and help differentiate a chronic from an acute process. The diagnosis of nonocclusive mesenteric ischemia or low flow states can be suggested by abnormal flow patterns within the splanchnic system if the studies are done after shock has been corrected.

Occasionally, each of these radiologic evaluations can provide specific information that might raise the issue of some other diagnosis. For example, kidney-ureter-bladder (KUB) tests might reveal unexpected gallstones or free intraperitoneal air; barium studies might reveal evidence for diverticulitis; or angiograms might reveal internal hernia or midgut volvulus. These occasional "incidental" findings are used by some to justify the use of angiograms, though the incidence of negative studies can be 15 to 25 per cent. A better justification is the need for early diagnosis and treatment of mesenteric ischemia; this need can be met adequately by no other diagnostic maneuver.

Other Diagnostic Procedures

Mention has already been made of the observation that persistent metabolic acidosis existing after shock has been corrected suggests mesenteric ischemia.

Some have suggested that angiographic abnormalities occurring after pharmacologic treatment (especially intra-arterial medication) can provide diagnostic and/or prognostic information. However, these observations are not definitive except in the circumstances of a postóperative recurrence of arterial occlusion or when an intra-arterial catheter used for medication has changed position. These latter cases can be discovered only when repeat angiograms are obtained on a routine basis or as a result of the patient's condition.

Exploratory laparotomy, as a time-honored diagnostic tool for the "surgical abdomen" or for peritonitis, has been applied to cases of mesenteric ischemia. Unfortunately, its use in these problems produces many difficulties. Even when mesenteric ischemia can be identified, its cause is seldom clear and thus treatment is poor. Confounding the surgeon is the fact that the mucosa can be infarcted while the serosa may remain normal. Venous occlusion may be suggested by an edematous mesentery, or arterial embolism by a single distal occlusion. However, in the vast majority of cases one cannot distinguish, at the operating table, between arterial embolism, arterial thrombus, venous occlusion and nonocclusive mesenteric ischemia. This indecision leads to treatment troubles: Does one resect all the gut, remove an embolus, or do a bypass graft?

Therapeutic Tests

Following either arterial embolectomy or bypass graft for arterial thrombosis, the majority of surgeons would consider a routine "second-look" operation as part of the definitive treatment, while others might consider it a therapeutic test. The principle of the routine second-look operation, done in all patients who have had an embolectomy and/or arterial bypass, is that resection of nonviable bowel is best accomplished 6 to 24 hours after revascularization has occurred. Resection accomplished during the first operation can remove only the grossly diseased bowel. Since in extensive mesenteric ischemia it is essential to preserve every centimeter of viable bowel, the definitive decision about resection should be accomplished during the second look. The second look can be considered a therapeutic trial because at this time the success of the corrective vascular surgery can be assessed.

In venous occlusive disease, resection of the involved bowel with postoperative anticoagulation is the treatment of choice. Thus, while a second look has been mentioned, it is seldom applied. Likewise in elective surgery for abdominal angina, the therapeutic test of second look is not applied.

Pharmacologic vasomotor manipulation of the splanchnic circulation, done through the intraarterial catheter, is considered by some a therapeutic test. If it produces relief of the splanchic vasoconstriction or is associated with relief of pain and absence of peritoneal findings, it can be considered definitive treatment. There are some who will not operate upon the patient with nonocclusive mesenteric ischemia if arterial medications are successful as manifested by relief of pain and the absence of peritonitis. Indeed, in a few selected cases, patients with mesenteric artery emboli who had adequate collaterals, shown by angiographic techniques with these collaterals remaining open under pharmacologic treatment, have been treated without operation. For the majority of patients, however, such pharmacologic treatment is a preoperative procedure. Surgery is then performed for acute extensive mesenteric ischemia, as described already: immediate operation and a second look for aterial occlusive phenomena; immediate operation for venous occlusive phenomena; and delayed operation following the principle of the second look for patients with nonocclusive mesenteric ischemia.

Potential Errors and Pitfalls in the Diagnosis

Throughout the clinical history of mesenteric ischemia, the most frequent error has been failure to consider the diagnosis in a patient complaining of severe abdominal pain but having minimal findings on examination of the abdomen. Such an error is easily made when the patient has radiologic phenomena suggesting small bowel obstruction or when the patient has the problems of volume abnormalities with less pain.

The second most common pitfall is to approach the patient as if the pain and associated abdominal findings justified the presence of "a surgical abdomen" for which an exploratory laparotomy is essential. This pitfall is particularly enticing if one forgets that the pathologic process can be extensive on the mucosal side in spite of the presence of a normal serosa as visualized by the operating surgeon. A third error in the diagnosis is to deny the need for an aggressive angiographic approach early in the disease, thus missing an opportunity for precise diagnosis of mesenteric ischemia and, equally important, of its specific etiology.

SEGMENTAL ISCHEMIA

Presenting Signs and Symptoms

Very rarely will a patient with segmental ischemia involving the small bowel be identified. Such patients have the presenting signs, symptoms, and history consistent with intraperitoneal inflammatory disease and are almost always treated as if they had appendicitis, diverticulitis, or cholecystitis. Not until the time of operation is a small segment of infarcted bowel found and the diagnosis considered for the first time. Only in patients who have had similar episodes of small bowel segmental infarction in the past is small bowel ischemia high among the possible differential diagnoses. For these reasons and for practical purposes, the significant clinical entity of segmental ischemia is synonymous with ischemic colitis.

Ischemic colitis presents as a bloody diarrhea with abdominal pain. However, because the pain is not a prominent symptom, these circumstances are seldom confused with extensive mesenteric ischemia. The degree of diarrhea and the degree of blood with the diarrhea are highly variable. Acute bleeding—to the extent that transfusions are necessary—can occur, but severe bleeding requiring emergency resection has not been observed in ischemic colitis. Peritoneal signs, if present at the onset, are minimal and localized. There are very rare cases of fulminant ischemic colitis in which transmural infarction occurs over the course of hours. Such patients manifest a rampant and progressive peritoneal process and are operated upon because of general peritonitis; the specific disease process, ischemic colitis, is found intraoperatively. Such a fulminant course can occur spontaneously, but it is seen more commonly in patients with evidence of ischemic colitis who have had a procedure in which the inferior mesenteric artery has been ligated (such as an extensive resection of left colon for cancer, or resection of an abdominal aortic aneurysm). The history of associated conditions with ischemic colitis is not as significant as in the extensive bowel ischemia entity. Such patients, however, may have been observed for colonic obstruction or had previous surgery, particularly that which interfered with the collateral circulation between the inferior mesenteric system and the superior mesenteric system.

Course and Complications

An extensive classification of ischemic colitis by etiology or associated conditions has been suggested, but the only clinically relevant classification is related to the degree or duration of peritoneal findings. Mild cases, which account for the majority, have transient episodes of bloody diarrhea, minimal additional findings, and no residual. The moderate process is more indolent and has definite signs of peritoneal inflammation. A severe case may be similar to the fulminant cases already described or it may be a "moderate" process that persists for weeks. Chronic problems are those presenting with evidence of a stricture but without acute bloody diarrhea. These are presumed to be secondary to an attack of ischemic colitis in the past.

The outstanding observation with ischemic colitis is its rapidly changing findings, particularly of the mucosal lesions. Indeed, the progression of the mucosal lesion as seen endoscopically or with barium enema differentiates ischemic colitis from many of the other conditions that might produce lesions in the mucosa. However, the course of an episode of ischemic colitis is determined by the physical findings within the abdomen, not by mucosal abnormalities.

The mild form of ischemic colitis is characterized by a course lasting a few days with bloody diarrhea, with minimal evidence of peritonitis, and with no systemic symptoms. It progresses to healing without residual and without recurrence. In the moderate form, patients are apt to have more evidence of peritoneal disease, but more importantly they have prolongation of their disease process beyond a few days. During this time they may have some mild systemic evidence of an inflammatory process, but they are not severely ill.

The severe form of ischemic colitis can take one of two courses. Very rarely it will be fulminant with rapid progression to transmural involvement and therefore to generalized peritonitis. More often, the severe form manifests itself as distinct peritoneal inflammation with a protracted course extending 2 weeks or longer. There is clear evidence of the inflammatory process manifest by fever, elevated white blood cell counts, and localized evidence of peritonitis. The rarest of all kinds appears to be the chronic form, which presents as a colonic stricture with partial and usually mild colonic obstruction. Unlike other strictures, they do not progress either to functional obstruction or to an anatomic defect.

Physical Examination

The emphasis in the diagnosis of ischemic colitis is on demonstrating mucosal lesions because this element differentiates the entity from many others. Physical examination does not reveal the same level of catastrophic systemic phenomena as seen with extensive mesenteric ischemia. It may reveal minimal abdominal distension and mild localized peritonitis. The diagnosis is established when on endoscopic evaluation of the colon the classic mucosal ulcerations and/or hemorrhagic bullae reflecting the hemorrhagic edema of the submucosa appear. Barium enema studies may also show the ulcerations and/or the submucosal edema seen as "thumbprinting."

The lesions of ischemic colitis are characteristically stable in location and in extent of involvement throughout any one acute attack, a feature that may differentiate these problems from other ulcerative phenomena of the colon. However, as already mentioned, within the involved area the lesions are characterized by rapid change in their character. There is no correlation between the findings in the mucosa and in the severity of the clinical illness as represented by peritoneal and/or systemic findings. Neither is there correlation between mucosal findings and associated phenomena, including those of atherosclerosis.

Laboratory Evaluation

Patients with ischemic colitis may have a slightly increased white blood cell count and a shift to the left. This finding is not of diagnostic importance because the process can occur without any laboratory abnormalities whatsoever. All other laboratory data are normal. In the presence of such an ulcerative, bloody diarrheal disease, most experts believe it is important to rule out the specific causes of colitis by examination and culture of the stool.

Radiologic Evaluation

All agree that the barium enema establishes the presence and extent of ischemic colitis and may show ulcerative phenomena and/or the characteristic submucosal edema called "thumbprints." Skip areas are lacking, and no transmural involvement is seen. Very rarely, a patient who is being evaluated for colonic obstruction may have prominent barium enema evidence of ischemic colitis that overshadows an associated partially obstructive colonic cancer. Careful appraisal of all findings should prevent this error. An ischemic stricture is characterized by a long, tapering defect and can be differentiated from carcinoma by endoscopic evaluation. Occasionally, the ischemic process in the colon is associated with an irregular and large diverticulum. Although original data suggested the importance of angiographic documentation of arterial obstruction in patients with ischemic colitis, it is now clear that proper management does *not* require angiographic evaluation.

Other Diagnostic Tests

Visualization of the ulcerative phenomena and/or of the hemorrhagic bullae establishes the diagnosis, but repeat studies showing change over only a few days may be essential to differentiate this process from some of the other ulcerative or hemorrhagic diseases. However, such repeat studies may not be essential for the diagnosis. The majority of patients have been securely diagnosed on the basis of a single examination done during an acute episode. Since it is unclear what percentage of patients form strictures, most researchers suggest follow-up barium enema and/or endoscopic evaluation. Unfortunately, no data exist about the frequency or time course of this complication. Endoscopic evaluation is particularly important with stricture to rule out the possibility of carcinoma and thus exclude the need for exploratory laparotomy.

Therapeutic Tests

Careful observation for evidence of peritoneal inflammation and/or increasing diarrhea is considered by many as a therapeutic test that is very important for definition of the presence of ischemic colitis and its differentiation from the other lesions. Others stress that diagnostic tests showing the lesion confined to its original location are also important in differentiating ischemic colitis from the other types of colitis.

Potential Errors or Pitfalls in Diagnosis

The most critical potential error in ischemic colitis is confusion with other types of colitis, either the specific variety, for which definitive treatment is available, or the nonspecific chronic varieties, such as granulomatous or ulcerative colitis. This error is serious because ischemic colitis is a self-limited disease with few patients having a recurrence and none having the protracted illness characteristic of chronic forms of colitis. One should avoid any thought that the strictures associated with this lesion might suggest cancer and require early operation, an error that is easily avoided by endoscopic confirmation. In addition, these strictures do not progress functionally and their mere presence in no way warrants "early" surgery.

PERITONITIS AND INTRA-ABDOMINAL INFECTION

By Peter M. Lamont, M.B., F.R.C.S.
and Hiram C. Polk, Jr., M.D.
Louisville, Kentucky

Peritonitis, an inflammation of the peritoneal cavity, may occur as a result of primary bacterial infection; more commonly, however, it is secondary to rupture or inflammation of adjacent viscera. Peritoneal inflammation may be localized and may present with discrete symptoms and signs, or it may be generalized with nonspecific signs of a severe inflammatory process. If localized inflammation is not treated, it may spread throughout the peritoneal cavity. Generalized inflammation may lead to overwhelming bacterial invasion and septicemia combined with massive fluid loss and hypovolemic shock; or it may become localized and lead to the formation of an intra-abdominal abscess.

Primary peritonitis is rare, and prior to the widespread use of antibiotics was caused by the hematogenous spread of infection from a remote site, especially in children. For example, pneumococcal peritonitis may follow pneumococcal pneumonia or otitis media, and streptococcal peritonitis may follow cutaneous erysipelas. Primary peritonitis now occurs more often in debilitated patients and is associated with either nephrosis or ascites. The symptoms and signs are often indistinguishable from secondary peritonitis, and diagnosis is made only after laparotomy has excluded all other causes.

Secondary peritonitis is much more common and may arise from a multitude of causes. Acute infection of a viscus, such as appendicitis or diverticulitis, usually develops gradually, with signs becoming localized after the adjacent peritoneum becomes inflamed. As the inflammation spreads, however, the signs become more diffuse until perforation of the viscus supervenes, leading to bacterial dissemination throughout the peritoneal cavity and producing signs of generalized peritonitis. The rupture of a viscus, such as a perforated duodenal ulcer or in penetrating abdominal trauma, leads to the acute onset of severe and generalized signs of peritoneal inflammation. Although the initial irritation following rupture may be chemical from leakage of gastric acid, bile, pancreatic secretions, blood, or urine, secondary bacterial infection rapidly supervenes. An interruption of the blood supply to the intestine leads to gangrene of the bowel and permits bacteria to cross the dead bowel wall into the peritoneal cavity, giving rise to signs of peritonitis. In the case of intestinal strangulation, these signs are often preceded by those of intestinal obstruction. In the case of mesenteric vascular occlusion, a prompt diagnosis is extremely difficult to make because of the paucity of clinical signs; by the time the evidence of peritonitis supervenes, it is usually too late to restore nutrient blood flow to the bowel. Peritonitis developing in the postoperative period is especially difficult to diagnose, as its signs may be masked by the usual incisional pain and tenderness and the expected presence of a postoperative ileus.

In very young patients, the ability to localize intra-abdominal infection is poorly developed, and the infection of a viscus may result in the spread to generalized peritonitis more rapidly than in the adult. Likewise, in patients whose host defenses are impaired, such as those who are elderly or who are receiving steroid therapy, not only may infection be more rapidly disseminated throughout the peritoneum, but symptoms and signs may be very mild, leading to a bland, late presentation of insidiously developing ileus and abdominal distention.

HISTORY

Regardless of the cause, abdominal pain is the predominant presenting symptom of peritonitis and is usually followed by anorexia, nausea, and vomiting. The character of the pain is related to the underlying pathologic condition and should be carefully elucidated. An extremely sudden onset of excruciating, constant, generalized abdominal pain is highly suggestive of a perforated viscus. Indeed, the patient may often be able to specify exactly the time of onset. In contrast, pain caused by a visceral infection is usually more gradual in onset and is initially poorly defined, reflecting the embryologic origin of the viscus involved—foregut to the upper abdomen, midgut to the periumbilical region, and hindgut to the lower abdomen. As the inflammation reaches the peritoneal surfaces, the pain becomes better localized. The classical picture of acute appendicitis commences with central abdominal pain, which later moves to the right quadrant. Pain in the left lower quadrant suggests diverticulitis, and pain in the right upper quadrant or epigastrium suggests cholecystitis or pancreatitis. Occasionally, a perforated duodenal ulcer may initially drain down the right paracolic gutter and present with right lower quadrant pain, leading to a mistaken diagnosis of acute appendicitis.

The pain of peritoneal inflammation is constant, but colicky pain may predominate when obstruction of a hollow viscus is the underlying cause, as in obstructive appendicitis. As necrosis of the visceral wall occurs, however, the pain becomes constant, due to increasing peritoneal involvement. Curiously, complete gangrene is often associated with disappearance of the pain. Furthermore, progression from localized pain to generalized pain suggests rupture of an infected viscus. The presence and site of referred pain may have particular significance. Irritation of the diaphragm by blood or peritoneal fluid may give rise to shoulder tip pain, as may occur in ruptured ectopic pregnancy or pancreatitis. Biliary tract pain may be referred around the side into the back and right shoulder, whereas pancreatic pain may be referred to the back.

Particular attention should be paid to the patient's past medical history, as peritonitis is more often than not a complication of previously existing intra-abdominal disease. The sudden onset of severe, generalized abdominal pain in the patient with a history of dyspepsia strongly suggests a perforated peptic ulcer. In the older patient with a long history of altered bowel habit or chronic left lower quadrant pain, the presence of a perforated colonic diverticulum or a cancer is more likely.

PHYSICAL EXAMINATION

Patients with peritonitis typically have an elevated temperature and tachycardia. They are obviously in pain and may appear to be in shock and have pallor and sweating. Respirations are rapid and shallow with an absence of abdominal movement. The patient lies as still as possible because movement or coughing exacerbates the pain. The abdomen is extremely tender to palpation and, where the tenderness remains localized, the site and extent of the tenderness may be valuable guides to the diagnosis; these data are also of obvious help when planning the surgical approach.

Peritoneal inflammation gives rise to overlying muscle spasm or guarding, which persists despite the gentlest examination and/or effort to distract the patient. Guarding is a most reliable sign of peritoneal irritation. In generalized peritonitis, this phenomenon is associated with the typical board-like rigidity felt throughout the abdominal wall. Rebound tenderness is likewise a sign of peritoneal irritation and may be excruciatingly painful; consequently, only the gentlest examination or even finger percussion may be all that is required to elicit it. Rebound is deceptive, however, and may be elicited in the absence of peritoneal irritation (frequent false-positive observation). Referred tenderness, when present, is another positive sign of peritoneal inflammation. For example, in acute appendicitis, palpation in the left lower quadrant causes pain in the right lower quadrant. Inflammation of the posterior peritoneum may be detected by eliciting pain on passive extension of the hip, which stretches the psoas muscle. Likewise, pain on stretching the internal obturator muscle by rotation of the fully flexed hip is a sign of pelvic peritoneal inflammation.

In the early stages of peritonitis, the abdomen is not typically distended unless an obstruction has been present; however, bowel sounds are absent, and as the inflammation continues, progressive ileus and distention occur.

The presence of abdominal masses may be difficult to determine in the patient with severe tenderness and guarding, but there may be a palpable inflammatory mass surrounding an acutely inflamed gallbladder, appendix, or colonic diverticulum. Rectal examination may reveal a palpably tender pelvic appendix or a pelvic or paracolic abscess. Vaginal examination is essential in women and may exlude pelvic inflammatory disease or salpingitis.

LABORATORY EXAMINATION

Hematocrit, hemoglobin, and white blood cell count estimations are essential ancillary aids in the diagnosis of peritonitis. The hematocrit reflects the degree of plasma volume depletion that may occur when dehydration results from vomiting and intraperitoneal effusion. The white cell count is usually elevated, but it may be normal in the early stages of peritonitis; indeed, progressive elevation of the white cell count suggests progression of the septic process. Typically, there is a preponderance of neutrophils and young cellular forms. In the presence of severe, overwhelming sepsis, the white cell count may be abnormally low.

Serum electrolyte estimation is required in order to evaluate the patient's losses and to permit appropriate replacement during resuscitation. Estimates of serum amylase levels contribute to the evaluation of acute abdominal pain, but the results must be interpreted with care. An elevation is by no means pathognomonic of pancreatitis because it also may occur in intestinal infarction, obstruction, or even perforation. On the other hand, the amylase level may be normal in the very early or late stages of acute pancreatitis.

Urinalysis and urine microscopy also aid in excluding diabetes and urinary tract infections as causes of abdominal pain, although white cells may appear in the urine in the absence of bacteria when an inflamed organ such as the appendix lies against the ureter or bladder. The exclusion of urinary tract infection is very important in suspected peritonitis.

In the presence of severe epigastric pain, an electrocardiogram is useful to exclude acute myocardial infarction, which occasionally presents in this manner.

RADIOLOGIC EXAMINATION

Radiologic examination of an acute abdomen includes plain films of the abdomen with the patient both erect and supine and a posteroanterior chest film. Nonspecific signs of localized peritonitis include obliteration of the psoas shadow and the presence of a localized ileus. Free air under the diaphragm occurs in around 70 per cent of cases of perforated peptic ulcer. A massive amount of air beneath both diaphragms suggests colonic perforation. Occasionally, it may not be possible to obtain films with the patient erect because of the severity of the pain or the debility of the patient. In such cases, a lateral decubitus view may reveal air between the liver and the lateral abdominal wall. In generalized peritonitis, an ileus may be apparent on the abdominal films, with distended loops of both small and large bowel. Extensive radiologic investigations are not required when a diagnosis of peritonitis has been made on clinical assessment because the clinical diagnosis is generally a sufficient indication of the need for surgical exploration.

DIFFERENTIAL DIAGNOSIS

Many diseases that do not warrant operation may cause symptoms suggestive of peritonitis. Although these diseases are relatively uncommon, they can usually be distinguished by a careful history and examination along with the routine tests outlined earlier. Within the chest, lower lobe pneumonia, diaphragmatic pleurisy, rib fracture, pericarditis, and myocardial infarction may all present with abdominal pain, but abdominal physical signs are usually absent. Nerve root pain referred to the abdomen as a result of herpes zoster may be severe and can precede the development of skin vesicles by a day or two. Systemic diseases presenting with abdominal pain include diabetes mellitus with severe hyperglycemia, diffuse vasculitis, various hemolytic crises, and acute porphyria. In such cases, laparotomy occasionally is required to definitely exclude peritonitis from diagnostic consideration.

COMPLICATIONS

In the acute phase the principal complications of peritonitis are due to shock, which may result from overwhelming infection, or from the hypovolemia that occurs when body fluids are sequestered within the peritoneal cavity and intestine. Without prompt and effective resuscitation, the immediate effect is circulatory collapse and death. With partial, incomplete, or delayed resuscitation, the end result is acute renal failure due to tubular necrosis, followed in turn by respiratory and hepatic failure. Spread of the septic process to the portal venous system may lead to the onset of pylephlebitis and liver abscesses. Impaired respiratory capacity due to severe abdominal pain predisposes to atelectasis and subsequent respiratory infection.

Should the patient survive these potentially fatal processes, the principal late complication is intraperitoneal abscess formation, which is discussed next. Peritonitis also promotes intraperitoneal adhesion formation, predisposing the patient in later life to either an acute episode of intestinal obstruction or recurrent episodes of subacute obstruction.

INTRA-ABDOMINAL ABSCESS

Intra-abdominal abscesses may occur as a complication of peritonitis, but they also may develop following operations on the alimentary tract. In such cases, the abscesses are caused by intraoperative contamination or inadequate drainage of biliary, pancreatic, or intestinal anastomotic leakage. Abscesses may be single or multiple and are most commonly found below the diaphragm, along the undersurface of the liver, down the paracolic gutters, or within the pelvis. Although no distinct anatomic barriers exist between the various subphrenic spaces, inflammatory adhesions often localize collections of pus to one of several potential sites. On the right side, pus may accumulate between the liver and the diaphragm or below the liver either anteriorly or posteriorly in the hepatorenal pouch. On the left side of the falciform ligament, pus may accumulate either directly below the diaphragm or anterior to the stomach or within the lesser sac.

The cause of the abscess may give a clue to its potential site and vice versa. Appendicitis may produce a right posterior subhepatic, a right paracolic, or a pelvic abscess. Infection arising from the gallbladder, stomach or duodenum tends to settle in the right subdiaphragmatic or anterior subhepatic spaces, but may track downward into the right paracolic gutter. Pancreatitis leads to a lesser sac abscess. Trauma or surgery to the stomach, pancreas, or spleen may result in a left subdiaphragmatic abscess; diverticulitis may result in a left anterior subhepatic, a left paracolic, or a pelvic abscess. Inflammatory bowel disease may result in abscesses within entwined bowel loops.

Whatever the cause, the diagnosis and location of an intraperitoneal abscess remains a challenging clinical problem. The progress of such abscesses may be insidious and associated with few localizing signs. This is especially so in the postoperative patient. A painful operative wound or abdominal distention may make examination difficult, and the concomitant administration of antibiotic or analgesic preparations may mask the clinical features. Less than half of the patients have localized tenderness, and the abscess mass is only rarely palpable. The main indicators are unexplained fever and leukocytosis persisting in the postoperative period, with or without positive blood cultures. The onset of respiratory, renal, and hepatic failure is an ominous sign of occult uncontrolled sepsis; stress ulceration and gastric mucosal failure also are a part of this threatening process.

Because the history and examination are so unreliable, the clinican may need to use a variety of diagnostic aids to confirm or deny the presence of an intra-abdominal abscess in a patient with unexplained fever and poor postoperative progress. The first approach is to obtain plain chest and abdominal x-rays, which are of value in about half of the cases, and which may reveal a sympathetic pleural effusion, elevation or fixation of the diaphragm, a soft-tissue mass, a collection of extraluminal gas with a fluid level, displacement of viscera, loss of definition of retroperitoneal structures (e.g., psoas shadow), or a localized ileus. Oral or rectal contrast studies may be useful when intestinal anastomotic leakage is suspected, but the overall sensitivity of these studies in the diagnosis of abscesses is poor. Should conventional radiography fail to show an abscess, other investigative modalities that may be used are radionuclide scanning, gray-scale ultrasonography, and computed tomography (CT).

Gallium citrate (^{67}Ga), a radioisotope, has been found to accumulate within inflammatory foci. Abscesses are revealed as an abnormal accumulation on a whole body scan; ^{67}Ga, however, is excreted via the intestine, and intestinal accumulations may cause false-positive results, despite cleansing enemas that may be poorly tolerated by the patient. Autologous leukocytes labeled with indium 111 (^{111}In) also accumulate in abscesses, and they may be used as an alternative scintigraphic agent. Intestinal accumulation does not occur, and the scan may be obtained more rapidly and accurately than with ^{67}Ga. Owing to normal splenic sequestration of the radiolabeled leukocytes, however, care should be taken in interpreting left upper quadrant accumulations. Technetium 99m (^{99m}Tc) liver-spleen scans can be used to detect parenchymal abscesses, and they may also reveal the presence of a subdiaphragmatic abscess by showing downward displacement or indentation of the liver or spleen. In general, such scans are misleading and of little practical merit.

Gray-scale ultrasonography is a highly accurate method of locating intra-abdominal abscesses. These appear rounded with slightly irregular walls and contain weakly echogenic debris, provided the collection is 2 cm or greater in diameter. Fluid-filled bowel loops can be distinguished by real-time ultrasonography. Ultrasound may fail to locate intra-abdominal abscesses in obese patients or where excess intestinal gas, as in paralytic ileus, reflects the sound beam. The presence of open wounds, colostomies, drains, or dressings can also limit the completeness of the examination.

Computed tomography of the abdomen is not subject to the constraints listed earlier, and it is as accurate as ultrasonography. It is, however, more expensive and less widely available. An abscess appears on the CT scan as a low-density mass. Abnormal collections of gas within the lesion are found in about 50 per cent of patients; rim enhancement is another variable feature. Fluid-filled bowel loops are delineated by oral contrast medium that is administered before the examination.

Abscesses that appear on ultrasonography and CT, although well defined, are not absolutely specific, and other lesions must be considered in the differential diagnosis. These include hematomas, seromas, collections of bile or urine, intra-abdominal cysts, pancreatic pseudocysts, and, occasionally, neoplasms. Consequently, both ultrasonography and CT are being used increasingly to guide percutaneous needle aspiration of suspected lesions in order to immediately confirm the diagnosis. These imaging techniques provide such distinct morphologic details of the surrounding viscera that the route of needle aspiration may be precisely planned to avoid the important structures. Aspiration of pus permits immediate Gram stain and culture, and the needle track should be used to guide insertion of a percutaneous catheter for definitive drainage of the abscess.

Inevitably, there are patients in whom all of these investigations are negative but who continue to exhibit direct or indirect evidence of progressive intra-abdominal sepsis. Surgical exploration, recognizing the very real attendant risks, is often the only alternative. The advent of hemodynamic instability, positive blood cultures, or organ failure is associated with 50 per cent mortality and is an indication for a full and comprehensive diagnostic laparotomy. Such incisions must permit exposure of the entire abdomen; discovery of the first intra-abdominal abscess is less valuable than discovery (and drainage) of the last.

VIRAL HEPATITIS AND ITS DIFFERENTIAL DIAGNOSES

By Leonard B. Seeff, M.D.
Washington, D.C.

Hepatitis is the term applied to the disease of the liver that is characterized by inflammation and necrosis of liver cells. Unfortunately, there are no pathognomonic features that unequivocally identify the disease, so that the diagnosis depends on the accumulation of historical, clinical, physical, and biochemical findings that, taken together, suggest the presence of hepatocellular necrosis and direct attention toward a specific etiology. Indeed, a similar disease may result from infection by one of several viruses, from drug or chemical injury, and in conjunction with severe hepatic congestion and with certain metabolic disorders. It may be recognized as an acute, subacute, or chronic illness, and some forms of the disease may culminate with the development of cirrhosis and/or primary hepatocellular carcinoma (PHC). On a global basis, *hepatitis due to viral infection* represents the most common of the various etiologies and will therefore constitute the major portion of the discussion that follows.

Several viruses can affect the liver and induce hepatitis, the most common of which are the *hepatitis A virus* (HAV), responsible for what was previously known as infectious hepatitis and now as hepatitis A; the *hepatitis B virus* (HBV), which causes the disease formerly referred to as serum or post-transfusion hepatitis but is now known as hepatitis B; and the recently recognized putative viruses of *non-A, non-B* (NANB) hepatitis. Among the other viral agents that can produce a hepatitis-like illness are the delta antigen, the cytomegalovirus, the Epstein-Barr virus (EBV), and rarely, particularly in adults, the herpes simplex, varicella-zoster, measles, rubella, and coxsackie viruses. Because of their special importance, the discussion that follows will focus on the disease caused by the Hepatitis A, B, and NANB viruses.

GENERAL SIGNS AND SYMPTOMS

There are certain clinical features that characterize the different hepatitis viruses, but they are insufficiently distinctive to categorically identify the agents. Thus, the only means of establishing a definitive etiologic diagnosis is through *serologic analysis.* Indeed, it has been established that if total reliance is placed on the classically accepted epidemiologic approach to define the specific virus, as many as 25 per cent of the cases will be misidentified. Nevertheless, some distinguishing features do exist; these are described later in this article.

In general, viral hepatitis evolves through four phases.

1. During the *early prodromal phase,* which begins 3 to 4 weeks before jaundice appears, a serum sick-

ness–like syndrome may develop, characterized by fever, arthralgia, arthritis, rash, and, occasionally, angioneurotic edema. These features are noted most commonly during the incubation period of hepatitis B, less commonly preceding hepatitis NANB, and least commonly prior to hepatitis A. In most instances, these symptoms disappear as jaundice emerges but occasionally the joint manifestations persist through and even beyond the overt hepatic illness.

2. The *preicteric phase* is signaled by the development of nonspecific constitutional, respiratory, and gastrointestinal symptoms consisting of malaise, fatigue, myalgia, anorexia, nausea and occasionally vomiting, an aversion to food and cigarettes, coryza, headache, photophobia, fever, pharyngitis, and cough. The respiratory symptoms occur most commonly in persons with hepatitis A. Occasionally, patients experience right upper quadrant pain and some individuals develop mild diarrhea. Physical examination at this time reveals lymphadenopathy (particularly in the posterior cervical region); moderately tender hepatomegaly (usually no more than two finger breadths below the right costal margin); and in 5 to 10 per cent of instances, splenomegaly. Rarely, spider nevi can be identified. This phase lasts from 2 to 3 days to 2 to 3 months.

3. With the onset of the *icteric phase,* the fever declines and constitutional symptoms begin to wane, although pruritus may become apparent. As a result, physical findings may now include evidence of excoriation due to scratching.

4. The *convalescent phase* begins when jaundice subsides (after a few days to as long as 4 to 6 weeks), associated with improvement in strength, appetite and energy, and loss of olfactory and gustatory dysfunction. Lymphadenopathy disappears, and the liver and spleen become impalpable. Full recovery is usually achieved within 6 months after disease onset.

LABORATORY FINDINGS

Biochemical tests with diagnostic relevance include the serum enzymes, the flocculation tests, the serum bilirubin, and the prothrombin time. There are numerous enzymes that become abnormal during acute viral hepatitis, but none has diagnostic superiority over the aminotransferases (transaminases), namely AST (SGOT) and ALT (SGPT). These are the first biochemical tests to become abnormal (signaling the beginning of the illness and hence the end of incubation period) and the last to normalize. The activity of both of these enzymes may range from two to three times to as much as 200 times the upper limit of normal. Generally, both aminotransferases are increased in activity to approximately the same degree, or more frequently (in more than 50 per cent of instances) the ALT activity exceeds that of AST. This is in marked contrast to the enzyme changes of alcoholic hepatitis, a disease in which the AST value rarely exceeds 300 IU per liter, whereas the ALT is almost always lower by at least half. Helpful clues to the responsible viral agents can sometimes be gained from examining the timing of onset (incubation period), the rate of rise, and the rate and degree of decline of these enzymes, as will be discussed.

Other enzymes that are often measured in persons with viral hepatitis are alkaline phosphatase (ALP) and lactic dehydrogenase (LDH). Their importance rests on the fact that they are usually not considerably abnormal in patients with acute viral hepatitis. The exception is the so-called "cholestatic" form of viral hepatitis, in which moderate elevations in ALP activity may occur (to be discussed later). Otherwise, a combination of moderate to marked abnormalities of both the aminotransferases and the ALP should lead to the consideration of alternative diagnoses, such as cytomegalovirus- or EBV-related hepatitis, drug-induced hepatitis, or extrahepatic gallstone obstruction that may be associated with ascending cholangitis.

The flocculation tests, namely thymol turbidity and cephalin flocculation, were previously considered to be useful measurements prior to the availability of the serum enzymes. However, they are now relegated to obscurity because of their nonspecificity and lesser sensitivity than the aminotransferases.

Measurement of the serum bilirubin level obviously permits definition of the degree of jaundice. By convention, a serum bilirubin level of 2.0 to 2.5 mg/dl distinguishes icteric from anicteric hepatitis. Generally, in acute viral hepatitis the bilirubin value does not exceed 20 mg/dl, but when it does, this signifies relatively severe disease. However, values in excess of 20 mg/dl should also be a signal to evaluate the patient for hemolysis and its causes, for example glucose-6-phosphate dehydrogenase deficiency (see the article on hereditary anemias). The bilirubin level almost always returns to normal before the aminotransferases, but sometimes mild indirect hyperbilirubinemia may persist, often diagnosed later as the Gilbert syndrome.

The coagulation tests—the prothrombin and partial thromboplastin times—represent the most important measures of severity of acute hepatitis. In uncomplicated acute viral hepatitis, these tests are normal, whereas if they are markedly deviated from normal (i.e., activity of less than 30 to 50 per cent or more than 3 to 4 seconds prolonged), severe complications such as hepatic failure can be anticipated. Hypoglycemia occurs rarely in the uncomplicated case, but it is a common and potentially lethal manifestation of fulminant hepatitis.

Nonspecific biochemical abnormalities seen in viral hepatitis include mild anemia, leukopenia, and increased levels of serum iron, manganese, copper, zinc, and vitamin B_{12}. Gross measurement of the serum proteins usually does not identify major abnormality, although a rising serum globulin and falling serum albumin level should warn of impending chronic hepatitis.

SEROLOGIC MANIFESTATIONS

Hepatitis A

The HAV, an RNA virus, can be detected in stools using immune electron microscopy, but this test obviously has no clinical application. Experimental studies indicate that viral particles usually disappear from the stool as the serum aminotransferases reach their peak levels. There is no clinically available test for the hepatitis A antigen (not surprising in view of the very short viremic period), but fortunately, serum antibody (anti-HAV) of the IgM class develops early during the acute illness. This permits specific diagnosis using sensitive assays. IgM anti-HAV usually declines within 6 months, at which time only IgG anti-HAV can be detected. Thus, identification of the latter antibody implies past infection and its presence is of diagnostic benefit only in that it excludes hepatitis A as the cause for recent or current aminotransferase abnormalities.

Hepatitis B

Serologic changes during acute hepatitis B are much more complex (Table 1). Associated with HBV (a DNA virus) are three antigens, namely hepatitis B surface antigen (HBsAg), hepatitis B core antigen (HBcAg), and hepatitis B e antigen (HBeAg). The first two are linked to particles that can be seen by electron microscopy; the latter is a soluble antigen. Each provokes a separate and specific antibody response, anti-HBs, anti-HBc, and anti-HBe, respectively. The first serologic markers to be detected as the acute disease develops (preceding biochemical abnormalties and symptoms) are HBsAg and HBeAg. Concurrently, other markers such as DNA polymerase (DNAP) and HBV DNA appear, but commercial tests for them are not available. HBcAg cannot be detected in serum; however, within a short time after the appearance of HBsAg (usually days), anti-HBc can be found and this antibody generally persists for life. The enzymes then become abnormal; later, as symptoms appear, HBeAg disappears, to be followed by the appearance of anti-HBe, and HBsAg begins to decline in titer. In 90 to 95 per cent of instances, HBsAg disappears completely (from days to 6 months after initial appearance). When finally anti-HBs can be detected (weeks to months later), complete resolution has resulted.

Five to 10 per cent of patients continue to be carriers of HBsAg. In the early phases of the carrier state (lasting months to years), HBeAg is also positive. Since this antigen is a marker for high infectivity, these are the carriers who are primarily responsible for propagation of HBV. Spontaneous loss of HBeAg occurs at a rate of 10 to 15 per cent a year, whereas there is only a 1 per cent loss per year of HBsAg. Carriers, especially among Asian populations who are infected at birth, are at high risk for the development of cirrhosis and PHC.

A new agent has been recognized, called the delta (δ) antigen. This appears to be a defective RNA virus that requires HBsAg for its expression. It infects only those individuals who are already HBsAg-positive, and appears to enter the liver after first being encapsulated by HBsAg. Hepatitis B virus and δ antigen infections may occur concomitantly, in which case the disease resembles acute hepatitis B, or the δ antigen may infect the HBsAg carrier. Superinfection with the δ antigen is associated with reduction in titers of HBV markers, often with acute exacerbation of disease in HBsAg carriers, sometimes with fulminant hepatitis, and commonly with progression of chronic hepatic disease. At present, diagnosis of δ infection is available only through research laboratories by the detection of IgM and IgG anti-δ in serum, and δ antigen in liver tissue using immunofluorescent techniques. A commercial test will soon be available for this important antigen.

NANB Hepatitis

Despite intensive research, there are presently no serologic tests for this disease. Based on epidemiologic and chimpanzee transmission studies, there appear to be at least two separate NANB viral agents in this country, one producing an ultra-short incubation period disease (7 to 10 days), and the other with an incubation period intermediate between that of hepatitis A and B. Both resemble hepatitis B. A putative third virus exists in India, which appears to be water-borne and associated with disease much like that of hepatitis A. The only available test for NANB hepatitis currently is a biologic assay using chimpanzees. NANB has been transmitted to these primates by blood obtained from persons with both acute and chronic NANB hepatitis, thus identifying a carrier state.

HISTOPATHOLOGY

The liver biopsy from a patient with acute hepatitis displays varying degrees of hepatocellular necrosis,

Table 1. Serologic Responses in Acute Hepatitis B

HBsAg	HBeAg	DNAP HBV DNA	Anti-HBc	ALT	Anti-HBe	Anti-HBs	Interpretations
+	+	+	−	−	−	−	Very early incubation
+	+	+	+	−	−	−	Early incubation
+	±	±	+	+	−	−	Acute illness
−	−	−	+	±	+	−	Early convalescence
−	−	−	+	−	+	+	Late convalescence

Abbreviations: HBsAg = Hepatitis B surface antigen; HBeAg = hepatitis B e antigen; DNAP = DNA polymerase; HBV DNA = hepatitis B virus DNA; anti-HBc = hepatitis B core antibody; ALT = alanine aminotransferase; anti-HBe = hepatitis B e antibody; anti-HBs = hepatitis B surface antibody.

including acidophilic bodies, ballooning degeneration, lobular disarray, lymphocytic infiltration, Kupffer cell hyperplasia, and various pigments (lipofuscin, bile, iron in the latter phases). Depending on the stage or severity of the disease, there may be evidence of bridging necrosis or the presence of fibrous strands linking portal or central areas. Morphologic features that distinguish between the different viruses include the finding of the highly eosinophilic "ground-glass" cells in HBsAg carriers (but not in persons with acute hepatitis) which can be further accentuated by special stains (e.g., orcein, aldehyde fuchsin), and of lymph follicle–like infiltration of portal areas and sometimes the presence of parenchymal fat in persons with NANB hepatitis.

CLINICAL VARIANTS

Viral hepatitis occurs most commonly as an anicteric disease (80 to 90 per cent of cases), less frequently as icteric hepatitis, and rarely as cholestatic hepatitis.

By and large, the difference in clinical features between anicteric and icteric hepatitis (distinguished by the presence of overt jaundice) is in degree. Thus, anicteric hepatitis, the more common expression of the disease in children and immunocompromised hosts, is less likely than icteric hepatitis to be associated with overt symptoms. Also, there is a tendency for lesser degrees of severe biochemical test abnormality and of histologic hepatocellular necrosis, although markedly elevated enzyme levels may certainly occur in this setting. Death from fulminant hepatitis is extremely rare in persons with anicteric hepatitis, whereas this outcome results in approximately 0.5 to 1 per cent of those with jaundice, regardless of the causative viral agent. On the other hand, there is a greater likelihood that chronic hepatitis will evolve in persons with anicteric than with icteric hepatitis.

Chronic hepatic disease never follows acute hepatitis A, whereas 10 per cent of persons with acute hepatitis B and 10 to 60 per cent of those with acute NANB hepatitis progress to chronic hepatitis. Liver biopsies of such individuals may show features of chronic persistent hepatitis, chronic active hepatitis, or even cirrhosis. Rarely, persons with icteric hepatitis, usually hepatitis B, persist with clinical, biochemical, and histologic features of acute hepatitis for as long as one year. This entity is referred to as *unresolved* or *chronic lobular hepatitis,* and does not advance to cirrhosis.

Cholestatic hepatitis is the least common of the clinical variants and tends to occur in clusters, often as an epidemic. These individuals develop fever, severe pruritus, and marked elevations in the serum alkaline phosphatase, bilirubin, and cholesterol levels. Their liver biopsies show "pseudoglandular" transformation, marked cholestasis, and numerous acidophilic bodies. Complete recovery is the rule, even though the disease may be protracted.

The features that help to distinguish between hepatitis A, B and NANB are shown in Table 2. It must be stressed, however, that accurate identification depends on serologic characterization.

DIFFERENTIAL DIAGNOSIS

Infectious Mononucleosis and Cytomegalovirus Infection

These two ubiquitous viruses sometimes produce liver disease that resembles viral hepatitis. (See the articles on these topics.) Infectious mononucleosis, presumably caused by the EBV, is a common infection, as evidenced by the fact that as many as 90 per cent of young children have detectable EBV antibodies acquired most frequently as an asymptomatic infection. Clinically apparent disease is the common presentation among adolescents and young adults up to 25 years of age as well as the rare cases involving much older persons.

The overt disease is almost always associated with mild to moderate fever, malaise, anorexia, headache, and pharyngitis. Physical examination reveals a generalized lymphadenopathy, particularly in the cervical region; periorbital edema; palatal petechiae; hepatosplenomegaly; and in a small number of patients, a maculopapular rash. Although the liver is commonly involved (witness the high frequency of detectable aminotransferase abnormalities), jaundice is not common (< 10 per cent of cases). Diagnostic clues come from the finding of a marked lymphocytosis, the presence of atypical lymphocytes (as many as 60 per cent), moderate elevations in aminotransferase levels (rarely exceeding 1000 IU per liter, more commonly in the range of 500 IU per liter), moderate elevations in ALP levels (higher than usually seen in viral hepatitis), and a fairly distinct morphologic pattern of injury on liver biopsy. This consists of hepatocellular necrosis (which is generally less extensive than is seen in viral hepatitis), the presence of fewer acidophilic bodies, lobular disarray, many mitotic figures, Kupffer cell hyperplasia, and an infiltration of the liver, most often concentrated in the sinusoids, with numerous monocytes. Sometimes the infiltration resembles a granuloma, accounting in part for the elevated ALP levels.

The majority of persons recover within 2 to 6 weeks. Occasionally, the disease may be protracted but chronic hepatitis and/or cirrhosis does not appear to result. Definitive diagnosis can be made by identification of a positive Monospot and heterophile antibody test (the latter amplified by the addition of differential absorption with guinea pig kidney and beef red blood cells) and by examination of acute and convalescent phase serum for evidence of rising EBV antibody titers.

Cytomegalovirus infection also is common, the complement-fixing antibody being found in the majority of persons by 35 to 40 years of age. The virus may infect newborn infants producing hematologic abnormalities (hemolytic anemia, thrombocytopenia), hepatomegaly, cholestatic jaundice, brain damage, and even death. In older children and adults, the virus is transmitted via infected oral secretions, urine, and, less commonly, blood. Most children who acquire the infection are asymptomatic. Symptomatic disease in older persons (post-perfusion syndrome, post-transfusion hepatitis—accounting for approximately 20 per cent of all such cases, immunologically compromised

Table 2. Comparative Features of Hepatitis Types A, B, and NANB

Characteristics	Hepatitis A	Hepatitis B	Hepatitis NANB
Clinical			
Age group	Mainly young	All ages	All ages
Onset	Abrupt	Insidious	Insidious
Incubation period	30–38 days	41–108 days	35–140 days
Symptoms			
Fever	Common before jaundice	Rare	Rare
Anorexia, N & V*	Usual	Usual	Usual
Jaundice	Rare in children	More common than hepatitis A	Less common than hepatitis B
Laboratory			
Enzyme increase—rate	Rapid	Slow	Slow
Enzyme increase—duration	3–18 days	35–200 days	Similar to hepatitis B
IgM	↑↑	↑	↑
Thymol turbidity	↑↑	↑	?
HBV markers (HBsAg)	–	+	–
Anti-HAV(IgM)	+	–	–
Virus	RNA	DNA	?
Viral Location			
Blood	Early prodrome	Early prodrome—to lifelong	Like hepatitis B
Feces	Early prodrome	No	–
Saliva	Probably not	Yes	?
Outcome			
Mortality	<1%	1–3%	1–3%
Chronic hepatitis	No	Yes ±10%	Yes ±50%
Carrier	No	Yes	Yes
Transmission			
Oral	+	+	?
Percutaneous	±	+	+
Household contact	+	±	?
Sexual contact	+	+	?
Transfusion	–	+	+
Drug abuse	+	+	+
Dialysis, transplant	–	+	+
Health care workers	–	+	+
Perinatal	–	+	+
Secondary cases	Common	Rare	Rare
Susceptible animals			
Marmosets	+	–	–
Chimpanzees	+	+	+
Tissue culture	+	–	–

*Nausea and vomiting.

persons) closely resembles infectious mononucleosis with fever, malaise, anorexia, nausea, and vomiting. Rarely, jaundice is noted and hepatosplenomegaly, but not lymphadenopathy, is common. The heterophile test is negative in this disease. Liver biopsy in infants demonstrates widespread necrosis in which the classical "owl's eye" inclusion bodies are found. Older persons show morphologic features indistinguishable from those of infectious mononucleosis.

Drug Toxicity

Adverse reactions to drugs may produce the entire spectrum of liver disease, ranging from acute and chronic hepatitis to obstructive jaundice with, in between, variable features of both. The mechanism of injury may be that of intrinsic drug toxicity (such as may occur with carbon tetrachloride, phosphorus, acetaminophen, and salicylates) or of host idiosyncrasy, the latter occurring as a result of hypersensitivity or metabolic derangement. Among the drugs that produce cytotoxic (hepatitis-like) reactions ascribable to hypersensitivity are the sulfonamides, para-aminosalicylic acid (PAS), halothane, methoxyfluorane, alpha-methyldopa, and phenytoin, whereas metabolic idiosyncrasy is the presumed mechanism for toxicity from isoniazid, iproniazid, cinchophen, ibuprofen, dantrolene, propylthiouracil, and phenylbutazone. A problem that is being increasingly recognized is that therapeutic doses of acetaminophen, normally quite safe, may lead to severe hepatotoxicity and even death when used by persons who are chronic alcoholics. Chronic ethanol ingestion appears to divert the metabolism of acetaminophen to a pathway that produces a toxic metabolite.

A number of drugs are known to cause both acute and chronic hepatitis. These include oxyphenisatin, nitrofurantoin, alpha-methyldopa, isoniazid, dantrolene, acetaminophen, sulfonamides, propylthiouracil, and acetylsalicylic acid. Of note is that chronic drug-related hepatitis affects females predominantly and in some instances resembles the autoimmune or "lupoid" form of chronic active hepatitis.

There are relatively few clinical features that distinguish drug-induced hepatitis from viral-induced hepatitis. Clinically, a history of drug ingestion is mandatory and the finding that the serologic markers of hepatitis are negative is helpful. Examination of the liver biopsy may also provide clues. Thus, drugs that are intrinsically toxic usually produce zonal necrosis, whereas drugs that cause injury through hypersensitivity frequently provoke an eosinophilic or granulomatous response in the liver. Other features that characterize hypersensitivity-related injury include a low incidence of toxicity; a lack of dose dependence; a short sensitization period between initial ingestion and onset of injury (1 to 5 weeks); recurrence of injury on drug readministration; and associated rash, fever, and systemic eosinophilia, occasionally associated with blood dyscrasias. Even if there are no clues to suggest drug toxicity, it is prudent for a person with acute hepatitis to discontinue all drugs that are not absolutely essential and to refrain from further use of established hepatotoxic drugs if no other specific etiology can be established, since readministration of such drugs occasionally causes death.

"Congestive" and "Ischemic" Hepatitis

Liver abnormalities of variable degree may result from both right-sided and left-sided ventricular failure as well as following recovery from shock. It is well known that persons with right-sided failure have, as one of their clinical manifestations, hepatomegaly that is often tender to palpation. Many of these patients have minor deviations in the liver-related chemical tests, which include an increase in serum bilirubin levels, usually the unconjugated fraction (the total rarely exceeding 3 mg/dl), impaired bromsulphalein (BSP) excretion, mild to moderate prolongation of the prothrombin time, and, in most instances, slight increases in the aminotransferase levels. Rarely, the values may exceed 500 and even 1000 IU per liter, accompanied by jaundice, thus simulating viral hepatitis. Liver biopsy findings show dilatation of the central veins and surrounding sinusoids, often containing many red blood cells, rarely, centrizonal necrosis, and if there has been long-standing congestion, pericentral fibrosis and even fibrous linkage of central veins, producing a morphologic picture of "congestive" or "cardiac" cirrhosis. The distinction of "cardiac" hepatitis from viral hepatitis can often be inferred by noting the rapid decline in aminotransferase levels that accompanies improvement in cardiac function.

More recently, it has become apparent that nonhypotensive patients with severe left-sided failure, often without evidence of right-sided failure, may develop overt liver disease resembling both clinical and biochemical features of acute viral hepatitis. This entity has been referred to as "ischemic" hepatitis. Many of the reported patients have had deep jaundice and aminotransferase levels rising to well above 1000 IU per liter. Diagnosis depends on the recognition of left-sided failure, the identification of distinct central hepatic necrosis on liver biopsy, and rapid improvement of the abnormal tests with treatment of the underlying heart disease. The basis for these manifestations is believed to be hypoperfusion with hypoxemia in the centrizonal region of the liver. It is important to recognize this entity and refrain from vigorous efforts to treat right-sided failure (e.g., with diuretics), since this may aggravate the hypovolemia and perhaps worsen the liver disease. Similar manifestations may ensue following an episode of shock or prolonged hypotension.

Alcoholic Hepatitis

While the clinical features of alcoholic hepatitis bear a superficial resemblance to acute viral hepatitis, closer inspection defines quite distinct differences. Thus, the disease develops on a background of long-continued alcoholism associated usually with a marked increase in alcohol intake in the weeks just preceding the development of the overt liver disease. Furthermore, many cases occur in persons with already established chronic liver disease who may therefore have the accompanying physical findings of spider nevi, malnutrition, weight loss, gynecomastia, a collateral venous pattern, testicular atrophy, occasionally Dupuytren's contractures, as well as the features of portal hypertension (splenomegaly, ascites, peripheral edema). The most important items that distinguish alcoholic from viral hepatitis include the presence of an enlarged and usually tender liver due to fatty infiltration; fever; the laboratory features of anemia, leukocytosis and thrombocytopenia; aminotransferase abnormalities consisting of an AST elevation that rarely exceeds 300 IU per liter and an abnormal ALT value (in approximately 50 per cent of the cases) whose height is less than half that of the AST; a moderate elevation in ALP levels; moderate to marked prolongation of the prothrombin and partial thromboplastin times; and, often, hypoalbuminemia and hyperglobulinemia. In addition, the serum bilirubin value is often markedly increased. However, definitive diagnosis is established by liver biopsy if this is permitted by acceptable measures of coagulation. The liver biopsy will show the presence of fat, focal necrosis with a polymorphonuclear leukocyte response, the presence of alcoholic hyalin (Mallory bodies), necrosis with cell drop-out in the central areas, and varying degrees of fibrosis and/or cirrhosis.

Metabolic Disorders

Metabolic diseases that may emulate both acute and chronic hepatitis include Wilson's disease (hepatolenticular degeneration) (see related article) and alpha$_1$-antitrypsin deficiency. It is essential to recognize Wilson's disease, since this serious, potentially lethal disorder responds well to treatment. Wilson's disease is a genetic disorder of copper transport and storage, resulting in copper deposition in various tissues such as the brain, liver, cornea, and kidney, ultimately producing dysfunction of these organs. With regard to the liver, variable forms of disease may ensue, including what appears to be acute viral hepatitis, chronic active hepatitis, and cirrhosis. Since the disease affects young persons (usually less than 25 years of age), it should always be a considered diagnosis in young individuals with hepatic disease. Unfortunately, accompanying neurologic abnormality is not inevitably present, but if it is, the diagnosis should be rigorously pursued. Helpful findings include the presence of Kayser-Fleischer rings in the cornea identified by slit-lamp examination, a lowered serum ceruloplasmin level, and increased copper levels in the liver. Additional information can be derived from the study of the kinetics of radiolabeled copper and of its rate of excretion in the urine. However, none of these tests is infallible in the diagnosis of Wilson's disease, since each of them may be falsely positive or falsely negative under certain circumstances. The liver biopsy may provide clues exclusive of increased copper deposition, namely the presence of fat, Mallory bodies, glycogen nuclei, and macronodular cirrhosis.

CIRRHOSIS OF THE LIVER

By Arun Samanta, M.D.
East Orange, New Jersey
and Thomas W. Kiernan, M.D.
Huntington, West Virginia

The liver architecture in cirrhosis is, by definition, distorted by parenchymal nodules separated by fibrous bands. The clinical manifestations of this disease are partly due to the etiologic mechanisms that ultimately result in cirrhosis. However, disordered hepatocyte function due to this disease and the deranged hepatic hemodynamics that result from lobular distortion are the main reasons for the general nonspecific symptoms and signs characteristic of cirrhosis.

PATHOGENESIS

Cirrhosis always results from a precursor lesion characterized by liver cell necrosis and often leukocyte infiltration. A variety of causes are responsible (Table 1). Alcoholic hepatitis, for example, results in cirrhosis in nearly one third of those afflicted. The direct effect of ethanol or acetaldehyde (its first metabolite) and/or cell-mediated immune mechanisms reactive to alcoholic hyaline (a product of hepatocyte injury) have been implicated in the pathogenesis of this hepatitis. Sensitized lymphocytes to the hyaline appear to elaborate a fibrogenic factor, resulting in the increased fibrogenic activity of hepatic fibroblasts. These cells deposit collagen in areas of injury, subsequently leading to hepatic fibrosis (centrilobular) and cirrhosis.

In chronic active hepatitis, continued injury around the limiting plate of the portal triad leads to fibrosis in portal-portal and portal-central areas of the hepatic lobule. A cell-mediated immune response to liver-specific lipoprotein may be responsible for continued liver cell necrosis and subsequent fibrosis. Common causes of chronic hepatitis include the hepatitis viruses type B and type non-A, non-B.

Other hepatic disorders characterized by cirrhosis, and for which the exact mechanisms of injury are less clear, include cryptogenic cirrhosis, primary biliary cirrhosis, Indian childhood cirrhosis, and sarcoid cirrhosis.

Congestive cirrhosis has resulted from prolonged congestive heart failure, diseases of the hepatic veins (Budd-Chiari and veno-occlusive disease), and sickle cell disease. Secondary biliary cirrhosis is due to prolonged obstruction of the extrahepatic biliary ducts. Cystic fibrosis has been associated with cirrhosis because of bile ductular obstruction by mucus. Cirrhosis may characterize congenital syphilis or hereditary hemorrhagic telangiectasia.

Drugs and chemicals have induced cirrhosis. Cirrhosis may follow use of some drugs predictably (e.g., methotrexate). Halothane and monoamine oxidase inhibitors are some common drugs that uncommonly and unpredictably result in cirrhosis (Table 2).

Abnormalities of inborn metabolism are clearly im-

Table 1. Etiologic Disorders in Cirrhosis

Alcoholic hepatitis
Chronic active hepatitis
Hepatitis virus, type B
Hepatitis virus, type non-A, non-B
Idiopathic
Drug-induced hepatitis
Predictable agents, e.g., methotrexate
Unpredictable agents, e.g., halothane
Toxic and chemical exposure
Congestive cirrhosis
Congestive heart failure
Budd-Chiari syndrome
Venoclusive hepatitic venous disease
Sickle cell disease
Secondary biliary cirrhosis (i.e., chronic biliary tract obstruction)
Incomplete biliary cirrhosis following cystic fibrosis
Congenital syphilis
Hereditary hemorrhagic telangiectasia
Inborn errors of metabolism
Iron storage disease
Wilson's disease (copper storage disease)
Type IV glycogen storage disease
Alpha-1-antitrypsin deficiency
Galactosemia
Tyrosinosis
Hereditary fructose intolerance
Thalassemia
Hypermethioninemia
Unknown causes
Primary biliary cirrhosis
Cryptogenic cirrhosis
Sarcoid cirrhosis
Indian childhood cirrhosis
Intestinal bypass surgery

plicated in cirrhosis. Wilson's disease (copper storage) and iron overload (hemochromatosis) are examples. Galactosemia, type IV glycogen storage disease, tyrosinosis, hereditary fructose intolerance, alpha$_1$-antitrypsin deficiency, hypermethioninemia and thalassemia are others. Intestinal bypass surgery for obesity commonly leads to fatty liver degeneration, but it may also occasionally lead to cirrhosis. The list of causes is obviously long and broadly based. However, a careful clinical understanding of these predisposing disorders is essential, since treatment is directed at the mechanism leading to cirrhosis.

NOMENCLATURE

The varieties of cirrhosis have been classified using anatomic description or specific cause. The liver has been described anatomically using the terms *macronodular* (when nodules are generally larger than 1 cm in diameter), *micronodular* (when nodules are generally smaller), and *mixed nodular.* Many specific disorders, however, may be manifested by one or more of these three anatomic types. Attempts at defining cirrhosis according to cause have led to long lists of names for specific entities. Cirrhosis due to viral hepatitis type B, for example, has been called posthepatitic cirrhosis, postcollapse cirrhosis, and postnecrotic cirrhosis, among other names. The Fogarty International Congress on Nomenclature of Diseases of the Liver and Biliary Tract (1975) has advocated defining each cirrhotic entity according to its specific cause (Table 1).

CLINICAL ASPECTS

History

Constitutional symptoms caused by cirrhosis are usually reflective of abnormal liver cell function. Nonspecific entities such as malaise, fatigue, lethargy, anorexia, and nausea are common. Other symptoms reflect the activity of concomitant inflammation. Fever, chills, and abdominal pain are examples. Other more specific symptoms may result from liver cell dysfunction: jaundice, pruritus, diarrhea, dark urine, and light acholic stools. Hematemesis, melena, and abdominal swelling (ascites) may be associated with aberrant hepatic hemodynamics attendant on cirrhosis.

Specific symptoms may reflect the unique clinical entity leading to cirrhosis. Wilson's disease, for example, may present with its neurologic symptoms. Iron storage disease may have symptoms related to the complicating diabetes mellitus or cardiomyopathy. An accurate knowledge of the extrahepatic manifestations of the many preceding disorders leading to cirrhosis is helpful (Table 3).

The factors of age and sex may direct the clinician's attention to specific causes. Wilson's disease, for example, is more commonly symptomatic during adolescence, whereas primary biliary cirrhosis is characteristically a disease of middle-aged women.

Alcohol consumption and medication use are important historical clues. Awareness of the patient's occupation and responsibilities may lead to discovery of toxin or chemical exposures (e.g., munition worker exposed to trinitrotoluene).

A family history of liver disease is common in Wilson's disease and iron storage disease. A history of hepatitis or exposure to parenterally administered illicit drugs might uncover the cause for chronic hepatitis. Arthralgia, and a history of hives, hematuria, or rash may suggest chronic active hepatitis.

Patients with cirrhosis, on occasion, are totally asymptomatic. The clinician must have a high index of suspicion in order to uncover it.

Table 2. Drugs Associated with Cirrhosis

Cinchophen (and derivatives)
Arsenicals
Methotrexate
Chlorpromazine
Oxyphenisatin
Monoamine oxidase inhibitors
Halothane
Isoniazid

Physical Examination

The clinician has three goals in his physical examination of the patient with cirrhosis:

1. To define the character of the liver.
2. To identify nonspecific complications.
3. To identify the extrahepatic manifestations of causative mechanisms.

The cirrhotic liver is frequently enlarged because of concomitant progressive hepatocellular necrosis and degeneration, reactive edema, and leukocytic infiltration. When the causative disorder has become quiescent or arrested (naturally or through definitive treatment), liver size will decrease. (Usual liver size in the adult is defined by percussion, with relative dullness demarcating the upper and lower borders of the liver. Percussion is performed in the right midclavicular line [RMCL] and midsternal line [MSL]. The normal sizes are 15 ± 2 cm RMCL and 4 ± 2 cm MSL.) The cirrhotic liver has a fine to grossly nodular surface. This latter characteristic may not be well elicited in obese patients or in patients with large ascites. A bruit may be heard over the liver. It is best heard just to the right of the xiphoid process. Alcoholic hepatitis, hepatocellular carcinoma, and arteriovenous fistulas may also be associated with this sign.

Extrahepatic findings owing to cirrhosis involve many systems. Jaundice may be noted on careful inspection of the conjunctivae, sclerae, underside of the tongue, soft palate, and skin. Gynecomastia, facial hair loss, a female escutcheon, and testicular atrophy are due in part to abnormalities in sex hormone metabolism. Peripheral cyanosis, clubbing, abdominal collateral veins, palmar erythema, arterial spider veins, and tachycardia are due to disordered pulmonary, splanchnic, and cardiovascular hemodynamics. Peripheral edema and ascites (characterized by flank bulging, shifting dullness, or a fluid wave) demonstrate disordered splanchnic hemodynamics and abnormal sodium and water clearance. Acholic stools

Table 3. Clinical Clues to Etiology of Cirrhosis*

Etiology	History	Physical	Investigations†
Alcoholic hepatitis	Alcohol consumption	Large parotids; myopathy; Dupuytren's contracture; testicular atrophy; neuropathy	SGOT > SGPT; polymorphonuclear leukocytosis
Chronic active hepatitis	Illicit drugs; transfusions; previous acute hepatitis	Multiorgan involvement: rash, arthritis, thyroiditis, colitis, etc. Endocrine: hypercorticism, hirsutism	Positive HBsAg; elevated gamma globulin
Primary biliary cirrhosis	Female sex; middle age; pruritus before icterus	Xanthomata; CRST syndrome; finger clubbing	Elevated IgM; antimitochondrial antibody
Iron storage disease	Positive family history	Signs of pseudogout; cardiomyopathy; diabetes; bronze skin; testicular atrophy	Elevated serum ferritin
Wilson's disease	Family history of liver or neurologic disease; childhood or adolescence onset	Kayser-Fleischer rings; osteochondritis dessicans; CNS and basal ganglia disorder	Low serum ceruloplasmin
Cryptogenic cirrhosis	Affects mostly women	Associated diseases: arthritis, thyroiditis, nephritis, etc.	Elevated gamma globulin; positive antinuclear antibodies

*Partial assessment of selected etiologies.
†Excluding biopsy.
Abbreviations: CRST = Calcinosis, Raynaud's phenomenon, sclerodactyly, telangiectasia, SGOT = aspartate aminotransferase; SGPT = alanine aminotransferase.

may be due to biliary duct gallstones. Melena or a bloody nasogastric aspirate may reflect bleeding esophageal varices. Altered mentation, asterixis, lethargy, stupor, and coma characterize portasystemic encephalopathy. White nailbeds seem to reflect low serum albumin levels.

Specific attention to the physical clues for the underlying mechanisms for cirrhosis is essential. Kayser-Fleischer corneal rings, a grossly flapping tremor, and a spastic gait should alert the clinician to Wilson's disease. The other entities causing cirrhosis can be identified similarly by examining the patient for specific telltale signs suggestive of the diseases (Table 3).

LABORATORY PROFILES

Biochemical Tests

Enzyme assays such as SGOT (aspartate aminotransferase) or SGPT (alanine aminotransferase) are nonspecific assays of cellular injury. Alkaline phosphatases may vary from normal to markedly abnormal (twofold to sevenfold elevation) in the absence of biliary obstruction. This test suffers, however, by its lack of hepatic specificity. Serum protein determinations demonstrate ordinarily a high gamma globulin and a normal or low serum albumin. Specific abnormalities of immunoglobulins may be helpful in primary biliary cirrhosis, in which a marked elevation of IgM is noted. Specific tests reflective of collagen turnover, such as urinary hydroxyproline levels, are too unreliable to be of assistance. Serum bile acids (fasting or 2-hour postprandial levels) and indocyanine green dye clearance may assist the clinician when biochemical tests are equivocally abnormal and cellular function is to be assessed. Serum cholesterol levels are high in primary biliary cirrhosis and obstructive biliary disease. These findings are also too nonspecific to be very useful. Ceruloplasmin levels are low in Wilson's disease. Ferritin levels are elevated in iron storage disease.

Serologic Tests

Serologic tests are helpful only in defining causative mechanisms of cirrhosis. Specific tests for hepatitis B surface antigen and alcoholic hyaline are useful for defining specific entities. Cellular (organelle-specific) antibodies, like smooth muscle and antinuclear antibodies, are noted in chronic active hepatitis, but none is pathognomonic. An antimitochondrial antibody is found in 90 per cent of patients with primary biliary cirrhosis, although it may be found in chronic active hepatitis and obstructive biliary disease less commonly.

LIVER BIOPSY

Liver biopsy is required for the definitive diagnosis of cirrhosis. Blind percutaneous biopsies with the Menghini needle are frequently misleading because of shattered biopsy specimens. Better samples are cut with the Vim-Silverman needle. Random sampling error may prevent the pathologist from diagnosing cirrhosis in 10 per cent of patients. Specific biopsy can be done incidentally during laparotomy for other conditions, or with the assistance of the peritoneoscope. Regenerative nodules or pseudolobules or both characterize cirrhosis. Specific stains for iron, copper, viral antigens, and cellular inclusions may assist in defining the cause.

RADIOLOGY

Routine radiologic procedures are usually not of benefit in the evaluation of the cirrhotic liver (see Complications).

RADIONUCLIDE SCANNING

Liver scanning with technetium 99m–labeled sulfur colloid shows a diffuse patchy uptake over the liver, which is often difficult to distinguish from multiple small defects of the liver. Usually the spleen is notably enlarged. Uptake of hepatic-bypassed colloid is noted in the vertebral spine.

HEMATOLOGY

Peripheral smears may demonstrate microcytic, normocytic, or macrocytic red cells. Iron deficiency may characterize the alcoholic who has recurrent gastrointestinal bleeding. Depleted folic acid stores in alcoholic cirrhosis may result in a macrocytic anemia with megaloblastic changes in the bone marrow. Ringed sideroblasts may be seen on occasion.

Macrocytes and "spur" cells may also be noted on a blood smear. Disordered cholesterol-lecithin relationships in the red cell stroma are accountable. At times, hemolytic anemia may result because of high ratio of red cell cholesterol to lecithin. Hemolytic anemia has been noted for other reasons in Wilson's disease and primary biliary cirrhosis.

Pancytopenia may be a reflection of hypersplenism, the effect of iron or folate deficiencies, or the direct effect of alcohol.

Cirrhotic patients are prone to ecchymoses and bleeding. Impaired protein synthesis results in decreased levels of Factors II, V, VII, IX, and X. Diminished platelet counts may be due to hypersplenism or the effects of alcohol. Fibrin split products are elevated in the blood of cirrhotics because of impaired extraction by the liver. Clinical coagulopathy caused by these latter products is often not clinically apparent. Cirrhotic ascitic fluid has been shown to have elevated levels. The displacement of this fluid into the systemic circulation through a peritoneojugular surgical shunt, however, may result in increased systemic levels leading to disseminated intravascular coagulopathy.

URINALYSIS

Urinalysis is not ordinarily abnormal in cirrhotics. One third may have a "proximal" renal tubular acidosis with a persistently alkaline urine pH. Urine potassium and calcium levels may be elevated in this condition.

COMPLICATIONS

Jaundice in cirrhosis is ordinarily due to impaired hepatocellular function. Cirrhotics are prone to pigmented (calcium bilirubinate) stones, which may cause biliary obstruction. Ultrasound of the gallbladder and biliary tract and a flat plate of the abdomen may be helpful screening techniques. Technetium 99m labeled HIDA [N,*a*-(2,6-dimethylphenylcarbamoylmethyl) iminodiacetic acid] or PIPIDA [N,*a*-(p-isopropylacetanilide) iminodiacetic acid] can be used to obtain hepatobiliary imaging and rule out obstruction; however, the imaging may be poor in severely jaundiced patients. Often a careful evaluation using percutaneous transhepatic cholangiography or endoscopic retrograde cholangiography is indicated. Alteration in bile composition may also lead to steatorrhea in cirrhosis.

Gastrointestinal bleeding in a cirrhotic patient is commonly due to bleeding esophageal varices. In alcoholic cirrhotics acute gastritis, peptic ulcer, esophagitis, and esophageal mucosal tears need to be considered. Early upper gastrointestinal fiberoptic endoscopy or celiac angiography or both may help to define the bleeding lesion. Hepatic vein cannulation may be helpful afterward in assessing portal hypertension. The wedge pressure is frequently a reflection of portal pressure in patients with postsinusoidal portal hypertension. Direct cannulation of the portal vein by umbilical catheterization is feasible for this evaluation in some large centers. Direct portography can then be carried out.

Ascites is characteristic of severe cirrhosis. Peritoneal fluid should be routinely assessed for bacteria, mycobacteria, fungi, and neoplastic cells. The fluid is ordinarily transudative (specific gravity less than 1.015 and fluid protein less than 2.5 gm/dl.) In 10 per cent of patients the fluid may be exudative. Peritoneoscopy with peritoneal biopsy may be indicated for fluid of uncertain origin.

Portasystemic encephalopathy is characterized in cirrhosis by a disordered mentation subsequently evolving into stupor and coma. Asterixis is noted in one phase only of the staging of this problem. Hepatic fetor is irregularly present. A careful evaluation for an inciting cause such as infection, gastrointestinal bleeding, hypovalemia, constipation, dietary protein intolerance, hypokalemia, renal failure, alkalosis, and use of sedatives, narcotics, or other drugs may be made for definitive treatment. Hypophosphatemia may aggravate this disorder. Treatment of the underlying causes of the liver disease is also pertinent.

Functional failure of the kidneys can be seen in cirrhosis. Sodium retention may be noted in the low daily output of urine sodium. As free water clearance becomes further impaired, urine volume and serum sodium decrease, as creatinine and blood urea nitrogen (BUN) progressively rise. When kidney failure is due to hepatocellular disease alone, the prognosis is poor. When an aggravating problem such as a treatable infection can be defined, the prognosis is still poor, but less grave.

Serum electrolyte patterns are commonly abnormal in cirrhosis. Impaired sodium and free water clearance may lead to hyponatremia. Hypokalemia is a complication of the secondary elevations of aldosterone. Magnesium and zinc depletion syndromes may result from an increased clearance of these electrolytes before functional renal failure ensues.

Cirrhosis may lead to disordered systemic as well as splanchnic hemodynamics. Cirrhosis results in intrapulmonary shunts leading to low arterial P_{O_2}. A decrease in peripheral resistance may lead to resting tachycardia and low systolic and a wide pulse pressure. High output cardiac failure may complicate cirrhosis, especially in patients undergoing portasystemic shunts.

Osteomalacia may complicate primary biliary cirrhosis. In the same patients an alteration in 25 hydroxylation of vitamin D_3 may play a part, but malabsorption of vitamin D may occur because of disordered bile composition. Vitamin A deficiency may be noted at times.

Cirrhotic patients are prone to systemic bacterial infections. Deranged humoral and cell-mediated immune responses are the likely causes. Infection may result in fever or hypothermia. Coliform bacteria, pneumococci, and *Mycobacterium tuberculosis* are common agents. Spontaneous septicemia and peritonitis are two complications carrying a grave prognosis.

The hepatic biotransformation of many drugs is impaired in cirrhosis, as a result of decreased functional parenchymal mass and intrahepatic shunting of splanchnic blood bypassing the liver cell. Toxic levels of drugs, such as theophylline and lidocaine, can occur with routine dosage. The central nervous system is also peculiarly sensitive to the depressant effects of sedatives, narcotics and analgesics, and other drugs (e.g., cimetidine and diphenoxylate).

Whenever a cirrhotic patient's condition begins to deteriorate (e.g., weight loss, apathy, progressive jaundice), the clinician should be suspicious of an underlying hepatocellular carcinoma. This neoplasm has been described in patients with cirrhosis owing to hemochromatosis, chronic active hepatitis, and alcoholism. Hypercalcemia, inappropriate erythrocytosis, and hypoglycemia are some of the extraheptic manifestations of this cancer that should raise the clinician's index of suspicion. Hepatic arteriography may allow a vascular blush to demarcate this lesion. Computerized axial tomography may also help to define a neoplasm.

GALLBLADDER AND BILE DUCTS

By Avram M. Cooperman, M.D.
New York, New York

Of individuals over the age of 40, 20 per cent are affected by biliary disorders. Cholecystectomy is the most commonly performed operation in the United States (500,000 per year). The spectrum of biliary pathology is so varied that the presentations range from acute and obvious to nonspecific and subtle.

CHOLELITHIASIS AND CHOLECYSTITIS

Clinical Presentation

The symptoms of all biliary disorders are similar. *Nonspecific symptoms* include indigestion, flatulence, pyrosis, and a change in fatty food tolerance. Episodes of pain, colic, and jaundice may be absent. These nonspecific symptoms usually warrant gastrointestinal studies, at which time gallstones are found as incidental findings. "Classic" biliary symptoms include sharp, abrupt onset of right upper quadrant pain (it frequently begins in the midline), nausea, and vomiting. While *biliary colic* is the common term, it is a misnomer since the pain is almost always sharp and steady, and may last from 1 to 10 hours. When the pain resolves, there is residual soreness and hyperesthesia in the right upper quadrant that lasts several hours. Between nonspecific and classic presentations are a multitude of presentations comprising elements of both. These are difficult management decisions. When stones obstruct the common bile duct, chills, fever (102 to 104°F), and jaundice are additional symptoms. When obstruction in the bile duct raises ductal pressures above those in the hepatic sinusoids, biliary bacteremia occurs. This explains why cholangitis, septic shock, and hypotension develop.

Less commonly, common duct stones obstruct the distal bile duct without causing pain, chills, or fever. In this circumstance a stone may obstruct the bile duct, causing cholestatic jaundice *without* other symptoms (silent stone).

Physical Findings

Physical findings vary, but they are usually localized to the area over the gallbladder. Direct tenderness and localized rebound tenderness in the right upper quadrant are common. When the gallbladder descends beneath the rib cage on deep inspiration, it may be palpated. An enlarged palpable gallbladder (hydrops) indicates cystic duct obstruction or periampullary neoplasm.

Laboratory Tests

Initial laboratory tests reflect acute inflammation. An elevated white blood cell count is supportive, but does not correlate with the physical findings or temperature elevation. Liver function tests may be normal, or there may be elevated serum enzymes, particularly of alkaline phosphatase (the earliest sign of bile duct obstruction). Serum bilirubin may also be increased. At times there may be confusion between hepatitis and gallstones on the basis of laboratory tests alone.

Roentgenographic Tests

The greatest advance in biliary diseases has been simplification of the differential diagnosis. Before direct imaging of the biliary tree was possible the differential diagnosis of jaundice was a polemic. This is an issue of the past.

For acute (or chronic cholecystitis, a plain roentgenogram of the abdomen is helpful. Gallstones may be visualized less than 10 per cent of the time (when calcifications are present), and a gas cleft may occasionally be seen in noncalcified stone (Mercedes-Benz sign).

An ultrasound study is the next diagnostic test. Its accuracy is 85 per cent. The value of ultrasonography is in detecting gallstones; it does not diagnose a diseased gallbladder without stones, nor are there other direct findings of cholecystitis.

If time is of the essence and the diagnosis in doubt, a radioisotope scan is next done. "HIDA" is an acronym for a group of studies that use technetium-labeled iminodiacetic acid. These materials are injected intravenously, are bound transiently to transferrin, and are then taken up by hepatocytes. They are excreted into the bile canaliculi and follow the course of bile flow. If the cystic duct is obstructed, this test provides presumptive evidence of acute cholecystitis, since the gallbladder will not visualize. Delayed bile excretion and intraluminal or mural defects in the common duct are also shown. HIDA scans are inaccurate for patients who have fasted for 48 hours (because the gallbladder does not contract as well), for patients on total parenteral nutrition, and for some patients with pancreatitis (particularly when food has been withheld). This remarkable "change in order" of diagnostic tests has relegated the oral cholecystogram to a lower priority and intravenous cholangiography to a seldom used test.

The oral cholecystogram has a role in delineating mucosal disease. Failure to visualize after a single dose of contrast medium is followed one day later by a repeat study. Nonvisualization or poor visualization of the gallbladder indicates a diseased viscus. When jaundice or intraductal pathology is suspected, an endoscopic or percutaneous study is indicated. The oral cholecystogram is safe and accurate. Because the test may take 48 hours to perform it can not be used in an urgent situation. Other prerequisites are absence of jaundice, normal intestinal absorption, normal liver function, and a willing patient. Since after excretion the water-soluble dye is not absorbed by the gallbladder, the viscus is visualized. Nonvisualization on two consecutive days implies (with 95 per cent accuracy) a diseased gallbladder or an obstructed cystic duct.

When jaundice is present or if intraductal pathology is suspected, endoscopic or percutaneous cholangiography is indicated. Both techniques provide diagnostic and therapeutic potential. The choice of procedure depends on the expertise available at an institution. Endoscopic retrograde cholangiopancreatography (ERCP) is safe (it avoids a puncture), visualizes both the bile duct and pancreatic duct, and provides an opportunity for decompression as well. The percutaneous technique involves a small but definite risk; however, it serves as an excellent diagnostic and therapeutic test.

Course

The natural history of cholelithiasis and cholecystitis is one of mild disease and chronicity. Statements that indicate 50 per cent of patients develop symptoms are accurate but do not take time into account. More recent studies report that 2 per cent of gallstone patients per annum develop symptoms. Thus the 50 per cent figure is correct when enough years are taken into account. Most episodes of cholecystitis are mild and resolve with nonspecific measures. This is true for 95 per cent of patients. Symptomatic cholecystitis poses no difficulties; asymptomatic cholecystitis is more controversial. What is certain is the higher incidence of choledocholithiasis in elderly patients, which increases the risk and complication rate of gallstones.

Complications

The complications of gallstones are many and include:

Gallstone Ileus. Erosion of gallstones into the duodenum, transverse colon, or stomach is uncommon; however, it is not a rare finding in elderly patients with intestinal obstruction (20 per cent of nonstrangulating obstruction in patients over age 65). The stone (usually > 3.5 cm) erodes through the gallbladder into a hollow viscus, where it migrates and obstructs. A history of intermittent and then complete bowel obstruction in a patient with known gallstones suggests this diagnosis. A plain film of the abdomen shows air in the biliary tree and small bowel obstruction.

Emphysematous Cholecystitis. Air within the gallbladder is secondary to overwhelming sepsis with gas production from anerobic or gas-forming aerobic organisms. This is uncommon; it is recognized on the plain roentgenogram because of air in the gallbladder wall. It is not more common in diabetics.

Empyema. Complete obstruction of the cystic duct with suppuration in the gallbladder results in empyema. This complication occurs in 8 per cent of patients with acute cholecystitis. It should be suspected when acute cholecystitis does not subside within 24 to 48 hours, when fever persists longer than 72 hours, and/or when tenderness persists in the right upper quadrant.

Common Duct Stones. Ten per cent of patients with gallstones have common duct stones. Since most common duct stones are discovered because of symptoms (chills, fever, or jaundice), it is difficult to know the natural history and course. Most common duct stones originate in the gallbladder and migrate through the cystic duct (secondary stones). Some stones develop primarily in the duct (primary stones) and are thought to be secondary to stenosis of the sphincter. Most common duct stones are residual and result from incomplete extraction of the stones at the first operation. These are diagnosed by postoperative "T" tube cholangiograms, which should be done routinely. Occasionally, bacterial proliferation behind a common duct stone that is completely impacted produces pus in the bile duct. *Suppurative cholangitis* is manifest by chills, fever, and toxicity and requires urgent (operative or nonoperative) ductal decompression.

Cancer of the Gallbladder. Less than 1 per cent of patients with gallstones develop cancer of the gallbladder, but 80 to 90 per cent of patients with gallbladder cancer have stones. Gallbladder cancer is three times as common in women. When discovered as an incidental finding at cholecystectomy, there is a reasonable chance for survival (greater than 50 per cent in favorable cases). When gallbladder cancer is symptomatic, the 5-year survival is nil. Jaundice, a nontender palpable gallbladder, and systemic manifestations of malignancy herald a very poor prognosis. There are no specific diagnostic tests for this malignancy. Calcifications in the gallbladder wall seen on plain abdominal roentgenograms are associated with some malignancies. Despite an association between gallbladder cancer and cholelithiasis, prophylactic cholecystectomy is not warranted for this reason alone.

Hyperplastic Cholecystoses. This represents a group of benign degenerative lesions in which there is excessive proliferation of gallbladder mucosa. The lesions appear as filling defects on oral cholecystogram, usually as incidental findings. These persistent filling defects on oral cholecystogram are usually accompanied by nonspecific digestive symptoms.

Postcholecystectomy Syndromes. After cholecystectomy, 5 per cent of patients remain with unrelieved symptoms. Complete re-evaluation of the gastrointestinal system must be done to be certain that other disorders of the stomach, intestine, colon, or esophagus are not overlooked.

Biliary diseases, including stones, strictures, and sphincter abnormalities, should be investigated. HIDA scans, ERCP, and manometrics of the sphincter offer new diagnostic modalities that define this area. Since personal experiences tend to dominate selection of studies in this field (there is little objective evidence), mine follow: If routine barium roentgenograms are normal, the patient is examined during an acute attack, laboratory tests are drawn, and a HIDA scan is ordered. Delayed flow or dilatation of the duct above the sphincter suggests a sphincter disorder. Manometrics done at the time of endoscopy are difficult to evaluate. The state of the art is evolving, but it is not yet precise.

COMMON BILE DUCT

Pathologic conditions involving the common bile duct are tumors, strictures, and stones.

Benign Tumors. Benign tumors of the bile duct are uncommon and include papillomas and adenomas. Intermittent colic and jaundice are the presenting signs. Since common duct stones are much more common than benign tumors, this is the usual initial diagnosis. HIDA scan will demonstrate a filling defect, and an ERCP will show a different configuration from a stone. Surgery confirms the diagnosis.

Strictures. Benign and malignant strictures of the bile duct are problems with significant consequences. Benign strictures are most commonly iatrogenic and follow unsuspected bile duct injuries during cholecystectomy. The presentation of chills, fever, and jaundice prompts investigation; HIDA scan, ultrasound, and then ERCP should pinpoint the site and nature of the obstruction. Percutaneous transhepatic cholangiography (PTC) is used instead of ERCP at many institutions. It is effective when bile ducts are dilated and has therapeutic benefit, since intubation and dilatation of the stricture are practiced today.

Bile Duct Cancer. Cancers of the bile duct are increasing in incidence at an alarming rate. Once considered rare, they are common in large referral centers and industrial areas (particularly the rubber industry). Jaundice that rapidly progresses, without colic, and pruritus are the most common symptoms. Weight loss and gas pain accompany these and are late signs. Of bile duct tumors, 40 per cent are located in the upper third of the duct, 40 per cent are in the lower third, and 20 per cent are in the middle third. Cholangitis is less common with bile duct cancer because the obstruction is progressive, gradual, and near total at presentation.

Laboratory tests reflect high-grade obstruction. Elevated levels of bilirubin (usually greater than 10 mg/dl) and alkaline phosphatase support this. Imaging of the liver and biliary tract by ultrasound or computed tomography (CT) demonstrates whether liver metastases are present, the level of obstruction, and the presence of ascites. A HIDA scan will quantitate and fractionate flow from each lobe of the liver. An ERCP or PTC delineates multicentricity and provides drainage. An angiogram is done next to demonstrate encasement of the hepatic artery or portal vein and intrahepatic metastases in order to assess operability.

SCLEROSING CHOLANGITIS

Primary sclerosing cholangitis presents in the third to fifth decade of life, more often in males, with symptoms similar to other causes of ductal obstruction (pruritus, cholangitis, jaundice). In addition to its association with a younger age group, an association with ulcerative colitis (20 to 30 per cent) is certain. Physical examination, laboratory tests, and roentgenographic studies are exactly as outlined for bile duct cancer.

The course of sclerosing cholangitis is variable. It may remain mild and inactive for years or may progress to malignancy, cirrhosis, liver failure, or bleeding esophageal varices.

HEPATIC AND PERIHEPATIC ABSCESS

By Henry A. Pitt, M.D.
Jonathan Hiatt, M.D.
and Jesse E. Thompson, Jr., M.D.
Los Angeles, California

In reporting a patient with a pyogenic hepatic abscess managed at the Guy's Hospital, London, in 1902, Taylor wrote that "the chief aid to the diagnosis . . . is knowledge that it may occur. . . . " More than 80 years later, this statement remains true. To establish a diagnosis of hepatic or perihepatic abscess, these disease entities must first be considered. However, today's clinician who includes these diagnoses in a differential has the advantage of being able to employ several diagnostic modalities that were not generally available even a decade ago. Fortunately, the widespread availability of ultrasound (US), computed tomography (CT), newer radionuclides, and CT- or US-guided percutaneous aspiration has resulted in both earlier diagnosis and improved survival.

Although *pyogenic hepatic abscess, perihepatic abscess,* and *amebic liver abscess* are three separate disease processes, many of the same modalities are employed in establishing the diagnosis for each. Therefore, in an effort to avoid repetition, the following discussions will focus on the diagnostic tests presently available and only clear differences of application to pyogenic hepatic, perihepatic, or amebic liver abscesses will be highlighted. A brief discussion of changing trends in incidence and current concepts of etiology follows next.

INCIDENCE

Autopsy and hospital admission data suggest that the incidence of pyogenic hepatic abscess has changed very little during the 20th century. The incidence of perihepatic abscess as a complication of appendicitis has also remained unchanged significantly since the preantibiotic era. However, the relative incidence of perihepatic abscesses resulting from gastrointestinal surgery and abdominal trauma has increased dramatically over the past 50 years. Although comparable data are not readily available, the absolute increase in the number of patients undergoing abdominal operations and sustaining abdominal trauma suggests that the incidence of perihepatic abscesses may have increased in recent years.

The incidence of amebic liver abscess, on the other hand, has definitely been increasing in Louisiana, Texas, Southern California, Chicago, and other areas where there are large numbers of immigrants from countries where amebiasis is endemic, such as Mexico and Southeast Asia. Very few amebic abscesses are seen in our indigenous population with the exception of patients in mental institutions, American Indians who remain on reservations, some military personnel, and other people who have recently traveled to an endemic region. In addition, there have been recent reports of amebic liver abscess in those homosexual men in whom intestinal amebiasis is epidemic.

ETIOLOGY

Pyogenic Liver Abscess. The majority of pyogenic liver abscesses are caused by infection in the biliary or intestinal tracts. Prior to the introduction of antibiotics, appendicitis and other intra-abdominal infections that transmitted bacteria to the liver via the portal vein were the leading causes of pyogenic hepatic abscess. However, comparison of 16 series (525 cases) published since 1970, with the collected series (622 cases) by Ochsner and colleagues reported in 1938, reveals a dramatic increase in the relative incidence of abscesses caused by ascending cholangitis (Fig. 1). In the recently collected series, 35 per cent of patients had a biliary etiology and 40 per cent of these patients had an underlying malignancy. The relative incidence of pyogenic abscesses resulting from systemic bacteria, direct extension, and trauma and those in which no etiology could be determined has remained relatively constant.

Perihepatic Abscess. Similarly, the etiology of perihepatic abscesses has been changing as the 20th century has progressed. In the first two decades, perforated ulcer, perforated liver abscess, and appendicitis were the leading causes of perihepatic abscesses. From 1920 to 1940, appendicitis became the leading cause, with perforated ulcers second and biliary tract disease third. Between 1940 and 1960, perihepatic abscesses occurred most frequently after peptic ulcer surgery. In the past two decades, these upper abdominal abscesses have occurred most often after biliary, gastric, or colonic surgery. In recent years, abdominal trauma has become the second most common cause while appendicitis remains third as a cause for perihepatic abscess.

Bacteriology of Pyogenic Hepatic and Perihepatic Abscesses. Most pyogenic hepatic and perihepatic abscesses will harbor a mixed flora of aerobes and anaerobes. *Escherichia coli* is the aerobic organism isolated most frequently from pyogenic ab-

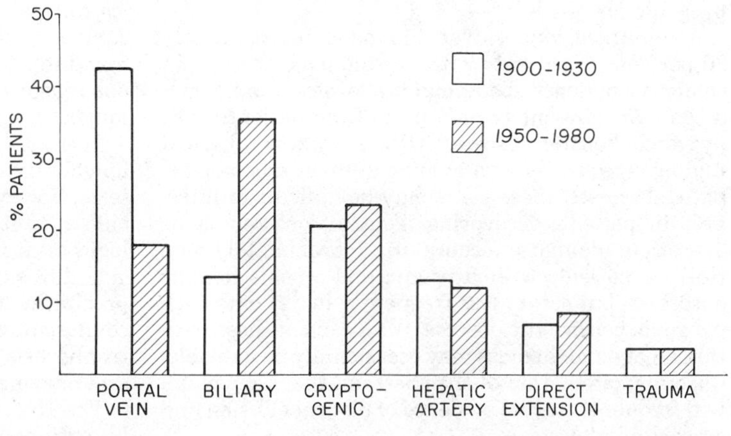

Figure 1. Changing trends in the etiology of pyogenic hepatic abscess. (From Pitt, H. A.: Liver abscess. In Shackelford, R.T., and Zuidema, G. D. (eds.): *Surgery of the Alimentary Tract,* volume 4. Philadelphia, W. B. Saunders Company, 1983.)

scesses in and around the liver. Aerobic, microaerophilic, and anaerobic streptococci are the species cultured next most often from liver abscesses. These organisms and a variety of gram-negative aerobes are also frequently isolated from perihepatic abscesses. *Bacteroides* species are found in approximately 10 per cent of liver abscesses but are isolated with greater frequency from perihepatic abscesses, especially those developing after appendicitis, diverticulitis, and colon surgery or trauma.

Amebic Liver Abscess. Amebiasis has a worldwide distribution, with the highest prevalence in subtropical and tropical climates and in areas with poor sanitation. In the continental United States, the prevalence of amebiasis in southern states is nearly double that found in northern states. *Entamoeba histolytica* in the cystic form gains access to the body by oral ingestion of contaminated material, usually water. These cysts pass into the intestine, where they develop into trophozoites. The trophozoites multiply in the lumen of the large intestine, especially the cecum. When tissue invasion occurs, the result may be hemorrhage, perforation, an enterocolic or cutaneous fistula, amebic appendicitis, or an ameboma. Amebic trophozoites may also enter the mesenteric venules or lymphatics and may be carried to the liver. Fortunately, amebic liver abscess occurs in only 3 to 7 per cent of all patients with amebiasis. (See the article on this topic.)

SYMPTOMS AND PHYSICAL FINDINGS

Most patients with pyogenic hepatic abscess present with symptoms of less than 2 weeks' duration. Although an occasional patient will present acutely in septic shock, in approximately one third of patients symptoms will be mild and will have been present for from 1 month to longer than a year. Fever and pain are the most common presenting symptoms of patients with an abscess in or around the liver. Although fever is the most frequent symptom among patients with a pyogenic abscess, pain is the most common symptom in patients with an amebic abscess. Other symptoms, such as nausea, vomiting, anorexia, malaise, and weight loss, occur less often. Diarrhea is seen in only 20 per cent of patients with amebic liver abscess and occurs even less frequently in those with pyogenic abscesses.

An enlarged, tender liver is found in approximately 80 per cent of patients with amebic liver abscess. In comparison, upper abdominal tenderness and hepatomegaly are present in only half of the patients with pyogenic hepatic abscess. Although these physical findings frequently also accompany pyogenic perihepatic abscesses, these signs may be difficult to interpret in patients recovering from major trauma or operation. Jaundice occurs in approximately one third of patients with pyogenic and amebic hepatic abscesses, but occurs less frequently in patients with pyogenic perihepatic abscess. With each of these entities, an abdominal mass may occasionally be palpable. Careful examination of the chest, on the other hand, will frequently reveal evidence of pleural effusion and associated atelectasis.

LABORATORY STUDIES

Approximately 70 per cent of patients with hepatic and perihepatic abscesses will present with leukocytosis with polymorphonuclear leukocytes predominating. Eosinophilia is rare, even in patients with amebic liver abscesses. A mild anemia is also present in approximately one half of patients with hepatic and perihepatic abscesses. Hematocrit levels of less than 30 per cent, however, are unusual. Elevations of alkaline phosphatase are seen in nearly 50 per cent of these patients, and mild elevations of serum transaminase levels are found in approximately a third of patients with hepatic or perihepatic abscesses. Significant elevations of transaminase and white blood cell levels have both been correlated with a poor prognosis.

Reviews of recent series of pyogenic hepatic abscesses, many of which are secondary to extrahepatic biliary obstruction, suggest that up to 40 per cent of these patients will have an elevated serum bilirubin. In comparison, mild increases in bilirubin are seen in approximately 30 per cent of patients with amebic liver abcess and in less than 10 per cent of patients with perihepatic abscesses. Hypoalbuminemia is present in approximately 55 per cent of patients with pyogenic abscesses and in approximately 45 per cent with amebic abscesses. Both hypoalbuminemia and hyperbilirubinemia tend to be prognosticators of a poor outcome.

While isolation of one or more bacteria from a patient's blood or from the abscess itself confirms the etiology of pyogenic abscesses, specific documentation of infection with *E. histolytica* may be more difficult. The modalities available for confirming a clinical suspicion of an amebic liver abscess are examination of aspirated abscess contents or stool specimens for trophozoites and amebic serology. The advisability and efficacy of aspiration of amebic liver abscesses will be discussed in a separate section.

Stool testing requires the precise coordination of several steps, including collection of a fresh specimen, transportation to the laboratory, proper preservation and storage, and availability of personnel trained in the identification of enteric pathogens. Examination of several stools may be necessary because excretion of cysts and trophozoites may be intermittent. Furthermore, a number of substances, including antibiotics, antiparasitic drugs, laxatives, antacids, radiologic contrast media, enemas, and antidiarrheal drugs, may interfere with stool examination. For these various reasons, amebae are not found in the stool of the majority of patients with an amebic liver abscess.

Perhaps the best way to confirm the diagnosis of an amebic liver abscess is with serologic testing. Many tests, however, are on the market, and each has specific advantages and limitations. The available serologic tests include indirect hemagglutination (IHA), gel diffusion precipitin (GDP), cellulose acetate precipitin (CAP), indirect immunofluorescence (IF), counterimmunoelectrophoresis (CIE), immunoelectrophoresis, complement fixation, latex agglutination, and enzyme-linked immunosorbent assay (ELISA).

The IHA test is the most widely available and can be obtained through state health departments, the

Centers for Disease Control, and some private laboratories. Both the IHA and GDP tests are very sensitive and specific, but have the disadvantage of requiring several days for results to become available. Furthermore, both of these tests will be positive in 85 to 90 per cent of patients with amebic colitis, and the IHA will frequently remain positive for many years following invasive amebiasis. On the other hand, in two thirds of patients the GDP will become negative within 6 months.

Unlike the IHA and GDP tests, the CAP, IF, and CIE can yield results within a few hours. Results with these tests are encouraging, but comparison studies with IHA or GDP in a large population of patients with amebic abscesses have not been reported. Because so many tests are available and are still being evaluated, physicians caring for a patient with a suspected amebic liver abscess should contact the clinical laboratory of their hospital to determine which tests are available and how they should be interpreted.

ROENTGENOGRAPHIC STUDIES

Roentgenograms of the chest are abnormal in approximately half of patients with a pyogenic hepatic abscess and in two thirds of patients with an amebic or subphrenic abscess. The most common radiologic findings are elevation of the right hemidiaphragm, right lower lobe atelectasis, and a right pleural effusion. Fluoroscopy will also reveal decreased diaphragmatic motion in many of these patients. These findings, of course, are suggestive but nonspecific. Similarly, plain abdominal films and barium studies may show hepatomegaly or displacement of the stomach or colon by an enlarged liver. The one finding on plain abdominal x-rays, however, that may be diagnostic is the presence of gas within the abscess. Approximately 10 to 20 per cent of patients with a pyogenic liver abscess and 35 to 45 per cent of patients with a perihepatic abscess will have gas in the abscess on plain abdominal films. In comparison, gas is not normally observed in patients with an amebic abscess and, if seen, may suggest secondary bacterial contamination.

Cholangiography has assumed increasing importance in the diagnosis of patients with pyogenic hepatic abscesses, since the percentage of patients with biliary obstruction as the cause for abscess formation has been increasing. Oral cholecystography (OCG), however, is perhaps the least rewarding means of biliary visualization in these patients, many of whom are jaundiced or are vomiting. Likewise, intravenous cholangiography (IVC) will frequently not visualize or will provide inadequate anatomic information. Furthermore, both OCG and IVC have been reported to give false-positive nonvisualization in patients with amebic liver abscesses who were not jaundiced and who were not vomiting.

Direct cholangiography, on the other hand, is extremely useful in defining the site and cause of biliary obstruction and occasionally will outline the abscess cavities (Fig. 2). Performance of endoscopic retrograde cholangiography (ERC) or percutaneous transhepatic

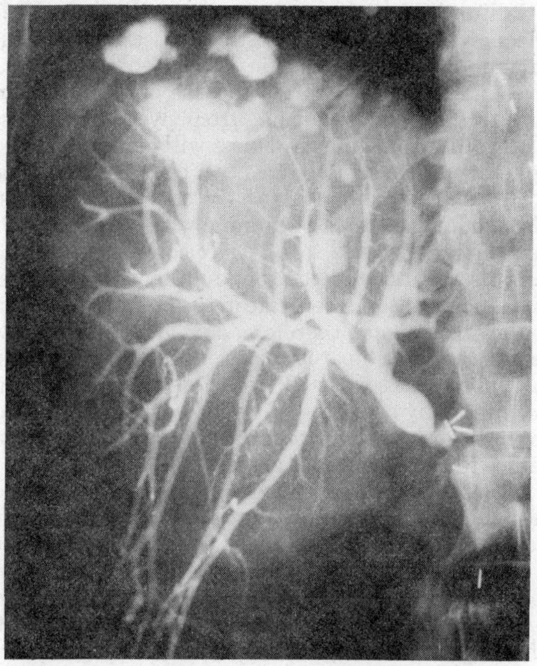

Figure 2. Percutaneous transhepatic cholangiogram demonstrating multiple abscess cavities in communication with the biliary tree in a patient with a stenotic choledochojejunostomy. (From Pitt, H. A.: Liver abscess. In Shakelford, R. T., and Zuidema, G. D. (eds.): *Surgery of the Alimentary Tract,* volume 4. Philadelphia, W. B. Saunders Company, 1983.)

cholangiography (THC), however, in patients with suppurative cholangitis and multiple liver abscesses may be quite hazardous. Increased intrabiliary pressure may only exacerbate the septic process, and urgent laparotomy may be necessary. What role endoscopic sphincterotomy or percutaneous transhepatic drainage should play in these patients has not been clearly defined and is beyond the scope of this discussion. Of course, ERC and THC are generally not helpful and, therefore, are usually not indicated in most patients with amebic or perihepatic abscesses.

RADIONUCLIDE STUDIES

One of the first steps toward eliminating delay in diagnosis and improving survival in patients with hepatic and perihepatic abscesses was the clinical introduction of hepatic scanning in the 1960s. Technetium sulfur colloid (^{99m}Tc), gallium citrate (^{67}Ga), and indium (^{111}In) labeled white blood cell scans are presently being employed for detection of hepatic and perihepatic abscesses. The ^{99m}Tc scan demonstrates decreased uptake by many space-occupying lesions, including benign tumors and cysts as well as malignancies and abscesses. By combining the ^{99m}Tc liver-spleen scan with a lung scan, separation of functioning parenchyma of these organs by a hepatic or perihepatic abscess can be demonstrated. A large cyst or tumor, however, may give the same picture.

Gallium citrate concentrates normally in the liver, spleen, bone, and gastrointestinal tract, as well as in inflammatory and neoplastic tissue. Recently, several investigators have reported the use of gallium scanning to differentiate amebic from pyogenic abscess. With gallium, an amebic abscess will demonstrate peripheral uptake around a central cold area, whereas a pyogenic abscess will have increased uptake throughout the abscess. Scanning with ^{67}Ga, however, frequently requires 2 to 3 days to complete, a significant disadvantage in the septic patient. In addition, gallium may also concentrate in the operative bed and healing wound and, therefore, may give false-positive results in the postoperative patient in whom a perihepatic abscess is suspected. For these reasons, gallium scanning may be better suited to work-up of fever of unknown origin than to evaluation of the septic patient with an abdominal abscess.

Autologous leukocyte labeling with indium oxine is the newest radiopharmaceutical imaging technique. Neutrophils are separated from a 50-ml blood sample, are labeled with ^{111}In, and are reinfused. Scans are done 18 hours later. This isotope will concentrate in liver, spleen, bone, and any inflammatory tissue to which leukocytes migrate. Early reports suggest that this test is highly accurate in detecting pyogenic and amebic hepatic abscesses as well as perihepatic abscesses (Fig. 3). To what degree this test will have problems with false-positive results in the early postoperative period has not yet been determined. Other theoretical and real limitations include:

1. Complexity of the preparation process.
2. Unreliability in chronic abscesses without an active inflammatory component.
3. False-negative results in patients with altered leukocyte function.

Although the new ^{99m}Tc pyridoxylidene-glutamate and *N*-substituted iminodiacetic acid (IDA) scans are quite useful in the diagnosis of acute cholecystitis, they generally should not be considered in the diagnosis of hepatic or perihepatic abscess. The exceptions to this statement, however, may be the patients who develop a subhepatic abscess as the result of gangrenous cholecystitis or a postoperative biliary leak. In summary, a decade ago liver scans provided a means for early detection of hepatic and perihepatic abscesses that was not previously available. This technique is useful in defining location, size, and number of abscesses as well as for follow-up. Liver scans, however, will not detect small abscesses less than 2 cm in diameter. Furthermore, the role of liver scanning in patients with hepatic abscesses has changed now that ultrasound and CT are available.

ULTRASONOGRAPHY

With improvements in ultrasound technology, delineation of liver lesions as small as 2 cm, the same resolution as with liver scanning, is now possible. In the detection of liver abscesses, however, ultrasonography has two distinct advantages over isotope scanning: there is no ionizing radiation, and it can distinguish fluid-filled from solid masses. In most cases, therefore, ultrasound will be able to differentiate abscesses from tumors. On the other hand, air, bone, and barium are echo-impermeable and represent the major obstacles to ultrasound examination. In addition, incisions, stomas, dressings, and appliances may limit the surface area available for contact. Considerable skill and experience are also important for the production and interpretation of scans.

Numerous reports have documented that ultrasound is 80 to 90 per cent accurate in diagnosing abscesses in and around the liver. The clinician should be aware, however, of several situations in which ultrasound may be inaccurate or misleading:

1. Ultrasound cannot easily visualize the dome of the right hepatic lobe and may miss lesions in this area.
2. Multiple microscopic abscesses, such as those generally found with ascending cholangitis, may not be appreciated.

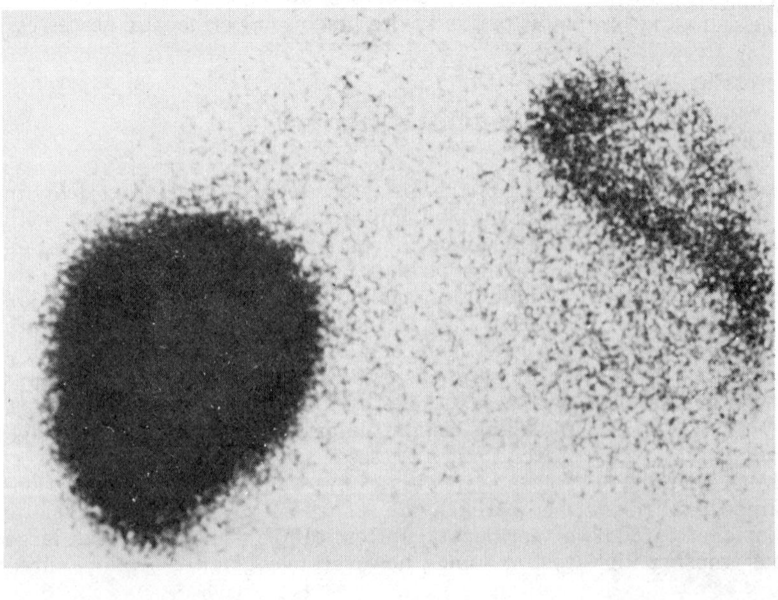

Figure 3. ^{111}Indium-labeled leukocyte scan demonstrating uptake by a large right subhepatic abscess, with some uptake also seen in the spleen. (Courtesy of Naomi Alazraki, M.D., VA Medical Center, Salt Lake City.)

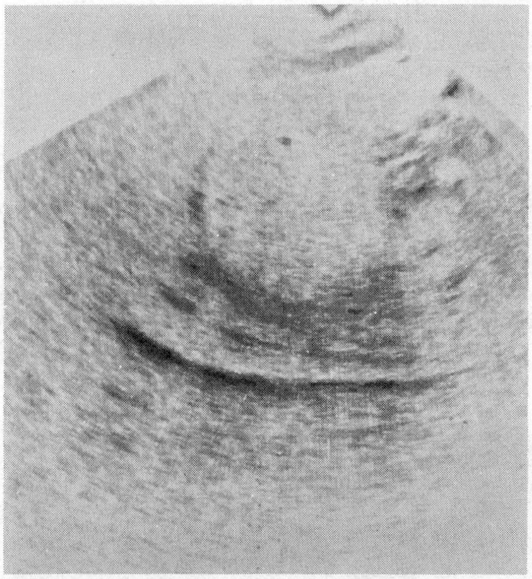

Figure 4. Sagittal abdominal ultrasound demonstrating a large amebic abscess in the right hepatic lobe. The abscess has homogeneous, fine echoes; a smooth wall; and some distalsonic enhancement. (From Pitt, H. A.: Liver abscess. In Shackelford, R. T., and Zuidema, G. D. (eds): *Surgery of the Alimentary Tract,* volume 4. Philadelphia, W. B. Saunders Company, 1983.)

3. Fatty infiltration may produce a markedly ecogenic liver resulting in failure to detect a small abscess.
4. The left subphrenic space may be difficult to image sonographically because of contiguous bony ribs and air-filled lung.
5. Fluid collections must be differentiated in the right subhepatic area from bowel or the gallbladder and in all perihepatic spaces from hematomas or loculated ascites. The demonstration of peristalsis with real-time ultrasound, cholecystography or scintigraphy, or percutaneous aspiration may be necessary to make these distinctions.

Recent reports by several ultrasonographers have suggested that amebic abscesses may be differentiated from pyogenic liver abscesses and other liver lesions by distinct ultrasonographic findings. These features include:

1. A smooth wall.
2. Internal echoes that are less dense than surrounding normal liver.
3. Contiguity with the liver capsule.
4. Slight distal sonic enhancement.

Several of these features are well demonstrated in Figure 4. In summary, despite certain limitations, ultrasound is safe and may be very useful in differentiating abscesses from tumors, in guiding percutaneous aspiration, and in following patients with amebic abscesses, the majority of whom do not require drainage.

COMPUTED TOMOGRAPHY

Extremely sensitive and specific for location of abnormal fluid collections, CT has the advantage over both liver scanning and ultrasonography of being able to detect intrahepatic lesions as small as 0.5 cm. This advantage may be very important in patients with multiple small (< 2 cm) pyogenic abscesses. Most amebic abscesses and perihepatic abscesses, however, are solitary and of sufficient size to be easily detected by ultrasound. Further potential advantages of CT include easy visualization of the entire liver and perihepatic areas, accurate interpretation of fatty infiltration of the liver, and immediate results. In addition, contrast agents may be given orally or intravenously to delineate vascular, biliary, or gastrointestinal structures.

Recent comparative studies suggest that CT may be the most accurate (85 to 95 per cent) diagnostic modality presently available for the detection of pyogenic hepatic and perihepatic abscesses. The only potential disadvantages of CT are these:

1. Interference by retained barium and metal clips.
2. Occasional difficulty in differentiating abscesses from neoplasms or cysts.
3. The immobility and expense of the equipment.

Despite the added cost, the advantages, in terms of accuracy, make CT the initial procedure of choice in patients suspected of having a pyogenic hepatic or intra-abdominal abscess. In addition, CT may be quite useful in the localization of abscesses for diagnostic or therapeutic aspiration (Fig. 5).

PERCUTANEOUS ASPIRATION

Until recently, most authorities have not recommended diagnostic aspiration of pyogenic hepatic or perihepatic abscesses. With the advent of ultrasound and CT-guided aspiration and percutaneous drainage, however, this diagnostic option has become safer and now must be considered in selected patients. While percutaneous aspiration and drainage may obviate the need for operation, this technique is not applicable in many patients with pyogenic abscesses in or around the liver. The fluid collection, of course, should be unilocular and accessible via a safe drainage approach. Furthermore, in case of failure or complications, the patient must be prepared for surgery prior to aspiration, and surgical consultation is mandatory in every case.

The main reasons to aspirate an amebic liver abscess are as follows:

1. To establish the diagnosis when the results of serologic tests and noninvasive procedures are unclear.
2. To reduce the likelihood of rupture of a large abscess.

Even before the advent of ultrasound or CT-guided aspiration, most experts had found diagnostic aspiration of amebic abscesses to be safe. As with stool testing, however, recovery and identification of trophozoites or cysts may not be reliable. In addition, aspiration may lead to bacterial superinfection or bleeding complications. Since the majority of patients with an amebic liver abscess respond to amebicidal drugs and do not require drainage, most experts would consider aspiration only if the patient did not respond to adequate medical management, if the abscess is adjacent to the pericardium, or if there is suspicion that the abscess may be secondarily infected with bacteria. Similarly, percutaneous drainage of amebic abscesses is rarely indicated.

Several recent studies suggest that percutaneous drainage of pyogenic hepatic and perihepatic abscesses can be successful in selected patients (Fig. 6). It must be remembered, however, that these are reports of selected patients; the authors stress that adequate drainage must be achieved, and this method may not be suitable for many patients with pyogenic abscesses. The categories of patients in whom percutaneous drainage should not be employed include:

1. Those with multiple abscesses.
2. Those with ascites.
3. Those having liver abscesses with a biliary etiology requiring surgery.
4. Those for whom there is an unknown etiology for the abscess.

One or more of these categories, unfortunately, may apply to many patients with pyogenic hepatic or perihepatic abscesses. Nevertheless, percutaneous drainage may be successful in 75 to 90 per cent of selected patients with pyogenic abscesses and has become an acceptable technique when physicians, radiologists, and surgeons cooperate in the selection and care of these patients.

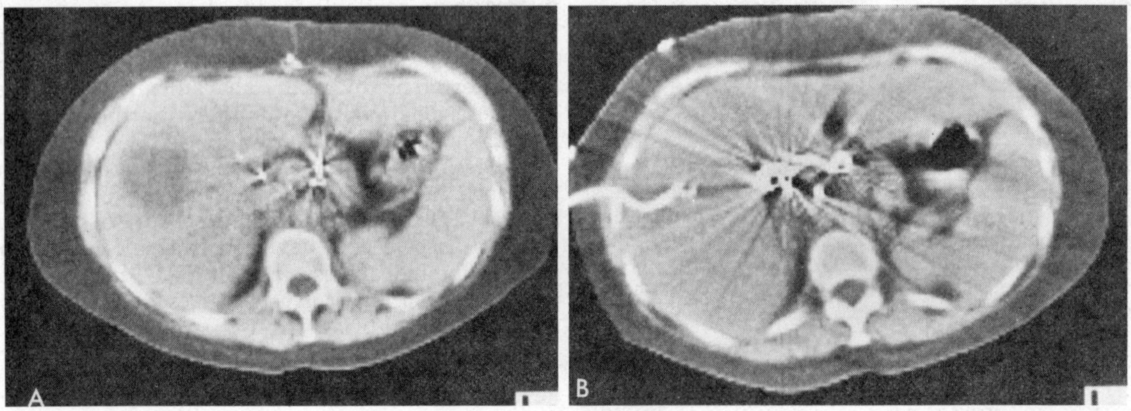

Figure 5. (*A*) Computed tomogram demonstrating a liver abscess in the right lobe. (*B*) Computed tomogram after 4 weeks demonstrating complete resolution of the cavity. The drainage catheter appears white within the liver. (From Pitt, H.A.,: Liver abscess. In Shackelford, R.T., and Zuidema, G.D. (eds.): *Surgery of the Alimentary Tract*, volume 4. Philadelphia, W. B. Saunders Company, 1983.)

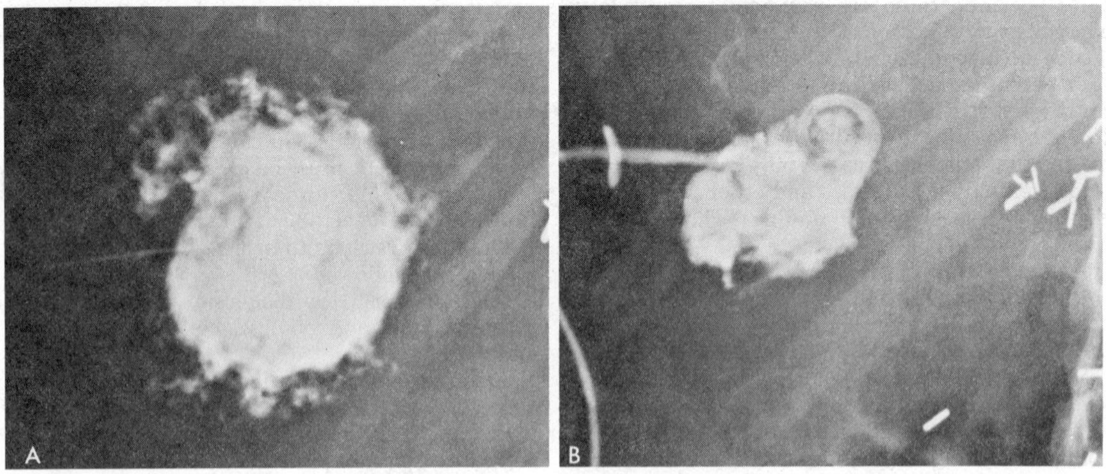

Figure 6. (*A*) Percutaneous aspiration with injection of contrast material into an abscess in the right hepatic lobe. (*B*) Sinogram performed 2 weeks later via the percutaneously placed drainage catheter demonstrating a decrease in the size of the cavity. (From Pitt, H.A.: Liver abscess. In Shackelford, R.T., and Zuidema, G.D. (eds.): *Surgery of the Alimentary Tract*, volume 4. Philadelphia, W.B. Saunders Company, 1983.)

ACUTE AND CHRONIC PANCREATITIS

By Avram M. Cooperman, M.D.
New York, New York

Acute and chronic inflammatory diseases of the pancreas are due to exogenous and endogenous agents. The course is variable, from benign and self-limiting to fulminant and rapidly fatal. Pancreatitis is classified as *acute* (glandular function and histology revert to normal after an episode), *acute relapsing* (quiescent periods between exacerbations), *chronic,* and *chronic relapsing.* Chronic pancreatitis implies irreversible (structural, secretory, and functional) changes and follows long-standing insults to the pancreas.

The causes of pancreatitis are multiple. In the United States 80 per cent of patients have gallstones or consume alcohol excessively. Gallstones have been associated with pancreatitis for more than 80 years, and isolation of stones from feces of patients with gallstone pancreatitis suggests transient obstruction of the ampullary sphincter as the mechanism. A cause-and-effect relation between alcohol and the pancreas is less clear. Inspissated, or thickened, pancreatic secretions and/or stenosis of the sphincter are two mechanisms of alcohol injury. What is certain is the long period (6 to 10 years) that precedes the onset of clinical pancreatitis. This suggests that in many patients with alcoholic pancreatitis there are irreversible changes preceding the first attack. Less common causes of pancreatitis include trauma (with disruption of the pancreatic duct), viral infections, drugs (thiazides, steroids), scorpion venom, vascular disease, hereditary factors, and congenital anomalies of the pancreatic duct.

ACUTE PANCREATITIS

Clinical Presentation

The clinical course and presentation of acute pancreatitis is variable, but almost always includes severe abdominal pain and, less often, nausea and vomiting. The pain is classically abrupt in onset, midline and deep in location, and steady in nature. Upper abdominal tenderness and guarding are usually present. Tachycardia and postural hypotension may be secondary to pain or fluid loss. These physical findings are nonspecific and are present with other acute intra-abdominal conditions. Differentiating acute pancreatitis from other acute disorders that require urgent surgery is crucial. Therefore, a precise diagnosis of pancreatitis is important. For this reason, laboratory and roentgenographic tests are needed.

Laboratory Tests

Serum amylase is elevated in more than 95 per cent of patients with acute pancreatitis, but amylase may be elevated in 5 per cent of patients with other acute intra-abdominal conditions. It has been suggested that more precise diagnosis is possible by using the amylase:creatinine clearance ratio. Although this test has a large number of advocates, limitations and controversy exist such that others (myself included) are skeptical of its value. Urine amylase, serum lipase, and plasma methemoglobin levels are of complementary value. Hyperlipidemia may be present, but the finding is of limited diagnostic importance.

Roentgenographic Tests

Direct and indirect imaging tests of the pancreas have improved the diagnostic accuracy in pancreatitis. Before the advent of ultrasound and computed tomography (CT), the secrets of the pancreas were obscured by the retroperitoneum; although it is still a mysterious organ, these tests have rendered the pancreas less of an enigma.

Plain roentgenograms of the chest and abdomen are of indirect value in 80 per cent of patients. Findings include segmental ileus (sentinel loop), dilatation of the transverse colon (colon cut-off sign), and obliteration of the psoas muscle shadow. Plain roentgenograms may be of great value in eliminating other acute causes such as perforated viscus or mechanical small bowel obstruction.

Ultrasonography has found an expanding role in the diagnosis of acute pancreatitis. Precise definition of the pancreas can be shown, and the common bile duct and gallbladder also can be visualized. Portable sonogram units allow this to be done at the bedside in critically ill patients. The limitation is surrounding bowel gas, which is common in severe acute pancreatitis. Images produced with CT are more precise; however, cost, length of time to do the test, importability of the machine, and more frequent "down" time for repairs make ultrasound a better first test.

Invasive Tests

Diagnostic paracentesis is of minimal diagnostic benefit. Peritoneal lavage with amylase determinations in recovered fluid is also of limited value. Endoscopy and endoscopic retrograde cholangiopancreatography (ERCP) are rarely required in acute pancreatitis. They are of great value in gallstone pancreatitis (suspected or proved), particularly when the pancreatitis is progressive and relief of duct obstruction is a consideration. ERCP is reasonably safe in acute pancreatitis, particularly since complete pancreatic duct obstruction almost always exists. Identification of an impacted bile duct stone by endoscopy or a penetrating ulcer may be an additional benefit of endoscopy.

Finally, laparotomy has a limited but definite role, particularly when a suspicion of a correctable cause is present. Mesenteric infarction and small bowel volvulus or obstruction are diagnostic difficulties.

Course

The course of acute pancreatitis is *generally* mild and self-limited. In 85 per cent of patients, spontaneous resolution occurs within 24 to 48 hours. Identification of the remaining 15 per cent with severe disease is important from a prognostic, diagnostic, and therapeutic standpoint. This high-risk group is identified by the presence of three or more of the following factors present on admission:

1. Age greater than 55 years.
2. White blood cell count greater than 16,000 per cu mm.
3. Blood glucose greater than 200 mg/dl.
4. Lactate dehydrogenase (LDH) greater than 350 U/liter.
5. Serum glutamic oxalacetic transaminase (SGOT) greater than 250 U/liter or developing during the first 48 hours.
6. Hematocrit fall after hydration greater than 10.
7. A blood urea nitrogen (BUN) increase more than 5 mg/dl.
8. Serum calcium level below 8 mg/dl.
9. Arterial Po_2 less than 60 mm Hg.
10. Base deficit greater than 4 mEq/liter.
11. Estimated fluid sequestration greater than 6000 ml.

While not all patients with three or more signs have a high mortality, the fact that more than 50 per cent of patients may die when five or more signs are present makes these prognostic signs of value in identifying the high-risk group.

CHRONIC PANCREATITIS

Chronic pancreatitis is a progressive irreversible inflammatory disease of many causes and presentations.

Etiology

Alcohol is the main contributing factor in 75 per cent of patients. The average pain-free interval and life expectancy after starting heavy drinking is 6 and 24 years, respectively. Not all heavy drinkers develop pancreatitis, since adequate nutrition may be protective. Trauma to the pancreas, particularly following blunt injury, may lead to pseudocyst formation and then persistent left upper quadrant pain. Traumatic disruption of the pancreatic duct is the cause. Congenital anatomic abnormalities, particularly of the ampullary sphincter, play a more important role in the etiology today. Objective data remain to be defined to establish this diagnosis.

Clinical Presentation

Recurrent or acute epigastric pain similar in character, setting, and location to acute pancreatitis is the common presentation. Alcoholism, drug addiction, and psychological problems frequently confuse the diagnosis. Previous bouts make patients aware of the diagnosis, but care must be taken to exclude other causes of acute abdominal pain. In some instances abdominal pain is absent and weight loss, steatorrhea, and malabsorption with or without diabetes mellitus may be the only presentation. A third presentation is due to mechanical complications of pancreatitis. These include duodenal obstruction, obstructive jaundice, gastrointestinal hemorrhage, pancreatic pseudocysts, and pancreatic ascites.

Laboratory Tests

When the presentation is acute and the diagnosis is unknown or in doubt, the evaluation is identical to that for acute pancreatitis. Levels of serum amylase may be less reliable, since the pancreatic parenchyma may be fibrosed and secretory activity may be minimal.

In the chronic setting, tests of malabsorption are indicated when steatorrhea is suspected. A 72-hour stool collection for fecal fat is initiated. Secretin stimulation with duodenal intubation helps quantitate the secretory response of the exocrine pancreas. An oral glucose tolerance test may allow quantitation of islet cell mass, but this test is not of practical value.

Roentgenographic Tests

A flat film of the abdomen may show pancreatic calcifications, a definite sign of chronic pancreatitis. Sonography and/or CT may show the size of the pancreas and the pancreatic duct (if it is dilated). A barium swallow roentgenogram evaluates encroachment on the duodenal bulb if obstruction is suspected. The "best" diagnostic test in our experience is ERCP. Precise definition of the pancreatic duct radicles and changes in the major pancreatic ducts are clearly shown.

Complications

Pancreatic Pseudocysts. See the article on Pancreatic Cysts and Neoplasms.

Duodenal Obstruction. Compression of the descending duodenum by a chronic inflammatory mass or fat necrosis is infrequent. Symptoms of gastric retention (nausea, vomiting, fullness) suggest this complication, which is diagnosed by barium studies or endoscopy.

Cholestatic Jaundice. When this is due to obstruction of the distal common bile duct in the head of the pancreas, it is usually caused by chronic fibrosis. Rarely, a pseudocyst may obstruct the duct. Elevations of serum alkaline phosphatase may precede jaundice by weeks or months. An ERCP proves the diagnosis.

Gastrointestinal Bleeding. Acute or chronic gastrointestinal bleeding associated with pancreatitis may be due to duodenal ulcer or gastric erosions. Specifically, obstruction of the splenic vein in chronic pancreatitis may cause gastric varices. The diagnosis is suspected at endoscopy and confirmed by a selective arteriogram or splenoportogram.

Pancreatic Ascites. Leakage of an obstructed pancreatic duct or a pseudocyst allows amylase-rich fluid to collect in the peritoneal cavity, causing pancreatic ascites. The diagnosis is suggested by a peritoneal tap recovering amylase-rich fluid. A sonogram will resolve the issue of a pseudocyst, and ERCP will demonstrate the leakage.

CONCLUSIONS

Acute and chronic pancreatitis overlap in definition, presentation, and course. For most patients, the natural history and course are mild and spontaneous resolution is the rule.

Direct imaging tests of the pancreas, ultrasound, ERCP, cholangiopancreatography, and CT display intrinsic abnormalities of the upper abdomen that are associated with pancreatitis.

Specific complications of pancreatitis lend themselves to precise diagnosis. A better understanding guides treatment.

PANCREATIC CYSTS AND NEOPLASMS

By Avram M. Cooperman, M.D.
New York, New York
and Robert E. Hermann, M.D.
Cleveland, Ohio

Pancreatic cysts and neoplasms include a variety of benign and malignant lesions that have multiple presentations and causes. Pancreatic cysts include pseudocysts, retention cysts, congenital cysts, and cystadenomas. Solid tumors include carcinoma and both functional and nonfunctional islet cell tumors.

PSEUDOCYSTS

Cystic accumulations of fluid rich in pancreatic enzymes that develop after pancreatitis, carcinoma, and trauma characterize nonepithelial-lined pancreatic pseudocysts.

Symptoms and Signs

Regardless of the cause of a pseudocyst, the presenting symptoms and signs are similar. Epigastric pain or fullness, anorexia, and weight loss are very common. In 30 to 50 per cent of patients, the pseudocyst is palpable and detected by the patient as well as the examiner. In 10 per cent of patients, atypical features exist. These include jaundice (from compression of the bile duct or associated pancreatitis in the head of the gland), gastrointestinal hemorrhage (from varices secondary to splenic vein thromboses or erosion into adjacent viscera), and *pancreatic* ascites (secondary to leakage of the cyst or pancreatic duct). Unusual presentations may occur; these include mediastinal, cervical, intrasplenic, or pelvic locations.

Diagnosis

A number of tests are available to diagnose pseudocysts. A plain roentgenogram of the abdomen may show displacement of contiguous viscera (secondary to fluid in the cyst). Indirect evidence may be further provided by a barium roentgenogram of the stomach or an intravenous pyelogram, both of which have limited value today. Direct visualization of the pseudocyst is provided by ultrasound (US) or computed tomography (CT). Cost alone favors ultrasound if personnel with expertise are available to interpret the scan correctly. A further advantage of these techniques is that the cyst may be followed to maturation or resolution. In some instances, particularly when pain is out of proportion to the findings or when chronic pancreatitis is present, endoscopic retrograde cholangiopancreatography (ERCP) may define associated duct abnormalities should surgery be contemplated. Sepsis secondary to infection of the pseudocyst is rare, but the fear of this complication has limited ERCP. Since percutaneous drainage and aspiration of pseudocysts is finding a definite place in treatment, more ERCPs will be done to exclude ductal obstruction.

Course

Until recently, the natural history of pseudocysts was difficult to plot because small lesions are difficult to detect and follow. With ultrasound, 50 per cent of patients with severe bouts of pancreatitis are shown to have cystic collections of fluid in the lesser sac. Many are asymptomatic. Approximately 25 to 40 per cent of these "pseudocysts" resolve spontaneously, usually within 6 weeks after diagnosis.

TRUE CYSTS

Benign cystic lesions that have columnar or cuboidal epithelium (retention or congenital) are very uncommon and are definitely diagnosed only at surgery. They may be unsuspected when pancreatitis or trauma does not precede the development of a cystic mass or when associated hepatic and renal cysts coexist in children.

CYSTADENOMA OR CYSTADENOCARCINOMA OF THE PANCREAS

Approximately 10 per cent of cystic lesions of the pancreas are neoplastic cysts, most frequently cystadenoma or cystadenocarcinoma.

Symptoms and Signs

In the absence of abdominal pain or pancreatitis, the insidious onset of abdominal discomfort, fullness, and a mass suggests cystadenoma or cystadenocarcinoma. About 400 cases have been reported, with a striking predominance in women (nine times as common) compared with men. A palpable epigastric mass or left upper quadrant fullness is the most common finding.

Diagnosis

As with pancreatic pseudocysts, a variety of indirect tests are available to establish the diagnosis of a cystic lesion. Cost efficiency limits indiscriminate use of all these examinations. Availability and expertise dictate what is possible at each institution. Ultrasound or CT scan may establish the size of the cyst, its relationship to contiguous organs, the part of the pancreas involved (head, body, tail), and the presence of both solid and cystic components.

Barium studies to delineate gastric, duodenal, and transverse colon anatomy may confirm the US or CT images and help the surgeon determine the operative approach.

Course

Slow, progressive increase in size of the mass is common. Hepatic metastases occur late and usually after multiple attempts to remove the cyst.

SOLID PANCREATIC NEOPLASMS

Solid pancreatic neoplasms unfortunately mean cancer in over 90 per cent of patients. This neoplasm is now the fourth most common malignant tumor and is increasing in frequency for unknown reasons. Since 90 per cent of patients will succumb within 48 months after the condition is diagnosed, it is important to establish a diagnosis rapidly and with a minimum of tests.

Adenocarcinoma arising from ductular epithelium accounts for over 90 per cent of the lesions. It arises in the head of the gland in 70 per cent, in the body in 20 per cent, and in the tail of the pancreas in 10 per cent.

Tumors of the Head of the Pancreas

Lesions in the head of the pancreas produce jaundice or gastrointestinal hemorrhage, while lesions in the body and tail cause pain (retroperitoneal nerve invasion) and, much less frequently, jaundice.

Since four lesions arising at or near the ampulla of Vater may mimic each other, differentiation between them is frequently difficult, both preoperatively and intraoperatively. These tumors include cancer of the head of the pancreas, of the distal common bile duct, of the duodenum, or of the ampulla of Vater. All have similar presenting symptoms and signs. Persistent and progressive jaundice is the hallmark of cancer of the head of the pancreas, usually accompanied by pain and significant weight loss, 15 lbs (7 kg) or more. Less frequently, gastrointestinal hemorrhage secondary to duodenal ulceration or duodenal obstruction are associated features.

Signs

Aside from icterus, nonspecific signs are frequently found. A dilated and palpable gallbladder (Courvoisier's sign) implies obstruction below the cystic duct, usually owing to a periampullary malignancy. A palpable, enlarged liver may indicate nonspecific enlargement or intrahepatic metastases. Signs of metastases, including periumbilical nodules (Sister Mary Joseph's sign) or left supraclavicular nodes (Virchow's node), indicate distant metastases.

Laboratory Tests

Because jaundice is progressive and intense, the level of serum bilirubin is frequently greater than 10 mg/dl at the time of diagnosis. Almost all of this is conjugated. Proportionate, or at times significantly higher, levels of alkaline phosphatase denote biliary obstruction. Modest elevations of transaminase may also be occasionally seen.

Roentgenographic Tests

Specific imaging of the pancreas and biliary tree has altered the diagnostic approach to pancreatic cancer. Only a few years ago, indirect measures made the preoperative diagnosis uncertain.

When a periampullary cancer is suspected, imaging by US or CT will disclose a mass, dilated bile ducts, and the possible presence of liver metastases.

Endoscopy and ERCP are done next. Medial encroachment on the duodenal wall by a pancreatic mass and complete obstruction of the main pancreatic duct are the findings in 99 per cent of patients with pancreatic cancer. A normal or nonobstructed duct pattern is seen in less than 1 per cent of cases. An additional value of ERCP is the placement of an endoscopic stent, which serves as a means to decompress the liver and to provide a prognostic guide.

If ERCP is unsuccessful or if the technique is not available at an institution, percutaneous transhepatic cholangiography with or without stent insertion is done next. Catheters can be advanced into the duodenum beyond the tumor.

Until recently, surgery was the only way to decompress the liver when malignant jaundice was present. Now nonoperative measures are the equal of surgical procedures in many instances. Therefore, it is vital to *assess* resectability preoperatively since some patients may be spared surgery. Selective pancreatic arteriography is now done routinely. When major vessel encasement is present (hepatic artery or mesenteric vein) the tumor is not surgically curable. If gastric outlet obstruction is not present, I prefer to decompress the liver nonoperatively. Thus, angiography plays a more important role.

"HIDA" (technetium 99m iminodiacetic acid) scans have a role in assessing bile flow before and after stenting.

Course

The natural course of cancer of the head of the pancreas is progressive and inexorable. Fewer than 10 per cent of patients undergo pancreaticoduodenal resection because regional, distant, or contiguous spread of tumor precludes attempts at curative resection. Decompression of an obstructed bile duct and liver by a biliary enteric bypass relieves jaundice, but it is unclear whether survival is significantly prolonged by these operations. Hepatic metastases, ascites, anorexia, or gastrointestinal hemorrhage secondary to obstructed mesenteric and portal veins are the usual causes of death, almost always within 5 years. Resection of the head of the pancreas, distal bile duct, duodenum, gallbladder, and distal stomach (Whipple operation) can be done in fewer than 10 per cent of patients, with an operative mortality that ranges from 5 to 30 per cent. This rate makes it important to accurately diagnose the tumor by biopsy or cytologic diagnosis.

Cancer of the Body and Tail of the Pancreas

Malignant tumors of the body and tail of the pancreas are fatal in 100 per cent of cases unless discovered by serendipity at surgery done for other reasons.

Symptoms and Signs

Weight loss and midepigastric pain boring through or radiating into the back are the hallmarks of cancer of the body and tail of the pancreas. Deep vein phlebitis of the lower extremity, which may be recurrent and migratory, is frequently associated with adenocarcinoma of the body of the pancreas. Pain relieved by leaning forward is characteristic of retroperitoneal involvement.

Cancer of the body of the pancreas is nonpalpable in nearly all patients. Since metastases are frequent, hepatomegaly and cervical nodes should be sought. Arterial bruits or venous hums in the left upper quadrant denote compression of the splenic artery and vein.

Diagnosis

Ultrasound or CT scan provides direct imaging of the pancreas, bile ducts, and liver and in time should prove to be the most sensitive noninvasive test to establish the diagnosis. Angiography (encasement of vessels) and ERCP (abrupt blockage of mid-duct) may help in atypical presentations and may provide strong indirect evidence of cancer.

Peritoneoscopy or laparotomy with biopsy of metastases will establish the diagnosis and determine resectability. Unfortunately, discovery of a resectable tumor is a rare circumstance.

Course

Treated or untreated cancer of the body and tail of the pancreas runs an inexorable course, leading to death within months to years. Ascites, jaundice (frequently owing to liver metastases), and back pain (secondary to retroperitoneal perineural invasion) are ominous late signs. Resectability is quite uncommon unless the tumor is discovered by chance at the time of laparotomy done for other reasons. We have never encountered a resectable lesion at laparotomy with the preoperative diagnosis of cancer of the body or tail of the pancreas.

ISLET CELL TUMORS

A third type of pancreatic neoplasm, usually solid and only rarely cystic, is the islet cell tumor. This tumor most often presents because of overproduction of one or more hormones which cause hypoglycemia (excess insulin), duodenal or marginal ulcers (gastrin), or watery diarrhea (vasoactive intestinal polypeptide or other members of the secretin family).

Hyperinsulinism

Overproduction of insulin by benign (90 per cent), malignant (10 per cent), or hyperplastic (less than 2 per cent) islet cell tumors frequently causes considerable confusion for patients who suffer from hypoglycemia and for physicians trying to establish the diagnosis.

Symptoms

Dizziness, weakness, palpitations, sweating, confusion, convulsions, and coma are the spectrum of symptoms experienced by hypoglycemic patients. As suggested by Whipple and Frantz, symptoms may be caused by exercise or fasting; the glucose level at the time of symptoms is 50 mg/dl or less, and symptoms abate with administration of glucose.

Diagnosis

Today the diagnosis of hyperinsulinism is facilitated by techniques that measure serum insulin by radioimmunoassay. Elevated levels or inappropriately elevated levels proportionate to plasma glucose have eased the diagnosis in most patients. A fast for 48 to 72 hours under observation still remains a reliable method for inducing symptoms. Provocative tests using leucine, tolbutamide, glucagon, and arginine are infrequently used. Measurement of proinsulin and C peptide are newer assays that help establish the diagnosis of organic hyperinsulinism. Proinsulin levels are elevated in insulinoma patients even when total insulin levels are normal. C-peptide concentrations of insulin reflect endogenous pancreatic output and may be used to exclude exogenous causes of hyperinsulinism.

Preoperative Localization

Having established a diagnosis of hyperinsulinism, preoperative localization by angiography reassures physicians, surgeons, and patients that a tumor may be found. Selective splenic artery catheterization with magnification views of the pancreas is available in most hospitals. Accurate localization is possible in 50 to 85 per cent of cases. More recently in a few institutions, transhepatic catheterization of the splenic vein with determination of insulin concentrations can localize the hyperfunctioning segment of pancreas.

Course

Since 90 per cent of insulin-producing lesions are benign and single, symptoms are usually due to excess production of insulin and not to metastases. While some individuals, not suspecting the diagnosis, eat frequently to avoid hypoglycemic episodes, the risks of central nervous damage from hypoglycemia are real in most patients and surgery is the wisest treatment.

Gastrinoma (Zollinger-Ellison Syndrome)

Some islet cell tumors produce gastrin, a hormone that causes excessive and significant quantities of gastric acid and pepsin. As a result, duodenal mechanisms that neutralize acid are overcome and ulcerations of the duodenum and jejunum are produced.

Symptoms and Signs

When first described in 1955 in patients with recurrent or ectopic ulcerations, marked gastric acid secretion in patients with non–beta cell tumors established the diagnosis. Today, nearly 30 per cent of these patients present with ordinary symptoms of duodenal ulcer disease present for one or more years, and 20 per cent have ulcer symptoms of more than 5 years' duration. One third have associated endocrine abnormalities such as hyperparathyroidism, renal stones, and adrenal or pituitary tumors.

Diagnosis

Elevated basal levels of serum gastrin two or more times normal or basal acid output greater than 15 mEq per hour make the diagnosis. In uncertain cases, secretin (1 mg/kg) or calcium (5 mg/kg) infusion should result in doubling of serum gastrin. Angiography may localize the lesion if present in the pancreas. Unfortunately, the test is of less value than with hyperinsulinism, since 50 per cent of benign lesions are multiple and two thirds of the malignant lesions have metastasized before diagnosis.

Course

Untreated or incorrectly treated, the disease terminates fatally from surgical complications or complications of the ulcer. The efficacy of such histamine receptor antagonists as cimetidine (Tagamet) has been documented in about 25 per cent of patients treated for periods of up to 3 years. If metastases are present, half the patients will succumb within 5 years.

Watery Diarrhea Syndrome

Even less frequent than insulinoma and gastrinoma is the syndrome known as pancreatic cholera, watery diarrhea, or Verner-Morrison syndrome.

Symptoms and Signs

Although this too is a spectrum of a disease presentation, nearly half the patients have profuse watery diarrhea in excess of 4 to 6 liters per day, hypokalemia, and hyperglycemia. Less frequently, hypercalcemia and flushing are associated findings.

Diagnosis

Common causes of diarrhea must be excluded. Inflammatory bowel disease (Crohn's disease and ulcerative colitis), laxative abuse, and functional diarrhea should be sought, as they are most common. Sigmoidoscopy and barium studies of the gastrointestinal tract help exclude some of these. Angiography may localize a pancreatic or extraperitoneal tumor. Perhaps the best diagnostic tests are serum radioimmunoassays for peptides of the "secretin" family.

If elevated levels of secretin, glucagon, and vasoactive intestinal polypeptide (VIP) are documented by reliable radioimmunoassay, this diagnosis must be strongly suspected.

Course

Untreated and undiagnosed, the metabolic effects of uncontrolled diarrhea may be fatal. Excision of benign or malignant pancreatic or extrapancreatic tumors may cure or relieve the diarrhea. Malignant tumors prove fatal, usually because of hypokalemia, dehydration, or uncontrolled electrolyte and fluid disturbances.

CYSTIC FIBROSIS

By Carol Cheney, M.D.
La Jolla, California
and Ivan R. Harwood, M.D.
San Diego, California

SYMPTOMS AND DEFINITIONS

Cystic fibrosis (CF) is a multisystem disease affecting all exocrine glands, with clinically significant involvement of the respiratory tract, pancreas, gastrointestinal tract, reproductive tract, and exocrine sweat glands.

The clinical syndrome was first identified in the 1930s and, over the years, has carried various names, including "mucoviscidosis," "pancreatic achylia," "fibrocystic disease of the pancreas," and "pancreatic fibrosis." Like those names that have been discarded, "cystic fibrosis" does not describe the breadth of multisystem involvement that characterizes the disease, but this is the name that is generally used in the United States.

Cystic fibrosis is an inherited disease, transmitted as an autosomal recessive. In the Caucasian American population, the carrier rate approximates 1 in 20 and the frequency of affected births is 1 in 1500 to 2000. CF is much less common in other racial groups, with an incidence of about 1 in 17,000 in American Blacks and 1 in 90,000 in Hawaiian Orientals. Because the basic genetic and biochemical defects responsible for the manifestations of CF have not been identified, approaches to prenatal diagnosis have been indirect. At present, no adequate test has been developed for either heterozygote detection or prenatal diagnosis.

There are ongoing investigations of several techniques believed to have promise of providing prenatal diagnosis; however, none seems to be reproducible or specific enough for clinical use. Several methods of screening newborn populations are in limited use, primarily in Europe. When field tested in the United States, they have had an unacceptably high level of both false-positive and false-negative results.

CLINICAL PRESENTATIONS

There is a great spectrum of the severity of disease and, consequently, of the mode of presentation. In general, the patterns of presentation can be predicted from a knowledge of the pathophysiologic process, which involves obstruction of the exocrine glands and of the organs into which they deliver their products by secretions that are abnormally thick and viscid.

Most presenting symptomatology involves the respiratory and/or gastrointestinal tract. In the respiratory tract, abnormal secretions and chronic infection at the bronchial level produce a bacterial bronchiolitis and consequent symptoms of small airway infection and obstruction. In the gastrointestinal tract, the primary manifestations are the result of blockage of small pancreatic ducts producing pancreatic insufficiency in more than 85 per cent of the patients.

Neonatal and Infancy

Respiratory symptoms may be manifested in the neonatal period, and gastrointestinal problems can occur in utero with thick meconium causing obstruction and perforation of the small bowel. The abnormality in the sweat glands—failure to reabsorb sodium and chloride in the sweat—is present at birth and is the basis for the diagnostic sweat test.

Approximately 15 per cent of the patients with CF present within the first 48 hours of life with meconium ileus, an obstruction of the small bowel with abnormal meconium that is thick and tenacious because of the absence of adequate pancreatic proteolytic enzymes. This is manifested as intestinal obstruction with symptoms of emesis, abdominal distention, and often failure to pass normal meconium.

Radiographically, dilated loops of small bowel are seen and there is a "ground-glass" appearance to the lower mid-abdomen. Prenatal rupture of the bowel can produce a sterile peritonitis and peritoneal calcifications, seen on radiograph, in addition to the symptoms of obstruction. Prolonged neonatal jaundice may be seen, reflecting extrahepatic and intrahepatic bile stasis.

In the first 12 to 18 months of life, these infants may present with a picture of respiratory distress that is clinically distinguishable from bronchiolitis due to other causes, principally viral. The signs and symptoms are hyperinflation (which is always present), coughing, wheezing, cyanosis, and hypoxia. These may be associated with failure to thrive and with malnutrition. This syndrome is most often seen in infants under 9 months of age and is important to recognize because of the life-threatening nature of this presentation and the typical need for prolonged hospitalization for treatment of the stubborn bacterial bronchiolitis. The organisms most commonly seen in this group of infants are *Pseudomonas aeruginosa, Klebsiella pneumoniae,* and *Escherichia coli;* also seen, but less frequently, is *Staphylococcus aureus.*

A syndrome of hypoproteinemia, edema, and bleeding is the presenting manifestation in a small but significant number of infants with cystic fibrosis. It generally occurs in infants under 1 year of age and is almost always seen in those who are fed breast milk or soybean-based formulas. Affected infants are usually edematous; have hypoprothrombinemia, which manifests as easy bruising and prolonged bleeding from injection sites; and are often anemic. In many instances, the syndrome will be misdiagnosed as child abuse. Any infant with this triad of symptoms should be treated for cystic fibrosis. Resolution of these symptoms occurs with an appropriate formula and pancreatic enzyme replacement.

Because of the inability of the sweat glands to reabsorb sodium, patients with cystic fibrosis lose approximately ten times the normal amount of sodium chloride through their sweat. This may contribute to a syndrome in infancy characterized by hypochloremia and presenting as progressive loss of appetite, development of persistent vomiting, weight loss, and weakness. Serum electrolytes will show a severe hypochloremia and hyponatremia with consequent elevation of serum bicarbonate. Chloride values have been known to fall below 50 mEq/liter in severely affected infants. Older children and adults may manifest this syndrome as a more classic heat stroke, which is also often associated with vomiting.

Infants and Young Children

In infancy, after the neonatal period, the most common presentation is failure to thrive—generalized malnutrition, usually resulting from the combination of malabsorption on the basis of pancreatic insufficiency and pulmonary infection. This failure to thrive is manifested by poor weight gain in the face of a voracious appetite; large, loose foul-smelling stools; and often recurrent respiratory infections.

In addition to malnutrition, malabsorption is characterized by bulky, greasy, and malodorous stools, and chronic diarrhea may be the presenting symptom. The bulky stools may be associated, in up to 20 per cent of the children, with rectal prolapse. This symptom tends to resolve with pancreatic enzyme replacement.

Older infants and children commonly present with chronic or recurrent respiratory symptoms. The most common complaints are recurrent or chronic cough; wheezing is frequently seen. It is not at all unusual for these children to be misdiagnosed and treated as allergic or asthmatic for long periods of time before recognition of the etiology of the symptoms. Frequent episodes of respiratory infection are often associated with bronchospasm. One clue to the diagnosis of CF in such patients is the presence of digital clubbing. With the exception of severe congenital heart disease, clubbing in childhood is virtually unique to CF.

Adolescents and Adults

The presentation of cystic fibrosis in patients first diagnosed in adolescence or adulthood is predictably more subtle. Like children, they may present with recurrent respiratory tract infections, "asthma," or malabsorption. In patients with a picture of recurring bronchitic infections, the appearance of the characteristic mucoid Pseudomonas should prompt consideration of CF. Pansinusitis is nearly universal in older patients with cystic fibrosis, and although often asymptomatic, it may be a presenting symptom. Nasal polyposis becomes more common with advancing age in CF, occurring in nearly half of all adults. Thus, the presence of nasal polyps, in children especially or in adolescents or young adults, in the absence of a classic history of atopy, should raise a strong suspicion of CF. Finally, 95 per cent of males with CF are sterile as the result of abnormal development of the vas deferens and epididymis. Thus, an infertility evaluation may prompt initial consideration of the diagnosis.

COURSE

The overall course of CF is largely determined by that of the pulmonary involvement, which is ultimately responsible for more than 95 per cent of the mortality in this disease. Early in the course, small airways become obstructed with viscid secretions and an infectious bronchiolitis results. With time there is involvement of progressively larger airways, with a sequential development of bronchiolectasis, bronchiectasis, and eventual destruction and fibrosis of the pulmonary parenchyma. The result is obstructive pulmonary disease with marked hyperinflation. There is a parallel progression of abnormalities in the results of pulmonary function tests.

The first changes in pulmonary function reflect small airway obstruction and hyperinflation, first seen as a decrease in end expiratory flow rates, generally not responsive to bronchodilators. The amount of hyperinflation is most easily quantified in the residual volume to total lung capacity ratio (RV:TLC), which increases early and again does not usually normalize with bronchodilator therapy. The progression of the disease is measured by the progressive deterioration in these parameters, with the amount of trapped air increasing until 75 to 85 per cent of total lung capacity is residual volume and the vital capacity decreases accordingly. At this degree of pulmonary dysfunction, respiratory failure and death ensue rapidly if there is no response to treatment.

Progression of the pulmonary disease is punctuated by episodes of clinical bacterial infection characterized by increased cough and sputum production, low-grade fever, deterioration of pulmonary function, and progressive inability to maintain weight. Early in the course of their disease, most patients become infected with *S. aureus.* Although this organism can be effectively controlled by oral antibiotic therapy, it is almost invariably replaced by *Pseudomonas aeruginosa,* an organism that, once established, cannot be eradicated.

Over the past 30 years there has been a dramatic improvement in the prognosis of children born with CF. The combination of early diagnosis and aggressive treatment of the nutritional and pulmonary problems has resulted in prolongation of life such that in large centers as many as 40 to 50 per cent of patients are over 18 years of age. The median age of survival continues to rise annually and is now into the third decade.

The clinical course of CF, like its initial presentation, may vary greatly from patient to patient. When large numbers of patients are studied, there is overall about a 3 per cent decrement in forced expiratory volume at 1 second (FEV_1) per year.

Several clinical features that are useful in predicting prognosis have been identified. Female patients generally do less well than do males, a fact that is well recognized but poorly understood. Those patients with the most extensive evidence of disease at presentation (i.e., involvement of both lungs and gastrointestinal tract and/or abnormal chest x-ray) do less well than those with a single-system presentation and those with normal radiographic findings. Predictably, those patients who are able to maintain positive caloric balance and ideal weight do better than those who are malnourished.

In the early stages of CF, patients appear quite healthy. Between episodes of clinical infection, they may have no functional impairment, may be free of cough, and may have normal pulmonary function. Infections can be effectively treated with restoration of the previous state of good health. Eventually, however, recurrent infections take their toll, and the patient suffers a slowly progressive pulmonary disability. As destructive changes progress and Pseudomonas becomes established, treatment of infection no longer eradicates the infection or restores the pulmonary function to previous levels. Ultimately, the disease progresses to produce respiratory failure and death.

PHYSICAL EXAMINATION

Features of the physical examination vary with the clinical condition. The patient may appear malnourished and pale, with muscle wasting and little subcutaneous fat. Frequently, however, especially in the early stages of the disease, patients may not be unusually thin and are occasionally even obese.

Examination of the nose will often reveal polyps, and there may be some tenderness over the sinuses. The most characteristic feature of the patient with established pulmonary disease is a chronic productive cough. The chest will be hyperexpanded, with increased anteroposterior diameter and flattened diaphragms. Auscultatory findings are very nonspecific —rales, rhonchi, and wheezes, either diffuse or localized, may all be heard.

There may be a striking amount of pulmonary disease radiographically and by pulmonary function measurement with normal auscultatory findings, and there can be significant clinical worsening in a patient with no change in those findings. Because the auscultatory findings are not particularly helpful in following the patient with cystic fibrosis, the data provided by the pulmonary function laboratory are an integral part of the examination. In most centers, minimum pulmonary function measurements such as forced vital capacity (FVC) and FEV_1 are done routinely at each patient encounter. Pulmonary function tests provide objective data about the patient's status, response to therapy, and progression of disease that are vital to management.

The abdomen may be protuberant, especially if pancreatic enzyme replacement is inadequate. Splenomegaly may be present in those patients with biliary cirrhosis and portal hypertension. The liver is generally normal in size, but may be palpable because of displacement by the hyperinflated lungs. Inguinal hernias occur with increased frequency in males. Examination of the extremities will generally reveal digital clubbing, and there may be peripheral cyanosis if the pulmonary disease is severe.

COMPLICATIONS

Pulmonary Complications

Pulmonary complications occur in the late stages of the disease. Parenchymal destruction and the consequent formation of bullae predispose to the development of *pneumothorax.* These bullae may be small and even asymptomatic, but generally they require tube thoracostomy and at times operative pleural abrasion to prevent recurrence.

Hemoptysis is a relatively common complication and is usually related to episodes of increased infection. It may be minimal and require no therapy, or it may be massive and even fatal. Massive hemoptysis (greater than 100 ml of blood in 1 hour) requires hospitalization and possibly transfusion. Bronchoscopy and, at times, therapeutic bronchial artery embolization may be required to localize and treat the site of bleeding.

Cor pulmonale is a direct consequence of the respiratory failure in the preterminal phases of the disease. Chronic severe hypoxia results in pulmonary arterial constriction and right heart failure. Although patients may notice mild facial or peripheral edema, many of the usual clinical features of right heart failure (enlarged right ventricle on chest x-ray, right ventricular hypertrophy on electrocardiogram, and accentuated P_2 on cardiac auscultation) may be obscured by the alteration in thoracic anatomy consequent to the patient's massive hyperinflation. Physiologic parameters—such as marked hypoxia (Po_2 less than 50 mm Hg), hypercarbia (Pco_2 greater than 50 mm Hg), and markedly decreased vital capacity (less than 40 per cent of predicted)—tend to be more reliable indicators of cor pulmonale in this setting.

Gastrointestinal Complaints

There is a broad spectrum of gastrointestinal complications in cystic fibrosis. *Meconium ileus equivalent* is a fairly common syndrome characterized by intermittent and partial small bowel obstruction resulting from failure to pass thick, inspissated stool. Although surgical intervention was frequently required in the past, the use of hypertonic enemas has nearly eliminated the need for laparotomy in this setting. Intussusception can also occur, resulting from a bolus of thick, retained feces in the small bowel which serves as a "lead point." This complication, likewise, generally can be managed conservatively. Unlike the pulmonary complications, these obstructive gastrointestinal problems are not limited to the late stage of the disease but can occur at any point in its course.

Hepatobiliary disease is relatively common in CF. The use of sensitive screening measures will reveal cholelithiasis and/or a thickened contracted gallbladder in as many as 30 per cent of patients, some of whom will develop symptomatic cholecystitis. A form of biliary cirrhosis, generally anicteric and asymptomatic, occurs in about 5 per cent of patients with CF, although 20 to 40 per cent may have abnormalities in hepatic function. Most commonly, there is an isolated elevation of the alkaline phosphatase, although mild elevation of the transaminases may be seen. Uncommonly, the hepatic disease may progress to produce portal hypertension and esophageal varices.

Acute pancreatitis occurs occasionally, generally in older children or adolescents with some residual pancreatic function. As the average age of patients with cystic fibrosis increases, there is a rising incidence of clinical *glucose intolerance,* occurring in up to 20 per cent of the adult population. The diabetes of CF is a secondary process, resulting from "strangulation" of the pancreatic islets by the fibrotic exocrine pancreas. Some insulin-secreting capacity is generally retained and, like other forms of secondary diabetes, the diabetes of CF tends to be relatively mild and ketosis resistant. As mentioned, male patients are nearly always aspermic. Female patients also have decreased fertility, probably due in large part to the abnormally viscid nature of the cervical mucus. As in many chronic diseases of childhood, puberty tends to be delayed but sexual maturation and function are otherwise normal in both men and women.

Drugs and Medications

Because of the large number of drugs used to treat patients with cystic fibrosis, there are, unfortunately, a number of potential iatrogenic complications. Oral antibiotics are used frequently and often continuously. Tetracycline, if used in young children, causes staining of the teeth, may retard bone growth, and can precipitate pancreatitis.

Chloramphenicol can cause optic and peripheral neuritis as well as the well-recognized bone marrow suppression. Chronic oral antibiotics may suppress the normal gut flora and result in bleeding due to vitamin K deficiency. In the later stages of CF, treatment for Pseudomonas infection is required and one may see renal or otic toxicity due to the aminoglycosides and abnormal platelet function or sodium overload due to semisynthetic penicillins. Finally, patients occasionally become overly "health conscious" and may medicate themselves with toxic doses of fat-soluble vitamins, minerals, and other substances.

Psychosocial Complications

As one might expect, these are frequent. From infancy, many children with CF see themselves as different from peers and siblings, and parents may tend to overprotect. These children often have physical stigmata, such as small size, decreased exercise tolerance, frequent cough, and delayed puberty, which attract teasing from peers and schoolmates. Adolescent and young adult years have the preceding problems, accentuated by increased concern about body image and the additional stresses of career planning and consideration of marriage.

Generally, patients and families cope exceedingly well, considering the magnitude of the problems, but the best care programs will take into consideration the stresses and, by patient and family education and special programs, will work to reduce the negative effect of these difficulties.

LABORATORY PROCEDURES

Sweat Test

Because the primary defect in cystic fibrosis is not understood, diagnosis is based on one of its clinical features—the universal abnormalities in sweat electrolytes. The sweat test is performed by first inducing sweat production with pilocarpine iontophoresis. Sweat is then collected and the specimen weighed to ensure an adequate collection (at least 100 mg). The chloride content is then measured. When the chloride content is greater than 60 mEq/liter, the results are diagnostic of cystic fibrosis. Intermediate values of 50 to 60 mEq/liter are suggestive but not diagnostic and bear repetition. The normal sweat chloride content rises somewhat with age, but the normal adult distribution does not significantly overlap with that of CF patients and the sweat test remains applicable in adulthood. The sweat test is normal in heterozygotes. Although there are other disease processes (e.g., untreated adrenal insufficiency or hypothyroidism, ectodermal dysplasia, nephrogenic diabetes insipidus, and some glycogen storage diseases) that elevate the sweat chloride, differentiation from CF rarely presents a clinical problem. By far the most important source of diagnostic error is improper technique in performing the sweat test. Screening or nonquantitative systems that have been used are clearly less accurate, and even a quantitative chloride method may produce inaccurate results if not performed by a technician expert in the procedure. Results obtained in hospitals or clinics that perform sweat tests infrequently are notoriously unreliable. Patients suspected of having CF should therefore be referred directly to one of the 120 designated centers supported by the Cystic Fibrosis Foundation for testing.

Other Evaluations

The sweat test is the only test diagnostic for cystic fibrosis. Various studies of pancreatic function may be used to evaluate the presence or extent of pancreatic insufficiency, but they do not play a significant role in the initial diagnosis of the disease. Efforts at developing a useful test for neonatal screening have thus far not identified a measure with an acceptably low rate of false-positive and false-negative results.

Laboratory measures are also helpful in monitoring the course of the patient with cystic fibrosis. We have already alluded to the use of serial pulmonary function tests. Serial chest radiographs also provide useful information about the progression of the disease. The x-ray in CF demonstrates thickening of the bronchial wall shadows, areas of hyperinflation (especially in the upper lung fields), and frequent hilar enlargement. With progression of disease, there is further hyperinflation, manifested by sternal bowing and flattening of the diaphragm; bullae may be seen. Retained secretions and plugging by mucus result in areas of atelectasis and patchy infiltration. It is not uncommon, as the disease progresses past the earliest stages, for the radiograph to look substantially "sicker" than the patient.

Finally, periodic laboratory evaluation is used to monitor for the complications of both therapy and the disease. Thus blood counts are measured in patients on chloramphenicol and drug levels in those on tobramycin. Periodic screening is done for glucose intolerance and hepatic disease.

PITFALLS IN DIAGNOSIS

Much of the dramatic improvement in life expectancy that has been achieved in CF can be attributed to early diagnosis and institution of appropriate therapy. Probably the major error on the part of physicians in making the diagnosis of CF is the failure to consider it. Cystic fibrosis, as we have emphasized, has a great spectrum of clinical presentations and can therefore mimic many other diseases. Underestimating the extent or progression of the pulmonary disease on the basis of auscultatory findings is a frequent pitfall.

Once the diagnosis is entertained, the patient should be referred to a designated CF center for sweat testing. In this way, accurate results can be assured. Should the diagnosis be confirmed, the patient and the family can then be counseled by a team experienced in the care of patients with cystic fibrosis and an appropriate course of therapy begun early.

DIAPHRAGMATIC HERNIAS

By F. Henry Ellis, Jr., M.D., Ph.D.
Burlington, Massachusetts

Herniation of abdominal viscera through defects in the diaphragm, whether naturally occurring or the result of trauma, includes a variety of acquired and congenital conditions. Not only are there anatomic differences between the various types of diaphragmatic hernias, but symptoms and treatment vary from one type of hernia to another. It is important, therefore, that an accurate diagnosis be made. To facilitate this goal, descriptions will cover the various diaphragmatic hernias. Certain common diagnostic techniques will be outlined, and their use in differentiating one diaphragmatic hernia from another will be elucidated.

CLASSIFICATION

A classification of diaphragmatic hernias is presented in Table 1 and in Figure 1.

Hiatal Hernias

Esophageal hiatal hernias not only are the most common hernias of the diaphragm but also are among the more common abnormalities affecting the upper gastrointestinal tract. *Sliding esophageal hiatal hernias* account for 90 per cent of hernias occurring through the esophageal hiatus. In this condition, the esophagogastric junction is displaced through the esophageal hiatus into the chest. These hernias are "sliding," in that the stomach can be demonstrated to move in and out of the thorax, and the hernia has a partial parietal peritoneal sac whose posterior wall is formed by the stomach. Symptoms are uncommon, and when they do occur, they are related to hypotension of the lower esophageal sphincter (LES).

In a *paraesophageal hiatal hernia,* the esophagogastric junction is often in its normal position but the fundus of the stomach and successively greater portions of the greater curvature rotate into the thorax through the hiatus alongside the esophagus. Rotation may continue in a counterclockwise manner and present as a totally intrathoracic "upside-down" stomach. The symptoms are directly related to the mechanical aspects of the hernia.

Table 1. Classification of Diaphragmatic Hernias

Hiatal hernias
Sliding esophageal
Paraesophageal
Combined forms
Short esophagus
Congenital hernias
Posterolateral (Bochdalek)
Retrocostal (Morgagni)
Traumatic hernias
Miscellaneous hernias
Postinflammatory
Parahiatal
Eventration
Intrapericardial

Not all paraesophageal hernias are pure. *Mixed forms* occur in which a sliding element exists, with migration of the esophagogastric junction into the posterior mediastinum in association with a large paraesophageal element. In the combined form, symptoms characteristic of both the sliding hernia and a paraesophageal entity may be present.

The esophagus may become shortened in response to long-standing reflux with esophageal ulceration, scarring, and fibrosis, leading in many instances to stricture formation either at the esophagogastric junction or at a higher level, as in the columnar epithelium-lined lower esophagus (Barrett). The *shortened esophagus hiatal hernia,* once considered to be congenital, is now correctly believed to be an acquired condition in almost every instance. It represents failure of treatment of reflux secondary to a hypotensive LES.

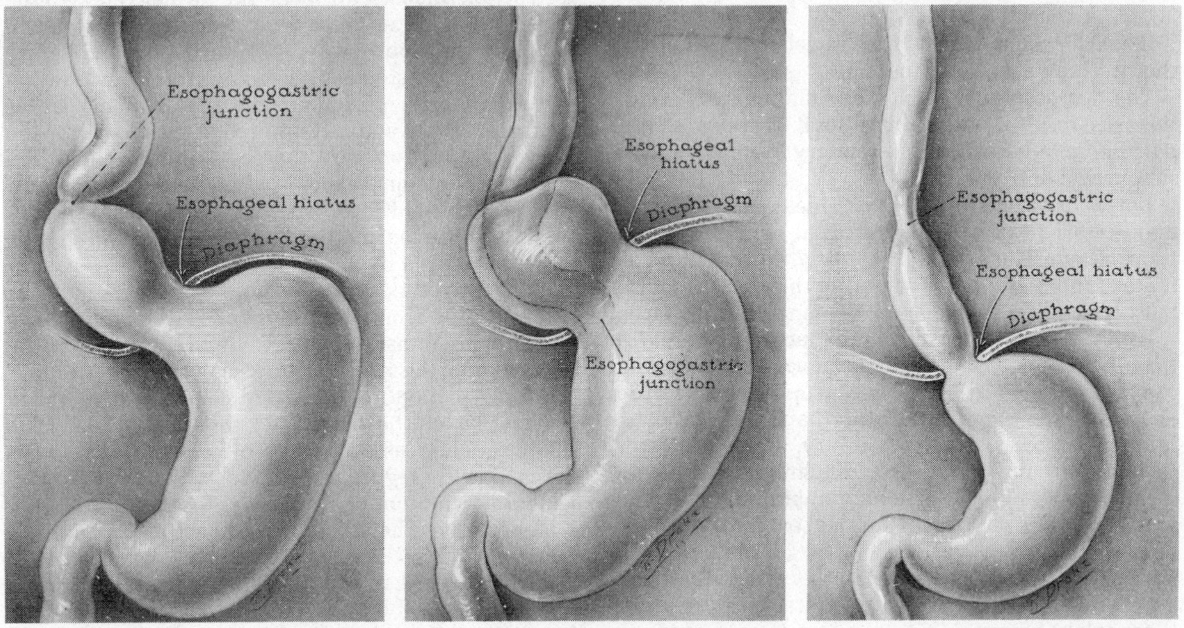

Figure 1. Types of diaphragmatic hernias occurring through the esophageal hiatus. (*Left*) Sliding esophageal hiatal hernia. (*Middle*) Paraesophageal hiatal hernia. (*Right*) Shortened esophageal hiatal hernia. (From Mobley, J.E., and Christensen, N.A.: Esophageal hiatal hernia: Prevalence, diagnosis, and treatment in an American city of 30,000. Gastroenterology 30:5, 1956. Reprinted with permission of the Williams & Wilkins Company, Baltimore.)

Congenital Hernias

A congenital hernia through the *posterolateral aspect* of the diaphragm (pleuroperitoneal canal or foramen of Bochdalek) is the most common diaphragmatic hernia found in infants and newborns. It occurs posterolaterally where the diaphragm develops normally from fusion of several anlagen completing separation of the thoracic and abdominal cavities. Failure of complete fusion of the pleuroperitoneal folds during the first trimester of gestation is considered to be the basic defect in this type of diaphragmatic hernia. Such a hernia may or may not have a hernial sac, depending on whether failure of fusion occurs during the initial or late stage of development; usually, however, the sac is absent.

The second most common type of congenital diaphragmatic hernia, variously known as anterior diaphragmatic, parasternal, retrosternal, or retrocostal hernia, is best known by its eponym, *foramen of Morgagni.* This hernia, probably the result of a congenital defect in the fusion of the sternocostal elements of the diaphragmatic anlagen, is uncommonly diagnosed in infants and children. The majority of hernias of this type are identified in adults, with most of them occurring on the right side.

Traumatic Hernias

Traumatic rupture of the diaphragm is usually the result of severe external trauma rather than a penetrating injury. The lesion usually presents as a linear tear radiating out from, but usually not involving, the diaphragmatic crus and is more common on the left than on the right side.

Miscellaneous Hernias

Listed for completeness are a variety of rare hernias that need no special discussion.

The decreasing frequency of inflammatory conditions has resulted in the almost total disappearance of *postinflammatory hernias* secondary to empyema or a subphrenic abscess.

Rarely, a hernia has all the clinical and diagnostic manifestations of a paraesophageal hernia, but will prove at operation to be *parahiatal,* in that the herniated fundus enters the chest, not through the hiatus but through a separate opening alongside the hiatus.

Unilateral elevation of the diaphragm, or *eventration,* may be on a congenital or an acquired basis and can present at any age. This usually results from anomalous development of the diaphragm or of its innervation or as a result of injury, at birth or later, to the phrenic nerve and diaphragm. Although, strictly speaking, this is not a diaphragmatic hernia, it may be difficult without surgical exploration to differentiate such elevations of the diaphragm from traumatic rupture, a large intrathoracic paraesophageal hiatal hernia, or a congenital posterolateral (Bochdalek) hernia.

Even less common are *intrapericardial diaphragmatic hernias* or *central tendon hernias.* They may be congenital or traumatic in origin and involve a communication between the peritoneal and pericardial cavities, probably as a result of a defect of the septum transversum. Most intrapericardial hernias occur in adults.

GENERAL DIAGNOSTIC CONSIDERATIONS

Clinical Evaluation

In this era of proliferation of specialized diagnostic techniques, the importance of the patient's clinical history is often overlooked. Useful clues to precise diagnosis can be obtained by careful attention to the patient's symptoms. Since esophageal hiatal hernias are the most common diaphragmatic hernias, certain symptomatic features of esophageal disease should be emphasized. Dysphagia, regurgitation, and heartburn are by far the most frequent symptoms of esophageal disease.

Dysphagia. Dysphagia refers to a sensation of obstruction or sticking of ingested material. It should be distinguished from *odynophagia,* which, if correctly used, refers to the sensation of painful swallowing. When discussing the symptom of dysphagia with a patient, it is important to elicit information regarding the type of ingested material that leads to dysphagia. Organic strictures—the result of failed management of hypotensive LES—usually cause dysphagia for solid foods first; dysphagia for liquids is a late development. Dysphagia may be associated with pain as the ingested material passes through the strictured area. Some patients with a hypersensitive mucosa will experience pain as the bolus passes over the sensitive area; the sensation is one of material passing over a raw area.

Regurgitation. Regurgitation and reflux are often used synonymously, although the former refers to the projection of material from the esophagus or stomach back into the mouth, whereas reflux is used to signify flow only from stomach to esophagus. In evaluating these symptoms, it is important to determine whether the material has actually entered the stomach, for the site of obstruction may thereby be determined. Patients with esophageal obstruction are prone to regurgitate undigested food, whereas the regurgitation of partially digested material or unneutralized gastric contents reflects hypotension of the LES with gastroesophageal reflux. Both of these symptoms must be differentiated from vomiting, and patients often use these terms indiscriminately. Reflux and regurgitation are effortless events, whereas vomiting is a powerful projection of gastric contents by reflex contraction of the abdominal muscles. Vomiting is also frequently associated with nausea, which is not the case with regurgitation and reflux. Vomiting is seldom a symptom of esophageal disease.

Heartburn The symptom of heartburn is hard to describe, and patients vary in their description of it. Heartburn refers to a substernal or epigastric burning sensation caused by the reflux of acid or bile or both from the stomach into the lower esophagus. It is not a painful sensation. Sometimes it radiates to the neck, angles of the jaw, and ears, and even into the arms.

Radiography

Radiographic examination of the upper gastrointestinal tract is almost always performed by means of an x-ray image intensifier, which has the advantages of delivering reduced amounts of radiation to the patient and of providing better delineation of details without requiring adaptation to the dark. Spot films may be made during fluoroscopy, but information of chief value is obtained during the passage of the ingested material through the esophagus. Photographing the fluoroscopic images on a film, as in cinefluoroscopy, or by tape provides the additional advantage of facilitating review of the study at the physician's leisure and adds considerably to the value of the examination.

Different contrast materials may be employed, including barium sulfate or iodinated contrast medium in aqueous solution, such as meglumine diatrizoate (Gastrografin). The former is the material of choice because it is nontoxic and nonabsorbable. The concentration of barium may be varied, depending on the information one wishes to obtain.

Radiographic examination of the esophagus is most useful in identification of either intrinsic or extrinsic points of obstruction and in identifying some abnormalities of motor function of the esophagus, although it is less accurate in this regard than tests to be described subsequently. It is also frequently used to identify the presence or absence of gastroesophageal reflux, although it is a less sensitive test of reflux than are some others because if sufficiently vigorous maneuvers are employed by the radiologist, reflux can be demonstrated in normal individuals as well as in those with true hypotension of the LES. It is important, however, that the radiologist be reminded to examine the patient for reflux because often this is not routinely included in the usual radiographic examination of the upper gastrointestinal tract.

Endoscopy

An equally important part of the evaluation of the patient suspected of having esophageal disease is endoscopy. The flexible fiberoptic instrument is preferred when diagnosis is the purpose of the study; rigid esophagoscopy is reserved for the management of impacted foreign bodies. I prefer the Olympus fiberoptic esophagoscope, which may include a teaching attachment and a camera mounted on the eyepiece. The examination is well tolerated by the patient, and prolonged examination of the entire esophagus is possible. The use of this technique facilitates the performance of esophageal dilation and the securing of biopsy material and cytologic material for histologic examination.

Esophageal Manometry

Esophageal manometry has provided the most important technical advance in the diagnosis of esophageal disease. Basically, the method consists of measuring pressures at different points in the esophagus by the use of intraluminal catheters connected by means of appropriate transducers to a recording mechanism. Catheters made of polyethylene or polyvinyl minimize distortion of the transmitted pressures, which may be recorded either directly using a transducer-tipped catheter or, more commonly, by perfused catheters. The use of a constantly infused system has proved to be more accurate and reproducible than other methods. Side holes 5 cm apart provide the simultaneous measurement of pressures at three different sites in the esophagus when a three-catheter system is employed.

The technique employed in the laboratory of the Lahey Clinic involves the use of three polyvinylchloride tubes with side openings 5 cm apart cemented together (Arndorfer Medical Specialties, Greendale, Wisc.) and connected to pressure detecting units (Hewlett-Packard Company, Medical Products Group, Model 1280 transducer, Waltham, Mass.), which in turn are connected to a sensitive recording device (Hewlett-Packard, Model 7758). Distilled water is infused through these open-tipped catheters at a rate of 1.14 ml/minute using a special pumping system (Arndorfer). The catheters are inserted either transnasally or transorally into the patient's stomach.

The examination consists of two parts. First, resting intraluminal pressures are measured by gradually withdrawing the catheter through the LES, the body of the esophagus, and the upper esophageal sphincter (UES). The LES is evaluated by two separate pull-through recordings, the second of which is conducted rapidly with the patient holding his breath to obtain more reproducible pressures; these pressures are averaged to provide the definitive recorded pressure at the LES.

After this portion of the study, the deglutitory response of the esophagus and its sphincters is evaluated. After repositioning the catheter system, it is withdrawn by 1 cm intervals to more proximal sites and the response of the recorded pressures to a swallowing effort is recorded. Wet instead of dry swallows are preferred because more than 95 per cent of them elicit a complete peristaltic sequence, compared with a lower percentage when dry swallows are used.

pH Reflux Test

The most sensitive test of gastroesophageal reflux is the pH reflux test. This test is performed by placing 300 ml of 0.1N hydrochloric acid (HCl) in the patient's stomach. A pH electrode (Beckman Instruments, Inc., Glass electrode 39042 and Reference electrode 5DU40249, Fullerton, Cal.) is then placed 5 cm proximal to the LES, previously identified by esophageal manometry. The pH at this level is monitored with the patient resting quietly in the supine position and then while performing various maneuvers that increase intragastric pressure, including deep breathing and the Valsalva and Müller maneuvers. A decrease in esophageal pH to less than 4 is considered positive evidence of gastroesophageal reflux.

When these maneuvers are performed in a physiologic fashion and not in an unnatural way, a high correlation will be found between symptomatic reflux and this objective test. False-positive results may occur, but they are less frequent in my experience than with any other method that attempts to provide objective confirmation of the presence or absence of gastroesophageal reflux.

Acid-Clearing Test

Used in patients with documented evidence of gastroesophageal reflux, this test measures the efficiency of the esophagus in clearing any regurgitated gastric contents. As in the previous test, the pH probe is placed 5 cm above the high-pressure zone, and a bolus of 15 ml of 0.1N HCl is introduced into the esophagus 10 cm proximal to the electrode. The patient is then asked to perform repeated dry swallows at 30-second intervals while the pH is monitored constantly. Normal individuals and those with hiatal hernia but without symptoms are normally able to clear the acid from the distal esophagus within ten swallows. If acid clearance of the distal esophagus is delayed, it is presumed that refluxed gastric contents would remain in contact with the lower esophagus for a prolonged time with the likelihood of the ultimate development of esophagitis being high. Accordingly, a prolonged acid-clearing test is considered an abnormal finding and reflects potentially poor prognosis in terms of the development of esophagitis and its complications. Endoscopic examination should be performed in such instances; a close correlation exists between endoscopic evidence of esophagitis and a positive acid-clearing test.

Other Tests

Acid Perfusion Test. The acid perfusion test was originally designed as a test for esophagitis and as a means for differentiating pain of esophageal origin from that of angina pectoris. With the patient sitting in a chair, a tube is introduced into the middle part of the esophagus, and a solution of 0.9 per cent sodium chloride or 5 per cent glucose is perfused through it at a rate of 10 ml/minute for 15 minutes. After the control period, the perfusion solution is switched to 0.1N HCl and continued for 30 minutes or until the patient complains of pain. The test is negative if HCl does not produce symptoms, if the pain elicited by the infusion is different from the spontaneous symptoms, or if the sodium chloride or glucose solution reproduces the patient's symptoms. Although conceivably a useful screening test in patients with bizarre retrosternal or upper abdominal pain, the high incidence of false-negative and false-positive tests in my experience relegates this test to one of lesser value in evaluating potential patients with esophageal disease.

24-Hour pH Monitoring of Distal Esophagus. To introduce more reliability into the objective identification of gastroesophageal reflux, the pH of the distal esophagus may be monitored continuously over many hours. The technique consists of positioning a pH electrode 5 cm above the LES. Changes are constantly recorded over a 24-hour period, and the patient is asked to record any change in symptoms that may occur during the period of pH monitoring. The final record is analyzed by the percentage of time in which the patient is in the upright and supine positions. In addition, the number of single reflux episodes, the number of episodes greater than 5 minutes, and the duration of the longest episode are recorded; an overall score is computed and recorded for the 24 hours.

Although this technique provides far more detailed information than any of the others described, it requires hospitalization and the prolonged presence of an indwelling tube, which is not always comfortable for the patient. This technique is not widely used, although it may find greater use when monitoring equipment not requiring hospitalization becomes available.

Scanning Techniques. The use of radioactive scanning in diagnosing esophageal disease is a relatively new development, and its role has yet to be determined. Sodium pertechnetate (^{99m}Tc) scanning has been used to identify the mucosal changes in patients with Barrett's esophagus. Scintiscanning also has been suggested as a safe and sensitive noninvasive method of detecting and quantitating gastroesophageal reflux. These techniques are in the investigative stages, but they may be applied more widely in the future.

DIAGNOSIS OF SPECIFIC CLINICAL CONDITIONS

This section deals in detail with the methods of diagnosis of only those conditions that are most commonly encountered clinically.

Sliding Esophageal Hiatal Hernia

Symptoms develop in only a minority of patients with a sliding esophageal hiatal hernia, and when they do develop, they are the result of a hypotensive LES. The characteristic symptoms are those of substernal pain, heartburn, and regurgitation, with accentuation of the symptoms by bending and reclining. In some instances, nocturnal regurgitation may occur with symptoms of aspiration, including cough and wheezing, which may lead to an incorrect diagnosis of asthma.

It is important that the diagnosis of gastroesophageal reflux be made before the development of major complications because after their development treatment becomes difficult. Bleeding from ulcerative esophagitis is rare. A more common complication is ulcerative esophagitis leading to stricture formation and esophageal shortening. Dysphagia to solid foods progressing to inability to ingest soft foods and finally liquids, after a long-standing history of heartburn and regurgitation, is a classic symptom of esophageal stricture. The stricture occurs at the esophagogastric junction, or—if there is cephalad migration of the junctional epithelium—a columnar epithelium-lined lower esophagus (Barrett's esophagus) may develop with a stricture at a higher level, even as proximal as the aortic arch. The symptoms of a Barrett's esophagus with stricture are similar to those exhibited by patient in whom the stricture occurs at the esophagogastric junction, since patients are not always able to localize accurately the site of obstruction. Barrett's esophagus, however, is unique in that it is a precancerous lesion and, if untreated, adenocarcinoma will develop in the columnar epithelium-lined lower esophagus in approximately 8 to 10 per cent of patients.

If a sliding esophageal hiatal hernia is suspected on clinical grounds, the diagnosis can be confirmed by radiography, which will disclose a pouch of stomach of variable size above the diaphragm, protruding through the esophageal hiatus with the esophagogastric junction lying well within the chest. The presence or absence of reflux can be determined in some cases by maneuvers carried out by the radiologist at fluoroscopy, although other objective measures of the presence or absence of reflux are more sensitive. Endoscopic examination of the esophagus may reveal linear esophagitis or esophageal ulceration. In the absence of a history of ingestion of caustic material, this is excellent supportive evidence of gastroesophageal reflux. The absence of such findings, however, does not preclude the diagnosis of reflux. It has been reported that the pathologic examination of biopsy specimens of the esophageal wall, even in the absence of macroscopic evidence of esophagitis, may be useful in diagnosing the presence of gastroesophageal reflux. By measuring the thickness of the esophageal epithelium in reference to the length of the mucosal papillae, an interested pathologist can be of considerable help. In normal patients, the papillary length is less than 60 per cent of the epithelial thickness measured from the base of the papilla to the luminal surface. In patients in whom the papillary length covers more than this amount, gastroesophageal reflux is considered to be present.

Probably the most sensitive objective test for the presence of gastroesophageal reflux is the pH reflux test. The acid perfusion test is widely used and may be helpful in differentiating substernal pain of cardiac origin from that of esophageal origin, but the test has a high incidence of false-negative and false-positive results. Another laboratory test of help in determining the significance of gastroesophageal reflux in any given patient is the acid-clearing test, which measures the efficiency of the esophagus to clear regurgitated material. If acid clearance is delayed, it constitutes a potentially poor prognosis in terms of the development of the complications of esophagitis.

Paraesophageal Hiatal Hernia

A patient with a paraesophageal hiatal hernia in its pure form exhibits symptoms totally different from those symptoms exhibited by a patient with a symptomatic sliding esophageal hiatal hernia. In the latter condition, a disturbance in esophageal physiology results in reflux with its accompanying symptoms. In the paraesophageal hernia, the symptoms are all explainable on a strictly mechanical basis as a result of the anatomic defect that characterizes the condition. The most common symptom is chronic, recurrent, asymptomatic occult gastrointestinal blood loss anemia. The patient, usually an elderly, obese woman, will complain of weakness, fatigue, and feelings of faintness; laboratory studies will disclose the unexplained anemia. Blood loss may occur either from a riding ulcer or gastritis when the hiatus impinges on the herniated stomach or, as is more likely, from venous congestion of the mucosa in the supradiaphragmatic stomach pouch with a slow but constant ooze of blood into the gastric lumen.

The next most common symptom is that of pain, usually located substernally and increasing in severity after meals. Vomiting may develop as a result of obstruction of the esophagogastric junction from marked dilatation of the herniated stomach. When the symptoms of pain become constant, the diagnosis of an incarcerated paraesophageal hernia must be considered. With further herniation and counterclockwise rotation of the herniated gastric pouch, volvulus may develop and result in the most serious complications of this hernia, namely, strangulation, gangrene, and perforation, a complication that is often lethal. Only in the mixed forms in which a sliding esophageal hiatal hernia coexists will the patient complain of symptoms of gastroesophageal reflux.

The diagnosis may be obvious from a plain radiograph of the thorax, which will disclose an air-fluid level behind the heart, a finding almost diagnostic of a paraesophageal hiatal hernia. Contrast radiography of the upper gastrointestinal tract will confirm the clinical suspicion and demonstrate a varying amount of stomach in the chest, often with marked narrowing at the level of esophageal hiatus. Further studies are not indicated because once the diagnosis has been confirmed by radiography, surgical treatment is mandatory.

Congenital Diaphragmatic Hernias

Herniation of abdominal contents through the posterolateral aspect of the diaphragm (foramen of Bochdalek) often presents as an acute respiratory emergency at or shortly after birth, depending in part on the amount of abdominal viscera herniated into the thorax but also on the degree of intrinsic congenital pulmonary insufficiency present. Only rarely do such hernias remain undetected until late childhood or adult life. Although severe respiratory insufficiency may be apparent at birth, an infant may appear to be normal initially and may not have symptoms until the ingestion of air and food causes distention of the herniated hollow viscera. Labored respiration with associated negative intrathoracic pressure may further increase the mass of abdominal organs herniated into the chest.

Physical examination reveals cyanosis and a greatly increased respiratory rate and effort. The affected hemithorax, usually the left, is dull on percussion with evidence of a shift of mediastinal structures to the right. The abdomen is characteristically scaphoid. Auscultation over the left chest fails to reveal breath sounds but rather reveals the characteristic sounds of intestinal origin.

The diagnosis is almost always apparent on standard radiographs of the thorax, which often clearly demonstrate gas-filled intestines. In rare instances, it is difficult to differentiate this process from various inflammatory conditions of the lung, enterogenous cyst, duplication, pneumothorax, lobar emphysema, or other anomalies. Under such circumstances, it is desirable to have the patient, usually an infant, ingest an appropriate nonirritating contrast medium.

The high incidence of associated congenital anomalies should be appreciated, particularly those of the gastrointestinal tract, including abnormalities of rotation and attachment, perhaps with associated peritoneal bands, all of which may affect intestinal patency or predispose to a volvulus. When symptoms develop later in life, gastrointestinal rather than respiratory symptoms predominate. Abdominal pain is present in approximately half the patients. Vomiting, dyspnea, and chest pain occur occasionally, and obstruction is rare.

Most patients with hernias of the foramen of Morgagni are asymptomatic, only about a third having symptoms related to the hernia. These, when present, are predominantly gastrointestinal in origin with upper abdominal or subcostal discomfort, fullness, cramping, and occasional vomiting. Some patients may present a history suggestive of partial obstruction of the large bowel. Respiratory distress, secondary to a hernia of the foramen of Morgagni, is uncommon in the adult, but in infants cardiorespiratory symptoms may predominate. In contrast to some of the other hernias through the diaphragm, complications in hernias of the foramen of Morgagni are uncommon.

The diagnosis is usually suggested by a routine radiograph of the thorax, which may show a rounded shadow of variable size in the right cardiophrenic angle. Lateral views will localize this shadow anteriorly very near the anterior chest wall. The presence of gas-containing bowel is diagnostic of the condition, which may be confirmed by the demonstration of colon within the mass or of angulation of the transverse colon toward the defect after a barium enema. Radiographic examination of the upper gastrointestinal tract is usually diagnostically less rewarding.

Traumatic Diaphragmatic Hernia

The majority of traumatic diaphragmatic hernias are on the left side, and the symptoms are related in great measure to the type and amount of herniated abdominal viscera present in the thorax. The symptoms may vary from none at all to life-endangering problems coincident with a severe injury. Late complications may include gastrointestinal hemorrhage and obstruction. With massive herniation, rapidly progressive cardiorespiratory distress can pose a life-threatening situation. Auscultation over the lower part of the left chest will often reveal the classic sounds of gastrointestinal activity.

A radiograph of the thorax made shortly after injury that demonstrates abnormal shadows above the left diaphragm, such as a gas-filled or homogeneous area combined with a shift of the mediastinum to the opposite side, is extremely suggestive of a ruptured diaphragm. Prompt confirmation of the diagnosis can be obtained by passage of a nasogastric tube, which also prevents progressive distention of the stomach. Occasionally, radiographic examination of the gastrointestinal tract is required for diagnosis.

Although a traumatic diaphragmatic hernia may be discovered soon after injury, occasionally it will not be diagnosed until long afterward because the patient was asymptomatic during the interval between the trauma and the diagnosis. Under such circumstances, the diagnosis is usually made after routine radiography of the thorax discloses the presence of abdominal viscera in the left hemithorax. Similar diagnostic maneuvers are required regardless of the timing of the diagnosis.

Section Eight

METABOLIC DISEASES

DIABETES MELLITUS

By John K. Davidson, M.D., Ph.D.
Atlanta, Georgia

DEFINITION

Diabetes is heterogeneous in origin and may be associated with any of the 122 conditions listed in Table 1. These include diseases of the pancreatic beta cells, hormonal excess and deficit states, insulin receptor abnormalities, side effects of drugs and chemical agents, genetic syndromes, and malnutrition. When fasting hyperglycemia is initially detected, about 95 per cent of affected North Americans are overweight and have non–insulin-dependent diabetes mellitus (NIDDM); about 5 percent are not overweight and have insulin-dependent diabetes mellitus (IDDM).

The criteria for diagnosing diabetes mellitus are listed in Table 2. The *most effective routine* for detecting those (nonpregnant) who have diabetes but do not know it, is noted in Table 3.

ETIOLOGY AND PATHOGENESIS

Homeostatic mechanisms interact to maintain the fasting plasma glucose level within a narrow range (60 to 130 mg/dl). One hormone (insulin) decreases the plasma glucose level, whereas six "contrainsulin" hormones (somatotropin, adrenocorticotropin, cortisol, epinephrine, glucagon, and thyroxin) increase it. Each hormone is secreted as needed to maintain normoglycemia. On the surface of hormone-responsive cells, each hormone combines with its specific receptor. This interaction initiates a train of postreceptor enzymatic and biochemical events. These lead to anabolism due to increased secretion of insulin and growth hormone during the fed state resulting in synthesis and storage of glycogen from glucose in liver and muscles, of protein from amino acids in many tissues but especially in muscles, and of triglycerides in adipose tissues from fatty acids and glucose. Or they lead to catabolism from increased secretion of the contrainsulin hormones during the fasted state. The latter involves breakdown of glycogen to glucose in liver and muscle, of proteins to amino acids in muscle and other tissues with transport to the liver for conversion to glucose (gluconeogenesis) or ketoacids, and of triglycerides to fatty acids and glycerol in adipose tissue with transport to the liver for conversion to ketoacids and glucose, respectively, or to muscle for use as an energy source.

The lean, normoglycemic adult secretes about 33 units of insulin each day. In the overfed, overweight individual, the plasma glucose rises slightly, the pancreatic beta cell mass increases, and insulin secretion can increase almost fourfold (to 120 units per day) in the very obese nondiabetic adult. The abnormally high insulin level down-regulates the number of insulin receptors on the surface of insulin responsive cells (receptorpenia), and formerly insulin-sensitive tissues become resistant to the glucose-lowering effects of even large amounts of endogenous and exogenous insulin. Eventually, glucose intolerance, which progresses to fasting hyperglycemia and NIDDM, results. All of these metabolic consequences of being overweight can revert to normal with sufficient therapeutically induced weight loss.

There is an increased need for insulin during the growth spurts of pregnancy and puberty and in the presence of excessive amounts of exogenously administered or endogenously produced somatotropin, adrenocorticotropin, cortisol, epinephrine, glucagon, or thyroxine. Thus, pregnancy, puberty, acromegaly, Cushing's syndrome, pheochromocytoma, glucagonoma, or hyperthyroidism may produce sufficient metabolic stress to cause an abnormal glucose tolerance test (GTT) or fasting hyperglycemia.

If the pancreatic beta cell mass is reduced below a critical level by damage or destruction, insulin production will fall (sometimes to less than 3 units per day). Fasting hyperglycemia and persistent catabolism leading to fatal diabetic ketoacidosis or a hyperglycemic hyperosmolar state will ensue unless insulin therapy is initiated. This condition is known as insulinopenic, or IDDM. Cellular insulin receptors are above normal in numbers, and the tissues are sensitive to exogenous insulin.

PRESENTING SYMPTOMS AND SIGNS

Subjective Findings

When initially detected, most individuals are asymptomatic. Subjective findings that may be present include a history of unexplained weight loss, polyuria, polydipsia, polyphagia, weakness, pruritus, dry mouth, leg cramps or pains, burning feet, family history of diabetes, large babies (more than 9 pounds), complications of pregnancy (abortions, toxemia, hydramnios, or stillborns who have congenital defects or large islets on autopsy), reactive hypoglycemia, vascular disease, and impotence.

Table 1. Conditions That May Be Associated with Fasting Hyperglycemia or an Abnormal Glucose Tolerance Test

Pancreatic Beta Cell Disease

Transient diabetes in newborn, congenital absence of islets, viral infection, cystic fibrosis, hemochromatosis, chronic pancreatitis, trauma, neoplasm, bacterial and fungal infections, surgical removal

Hormone Excess

Endogenous

Pheochromocytoma; glucagonoma; somatostatinoma; aldosteronoma; acromegaly; hyperthyroidism; tumors producing excess amounts of glucocorticoids, progestins, or estrogens; hypothalamic lesions

Exogenous

Adrenocorticotropin, glucagon, cortisone, cortisol, prednisone, somatotropin, thyroid hormones, calcitonin, estrogens, medroxyprogesterone (in oral contraceptives), prolactin, epinephrine, norepinephrine

Hormone Deficit

Isolated growth hormone deficiency (type 1, type 2), multitropic pituitary deficiency, Laron dwarfism, hypothalamic lesions, hypoparathyroidism with hypocalcemia

Insulin Receptor Abnormalities

Congenital lipodystrophy with virilization and acanthosis nigricans, immune disorder with insulin-receptor antibody

Drugs and Other Chemical Agents

Diuretics and Antihypertensive Agents

Thiazides, furosemide, metalazone, diazoxide, clonidine, chlorthalidone, bumetamide, clopamide, chlorexolone, ethacrynic acid (hyperglycemia response may be independent of fluctuations in serum K^+)

Psychoactive Agents

Chlorprothixene, haloperidol, lithium carbonate, chlorpromazine, perphenazine, amitriptyline, desipramine, doxepin, imipramine, nortriptyline, marijuana

Neurologically Active Agents

Diphenylhydantoin, isoproterenol, levodopa, buphemine, fenoterol, propanolol

Analgesics

Indomethacin, acetaminophen, aspirin, morphine

Antineoplastic Agents

Alloxan, L-asparaginase, streptozotocin, cyclophosphamide, megestrol acetate

Miscellaneous

Isoniazid, nicotinic acid, carbon disulfide, cimetidine, edetic acid, ethanol, heparin, mannoheptulose, nalidixic acid, nickel chloride, niridazole, pentamidine, phenolphthalein, rodenticide (Vacor), thiabendazole

Genetic Syndromes

Glycogen storage disease type 1, acute intermittent porphyria, hyperlipidemia, hyperglycerolemia, ataxia telangiectasia, myotonic dystrophy, Mendenhall's syndrome, lipoatrophic syndromes, optic atrophy with diabetes mellitus, diabetes insipidus with nerve deafness, muscular dystrophies, late-onset proximal myopathy, Huntington's chorea, Machado's disease, Herrman syndrome, Friedreich's ataxia, Alstrom syndrome, Laurence-Moon-Biedl syndrome, Pseudo-Refsum's syndrome, Prader-Willi syndrome, achondroplasia, steroid-induced ocular hypertension, epiphyseal dysplasia and infantile-onset diabetes, Down's syndrome, Turner's syndrome, Klinefelter's syndrome

Malnutrition

Overnutrition with excess body weight, undernutrition with semistarvation

Pregnancy

See Table 2

Objective Findings

Physical findings that may be present include above-ideal body weight; visual abnormalities (changing visual acuity, cataracts); microangiopathy (retinopathy, glomerulosclerosis); arteriopathy (cerebral, coronary, peripheral); hypertension; neuropathy (peripheral, spinal cord or roots, autonomic with postural hypotension, gastric atony, diarrhea or constipation, fecal incontinence and/or urinary bladder atony, cranial nerve damage); amyotrophic lateral sclerosis; genitourinary abnormalities (Candida vulvovaginitis, Candida balanitis, bacterial bladder or kidney infection, renal failure, nephrotic syndrome); Dupuytren's contracture; xanthomatosis; skin abnormalities (necrobiosis lipoidica diabeticorum, granuloma annulare, alopecia, pyogenic or fungal infections); foot abnormalities (dermatophytosis, onychomycosis,

Table 2. Criteria for Establishing the Diagnosis of Diabetes Mellitus

Nonpregnant Adults and Children	Number of Measurements				
Fasting plasma glucose ⩾140 mg/dl (7.8 mmol/liter)	3	2	1		
Random plasma glucose ⩾200 mg/dl (11.1 mmol/liter)		+ 1	+ 1		
Postprandial plasma glucose ⩾200 mg/dl (11.1 mmol/liter)			+ 1		
GTT sum (fasting +1 +2 +3 hours) ⩾800 mg/dl (>44.6 mmol/liter)	↓	↓	↓	2 ↓	
	Diabetes mellitus	Diabetes mellitus	Diabetes mellitus	Diabetes mellitus	
GTT sum 601 to 800 mg/dl (33.5–44.6 mmol/liter)					1 ↓ High normal

For *pregnant women (gestational diabetes)*: The upper limits of normal for a glucose tolerance test (after 100 gm glucose at time 0) during pregnancy (O'Sullivan criteria) are:

Fasting	1 Hour	2 Hours	3 Hours
105 mg/dl (5.8 mmol/liter)	190 mg/dl (10.6 mmol/liter)	165 mg/dl (9.2 mmol/liter)	145 mg/dl (8.1 mmol/liter)

Two or more levels above the upper limits = diabetes mellitus; one level above the upper limits = borderline.

Abbreviation: GTT = Glucose tolerance test.

Table 3. Sequential Testing Routine to Detect (Nonpregnant) Individual with Unknown Diabetes

1. Screen yearly (using polarographic glucose analyzer) by quantitative RUG*
   a. If 3 to 25 mg/dl (~97%), STOP. Diabetes has been ruled out.
   b. If > 25 mg/dl, go to 2. immediately.
2. Random venous plasma glucose
   a. If > 200 mg/dl and symptomatic, initiate therapy.
   b. If > 140 mg/dl and asymptomatic, go to 3.
3. Fasting venous plasma glucose
   a. If > 140 mg/dl × 2, initiate therapy.
   b. If < 140 mg/dl, go to 4.
4. GTT (Nonmedicated, diet-prepped, ambulatory)
   a. Sum > 800 mg/dl = diabetes mellitus.
   b. Sum 601 to 800 mg/dl = high normal (nondiabetic) GTT.
   c. Sum ⩽ 600 mg/dl = nondiabetic
   d. If RUG > 25 mg/dl and 1 hour GTT urine glucose > 80 mg/dl, = renal glucosuria.

*One hundred per cent sensitivity and 99.3 per cent specificity in detecting individuals who have a GTT sum (fasting plus 1-, 2-, and 3-hour post-100 gm glucose load) greater than 800 mg/dl. In those with RUG greater than 25 mg/dl, 75 per cent have diabetes mellitus (GTT sum > 800 mg/dl), and 25 per cent have renal glucosuria (RUG > 25 mg/dl, 2 hour GTT urine glucose > 80 mg/dl) on follow-up testing.

Abbreviations: RUG = Random urine glucose; GTT = glucose tolerance test.

trophic ulcers, arterial insufficiency, gangrene); periodontal disease; and many infections, including tuberculosis and mucormycosis.

Laboratory findings that may be present and that may lead to the diagnosis of diabetes mellitus include: random urine glucose (RUG) >25 mg/dl, random fasting venous plasma glucose >140 mg/dl, 2 hours after 100 grams of carbohydrate venous plasma glucose >175 mg/dl, hyperlipidemia, hyperlipoproteinemia, azotemia, hyperuricemia, and albuminuria.

DETECTING UNDIAGNOSED DIABETES MELLITUS AND CONFIRMING THE DIAGNOSIS

The preferred sequential testing technique for detecting the undiagnosed nonpregnant individual with diabetes mellitus is noted in Table 3. About 75 per cent of those being screened for diabetes who have a RUG >25 mg/dl have diabetes mellitus on follow-up testing; the other 25 per cent have a "high normal" GTT or renal glucosuria. Essentially, none of those with a normal RUG (3 to 25 mg/dl) will have a GTT sum >800 mg/dl (diabetes mellitus) on follow-up testing. For detecting the undiagnosed nonpregnant individual with diabetes mellitus, a RUG >25 mg/dl has 100 per cent sensitivity, 99.3 per cent specificity, and 75 per cent predictive value.

If the patient gives a history of symptoms that suggest reactive hypoglycemia between 2 and 5 hours after meals (which may occur in early diabetes), the GTT should be extended from 3 hours to 6 hours. The time of all symptoms and signs occurring during the test should be recorded by the patient so that the physician can determine whether or not these correlate with plasma glucose levels. Symptomatic reactive hypoglycemia in the adult almost never occurs at a plasma glucose nadir higher than 50 mg/dl and may not occur with plasma glucose levels as low as 30 mg/dl. If characteristic symptoms of hypoglycemia occur between routine sampling times, an additional plasma glucose measurement should be done at the time of symptoms.

COURSE AND COMPLICATIONS

Diabetes begins as an asymptomatic disease with abnormal glucose tolerance that progresses to sustained fasting hyperglycemia with persistent glucosuria, and eventually to characteristic subjective and objective findings. If undiagnosed, this sequence of events in IDDM (and occasionally in NIDDM) will terminate in diabetic ketoacidosis or a hyperglycemic hyperosmolar state and death.

In NIDDM, diet and exercise therapy with reduction to ideal body weight can attain and sustain normoglycemia. In IDDM, therapy with diet, exercise, and insulin can attain and sustain near-normoglycemia in many individuals who routinely monitor their blood glucose levels at home and make indicated adjustments in their insulin, diet, and exercise patterns on a daily basis. There is evidence that these therapeutic interventions will prevent the acute complications, and may prevent, delay the appearance of, or even reverse the vascular problems specific to the diabetic state (microangiopathy).

Atherosclerosis (macroangiopathy or arteriopathy) occurs with greater frequency in diabetics than in nondiabetics. It is related more to the age of the individual and is limited to well-defined risk factors (hypertension, obesity, hyperlipidemia, smoking). There is little evidence that atherosclerosis is arrestable, but control of hypertension, obesity, hyperlipidemia, and discontinuation of smoking appear to be worthwhile efforts in delaying progression of vascular damage.

The nature of the two acute complications (diabetic ketoacidosis and hyperglycemic hyperosmolar state) and the four chronic complications of diabetes (retinopathy, nephropathy, arteriopathy, and neuropathy) are described next.

Acute Complications

Diabetic ketoacidosis may be *mild* (CO_2 content >20 mEq/liter); *moderate* (CO_2 content 11 to 20 mEq/liter); or *severe* (CO_2 content ≤10) mEq/liter). *A hyperglycemic hyperosmolar state* is present if the serum osmolality is greater than 350 mOsm/kg. It may occur in the presence or absence of diabetic ketoacidosis. Patients may be hypotensive, markedly dehydrated, and in shock. Adults may have lost as much as 12 liters of water, 800 mEq sodium, and 800 mEq of potassium. The death rate from appropriately treated, uncomplicated severe diabetic ketoacidosis is about 1 per cent; from complicated (major vascular occlusions, severe infections), severe diabetic ketoacidosis it is about 10 per cent; and from the hyperglycemic hyperosmolar state it is about 25 to 50 per cent. These problems are genuine medical emergencies. Although treatment is not discussed here, the diagnostic routine should be completed within a few minutes, and therapy with insulin, water and electrolytes started immediately.

Chronic Complications

Retinopathy

Prevalence is routinely correlated with duration of diabetes: 7 per cent in those having the disease less than 10 years, 26 per cent in diabetics of 10 to 14 years' duration, and 63 per cent in those who have been diabetic more than 15 years. Of the diabetic population, 25 per cent have some form of retinopathy, and 5 per cent have the most severe form (proliferative retinopathy). Retinopathy is now the leading cause of blindness in the 20- to 64-year-old age group in the United States.

Preproliferative diabetic retinopathy ("nonproliferative" or "background") is characterized by abnormal retinal vascular permeability (may be demonstrated by fluorescein angiography), and intraretinal hypoxia or ischemia (which leads to retinal and macular edema, the most common cause of decreased vision in preproliferative retinopathy). Ophthalmoscopic examination may reveal microaneurysms, blot intraretinal hemorrhages, cotton-wool spots, and/or hard exudates. If vision decreases significantly, the ophthalmologist should examine the macula with a biomicroscope and a contact or Hruby lens.

Proliferative diabetic retinopathy is the growth of newly formed fibrovascular tissue in response to underlying retinal ischemia. It may also develop secondary to sickle cell anemia, retinal vein obstruction, or retrolental fibroplasia. Small capillary networks grow into the vitreous in response to the angiogenesis factor secreted by the ischemic retina, which can diffuse as far anteriorly as the iris and cause proliferation of new capillaries (rubeosis iridis). The preretinal membrane is incomplete near the optic disc, and proliferation of new vessels is prone to occur there, although new vessel formation may occur over any portion of the hypoxic retina. These vessels are very fragile and are prone to break and bleed into the preretinal space or the vitreous, with a resulting marked loss of vision or legal blindness (visual acuity <5/100). Growth of fibrous tissue into the vitreous and its subsequent contraction leads to traction detachment of the retina.

Macular edema and proliferative retinopathy can be successfully treated with argon laser photocoagulation. The National Eye Institute's Diabetic Retinopathy Study reported that the rate of severe visual loss (to <5/200) in proliferative and severe preproliferative diabetic retinopathy was reduced by 61 per cent following argon laser photocoagulation.

Vitrectomy (surgical removal of the vitreous and replacement by a clear solution) has relieved blindness in about half the treated cases. It is indicated for severe vitreous hemorrhage that has not cleared spontaneously and for traction retinal detachment which threatens macular vision.

Nephropathy

In early diabetes, the glomerular filtration rate is increased and the kidneys are enlarged. Both can be reduced by optimal control of the plasma glucose level. After a number of years of hyperglycemia, autopsy or biopsy criteria that confirm the presence of nephropathy include the following:

1. The glomerular basement membrane becomes thickened, the mesangial matrix increases diffusely, and nodular lesions within the glomerulus may develop.
2. A "fibrin cap" (amorphous eosinophilic crescent-shaped material at the periphery of the glomerular lobule) and/or a "capsular-drop" (small rounded eosinophilic mass on the inside of Bowman's capsule) may be present.
3. Atherosclerosis and hyalinization of the arterioles with fibrosis of the interstitial tissue are present, often with inflammatory cells.

It is usually possible to diagnose diabetic nephropathy, without biopsy, with the following data base:

1. Clinical diabetes or abnormal GTT.
2. 24-hour urine protein concentration >3 gm/day.
3. Presence of diabetic retinopathy (with a possible need for fluorescein angiography).

Five other renal problems should be considered in a proteinuric or azotemic diabetic:

1. Urinary tract infection (atonic bladder, bladder neck obstruction from hyperplastic prostate, stones).
2. Hypertension (present in up to 50 per cent of those with diabetes).
3. Renal papillary necrosis (hematuria, flank pain, urinary tract infection).
4. Renal infarction (hematuria, flank pain).
5. Poststreptococcal glomerulonephritis (which usually follows a chronic streptococcal infection of the skin of a leg or finger).

Progressive renal failure may go through several stages, and it is essential to adjust medical management to the patient's changing needs:

1. Hypertension demands vigorous treatment.
2. Insulin therapy must be adjusted (usually downward and in terminal renal failure perhaps to no insulin) based on *plasma glucose measurements,* since there may be no glucosuria at high plasma glucose levels.
3. In the nephrotic syndrome it is common practice to give more dietary protein to compensate for urinary loss (which may reach 20 gm/day), to limit sodium intake, and to use diuretic therapy (furosemide) as appropriate.
4. In progressive azotemia (blood urea nitrogen >100 mg/dl, creatinine >5 mg/dl) it is necessary to restrict protein intake to 0.2 to 0.3 gm/pound ideal body weight per day plus the number of grams lost in the urine. If sodium or potassium or water cannot be excreted satisfactorily, intake must be restricted as indicated, and many drugs should be given in greatly reduced doses because of decreased renal excretion.

In end-stage diabetic glomerulosclerosis, hemodialysis or peritoneal dialysis work well for most patients for 2 to 3 years. During dialysis, dietary protein intake is increased to 0.5 to 0.9 gm/pound ideal body weight per day to replace amino acids lost in the dialysate. It is estimated that by the mid-1980s diabetics will make up more than half of those being treated by dialysis. Kidney transplantation offers the best chance for prolonged survival and a return to a comfortable productive life. Present 3-year survival in related-donor graft recipients in the best medical centers is 75 per cent. In some patients, function of the transplanted kidney has remained excellent for 10 years, though these kidneys are developing the classic pathologic findings associated with diabetic nephropathy.

Arteriopathy

Coronary Atherosclerosis. This condition accounts for about 70 per cent of the deaths in those who have diabetes, due to arrhythmia or asystole with sudden death, or myocardial infarction. It is estimated that at least 15 per cent of the initial myocardial infarctions in those with diabetes are painless because of autonomic neuropathy with decreased visceral pain sensation, and that two to three times as many of the initial infarcts in those with diabetes terminate fatally compared with those who do not have diabetes. Otherwise the clinical presentation of myocardial infarction and angina pectoris in the diabetic is similar to that in the nondiabetic. About 17 per cent of diabetic patients with congestive heart failure but without previous symptoms have "clean coronaries" on angiography. This has been termed "diabetic cardiomyopathy" and has been attributed to microangiopathy in the myocardium. At the Mayo Clinic, 5-year survival of diabetic patients after the initial myocardial infarction was 85 per cent; 3-year survival after onset of congestive heart failure without antecedent clinical heart disease was 44 per cent.

Cerebral Thrombosis. Cerebral thrombosis is about two times as prevalent in the diabetic as in the nondiabetic population. Its clinical presentation and treatment do not differ in the two groups.

Peripheral Vascular Disease. The macrovascular lesions in the lower limbs of diabetics are more diffuse and extensive and involve distal blood vessels (tibial and peroneal) more frequently than in nondiabetics. It is estimated that peripheral vascular disease is 40 times as prevalent in the diabetic as in the nondiabetic population, and that about 25 per cent of those with diabetic peripheral vascular disease also have peripheral neuropathy.

The first subjective finding may be intermittent claudication, or pain in the calf, thigh, or buttock after walking that is relieved by rest; this may progress to pain even at rest. Objective findings may include absent pulses, tight shiny skin, hair loss, hypertrophy of toenails, delayed venous filling and delayed capillary flush when the leg returns to the dependent position after several minutes elevation, localized pallor and/or cyanosis, callus formation, muscle atrophy, ulceration, gangrene, diminished sensation, and absent reflexes.

The average blood flow to the lower extremity in the normal individual during rest is 300 to 600 ml/minute. This increases fivefold to tenfold during exercise and following release of an inflated cuff on the thigh (reactive hyperemia). Blood flow is lower in patients with diabetes, and the response to exercise and occlusion greatly reduced.

Noninvasive tests are available to evaluate the circulation in the lower extremities: Doppler ultrasonography, and plethysmography (the photo pulse type being the most sensitive). The ratio of systolic ankle to brachial pressure is expressed as the ischemic index (normal = 1.0–1.1). Segmental pressures may be measured by Doppler ultrasonography; even mild vascular occlusion can be detected by a pressure drop across the diseased segment. In the mildest form of disease, the pressure drop may be evident only following reactive hyperemia or exercise. Pulsatile flow produces volume changes that can be detected by plethysmography measurements over toes, feet, calf, or thigh. Pulse return time following compressive occlusion of the calf by an inflated cuff is characteristically prolonged in the presence of atherosclerotic occlusion. Arteriography has significant morbidity (0.3 to 14 per cent) and mortality (0.05 per cent) and it should be avoided if the patient has diminished renal function, since acute tubular necrosis and anuria may develop. It is reserved for patients who are candidates for surgical bypass or balloon catheter angioplasty of an occluded segment or narrowed collateral in an attempt to relieve severe claudication or to permit healing of an ischemic, necrotic lesion.

When gangrene develops and the ankle ischemic index is less than 0.5 ($\leq$55 mm Hg systolic pressure), healing distal to the ankle usually does not occur.

When segmental pressures are known and angiographic studies are available, the site of amputation can be selected so that satisfactory wound healing takes place.

Neuropathy

Prevalence of neuropathy varies in different populations depending on sensitivity of the tests used to detect it. It is clinically evident with symptoms (e.g., pain, paresthesias) in about 30 per cent of individuals with diabetes $\geq$10 years' duration. Any nerve or combination of nerves may be affected: cranial, somatosensory, mononeuropathy, amyotrophy, or autonomic (atonic bladder, gastroparesis, diarrhea or constipation, postural hypotension, gustatory sweating, and abnormal pulse rate responses to the erect stance and Valsalva maneuver). Motor and sensory nerve conduction velocity is reduced, cerebrospinal fluid protein is increased, and there is evidence of denervation and fasciculation on electromyography. Pathologically the nerves show segmental demyelinization, axonal degeneration, and basal lamina thickening. There is evidence of accumulation of sorbitol, fructose, and glucose in the osmotically disrupted axon, a defect of myelin synthesis, myoinositol deficiency, and accelerated Schwann cell death.

The differential diagnosis should consider degenerative disc disease, cord tumor, alcoholic neuropathy, uremic neuropathy, heavy metal(s) toxicity, pernicious anemia, hypothyroidism, Paget's disease of the spine, and syphilis.

The neuropathic foot should be kept clean, lubricated, and free of fungal infections; tight shoes, trauma, excessive heat, and cold should be avoided. Neuropathic ulcers should be healed by conservative measures including bed rest, protective plastazote or special shoes, local debridement, and systemic antibiotic therapy for infection (including localized osteomyelitis). If circulation is adequate, amputation can almost always be avoided.

A THERAPEUTIC TEST TO IDENTIFY NIDDM AND IDDM WHEN THE DIAGNOSIS IS IN DOUBT

Insulin therapy is indicated in certain individuals:

1. Those who are at or below ideal body weight and who have a fasting plasma glucose consistently above 140 mg/dl.
2. Those who are pregnant and meet the criteria given in Table 2 (to protect the fetus).
3. Those who are in ketoacidosis and/or a hyperglycemic hyperosmolar state regardless of body weight.

The vast majority of those who are above ideal body weight and have no history of ketoacidosis have NIDDM, whereas the vast majority of those who are at or below ideal body weight and/or have a history of ketoacidosis have IDDM. Since many individuals with NIDDM are being treated inappropriately with insulin, a therapeutic test to identify these individuals has been developed. It is carried out as follows:

1. Nonpregnant individuals who are significantly overweight, who have no history of ketoacidosis, and who are not on insulin therapy may be fasted and monitored every 2 days as outpatients.
2. Those on inappropriate insulin therapy are hospitalized, and plasma glucose and the serum CO_2 content are monitored daily for 10 to 12 days.
3. Insulin therapy is discontinued abruptly, and the patient is fasted totally for 7 days if there are no contraindications (pregnancy, diabetic ketoacidosis or hyperglycemic hyperosmolar state, myocardial infarction within last 6 weeks, unstable angina, transient ischemic attacks, incipient gangrene, renal failure, gout, suicidal tendency).
4. The plasma glucose returns to normal or near-normal and the CO_2 content does not fall below 15 mEq/liter in those who have NIDDM; the plasma glucose does not return to normal and the CO_2 content falls below 15 mEq/liter in those who have IDDM.
5. Insulin therapy should be restarted immediately in those who have IDDM. In those who have NIDDM, weight loss should continue until ideal body weight is attained on a 500- to 1000-calorie diet containing only skim milk, vegetables, and fruits, plus supplementary vitamins and minerals if the diet continues for more than 4 weeks.

Available data suggest that 1 to 2 per cent of those with NIDDM progress to acquiring IDDM each year. Many with NIDDM who attain ideal body weight revert to showing a normal GTT, which in some individuals has been noted to last for more than 10 years of follow-up.

POTENTIAL ERRORS AND PITFALLS

The most frequent causes of making an erroneous diagnosis of diabetes mellitus are the following:

1. Failure to prepare the patient with an adequate intake of carbohydrate (300 gm/day for 3 days) prior to the test.

2. Failure to recognize that many chronic diseases and acute illnesses may be associated with an abnormal GTT.

3. Failure to discontinue hormones and other medications (which may elevate the plasma glucose level) for at least 3 days prior to the GTT.

4. Improper laboratory testing.

5. Use of GTT criteria that are too sensitive and nonspecific and that result in many false-positive diagnoses, thus erroneously increasing the perceived prevalence of diabetes mellitus in a given population.

Studies of an unselected population being screened for diabetes mellitus which compared the prevalence of diagnosed diabetes using different GTT criteria (Table 4) have shown that British Diabetic Association GTT criteria diagnose diabetes 7.7 times as frequently as fasting plasma glucose criteria >140 mg/dl, and 7.2 times as frequently as GTT sum criteria >800 mg/dl. Fajans-Conn criteria (using GTT 1-hour level of 195 mg/dl as the upper normal limit) diagnose diabetes 6.3 times as frequently as fasting plasma glucose criteria >140 mg/dl, and 6.0 times as often as GTT sum criteria >800 mg/dl. A 4-year follow-up of the GTT sum "high normal" group (601 to 800 mg/dl) revealed that 67 per cent had reverted to a GTT sum <600 mg/dl, 29 per cent were still high normal (sum 601 to 800 mg/dl), 4 per cent had a GTT sum >800 mg/dl, and none had a fasting plasma glucose >140 mg/dl. This study confirms the impressions of a number of other investigators that GTT criteria that are too sensitive and that are nonspecific erroneously diagnose diabetes mellitus (false-positive diagnoses) in many individuals who do not have it.

Since an erroneous diagnosis of diabetes can lead to psychological problems, inappropriate drug and/or diet therapy, and unemployability and uninsurability, great care should be taken to avoid error.

Table 4. Criteria for Interpretation of Oral Glucose Tolerance Tests in Nonpregnant Individuals

Source	Prevalence of Diabetes*
British Diabetic Association[1]	
Diabetes mellitus if:	
30, 60, or 90 min. above 120 mg/dl plus 120 min. above 140 mg/dl	12.3%
Fajans-Conn[2]	
Diabetes mellitus if:	
60 min. above 185 (195) mg/dl	
Plus 90 min. above 165 mg/dl (1 hr > 185)	12.3%
Plus 120 min. above 140 mg/dl (1 hr > 195)	10.1%
Borderline if:	
One or two of the above	
Nondiabetic if:	
None of the above	
USPHS Wilkerson Point System[3]	
Fasting above 130 mg/dl = 1 point	
60 min. above 195 mg/dl = ½ point	
120 min. above 140 mg/dl = ½ point	
180 min. above 130 mg/dl = 1 point	
Diabetes mellitus with 2–3 points	6.0%
Equivocal with ½–1½ points	
Nondiabetic with 0 points	
National Institutes of Health Diabetes Data Group[4]	
Diabetes mellitus if:	
Fasting above 140 mg/dl (three occasions)	1.5%
or 120 min. above 200 mg/dl plus at least one of 30, 60, or 90 min. above 200 mg/dl	5.8%
Impaired glucose tolerance if:	
One of 30, 60, or 90 min. above 200 mg/dl and 120 min. between 140–199 mg/dl	5.4%
Andres[5]	
Diabetes mellitus if 120 min. sample is:	
Age 20 above 180 mg/dl	
30 — 190	
40 — 200	
50 — 210	
60 — 220	
70 — 230	
80 — 240	3.4%

Table continued on following page

Table 4. Criteria for Interpretation of Oral Glucose Tolerance Tests in Nonpregnant Individuals (Continued)

Source		Prevalence of Diabetes*
European Diabetes Epidemiology Study Group[6]		
Diabetes mellitus if:		
One of the following		
30 min. above 285 mg/dl		
60 min. above 255 mg/dl		
90 min. above 255 mg/dl		
And 120 min. above 200 mg/dl		2.5%
Nondiabetic if:		
30, 60 and 90 min. less than 185 mg/dl and 120 min. less than 140 mg/dl.		
Borderline:		
Between the above values		
Siperstein[7]		
Diabetes mellitus if:		
60 min. above 260 mg/dl and 120 min. above 220 mg/dl		1.6%
Sum of Values[8]		
Sum fasting, ½-, 1-, and 2-hour glucose values		
Diabetes mellitus if:		
Sum is greater than 800 mg/dl		1.6%
Equivocal if:		
Sum is 501–800 mg/dl		
Nondiabetic if:		
Sum is less than 500 mg/dl		
Sum (Emory University)[9]		
Values for plasma glucose in GTT (Mean + 3 standard deviations)		
Fasting 130 mg/dl		
60 min. 265 mg/dl		
120 min. 230 mg/dl		
180 min. 185 mg/dl		
Sum fasting, 1 hr., 2 hr. and 3 hr. values		
Diabetes mellitus if:		
Sum is greater than 800 mg/dl	*Sum > 800	1.6%
High Normal if:	Sum > 750	2.3%
Sum is 601–800 mg/dl	Sum > 700	3.2%
Nondiabetic if:	Sum > 650	6.6%
Sum is less than 600 mg/dl	Sum > 600	10.2%

*Per cent prevalence of diabetes by the different diagnostic criteria was determined on 450 individuals aged 15–80 years who were not known to have diabetes and who had a normal random urine glucose (3–25 mg/dl). In the Emory University study, the prevalence of diagnosed diabetes mellitus increased more than sixfold as the cutpoint was lowered from > 800 mg/dl (1.6%) to > 600 mg/dl (10.2%).

1. Fitzgerald, M.G., and Keen, H.: Br. Med. J., 1:1568, 1964.
2. Fajans, J.J., and Conn, J.W.: Ann. N.Y. Acad. Sci., 82:208, 1959.
3. Wilkerson, H.L.C., Hyman, H., Kaufman, M., et al.: N. Engl. J. Med., 262:1047, 1960.
4. National Diabetes Data Group: Diabetes, 28:1039, 1979.
5. Andres, R.: Med. Clin. North Am., 55:835, 1971.
6. European Diabetes Epidemiology Study Group (EDESG): Diabetologia, 6:453, 1970.
7. Siperstein, M.D.: The glucose tolerance test. In Stollerman, G.H. (ed.): *Advances in Internal Medicine.* Chicago, Year Book Medical Publishers, Inc., 1975, p. 297.
8. Danowski, T.S., Aarons, J.H., Hydovita, J.D., and Wingert, J.P.: Diabetes, 19:524, 1970.
9. Davidson, J.K.: Fed. Proc., 40:741 (abstr. 2917), 1981.

HYPOGLYCEMIA

By John K. Davidson, M.D., Ph.D.
Atlanta, Georgia

The mean plasma glucose level in normal humans fasted overnight is 92 mg/dl (range 78 to 115 mg/dl). In such individuals, the glucose level fluctuates over a remarkably narrow range, rising modestly after feeding and falling modestly during fasting. When glucose production (primarily from glucose absorbed from the gastrointestinal tract after feeding and from liver gluconeogenesis during fasting) lags behind glucose utilization (primarily to provide substrate for energy production during exercise, or to be stored as glycogen when insulin levels are inappropriately elevated) for a significant period of time, hypoglycemia results.

The lowest level of plasma glucose that can be regarded as normal varies from person to person. Some patients are symptomatic when the plasma glucose falls as low as 50 mg/dl, whereas some are asymptomatic when the plasma glucose falls as low as 30 mg/dl. Thus, the level from 3 to 5 hours after a glucose load may fall as low as 35 mg/dl in some asymptomatic individuals, and during fasting the level may fall as low as 30 mg/dl in some asymptomatic females.

Because prolonged or repeated hypoglycemic episodes can result in permanent brain damage and death, it is prudent, as a general rule, to regard all patients with measured plasma glucose levels <50 mg/dl as having hypoglycemia until proven otherwise. Individuals who have a plasma glucose level of 30 to 50 mg/dl and who are asymptomatic when initially seen should be classified as hypoglycemia suspects. They should be carefully studied to determine whether symptomatic fasting hypoglycemia or symptomatic reactive hypoglycemia develops after a glucose load.

RECOGNITION

Symptoms and signs similar to those of hypoglycemia frequently occur in emotionally disturbed patients (e.g., anxiety, depression, psychosis, hyperventilation syndrome). Thus, a diagnosis of symptomatic hypoglycemia cannot be confirmed unless the timing of symptoms and signs coincides with the lowest plasma glucose levels. One should avoid an erroneous diagnosis of hypoglycemia because of improper blood specimen collection, preservation, or analysis ("desk-top hypoglycemia"). Many patients with diabetes, especially those with neuropathy, have severe hypoglycemic episodes which neither they nor their peers recognize, and many patients with insulin-producing tumors have been confined to mental institutions because hypoglycemia was not suspected.

More than 95 per cent of hypoglycemia episodes seen in most emergency departments occur in patients known to have diabetes mellitus that is being treated with insulin or sulfonylurea. About two thirds of those affected have not eaten appropriately. Hypoglycemia of brief duration may cause cerebral malfunction that can result in accidental injury or jail confinement, and more prolonged hypoglycemia (usually 4 or more hours) may result in irreversible brain damage with paralysis and/or imbecility, or death. In a 2-year audit (1973–1975) of 240 cases of hypoglycemia observed in the Grady Memorial Hospital Emergency Clinic, Atlanta (see Table 5), eight (3.3 per cent) terminated fatally. Thus, all cases of hypoglycemia should be regarded as true medical emergencies that require prompt confirmation by a stat plasma glucose measurement and immediate treatment with oral or intravenous glucose. The plasma glucose level can be measured accurately within 1 minute using the glucose oxidase procedure in a polarographic glucose analyzer. If such an analyzer is not readily available, the blood glucose level may be estimated within 2 minutes using visually read color development on a Chemstrip bG or a Visadex Strip, or meter-read on a digital meter: Accucheck (Chemstrip bG); Dextrometer (Dextrostix); or Glucoscan II (Glucoscan Test Strips).

PATHOGENESIS

An understanding of the pathogenesis of symptomatic hypoglycemia (Table 1) facilitates data base collection and therapy. Over 95 per cent of cases of hypoglycemia seen in a busy emergency department are exogenous in origin. Causes of exogenous hypoglycemia in patients being treated for diabetes mellitus are listed in Table 2, and some drugs that can lower the plasma glucose and precipitate hypoglycemia in patients being treated for diabetes mellitus are listed in Table 3. Alcohol-induced hypoglycemia should be considered in the differential diagnosis. Reactive hypoglycemia of early diabetes,

Table 1. Symptomatic Hypoglycemia: Pathogenesis and Findings

1. Adrenal medulla overactivity with hyperepinephrinemia
   Subjective: Anxiety, palpitation, occasionally angina pectoris
   Objective: Perspiration, pallor, hypothermia, tachycardia, hypertension, cardiac arrhythmias, dilated pupils
2. Neurologic dysfunction
   Initially, the higher cortical centers malfunction because the glucose supply is insufficient to maintain normal metabolic activity. Oxygen utilization decreases. Later, centers in the midbrain and medulla are similarly affected. In fatal reactions there is cerebral edema, multiple petechial hemorrhages, and widespread necrosis of cortical ganglion cells. Prolongation of hypoglycemia (usually 4 or more hours), not depth to which the plasma glucose falls, is responsible for irreparable brain damage.
   Subjective: Headache, blurring of vision, transient diplopia, paresthesias, hunger, nausea, fatigue, drowsiness, irritability, vertigo
   Objective: Mental confusion, bizarre behavior, speech difficulties, irrational agitation, combativeness, delirium, vomiting, lethargy, somnolence, aphasia, tremor, ataxia, nystagmus, paralysis, seizures, coma, Babinski reflexes, shallow respiration, bradycardia

Table 2. Causes of Hypoglycemia in Patients Being Treated for Diabetes Mellitus

1. Inadequate carbohydrate intake
2. Vigorous exercise
3. Insulin therapy
   a. Excess insulin dose
      (1) Erroneously prescribed
      (2) Failure to match insulin potency with correct syringe (i.e., each should be 100 units/ml)
      (3) Visual failure with inability to measure correct dose
   b. Failure to reduce insulin dose when need for insulin decreases
      (1) During reduction of body weight
      (2) Endocrine deficiency
         (a) Hypopituitarism
         (b) Adrenal cortical insufficiency
      (3) Reduction in dose of corticosteroid
      (4) Decreased rate of insulin degradation due to kidney failure or liver failure
      (5) After recovery from stressful situations
         (a) Infection
         (b) Pancreatitis
         (c) Acutely decompensated diabetes
         (d) Surgery
      (6) At termination of pregnancy
4. Sulfonylurea therapy (tolbutamide, tolazamide, chlorpropamide, acetohexamide, glyburide, glipizide)
   a. Excess dose
   b. Diminished degradation or excretion, as in kidney failure
   c. Potentiation by other drugs (see Table 3) that displace sulfonylureas from albumin-combining sites
   d. Attempted suicide or homicide
5. Ethanol, drugs, and toxins that lower plasma glucose level

due to delayed hyperinsulinemia following a meal or glucose load, and hypoglycemia in infants of diabetic mothers, due to beta cell hyperplasia and transient hyperinsulinemia following birth, are seen occasionally. Other causes of endogenous reactive and endogenous fasting hypoglycemia are rarely seen.

Table 4 indicates the subjective and objective information that should be obtained as well as the considerations necessary to determine whether the hypoglycemia is exogenous, endogenous reactive, or endogenous fasting.

Table 5 shows the results of an earlier audit we carried out on 240 known diabetic patients with hypoglycemia. In two thirds the cause of hypoglycemia was inadequate food intake.

The following outlines our approach to assessment and management of patients with hypoglycemia.

1. Initial (in Emergency Department): Initiate immediately after drawing stat venous plasma glucose:

a. If the patient is able to swallow, give oral glucose, candy, a cola beverage, orange juice, or food.

b. If the patient is unable to swallow give intravenous (IV) glucose (25 gm), or glucagon (1 mg) subcutaneously or intramuscularly.

c. Observe until there is complete recovery, repeat plasma glucose, and give additional food.

d. If there is *prompt* recovery, reinstruct on and/or revise as indicated: diet, insulin, and/or exercise. Omit ethanol, drugs, and toxins.

e. If there is *delayed* recovery, neurologic damage, or uncertain etiology of hypoglycemia, hospitalize.

2. Evaluation in hospital:

a. Abnormalities to be sought:

If there is endogenous reactive hypoglycemia, perform an oral 6-hour glucose tolerance test (GTT) after giving 300 gm carbohydrate per day diet for 3 days prior to the test. The oral GTT is abnormal in early diabetes and may be abnormal after gastrointestinal surgery (IV GTT normal). Possibly do a fructose tolerance test to confirm hereditary fructose intolerance.

If there is endogenous fasting hypoglycemia, prescribe up to a 72-hour fast with plasma glucose measurement every 6 hours and terminate if hypoglycemia occurs. Hyperinsulinemia is confirmed if immunoreactive insulin is >6 μU/ml serum, and plasma glucose <40 mg/dl. That the hyperinsulinemia is endogenous, as occurs with an insulinoma or other endogenous hyperinsulinemic states, may be confirmed by finding elevated C-peptide levels in serum and/or urine plus elevated plasma insulin levels. Also, in the C-peptide suppression test, C-peptide levels do not fall appropriately with IV insulin infusion (0.1 U/kg body weight). A decrease in C-peptide level is a result of the feedback control of a low plasma glucose level on insulin and C-peptide secretion in normals, but this effect is absent or decreased in those with insulinomas.

Exogenous insulin administration, with suicidal or homicidal intent, results in a high insulin level (sometimes antibodies to beef and/or pork insulin are present) and a low C-peptide level. Perform selective angiography to localize 80 per cent of insulinomas prior to surgical removal.

When indicated, collect data to evaluate the rarely occurring problems listed under Assessment, (b) Endogenous reactive? and (c) Endogenous fasting? in Table 4. These data may include various biochemical,

Table 3. Some Drugs That Lower the Plasma Glucose Level in Patients Being Treated for Diabetes Mellitus

1. Potentiation of sulfonylureas
   a. Barbiturates
   b. Bishydroxycoumarin
   c. Chloramphenicol
   d. Monamine oxidase inhibitors
   e. Phenylbutazone
   f. Salicylates
   g. Sulfonamides
   h. Thiazides
2. Increased insulin production
   a. Alpha adrenergic blockers
   b. Beta adrenergic stimulators
   c. Monamine oxidase inhibitors
3. Decreased hepatic glycogenolysis
   a. Propranolol
4. Mechanism unknown
   a. Antihistamines
      (1) Antazoline phosphate
      (2) Tripelennamine hydrochloride
   b. Morphine
   c. Probenecid
   d. Propylthiouracil
   e. Tuberculostatic drugs
      (1) Isoniazid
      (2) Aminosalicylic acid

Table 4. Disease Process Standard for Recognition and Assessment of Hypoglycemia
Problem Statement: Hypoglycemia (Subsets: Exogenous, Endogenous Reactive, Endogenous Fasting)

Recognition (Defined Data Base)

Subjective

1. Neurologic dysfunction: headache, blurring of vision, transient diplopia, paresthesias, hunger, nausea, fatigue, drowsiness, irritability, vertigo
2. Hyperepinephrinemia: anxiety, palpitation, occasionally angina pectoris
3. Known diabetes mellitus
4. Insulin therapy: type, dose, time
5. Sulfonylurea therapy: type, dose
6. Diet prescription: calories, grams of protein, carbohydrate, and fat, division
7. Missed food: time
8. Vigorous exercise: time
9. Level of control of diabetes
10. Previous hypoglycemia
11. Weight loss
12. Duration of symptoms (minutes)
13. Drugs: salicylates, steroids, other
14. Ethanol
15. Toxins
16. Gastrectomy

Objective

1. Neurologic dysfunction: mental confusion, bizarre behavior, speech difficulties, irrational agitation, combativeness, delirium, vomiting, lethargy, somnolence, aphasia, tremor, ataxia, nystagmus, paralysis, seizures, coma, Babinski reflexes, shallow respiration, bradycardia
2. Hyperepinephrinemia: perspiration, pallor, hypothermia, tachycardia, hypertension, cardiac arrhythmias, dilated pupils
3. Venous plasma glucose < 50 mg/dl (absolute requirement)

Assessment

Exogenous Hypoglycemia?

1. Insulin
2. Sulfonylurea
3. Insulin or sulfonylurea plus missed meal and/or strenuous exercise
4. Ethanol
5. Drugs (see Table 3)
6. Toxins (such as hypoglycin in Jamaican vomiting sickness)

Endogenous Reactive Hypoglycemia?

1. Early diabetes mellitus (3- to 6-hour post-glucose load during glucose tolerance test)?
2. Dumping syndrome (postgastrectomy)?
3. Physiologic post-meal or post-glucose load (rule out anxiety, depression, psychosis)
4. Hereditary fructose intolerance (post-fructose load)
5. Galactosemia (after infant ingests lactose or galactose)

Endogenous Fasting Hypoglycemia?

1. Malnutrition
2. Hyperinsulinemia (benign adenoma—single or multiple, microadenomatosis, carcinoma, nesidioblastosis)
3. Nonpancreatic tumors (mesenchymal retroperitoneal or mediastinal, hepatoma, adrenocortical carcinoma, lymphoma, gastrointestinal, other)
4. Severe liver disease (e.g., cirrhosis, congestive heart failure, viral destruction)
5. Severe kidney disease (renal failure)
6. Endocrine abnormalities (hypopituitarism, adrenal cortical insufficiency, congenital adrenal hyperplasia, epinephrine deficiency, hypothyroidism, cretinism)
7. Hypothalamic disease
8. Liver glycogenosis due to deficiency of liver enzymes that produce glucose from liver glycogen stores (types I, II, VI, IX) and other hereditary enzyme deficiencies (glycogen synthetase, fructose 1-6 diphosphatase, pyruvate-carboxylase, phosphoenol pyruvate carboxykinase)
9. Glycerol intolerance
10. Hereditary defects in amino acid metabolism (maple syrup urine disease, propionic acidemia, methylmalonic acidemia, tyrosinosis, phenylketonuria, type 2 glutaric-acidemia, hydroxymethylglutaric acidemia)
11. Ketotic hypoglycemia (due to hepatic glycogen depletion in 30 to 50% of cases secondary to inadequate amino acid precursors for gluconeogenesis, especially alanine; cause of 50 to 70% of cases unknown)
12. Reye's syndrome
13. Somatomedin deficiency (Laron dwarf)
14. Transient neonatal hyperinsulinemia in infant of diabetic mother (usually when mother's diabetes has been poorly controlled)
15. Idiopathic in neonate

Table 5. Causes of 240 Consecutive Cases of Hypoglycemia in Patients Known to Have Diabetes Mellitus*

Cause	%
Inadequate food (carbohydrate) intake	66%
Excess insulin dose	12%
Sulfonylurea therapy	12%
Strenuous exercise	4%
Ethanol intake	4%
Other (kidney failure, liver failure, decrease in corticosteroid dose)	2%

*Based on data from Grady Memorial Hospital, Emergency Clinic, Atlanta, 1973–1975.

enzymatic, hormonal, and histologic examinations, depending on the problem(s) being considered in the differential diagnosis.

b. Residual effects of prolonged and/or severe hypoglycemia:

Evaluate residual neurologic damage: electroencephalogram (EEG), motor, sensory, cerebellar, judgment, memory, intelligence score, and cranial nerves. Evaluate the electrocardiogram (ECG) and cardiac status.

c. Predischarge examinations:

Were precipitating factors identified and appropriately treated? Were precautions taken to avoid recurrence?

d. Management after hospital discharge:

If indicated, revise diet, insulin therapy, or exercise pattern. Patient should carry candy at all times. Prescribe a snack 60 minutes before hypoglycemia is prone to occur. Prescribe for and instruct relatives on the use of glucagon if there is a recurrence of hypoglycemia and if the patient is unable to swallow. Give a diabetes identification card, bracelet, or necklace. Caution about driving motor vehicles and working around dangerous machinery and in unprotected high places. Arrange continuing follow-up in an ambulatory care facility such as a diabetes clinic or physician's office.

HEREDITARY DISORDERS OF CARBOHYDRATE METABOLISM

By Julian C. Williams, M.D., Ph.D.
and R. Rodney Howell, M.D.
Houston, Texas

Genetic abnormalities in carbohydrate metabolism have played an important role in the emergence of the concept of a molecular basis of disease. Pentosuria was one of the diseases utilized by Garrod in 1909 to formulate the principle of inborn errors of metabolism. Von Gierke's disease, or glucose-6-phosphatase deficiency, was delineated in 1952 as the first hepatic enzyme defect in humans. In 1963 the concept of lysosomal storage disease was based on the discovery of alpha-glucosidase deficiency as the molecular error in Pompe's disease. This article addresses established transport or enzymatic protein abnormalities that result in defects of carbohydrate metabolism.

The hereditary disorders of carbohydrate metabolism may be categorized in the following manner:

1. Transport defects.
2. Pentosuria.
3. Disorders of fructose metabolism.
4. Inborn errors of galactose metabolism.
5. Glycogen storage diseases.
6. Defects of pyruvate metabolism.

Deficiencies of a number of enzymes of anaerobic glycolysis (hexokinase, glucose-phosphate isomerase, phosphofructokinase, aldolase, triosephosphate isomerase, phosphoglycerate kinase, 2,3-diphosphoglyceromutase and phosphatase, pyruvate kinase, and lactate dehydrogenase) have been reported in mature erythrocytes (Fig. 1). All, except lactate dehydrogenase and 2,3-diphosphoglyceromutase and phosphatase deficiencies, are associated with hemolytic syndromes. Clearly, total enzyme deficiency in more critical organs would be lethal. Two deficiencies, glucose-6-phosphate dehydrogenase and 6-phosphogluconate dehydrogenase, of aerobic glycolysis or the pentose phosphate shunt, are also known to cause hemolysis. These disorders are inherited as autosomal recessives except phosphoglycerate kinase and glucose-6-phosphate dehydrogenase, whose loci are located on the X chromosome.

With the exception of alpha-glucosidase deficiency, all of these disorders involve nonlysosomal proteins and are considered defects in intermediary metabolism. Lysosomal enzyme deficiencies involving carbohydrate moieties are covered in other articles.

TRANSPORT DEFECTS

These are congenital abnormalities of specific disaccharidase or transport proteins of the small intestine brush border and renal tubules.

Glucose-Galactose Malabsorption

This rare, autosomal recessive inherited condition is due to a defect in the glucose-galactose transport protein and presents in the neonatal period with diarrhea, dehydration, and failure to thrive. Symptoms are induced by all enterally delivered forms of carbohydrate except fructose. Glucose and galactose are present in stools. Bacterial action results in an acid stool pH. Glucosuria in the range of 250 to 1000 mg/dl occurs. In vitro incubation of an intestinal biopsy fails to concentrate glucose, establishing the diagnosis. Unlike disaccharidase deficiencies, an oral glucose-galactose tolerance test fails to increase blood glucose levels. Treatment consists of eliminating all carbohydrate except fructose from the diet.

Sucrase-Isomaltase Deficiency

Symptoms usually appear at 2 to 3 months of age when sucrose-containing foods such as fruits or prepared baby foods are added to the diet. Symptoms consist of watery diarrhea, flatulence, and crampy abdominal pain. This disorder resembles lactose intolerance except that it is induced by table sugar rather than milk sugar. Recent estimates of the incidence of this autosomal recessive inherited condition indicate 2 per 1000 in North America, but as high as 10 per cent in Greenland Eskimos.

Symptoms are due to the absence of the disaccharidase necessary to hydrolyze sucrose and isomaltose. This results in accumulation of these compounds in the intestinal lumen and its resultant osmotic diarrhea. Diagnosis is made by an oral sucrose tolerance test, hydrogen breath test, or enzymatic assay of an intestinal biopsy.

Lactose Intolerance

Lactose, or milk sugar, is hydrolyzed by the enzyme lactase (β-galactosidase) in the brush border. There are three major forms of lactose intolerance:

1. Congenital lactase deficiency.
2. Delayed onset lactase deficiency.
3. Acquired deficiency due to damage of the intestinal brush border.

Congenital lactase deficiency presents in infancy with severe watery diarrhea, lactosuria, and failure to thrive upon exposure to lactose. Lactose, a reducing

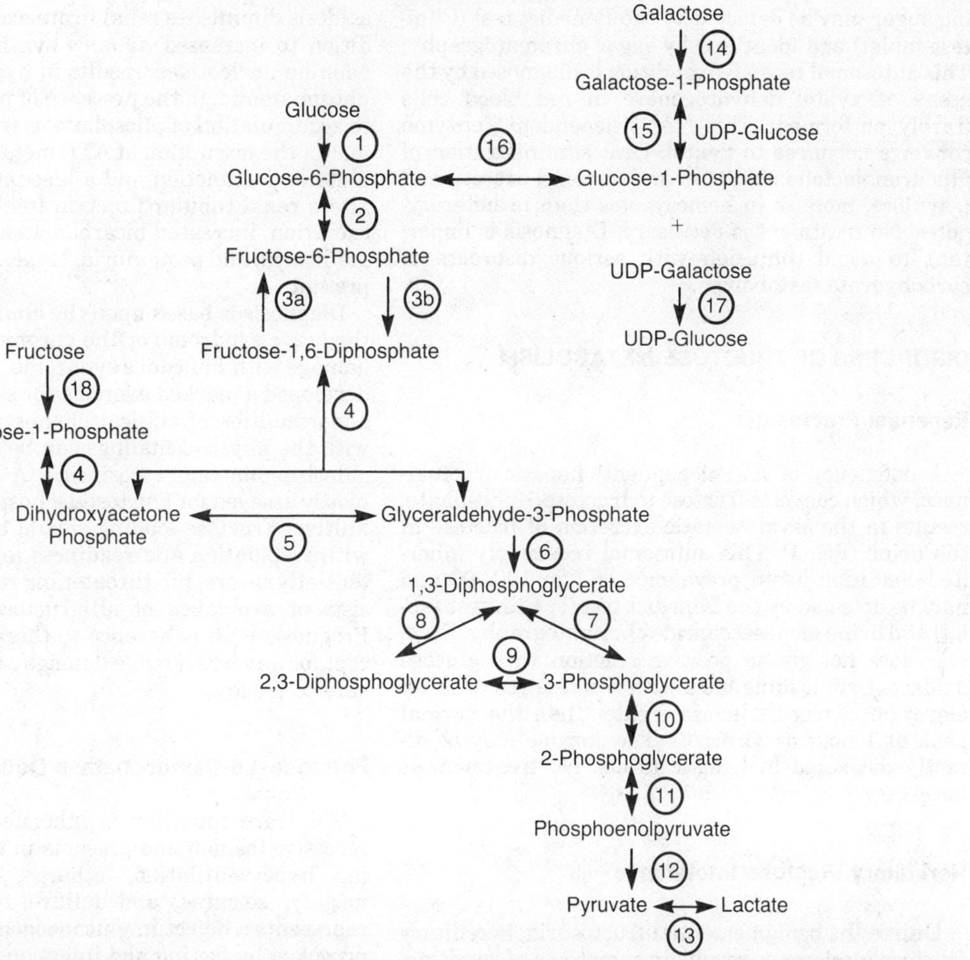

Figure 1. Glucose, galactose, and fructose metabolism. (*1.*) Hexokinase. (*2.*) Glucose phosphate isomerase. (*3a.*) Frustose-1,6-diphosphatase. (*3b.*) Phosphofructokinase. (*4.*) Fructose phosphate aldolase. (*5.*) Triosephosphate isomerase. (*6.*) Glyceraldehyde-3-phosphate dehydrogenase. (*7.*) Phosphoglycerate kinase. (*8.*) Diphosphoglyceromutase. (*9.*) Diphosphoglycerate phosphatase. (*10.*) Phosphoglyceromutase. (*11.*) Enolase. (*12.*) Pyruvate kinase. (*13.*) Lactate dehydrogenase. (*14.*) Galactokinase. (*15.*) Galactose-1-phosphate uridyltransferase. (*16.*) Phosphoglucomutase. (*17.*) UDP-Galactose-4-epimerase; UDP = uridine diphosphate. (*18.*) Fructokinase.

sugar, will give a positive Clinitest reaction. Oral lactose tolerance tests should be avoided because of resulting severe dehydration. Demonstration of lactase deficiency in an intestinal brush border biopsy is diagnostic. The mode of inheritance is unclear in this rare disorder and treatment consists of elimination of lactose from the diet. A few infants present with a severe toxic response to lactose, which includes diarrhea, emesis, lactosuria, aminoaciduria, and renal tubular acidosis. Intestinal lactase activity is normal, either initially or after the toxic episode, and the mechanism of this disorder is not understood.

Delayed-onset lactase deficiency appears between childhood and the adolescent years. Its incidence varies from 5 to 20 per cent of North American whites, 70 to 75 per cent of North American blacks, 74 per cent of Mexicans, and 87 to 97 per cent of Orientals. It seems that loss of, or a severe decrease in, intestinal lactase activity after childhood is normal in humans and that only in certain races has a mutation (possibly autosomal dominant) occurred that preserves this enzyme. Symptoms vary widely and range from none to nausea, abdominal distention, cramping pain, flatulence, and watery diarrhea. Diagnosis may be established by lactase assay of an intestinal biopsy, oral lactose tolerance test, or a hydrogen breath test. Treatment consists of eliminating lactose from the diet.

Secondary lactase deficiency occurs commonly, especially in children, with gastroenteritis, intractable diarrhea, celiac sprue, cystic fibrosis, inflammatory bowel disease, malnutrition, and intestinal surgery. Enzyme activity recovers after treatment of the primary condition.

PENTOSURIA

Essential pentosuria is a benign disorder occurring primarily in Jewish and Lebanese populations with a prevalence of 1 to 2 per 5000. There are no symptoms, and the only sign is the excretion of 1 to 4 grams per day of the pentose L-xyulose in the urine. The reducing sugar may be detected by the Benedict test (Clinitest tablet) and identified by sugar chromatography. This autosomal recessive condition is diagnosed by the assay of xylitol dehydrogenase in red blood cells (rarely performed). This NADP-dependent* enzyme converts L-xylulose to xylitol. Oral administration of glucuronolactone results in an increased excretion of L-xylulose, more so in homozygotes than in heterozygotes. No treatment is necessary. Diagnosis is important to avoid confusion with serious disorders of carbohydrate metabolism.

DISORDERS OF FRUCTOSE METABOLISM

Essential Fructosuria

A deficiency of ATP-dependent† hepatic fructokinase, which converts fructose to fructose-1-phosphate, results in the asymptomatic excretion of fructose in the urine (Fig. 1). This autosomal recessively inherited condition has a prevalence of 1 in 130,000 and may be detected by the Benedict test (or Clinitest tablet) and urine monosaccharide chromatography. Fructose does not give a positive reaction with glucose oxidase. Oral loading tests with fructose result in an elevation of blood fructose greater than the normal peak at 1 hour of 25 mg/dl. The enzyme may be directly measured in hepatic tissue. No treatment is necessary.

Hereditary Fructose Intolerance

Unlike the benign essential fructosuria, hereditary fructose intolerance results in symptoms of vomiting, gastrointestinal hemorrhage, disseminated intravascular coagulation, hypotension, tachycardia, sweating with tremulousness, seizures, and coma that may result in death. Chronic exposure leads to hypotonia; failure to thrive; hepatosplenomegaly with jaundice, ascites and cirrhosis; and Fanconi's syndrome.

This condition is inherited in an autosomal recessive fashion and is due to a mutation in fructose-1-phosphate aldolase (aldolase B) (Fig. 1). Although once thought to be very rare, it may be more common, with its incidence in Switzerland found to be 1 in 20,000. The enzyme is found in the liver, renal cortex, and small intestine. Three aldolases (A, B, and C) occur in humans and differ in their tissue distribution as well as in their activities against the two natural substrates: fructose-1,6-diphosphate (FDP) and fructose-1-phosphate (FIP). Aldolase B normally has a FDP: FIP ratio of 1.0:1.3 and is 2.5:20 in affected patients with a greatly diminished total activity. Decreased activity of this enzyme results in accumulation of the toxic intermediate fructose-1-phosphate which inhibits fructokinase, resulting in fructosemia and fructosuria, It also inhibits phosphorolysis of glycogen to glucose-1-phosphate, causing hypoglycemia. Lactic acidosis diminishes renal urate excretion. This, in addition to increased *de novo* synthesis of urate from adenine nucleotides, results in hyperuricemia. Hypophosphatemia, in the presence of phosphaturia, is due to accumulation of phosphate as fructose-1-phosphate and in the disruption of ATP metabolism. This causes platelet dysfunction and a bleeding diathesis. It also alters renal tubular function to elicit decreased acid excretion, increased bicarbonate loss, aminoaciduria, mellituria, and proteinuria. Hypokalemia may also be present.

Diagnosis is based upon the clinical presentation of the acute syndrome or the chronic picture of hepatic damage with Fanconi's syndrome. Most patients have developed a marked aversion for sweets. The multiple abnormalities of clinical chemistries in conjunction with the physical findings can be confused only with galactosemia and tyrosinosis. A liver or intestinal biopsy assayed for fructose-1-phosphate aldolase is definitive. Fructose loading should be undertaken only with trepidation and readiness to counteract the potentially severe, life-threatening results. Therapy consists of avoidance of all fructose-containing foods. Prognosis with adherence to therapy is excellent except for any irreversible damage caused by prior exposure to fructose.

Fructose-1,6-Diphosphatase Deficiency

This rare condition is inherited in an autosomal recessive fashion and presents in infancy with vomiting, hyperventilation, lethargy, hypotonia, hepatomegaly, seizures, and failure to thrive. Since it represents a defect in gluconeogenesis, symptoms are provoked by fasting and infection. Hypoglycemia is a prominent feature. Many of the symptoms are due to hypoglycemia, ketosis, and lactic acidosis, which promptly remit with infusion of glucose and bicarbonate. Recurrent episodes of hypoglycemia result in mental retardation.

The disorder is due to a deficiency of fructose-1,6-diphosphatase, a key enzyme in gluconeogenesis which converts fructose-1,6-diphosphate to fructose-6-phosphate (Fig. 1). Thus, in its absence, generation of glucose from pyruvate and amino acids is interrupted; the result is hypoglycemia. Metabolic compensation leads to mobilization of free fatty acids, ketosis, and hepatic triglyceride storage. Excess pyruvate causes lactate accumulation.

Diagnosis is most accurately established by measurement of the relevant enzyme in liver, kidney, or intestinal tissue. The defect may be suspected by the failure to elevate glucose levels upon infusion of gluconeogenic precursors or by a provocative fast. Both of these types of test may produce dangerous changes in sensorium and metabolic homeostasis. Treatment consists of avoiding fasting by means of frequent feedings and/or a continuous nocturnal nasogastric drip. Fructose and sorbitol should be avoided and dietary fat partially restricted. In a small percentage of patients, folic acid increases residual enzyme activity. With therapy, prognosis is good if episodic deterioration during infection is not lethal.

*NADP = Nicotinamide adenine dinucleotide phosphate.

†ATP = Adenosine triphosphate.

INBORN ERRORS OF GALACTOSE METABOLISM

Galactokinase Deficiency

Galactokinase catalyzes the conversion of galactose to galactose-1-phosphate (Fig. 1). In its absence, galactose is elevated in the blood and urine. Nuclear cataracts develop as a result of the conversion of galactose to galactitol. Unless treated early by elimination of galactose from the diet, the cataracts are irreversible. This condition is inherited as an autosomal recessive, and the incidence is about 1 in 40,000.

Asymptomatic patients with early cataracts should be screened for galactokinase deficiency. Degenerative central nervous system disease has been seen in one adult patient and is felt to be coincidental. An oral galactose tolerance test results in elevation of blood galactose levels and excretion of galactose in the urine. No rise in blood glucose occurs, and gastrointestinal symptoms are absent. Galactosuria is indicated by a positive reducing substance test that is negative to glucose oxidase. Sugar chromatography will specifically identify the substance as galactose. Diagnosis is established by finding a deficiency of red blood cell galactokinase in the presence of normal galactose-1-phosphate uridyltransferase.

UDP-Galactose-4-Epimerase Deficiency*

This very rare deficiency has only been described in eight European patients. It results in an abnormal Guthrie newborn screening test due to an elevated erythrocyte galactose-1-phosphate, not an increase in galactose (Fig. 1). Galactosuria is not present. There are no symptoms. Erythrocyte and leukocyte UDP-galactose-4-epimerase activity is decreased, but it is normal in fibroblasts and liver. This defect in conversion of UDP-galactose to UDP-glucose is inherited as an autosomal recessive.

Galactosemia

Classic galactosemia is due to the deficiency of galactose-1-phosphate uridyltransferase (Fig. 1). It is inherited in an autosomal recessive fashion, and the incidence is approximately 1 in 50,000. In this condition, galactose-1-phosphate is not converted to UDP-galactose and thus accumulates intracellularly. This toxic intermediate results in hepatic and renal damage, nuclear cataracts, and mental retardation.

Soon after beginning milk ingestion, infants develop emesis, hypoglycemia, seizures, pseudotumor cerebri, jaundice, hepatomegaly, ascites, edema, failure to thrive, and cataracts. Progressive liver damage results in unconjugated hyperbilirubinemia, hypoproteinemia, and clotting abnormalities. Renal tubular dysfunction is manifested by glucosuria, aminoaciduria, and proteinuria. Death may result in a few weeks, frequently from *Escherichia coli* sepsis.

*UDP = Uridine diphosphate.

Cataracts develop in survivors. With treatment by exclusion of galactose (mainly occurring in milk products) from the diet, the renal and liver damage usually reverse dramatically. The patient is often left with cataracts and some learning disability.

This disease is detectable by the Guthrie bacterial screening test for elevated blood galactose. This test is required in the newborn period in many states. Early detection and treatment results in avoidance of most, if not all, of the symptoms. Strict adherence to the diet prognosticates an excellent outcome. Diagnosis is based upon the clinical picture, galactosemia, galactosuria, and measurement of the deficient enzyme in erythrocytes. Galactose tolerance tests should not be performed because of provocation of severe symptoms. Prenatal diagnosis is possible on fibroblasts obtained by amniocentesis.

GLYCOGEN STORAGE DISEASES

Glycogen storage disease (GSD) causes abnormalities of muscle and/or hepatic tissue due to hereditary deficiencies of one of the enzymes required for synthesis or degradation of glycogen. This results in the accumulation of glycogen in one or more tissues. The central homeostatic role of glycogen as the sole source of readily available energy explains the multiple clinical and secondary metabolic effects arising from blocks in its anabolic and catabolic pathways. Clinically, these disorders can be divided into two primary groups, hepatic and muscular, according to their predominant symptomatology. Due to inconsistencies in various authors numbering these diseases as Type I, Type II, and so on, we will refer to them by the known enzymatic defect.

Hepatic Forms

All of these disorders occur with an incidence of approximately 1 in 100,000 live births, except brancher deficiency (1 in 500,000). With the exception of phosphorylase b kinase, all of the glycogen storage diseases, both hepatic and muscular forms, are inherited as autosomal recessives.

Glucose-6-Phosphatase Deficiency

Also known as Type I, von Gierke's disease, or hepatorenal GSD, this condition presents in childhood with proportionate short stature and massive hepatic enlargement due to storage of glycogen and lipid (Fig. 2). Radiographic examination reveals bilateral renal enlargement. Other clinical findings include xanthomas of the extensor surfaces of the extremities; tophaceous gout in older patients; and discrete, yellowish plaques surrounding the optic macula. Frequent epistaxis and easy bruising are also common. Older patients develop multiple benign hepatic adenomas and, very rarely, hepatic carcinoma.

Abnormal laboratory data include hypoglycemia after minimal fasting, lactic acidosis, hyperuricemia, and elevations of free fatty acids, triglycerides, and cholesterol. Because glucose-6-phosphatase is necessary to release free glucose in the circulation, injection of glucagon or epinephrine raises the blood glucose level only modestly. This slight rise is due to the ability of debrancher enzyme to release a small amount of free glucose from glycogen branch points. The specific diagnosis is established by measurement of glucose-6-phosphatase activity in a liver biopsy. Type Ib GSD refers to patients with clinical glucose-6-phosphatase deficiency in whom measurement of the enzyme is normal in frozen tissue. It has been shown that the enzyme is defective in fresh tissue and that the primary abnormality is due to the organization of the enzyme in the microsomal membranes of the hepatic parenchymal cell.

In recent years, very successful treatment of this condition has been achieved by the use of continuous nocturnal nasogastric feeding. Avoidance of hypoglycemia prevents the secondary hormonal changes that induce the secondary metabolic abnormalities. Normal growth in children, resolution of xanthomas, and amelioration of the bleeding diathesis occur with treatment. It is not known whether this treatment will decrease the formation of hepatic adenomas, although there are suggestions that treatment may reduce their size.

Debrancher Enzyme Deficiency

Debrancher enzyme deficiency (Type III GSD) manifests in childhood as a clinically milder form of von Gierke's disease (Fig. 2). Hypoglycemia is less severe, as is growth retardation. Although hypertriglyceridemia may be present, xanthomas are very rare. Hyperuricemia and gout do not occur. The hepatomegaly, mild inflammatory disease, and minimal cirrhosis present in young children frequently remit after puberty. The kidneys are not enlarged. The aberrant function of debrancher enzyme results in the synthesis of glycogen with short outer chains in multiple tissues. Muscle, in particular, may show clinical effects of wasting and weakness. Recently, a group of adult patients has been recognized who, although apparently normal in childhood, develop a progressive myopathy. Some have congestive heart failure and cardiac myopathy and hypertrophy.

Glycogen with an abnormal structure is increased in liver, and debrancher enzyme deficiency is present. The enzyme may also be assayed in multiple tissues such as leukocytes, muscle, and cultured fibroblasts. As discordance of enzyme activity in the other tissues versus the liver is common, a liver biopsy is definitive. Treatment, if necessary, is for the hypoglycemia and growth failure by means of continuous nocturnal nasogastric feeding. It is not known whether this will alter the course of the adult myopathy.

Brancher Deficiency

Brancher deficiency (Andersen's disease, amylopectinosis, Type IV GSD) presents as liver failure in early infancy (Fig. 2). Initial hepatomegaly progresses rapidly to jaundice, ascites, cirrhosis, and failure to thrive. There is no treatment, and death usually occurs in the second year of life. Diagnosis is established by measurement of brancher enzyme in liver, leukocytes, or fibroblasts, allowing accurate prenatal diagnosis. Glycogen content is normal or elevated with an abnormal structure due to the presence of long outer chains and few branch points.

Hepatic Phosphorylase Deficiency

Hepatomegaly with increased liver glycogen levels and very mild or no hypoglycemia is encountered in patients with hepatic phosphorylase deficiency (Fig. 2). No other symptoms are usually present, nor is any treatment required. The enzyme defect is only partial. Detailed enzymatic study of these patients revealed a subset in whom the deficiency was present only in males and inherited as an X-linked recessive. These patients were found to have a deficiency of phosphorylase b kinase, an enzyme necessary for activation of phosphorylase. Affected patients (hemizygotes) manifest hepatomegaly and lymphocytic infiltration on liver biopsy. Liver enzymes are mildly elevated. No other symptoms are present, and treatment is unnecessary. Heterozygotes (females) may have modest

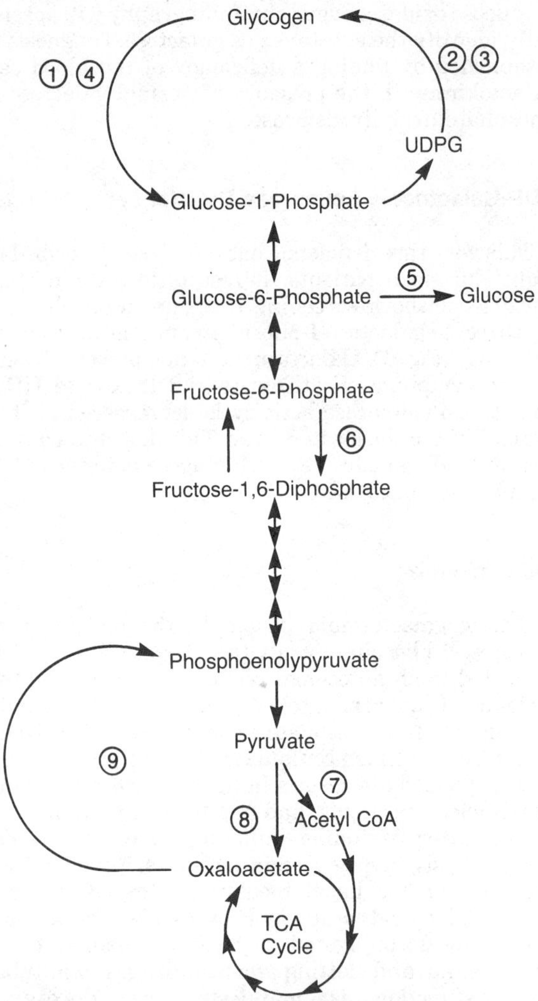

Figure 2. Glycogen metabolism and gluconeogenesis. (*1.*) Phosphorylase. (*2.*) Glycogen synthetase. (*3.*) Branching enzyme. (*4.*) Debranching enzyme. (*5.*) Glucose-6-phosphatase. (*6.*) Phosphofructokinase. (*7.*) Pyruvate dehydrogenase. (*8.*) Pyruvate carboxylase. (*9.*) Phosphoenolpyruvate carboxykinase.

hepatomegaly. Hepatic phosphorylase deficiency is most accurately assessed using liver tissue. Leukocytes, fibroblasts, or a hepatic biopsy may be assayed for phosphorylase b kinase.

Muscular Forms

The glycogen storage diseases already described rarely have clinically apparent muscle dysfunction except in older patients with Type III disease and children with brancher deficiency.

Pompe's Disease

Pompe's disease (lysosomal alpha-glucosidase deficiency, Type II GSD) is a devastating, untreatable illness presenting at birth or in the first few months of life with hypotonia, muscle weakness, and cardiomegaly. Massive biventricular hypertrophy with large QRS voltages and a short PR interval are present. Cardiac and respiratory muscle dysfunction inexorably progresses to death by 2 years of age.

This disorder is the only glycogen storage disease due to an abnormality of a lysosomal enzyme. Its incidence is approximately 1 in 100,000. The pathophysiology results from progressive lysosomal enlargement and concomitant disruption of muscle fiber structure. The enzyme alpha-glucosidase is deficient in all tissues, and glycogen accumulation results. Care must be used in assessing enzyme activity due to the presence of cytosolic alpha-glucosidases with neutral pH optima which may overlap the acid pH optimum of the lysosomal enzyme. This is particularly true in leukocytes and kidney tissue.

Alpha-Glucosidase Deficiency

An adult form of alpha-glucosidase deficiency (acid maltase deficiency) is recognized. Presenting in the second, third, or fourth decades of life with muscle weakness, it is characterized by a chronic wasting myopathy without cardiac involvement. The same lysosomal alpha-glucosidase is absent in all tissues, as in Pompe's disease; however, glycogen accumulation occurs only in clinically affected striated muscles. The few cases that have presented in childhood with mild cardiac symptoms may represent genetic compound heterozygotes of the infantile and adult forms. As in Pompe's disease, there is no treatment and death usually results from respiratory failure and/or pneumonia. Prenatal diagnosis of all the clinical forms of alpha-glucosidase deficiency is possible by measurement of enzyme activity in amniotic cells.

Muscle Phosphorylase Deficiency

Also called McArdle disease, muscle phosphorylase deficiency is quite rare, occurring about 1 in 500,000 live births (Fig. 2). Symptoms appear after puberty, when patients manifest painful muscle cramps and myoglobinuria after strenuous exercise. Renal failure may result if the myoglobinuria is severe. As this enzyme is necessary to convert muscle glycogen to glucose-1-phosphate and subsequently lactate via glycolysis, these patients fail to generate lactate in a forearm ischemic exercise test. Exercise under anaerobic conditions induces transient contractures which are electrically silent by electromyographic (EMG) monitoring. No other symptoms are present initially, and the only treatment is avoidance of strenuous exercise. In the fourth and fifth decades of life, many patients develop chronic muscle weakness and wasting.

Diagnosis in this clinical setting is confirmed by a muscle biopsy demonstrating increased glycogen concentration of normal structure present as subsarcolemmal blebs and absence of muscle phosphorylase activity. McArdle's disease should be differentiated from muscle phosphofructokinase deficiency, which presents in a clinically identical manner with the addition of a mild hemolytic anemia (Figure 2). Phosphofructokinase activity measurement in muscle or erythrocytes permits diagnosis of this very rare condition.

DISORDERS OF PYRUVATE METABOLISM

There are three hereditary enzyme deficiencies affecting the flow of glucose-derived substrate into and out of the tricarboxylic acid cycle. All are associated with lactic acidosis. Two of these disorders, pyruvate dehydrogenase and pyruvate carboxylase deficiency, have been reported in some, but not all, patients with Leigh's encephalopathy. Further investigation is necessary to determine whether a causal relationship exists.

Phosphoenolpyruvate Carboxykinase (PEPCK) Deficiency

Absence of this enzyme results in an inability to convert oxaloacetate to phosphoenolpyruvate, the second step in the gluconeogenic pathway (Fig. 2). Onset is usually soon after birth, and survival is brief. The symptoms are hypoglycemia, seizures, hypotonia, hepatomegaly with jaundice, macroglossia, and mental retardation. Chemical abnormalities include lactic acidosis, ketosis, hypercholesterolemia, and hypertriglyceridemia. The only theoretically effective treatment is glucose infusion, but the hypoglycemia is usually refractory. Diagnosis is established by assay of PEPCK in liver. The extreme rarity of this disease precludes determination of its incidence and mode of inheritance, although parents of affected infants are clinically normal.

Pyruvate Dehydrogenase Deficiency

Clinical presentations of this disorder may be classified into two major groups (Fig. 2). Severe deficiencies have early onset psychomotor retardation with cortical and optic atrophy, poor coordination, and hyperactive reflexes in the presence of muscular hypotonia. Death occurs in the first decade of life. In the milder variant, intellectual function is preserved; however, episodic ataxia and encephalopathy occur with exacerbations, frequently associated with infection. Chronic mild motor dysfunction and optic atrophy may also be present.

Elevated blood levels of lactate, pyruvate, and alanine are present. Infection and a high-carbohydrate diet worsen these abnormalities. Diagnosis is established by determination of pyruvate dehydrogenase in liver, brain, muscle, or fibroblasts. The extreme difficulty of accurately measuring this complicated enzyme precludes its assay except in a few specialized laboratories.

This rare disorder is inherited as an autosomal recessive. Treatment is symptomatic and dietary in that some patients have improved on a high-fat diet.

Pyruvate Carboxylase Deficiency

Pyruvate carboxylase catalyzes the conversion of pyruvate to oxaloacetate, the first step of gluconeogenesis (Fig. 2). The few patients described have lactic acidosis, pyruvicacidemia, hyperalaninemia, hypoglycemia, and ketosis. Onset is early in infancy with seizures, posturing, psychomotor retardation, and hypotonia. Hepatomegaly may be present. Deterioration is rapid with death resulting in the first few years of life. Symptoms are exacerbated by catabolic events such as fasting and infection. Although high-protein diets and pharmacologic doses of vitamin B_6 and thiamine have been utilized, there is no effective treatment of this autosomal recessive disorder.

Enzymatic proof of the existence of this disease in a given patient is extremely difficult because of the instability of the enzyme in biopsy specimens and the complexity of the assay. It may be accurately measured if liver, kidney, or brain biopsy tissues are frozen in liquid nitrogen within 20 seconds of interruption of its blood supply. Because of these technical limitations, measurement in fibroblasts is more practical. The diagnosis may also be suggested in the proper clinical setting by the appearance of ketosis during the performance of an intravenous glucose tolerance test. This is thought to be due to saturation of the tricarboxylic acid and overflow of acetyl CoA derived from glucose into ketone body synthesis.

MUCOPOLY-SACCHARIDOSES

By Julian C. Williams, M.D.
and R. Rodney Howell, M.D.
Houston, Texas

The genetically determined abnormalities of mucopolysaccharide metabolism are known collectively as the mucopolysaccharidoses (MPS) (Table 1). Affected patients appear normal at birth, but with the passage of time accumulation of mucopolysaccharide in the tissues leads to functional impairment, particularly of the ocular, cardiac, skeletal, and central nervous systems. The term mucopolysaccharidoses encompasses those systemic disorders in which excessive mucopolysaccharides (glycosaminoglycans) are excreted in the urine (mucopolysaccharidurias) as well as those in which the defect can be detected only by studying cellular metabolism. Definitive diagnosis relies on the assay of enzymes involved in mucopolysaccharide degradation, yet features of several of the types are sufficiently distinctive to permit diagnosis on clinical grounds.

SIGNS AND SYMPTOMS

Six distinctive conditions associated with mucopolysacchariduria are recognized. In each type, there exist at least two subgroups, defined on either clinical or biochemical criteria (see Tables 2 and 3). Specific enzymatic deficiencies have been identified for each of the diseases.

Infants with mucopolysaccharide storage disorders grow excessively during intrauterine life and may continue to do so for the first year or so after birth. Thereafter, retardation of linear growth characterizes patients with the Hurler, Hunter, Morquio, and Maroteaux-Lamy syndromes. Dwarfing is variable in β-glucuronidase deficiency, minimal in Sanfilippo's syndrome, and absent in the Scheie syndrome.

There is widespread accumulation of mucopolysaccharides in the tissues. As a result the facial features coarsen, evolving into the typical facies with thick pouting lips, enlarged tongue, prominent forehead, and depressed nasal bridge. These features are well established in the Hurler, Hunter, and Maroteaux-Lamy syndromes within the first few years of life. Patients with the Morquio, Sanfilippo, and Scheie syndromes do not exhibit these gargoyle-like features. Wide spacing of the teeth occurs in all mucopolysaccharidoses. Noisy breathing with constant rhinorrhea develops early and may persist throughout life. Repeated ear infections with subsequent hearing loss are common. Likewise, umbilical, inguinal, and abdominal wall hernias appear during the first year of life and frequently recur after surgery. Tissue storage of mucopolysaccharides explains the cardiac murmurs, hepatosplenomegaly, and thickened skin. There is usually an abundance of fine lanugo-like hair, most prominently over the back and extensor surfaces of the extremities, especially in the Sanfilippo syndrome. Cutaneous nodules may be present along the inferior border of the scapulas in the Hunter syndrome.

Clouding of the cornea occurs in each type except the Hunter and Sanfilippo syndromes. Slit-lamp examination may be required to appreciate the clouding, especially early in its development. Simultaneously, retinal degeneration is in progress, although this process may be largely obscured by the corneal clouding. Blindness may result as a combination of the two processes.

Skeletal changes commonly first attract attention in these disorders. As the infant learns to sit alone, a gibbus (cat-back) deformity of the thoracic or lumbar spine becomes apparent. Soon after, limitation of joint mobility appears and becomes progressively more disabling. The upper extremities and shoulder girdle are affected to a greater degree than the lower extremities. The hands become stiff and fixed in a claw-like

Table 1. Synonyms Used in the Mucopolysaccharidoses (MPS) and Related Metabolic Disorders

Common Name	Other Names Used
Hurler syndrome	MPS I–H (formerly MPS 1), gargoylism, Hurler-Pfaundler syndrome
Scheie syndrome	MPS I–S (formerly MPS V)
Hunter syndrome	MPS II (mild and severe subtypes)
Sanfilippo syndrome	MPS III (A, B, C, and D subtypes), polydystrophia oligophrenia
Morquio syndrome	MPS IV (A and B subtypes), Morquio-Ullrich syndrome, Brailsford syndrome, chondro-osteodystrophy, keratansulfaturia
Maroteaux-Lamy syndrome	MPS VI (mild and severe subtypes), polydystrophic dwarfism
β-Glucuronidase deficiency	MPS VII, Sly syndrome
I-Cell disease	Mucolipidosis II
Pseudo-Hurler syndrome	Mucolipidosis III, pseudopolydystrophy

position. Carpal tunnel syndrome may occur from compression at the wrist. Severe changes of this nature affect patients with the Hurler and Maroteaux-Lamy syndromes; lesser changes are noted in the Hunter, β-glucuronidase deficiency, and Scheie syndromes, and only minimal changes are noted in the Sanfilippo syndrome. The skeletal changes in Morquio's syndrome, while severe, are quite different in nature from those in the other mucopolysaccharidoses. The chest commonly has a pectus carinatum (pigeon breast) deformity in addition to flaring of the lower rib cage; the vertebral column may be kyphotic, usually with some degree of scoliosis; and the knees are in valgus position. The joints are not stiff; some, particularly the wrists, are lax. Most importantly, in the Morquio, Hurler, and Maroteaux-Lamy syndromes, the odontoid process may be hypoplastic. This, coupled with ligamentous laxity, allows dislocation of C1 on C2 with compression of the cervical spinal cord.

Patients with the Hurler, Hunter, β-glucuronidase deficiency, and Sanfilippo syndromes develop moderate to profound mental retardation. This tends to be milder in the Hunter and β-glucuronidase deficiency syndrome. During the initial months following birth, this may be mild or absent altogether but it always becomes obvious prior to school age. The Scheie, Morquio, and Maroteaux-Lamy syndromes, as well as one variant of the Hunter syndrome, are exempt from the central nervous system deterioration, at least during the childhood years. Hydrocephalus and/or cervical cord compression due to pachymeningitis may occur in the Hunter, Hurler, and Maroteaux-Lamy syndromes.

Cardiac disease, due to deformation of the aortic and mitral valves resulting in stenosis and/or regurgitation, is common in all of the mucopolysaccharidoses except the Sanfilippo syndrome. Arteriosclerosis is also prominent. The combination of these factors is frequently the cause of death.

ROENTGENOGRAPHIC FINDINGS

Roentgenographic findings in the Hurler syndrome include scaphocephaly, dense calcification at the base of the skull, enlarged or shoe-shaped sella turcica, anterior beaking of the vertebral bodies, widening of the diaphysis of the long bones, and expansion of the shafts of the ribs and clavicles. The phalanges are shortened and broad with constriction of the ends. These changes of dysostosis multiplex characterize the mucopolysaccharidoses. In degree, the Hurler and Maroteaux-Lamy syndromes are characterized by severe involvement, and the Hunter and Scheie syndromes by less involvement, with particular absence of gibbus deformity. The least effect is seen in the Sanfilippo syndrome, but striking thickness of the calvarium is exhibited. In the Morquio syndrome the roentgenologic changes predate clinical abnormalities and include odontoid aplasia or hypoplasia, kyphosis, and platyspondyly with increased intervertebral distances; degeneration of the femoral heads; widening of the ribs; proximal pointing of the metacarpals; and generalized osteoporosis. The skull is normal.

GENETICS

All but one of the known mucopolysaccharidurias are inherited as autosomal recessive disorders (Table 2). The Hunter syndrome follows an X-linked pattern of transmission. Allelic subgroups probably exist, which in part explain the remarkable heterogeneity seen within the six groups.

CLINICALLY RELATED DISORDERS

Numerous patients have been described with clinical and roentgenologic features suggestive of the mucopolysaccharidoses but who lack the biochemical abnormalities necessary for diagnosis of the disorders just described. From this heterogeneous group, several specific entities have been delineated. Others remain as diagnostic enigmas.

Mannosidosis, fucosidosis, and generalized gangliosidosis are storage disorders that have clinical features, particularly visceral, in common with the Hurler syndrome. Likewise, the mucolipidoses share clinical features with the mucopolysaccharidoses. Mucolipidosis II (I-cell disease) is characterized by severe Hurleroid features present at birth and inclusions in all cells of the body. Patients with mucolipido-

Table 2. Classification of the Mucopolysaccharidoses (MPS)

Disorder	Genetics	Clinical Features
Hurler syndrome (MPS–I)	AR	Excessive growth in infancy followed by severe dwarfing thereafter, hernias, hepatosplenomegaly, progressive clouding of cornea, limitation of joint mobility, deterioration of mental function and coarsening of facial features, rhinorrhea, hydrocephalus, deafness, cardiac murmurs, death usually in first decade of cardiorespiratory causes
Scheie syndrome (MPS I–S)	AR	Progressive clouding of cornea and joint limitation, aortic insufficiency, normal intelligence, normal stature
Hurler-Scheie compound (MPS I–H/I–S)	AR	Features intermediate between Hurler and Scheie syndromes
Hunter syndrome (MPS II) Severe	X	Dwarfing, deafness, retinal degeneration, hepatosplenomegaly, hernias, progressive limitation of joint mobility and deterioration of mental function, cardiac murmurs, clear cornea, cutaneous nodules, death usually in the second decade
Mild		Same general features as severe Hunter syndrome, but mental deterioration much slower, survival well into adult life
Sanfilippo syndrome A (MPS III–A) B (MPS III–B) C (MPS III–C) D (MPS III–D)	AR	Clear cornea, severe deterioration of mental function prior to school age, minimal organomegaly and shortening of stature, no differences in clinical features between the various types
Morquio syndrome (MPS IV) Morquio A	AR	Severe dwarfing, pectus carinatum, kyphoscoliosis, genu valgum (prominent joints, some of which may be lax), corneal clouding, normal intelligence, may have cervical cord compression because of cervical spine dislocation, thin enamel
Morquio B		Similar to Morquio A syndrome, but dysostosis multiplex is milder and enamel is normal
Maroteaux-Lamy syndrome (MPS VI) Severe	AR	Normal or excessive growth during infancy followed by severe dwarfing, limitation of joint mobility, corneal clouding, coarsening of facies, hepatosplenomegaly, hernias, cardiac murmurs, deafness, normal intelligence
Mild		Skeletal features and growth retardation less prominent than in severe Maroteaux-Lamy syndrome
β-Glucuronidase	AR	Variable features including coarse facies, hepatosplenomegaly, hernias, corneal clouding, dysostosis multiplex and mental retardation

Abbreviations: AR = Autosomal recessive; X = X-linked recessive.

sis III (pseudo-Hurler polydystrophy) have mild facial and cerebral manifestations but develop corneal clouding and joint stiffness. None of these disorders is characterized by massive urinary mucopolysaccharide excretion, although cells from patients with mucolipidosis II and mucolipidosis III accumulate sulfated mucopolysaccharides (Table 3).

LABORATORY STUDIES

Several simple screening tests for detecting increased concentrations of mucopolysaccharides in the urine are commonly used.

The simplest of these is the so-called *toluidine blue spot test.* In this test, fresh urine is spotted directly on filter paper. The filter paper is subsequently stained with toluidine blue, decolorized, and examined for the presence of purple spots that would indicate the presence of mucopolysaccharides, which stain metachromatically.

Another widely used screening test is the *acid albumin test.* In this procedure, excess mucopolysaccharides present in urine are precipitated in the presence of an acidified albumin solution. The presence of turbidity can be visually estimated or measured with a spectrophotometer. The *cetyltrimethylammonium bromide test* for screening urine has a similar basis, in that mucopolysaccharides are precipitated, and this is usually estimated visually.

Although inclusions that stain metachromatically may be identified in lymphocytes and cultured fibroblasts, especially in the β-glucuronidase deficiency and Maroteaux-Lamy syndromes, these findings are variable and should not be relied upon for diagnosis of the mucopolysaccharidoses or for distinguishing one type from another.

METHODS FOR BIOCHEMICAL DIAGNOSIS

Mucopolysaccharide Analysis. In those patients who have positive urine mucopolysaccharide screening tests, additional tests should be done to assess both the amount and the type of mucopolysaccharide excreted. Certain laboratories have also demonstrated that the urinary mucopolysaccharides, in addition to being present in increased concentrations in urine, have a larger average molecular weight. The type of mucopolysaccharide can be determined by electrophoresis and by chemical analysis.

Cell Culture. A useful screening test for preliminary identification of the presence of an enzymatic defect in the degradation of mucopolysaccharides is measurement of radioactive sulfate accumulation. Specific biochemical study of fibroblasts (cultured from skin biopsies) offers a set of reliable procedures for differentiating mucopolysaccharidoses from each other, from mucolipidoses, and from other clinically related conditions. This is accomplished by measurement of the relevant enzyme. These assays can also be performed on leukocytes isolated from peripheral blood. The test of choice is determined not only by the biochemical characteristics of the disorder at risk but also by the relative difficulty of the available methods and by the specialized expertise of the testing laboratory. These enzymatic assays are available in only a few specialized centers. A summary of presently available methods is presented in Table 3.

Prenatal Diagnosis. Estimation of fetal urinary mucopolysaccharide excretion by analysis of mucopolysaccharide in amniotic fluid is an unreliable procedure for prenatal diagnosis and is prone to false-negative results. Thus, prenatal detection of the mucopolysaccharidoses as well as that of the mucolipidoses requires the time-consuming process (about a month) of culturing cells found in amniotic fluid. By the use of such cultured cells, prenatal diagnosis has been accomplished or is theoretically possible in each of the mucopolysaccharidoses.

Heterozygote Detection. When an enzyme deficiency disease is inherited in an autosomal recessive manner, the carrier usually has roughly half the normal level of activity. Thus, carrier detection is possible only when a partial enzyme deficiency can be reliably determined. Because of the wide range of normal values, substantial overlaps between the carrier and unaffected states exist in all of the mucopolysaccharidoses and absolute determination of the carrier state is difficult.

Because of the special rules governing the activity of X-chromosomes, the heterozygote in X-linked disorders (of which the Hunter syndrome is the only one under consideration here) is in effect a mosaic of normal and abnormal cells. Carrier detection by cloning two populations of fibroblasts is possible but complicated by the chance that one type of cell may have a selective advantage over the other. Thus, whereas the finding of clones with the biochemical characteristics of Hunter cells unambiguously demonstrates the carrier state, the absence of such clones does not guarantee normality. Female relatives of Hunter patients should still be counseled on the basis of their statistical risk of carrying the Hunter gene.

Table 3. Biochemical Diagnosis of the Mucopolysaccharidoses

Syndrome	Abnormal Sulfate Accumulation in Cultured Fibroblast	Urine Excretion of Mucopolysaccharides	Primary Enzyme Deficiency
Hurler, Scheie, and Hurler/Scheie compound	+	Dermatan sulfate Heparan sulfate	α-L-iduronidase
Hunter	+	Dermatan sulfate Heparan sulfate	Iduronate sulfatase
Sanfilippo			
A	+	Heparan sulfate	Heparan N-sulfatase
B	+	Heparan sulfate	N-acetyl-α-D-glucosaminidase
C	+	Heparan sulfate	Acetyl CoA:α-glucosaminide-N-acetyl-transferase
D	+	Heparan sulfate	N-acetyl-α-D-glucosaminide-6-sulfatase
Morquio			
A	–	Keratan sulfate	N-acetylgalactosaminide-6-sulfatase
B	–	Keratan sulfate	β-galactosidase
Maroteaux-Lamy	+	Dermatan sulfate	Arylsulfatase B (N-acetylgalactosaminide-4-sulfatase)
β-glucuronidase deficiency	+	Dermatan sulfate Heparan sulfate	β-glucuronidase
I-cell disease	+	–	UDP-GlcNAc:glycoprotein N-acetylglucosaminyl-1-phosphotransferase
Pseudo-Hurler	+	–	UDP-GlcNAc:glycoprotein N-acetylglucosaminyl-1-phosphotransferase

Abbreviations: UDP = Uridine diphosphate; GlcNAc = N-acetylglucosamine.

DISORDERS OF LIPID TRANSPORT

By Ernst J. Schaefer, M.D.
New York, New York
and Robert I. Levy, M.D.
Boston, Massachusetts

LIPOPROTEIN COMPOSITION AND METABOLISM

Abnormalities of plasma lipids are common in Western society. Plasma lipids (free and esterified cholesterol, phospholipids, and triglycerides), in conjunction with various proteins, known as apolipoproteins (apo), are transported in the bloodstream as spherical particles known as *lipoproteins.* The density of lipoproteins in plasma depends on their relative content of protein and lipid, while the electrophoretic mobility is determined by their net charge. Characteristics of plasma lipoproteins are given in Table 1.

Chylomicrons, synthesized in the intestine in response to fat feeding, and very low density lipoproteins (VLDL) produced by the liver are the major triglyceride-carrying lipoproteins. Low-density lipoproteins (LDL) are the major cholesterol-carrying lipoproteins. High-density lipoproteins (HDL) are relatively rich in protein and appear to serve as a vehicle to remove cholesterol from peripheral tissues and the arterial wall. Marked chylomicron elevation in fasting plasma has been associated with an increased risk of pancreatitis, whereas increased LDL, increased abnormal beta migrating VLDL, and decreased HDL have been independently associated with premature coronary artery disease (CAD).

The major distinguishing features of plasma lipoproteins are their varying lipid and protein (*apolipoprotein*) content. Characteristics of apolipoproteins are shown in Table 2. ApoA-I and apoA-II are the major proteins of HDL; apoB-100 is the major protein of LDL. The C apolipoproteins and apoE are protein constituents of triglyceride-rich lipoproteins (chylomicrons and VLDL) and HDL and play an important role in lipoprotein metabolism.

An understanding of normal lipoprotein metabolism is crucial to elucidating the metabolic defects in various dyslipidemic states. Newly formed intestinal chylomicrons contain various apolipoproteins, including apoB-48; these particles pick up the C apolipoproteins and apoE. Chylomicron triglycerides in the plasma are hydrolyzed by lipoprotein lipase (LPL, activated by apoC-II) to form fatty acids and glycerol. VLDL tryglycerides may also be hydrolyzed by another enzyme, *hepatic lipase.* In this process phospholipids and apolipoproteins are transferred to HDL. Deficiency of lipoprotein lipase or its activator protein (apoC-II) results in marked hypertriglyceridemia with chylomicron accumulation. Following lipolysis, cholesterol ester-rich chylomicron "remnants," containing apoB-48 and apoE, are taken up by the liver via an apoE receptor–mediated process. Abnormalities of apoE result in accumulation of chylomicron remnants as seen in Type III hyperlipoproteinemia (broad beta disease).

The liver produces VLDL containing apoB-100 as well as other apolipoproteins. Like chylomicron triglyceride, VLDL triglyceride is hydrolyzed by lipoprotein lipase, and some VLDL lipid and protein constituents are transferred to HDL. In the process, VLDL is catabolized to form LDL, which contains apoB-100 as its predominant protein constituent. LDL is removed from the circulation and is catabolized by peripheral cells and the liver by an apoB receptor–mediated process. When LDL binds to its receptor and is internalized, the activity of β-hydroxy-β-methylglutaryl-CoA (HMG CoA) reductase, the rate-limiting enzyme in intracellular cholesterol synthesis, is suppressed. If a defect in the LDL receptor is present, LDL accumulates in the plasma (Type II hyperlipoproteinemia).

HDL can be formed by direct synthesis in the intestine or liver, or, as previously mentioned, as a result of VLDL or chylomicron lipolysis. In addition, HDL can pick up free cholesterol in the periphery, cross back into the plasma space, and serve as a vehicle to transport lipid from the periphery to the liver. Free cholesterol in plasma is converted to cholesterol ester by the enzyme lecithin:cholesterol acyltransferase (LCAT), while phospholipid and triglyceride on lipoproteins in plasma are hydrolyzed by the enzyme hepatic lipase.

APPROACH TO THE PATIENT

In screening subjects for disorders of lipid transport, it is crucial to obtain measurements of plasma or serum cholesterol, triglycerides, and HDL cholesterol on samples after a 12- to 14-hour fast. When the fast-

Table 1. Plasma Lipoproteins

Lipoprotein Class	Density Range (gm/ml)	Electrophoretic Mobility	Composition (Weight %) Protein	Triglyceride	Cholesterol Free	Cholesterol Ester	Phospholipid
Chylomicrons	< 0.94	Origin	1–2	80–95	1–3	2–4	3–6
VLDL	0.94–1.006	Pre-beta	6–10	45–65	4–8	16–22	15–20
LDL	1.006–1.063	Beta	18–22	4–8	6–8	45–50	18–24
HDL	1.063–1.21	Alpha	45–55	2–7	3–5	15–20	26–32

Abbreviations: VLDL = Very low density lipoproteins; LDL = low-density lipoproteins; HDL = high-density lipoproteins.

Table 2. Apolipoproteins

Apolipoprotein	Lipoprotein Density Class	Approximate Plasma Concentration (mg/dl)	Approximate Molecular Weight (Daltons)	Function
A–I	HDL	120	28,000	Cofactor—LCAT Structural role in HDL
A–II	HDL	35	17,000	Cofactor—HL Structural role in HDL
B–100	VLDL, LDL	100	250,000	Binding protein cell receptor; structural role in VLDL, LDL
B–48	Chylomicrons, VLDL	?	?	Structural role in chylomicrons
C–I	Chylomicrons, VLDL, HDL	7	6,500	Cofactor—LCAT
C–II	Chylomicrons, VLDL, HDL	4	10,000	Cofactor—LPL
C–III	Chylomicrons, VLDL, HDL	13	10,000	Cofactor—lysosomal sphingomyelinase, inhibitor—LPL
E_{1-3}	Chylomicrons, VLDL, HDL	5	35,000	Binding protein-cell receptor

Abbreviations: HDL = High-density lipoproteins; VLDL = very low density lipoproteins; LDL = low-density lipoproteins; LCAT = lecithin:cholesterol acyltransferase; LPL = lipoprotein lipase; HL = hepatic lipase.

ing plasma triglyceride concentration is below 400 mg/dl, the following formulas can be used to calculate VLDL and LDL cholesterol:

VLDL cholesterol = triglyceride/5

LDL cholesterol = total cholesterol − (VLDL cholesterol + HDL cholesterol).

It should be noted that this formula does not apply when Type III hyperlipoproteinemia (broad beta disease, as determined by lipoprotein electrophoresis) is present, since VLDL in these patients is very rich in cholesterol. Usually, if values are within the normal range (5th to 95th percentile), as shown in Table 3, no further lipoprotein work-up is required.

Normal Levels of Serum or Plasma Cholesterol, Triglycerides, and HDL Cholesterol

It is difficult to define the normal or safe level of serum cholesterol, since prospective studies have shown that the incidence of coronary heart disease rises in linear fashion with the level of total and LDL cholesterol in plasma, and values that are within the normal ranges (5th to 95th percentile) in the United States as defined statistically are higher than those found among comparable individuals in populations with a low incidence of CAD.

The optimal serum cholesterol for the middle-aged American is probably 200 mg/dl, or less. For practical purposes, hypercholesterolemia is defined as a value above the 95th percentile for the population, which in Americans ranges from 203 mg/dl in individuals less than 20 years old, to 303 mg/dl in individuals more than 60 years old. However, these limits are clearly excessive because of the known cardiovascular risk of cholesterol values at these levels, and a convenient rule of thumb is that any level of serum cholesterol higher than 200 mg/dl plus the person's age should be considered elevated. Even these limits may be too high. In contrast to serum cholesterol, it is not clear that serum triglycerides are independent risk variables. Triglyceride levels, like cholesterol, do vary with age, and it is reasonable to consider a serum triglyceride concentration of greater than 250 mg/dl as abnormal.

As previously indicated, even more information can be obtained about coronary risk by viewing the plasma cholesterol in terms of the units of lipid transport—the lipoproteins—than by a simple measurement of total cholesterol. Sixty to 75 per cent of total plasma cholesterol is transported on LDL. Therefore at all ages the total plasma cholesterol is usually a reflection of LDL cholesterol values. In fact, the observed direct relationship between the total plasma cholesterol and CAD is due to the powerful direct relationship between LDL cholesterol and CAD. HDL, which normally accounts for only 20 to 25 per cent of the total plasma cholesterol, is inversely associated with cardiovascular risk. HDL cholesterol levels are positively correlated with exercise and moderate alcohol intake and inversely related to cigarette smoking, obesity, and the use of progestin-containing oral contraceptives. Some drugs used in the treatment of hypertension (thiazide diuretics and beta-blockers) cause increases in plasma triglycerides and decreases in HDL values.

Studies show CAD prevalence at HDL levels of 30 mg/dl to be more than double that at 60 mg/dl, and familial excesses of HDL (hyperalphalipoproteinemia) or deficiency of LDL (hypobetalipoproteinemia) has been associated with decreased CAD risk and longevity. These findings provide a cogent reason to determine whether borderline elevated plasma cholesterol levels are due to increases in LDL or the "benevolent" HDL.

Table 3. Plasma Lipid and Lipoprotein Cholesterol Concentrations*

	Plasma Cholesterol (mg/dl)			Plasma Triglyceride (mg/dl)			VLDL Cholesterol (mg/dl)			LDL Cholesterol (mg/dl)			HDL Cholesterol (mg/dl)		
Percentiles†	*5*	*50*	*95*	*5*	*50*	*95*	*5*	*50*	*95*	*5*	*50*	*95*	*5*	*50*	*95*
Age (Years)							Males								
0–14	114	155	203	29	54	59	0	8	22	63	92	132	37	55	74
15–24	113	161	218	37	78	201	1	12	28	62	97	147	30	46	63
25–34	133	184	254	48	100	266	3	17	48	70	120	185	28	45	63
35–44	146	200	270	54	118	321	3	20	56	81	133	189	27	43	67
45–54	158	210	277	58	124	324	5	22	62	89	142	202	28	45	64
55–64	156	211	276	58	119	289	3	18	49	83	144	210	28	48	74
65+	151	186	274	57	112	267	0	16	45	88	144	210	30	49	78
							Females								
0–14	112	159	205	32	61	131	1	10	24	68	96	140	36	59	73
15–24	120	157	216	36	65	131	2	11	24	60	96	135	35	51	73
25–34	128	170	216	38	67	151	0	10	25	67	106	151	37	55	78
35–44	140	187	252	40	78	191	1	13	35	76	118	174	33	54	87
45–54	152	233	285	46	93	233	0	14	38	80	134	215	33	58	89
55–64	172	228	300	52	102	262	1	16	51	95	150	234	36	59	91
65+	169	228	303	60	112	243	0	14	52	96	151	223	33	60	91

*Based on Lipid Research Clinics population studies in the United States and Canada in 24,425 white males and 18,108 white females (non–sex hormone users) for plasma cholesterol and triglyceride values, and in 3524 white males and 2545 white females (non–sex hormone users) for lipoprotein concentrations as derived from NIH publication No. 80–1527, 1980. All subjects were sampled in the fasting state. Five-year age spans were combined to the above age spans utilizing the lowest 5th percentile and highest 95th percentile for each age span. The lowest 5th percentile and highest 95th percentile for all age and sex groups in mg/dl are: cholesterol, 112–303; triglyceride, 29–34; VLDL cholesterol, 0–62; LDL cholesterol, 60–234; and HDL cholesterol 27–91.

†The figures 5, 50, and 95 are population percentiles; values between the 5th and 95th percentiles are considered to be within the normal range.

Abbreviations: VLDL = Very low density lipoprotein; LDL = low-density lipoprotein; HDL = high-density lipoprotein.

Laboratory Methods

Plasma cholesterol is generally determined by colorimetric or enzymatic methods. HDL cholesterol is usually measured after the removal of VLDL and LDL from plasma by precipitation techniques. It is important that samples be stored at 4°C and be processed within 5 days to minimize exchange of lipids between lipoproteins; otherwise, erroneous results will be obtained for HDL cholesterol. In addition, turbid supernates following precipitation cannot be used for HDL cholesterol determination. Supernates can generally be cleared by diluting the sample 1:1 with 0.15 mol/liter NaCl and repeating the precipitation. Alternatively, one can use a 0.22-μm filter (Millipore Corp.). The plasma triglyceride concentration generally is assayed by determining the glycerol content of the plasma following triglyceride hydrolysis by lipase.

Lipoprotein electrophoresis on serum or plasma is useful only to help verify the diagnosis when hyperlipidemia exists and should always be accompanied by measurement of plasma triglyceride, plasma total cholesterol, and HDL cholesterol values. Electrophoresis is not a screening test and should be done only if triglycerides or cholesterol levels are elevated or abnormally low. It is important to realize that significant variability can exist between results obtained from various laboratories. Be sure of the accuracy and precision of the determinations as done by your laboratory.

Patients with abnormal values may require the following additional tests for definitive diagnosis:

1. High-resolution agarose lipoprotein electrophoresis.
2. Lipoprotein quantitation by ultracentrifugation.
3. Measurement of free to total cholesterol ratio.
4. Measurement of post-heparin lipoprotein lipase and hepatic lipase.
5. Measurement of plasma apoA-I, apoB, apoB-100, apoB-48, apoC-II, apoC-III, and apoE.
6. Apolipoprotein isoform analysis by isoelectric focusing.
7. Measurement of betasitosterol or cholestanol by gas liquid chromatography.
8. Fibroblast LDL receptor studies.

These latter tests are generally only available in specialized lipid research laboratories.

Secondary Hyperlipidemia

Prior to diagnosing primary disorders of lipid metabolism, secondary causes of dyslipidemia should be excluded. Causes of significant hypercholesterolemia due to increased LDL levels include a high-cholesterol, high saturated fat diet; thyroid disease; liver disease; nephrosis; porphyria; glycogen storage disease; and dysproteinemia. In obstructive liver disease, marked elevations of free cholesterol and phospholipid associated with accumulation of an abnormal

LDL called lipoprotein-X occur due to acquired deficiency of the enzyme LCAT. Significant hypertriglyceridemia has been associated with uncontrolled diabetes mellitis, systemic lupus erythematosus, renal failure, lipodystrophy, excessive alcohol ingestion, and various medications (estrogens, beta-blockers, and hydrochlorothiazide). Since primary forms of dyslipidemia in general are genetic disorders, the entire family should be screened if an abnormality is found.

Classification of Patients

Patients with lipid disorders can be classified utilizing plasma cholesterol, triglyceride, and HDL cholesterol values into the following simple categories:

1. Hypertriglyceridemia only.
2. Hypercholesterolemia and hypertriglyceridemia.
3. Hypercholesterolemia only.
4. Decreased HDL with normal plasma lipids.

A more sophisticated classification was developed at the National Institutes of Health based on which lipoprotein class was elevated (lipoprotein phenotyping) utilizing the following terminology:

1. Type I hyperlipoproteinemia (HLP), characterized by increased chylomicrons.
2. Type IIa HLP, with increased LDL.
3. Type IIb, with increased VLDL and LDL.
4. Type III, with increased VLDL of abnormal electrophoretic mobility-beta VLDL.
5. Type IV HLP, with increased VLDL.
6. Type V HLP, with increased chylomicrons and VLDL.

This classification has served as a useful framework for the diagnosis of hyperlipidemic states. Representative lipid values in various dyslipidemic states are shown in Table 4. It has become clear that lipoprotein phenotypes do not always correspond to genotypes, since kindreds have been reported with family members having several different lipoprotein phenotypes. Therefore, for definitive diagnosis of genetic dyslipidemias, family screening studies and additional biochemical assays as previously mentioned are essential. A summary of disorders of lipid transport is shown in Table 5. In the future these disorders increasingly will be classified by their unique metabolic defect.

HYPERCHYLOMICRONEMIA STATES (TYPES I AND V HLP)

These patients have severe hypertriglyceridemia (generally in excess of 1000 mg/dl) in the fasting state and are at increased risk of developing pancreatitis. Significant chylomicronemia is present in the fasting state.

Lipoprotein Lipase Deficiency

Patients with this uncommon disorder have a marked deficiency of lipoprotein lipase as determined in post-heparin plasma. This autosomal recessive disorder often presents in childhood or early adult life with bouts of recurrent abdominal pain and pancreatitis. These patients may develop lipemia retinalis, eruptive xanthomas, and hepatosplenomegaly. They are usually not obese, diabetic, or hyperuricemic and do not appear to be at increased risk for premature CAD. (An acquired variant of this disorder occurring in systemic lupus erythematosus or other autoimmune disorders is due to a circulating inhibitor of lipoprotein lipase.) Typical plasma lipid and lipoprotein cholesterol values are shown in Table 4. These patients usually have Type I hyperlipoproteinemia and significantly decreased LDL and HDL cholesterol values.

Apolipoprotein C-II Deficiency

Clinically these rare patients present with a similar clinical picture as subjects with lipoprotein lipase deficiency. Instead of being deficient in lipoprotein lipase, they lack the activator protein for this enzyme, namely apoC-II. They have been reported to usually have a Type V phenotype on lipoprotein electrophoresis (increased chylomicrons and VLDL). This disorder has an autosomal recessive mode of transmission.

Type V HLP

While Type V HLP is frequently seen in association with diabetes, alcoholism, or kidney disease, in some patients it is a primary disorder. Type V subjects generally do not present until adulthood and may develop hepatosplenomegaly, eruptive xanthomas, and lipemia retinalis as well as recurrent pancreatitis. These patients are often obese, hyperuricemic, and diabetic. They do not have lipoprotein lipase or apoC-II deficiency. Typical lipid values for Type V HLP patients are shown in Table 4. A significant percentage of these patients (about 70 per cent) are heterozygotes or homozygotes for the apoE4 isoform of apoE. (Most normal subjects are heterozygotes or homozygotes for apoE3.) ApoE isoforms can be determined when VLDL protein is subjected to isoelectric focusing (pH range 4 to 6), and six possible apoE phenotypes exist in the normal population: E2, E2/3, E3, E3/4, E2/4, E4. ApoE has been shown to be a crucial protein for receptor-mediated liver uptake of chylomicron remnants, and abnormalities of apoE have been associated with a number of dyslipidemic states.

INCREASED BETA VLDL (TYPE III HLP)

Apolipoprotein E2 Homozygosity

Patients with primary Type III hyperlipoproteinemia have combined elevations of both cholesterol and triglyceride, owing to a marked increase in cholesterol-rich VLDL that has beta mobility on lipoprotein electrophoresis instead of the usual pre-beta mobility. In addition, these patients generally have a VLDL cholesterol to plasma triglyceride ratio ≥ 0.30 in contrast to normal subjects in whom this ratio is

Table 4. Plasma Lipid and Lipoprotein Cholesterol Concentrations in Dyslipidemic Subjects*

	Plasma Cholesterol (mg/dl)	Plasma Triglyceride (mg/dl)	VLDL Cholesterol (mg/dl)	LDL Cholesterol (mg/dl)	HDL Cholesterol (mg/dl)
Normals (n = 1088)	189 ± 1	87 ± 1	16 ± 1	123 ± 1	50 ± 1
Hyperlipoproteinemic subjects					
Type I (n = 12)	324 ± 57	3316 ± 677	285 ± 57	22 ± 2	17 ± 2
Type II (n = 454)	354 ± 4	135 ± 4	24 ± 1	286 ± 9	44 ± 1
Type III (n = 66)	441 ± 54	694 ± 60	292 ± 19	111 ± 7	38 ± 2
Type IV (n = 299)	251 ± 4	438 ± 24	78 ± 4	132 ± 2	37 ± 1
Type V (n = 95)	373 ± 19	2071 ± 213	274 ± 22	72 ± 4	27 ± 1
Hypolipoproteinemic subjects					
Abetalipoproteinemia (n = 4)	41 ± 4	20 ± 3	1 ± 0	2 ± 1	38 ± 2
Tangier disease (n = 11)	65 ± 4	200 ± 31	21 ± 4	42 ± 13	2 ± 1

*Mean values ±SEM, VLDL represents 1.006 gm/ml, and therefore includes chylomicrons when present, as in types I and V hyperlipoproteinemia.
Abbreviations: VLDL = Very low density lipoprotein; LDL = low-density lipoprotein; HDL = high-density lipoprotein.

Table 5. Lipid Transport Disorders

Increased Chylomicrons (Types I, V HLP)	Increased VLDL (Type IV HLP)	Increased Beta VLDL (Type III HLP)	Increased or Abnormal LDL	Chylomicron, VLDL, LDL Deficiency	HDL Deficiency
Lipoprotein lipase deficiency	Familial hypertriglyceridemia	Apolipoprotein E2 phenotype (variants)	Familial combined hyperlipidemia	Abetalipoproteinemia	Tangier disease
Apolipoprotein C–II deficiency	Familial combined hyperlipidemia	Apolipoprotein E deficiency	Familial hypercholesterolemia (LDL receptor abnormalities)	Hypobetalipoproteinemia	HDL deficiency with planar xanthomas
Apolipoprotein E4 phenotype		Hepatic lipase deficiency	Beta sito-sterolemia	Normotriglyceridemic abetalipoproteinemia	Apolipoprotein A–I and C–III deficiency
			CTX		Apolipoprotein A–I absence
					LCAT deficiency
					Fish eye disease
					Hypoalphalipoproteinemia
					ApoA–I Milano

Abbreviations: VLDL = Very low density lipoproteins; HDL = high-density lipoproteins; LDL = low-density lipoproteins; LCAT = lecithin:cholesterol acyltransferase; CTX = cerebrotendinous xanthomatosis.

less than 0.25. On lipoprotein electrophoresis of their whole plasma or serum, these subjects often have a broad beta lipoprotein band. These patients may have tubo-eruptive xanthomas on their elbows, knees, and buttocks and palmar xanthomas; are at increased risk for premature CAD and peripheral vascular disease; and frequently have glucose intolerance and hyperuricemia. The disease usually does not present until adulthood.

Type III HLP may occasionally be seen in patients with hypothyroidism or dysproteinemia. Most patients with Type III hyperlipoproteinemia, however, are apoE2 homozygotes, but often have additional factors predisposing to hyperlipidemia such as obesity. Males often present with Type III HLP and xanthomas approximately 10 to 15 years earlier (age 25 to 40 years) than do females.

Apolipoprotein E Deficiency

A black kindred from southern Virginia was recently described in which four siblings had significantly elevated plasma cholesterol and mild triglyceride elevations associated with marked VLDL elevations. Their lipoprotein electrophoresis was consistent with Type III hyperlipoproteinemia (broad beta disease), and their mean VLDL cholesterol to plasma triglyceride ratio was approximately 1.0. Three of the four siblings had evidence of premature

CAD. All had tubo-eruptive xanthomas. The mode of inheritance was autosomal recessive. ApoE was undetectable in the plasma of all homozygotes, and apoB-48 and apoA-IV were noted in the VLDL, IDL, and LDL fraction. Obligate heterozygotes had normal lipoprotein levels. Observations in these patients support the concept that apoE is crucial for hepatic uptake of chylomicron remnants.

Hepatic Lipase Deficiency

A Canadian kindred was recently reported in which the proband was a 38-year-old male with angina pectoris and tubo-eruptive and palmar xanthomas. Serum cholesterol levels ranged between 260 and 1495 mg/dl and triglycerides between 395 and 8200 mg/dl. The patient was noted to have Type III HLP with a marked increase in beta VLDL; however, his VLDL was not cholesterol-enriched, and the VLDL cholesterol to plasma triglyceride ratio was normal. LDL and HDL were reported to be enriched in triglyceride and phospholipid (phosphatidyl-choline), and HDL_2 was increased in concentration. The VLDL apoE phenotype was normal, and the patient and one brother were found to have marked post-heparin hepatic lipase (HL) deficiency. The proband's two sons had HL values that were 15 per cent and 45 per cent of normal, respectively.

INCREASED VLDL (TYPE IV HLP)

This form of hyperlipoproteinemia is quite common and generally presents in adulthood. These patients frequently are obese, diabetic, and hyperuricemic. They usually do not have xanthomas. Type IV HLP is often secondary to moderate alcohol ingestion and can be produced by stress, oral contraceptives, thiazides, or beta-blockers. Two different genetic patterns have been observed in primary Type IV HLP kindreds: (1) familial combined hyperlipidemia (to be discussed subsequently), and (2) familial hypertriglyceridemia.

Familial Hypertriglyceridemia

Patients with this common autosomal dominant disorder have moderate hypertriglyceridemia with increased VLDL, normal LDL, and generally decreased HDL concentrations. They do not have lipoprotein lipase, hepatic lipase, or apoC-II abnormalities, nor do they have abnormalities of VLDL apoE isoforms. Typical lipid values for these patients with the Type IV HLP phenotype are shown in Table 4. It has been recently suggested that unlike Type IV subjects with familial combined hyperlipidemia, these patients have normal LDL protein (apoB) to cholesterol ratios and may not be at greatly increased risk for premature CAD. The lipoprotein abnormality generally does not present until adulthood, and these patients usually do not have xanthomas. The molecular defect in familial hypertriglyceridemia is not known. These patients often have increased VLDL production as well as delayed catabolism.

INCREASED OR ABNORMAL LDL

Familial Combined Hyperlipidemia

This relatively common autosomal dominant disorder is characterized by the finding of several types of hyperlipidemia within the same kindred. Approximately 33 per cent of those affected will have only hypercholesterolemia (increased LDL, Type IIa phenotype), 33 per cent will have only hypertriglyceridemia (increased VLDL, Type IV phenotype), and 33 per cent will have both hypercholesterolemia and hypertriglyceridemia (increased VLDL and LDL, Type IIb phenotype). Rarely patients in these kindreds may have the Type V HLP phenotype. Approximately 11 to 20 per cent of myocardial infarction survivors under age 60 years will have this disorder. Xanthomas are very rare in these patients. Individuals with this disorder are at significantly increased risk for premature CAD. The precise molecular defect in this condition is unknown, but these patients are often overweight and appear to have increased VLDL and LDL production.

Familial Hypercholesterolemia

Patients with this common autosomal dominant disorder, which presents in childhood, have hypercholesterolemia associated with increased LDL levels and generally have normal VLDL concentrations (Type IIa phenotype), but may have increased VLDL levels (Type IIb phenotype). It is estimated that the frequency of heterozygotes in the population is 1:500, while homozygotes are exceedingly rare. Heterozygotes account for approximately 3 to 6 per cent of myocardial infarction survivors under age 60 years and may develop CAD in the third to fifth decade of life. Males with this disorder often manifest CAD 10 to 12 years earlier than females. The risk of premature CAD in these subjects appears to be greatly exacerbated by the presence of other risk factors such as smoking or hypertension. Heterozygotes may develop arcus and tendinous xanthomas, and their cholesterol levels are usually significantly higher than in patients with familial combined hyperlipidemia. Homozygotes have plasma cholesterol levels which are usually over 600 mg/dl; they develop planar and tuberous xanthomas of the extensor surface on their hands, elbows, buttocks, and knees, as well as tendinous xanthomas; and frequently they develop premature and often fatal CAD in their teens.

The defects in these kindreds appear to be due to either the absence of LDL binding to skin fibroblasts (LDL receptor negative), a marked decrease in LDL binding (LDL receptor defective) or normal binding, but lack of internalization of LDL into the cell (internalization defect). These states may correlate with absence of the receptor itself, an abnormal receptor, or a post-receptor defect. Homozygotes may be homozygotes for a single defect or heterozygotes for two distinct defects. The LDL receptor pathway appears to be crucial for regulating cellular cholesterol homeostasis and LDL metabolism. Patients with this group of diseases have delayed catabolism of LDL. Synthesis of LDL may be increased as well.

Betasitosterolemia

Patients with this very rare disorder have normal lipids or moderate hypercholesterolemia and increased levels of plant sterols within VLDL and LDL (mainly betasitosterol) as determined by gas liquid chromatography. These patients absorb plant sterols as well as cholesterol in the intestine, while normal subjects absorb only cholesterol. They develop tendinous and tuberous xanthomas filled with betasitosterol and may develop premature atherosclerosis. Why these patients hyperabsorb plant sterols is unknown. The diagnosis should be considered in patients with tendinous xanthomas and normal serum cholesterol or modest hypercholesterolemia.

Cerebrotendinous Xanthomatosis (CTX)

This rare autosomal recessive disorder should also be considered when a patient presents with normal plasma lipid levels and tendinous xanthomas. CTX patients may have mental retardation secondary to xanthomas in the brain. These patients have markedly increased cholestanol levels in their plasma lipoproteins as determined by gas liquid chromatography. (Normally, only trace amounts are present.) VLDL and LDL levels are usually normal, while HDL levels are decreased. These patients have been reported to have a block in bile acid production, and oral administration of chenodeoxycholate reduces their plasma cholestanol levels to near normal values.

HDL DEFICIENCY

HDL levels are significantly lower in males than females in all postpubertal age groups. Decreased HDL levels have been associated with a sedentary lifestyle, obesity, cigarette smoking, and hypertriglyceridemia.

Of all the disorders characterized by HDL deficiency, only hypoalphalipoproteinemia may be common enough to serve as a relatively significant cause of premature CAD in the population. Determination of plasma apoA-I concentrations, as well as analysis of apoA-I isoforms, is extremely helpful in the diagnosis of the various disease states.

Tangier Disease

Homozygotes with this autosomal recessive disorder have hypocholesterolemia and mild hypertriglyceridemia associated with mildly increased chylomicrons and VLDL, decreased LDL, and marked HDL deficiency in the fasting state. Typical values for these parameters are shown in Table 4. These patients have cholesterol ester deposits in reticuloendothelial cells (causing orange tonsils, hepatosplenomegaly, and lymphadenopathy), develop mild corneal opacification, and may have transient peripheral neuropathy, as well as premature CAD over the age of 40 years. They have marked reductions of plasma apoA-I (1 to 2 mg/dl, normal 120 mg/dl) and apoA-II (2 to 4 mg/dl, normal 30 to 35 mg/dl), and have hypercatabolism of these apolipoproteins. The disease has recently been shown to be due to an apoA-I variant (apoA-$I_{Tangier}$) that differs from normal apoA-I in terms of its molecular weight, amino acid composition, and in vivo kinetic behavior. Heterozygotes have HDL values which are 50 per cent of normal and often have mild elevations of triglyceride (VLDL) as well. The disease derives its name from the Chesapeake Bay island home of the original kindred. Homozygotes may be protected from strikingly premature CAD by their decreased LDL levels.

HDL Deficiency with Planar Xanthomas

The proband in this kindred was a 54-year-old white Swedish female with angina pectoris and a long history of widespread yellow discoloration of her skin, especially around the eyes and in the groin. Examination of her lipoproteins revealed normal VLDL and LDL levels and marked HDL deficiency (1 per cent of normal). Her mean plasma apoA-I and apoA-II concentrations were reduced at 2 and 15 mg/dl, respectively. Apolipoprotein C-III and E levels were normal. The proband's mother had similar skin discoloration and died at age 72 years following a cholecystectomy. Three of six cousins had reduced HDL values. Additional findings in the proband included corneal infiltration, hepatosplenomegaly, normal tonsils, and yellow discoloration of the soft palate of the mouth. Biopsy of skin and rectal mucosa revealed triglyceride as well as free and esterified cholesterol deposition. This disease differs from Tangier disease in three major respects: normal tonsils, the presence of planar xanthomas, and normal LDL levels. The disease may be due to an abnormal apoA-I.

Familial Deficiency of Apolipoproteins A-I and C-III

Two white sisters from Detroit, Michigan, aged 33 and 31 years with severe CAD and yellowish plaques on the eyelids, neck, and trunk since adolescence were noted to have decreased VLDL, normal LDL, and markedly decreased HDL concentrations (mean HDL cholesterol 6 mg/dl). Mean apoA-I concentrations were 0.0059 mg/dl (normal, 121) while apoA-II levels were about 50 per cent of normal by radioimmunoassay. ApoC-III was not detectable in the plasma of either patient by electroimmunoassay. The parents and offspring had decreased HDL cholesterol and apoA-I concentrations. Both patients were noted to have mild corneal opacification. The ratio of free to esterified cholesterol was normal and LCAT activity was 40 per cent of normal.

Apolipoprotein A-I Absence

The proband in this kindred from Alabama was a 45-year-old white female with normal tonsils, no xanthomas, mild corneal opacifications, and severe diffuse CAD. Lipoprotein analysis revealed decreased

VLDL, normal LDL, and markedly decreased HDL levels. ApoA-I was not detectable in the proband's plasma by radioimmunoassay, and apoA-II levels were 10 per cent of normal. Apolipoprotein C-I and C-II levels were reduced, while apoB concentrations in plasma were mildly elevated. The patient had an increased apoB : cholesterol ratio within LDL. Three offspring and one brother had HDL cholesterol and apoA-I values that were 50 per cent of normal. The ratio of free to esterified cholesterol was normal, and LCAT activity was 40 per cent of normal. The defect in this disease appears to be due to an inability to synthesize apoA-I. Recent data suggest that this kindred may also have apoC-III and apoD deficiency.

Familial LCAT Deficiency

This rare autosomal recessive disorder is generally characterized by moderate hypercholesterolemia (107 to 600 mg/dl), almost solely due to free cholesterol, and hypertriglyceridemia (105 to 1800 mg/dl). On lipoprotein electrophoresis there is a broad band from the origin to the beta region. Pre-beta and alpha lipoproteins are not detected. The patients have increased levels of abnormal triglyceride and free cholesterol enriched VLDL and LDL, and marked HDL deficiency. They have striking reductions in plasma LCAT activity, due either to reduced LCAT mass or to functionally abnormal enzyme. Within LDL and HDL, lipoprotein particles on electron microscopy appear as stacked discs instead of spheres. These patients develop severe corneal opacification and anemia and often develop premature atherosclerosis and renal failure.

Fish Eye Disease

Three Swedish kindreds have been described with marked corneal opacification, increased triglyceride levels, and HDL levels about 10 per cent of normal. HDL composition, LCAT activity, and the ratio of free to esterified cholesterol were all normal in these patients. The patients had normal tonsils and reticuloendothelial tissues. Atherosclerosis was present in some members of these kindreds. The cause of the defect is unknown.

Hypoalphalipoproteinemia

Evidence for autosomal dominant inheritance of low HDL levels has been reported in a large kindred with a high prevalence of CAD. Other studies tend to support this view. VLDL and LDL values are generally normal. The defect in this disorder is not yet known.

ApoA-I$_{Milano}$

An Italian kindred from Milano was reported in which the proband had mild hypertriglyceridemia and significant HDL deficiency. The proband's apoA-I was found to be abnormal in that it contained cysteine and therefore formed apoA-I:apoA-I and apoA-I:apoA-II dimers in plasma. The wife of the proband had normal lipoproteins, while two of the three offspring of the proband had reduced apoA-I and HDL cholesterol levels. The genetics of this disorder remain to be clarified. No premature CAD in this kindred has been detected.

DEFICIENCIES OF CHYLOMICRONS, VLDL, AND LDL

Reduced levels of total cholesterol, LDL cholesterol, and VLDL cholesterol may be seen in cachexia, cystic fibrosis, pancreatic disease, severe bacterial infection, and malabsorption.

Abetalipoproteinemia

Patients with this rare autosomal recessive disorder have marked hypocholesterolemia and hypotriglyceridemia, associated with virtual absence of chylomicrons, VLDL, and LDL from their plasma. Typical lipid values are shown in Table 4. These patients have acanthocytosis, deficiency of the fat-soluble vitamins (A, D, E, and K) in plasma, fat malabsorption, and lipid-laden intestinal epithelial cells on small bowel biopsy; they may develop spinocerebellar ataxia and retinitis pigmentosa. Obligate heterozygotes have normal lipoprotein values and no clinical manifestations. The molecular defect appears to be due to inability to synthesize both apoB-100 and apoB-48.

Hypobetalipoproteinemia

This disorder is very similar to abetalipoproteinemia in its clinical and laboratory manifestations for homozygotes except that heterozygotes have VLDL and LDL levels that are about 50 per cent of normal. Homozygous hypobetalipoproteinemia may also be a somewhat less severe condition clinically with regard to neurologic and visual impairment than abetalipoproteinemia. A similar molecular defect exists with regard to the B apolipoproteins. Heterozygotes usually have no clinical sequelae, may have enhanced longevity, and have decreased LDL synthesis.

Normotriglyceridemic Abetalipoproteinemia

One female subject with this disorder has been reported who presented with mild mental retardation and vitamin E deficiency. In the fasting state her plasma lipid and lipoprotein cholesterol levels were similar to those of patients with abetalipoproteinemia, but after a fat load her plasma triglyceride levels rose to as high as 200 mg/dl and chylomicrons were clearly present. The molecular defect in this disease appears to be an inability to synthesize apoB-100, whereas apoB-48 production is unimpaired. These two forms of apoB can be detected by subjecting chylomicron and VLDL protein to 3.5 per cent acrylamide SDS gel electrophoresis.

CONCLUSION

Significant advances have been made in the last few years with regard to our understanding normal lipid transport and the pathogenesis of the various forms of dyslipidemia. Apolipoprotein, enzyme, and receptor analysis is assuming an increasingly important role in diagnosing disorders of lipid transport, which predispose patients to either pancreatitis (chylomicronemia, Types I and V HLP), premature coronary artery disease (increased VLDL, beta VLDL, LDL, or decreased HDL) or severe fat malabsorption and neurologic disease (abetalipoproteinemia or hypobetalipoproteinemia).

SPHINGOLIPIDOSES

By William G. Johnson, M.D.
New York, New York

The sphingolipidoses are disorders in which sphingolipids are stored because of a genetically determined deficiency of an enzyme required for their breakdown (Fig. 1). For each enzyme deficiency, an increasing range of clinical phenotypes is becoming known, each phenotype related to a different type or degree of genetic damage to that enzyme's activity. Hexosaminidase deficiency, for example, may be suspected in patients from infancy to middle age with a wide range of neurologic diseases. When a patient's enzyme deficiency is known, it is usually possible to do accurate patient diagnosis, prenatal diagnosis, carrier testing, and genetic counseling.

Evaluation of these patients includes (1) biochemical testing, (2) electrophysiologic, roentgenographic, and cerebrospinal fluid studies, and (3) appropriate morphologic examination of biopsies. It is important that even apparently typical cases be carefully evaluated, since variants (often genetic compounds) are commonly encountered and these complicate management and prenatal diagnosis.

The finding of a specific enzyme deficiency must be put in perspective with the clinical history and confirmatory tests. If only a single enzyme activity was measured on a specimen, an apparent deficiency may be merely a sample artifact. An enzyme may appear deficient because of a secondary hormonal or metabolic effect as in the diminished hexosaminidase A (HEX A) fraction in pregnancy or diabetes. A genetically determined enzyme deficiency in a single tissue may be a harmless polymorphic variant, as in the partial alpha-L-fucosidase deficiency in serum. Even a severe, genetically determined enzyme deficiency may be occasionally seen without disease. A few asymptomatic adults with severe deficiencies of sulfatase A, hexosaminidase A, or hexosaminidase A and B have been found, usually in families of patients with that enzyme deficiency. Although some may be presymptomatic, others appear to be genetic compounds with an enzyme that functions adequately in vivo but not in the test tube with artificial substrates.

CLINICAL PRESENTATIONS

G_{M2} Gangliosidoses (Hexosaminidase Deficiencies)

Signs and symptoms are nearly always confined to the nervous system. In infants, encephalopathy develops at 4 to 6 months with slowing, and later regression, of development, visual deterioration, myoclonic seizures, dementia, and death before the age of 5 years. Signs include macular cherry-red spot (whitish perimacular lipid deposits surrounding the cherry-red macula), accentuated sound-startle response, and, after age 2 years, macrocephaly. At least three types of hexosaminidase deficiency give this phenotype:

1. Classical Tay-Sachs disease (an alpha-locus deficiency).
2. Classical Sandhoff disease (a beta-locus deficiency).
3. The AB variant (an activator-locus deficiency).

The same basic picture of encephalopathy may develop in the late infantile or juvenile period; however, since the children have usually begun walking, gait difficulty, usually ataxia, is part of the picture. Cherry-red spot is usually absent in the later-onset phenotypes. In the juvenile or adolescent, cerebellar ataxia may be the presenting feature, often with spinal muscular atrophy as a major or minor feature. Features of encephalopathy may be present, or they may develop later.

In adolescents or young adults, slowly progressive spinal muscular atrophy may be the presenting feature. A cerebellar syndrome may be present, or it may develop; however, features of encephalopathy are not usually prominent. These late-onset phenotypes may occur with either alpha- or beta-locus disorders, and probably with activator-locus disorders too.

G_{M1}-Gangliosidosis, Generalized Gangliosidosis, Landing's Disease (Deficiency of Ganglioside Beta-Galactosidase)

In the infantile form, signs of encephalopathy develop soon after birth. Macular cherry-red spot is present in about half the cases. Hepatomegaly and, to some extent, splenomegaly develop. Coarse features, frontal bossing, joint stiffness and deformity, and often faint corneal haze are seen, changes reminiscent of the mucopolysaccharidoses. Patients survive less than 2 years.

A late infantile form presents as a primarily neurologic disorder with progressive dementia, seizures, ataxia, and spasticity. Later-onset forms have been seen, but some of them were in fact sialidoses, since the beta-galactosidase deficiency was accompanied by, and apparently secondary to, a more severe and consistent deficiency of sialidase.

A late-onset form strikingly similar to Morquio syndrome (classified as MPS IV-B or Morquio Type B) is characterized primarily by severe skeletal involvement.

Fabry Disease, Angiokeratoma Corporis Diffusum (Deficiency of alpha-Galactosidase)

The presenting feature in childhood or adolescence is usually either the neuropathy with burning pains in feet and hands, paresthesias, and anhydrosis; or the characteristic skin lesions, which are purple, macular, or maculopapular hyperkeratotic lesions seen over the groin, buttocks, scrotum, and umbilicus. Although stroke, limb edema, myocardial involvement, or faint corneal haze may occur, the most serious problem is usually renal failure in the third or fourth decade. Fabry disease is X-linked (incompletely) recessive. The full syndrome is seen in males (hemizygotes). Heterozygous females are sometimes affected, usually more mildly.

Gaucher Disease (Glucocerebrosidase Deficiency)

At least four phenotypes are known. Brain is involved in the infantile form (also called Type 2). Stridor, trismus, difficulty in sucking and swallowing, strabismus, spasticity, hyperreflexia, opisthotonus, head retraction, and developmental regression develop early in the first year with hepatosplenomegaly. Death occurs before 2 years of age.

A heterogeneous group of patients have juvenile onset of nervous system disease (Type 3) with mental defect (retardation or dementia), seizures, incoordination, and tics, with onset in childhood or adolescence. Splenomegaly varies from mild to massive.

So-called adult Gaucher disease (Type 1) is characterized by lack of nervous system involvement. Despite its name, splenomegaly may be noticed in young children and may become massive. Signs of hypersplenism, especially bleeding due to thrombocytopenia, and painful bony involvement constitute the major clinical complications. Occasionally, multiple

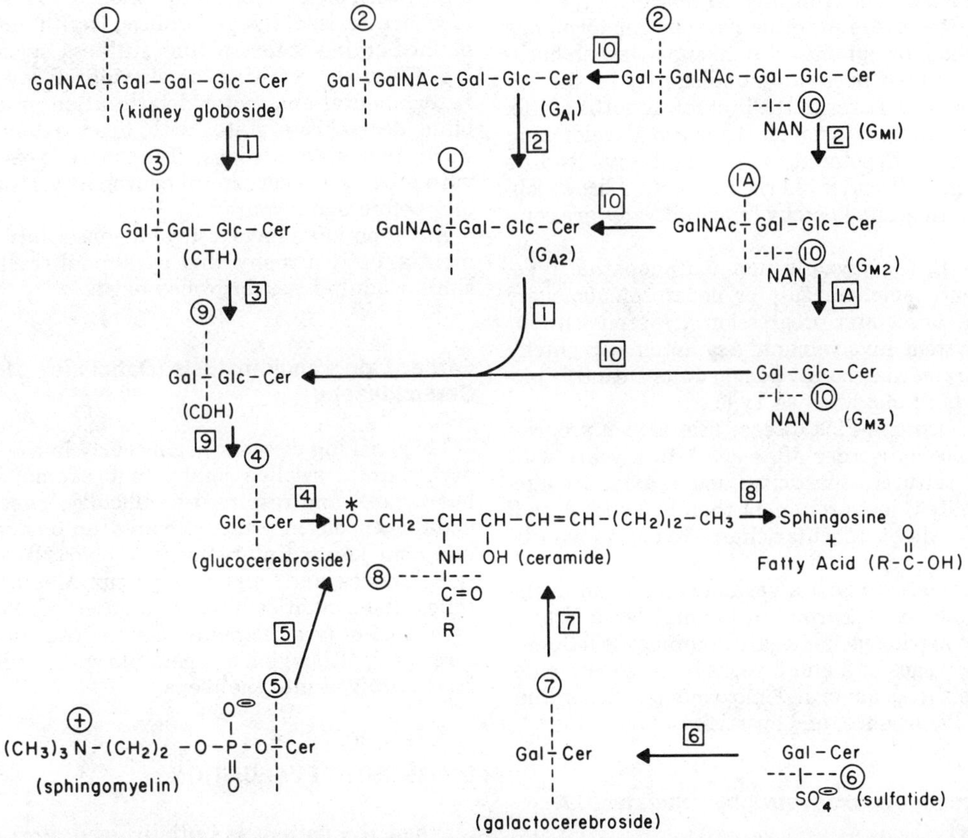

Figure 1. Degradation of the major sphingolipids by lysosomal hydrolase enzymes. Cer = Ceramid; Glc = glucose; Gal = galactose; GalNAc = N-acetylgalactosamine; NAN = N-acetylneuraminic acid; * = point at which glucose, or galactose, or phosphorylcholine is attached to ceramide, G_{M1} = G_{M1}-ganglioside; G_{M2} = G_{M2}-ganglioside; G_{M3} = G_{M3}-ganglioside; G_{A1} = asialo-G_{M1}-ganglioside (gangliotetraosylceramide); G_{A2} = asialo-G_{M2}-ganglioside (gangliotriaosylceramide); CTH = ceramide trihexoside (globotriaosyl ceramide); CDH = ceramide dihexoside (lactosylceramide).

Solid arrows and numbers in squares show enzyme reaction pathways; broken lines and numbers in circles show position of bond broken by enzyme reaction. 1 = hexosaminidases A and B; IA = hexosaminidase A only (with activator); 2 = G_{M1}-ganglioside beta-galactosidase; 3 = alpha-galactosidase (ceramide trihexosidase); 4 = cerebroside beta-glucosidase (glucocerebrosidase); 5 = sphingomyelinase; 6 = sulfatase A (arylsulfatase A); 7 = cerebroside beta-galactosidase (galactocerebrosidase): 8 = ceramidase; 9 = lactosylceramide beta-galactosidase; 10 = monosialoganglioside neuraminidase.

myeloma may be a late complication. This form is most common in patients of Ashkenazi Jewish background.

In a few cases, otherwise compatible with the diagnosis of adult Gaucher disease, there has been central nervous system involvement, including seizures and dementia. These patients probably have a fourth distinct phenotype.

Niemann-Pick Disease (Sphingomyelinase Deficiency in Some Types Only)

This name is given to a heterogeneous group of diseases that have in common tissue storage of the sphingolipid sphingomyelin. Types A and B in the Crocker and Farber classification have sphingomyelinase deficiency. In Types C and D the basic defect is unclear; they may not be related at all to Niemann-Pick disease, but no better name is at hand. Partial and variable sphingomyelinase deficiency has been reported in Types C and D. A sphingomyelinase isozyme has been reported deficient in Types C and E. Heat-labile sphingomyelinase deficiency has been reported as Type F in a disorder clinically resembling Type B.

Type A, the severe infantile neuropathic form, has a predilection for patients of Ashkenazi Jewish background. Transient neonatal jaundice may be the initial abnormality. Later in the first few months of life, hepatosplenomegaly is noted. Dementia, developmental regression, hypotonia, and weight loss lead to death by age 2. Macular cherry-red spots, a brownish-yellow skin tinge, and patchy lung infiltrates are common.

In Type B, the juvenile non-neuronopathic type, asymptomatic splenomegaly or hepatosplenomegaly of variable onset and progression are seen without nervous system involvement. Asymptomatic patchy lung infiltrates may occur. Some adults with this picture have been classified as Type E.

Type C Niemann-Pick disease begins as a progressive neurologic disorder after age 1 to 2 years with dementia, seizures, spasticity, and ataxia. Hepatosplenomegaly is less prominent than in Types A or B and may be slight. Macular cherry-red spots may be seen.

Type D, the Nova Scotia variant, was found in the inbred Acadians of Yarmouth County, Nova Scotia. Prominent hepatosplenomegaly in infancy is followed between the ages of 2 and 5 years by progressive dementia, seizures, abnormal movements, incoordination, gait disturbance, and spasticity.

Metachromatic Leukodystrophy (Sulfatase A Deficiency)

At least four phenotypes have been described. Late-infantile metachromatic leukodystrophy (MLD) begins, usually in the second year of life, with difficulty walking due to flaccid hypotonic paraparesis, spastic paresis, or even ataxia. Later dementia and dysarthria occur, and tendon reflexes are lost. Patients die in a vegetative state, quadriplegic, with bulbar and pseudobulbar palsies and optic atrophy, usually between ages 4 and 8 years.

A heterogeneous group of patients with juvenile MLD has a similar clinical picture with later onset (usually ages 3 to 10 years) and slower progression. These may present with emotional, intellectual, or gait disorders.

An adult phenotype presents with psychiatric disorder or progressive dementia in the third or fourth decade. Seizures, ataxia, or hyperreflexia may be found; neuropathy is not usually clinically apparent.

A fourth phenotype is that of multiple sulfatase deficiency (MSD). The neurologic disorder resembles that of late-infantile MLD, though onset may be earlier and early development slow. However, patients develop skeletal changes resembling those of the mucopolysaccharidoses, mildly coarsened facial features, icthyosis, and in some cases seizures and hepatosplenomegaly.

Krabbe Leukodystrophy, Globoid Cell Leukodystrophy (Deficiency of Cerebroside beta-Galactosidase)

Krabbe leukodystrophy nearly always begins in infancy, with onset at age 3 to 6 months. The condition is characterized by generalized irritability, unexplained crying or fevers, limb stiffness, seizures, feeding difficulty, vomiting, or slowing of development. Later, mental and motor deterioration progress to a blind decerebrate state, with head extended backward, and optic atrophy. Tendon reflexes decrease with progressive peripheral neuropathy. Death is usually before age 2 years.

A few patients have a juvenile-onset form with dementia, optic atrophy, and pyramidal tract signs. A similar adult-onset form may exist.

Farber Lipogranulomatosis (Deficiency of Acid Ceramidase)

This striking disorder begins early in the first year with painful swollen joints, limb edema, vomiting, hoarseness, and respiratory difficulty. Subcutaneous nodules appear at pressure points, on tendon sheaths and near joints. Enlargement of heart, liver, spleen, lymph nodes, and tongue may occur. Mental defect or reflex abnormalities have been observed. Pulmonary involvement (granulomata) usually leads to death before age 2, although a few patients with a milder form have survived into the teens.

DIAGNOSTIC EVALUATION

When the patient is initially seen, it is not clear whether the cause of the clinical syndrome is a sphingolipidosis, another genetic-metabolic disease, or a nongenetic disorder. We have classified our evaluation for suspected genetic-metabolic disease into (1) history and examination, (2) family history and genetic evaluation, and (3) laboratory evaluation. This discussion focuses on testing for the sphingolipidoses; obviously, a wider group of metabolic screening tests is appropriate for most patients with suspected genetic-metabolic disease.

History and Examination

If the clinical disorder was present at birth or if it began abruptly after meningitis or encephalitis, and if the clinical defect has been nonprogressive for many years, the chances are small that a sphingolipidosis is the cause.

A clinical disorder confined to the nervous system suggests a G_{M2}-gangliosidosis (nearly all types), late-infantile G_{M1}-gangliosidosis, metachromatic leukodystrophy, or Krabbe leukodystrophy; some patients with Niemann-Pick disease Type C have little organ enlargement.

Isolated splenomegaly, often with thrombocytopenia or bleeding diathesis, suggests the "adult type" (Type 1) of Gaucher disease. Hepatomegaly is prominent in Niemann-Pick disease and in Farber disease, although splenomegaly may also occur. Hepatosplenomegaly is seen in infantile G_{M1}-gangliosidosis, infantile Gaucher and Niemann-Pick diseases, and multiple sulfatase deficiency, as well as early-onset sialidoses, Wolman disease, and other lysosomal storage diseases.

Skeletal changes of mucopolysaccharidosis are seen (clinically and roentgenographically) in infantile G_{M1}-gangliosidosis and multiple sulfatase deficiency, as well as in sialidoses and other mucolipidoses.

Characteristic skin lesions (angiokeratomata) are seen in Fabry disease; similar lesions may occur in fucosidosis and sialidosis. Characteristic skin nodules and arthritis are seen in Farber disease. Ichthyosis is noted in multiple sulfatase deficiency. Increased skin pigmentation may occur in Gaucher or Niemann-Pick disease or in adrenoleukodystrophy.

Macular cherry-red spot is seen in early onset G_{M2}-gangliosidoses, infantile G_{M1}-gangliosidosis, some forms of sialidosis, and Niemann-Pick disease Type A and occasionally Type C. Perifoveal grayish deposits have been seen in metachromatic leukodystrophy and Farber disease. A typical cherry-red spot in juvenile G_{M2}-gangliosidosis may "degenerate" into a brownish macular and perimacular deposit. Pigmentary retinal degeneration is seen in the closely related neuronal ceroid lipofuscinoses, as well as Refsum disease, Bassen-Kornzweig disease, and Kearns-Sayre syndrome. Tortuous retinal vessels may be seen in Fabry disease. Corneal clouding may occur in infantile G_{M1}-gangliosidosis and Fabry hemizygotes or heterozygotes, as well as in patients with mucopolysaccharidosis or mucolipidoses. Optic atrophy occurs in both Krabbe and metachromatic leukodystrophies and in some other sphingolipidoses.

Lymphedema of the legs or stroke may occur in Fabry disease.

Family History and Genetic Evaluation

If the family history shows apparently dominant transmission of the same defect over three consecutive generations, the likelihood of sphingolipidosis is small. Fabry disease, the only X-linked sphingolipidosis, has a characteristic pedigree pattern. All of the other sphingolipidoses have autosomal recessive inheritance. Characteristically, multiple affected sibs, both male and female, are born from normal parents. Increased frequency of parental consanguinity is seen in rare recessives and this should be inquired after. Alpha-locus hexosaminidase deficiencies, adult Gaucher disease (Type 1), and Niemann-Pick disease Type A have predilection for patients of Ashkenazi Jewish background. (See article on Approach to Genetic Disease.)

It is important to document the carrier state in the patient's family members when this is possible. This helps confirm the patient's diagnosis. It also helps to detect genetic compounds. It is important to complete thorough documentation of the patient's enzyme deficiency, and the carrier state in parents, in cultured skin fibroblasts well before prenatal diagnosis is contemplated.

Laboratory Evaluation

The laboratory evaluation (Table 1) for suspected sphingolipidosis consists of three parts:

1. Biochemical study of blood, urine, and cultured skin fibroblasts.
2. Electrophysiologic and roentgenographic studies.
3. Light and electron microscopic study of biopsy material.

Most of the sphingolipidoses can be readily diagnosed by means of noninvasive (Group 1) studies. Three kinds of specimens are useful: blood, urine, and cultured skin fibroblasts. It is important to check the requirements of the laboratory performing the assays *before* any specimens are taken.

Biochemical Studies

Blood Studies. Nearly all of the sphingolipid hydrolases can be determined in blood. For some enzymes, however, there is better discrimination between patients and controls, or between heterozygous carriers and controls, in cultured skin fibroblasts. Some enzymes are more readily determined in blood leukocytes than in serum (or vice versa). Some enzymes can conveniently be determined together in a single leukocyte preparation. Others require a special extraction procedure and a separate blood sample for their determination.

Ten lysosomal hydrolase enzymes, all relatively active and easily measured in blood using artificial substrates, can be determined together as a lysosomal battery screening test: hexosaminidase (A and B), beta-galactosidase, alpha-galactosidase, sulfatase A, alpha-mannosidase, alpha-L-fucosidase, alpha-glucosidase, alpha-N-acetylglucosaminidase, beta-glucuronidase, and acid phosphatase. These include four of the sphingolipidoses discussed (Table 1).

A lysosomal battery ordinarily requires 1 ml serum and leukocytes from 10 ml plasma. For the serum sample, a single 7-ml clotted Vacutainer tube is filled (or half-filled) and conveyed to the laboratory cooled with crushed ice. Serum may be separated and stored frozen (–70°C) if a series of samples is to be collected and shipped together. Plasma, however, should be collected (usually with citrate or EDTA) on the same day or the day before it is used to prepare a leukocyte

Table 1. Laboratory Evaluation for Suspected Sphingolipidoses

Disorder	Characteristic Clinical Features	Enzyme Deficiency*	Enzyme Diagnosis in	Confirmatory Tests
G_{M2}-gangliosidoses	Dementia, myoclonic seizures, blindness, and macular cherry-red spots predominate in *early-onset forms*; cerebellar ataxia and spinal muscular atrophy predominate in *late-onset forms*. Ashkenazi Jewish predilection (alpha-locus forms)	Hexosaminidase (#1, 1A) a. Alpha-locus disorders: Hexosaminidases A (and S) (Tay-Sachs disease and variants) b. Beta-locus disorders: Hexosaminidases A and B (Sandhoff disease and variants) c. Activator-locus disorders: Hexosaminidase A activator (AB-variant)	a. Serum, leukocytes, cultured skin fibroblasts, urine b. Serum, leukocytes, cultured skin fibroblasts, urine c. Cultured skin fibroblasts	Membranous cytoplasmic bodies in rectal ganglion cells (all types) Excess urinary oligosaccharides in beta-locus disorders
G_{M1}-gangliosidoses	*Infantile form* gives encephalopathy, hepatosplenomegaly, bone and joint involvement, often cherry-red spots; in a *late-infantile* form, encephalopathy predominates; in a later onset form (*Morquio type B*), skeletal involvement predominates	G_{M1}-ganglioside beta-galactosidase (#2)	Leukocytes, cultured skin fibroblasts	Excess urinary oligosaccharides in characteristic pattern
Fabry disease	Purple 1- to 3-mm macular-maculopapular skin lesions, painful neuropathy, renal disease; X-linked (incompletely) recessive inheritance; vascular involvement may occur (lymphedema, stroke)	Alpha-galactosidase A (#3)	Plasma or serum, leukocytes, cultured skin fibroblasts	Characteristic histologic and histochemical appearance of biopsied skin lesions
Gaucher disease	*Infantile form:* severe hepatosplenomegaly and severe encephalopathy; *juvenile form:* milder nervous system involvement, variable splenomegaly; *"adult" form* (may begin in childhood): splenomegaly (thrombocytopenia), bone involvement, nervous system unaffected, Ashkenazi Jewish predilection	Cerebroside beta-glucosidase (glucocerebrosidase) (#4)	Cultured skin fibroblasts, leukocytes	Characteristic foam cells in bone marrow

Niemann-Pick disease	*Type A:* severe infantile hepatosplenomegaly and severe encephalopathy, often cherry-red spots, Ashkenazi Jewish predilection, *Type B:* hepatosplenomegaly in childhood without encephalopathy; *Type C:* childhood encephalopathy with variable organ enlargement; *Type D:* infantile hepatosplenomegaly and childhood encephalopathy in Nova Scotia Acadians; *Type E:* adult organ enlargement without nervous system involvement; *Type F:* resembles Type B but with heat-labile sphingomyelinase	Sphingomyelinase (#5) (Deficient in types A, B, and F only; often partially deficient in "type C"; heat-labile in type F)	Cultured skin fibroblasts, leukocytes (Types A, B, and F only)	Characteristic foam cells in bone marrow (all types) Types C and D: Characteristic membranous bodies by electron microscopy in rectal, skin, or conjunctival biopsy Types C, D, and E: Elevated sphingomyelin in liver biopsy
Metachromatic leukodystrophy	*Late infantile form:* dementia, spasticity, optic atrophy, neuropathy; *juvenile forms:* similar but later onset; *adult form:* dementia predominates; *multiple sulfatase deficiency:* infantile neurologic deterioration with seizures, ichthyosis, and mucopolysaccharidosis-like face and bone changes	a. Sulfatase A (sulfatide sulfatase) (#6) (late-infantile, juvenile, and adult forms) b. Sulfatase A activator (usually resembles juvenile form clinically) c. Sulfatase A and at least ten other sulfatases (multiple sulfatase deficiency)	a. Serum, leukocytes, cultured skin fibroblasts, urine b. Cultured skin fibroblasts c. Cultured skin fibroblasts	Metachromatic cells and demyelination by light microscopy, tuffstone bodies by electron microscopy in myelinated nerve from skin or sural nerve biopsy
Krabbe leukodystrophy	*Infantile* encephalopathy, seizures, optic atrophy, neuropathy; rare later-onset forms	Cerebroside beta-galactosidase (#7) (galactocerebrosidase)	Serum, leukocytes, cultured skin fibroblasts	Demyelination and needle-like inclusions by electron microscopy on nerve biopsy
Farber disease	Early infantile painful arthropathy; subcutaneous nodules near joints, tendon sheaths, and pressure points; hoarseness; often hepatomegaly	Acid ceramidase (#8)	Cultured skin fibroblasts, leukocytes	Characteristic light and electron microscopic picture of biopsied skin lesions

*Numbers in parentheses refer to reactions in Figure 1.

pellet for assay. This blood must *not* be frozen, but should be conveyed to the laboratory on crushed ice. For shipping, a large styrofoam container (1 to 2 cubic feet contents) containing well-labeled blood tubes and crushed ice (not dry ice or "freezer-paks") in separate sealed plastic bags is sent by overnight carrier to arrive by the middle of the following day.

Certain other lysosomal hydrolase enzyme measurements require an entire leukocyte pellet, or a separate extraction procedure, or are better determined in fibroblasts. These include four of the sphingolipidoses (Table 1). In addition, the activator-deficient forms of G_{M2}-gangliosidosis and metachromatic leukodystrophy require study of cultured skin fibroblasts.

Urine Studies. Patients with the various forms of G_{M1}-gangliosidosis excrete excess urinary oligosaccharides (as do patients with other forms of the so-called mucolipidoses). The characteristic pattern of urinary oligosaccharides can be demonstrated by thin-layer chromatography or liquid chromatography using 1 ml of urine brought or shipped to the laboratory on wet ice or frozen. The excessive urinary mucopolysaccharides found in multiple sulfatase deficiency can be demonstrated by screening tests using 1 to 5 ml of urine or by more definitive quantitative and qualitative testing using a 25- to 100-ml aliquot of 24-hour urine of known volume delivered as described.

Fibroblast Studies. Skin biopsy is probably the most useful single diagnostic procedure. All of the sphingolipidoses (except Niemann-Pick disease, types C, D, and E) can be diagnosed by enzyme assay in cultured skin fibroblasts. The piece of skin should be divided sterilely immediately after biopsy: half is placed in a sterile solution for culture (usually minimal essential medium plus 10 per cent fetal calf serum, most easily obtained from a hospital laboratory growing cells from amniocentesis fluid for chromosome study), the other half is fixed in buffered glutaraldehyde solution for electron microscopy (EM).

Skin biopsy, a simple painless procedure, may be done at the same time as muscle or nerve biopsy. As a separate procedure (routinely done by medical geneticists and dermatologists), a sterile 3.5-mm disposable punch is used to remove a full-thickness plug from skin that has been carefully cleaned and infiltrated with intradermal xylocaine. Any bleeding is stopped with direct pressure of a sterile gauze pad or a sterile swab with Monsel's solution (ferric subsulfate) or aluminum chloride solution. A suture may or may not be used. The usual location is the volar forearm or shoulder; buttock or anterior thigh may be used with a small infant. Skin plugs for culture or EM may be shipped directly cooled with wet ice. Preconfluent cultures are shipped at room temperature in sealed flasks filled with medium, protected from temperature extremes by a styrofoam container. Harvested fibroblast pellets may be shipped on dry ice with control fibroblasts grown under identical conditions.

Electrophysiologic, Roentgenographic, and Cerebrospinal Fluid Studies

These studies are nonspecific, but are often very helpful. Decreased nerve conduction velocities indicating demyelinating neuropathy are helpful in Krabbe leukodystrophy and metachromatic leukodystrophy.

Electromyography (EMG) provides a useful indication of denervation from neuropathy (leukodystrophy or Fabry's disease) or anterior horn cell disease (hexosaminidase deficiencies).

Electroretinogram (ERG) is abolished in patients with the neuronal ceroid lipofuscinoses (disorders clinically similar to G_{M2}-gangliosidoses) and other patients with pigmentary retinal degeneration. The ERG may be abnormal in disorders with cherry-red spot or milder retinal involvement (late-onset hexosaminidase deficiency). Visual evoked responses are helpful to document optic atrophy, as in the early-onset leukodystrophies.

Roentgenographic changes of mucopolysaccharidosis, especially beaked ovoid vertebrae on lateral spine films, are helpful in diagnosis of G_{M1}-gangliosidosis and multiple sulfatase deficiency. Calcified adrenal glands on abdominal films are seen in Wolman disease.

Elevated cerebrospinal fluid (CSF) protein is also a helpful though nonspecific finding in the early-onset leukodystrophies. Interestingly, some patients with late-onset hexosaminidase deficiency have had oligoclonal bands in CSF.

Biopsies

Although nearly all the sphingolipidoses are diagnosable by specific enzyme testing, biopsies remain useful for five reasons:

1. Skin biopsies are routinely required as a source of cultured skin fibroblasts.
2. The enzyme deficiencies in some sphingolipidoses, such as Niemann-Pick disease types C and D, are unknown. The only method of diagnosis is by demonstration of stored sphingomyelin (and other phospholipids) in tissue together with the characteristic clinical, histologic, and ultrastructural features.
3. In some sphingolipidoses, such as the AB variant (where a HEX A activator is deficient) or the metachromatic leukodystrophy variant with activator deficiency (where a sulfatase A activator is deficient), specific biochemical testing is difficult, time-consuming, and expensive; such testing is most clearly warranted after clear ultrastructural evidence of the disorder is obtained by rectal or sural nerve biopsy, respectively.
4. Related disorders in the differential diagnosis, such as the neuronal ceroid lipofuscinoses, the progressive myoclonus epilepsies, or the neuraxonal dystrophies, may be diagnosed only by biopsy.
5. Biopsy is useful to confirm that an enzyme deficiency found (even a genetically transmitted one) is really the cause of the patient's disease.

Rectal biopsy remains useful both as a screening test and confirmatory test because it is the simplest and safest source of nerve cell bodies for electron microscopy. In the G_{M2}-gangliosidoses, ganglion cells alone are filled with membranous cytoplasmic bodies, although some axons and Schwann cells may show abnormalities. The sample should be taken at least 3 cm in from the mucocutaneous junction to avoid the aganglionic zone. The biopsy should be mucosal-submucosal (not deep into the muscularis) and directed posteriorly toward the sacrum to avoid the risk of perforation. Careful handling, positioning, and embedding of the specimen are essential, since submucosal ganglion cells are sparse.

Sural nerve biopsy remains useful in the leukodystrophies. It may be done at the ankle with skin biopsy or at the calf with skin and muscle biopsy. If metachromatic leukodystrophy is clinically suspected but enzyme measurements with artificial substrates fail to show clear sulfatase A deficiency, nerve biopsy may still show demyelinating neuropathy with metachromatic changes and the characteristic tuffstone bodies by EM. With Krabbe leukodystrophy, the characteristic ultrastructural needle-like inclusions in nerve are useful in confirming the enzyme deficiency.

Ultrastructural study of the *skin biopsy* is particularly useful, since sweat glands, hair follicles, blood vessels, and some myelinated nerve fibers can be seen. Schwann cells of myelinated nerve fibers will show changes in leukodystrophies as discussed. Widespread, intracellular, punched-out lysosomal membranous and vesicular bodies are seen in Niemann-Pick disease, type C. The neuronal ceroid lipofucinoses have curvilinear bodies in multiple cell types in skin. Electron microscopy of biopsied skin is the simplest diagnostic test for Lafora disease (a form of recessive progressive myoclonus epilepsy), which has characteristic inclusions in sweat gland duct cells (only) of skin.

Bone marrow aspirate can be examined by both light and electron microscopy. This is a generally useful screening procedure because many lysosomal diseases have foam cells or otherwise distinctive abnormal storage cells in the marrow. This remains especially useful for Gaucher disease and Niemann-Pick disease, especially the forms without sphingomyelinase deficiency. Likewise on the *peripheral smear,* many lysosomal diseases will produce vacuoles or abnormal granules in lymphocytes or monocytes, making this a simple and useful though nonspecific and nondefinitive screening test.

Conjunctival biopsy is also a useful nonspecific source of tissue for screening ultrastructural studies.

Muscle biopsy, often obtained for study of disorders affecting the lower motor neuron, provides another useful source of tissue in which nonspecific lysosomal bodies may be seen in the sphingolipidoses.

Finally, the *placenta* should not be overlooked as a source of tissue for ultrastructural or biochemical study in the neonate; a few cases of G_{M1}-gangliosidosis, Niemann-Pick disease, and congenital sialidosis will be identified in the neonate.

GENETIC DEFECTS OF AMINO ACID METABOLISM AND TRANSPORT*

By Irvin A. Kaufman, M.D.
and William L. Nyhan, M.D., Ph.D.
San Diego, California

Disorders of amino acid metabolism and transport are hereditary conditions, all but one of which described to date are transmitted as autosomal recessive traits. Parents of affected children are asymptomatic heterozygous carriers of the mutant gene. In most populations the frequency of the carrier state is relatively high, whereas the chance that two nonconsanguineous carriers will mate is small. In any pregnancy the chance is one in four that two carriers will produce an affected child. For the most part, these disorders result from a defect in a single enzyme. Thus they are classic inborn errors of metabolism as first described by Garrod, the founder of the science of modern biochemical genetics.

These disorders include conditions in which the metabolic defect is generalized throughout the body and those in which the abnormality is specific to a single tissue or transport function. *Aminoaciduria* is the hallmark of most of these disorders. However, in some, such as albinism, the defect is so localized that there is no evidence of altered metabolism in urine or blood. Aminoaciduria can result from inefficient metabolism of amino acids, leading to elevated levels in the blood, which then exceed the renal capacity for reabsorption and overflow into the urine. Alternatively, aminoaciduria can be the result of defects in renal tubular transport. In these conditions, plasma concentrations of amino acids are normal or low. There are also the no-threshold aminoacidurias, such as argininosuccinicaciduria. In these situations the compound is excreted so efficiently or reabsorbed so inefficiently that elevated concentrations are not found in blood, even though the basic mechanism for the aminoaciduria is a defect of cellular metabolism.

DISORDERS OF AMINO ACID METABOLISM

Clinical manifestations vary widely (Table 1). Some are biochemical abnormalities in which there are no clinical consequences at all, whereas in others life-threatening illnesses may manifest themselves from the moment of birth. With few exceptions, the manifestations of these diseases are not specific. Many interfere with the development of the central nervous system, causing mental retardation. Seizures may occur with or without other neurologic signs. Many of the disorders of amino acid metabolism and transport have been discovered by screening populations of retarded individuals.

An increasing number of disorders of amino acid metabolism are recognized to produce severe illness and death in early life. They should be considered in very ill newborns with unexplained acidosis, hyperammonemia, convulsions, coma, or hypotonia. Early recognition and diagnosis are important, as these diseases that present with overwhelming illness in the newborn period do not necessarily cause mental retardation.

When large populations of patients with established symptoms—for instance, populations with mental retardation—are screened for aminoaciduria, the incidence of positives is small, approximately 0.2 per cent. Screening is nevertheless important, because the recognition of an affected child alerts the physician to the possibility of further cases in a family. Many of these disorders are susceptible to programs of prenatal diagnosis and carrier detection once an index case has been diagnosed.

Because some of these disorders are associated with no obvious abnormality of development or intelligence, it is possible that other inborn errors of metabolism occur in populations of children who have never been screened. With current technology and the growing recognition that the metabolic screening of newborns is a worthwhile public health measure, it is likely that we will be able to establish the true incidence and significance of many more inborn disorders of metabolism.

Phenylketonuria

Phenylketonuria (PKU) is the result of a metabolic defect in which phenylalanine cannot be converted to tyrosine and phenylpyruvic acid is excreted in the urine. With the advent of large-scale screening of newborn infants, it has become evident that a variety of phenylalaninemias exist in addition to what has come to be known as classic phenylketonuria.

The most important clinical characteristic in classic phenylketonuria is mental retardation. Most untreated patients have a severe degree of mental deficiency, with intelligence quotients under 30. However, a few untreated phenylketonuric patients have been reported with borderline intelligence. Phenylketonuric infants appear normal at birth. Symptoms occur in over half of them early in life. Vomiting has been severe enough to lead to surgery for pyloric stenosis. Irritability, an eczematoid rash, or a peculiar odor may also be present in the early months. General physical development is usually normal. These children are fair-haired, fair-skinned, and blue-eyed in over 90 per cent of the cases. However, dark skin, hair, or irides do not exclude the diagnosis. Minor anomalies such as epicanthal folds may be seen in an appreciable number of patients with this disorder or with other inborn errors of metabolism.

Neurologic findings are not prominent. A third of the patients have none, whereas minimal signs, such as hyperactivity of deep tendon reflexes or mildly hypertonic muscles, occur in another third. More

*Supported by a grant from Maternal and Child Health Services MCJ-004007.

Table 1. Inborn Errors of Amino Acid Metabolism

Disorder	Enzyme Defect	Manifestations
Albinism	Tyrosinase (melanocyte granules)	Lack of pigment, local or universal—skin, hair and eyes
Alkaptonuria	Homogentisic acid oxidase	Dark urine, reducing substance; ochronosis; arthritis
Argininosuccinic aciduria	Argininosuccinase	Trichorrhexis nodosa, seizures, hyperammonemia, MR*
Citrullinemia	Argininosuccinate synthase	Mental retardation, hyperammonemia, death†
Cystathioninuria	Cystathionase	Mental retardation; may be normal
Ethylmalonic aciduria	Multiple acyl CoA dehydrogenases, exact defect unknown	Coma, hypoglycemia, hyperammonemia
Glutaric aciduria I	Glutaryl CoA dehydrogenase	Spasticity, neurologic deterioration progressing to death
Glutaric aciduria II	Multiple acyl CoA dehydrogenases, exact defect unknown	Acidosis, hypoglycemia and death
Hawkinsinuria	4-Hydroxyphenylpyruvic acid dioxygenase	Acidosis, failure to thrive
Histidinemia	Histidase	Speech retardation, $FeCl_3$, may have MR
Homocystinuria	Cystathionine synthase	Ectopia lentis, thromboembolism, failure to thrive, MR
γ-Hydroxybutyric aciduria	Succinic semialdehyde dehydrogenase	MR, seizures
3-Hydroxy-3-methylglutaric aciduria	3-Hydroxy-3-methylglutaric CoA lyase	Acidosis, coma, apnea, hypoglycemia
Hyperammonemia	Carbamylphosphate synthetase, ornithine transcarbamylase	Episodic coma, MR
Hyperhydroxyprolinemia	Hydroxyproline oxidase	Small kidneys, hematuria, MR, may be normal
Hyperlysinemia	Lysine α-ketoglutarate reductase	Convulsions, hypotonia, growth retardation
Hyperprolinemia	Proline oxidase, Δ-pyrroline-5-carboxylic acid dehydrogenase	Nephropathy, deafness, MR, may be normal
Hypersarcosinemia		MR, vomiting, failure to thrive
Hypervalinemia	Valine transaminase	Death,† MR
Isovaleric acidemia	Isovaleryl CoA dehydrogenase	Odor, convulsions, coma, MR, death†
Maple syrup urine disease	Branched-chain keto acid decarboxylase	Urinary odor, coma, flaccidity, opisthotonus, death,† MR
β-Methylcrotonylglycinuria	β-Methylcrotonyl CoA carboxylase	Failure to thrive, dermatosis, ketosis, acidosis, death†
α-Methyl-β-hydroxybutyric acidemia	α-Methylacetoacetyl CoA thiolase	Intermittent acidosis, ketosis, MR
Methylmalonic acidemia	Methylmalonyl CoA mutase	Recurrent vomiting, ketosis, coma, failure to thrive, pancytopenia, death,† MR
Multiple carboxylase deficiency	Holocarboxylase synthetase biotin transport defect	Skin rash, vomiting, alopecia, seizures
Nonketotic hyperglycinemia		Convulsions, cerebral palsy, MR, death†
Oxalosis	Glyoxylate carboligase	Renal calculi, renal failure
Phenylketonuria	Phenylalanine-hydroxylase	Blond hair, blue eyes, eczema, $FeCl_3$, MR, urinary reducing substance
Propionic acidemia	Propionyl CoA carboxylase	Recurrent vomiting and ketosis, thrombocytopenia, neutropenia, osteoporosis, death,† MR
Pyroglutamic acidemia	Glutathione synthetase	Chronic acidosis, ataxia, MR
Tyrosinosis (Medes) Tyrosinosis	*p*-Hydroxyphenylpyruvic acid oxidase	Hepatic cirrhosis, renal Fanconi syndrome

In each instance it is recognized that there may be heterogeneity in which multiple forms of a defective enzyme may lead to different phenotypic manifestations. For instance, in the decarboxylation of the branched-chain keto acids a complete deficiency leads to classic maple syrup urine disease; a different level of defect leads to a milder disease known as intermittent branched-chain ketoaciduria. In this table only one form has been listed.

*MR indicates mental retardation.

†The disorders designated as causing death are those in which a rapid fulminating course often complicates early infancy.

severely involved patients may have manifestations of spastic cerebral palsy. Seizures occur in about a fourth of the patients, usually those most severely retarded. Electroencephalographic abnormalities have been described in approximately 80 per cent of patients, and pneumoencephalograms may reveal cortical atrophy.

Autopsy reports on affected children show lack of myelinization in the central nervous system. The absence of these findings in patients studied after 21 years of age suggests that the formation of myelin is delayed or inhibited by the chemical abnormality and is consistent with the idea that the manifestations of phenylketonuria are those of an intoxication.

Phenylalanine is normally converted to tyrosine in the first step of its oxidative metabolism. The tyrosine formed is then oxidized, ultimately forming acetoacetate and fumarate, which are readily converted to carbon dioxide and water. The fundamental defect in phenylketonuria is the absence of phenylalanine hydroxylase. With a block in phenylalanine hydroxylase, tyrosine becomes an essential amino acid and alternate pathways are used to metabolize phenylalanine, which along with its metabolic products accumulates in body fluids. These compounds are normal metabolites present in abnormal amounts. Plasma concentrations of phenylalanine range from 6 to 80 mg/dl in patients with phenylketonuria, in contrast to values approximating 1 mg/dl in controls. Most patients with classic phenylketonuria have concentrations well over 30 mg/dl throughout infancy. There is a roughly linear relation between levels of phenylalanine in the blood and the urinary excretion of phenylpyruvic acid.

The disease occurs in 1 out of every 10,000 to 20,000 persons. It is an autosomal recessive character, equally represented in both sexes. Many heterozygotes may be recognized by the measurement of plasma concentrations of phenylalanine and tyrosine after oral loading with phenylalanine, but there is overlap with the normal population and a normal phenylalanine tolerance curve does not exclude heterozygosity.

Successful prevention of the clinical manifestations of the disease by restriction of the dietary intake of phenylalanine has provided strong support for the concept that the clinical disease represents an intoxication produced by the abnormal chemical milieu in which these patients must live and develop. Palatable preparations such as Lofenalac (Mead Johnson) make long-term treatment economically feasible. Dietary therapy readily lowers levels of phenylalanine in the blood, and concomitantly phenylpyruvic acid and its metabolic products disappear. Clinical improvement in neurologic findings, in behavior, and in the electroencephalogram is observed. Eczematoid lesions heal and increase in pigmentation occurs. Patients tolerate the diet well, but the management of an infant on a low-phenylalanine diet is not easy. Phenylketonuric infants often vomit or refuse feedings. Infections may complicate their metabolic state. Management should be under the direction of an experienced physician with the laboratory facilities for the routine accurate determination of the serum concentration of phenylalanine. All infants, including those with phenylketonuria, require a certain amount of phenylalanine. These minimal essential quantities are known and should be employed in management.

The major criterion for undertaking dietary therapy is its effect on mental capacity. In general, the diet is effective in preventing mental deficiency and neurologic abnormalities, if started in the first weeks of life. A loss of 5 IQ units for each 10 weeks that treatment is delayed has been calculated. This figure is certainly only approximate, but it provides a strong argument for early diagnosis and the early institution of dietary therapy. Treatment of patients for the first time after the age of 3 years is without effect on mental development. Therapy may be of use in the clinical management of older patients because of beneficial effects on eczema, seizures, or uncontrollable behavior even in the absence of effects on intelligence.

It has now become routine in the United States and most of the developed countries of the world to test all newborn infants in the population in order to recognize patients with phenylketonuria as early as possible. Urine tests are of limited value for this purpose, for phenylpyruvic acid is not detected until plasma phenylalanine levels exceed 15 to 20 mg/dl, and may be absent from the urine of phenylketonuric patients for 1 to 2 months. Current screening procedures employ an assay for the concentration of phenylalanine in a drop of blood spotted on a piece of filter paper. Levels of phenylalanine above 6 mg/dl are considered positive. Once the physician is confronted with a positive screening test, he must then make a diagnosis.

The first step in diagnosis is the quantitative analysis of the concentrations of phenylalanine and tyrosine in the blood. Most infants turned up in the screening programs simply have a delayed maturation of amino acid metabolizing enzymes, and their tyrosine concentrations are very high. These infants can then be excluded and followed expectantly. On a normal diet the patient with classic phenylketonuria generally has a very rapid rise in the serum concentration of phenylalanine to levels well over 30 mg/dl, whereas the concentration of tyrosine is low. We like to admit infants with elevations of serum phenylalanine without tyrosine to the hospital to study them while they are receiving known daily intake of phenylalanine. We initiate dietary therapy in patients who have high concentrations of phenylalanine in the blood and excrete its metabolites in urine.

When the baby is 3 to 4 months old, we readmit to the hospital and challenge with a 3-day phenylalanine load. An infant with classic PKU will experience a steady rise in serum phenylalanine concentration to a level over 30 mg/dl. Metabolites will appear in the urine. These methods reliably distinguish patients with hyper-phenylalaninemia who do not need dietary treatment from patients with PKU who do.

A number of patients have recently been described with hyper-phenylalaninemia and normal phenylalanine hydroxylase activity. These patients have presented with progressive cerebral symptoms in spite of adequate dietary treatment, with serum phenylalanine levels maintained in a range usually associated with a good prognosis. They have been found to have defects in the synthesis of tetrahydrobiopterin, the cofactor for phenylalanine hydroxylase, or in the enzyme dihydropteridine reductase, which regenerates tetrahydrobiopterin from the quinonoid dihydrobiopterin that results from the phenylalanine hydroxylase reaction. Thus, each of these newly described defects results in the inability to convert phenylalanine to tyrosine, even though the phenylalanine hydroxylase apoenzyme is normal.

Tetrahydrobiopterin is also the cofactor for the hydroxylation of tryptophan and tyrosine. Thus its deficiency should interfere with the synthesis of serotonin, dihydroxyphenylalanine (dopa), and norepinephrine. Data have been obtained that indicate that this is the case, since levels of 5-hydroxyindoleacetic acids, vanillyl-mandelic acids, and homovanillic acid in the urine were considerably lower than normal.

Involved patients have had marked hypotonia, as well as spasticity and dystonic posturing. Some have seizures, myoclonus, and electroencephalographic abnormalities. Drooling is common. The delay in psychomotor development is usually profound.

The diagnosis of dihydropteridine reductase deficiency can be confirmed by assay of the enzyme in biopsied liver or cultured fibroblasts. The defective biosynthesis of tetrahydrobiopterin can be made by assay of the pattern of excretion of pterins in the urine. It can also be made by quantitative assay of tetrahydrobiopterin in the plasma, especially after the administration of a phenylalanine load. Phenylalanine leads to a dramatic increase in the level of tetrahydrobiopterin in normal individuals and in those with PKU or with dihydropteridine reductase deficiency, but there is no change in patients with defective biopterin synthesis.

The administration of tetrahydrobiopterin, which is currently available from investigators in Switzerland, leads to a prompt decrease to normal of serum concentrations of phenylalanine in patients with reductase and synthesis defects while the patient is receiving a normal diet. However, there is some question from animal experiments as to whether any administered tetrahydrobiopterin can get into the brain. Thus it is recommended that patients with these abnormalities be treated with biogenic amine precursors, such as 5-hydroxytryptophan and dopa, that do not require hydroxylation.

Tyrosinosis

Tyrosinemias are much more common than phenylalaninemias. In addition to the tyrosinemias that result from delayed maturation of tyrosine metabolizing enzymes and are particularly common in premature infants, tyrosinemia occurs in scurvy and many forms of liver disease. There are three disorders known as tyrosinosis.

In the form first described, tyrosinosis is an extremely rare metabolic disorder characterized by the excretion of p-hydroxyphenylpyruvic acid in the urine. There are probably no clinical manifestations of this metabolic abnormality, although the patient initially described had myasthenia gravis. These patients have a reducing reaction to the urine, which is due to the excretion of p-hydroxyphenylpyruvic acid. Patients with liver disease excrete abnormal quantities of this keto acid, but levels found in tyrosinosis were nearly ten times the highest values observed in liver disease. The metabolic abnormality of tyrosinosis could result from a deficiency of p-hydroxyphenylpyruvic acid oxidase. Exogenously administered, homogentisic acid is metabolized normally.

A much more common form of tyrosinosis is manifested by abnormalities in hepatic and renal function. Symptoms may begin early in infancy with an acute rapid course to demise or may progress more chronically. Although the disease has been described in two forms, acute and chronic, both have occurred in the same family, suggesting that a single disease is involved. Most patients have presented with failure to thrive and hepatosplenomegaly. The livers of these patients are cirrhotic, and icterus, ascites, and hemorrhage often ensue. They also develop a renal tubular acidosis of the Fanconi type, with glycosuria, hyperphosphaturia, and generalized amino-aciduria. Clinical rickets and typical roentgenographic changes may develop.

Biochemical alterations include elevated plasma concentrations of tyrosine, usually in the range of 3 to 12 mg/dl, and the excretion of tyrosyl compounds in the urine. Methionine concentrations in the plasma are also usually elevated. Hypoglycemia may occur with liver failure. Coagulation defects are common. Study of the enzymes of liver obtained at biopsy has indicated a deficiency of *p*-hydroxyphenylpyruvic acid oxidase, but it has not been established that this is the primary expression of the abnormal gene.

Succinyl acetone has recently been identified in the urine of these patients, and defective activity of maleylacetoacetate oxidase has been reported.

Genetic transmission appears to be that of an autosomal recessive. A particularly high frequency (0.67 per 1000 births) has been observed in a French-Canadian isolate. Frequency data are not available for other populations.

Treatment has been undertaken with diets low in both phenylalanine and tyrosine. Some patients have responded quite favorably in both the clinical and chemical features of the disease. Others have not.

Another form of tyrosinemia has been described in which the activity of tyrosine aminotransferase is deficient in the soluble cytoplasm of the liver. None of the patients with this disorder has had any evidence of hepatic or renal damage. One patient described in detail had multiple congenital anomalies, severe mental retardation, and self-mutilative behavior. He had corneal ulcers early in life and erythematous papular lesions on the palms and soles. Plasma concentrations of tyrosine ranged from 20 to 60 mg/dl.

A number of other patients have been reported. Some, but not all of them, have had marked retardation of mental development. All have had corneal lesions and lesions on the palms and soles that were either erythematous or keratotic.

Tyrosine aminotransferase activity is found in the mitochondria and in the cytoplasm. Only the cytoplasmic enzyme is deficient.

Hawkinsinuria

Hawkinsinuria is an unusual metabolic disease, in that it is an autosomal dominant trait with clinical expression in the heterozygote, at least in infancy. Its pathogenesis appears to result from the accumulation of a compound that produces illness by reaction with a variety of body constituents as well as the reaction with glutathione, which leads to the characteristic sulfur-containing amino acid that was named hawkinsin. Such mechanisms could explain how inborn metabolic defects could lead to teratogenesis. The new sulfur-containing amino acid isolated in this disorder is (2-L-cystein-S-yl-1,4-dihydroxycyclohex-5-en-1-61)-acetic acid, a name so complicated that it was named hawkinsin after the family in which it was first found.

The metabolic pathway affected in this disorder involves the degradation of tyrosine. The first step in this pathway is the transamination to *p*-hydroxyphenylpyruvic acid. The further metabolism of this compound to homogentisic acid is a complicated series of reactions that may involve a number of discrete enzymes. An enlarging group of disorders in which the fundamental defect is at this step is assisting in the unraveling of this complex set of reactions.

Clinical disease in hawkinsinuria has been reported in two infants who had acidosis and failure to thrive. Symptoms began after being weaned from breastfeeding. They developed severe metabolic acidosis with tachypnea, irritability, and failure to thrive. An unusual compound found in their urine was later identified as hawkinsin. The mother of the first patient and four members of the second patient's family had the metabolic disorder, but they were unsymptomatic. All had been breast fed for 6 to 12 months. This protective effect may simply represent the effects of a low-protein intake. Further, it appears that most patients, regardless of early symptoms, are asymptomatic later in life. So protection may be necessary only in infancy.

It has been postulated from the metabolites observed that the fundamental defect is in the enzyme 4-hydroxyphenylpyruvic acid dioxygenase, which has not been measured directly.

The early life histories of many family members that were asymptomatic suggest that long-term ingestion of breast milk in infancy may be protective. Ascorbic acid is effective in infants with transient tyrosinemia in removing concentrations of tyrosine. It appears to protect the enzyme 4-hydroxyphenylpyruvic acid dioxygenase. Accordingly, the second infant was treated with breast milk and ascorbic acid up to 1000 mg per day. On this regimen, symptoms abated and he thrived. The unusual odor disappeared. By 13 months he tolerated normal feedings.

Alkaptonuria

Alkaptonuria results from a defect in the enzyme homogentisic acid oxidase. It is characterized by a dark color of the urine.

In this disorder fresh urine appears normal, but, on standing and particularly after alkalinization, oxidation of homogentisic acid proceeds and a dark brown or black pigment appears in the urine. This permits the condition to be recognized very early in life. However, the diagnosis is usually first made in adult life through routine urinalysis or in the investigation of arthritis. The urine also gives a positive test for reducing substance and a positive ferric chloride test. Testing for glucose with glucose oxidase sticks is negative.

Persons with this condition are usually asymptomatic in childhood. After the third decade, deposition of brownish or bluish pigment is seen, particularly in the ears and sclerae. The deposition of pigment, which may be extensive in fibrous tissues, is referred to as *ochronosis.* Ochronotic arthritis occurs later. Symptoms may resemble those of rheumatoid arthritis or osteoarthritis. Some degree of limitation of motion is usually seen, and complete ankylosis is not uncommon. Degeneration in the intervertebral discs may be striking. The condition is inherited as an autosomal recessive character.

Although homogentisic acid is excreted in large quantities in the urine, blood levels of the compound are not detectable. This disorder is a classic example of the no-threshold metabolic disorders.

The original suggestion of Garrod that the disorder resulted from an absence of the enzyme in the liver that catalyzed the oxidation of homogentisic acid was confirmed by La Du and colleagues, who found the enzyme catalyzing the conversion of homogentisic acid to maleylacetoacetate to be absent in biopsied liver from an alkaptonuric patient.

Albinism

Albinism is an inherited metabolic defect confined to the melanocyte, in which this cell cannot form melanin.

Albinism occurs in all races of man. Universal albinism, in which melanin is absent from the pigment cells of the skin, hair, and retina, is readily recognized. A variety of localized forms occur in which the defect is confined to an area of skin, the eyes, or a white forelock of hair. The skin in universal albinism is milk-white; the hair is white or yellow and, in Caucasians, very fine. The iris is generally blue. The pupil is red in children, but usually becomes black in adulthood. Photophobia and horizontal nystagmus are characteristic, and visual acuity is nearly always decreased. The skin is very sensitive to sunlight, and these patients have a propensity to develop skin cancers.

Universal albinism is inherited as an autosomal recessive character, although more than one gene produces the disorder. Normally pigmented children have occurred in a family in which both parents were albinos. Localized forms of albinism may be inherited as dominant, recessive, or—as in the case of ocular albinism—sex-linked characters.

A few patients have been reported in whom universal albinism has been associated with prolonged bleeding time and peculiarly pigmented reticuloendothelial cells in the marrow, lymph nodes, and liver.

Melanin is a polymer that exists in nature in high molecular weight. It is a brown or black insoluble material contained in the melanin granules of the melanocytes, where the entire transformation from tyrosine takes place. These granules can be demonstrated with the electron microscope and have been shown to be present, but without melanin, in albinism. The enzyme tyrosinase is a copper-containing oxidase that catalyzes the first two steps in the conversion of tyrosine to melanin. The first step, the conversion of tyrosine to 3,4-dihydroxyphenylalanine, is the limiting step, for the second step and most of the rest of melanogenesis may proceed nonenzymatically. Tyrosinase has been demonstrated in tissues radioautographically, and shown to be absent in the usual form of albinism.

Tyrosinase can be demonstrated by incubating hair roots with tyrosine. It is now clear that there are tyrosinase positive as well as tyrosinase negative forms of universal albinism. The tyrosinase-positive patients have creamy rather than milk-white skin; the hair may be yellow and tends to darken with age. These patients have severe visual defects, but less so than the tyrosinase negative albinos, most of whom ultimately become legally blind.

Histidinemia

Histidinemia is a disorder of metabolism in which large amounts of histidine are found in blood and urine. The condition must be included in the differential diagnosis of phenylketonuria, for the urine is positive when examined with ferric chloride.

The condition may occur without clinical manifestations, but more than half of reported patients have had speech retardation. Mental deficiency and growth retardation have also been observed in individual patients. Relatively fair hair and blue eyes have been common.

In histidinemia elevated concentrations of histidine have been demonstrated in the plasma, urine, and cerebrospinal fluid. Imidazole-pyruvic acid is excreted in the urine and is responsible for the positive ferric chloride test. Many patients also have elevations of alanine in the plasma.

Deficiency of histidase has been demonstrated by direct assay of the enzyme in skin. When histidine cannot be converted to urocanic acid, it is converted to imidazolepyruvic acid and its derivatives, much as phenylalanine is metabolized in phenylketonuria.

Maple Syrup Urine Disease: Branched-Chain Ketoaciduria

In this syndrome major cerebral symptoms appear very rapidly in the newborn period, and there is an odor in the urine reminiscent of maple syrup. The branched-chain amino acids, leucine, isoleucine, and valine, are present in high concentration in the blood and urine, and the keto acid analogues are found in the urine.

Infants with maple syrup urine disease appear well at birth. In the typical case, symptoms begin at 3 to 5 days of life and progress rapidly to death. Early manifestations include feeding difficulty, vomiting, and irregular respirations. The infant then develops progressive neurologic symptoms, including convulsions, opisthotonos, and generalized muscular rigidity with or without flaccidity.

Severe hypoglycemia has occasionally been observed. Slight cortical atrophy has been seen on pneumoencephalography. In patients surviving past the first year, defective myelinization similar to that of phenylketonuria has been reported.

A few patients have been described in whom milder forms of the disease have occurred with characteristic biochemical abnormalities. The conditions in these patients are known as intermittent or variant branched-chain aminoaciduria and appear to represent distinct alterations at the same locus as that of classic maple syrup urine disease. Ataxia and repeated episodes of lethargy progressive to coma have been seen without mental retardation. These episodes have been induced by infection and by surgery with anesthesia, and they have responded to the removal of milk from the diet and the substitution of parenteral fluid therapy.

A disorder of branched-chain keto acid decarboxylation has been described by Scriver and colleagues in which the abnormal accumulation of amino acids in blood was completely reversed by the administration of thiamine. The patient described was retarded and had an abnormal electroencephalogram, but had not had any of the life-threatening crises typical of maple syrup urine disease. The therapeutic dose of thiamine hydrochloride was 10 mg per day.

The characteristic that permits any form of branched-chain ketoaciduria to be distinguished from other cerebral degenerative diseases of infancy is the characteristic odor of maple syrup to the urine, skin, or hair. The odor may become evident after 1 or 2 days of life and persist thereafter, but considerable variation in intensity has been observed and in some specimens the odor cannot be detected. Freezing the urine intensifies the odor in an oil at the top of the specimen. Keto acids may be recognized in the urine by the yellow precipitate that forms on the addition of 2,4-dinitrophenylhydrazine.

The branched-chain ketoacidurias all appear to be transmitted as autosomal recessives.

Maple syrup urine disease is an abnormality in the metabolism of the branched-chain amino acids, resulting in increased quantities of leucine, isoleucine, and valine in the plasma and urine.

The catabolism of leucine and the other branched-chain amino acids is initiated by transamination to form the keto acids, α-ketoisocaproic acid, and the corresponding derivatives of isoleucine and valine. This is followed by decarboxylation to coenzyme A derivatives.

The presence of the keto acid derivatives of leucine, isoleucine, and valine in the urine and the absence of the decarboxylation products suggested a block in the oxidative decarboxylation of the keto acids. This can be demonstrated both in leukocytes and in fibroblasts in culture. In patients with intermittent branched-chain ketoaciduria there is a partial defect in this decarboxylation reaction. In thiamine-responsive patients, treatment with thiamine permits oxidative decarboxylation of leucine at a rate 40 per cent of normal.

Experience has now been accumulated in the dietary therapy of maple syrup urine disease, using a synthetic diet made up of individual amino acids, in which the intake of leucine, isoleucine, and valine is closely controlled. Plasma concentrations of the branched-chain amino acids can in this way be maintained within normal limits. Therapy is very difficult and may require prolonged hospitalization; most patients have had permanent brain damage before treatment was started. Experience with siblings of previous cases, in whom very early diagnosis is possible, and with at least one patient detected by a neonatal screening program, indicates that a normal IQ may be achieved.

Hypervalinemia

Hypervalinemia has been described in a single patient who was both mentally and physically retarded. Vomiting and difficulty with feeding were prominent findings early in infancy. He was treated with a diet low in valine, with concomitant lowering of the plasma concentration of valine, improvement in weight gain, and reduction of vomiting and hyperactivity.

The plasma concentration of valine was as high as 10 mg/dl, and there was increased excretion in the urine. A defect has been documented in the leukocyte in the transamination of valine.

Propionic Acidemia

Propionic acidemia is a disorder of branched-chain amino acid metabolism in which elevated concentrations of propionate are found in body fluids. These patients also have elevated concentrations of glycine. A number of disorders of amino acid metabolism present with abnormal concentrations of glycine in body fluids. These include nonketotic hyperglycinemia, propionic acidemia, and methylmalonic aciduria. Isovaleric acidemia may also present with hyperglycinemia. All these disorders present clinically with overwhelming illness in early infancy. Patients with propionic acidemia and methylmalonic acidemia have what has been called the ketotic hyperglycinemia syndrome.

This syndrome is characterized by recurrent episodes of metabolic acidosis and massive ketosis, similar to that observed in diabetic coma. These patients may also have neutropenia, thrombocytopenia, and osteoporosis severe enough to lead to pathologic fracture. Mental retardation occurs except in cases in which there are early diagnosis and effective dietary therapy. Symptoms have begun as early as 18 hours after birth, with vomiting, acidosis, and ketonuria. Death has occurred with intractable acidosis, and it seems probable that other patients may have died unrecognized early in life. Convulsions and electroencephalographic abnormalities may be found.

The disease is transmitted as an autosomal recessive.

The diagnosis can be suspected clinically. It should be documented chemically. In our hands the most useful determination in the initial documentation of the diagnosis is the detection of methylcitric acid in the urine. This unique metabolite is found only in the presence of disorders of propionate metabolism, such as propionic acidemia and methylmalonic acidemia. It is present in large amounts and is quite stable; thus it is suitable for the diagnosis in a specialized laboratory distant from the patient. Propionic acid, by contrast, is highly volatile. It should be measured in the blood, but it is not the most reliable approach to the initial diagnosis. The danger is that the propionic acid may disappear from the blood after the blood has been removed from the patient. The chemical diagnosis may be suggested by the detection of elevated concentrations of glycine in the blood or urine. Examination of the urine by paper chromatography may be helpful and is often the first test that suggests the diagnosis. However, the amounts of glycine excreted in normal urine are large, and a prominent glycine spot is so commonly encountered that it is easy to miss a hyperglycinuria with the methods usually employed in screening the urine for amino acids. The plasma concentrations of glycine are nearly always elevated, often approximating ten times those of controls. However, a normal concentration of glycine, especially in a very sick infant, does not rule out a diagnosis of propionic acidemia. We have recently been able to detect propionic acidemic fetuses in utero by the identification of methylcitrate by gas chromatography-mass spectrometry in the amniotic fluid. Restriction of the dietary intake of protein in these patients was found to reduce the frequency and severity of attacks of ketosis and acidosis. Ketosis could be produced by the administration of leucine, isoleucine, threonine, valine, or methionine, as well as by natural stresses such as infection. The metabolic defect is in the enzyme propionyl CoA carboxylase, which catalyzes the formation of methylmalonyl CoA from propionyl CoA.

This defect explains the intolerance of these patients to isoleucine, methionine, valine, and threonine, for they are all metabolized through this pathway. The defect can be demonstrated in leukocytes and in cultured fibroblasts and amniotic fluid cells.

Diets in which the amounts of the amino acids listed above are restricted are tolerated by patients with the disease. At least two infants have now been diagnosed early in infancy and raised with these dietary principles in mind. Both have passed the age of 15 years and appear to have normal intelligence.

Methylmalonic Acidemia

At least three different disorders present with methylmalonic acidemia. They have similar clinical manifestations to those of the ketotic hyperglycinemia syndrome. Episodes of ketoacidosis may begin very early in life and lead to coma and death. Neutropenia, thrombocytopenia, and osteoporosis are prominent manifestations. Mental retardation has been observed in surviving patients.

Infections are common and may precipitate life-threatening ketoacidosis. Some patients have had chronic monilial infection. The bone marrow is not megaloblastic. Growth retardation is striking.

Methylmalonic acid is normally formed from methylmalonyl CoA, which is the product of the propionyl CoA carboxylase reaction. Methylmalonyl CoA is converted by methylmalonyl CoA mutase to succinyl CoA, which can then be metabolized through the citric acid cycle. The amino acids isoleucine, valine, methionine, and threonine are catabolized along this pathway, and they are all precursors of methylmalonic acid in man. The mutase enzyme has a B_{12} coenzyme. Patients have been treated with vitamin B_{12} in large doses. Some have responded and some have not, thus delineating two forms of the disease. Patients who do not respond to B_{12} may be successfully treated with diets low in threonine, isoleucine, valine, and methionine. In a third form of methylmalonic acidemia, increased quantities of homocystine and cystathionine were found in the urine. In this condition there is a defect in the activity of tetrahydrofolate methyltransferase and a defect in the accumulation of coenzymatically active derivatives of vitamin B_{12}. The B_{12} responsive individuals who have no problem with sulfur amino acid metabolism have a defect in the conversion of B_{12} to deoxyadenosyl B_{12}.

Multiple Carboxylase Deficiency: 3-Methylcrotonylglycinuria

A new disorder of branched chain amino acid metabolism was first recognized through the identification of 3-methylcrotonylglycine and 3-hydroxyisovaleric acid in the urine. These findings are consistent with a defect in 3-methylcrotonyl CoA carboxylase, an integral step in the catabolism of leucine. More recently it has been found that methylcitric and hydroxypropionic acids are excreted by these patients and that there is defective activity of propionyl CoA carboxylase as well as of 3-methylcrotonyl CoA carboxylase. Thus the disorder is now referred to as a multiple carboxylase deficiency. These observations are consistent with the early clinical observation that patients with multiple carboxylase deficiency respond to pharmacologic doses of biotin. Thus it appeared that the fundamental defect involved the metabolism, transport, or availability of biotin.

It is now clear that there are two distinct forms of multiple carboxylase deficiency. The most commonly encountered form presents as life threatening acidotic illness in the early days of life, and it has now been shown to be due to a defect in the enzyme holocarboxylase synthetase, which is essential for the attachment of biotin to the inactive apocarboxylase enzymes. The other disorder usually presents later in infancy with more indolent symptoms in which neurologic abnormalities accompany those of the skin and hair. This disorder appears to be due to defective activity of biotinidase, an enzyme detectable in serum. Infants who present with metabolic acidosis and ketosis have persistent vomiting and an extensive skin rash. Treatment with biotin leads to dramatic clinical improvement, and the abnormal metabolites disappear from the urine.

The skin lesions are a characteristic feature of this disorder. The picture is that of a bright, red, total body eruption with generalized scaling and with weeping in the intertriginous areas. Secondary infection with monilia is common, but the eruption occurs in very striking presentation, independently of monilia. In addition there is alopecia totalis. These ectodermal features are those observed in man and animals deficient in biotin.

The later infantile form of multiple carboxylase deficiency, unlike the neonatal form, tends to have significantly low levels of biotin in the plasma, and levels in the urine may be even more impressively reduced. This disorder has been referred to as biotin dependency, or biotin dependent multiple carboxylase deficiency. The neonatal form may best be distinguished by referring to it as holocarboxylase synthetase deficiency. The later, biotin-dependent form, may present as early as 3 months with dermatologic manifestations or as late as 4 years. Onset has been reported with seizures at 3 months of age. The alopecia, once begun, is progressive to alopecia totalis. The involvement of the skin tends to be patchy, as opposed to the total body eruption seen in the neonatal form. Development may be delayed. Ataxia may develop, severe enough to interfere with walking. Episodic acidosis may be seen at times of acute infection. Such a patient may develop coma, hypothermia, massive hypotonia, and absent reflexes. Immunodeficiency has been reported with abnormalities in function of both T and B cells. Death from the disease has been reported at 9 months and at 3 years of age. Evidence of immunodeficiency has also been observed in holocarboxylase synthetase deficiency, characterized by decrease in T cell number and reactivity.

The index features of the disease, the excretions of 3-methylcrotonylglycine and 3-hydroxyisovaleric acid, may be quite variable in degree. Studies on the carboxylases in various tissues may elucidate the two syndromes in any given patient. The activities of all three carboxylases including pyruvate carboxylase are defective in leukocytes of both types of patients. They become normal within a few days of biotin therapy. On the other hand the activities of the carboxylases in fibroblasts are very low in media containing 5 mg/ml or less of biotin in holocarboxylase synthetase deficiency, while in the late chronic disease carboxylase activities in fibroblasts are normal. In both diseases normal activity is found in fibroblasts grown in the presence of large amounts of biotin.

The disorders are both transmitted as rare autosomal recessive traits. Consanguinity has been documented in both types of multiple carboxylase deficiency.

Patients are exquisitely sensitive to exogenous biotin. The usual dose employed has been 10 mg/day. Doses as low as 5 mg/day have been employed in the late chronic form. It may be expected that with further experience heterogeneity in this condition, as well as its response to biotin, will be observed. In response to treatment, the levels of organic acid metabolites usually decrease to normal in the late chronic form but remain somewhat elevated in patients with holocarboxylase synthetase deficiency.

The clinical response is dramatic. The skin lesions disappear, and the hair begins to grow. Abnormalities of the electroencephalograph (EEG) and computed tomographic (CT) scan have been documented to disappear. Convulsions not controlled with the usual anticonvulsant therapy have disappeared. Lethargy, hypotonia, and ataxia disappear. Some persisting neurologic abnormalities have been observed, probably a function of the length of time before diagnosis and the initiation of treatment.

Alpha-Methyl-Beta-Hydroxybutyric Aciduria-Thiolase Deficiency

This disorder of isoleucine metabolism has been reported in four patients. The patient of Daum and colleagues was first admitted in coma after an upper respiratory infection and was found to have severe metabolic acidosis. Thereafter he had multiple episodes of recurrent ketosis and acidosis. The second patient was studied at 4 years of age because of vomiting and ketonuria. Her sister had died at 12 months of age in a similar episode. The patient had normal intelligence, but an older brother who had the same disease was retarded.

These patients were all typical examples of the ketotic hyperglycinemia syndrome. However, the concentration of glycine in the blood was never elevated. In contrast, the patient of Keating and colleagues had the ketotic hyperglycinemia syndrome in its complete expression. In addition to recurrent episodes of ketosis and acidosis, this patient was operated on for pyloric stenosis. She also had neutropenia, thrombocytopenia, and osteoporosis. Large amounts of glycine were found in the blood and urine.

Alpha-methyl-beta-hydroxybutyric acid and alpha-methylacetoacetic acid were found in the urine of these patients. Isoleucine was converted imperfectly to carbon dioxide, whereas labeled propionate and methylmalonate were oxidized normally. These observations suggested that the defect in these patients is in the beta-ketothiolase that converts alpha-methylacetoacetyl CoA to propionyl CoA and acetyl CoA.

Isovaleric Acidemia

Isovaleric acidemia is a disorder of the catabolism of leucine that usually presents with severe illness in early life.

Vomiting and acidosis are prominent, and patients have a characteristic pungent or cheesy odor. Shortly after onset, neurologic abnormalities including tremors or convulsions ensue and deep coma may develop. Death occurs within a few weeks after birth in more than half the patients.

In infants who survive the initial attack, there are recurrent episodes of vomiting, acidosis, and ataxia, progressing to lethargy and coma. Acute episodes often occur with infections or following surgery. The odor is more likely to be appreciated during an episode of acute illness, but it may be absent. Some degree of mental retardation has been a common sequel. Patients with isovaleric acidemia also may have leukopenia, thrombocytopenia, and anemia.

Isovaleryl CoA is the product of the branched-chain decarboxylase reaction in the catabolism of the keto-acid of leucine. It is catabolized in a dehydrogenase reaction to beta-methylcrotonyl CoA. The compound responsible for the unusual odor in this disease is isovaleric acid. Its concentration in the serum is elevated even during remission. During acute episodes, levels may be enormous, up to 10 millimolar. Isovaleric acid is excreted in the urine conjugated with glycine, and this compound may be excreted in amounts up to 3 gm/day. Normal individuals excrete less than 2 mg/day. Assay for urinary isovalerylglycine is the most reliable approach to the biochemical detection of this disease. Beta-hydroxyisovaleric acid is also found in the urine, and elevated levels of glycine may be found in the blood or urine. The molecular defect is in the activity of isovaleryl CoA dehydrogenase.

Treatment of the acute episode involves the vigorous use of parenteral fluids containing glucose and electrolytes. The acidosis may require sodium bicarbonate or sodium lactate. Exchange transfusion or peritoneal dialysis may be indicated. Chronic treatment requires the restriction of the dietary intake of leucine by lowering the intake of protein until the amounts of leucine ingested are those just necessary for growth. The observed conjugation of isovaleric acid with glycine has suggested the possibility that exogenous glycine may have a place in treatment.

3-Hydroxy-3-Methylglutaric Aciduria

This is a disorder of leucine metabolism that leads to overwhelming illness early in life. The pattern is that of an organic aciduria with metabolic acidosis, coma and apnea. Hypoglycemia is severe, and ketosis is absent. The disorder may easily be mistaken for Reye's syndrome.

3-Hydroxy-3-methylglutaric acid is an intermediate in the catabolism of leucine. 3-Hydroxy-3-methylglutaryl CoA is cleaved in the lyase reaction to form acetyl CoA and acetoacetic acid. This is a key reaction in the formation of ketone bodies.

Nine patients have been reported since 1976. Hypoglycemia is profound, and hyperammonemia is common. Episodes of severe acidosis and hypoglycemia leading to deep coma begin in infancy. Persistent vomiting is often the first symptom. Patients then develop lethargy progressive to coma, pallor, hypotonia, dehydration, and apnea. In the absence of artificial ventilation, death ensues. Some patients have had convulsions. Most but not all patients have hepatomegaly. No patients have had ketonuria at times of acute illness. This property serves to distinguish them from patients with other organic acidurias, such as propionic acidemia or methylmalonic acidemia.

The disorder is transmitted as an autosomal recessive trait. In several families the parents have been consanguineous. Intermediate activities of the enzyme 3-hydroxy-3-methylglutaryl CoA lyase have been documented in fibroblasts derived from parents. Prenatal diagnosis has been accomplished by analysis of the metabolites in maternal urine.

Management of the patient should be considered

under both long-term management and treatment of the acute crisis. The latter is an emergency, and care must be devoted first to measures of general support, such as assisted ventilation and repair of deficits of fluid and electrolytes and elevation of the blood concentration of glucose. Exchange transfusion or peritoneal dialysis may be necessary.

Long-term management rests largely on the avoidance of long fasts, especially during intercurrent illness. Frequent feedings of a high-carbohydrate diet are advisable, and supplementation with glucose polymers is convenient, especially in intercurrent illness. Restriction of the intake of fat and protein appears useful.

Nonketotic Hyperglycinemia

Patients with nonketotic hyperglycinemia usually have severe seizure disorders. Convulsions or lethargy have been observed from birth. One patient had almost continuous status epilepticus for his first year of life. This disease also can produce overwhelming illness in the neonatal period, and death in the first year of life is common.

Most patients have had very severe mental retardation in which there was little functional cortical activity. Two had irritability and microcephaly. Hypertonicity and hypotonicity have been observed, often in the same patient. Hyperreflexia is the rule. Porencephaly and ventricular dilatation have been seen on pneumoencephalography. Electroencephalograms were very abnormal.

Plasma concentrations of glycine were elevated in a range of about 5 to 12 mg/dl. The amounts of glycine in the urine were also increased, and the glycine content of the cerebrospinal fluid and its ratio to that of the plasma in this disorder appear to exceed those of any other condition. Neutropenia has been observed in only one patient.

A defect has been found in vivo in the conversion of carbon 1 of glycine to CO_2 and of carbon 2 of glycine to carbon 3 of serine. This was consistent with a defect in an enzyme catalyzing the conversion of glycine to CO_2 and hydroxymethyl-tetrahydrofolic acid. Defective activity of the glycine cleavage enzyme has now been demonstrated in liver and brain.

Sarcosinemia

Sarcosine is the N-methyl derivative of glycine. It is formed from dimethylglycine, which may be a product of betaine or choline. Although sarcosine is not normally present in blood or urine in amounts sufficient to be detected, sarcosinuria is occasionally found after the ingestion of lobster or other foods.

Seven patients have been reported with sarcosinemia. Three had subnormal intelligence. The others had shortness of stature. Sarcosine concentrations in the blood ranged from 0.5 to 6.8 mg/dl. Urinary excretion of sarcosine was as high as 168 mg per 24 hours in a patient less than 1 year of age and 500 mg per 24 hours in a 2 year old. A deficiency of hepatic sarcosine dehydrogenase has been postulated.

Hyperoxaluria and Oxalosis

Primary hyperoxaluria is a metabolic disorder in which large amounts of oxalate are excreted in the urine, leading to calcium oxalate lithiasis and nephrocalcinosis. When extrarenal deposits of calcium oxalate ensue, the condition is known as oxalosis.

There are reports of 20 to 30 patients, in most of whom the diagnosis was not established during life. An early onset of symptoms of urolithiasis, hematuria, passage of calculi, and colic, as well as nephrocalcinosis, urinary tract infections, and extrarenal deposits, is sufficiently characteristic to warrant investigation for the presence of oxalate in the urine. Renal failure is common, and the mean age at death in 16 cases was 4 years. Attempts at treatment have not been effective.

The disorder is caused by a rare recessive gene.

Oxalic acid is a dicarboxylic acid that forms a calcium salt of very low solubility. It may be formed from glyoxylic acid, which may be formed from glycine, or glycolic acid. It may also be a metabolite of ascorbic acid. In hyperoxaluria, levels of oxalate excretion may reach 30 times those of control subjects. The site of the defect appears to be the metabolism of glyoxylic acid, in a carboligase enzyme which catalyzes the reaction of glyoxylate and alpha-ketoglutarate to alpha-hydroxy-beta-ketoadipate.

Hyperprolinemia and Hydroxyprolinemia

Hyperprolinemia was first recognized in a family in which cerebral dysfunction, renal anomalies, nephropathy, and deafness occurred in various members. The initial patient presented at 2 years with congenital renal hypoplasia, deafness, convulsions, and mental retardation. He was found to have hyperprolinemia, as were three female siblings, all of whom had EEG abnormalities. Another of the siblings had renal hypoplasia, nerve deafness, hematuria, and electroencephalographic abnormalities. Neither her proline levels nor those of the father were abnormal. Hematuria and deafness occurred frequently in the mother's family in a pattern suggesting dominant inheritance.

In affected persons plasma concentrations of proline were between 7.9 and 20.1 mg/dl. Proline was not elevated in the cerebrospinal fluid. In the urine, proline and hydroxyproline, which are not found in the urine after the neonatal period, were prominent, and in some instances glycine excretion was increased.

The infusion of proline into normal adults produced a hydroxyprolinuria and glycinuria as well as prolinuria, indicating that the urinary findings are secondary to the basic defect in the metabolism of proline.

Hydroxyprolinemia has been described in a mentally retarded girl who also had increased numbers of leukocytes and erythrocytes in the urine and roentgenographically small kidneys. Shortness of stature was also observed. Her mother was also mentally retarded, but had no hydroxyproline abnormality.

Thus both hyperprolinemia and hydroxyprolinemia have been associated with mental deficiency and nephropathy. In involved families, members with the metabolic abnormality have had no clinical defect and vice versa. Therefore, it is probable that these abnormalities of amino acid metabolism are simply biochemical phenotypes without clinical disease.

It is now known that there are two forms of hyperprolinemia: Type I, in which there is a deficiency of proline oxidase, and Type II, in which the next enzyme on the degradative pathway, Δ'-pyrroline-5-carboxylic acid dehydrogenase, is deficient. In hydroxyprolinuria a defect in hydroxyproline oxidase has been reported.

Cystathioninuria

Cystathioninuria was first reported in two adults with mental deficiency. It has also been observed in patients with thrombocytopenia and endocrinopathy, as well as in persons with no disease. It is possible that the biochemical defect is coincidental. The first patients were 64 and 44 years of age when the disease was recognized. Developmental retardation was present from birth. One was otherwise normal except for talipes calcaneovalgus. The other had acromegaly, small ears, deafness, and facial clefts. The abnormal aminoaciduria has generally been found in the course of routine screening. Cystathioninuria also occurs in a secondary fashion in patients with neuroblastoma, hepatoma, galactosemia, or other forms of hepatocellular disease.

Cystathionine is an intermediate in the formation of cysteine and homoserine from methionine and serine. Cystathionine is normally cleaved to form cysteine and α-ketobutyrate. The compound is not usually found in the urine, but in patients as much as 500 to 1300 mg is excreted each day. Cystathionine is not usually detected in the blood. Pyridoxine (vitamin B_6) administration may lead to a decrease in cystathionine excretion. High doses of vitamin B_6 have been used to maintain urine concentrations of cystathionine near zero.

The enzyme cystathionase has been found to be defective in the liver of patients with cystathioninuria, and the in vitro addition of large amounts of pyridoxine corrected the defect.

The disorder is transmitted as an autosomal recessive trait.

Homocystinuria

Homocystinuria is a disorder of the metabolism of the sulfur-containing amino acids. Homocystinuria is especially prevalent in Ireland, where a frequency of 0.7 per 100,000 population has been estimated.

Most patients described have been mentally retarded. Many have had marked failure to thrive. They have been thin and hypertonic. Some had died before a year of age. Less severely affected patients have had mental deficiency without systemic disease. Ectopia lentis is the most characteristic feature of the disease and may be the only manifestation. Cataracts and glaucoma have also been seen. The hair is usually fair and sparse, the complexion fair, and the eyes blue. A malar flush and livedo reticularis are characteristic. Most patients have had skeletal abnormalities, such as genu valgum, pes cavus, or pectus excavatum or carinatum. Osteoporosis is common, and patients are frail and thin. They are frequently mistaken for patients with the Marfan syndrome and vice versa, but in homocystinuria the joints tend to be limited in mobility rather than hypermobile.

Spontaneous thromboembolic phenomena are prominent in homocystinuria and often the cause of death. Occlusion of coronary, renal, or cerebral arteries or veins may lead to major complications such as hemiplegia or renal hypertension as well as death. Pulmonary embolism is a frequent terminal complication. Many patients have convulsions, and the electroencephalogram is usually abnormal. Classic tests of clotting function have been normal, but platelets from these patients have shown unusual adhesiveness. Furthermore,the addition of homocystine to normal blood causes the platelets to become sticky.

Homocystine is an intermediate in the metabolism of methionine. After the conversion of methionine to S-adenosylmethionine, demethylation yields S-adenosylhomocysteine, which is cleaved to homocysteine. This compound is normally combined with serine in the presence of cystathionine synthase to form cystathionine. Free homocysteine condenses to form the disulfide homocystine, as cysteine does to form cystine.

The presence of homocystine in the urine may be the only readily detectable abnormality in these patients, but the compound should be detectable in the blood and levels of methionine are usually elevated. The amounts of homocystine excreted in the urine of these patients usually exceed 20 mg/day and can be increased by the oral administration of methionine. The mixed disulfide of cysteine and homocysteine is also present in the urine. Screening of urine for the presence of homocystine can be carried out by the addition of cyanide and nitroprusside.

The enzymatic defect in the most common form of homocystinuria is in cystathionine synthase. The enzyme defect can be demonstrated using biopsied liver or cultured fibroblasts or amniotic fluid cells. The disorder is transmitted as an autosomal recessive trait. Heterozygotes have reduced levels of activity of cystathionine synthase.

Experience with treatment provided the first evidence of genetic heterogeneity in homocystinuria, for some patients respond to the administration of large doses (100 to 500 mg/day) of pyridoxine and some do not. Patients who respond to pyridoxine should be treated with this vitamin. Those who do not respond to pyridoxine may be treated with a diet in which methionine is restricted and a supplement of cystine is added. There is accumulating evidence for clinical benefit from each of these forms of therapy.

Homocystinuria may result from defects other than that of cystathionine synthase. The disorder in which homocystinuria coexists with cystathioninuria and methylmalonic aciduria tends to lead to overwhelming illness and death early in life, as does the usual form of methylmalonic aciduria. Enzyme assay in these patients reveals abnormally low activity of N^5-methyl-tetrahydrofolate-homocysteine methyl transferase. In this reaction 5-methyltetrahydrofolate is demethylated to tetrahydrofolate, yielding the methyl group for the conversion of homocysteine to methionine. The defect is not in the apoenzyme of the methyltransferase; it is in the conversion of hydroxy B_{12} to methyl B_{12} and to adenosyl B_{12} that serves as cofactor for methylmalonyl-CoA mutase. The underlying defect is probably in the uptake or reduction of B_{12}.

A different form of aberrant B_{12} metabolism leads to homocystinuria because of the role of B_{12} in the activity of methyltransferase. These patients have a familial selective B_{12} malabsorption, with a megaloblastic anemia. They excrete methylmalonic acid as well as homocystine, and all these findings disappear on treatment with parenteral B_{12}.

Three patients have been described in whom homocystinuria was due to deficiency of $N^{5,10}$-methylene tetrahydrofolate reductase. These patients had ten times normal concentrations of methionine and normal concentrations of B_{12}. They did not have methylmalonic aciduria. The defect in $N^{5,10}$-methylene tetrahydrofolate reductase leads to a deficiency in methyltetrahydrofolate, which is the methyl donor in the methyl transferase reaction that converts homocysteine to methionine.

Argininosuccinic Aciduria

Argininosuccinic aciduria is one of a group of metabolic defects involving enzymes of the urea cycle.

A number of patients have been reported and two clinical forms have been distinguished. One is an overwhelming neonatal illness that leads to early death. The late-onset form of the disease is marked by severe mental deficiency, generalized seizures, EEG abnormalities, and ataxia. Hepatomegaly is common. A certain number of patients have short, brittle hair that seldom needs cutting, diagnosed as trichorrhexis nodosa. The biochemical findings of this disease may be found in patients in whom mild mental deficiency is the only clinical abnormality.

Argininosuccinic acid is formed from citrulline and aspartic acid and is not normally found in body fluids. Argininosuccinic aciduria represents a failure in the cleavage of this compound to arginine and fumaric acid, which is catalyzed by argininosuccinase. This enzyme is defective in argininosuccinic aciduria. Correlation of the severity of the clinical disease and molecular abnormality has not yet been made.

Low plasma concentrations of argininosuccinic acid and its very high urinary excretion in this condition are consistent with very efficient renal clearance. Thus this disorder is among the no-threshold aminoacidurias. High concentrations of argininosuccinic acid are found in the cerebrospinal fluid. Therefore, it has been suggested that the enzyme defect is present in the brain and that argininosuccinic acid produced in the brain may produce cerebral symptoms. These patients develop postprandial elevation of blood ammonia and signs of ammonia toxicity. Dietary protein restriction has been employed in treatment. Supplementation with arginine permits the operation of a shortened cycle in which waste nitrogen normally excreted as urea is excreted as argininosuccinate.

Citrullinemia

Citrullinemia is a disorder of urea cycle metabolism that was originally recognized through screening survey of the urine of mentally retarded children for amino acids. It is now apparent that there are at least three forms of citrullinemia, and there is a correlation between the severity of the clinical disease and the nature of the molecular defect.

The acute neonatal form of citrullinemia has been reported in a number of patients. Of these, most have died at less than a week of age. Most diseases that present with acute overwhelming illness in the neonatal period are probably much more common than reports in the literature would suggest. The picture is that of death in coma with respiratory arrest. Blood concentrations of ammonia are very high.

Patients with the second form of citrullinemia have episodic vomiting and postabsorptive elevation in blood ammonia. Severe vomiting, coma, and seizures may develop. Microcephaly with severe mental deficiency is the rule.

The third form of citrullinemia has been reported in only one patient, a boy who may be clinically normal. He was admitted to the hospital because of aspiration and tachypnea, and he was found to have citrullinemia on a routine screen. No hyperammonemia was demonstrated, even postprandially.

The metabolic block in this disease is in the formation of argininosuccinic acid from citrulline. Argininosuccinic acid synthase has been found to be deficient in liver and in fibroblasts cultured from the skin. The disorder is inherited as an autosomal recessive trait. Molecular heterogeneity is evident in the levels of activity of argininosuccinic acid synthase, virtually absent in patients with the acute neonatal form, and considerably greater in the third or benign form.

The acute hyperammonemic episodes that characterize the neonatal forms of citrullinemia and ornithine transcarbamylase deficiency and that occur in some argininosuccinic aciduria and carbamylphosphate synthetase deficiency may be treated successfully with exchange transfusion, hemodialysis, or peritoneal dialysis. Arginine therapy is also of interest in this condition. More long-term therapy has been employed using a mixture of the keto acids or hydroxy acids of a number of essential amino acids. This form of treatment has been successful in bringing ammonia levels to normal and permitting the intake of sufficient quantities of protein to permit normal growth and development. The use of sodium benzoate and phenylacetate to promote waste nitrogen excretion as hippurate and phenylacetyl glutamine has represented a considerable advance in management.

Carbamyl Phosphate Synthetase Deficiency

The first step at which a defect in the urea cycle leads to hyperammonemia is that of carbamyl phosphate synthetase. This enzyme catalyzes the formation of carbamyl phosphate from NH_4^+ and HCO_3^- and thus provides a branch point to pyrimidine biosynthesis as well as urea synthesis. Clinical manifestations are those of ammonia intoxication. Episodic vomiting, lethargy, and stupor or coma may be seen as early as 10 days of age. Most patients described have been reported, and elevated concentrations of ammonia are found. Assay of the enzyme requires liver tissue. Therapy with benzoate and arginine is useful.

Ornithine Transcarbamylase Deficiency

Carbamyl phosphate reacts with ornithine in the presence of ornithine transcarbamylase to form citrulline. Assay of this enzyme also requires liver.

A number of patients have been described with deficiency of this enzyme. The gene is on the X chromosome. Involved males have usually died in the newborn period. Symptoms have begun with vomiting and lethargy, progressing to coma. Activity of the enzyme in liver was less than 2 per cent of normal. Female patients have had a more indolent course. Mental deficiency, episodic vomiting, hypotonia, and lethargy have been prominent. Some patients have had seizures. Concentrations of ammonia were elevated. Increased amounts of orotic acid are found in the urine in this condition as well as in citrullinemia. Therapy with benzoate and arginine is useful.

Argininemia

A small number of patients with argininemia have been described. Like other patients with hyperammonemia, they may present with vomiting and retarded mental and motor development. Characteristic of argininemia is the degree of spastic quadriparesis. Two had seizures, and one had an abnormal electroencephalogram. Hepatomegaly with abnormal liver function tests has been observed.

The blood ammonia is markedly elevated both in the fasting state and postprandially. There is a pattern in the urine similar to that seen in cystinuria, with increased excretion of cystine, lysine, and ornithine, as well as arginine. Citrulline may also be excreted in abnormal quantities. The concentration of arginine in the plasma is elevated 6 to 15 times, and the cerebrospinal fluid concentration may also be increased. Orotic acid is also found in large amounts in the plasma. Arginase assays were performed on the erythrocytes of the patients, and the activity was greatly reduced or unmeasurable. Treatment with a low-protein diet may be effective.

Ornithinemia

Three types of ornithinemia have been reported. In one, mental retardation, prolonged icterus, and EEG abnormalities were associated with increased concentrations of ornithine in the blood. There was a generalized aminoaciduria but not hyperammonemia or homocitrullinuria.

In another disorder there were mental retardation, ataxia, and hyperammonemia, along with homocitrullinuria. A defect has been postulated in ornithine transport into the mitochondria.

The most common of the ornithinemias is gyrate atrophy of the choroid and retina. The activity of ornithine-δ-transaminase is deficient. Treatment with pyridoxine may be effective.

Hyperlysinemia

A number of different inborn errors of metabolism present with elevated concentrations of lysine in the blood. One of these is due to a deficiency of lysine: α-ketoglutarate reductase. The first child described with this disorder had mental retardation and delayed physical development, but two subsequent children were mentally and physically normal. Consanguinity has been observed. Concentrations of lysine were elevated in the blood, with levels generally exceeding 10 mg/dl. The product of the reductase enzyme is saccharopine. This pathway is the major route of lysine catabolism. The enzyme defect is demonstrable in cultured fibroblasts.

Saccharopinuria has been found in two patients as a result of routine screening of mentally retarded individuals. Plasma lysine was elevated in both. This abnormality is due to a defect in saccaropine dehydrogenase.

An alternate pathway for the catabolism of lysine is through pipecolic acid. A patient has been described who appeared to have a defect in this pathway because large amounts of pipecolic acid were found in the plasma and urine. Concentrations of lysine were not elevated. This child died of a progressive neurologic disease associated with hepatomegaly.

Another disorder has been described under the heading of lysinuric protein intolerance in which there is episodic ammonia intoxication and coma. Such a patient could be clinically indistinguishable from those described under hyperammonemia. Patients described from Finland as having "familial protein intolerance" all had hyperammonemia and hyperlysinuria.

Glutaric Aciduria, Type I

Glutaric aciduria was first described in two siblings with a neurodegenerative disorder, one of whom had a tendency to a compensated metabolic acidosis. A specific defect has been found in glutaryl CoA dehydrogenase.

Glutaryl CoA is an intermediate in the catabolism of lysine, tryptophan, and hydroxylysine. The dehydrogenase that converts glutaryl CoA to glutaconyl CoA is a mitochondrial FAD-dependent enzyme found in liver and kidney.*

The first two patients reported were siblings. The youngest had developed normally for 3 months, when she developed irritability and progressive neurologic deterioration. At 1 year of age she had generalized

*FAD = Flavin-adenine dinucleotide.

spasticity, tonic neck posturing, clenched fists, and scissoring. Her brother was well for 7 months when neurologic deterioration began. At 2 years the physical findings were identical to those described for his sister. The serum bicarbonate concentration ranged from 7.5 to 15.7 mEq/liter. Two other siblings with glutaric aciduria had dystonic cerebral palsy. The disorder is progressive to death.

The cardinal chemical feature is massive glutaric aciduria.

Intact leukocytes metabolized C-labeled glutaric acid to CO_2 normally, but leukocyte lysates were completely defective in the conversion of C-labeled glutaryl CoA to CO_2. These observations are consistent with a deficiency of glutaryl CoA dehydrogenase. Inheritance appears to be autosomal recessive.

Treatment with a low-protein diet has been reported to be beneficial. Treatment with riboflavin, the coenzyme for glutaryl CoA dehydrogenase, has also been followed by substantial reduction in glutaric aciduria. Slight clinical improvement was reported. Three patients were treated with 4-amino-3-(4-chlorophenyl)butyric acid (Lioresal), a GABA* analog, with considerable improvement in symptomatology. The use of all 3 modalities—diet, riboflavin, and the GABA agonists—are recommended in treatment.

Glutaric Aciduria, Type II

Glutaric aciduria, Type II, was first described in an infant with severe hypoglycemia and profound metabolic acidosis without ketosis. The disorder is characterized by overwhelming illness in the neonatal period, and it has been uniformly fatal. Organic acid analysis revealed the accumulation of a wide variety of organic acids, including lactic and ethylmalonic acids, as well as glutaric acid. A number of dicarboxylic acids and hydroxy acids occur in the urine, and there are elevated levels of a number of short-chain acids in the blood. There is a generalized defect in the activity of many acyl CoA dehydrogenases.

Glutaric aciduria, Type II, presents in the neonatal period with life-threatening illness. Several patients were noted to have a "very disagreeable sweaty-feet odor." Most had convulsions. Persistent metabolic acidosis in spite of therapy with parenteral fluids and $NaHCO_3$ is characteristic. Hypoglycemia is observed regularly, but ketosis is absent. Hyperammonemia was a feature in all patients. Fatty infiltration of the liver was a consistent postmortem finding. One patient who survived to 7 weeks developed edema, cardiomegaly, bradycardia, and ultimately ventricular tachycardia, and was thought to have a cardiomyopathy. There was fatty infiltration of the myocardium as well as the liver at autopsy.

Dysmorphic features were prominent in one patient. These included low-set, malrotated ears and semilunar folds below the eyes. Polycystic kidneys were found at autopsy. The patient also had a disproportionately large head, a high forehead, a depressed nasal bridge, and a short anteverted nose. There were single horizontal palmar creases. He also had an interventricular septal defect.

In patients with glutaric aciduria, Type II, the conversion of ^{14}C-labeled glutaric acid to $^{14}CO_2$ by intact fibroblasts derived from a patient was about 15 per cent of the level observed in control fibroblasts. The oxidations of labeled valine, leucine, isoleucine, 2-ketovaleric acid, and 2-ketoisocaproic acids to CO_2 were also abnormally low. These observations are consistent with a general defect in the acyl CoA dehydrogenases for butyryl CoA, isovaleryl CoA, and 2-methylbutyryl CoA as well as that for glutaryl CoA.

The first patient reported was the fourth child of healthy Turkish parents in whom there was no known consanguinity. The first child in that family, also a male, died a few hours after birth. The next two, both girls, were well. The pedigree of the second family indicated all of the males were involved and all of the females normal. Two additional male patients have been reported. These observations suggest the possibility of an X-linked recessive mode of inheritance, but do not rule out an autosomal recessive mode. Two female patients have been reported. While there were some features distinct from the other cases, this weakens the case for X-linked inheritance, but there may well be heterogeneity. The dysmorphic form especially appears likely to represent a distinct disease.

No successful treatment has been reported.

Ethylmalonic Aciduria

Ethylmalonic aciduria was described in a 4-year-old girl who presented with episodic coma, hypoglycemia, and hyperammonemia. The metabolites 2-ethylmalonic acid, adipic acid, and N-hexanoylglycine were found in the urine. Defective activity has been presumed in multiple acyl CoA dehydrogenases and has been demonstrated in the case of butyryl CoA dehydrogenase and isovaleryl CoA dehydrogenase. The exact molecular defect is not known.

The first patient appeared well until 7 weeks of age, when, after a brief period of poor intake, she had episodes of tonic seizures. A sister had died on the third day of life, presumably of sepsis, although autopsy showed only hepatomegaly and fatty infiltration of the liver. The patient had two other episodes of lethargy progressive to coma and convulsions at 1 and 4 years of age, associated with marked hypoglycemia, ketoacidosis, and hyperammonemia. The SGOT and lactic dehydrogenase were also elevated. At 9 years of age, this patient showed normal intelligence. She continued to have episodes of illness with acidosis.

The hallmark of this disorder is the finding of 2-ethylmalonic acid on organic analysis of the urine. This compound may also be found in glutaric aciduria, Type II, but in patients with that disease large amounts of glutaric acid are regularly found, as are large amounts of isobutyric and isovaleric acid, and most patients with that disease have died in the first days of life.

Challenge tests by oral loading with medium-chain triglycerides (MCT) produced vomiting and lethargy

*GABA = Gamma-aminobutyric acid.

within 45 minutes. The excretion of ethylmalonic acid increased more than 20 times from baseline levels. The data available suggest that ethylmalonic aciduria is a multiple acyl CoA dehydrogenase deficiency.

The disorder is doubtless autosomal recessive. Fibroblasts derived from the parents oxidized ^{14}C-butyrate at intermediate rates, consistent with heterozygosity. In view of the dramatic response to MCT, a low-fat diet was tried. The amounts of organic acids in the urine decreased but clinical improvement was less obvious. Treatment with glycine failed to alter the biochemical status, but subjective improvement was reported.

Hyper-Beta-Alaninemia and Carnosinemia

Hyper-β-alaninemia has been reported in a single infant who died very early in life. Symptoms were those of somnolence, hypotonia, and intermittent seizures, which could not be controlled with the usual anticonvulsant therapy. Deep tendon reflexes were depressed.

β-Alanine was found to be elevated in the blood, urine, and cerebrospinal fluid. Large amounts of taurine and β-aminoisobutyric acid were also found in the urine. γ-Aminobutyric acid was present in the plasma, urine, and cerebrospinal fluid. The concentration of γ-aminobutyric acid in brain tissue obtained post mortem was markedly increased.

Carnosine is the dipeptide of β-alanine and histidine. It is normally present in high concentrations in muscle and thus is a common dietary constituent. It is not normally found in the blood. Seven patients have been reported with carnosinemia. Five had progressive neurologic degeneration with onset early in infancy. They also had seizures and electroencephalographic abnormalities. However, two persons have been described in whom the biochemical abnormality was present without detectable clinical manifestations. Carnosinase activity, normally present in the serum, is absent in patients with carnosinemia.

Carnosinemia should be distinguished from normal dietary carnosinuria. Patients with carnosinemia have persistent carnosinuria while receiving a carnosine-free diet. They do not have 1-methylhistidine in the urine. Normal persons receiving a meal rich in protein, such as white meat of chicken, excrete anserine and β-alanyl-1-methylhistidine, and the urine always contains 1-methylhistidine.

Pyroglutamic Acidemia

Pyroglutamic acidemia was first described by Eldjarn and colleagues in Norway in 1970. A second patient was observed in Sweden. Metabolic acidosis is a consistent feature of this disorder. The first patient with this disorder was mentally retarded and ataxic. At the age of 16 years he began to have episodes of violent vomiting. His metabolic acidosis was first noted when he was admitted to the hospital for repair of a hiatal hernia, and it became life-threatening in the postoperative period. Over a 3-year period of study, he was admitted to a hospital five times, always revealing a chronic acidosis without acute exacerbations. It is not clear that any of his clinical manifestations were related to his pyroglutamic acidemia. The second patient developed a severe metabolic acidosis on the third day of life. This was correctable with $NaHCO_3$, but she had exacerbations of acidosis whenever alkali therapy was discontinued. This patient had no other abnormalities, and at 14 months of age her physical and intellectual development were normal.

Pyroglutamic acid is 2-pyrrolidone-5-carboxylic acid. Glutamine cyclizes readily to pyroglutamic acid in aqueous solutions at physiologic pH. The compound does not react with ninhydrin. Therefore it is not detectable using routine methods of screening the urine for amino acids. It has been found using gas liquid chromatography.

The first patient excreted 30 to 40 grams of pyroglutamate in the urine in 24 hours. Serum concentrations were as high as 50 to 60 mg/dl or 4 to 5 mEq/liter. This would account for the acidosis. In the second patient, 6 to 7 grams of pyroglutamate was excreted each day in the urine.

The kidney appears to be the site of formation of pyroglutamate. A relationship has been suspected between renal ammonia production and pyroglutamate formation. It is generally accepted that the amide nitrogen of glutamine is the source of renal NH_4^+. Spontaneous deamination of glutamine in aqueous solutions yields predominantly pyroglutamate, not glutamate. Furthermore, there is generally a close parallel in patients with pyroglutamic aciduria between the amounts of pyroglutamate and ammonia in the urine. Pyroglutamate is formed in the enzymatic hydrolysis of gamma-glutamyl peptides.

The molecular defect is in the enzyme glutathione synthetase. Pyroglutamic aciduria results from the accumulation of α-glutamyl cysteine which is a substrate for the cyclotransferase that forms pyroglutamic acid, as well as for the defective enzyme.

γ-Hydroxybutyric Aciduria

γ-Hydroxybutyric acid and succinic semialdehyde have been found in the urine of four patients with mental and motor retardation. γ-Hydroxybutyric acid has been developed as an intravenous anesthetic designed to serve as an analogue of γ-aminobutyric acid capable of crossing the blood-brain barrier. This metabolic abnormality provides a unique example of the accumulation of a compound of known neuropharmacologic activity.

The key intermediate in the relevant pathway is succinic semialdehyde which is the direct product of the transamination of γ-aminobutyric acid. The transamination is active in brain as well as liver. γ-Aminobutyric acid is derived from glutamic acid by decarboxylation. Succinic semialdehyde is normally converted to succinic acid in a reaction catalyzed by succinic semialdehyde dehydrogenase. The further oxidation of succinic acid takes place in the citric acid cycle. The reduction of succinic acid semialdehyde to γ-hydroxybutyric acid is normally a minor metabolic pathway. It would become more important in the presence of accumulation of succinic semialdehyde.

γ-Hydroxybutyric acid has been known to have neuropharmacologic effects since its introduction in 1960 as an intravenous anesthetic. It was hoped that it would serve as an effective analogue of γ-aminobutyric acid, which could cross the blood brain barrier. In animals the compound produced EEG changes at serum levels consistent with those found in the patients. In the presence of even higher levels, generalized seizures occur. These findings precluded the use of the compound as a drug in man.

Succinic semialdehyde dehydrogenase is not detectable in normal fibroblasts. However, it is active in lymphocytes. The level of activity has now been assayed in freshly isolated peripheral blood lymphocytes, and this is the site of the defect in γ-hydroxybutyric aciduria. The disorder appears to be autosomal recessive. No effective treatment has been developed to date.

DISORDERS OF AMINO ACID TRANSPORT

Hartnup Disease

Hartnup disease is an unusual disorder in which the transport of certain amino acids, particularly tryptophan, is abnormal in the intestine and in the renal tubule. It was named for the first family described, in which four of the eight children of parents who were first cousins were affected. The constant feature of the disease is the aminoaciduria.

Clinical characteristics are intermittent and variable. Patients may develop a pellagra-like, photosensitive, red, scaly eruption on the exposed skin. In addition, they have cerebellar ataxia occurring in attacks of variable severity, which are completely reversible. Other patients have had psychiatric abnormalities similar to those observed in pellagra. Mental retardation is common but not uniform. Attacks have been precipitated by infection. Transmission is as an autosomal recessive character.

Patients may be recognized even in the absence of symptomatology by the aminoaciduria. It is renal in type, with plasma concentrations of amino acids normal or decreased. The following amino acids are excreted in five to ten times the usual amounts: threonine, serine, asparagine, glutamine, alanine, valine, isoleucine, leucine, tyrosine, phenylalanine, histidine, and tryptophan. This is a large group of amino acids, but the pattern is striking. It differs from the commonly encountered generalized aminoaciduria in that the excretion of glycine, glutamic acid, and lysine are normal, and that there is no free proline or hydroxyproline in the urine. The urine in this condition is also characterized by the presence of a number of indolic derivatives of tryptophan, including indican. These patients respond to an oral load of tryptophan with increased excretion of indican and indolic acids. Tryptophan loading after sterilization of the intestinal flora with antibiotics resulted in no increase in indole excretion, and unabsorbed tryptophan accumulated in the feces. These observations indicate that there is a defect in the absorption of tryptophan in the cells of the intestine as well as in the kidney. The indoles found in the urine in this disease are secondary to the action of intestinal bacteria on unabsorbed tryptophan.

Most patients have been treated with nicotinamide. It is not certain that improvements observed in cutaneous and neurologic manifestations with treatment were not spontaneous, but treatment is recommended.

Cystinuria

Cystinuria is an inherited defect in renal tubular function in which the reabsorption of cystine, lysine, arginine, and ornithine is impaired. The abnormality is of clinical significance because of the insolubility of cystine which can form stones when present in the urine in high concentration. The excretion of the other three amino acids does not influence the health of the patient.

Patients with cystinuria generally develop calculi some time before the age of 30 years. Some have large numbers of calculi requiring surgical removal for relief of colic or obstruction. Repeated infections of the urinary tract and renal failure are common. The stones represent aggregations of cystine varying from tiny sands or gravel to staghorn calculi filling the renal pelvis or huge calculi of the bladder. This disorder should be distinguished from cystinosis or the Lignac-de Toni-Fanconi syndrome, in which glycosuria, generalized aminoaciduria, phosphaturia, and renal rickets are associated with deposits of cystine in tissues. Such patients do not have abnormal amounts of cystine in the urine.

In cystinuria the concentrations of cystine and the other amino acids in the blood are not elevated. The clearance of cystine, lysine, arginine, and ornithine is markedly elevated. There is also a disorder of intestinal absorption, in some patients with cystinuria, involving the amino acids cystine, lysine, arginine, and ornithine. Inefficiently absorbed lysine, arginine, and ornithine are converted by intestinal bacteria to the diamines, cadaverine and putrescine, which may be detected in the urine.

Genetic studies indicate that there are at least three forms of cystinuria in which the homozygotes are clinically indistinguishable. They are now designated Types I, II, and III. In Type I the heterozygotes are detectable only by studies of the intestinal transport of cystine or the dibasic amino acids. This is the most common form, accounting for almost two thirds of all carriers. Type I homozygotes, of course, also have the intestinal transport defect. In Types II and III the heterozygotes excrete increased amounts of cystine and lysine in the urine. Type II differs from Type III in that in the former an oral load of cystine appears not to be absorbed into the blood and lysine transport is altered in intestinal cells in vitro. The three genes are allelic, and double heterozygotes have been observed who carry two different abnormal genes and thus have clinical manifestations of homozygous cystinuria.

Cystinuria is relatively common, occurring about once in every 20,000 live births. The condition can be screened for, using the simple cyanide nitroprusside test. Confirmation of the diagnosis requires a quantitative assay of cystine content of the urine.

Treatment of cystinuria is aimed at the prevention of urinary lithiasis. Crystallization and stone formation can be minimized by increasing urine volumes or by increasing cystine solubility. However, very large amounts of oral fluids are required, and in practice very few adults and almost no children will drink enough to prevent stones. Alkalinization sufficient to promote the solubility of cystine requires a urine pH of over 7.6, which is not achievable physiologically. Penicillamine therapy has therefore brought about a real advance in the management of this disease. Penicillamine forms a mixed disulfide with cysteine that is considerably more soluble than cystine. Oral administration of penicillamine to cystinuric patients can reduce the cystine content in the urine to levels at which stones do not form.

Two conditions related to cystinuria are hyperdibasic aminoaciduria and hypercystinuria. In the former, the dibasic amino acids, lysine, ornithine, and arginine, are excreted in large amounts because of a renal tubular absorptive defect, but cystine excretion is normal. Lysine transport in the intestine appears also to be abnormal. The trait is inherited as a dominant and appears to have no clinical manifestations. In hypercystinuria, cystine is excreted in the urine in increased amounts because of a specific tubular transport defect, whereas the excretion of the dibasic amino acids is normal. The amounts of cystine in the urine in this condition are only 25 per cent of those found in cystinuria. Clinical manifestations have not been observed, but the disorder has been observed in only one family. The existence of these two conditions indicates that more than one transport system is involved in the excretion of cystine and the dibasic amino acids.

Iminoglycinuria

Renal iminoglycinuria appears to be a benign chemical abnormality in which there is no clinical abnormality. There is selective impairment in the shared transport system for proline, hydroxyproline, and glycine. Net renal tubular reabsorption of the amino acids is about 80 per cent of normal and that of glycine is about 60 per cent of normal. An intestinal transport defect for the same amino acids has been observed in some families but not in others.

In most heterozygotes there is impaired renal tubular transport of glycine. Thus these individuals may present with tubular hyperglycinuria. It is thought that this accounts for patients with glycinuria reported as having a dominantly inherited condition. On the other hand, some heterozygotes may have no glycinuria. These observations and those on intestinal transport suggest that there is more than one allelic mutation responsible for iminoglycinuria.

GOUT

By Thomas E. Weiss, M.D.
and Richard K. Lange, M.D.
New Orleans, Louisiana

SYNONYM

Podagra, crystalline arthritis (uric acid).

DEFINITION

In past centuries, the term gout meant a drop of diseased "humours." It was assumed that this applied primarily to the involved joint. Gout is now considered a metabolic disease occurring in paroxysms, with painfully inflamed joints, deposits of uric acid crystals in the joints and fibrous parts about the joints, and usually an elevated serum uric acid. It is usually monoarticular.

The disease may be primary or secondary. Primary gout is an inborn defect of purine metabolism resulting from an overproduction of uric acid, reduced excretion of uric acid, or a combination of both. Some hyperuricemic patients have a specific genetic defect with excessive uric acid production caused by the absence of the enzyme hypoxanthineguanine phosphoribosyltransferase (HGPRTase). When this genetic defect is total, the tragic Lesch-Nyhan syndrome exists in the youthful patient. Sometimes this defect is only partially evident.

Secondary gout is characterized by clinical manifestations that generally resemble primary gout, but the entity is secondary to an associated primary disease that results in the hyperuricemia. This type of gout most often occurs in the myeloproliferative diseases, particularly polycythemia vera and multiple myeloma. It occurs less commonly with chronic leukemia, hemolytic anemia, Cooley's anemia, and malignant lymphoma. Excessive use of diuretics, lead poisoning, and other agents that alter the renal excretion of uric acid may result in gout. Cytotoxic agents and radiation therapy with marked cellular destruction may be a causative factor. Women with secondary gout may have renal calculi and tophi before the first gouty attack.

The clinical picture in either primary or secondary gout may be an acute attack of synovitis, an interval phase between attacks (without gouty arthritis or tophi) or a chronic phase of tophaceous gouty arthritis. Hyperuricemia alone does not signify gout, but may indicate long-term exposure to heavy metals, especially lead toxicity. This toxicity results in enhanced net renal absorption and possibly chronic volume depletion. Other heavy metals, such as copper, mercury, and platinum as well as lead, may cause interstitial renal pathology and then renal failure. This kidney involvement may be more important than uric acid deposits in the renal parenchyma and tubular system.

PRESENTING SIGNS AND SYMPTOMS

The common picture of acute gout occurs in a middle-aged male who experiences monoarticular arthritis where the involved joint is swollen, red, warm, and exquisitely tender. About 95 per cent of patients are males. Rarely does gout occur in premenopausal women, but it is seen much more frequently in postmenopausal women, possibly with the same frequency as in males. When the condition does occur in premenopausal women, it is usually associated with a strong family history of gout. Diuretic therapy has a high correlation with gouty attacks in menopausal females.

The typical initial attack involves the first metatarsophalangeal joint or a large articulation. Between acute attacks the involved joint sites are grossly normal, completely comfortable, and able to be used freely. Often such an initial acute attack occurs during the night or early morning. While about 60 per cent of these first attacks are in the base of the great toe, this classical site usually becomes involved in about 90 per cent of patients. It is important to differentiate between this site of involvement and swelling in the interphalangeal joint of the great toe. Often the patient is first aware of acute classical gout (podagra) when the foot is placed on the floor upon arising from a comfortable night's sleep. If awake, a patient who has experienced several acute attacks may be aware of a vague discomfort or detectable sensation at the joint site that will then become very painful and fully involved with acute gout. This may precede the apogee of pain by 2 to 24 hours and become a "patient warning sign of acute gout." It is of diagnostic significance, and although it does not occur in all patients, it frequently aids the patient in initiating the correct diagnosis and early therapy. The swollen, red skin over the bunion joint often desquamates after the acute attack begins to subside. This too can be a helpful diagnostic sign.

Although no joint is immune to attacks of gout, the shoulders, hips, and axial skeleton are seldom involved with acute gouty synovitis, but may be the sites of advanced tophaceous gout.

A precipitating factor is not apparent in most acute attacks of gout, but trauma to the site or a stressful situation may precede the attack. With the increased interest in weight loss by exotic diets and other dietary fads, there may be a rather marked weight loss and a drastic rise in the serum uric acid level that is followed by an attack of acute gout. The current interest in exercising, particularly jogging, may result in minor soft-tissue injuries that may be a precipitating factor in a person subject to acute gout. Postoperative gout is not unusual in the hospital population and can be confused with cellulitis and phlebitis.

Myocardial infarction is sometimes followed by acute gout. Frequently, patients who have had a myocardial infarction are overweight and their caloric intake is restricted as a therapeutic aid. Hyperuricemia may be more marked in this phase of hospitalization and cardiac treatment.

Thiazide diuretics and furosemide may be associated with uric acid retention and acute gout. While injections of adrenocorticotropic hormone (ACTH) may be very helpful in relieving a resistant bout of acute or subacute gout, it should be remembered that withdrawal of either ACTH or adrenal steroids that have been given for therapy may be followed by another acute gouty attack.

COURSE

Hyperuricemia, a biochemical abnormality, may occur in the second decade of life and continue thereafter. With automated serum chemistry determinations that are frequently obtained on general examinations, the uric acid elevations are noted more frequently. The presence of an elevated serum uric acid level alone is not sufficient reason for therapy. The uric acid level varies according to sex, age, and certain genetic tendencies, as well as renal status. Laboratory normals reflect that the exact figure for serum uric acid, which indicates hyperuricemia, varies from 6 to 9 mg/dl. The saturation point of monosodium urate in serum at 37°C is approximately 6.4 mg/dl, which could be accepted as a crucial serum level, but most colorimetric methods give readings of 0.5 to 1.0 mg/dl above enzymatic methods for uric acid. Therefore, it would be practical to assume that hyperuricemia exists if the serum level is above 8.0 mg/dl if the former are used.

It is estimated that 5 to 20 per cent of Americans, or 6.5 to 13 million people in the United States, have hyperuricemia. Of hospital populations, 25 per cent have hyperuricemia, but there are other reasons for their hospitalization. With the increased influx of Asiatics and Orientals, it should be appreciated that some of these Pacific groups, particularly from the Philippines, do exhibit a serum uric acid level that may be above American norms.

There is no typical pattern of subsequent attacks, and the second attack of acute gout may occur 2 to 10 years following the first. The higher the hyperuricemia, the greater the frequency of acute attacks and development of tophi. The passage of uric acid stones may precede an initial attack of acute gouty synovitis, but fewer than 1 per cent of patients having their initial attack of acute gout have tophi.

The sites of gouty attacks are seldom symmetric and are usually found in the joints of the lower extremities. Those unusual cases of acute gout that tend to occur with some frequency and follow an acute polycyclical pattern may resemble rheumatoid arthritis, and at this point it is important that a specific diagnosis be made.

While the serum uric acid level of a few patients in the early stage of gout may be normal, it usually rises to an elevated level after a few attacks of gout. Some

50 to 60 per cent of untreated gouty patients develop tophi within 15 years of their first attack of gout. Those patients with normal serum uric acid levels may have an enlarged miscible pool of uric acid. The measurement of this is rather complex and cannot be carried out by routine laboratory procedures.

The most important sources of uric acid in the body are purines from the diet and the de novo synthetic pathway of purines to uric acid. Dietary intake rarely causes sustained hyperuricemia. The synthesis of uric acid is complicated, but the most important part is the final stage, at which hypoxanthine is degraded to xanthine and then uric acid. Xanthine oxidase is the catalyst for this important change. Fortunately, the drug allopurinol blocks this enzyme, thereby reducing the amount of serum uric acid produced. It is recognized, then, that this can be a part of therapy in selected patients.

Uric acid is eliminated from the body via the intestinal tract (approximately 200 mg/day by intestinal uricolysis). Normal renal excretion accounts for the greater disposal from the body, usually around 600 mg in a 24-hour period, but this may be greater when larger amounts of serum uric acid are present. There is first complete filtration of uric acid at the glomerulus, then about 98 per cent is reabsorbed in the proximal tubules. This uric acid is then secreted by the lower section of the tubules, and finally there is reabsorption of the uric acid. Alterations of this physiologic function at any of these levels by toxic agents, disease or drugs will alter the renal handling of uric acid.

The purine de novo synthetic route and the renal excretory pathways are the most important physiologic features that determine the serum uric acid levels and the uricosuria. Current evidence suggests that gout alone rarely causes depression of renal function and that nephropathy seen in patients with gout is probably associated with intrinsic kidney disease and/or the complications of hypertension. Consequently, in evaluating hyperuricemia, it is important to evaluate the cardiovascular and renal status accurately, and, if possible, direct treatment to these sites, as well as the gout pathology.

There has been a marked reduction in the occurrence of gouty nephropathy and azotemia in the past 20 years. Also, tophi are seen far less frequently now than they were 20 to 30 years ago. This reduction in tophi is evident in both non-nephropathic and nephropathic gout. It has been observed that currently about 18 per cent of patients with the former type of gout have tophi, whereas about 37 per cent of patients with the latter type do. Patients with chronic, recurring, acute, or subacute gouty attacks often have persistent, chronic joint pains that may require therapy and that can be mistaken for rheumatoid arthritis.

Some acute attacks of gouty synovitis may respond partially to therapy. This may be followed by a repeated flare-up in the same joint or another articulation may become the site of acute arthritis. If the patient is not given colchicine as a prophylactic agent and the attack is not fully treated, even beyond the stage of partial regression of the inflammation, there may be repeated flares that will be misleading and become a diagnostic challenge as well as a therapeutic problem. In evaluations of patients with gout, a history of excessive alcohol consumption, associated liver disease, peptic ulcers, and renal disease is important. In the southeastern part of the United States, "bootleg" liquor produced with a make-shift still containing some lead parts has been found responsible for a fair number of patients with gout. This is thought to be secondary to lead nephropathy, which leads to reduced uric acid excretion and then gout. This may be significant in patients with low incomes who consume bootleg alcohol. These problems are significant in evaluating the status of gout and decision making regarding future therapy.

The use of nonsteroidal anti-inflammatory drugs may depend on underlying health problems. The use of such drugs may be contraindicated in the presence of renal or hepatic disease or congestive heart failure. Recent studies suggest avoidance of the concurrent use of triamterene (Dyrenium) and indomethacin.

PHYSICAL EXAMINATION

A patient suffering from acute gout may be practically immobilized because of fear of irritating the involved extremity. With this come apprehension and impatience and often a request for immediate relief. The patient frequently is febrile. The temperature may reach 102°F. Tachycardia can also be present at these times, but usually within 2 or 3 days the fever and tachycardia and systemic symptoms subside. A patient with classical gout is frequently an obese, plethoric, middle-aged male who is unable to bear weight on an involved joint. These patients classically are first seen with a split shoe or cut slipper in place of the regular footwear and using a cane awkwardly to prevent painful weight bearing. The attack occurs so suddenly that they are willing to cut a pair of shoes or slippers to relieve any pressure on the involved foot joint. Initially, the involved joint is only slightly puffy and tender, but within several hours the site becomes pink, edematous, and swollen, and in a few days may become purplish and dusky. The site is exquisitely sensitive to any pressure, and is warm, dry, usually tight, and sometimes shiny. Articular effusion is frequently present, and while it can also be noted in some involved bunion joints, it is readily detectable in larger joints such as the knees. Here the swelling extends beyond the joint margins, and aspiration of this joint is easily carried out. The acute attack may cover a 2- to 10-day period, but the site will become less painful, less swollen, and less sensitive as the attack subsides. Desquamation of the site occurs in the phase of clearing of the joint swelling and inflammatory process. Seventy per cent of these patients experience the initial attack of acute gout in the first metatarsophalangeal joints. Subsequent attacks may involve the same or opposite joints. This is also true when the initial attack is in the wrist. The follow-up attack would frequently be in the same site, and subsequent attacks would be in the opposite joint. The olecranon and prepatellar bursae may become enlarged, red, bulbous, and hot and quite tender. The adjoining elbow joint moves without too much discomfort. Once the joint inflammation subsides completely, the joint is completely functional and comfortable and can be used in a normal manner, and there is seldom, if ever, a chronic effusion during the first 10 to 15 years of acute recurring gout. Further progression of the gouty attacks may result in a low-grade effusion and reduced range of motion of the articulation involved.

When gouty tophi are found, they are often located on the helix of the ears, in the olecranon and prepatellar bursae, and over the extensor surfaces of the fingers and knees. They usually denote long-standing disease. Tophi are found in less than 1 per cent of patients experiencing their first attack of gout. Tophi are painless, firm, and movable. They may vary from a lesion that is 1 or 2 mm in size to one that can be 2 to 3 cm across. Rarely they may drain chalky, toothpaste-like crystal and amorphous urate salts. Fortunately, infection seldom seems to occur, though this is a possibility and should be kept in mind. The tophaceous deposits may restrict joint motion or cause pain with weight bearing. Particularly around the olecranon bursa, the tophi can be confused with rheumatoid arthritis nodules and calcinosis in the skin or subcutaneous tissue and may also be confused with sarcoidosis and xanthomas. Nerves at the wrists have been entrapped by urate tophi, and the presenting picture is one of the carpal tunnel syndrome.

COMMON COMPLICATIONS

The most serious musculoskeletal disability is progressive, disabling chronic gouty arthritis with loss of function of the joints required for everyday living. The most important extraskeletal complication is kidney damage. Some gouty kidneys contain urate deposits within the interstitial tissues, but other pathologic changes may be associated with gout. Fortunately, there is infrequent occurrence of severe uremia. Urate urolithiasis occurs in about 20 per cent of patients with primary gout, which would be compatible with the number of patients who have an increased excretion of uric acid. On rare occasions, the renal pelvis may become mechanically blocked with uric acid sludge. This usually occurs in secondary gout associated with excessive cellular breakdown, most frequently seen in patients who are treated with cytotoxic and/or irradiation therapy. These patients may be hyperuricemic before the treatment, have had a very minute fluid daily intake, and may also be afflicted with serious obesity and low-grade renal function. Ischemic heart disease, diabetes mellitus, and hypertension are frequently found along with gout, but the significance of the association is not fully understood.

Drug interactions are important in the therapy of gout. This includes the initial evaluation, the therapeutic approaches to treatment of acute gout, and subsequent management of hyperuricemia and tophaceous gout.

LABORATORY FINDINGS

Confirmation of the diagnosis of gout is usually dependent upon laboratory findings. This may be either the histologic diagnosis of a tophus or the demonstration of one major criterion; that is, the finding of monosodium urate monohydrate microcrystals in joint fluid or bursa during an attack. More than 95 per cent of patients with gout eventually have an elevated serum uric acid level. Using colorimetric procedures, the serum uric acid concentration is found to be between 3 and 7 mg/dl for the adult male, yet 2 to 5 per cent of the male population accepted as normal may have higher serum uric acid concentrations. Premenopausal women usually have serum urate levels 1 mg/dl below those of males of the same age. The blood urea nitrogen and the creatinine rise with renal failure, but these changes may be subtle and slow. A young male with hyperuricemia and a strong family history of gout or urate kidney stones should be considered a candidate for future gout.

Liver function studies should be obtained for baseline data. Many medications utilized in gout therapy may affect the liver—in particular, allopurinol, and, to a lesser extent, the nonsteroidal anti-inflammatory drugs. Liver functions need monitoring if allopurinol therapy is utilized.

The normal 24-hour urinary uric acid excretion on a low-purine intake is about 600 mg. The urine pH is often low (5.0 to 5.5). There is elevation of the erythrocyte sedimentation rate, and the white blood cell count is increased in many patients with acute gout. This is not a necessary finding, but would be compatible with the inflammation.

Albuminuria is a common manifestation of urate nephropathy, occurring in 20 to 40 per cent of patients. The albuminuria may be intermittent or mild.

A deficiency of hypoxanthine-guanine phosphoribosyltransferase, which can be a factor in the cause of hyperuricemia, can be determined by calculating the ratio of urinary uric acid to urinary creatinine. This screening test notes that in the complete syndrome the ratio exceeds 2.0, whereas in the partial expression of the abnormality (also in leukemia and von Gierke's disease) values exceed 0.75.

The most direct method of diagnosing gout is identification of urate crystals from joint, bursa, or tophus. Examination of fluid aspirated from an acute gouty joint will usually demonstrate needle-like crystals within a leukocyte, but from a subacute joint only a few crystals may be identified. The crystals can be identified by using a polarizing light microscope with a first-order red compensator, which demonstrates the strongly negative birefringent optical properties of urate crystals. This equipment is available in clinical laboratories of most large hospitals. The percentage of positive findings varies according to the interest of the examiner, but one should not expect 100 per cent positive findings; yet when done properly, the procedure has a high yield for positive diagnoses in gouty patients. The fluid from acute gouty joints may appear grossly to be cloudy or, more rarely, milky. A poor mucin clot and 10,000 to 15,000 white blood cells per cu mm with 75 per cent neutrophils are typical of joint fluid from an acute gouty joint. The joint fluid glucose concentration, compared with the serum glucose, is normal, and culture is negative for microorganisms. Liver function studies should be closely scrutinized. It is advisable that serum uric acid levels be obtained on all known patients with gout, as well as those suspected of having the malady. The initial information obtained should include liver function studies, because many medications used in gout therapy and also for the relief of pain may affect the liver. Allopurinol and to a lesser extent the nonsteroidal anti-inflammatory drugs are rather frequent offenders in this area.

ROENTGENOGRAPHY

Gout is never diagnosed by radiographs. This is particularly true of the early attacks, for changes are seldom found in the joints during the first several attacks of gout. Uric acid and urate salts are translucent to x-rays. Unless calcium is present in the tophus, the involved area appears clear. There is rarely a uric acid deposit next to the edge of the joint sufficient to form an area of osteoporosis that is typical of gout unless the patient has suffered from the disease for a number of years.

Nonspecific soft-tissue swelling is found as an early roentgenographic change in acute gouty joints. The small tophaceous lesions on the edges of the bony structures are actually bubble-like erosions and are seen only after several attacks of gout in one localized area. Similar lesions may be seen in rheumatoid arthritis, but their location is not always as classical as that of gout. Renal calculi may be demonstrated in 6 per cent of patients with gout who undergo x-rays, but it must be remembered that the uric acid stone is also translucent and requires the use of contrast dye for the pyelogram. Radioisotope joint scans show marked localization at the site of the acute gout. The localization subsides quickly following therapy. Ultrasound of a renal structure or the ureter may demonstrate a stone, but the composition, of course, is not identifiable with this method.

The preliminary criteria for classification of acute arthritis of primary gout are given in Table 1.

Table 1. Classification of Acute Arthritis of Primary Gout*

Major Criteria

1. Monosodium urate monohydrate microcrystals in joint fluid during attack
2. Tophus (proved)

Minor Criteria

1. Maximum inflammation developed within 1 day
2. More than one attack of acute arthritis
3. Monoarthritis attack
4. Redness observed over joints
5. First metatarsophalangeal joint painful or swollen
6. Unilateral first metatarsophalangeal joint attack
7. Unilateral tarsal joint attack
8. Tophus (suspected)
9. Hyperuricemia
10. Asymmetric swelling within a joint on x-ray examination
11. Subcortical cysts without erosions on x-ray examination
12. Joint fluid culture negative for organisms during attack

*Classification as the acute arthritis of primary gout requires one major criterion or any six of the 12 minor criteria. From the American Rheumatism Association, 1977.

THERAPEUTIC TESTS

Acute joint inflammation and systemic symptoms of gout may be relieved in 80 to 90 per cent of patients who receive a full therapeutic dose of colchicine. It is essential that this colchicine be administered as early as possible when the acute attack begins. The first oral dose is 1 mg; then 0.5 mg is given every 2 hours until relief of symptoms or gastrointestinal toxicity occurs. Some therapists prefer intervals of 1 hour between doses, but occasionally this causes gastrointestinal tract upset before sufficient drug is absorbed to be effective. Usually, symptomatic benefits are noted 6 to 12 hours after the complete therapeutic dose of colchicine is given, and the favorable change is significant in 48 to 72 hours. Customarily it is preferred not to give over 10 to 12 doses, but should diarrhea occur before that, the drug should be discontinued immediately and the patients should be forewarned and possibly given some antidiarrhea drug, such as paregoric, or they will be miserable from this phase of treatment.

A diagnostic test with a therapeutic dose of intravenous colchicine may be used if it is administered carefully and properly diluted. The intravenous injection of up to 3 mg of colchicine over a 5-minute period is the initial dose. As the agent can be very sclerosing, it should be certain that this is given directly into a vein and injected slowly. To avoid a recurrence of acute symptoms, 0.5 mg of intravenous colchicine may be given in 6 to 8 hours once or twice daily, not over 5 mg total dosage. Oral colchicine can be given for the same reason in doses of 0.5 mg once or twice daily after the initial dose has been administered. Diarrhea may occur after the intravenous colchicine injection but possibly not as frequently. Occasionally, patients suffering from calcific gout or sarcoid arthritis will be relieved of their symptoms, but usually other clinical and laboratory findings will differentiate these conditions from gout. The exact acuity of these therapeutic tests has been questioned, but clinical trial is often indicated and a favorable experience can be very convincing.

PITFALLS IN DIAGNOSIS

The diagnostician is prompted to think of gout when hyperuricemia is discovered on the serum chemical analysis, but it may be found in many other conditions or diseases, including psoriasis, renal failure, heavy metal poisoning, hyperparathyroidism, diabetes mellitus, obesity, strenuous dieting, myeloproliferative and lymphoproliferative disorders, glycogen storage disease (Type I), sarcoidosis, Down's syndrome, hypertension, and alcoholism. Thiazide, furosemide, ethacrynic acid, levodopa, ethambutol, and small doses of aspirin (1200 to 1800 mg/day) may cause hyperuricemia that is completely asymptomatic. The consumption of a large amount of aspirin can serve as a uricosuric agent with lowering of the serum uric acid level. Often though, this causes gastric irritation and cannot be sustained for any long periods of time. Glycopyrrolate (Robinul) may lower serum uric acid levels by altering its renal excretion. By reducing the serum uric acid, such drugs may introduce a diagnostic error in patients who without these drugs would have hyperuricemia.

Moderately large doses of ascorbic acid (4 gm) may increase uric acid excretion and decrease serum uric acid levels. This may also contribute to renal stone formation. Also ascorbic acid may alter the colorimetric assay of serum uric acid causing a false elevation in the reading.

The routine use of radiocontrast agents in the evaluation of a patient's kidneys may temporarily reduce the serum uric acid and increase the urine uric acid excretion for 5 to 6 days. This may result in errors in diagnosis as well as in the therapeutic approach. Intravenous pyelogram studies must be done selectively and closely followed in patients with significant hyperuricemia to avoid further renal complications.

Infection or cellulitis in or about an articulation and acute thrombophlebitis near a joint may suggest acute "gouty arthritis," particularly when it occurs explosively and postoperatively.

Locally inflamed bunion joints may be differentiated from podagra by careful x-ray studies or a therapeutic test dose of colchicine if it is not possible to aspirate fluid from the bursa and study it for monosodium urate crystals.

Chondrocalcinosis (pseudogout) is often associated with episodes of acute arthritis that often occur in the knees but may involve the small joints. This condition is seen more frequently in females than in males, and it usually occurs in middle-aged or older patients. Often there is chronic polyarticular disease. The attack is seldom as severe as uric acid gout. The diagnosis is reinforced by radiologic chondrocalcinosis and then confirmed by the presence of calcium pyrophosphate crystals in the synovium and synovial fluid of acute pseudogout. The calcium pyrophosphate crystals are weakly positive birefringent under polarized light. Again, this particular type of crystalline arthritis depends upon special microscopic studies for verifying the diagnosis.

Acute attacks of palindromic rheumatism that occur explosively are associated with a very painful monarticular arthritis, are probably a modified version of early acute rheumatoid arthritis, and may simulate acute gout. These attacks are usually quite brief, disappear completely, and are not associated with hyperuricemia. The joint fluid from these patients does not contain crystals.

Olecranon bursitis of rheumatoid arthritis with nodules sometimes requires a biopsy of the nodule to differentiate it from gout. A gouty tophaceous lesion on biopsy will present with uric acid crystals. In England, a few urate crystal tophi have been found without gout or acute inflammation.

A patient with septic arthritis will initially have an acutely swollen, very painful joint. Joint aspiration with smear and culture will reveal the causative agent. Although the Gonococcus organism may be difficult to isolate in some of these patients, the presence of cutaneous hemorrhagic lesions typical of neisserian infection is helpful in diagnosis. If there is a question of gout or gonococcal arthritis involving one joint, it would be wise to treat the joint as an infected joint until the diagnosis can be proved. In this way, acute joint destruction from septic involvement can be avoided. The fluid of such a joint will usually have a low glucose content, but it is important that this level of glucose be compared with the serum glucose so that an exact reading may be obtained. Traumatic arthritis may be confused with gout, but usually the degree of injury and the history identify the cause.

A recurrence often follows inadequate therapy of the acute attack of gout or failure to continue daily prophylactic colchicine following an acute attack. The initial administration of a uricosuric drug (probenecid or sulfinpyrazone) or allopurinol (Zyloprim) without daily colchicine (0.5 mg) results in an acute flare-up in 30 per cent of these patients. Attacks of gout tend to recur in a rebound pattern. This also follows with withdrawal of ACTH or after the intramuscular injection of high-potency adrenal steroids. Acute polycyclic gout may require more than general administration of a round of colchicine and/or an anti-inflammatory agent. The failure of an acute attack of gout to respond fully to conventional therapy can cause confusion in diagnosis and treatment.

Reduced range of joint motion and chronic pain mark chronic gouty arthritis. If a patient with this condition is seeing a physician for the first time, it may easily be confused with one of the other arthritic problems.

Probenecid and sulfinpyrazone may be very effective in lowering serum uric acid levels, but the effect may be blocked by the concurrent administration of salicylates or citrates, producing faulty therapeutic results.

The microscopic study of tissues for urate crystals requires that the specimens be fixed in absolute ethanol. A formalin solution, which is used routinely, may dissolve the crystals, thereby leaving a blank space at the tissue site and may confuse the correct diagnosis.

THE PORPHYRIAS

By Herbert L. Bonkovsky, M.D.
White River Junction, Vermont

NORMAL HEME METABOLISM

The porphyrias are diseases, usually inherited, caused by severe defects in heme biosynthesis. They are expressed clinically in two major ways: by attacks of neurologic dysfunction, and by photosensitivity. In some types of porphyria, only one or the other of these manifestations occurs, whereas in others both types may occur, either concurrently or independently.

The Heme Biosynthetic Pathway

Understanding the porphyrias and the methods used for their diagnosis requires knowledge of the heme biosynthetic pathway, which is summarized in Figure 1.

Heme is synthesized from the building blocks succinyl CoA, glycine and iron. The specific precursors of

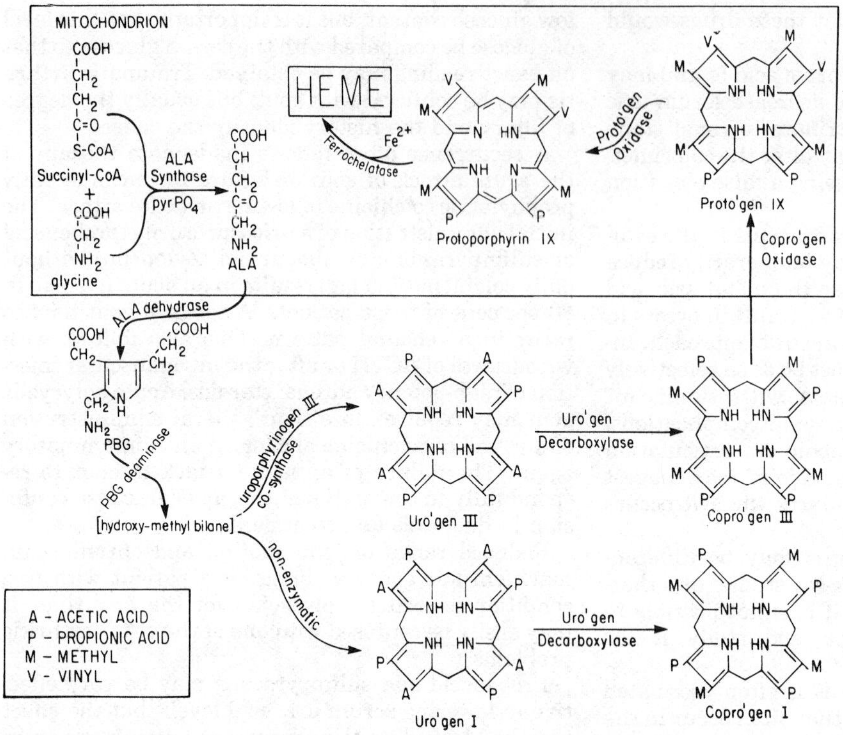

Figure 1. The heme biosynthetic pathway, showing structures of the intermediates and cellular compartmentalization of the enzymes. ALA = 5-aminolevulinic acid; copro'gen= coproporphyrinogen; PBG = porphobilinogen; proto'gen = protoporphyrinogen; uro'gen = uroporphyrinogen. (From Bonkowsky, H.L.: Porphyrin and heme metabolism and the porphyrias. In Zakim, D., and Boyer, T. (eds.) *Hepatology: A Textbook of Liver Disease.* Philadelphia, W. B. Saunders Company, 1982.)

heme are 5-aminolevulinic acid (ALA), the monopyrrole porphobilinogen (PBG), a series of tetrapyrrolic porphyrinogens with decreasing numbers (from 8 to 2) of carboxylic acid side chains, and finally protoporphyrin and Fe^{2+}. Only porphyrinogens belonging to the III isomer series are converted to heme. Normally, very little porphyrinogen of the I series is formed.

Defective activity of one of the enzymes of the heme synthetic pathway is the primary cause of each type of porphyria (Table 1). As might be expected, such defects may lead to the accumulation of heme precursors proximal to the defective enzyme. In some instances, the rate and severity of this accumulation are markedly increased owing to secondary increases in activity of ALA synthase, the first and normally rate-limiting enzyme of the pathway. In the liver, for example, there is much evidence to support the model shown in Figure 2, wherein a *regulatory heme pool* exerts end-product negative feedback repression on ALA synthase. A partial block in normal heme synthesis, an increased need for heme to synthesize hemoproteins, especially cytochrome P450, or an increased rate of breakdown of hepatic heme or hemoproteins will deplete the regulatory heme pool, de-repress ALA synthase, and tend to restore the regulatory heme pool to normal. The more severe the block in synthesis, the greater the increase in ALA synthase required to restore the rate of heme synthesis to normal.

Porphyrins and Porphyrin Precursors

Among the porphyrins, only protoporphyrin IX serves as a precursor for heme (Fig. 1). All other tetrapyrrolic precursors are porphyrinogens, which are the reduced forms of porphyrins. These porphyrinogens are colorless and nonfluorescent, whereas the porphyrins are red to purple in color and exhibit intense red fluorescence when excited by light with a wavelength around 400 nm. Although in several of the porphyrias, it is actually the porphyrinogens that accumulate, they are readily oxidized to their corresponding porphyrins. Such oxidation may occur within the body or in plasma, urine, or feces after their removal from or excretion by the patient.

The porphyrins also differ markedly in their solubility characteristics. Those with many carboxylic acid side chains (e.g., uroporphyrin) are water-soluble and mainly excreted in the urine, whereas those with few carboxylic acid side chains (e.g., protoporphyrin) are lipid-soluble and excreted via the bile into the feces. Those with intermediate numbers of carboxylic acid side chains (e.g., coproporphyrin) are excreted by both routes, and the relative amounts excreted may vary. In the presence of cholestasis, for example, relatively more coproporphyrin is excreted in the urine.

The methods in common clinical use for separating porphyrins depend on differences in solubility and employ solvent extraction and partition techniques. They yield fractions, called "uro-," "copro-," and "protoporphyrin," that in fact contain a mixture of closely related porphyrins. Usually, but not always, each consists mainly of the porphyrin for which it is named. Thin-layer or high-performance liquid chromatographic methods of separation of porphyrin free acids or their methyl esters have been developed. These methods can separate and quantitate each individual porphyrin (e.g., 8,7,6-COOH groups) and can also separate the I and III isomers. These newer methods, however, are not usually needed for clinical diagnosis.

Porphyrins are intensely photoactive and cause the photosensitivity reactions that are one of the clinical hallmarks of the porphyrias. However, for some reason, the damage caused by uro- or coproporphyrin is quite different from that caused by protoporphyrin. Unlike photosensitivity, the pathogenesis of the neurologic manifestations of acute porphyria remains less well understood. However, evidence is growing that ALA plays an important role in causing at least some of the neurologic manifestations of acute porphyria.

Screening Tests

Rapid presumptive diagnosis of the porphyrias is aided by the use of a few simple tests.

Porphyrins in Urine

Talc Test. Adjust the pH of 10 ml of urine to about 4.0 by adding 1 ml 1M sodium acetate, pH 3.7. Add 0.1 gm talc (Riedel de Haen) and shake vigorously. Centrifuge for 10 minutes at about 1000 g, and examine the talc under a Wood's lamp. Distinct pink or red fluorescence of the talc is positive.

Amyl Alcohol Test. Adjust the pH of 4 ml of urine as described earlier. Add 1 ml amyl alcohol, shake, and allow phases to separate. Examine with a Wood's lamp. Pink or red fluorescence in the upper, organic layer is positive.

A positive result with either test suggests the presence of increased porphyrins in the urine, which may be due to porphyria or other conditions. Therefore, all positives should be confirmed by a procedure that quantitates both uro- and coproporphyrin fractions. Occasionally, nonporphyrins will fluoresce, causing false-positive reactions. False-negative results may also occur because of an insufficent concentration of porphyrin in the urine sample tested (e.g., very dilute urine) or because of the presence of compounds that quench porphyrin fluorescence.

Porphyrins in Erythrocytes

One of the following tests is ordinarily used, depending upon the equipment available:

Acid Extraction. Collect blood in heparin under subdued light and keep in the dark. Mix 0.1 ml of blood with 2.5 ml of a mixture of peroxide-free ether (or ethyl acetate) plus glacial acetic acid (4:1, volume:volume [v:v]). Break up the red blood cells

Table 1. Classification of Porphyrias*

	Synonyms	Primary Enzymatic Defect	Inheritance
Acute† hepatic porphyrias			
Acute intermittent porphyria	Swedish porphyria Pyrroloporphyria	Porphobilinogen deaminase	Dominant
Hereditary coproporphyria		Coproporphyrinogen oxidase	Dominant
Variegate porphyria	South African porphyria	Protoporphyrinogen oxidase Ferrochelatase ?	Dominant
Porphyria due to deficiency of delta-aminolevulinic acid (ALA) dehydrase		ALA dehydrase	Recessive
Porphyria cutanea tarda	Chronic hepatic porphyria, type D Symptomatic porphyria	Uroporphyrinogen decarboxylase (heterozygous)	Sporadic or dominant
Protoporphyria	Erythrohepatic protoporphyria Erythropoietic protoporphyria	Ferrochelatase	Dominant
Hepatoerythropoietic porphyria		Uroporphyrinogen decarboxylase (homozygous)	Recessive
Erthropoietic porphyria			
Congenital erythropoietic porphyria	Günther's disease	Uroporphyrinogen III cosynthase ? Increased porphobilinogen deaminase ?	Recessive

*From Bonkowsky, H.L.: Porphyrin and heme metabolism and the porphyrias. In Zakim, D., and Boyer, T. (eds.): *Hepatology: A Textbook of Liver Disease.* Philadelphia, W.B. Saunders Company, 1982, p. 366.
†As used in this classification, the term "acute" refers to the fact that acute attacks of neurovisceral dysfunction may occur in these diseases. The underlying genetic defect, however, is present throughout life.

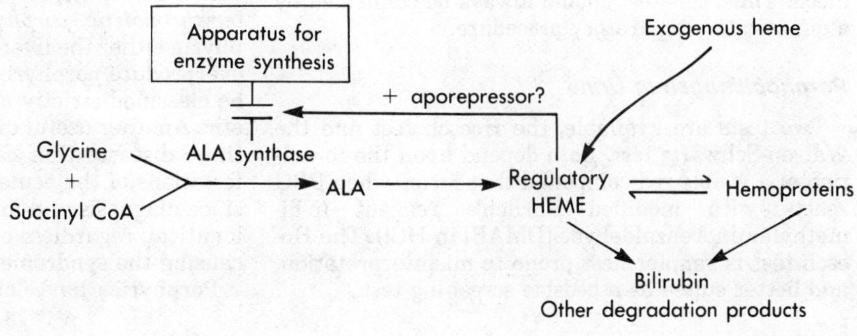

Figure 2. Regulation of hepatic heme synthesis. (From Bonkowsky, H. L.: Porphyrin and heme metabolism and the porphyrias. In Zakim, D., and Boyer, T. (eds.): *Hepatology: A Textbook of Liver Disease.* Philadelphia, W. B. Saunders Company, 1982.)

with a glass rod and shake vigorously. After the phases have separated, transfer the supernatant to a glass tube and extract with 1.0 ml of 3M HCl. Again, centrifuge briefly or allow phases to separate by gravity and examine the lower (aqueous acid) layer with a Wood's lamp. Distinct pink to red fluorescence is positive.

This test is positive in erythropoietic porphyria, usually in protoporphyria, and often in lead poisoning or iron deficiency anemia in which zinc protoporphyrin is increased in erythrocytes. Treatment with acid removes zinc readily, leaving free protoporphyrin. Erythrocyte porphyrins are usually normal in the hepatic porphyrias, but the elevated levels in plasma in patients with severe skin lesions may lead to a positive result in this test.

Fluorescence Microscopy. Mix a drop of freshly obtained heparinized blood with two drops of normal saline on a glass slide. Cover with a cover slip and examine for porphyrin fluorescence (excitation = 380 to 450 nm, emission = 580 to 650 nm). A positive test is the presence of numerous fluorescent erythrocytes. Normally, only rare fluorescent cells are seen. The major pitfall here is that the fluorescence of protoporphyrin fades rapidly, especially when, as is usual, a mercury vapor lamp is used. (Fluorescence of protoporphyrin lasts a minute or more when a 100-watt iodine-tungsten quartz lamp is used.)

A positive result with either test should be confirmed by quantitative determination of porphyrin in separated erythrocytes and plasma. Zinc protoporphyrin, but not free protoporphyrin, can be extracted from erythrocytes with neutral ethanol, permitting clear differentiation between increased free protoporphyrin and increased zinc protoporphyrin.

Porphyrins in Stool

To a portion (1 to 2 gm) of stool add 2 ml of a solution of amyl alcohol, glacial acetic acid, and ether (1:1:1, v:v:v). View under a Wood's lamp, looking for red fluorescence. If such fluorescence is seen, add 2 ml of 1.5M HCl and shake vigorously. A positive test is shown by the appearance of red fluorescence in the aqueous acid (lower) phase. Chlorophyll, which also fluoresces red, remains in the organic (upper) phase. This test is difficult to interpret because some samples from nonporphyric, especially constipated, subjects may be positive. Then too, most of the protoporphyrin in normal stool is derived from bacterial action on heme compounds in the diet rather than protoporphyrin secreted in the bile. Gastrointestinal bleeding often causes increased fecal protoporphyrin that is not invariably accompanied by a positive test for occult blood. Thus, this test should always be confirmed by a quantitative separatory procedure.

Porphobilinogen in Urine

Two tests are available, the Hoesch test and the Watson-Schwartz test. Both depend upon the formation of a visible red compound that forms when PBG reacts with modified Ehrlich's reagent (p-dimethylaminobenzaldehyde [DMAB] in HCl). The Hoesch test is simpler, less prone to misinterpretation, and better suited as a bedside screening test.

Hoesch Test. Prepare a solution of 2.0 gm DMAB in 100 ml of 6M HCl. To 1 to 2 ml of this reagent add 1 to 2 drops of urine. A positive test is shown by the immediate development of a cherry-red color at the top of the solution as the urine contacts the reagent.

Watson-Schwartz Test. The DMAB solution in this case is 0.7 gm dissolved in 150 ml of concentrated HCl plus 100 ml of water. Add 1 ml of urine to 1 ml of this reagent. An immediate red color suggests the presence of excess PBG. Neutralize the mixture by adding 2 ml of saturated sodium acetate; formation of a red color only at this stage, or marked deepening of the color, suggests the presence of urobilinogen. Add 3 ml of chloroform and shake vigorously. A positive test for PBG is a red color in the aqueous (upper) phase. In contrast, the urobilinogen chromophore partitions into the organic (lower) phase. Positive results may be further confirmed by re-extracting the aqueous phase (in a second tube) with an equal volume of n-butanol. The PBG chromophore remains in the aqueous (now lower) phase.

As shown in Table 2, a number of substances will give a red color with Ehrlich's reagent. The possibility of a red pH indicator should be checked by reacting the urine with 6M HCl not containing DMAB. Urobilinogen should not lead to confusion, and most of the other compounds listed will also be extracted into chloroform or n-butanol. However in some subjects, indoles, methyldopa metabolites, or other substances may remain in the aqueous phase. Therefore, all positive tests should be confirmed by quantitative determination of PBG, preferably with simultaneous measurement of ALA as well. An additional pitfall is that, especially at acid pH, PBG rapidly polymerizes nonenzymatically to form uroporphyrin or porphobilin. Therefore, relatively small increases in PBG may be missed, especially if the urine is not tested promptly. Usually, neither the Watson-Schwartz test nor the Hoesch test is positive unless concentrations of PBG exceed about 10 mg/liter. (The normal upper limit is about 2.5 mg/liter.)

CLASSIFICATION OF THE PORPHYRIAS

Most of the porphyrias were described clinically before the normal pathway of heme biosynthesis had been elucidated. Accordingly, they are not generally named for the primary enzymic defects now known to cause them. As shown in Table 1, several of the diseases have alternative names. One useful method of classification, followed in Table 1, is according to the major site of overproduction of heme precursors, either the liver (*hepatic porphyrias*) or the bone marrow (*erythropoietic porphyrias*). However, in protoporphyria either the liver, the bone marrow, or both may overproduce porphyrin. Thus, protoporphyria cannot be classified strictly as either hepatic or erythropoietic. Another useful distinction can be made between those diseases that can cause the neurologic manifestations of the acute attack and those that cannot, since diagnosis and management of such attacks are identical, regardless of the specific type of porphyria causing the syndrome.

Porphyrias have long been classified as *manifest*

Table 2. Substances Giving a Red Color in Screening Tests for Porphobilinogen

pH Indicators That Turn Red in Acid Solution*
Phenazopyridinium chloride (Pyridium)
Methyl red
Urosein
Substances Reacting with Ehrlich's Reagent
Porphobilinogen
Urobilinogen
Metabolites of
Cascara sagrada bark extract
Levomepromazine
Methyldopa
Sedormid
Phylloerythrinogen
Indoles
Pyrrole mono- and dicarboxylic acids

*Can be detected by use of hydrochloric acid not containing Ehrlich's reagent in the Watson-Schwartz or Hoesch Test.

(i.e., with clinical manifestations) or *latent* (i.e., with overproduction of heme precursors but lacking clinical manifestation). The advent of methods for testing for specific enzymic defects has revealed a third category of affected persons, namely, the *carrier state.* Carriers lack both clinical features and overproduction of heme precursors, but demonstrate the underlying genetic defect in enzymic activity. The existence of the carrier state (1) proves that defective enzymic activities are themselves not sufficient to produce clinical porphyria and (2) makes it necessary to measure enzyme activities in order to fully diagnose some porphyric kindreds.

As shown in Table 1, most of the porphyrias are inherited. However, porphyria cutanea tarda (PCT) is often acquired, occurring sporadically in subjects with no family history. Even here, however, an inherited form of the disease also exists and in some populations may predominate.

PCT is probably the most common form of porphyria, followed by protoporphyria. Acute intermittent porphyria (AIP) is the most commonly recognized form of acute porphyria except in South Africans of Dutch extraction, in whom variegate porphyria (VP) is highly prevalent. Hepatoerythropoietic porphyria is an extremely rare disorder that apparently represents very severe, probably homozygous, deficiency in activity of uroporphyrinogen decarboxylase. Congenital erythropoietic porphyria (CEP) is also very rare.

ACUTE HEPATIC PORPHYRIAS

Four distinct forms of hepatic porphyria may produce severe neurologic manifestations: AIP, hereditary coproporphyria, VP, and porphyria due to a genetic deficiency of ALA dehydrase. An acute porphyric syndrome, accompanied by an acquired severe deficiency of ALA dehydrase, may also occur in lead poisoning and hereditary tyrosinemia. Clinically, the neurologic manifestations are identical in all these disorders and specific diagnosis depends upon chemical determinations.

The Acute Attack

The typical patient is a woman in her 20s who develops severe colicky abdominal pain during the luteal phase of her menstrual cycle. The pain may abate as menses begin, only to recur during later menstrual cycles. The acute attack may also worsen and involve the following:

1. The autonomic nervous system, with tachycardia, supine hypertension, and orthostatic hypotension.
2. The peripheral nervous system, usually with mainly motor deficits.
3. The central nervous system, with bulbar involvement, delirium, seizures, and coma.

The relative frequencies of the more common manifestations are listed in Table 3.

As listed in Table 4, several other factors besides the luteal phase of the menstrual cycle are known to precipitate or worsen acute porphyric attacks. Among these, drugs and chemicals are most important. In men, for example, the most common recognizable precipitating event is barbiturate ingestion. Several patients with unrecognized disease have been worsened or killed by barbiturates administered intra- or perioperatively, during ill-advised surgical procedures undertaken because of abdominal pain.

As shown in Table 5, drugs fall into three categories with respect to acute porphyria:

1. Those that have been reported to exacerbate disease.
2. Those that are theoretically risky, although not yet reported to have exacerbated disease.
3. Those believed to be safe, based both upon clinical experience and theoretical considerations.

(A fourth large category, namely drugs of unknown status, might be added.) In general, the "risky" drugs are those that tend to deplete the hepatic regulatory heme pool (Fig. 2), including all inducers of cytochrome P450.

Laboratory Findings and Chemical Features

Routine laboratory determinations (hemogram, urinalysis, erythrocyte sedimentation rate, electrolytes, blood urea nitrogen, serum amylase, liver function tests) are usually normal, helping to exclude other causes of abdominal pain. Patients may have hyponatremia, which in some is related to the syndrome of inappropriate secretion of antidiuretic hormone (SIADH). Serum thyroxine (T_4) is often elevated owing to increased concentrations of thyroid-binding globulin; the free T_4 is normal. Serum cholesterol and low-density lipoproteins (LDL) concentrations are often increased.

The most useful laboratory test to aid in rapid diagnosis of symptomatic acute porphyria is one of the qualitative tests for PBG in the urine. Regardless of whether one is dealing with AIP, hereditary coproporphyria, or VP, the test for PBG will be strongly positive. It is essential to recall that PBG, a monopyrrole, is *not* a tetrapyrrolic porphyrin (see the structures in Fig. 1); therefore, it is not adequate to request a urine porphyrin-screen. Furthermore, in the genetic or acquired severe deficiencies of ALA dehydrase, urinary

Table 3. Clinical Features of Manifest Acute Intermittent Porphyria Necessitating Hospitalization (Percentages of Patients with Symptoms and Signs)*†

Symptom	Per Cent	Sign	Per Cent
Abdominal pain	95	Tachycardia (heart rate > 100/min at rest)	80
Extremity pain/paresthesias	50	Dark urine	74
Constipation	48	Peripheral motor deficit	60
Nausea, vomiting	43	Bulbar involvement	46
Back pain	29	Mental confusion/hallucinations	40
Chest pain	12	Hypertension (diastolic pressure > 90 mm Hg)	36
Diarrhea	5	Absent reflexes	29
		Peripheral sensory deficit	26
		Postural hypotension (> 20 mm Hg pressure reduction in upright position)	21
		Palpable dilated loops of bowel	21
		Seizures	20
		Bladder distention	12
		Coma	10
		Dyshydrosis	12
		Fever (no apparent cause)	9
		Fecal impaction	6

*From Bonkowsky, H.L.: Porphyrin and heme metabolism and the porphyrias. In Zakim, D., and Boyer, T. (eds.): *Hepatology: A Textbook of Liver Disease.* Philadelphia, W.B. Saunders Company, 1982, p. 368.
†Findings in variegate porphyria and hereditary coproporphyria are similar.

Table 4. Factors That May Precipitate or Worsen Attacks of Acute Porphyria

Drugs and chemicals (see Table 5)
Luteal phase of menstrual cycle
Diminished intake of food, especially carbohydrates
Infection
Emotional and other stress

PBG is normal or nearly normal, whereas urinary ALA is markedly increased. Thus, if the index of suspicion of acute porphyria is high but the PBG-screening test is normal, urine should be sent for quantitative ALA and PBG determination.

Differential Diagnosis

During acute attacks, the differentiation between AIP, hereditary coproporphyria or VP is of little practical importance, since management is the same for all. Photosensitivity-induced skin lesions do not occur in AIP and are rare in hereditary coproporphyria (unless there is intercurrent cholestasis from some other cause); however, they occur in most patients with VP who have acute attacks. The skin lesions in VP or hereditary coproporphyria are indistinguishable from those caused by PCT. Skin lesions do not occur in the diseases due to deficiency of ALA dehydrase (lead poisoning, hereditary tyrosinemia, genetic severe deficiency).

Specific diagnosis rests upon quantitative determination of urinary and fecal heme precursors. Table 6 summarizes the usual chemical findings in latent and manifest porphyrias. As shown, AIP, hereditary coproporphyria, and VP can usually be distinguished by the stool porphyrin patterns: normal in AIP, mainly coproporphyrin in coproporphyria, mainly protoporphyrin in VP.

Evaluation of Latent Cases and Kindreds

Between acute attacks of disease or among patients who have never had an acute attack, urinary excretion of ALA and PBG may be normal. This occurs most often in hereditary coproporphyria or VP. Diagnosis then rests upon family history, quantitative urinary and fecal porphyrin excretions, and assays of specific enzymes in the heme pathway.

The test for PBG deaminase, the enzyme that is defective in AIP, is carried out most conveniently on erythrocytes, whereas those for the mitochondrial oxidases of coproporphyrinogen and protoporphyrinogen, deficient in hereditary coproporphyria and VP respectively, require leukocytes, cultured fibroblasts or other mitochondria-bearing tissue. Studies of kindreds of known patients have shown that, especially in AIP, genetic carriers with normal heme precursor excretions are common, accounting for one third of all subjects with the gene defect.

Thus, thorough diagnostic evaluation of kindreds optimally includes these enzyme assays in addition to excretory data. Unfortunately, the enzyme assays for the mitochondrial oxidases are complicated and are done in only a few research laboratories. Even the assay for PBG deaminase in erythrocytes requires careful interpretation, since it is affected by many variables (e.g., age of patient, age of erythrocytes, handling and storage of erythrocytes) and since some patients with AIP have been described with normal deaminase activities.

PORPHYRIA CUTANEA TARDA

Clinical Features

Patients usually seek medical help in mid- or late summer because of vesicles, bullae, and sores on the dorsa of the hands. The vesicles and bullae contain a

Table 5. Drugs and Chemicals in Acute Hepatic Porphyrias*

Reported to Exacerbate Disease†	Theoretically Risky	Believed to be Safe
Barbiturates		
Bemegride	Allyl-containing compounds	Aspirin
Chloramphenicol		Atropine
Chlordiazepoxide	Clonazepam (large doses)	Bromides
Chlorpropamide	Clonidine	Calcium salts
Chloroquine	Hydralazine	Chlorpromazine
Danazol	Methychlorthiazide	Chloral hydrate
Diazepam	Pargyline	Corticosteroids
Ergot preparations	Phenoxybenzamine	*d*-Tubocurarine
Estrogens	Spironolactone	Cyclopropane
Ethanol Excess		Dicumarol
Eucalyptol (in mouthwash)		Droperidol
Glutethimide	All agents known to induce cytochrome P450 or to increase hepatic heme turnover	Ether
Griseofulvin		Gallamine
Halothane		Guanethidine
Hydantoins		Mefenamic acid
Imipramine		Meperidine
Ketamine		Methadone
Meprobamate		Morphine
Methyldopa		Neostigmine
Methyprylon		Nitrous oxide
Methsuccimide		Paraldehyde
Nikethamide		Penicillin
Oral Contraceptives		Pentamethonium
Pentazocine		Procaine
Phensuccimide		Promazine
Phenylbutazone		Promethazine
Progestagens		Propoxyphene
Pyrazinamide		Propranolol
Pyrazolone derivatives		Reserpine
Sulfonamides		Succinylcholine
Theophylline derivatives		Tetracycline
Tolbutamide		Vitamins A, B, C, D, and E
Troxidone		
Valproate		

*From Bonkowsky, H.L.: Porphyrin and heme metabolism and the porphyrias. In Zakim, D., and Boyer, T. (eds.): *Hepatology: A Textbook of Liver Disease.* Philadelphia, W.B. Saunders Company, 1982, p. 370.

†Among agents reported to exacerbate disease, those in italic type are incriminated most often. Those listed as Theoretically risky have not been incriminated clearly in humans, but experimental studies indicate they have potential for damage. Those believed to be safe have been used in humans without ill effects, are not theoretically risky, and have not been reported to exacerbate porphyria.

serous fluid high in porphyrin concentration. Such lesions break down to form sores that heal very slowly, usually with scarring and hypo- or hyper pigmentation. Abrasions and chronic sores occur after trivial damage to the skin and there is a marked increase in skin fragility.

The typical patient is a middle-aged man who drinks substantial quantities of alcohol. Overt diabetes mellitus or milder degrees of glucose intolerance are common. There may also be evidence of skin damage about the ears, head, and neck; and temporal hirsutism is frequent. The disease is being reported with increasing frequency in young women taking oral contraceptives and in patients undergoing chronic hemodialysis.

Patients with PCT usually have evidence of liver disease. In most, alcohol or some other etiologic agent can be incriminated as an inciting stimulus for development of both liver disease and PCT. In some, however, no cause for the liver disease can be found, other than the abnormal deposition of porphyrins, and it may be that the stored porphyrins themselves are hepatotoxic. In addition to the skin lesions, patients often have hepatomegaly and sometimes splenomegaly as well. Testicular atrophy, Dupuytren's contractures, palmar erythema and other peripheral stigmata of liver disease may occur, but are of little diagnostic aid.

Patients usually have a history of heavy alcohol intake and/or of estrogen use. Positive family history is usually lacking, although careful study of family members may reveal subclinical evidence of abnormal porphyrin metabolism in some kindreds.

Laboratory Findings and Chemical Features

Routine hemogram and urinalysis as a rule are normal, although glycosuria may be present. Some (usually modest) elevation of liver function tests (SGOT, SGPT, serum alkaline phosphatase) is the rule. Patients are rarely icteric. Serum ferritin and saturation of serum transferrin are commonly increased, and liver biopsy reveals moderate siderosis. There is also mild to moderate hepatic inflammation and fibrosis. Spotty hepatocellular necrosis and fatty change are common. Unfixed liver tissue fluoresces brightly, owing to a marked increase in uro- and 7-carboxyl-porphyrin content.

The key screening test is for urinary porphyrins; this should be strongly positive, since patients rarely have symptoms unless they are excreting more than 800 μg of urinary porphyrin per day. It is essential to obtain quantitative confirmation of a positive screening test. As shown in Table 6, the urinary uroporphyrin will be markedly increased, usually several fold above the coproporphyrin.

Differential Diagnosis

Quantitative stool and erythrocyte porphyrins should also be carried out in all cases of presumed PCT. Stool porphyrins should be done to help exclude VP or the rare case of hereditary coproporphyria and intercurrent liver disease that presents with skin lesions. In both manifest hereditary coproporphyria and VP, urinary PBG may sometimes polymerize to the extent that urinary uroporphyrin concentrations will resemble those in PCT. It is therefore useful to measure urinary ALA and PBG, as well as porphyrins, since even after such nonenzymatic polymerization, excess concentrations of ALA and PBG usually persist. The increase in fecal "coproporphyrin" observed in PCT is mainly due to the presence of compounds of the isocoproporphyrin series. Such compounds accumulate only when activity of uroporphyrinogen decarboxylase is decreased. Thus, measurement of the ratio of isocoproporphyrin/coproporphyrin can aid in distinguishing PCT from other cutaneous porphyrias in difficult cases. In PCT the ratio is greater than 0.5, whereas it is less than 0.5 in hereditary coproporphyria or VP. Measurement of erythrocytic porphyrins will distinguish PCT from the

Table 6. Usual Chemical Findings in the Porphyrias*

	Urine (mg/gm Creatinine)		Urine (μg/gm Creatinine)		Feces (μg/gm Dry Weight)			Erythrocytes (μg/dl Packed Erythrocytes)		
	ALA	*PBG*	*Uro*	*Copro*	*Uro*	*Copro*	*Proto*	*Uro*	*Copro*	*Proto*
Normal values†	< 3	< 2.5	10–60	50–250	0–5	Tr–50	Tr–120	0–1	0–20	15–60
Acute hepatic porphyrias										
Acute intermittent porphyria										
Latent	↑	↑	N	N	N	N	N	N	N	N
Manifest	↑↑	↑↑	↑	↑	N	N	↑	N	N	N
Hereditary coproporphyria										
Latent	N	N	N	↑↑	N	↑	N	N	N	N
Manifest	↑↑	↑↑	↑	↑↑	N	↑↑	↑	N	N	N
Variegate porphyria										
Latent	N	N	N	↑	N	↑	↑	N	N	N
Manifest	↑↑	↑↑	↑	↑↑	N	↑	↑↑	N	N	N
ALA dehydrase deficiency	↑↑	↑	N	↑↑	N	N	N	N	N	↑↑
Porphyria cutanea tarda										
Latent	N	N	↑	N	↑	N	N	N	N	N
Manifest	N	N	↑↑	↑	↑	↑	N	N	N	N
Protoporphyria										
Latent	N	N	N	N	N	N	↑	N	N	↑
Manifest	N	N	N	N	N	N	↑↑	N	N	↑↑
Hepatoerythropoietic porphyria	N	N	↑↑	↑	↑	↑	↑	N	N	↑
Erythropoietic porphyria										
Congenital erythropoietic uroporphyria	N	N	↑↑	↑	↑↑	↑↑	N	↑↑	↑	↑

*From Bonkowsky, H.L.: Porphyrin and heme metabolism and the porphyrias. In Zakim, D., and Boyer, T. (eds.): *Hepatology: A Textbook of Liver Disease.* Philadelphia, W.B. Saunders Company, 1982, p. 364.

† As used in the author's laboratory.

With the methods usually employed, "uroporphyrin," "coproporphyrin," and "protoporphyrin" are not strictly separated and identified. Each fraction may contain a mixture of closely-related porphyrins that can be separated completely by thin-layer or high-performance liquid chromatography. Nevertheless, the classic solvent extraction procedures remain satisfactory for clinical purposes.

This table is intended only as an approximate guide. In some instances (e.g., acute hepatic porphyria due to ALA dehydrase deficiency, hepatoerythropoietic porphyria), data are derived from only a few cases. There is variability from patient to patient, and exceptions to these general patterns may occur.

Abbreviations: ALA = Delta-aminolevulinic acid; copro = coproporphyrin; N = normal; PBG = porphobilinogen; proto = protoporphyrin; uro = uroporphyrin; Tr = trace.

Symbols: ↑ = Increase; ↑↑ = marked increase.

Table 7. Conditions Other Than Porphyrias That Cause Abnormalities in Porphyrins and Porphyrin Precursors

Condition	Urine	Feces	Erythrocytes
Gastrointestinal bleeding	Normal	Increased proto	Normal
Hematologic disorders			
Hemolytic and sideroblastic anemias	Normal or increased copro	Normal	Increased copro, proto
Iron deficiency	Normal	Normal unless GI bleeding	Increased proto*
Hodgkin's disease, leukemias	Normal or increased copro	Normal	Normal or increased proto
Liver diseases			
Alcoholic liver disease (fatty liver, alcoholic hepatitis, cirrhosis)	Increased copro (mainly I)	Normal	Normal
Cirrhosis of other cause	Increased copro (mainly I)	Normal	Normal
Impaired biliary secretion	Increased copro (mainly I)	Normal	Normal
Hereditary tyrosinemia	Increased ALA	Normal	Normal
Miscellaneous systemic diseases and infections†	Increased copro	Normal	Normal
Toxins			
Alcohol abuse	Increased copro (Mainly III)	Normal	Normal (or increased copro, proto‡)
Benzene and related aromatic hydrocarbons	Increased copro	Normal	Normal
Carbon tetrachloride and related compounds	Increased copro	Normal	Normal
Lead	Increased ALA and copro Normal or slightly increased PBG	Normal	Increased proto*
Other heavy metals	Increased copro	Normal	Normal

* The increase is actually in the zinc chelate of protoporphyrin, but the acid extraction tests in common use remove zinc from the complex, leading to an apparent increase in "free" protoporphyrin.
† Examples include diabetes mellitus, myocardial infarction, pregnancy, severe infections, and starvation.
‡ If sideroblasts are present.
Abbreviations: ALA = Delta-aminolevulinic acid; copro = coproporphyrin; proto = protoporphyrin; PBG = porphobilinogen; GI = gastrointestinal.

rare case of congenital erythropoietic porphyria that does not present until adulthood.

The differential diagnosis of PCT also includes polymorphous light eruptions of diverse, often obscure etiology, in which urinary porphyrins are normal. Subjects with secondary porphyrinurias (Table 7) do not have skin lesions, and they overexcrete coproporphyrin rather than uroporphyrin.

Evaluation of Latent Cases and Kindreds

Although in some recent studies, especially from the United States, a genetic defect in uroporphyrinogen decarboxylase has been demonstrated in kindreds of patients with PCT, few of the relatives so affected have had clinical disease or porphyrin overexcretion. Also, the assay for uroporphyrinogen decarboxylase is rather difficult and not performed routinely in clinical laboratories. Thus, measurement of urinary porphyrins in relatives at risk must usually suffice. Those should be cautioned not to ingest estrogens or excessive quantities of iron or alcohol and should be reevaluated periodically.

PROTOPORPHYRIA

Clinical Features

The typical patient is an infant or small child who develops erythema, itching, and urticaria in the spring, following brief exposure to the sun. This is caused by an immediate kind of photosensitivity, different from that just described for PCT or VP. Patients often become more tolerant of sunlight as summer unfolds because of increased cutaneous melanin formation. However, they rarely "outgrow" their photosensitivity, and a delay of onset of symptoms until adulthood is likewise rare. A positive family history is usual but by no means universal.

The affected skin is mainly on the bridge of the nose, the cheeks, and over the second and third knuckles of the hands. Repeated damage and healing leads eventually to shallow scars and lichenification.

Usually the disease is benign. The most frequent complication is pigmented gallstones, composed largely of protoporphyrin. Cholestasis due to any cause may produce exacerbations of disease because of compromise of hepatic protoporphyrin secretion. Rarely, the deposition of protoporphyrin in the liver may lead to progressive and fatal cirrhosis and liver failure. In such cases the liver appears black and contains high concentrations of protoporphyrin.

Laboratory Findings and Chemical Features

Routine laboratory tests are normal or show a mild anemia with microcytosis and normochromia or hypochromia. Tests of liver function are usually normal, although the presence of gallstones or fibrosis or cirrhosis may lead to the changes to be expected in these disorders, regardless of cause.

The key to diagnosis is the demonstration of excess protoporphyrin in erythrocytes, feces, or both. A substantial increase in the concentration in erythrocytes should be present in all patients with active skin disease; isolated increases in fecal excretions have been reported in relatives of clinically affected persons. In severe disease, plasma protoporphyrin is also increased substantially. Great care must be exercised in measuring plasma protoporphyrin because of its marked instability to light.

It must be remembered that virtually no protoporphyrin is excreted in the urine. Therefore, urinary porphyrin excretion is normal in protoporphyria, and the diagnosis will be missed if only a urinary porphyrin screen is done.

Differential Diagnosis

Affected children are often thought to be suffering from an allergic dermatitis. Inability to identify an allergen and the relative paucity of objective skin changes may lead to a mistaken diagnosis of a functional disorder.

Increased erythrocytic protoporphyrin has also been described in the porphyria due to genetic deficiency of ALA dehydrase and in hepatoerythropoietic porphyria (Table 6). Clinically, these disorders are usually readily distinguished from protoporphyria.

In all instances, urinary heme precursors should point to the correct diagnosis. Other conditions that may cause elevated erythrocytic protoporphyrin (Table 7) exhibit no photosensitivity and show increased zinc protoporphyrin rather than free protoporphyrin. In VP, although fecal protoporphyrin is increased, so is fecal coproporphyrin; erythrocytic porphyrins are normal.

Evaluation of Latent Cases and Kindreds

Blood relatives of known patients should be tested for fecal and erythrocytic protoporphyrin levels. These tests will detect most affected persons and virtually all those who are at risk for developing clinical disease. In analogy to other forms of porphyria, however, some persons carrying the genetic defect for protoporphyria have normal production and concentrations of protoporphyrin. Such genetic carriers can be detected only by assay of ferrochelatase activity, generally carried out using cultured skin fibroblasts or leukocytes. Indirect methods, depending upon the generation of protoporphyrin from ALA, have also been described, but none is available on a routine basis. Even if they were, their routine use would not be warranted.

RARE FORMS OF CUTANEOUS PORPHYRIA

Hepatoerythropoietic Porphyria

Clinical Features

This disease has been described thus far in fewer than ten cases. It usually manifests within the first year of life with severe photosensitivity, indistinguishable from that seen in PCT or VP, except that it occurs in infants. Facial hypertrichosis develops in childhood. Later, scarring, which may produce scleroderma and acrosclerosis, develops. Photosensitivity tends to lessen as patients grow older, but evidence of liver disease supervenes. Usually, this takes the form of relatively mild, nonspecific hepatitis.

Laboratory Findings and Chemical Features

Adults typically have mild, normochromic anemia. Serum transaminases, gamma-glutamyl transferase, and bromsulphalein (BSP) or indocyanine green (ICG) retention are often increased mildly in adults. Abnormalities in porphyrins resemble those seen in PCT with the additional feature that erythrocytic protoporphyrin is also increased. The PCT-like picture is due to the fact that the basic defect in hepatoerythropoietic porphyria is a severe deficiency in the activity of hepatic uroporphyrinogen decarboxylase, the enzyme that is also, but less severely, affected in PCT. Ordinarily, the two diseases are readily distinguished by the differences in severity and age of onset. However, they in fact form a spectrum of clinical disease that depends upon the severity of the defect in uroporphyrinogen decarboxylase activity. The cause of the increased erythrocytic protoporphyrin in hepatoerythropoietic porphyria is unknown.

Congenital Erythropoietic Porphyria

Clinical Features

This rare disease (fewer than 70 cases reported) usually presents in children younger than 3 years of age. Typically they have severe photosensitivity, with changes as described for PCT or hepatoerythropoietic porphyria. Patients may also present with red urine, owing to massive porphyrinuria. Splenomegaly is common, and the deciduous and permanent teeth fluoresce bright-red (erythrodontia) when exposed to a Wood's lamp, owing to the avid adsorption of porphyrin by calcium phosphate. Severe mutilation of the hands, ears, and face is common as patients age.

Laboratory Findings and Chemical Features

There is often evidence of hemolysis, sometimes with anemia. The major abnormality in porphyrins is a marked increase in uroporphyrin I in red blood cells and urine. Coproporphyrin I is also increased somewhat in red cells and urine and predominates in the feces (Table 6).

Differential Diagnosis

Congenital erythropoietic porphyria is readily distinguished from protoporphyria by the fact that urinary porphyrins are markedly increased only in the former. Differentiation from other cutaneous porphyrias is based upon the fact that only in congenital erythropoietic porphyria is there markedly increased erythrocyte uroporphyrin.

CONDITIONS OTHER THAN PORPHYRIAS THAT CAUSE ABNORMALITIES IN PORPHYRIN METABOLISM

A large variety of pathologic conditions besides the porphyrias may cause abnormalities in porphyrin and heme metabolism. Some of these (e.g., lead poisoning, hereditary tyrosinemia) have already been discussed, and the major ones are summarized in Table 7. Photosensitivity is not a feature of any of these disorders. Those related to hepatic disease are characterized principally by relatively mild increases in urinary coproporphyrin excretion. Those related to hematologic disorders principally increase erythrocytic protoporphyrin (often actually zinc protoporphyrin).

The abnormalities in porphyrin metabolism may be quite helpful in diagnosis of these disorders (e.g., lead poisoning, Rotor's syndrome). The major pitfall is to conclude erroneously that such patients suffer from a porphyria. This is best avoided by quantitation of fecal, urinary, and erythrocytic porphyrins and of urinary ALA and PBG. The clinical and chemical findings should be used in conjunction with the data of Tables 6 and 7 to arrive at the proper diagnosis.

HEPATOLENTICULAR DEGENERATION (WILSON'S DISEASE)

By Irmin Sternlieb, M.D.
and I. Herbert Scheinberg, M.D.
Bronx, New York

SYNONYMS

Hepatocerebral degeneration, Konovalov-Wilson's disease, progressive lenticular degeneration.

DEFINITION

Wilson's disease is an inherited disorder of copper metabolism, characterized by excessive accumulations of copper in the liver, central nervous system, kidneys, eyes, and other organs. Although the inherited defect is present from birth, significant pathologic changes and clinical manifestations do not appear before the age of 5 years and are sometimes delayed until the fifth decade. The metabolic defect that leads to the accumulation of copper is inherited in autosomal recessive fashion. Consequently, the affected homozygote inherits one member of a pair of abnormal alleles from each heterozygous parent. Moreover, each sibling of a patient has one chance in four, *a priori*, of being a homozygote. Rarely does one encounter Wilson's disease in consecutive generations as the child of a patient—the abnormal homozygote—who has married a heterozygous carrier. Recent data suggest the carrier frequency in the general population to be about 1 in 90; the prevalence of patients, 1 in 30,000.

The abnormal gene for Wilson's disease is ubiquitous, affecting all races and ethnic groups. Apparent differences in prevalences of Wilson's disease in various populations are primarily due to the degree of diagnostic sophistication; real increases in incidence occur in isolated inbred populations.

The fundamental pathophysiologic disturbance in Wilson's disease is a defect in the excretion of copper from the liver into the intestine via the bile. Copper consequently accumulates progressively in the liver, causing toxic changes. When the capacity of the liver to retain copper is exceeded, the metal diffuses, or is released, into the blood and is then distributed to other organs. Although not always clinically detectable, pathologic changes in the liver occur before those in the central nervous system and kidneys and before copper deposits in Descemet's membrane of the cornea become visible as Kayser-Fleischer rings.

PRESENTING SIGNS AND SYMPTOMS

The patient with Wilson's disease may present with hepatic, neurologic, psychiatric, renal, skeletal, or endocrine manifestations, or any combination of these. The onset of hepatic disease may be acute and brief, mimicking acute hepatitis or it may progress rapidly downhill, suggesting fulminant hepatitis. In other patients the onset may be more insidious, with the slow development of hepatic insufficiency, resembling the course of chronic active hepatitis or cirrhosis. In some patients, portal hypertension with splenomegaly, hypersplenism, or bleeding from esophageal or gastric varices may be the first indication of the presence of liver disease. Physicians should suspect Wilson's disease in asymptomatic subjects with persistent transaminasemia of unknown cause. Delayed puberty in boys or primary or secondary amenorrhea may also be the first signs of Wilsonian liver disease, as may bleeding and easy bruising due to deficiencies of fibrinogen or factors II, V, VII, or X.

The neurologic signs and symptoms of Wilson's disease tend to appear during the second or third decade of life, somewhat later than the hepatic manifestations. Any combination of resting or intention tremors; diminished dexterity; dysarthria; drooling; spastic rigidity of the mouth, arms, or legs; unsteady gait; or choreiform movements may be encountered. The neurologic onset is usually insidious and, if untreated, progressive. Kayser-Fleischer rings are *always* present if an untreated patient exhibits neurologic abnormalities caused by Wilson's disease.

The predominant initial abnormality is psychiatric in perhaps 20 to 30 per cent of patients. There may be a sudden or insidious deterioration of the quality of school work; an inability to concentrate or read; memory loss; confusion due to chronic or acute attacks of anxiety; paranoid delusions; manic-depressive disease; severe depression; schizophrenia; dementia; or, most commonly, impulsive, inappropriate, or antisocial behavior with temper tantrums, exhibitionism, voyeurism, sexual promiscuity, lying, thievery, alcoholism, or use of illicit drugs. Patients are rarely diagnosed when they exhibit only psychiatric manifestations, in part because the psychiatric abnormalities—or the results of their nonspecific treatment—may mask the neurologic disturbance.

Gross or microscopic hematuria, mimicking glomerulonephritis in children; mild renal tubular acidosis; renal calculi; or nephrocalcinosis may be the first manifestation of Wilson's disease. Skeletal changes—principally osteoporosis, spontaneous fractures, rickets, osteomalacia, osteoarthritis, osteochondritis dissecans, or chondromalacia patellae—are found infrequently in patients in North America, and may be caused in part by renal tubular loss of calcium and phosphorus. Cardiac and pancreatic abnormalities have been reported, but are rare and not of clinical significance.

DIAGNOSTIC LABORATORY ABNORMALITIES

Deficiency of Ceruloplasmin. Ninety-five per cent of patients with Wilson's disease have less than 20 mg/dl of this blue copper-protein. The normal concentration lies between 20 and 40 mg/dl. About 25 per cent of patients have no detectable ceruloplasmin in their serum. Since this protein binds irreversibly in vivo a constant 0.3 per cent of copper, deficiency of ceruloplasmin is reflected in a reduction in ceruloplasmin-copper, but not always in a significant reduction in total serum copper, since the sera of untreated patients contain more nonceruloplasmin copper than the 5 to 10 μg/dl found normally. A temporary stimulus to synthesis of ceruloplasmin, caused by activity of the inflammatory process in the liver or by an excess of circulating estrogens, may elevate a typically Wilsonian concentration of ceruloplasmin into the low normal range, 20 to 30 mg/dl.

About 10 per cent of heterozygous carriers of one Wilson's disease gene also exhibit hypoceruloplasminemia. Therefore, a reduced concentration of ceruloplasmin is not a sufficient criterion for the diagnosis of Wilson's disease and there will be about 30 hypoceruloplasminemic heterozygotes for one patient with Wilson's disease. The disease never develops in heterozygotes, and they must not be treated with penicillamine.

Excess of Hepatic Copper. In untreated Wilson's disease, hepatic concentrations of copper exceed 250 μg/gm dry tissue (normal, 20 to 50 μg/gm). The intracellular distribution of copper changes with the stage of the disease: during early phases, it is diffuse in the cytoplasm, while late in Wilsonian cirrhosis it is concentrated in hepatocellular lysosomes. Only in the latter situation is the excess copper demonstrable by routine histochemical stains. Since concentrations of copper indistinguishable from those in Wilson's disease are seen in some patients with primary or secondary biliary cirrhosis or chronic cholestasis, an elevation of the hepatic copper concentration alone, is—like hypoceruloplasminemia—not a sufficient diagnostic criterion.

Excess of Urinary Copper. The majority of symptomatic patients with Wilson's disease excrete more than 100 μg of copper in a 24-hour urine collection (normal, 30 μg). Considerably larger amounts are excreted when necrosis of the liver results in the release of large amounts of copper from hepatic stores. Asymptomatic patients may not exhibit hypercupriuria.

Decreased Incorporation of Radiocopper into Ceruloplasmin. In normal subjects, orally administered radiocopper is promptly incorporated into ceruloplasmin. Little or no incorporation of the isotope is demonstrable in patients with Wilson's disease, even in the 5 per cent with low normal concentration—20 to 30 mg/dl—of ceruloplasmin in serum.

Liver Histology. Under the light microscope, any combination of these—microvesicular fat; an inhomogeneous, eosinophilic cytoplasm; glycogen-filled or irregularly sized nuclei; collapse of periportal reticulum: or deposition of periportal or intralobular collagen—in a young person who has not been exposed to alcohol or exogenous toxins supports the diagnosis of Wilson's disease. At this early stage, attempts to stain copper are usually negative, in spite of the marked increase in hepatic copper content. Staining may be positive, however, during the stage of chronic active hepatitis and in patients with established cirrhosis, in whom hepatocellular lysosomal copper deposits are present throughout certain nodules. The histologic appearance of this phase of Wilson's disease is not distinguishable from other forms of chronic active hepatitis.

Liver Ultrastructure. The earliest stages of Wilson's disease are characterized by the occurrence of pathognomonic mitochondrial changes in hepatocytes. These electron microscopic changes disappear with the progression to cirrhosis. Electron-dense, copper-containing lysosomal granules are prominent in the hepatocytes of patients with advanced Wilsonian liver disease.

DIAGNOSIS

Two tests should be performed in every subject suspected of suffering from Wilson's disease: (1) a slit-lamp examination for Kayser-Fleischer rings and (2) a determination of the concentration of ceruloplasmin in serum. In addition, a liver biopsy for quantitative measurement of hepatic copper content and light microscopic examination; a measurement of the 24-hour urinary copper excretion; and a test of radiocopper loading may be required for confirmation of the diagnosis.

In any individual, the demonstration of the presence of corneal Kayser-Fleischer rings and of a serum ceruloplasmin concentration of less than 20 mg/dl of serum suffices to make the diagnosis.

In many patients, however, confirmation of the diagnosis is more difficult: Kayser-Fleischer rings may not have formed in young patients; patients with active liver disease may exhibit a temporary rise of their serum ceruloplasmin concentrations into the low normal range (20–30 mg/dl); in some patients with non-Wilsonian fulminant hepatitis and a generalized inability to synthesize serum proteins, there may be ceruloplasmin deficiency; a few patients with long-standing cholestatic syndromes may exhibit Kayser-Fleischer rings; in instances of primary biliary cirrhosis or cholestatic syndromes elevated hepatic copper concentrations may overlap those encountered in patients with Wilson's disease, and 24-hour urinary copper excretion may exceed 100 μg. A diagnosis of Wilson's disease inescapably means a commitment to life-long therapy—a treatment that carries justifiable risks for this lethal disease but to which patients without Wilson's disease must not be subjected. Diagnostic procedures to be followed depend on the patient's mode of presentation.

Patients Presenting with Manifestations of Liver Disease. Signs and symptoms of liver disease may appear as early as age 5 years or may be delayed until the patient reaches 35 years. In children or young adults, acute hepatitis, particularly if associated with even mild hemolytic anemia, should raise suspicion of Wilson's disease, as should a clinical picture of fulminant hepatitis, chronic active hepatitis, or cirrhosis of unknown etiology.

There may be difficulty in diagnosing patients with a hepatic presentation because ceruloplasmin is an acute phase reactant; thus, the ceruloplasmin concentration of a Wilsonian patient with active liver disease may rise above 20 mg/dl; and because cholestasis may impair hepatic excretion of copper, a non-Wilsonian patient may have a concentration of copper in the liver equal to that seen in Wilson's disease. But the diagnosis of Wilson's disease is certain in a patient with hepatic manifestations if the serum ceruloplasmin concentration is less than 20 mg/dl and Kayser-Fleischer rings are present.

If liver disease of unknown etiology is associated with a serum ceruloplasmin concentration of between 20 and 30 mg/dl, a liver biopsy should be performed. Two specimens, one for quantitative copper determination and a second for light microscopic examination, should be obtained. If biopsy is contraindicated because of clotting abnormalities, for example, the diagnosis can usually be established or ruled out by a radiocopper loading test, which is of differential diagnostic value only in patients with normal concentrations of serum ceruloplasmin.

Patients with Central Nervous System Manifestations. The certain absence of Kayser-Fleischer rings excludes the diagnosis of Wilson's disease in a patient with neurologic manifestations who has not been previously treated with penicillamine, Trien, or British Anti-Lewisite. In more than 95 per cent of patients whose neurologic or psychiatric symptomatology is due to Wilson's disease, the serum ceruloplasmin concentration will be less than 20 mg/dl. If Kayser-Fleischer rings are present and the serum ceruloplasmin is greater than 20 mg/dl, the diagnosis of Wilson's disease is probable but should be confirmed by hepatic biopsy or a radiocopper incorporation test.

Asymptomatic Patients. When Wilson's disease is suspected, as it must be in any asymptomatic sibling and should be in any other blood relative, the following should be performed:

1. Determination of the serum ceruloplasmin concentration.
2. Physical examination, with particular attention to abnormalities in the size and consistency of the liver and spleen, and to the neurologic status.
3. Corneal slit-lamp examination.
4. In children, measurement of serum aminotransferase (transaminase) levels.

If, in such an individual, the serum ceruloplasmin concentration is less than 20 mg/dl, a hepatic biopsy sample should be obtained. If its copper concentration is greater than 250 μg/gm dry tissue, the diagnosis of Wilson's disease is confirmed. Light microscopy will almost always reveal histologic abnormalities in a section of such a liver biopsy specimen.

If the ceruloplasmin concentration of such an asymptomatic subject is greater than 20 mg/dl, without any characteristic abnormality in the history, physical, or slit-lamp examinations or of the serum aminotransferase levels, no further diagnostic procedures need to be performed and the patient can be assumed not to have Wilson's disease until, if ever, periodic examinations reveal a sign or symptom of the illness. Then the procedures to be followed are the same as for the hepatic patient with a ceruloplasmin concentration of $>$ 20 mg/dl.

A decreased concentration of serum ceruloplasmin in a healthy individual in whom all of these tests are negative suggests that the subject is a heterozygous carrier of one abnormal Wilson's disease gene.

DIAGNOSTIC PITFALLS

The major pitfall is failure to think of the possibility of Wilson's disease in a young patient with hepatic, neurologic, or psychiatric manifestations of unknown etiology. Caution is necessary, in addition, in interpreting analytic results obtained from laboratories that rarely perform serum ceruloplasmin or copper determinations, and in results of urinary copper analyses made on collections obtained without copper-free precautions or those collected while the patient is taking penicillamine.

IRON STORAGE DISEASE

By Don M. Samples, M.D.
New Orleans, Louisiana

SYNONYMS

Idiopathic hemochromatosis (IHC), hereditary or primary hemochromatosis, pigmentary cirrhosis, bronzed diabetes.

Erythropoietic hemochromatosis, iron-loading anemias, secondary hemochromatosis.

DEFINITION

Hemochromatosis is a disorder of iron overloading, in which the excess iron is deposited in parenchymal tissues, ultimately causing cell damage, fibrosis, and impaired function, particularly of the liver, pancreas, and heart. In contrast, increased deposition of iron in the reticuloendothelial tissues (*hemosiderosis*) is relatively innocuous and is not included in the definition.

In adults, total body iron is relatively constant at about 4 grams. In IHC, excessive iron is absorbed irrespective of the need for iron. This excess may be as much as 3 to 5 mg per day, resulting in the accumulation of 25 to 60 grams of total body iron over 30 to 50 years. Idiopathic hemochromatosis (IHC) is an inherited, autosomal-recessive disease; the gene is closely linked to the histocompatibility antigen HLA A-3, located on chromosome 6.

Erythropoietic hemochromatosis occurs in patients with hyperplastic bone marrow and ineffective erythropoiesis. The excess iron stores result not only from transfusion but also from increased iron absorption secondary to the ineffective erythropoiesis, as in thalassemia major and, less frequently, in sideroblastic anemia. Prolonged excessive iron consumption and parenteral iron administration, either as medicinal iron or as blood transfusions, usually result in hemosiderosis. Although "secondary" hemochromatosis has been observed in some patients receiving excessive iron, it is likely that most had IHC as their basic disorder.

PRESENTING SIGNS AND SYMPTOMS

Clinical manifestations of IHC are four times more common in males and occur at an earlier age, 40 to 60 years, than in females. The classic triad of cirrhosis, diabetes mellitus, and pigmentation characterizes advanced IHC.

The predominant clinical picture may include liver failure with hepatosplenomegaly, ascites, jaundice, and spider angiomas. Two thirds of the patients have diabetes, which is the presenting feature in one third of this group. Most diabetics with IHC require insulin, and the usual complications of diabetes do occur. The pigmentation of the skin is usually caused by melanin deposition, but there may be increased amounts of iron present in 50 per cent of such patients.

Less specific symptoms, such as weight loss and fatigue, may be present for years before the diagnosis is made. Nausea, vomiting, abdominal pain (usually right upper quadrant), and even diarrhea may be prominent. Sexual impotency, testicular atrophy, and loss of body hair are common. Arthropathy affects approximately 50 per cent of the patients and may be the presenting feature. The metacarpophalangeal, proximal interphalangeal, wrist, knees, and spine joints are the most commonly involved. Some patients have chondrocalcinosis, which can be associated with attacks of acute synovitis. Cardiac manifestations of refractory myocardial failure and arrhythmias may occur at an unusually early age. Most patients who are untreated die of hepatic or cardiac complications within a few years of onset of symptoms. Hepatoma may develop in 10 per cent of patients.

Erythropoietic hemochromatosis (EHC) is characterized by the same signs and symptoms as IHC, though it occurs in children with thalassemia major and in adults with long-standing refractory anemia, particularly sideroblastic anemia.

LABORATORY DIAGNOSIS

The laboratory diagnosis of IHC requires demonstration of iron overload in parenchymal tissue (usually liver) and exclusion of causes of secondary hemochromatosis, e.g., thalassemia major and cirrhosis with iron overload. In IHC, the serum iron usually is greater than 200 μg/dl, and the serum transferrin saturation is greater than 80 per cent in males and 70 per cent in females. The transferrin saturation may also be increased in liver disease, various erythrocyte disorders, and iron therapy. The serum ferritin reflects total body iron stores and values greater than 300 ng/ml in males and 200 ng/ml in females indicate increased stores and should be evaluated further. Most patients with IHC have values greater than 500 (500 to 10,000) ng/ml. However, in premenopausal females and young males the serum ferritin may be only marginally elevated. The ferritin may be inappropriately high in patients with infection, malignancy, or hepatocellular necrosis but without iron overload.

Parenchymal iron overload may be estimated by measuring the 24-hour urinary iron excretion after the intramuscular injection of 0.5 grams of deferoxamine, an iron-chelating agent. In the absence of renal dysfunction or ascorbate deficiency, patients with IHC will excrete greater than 5 mg of iron; those with increased reticuloendothelial iron stores, less than 3 mg; and normals, less than 2 mg.

Estimation of hepatic iron is the definitive test for confirmation of iron overload. Hemosiderin stains with Prussian blue, and the amount of iron is graded from 0 to 4, with grades 2 to 4 indicating increased iron stores. Hepatic iron can be quantified. Normals have less than 100 μg/100 mg dry weight, Patients with untreated IHC have values of 1,800 to 5,000 μg/100 mg dry weight; those with the precirrhotic phase of IHC and females have lower values. Unusually high values can occur in patients who have alcoholic cirrhosis and small livers, although total hepatic iron content is only slightly increased. These patients can be differentiated from those with IHC by the deferoxamine chelation test and by quantitative phlebotomy in which each 500 ml removes approximately 250 mg of iron. Iron deficiency is noted in normal adult males after removal of 1.5 to 2 gm of iron, in patients with cirrhosis after removal of less than 5 gm of iron, and in those with IHC greater than 20 gm of iron.

Because IHC is an heritable disorder, it is important to screen relatives for precirrhotic hemochromatosis. Recommendations include:

1. All first-degree relatives over the age of 10 should have determinations of serum iron, transferrin saturation, and serum ferritin.
2. If any one of the tests is abnormal, a liver biopsy should have determinations of serum iron, transferrin saturation,and serum ferritin.
3. Serial screening tests over a number of years are recommended, as normal values do not preclude the later development of iron overload and cirrhosis. Human leukocyte antigen (HLA) typing may identify relatives at risk. A sibling who shares two HLA haplotypes with the proband is at high risk of developing iron overload. If one offspring has evidence of the disease, this may allow identification of all haplotypes associated with the disease and aid in the diagnosis of other offspring at high risk.

RICKETS AND OSTEOMALACIA

By Donald Fraser, Ph.D., M.D.
and Sang Whay Kooh, Ph.D., M.D.
Toronto, Canada

DEFINITIONS

The terms rickets and osteomalacia describe histopathologic lesions.

Osteomalacia refers to the skeletal condition in which there is generalized failure of bone minerals to be deposited promptly in the recently formed protein matrix of bone. A coarse texture of the trabeculae and pseudofractures are characteristic radiographic features. Deformities may sometimes be present.

Rickets is the pediatric counterpart in which the mineralization defect is also present in the metaphyseal regions of the long bones and at the zones of provisional calcification of the growth plates. Usually, but not always, there are deformities. Growth is impaired in long-standing cases.

WHEN SHOULD THE DIAGNOSIS OF RICKETS OR OSTEOMALACIA BE CONSIDERED?

There are many different forms of rickets and osteomalacia. The physician should entertain the possibility of rickets or osteomalacia in individuals with the following manifestations:

1. Skeletal deformities, especially bow-legs (genu varum), knock-knees (genu valgum), and enlargement of the costochondral junctions.
2. Convulsions with associated hypocalcemia.
3. Generalized bone pain, muscle weakness.
4. Patients with chronic renal failure, hepatobiliary obstruction, and chronic steatorrhea.
5. When a routine plasma screening assessment unexpectedly reveals abnormal values for calcium, inorganic phosphate, or alkaline phosphatase.
6. When a radiograph conducted for another condition reveals features of rickets or osteomalacia in the bones.

WHICH SIGNS OF RICKETS AND OSTEOMALACIA SHOULD BE ANTICIPATED AT VARIOUS AGES?

In general, skeletal deformities are absent during early infancy. They tend to be most marked at the time of weight bearing in the infant and toddler. If the pathology cannot be corrected by treatment, deformities and stunted stature become progressibely more severe with time.

At Birth. In the developed countries, nutritional rickets does not occur at birth. Similarly, in the hereditary forms, bone lesions are not apparent at the time of delivery, though biochemical changes in plasma can occur in the neonatal period.

Two to Six Months. Convulsions due to hypocalcemia are the usual presenting feature; tetany occurs rarely. The skull bones are often involved. Craniotabes (a "ping-pong" sensation) may be palpable. Generalized osteopenia and disappearance or smudging of the usually distinct margins of the cranial bones are characteristic early radiographic signs. Enlargements of the costochondral junctions are common, but deformities of the long bones are rare.

Six to Eighteen Months. Enlargements are present at the ends of the long bones and particularly at the costochondral junctions. Knock-knee deformity and a rolling or waddling gait are the usual features if the patient has started to walk. The lower anterior thorax may develop Harrison's sulci. Tetany and convulsions are rare. Radiographic signs of rickets are best seen in anteroposterior views of the knees and wrists. Signs consist of increased thickness of the growth plates, fraying of the metaphyses of the long bones, and a coarse texture of the trabecular architecture.

Beyond 1 Year. Skeletal deformities and stunted growth are common features. Genu varum occurs if onset is before 3 years of age, and genu valgum tends to occur if onset is after 3 years of age (as in chronic renal failure). The forehead may be prominent (frontal bossing), and the skull may be long and narrow (dolicocephaly). Typical radiographic signs are present in the long bones. Premature sagittal synostosis may occur.

Adult. Physical signs and symptoms may be absent. The patient may complain of generalized dull aching pain in the bones during weight bearing and prolonged physical activity; sometimes there may be localized bone pain and tenderness at the site of a pseudofracture. Deformity of the lower limbs may develop gradually, and early onset of osteoarthritis is common. Radiographic signs are usually limited to coarse texture of the trabeculae. Pseudofractures of the femora, pubic and ischial rami, ribs, and scapulae are diagnostic when present. Radiographic density of the bones is usually decreased, but may sometimes be increased if long-standing vitamin D refractory rickets was present in childhood.

ESTABLISHING THE SPECIFIC FORM OF RICKETS OR OSTEOMALACIA

When rickets or osteomalacia is identified in a patient, it is essential to establish the exact diagnosis in order to define therapy, to establish prognosis, and to offer genetic counseling. The diagnosis can usually be made with two or three visits to the doctor's office. We employ a system of classification based on pathophysiologic principles in which patients are categorized into one of three main groups.

1. Those associated with calcipenia (impaired cell transport and availability of calcium).
2. Those with phosphopenia.
3. Those with a defect in calcifiability of matrix.

The classification of the more than 15 forms of rickets into the three general categories is shown in Table 1.

Table 1. Pathophysiologic Classification of Rickets and Osteomalacia

Calcipenia
- Vitamin D deficiency (deficient vitamin D intake plus lack of sunlight)
- Impaired vitamin D absorption
  - Hepatobiliary disease
  - Chronic intestinal diseases
  - Pancreatic insufficiency
- Impaired vitamin D metabolism
  - Anticonvulsant rickets and osteomalacia
  - Vitamin D dependency rickets, type I (VDDR I)
  - Renal osteodystrophy
- Impaired end-organ response to 1,25-dihydroxyvitamin D
  - Vitamin D dependency rickets, type II (VDDR II)
- Rickets due to calcium deficiency

Phosphopenia
- Deficient phosphate intake
- Defective renal phosphate conservation
  - X-linked hypophosphatemia (XLH)
  - Autosomal dominant hypophosphatemia
  - Fanconi syndrome
    - With cystinosis
    - Without cystinosis
    - Due to nephrotoxic agents (e.g., lead, outdated tetracycline)
  - Tumor-induced hypophosphatemia
  - Miscellaneous causes of renal phosphate loss
    - Hereditary tyrosinemia
    - Oculo-cerebro-renal (Lowe's) syndrome
    - Wilson's disease
    - Distal renal tubular acidosis

Defective Matrix Calcifiability
- Hypophosphatasia

FORMS OF RICKETS ASSOCIATED WITH CALCIPENIA

A main factor that maintains normocalcemia and stimulates calcium transport is vitamin D. Almost all forms of calcipenic rickets (exception calcium deficiency rickets) are attributable to some defect in the vitamin D system: deficient intake or absorption, impaired conversion through 25-hydroxyvitamin D (25-OHD) to 1,25-dihydroxy D(1,25[OH]$_2$D), or impaired response of target tissues to the latter highly active hormonal form.

Vitamin D Deficiency

Vitamin D deficiency rickets is due to lack of adequate dietary intake of the vitamin plus insufficient sunlight exposure to generate endogenous vitamin D in the skin. In North America practically all dairy milk and commercial infant formulas are enriched with vitamin D. However, breast milk and other foods contain little vitamin D. Breast-fed infants and children consuming strictly vegetarian diets who do not receive proprietary vitamin D supplements are candidates for developing vitamin D deficiency rickets. Three clinical stages of vitamin D deficiency can be distinguished.

Plasma 25-hydroxyvitamin D (25-OHD) is the best biochemical measure of vitamin D nutrition. It is low or undetectable in all stages of vitamin D deficiency (normal plasma 25-OHD, 19 to 40 nmol/liter in our laboratory). During the early stages of vitamin D deficiency, plasma 1,25(OH)$_2$D is often normal or supranormal and this determination thus tends not to be helpful for diagnosis.

Stage I (Age 2 to 5 Months). This stage is manifested by impaired intestinal calcium absorption and diminished calcium mobilization from bone. The result is hypocalcemia. Plasma inorganic phosphate and alkaline phosphatase are not usually abnormal at this stage, there are no deformities, and radiographic lesions are minimal. The presenting sign is convulsions, rarely tetany. The Trousseau test is positive. Low plasma 25-OHD and lack of hyperphosphatemia distinguish Stage I vitamin D deficiency from congenital hypoparathyroidism.

Stage II (Age 5 to 12 Months). Hypocalcemia of Stage I stimulates parathormone (PTH) secretion, and in Stage II the plasma calcium becomes normal or nearly normal. However, the secondary hyperparathyroidism causes hyperphosphaturia with resultant hypophosphatemia; it also causes generalized aminoaciduria. Classical deformities and radiographic signs are present in this stage. Convulsions and tetany are absent, and the Trousseau test is negative. Plasma calcium is normal or nearly normal, phosphate is low, and alkaline phosphatase is elevated. Generalized aminoaciduria is present. Plasma 25-OHD is low or undetectable, and PTH is elevated.

Stage III (Age 5 to 18 Months). When vitamin D stores are severely depleted, the consequent severe rachitic lesions make the patient less sensitive to the plasma calcium–raising action of PTH. Hypocalcemia returns during this advanced stage of depletion, while PTH-stimulated hypophosphatemia and aminoaciduria persist. Deformities and radiographic signs are prominent. Convulsions or tetany may occur, and the Trousseau test may be positive. Plasma calcium and inorganic phosphate are low, alkaline phosphatase is elevated, and generalized aminoaciduria is present. Plasma 25-OHD is low; PTH is elevated.

Impaired Vitamin D Absorption

Hepatobiliary Rickets. Rickets occurs sometimes, and osteomalacia occasionally, in patients with chronic hepatobiliary disease. The biochemical features and the skeletal lesions are similar to those in vitamin D deficiency. Bile salts are required for efficient vitamin D absorption, and the mechanism of rickets appears to be malabsorption of the vitamin rather than its defective conversion to 25-OHD by the damaged liver.

Intestinal and Pancreatic Disease. *Chronic intestinal malabsorption* and *pancreatic insufficiency* can occasionally result in rickets or osteomalacia by causing impairment of vitamin D and probably of calcium absorption. However, rickets rarely occurs in celiac disease.

Impaired Vitamin D Metabolism

To exert biologic activity, vitamin D must be hydroxylated by the liver to 25-OHD, which in turn must be hydroxylated by the kidney to $1,25(OH)_2D$: Several rachitic and osteomalacic syndromes have been identified with impaired vitamin D metabolism.

Anticonvulsant Rickets or Osteomalacia. Phenobarbital and phenytoin (Dilantin) can alter hepatic metabolism of vitamin D and cause decreased plasma levels of 25-OHD. The manifestations include hypocalcemia and rickets or osteomalacia. Only a small proportion of patients on long-term, high-dose anticonvulsants develop hypocalcemia and bone lesions—principally those patients whose vitamin D intake is only marginally adequate.

Autosomal Recessive Vitamin D Dependency Rickets, Type I (VDDR I). Also known as pseudovitamin D deficiency rickets. VDDR I (Table 2) is due to an inherited defect in the specific renal 1-hydroxylase that converts 25-OHD to $1,25(OH)_2D$. Plasma 25-OHD is normal, and plasma $1,25(OH)_2D$ is very low or undetectable. The disease usually manifests before 6 months of age. It resembles Stage III vitamin D deficiency and is characterized by hypocalcemia, hypophosphatemia, severe deformities, secondary hyperparathyroidism, and generalized aminoaciduria in spite of a vitamin D intake that would ordinarily prevent rickets. Enamel hypoplasia is always present in the permanent incisors because of the hypocalcemia during tooth formation in infancy. A feature of diagnostic importance is complete healing of the biochemical and skeletal lesions with massive doses of vitamin D (1000 to 1600 IU/kg/day) or physiologic doses of $1,25(OH)_2D_3$ (approximately 0.01 μg/kg/day).

Renal Osteodystrophy. Chronic renal failure causes complex derangements of calcium and phosphate transport. Osteodystrophy soon develops; the lesions include elements of rickets, osteomalacia, secondary hyperparathyroidism (erosion of cortices of phalanges and metaphyses of long bones), and sometimes osteosclerosis. Plasma 25-OHD levels are normal, and $1,25(OH)_2D$ may be normal, reduced, or occasionally undetectable. Plasma calcium levels are usually normal, but inorganic phosphate, PTH, and creatinine levels are elevated. Acidosis is often present. The usual signs and symptoms of renal insufficiency are also present.

Impaired End-Organ Response to 1,25-Dihydroxyvitamin D

This is an extremely rare, often familial, condition. As in VDDR I, patients have hypocalcemia, hypophosphatemia, aminoaciduria, normal 25-OHD and raised PTH levels, and severe rickets of early onset. However, in contrast to VDDR I, plasma $1,25(OH)_2D$ levels are raised, often five to ten times normal. The pathogenesis is refractoriness of target organs to $1,25(OH)_2D$. A striking feature in the majority of patients is alopecia totalis developing during the first year of life.

Calcium Deficiency Rickets

Diets markedly deficient in calcium can occasionally cause rickets. The features are those of Stage III vitamin D deficiency, but the level of plasma 25-OHD is normal.

RICKETS ASSOCIATED WITH PHOSPHOPENIA

Deficient Phosphate Intake

Phosphate is plentiful in the normal diet, and intestinal absorption is ordinarily efficient. Deficient intake of phosphate with resultant hypophosphatemia and bone disease is encountered mainly in premature infants with inability to ingest adequate amounts of formula and in patients of any age maintained for prolonged periods on total parenteral nutrition (TPN). Occasionally, osteomalacia has been observed in patients receiving large amounts of aluminum hydroxide, a phosphate-binding gel.

Defective Renal Phosphate Conservation

Renal handling of phosphate is an important determinant of the plasma inorganic phosphate level. Renal tubular reclamation of phosphate is ordinarily very efficient. Impairment of phosphate conservation by the renal tubules leading to hypophosphatemia is usually due to genetic abnormalities that cause isolated phosphate or multifactorial losses in the urine. Other causes are hyperparathyroidism and nephrotoxic agents. Chronic hypophosphatemia can cause phosphopenic rickets.

Familial Vitamin D Refractory Rickets

X-linked (dominant) hypophosphatemia (XLH) is the most common type of phosphopenia rickets (Table 2). *Autosomal dominant hypophosphatemia* is a less common condition, with similar hypophosphatemia

Table 2. Features of the Common Genetic Types of Vitamin D Refractory Rickets

	Vitamin D Dependency Type I (VDDR I)	X-Linked Hypophosphatemia (XLH)	Fanconi Syndrome (Includes Cystinosis)
Genetics	Autosomal recessive	X-linked dominant	Cystinosis and other forms; autosomal recessive
Age of onset of physical signs	3–12 months	9–18 months (hypophosphatemia presents shortly after birth)	Infancy, childhood, adulthood
Presentation	Tetany or convulsions, severe deformities, irritability, weakness; enamel hypoplasia of permanent teeth	Bow legs, stunted, stocky, strong; females less severe and may have no deformities; no enamel changes	Infancy: failure to thrive, polyuria Childhood: short stature, rickets, and polyuria Cystinosis also shows cystine deposits in cornea, rectal mucosa, bone marrow, and cultured skin fibroblasts
Radiographic appearance	Severe rickets, thin cortices, tendency to osteoporosis	Mild to moderate chronic rickets with coarse trabecular pattern and thick cortices; females may have normal radiographs but abnormal histology	Mild to severe rickets and osteoporosis
Plasma			
Calcium	↓	Normal	Normal or ↓
Phosphate	↓	↓↓	↓, late normal or ↑
Alkaline phosphatase	↑↑	↑	Normal or ↑
25–OHD	Normal	Normal	Normal
$1,25(OH)_2D$	0 or ↓↓	Normal	Normal
Parathormone	↑	Normal	Normal or ↑
Electrolytes	Normal	Normal	Hypokalemia and acidosis
Creatinine	Normal	Normal	Early normal; late ↑
Urine			
amino acids	Generalized ↑	Normal	Generalized ↑
Prognosis	Normal life expectancy, but lifelong therapy required; with treatment, should readily achieve normal calcium and phosphate homeostasis, bone mineralization, and growth	Normal life expectancy; probably requires lifelong therapy; males and many females may remain stunted and deformed	Cystinosis Infant (Type I): severe uremia by age 10 years Adolescent (Type III): good life expectancy Other forms of Fanconi: variable.

Symbols: ↑ = Increase; ↑↑ = marked increase; ↓ = decrease; ↓↓ = marked decrease.

but less severe physical defects. Both this condition and XLH have been referred to as familial vitamin D refractory (or resistant) rickets.

A low plasma inorganic phosphate (Pi) concentration is the constant feature of these two genetic forms of rickets and is present from early infancy. Serum calcium levels are normal. Raised plasma PTH and generalized aminoaciduria—hallmarks of the rachitic syndromes associated with calcipenia—are absent. The level of plasma 25-OHD is normal, and the $1,25(OH)_2$ D level lies within the normal range.

The patient with XLH usually has deformities and is of short stature. The deformities are less severe than those of VDDR I or II and are later in onset, becoming evident between 9 and 15 months of age. The severity of the physical abnormalities varies greatly. The child usually develops into a strong, stocky adult with varying degrees of genu varum, short stature, and dense but osteomalacic bones. Males tend to be more affected (lyonization); even without treatment some hypophosphatemic females have no physical or radiographic abnormalities. Male-to-male inheritance does not occur. In autosomal dominant hypophosphatemia, deformities tend to be less severe and there is no sex difference. Enamel hypoplasia is not a feature in either form.

The diagnostic feature of both conditions is hypophosphatemia. However, to establish hypophosphatemia, one must take into account the patient's age and sex because these factors greatly influence the normal plasma inorganic phosphate level (Fig. 1). A plasma inorganic phosphate level of 1.5 mmol/liter (4.5 mg/dl) is abnormally low for a newborn infant but abnormally high for a 50-year-old man. Diminished per cent tubular reabsorption of phosphate (per cent TRP) is present even at the low plasma phosphate concentrations.

Fanconi Syndrome

The several genetically distinct conditions included under this syndrome are described in Table 2. All have a multifactorial disturbance of proximal renal tubule function characterized by phosphaturia, generalized aminoaciduria, proteinuria, glycosuria, and usually hypokalemia and renal acidosis. The resultant hypophosphatemia leads to rickets. *Cystinosis* is by far the most common form, but Fanconi syndrome without disordered cystine metabolism occasionally occurs.

Tumor-Induced Hypophosphatemia

In rare instances, hypophosphatemic rickets or osteomalacia occurs in association with certain benign mesenchymal tumors, often of vascular type. Tubular reabsorption of phosphate is decreased. Plasma 25-OHD is normal; $1,25(OH)_2D$ is undetectable. Hypo-

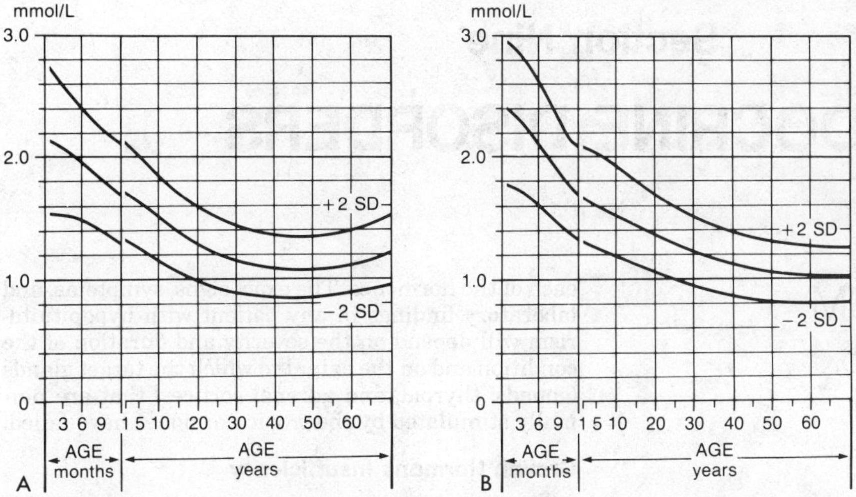

Figure 1. Age-related values of normal plasma inorganic phosphate in females (*A*) and males (*B*). The curves depict the mean and 95 per cent population limits. Values reported in mg/dl can be converted to mmol/liter by multiplying by 0.323. (Data for infants aged 0 to 6 months are from Owen, G. M., et al.: Pediatrics, 31: 495, 1963; data for subjects 1 year of age and older are from Greenberg, B. G., et al.: J. Clin. Endocrinol. Metab., 20: 364, 1960.)

phosphatemia and the bone lesions are cured if the tumor is removed. Chronic hypophosphatemia occurs in some patients with metastatic prostatic carcinoma.

Miscellaneous Causes of Renal Phosphate Loss

Many functions of the proximal renal tubule cells may be damaged by toxic substances (e.g., lead, outdated tetracycline). Rickets occasionally is seen. *Distal renal tubular acidosis* may also cause rickets or osteomalacia.

In hereditary *tyrosinemia* and *oculo-cerebro-renal (Lowe's) syndrome,* the many functions of the proximal tubules are impaired as part of inborn errors of metabolism affecting many organs. As in cystinosis, the resultant hypophosphatemia and renal acidosis can cause rickets.

DEFECTIVE MATRIX CALCIFIABILITY

Hypophosphatasia is an uncommon autosomal recessive disturbance of bone mineralization. Measurements of plasma calcium and inorganic phosphate are normal, but hypercalcemia is often present in severely affected infants. The rickets-like lesions are due to impaired calcifiability of bone matrix and cartilage. Biochemical abnormalities of diagnostic importance are raised plasma and urine levels of phosphorylethanolamine and very low plasma alkaline phosphatase activity (whence the name hypophosphatasia). Elevated plasma and urine concentrations of pyrophosphate have been observed and probably are of pathogenetic significance.

The disease varies greatly in the clinical manifestations and age of presentation. The most severely affected patients have defective skeletal mineralization in utero. At the time of delivery, the bones are short, thin, deformed, and frequently fractured, and the calvarium is virtually uncalcified. Such patients die in the neonatal period. The diagnosis of osteogenesis imperfecta is often mistakenly made for these patients.

More commonly, skeletal abnormalities are first recognized during the early months of life or during the second year. Patients have prominent rickets-like deformities with costochondral beading, enlargement at the ends of the long bones, and frequently stunted growth. Characteristically, the skull is small in circumference with a bulging anterior fontanelle, which is evidence of increased intracranial pressure. Radiographically, lack of mineralization along the edges of the calvarial bones may be misinterpreted as separation of the sutures. Radiographs show defective metaphyseal mineralization that is not dissimilar from that of rickets, but in addition there are characteristic projections of poorly mineralized cartilage extending into the diaphyses. In less severely affected patients, premature loss of deciduous teeth at 2 or 3 years of age is frequently the presenting sign. Genu varum or valgum is evident. Craniosynostosis usually develops. Rickets tends to be most active in the first months of life and tends to become less marked as the child grows older.

Occasionally, patients present initially in adult life with deformities and radiographic lesions similar to those of hereditary hypophosphatemic osteomalacia. The short stature usually observed indicates that unrecognized defects in bone mineralization were present before puberty.

Section Nine

ENDOCRINE DISORDERS

HYPOPITUITARISM

By Raymond V. Randall, M.D.
Rochester, Minnesota

SYNONYMS

Anterior pituitary insufficiency, anterior pituitary failure, Simmonds' disease, Sheehan's syndrome, panhypopituitarism, hypophyseal cachexia.

DEFINITION

Hypopituitarism is an endocrine syndrome characterized by deficiency of one or more of the hormones secreted by the anterior lobe of the pituitary gland: growth hormone (GH), prolactin (PRL), gonadotropin hormones (follicle-stimulating hormone or FSH, and luteinizing hormone or LH), thyrotropic hormone (TSH), and adrenocorticotropic hormone (ACTH). Beta-lipotropin (β-LPH) is secreted in unison with ACTH, but it will not be mentioned further in this discussion since the exact role of beta-lipotropin in the endocrine system is not known at this time.

The term "unitropic failure" is used when there is a deficiency of a single hormone secreted by the anterior lobe of the pituitary. The term panhypopituitarism, although by definition synonymous with failure of both the anterior lobe and the neurohypophysis, is, by common usage, used to denote only a deficiency of all hormones of the anterior lobe.

Although Simmonds' original description included a patient in whom anterior pituitary insufficiency developed after delivery, the term "Sheehan's syndrome" specifically designates hypopituitarism in mothers secondary to pituitary necrosis at parturition, which is usually, but not always, associated with shock, hemorrhage, or sepsis.

The term "Simmonds' disease" is synonymous with hypopituitarism from any cause.

Table 1 provides a classification of causes of anterior pituitary failure.

CLINICAL PICTURE

The signs, symptoms, and physical and laboratory findings in hypopituitarism result from decreased production or lack of one or more of the hormones produced by the anterior lobe. Hence, the clinical picture of hypopituitarism is best described by reviewing the contributions made to this syndrome by the lack of each of the hormones. The exact signs, symptoms, and laboratory findings in any patient with hypopituitarism will depend on the severity and duration of the condition and on the extent to which the target glands (gonads, thyroid, and adrenal cortices) that are normally stimulated by the tropic hormones have failed.

Growth Hormone Insufficiency

Although many physiologic functions have been ascribed to or have been associated with the elaboration of growth hormone, impaired linear growth (dwarfism) is the one significant finding noted with impaired production of growth hormone in humans who have not yet reached adult stature. Once a person has obtained adult stature, a lack of growth hormone alone seems to have no significant clinical sequelae, although it can contribute to the hypoglycemia that may occur in patients with severe pituitary insufficiency who are especially deficient in production of ACTH.

Prolactin Insufficiency

It is still not clear what role prolactin deficiency plays in hypopituitarism. Physiologic amounts of prolactin seem to be essential for normal function of the gonads in both sexes, but exactly how lack of prolactin contributes to infertility seen in patients with panhypopituitarism is not clear at this time.

Gonadotropin Insufficiency

In children, the lack of gonadotropins (FSH and LH) leads to failure of the gonads to develop normally or to secrete the hormones essential for sexual maturation and some of the somatic changes of puberty. The sexual changes of puberty do not occur, and secondary sexual characteristics such as thelarche or growth of the breasts, menarche, growth of sexual hair, maturation of the voice, and development of adult female habitus fail to take place. In males, growth of genitalia, sexual hair, maturation of the voice, adult male habitus, and spermatogenesis all fail to appear. If other hormones of the pituitary gland are elaborated normally in the absence of gonadotropins, linear growth will continue beyond the usual time and a eunuchoid habitus will develop. The exact findings depend upon the timing of gonadotropin failure. For example, an adolescent may be partially through puberty, but if gonadotropic failure intervenes, puberty will not be completed. Thus, an adolescent female may develop normal breasts and sexual hair and attain full growth but may fail to have menarche. If neither growth hormone nor gonadotropins are produced, both sexual and somatic retardation will take place.

When gonadotropic failure occurs in an adult in whom sexual maturation has already taken place, the clinical picture differs from that seen in developing adolescents.

In men the earliest evidence of gonadotropic failure is impotence and loss of libido. Concurrently or shortly thereafter, there will be prostatic atrophy—a sensitive index of testicular failure—and later a decrease in the rate of growth of the beard. In women, there will be loss of libido and irregular menses or amenorrhea. The nipples may lose their pigmentation, but significant atrophy of the breasts is uncommon. In both sexes hot flashes may be present during the onset of gonadotropic insufficiency, and failure of the gonads is accompanied by thinning or loss of axillary and pubic hair as well as hair from the trunk, arms, and legs. The lateral portions of the eyebrows become sparse. The skin becomes atrophic, pale, and thin, and the complexion may acquire a pasty, yellowish tinge.

Thyrotropin Failure

In some patients with hypopituitarism, which includes thyrotropin failure, the typical characteristics of primary myxedema, such as myxedematous skin, myoedema, slowed tendon reflexes, and hypercholesterolemia may develop. The term "pituitary myxedema" is usually used to describe this clinical picture. However, the majority of patients with thyrotropin failure do not develop these findings even though the thyroid failure is severe and of long duration. The failure of most patients with pituitary insufficiency to develop findings associated with primary myxedema may be because failure of other endocrine glands may alter the response of the body to the lack of thyroid hormone, or, more likely, because in pituitary insufficiency the anterior lobe often continues to elaborate small amounts of the tropic hormones, including TSH, unless the anterior pituitary has been completely destroyed.

Regardless of whether the characteristic features of myxedema develop, as the thyroid fails the patient experiences intolerance to cold, decreased perspiration, and some dryness of the skin. Patients with unitropic thyrotropin failure usually develop the classic findings associated with primary myxedema.

Adrenocorticotropin Failure

Failure of the anterior lobe to elaborate ACTH in turn leads to failure of the adrenal cortices to elaborate their hormones, which results in generalized weakness, decreased resistance to infection, and inability to cope with stress in a normal fashion. Failure of the adrenal cortices also plays a partial role in the loss of sexual hair and paleness of the skin.

Hypoglycemia is occasionally found in patients with severe hypopituitarism. Although several factors play a role in the development of hypoglycemia in such patients, it is primarily the result of adrenocortical failure and is readily prevented by the administration of adrenocortical steroids.

Table 1. Classification of Causes of Anterior Pituitary Failure

Idiopathic

Secondary

Trauma
- Accident
- Operation

Therapeutic Ablation
- Operation
- Irradiation

Neoplasm
- Primary tumor
  - Pituitary adenoma
  - Pituitary carcinoma
  - Pituitary sarcoma
  - Craniopharyngioma
  - Meningioma
  - Epidermoid cyst
  - Dermoid cyst
  - Germ cell tumor (ectopic pinealoma)
  - Glioma
  - Chordoma
  - Hamartoma
  - Granular cell tumor (myoblastoma)
  - Sphenoid sinus tumor
  - Miscellaneous
- Metastasis

Vascular Disease
- Postpartum necrosis (Sheehan's syndrome)
- Hemorrhage
- Thrombosis
- Aneurysm
- Vasculitis

Infectious Disease
- Abscess
- Granulomatous disease
- Meningitis
- Aqueductal stenosis

Systemic Disease
- Sarcoidosis
- Histiocytosis X
- Hemochromatosis
- Lymphoma, leukemia, and related diseases
- Autoimmune endocrine failure

Developmental Anomaly
- Aqueductal stenosis
- Arachnoid cyst
- Basal encephalocele
- Intrasellar (Rathke's cleft) cyst

GENERAL CONSIDERATIONS

Symptoms such as apathy, fatigue, and lack of stamina cannot be ascribed to failure of any specific hormone of the anterior pituitary or disorder of any specific target gland and probably are the result of the generalized debility that comes with advanced hypopituitarism. Some patients may also have vague but debilitating, nonspecific muscular and joint aches without objective evidence of joint changes. Most of these symptoms are helped by the administration of physiologic amounts of adrenocortical hormones.

Unitropic failure may be idiopathic or familial, and in most instances it is not clear whether the primary defect lies in the anterior pituitary lobe or in the hypothalamus. Frequently, what appears to be unitropic failure in an adolescent or adult may actually be the first manifestation of a lesion that will grow and cause progressive anterior pituitary failure.

When hypopituitarism results from a tumor in or around the sella turcica, there may be symptoms and findings related to pressure caused by the space-occupying lesion. An early finding is often involvement of the optic chiasm with visual field defects. As time goes on, the visual field defects may become more extensive, and optic atrophy may develop. Headaches of a nonspecific nature are a frequent complaint. Less common findings are paresis of the extraocular muscles, anosmia, and increased intracranial pressure with papilledema secondary to pressure on the third ventricle. Encroachment upon the neurohypophysis may result in diabetes insipidus.

COURSE

With progressive hypopituitarism there is usually first a loss of production of growth hormone followed by loss of production of gonadotropins, TSH, and finally ACTH. It is not clear at what point in this sequence failure of prolactin production takes place. The sequence of loss of hormones in the anterior lobe is not constant, and at times the adrenal cortices may fail before the thyroid gland, and either of these glands may fail before the gonads, although it is unusual for them to do so. In most instances of progressive hypopituitarism, however, there is almost always failure to elaborate growth hormone before other hormones become deficient.

When hypopituitarism results from metastatic tumor or systemic disease, such as sarcoidosis or histiocytosis X, the clinician can expect to find the signs, symptoms, and physical findings typically associated with these conditions.

Hypopituitarism may be caused by a hyperfunctioning pituitary adenoma. The most common association is that of pituitary insufficiency in conjunction with a prolactin-producing pituitary adenoma. This is more likely to be found in men than in women, since these tumors are characteristically diagnosed at an earlier stage in women. Less commonly, hypopituitarism may be associated with a pituitary adenoma producing excessive growth hormone (acromegaly), gonadotropins, or TSH. It is unusual for hypopituitarism to be found in association with a pituitary tumor producing excessive ACTH (Cushing's disease) because the condition is usually diagnosed and treated before the pituitary tumor becomes large enough to cause anterior pituitary failure.

When hypopituitarism is associated with a nonfunctioning chromophobe adenoma (null cell adenoma), a growth hormone–producing tumor (acromegaly), or a prolactin-producing adenoma, the presence of multiple endocrine neoplasias (MEN syndrome) with adenomas of other endocrine glands, particularly the parathyroids and islets of the pancreas, must be considered.

PROGNOSIS AND COMMON COMPLICATIONS

Generally, hypopituitarism is slowly progressive and may be compatible with life for many years. However, untreated patients with hypopituitarism are sensitive to undue physical stress, and relatively mild febrile illnesses or surgical procedures may precipitate a pituitary crisis manifested by progressive weakness, hypotension, collapse, and, if untreated, death.

Pituitary apoplexy (abrupt pituitary insufficiency) may be precipitated by hemorrhage into a pituitary tumor or by pituitary necrosis secondary to postpartum shock, hemorrhage, or sepsis. In rare instances it may be precipitated by hemorrhage into a normal pituitary gland, usually in patients with diabetes mellitus. Pituitary apoplexy, if not recognized and treated promptly, frequently results in death.

DIAGNOSTIC STUDIES

Endocrine Findings

In hypopituitarism there will be a decrease or lack of secretion of growth hormone, prolactin, the gonadotropins, TSH, and ACTH, and a secondary decrease in the secretions of the target glands, namely the gonads, thyroid, and adrenal cortices. There are techniques available to measure each of the hormones of the anterior pituitary and to measure the hormones secreted by the target endocrine glands. There also will be a lack of pituitary reserve—that is, failure of the anterior pituitary to produce its hormones when challenged to do so by various tests.

When failure of one or more of the target glands is demonstrated, whether the cause is primary failure of the target gland or failure secondary to hypopituitarism must be determined. If there has been primary failure of the target gland, the production of its tropic hormone should be increased by the anterior pituitary in an attempt to compensate for the falling level of the target gland's hormone or hormones. Also , the target gland should not respond to the administration of exogenous tropic hormone because it is unable to respond to the endogenous increase of that hormone. On the other hand, if secondary or pituitary failure of the target gland has occurred, production of the tropic hormone by the pituitary should be decreased or absent, and the target gland should respond to the administration of this hormone.

When there is primary failure of one or more of the target glands, usually a clear-cut separation is found between the increased values of the tropic hormone or hormones and normal values. On the other hand, measuring tropic hormones, growth hormone, and prolactin often is not helpful when trying to distinguish between secondary (pituitary) failure and normal because usually no clear-cut differentiation can be made between low, but normal and abnormally low values of these various hormones. Under such circumstances, stimulation or provocative tests may be helpful in determining whether the pituitary is capable of producing the hormone(s) in question.

The following discussion will review currently used methods of assessing function of the anterior pituitary and its target glands.

Evaluation of Growth Hormone Production

Plasma growth hormone is measured by radioimmunoassay. When hypopituitarism is suspected, measurement of basal growth hormone is frequently not helpful because the values may be low or undetectable in normal persons. On the other hand, useful information can be obtained by measuring the ability of the pituitary to increase its output of growth hormone after administration of insulin, arginine, L-dopa, or propranolol and glucagon.

The stress of insulin-produced hypoglycemia normally results in a secretion of a number of hormones, including growth hormone, ACTH, prolactin, cortisol, and catecholamines. The test is performed after an overnight fast and after measuring plasma glucose level to make certain that the patient is not hypoglycemic before the test is begun. Blood is drawn for baseline growth hormone and glucose values. The patient is then given an intravenous injection of 0.1 U of regular insulin per kilogram of body weight, and specimens for growth hormone and blood glucose measurements are obtained at half-hourly intervals for 2 hours following the administration of insulin. In satisfactory tests the values for blood glucose fall to 50 per cent or less of the fasting level. Failure of growth hormone values to increase more than 5 ng/ml or to a level greater than 10 ng/ml is evidence of growth hormone deficiency and lack of growth hormone reserve. The dose of insulin used is capable of evoking fatal hypoglycemia, particularly if the adrenal cortices are severely hypofunctioning. If such is suspected, the test should be omitted or the dose of insulin reduced to 0.05 U/kg body weight. All patients undergoing an insulin hypoglycemia test must be watched carefully, and the attendant must be prepared to administer 50 per cent dextrose intravenously if serious manifestations of hypoglycemia develop. At the end of the test it is prudent to give the patient 25 gm of dextrose intravenously or glucose orally. During the test an indwelling intravenous needle, kept open by a slow drip of isotonic saline solution, will facilitate the administration of dextrose if it is suddenly needed. The test is contraindicated in patients with a convulsive disorder or ischemic cardiovascular disease.

Some patients who have normal growth hormone reserve may fail to respond to insulin hypoglycemia, and one of the other stimulation tests mentioned earlier should be performed when it is important to know whether growth hormone reserve is normal. The reader should consult one of the standard textbooks on endocrinology for details about these tests since space limitations prohibit giving details here.

Evaluation of Prolactin Secretion

Evaluation of prolactin secretion is made by measuring serum prolactin under basal conditions. The normal values in our laboratories are up to and including 20 ng/ml for men and 23 ng/ml for women. No clear-cut differentiation can be made between low normal and abnormally low prolactin values. Since the prolactin values normally rise during sleep, especially toward the end of sleep, and may not fall to baseline until 30 minutes or so after awakening, blood for baseline prolactin values should not be obtained immediately upon the patient's awakening. Patients who are taking estrogens, birth control pills, or tranquilizers, or who are under stress, may have an elevation of basal prolactin values (see article on Hyperprolactinemia).

Prolactin reserve is tested by the thyrotropin releasing hormone (TRH) test. TRH stimulates the release of both TSH and prolactin. The procedure is performed with the patient fasting and at rest. A blood sample is obtained for basal prolactin determination and 400 μg of TRH is administered intravenously as a bolus. Blood samples are obtained again at 30 and 60 min. The response in the normal person varies with age, sex, and basal prolactin level. In general, the prolactin values should rise more than 100 per cent above baseline.

Evaluation of Gonadal Function

In gonadal failure secondary to hypopituitarism, values for the following laboratory tests are decreased or zero in both sexes: urinary pituitary gonadotropins, serum FSH and LH, and urinary and serum estrogens. In the male, serum testosterone and urinary 17-ketosteroids will be decreased. Approximately one third of the urinary 17-ketosteroids in the male are produced by the adrenal cortices.

In primary gonadal failure, values for urinary estrogens and serum estrogens or testosterone will be decreased or absent, but the values for urinary pituitary gonadotropins and serum FSH and LH will be increased above normal.

In secondary gonadal failure, the gonads will respond to the administration of human pituitary gonadotropins, but they will fail to do so in primary gonadal failure. The cost and limited supply of human pituitary gonadotropins have precluded their use in routine diagnostic work of this type.

Tests of pituitary gonadotropin reserve are performed by administering gonadotropin releasing hormone (GnRH), which stimulates the release of both FSH and LH.

Evaluation of Thyroid Function

In either primary or secondary thyroid failure, values for basal metabolic rate, total and free thyroxine, and uptake of radioiodine by the thyroid are decreased. The concentration of TSH in the blood is elevated in primary thyroid failure, and the measurement of TSH is helpful in differentiating primary from secondary thyroid failure. However, the determination of TSH level is not helpful in distinguishing the euthyroid state from secondary thyroid failure because the distinction between low but normal and abnormally low values is not clear-cut.

Pituitary reserve in relation to TSH can be evaluated by administering TRH as described in the section on evaluation of prolactin secretion. Normally there should be 100 per cent rise or more in TSH level following administration of TRH. In the presence of primary hypothyroidism the response is exaggerated and prolonged. The TRH test has replaced the test whereby the uptake of radioiodine was measured before and following the administration of TSH. In the latter test, exogenous TSH stimulates the thyroid in secondary failure but fails to do so in primary failure.

Evaluation of Adrenocortical Function

In both primary and secondary adrenal failure, plasma cortisol, urinary 17-ketosteroids, and urinary ketogenic steroid levels are decreased or absent. ACTH is increased in the blood in patients with primary adrenal failure, but this is not usually helpful in distinguishing secondary failure from normal because the distinction between low but normal and abnormally low value for ACTH is not clear-cut.

When doubt exists in distinguishing primary from secondary adrenocortical failure, the differentiation can be made by administering exogenous ACTH. Baseline values of plasma cortisol or corticosteroids are measured at 8 A.M. and 4 P.M., and for urinary ketogenic steroids in a 24-hour urine specimen. The patient is then given 25 IU of ACTH intravenously in 500 ml of isotonic saline solution over 8 hours (8 A.M. to 4 P.M.) daily for 3 days or 40 IU of ACTH gel (Acthar) intramuscularly every 12 hours for 3 days. On the third day, values for plasma cortisol or corticosteroids and urinary ketogenic steroids are again determined. If the adrenal cortices respond normally to stimulation, the values measured should increase two times or more, or if the baseline values are near zero, the values after stimulation should be well within the normal range. The measurement of urinary 17-ketosteroids in the ACTH test is not crucial since the value often will not increase significantly even though the values for plasma cortisol and urinary ketogenic steroids respond normally. (*Caution:* The physician should be familiar with the anaphylactoid reactions and other serious toxic effects that may occur during the administration of ACTH.)

Pituitary reserve, with regard to the production of ACTH, is determined by performing an insulin hypoglycemia test (see details in the section on Evaluation of Growth Hormone Production). During the test, a blood sample for baseline plasma cortisol or corticosteroid determination is obtained and then at half-hourly intervals for 2 hours following the administration of insulin. Normally plasma cortisol or corticosteroid values should rise to greater than 20 μg/dl or by at least 7 μg/dl.

Electrolytes

Patients with hypopituitarism usually have essentially normal aldosterone levels because the production of aldosterone is primarily under the influence of the renin-angiotensin system; they do not have the hyponatremia, hypochloremia, and hyperkalemia found in some patients with primary adrenal failure. However, when patients with hypopituitarism become acutely ill, especially when vomiting and diarrhea are present, hyponatremia and hypochloremia may develop. Likewise, patients with severe hypo-pituitarism may be unable to excrete a water load normally and are subject to water intoxication, a situation that is readily prevented by the administration of physiologic amounts of adrenocortical steroids.

On rare occasions I have seen patients with hypopituitarism, usually secondary to a lesion in the hypothalamus, who are unable to retain sodium and chloride normally. These usually have been relatively young patients who have needed an electrolyte-retaining hormone (fludrocortisone) to maintain electrolyte balance. Also, I have had a few adult patients who, because of their occupation, perspire excessively and may become hyponatremic, a situation that is corrected by the administration of additional salt, and which may also require the administration of an electrolyte-retaining hormone, such as fludrocortisone.

Blood Glucose

Typically the blood glucose level is normal in patients with hypopituitarism. However, as noted earlier, some patients may develop hypoglycemia, a situation that is readily prevented by administering physiologic amounts of adrenocorticosteroids. The finding of hypoglycemia in a patient with a pituitary adenoma should alert one to the possible presence of multiple endocrine neoplasias (MEN syndrome) or an insulin-secreting islet cell adenoma(s).

Peripheral Blood

The hemoglobin level and erythryocyte count are normal in patients with mild hypopituitarism. However, with prolonged or severe hypopituitarism, moderate or severe normochromic, normocytic anemia may develop, especially in male patients. This anemia responds readily to hormonal replacement. A mild eosinophilia of 5 to 8 per cent may be present in hypopituitarism and responds to the administration of physiologic amounts of adrenocortical hormones.

Urinalysis

The results of routine urinalyses are normal in hypopituitarism. However, if diabetes insipidus is present, the specific gravity of the urine will be low and the daily volume of urine will be increased. Occasionally a patient with diabetes insipidus, particularly when it develops following surgery for a tumor in or around the pituitary, may develop diabetes insipidus without a compensating thirst drive. Such patients will excrete a dilute urine with an essentially normal volume. If the situation is not recognized and corrected by the administration of antidiuretic hormone and adequate amounts of fluid, the patients may develop hypernatremia, hyperosmolality, and even stupor or unconsciousness.

Imaging

Imaging studies should be obtained in all patients suspected of having hypopituitarism. The majority of patients who have an intrasellar pituitary tumor will have enlargement or erosion of the sella, which is usually evident on plain roentgenograms of the skull. It is important to remember that a normal sella on plain roentgenograms of the skull does not rule out an intrasellar tumor. Small abnormalities in the contours of the sella may be better appreciated by polytomograms with anteroposterior and lateral views taken serially every 3 mm.

Bilateral carotid angiography with magnification and subtraction views may reveal tumors as small as 3 or 4 mm in diameter, which cannot otherwise be seen, and this technique is also helpful when an aneurysm is suspected. However, in the past several years computed tomographic (CT) scanning with serial axial and coronal views obtained during the infusion of contrast medium using one of the newer fourth generation scanners has proved to be the most successful method to date of detecting pituitary adenomas. Approximately 85 per cent of such tumors can be detected, and small suprasellar lesions can also be detected by this technique. It is no longer necessary to do pneumoencephalographic studies in patients suspected of having a sellar or suprasellar lesion.

Nuclear magnetic resonance (NMR) scanning is just beginning to be used in the detection of intrasellar and suprasellar lesions at the time of this writing, but it holds great promise and may prove to be more sensitive than current CT scanning.

Examination of Visual Fields

The visual fields should be charted accurately by tangential screen or perimetric examination in all patients suspected of having hypopituitarism. Typically, the earliest visual field defect of a chiasmal lesion from a pituitary tumor is loss of vision in the upper, outer quadrant of each eye. If the lesion progresses, total bitemporal hemianopia will subsequently develop, and later only an island of vision will remain in the nasal portion of each eye. Even these islands may be affected if the tumor continues to grow.

Electroencephalography and Echoencephalography

In general, electroencephalography and echoencephalography are of little help in establishing a diagnosis of an intrasellar or suprasellar tumor.

THERAPEUTIC TRIALS

As a rule, administration of hormonal replacement therapy as a therapeutic trial is not justified in patients suspected of having hypopituitarism. Since this syndrome is so complex and since, with rare exceptions, the patients must take replacement therapy for the remainder of their lives, the diagnosis should be confirmed by appropriate endocrine tests and other studies already reviewed rather than be based on a therapeutic trial of hormonal replacement therapy, which may be difficult or impossible to evaluate.

PITFALLS IN DIAGNOSIS

The major pitfall in dealing with a patient with hypopituitarism is to establish the diagnosis of hypopituitarism and then, upon failing to find an etiologic factor, to assume that it is idiopathic in origin. Almost without exception, especially in adults, hypopituitarism that is not unitropic is secondary to another condition rather than idiopathic. It should be emphasized that in hypopituitarism, as in diabetes insipidus, evidence of pituitary dysfunction may precede by months or years other manifestations of an underlying tumor or other lesion in or around the sella or manifestations of some systemic disease. In my experience the temporal hiatus has been as long as 10 to 12 years in some instances.

When a diagnosis of unitropic failure, especially gonadotropic failure, has been made in an adult, it should be kept in mind that this may be merely the first manifestation of what may ultimately progress to panhypopituitarism. In such instances, the pituitary gland will usually fail to elaborate normal amounts of growth hormone in response to an adequate stimulus, such as insulin-induced hypoglycemia.

The possibility of hypopituitarism should be considered and CT scans of the sellar and suprasellar regions should be obtained in all young women who have never undergone menarche or who have menstruated and subsequently experienced amenorrhea not caused by pregnancy. These patients should also have a determination of serum prolactin level to rule out the possibility of hyperprolactinemia.

It has occasionally been stated that the differentiation of hypopituitarism from anorexia nervosa is so obvious that it is not necessary to mention the latter condition in discussing hypopituitarism. Nonetheless, the fact remains that all too frequently a diagnosis of hypopituitarism is made in patients with anorexia nervosa, and consequently institution of appropriate therapy for anorexia nervosa has been unnecessarily delayed. In actuality, patients with advanced anorexia nervosa have what can be regarded as partial, physiologic failure of the anterior lobe of the pituitary as the result of starvation. Gonadotropins are no longer secreted and menses cease. The basal metabolic rate may be as low as –40 to –50, although the thyroid is functioning normally. 17-Ketosteroids may be absent from the urine and the amount of ketogenic steroids in the urine may be decreased, although the plasma cortisol or corticosteroid levels remain normal, or, in some instances, are increased. Consequently, it is apparent why anorexia nervosa may sometimes be misdiagnosed and called hypopituitarism. Patients with anorexia nervosa are almost invariably young females. There may be slight loss of sexual hair, but the axillary and pubic hair is rarely lost completely. A fine lanugo-like hair may appear over the face and trunk. Important is the fact that patients with anorexia nervosa lead active lives despite extreme emaciation. Patients with hypopituitarism who are ill enough to become severely emaciated are usually totally disabled and unable to do more than exist. Extreme emaciation in a young female who is mentally and physically active should suggest the presence of anorexia nervosa rather than anterior pituitary failure.

EMPTY SELLA SYNDROME

By Barbara A. Baker, M.D.
Tulsa, Oklahoma
Stephen F. Hodgson, M.D.
and Raymond V. Randall, M.D.
Rochester, Minnesota

DEFINITION

The dural reflections that form the diaphragma sellae usually provide a covering for the sella turcica, which is traversed only by the pituitary stalk. Occasionally, however, the arachnoid membrane and cerebrospinal fluid may protrude or enter into the sella. When this occurs, the pituitary gland may be compressed in a posterior and inferior direction against the sella floor, and the sella itself may become enlarged and undergo bony remodeling. Gross anatomic inspection of the sella then gives the impression that the sella is "empty." An empty sella may occur for two reasons.

1. A congenital deficiency or absence of the diaphragma sellae may allow the suprasellar arachnoid membrane to herniate directly into the sella. The resulting transmission of cerebrospinal fluid pressure then results in pituitary compression and bony remodeling. This is known as the *primary* or *idiopathic empty sella syndrome.*
2. Volume reduction of intrasellar contents, whether by operation, irradiation, or infarction and necrosis of tissue, allows collapse of the suprasellar arachnoid membrane into the sella (and occasionally other structures as well, such as the optic chiasm). This pathologic condition is known as the *secondary empty sella syndrome.*

Changes compatible with a diagnosis of the primary empty sella syndrome have been demonstrated in 5.5 to 6.7 per cent of autopsy series.

PRESENTING SIGNS AND SYMPTOMS

Most patients in whom a diagnosis of a primary empty sella syndrome is made are middle-aged, multiparous females. However, the diagnosis has been made in both sexes and at all ages. Presenting complaints are usually nonspecific and may include headache, sinus problems, or fatigue. Physical examination reveals a high prevalence of obesity and often mild hypertension. Evidence of endocrine gland dysfunction is usually absent. Visual field defects are found rarely, and these may be associated with increased or normal intracranial pressure. Cerebrospinal fluid rhinorrhea may occur and may occasionally result in the development of meningitis.

DIAGNOSIS

Standard head roentgenograms reveal the empty sella to be moderately enlarged, with a symmetric and rounded or globular contour. The clinoid processes are not displaced, and the dorsum sellae is not straightened, in contrast to changes often seen with expanding intrasellar tumors. Although bony remodeling of the sella is usually symmetric, a "double floor" contour may occasionally be seen on lateral projections. Pneumoencephalography was previously used to demonstrate an empty sella, but it is now accepted that computed tomographic (CT) scanning provides a reliable, noninvasive method of making this diagnosis. We use the following computed tomographic findings for the diagnosis of an empty sella:

1. An area of low attenuation (cerebrospinal fluid) extends from the suprasellar cistern to below the level of the diaphragm into the sella.
2. After injection of contrast medium, the pituitary stalk can be seen to extend down to a flattened pituitary gland in the posterior inferior portion of the sella.
3. The optic chiasm lies lower than usual and may dip below the level of the diaphragm.

LABORATORY RESULTS

Routine laboratory tests are unaffected by the presence of an empty sella. The pituitary gland, although distorted in shape, remains histologically and functionally normal, while retaining its susceptibility to other pathologic processes. Associated endocrine abnormalities are rare.

DIFFERENTIAL DIAGNOSIS

The empty sella syndrome may mimic a subarachnoid cyst, and, more importantly, a pituitary tumor. Although the history and physical examination may suggest the presence of a functioning pituitary tumor, CT scanning of the head should allow differentiation of the two conditions. However, pituitary tumors and an empty sella may coexist. Visual field defects may be seen when an expanding intrasellar tumor compresses the optic chiasm, with development of a secondary empty sella syndrome with prolapse of the optic chiasm into the sella, or rarely with a primary empty sella syndrome. Here again, CT scanning of the head aids in making the correct diagnosis.

TREATMENT AND FOLLOW-UP EXAMINATION

The primary and secondary empty sella syndromes usually require no treatment. Surgery is indicated, however, to correct cerebrospinal fluid rhinorrhea or to halt progressive visual loss occurring with secondary empty sella syndrome.

All patients with an empty sella syndrome, primary or secondary, should be examined periodically. Examination should include an assessment of sellar size, endocrine evaluation, funduscopic examination, inquiry about possible cerebrospinal fluid rhinorrhea, and plotting of the visual fields.

DIABETES INSIPIDUS

By Ronald Skowsky, M.D.
Long Beach, California

DEFINITION

Diabetes insipidus (DI) is a disease characterized by excessive polyuria and subsequent polydipsia, which results from a relative or absolute deficiency of secretion or end-organ resistance to the action of the antidiuretic hormone (ADH), arginine vasopressin (AVP).

CAUSES

Diabetes insipidus can be classified by etiology and therapeutic responsiveness to exogenous vasopressin into *central or neurogenic diabetes insipidus* (vasopressin-sensitive) and *nephrogenic diabetes insipidus* (vasopressin-resistant) (Table 1). In approximately 50 per cent of patients with neurogenic DI, no cause is apparent, and these patients are classified in the idiopathic category, although the cause is believed to be central in origin. Conversely, fewer than 1 per cent of subjects exhibit AVP deficiency on an hereditary basis, usually by an autosomal dominant mode of inheritance, but occasionally via an X-linked recessive transmission. Recently, a syndrome complex has been described comprising diabetes insipidus, diabetes mellitus, optic atrophy, and high-tone deafness; this has been designated the *DIDMOAD syndrome* and is transmitted by an autosomal recessive mode.

Secondary causes of neurogenic DI include a large number of pituitary and suprasellar lesions: chromophobe adenoma, craniopharyngioma, glioma, pinealoma, and cysts. Carcinomas of the breast and bronchus are the most common metastatic tumors to produce DI in adults. Infiltrative central nervous system diseases that commonly lead to neurogenic DI include histiocytosis X, tuberculosis, sarcoidosis, syphilis, Hodgkin's disease, and leukemia. DI may also develop following viral or bacterial meningitis or encephalitis, especially in the pediatric age group.

Basal skull fractures or other forms of severe head trauma may lead to the onset of neurogenic DI. Not uncommonly, the disorder will develop following neurosurgical intervention for pituitary or suprasellar lesions. In some patients with preoperative adrenocorticotropic hormone (ACTH) deficiency, symptoms of polyuria and polydipsia may be minimal until postoperative corticosteroid therapy induces complete clinical expression of the disorder. Neurosurgical high sectioning of the hypophyseal stalk and median eminence damage during hypophysectomy will produce a characteristic triphasic response. The initial phase consists of severe polyuria and polydipsia of about 1 week's duration (secondary to removal of the stored AVP within the neurohypophysis), followed by a second week of antidiuresis (reflecting leakage of AVP from the surgically sectioned neurons). Following this phase, temporary or permanent DI may occur depending on the extent of the surgery.

Miscellaneous causes for neurogenic DI include central nervous system injury from vascular aneurysms, sickle cell disease, and, occasionally, high-pressure hydrocephalus.

Nephrogenic DI generally refers to the rare familial disorder believed to be transmitted by an X-linked dominant inheritance with variable penetrance and characterized by a vasopressin-resistant polyuric state. Other genetic diseases that may present with clinical nephrogenic DI are sickle cell disease and nephronophthisis. However, renal unresponsiveness to AVP is more commonly seen following a variety of chronic renal disorders, including pyelonephritis, medullary cystic disease, uric acid or analgesic nephropathy, obstructive uropathy, myeloma, and Sjögren's syndrome, and following renal transplantation. Hypercalcemia and hypokalemia are also frequently encountered conditions associated with renal tubular resistance to AVP. Finally, lithium and demeclocycline appear to be drugs that will induce states of renal AVP unresponsiveness depending on dosage given.

PATHOPHYSIOLOGY

Vasopressin secretion is normally regulated by a finely tuned system of osmoreceptors and baroreceptors. Hypothalamic osmosensitive cells in the perinuclear zone of the supraoptic nucleus, the major site of AVP synthesis, are sensitive to small changes in plasma osmolality. Lowering the plasma osmolality by oral water ingestion to a mean of 281.7 mOsm/kg

Table 1. Classification of Diabetes Insipidus

Neurogenic (Central) Diabetes Insipidus

I. Primary
- Idiopathic
- Hereditary

II. Secondary
- Tumors: Pituitary, hypothalamic, and metastatic
- Infiltrative disease
- Inflammatory disease
- Post-traumatic
- Postneurosurgical
- Miscellaneous

Nephrogenic Diabetes Insipidus

I. Primary: Hereditary

II. Secondary
- Chronic renal disease
- Drugs
- Hypercalcemia
- Hypokalemia
- Sickle cell disease

will suppress AVP release and produce a maximum diuresis, whereas infusion of hypertonic saline can raise the plasma osmolality to a mean of 287.3 mOsm/kg, the osmotic threshold for AVP release in normal subjects.

Hemodynamic changes, monitored via baroreceptors within the vascular system, are the second major control mechanism regulating AVP secretion. A decrease in mean arterial blood pressure stimulates carotid and aortic arch arterial baroreceptors to augment AVP release. In a similar fashion, a drop in circulating plasma volume decreases the tonic inhibitory impulses from left atrial stretch receptors to the hypothalamus and increases AVP secretion. Thus, the intact subject will attempt to reestablish a normal circulating blood volume and homeostasis at the expense of plasma hypotonicity.

Finally, there appears to be a multitude of nonosmotic, nonhemodynamic mechanisms for augmenting AVP secretion. Such factors include pain, psychologic stress, emesis, and a variety of drugs, including the monoamine and endorphin neurotransmitters. Appreciation of these variables is important in the diagnostic evaluation of the patient with presumed diabetes insipidus, since the defect in AVP secretion may lie at a number of sites along physiologic or anatomic pathways regulating AVP synthesis or secretion in response to osmoregulatory or hemodynamic mechanisms or both. At least four types of neurogenic DI can be distinguished clinically or by sophisticated testing (discussed under Diagnostic Tests):

1. Severe absence of AVP release following osmotic and hemodynamic stimuli.
2. Partial absence of AVP release following osmotic and hemodynamic stimuli.
3. Absence of AVP release following osmotic stimuli but responsive to hemodynamic stimuli.
4. Adequate AVP release only after abnormally high osmotic stimuli (i.e., elevated osmotic threshold), usually in the presence of hypodipsia.

DIAGNOSTIC TESTS

The differential diagnosis of nonglucosuric polyuria, in the absence of diuretic-induced natriuresis, is generally between neurogenic DI, nephrogenic DI, and primary polydipsia (a compulsive and excessive intake of water, usually observed in a subject with a background of psychiatric disorder). The diagnostic studies described attempt to reproduce osmotic or hemodynamic stimuli for AVP secretion, which are reflected by end-organ effects of AVP on renal concentration, or via direct immunologic quantitation of plasma AVP. The results of the tests described, however, must be interpreted with some degree of caution. Persistent polyuria, in and of itself, will "wash out" the renal medullary concentration gradient and will lower the maximal urine concentration achieved following dehydration or administration of exogenous vasopressin. In addition, patients with partial neurogenic DI possess an augmented sensitivity to low levels of vasopressin, which may obscure results obtained during prolonged dehydration. Thus, a single diagnostic study may not always reliably predict the correct diagnosis.

DEHYDRATION TEST

Fluid deprivation for 8 hours or longer should normally induce a fall in urine volume and a progressive rise in urine osmolality to between 600 and 1200 mOsm/kg, which should not be further increased by exogenous administration of vasopressin. Patients are placed on complete fluid restriction for periods of 12 to 16 hours (less if the severely polyuric subject experiences a weight loss of more than 3 per cent during testing) until hourly urine measurements of osmolality stabilize, indicated by an increase of less than 30 mOsm/kg for at least three successive hours. A plasma sample is obtained for osmolality to ensure that the dehydration testing was sufficient to raise plasma osmolality above 290 mOsm/kg, and the patient then receives either aqueous vasopressin (Pitressin), 5 units subcutaneously, or desmopressin (DDAVP), 20 μg intranasally. Urinary osmolality is again measured 30 and 60 min later. The normal response is a rise in urine osmolality greater than that of plasma osmolality following dehydration, and a fall or rise by less than 9 per cent after vasopressin administration.

In severely polyuric patients who have complete inability to concentrate the urine following fluid deprivation, this single study along with the renal response to exogenous vasopressin will be sufficient to establish the diagnosis of severe neurogenic or severe nephrogenic DI and to exclude the diagnosis of primary polydipsia. However, in patients who demonstrate ability to increase urine concentration to some degree during dehydration, further studies are required to reliably exclude primary polydipsia (or possibly partial nephrogenic DI) even though the majority (75 per cent) of this group will have partial neurogenic DI.

These patients, who demonstrate elevation of urine osmolality greater than 9 per cent following fluid deprivation, should have plasma samples obtained following the dehydration study (and before administration of exogenous vasopressin) for vasopressin measurement. If fluid deprivation failed to cause elevation of plasma osmolality above 292 mOsm/kg, vasopressin determination alone may not reliably distinguish partial DI from primary polydipsia, and the patient should undergo a hypertonic saline infusion (described later in this article) with additional plasma AVP samples.

Prolonging the dehydration test in severely polyuric patients carries the risk of iatrogenic induction of hypovolemic shock, and body weights should be obtained during the procedure, especially in the pediatric age group. On occasion, development of mild hypovolemic orthostatic hypotension is desirable to correctly diagnose the rare neurogenic DI patient with a disturbance in osmoregulation but intact baroreceptor regulation of AVP. In such a patient, dehydration testing alone will fail to increase urinary concentration or plasma AVP, whereas a mild decrease in mean arterial blood pressure will augment vasopressin secretion.

In addition, polyuric patients with DI secondary to an elevated osmotic threshold may demonstrate relatively normal urinary concentration following dehydration. However, the plasma osmolality at this point (prior to exogeneous vasopressin administration) will be markedly elevated (295 to 300 mOsm/kg), and the correct diagnosis can be ascertained. These patients usually have a severe impairment of the thirst center and are unaware of their hyperosmolar state. If fluids are forced upon these patients, the fall in plasma osmolality to "normal" levels will suppress AVP secretion and they will manifest clinically significant polyuria.

HYPERTONIC SALINE INFUSION

Osmoreceptor integrity can be evaluated by quantitating the change in renal concentration and plasma AVP levels following induction of a hyperosmolar state via hypertonic saline infusion. The osmotic threshold for AVP release can be measured by intravenously infusing into a large antecubital vein of the recumbent patient 5 per cent sodium chloride at a rate of 0.5 ml/kg/min for 2 hours. Blood and urine samples are obtained at 15-min intervals for quantitation of plasma and urine osmolality and plasma AVP. Plasma osmolality and plasma AVP will normally rise during the infusion. The osmotic threshold for AVP release (normal, 285 to 292 mOsm/kg) can be interpolated from a simple regression slope as that point when free water clearance first falls 2 standard deviations below the mean basal level. Patients with severe neurogenic DI will show an absent threshold, but subjects with an elevated osmotic threshold will be above the normal range. The hypertonic saline infusion with simultaneous AVP measurement is also recommended to separate partial neurogenic DI from primary polydipsia in the rare situation when dehydration alone fails to elevate the plasma osmolality sufficiently highly to produce significant elevations in plasma AVP.

PLASMA ARGININE VASOPRESSIN MEASUREMENT

Radioimmunoassay quantitation of plasma AVP is at present available from a number of commercial laboratories. However, care must be exercised in interpretation, since marked differences exist in sensitivity, specificity, and reference standards used for reporting results. AVP values should be evaluated with concurrent plasma osmolalities and reported with a nomogram previously established with the particular reference laboratory.

Isolated plasma AVP determinations are unlikely to be confirmatory in the 25 per cent of polyuric subjects in whom the dehydration test is nondiagnostic between partial neurogenic DI and primary polydipsia; repetitive AVP sampling during prolonged dehydration or hypertonic saline infusion may be necessary. Repeated very low plasma AVP levels in the presence of marked plasma hyperosmolality strongly suggests neurogenic DI. In addition, plasma AVP levels in nephrogenic DI tend to be normal or elevated for the concurrent plasma osmolality.

PITFALLS IN DIFFERENTIAL DIAGNOSIS

1. Chronic polyuria (whether secondary to diabetes insipidus or caused by compulsive water ingestion) will produce a decrease in the maximal concentrating capacity of the kidney.
2. Patients with neurogenic DI and low levels of endogenous AVP show an increased sensitivity in renal concentration to doses of exogenous vasopressin, which can confuse the distinction between partial neurogenic DI and primary polydipsia.
3. Basal plasma AVP and basal plasma osmolality determinations are not diagnostic.
4. Patients with an elevated osmotic threshold for vasopressin release may present with a relatively normal renal response to dehydration (but will demonstrate a markedly elevated plasma osmolality).
5. Therapeutic trials with exogenous vasopressin to distinguish the cause of polyuria will not always be diagnostic, since compulsive water drinkers may also respond with a fall in urine volume.

ACROMEGALY

By John A. Linfoot, M.D.
Berkeley, California

SYNONYM

Hypersomatotropism.

DEFINITION

Acromegaly is an uncommon endocrinopathy resulting from the hypersecretion of growth hormone (GH). Excessive GH secretion originates usually from an adenoma of somatotropic cells of the anterior lobe of the pituitary, occasionally from hyperplasia of pituitary somatotropic cells, and rarely from ectopic or nonpituitary tumors producing GH or GH releasing factors.

A combination of clinical findings, light microscopy, and immunocytochemical staining is required to classify pituitary tumors in acromegaly and gigantism. The use of hematoxylin and eosin staining of pituitary tumors reveals the presence of typical eosinophilic cells in the majority of acromegalic patients. Ultrastructural studies typically will demonstrate high-density granules in the eosinophilic cells, usually ranging from 160 to 342 nm in size. Size of the hormone granules is determined by functional factors, such as rates of hormone synthesis and release. Immunocytochemical stains using specifically tagged anti-growth hormone or anti-prolactin antibodies frequently reveal both GH and prolactin (PRL) in many tumors. Acromegaly can be associated with tumors composed of purely eosinophilic cells, mixed GH and PRL cells, or stem cells. Staining characteristically reflects tumor secretory activity, the larger, more actively secreting tumors showing the fewest secretory granules. The correlation between tumor cell characteristics, secretory activity, and tumor growth characteristics (invasiveness) is still unclear. Pituitary tumors are locally invasive but rarely metastasize.

On the basis of histologic studies, Jules Hardy, from his extensive surgical experience on the anterior hypophysis, reported a surprisingly consistent anatomic distribution of functioning pituitary microadenomas. Acidophilic tumors associated with acromegaly or gigantism are inferior-lateral, which explains the usual asymmetric expansion of the sella turcica.

Studies employing tissue cultures of biopsy material from pituitary tumors have demonstrated that most tumors secrete GH as well as PRL into the media, but because of certain in vitro behaviors of these cells, the PRL-secreting cells tend to predominate after a period of time and thus results of these studies may not correlate with the clinical activity of pituitary tumors. Approximately 40 per cent of my acromegalic patients have hyperprolactinemia. The coexistence of separate GH and PRL cell adenomas in the same patient has been described. The overall incidence of "double" adenomas or mixed adenomas may be higher than is currently recognized.

The incidence of acromegaly in families is rare. Familial endocrine neoplasia and hyperplasia are usually divided into two patterns. *Multiple endocrine adenomatosis (MEA) type 1* is a syndrome characterized by multiple endocrine tumors involving the parathyroids, pituitary, pancreatic islets, and adrenal cortex. MEA type 1 is an uncommon syndrome in my series of 303 patients with acromegaly. Only the incidence of hyperparathyroidism was increased in this series; it probably represents a separate form of multiple endocrine tumors that should not be classified as MEA type 1 or type 2. The second pattern, *MEA type 2 (Sipple's Syndrome)* is characterized by medullary thyroid carcinoma, pheochromocytoma, and parathyroid tumors and is not associated with acromegaly and gigantism.

CLINICAL SIGNS AND SYMPTOMS

The symptoms that cause the patient to see a physician are varied. In women, cessation of menstruation is most common and may or may not be associated with galactorrhea. Headache is an early symptom; backache, disturbance of vision, goiter, muscle atrophy, generalized weakness, deepening of the voice, paresthesias, and many other symptoms have been described. In advanced cases, symptoms of hypopituitarism due to loss of one or more tropic hormones may predominate.

A history of change in glove, ring, or shoe size can be elicited from all patients. Other signs of soft tissue enlargement are reflected in the large, moist, doughy hand (a diagnostic finding), and the generalized coarsening of facial features with furrowing of the brow, widening of the jaw, enlargement of the lips and tongue, partial thickening of the facial folds, and enlargement and broadening of the nose. Weight gain and acral changes are more prominent in the postpubertal acromegalic patient; linear growth can occur only in the prepubertal patient and results in gigantism. Increasing bra size without change in cup size or decreased cup size is a common symptom in women.

COURSE

Acromegaly is characterized by disproportionate enlargement of the face, hands, and feet that occurs in adulthood after linear growth has ceased. It is thought to reduce life expectancy, and indeed in some studies 50 per cent of 100 patients died before the age of 50 years; 89 per cent died by age 69 years. The leading cause of death is cardiovascular disease. Acromegaly is a debilitating disease; however, with early diagnosis and individualized treatment the disease may be arrested and life may be prolonged.

COMMON COMPLICATIONS

Acromegaly and its associated complications produce a variety of morbid deformities and show multiple x-ray abnormalities. Some abnormalities of the sella turcica are found in at least 90 per cent of patients. Prognathism due to widening of the angle of the jaw, enlargement of sinuses, and prominent external occipital protuberance are other x-ray abnormalities of the skull that are frequently found. An increase in the soft tissues of the extremities is best quantitated by measurement of heel pad thickness, defined as the shortest distance between the calcaneus and the plantar surface of the skin. Standardization of the measurement and support of the foot are technical requirements for valid measurements. Normal heel pad thickness averages 17.8 mm (range, 13 to 21 mm); Acromegalic patients show an average of 25.6 mm (range, 17 to 30 mm). Although obesity and other local factors may influence heel pad thickness in otherwise normal subjects, values above 18 mm in females and 21 mm in males are highly indicative of acromegaly. This measurement has been found to be superior to measurement of skin fold thickness and other parameters of soft tissue change in acromegaly.

Other x-ray findings, including tufting of the phalanges, increase in the sesamoid index (the product of the smallest and largest perpendicular diameters of the sesamoid metatarsal bone), and calcification of the anterior margins of the spinal vertebrae, are indicative of the existence of acromegaly. Widening of the joint spaces and protrusion of the chest are less specific radiographic findings. Thickening of the cranial bones as well as cortical thickening of the appendicular bones are typical of acromegaly.

Osteoarthritis, especially involving the hips and knees, is the cause of considerable disability in acromegaly, since degenerative arthritic changes develop at a young age and are often more advanced in these patients.

A common finding is proximal muscle weakness, which typically presents as difficulty in arising from a chair. It is now clear from a variety of reports that proximal muscle weakness of myopathic or neuropathic origin is common in acromegaly and exists in probably 50 per cent of patients. These findings suggest that a patchy myopathic process is present in the proximal muscles of acromegalic individuals, even in patients without clinical symptoms or demonstrable muscle weakness.

A number of symptoms result from involvement of sellar or parasellar structures. Headache is one of the more frequent complaints in acromegaly, affecting 75 to 87 per cent of patients. Often violent, it does not respond well to commonly used analgesic drugs. Headache may result from increased traction on dural structures, expansion of intrasellar mass, or bony overgrowth and traction on periosteal nerve endings. The typical headache varies location but often is bitemporal, occasionally vertical, but may be frontal or occipital or both. The patients with headache often have photophobia, but photophobia is also common (40 to 50 per cent) in the absence of headache. The cause of photophobia is unknown.

Peripheral neuropathies are also observed in acromegaly, the most common of which are acroparesthesias along the median nerve distribution or carpal tunnel syndrome. Improvement in the acroparesthesias occurs dramatically with treatment of acromegaly. In my experience, improvement often occurs before the GH level returns completely to normal. Other, less common peripheral nerve lesions include a proximal neuropathy or hypertrophic neuropathy that occurs exclusively in acromegaly.

The early diagnosis of a pituitary tumor reduces the frequency of visual field and extraocular motor abnormalities. Visual complaints, a late manifestation of pituitary tumors, are noted significantly less frequently now than in earlier series. The proximity of the optic chiasm to the pituitary makes it susceptible to compression from lesions originating within the sella turcica and extending superiorly to encroach on the chiasm as well as on the optic nerves and tracts. Depending on the location of the optic chiasm, great variability can be observed in visual field defects in patients suffering from chiasmal syndromes. Suprasellar tumor extension will usually produce bitemporal hemianopia, but variable field cuts, including complete blindness, can occur. Conformational field defects reflect advanced changes; tangent screen examination using a small (1 mm) white or red object will pick up more subtle change. Lateral tumor extension into the cavernous sinus will cause diplopia owing to damage to the cranial nerves, particularly the extraocular motor nerves.

Although voice change and visible laryngeal enlargement are common, acromegaly of the larynx, a severe complication, is rare. The possibility of laryngeal stricture and upper airway pathology should be borne in mind when anesthetizing acromegalic patients undergoing surgery. Thyromegaly or substernal goiter will rarely cause obstruction in these patients.

In addition to high prevalence of coronary artery disease and hypertensive heart disease in acromegaly, a few patients have a specific, potentially reversible cardiomyopathy, probably related to prolonged acromegaly or to very high GH concentrations. The reversibility of this process, observed in the ultrastructure of skeletal muscle, would suggest that lowering of GH may have reversible effects on cardiac muscle. The exact cause of hypertension in acromegaly is unknown. Typically, acromegaly is associated with low-renin hypertension. The increased plasma and blood volume are contributing factors to the hypertension in acromegaly and may explain the renin-angiotensin abnormalities of this condition. Acromegaly associated with hyperaldosteronism secondary to an adrenal adenoma has been reported, but in my experience this is a rare cause of hypertension.

Overt diabetes is seen in 15 per cent of patients; glucose intolerance during a standard oral glucose tolerance test is seen in approximately 50 per cent. Fasting GH levels do not correlate well with the diabetic state, nor do aging, obesity, family history of diabetes, age at onset of acromegaly, or duration of clinically active disease. I have observed microangiopathic diabetic complications in only two of my acromegalic patients, both of whom developed mild, nonproliferative retinopathy. Microangiopathy is infrequent, but the significance is difficult to interpret, since there may be a difference between the diabetic state in acromegaly and genetic diabetes mellitus.

A variety of dermatologic manifestations accompany acromegaly. The skin tends to be coarse and leathery, with exaggeration of the skin pores and markings. Local hypertrophy of the subcutaneous fibrous tissue gives rise to multiple warts (fibroma molluscum) that occur in about 25 per cent of patients. Hypertrichosis is also present in some female subjects. Perspiration may be related to hypertrophy of the sweat glands, and hyperhydrosis clears dramatically with treatment.

PHYSICAL EXAMINATION

Acral changes tend to be more pronounced in male than in female patients. Typically, in my experience, patients will not be diagnosed until symptoms have been present for at least 10 years. The most helpful examination is to review serial photographs, noting particularly changes in facial features. Such a chronologic review (Fig. 1) will be sufficient to confirm the extent and rapidity of acral change in a given patient. The patient in Figure 1 thought that her marriage and the raising of her family caused these changes in her appearance; however, further studies confirmed that this was active acromegaly and not "the hard life of a married woman."

On physical examination, coarsened features, thick hyperhidrotic skin, and furrowed brow should suggest a diagnosis of acromegaly. The puffy, doughy hands, tufted fingers, bulbous toes, and thickened soles and heel pads are also important features. Chest deformity with a dorsal kyphosis and increased anteroposterior diameter is seen in all advanced cases. The fibromas are typically seen in intertriginous areas or on the neck, where friction from garments occurs. Palpable organomegaly is surprisingly infrequent in these patients.

METABOLIC ABNORMALITIES

Hyperphosphatemia, with a serum phosphorus level greater than 4.5 mg/dl on most chemistry panels, is a frequent finding in my series as well as in others. Prior to the availability of radioimmunoassay (RIA) measurements for GH, hyperphosphatemia was used as an indicator of activity for acromegaly, although it was present in only half of the patients. An increase in tubular reabsorption is probably responsible for decreased excretion and increased plasma phosphorus levels in acromegaly. Glomerular filtration rate (endogenous creatinine clearance) is elevated in many patients. Altered phosphorus metabolism in acromegaly can be accentuated by performing an insulin tolerance test, in which there is smaller decrease than normally in plasma phosphorus despite production of marked hypoglycemia. The normal diurnal rhythm in plasma phosphorus levels (higher levels at 9 A.M. than at 4 P.M.) is reversed in acromegaly. For reasons that are not entirely clear, elevation of phosphorus level is more common in America than in Great Britain.

Hypercalciuria and increased hydroxyproline excretion result from the direct effects of GH on kidneys, bone, and cartilage. Even in the absence of hyperparathyroidism, serum calcium levels in acromegaly are characteristically in the upper normal range. After successful treatment, the levels of calcium decline but remain in the normal range.

It is well established that patients with acromegaly have a high frequency of altered carbohydrate metabolism, characterized by impaired glucose tolerance, hyperinsulinism, insulin resistance, and clinical diabetes. Hyperglucagonemia has also been described. Since high plasma glucose and plasma insulin levels are known to be associated with elevated serum triglyceride concentrations, and since GH has a marked lipolytic activity and increases plasma free fatty acid turnover, it is reasonable to suspect that hypertriglyceridemia might be common and related to the high incidence of cardiovascular disease observed in these patients. Data relating to this matter are conflicting; only occasional cases of gross hyperlipidemia and cutaneous xanthomatosis have been reported. Other authors do not see abnormal lipid patterns in acromegaly and in my early studies of low-density lipoprotein (LDL) and high-density lipoprotein (HDL) levels in fasting blood samples, no characteristic pattern was seen. The mean serum cholesterol level in acromegalic patients tends to be lower, and the mean serum triglyceride levels tend to be higher, than the levels in an age-matched normal population. Overall, the incidence of hypercholesterolemia is similar to that of the general population, whereas the incidence of hypertriglyceridemia was almost three times higher. Serum triglyceride concentrations do not correlate with relative body weight, serum GH level, insulin levels, glucose tolerance, or insulin response to oral glucose. However, as a group, patients with the highest plasma insulin response to oral glucose tend to have higher triglyceride levels. Lowering of triglyceride levels was achieved with successful lowering of GH levels. These observations are valid only when diabetes and secondary tropic hormone deficiencies are excluded. Further studies of lipid metabolism are clearly indicated in acromegaly.

Increased plasma and red blood cell volumes may contribute to several abnormalities observed in acromegaly. Several investigators suggest that acute hypervolemia may be responsible for increases in urinary calcium level, cardiac output, and renal plasma flow, and that hypervolemia may also antagonize the stimulation by GH of renal sodium and phosphate reabsorption. However, the lack of inhibition of the renin-angiotensin-aldosterone system in normotensive acromegalics and the urinary sodium decrease in response to sodium restriction are in favor of an adaptation to the chronic increase of vascular volume.

The finding of elevated serum creatine kinase in some patients supports the electromyographic evidence of myopathy and points to an abnormal permeability of necrotic muscle fibers, which are seen in biopsy specimens. Electromyography may show significant reduction in the duration of the motor neuron action potential, indicating the fallout of muscle fibers from motor units or failure of certain fibers to contribute to the electrical activity of the motor unit to which they belong. If we conclude that a direct toxic effect of GH on skeletal muscles occurs in acromegaly, it is likely that toxic effects will be seen in cardiac muscles as well, which seems, to be an apt explanation for the cardiomyopathy of acromegaly.

HORMONE SECRETION IN ACROMEGALY

Since the isolation of GH and the subsequent demonstration of its biologic activity in humans, extensive work has been carried out in the characterization of this hormone as well as in its normal physiology. It is now generally agreed that GH appears to exist in multiple forms, both in the pituitary and in the blood stream, in which it is present in a free or unbound form. Although GH is about 100 times more abundant than PRL in the pituitary, it tends to have lower concentration than PRL in the peripheral blood. The half-life of GH is about 20 minutes; the hormone is subsequently degraded in the liver and kidneys. Growth hormone has no specific target organ; it acts on many tissues. Although in vitro studies show direct action of GH on skeletal muscle, adipose tissue, liver, aortic media, and bone marrow, promotion of skeletal growth appears to be mediated indirectly by somatomedins (originally called sulfation factor), which are small peptides (molecular weight, ~6000) produced in the liver and which circulate bound to a specific carrier protein. Somatomedin C, which is chemically and immunologically identical to insulin-like growth fac-

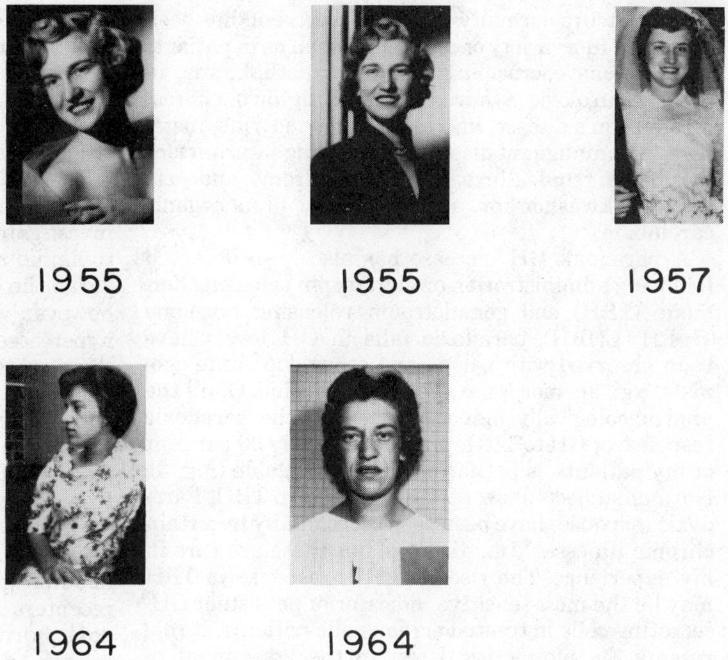

Figure 1. Development of progressive acral changes in a young woman with active acromegaly. Prominent early symptoms included headache, menstrual irregularity, hyperhydrosis, and enlarged feet and fingers requiring enlargement of wedding rings and change in shoe size from 6D to 8EEE.

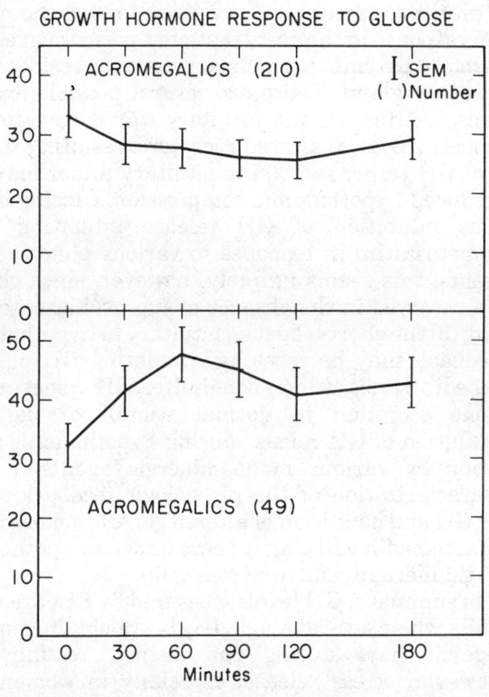

Figure 2. Serum growth hormone (GH) responses in patients with active acromegaly during a standard glucose tolerance test. Lack of GH suppression below 5 ng/ml is typical of acromegaly. Some patients will have a paradoxical rise in growth hormone.

tor (IGF-2), is the most important serum growth factor to measure in acromegaly.

Early studies of GH using RIA suggested that GH secretion in acromegaly may be autonomous and unresponsive to the usual physiologic and pharmacologic stimuli. If this were the case, single measurements of GH could easily distinguish pathologic hypersomatotropinism from altered physiologic states; in clinical practice this does not hold true.

DIAGNOSTIC TESTS

In normal subjects, GH level rises and falls throughout the day, which is in part related to food intake as well as exercise. The levels are higher in female than in male individuals, and the levels in females frequently overlap those observed in acromegaly. The greatest physiologic rise occurs at the onset of sleep. Hourly serum GH sampling shows that GH levels may vary markedly during a 24-hour period in acromegalic patients and may fluctuate as much as 20-fold; levels ranging from 6 to 531 ng/ml have been observed in a single acromegalic patient throughout a day. In acromegalic patients, GH peaks may occur during exercise as well as postprandially, but the characteristic GH peak following the onset of sleep is not observed. Numerous studies have shown that the total concentration of GH is altered in these states and that abnormalities in normal physiologic and pharmacologic GH secretion are present.

Because of the lability of GH in normal subjects as well as in acromegalic patients, administration of various pharmacologic agents is required for adequate assessment of GH hypersecretion. The most practical, definitive, and confirmatory test for acromegaly is measurement of plasma GH after glucose administration using a standard 3-hour 75 to 100 gm glucose load. Typically the elevated fasting GH level will not be suppressed below 5 ng/ml at any time during the test (Fig. 2). In 20 per cent of acromegalic patients, a paradoxic rise will occur beginning at 30 min after administration of glucose. Glucose intolerance and, when indicated, insulin secretion can be measured simultaneously during this procedure. The paradoxic response of GH to glucose is not unique to acromegaly, since it occurs normally in the newborn and has been described in a variety of conditions, such as in patients with lesions encroaching on the hypothalamus; in other neurologic syndromes, Huntington's chorea, and Wilson's disease; and in certain endocrine, metabolic, and malignant disorders, including intermittent porphyria, renal failure, Turner's syndrome, anorexia nervosa, kwashiorkor, and breast and bronchogenic carcinoma.

A paradoxic GH increase has also been observed following administration of thyrotropin releasing hormone (TRH) and gonadotropin releasing hormone (GnRH, LHRH); paradoxic falls in GH levels have been observed with L-dopa and other dopamine agonists, e.g., apomorphine and bromocriptine. Of all the pharmacologically induced responses, the paradoxic response of GH to TRH, present in nearly 90 per cent of my patients, is perhaps the most valuable (Fig. 3). Normal subjects show no GH response to TRH. Paradoxic responses have been seen occasionally in certain chronic illnesses, e.g., diabetes, but these are rare in my experience. The rise of GH in response to TRH may be the most sensitive indicator of persistent GH-secreting cells in treated acromegalic patients; it represents the most critical test in the assessment of treatment, with normalization or lessening of the GH response being associated with a favorable response to treatment. The mechanism of the paradoxic response is uncertain but probably represents altered membrane receptors on the tumor cells.

Insulin-induced hypoglycemia, a physiologic stimulus, is the basis for an important pharmacologic stimulus for GH, PRL, and ACTH secretion. Hypoglycemia produced no change in GH secretion in 40 per cent and produced a slight but variable increase in 60 per cent of my patients. The presence of insulin resistance (less than 50 per cent fall in glucose after intravenous injection of 0.1 unit of regular insulin per kilogram body weight) or lack of GH rise after adequate hypoglycemia is a sign of active acromegaly. Loss of insulin resistance and normalization of GH level occur with successful treatment. In general, the responses to stimuli are reproducible in a given patient.

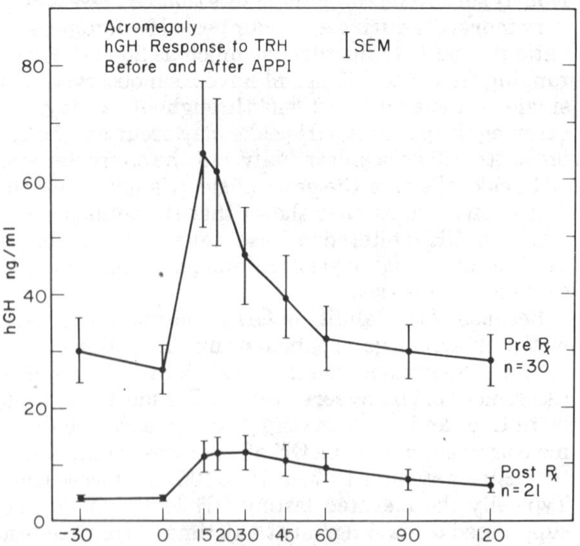

Figure 3. Paradoxical growth hormone (GH) response to thyrotropin-releasing hormone (TRH). Normal subjects do not show this rise in GH during provocative testing with TRH. This is the most consistent paradoxical rise in my series of patients. APPI = Alpha particle pituitary radiation.

The ultimate functional relationship between the hypothalamus and the pituitary has prompted many investigators to hypothesize that a defect in hypothalamic regulation of GH releasing factor may underlie the development of acromegaly. The difficulty, however, with a proposed hypothalamic cause for GH hypersecretion in either acromegaly or gigantism is the need to explain the origin of the pituitary adenomas that are characteristically found in these disorders. Such adenomas may be present in a microadenomatous stage, with small foci of somatotropes responding preferentially to excessive somatotropin releasing factor with hyperplasia and, eventually, adenoma formation. Similar changes have been observed in other endocrine organs, such as nodular goiter of the thyroid. Altered membrane receptors in the tumor cells may explain the paradoxic hormone responses as well as contribute to the growth or proliferation of tumor cells.

The loss of paradoxic response following treatment of pituitary tumors and reversion toward the normal GH response in the post-treatment period suggest that in many patients the primary disorder resides in the pituitary gland. There are several possible explanations for this: (1) the pituitary tumor somatotropes probably possess altered receptors, resulting in aberrant GH responses; (2) the pituitary tumor may have produced hypothalamic compression, causing continuous inhibition of GH release inhibiting factor (somatostatin) in response to various pharmacologic agents; this seems unlikely, however, since changes are observed in the absence of suprasellar extension; and, (3) the short-loop (i.e., pituitary to hypothalamus) feedback may be reset by circulating GH or somatomedin levels, which could alter GH releasing hormone secretion to normal stimuli or paradoxic inhibition of GH release during hypothalamic stimulation by various monoaminergic agents. Further characterization of the physiologic feedback system for GH and definition of altered generation or effect of somatomedin will clarify these important pathophysiologic mechanisms in acromegaly.

In summary, GH levels measured by RIA are worthwhile when several single levels are obtained on subsequent days during the fasting, resting state. However, stress release, especially in women, may produce levels that overlap with levels seen in acromegalic patients. Lack of suppression to hyperglycemia during a standard glucose tolerance test, a paradoxic response to TRH (a paradoxic response to GnRH occurs less predictably), and an anomalous GH response to dopaminergic drugs are the most reliable tests for evaluating hypersomatotropism in acromegaly. The somatomedin C assay by RIA appears to eliminate some of the problems of overlap that have been seen between active and inactive acromegalic patients. The measurement of somatomedin level may be of benefit because it is less influenced by GH fluctuations throughout the day and may be a better indicator of growth activity than is GH level measured by RIA. However, the fact that somatomedin levels have been found to be present in the absence of demonstrable GH and the fact that limited in vivo data indicate that somatomedins stimulate linear growth should add a note of caution to the exclusive use of this measurement in the diagnosis and evaluation of treatment of acromegaly. Somatomedins are age-dependent, with higher levels observed in younger children.

Somatostatin measurements are of no value in clinical management of acromegaly. The wide distribution of somatostatin throughout the brain and spinal cord suggests a more important role as a functional neurotransmitter and neuromodulator rather than as a neurohormonal inhibitor of GH secretion.

The first direct measurement of beta-endorphin in extracted serum in my laboratory has demonstrated that beta-lipotropin and beta-endorphin levels are elevated in the serum and cerebrospinal fluid of many acromegalic patients. Other studies have shown that opiate blockade with naloxone causes a rise in GH level in normal subjects. The role of opiomelanocorticotropin peptides in acromegaly is currently unknown.

RADIOLOGIC DIAGNOSIS

Although some abnormality of the sella turcica is present in more than 90 per cent of patients with pituitary adenomas, subtle changes may not be apparent on plain skull films and may be detected only when tomography is employed. This is especially true in the case of pituitary microadenomas measuring less than 10 mm, in which the sellar volume is normal. It is therefore extremely important to perform thin-section central axial tomography in the majority of patients. New generation computed tomographic (CT) scans will also detect the degree of suprasellar as well as inferior and lateral extension and thus characterize the invasiveness of the tumor. In addition, the presence of an empty sella can be recognized. This information is important in classifying the tumors; the presence or absence of invasiveness determines the prognosis and therapeutic response in most patients. Carotid angiography is less helpful in evaluating suprasellar extension or presence of microadenoma, but other observers have detected tumor blush and small vascular changes. Lateral tumor extension can be detected by carotid arteriography; however, extensive tumor invasion is usually necessary before carotid displacement is observed. Digital subtraction angiography has largely replaced carotid angiography. Cavernous sinus venography better delineates lateral tumor invasion. CT scans, with newer scanners capable of producing thin-section coronal projections, show lateral extensions and can provide the most information, so that other studies may not be required. Complex motion tomography is seldom necessary. Small suprasellar extensions may not be detected on CT scans and are best assessed with metrizamide. Pneumoencephalography with polytomography is rarely employed. Third- and fourth-generation CT scans and digital subtraction angiography have replaced the more invasive procedure.

PITFALLS IN DIAGNOSIS

The ectopic production of GH from nonpituitary tumors has been described, as has acromegaly attributable to the presence of excess ectopic release of a GH releasing factor from lung or pancreatic tumors. After evading isolation for many years, GH releasing hormone has recently been isolated and purified from a malignant pancreatic tumor excised from a patient with acromegaly. A GH releasing factor containing 44 amino acids was found to have full biologic activity (selective stimulation of GH release) in vivo and in vitro and is identical in biologic activity and similar in physiochemical properties to still uncharacterized GH releasing factor in mammalian hypothalamic extracts. Thus, in the patient with a normal sella and GH excess, an ectopic tumor source should be considered as a cause for acromegaly.

HYPERPROLACTINEMIA

By Elizabeth A. Cowden, M.D.
and Henry G. Friesen, M.D.
Winnipeg, Manitoba, Canada

DEFINITION

Hyperprolactinemia is the biochemical finding of circulating prolactin concentrations that are above a defined normal range. This entity has become increasingly recognized with widespread availability of sensitive and specific homologous human prolactin (hPRL) radioimmunoassays, which were first described in the early 1970s.

Although there are characteristic clinical features that may be attributed to hyperprolactinemia, and these will be discussed, clearly many of the findings on physical examination and in history taking in the patient with hyperprolactinemia reflect the underlying cause of the biochemical abnormality. So too will the natural history and complications of the condition reflect the underlying cause and not hyperprolactinemia per se.

ETIOLOGY

Hyperprolactinemia may occur both physiologically and pathologically (Table 1). Greater appreciation of the control mechanisms involved in prolactin secretion has demonstrated that many examples of hyperprolactinemia result from alterations in these normal control pathways. For example, hyperprolactinemia may result from (1) disruption of the normal dopaminergic inhibitory control on PRL secretion (by prolactin inhibiting factor or PIF) (head injury); (2) activation of intrinsic or extrinsic prolactin releasing factors (PRF) (hypothyroidism); and (3) inactivation of the usual inhibitory feedback control that PRL exerts over its own secretion (prolactinoma).

Table 1. Classification of Hyperprolactinemia

Physiologic
- Newborn
- Pregnant women
- Nursing mothers
- Stress-induced
- Diurnal variations

Pharmacologic
- Dopamine receptor blockers (e.g., phenothiazines, metoclopramide)
- Dopamine depleting agents (e.g., alpha-methyldopa, reserpine)
- Other agents (e.g., estrogens, thyrotropin-releasing hormone)

Pathologic
- Hypothalamic disorders
- Pituitary disorders
- Hypothalamic-pituitary disease
- Stalk irritation (e.g., head injury)
- Primary hypothyroidism
- Renal disease
- Ectopic production of prolactin
- Idiopathic

However, even in healthy individuals several factors may affect prolactin status, and appropriate interpretation of a given result demands adequate locally obtained data in relation to factors such as sex, reproductive status, age, circadian rhythm, pulsatility of secretion, and drug ingestion. It is particularly important that each center be able to provide its own control data since, although there is a recently available international reference preparation for hPRL, as yet there has been no standardization of either reagents or methods for hPRL radioimmunoassays. Hence, results from different laboratories may not be comparable.

In general, mean basal prolactin levels are higher in women than in men, though there is a considerable overlap in their ranges. The relationship between prolactin and estrogen levels in pregnancy is well known, and the stimulant effect of estrogens on prolactin secretion has also been demonstrated experimentally. However, it is of interest that in postmenopausal women there is a small but significant fall in prolactin levels, which may well be estrogen-related, since no similar fall is seen in aging men. The importance of age as a factor that may affect basal prolactin status is emphasized by the well-recognized finding of hyperprolactinemia in neonates, which is as yet unexplained. Its presence, however, may be a possible cause of the "witch's milk" sometimes seen in the newborn.

A diurnal variation in prolactin secretion occurs with maximum levels of prolactin in the blood reached during sleep, in the early hours of the morning. However, prolactin levels may still be significantly elevated between 6:00 and 8:00 A.M.—a common time for blood sampling in hospitalized patients. There also exists a diurnal variation in prolactin secretion during waking hours, with higher prolactin levels in the early morning and a trend toward higher levels again in the evening. The ideal sampling time therefore would be 9:00 A.M. to noon, when prolactin levels are at their nadir.

In both male and female individuals there is a modest individual variation in prolactin secretion from day to day in the same subject. The effect is more marked in women, but it occurs in both sexes and, because of this, sampling on several different days may be of more value in the confirmation of significant hyperprolactinemia than the usually advocated repeated sampling over a short period via an indwelling intravenous cannula.

Again, from the practical viewpoint, it is important to recognize that hPRL is a "stress hormone," not just in circumstances such as major surgery or insulin-induced hypoglycemia but in the more common circumstances of psychic stress, such as hospital attendance or pelvic examination in a woman. Some have even suggested that venipuncture per se is sufficient stress to cause hyperprolactinemia, although this has been difficult to substantiate. Nevertheless, it is clearly necessary to demonstrate persistently elevated prolactin levels before attributing any clinical abnormality to hyperprolactinemia.

Drug-induced hyperprolactinemia may be viewed as physiologic and is perhaps one of the most common causes of elevated prolactin levels seen in clinical practice. A selection of the most frequent offending agents is given in Table 2. With long-term therapy, the degree of hyperprolactinemia induced is often modest (many patients will have levels less than twice the upper limit of normal), and none of the characteristic clinical signs or symptoms of hyperprolactinemia may be present.

When secondary causes of hyperprolactinemia have been excluded, the presence of a prolactin-secreting tumor of the pituitary, a "prolactinoma," should be suspected, since these are now recognized as the most common of all pituitary tumors. Prolactinomas may vary in size from less than 10 mm (microadenoma) to very large indeed (macroadenoma), with para- and suprasellar extension of the tumor mass. In general, if the basal prolactin level is very high (greater than 100 ng/ml), the likelihood of pituitary tumor is similarly high, but the overall correlation between tumor size and basal prolactin level is poor, hence, basal prolactin level alone is not an adequate diagnostic test.

CLINICAL PRESENTATION

Appreciation of pathologic prolactin secretion has advanced considerably since the early recognition that not all patients who have elevated prolactin levels have galactorrhea and, conversely, that patients with profuse galactorrhea may have normal prolactin concentrations.

Irrespective of its underlying cause, hyperprolactinemia in women has been associated with the char-

Table 2. Drugs That May Cause Hyperprolactinemia

Estrogen-containing oral contraceptives	Imipramine
Chlorpromazine	Amitriptyline
Fluphenazine	Haloperidol
Metoclopramide	Methyldopa
	Reserpine

acteristic triad of amenorrhea, infertility, and, in about 30 per cent of patients, galactorrhea. Thus, hyperprolactinemia is particularly common in infertile patients. However, it is also important to remember that hyperprolactinemia, although classically associated with amenorrhea, may also result in oligomenorrhea and even rarely in perfectly regular but anovulatory cycles. Hence, it is not wise to assume that a patient who is having regular menstrual bleeding is necessarily ovulating and therefore cannot have excessive prolactin secretion.

Women who are hyperprolactinemic are usually estrogen-deficient, both because of impaired cyclic release of GnRH from the hypothalamus and because of impaired gonadotropin function at the gonadal level. This lack of estrogen output may itself give rise to symptoms of dyspareunia, lack of libido, and flushing attacks in the patient whose underlying problem is hyperprolactinemia.

Men are not exempt from hyperprolactinemia, owing to such factors as drug therapy, hypothyroidism, and prolactinoma, and the usual symptoms are loss of potency and lack of libido. Both of these symptoms usually result from very low testosterone levels induced by elevated circulating prolactin levels. Prolactin-secreting pituitary tumors in men are unfortunately rarely diagnosed when they are small; for this reason, visual field defects as a result of suprasellar pituitary tumor and persistent headache are common presenting complaints in men. The reason for the distressingly late diagnosis in male patients is perhaps partly due to reticence on the part of the patient concerning complaints of sexual dysfunction and partly to a cavalier attitude of the physician's that impotence is always psychogenic and does not require endocrine assessment.

STRATEGY FOR THE ASSESSMENT OF PROLACTIN STATUS

Following is a suggested strategy that may be adopted for the assessment of prolactin status in individuals with clinical presentations suggestive of hyperprolactinemia.

1. Draw blood sample, under resting basal conditions, ideally between 9 A.M. and noon, although sampling between 9 A.M. and 5 P.M. is acceptable.
2. If an elevated prolactin level is demonstrated, compared with appropriate age- and sex-related control subjects, exclude the following:
   a. Drug therapy (including oral contraceptives).
   b. Pregnancy.
   c. Primary hypothyroidism.
   d. Chronic renal failure.
   e. Hypothalamic-pituitary disease.

   Relate level to appropriate reference ranges in groups *a* to *d*.
3. Repeat sample:
   a. If both levels are greater than 25 ng/ml, this is unlikely to be due to stress.
   b. If both levels are greater than 50 ng/ml, this is likely to be due to a pituitary tumor.
4. For confirmation of a suspected prolactin secreting tumor, further investigation may involve
   a. *Radiologic assessment*

   Until recently, the diagnosis of pituitary tumors had relied on radiologic studies that even experienced neuroradiologists find notoriously difficult to interpret because the anatomy of the fossa varies and the characteristic radiologic changes associated with microadenomas are subtle. Suffice it to say that pituitary fossa tomography, even in the best centers, has significant false-negative and false-positive rates in the detection of pituitary microadenomas; hence, it is not the ideal tool for the diagnosis of small prolactinomas.

   Perhaps the most reliable radiologic tool that is currently available is contrast-enhanced computed tomography (CT) of the pituitary fossa with the most up-to-date (sixth generation) equipment. There is no doubt that this technique offers the best opportunity of visualizing even 2- and 3-mm lesions, but the rate of false-positive and false-negative examinations remains to be determined.

   b. *Dynamic tests of prolactin secretion*

   Although it has been demonstrated that suppression tests using agents such as L-dopa, bromocriptine, and nomifensine may be of little value in differentiating hyperprolactinemia of various types, tests of prolactin reserve by stimulation (TRH, metoclopramide) may be of greater value in identifying patients in whom hyperprolactinemia is attributable to prolactinoma. Characteristically, in patients who are pregnant, hypothyroid, or on drug therapy, prolactin response to pharmacologic stimulation occurs, despite an elevated basal level, whereas in patients who harbor prolactinomas the response is abolished. The false-positive rate for TRH and metoclopramide stimulation is low, but the false-negative rate is as yet undocumented. An additional characteristic of prolactinomas is loss of the normal nocturnal peak in prolactin secretion, akin to the loss of the diurnal rhythms of cortisol and growth hormone in Cushing's syndrome and acromegaly, respectively. Any of these dynamic tests would be of particular value in the investigation of patients with normal radiological studies and modestly elevated basal prolactin levels.

RECENT ADVANCES

Until recently, only estimates of prolactin *concentration* in human serum have been possible by means of sensitive radioimmunoassays. It has not been feasible to study *biologic activity,* since available bioassays for serum prolactin were not sufficiently sensitive to detect normal circulating levels of the hormone. Radioimmunoassays alone of course usually serve well, but unusual cases are encountered from time to time in which it would be of considerable interest to compare the ratio of biologic to immunologic activity—e.g., in hyperprolactinemia with no obvious reproductive dysfunction, and in normoprolactinemic galactorrhea.

With the use of the recently described Nb2 lymphoma cell bioassay for lactogenic hormones, it is now possible to assess prolactin bioactivity in human serum. This assay involves specific stimulation of growth of a rat lymphoma cell line in suspension culture by all lactogenic hormones, including human prolactin, and it represents a useful recent advance in the laboratory assessment of prolactin status.

HYPERTHYROIDISM

By Monte A. Greer, M.D.
and Michael R. McClung, M.D.
Portland, Oregon

DEFINITION

Hyperthyroidism is a disorder in which there is an excessive amount of thyroid hormone in the body. Although the known metabolically active thyroid hormones, thyroxine (T_4) and tri-iodothyronine (T_3), may both be present in excess in individual patients, supranormal levels of only one or the other of these hormones may be present. The clinical signs and symptoms vary considerably among afflicted individuals and are related to the degree of elevation of plasma thyroid hormone concentrations, the tolerance of the patient to excessive thyroid hormone, the duration of the disease, and the age of the patient. In general, signs and symptoms decrease in intensity with increasing age.

ETIOLOGY

Various causes of hyperthyroidism are listed in Table 1. Graves' disease is a more common cause of thyrotoxicosis in the United States than all other possible causes combined. It can occur at any age, but a first attack is seen most frequently in young women less than 30 years old. Graves' disease is part of the spectrum of autoimmune thyroid disease. The pathogenesis of this disease is uncertain, but current consensus is that the hyperthyroidism is due to the presence of immunoglobulins that directly stimulate the growth and activity of the thyroid gland.

Toxic nodular goiter, with single or multiple nodules, is believed to arise from one or more clones of thyroid cells that are independent of control by thyrotropin. If the mass of autonomously functioning tissue becomes large enough (usually in excess of 2 cm in the case of single nodules), hyperthyroidism is produced.

Hyperthyroidism can also be caused by release of excessive amounts of thyroid hormone from low-grade chronic destruction of parenchymal tissue caused by lymphoid thyroiditis or, with a more massive acute release of thyroid hormone, by subacute granulomatous thyroiditis.

PRESENTING SIGNS AND SYMPTOMS

These vary considerably with individual patients, but the most common are listed in approximate order of frequency in Table 2. The most frequent complaints are nervousness, tremor, palpitation, weight loss, heat intolerance, and an unusually irritable disposition. Physical fatigue is also often noted, although the patients may have an increased desire to be actively involved in physical or mental activity. Angina pectoris, congestive heart failure, or atrial fibrillation may appear for the first time or be accentuated by the development of hyperthyroidism. Atrial fibrillation in particular is often the presenting sign that leads to the diagnosis of hyperthyroidism in elderly patients.

Gastrointestinal problems typically include weight loss despite an increase in appetite and food intake, increased stool frequency (often four or more per day) without diarrhea, and softer stools. In many older hyperthyroid patients, appetite may be decreased or constipation may be a complaint. In rare individuals, particularly teenaged girls, weight may increase because the appetite is stimulated to a greater extent than the metabolic wasting of calories.

The characteristic neuromuscular manifestation is a fine rapid hand tremor and general rapid darting movements. In some patients, muscle atrophy is present. Weakness of the legs may be noted, resulting in difficulty in climbing stairs or in arising from a sitting position. Motor coordination is sometimes impaired, and rarely choreoathetoid movements are seen. Both hypokalemic periodic paralysis (in patients of Asian extraction) and myasthenia gravis occur with increased frequency in patients with Graves' disease. The affect of the hyperthyroid patient is often abnormal. He or she may be anxious, irritable, and short-tempered or depressed. Elderly patients who demonstrate a flat affect and who lack the hyperkinetic features of younger thyrotoxic patients are said to have "apathetic hyperthyroidism." Neurotic behavior and even frank psychotic manifestations can occur and may dominate the clinical picture.

Ocular complaints are primarily limited to patients with Graves' disease and are related to the infiltra-

Table 1. Etiology of Hyperthyroidism

- I. *Endogenous*
  - A. Thyroid hormone overproduction
    - 1. Humoral thyroid stimulators
      - a. Thyroid stimulating immunoglobulins (Graves' disease)
      - b. Human chorionic gonadotropin (choriocarcinoma)
      - c. Thyroid-stimulating hormone (pituitary tumors)
    - 2. Toxic nodular goiter
      - a. Single nodule
      - b. Multinodular
  - B. Follicular disruption
    - 1. Thyroiditis (viral, autoimmune, radiation)
- II. *Exogenous*
  - A. Iatrogenic
  - B. Surreptitious

Table 2. Common Signs and Symptoms of Thyrotoxicosis

Nervousness	Forceful cardiac impulse
Tremor	Fatigue
Increased perspiration	Weakness
Heat intolerance	Increased appetite
Goiter	Weight loss
Eye signs	Increased stool frequency
Palpitation	Brisk reflexes
Tachycardia	

tive ophthalmopathy that occurs in approximately 30 to 50 per cent of patients with this condition. The suspicion that Graves' disease may exist is often first aroused when the patient's friends or relatives (less commonly the patient) note that the patient's eyes are much more prominent and "staring" than previously. Common symptomatic complaints are pain in the eyes, photophobia, lacrimation, and blurred or double vision.

PHYSICAL FINDINGS

A variety of physical findings may be detected in hyperthyroidism. Other than those specifically related to Graves' disease, they may not be specific. The signs that correlate most highly with thyrotoxicosis are weight loss, thyroid enlargement, hyperkinesis, fine tremor of the extended fingers, tachycardia, and atrial fibrillation.

The skin is typically smooth and velvety, and the palms are warm and moist. The cardiac impulse is forceful and rapid. The thyroid gland is almost always visually or palpably enlarged. In Graves' disease, the gland is not often tender, but it is usually diffusely enlarged with a consistency of soft rubber, although it may be very firm or woody. Although the thyroid in Graves' disease is usually symmetrically enlarged, one lobe may be larger than the other (both lobes being enlarged), or hypertrophy may be limited to a single lobe. The goiter in Graves' disease may also be irregular rather than smooth, or may even be nodular.

In large hyperplastic thyroids of Graves' disease, in which there is a marked increase in thyroid blood flow, a bruit and thrill may be detected. However, these findings are not specific for Graves' disease, but only for a marked increase in blood flow. The enlarged hyperplastic glands of patients with hypothyroidism caused by a biosynthetic defect in thyroid hormone formation may also have a thrill and bruit.

Thyroid glands with autonomously functioning nodules producing hyperthyroidism are usually firmer than those in Graves' disease, and one or more distinct nodules are usually palpable. There is no pathognomonic physical characteristic that distinguishes hyperfunctioning glands from nontoxic nodular goiters.

There is characteristically a rapid, bounding pulse due to an increase in systolic and decrease in diastolic blood pressure, with a resultant increase in pulse pressure. Atrial fibrillation is frequent in older patients. The precordium is often hyperdynamic, and cardiomegaly may be noted. However, congestive heart failure is uncommon except in elderly hyperthyroid patients with an underlying heart condition. A systolic murmur may be heard over the entire precordium. Rarely, a rough sound may be heard at the upper left border of the sternum (Means-Lerman scratch), which resembles a friction rub. Although the cardiac changes are not specific for thyrotoxicosis, this diagnosis should be entertained in any patient who develops artrial fibrillation or congestive cardiac failure without known pre-existing heart disease.

The eye findings in Graves' disease are usually divided into those due to thyrotoxicosis per se, resulting from increased responsiveness to catecholamines (noninfiltrative ophthalmopathy), and those that are specifically due to the underlying pathophysiology of Graves' disease (infiltrative ophthalmopathy). Signs of noninfiltrative ophthalmopathy include retraction of the upper eyelids, stare, decreased blinking, and lid lag. Infiltrative ophthalmopathy is due to lymphatic inflammation, mucopolysaccharide infiltration, and edema of the retrobulbar tissue and extraocular muscles. There is vascular hyperemia of the conjunctivae (conjunctival edema or chemosis), failure of the upper lid to completely cover the eyeball (lagophthalmos), photophobia, diplopia, inability to maintain conjoint movement of the eye muscles, and proptosis. The exophthalmos is usually bilateral, but it may be unilateral. Proptosis is usually measured from the edge of the lateral bony orbit to the farthest anterior protrusion of the cornea with the patient looking straight ahead. Quantification of proptosis can be done with a ruler, although simple specialized tools, such as a Luedde exophthalmometer, make this much easier.

LABORATORY FINDINGS

Since the clinical syndrome of hyperthyroidism results from excess concentrations of circulating and tissue thyroid hormones, it seems logical that the first line of confirmatory laboratory tests should be direct measurements of circulating thyroid hormones.

Serum Total Thyroxine (T_4)

Total serum level of T_4 is currently the most widely available thyroid function test. Results can be available in 24 hours. The normal range is 4 to 12 μg/dl. An elevated value is usually an indication of thyrotoxicosis, but because T_4 is largely (99.95 per cent) bound to thyroid hormone–binding globulin (TBG), such a value may be due to an increased concentration of binding protein. Elevations of TBG that result in a secondary elevation of total serum T_4 levels occur in pregnancy, in liver disease, as a result of estrogen therapy or chronic narcotic drug usage, and on a genetic basis. It is therefore essential in these circumstances to obtain a measure of thyroid hormone binding before making a diagnosis of hyperthyroidism on the basis of T_4 level alone.

A normal T_4 level does not exclude a diagnosis of thyrotoxicosis since approximately 5 per cent of hyperthyroid patients have preferential T_3 secretion (T_3-toxicosis). The converse situation of elevated T_4 levels with normal T_3 concentrations (T_4-toxicosis) has also been described, particularly in elderly patients with severe nonthyroid illnesses.

Thyroid-Binding Proteins and the Free T_4 Index (FTI)

The most commonly employed method for assessing thyroid hormone binding is the T_3 resin uptake test. This procedure determines the number of unoccupied thyroid hormone–binding sites in serum. Radioiodine-labeled T_3 is added to the patient's serum and incubated with a nonspecific receptor (resin), which competes for labeled T_3 with the unoccupied binding sites in the patient's serum. The T_3 resin uptake varies inversely with the number of unoccupied thyroid hormone binding sites in the patient's serum. Thus, when there are excess binding sites in the patient's serum owing to a high TBG level, the T_3 uptake will be low, whereas with a diminished number of binding sites because of either TBG deficiency or hyperthyroidism with consequent saturation of sites, the T_3 uptake will be high.

From separate measurements of serum T_4 and T_3 resin uptake (T_3RU), a free T_4 index (FTI) may be calculated by multiplication. Such an index is directly proportional to the free T_4 concentration in the serum and is a means of correcting total T_4 levels for changes in thyroid hormone binding.

Serum Free Thyroxine (FT_4)

A simple, direct assay for free thyroxine is now available and may ultimately replace the separate use of total T_4 and T_3RU. This test estimates the putative active portion of serum T_4 that is not bound to plasma proteins. The normal range for the serum FT_4 concentration is approximately 0.7 to 2 ng/dl. In most instances there is good linear correlation between the FT_4 and the FTI when plotted against each other in patients with thyroid-binding protein variations and in those who have thyroid dysfunction.

Serum Total Tri-iodothyronine (T_3)

Serum total T_3 concentration can also be measured by radioimmunoassay (RIA). In view of the disproportionate increase in T_3 secretion in most patients with thyrotoxicosis, little overlap has been observed in total T_3 levels between euthyroid and hyperthyroid patients. The T_3 values in euthyroid subjects fall typically in the 90 to 230 ng/dl range. Serum T_3 levels tend to decrease with age because of a reduced rate of extrathyroidal conversion of T_4 to T_3, and they are often reduced with severe nonthyroidal illness, malnutrition, or acute loss of body weight. To minimize the cost of laboratory evaluation, we prefer to confirm the presence of hyperthyroidism with the FT_4, reserving the use of T_3 RIA to those few patients who do not have elevated serum T_4 concentrations but in whom the clinical suspicion of hyperthyroidism persists. The incidence of T_3 toxicosis is about 5 per cent and is higher in areas where dietary iodine intake is suboptimal.

Serum Thyroid-Stimulating Hormone

Pituitary secretion of TSH will be almost completely suppressed if hyperthyroidism is caused by Graves' disease, toxic nodules, or any disorder other than inappropriate thyrotropin secretion, such as from a pituitary tumor. Thus, plasma TSH levels should be below normal limits in hyperthyroidism and provide a rapid and simple screening test. Unfortunately, until very recently commercial assays were insufficiently sensitive to distinguish between low but normal and subnormal plasma TSH levels. With the advent of highly sensitive assays, plasma TSH determinations may replace T_4 and T_3 as the primary screening test for thyrotoxicosis.

Thyrotropin-Releasing Hormone Stimulation Test

In 5 to 10 per cent of patients suspected of having hyperthyroidism, either the clinical findings or usual screening laboratory results are insufficiently clear to permit a definite diagnosis. In these patients, the thyrotropin-releasing hormone (TRH) stimulation test is often of diagnostic benefit.

This test employs TRH to stimulate the release of TSH from the pituitary gland. Serum TSH is determined before and 30 minutes after a bolus intravenous injection of 500 μg of TRH. In euthyroidism, the rise in serum TSH is generally greater than 4 microunits/ml and the 30-minute level is at least 100 per cent more than the baseline value. By contrast, in hyperthyroid patients there is no increase in serum TSH level. The TRH test is used primarily to exclude rather than positively diagnose hyperthyroidism. A normal increment in serum TSH and TRH administration is inconsistent with the hyperthyroid state. A blunted or flat response is consistent with, but not proof of, the diagnosis of hypothyroidism. A blunted response may also be observed in a small proportion of normal individuals and in some patients with ophthalmic Graves' disease or nodular goiter who do not appear to be hyperthyroid.

Thyroid Radioactive Iodine Uptake (RAIU) and Imaging Procedures

With the advent of reliable and specific assays of circulating thyroid hormones, the need for measuring the thyroidal radioactive iodine uptake (RAIU) in the investigation of hyperthyroidism has greatly diminished. However, the 24-hour RAIU test continues to be useful in two specific circumstances: (1) in determining the cause of the hyperthyroidism in order to institute appropriate therapy, and (2) in demonstrating satisfactory iodine uptake before administering a therapeutic dose of radioiodine.

It is useful to subdivide hyperthyroid patients into those with relatively high RAIU and those with very low RAIU. Causes of hyperthyroidism with a 24-hour RAIU greater than 12 to 15 per cent include Graves' disease, toxic multinodular goiter, toxic autonomously functioning thyroid adenoma, TSH-producing pituitary adenoma, and trophoblastic tumors. By contrast, a 24-hour RAIU of less than 3 per cent is characteristic of silent thyroiditis, the hyperthyroidism due to exogenous thyroid hormone or iodine, struma ovarii, and metastatic follicular thyroid carcinoma.

Thyroid scanning procedures with ^{123}I, technetium-99m, or ^{131}I are not tests of thyroid function but are used to evaluate the distribution of functioning tissue within the thyroid. These tests are not of value in determining whether a patient is hyperthyroid, although they may be useful in differentiating toxic nodular goiter from Graves' disease.

Serum Thyroglobulin (TG)

A small amount of thyroglobulin is normally secreted from the thyroid, chiefly via the rich lymphatic network surrounding each follicle, and can readily be detected with current RIA techniques. This test is particularly valuable in differentiating thyrotoxicosis factitia due to surreptitious ingestion of thyroid hormone by the patient from other forms of thyrotoxicosis in which there is a very low thyroid radioiodine uptake (silent thyroiditis, a very high body iodide pool from iodine-containing contrast media, metastatic thyroid carcinoma, and so forth). Oral ingestion of any form of thyroglobulin, such as desiccated thyroid, results in degradation of the TG in the gastrointestinal system. No significant blood concentration of TG is produced. T_4 and T_3 preparations do not have thyroglobulin contamination. Thus, a thyrotoxic patient with a very low or undetectable thyroid radioiodine uptake and serum thyroglobulin and high plasma thyroid hormone concentrations almost surely has thyrotoxicosis factitia. One caveat is that TG cannot be accurately measured in the presence of high titers of anti-thyroglobulin antibodies.

Plasma Iodide

This test is useful in distinguishing between various diagnostic alternatives in patients with thyrotoxicosis and a low thyroid radioiodine uptake. Normal values are below 1 μg/dl. Values greater than 5 μg/dl indicate iodine contamination of the body iodide pool, usually by the prior use of iodine-containing materials for x-ray contrast studies or from high iodide therapy in patients with chronic pulmonary problems.

FLOW PLAN FOR DIAGNOSTIC WORK-UP

The systematic plan which we find useful in the diagnosis of suspected hyperthyroidism is shown in Figure 1.

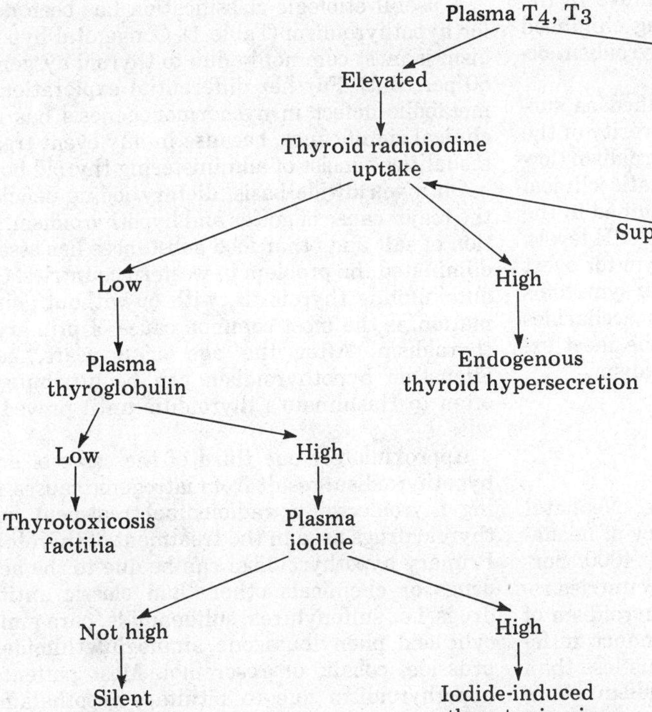

Figure 1. Evaluation of suspected hyperthyroidism.

HYPOTHYROIDISM

By Ludo De Keyser, M.D.
and Andre Van Herle, M.D.
Los Angeles, California

DEFINITIONS AND CLASSIFICATIONS

Hypothyroidism is a syndrome that results from a deficient production of thyroid hormones or, very rarely, from decreased action of these hormones. Since normal secretion of thyroid hormones depends upon the integrity of the hypothalamic-pituitary-thyroid axis, lesions at any level of this feedback system may result in hypothyroidism.

Primary hypothyroidism refers to a primary, intrinsic lesion of the thyroid gland and is characterized by decreased levels of thyroid hormones T_4 and T_3 in peripheral blood, compensatory elevated serum levels of thyroid-stimulating hormone (TSH), and an exaggerated TSH response to exogenous thyrotropin-releasing hormone (TRH). Secondary hypothyroidism results from a pituitary lesion leading to deficient TSH production and hence deprivation of the thyroid from its normal TSH stimulation. Tertiary hypothyroidism indicates deficient hypothalamic TRH production and subsequent low TSH and peripheral thyroid hormone levels. Most cases of hypothyroidism fall in the category of primary hypothyroidism, whereas fewer than 5 per cent of all cases are caused by pituitary-hypothalamic disease.

Hypothyroidism may be a congenital or an acquired disorder. The age of its onset results in distinct clinical pictures: cretinism indicating thyroid failure in the newborn, juvenile hypothyroidism during childhood or adolescence, and finally adult hypothyroidism occurring in adulthood.

Whether the hypothyroidism is classified as subclinical, mild, or overt depends on the severity of the signs and symptoms. Subclinical hypothyroidism (low thyroid reserve) refers to an asymptomatic clinical state in which T_4 and T_3 levels are maintained in the normal range at the expense of increased TSH levels. The term myxedema is a common synonym for overt hypothyroidism and refers to a complex of symptoms resulting from the deposition of mucopolysaccharides in various tissues. Myxedema coma is the most extreme clinical presentation of hypothyroidism.

EPIDEMIOLOGY

Hypothyroidism is not a rare disease. Neonatal screening programs indicate the frequency of neonatal hypothyroidism in live births to be 1:4000. Surveys of the adult population in western countries reveal an overall incidence of overt hypothyroidism of about 0.8 per cent with a clear predominance in female subjects (2 per cent in women versus less than 0.1 per cent in men). Although hypothyroidism occurs at any stage of life, its incidence increases with age: it is most prevalent in the age group of 30 to 60 years, and it is more commonly seen in postmenopausal women.

Table 1. Etiology of Hypothyroidism

I. Primary Hypothyroidism
  A. Congenital
    1. Thyroid dysgenesis
      a. Aplasia
      b. Hypoplasia
      c. Ectopia
    2. Dyshormonogenesis
    3. Maternal antithyroid medication
    4. Maternal iodine deficiency
  B. Acquired
    1. Endemic hypothyroidism
      a. Iodine deficiency
      b. Food goitrogens
    2. Autoimmune thyroiditis (Hashimoto's disease)
    3. Iatrogenic
      a. Antithyroid drugs and chemicals
      b. Radioiodine therapy
      c. Thyroidectomy
      d. External radiation
    4. Infiltrative disease of the thyroid, e.g., sarcoidosis, amyloidosis, cystinosis)
    5. Riedel's thyroiditis
    6. Subacute thyroiditis end stage (rare)
    7. Graves' disease end stage (rare)
    8. Primary or metastatic thyroid tumors (rare)
II. Secondary Hypothroidism: Pituitary disease
III. Tertiary Hypothyroidism: Hypothalamic disease
IV. Peripheral Hypothyroidism: Resistance to the action of thyroid hormones (rare)

ETIOLOGY

A useful etiologic classification has been designed for hypothyroidism (Table 1). Congenital hypothyroidism is most commonly due to thyroid dysgenesis ($\approx$ 80 per cent). Further differential exploration of the metabolic defect in dyshormonogenesis has no real clinical significance, because in any event treatment modalities consist of administering thyroid hormone.

On a worldwide basis, dietary iodine deficiency is the major cause of goiter and hypothyroidism. Iodination of salt and other food substances has essentially eliminated the problem in western countries. Chronic autoimmune thyroiditis, with or without goiter formation, is the most common cause of primary hypothyroidism. After the age of 8 years, acquired idiopathic hypothyroidism can be attributed most often to Hashimoto's thyroiditis until proved otherwise.

Approximately one third of the cases of acquired hypothyroidism result from iatrogenic causes, including thyroidectomy, radioiodine treatment, or antithyroid drugs used in the treatment of thyrotoxicosis. Primary hypothyroidism can be due to the action of drugs or chemicals other than classic antithyroid drugs, i.e., sulfonylurea, sulfonamide, para-aminosalicylic acid, phenylbutazone, aminoglutethimide, nitroprusside, cobalt, or resorcinol. Most patients with hypothyroidism due to pituitary-hypothalamic disease have other hormonal deficiencies, although monohormonal deficiency does exist. Recognition of associated adrenocorticotropic hormone (ACTH) deficiency is critical because thyroid replacement without preceding corticosteroid therapy can precipitate acute adrenal insufficiency.

SYMPTOMS

Since thyroid hormones impact on a number of physiologic and biochemical processes, almost every organ system is affected in hypothyroidism, resulting in widespread clinical manifestations. The symptoms can develop very insidiously, and quite often they go unnoticed by the patient or relatives. Both classic and atypical clinical presentations can occur, with a spectrum of severity ranging from an asymptomatic subclinical form to myxedema coma.

A goiter in the neck area is a common finding in hypothyroidism except when the disorder occurs following ablative therapy (radioactive iodine or surgery), or in atrophic thyroiditis, congenital athyreotic cretinism, lingual thyroid, and pituitary-hypothalamic hypothyroidism.

The degree and the duration of the thyroid hormone deficiency, as well as the age of onset, determine to a certain extent the resulting clinical picture.

Cretinism

Most hypothyroid infants are of normal length and weight at birth and have few, if any, signs of hypothyroidism (only 3 per cent of hypothyroid newborns detected by neonatal screening programs were clinically suspected of having the disease). Subtle manifestations of hypothyroidism develop during the first 3 to 6 weeks of life, while the more classic features of cretinism appear by 3 to 6 months. It is questionable whether or not breast-feeding may delay the onset of symptomatic hypothyroidism.

The irreversibility of the neurologic impairment of cretinism necessitates the earliest possible diagnosis (hence, the usefulness of the neonatal screening programs). When therapy is started before 2 months of age, normal mental and intellectual development may ensue.

Signs that should alert the physician include persistence of the physiologic icterus (longer than 3 days in term infants), respiratory distress in a full-term infant, somnolence, feeding problems, dry skin, a hoarse cry, constipation, and an umbilical hernia larger than 0.5 cm. Later on, the growth retardation and progressive, irreversible reduction in mental capacity become apparent. Other symptoms and signs of cretinism include lethargy, increased trunk-limb ratio, large head with large fontanelles, sparse hair, puffy face, flat nasal bridge, thick neck, protruding tongue, and dry, cold, mottled skin. Goiter (depending on the cause of the hypothyroidism), bradycardia, distended abdomen, umbilical hernia, hypotonia, muscular weakness, and hyporeflexia may also be present.

Juvenile Hypothyroidism

Beyond the second year of life hypothyroidism is not associated with irreversible mental retardation. Growth abnormalities are prominent, however, and the child may appear as a dwarf with an increased trunk-to-limb ratio. Bone age is retarded in relation to chronologic age. All of the symptoms of adult hypothyroidism may be present, but the full picture of adult myxedema is rarely seen.

Adult Hypothyroidism

In the typical case, the patient complains of decreased appetite, slight weight gain, fatigue and loss of energy, and decreased intellectual capacities. Other symptoms include hoarse voice, intolerance of cold, acroparesthesia, constipation, depression, headache, hearing loss, dyspnea, muscle aching and stiffness, decreased libido, impotence, and menstrual abnormalities (particularly menorrhagia).

Clinical findings may include dry, brittle hair with loss of hair on the scalp and the lateral aspects of the eyebrow; brittle nails; and pale, cold, dry, scaling skin with yellow appendages attributable to hypercarotenemia. Facial puffiness and periorbital edema are found, with nonpitting edema above the dorsum of the hands and feet and in the supraclavicular area. Also commonly present are hoarseness, goiter, bradycardia, faint cardiac sounds, cardiac enlargement, diastolic hypertension, and delayed relaxation of knee and ankle jerk reflexes. Other, less common clinical findings are effusions into pleural, pericardial, and peritoneal spaces; nerve entrapment syndrome similar to carpal tunnel syndrome; and vitiligo, the latter in association with autoimmune thyroiditis.

Severe hypothyroidism may progress to myxedema coma, which is usually precipitated by another stressful illness. It is manifested by a comatose state, hypothermia, hypotension, hypoglycemia, hyponatremia, and respiratory failure. Rapid and intensive therapy is mandatory in this potentially lethal condition.

COURSE AND PROGNOSIS

In most patients, hypothyroidism develops insidiously owing to slowly progressive thyroid failure. More rapid development of the hypothyroid state occurs after discontinuation of thyroid replacement therapy in hypothyroid patients who have undergone surgery or radioactive iodine treatment, or both.

The prognosis depends on the degree of thyroid hormone deficiency. Several recent reports indicate an increased incidence of coronary atherosclerosis in untreated subclinical hypothyroidism. Fatal outcome may occur in the untreated patient after several years and result from intercurrent infection, respiratory failure, or myxedema coma.

DIAGNOSIS

When the manifestations of hypothyroidism are blatant, the diagnosis is usually simple. Mild cases may be overlooked clinically quite easily, however. Since the symptoms of hypothyroidism usually develop insidiously, the diagnosis relies primarily on the suspicion of the clinician and confirmatory evidence by sensitive thyroid function testing. A clinical diagnosis of hypothyroidism should always be confirmed or documented by laboratory investigation, since in most cases lifelong therapy with thyroid hormones will be necessary. This holds particularly true for newborns, in whom only 3 per cent of cases detected by neonatal screening were clinically suspected, and any delay in diagnosis can result in irreversible neurologic damage.

Thyroid Testing

T_4 and T_3. Characteristically, hypothyroidism results in a decrease of total and free T_4 and T_3, reverse T_3 (rT_3), and T_3 resin uptake. Whereas a serum T_4 radioimmunoassay (RIA) of less than 2.5 μg/dl is a sensitive and specific index for hypothyroidism, T_3 RIA is frequently in the normal range in milder cases. Conversely, serum T_3 level may be low in euthyroid patients with systemic illness and does not reflect the hormonal balance of the patient. The important clinical corollary is that serum T_3 levels are unreliable in discriminating between the hypothyroid and the euthyroid states. The T_3 resin uptake test is not a sensitive test in hypothyroidism, but it is useful in calculating free T_4 and T_3 indices; the latter is required to detect low T_4 levels based on thyroid-binding globulin (TBG) deficiency.

TSH Level. The TSH level, on the other hand, is a highly sensitive index in the diagnosis of primary hypothyroidism. Basal TSH level is elevated as a consequence of negative feedback in primary hypothyroidism, although it is low in the rare cases of pituitary-hypothalamic hypothyroidism. TSH level is the earliest biochemical marker of impending thyroid failure. A rise in serum TSH level may be observed when hypothyroidism develops before the patient has any symptoms and before any other measurable disturbance in thyroid function has occurred. It is the test of choice to confirm or exclude primary hypothyroidism in the face of low or borderline T_4 or free T_4 index (FT_4I), since a normal TSH level excludes a diagnosis of primary hypothyroidism.

The degree of TSH elevation varies from a slight increase to values as high as 2000 microunits/ml; extremely high values do not necessarily correlate with the duration or the severity of the deficiency in thyroid function. In general, serum TSH levels greater than 10 microunits/ml can be used as a cut-off point for diagnosis.

TRH Testing. TRH testing may be useful to clarify borderline elevated basal TSH values. In primary hypothyroidism the response to TRH is exaggerated and peak serum TSH levels usually exceed 30 microunits/ml (at 30 min). The TRH test is also useful in differentiating secondary from tertiary hypothyroidism; indeed, no TRH response is seen in cases of pituitary disease (secondary hypothyroidism), whereas in hypothalamic disease (tertiary hypothyroidism) the response to TRH is normal in magnitude and normal or delayed in time course.

Thyroid Antibodies. When present, these suggest autoimmune thyroiditis as the cause of hypothyroidism, but they give no information about the patient's metabolic status. Antimicrosomal antibodies are positive at a titer of more than 1:100 and antithyroglobulin antibodies at a titer of more than 1:5, measured by hemagglutination techniques.

Radioactive Iodine Uptake. Thyroid uptake of radioactive iodine-131 usually is reduced in hypothyroidism of any type. The value of this test has been questioned because of the high iodine content in the average American diet. The normal values for iodine uptake actually overlap with those seen in hypothyroidism.

Other Tests. Tests of peripheral tissue function, such as basal metabolic rates, Achilles tendon reflex time, serum lipid levels, and serum enzyme concentrations, are nonspecific and less sensitive and play little role in the diagnosis of suspected hypothyroidism.

It is recommended that in neonatal screening studies (North American), all samples be analyzed for T_4 with a follow-up TSH determination on sera when a value lower than 6 μg/dl is found. Optimal time for blood sampling is between 3 and 7 days. Both TSH and T_4 can be measured in the eluate of blood spots on filter paper.

Other Laboratory Findings

A variety of nonspecific abnormalities may develop secondary to the hypothyroid state. Hypercholesterolemia may occur in primary hypothyroidism, but not in pituitary-hypothalamic disease; there may be increased creatine kinase (CK), transaminase (SGOT, AST) and lactate dehydrogenase (LDH) levels. In children, the serum alkaline phosphatase (ALP) level does not display the usual increase associated with active growth.

Hyponatremia may be present. There may be a mild anemia, mostly normocytic normochromic, due to decreased production of erythropoietin. Macrocytic anemia may occur owing to vitamin B_{12} malabsorption, and microcytic anemia may be secondary to iron deficiency (defective absorption or menorrhagia). Achlorhydria is common in primary hypothyroidism and is found along with impaired vitamin B_{12} absorption and pernicious anemia.

A decreased 24-hour urinary excretion of 17-ketosteroids and 17-hydroxycorticosteroids is due to a decreased turnover of cortisol. Cortisol levels are usually normal, however.

Other findings include increased prolactin secretion, which may result in galactorrhea. Oral glucose tolerance tests characteristically demonstrate a flat glucose response with delayed insulin release. Sinus bradycardia, prolonged PR interval, low voltage, and flattened or inverted T-waves are frequently observed on electrocardiography (ECG).

Pitfalls in Diagnosis

Nonthyroidal Illnesses (NTI). These include a wide variety of acute and chronic conditions that can cause low T_3, T_4 levels. It is believed that such findings occur as adaptive mechanisms to conserve protein and reduce caloric expenditure. As such, these conditions do not require therapy, unlike the true hypothyroid state. The differential diagnosis is based on the measurement of serum rT_3 levels, which are normal or high in nonthyroidal illness and low in hypothyroidism, and on the serum TSH level, which is rarely elevated in nonthyroidal illness.

TBG Deficiency. Serum T_4 level may be reduced in cases of congenital or acquired thyroxine-binding globulin (TBG) deficiency or by agents that compete for the TBG-T_4 binding, such as salicylates and phenytoin. The T_3 resin uptake test indicates an increased number of unoccupied T_4 binding sites so that the free T_4 index is normal; also, TSH levels are normal.

Acquired causes of TBG deficiency include use of androgens, high doses of corticosteroids, asparaginase, malnutrition, nephrosis, and cirrhosis.

Transient Hypothyroidism. This can occur in different clinical settings, such as in the neonatal period owing to maternal exposure to iodine or goitrogens either antepartum or in the postnatal period (breast feeding); in the first months after radioactive iodine or surgical treatment of thyrotoxicosis; in the evolution of subacute thyroiditis; in the period following the discontinuation of prolonged thyroid hormone therapy in euthyroid subjects; and in the postpartum period in patients with chronic autoimmune thyroiditis, with a return to the euthyroid state 5 to 10 months post delivery.

Continuation of Treatment. To evaluate the need for continuation of therapy in patients already receiving thyroid hormone, but without reliable previous diagnosis, treatment can be stopped for about 5 weeks. At that time, levels of T_4 will be low and of TSH clearly elevated in the case of true hypothyroidism, while those values will be normal in euthyroid subjects.

Another method by which hypothyroidism can be ruled out in subjects who are taking thyroid hormone supplements is to switch to T_3 (Cytomel) in a dosage of 100 μg/day orally for 4 weeks, after which serum T_4 levels are measured. In the euthyroid subjects, the mean serum T_4 level was found to be 2.6 ± 0.36 μg/dl (range, 1.3 to 3.7 μ/dl). In hypothyroidism T_4 values were undetectable (less than 0.625 μg/dl).

In summary, the diagnosis of hypothyroidism is usually based on clinical suspicion and further confirmatory evidence from laboratory tests. In the neonate and in patients with low thyroid reserve, laboratory screening tests point toward a correct diagnosis. Clinical findings may be absent or subtle. In patients who were arbitrarily started on thyroid hormone therapy, discontinuation of their medication and subsequent tests will usually reveal those patients with true hypothyroidism.

THYROIDITIS

By William T. Cave, Jr., M.D.
Rochester, New York

"Thyroiditis" is a general, nonspecific term used to characterize any inflammatory or infiltrative process in the thyroid. It may occur rarely as a pathologic manifestation of a wide variety of systemic diseases, such as syphilis, typhoid, tuberculosis, echinococcosis, sarcoidosis, mycosis, and amyloidosis. In this article, however, the types of thyroiditis that will be discussed are those in which the thyroid alone is the predominant focus of the disease. These will be presented in order of their clinical frequency and will be classified as follows: (1) Hashimoto's thyroiditis, (2) subacute thyroiditis, (3) silent thyroiditis, (4) acute suppurative thyroiditis, and (5) Riedel's thyroiditis.

At the present time, the exact causes of several of these types of thyroiditis are unknown. As a result, their classification as separate disease entities rests primarily on their relatively distinctive epidemiologic, clinical, and pathologic characteristics. Generally, these classification criteria are well accepted, but it should be recognized that some investigators believe that cases classified as silent thyroiditis may actually be atypical cases of subacute thyroiditis. In this article I have chosen to consider silent thyroiditis as a separate syndrome because its unique clinical and pathologic features commonly pose enough diagnostic difficulties to warrant additional discussion.

HASHIMOTO'S THYROIDITIS

Synonyms

Autoimmune thyroiditis, struma lymphomatosa, lymphocytic thyroiditis, lymphoid goiter, chronic thyroiditis.

Definition

Hashimoto's thyroiditis is a chronic, progressive disease that is presumed to be the result of an autoimmune disorder. It is the most common form of thyroiditis and is a frequent cause of thyroid enlargement and hypothyroidism. Most patients with this disease have circulating autoantibodies to one of several distinct thyroid antigens together with histologic evidence of lymphocytic infiltration, fibrosis, and follicular cell hypertrophy.

Presenting Signs and Symptoms

Hashimoto's thyroiditis occurs predominantly in adult women (female-male ratio, 4:1 to 20:1) during the fourth to fifth decades of life. No age group is exempt, however, as it is also a major cause of nontoxic goiter in childhood and adolescence. In over one third of patients, a family history of Hashimoto's thyroiditis, Graves' disease, hypothyroidism, or goiter can be elicited, and recent evidence suggests that there is a significant association of the human leukocyte antigen HLA-DRw3 with this disease.

Although the clinical presentation of Hashimoto's thyroiditis can be quite varied, its presence in most patients is heralded by diffuse thyromegaly. This thyroid enlargement normally occurs in a gradual and asymptomatic fashion, but occasionally it may advance rapidly and produce neck discomfort. Symptoms of subtle or overt hypothyroidism, such as fatigue, cold intolerance, dry skin, and menorrhagia, can also be obtained in 20 per cent or more of patients when first seen. Sometimes these symptoms may be precipitated by the inadvertent administration of iodine-containing medications from whose antithyroid effects the diseased gland cannot escape. In other less typical cases of Hashimoto's thyroiditis, hypothyroidism may occur in the absence of thyromegaly and, in a small number of patients (2 to 10 per cent), Hashimoto's thyroiditis may coexist with hyperthyroidism.

Course

The course of Hashimoto's thyroiditis can be quite variable, but normally the follicular elements of the thyroid continue to undergo gradual fibrous atrophy and to lose their functional capacity. In the early stages of the disease, these changes are often accompanied by increasing thyromegaly, but as the fibrosis progresses the gland usually decreases its size somewhat and becomes hard and irregular. Patients who are euthyroid or hyperthyroid when first seen eventually tend to develop clinical and laboratory features of hypothyroidism.

Complications

There are usually no major complications of this disorder as long as the patient is maintained in a euthyroid state with supplemental thyroid hormone as needed. It should be recognized, however, that certain other autoimmune diseases (Table 1) do occur more frequently in patients with Hashimoto's thyroiditis than in the normal population. The term Schmidt's syndrome is used specifically to denote the association of autoimmune adrenal failure with hypothyroidism due to Hashimoto's thyroiditis.

Physical Examination

As noted previously, a moderate-sized goiter (two to four times normal) is commonly found as the initial manifestation of this disease. It is frequently first observed during an examination for some other complaint. The thyroid enlargement is usually symmetric and involves both lobes as well as the pyramidal lobe if the latter is present. The gland tends to be firm in consistency and moves freely on swallowing. Frank nodularity is rare, but a slight diffuse irregularity of the surface is common. The typical manifestations of hypo- or hyperthyroidism, which may also be present are described in detail elsewhere. (See articles on these topics.)

Table 1. Disorders Associated with Hashimoto's Thyroiditis

Pernicious anemia
Addison's disease
Diabetes mellitus
Myasthenia gravis
Rheumatoid arthritis
Premature ovarian failure
Hypoparathyroidism
Chronic active hepatitis
Sjögren's syndrome
Systemic lupus erythematosus

Laboratory Procedures

The laboratory studies most useful in the diagnosis of Hashimoto's thyroiditis are those chiefly limited to the indices of thyroid function and specific immunologic tests. The vast majority of patients (more than 90 per cent) will have evidence of elevated titers of circulating antithyroid antibodies if both the thyroglobulin and microsomal antigens are tested. Although mild elevations in these antibody titers can also occasionally be observed in other thyroid diseases, high titers are virtually diagnostic of autoimmune thyroid disease.

The results obtained on routine thyroid function studies will depend primarily on the stage of the disease process. They can be found to range anywhere from frankly hypothyroid values to the hyperthyroid values seen in "Hashitoxicosis." In the initial stages of the disease, however, these tests will usually demonstrate only a mild inability of the diseased gland to incorporate iodine into thyroid hormone. Such abnormalities as an elevated serum butanol nonextractable iodine (iodoalbumin) level and a mildly elevated thyroid-stimulating hormone (TSH) level will be found along with a normal or low normal free thyroxine (T_4) level. An exaggerated TSH response to thyrotropin-releasing hormone (TRH) is also frequently demonstrable at this time. Later, however, after continued progression of the disease, more dramatic evidence of hypothyroidism will become apparent; the free T_4 level will be unquestionably low and the serum TSH level will be clearly elevated.

Standard isotopic studies of thyroid function also vary significantly with the stage of the disease. At the beginning, when there is only minimal evidence of dyshormonogenesis, ^{99}Tc pertechnetate, a tracer that is trapped by the thyroid but not organically incorporated into hormone, will usually be rapidly accumulated and give a relatively clear image. Later on, after significant fibrosis has occurred, the uptake pattern often changes and becomes more patchy, similar to that seen in multinodular goiter. Likewise, the radioiodine uptake value tends to be somewhat increased early in the course of the disease in response to the TSH elevation that is present, but, as the available functioning tissue diminishes, it also will be seen to fall. A perchlorate discharge test, although rarely needed for diagnosis, can often nicely illustrate the intrathyroidal defect in the organification of iodine that is characteristically present in this disease.

Other Diagnostic Procedures

Normally the laboratory tests listed previously are sufficient to establish the diagnosis. When there is some concern that a neoplastic lesion is present, however, the situation can often be clarified by a fine-needle aspiration biopsy or an open biopsy under general anesthesia.

Pitfalls in Diagnosis

The diagnosis of the classic forms of Hashimoto's thyroiditis can usually be made without difficulty if high levels of antithyroid antibodies are present. In the absence of this finding, evidence of hypothyroidism will usually be sufficient to exclude nontoxic goiter and neoplasia from diagnostic consideration. In euthyroid patients, well-defined nodules generally indicate the presence of a multinodular goiter, but when a nodule is solitary and carcinoma is a serious consideration, a biopsy may be required to resolve the question definitively. In euthyroid adolescent patients, differentiation of Hashimoto's thyroiditis from diffuse nontoxic goiter may be especially difficult in the absence of markedly elevated antithyroid antibody titers; in practical terms, however, this distinction may not be absolutely necessary, as thyroid hormone replacement usually provides equally effective treatment in both conditions.

SUBACUTE THYROIDITIS

Synonyms

De Quervain's thyroiditis, viral thyroiditis, granulomatous thyroiditis, giant cell thyroiditis, pseudotuberculous thyroiditis, acute nonsuppurative thyroiditis.

Definition

Subacute thyroiditis is a self-limited inflammation of the thyroid that is presumed to be of viral origin. It is characterized clinically by abnormalities in iodine metabolism and is distinguished histologically by the presence of disrupted thyroid follicles, giant cells, polymorphonuclear cell infiltration, and fibrosis. It is the second most common form of thyroiditis.

Presenting Signs and Symptoms

Consistent with its presumed viral etiology, subacute thyroiditis often occurs in a seasonal or geographic pattern. It has been specifically associated with mumps virus, coxsackie virus, influenza virus, adenovirus, and echovirus infections. It is most frequently observed in women (female-male ratio, 3:1 to 6:1) during their second to fifth decades of life and is rarely found in young children.

Patients acquiring this disease usually complain of the gradual or sudden onset of pain in the region of the thyroid, which may radiate to the neck and ears. It is often initially accompanied by symptoms of mild hyperthyroidism and such nonspecific inflammatory symptoms as chills, fever, malaise, myalgias, and arthralgias. In atypical cases, however, symptoms of pain and acute inflammation may be relatively insignificant and only thyromegaly or mild thyrotoxicosis may mark the presence of this disease.

Course

In the initial phase of subacute thyroiditis, the acute inflammatory symptoms noted earlier are usually found together with clinical features of hyperthyroidism resulting from the excessive release of stored colloid from the gland. Usually these acute-phase symptoms will begin to remit after 3 to 6 weeks, and following a brief period of euthyroidism they will be replaced by complaints of lethargy and fatigue. The thyroid at this stage has become virtually depleted of stored hormone, and new hormone synthesis is severely limited by the disruption of the parenchyma by the inflammatory process. Overt hypothyroid symptoms will remain for several weeks in more than 25 per cent of these patients, but as the gland begins to recover function, their symptoms gradually improve and they ultimately become euthyroid again.

Although widely variable, the full course of the disease is usually of 2 to 5 months' duration. Recurrences do occur in about one fifth of patients, however, and may significantly prolong the return to complete recovery. In more than 90 per cent of patients with subacute thyroiditis, complete restoration of normal thyroid function is observed, but, rarely, permanent myxedema secondary to complete destruction of the thyroid does occur.

Physical Examination

On physical examination, the thyroid is usually found to be diffusely enlarged, firm, tender, and without associated cervical adenopathy. Occasionally, however, the process may seem to be initially restricted to one lobe. Clinical manifestations of overt hyperthyroidism are frequently detected early in the course of the disease.

Laboratory and Radiologic Procedures

The laboratory values, like the clinical symptoms, vary greatly throughout the course of the disease. During the initial stage, features of inflammation and hyperthyroidism are dominant. The erythrocyte sedimentation rate (ESR) is usually greater than 50 mm/hour by the Westergren method, and the free T_4, T_3, thyroglobulin, and iodine values are elevated significantly. A reduction in TSH release from the pituitary can also be demonstrated during this stage, and since this further impairs the ability of the damaged follicular cells to synthesize hormone, the radioiodine uptake often falls to values less than 5 per cent.

Once all of the stored hormone has been released from the disrupted follicles, however, this hyperthyroid stage begins to disappear and, owing to the inability of the gland to adequately synthesize new hormone, a transient stage of hypothyroidism ensues.

It is during this stage that the previously suppressed TSH level starts to recover gradually and TSH begins to stimulate increased hormone synthesis in the regenerating follicle cells. The radioiodine uptake values will be seen to increase at this point, and the thyroid image on ^{99m}Tc pertechnetate scanning will once again become clearly visible. At the end of this recovery stage, all parameters of thyroid function will have returned to normal.

Pitfalls in Diagnosis

In the initial phase, subacute thyroiditis may be misdiagnosed as pharyngitis because of the sore throat that is often the presenting complaint. However, once a thyroidal basis has been considered, the laboratory tests should establish the diagnosis. Sometimes an acute hemorrhage into a thyroid nodule or cyst may produce symptoms of local pain and tenderness that a mimic those of subacute thyroiditis, but usually the presence of a normal ESR and radioiodine uptake will resolve this question. Finally, in rare cases of subacute thyroiditis, where pain and tenderness are absent, the rapid formation of a goiter may be erroneously attributed to a neoplastic process. Normally, appropriate laboratory studies will establish the correct diagnosis, but if these are inconclusive, definitive information can be obtained by fine-needle aspiration biopsy.

SILENT THYROIDITIS

Synonyms

Painless thyroiditis, hyperthyroiditis, chronic lymphocytic thyroiditis with spontaneously resolving hyperthyroidism, transient goitrous hyperthyroidism.

Definition

Silent thyroiditis has been defined as a spontaneously resolving form of thyroiditis that is associated with thyrotoxicosis. Histologically the thyroid glands of these patients demonstrate a diffuse or focal lymphocytic thyroiditis. Many consider this syndrome to be a variant of subacute thyroiditis, but its different histologic features and apparently distinctive epidemiology have led others to classify it as a separate disease entity.

Presenting Signs and Symptoms

The age and sex distribution of this syndrome is reported to be similar to that observed in subacute thyroiditis, but a unique feature of silent thyroiditis is that approximately 10 per cent of cases occur in new mothers within 1 to 6 months after delivery. Characteristically, patients with this disorder present with typical symptoms of hyperthyroidism, such as weight loss, fatigue, heat intolerance, and diaphoresis, but they give no history of antecedent viral infection or thyroid tenderness. It is generally impossible by history or physical examination alone to distinguish patients with silent thyroiditis from those with toxic diffuse goiter.

Course

As in subacute thyroiditis, the cause of the thyrotoxicosis observed in this syndrome is the excessive release and proteolysis of stored thyroglobulin from the disrupted thyroid follicles. The condition usually resolves spontaneously within 2 to 5 months, but it may on occasion last for as long as 10 months. Before full recovery, approximately 25 to 30 per cent of patients will experience a 2- to 4-week hypothyroid phase. Permanent hypothyroidism is rare, but recurrent episodes of hyperthyroidism may occur in as many as 10 per cent of patients.

Physical Examination

The most common findings on physical examination are tachycardia, resting tremor, and hyperactive reflexes. In approximately 50 per cent of patients, thyromegaly (up to two to three times normal size) will also occur. The gland usually feels firmer than normal on palpation, but tenderness is not present. As the syndrome begins to resolve, the thyroid enlargement will diminish, and in over half of patients the gland will return to normal size.

Laboratory Procedures

The typical patient with silent thyroiditis will have elevated free T_4 and T_3 levels together with low TSH levels that are unresponsive to exogenous TRH. These patients will also have radioiodine uptakes that are uniformly suppressed to 3 per cent or below, but, unlike the situation in subacute thyroiditis, the ESR will be normal or only slightly elevated. Later in the course of the disease, evidence of transient hypothyroidism may be observed. Permanent hypothyroidism is extremely uncommon, but abnormal TRH responses consistent with loss of thyroid reserve and persistent low antithyroid antibody titers have been reported in some patients.

Pitfalls in Diagnosis

In the absence of exophthalmos and pretibial myxedema, it may be very difficult on the basis of history and physical examination to differentiate patients with Graves' disease from those with silent thyroiditis. The radioiodine uptake, however, should be clearly depressed in silent thyroiditis and normal or elevated in Graves' disease. Occasionally, an artifactually low radioiodine uptake due to acute iodine loading may occur in a patient with Graves' disease, but usually, once the iodine is cleared, the uptake will again return to an elevated level.

It may also, at times, be difficult to differentiate patients with factitious thyrotoxicosis from those with silent thyroiditis. However, thyromegaly is not usually present in those surreptitiously taking thyroid hormone, and the thyroids of these patients should respond normally to exogenous TSH stimulation.

ACUTE SUPPURATIVE THYROIDITIS

Synonyms

Pyogenic thyroiditis, infectious thyroiditis.

Definition

Acute suppurative thyroiditis is an extremely rare condition that results from bacterial or fungal infection of the thyroid. Most commonly it is caused by the direct extension of a local infection in the neck, but it can also occur as the result of metastatic seeding during septicemia. The introduction of antibiotics has virtually eradicated this condition from usual medical practice.

Presenting Symptoms

Patients with acute suppurative thyroiditis usually present with systemic symptoms of sepsis, such as fever, chills, malaise, tachycardia, and diaphoresis. They typically complain of severe pain or tenderness in the region of the thyroid that is often aggravated by extension of the neck or swallowing and alleviated by neck flexion.

Course

In the absence of antibiotic therapy, the infection may progress to abscess formation and involve other adjacent structures in the neck. Permanent hypothyroidism can ensue if local damage to the gland is severe enough; however, appropriate antibiotic therapy will usually cause the thyroiditis to subside and preserve normal thyroid function. Occasionally, incision and drainage of the lesion may also be required if an abscess has already formed.

Physical Examination

On physical examination most patients appear acutely ill and have temperatures between 38° and 40°C. The thyroid region of the neck is frequently swollen and warm, and the thyroid glands are exquisitely tender to palpation. A search for possible primary sources of bacterial infection outside the thyroid should always be made.

Laboratory Findings

Patients with acute suppurative thyroiditis characteristically have normal circulating thyroid hormone levels and radioiodine uptakes, but their scans may show decreased function in the most actively involved regions. They usually have elevated ESR and leukocytosis. The specific bacteriologic diagnosis can often be made by needle aspiration of the thyroid.

RIEDEL'S THYROIDITIS

Synonyms

Ligneous thyroiditis, invasive fibrous thyroiditis, chronic sclerosing thyroiditis, Riedel's struma, struma fibrosa, chronic productive thyroiditis.

Definition

Riedel's thyroiditis is an extremely rare disease of unknown cause in which all or a portion of the thyroid and surrounding tissues become invaded with dense fibrous tissue. On histologic examination, perivascular inflammation is often found accompanying this fibrotic process. Some patients also have evidence of associated retroperitoneal and mediastinal fibrosis.

Presenting Symptoms

Riedel's thyroiditis predominantly occurs in women (female-male ratio, 2:1 to 4:1) between the ages of 30 and 60 years. It frequently begins as an asymptomatic thyroid enlargement, but as the course of the disease progresses it produces increasingly severe symptoms of neck compression, leading to complaints of dyspnea, dysphagia, hoarseness, and even dysphonia.

Course

The outcome of this disease is variable. The fibrotic process occasionally halts spontaneously and may even regress, but more commonly it progresses in an unremitting fashion. If the compressive symptoms become severe enough, a wedge resection of the isthmus can be performed. This procedure will usually be sufficient to alleviate most of the major symptoms and allow the process to subsequently pursue a relatively benign course. Only rarely will a second operation be required. Hypothyroidism, although uncommon, may ultimately occur if the whole gland becomes extensively involved.

Physical Examination

On palpation, the thyroid gland is often noted to be moderately enlarged, and the involved areas, which may be found in one or both lobes, usually feel stony and hard. The compressive effects often seem disproportionately severe for the size of the goiter. Regional lymph node enlargement is uncommon.

Laboratory Procedures

Unless the whole gland becomes overwhelmingly involved, most of the thyroid function studies in these patients remain within the normal range. The thyroid scan, however, will often show reduced isotope uptake in the regions where fibrosis is most severe. Antithyroid antibody titers are generally reported to be absent or very low in this condition.

Other Diagnostic Procedures

The slowly progressive nature of this disorder will usually distinguish it from the more rapidly progressive forms of sclerosing undifferentiated thyroid carcinoma, but, as noted previously, surgical intervention may be necessary for both therapeutic and diagnostic considerations.

THYROID TUMORS

By Paul W. Ladenson, M.D.
Baltimore, Maryland
and E. Chester Ridgway, M.D.
Boston, Massachusetts

The thyroid nodule or tumor represents an extremely prevalent clinical endocrine disorder. It poses a challenging diagnostic dilemma, since (1) clinically significant thyroid cancer is present in only a small fraction of these very common nodules and (2) surgical excision of all nodules, although clearly diagnostic and frequently curative, is associated with morbidity and expense.

HISTORY

Historical information modifies the form, pace, and extent of the laboratory evaluation of a thyroid nodule. The patient's age and sex alter the clinician's index of suspicion. Thyroid nodules are more likely to be malignant in the young (under 20 years old) and when newly present in the elderly. Although thyroid cancer occurs three times more frequently in women, benign thyroidal disorders, such as multinodular goiter and autoimmune thyroiditis, are even more common in women (eight times). A thyroid nodule in a male patient, therefore, is relatively more likely to be malignant. A history of head, neck, or upper thoracic radiation therapy in childhood or adolescence must be carefully sought, since thyroidal irradiation, especially less than 2000 rad, has been clearly associated with an increased incidence of both benign and malignant thyroid neoplasms. In addition to questioning the patient, information must often be sought from parents, pediatricians, and hospital or office radiology records. The indications for this therapy in the 1940s and 1950s included recurrent tonsillitis, adenoiditis, otitis, mastoiditis, thymic enlargement, hemangiomas, ringworm, acne, and other dermatologic conditions. A positive history of irradiation should prompt a particularly expeditious and definitive diagnostic evaluation.

Several characteristics of the nodules should be explored in the history. It is important to define the pattern of enlargement. A gland that has stayed stable in size for a long time, or very rapid enlargement (e.g., hours or a few days), is relatively reassuring, whereas an intermediate pattern of growth (e.g. weeks or months) is more consistent with a neoplasm. Unfortunately, a clear delineation of the thyroid nodule's temporal development often cannot be obtained.

Inquiry should be made about associated local symptoms. Capsular invasion, nerve entrapment, or involvement of extrathyroidal tissue by a thyroid malignancy can produce local pain in the neck or pain radiating to the jaw or ear. Acute pain can also be seen, however, during the hemorrhagic degeneration of a benign adenomatous goiter; and exquisite thyroid tenderness is characteristic of subacute thyroiditis. Therefore, thyroidal pain that is prolonged beyond the expected duration seen with hemorrhagic degeneration in adenomatous goiter (less than 2 weeks) or subacute thyroiditis (less than 3 months) should prompt concern. Persistent or progressive dysphagia, dyspnea, or hoarseness may reflect esophageal, tracheal, or recurrent laryngeal nerve compression, respectively, by a thyroid cancer. These symptoms are not, however, pathognomonic of cancer, and each may also be seen with benign causes of thyroidal enlargement, particularly large multinodular goiters. Hemoptysis is a less well appreciated symptom of tracheal invasion by thyroid cancer.

Symptoms of thyroid hormone excess or deficiency are relatively reassuring. Malignant nodules do not usually cause, and are not associated with, hyperthyroidism or hypothyroidism. By contrast, benign hyperfunctioning follicular adenomas may produce hyperthyroidism (Plummer's disease), and hypofunctioning thyroid nodules may be seen with either multinodular goiter or autoimmune thyroiditis. (See article on Thyroiditis.) The interviewer should also seek information on symptoms suggestive of medullary carcinoma of the thyroid or its associated endocrine neoplasms. Occasionally diarrhea is the sole complaint associated with calcitonin excess. Since medullary cancer is associated with hyperparathyroidism and with pheochromocytoma in the multiple endocrine neoplasia type 2 syndrome (MEN type 2), symptoms indicative of these disorders should also be specifically probed.

The patient should be questioned about symptoms indicative of metastases to or from the thyroid gland. Primary nonthyroidal neoplasms, e.g., involving the breast, colon, kidney, and other structures, may spread to the thyroid and present as a nodule. Complaints suggesting these malignancies should be reviewed. Since thyroid cancers themselves metastasize principally to regional lymph nodes in the neck or the lungs and bone (see later discussion), inquiry should be made about other neck masses, dyspnea, cough, hemoptysis, bone pain, and hypercalcemic symptoms.

Finally, the history should elucidate the degree to which the thyroid nodule has evoked patient anxiety and cosmetic concern. These factors as well as the ease and reliability of follow-up care should influence both the diagnostic approach and the decision about surgical excision of a thyroid nodule. Seldom does the history yield information that by itself necessitates or excludes surgical excision.

The family history, although of interest, generally provides no information that is decisive in defining the subsequent diagnostic work-up. The familial occurrence of multinodular goiter or autoimmune thyroid disease is mildly reassuring but does not obviate the need for further studies. A family history of medullary carcinoma of the thyroid or its accompanying MEN type 2 features is certainly significant and should prompt special laboratory procedures to consider this diagnosis (see later discussion). Other forms of thyroid cancer, with only a few reported exceptions, are not familial.

PHYSICAL EXAMINATION

The sensitivity of physical examination in the detection of thyroid nodules is directly related to the skill, experience, and thoroughness of the examiner. Even with careful technique, it is clear that many thyroid nodules, particularly those less than 1 cm in diameter, may not be detected. The isthmus of the thyroid gland normally lies over the second to fourth tracheal rings with its upper border just beneath the lower extent of the thyroid cartilage (Fig. 1*A*). The lobes of the gland extend laterally and posteriorly, occupying a space bounded medially by the tracheoesophageal groove and laterally by the sternocleidomastoid muscles (Fig. 1*B*). Since the posterior capsule of the gland is continuous with the pretracheal fascia, the normal thyroid gland moves freely with deglutition. Examination of the thyroid should begin with observation of the anterior neck during swallowing. A cup of water is an indispensable aid in the thyroid examination to facilitate repeated swallowing by the patient. The isthmus of the gland should be localized by palpation, taking care to differentiate glandular tissue from the normally harder adjacent and underlying cricoid cartilage and smaller tracheal rings. The lateral lobes can be individually palpated with firm probing lateral to the trachea during deglutition. The lateral lobes can also be displaced from their recesses by gentle deviation of the trachea with the thumb of the opposite hand. This process should be repeated during swallowing. Normally the lateral lobes of the gland are less than 5 cm in length. Mild asymmetry is common, with the right lobe usually larger than the left. The gland is normally smooth and has a soft to firm consistency, feeling quite similar to the ear lobe.

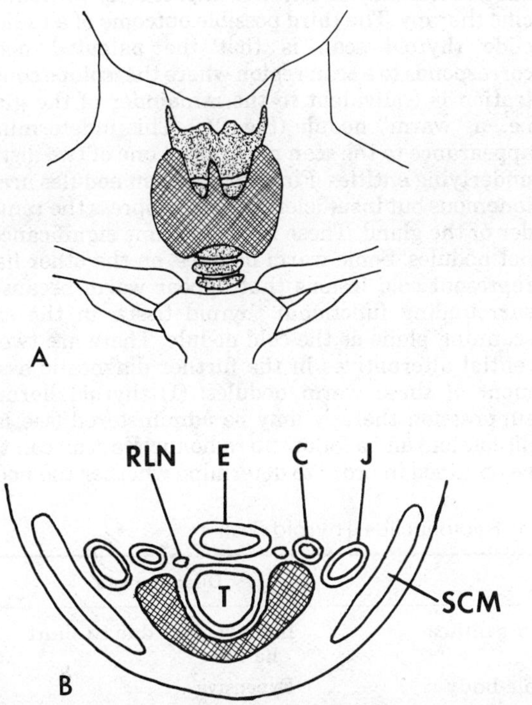

Figure 1. Diagrammatic representation of the anatomic relationships of the normal thyroid gland. In the anterior view (*A*), the isthmus of the gland lies inferior to the thyroid cartilage. A pyramidal lobe may project superiorly from the isthmus. In a cross section of the anterior neck (*B*), the position of the lateral lobes in relationship to the trachea (T), esophagus (E), carotid artery (C), jugular vein (J), sternocleidomastoid muscles (SCM), and recurrent laryngeal nerve (RLN) is shown.

The size, symmetry, contour, consistency, and mobility of the thyroid nodule and extranodular thyroid tissue should be defined. The dimensions of the thyroid nodule should be determined as precisely as possible to provide an accurate baseline for subsequent comparisons. One approach is to cover the skin overlying the nodule with paper adhesive tape, mark the margins of the nodule, and save the tracing for future reference. Classically the malignant thyroid nodule is an irregular, hard mass fixed to adjacent structures, with associated regional lymphadenopathy. However, the spectrum of size, contour, and consistency for benign and malignant thyroid lesions shows considerable overlap. Regrettably, no combination of physical features of the nodule alone is sufficient to exclude malignancy.

A careful examination of extranodular thyroid tissue is important in the clinical assessment of the thyroid nodule. A solitary thyroid nodule is more likely to be malignant than one of several nodules since the latter suggests the possibility of benign multinodular goiter. However, any single nodule or region within such a gland that has recently enlarged or has been associated with local symptoms, a so-called dominant nodule, deserves the same diagnostic attention as a solitary nodular lesion. If extranodular tissue is diffusely enlarged, gritty, and firm, autoimmune thyroiditis may be present. If the remainder of the gland is atrophied or nonpalpable, the nodule may represent a benign hyperfunctioning adenoma.

Physical examination for possible regional involvement by thyroid cancer should be performed. The presence of anterior cervical or supraclavicular lymphadenopathy, hoarseness with confirmation of vocal cord paralysis by indirect laryngoscopy, tracheal deviation, and stridor all suggest, but do not establish, the presence of malignancy. The general examination should be directed to reveal signs of hyperthyroidism or hypothyroidism (see articles on these topics); signs of metastatic thyroid cancer or primary nonthyroidal malignancy which might secondarily involve the thyroid; and signs consistent with MEN type 2 or 2a syndrome (i.e., hypertension or mucosal neuromas).

LABORATORY ASSESSMENT

Serum Thyroid Function Tests

In virtually every patient, occult hyperthyroidism or hypothyroidism should be excluded by measurement of the serum concentrations of thyroid hormones and pituitary thyrotropin (TSH). Normal serum thyroxine (T_4), free T_4, and triiodothyronine (T_3) levels, for most practical purposes, rule out significant thyroid dysfunction. Since an isolated elevation of the serum TSH level may occur in autoimmune thyroiditis in the setting of subclinical hypothyroidism, this parameter should also be assessed.

Other blood tests should be employed only selectively. A basal serum calcitonin level as well as determinations of the calcitonin level following calcium or pentagastrin stimulation (see later discussion) may be required if the clinical evaluation suggests medullary carcinoma or MEN type 2. Measurements of anti-thyroid antibodies (i.e., antimicrosomal, anticolloidal, or tanned red cell thyroid antibodies) may be of value in revealing the diagnosis of autoimmune thyroiditis when there is diffuse enlargement of the gland. Serum thyroglobulin determination has proved disappointing in the differentiation of benign from malignant nodules. This test is primarily useful in the follow-up of patients with metastatic thyroid cancer.

Radionuclide Thyroid Scan

The thyroid scan plays a central role in diagnostic evaluation of the thyroid nodule. First, it defines a group of "cold" or hypofunctioning nodules, which include most thyroid cancers. In addition, the scan identifies autonomously functioning ("hot") thyroid nodules, which are benign. It also augments the physical examination in recognizing the multinodular goiter. Finally, the thyroid scan may be useful for the initial screening of patients with a history of neck irradiation even in the absence of palpable abnormality.

The relative merits of the radioisotopes commonly employed for thyroid imaging are summarized in Table 1. Iodine-123 (^{123}I) is the agent of choice because of its low associated radiation burden and its ability to assess two distinct steps in thyroid hormone biosynthesis. However, convenience often necessitates the use of technetium-99m (^{99m}Tc) as an alternative. Thyroid cancers have rarely been reported to concentrate ^{99m}Tc, and this potential for occasional misdiagnosis must be remembered if the agent is employed.

There are, in general, three possible outcomes of the radionuclide thyroid scan (Fig. 2). Proper interpretation of the study requires accurate localization of the palpated nodule on the scan image. First, the nodule may overlie a region of decreased radionuclide activity, i.e., a cold nodule (Fig. 2*A*). Although the majority of such lesions will be benign, further diagnostic evaluation is essential for cold lesions, since it is among these nodules that most malignancies will be found. Alternatively, the nodule may concentrate the radioisotope and the remainder of the gland may be suppressed, i.e., a hot nodule (Fig. 2*B*). In this circumstance the autonomous production of thyroid hormones by a follicular adenoma results in the inhibition of pituitary TSH secretion, which in turn decreases extranodular radioisotopic uptake. Although a few exceptions have been reported, hot nodules can, for practical purposes, be considered benign. In the absence of clinical or chemical hyperthyroidism, such hot nodules may be followed expectantly without specific therapy. The third possible outcome of a radionuclide thyroid scan is that the palpated nodule corresponds to a scan region where the isotope concentration is equivalent to the remainder of the gland, i.e., a "warm" nodule (Fig. 2*C*). This indeterminant appearance to the scan may reflect one of two distinct underlying entities. First, some warm nodules are autonomous but insufficiently so to suppress the remainder of the gland. These have the same significance as hot nodules. Some warm nodules, on the other hand, represent cold lesions that appear warm because of surrounding functional thyroid tissue in the same scanning plane as the cold nodule. There are two potential alternatives in the further diagnostic assessment of these warm nodules: (1) thyroid hormone suppression therapy may be administered (see later discussion) and a follow-up radionuclide scan can then be obtained in order to determine whether the nodule

Table 1. Comparison of Isotopes for Radionuclide Thyroid Scan

Isotope	Advantages	Disadvantages
Iodine-123 (^{123}I)	Tests trapping (T) and organification (O) functions	Inconvenient due to short half-life
	Low thyroidal and whole-body radiation dose*	Expensive
Technetium-99m (^{99m}Tc)	Convenient, inexpensive	Tests trapping only
	Low thyroidal radiation dose	Higher whole-body radiation dose
Iodine-131 (^{131}I)	Tests both T and O Convenient	Higher thyroid (and whole-body) radiation dose

*Delay in ^{123}I utilization increases the relative quantity of longer-lived radiocontaminants, e.g., ^{124}I, negating this advantage.

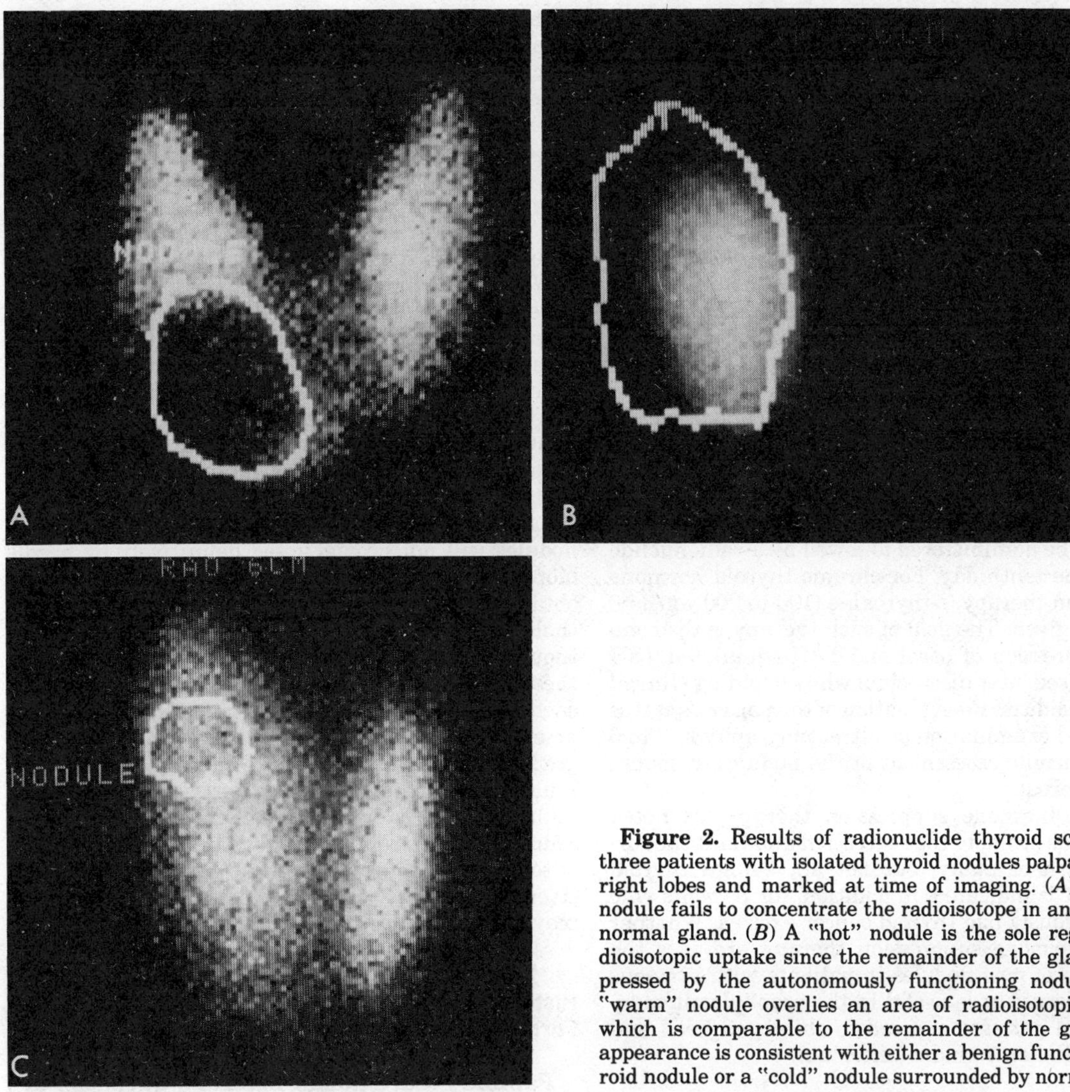

Figure 2. Results of radionuclide thyroid scanning in three patients with isolated thyroid nodules palpated in the right lobes and marked at time of imaging. (*A*) A "cold" nodule fails to concentrate the radioisotope in an otherwise normal gland. (*B*) A "hot" nodule is the sole region of radioisotopic uptake since the remainder of the gland is suppressed by the autonomously functioning nodule. (*C*) A "warm" nodule overlies an area of radioisotopic activity, which is comparable to the remainder of the gland. This appearance is consistent with either a benign functional thyroid nodule or a "cold" nodule surrounded by normal tissue.

is, in fact, autonomously functioning and nonsuppressible; or (2) the lesion may be managed in the same manner as a cold nodule (see later discussion).

Ultrasonography of the Thyroid

High-resolution ultrasonographic examination of the thyroid gland may be helpful in further establishing the nature of certain thyroid nodules. With this technique, it is often possible to identify other clinically undetected nodules in a multinodular goiter. Ultrasonography can clearly categorize thyroid nodules as solid, purely cystic, or complex cystic lesions that include solid elements. Small, simple cysts are almost invariably benign. However, ultrasonography is unfortunately not sufficiently specific to exclude thyroid malignancy in most other thyroid nodules. Complex cysts, or even simple cysts with a diameter greater than 4 cm, may occasionally represent malignant lesions. Although follicular adenomas are often surrounded by a thin lucent halo, cancer cannot be excluded on this basis alone. For these reasons, diagnostic ultrasound should be selectively employed in the primary evaluation of patients with a thyroid nodule. It may be effectively used to monitor the effects of thyroid hormone suppression therapy on nodule size (see later discussion).

Thyroid Hormone Suppression or Therapeutic Trial

The rationale underlying the administration of thyroid hormones in the differential diagnosis of hypofunctioning thyroid nodules is that benign, TSH-dependent lesions will decrease in size while thyroid cancers will continue to enlarge. Unfortunately, this approach is not specific enough to be recommended as the sole diagnostic maneuver for most thyroid nodules. Hot nodules, although benign, would not be expected to regress with thyroid hormone therapy. Furthermore, iatrogenic hyperthyroidism may be caused by the combination of exogenous therapy and the autonomous production of thyroid hormones by the hot nodule. Among cold nodules, it is true that many that are benign will shrink and many that are malignant will grow further under suppression therapy. However, a significant number of benign lesions will also remain stable or enlarge, and apparent temporary regression of thyroid cancers has occasionally been reported. Despite its limitations as a primary diagnostic modality, thyroid hormone suppression therapy may be employed, as noted previously, for the differentiation of warm nodules into the hot or cold category. In addition, it proves useful occasionally in the evaluation of a dominant nodule within a multinodular gland. Finally, this treatment method can be recommended for the follow-up of a radionuclide scan abnormality unassociated with a palpable nodule in the irradiated patient. In this circumstance, therapy may shrink extranodular tissue and make the nodule accessible to physical examination and biopsy.

For short-term thyroid hormone administration in preparation for a radionuclide scan, either T_3 (25 μg three times a day for 10 days) or T_4 (3 mg as a single dose), can be administered followed by a radionuclide scan on the tenth day. For chronic thyroid hormone suppression therapy, L-thyroxine (100 to 200 μg/day) should be given. The goal of such therapy is the complete suppression of basal and TRH-stimulated TSH secretion (see later discussion) while avoiding clinical hyperthyroidism. Re-evaluation of the patient's status by physical examination or ultrasonography in 3 to 6 months permits assessment of the nodule's response to this approach.

Thyroid hormone suppression therapy, as noted earlier, does promote the regression and limit the further growth of many, but not all, benign thyroid nodules. It is indicated, in addition, for patients who have previously had thyroid cancer excised. Whether thyroid hormone suppression therapy prevents the emergence of new nodules in patients with previous nodular disease or is useful in the prophylactic management of patients exposed to childhood head and neck irradiation remains uncertain.

Biopsy of the Thyroid Nodule

The application of needle biopsy techniques to the thyroid nodule has represented a significant advance in their differential diagnosis. Several techniques, each with distinct advantages and pitfalls, have been employed (see Table 2). Cutting-needle biopsy yields specimens of sufficient size to allow a histopathologic interpretation, but it is also the most difficult technique to master and is associated with more risk. At the other end of the spectrum, fine-needle aspiration biopsy is technically simpler, but generally it provides only cytologic specimens that require special expertise to evaluate and that more frequently result in indeterminant diagnoses.

With needle biopsy specimens, the majority of cases of benign follicular and colloidal adenomas or autoimmune thyroiditis can be diagnosed. Patients with these lesions, which represent the most frequent causes of thyroid nodules, can therefore avoid the morbidity and cost of surgery. Patients with malignant nodules identified by this technique benefit from the preoperative planning of subsequent surgery. Tumor seeding of the needle tract with these techniques has not proved to be a problem. A minority of thyroid nodules will not be diagnosed definitively by needle biopsy. When an inadequate tissue sample has been obtained, the biopsy may be repeated. Certain histopathologic appearances, however, remain suggestive, although not diagnostic, of malignancy. In general, these lesions should be excised. Cellular adenomas, such as the microfollicular adenoma, fetal adenoma, or embryonal adenoma, may in fact represent low-grade follicular carcinomas. Similarly, lymphocytic infiltration of the gland may be seen with autoimmune thyroiditis or thyroidal lymphoma. In the absence of other evidence suggesting the presence of autoimmune thyroiditis—e.g., hypothyroidism or strongly positive antithyroid antibodies—excision may be required in this circumstance as well.

Histologic Types of Thyroid Malignancy: Further Diagnostic Assessment

Papillary Carcinoma. Papillary carcinoma and mixed papillary-follicular carcinoma of the thyroid are the most common forms of thyroid cancer, accounting for two thirds of all thyroid malignancies. In general, these tumors are indolent in their growth and spread to regional lymph nodes or undergo local invasion. In the elderly, papillary cancer may be more

Table 2. Comparison of Thyroid Needle Biopsy Techniques*

	Fine Needle Aspiration	Aspiration Needle Biopsy	Cutting Needle Biopsy
Needle size	22–27 gauge	16–18 gauge	14 gauge
Expertise required	+	++	+++
Potential morbidity	0	+	++
Adequate specimens obtained	85%	60%	90%
Difficulty of pathologic interpretation	+++	++	+
Smallest nodules feasible for biopsy	0.5 cm	1.0 cm	1.5 cm

*Adapted from Hamburger, J.I., Miller, J.M., and Kini, S.R.: *Clinical Pathological Evaluation of Thyroid Nodules Handbook and Atlas*. Detroit, 1979, p. 84.

aggressive and pulmonary metastases may occur. For the most part, these forms of thyroid cancer fail to concentrate significant quantities of radioactive iodine.

There is considerable controversy regarding the most appropriate surgical management of this disease. The more limited surgical approach is a unilateral lobectomy when the contralateral lobe is grossly normal. Other surgeons recommend a total lobectomy on the affected side with a subtotal or near total resection of the opposite lobe to eradicate microscopic foci of cancer that may be present there. The role of postoperative radioactive iodine ablation also continues to be vigorously debated. A preoperative radionuclide scan suggesting bilateral disease might favor a more aggressive surgical approach or radioactive iodine therapy, or both. If complete ablation of thyroid tissue is desired, repeated radionuclide scanning may be employed to assess the efficacy of such therapy (see later discussion). Since long-term L-thyroxine suppression therapy is indicated for patients with papillary carcinoma, measurements of serum thyroxine level, free thyroxine index, and the basal and often the TRH-stimulated TSH levels are required to monitor thyroid hormone treatment. Determination of serum thyroglobulin concentration is useful in the follow-up of residual or recurrent tumor when the serum thyroglobulin concentration exceeds 10 ng/ml. In addition, ultrasound examination of the neck and chest x-ray often prove valuable in the assessment of residual tumor tissue.

Follicular Carcinoma. In follicular carcinoma, which represents approximately one fifth of thyroid cancers, the cancerous tissue retains the general histologic features of normal thyroid architecture as well as the ability to concentrate iodine and synthesize iodothyronines. Follicular cancer spreads by capsular invasion and by hematogenous metastatic spread to the lungs, bone, and liver. Regional lymph nodes are less commonly involved than in papillary tumors. The prognosis for patients with this disease worsens with increasing tumor size, greater degrees of vascular invasion, increasing patient age, and greater extent of distant metastases.

Small (less than 1 cm) follicular cancers without capsular invasion or metastatic disease may, like small papillary tumors, be successfully treated with lobectomy or subtotal thyroidectomy and thyroid hormone suppression therapy. Surgery in most patients with follicular thyroid cancer, however, is directed toward the primary resection of both tumor tissue and as much normal thyroid tissue as can safely be accomplished. This approach maximizes the likelihood of subsequent radioactive iodine uptake by residual or metastatic follicular carcinoma tissue. Radioactive iodine scanning is, therefore, particularly important in the postoperative follow-up of patients with follicular carcinoma. Following surgery, 1 to 10 mCi ^{123}I or ^{131}I may be administered in order to determine the completeness of thyroidectomy. If residual thyroid tissue is visualized in the neck, 30 to 100 mCi ^{131}I is administered. Following radioactive iodine ablation therapy, the scanning is repeated after 4 to 12 months to determine if distant metastases are present. In patients on chronic L-thyroxine suppression therapy, T_4 is routinely discontinued 4 to 6 weeks prior to ^{131}I administration. In order to prevent intercurrent hypothyroidism, T_3 (25 μg two or three times daily until 10 to 14 days before radioactive iodine is administered) may be given. Tracer doses of ^{131}I for the purpose of identifying metastases are administered in a dose of 1 to 5 mCi with total body scanning at 1 to 7 days. Quantitative determination of radioactive iodine uptake in metastases permits estimation of the subsequent local therapeutic radiation dose. In addition, the serum thyroglobulin concentration, chest x-ray, bone x-rays, and bone scans may prove useful in the follow-up of patients with follicular carcinoma of the thyroid.

Anaplastic Carcinoma of the Thyroid. Anaplastic carcinoma of the thyroid represents one of the most aggressive malignancies in humans. These undifferentiated tumors occur primarily in the elderly as a rapidly enlarging thyroid nodule or diffuse enlargement of the entire gland. Surgery, radiation therapy, and chemotherapy have all been employed, with only occasional success. The rapid clinical progression of these tumors usually obviates the need for more sophisticated laboratory methods in monitoring the status of patients with anaplastic carcinoma. Since anaplastic carcinoma fails to concentrate radioactive iodine, radionuclide scanning has little role in the diagnosis, treatment, or follow-up of this lesion.

Medullary Carcinoma of the Thyroid. Medullary carcinoma of the thyroid arises from the parafollicular or C cells of ultimobranchial body origin. These tumors are frequently familial and may or may not be associated with other features of the MEN type 2 syndrome. They may spread via local lymphatics or, less frequently, metastasize hematogenously. Most medullary cancers behave indolently, although a minority may exhibit a more rapid, aggressive growth pattern. Therapy involves the resection of primary and locally metastatic tumor tissue and, in most circumstances, a total or near total thyroidectomy in view of the high incidence of multifocal and bilateral disease. Measurement of the serum calcitonin level is useful, not only in the preoperative diagnosis of this tumor, but also in the postoperative follow-up of medullary cancer patients with residual or recurrent disease. In addition, the serum calcitonin concentration should be employed to screen relatives of a patient with medullary carcinoma. When there is known familial disease, it has been demonstrated that measurement of not only the basal serum calcitonin concentration but also calcitonin levels following calcium or pentagastrin stimulation is useful in the identification of early malignant lesions. These stimulation test protocols involve the administration of calcium (5 mg/kg/4 hours intravenously) with serum samples for calcitonin being obtained at 0, 30, 60, 90, 120 and 240 minutes; alternatively pentagastrin (0.5 μg/kg) may be given intravenously with sampling at 0, 1, 2, 3, 6, and 9 minutes. Some patients with medullary carcinoma of the thyroid may also secrete carcinoembryonic antigen (CEA), adrenocorticotropic hormone (ACTH), or other hormonal peptides, which can be monitored in the follow-up of these individuals.

Lymphoma of the Thyroid. Thyroidal lymphoma, previously thought to represent a distinct class of "small cell" thyroid cancer, is an unusual thyroid tumor that may occur in isolation or in the presence of disseminated extrathyroidal lymphoma. Clinically, patients typically present with a diffusely enlarging goiter that histologically is composed of lymphocytes and atypical reticulum cells. On these grounds, the potential for confusion with autoimmune thyroiditis exists. Patients with lymphoma, however, are not usually hypothyroid, nor do they typically have an elevation of the serum TSH level (subclinical hypothyroidism) or a high titer of antithyroid antibodies. Furthermore, they are more likely to experience local compressive symptoms or signs due to rapid thyroidal enlargement. An open or excisional biopsy, or both, is occasionally required to distinguish these two disorders. The diagnosis of thyroidal lymphoma is very important to establish since (1) further radiologic and biopsy procedures are indicated to identify possible extrathyroidal disease, and (2) specific therapeutic options, i.e., external radiation and chemotherapy, are indicated for this particular form of thyroid malignancy.

PRIMARY HYPERPARATHYROIDISM

By Robert K. Rude, M.D.
and Frederick R. Singer, M.D.
Los Angeles, California

DEFINITION

Primary hyperparathyroidism encompasses those disorders of the parathyroid gland characterized by an excessive and inappropriate secretion of parathyroid hormone (PTH), resulting in hypercalcemia. Primary hyperparathyroidism is caused by a solitary adenoma in one parathyroid gland in about 80 per cent of cases and by multiple adenomas in a small percentage of cases (less than 5 per cent). Chief cell hyperplasia of all four parathyroid glands, which is frequently a hereditary trait, accounts for about 15 per cent of cases and parathyroid carcinoma is responsible for less than 3 per cent of all cases.

SIGNS AND SYMPTOMS

The signs and symptoms that may be present in patients with primary hyperparathyroidism are quite variable, as shown in Table 1. They are nonspecific but presence of any one, or a constellation of a number of them, should alert the physician to the possibility of this diagnosis.

The clinical expression of primary hyperparathyroidism has changed since the introduction of multiphasic biochemical testing. In the majority of patients (60 per cent), hypercalcemia is discovered in the absence of symptoms or complications due to the hypercalcemia. In some patients subtle elevations in the serum calcium concentration or only intermittent hypercalcemia presents a diagnostic dilemma.

When symptoms are present, perhaps the most common, although the most vague, are those related to the neuromuscular system. Patients frequently complain of fatigue, malaise, and muscle weakness. Depression, apathy, and inability to concentrate may also be prominent symptoms.

Renal colic secondary to calcium-containing renal calculi is a serious complication of primary hyperparathyroidism. Primary hyperparathyroidism should be considered in any patient with renal stones. Frequency, urgency, and dysuria may be due to renal stones or to superimposed urinary tract infection.

Hypercalcemia may induce a mild nephrogenic diabetes insipidus and therefore thirst, polydipsia, and polyuria may be prominent complaints. Other, less common gastrointestinal complaints include anorexia, nausea, and vomiting.

Metastatic calcification may be a serious complication of chronic hypercalcemia. Diffuse nephrocalcinosis leading to impairment of renal function is the most serious. Other sites of metastatic calcification include the eye (cornea and conjunctiva) and vascular tissue.

Osteitis fibrosa is not encountered today as a serious clinical problem, although it was in the past. Earlier diagnosis has led to appropriate treatment prior to the development of severe bone pain, cystic bone changes, or pathologic fractures. Perhaps the greatest skeletal problem is the development of diffuse osteoporosis. Since many patients with primary hyperparathyroidism are postmenopausal women, the excessive secretion of PTH worsens an already accelerated bone mineral loss and may lead to vertebral crush fractures.

Joint pain may also be a prominent feature of primary hyperparathyroidism. The causes of this may include pseudogout, gout, subchondral erosion, and periarticular calcification.

The incidence of hypertension is higher in patients with primary hyperparathyroidism than in the general population. In some patients the hypertension is reversed by parathyroidectomy.

COURSE

The clinical course of patients with primary hyperparathyroidism is unpredictable. Patients may be asymptomatic and remain so for years following the

Table 1. Signs and Symptoms of Primary Hyperparathyroidism

Systemic:	Fatigue, weakness, malaise
Musculoskeletal:	Arthralgia, bone pain, joint effusion, muscle weakness, myalgia
Neuropsychiatric:	Impaired concentration, lethargy, confusion, depression, obtundation, coma, hyporeflexia
Genitourinary:	Polyuria, nocturia, renal colic
Gastrointestinal:	Anorexia, nausea, vomiting, polydipsia, constipation, peptic ulcer disease
Cardiovascular:	Hypertension
Ophthalmologic:	Conjunctival and corneal calcification

diagnosis of this disorder. In other patients the signs and symptoms discussed earlier may become prominent. It is at present impossible to predict which patients will have the most serious problems. In general the higher the serum calcium concentration, the more likely is the possibility that morbid events will result as a consequence of the hypercalcemia.

COMPLICATIONS

Complications of primary hyperparathyroidism are outlined under Signs and Symptoms. The most serious include renal stones and nephrocalcinosis leading to renal failure and osteitis fibrosa, with bone pain, cystic bone changes, and pathologic fractures. Other, less specific but more common, serious complications include osteoporosis, hypertension, and joint pain.

PHYSICAL EXAMINATION

The physical examination in most patients with primary hyperparathyroidism is unremarkable. Proximal muscle weakness may be noted on muscle strength testing. Loss of mental awareness is clinically apparent only with rapidly developing hypercalcemia. Corneal calcification (band keratopathy) may be present in up to one third of patients with chronic hypercalcemia but most often is demonstrable only by slit-lamp examination. Conjunctival calcium deposits may also be observed in chronic hypercalcemia. An acute or rapid elevation in the serum calcium concentration may result in marked conjunctival injection with tearing.

Other physical findings that are even less common include joint effusions and loose teeth. Rarely, a parathyroid carcinoma or a large adenoma may be palpable in the neck.

LABORATORY PROCEDURES

The diagnosis of primary hyperparathyroidism is made on the basis of laboratory examination. A direct measurement of the simultaneous concentrations of calcium and immunoreactive parathyroid hormone (iPTH) in the serum, or an assessment of various biologic effects of parathyroid hormone (PTH) on its end organs, is the major direction of the laboratory evaluation.

Serum Calcium. Calcium in the plasma exists in three forms: the protein-bound fraction, an ionized fraction, and a small fraction complexed to citrate and other plasma anions. Forty per cent of the total serum calcium is bound to plasma proteins (chiefly albumin), whereas about 10 per cent is complexed to anions. The remainder, about 50 per cent, is free ionized calcium. It is an increase in the ionized fraction that results in the signs and symptoms of hypercalcemia discussed earlier.

Measurement of the total serum calcium concentration is the most readily available and least expensive means of determining if hypercalcemia is present. The serum calcium concentration must always be evaluated concomitantly with the serum albumin concentration. One gram of albumin per deciliter of serum will bind about 0.8 mg/dl of calcium. Any change in the serum albumin concentration will therefore result in a corresponding change in the total serum calcium concentration. Ionized serum calcium will remain unchanged. When the serum albumin concentration deviates from normal, the appropriate "correction" of the serum calcium concentration must be made to assess whether or not hypercalcemia is present, and if so, to what degree. Once the serum albumin concentration has been accounted for, two to three determinations of the serum calcium concentration should be made to document the presence of hypercalcemia. The upper limits of normal for the total serum calcium concentration may vary among laboratories. Usually any patient with a serum calcium concentration consistently above 10.1 mg/dl is considered to have hypercalcemia.

A direct determination of the ionized serum calcium concentration can be made using a special calcium ion selective electrode. This measurement is usually made after the serum has been corrected to a pH of 7.4. Since ionized and protein-bound fractions of the serum calcium are directly affected by pH, any deviation of the plasma pH from pH 7.4 will alter the concentration of ionized calcium. The ionized calcium concentration will change inversely with pH. For each 1.0-unit pH change there will be a 1.68 mg/dl inverse change in the serum ionized calcium concentration. The mean normal ionized concentration is about 4.7 mg/dl, with a range of normal of 4.4 to 5.1 mg/dl.

Immunoreactive Parathyroid Hormone. Direct determination of the concentration of PTH by radioimmunoassay is probably the best test of parathyroid function. Each laboratory measuring iPTH has determined a normal range. Although most normal individuals have measurable quantities of PTH in the circulation, some (10 to 20 per cent) may have undetectably low levels owing to lack of assay sensitivity. If the serum calcium concentration is increased by a calcium infusion intravenously or by hypercalcemia induced by pathophysiologic processes other than parathyroid hormone excess, iPTH concentration should become undetectable or low. Therefore, it is of utmost importance that the iPTH concentration be assessed concomitantly with serum calcium concentration. An elevated iPTH concentration in the presence of hypercalcemia makes the diagnosis of primary hyperparathyroidism. Even an iPTH concentration in the normal range in the face of hypercalcemia suggests the diagnosis of primary hyperparathyroidism, since PTH secretion should be suppressed if the hypercalcemia is caused by any other pathophysiologic process (except the rare occurrence of ectopic PTH production by a tumor). It is in this area that the assay for iPTH is imperfect.

Most commercial laboratories use an antiserum against PTH that is directed toward the carboxy-terminal, biologically inactive region of the PTH molecule. Such an assay will measure not only intact PTH but carboxy-terminal fragments of PTH as well. This assay will give a good separation of patients with primary hyperparathyroidism from normal subjects. The half-life of the carboxy-terminal fragments is long, and they are cleared by the kidney. Any decrease in glomerular filtration rate, as may be found in chronic hypercalcemia, will cause accumulation of this immunoreactive species of PTH. The suppressed parathyroid gland in hypercalcemic disorders other than PTH excess, although it does not secrete intact PTH, may continue to release these inactive fragments of PTH. It is common therefore to find "normal" concentrations of iPTH in situations such as the hypercalcemia of malignancy when a carboxy-terminal–specific PTH radioimmunoassay is utilized. In this case, a PTH radioimmunoassay directed toward the amino-terminal, biologically active end of the PTH molecule will better separate patients with primary hyperparathyroidism from patients with hypercalcemia due to other causes.

Urinary Cyclic AMP Excretion. PTH is thought to elicit its biologic effect at its end organs (kidney and bone) primarily via the intermediary action of cyclic AMP. The excretion of cyclic AMP in the urine has been used as a biologic index of PTH secretion. The mean excretion rate of urinary cyclic AMP in patients with primary hyperparathyroidism is higher than that of normal subjects, although much overlap is seen. If plasma cyclic AMP concentration is determined at the time the urine collection is made, the nephrogenous component of urinary cyclic AMP can be calculated. This nephrogenous component accounts for about 50 per cent of total cyclic AMP excreted into the urine and is principally attributable to the effect of PTH on the kidney. Nephrogenous cyclic AMP can be calculated by the following equation:

$$\begin{gathered}\text{Nephrogenous cyclic AMP} = \\ \text{Total urinary cyclic AMP } (\mu\text{mol/gm creatinine}) \times \\ \text{Serum creatinine (mg/dl)} - \\ \text{Plasma cyclic AMP (nmol/dl)}\end{gathered}$$

Utilizing this parameter, a much better separation of patients with primary hyperparathyroidism from normal subjects is obtained. In general, cyclic AMP excretion in the urine is low in hypercalcemia from most other causes. The exception to this is in patients with malignancies. Cancer patients who have either normal or elevated serum calcium concentrations may have elevated, normal, or low urinary or nephrogenous cyclic AMP excretion. The cause of the increase in urinary cyclic AMP excretion is unknown. Therefore, although a suppressed urinary cyclic AMP excretion is evidence against a diagnosis of primary hyperparathyroidism, an elevated urinary excretion rate of cyclic AMP does not exclude malignancy as a cause of the hypercalcemia. In most patients with hypercalcemia and malignancy, however, the tumor is usually clinically apparent.

Calcium Load Test. Some patients may have a slight elevation in the serum calcium concentration or are only intermittently hypercalcemic, and determination of iPTH and urinary cyclic AMP may not be diagnostic. While this group of patients may merely be placed under observation, the potential problem of rapidly developing osteoporosis, with crush fracture in postmenopausal women, must be considered. In addition, the occurrence of renal calculi makes the diagnosis of absorptive idiopathic hypercalciuria a possibility. The application of an oral calcium load test may aid in the diagnosis of mild primary hyperparathyroidism or idiopathic hypercalciuria.

This test examines the serum calcium concentration and urinary calcium and nephrogenous cyclic AMP excretion before and following an oral calcium load. After a 2-hour fasting urine specimen is collected for cyclic AMP, calcium, and creatinine determinations, and a blood specimen is collected for calcium, cyclic AMP, and creatinine measurements, 1 gm of calcium is given by mouth. Two additional 2-hour urine specimens are obtained, and another blood specimen is taken for calcium, cyclic AMP, and creatinine determinations during the last 2-hour urine collection period.

The mean rise in the serum calcium concentration following calcium ingestion in normal subjects has been reported to be 0.2 mg/dl, and the rise in urinary calcium during the last urine collection has been less than 0.21 mg calcium/dl glomerular filtrate (GF). Patients with primary hyperparathyroidism (60 per cent) and idiopathic hypercalciuria, however, have been shown to display a mean rise in the serum calcium concentration of about 1.0 mg/dl and a mean increase in urinary calcium level greater than 0.3 mg/dl GF, which represent manifestations of intestinal hyperabsorption of calcium. Nephrogenous cyclic AMP excretion in normal subjects usually falls from a mean of 2.0 nmol/dl GF to 0.9 nmol/dl GF (less than 1.5 nmol/dl GF). Patients with idiopathic hypercalciuria have a fall in nephrogenous cyclic AMP excretion comparable to normal rates. Because PTH secretion is not under normal negative calcium feedback control in primary hyperparathyroidism, nephrogenous cyclic AMP excretion does not usually fall normally in these patients. Most nephrogenous cyclic AMP excretion rates in primary hyperparathyroidism fall less than in the normal subjects and patients with idiopathic hypercalciuria (minimum value, greater than 1.5 nmol/dl GF).

Other Biochemical Markers. PTH influences acid-base status in that it acts to increase urinary bicarbonate excretion. In PTH excess states, such as primary hyperparathyroidism, a mild hyperchloremic metabolic acidosis may be noted. By contrast, in hypercalcemic disorders from other causes, when endogenous PTH secretion is suppressed a mild hypochloremic metabolic alkalosis may be observed. If the patient has been on diuretic therapy or has had vomiting or diarrhea, the metabolic alkalosis may be secondary to these events and does not exclude the possibility of primary hyperparathyroidism.

PTH also lowers the renal tubular threshold for phosphate, and hypophosphatemia is commonly encountered in primary hyperparathyroidism. An increase in the amount of calcium filtered and excreted by the kidney may also increase urinary PO_4 excretion, and hypophosphatemia is frequently observed in other hypercalcemic states as well. For this reason the serum PO_4 concentration is not a useful index of PTH overactivity. Similarly, the determination of the renal phosphate threshold may not distinguish primary hyperparathyroidism from other causes of hypercalcemia.

Serum alkaline phosphatase activity may reflect an increase in osteoblastic bone formation, as may be seen in patients with primary hyperparathyroidism. It is a nonspecific marker of increased bone turnover and may be observed to be elevated in disorders in which bone resorption is a factor in hypercalcemia. This test is not useful in the differential diagnosis of hypercalcemia.

Urinary calcium excretion is usually elevated in patients with primary hyperparathyroidism. The effect of PTH on the kidney is to increase fractional calcium reabsorption. However, since the filtered load is high, a net increase in renal calcium excretion occurs. Other hypercalcemic conditions also are associated with hypercalciuria, but probably of a greater degree than that seen in primary hyperparathyroidism at any comparable serum calcium concentration. An exception is *familial hypocalciuric hypercalcemia,* an autosomal dominant disorder. This disorder is characterized by hypercalcemia, hypermagnesemia, and low urinary excretion of calcium and magnesium. Since this condition is frequently misdiagnosed as primary hyperparathyroidism, urinary calcium excretion should be determined in all patients suspected of having primary hyperparathyroidism. If the urinary calcium excretion is less than 150 mg/day, familial hypocalciuric hypercalcemia should be considered a diagnostic possibility.

RADIOLOGIC EVALUATION

Routine x-rays are infrequently helpful in the evaluation of a patient with primary hyperparathyroidism. While the effects of PTH excess on bone ("salt and pepper" skull, subperiosteal resorption, and bone cysts) are well recognized, the patient of today is usually evaluated well before these changes occur.

Chondrocalcinosis may involve articular cartilage, most commonly the knee, wrist, and lateral clavicle. This radiologic finding may or may not be associated with pseudogout.

Nephrocalcinosis may be a "silent" complication of primary hyperparathyroidism until either recurrent urinary tract infections or chronic renal failure develops. The finding of renal calcification on a plain film x-ray of the abdomen demands surgical intervention for cure of the primary hyperparathyroidism. Renal calculi may also be seen on plain x-ray films of the abdomen or by intravenous urogram. Any symptom of urinary tract infection or renal colic in patients with suspected primary hyperparathyroidism should be evaluated radiologically.

OTHER DIAGNOSTIC PROCEDURES

Selective venous catheterization may be utilized for localization of abnormal parathyroid tissue. This is accomplished by obtaining blood specimens at various sites in the neck and mediastinum, followed by radioimmunoassay for PTH. A stepwise increase in iPTH concentration over the peripheral vein level would localize the site of the abnormal parathyroid tissue. This test is usually indicated only in those patients who have had negative results on exploration of the neck for primary hyperparathyroidism.

Computed tomography (CT) and ultrasonography may also be of value for parathyroid localization. Their application appears most useful in finding parathyroid adenomas in the anterior mediastinum.

THERAPEUTIC TESTS

The hydrocortisone suppression test (120 mg hydrocortisone per day for 10 days) may be needed infrequently to aid in separating patients with primary hyperparathyroidism from those with hypercalcemia secondary to sarcoidosis. The latter disorder is sensitive to the hydrocortisone, whereas the serum calcium concentration will rarely fall in patients with hyperparathyroidism.

HYPOPARATHYROIDISM

By C. Conrad Johnston, Jr., M.D.
and James W. Edmondson, M.D.
Indianapolis, Indiana

Hypoparathyroidism can be defined as a group of disorders of calcium homeostasis in which there is either deficiency of or resistance to parathyroid hormone. Table 1 lists the major entities now recognized as hypoparathyroid states. Of those disorders in which parathyroid hormone secretion is deficient, postoperative hypoparathyroidism is most common, accounting for at lesat three quarters of all cases of chronic hypoparathyroidism. Transient hypoparathyroidism may be seen in the newborn offspring of mothers with primary hyperparathyroidism and may also follow the successful removal of a parathyroid adenoma.

The states of parathyroid hormone resistance represent a more complex group of disorders of which pseudohypoparathyroidism is the most prevalent example. While some patients with pseudohypoparathyroidism have distinct somatic features that lead to easy recognition, many patients with this form of the disease lack these traits and require identification by biochemical procedures. It is also possible to distinguish several biochemical variants of pseudohypoparathyroidism. Recognition of the pathogenesis of pseudohypoparathyroidism has fostered understanding of the molecular basis for the actions of parathyroid hormone.

CLINICAL FEATURES

Absence of and biologic resistance to parathyroid hormone leads to hypocalcemia and hyperphosphatemia. Most of the clinical features of the hypoparathyroid states can be traced to these biochemical abnormalities. Table 2 is a compilation of frequently encountered clinical features. Neuromuscular irritability underlies the most obvious clinical feature of hypoparathyroidism and is predominantly the consequence of depression of blood levels of ionized calcium. Although not specific for hypoparathyroidism, Chvostek's and Trousseau's signs can be helpful markers for the presence of hypocalcemia and tetany. Another feature is calcification of the basal ganglia, which can be detected easily by computed

Table 1. Differential Diagnosis of Hypoparathyroidism

A. **Absent or Inadequate Parathyroid Hormone Secretion**
1. Idiopathic hypoparathyroidism
2. Postoperative hypoparathyroidism
3. Destruction of parathyroid glands by ^{131}I therapy for thyroid disease or by hemochromatosis or metastatic disease
4. Neonatal hypoparathyroidism: premature infant syndrome, maternal hyperparathyroidism
5. Hypomagnesemia (inadequate secretion and resistance)

B. **Hypersecretion of Parathyroid Hormone Secondary to End-Organ Resistance**
1. Pseudohypoparathyroidism (Types Ia, Ib, II, and possibly other forms)
2. Parathyroid hormone antibodies (secondary to administration of hormone)
3. Selective 1,25-dihydroxyvitamin D deficiency

tomographic (CT) scanning of the cerebrum and may be clinically apparent as an extrapyramidal syndrome.

Although many patients with pseudohypoparathyroidism may be clinically indistinguishable from others with different forms of the disease, one form of pseudohypoparathyroidism is clinically unique and is characterized by short stature, a round face, and shortening of the metacarpal bones. This variant of pseudohypoparathyroidism has been designated *Albright's hereditary osteodystrophy.* Patients with this and other forms of pseudohypoparathyroidism may also manifest features of typical hypoparathyroidism (see Table 2).

CAUSES AND COMPLICATIONS

Prior to the routine availability of serum calcium measurements, patients with hypoparathyroidism sometimes escaped detection for many years. If untreated, hypoparathyroidism is more likely to result in soft tissue calcification, cataract formation and symptomatic hypocalcemia. A common complication attending treatment of hypoparathyroidism is the development of vitamin D intoxication with hypercalcemia, further worsening of tissue calcification, and development of kidney damage and azotemia.

LABORATORY TESTING

The sine qua non for the diagnosis of hypoparathyroidism is the demonstration of hypocalcemia together with hyperphosphatemia. The laboratory evaluation must then begin with measurements of serum total calcium and inorganic phosphorus levels. Nearly 50 per cent of serum calcium is protein-bound, primarily to albumin; thus, measurement of serum albumin concentration is required before true hypocalcemia can be presumed to be present. Since there is no good method for calculation of serum ionized calcium concentration within the range of concentrations usually found, it may be necessary to measure this ion directly in patients with depressed total calcium concentrations, hypoalbuminemia, and symptoms consistent with hypocalcemia. Measurement of serum alkaline phosphatase may also be helpful in the evaluation of the hypocalcemic patient, since patients with hypoparathyroidism usually have normal concentrations, while those with osteomalacia, another disease associated with hypocalcemia, usually also have hyperphosphatasia. Serum magnesium level should be measured to identify hypomagnesemic hypoparathyroidism. Measurement of serum immunoreactive parathyroid hormone concentration also may be of value, and at present this is the most readily available means of distinguishing patients with typical hypoparathyroidism from those with pseudohypoparathyroidism, for in the latter state elevated levels of this hormone are demonstrable.

Radiographic evaluation of patients with hypoparathyroidism has more limited diagnostic utility but is of value for documenting the presence of basal ganglion calcification and for identifying other sites of soft tissue calcification. Patients with somatically identifiable pseudohypoparathyroidism may also exhibit radiographic shortening of the metacarpals (brachydactyly). These subjects and other patients with pseudohypoparathyroidism may also show the skeletal changes of hyperparathyroidism—e.g., subperiosteal resorption, brown tumors, and other features.

SPECIAL DIAGNOSTIC PROCEDURES

The Ellsworth-Howard test had earlier been available to aid in differentiating patients with typical hypoparathyroidism from those with pseudohypoparathyroidism. In this test, parathyroid extract is infused intravenously in anticipation of a biochemical response to parathyroid hormone— e.g., increased serum calcium concentration or enhanced

Table 2. Clinical Features of Hypoparathyroidism

Neuromuscular:
- Tetany
- Chvostek's sign
- Trousseau's sign
- Carpopedal spasm

Ectodermal
- Brittle nails with transverse ridging
- Dry skin and hair
- Maleruption of dentition
- Hypoplasia of dental enamel

Ocular
- Cataract formation
- Papilledema

Central Nervous System
- Seizures (grand mal, petit mal, and focal)
- Extrapyramidal disturbances with basal ganglion calcification (parkinsonism, choreathetosis)
- Psychosis
- Impaired memory
- Pseudotumor cerebri

Cardiovascular
- Impaired cardiac output
- Hypotension
- ECG changes (prolonged QT interval)
- Digitalis resistance

Other:
- Soft-tissue calcification

urinary inorganic phosphorus or cyclic adenosine monophosphate (cyclic AMP) excretion. At present, parathyroid extract is not available for routine clinical use, and distinction between hypoparathyroidism and pseudohypoparathyroidism rests on measurement of the parathyroid hormone concentration.

DIFFERENTIAL DIAGNOSIS

If chronic hypocalcemia with hyperphosphatemia is found, some form of hypoparathyroidism is likely to be present. Other problems that must be considered include osteomalacia, hypoalbuminemia, acute pancreatitis and chronic renal insufficiency. In most circumstances, these states are easily distinguishable from hypoparathyroidism.

ACUTE ADRENOCORTICAL INSUFFICIENCY

By John C. Laidlaw, M.D.
Hamilton, Ontario, Canada

SYNONYMS

Acute hypoadrenocorticism, acute adrenal cortical deficiency.

DEFINITION

Acute adrenocortical insufficiency results when an individual's requirements for either cortisol (hydrocortisone) or aldosterone or for both exceed the amount produced by the adrenal cortex plus the amount of glucocorticoids or mineralocorticoids that the patient may be receiving. Acute adrenocortical insufficiency occurs most commonly when acute stress (acute medical illness, trauma from surgery or other cause) supervenes in patients who are receiving pharmacologic doses of glucocorticoid for some other reason and in whom the dose of glucocorticoid is not increased during the period of stress. In these patients the pituitary-adrenal axis is suppressed by the exogenous glucocorticoid, and cortisol, although not aldosterone, deficiency may develop in times of stress.

Acute adrenocortical insufficiency may also occur in the presence of acute stress in a patient with unrecognized chronic adrenal insufficiency. This may be primary (Addison's disease, congenital adrenal hyperplasia) or secondary to disease of the hypothalamus or anterior pituitary. Alternatively, the patient may have been receiving replacement therapy for chronic adrenocortical insufficiency, but the dose of glucocorticoid or mineralocorticoid was not increased at the time of stress.

Finally, and rarely, acute adrenocortical insufficiency may result from adrenal hemorrhage due to anticoagulant overdose or may be associated with overwhelming septicemia (Waterhouse-Friderichsen syndrome).

PRESENTING SIGNS AND SYMPTOMS

There is often evidence of the "stress" that precipitated the acute adrenocortical insufficiency, namely, recent trauma from surgery or other cause, or an acute infection. In mild or early states of acute insufficiency, nonspecific symptoms such as malaise, lassitude, nausea, and lightheadedness in the upright posture usually predominate. As the insufficiency advances, fever, vomiting, and diarrhea may appear. Later, dehydration, shock, and coma may ensue, particularly if a combined deficiency of cortisol and aldosterone is present. At this stage, the condition may be rapidly fatal.

PHYSICAL EXAMINATION

In mild or early insufficiency, orthostatic hypotension may be the only physical sign. Later the patient may show fever, signs of dehydration, hypotension in the recumbent position, and a thready pulse. Irritability, confusion, and stupor are ominous signs requiring energetic administration of glucocorticoids and glucose-saline solution by intravenous infusion. If unrecognized chronic primary adrenal insufficiency (Addison's disease) has antedated the acute insufficiency, the patient's heart may be small, and excessive brown (melanin) pigmentation of skin and oral mucosa may be present. In contrast, when the underlying chronic adrenocortical insufficiency is secondary to hypopituitarism, the skin is pale. In infants and children in whom the underlying chronic insufficiency has been due to congenital adrenal hyperplasia, the girls may show pseudohermaphroditism and the boys, macrogenitosomia praecox. In the Waterhouse-Friderichsen syndrome there is usually widespread purpura, cyanosis, high fever, and profound shock.

LABORATORY FINDINGS

The hematocrit may be elevated by dehydration. The leukocyte count may be normal or increased, and there is a tendency to lymphocytosis and eosinophilia. Serum sodium and potassium concentrations are normal in mild insufficiency, but in severe insufficiency, particularly of aldosterone, hyponatremia and hyperkalemia occur. Dehydration and hypotension lead to prerenal impairment of renal function with elevation of blood urea nitrogen and serum creatinine concentrations, and even metabolic acidosis. Fasting blood glucose concentration is often low.

Plasma cortisol levels are usually low. In the presence of an acute stress, however, they may be normal, not increased as they would be in normal subjects in this situation. *In any event when the presence of acute adrenocortical insufficiency is suspected, do not await the results of plasma cortisol determinations before in-*

stituting glucocorticoid therapy. Such determinations take at least several hours, and in the interim period the untreated insufficiency may progress to a serious degree.

Attempts to document the presence of an underlying primary adrenocortical insufficiency by means of an adrenocorticotropic hormone (ACTH) test or the presence of ACTH deficiency by a metyrapone or an insulin tolerance test should be deferred until the state of acute insufficiency has been relieved.

COMMON COMPLICATIONS

Dehydration and hypotension may lead to oliguria and even severe renal failure. Psychosis may occur in severe acute insufficiency. The hyperkalemia and hyponatremia of aldosterone deficiency may give rise to cardiac arrhythmias and sudden death.

PITFALLS IN DIAGNOSIS

It should be emphasized that large doses of glucocorticoid may aid in the relief of shock from a number of causes (e.g., gram-negative septicemia). Hence, it should not be concluded that such patients have an underlying chronic adrenocortical insufficiency without performing one or more of the tests described.

CHRONIC ADRENAL INSUFFICIENCY

By Terence D. Wingert, M.D.
and Patrick J. Mulrow, M.D.
Toledo, Ohio

Chronic adrenal insufficiency may be primary, resulting from disease of the adrenal gland, or secondary to pituitary disease. In both primary and secondary adrenal insufficiency the presenting signs and symptoms may be subtle in the unstressed patient, and a high index of suspicion is necessary to make the diagnosis.

DEFINITION

Primary adrenal insufficiency is defined as an absolute or partial deficiency of glucocorticoids, mineralocorticoids, and adrenal androgens as a result of intrinsic adrenal disease. It can be subdivided into those disorders in which the dominant feature is glucocorticoid deficiency and those in which there is lack of mineralocorticoids only.

Glucocorticoid-deficient states can be congenital or acquired. The congenital causes include congenital adrenal hyperplasia, adrenoleukodystrophy and its variant adrenomyeloneuropathy, X-linked adrenal hypoplasia, and congenital adrenocortical unresponsiveness to adrenocorticotropic hormone (ACTH). Congenital adrenal hyperplasia is a group of syndromes in which there is an inborn error in adrenal enzyme synthesis that results in cortisol deficiency and varying degrees of androgenization. We will not discuss these syndromes further as they are covered elsewhere in this book. (See article on Congenital Adrenal Hyperplasia.) Adrenoleukodystrophy and adrenomyeloneuropathy are diseases that involve the nervous system as well as the adrenal cortex. X-linked adrenal hypoplasia and congenital adrenocortical unresponsiveness to ACTH usually present very early in childhood. Addison's disease is a term now used to define adrenal insufficiency from any acquired cause that leads to destruction of the adrenal cortex.

Hypoaldosteronism can also be a congenital or an acquired disorder. Congenital deficiency of aldosterone is usually manifested in infancy and is the result of an enzyme block. A similar syndrome, called pseudohypoaldosteronism, also occurs; in this disorder there is a congenital deficiency in receptors in the kidney for aldosterone. The secretion of aldosterone is normal or increased, but the kidney is unable to respond. Acquired hypoaldosteronism is a condition associated with a low plasma renin activity that is often described as the hyporeninemic hypoaldosteronism syndrome. It is frequently accompanied by hyperkalemia. The syndrome occurs primarily in adults and is by far the most common cause of hypoaldosteronism. The typical patient is an elderly diabetic individual with mild renal insufficiency.

Secondary adrenal insufficiency results in a loss of glucocorticoid and androgen production by the adrenal gland due to a reduction of ACTH secretion. Basal aldosterone is preserved in secondary adrenal insufficiency, since the main control of aldosterone secretion is the renin-angiotensin system.

PATHOGENESIS

Adrenoleukodystrophy and adrenomyeloneuropathy are disorders that are thought to be due to a metabolic defect in long-chain fatty acid metabolism. The exact enzymatic basis for this abnormality remains unknown. Adrenoleukodystrophy is a disease of childhood characterized by rapdily progressive neurologic deficits resulting in blindness, quadriparesis and dementia. Adrenomyeloneuropathy occurs in adulthood and is characterized by slowly progressive paraparesis and distal symmetric polyneuropathy. Both have adrenal insufficiency. Adrenoleukodystrophy and adrenomyeloneuropathy have been described in the same kindred. At the present time the disease is thought to be inherited as a single X-linked genetic defect that results in a varying spectrum of clinical presentations.

Congenital X-linked adrenal hypoplasia is a syndrome that presents at varying times, usually in the first year of life. There are several types of X-linked congenital adrenal hypoplasia that have been delineated based on the time of presentation. In Type 1, infants present at birth with signs and symptoms of adrenal insufficiency. It is believed that these patients have a true aplasia of the adrenal glands. Type 2 consists of patients who are well at birth and appear to have normal adrenal function at that time; the secretory function of the fetal adrenal is believed to be normal. Symptoms develop at 1 to 3 weeks of life when the fetal adrenal tissue is involuting and there is no organogenesis of the adult zone of the adrenal gland. Type 3 includes those infants who present several months after birth with adrenal insufficiency, which suggests that the adult zone of the adrenal gland functions initially but later loses function. Patients with congenital adrenal hypoplasia have loss of both glucocorticoid and mineralocorticoid function.

Congenital adrenal unresponsiveness to ACTH is characterized by symptoms of glucocorticoid deficiency but not mineralocorticoid deficiency. The primary abnormality is thought to be a defect at the ACTH receptor or postreceptor site in the adrenal gland. Although aldosterone secretion is normal, aldosterone response to ACTH is absent. The inheritance of this syndrome appears to be autosomal recessive.

In Addison's disease there is destruction of adrenal tissue that results in all three zones of the adrenal cortex being destroyed, with the subsequent reduction of glucocorticoid, mineralocorticoid, and adrenal androgen secretion. Historically, tuberculosis of the adrenal was the most common cause of Addison's disease and was the classic form described by Thomas Addison in 1849. At the present time, idiopathic adrenal atrophy accounts for most cases of Addison's disease. The evidence suggests that idiopathic atrophy of the adrenals represents an autoimmune destruction, as antiadrenal antibodies are commonly found, and the adrenal disease often presents with other endocrine gland hypofunction such as Hashimoto's thyroiditis, diabetes mellitus, pernicious anemia, and gonadal atrophy. Adrenal insufficiency, hypoparathyroidism, and candidiasis is a familial syndrome observed in children.

Other processes that can lead to destruction of the adrenal glands and the clinical presentation of Addison's disease include fungal infections endemic to certain geographic areas, granulomatous destruction of the adrenal gland, amyloidosis, hemochromatosis, and metastatic carcinoma. Adrenal hemorrhage has recently been recognized as a cause of primary adrenal insufficiency. It usually is anticoagulant-related and is seen in patients with shock. The hypotension produces necrosis of the corticomedullary junction of the adrenal gland. In a setting of stress and anticoagulant therapy, a hypotensive episode with subsequent necrosis could lead to hemorrhage of the adrenal gland when resolution of hypotension is followed by reperfusion. Adrenal hemorrhage may occur spontaneously in children. Primary adrenal insufficiency also follows adrenalectomy for Cushing's disease, breast carcinoma, or treatment with mitotane (o,p'–DDD), a drug that destroys the zona fasciculata and zone reticularis, leading to glucocorticoid deficiency.

Congenital hypoaldosteronism is very rare, but acquired hypoaldosteronism is quite common in adults. This acquired deficiency is often seen in association with diabetic nephropathy or other causes of mild renal insufficiency. The exact pathogenesis is not understood, but the disorder is mainly due to an impairment of renin secretion. Nonsteroidal anti-inflammatory drugs may inhibit renin release and produce the syndrome.

Secondary adrenal insufficiency is most commonly due to destruction of the pituitary from pituitary adenomas and is usually associated with deficiencies of several pituitary hormones. A number of other diseases can cause deficiency of pituitary hormone secretion and are discussed in detail elsewhere (see article on Hypopituitarism). Chronic exogenous glucocorticoid treatment may suppress the pituitary-adrenal axis and result in adrenal atrophy. Occasionally, adrenal hypofunction persists for several months after the steroid therapy is discontinued.

PRESENTING SIGNS AND SYMPTOMS

Patients with chronic, primary adrenal insufficiency that involves both glucocorticoids and mineralocorticoids present with weight loss, dehydration, anorexia, nausea and vomiting, fatigue, muscle wasting, hypoglycemia, and postural dizziness. These symptoms are nonspecific and can be seen in other disorders. A more classic sign is darkening of the skin. Typically the pigmentation is most conspicuous on the exposed parts of the body, such as the face and hands. The pigmentation on the hands is most marked over the knuckles and the creases of the palms. It is also prominent on the nipples, in the axilla, and on areas subject to pressure. Pigmentation of the buccal mucosa is less prominent, but when present it is patchy and blue-black in color. Another important clinical sign is postural hypotension, which is present in most patients.

The syndrome of congenital adrenocortical unresponsiveness to ACTH shows the same cutaneous pigmentation, muscular weakness, and hypoglycemia but is also associated with convulsions and feeding problems early in life. In patients with this disorder, dehydration is less likely to be found, as aldosterone secretion is normal.

Those patients with chronic aldosterone insufficiency generally present with hyperkalemia without clinical manifestations but may have sufficient sodium wasting to develop hypovolemia and hypotension.

The striking clinical difference noted in secondary adrenal insufficiency is lack of increased pigmentation. Indeed, many of these patients lose their ability to tan from sun exposure. Another distinguishing clinical feature is the absence of postural hypotension in most patients. Since basal aldosterone level is normal, these patients do not become volume depleted.

LABORATORY FINDINGS

Routine laboratory studies that are suggestive evidence for primary adrenal insufficiency include hyponatremia and hyperkalemia. The serum sodium level is seldom less than 120 mEq/l and the serum potassium is seldom greater than 7.0 mEq/l. The hyponatremia is accompanied by an elevated urinary sodium excretion. Other routine laboratory findings include an elevated blood urea nitrogen (BUN), a low glucose level, mild acidemia with the bicarbonate concentration usually between 15 and 20 mEq/l, and occasionally an elevated serum calcium level. The routine complete blood count shows a mild normocytic, normochromic anemia, increased number of eosinophils, and a relative lymphocytosis.

To confirm a diagnosis of primary adrenal insufficiency, laboratory studies should document low cortisol production and an increased plasma ACTH concentration, or a failure of cortisol secretion to increase after ACTH administration. The plasma cortisol and ACTH levels should be measured simultaneously, preferably in the morning to avoid confusion from the diurnal rhythm of ACTH and cortisol. A cortisol level that is very low while the ACTH level is very high represents a state in which the adrenal cortex is unable to respond to ACTH. There are still some difficulties with measurement of plasma ACTH levels, and the clinician must be familiar with the work of the laboratory doing the measurement. At the present time, an ACTH infusion test should still be performed in every patient in whom the diagnosis is not obvious to document a failure to respond to exogenous ACTH.

Older measurements of nonspecific urinary steroid metabolites have given way to newer specific plasma steroid immunoassays; however, measurement of urinary 17-hydroxycorticosteroids by the Porter-Silber method continues to have a place in the laboratory evaluation of the adrenal. This test measures some of the end products of cortisol metabolism in a relatively simple and reproducible way. When the urinary 17-hydroxycorticosteroids are low, chronic adrenal insufficiency is present.

Ideally, we would like to diagnose chronic adrenal insufficiency before it has advanced to complete failure and the patient has lost the ability or reserve to meet the stresses of everyday life. This requires dynamic endocrine testing. The first test usually performed is the ACTH stimulation test. The rapid ACTH test is easy to perform, without discomfort to the patient, and reliably predicts the integrated hypothalamic-pituitary-adrenal response. Some have believed that corticotropin administration tests only the function of the adrenal cortex and not the hypothalamic-pituitary part of the axis. With the rapid ACTH test, the adrenal cannot respond unless it has previously been primed by the central part of the axis. It is performed by administering 0.25 mg of synthetic ACTH after determining baseline cortisol level and repeating the cortisol measurement at 60 min after injection. This stimulated plasma cortisol level should be greater than 20 μg/dl and have an increment of greater than 10 μg/dl over the baseline. A patient with a borderline result should have further evaluation of the hypothalamic-pituitary-adrenal axis.

If there is no response to the rapid ACTH test, a longer ACTH stimulation is done to determine if the chronic adrenal insufficiency is primary or secondary in orgin. This test is performed by infusing 0.25 mg of ACTH over 8 hours or administering 80 units of ACTH gel intramuscularly. Again, the plasma cortisol level at the end of 8 hours should be two to three times the baseline, with an absolute value greater than 20 μg/dl.

In certain cases of chronic secondary adrenal insufficiency, the adrenal gland is sluggish and a more prolonged ACTH stimulation is necessary. A prolonged ACTH test is done by measuring the urinary 17-hydroxycorticosteroids on the second day of a 48-hour infusion of ACTH (40 units of ACTH in 500 ml of normal saline over 12 hours for four consecutive periods), and the result should be greater than 10 mg/24 hours. Patients with primary adrenal insufficiency do not respond to prolonged infusion whereas those with secondary adrenal insufficiency do.

Insulin-induced hypoglycemia is uncomfortable for the patient and requires strict physician supervision throughout the test, which makes it time-consuming, but it is the most acceptable test of the response of the hypothalamic-pituitary-adrenal axis to stress. Blood sampling is performed at 0, 30, 45 and 90 minutes after an intravenous injection of rapid-acting insulin in doses 0.05 to 0.15 units/kg body weight. For the test to be interpretable, the plasma glucose level must fall to less than half of the baseline and ideally to less than 40 mg/dl. A normal response is for the plasma cortisol to have an increment of 5 μg/dl and a maximum level greater than 20 μg/dl. Replacement doses of adrenal steroids are not given on the morning of testing. The metyrapone test is rarely done; it is not a reliable indicator of the response to stress, as it merely assesses the feedback mechanism.

Radiologic examinations that should be performed for primary adrenal insufficiency include an abdominal x-ray to search for adrenal calcifications, often suggestive of adrenal tuberculosis. A tuberculin skin test may also be helpful. If secondary adrenal insufficiency is suspected, skull x-rays, sellar tomograms, and a computed tomographic (CT) scan of the pituitary area may be indicated.

A diagnosis of hypoaldosteronism can be made when the plasma aldosterone level is low while the plasma renin level is high. In patients suspected of having hyporeninemic hypoaldosteronism, stimulation of the renin-angiotensin-aldosterone system should be attempted. The furosemide (Lasix) stimulation test is the most commonly used method. Furosemide, 40 mg, either orally or intravenously, is administered and the patient ambulates for 2 to 4 hours before blood is drawn for measurement of plasma renin activity and aldosterone. Low levels despite stimulation with volume depletion and upright posture confirm the diagnosis.

PITFALLS IN DIAGNOSIS

The most common pitfall in diagnosing chronic adrenal insufficiency is not to consider the diagnosis at all. The nonspecific symptoms and physical signs often are ascribed to stress or to a temporary illness, such as influenza. The mild hyperkalemia or hyponatremia, if present, may be overlooked. With a high index of suspicion and the use of dynamic endocrine screening tests, the diagnosis of chronic adrenal insufficiency can readily be made.

CUSHING'S SYNDROME

By Peter H. Forsham, M.D.
and J. Blake Tyrrell, M.D.
San Francisco, California

DEFINITION

Cushing's syndrome is induced by chronic overproduction of cortisol and related glucocorticoids by the adrenal cortex. Excess and long-term administration of glucocorticoid or adrenocorticotropic hormone (ACTH) may produce an identical iatrogenic variety of the syndrome. The excess glucocorticoid production may derive either from excess ACTH production by the anterior pituitary (Cushing's disease) or by production in ectopic sites by ACTH-producing tumors (Cushing's syndrome), or it may derive directly from andrenocortical overactivity in an andrenocortical adenoma, rarely in a nodular hyperplasia or in a carcinoma. Cushing's syndrome must be suspected in any patient revealing inappropriate truncal obesity and a moon face, muscle weakness, hypertension, purplish cutaneous striae, purpura, hirsutism, or glycosuria.

INCIDENCE

Cushing's syndrome is found in approximately 1 in 5000 hospital admissions; most cases arise between the ages of 20 and 50 years. Specifically, Cushing's disease, as opposed to the syndrome, is the most frequent type, constituting about 70 per cent of reported cases. It is more common in women than in men (ratio, 5:1). Cushing's syndrome may result from adenoma or carcinoma of the adrenals. It occurs in about two per million population per year with a mean age of about 40 years at onset. Adrenal adenomas are much more common in females than in males, as are adrenocortical carcinomas. Considering all types of tumors of the adrenal cortex, however, including nonsecreting ones, the overall incidence is higher in males.

CLASSIFICATION

Cushing's syndrome refers to the clinical manifestation produced by hypercortisolism irrespective of its cause. These are listed in Table 1. In fact, with the widespread use of glucocorticoids in therapy, iatrogenic Cushing's syndrome is more frequent than the spontaneous type.

Cushing's disease with bilateral adrenocortical hyperplasia due to ACTH excess of pituitary origin is the most common type (70 per cent). Most of these are due to pituitary *microadenomas.* The pituitary microadenomas may be intrapituitary and vary in size from 2 to 10 mm in diameter. The histology is predominantly that of a chromophobe adenoma, rarely a basophilic adenoma, and occasionally mixed. Although usually benign and small, they may on rare occasion expand above the tegmentum sellae and produce changes in the visual fields (bilateral hemianopia). There are rare cases of chromophobe-basophilic pituitary hyperplasia, presumably due to excess corticotropin-releasing factors. Sellar enlargement, so common for other pituitary tumors, is found in less than 8 per cent of cases, representing macroadenomas.

The *ectopic ACTH syndrome* with bilateral adrenocortical hyperplasia is responsible for Cushing's syndrome in about 17 per cent of cases and is due to the production of ACTH or a related abnormal polypeptide by various carcinomas. The most common is oat cell carcinoma of the lung, accounting for some 50 per cent of cases. There is a 3:1 preponderance of males, which is beginning to change with increased smoking by women.

Recently, all lung cancers of varying types were shown to have significant concentrations of ACTH, which is mostly in the form of "big ACTH" or the large precursors of the more biologically active ACTH. Yet only 2 per cent of patients with lung cancer show overt Cushing's syndrome.

Some lung and pancreatic tumors have been found to produce corticotropin-releasing hormone (CRH) and related polypeptides, so that patients with ectopic ACTH have a high circulating level of ACTH in spite of high levels of cortisol, which would normally suppress pituitary ACTH as well as, in some cases, the ACTH from the ectopic tumor.

Other sites of ectopic excess ACTH production are shown in Table 2.

ADRENAL TUMORS

Adrenal cortical adenomas are characterized by hypersecretion of predominantly cortisol, and circulating plasma ACTH levels are suppressed. This typically leads to hypoplasia of the contralateral adrenal cortex, a significant diagnostic finding. The symp-

Table 1. Etiology of Cushing's Syndrome

	Approximate Incidence (Per Cent)
ACTH-dependent	
Cushing's disease	66
Ectopic ACTH syndrome	17
ACTH-independent	
Adrenal adenoma	10
Adrenal carcinoma	7
Total	100

ACTH = Adrenocorticotropic hormone.

Table 2. Tumors Responsible for the Ectopic ACTH Syndrome

Oat cell carcinoma of the lung (50% of cases)
Thymoma
Carcinoid tumors (lung, gut, pancreas, ovary)
Pancreatic islet cell tumors
Medullary carcinoma of the thyroid
Pheochromocytoma and related tumors

toms are usually those of Cushing's disease, since only cortisol is in excess, and there is no increase in either androgens or aldosterone.

Adrenocortical carcinomas are relatively more common in children. The hypersecretion involves adrenal cortical steroids in general. Thus, cortisol and adrenal androgen levels are always elevated, and there may be increased secretion of aldosterone, deoxycorticosterone, or estrogens. Not only are plasma and urinary cortisol levels markedly elevated, but in addition levels of dehydroepiandrosterone (DHEA) (free and sulfated) and urinary 17-hydroxysteroids and 17-ketosteroids are elevated as well. Features of androgen excess predominate, with or without virilism in women. (Unlike pure Cushing's disease, with adrenal carcinomas hypertension and hypokalemia are marked, owing to the excess of aldosterone and its precursors as well as deoxycorticosterone.)

The tumors are not always in the adrenal cortex but may be located in the ovaries, testes, or perirenal areas that orginated as embryonic remnants.

SYMPTOMS AND SIGNS

Obesity

This most common manifestation (see Table 3) is associated with initial weight gain that tends to level off. It affects the cheeks, the neck and the abdomen, with sparing of the extremities. Central obesity is most common in children. A red, round (moon) face is striking. Fat pads are found in the supraclavicular and dorsal cervical areas producing what is known as the "buffalo hump." Obesity is rarely absent; if it is it usually spares the patients with carcinoma or malnutrition but leaves the telltale red cheeks.

Skin Changes

These are typical of the disease. Red cheeks, caused by atrophy of the skin revealing the subcutaneous blood vessels, are combined with easy bruisability over the entire body. The purpura is caused mainly by increased fragility of small blood vessels and their inability to constrict when traumatized. This is because of poor perivascular muscle owing to a negative nitrogen balance produced by excess cortisol. Striae occur in up to 75 per cent of patients. They are most marked on the abdomen, but they also occur on the thighs, buttocks, arms, axillae, and breasts. They are red to purple and depressed below the skin surfaces; this can be felt by pressing the finger over the striae. The depression results from loss of underlying connective tissue. These striae should not be confused with the white ones that occur in rapid growth situations, such as on the breasts of young girls at puberty, radiating from the areola, or on the thighs or buttocks of people becoming rapidly obese. In addition, wound healing is very poor.

Melanin pigmentation is not found in Cushing's disease at all; however, it may be present in carcinoma or in the ectopic ACTH syndromes, and it is characteristic of Nelson's syndrome, in which an ACTH-producing tumor follows total adrenalectomy (which was formerly performed for treatment of Cushing's disease).

Patients with Cushing's syndrome and a defective immune defense system are prone to mucocutaneous infections, including tinea versicolor, candidiasis, and nail involvement (onychomycoses).

Hirsutism

Hirsutism is found in some 80 per cent of patients. It is most noticeable in women who develop facial hirsutism in male pattern of distribution; however, hair growth is generalized over the abdomen, breasts, chest, and upper thighs. Hirsutism is commonly associated with seborrhea and acne. Virilization involving genital hirsutism is associated with definite enlargement of the clitoris only in adrenal carcinoma and then in no more than 20 per cent of cases. Menstrual disorders are common; after initial hypermenorrhea, amenorrhea then follows. In men there is decreased fertility with soft testes and lack of libido.

Hypertension

Hypertension occurs in 85 per cent of cases and involves elevation of diastolic pressure in over 50 per cent and of systolic pressure in practically all patients. It is associated with increased atherosclerosis. The cause of death in untreated Cushing's syndrome

Table 3. Clinical Features of Cushing's Syndrome in Order of Frequency

	Frequency (Per Cent)
Obesity	94
Facial plethora	84
Hirsutism	80
Menstrual disorders	78
Hypertension	85
Muscular weakness	58
Back pain	58
Striae	52
Acne	40
Psychologic symptoms	40
Bruising	36
Congestive heart failure	22
Edema	18
Renal calculi	16
Headache	14
Polyuria-polydipsia	10
Hyperpigmentation	6

is due to cardiovascular pathology in 45 per cent of cases.

Muscle Weakness and Osteoporosis

The muscles are weak and atrophic. The quadriceps femoris group is so weakened in advanced Cushing's syndrome that the patient cannot rise from a chair while extending the arms above the head. This is due to generalized excessive catabolism. Cushing's syndrome is invariably accompanied by severe osteoporosis associated with back pain. Rib fractures are frequent, and compression fractures of the vertebral bodies occur in the lumbar and thoracic areas. Using improved radiologic methods, the incidence of osteoporosis may be put at 80 per cent, and that of various bone fractures at about 30 per cent. Renal calculi secondary to hypercalciuria, with or without renal colic, are found in 16 per cent of cases.

Thirst and Polyuria

These frequently are found as a result of hyperglycemia and diabetes mellitus, which occur in about 20 per cent, whereas 80 per cent show only an abnormal glucose tolerance test. The polyuria is also partly due to the natural antagonism of cortisol to pituitary antidiuretic hormone.

Psychologic Disturbances

These occur in over two thirds of all patients. Patients always show increased irritability and emotional instability. Euphoria is dominant, and patients may become manic. Sleep disorders are manifested by insomnia or early awakening with great anxiety. Depression and poor memory and concentration may also be seen.

The psychiatric syndrome may advance to frank psychosis with delusions, hallucinations, and, rarely, paranoia. Suicide must be guarded against in these patients. Reduction of excess cortisol levels leads to remission in all of these psychotic disorders except in a few patients in whom the mental disease persists after establishment of a normal cortisol level.

Some of the less frequent symptoms and signs of Cushing's syndrome are given in Table 3. Of these, congestive heart failure is the most noteworthy and responds rapidly to adequate diuresis and blood pressure lowering medications.

GENERAL LABORATORY FINDINGS

A tendency to polycythemia is noted. Total white blood cell count is slightly elevated. The percentage of lymphocytes is subnormal, eosinophil levels are depressed or absent, and the total eosinophil count is less than 100 cu mm. Electrolyte balance rarely shows an alkalosis with a low serum potassium level; this is found especially in the ectopic ACTH syndrome or with adrenal cortical carcinoma.

Serum calcium level is normal; serum phosphorus level is low; hypercalciuria is present in nearly half of the cases.

Fasting hyperglycemia may be present in up to 15 per cent of patients, but postprandial hyperglycemia is more common. Glucose tolerance tests (totally unnecessary) will reveal elevation in glucose levels in 80 per cent of cases, but fasting blood glucose level remains normal because of increased hyperinsulinism in the presence of excess cortisol.

Electrocardiography may reveal hypertensive, ischemic, and low potassium changes of no specific diagnostic value.

Routine x-ray studies may reveal vertebral compression fractures, greenstick rib fractures, renal calculi, and various degrees of cardiomegaly. Routine anteroposterior and lateral skull films rarely reveal sellar enlargement, but CT scans often reveal a microadenoma, if present.

TESTS TO ESTABLISH PRESENCE OF CUSHING'S SYNDROME

Dexamethasone Suppression Test (1 mg)

In this test 1 mg of dexamethasone is administered by mouth at 11:00 P.M., and blood is drawn for plasma cortisol determinations at about 8:00 A.M. with minimal exertion by the patient. A plasma cortisol level of less than 5 μg/dl eliminates Cushing's syndrome for all intents and purposes. A plasma cortisol level above 10 μg/dl makes the diagnosis almost certain. The gray area between 5 and 10 μg/dl requires a repeat test under resting conditions.

False-positive responses may be obtained in obesity, in which case 2 mg of dexamethasone may be necessary. High-estrogen states such as occur in patients taking oral contraceptives or receiving estrogen therapy in general or during pregnancy also produce false-positive results. Estrogens artificially increase plasma cortisol by raising the level of cortisol binding globulin (CBG). Levels of 40 to 80 μg/dl of cortisol may be found with the overnight 1-mg dexamethasone suppression test, but when compared with the level on a previous day without treatment, a normal 60 per cent decrease may be seen. Alternatively, the test can be repeated after the patient has discontinued taking estrogens for at least 2 months.

Acute or chronic illness may cause elevation of glucocorticoid secretion naturally, and the secretion may not be suppressible by 1 mg of dexamethasone. The study must be repeated after the acute illness or chronic stress is over. In a few patients with chronic and acute alcoholism, all tests for Cushing's syndrome may be positive, and the tests must be repeated when the patient has stopped drinking alcohol.

Endogenous depression leads to increased cortisol secretion with all of the chemical signs of Cushing's syndrome, including a positive dexamethasone suppression test. Such patients can be differentiated from those with true Cushing's syndrome of any type because they will show an increase in plasma cortisol levels in response to insulin-induced hypoglycemia, which patients with Cushing's syndrome do not do.

Drugs such as phenytoin, phenobarbital, and primidone may cause falsely low results for the dexamethasone suppression test, suggesting Cushing's syndrome. The patient should have discontinued taking all such drugs for at least 1 week before the test is performed.

24-Hour Urinary Free Cortisol Level

This is the most specific test of all for the diagnosis of Cushing's syndrome. A 24-hour sample is collected on an outpatient basis, being careful to instruct the patient to void first and then collect every drop of urine, including that voided the same time the next day. For stability, addition of one tablespoon of white vinegar to the specimen container in case no other preservative is available is advisable. A free urinary cortisol test requires an accurate 24-hour collection. Urine creatinine level may be measured at the same time; in women it should be of the order of 600 mg per day, in men 1000 mg per day, both lower than those found in normal subjects because of the reduced muscle mass. If there is a marked deviation from these values, the urine was not collected properly over 24 hours and cortisol values must be corrected.

There are no false-positive or false-negative results with this test. Whereas obesity will result in high levels of urinary 17-hydroxycorticoids, free urinary cortisol level is normal in obesity.

TESTS TO ESTABLISH SPECIFIC TYPES OF CUSHING'S SYNDROME

Cushing's Disease

This disorder is characteristically found in women between 20 and 50 years old, is slowly progressive, and is associated with obesity with specific fat distribution but with limited manifestations of androgenicity, such as acne and hirsutism. Finding a high urinary free cortisol level (above 100 μg per 24 hours) strongly suggests the diagnosis. ACTH excess due to an adrenal or other carcinoma may be ruled out with the *5-mg overnight dexamethasone suppression test.* It will show a 50 per cent reduction in plasma cortisol level compared to a previous day. Plasma ACTH determinations are used only to rule out other causes of Cushing's syndrome. Although values tend to be high in these conditions, they overlap with the normal range (20 to 100 pg/ml) and values in Cushing's disease (40 to 200 pg/ml).

Ectopic ACTH Syndrome (Systemic Carcinoma)

This is found predominantly in men, with a maximum incidence between 40 and 60 years of age. Weakness, hypertension, and diabetes predominate. Hyperpigmentation, hypokalemia, and alkalosis are common, together with weight loss and anemia. A rapid onset of the syndrome is characteristic, with marked elevation in both glucocorticoids and androgens. Search for a primary systemic tumor must be pushed hard. With ectopic ACTH syndrome due to bronchial carcinoids and other, more benign tumors (benign systemic tumor) the onset of the disease is much slower, and differentiation from ordinary pituitary-dependent Cushing's disease is difficult.

The 1-mg dexamethasone overnight suppression test will show *non-suppression of ACTH secretion*, and plasma ACTH levels will be very high, from 200 to 10,000 pg/ml; only rarely are values below 200 pg/ml noted. Even with the 5-mg dose overnight dexamethasone suppression test, there will be no lowering of plasma cortisol level. In 90 per cent of cases a primary malignant tumor has been found, and unlike all other cases of Cushing's syndrome anemia will be present.

A problem in diagnosis of ACTH-dependent Cushing's syndrome is *episodic hypercortisolism,* which causes spontaneous fluctuations from day to day in plasma cortisol levels. Repeated testing and highly specialized catheterization studies to ascertain high ACTH levels in various parts of the venous system are necessary to establish the source of ACTH in these very few cases.

Adrenal Adenoma

In this syndrome, glucocorticoid excess predominates greatly over androgenic excess, and thus the signs of hyperandrogenicity are few and mild. The 24-hour urinary free cortisol level will be much above 100 μg/24 hours. Morning ACTH levels will be below 20 pg/ml as a rule. The perirenal CT scan will show an adrenal tumor on one side and only fat on the other.

Adrenocortical Adenocarcinoma

Adrenal carcinomas produce a rapid onset of excessive glucocorticoid, androgen, and mineralocorticoid secretion and are rapidly progressive and fatal. Both cortisol and androgens (17-ketosteroids) are elevated. Hypokalemia, abdominal pain, and a palpable mass in the costovertebral angle are common. Pulmonary and liver metastases occur early. Cushingoid symptoms, together with hyperandrogenicity and little catabolic evidence, suggest this diagnosis. A low plasma ACTH level, less than 20 pg/ml, is highly suggestive. The diagnosis is made by perirenal CT scan, as with an adenoma. A more irregular outline of the mass will suggest a carcinoma.

PITFALLS IN DIAGNOSIS

Laboratory tests are 90 per cent successful, provided that collection of the plasma or urine specimen is accurate and the specimen is adequately preserved by refrigeration. Also, the patient should have discontinued taking drugs for at least 2 days before testing.

Obesity must be ruled out as the sole cause of the symptoms and signs noted. Patients with severe mental depression and anxiety must be identified initially, since they have many of the signs of and positive test results for Cushing's syndrome. Patients taking glucocorticoids surreptitiously, often individuals from the medical professions, usually have no hirsutism and show a rapid decrease in urinary free cortisol level after being in hospital without the drug for a few days. Such patients can be protected from collapse by being given 2 mg of dexamethasone every morning.

DETECTION OF PITUITARY ADENOMAS

This is carried out by high resolution computed tomographic (CT) scanning of the sella turcica. Pituitary adenomas as small as 2 to 5 mm in diameter can be detected. While this is successful with only 85 per cent of all microadenomas, it is still the method of choice to finalize the diagnosis. If the endocrine tests strongly suggest the presence of hypercortisolism, a pituitary transsphenoidal exploration must be carried out regardless of negative CT/scans. Oftentimes a tumor is found that was not detected by scanning. On the other hand, pituitary exploration based on a positive high-resolution CT scan may, in up to 5 per cent of patients, fail to reveal a pituitary adenoma. In that case, total hypophysectomy should be performed, followed by treatment for Addison's disease and with thyroxine.

Macroadenomas may be seen on a lateral film of the sella turcica, which reveals slight ballooning and depression of the floor on one side. A definite demonstration of this can be made by a polytomogram. This may show erosion of the floor with invasion of the sphenoid sinus, whereas the CT scan will document suprasella extension or the presence of a partially empty sella turcica.

LOCALIZATION OF ADRENAL MASSES

An ultrasonogram of the renal region will clearly demonstrate one of three conditions: a unilateral tumor with contralateral atrophy; a unilateral tumor with a smaller contralateral adrenal; or small adrenals resulting from an extra-adrenal tumor in the testis or ovary that is not in the field of the scan.

CONCLUSIONS

During a period of over 35 years of active research on pituitary-adrenal pathophysiology in humans, we have witnessed an enormous increase in the complexity of the field. Yet with concurrent advances in diagnostic methodology, precise diagnosis has become ever more simplified and definitive. The breakthrough came with the early recognition that contrary to Cushing's belief that the disease named after him was of pituitary origin, the adrenal cortical hormones are the final culprit. The ability to estimate their levels accurately in body fluids opened up a new era. Then development of the immunoassay of ACTH completed the hormonal diagnostic armamentarium. As the rather primitive radiology of the pituitary and the adrenals was replaced by CT scans and sonography, it became possible to localize the responsible tumors and hyperplastic glands. Joining this with the now highly specific hormonal determinations, an accurate diagnosis can be achieved in over 90 per cent of pituitary-adrenal problems. Most of the procedures are noninvasive and can bring no harm to the patient.

PRIMARY ALDOSTERONISM

By James C. Melby, M.D.
and George T. Griffing, M.D.
Boston, Massachusetts

DEFINITION

"Primary aldosteronism" is a generic term for disorders in which chronic aldosterone excess is independent of the renin-angiotensin system, resulting in hypertension and, usually, hypokalemia. Estimates of the incidence of primary aldosteronism vary from 0.5 to 2.0 per cent of the hypertensive population, with a prevalence of 115,000 to 460,000 cases in the United States at present. The peak age distribution of diagnosis is between the third and fifth decades, with more women being affected than men in a preponderance of 3:1.

Aldosterone overproduction results in hypertension, potassium and magnesium depletion, and suppression of plasma renin activity. Hypersecretion of aldosterone is semiautonomous in primary aldosteronism, with the exeception of patients with glucocorticoid-remediable hyperaldosteronism. Primary aldosteronism is usually due to an aldosterone-producing solitary adenoma (Conn's syndrome), but it may also be due to bilateral micronodular or macronodular hyperplasia of the adrenal cortex (idiopathic hyperaldosteronism) or, rarely, aldosterone-producing adrenocortical carcinoma (Table 1).

PATHOPHYSIOLOGY

Aldosterone stimulates active sodium transport in the distal convoluted tubule and collecting duct cells of the kidney. With enhanced sodium resorption, reciprocal movement of potassium and hydrogen ions into urine occurs leading to potassium depletion. Increased sodium resorption by the kidney leads to expansion of extracellular fluid volume and elevated total body sodium content. Expansion of the extracellular fluid volume and intravascular volume exceeds 2 l, and the volume may expand by 4 l. This expansion of the extracellular fluid volume is limited by the renal counter-regulatory mechanism of inhibition of proximal tubular sodium resorption, a phenomenon which has been referred to as mineralocorticoid "escape."

Expansion of intravascular blood volume, and perhaps altered cation metabolism per se (K^+, Mg^{++} depletion), leads to development of hypertension. Many, but not all, patients with primary aldosteronism ex-

Table 1. Classification of Primary Aldosteronism (Surgical Cases)

	Frequency (Per Cent)
Aldosterone-producing adenoma (Conn's syndrome)	~65
Idiopathic hyperaldosteronism (bilateral adrenocortical hyperplasia)	~34
Aldosterone-producing adrenocortical carcinoma	<1
Glucocorticoid-suppressible aldosteronism	<1

hibit increased extracellular fluid volume, increased exchangeable sodium, and high cardiac output. Increased extracellular fluid volume and exchangeable sodium directly suppress juxtaglomerular cell activity in the kidneys, with resultant low plasma renin activity (PRA).

CLINICAL FEATURES OF PRIMARY ALDOSTERONISM

All the signs and symptoms of severe, long-standing hypertension have been observed in patients with primary aldosteronism. There is no clinical feature of the hypertension of primary aldosteronism that is distinctive. The most obvious biochemical manifestation of primary aldosteronism is hypokalemia due to excessive renal potassium wastage. Spontaneous hypokalemia with primary aldosteronism is observed in 80 to 90 per cent of patients, and easily provokable hypokalemia is seen in the remainder. The degree of hypokalemia is related, in part, to sodium intake. More than 50 per cent of hypertensive patients who exhibit hypokalemia have primary aldosteronism. Sodium restriction leads to potassium retention and improves hypokalemic manifestations. Conversely, sodium excess promotes renal potassium wastage in primary aldosteronism and can lead to profound hypokalemia. A substantial portion of patients with spontaneous hypokalemia admit to no symptoms. Nocturnal polyuria and polydipsia are common signs of potassium deficiency. Neuromuscular manifestations, including weakness, paresthesias, intermittent paralysis, visual disturbances, and frank tetany, may wax and wane with variations in potassium balance. In addition, cardiac arrhythmias, potentiation of digoxin toxicity, and sudden death may be associated with hypokalemia in this disorder. Abnormal glucose tolerance associated with insulinopenia is demonstrable in over half the patients, and frank diabetes mellitus may be precipitated in patients genetically susceptible to this disease.

Solitary Aldosterone-Producing Adenoma (Conn's Syndrome)

The most common adrenal lesion responsible for the primary aldosteronism syndrome in surgical cases is a solitary adrenocortical adenoma (65 per cent of cases). The biochemical manifestations are more pronounced in Conn's syndrome; aldosterone biogenesis by the adenoma appears to be only partially autonomous in that plasma aldosterone concentrations still exhibit a circadian rhythm paralleling plasma cortisol and ACTH levels. The diagnosis of primary aldosteronism is made by demonstrating inappropriately raised blood aldosterone concentrations and urinary aldosterone metabolite excretion in the presence of low PRA, both before and after acute induction of negative sodium balance. Following diagnosis, the adrenal lesion must then be identified and localized. If the adrenal lesion is unilateral, treatment is surgical. Unilateral adrenalectomy for the removal of a solitary adenoma results in the disappearance of hypertension for a year or more in 70 per cent and permanently in 50 per cent of patients. Bilateral total adrenalectomy for micronodular or macronodular hyperplasia of the adrenals (idiopathic hyperaldosteronism), on the other hand, results in the disappearance of hypertension in only one third of patients so treated.

Bilateral Adrenocortical Hyperplasia (Idiopathic Hyperaldosteronism)

In this form of primary aldosteronism (idiopathic hyperaldosteronism), both adrenal glands are involved with diffuse micronodular or macronodular changes, or both, in the presence of hyperplasia of the zona glomerulosa. The nodules secrete excessive amounts of aldosterone with resultant arterial hypertension, potassium depletion, and suppression of PRA. Of all patients with primary aldosteronism, perhaps 40 to 60 per cent have the idiopathic type; their biochemical abnormalities may not be as pronounced as in Conn's syndrome; the hypokalemia may be less severe; and the suppression of plasma renin activity may be incomplete. Activation of aldosterone biogenesis by small increments in PRA occurs when these patients stand after prolonged recumbency, and no parallelism can be demonstrated between their plasma aldosterone and cortisol concentrations. Although the cause of idiopathic hyperaldosteronism is unknown, a newly described aldosterone-stimulating factor may be causative. It can be demonstrated that these patients have elevated urinary levels of an aldosterone-stimulating glycoprotein that is approximately 31,000 daltons. This molecule has not been characterized.

Idiopathic hyperaldosteronism differs only in degree from a more ambiguous entity entitled "indeterminate" or "evolving" primary aldosteronism. Fourteen per cent of patients with essential hypertension can be demonstrated to have suppressed PRA and aldosterone levels that are inappropriate for this PRA. The average level of plasma aldosterone is above 13 ng/dl, and urinary aldosterone excretion is normal or slightly elevated in these patients. Furthermore, these patients respond with a lowering of blood pressure when given inhibitors of aldosterone biogenesis, and this antihypertensive response is greater than in other patients with essential hypertension.

Congenital or Juvenile Aldosteronism

Primary aldosteronism in the young is rare (and it is very similar to idiopathic hyperaldosteronism). Usually it is associated with bilateral adrenal glomerulosa hyperplasia, and it may have a familial occurrence. Diagnostic procedures are similar to those for the other forms of primary aldosteronism.

Aldosterone-Producing Adrenocortical Carcinoma

Adrenocortical carcinoma is a rare cause of primary aldosteronism. No more than one dozen cases have been reported, with the incidence in a large series of about 1 per cent of patients with primary aldosteronism. Tumors are often large and identifiable by excretory urography. Other adrenocortical steroids may be secreted by the tumor.

Glucocorticoid-Remediable Hyperaldosteronism

This rare form of primary aldosteronism is associated with bilateral micronodular adrenocortical hyperplasia and is characterized by relief of hypertension and induction of positive potassium balance by administration of glucocorticoids. Dexamethasone-responsive hyperaldosteronism apparently is due to small but measurable increments in plasma ACTH levels without concomitant excessive cortisol secretion. Management involves long-term suppression of ACTH by the administration of small doses of dexamethasone or other long-acting glucocorticoids.

DIAGNOSIS

Primary aldosteronism should be suspected in hypertensive patients who have spontaneous hypokalemia. Also suggestive is development of hypokalemia with diuretic therapy and its persistence after diuretics are stopped, or development of hypokalemia after ingestion of large amounts of sodium chloride. Some patients with primary aldosteronism have normal potassium levels, and this is usually due to sodium depletion associated with dietary sodium restriction.

Therefore, a salt-loading maneuver may be used as a provocative screening test for aldosteronism in hypertensive patients with persistently normal serum potassium levels. When aldosterone secretion is suppressed by salt ingestion in healthy subjects, the distal tubular stimulus to sodium resorption is quickly dissipated, whereas patients with autonomous aldosterone secretion exhibit continued distal tubular sodium resorptive activity in response to a marked increase in the filtered sodium load. Ingestion of sodium in excess of 200 mEq per day (nine 1-gm sodium chloride tablets per day plus dietary sodium) for 4 days does not influence the serum potassium level in the absence of aldosteronism. Patients with aldosteronism exhibit a reduction of serum potassium level to below 3.5 mEq/liter.

In patients suspected of having primary aldosteronism, confirmation of the diagnosis is established by the combination of renin suppression associated with aldosterone excess. Before any tests are undertaken, however, diuretics should be discontinued for 4 weeks and spironolactone for 6 weeks. Antihypertensive sympathetic inhibitors should be discontinued 1 week before patients are studied.

The patient is then admitted to the hospital on a regimen of approximately 130 mEq of sodium per day. The diagnosis of primary aldosteronism is confirmed if the urinary excretion of the aldosterone metabolite is increased in the presence of suppressed PRA (Table 2).

Once the diagnosis of primary aldosteronism has been established, its cause must be determined. The two major causes of primary aldosteronism are (1) aldosterone-producing adenomas and (2) idiopathic hyperaldosteronism. It is important to distinguish these two entities, since their treatments differ markedly. Aldosterone-producing adenomas can be cured by unilateral adrenalectomy, but idiopathic hyperaldosteronism requires medical therapy with aldosterone antagonists. A number of noninvasive and invasive tests are available to differentiate these two disorders (Table 3). Measurements of supine and 4-hour upright plasma aldosterone levels can differentiate these two entities in 90 per cent of patients. Plasma aldosterone measurements made on blood specimens obtained at 8:00 A.M. and noon during the initial studies can be evaluated (see Table 2). In patients with an aldosterone-producing adenoma, plasma aldosterone levels parallel the cortisol and ACTH circadian variations and are, therefore, significantly lower at noon than 8 A.M. Plasma 18-hydroxycorticosterone is sometimes measured with aldosterone. Although its level parallels that of aldosterone, 18-hydroxycorticosterone level is disproportionately elevated (>100 ng/dl) in aldosterone-producing adenomas and this may, therefore, be a more sensitive test.

Adrenal Scintigraphy

Adrenal imaging with NP-59 iodocholesterol (^{131}I-6β-iodomethyl-19-norcholesterol) gives a functional assessment of this disorder, and it can accurately diagnose aldosterone-producing adenomas (APA) in 90 per cent of cases. NP-59 accumulates rapidly in the adrenals, permitting scintigraphy within 1 day of administration. However, adrenal scanning is usually performed after 5 days of dexamethasone pretreatment to reduce ACTH-induced adrenal steroidogenesis.

Asymmetric uptake between the two adrenals during suppression scintiscans is obvious in patients with solitary aldosterone-producing adenomas at 5 days after the tracer is injected. No lateralization is observed in patients with bilateral micronodular or macronodular hyperplasia. NP-59 will supplant adrenal vein catheterization for diagnosis and localization in primary aldosteronism. Adrenal venous aldosterone measurements can be obtained when the results of scintigraphy are ambiguous.

Table 2. Confirmation of Primary Aldosteronism

Discontinue spironolactone (6 weeks), diuretics (4 weeks), and sympathetic inhibitors (1 week).

Unrestricted sodium intake prior to admission (1 week).

Day 1: Admit patient to hospital on liberal sodium intake (> 100 mEq/day). Replace potassium deficit and keep patient recumbent overnight.

Day 2: Draw blood for supine (8:00 A.M.) and 4-hour upright (noon) determinations of plasma aldosterone level, plasma renin activity,* and 18-hydroxycorticosterone levels. Start 24-hour urine collection (8:00 A.M.) for aldosterone or tetrahydroaldosterone determination.†

Day 3: Complete 24-hour urine collection (8:00 A.M.).

*Plasma renin activity (PRA) can also be measured following diuretic stimulation (e.g., furosemide [Lasix], 40 mg P.O.).

†Plasma potassium level should be normal before performing this test.

Adrenal Venous Aldosterone Sampling (Adrenal Venous Catheterization)

Selective adrenal venous sampling for aldosterone is the most accurate test in the differential diagnosis of primary aldosteronism, the usefulness of which depends on the proficiency of the radioangiographer. If the right adrenal vein is routinely entered, the accuracy of comparative adrenal venous aldosterone levels in determining the presence of either an aldosterone-producing adenoma or idiopathic hyperaldosteronism exceeds 95 per cent. Most often, aldosterone levels on the side of a unilateral adenoma are 20 times higher than those in the venous blood from the contralateral gland. Adrenal venography should not be attempted when obtaining specimens for aldosterone measurement because of the high incidence (10 per cent) of corticomedullary hemorrhage due to excessive volumes of dye solution.

The adrenal venous aldosterone concentration is normally 100 to 400 ng/dl. In aldosterone-producing adenoma, the ipsilateral adrenal venous aldosterone concentration is 1000 to 10,000 ng/dl, and more importantly the ratio of ipsilateral to contralateral aldosterone concentrations is usually greater than 10:1. Correct placement of the catheter in the adrenal vein is essential in this procedure. This can be best evaluated by obtaining ACTH-stimulated simultaneous selective adrenal vein cortisol levels. An aldosterone ratio of 10:1 in the presence of bilateral ACTH-induced cortisol responses is diagnostic of an aldosterone-producing adenoma.

Table 3. Localization Tests for Primary Aldosteronism

	Accuracy (Per Cent)
Postural plasma aldosterone and 18-hydroxycorticosterone levels	~ 90
Adrenal iodocholesterol (NP–59) scintigraphy	~ 80
Adrenal CT scanning	?
Adrenal ultrasound	?
Adrenal venous aldosterone sampling	~ 95

PROGNOSIS AND TREATMENT

For treatment of aldosterone-producing adenomas, unilateral adrenalectomy is highly successful when carried out with a posterior incision made through the bed of the twelfth rib. One year postoperatively, 70 per cent of patients are normotensive, but by 5 years postoperatively, only 53 per cent remain normotensive. The restoration of potassium balance, however, is permanent. In idiopathic hyperaldosteronism, bilateral adrenalectomy relieves hypertension in only 33 per cent of cases and has all but been abandoned. Potassium-sparing diuretics, especially amiloride and spironolactone, are effective in restoring potassium balance, and in 50 per cent of the patients also act as anti-hypertensive agents. The remaining 50 per cent of patients require additional antihypertensive drugs.

SECONDARY ALDOSTERONISM (HYPERRENINEMIC HYPERALDOSTERONISM)

"Secondary aldosteronism" is the term used to describe excessive production of aldosterone by the adrenal zona glomerulosa, activated by stimuli outside the adrenal. With the exception of a single entity, the rare syndrome of glucocorticoid-suppressible aldosteronism, secondary aldosteronism results from excessive, prolonged stimulation of angiotensin II production. In general, secondary aldosteronism is characterized by elevated plasma renin activity, plasma angiotensin II levels, and plasma aldosterone concentrations. Aldosterone hypersecretion is appropriate for the degree of activation of the renin-angiotensin system. The heightened activity of the renin-angiotensin system in secondary aldosteronism most often is secondary to events causing reduction of the effective blood volume and extracellular fluid volume, with increasingly negative sodium balance. Secondary aldosteronism must be viewed as a physiologic counterregulatory response to these events, although manifestations of aldosterone overproduction are predominant. Disorders associated with secondary aldosteronism are listed in Table 4.

Secondary aldosteronism is a concomitant of sodium depletion in pregnancy. With sodium depletion, there are increased circulating levels of angiotensin II and increased adrenocortical sensitivity to angiotensin II. Increased renin secretion results, in part, from negative sodium balance, and it is also accompanied by elevated levels of plasma renin substrate, induced by elevated estrogen levels. In pathologic states, secondary aldosteronism leads to varying degrees of potassium depletion and, when edema is present, to positive sodium balance. When secondary aldosteronism accompanies hypertensive disorders in which volume contraction and negative sodium balance coexist, renin hypersecretion is reactive or secondary. On the other hand, the increased

Table 4. Hyperaldosteronism Associated with Elevated Plasma Renin Activity (Hyperreninemic or Secondary Hyperaldosteronism)

A. Without Hypertension
1. Nephrotic syndrome
2. Hepatic cirrhosis with ascites
3. Pregnancy
4. Bartter's syndrome
5. Congestive cardiac failure

B. With Hypertension
1. Primary hyperreninism
   a. Juxtaglomerular cell tumor
   b. Wilms's tumor
2. Secondary hyperreninism
   a. Accelerated hypertension
   b. Essential hypertension (10%)
   c. Hypertension treated with diuretics
   d. Oral contraceptive–induced hypertension
   e. Pregnancy

synthesis and release of renin by renin-producing tumors are primary effects and are unresponsive to alterations in either extracellular fluid volume or sodium balance.

Hypertension precipitated by administration of estrogen-containing oral contraceptives is frequently hyperreninemic, although not necessarily renin-dependent. It is estimated that in over 15 per cent of the adult hypertensive population, elevated plasma renin activity and hyperaldosteronism can be demonstrated. A majority of the patients have moderately severe or accelerated hypertension, the level of which is determined more by elevated peripheral arteriolar resistance than by any other determinant of blood pressure. Using angiotensin II blockade with a converting enzyme inhibitor, captopril, these hyperreninemic patients respond with a significant reduction in blood pressure.

CONGENITAL ADRENAL HYPERPLASIA

By John S. Parks, M.D., Ph.D.
Atlanta, Georgia

DEFINITION

Congenital adrenal hyperplasia refers to several distinct diseases, which are inherited in an autosomal recessive manner, involve defects in specific steroid biosynthetic enzymes, and are accompanied by hyperplasia of the adrenal cortex. Although each disease is present during fetal life, the timing and nature of presentation are dependent on which enzyme is defective, the severity of the defect, and the sex of the affected individual. The pathways of aldosterone, cortisol, and sex steroid biosynthesis are shown in Figure 1, while the distinguishing characteristics of the various enzyme deficiencies are given in Table 1.

Deficiency of adrenal 21-hydroxylase is the most familiar form. It accounts for approximately 90 per cent of all cases of adrenal hyperplasia. The incidence of the disease may be as high as 1:3000 among Caucasians in the United States and 1:250 among Yupik Eskimos in Alaska. Recent studies have shown the mutations responsible for deficiency of 21-hydroxylase are located near the HLA gene complex on human chromosome 6. The enzyme is required for synthesis of aldosterone and cortisol, but it is not required for the production of testosterone or estradiol. Inefficient production of cortisol evokes an increase in adrenocorticotropic hormone (ACTH), which results in adrenal hyperplasia and an overflow of metabolites into the pathway leading to testosterone. Excessive androgen production results in prenatal virilization of the external genitalia in genetic females and progressive virilization of both male and female patients during childhood. Hydrocortisone replacement meets the need for glucocorticoids and removes the stimulus to androgen production. More than 30 per cent of individuals with deficiency of 21-hydroxylase have a severe, salt-losing variant in which production of aldosterone is inadequate to permit survival without appropriate treatment. They generally require replacement with a mineralocorticoid, such as 9α-fluorohydrocortisone, as well as hydrocortisone.

Deficiency of 11β-hydroxylase also produces prenatal virilization of female subjects and postnatal virilization of both male and female patients. However, this disorder does not result in salt loss. The enzyme is one step farther down on the pathways to aldosterone and cortisol synthesis. There is overproduction of 11-deoxycortisol, which exerts a salt-retaining effect and eventually causes hypertension. Treatment with hydrocortisone inhibits production of 11-deoxycortisol and adrenal androgens. The mutation responsible for this disorder is distinct from that for 21-hydroxylase deficiency and is not linked to the HLA gene complex.

Three other types of congenital adrenal hyperplasia also interfere with cortisol biosynthesis. They each involve enzymes that are shared by gonadal and adrenal tissue, so they cause undervirilization of the male fetus and incomplete pubertal development in both male and female subjects.

Cholesterol desmolase acts at a very early stage in the pathways to aldosterone, cortisol, and sex steroid synthesis. With deficiency of this enzyme, the features of mineralocorticoid and glucocorticoid deficiency predominate. Biochemically, the condition is characterized by a paucity of all steroid metabolites.

Deficiency of 3β-hydroxysteroid dehydrogenase (3β-HSD) impairs production of aldosterone, cortisol, testosterone, and estradiol. There is overproduction of $\Delta5$ metabolites, which include the weak androgen dehydroepiandrosterone (DHEA). The result is mild virilization of the female fetus, undervirilization of the male fetus, and postnatal salt loss. Undertreatment during childhood is associated with progressive virilization. Male patients with this disorder are sterile despite treatment.

The enzyme *17α-hydroxylase* is required for cortisol, testosterone, and estradiol production, but it is not needed for aldosterone production. With a block at this point, there is undervirilization of the male fetus

Table 1. Clinical and Laboratory Features of Congenital Adrenal Hyperplasia

Ambiguous Genitalia		Salt Loss	High BP	Postnatal Viriliza-tion	Enzyme Deficiency	Urinary Metabolites			Circulating Hormones		
Female	*Male*					*17-KS*	*17-OH*	*PT*	*17-OHP*	*Δ4*	*Testo-sterone*
					21-Hydroxylase						
+	0	+	0	+	Salt-losing	↑↑	N	↑↑	↑↑	↑↑	↑
+	0	0	0	+	Non-salt-losing	↑↑	N	↑↑	↑↑	↑↑	↑
0	0	0	0	+	Late onset	↑	N	↑	↑	↑	↑
+	0	0	+	+	11β-Hydroxylase	↑	↑*	↑	↑	↑↑	↑
0	+	+	0	0	Cholesterol desmolase	↓↓	↓↓	↓↓	↓	↓	↓
+	+	+	0	+	3β-HSD	↑†	↓↓	↑	N	N	↑
0	+	0	+	0	17α-Hydroxylase	↓↓	↓↓	↓	↓	↓	↓

*Mostly tetrahydrodeoxycortisol.
†Mostly Δ5-17-ketosteroids.
Abbreviations: BP = Blood pressure; 17-KS = 17-ketosteroids; 17-OH = 17-hydroxysteroids; PT = pregnanetriol; 17-OHP = 17-hydroxyprogesterone; Δ4 = Δ4-androstenedione; N = normal.

and lack of spontaneous pubertal development in both male and female patients. Overproduction of corticosterone meets physiologic needs for glucocorticoids, but it causes salt retention and leads to hypertension. Cortisol replacement corrects the elevation in blood pressure.

PRESENTING SIGNS AND SYMPTOMS

Infants. The earliest sign of congenital adrenal hyperplasia is ambiguity of the external genitalia. Subjects with 21-hydroxylase deficiency who are genetic females show varying degrees of intrauterine virilization. This ranges from a mild degree of clitoral enlargement and posterior fusion of the labia minora to a large phallus with a phallic urethra and a scrotum that is empty but otherwise normal in appearance. Many female patients with the disease occupy an intermediate position, with some phallic enlargement, chordee, and hypospadias with a single urethrogenital opening. Fusion of the urethrolabial and labioscrotal folds reflects production of adrenal androgens during a critical period between 8 and 12 weeks of fetal life, while clitoral enlargement can occur at any time in late fetal or postnatal life. Male subjects with the common form of congenital adrenal hyperplasia are indistinguishable from other male infants at birth. The contribution of adrenal androgens adds little to the powerful effect of fetal testicular function. Prenatal virilization tends to be less severe in female subjects with 11β-hydroxylase or 3β-HSD deficiency and does not occur in those with cholesterol desmolase or 17α-hydroxylase deficiency. Subjects with 3β-HSD or 17α-hydroxylase deficiency who are genetic males also present with genital ambiguity, and their testes may be either palpable or undescended.

Salt loss with dehydration constitutes another common presentation in infants with congenital adrenal hyperplasia. The typical history is of an infant who was well in the nursery, but returns at 1 to 3 weeks of age with a history of refusing feedings, continuing urination, and increasing lethargy. Without intervention, the course will progress to hypovolemic shock and death.

Children. The hallmark of non-salt-losing 21-hydroxylase or of 11β-hydroxylase deficiency during childhood is progressive virilization. Signs of this process may appear as early as the second year of life. The adrenal androgens stimulate somatic growth, so an affected child will be unusually tall for age and genetic background. There may be unusually prominent musculature, acne, and a deep voice. Female patients will show clitoral enlargement and sexual hair. Male patients show phallic enlargement and pubic hair, but the testes tend to be smaller than normal for chronologic age and strikingly small in light of other signs of pubertal development. Early breast development is unusual in boys and girls with these forms of congenital adrenal hyperplasia. In some children, signs of acute adrenal insufficiency during stress are the presenting features, and signs of virilization may be recognized only upon close examination. Unexplained hypertension may accompany virilization in children with 11β-hydroxylase deficiency or be an isolated finding in children with 17α-hydroxylase deficiency.

Adolescents and Adults. Some persons with congenital adrenal hyperplasia escape detection until late in life. Delay in diagnosis does not necessarily reflect mildness of disease. An extreme case was described by De Crecchio in 1865. A deceased male subject was found to have a penis with first degree hypospadias and no palpable gonads. Dissection disclosed a vagina, uterus, fallopian tubes, ovaries, and very large adrenals. In retrospect, this subject was probably a genetic female with non-salt-losing 21-hydroxylase deficiency. A more typical case would be a female individual who was large for age through early and mid-childhood but short at the time of examination because of early cessation of growth. Leg length would be short relative to body length. Pubic and axillary hair would have been present since childhood, but there would be minimal breast development and irregular or no menses. Although clitoromegaly would be present, there might be no signs of early fetal virilization. Some women show no features of virilization until adolescence or early adulthood but nevertheless have hormonal findings consistent with 21-hydroxylase deficiency. The terms late-onset and acquired adrenal hyperplasia have been applied to this entity. The mutation responsible for this condition also appears to be linked to the HLA gene complex, but it is probably a different mutation, since late-onset and classic 21-hydroxylase deficiencies do not occur in the same families.

Older male patients with 21-hydroxylase deficiency may present with testicular masses. These masses represent hypertrophied adrenal rest tissue located adjacent to the testis, and they will regress with hydrocortisone treatment. Otherwise, testicular size and function tend to be normal. The effects of adrenal androgens are not sufficient to preclude eventual growth of the testis and normal spermatogenesis. Male patients with partial defects in 3β-HSD may present with gynecomastia at puberty. The presence of hypospadias differentiates this disease from more common causes of gynecomastia. Male and female individuals with 17α-hydroxylase deficiency combine the features of lack of pubertal development and presence of hypertension.

LABORATORY FINDINGS

Nonspecific Findings. Determination of genetic sex is mandatory in all cases of genital ambiguity without palpable testes. In this setting, chromatin positivity and a 46,XX karyotype point to the likelihood of 21-hydroxylase deficiency and the potential for life-threatening salt loss. Vaginograms are useful during the neonatal period in confirming the presence of a uterus and in defining the site of connection between vagina and urethra. Intravenous pyelograms do not provide comparable information and are hazardous in that osmotic diuresis may contribute to hypovolemia and shock. Diminished serum sodium and CO_2 content and elevated potassium level are characteristic of dehydration due to 21-hydroxylase, 3 β-HSD, or cholesterol desmolase deficiencies. Hypoglycemia is rarely a presenting sign of congenital adrenal hyperplasia, but it is fairly common in treated children who do not receive sufficient hydrocortisone at times of stress. The child with late-diagnosed congenital adrenal hyperplasia will have a bone age that is markedly advanced in comparison to height age as well as to chronologic age.

Steroid Hormones. Laboratory diagnosis of congenital adrenal hyperplasia involves measurement of two types of steroid metabolites—those that accumulate proximal to the enzymatic block and those that are produced in excess as a result of the flow of the first category of compounds into alternate pathways. Assays may be done on serum or urine specimens. In 21-hydroxylase deficiency, serum 17-hydroxyprogesterone levels are abnormally high as the result of an inability to convert this compound to deoxycortisol. Δ4-androstenedione, which is one step away from 17-hydroxyprogesterone, is also elevated. Urinary pregnanetriol represents a metabolite of 17-hydroxyprogesterone, and 17-ketosteroid excretion also reflects increased production of Δ4-androstenedione.

There has been a tendency to switch to diagnostic measurements of circulating hormones by radioimmunoassay because of the greater ease of specimen collection at any age and because of a clearer discrimination between normal and abnormal values in the newborn period. Serum testosterone level is low in male infants with 21-hydroxylase deficiency in the newborn period, but it is markedly elevated for age in

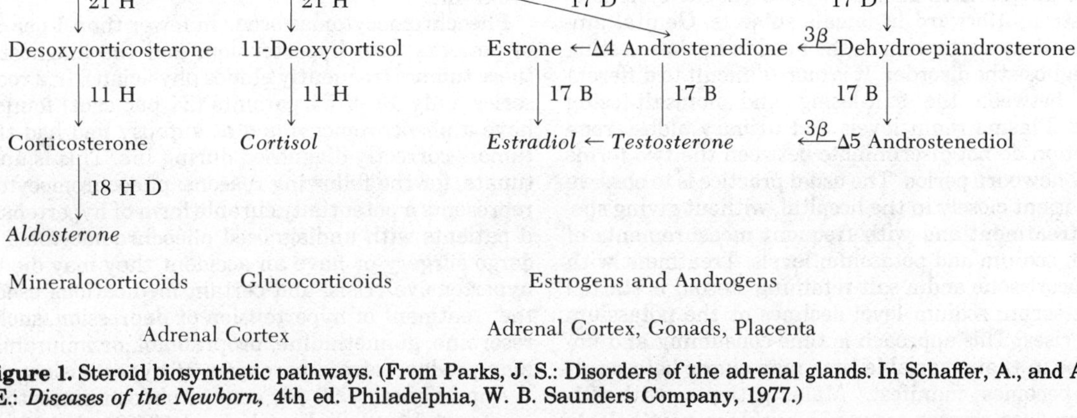

Figure 1. Steroid biosynthetic pathways. (From Parks, J. S.: Disorders of the adrenal glands. In Schaffer, A., and Avery, M. E.: *Diseases of the Newborn*, 4th ed. Philadelphia, W. B. Saunders Company, 1977.)

older infants and children. Abnormally high levels of these hormones suggest, but do not prove, the diagnosis of congenital adrenal hyperplasia. This requires demonstration that hormone levels decline to the normal range following the initiation of hydrocortisone treatment.

The other types of congenital adrenal hyperplasia show hormonal abnormalities that are predictable from knowledge of the sites of the defects. Deficiency of 11β-hydroxylase results in a less dramatic elevation of the same compounds that are abnormally high in 21-hydroxylase deficiency. There is, in addition, diagnostic elevation of serum 11-deoxycortisol levels and an accompanying increase in urinary excretion of tetrahydrodeoxycortisol. Deficiency of 3β-HSD is difficult to diagnose biochemically. There is an increase in the excretion of 17-ketosteroids, and with gas-liquid chromatography or other specialized techniques this can be shown to be due to an increase in Δ compounds. Serum levels of 17-hydroxypregnenolone are increased. Beyond the neonatal period, there is peripheral conversion of this compound to 17-hydroxyprogesterone and increased urinary excretion of pregnanetriol. Testosterone levels are normal in pubertal and adult men with this condition, but there is a marked elevation of androstenediol. Serum levels of most steroid hormones are abnormally low in patients with 17α-hydroxylase deficiency, but corticosterone level is elevated. Cholesterol desmolase deficiency produces a paucity of all measurable steroid hormones.

HLA Typing. HLA typing can be used to track the transmission of mutant 21-hydroxylase genes through a family. The technique is of practical usefulness in determining which of an affected child's siblings are carriers of the disease as well as in prenatal diagnosis in subsequent pregnancies. There is linkage disequilibrium or a statistical association between 21-hydroxylase deficiency and the HLA-Bw47 allele. This antigen is present in fewer than 1 per cent of the normal population, but has been found in 6 to 50 per cent of Caucasian patients with the disease. The haplotype A3, Cw6, Bw47, BfF, DR7 appears to be a specific marker for one type of 21-hydroxylase mutation.

PITFALLS IN DIAGNOSIS

The diagnosis of 21-hydroxylase deficiency is usually straightforward in female subjects. Genital ambiguity draws attention to the need to initiate testing to diagnose the disorder. It is more difficult to differentiate between the salt-losing and non-salt-losing forms. Plasma renin levels and urinary aldosterone excretion do not discriminate between the two forms in the newborn period. The usual practice is to observe the patient closely in the hospital, without giving specific treatment and with frequent measurements of serum sodium and potassium levels. Treatment with hydrocortisone and a salt-retaining steroid is started when serum sodium level declines or the potassium level rises. This approach is time-consuming and imprecise in that a variable time may elapse before salt loss becomes manifest. Male patients with 21-hydroxylase present more of a problem, particularly if they are the first children with the disorder in a family. There is nothing remarkable about them at birth. Salt-losers may die without medical attention, or a physician may fail to consider congenital adrenal hyperplasia in the differential diagnosis of their hyponatremic, hyperkalemic dehydration. Non-salt-losers may be well advanced in somatic growth and skeletal maturity before their disorder is recognized. Routine newborn metabolic screening, with assay of 17-hydroxyprogesterone levels in capillary blood samples spotted on filter paper, provides a solution to both types of problem.

PHEOCHROMOCYTOMA

By Jerome M. Feldman, M.D.
Durham, North Carolina

SYNONYMS

Chromaffinoma, catecholamine-secreting paraganglioma.

DEFINITION

Pheochromocytomas are tumors composed of chromaffin cells that originate from neuroectodermal tissue. The hallmark of pheochromocytomas is the production of catecholamines such as dopamine (DA), norepinephrine (NE), and epinephrine (E). Ninety per cent of pheochromocytomas arise from adrenal medullary tissue and are thus located in the adrenal gland. The remaining 10 per cent arise from sympathetic nervous system tissue located outside the adrenal gland. These tumors can be found along the aorta in both the abdomen and the thorax. In addition, catecholamine-secreting tumors called chemodectomas can arise from the chemoreceptor system, such as the carotid or aortic bodies and the glomus jugulare in the neck. Neuroblastomas, which are usually found in children, and ganglioneuromas, found in both children and adults, occasionally produce enough catecholamines to result in a pheochromocytoma-like syndrome.

Pheochromocytomas occur in fewer than 1 per cent of patients with hypertension, and the diagnosis of these tumors frequently eludes physicians. In a recent series, only 13 of 54 patients (24 per cent) found to have a pheochromocytoma at autopsy had had their tumors correctly diagnosed during life. This is unfortunate, for the following reasons: pheochromocytoma represents a potentially curable form of hypertension; if patients with undiagnosed pheochromocytoma undergo surgery or have an accident they may die of a hypertensive crisis; and certain medications used in the treatment of hypertension or depression, such as reserpine, guanethidine, propranolol, or imipramine, may produce severe paroxysm of hypertension.

Approximately 90 per cent of pheochromocytomas are located in the adrenal glands. The rule of 10 per cent is a handy way to recall some information on pheochromocytomas; 10 per cent occur in both adrenal glands (are bilateral), 10 per cent are extra-adrenal, and 10 per cent are malignant.

PRESENTING SIGNS AND SYMPTOMS

The diagnosis of possible pheochromocytoma is usually suggested by the finding of hypertension. In half the patients the bouts of hypertension are intermittent, whereas in the other half of patients the hypertension is sustained. In the patients with intermittent hypertension, the blood pressure elevation is frequently associated with pounding headaches, profuse sweating, nervousness, anxiety, a feeling of impending doom, and pallor of the skin. Rarely a patient will have flushing associated with the attacks. In some cases the attack is provoked by exercise, sexual activity, or hyperventilation. In the case of a pheochromocytoma in the bladder, it may be provoked by micturition, and in certain cases, an intra-abdominal pheochromocytoma causes an attack after abdominal palpation. Attacks can fortuitously follow injuries, general anesthesia, or administration of medications that discharge catecholamines, such as reserpine, guanethidine, imipramine, or desipramine. Beta-adrenergic blocking agents such as propranolol may cause hypertensive attacks by blocking the vasodilating beta-adrenergic receptors and leaving the vasoconstricting alpha-adrenergic receptors unopposed. Other clinical manifestations include abdominal or chest pain, weakness, fatigue, weight loss, dyspnea, heat intolerance, visual disturbances, constipation, grand mal seizures, and fever of unknown origin.

In the 50 per cent of patients in whom the hypertension is sustained, there may be no episodic attacks. These patients may have a picture identical to that of patients with essential hypertension. There are also some patients with functioning pheochromocytomas who have neither episodic nor sustained hypertension.

COURSE

In general, the recommended therapy for pheochromocytomas is surgical removal. Thus, there are no long-term longitudinal studies of patients with benign pheochromocytomas. It is generally believed that these tumors continue to grow, and their increased size makes resection more difficult. The malignant pheochromocytomas metastasize to lymph nodes, liver, and bone. In patients with multiple endocrine neoplasia (MEN) Type II or III, the patients may succumb to metastatic medullary carcinoma of the thyroid. In patients with von Recklinghausen's neurofibromatosis, neurofibrosarcomas or malignant schwannomas may lead to the patient's death.

COMMON COMPLICATIONS

Because of the diabetogenic effects of catecholamines, many patients with pheochromocytomas eventually develop diabetes mellitus. Because of the extreme surges in blood pressure, they may have cerebrovascular accidents. In addition they suffer from all of the long-standing complications of arterial hypertension, such as hypertensive cardiovascular disease with congestive heart failure and nephrosclerosis with renal insufficiency and failure. They may develop congestive heart failure from a catecholamine myocarditis. Finally, some patients are incapacitated by "anxiety attacks" that are incorrectly attributed to psychogenic factors.

PHYSICAL EXAMINATION

Examination of most patients harboring pheochromocytomas reveals either sustained or intermittent hypertension. Frequently the patient who has intermittent hypertension is normotensive when seen by the physician. In some cases, patients who give histories suggestive of hypertension can be taught to do home blood pressure monitoring so that they can obtain an accurate blood pressure prior to coming to the office.

Because of their contracted extracellular fluid volume, the majority of patients with functioning pheochromocytomas have orthostatic hypotension. They may be observed to have profuse sweating during the physical examination even though the room is not particularly warm. If observed during an attack, their faces may demonstrate pallor or, less frequently, flushing that is suggestive of the carcinoid syndrome. They may also appear to have anxiety problems rather than physical origins for their complaints. The majority of patients either have weight loss or maintain their weight; however, weight gain is occasionally seen in a patient with pheochromocytoma. In addition to sweating, the patient may have a tremor of the fingers suggesting hyperthyroidism. Body temperature may be intermittently elevated with no explanation found for the fever. Patients with von Recklinghausen's neurofibromatosis may have palpable neurofibromas or café au lait spots. The patient with medullary carcinoma and MEN Type II or III may have a nodule in the thyroid gland. Patients with pure epinephrine-secreting pheochromocytomas may present with hypotension or circulatory shock. This is quite uncommon in my experience, and most patients with pheochromocytomas that secrete predominantly epinephrine also have intermittent or sustained hypertension.

LABORATORY PROCEDURES

The diagnosis can be made in over 90 per cent of patients with appropriate urinary and blood tests for catecholamines and their metabolites. I have found that the most useful tests are measurements of the 24-hour urinary excretion of 3-methoxy-4-hydroxymandelic acid (vanillylmandelic acid, VMA), norepinephrine, and epinephrine. It is essential that these analyses be performed by a reliable laboratory using sound analytic techniques.

The spectrophotometric method of Pisano et al. for

measuring VMA has consistently been the most reliable technique over the years. However, excellent methodology is also now available with high-performance liquid chromatography (HPLC). Some of the colorimetric kits have been less reliable, with a high frequency of artifactual drug interference. Normal values for catecholamines and their metabolites are given in Table 1.

Measurement of urinary NE and E by fluorometric techniques has also been valuable in diagnosing pheochromocytomas. Recently, highly specific radioenzymatic methods in which DA, NE, and E are converted to radioactive O-methylated derivatives with the enzyme catechol-O-methyltransferase (COMT) have become available.

Measurement of urinary metanephrines is useful if performed by a technique such as high-performance liquid chromatography. The colorimetric method for metanephrines frequently gives misleading results because of the high incidence of false-positive tests due to interference by medications.

Occasionally malignant pheochromocytomas secrete almost exclusively DA, and DA is metabolized to homovanillic acid (HVA) rather than VMA; thus, affected patients may have normal urinary excretion of VMA, E, and NE. Such tumors can be detected by measuring urinary DA and HVA or plasma DA concentration.

Recently, sensitive and specific radioenzymatic assays have been developed for measuring NE, E, and DA in small amounts of peripheral plasma. Some physicians believe that such plasma measurements are preferable to studies of urinary excretion. I have noted a significant number of patients with surgically proved pheochromocytomas who had normal plasma NE levels but elevated urinary VMA and catecholamine levels. This may occur because some pheochromocytomas secrete catecholamines only intermittently, and the secreted catecholamines rapidly leave the vascular compartment. Another problem is that the sympathetic nervous system probably plays some role in essential hypertension, and as many as 40 per cent of patients with moderate to severe hypertension have elevated plasma NE concentration. Some investigators have tried to circumvent this problem by observing the NE response to pentolinium or clonidine. In response to these agents the plasma NE concentration of patients with essential hypertension falls to normal, whereas the plasma NE level of patients with pheochromocytomas remains elevated. However, urinary excretion of VMA, E, NE, and metanephrines is almost always within the normal range in patients with essential hypertension who do not have pheochromocytomas, and I believe that analysis of urine for these substances remains the most useful technique in the diagnosis of pheochromocytomas.

We have developed methods of measuring NE in platelets by converting NE to E using the enzyme phenylethanolamine-*N*-methyltransferase (PNMT). The advantage of this method is that the NE is concentrated in the platelets during episodes of hypertension and levels remain elevated even between attacks, when plasma NE concentration has fallen to normal. It takes a finite period of time for the NE to be concentrated in the platelets; therefore, the elevated plasma NE levels induced by stress of seeing a physician or having a venipuncture are usually associated with normal platelet NE concentration. However, 27 per cent of patients with moderate to severe hypertension have elevated platelet NE concentrations. The platelet NE concentration in these patients returns to normal when their blood pressure is reduced; in contrast, the platelet NE concentration of patients with pheochromocytomas remains elevated even when they are normotensive. Thus, platelet NE level is a screening test for pheochromocytoma, and patients with elevated values must be followed up with measurements of urinary VMA and catecholamine levels. Another group has found that the COMT method can be used to measure NE and E levels in platelets. As yet neither test is commercially available.

Table 1. Normal Values for Catecholamines and Their Metabolites

Urinary Catecholamines	
Vanillylmandelic Acid (Vanillin Method)	< 7 mg/24 hours
Metanephrines	< 1.6 mg/24 hours
Norepinephrine (Fluorometric Method)	20–50 μg/24 hours
Epinephrine (Fluorometric Method)	5–25 μg/24 hours
Homovanillic Acid	2–11 mg/24 hours
Dopamine (COMT Method)	200–460 μg/24 hours
Norepinephrine (COMT Method)	15–40 μg/24 hours
Epinephrine (COMT Method)	5–40 μg/24 hours
Plasma Catecholamines	
Dopamine (COMT Method)	< 5–65 pg/ml
Norepinephrine (COMT Method)	65–219 pg/ml
Epinephrine (COMT Method)	15–55 pg/ml
Platelet Norepinephrine (PNMT Method)	0.05–0.90 pmol/mg platelet protein

Abbreviations: COMT = Catechol-O-methyltransferase; PNMT = phenylethanolamine-N-methyltransferase.

Patients with pheochromocytomas may have modest elevations in hemoglobin and hematocrit. These are relative increases due to a decreased plasma volume secondary to the vasoconstricting effects of catecholamines. A small number of patients with pheochromocytomas have absolute increases in hemoglobin and hematocrit values due to release of erythropoietin by the pheochromocytomas. Erythropoietin stimulates red blood cell formation in the bone marrow. This distinction can be made by measuring the red cell mass with ^{51}Cr-labeled red cells or measuring the plasma volume with ^{131}I-labeled serum albumin. The plasma volume expands after adequate preoperative therapy with phenoxybenzamine, correcting the relative increases in hemoglobin and hematocrit; the absolute increase in hemoglobin and hematocrit values is corrected after surgical removal of the erythropoietin-producing pheochromocytoma.

Because of the diabetogenic effects of catecholamines, patients harboring pheochromocytomas may have fasting hyperglycemia or, more frequently, an abnormal glucose tolerance test. Unlike the situation with idiopathic diabetes mellitus, the glucose intolerance is frequently ameliorated by phenoxybenzamine or surgical resection of the pheochromocytoma.

Because of tremor, weight loss, diaphoresis, and anxiety, hyperthyroidism is sometimes a diagnostic consideration. Serum thyroxine (T_4), triiodothyronine resin uptake (RT_3U), and ^{131}I thyroid uptake are usually within normal limits.

RADIOLOGIC EVALUATION

In the case of a medium to large sized pheochromocytoma the tumor may be visualized with a plain abdominal x-ray because of calcification. Intravenous pyelography (IVP) with nephrotomography may also be helpful in localizing the tumor because of downward displacement of the kidney by the tumor. However, the most significant advance in the diagnosis of pheochromocytomas has been the development of ultrasonography and computed tomography (CT scan). Both of these techniques are said to detect 90 per cent of pheochromocytomas. At my medical center we prefer the CT scan. In the majority of patients, normal-sized adrenal glands can be visualized on CT; however, in some patients with inadequate perirenal fat, normal adrenal glands are not visualized. If the adrenal glands are visualized and appear normal in size and configuration, this usually excludes an adrenal location of a pheochromocytoma 1 cm or larger in diameter. Certainly, small extra-adrenal pheochromocytomas can be missed with both ultrasonography and CT.

An exciting new development in localization of pheochromocytomas is scintigraphic localization with ^{131}I-meta-iodobenzylguanidine (^{131}I-MIBG). ^{131}I-MIBG is a radioactive analogue of NE and is taken up by chromaffin tissue anywhere in the body. This technique appears to be useful in localizing small adrenal pheochromocytomas, extra-adrenal pheochromocytomas, multiple pheochromocytomas, and even adrenal medullary hyperplasia. The scans can be performed by any nuclear medicine laboratory. At the present time ^{131}I-MIBG, which was developed at the University of Michigan Medical Center, is not yet commercially available. However, in the near future this promising technique will probably be available throughout the United States.

Arteriography, adrenal venography, vena caval catheterization for determination of plasma catecholamine concentrations, and retroperitoneal carbon dioxide insufflation are four techniques that have been used in the past for localizing pheochromocytomas. These techniques involve definite risks, and they can on occasion be misleading; in general they have been supplanted by ultrasonography, CT scans, and ^{131}I-MIBG scans. Carbon dioxide insufflation should not be performed, while the other three techniques should be used only under special circumstances when the noninvasive tests have not furnished the necessary information. Invasive techniques should not be used until adequate alpha-adrenergic blockade has been established with phenoxybenzamine. Phentolamine, nitroprusside, propranolol, and NE should be available in the procedure room to abort any dangerous changes in blood pressure or heart rate and/or rhythm.

OTHER DIAGNOSTIC PROCEDURES

Prior to the availability of sensitive and specific biochemical tests for excessive catecholamine production, provocative and suppressive tests were used for the diagnosis of pheochromocytoma. Provocative tests were used in patients who had good histories for intermittently secreting pheochromocytomas, but who had normal blood pressures when seen by their physicians. In these tests the patient's blood pressure response to intravenous injection of histamine or glucagon or the intravenous infusion of tyramine was compared to his or her response to the nonspecific blood pressure effects of the cold pressor test. I would not recommend the tyramine infusion or histamine injection test, as a pharmaceutical preparation of tyramine is not commercially available, and injection of histamine can lead to unpleasant side effects and a dangerous rise in blood pressure. The glucagon provocative test may be useful in the rare patient in whom the diagnosis of pheochromocytoma cannot be made by biochemical tests. However, a substantial number of patients with surgically proved pheochromocytomas have had negative glucagon provocative tests. The standard test is performed by rapidly injecting 1 mg of crystalline glucagon (Lilly) in 1 ml of diluent intravenously and recording the blood pressure every 30 sec for the first 5 minutes and then every minute for the following 5 minutes. The rise in blood pressure is usually noted in the first 3 min and consists of a 35 mm systolic, 25 mm diastolic pressure increase over the baseline. Occasionally 1 mg of glucagon has provoked a dangerous rise in blood pressure in a patient with a pheochromocytoma. Thus, if there is a strong suspicion of a pheochromocytoma I suggest that the test first be done with 0.5 mg of glucagon; if negative, it can be followed later by the full 1 mg of glucagon. Nitroprusside, phentolamine, and propranolol should be available in the testing room in case there is an untoward response. The test can be made more specific by drawing samples of blood for plasma catecholamine determinations at 0, 3, 5, and 10 minutes to see if the change in blood pressure is accompanied by an increase in plasma catecholamine levels. It should be mentioned that patients harboring unsuspected pheochromocytomas may have dangerous and unanticipated increases in blood pressure when glucagon is used in radiologic examinations (barium enema, CT), endocrine testing (provocative test for insulinoma), or tests of the inotropic effect of glucagon on the heart.

The only suppressive test that is sometimes used is observing the effect of phentolamine mesylate (Regitine) on the hypertensive patient's blood pressure. Although this test has been supplanted by more specific biochemical tests, there is one situation in which it is still useful. This is prior to initiating conventional antihypertensive therapy in patients with life-threatening hypertension, such as malignant hypertension. The standard phentolamine test is performed by starting an intravenous infusion and taking baseline blood pressures until they are stable. One tester is needed to take blood pressures while the other tester injects the phentolamine intravenously on a prearranged signal of which the patient is unaware. Blood pressures are recorded every minute for 10 minutes. A positive test consists of a drop in blood pressure of 35 mm systolic, 25 mm diastolic. Although the standard dose of phentolamine used in this test is 5 mg, some patients with pheochromocytoma have a striking fall in blood pressure with this dose. Thus, it is prudent to use 1 mg of phentolamine first; if the response to 1 mg is negative after 10 minutes, repeat the test with the standard 5 mg of phentolamine. Unfortunately a number of false-positive results occur with this test owing to concomitant illness (recent cerebrovascular accident, dehydration) or medications (reserpine and other antihypertensives, ethambutol), which limit its usefulness. However, if a pheochromocytoma is uncovered as the cause of severe hypertension, effective therapy can be undertaken with additional phentolamine followed by phenoxybenzamine. Again, nitroprusside, propranolol, and NE should be readily available in the testing room in case of dangerous alterations in blood pressure.

THERAPEUTIC TESTS

In the majority of patients the diagnosis of pheochromocytoma can be made or ruled out with appropriate biochemical tests. Occasionally in a patient with short recurring attacks the diagnosis may be suspected but not proved. In such cases a therapeutic trial with phenoxybenzamine, 20 to 40 mg/day divided into two or three doses, may be helpful. Most patients with hypertension not due to pheochromocytoma have only a minimal reduction in supine blood pressure from phenoxybenzamine, although they may have a greater orthostatic fall in blood pressure from the drug; patients with pheochromocytoma usually have a dramatic fall in supine and standing blood pressure from the drug. In addition, they will report a decrease in the frequency and intensity of their episodic attacks. Prazosin (Minipress) is also effective in treating the hypertension of patients with pheochromocytoma. However, prazosin is also effective in essential hypertension and should not be used in place of phenoxybenzamine in the therapeutic trial.

POTENTIAL ERRORS AND PITFALLS IN DIAGNOSIS

I am impressed with the substantial number of patients I have seen with pheochromocytomas who had no clinical features that distinguished them from patients with essential hypertension. The greatest pitfall is therefore not considering pheochromocytoma in the differential diagnosis. Every patient with newly diagnosed hypertension should have urine analyzed for VMA and either metanephrines or catecholamines by a laboratory with excellent technical facilities and experience prior to initiation of antihypertensive therapy. These determinations should be done prior to resection of adrenal masses, even if the patient is normotensive and denies a history of hypertension or "spells." The tests should also be done prior to thyroid surgery in patients who are suspected of having medullary carcinoma of the thryoid or who have a family history of multiple endocrine neoplasia Type II or III. If the patients are found to have both medullary carcinoma of the thyroid and pheochromocytoma, the pheochromocytoma should be removed prior to thyroid surgery to avoid severe hypertension. Finally, any patient with a history of hypertension following general anesthesia or trauma should be screened for pheochromocytoma.

There are a number of pitfalls in the biochemical diagnosis of pheochromocytoma. Fluorescent medications and vitamins, such as alpha-methyldopa (Aldomet), quinidine, and riboflavin, can falsely elevate catecholamine levels when fluorometric methods are used for catecholamine analysis. Coffee, vanilla, and other food ingredients can falsely elevate VMA when determined by colorimetric (but not by the vanillin) method of analysis. Medications such as L-dopa and aspirin that are metabolized to potent reducing agents (3,4-dihydroxyphenylacetic and gentisic acid, respectively) cause an artifactual decrease in VMA excretion in patients with pheochromocytomas even with the vanillin method. L-Dopa therapy causes a true increase in HVA excretion; in addition, numerous drugs interfere with metanephrine determination by colorimetric (but not high-performance liquid chromatography) methods of analysis. Plasma catecholamine measurements may be elevated by the stress of seeing a physician or venipuncture and are elevated in some patients with essential hypertension; also, plasma catecholamines may be within normal limits in some patients with intermittently secreting pheochromocytomas.

Recall that even though a patient has another apparent cause for secondary hypertension, a pheochromocytoma may also be present. For example, compression of a renal artery by an extra-adrenal pheochromocytoma sometimes causes a picture of renovascular hypertension. Patients with pheochromocytomas can have elevated basal and furosemide-stimulated plasma renin levels (greater than 5 ng/ml), suggesting renovascular hypertension. Thus a post-furosemide renin activity of this magnitude is not diagnostic of renovascular hypertension. This exclusion can be made only with appropriate measurements of catecholamine excretion. The mechanism of the elevated renin levels in patients with pheochromocytoma is probably the contracted plasma volume and stimulation of renin release by catecholamines. Renal arteriography would certainly be potentially dangerous in a patient with a pheochromocytoma who has not been treated with phenoxybenzamine.

A number of other problems can mimic pheochromocytoma clinically, but they can usually be excluded by appropriate history and biochemical tests. Patients taking monoamine oxidase inhibitors such as pargyline hydrochloride (Eutonyl), tranylcypromine

(Parnate), or phenelzine (Nardil) can have hypertensive episodes after ingesting foods and beverages such as cheddar cheese, pickled herring, or Chianti wine or after receiving medications such as sympathomimetic amines. Patients taking beta-adrenergic blocking agents such as propranolol (Inderal) for angina pectoris or essential hypertension can have severe hypertensive episodes after receiving conventional doses of epinephrine for bronchial asthma. Patients who suddenly discontinue antihypertensive agents such as clonidine can have severe rebound hypertension. In addition, some patients have a form of autonomic epilepsy that can mimic pheochromocytoma because of sympathetic nervous system overactivity. Surreptitious ingestion or injection of E or NE has been reported in mentally disturbed individuals who are trying to feign a pheochromocytoma. This can usually be suspected because the urinary catecholamine levels are disproportionately higher than the urinary VMA. Finally, there is a group of patients with essential hypertension who have episodic attacks that mimic pheochromocytoma. The diagnosis of pheochromocytoma can be excluded only by appropriate biochemical tests.

CARCINOID TUMOR AND CARCINOID SYNDROME

By John S. Kaufmann, M.D., Ph.D.
Winston-Salem, North Carolina

SYNONYMS

Carcinoid tumor, argentaffinoma, carcinoid syndrome, malignant carcinoid syndrome, functional carcinoid, argentaffinosis, carcinoid spectrum, Björck-Thorson syndrome.

DEFINITION AND PATHOLOGY

The carcinoid tumor is a neoplasm arising from neuroectodermal cells that normally are incorporated into primordial gut structures during embryonic development. Thus, primary carcinoid tumors most frequently occur in any structural derivative of the embryonic foregut, midgut, or hindgut. The embryonic foregut gives rise to elements of the bronchopulmonary tree, the proximal gastrointestinal tract as far as the jejunum, the thyroid gland, thymus, pancreas, and biliary tract. Midgut components include jejunum, ileum, cecum and appendix, and ascending colon; the remainder of the colon and rectum are derived from the hindgut. In addition to these general sites, carcinoids may occur in gonadal teratomas and, rarely, in embryonic cell rests presumably originating from enterochromaffin derivatives of pluripotential cells.

A clear distinction must be made between the carcinoid tumor and carcinoid syndrome. The carcinoid tumor is a neoplasm, the diagnosis of which depends upon histopathologic criteria. The diagnosis of carcinoid syndrome is based upon the identification of certain functional abnormalities caused by one or more biologically active compounds released into the systemic circulation by a carcinoid tumor. The typical gastrointestinal tract carcinoid originates from enterochromaffin cells in the basal layer of the mucosa; extends slowly into the submucosal region, eventually invading the muscularis; and subsequently spreads locally, then regionally, and finally to distant sites by both lymphatic and vascular routes. The histologic appearance of a carcinoid tumor usually belies its malignant potential, and few anaplastic or mitotic cells are present. The cells commonly are round or polygonal and uniform in appearance with central nuclei and acidophilic cytoplasmic granules. They may appear as pseudoacinar or rosette clusters and in cords or ribbons with a variable amount of stroma. Some tumors contain large amounts of fibrous tissue, and the surrounding structures may display a marked desmoplastic reaction. Typically, few tumors 1.0 cm or less in diameter metastasize, whereas the vast majority of primary tumors over 2.0 cm in diameter are associated with metastatic spread. Thus, the gross size and degree of invasiveness of carcinoid tumors are more reliable indicators of the degree of malignancy than are histologic criteria.

The cells of typical carcinoid tumors demonstrate an affinity for chromium salts (and therefore are chromaffin-positive) in a manner similar to adrenal medullary and ganglionic neuronal cells. These cells also contain dense granules identified histochemically by their ability to precipitate silver salts. Most of the tumors of midgut origin and some foregut tumors have cellular granules that react directly with silver salts and therefore are said to be argentaffin-positive. The remainder of the tumors react variably with silver salts but only in the presence of an added reducing agent. This reaction identifies cells said to be argyrophilic (all argentaffin-positive cells are argyrophilic). In the past, staining for argyrophilicity usually has been negative for hindgut tumors, and as a consequence a positive correlation could be made between the functional capacity of tumors and the type and degree of avidity for silver salts. More recently, however, improved sensitivity for argyrophilicity has been achieved (e.g., use of the Churukian-Schenk staining technique) as a result of which virtually all carcinoids including tumors can be successfully identified. Thus, histochemical demonstration of argyrophilicity by intracellular granules corroborates the diagnosis of carcinoid but cannot be used to predict a tumor's site of origin or its endocrine functional capacity.

The carcinoid tumor is not a common malignant neoplasm, and only 5 to 6 per cent of the more than 4000 reported cases of carcinoid tumor have been associated with the carcinoid syndrome and its variants. The vast majority (80 per cent) of these cases of carcinoid syndrome have been caused by primary tumors of the ileocecal region of the gastrointestinal tract with hepatic metastases. Tumors originating in the colon and bronchopulmonary tree have accounted for an additional 5 per cent each, while the remainder have arisen from nonbronchial foregut structures or teratomas of the gonads. Except for some of the bronchial and gonadal tumors that have systemic venous drainage, carcinoids that give rise to the functional syndrome are almost always metastatic to the liver and possibly other sites. This phenomenon reflects the ability of the liver to inactivate the humoral substances released into the hepatic portal system by most primary gastrointestinal carcinoids, thereby precluding the appearance of symptoms until hepatic metastases subsequently release the compounds into hepatic venous blood. Approximately one fourth of the jejunoileal carcinoids appear to have a multicentric origin and occasionally rectal carcinoids are manifested in this manner. There is also a strikingly high association between functional carcinoid tumors and the occurrence of other malignant neoplasms, for approximately one fourth of the patients with carcinoid syndrome develop a different neoplasm during the course of the disease.

Some foregut carcinoids (and very rarely, hindgut tumors) have been associated with other neoplasms having ectopic endocrine function. Such malignancies as oat cell carcinoma, duodenal islet cell tumor, and medullary carcinoma of the thyroid share histologic similarities with carcinoid, and at times it is virtually impossible to distinguish one from the other. An increasing number of foregut tumors have been shown to secrete any of several polypeptide hormones, including adrenocorticotropic hormone (ACTH), calcitonin, glucagon, insulin, gastrin, and vasoactive intestinal polypeptide. These tumors usually secrete lesser amounts of tryptophan derivatives and may produce one of the "variants" of carcinoid syndrome, reflecting excessive ectopic secretion of one or more polypeptide hormones. In addition, there is an increased incidence of carcinoid tumors in patients with multiple endocrine adenomatosis (e.g., parathyroid adenomas and pancreatic adenomas associated with Zollinger-Ellison syndrome). These observations suggest that the various endocrinologically active tumors share a common neural crest stem cell origin but subsequently manifest a variable expression during development.

TUMOR PHARMACOLOGY AND ENDOCRINE FUNCTION

Serotonin (5-Hydroxytryptamine; 5-HT). One of the most constant features of carcinoid tumor cells is their ability to take up dietary tryptophan and by the action of tryptophan hydroxylase form 5-hydroxytryptophan (5-HTP). With the exception of most foregut tumors, carcinoid neoplasms also contain the enzyme aromatic L-amino acid decarboxylase, which catalyzes the formation of serotonin from 5-HTP. Serotonin is stored with ATP in intracellular granules that resemble those of many neurosecretory cells. A number of stimuli, both physical and chemical, are able to effect release of serotonin into the venous blood. Normally, blood platelets take up most of the circulating serotonin, which is produced primarily by enterochromaffin cells of the gastrointestinal tract. Serotonin released from any source eventually is metabolized by the monoamine oxidase–aldehyde dehydrogenase system to 5-hydroxyindoleacetic acid (5-HIAA). Indeed, the urinary excretion of excessive amounts of 5-HIAA is the diagnostic hallmark of carcinoid syndrome.

Serotonin can cause bronchoconstriction and gastrointestinal hypermotility. Its cardiovascular effects are complex and, despite its direct vasoconstrictive property, its ability to decrease cardiac output indirectly and cause vasodilatation in skeletal muscle often results in a net decrease in blood pressure. Serotonin's ability to decrease glomerular filtration rate may contribute to edema formation in some patients. Initially serotonin was thought to be the primary effector of the carcinoid flush; however, subsequent studies have failed to support this concept. Serotonin may play a significant role in the development of endocardial fibrosis seen in many carcinoid patients but this role has not been confirmed. Evidence does exist, however, to suggest that serotonin plays a causative role in the diarrhea of carcinoid syndrome. Parachlorophenylalanine, a tryptophan-hydroxylase inhibitor, has been used experimentally in humans, and its use results in a 50 per cent reduction in the overall severity of diarrhea in carcinoid patients.

Kinins. More recently carcinoid tumors have been demonstrated to contain large amounts of kallikrein, an enzyme that forms kinins from endogenously available kininogens in plasma. The two major kinins are bradykinin and lysylbradykinin. These compounds are potent vasodilators and constrictors of bronchial and gastrointestinal smooth muscle. It is now thought that kinins are the mediators of carcinoid flush in many instances. The activation or release of kallikrein from tumors (thus leading to the carcinoid flush) can be brought about by numerous physical and pharmacologic mechanisms. Specifically, beta-adrenergic agonists are able to cause carcinoid flushing attacks in exceedingly small doses (as little as 0.5 μg intravenously). Likewise, kallikrein activation can result from diverse stimuli, including excessive emotion, ethanol ingestion, intake of certain foods, exercise, intravenous administration of calcium salts, and tumor manipulation. Although the role of kinins has been established in the carcinoid flush in some patients, its importance in others is of lesser degree. Kinins probably function in some additive or synergistic manner during episodes of bronchoconstriction, diarrhea, and edema formation.

Histamine. Histamine is formed by the decarboxylation of dietary histidine and is found primarily in gastric carcinoids. It also is stored in granular form, and its release from carcinoid tumors can lead to flushing, hypotension, lacrimation, and tachycardia. Whether the increased incidence of peptic ulceration in patients with gastric carcinoid is causally related to excessive histamine production by the tumor has not been resolved. Administration of pentagastrin will cause release of histamine from gastric carcinoids, and the combined use of H_1 and H_2 histamine antagonists effectively prevents histamine's deleterious actions.

In addition to the desmoplastic response of tissues to invasive carcinoid tumors, at least 50 per cent of patients with carcinoid syndrome have a unique endocardial fibrosis that most commonly involves the right cardiac chambers and valvular structures. Its proclivity for the right side of the heart and its progressive development suggest that this abnormality results from one or more humoral substances secreted by a carcinoid tumor.

Non-appendiceal intra-abdominal carcinoids seldom produce symptoms until significant local invasion or metastasis has occurred. Although intussusception has occurred in carcinoid patients, luminal encroachment and pseudopolyp formation are not characteristic of the tumor. Conversely, invasion of the muscularis layer to the serosal surface is common and the frequent consequential muscular hypertrophy and desmoplastic reaction may lead to kinking of bowel loops, with subsequent obstructive symptoms.

PRESENTING SIGNS AND SYMPTOMS OF CARCINOID TUMORS

Most patients with carcinoid tumors are asymptomatic. Nonfunctional carcinoid tumors are frequently incidental findings during surgical procedures or during diagnostic studies done for other suspected conditions. The tumors may produce signs or symptoms because of encroachment on adjacent tissues in specific locations. Thus, bronchial carcinoids not uncommonly produce effects related to mucosal erosion or obstruction, and appendiceal carcinoids, which constitute 40 per cent of all such tumors, frequently lead to signs and symptoms of acute appendicitis. Although hepatic metastases are common in carcinoid patients, widespread metastases are relatively infrequent. When dissemination does occur, however, metastases may involve such structures as bone, brain, pancreas, lungs, and other organs. Although most patients with carcinoid syndrome have metastatic disease, widespread metastases can occur without the functional syndrome being seen. Cachexia, hypoalbuminemia, anemia, infection, and other features common to most advanced malignancies likewise may occur in nonfunctional carcinoid tumors late in the course of the disease.

Production of Polypeptides. As indicated earlier, foregut tumors may elaborate a variety of polypeptide hormones, including ACTH, insulin, gastrin, glucagon, and calcitonin. Tumors associated with increased ACTH production have been noted to cause hyperadrenocorticism; however, the direct and indirect endocrine effects of other polypeptide hormones from foregut tumors have not been adequately evaluated.

Miscellaneous. The levels of prostaglandins and other arachidonic acid derivatives have been noted to be elevated in selected cases of carcinoid tumor, but their precise role in the genesis of the pathophysiologic features of carcinoid syndrome is unknown. Dopamine and other catecholamines have been found in a number of carcinoid tumors, and a presumptive role in modulation of bradykinin and possibly amine release has been inferred but not documented.

SIGNS AND SYMPTOMS OF CARCINOID SYNDROME

General Symptoms. In the earlier discussion of the pathologic aspects of carcinoid tumors, a brief description of some of the pathophysiologic consequences of any invasive or metastatic neoplasm was presented. Although few patients are seen initially because of symptoms related to tumor spread per se, a rare patient may present with significant weight loss, anemia, or other constitutional symptoms of nonspecific nature. Therefore, the following discussion will be limited largely to a description of signs and symptoms of importance in the diagnosis of carcinoid syndrome.

The most frequent signs and symptoms associated with carcinoid syndrome are cutaneous flushing (75 to 90 per cent), diarrhea (60 to 75 per cent), evidence of cardiac valvular dysfunction (40 to 50 per cent), bronchoconstriction (15 to 20 per cent), other cutaneous manifestations (5 to 15 per cent), and edema (10 to 40 per cent).

Flushing Attacks. The flushing attacks of carcinoid syndrome vary considerably, not only in frequency, duration, and severity, but also in cutaneous discoloration and association with other symptoms. Typically, midgut carcinoids that are metastatic to the liver release substances such as bradykinin, which cause a diffuse flush over the face, neck, and upper chest region and less commonly over more distal points. The flush may be erythematous to violaceous in color and may last from 2 to 15 min, recurring as often as several times per hour. Flushes may or may not be associated with abdominal cramping and diarrhea. Patients who have experienced flushing attacks for a long period of time may develop an increasingly constant cyanotic discoloration associated with telangiectases, especially over the face, and more rarely a suffusion of the conjunctivae. Functional foregut tumors, especially those arising in the bronchi, are apt to produce prolonged flushes, which may last several days, often involving the entire body and being associated with profuse lacrimation, facial edema, and hypotension. The histamine-secreting gastric carcinoids may produce a unique, bright red, sharply delineated, patchy type of flushing not uncommonly precipitated by ingestion of food. Flushing attacks are not life-threatening situations; however, they may be virtually incapacitating in individual patients, especially those with bronchial carcinoids.

Diarrhea. Gastrointestinal hypermotility, abdominal cramping, and episodes of diarrhea are usually superimposed on a chronically excessive number of stools per day. Acute bouts of diarrhea may result in severe dehydration and electrolyte imbalance. Some patients develop malabsorption syndrome, which may add significantly to pre-existing or tumor-related nutritional problems.

Cadiac Valvular Dysfunction. Over 50 per cent of patients with full-blown carcinoid syndrome will have evidence of cardiac dysfunction. Cardiac decompensation secondary to cardiac valvular abnormalities is one of the leading causes of death in patients with carcinoid syndrome; however, this complication usually occurs later in the course of the disease. The primary cause of cardiac dysfunction is the development of an endocardial fibrosis that is unique in that it occurs on the endothelial surface but does not involve tissues beyond the internal elastic lamina. The fibrous tissue appears histologically as young collagen, and this desmoplastic reaction involves and distorts the papillary muscles, chordae tendineae, and valvular cusps, especially those in the right heart chambers. The most frequently encountered valvular lesions are tricuspid insufficiency and pulmonic stenosis. Rarely the adjacent vena caval inflow tract and left heart chambers are also involved. Thus, murmurs associated with these valvular lesions may be audible and should be documented early in the course of the disease. It is not known why some patients develop such heart lesions while others do not. The distribution of the lesions suggests that one or more humoral substances lead to endocardial fibrosis at sites where maximal blood turbulence occurs.

Bronchoconstriction. Attacks of bronchospasm occur with moderate frequency in some patients with carcinoid syndrome. The severity of the attacks is usually moderate, but those associated with foregut tumors, especially bronchial carcinoids, may be quite severe and prolonged.

Other Cutaneous Manifestations. In addition to the telangiectasia that may be present over the malar regions, a yellow-brown to orange-brown, mottled discoloration may appear over the upper body and in those areas exposed to sunlight. These skin changes resemble those seen in pellagra and may, in part, be related to niacin deficiency caused by the abnormally high degree of tryptophan utilization by the tumor in the formation of serotonin.

Edema. Mild degrees of edema are not uncommon in carcinoid patients. Usually this occurs to a greater degree later in the course of the disease and may be related to cardiac decompensation, hepatic failure, or hypoalbuminemia. Localized facial edema and conjunctival suffusion, however, may be seen early in the course of the disease in patients with bronchial carcinoids and results presumably from increased capillary permeability secondary to tumor secretions.

Other Manifestations. Rarely patients present with signs and symptoms suggestive of arthropathies, localized fibrotic processes (Peyronie's disease), possible intestinal obstruction, abdominal crises associated with tumor necrosis, peptic ulceration, and other manifestations.

COURSE

The prognosis for patients with carcinoid tumors not associated with carcinoid syndrome has been alluded to in earlier discussion. Carcinoids of the appendix and nonfunctioning carcinoids of the bronchus have very good prognoses consequent to early discovery and surgical removal. Nonmetastatic bronchial carcinoids and gonadal carcinoids associated with the carcinoid syndrome may produce symptoms prior to metastasis and therefore represent potential surgical cures. This group of patients, therefore, has a far better prognosis than the remaining patients with carcinoid syndrome, who almost invariably have metastatic disease. This latter group of patients has a mean survival of 3 to 5 years; however, a significant number of them may live 10 to 20 years after diagnosis is made. Severity of symptoms and characterization of tumor malignancy by its primary location and secretory products do not accurately predict long-term survival in the individual patient. Conversely, such information is quite valuable as a basis on which a therapeutic program to diminish the severity and duration of incapacitating symptoms can be formulated. The immediate causes of death in patients with carcinoid syndrome include congestive heart failure, generalized neoplastic disease with cachexia, hepatic failure, complications of bowel obstruction or perforation, cardiovascular collapse, and postsurgical complications.

PHYSICAL EXAMINATION

General Appearance and Vital Signs. Most patients will appear normal when first seen; however, those with advanced malignancy may demonstrate general cachexia. Patients with carcinoid syndrome may have flushing attacks when examined and many become hypotensive during these episodes. Orthopnea and evidence of peripheral edema may be present, especially in patients with decompensated carcinoid heart disease or hypoalbuminemia.

Skin. If an acute flushing attack occurs during the initial examination, the previously described red-violaceous discoloration may be a prominent feature. Patients with functional bronchial carcinoids may demonstrate, in addition to the flush, a profound degree of lacrimation, perspiration, parotid and submandibular glandular swelling, and facial edema with conjunctival suffusion. The appearance of a sinuously demarcated, bright red, splotchy discoloration over the face often heralds a functional gastric carcinoid. Previously described cyanosis, mottled brown discoloration and facial telangiectases may be present if the patient is seen late in the course of carcinoid syndrome.

Cardiorespiratory Findings. Evidence of bronchospasm may be present, especially with functioning foregut carcinoids. Signs of cardiac decompensation more frequently are related to diseases of the right heart. Gallop rhythms may be present during late stages of cardiac failure, and a variety of murmurs can be heard, depending upon the nature and extent of valvular involvement by endocardial fibrosis. The most frequent lesions are tricuspid insufficiency and pulmonic stenosis, and a holosystolic murmur heard over the lower left sternal border may be coupled with a more harsh murmur in the second left intercostal space with these respective lesions. Venous pulsations usually reflect a very prominent V wave and, more rarely, if significant tricuspid stenosis is present, a perceptible A wave may be present. Not uncommonly a precordial lift along the left sternal border may be felt in patients with significant disease. Although the left heart chambers may rarely be involved, mitral valvular disease, if present, is generally mild.

Abdomen. Generally only patients with carcinoid syndrome will have significant abdominal findings; however, patients with appendiceal carcinoids may have right lower quadrant tenderness and other signs associated with appendicitis. Hepatomegaly is not uncommon in carcinoid syndrome patients and usually results from metastatic disease, more frequently involving the right lobe of the liver. Superimposed right heart failure contributes significantly to the finding of hepatomegaly especially late in the course of the disease. The liver therefore may be diffusely enlarged, with palpable masses accompanied by moderate tenderness and an occasional audible friction rub. Diffuse abdominal tenderness may be present chronically. Episodes of acute abdominal pain and severe tenderness may occur secondary to necrosis of tumor masses. A significant fraction of patients will have a palpable abdominal mass, which most often is not the primary carcinoid tumor but usually represents a metastatic lesion, a fibrotic mass of intestinal loops, or a concurrent histologically different neoplasm of the digestive tract. Auscultation of the abdomen will often detect the hypermotility characteristic of carcinoid syndrome. Carcinoids of the ovary are most often part of a much larger ovarian teratoma that is usually detectable by bimanual palpation during the pelvic examination.

Miscellaneous. Patients with carcinoid arthropathy usually do not display evidence of an inflammatory process and will demonstrate only limitation of motion, most frequently in the small joints of the hands. A variety of other cutaneous manifestations have been described, including some suggestive of scleroderma, but the true nature and specificity of these lesions related to carcinoid are unknown. The rare testicular carcinoids are usually easily palpable, but primary lesions of the testes are seldom associated with carcinoid syndrome. As indicated earlier, physical signs suggestive of hyperadrenocorticism may be present in patients with foregut carcinoids and ectopic ACTH production. Generalized muscular weakness, more prominent over the larger truncal muscles, occurs in some patients, but its cause is unknown. Patients also have been reported to have abnormalities in affective behavior, but specificity for carcinoid syndrome and putative relationship to tumor secretions are undocumented.

COMMON COMPLICATIONS

Most complications commonly seen in carcinoid patients have been discussed in earlier sections. The major complications include right heart decompensation; hepatic failure secondary to metastatic disease or heart failure; peptic ulceration with or without perforation; bowel obstruction; severe hypotension; abdominal crises usually related to spontaneous or cancer chemotherapy–related tumor necrosis; complications related to increased incidence of secondary malignancies; niacin deficiency secondary to tumor utilization of dietary tryptophan; and steatorrhea and fluid and electrolyte imbalances related to diarrhea. In addition, the excessive desmoplastic reaction to carcinoid secretions may become life-threatening. In this regard, several instances of retroperitoneal fibrosis resulting in ureteral obstruction and renal failure have been reported in carcinoid patients.

Unfortunately, a number of significant complications in patients with carcinoid syndrome are iatrogenic. Patients who present with signs and symptoms of bronchoconstriction have been inadvertently treated with beta-adrenergic agonists, which in these particular patients led to additional, massive release of tumor secretions and worsening of the bronchoconstriction and marked hypotension. In addition, the administration of curare-like drugs, morphine and similar narcotics, and a variety of volatile anesthetic agents during both anesthesia induction and postsurgical care have led to massive release of biologically active compounds from carcinoid tumors, with ensuing carcinoid functional crises.

LABORATORY FINDINGS

As indicated earlier, most patients with uncomplicated carcinoid will have normal laboratory profiles for routine studies of blood chemistries, hemogram, and urinalyses. The single most important diagnostic test is the quantitative assay of urinary 5-HIAA. Carcinoid patients will usually excrete in excess of 30 mg/24 hours and may have values up to 800 or 1000 mg/24 hours. Patients with foregut tumors, which have a relative lack of aromatic L-amino acid decarboxylase, tend to have somewhat lower urinary excretion of 5-HIAA and serotonin, but will have quite elevated levels of 5-HTP. Elevated levels of histamine and histamine metabolites will be present in most patients with gastric carcinoid. All tumors that are biopsied or tumor masses that are removed surgically should be frozen and saved for assay of serotonin and other biologically active substances, depending upon the availability of the assays in question. Such information is not merely academic but can serve as a basis for the rational design of therapy in individual patients. As indicated earlier, during advanced stages of carcinoid syndrome abnormalities in hepatic function appear to reflect both obstructive and parenchymal hepatic damage. This factor, added to decreased intake and increased tumor utilization of tryptophan and other protein precursors, may lead to clinically significant hypoalbuminemia. Careful evaluation and follow-up of serum electrolytes may be necessary in order to avoid complications associated with hypokalemia, acidosis, or hyponatremia. In addition to these derangements resulting from diarrhea, some patients develop overt steatorrhea and malabsorption. Hypovitaminoses, both water soluble and fat-soluble, thus may be present, and it may become necessary to quantify the degree of malabsorption by use of appropriate tests, such as quantitative assay for stool fat, D-xylose absorption, vitamin A absorption, and others. Specific tests designed to identify and quantify any of the several ectopic polypeptide hormones secreted from foregut tumors should be done when indicated and when such test capability exists.

GENERAL DIAGNOSTIC APPROACH AND RADIOLOGIC STUDIES

As outlined earlier, the diagnosis of carcinoid syndrome depends on the identification of certain clinical abnormalities associated with a functioning carcinoid tumor and evidence of tumor secretory capability by the finding of elevated urinary 5-HIAA or other tryptophan metabolites, or of both. Once this is established, it is mandatory that all necessary steps be taken to determine the primary tumor site or, more specifically, to exclude with certainty that a curable ovarian, testicular, or bronchial carcinoid is not being overlooked. Most carcinoid tumors leading to the syndrome, of course, are metastatic to the liver and therefore are generally considered to be incurable. Because a significant number of patients live for prolonged periods with metastatic disease, it is incumbent upon the attending physician to ensure that adequate evaluation of the individual patient's status be done. Only then can rational decisions be made concerning the feasibility of palliative surgical removal of large tumor masses or cardiac valvulotomy and prosthetic valvular replacement. In order to achieve these goals a complete assessment of the location and extent of hepatic and extra-hepatic metastases is necessary by use of appropriate scanning and arteriographic methods. In addition to this evaluation of tumor mass, a concurrent evaluation of general hepatic and cardiac function must be undertaken to determine if corrective measures are required prior to any tentative surgical intervention. Such extensive evaluation should not be viewed as heroic in nature, for a number of patients have enjoyed a greatly enhanced quality of life as a result of such procedures, despite the fact that no hope of cure was present.

PITFALLS IN DIAGNOSIS

In previous sections, categories of potential differential diagnostic problems related to carcinoid syndrome were mentioned. It is apparent that virtually any other tumor that might arise in structures also commonly involved by carcinoids should be considered in the differential diagnosis of this disease. Other causes of cardiac and hepatic failure should be excluded, as should instances of recent-onset asthma; angioneurotic edema and other anaphylactoid-type reactions; nontropical sprue and additional causes of diarrhea and malabsorption; and other causes of ectopic hormone production. Careful screening of a patient's dietary habits and drug intake should be made to exclude causes of false-positive and false-negative abnormalities in urinary 5-HIAA excretion.

The classic carcinoid syndrome is not usually a difficult diagnosis, but the diagnostic evaluation of individual patients and the application of such information in the design and implementation of a rational and optimal therapeutic program is both demanding and rewarding.

Section Ten

NERVOUS SYSTEM AND MUSCLE

MIGRAINE AND ITS VARIANTS

By J. M. S. Pearce, M.D., F.R.C.P.
Hull, England
and C. G. Clough, M.R.C.P.
Birmingham, England

DEFINITION

The word migraine is derived from the term hemicrania first introduced in an account of the disease by Galen (A.D. 131 to 201). It comprises a wide variety of symptoms, the most common being paroxysmal headache. Many diagnostic criteria for migraine have included as necessary elements for diagnosis the occurrence of accompanying neurologic features or the response of headache to ergotamine. Such dogmatism is unwarranted, leading to the elimination of the correct diagnosis for many migraine patients. Vahlquist's definition is one of the more useful: Paroxysmal headaches separated by intervals of freedom from pain plus at least two of the following four points: (1) unilateral headache, (2) nausea, (3) visual or sensorimotor aura, and (4) family history.

A distinction is made between common and classic migraine, although many sufferers have both types of attack. Those attacks that have associated visual or cerebral symptoms or signs are termed *classic;* those without focal neurologic disturbance are termed *common* migraine. The second condition is much more frequently encountered. Variants of migraine are listed in Table 1.

CLINICAL FEATURES

Various studies have put the incidence of migraine in the population as between 15 and 25 per cent, females being affected more often than males in a ratio of 3:2. Many patients have infrequent attacks, some three to four in a lifetime. At the other end of the spectrum a minority can have regular attacks, say five or six per month, and occasional times when anxiety factors can result in an almost continuous headache. Seventy per cent of patients have a family history, especially those with classic migraine. Migraine is said to affect intelligent people more commonly than others, but this may be a false impression; it does seem that sufferers more often than not have obsessional or neurotic personality traits and are prone to anxiety. Indeed, this element is an important factor in precipitation of attacks and a high attendance rate for consultations. The symptoms of a classic attack can be usefully divided into stages.

Prodromal Features. For hours up to a day before the attack, some patients may describe feelings of elation, yawning, or euphoria. Others become drowsy and lethargic or even depressed. Clear-cut tension headache may precede migraine attacks and merge into the vascular headache. Weight gain and fluid retention are fairly common.

Aura. This refers to the neurologic warning of the headache that distinguishes classic from common migraine. These symptoms may be due to intracerebral oligemia leading to focal ischemia or to depression of cortical neuronal activity. This results in focal negative or positive phenomena. It is believed that this is followed by a period of vasodilation that produces distention of sensitive pain fibers in the arteries, arterioles, and veins, thus resulting in headache. This is corroborated by the dilation of extracranial vessels and relief from headache experienced by many patients on compression of these vessels.

The aura usually occurs before headache and lasts 10 to 40 minutes, although headache sometimes can accompany it. This fact plus the observation that a focal deficit can occur on the same side as headache suggests that oligemia and vasodilation are not mutually exclusive and may occur in different parts of the brain at the same time. The most common aura is visual, occurring in up to 30 per cent of migraine patients. Occipital auras frequently take the form of flashing lights or stars (*photopsiae*). These occur in the periphery of the visual field, but can expand to involve the central vision or vice versa. They are frequently colored, but can be black and white and tend to scintillate. Some patients notice a small paracentral area often described as a filament of a light bulb. Various geometric shapes and zigzag lines known as fortification spectra (*teichopsiae*) may occur in one half of the visual field.

Other, more complex hallucinations result from ischemia of the optic radiation in the temporal lobes. These are often of bright primary colors and may produce the illusion of a person, animal, or object. Negative effects of ischemia result in scotomas. These can progress to result in complex fragmented or altitudinal visual field defects. Those scotomas involving one eye can be "thrown" by eye movements and are caused by the ischemic retina; indeed, permanent scotomas due to retinal artery occlusion as a complication of migraine have been reported.

Table 1. Migraine and Variants

Classical—With visual, sensory, or speech disorder

Common—Without such focal neurologic accompaniments

Variants

1. Cluster headache (periodic, chronic)
2. Facial migraine (syn. lower half headache)
3. Ophthalmoplegic migraine
4. Hemiplegic migraine, including hemisensory attacks
5. Basilar artery migraine

Disturbance of parietal lobe function results in disorders of perception (*metamorphopsia*). Objects may appear large (*macropsia*) or small (*micropsia, Lilliputian syndrome*) and the limbs and hands may feel blown up to gigantic size. Visual agnosia is uncommon but can occur, so that patients cannot recognize objects or understand their use. Ischemia of the motor and sensory cortex occurs and usually results in feelings of heaviness or vaguely defined numbness and tingling in contralateral limbs. The arm or leg on that side will feel clumsy or useless, although true hemiplegia is rare. When patients first seek medical help, they are understandably alarmed at the symptoms and may think they are developing a stroke. Sensory symptoms such as "pins and needles" occur most frequently around the mouth and tongue and may spread to the arm and rarely to the leg. If the dominant hemisphere is involved, dysphasia will result. This is usually mild and expressive in type so that patients experience difficulty in getting the right word out. Word blindness and dysgraphia can occur. All of these auras disappear in 10 to 60 minutes. Very rarely, permanent sequelae betoken infarction that is confirmed by computed tomographic (CT) scanning.

Headache. Headache may commence during the aura or after. In common migraine, headache may be the only symptom and can occur out of the blue. It is usually unilateral, as the term hemicrania implies. However, it may change sides from attack to attack and can involve both sides at once, spreading to the whole cranium. Headache is described as aching and throbbing like a hammer banging inside the head, or the pain can have a burning intensity. It gradually builds up so that it reaches a peak at 1 to 2 hours. It may be just an inconvenience to some, while others have extremely severe, prostrating pain with photophobia, resembling the symptoms of a subarachnoid hemorrhage. Most patients have anorexia and nausea; some feel very ill and have marked pallor, sweating, nausea, and vomiting. These last two symptoms occur in 50 per cent of all sufferers and are associated with gastric stasis and slowing of the gastrointestinal motility. Other patients have diarrhea. Polyuria may be noticed, as may tenderness over the scalp or the temporal arteries. The majority of sufferers who cannot work during their attacks will find a quiet, soothing darkened room and lie still or sleep until it is over. The slightest noise or movement may make headache worse, and some may find normal sounds and smells exaggerated and unpleasant. Headache can last from 1 to 2 hours or up to 48 hours, and as it dies down many patients are left with a feeling of lifelessness and fatigue; they may feel washed out for the next day. Victims of migraine seek repose; those with cluster headache wander restlessly.

PRECIPITATING FACTORS

Many attacks come for no particular reason. Patients will report many different factors that they believe bring on attacks. Most of these will be casual rather than causal relationships. However, it is worthwhile to record every patient's precipitating factors and to inquire routinely about certain known common precipitants (Table 2).

The most common precipitating factor is emotional disturbance, and anxiety and stress may result in both tension headache and migraine. Anxiety and depression also result in sleeplessness and fatigue that can trigger attacks, thus initiating a vicious circle that can lead to almost continuous headache—a crossbreed of tension and migraine. Let-down headaches may follow periods of tension, for example, following interviews. This commonly affects the vigorous business or professional person who, following periods of stress at work, finds weekends or holidays marred by attacks of headache. As migraine sufferers tend to be obsessional, breaking their fixed routine may well precipitate attacks.

Much emphasis has been placed on diet in causing migraine. Certainly different foodstuffs can provoke an attack in susceptible persons; however, this provocation is not as common as once thought. Foods such as cheese and herring that contain tyramine are frequently implicated, as is chocolate, which contains the related amine phenylethylamine. Missing meals or fasting for whatever reason can promote attacks. Sunlight, bright lights, or glare from a reflective surface also provides a trigger; hence many sufferers resort to wearing tinted glasses, although this usually denotes emotional insecurity rather than light-induced migraine. Endocrine factors are certainly important, although the explanations of their effects are somewhat vague. Many women report an association of migraine with menstruation and some a reduced or increased frequency of attacks at the onset of menopause; attacks commonly remit in pregnancy. The approach to this problem should be empirical rather than guided by theoretic considerations.

INVESTIGATIONS

The diagnosis of migraine is made on the basis of history, and this should be confirmed by an absence of

Table 2. Precipitants of Migraine

Common	Less Common
Anxiety states	Alcohol
Relaxation—vacation or weekends	Hunger or fasting
Excess or lack of sleep	Dietary idiosyncrasies
Menstruation, menopause, use of oral contraceptive pill	High humidity
Bright lights	
Travel	

findings on clinical examination. Usually no further tests are necessary. Only rarely is it necessary to exclude subarachnoid hemorrhage by lumbar puncture when the patient presents with a very severe headache of acute onset.

Complicated migraine has been investigated extensively by several workers in the past, using carotid angiography. They have seldom found it rewarding, arteriovenous malformations being rarely discovered. Carotid angiography is thus not indicated in the investigation of migraine without clinical signs. If migraine is complicated by focal epilepsy, by fits at the height of an attack, or by subarachnoid hemorrhage, CT scanning and angiography will be necessary. Similarly, the electroencephalogram (EEG) is a virtually useless diagnostic aid, although it is frequently requested. Associated disorders discovered at clinical examination—for example, hypertension—can be aggravating factors and should be investigated and treated in their own right.

VARIANTS

Cluster Headache. This is known under many synonyms—periodic migrainous neuralgia, histamine headache, ciliary neuralgia, Horton's syndrome, sphenopalatine neuralgia, autonomic facial cephalgia, Harris's neuralgia. Usually it has been regarded as a variant of migraine. However, it is a separate entity and differs in several important aspects. It is important that the condition not be misdiagnosed, as treatment can have a dramatic effect in improving the life of sufferers—this can be an almost unbearable disease. Cluster headache occurs in both sexes; however, it is much more common in men. Age of onset is between 20 and 40 years, and there is usually no previous history of migraine or family history of cluster headaches.

As the name implies, headaches occur in clusters or in runs typically up to two to three per day for 1 to 4 months at a time. Remissions then can last for a few months or even years. Classically, paroxysms of headache occur at exactly the same time each day. Patients report they are awakened by headache in the early hours of the morning so regularly that they can set their clocks by it—hence "alarm clock headache." Headaches last 30 minutes to 2 hours and are of a very intense, boring, aching, or burning nature. In fact, some consider it the worst pain known to humans; some patients contemplate suicide. The patient is restless, not bedfast.

This pain is situated around one orbit or supraorbitally and is confined to that orbit for the duration of the cluster headache, although it may move to the other eye in further bouts. There can be radiation of pain to the nose, cheek, or teeth of the upper jaw, sometimes to the lower jaw and neck.

Commonly, there is watering and redness of the eye on the side of the headache, although these are not invariable signs. The nostril on that side may also be blocked or feel stuffy. The face may appear red and puffy, and there may be tenderness over a prominent temporal artery. Autonomic involvement may be signaled by miosis, ptosis, and sweating on the affected side. Horner's syndrome occurs in 18 per cent of patients and occasionally persists after the attack. Precipitating factors are rare, although alcohol, nitrites, and histamine have been proved to trigger attacks.

The features of this headache are so characteristic that the diagnosis should be made from the history and no further investigation is necessary. The periodicity of attacks, their intense nature, and the associated signs should clearly distinguish this syndrome from tic douloureux and other causes of facial pain. Chronic cluster headache can develop. This is rare and refers to attacks that have become continuous, with no periods of remission.

Facial Migraine. This refers to variants of migraine affecting the facial vasculature. It has all the typical features of migraine: periodicity, length of attacks, and associated features.

Lower-half headache is a unilateral pain affecting the lower face below the ear. There are two maximum sites of pain, one in the orbit and at the base of the nose, the other posterior to the mastoid process in the temporal bone. The pain is dull, bursting, and nagging, and it may sometimes have a throbbing component. Occasionally it may spread to the neck and shoulder and rarely may radiate into the arm.

Other types of facial migraine have similar qualities, with deep, boring pains in the orbit and cheek; lacrimation and nasal secretion are common, although not invariable, features. Sometimes the temporal artery is affected, with visible swelling and tenderness.

Carotidynia is an episodic throbbing pain in the neck related to a tender carotid artery. Pressure over this causes more pain, but firm pressure may completely relieve symptoms.

Facial migraine is distinguished from trigeminal neuralgia by the fact that the latter is characterized by short, sharp, lancinating pains. Facial migraine occurs in younger patients, is seldom confined to the distribution of the trigeminal nerve, and does not have the trigger areas with precipitation of pain by talking and washing so characteristic of trigeminal neuralgia. Atypical or psychogenic facial pain can occur in the maxillary area on one or both sides of the face. It typically affects young women, who will describe the pain as unbearable and yet remain impassive. In highly colored terms the pain will be described as burning, deep, or as if the skin were crawling or being torn from the skull. It is different from that of migraine because it is continuous and sometimes spreads to other areas of the face and neck.

Ophthalmoplegic Migraine. This variant affects both sexes equally and can occur in people who have had previous common or classic migraine, although it often presents in childhood. This headache is of a boring rather than throbbing nature and is periorbital, almost always occurring on the same side. It lasts from 12 to 36 hours and, as it is fading, is accompanied by ptosis and double vision. Headache then disappears and complete closure of the eye can be a sequel. Third-nerve lesions occur in more than 80 per cent of patients. In up to 12 per cent of patients, sixth-nerve lesions are reported and fourth-nerve lesions in a minority. An internal ophthalmoplegia may accompany the external ophthalmoplegia, with a fixed or reacting dilated pupil. The ocular palsy persists for 1 to 4 weeks. Attacks may recur at infrequent intervals.

The differential diagnosis from internal carotid or posterior communicating aneurysms that compress the third nerve can at times be difficult. If the clinical course is not typical, angiography and CT scanning should be performed to exclude a lesion that can be surgically corrected. Angiography is deferred until the attack has resolved, if possible, because complications such as fatal carotid thrombosis have been reported when this is performed during the attack.

Hemiplegic Migraine. Sporadic focal symptoms in migraine are not uncommon. Up to one third of migraine patients will experience hemisensory symptoms or hemiparesis on at least one occasion. This is usually part of the aura and lasts only about an hour. Rarely, symptoms will persist for up to 24 hours and sometimes for a week after the attack. This usually means infarction of cerebral cortex has taken place. Sensory symptoms are more common, with tingling and "pins and needles" affecting the face, arm, and leg, or characteristically felt around both sides of the tongue and around the lips. Complete hemiplegia is rare; much more frequently feelings of heaviness are present in the arm and rarely the leg.

Familial hemiplegic migraine is a similar but separate entity and is quite rare. In contrast to sporadic hemiplegic migraine, the weakness will always recur on the same side and may outlast the headache. There is always a family history, suggesting an autosomal dominant inheritance, and within that family hemiplegia always occurs on the same side.

Basilar Migraine. Basilar migraine results from involvement of the basilar artery with ensuring symptoms of brain stem ischemia. Symptoms of brain stem involvement are common in many patients with common or classic migraine. These are described as feelings of dizziness or lightheadedness. Distinguishing features of basilar migraine are vertigo, double vision, dysarthria, and ataxia. These symptoms usually occur as an aura prior to the headache; thus the diagnosis should become clear. Paresthesia may involve the arms and face classically in a perioral fashion. Involvement of the occipital poles results in hemianopia or blindness in both eyes. At the height of an attack of basilar migraine, syncope commonly occurs. Simple vasovagal-initiated syncope can happen to some migraine sufferers because of headache and autonomic disturbance. Prolonged unconsciousness or maintenance of an erect position may even result in an anoxic fit, although this may require investigation on its own account.

Childhood Migraine. Children can present with straightforward migraine and this diagnosis should not be a problem if a history of paroxysmal unilateral headache can be elicited. More often, abdominal symptoms predominate. In the past, these attacks have been labeled by pediatricians as cyclical vomiting, periodic syndrome, or childhood acidosis. If a careful history is taken, more often than not a child will describe headaches as well as the other, more obvious distressing symptoms. Thus it is clear that this is a migraine variant. Attacks may follow exercise. The child appears pale, sweats, and complains of pains in the abdomen. Nausea and vomiting are common accompaniments, and sometimes diarrhea or constipation occurs.

These patients appear to have an acute abdomen and are often suspected of having appendicitis. Fever and leukocytosis can occur, but diagnosis can be made if there is a history of periodic attacks with good health in between, along with a family history of migraine. Attacks tend to be short, but may last for 24 hours. Patients appear pale, irritable, and tired. They then become moody or lethargic for the duration of the attack. Childhood migraine has a good prognosis; up to 50 per cent of the children recover completely and have no further problems. Others have attacks of sickness or develop symptoms of adult migraine as they reach adolescence.

PITFALLS IN DIAGNOSIS

As stressed, history and examination will establish the diagnosis of migraine in the majority of patients. Difficulty often arises when headache or neurologic deficit presents acutely. In this case other conditions may need to be excluded.

Acute Headaches

Subarachnoid Hemorrhage. The onset of headache is more abrupt than in migraine, likened to being "struck on the back of the head or neck with a baseball bat." Loss of consciousness is common, as is associated vomiting. Patients can usually distinguish the severity of this headache from their ordinary headaches; they will be markedly photophobic and have a stiff neck; they will need to lie quietly in a darkened room. Any patient who presents for the first time with such a history should have a CT scan, followed by lumbar puncture if necessary.

Meningitis. Meningitis is less easily confused with other causes of headache. In this case, headache is of gradual onset and is generalized. Pyrexia and neck stiffness usually distinguish these patients.

In patients with chronic or recurring headache, migraine has to be distinguished from other conditions (Table 3).

Recurrent or Chronic Headache

Tension Headache. This is the most common of all headaches. It is produced at times of stress, although this factor may not be apparent. Its character is described as a tight band around the head, as if it were in a vise or a heavy weight were pressing on top of the head. Pain tends to lack the throbbing quality of migraine and is rarely unilateral. Autonomic disturbance can occur, with feelings of nausea and occasionally vomiting. It should be remembered that migraine sufferers commonly have tension headaches as well, either separate from or precipitating migraine attacks. In the latter instance, a vicious circle of tension and migraine headache can arise, with tension precipitating migraine, resulting in more stress, and so on. It is important to distinguish the two components in the history and to treat both.

Recent work has attempted to blur the distinction between tension headache and migraine, claiming that the latter is but a severe variety of the former and that the accompanying vomiting and prostration indicate only reactions to the severity of the pain. Electromyographic (EMG) studies show muscle contraction in migraine attacks as well as in tension headache. These interesting findings, however, do not explain the demonstrable oligemia that characterizes the migraine attack—as elegantly shown by Danish workers using cerebral blood flow studies. For clinical purposes the distinction remains valid and has implications for treatment, which remains different for the two conditions.

It is important to recognize ergotamine-induced headache, which usually occurs in nervous patients whose migraine has become more frequent. These patients may resort to using more and more ergot and finally present with daily headaches accompanied by nausea and malaise, relieved only by further doses of ergotamine. Although signs of ergotism are rare, it is vital to realize that chronic ergotamine overdosage leads to throbbing headache and sickness; the proof and cure for this situation are found in admitting the patient to hospital, total withdrawal of ergotamine, and a few days' sedation. It is rare to encounter failure with this regimen.

Post-traumatic Headache. This more often follows minor than major head injury. It is seldom seen in sports injuries and is strongly associated with an unsettled compensation claim for injury at work or in road accidents. The pain is at the site of any scar or is diffuse and of the tension type. There are no neurologic signs; it is surprisingly rare as a lasting complaint in those who have been unconscious for 24 hours or more. Although its mechanism is disputed by purists, its recognition is not difficult. Migraine preceding head trauma may be apparently aggravated by it, although probably not by organic mechanisms. Injury to the head is *not a cause* of migraine.

Sinusitis. This can sometimes cause a dull facial pain over the frontal or maxillary sinuses. Local tenderness is present. X-ray may help to confirm the diagnosis. Chronic sinusitis is often implicated in causing recurrent headaches, but this is seldom the case.

Acute Glaucoma. This can produce acute, severe orbital pain associated with vomiting and deterioration of vision in that eye. The eye will feel rock-hard, with central injection and clouding of the cornea. This can be assessed roughly by digital palpation and by tonometry prior to urgent treatment.

Skull Lesions. Paget's disease of bone or metastases in the skull can cause chronic or recurring headaches of either localized or generalized distribution. Radiology shows the cause.

Temporal Arteritis. Temporal arteritis is not an uncommon cause of headache after the age of 65 years. The onset of headache is gradual. It is constant, can be relieved by simple analgesics, and generally presents with other features such as nocturnal sweating, malaise, and thickened, pulseless, tender temporal arteries. If this diagnosis is suspected, it is a simple matter to check the erythrocyte sedimentation rate (ESR), which will be raised, or, if necessary, perform temporal artery biopsy. If this condition is missed, the grave consequences of retinal ischemia can ensue. It is important not to be misled by a *single* normal or marginally raised ESR. If clinical doubt persists ESR is measured three times within 48 hours, and a biopsy should be done if the results remain equivocal. Headache is variable, sometimes intermittent, and occasionally absent in the presence of fever, malaise, polymyalgia, or masseter claudication; each of these features should lead to biopsy in the elderly subject and to the prompt initiation of steroid therapy.

Cervical Spondylosis. This can produce headache in the middle-aged, which can aggravate or simulate migraine. It can lead to an occipital ache radiating to the top of the head downward into the shoulder or arms or around into the jaw. Pain can be intermittent and unilateral, although it is rarely associated with systemic upset. On examination one should look for restriction of neck movements or signs and symptoms of root or cord compression. Radiology is seldom helpful, and if both conditions coexist, each may require treatment.

Raised Intracranial Pressure. Raised intracranial pressure due to a tumor or subdural hematoma produces a headache that initially occurs every morning. It has a generalized distribution, may be associated with effortless vomiting, and is made worse by coughing, sneezing, bending, or defecation. Eventually the headaches become constant, and usually at this stage changes of personality, epilepsy, or focal signs supervene, and papilledema may be discovered. Rare causes of episodic headache are intermittent obstructive hydrocephalus secondary to a colloid cyst of the third ventricle and tumors obstructing the fourth ventricle. These produce a severe headache and vomiting due to raised intracranial pressure, and will classically be precipitated and relieved by sudden changes of posture. CT scanning and ventriculography may be required in these rare cases.

Transient Ischemic Attacks. The neurologic symptoms of the aura of migraine can be indistinguishable from transient ischemic attacks. By definition, the latter resolve within 24 hours and they are not usually accompanied by headache, although mild

Table 3. Pitfalls in Diagnosis

Other Acute Headaches
Subarachnoid hemorrhage
Acute meningitis
Recurrent or Chronic Headaches
Tension headache
Post-traumatic headache
Trigeminal neuralgia
Atypical facial pain
Acute sinusitis
Acute glaucoma (closed-angle type)
Skull lesions: Paget's disease, metastases
Temporal arteritis
Cervical spondylosis
Raised intracranial pressure
Tumor
Subdural hematoma
Hydrocephalus
Focal cerebral lesions—TIAs*
Paroxysmal or accelerated hypertension
Cluster headache
Other migraine variants

*TIA = Transient ischemic attack.

contralateral head pain can occur. The onset of focal neurologic symptoms and signs such as those described should always be considered as transient ischemic attacks in older patients who have no previous history of classic migraine or in patients without headache and investigated accordingly, if necessary by means of angiography.

Paroxysmal Hypertension. This will produce severe headache that often can mimic migraine. It can be due to a pheochromocytoma, to a reaction to monoamine oxidase inhibitors, or to ingestion of tyramine in cheese. Demonstration of pallor, tachycardia, and a greatly raised blood pressue during an attack will establish the diagnosis.

Headache is not a symptom of uncomplicated hypertension. In malignant or accelerated hypertension (with grade 3 or 4 retinopathy, proteinuria, and diastolic pressure of over 130), raised pressure headaches in the mornings, relieved by change of posture and analgesics, do occur in some patients, and demand urgent investigation and treatment in hospital.

NEURALGIAS OF THE TRIGEMINAL, GLOSSOPHARYNGEAL, AND FACIAL NERVES

By John M. Tew, Jr., M.D.
and Harry Van Loveren, M.D.
Cincinnati, Ohio

TRIGEMINAL NEURALGIA (TIC DOULOUREUX, FACIAL NEURALGIA)

Definition

Trigeminal neuralgia is a condition of paroxysmal facial pain provoked by cutaneous stimuli to trigger points in the orofacial regions and radiating in the distribution of the trigeminal nerve.

Presenting Symptoms

There are five features that distinguish tic douloureux from other painful conditions of the face:

1. Pain, paroxysmal in character, is the only symptom.
2. The pain is confined to the distribution of the trigeminal nerve.
3. The pain is preceded by cutaneous stimuli, such as touch, talking, moving the tongue, or even a light breeze blowing against the face. Shaving, brushing the teeth, or even eating becomes impossible for victims during an attack of tic douloureux.
4. The pain never crosses the midline. Although 1 per cent of patients develop bilateral tic douloureux, the condition rarely occurs simultaneously on both sides of the face.
5. The disorder is subject to exacerbations and remissions. Because of this characteristic, support has been given to many forms of treatment. However, almost invariably the pain recurs after increasingly short periods of remission, only to persist longer and cause more suffering.

Physical Findings

During periods of remission, the physical and neurologic examination is normal. The slightest evidence of altered sensation, facial paralysis, or hearing loss should suggest that a neoplasm, vascular anomaly, or compressive lesion may be present. Appropriate diagnostic studies are mandatory.

If the examination is conducted during an episode of pain, the face is frequently immobile, hygiene may be disregarded, and the face is protected from any touch. If the patient permits it, sensory examination will elicit paroxysms of pain on stimulation of trigger sites, principally around the nose, lips, and eyebrows, even by the most gentle touch. Calibrated testing may demonstrate decreased sensation, a feature that suggests fatigue or metabolic exhaustion of the ganglion cells. Autonomic features, such as tearing, rhinorrhea, and redness of the face may accompany attacks of pain in some patients and lead to confusion with cluster or migraine headaches.

Suffering associated with tic douloureux is highly variable. The paroxysmal pain in the early stages is usually mild and is frequently confused with pain of dental origin. This feature leads the victim to seek dental care and, in many circumstances, results in multiple dental extractions, revision of occlusion, and explorations of the paranasal sinuses. As the attacks become more severe, the pain is variously described as "stabbing," "jabbing," or "like a hot poker," and it may even become constant, as if the face were "on fire." During the attacks of extreme pain, victims may attempt suicide because analgesics and narcotics are ineffective.

Natural History

Remissions and exacerbations are common, but spontaneous cure rarely occurs. The disease rarely develops in patients less than 40 years of age. However, I have seen cases in three patients younger than 20 years old. There is a predilection for females, the pain is more common on the right side, and a familial disposition is recognized. The incidence is approximately 1 in 25,000 persons.

In time, the condition worsens, the pain often overcomes medical therapy, and the neuralgia recurs after peripheral nerve destruction. It responds to interruption of the nerve proximal to the gasserian ganglion, with cure or protracted remission.

Laboratory Diagnosis

The correct diagnosis of tic douloureux is based almost entirely on the history and the patient's description of the classic features of an attack of pain.

Laboratory studies are useful in identifying certain conditions that may cause trigeminal neuralgia. Skull x-rays are of value in the assessment of basilar impression, osteoporosis, Paget's disease, and other bony disorders that may be associated with compression of the trigeminal nerve.

Tumors in the posterior fossa may cause trigeminal neuralgia–like symptoms. Facial neuralgia due to tumors is generally constant rather than intermittent, and there is a major detectable neurologic deficit, which distinguishes this disorder from classic tic douloureux. Computed tomography of the brain and base of the skull will effectively demonstrate most brain tumors. The pain in these patients is almost always relieved following removal of the tumor.

Neurovascular compression of the trigeminal root by aberrant arteries or veins is probably a cause of trigeminal neuralgia in some patients. Unfortunately, angiography is not helpful in identifying those patients who have significant neurovascular compression and therefore it is not performed routinely. Surgical decompression of the trigeminal nerve is reserved for selected patients.

Multiple sclerosis is likewise primarily a clinical diagnosis. Spinal fluid analysis may provide supportive evidence of this disease if there is elevation of the gamma globulin fraction or oligoclonal IgG. Elevated cerebrospinal fluid protein level is more suggestive of tumor.

Differential Diagnosis

The differentiation of more obscure forms of facial pain may be quite difficult at times; among the conditions to be considered are (1) atypical facial pain, (2) symptomatic lesions, (3) dental neuralgia, (4) cluster migraine, (5) temporomandibular joint disease, (6) multiple sclerosis, and (7) other cranial neuralgias.

Atypical facial pain is a descriptive term contrived to include all the conditions that are not "classic" idiopathic trigeminal neuralgia. This diagnosis is basically one of exclusion; however, certain features of the history are found in most patients. The pain is gradual in onset, is constant rather than paroxysmal, and is often described as burning, boring, or aching in character. The pain frequently radiates across the midline and outside the trigeminal nerve distribution. This condition tends to occur in younger persons and tends to be associated with depression or serious neurosis. Patients with atypical facial pain seldom appear to suffer, rub the face frequently, and rarely identify trigger points. Unlike tic douloureux, the pain is seldom alleviated by carbamazepine (Tegretol). The physical examination is normal, although the patient with chronic pain may already have been subjected to a series of procedures (nerve destruction, dental extraction, sinus exploration), which may have made the condition worse. Differentiation is critical because destructive procedures on the nervous system invariably aggravate the pain. Psychotropic drugs and counseling are probably the only effective approaches to this problem.

Symptomatic lesions, such as neoplasms, multiple sclerosis, vascular anomalies, and compressive lesions, may cause a tic-like pain, but in most instances there are distinguishing features, such as constancy of pain or presence of focal neurologic deficits. The appropriate laboratory tests should confirm the diagnosis.

Dental neuralgia is occasionally a perplexing problem, since most patients with facial pain have undergone a considerable number of dental procedures. These patients may be uncertain which came first, the pain or a dental procedure that may have injured a peripheral nerve and caused a painful neuralgia. Pain of dental origin is more likely to be constant, burning, limited to the distribution of a dental nerve, and associated with some sensory deficit in the distribution of that nerve. The pain should be eliminated by local injection with anesthetics, but resection of the nerve may fail to provide permanent relief.

Cluster migraine (Horton's cephalgia, red migraine) may be confused with tic douloureux because of its paroxysmal character, radiation into the trigeminal distribution, and association with autonomic phenomena. However, the disorder can be distinguished by familial occurrence; by attacks that are throbbing, constant in severity, and progressive in nature, developing in a crescendo fashion to termination suddenly after 30 to 45 minutes; by the absence of trigger sites; and by provocation by alcohol and certain foods. Interestingly, some patients whose condition cannot be diagnosed with certainty may respond partially to drug treatment and satisfactorily to surgical approach. Their disease has been called *cluster tic douloureux.*

Temporomandibular joint disease should never be confused with tic douloureux because the pain caused by malocclusion or arthritis of the temporomandibular joint does not resemble tic pain, is focal in nature, and can be reproduced by manipulation of the jaw. The diagnosis is confirmed by radiographic changes of the temporomandibular joint.

Multiple sclerosis may be associated with painful neuralgia that is indistinguishable from tic douloureux. The physical examination should indicate evidence of neurologic abnormalities, such as ataxia, nystagmus, or sensory deficits. The history may indicate previous episodes of neurologic disturbance in an otherwise normal patient.

VAGOGLOSSOPHARYNGEAL NEURALGIA

Vagoglossopharyngeal neuralgia is a painful condition associated with a disorder of the ninth or tenth cranial nerves or of both nerves. This disease is rare in comparison to trigeminal neuralgia, occurring in a ratio of about 1:100. The characteristics of the pain are identical to those of trigeminal neuralgia, but the localization of the pain is different. The pain frequently radiates into the pharynx, throat, tonsillar fossa, base of the tongue, and inner ear. The trigger mechanism may be pressure on the ear or swallowing. If pain occurs solely in the ear and mastoid region, it is difficult to distinguish from trigeminal neuralgia. Trigger points are frequently elicited in the tonsillar fossa and pharynx. Cessation of the pain following application of cocaine to this area is diagnostic of this disorder.

A dangerous feature of vagoglossopharyngeal neuralgia is the occasional occurrence of syncope, bradycardia, hypotension, and cardiac arrest. These symptoms are probably mediated through fibers of the carotid sinus (nerve of Herring), which causes a reflex increase in vagal tone via the vagus nerve. These attacks may be initiated by stimulation of any structure within the sensory distribution of the glossopharyngeal or vagus nerve. The stimulus is often as subtle as coughing or swallowing. Carotid sinus massage itself will not induce such an attack, thus distinguishing this disorder from carotid sinus syndrome.

Vagoglossopharyngeal neuralgia and vagoglossopharyngeal syncope often respond to carbamazepine (Tegretol), although surgical section of the nerves may be necessary if the condition becomes intractable.

GENICULATE NEURALGIA

Geniculate neuralgia is a rare, painful condition that involves the sensory branch of the facial nerve (the nervus intermedius of Wrisberg) and its sensory ganglion (the geniculate ganglion). The condition is characterized by paroxysmal, lancinating pain in the cutaneous distribution of the nervus intermedius, which includes the concha, tragus, antitragus, lobule, antihelix, external auditory canal, and a portion of the tympanic membrane. Paroxysms of pain are usually triggered by pressure anterior to the ear. Since the innervation of the auricle is complex, involving many cranial nerves, this is generally a diagnosis of exclusion and may account for failure of some patients to respond favorably to surgical procedures directed at the fifth, ninth, or tenth cranial nerve. Geniculate neuralgia may respond favorably to medical therapy, but on occasion section of the nerve of Wrisberg may be indicated.

VERTIGO

By John H. Per-Lee, M.D.
and Robert F. Kibler, M.D.
Atlanta, Georgia

Not all dizziness represents vertigo. The vertiginous patient is spatially disoriented and experiences movement distortion. True vertigo implies a subjective sense that the environment or the patient is moving when no motion is taking place, or a sense of spatial disorientation when the patient's head is in actual motion. Vertigo is accompanied by a feeling of environmental movement when the eyes are open and a feeling of patient movement when the eyes are closed.

Calorization of an ear with cold or warm water (do not do this if the eardrum is perforated) will reproduce the appropriate sense with which the patient might compare symptoms. Weakness, lightheadedness, eye spots, generalized numbness, tingling, and faintness suggest a nonvertiginous problem. Loss of balance, a sense of dysequilibrium or drunkenness, unsteadiness, falling, whirling, and a sense of being pushed strongly suggest vertigo.

Vertigo does not include a disturbance of consciousness. The clinician must be prepared to take the time to explore the patient's symptoms, since dizziness of an ill-defined nature and described by a patient in a variety of terms may occur in a primary vertiginous disorder. On the other hand, "dizziness" is a frequent complaint expressed by patients with vasovagal syncope, hyperventilation, visual impairment, and ataxia.

Balance coordination requires healthy *vestibular, proprioceptive,* and *oculomotor systems* integrated by an undisturbed *central nervous system.* The central nervous system has a great capacity to compensate for abnormal peripheral signals, but damage will initially cause symptoms. Turning vertigo occurs with damage only to the vestibular system—the labyrinthine end organ, vestibular nerve, or vestibular nuclei. Spatial disorientation occurs when damage affects any component of the larger three-system complex.

CLASSIFICATION

Up to a point, vertigo lends itself to an anatomic or functional classification. In any given clinical case, however, a clear understanding of the pathophysiology can be elusive.

Common classifications usually divide cause into anatomic categories of peripheral and central location. The disorders may then be classified according to function and pathology (Table 1).

HISTORY

It is necessary to discern a vertigo pattern, since most true vertigo occurs in one of three patterns: episodic, continuous, or induced only by a particular position or motion. Although this is not exclusively so, episodic peripheral vertigo at rest may be due to hydrops, transient ischemia, or metabolic abnormality. Viral neuropathy, trauma, and acute inflammations produce sustained vertigo. Dizziness from a previously or chronically diseased labyrinth or its central nervous system connections will likely be expressed as movement- or position-related vertigo. A labyrinthine fistula causes the same pattern.

Sustained vertigo is limited because the central nervous system can compensate for abnormal peripheral signals. This converts a sustained pattern to an episodic one, often of the position type, or suppresses vertigo altogether. It is important to know whether the vertigo is severe or mild. Of equal importance is the presence or absence of hearing loss. Tinnitus without hearing loss implicates the auditory system as well.

What other symptoms are present? Nausea implies that the dizziness is likely to be vertiginous. Otorrhea implicates the middle ear, mastoid, or both. Local ear pain implies a possible inflammatory process. Ear fullness and pressure are common with hydrops.

Table 1. Classification of Vertigo

Peripheral (Labyrinth and Vestibular Nerves)

I. Associated with Hearing Loss
- A. Inflammation
  - 1. Primary in the labyrinth
    - a. Viral labyrinthitis (nonsuppurative)
    - b. Bacterial labyrinthitis
    - c. Syphilis
    - d. Noninfective: Autoimmune disease (Cogan's syndrome)
  - 2. Primary in the perilabyrinth (middle ear, mastoid, etc.)
    - a. Bacterial otitis and mastoiditis causing:*
      - i. Labyrinthosis (induction of inflammation without infection)
      - ii. Labyrinthitis (direct infection)
      - iii. Bone erosion leading to otic capsular fistula with or without circumscribed labyrinthitis
    - b. Herpetic neuritis (herpes zoster)
- B. Trauma
  - 1. Transverse basilar skull fracture
  - 2. Concussion
  - 3. Barotrauma
    - a. Cochlear membrane rupture
    - b. Explosive decompression
  - 4. Acoustic trauma
  - 5. Surgical fistula
- C. Disordered endolymph production and resorption (endolymphatic hydrops)
- D. Neoplasms
  - 1. Labyrinth
    - a. Glomus tumor
    - b. Carcinoma
    - c. Proliferative processes (histiocytosis)

I. Associated with Hearing Loss (Continued)
- D. Neoplasms (continued)
  - 2. Internal auditory canal and cerebellopontine angle
    - a. Neurilemmoma
    - b. Primary cholesteatoma
    - c. Metastatic carcinoma
- E. Osteodystrophies: Otosclerosis
- F. Degenerative causes (with or without hearing loss)
  - 1. Macular
  - 2. Ampullar
- G. Drug-induced
- H. Vascular insufficiency
- I. Congenital (possible membrane rupture)

II. Not Associated with Hearing Loss
- A. Inflammatory: Vestibular neuronitis
- B. Benign positional vertigo
  - 1. Cupulolithiasis
  - 2. Damage of several causes: trauma, infection, degeneration
- C. Degenerative (see I.F.)
- D. Metabolic
- E. Drugs
- F. Vascular insufficiency
- G. Cervical disease

Central

I. Multiple Sclerosis

II. Vascular
- A. Transient ischemic attacks
- B. Cerebrovascular accidents

III. Neoplasms

IV. Seizures

V. Trauma

*Previous temporal bone fracture increases chance for labyrinth invasion.

Headaches may be extracranial or intracranial, and migraine can accompany peripheral or central vertigo. Diplopia, dysarthria, and peripheral sensory or motor symptoms suggest a brain stem locus. Cardiovascular disturbances expressed as hypertension, cerebrovascular accident, claudication, or visual symptoms alert the physician to the possibility of ischemia. The examiner hopes to uncover at least one localizing symptom or sign besides vertigo to place a lesion in the central nervous system. Suspicion of peripheral disease, especially when there are no auditory symptoms, depends first upon the vertigo pattern; then on knowledge of the patient's age, health, metabolic status, and drug ingestion; and finally on a history of previous ear disease or head and neck trauma.

PHYSICAL EXAMINATION

The physical examination seeks to document that the vestibular (peripheral or central) system is abnormal. Non-ocular spontaneous nystagmus, any positional nystagmus, or an induced abnormal nystagmus pattern indicates abnormality. Since light and visual fixation suppress peripheral nystagmus, use of 20-diopter glasses—or better, appropriate electronystagmography (ENG) equipment—will minimize suppressing factors. A standard approach is to observe for spontaneous nystagmus and instability with the *Romberg test* and heel-to-toe walking. A series of head accelerations with position change, the *Dix Hallpike test*, elicit positional nystagmus. Finally, vertigo is induced by a calorization process, and the results are used to compare the labyrithine response of each ear. Preferably, caloric-testing is done with warm and cold water and the results are recorded by ENG equipment. A simple screening procedure is as follows: Place 0.5 ml of ice water in the test ear for 30 seconds and note nystagmus intensity and duration. Do the same to the other ear. Nystagmus intensity and duration are compared and often it is possible to rule out hypoactivity or asymmetry of response. If the examiner cannot confirm abnormal vestibular function and still suspects a true vertiginous disorder, repetitive testing, especially when the patient has active vertigo, is helpful.

Prior to functional testing, evidence for middle ear and mastoid disease, including a labyrinthine fistula, should be sought. The clinician seeks evidence for vascular disease, especially by listening for neck and ear bruits; neurologic deficits with a cranial and peripheral neurologic examination; ocular disease; and objective confirmation of systemic disease suggested by the history. Measuring the blood pressure is important.

The auditory system should be studied thoroughly. Tuning forks, a masker for bone conduction tests, and a speaking tube are the bedside tools for the initial examination of auditory integrity. The tuning fork (250 and 500 cycles) will detect asymmetric hearing and suggest whether conductive or sensorineural loss, or both, are present. However, only accurate audiometry will quantify and truly differentiate conductive, cochlear, and retrocochlear losses. Evoked response audiometry refines knowledge of a patient's auditory nerve and brain stem function. The most common need in a vertiginous patient is to differentiate one ear from another and cochlear from retrocochlear disease.

The radiologist contributes to the diagnosis by demonstrating anatomic distortions, masses, and vascular disruptions. A computed tomographic (CT) scanner has become the most useful tool for this purpose. It clearly yields more information on average than conventional tomography or routine x-ray.

Selected laboratory studies round out the work-up. A search for anemia, thyroid disorder, diseases of glucose and fat metabolism, syphilis (FTA-ABS supported by a rapid plasma reagin test is most reliable), allergic diathesis, autoimmune phenomenon (sedimentation rate, antinuclear antibody tests, and others) are indicated when the history and physical examination suggest the need.

DIFFERENTIAL DIAGNOSIS

Peripheral Vertigo

Peripheral Vertigo with Hearing Loss

Inflammation. The most common inflammatory cause of vertigo is viral labyrinthitis. In this condition the end organ is infected. Symptom onset is abrupt. Vertigo and hearing loss usually are severe, unilateral, and of several days' duration, following which a gradual recovery of balance takes place. Residual positional vertigo is possible. The fate of the hearing varies from recovery to severe sensorineural loss. A prodromal respiratory illness commonly occurs. Absence of trauma rules out physical injury as a cause. The differential diagnosis in an elderly patient, especially one with a history of vascular disease or hypertension, includes a localized vascular occlusion or bleeding episode, especially if there is no history of prodromal respiratory disease.

Bacterial infection in the middle ear or mastoid can inflame the labyrinth. Erosion and direct invasion produce intense vertigo and destroy the hearing. An induced inflammation behind an intact membrane is more circumscribed, and the symptoms are likely to be less intense. However, in both instances vertigo is sustained. The possibility of bacterial otitis is supported by ear pain and otorrhea.

Suppurative labyrinthitis is uncommon today; it is seen only rarely, even in a specialist's office. More common are the vertiginous sequelae of a bony fistula produced by the erosion of a cholesteatoma, an occasional neoplasm, and rarely other inflammatory processes. Evidence of inflammatory mastoid disease, episodic positional vertigo, and a positive fistula test suggests a fistula. Circumscribed labyrinthitis with more insistent vertigo on movement accompanies an active chronic mastoid infectious lesion that is in contact with the membrane-covered fistula. A history of previous temporal bone trauma increases the likelihood that labyrinthitis will complicate bacterial otitis.

Autoimmune disease, with or without eye inflammation such as iritis or keratitis, is rare, although it may be more common than is thought. It produces sudden sustained vertigo and sensorineural hearing loss. It is usually bilateral, although it may be unilateral at first. If the patient has Wegener's granulomatosis or systemic vasculitis, the sedimentation rate will be elevated. However, isolated autoimmune ear disease is associated with a normal sedimentation rate and usually negative screening immunologic tests. Steroid therapy becomes a diagnostic tool.

Trauma. The history is the key to a diagnosis of trauma. In addition to balance disturbance and hearing loss, the symptoms and signs may include facial paralysis, bleeding from the ear, ossicular damage, and evident contusion. A transverse basilar skull fracture often traverses the petrous bone to damage the labyrinth. Coronal plane fractures usually spare the labyrinth. The labyrinth is also subject to concussion without fracture. Fracture-induced vertigo is sustained and usually severe. Vertigo from a concussion may or may not be severe. Also, hearing loss may not occur with concussion. Trauma often results in lasting positional and movement-induced vertigo.

Explosive noise of 180 decibels (dB) can perforate a tympanic membrane and injure the labyrinth. A history of trauma from an explosion is the key to the etiologic diagnosis. Vertigo lasts a few hours to days and is a function of the damage suffered.

Barotrauma can produce a perilymphatic fistula at the round or oval window and result in vertigo. The vertigo, initially at least, is usually sustained but will become movement-related. It is usually associated with hearing loss, which in turn is often fluctuant. A fistula may also follow stapedectomy.

Endolymphatic Hydrops. Episodic vertigo lasting a few minutes to several hours, ear fullness, tinnitus, and fluctuant hearing loss constitute the classic *syndrome of Meniere*. Disordered endolymph production and/or absorption result in endolymphatic hypertension. Fullness and tinnitus usually intensify as the hearing drops or vertigo recurs. As the disease progresses, the attacks may cease to be episodic. In addition, the hearing becomes permanently impaired but for some time fluctuates. Patients eventually experience chronic unsteadiness between acute vertiginous attacks. The process is bilateral in 15 to 30 per cent of cases, tending to the higher proportion when the process begins at an early age. The average patient is middle-aged, but the span is from youth to old age.

Episodic vertigo with fullness in the absence of hearing fluctuation also occurs and is called *vestibular hydrops*. On the other hand, fluctuant hearing loss and fullness may be found without vertigo; this is called *cochlear hydrops*. The causes of hydrops that should be considered include precursor inflammatory disease, syphilis, trauma, and otosclerosis. Disordered fat metabolism, glucose metabolism, and abnormal immunologic homeostasis are also suspect. Hydrops is the end point of several apparently unrelated processes, some of which are probably still to be discovered. A characteristic history confirmed by demonstrating fluctuant hearing loss makes the diagnosis of Meniere's syndrome.

Fluctuant hearing loss or episodic vertigo can occur in childhood. The clinical picture is similar to that of hydrops, and the problem is potentiated by congenital anatomic variations, including an enlarged cochlear aqueduct. Such anatomic configurations can occasionally be visualized with a CT scan.

Neoplasms. Tumors of the temporal bone are rare. A glomus tumor is generally recognized in the middle ear as a pulsatile red mass. Isolated carcinoma of the middle ear is unusual, but the tumor is visible on examination. Tumors, including metastatic carcinoma, are found in the temporal bone by roentgenography and confirmed by biopsy.

Primary mass lesions within the internal auditory canal mainly include acoustic neuroma, primary cholesteatoma, meningioma, and metastatic carcinoma. Initial symptoms reflect eighth nerve impairment. Tumors generally do not cause episodic dizziness unless they compromise labyrinthine circulation; unsteadiness is more common. The examiner's suspicion is aroused by eliciting characteristic patterns with audiometry, which measures auditory habituation and brain stem evoked response abnormalities. Confirmation requires x-ray visualization, usually with a CT scan. Small tumors may not be seen without air contrast.

Otosclerosis. Otosclerosis, commonly associated with conductive hearing loss, can produce sensorineural loss by encroaching on the membranous cochlea and vertigo by encroaching on the membranous labyrinth. Vertigo is usually episodic and may be part of a full Meniere's syndrome. Such a pattern, with the concomitant conductive hearing loss and the normal eardrum, suggests this diagnosis. Although otosclerosis causes Meniere's syndrome, it is not a common cause of hydrops.

Paget's disease and osteogenesis imperfecta may also encroach on the labyrinth and cause vertigo.

Degeneration. The labyrinth degenerates in time and can give rise to macular and ampullary dysequilibrium of aging. The patient with the former problem has trouble arising from bed in the morning but once having risen feels better. Ampullary dysequilibrium is a momentary unsteadiness with angular head movement seen in the elderly.

Ototoxic Drugs. Aminoglycocide antibiotics such as gentamicin and tobramycin and the diuretics ethacrynic acid and furosemide are toxic to the vestibular and cochlear end organs. Drug toxicity generally produces unsteadiness, which is enhanced by a dark environment. Appropriate dosage monitoring averts this complication, but a history of such drug treatment in the dizzy patient may be significant. Objective vestibular testing reveals bilateral hypofunction, and audiometry uncovers a sensorineural hearing loss.

Vascular Insufficiency. It is difficult to prove that vascular insufficiency causes episodic end-organ vertigo, but it is a suspected cause in the aged patient. There is no question that an acute vascular inner ear accident causes sustained vertigo with hearing loss. As expected, this occurs primarily in the elderly. Recall that viral labyrinthitis produces this same picture, so that the patient's age and history for vascular disease become important to the differential diagnosis.

Peripheral Vertigo Without Hearing Loss

It has already been stated that peripheral episodic vertigo can occur without hearing loss in vestibular hydrops and vascular insufficiency. Sustained vertigo also occurs without hearing loss. Vestibular neuronitis, presumably a viral neuropathy, is the chief cause. Vertigo begins suddenly. It produces disabling, whirling vertigo with nausea. It is associated occasionally with headache and lasts several days. There are no subjective or objective auditory changes. This disorder is generally a self-limited process and has been known to recur in the same patient.

Movement- or position-related vertigo is called *benign positional vertigo* and has multiple causes. Such vertigo classically is induced by position change or assumption of a particular position. It apparently results from previous trauma, inflammation, degeneration, or insult to the peripheral or central vestibular system. In the instance of peripheral disease, free otoconia, separated from the macular organs by injury, disease, or degeneration, flow into one of the ampullae, most commonly the posterior one, and stimulate the ampulla. Once the position is assumed, the vertigo has a short latency of about 15 seconds and a limited duration, usually of less than a minute; it is fatigable when the position is repetitively resumed. When the position is supine with the involved ear undermost this disorder is called by Schuknecht *cupulolithiasis.*

Finally, hypoglycemia and vestibulotoxic drugs can cause vertigo without hearing loss. The former possibility is suggested by a relationship to food abstinence and reinforced by results of a 5-hour glucose tolerance curve and appropriate chemical studies. Vestibulotoxic drugs produce chronic unsteadiness. An appropriate drug history plus bilateral loss of function on calorization helps to make the diagnosis.

Neck injuries, such as a whiplash, can damage proprioceptive receptors. Subsequent neck torsion may induce vertigo while the torsion stresses are in force. A history of injury plus appropriate position testing suggests the diagnosis.

Central Vertigo

Multiple Sclerosis

Although an isolated complaint of episodic vertigo is seldom a manifestation of central nervous system disease, there are certain disorders, such as multiple sclerosis, in which this may occur. Rarely, during an exacerbation multiple sclerosis patients have vertigo as their only complaint. However, unless the episode of vertigo is accompanied by other brain stem signs or symptoms, it should seldom be used in the diagnostic criteria for multiple sclerosis; there are too many other central nervous system causes of vertigo. In addition, an isolated episode of vertigo should not be used as evidence for a second attack in patients who have had only one prior episode of neurologic involvement, nor should it be used as evidence for lesion dissemination within the nervous system in a patient in whom the other signs and symptoms can be attributed to a single locus. In patients with well-established multiple sclerosis, an episode of vertigo lasting several days can be accepted as an exacerbation of the disease. It is not surprising that multiple sclerosis could cause isolated vertigo in view of the very discrete nature of the plaques, which may affect the vestibular nuclei or their connections without encroaching on other systems.

Vascular Disorders

Transient Ischemic Attacks. Recurrent episodes of vertigo may rarely be a manifestation of vertebral basilar ischemia; however, the patient should always be questioned closely about other brain stem symptoms. During an attack, the patient's attention may be so focused on the distressing vertigo that he or she fails to note other symptoms. The presence of tingling paresthesias, dysarthria, double vision, and weakness of an estremity with any one of the attacks of vertigo will help differentiate the vertigo from episodic vertigo of peripheral origin. Nausea, vomiting, blurred vision, and ataxia should not be used in this analysis, since they are frequent symptoms of vertigo of whatever cause. Certainly, the clinician should be reluctant to treat isolated episodic vertigo with anticoagulation unless a diagnosis of vertebral basilar insufficiency can be made on other grounds.

Cerebrovascular Accident. A syndrome identical to that of acute labyrinthitis has been described in patients with embolic infarction in the distal distribution of the posterior inferior cerebellar artery. The infarction involves the appropriate cerebellar hemisphere with extension into midline structures but spares the brain stem. Despite the cerebellar hemisphere involvement, there is no limb ataxia, but a gait ataxia develops as a result of involvement of the midline structures of the cerebellum. However, the ataxia is usually interpreted by the physician as secondary to the severe vertigo. The vertigo is presumably due to involvement of the connections between the floccular nodular lobe of the cerebellum and the vestibular nuclei of the brain stem. Such a possibility should always be entertained in a patient with a known embolic source, and a CT scan of the head is indicated.

Vertigo can be a prominent symptom in patients with infarctions of the brain stem secondary to vertebral basilar occlusions, particularly those involving the medulla and pons. Thus, vertigo is common when there is occlusion of a vertebral artery with infarction of the lateral medulla, the so-called *lateral medullary plate syndrome.*

Neoplasms

Most tumors that involve structures capable of generating vertigo grow slowly enough that accommodation occurs and vertigo is not a prominent symptom. For example, acoustic neuromas seldom cause episodic vertigo; usually the complaint is more one of unsteadiness than a true vertigo. On occasion, patients with brain stem gliomas may have vertigo that is so incapacitating that they lie rigidly in bed in one position and complain bitterly when placed in another. Vertigo is well described with lesions at the foramen magnum, such as meningiomas, vertebral aneurysms, and the Arnold-Chiari malformation. Often the vertigo is precipitated by head movements. Intermittent compression of the vertebral arteries is a possible mechanism in such cases.

Seizures

The relationship between vertigo and seizures is a controversial one. Some patients with severe vertigo may seem to lose consciousness momentarily, and in others the vertigo may be responsible for precipitating a seizure, so called *reflex epilepsy.* Induction of vertigo during cold caloric testing has been reported to precipitate a seizure. However, such seizures are not necessarily vertiginous in nature. Vertigo may be a manifestation of a seizure arising from the temporal lobe. The complaint is often vague and a sensation of true spinning is rare. Other symptoms occurring during the episode help establish its true nature.

Trauma

Vertigo-like dizziness is often a prominent part of the *post-traumatic syndrome,* which includes headache, depression, lack of concentration, and poor memory. The vertigo in some of these cases has a peripheral origin, but the suggestion that in others there are abnormalities in the brain stem evoked responses suggesting a brain stem origin has not been documented.

CEREBROVASCULAR DISEASE

By Konstantinos S. Polyzoidis, M.D.
and James H. Wood, M.D.
Atlanta, Georgia

The clinical term *stroke* is ambiguous, and therefore the differential diagnosis of patients with symptomatic cerebrovascular disease requires more precise definitions related to the pathophysiology. Overall, about 80 per cent of strokes are of ischemic and 20 per cent are of hemorrhagic nature. With respect to referral patterns, approximately 10 per cent of strokes are secondary to subarachnoid hemorrhage (SAH), while intracerebral hemorrhage accounts for 10 per cent and lacunar basal ganglionic and brain stem infarctions account for 15 per cent. Cardiac emboli are responsible for 20 to 30 per cent of strokes. The remaining 35 per cent are related to thrombosis or emboli secondary to large-vessel occlusive disease.

The etiologic organization of this article will aid in the clinical diagnosis of stroke type based upon clinical, laboratory, and radiologic findings.

Table 1. Causes of Cerebral Arterial Thrombosis

1. Atherosclerosis (obstructing the main artery or the orifice of a branch)
2. Lipohyalinosis
3. Vasculitis
   a. Primary arteritis: Periarteritis nodosa, granulomatous angiitis, Wegener's granulomatous, hypersensitivity angiitis, temporal arteritis, Takayasu's disease (idiopathic aortitis of the young), local carotid arteritis, rheumatic arteritis(?), cerebral thrombo angiitis obliterans
   b. Secondary to meningitis: Pyogenic (staphylococcus, streptococcus, pneumococcus, *Hemophilus influenzae*, etc.), tuberculous, syphilitic, fungous (cryptococcus, mucor, coccidioides, candida)
   c. Secondary to upper respiratory infection in children (postulated)
   d. Miscellaneous: Sarcoidosis, septic embolism, carotid arteritis secondary to cavernous sinusitis, drug addiction, Behçet's disease, trigeminal herpes zoster, malaria(?), typhus, schistosomiasis, nematode infestation
4. Hematologic disorders
   a. Thrombotic thrombocytopenic purpura
   b. Polycythemia
5. Trauma to head and neck
   a. Pressure of lateral process of atlas
   b. Cervical fracture-dislocation
6. Undetermined cause in young adult females (related or not related to contraceptive medication, pregnancy, and puerperium), young adult males, and children
7. Miscellaneous
   a. Mural thrombus in fusiform aneurysm
   b. Extension of thrombus in parent artery to block branch orifice, postoperative complication

Modified from Fisher, C.M.: The anatomy and pathology of the cerebral vasculature. By permission from Table 2, page 20, in *Modern Concepts of Cerebrovascular Disease* by John Stirling Meyer (ed.). Copyright 1975, Spectrum Publications, Inc., New York.

EPIDEMIOLOGIC RISK FACTORS

As with most illnesses, the most important aspect of diagnosing cerebrovascular disease is an accurate history. Epidemiologic studies have demonstrated correlations between blood pressure and risk of stroke for all age groups and both sexes. The efficacy of blood pressure control in reducing the rate of stroke supports the premise that hypertension is the most important risk factor. Solid evidence also exists for higher risk among patients with diabetes mellitus, arteriosclerotic or rheumatic heart disease, transient ischemic attacks (TIAs), amaurosis fugax, and blood hyperviscosity syndromes. Supportive evidence has implicated hyperlipidemia, obesity, cigarette smoking, and oral contraceptives as risk factors. The overall male-to-female ratio is 1.30, with that of myocardial infarction being about 4.0. More specifically, this sex ratio is 1.45 for cerebral infarction, 1.00 for intracerebral hemorrhage, and 0.66 for subarachnoid hemorrhage. Race, geographic distribution, meteorologic, and dietary factors appear to be contributory. Japanese persons residing in Japan or Hawaii have higher stroke rates than their counterparts living in California despite lower blood pressure levels.

ISCHEMIC CEREBROVASCULAR DISORDERS

Precise differential diagnosis of patients with acute ischemic neurologic deficits is needed for assessment of potential reversibility and of prognosis. The regional reduction of cerebral blood flow and oxygen delivery below that which is necessary for neuronal function is termed *focal cerebral ischemia.* More severe and prolonged deprivation results in irreversible alterations causing cell death or *infarction.* In addition to an inadequate blood supply through major afferent arteries, the presence of cerebral ischemia implies a concomitant failure of collateral perfusion to maintain neuronal metabolism. Focal cerebral ischemia has been associated with arterial thrombosis and embolization as well as myriad other disorders (Tables 1 through 3).

Clinical Evaluation

Ischemic disorders are defined to reflect their temporal course with respect to onset and resolution of neurologic deficits. Acute ischemic deficits related to the brain that resolve completely within 24 hours are termed *TIAs. Amaurosis fugax* refers to the transient loss of vision in one eye (transient monocular blindness) lasting several minutes. Deficits that persist longer than 24 hours but clear completely are termed *prolonged reversible ischemic neurologic deficits* (PRINDs or RINDs). *Progressing strokes* have a slow, continuous evolution or a stuttering clinical course over a few hours to a few days. Rapidly developed ischemic neurologic deficits that do not clear completely are termed *completed* or *established* strokes.

Symptoms such as hemiparesis with central facial paresis on the same side, hemisensory loss on the body and face, dysphasia, disturbances of cognitive functions, and amaurosis fugax or hemianopia are indicative of involvement of the carotid arterial system.

Dysfunction of the vertebrobasilar system is suspected in the presence of bilateral or alternating motor or sensory deficit, loss of balance, vertigo, diplopia, dysphagia, dysarthria, Horner's syndrome, and visual loss (cortical blindness or hemianopia). More than one of these symptoms are usually present. The diagnosis of vertebrobasilar insufficiency is not definitive on the basis of isolated drop attack, dizziness, transient global amnesia, or only one of the symptoms mentioned previously.

In addition to a detailed neurologic examination, careful cardiac, peripheral vascular, and pulmonary examinations are of particular importance. Apart from the routine assessment of the heart rate, bilateral brachial pressure, and cardiac rhythm, the blood pressure should be measured in the supine and standing positions when autonomic system disorders are suspected. Palpation of the carotid arteries should be very gentle to prevent dislodgment of embolic material from an atherosclerotic plaque or syncope in the case of a very sensitive carotid sinus. Palpation of the superficial temporal and facial arteries may be helpful in distinguishing between common and internal carotid artery occlusion, as well as in the diagnosis of temporal arteritis.

Typically, the bruit over the carotid bifurcation is systolic, is harsh, and radiates to the angle of the mandible. These bruits strongly suggest an underlying carotid stenosis and have been associated with higher than normal incidence of stroke, even in asymptomatic patients. Those systolic bifurcation bruits that are heard as faint and high-pitched and that extend into diastole indicate the presence of tight stenosis. The disappearance of a known bruit may indicate carotid arterial occlusion at the site of stenosis. Carotid bruits may also occur in patients with internal carotid arterial occlusion who have concomitant external carotid arterial stenosis. Bruits transmitted from the heart are usually bilateral and associated with cardiac murmurs. Cephalic bruits are common in children and are found in 10 to 25 per cent of patients with arteriovenous malformations (AVMs). Orbital bruits reflect increased blood flow in the ophthalmic artery as a collateral channel, or turbulent intracranial flow transmitted to the orbit.

Ophthalmoscopy is an important aid in the diagnosis of ischemic symptoms. Retinal emboli usually present in three varieties. Cholesterol emboli (Hollenhorst plaques) are seen as birefringent, orange-colored arterial obstructions that appear larger than the vessel diameter. These emboli do not usually break up and move distally. Cholesterol emboli are associated with atherosclerotic lesions in the arch or ipsilateral carotid artery. Bright white calcific emboli may be found in both eyes and signify calcific valvular disease in the heart. Platelet-fibrin emboli, appearing as filmy, whitish debris consistent with the arterial diameter, tend to lyse and move distally in the retina. Diffuse retinal ischemia due to carotid or ophthalmic obstructive disease may present, with a blotchy, "peppered" appearance of the retina. Central retinal arterial occlusion with monocular blindness may be the first ischemic symptom in elderly patients with temporal arteritis and may precede cerebral arterial occlusion.

The opacification of the retina and the central cher-

Table 2. Causes of Cerebral Embolism

A. Cardiac origin
   1. Atrial fibrillation and other arrhythmias in heart disease—rheumatic, atherosclerotic, hypertensive, congenital, thyrotoxic, and myopathic; rarely in electrocardioversion
   2. Rheumatic heart disease without arrhythmias—mitral stenosis, aortic stenosis
   3. Myocardial infarction with mural thrombus
   4. Acute and subacute bacterial endocarditis
   5. Cardiac valve prosthesis
   6. Complication of cardiac surgery and pump circulation
   7. Nonbacterial thrombotic endocardial vegetations (marantic endocarditis)
   8. Paradoxic embolism with congenital heart disease (and pulmonary arteriovenous fistula)
   9. Fibroelastosis
   10. Atrial myxoma
   11. Trichinosis

B. Local embolism from: (1) Sites of cervicocranial thrombosis (aorta and innominate, carotid, subclavian, vertebrobasilar, and middle cerebral arteries), platelet material, thrombus, atheromatous material, or cholesterol crystals; (2) complication of neck and thoracic surgery

C. Complication of arteriographic studies—cerebral or cardiac—with catheter or needle, blood clot, cotton fiber, broken catheter tips, reflux from monitoring catheter in radial or brachial artery

D. Thrombus in pulmonary veins

E. Fat

F. Air

G. Tumor

H. Miscellaneous: Incompatible blood transfusion, nucleus pulposus (spinal cord), capillary obstruction by malaria, microfilariasis

I. Embolism from undetermined site

From Fisher, C.M.: The anatomy and pathology of the cerebral vasculature. By permission from Table 3, page 24, in *Modern Concepts of Cerebrovascular Disease* by John Stirling Meyer (ed.).

Table 3. Ischemic Cerebrovascular Disease Not Clearly Thrombotic or Embolic

1. Unexplained strokes in adults
2. Migrainous accompaniments, transient and permanent
3. Dissection of carotid, basilar, and other cerebral arteries or extension of aortic dissection
4. Moyamoya disease
5. Vasospasm: Secondary to subarachnoid hemorrhage (ruptured saccular aneurysm, trauma, postcraniotomy, venous infarction), drug abuse, ergotamine
6. Undetermined type in children and young adults, male and female
7. Young female adults: Related to contraceptive medication, pregnancy, puerperium, or estrogen therapy
8. Systemic hypotension: Fainting, acute blood loss, myocardial infarction; Stokes-Adams attacks, carotid sinus sensitivity, traumatic or postoperative shock, gram-negative septicemia, postural hypotension, antihypertensive medication, low cerebral blood flow during open heart surgery, cough syncope
9. Tentorial, subfalcial, and foramen magnum herniation
10. Thrombocythemia, cryoglobulinemia, hyperviscosity, hemoglobinopathy
11. Acute hypertensive encephalopathy, eclampsia
12. Lupus erythematosus
13. Intrauterine and neonatal cerebral ischemia and anoxia
14. Miscellaneous: Fibromuscular dysplasia, complications of arteriography, trauma, dehydration (diarrhea, excessive diuresis), hypoglycemia, carotid kinking, regional enteritis, surgical occlusion, subclavian steal, large cerebral or dural AVMs, increased platelet reactivity in prebeta hyperlipoproteinemia, neck rotation, compression or constriction of arteries by tumor, homocystinuria, thrombosis within giant aneurysm, mural thrombus in basilar thrombus or fusiform aneurysm, radiation angiopathy, Behçet's disease, exertion, hypoimmune states, progeria, emotion (anger, fear), hypoxia, allergic reaction, delayed anoxic demyelination, lateral pressure of intracerebral hemorrhage, Binswanger's chronic progressive subcortical encephalitis, and stenosis of the lumbar spinal canal

From Fisher, C.M.: The anatomy and pathology of the cerebral vasculature. By permission from Table 4, page 28, in *Modern Concepts of Cerebrovascular Disease* by John Stirling Meyer (ed.). Copyright 1975, Spectrum Publications, Inc., New York.

ry-red spot are the classic signs of central retinal arterial occlusion, become apparent only after several hours, and persist for 2 or more weeks. The opacity is denser around the fovea and fades progressively toward the periphery. It disappears as the ganglion cells disintegrate and as the nerve becomes atrophic. Hemorrhages are not seen unless the vein is also obstructed. Branch retinal obstruction simulates that of the central retinal artery except that it involves only one sector (most commonly the temporal branches). A unilateral altitudinal visual field defect is associated with retinal branch arterial occlusions, but, if inferior, may indicate optic nerve ischemia.

Laboratory Tests

A complete hematologic profile should be obtained promptly. The rheologic importance of high hematocrit values and thrombocythemia is being increasingly recognized. Since infarct size correlates directly with hematocrit in patients with occluded internal carotid arteries, elevated blood viscosity secondary to the high hematocrit values may impede collateral perfusion to ischemic brain regions, thereby enhancing infarction. Elevated plasma fibrinogen levels and augmented platelet aggregation have been associated with cerebral infarction, again suggesting the importance of rheologic factors. Plasma protein quantitation, serum protein electrophoresis, and serum immunoelectrophoresis may detect proteinopathies associated with increased blood viscosity and impeded cerebral blood flow. Direct monitoring of blood viscosity and hemodilution may be indicated in patients with ischemic symptoms and hyperviscosity syndromes. Lipoprotein electrophoresis is helpful in patients suspected of having hyperlipidemia.

Erythrocyte sedimentation rate (ESR) determination is an urgent test in elderly patients with ischemic visual or cerebral symptoms, who are at risk for temporal arteritis. Temporal arterial biopsy may be required to establish this diagnosis. Patients suspected of having collagen vascular disease should undergo a lupus erythematosus blood smear (LE preparation), antinuclear antibody determination, and ESR. Serologic tests for syphilis are generally recommended.

Electrolytes, urea, glucose, cholesterol, and triglycerides in the serum should also be measured routinely. Hyperglycemia should be documented and treated, if present, since recent evidence suggests a detrimental effect of glucose in ischemic situations.

In black patients, a search for sickle cell anemia and sickle cell trait should be undertaken by smear testing for sickle cells and identification of abnormal hemoglobin by electrophoresis.

Cardiac Evaluation

An electrocardiogram is essential in the diagnosis of recent and remote myocardial infarction and cardiac arrhythmias, which are frequently associated with brain ischemia. Low cardiac output syndromes may cause cerebral hypoperfusion with symptoms due to ischemia in "watershed" regions. Twenty-four-hour Holter monitoring may be necessary for the identification of short-lasting alterations of the cardiac rhythm that impair ventricular filling. Echocardiography has considerable diagnostic value in detecting cardiac sources of emboli, such as mitral valve prolapse (Barnett's syndrome), valvular disease, vegetative endocarditis, atrial myxoma, mural thrombus, or ventricular aneurysm. This type of evaluation is especially indicated for patients with embolic symptoms in more than one cerebrovascular distribution or if calcific retinal emboli are visualized. Cardiac muscle enzymes may be the only means of revealing a recent myocardial infarction in a stroke patient.

Noninvasive Studies

Several noninvasive tests for the evaluation of carotid artery disease have been developed over the past several years; these are listed in Table 4. These noninvasive procedures offer direct assessment of the anatomy and physiology of the cervical carotid bifurcation, indirect monitoring of hemodynamic alterations distal to the carotid bifurcation affecting the superficial and deep orbital circulatory beds, and direct assessment of the cerebral perfusion. Direct carotid morphologic and indirect hemodynamic testing, in various combinations, are of value in detecting of hemodynamically significant stenosis but offer little help in identifying ulcerated plaques or minimal stenosis, or in distinguishing between occlusion and severe stenosis.

Only the direct measurement of regional cerebral blood flow offers noninvasive evaluation of the degree and vascular distribution of cerebral perfusion abnormalities. Normal mean values are about 55 ml/100 gm/minute but decrease with age. Deranged brain electrical activity occurs with depressions of cerebral blood flow to about 18 ml/100 gm/minute. The dilatatory or constrictive response of cerebral arterioles to induced alterations in the P_{CO_2} of arterial blood can be quantified using regional cerebral blood flow analysis, and reductions in this *cerebrovascular CO_2 reactivity* indicate regions of arterial dysfunction. The clinical usefulness of the technique consists in distinguishing between hemodynamic and embolic ischemia in patients with carotid occlusive disease, localizing an ischemic territory, showing hyperemia in migraine, and assessing the efficacy of medical or surgical management over a period of time.

In combination with digital subtraction angiography, these noninvasive procedures might be used in the screening of asymptomatic patients with carotid bruits or of candidates for cardiac or peripheral vascular operations. In patients with TIAs, conventional angiography is indicated regardless of the findings of the noninvasive testing.

An electroencephalogram (EEG) is essential in the differential diagnosis between TIAs and epilepsy. Alterations in computer-assisted analysis of EEG (Fourier Transform) have been shown to correlate with cerebral blood flow in patients with cerebral ischemia and may have usefulness in patient monitoring.

Radiologic Studies

Computed tomography (CT) allows direct visualization of the brain parenchyma and thus has revolutionalized the investigation of cerebrovascular disease, especially in differentiating among infarction, hemorrhage, and hemorrhagic infarction. In addition, the vascular distribution, multiplicity of infarcts, edema formation with mass effect, and, sometimes, cause of the insult can be assessed noninvasively. Both uncontrasted and contrast-enhanced CT scans are indicated to differentiate isodense subdural hematomas, tumors, AVMs, and aneurysms that may present as ischemic lesions. The presence of multiple or bilateral infarcts on CT may suggest proximal origins of emboli, usually a cardiac source. Although TIAs are not associated with structural changes, RINDs may cause evidence of infarction on CT despite resolution of clinical symptoms.

During the first 48 hours, only 50 per cent of all cerebral infarcts are detected. The rate increases to about 75 per cent after 7 to 10 days, possibly because of reduction of the amount of edema and progression of necrosis. In addition to age, the size of the infarct is important, since the reported overall detection

Table 4. Noninvasive Techniques for Evaluation of Cerebrovascular Disease

A. Direct assessment of morphology of carotid bifurcation
  1. Doppler ultrasonic scanning
  2. Real-time B-scan imaging
  3. Audiofrequency analysis of bruits and phonoangiography

B. Indirect assessment of hemodynamic condition distal to carotid bifurcation
  1. Ophthalmodynamometry
  2. Oculoplethysmography
  3. Thermography
  4. Directional Doppler flow studies
  5. Arm-to-retina circulation time

C. Direct assessment of regional cerebral blood flow
  1. Xenon–133 inhalation and washout technique of Obrist
  2. Stable-xenon computed tomography
  3. Single-photon–emission tomography (experimental)
  4. Positron-emission tomography (experimental)

rates are 0 to 32 per cent for small and 40 to 81 per cent for medium-sized pathologically proven infarcts.

The initial isodense appearance of brain infarction may be caused by metabolic factors, although CT density values may increase, depending upon whether or not hemorrhage is present. Owing to variations in normal CT attenuation values, the density of the lesion is best described in percentage of difference with respect to the adjacent brain tissue. As the pathologic process matures, the infarct will appear as a focal, hypodense area. Older lesions appear as cystic, well-circumscribed lesions, with density values approaching those of cerebrospinal fluid, and dilation of adjacent cerebrospinal fluid spaces. A hyperdense lesion of the cortex with hypodensity in the white matter is characteristic of hemorrhagic infarction on uncontrasted CT scans.

Classically, infarcts are visualized on CT scans within the region of distribution of a major cerebral artery, with considerable variation in shape. Watershed infarcts are located at the boundary zone between terminal branches of two major cerebral arteries, in the convexity or adjacent to the lateral ventricles.

Pathologic studies have shown that the swelling around the infarct peaks by the fourth to seventh day. After about 3 weeks the necrotic tissue tends to occupy less space than the previous brain parenchyma. Presence of mass effect in the CT scan after that period should raise questions about the correctness of the diagnosis. Evidence of mass effect includes shift of the midline structures, compression of a ventricle, effacement of sulci, and obliteration of the subarachnoid space.

Intravenous contrast injection may allow the depiction of small infarcts. Enhancement of the infarcted area has been seen in about 80 per cent of the cases during the third week. Such enhancement is rare prior to the third day, reaches maximum during the third week, and becomes uncommon after the second month. It may represent breakdown of the blood-brain barrier, neovascularity, or luxury perfusion.

The response to treatment or the natural history can also be monitored with serial CT scanning.

Static radionuclide scanning becomes positive only after a delay of several days in the acute phase of stroke and becomes normal several months later, diminishing its usefulness in diagnosis and serial evaluations. Differentiation among hemorrhage, infarction, and hemorrhagic infarction is not possible. The dynamic study provides information regarding the patency of the major cervical vessels and gross cerebral perfusion. The detail and accuracy of the information are rarely sufficient for clinical use.

Early cerebral angiography enables definitive diagnosis to be made in many cases and thus may alter the course of therapy; however, it should only be performed if surgery is contemplated. This invasive procedure, usually performed by femoral catheterization, carries a 1.5 per cent risk of ischemic complications and has an overall 0.5 per cent permanent morbidity rate.

The resolution provided by cerebral angiography in the investigation of vascular abnormalities is unparalleled by any other presently available technique. Bilateral carotid and aortic arch studies should be performed in patients with anterior cerebral circulation ischemic symptoms. If an internal carotid artery occlusion is found, adequate visualization of the superficial temporal artery is necessary if cerebral arterial bypass surgery is contemplated. If a common carotid occlusion is observed, late views will be needed to assess reconstitution of the superficial temporal artery from facial and scalp collaterals to assess the possibility of saphenous vein interposition grafting of the common carotid artery to the external carotid artery in preparation for subsequent cerebral arterial bypass surgery. If ischemic symptoms suggest vertebrobasilar pathology, vertebral angiography is necessary for precise diagnosis and more appropriate therapy.

Combined with magnification, subtraction techniques will demonstrate ulcerated or smooth atherosclerotic plaques, tandem intracranial lesions, vessel occlusions, and the pattern of collateral circulation. Incidental intracranial aneurysm, AVM, venous thrombosis, and vasculitis may be detected. Disappearance of embolic material is not an uncommon cause of lack of intracranial angiographic findings among stroke patients. Cerebral angiography, however, provides only indirect and nonspecific evidence of intraparenchymal pathologic processes, such as hematoma or infarction. Infarction may be inferred by the demonstration of mass effect, arterial branch occlusion or narrowing, luxury perfusion, or collateral circulation with retrograde filling of distal arteries. An intracerebral hematoma may remain undetected unless it produces significant mass effect.

Intravenous digital subtraction angiography, in its current state, cannot match the resolution of conventional angiography and is deficient in assessing intracranial arterial lesions or collateral circulation. When combined with cerebral blood flow analysis, this noninvasive radiographic study is useful in screening asymptomatic patients with cervical bruits. Since the total dose of contrast material is similar to that used in conventional cerebral angiography, renal function should be evaluated. Digital arterial subtraction angiography requires femoral catheterization but needs only about 20 per cent of the contrast medium used in either of the other types of angiography. This invasive arterial study allows reasonable definition of intracranial circulation and may be the preferred method of studying patients with vertebral ischemic disease.

INTRAPARENCHYMAL BRAIN HEMORRHAGE

The term *intraparenchymal hemorrhage* describes the extravasation of blood into brain tissue. The most common causes include systemic hypertension, saccular aneurysm, AVM, trauma, bleeding tendency, hemorrhage into a brain tumor, septic embolism and mycotic aneurysm, arteritis, and cerebral venous thrombosis (Table 5).

The hypertensive brain hemorrhages constitute the majority and are distributed as follows: 55 per cent in the putamen, 15 per cent in the subcortical white matter, 10 per cent in the thalamus, 10 per cent in the pons, and 10 per cent in the cerebellum. Their inci-

Table 5. Causes of Intraparenchymal Brain Hemorrhage

1. Hypertensive intracerebral hemorrhage, hypertensive hemorrhage under unusual circumstances, vasopressor drugs, methamphetamine use
2. Ruptured saccular (developmental) aneurysm
3. Ruptured arteriovenous malformation
4. Trauma: Cerebral contusion, subdural hemorrhage, extradural hemorrhage, intracerebral hematoma, delayed apoplexy
5. Abnormal bleeding tendency: Excessive therapeutic anticoagulant, thrombocytopenia associated with anticancer drugs and immunosuppressive agents, leukemia, liver disease, hemophilia, Christmas disease, thrombotic thrombocytopenic purpura, aplastic anemia, hypofibrinogenemia, hyperfibrinolysis, snake venom poisoning
6. Hemorrhage into primary and secondary brain tumor
7. Septic embolism and mycotic aneurysm
8. Hemorrhagic infarction
9. Secondary brain stem hemorrhage in tentorial compression
10. Cerebral venous thrombosis
11. Miscellaneous: Early-life carotid occlusion, moyamoya, hepatic disease, exertion, lipohyalinosis without hypertension, carotid–cavernous sinus fistula, cerebral lupus erythematosus, the arteritides (polyarteritis, granulomatosis, aspergillosis), Osler-Rendu-Weber disease, multiple uremic hemorrhages, brain purpura, acute hemorrhagic leukoencephalopathy, post-traumatic aneurysm, migraine, Wernicke-Korsakoff encephalopathy, teratomatous malformation
12. Undetermined cause: Normal blood pressure and no obvious angioma

Modified from Fisher, C.M.: The anatomy and pathology of the cerebral vasculature. By permission from Table 5, page 29, in *Modern Concepts of Cerebrovascular Disease* by John Stirling Meyer (ed.). Copyright 1975, Spectrum Publications, Inc., New York.

dence is decreasing, primarily because of improved antihypertensive treatment. Vigorous and detailed pathologic examination at autopsy or of the surgically removed clot has been reported to demonstrate vascular dysplasias in the majority of cases clinically diagnosed as hypertensive hemorrhages.

The clinical onset with headache and decreasing level of consciousness favor hemorrhage, although headache in alert patients has also been associated with cerebral embolism. The symptoms and findings depend upon the location and size of the clot. Subcortical hematoma may cause contralateral motor or sensory loss, or both, and gaze preference toward the side opposite of the hemiparesis without visual loss. Thalamic lesions produce a similar picture with initial contralateral hemisensory loss, followed by hemiparesis as the internal capsule becomes involved, as well as the addition of upper gaze paresis, small reactive pupils, and impaired level of consciousness. Putaminal hemorrhage may result in smooth and steadily progressive contralateral hemiparesis accompanied in some cases by hemisensory loss and hemianopia. Pontine hemorrhages lead rapidly to coma, with pinpoint, minimally reactive pupils, impairment of ocular movements, and spastic quadriparesis.

CT scanning without contrast administration shows the exact location and size of the hematoma and can be performed rapidly to allow urgent neurosurgical intervention if necessary. Contrast-enhanced scan and cerebral angiography are indicated when an aneurysm or vascular malformation is suspected with an atypically located hemorrhage.

Arteriovenous malformations may present with parenchymal or subarachnoid hemorrhage. The clinical picture is not as dramatic as with aneurysmal rupture, and vasospasm is uncommon. Individuals affected are younger (second to fourth decades) than those with hemorrhages of different causation. Seizures, headaches, progressive neurologic deficit, congestive heart failure (usually in children), and pseudotumor cerebri are also possible presenting features. AVMs range from small, cryptic dysplasias to giant malformations involving the entire hemisphere. Most AVMs occur in the cerebral hemisphere. Ten per cent occur in the basal ganglia and internal capsule and 6 per cent in the posterior fossa. Their incidence is about one tenth that of aneurysms and the sexes are equally affected.

CT scans may demonstrate a hematoma, calcifications, or encephalomalacia adjacent to the AVM. The serpentine vascular channels usually become apparent with contrast injection, although angiography is a necessary procedure for proper management. External carotid injections may also be needed for complete angiographic assessment of AVMs, especially if the patient is a candidate for embolization procedure.

SUBARACHNOID HEMORRHAGE

Hemorrhage contained within the subarachnoid space (SAH) is most commonly caused by the rupture of an intracranial aneurysm, if trauma is excluded. According to the Cooperative Study (1969), intracranial aneurysm accounted for 51 per cent, hypertensive arteriosclerotic disease for 15 per cent, AVMs for 6 per cent, and multiple or miscellaneous causes for 6 per cent of the patients with SAH whenever studied. No cause was identified in 22 per cent of cases. Substantial improvement in angiographic techniques since that study was published has resulted in more frequent demonstrations of the cause of bleeding (Table 6). At present, only about 7 per cent of patients with SAH have normal cerebral angiograms.

Blood within the subarachnoid space produces signs of meningeal irritation, such as severe headache, photophobia, and stiff neck. Half of the patients with ruptured aneurysm present with these symptoms in combination with some degree of cloudiness of the sensorium. The hallmark symptom is the characteristic explosive headache. Occasionally atypical headaches may be the only manifestation, possibly representing limited hemorrhages described as "warning leaks." Prompt recognition of the entity is of extreme importance, since results of surgical treatment are superior in this group of patients. One fifth of the patients present with sudden loss of consciousness. Other presenting symptoms include convulsions, nausea, vomiting, focal neurologic deficits, such as motor paralysis or cranial nerve involvement, and brain stem dysfunction. Usually the clinical neurologic deficits may predict the location of the ruptured aneurysm (Table 7).

Patients with SAH secondary to aneurysmal rupture are routinely graded according to the classification of neurologic signs and symptoms shown in Table 8. Surgical mortality is directly related to preoperative clinical grade.

Ruptured aneurysms, like AVMs, may cause intracerebral, intraventricular, or, uncommonly, subdural hematoma and may be associated with progressive signs of transtentorial herniation, thus constituting a neurosurgical emergency. At times, unruptured aneurysm may be manifested clinically as a space-occupying lesion compressing the cranial nerves involved in vision or eye movements.

Neurologic deterioration of the condition of patients with ruptured aneurysms is usually due to rebleeding, delayed ischemia secondary to cerebral vasospasm, or hydrocephalus. Other causes include hypoxia of neurogenic pulmonary edema or blood electrolyte disturbances due to hypothalamic dysfunction. Cardiac arrhythmias and even infarction may occur.

Lumbar Puncture

To avoid deterioration of the patient's condition due to shifts of intracranial contents, lumbar puncture should be performed only after CT scanning. This invasive procedure should be performed in patients with suggestive history of intracranial hemorrhage and nondiagnostic CT scans. Lumbar puncture should be avoided in patients with blood dyscrasias or known spinal cord AVMs as well as in those receiving anticoagulants.

By definition, the presence of a single erythrocyte in the cerebrospinal fluid technically is SAH; however, 100 erythrocytes per cu mm are considered diagnostic of clinical SAH. The number of erythrocytes in lumbar cerebrospinal fluid does not always correlate with that contained in the cephalic subarachnoid cerebrospinal fluid. The cerebrospinal fluid will be uniformly blood-tinged, pink to red, in the majority of symptomatic patients at the time of initial puncture. Occasionally, blood from an intracranial bleeding source will not extend to the lumbar subarachnoid space for 6 to 12 hours, and sometimes intraparenchymal bleeding will not extravasate into the subarachnoid space.

Normally, cerebrospinal fluid is clear and colorless; however, it may contain as many as 500 erythrocytes per cu/mm and appear clear. Gross evidence of bleeding (more than 4000 erythrocytes per cu/mm) may disappear within 24 hours but usually persists for 7 to 14 days. If the cerebrospinal fluid is bloody, the specimen should be centrifuged and the supernatant examined for the presence of any color.

The differentiation of trauma-induced cerebrospinal fluid hemorrhage from true SAH is important in diagnosis. Traumatic punctures will be associated

Table 6. Causes of Subarachnoid Hemorrhage

Common Causes

1. Traumatic
2. Spontaneous
    a. Intracerebral hemorrhage with rupture into the subarachnoid space
    b. Primary
        1. Ruptured berry aneurysm
        2. Bleeding arteriovenous malformation
        3. Ruptured mycotic aneurysm

Rare Causes

1. Developmental defects including pseudoxanthoma elasticum, Ehlers-Danlos syndrome, Sturge-Weber disease, hereditary hemorrhagic telangiectasia, telangiectasia pontis
2. Infections: Herpes simplex encephalitis, acute hemorrhagic leukoencephalitis, brain abscess, tuberculous meningitis, syphilitic vasculitis
3. Neoplasm: Primary or metastatic brain tumor; hemangioblastoma of the cerebellum or brain stem
4. Blood dyscrasias: Leukemia, Hodgkin's disease, thrombocytopenia, sickle cell anemia, hemophilia, aplastic anemia, pernicious anemia
5. Vasculitis: Polyarteritis nodosa, anaphylactic purpura
6. Arteriosclerosis: Rupture of arteriosclerotic vessel
7. Iatrogenic: Anticoagulant therapy

From Gilroy, J., and Holliday, P.L.: *Basic Neurology.* New York, Macmillan Publishing, 1982, pp. 142.

Table 7. Signs and Symptoms of Aneurysms According to Site of Origin

Origin of Aneurysm	Structure Involved	Signs and Symptoms
Internal carotid, cavernous portion	Compression of cranial nerves 3, 4, and 6; compression of ophthalmic division of cranial nerve 5; compression of pituitary; rupture into cavernous sinus producing an AV fistula	Mydriasis, diplopia, ptosis, trigeminal neuralgia, atypical facial pain, hypopituitarism, noise in the head
Internal carotid, supraclinoid portion	Compression of optic nerve, compression of optic chiasm, compression of cranial nerve 3	Visual failure, optic atrophy, visual field defects, mydriasis, diplopia, ptosis
Ophthalmic artery	Compression of optic nerve, compression of pituitary	Visual failure, optic atrophy, hypopituitarism
Middle cerebral artery	Irritation of the cortex	Usually causes few signs and symptoms before rupture; partial seizures
Anterior cerebral artery	Compression of optic chiasm, compression of olfactory tract	Visual field defects, unilateral anosmia
Posterior communicating artery	Compression of cranial nerve 3 or 6	Mydriasis, diplopia, ptosis, diplopia
Posterior cerebral artery	Compression of the midbrain	Usually causes few signs and symptoms before rupture; hydrocephalus, stupor, akinetic mutism
Basilar artery	Compression of cranial nerve 5 or 7, compression of midbrain	Trigeminal neuralgia, atypical facial pain, facial paralysis, hydrocephalus
Vertebral artery	Compression of cranial nerves 9 and 10, compression of brain stem	Paralysis of the palate, pharynx, dysphagia, vertigo, ataxia, vomiting

From Gilroy, J., and Holliday, P.L.: *Basic Neurology*. New York, Macmillan Publishing, 1982, pp. 142.

Table 8. Classification of Patients with Intracranial Aneurysms According to Surgical Risk

Grade	Criteria
0	Unruptured aneurysm
I	Asymptomatic, or minimal headache and slight nuchal rigidity
Ia	No acute meningeal or brain reaction, but fixed neurologic deficit
II	Moderate to severe headache, nuchal rigidity, no neurologic deficit other than cranial nerve palsy
III	Drowsiness, confusion, or mild focal deficit
IV	Stupor, moderate to severe hemiparesis, possibly early decerebrate rigidity, and vegetative disturbances
V	Deep coma, decerebrate rigidity, moribund appearance

From Hunt, W.W.: Timing of surgery for intracranial aneurysm. In Wilkins, R.H. (ed.): *Cerebral Arterial Spasm*. © 1980, The Williams & Wilkins Company, Baltimore, p. 460.

with a decline in the number of erythrocytes as more cerebrospinal fluid is serially drained from the spinal needle, and the proportion of leukocytes to erythrocytes will be similar to that in blood—about 2 leukocytes per 1000 erythrocytes. Crenated erythrocytes, if present, do not indicate an earlier bleeding episode. After cerebrospinal fluid centrifugation, if the supernatant exhibits yellow discoloration (*xanthochromia*), true SAH likely antedated the puncture. Xanthochromia appears in the cerebrospinal fluid supernatant within 2 hours after SAH in a few cases, within 6 hours in 70 per cent of cases, and within 12 hours in 90 per cent of cases after the onset of clinical symptoms. Traumatic puncture is suspected if a clot forms in the specimen vial, usually with an erythrocyte count exceeding 200,000 per cu mm. Bleeding from any source will elevate the cerebrospinal fluid protein content about 1 mg/1000 erythrocytes. If the actual total protein level exceeds the sum of this calculated protein elevation and the upper limit of normal cerebrospinal fluid protein, true SAH has likely occurred. The presence of cerebrospinal fluid leukocytosis—e.g., leukocyte/erythrocyte ratios greater than that in blood (2 leukocytes/1000 erythrocytes)—indicates the SAH had occurred at least 24 hours before the CSF sampling.

Following SAH, the glucose concentrations in cerebrospinal fluid may be low (*hypoglycorrhachia*). Generally, the ratio of cerebrospinal fluid to blood glucose levels is less than 0.6 in SAH.

Radiologic Studies

CT scanning before and after intravenous contrast injection should be performed immediately upon presentation of a patient suspected of having SAH. This noninvasive study may provide the initial diagnosis; information on the extent, location, and cause of the SAH; and the means of detecting complications of SAH, such as brain infarction and hydrocephalus.

Accuracies of 78 to 95 per cent in the detection of SAH on CT have been reported in patients who are scanned within 5 days after the rupture of their aneurysm. Seven days after the ictus, CT may be unreliable in demonstrating SAH. SAH in sulci and fissures and along the tentorium is seen on uncontrasted CT scans as a thin, flat plate of high-density blood. When such a collection of blood lies parallel to the CT plane, it may be difficult to visualize as an area of increased density because of the "partial-volume phenomenon." A small SAH is more easily recognized if it lies perpendicular to the CT plan—e.g., along the falx—than if the blood lies in the basilar cisterns parallel to the CT plane (CT without contrast should be performed first, since contrast enhancement of the falx and tentorium may mask thin collections of blood adjacent to these structures). Small amounts of blood may be easily identified in the sylvian fissure, perimesencephalic (ambient) cistern, and deep cerebral sulci (Fig. 1).

CT is useful in localizing the site of hemorrhage in patients with SAH, in determining which of multiple aneurysms has bled, and in lateralizing the bleeding site so that angiography can first study those vessels most likely to be responsible for bleeding.

Some patterns of CT findings are characteristic of particular bleeding sites, although overlap of appearance occurs. Anterior communicating artery aneurysms almost invariably bleed into the suprasellar cisterns and frontal interhemispheric fissure. Blood from anterior communicating artery aneurysms is also frequently visualized around the upper brain stem and in the sylvian fissures. Internal carotid and posterior communicating artery aneurysms may produce a similar CT picture, but with aneurysms of the posterior communicating artery, the sylvian fissure is more frequently involved than the interhemispheric fissure. Middle cerebral artery aneurysms invariably bleed into the sylvian fissure, most often unilaterally.

Findings that are more characteristic of aneurysmal locations are:

1. Septal hematoma that occurs with rupture of anterior communicating artery aneurysms.
2. Frontal hematoma, seen most often with aneurysms of the anterior communicating artery, internal carotid artery, and rarely middle cerebral artery.
3. Sylvian fissure hematoma associated with temporal lobe hematoma, which suggests ipsilateral rupture of an aneurysm of the middle cerebral, internal carotid, or posterior communicating artery. Intraventricular hemorrhage can be seen with ruptured aneurysms originating from any major cerebral artery.

Vertebral artery aneurysms produce maximal SAH in the infratentorial cisterns and fourth ventricle, and not infrequently reflux small amounts of blood up toward the aqueduct and into the third and lateral ventricles. Basilar tip aneurysms produce maximal SAH in the tentorial cisterns. Other localizing CT findings of basilar tip aneurysms include focal interpeduncular cisternal subarachnoid hematoma, demonstration of a hypothalamic hematoma, isolated bleeding into the third ventricle, or actual visualization of the aneurysm within the interpeduncular cistern.

Important correlations have been found between the CT extent of SAH and the clinical grade and the degree of vasospasm. Among patients studied by CT within 4 days after the ictus, the absence or the presence of only minimal amounts of SAH is associated with a continual good clinical status (in 89 per cent) and the absence or the presence of only minimal vasospasm (in 71 per cent); whereas the presence of moderate to severe SAH on CT is associated with poor clinical status (in 50 per cent) and the presence of severe vasospasm (in 70 per cent).

Intravenous contrast administration with subsequent CT scanning demonstrates the aneurysm in 30 per cent of cases and may reveal an AVM. However, its use is limited by the density of the SAH or hematoma surrounding the aneurysm. Over the first 2 to 3 weeks after SAH, "meningeal hyperemia" may be responsible for the enhancement that is observed in the basal cisterns and cortical sulci. This subarachnoid enhancement may permit the diagnosis of SAH in the absence of evidence of cisternal blood on precontrast CT scans. This enhancement is associated with an increased incidence of hydrocephalus, but it does not correlate with clinical grade, arterial spasm, site of bleed, or temporal relation to the ictus.

Serial CT scanning has diagnostic value in SAH

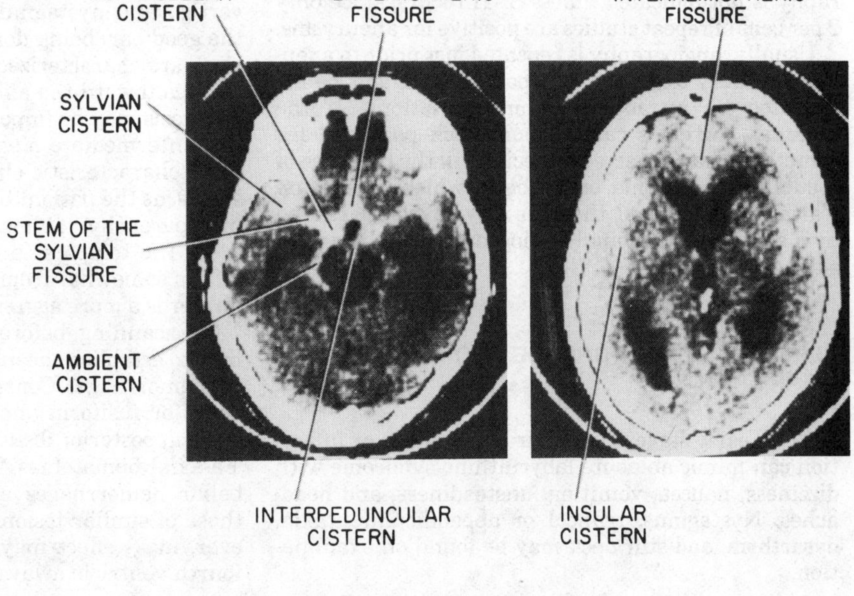

Figure1. Main subarachnoid cisterns and fissures in patient with subarachnoid hemorrhage from ruptured aneurysm. (From Kistler, J. P., Crowell, P. M., Davis, K. R., Heros, R., Ojemann, R. G., Zervas, N., and Fisher, C. M.: The relationship of cerebral vasospasm to the extent and location of subarachnoid blood visualized by CT scan: A prospective study. Neurology, 33:424, 1983.)

patients whose conditions deteriorate clinically, because aneurysmal rebleeding and hydrocephalus are easily identified on CT. Ventricular enlargement will be observed in about 12 per cent of patients, but only 7 per cent will require cerebrospinal fluid shunting. The noninvasive combination of an unchanged CT scan and worsening cerebral blood flow would suggest vasospasm and may obviate the need for repeat cerebral angiography. Serial CT evaluations may detect the presence of ischemic infarction caused by vasospasm and will allow demonstration of the resolution of intracranial blood collections.

Cerebral angiography is the definitive procedure in the diagnosis of SAH. Resolution permitting the demonstration of vasospasm and relationships of the lesion to neighboring vasculature is enhanced by obtaining oblique and basal as well as conventional views and by employing magnification and subtraction techniques.

All patients with SAH should undergo a complete four-vessel cerebral angiogram because 20 per cent of aneurysm patients have multiple aneurysms, and patients with AVMs require full evaluation of feeding arteries and draining veins. Patients with AVMs also require angiography of the external carotid circulation.

In the presence of multiple intracranial aneurysms, angiographic findings suggesting which aneurysm has bled include the following:

1. Extravastion of contrast material through the aneurysm wall (the most reliable, yet rare, sign).
2. Localized irregularity or loculation along aneurysm dome ("Murphy's teat").
3. Relative aneurysm size (the larger aneurysm is most likely to have ruptured).
4. Localized vasospasm (the least reliable sign).

Obviously, localization of blood on CT will help to differentiate the bleeding aneurysm.

Usually, early angiography of patients with SAH is preferred in order to make the diagnosis. Cerebral angiography does not precipitate rebleeding. Although nonvisualization of an existing intracranial aneurysm probably represents the most common explanation for normal angiography, repeat panangiography is not indicated unless SAH recurs, since only 2 per cent of repeat studies are positive for aneurysms.

Usually, angiography is repeated just prior to aneurysm surgery to detect vasospasm that might be aggravated by intraoperative manipulations. If the patient's SAH has caused more back pain and leg symptoms than expected (especially in the presence of a cutaneous angioma of the back, which blushes on Valsalva maneuvers), the ictus may have been caused by a spinal AVM. Spinal angiography is indicated in such cases.

CEREBELLAR HEMORRHAGE AND INFARCTION

At an early stage, cerebellar hemorrhage or infarction can mimic an acute labyrinthine syndrome with dizziness, nausea, vomiting, unsteadiness, and headaches. Nystagmus, truncal or appendicular ataxia, dysarthria, and stiff neck may be found on examination.

At the intermediate stage, patients present with drowsiness, irritability, diplopia, and clinical signs of mild hemiparesis—peripheral facial palsy, contralateral gaze deviation, and Horner's syndrome (small reactive pupils, especially when examining the patient in a dimly lit room). The late stage is characterized by stupor or coma with decerebrate or decorticate posturing, pinpoint reactive pupils, respiratory changes secondary to brain stem dysfunction, and cardiovascular instability. Because of the tendency to worsen progressively, patients with acute onset of the classic triad of ipsilateral appendicular ataxia, peripheral facial palsy, and gaze palsy should be evaluated for cerebellar hemorrhage on an emergent basis. A history of hypertension is present in two thirds of all patients with spontaneous cerebellar hemorrhages and in 40 per cent of patients with cerebellar infarction, which in the vast majority of the cases is secondary to occlusion of the vertebral or posterior inferior cerebellar artery. Chiropractic neck manipulation is being increasingly recognized as a causative factor of vertebral artery occlusion and cerebellar infarction. Embolism, most commonly of cardiac origin, is implicated in 50 per cent of cases of cerebellar infarction.

The clinical presentation reflects the degree of brain stem dysfunction either because of compression by a hemorrhagic or swollen cerebellum, or because of concomitant infarction (as in the case of the lateral medullary syndrome). Compression of the brain stem with obstruction or kinking of the aqueduct may lead to the rapid development of noncommunicating hydrocephalus, resulting in a dramatic rise of pressure within the supratentorial compartment, which, transmitted transtentorially, further impairs the brain stem function.

An early prominence of unsteadiness of gait, repeated falls, and ataxia in addition to the degree of headache will help to differentiate cerebellar from subarachnoid hemorrhage. However, nuchal rigidity, nausea, vomiting, dizziness, and headache are findings common to both entities, since blood can leak into the subarachnoid space after a cerebellar infarction or hemorrhage. Patients with acute labyrinthitis have a tendency to fall toward the affected side, with vertigo and nystagmus (the fast component toward the good ear) being dominant features. Cerebellar lesions are characterized by the rapid phase of the nystagmus toward the affected side, but this differential diagnosis may be impossible only on clinical grounds. The intermediate stage, as described earlier, has a more characteristic clinical presentation. In the late stages, as the patient becomes comatose, other sites of intraparenchymal hemorrhage should also be considered. The temporal profile of cerebellar hemorrhage differs somewhat from that of infarction, in that the former is a more aggressive, rapidly expanding lesion.

CT scanning before contrast administration will help to establish the diagnosis of cerebellar infarction or hemorrhage. Contrast-enhanced CT may detect berry or fusiform aneurysms of the vertebrobasilar system, posterior fossa AVMs, tumors, or isodense extra-axial hematomas. The CT characteristics of cerebellar hemorrhages and infarctions are similar to those of similar lesions elsewhere in the brain; however, mass effect may be detected by a shift of the fourth ventricle away from the lesion. Acute obstructive hydrocephalus may be visualized as symmetric enlargement of the third and lateral ventricles with periventricular hypodensity reflecting transependymal cerebrospinal fluid absorption. CT scanning should be done on an emergency basis in any patient suspected of having cerebellar hemorrhage or infarction, because prompt surgical posterior fossa decompression or ventriculostomy may yield dramatic improvement even in comatose patients.

Lumbar puncture is contraindicated in patients having posterior fossa signs unless the CT is normal. The performance of vertebral angiography would only delay the appropriate management of a patient with a typical cerebellar hemorrhage. Angiography is useful in young patients, in patients in whom an AVM or vascular tumor is suspected, and in stable patients with an inconclusive CT scan, in whom a cerebellar infarction secondary to occlusive vertebrobasilar disease is suspected.

VENOUS THROMBOSIS

Thrombosis of the cerebral venous channels is usually confined to the superficial draining system (with the exception of occlusion of the vein of Galen), which may occur in children and be devastating, and occlusion of the cavernous sinus. Because of an abundance of anastomotic channels, damage to the cerebral parenchyma is uncommon.

Factors causing intracranial venous thrombosis are listed in Table 9. The most commonly encountered process is sepsis of the middle ear, mastoid, and paranasal sinus causing thrombophlebitis of the mucosal veins. This infection spreads to the emissary veins, the cranial sinuses, and the cerebral veins, although the latter are usually affected by subdural empyema or purulent meningitis.

The majority of the cases remain asymptomatic. Although thrombosis or surgical ligation of the anterior half of the superior sagittal sinus usually has no sequelae, two clinical syndromes may occur.

When the posterior half of the superior sagittal sinus or the dominant lateral sinus, which is usually the right, is occluded, drainage of cerebral blood is impaired. Absorption of cerebrospinal fluid is also hindered. Both lead to increased intracranial pressure in the form of pseudotumor cerebri (benign intracranial hypertension). Headache, nausea or vomiting, and visual disturbances are the classic symptoms. Diplopia and transient drowsiness may occur. The only clinical finding, with the exception of the occasional sixth-nerve palsy, is papilledema with normal visual acuity in a neurologically normal and usually fully alert patient. The size of the cerebral ventricles is found to be normal or small on the CT scan. The cerebrospinal fluid is normal in composition but under high pressure.

Table 9. Causes of Intracranial Venous Thrombosis

Trauma	Head injury (penetrating and closed injuries)
Infection	Middle ear, mastoid, and paranasal sinus infection
Endocrine imbalance	Pregnancy Puerperium Oral contraceptives
Dehydration	Diarrheal illness in children Hyperosmolar diabetic coma Ulcerative colitis
Hematologic disorders	Thrombocytosis Sickle cell anemia Hemolytic anemia Paroxysmal nocturnal hemoglobinuria Cryoglobulinemia
Propagation	Spread from an extracranial venous thrombosis following jugular venous canalization
Impaired cerebral circulation	Cerebral arterial occlusion Anesthesia in seated position Congestive cardiac failure Congenital webs in sagittal sinus
Tumor	Compression of intracranial venous channel, particularly parasagittal meningioma

From Burrow, D.D., and Toole, J.F.: Pathophysiology and clinical evaluation of ischemic vascular disease. In Youmans, J.R. (ed.): *Neurological Surgery*. Philadelphia, W.B. Saunders Company, 1982, pp. 1511–1558.

Displaying different presentation, cortical vein thrombosis may result in congestion, edema, and hemorrhage from vessel rupture, which can be intracerebral, subarachnoid, or subdural in location. Only 5 to 10 per cent of patients develop frank hemorrhages; however, 60 per cent present with focal seizures. In addition to cortical venous infarction, anoxic encephalopathy and herpes simplex encephalitis are the disease processes that cause bilateral epileptic foci. About half of the patients with cortical vein thrombosis have low-grade fever and headache, making differentiation from meningitis important. Cloudiness of the sensorium is frequent.

Following uncontrasted and contrast-enhanced CT for the detection of intraparenchymal venous hemorrhagic infarctions and exclusion of brain abscess or subdural empyema, lumbar puncture will rule out purulent meningitis by yielding sterile cerebrospinal fluid with moderate leukocytosis. Cerebral venous or sinus thrombosis may be documented noninvasively by employing intravenous digital subtraction angiography.

ACUTE BACTERIAL MENINGITIS

By Peter A. Rice, M.D.
Boston, Massachusetts

Bacterial meningitis is a life-threatening infection that must be recognized early in order to avert a catastrophic result. Prior to the advent of effective antimicrobial therapy, this infection was almost always uniformly fatal; however, with prompt recognition and correct antimicrobial therapy and supportive care both the case fatality rate and neurologic sequelae can be greatly reduced. In order to make a rapid diagnosis, the clinician must suspect bacterial meningitis in patients with fever and altered mental status; meningeal signs are usually although not invariably present.

A lumbar puncture must be performed promptly in patients suspected of having bacterial meningitis both for confirmation of the diagnosis and to provide a guide to initial antimicrobial therapy, which can only come from the evaluation of cerebrospinal fluid. Patients who have a questionable clinical diagnosis of bacterial meningitis and who have signs of increased cerebrospinal fluid pressure accompanied by focal neurologic signs may need alternative neurologic evaluation in the form of brain scan, computed tomography (CT), or angiography performed immediately to exclude other neurologic disorders in which lumbar puncture may be contraindicated. However, if these ancillary studies do not rapidly provide an alternative diagnosis, the lumbar puncture must be performed even in the face of increased cerebrospinal fluid pressure.

The overwhelming majority of cases of acute bacterial meningitis in patients older than 2 months of age are caused by three pathogens. *Hemophilus influenzae* type b is the most common, followed by *Neisseria meningitidis* and *Streptococcus pneumoniae.* Together these species account for more than 95 per cent of all cases. "Unusual" organisms account for the remaining 5 per cent or less.

ASSESSMENT OF THE PATIENT SUSPECTED OF HAVING BACTERIAL MENINGITIS

The age of the patient dictates which bacterial species (or subspecies) is likely to be the cause of meningitis. *Hemophilus influenzae* type b is the predominant pathogen in children through 4 years of age, *N. meningitidis* is common under the age of 20 years, and *S. pneumoniae* is common at all ages greater than 2 months and is the most common pathogen in adults. Other organisms predominate in neonates and also cause bacterial meningitis in compromised hosts (Table 1).

Associated findings or illnesses are important considerations in judging the most likely pathogen responsible for bacterial meningitis, and these must be sought rapidly in patients being assessed for possible meningitis. A congenital abnormality of the central nervous system such as meningomyelocele will more frequently be associated with meningitis caused by *Staphylococcus aureus,* group A and group D streptococci, and enteric bacilli. Trauma to the head (not necessarily penetrating), resulting in an inapparent fracture of the skull or cribriform plate or a dural tear, can be associated with pneumococcal meningitis, either shortly after the trauma or at varying intervals thereafter. Often patients with such injuries will develop minimal symptoms early in the course of their disease and it is important to consider the diagnosis of bacterial meningitis despite the patient's relative well-being. Penetrating trauma to the skull (including neurosurgery) may result in meningitis caused by Staphylococcus or enteric bacilli. Such infections caused by gram-negative organisms may also develop at a slow pace (like pneumococcal meningitis in patients with nonpenetrating head trauma) and early clues may be sparse; hence the clinician must be watchful for subtle indications of this disease. Often the strains causing these infections (Staphylococcus or enteric gram-negative bacilli) are responsible for infection or colonization at other sites, such as wound infections, catheter infections, or urinary tract infections. Intracranial foreign bodies, such as ventriculoatrial shunts for relieving hydrocephalus, may become infected with *Staphylococcus epidermidis* and less commonly with *Staphylococcus aureus* or diphtheroids. Ven-

Table 1. Bacterial Causes of Acute Meningitis

Organisms	Neonates	Children	Adults
Gram-positive	Group B streptococci Other streptococci Staphylococci *Listeria monocytogenes* *Streptococcus pneumoniae*	*Streptococcus pneumoniae* Other streptococci	*Streptococcus pneumoniae* Other streptococci Staphylococci *Listeria monocytogenes*
Gram-negative	*Escherichia coli* Klebsiella Proteus Pseudomonas *Hemophilus influenzae*	*Hemophilus influenzae* type b *Neisseria meningitidis* *Hemophilus parainfluenzae* Gram-negative enteric* organisms	*Neisseria meningitidis* Acinetobacter* Klebsiella* Pseudomonas* *Hemophilus influenzae*

* Rare; occurs in the compromised host or after neurosurgery.

triculoperitoneal shunts may also be infected with these organisms or with enteric bacilli.

Infections associated with bacteremia, especially endocarditis, may be associated with meningitis. However, meningitis resulting from endocarditis infrequently yields an organism either on Gram's stain or culture of cerebrospinal fluid (CSF); for this reason, bacteriologic diagnosis usually depends upon results of blood cultures. Upper respiratory infections, particularly otitis, mastoiditis, and sinusitis, may serve as foci for meningeal spread of Hemophilus, *Streptococcus pneumoniae*, and infrequently Staphylococcus; these foci may require surgical drainage in addition to specific antimicrobial therapy. Pneumococcal pneumonia may be accompanied by bacteremia and meningitis, particularly in elderly or debilitated patients. Immunocompromised hosts, especially those with malignancies or disease states that are being treated with immunosuppressive drugs, are susceptible to bacterial meningitis caused by a variety of bacterial agents, including *Listeria monocytogenes,* enteric bacilli, and *Hemophilus influenzae* (even in adults), plus agents commonly associated with bacterial meningitis in a usual setting.

OTHER CONDITIONS TO BE CONSIDERED

Nonbacterial meningitis or meningoencephalitis may mimic bacterial meningitis; these infections may be caused by viruses, spirochetes, protozoa, mycobacteria, and fungi.

"Aseptic" or viral meningitis is typically self-limited and is characterized by CSF lymphocytosis, normal glucose levels, and modest elevation in CSF protein levels. These infections are usually caused by enteroviruses (echovirus and coxsackievirus), particularly in the summer months. Herpes simplex and several other diseases associated with aseptic meningitis, such as syphilis and leptospirosis, may require specific therapy. Occasionally, partially treated bacterial meningitis may have a CSF profile compatible with aseptic meningitis. Conversely, viral meningitis may initially cause predominance of polymorphonuclear leukocytes in CSF and occasionally (with mumps, herpes simplex, and lymphocytic choriomeningitis) a low CSF glucose level.

Toxoplasmosis, trichinosis, and cysticercosis may cause meningitis with a lymphocytic profile (cysticercosis produces a low CSF glucose level as well).

Amebic meningoencephalitis (caused by fresh water free-living Hartmanella and Naegleria species) may produce a purulent CSF with a predominance of polymorphonuclear leukocytes and low glucose level.

Tuberculous meningitis may cause a fulminant meningitis with a CSF pattern highlighted by a predominance of lymphocytes and low glucose level. Particularly in children with miliary tuberculosis, findings on chest x-ray may be negative and diagnosis may ultimately rest on culture of the CSF although biopsy and acid-fast stains of liver and bone marrow may yield a prompt diagnosis. Acid-fast stains of CSF should be performed, but these are usually negative.

Cryptococcal, candidal, and coccidioidal meningitis may also mimic bacterial meningitis, but, as in tuberculous meningitis, these may be difficult to diagnose immediately. Therapy for tuberculosis or fungal meningitis may have to be presumptive, pending results of cultures and stains of tissue that cannot be performed immediately. In particular, nonbacterial meningitis in an immunocompromised host may dictate a presumptive diagnosis (such as varicella, herpes simplex, *Toxoplasma gondii,* or *Cryptococcus neoformans*) and therapy, if warranted.

Parameningeal infection, including brain abscess, may mimic bacterial meningitis and should be considered in the evaluation of a patient with fever and CSF pleocytosis because antimicrobial therapy would differ from that for most types of meningitis. In addition, surgical drainage, if possible, is needed in all cases of parameningeal infection. Brain abscess may produce neurologic signs of a mass lesion but can present with only fever, headache, spinal fluid pleocytosis, and no focal neurologic signs. A low CSF glucose level (less than one half of simultaneously obtained blood glucose level) suggests rupture or leak of the abscess. Other examples of parameningeal foci include vertebral osteomyelitis, retropharyngeal abscess with spinal epidural abscess, and subdural empyema (over the skull); all require prompt surgical drainage (for bacteriologic diagnosis and therapy) and specific antimicrobial therapy.

The preliminary diagnosis of bacterial meningitis or even of central nervous system infection may in some instances be incorrect despite CSF patterns that are highly suggestive. In particular, chemical meningitis caused by hemorrhage, spinal anesthesia, contrast media, detergents, and keratin from dermoid tumors may rarely produce a purulent CSF with a predominance of polymorphonuclear leukocytes and low glucose level. A number of other unusual diseases may also produce a similar CSF profile: cerebritis caused by systemic lupus erythematosus, Behçet's syndrome, Mollaret's meningitis (in the initial phase), Harada's disease, Vogt-Koyanagi disease, and hypersensitivity meningitis caused by drugs (sulfonamides). Carcinomatous meningitis may also result in a low CSF glucose level; in this disorder, however, lymphocytes usually are the predominant cell type.

Another important class of diseases to be considered in the initial assessment of a patient with suspected bacterial meningitis is intracranial hemorrhage. Although focal neurologic signs and minimal fever may suggest this possibility, the most important distinguishing points will be the clinical setting and ancillary features of the patient's history and physical examination. Patients strongly suspected of having intracranial hemorrhage should not have an initial lumbar puncture, but their neurologic evaluation should proceed rapidly (brain scans, CT, arteriograms), and the decision to perform a lumbar puncture to evaluate the possibility of meningitis should be made in these patients after hemorrhage or a mass lesion has been excluded. If a patient has signs of increased CSF pressure but needs a lumbar puncture because the suspicion of meningitis is strong, certain precautions should be taken to minimize the possibility of brain herniation. Perform the lumbar puncture with a small-bore needle (20 to 22 gauge), and be prepared to treat herniation (opening pressure levels greater than 350 mm H_2O). The lumbar puncture needle should not be removed, and the stylet should be reinserted. Mannitol should be administered intravenously in a dose of 1.5 to 2 gm/kg body weight as 500 mls of a 20 per cent solution until the CSF pressure is less than 200 mm H_2O. The pressure should be controlled, if indicated, with mannitol or steroids, or both, after the lumbar puncture needle is removed.

ASSESSMENT OF THE CEREBROSPINAL FLUID

Cerebrospinal Fluid Cell Count

There may be considerable variation in the CSF cell count in bacterial meningitis at the time of diagnosis, with counts ranging from 0 to greater than 50,000. Two thirds of patients will have counts greater than 1000 white cells per cu mm, and polymorphonuclear leukocytes will predominate. A differential cell count in the CSF of less than 70 per cent polymorphonuclear leukocytes reduces the likelihood of bacterial meningitis, even if the patient has been taking antimicrobials. In early or overwhelming infection, as few as 3 or 4 white cells per cu mm may be all that are present; in these instances, however, the chemical analyses may be diagnostic and Gram's stains are often positive.

Cerebrospinal Fluid Glucose and Protein Levels

A normal glucose level in the CSF ranges between one half to two thirds the value of blood simultaneously obtained. Bacterial meningitis characteristically is associated with a low CSF glucose. In addition, the concentration of protein in CSF is nearly always elevated (i.e., greater than 50 mg/dl), and often parallels the severity of the disease. High levels of protein that persist during the course of therapy while other parameters are otherwise improving may indicate the presence of suppurative complications. The glucose level in the CSF may be measured as artificially low if red and white cells, which continue to utilize glucose, are not separated from the CSF. In addition, protein levels may be elevated if large numbers of red cells lyse in the CSF. As a guide, consider that the protein level will be elevated by 1 mg/ml for each 1000 cells per cu mm in a specimen that has not been centrifuged. The glucose determination in an old specimen is unreliable even if all the cells are removed from the CSF. A 3 to 4 mg/dl per hour decrease in the level of CSF glucose will occur at room temperature.

The results of standard laboratory tests in neonates tend to be misleading. For example, peripheral leukocyte counts are normally elevated in the first days of life and the CSF of healthy babies may contain white blood cells and increased concentrations of protein (Table 2). This is not to say that these examinations are not important in the total evaluation of the sick neonate.

Table 2. Cerebrospinal Fluid Findings in Normal Neonates

Laboratory Value	Term Infant	Preterm Infant
White Blood Cell Count (cells/cu mm)		
Mean	8.2	9.0
Standard deviation	7.1	8.2
Range	0–32	0–29
Percentage of polymorphonuclear leukocytes	61.3	57.2
Protein (mg/dl)		
Mean	90	115
Range	20–170	65–150
Cerebrospinal Fluid/Blood Glucose (%)		
Mean	81	74
Range	44–248	35–105

The physician must be aware that 0 to 32 white blood cells per cu mm (mean, 8 cells per cu mm) may be found in normal babies 1 to 10 days of age and that 60 per cent or more of these cells are polymorphonuclear leukocytes. The percentage of CSF glucose to blood glucose is greater in newborn infants than in older infants and children, and ranges from 44 per cent to greater than 100 per cent. The spinal fluid protein content is elevated during the neonatal period and is higher in premature than in full-term infants. Thus, results of the CSF examination in neonates suspected of having meningitis must be interpreted with reference to the values found in noninfected babies.

Gram's Stain of the Cerebrospinal Fluid

Gram's staining of the CSF is essential in the evaluation of the patient suspected of having bacterial meningitis. The Gram's stain will be positive if greater than 10^5 to 10^6 organisms per milliliter of uncentrifuged CSF are present. Centrifugation will facilitate visualization of the organisms and should be performed for 20 to 30 minutes (2000 to 3000 rpm) in a standard bench top centrifuge. The sediment thus obtained is suspended in a drop of CSF; this suspension is then placed on a microscope slide and allowed to air dry (the specimen should not be heat fixed). If the suspension is thin, layer several drops one on top of the other on the slide to further concentrate the specimen. In nearly 85 per cent of cases of bacterial meningitis, a Gram-stained smear will be positive for the etiologic agent. When antibiotics have been administered prior to obtaining a specimen for culture, a positive Gram's stain may be seen in conjunction with a negative culture.

Culture of the Cerebrospinal Fluid

Bacteriologic culturing of the CSF should include direct plating of the specimen onto solid media and broth inoculation. The CSF should be inoculated onto blood agar and chocolate blood agar (with 1 per cent Supplement B or Iso-vitalex). Staphylococcal streaking of a blood agar plate may not assist in the isolation of small numbers of *H. influenzae* type b and should not be used. If sufficient numbers of organisms are present, slide agglutinations for *H. influenzae* type b and Quellung reactions for *S. pneumoniae* will assist in establishing a specific diagnosis. The Quellung reaction permits assessment of capsular swelling when antiserum is added to organisms visible on a wet mounted slide.

Interpretation of Cerebrospinal Fluid Findings

All the available data must be considered in the accurate analysis of CSF. No single laboratory test, except the culture of CSF, can verify or exclude the diagnosis of acute bacterial meningitis. For example, leukocyte counts in the CSF exceeding 1000, differential counts that yield more than 75 per cent polymorphonuclear leukocytes, glucose concentrations less than 40 mg/dl, and protein concentrations above 50 mg/dl strongly suggest a diagnosis of bacterial meningitis. In a recent study of patients of all ages with meningitis, carried out prospectively, 19 per cent had an initial CSF glucose level greater than 60 mg/dl, 9 per cent had initial CSF protein levels less than 50 mg/dl, and 36 per cent had initial CSF white cell counts of less than 1000 cells per cu mm. Occasionally, CSF cell counts that exceed 1000 per cu mm, with differential counts containing greater than 75 per cent polymorphonuclear leukocytes, can initially be encountered in viral meningitis, particularly those caused by enteroviruses. In these cases, repeat lumbar punctures will be useful and a significant reduction in the proportion of polymorphonuclear leukocytes in CSF in nearly 90 per cent of patients with viral meningitis will be seen 6 to 8 hours after a repeat lumbar puncture is performed.

Numerous other infectious and noninfectious diseases of the central nervous system can cause the appearance of polymorphonuclear leukocytes or lymphocytes in the CSF, and some may also lower the glucose. Protein levels may be moderately elevated in diabetes, alcoholism, connective tissue disorders, demyelinating syndromes, and central nervous system abscess. Cerebrospinal fluid protein levels may be extremely high in chronic meningitis. Guillan-Barré syndrome, chronic subdural hemorrhage, or spinal subarachnoid block. Careful analysis of the history in each of these cases, coupled with the clinical features and a consideration of the abnormalties of cells, glucose and protein levels, and results of Gram's stain nearly always leads to the correct diagnosis. Table 3 summarizes these differential characteristics.

An often encountered problem confronting the clinician is that of a grossly bloody spinal fluid. The distinction between a traumatic lumbar puncture and a subarachnoid hemorrhage may complicate the diagnosis of bacterial meningitis. In addition, blood alone in sufficient quantities may cause a chemical meningitis with a pleocytosis consisting principally of polymorphonuclear leukocytes. In addition, the CSF glucose level may be low (i.e., 20 to 30 mg/dl) and the protein content may be elevated. The first and fourth tubes of CSF collected from the patient should both be sent for cell count to assess clearing of red cells from the first tube to the fourth. If the fluid contains blood as a result of a traumatic tap, the cell count should contain the same red to white cell ratio as peripheral blood. For example, a count of 5,000,000 red cells and 10,000 white cells gives a ratio of 500 red cells per white cell. Therefore, a CSF red cell count of 86,000 justifiably could have 172 white cells with a percentage of polymorphonuclear leukocytes similar to that in the blood. It is important to centrifuge and remove red cells, as mentioned earlier, since their presence may spuriously reduce the CSF glucose level and increase the protein content. In addition to subarachnoid hemorrhage and traumatic lumbar punctures, red cells may commonly occur with septic or bland emboli, mycotic aneurysms, and herpes simplex encephalitis.

Occasionally, the CSF values will not be diagnostic. There may be a significant pleocytosis, usually in the hundreds, with a polymorphonuclear leukocyte percentage of 40 to 50 per cent. The level of CSF glucose may also be equivocal, falling to a level between 40 and 60 per cent that of the simultaneously obtained blood. The CSF protein is elevated occasionally and the Gram stain shows no organisms. Although these findings are not specific for bacterial meningitis, these CSF findings may be consistent with a number of other diseases. Among those to be considered are chronic meningitis, tumor or parameningeal foci (i.e., epidural abscess, subdural hematoma, sinusitis, mastoiditis, or adjacent osteomyelitis of the skull or spine). Of great importance is the possibility of brain abscess, which typically has these CSF findings.

It is greatly debated whether prior antibiotic therapy can alter CSF findings to the extent that bacterial meningitis will not be recognized. In some settings, as many as 30 to 50 per cent of patients who present with bacterial meningitis have received at least some antimicrobial agent. Prior treatment appears to decrease the yield of positive cultures, but otherwise it has little effect. In addition, patients who have received partial treatment before the diagnosis of bacterial meningitis is made have as good a prognosis for recovery as those who are untreated prior to diagnosis. Thus, prior therapy may confuse the clinical picture, but should not be otherwise detrimental to the individual patient.

ADDITIONAL DIAGNOSTIC LABORATORY TESTS

Blood cultures should be obtained because of the frequently associated bacteremia that occurs with bacterial meningitis. Over 50 per cent of patients with bacterial meningitis caused by *H. influenzae* type b, *S. pneumoniae*, and *N. meningitidis* have concomitantly positive blood cultures. Occasionally, blood cultures are positive when CSF cultures fail to yield organisms.

When paracranial infections or infections resulting from trauma are suspected, radiographic studies of the skull, mastoid processes, and sinuses may be helpful. Tomography of the ethmoid and sphenoid sinuses may be the only way to visualize these important

Table 3. Cerebrospinal Fluid Profiles in Meningitis

	Purulent	Lymphocytic (Low Glucose Type)	Lymphocytic (Normal Glucose Type)
Predominant Cells (Adults)*	Polymorphonuclear Leukocytes	Lymphocytes	Lymphocytes
Glucose Level†	Low	Low	Normal
Protein Level (Normal, 50 mg/dl)	Increased	Normal or Increased	Normal or Increased
Causes of Meningitis	I. Infections A. Common: Bacterial B. Uncommon §1. Viral (early phase only; up to 85% PMNs)‡ §2. Embolic cerebral infarction (bacterial endocarditis) 3. Certain parameningeal infections §a. Subdural empyema b. Cerebral abscesses with leakage into ventricular system §c. Cortical venous thrombophlebitis or phlebitis of major dural venous sinuses‡ 4. Amebic meningoencephalitis (Naegleria or Hartmanella) 5. Tuberculous (rare and only very early in the disease) 6. Acute hemorrhagic encephalitis II. Noninfectious Causes (rare) A. Chemical: hemorrhage; spinal anesthesia; contrast media; detergents; keratin from dermoid tumors; craniopharyngiomas §B. Unusual diseases‡: Behçet's syndrome; Mollaret's meningitis (in initial phase); Harada's disease; Vogt-Koyanagi disease §C. Hypersensitivity: Sulfonamides	I. Infections A. Common 1. Tuberculous 2. Fungal a. Cryptococcal b. Coccidioidal c. Histoplasmal B. Uncommon 1. Bacterial a. Common agents *partially treated with antibiotics* b. Spirochetal i. Leptospiral ii. Syphilitic iii. Lyme disease c. Uncommon agents (e.g., *Listeria monocytogenes*) 2. Viral a. Mumps (about 10% of cases) b. Lymphocytic choriomeningitis (occasionally) c. Herpes simplex meningoencephalitis 3. Cysticercosis II. Noninfectious Causes A. Malignancy 1. Metastatic carcinoma 2. Leukemia, lymphoma B. Sarcoidosis of meninges C. Subarachnoid hemorrhage	I. Infections A. Common 1. Viral meningitis or encephalitis 2. Post-infectious encephalomyelitis B. Uncommon 1. Bacterial: Common agents *partially treated with antibiotics* 2. Parameningeal infection a. Abscess: brain, epidural, subdural b. Epidural infection associated with mastoiditis, sinusitis of ethmoid, frontal, or sphenoid sinuses c. Thrombophlebitis of cortical veins and dural venous sinuses 3. Early phase of fungal and tuberculous meningitis 4. Parasitic disease a. Trichinosis b. Toxoplasmosis

* Normal, less than 5 cells per cu mm, with only mononuclear leukocytes present. See Table 2 for data for neonates.

† Normal = one half to two thirds of simultaneously obtained blood glucose level.

‡ Lymphocytes may also be seen with these entities.

§ Cerebrospinal fluid glucose level is usually normal.

since thrombosis or cerebritis may produce nonspecific changes; however, if structural lesions are being sought, a positive scan may be helpful. It is hoped that with the advent of CT scanning many diagnostic dilemmas will be solved.

Many special diagnostic techniques have appeared recently, and most probably are not useful. However, because the frequently observed symptoms, signs, and laboratory data for central nervous system infections occasionally are nonspecific, interest has been generated in a variety of laboratory examinations that distinguish bacterial causes from those caused by other agents.

Endotoxin assays have proved to be cheap, practical, and reliable for the diagnosis of meningitis due to gram-negative organisms (including *H. influenzae* and *N. meningitidis*) in older infants, children, and adults. False-positive results do not occur in carefully controlled assays performed with pyrogen-free reagents; however, false-negative results do occur in one third of culturally proved cases of gram-negative meningitis in neonates.

Counterimmunoelectrophoresis (CIE) and agglutination employing latex particles with specific antibody affixed appear to be sensitive methods for diagnosing *H. influenzae* type b infection and to be less so for meningitis caused by *N. meningitidis* or *S. pneumoniae*. The use of these methods appears most promising in directing initial therapy when Gram-stained slides show no organisms and when the patient has been treated with antibiotics prior to obtaining a CSF specimen. Volatile acids, particularly lactic acid, have been examined in the CSF by gas-liquid chromatography (GLC). Increases in CSF lactic acid concentration appear to be specific for bacterial meningitis. Increases do not correlate with other elements of inflammation, such as total number of white blood cells or protein concentration. As yet, volatile acids have not been studied in detail, but the ease and availability of GLC make this procedure promising for future investigation.

BRAIN ABSCESSES

By Javad Hekmatpanah, M.D.
Chicago, Illinois

A brain abscess is a purulent intracranial mass. Because it results from an infectious process and is a space-occupying lesion, its signs and symptoms are related to both of these processes. Similarly, management of a brain abscess is basically related to treatment of the infection and to elimination of the mass.

Bacteria causing the abscess reach the brain from almost any infectious foci in the body, but brain abscesses most commonly occur in association with one of the following four conditions:

1. Infections that are in the immediate vicinity of the brain, such as those involving the ears, paranasal sinuses and scalp, and osteomyelitis of the skull.
2. Infections involving the thorax, such as those occurring in the lungs and in the mediastinum, especially when there is bronchiectasis.
3. Bacteremia.
4. Direct implantation of bacteria in the brain, either through penetrating sharp objects and foreign bodies, such as bullets, or, in rare instances, after an intracranial operation.

The incidence of the brain abscess is higher in patients with congenital heart disease with septal defects, and it is probably higher in patients with diabetes, in patients taking immunosuppressive drugs for prolonged periods of time, and in addicts taking drugs through nonsterile injections.

Although great advances have been made in surgical techniques and a large number of antibiotics are available, the mortality rate of the brain abscess remains high. Mortality figures up to 30 per cent are still appearing in the literature. There are several reasons for such a high mortality rate, but the main reasons are without doubt delay or error in diagnosis. This is unfortunate, since now all that is required is to suspect the possibility of an abscess; recent scanning techniques have simplified the diagnosis.

CLINICAL PRESENTATION

The reason that a brain abscess may not be suspected stems, in part, from the fact that it presents different symptoms and signs during its various stages of development. When the pathogenic bacteria settle in the brain, three stages of pathophysiologic alterations take place. These are the periods of local cerebritis, encapsulation, and liquefaction and expansion.

Period of Local Cerebritis

During this period, the primary somatic responses to infection, such as chills, fever, malaise, tachycardia, and leukocytosis, are present, as they are in infections elsewhere in the body. Cerebral swelling occurs around the area of cerebritis, causing a rise in intracranial pressure. Various degrees of meningitis or meningeal reaction also occur, especially around the area of cerebritis. These will cause headaches, nuchal rigidity, and organic mental changes. Based on the location of cerebritis, specific focal or generalized seizures and local neurologic abnormalities may occur. If a spinal tap is done, it often shows elevated pressure and increases in white cells and protein. The glucose level in cerebrospinal fluid may be low, and bacteria may or may not be present in the culture.

Period of Encapsulation

About 1 week after the onset of cerebritis a capsule begins to develop around the area of local cerebritis. It usually takes about 2 weeks for a thick capsule to develop. As the capsule separates the area of cerebritis from the rest of the brain, the somatic response to the infection declines. The temperature might return to near normal but often will fluctuate. The white blood cell count may decline, and the patient may actually feel better. Although it is not recommended, a spinal tap would show a decline in the white blood cell count, but the protein content and the pressure might still be elevated.

Period of Liquefaction and Expansion

As the abscess becomes walled off, its center becomes necrotic and liquefied; also, various degrees of expansion may take place. During this period the signs and symptoms of infection further decline, but the patient continues to have signs of an intracranial mass. Based on the size and location of the abscess, various degrees of ventricular obstruction may occur, causing a further rise in intracranial pressure. Other signs of raised intracranial pressure, such as sixth nerve palsy, third nerve palsy, drowsiness, or coma, may develop. The disturbances of consciousness could, of course, develop even at early stages of the brain abscess if cerebritis is massive.

EPIDURAL AND SUBDURAL ABSCESSES

Infection from paranasal sinuses may erode the skull or the orbit, causing epidural, subdural, or retro-orbital abscesses. In a patient with unilateral swollen eyelid, chemosis, ophthalmoplegia, fever, and leukocytosis, orbital infection should be considered. In such a patient, extension of the infection and the pus to the epidural and subdural regions should be kept in mind, especially when the patient is drowsy or disoriented. This is an emergency condition; evaluation through x-ray studies must be done immediately and the diagnosis confirmed, followed by antibiotic therapy and surgical drainage of the pus. At times, combined or multiple operations are needed to drain pus from the orbit, sinuses, and epidural and subdural regions. Epidural and subdural abscesses often take the form of multiple pocket formations. If these pocket formations are not adequately drained, symptoms are likely to remain. Chronic infection of the sphenoid sinus might erode the floor of the sella turcica and cause an abscess in the sella and the pituitary region. In such patients vision may rapidly decline. Here, too, immediate evaluation and management should be considered.

RADIOLOGIC DIAGNOSIS OF BRAIN ABSCESS

Skull X-rays

Except when it is old and calcified, a brain abscess cannot be detected on simple skull films. Osteomyelitis, opacification or fluid level in sinuses, and fracture on the skull films, however, may help to indicate the possibility of an associated brain abscess.

Cerebral Angiography

Angiography often shows evidence of an avascular mass, but on rare occasions the neovascularization of the wall of the abscess may appear as a circular "stain" on the late angiographic films. Whereas epidural and subdural abscesses can be detected by angiography, the picture is identical to that of a hematoma in this region, unless it is associated with a specific stain. The stain here is composed of a flat, fine vascular pattern on the surface of the abscess.

Isotope Scan

Isotope scans show a circular uptake and are more helpful than angiography in revealing a cerebral abscess (Fig. 1). These scans may not detect abscesses located low in the temporal region, in the base of the skull, in epidural, or in subdural regions.

Computed Tomography

Computed tomography (CT) is the best radiologic technique for diagnosis of brain abscess. It shows a mass with the enhancing ring of the capsule (Fig. 2). CT scan also reveals the area and the extent of the swelling around the abscess, and the exact location, the size, and the number of abscesses. These data, together with the determination of proximity of the abscess to the ventricular wall, presence or absence of hydrocephalus, and determination of ventricular shift, all provide important information for managing the abscess judiciously and effectively.

PITFALLS IN DIAGNOSIS OF BRAIN ABSCESS

During the period of cerebritis it would not be unusual for an abscess to be mistakenly diagnosed as meningitis. At this stage such a diagnosis is seldom harmful since the patient is likely to receive antibiotic

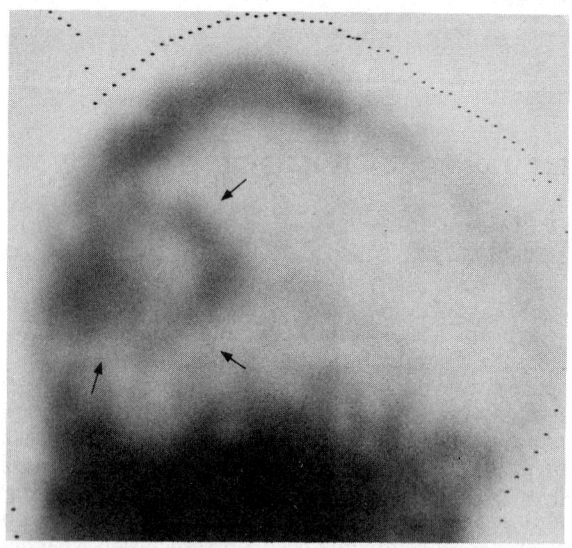

Figure 1. Isotope scan of a young child with an abscess in the occipital region (arrows). This patient had been treated for presumed meningitis for several weeks. Although the signs of infection had decreased, he began to develop signs of increased intracranial pressure.

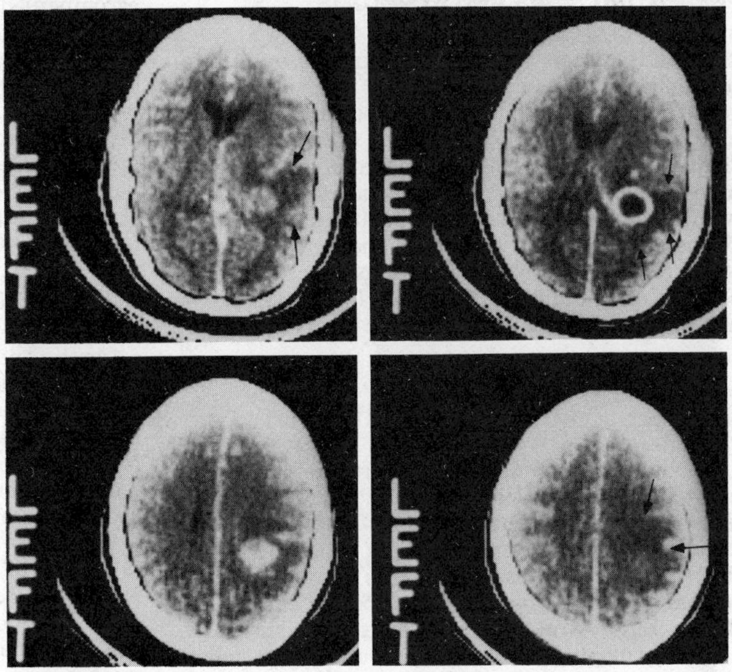

Fig 2. CT scan in a 20-year-old patient with a brain abscess. She had congenital heart disease. Note extensive edema around the abscess (arrows). This is a postinfusion scan showing the capsule of the abscess as a dense ring.

therapy. Indeed, it is possible that at this stage an abscess can be completely eradicated by antibiotic therapy without its presence being suspected. But with a large abscess, if the assumed diagnosis of meningitis is maintained, the patient would have partially improved but would not recover satisfactorily in spite of presumably adequate treatment for meningitis. In such a condition it is mandatory to establish a definitive diagnosis through radiologic techniques, preferably the CT scan. In later stages, after encapsulation of the abscess, the symptoms of infection might diminish or completely disappear, and the brain abscess might be mistaken for a brain tumor, especially if history of earlier illness is not obtained. Although the correct diagnosis will eventually be made at surgery, the operations performed may not necessarily be the best that would have been considered if the correct diagnosis had been made. Hence, if a patient suspected of having a brain tumor has an associated condition capable of sending bacterial emboli to the brain, the possibility of a brain abscess should be considered. Finally, at times the correct diagnosis is impossible until surgery takes place. This is particularly true in patients with brain abscess who also have a known malignancy, such as leukemia, or in patients with an infected tumor of the lungs or in the vicinity of the brain.

POOR OUTCOME OR FAILURE IN TREATMENT OF BRAIN ABSCESS

Although at times a small brain abscess may calcify, with or without antibiotic therapy, and cause little or no problem, an inadequately treated abscess often causes serious neurlogic disabilities and death. The abscess may rupture into the subarachnoid region or into the ventricle, resulting in severe meningitis or ventriculitis and death. Multiple abscesses of the brain or abscesses associated with multiple pocket formations in the epidural or subdural region may continue to be symptomatic if treated inadequately. Indeed, sometimes all treatments will be ineffective because of numerous pocket formations and severe extent of the disease.

ASEPTIC MENINGITIS AND VIRAL MENINGITIS

By Donald M. McLean, M.D.
Vancouver, British Columbia, Canada

SYNONYMS

Acute lymphocytic meningitis, benign lymphocytic choriomeningitis, nonbacterial meningitis, serous meningitis, viral meningoencephalitis.

DEFINITION

Acute viral inflammation of the meninges, principally affecting the pia and arachnoid membranes, induces elaboration of excess cerebrospinal fluid (CSF), which is rich in leukocytes, principally lymphocytes, but the glucose and protein contents remain virtually unchanged. Headache and neck stiffness, usually accompanied by vomiting and fever, constitute the usual range of clinical manifestations. Mumps virus and enteroviruses are the common causative agents in aseptic meningitis.

PRESENTING SIGNS AND SYMPTOMS

There is sudden onset of severe frontal or parietal headache, usually accompanied by vomiting, and fever of 38 to 40°C (100 to 104°F). Neck and spine stiffness are noted shortly thereafter. Convulsions may signify the onset in about 15 per cent of children with mumps meningitis and in somewhat fewer patients with enteroviral meningitis. Usually medical attention is sought 12 to 24 hours after onset, at which time lumbar puncture is performed to reveal clear to cloudy CSF containing 30 to 3000 leukocytes per cu mm or more, the majority of which are lymphocytes.

COURSE

In mumps meningitis, temperature elevations above 38°C (100°F) usually persist for 2 to 4 days, but in 25 per cent of patients fever may persist 5 to 7 days. Abatement of symptoms, including headache, vomiting, and neck stiffness, often occurs within 6 hours of lumbar puncture when this is performed early in the illness. Enteroviral meningitis runs a similar course.

Mumps meningitis has been encountered during all months of the year, with an increased incidence during winter and spring. Enteroviral meningitis usually occurs only during summer and autumn.

PHYSICAL EXAMINATION FINDINGS

Obvious neck stiffness is usually accompanied by the tripod sign. Kernig's or Brudzinski's signs, or both, are positive. Usually the skeletal musculature shows normal power and tone. In mumps meningitis, the incidence of illness in males exceeds that in females by 2:1 or greater, but in enteroviral meningitis the sex ratio is 1:1.

COMMON COMPLICATIONS

Mumps meningitis may develop from 6 days before to 14 days after the onset of swelling of the parotid or submandibular salivary glands or both, but 25 to 33 per cent of patients with virologically confirmed disease may exhibit meningitis without parotitis. Meningitis may be accompanied by other systemic manifestations of mumps virus infection, including pancreatitis when there is severe upper midline abdominal pain accompanied by a transient increase of serum amylase, unilateral or bilateral orchitis, or oophoritis manifested by lower abdominal pain. Hyperpyrexia may be accompanied by temporary mental confusion. Transient monoplegia or quadriplegia has been observed occasionally. Dehydration and electrolyte imbalance may result from protracted vomiting.

Enteroviral meningitis, especially that caused by echovirus-9, may be accompanied by a maculopapular rash in 33 per cent of patients. This rash shows a peripheral distribution, and is noted especially on the palms, but in contradistinction to measles it is not accompanied by nasal and conjunctival inflammation and discharge. Enteroviral meningitis caused by coxsackievirus group B may be accompanied by pleurodynia (sharp chest pain on deep inspiration plus a pleural friction rub), pericarditis (pericardial pain plus pericardial friction rub), serous peritonitis or mesenteric adenitis (severe generalized abdominal pain and tenderness), or severe myalgia affecting the skeletal musculature.

CLINICAL LABORATORY FINDINGS

Cerebrospinal fluid findings pathognomonic of aseptic meningitis:

1. Total leukocyte count 30 to 3000 per cu mm or more, of which 70 to 99.9 per cent are lymphocytes. Many patients with mumps meningitis show CSF leukocyte counts above 500/cu mm, but this is less common in enteroviral meningitis.
2. Glucose content normal (70 to 120 mg/dl).
3. Protein content usually normal at 30 to 40 mg/dl, but occasionally as high as 100 mg/dl.
4. Chloride content normal.
5. No microorganisms seen on Gram-stained smears.
6. Virions of mumps may be observed frequently in CSF from patients with mumps meningitis by electron microscopic examination after negative staining with phosphotungstic acid.

Additional findings in patients with complications may include the following:

1. Moderately diffusely abnormal electroencephalograms in patients with hyperpyrexia and temporary confusion or convulsions.
2. Inversion or flattening of the T waves in electrocardiographic leads V_3 to V_5 is noted regularly in pericarditis.

CAUSATIVE ORGANISMS

Most cases of aseptic meningitis are due to infections with two major groups of viruses, paramyxoviruses and picornaviruses. Within the paramyxovirus group, mumps virus is the sole virus serotype regularly associated with aseptic meningitis, but measles virus is an uncommon yet extremely important cause of encephalitis that may include meningeal involvement. Within the picornavirus group, comprising more than 60 serotypes, at least 14 virus serotypes are associated regularly with outbreaks of aseptic meningitis. These include echovirus types 4, 6, 9, 16, and 30, coxsackievirus types A9 and B1 through B5, and, less frequently, poliovirus types 1 through 3. Occasional cases of aseptic meningitis have resulted from infection with most of the other echovirus serotypes, particularly types 2, 3, 5, 7, 11, 14, 18, 19, 20, 21, 31, and 33, plus coxsackievirus B6. Usually during an epidemic, one enterovirus serotype becomes dominant, and a wide variety of other serotypes affect relatively few patients.

Viruses within other groups have been associated infrequently with aseptic meningitis. Adenovirus types 3 and 5 have been recovered from the CSF of patients with meningeal signs. Herpes simplex virus types 1 and 2 may occasionally induce disease of the central nervous sytem, which is usually manifested as encephalitis rather than meningitis. Arbovirus infections within the central nervous system usually induce encephalitis concomitantly with meningitis. North American arboviruses include infections by the alphaviruses (eastern and western equine encephalomyelitis), the flaviviruses (St. Louis encephalitis and Powassan virus), the Bunyaviruses (California encephalitis) and the orbiviruses (Colorado tick fever).

VIROLOGIC LABORATORY DIAGNOSIS

The cerebrospinal fluid constitutes the single most important specimen source for establishing a definitive virologic diagnosis by laboratory techniques. Optimal rates of virus isolation or identification by other means are achieved when CSF is collected within 1 day after onset of meningitis. Virus isolation may be achieved in 33 per cent of cases of mumps meningitis and about 20 per cent of cases of enteroviral meningitis by inoculation of primary monolayer tissue cultures of monkey kidney cells. Direct electron microscopic examination of uncentrifuged CSF after negative staining with phosphotungstic acid will reveal the pleomorphic enveloped mumps virions about 200 nm in diameter with helical nucleocapsids, in about the same proportion of cases of mumps meningitis whose CSF yields virus. Visualization of naked 27-nm icosahedral enterovirus virions in CSF of enteroviral meningitis is facilitated by addition of antiserum to the particular virus serotype before examination of negatively stained preparations, thereby also proving a rapid means of serologic identification of the causative virus. Enteroviruses attached to the surface of leukocytes in CSF have been identified serologically by specific immunofluorescence, after addition of homotypic fluorescein-labeled antiserum.

Since virus excretion occurs regularly in feces and to a lesser extent in throats of patients with enteroviral meningitis, isolation of virus from either of these specimens provides good presumptive evidence regarding the viral causation in at least 40 per cent of patients.

Collection of paired serum samples is essential for virologic diagnosis by serologic techniques. The first sample should be collected upon initial contact with the patient, and the second sample should be obtained not less than 24 hours after defervescence and abatement of meningeal signs. The interval between serum collections therefore is usually 3 to 7 days, but it may be longer in some instances. In mumps meningitis, diagnosis is established by demonstration of rising antibody titers in hemagglutination inhibition (HI) tests using a recent CSF mumps virus isolate, or in complement fixation (CF) tests using the nucleocapsid or soluble (S) antigen. In enteroviral meningitis, rising antibody titers are demonstrated by tissue culture neutralization (NT) tests or by enzyme immunoassay (ELISA) tests.

PITFALLS IN DIAGNOSIS

Aseptic meningitis must be distinguished clearly from the following clinical conditions: (1) encephalitis, (2) purulent (bacterial) meningitis, (3) tuberculous meningitis, (4) leptospirosis, (5) leukemic infiltrations of the central nervous system, and (6) space-occupying lesions such as cerebral abscesses, neoplasms, or hydatid cysts.

1. *Encephalitis* is usually manifested by hyperpyrexia with temperatures of 40 to 42°C (104 to 107.5°F), accompanied by twitchings or convulsions, depression of the level of consciousness to stupor or coma, upgoing plantar reflexes, and occasionally spastic paresis of the skeletal muscles. This condition occurs rarely in mumps or enteroviral infections, but viruses found more commonly in association with encephalitis include those of herpes simplex and measles, and certain arboviruses.

2. *Purulent meningitis* has an equally sudden onset, accompanied by high fever and gross neck stiffness. The CSF contains numerous polymorphonuclear leukocytes, a grossly elevated protein level, and a glucose level from 0 to 50 mg/dl. Gram-stained smears may reveal bacteria intracellularly or extracellularly, and cultivation of bacteria such as *Neisseria meningitidis, Diplococcus pneumoniae,* or *Hemophilus influenzae* type b confirms the diagnosis.

3. *Tuberculous meningitis* may develop insidiously, and may present with clouding of consciousness, vomiting, and gross neck stiffness. Positive Mantoux reactions, together with lymphocytosis of CSF that shows a low glucose content, an elevated protein level, and a pellicle upon standing overnight, suggest the diagnosis of tuberculous meningitis, which is confirmed by cultivation of *Mycobacterium tuberculosis* or observation of acid-fast rods in smears of pellicles stained by the Ziehl-Neelsen method.

4. *Leptospirosis* is diagnosed by the isolation of Leptospira on appropriate artificial media, from CSF or blood of patients living in regions of high incidence of this infection in wild or domestic animals.

5. *Leukemic infiltrations* of the central nervous system usually show large numbers of abnormal leukocytes in CSF.

6. *Space-occupying lesions* are usually detected by a combination of diagnostic procedures, including electroencephalography, echoencephalography, x-ray of the skull, air encephalography, and computed tomography (CT).

ACUTE VIRAL ENCEPHALITIS

By Paul Brown, M.D.
Bethesda, Maryland

DEFINITION

The term viral encephalitis describes a clinical syndrome characterized by an acutely altered state of consciousness that is usually accompanied by fever, headache, and a variety of neurologic signs, caused by a viral-induced process of inflammation and neuronal destruction.

Strictly speaking, encephalitis refers to inflammation restricted to the brain, myelitis to inflammation of the spinal cord, and encephalomyelitis to combined brain and spinal cord inflammation. Since each of these descriptive illnesses can be caused by the same viruses, the term encephalitis will be understood throughout this article to represent these variants, as well as encephalitis associated with meningitic inflammation (meningoencephalitis).

It must also be pointed out that the usual pathologic features of diffuse perivascular round cell infiltrates, microgliosis, and neuronal degeneration are not inflexible criteria of viral encephalitis, since the so-called postinfectious encephalitides, in which an immune mechanism rather than direct viral damage may be responsible for disease, are instead usually characterized by perivenular demyelination of the white matter.

CLINICAL PRESENTATION

Encephalitic illness may present as but one infrequent aspect of a systemic disease, such as measles or varicella, or it may be the sole manifestation of illness, as with herpes simplex and many arbovirus infections. When encephalitis complicates a systemic illness, it more often than not occurs after more characteristic features of the illness have become evident. When encephalitis is itself the major presenting illness, a minor, often influenza-like prodrome of headache, myalgia, malaise, and pharyngitis or upper respiratory symptoms may occur in the days or week before neurologic symptoms cause the patient to seek medical help.

The onset of neurologic symptoms is usually abrupt. These almost always include an altered state of consciousness—lethargy, drowsiness, or stupor—and often, if consciousness is not too depressed, confusion, disorientation, hallucinations, or some form of bizarre or at least uncharacteristic behavior. Fever, headache, stiffness of the neck, nausea, and vomiting are common complaints. Convulsions are especially frequent in children, in whom they can be the sole presenting symptom.

There may or may not be abnormalities other than those just described; what is seen will depend on the extent of inflammation and the areas of the central nervous system that are involved. Almost every neurologic sign, or combination of signs, has been described in individual case reports of patients with viral encephalitis: Cerebral hemisphere involvement is evidenced by psychic abnormalities, disturbances of higher cortical function, seizures, long-tract signs, and sensory losses; cerebellar or basal ganglia involvement by movement disorders; brain stem involvement by cranial nerve deficits, long-tract signs, and ataxia; and spinal cord involvement by flaccid paralyses, loss of tendon reflexes, bladder and bowel dysfunction, and variable sensory deficits.

DIFFERENTIAL DIAGNOSIS

To the patient who presents the clinical syndrome of acute viral encephalitis, diagnosis of a viral cause is of far less urgency than exclusion of nonviral causes, because most of the nonviral causes can be treated. To be misled by an imperfectly treated bacterial meningitis, a subdural hematoma resulting from inapparent head injury, or a case of salicylate intoxication can be one of the most costly mistakes in clinical medicine. Central nervous system damage is tragic under any circumstances, and preventable damage is inexcusable.

For this reason, discussion of viral encephalitis begins, rather than ends, with a consideration of differential diagnosis. In Table 1 are listed a number of conditions that can present a picture clinically indis-

Table 1. Nonviral Conditions That Can Be Mistaken for Acute Viral Encephalitis

Infections

Bacteria: Especially very early or imperfectly treated meningitis or brain abscess, and parameningeal infections such as epidural abscess or petrositis; the ordinarily chronic illnesses caused by mycobacteria and spirochetes, especially leptospirosis, can also on occasion present acutely; endocarditis with embolization; *Mycoplasma pneumoniae*; *Brucella melitensis*

Fungi: Coccidioides, Cryptococcus, Blastomyces, Histoplasma, Nocardia, and Candida species

Rickettsiae: Most species can produce CNS symptoms; Rocky Mountain spotted fever can be particularly difficult to distinguish from Colorado tick fever, especially when partially treated

Protozoa: "Fresh water" amoebae (Naegleria); *P. falciparum* malaria in travelers, which can be overlooked in temperate zones; Toxoplasma

Metazoa: *Taenia solium* (cysticercosis), Echinococcus, Angiostrongylus, Trichinella, Schistosoma, Paragonimus (lung fluke), all typically chronic systemic diseases, can have unexpectedly abrupt onset of CNS symptoms, especially seizures; travel history essential

Intoxications

Numerous causes, the most important of which are salicylates, barbiturates, and heavy metals, especially acute lead poisoning; tick paralysis (removal of tick is curative)

Head Trauma, Subdural or Epidural Hematomas

Endocrine/Metabolic Disorders

Most important are acute sodium, calcium, or carbohydrate imbalance, especially in association with bacterial infection; porphyria; pheochromocytoma

Other Causes

Sarcoid, hyperglobulinemia, hypersensitivity syndromes, collagen diseases, and some neoplasms, including leukemia and lymphomas; acute psychotic states tinguishable from that of acute viral encephalitis. Many of these conditions can be conclusively diagnosed within an hour or two of the patient's admission, from careful attention to details of the history (even if obtained from others), physical examination, and appropriate laboratory studies. Examination of the cerebrospinal fluid is particularly important and should always include cell counts and identification, smears of the centrifuged sediment stained by the Gram, Geimsa, and Ziehl-Neelsen methods, India ink preparations, and darkfield microscopy. Fluid should also be cultured for aerobic and anaerobic bacteria, fungi, and mycobacteria.

Sometimes further investigation will be required as the clinical course unfolds, and the possibility of nonviral illness must be repeatedly questioned until a diagnosis of viral encephalitis has been established beyond any reasonable doubt. *The whole of the following discussion of particular viruses that cause encephalitis is of far less moment than the successful discrimination between viral encephalitis and other, treatable conditions. The single exception to this statement is the urgency for diagnosis of herpes simplex encephalitis, which can now also be treated.*

LABORATORY TESTS

General laboratory studies, ordinarily of little diagnostic help in patients with viral encephalitis, can occasionally suggest the cause of illness in patients whose encephalitis represents but one manifestation of systemic disease. For example, examination of the blood will usually reveal atypical lymphocytes in patients with infectious mononucleosis; urinalysis can reveal characteristic cells of cytomegalic inclusion disease; and elevated amylase or transaminase levels can point to enteroviruses as the cause of associated encephalitis (amylase is almost never elevated in mumps in the absence of clinically apparent parotitis).

Lumbar puncture in most patients will reveal an opening pressure that is normal or slightly increased, a clear spinal fluid with increased numbers of white cells, most often in the range of 50 to 500 cells per cu mm, a slightly to moderately elevated protein concentration, and a normal glucose concentration. Occasionally, the initial spinal tap will yield entirely normal fluid or only a marginal elevation of protein, but a repeat tap a day or two later will almost always be abnormal. Very early in the illness there is often a predominance of polymorphonuclear cells; but as the illness progresses, mononuclear cells become the dominant or exclusive cell type, and the protein level will often rise as the total cell count falls.

Certain findings can point to one or another viral cause; red cells as well as white cells in the cerebrospinal fluid suggest infection by either California encephalitis or herpes simplex viruses; persistence of significant numbers of polymorphonuclear cells with relatively high total cell counts is suggestive of eastern equine encephalitis; and in encephalitis caused by infectious mononucleosis, a careful examination is occasionally rewarded by the discovery of atypical lymphocytes.

The *electroencephalogram* (EEG) is almost always abnormal in patients with encephalitis. A variety of alterations can occur, but usually there is seen a diffuse slow-wave activity, either delta or theta, with disruption of normal rhythms, and sometimes periodic high-amplitude bursts, or spike and wave complexes. The EEG is most valuable in those patients who present clinically with a focal neurologic deficit: in the absence of severe depression of consciousness, generalized EEG dysrhythmias (with or without associated localized abnormalities) lead one away from alternative diagnoses, such as tumor, abscess, or hematoma.

In exceptional circumstances, it may be necessary to obtain a brain scan, computed cranial tomograms, pneumoencephalogram, or arteriogram, or even to resort to surgical exploration to differentiate mass lesions from viral encephalitis presenting with a focal deficit.

CLINICAL COURSE

The evolution of viral encephalitis may run the gamut from a short-lived benign course to a devastating illness either leaving serious permanent neurologic deficits or ending in death. Although certain viruses ordinarily cause a very mild illness (mumps, California encephalitis) and others are notorious for their severity (herpes simplex, eastern equine encephalitis), a complete spectrum of symptomatic disease has been described for every one of the viruses associated with encephalitis. Two complications that may occur during the course of the disease deserve special mention, as they may occur rapidly and unexpectedly and require immediate recognition to support or correct: a salt-wasting syndrome resulting from hypothalamic involvement, and interference with temperature or respiratory control centers owing to brain stem involvement.

The acute phase of encephalitic illness ordinarily lasts not more than a few days to a week, and its resolution can be either abrupt, as is characteristic of rubella and some of the arbovirus infections, or gradual, as often occurs in patients recovering from herpes simplex infections. Neurologic deficits may, however, continue to diminish over a period of weeks to months, so that patients who remain to some degree disabled on discharge from the hospital may be encouraged to expect further recovery in the future.

EPIDEMIOLOGY

Surveillance of acute viral encephalitis in the United States by the Centers for Disease Control (CDC) indicates that in only about one third of reported cases has the specific viral cause been identified, and that well over half of these have been caused by St. Louis encephalitis and mumps viruses. St. Louis encephalitis, herpes simplex, and varicella viruses have been responsible for over 80 per cent of the deaths, and eastern equine, herpes simplex, and herpes zoster encephalitides have had the poorest prognoses (proportion of fatal to total cases). *From an overall viewpoint of numbers of cases, numbers of deaths, and mortality rates, herpes simplex remains the most consistently occurring and gravest of all the acute viral encephalitides seen in the United States.*

The incidence of arbovirus and enterovirus infections varies broadly from year to year. Some years there are but a handful of cases nationwide for one or another of these viruses, whereas in other years encephalitic activity is of epidemic proportions. California encephalitis and coxsackievirus encephalitis have generally shown the least yearly variability. The number of cases of encephalitis associated with measles, mumps, and rubella continues to decline in tandem with the reduced incidence of these diseases following successful immunization programs begun within the last 20 years.

This summary of the overall United States experience in recent years should be supplemented by current information obtained from the health department of the state or country in which the physician is practicing, because an awareness of increased local activity of one or another virus can be useful to the clinician in balancing probabilities of viral diagnosis. When combined with knowledge of the seasonal, geographic, and age group occurrence of disease, the clinical setting of an individual case of encephalitis can often furnish enough further information to make possible an informed guess about the correct viral etiology.

SPECIFIC VIRUS DIAGNOSIS: CLINICAL ASPECTS (TABLE 2)

Table 2 characterizes the encephalitic illnesses most commonly encountered in the United States caused by the following viruses:

Herpes simplex virus
St. Louis encephalitis virus
Western equine encephalitis (WEE) virus
California Encephalitis (CE) virus
Enteroviruses
Varicella virus
Mumps virus
Measles virus

Less common causes of acute viral encephalitis are described in the following paragraphs.

Other Arboviruses

Eastern equine encephalitis (EEE) occurs sporadically during the summer and fall along the Atlantic and Gulf coastal states and as far south as Argentina. Limited epidemics have occurred in Louisiana, Massachusetts, New Jersey, Jamaica, and the Dominican Republic, usually in association with horse epizootics. The virus is transmitted by mosquitoes, has by far the highest rate of overt to subclinical infection (1 in 5 to 50 cases), and is characteristically the most devastating of all the arbovirus encephalitides, with a predilection for older adults and children, especially infants. Onset is sudden, with high fever, seizures, and frequent focal signs, progressing to coma and death within 3 to 5 days. A predominantly polymorphonuclear response is seen in both the cerebrospinal fluid and blood. Adults recover far more frequently than children, in whom survivors are usually left with neurologic sequelae.

Venezuelan equine encephalitis (VEE) occurs in South and Central America, and has been seen in the United States only in Texas, California, and Florida, where it is endemic in the Everglades. The virus is mosquito-borne, affecting horses as well as humans, and because of its tropical and subtropical distribution it may occur at almost any time of year. As with other equine encephalitides, the people most often affected are less than 15 or over 50 years of age. Prodromal febrile illness is not uncommon, and may show a biphasic course, with encephalitic symptoms appearing several days to a week after the prodrome. The severity of the illness has varied widely in different epidemics, as well as in sporadic cases.

Colorado tick fever occurs in the western United States in correspondence with the distribution of its vector, the wood tick. Disease is transmitted only in spring and summer, and has occasionally appeared in vacationers returning to their homes far from the endemic region. Typically, after an incubation period of 3 to 6 days, the illness presents a biphasic course of influenza-like symptoms, but with leukopenia and occasionally splenomegaly and rash. Encephalitis is an uncommon complication, occurring almost exclusively in children.

Powassan encephalitis has to date been described in only a few individuals (mostly young children) living in eastern Canada, New York state, and Pennsylvania, although the causative virus has been isolated from ticks in the New England states and Colorado, and from both ticks and mosquitoes in the Pacific maritime region of Russia (Primorsky Krai), where serologic studies indicate a silent human infection rate of 8 to 9 per cent in the general population. Transmission by ticks has occurred only in summer, and the resulting encephalitis is generally not distinguished by any unusual clinical features, although in one recent case the patient presented with temporal lobe signs suggesting herpes simplex infection. There have been two deaths, and in two of the three other patients who recovered, a dual infection with echoviruses was also documented.

Other arbovirus infections that can cause encephalitis do not occur in North America, except in travelers who have been infected and then returned from endemic regions in other parts of the world. These include Japanese (Asia and the western Pacific), tick-borne (U.S.S.R), and Murray Valley encephalitides (Australia and New Guinea), louping ill (Great Britain), West Nile encephalitis (Egypt and the Near East), and yellow fever (South America and Africa).

Other Herpes Viruses

Epstein-Barr (EB) virus is responsible for classic, heterophil-positive infectious mononucleosis, which is occasionally complicated by neurologic disease. Encephalitis may supervene at any time during the course of illness, and rarely may be the presenting feature. EB virus may also cause encephalitis or transverse myelitis in patients without the clinical syndrome of infectious mononucleosis, and who may furthermore not have detectable hetrophil antibody. The majority of patients are older adolescents or young adults, who acquire the virus of mononucleosis by oral contact. The incubation period is from 1 to 2 months in adults, and about half as long in children, and the clinical course is usually benign, although deaths have been reported. Diagnosis is simplified when the typical syndrome of infectious mononucleosis occurs in conjunction with an elevated heterophil antibody titer and atypical lymphocytes, particularly when they are also found in cerebrospinal fluid. In their absence, diagnosis must be made by demonstration of fourfold or greater changes in antibodies to one or more of the EB virus antigens.

Cytomegalovirus (CMV) infection can be devastating, as in the congenital form, in which chronic encephalitis may pro-

Table 2. Characteristics of the Most Frequently Encountered Viral Encephalitides in the United States

Causative Virus	Seasonal Occurrence and Geographic Distribution	Transmission	Ages Affected	Incubation Period	Distinctive Features
Herpes simplex	Year-round occurrence, with worldwide distribution	Human-to-human salivary contact in primary infection; reactivation of latent herpes thereafter	All ages, but less common in 20–40 year age group	?	Frequent upper respiratory infection prodrome, frontotemporal lobe localization with personality change, seizures, red cells in CSF; usually severe, often prolonged clinical course, *diagnosis by brain biopsy*
St. Louis encephalitis (SLE)	Summer/fall occurrence; sporadic cases nationwide; endemic in central and southwestern U.S. and in California; rural predominance in west, urban/suburban elsewhere	Mosquitoes	Adults more often than children	5–15 days	Abrupt onset of prodromal illness followed by usually benign neurologic course, with often abrupt remission in 5–10 days; tends to be more severe in adults, with up to 30% mortality in epidemics
Western equine encephalitis (WEE)	Summer/fall occurrence; almost all U.S. cases occur west of Mississippi River; also occurs in Canada and Brazil	Mosquitoes	Most often in young children and older adults	5–15 days	Clinically similar to SLE, but more severe in infants than in adults; up to 15% mortality in epidemics
California encephalitis (CE)	Summer/fall occurrence; sporadic cases in North and South America and Europe: endemic in north-central and Middle Atlantic states; rural predominance	Mosquitoes	Almost always under 15 yrs, especially in 5–9 year age group	5–15 days	Prodrome is common; focal deficits (often frontotemporal) in up to 40% of patients, and 50% present with seizures; sometimes red cells in CSF; fatalities are rare
Enteroviruses (echovirus and coxsackievirus)	Year-round occurrence, with summer/fall outbreaks; worldwide distribution	Human-to-human fecal/skin/oral contamination	All ages, but somewhat more common in children	2–5 days	Usually benign course; often the only symptom, but can be associated with an array of systemic syndromes, including pleurodynia, peri- and myocarditis, orchitis, gastroenteritis, herpangina, exanthems
Mumps	Year-round occurrence, with winter/spring outbreaks; worldwide distribution	Human-to-human respiratory droplets	All ages, but mostly in children	ca.18 (12–26) days	Occurs in about 1 per 400 cases, usually benign course; may precede, accompany, or follow parotitis (orchitis, pancreatitis in adults), or may be only symptom
Varicella	Year-round occurrence, with winter/spring outbreaks; worldwide distribution	Human-to-human respiratory droplets	Almost always in children	13–17 days	Occurs in about 1 per 2000 cases, frequently serious illness; usually follows rash by 4–8 days, but may accompany or precede it; transverse myelitis and cerebellar ataxia syndromes are distinctive
Measles	Year-round occurrence, with winter/spring outbreaks; worldwide distribution	Human-to-human respiratory droplets	Mostly children	ca.10 (8–13) days	Occurs in about 1 per 1000 cases, often serious illness; onset usually 4–5 days after rash, can occur coincidentally or even before; delayed, subacute form (SSPE)

duce microcephaly and developmental retardation or death; or it may be entirely asymptomatic, as is usual in acquired infection in children and adults. The virus can produce a heterophil-negative clinical syndrome of infectious mononucleosis, and is seen most often in a setting of altered immunity resulting from the acquired immunodeficiency syndrome (AIDS), leukemia, lymphoma, or renal transplantation, and in postperfusion patients. Encephalitis in these patients is a distinctly rare complication with a usually benign outcome.

Herpes zoster is the same virus as that causing varicella, but is discussed separately because of the distinct clinical syndromes produced. The manifestations of herpes zoster represent reactivation of latent virus acquired during primary varicella infection, and, although seen occasionally in children and young adults, occur most often in middle and late adult life. Like CMV, herpes zoster shows a predisposition to affect patients with leukemia, lymphoma, and other states with altered immunity. The cutaneous eruption of segmentally distributed vesicles is distinctive, but may be preceded by several days of radicular dysesthesia or pain. Encephalitis is an unusual complication, which in the majority of cases begins 2 to 8 days after the onset of the cutaneous eruption, and is often serious or even fatal.

Herpesvirus simiae (B virus) is the monkey counterpart of herpes simplex in humans, and exists as a latent infection in from 20 to 100 per cent of normal colonized monkeys. Its importance to humans lies in the usually fatal encephalitis that follows infection from bites or, less commonly, simple exposure of traumatized skin to saliva or infected monkey tissue culture preparations. The incubation period is ordinarily between 10 and 20 days, and may be terminated by gastrointestinal symptoms or pneumonitis before the onset of neurologic signs. The rare patient who recovers is almost always left with severe neurologic residua.

Miscellaneous Viruses

Lymphocytic choriomeningitis (LCM) virus is endemic in certain smaller rodents, especially the common field mouse, which through its secretions may contaminate human dwellings and, especially during the cooler months, result in inhalation infection. Pet and laboratory hamsters, as well as mice, have also been responsible for human disease. Infection is most often clinically inapparent, but after an incubation period of 1 to 2 weeks it can produce an influenzal or meningitic illness and, less commonly, encephalitis. An influenzal prodrome is seen in about half the patients with encephalitis, who may show a biphasic course with associated features of arthritis, orchitis, or pneumonitis. Recovery is usually complete, although a few deaths have been reported.

Rubella is associated with encephalitis in probably not more than one in every 5000 to 10,000 cases, and appears to complicate adolescent or adult infection more often than the usual childhood disease. As with other exanthems, neurologic signs usually appear a few days after onset of the rash, but may occur coincidentally or even precede it. Onset is usually abrupt and the clinical course rapid, with recovery or death occurring within a few days of onset. Delayed subacute sclerosing panencephalitis (SSPE)-like illness may rarely follow congenital or infantile infections.

Adenovirus encephalitis is a rare but often fatal complication of this common virus infection, usually identified only during epidemics, and occurring almost exclusively in children with severe respiratory illness. Adenoviruses have been implicated as well in numerous sporadic cases of encephalitis, but in most such patients the diagnosis has not been secured by virus isolation from cerebrospinal fluid or central nervous system tissues.

Rabies, smallpox, and poliomyelitis (see articles on rabies and poliomyelitis) have all but disappeared as human diseases in the United States during the past decade.

SPECIFIC VIRUS DIAGNOSIS: LABORATORY ASPECTS

The physician who wishes to identify a specific virus as the cause of encephalitis must often be prepared to await the results until after the patient's illness has been resolved, and it may seem gratuitous to make the effort when the outcome will in all likelihood have no effect on ability to care for the patient. Yet the interests of public health as well as the inherent satisfaction of establishing a diagnosis merit the additional attention required to collect and arrange for transportation of appropriate diagnostic specimens.

As quickly as possible after the patient is first seen, samples of heparinized or defibrinated blood, cerebrospinal fluid, urine, and nasopharyngeal and rectal swabs should be obtained for attempted viral isolation. (Not all these specimens may be needed in a particular case, but it is preferable to allow the laboratory to make that choice.) The swabs should be immersed in tissue culture media, infusion broth, or isotonic saline containing antibiotics and 10 per cent protein. *All these specimens should be kept refrigerated and sent or, preferably, taken the same day to the nearest viral diagnostic laboratory together with a very brief clinical summary.* If there is unavoidable delay of more than a day, all specimens except the whole blood should be stored frozen until delivery can be arranged.

A serum sample should also be obtained and kept frozen until a second sample can be obtained 2 to 3 weeks later. This may be done most conveniently on the occasion of a follow-up clinic visit. Both serum samples should then be sent to the laboratory, which will test them together for antibodies to appropriate viruses.

If all these things are done properly, an exact viral diagnosis may be expected in nearly three quarters of patients with viral encephalitis. Desultory efforts will be rewarded with correspondingly less success. Virus isolation from cerebrospinal fluid or blood, together with a fourfold or greater rise in serum antibody titers to the same virus, establishes a specific diagnosis. A somewhat less certain but still probable diagnosis is provided by virus isolation from the cerebrospinal fluid or blood in the absence of an antibody rise; or by a rise in antibody titer in the absence of virus isolation, or isolation from elsewhere in the body. Virus has been most readily obtained from patients with encephalitis caused by enteroviral infections, and much less often from other encephalitides, so that serologic diagnosis remains the most practical and often the only means by which a specific viral cause can be determined.

Herpes simplex encephalitis presents an urgent and rather special diagnostic problem, because isolation of the virus from cerebrospinal fluid or blood is extremely rare, and a rise in serum antibody levels does not always occur even in proved cases; moreover, antibody fluctuations have been documented in association with encephalitis from other causes. Diagnosis therefore depends on the identification of virions (electron microscopy), viral antigen (fluorescence microscopy), or infectious virus (inoculation of mice and tissue culture) in affected brain tissue. *Biopsy should be performed without delay in any patient suspected of having encephalitis due to the herpes simplex virus.*

POSTINFECTIOUS ENCEPHALITIS

Certain viral infections, as well as vaccination and antirabic treatment, can result in a form of disease called postinfectious or postvaccinal encephalitis. Viruses most commonly implicated are those of measles, mumps, and varicella, whereas cases caused by smallpox, rubella, influenza, dengue, and yellow fever are comparatively rare.

A distinction between encephalitis resulting from direct viral invasion of the central nervous sytem and postinfectious encephalitis caused by an abnormal host-virus interaction is usually impossible to make on clinical grounds alone. Typically, onset of neurologic symptoms is abrupt and follows by several days the major systemic manifestations of the infection, but may occur simultaneously or, rarely, even before they have appeared. Postvaccinal encephalitis usually develops about 10 days after primary vaccination, with a range of from 2 to 24 days. Encephalitis occurring during the course of antirabic treatment usually appears from 1 to 3 weeks after the first dose of vaccine.

The clinical course of encephalitis is usually not distinctive, except for the comparative frequency of encephalomyelitis following antirabic treatment, cerebellar and transverse myelitis syndromes in varicella encephalitis, and trismus and myoclonus in postvaccinal encephalitis. Changes in the cerebrospinal fluid are similar to those described for acute viral encephalitis: lymphocytic pleocytosis, slightly increased protein, and normal glucose concentrations. Recovery or death usually occurs within 1 to 2 weeks after onset, with the mortality rate particularly high (40 to 60 per cent) in postvaccinal encephalitis.

Diagnosis depends on microscopic examination of central nervous system tissue, which reveals perivenular demyelination confined mainly to the white matter, variable thrombosis and hemorrhage, diffuse gliosis, and only minimal degeneration or necrosis of neurons.

SUBACUTE AND CHRONIC VIRAL ENCEPHALITIS AND ENCEPHALOPATHY

By Paul Brown, M.D.
and David M. Asher, M.D.
Bethesda, Maryland

DEFINITION

The terms subacute and chronic viral encephalitis or encephalopathy describe central nervous system virus infections that evolve over a period of months to years, with inflammatory neuropathology either present (encephalitis) or absent (encephalopathy). Two of these diseases are due to slowly progressive infections by "unconventional" viruses (Creutzfeldt-Jakob disease and kuru), and four are due to unusually delayed manifestations of persistent infections by conventional viruses (progressive multifocal leukoencephalopathy, subacute sclerosing panencephalitis, subacute rubella panencephalitis, and chronic tick-borne encephalitis). Table 1 summarizes some features of the three diseases most often seen in the United States.

CREUTZFELDT-JAKOB DISEASE

Originally described by Creutzfeldt and Jakob in the early 1920s in a group of six cases (of which only two conform to its present definition as a spongiform encephalopathy), the disease known as Creutzfeldt-Jakob disease (CJD) was shown by Gibbs, Gajdusek, and co-workers in 1968 to be transmissible by inoculation to chimpanzees and in subsequent years to be transmissible to numerous species of Old and New World monkeys, sheep, goats, cats, and rodents. CJD is now appropriately termed a transmissible virus dementia.

Frequency and Occurrence

The annual incidence of CJD in metropolitan areas is approximately one case per million inhabitants and it may be lower in rural areas. CJD is predominantly a disease of late middle age, the great majority of cases occurring between the ages of 55 and 75 years, with a peak incidence in the early 60s. However, autopsy-verified CJD has been documented in eight patients under the age of 30 years (the youngest was 16 years old), and several cases have been reported in patients over the age of 80.

Clinical Presentation

Prodromal symptoms of asthenia, weight loss, or disordered sleep patterns, beginning weeks to months before the onset of neurologic signs, can be elicited in over one third of patients. A gradually progressive mental deterioration is the most common presentation, usually in the form of simple memory loss, errors in judgment, mood change (often depression), or uncharacteristic behavior. Less often, mental deterioration takes the form of higher cortical function deficits, such as aphasia or apraxia, and sometimes there are episodes of frank confusion. In about half the patients, cerebellar or visual signs dominate the clinical presentation, with only moderate to minimal mental deterioration. Often, this type of presentation is comparatively rapid; indeed, the sudden onset of vertigo, diplopia, ataxia, and even paralysis or paresthesia occurs in up to 20 per cent of patients, often leading to a mistaken initial diagnosis of cerebrovascular accident. The frequencies of presenting symptoms in a recent series of 225 consecutive, verified cases of CJD are summarized in Table 2.

Table 1. Summary of Three Types of Subacute or Chronic Virus Encephalitis/Encephalopathy Most Often Seen in the United States

	Creutzfeldt-Jakob Disease	Progressive Multifocal Leukoencephalopathy	Subacute Sclerosing Panencephalitis
Usual Age at Onset (Range)	55–75 years (16–85)	45–65 years (5–85)	5–15 years (1–50)
Male/Female Ratio	1:1	3:2	2:1
Predisposing Setting	Family history of presenile dementia (about 10%)	Immune deficiency (especially leukemias and lymphomas)	Preceding measles infection (especially before age 2 years)
Usual Duration of Illness (Range)	2–5 months (1 month–14 years)	3–6 months (1 month–10 years)	1–3 years (2 months–10 years)
Clinical Signs and Symptoms			
Mental	+	+	+
Visual	+	+	+
Cerebellar/Extrapyramidal	+	Uncommon	+
Pyramidal	+	+	Uncommon
Myoclonus	+	–	+
Laboratory Diagnostic Clues	Periodic EEG activity	Multifocal lucent lesions by computed tomography	Antibody to measles virus in CSF; periodic EEG activity

Clinical Evolution

Disease progression is usually relentless. Mental deterioration and mood alteration evolve into a state of dementia, confusion, and mutism; visual deterioration continues to cortical blindness, often with hallucinations; and motor impairments progress to increasingly severe incoordination, marked oppositional rigidity, and abnormal movements (usually myoclonic, but often trembling and sometimes choreoathetoid or complex). The frequencies of symptoms occurring during the evolution of CJD are presented in Table 3.

The mean duration of illness is approximately 8 months, but this average is unduly influenced by 5 to 10 per cent of patients with illnesses lasting more than 2 years in whom there is often an initial stable or slowly progressive stage of memory loss, depression, or personality change, followed by a second, rapidly advancing cascade of mental and physical deterioration. The majority of patients die within 6 months, most often within 2 to 3 months of the onset of illness. There are no reported recoveries.

Laboratory Diagnosis

The *electroencephalogram* (EEG) is an extremely valuable diagnostic aid and not infrequently suggests the correct diagnosis. The EEG may be normal very early in the course of illness, but invariably it becomes abnormal as the disease progresses. The earliest tracings usually show little more than nonspecific slow-wave activity, but in the majority of patients they evolve into some form of periodic activity, either as bursts of high-voltage slow waves (Fig. 1*A*), which are evocative but may also be seen in a number of other disorders, including Alzheimer's disease, or as a distinctive sharp, triphasic, periodic pattern occurring at a frequency of 1 to 2 cycles per second (Fig. 1*B*), often but not invariably associated with myoclonic jerking. If serial tracings are taken during the course of disease, it is not uncommon to observe the progression from slow waves to slow-wave bursts to periodic triphasic waves in a single patient. Terminally, these patterns may be replaced by nonspecific diffuse, low-voltage slow-wave activity.

Other laboratory tests are generally unrevealing. The cerebrospinal fluid is normal, with at most a slight increase in protein concentration. Results of examination by pneumoencephalography, computed tomography, arteriography, and radionuclide scanning may be normal or show slight to moderate cerebral atrophy. No immunologic response, humoral or cellular, to the virus responsible for CJD has yet been demonstrated.

Neuropathologic examination and disease transmission to experimental animals remain the ultimate laboratory diagnostic procedures. The gross appearance of the brain is usually unremarkable or shows a modest degree of cerebral atrophy. Microscopic examination of either biopsy or autopsy tissue reveals a triad of spongiosis, gliosis, and neuronal loss, mostly

Table 2. Frequency of Presenting Symptoms in 225 Consecutive Verified Cases of Creutzfeldt-Jakob Disease

Symptom Category	Percentage	
Mental deterioration	65	
Dementia		34
Behavioral abnormalities		31
Higher cortical function		17
Cerebellar-visual	48	
Cerebellar		35
Visual		19
Vertigo		7
Headache	8	
Sensory	4	
Pyramidal	3	
Extrapyramidal	2	
Abnormal movements	1	

Table 3. Frequency of Symptoms Occurring During Clinical Course of 225 Consecutive Verified Cases of Creutzfeldt-Jakob Disease

Symptom Category	Percentage	
Mental deterioration	100	
Dementia		92
Behavioral abnormalities		49
Higher cortical function		41
Movement disorder	91	
Myoclonus		88
Other		32
EEG periodicity	80	
Triphasic 1–2 cycles per second		55
Extrapyramidal	66	
Cerebellar	64	
Visual	47	
Pyramidal	43	
Headache	14	
Lower motor neuron	11	
Sensory	10	
Vertigo	9	
Seizures	9	
Cranial nerve	2	

confined to gray matter and occurring in an irregular but diffuse distribution. Transmission of the virus is most easily accomplished by intracerebral inoculation of a 10 per cent saline homogenate of frozen cerebral tissue into squirrel monkeys. In this host, the average incubation period is 2 years, and the average duration of illness is 1 month.

Differential Diagnosis

The combination of mental deterioration, multifocal neurologic signs (especially visual, cerebellar, and extrapyramidal disorders), myoclonus, and a typical periodic triphasic EEG pattern evolving over a period of several months in a late middle-aged patient virtually assures a diagnosis of CJD. Nevertheless, this "typical" picture of CJD has in rare instances been exactly imitated by Alzheimer's disease, primary brain tumors and occult metastatic carcinomas, severe thiamine deficiency, and, in young patients, subacute sclerosing panencephalitis.

When CJD begins suddenly with an episode of confusion, diplopia, vertigo, paresis, or incoordination, an initial diagnosis of cerebrovascular accident or multiple sclerosis may be made. In patients with a more prolonged course, the early appearance of "pill-rolling" tremors and rigidity, or of significant muscular atrophy associated with paresis and fasciculations, may suggest Parkinson's disease or amyotrophic lateral sclerosis. In other patients with a prolonged clinical course dominated by mental or affective abnormalities, in whom neurologic signs are minimal or absent, the differential diagnosis will include Alzheimer's or Pick's disease, multi-infarct dementia, and alcoholic or nutritional deficiency syndromes. In particular, only by neuropathologic examination may it be possible to distinguish between CJD of long duration and Alzheimer's disease with neurologic signs (including myoclonus).

Infectivity and Precautions

It is not known how the disease is naturally acquired. Iatrogenic transmission has been documented to follow corneal transplantation and intracerebral stereotactic electrode placement, and it is suspected to have occurred as a consequence of neurosurgery in a few other patients. Incubation periods in these cases have been between 16 and 20 months, but incubation periods in "natural" transmission (however it occurs) may be as long as 20 years. Approximately 5 to 10 per cent of cases in some series occurred in familial patterns suggestive of autosomal dominant transmission, but in the great majority of cases no contact has been established between any one patient and another.

Notwithstanding the negative epidemiologic evidence regarding disease transmission by conventional routes, including the absence of any increased risk among spouses, friends, and medical and paramedical personnel caring for CJD patients, concern has been expressed about precautionary measures to prevent disease.

The cardinal precaution is to avoid autoinoculation by needles, scalpels, and other instruments that have been contaminated by the patient's tissues (brain, spinal fluid, visceral organs, and possibly blood). Secretions, excretions, skin and mucosal surfaces, and expired air are not known to be infectious and require no special precautions. Contaminated material should be steam autoclaved for 1 hour at a temperature of at least 121°C, or, when autoclaving is impractical, immersed for 1 hour in either 5 to 10 per cent sodium hypochlorite (household bleach) or 1 *N* NaOH, both of which provide excellent chemical disinfection.

KURU

This progressive, fatal infection of the central nervous system is included for its historical importance as the first human disease shown to be due to a "slow," or unconventional, virus. Geographically confined to the Fore linguistic group in the Eastern Highlands of Papua New Guinea and predominantly a disease of children and young adult women, kuru was first described by Gajdusek and Zigas in 1957, and it was subsequently shown by Gajdusek and co-workers in 1965 to be transmissible to the chimpanzee after an incubation period of more than a year.

The word "kuru" in the Fore language means shivering or trembling and accurately describes one of the cardinal symptoms of the disease, which begins with a subtle instability of gait that steadily progresses to a dramatic picture of generalized incoordination with coarse trembling or jerking movements, hyperreflexia, dysarthria, oculomotor deficits, strabismus, and dysphagia. Apart from an inappropriately sanguine mood, mental abnormalities are either minimal or absent throughout the entire course of illness, which terminates in death from malnutrition, dehydration, and infection within 9 to 12 months of onset. Laboratory investigations are unrevealing, but the distinctive clinical picture is sufficient to make the correct diagnosis, which is verified by the neuropathologic findings of spongiosis, gliosis, neuronal loss,

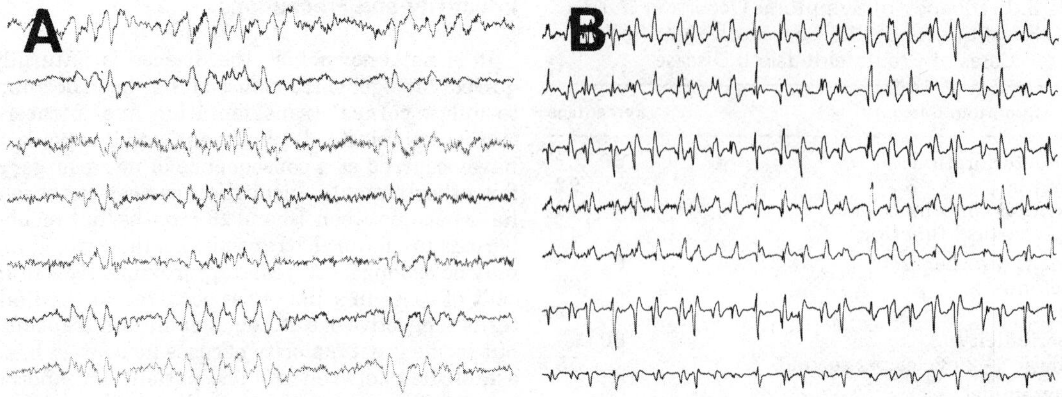

Figure 1. Abnormal electroencephalograms in patients with Creutzfeldt-Jakob disease. *A.* Periodic bursts of high-amplitude slow-wave activity. *B.* Periodic 1–2 cycles per second triphasic slow-wave activity.

and amyloid plaques occurring throughout the cerebral cortex and cerebellum.

It has been speculated that at some time in the past a sporadic case of Creutzfeldt-Jakob disease may have occurred in a member of the Fore linguistic group, and that by the practice of ritual cannibalism the virus became rapidly and widely transmitted to produce an altered clinical illness of epidemic proportions in these people. The incidence of disease has been steadily declining in the 20 years since cessation of the practice of cannibalism, and the disease appears to be nearing complete extinction.

PROGRESSIVE MULTIFOCAL LEUKOENCEPHALOPATHY

Described as a clinical entity by Åström in 1958, and later suspected to have a viral origin on the basis of electron microscopic visualization of virions in oligodendrocytes, this multifocal demyelinating disease finally yielded to persistent virologic investigation in 1971 with the independent isolations by Padget and Weiner and their colleagues of papovaviruses in affected brain tissue from three patients.

Frequency and Occurrence

The true incidence of progressive multifocal leukoencephalopathy (PML) is unknown, but nearly 200 cases have been reported in the 25 years since its original description. Its predominant occurrence in the 45 to 65 year age group reflects the age range of the diseases on which it is superimposed, and cases have also been reported in a child, in an adolescent, and in elderly persons. Males are affected slightly more often than females (3:2 sex ratio).

The great majority of cases occur in individuals with chronic systemic diseases associated with impaired immune responses, most frequently the lymphoproliferative disorders of chronic lymphocytic leukemia, lymphosarcoma, and Hodgkin's disease; less often with myeloproliferative disorders, non-neoplastic granulomatoses, such as Whipple's disease, sarcoidosis, or tuberculosis; and the connective tissue diseases rheumatoid arthritis, systemic lupus erythematosus, and polymyositis. Cases have also been reported in patients with congenital combined immunodeficiency disease, carcinomatosis, and long-term corticosteroid-treated asthma and in immunosuppressed renal transplant patients. Indeed, any disorder in which an immune deficiency occurs, whether congenital, acquired, or iatrogenic, may provide a suitable setting for opportunistic papovavirus invasion of the central nervous system. Among the handful of patients in whom PML occurred in the absence of a clinically evident immunodeficiency state, some were shown by laboratory investigation to have had more subtle immunologic abnormalities.

Clinical Presentation

The onset of PML usually follows by several years the onset of the underlying chronic disease; is almost always insidious; and usually begins with paresis or hemiparesis, mental deterioration (including memory loss, deficits of higher cortical function, or personality change), visual loss, or sensory abnormalities. In approximately 10 per cent of patients, PML presents as a focal cerebral mass lesion (usually frontoparietal or temporal), and in another small proportion of patients, the clinical presentation is confined to signs of cerebellar or brain stem damage, including ataxia, dysarthria, vertigo, nystagmus, diplopia, and cranial nerve abnormalities.

Clinical Evolution

The illness is usually relentlessly progressive, although in a few patients the clinical course may wax and wane, stabilize, or even remit. Eventually, mental deterioration progresses to overt dementia and coma amid a panoply of increasingly severe and multifocal neurologic deficits. Movement disorders are rare, however, and myoclonus has never been reported.

Unusually rapid illnesses of less than a month, and extraordinarily prolonged courses of 10, 20, or even 30 years have been reported, but after a steady progression of symptoms most patients die within 3 to 6 months of onset. Some of the longest durations of the disease have been recorded in the small group of patients without demonstrable immunodeficiency diseases.

Laboratory Diagnosis

Cerebrospinal fluid is usually normal. In some patients, slight elevations in pressure, cells, or protein have been described as isolated abnormalities. The EEG, although almost always abnormal, shows only nonspecific focal or diffuse polymorphous slow-wave activity, and never paroxysmal or periodic electrical patterns. Conventional radiographic techniques are not usually helpful, but computed tomography has in some cases identified a distinctive pattern of asymmetric patchy areas of low density that has suggested the correct diagnosis.

Demonstration of serum antibody to the causative papovavirus (in all but two cases the JC virus, the initials of the patient from whom the virus was first isolated) is not helpful, since the virus causes inapparent childhood infections in over 70 per cent of the general population, with antibody persisting throughout life. Thus, in the absence of cerebrospinal fluid antibody (which has never been detected), diagnosis can only be based on an unusually high serum antibody level in a single specimen (reported once), or on a significant rise of antibody in serial specimens taken during the course of illness (also reported only once). The rarity of such observations may in part be due to a damping effect on antibody production exerted by the associated underlying immunodeficiency disorders.

Diagnosis must therefore await neuropathologic examination, which shows a characteristic picture of multiple areas of demyelination associated with abnormal virus-laden oligodendrocytes and, often, giant astrocytes. Perivascular lymphocytic infiltration is uncommon, and when it occurs it is usually confined to the foci of demyelination.

Virus antigen in the infected oligodendrocytes can be demonstrated by immunofluorescence microscopy, and with more difficulty infective virus can be isolated in explant tissue cultures. In two of the original three patients, in whom the source of infection remains obscure, the causative virus was identified as SV-40, normally a latent virus of monkeys. In the other original case and all subsequent cases, the causative virus has been JC virus, which apparently remains latent after primary childhood infection, and then rarely, in an immunodeficient host, invades and replicates in the central nervous system to produce PML.

Differential Diagnosis

The appearance of neurologic symptoms in any patient with a chronic systemic disease associated with impaired immunity should immediately call to mind the diagnosis of PML. The most important alternative diagnoses to investigate are central nervous system involvement by the underlying disease, e.g., leukemia, sarcoidosis, systemic lupus erythematosus, and so forth, and central nervous system infection by other opportunistic organisms, particularly Cryptococcus, which may also complicate PML in such chronically ill hosts. In patients whose symptoms suggest a mass lesion, PML must be differentiated from tumors, hematomas and other pathologic vascular events, and abscesses.

Diagnosis of PML is most difficult in patients without known immunodeficiency-associated disorders, and because of the multifocal nature of the disease, it may be mistaken for a wide variety of neurologic illnesses, including three of the diseases described in this chapter—CJD and late-onset measles or rubella panencephalitis. The absence of movement disorders (especially myoclonus) and EEG periodic activity will eventually exclude CJD, and the absence of central nervous system antibody to measles or rubella will exclude the two panencephalitic diseases.

SUBACUTE SCLEROSING PANENCEPHALITIS

This chronic encephalitis is caused by a persistent measles virus infection. It was first clearly described and a viral etiology postulated by Dawson. Greenfield recognized that it was identical to the chronic encephalitides described by several European neuropathologists and suggested the name subacute sclerosing panencephalitis (SSPE), now generally used. Bouteille and co-workers recognized measles virions in brain cells of SSPE, and virus isolation was accomplished in 1969 by Horta-Barbosa et al. and by Payne et al.

Frequency and Occurrence

SSPE is a rare disease that occurs throughout the world. Data for the United States have been compiled for cases with onset in 1956 or later by an SSPE Registry (now located at the Medical College of Georgia). The disease has been recognized in patients aged 2 months to more than 50 years, but it primarily affects older children and young adolescents. Eighty-five per cent of cases had onset between 5 and 14 years of age. Only about 1 per cent of cases began after age 17 years, and some adult cases have not been well documented. The risk of SSPE for boys is more than twice that for girls and is higher for farm children than city children. SSPE is especially common in the southeastern part of the United States, and incidences significantly higher than average are also found in the Ohio River Valley and in some New England states. Acquisition of measles before the age of 18 months seems to increase the risk of SSPE substantially. Exposure to birds and other animals has been reported with abnormal frequency in histories of patients with SSPE.

Mean annual incidence rates of SSPE in the United States have fallen markedly since 1960—from 0.61 cases per million persons under age 20 years to an estimated 0.06 cases in 1980. This drop roughly parallels the progressive decline in annual numbers of measles cases diagnosed since the introduction of live attenuated measles vaccine in the United States in 1963 (Fig. 2). The risk of SSPE has been estimated at 8.5 SSPE cases per million cases of measles for a 6-year period during which the estimated risk after measles vaccination was only 0.7 cases per million doses of vaccine. It is anticipated that SSPE will become increasingly rare in North American children, but will continue to occur in other areas of the world where measles remains unchecked.

Clinical Presentation

Children with SSPE generally have a history of typical measles from which they had made full recovery several years before the onset of neurologic disease. The mean interval between measles and onset of SSPE in the United States was about 7 years, but recently it has increased to about 10 years. Measles may have been either mild or severe. Some patients with SSPE have had measles pneumonia, but none has had a history of typical measles encephalitis. The onset of SSPE is usually insidious, marked by subtle changes in behavior and deterioration of school work, followed soon afterward by frank dementia. There is no fever, photophobia, or other findings of acute encephalitis except for occasional complaints of headache. Diffuse neurologic disease becomes progressively more severe, frequently with myoclonic jerks or other abnormal movements, convulsions, cerebellar ataxia, and variable dystonias. Retinopathy and optic atrophy may appear, sometimes even before the behavioral changes.

Clinical Evolution

Dementia progresses to stupor and coma, often with autonomic insufficiency. Total duration of illness may be as short as a few months, but most patients survive for 1 to 3 years after diagnosis, with a mean of about 18 months. Occasionally patients have shown spontaneous improvement and have lived for more than 10 years. It has been reported that treatment with inosiplex may have increased the number of patients with prolonged survival. Other treatments have been ineffective. Information on current therapeutic trials should be sought through the SSPE Registry.

Laboratory Diagnosis

The blood is normal except for elevated titers of antibodies to measles virus. Examination of the spinal fluid is most useful for establishing the diagnosis of SSPE. Cell content of the cerebrospinal fluid is generally normal, although stained sediments are reported to show plasma cells. Total protein content is normal or only slightly elevated; however, the gamma globulin fraction is greatly elevated, resulting in a paretic type of colloidal gold curve. The immunoglobulin is mainly IgG, and when the cerebrospinal fluid is examined by gel electrophoresis discrete "oligoclonal" bands of immunoglobulin are observed. Antibodies to measles virus, not normally found in unconcentrated cerebrospinal fluid, make up most of the immunoglobulin increase, and these may often be detected in dilutions of 1:8 or more. The complement-fixation test is especially useful for demonstrating cerebrospinal fluid antibodies, but hemagglutination inhibition and other serologic tests, including enzyme-linked immunosorbent assay (ELISA), are also satisfactory. Whatever serologic test is selected, it should be performed in an experienced quality-controlled laboratory. The normal ratio of titer in serum to titer in cerebrospinal fluid is reduced (below 200) for measles antibodies, while serum–cerebrospinal fluid ratios are normal for other viral antibodies and for albumin, indicating that the increased amounts of spinal fluid antibodies in SSPE result from local synthesis and that the blood-brain barrier is normal.

The EEG is also useful in establishing the diagnosis of SSPE. Most patients eventually have a "suppression-burst" pattern of high-amplitude slow waves recurring at intervals of 3 to 5 seconds on a slow background; however, that pattern is not unique to SSPE. The pneumoencephalogram or computed tomogram may show variable cortical atrophy and ventricular enlargement, and there may be focal or multifocal low-density lesions in white matter.

Brain biopsy is no longer needed to diagnose SSPE, but when performed it shows mild inflammation of meninges and panencephalitis, with cuffs of plasma cells and lymphocytes around blood vessels and increased numbers of glia throughout gray and white

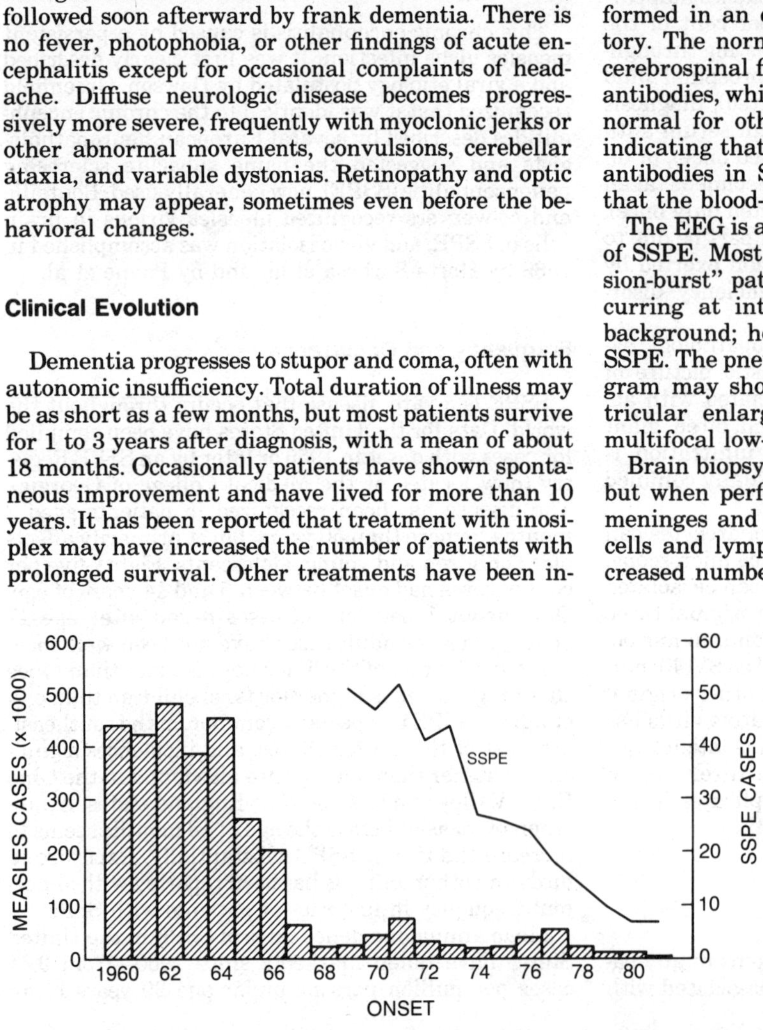

Figure 2. Measles cases reported to the Centers for Disease Control and subacute sclerosing panencephalitis (SSPE) cases reported to the SSPE Registry for the United States by year. The actual number of cases of measles that occurred is estimated to have been about ten times the number of reported cases. (From the Morbidity and Mortality Weekly Report, Centers for Disease Control.)

matter. Neuronal loss may not be marked until late in the course of illness. The "Cowdry type A" inclusion bodies noted by Dawson may be seen in hematoxylin and eosin stained sections within nuclei of neurons, astrocytes and oligodendrocytes, but they are sometimes difficult to find. By electron microscopy the inclusions are seen to contain viral nucleocapsid tubules, and measles viral antigens can be demonstrated by labeled-antibody techniques within inclusions as well as in cells without inclusions. The same findings of inclusion-body panencephalitis are present throughout the brain at autopsy, sometimes with the lesions being unevenly distributed.

Isolation of measles virus from brain tissue has been achieved by "cocultivating" viable brain cells together with cells known to be susceptible to measles virus and then propagating the mixed cultures for several serial passages. Persistence of measles virus infection in the cultures can be demonstrated by labeled-antibody techniques before complete virus appears. However, many specimens have failed to yield complete virus, even though measles antigens were found to persist in cultures.

Differential Diagnosis

In the diagnosis of SSPE, as for other slow viral infections, the most important thing is to rule out potentially treatable illnesses, such as bacterial infections and tumors. The diverse cerebral storage diseases and nonstorage poliodystrophies, leukodystrophies, and demyelinating diseases of childhood can also produce progressive dementia with seizures and paralysis resembling SSPE. Early in the course of illness, SSPE must be distinguished from atypical acute viral encephalitides. Other slow viral infections, such as CJD and progressive rubella panencephalitis, must be considered in the appropriate age groups. The presence of a typical EEG pattern is suggestive of SSPE, as are unusually high levels of measles antibodies in serum. The diagnosis is practically confirmed if measles antibodies are detected in cerebrospinal fluid.

Infectivity and Precautions

The persistent measles infection in SSPE is not productive of complete virus particles. Patients with SSPE therefore pose no hazard of infection to others, and no special precautions need be taken.

PROGRESSIVE RUBELLA PANENCEPHALITIS

Progressive rubella panencephalitis (PRP) is an exceedingly rare chronic encephalitis, associated with persistent rubella virus infection. PRP was first reported by Lebon and Lyon in 1974 and fewer than 20 cases have been recognized since then. Rubella virus was isolated from the brain of a patient with PRP by Cremer et al. in 1975, and from blood by Wolinsky et al. All patients have been boys who were between the ages of 8 and 19 years at onset; most had typical stigmata of the congenital rubella syndrome, including cataracts, deafness, and mental retardation, but two apparently had childhood rubella from which they made full recovery. If the incidence of congenital and acquired rubella continues its recent dramatic decline (down 82 per cent from 1979 to 1981) PRP should soon become even more rare in the United States.

The onset of PRP resembles that of SSPE, with insidious changes in behavior and deterioration in school performance, followed by frank dementia and other signs of multifocal brain disease, including seizures, cerebellar ataxia, and spastic paralysis. Myoclonus and other abnormal movements may occur, but these are not as common as in SSPE. Retinopathy, similar to that of acute rubella, and optic atrophy may occur. The course of illness in PRP is similar to that in SSPE, progressing to coma, spastic paraplegia, brain stem involvement, and death in 2 to 5 years.

Laboratory Diagnosis

The peripheral blood is normal except for elevated titers of antibodies to rubella virus. The cerebrospinal fluid shows normal or slightly elevated cell content; protein is slightly elevated, with marked increase in globulin, which may make up more than 50 per cent of total protein. Oligoclonal electrophoretic bands of globulin are found in spinal fluid of PRP patients; the bands are similar to those in SSPE, but consist of antibodies to rubella virus antigens. Antibodies to rubella virus are readily detectable in cerebrospinal fluid, often at dilutions of 1:8 or higher. The complement-fixation, hemagglutination-inhibition, and ELISA techniques are satisfactory for testing spinal fluid. Most of the rubella antibodies in the cerebrospinal fluid are IgG, although some IgM antibodies have also been detected early in the course of PRP. The serum–cerebrospinal fluid ratio of antibody titers to rubella virus is reduced, while ratios of titers to measles and other viruses are normal.

The EEG shows generalized slowing with occasional high-voltage activity, but the clear-cut suppression-burst pattern of SSPE has not been seen in PRP. Computed tomograms and pneumoencephalograms may show enlargement of all ventricles, especially the fourth, with prominent atrophy of the cerebellum.

Histopathologic changes in brains of patients with PRP are similar to those in SSPE, with cuffs of lymphocytes and plasma cells around blood vessels, glial nodules in the cortex, some loss of neurons, and an increase in astrocytes throughout gray matter and even of more severe proportions in the white matter. The histopathology of PRP differs from that of SSPE in two important respects: in PRP no inclusion bodies have been recognized, and deposits of periodic acid–Schiff (PAS)-staining material are found around vessels in subcortical white matter.

Rubella virus was isolated from brain cell cultures of one patient with PRP by cocultivation with susceptible cells as well as by propagation of explanted cells alone. Several similar attempts at isolation from brain tissues of other patients were not successful. Rubella virus has also been isolated from separated blood lymphocytes of a patient with PRP by cocultivation with susceptible cells.

Differential Diagnosis

Differential diagnosis of PRP is the same as that for SSPE. The stigmata of congenital rubella syndrome or history of German measles suggests PRP. Elevated levels of rubella antibodies in serum, and presence of oligoclonal bands of gamma globulins and rubella antibodies in the spinal fluid, with reduction of normal serum-cerebrospinal fluid rubella antibody ratio, should establish the diagnosis of PRP. Isolation of rubella virus from blood lymphocytes may be attempted. Brain biopsy is not needed.

Patients with PRP pose no substantial risk of infection to others, although it seems reasonable to avoid exposing rubella-susceptible persons to blood of patients with PRP. Virus has not been detected in urine, and secretions have apparently not been studied.

CHRONIC TICK-BORNE ENCEPHALITIS

The virus of tick-borne encephalitis (TBE), a member of the flavivirus group of small enveloped RNA viruses, usually causes an acute meningoencephalomyelitis, also called Russian spring-summer encephalitis, which may be of variable severity. A few patients—in some series as many as 20 per cent—recover from acute encephalitis only to develop new signs of progressive neurologic disease months or even years later. Most cases of chronic progressive TBE have been reported from the Soviet Union, but two typical patients have been described in Japan. Chronic progressive TBE is characterized by (1) movement or seizure disorders of which *epilepsia partialis continua* (Kozhevnikov's epilepsy) is the most common, (2) paralytic disorders, often with brain stem involvement, or (3) mixed syndromes. The seizure and movement disorders may stabilize or remit, but the progressive paralytic syndrome is usually fatal. The cerebrospinal fluid in chronic TBE may contain elevated levels of antibodies to TBE virus. Brain tissue shows panencephalitis without inclusion bodies or virus-like structures by electron microscopy. Isolation of TBE virus has occasionally been reported from brain tissue or cerebrospinal fluid of patients with chronic syndromes, but most attempts have failed to isolate the virus.

CHRONIC ENCEPHALITIS OF UNKNOWN ETIOLOGY

Patients with similar types of chronic encephalitis not associated with any known viral infection have been recognized throughout the world. In North America a syndrome of seizures, spastic paralysis, and mental retardation associated with chronic encephalitis was described by Rasmussen and colleagues in children, adolescents, and young adults. Patients had no history of preceding acute encephalitis. Computed tomography or pneumoencephalography of patients with Rasmussen's encephalitis may show cerebral cortical atrophy or ventricular dilatation, and when brain tissue is resected a panencephalitis without inclusion bodies or virus-like particles is found. Efforts to isolate viruses have been unsuccessful, and the etiologic agent remains unknown.

POLIOMYELITIS

By Harry T. Wright, Jr., M.D., M.P.H.
Los Angeles, California

SYNONYMS

Essential paralysis of childhood, debility of the lower extremities, infantile paralysis, acute anterior poliomyelitis, polio, Heine-Medin disease.

DEFINITION

Poliomyelitis is an acute infectious and communicable disease that affects the central nervous system and may result in paresis and paralysis. The word comes from the Greek words *polios,* meaning gray, and *myelos,* meaning the marrow.

INFECTIOUS AGENT

There are three immunologically distinct types of poliovirus: types 1, 2, and 3, known originally as Brunhilde, Lansing, and Leon viruses. These viruses are picornaviruses (from Latin *pico,* meaning small, and *rna* for ribonucleic acid), are 25 to 30 nm in size, contain ribonucleic acid, and are of worldwide distribution.

The virus enters through the mouth, localizes in the oropharynx and portions of the intestinal tract, where it multiplies, and then travels to regional lymph nodes and to the blood stream. Although the polioviruses affect principally the central nervous system, they are not commonly found in the cerebrospinal fluid of humans.

High concentrations of virus are excreted in the stools for up to 8 weeks after the onset of abortive, nonparalytic, or paralytic disease. Virus has been found in pharyngeal swabs taken in the first week of illness but is not often found thereafter.

Although the exact pathways taken by the virus from the infected to the susceptible person have not been clearly defined, it would appear that the principal mode of spread is through intimate human contact.

EPIDEMIOLOGY

Poliomyelitis is almost certainly an ancient disease, probably endemic for centuries in the Western civilizations. Atrophy of an extremity has been recorded in stone by the Egyptians as early as 1600 B.C.

A dramatic change occurred in the expression of this disease with the first appearance of large epidemics toward the end of the 19th century in Scandinavia and the United States. Subsequently increasingly severe epidemics were observed elsewhere in North America and Europe, Australia, and New Zealand.

In underdeveloped countries, where populations live with poor sanitation and heavy fecal pollution, serologic investigations have shown that polioviruses are widely disseminated. Infections occur in infancy. In almost 100 per cent of children, antibodies develop in the first few years of life, resulting in a highly immune population. In countries with higher standards of living, exposure is limited, infection occurs later in life, large proportions of the population remain susceptible, and severe epidemics affecting older children and young adults may result from the introduction of virulent strains of virus.

The reservoir of infection is human; animals are not yet known to harbor the infection under natural conditions. In households, exposure of susceptible persons to an infected family member results in an infection rate of almost 100 per cent in children and slightly less in young adults. Children under 2 years of age easily disseminate virus, probably because of their well-known habits of fecal contamination.

The patient is infectious several days before the first symptoms appear. The disease, although highly infectious, results in a clinically recognizable disease so infrequently that it is possible to determine communicability only by isolation of the virus from stools of exposed persons.

The virus has been recovered from the pharynx from 5 days before to 14 days after the first sign of illness. The virus has been recovered from stools of nearly all patients with known disease. It has been detected from several weeks before the onset of paralysis to almost 6 months after so-called abortive illness. Viruses have been recovered also from healthy carriers.

HOST FACTORS

Certain host factors are known to predispose nonimmune individuals to more severe and extensive paralytic disease when infected with a virulent poliovirus.

Age has a definite effect on the incidence and severity of paralysis. Reports in the literature indicate attack rates during an epidemic are several times higher among adolescents and adults than among children. Among nonfatal cases, the average extent of paralytic involvement increases with age, as does the frequency of severe bulbar and respiratory involvement.

Nonspecific factors, such as stress, significant fatigue, strenuous exercise, or pregnancy, all increase the risk of paralytic disease. Tonsillectomy and adenoidectomy are both known to increase the risk of paralysis, particularly of the severe bulbar and spinobulbar forms. Finally, if poliomyelitis occurs within 1 month after an injection of any kind of antigen, there is increased likelihood that paralysis will occur in the injected extremity.

CLINICAL MANIFESTATIONS

The manifestations of severe poliomyelitis are usually apparent, since paralysis is a condition which is quite obvious. However, most infections with poliovirus cause no symptoms at all. Even when infections becomes manifest, the symptoms are quite variable and may be quite different from the classic picture of paralysis.

Poliomyelitis has two main phases, the minor illness and the major illness. The minor illness is also called abortive poliomyelitis. The major illness may have two stages: the meningitic or nonparalytic stage, and the paralytic stage.

Incubation Period

When definite exposure is known, the incubation period of the major illness appears to be between 1 and 2 weeks. The interval from the time of infection to the minor illness may be 3 to 5 days. Virus multiplication after the administration of live vaccine occurs within 24 hours and the virus may have spread to contacts in 3 days.

The Minor Illness (Abortive Poliomyelitis)

Abortive poliomyelitis or minor illness starts abruptly and lasts from a few hours to a few days. Symptoms are nonspecific. Malaise is the most common symptom, along with fever, sore throat, headache, nausea, anorexia, vomiting, and abdominal pain. Except for slight redness of the throat, there are usually no remarkable physical findings.

This phase of disease differs in no significant detail from any number of acute communicable diseases. If no further manifestations appear, the diagnosis of poliomyelitis cannot be made unless the season of the year, prevalence of the disease, and virologic-epidemiologic evidence support the diagnosis of abortive poliomyelitis. Symptoms subside, the patient feels better, and the illness appears to be roughly terminated for most of the patients in 24 to 36 hours.

A biphasic course is observed in some patients. A minor illness appears, but there is improvement over 1 to 4 days or more before onset of the major illness becomes obvious. This biphasic course has been called "the dromedary phenomenon."

The Major Illness

The major illness may occur without any preceding minor illness, it may follow a few days of apparent well-being after the minor illness, or the minor illness may merge into the major without any interval.

Nonparalytic Poliomyelitis. Symptoms encountered during the minor illness reappear and are exaggerated. The fever may be slightly higher, frontal headache is a fairly constant complaint, and nausea progresses to vomiting. The headache may be fairly severe, but it is never intolerable, as it is in bacterial meningitis. The patient appears more ill than the temperature or clinical findings would suggest. Pain in the limbs is common, but it is usually mild. There is a strained, anxious expression of the face. Hypersensitivity may be present to such a degree that even touching the skin may irritate the patient. Hyperhidrosis, or increased sweating, is commonly seen, particularly about the head and neck. In some patients evidence of cerebral involvement is insignificant, whereas in other patients there is development of a stiff neck and a stiff spine. At this stage, the cerebrospinal fluid usually shows pleocytosis with a slightly elevated protein level.

Muscle pain is usually present early in the major illness, and it can persist for weeks. Pain may be excruciating, especially at night; it is most often felt in the back, flanks, and legs. The pain is characteristically relieved by motion. Pain and tenderness may be accompanied by spasm or increased muscle tone. The spasm may remain for weeks or months.

Paralytic Poliomyelitis. Paralytic poliomyelitis often begins as nonparalytic poliomyelitis with an initial phase similar to that of the abortive or minor illness. After a period of well-being lasting from 1 to 7 days, the same symptoms may return in more severe form, with evidence of central nervous system invasion. Paralysis may occur in 1 to 2 days. Although paralysis may be the first sign of the major illness, the meningitic phase usually lasts for a day or two before the first signs of paralysis are seen. Rarely paralysis may develop without any preceding illness at all.

The onset of paralysis is usually preceded by stiffness of the neck and back. This is demonstrated by the tripod sign: the patient is unable to sit up straight and needs to brace the body with arms extended backward. The patient is apprehensive and restless and may be stuporous or drowsy. Kernig's and Brudzinski's signs are positive. Loss of superficial abdominal and cremasteric reflexes may precede paralysis of the legs. The tendon reflexes usually show hyperactivity at first and then become diminished or absent. Pain in the legs or arms, tremors of the arms, and hyperesthesia may be predictors of paralysis. The paralysis is of lower motor neuron type. There is flaccidity of the affected muscles accompanied by loss of deep tendon reflexes.

Power of the muscles of the upper extremity can be assessed by testing the grip, pronation and supination of the forearm, flexion and extension at the elbow, and abduction and adduction of the shoulder. The strength of the flexors of the neck can be estimated by asking the patient to lift the head against the resistance of the examiner's hand on the patient's forehead; the extensors are tested by pressing the head back against the resistance of the examiner's hand on the back of the patient's head.

Weakness of the abdominal muscles can be determined by feeling with the hand for the tightening of the rectus muscles in lifting the head off the bed or blowing the nose. The action of the diaphragm can be tested by noting whether the hand on the abdomen is lifted or sucked inward on inspiration. The action of the intercostals can be assessed by noting the movements of the chest wall with breathing. Inability to bend the foot up or down against resistance, to raise the leg off the bed, to bend the knee or to keep it straight against resistance, or to bring the leg down on the bed against resistance are all evidences of paralysis that can be elicited without much disturbance to the patient.

If paralysis occurs at all, it usually develops in the first week of major illness. Sometimes paralysis appears as early as the first day, or it may be delayed until the seventh to the tenth day. Weakness often progresses gradually for 2 or 3 days before paralysis develops. Seldom does paralysis emerge or progress after the temperature has returned to normal.

The distribution of paralysis in poliomyelitis is characteristically asymmetric. The legs are more vulnerable than the arms. The sites of paralysis vary, but the large muscle groups of the arms and legs generally show more involvement than do the small muscles of the hands and feet. In the leg, the muscles most frequently involved are the anterior tibial, peroneal, quadriceps, and hamstring. In the arm, the shoulder girdle, especially the deltoid, is commonly affected. Various chest deformities may result from paralysis of the shoulder and thoracic muscles. The severity of paralysis is characteristically variable in degree and spotty in distribution, depending on the number of damaged nerve cells. Difficulty in breathing indicates weakness of the diaphragm, intercostal muscles, or both; alternatively, it may originate in the medulla.

Paralysis of the muscles of respiration results from damage to many nerve cells in the cervical and thoracic segments of the spinal cord. It causes much anxiety in the patient, who becomes restless and wakeful. The voice grows weak, cough becomes ineffective, and the patient has difficulty in holding the breath or in counting up to ten in one breath. Respirations become shallow and rapid. Unless some form of mechanical aid to respiration is provided, the patient will suffocate. Respiratory paralysis seldom appears early and may occur quite late in the disease. Although it is always a serious manifestation, it may persist for several days yet result in complete recovery. Paralysis of the diaphragm results in breathing that is wholly thoracic. On inspiration the abdominal wall is retracted instead of protruded. Urinary retention and constipation are fairly common but usually transitory. Paralysis of the bladder is a very common symptom.

After the fever subsides, the spread of weakness or paralysis stops. For a period of days or weeks there may be little visible change. Spontaneous improvement then occurs, as shown by returning of the reflexes and muscle strength. The return of muscle power usually reaches its limit in about 18 months to 2 years. Thereafter, residual paralysis is likely to be permanent.

Sensory disturbances are generally absent, except in the acute phase. Atrophy of paralyzed muscles occurs after 1 or 2 months. The paralyzed extremity is smaller than the unaffected limb. Circulation is poor and growth is arrested in the whole limb, which eventually becomes shorter.

Polioencephalitis. In polioencephalitis the main symptom is disturbance of consciousness. This is one of the less common manifestations of poliomyelitis and therefore is often misdiagnosed. Encephalitic patients have hyperpyrexia, cerebellar signs, delirium, stupor, or coma. As most of the signs of polioencephalitis can be produced by hypoxia or hypercapnia, polioencephalitis should not be diagnosed unless the signs of supramedullary involvement fail to subside despite correction of abnormal blood gases. Seizures are so uncommon in patients with encephalitis caused by poliovirus that the occurrence of a seizure makes the diagnosis unlikely.

In a child it is usually impossible to detect evidence of flaccid limb paralysis. There may, in fact, be spasticity of limbs, increased tendon reflexes, and other signs of upper motor neuron or cerebral lesions so that it is impossible to distinguish the condition from acute disseminated encephalomyelitis. The condition is usually fatal within a few days of onset.

In older patients the main symptoms may be intense headache, meningismus, vomiting, ataxia, speech difficulties, and confusion. The patient is often extremely restless and difficult to control. Sometimes coma supervenes and the patient may die within a few days. More often he or she becomes drowsy and stuporous for several days, although sometimes the hyperexcitability persists and the patient is unable to sleep or rest. A variety of neurologic signs may be found at this stage, including ocular or facial paralyses, spasticity or incoordination of limbs, and exaggerated tendon reflexes or ankle clonus.

Bulbar Poliomyelitis. Bulbar poliomyelitis is characterized by damage to the motor nuclei of the cranial nerves and other vital zones in the medulla concerned with respiration and circulation. It may occur in the absence of clinically recognized involvement of the spinal cord. Although bulbar poliomyelitis is potentially the most life-endangering form, it is not always fatal. Moreover, if the patient survives the acute stage, recovery from cranial nerve paralysis is usually complete.

Patients with damage to the tenth nerve may develop weakness or paralysis of the soft palate, the pharynx, and vocal cords. A nasal tone to the voice or hoarseness may be the first sign. A child may refuse to eat or drink because swallowing is difficult. It is important to recognize accumulation or pooling of secretions in the throat. There may be regurgitation through the nose. Laryngeal stridor, a dangerous sign, may occur.

The most ominous form of bulbar poliomyelitis results from spread of infection to the respiratory and vasomotor centers. Damage to the respiratory center causes breathing to become irregular in rhythm and depth. Respirations are shallow and are associated with periods of apnea. The pulse rate and temperature become higher. The blood pressure, at first elevated, may drop rapidly to shock levels. The patient becomes confused, delirious, and comatose, and then respirations stop. When the vasomotor center is involved, the pulse becomes extremely rapid, irregular, and difficult to palpate. The blood pressure fluctuates from high to low levels with a small pulse pressure. The patient shows marked anxiety and restlessness. The skin, which is cold and clammy, has a dusky red appearance that progresses to mottled cyanosis. The heartbeat usually becomes inaudible before breathing stops.

The Landry type of ascending paralysis has been seen in outbreaks of poliomyelitis. It is characterized by paralysis ascending from the lower extremities to the trunk, arms, and muscles of respiration, and upward to involve vital centers in the medulla. The outcome is often fatal. A descending type of paralysis also may occur.

COMMON COMPLICATIONS

When paralysis is limited to the muscles of the limbs and trunk, complications are mainly of an orthopedic nature. They are due to muscle weakness and imbalance or to failure of growth. When the patient has respiratory embarrassment due to pharyngeal or respiratory paralysis, innumerable complications may occur. Ventilatory insufficiency is the immediate, life-threatening complication of spinal poliomyelitis. Significant arm and shoulder weakness should alert the clinician to the possibility of impending diaphragmatic and intercostal muscle weakness.

Irregularities of the rate, depth, and rhythm of breathing suggest ventilatory failure as the result of the involvement of the medullary respiratory center. The prognosis is ominous.

Pharyngeal paralysis results in difficulty in swallowing and an accumulation of secretions in the oropharynx, leading to aspiration and ventilatory obstruction. Hypoxia, hypercapnia, and shock may also be present.

Acute urinary retention lasting from a few hours to many weeks is a frequent complication of paralytic poliomyelitis. Most patients who have weakness in the lower extremities develop transient urinary retention. Urinary output should be monitored carefully, and if the patient fails to void after adequate hydration, diagnostic catheterization should be performed. If retention is detected and the patient continues to be unable to void, recatheterization should be done at 8-hour intervals on an "in and out" basis several times before an indwelling catheter is inserted. The urinary retention frequently lasts less than 24 hours, and it is desirable to avoid problems associated with the insertion of an indwelling catheter whenever possible.

Circulatory complications characterized by shock, hypotension, or hypertension occur. Hypertension may occur in half of the patients with poliomyelitis, but it is usually gone within 1 week unless the patient needs a respirator. Specific lesions of the myocardium may occur in the acute stage of the disease and be associated with these complications or they may be related to other causes of paralysis.

Gastrointestinal complications include constipation, acute dilatation of the stomach, and gastric and duodenal ulceration often resulting in massive gastrointestinal hemorrhage. Ulcers are common in patients who are managed with mechanical aids to ventilation.

Other common complications of the paralytic process that may occur include atelectasis, pneumonia, and thrombophlebitis with pulmonary embolism.

Kidney stones sometimes occur in patients kept immobilized for long periods of time and may be related to decalcification of bone from disuse, resulting in increased levels of serum and urinary calcium.

DIAGNOSTIC STUDIES AND LABORATORY FINDINGS

The diagnosis of poliomyelitis depends on collecting as much information as possible about the patient. The presence of an epidemic, contact with another person with poliomyelitis among close associates, and significant clinical and laboratory findings all help to make the diagnosis. The finding of virus in pharyngeal secretions or in the stools is helpful but does not confirm the diagnosis, since there are carriers among both healthy individuals and those with other illnesses.

Paralytic poliomyelitis has become a rare disease in recent years. A total of 16 cases of paralytic poliomyelitis was reported from the Centers for Disease Control for 1980 and 1981. If a patient has the paralytic poliomyelitis syndrome, the physician should consider recent ingestion of oral poliovirus vaccine (OPV), contact with an OPV recipient, or recent entry to the United States from an area endemic for poliomyelitis as the source.

Routine Laboratory Studies

No specific abnormalities are found in the routine laboratory studies of patients with poliomyelitis. Urinalysis and blood chemistry determinations may be abnormal, indicating disturbances in the fluids and electrolytes due to dehydration, vomiting, and fever. Blood gases may be abnormal as a result of ventilatory failure due to respiratory failure.

Cerebrospinal Fluid Findings

There is nothing pathognomonic about the cerebrospinal fluid findings in poliomyelitis. In the minor illness, or abortive form, the cerebrospinal fluid usually is normal. If the examination is repeated in several days, increased amounts of cells or protein may be observed. The cerebrospinal fluid remains normal throughout the disease in about 10 per cent of patients.

In the major illness cerebrospinal fluid examination reveals pleocytosis (15 to 500 cells/cu mm), mostly lymphocytes, although polymorphonuclear cells may predominate early. The protein level may remain normal during the first week of illness (25 to 150 mg/dl) but it rises during the second and third weeks (100 to 400 mg/dl). Paralyzed patients generally show higher levels of cerebrospinal fluid protein than do nonparalytic patients. Glucose and chloride values remain normal throughout. Bacterial cultures are sterile.

Viral Studies

Polioviruses can be readily isolated and identified with modern tissue culture techniques. They can be isolated from blood early in the course of illness, but only rarely have they been recovered from cerebrospinal fluid specimens. Virus can usually be grown in tissue culture from pharyngeal or throat swabs in the first week of the acute stage of the illness. From the feces, virus has been recovered for at least 3 weeks and often up to 2 months.

Throat swabs and rectal swabs should be collected, placed in a virus-holding medium, and stored at −20°C to −70°C until specimens can be inoculated into primary rhesus monkey kidney tissue cultures. Polioviruses in clinical specimens may produce detectable cytopathic effects as early as 24 hours after inoculation of the tissue cultures, although longer incubation is frequently necessary. Cytopathogenic agents are identified as specific poliovirus types by neutralization with type-specific hyperimmune sera.

In addition to specimens for virus isolation, patients should have an acute serum sample drawn and stored for serologic tests at the time the diagnosis is first suspected. A convalescent serum should be obtained 2 to 3 weeks later. These sera are separated from the clots and stored frozen until tested. It is important that the serologic test be performed on the acute and convalescent samples simultaneously. Serologic confirmation of a poliovirus infection is obtained by demonstrating a fourfold or greater rise in neutralizing or complement-fixing antibody against a prototype strain of one of the three poliovirus types.

In recent years it has become possible to distinguish wild strains of poliovirus from those that are vaccine-derived. Laboratory tests that have been developed to help distinguish these wild poliovirus strains include: (1) temperature-marker test, (2) modified Wecker intratypic serodifferentiation test, (3) van Wezel test, (4) polypeptide analysis, and (5) oligonucleotide "fingerprinting" analysis. These tests are available in the United States at the Centers for Disease Control.

DIFFERENTIAL DIAGNOSIS

On clinical grounds alone it has been difficult at times to distinguish nonparalytic and preparalytic poliomyelitis from aseptic meningitis due to some other agent.

Paralytic poliomyelitis has been confused with infectious polyneuritis (Guillain-Barré syndrome). In contrast to poliomyelitis, the distribution of paralysis in the Guillain-Barré syndrome is symmetric; sensory changes, including loss of sensation, occur frequently. The cerebrospinal fluid shows a normal cell count and high protein content (albuminocytologic dissociation) early in the disease, and recovery is usually rapid and complete.

Paralysis caused by postdiphtheritic polyneuritis and by transverse myelitis has been mistaken for poliomyelitis. Patients may present with pseudoparalysis, resulting in unwillingness to move an extremity because of pain and tenderness. Pseudoparalysis may mimic poliomyelitis yet have a specific cause, such as osteomyelitis, acute rheumatic fever, trichinosis, or scurvy. Hysterical paralysis is not uncommon during poliomyelitis epidemics.

Acute myelitis or encephalomyelitis may be the first manifestation of multiple sclerosis. Certain other neurologic conditions that have been confused with poliomyelitis include cerebrovascular accidents, syringomyelia, hematomyelia, myelitis resulting from infection with bacteria, infections with acid-fast bacteria or fungi, epidural abscess, neoplasms of the brain and spinal cord, and acute anterior myelitis associated with non-poliovirus enteroviral infections.

RABIES

By Richard W. Emmons, M.D., Ph.D.
Berkeley, California

SYNONYMS

Hydrophobia, rage, rabia, lyssa.

DEFINITION

Rabies is an acute, infectious zoonotic disease which is almost invariably a rapidly fatal encephalomyelitis. It is caused by a virus in the genus Lyssavirus of the family Rhabdoviridae. Closely related viruses (Lagos bat, Duvenhage, and Mokola viruses) have been described from Africa but their origins, ecology, and significance for humans are not well understood as yet. Rabies virus strains, and the clinical disease in humans, are essentially identical throughout the world.

ECOLOGY

Rabies virus in the saliva of a rabid animal is usually inoculated by bite. Rarely it may also gain access by contamination of mucous membranes or nasal mucosa with saliva or infected neural tissue (licking by an animal, aerosols in certain bat-inhabited caves, or laboratory accidents). Human-to-human transmission via corneal transplant has been documented several times.

Rabies is relatively rare in humans, but is common in certain wildlife species and domestic animals (primarily dogs) in much of the world, so that rabies exposure is a common and serious threat. The few rabies-free areas of the world include Australia, New Zealand, Japan, Taiwan, Hawaii, various other Pacific Islands, the United Kingdom and Ireland, some West Indies islands, parts of the Scandinavian countries, and some other islands and small countries.

The usual wildlife hosts include skunks, insectivorous bats, foxes, and raccoons in the United States; vampire bats in Central and South America; mongooses in the Asian subcontinent and some Caribbean islands; arctic foxes in the North Polar zone; and foxes, wolves, jackals, and other carnivores and viverrids in Europe, Asia, and Africa. Domestic species such as cows and horses acquire rabies from bites by wildlife hosts, but they do not perpetuate the virus cycle and almost never have transmitted rabies to humans. Rodents and rabbits are almost never found to be positive and have not been proved to transmit the disease to humans. The domestic dog is the most significant host as a source of exposure or actual transmission of the disease to humans throughout the world. The domestic cat is also involved, although to a lesser extent.

PRESENTING SIGNS AND SYMPTOMS

The incubation (latent) period varies from 9 days to more than a year, but it is usually 1 to 3 months. Severe, multiple, or head, face, or hand bites seem to pose a higher risk and to be associated with a shorter incubation period. The site and state of the virus during this latent period is uncertain, but it may be in muscle cells at the bite site. After gaining access to the peripheral afferent nerves, the virus moves rapidly to the central nervous system, disseminates widely through the brain, then spreads peripherally to various highly innervated tissues, including salivary glands, lacrimal glands, corneal epithelial cells, various internal organs, and the skin.

There is gradual onset of a prodromal phase, which lasts 2 to 10 days and probably represents beginning viral infection of the central nervous system. Vague and fluctuating symptoms of headache, malaise, lethargy, chills, sore throat, myalgia, tightness in the chest, anorexia, nausea and abdominal pains, vomiting, vertigo, and dyspnea may occur. Slight to moderate fever is noted in one third to one half of cases, and tachycardia is common. Restlessness, insomnia, a sense of anxiety, and other psychologic abnormalities may be seen. The patient or family may not recall, or may not have been aware of, significant animal exposure, adding to the difficulty of assessing this prodromal illness. The earliest specific symptom that suggests rabies is an abnormal sensation (pain, burning or sensation of cold, pruritus, tingling, other paresthesias or numbness), usually at the bite site or in the bitten extremity and noted in 30 to 80 per cent of cases.

On suspicion of rabies, the patient should be hospitalized for observation, diagnostic testing, and medical management. Appropriate isolation precautions should be used to protect hospital personnel.

COURSE

An acute neurologic phase lasting a few days to a week usually follows. There is general excitation and stimulation of the nervous system, with hyperactivity, irritability, volubility, emotional instability, apprehension, muscle fasciculations or tics, and generally increased reflex activity of the musculature. There is often hypersensitivity to noise, bright lights, pressure of bedclothes, and other stimuli. Disorientation, hallucinations, increasing agitation, shouting, thrashing, and episodes of running, biting, and other bizarre behavior may be noted. These episodes are interspersed with periods of relative calm and lucid, cooperative demeanor. In about half of the cases, attempts to drink liquids result in painful, reflex spasms of the pharnyx and larynx, choking, and gagging, so that the patient avoids fluids. Even the sight, sound, or mention of water may elicit this response (hydrophobia). A draft of air blowing on the face may have a similar effect (aerophobia). Hypersalivation and the inability to swallow lead to drooling or repeated spitting by the patient. Hoarseness or complete loss of voice may occur. Incontinence of urine or feces, cardiac arrhythmias, hyperventilation, fluctuating fever, blood pressure changes, and other signs of autonomic nervous system instability may also occur.

Despite these manifestations of severe encephalitis, ability of the patient to communicate and respond to requests and questions is often preserved until late in the course. The excitation phase may continue, with focal or generalized seizures and early death; or a depressive phase may ensue, often beginning with weakness in the bitten limb progressing as an ascending paralysis and ending with stupor, coma, and respiratory and bulbar paralysis. Sometimes the paralytic form dominates the clinical picture from the start and mimics the Landry-Guillain-Barré syndrome. This has been noticed especially following vampire bat bite or in patients given a partial (unsuccessful) course of postexposure immunizations. The patient may survive in a comatose state for 2 to 3 weeks even without special treatment, but modern intensive care has maintained some patients for months.

In the rare cases of presumed or proven recovery from rabies, improvement began after a week or so in coma, and slow, progressive return of neurologic function followed. However, only one case associated with complete recovery has been documented by modern diagnostic criteria.

COMMON COMPLICATIONS

Numerous complications may occur during the course of the disease and may be the immediate cause of death. Increased intracranial pressure is common, owing to the cerebral edema that results from inflammation of the brain or hypoxia. Other complications include hypothalamic dysfunction with inappropriate secretion of antidiuretic hormone or diabetes insipidus; autonomic dysfunction with hypotension, cardiac arrhythmias, high fever, or hypothermia; respiratory depression, hypoxemia, atelectasis, and pneumonia; and paralytic ileus, bladder paralysis, gastrointestinal bleeding, renal failure, metabolic acidosis, and other electrolyte imbalances. Anticipating, preventing, and promptly overcoming these complications may result in complete recovery of additional cases of rabies, since the direct viral damage to neurons may not be the most important pathologic effect.

PHYSICAL EXAMINATION

Most of the significant physical findings have already been mentioned. In general, these are not very helpful or specific, and merely reveal an acute encephalitis. Increased salivation, lacrimation, and excessive perspiration are common. Tachycardia often occurs early, and bradycardia and arrhythmia late in the course. The fever is low to moderate and fluctuating. Respirations may be shallow, and Cheyne-Stokes respiration is common. The pupils may be dilated early in the course; later there is loss of corneal reflex, and the pupils may be constricted, unequal, and poorly reactive to light. Nystagmus, diplopia, strabismus, and vertigo may be present. Initially there are increased muscle reflexes and tics, generally increased muscle tone, stiffness of the neck, and a positive Babinski test, but Kernig's and Brudzinski's signs are not seen. Later, reduced reflexes; weakness of various muscle groups; diminished sensation to pinprick, heat, and cold; paralysis; and finally a comatose state ensue.

LABORATORY PROCEDURES

Initial work-up will reveal moderately increased cerebrospinal fluid pressure with slight increase in protein levels, and only a few to a moderate number of mononuclear cells in the fluid. The peripheral blood leukocyte count is usually somewhat elevated, with an increase in the percentage of polymorphonuclear cells. The urine may show slight albuminuria.

When the diagnosis of rabies is considered, appropriate specimen collection should be instituted promptly to verify the diagnosis and help in case management. Periodic serum and cerebrospinal fluid samples can be tested for antibody titers against rabies or other viruses that cause encephalitis. Stool or rectal swabs, throat swabs or throat washings, and cerebrospinal fluid samples should be inoculated into cell culture systems to detect various other encephalitis-causing viruses. Multiple throat swabs or throat washings, saliva samples, and cerebrospinal fluid samples should be inoculated into suckling and adult mice to detect rabies virus. The virus has also been detected in material from eye swabs, tracheal aspirates, urine sediment, skin biopsy specimens, and brain biopsy specimens in a few cases. Rapid immunofluorescence staining can sometimes detect rabies virus antigen in corneal cell preparations, skin biopsy samples, or brain biopsy specimens many days before virus isolation can be achieved. At autopsy, brain and spinal cord tissue from a variety of sites, salivary glands, and various other organs may be tested by immunofluorescence staining and virus isolation procedures. These specimens should be collected aseptically, using separate instruments for each specimen to avoid cross contamination between them. Fresh, unfixed tissue samples are needed for these tests. Formalin-fixed, paraffin-embedded tissues can be tested by a special immunofluorescence staining method, but this is still experimental and not routinely available.

POTENTIAL ERRORS AND PITFALLS IN DIAGNOSIS

Various diseases may mimic some of the acute encephalitic or paralytic manifestations of rabies, but they can be ruled out by appropriate history, clinical evaluation, and laboratory tests. These include herpes simplex encephalitis; mumps meningoencephalitis; herpesvirus simiae (B virus) encephalomyelitis (acquired from rhesus or cynomolgus monkey bite or exposure to infected tissues); *Pasteurella multocida*, tularemia, rat-bite fever, or cat-scratch disease (all acquired from animal bite or contact); acute poliomyelitis; enteroviral encephalitis (coxsackievirus A or B or echoviruses); arboviral encephalitis (most commonly western equine encephalomyelitis, eastern equine encephalomyelitis, St. Louis encephalitis, and California encephalitis in the United States, and various other mosquito- or tick-transmitted viruses in other countries); tick-bite paralysis; acute infective polyneuritis; Landry-Guillain-Barré syndrome; and tetanus, botulism, and postvaccination or postinfectious encephalitides (e.g., following measles, varicella, herpes zoster, influenza, and other diseases).

Patients with rabies hysteria may have some symptoms and signs of rabies (anxiety, restlessness, irritability and aggressiveness, pain at the site of the bite, simulated hydrophobia and convulsions, and bizarre behavior). These do not progress, however, and laboratory findings are negative. Response to psychiatric or other treatment is usually prompt.

Neurologic reactions to postexposure treatment with rabies vaccine are rare but may initially simulate rabies encephalitis. They usually occur within 2 weeks of beginning treatment and gradually resolve. When postexposure treatment has been started but has failed to abort the disease, it may be difficult or impossible in serologic tests to distinguish between passively administered antibody or antibody response to the vaccine, on the one hand, and antibody produced by the patient in response to the infection, on the other hand. In the latter case, antibody in serum or cerebrospinal fluid is usually not detectable for 1 week or more following onset of symptoms. It may be difficult to detect rabies antigen in corneal cell preparations, skin biopsy specimens, or brain biopsy samples owing to sparse or irregular distribution of virus; alternatively, false-negative results may be obtained by the laboratory. A false-positive result in the immunofluorescence staining test is another pitfall to be avoided.

TETANUS

By Wesley Furste, M.D.
George W. Paulson, M.D.
and Robert J. Fass, M.D.
Columbus, Ohio

SYNONYM

Lockjaw.

DEFINITION

Tetanus, a severe and dreaded infectious complication of wounds, is caused by the toxin-producing *Clostridium tetani.* This disease is characterized by tonic spasms of the voluntary muscles, by a tendency toward episodes of respiratory arrest, and by a mortality rate of about 50 per cent worldwide. Although tetanus is uncommon in developed countries, the World Health Organization has estimated as recently as 1981 that about 1,000,000 tetanus deaths, including about 900,000 from neonatal tetanus, occur per year throughout the world. Figure 1 shows the incidence of tetanus in the United States.

ETIOLOGIC AGENT

Clostridium tetani is a ubiquitous, large, motile anaerobic, spore-forming, gram-positive bacillus without a capsule. It is an obligate anaerobe and can be cultivated on artificial media in the absence of atmospheric oxygen. Characteristic spherical terminal spores are produced, which are highly resistant; if protected from direct sunlight, they can survive for many years. Tetanus spores are often present in the intestinal contents of humans and animals and have been found in soil and street dust in many parts of the world. Under suitable conditions of growth, *C. tetani* elaborates a powerful exotoxin. Following invasion by the specific microorganism and production of the specific neurotoxin, the central nervous system is altered, with hyperexudation. Tetanus is thus a toxi-infection, being neither simply a toxic state nor solely an infection.

PATHOGENESIS

Clostridium tetani is carried into human tissues by contamination of a wound. A variety of lesions, both large and small, may offer a suitable haven for growth: lacerations, compound fractures, gunshot wounds, septic abortions, and lesions produced by nails, slivers, and human and animal bites. For example, tetanus with death resulted when a 49-year-old woman was bitten by a pet rooster. Cases have resulted from the use of unsterile surgical supplies and unsterile biologic materials. Infections of the postpartum uterus and the umbilical stump (tetanus neonatorum) were once common but now can be rare with proper tetanus toxoid immunization of the mother and use of aseptic obstetric technqiues. Cultural habits can be important etiologic considerations; the practices of rubbing the umbilical cord with dirt or dung, piercing of earlobes, or, in the United States, "skin popping" of contaminated heroin, may be responsible for tetanus. *Clostridium tetani* is so ubiquitous in the human environment that almost any contaminated wound may contain the organisms; hence, tetanus may occur wherever humans live.

The mere fact that *C. tetani* is present does not necessarily mean that the patient has tetanus or that it will develop. In a wound, the organism will proliferate only in the presence of an oxidation-reduction potential far lower than that existing in normal living tissue. Once the organism begins to grow, it produces an exotoxin. This neurotoxin is known to block release of inhibitory amino acids, such as glycine; although peripheral synapses can be affected, the major effect is to produce central disinhibition with increase in reflex excitability of all spinal efferents.

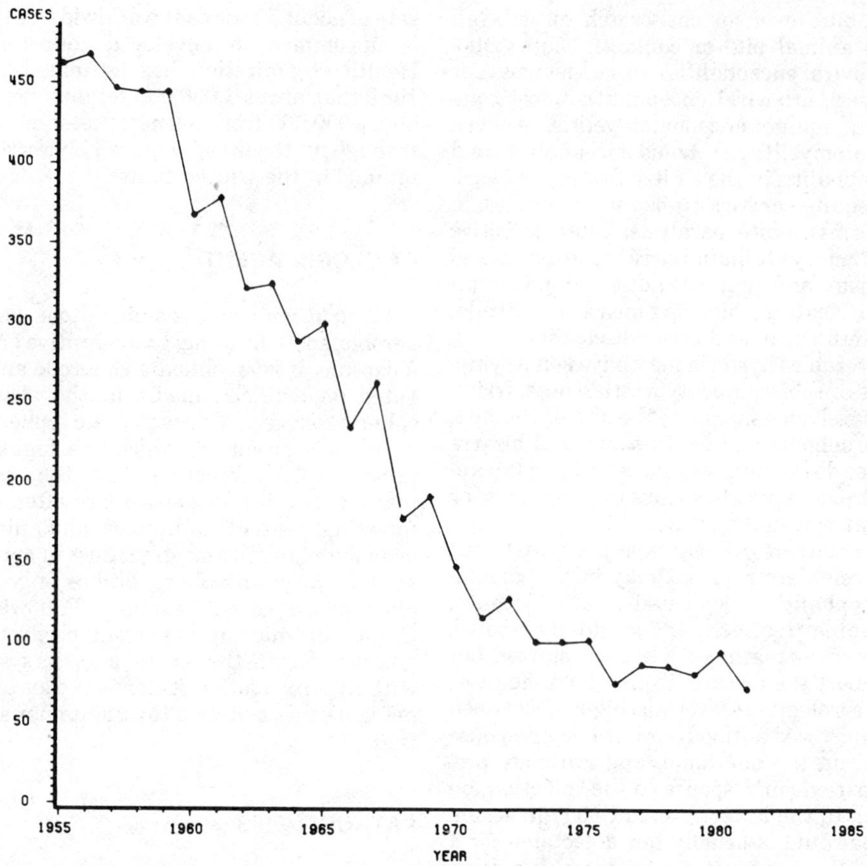

Figure 1. Reported cases of tetanus, by year, in the United States, 1955–1981. The number of cases has been stable since 1976. The lack of further decline in the number of tetanus cases may reflect continued, inadequate vaccination coverage of the older portion of the population. (Courtesy of Centers for Disease Control, Public Health Service, U.S. Department of Health and Human Services. Annual Summary 1981, *Morbidity and Mortality Weekly Report* 30:87, 1982.)

PRIOR HISTORY IN SUSPECTED TETANUS

The amount of the very potent tetanus toxin necessary to produce tetanus is so small that it will not incite an active antibody level high enough to prevent a second attack of tetanus. Consequently, tetanus is a nonimmunizing disease; hence, a history of tetanus does not rule out the possibility of a second attack of tetanus.

If a patient has had a traumatic wound during the previous days or few weeks, tetanus should be considered. In these days of numerous automobile collisions, burns, occasional airplane crashes, and other accidents, deep wounds are caused in which tetanus toxin can be produced. Tetanus has occurred as a complication of wounds of all sizes, including lacerations, compound fractures, burns, abrasions, and even hypodermic injections in drug addicts. Not uncommonly, tetanus may develop in a neglected or forgotten trivial wound considered by the patient not important enough to require a visit to the physician, and it may even occur in persons in whom a wound of entry of the organism cannot be demonstrated. Since many patients with tetanus will not have an obvious wound and since tetanus is a toxic state, a diagnosis can be made in the absence of cultural proof.

The incidence of tetanus caused by contaminated catgut or surgical instruments has fortunately become very low. Rarely tetanus has occurred after operations on the intestinal tract, which has been a source of the *C. tetani* organisms.

Definite proof that a wounded person has previously had adequate tetanus toxoid immunization is reassuring and—according to follow-up studies on World War II veterans—just about eliminates the possibility of tetanus if a booster dose of tetanus toxoid is given to a wounded patient. The efficiency and safety of tetanus toxoid as a prophylactic agent were proved by the World War II experiences of the United States Army. Twelve cases of tetanus occurred in a series of 2,734,-819 hospital admissions for wounds and injuries for an incidence of 0.00044 per cent. Of these 12 patients, only 4 had been given adequate basic immunization plus emergency stimulating toxoid injections.

Unfortunately, not all civilians have adequate active tetanus immunization; hence, if wounded, they may develop tetanus. Older women who have not received tetanus toxoid as infants, as children, as adults, or as members of the armed forces are particularly vulnerable. Figure 2 shows the relationship between age and tetanus incidence.

INCUBATION PERIOD

The incubation period may be as short as 1 day or as long as 54 days. Prognosis is generally better when the incubation period is longer. The longer incubation periods are particularly likely to occur when the patient has received partial protection from human or equine antitoxin or when secondary surgical revision or manipulation of wounds, especially war wounds, is performed. Rarely, when a scar of a wound has of necessity been surgically explored, tetanus has occurred many years after the time of the primary wound.

CLINICAL MANIFESTATIONS

The disease almost always appears in a general form (Fig. 3), but it may occasionally appear as local tetanus. Uncommon in humans, local tetanus may start in the muscles near the infection, probably because of the path of ascent of the neurotoxin, or in the facial muscles, particularly if the ear or jaw is the source. With local tetanus, usually general symptoms occur sooner or later, but then the disease is likely to be milder and less often fatal than the general type usually seen.

In the more familiar general form, the earliest indications of tetanus infection usually become evident from 1 to 2 weeks after injury. The severity of the clinical picture and the mortality rate are roughly inversely proportional to the duration of the incubation period.

Some patients have prodromal symptoms of restlessness and headaches. In others, the first symptoms are those stemming from the developing muscular rigidity, with vague discomfort in the jaws, neck, or lumbar region. At an early stage, spasm of the muscles of mastication causes trismus and difficulty with chewing, i.e., lockjaw. Sustained contraction of the facial muscles produces a distorted grin (risus sardonicus). Figure 3 demonstrates risus sardonicus and carpopedal spasm as well as opisthotonos. Spasm of the pharyngeal muscles makes swallowing difficult. Stiff neck and opisthotonos are also among the early signs. Progressively, other muscle groups become involved, with tightness of the chest and rigidity of the abdominal wall, the back, and the limbs. Generalized tonic convulsions are frequent and exhausting. Any sudden jar or sound, such as a hypodermic injection or the fall of a broom outside the patient's door, will excite such generalized convulsions. Generally speaking, touch or position change is more likely to trigger the convulsions than is stimulation by light or sound. In association with these convulsions, spasm of the laryngeal and respiratory muscles is present, sometimes with a resulting respiratory arrest and possibly fatal acute asphyxia. Respiratory complications are the most common cause of death; and, in neonatal tetanus in particular, the inability to swallow and aspiration can lead to a rapid demise.

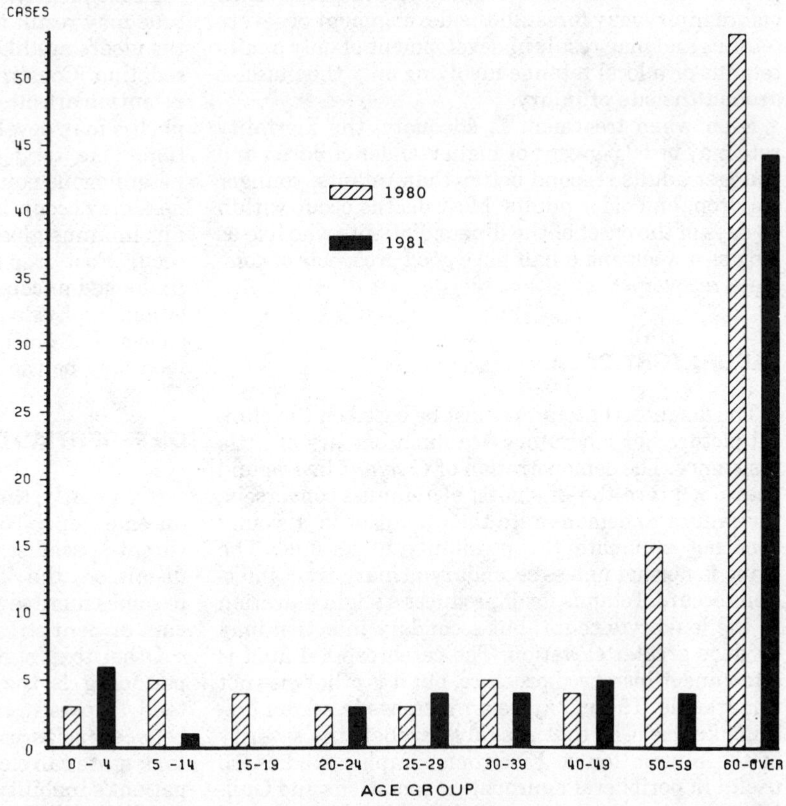

Figure 2. Reported cases of tetanus by age group, in The United States, 1980 and 1981. Cases with unknown ages are excluded. The largest number occurs in those older than the 60-year-old age group, suggesting inadequate immunization against tetanus in this group. (Courtesy of Centers for Disease Control, public health service, U.S. Department of Health and Human Services. Annual Summary 1981, *Morbidity and Mortality Weekly Report* 30:88, 1982.)

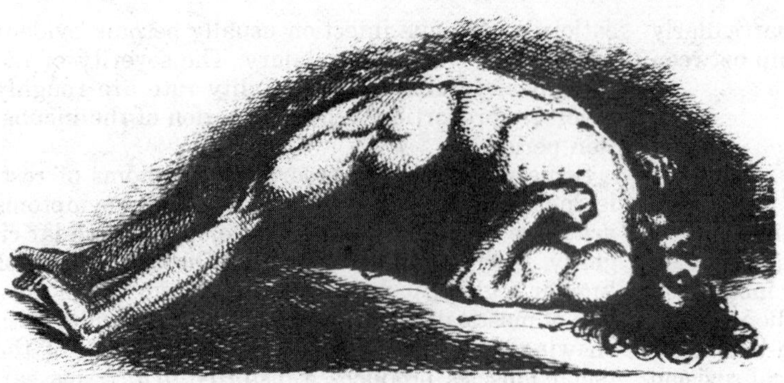

Figure 3. Tetanus as depicted by Sir Charles Bell during the middle of the 19th century. (Courtesy of United States National Library of Medicine.)

The patient is mercilessly mentally clear throughout the course of the disease and suffers great pain from the muscular spasms. The pulse rate is elevated, and there is profuse perspiration. Vegetative disturbances, including increased or decreased blood pressure and even respiratory irregularities, can originate from the effects of the toxin on the medulla, but the major neurologic findings are hyperactive reflexes, clonus, and the stimulus-sensitive myoclonus or spasms. Sensory changes are absent. Fever may or may not be present.

If the patient survives, the intensity of the muscular contractions begins to diminish during about the second week. Even with adequate treatment, improvement may be slow; contractions can continue for over a week. Complete recovery may take several months.

Occasionally, mild cases occur in which there is only moderate muscle rigidity without tetanus seizures. The administration of tetanus antitoxin to a person who has not had tetanus toxoid prophylaxis before injury may forestall the development of severe tetanus and may result in development of only a mild tetanus or a local tetanus involving only the muscles around the site of injury.

Even when treatment is adequate, the mortality rate may be 50 per cent or higher. Older children and younger adults respond better than infants, younger children, and older adults. Most deaths occur within 10 days of the onset of the illness. Patients who live as long as a week and a half have good prospects of complete recovery.

LABORATORY DATA

The diagnosis of tetanus must be based on the clinical picture, for laboratory examinations are of little assistance. The demonstration of *C. tetani* in a wound does not prove the diagnosis of tetanus; conversely, the failure to demonstrate the organism in a wound does not eliminate the possibility of tetanus. The urine is normal unless secondary urinary tract infections occurs. Tetanus itself produces a slight elevation in the leukocyte count, but secondary infection may produce greater elevation. The cerebrospinal fluid is often under increased pressure, but it is otherwise not remarkable. There may be an increase in serum creatine kinase (CK) that roughly parallels the severity of the muscle tonus. Electromyographic studies, so useful in peripheral neuropathic conditions and Guillain-Barré syndrome, are of little value in tetanus. Electroencephalograms may be useful in estimating the extent of cerebral involvement, especially in patients who have had hypoxia. The activity recorded on electroencephalograms is not specifically diagnostic of tetanus, but serial electroencephalograms at the proper time during the course of the disease may be of considerable importance in the long-range evaluation and care of the patient and in respect to liability problems.

COMMON COMPLICATIONS

Complications and death in early tetanus are almost solely due to respiratory difficulty and can often be avoided by adequate control of the muscle spasms. Pulmonary atelectasis may be followed by pneumonia, which is especially to be dreaded, for it seriously lessens the chances of recovery. Traumatic glossitis is seen frequently. Compression fractures of the vertebrae may result from the convulsive seizures. Decubitus ulcers are likely to occur in patients under heavy sedation. Constipation, fecal impaction, and urinary retention are often encountered. Cystitis and pyelonephritis may develop in patients requiring catheterization. One to 3 weeks after the administration of heterologous equine or bovine antitoxin, serum sickness may occur. If homologous human antitoxin (tetanus immune globulin) is given, such sickness will not occur. Foot drop and muscle contractures may follow prolonged unconsciousness with the limbs in poor position. Asphyxia from respiratory or laryngeal muscle spasm or from aspiration of secretions, vomitus, or food may be the immediate cause of death.

DIFFERENTIAL DIAGNOSIS

Frequently, the tetanus patient has been seen by (1) an emergency room physician, (2) an ear, nose, and throat specialist, or (3) a dentist, each of whom has dismissed the patient. Then, when the tetanus becomes more severe, the patient returns to the physician or dentist.

Other toxic states rarely mimic tetanus; strychnine poisoning is the classic example. Whereas spasms tend to persist in tetanus, the muscles are relaxed between seizures in strychnine poisoning, and this toxic state can clear rapidly. Rabies is indicated by the patient's inability to swallow as an early symptom, by drooling of saliva, and by spasms of the muscles of deglutition. Hypocalcemia, especially in the neonate, may produce rigidity but usually not the severe sensitivity of tetanus. Tetany, when related to parathyroid dysfunction, is rarely severe and may affect only the upper limbs. Laboratory studies will clarify these problems. The remarkably common acute dystonic reaction secondary to phenothiazines can be diagnosed by history as well as by the rapid response to treatment. Toxicity secondary to penicillin or haloperidol use may produce a tetanus-like condition. Heterologous serum sickness can be confused with early tetanus.

In addition to such toxic problems, infectious states can produce some increased tone, particularly meningitis or encephalitis. In these conditions, tremor or myoclonus can also occur, but they usually have more cerebral involvement than tetanus and can be diagnosed by cerebrospinal fluid examination.

Local infections of the jaws or tumors and infections of the oropharynx will rarely lead to diagnostic confusion. Growth of a primary or secondary tumor is rarely missed, although we have seen one patient with severe trismus due to pressure of a large craniopharyngioma on the trigeminal region.

The spasms of a localized group of voluntary muscles caused by soft tissue or bone injuries may simulate local tetanus.

Hysteria or malingering can be confusing in all branches of medicine. One unusual patient presented such a picture in order to remain near a ward nurse and be with her, particularly at night. In such cases, the electroencephalogram can be of value. Hyperventilation syndrome, with concomitant carpopedal spasm, is usually brief and readily identified. The rigidity of parkinsonism, Jakob's disease, or the "stiff man" syndrome will not be confused with tetanus because of the long course and distinctive clinical pattern in each of these entities. Neonatal tetanus, though uncommon in developed countries, may be confused with many serious conditions of the neonate, such as meningitis, sepsis, hypocalcemic tetany, hypomagnesemia, metabolic alkalosis, and intracranial hemorrhage. Newborn infants of drug-addicted mothers may temporarily present a clinical picture suggesting tetanus.

While diagnostic efforts are under way, the response of the spasms to adequate therapy will help not only with diagnosis but also with prognostication. This toxi-infection must first be suspected in order to be diagnosed and may appear when least suspected.

BOTULISM

By Michael Cherington, M.D.
Denver, Colorado

DEFINITION

Botulism is a paralyzing disease caused by the most toxic substance known to humans. The toxin is produced by the bacterium *Clostridium botulinum*, and has been estimated to cause death in humans in doses as small as 0.1 to 1.0 μg. Eight immunologically distinct toxins have been identified (A, B, C_1, C_2, D, E, F, and G). Human botulism is almost always due to type A, B, or E. When contaminated seafood is found to be the responsible food, the toxin present is often type E. Types C and D toxins may not be absorbed by the human gastrointestinal tract.

Botulism toxin is heat labile and thus is often destroyed by cooking. By contrast, the spores of *C. botulinum* are heat-resistant. When spores are present in food, actively multiplying bacilli produce the toxin at room temperature and under anaerobic conditions at a pH of 6 or above. The toxin causes paralysis of skeletal muscles by interfering with the release of acetylcholine.

PRESENTING SIGNS AND SYMPTOMS

The clinical features of botulism have a characteristic presentation. The symptoms usually occur within 12 to 36 hours after ingestion of contaminated food. The signs and symptoms begin in the cranial nerve territory, with blurring of vision, dysarthria, and dysphagia. The signs then descend as a result of involvement of the extremities. This distinguishes botulism from the Guillain-Barré syndrome, which is characterized by ascending paralysis. Prominent features of botulism include external ophthalmoplegia and paralysis of the tongue. It would be most unusual, if not unique, for a patient to have paralysis of the limbs without some evidence of ophthalmoplegia. The pupils, however, are usually normal, particularly early in the disease.

CLINICAL COURSE

Weakness of skeletal muscles progresses until it reaches a plateau in about 4 or 5 days. Respiratory paralysis can follow and is often fatal unless dealt with. Alertness, mentation, and the sensory system remain normal. Symptoms of parasympathetic dysfunction may include dryness of the mouth and eyes and gastrointestinal ileus. Recovery, if it occurs, is prolonged but nearly total.

LABORATORY FINDINGS

Laboratory confirmation usually requires the detection of toxin in the patient's serum or stool, or in the contaminated food. Mouse toxicity tests with antiserum neutralization are most useful. Specimens that should be examined include serum, gastric contents, feces, exudates from wounds, and the contents of suspected jars or cans. The Centers for Disease Control in Atlanta, Georgia, along with the State Health Department, can be most helpful in the collection of these materials and in their testing. Radioimmunoassay tests may be practical in the future.

In many patients, particularly those who are not studied early, results of laboratory studies may be negative. It is particularly in these cases that electrophysiologic studies can be of much help to the clinician. The expected findings in botulism may be summarized as follows:

1. Motor conduction velocities are normal; sensory nerve amplitudes and latencies are also normal.

2. There is almost always a small evoked muscle action potential in response to a single supramaximal nerve stimulation *if* the tested limb is clinically affected; conversely, the amplitudes are normal in about 15 per cent of patients.

3. Post-tetanic facilitation is similar to, but less notable than, that seen in Lambert-Eaton syndrome. Whereas facilitation is always found in patients with Lambert-Eaton syndrome, 38 per cent of patients with botulism lacked evidence of facilitation. Evidence of facilitation is seen more often (84 per cent of patients) in type B botulism. The degree of facilitation in botulism is usually between 30 and 100 per cent; by contrast, in Lambert-Eaton syndrome facilitation is often twofold or more.

4. The decremental response of muscle action potential to slow rate of stimulation is absent or minimal (less than 8 per cent).

5. Needle electromyographic studies reveal an increased number of brief, polyphasic motor unit action potentials. These changes are found in muscles that are clinically affected. Single fiber electromyographic studies reveal increased jitter and blocking. Jitter is frequency-dependent and decreases with higher innervation frequency. Fiber density values are lowered.

REYE'S SYNDROME

By Timothy Patrick Bohan, M.D., Ph.D.
and Charles R. Roe, M.D.
Durham, North Carolina

SYNONYMS AND DEFINITION

In 1963 Reye and associates in Australia and Johnson and associates in the United States described a distinct clinical and pathologic entity characterized by encephalopathy and fatty infiltration of the viscera. Reye's syndrome is currently defined as an acute noninflammatory encephalopathy with concurrent fatty infiltration of the viscera and hepatocellular dysfunction. The diagnosis of Reye's syndrome requires the exclusion of other causes of encephalopathy and liver dysfunction as well as drug intoxication and inborn errors of metabolism.

Although Reye's syndrome has been described in young adults, it usually occurs in children. Sixty per cent of patients are 5 to 14 years of age, and 35 per cent are younger than 5 years of age. Of the remaining 5 per cent, most are younger than 20 years of age. Boys and girls are affected in equal numbers and over 90 per cent of patients are Caucasians. Although Reye's syndrome occurs year round, there is a higher incidence during the season of influenza, late winter and early spring. In the United States during the last 10 years, there have been 500 to 1000 cases per year with the higher incidence occurring in years with influenza B outbreaks. Several epidemiologic studies have demonstrated an association of Reye's syndrome with administration of aspirin during the antecedent illness. Some believe this indicates a causative role for aspirin in Reye's syndrome.

PRESENTING SIGNS AND SYMPTOMS

Prior to developing Reye's syndrome most patients are in good health and have had normal growth and development. The illness is biphasic, with the initial phase being a viral infection. In over 50 per cent of patients this is a respiratory infection. Although it is most commonly due to influenza A or B virus, it may also result from many of the other viruses that can infect the respiratory tract. Thirty per cent of patients have varicella, and 10 per cent have viral gastroenteritis. During, or shortly after, recovery from the initial illness, the child develops lethargy, irritability, and vomiting with little or no fever. Vomiting is the cardinal presenting symptom. Initially the patient's condition may fluctuate between lethargy and a hyperexcitable state with delirium and increased activity of the sympathetic nervous system (e.g., sweating, tachycardia, and pupillary dilation). There are also bilateral upper motor neuron lesions as indicated by hyperreflexia and bilateral Babinski signs. The neurologic signs may fluctuate, but they are always symmetric and nonfocal. Although a computed tomographic (CT) scan may show cerebral edema, neither papilledema nor a bulging fontanelle may be present initially.

The remainder of the physical examination is unremarkable. Skin lesions may be present if the preceding viral illness had an accompanying exanthem. Even with significant liver dysfunction, hepatomegaly may not be present.

COURSE

The progressive cerebral dysfunction is accompanied by cerebral edema and increased intracranial pressure. Cerebral dysfunction progresses in a rostrocaudal pattern that is in some ways similar to the pattern in patients with increased intracranial pressure from other causes. For prognostic reasons as well as for monitoring the progression of the disease, it is helpful to stage the severity of the illness. Several clinical staging systems exist as well as one based on the electroencephalogram (EEG). For clinical staging one can use a five-stage system (Table 1) similar to that of Lovejoy et al., whereas for EEG staging the system of Aoki and Lombroso (Table 2) is useful. Clinical staging is easier for continuous monitoring, whereas the EEG-based system has more prognostic value. EEG deterioration often precedes clinical deterioration.

The clinical course and prognosis depend on several factors, which include the stage of the disorder at the time of diagnosis, the speed and degree of progression, the age of the patient, the duration of the coma, and the degree and persistence of the intracranial hypertension. Other important prognostic factors are the severity of the acute complications and results of cer-

Table 1. Clinical Staging of Reye's Syndrome

	Stage 1	Stage 2	Stage 3	Stage 4	Stage 5
Level of Consciousness	Vomiting, lethargic and drowsy, but still responsive to command	Disoriented with mild delirium alternating with combative behavior; verbalizes inappropriately; unresponsive to command	Obtunded or comatose	Comatose	Comatose
Response to Pain	Normal	Purposeful	Decorticate	Decerebrate	Absent
Ventilatory Pattern	Normal to increased	Hyperventilation	Hyperventilation and possible Cheynes-Stokes breathing	Hyperventilation; irregular pattern or absent	Absent
Pupillary Reaction	Normal	Dilated and briskly responsive	Dilated and briskly responsive	Dilated and slowly responsive or even unresponsive	Absent
Reflexes					
Babinski	±	Present	Present	Present	Present or no response
Doll's eyes	Present	Present	Present	Absent	Absent
Response to caloric stimulation	Present	Present	Present	Dysconjugate	Absent
Corneal	Present	Present	Present	Possibly absent	Absent

tain laboratory tests. As one would expect, the prognosis is poorer with presentation in a more advanced stage and with rapid neurologic deterioration. In recent years, owing to earlier diagnosis and better treatment, the prognosis is better. In the past, many patients had reached an advanced stage by the time of diagnosis and a significant number died. Now most patients have Stage 1 or 2 disease at the time of diagnosis and have either minimal or no progression. Once neurologic improvement begins, relapse is unlikely. In patients who survive, the encephalopathy characteristically persists for 24 to 96 hours. In general, those who reach only Stage 2 survive, those who reach Stage 3 or 4 may have a 50 per cent morality rate, and those reaching Stage 5 have an 80 per cent mortality rate. The recent improvement in mortality rate, which is now 20 to 30 per cent, is primarily due to increased survival in older children. In children under the age of 3 years the mortality rate remains 50 per cent or greater. With more advanced stages of the disease (Stages 3 to 5) intracranial hypertension may exceed 20 cm of water and require more aggressive therapy (e.g., osmotic diuretics).

COMMON COMPLICATIONS

Except for shock, which may occur with Stage 5, acute complications in Reye's syndrome are essentially limited to the nervous system, specifically seizures and altered respiratory rate. Seizures, which may be tonic-clonic, multifocal, or myoclonic, usually do not occur until there are signs and symptoms of brain stem dysfunction (i.e., Stages 3 to 5). Consequently, they carry a poor prognosis. Surprisingly, there may be no EEG evidence of seizure discharges even when there are clinical convulsions. In children under the age of 3, seizures are more common and often occur during Stage 1 or 2. Seizures usually cease once recovery occurs. The respiratory abnormalities are more pronounced with more advanced stages of the disease (Table 1). Hyperventilation occurs in the early stages, Cheynes-Stokes respiration in Stage 3, more irregular patterns in Stage 4, and finally cessation of spontaneous respiration in Stage 5. Apnea and periodic breathing are more common in infants and may occur during Stages 1 and 2.

Although as a group the patients have a favorable neurologic prognosis, long-term neuropsychologic sequelae can occur, particularly in the more severely ill and in the younger patient. Indicators of the severity of the illness include duration of coma, highest stage reached, and the degree and persistence of the intracranial hypertension. If the coma lasts longer than 96 hours, there is a significant incidence of neurologic sequelae regardless of the age of the patient. Patients under 3 years old, and particularly infants under 1 year of age, have a 40 to 60 per cent incidence of pronounced developmental and even gross motor handicaps. In older children with apparent recovery, careful follow-up may reveal a significant proportion with psychological problems. The most common problems are transient anxiety reaction, possibly related to the illness, mild attention deficits, hyperactivity, and occasional mild dysarthria.

LABORATORY FINDINGS

Laboratory studies are essential for differentiating Reye's syndrome from other causes of acute encephalopathy, particularly viral encephalitis. More rarely, Reye's syndrome could be confused with other forms of acute liver failure as well as with intoxications and inherited metabolic disorders.

A brain CT scan may show cerebral edema but will otherwise be nonfocal, thereby ruling out a structural lesion. Lumbar puncture should be performed and may demonstrate either a normal or elevated pressure. Lumbar puncture is not contraindicated by the possibility of elevated cerebrospinal fluid pressure. The cerebrospinal fluid protein and glucose levels will be normal unless there is significant systemic hypoglycemia, in which case there will be hypoglycorrhacia. Most important, there should be no more than 8 white cells per cu mm and these should all be lymphocytes.

Table 2. Electroencephalographic Staging in Reye's Syndrome

Stage	Background Activity	Age (Years)
1	Predominant theta and less alpha	Over 10
	Predominant theta and less delta	5–10
	Predominant delta and less theta	Under 5
2	Predominant theta and less delta	Over 10
	Predominant delta and less theta	5–10
	Predominant delta and little theta	Under 5
3	Diffuse high voltage rhythmic or arrhythmic delta activity with little or no theta	All ages
4	(a) Diffuse, mostly low voltage (less than 50 μV) delta activity with little or no theta activity	All ages
	(b) Burst-suppression activity	All ages
5	Nearly isoelectric activity	

Reye's syndrome can be differentiated from other forms of liver failure by the characteristic pattern of laboratory values (Table 3), which indicate that in Reye's syndrome there is predominantly mitochondrial damage. A bilirubin level greater than 2.5 mg/dl indicates that the liver dysfunction is due to some condition other than Reye's syndrome. In addition, the prolonged prothrombin time may reflect an insufficient amount of Vitamin K. A serum amylase reading should be obtained to rule out pancreatitis. The concentration of serum glucose is usually normal except in children under 5 years old, who may have marked hypoglycemia. Arterial blood gas measurements may show both a respiratory alkalosis due to hyperventilation, and a metabolic acidosis due to presence of lactic acid and other organic acids.

A liver biopsy obtained during the acute illness shows diffuse small-droplet fatty infiltration of the liver parenchyma. The mitochondria characteristically are spherical or ameboid in shape with swollen matrixes, loss of cristae, and dense bodies. Less commonly seen are proliferation of endoplasmic reticulum, increased numbers of peroxisomes, and empty Golgi membranes. Although a liver biopsy may confirm a diagnosis of Reye's syndrome, it is usually not

Table 3. Biochemical Criteria for Reye's Syndrome

	Degree of Abnormality
Blood ammonia	At least twice normal
Serum transaminases	2–3 times normal
Prothrombin time	> 1.3 times control
Bilirubin	< 2.5 mg/dl

necessary. In addition to the risk of bleeding, diagnostic electron micrographs may not be available for several days. Furthermore, it is not certain that inborn errors of metabolism can be excluded by electron microscopy.

In addition to clarifying the diagnosis, laboratory studies have prognostic importance and are helpful in following the course of the disease. Children with a peak serum ammonia concentration more than five times normal have not only a higher mortality rate but also a higher incidence of neurologic sequelae. The peak ammonia concentration usually occurs within 4 hours of admission and correlates with overall severity of the disease. However, serial ammonia concentrations do not correlate with the degree of coma. The ammonia may decrease toward normal values with persisting coma. Serum lactic acid concentration does, however, correlate with the degree of the coma. Additionally, serum hepatic and muscle enzyme concentrations—serum glutamic-oxaloacetic transaminase (SGOT), serum glutamic-pyruvic transaminase (SGPT), and creatine kinase (CK)—may be valuable predictors of outcome. Primary liver involvement (elevated transaminases with SGPT greater than SGOT and near normal levels of CK), or primary muscle involvement (an elevated CK and normal to only mildly elevated transaminases with SGOT greater than SGPT), suggests the patient will survive. Dual organ involvement (elevation of CK and transaminases with SGPT greater than SGOT) suggests that the patient will die.

POTENTIAL ERRORS AND PITFALLS

Drug intoxications and inborn errors of metabolism must be distinguished from Reye's syndrome. The intoxications that can mimic Reye's syndrome are listed in Table 4 and should be excluded. Intoxications by salicylate and valproic acid are those most commonly confused with Reye's syndrome. Serum salicylate level should always be determined. In Reye's syndrome the serum salicylate level is in or below the therapeutic range (less than 20 mg/dl).

Recently, valproic acid has been associated with a number of cases of a Reye's syndrome–like disorder with vomiting and altered mental status, but no jaundice. This rare complication, from which most patients recover, can occur even when the serum concentration of valproic acid is within the therapeutic range. To date, 80 per cent of the patients with severe toxicity have been under the age of 20 years. Most cases occur within the first 12 months of therapy. Although both serum transaminases and ammonia are usually elevated, stupor and coma can occur with normal levels of transaminases and only hyperammonemia. Patients taking valproic acid can also develop an asymptomatic hyperammonemia, which appears to be related to a deficiency in carnitine. Although in the United States there have been over 20 deaths in patients taking valproic acid, these patients apparently had a different problem with jaundice and hepatic necrosis rather than a Reye's syndrome–like condition.

Rare inborn errors in metabolism should be considered in the differential diagnosis of Reye's syndrome. These should be considered specifically in (1) children under the age of 3 years; (2) children with previously abnormal growth or development; (3) children with "recurrent" Reye's syndrome; and (4) children with a family history of Reye's syndrome.

The work-up for inherited metabolic disorders should be focused on these disorders, which can mimic Reye's syndrome (Table 5). Certain routine laboratory tests may be helpful in suggesting a particular type of disorder. The combination of thrombocytopenia and hyperammonemia suggests propionic or methylmalonic aciduria, whereas an extremely elevated ammonia concentration (greater than 1000 μg/dl) suggests a primary urea cycle defect. A complete evaluation for inborn errors of metabolism should include measurement of serum amino acids, urinary organic acids, and serum and urinary total and free carnitine levels. The organic acids and carnitine measurements, which are only available in specialized laboratories, not only allow differentiation of inherited disorders from Reye's syndrome but are also diagnostic. The carnitine values are important to diagnose both systemic carnitine deficiency and organic acidurias that may be complicated by secondary carnitine deficiency.

Table 4. Some Intoxications that Can Masquerade as Reye's Syndrome

Salicylism
Valproic acid (Depakene) intoxications
Chlordane intoxications
"Outdated" tetracycline intoxications
Phenformin intoxications
Pyrrolizidine (Senecio) intoxications
Methyl bromide intoxications
Jamaican vomiting sickness
Isopropyl alcohol intoxications

In summary, patients presenting with the signs and symptoms of Reye's syndrome represent a heterogeneous group, which includes those with genetic disorders and intoxications. Selection of appropriate therapy requires accurate diagnosis.

Table 5. Inborn Errors of Metabolism that Can Masquerade as Reye's Syndrome

Propionic acidemia
Methylmalonic aciduria
Primary urea cycle defects
Systemic carnitine deficiency
Primary lactic acidosis
3-Hydroxy-3-Methylglutaric aciduria
Glutaric aciduria type II
Suberylglycinuria
Defect in fatty acid oxidation

METABOLIC ENCEPHALOPATHY

By Simon Horenstein, M.D.
St. Louis, Missouri

DEFINITION

The terms metabolic, exogenous, or secondary encephalopathy and metabolic coma are applied to disorders of the brain of diverse origin, including endogenous and endocrine diseases, exogenous toxins and drugs, and some physical agents. These states are characterized by altered consciousness, impaired mental function, disordered posture and movement, and recently acquired toxic, biochemical, and electroencephalographic abnormalities. These conditions usually result from intoxications or diseases that alter metabolism outside the central nervous system and affect the latter only secondarily. Endogenous derangements of cerebral metabolism that appear to result from disorders of nerve cells independent of changes in function of extraneural organs will not be considered here. This article will emphasize those disorders that occur commonly, require urgent treatment, and may result in irreversible damage to the nervous system. Table 1 lists the common forms of metabolic encephalopathy and the approaches to their diagnosis.

The major features of metabolic encephalopathy—disturbance of consciousness, impairment of mental function, disorder of posture and movement, and abnormalities of body chemistry and electrographic function—are present to varying degrees in each patient. Except for an acute confusional disorder followed by coma within 7 to 9 seconds consequent upon abrupt and complete anoxia, these conditions begin slowly and evolve over the course of minutes (e.g., hypoglycemia), hours (e.g., hepatic encephalopathy), or days (e.g., uremic encephalopathy). The abrupt onset of coma in the absence of hypoxia is more likely to reflect an intracerebral catastrophe, such as brain hemorrhage or an epileptic disorder. Metabolic encephalopathy of endocrine or endogenous type almost always emerges from a background of clear-cut, previously known, and easily recognized systemic disease. It frequently occurs while the patient is under medical observation in hospital and often is the direct result of drugs or other treatments that have recently been administered. As a general rule, the development of a neurologic syndrome in a patient suffering a non-neurologic disease should suggest that the former is caused by the non-neurologic disease or its treatment.

CAUSES OF METABOLIC ENCEPHALOPATHY

The most frequent clinical disorders that predispose to metabolic brain disease are (1) exposure to exogenous poisons—in particular, medically or self-prescribed sedative or tranquilizing drugs, or substances used for recreational purposes; (2) metabolic acidosis; (3) liver disease, (4) kidney disease, (5) lung disease, (6) endocrine disorders; (7) hypoxic hypoxia; (8) ischemic hypoxia; (9) hypoglycemia; (10) derangements of ionic equilibrium or serum osmolality; or (11) exposure to physical agents, notably heat (Fig. 1).

The ease with which any given patient may develop encephalopathy, regardless of cause, and the rate at which it evolves are not uniform but appear to depend upon the nature and degree of metabolic derangement. They seem, moreover, to be proportional to the age of the patient; the quality of general health; the nature, severity, and duration of pre-existing or associated brain lesions; the concomitant administration of medication; and the nature of the environment in which the illness is evolving. Rapid changes in acid-base equilibrium may result in asymmetric fluid or ion shifts in various tissue compartments. These in turn serve to maintain, enhance, or sustain confusion and are likely to complicate the course and treatment of renal disease. The resulting confusion or coma may indicate the development of secondary water intoxication.

Younger age is a factor that often affords protection against the effects of hypoxia. Alternatively, elderly patients may develop symptoms of drug intoxication at relatively lower doses and blood levels than younger people (e.g., bromism). Differential metabolism of benzodiazepines predisposes the elderly to drug-induced confusion. It is believed that derangements secondary to or associated with congestive heart failure, chronic obstructive pulmonary disease, or diabetes mellitus may be additive to those induced by biochemical abnormalities or endocrine organ failure. Such a concatenation of events compounds the effects of each, thus resulting in neurologic disease earlier or to a greater degree than might have occurred were the person not suffering such complicated illness.

In any disorder that might affect behavior, a nervous system which has been influenced by intrinsic or endogenous disease has less "behavioral reserve." A common example is the ease with which patients with senile dementia may become severely confused when subjected to minor degrees of fever, hypotension, or dehydration. Manageable and hence therapeutically significant factors include care in the use of sedative, hypnotic, analgesic, anticholinergic, or stimulant drugs in treating behavioral disorders, as they may worsen other effects of metabolic derangement. The occurrence of progressive confusion and stupor in a hospitalized patient who was alert at admission most often reflects adverse reaction to medication or some other aspect of care. The environment in which a confusional illness is occurring determines to an important degree the extent of the mental disorder. A quiet room in which the patient sees hardly more than bare walls and hears little save indistinct or muffled sounds may result in "perceptual isolation," with hallucinosis and disorientation. It may include prolonged periods of sleep, which lead to further disorientation. Patients recovering from drug withdrawal delirium or hepatic or uremic encephalopathy may benefit from the provision of a lamp, short but frequent visits, familiar objects to look at or handle, and protection

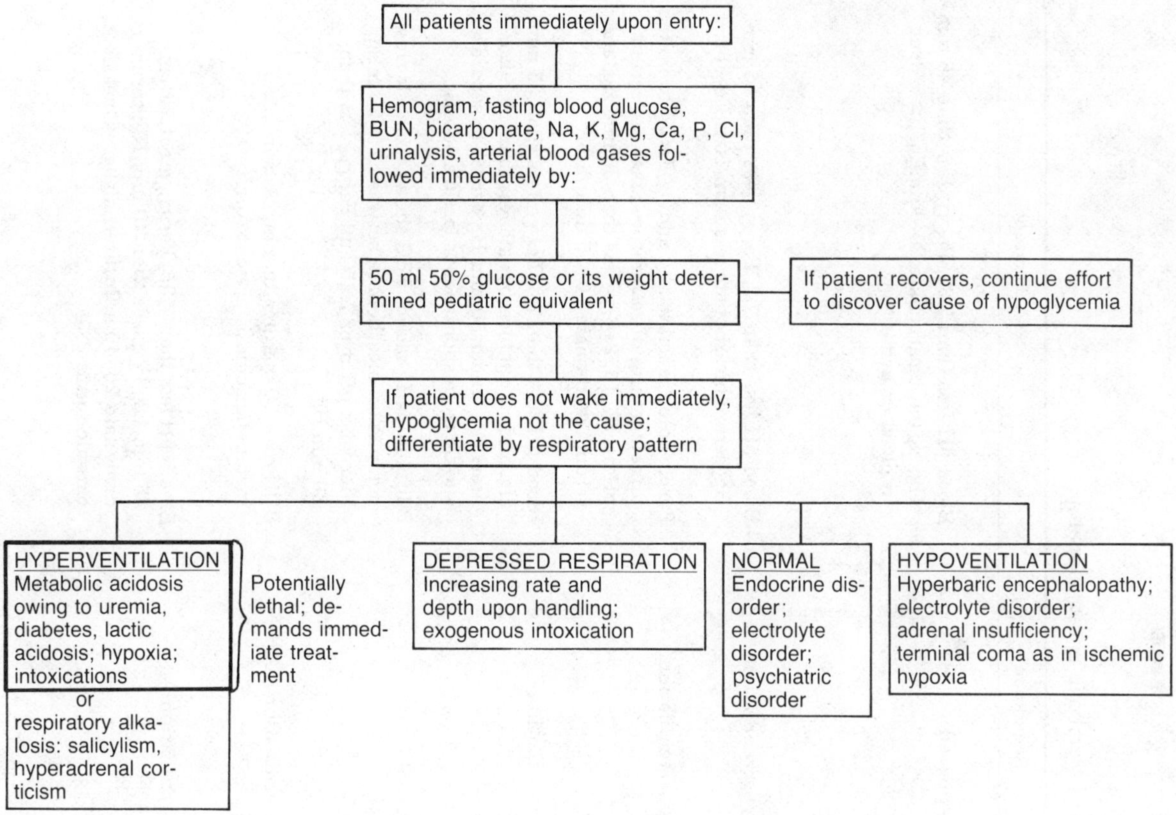

Figure 1. Detection of treatable forms of metabolic encephalopathy.

from indistinct sounds, as these measures alone may lessen the confusion and materially reduce the "encephalopathy."

MANIFESTATIONS

Disturbances of Consciousness

The disturbance of consciousness that occurs in metabolic brain disease may be expressed as either delirium or stupor and appears to result from affection of the cerebral cortex, the reticular formation, or both. Environmental factors additionally may determine moment-to-moment changes in the severity of the delirium or stupor independently of any change in the underlying disorder. Thus, it often happens that with very little change in body chemistry, oxygenation, or cerebral perfusion, rapid fluctuations between delirium and stupor may occur as a patient is stimulated, examined, or subjected to such nursing procedures as bathing.

Confusion is the common denominator of both delirium and stupor. It is a term that is applied to that disturbance of mental function in which an individual's orientation to self and environment is grossly altered despite the preservation, to any degree, of other mental or intellectual functions, such as the ability to calculate or identify persons or objects. It usually is acute and transient. The major functions affected are the senses of time (including the knowledge of the date and the ability to estimate elapsed time) and place. Personal disorientation is a later and more extreme aspect of confusion and may be so severe that the patient does not know whether he or she is dressed. It is, however, rare that patients forget their own names. Loss of memory for one's own name and preservation of other aspects of orientation and mental function is highly suggestive of a psychogenic disorder. When confusion is accompanied by drowsiness or lethargy, the patient is said to be stuporous. The patient usually appears drowsy or may be found asleep. It may be difficult to rouse the patient, or, once alerted, he or she may be unable to maintain an attentive state. Occasionally the stuporous patient will become agitated when disturbed.

A state of confusion accompanied by agitation, sleeplessness, and excessive attentiveness to any novel stimulus is called delirium. In this hyperactive state the patient may be sweaty, wide-eyed, tremulous, and readily startled; often there is active hallucination. The hallucinations may be auditory, especially in drug-withdrawal states. When they are, their content is commonly offensive and obscene, provoking in turn additional agitation and terror. Visual hallucinations may range from a moving spot in the periphery of the field which the patient endlessly pursues but never quite catches, to intensely perceived specters at which he or she stares fixedly. The former is characteristic of drug-withdrawal delirium, such as from alcohol, and the latter often accompanies intoxication, as with anticholinergic drugs. Somatic hallucinations, such as the sensation that ants are crawling on or beneath the skin or that someone else is sharing the bed, are less often encountered.

Table 1. Differentiation of Common Forms of Metabolic Encephalopathy

Type	Features	Respiration	Laboratory
I. Exogenous poisons	Known user; flask or container found		
	a. Stupor or coma—often "sleep-like"; pupils may be small and reactive (opiates) or fixed and large (glutethimide, anticholinergics); odor of alcohol may be present; hypothermia with barbiturates, phenothiazine; nystagmus, ocular palsy with thiamine deficiency in alcoholic	a. Depressed	Blood pH less than 7.35, Pa_{CO_2} less than 45 mm Hg; serum bicarbonate 20–30 mEq/liter; drug in blood or urine
	b. Methyl alcohol, ethylene glycol, decomposed paraldehyde odor on breath or body in a stuporous or comatose person	b. Hyperventilation	Blood pH less than 7.3, Pa_{CO_2} less than 35 mm Hg; serum bicarbonate less than 10 mEq/liter
	c. Salicylates—fever; stupor or coma, often in a child; if awake, may complain of dizziness or ringing in ears; history of chronic salicylate usage	c. Hyperventilation	Purple color generated by adding $FeCl_3$ to boiled urine; features of respiratory alkalosis; serum pH over 7.45, Pa_{CO_2} less than 30 mm Hg, and serum bicarbonate 10–15 mEq/liter
II. Metabolic acidosis	Acute coma in uremia, diabetes (ketoacidosis or lactic acidosis), anoxia, intoxication (see I.b)	Hyperventilation	Blood pH less than 7.3, Pa_{CO_2} less than 35 mm Hg, and serum bicarbonate less than 10 mEq/liter; P_{O_2} under 50 mm Hg serves to separate anoxic from spontaneous lactic acidosis
III. Hepatic encephalopathy	Signs of liver diseased marked; asterixis, myoclonus prominent; may be decerebrate in deep coma	Hyperventilation	Bilirubin, NH_3 raised; EEG shows triphasic slow complexes; bicarbonate between 15–25 mEq/liter with pH over 7.45 and Pa_{CO_2} less than 30 mm Hg
IV. Uremic encephalopathy	Known renal disease; reflexes often reduced; uremic odor and frost; asterixis, myoclonus, seizures prominent	Hyperventilation	BUN over 50 mg/dl; albumin, casts in urine, metabolic acidosis present (q.v.)
V. CO_2 narcosis or hypercarbic encephalopathy	Deformed, emphysematous chest; rales; cyanosis; clubbed fingers; occasional papilledema; often obese; slow respiratory rate	Hypoventilation	Blood pH less than 7.35; Pa_{CO_2} greater than 45 mm Hg; P_{O_2} less than 40 mm Hg; serum bicarbonate 20–40 mEq/liter, higher values in chronic forms

VI. Endocrinopathies: pituitary, thyroid, parathyroid, adrenal, pancreatic	Deep coma possible, especially in myxedema, but not the rule; signs of primary endocrine disorder often prominent or known; usually not primary presentation of underlying disorder; common clinical causes are abandonment of replacement therapy, especially in myxedema and stress or steroid withdrawal in first- or second-degree adrenal insufficiency	Respiration usually normal except in adrenal insufficiency where hypoventilation prominent	Hormonal abnormality on specific testing, skull x-ray abnormal in pituitary disease; renal stones in hyperparathyroidism; metabolic alkalosis (pH over 7.45, Pa_{CO_2} under 55 mm Hg, and serum bicarbonate over 30 mEq/liter with hypokalemia) in hyperadrenal corticism
VII. Hypoxia or anoxia	Cyanotic; cherry red (CO poison); purplish lips (methemoglobinemia); occurs with pulmonary disease, oxygen-poor environment (anoxic form), anemia or hemoglobin inactivation (CO poisoning or methemoglobinemia)	Hyperventilation	Hypoxic form—P_{O_2}, O_2 saturation low; anemic form—P_{O_2} normal, saturation low or normal; toxic form—CO hemoglobin, methemoglobin in blood
VIII. Ischemia (defective oxygen delivery plus accumulation of metabolic by-products)	Results from any condition which may lower cerebral blood flow, especially cardiac arrhythmia, myocardial or pulmonary infarction, shock, sepsis, congestive heart failure, vasospasm in hypertensive or lead encephalopathy, fat embolism to lung	Usually hyperventilation, but breaths may be shallow; arrest of respiration may occur	P_{O_2}, O_2 saturation may be normal; ECG abnormal; enzymes elevated in serum; P_{O_2}, CO_2 decreased, lung scan positive in pulmonary embolism; raised intracranial pressure and CSF protein in lead intoxication; hypertension; fat globules in urine and sputum in fat embolism
IX. Hypoglycemia	Vast majority in diabetics receiving oral agents or insulin; may be abrupt or slow; usually recurrent; delirium-stupor, focal weakness, focal or generalized seizures, reversed rapidly by 50 ml 50% glucose IV	Central neurogenic hyperventilation or Cheyne-Stokes respiration	Blood sugar less than 30 mg/dl
X. Derangements of ionic equilibrium or serum osmolality	Delirium, stupor, weakness, seizures; may be seen following diuresis, excess water intake, especially after tap-water enema or use of "water" diuresis, feeding of excess electrolyte, or hyperglycemia in diabetic or burned patients without ketosis; hypercalcemia may be seen in bone-destructive or chronic renal disease	Unaltered or hypoventilation	Na, K, Ca, Mg lowered or raised with corresponding abnormality of serum osmolality (less than 260 mOsm/kg or more than 320); ECG in hypokalemia shows sagging ST segment, depressed T waves, elevated U waves

Stupor suggests a metabolic encephalopathy of hepatic or endocrinopathic origin, whereas delirium is more likely to be present with milder degrees of hypoxia, uremia, or withdrawal from drugs of both therapeutic and recreational variety. If the metabolic encephalopathy is associated with deficiency of a vitamin or other nutritional factor, the heightened energy requirements of the delirium may seriously and rapidly deplete the patient's remaining stores of the deficient factor. A new or heightened neurologic deficit may emerge. It is likely to be focal and to reflect neuronal failure, maximal in regions most dependent on the deficient substance. The distribution of lesions in the mamillary bodies, walls of the third and fourth ventricles, and about the aqueduct of Sylvius in Wernicke-Korsakoff disease is an example of the greater dependence of these structures on thiamine. Delirium or stupor may then be followed by greater impairment of consciousness, leading ultimately to deep coma. In these states, signs of destruction of the brain stem (loss of pupillary and vestibular reflexes) may be present.

Intellectual Changes

The intellectual changes of metabolic brain disease, especially when chronic, recurrent, and mild enough to sustain detailed examination, are often variable but may become irreversible. The chief disorders are likely to be of memory, attention, and emotional control. Other aspects of intellect, such as abstracting and planning ability, perceptual and cognitive function, calculation, reasoning, and the use of language, may be affected, although not necessarily in proportion to the memory disorder. The latter may be one in which recollection of past and recent events is lost, leaving intact very short-term or "scratch-pad" memory. Alternatively, it may spare many components of past memory but severely impair recall of recent events. When the genesis of the disorder or the history of the illness is unknown, the finding of any severe deficit in memory or cognitive function may mislead the physician into thinking the patient has a primary dementing disorder, such as Alzheimer's disease. The diagnostic clue inevitably resides in the fact that an extraneural illness accompanies metabolic encephalopathy, while the patient who has Alzheimer's disease alone is usually in good physical health. Profound disorder of intellect without intense confusion is not a feature of metabolic encephalopathy. When confusion is disproportionately intense, it may mean that a recently acquired metabolic encephalopathy has superimposed upon some other disease of the brain—e.g., pre-existing senile dementia or the cumulative effects of multiple small infarcts.

Although acute confusional states tend to subside, many who have suffered episodes of metabolic encephalopathy are left with permanent intellectual change. This is particularly likely to occur in conditions such as hypoglycemia, ischemia, and hypoxia. Moreover, since they tend to recur, cumulative damage to the brain often results in an apparently progressive dementia. In other conditions, such as hepatic encephalopathy, the change in mental state fluctuates with variations in the amount of toxic materials (e.g., ammonia) present in the blood or in the cells of the brain. Improvement in mental function after admission to hospital despite lack of specific treatment should raise the suspicion that the patient has been exposed to an exogenous or self-administered toxin, such as barbiturates, scopolamine, or various street drugs, or has failed to conform to the stringencies of treatment, as may happen in the course of thyroid disease when noncompliance may lead to the development of myxedema encephalopathy.

The lasting intellectual loss in chronic metabolic encephalopathy is likely to be subtle, variable in its expression, and marked by major disorders of conative function, in which planning, execution, judgment, and abstracting capacities are impaired, while language function, vision, and perception are better preserved. The behavioral outcome in any case appears to depend upon interaction among three sets of forces. The first is anatomic. Thus, lesions which involve the hippocampus, as in hypoxia, cause severe impairment of memory. The second is the mass of the lesion or lesions. Thus, the degree and extent of pathology affect the totality of behavior independently of the density of focal processes. This may be seen by comparing behavioral disintegration in hypoglycemia with its preservation after capsular infarction with hemiplegia. The third is the nature of the premorbid personality, including the patient's special skills, intelligence, habitual reaction patterns, and personality.

Motor Disturbances

Motor derangements occur regularly in both chronic and acute forms of metabolic encephalopathy but are not present to the same degree in every patient or on the two sides of the body. Their existence may be a clue to the presence of metabolic brain disorder. They may be divided into those that impair the use and posture of the limbs, face, and trunk, and those that express themselves as autonomic abnormalities, especially involving the reactions of the pupils and the pattern of breathing.

Restlessness. The most common of the motor abnormalities is restlessness. This is seen in delirious or agitated patients. Each novel stimulus catches the attention of the patient who, owing to imperception of its nature, commonly responds excessively. The random occurrence of unclear or indistinct events in the environment, coupled with inability of the patient to sustain interest in them, appears to be a necessary condition for such hyperactivity.

Myoclonus. Myoclonus may be observed in nearly all forms of metabolic encephalopathy. It may be "bulbar" and appear as an abrupt, bilateral, and symmetric movement marked by flexion of the neck, trunk, and limbs. Each episode may occur singly or may be repeated and become self-sustaining. Bulbar myoclonus resembles the common and normal startle reaction seen when a preoccupied individual is touched suddenly, but it differs in that it does not habituate. Thus, the normal startle reaction can rarely be evoked more than twice, but stimulus-sensitive myoclonus may be elicited repeatedly. Focal, segmental, or isolated myoclonus is somewhat more common than the bulbar form. It may occur in multiple foci simultaneously and is less likely to be provoked by sound, light, or touch. It often bears a close relationship to muscle contraction, occurring at the beginning or end of movement. Each focus generally remains restricted to a muscle or a muscle segment, although many parts may be involved. Such myoclonus rarely becomes generalized and is only infrequently the precursor of a generalized convulsion.

Multifocal myoclonus is quite common, and careful bedside evaluation should disclose the fact that several foci are active simultaneously. Myoclonus may occasionally be seen as a duplicated or repeated contraction of very brief duration. Occasionally a whole muscle is involved, leading to joint displacement. Each twitch is quite brief, although occasionally a focus of myoclonus may become sustained, producing continuing localized contraction of a body segment, such as the pectoralis major muscle or a quadrant of the abdominal wall. This is called "status epilepticus partialis continua." When confined to one part or side of the body, it may indicate localized brain disease. A simultaneously recorded electroencephalogram may contain low-voltage slow or fast waves or disclose multiphasic bursts of high-amplitude, sharp and slow activity, neither of which need coincide with the movements.

Myoclonus regardless of form usually does not subside upon anticonvulsant drug administration and may persist when the patient is asleep. It may continue into the recovery period. It is an early and frequent phenomenon after drug withdrawal, especially of alcohol and barbiturates, and a relatively late although persistent one in uremia. In many forms of chronic metabolic encephalopathy, such as that associated with liver disease, its variations provide a sensitive indication of fluctuations in the underlying process. Myoclonus appears to indicate disorganization in the pattern of neuronal activation. It is not an "epileptic" phenomenon and appears to result from disease at any anatomic level, including the spinal cord.

Asterixis. Asterixis, often called "liver flap" or "metabolic flap," is an intermittent irregularity of sustained effort which occurs in numerous forms of metabolic encephalopathy. It is totally unrelated to any other disorder of movement and is involuntary rather than the result of inattentiveness. Most patients are unaware of its presence and cannot restrain it when attention is called to it. It occurs as a violation of reciprocal innervation when for a brief time simultaneous inhibition of protagonistic and antagonistic muscles occurs. This event is seen clinically as a lapse of posture. The quick restitution to the erstwhile posture that follows completes the "flap." Asterixis may be seen in any muscle group, including the tongue, face, or eyebrows. It may be asymmetric and is not seen to the same extent in all affected areas or at all times. In uremia and hepatic insufficiency it appears early and frequently. It is most readily detected by asking the patient to maintain a part of the body in a fixed attitude, e.g., extending the wrist and fingers. Since many patients with asterixis are drowsy or stuporous, the physician must ensure that the patient is sufficiently awake and alert to comply. It is possible to recognize the flapping tremors of asterixis even when the patient is drowsy. The torpid patient may be asked to squeeze the physician's fingers firmly and steadily. When asterixis is present, irregular relaxation and contraction may be felt. Another technique is to ask the patient to squeeze the bulb of a sphygmomanometer, in which case variations in the pressure can be seen. Asterixis may also be superimposed upon the grasp reflex.

Tremor. Either static or kinetic tremor is common in metabolic encephalopathy and may persist into recovery. It is usually rapid and of moderate amplitude, and hence easily seen. It ordinarily appears on both sides of the body and tends to be symmetric. The tremor in metabolic encephalopathy is usually not observed at rest and therefore is readily distinguished from that of paralysis agitans or a complication of the use of phenothiazine drugs. It may occur during the active phase of movement (kinetic) or after movement has been completed and the limb is being maintained in a fixed position (static). Like asterixis, it disappears in coma. When permanent, it suggests some fixed alteration of brain function. Anatomic studies have failed to implicate any single part of the brain. The tremor may represent either the result of diffuse structural changes or permanent impairment of some unidentified forebrain transmitter mechanism.

Other Disturbances

Focal Weakness. Persistent focal weakness or lateralized reflex abnormalities are usually not parts of metabolic encephalopathy. Either may be present, however, when the onset has been abrupt, especially in the newborn and in hypoglycemia at any age. Such asymmetry, despite examples to the contrary, need not indicate associated cerebrovascular disease or structural brain pathology. Nevertheless, asymmetry of abnormalities in a patient who is presumed to have metabolic encephalopathy should alert the examiner to the possibility that an additional process is present. Suspicion of the latter should be high when focal or lateralized defects are profound while the confusional or "encephalopathic" component is mild, or if they persist after the mental irregularity has been corrected.

Speech Disorders. Impaired ability to name objects, read with comprehension, compose a paragraph, or sustain conversation are common features of metabolic encephalopathies along with other brain disorders. Speech is usually fluent. Comprehension of spoken language and the ability to repeat test phrases are preserved. Loss of speech, failure to comprehend simple commands, and homonymous visual field defects are not seen in metabolic encephalopathy, except when a focal lesion is also present.

Asthenia. Generalized weakness or asthenia may occur, and there may be enhanced stretch reflexes. Spasticity, i.e., exaggeration of shortening and lengthening reactions in muscles, does not occur. Grasp reflexes, perioral prehensile movements upon tactile stimulation of the lips or cheek, sustained plantar flexion and inversion at the ankle after stroking the sole, or extensor plantar responses are common. Varying degrees of apparently willed resistance to passive limb manipulation (countermovements or gegenhalten) may be seen in the early stages of metabolic encephalopathy.

Seizures. Seizures sometimes occur, but fortunately they are not very frequent and usually are generalized. They are peculiar to no form of metabolic encephalopathy and have been seen in all types. Focal convulsion may occur in the newborn infant or very elderly patient with metabolic encephalopathy. Such occurrence in the adult or when there is no derangement of mental state should raise the possibility of focal brain disease. Decisions regarding additional diagnostic studies should be based on the issues requiring definition.

Stupor. With progressive disintegration of brain function, the patient will lapse more deeply into stupor. As this happens, tonic forces acting upon the diencephalon dominate. The patient now has the upper limbs flexed and the lower limbs extended. Doll's eye movements (oculocephalic reflexes) become exaggerated. These may be elicited by turning the head from side to side or up and down. The eyes will seem to remain fixed on a point in space and thus appear to move in a direction opposite to that in which the head has been turned. The patient shows defensive movements against painful or noxious stimuli by attempting to remove them with the hand. As the encephalopathic process worsens, however, the patient may lapse into coma from which he or she cannot be roused. A posture in which the spine and limbs are extended firmly at the hips and shoulders may then be taken. Relatively lesser degrees of heightened muscle tone are found more distally in the limbs, the fingers usually remaining loosely flexed. Painful or noxious stimulation enhances the posture, and the patient does not try to remove noxious stimuli. As the patient further declines into coma, the limbs may become flaccid, and painful stimulation now may lead to flexion of the lower limb. A characteristic feature of intoxications, especially with benzodiazepines, barbiturates, meprobamate, chloral hydrate, and glutethimide, is improvement in the neurologic examination upon handling the patient. This may be documented by improvement in the electroencephalogram upon stimulation, as the diffuse synchronous slow waves of coma tend to become faster and the record displays local features (desynchronization).

Pupillary Responses. Autonomic function may also be affected in metabolic encephalopathy. The reactions of the pupils to light are preserved except following the use of drugs, which themselves affect the pupils. Morphine, heroin, and other opiates cause them to become small or pinpoint, although they are still reactive. The pupils will dilate upon the administration of nalorphine or other opiate antagonist. Glutethimide causes slightly dilated but usually fixed pupils. Scopolamine, atropine, or other anticholinergic drug poisoning is marked by widely dilated and fixed pupils. Prolonged hypoxia may be associated with unreactive and unequal pupils of any size. The persistence of pupillary abnormalities following hypoxia usually indicates necrosis of one or more portions of the brain stem, ordinarily adjacent to the aqueduct of Sylvius in the midbrain tegmentum.

Body Temperature and Blood Pressure Changes. Body temperature regulation may be altered in metabolic encephalopathy. It is often reduced in hypothyroidism, after hypoglycemia, or following the ingestion or administration of barbiturates, anticholinergic drugs, salicylates, and combinations of antihistamines, phenothiazines, or meperidine. Agitated delirium, such as that associated with drug withdrawal, results in marked increase in energy requirements and heat production. It is usually accompanied by some elevation of blood pressure, tachycardia, and profuse perspiration. Blood pressure regulation may be unstable, and in the case of agitated delirium, treatment designed to calm the patient may result in a marked fall in blood pressure even though the patient is lying flat. Orthostatic postural hypotension of the central type may accompany encephalopathy caused by drug ingestion, thiamine deficiency, hypoglycemia, or hypoxia. The orthostatic postural hypotension following the hypoxia may persist for several days and expose the patient to additional risk of ischemic brain damage. If the hypotension is of the "centrally" mediated variety, compensatory phenomena, such as faintness, blurred vision, tingling lips and fingers, pallor, and tachycardia, will be absent. The only warning other than fainting will be rapidly falling blood pressure.

Respiration. Respiration is the most significant autonomic function affected in metabolic encephalopathy. A differential scheme of the respiratory abnormalities found in common clinical comas will be found in Table 1. Its usefulness is limited to those conditions in which the patient is free of pre-existing abnormality of the lung or chest wall. The latter or the simultaneous operation of multiple encephalopathic mechanisms further limits the utility of the diagnostic scheme. In any approach to decompensation of brain function, respiratory patterns reflect physiologic derangements rather than specific disease states. The chief use of such a table is in helping to identify those forms of encephalopathy associated with metabolic acidosis, a potentially lethal state requiring prompt treatment.

The pattern of respiration in metabolic disorders depends on the degree to which systemic acid-base regulation has been disordered, the direction in which it is changing, the extent to which chemoreceptors are functioning, and the functional and structural integrity of the brain stem. Acidosis may occur in metabolic comas associated with uremia, diabetes (both ketoacidotic and lactic acidotic), hypoxia, or various forms of drug intoxication. Hyperventilation is the typical respiratory abnormality. In this condition the serum pH is less than 7.3 and the serum bicarbonate level is low (10 mEq/liter or less). The Pa_{CO_2} is less than 35 mm Hg. Hyperventilation may also occur in respiratory alkalosis, but in that condition the serum pH is elevated and the bicarbonate level will be between 15 and 30 mEq/liter. Respiratory alkalosis commonly occurs in hepatic coma, certain forms of cardiopulmonary disease, salicylate poisoning, and bacterial endotoxic shock or sepsis; it is a complication of central neurogenic hyperventilation.

Hypoventilation may result from either metabolic alkalosis or respiratory acidosis. The former is associated with a serum pH over 7.45. The serum bicarbonate level exceeds 30 mEq/liter. Metabolic alkalosis does not ordinarily lead to severe encephalopathy. It occurs as a complication of diuretic therapy, hypokalemia of any cause, primary hyperaldosteronism, hyperadrenal corticism, and loss of gastric hydrochloric acid (HCl) after prolonged vomiting. These conditions are usually self-evident or readily discovered. Respiratory acidosis is associated with serum pH of less than 7.35 and marked elevation of Pa_{CO_2}. The latter invariably is greater than 45 mm Hg and is usually over 55 mm Hg. Serum bicarbonate level is often elevated but cannot be relied upon in diagnosis, as it also may be normal, especially after partial treatment. The Pa_{O_2} is usually depressed. Respiratory acidosis usually reflects chronic pulmonary disease, peripheral respiratory failure secondary to neuromuscular disorder of acute (infective polyneuritis) or chronic (late muscular dystrophy) type, or poisoning with a depressant drug. When infective polyneuritis is the cause, the physical habitus and signs of chronic pulmonary disease or the pickwickian syndrome are usually present. The hypoventilating patient is usually violaceous. The neuromuscular causes of peripheral failure are also readily apparent. Hypoxia may complicate hypercarbia in cases of peripheral respiratory failure secondary to neuromuscular disorders or depressant drug poisoning.

DIFFERENTIATION FROM OTHER DISORDERS

Metabolic encephalopathy is usually obvious, as it most often occurs in the context of some extraneural disease. It can usually be recognized quickly, although it may be confused with endogenous depression, mental retardation, primary dementia, encephalopathies of other causes, stroke, or intracranial mass lesions, especially bilateral subdural hematoma.

Depression and Mental Retardation

Metabolic encephalopathy is usually readily distinguished from depression and mental retardation because the thinking, behavior, and state of consciousness of the patient with metabolic encephalopathy have only recently become deranged, and the patient had earlier sought treatment for the underlying systemic disease. The mood of the patient with metabolic encephalopathy is usually labile rather than steadily depressed. Incontinence is rare in depression and common in diffuse brain disease. There is evidence of prior mental attainment which exceeds that to be expected in retardation. This may be established on mental state examination by noting the breadth of vocabulary retained, ability to calculate, and a rich fund of information. The adult retardate retains both the simplicity of affect and the immature intellect of the juvenile retarded person. Ordinarily the individual cannot perform the operations of mental arithmetic. The patient's fund of knowledge is limited to the trivialities of the immediate environment. He or she cannot comprehend the command to reverse the order in which digits are spoken, although the patient may be able to repeat up to six digits. The myoclonus, changes in reflexes, movement, posture, altered pupillary function, and respiratory rate and rhythm that are so likely to be part of metabolic encephalopathy do not occur in mental retardation or depression. Conversely, recent or recurrent decline in mood identifies the depressed patient. Knowledge of the onset of the disorder is as important in the recognition of depression as in systemic disease in metabolic encephalopathy. Despite psychomotor retardation, which may block responses, the depressed person is clearly alert, is without confusion or intellectual or neurologic abnormality, and almost never is incontinent without local cause. The retarded person is ordinarily alert and responsive but dull. The neurologic examination is normal except for evidence of growth disturbance with or without movement disorder in the case of patients whose mental retardation arose from an encephaloclastic illness. This is not to say, however, that metabolic brain disorder cannot be superimposed upon either depression or mental retardation, especially when patients are given drugs aimed at modifying behavior.

Hysteria and Schizophrenia

Stupor or coma attributable to hysteria is easily differentiated because of the patient's apparent well-being, history of prior emotional disorder, multiple mysterious illnesses, and ready response to suggestion. In hysterical states in which the patient remains responsive, the primary disorientation involves the patient's own name and where he is, leaving intact major intellectual functions. Metabolic parameters are usually normal in hysterical or other psychogenic states, although sustained hyperventilation may cause hypocapnia. The mental state in schizophrenia is marked by a thought disorder with paranoid and delusional features. Hallucinations are highly systematized, continual, and often pleasurable. The neurologic examination is either normal or marked by inconsistencies, which help disclose the nature of the disorder. Asterixis or myoclonus is never present. Some tremor may be seen in anxiety, but it fluctuates with the emotional state. Schizophrenic patients may assume and maintain postures or attitudes, but with inconsistency.

Primary Brain Disorders

Alzheimer's or Pick's disease; dementia following cerebral trauma, infarction, or infection; and endogenous disorders of brain metabolism that may be associated with extraneural metabolic abnormalities (Wilson's disease, cerebral lipidoses) should be thought of as primary disorders of the brain. They can readily be separated from those cases in which metabolic encephalopathy complicates disease that is primary outside the nervous system. The history is generally longer and often subtler. Similar diseases may have occurred in other family members. Except for certain infantile conditions such as galactosemia, the patients are alert. Stigmata such as the Kayser-Fleischer ring or sebaceous adenoma may be present. Grave acute biochemical disorders, such as hypoglycemia, hypoxia, metabolic acidosis, or renal or hepatic failure, are usually absent early when neurologic manifestations are emerging. In most cases of primary brain disorder the patient ordinarily displays more loss of intellect, and less agitation and personal disorientation. The major defects are of memory, affect, language, and cognitive and conative function. Autonomic and respiratory disorders usually are absent. Motor disorders occur late in Alzheimer's disease and senile dementia, although they are prominent early in Huntington's and Wilson's diseases. Myoclonus, although present in Huntington's disease, is usually less important than choreoathetosis, and asterixis is usually absent in Wilson's disease.

Vascular Brain Disorders

Cerebral infarction, hemorrhage, or arterial insufficiency may be confused with metabolic encephalopathy when a short-lived disturbance of behavior is present. Transient global amnesia is a memory disorder of sudden onset and short duration. Since most of these states are transient, their rapid resolution often answers the question of their nature. Seizures, myoclonus, and asterixis are unusual. Blood chemistry results are usually normal or but slightly altered. The conditions are usually of sudden onset and characteristically form in a patient with little or no prior mental disorder.

Infections

Chronic infections may present with myoclonus, loss of intellectual function, seizures, headache, and stiff neck. The frequency of the latter three symptoms and the absence of asterixis or respiratory or other autonomic abnormality should lead away from consideration of metabolic encephalopathy. Spinal fluid examination usually settles the issue.

Intracranial Mass Lesions

Intracranial mass lesions (abscess, hematoma) or tumors of the brain may be difficult to differentiate, especially when caused by a bilateral and more or less symmetric disorder, such as subdural hematoma occurring in an elderly or alcoholic patient. Intracranial space-occupying lesions may cause the patient to be stuporous or tremulous and display many of the postural and motor changes observed in metabolic encephalopathy. Metabolic derangements may be present, especially if the brain lesion is metastatic and the primary tumor produces a polypeptide that results in hyponatremia or hypoglycemia. Treatment of the hypoglycemia may result in apparent worsening of the neurologic disorder. Autonomic and ventilatory disorders and asterixis are usually absent, whereas focal seizures, lateralized neurologic deficits, headache, and loss of pulsations in the central retinal veins owing to intracranial hypertension are common features of these progressive illnesses. There is often evidence of cancer elsewhere or a history of recent trauma followed by altered behavior. Signs of injury may be found on the body or head. If the intracranial mass lesion has arisen in the posterior fossa, there are usually abnormalities of eye movement or of some of the lower cranial nerves, phenomena which are rarely encountered in metabolic disorders except in the context of chronic malnutrition with alcoholism. There is usually no evidence of significant or recently decompensated extrinsic disease except cancer, and the blood chemistry results are usually normal or nearly so. The performance of diagnostic procedures such as computed transverse tomography may be required to resolve doubtful cases. In view of the importance of appropriate treatment for both metastatic cancer and subdural hematoma, this should not be delayed once the suspicion has arisen.

APPROACH TO DIAGNOSIS

History and Physical Examination

The successful diagnosis of metabolic encephalopathy requires thorough attention to the history and physical examination and a reasonable amount of shrewdness in using clinical clues. Drug ingestion should be suspected if a previously physically well but psychologically disturbed patient has been brought to hospital, having been discovered in stupor or coma. Since most patients with metabolic encephalopathy have developed it in the context of recognizable antecedent extraneural disease, diagnosis in the known case is not difficult. The history and general physical examination in unknown cases should focus on data that might indicate underlying hepatic, renal, cardiac, endocrine, or pulmonary disease. In hepatic encephalopathy, for example, signs of gross decompensation of liver function, such as jaundice, ascites, spider nevi, periumbilical venous distention or hum, hemorrhoids, and palmar erythema, are evident. The uremic patient is likely to be hypertensive, may display some degree of albuminuric retinopathy, and frequently has had one or several seizures. Patients with cerebral ischemia or hypoxia secondary to heart disease often have hypertensive stigmata, cardiac enlargement, an arrhythmia, or signs of congestive failure. Pulmonary disease is usually evident, owing to rales, an abnormal chest configuration, cyanosis, or obesity.

The neurologic signs which are most critical in diagnosis, in differentiation of the clinical forms, and in assessing the risks of irreversible damage to the brain are, in order of importance:

1. The pattern of respiration.
2. Nature and depth of the disorder of consciousness and accompanying mental and intellectual abnormalities.

3. Seizures, grasp reflexes, myoclonus, asterixis, focal neurologic deficit, and the posture of the limbs.
4. The nature of pupillary response to light.

In metabolic encephalopathy, the neurologic signs do not usually point to a single anatomic locus but do localize the site in focal diseases of the brain that cause local destruction. Moreover, they define the physiologic state of the patient but rarely disclose the cause of the encephalopathy. The hemogram, fasting blood sugar, bilirubin, blood urea nitrogen, serum bicarbonate, electrolytes, (including Na, K, Mg, Ca, P, and Cl), and arterial blood gases should be measured or determined as soon as the patient is seen during the initial examination. When there is evidence of liver disease on physical examination or when the bilirubin level is found to be elevated, serum ammonia level should be determined. In the event that any abnormality of respiratory rhythm is observed, especially in the presence of any form of hyperventilation, arterial blood gases, and pH should be measured at the end of the apneic phase. Whenever there is the least suspicion that the patient might have ingested a drug, blood and urine samples should be obtained for multiple drug screening. Respiratory alkalosis combined with metabolic acidosis, especially in a child, may indicate salicylate ingestion, which may in turn be verified by adding $FeCl_3$ to boiled urine and observing purplish discoloration. An electrocardiogram should be obtained in every case. The chest should be examined by x-ray.

Signs of possible head injury should be noted. In the event that head injury seems possible, a lateral film of the cervical spine and computed tomography (CT scan) are indicated. The cervical spine x-ray must display all seven vertebrae. In the absence of CT scan, skull x-ray may be obtained. In cases of trauma, especially when the chest has been involved, hypoxia secondary to traumatic pleural effusion or pulmonary contusion should not be confused with respiratory depression occurring as a primary effect of brain or concomitant cervical spinal cord injury. Urinalysis should be obtained in comatose patients, by catheterization if necessary. It is my practice to examine the cerebrospinal fluid from every patient who is febrile or has unexplained resistance to neck flexion, as the diagnosis and treatment of bacterial meningitis should not be delayed. Every deeply stuporous or comatose adult should receive 50 ml of 50 per cent glucose as soon as the blood has been drawn and before detailed examination, as hypoglycemic coma should be reversed as quickly as possible. This amount of glucose will do nothing to obscure the diagnosis or treatment of any other condition.

Electroencephalography

The electroencephalogram may be useful, as in some forms of metabolic stupor more or less characteristic wave patterns are seen. Performing electroencephalography should not, however, take priority over examination of the blood, urine, or spinal fluid, nor should it delay radiologic study of the skull and chest. In acute metabolic comas or encephalopathies, the electroencephalogram is not particularly helpful in diagnosis, although it may be useful in identifying more chronic states, following the course of the illness, detecting episodic phenomena, or quantifying the effect of treatment. In general, the electroencephalogram in all forms of metabolic encephalopathy is characterized by generalized and more or less symmetric slow waves. As consciousness becomes degraded, the record becomes slower and increasingly synchronous and symmetric. The pattern is often quite severely affected in diabetic, hypoglycemic, uremic, and hepatic encephalopathies. Among these, the electroencephalogram in hepatic coma is most likely to be helpful. Triphasic periodic slow waves appear symmetrically, bilaterally, and frontally most of the time and extend caudally as the process worsens. The distribution of such waves in the posterior parts of the head bears a direct relationship to the severity of the process. There may be relatively well-preserved posterior alpha activity when the frontal region is quite abnormal. Uncommonly in hepatic encephalopathy the slow activity begins occipitally or temporally. In both hypoglycemia and diabetic acidosis, the diffusely slow pattern on the electroencephalogram becomes normal upon correction of the underlying abnormality. In hypoglycemia, the resolution is so rapid that infusion of glucose during recording usually results in reversion of the record to normal within less than 1 minute. In hypoadrenal, hypo-osmolar, and hyponatremic states, the electroencephalogram is usually slow, with little or no activity faster than 7 Hz. The finding of activity faster than 12 Hz should make the physician doubtful that the encephalopathy results from one of these causes. Myxedema and hypopituitarism with secondary myxedema are also associated with slowing to less than 7 Hz. Hypercalcemia and hypocalcemia may both be associated with slow patterns. The latter condition additionally may cause paroxysmal discharges. The electroencephalogram may also be slowed in other electrolyte disorders and in porphyria. For the most part, the electroencephalogram reflects function rather than a specific illness.

Radionuclide Brain Scanning

The radionuclide brain scan has little place in the diagnosis of acute metabolic encephalopathy, especially when the patient is comatose, but it may be of great value in chronic cases, particularly when such conditions as tumor or subdural hematoma are considerations.

Computed Tomography

The advent of computed tomography (CT) has revolutionized the management of the comatose patient since the procedure is safe and rapid. It permits the diagnosis of tumor, hemorrhage, brain edema, infarction, and subdural or epidural hematoma with minimal manipulation and usually without lumbar puncture. Most conditions can be recognized without contrast enhancement. CT is the imaging procedure of choice at this time.

PARTICULAR FORMS OF METABOLIC ENCEPHALOPATHY

When metabolic encephalopathy is associated with hypoxia, it results from a fall in the arterial oxygen partial pressure (hypoxic hypoxia), the oxygen-carrying capacity of the blood (anemic hypoxia), or reduction of cerebral blood flow (stagnant or ischemic hypoxia). Rarely does the hypoxia result from histotoxic causes (e.g., cyanide). When hypoxia is chronic, the condition may be characterized by delirium or stupor, confusion, hallucination, and seizures. The pupils are usually small but reactive, and breathing is periodic. When the hypoxia is acute and severe, consciousness is lost within a few seconds, and seizures and myoclonus are common along with abnormal postures. The arterial oxygen tensions will be low, as will the venous, indicating maximal extraction of oxygen by the tissues. Hypoxia as a consequence of chest disease requires specific treatment. Hypoxic encephalopathy may complicate pneumonia, neuromuscular disease, spinal cord injury, and a variety of other conditions. It often begins with headache followed by restlessness and hallucinosis. Common causes of ischemia are reduced cardiac output, intracranial vaso-occlusive or vasospastic conditions that reduce cerebral blood flow by raising cerebral vascular resistance, and raised intracranial pressure. Cerebral ischemia occurs when the cerebral perfusion pressure (CPP) is less than 50 torr. It may be calculated at the bedside by subtraction of the spinal fluid pressure in mm Hg from the systemic arterial pressure. Where the spinal fluid pressure (pCSF) is unknown and pulsations are present in the central retinal vein, the pCSF may be assumed to be less than 180 mm CSF or 13.29 mm Hg. (Sp. gv. of Hg is 13.546; 180/13.546 = 13.29.)

The flow calculation is made as follows:

$$\text{CPP} = \frac{(\text{Systolic BP} + 2 \text{ Diastolic BP})}{3} - \text{pCSF mm Hg}$$

Thus, where the blood pressure is 100/85, the perfusion becomes:

$$\text{CPP} = \frac{100 + 170}{3} - 13.29 = 76.71 \text{ mm Hg}$$

assuming cerebrospinal fluid pressure to be no higher than 13.29 mm Hg.

Hypoglycemia as a cause of encephalopathy, stupor, or coma is usually readily evident, as the patient commonly is known to have diabetes and to be receiving insulin. Often the patient is an elderly person who has been using an oral agent. The long-acting insulins appear far more likely to cause trouble in patients who eat poorly and are ill nourished, with inadequate carbohydrate reserves. The hypoglycemic patient is usually confused and may display delirium or stupor, lasting several minutes or hours, before lapsing into coma. Abnormal postures and movements may precede deeper coma when limb extension may be seen. Some hypoglycemic patients develop sharply focal or lateralized neurologic signs, and others have either focal or generalized convulsions.

Metabolic acidosis announces itself by hyperventilation. Its presence is readily confirmed by laboratory studies (Table 1). Although it is not the most frequent cause of metabolic encephalopathy in patients brought to an emergency room, it can be lethal or leave permanent cerebral residuals, and hence should be recognized and treated promptly to prevent neuronal loss. Patients presenting with metabolic coma of acute onset are best regarded as suffering hypoxia, hypoglycemia, or metabolic acidosis until proven otherwise. Physical examination, blood gas determination, and glucose and serum electrolyte measurement should lead quickly to the correct diagnosis and treatment.

Hepatic encephalopathy may appear as an apathetic stupor or agitated delirium and include any variety of abnormalities of consciousness, mental state, or posture. Respiratory alkalosis with hyperventilation is seen commonly in such patients when they are stuporous. Grasp reflexes are usual, and the disorder is frequently associated with asterixis. In chronic hepatocerebral disease, gross and often irreversible abnormalities of mental state may be accompanied by choreoathetosis. The serum ammonia level is usually raised, and the chemical changes of respiratory alkalosis are present. The serum ammonia level does not always parallel the neurologic state. The cerebrospinal fluid is normal and does not contain bilirubin unless there has been a meningeal disorder that alters the blood-brain barrier or the serum bilirubin level has been over 5 mg/dl for several days.

Uremic encephalopathy may present as coma and is ordinarily associated with hyperventilation and metabolic acidosis. It is one form of metabolic encephalopathy in which the tendon reflexes may be diminished or absent owing to associated uremic polyneuropathy. The clinical signs are stupor proceeding to coma, shifting focal neurologic deficits, widespread myoclonus, and convulsions, although in the early stages agitation and delirium may be present. The common laboratory findings in addition to those of serum acidosis include varying degrees of azotemia, the level and rate of change of which appear to have little to do with the mental or neurologic disorder. It would seem that intracellular metabolic changes are not wholly reflected by the serum values of the blood urea nitrogen (BUN). The cerebrospinal fluid appearance, pressure, and content are usually normal. Uremic meningitis occurs occasionally, the spinal fluid containing up to 500 cells per cu mm of mixed type. Such patients often have a stiff neck. Elevation of spinal fluid pressure is not part of uremic encephalopathy. Its presence usually indicates some other process, such as hypertensive encephalopathy or water intoxication complicating renal dialysis. The latter may be inferred from the finding of hyponatremia or identified by serum osmolality of less than 260 mOsm/kg. Since the patient is usually hypertensive, the problem of differentiating uremic encephalopathy from hypertensive encephalopathy is significant, as the therapies are quite different. An associated peripheral neuropathy is absent in hypertension, and the reflexes are more likely to be exaggerated. The BUN is invariably quite high in uremia. This is less often the case in hypertensive encephalopathy. Multifocal myoclonus and asterixis are common in uremia but unusual in hypertensive encephalopathy. Fleeting focal neurologic deficits, papilledema, unilateral or bilateral hemianopia, raised cerebrospinal fluid pressure and protein levels, and diastolic blood pressure over 120 mm Hg are the key clinical features of hypertensive encephalopathy.

Hypercarbic encephalopathy or CO_2 narcosis ordinarily emerges from a background of chronic pulmonary disease. It frequently evolves slowly and runs a relapsing course characterized by hypoventilation; dull diffuse headache with or without intermittent drowsiness, especially after meals; papilledema; and the blood chemical changes of respiratory acidosis. Most patients are cyanotic. Myoclonus and asterixis are common, as is muscular irritability. Cerebrospinal fluid pressures may be very high, but the cell counts and protein contents are ordinarily normal. Acute decompensation of pulmonary function and the development of stupor are likely to follow respiratory infection or the administration of sedative or hypnotic drugs.

Many patients with chronic encephalopathy use drugs that modify behavior or in other ways cause cumulative toxicity that obscures the clinical picture. Diazepam is an important example, as it is metabolized more slowly in the elderly and is the source of at least two active by-products. Additionally, other factors may be present, such as cerebrovascular disease or senility.

Alteration of, or rapid changes in, the ionic environment or acid-base equilibrium may also alter the function of the nervous system, producing changes in alertness, muscle strength, orientation, and posture. When the ionic content of the serum has fallen, it is said to have become hypo-osmolar. Water then flows into the electrolyte-rich brain, resulting in swelling, stupor, headache, disorientation, and even coma with tentorial or cerebellar tonsillar herniation. Water flows from the brain when the serum electrolyte content becomes increased relative to that of the brain.

Dehydration may also be associated with delirium and agitation. If extreme, it can result in subpial hemorrhage, seizures, coma, and death. The latter events are more common in infants but also are risks of the treatment of cerebral edema by osmolar diuresis. As a general rule, neurologic symptoms occur when there are sudden shifts in serum osmolality, regardless of the initial level, as slow shifts are compensated for by incompletely understood mechanisms, thus enabling the patient to tolerate quite abnormal levels of osmolality. Neurologic symptoms may thus result from abrupt shifts during the course of treatment. Serum osmolality may be calculated from clinical chemical data as follows:

$$\text{mOsm/kg} = 2(\text{Na} + \text{K}) + \frac{\text{glucose}}{18} + \frac{\text{BUN}}{2.8}$$

The normal range is 285 to 295 mOsm/kg. There may be slow restoration of compartmental equilibrium so that the neurologic recovery may lag behind that of the serum.

Hyperosmolar states result from water depletion, as may occur in diarrhea or from less water intake than required by the amount of solutes consumed. The osmolality may exceed 320 to 330 mOsm/kg, and the fluid deficit 10 liters. "Hyperglycemic hyperosmolar nonketotic coma" usually occurs in elderly, untreated, neglected diabetics or in patients after severe burns. The blood glucose may exceed 1000 mg/dl and is always above 400, thus adding 25 to 55 mOsm/kg to the serum values. The patients are usually stuporous rather than comatose. Convulsions often are present. Symptoms remit upon initial hydration with isotonic saline followed by small amounts of insulin and subsequent adjustment of the fluid and electrolyte regimen. Too rapid treatment may lead to cerebral water intoxication and convert a stuporous confused patient to one in lethal coma owing to brain swelling.

Hypo-osmolar states, or "water intoxication," result from hyponatremia and are often the consequence of overzealous treatment of hyperosmolar states. The accumulation of fluid in the brain is followed by decreased intracellular potassium and extracellular sodium levels. When serum osmolality falls below 260 mOsm/kg, these ionic shifts enhance neuronal excitability, which is believed to result in seizures, stupor, delirium, and coma. The clinical conditions that result in this state most commonly include the replacement of sodium-containing body fluid by water; the use of diuretics, especially in the elderly; and severe renal disease. Tap-water enemas used in the preparation of infants or aged patients for x-ray studies or the treatment of fecal impaction may be institutional causes of water intoxication. Less commonly, inappropriate antidiuretic hormone secretion, adrenal insufficiency, hypothyroidism, excessive ingestion of water as part of an emotional illness, and renal dialysis are responsible.

Hypercalcemia occurring in various conditions, including chronic renal disease, sarcoidosis, and metastases to bone, may present with a chronic dementia of nonspecific type, headache, and occasionally delusions of persecution. Moreover, in conditions such as chronic renal disease, which vary in severity, symptoms may remit and relapse. Primary or secondary *hypocalcemia* may also present with apparent chronic dementia, recurrent seizures, especially in children, and papilledema. Both of these conditions should be identifiable through initial blood chemistry studies.

It often happens that the diagnosis of the specific form of metabolic encephalopathy remains unclear, as the disorder in any given patient commonly results from the concatenation of multiple concurrent causes. This is especially likely to be the case with an elderly patient whose brain bears the burdens of senile or vascular disease, anoxia, and the accumulation of tissue metabolites secondary to ischemia. The important rule in metabolic encephalopathy regardless of severity is to recognize that a neurologic disorder characterized by altered consciousness and impaired mental and motor function may belong to a class of illness that is metabolic and separate from structural disease. In each case the potentially lethal factors should receive first diagnostic and therapeutic consideration: hypoxia, hypoglycemia, and metabolic acidosis. In the presence of fever, intracranial infection must be excluded. When nystagmus or ocular palsy is present, thiamine deficiency should be considered. If these principles are kept in mind, the reversible lethal causes will be dealt with early, leaving adequate time to refine the diagnosis in safety.

TRAUMA OF THE CENTRAL NERVOUS SYSTEM

By Suzie C. Tindall, M.D.
Atlanta, Georgia

Central nervous system trauma constitutes a major cause of morbidity and mortality in the United States each year. Motor vehicle accidents account for the majority of injuries to the head and spine, but falls, assaults, gunshot and stab wounds, and occupational and sporting accidents are responsible for many more. Although in the majority of cases the traumatic cause of the problem is easily recognized, in others a high index of suspicion is necessary in order to arrive at a correct diagnosis. When confronted with a patient who has suffered central nervous system trauma, the physician is often called upon to simultaneously provide acute emergency management, recognize and treat assorted associated injuries, and rapidly arrive at a specific diagnosis of the type of head or spine injury so as to render rapid and effective treatment. Under such circumstances it is advantageous to have in mind a clear and logical sequence of steps to follow at the outset.

For purposes of organization, the following discussion will consider head injury (injury to the brain and its coverings) and spinal injury (injury to the spinal cord and the bony spine) separately. However, it is well to remember that 3 to 10 per cent of all patients with severe head injuries will have an associated injury of the cervical spine.

HEAD INJURY

A simple classification of head injury is listed in Table 1. Although each type of injury may occur as an isolated entity, it is not unusual to see two or more such injuries in any individual patient. Scalp injuries such as lacerations, abrasions, avulsions, or hematomas are usually easily recognized upon careful inspection of the scalp. Prior to closure, the depths of all scalp lacerations should be palpated so as to discover any associated depressed skull fracture. If a depressed skull fracture is suspected, either because of findings on palpation or consideration of the mechanisms of injury, it may be confirmed by visualizing a double density shadow on plain skull film. However, not all depressed skull fractures can be demonstrated on plain skull x-rays, and it is my practice to investigate all suspected depressed fractures using a computed tomographic (CT) scan with bone window settings. Linear or nondepressed skull fractures may not be apparent clinically and if present as an isolated consequence of head injury will be of little therapeutic significance. Consequently, "routine" skull films in victims of head trauma are not recommended and do not prove to be cost-effective. Basilar skull fractures through the frontal, sphenoid, or temporal bone are best suspected clinically, noting periorbital ecchymoses ("raccoon sign"), retromastoid hemorrhage ("Battle's sign"), hemotympanum, or cerebrospinal fluid rhinorrhea or otorrhea. No diagnostic study is as sensitive as the clinical examination in confirming basilar skull fracture.

Intracranial consequences of closed head injury include concussion, which is a clinical syndrome of loss of consciousness in the absence of gross traumatic pathology. Axial stretching or primary neuronal injury may result from the vector forces of cranial impact. In both of these instances, CT scanning may be unrevealing. Whereas the loss of consciousness associated with concussion is brief, primary brain stem injury from axonal stretching may result in a very protracted comatose state. Cerebral edema may occur diffusely, particularly in younger individuals, and is often associated with an elevation in intracranial pressure. More focal cerebral edema may accompany any of the hemorrhagic intracranial lesions associated with closed head injury.

Acute epidural hematoma (Fig. 1) is a focal collection of blood, usually arterial, between the dura and the inner table of the skull. It is frequently located immediately beneath the point of traumatic impact, usually in the region of the middle meningeal artery. Classically, acute epidural hematoma is associated clinically with a lucid interval—the patient is either stunned or rendered transiently unconscious at initial injury, only to awake and appear normal for several hours prior to a rapid decline in level of consciousness. CT scanning in acute epidural hematoma will reveal a high-density lenticular-shaped lesion because of the tendency of the dura to resist stripping from the inner table of the skull.

Acute subdural hematoma (Fig. 2) is a collection of blood between the dura and brain surface. It may be remote from the point of traumatic impact and is usually due to tearing of a vein bridging the cortical surface to an intracranial venous sinus. A smaller percentage of acute subdural hematomas are second-

Table 1. Classification of Head Injury

Scalp injuries
Skull fractures
Nondepressed
Depressed
Intracranial injury—closed
Concussion
Without hematoma
Axial stretch
Cerebral edema
With hematoma
Epidural hematoma
Subdural hematoma
Intracerebral hematoma
Intracranial injury—open
Gunshot wounds
Other penetrating objects
Miscellaneous
Arterial injuries
Traumatic aneurysms
Carotid cavernous fistulas
Traumatic cerebrospinal fluid fistulas

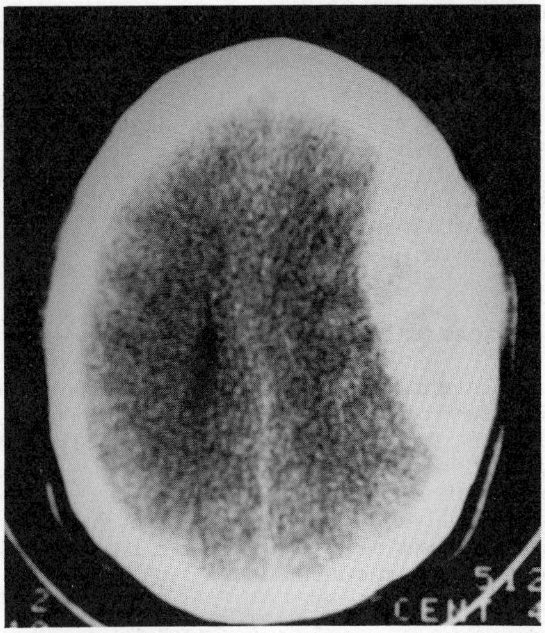

Figure 1. Acute epidural hematoma.

ary to arterial bleeding from a damaged cortical artery. CT scanning shows a crescent-shaped high-density area conforming to the cortical surface and frequently covering much of the surface of the frontal, parietal, and occipital lobes. This lesion is usually associated with a considerable shift of the midline brain structures and, in the event of transtentorial herniation, dilatation of the contralateral lateral ventricle may be noted.

Favored locations for *traumatic intracerebral hematomas* (Fig. 3) are the low anterior frontal poles, anterior temporal lobe tips, and the occipital poles. They appear as irregular high-density lesions on CT scans and may also be associated with considerable shifts of normal intracranial structures.

Penetrating intracranial injury, such as that from gunshot wounds, knives, nails, and similar instruments, is usually self-evident by history and brief patient inspection. Skull films and CT scanning are mandatory in all such injuries to correctly localize in-driven objects and skull bone fragments as well as to localize any associated hemorrhagic lesions.

Traumatic intracerebral arterial aneurysms are rare and, because angiography is no longer routinely used in the evaluation of the head-injured patient, they are usually discovered only when the patient suffers a subarachnoid hemorrhage sometime after the primary head injury. Carotid cavernous fistulas are due to tearing of the carotid artery within its intercavernous portion with the creation of a direct arteriovenous shunt. Clinically the patient usually notices an audible bruit and demonstrates a proptotic, chemotic eye. Progressive unilateral visual loss and extraocular muscle palsy may follow. Post-traumatic cerebrospinal fluid fistulas manifested as otorrhea or rhinorrhea are usually the consequence of basilar skull fracture. Although most of these promptly seal, those that persist are best localized using a combination of coronal CT imaging and metrizamide cisternography.

Facial fractures and soft-tissue injuries, thoracic and abdominal trauma, and long bone fractures frequently accompany head injury and may contribute significantly to the morbidity and mortality in head-injured patients.

Basic Approach to the Head-Injured Patient

The major causes of morbidity and mortality in severely head-injured people are the following:

1. Irreversible parenchymal damage in vital cerebral areas, such as the brain stem.
2. Uncontrolled intracranial hypertension with cerebral shifts and herniation secondary to either sizable intracranial hematoma or diffuse cerebral swelling.
3. An intercurrent systemic medical complication, such as hypoxia, hypotension, or acidosis.

Prompt, appropriate emergency management, accurate diagnosis, and rapid treatment can produce favorable results in causes 2 and 3.

In most instances the fact that the patient has suffered a head injury is readily apparent by history. However, the possibility of head injury should always be considered in the differential diagnosis of the patient who presents with confusion or coma of undetermined cause. Likewise, altered level of consciousness should never be attributed simply to intoxication or metabolic causes unless the examiner can be sure, either on clinical grounds or, in most instances, with the support of appropriate diagnostic studies, that no focal intracranial lesion exists.

The first consideration when confronted with a seriously head-injured patient is to establish and maintain an airway with good oxygenation. All patients

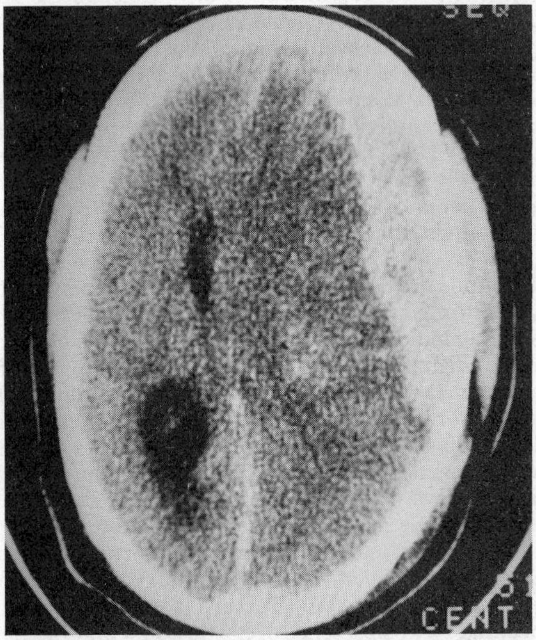

Figure 2. Acute subdural hematoma.

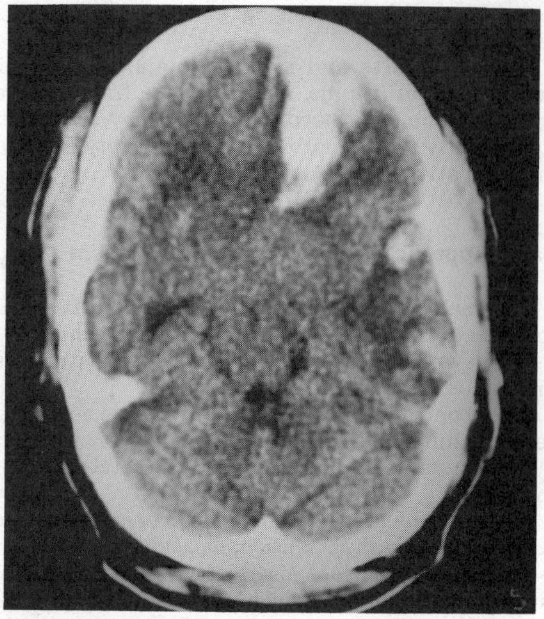

Figure 3. Traumatic intracerebral hematomas.

who are comatose should be intubated, and in order to help reduce any possible elevated intracranial pressure, hyperventilation to P_{CO_2} of 25 mm Hg is rapidly performed. Hypotension is then treated. Hypotension is unusual in isolated head injury unless blood loss from a scalp laceration has been excessive, and its presence should prompt a complete evaluation of the thorax, abdomen, and long bones to determine the source of blood loss. A lateral cervical spine film should be taken and evaluated prior to any manipulation of the patient's neck. After emergency stabilization, a rapid patient assessment is performed.

This patient evaluation should first include an assessment of the patient's level of consciousness. The Glasgow Coma Scale (Table 2) is the internationally accepted scale for evaluating level of consciousness in the head-injured patient. The patient's postresuscitation Glasgow Coma Score (GCS) should be recorded with the individual categories delineated—i.e., (E2/M4/V1) = 7. The scalp and skull are then checked thoroughly for evidence of traumatic laceration, contusion, hematoma, abrasion, fracture, or entrance and exit wounds from a penetrating object. If necessary, a questionable area of the scalp may need to be shaved. The pupils are each checked for size and reactivity to light. Pupillary asymmetry is a troublesome finding, as it may indicate early third nerve compression from uncal herniation secondary to an expanding intracranial mass lesion. Spontaneous eye movements or gaze preference are noted, and after the cervical spine film has been checked to rule out a fracture-dislocation, horizontal eye movements are evaluated with the doll's-eye maneuver. Corneal reflexes are tested. Abnormalities in eye movements, altered pupillary reflexes or size, and alterations in the corneal reflexes may suggest primary brain stem injury. A search for evidence of basilar skull fracture is made by quickly checking for the presence of Battle's sign and raccoon eyes, and the tympanic membranes are checked for integrity and hematotympanum using the otoscope. The patient's motor performance has already been evaluated in determining the GCS, but a rapid check of postural tone in each extremity, a check for symmetry of reflexes, and evaluation of the plantar responses may prove helpful in localizing a focal deficit.

In the patient with a more minor injury this examination can be expanded to include a detailed evaluation of the mental status, gait, coordination, and sensory systems.

Indications for Hospitalization

All patients who, at the time of evaluation in the emergency room, show any alteration in level of consciousness, focal neurologic findings, evidence of basilar skull fracture, or depressed skull fracture should be hospitalized for observation. If the history suggests the possibility of an epidural hematoma, the patient should be observed for at least several hours, even if alert upon initial examination.

Indications for Further Diagnostic Studies

Anteroposterior and lateral skull films are obtained in any patient suspected of having a depressed skull fracture by the nature of the blow to the head and the instrument with which it was delivered, or in any patient who has suffered a penetrating injury.

CT scanning is the backbone of the diagnostic armamentarium in evaluation of the head-injured patient. It is a noninvasive study when performed without the injection of contrast agent, and it rapidly determines if surgically significant post-traumatic intracranial lesions are present. No longer is there a place for prolonged observation awaiting signs of herniation, such as a dilated pupil or of focal neurologic deficit, prior to investigating the head-injured patient. Any patient with a score of 5 or less on the best motor response section of the Glasgow Coma Scale should have an emergency CT head scan immediately after

Table 2. Glasgow Coma Scale

Eye Opening		
Spontaneous	E	4
To speech		3
To pain		2
Nil		1
Best Motor Response		
Obeys	M	6
Localizes		5
Withdraws		4
Abnormal flexion		3
Extensor response		2
Nil		1
Verbal Response		
Oriented	V	5
Confused conversation		4
Inappropriate words		3
Incomprehensible sounds		2
Nil		1

Coma Score (E + M + V) = 3 to 15

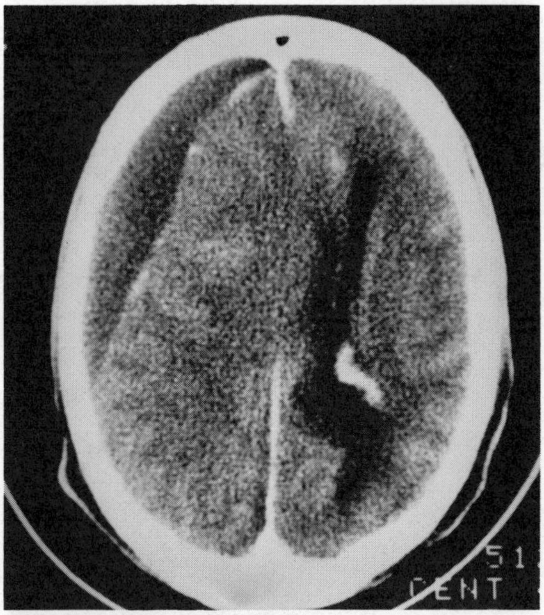

Figure 4. Chronic subdural hematoma.

stabilization. Patients with penetrating intracranial injuries and suspected depressed skull fractures also merit a rapid scan. Less severely injured patients can be scanned at the discretion of the evaluating physician. I frequently caution house staff, "It's better to be safe than sorry."

The importance of serial CT scanning in the head-injured patient has been emphasized as a means of detecting delayed intracerebral hematomas and post-traumatic hydrocephalus. Consequently, failure of a patient to improve or neurologic deterioration, or both, is a definitive indication for repeat CT scanning.

Arteriography, formerly the mainstay of diagnostic evaluation in head injury, has limited application these days. It is indicated if major arterial injury is suspected or to better delineate an equivocal abnormality on CT scan, such as a suspected bilateral subdural hematoma.

Lumbar puncture is contraindicated in the diagnostic evaluation of head-injured patients, as it yields little useful information and in addition it may exacerbate intracranial shifts and can precipitate transtentorial herniation.

Recognition of the Sequelae of Head Injury

It has recently been well shown that even mild head injury may be associated with a significant intellectual morbidity. Certainly, the survivors of major head injury frequently suffer from permanent neurologic deficits involving the higher cortical functions and the motor, cerebellar, and sensory systems. Cranial nerve damage may manifest itself as anosmia, unilateral or bilateral blindness, extraocular muscle palsies, facial paralysis, hearing loss, or difficulties with swallowing. Post-traumatic epilepsy develops in a significant number of head-injured victims.

The postconcussive syndrome may follow any minor or major head injury and is characterized by headaches, difficulties with concentration, dizziness, memory disturbances, irritability, tinnitus, and various other psychomotor difficulties. Resolution of the syndrome is gradual.

Two sequelae of head injury that are readily treatable and frequently misdiagnosed until late in their course are chronic subdural hematoma and post-traumatic hydrocephalus. A history of trauma may not be readily obtainable in the patient harboring a chronic subdural hematoma who presents with progressive confusion and intellectual deterioration, gait disturbance, and, late in the course, evidence of focal hemiparesis. Post-traumatic hydrocephalus may present in a similar fashion but is not often associated with focal neurologic deficit. Both are easily diagnosed on CT scanning. The chronic subdural hematoma will be seen as a lucent, fluid-filled area overlying the brain associated with significant shift of midline structures (Fig. 4), and post-traumatic hydrocephalus will result in dilatation of the entire ventricular system.

SPINE INJURY

A simple classification of spine injury is presented in Table 3. Each of these injuries may or may not have associated injury to the spinal cord and subsequent neurologic deficit. Some of the lesions are more likely to have associated neurologic deficit than others. It is easiest to think of the various types of spinal injury according to anatomic location.

Because of the unusual anatomy and function of the atlas and the axis, injuries to this area are unique and classified separately. Jefferson's fracture is a fracture (usually more than one) of the ring of C1 vertebra. It is the result of an axial loading injury, is rarely associated with neurologic deficit, and is usually a stable injury, by which is meant that left alone it will not have a propensity for subluxation or dislocation. Injuries to the odontoid complex may be fractures or liga-

Table 3. Classification of Spinal Injury

Cervical	
C1–C2	Jefferson's fracture
	Odontoid fracture
	Hangman's fracture
C3–T1	Fracture-dislocation
	Ligamentous injury
	Facet injury
	Jumped facet
	Fractured facet
	Central cord of spondylosis
	Acute central disc rupture
Thoracolumbar	
Compression fracture	
Burst fractures	
Fracture-dislocation	
Acute central disc rupture	
Penetrating	
Gunshot	
Knife	
Other	

mentous tears, and in either instance they result in an unstable situation in which the arch of C1 rides forward over the body of C2 (Fig. 5). These injuries are usually not associated with neurologic deficit unless left untreated. A Hangman's fracture is a fracture through the pedicles of C2 causing a separation of the C1–2 complex from the laminal arch of C2 and the remainder of the spine. Patients suffering this injury usually die immediately or suffer no neurologic deficit. The fracture should be considered unstable.

Injuries to the remainder of the cervical spine include the fracture-dislocation injury so common as a result of diving and automobile accidents. In this injury, the vertebral body or disc anteriorly and the laminal arch or facets posteriorly are fractured or torn, thus allowing the upper part of the spine to ride forward or backward upon the lower part. These injuries are associated with a very high incidence of severe neurologic deficit. Purely ligamentous injury may result in spinal instability and associated neurologic deficit. In such instances no specific fracture may be demonstrable on plain films and at times flexion and extension views are required for diagnosis (Fig. 6). Injuries to the facets, either ligamentous or fracture, may result in cervical instability in the form of subluxation or abnormal rotation. Facet injuries are a common cause of purely radicular neurologic deficit from spinal cord injury. A sudden hyperextension injury in a patient with pre-existing cervical spondylosis (Fig. 7) due to degenerative arthritis may on occasion result in a distinct neurologic syndrome—the central cord syndrome—in which the hands and arms are weaker than the legs. X-rays in such a situation will reveal only the degenerative arthritic changes and no fracture or dislocation. Rarely, trauma will cause central herniation of a cervical disc, leading to an acute or rapidly progressive quadriparesis, and in such circumstances x-ray examination will not show pathology sufficient to explain the extensive neurologic deficit. Laterally herniated cervical and lumbar discs will not be considered in this discussion.

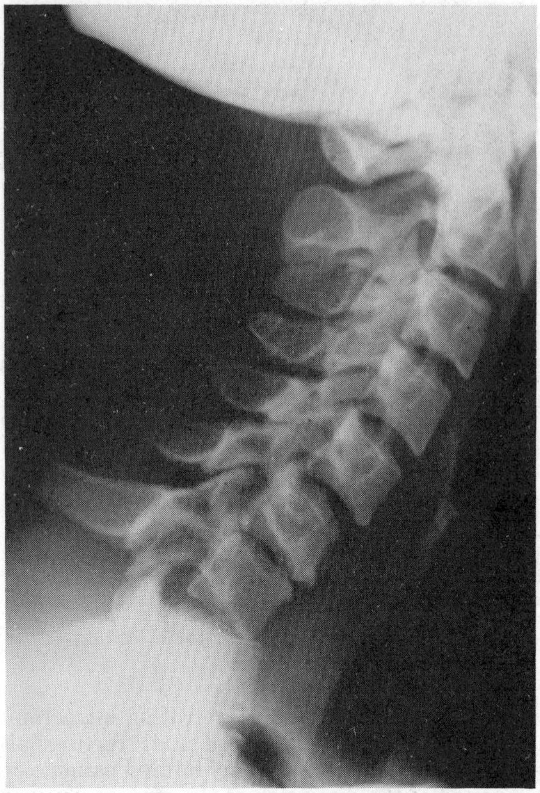

Figure 6. Cervical instability at the C_7 - T_1 level due to ligamentous injury. This patient had no neurologic deficit but did complain of neck pain after an automobile accident. The patient was initially discharged from an emergency room because films did not reveal a fracture. When he returned complaining of persistent neck pain, flexion and extension films were obtained and showed the ligamentous injury with instability.

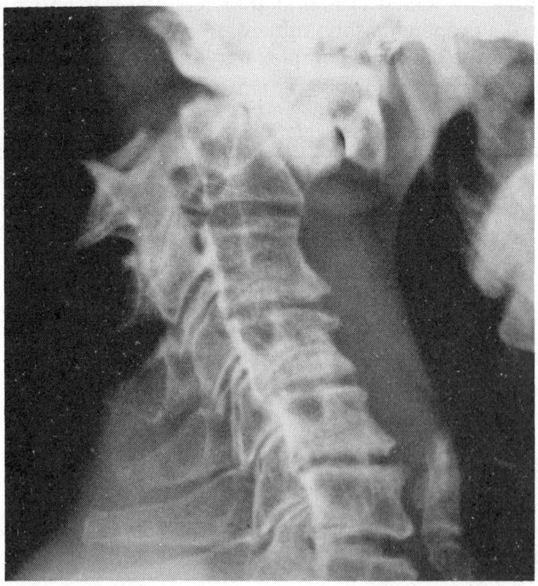

Figure 5. Odontoid fracture with C_1 on C_2 dislocation. Several weeks prior to examination, the patient had been hit by a car. At the time of examination, the patient complained of neck pain but was otherwise neurologically intact.

Traumatic compression fractures, burst fractures, and fracture-dislocations of the thoracolumbar spine require a great deal of traumatic force and are usually the result of automobile or industrial accidents. They are associated with varying degrees of neurologic deficit depending upon their severity and spinal level. Compression fractures in the older individual may occur with less severe trauma and are frequently associated with osteoporosis. In such circumstances, neurologic deficit is uncommon. The possibility of a pathologic fracture, i.e., one associated with cancerous involvement of the vertebra, should be considered whenever a compression fracture is encountered in a patient over 45 years of age. Acute central thoracic disc rupture is rare. The diagnosis is sometimes difficult to make because trauma will not be a prominent part of the history, and the patient may present with back pain and progressive paraparesis of a combined upper and lower motor neuron type. Acute central disc rupture in the lumbar canal also presents with back pain and a progressive lower motor neuron paraparesis.

Acute penetrating injuries to the spinal area are almost never unstable injuries and are associated with varied neurologic deficits, depending upon the anatomic point of penetration of the missile and, in the case of bullet wounds, upon the caliber and speed of the bullet.

Evaluation and Emergency Management of the Spinal Injury

Any patient suspected of having a spinal injury, no matter how minor, should be immobilized until such time as he or she has been adequately evaluated and a significant injury ruled out or the injury determined to be stable. Immobilization is one of the few interventions that have been shown to positively affect the course of the spine-injured patient. In most instances the fact that the patient has suffered a spinal cord injury will be quickly evident on the basis of the neurologic examination. Any patient who has spinal pain following trauma should have an x-ray examination to rule out fracture; if this is normal, a flexion and extension view may be required to demonstrate the pathologic lesion. A high index of suspicion is sometimes necessary to diagnose spinal injury in a patient who, for whatever reason, is uncooperative, confused, or comatose, or in whom the history of prior trauma is not clear.

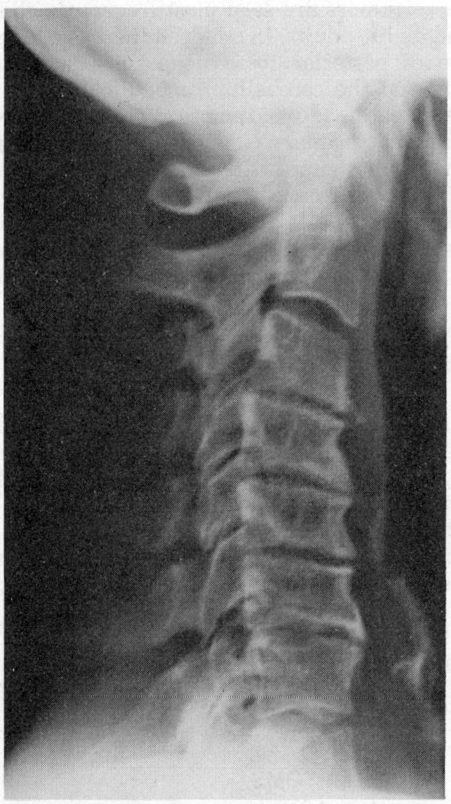

Figure 7. Cervical spondylosis in a patient who suffered a central cord injury with acute cervical hyperextension. Despite the major neurologic deficit in this patient, the films reveal only changes of degenerative arthritis and no acute fractures or dislocations.

Like the head-injury patient, the patient with spinal injury must be evaluated and treated for associated injuries immediately after immobilization, particularly if such injuries are responsible for respiratory compromise or hemorrhagic shock. The neurologic evaluation of the patient will then follow.

A quick check of the patient's mental status will establish whether or not he or she is alert, oriented, and able to follow commands. If the patient is confused, the first parameter to check is arterial oxygenation, as hypoxia is a common cause of confusion in the patient with a cervical spinal cord injury. Associated head injury and drug or alcohol intoxication may also be causes for confusion. The patient is questioned regarding spinal pain, and the position of pain may help to grossly localize the level of injury. With the patient supine, an attempt is then made to localize the level of the injury, first by testing the motor system and then by checking the sensory system. A functional level is determined bilaterally—that is, the lowest level of functional muscle contraction or sensory preservation to pain. Table 4 outlines the motor and sensory findings for each functional level. Joint position sense is then tested in all extremities to evaluate the function of the posterior columns. Reflex testing is not reliable during the acute stages of spinal cord injury, when spinal shock may be present. Moreover, all injuries should be considered incomplete until spinal shock resolves and the bulbocavernous reflex returns. With resolution of spinal shock, reflexes below the level of injury will become hyperactive in the case of upper motor neuron injury to the cervical or thoracic cord and the Babinski responses will become extensor. The bladder will become small and spastic. Spinal injuries in the lumbar area will involve the cauda equina and cause depressed or absent reflexes in the legs, and the bladder will become large and atonic. Injuries at the T12 to L2 levels may result in combined upper and lower motor neuron signs due to injury of both the conus medullaris and upper cauda equina. Mention should be made of the neurologic findings in the central cord syndrome, which, as noted earlier, is usually due to cervical hyperextension injuries in patients with pre-existing cervical spondylosis (Fig. 7). In these patients, the hands and arms are weaker than the legs, and the patient may have paresthesias and loss of sensation limited to the hands.

A carefully recorded initial examination is invaluable for future references, and the results of this examination will direct attention to the level of the spine that will require radiographic investigation.

Radiologic Investigation in Spinal Injury

Plain x-rays in the anteroposterior and lateral positions are the best initial diagnostic studies in patients with spinal injury. Frequently these are all that are required to adequately visualize the fracture or dislocation and to plan treatment. A systematic method of evaluating each spinal film is most helpful so that a subtle finding is not missed. For instance, when reviewing a lateral cervical spine film, examine the following structures in order of mention: the C1–2 complex; the soft tissues anterior to the spine; the lines of

Table 4. Neurologic Evaluation of Spinal Injury Levels

Functional Level	Motor Intact	Sensory Intact
C4	Diaphragm	Above top of shoulder
C5	Deltoid	Lateral upper arm
C6	Biceps, wrist extensors	Lateral forearm, thumb, and index finger
C7	Triceps, wrist flexion	Middle finger
C8	Finger flexion	Medial forearm, ring, and small finger
T1	Interossei—finger adduction and abduction	Medial upper arm
T2–10	± Upper abdominals	By dermatomal sensory
T10–12	± Lower abdominals	By dermatomal sensory
T12–L3	Iliopsoas, quadriceps	Anterior thigh
L4	Tibialis anterior	Medial foot
L5	Foot dorsiflexors	Dorsum of foot
S1	Toe and foot plantar flexion	Lateral and sole of foot
S2	Hamstrings	Posterior thigh
S3–5	Anal sphincter	Perianal

the anterior and posterior longitudinal ligaments; the integrity of vertebral bodies; the pedicles and facets; the laminal arches and spinous processes. At times polytomography or CT scanning will help to better delineate fractures and foreign bodies or bone within the spinal canal.

When the plain films fail to demonstrate spinal pathology, a controlled flexion and extension view of the area of the spine with questioned injury may be obtained. A physician should be present for supervision of such filming, and the flexion or extension maneuvers should be halted if the patient reports pain or there is increased neurologic deficit.

The role of myelography in patients with spinal injury has always been controversial. Now, with the introduction of water-soluble contrast agents and computer-assisted metrizamide myelography, even wider myelographic alternatives are available. Some possible indications for such studies would include the presence of a neurologic deficit out of proportion to the findings on plain films or a progressing neurologic deficit despite immobilization.

INTRACRANIAL NEOPLASMS

By Eugene A. Quindlen, M.D.
Mobile, Alabama

With the advent of computed tomographic (CT) scanning of the head, the diagnosis of brain tumors has been made considerably easier for the practitioner and patient alike. However, the problem of selecting patients for this procedure still remains a matter of clinical judgment. In addition, some of the common presenting symptoms and signs of intracranial neoplasms, such as headache and seizures, are frequently seen in clinical practice, and sound clinical judgment should be exercised in referring patients for neuroradiologic evaluation, including CT scan.

Although intracranial neoplasms may occur at any age, these tumors are seen most frequently children and middle-life adults. In children there is a high percentage of posterior fossa neoplasms, such as astrocytoma of the cerebellum, medulloblastoma, and ependymoma. In adults, tumors of glial origin are the most frequent primary tumor, with half of these tumors being malignant astrocytomas (glioblastomas). As patients with cancer survive for longer periods beyond their initial diagnosis, the practitioner is encountering more metastatic cerebral tumors. In this regard, breast and lung cancer are the most frequent.

COURSE

The symptomatic course of patients with brain tumors tends to be an indolent or slowly progressive one, with symptoms developing over a period of weeks to months. The patient, however, may indicate a very short course of symptoms upon presentation, neglecting to mention early symptoms, such as transient periods of weakness, numbness, small focal motor seizures, or confusion. In contrast, some tumors, such as midline posterior fossa tumors or intraventricular tumors, can produce an abrupt onset of symptoms when they cause obstructive hydrocephalus.

SIGNS AND SYMPTOMS

The patient with an intracranial tumor can present with nonspecific or generalized signs and symptoms, with focal neurologic complaints, or with a constellation of symptoms including both types.

Generalized Signs and Symptoms

The most common generalized symptom is headache. The patient may describe chronic intermittent or daily headaches that can be related to any part of the cranium but often are global or frontal in location. The headaches may be more frequent in the morning, just after awakening, becoming less severe as the day wears on. They may be described as aching or throbbing in character. Initially they may be relieved by aspirin or other analgesics, but later may become refractory to symptomatic treatment.

When a patient first presents with headache, many other conditions are considered that are more common than an intracranial tumor. These conditions include tension headache, migraine headache, sinusitis, allergic rhinitis, need for ocular refraction, and systemic hypertension. Usually a complete physical examination, including neurologic examination, will help to direct the physician to the correct diagnosis.

When a patient has intractable headaches for which no specific cause can be found, a CT scan without and with intravenous contrast agent should be performed to rule out intracranial pathology. Other diagnostic tests may also be required, as described later (Figs. 1 and 2).

If a patient presents with severe headache of sudden onset with or without neurologic complaints, followed by meningismus, photophobia, and drowsiness, the most likely diagnosis is subarachnoid hemorrhage, usually due to a cerebral aneurysm or possible arteriovenous malformation. Rarely, a primary intracranial tumor will present in such a fashion, with bleeding into the formerly asymptomatic tumor. More commonly, however, subarachnoid hemorrhage is associated with certain metastatic tumors that have a propensity for hemorrhage. This would include metastatic melanoma, choriocarcinoma, or hypernephroma.

Another nonspecific symptom or sign is that of behavioral or mental changes. The patient is often brought to the physician by family members, who may relate any number of complaints, including confusion, drowsiness, depression, senility, emotional lability, or inappropriate behavior, such as paranoia, cursing, or lack of inhibition. A careful history is necessary to determine the onset of the changes, previous psychiatric illness, and other medical problems. The physician must determine if any of these general mental disturbances in fact represent specific neurologic deficits. Aphasia is often mistaken for generalized confusion, depression for drowsiness, and temporal lobe type or psychomotor seizures for emotional changes. Patients with nondominant hemisphere lesions may present with confusion as to their location even in familiar surroundings, may have a "dressing" apraxia, and may even deny that anything is wrong with them (anisognosia).

Changes in mental function are most often associated with frontal or temporal lobe tumors. The onset may be insidious and the changes gradual. The family of an older patient may assume that the patient is just gradually becoming senile. More rapid onset of behavioral changes points to a more rapidly expanding lesion or to raised intracranial pressure associated with obstructive hydrocephalus. In either case, these patients will require thorough neurologic and neuroradiologic investigation.

Another nonspecific symptom of an intracranial mass is seizure activity, which is the second most common symptom of tumor after headache. In some cases, focal seizures of the jacksonian type with clonic activity in an extremity will pinpoint the location of the lesion to the contralateral motor cortex. Likewise, olfactory or gustatory hallucinations or psychomotor seizures will indicate pathology in one of the temporal lobes.

More commonly, however, the patient will present with a generalized motor seizure with loss of consciousness and generalized tonic-clonic activity of the limbs. It is generally considered an axiom of neurology that a first-onset seizure in an adult indi-

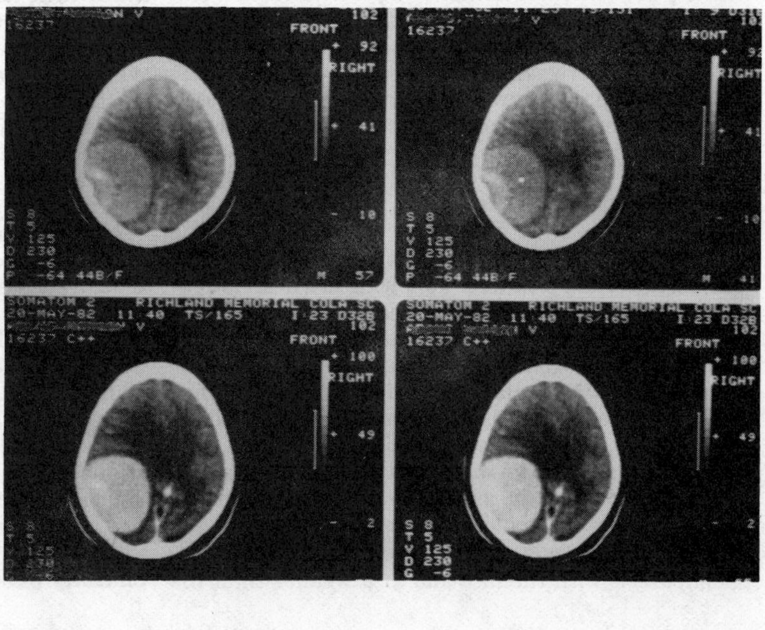

Figure 1. This CT scan without (upper) and with (lower) contrast was performed on a 39-year-old woman who had chronic headaches and sinusitis. The scan was obtained after usual medical therapy failed. A right visual field deficit was found on examination. The tumor has a homogeneous density, which enhances with contrast, and local hyperostosis of the skull is present indicating a meningioma. Removal of the tumor was followed by relief of her symptoms.

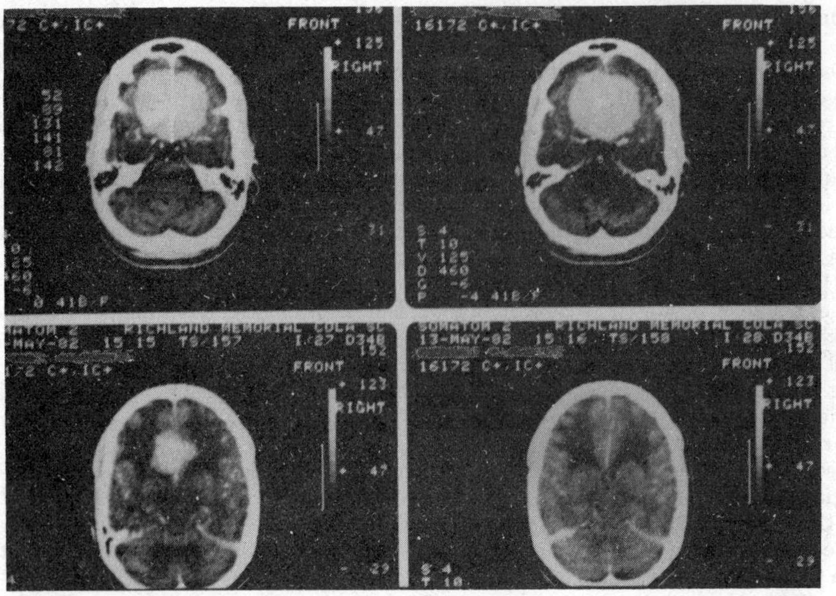

Figure 2. A 25-year-old woman with intractable headaches and progressive lack of spontaniety and interest in her usual activities underwent CT scanning. The scan shows the characteristic features of a meningioma in the floor of the anterior cranial fossa pressing on both frontal lobes. Removal of the tumor relieved the patient's headaches and produced return of her original personality.

cates a tumor until proven otherwise. However, other metabolic causes of generalized seizures must be excluded.

A prolonged postictal paresis (Todd's paralysis) or confusional state often suggests the presence of an intracerebral neoplasm as the cause of the seizure.

Focal Signs and Symptoms

Focal neurologic deficits may be more helpful in localizing the site of the patient's tumor. However, no focal sign is specific for neoplasm, and other diseases of the central nervous system must be considered. A careful neurologic examination is most valuable, since elicitation of additional signs may help to localize the area of dysfunction in the central nervous system. For example, a patient who presents with a left hemiparesis and is found on examination to have a left hemisensory deficit most likely has a lesion involving the right prerolandic and postrolandic cortex or subcortical white matter. On the other hand, a patient who has a left hemiparesis and a contralateral facial nerve or trigeminal nerve palsy most likely has a lesion in the right cerebellopontine angle compressing the ipsilateral cerebral peduncle and brain stem.

Symptom Constellations

Certain constellations of symptoms can suggest neoplasms in certain locations. Following is a description of the more common symptomatic complexes.

The insidious onset of dementia, lack of inhibition, and social unawareness, combined with frontal reflex signs (snout, touch, and grasp with loss of olfactory sense), most often suggests a bifrontal tumor, such as an olfactory groove meningioma. If the patient has frontal lobe signs alone with rapid onset of these signs and no loss of olfaction, an intrinsic glioma involving both frontal lobes would be suggested.

A patient who presents with a seizure and residual hemiparesis with the face and arm weaker than the leg would most likely have a posterior frontal lesion.

Paraparesis and urinary incontinence without any sensory deficit indicates a lesion in the parasagittal area involving the paracentral lobule. Such a lesion is usually a falx or parasagittal meningioma.

An expressive or motor aphasia with right hemiparesis suggests an opercular and left posterior frontal lesion. More posterior lesions in the left cerebral hemisphere can produce a sensory or Wernicke's aphasia when the parietal lobe is involved. Farther posteriorly, tumor involvement of the left parieto-occipital junction can produce dyslexia, dyscalculia, and right-left disorientation (Gerstmann's syndrome), and is usually the result of an intrinsic tumor in that region.

A patient who presents with a visual field defect which is homonymous hemianopia usually has a lesion in the opposite occipital lobe. There are often associated sensory changes or adjacent parietal lobe signs, such as hemineglect (feeling that half of the body does not exist), constructional apraxia, confusion in space (to nondominant hemisphere) or Gerstmann's syndrome (dominant hemisphere).

Visual field examination can be quite revealing and sometimes almost characteristic of the lesion involved. A homonymous superior quadrantopia indicates a lesion in the posterior temporal lobe that has interrupted the inferior optic radiation (Meyer's loop).

A bitemporal hemianopia almost always indicates a mass in the suprasellar-infrachiasmatic area. Although such a lesion could be a cerebral aneurysm, it most commonly is due to an enlarging pituitary tumor with suprasellar extension or a craniopharygioma, which is more commonly seen in children or young adults.

Tumors of the posterior fossa present with the fairly characteristic signs of ataxia, diplopia, or other cranial nerve signs, such as dysarthria, dysphonia, or difficulty in swallowing. The patients may have vertigo and often have nystagmus. Midline or vermis lesions produce a truncal ataxia; the patient has difficulty walking or wavers while sitting and has vertical nystagmus. Lateral cerebellar lesions produce appendicular ataxia with uncoordinated movements of the ipsilateral extremities. The third, fourth, and sixth cranial nerves can be affected with posterior fossa lesions producing diplopia.

Tumors in the posterior fossa often produce obstructive hydrocephalus due to compression of the fourth ventricle and resultant obstruction of cerebrospinal fluid flow. Because of this, the patient may present with a rapidly evolving course of headache, nausea, vomiting, and confusion. Papilledema is often present. The child with headache, nausea, and vomiting may be misdiagnosed as having viral gastroenteritis unless a careful neurologic examination including fundoscopy is performed.

Many endocrine syndromes are caused by tumors of the pituitary gland or tumors involving the hypothalamic area. Hypothalamic gliomas or hamartomas can lead to growth failure in young children or frank hypopituitarism. Craniopharygiomas can produce the same symptoms. In adults, Cushing's disease, acromegaly, hyperprolactinemia with amenorrhea-galactorrhea, and hypopituitarism can all be the result of pituitary tumors. Some of these tumors (microadenomas) are extremely small (2 to 5 mm) and may not be seen with conventional CT scanning techniques. Complete endocrine evaluation will be required, and if this indicates abnormal hormone production of pituitary origin, sellar exploration may be warranted.

A child or young adult with an intrinsic brain stem glioma presents with an insidious, intermittent course of clumsiness and diplopia extending over a period of weeks to months. Examination usually shows no papilledema, but lower cranial nerve palsies, quadriparesis, hemiparesis, or, at a minimum, hyperactive reflexes with Babinski responses will be present.

Tinnitus and slowly progressive unilateral deafness may be the only presenting signs of an acoustic neuroma—an extrinsic cerebellopontine angle tumor that slowly compresses the cranial nerves and brain stem. Neurologic examination may demonstrate a depressed corneal reflex and mild facial weakness on the same side as the hearing loss. As this slowly growing tumor enlarges, vertigo, ipsilateral ataxia, or hemiparesis may result. This tumor is often detected by the audiologist, who finds a hearing loss characteristic of sensorineural deafness along with characteristic changes in tone decay.

The ophthalmologist is often the first clinician to see a patient harboring a pineal gland tumor, since these patients present with diplopia, failure of upward gaze, and nystagmus (Parinaud's oculoglandular syndrome) and may have papilledema. In a more advanced stage, the patients can present with obstructive hydrocephalus with progressive headache, confusion, and vomiting.

DIAGNOSTIC EVALUATION

After a thorough history, physical examination, and neurologic examination, patients with suspected brain tumors are referred for CT scanning of the head. The CT scan has become the primary and initial diagnostic modality for the evaluation of patients with suspected intracranial neoplasms. This test has largely replaced lumbar puncture, electroencephalography (EEG), and pneumoencephalography in the diagnostic evaluation.

When requesting a CT scan, the practitioner should give radiologic colleagues sufficient clinical information, such as location of tumor or type of neurologic deficit suspected, so that an adequate CT scan can be performed. For patients with suspected tumors, the scan is performed without and with the infusion of intravenous contrast material. The contrast-enhanced CT scan can give valuable information as to the vascularity of the tumor or even its potential tissue type. Some tumors that cannot be seen on plain CT scan can be detected with contrast infusion. It is important to specify possible location of the tumor, since with modern CT scanners special thin sections through difficult-to-image areas (e.g., the orbit, sella, petrous bone, and foramen magnum) can often visualize lesions not seen on a routine scan. In addition, the new scanners can perform reconstruction of the image in any plane, which can be of additional localizing value.

For lesions extrinsic to the brain parenchyma, injection of metrizamide into the spinal subarachnoid space prior to CT scanning can detect lesions such as small acoustic neuromas or tumors near the base of the skull.

Cerebral angiography still remains a valuable adjunct to CT scanning in the evaluation of a suspected brain tumor and is especially useful before neurosurgical intervention. The type of neovascularity that can be seen on angiography may indicate the type of tumor, such as metastatic versus primary cerebral tumor. The recently introduced intravenous bolus digital subtraction angiography (DSA) provides yet another potential, but it is as yet not completely tested for assessment of vascular tumors.

Plain skull films can be helpful in evaluating patients with discrete masses of the calvarium, patients with metastatic tumors, and patients with tumors that tend to involve the bony calvarium, such as meningiomas and chordomas. Polytomography of the skull can delineate lesions of the base of the skull, sinuses, orbit, optic canals, and internal auditory canals in addition to providing precise definition of lesions affecting the sella, such as small pituitary tumors.

COMPLICATIONS

In general, with an expeditious evaluation and neurosurgical referral, most patients can avoid secondary complications of their tumors. Nonetheless, pulmonary emboli from deep vein thromboses, especially in bedridden patients, do occur. Aspiration pneumonitis may follow a seizure or vomiting occurring in the drowsy, obtunded patient, or may be due to inability to control normal pharyngeal reflexes in the patient with brain stem and cranial nerve compromise. Large supratentorial lesions with surrounding cerebral edema can produce uncal herniation with resulting compression of the brain stem and worsening of the patient's condition and prognosis. Temporal lobe lesions are most likely to produce this complication. High-dose corticosteroids have been found to reduce peritumoral edema (so-called oncogenic edema), and most patients are started on a regimen of dexamethasone, 4 to 10 mg either orally, intravenously or intramuscularly every 6 hours as soon as the diagnosis of brain tumor is made.

Seizures can be a problem at any time during a patient's course and may aggravate cerebral edema if the patient has prolonged generalized motor seizures. For this reason, patients are usually placed on prophylactic anticonvulsants, such as phenytoin or phenobarbital.

PITFALLS IN DIAGNOSIS

Although patients with intracranial neoplasms present with a history of slowly progressing signs and symptoms, some patients can present with a sudden onset of neurologic symptoms, such as aphasia, hemiparesis, or visual field deficit. The practitioner may diagnose the patient's difficulty as the result of a vascular event or stroke. However, this clinical diagnosis should be confirmed by performing a CT scan without and with contrast enhancement, since occasionally a patient may have a cerebral tumor with hemorrhage or vascular compromise of intracranial vessels. Patients who do appear to have had a cerebral infarct or hemorrhage should have a follow-up CT scan in 7 to 14 days to confirm the diagnosis of stroke as opposed to another lesion.

Patients with brain abscess may present with the characteristic signs of an intracranial mass lesion, such as headache, papilledema, and seizures. However, if the patient is also febrile, usually with confusion and drowsiness, the physician should suspect brain abscess as opposed to brain tumor. The diagnosis of brain abscess would prompt the immediate institution of intravenous antibiotics, a search for the primary source of infection (e.g., sinusitis, pulmonary abscess, cardiac septal defect, and endocarditis), and immediate neurosurgical intervention where appropriate (see article on brain abscesses).

EXPANDING INTRASPINAL LESIONS

By David Yashon, M.D.
Columbus, Ohio

DEFINITION

Expanding intraspinal lesions signify an adverse disease process which, by either gradual or rapid growth, compromises vital structures within the vertebral canal. Such an occurrence may be a secondary result of a lesion elsewhere, or it may arise primarily from anatomic structures comprising the bony spinal canal and its contained structures. Almost any category of disease process can result in an expanding intraspinal lesion with subsequent neurologic deterioration. Synonyms may be related to the actual etiologic factors that cause the intraspinal expanding lesion.

SIGNS AND SYMPTOMS

Signs and symptoms relating to expanding intraspinal lesions may vary according to the location within the spinal canal. If the lesion is at the foramen magnum, structures below that area will be involved, whereas if the lesion occurs in, for example, the lower thoracic area all areas above, relating to both motor and sensory function, will be spared. The etiology and biologic activity are also factors in signs and symptoms. At the level of the L1 vertebral body, signs and symptoms may be caused by involvement of the spinal cord or roots, or both. Below that level only root dysfunction occurs, and above only spinal cord dysfunction occurs. The exception to the latter occurs when a higher root is involved by a lesion in the area of the root entry zone, in which case root symptoms above that level may predominate. The biologic activity and etiology influence the speed of development of signs and symptoms. Malignant extradural tumors most often have a shorter course after initial complaints than do benign tumors and low-grade infections. A vascular lesion may have a sudden, devastating onset. In certain cases, hemorrhage or edema resulting from trauma may also cause rapid or immediate development of neurologically related signs and symptoms.

Extradural Lesions

These lesions are located outside the dura, but within the bony spinal canal. Lesions in this area include infections, either acute or chronic (streptococcal, staphylococcal, tuberculosis, or brucellosis). The vertebral column itself may be involved by infection, but these are rare lesions. Also included are herniated or extruded intravertebral discs, which occur most commonly in the lower lumbar area but are also seen in the thoracic and cervical areas. Metastatic tumors arise primarily in the lung, breast, gastrointestinal tract, kidney, or prostate. Meningiomas (5 to 10 per cent are extradural) and schwannomas (25 per cent are extradural) can be present also. Epidural bleeding may be associated with trauma, anticoagulant therapy, blood dyscrasias, systemic hypertension, lumbar puncture, and, in unusual cases, vascular malformations. Pneumoencephalography is very rarely carried out today, but this was a cause in the past.

In these areas, the initial and most common symptom is pain due to distortion of roots or periosteal structures in the bone that have a radicular distribution. The pain is often bilateral and is distributed in a girdle fashion around the trunk or in a radicular pattern, radiating to a leg or arm. The Valsalva maneuver, with coughing or straining, frequently aggravates the pain. The patient may be awakened at night because of stretching of the involved nerve roots when after several hours of recumbency the vertebral column (mostly owing to the discs) gradually elongates. Sensory symptoms such as numbness and paresthesias may also occur, either below the level of the lesion or in the root distribution. Pressure on the spinal cord tracts themselves gives rise to sensory symptoms below the level of the lesion, including numbness, hypalgesia, and anesthesia. A sensory deficit known as Brown-Séquard syndrome, or a variant thereof, may be due to pressure on the lateral spinothalamic tract and may occur two or more segments below the lesion opposite the side of the cord compression. Hypalgesia to pinprick is the foremost sign, and unilateral posterior column signs can occur.

Motor complaints may vary with the level of the lesion (just as may sensory complaints) with weakness or spasticity, or both. If the spinal cord is involved on a chronic basis, spasticity with increased reflexes and an upper motor neuron lesion can be found, with an extensor toe response. In acute extradural lesions, sometimes flaccidity occurs, and this can lead to diagnostic difficulties. Involvement of a root can result in weakness, decreased muscle tone in the distribution of the root, fasciculations, or diminished reflexes at the appropriate level. Combinations of both root-type disturbance and spinal cord disturbance can occur, and this can provide the clinician with a sense of dermatomal or myotomal level for diagnosis.

Bowel and bladder dysfunction may be seen with these lesions; complaints consist of difficulty in initiating urination and overflow incontinence with dribbling. Sometimes in upper motor neuron type lesions there is a sudden emptying of the bladder in its entirety. Constipation is a common early sign, and rectal examination may disclose a loss of tone and inability to constrict the muscles around the examining finger.

Intradural, Extramedullary Lesions

These lesions lie within the dural sac but external to the spinal cord and may involve nerve roots. Examples of this type of lesion are most schwannomas and meningiomas, some ependymomas (a glial tumor), and congenital or embryonic lesions, such as lipomas, dermoids, and epidermoids. In rare cases, hemorrhage may occur in this area.

The signs and symptoms relating to this type of lesion are primarily of the root initially, but as the lesion expands other structures can be involved, and almost any constellation of signs and symptoms may arise. Again, night pain is probably most common in this type of lesion. In long-standing tumors arising in the pediatric age groups, skeletal deformities and cutaneous manifestations may be found. On examination, café au lait spots, angiomas, atrophic skin, hypertrichosis, and sinuses and dimples of the skin may be seen.

Arteriovenous malformation and vascular anomalies occur most commonly as intradural-extramedullary lesions, but there may be an intramedullary component.

Intramedullary Lesions

These masses occur within the substance of the spinal cord itself and arise primarily from glial tissue. The lesions include primarily gliomas, which are usually low-grade, but in addition ependymomas, lipomas, dermoids and epidermoids, hydromyelia, and syringomyelia, as well as arteriovenous malformations occur. These lesions generally have a longer biologic course and pain is less often a symptom. Usually there is involvement of the long tracts of the spinal cord, and the manifestations are first motor, with sphincter disturbances coming later and sensory loss being variable. In the congenital lesions the skin deformities and cutaneous manifestations mentioned earlier may occur.

COURSE

The course of expanding spinal lesions varies according to the cause. In general, intradural, extramedullary lesions and intramedullary lesions are slower growing than extradural lesions. The course is gradually or rapidly progressive in vertebral lesions, to the point where severe neurologic deficit may occur, including paraplegia or quadriplegia. Sometimes in the case of an extramedullary lesion compression of the anterior spinal artery can occur, with sudden loss of neurologic function below the level of spinal cord infarction. Because touch, position sense, and vibration sense are located posteriorly, sometimes these are preserved, providing a hint to the diagnosis. By virtue of various diagnostic measures, the course can be interrupted by surgical intervention, and improvement may even occur.

PHYSICAL AND NEUROLOGIC EXAMINATION

The physical and neurologic examinations have been alluded to earlier. In the general physical examination, sources of metastatic lesions external to the vertebral column should be sought. The dermal and skeletal signs of a congenital lesion should be looked for. A thorough neurologic examination should be performed. A useful sign of involvement of bladder sensation is "catheter tug." In a normal individual when the catheter is pulled, severe pain is felt. When anesthesia supervenes, no pain is felt. The presence of pain sensation sometimes is the last sign of retained neurologic function in rapidly progressive spinal cord compression. Pinprick sensation is also important in determining the dermatomal sensory level, and sometimes very subtle changes may occur. It is important to compare lower areas with an area above the site of the lesion so that subtle differences in the quality of perception can be ascertained.

LABORATORY PROCEDURES

Routine blood chemistry studies and blood counts can reveal, or at least give hints to, the cause of the problem. A high white blood cell count may indicate infection, and an elevated acid or alkaline phosphatase level may be indicative of certain carcinomas. Examination of the cerebrospinal fluid is done in conjunction with the myelogram; however, in my opinion it is not very useful. In most cases of intramedullary or even extramedullary compression, the cerebrospinal fluid protein is elevated and all this implies is that there is a nonspecific lesion, which is already known because of the abnormal examination. A diminished cerebrospinal fluid glucose level can give a hint of intradural infection or carcinomatous meningitis. The Queckenstedt test is of almost no use in my opinion. A large intraspinal lesion with an opening only the size of a number 18 needle may accompany a normal Queckenstedt test. If in doubt, myelography should be performed and then the issue can be settled. False-negative Queckenstedt tests can occur with abdominal compression even in the face of a complete block. The cerebrospinal fluid protein electrophoretic pattern is of less importance when a space-occupying lesion is present. In lesions causing spinal blocks, the protein may reach over 1000 mg/dl with coagulation of the fluid on standing (Froin's syndrome) and xanthochromia. Cell blocks for cytologic examination may be useful in diagnosing metastatic tumors. Immunoelectrophoresis may be used in ruling out demyelinating diseases.

When bladder dysfunction occurs, a cystometrogram can give a quantitative estimation and may be helpful in marginal cases when the diagnosis is in doubt. An intravenous pyelogram and voiding cystogram sometimes may assist.

Electromyography is of use in diagnosing root or cauda equina lesions, but is of almost no use in diagnosing intraspinal lesions. It is helpful in ruling out a degenerative, nonexpanding spinal disease, such as amyotrophic lateral sclerosis, and in slowly progressive cases is probably a necessity.

RADIOLOGIC PROCEDURES

All patients should have appropriate x-rays of the area of the spine involved, and chest x-rays are useful since many tumors arise in the lung. Plain spinal x-rays can show destruction or erosion of bone, excess calcification, and changes in the size of the canal using established measurements. Sometimes the nature of the lesion can be determined by the plain x-rays. For example, metastatic tumors may lead to destruction of the vertebral body and pedicles, whereas more slowly growing intradural tumors and congenital lesions can lead to widening of the bony canal and intrapedicular distance. Oblique views can show widening and enlargement of the intravertebral foramina, as in certain neurofibromas. Destruction of the intravertebral disc, with or without kyphosis, is sometimes seen in conjunction with paravertebral masses and may indicate the rare case of tuberculosis or brucellosis.

Probably the most useful radiologic procedure is a myelogram performed with oil-soluble (Pantopaque) or water-soluble (Amopaque) contrast medium. Air tomography is sometimes utilized, but is less specific. Upper and lower limits of the lesion can be ascertained by instillation of contrast media via a spinal puncture laterally at C1 and another puncture in the lower lumbar area. The upper puncture is seldom necessary. Myelography should be carried out at a time and place where definitive surgical therapy can be performed, as occasionally deterioration occurs as a result of a lumbar puncture.

CT scanning of the spinal canal has been useful, and lateral reconstructions sometimes show the extent of the lesion. I have performed CT scanning almost routinely 4 to 6 hours after the introduction of Amopaque for an excellent display of intravertebral canal pathology.

Spinal cord arteriography carries some risks and is not routinely used to diagnose intraspinal lesions unless an arterial malformation is strongly suspected.

PITFALLS IN DIAGNOSIS

Confusion of degenerative or intrinsic spinal cord nonexpanding diseases, such as motor neuron disease (e.g., amyotrophic lateral sclerosis, multiple sclerosis, arachnoiditis, combined system disease, and others), with an expanding, surgically treatable spinal cord lesion is most dangerous. Subarachnoid hemorrhage from ependymomas of the terminal spinal cord and other expanding lesions can be confused with an intracranial source of bleeding. Papilledema has even been observed in spinal cord lesions with high levels of cerebrospinal fluid protein. In case of doubt, myelography is a relatively benign test, particularly when Amopaque is used. With this technique it is hoped that the cause will be revealed, which will permit appropriate treatment that will prevent further neurologic deterioration.

THE DEMENTIAS

By Ira Shoulson, M.D.
and Roger Kurlan, M.D.
Rochester, New York

DEFINITION

Dementia refers to intellectual failure and is usually accompanied by behavioral change. Intellectual function covers an array of mental operations but generally applies to cognition, memory, perception, language, and orientation. In contrast to mental retardation, in which the intellect was never normal, dementia is an acquired loss of intellect. Dementia is not a distinct diagnostic entity. The terminology is similar to the designations congestive heart failure or chronic renal failure. Accordingly, dementia arises from different causative factors and some causes are reversible.

CLASSIFICATION

Radiographic advances in computed tomography (CT), positron emission imaging, and nuclear magnetic resonance (NMR) are helping to better define functional-anatomic correlates of dementia. Recombinant DNA analysis, improved virologic detection, and monoclonal antibody techniques hold promise in clarifying the underlying causes of many idiopathic dementias. Notwithstanding these advances, the causes of many dementias remain obscure.

The dementias may be classified by cause, age of onset, attendant neurologic signs, or reversibility. At present it is most useful to classify the dementias on the basis of brain localization because the signs and symptoms generally reflect the locus of the brain affected and not the type of disease process. This classification has limitations because many dementias are progressive and involve extensive areas of the brain, so that strict categorization becomes meaningless. The ultimate worth of such a classification is to aid in early clinical recognition, allowing investigative and therapeutic efforts to proceed on a rational basis.

We classify dementias according to those that can be localized to the *cortical, subcortical,* or *axial* regions of the brain, in comparison with those that reflect more *global* brain involvement.

Cortical dementias are characterized by disturbances in cerebral association areas serving language, complex motor activity, and sensory interpretation. These disturbances result in *aphasias* (impairment of language), *apraxias* (disorders of learned complex movements), and *agnosias* (failure of perception). These cortical deficits may at first appear mild, but they evolve in the course of illness and eventually become conspicuous.

Subcortical dementias are characterized by a decline in cognitive powers but without evident loss of associative cortical processing. Aphasia, apraxia, and agnosia are not prominent in patients with subcortical dementias, who typically show deficits in attention, spontaneity, elaboration, organization, rapid mental processing, and memory. Features of basal ganglia disease frequently coexist.

Axial dementias are so designated because they involve the axial structures of the brain, such as the medial portion of the temporal lobes, hippocampus, fornix, mammillary bodies, hypothalamus, and medial thalami. It is these areas that are largely related to the registration of memory. The prominent feature of axial dementias is the marked and seemingly circumscribed disturbance in recent memory, which severely hampers learning a new task or retaining new information. Confabulation frequently results. Equally striking is the absence of those intellectual disturbances characteristically found in the cortical and subcortical dementias. In most instances of axial dementia, there are few overt behavioral abnormalities.

If the disturbance in intellectual function appears widespread, especially at end-stage disease, this classification loses its value and the term *global dementia* is applied. Some dementing illnesses may overlap into two or more categories. A small number of patients with dementia defy classification. However, this descriptive approach correlates surprisingly well with postmortem pathologic findings and provides a basis for further investigation and therapy. Despite its drawbacks, most common causes of dementia, including the diagnostic entities that follow, can be accurately viewed in the foregoing classification scheme (Table 1).

ALZHEIMER'S TYPE DEMENTIA

Synonyms

Alzheimer's disease, senile dementia, presenile dementia, senile dementia of the Alzheimer's type.

Definition

Alzheimer's type dementia (ATD) is a very common degenerative disorder, characterized by a progressive cortical dementia and associated behavioral changes. Pathologic alterations include diffuse cerebral atrophy, neuronal loss, senile plaques, and neurofibrillary tangles. Recent studies suggest that the nucleus basalis, a dense collection of subcortical cholinergic neurons that projects widely to the cerebral cortex, is the site of major pathologic change in ATD. Choline acetyltransferase, the synthesizing enzyme for acetylcholine, is reduced in amount in the cerebral cortex of patients with senile dementia and the reduction correlates well with the extent of intellectual impairment. The current view is that ATD primarily reflects a disruption of cholinergic pathways arising in subcortical structures and projecting to cortical regions. There is little basis for the artificial distinction between senile and presenile ATD. Pick's disease is clinically similar to ATD, but can usually be distinguished at pathologic examination. At present, there are insufficient clinical criteria for antemortem confirmation of Pick's disease.

Presentation

Behavioral changes often precede intellectual problems in ATD and include the following:

1. Accentuation of prior behavioral traits to the point of eccentricity.
2. An apathetic attitude, which precludes taking on novel ventures.
3. The inability to handle multiple mental operations, with a marked distractibility when required to do so.

Memory impairment is the earliest sign of intellectual deficit in most patients. As the cortical dementia evolves, well-developed aphasic, apractic, and agnostic syndromes typically emerge. Early language problems are usually manifested by word-finding difficulties, intrusion of words previously used, and

Table 1. Classification of Common Dementias

Cortical Dementias	**Subcortical Dementias (Continued)**
Alzheimer's type	Parkinson's disease
Multi-infarct	Normal pressure hydrocephalus
Creutzfeld-Jakob	Neoplastic
Metabolic	Head trauma
Infectious	**Axial Dementias**
Neoplastic	Korsakoff's psychosis
Subcortical Dementias	Normal pressure hydrocephalus
Huntington's disease	Herpes encephalitis
Progressive supranuclear palsy	Head trauma

gradual attrition of complex language capabilities, both in expression and in comprehension. Reading and writing eventually suffer, along with deterioration in spoken language. Practic disorders lead to confusion in carrying out the sequence of motor acts, such as cooking, dressing, and other accustomed tasks. Perceptual disorders are usually manifested by problems with construction and geographic orientation. Confusion at night is common because sensory input is lessened. Even minor changes in the patient's health or living situation, such as changes in medication or environment, may worsen intellectual functioning.

Course

The course of ATD is predictably progressive, usually extending over a period of 5 to 10 years from the initial emergence of symptoms. The patient rapidly loses gainful financial and domestic skills and eventually is no longer capable of caring for his or her own needs. Bronchopneumonia or other intercurrent illness is the usual immediate cause of death.

Physical Examination

Primary visual, motor, and sensory functions remain relatively intact throughout the course of ATD. Presence of focal neurologic deficits, such as hemiplegia and hemianopia, suggests that the appropriateness of the diagnosis must be questioned or that another pathologic process coexists. Muscle stretch reflexes are not greatly altered, and the plantar responses typically remain flexor. Seizures are rare, but widespread myoclonic jerks are occasionally observed. The so-called frontal release signs (e.g., snout, grasp, and palmomental reflexes) are primitive complex reflexes that may emerge as a consequence of lost cortical inhibition.

Laboratory Procedures

Computed tomography of the head may show diffuse cortical atrophy; however, the degree of cortical atrophy may not exceed that observed in many intellectually intact persons. For this reason, the head CT scan is not sufficiently sensitive or specific for the diagnosis of ATD. However, CT of the head is extremely helpful in excluding other causes of dementia, such as subdural hematoma, tumor, multiple cerebral infarctions, and hydrocephalus. The electroencephalogram (EEG) may show diffuse slowing, but this usually occurs in the advanced phases of the illness. Spinal fluid is usually normal, although total protein level may be slightly elevated. Neuropsychological testing is often useful in defining that the dementia is of a cortical variety. Serial testing may help in quantifying the extent and rate of intellectual decline.

Pitfalls in Diagnosis

Although reversible forms of dementia are infrequent, the specter of dementia—a failing mind in a healthy body—is so dreadful that a missed opportunity for treatment has immense implication for the patient and family. As will be discussed, the clinician is compelled to exercise utmost care in ruling out more reversible types of dementia. Therapeutic outcome in all types of dementia, including ATD, is largely related to the precision of diagnosis.

MULTI-INFARCT DEMENTIA

Definition

Multi-infarct dementia (MID) refers to impairment of intellectual function resulting from multiple cerebral infarctions. It is not synonymous with "arteriosclerotic dementia," a vague and probably rare entity.

Presentation

MID is recognized clinically by the accumulation of abrupt vascular episodes (strokes), generally in association with focal neurologic deficits. The cerebral infarctions may result from intracranial or extracranial atheromatous disease or from cardiac origins. The hypertensive patient is particularly prone to small lacunar infarctions, which may elude radiographic detection. Multiple lacunae may produce a picture of pseudobulbar paresis with its typical emotional lability, dysarthria, dysphagia, and hyperactive facial and mandibular reflexes. However, the degree of focal neurologic deficit may be small in comparison to the intellectual impairment. A cortical type of dementia will generally emerge, but some patients may show predominant subcortical features referable to infarctions in the basal ganglia and adjacent structures.

Course

MID is characterized by a stepwise progression in intellectual function reflecting the multiple occurrences of cerebral infarction. This is in contrast to the indolent course that characterizes most degenerative dementias.

Physical Examination

Cortical, subcortical, or mixed features of dementia may occur. The cortical infarctions are usually reflected by focal neurologic deficits, often in association with corticospinal tract signs, visual field loss, and cortical sensory disturbances. The pseudobulbar state may be present.

Laboratory Procedures

CT of the head usually shows multiple areas of cerebral infarction. However, small lacunar infarcts may not be visualized. Conventional angiography, digital subtraction, or noninvasive carotid artery imaging may detect remediable sources of cerebral embolization in extracranial vessels. Many patients have cardiac abnormalities, such as atrial fibrillation or cardiac valvular disease, which predispose to cerebral emboli. The electroencephalogram (EEG) may show focal slowing or discharging features referable to the areas of infarction.

Pitfalls in Diagnosis

"Cerebral arteriosclerosis" is a vague entity, commonly attributed as a cause of dementia. The clinical verification of MID is important because the degree of disability and the course may be favorably altered by therapy (e.g., antihypertensive drugs, anticoagulants, antiplatelet agents, vascular surgery).

CREUTZFELDT-JAKOB DISEASE

Synonyms

Jakob-Creutzfeldt disease, subacute spongiform encephalopathy.

Definition

Creutzfeldt-Jakob disease (CJD) refers to a clinical syndrome characterized by rapidly progressive and profound dementia, usually in association with extrapyramidal dysfunction, cerebellar ataxia, and periodic myoclonic jerks. The major neuropathologic changes occur diffusely in the cerebral and cerebellar cortices and consist of widespread neuronal loss and gliosis accompanied by a striking vacuolation or spongy state. A transmissible virus-like agent has been demonstrated to underlie the pathogenesis of this disease. Familial cases have been observed, and transmission has occurred in some isolated instances following neurosurgery and corneal transplantation. (The article on subacute and chronic viral encephalitis and encephalopathy provides additional information.)

Presentation

The early manifestations CJD vary, but changes in behavior and intellect are common, in association with abnormalities of motor, cerebellar, and visual functions. Delirious states may be seen in the early phases.

Course

CJD characteristically progresses at a steady and rapid pace. Myoclonic jerks involving various muscle groups eventually appear in nearly all patients. The myoclonic jerks tend to be initiated by a variety of sensory stimuli, but also occur spontaneously. Ataxia and dysarthria usually become prominent. Some patients develop parkinsonian features. Stupor and coma eventually supervene. The disease is invariably fatal, usually in less than 1 to 2 years from the time of onset.

Laboratory Procedures

The EEG is most helpful, changing over the course of the illness from diffuse slowing to high-voltage, synchronous sharp waves with periodic discharges followed by a "burst suppression" pattern. Blood and cerebrospinal fluid studies are generally normal, and proper care must be taken in the handling of spinal fluid and neural tissue. CT scan of the head shows no characteristic changes.

Pitfalls in Diagnosis

The EEG alterations described are not pathognomonic of CJD. Myoclonus is also observed in several other dementias, including ATD.

HUNTINGTON'S DISEASE

Synonyms

Huntington's chorea, hereditary chorea.

Definition

Huntington's disease (HD) is an autosomal dominant hereditary disorder characterized clinically by disordered movement, dementia, and a variety of behavioral disturbances. Penetrance is complete for those who inherit the HD gene, and spontaneous mutations have not been documented. Clinical manifestations reflect neuronal degeneration localized primarily to the caudate nucleus and putamen (neostriatum). Cortical regions are relatively unaffected. (This condition is also discussed in the article on extrapyramidal disorders.)

Presentation

Symptoms and signs of HD usually become evident in the third or fourth decade of life, but onset may appear as early as childhood or as late as the seventh or eighth decade. Initial clinical features may take the form of motor, behavioral, or intellectual disturbance. Involuntary choreic movements characteristically appear and may merge with dystonic posturing to produce choreoathetosis. Patients with early onset in childhood or adolescence may develop prominent parkinsonism and cerebellar dysfunction and show minimal if any chorea. Early behavioral disturbances commonly include personality change, apathy, irritability, seclusiveness, and depression. Some HD patients may show frank psychotic features with schizophrenic-like disorders.

The dementia of HD is characterized by progressive memory disturbance, difficulties in organization, and problems in changing from one cognitive task to another. This intellectual disarray results in early loss of gainful skills and eventual loss of financial and domestic abilities. The pattern of intellectual impairment in HD typifies that of a subcortical dementia. Although articulation is inevitably disturbed, central language functions remain preserved. Insight and orientation usually remain intact. Apraxias and agnosias appear rarely in the most advanced stages of illness.

Course

HD is an inexorably progressive disorder with the course of illness usually spanning 10 to 20 years from the onset of clinical features. In some patients the disease progresses at a faster rate than others. Self-care capacities eventually become compromised, and patients require progressively higher levels of care. The relatively high incidence of suicide in HD is partly attributed to preserved insight and the common occurrence of depression.

Physical Examination

Disordered movement is a characteristic feature of HD. While typically appearing hyperkinetic with chorea or choreoathetosis, the patient may also show parkinsonian and cerebellar features as the predominant movement disorder, especially in those patients with early onset and in the advanced phases of illness. Seizures are occasionally observed in HD patients in whom onset was in childhood or adolescence. Dysarthria and dysphagia become prominent and eventually result in serious communication problems and recurrent aspiration pneumonia. Although muscle stretch reflexes often become hyperactive and extensor plantar responses occasionally appear, weakness and sensory deficits do not develop. Visual acuity is not affected, but saccadic eye velocity becomes impaired and some patients may develop limited gaze and convergence.

Laboratory Procedures

The family pedigree is pivotal for the diagnosis of HD. At present, there are no diagnostic procedures that can reliably detect the HD gene prior to the onset of clinical signs. Although intellectual and behavioral changes may be the earliest manifestations of HD, the appearance of a movement disorder remains the most specific and reliable diagnostic indicator.

CT of the head will eventually show evidence of caudate nucleus atrophy in HD patients. However, this radiographic finding is frequently not present in the early phases of HD and is not by itself sufficiently specific for early diagnosis. Neither the EEG nor cerebrospinal fluid shows characteristic findings.

Pitfalls in Diagnosis

A complete and accurate family history is the most important aid in the diagnosis of HD and other hereditary dementias. (See article on the approach to genetic diseases.) Diseases associated with movement disorder and dementia and which also occur in hereditary patterns include Wilson's disease, spinocerebellar degeneration, choreoacanthocytosis, and myoclonus epilepsy. Because Wilson's disease is eminently treatable, this disorder requires appropriate exclusion in patients with undiagnosed movement disorder. Alzheimer's type dementia, Creutzfeldt-Jakob disease, and some variants of parkinsonism have been reported to occur in autosomal dominant patterns, but the genetic basis for these disorders has not yet been clarified.

A variety of drugs, especially antipsychotic agents, exert neuroleptic properties and can induce hyperkinetic and hypokinetic movement disorders. Delayed-onset dyskinesia (tardive dyskinesia) may mimic many of the clinical features of HD. A careful history of drug and toxic exposure is therefore essential in the evaluation of patients with movement disorders. The use of antipsychotic agents in individuals at risk for HD should be carefully weighed in view of the propensity for these drugs to induce movement disorders.

PARKINSON'S DISEASE

Synonyms

Paralysis agitans, idiopathic Parkinson's disease, primary Parkinson's disease, parkinsonism.

Definition

Parkinson's disease (PD) is a symptom complex consisting of tremor, rigidity, slowness and paucity of movement (bradykinesia, hypokinesia), and disorders of posture and balance. Clinical features and variants (e.g., progressive supranuclear palsy) are discussed in greater detail elsewhere (see article on extrapyramidal disorders). This discussion is restricted to the intellectual and behavioral changes that may accompany Parkinson's disease. Only a few studies have examined the prevalence of dementia among patients with Parkinson's disease. Interpretation of the literature is difficult because of the failure, in most studies, to clearly define dementia. Nevertheless, it is estimated that between 20 and 40 per cent of patients with Parkinson's disease show progressive intellectual decline.

Presentation

The clinical features of dementia in PD patients are not well delineated. However, certain deficits in intellectual function tend to be prominent in PD, including disturbances in visuospatial discrimination and in memory. Patients may appear apathetic or depressed and have difficulty with tasks that require a sequence of mental operations. These features of dementia can be loosely categorized as of subcortical type, but some PD patients may develop a profile of intellectual failure that is indistinguishable clinically and pathologically from ATD. Dementia is usually seen more frequently in patients with atypical parkinsonism, which is associated with symmetric motor involvement, minimal or absent tremor, poor response to antiparkinsonian therapy, and attendant autonomic, cerebellar, or spinal cord disturbances.

Course

Several investigations of PD have indicated a close relationship between the extent of bradykinesia and a decline in intellectual activity. Although dementia usually emerges as a sequela of advanced PD, it may also appear in the early phases of illness.

Pitfalls in Diagnosis

There appears to be a subgroup of patients with PD who also show clinical and neuropathologic signs of ATD. Since a high proportion of patients with PD develop depression at some point during the course of illness, a psychiatrically based pseudodementia may develop. In addition, various antiparkinsonian drugs may produce cognitive and behavioral changes that can mimic dementia.

KORSAKOFF'S PSYCHOSIS

Synonyms

Wernicke-Korsakoff syndrome, amnestic-confabulatory psychosis.

Definition

Korsakoff's psychosis refers to a serious sequela of nutritional deficiency in which retentive memory is prominently impaired out of proportion to other cognitive operations. Korsakoff's psychosis may appear in conjunction with or following Wernicke's syndrome, which is characterized by the clinical triad of ophthalmoplegia, ataxia, and mental confusion. Wernicke's syndrome is a consequence of thiamine deficiency and is observed primarily, although not exclusively, in alcoholics. Korsakoff's psychosis is typically associated with alcoholism and malnutrition, but it may stem from a variety of brain disorders involving the temporal lobes and diencephalon. The specific pathogenetic role of thiamine deficiency is more firmly established in Wernicke's syndrome than in Korsakoff's psychosis.

Presentation

Any of the clinical features of Wernicke's syndrome, alone or in combination, may be the initial manifestations of Korsakoff's psychosis. The ocular abnormalities consist of (1) horizontal and vertical nystagmus, (2) paresis of lateral rectus muscles, and (3) paresis of conjugate gaze. In advanced stages, there may be complete loss of ocular movements, and the pupils, which are typically spared, may become miotic and fixed. Ataxia of station and gait occurs with variable severity.

Some patients who develop Korsakoff's psychosis may show signs of alcohol withdrawal with a global confusional state. As confusion subsides, the striking change in memory becomes evident. The patient may have some degree of retrograde memory loss that extends back for weeks or years. This is usually a discontinuous loss with some islands of preserved memory. The memory disorder is usually so severe that it is almost impossible for the patient to retain new material. Confabulation is not a sine qua non for the diagnosis of Korsakoff's psychosis, but it is frequently present. This pattern of amnestic disturbance represents a type of axial dementia.

Course

The mortality rate in the acute phase of Wernicke's syndrome may approach 15 to 20 per cent. Fatalities are usually related to delirium tremens, associated infections, or hepatic failure. Patients who receive prompt and adequate doses of thiamine usually recover in a fairly predictable pattern. A dramatic restoration of ocular motility often begins within hours of thiamine administration. Failure of the ocular palsies to respond to thiamine should raise doubts concerning the diagnosis of Wernicke's syndrome. Ocular abnormalities recover completely within a week or two in most cases, but vertical nystagmus may occasionally persist for several months. Horizontal nystagmus is unique among the ocular signs in that it may remain as a permanent sequela. In contrast to the ocular signs, improvement of ataxia may be delayed for several weeks after thiamine treatment. Some patients do not recover completely but may have coexistent cerebellar dysfunction and are left with residual gait disturbances.

The symptoms of delirium and global confusion usually resolve over a period of weeks, but the circumscribed defects in memory and learning of Korsakoff's psychosis may become more evident. Only a small proportion of patients recover from the memory disorder once it becomes established.

Physical Examination

Patients may show signs of chronic alcoholism, malnutrition, and chronic hepatic failure. Ocular abnormalities may include nystagmus and gaze palsies. Signs of peripheral neuropathy are found in most patients with Wernicke's syndrome. Autonomic dysfunction, including tachycardia, postural hypotension, and fever, may indicate coexistent delirium tremens.

Laboratory Procedures

The cerebrospinal fluid is normal or shows only a modest elevation of protein content. Blood pyruvate level is consistently elevated before treatment with thiamine. Patients show a marked reduction in erythrocyte transketolase activity, an index of thiamine deficiency. Brain stem auditory evoked potentials and electronystagmography have been reported to be abnormal.

Pitfalls in Diagnosis

Although Wernicke's syndrome and Korsakoff's psychosis are usually associated with alcoholism, it is emphasized that a variety of metabolic insults and diseases may produce this clinical picture. These include prolonged parenteral nutrition, extensive burns, tumors, strokes, herpes simplex encephalitis, head trauma, and anoxia. A transient amnesic syndrome may be caused by temporal lobe epilepsy or the syndrome of transient global amnesia.

A more global form of dementia often results from chronic alcohol abuse and is not associated with oculomotor disturbances or isolated amnesic features. Although global alcoholic dementia has not been linked specifically to thiamine deficiency, it is usually associated with chronically poor nutrition.

NORMAL PRESSURE HYDROCEPHALUS

Definition

Normal pressure hydrocephalus (NPH) is a clinical syndrome consisting of intellectual impairment, gait disturbance, and sphincteric incontinence. This clinical triad is associated with radiographic evidence of communicating hydrocephalus and normal intracranial pressure. This constellation of clinical and radiographic findings is often a sequela of subarachnoid hemorrhage or meningitis, but in many instances is related to undetermined causes of disturbed cerebrospinal fluid dynamics.

Presentation

The dementia of NPH may appear as an axial type with prominent memory disturbance. This may be related to an enlarged third ventricle and involvement of the medial thalamic nuclei. Some patients may show prominent subcortical features in association with parkinsonism. The gait disorder of NPH is characterized by prominent hesitancy, small steps, and ataxia. Urinary and bowel incontinence classically accompany the gait disorder. These motor and autonomic disturbances may be related to compromise of the corticospinal tracts, which course near the dilated lateral ventricles.

Course

The clinical features of NPH are slowly progressive. Gratifying functional improvement and complete restoration of mental and motor functions may result from surgical shunting of ventricular fluid, but the outcome of shunting procedures remains difficult to predict.

Laboratory Procedures

CT of the head demonstrates widened ventricles, which are disproportionately enlarged in comparison with any cortical atrophy. Radionuclide cisternography reveals prolonged isotope distribution in the ventricles and delayed pericerebral diffusion. According to some investigators, the infusion of normal saline into the lumbar subarachnoid space at a rate of 0.76 ml per minute for 30 to 60 minutes produces a rise in pressure to greater than 300 mm of water that is not observed in normal individuals. Drainage of large amounts (15 to 25 ml) of cerebrospinal fluid by lumbar puncture may result in transient but dramatic clinical improvement in some patients with NPH. This type of clinical response may aid in predicting a beneficial response to ventricular shunting.

Pitfalls in Diagnosis

NPH is a potentially reversible cause of dementia. Patients who seem best suited to shunting are those with a brief duration of classic clinical features and those with an antecedent history of subarachnoid hemorrhage or meningitis. The head CT scan alone cannot reliably differentiate between NPH and other atrophic disorders.

PSEUDODEMENTIA

Synonyms

Functional dementia, psychiatric dementia, depressive pseudodementia.

Definition

Pseudodementia refers to intellectual impairment arising from a primary psychiatric disorder. The intellectual deficits resemble, at least in part, those features found in other dementias, but pseudodementia is potentially reversible if the underlying psychiatric disorder is amenable to treatment. Pseudodementia does not relate specifically to one psychiatric disorder, although it occurs most commonly in patients with affective disorders.

Presentation

Patients with pseudodementia usually exhibit a subcortical pattern of intellectual impairment in association with inattention, slowed mental processing, lack of spontaneity, poor motivation, and deficits in memory retrieval. Cortical dementias and circumscribed axial patterns are generally not seen.

Despite the similarity of symptoms between pseudodementia and more classic forms of dementia, there are clinical features that aid in differential diagnosis. A past history of affective disorder suggests a primary psychiatric disturbance. Performance on neuropsychological testing may be helpful in that patients with pseudodementia often show inconsistent performance from test to test and less severe objective deficits than are suggested by the history. Patients may make little effort to perform simple tasks, and "I don't know" answers are typical. Symptoms due to the associated psychiatric disorder are frequently present. Insomnia, anorexia, reduced libido, and crying spells may be seen in patients with depression. More blatant behavioral disturbances with delusionary patterns and paranoid ideation may occur in patients with underlying schizophrenic-like illness.

Laboratory Procedures

Formal neuropsychological testing may be useful in differentiating pseudodementia from other dementing illnesses. The dexamethasone suppression test (DST) has been reported to be abnormal in some patients with depression, but the clinical value of this test is controversial.

Neuropsychological testing is not infallible in discriminating "organic" and "functional" disorders. Confirmation of the diagnosis of pseudodementia may ultimately depend on an evaluation of pharmacotherapy, such as trials of antidepressant or antipsychotic medications.

Pitfalls in Diagnosis

Depressive and other psychiatric symptoms commonly occur in individuals with neuropathologically based dementias. Thus, the presence of psychiatric features does not preclude an underlying organic dementia. Moreover, pseudodementia and other dementing diseases may coexist in the same patient.

DIAGNOSTIC EVALUATION OF PATIENTS WITH DEMENTIA

For diagnostic purposes, the general phrases "dementia" and "organic brain syndrome" refer to those conditions in which the patient has intellectual failure of yet undetermined cause. However, specific clinical diagnosis can usually be made in the overwhelming number of patients presenting with intellectual decline. Identification of the underlying disease will have direct therapeutic importance for most patients.

All patients with presumed intellectual impairment should have the benefit of a complete clinical evaluation, based on a systematic and comprehensive history, physical examination, and laboratory assessment. Diagnostic evaluation is of obvious importance for potentially reversible disease processes (Table 2). In addition, the evaluation process will help to better focus on the needs and concerns of both patients and families and will ultimately improve care.

History

The most helpful and reliable historical information in evaluating dementia is usually obtained from relatives or friends, rather than directly from the patient. It is uncommon for the patient with dementia to initiate the clinical contact. If the patient initiates the clinical evaluation or is preoccupied with concerns of a memory problem, the examiner should be alerted to the possibility of a pseudodementia, particularly due to depression. The history may also provide a focus for the types of mental operations that appear to be most affected, suggesting a cortical, subcortical, or axial pattern of dementia.

The temporal course of the intellectual decline is a useful indicator of the underlying cause of dementia. A sudden, definable onset suggests more precipitous causes of dementia, such as multiple infarcts, head trauma, or infection. A more insidious onset is associated with degenerative disorders, such as Alz-

Table 2. Potentially Reversible Causes of Dementia

Intracranial Conditions
Neoplasms, subdural hematoma, hydrocephalus, epilepsy, multiple sclerosis, multiple infarctions

Infections
Syphilis, chronic meningitis, herpes simplex encephalitis, brain abscess, cysticercosis, Whipple's disease

Drugs

Heavy Metals
Mercury, arsenic, lead, thallium

Hereditary Disorders
Wilson's disease

Toxins
Organophosphates, carbon disulfide, toluene, trichlorethylene, carbon monoxide, alcohol

Deficiency States
Vitamin B_{12} deficiency, pellagra, folate deficiency

Endocrinopathies and Related Factors
Hypothyroidism, Cushing's disease, corticosteroid therapy, hypoglycemia, hypoparathyroidism, hyperparathyroidism, panhypopituitarism, Addison's disease, hyperthyroidism

Systemic Illnesses and Related Factors
Anemia, polycythemia vera, cardiac failure, pulmonary insufficiency, renal insufficiency, renal dialysis, portosystemic encephalopathy, hyperosmolarity, hyponatremia, porphyria, sarcoidosis, vasculitis

Psychiatric Illnesses (Pseudodementia)

heimer's or Huntington's disease. Some dementias are typically rapidly progressive, such as Creutzfeldt-Jakob disease or malignant brain tumor. The course of multi-infarct dementia may be slow but shows episodic, stepwise deterioration.

Inquiries should be made into possible drug, toxic, or infectious exposure and the patient's nutritional status. A history of prior psychiatric illness may provide important diagnostic clues. A complete family history is essential in the evaluation of all patients.

Mental Status Examination

A systematic examination of all cognitive functions should be performed and recorded. Orientation, memory, abstraction, judgment, perception, and language are mental operations that specifically need to be tested to give a quick appraisal of mental status.

Orientation is assessed by questions about person, place, and time. Memory is analyzed in terms of immediate, recent, and remote recall. Immediate memory is best tested by asking the patient to remember digit sequences, while recent memory is traditionally evaluated by observing the ability to retain three items after 5 minutes or similar tasks. Remote memory is assessed by referring back to past events. Abstraction may be tested by proverb interpretation. Judgment is best assessed by information from relatives as well as by the patient's judgment in hypothetical situations. Observing the ability to copy simple and complex figures is a reliable way to test perception. A quick survey of language ability can be done in the course of conversation, but observations should be made regarding spontaneous production of speech, complexity of speech, use of correct names, and comprehension. Simple tests of object recognition and naming should be performed. Subtle aphasic problems may be detected by noting the patient's ability to produce several words in one category, such as naming 10 flowers or 10 words starting with a certain letter.

In most instances, a systematic, comprehensive mental status examination should suffice for the formulation of a specific diagnosis. Formal neuropsychological testing may be necessary to clarify the cognitive profile, however, and may also be important in establishing a baseline for follow-up evaluation. Several brief rating scales of intellectual performance have been formulated in recent years and may prove useful.

Neurologic Examination

The formal neurologic examination of a patient with dementia may have important therapeutic as well as diagnostic implications. For example, abnormalities of gait may suggest parkinsonism or normal pressure hydrocephalus, both of which may be amenable to appropriate therapy. Altered tone or abnormal movements may indicate basal ganglia or cortical dysfunction. Focal sensorimotor deficits or prominent asymmetry of the muscle stretch reflexes may point to a more focal disease, such as stroke or tumor.

Certain diseases causing dementia are invariably associated with other neurologic signs. These include Huntington's disease (movement disorder), demyelinating disease (spasticity, pseudobulbar palsy, blindness), lipid-storage diseases (myoclonic seizures, blindness, spasticity, cerebellar ataxia), Creutzfeldt-Jakob disease (periodic myoclonus), and myoclonic epilepsy (diffuse myoclonus, generalized seizures, ataxia). Other disease entities that are often, although not invariably, associated with neurologic signs include multiple cerebral infarctions, brain tumor, cerebral trauma, and hydrocephalus.

General Physical Examination

The general physical examination is an essential part of the patient's evaluation. An accurate assessment of vital signs, cardiovascular condition, and pulmonary status is required. Many treatable causes of dementia may surface as a result of the general physical examination.

Laboratory Examination

The laboratory evaluation of the patient with dementia aids in diagnosis and in pinpointing appropriate therapies. CT of the head may show cortical atrophy, but is most important in excluding conditions such as tumor, subdural hematoma, hydrocephalus, multiple cerebral infarctions, and advanced Huntington's disease. Other tests considered essential in the laboratory investigation of the patient with dementia include metabolic screens for electrolytes, calcium, magnesium, hepatic and renal functions; serologic tests for syphilis; urinalysis; and chest x-ray. Screening tests for endocrine dysfunction, drug or heavy metal exposure, and vitamin deficiencies are necessary in most patients. The EEG may assist in the recognition of metabolic disorders or in the identification of focal processes. In certain patients, cisternography or angiography may be warranted.

Those diseases in which dementia is generally associated with clinical or laboratory signs of other medical diseases include hypothyroidism, Cushing's syndrome, syphilis, Wernicke-Korsakoff syndrome, subacute combined degeneration (vitamin B_{12} deficiency), hepatolenticular degeneration (Wilson's disease), bromism, and chronic barbiturate intoxication.

EPILEPSY AND OTHER CONVULSIVE DISORDERS

By J. Bruni, M.D.
Toronto, Ontario, Canada,

and B. J. Wilder, M.D.
Gainesville, Florida

DEFINITION

An epileptic seizure is defined as a transient neurologic dysfunction resulting from an excessive electrical neuronal discharge of gray matter. Isolated seizures are common manifestations of acute neurologic disorders or intoxications; the term epilepsy denotes chronicity and should be employed when referring to a disorder that is clinically manifested as repeated epileptic seizures over time.

INCIDENCE

Epilepsy represents one of the most common neurologic disorders, with an incidence that has been variously reported to range from 0.1 to 0.7 per cent. The highest incidence of epilepsy occurs among individuals of less than 1 year to 4 years of age . Of all new cases of epilepsy, 77 per cent occur before the age of 20 years. Epilepsy should not be considered a single disease entity since it may represent a symptom complex that indicates recurrent central nervous system dysfunction caused by a variety of different etiologic factors.

CLINICAL MANIFESTATIONS

The clinical manifestations of epilepsy in humans are numerous. These include disturbances of consciousness, abnormal movements, and changes in emotions, sensation, visceral function, or behavior. Seizures originating in local areas of the brain may produce disturbances of function indicative of the involved region. The seizure discharge can subsequently spread from focal abnormal areas into normal areas.

Epileptic activation can involve physiologically normal tissue by spreading directly from a contiguous area of brain or by projecting and propagating paroxysms of abnormal discharge along neural pathways to other distant brain or brain stem centers. This sequential activation can be clinically manifested by motor or sensory marches and changes in autonomic functions.

CLASSIFICATION

An accurate seizure classification is important for the evaluation of possible etiologic factors and subsequent therapy. Unanimity in terminology relating to seizures is also important for purposes of communication. Although a completely satisfactory classification of epileptic seizures is not available, the classification of epileptic seizures of the International League Against Epilepsy, based on clinical and electroencephalographic features, is most widely accepted. The main feature of this classification is the distinction between seizures that are generalized from the beginning and those that are partial or focal at the onset and which may become generalized later on (Table 1).

CAUSES OF EPILEPSY

Partial seizures that may or may not become generalized at a later time often have causes which can be determined. These include congenital anomalies, cerebral neoplasms, gliosis, vascular malformations, infectious processes, traumatic factors, or infarctions. Inborn errors of metabolism, progressive central nervous system degenerative diseases, and central nervous system storage diseases are uncommon causes of partial or generalized seizures.

The etiologic factors in primary generalized seizures are less well understood. Absence seizures (petit mal) and myoclonic and tonic-clonic (grand mal) seizures, in many instances, have genetic factors involved. Some studies have indicated that the trait for absence seizures and tonic-clonic seizures may be inherited as an autosomal dominant trait with incomplete penetrance. Alcohol or drug withdrawal, febrile seizures, and seizures as a result of renal, hepatic, or toxic factors should be considered in the differential diagnosis of seizures; however, they are not included in the classification of epileptic seizures.

Table 1. Classification of Seizures

I. **Partial (Focal, Local) Seizures**
   A. Simple partial seizures
      1. With motor signs.
      2. With somatosensory or special sensory symptoms.
      3. With autonomic symptoms or signs.
      4. With psychic symptoms (disturbance of higher cognitive functions).
   B. Complex partial seizures (psychomotor, temporal lobe)
      1. Simple partial onset followed by impairment of consciousness.
      2. Impairment of consciousness at onset.
   C. Partial seizures evolving to secondarily generalized seizures. (This may be generalized tonic-clonic, tonic, or clonic.)
      1. Simple partial seizures (A) evolving to generalized seizures.
      2. Complex partial seizures (B) evolving to generalized seizures.
      3. Simple partial seizures evolving to complex partial seizures evolving to generalized seizures.

II. **Generalized Seizures (Convulsive and Nonconvulsive)**
   A. Absence seizures (petit mal).
   B. Myoclonic seizures.
   C. Clonic seizures.
   D. Tonic seizures.
   E. Tonic-clonic seizures (grand mal).
   F. Atonic seizures.

III. **Unclassified Epileptic Seizures**

DIFFERENTIAL DIAGNOSIS OF SEIZURES

In the evaluation of a patient with a possible seizure disorder three main problems should be addressed.

1. Is the patient suffering from seizures?
2. What type of seizure is it?
3. What is the cause?

In establishing whether a patient presents with a seizure disorder, the history is of paramount importance. A careful history from both the patient and observers is important in order that a detailed description of the clinical event can be obtained. Seizures are generally brief and have stereotyped patterns. They may have characteristic auras, and convulsive manifestations may be evident. A short period of mental confusion is common with seizures in which consciousness is impaired. Other conditions that have to be distinguished from true epileptic seizures include migraine, hysterical seizures, syncope, hypoglycemia, and transient cerebral ischemia.

Syncope is characterized by generalized weakness and impaired consciousness that occurs relatively quickly, but generally not as rapidly as a convulsive seizure. Except in fainting due to Stokes-Adams attacks, the patient is nearly always upright, and there is usually a warning of "feeling bad," giddiness, blurring of vision, pallor, perspiration, and yawning. Harmful falls are unusual. Autonomic features include pupillary dilation, bradycardia, hypotension, and a weak pulse. Rarely, a few clonic jerks or urinary incontinence may be observed. The entire sequence lasts seconds or minutes, rarely longer (e.g., with aortic stenosis or hypoglycemia). The patient usually recovers fully with no headaches and no confusion. True seizures, on the other hand, are of swift onset, and an aura, if present, is generally brief. Occurrence is unrelated to posture, and duration is generally longer than a simple syncopal event. Injury and tongue-biting may occur during a convulsive seizure, and urinary or fecal incontinence may occur. In a convulsive seizure, cyanosis is frequently present, pallor is uncommon, and breathing may be stertorous. The most characteristic feature distinguishing a seizure from syncope is a period of postictal confusion. Postictally, the neurologic examination is usually normal, but an extensor plantar response may be present. If the seizure is due to focal cerebral pathology, lateralizing neurologic signs may be present.

In *hysterical seizures or pseudoseizures,* a relationship to psychological stress frequently can be documented. The "seizure" pattern is variable, involuntary movements are more organized and they can frequently be triggered, physical injury and urinary incontinence are rare, the seizures do not respond to anticonvulsant therapy, and patients generally return to consciousness quickly. There may be an emotional display. It is important to note, however, that a number of patients may have both epileptic seizures and pseudoseizures, and at times great difficulty may be encountered in distinguishing the two on clinical grounds alone.

Migraine headaches may have syncopal manifestations, and the visual symptoms may at times be mistaken for an epileptic visual aura. The history of headache with loss of consciousness is important in suggesting a diagnosis of migraine, and frequently a history of similar headaches is present in the absence of syncope. Rarely, a generalized tonic-clonic convulsion may be evoked by a migraine attack, although the pathophysiology is unclear.

Transient cerebral ischemic episodes may rarely present with episodic losses of consciousness; however, in these patients (usually elderly) other symptoms of cerebral ischemia can be elicited.

DIAGNOSIS OF GENERALIZED AND PARTIAL SEIZURES

Absence Seizures

The hallmark of the absence attack is a sudden interruption of ongoing activities, a blank stare, and possibly a brief upward rotation of the eyes with frequent eyeblinks. The attack lasts from a few seconds to half a minute and terminates abruptly, with no postictal confusion. Some absence seizures may have associated mild clonic components, changes in postural tone, or brief automatisms.

Tonic-Clonic Seizures

The hallmark of tonic-clonic seizures is the sudden occurrence of tonic contraction of muscles and a subsequent clonic phase, which lasts a variable period of time. There may be an initial cry, stridor, or moan. Postictally the patient is unconscious for a variable period of time and may complain of muscle soreness on awakening. Rarely purely tonic or clonic seizures may occur.

Myoclonic Seizures

Myoclonic jerks are sudden, short, shock-like contractions that may be generalized or confined to the face and trunk, to one or more extremities, or even to individual muscles or groups of muscles. Consciousness is maintained during these attacks.

Atonic Seizures

Atonic seizures are characterized by a sudden diminution of muscle tone which may be fragmentary, leading to a head drop with slackening of the jaw, the drooping of a limb, or a loss of all muscle tone, resulting in a fall. If consciousness is lost, this loss is usually of brief duration.

Partial Seizures

The manifestations of simple partial seizures can vary according to the site of origin of the epileptic discharge. Partial motor seizures may involve clonic activity of the face or an extremity. Consciousness is preserved. Partial sensory or somatosensory seizures may present with paresthesias; visual, auditory, or olfactory phenomena; autonomic symptoms; or psychic symptoms.

During complex partial seizures consciousness is impaired. There may be associated automatisms, such as chewing or swallowing; gestural, verbal, ambulatory automatisms; or automatisms of mimicry (e.g., fear). The automatisms that occur with complex partial seizures are generally more complex than those observed with some types of absence seizures. Postictally the patient may be confused for a brief period of time.

DIAGNOSTIC EVALUATION

The neurologic and physical examinations often are unrewarding in the diagnostic work-up of the seizure patient. However, physical examination sometimes reveals characteristic features of patients with certain disorders who often first seek medical attention because of the onset of seizures. Tuberous sclerosis, neurofibromatosis, Sturge-Weber syndrome, and other examples can be cited.

Neurologic Examination

The neurologic examination becomes critically important when certain specific factors cause seizures. Birth-related trauma may result in asymmetries in motor development, cranial bruits may indicate an arteriovenous malformation, and space-occupying lesions may result in changes in the fundi or in focal motor, sensory, or reflex changes.

In 50 per cent of patients an etiologic diagnosis can be established. In the pediatric age group, perinatal injury, infections, metabolic defects, and genetic factors can often be recognized. In adults, trauma, tumors, vascular causes, previous prolonged febrile seizures, and degenerative diseases are important causes of seizures.

Laboratory Investigation

In the initial outpatient investigation of the patient with seizures, a complete blood count, biochemical screen, VDRL test for syphilis, blood sugar, and calcium levels should be evaluated. The electroencephalogram (EEG) is an indispensable tool in diagnosis and achieves its greatest clinical usefulness in convulsive disorders. EEG patterns reflect the physiologic activity of the cerebral cortex. It is important to realize, however, that an abnormal EEG does not necessarily indicate clinical epilepsy and that a normal EEG does not exclude epilepsy. Some patients with clinically documented seizures have normal results on EEG, even after serial recordings, sleep recordings, and special activation techniques. The EEG is most frequently helpful in diagnosing absence seizures, in detecting focal versus a generalized abnormality, and in examining certain clinically silent areas of brain, such as the frontal regions. One of the routinely used activation techniques is hyperventilation, which may evoke generalized spike-wave discharges characteristic of absence seizures, or focal spike or sharp-wave discharges suggestive of a partial seizure disorder. Photic stimulation is of particular importance in relation to the evaluation of photosensitive seizures. In occasional circumstances, drug activation techniques with methohexital are employed. EEG evaluation can be supplemented with simultaneous video monitoring for the documentation of ictal events, thus allowing a strict correlation between EEG changes and clinical manifestations.

Other Studies

Routine skull x-rays should be obtained on seizure patients and, although usually normal, they can occasionally establish an etiologic diagnosis. Intracranial calcifications, pineal shifts, bony changes due to meningiomas, and changes of increased intracranial pressure may be observed. In adults with seizures of recent onset a chest x-ray should also be obtained to exclude a primary lung malignancy as a possible source of cerebral metastases.

Radionuclide scanning may detect intracranial tumors; however, recently it has been largely replaced by computed tomography (CT scanning). With CT scanning, not only tumors but also cerebral atrophy, hydrocephalus, cerebral hemorrhages, infarctions, subdural hematomas, cystic lesions, and arteriovenous malformations can be detected. CT scanning is most helpful in children with focal seizures, in patients with suspected mass lesions, and in patients who have adult-onset seizures. CT abnormalities are more frequently found in patients with partial seizure disorders as compared with the generalized seizure disorders.

Arteriography is occasionally employed in certain patients with mass lesions or arteriovenous malformations. Pneumoencephalography is generally not employed in the routine evaluation of seizure patients.

Cerebrospinal fluid examination is not necessary in every patient with a seizure disorder. Findings are usually normal in the patient with uncomplicated epilepsy. Abnormalities of pressure, protein, cells, or glucose content usually denote central nervous system disease. In some circumstances cerebrospinal fluid examinations should be performed to rule out central nervous system infection such as meningitis, which may present with fever and acute seizures.

NEONATAL SEIZURES, INFANTILE SPASMS, AND FEBRILE SEIZURES

Neonatal seizures occurring in the first month of life are often the presenting manifestation of serious neurologic disturbance. Because of an immature nervous sytem, seizure phenomena in the newborn differ from those in older children and adults. Causative factors that must be considered include infection, metabolic disorders such as hypoglycemia and hypocalcemia, congenital malformations, birth trauma, hypoxia, and drug withdrawal. Since many etiologic factors may be responsible, a careful prenatal and natal history is important, and a complete physical examination is mandatory. Laboratory evaluation should include examination of the cerebrospinal fluid for bacterial meningitis, as well as determination of blood glucose, serum electrolytes, and blood urea nitrogen levels. The EEG is generally of little use in establishing an etiologic diagnosis. Skull x-rays and CT scans are of value in the evaluation of the infant who has suffered a birth injury. Inborn errors of metabolism (e.g., aminoacidurias) can be diagnosed by appropriate screening procedures.

Infantile spasms denotes an epileptic syndrome complex of infancy associated with brief severe tonic seizures, massive myoclonus, and flexor and extensor spasms. No single etiologic factor has been discovered; however, many diverse pathologic processes have been implicated. The EEG findings have been described as hypsarrhythmia. The diagnosis is made on clinical and EEG findings.

Febrile seizures occur with greatest frequency during the first year of life and generally are self-limiting, with epilepsy developing later only in rare instances. In 85 per cent of patients, febrile seizures do not recur. With a first febrile seizure, efforts should be made to rule out a possible intracranial cause. However, in an uncomplicated febrile seizure, complete blood count, measurement of blood levels of electrolytes, calcium, and glucose, skull x-rays, and CT scans are rarely useful. The role of the EEG in the evaluation of febrile seizures is controversial; an abnormal EEG does not reliably predict the development of epilepsy in a patient with febrile convulsions.

EXTRAPYRAMIDAL DISORDERS

By Melvin D. Yahr, M.D.
New York, New York

Diseases of the basal ganglia, or extrapyramidal diseases, comprise a complex group of clinical disorders characterized primarily by abnormal involuntary movements (dyskinesias), alterations in muscle tone, and disturbances in bodily posture. The major clinical states included under this title are *parkinsonism, chorea, athetosis, dystonia,* and *hemiballism.* Those terms not only are used to denote particular disease entities but in a descriptive sense refer to constellations of symptoms that may occur in a variety of disorders, some intrinsic to the central nervous system, others of a generalized nature that involve the basal ganglia or their connections. They are distinguishable by the degree, form, and combination of the triad of symptoms noted earlier and are recognizable as disease entities by the age and mode of onset, the identification of particular etiologic and genetic factors, and the rate and manner of progression of symptoms.

Although much is known about the clinical aspects of extrapyramidal disorders, our information is deficient with regard to their fundamental anatomic, physiologic, and pathogenic bases. However, a growing body of information regarding biochemical alterations in the basal ganglia has provided considerable understanding of the mechanisms by which symptoms occur as well as suggested a rational approach to their treatment.

The most prominent biochemical feature of the basal ganglia is their particularly high content of putative neurotransmitter agents, notably acetylcholine (ACh), dopamine (DA), and gamma-aminobutyric acid (GABA). The substrates and enzyme systems for their production and degradation are found within the cellular components of the basal ganglia. In some instances these neurotransmitter agents are produced within the segment in which they have their action; in others, cellular elements in one area are responsible for their production and they are transported via connecting axons to another area where they produce their effects. Experimental evidence is available indicating that dopamine, for example, is produced in the pars compacta of the substantia nigra and is transported via a neuronal tract, the nigral-striatal pathway, to the caudate nucleus and putamen. Normal function in the basal ganglia appears to depend on an exquisite balance between these various neurotransmitter agents; i.e., they may be viewed neurophysiologically as being either inhibitory (DA and GABA) or excitatory (ACh) in nature. Disturbances in their homeostasis result in one or another of the symptoms that are generally attributed to this area of the brain. In general, dopamine deficiency allows for cholinergic hyperactivity and can be correlated with the akinetic-rigid disorders, such as parkinsonism. Dopamine hyperactivity, cholinergic hypoactivity, or both result in the hyperkinetic phenomena encountered in Huntington's chorea. To a considerable extent, present approaches to the treatment of basal ganglia disorders rely on the use of agents capable of re-establishing neurotransmitter balance.

PARKINSONIAN SYNDROME

James Parkinson first described the major manifestations of this syndrome in his "Essay on the Shaking Palsy" (1817): ". . . involuntary tremulous motion with lessened muscular power in parts not in action and even when supported; with a propensity to bend the trunk forward and to pass from a walking to a running pace." Parkinsonism, which is characterized by tremor, muscular rigidity, and loss of postural reflexes, is one of the most frequently encountered of all disorders of the basal ganglia and is a prominent cause of disability resulting from disease of all types. Its prevalence has been placed at close to 1 million patients in the United States, with the addition of 50,000 new cases each year. As a symptom complex, its occurrence has been noted in a number of disease processes, either as the sole manifestation or in association with other symptoms. However, in the vast majority of cases no definable cause has as yet been found; since the latter cases seem to have many features in common, particularly in regard to evolution, they have been designated as primary parkinsonism.

The cases in which definable processes are found are best classified as *secondary* or *symptomatic par-*

kinsonism. This separation into clinical groups cannot be construed as indicative of a difference in pathophysiology or even pathogenic mechanisms for the production of symptoms, since all cases of parkinsonism may well have a common origin. Indeed, from the standpoint of what is presently known about its chemical pathology, a deficiency of striatal dopamine is common to all types of parkinsonism. In some instances of parkinsonism, regardless of cause, cell loss is consistently found in the substantia nigra in association with other changes diffusely distributed in the corpus striatum and cortex.

No specific laboratory tests exist to aid in establishing the diagnosis of parkinsonism. Routine examination of blood, spinal fluid, and urine yields normal results. The disturbance in cerebral dopamine metabolism may result in a decrease in cerebrospinal fluid homovanillic acid (HVA); however, it has limited reliability in confirming the diagnosis. The electroencephalogram is usually normal, although diffuse slowing may be present and sleep recordings may be abnormal. CT scans of the head show no abnormalities in primary parkinsonism but are helpful in some of the secondary forms and in eliminating disorders whose symptoms mimic these conditions. CT scans should be done routinely as a screening procedure and as a baseline for future reference.

Primary Parkinsonism

Synonyms

Parkinson's disease, paralysis agitans.

Manifestations

The largest number of cases of parkinsonism fall into this category. The disease most frequently makes its onset between the ages of 50 and 65 years. A rarely encountered juvenile form has been described. The disease affects both sexes and all races. There is no evidence to indicate a hereditary factor, although a familial incidence is claimed by some authorities.

The disease begins insidiously; any of its three cardinal manifestations may appear alone or in combination. Tremor, usually in one or sometimes in both hands, involving the fingers in a pill-rolling motion, is the most common initial symptom. This is often followed by stiffness in the limbs, general slowing of movements, and inability to carry out normal and routine daily functions with ease. As the disease progresses, the face becomes "masklike," with a loss of eye blinking and failure to express emotional feeling. The body becomes stooped, the gait becomes shuffling with loss of arm swing, and the patient is unable to readily gain and maintain an erect posture. Speech becomes slow and monotonous. The patient tends to drool. The skin takes on an oily quality, and there is a tendency to seborrheic dermatitis.

Although paralysis agitans is invariably progressive, the rate at which symptoms develop and disability ensues is extremely variable. In some instances the disease is rapidly progressive and patients become disabled within 5 years of onset. More often, a slower, more protracted course of evolution of symptoms occurs and patients remain functional for extended periods of time.

The major neurologic findings are as follows:

1. lack of facial expression with diminished eye blinking but ready induction of blepharospasm when the frontalis muscle is tapped (Myerson's sign).
2. Tremor of the distal segments of the limbs at rest, accentuated by suspension but decreased during active movements and eliminated by sleep. The tremor is rhythmic, alternately affecting flexor and extensor muscles, and may involve upper or lower limbs, mouth, or head.
3. Muscular rigidity readily evident on passive movement of a joint and manifested by a series of interrupted jerks (cogwheel phenomenon) rather than a smooth-flowing, easy motion.
4. Bradykinesia, the tendency to slowness in the initiation of movement, and sudden unexpected arrests of volitional movements while carrying out purposeful acts. The parkinsonian patient appears disinclined to move, and in the middle of performing a routine function suddenly becomes "frozen" and unable to follow through the sequence of motion necessary to complete the action. This is especially evident in writing or feeding and can be striking when, in attempting to walk, the patient finds that the feet are suddenly "frozen to the ground." Rapid alternating movements of the extremities are slowed.
5. Postural abnormalities evident in the erect and sitting positions. The patient has a tendency to let the head fall forward on the trunk, and the body tends to fall forward or backward when the patient is seated on a stool unless supported. When pushed from in front or from behind in the erect position, the patient falls, and no attempt is made to stop the fall either by a step or by movements of the arms. There is a tendency for deformities of the trunk, hands, and feet to occur. Kyphotic deformity of the spine, causing a stooped posture, is a hallmark. There are ulnar deviations of the hand, flexion contractures of the fingers, and an equinovarus posture of the foot.

Secondary or Symptomatic Parkinsonism

Parkinson's syndrome occurs in numerous situations as the predominant clinical manifestation. Those most commonly encountered are indicated in Table 1.

Parkinson's syndrome is occasionally seen during the acute phase of several types of viral encephalitis, although permanent extrapyramidal residua are rare. The exception is the Parkinson's syndrome that developed following the epidemic of encephalitis lethargica from 1919 to 1926. Sporadic cases still occur occasionally.

Cerebral atherosclerosis with multi-infarction of the cerebrum produces a parkinsonism-like state. Lack of initiation of movement and gait disturbances occur with cerebral arteriosclerosis and are more properly classified as "pseudoparkinsonism." They rarely respond to therapeutic measures effective for Parkinson's disease.

Parkinsonism has been reported following poisoning with carbon monoxide. Chronic manganese intoxication, seen in several industrial situations, produces

Table 1. Causes of Secondary Parkinsonism

Infections: Postviral encephalitis
Atherosclerotic
Drug-induced
Toxins:
Carbon monoxide
Manganese
Meperidine analogue (MPTP)
Metabolic:
Parathyroid dysfunction
Anoxia
Tumors
Head trauma
Degenerative:
Parkinson's dementia complex (Guam)
Striatonigral degeneration
Progressive supranuclear palsy
Olivopontocerebellar atrophies
Parkinsonism with autonomic dystrophy (Shy-Drager syndrome, multisystem atrophy)

a Parkinson's syndrome accompanied by dystonia and mental changes. Parkinsonism may appear as a side effect of drugs that deplete or block the action of cerebral monoamines. Most commonly it appears as a side effect of various neuroleptic drugs, such as the phenothiazines and butyrophenones. Occasionally antihypertensive agents, such as reserpine and methyldopa, are the cause. Recently a meperidine analogue, MPTP (1-methyl-4-phenyl-1,3,5,6,-tetrahydropyridine), used intravenously by drug addicts, has induced an irreversible parkinsonian state.

Hypoparathyroidism is associated with calcification of the basal ganglia and may produce parkinsonism as well as chorea and athetosis. When calcification of the basal ganglia is not apparent on plain skull x-rays, computed tomography (CT) may demonstrate small calcific deposits in the basal ganglia.

Brain tumors in the region of the basal ganglia may present with a hemi-Parkinson's syndrome. Frontal lobe tumors also occasionally produce gait and movement abnormalities that may mimic parkinsonism.

A parkinsonian syndrome may be present to varying degrees as a component in several so-called degenerative diseases of unknown cause that involve multiple areas of the central nervous system: *progressive supranuclear palsy, olivopontocerebellar atrophy,* and the *Shy-Drager syndrome* are the most frequently encountered. In progressive supranuclear palsy the major abnormalities in addition to parkinsonian symptoms are subcortical dementia, pseudobulbar signs, and vertical gaze palsy. In olivopontocerebellar atrophy, cerebellar incoordination is an added feature. It also has a high familial incidence, and the recessive form is associated with a deficiency in the enzyme glutamate dehydrogenase. In the Shy-Drager syndrome, diffuse autonomic insufficiency in which postural hypotension is a major problem may precede or occur concomitantly with parkinsonism. In all of these syndromes the extrapyramidal findings respond somewhat to L-dopa (levodopa) therapy, whereas the other major neurologic abnormalities are unaffected.

Other disorders that may be confused with parkinsonism include myxedema, normal pressure hydrocephalus, hepatic encephalopathy, and depression. Postencephalitic and drug-induced parkinsonism are distinctive clinical entities that warrant additional description.

Postencephalitic Parkinsonism

One of the most prominent sequelae of the epidemic of encephalitis lethargica (von Economo's disease) that occurred between 1919 and 1926 was the parkinsonism syndrome. The syndrome developed after mild as well as severe encephalitis lethargica. Although in most instances it immediately followed the acute infectious process, in some patients prominent symptoms were not evident for intervals of up to 10 years. The causative agent of encephalitis lethargica was never established; however, studies suggest that it was produced by a virus with immunologic characteristics similar to those of influenza type A virus. The evolution and consequences of this form of parkinsonism differ from others, making its clinical recognition of importance.

Postencephalitic parkinsonism has a number of distinctive and unique features, including the following:

1. A history of encephalitis lethargica during the epidemic period 1919 to 1926. Since the pandemic of influenza occurred concurrently with encephalitis, it is essential that careful documentation be undertaken in differentiating these two infectious processes.
2. In addition to any or all of the parkinsonian symptoms indicated earlier, one or more of the following neurologic deficits may be found: hemiplegia, bulbar or ocular palsies, dystonic phenomena, tics, or behavioral disorders.
3. The parkinsonism itself is, as a rule, incompletely developed and has been static or slowly progressive over a period of years.
4. Episodes termed "oculogyric crises" may occur. These consist of attacks in which spasms of conjugate eye muscles occur so that the eyes are deviated upward, downward, or to one side for minutes or hours at a time.

As a general rule, patients with postencephalitic parkinsonism are more sensitive to L-dopa and less sensitive to anticholinergic drugs than patients with idiopathic parkinsonism. Lower doses of L-dopa and higher doses of anticholinergic drugs are therefore necessary for optimal results.

Drug-Induced Parkinsonism

The use of neuroleptic drugs as psychotherapeutic or antiemetic agents has resulted in the occurrence of a number of extrapyramidal syndromes: parkinsonism indistinguishable from that previously described, dystonic movements involving the tongue and face, and akathisia (a restless, fidgety state with a desire to be in constant motion) are those frequently encountered. Adults are more likely to develop parkinsonism and akathisia, whereas dystonic movements predominate in children. In some instances these reactions are dose-dependent; in others they are related to individual susceptibility. The symptoms usually disappear within a few days when the drugs are withdrawn but occasionally persist for months. In some subjects, permanent remnants of parkinsonian symptoms have been found years after elimination of the drugs.

Paradoxically, involuntary movements may make their initial appearance after withdrawal of neuroleptic agents. This condition, termed *tardive dyskinesia,* tends to occur in older patients who have been on neuroleptic drugs for extended periods of time during which they have shown signs of parkinsonism. The incidence is reportedly higher in postmenopausal women. Stereotyped, repetitious movements of lips, tongue, and mouth and choreiform movements of limbs and trunk characterize this disorder. It may diminish in intensity or disappear spontaneously after weeks or months, but in some patients it has persisted indefinitely. Phenothiazines are commonly associated with extrapyramidal side effects, although some nonphenothiazine tranquilizers, such as haloperidol (Haldol), also produce extrapyramidal reactions. In general, phenothiazines with a piperazine side chain produce the most severe extrapyramidal side effects: trifluoperazine (Stelazine) fluphenazine (Permitil, Prolixin), thiopropazate dihydrochloride (Dartal), prochlorperazine maleate (Compazine), and perphenazine (Trilafon).

ESSENTIAL TREMOR

Synonyms

Familial tremor.

Manifestations

This is a monosymptomatic condition in which tremor involves the hands or the head and face, or all three. The tremor is usually not present at rest, occurs with suspension of the limbs, and is more rapid than that encountered in parkinsonism. It is accentuated by emotional factors, may be worsened by volitional movement, and is usually suppressed by the use of alcohol. The age at onset is variable, but in most cases the disorder begins prior to the age of 25 years and tends to persist throughout life. Some progression of the intensity of tremor and spread to other bodily parts usually occur over the years, which may result in significant physical and social disability.

There is a strong familial incidence, with occurrence in several successive generations and members of the same family, but the genetic pattern of inheritance has not been determined. Some have suggested its transmission as an autosomal dominant trait. It is also unusually common in patients with torsion dystonia, the neuromuscular disorder described by Kugillens and Veilland, and in males with sex chromosome abnormalities. No specific pathologic lesion has been reported in the nervous system of people with this condition. On rare occasions it has been a prodrome of primary parkinsonism, and the suggestion has been made that the condition is one of its abortive forms. There is no specific effective therapy for controlling the tremor, although beta-adrenergic blocking agents, such as propranolol in doses up to 250 mg/day divided equally into three or four doses, are occasionally effective. Sedatives such as phenobarbital, 15 mg three times a day, or diazepam (Valium), 10 mg three times a day, may reduce the intensity of the tremor. Anxiety tremor and hyperthyroid tremor are quite similar in appearance and may be mistaken for essential tremor. It is of utmost importance to differentiate essential tremor from parkinsonism. By and large, the distinguishing characteristics are earlier age at onset; lack of severe progression, akinesia, rigidity, or postural abnormalities; and the strong family history of tremor.

SENILE TREMOR

Tremor is a frequent finding in the elderly, most often involving the upper limbs and head. It differs from parkinsonian tremor in that it is finer and more rapid and at first occurs only with voluntary movements. As time goes on, it becomes more constant and is also present while the limbs are at rest. There is no associated weakness or alteration in muscle tone. These features differentiate this form of tremor from parkinsonism. The cause in unknown. Since senile tremor has both cerebellar and extrapyramidal features, in that it occurs both at rest and with movement, the assumption is that some critical pathway linking these systems has undergone degeneration. There is no effective treatment, although mild benefit may be derived from sedatives or the use of diphenhydramine (Benadryl), 25 mg three times a day. Most patients accept this condition as another of the many changes that come with advancing years. Occasionally, patients have to be reassured that they do not have parkinsonism or some other progressive neurologic disorder.

THE CHOREAS

There are a number of disease entities that, although wholly unrelated etiologically, have choreiform movements as their major manifestation. In some, intimate relationships with infectious processes have been found, whereas in others, familial tendencies have pointed to a strong genetic component. In the light of newer concepts of inheritance, a common pathogenesis may exist for all. Considerable controversy exists as to the exact anatomic site from which movements of this type derive. Pathologic changes have been found in various components of the basal ganglia, many of which have their influence on the motor system via the pallidum. It is postulated that choreiform movements result from a loss of inhibition of the pallidum as a result of impaired afferent connections. Chorea is induced by biochemical agents that enhance dopaminergic activity at the striatal level when supersensitivity to this neurotransmitter exists. This most commonly occurs when the small-cell components of the caudate nucleus and putamen are involved.

The classification of chorea into separate entities is at present somewhat arbitrary and is based on age at onset, association with identifiable disease processes or familial tendency, and occurrence of other neurologic abnormalities. The major disorders in which chorea occurs are indicated in Table 2.

Choreic movements may be noted in any part of the body—e.g, limbs, face, hands, tongue, or trunk. They may at first appear to be a part of the natural pattern of coordinated movements but are soon noted to be completely random, jerking, aimless, and purposeless. They occur at rest, are accentuated by an attempt at volitional movement, and disappear during sleep.

Table 2. Conditions Associated with Chorea

Central Nervous System Infections	
	Encephalitic lethargica (von Economo's disease)
	Meningoencephalitis due to mumps, measles, EB virus, and other viruses
	Subacute sclerosing panencephalitis
	Parenchymatous neurosyphilis
Following Parainfectious Disease	
	Sydenham's chorea (poststreptococcal infection)
	Associated with other infections: pertussis, varicella, diphtheria
Autoimmune Disorders	
	Lupus erythematosus
	Henoch-Schönlein purpura
	Rheumatoid arthritis
	Polyarteritis nodosa
	Serum sickness reaction to tetanus antitoxin
	Lyme disease
Metabolic Disorders	
	Thyrotoxicosis
	Hypo- and hyperparathyroidism
	Hypocalcemia
	Hypoglycemia
Drug Intoxications	
	Atropine poisoning and other anticholinergic intoxications
	Anticonvulsants
	Amphetamines
	Levodopa
	Lithium
	Oral contraceptives
	Phenothiazine and related neuroleptic drugs
	Isoniazid
Genetic	
	Huntington's disease
	Cerebral lipidoses
	Acute intermittent porphyria
	Wilson's disease
	Ataxia-telangiectasia
	Lesch-Nyhan syndrome
	Acanthocytosis
	Glutaric acidemia
	Olivopontocerebellar atrophy, dominant form
Miscellaneous	
	Pick's and Alzheimer's diseases
	Senile chorea
	Benign familial chorea
	Polycythemia
	Beri-beri
	Pregnancy (chorea gravidarum)
	Cerebrovascular disease
	Arteriosclerotic vascular disease
	Meningovascular lues
	Brain tumor, primary or metastatic
	Trauma, subdural hematoma

*EB = Epstein-Barr (virus).

They may be very mild and may minimally affect normal function, or they may be so forceful and frequent as to be totally disabling. Facial grimacing and difficulty in speech, chewing, and swallowing occur when the muscles subserving these functions are involved. Interruption of voluntary movements by involuntary ones leads to incoordination. Frequently objects drop from the hands, walking is awkward and performed in an ungainly fashion, and a general appearance of incoordination is present.

Certain cardinal features can be found in almost all patients. These include:

1. Pronation of the forearm when the upper limbs are raised and extended.
2. Inability to sustain muscle contraction when the examiner grasps the patient's hand or when the patient protrudes the tongue so that it darts rapidly in and out of the mouth.
3. Abnormal posturing of hands in which the wrist is noted to be sharply flexed and the fingers hyperextended at the metacarpophalangeal joints.

There are no specific laboratory tests for chorea. The cerebrospinal fluid is normal. The electroencephalogram (EEG) may or may not show diffuse abnormalities that correlate with the severity of the disease. Unless there are associated disease processes that manifest themselves in abnormalities of blood count, chemistry, or sedimentation rate, these studies are normal. Computed tomography (CT) of the head may be helpful in identifying the underlying nature of the disease.

Acute Choreas

Considered as a symptom complex rather than as a specific disease entity, acute choreiform movements have been encountered as initial manifestations of a variety of conditions. There are few distinctive features of the movements themselves that indicate the underlying cause. It is, therefore, of utmost importance to thoroughly evaluate each patient with a view to uncovering the associated disease process. The more frequently encountered conditions are detailed.

Sydenham's Chorea

Also called St. Vitus dance and rheumatic chorea, Sydenham's chorea has as its outstanding clinical features involuntary movements, incoordination, muscle weakness, and emotional lability. Although the onset of symptoms may be abrupt and obvious, more often it is insidious and subtle. The most frequent initial complaints include clumsiness of the limbs, evidenced by dropping objects from the hands, or an awkward gait, particularly during emotionally tense situations. When these are coupled with irritability, poor performance in school, and generally fidgety behavior, frequently a hasty conclusion is reached, blaming the child or implying a psychiatric disorder.

The age at onset and the distinctive involuntary movements readily differentiate Sydenham's chorea from other disorders of the basal ganglia. This condition principally occurs between 7 and 14 years of age, with girls being affected more frequently than boys.

Rheumatic manifestations such as carditis, valvular disease, or joint involvement may occur prior to, coincident with, or following an attack of chorea. Tics and habit spasms may be confused with mild cases of Sydenham's chorea, but their movements are quite different, being stereotyped, repetitive patterns localized to a single group of muscles. *Huntington's chorea* rarely begins in childhood, and when it does is usually rigid in form rather than hyperkinetic. Furthermore, there is a strong familial tendency with associated dementia in Huntington's chorea. Movement disorders associated with cerebral palsy occur in childhood but have an athetoid element. The use of phenothiazines may induce abnormal movements, but the history of drug ingestion will differentiate these.

Sydenham's chorea is a self-limited disease, recovery occurring in 2 to 6 months. Recurrence, with as many as two or three attacks over a period of years, appears in almost one third of the patients. There is no specific therapy. Bed rest and reduction of external stimuli to a minimum, combined with sedative drugs (e.g, phenobarbital or chloral hydrate), are beneficial in controlling the severity of the movements. Paradoxically, the phenothiazines haloperidol and reserpine, although capable of inducing chorea, have also been shown to be effective in its control. Because of the high incidence of rheumatic valvular heart disease complicating acute chorea, prophylaxis with antimicrobial drugs over a long interval of time similar to that utilized in acute rheumatic fever is now recommended. If emotional symptoms are intense, psychotherapy may be in order. With recovery most patients show few, if any, neurologic sequelae.

Chorea Gravidarum

Chorea gravidarum occurs most commonly in the first pregnancy in women who have a previous history of chorea. A definite previous history of rheumatic fever can be obtained in approximately one third of patients. Since the incidence of rheumatic fever has declined, chorea gravidarum is now encountered only rarely. When it does occur, consideration must be given to other causes, such as lupus erythematosus or Huntington's disease. Characteristically, the movements appear in the first trimester and resolve spontaneously after a few months, although they may persist until after delivery. Chorea may recur in subsequent pregnancies.

Other Causes of Acute Chorea

Choreic movements localized to a body segment or generalized in nature may occur in association with system disease or be induced by pharmacologic as well as toxic agents. There are no characteristic features of the choreic state nor any fixed time course that might be helpful in diagnosis. Early recognition and institution of appropriate therapy for the basic disease most often eliminates the choreic movements, but in some instances they persist and require symptomatic treatment.

Lupus erythematosus is one of the more common causes of acute chorea, especially in middle-aged women. Chorea may occur as the initial manifestation or during the course of the illness. Not infrequently it is associated with other central nervous manifestations, such as convulsive seizure phenomena or behavioral disturbances. Autoimmune disorders, blood dyscrasias such as polycythemia, and endocrine disorders such as parathyroid or thyroid dysfunction must be considered when chorea is a prominent clinical manifestation.

Iatrogenic chorea induced by pharmacologic agents is most frequently seen in women taking oral contraceptive agents, in epileptics taking anticonvulsants, in psychiatric patients using neuroleptics, and in parkinsonian patients being treated with levodopa. In most instances, withdrawing the offending agents results in elimination of the choreic movements within a few days. On occasion, particularly with the use of neuroleptics, they have persisted for extended periods of time. Since their induction and persistence may be related to dosage level and duration of administration of the drug, early recognition and discontinuation of the offending agent is of prime importance.

Huntington's Chorea (Chronic Progressive Chorea, Hereditary Chorea)

Hereditary chorea is a progressive degenerative disease of the basal ganglia and cerebral cortex beginning in adult life and characterized by choreiform movements and mental deterioration. The inheritance of the disease is based on a single dominant autosomal gene. It may be transmitted by either sex, and both sexes are equally affected. The trait is transmitted from affected individual to affected individual so that those who escape being involved rarely transmit the disease. Only approximately 50 per cent of the offspring are affected. The disease is relatively rare, although its incidence may be high in geographic regions where affected families have resided for many generations. It was originally described by Huntington in 1872 in English immigrants living on Long Island. The disease has been reported in most areas of the world.

Pathologically, widespread degenerative changes with cell loss and reactive gliosis are found, primarily in the cerebral cortex and caudate nucleus. It has been demonstrated that glutamic acid decarboxylase activity and choline acetylase activity are reduced in the basal ganglia of patients with Huntington's chorea. This results in a deficiency of gamma-aminobutyric acid (GABA), an inhibitory transmitter substance in the brain, as well as depressed function of the excitatory transmitter acetylcholine. Disruption of the homeostatic relationship of these agents may underlie the choreic manifestions of this disorder.

The clinical manifestations consist of choretic movements, emotional disturbance, and intellectual deterioration which vary in degree, rate of appearance, and progression. The disease usually makes its appearance between the ages of 35 and 50 years, somewhat insidiously with any of the symptoms listed, but as a rule with abnormal movements. The movements, although similar to those of acute chorea, are usually more jerky but less lightning-like. They involve primarily the trunk and shoulder girdle and more often the lower limbs than the upper. This pattern of involvement tends to produce a dancing sort of gait, which is a prominent feature of the disease. In rare instances a parkinsonism-like rigidity rather than involuntary movements is encountered as the major manifestation. The mental deterioration is similar to that of any organic dementia, with progressive impairment of memory and intellectual capacity and inattention to personal hygiene. Emotional disturbances include heightened irritability, bouts of depression, and fits of violent behavior.

Rarely, Huntington's chorea appears in children. In such patients, rigidity and dementia predominate and chorea is minor. A high percentage of patients who acquire the disease in childhood have inherited it from their fathers rather than from their mothers.

With the typical triad of choreiform movements, dementia in adult life, and documentation of similar symptoms in family members, the diagnosis is readily evident. However, there is a tendency for families to deny the existence of mental disease, and it is sometimes difficult to obtain corroborative data even when the diagnosis is strongly suspected.

Few laboratory tests are helpful in establishing the diagnosis. The EEG is usually abnormal but nonspecifically so. Caudate atrophy may be demonstrable on CT scan in association with generalized cerebral atrophy, but this may not occur until late in the disease procress. Decreased levels of cerebrospinal fluid GABA levels, reflecting the decreased synthesis of this neurotransmitter, have been reported by some but are questioned by others.

Little difficulty occurs in differentiating hereditary chorea from acute chorea, but senile chorea may raise a problem. The latter, which presents late in life, involves few mental changes, if any, lacks a familial history, and is usually benign. Because of the dementia and similarity in age at onset, other diseases such as the presenile psychoses (Alzheimer's and Pick's diseases) may offer some difficulty, especially in instances in which choreiform movements are inconspicuous. CT scanning of the brain demonstrating selective atrophy of the caudate nucleus may help to establish the correct diagnosis in such instances. There is a tendency to overdiagnose hereditary chorea, applying this diagnosis to diverse neurologic disorders, such as cerebellar degenerations and familial tremors. The dire implications of Huntington's chorea require strict adherence to the diagnostic criteria.

There is no effective therapy. Theoretically, drugs that are capable of elevating GABA levels or enhancing the brain's cholinergic activity should be helpful. Although some, such as phenelzine sulfate and deanol, are undergoing trial, inadequate reports are available at present to comment on their use. Levodopa worsens chorea in affected individuals and may induce chorea in patients at risk. It has been suggested that this may be a useful provocative test for early identification of affected individuals prior to the onset of the disease. Ethical issues regarding the desirability of such a test have been raised in view of the psychological trauma imposed.

Huntington's chorea is relentlessly progressive, leading to total incapacity and inevitably death, usually within 15 years of onset. In the early stages, the patient can be managed at home with supervision and the use of phenothiazines (e.g., haloperidol or reserpine) to reduce the intensity of the movements and to control the behavior to some extent. As the disease advances, confinement to a psychiatric facility becomes necessary.

Senile Chorea

Infrequently, choreiform movements are encountered as an isolated symptom in persons over 60 years of age. As a rule, the movements are mild and may involve the limbs either unilaterally or bilaterally. Involuntary complex movements of the face, mouth, and tongue may occur in association with limb movements or as the only manifestations of this disorder. No associated mental disturbance occurs in such patients, and no family history indicative of Huntington's chorea can be obtained. In many instances the symptoms come on abruptly, are unilateral, and show little, if any, progression. This has suggested an underlying vascular lesion, which may be found in an exceptional case. More often than not the pathologic findings are similar to those of Huntington's chorea insofar as involvement of the caudate nucleus is concerned, but the cerebral cortex is spared. This has led to the contrary consideration that these cases are a variant of Huntington's chorea occurring sporadically. This form of chorea probably has several causes. As a rule, the symptoms are mild and the course so benign that therapeutic considerations are unimportant.

TICS (HABIT SPASMS)

A tic is a sudden, abrupt, rapid, purposeless, involuntary contraction of a muscle or group of functionally related muscles. Usually an irregular sequence of such contractions occurs that may result in eye blinking, head shaking, shrugging of the shoulder, or any sudden gesture of limbs or face. Tics may be voluntarily controlled for brief intervals, but such a conscious effort is usually followed by more intense and frequent contractions. Many persons experience minor transitory tic phenomena under periods of stress that are of no consequence. More persistent, sustained, and gross movements may be related to particular personality disturbances and may be amenable to psychotherapy. In some instances tics have occurred during the acute phase of encephalitis; these are thought to be an expression of extrapyramidal dysfunction. Tics in younger patients must be differentiated from chorea. Their patterned, predictable, and stereotyped character makes this distinction.

An unusual form of generalized tic (*maladie des tics, Gilles de la Tourette's disease*) involving facial twitching, continuous gestures associated with echolalia, foul language, and obsessional ideas is occasionally encountered in childhood. The disorder is progressive and sometimes associated with marked personality changes. However, a number of reports have appeared suggesting that haloperidol (Haldol) in divided dosage of 3 to 20 mg/day may be effective both in reducing the movement disorder and in overcoming the unfortunate verbal outbursts.

ATHETOSIS (MOBILE SPASMS)

This involuntary movement disorder is most frequently encountered in early infancy. Although in some respects it resembles chorea and although there are, in fact, transitional forms (so-called choreoathetosis), the athetotic movements are distinguishable by being slower, coarser, and more writhing. They occur when pathologic conditions involve the basal ganglia, primarily the pallidum, as well as additional motor pathways such as the corticospinal tract.

Athetosis is most often found in the heterogeneous group of conditions now lumped together under the term "cerebral palsy." More often than not, patients with cerebral palsy have marked alteration in muscle tone consisting of a combination of spasticity and rigidity. Their extrapyramidal movements may be widespread or limited and encompass a wide variety of dyskinetic phenomena. Congenital defects, anoxia or trauma at birth, and other degenerative conditions have all been implicated.

Some attempt has been made to identify specific entities based on clinicopathologic correlations. One such entity is *athetosis simplex* or *status marmoratus.* Autopsies in cases of this disorder, which exemplify all of the features of athetosis, show a distinctive marbled appearance of the basal ganglia, the result of an abnormal overgrowth of myelin sheaths and increased numbers of glial cells. The cause of this morphologic abnormality is unknown. Other cases have been grouped together on the basis of primary pathologic changes consisting of cell loss and failure of myelin sheath formation in the region of the basal ganglia, so-called *status demyelination.* Still other cases have been encountered in which abnormal deposits of pigments occur, or in which one of the lipidoses or another storage disease is found, with the predominant clinical picture of athetotic movements. Athetosis is infrequently encountered in adult life, but when it is, tumors, vascular insufficiency, malformations, and the effects of toxic agents have been found in the region of the basal ganglia.

Typical athetosis possesses the following features in varying degrees. One or both sides of the body are involved. The movements involve the upper limbs to a greater extent than the lower limbs and primarily their distal segments. The muscles innervated by the cranial nerves are invariably involved so that facial grimacing, writhing movements of the tongue, and disturbances in articulation and swallowing are encountered. Abnormal postures of the limbs are assumed. In the upper extremities, these consist of adduction and internal rotation at the shoulder, semiflexion at the elbow, flexion of wrist and metacarpophalangeal joints, and extension at interphalangeal joints. In the lower limbs the foot is maintained in internal rotation and plantar flexion with dorsiflexion of the toes. Superimposed on these abnormal postures are the athetotic movements described above. Muscle tone is increased during movement but hypotonic during relaxation, and some degree of weakness is usually found. The reflexes may be hyperactive, with abnormal toe responses. In many instances some degree of intellectual impairment may be found.

The abnormal movements and postural abnormalities are distinctive enough to make this condition readily recognizable. The age at onset, the admixture of other neurologic abnormalities, and the manner in which the symptoms progress identify the disease. Since most instances of athetosis appear in early infancy (before 1 year of age), diseases of the perinatal period are considered primarily. Athetosis occurring in later childhood or adult life may be a part of other extrapyramidal disorders—e.g., dystonia, chorea, or hepatolenticular degeneration. Less frequently, athetosis is a manifestation of a wide spectrum of neurologic disorders already mentioned in which the pallidum is coincidentally involved.

TORSION DYSTONIAS

The torsion dystonias comprise a group of movement disorders characterized by intense, irregular, sustained torsion spasms of the musculature with resultant marked abnormalities of bodily posture. The dystonic movements may be (1) focal, involving one bodily site such as foot or hand, (2) segmental, involving more than one site, in which proximal segments such as shoulder or pelvic girdle or both are prime sites, and (3) generalized, involving the limbs and trunk simultaneously. The pathophysiology and underlying morbid anatomy of this condition are unknown.

Three forms can be recognized based on genetic, clinical, and presumed causative factors. These consist of (1) inherited (autosomal recessive and autosomal dominant), (2) idiopathic, and (3) symptomatic types. The inherited and idiopathic forms are often referred to as primary dystonia in contrast to the symptomatic types, which are considered secondary.

Primary Dystonia

Inherited Types

The *autosomal recessive form* is found most often in Ashkenazi Jews, beginning between the ages of 5 and 15 years. Its onset is variable, but more frequently it begins with intermittent spasmodic inversion of the foot so that on walking, the child experiences difficulty in placing the heel on the ground. Bizarre stepping or a bowing gait may be noted when the dystonic movements affect the more proximal muscles of the leg or the spine. As the movements become more intense and the proximal musculature is more prominently involved, lordosis and tortipelvis appear. If the muscles of the neck and shoulder girdle are involved, torticollis is an early finding. Facial grimacing and difficulties in speech become evident as the muscles subserving these functions become involved. The continuous spasms over a period of time result in marked distortions of the body of a degree rarely seen in any other disease process. Although muscle tone and power appear to be normal, the involuntary movements interfere with function to such a degree as to make them useless. No changes in the tendon reflexes occur, and mentation remains normal.

The *autosomal dominant form* has its onset in early adult life and generally involves the axial musculature, with torticollis a frequent presenting symptom. In contrast to the recessive form, it remains more restricted in the regions of the body involved and is more slowly progressive. It has been found by some that plasma dopamine-hydroxylase activity is markedly elevated in the dominant form. This finding is strictly empiric and of questionable value in differentiating this type of dystonia from others.

In its early stages, dystonia musculorum deformans must be differentiated from other movement disorders in which dystonic phenomena may occur. The history and physical findings exclude hepatolenticular degeneration and epidemic encephalitis. The age at onset and the involvement of proximal musculature in the movements are enough to differentiate it from athetosis. Chorea is characterized by movements that are more rapid and of shorter duration than those of dystonia. Hysteria is often a consideration; if it is not positively established by the personality characteristics of the patient, the course of the disease will soon suggest the correct diagnosis.

There is extreme variability in the rate of progression and eventual disability of both forms of the genetically determined disorder. In their early phases there may be complete remission of symptoms or lack of progression of initial symptoms for long intervals of time. Because the natural history is subject to wide variations, evaluation of the effects of various therapeutic measures is difficult. As a rule, the earlier the age of onset the poorer the outcome with regard to severity and generalized nature of the dystonic process. Focal dystonia occurring in childhood and usually involving lower limbs will signify a progressive course. However, in adult life focal dystonia usually will involve upper limbs, be less progressive, and remain limited.

Idiopathic Types

Spasmodic Torticollis. The restriction of dyskinetic movements to neck muscles so that abnormal postures of the head result is the distinguishing characteristic of this symptom complex. Involuntary activity involves the sternocleidomastoid, trapezius, and scalenus muscles in sustained contractions that result in slow, twisting, turning movements of the head (torticollis) or, less often, forward flexion (anterocollis) or forceful extension (retrocollis). In most instances there is bilateral involvement, and the resultant postural deformity is maintained for varying lengths of time. The muscles of the neck appear under tension, and the continual muscular activity may lead to some degree of hypertrophy, especially evident in the sternocleidomastoid muscles. Similar activity may spread to facial and brachial musculature. The amount of active motion or static postural deformity is extremely variable.

Spasmodic torticollis has variably been described as a psychogenic disorder, a limited form of dystonic musculorum deformans, or a compensatory postural defect in persons with congenital ocular muscle imbalance or defects of the cervical spine or musculature. Hyperthyroidism has been present in a few patients. In some instances the torticollis has occurred as a part of a wide spectrum of extrapyramidal disorders that follow encephalitis lethargica. There is no information at present regarding either its pathophysiology or its pathology.

The disorder has been encountered at all ages but most frequently makes its appearances during the third to sixth decades of life. The course is extremely variable, being transitory and remitting after a few months in some patients and relentlessly progressive and leading to incapacity in others. Some patients reach a static phase in which movements cease or are minimal and a minor postural deformity of the head persists.

The evaluation of this condition includes a search for ocular and vertebral signs, major psychiatric disturbances, and other neurologic conditions with which it may be associated. Definable conditions account for only a small percentage of cases. In most, no underlying cause is uncovered.

Cranial Dystonias. Blepharospasm, oromandibular dystonia, and laryngeal and pharyngeal dystonia all fall into the category of cranial dystonias. They all occur in adult life, usually in the fifth or sixth decade, their cause is unknown, and they are resistant to most therapeutic measures. Each is characterized by intermittent spasms of selected groups of muscles, which markedly interfere with function. As a rule they remain localized but in some instances occur in combination. For example, the combination of oromandibular dystonia with blephorospasm is referred to as *Mieg's syndrome.* All of these conditions must be differentiated from drug-induced and tardive dyskinesias as initial manifestations of more generalized neurologic disorders and psychiatric conditions.

Writer's Cramp. Spasms of the muscles of the hand and forearm occurring during the act of writing characterize this disorder. A typical posture results with pen grasped tightly and the distal segment of digits extended, the forearm pronated and the wrist flexed. Tremor of the limb ensues as when script writing is attempted. Surprisingly, symptoms are less profound when writing is attempted in the standing position, such as writing with chalk on a board. In most individuals, symptoms remain limited to writing but in some patients may go on to involve other coordinated acts, such as using a key to open a door.

Conditions akin to writer's cramp have been associated with other skilled acts usually linked to occupational activities. Hence, typist's cramp, violinist's or cellist's cramps, and so forth, have been described. All seem to fall into a similar category for which cause and effective therapy are unknown.

Secondary Dystonia

A long list of conditions have been identified as causing dystonia. As a rule these conditions produce focal dystonic movements or postures that more frequently affect the upper limbs and particularly the

Table 3. Causes of Secondary Dystonia

Genetic
Wilson's disease
Huntington's disease
Hallervorden-Spatz disease
GM-1-gangliosidosis
Viral encephalitis
Arteriovenous malformation
Tumors
Drugs
Toxins—heavy metals

hand. This is especially so for destructive lesions, such as tumors or arteriovenous malformations of the brain. When focal dystonia is encountered in an adult, it is imperative that complete study be undertaken for causative factors. In addition to giving consideration to a long list of genetically determined disorders, drug-induced and toxic factors must be considered. Table 3 is included as a guide to identifiable conditions.

HEMIBALLISMUS

Hemiballismus is a rather violent involuntary movement that occurs when lesions involve the contralateral subthalamic nucleus, the corpus Luysii. Although a variety of pathologic processes such as tumor and infectious diseases have been found as underlying causes, most cases result from vascular lesions, either hemorrhagic or occlusive. In consequence, they are encountered in older patients, sometimes after a transitory hemiparesis. The event leading to the onset of this movement disorder often is an acute cerebrovascular accident with weakness or sensory deficit, or both.

As the neurologic signs clear or at a variable interval afterward, the ballistic movements begin. The movements do not occur during sleep, are localized to one side of the body, and involve the limbs in a forceful throwing movement, a result of almost continuous activity of the proximal musculature. Initially, their violence may exhaust and incapacitate the patient to such an extent that death may ensue. However, in most instances, the initial intensity decreases gradually so that they become tolerable, and in approximately 6 to 8 weeks the movements stop spontaneously. Surgical measures, such as thalamotomy, are rarely needed for control. In this regard, it is interesting to note that hemiballismus has occurred following attempted thalamotomy for other extrapyramidal disorders when poor localization for lesion placement has occurred. In such instances, the surgeon has inadvertently placed a lesion in the region of the corpus Luysii.

WILSON'S DISEASE

Wilson's disease (hepatolenticular degeneration) is an inherited disorder of copper metabolism in which degenerative lesions of the basal ganglia and cirrhosis of the liver occur. It is named after the English neurologist who described the clinical and pathologic manifestations of the disease in 1912.

Copper is widely distributed in all body tissues. It is most concentrated in the liver, central nervous system, and kidney. The highest concentrations of copper in the brain are found in two pigmented nuclei, the locus ceruleus and the substantia nigra. Copper in humans is obtained by oral ingestion; it is present in many foods and in drinking water. Most serum copper is bound to ceruloplasmin, an alpha$_2$-globulin; less than 5 per cent is bound to albumin. Not all the physiologic functions of copper are known. It is involved in the control of cellular cytochrome oxidase activity, and it may have other specific functions in neural metabolism.

In Wilson's disease the major defect is inability of the liver to adequately synthesize ceruloplasmin. This results in an excess of unbound serum copper, which then becomes deposited in the liver, brain, kidneys, and cornea. In the brain, necrosis with cavitation of the putamen may occur. Lesser changes take place in the caudate nucleus, globus pallidus, thalamus, and cortex. An astrocytic gliosis of Alzheimer type II cells, with eccentric, large nuclei, called Opalski cells, has also been described. The liver shows changes typical of postnecrotic cirrhosis.

Wilson's disease is inherited in an autosomal recessive manner. There is no racial or sexual predilection. Many affected individuals have consanguineous parents or come from areas where consanguinity is common. The age at onset is variable. Although abnormalities of copper metabolism exist from birth, symptoms of the disease usually appear between 10 and 40 years of age.

The first symptoms usually develop gradually. They include involuntary movements, dysarthria, and mental abnormalities. The most common involuntary movement is a coarse, flapping tremor of the arms, often characterized as "wing-beating." Dystonia, chorea, and athetosis have all been described. The involuntary movements may be present at rest and are worsened with attempts at holding the posture. Spasticity with hyperactive tendon reflexes and extensor plantar reflexes is common, as are generalized rigidity and bradykinesia. Mild lower motor neuron wasting is a rare finding.

Mental abnormalities are quite variable and range from minor personality changes to severe progressive dementia. In one series, approximately 60 per cent of patients presented with psychiatric manifestations. Patients are often misdiagnosed as having schizophrenia. Seizures have also been reported.

Signs of hepatic disease may appear at any stage of the disease. Jaundice, hepatosplenomegaly, or chronic hepatitis may be the presenting problem, particularly in children. Episodes of acute hemolytic anemia and impaired renal tubular function may also develop. In patients with long-standing disease, aminoaciduria may occur secondary to defective renal tubular reabsorption.

The most unique finding in Wilson's disease is a brownish-green ring of pigmentation at the limbus of the cornea, known as a Kayser-Fleischer ring. This is caused by copper deposition in Descemet's membrane, one of the inner layers of the cornea. The ring may be incomplete; it is usually most marked superiorly and inferiorly. The ring may be detected by inspection, but slit-lamp examination is necessary to ascertain that pigmentation is absent. The Kayser-Fleischer ring is nearly always present when neurologic disease has developed, although it may fade or disappear with penicillamine therapy.

The course of untreated Wilson's disease is usually one of progression, although spontaneous remissions occasionally occur. The duration of the disease from onset to complete disability and death is quite variable. Patients may survive for 15 years or more. Death may be due to chronic hepatic failure or intercurrent infections. The introduction of penicillamine therapy has, however, radically changed the prognosis. Patients treated before permanent hepatic or brain damage takes place have an excellent prognosis.

SPINOCEREBELLAR DEGENERATIONS

By Gary S. Pearl, M.D., Ph.D.
Atlanta, Georgia

Also known as spinocerebellar ataxias and hereditary ataxias, the spinocerebellar degenerations are a heterogeneous group of neurologic disorders characterized clinically by chronic progressive ataxia and pathologically by degeneration of some portion or portions of the cerebellar afferent system at the spinal or brain stem level, the cerebellar parenchyma, or the cerebellar nuclei and efferent pathways. Differences in the predominant site of pathologic involvement, as well as differences in associated clinical and pathologic abnormalities, have led to a multitude of classifications with varying terminology for different forms of spinocerebellar degeneration. Further, there has also been some disagreement as to which disorders fall into this general category. In any case, it is important to consider Greenfield's statement, "It is commonplace that no differential diagnosis between the various forms of cerebellar atrophy is possible during life," when evaluating patients with one of these abnormalities. This is particularly true since spinocerebellar degenerations of the same general type may differ clinically or pathologically when they occur in different families or even within a single family.

A concise, simplified classification schema based on that of Greenfield is presented in Table 1. Each of the disorders listed, other than ataxia-telangiectasia, probably represents a group of similar or related disease processes. Other forms that have been described probably represent variants of or transitions between these major classes.

FRIEDREICH'S ATAXIA

Synonyms. Friedreich's disease, heredofamilial spinal ataxia.

Definition. Friedreich's ataxia, the most common and most stereotyped of the spinocerebellar degenerations, is an autosomal recessive disorder characterized by degeneration of the dorsal columns, lateral corticospinal tracts, dorsal, and to a lesser extent ventral spinocerebellar tracts; Clarke's column in the spinal cord; the dorsal roots and ganglia; and large myelinated axons in peripheral nerves.

Presenting Signs and Symptoms. Patients with Friedreich's ataxia generally present with neurologic dysfunction before puberty, with most presenting between 8 and 10 years of age; only rarely does the disease develop after 20 years of age. Gait ataxia is usually the first manifestation, although weakness or easy fatigability may precede the gait ataxia. The gait ataxia may present as difficulty in walking in a child who is already able to walk or, more commonly, as slowness in learning to walk or a clumsy gait in a child just beginning to walk. Kyphoscoliosis or pes cavus may also be an early manifestation of the disease and may even be seen in otherwise unaffected relatives of patients with Friedreich's ataxia.

Course. The course is generally progressive without remission. The ataxia progresses from predominantly involving the lower extremities to involvement of the upper extremities and trunk as well. The gait ataxia generally progresses to an inability to walk within 5 years. Dysarthria, characterized by slow, slurred, and explosive speech, is eventually present in all patients. Pes cavus or progressive kyphoscoliosis, or both, usually develops within 2 years of the onset of neurologic disease. Patients become hypotonic, with distal weakness predominantly involving the legs. Sensory abnormalities with loss of position and vibratory sensation and occasionally paresthesias become evident, primarily in the lower extremities. Some patients may also develop choreiform movements, optic atrophy, partial deafness, or vertigo during the course of their illness. Hypertrophic cardiomyopathy is a frequent component of the disease, and many patients show some signs of cardiac failure. The overall course is slowly progressive, with a mean duration of approximately 25 years, and death is usually secondary to cardiac failure or infection.

Physical Examination. Physical findings are dependent on the stage of the disease process when the patient is being evaluated. Early findings include gait ataxia which may be associated with pes cavus, truncal ataxia, and dysarthria. Later, there is marked dysmetria in the lower extremities with poor performance of heel-to-shin testing and a lesser defect on finger-to-nose testing of the upper extremity. Gait abnormalities are often marked, with severe ataxia and spasticity. The lower extremities are often weak and hypotonic, and there are markedly decreased or absent tendon reflexes and extensor plantar reflexes. The upper extremities are less affected and tendon reflexes may only be mildly decreased. Dysarthria, nystagmus, choreiform movements, intention tremor, and titubation are frequently observed. Sensory testing reveals impairment of tactile discrimination and vibratory and position sense in the legs and, in later stages of the disease, in the arms as well. Cardiac examination frequently demonstrates a systolic ejection murmur or diastolic third or fourth heart sound.

Table 1. Classification of Spinocerebellar Degenerations

Disorder	Onset	Major Site of Involvement
Friedreich's ataxia	Juvenile	Peripheral nerve, spinal cord
Olivopontocerebellar atrophy	Adult	Brain stem, cerebellum
Cerebellar cortical degeneration	Adult	Cerebellum
Ataxia-telangiectasia	Juvenile	Cerebellum, immune system

Laboratory Findings. The glucose tolerance test is abnormal in up to 40 per cent of patients with Friedreich's ataxia, and clinical diabetes mellitus occurs in approximately 10 to 20 per cent of patients. Pyruvate dehydrogenase activity is reported to be impaired in many patients with Friedreich's ataxia, with the major abnormality being a decrease in lipoamide dehydrogenase activity. Defects in pyruvate carboxylase and mitochondrial malic enzyme activity have also been reported. The significance of these findings in the differential diagnosis of Friedreich's ataxia is uncertain at present, but may be of greater importance in the near future.

Radiologic Evaluation. Chest x-ray shows cardiomegaly in approximately 30 per cent of patients. Spine x-rays may be helpful in demonstrating and evaluating kyphoscoliosis. Computed tomographic (CT) scanning of the head is generally normal.

Other Diagnostic Procedures. Electrophysiologic studies may be helpful in diagnosis. The electrocardiogram is abnormal in almost all patients, although it may be normal initially, becoming abnormal at a later stage. Frequent abnormalities include ST-T wave changes, evidence of right ventricular hypertrophy, and atrial tachyarrhythmias. The electroencephalogram (EEG) may be normal or may show mild nonspecific abnormalities. Nerve conduction studies in sensory nerves generally show an absence of action potentials in the legs, with decreased amplitude and velocity in the arms. Motor nerve conduction studies and electromyography (EMG) are generally normal. Sensory evoked potentials (SEP) show severe bilateral abnormality, while brain stem auditory evoked potentials (BAEP) are usually normal. Peripheral nerve biopsy, which is rarely necessary, shows a loss of large myelinated axons with preservation of unmyelinated axons.

Pitfalls in Diagnosis. Classic cases of Friedreich's ataxia generally provide no difficulty in diagnosis; however, abortive or atypical forms are often seen. The presence of infrequently associated abnormalities, such as optic atrophy or pigmentary degeneration of the retina, should not rule out the diagnosis. Syndromes of different pathogeneses may share some of the clinical and pathologic features of Friedreich's ataxia and have even been classified with it in the past. The *Roussy-Levy syndrome (hereditary arreflexic dystasia)* is characterized by mild gait ataxia, loss of tendon reflexes in the legs, kyphoscoliosis, and pes cavus in association with marked wasting of muscles in the distal legs. However, dysarthria and nystagmus are not present, and there is a prominent neuropathic component with hypertrophic neuropathy and onion-bulb formation. Motor nerves show decreased nerve conduction velocity, and there is evidence of denervation on EMG and muscle biopsy. This disorder is probably best classified with the hypertrophic neuropathies.

Several disorders of lipid metabolism may also have features of Friedreich's ataxia. *Abetalipoproteinemia (Bassen-Kornzweig syndrome)* is characterized by the onset of gait and limb ataxia at 5 to 10 years of age, with progression of neurologic findings to include dysarthria, hyporeflexia, nystagmus, loss of position and vibratory sensation, and extensor plantar reflexes. Pes cavus, cardiomyopathy, and pigmentary retinal degeneration are also seen. Abetalipoproteinemia is differentiated from Friedreich's ataxia by the presence of malabsorption of fat with steatorrhea, acanthocytosis on peripheral blood smear, decreased serum cholesterol level, and absent beta-lipoproteins. *Refsum's disease (hereditary ataxic polyneuritis)* is an autosomal recessive disorder characterized by increased serum and tissue phytanic acid. It presents in the first or second decade of life with gait ataxia and visual disturbance. It progresses to marked gait ataxia, limb ataxia, nystagmus, pigmentary retinal degeneration, sensorineural hearing loss, sensory deficits, and cardiac arrhythmias. Pes cavus and scoliosis may also be present. However, significant involvement of the upper extremities, a hypertrophic neuropathy with decreased nerve conduction velocities and denervation on EMG, ichthyosis, increased serum lipid levels, and phytanic acid accumulation distinguish it from Friedreich's ataxia. Features of Friedreich's ataxia may also be seen as a component of several other metabolic diseases, including forms of *hexosaminidase deficiency,* particularly in adults, *gamma-glutamyl-cysteine synthetase deficiency, aminoacidurias,* and adult *metachromatic leukodystrophy.* These can be ruled out with appropriate metabolic tests and by the presence of other associated features. Posterior fossa neoplasms may present with ataxia, but they are generally demonstrable with CT scanning.

OLIVOPONTOCEREBELLAR ATROPHY

Definition. Olivopontocerebellar atrophy (OPCA) consists of a group of disorders characterized by degeneration of the lateral corticospinal tracts, the dorsal spinocerebellar tracts, the dorsal columns, and Clarke's columns in the spinal cord, as well as cranial nerve nuclei V, VII, XII, the inferior olivary nuclei, the pontine nuclei, the middle cerebellar peduncle, and the cerebellar cortex. Some authors have subclassified OPCA into several types depending on whether the disorder was autosomal dominant (Menzel type) or sporadic (Dejerine-Thomas type) and on the basis of associated abnormalities in other portions of the nervous system. The latter subclassification is unnecessary because of the variability in clinical features from family to family and even within a single family.

Presenting Signs and Symptoms. OPCA may be inherited in an autosomal dominant or, rarely, in an autosomal recessive fashion. It frequently occurs sporadically. Patients generally present with gait and limb ataxia involving predominantly the lower extremities, with a mean age of onset in the fourth decade for hereditary cases and in the fifth to sixth decade for sporadic cases.

Course. OPCA is a slowly progressive disorder with a duration of approximately 20 years. Neurologic abnormalities progress from gait ataxia to an inability to stand without support; severe dysarthria with slow, slurred, scanning speech; and ataxia of the upper extremities with intention tremor. Patients often develop parkinsonian features, with rigidity, bradykinesia, and resting tremor. Sphincter dysfunction may be a late complication. In some cases, ophthalmoplegia or dementia may also be a prominent feature, whereas retinal degeneration, optic atrophy, or autonomic dysfunction, such as orthostatic hypotension, may occur in other cases, with ophthalmoplegia and optic atrophy being more common in heredofamilial cases. In general, strength, sensation, and cognition are preserved, and death usually occurs in the sixth or seventh decade as a result of respiratory infection.

Physical Examination. The physical examination is dominated by evidence of cerebellar dysfunction, which may differ depending on the point in the time course when the patient is evaluated. Early, there may be only leg ataxia and an abnormal gait. Later in the disease there may be four-limb ataxia with dysmetria and dysdiadochokinesis, severe dysarthria, and intention tremor. Nystagmus may be present. Tendon reflexes are generally normal or hyperactive, and plantar reflexes are often extensor. Choreiform movements may also occur. If parkinsonian features supervene, rigidity, bradykinesia, facial impassivity, and resting tremor will be observed. Although sensory examination is usually normal, some patients may have signs of dorsal column disease with impaired position and vibratory sensation. Mentation is usually normal, although dementia may be present in some patients. Retinal degeneration, ophthalmoplegia, optic atrophy, or signs of cranial nerve dysfunction may occur, and these variations may be characteristic within a family.

Radiologic Evaluation. CT scan may demonstrate cerebellar and brain stem atrophy with enlargement of cerebellar sulci, the fourth ventricle, the cisterna magna, and the superior cerebellar, quadrigeminal, prepontine, and ambient cisterns. Cerebral cortical sulci and the lateral ventricles may also be enlarged in some cases, indicating cerebral cortical atrophy.

Other Diagnostic Procedures. BAEP is frequently abnormal, with small and delayed peaks, whereas SEP is usually normal or only mildly abnormal.

Pitfalls in Diagnosis. It is often difficult or even impossible to clinically differentiate OPCA from some cases of cerebellar cortical degeneration. However, since treatment is not available for either at the present time, differentiation during life is not of great importance. The variation in clinical signs between or even within families may create some confusion in diagnosis, but it is not significant when determining genetic pedigrees. The presence of progressive cerebellar ataxia in middle age with other associated abnormalities suggests OPCA. When parkinsonian features are prominent, diagnosis may be difficult, but the presence of cerebellar dysfunction will suggest OPCA with extrapyramidal involvement. The designation "Marie's ataxia" should no longer be considered appropriate, since this term refers to a very heterogeneous group of disorders, including different variants of OPCA and cerebellar cortical degeneration.

CEREBELLAR CORTICAL DEGENERATION

Synonyms. Cerebello-olivary atrophy, parenchymatous cerebellar degeneration (Holmes type), delayed cortical cerebellar atrophy (Marie-Foix-Alajouanine type), lamellar cerebellar atrophy, late corticocerebellar atrophy.

Definition. This group of disorders is characterized by marked degeneration of the cerebellar cortex with or without degeneration of the inferior olivary nuclei. Clinical features are generally restricted to those of cerebellar dysfunction in classic cases; however, variations are frequently seen.

Presenting Signs and Symptoms. Patients generally present in the fifth or sixth decade with gait ataxia and progressive ataxia of the lower extremities. At the time of presentation, upper extremity coordination and speech are generally intact.

Course. The condition progresses from lower extremity ataxia to ataxia involving the upper extremities as well. Dysarthria develops, characterized by scanning, slurred, and explosive speech. Nystagmus may occur in some patients. In general, mentation and sensation remain intact, although some patients do develop sensory loss, reflecting dorsal column dysfunction or dementia. Rarely, patients may develop some parkinsonian features. The disorder is slowly progressive, with a duration of 15 to 20 years and with the cause of death generally being respiratory infection.

Physical Examination. Early in the disease process, patients have a wide-based, ataxic gait, with ataxia and intention tremor of the lower extremities and truncal ataxia. Later in the course, the upper extremities become involved with dysmetria, dysdiadochokinesis, and intention tremor. Titubation of the head may also be present. Some patients may have nystagmus, but this is often a late finding. Dysarthria is commonly present. Tendon reflexes may be normal or hyperactive, although ankle jerks may be hypoactive late in the disease. An extensor plantar response may be seen in some patients. Sensation is generally intact, but some patients may have mildly impaired position and vibratory sensation in the legs. Mentation is usually intact, although dementia may occur in some patients. Similarly parkinsonian features may rarely occur, but these are usually mild.

Radiologic Findings. CT scan shows cerebellar atrophy with enlargement of cerebellar sulci and the fourth ventricle.

Pitfalls in Diagnosis. Cases of cerebellar cortical degeneration may be impossible to distinguish clinically from OPCA, particularly if a variant with extracerebellar manifestations is seen. Although dyssynergia cerebellaris myoclonica (Ramsay Hunt syndrome) has been considered by some to be a distinct entity characterized by progressive cerebellar dysfunction with seizures and myoclonus, it is probably heterogenous, including some cases of Friedreich's ataxia and cerebellar cortical degeneration, as well as some other causes of cerebellar degeneration. It is important to distinguish the idiopathic form of cerebellar cortical degeneration from acquired cerebellar cortical degeneration. The latter is most often associated with chronic ethanol abuse, neoplasms, or chronic anticonvulsant therapy, particularly with phenytoin. Alcoholic cerebellar cortical degeneration generally occurs after years of ethanol abuse and may be related to nutritional deficiency. It is characterized by a subacutely progressive course over weeks to months, but may remit with improved nutrition and abstention from alcohol. In addition to a history suggesting an alcoholic basis, the clinical findings may suggest this entity. Patients generally show a marked ataxia of the lower extremities and trunk with an ataxic gait and stance that worsens with postural changes. By contrast, the upper extremities are only mildly involved and dysarthria is mild or absent. CT scan shows atrophy localized to the midline with enlargement of the cerebellar vermian sulci and superior cerebellar cistern. Cerebellar cortical degeneration in association with anticonvulsant therapy is distinguished by a history of anticonvulsant use, often extending over decades. Although acute intoxication, which is characterized by gait ataxia, dysarthria, and nystagmus, is reversible with discontinuation of the drug, chronic use may lead to irreversible gait ataxia, intention tremor, dysarthria, nystagmus, and hypotonia. Paraneoplastic cerebellar cortical degeneration may occur before or after the first clinical signs of a neoplasm and is most often associated with carcinoma of the lung, breast, or ovary in adults and with neuroblastoma in children. It is characterized by a rapidly progressive ataxia beginning with an ataxia of gait and progressing to involve all extremities and the trunk. Dysarthria also develops. Nystagmus, ophthalmoplegia, and opsoclonus may also be present. In patients with an acute to subacute progressive ataxia, particularly in adults, an occult malignancy should be sought.

ATAXIA-TELANGIECTASIA

Synonym. Louis-Bar syndrome.

Definition. Ataxia-telangiectasia is a well-characterized, autosomal recessive, multisystem disorder with features of neurologic, vascular, endocrine, and immune dysfunction. Classic features include cerebellar dysfunction, oculocutaneous telangiectasia, and recurrent sinopulmonary infections.

Presenting Signs and Symptoms. The most common clinical presentation is gait ataxia when a child first learns to walk during infancy, although some patients may present first with ocular telangiectasia or a side-to-side head tremor.

Course. The course of the neurologic disease is characterized by progression of cerebellar dysfunction from gait ataxia to a four-limb ataxia with dysarthria, coarse nystagmus, and oculomotor dyspraxia. Intellectual development may be arrested during childhood, with some individuals showing mild mental retardation. Later in the course, choreoathetosis and myoclonic jerks are common, and some patients develop distal weakness.

The non-neurologic manifestations also progress during the course of the disease. Telangiectasia generally develop first in the bulbar conjunctiva at 3 to 5 years of age, with subsequent development on the ears, nose, cheeks, anterior neck, and antecubital and popliteal fossae. Body development and the development of secondary sexual characteristics may be retarded. Recurrent sinopulmonary bacterial infections are a prominent feature, often commencing at 3 to 8 years of age, although they may have an earlier onset. These may lead to chronic bronchitis or bronchiectasis and chronic pulmonary insufficiency. Patients generally die by the third decade, although some may survive longer, with the cause of death usually pulmonary disease, infection, or neoplasm. In fact, the frequency of neoplasms, in particular those of lymphoreticular origin, is increased in ataxia-telangiectasia.

Physical Examination. Characteristic physical findings include those of neurologic dysfunction, pulmonary disease, and oculocutaneous telangiectasia. Early in the disease, only gait ataxia may be seen. Later, four-limb ataxia with intention tremor and dysmetria, coarse nystagmus with ocular dyspraxia, and dysarthria are seen. Tendon reflexes may be hyperactive early in the course, but often become hypoactive later. Plantar reflexes may be extensor. Patients may be hypotonic and, although strength and sensation are normal earlier in the course, some may develop distal weakness or impairment of position and vibratory sensation later in the disease. Patients may also demonstrate choreoathetoid movements and myoclonic jerks late in the disease process and some may show mild retardation of intellectual development.

Telangiectasias are generally seen in the bulbar conjunctiva, in exposed areas of skin and on surfaces exposed to friction. Many children have short stature, and progeric changes are frequently present in the hair and skin. Tonsillar lymphoid tissue is generally decreased. Patients may also have chronic bronchitis or bronchiectatic findings on pulmonary examination.

Laboratory Findings. Abnormalities of immune testing are frequent, as most patients have decreased serum and secretory IgA, decreased serum IgE, or low molecular weight IgM in the serum. Approximately one third of patients have lymphocytopenia associated with a decrease in T-helper lymphocytes, and many patients have an impaired antibody response to several antigens that may be tested. Cell-mediated immunity is also impaired, with most patients failing to respond on skin testing to common antigens. Almost all patients have an elevation in serum alpha-fetoprotein, with levels often between 100 and 300 ng/ml. Mild increases in serum alanine aminotransferase, aspartate aminotransferase, and alkaline phosphatase may also be present. Glucose intolerance is common, associated with insulin resistance and elevated fasting insulin levels.

Radiologic Findings. Chest x-ray may demonstrate chronic pulmonary disease. CT scan of the head may show diffuse cerebellar atrophy with enlargement of sulci and the fourth ventricle.

Pitfalls in Diagnosis. When the syndrome is fully developed, there should be no difficulty in diagnosis. However, early in the disease, findings may resemble those in Friedreich's ataxia. Family history, the development of cutaneous telangiectasia, increased alpha-fetoprotein, and the lack of skeletal abnormalities in ataxia-telangiectasia may serve to differentiate the two diseases. Since progressive ataxia may be seen in several metabolic diseases or in posterior fossa neoplasms, these should be ruled out, as described for Friedreich's ataxia.

MULTIPLE SCLEROSIS AND OTHER DISEASES OF THE WHITE MATTER

By Charles M. Poser, M.D.
Boston, Massachusetts

Diseases of the myelin sheath comprise two major categories: the *demyelinating* or *myelinoclastic* diseases and the *dysmyelinating* diseases.

The first group (the demyelinating diseases) includes conditions in which the myelin sheath has developed normally and has a completely normal metabolic maintenance system, but in which the sheath appears to be the primary target of various conditions. In this group, two major subgroups are recognized: the first one is a disease of unknown etiology and pathogenesis called multiple sclerosis, and some of its variants. The second group consists of the complications of various infections, principally viral, and vaccinations, which result from a misdirection of the immune response that has been activated by the infection or vaccination. As a result, both humoral and cellular (delayed) immune factors cause the myelin sheath of either the central or the peripheral nervous systems, or of both, to become inflamed, edematous, or destroyed.

In the second major group, the dysmyelinating diseases, an inborn error of metabolism causes a disturbance of myelinogenesis. In some cases, the dysmyelination results from a metabolic failure of the myelin maintenance system after normally formed myelin has been laid down.

The dysmyelinating diseases are of many types and include such disparate conditions as the leukodystrophies (which will be discussed later); the gangliosidoses, such as Tay-Sachs disease; several aminoacidopathies, such as phenylketonuria and maple syrup urine disease; and probably other metabolic disturbances which in one way or another interfere with the normal development of myelin.

It should be pointed out that destruction of myelin is a nonspecific result of almost any injury to the nervous system and can be seen following physical trauma or vascular insults, with infections and neoplasms, or as a result of various intoxications. The conditions considered here are those in which such causes and factors are not recognized. Two conditions, *central pontine myelinolysis* and *Marchiafava-Bignami* disease, have been included because they fulfill the criteria of being primary diseases of myelin, although they are not easily classifiable as either variants of multiple sclerosis or instances of postinfectious or postvaccinal reactions of the nervous system.

The conditions to be described here affect primarily, but not exclusively, the central nervous system. While multiple sclerosis is a disease restricted to the central nervous system, the leukodystrophies characteristically also involve the peripheral nerves; the postinfectious or postvaccinal reactions may be restricted to the central nervous system (encephalomyelitis), or peripheral nervous system (Guillain-Barré syndrome) or may involve both to varying degrees.

The following conditions will be discussed:

A. The Myelinoclastic (Demyelinating) Diseases
   1. Multiple sclerosis
   2. Myelinoclastic diffuse sclerosis
   3. Post-infectious and postvaccinal encephalomyelitis (disseminated vasculomyelinopathy)
   4. Transverse myelitis
   5. Central pontine myelinolysis
   6. Marchiafava-Bignami disease
B. The Dysmyelinating Diseases—the Leukodystrophies
   1. Metachromatic leukodystrophy
   2. Globoid cell leukodystrophy
   3. Adrenoleukodystrophy
   4. Spongy sclerosis

THE MYELINOCLASTIC DISEASES

Multiple Sclerosis

Multiple sclerosis (MS) is a disease that affects the central nervous system exclusively. It is somewhat more frequent in women, and attacks young adults. The common age of symptomatic onset is in the third and fourth decades; it is quite rare before the age of 10 and after the age of 60 years. The disease attacks myelin, sparing the axon itself, and is associated with a inflammatory glial reaction. It involves predominantly white matter, although plaques not infrequently extend into adjacent gray matter. The lesions are usually quite small, the diameter rarely exceeding

4 to 5 mm, although larger plaques may be seen as well.

It is often difficult to reconcile the clinical manifestations of the disease with the distribution of plaques found at postmortem examination. Many of the plaques affect what are known as silent areas of the brain, in particular the subcortical white matter, whereas others, despite their location in what appear to be anatomically and physiologically critical areas, remain asymptomatic. Thus, while it is true that in roughly two thirds of the patients the disease is characterized by remissions and exacerbations, these symptomatic manifestations may represent only the tip of the iceberg, the disease progressing relentlessly and unremittingly in areas that remain clinically silent.

MS has a striking geographic distribution, with a high incidence directly proportional to latitude, being significantly more common in Canada, the northern United States and northern Europe. This apparent geographic predilection can probably best be translated into a genetic predisposition in individuals of Germanic origin (including Scandinavian and Anglo-Saxon). MS does occur in American Blacks, although with less frequency than in nonblacks and again reflecting the geographic region in which the individual resides. It is much rarer in Orientals and is essentially unknown in African Blacks.

Diagnostic Criteria

The diagnosis of MS remains a clinical one, since there are no reliable pathognomonic diagnostic laboratory tests. Recently described laboratory procedures, in particular the measurement of evoked responses, and availability of tissue imaging have expanded the diagnostic facilities. The former, which are considered to be extensions of the neurologic examination, have proved to be extremely useful in demonstrating additional lesions, many of which have been and remain asymptomatic. Despite these advances, the diagnosis still depends very much upon the classic description of the disease—i.e., its distribution in time and in space.

New diagnostic criteria to be used as guidelines for research protocols, but also applicable to the clinical situation, have recently been introduced.*

According to these criteria, MS is classified into four groups: clinically definite, laboratory-supported definite, clinically probable, and laboratory-supported probable.

Clinically definite MS is characterized by one of these conditions:

1. Two attacks and clinical evidence of two separate lesions.
2. Two attacks, clinical evidence of one lesion, and paraclinical evidence of another lesion.

Laboratory-supported definite MS can be defined by one of these situations:

1. Two attacks and either clinical or paraclinical evidence of one lesion, and the presence of cerebrospinal fluid oligoclonal bands or of increased intrathecal immunoglobulin G (IgG) production.
2. One attack plus clinical evidence of two separate lesions, and oligoclonal banding or increased IgG production.
3. One attack, clinical evidence of one lesion, and paraclinical evidence of another separate lesion, as well as the presence of oligoclonal bands or of increased intrathecal IgG production.

Clinically probable MS is based on one of these situations:

1. Two attacks and clinical evidence of one lesion.
2. One attack and clinical evidence of two separate lesions.
3. One attack and clinical evidence of one lesion and paraclinical evidence of another lesion.

Finally, *laboratory-supported probable MS* is based on the occurrence of two attacks and the presence of cerebrospinal fluid oligoclonal bands or increased intrathecal production of IgG.

Attacks (bouts, episodes, exacerbations) consist of the occurrence of one or more symptoms of neurologic dysfunction lasting more than 24 hours. Clinical evidence is defined as signs of neurologic dysfunction demonstrable by neurologic examination, whereas paraclinical evidence of a lesion consists of the demonstration by means of various tests and procedures of the existence of a lesion of the central nervous system that has not produced signs of neurologic dysfunction, but which may or may not have caused symptoms in the past. A remission is defined as a definite improvement of signs, symptoms, or both, that have been present for at least 24 hours; a remission should last at least one month. To be considered evidence for the diagnosis, the manifestations of the disease must be shown to be characteristic of MS and not attributable to another condition. A disease that has progressed steadily from onset, without reliable evidence of exacerbations or remissions, with manifestations reflecting a single lesion, and with lack of paraclinical evidence of a lesion elsewhere in the central nervous system is not to be classified as MS for research purpose, even in the presence of oligoclonal bands or increased IgG production in the cerebrospinal fluid.

Put in a simpler fashion, patients who exhibit clinical or paraclinical evidence, by neurologic signs or well-documented symptoms, of lesions affecting separate parts of the central nervous system, and who have had at least two clearly separate episodes of neurologic dysfunction that cannot be explained on any other basis, should be considered highly suspect of having MS, provided that other conditions that produce similar distribution in time and space have been adequately ruled out.

Signs and Symptoms

MS appears to show a predilection for certain portions of the nervous system, such as the optic nerves and chiasm, the brain stem and cerebellum, and the spinal cord.

Examination of the clinical course of 111 autopsy-

*Poser, C., Paty, D., Scheinberg, L., et al.: New diagnostic criteria for multiple sclerosis: Guidelines for research protocols. Ann. Neurol., 13:227, 1983.

proved cases of MS revealed involvement of the pyramidal tracts in nearly 100 per cent of the cases, of the ocular system (disturbances of visual acuity or of ocular motility, or of both) in 85 per cent, disturbances of micturition in 82 per cent, nonequilibratory signs or symptoms in 80 per cent, diminution of vibratory or position sense or of both in 71 per cent, sustained nystagmus in 70 per cent, paresthesias in 66 per cent, dysarthria in 55 per cent, gait ataxia in 55 per cent, and mental or cognitive disturbances in 50 per cent.

Certain sign and symptom combinations, while definitely not pathognomonic, are quite characteristic of the disease. These include diplopia due to internuclear ophthalmoplegia; acute optic or retrobulbar neuritis, which if it occurs asymptomatically is detected only by the presence of monocular color blindness; numbness or paresthesias without objective evidence of decreased sensation; absence of abdominal reflexes, particularly if unilateral; decreased vibratory sense; and Lhermitte's sign (a sensation of electric shock running down the middle of the back when the head is flexed forward). Other symptoms that are quite suggestive are the presence of typical trigeminal neuralgia in an individual under the age of 40 years or idiopathic vertigo in a young individual. Mental and cognitive changes are much more common in MS patients than is suspected, but the latter must usually be demonstrated by specific neuropsychologic examination. Fatigability is an extremely common and distressing symptom in MS, but one which unfortunately is often erroneously ascribed to depression.

Early in its course, when it is most important to correctly identify the reason for neurologic problems, the diagnosis of MS may be quite difficult. This is particularly true when the physician is unfamiliar with the often transient and bizarre manifestations of the disease and is inexperienced in separating functional disturbances from symptoms and signs of neurologic dysfunction. The proliferation of medical information for lay persons has resulted in a heightened awareness of the symptoms of diseases such as MS and along with this a commensurate rise in the anxiety level associated with what often turn out to be completely insignificant discomforts. MS is probably as frequently diagnosed when it is not present as when it is. It should be stressed that MS does not involve the peripheral nervous system, so the presence of such lesions militates against that diagnosis; on the other hand, the third, fifth, and seventh cranial nerves may be involved, as they course through the brain stem.

One of the major problems with the clinical diagnosis of MS is that the symptoms not only are transient, often lasting only minutes, but in addition are often difficult to reconcile with anatomic reality. There is a very natural and common tendency on the part of many patients to subconsciously exaggerate or extend their symptoms: thus, an individual with double vision may complain of triple or quadruple vision; numbness of one arm may be subconsciously extended to the entire side of the body. These complaints tend to ignore anatomic and physiologic boundaries and confuse the examining physician. The superimposition of hysterical manifestations is extremely common in MS and complicates the differential diagnosis.

Ancillary Clinical Procedures

The Hot Bath Test. Increasing body temperature produces conduction block in myelinated nerve fibers. In axons that have been completely or partially denuded of their myelin sheath, such elevation of body temperature may produce the typical signs and symptoms of MS. To perform the hot bath test, the patient is immersed in a bath with the water at a temperature of 40° to 41° C. The elevation of body temperature may then either produce new signs and symptoms or reproduce signs and symptoms that had been experienced previously. These most often include diminution of visual acuity, diplopia, cerebellar incoordination, hyperreflexia, and Babinski signs. The patient should not be left unattended, the test should not be prolonged beyond 10 to 15 minutes, and care must be taken that the severe peripheral vasodilatation does not result in hypotension. Fortunately, whatever neurologic disturbances are revealed by the test disappear immediately upon cooling. These tests, however, should never be performed in a patient who has what appears to be having an active exacerbation. It is, of course, usually not necessary under those circumstances anyway.

Detection of Monocular Color Blindness. By using Ishihara or AO-pseudoisochromatic plates, monocular color blindness (red-green) can often be detected. This provides excellent evidence that the patient has suffered a previous optic or retrobulbar neuritis. It should be remembered that monocular color blindness is never noted by the patient except by the fortuitous circumstance of closing one eye at the appropriate time.

Psychophysiological Ophthalmologic Procedures. A number of sophisticated physiologic and psychophysiologic ophthalmologic procedures exist that are quite useful when they are available. These include determination of contrast sensitivity, flicker-fusion and flight of color tests, determination of speed of saccade initiation, and several others.

Laboratory Studies

Neurophysiologic Studies. A variety of evoked response studies have been devised that have proved to be extraordinarily useful in detecting the presence of lesions in other parts of the nervous system, some of which may or may not have been symptomatic. Among the most useful tests are the visual evoked responses, which are elicited either by flashes of light or by pattern reversal of black and white squares. Delays in the evoked potentials recorded in the occipital cortex as well as changes in wave form and differences in amplitude between the two sides are common abnormalities; however, increased latency is by far the most useful and reliable. Although visual evoked responses are practically always abnormal in patients with a history of optic or retrobulbar neuritis, their real value lies in the fact that in patients with definite MS, they are abnormal in as many as 75 per cent of individuals who have never had any historical or physical evidence of involvement of the visual system. In this group of patients, abnormal results are found in from 68 to 100 per cent. Another valuable procedure is elicitation of somatosensory evoked responses by stimulation of the tibial or the median nerve. The average percentage of individuals with MS who have delays in these responses and who have had no signs or symptoms of lesions in the spinal cord is 67 per cent. The number of individuals with alterations of the brain stem auditory evoked responses averages 41 per cent, again in patients who have never had any indication of involvement of brain stem structures. Other procedures, such as the Kimura blink reflex and trigeminal evoked responses, are less useful.

When several of these neurophysiologic tests are done on a single patient, the yield is most remarkable: in one series, at least one clinically unsuspected lesion was discovered in nearly half the patients when pattern reversal visual, brain stem auditory, and somatosensory evoked responses were measured in each patient. In another series, when the blink reflex was added, one such unsuspected lesion was found in 63 per cent of patients.

It must be pointed out that abnormalities of evoked responses are not specific for MS, and great care must be applied in interpreting these results. For example, a refractive error of more than 20/200 may produce abnormalities of visual evoked responses, as can retinal disease, Parkinson's disease, and the use of such drugs as the phenothiazines and haloperidol. The great advantage of these tests is that they are completely noninvasive, are harmless, and have a relatively high yield.

Cerebrospinal Fluid Examination. The presence of an elevated number of white blood cells in the cerebrospinal fluid (above 5/cu mm) is highly significant. Although this finding of lymphocytosis of the cerebrospinal fluid has often been interpreted as a sign of activity, it is highly unreliable. Cerebrospinal fluid protein level is rarely if ever elevated in MS, and a cerebrospinal fluid protein content above 100 mg/dl should cast doubt upon the diagnosis.

The demonstration of increased IgG production (usually above 13 to 15 per cent of the total protein) is present in roughly 60 to 65 per cent of patients with MS. This, however, is not specific for MS and may be found in a number of other conditions, including neurosyphilis, subacute sclerosing panencephalitis, several viral infections of the nervous system, and other disturbances of the immune system affecting the nervous system, such as postinfectious and postvaccinal encephalopathies, the Guillain-Barré syndrome, and similar disorders. Agar electrophoresis demonstrates presence of oligoclonal IgG bands (when the test is properly carried out) in more than 90 per cent of patients with MS. This test likewise is not specific; oligoclonal IgG bands may be found, although less frequently, in all the conditions just listed. These two tests, in particular the presence of oligoclonal bands, become exceedingly valuable confirmatory evidence for the diagnosis when coupled with the appropriate clinical findings.

The demonstration in cerebrospinal fluid of myelin basic protein cannot be considered as diagnostic of MS since it is a completely nonspecific index of the destruction of myelin, regardless of cause. It may be useful in some instances as an indicator of activity of the disease.

Immunologic Tests. It has been demonstrated in large groups of MS patients of Germanic origin (in Scandinavia, England, the United States, and Canada) that histocompatibility antigens HLA-A3, HLA-B7, and in particular HLA-Dw2 are present in a statistically highly significant number of individuals compared with control groups. However, careful studies carried out in twin pairs as well as in families with more than one individual with MS have clearly demonstrated that this test has absolutely no value whatsoever in predicting the occurrence of the disease in families or in blood relatives of an individual already affected by the disease. The other immunologic procedure which has reached some degree of totally unwarranted popularity is a demonstration of rosette formation by lymphocytes of MS patients when exposed to epithelial cells that have been infected with measles virus. This is also a nonspecific test that has no diagnostic value whatsoever.

Tissue Imaging. Computed tomography (CT) has introduced a new dimension in the diagnosis of MS. Areas of low density in cerebral white matter, and in particular the classic periventricular areas, can yield results on CT that may be quite helpful in supporting a clinical diagnosis. Ventricular enlargement or cerebral atrophy is too nonspecific to be of any value. The low yield of this procedure can be increased by the use of contrast medium to enhance results, and it is the presence of such enhancement that makes the test valuable. The yield can be quite dramatically increased even further (although the risks of the procedure are commensurately increased as well) by administering a double dose of contrast agent and delaying the procedure for 1 or 1½ hours. This so-called DDD CT scan provides the highest yield: in some series well over half of patients have lesions demonstrated by this technique. At this time, the sensitivity of CT scanning is still not high enough to reliably demonstrate lesions in optic nerve, brain stem, or spinal cord, although claims to that effect have been made.

The newer procedure of nuclear magnetic resonance promises to demonstrate lesions with even greater facility than CT scanning. The few published articles reveal large numbers of lesions demonstrable in areas such as the brain stem and spinal cord.

Differential Diagnosis

Optic or Retrobulbar Neuritis. Optic or retrobulbar neuritis is often considered to be the first manifestation of MS. Although it is true that other causes for this condition are extremely rare, a number of studies have demonstrated that other lesions of the central nervous system simply never develop in such patients even after very long follow-ups. The results vary tremendously, from 13 to 87 per cent, depending on the series and the techniques used for the detection of other lesions. In general, however, it is a reasonably safe assumption to state that anywhere from one fourth to one third of patients with acute optic or retrobulbar neuritis will eventually develop MS.

Acute Transverse Myelitis. Although acute transverse myelitis does indeed occur during the course of MS, it is much less frequent than generally believed. Similarly, whereas it is believed that patients who present with acute transverse myelitis without any previous episodes of neurologic dysfunction will develop MS, several well-documented series reveal that only approximately 6 to 8 per cent of such patients will eventually develop signs and symptoms, or paraclinical evidence, of involvement of other parts of the central nervous system. It should also be pointed out that when the appropriate electrodiagnostic studies are carried out in patients with acute transverse myelitis, in a surprisingly high number of them (between 40 and 60 per cent), evidence of involvement of roots and peripheral nerves can be demonstrated, which essentially rules out MS as a cause for the illness.

Acute Disseminated Encephalomyelitis (ADEM) (Acute Disseminated Vasculomyelinopathy). This is the most troublesome of problems in differential diagnosis from an acute attack of MS. In fact, it is impossible to differentiate between the first attack of MS and an attack of ADEM unless electrodiagnostic studies clearly reveal the presence of root or peripheral nerve involvement. Although in most instances ADEM is a monophasic illness, there are now well-documented cases of recurrences of the disease as well as some with progressive evolution over a period of several weeks, even months. Clinically, as well as by means of laboratory procedures, the conditions are indistinguishable. Eliciting a history of a precipitating event, such as a viral infection or especially a vaccination of any kind, may help in differentiating ADEM from MS. Thus, a patient with coincidental optic neuritis and transverse myelitis, a condition often referred to as *Devic's disease,* can represent ADEM equally as well as MS. Similary, the fact that a patient with acute transverse myelitis can be shown to have a delay of pattern-reversal visual evoked responses is not a guarantee that MS is present since the same situations may obtain in ADEM. In fact, only prolonged observation on followup can provide a clue to the true nature of the illness.

Other Conditions. Any conditions that will produce involvement of separate parts of the nervous system must be differentiated from MS. In particular, these include the collagenoses, such as lupus erythematosus, other vasculitides, and sarcoidosis.

Conclusion

The diagnostic accuracy for MS has been quite markedly enhanced by the increasing availability of evoked response tests, reliable examination of the cerebrospinal fluid for IgG production and the presence of oligoclonal IgG bands, and contrast enhancement of lesions on CT scanning. Nevertheless, since none of these results is truly specific for MS, their significance and usefulness can be evaluated only in terms of the clinical presentation.

Myelinoclastic Diffuse Sclerosis

Definition. This is an extremely rare disorder also known as *Schilder's disease,* 1912 type. It is characterized by the destruction of myelin in large, usually asymmetric areas of the subcortical white matter and must be considered a variant of MS, sharing with it the postulated pathogenesis and cause, both of which are still unknown. For unknown reasons, it occurs much more frequently in children, although in adults it is more likely to take the form of what is known as transitional or disseminated-diffuse sclerosis, characterized by a combination of very large areas of sclerosis typical of subcortical demyelination with scattered plaques of MS. It is probable that many of the cases diagnosed as myelinoclastic diffuse sclerosis in the past, in particular those occurring in boys, are instances of adrenoleukodystrophy.

Course and Clinical Findings. The child invariably demonstrates normal development, usually until late childhood, when the disease starts. The first manifestation usually consists of intellectual deterioration followed by increasing spasticity, blindness, and deafness. Other signs, such as convulsive seizures, papilledema, ophthalmoplegia, nystagmus, hemiparesis, bladder disturbances, and changes in personality, may all occur. In the very rare adult form, psychiatric manifestations are common presenting symptoms. The course is that of subacute or chronic mental and neurologic deterioration, with the usual duration of the disease between 2 and 5 years.

Laboratory Findings. The findings in spinal fluid are identical to those already described in multiple sclerosis, with occasional elevation of cerebrospinal fluid IgG levels and the presence of oligoclonal bands. The electroencephalogram, (EEG) may show a large slow-wave focus corresponding to the area of myelinoclasia. CT scan will reveal the large areas of attenuation of white matter, usually asymmetric and multiple, and most characteristically surrounded by an area of enhancement.

Differential Diagnosis. In some instances, the combination of papilledema and focal neurologic signs may suggest an intracranial tumor, although supratentorial neoplasms are rare in this age group. Adrenoleukodystrophy without clinical signs of adrenocortical insufficiency, metachromatic leukodystrophy, and subacute sclerosing panencephalitis are the main disorders in the differential diagnosis. Presence of normal plasma cortisol levels after ACTH stimulation should help rule out adrenoleukodystrophy; a normal level of cerebrospinal fluid protein along with elevation of IgG level should rule out metachromatic leukodystrophy; while subacute sclerosing panencephalitis should be ruled out on the basis of the EEG and the invariable and very striking elevation of both cerebrospinal fluid IgG and antimeasles antibody titers in serum and cerebrospinal fluid.

Postinfectious and Postvaccinal Encephalomyelitis (Disseminated Vasculomyelinopathy)

Definition. Both of these conditions have been grouped under the generic designation *disseminated vasculomyelinopathy* in order to stress the involvement of the blood vessels as well as the myelin sheath. In fact, involvement of the myelin sheath is not an obligatory component of these reactions, which are primarily, and often exclusively, inflammatory in nature. They are generally classified as autoimmune disorders since they result from what must be considered an abnormal response of the individual's immune system, which is misdirected against its own nervous system.

Any part of the nervous system, from brain to peripheral nerve, may become involved. Since the nature, severity and particular anatomic location of the response are the result of the individual's genetic makeup and immunologic experience, the variability in presentation of this illness is easily appreciated.

Encephalitis, optic neuritis, brain stem encephalitis, cerebellitis, myelitis, brachial plexitis, radiculitis, polyneuritis, or mononeuritis may all occur singly or in various combinations and permutations. In fact, conditions ranging from an isolated fourth cranial nerve paresis to a lumbosacral plexitis, a myeloradiculitis, or an acute cerebellitis have all been reported. The nature of the precipitating viral infection seems to have little to do with the localization of the illness to a particular part of the nervous system, with the possible exception of varicella, which appears to be followed more often than not by an acute cerebellitis.

When vaccines are responsible, vaccination against rubella appears to produce a relatively specific myeloradiculopathy, which expresses itself clinically by either a brachial or a lumbosacral plexitis; vaccination against swine influenza has produced a predominant, but not exclusive, involvement of the peripheral nervous system resulting in the Guillain-Barré syndrome. In general, however, the nature of the vaccine, be it killed or live-attenuated, plays no role in determining the localization of the reaction to any particular part or parts of the nervous system, nor does it affect the type and severity of the pathologic reaction: antirabies vaccination, for example, may cause an acute hemorrhagic leukoencephalopathy, a transverse myelitis, or simply a lymphocytic meningitis.

It should be pointed out that involvement of the central nervous system, whether of the brain or spinal cord, may mask involvement of the peripheral nervous system, which will then be detected only by means of electrodiagnostic studies. Conversely, severe peripheral nervous system involvement may obscure involvement of the spinal cord.

Presenting Signs and Symptoms. Symptoms most often appear within 2 or 3 weeks after a viral infection or an immunization. It may be impossible to distinguish between an acute viral encephalitis and postviral encephalitis, particularly since the two may be coincidental or may follow each other without the classic quiescent interval. In some instances, however, the onset of illness may occur weeks or even months afterward. An acute exacerbation may follow a slowly progressive or even smoldering condition lasting for weeks or months. An acute exacerbation may also occur after a subclinical illness that has lasted for months.

Although these illnesses are as a rule monophasic, progressive over a matter of weeks, development of new symptoms weeks after the onset as well as a relapsing chronic course have also been reported. Presenting signs and symptoms obviously reflect involvement of the particular part or parts of the nervous system. Fever, headache, and stiff neck may be present. In the encephalitic form, convulsions and alterations of consciousness are not uncommon; when the spinal cord is primarily involved, the signs of an acute transverse myelitis may be present.

Physical Examination. Findings on physical examination relate to the particular areas of the nervous system that are involved. Signs of meningeal irritation are common. Weakness ranges from a hemiparesis to paraplegia or tetraplegia or to the flaccid, fairly symmetric weakness of peripheral neuropathy of the Guillain-Barré type. Ataxia and other cerebellar signs, such as dysmetria, intention tremor, and nystagmus, may be prominent. Brain stem involvement manifested by internuclear ophthalmoplegia, other extraocular movement disturbances, and bilateral facial weakness, loss of taste sensation, dysarthria, and dysphagia may all be present. Sensory complaints usually are more severe than objective sensory deficits, although purely sensory neuropathies have been reported as variants of the Guillain-Barré syndrome.

Laboratory Findings. Cerebrospinal fluid leukocytosis is quite common early in the course and there may even be a predominance of polymorphonuclear cells. Elevation of spinal fluid protein to a mild degree is very common. When the elevation becomes exaggerated it tends to indicate involvement of the spinal nerve roots, as in the Guillain-Barré syndrome. Elevated cerebrospinal fluid IgG levels are found in 20 to 25 per cent of cases, as is the presence of oligoclonal IgG bands.

Electrodiagnostic tests, in particular nerve conduction velocities and somatosensory evoked responses, are very important in order to determine if peripheral nerve involvement is present when central nervous system signs and symptoms appear to predominate. Electroencephalography, radionuclide brain scanning, and CT scanning are usually of little help.

Differential Diagnosis. The major problem lies in differentiating the acute and recurrent forms of this illness from MS. The demonstration of peripheral nerve involvement either clinically or by electrodiagnostic procedures is of major importance. Elevation of cerebrospinal fluid protein above 100 mg/dl, which is not uncommon in this illness, is extremely rare in MS. Involvement of certain cranial nerves, in particular the seventh, with lesions of the chorda tympani producing loss of taste, is clear indication of peripheral nerve involvement and is extremely rare in MS.

In some instances, CT scanning may reveal cerebral lesions, even some with ring-like enhancement, which are indistinguishable from the appearance of brain abscess or malignant tumor. Differentiation from acute viral encephalitis, especially herpes simplex encephalitis, may be extremely difficult unless the classic temporal lobe involvement of the latter can be demonstrated by EEG or CT scanning, or by both.

Transverse Myelitis

Definition. The term transverse myelitis (TM) should be restricted to an acute, inflammatory lesion that produces a functionally complete or nearly complete transection of the spinal cord. The inflammation usually involves both the gray and the white matter. As a rule, it is limited longitudinally to one to three segments, although it has sometimes spread progressively upward, in which case it is known as ascending myelitis. The disease follows a variety of infections, usually viral, or all kinds of vaccinations. In many cases, the preceding infection cannot be identified, because it has been either subclinical, not recognized, or forgotten. TM should be considered as simply a limited postinfectious or postvaccinal encephalomyelitis. Postvaccinal TM has been reported with nearly all vaccines used, both live-attenuated or killed, in all age groups. In many instances, electrodiagnostic studies will reveal the presence of coincidental involvement of spinal roots and peripheral nerves, thus indicating that the TM is in fact a myeloradiculoneuropathy.

Acute TM may represent the first episode of MS although the latter diagnosis is made in only 6 to 8 per cent of cases. Similarly, acute TM is quite unusual during the course of established MS.

The combination of TM and optic neuritis has in the past been referred to as neuromyelitis optica or Devic's disease. Such a classification is no longer warranted: involvement of both the spinal cord and the optic nerve may and do frequently occur as postinfectious or postvaccinal complications and, therefore, neuromyelitis optica cannot simply be considered as equivalent to MS. All it means is that both anatomic structures are involved by a similar disease process.

Presenting Signs and Symptoms. A history of an antecedent viral infection may not be obtainable. It may be necessary to inquire about the possibility that such an infection (or a vaccination) may have taken place more than the traditional 4 to 6 weeks previously. Systemic manifestations, such as low-grade fever, malaise, headache, and so forth, may occur, but the neurologic disease may be ushered in without such prodromes. Nuchal rigidity and pain, either in the neck or as a girdle-like sensation in the thoracic region, are frequently present. The initial spinal cord symptoms usually consist of paresthesias involving the feet and legs associated with progressive weakness of the legs. Urinary retention or incontinence is often present early.

Physical Examination. Early (but very rarely) in the course there may be some degree of spinal shock, depending to some extent on the speed with which the disease has developed, with characteristic areflexic flaccid paraparesis or paraplegia. This rapidly changes into spastic involvement of the legs with hyperactive reflexes and Babinski signs. Sensory loss to all modalities of varying degrees is found with the establishment of a sensory level. Bowel and bladder symptoms are common. The bladder, which originally is large and atonic, becomes small and hypertonic.

Course. The course of TM is extremely variable in that after reaching peak in a matter of hours or in 1 to 2 weeks, either complete or almost complete recovery may occur or severe paraplegia may remain.

Laboratory Findings. The acute clinical course is so characteristic that contrast myelography is rarely if ever indicated. In some cases, however, the acute swelling of the spinal cord will produce a myelographic block that may cause an elevation of the cerebrospinal fluid protein level. In the abscence of a myelographic block, marked elevation of the cerebrospinal fluid protein level strongly suggests the coincidental involvement of spinal roots, which may be masked by the myelitic involvement. Electrodiagnostic studies, including electromyography, nerve conduction velocity studies, and somatosensory evoked responses, may be indicated to discover if the peripheral nervous system is also involved, as is often the case. The cerebrospinal fluid white cells, usually lymphocytes, may be elevated (up to 100 per cu mm). In 20 to 25 per cent of cases elevation of cerebrospinal fluid IgG level may be found, and oligoclonal IgG bands may be observed.

Differential Diagnosis. The most commonly and erroneously made diagnosis is that of thrombosis of the anterior spinal artery. This is not only a very rare condition, but in addition it is characterized by sparing of the posterior columns; thus, impairment of vibratory and position sense below the level of the lesion should quickly rule out such vascular causation. In the absence of a history of trauma, it is rare for extrinsic compressive lesions, such as tumors, empyemas, or hematomas, to occur with so rapid a course.

Central Pontine Myelinolysis

Definition. Central pontine myelinolysis (CPM) is an acute, limited demyelinating condition restricted to the base of the pons. It invariably is associated with some other serious, often life-threatening, disease or condition resulting in malnutrition and debilitation.

Presenting Signs and Symptoms. Although the majority of patients have had severe, chronic alcoholism, the disease has also been found in conjunction with chronic renal failure characterized by severe degree of weight loss or prolonged periods of nausea and vomiting; hepatic failure; advanced stages of lymphoma or carcinoma; severe bacterial infection; dehydration; electrolyte disturbances; acute hemorrhagic pancreatitis; and even pellagra. In many patients the lesion, which as a rule does not encroach upon the pontine tegmentum, remains clinically silent. Whenever a patient who is gravely ill with a general medical disease (particularly an alcoholic patient) develops a quadriplegia, pseudobulbar palsy, and pseudo-coma over a period of several days, the clinical diagnosis of CPM should be considered. In addition, confusion, cranial nerve dysfunction, weakness of limbs, reflex changes, and hypotension may be present. Theoretically, since the disease involves only the myelin sheath, it is completely reversible, and this has now been successfully demonstrated by means of CT scanning (see later discussion). Another important characteristic of the disease is that in the vast majority of cases it seems to have resulted from, or followed, rapid correction of a severe hyponatremia from various causes.

Course and Physical Findings. The clinical picture may range from areflexic, flaccid quadriplegia to spastic quadriparesis with dysarthria, dysphagia, and facial weakness. Mutism with paralysis, a form of the "locked-in" syndrome, may occur but represents another interpretation of the paralytic stage of pseudocoma. Pupillary reflexes, movements of the eyes and lids, corneal reflexes, and facial sensations are spared, although conjugate eye movements may become limited. Although in most instances the correct diagnosis was made post mortem, there are now several well-documented cases of complete clinical recovery.

Laboratory Findings. An initial severe hyponatremia that is rapidly corrected provides an important clue for the diagnosis. High-resolution CT scanning has now demonstrated the typical low-density lesion in the central pons with or without slight peripheral enhancement. Some authors have reported delays in brain stem auditory evoked response. Cerebrospinal fluid myelin basic protein may be elevated, a nonspecific finding of destruction of the myelin sheath which nevertheless may prove useful in relation to the patient's medical background and the clinical history and findings. CT scans, however, may be normal and remain so throughout the course of the illness.

Differential Diagnosis. The correct diagnosis should be considered in a debilitated, particularly an alcoholic, severely hyponatremic individual. Disease of the basilar arterial system may mimic the clinical picture, but the onset is usually more rapid and more dramatic and also as a rule involves the tegmentum as well as the base of the pons. Some of the toxic and metabolic disturbances may mimic the confusion, cranial nerve dysfunction, and reflex changes that may be seen in CPM. Postinfectious, postvaccinal, or paraneoplastic inflammatory reactions of the brain stem may also present with similar clinical findings.

Marchiafava-Bignami Disease

Definitions. Marchiafava-Bignami disease (MBD) is a demyelinating disease that affects primarily the medial portion of the corpus callosum but not infrequently may extend into other areas of white matter, including the anterior commissure, the subcortical frontal white matter, and even the brachium pontis.

The lesions are almost invariably symmetric. The condition was for many years believed to occur only in middle-aged or elderly Italian men who drank large quantities of Italian red wine. This is no longer believed to be the case, although alcoholism and malnutrition remain in the background of practically all cases.

Presenting Signs and Symptoms. The clinical diagnosis is extremely difficult to make for several reasons, the most common being that signs and symptoms of chronic alcoholism or alcohol withdrawal may mask symptoms more directly attributable to the disease. Similarly, bilaterally symmetric involvement of frontal lobe white matter may cause the patient to present with frontal lobe syndromes or signs and symptoms suggestive of Alzheimer's disease. Acute impairment of consciousness or nonspecific dementia may be the presenting picture.

Course and Physical Findings. Most of the patients have been middle-aged or elderly, severely alcoholic men. The clinical features are very variable: stupor or coma, convulsive seizures, dysarthria, unsteadiness, aphasic disorders, and other signs have been noted. So far as is known, the disease invariably is progressive and fatal.

Laboratory Findings. No specific abnormalities have been reported, but the CT scan may show a low-density lesion involving the corpus callosum.

Differential Diagnosis. The Wernicke-Korsakoff syndrome and acute ethanol withdrawal are much more likely diagnoses in chronic alcoholics with dementia or alterations of the state of consciousness. Subdural hematoma must always be kept in mind.

THE DYSMYELINATING DISEASES

The leukodystrophies are the prototypes of dysmyelinating diseases. The nomenclature and classification of the leukodystrophies is unnecessarily confusing. Some of the conditions that are usually included in this category are subjects of controversy, not only regarding their existence as separate disease entities, but also in terms of nosology. Because of their extreme rarity, conditions such as fibrinoid leukodystrophy (Alexander's disease), Pelizaeus-Merzbacher's disease, and other so-called sudanophilic or orthochromatic leukodystrophies will not be discussed.

Four entities will be considered here: metachromatic and globoid cell leukodystrophies, spongy sclerosis, and adrenoleukodystrophy. The first two have much in common in terms of pathology: there is widespread if not complete absence of myelin from all parts of the nervous system with the exception of the subcortical U-fibers, which appear to be normally myelinated. Peripheral neuropathy is a prominent component of these two conditions. In each of them a single enzyme defect has been identified, which although it fails to provide a complete explanation for the observed pathologic manifestations, remains an extremely useful diagnostic and genetic marker. In spongy sclerosis, in addition to the widespread dysmyelination, another condition—spongiform degeneration of the subcortical white matter, especially in the area of the U-fibers—is very prominent; this may be a parallel phenomenon, unrelated to the dysmyelination. Spongy sclerosis occurs as a result of a very large number of metabolic disturbances. Finally, adrenoleukodystrophy and its phenotypic variants may be of two types, a myelinoclastic type and a dysmyelinating type. Adrenal insufficiency is a requirement for diagnosis. Adrenoleukodystrophy differs from other leukodystrophies in that inheritance in most instances is x-linked rather than autosomal recessive.

Metachromatic Leukodystrophy

This condition (also known as sulfatide lipidosis) is inherited in an autosomal recessive manner and, in addition to the widespread dysmyelination involving both central and peripheral nervous systems, is characterized, by the accumulation in the brain parenchyma, neurons, and phagocytes of large amounts of cerebroside sulfate (sulfatide). The term metachromatic relates to the fact that this sulfatide produces either a reddish color when stained with a toluidine blue or thionine stain or a brownish color when stained with acetic acid–cresyl violet solution. A deficiency or absence of the enzyme arylsulfatase-A has been identified as the cause for the accumulation of the characteristic sulfatide. In addition to the accumulation of sulfatide in brain and to a much lesser extent in peripheral nerve, sulfatide is also found in the testes, the wall of the gallbladder, the pituitary capsule, and the renal tubules.

Four types of the illness are recognized, based upon the age at onset, each with minor quantitive variation in the enzyme activity: congenital, infantile, juvenile, and adult forms. The infantile type is by far the most common.

Course and Clinical Features. Except in the rare congenital form, the affected child invariably develops completely normally for months or even years. Age of onset is usually between 1 and 4 years, the first symptoms appearing in most cases between the ages of 12 and 18 months. The illness is associated with the reduction or absence of tendon reflexes and with weakness and hypotonia (reflecting the presence of peripheral neuropathy), which is then followed by the superimposition of nystagmus, cerebellar and Babinski signs, dementia, tonic seizures, optic atrophy, and spastic quadriparesis. The disease is invariably fatal.

In the juvenile and adult forms, the features of the disease are much less characteristic. The older the patient, the greater the tendency for mentation and behavioral disorders to dominate the clinical picture, which makes recognition difficult since it frequently presents as a psychiatric illness. The suggestion has been made that a routine search for metachromatic leukodystrophy should be carried out among patients with neuropsychiatric symptoms who show unusual psychoses, presenile dementias, or nonspecific disturbances of motor coordination and who are also found by electrodiagnostic studies to be suffering from peripheral neuropathy. In some of the infantile cases, a grayish discoloration of the macula has been described, although a more classic cherry-red spot has also been reported in several instances.

Laboratory Findings. The cerebrospinal fluid protein level is almost invariably significantly elevated, usually above 100 mg/dl. Radiologically, the CT scan shows a characteristic attenuation, i.e., low-density appearance of the entire cerebral and cerebellar white matter; this is a nonspecific finding noted in all leukodystrophies. Because of involvement of the gallbladder wall, cholecystography may be useful in demonstrating a nonfilling gallbaldder in the child, a highly significant finding.

Electroencephalography is frequently abnormal, but findings are nonspecific. On the other hand, marked reduction in the conduction velocity of peripheral nerves becomes of great importance when combined with the obvious signs of cerebral involvement. Similarly, increased latencies of visual and auditory brain stem evoked responses can be strongly supportive of the diagnosis.

The specific diagnosis, which in the past was based on tissue biopsy (brain, peripheral nerve, kidney), no longer depends on such procedures. Instead, the biochemical identification of the disease is based on the ability of the enzyme arylsulfatase-A to split nitrocatecholsulfate, nitrocatechol giving a red color when dissolved in an alkaline medium. Deficiency of arylsulfatase-A can be demonstrated in blood leukocytes or cultured fibroblasts. There is also a method for measuring arylsulfatase-A by sepharose column chromatography. The same techniques can be used for the detection of heterozygotes and for examination of cells in amniotic fluid for prenatal diagnosis.

Differential Diagnosis. The other leukodystrophies (globoid cell and spongy sclerosis) as a rule occur in the first 6 months of life, as opposed to the later onset of metachromatic leukodystrophy. Adrenoleukodystrophy is usually characterized by a concomitant adrenal insufficiency and occurs in late, rather than early, childhood. Subacute sclerosing panencephalitis is easily differentiated on the basis of the characteristic EEG and the almost invariable presence of very high levels of IgG in cerebrospinal fluid, which is never seen in metachromatic leukodystrophy.

Globoid Cell Leukodystrophy

Globoid cell leukodystrophy is frequently referred to as Krabbe's disease. It is characterized by the accumulation of large epithelioid and globoid cells, both in the parenchyma and in the periadventitial tissues, in addition to the extensive dysmyelination of the central and peripheral nervous systems. The globoid cells have been found to contain galactocerebroside and the deficiency of beta-galactosidase has been identified as the characteristic enzymatic disturbance. In this condition as well, this particular enzyme deficiency does not account for the many abnormal pathologic and biochemical features of the disease, but it remains a useful clincal and genetic marker. Globoid cell leukodystrophy appears to be transmitted as an autosomal recessive trait.

Course and Clinical Findings. The disease affects infants and has its onset in the first few months of life, preceded by quite normal early development and maturation. The clinical evolution of the disease usually consists of three stages, the first being characterized by irritability and sensitivity to light and noise, which bring on violent tonic spasms. Mental and motor development stagnates, and muscle tone becomes increased while reflexes tend to disappear. In the second stage, the children become opisthotonic; myoclonic jerks, hypotonic fits, and other atypical seizures occur. Optic atrophy and blindness also take place while reflexes are being lost. Spasticity results in severe quadriparesis. Death is inevitable after an illness that lasts approximately 2 years.

Laboratory Findings. The cerebrospinal fluid protein level is usually markedly elevated. The CT scan reveals the typical symmetric low-density appearance of the white matter, which is characteristic for all leukodystrophies. EEG is abnormal but nonspecific, whereas nerve conduction times are usually abnormal and reflect the presence of the peripheral neuropathy. The specific diagnosis can be made on the basis of the deficiency of galactocerebrosidase in serum, leukocytes, and skin fibroblasts. Similar techniques are used for the identification of heterozygotes as well as in prenatal diagnosis.

Differential Diagnosis. The major problem is differentiation from spongy sclerosis. In the latter, however, marked enlargement of the head is a striking clinical finding; this does not occur in globoid cell leukodystrophy. Conversely, elevation of spinal fluid protein level does not occur in spongy sclerosis. It is difficult, if not impossible, to differentiate globoid cell leukodystrophy clinically from the infantile form of metachromatic leukodystrophy or from some of the gangliosidoses with onset in early infancy.

Adrenoleukodystrophy

The disease is also known as *melanodermic diffuse sclerosis* or *Addison-Schilder's disease.* A number of conditions that represent simple anatomic variants have now been reported under the names of *adrenomyeloneuropathy* and *adrenoleukomyeloneuropathy.* Other variants of this leukodystrophy, such as myeloneuropathy, peripheral neuropathy, or primary Addison's disease, may occur among blood relatives of a patient with the complete phenotype. Adrenoleukodystrophy is generally believed to be inherited as an X-linked recessive condition, but unquestionable cases have now been reported in women.

The disease may be expressed in two forms: one in which there is a disturbance of myelinogenesis, resulting in true dysmyelination; and another in which there appears to be a disturbance of the myelin maintenance system, resulting in a condition that is closer to the myelinoclastic diseases. A peripheral neuropathy is often present.

It is the association with adrenocortical insufficiency that separates this leukodystrophy from the others. This adrenal insufficiency, however, need not be manifested clinically and in fact may not even be detectable by chemical means.

Biochemically, the condition is characterized by the fact that the fatty acid moiety of cholesterol esters contains a substantially higher proportion of very long chain (C25 or C26) fatty acids.

Course and Clinical Findings. The disease usually starts during the first decade of life, although it has been reported with onset as late as the fifth and sixth decades. The initial manifestations are usually those of behavioral disturbances, followed by changes in gait and loss of vision. In general, the clinical manifestations reflect progressive cerebral degeneration. Convulsive seizures are rare early in the disease, but occur in almost half of the patients at a later date. Spastic quadriparesis with blindness is the usual end result, with death occurring anywhere between 1 and 5 years after onset.

The presence of a positive family history as well as the characteristic clinical signs of Addison's disease (when they are present) clearly point to the diagnosis. Signs and symptoms of hypoadrenalism are present in approximately one third of patients.

Laboratory Findings. The results of adrenocorticotropic hormone (ACTH) stimulation tests will frequently reveal a diminished plasma cortisol response in most patients even in the absence of clinical manifestations of Addison's disease. CT scanning may reveal either the diffuse low-density appearance of the white matter characteristic of leukodystrophy or the more irregular, asymmetric, evenly contrast-enhancing lesions characteristic of myelinoclastic disease. EEG is nonspecifically abnormal, nerve conduction velocities may be elevated, and cerebrospinal fluid protein level is very frequently elevated. Elevation of the cerebrospinal fluid IgG level as well as the presence of oligoclonal IgG bands has also been reported in the myelinoclastic form of the disease. The use of adrenal, brain, or sural nerve biopsy has now been replaced by electron microscopic examination of skin fibroblasts in tissue culture or of skin or conjunctival biopsy specimens, revealing distinctive cytoplasmic inclusions, which are pathognomonic for the disease. There is also a new method for the measurement of the saturated very long chain fatty acids, which can be found in the plasma of such patients. In cultured skin fibroblasts, an increased C26:C22 fatty acid ratio can also be demonstrated.

Differential Diagnosis. The early presentation of behavior abnormalities may lead to an erroneous psychiatric diagnosis. The asymmetric manifestations may also call to mind the possibility of other progressive neurologic conditions. True myelinoclastic diffuse sclerosis must also be considered, although it would appear to be rarer than adrenoleukodystrophy, particularly in boys. Subacute sclerosing panencephalitis must also be considered and, because of the similarities in cerebrospinal fluid findings, may have to depend upon the characteristic EEG findings of subacute sclerosing panencephalitis as well as the demonstration of increasing titers of antimeasles antibodies in serum and cerebrospinal fluid.

Spongy Sclerosis

Spongy sclerosis was originally described under the term infantile idiocy with spongy degeneration of the neuraxis. This is also frequently referred to in the American literature as *Canavan's disease.*

Spongy sclerosis is a classic leukodystrophy in that there is almost complete absence of myelin in the central nervous system, but in addition there is a very noticeable degeneration of the deeper layers of the cortex and the superficial layers of the white matter —i.e., the area of the U-fibers. It differs from the other leukodystrophies in that the condition has been described in a large number of otherwise identified conditions, which include phenylketonuria, maple syrup urine disease, and several other aminoacidopathies; in a unique disturbance of ganglioside synthesis termed hematosidosis; and in a number of idiopathic conditions. It has also been found in a peculiar form of glycogen storage disease, as well as in the condition referred to as ophthalmoplegia plus (ragged red fiber myopathy). It would appear, therefore, to be a manifestation of a number of quite different metabolic disturbances. The spongy degeneration on the one hand, and the dysmyelination on the other, may represent either two causally unrelated phenomena or disparate manifestations of a common metabolic disturbance; clearly, the dysmyelination is *not* the result of the spongy degeneration.

Because this disease is found in patients suffering from such a wide variety of metabolic disturbances, no single enzyme deficiency can be implicated to explain all cases. There may be two types of the idiopathic form of the disease, although the infantile (as opposed to the juvenile) form is by far the more common of an extremely rare disease, fewer than 100 cases having been recorded in the literature. In the majority of the idiopathic infantile cases the patients are of Jewish extraction, a feature that is unique among the leukodystrophies.

Course and Clinical Findings. The disease may occur shortly after birth, but more usually it follows 3 to 6 months of completely normal development. Onset is usually within the first 9 months of life. Death occurs at an average age of 18 months.

Initially, the infant quickly becomes sluggish and hypotonic; head enlargement becomes quite noticeable by the age of 4 months, at which time the arrest of psychomotor development is already obvious. A hyperextension resembling decerebrate and decorticate posturing becomes superimposed on the generalized hypotonia; blindness occurs; choreoathetoid and myoclonic seizures are frequent; eventually generalized spasticity supervenes.

Laboratory Studies. The CT scan can be extremely helpful in actually making the specific diagnosis by revealing both the widespread low-density appearance of the white matter and the spongy degeneration of the gray matter junction. Specific enzymatic or biochemical disturbances are useful in identifying the underlying disease when indicated by associated features in the nonidiopathic cases.

Differential Diagnosis. The disease is impossible to differentiate from Alexander's disease (fibrinoid leukodystrophy), which is also characterized by megalencephaly. Because of the frequent occurrence in Jewish children, GM_2 gangliosidosis (Tay-Sachs disease) must be considered, but this disorder can usually be distinguished from spongy sclerosis by the characteristic macular cherry-red spot.

PERIPHERAL NEUROPATHY

By Elmo F. Masucci, M.D.
Washington, D.C.

DEFINITION

Peripheral neuropathy is a disorder involving peripheral motor, sensory, and autonomic neurons. The clinical picture is usually characterized by muscle weakness with or without atrophy, sensory impairment, and decreased to absent tendon reflexes. Autonomic manifestations may or may not be present. There are two clinical categories: polyneuropathy, in which there is bilateral, symmetric involvement, and mononeuropathy, characterized by isolated lesions of individual peripheral nerves. Multiple mononeuropathy or mononeuritis multiplex refers to involvement of multiple nerves, usually in an asymmetric fashion. Polyneuropathies are frequently associated with agents or disorders that act diffusely on the peripheral nervous system, such as toxins, deficiency states, metabolic disturbances, inflammatory states, infections, and genetically determined abnormalities. The mononeuropathies are the result of processes that produce local damage, including mechanical injury; thermal, electrical, or radiation injury; vascular lesions; infiltrative processes; and tumors.

Most frequently, polyneuropathies are characterized by sensorimotor involvement. Occasionally they may be predominantly motor or predominantly sensory, and in some instances they may be completely motor or sensory. In sensorimotor neuropathies, the weakness is usually maximal distally in the arms and legs; tendon jerks are decreased to absent in the lower limbs before the upper limbs and in the ankles before the knees; and distal sensory changes are of "glove-and-stocking" distribution. The lower extremities (longest peripheral nerves) are usually involved before the upper extremities. In some instances, the earliest manifestations develop in the upper limbs; lead neuropathy usually begins with a bilateral wrist drop. Symptoms of vitamin B_{12} deficiency may begin in the hands, and primary familial amyloid neuropathy frequently begins with symptoms referable to the hands when the carpal tunnel syndrome is present. Occasionally a proximal rather than a distal distribution of motor involvement may be observed. Proximal motor involvement may occur in acute idiopathic polyneuritis, polyneuropathy secondary to infectious mononucleosis, and acute intermittent porphyria. Proximal sensory deficits are much less common and may be seen in acute intermittent porphyria.

Pathologic classifications of peripheral neuropathy are based on the nature of the fiber degeneration, the site of the pathologic change, and the specific histologic abnormality (necrotizing panarteritis with occlusion and focal infarction of nerve in polyarteritis nodosa; lymphocyte and plasma cell infiltration in spinal roots, nerves, and sympathetic ganglia and perivenous myelin destruction in acute idiopathic polyneuritis and infectious mononucleosis; amyloid deposition in connective tissue and vessel walls in amyloid polyneuropathy; and demyelination without inflammatory reaction in diphtheritic polyneuropathy). The three major types of fiber degeneration are *wallerian degeneration, segmental demyelination,* and *axonal degeneration.* In segmental demyelination (acute idiopathic polyneuritis, porphyria, compression, and ischemia) there is focal degeneration of the myelin sheath with sparing of the axon. Degeneration of both axon and myelin sheath may occur either distal to axonal interruption, as in wallerian degeneration (trauma or disease), or as a "dying-back" process (axonal degeneration), characteristic of the more generalized, metabolically determined polyneuropathies (alcoholic and uremic polyneuropathies).

It is not possible to differentiate the many disorders that affect the peripheral nerves on the basis of these three pathologic processes, but knowledge of the effects of certain diseases on the various types and sizes of nerve fibers combined with the topography of the lesion and course of the illness is frequently helpful in differential diagnosis.

PRESENTING SIGNS AND SYMPTOMS

Motor Involvement

Temporary weakness or paralysis may be caused by toxins, cooling, or anesthetics, but persistent impairment of motor function indicates the occurrence of segmental demyelination, axonal interruption, or motor neuron destruction. Most commonly the feet and legs are affected first and most severely involved, and later the hands and forearms become involved. Frequently only the lower extremities are affected. Most of the nutritional, metabolic and toxic neuropathies follow this pattern. Trunk and neck muscles may be involved, often leading to respiratory impairment, as in acute idiopathic polyneuritis. Muscle atrophy progresses slowly over several months, as the result of disuse in the demyelinative neuropathies and disuse and denervation in neuropathies characterized by axonal degeneration and motor neuron destruction. In contradistinction to the acute demyelinative neuropathies, in which atrophy does not parallel the disease process, the chronic neuropathies are characterized by parallel development of paralysis and atrophy. Loss of denervated muscle fibers begins in 6 to 12 months. Motor function and muscle volume may be completely restored if reinnervation takes place within a period of 1 year.

Tendon Areflexia

Decreased or absent tendon reflexes are the characteristic findings in most polyneuropathies. Reflexes may be diminished out of proportion to weakness. In small fiber neuropathies, the tendon reflexes in some instances may be retained despite the loss of pain and temperature sensation and autonomic function. In some neuropathies, such as that due to amyloidosis, loss of tendon reflexes is common but may not occur until the late stage, leading to an erroneous diagnosis because of the presence of a distal sensory loss unaccompanied by reflex involvement. Superficial abdominal and cremasteric reflexes are frequently absent or diminished in acute idiopathic polyneuritis. Tendon reflexes are lost first distally, and later, in more advanced cases, generally. Decreased or absent deep tendon reflexes may be observed in various forms of myopathy, in certain stages in the course of multiple sclerosis, in a large percentage of patients with subacute combined degeneration of the spinal cord secondary to pernicious anemia, in Friedreich's ataxia, and in lesions of the cauda equina.

Sensory Loss

In the polyneuropathies sensation is usually deficient in the distal portions of the limbs, the feet and legs being more severely involved than the hands and forearms. Most commonly, all sensory modalities are affected; however, dissociated sensory impairment may occur. One sensory modality may be disturbed more than another, or superficial sensation may be affected more than deep sensation. In diabetes mellitus, vibratory sense may be more involved than position and touch senses. In hereditary sensory neuropathy, certain primary familial amyloid neuropathies, and Tangier disease, pain and temperature sensation may be affected with sparing or lesser involvement of touch, pressure, vibratory, and position sensation. Friedreich's ataxia is characterized by loss of joint position and vibration sensation and impaired touch-pressure sensation, with preservation of pain and temperature sense.

Paresthesias, Dysesthesia, Hyperpathia, and Pain

Paresthesias, in the form of tingling, electric, pins-and-needles sensations, are a frequent accompaniment of a sensory or a sensorimotor neuropathy, and are usually marked in the hands and feet. In some neuropathies, pain is the predominant complaint. The pains may be aching, sharp-cutting, or crushing. Perversion of sensation (dysesthesia) in the form of tingling or burning pain precipitated by a tactile stimulus is also common. Such a stimulus frequently results in a sensation that radiates unnaturally and persists for a period of time after the stimulus is withdrawn (hyperpathia). Paresthesias and dysesthesias are common in one type of alcoholic beriberi with its characteristic "burning feet," Fabry's disease, herpes zoster, some cases of diabetes, and some types of vascular neuropathy. An intense form of pain typifies the causalgia seen in partial lesions of the ulnar, median, posterior tibial, or peroneal nerve. A painful single-root syndrome may develop in diabetic polyneuropathy and may simulate herniated intervertebral disc pain or a tumor affecting a nerve root. Myelography may be necessary for the differential diagnosis.

Sensory Ataxia and Tremor

Sensory ataxia in the limbs may result from impairment of proprioceptive sensation. When the upper limbs are affected, this may be reflected in the occurrence of pseudoathetoid movements of the fingers when the hands are held outstretched and the eyes are closed. Tremor of the outstretched hands and limb ataxia may be observed in neuropathies such as acute idiopathic polyneuritis, hereditary hypertrophic neuropathy, and chronic relapsing demyelinating neuropathy in the absence of detectable loss of postural or movement sensation. The explanation for this is uncertain.

Deformity and Trophic Changes

Chronic neuropathies that occur before cessation of the growth period may give rise to foot, hand, and spinal deformity. Foot and spinal deformities are not uncommon in hypertrophic neuropathy. Clawhand and clawing of the toes may occur in a neuropathy that begins at any age, but the presence of pes cavus or a spinal deformity, usually kyphoscoliosis, indicates an onset in childhood.

The main trophic disturbance resulting from interruption of motor nerves is denervation atrophy of muscle. Sensory impairment in the form of analgesia may result in increased susceptibility of distal parts to pressure sores, burns, or other forms of injury as well as infection. The skin of the anesthetic limb becomes tight and shiny, nails become curved and ridged, and subcutaneous tissues become thickened. Subcutaneous infections may result in loss of digits, and in sensory neuropathies fingers and toes may be lost even when pain is not present. Ischemia and gangrene may occur in diabetic polyneuropathy, whereas Charcot arthropathy may be observed in familial neuropathies in which analgesic joints are subjected to trauma.

Autonomic Involvement

Anhidrosis and orthostatic hypotension are the two most common manifestations of a disorder of autonomic nerves and may be the presenting or major features of some polyneuropathies. They are most commonly seen in the hereditary polyneuropathies, particularly the amyloid variety, diabetic polyneuropathy, some congenital types, purely autonomic neuropathies, and the Shy-Drager syndrome.

Nerve Thickening

Palpable or visible enlargement of nerves may be observed in a number of polyneuropathies and may be helpful in the diagnosis of a particular variety of neuropathy. Nerve thickening may be a conspicuous feature of leprous neuropathy in lepromatous leprosy and is most easily detectable in the great auricular nerve in the neck, the supraclavicular nerves over the clavicles, the ulnar nerve at the elbow, the common peroneal nerve at the neck of the fibula, and the superficial peroneal nerve at the ankles or on the dorsa of the feet.

Nerve thickening may also be an important manifestation of hypertrophic neuropathies, both the inherited and the acquired forms. It is more conspicuous in the recessively inherited Dejerine-Sottas variety than in the dominantly inherited hypertrophic form of peroneal muscular atrophy. Nerve enlargement may also be observed in idiopathic polyneuritis, chronic relapsing polyneuropathy, amyloid neuropathy, acromegaly, and neurofibromatosis.

MONONEUROPATHIES

Unlike the generalized polyradiculoneuropathies that produce diffuse involvement of the peripheral nervous system, the mononeuropathies and multiple mononeuropathies represent focal or multifocal manifestations of disease. They produce motor weakness and sensory deficits in the distribution of the affected nerves. It is important in the initial evaluation of the patient to determine whether a mononeuropathy which is usually due to local causes or a more generalized polyneuropathy is present, since the diagnostic work-up is dictated by the clinical impression. On the other hand, mononeuritis multiplex and generalized polyneuropathies frequently have similar causes.

Mononeuropathies usually result from damage to peripheral nerve trunks, plexuses, and spinal nerves by various forms of trauma, contusion, laceration and traction, or compression (entrapment and compression neuropathies). Dysfunction may also result from electrical, radiation, vascular, metabolic, granulomatous, or neoplastic processes.

The common brachial and crural mononeuropathies would include those involving the brachial plexus; long thoracic, suprascapular, and axillary nerves and the nerves supplying the forearm and hand muscles; the lateral femoral cutaneous nerve (meralgia paresthetica); femoral and sciatic nerves, lumbosacral plexus; and the nerves supplying leg and foot muscles.

Entrapment and Compression Neuropathies

Carpal Tunnel Syndrome

Compression of the median nerve in the carpal tunnel results in manifestations of numbness and pain in the thumb, palm, and the first three fingers. Extreme flexion may reproduce the painful numbness. Opponens pollicis muscle weakness may be present, but thenar muscle atrophy is a late sign. The sensory symptoms may be accompanied by a sensory deficit involving the palmar surface of the thumb and first finger. Tinel's sign is usually present.

The differential diagnosis should include any lesion producing irritation of the fifth to the eighth cervical nerve roots, such as protruded cervical discs, cervical spondylosis and cervical nerve root injury, brachial plexus involvement, and brachial neuritis. The presence of Tinel's sign, a positive wrist flexion test, and objective sensory findings limited to the median nerve distribution distal to the wrist favors the diagnosis of the carpal tunnel syndrome.

Tardy Ulnar Nerve Palsy

Compression in the ulnar groove may produce weakness of the opponens and abductor muscles of the little finger, the interossei, and the last two lumbricals. The sensory deficit involves the little finger and the ulnar half of the ring finger.

Acute Radial Nerve Palsy

This type of palsy most commonly occurs in alcoholics (whose nerves are already damaged) who fall asleep with the arm against a hard surface, creating pressure ischemia of the radial nerve. The muscle paralysis includes the brachioradialis (weakness of elbow flexion), the supinator, wrist and finger extensors, and thumb extensors.

Tarsal Tunnel Syndrome

Compression of the posterior tibial nerve results in symptoms of intermittent burning pain, tingling, and numbness in the foot, particularly the toes and distal sole of the foot if the medial or lateral plantar branches are involved. Sensory deficits occur within the distribution of the branch or branches involved. Weakness of toe flexion and atrophy of the abductor hallucis muscle may be present.

Nerve Conduction Studies in Mononeuropathies

Diagnosis of the entrapment and compression neuropathies can be established by determining the location of the block through nerve conduction velocity measurements.

MONONEUROPATHY MULTIPLEX

This disorder is characterized by involvement of two or more nerve trunks, usually in an asymmetric fashion. The dysfunction develops in several individual nerve trunks at different times. Occasionally there is diffuse and marked involvement of all the nerves of a particular body part (lower extremity) with very minimal involvement (reflexes only) of the opposite extremity. Diabetes is the most common cause of this syndrome and can produce either a femoral neuropathy with anterior thigh pain followed in several days by involvement of most muscles innervated by this nerve, or a multinerve asymmetric neuropathy involving several extremities.

There are many additional causes of this syndrome, including polyarteritis nodosa and other connective tissue diseases, certain blood dyscrasias, sickle cell anemia, acute idiopathic polyneuritis, amyloidosis, macroglobulinemia, the hypertrophic neuropathy of Dejerine-Sottas, rheumatoid arthritis, sarcoidosis, carcinomatous neuropathy, leprosy, vitamin deficiencies, porphyrinuria, alcohol, and the intoxication with the heavy metals lead and arsenic.

Diabetes mellitus and the collagen-vascular diseases can result in either a mononeuropathy or mononeuropathy multiplex. The mononeuropathy multiplex form of polyarteritis nodosa occurs more commonly than the more generalized polyneuropathy. Acute brachial neuritis (neuralgic amyotrophy, Parsonage-Turner syndrome) is neuropathy that may involve the lower cervical roots (particularly the fifth and sixth) and the trunks of peripheral nerves in the form of a mononeuropathy (long thoracic, suprascapular, or circumflex nerve) or a multiple mononeuropathy. The syndrome is characterized usually by the sudden onset of shoulder or upper arm pain on one or both sides, followed sequentially by weakness in 1 to 4 days and then muscle atrophy. The weakness is usually more widespread than that produced by a single cervical root compression, so that myelography to rule out a cervical disc herniation is seldom necessary.

Frequently, despite a complete diagnostic work-up, the cause of mononeuritis multiplex cannot be determined.

Clinical Clues to the Possible Cause of a Peripheral Neuropathy

Abnormalities observed in the skin or mucosae may serve as clinical clues to a possible toxic cause for the peripheral neuropathy. Acute alopecia is highly suggestive of thallium poisoning. Gingival margin pigmentation is seen in chronic lead poisoning. Skin pigmentation may occur in a number of chronic heavy metal intoxications. Transverse white lines in the nails (Mee's lines) occur in arsenic or thallium poisoning. Skin or mucosal changes may be observed in inherited diseases, including ichthyosis in Refsum's disease, angiokeratomata in Fabry's disease, and curly hair in giant axonal neuropathy. Addisonian pigmentation should suggest adrenomyeloneuropathy. Depigmented, anesthetic patches are characteristic of leprosy. Retinitis pigmentosa may be observed in inherited neuropathies, such as the Bassen-Kornzweig syndrome and Refsum's disease. Nerve thickening may be a major manifestation of hypertrophic, chronic relapsing, and amyloid neuropathies.

Major clinical signs may be of considerable value in the differential diagnosis of neuropathies. Cranial nerve abnormalities are uncommon in alcoholic, arsenical, and most toxic neuropathies, except in advanced cases. The presence of a polyneuropathy with cranial nerve involvement should suggest entities in which cranial nerve abnormalities are common, such as diabetes, sarcoidosis, porphyria, periarteritis nodosa, acute idiopathic polyneuritis (including the Fisher variant), meningeal carcinomatosis, and neuropathies secondary to stilbamidine and furaltadone. Motor neuropathies are characteristic of vasculitis, diabetes, intoxications such as with lead and nitrofurantoin, and acute idiopathic polyneuritis. Autonomic disturbances accompanying a neuropathy should suggest diabetes, porphyria, acute idiopathic polyneuropathy, amyloidosis, alcoholic neuropathy, or the Riley-Day syndrome. The thickened peripheral nerves seen in the hypertrophic neuropathies should call to mind Refsum's disease, Dejerine-Sottas polyneuropathy, amyloidosis, Charcot-Marie-Tooth disease, leprosy, and the entrapment neuropathies.

POLYNEUROPATHIES

Idiopathic Polyneuritis (Acute Inflammatory Demyelinating Polyradiculoneuropathy)

Idiopathic polyneuritis is an acute or subacute, usually progressive, sensorimotor neuropathy initially manifested by muscle weakness or pain or by combinations of motor and sensory disturbances, with variable modes of spread: ascending, descending, or spread only within the confines of extremities initially involved. Bilateral proximal and distal muscle involvement usually is present, and there is an affinity for involvement of particular muscle groups. Tendon reflexes are invariably absent or diminished, and cranial nerves may or may not be involved. Predominantly motor, sensory, cranial, and autonomic varieties may occur. Cerebrospinal fluid protein values are usually elevated, and fewer than 10 mononuclear white cells per cubic millimeter are present. Occasionally there may be a modest increase in number of mononuclear cells or a normal protein level. Complete functional recovery occurs in most but not all patients. Improvement usually occurs within weeks but may extend over months or even years. Severe respiratory, pulmonary, and other complications leading even to death occur in an appreciable number of patients. Studies of motor nerve conduction velocity performed near the peak of the illness will show reduced conduction times in most patients. When peripheral conduction times are normal, slow F-wave conduction velocities are of value in indicating nerve fiber demyelination in proximal roots or the brachial plexus. Segmental demyelination combined with lymphocytic inflammatory infiltrates on sural nerve biopsy is diagnostic but is seldom necessary.

Differential Diagnosis in Idiopathic Polyneuritis

In the differential diagnosis, such entities as acute polymyositis, acute intermittent porphyria, infectious mononucleosis, tick paralysis, botulism, paralytic stage of acute poliomyelitis, periodic paralysis, and diphtheritic polyneuropathy should be considered.

In *acute polymyositis,* reflexes are usually preserved, and the cerebrospinal fluid protein levels are not elevated. Electromyography, nerve conduction studies, creatine kinase levels, and muscle biopsy should enable the clinician to distinguish between polymyositis and idiopathic polyneuritis.

Sensory disturbance, ascending spread of the weakness of paralysis, and elevated cerebrospinal fluid protein levels are uncommon in *acute intermittent porphyria* with peripheral neuropathy. Abdominal complaints, convulsive seizures, and mental manifestations are frequent. The peripheral neuropathy may be symmetric or may take the form of a mononeuropathy multiplex, progressing slowly over a period of weeks or months. The urine and stool are usually positive for porphobilinogen, and the uroporphyrinogen-l-synthetase (erythrocyte) level is decreased about 50 per cent. (See article on the porphyrias.)

The polyneuritis that accompanies *infectious mononucleosis* is clinically quite similar to idiopathic polyneuritis. In most patients, the prodromal systemic manifestations permit the diagnosis to be made. The prodrome is usually followed or associated with the onset of the polyneuritis. However, neurologic symptoms may be the only manifestation of the disease. The presence of meningeal signs or encephalitis should suggest the possibility of infectious mononucleosis. A positive heterophil antigen reaction is diagnostic. (See article on infectious mononucleosis.)

Tick paralysis is characterized by weakness of the lower extremities, which can be followed by flaccid paralysis of the extremities, trunk, and bulbar muscles within 24 to 48 hours. Death may occur. Tendon reflexes are absent and sensation is preserved. Flaccid paralysis in an individual living close to a tick-infested area should suggest the diagnosis.

Botulism resembles the descending form of idiopathic polyneuritis. Difficulty in converging the eyes followed by ptosis and extraocular muscle paralysis are early manifestations. Weakness of the jaw and difficulty in swallowing are soon followed by weakness of the extremities. Involvement of several members of a family or group with or without preceding gastrointestinal complaints should suggest the possibility of botulism (see article on this topic).

The paralytic stage of *acute poliomyelitis* is usually characterized by asymmetric or spotty weakness of one or more limbs. Symmetric four-limb paresis or paralysis is not common but does occur. In contrast to idiopathic polyneuritis, the cerebrospinal fluid cell count is almost always increased, with the highest counts in the preparalytic stage. Cell counts less than 10/cu mm are occasionally seen. In poliomyelitis the cells decrease rapidly in numbers while the protein level rises so that the spinal fluid in the second week will mimic that of acute idiopathic polyneuritis (see article on poliomyelitis).

The clinical course of *diphtheritic polyneuritis* might resemble the descending variety of idiopathic polyneuritis in that palatal weakness and blurring of vision are usually the first symptoms. Within a few days or weeks, other cranial nerve and peripheral nerve involvement occurs, manifested by paralysis of pharyngeal, facial, external ocular, and extremity muscles. Palatal and ciliary muscle weakness with blurring of vision due to paralysis of accommodation is rarely seen in idiopathic polyneuritis and represents a clue to the possible presence of diphtheria (see article on diphtheria).

Periodic paralysis might be mistaken for acute idiopathic polyneuritis. The differential diagnosis usually depends on a history of similar attacks, the short duration of the attack (a few hours to 24 to 48 hours), the frequent association of attacks with a meal high in carbohydrates the evening before the attack, the absence of signs and freedom from symptoms between attacks, and the high or low serum potassium level usually associated with most attacks (see article on the periodic paralyses).

Diabetic Polyneuropathy

Diabetic neuropathy can be manifested in a variety of forms or clinical syndromes, including distal symmetric, primarily sensory polyneuropathy; symmetric proximal motor neuropathy; autonomic neuropathy; painful, asymmetric mononeuropathy multiplex; diabetic ophthalmoplegia; and acute mononeuropathy. Combinations of these forms frequently coexist, and overlapping of the various forms is common.

Numbness, tingling, and mild pain involving the feet and legs together with diminished Achilles tendon reflexes are the characteristic manifestations of the *distal symmetric, primarily sensory neuropathy.* Mild muscle weakness, deep ulcerations, and neuropathic joints are present occasionally.

Symmetric proximal motor neuropathy occurs most commonly in elderly diabetic individuals. The findings usually consist of bilateral proximal and pelvic girdle weakness, wasting, absent patellar reflexes, pain, and weight loss. Autonomic signs are frequently present. Overlapping signs between this variety and the asymmetric mononeuropathy multiplex form suggest a range of manifestations and a common basis for both varieties.

Sexual impotence, atonic bladder, nocturnal diarrhea, and impaired sweating and vascular reflexes are the usual manifestations of the *autonomic variety of neuropathy.* Postural hypotension may be seen in some cases.

Painful, asymmetric mononeuropathy multiplex is the variety that frequently goes unrecognized or is misdiagnosed. It occurs in elderly individuals with mild or latent diabetes. In some cases, even the glucose tolerance test remains negative for 1 year or more after onset of symptoms. The syndrome is characterized by deep burning or tearing pain, worse at night, involving the lower back, hip, thigh or knee, and pelvic girdle; weakness; and atrophy with occasional distal muscle weakness. Sensory impairment is mild to moderate and may be manifested by either a multiple nerve or a root distribution. The patellar reflex is usually absent on the affected side. Vesical and anal sphincters may be affected.

The occurrence of ocular palsies in diabetes (such as *diabetic ophthalmoplegia*) is not uncommon. Most frequent are isolated third or sixth nerve lesions. Bilateral sixth, bilateral third, and combinations of unilateral and bilateral third, fourth, and sixth nerve involvement also occur. Cases have been described in which as many as six or seven cranial nerves have been affected. Third nerve involvement with sparing of the pupil, with or without frontal or orbital pain, is suggestive of a diabetic etiology. Ophthalmoplegias, including recurrent ocular palsies, are not uncommonly the only presenting signs in patients with unrecognized diabetes.

The *acute mononeuropathy* form most commonly involves the femoral nerve. Acute onset of pain in the thigh and medial side of the leg is associated with weakness of the quadriceps and iliopsoas muscles. The patellar reflex may be absent.

The ataxic or pseudotabetic form of neuropathy consists of lancinating pain, sensory ataxia, mild weakness, and bowel and bladder signs simulating tabes dorsalis.

Low nerve conduction velocity with no clinical evidence of neuropathy is characteristic of the asymptomatic variety of neuropathy.

The cerebrospinal fluid protein level may be elevated (50 to 200 mg/dl) in all varieties of diabetic neuropathy. Increased protein levels may be present also in diabetic individuals with no clinical evidence of neuropathy.

Third-nerve palsies with uninvolved pupils, recurrent cranial nerve palsies, painful femoral nerve mononeuropathy simulating a ruptured lumbar intervertebral disc syndrome, or a painful lower extremity mononeuropathy multiplex should alert the clinician to a possible diabetic etiology.

Alcoholic Polyneuropathy

The typical alcoholic neuropathy is insidious in onset, is chronic in nature, and involves distal lower extremities with weakness, wasting, and a mild sensory deficit including all sensory modalities. There may be tenderness, pain, and paresthesias involving the calves. Achilles tendon reflexes are usually absent and patellar reflexes may be affected. Distal vasomotor and sudomotor manifestations are usually present.

In some cases of alcoholic neuropathy, an acute onset and rapid progression of weakness may occur. Pain, calf tenderness, and paresthesias are prominent in this variety.

Cranial nerves are not involved except in severe neuropathies, when manifestations of vagus nerve involvement may occur.

Spinal fluid studies are normal in most cases.

Vascular Neuropathies

Neuropathy is not an uncommon complication of such vasculitides as polyarteritis nodosa, rheumatoid arthritis, and Wegener's and other granulomatoses, but it does not occur as frequently in Sjögren's syndrome and cranial arteritis. Manifestations may be expressed in the form of a mononeuropathy, but a characteristic multiple mononeuropathy due to a necrotizing angiopathy is more common. Signs and symptoms usually develop within the distribution of the peroneal or ulnar nerve. Other limb nerves may subsequently be affected. Diffuse, symmetric polyneuropathy may also occur.

Polyarteritis Nodosa

A mononeuropathy multiplex is characteristic of polyarteritis nodosa, but an acute, diffuse, symmetric polyneuropathy may occur. Spinal and cranial nerves may be involved. Motor point muscle biopsy, including nerve, is useful in confirming the clinical impression.

Genetic Neuropathies

The genetic neuropathies are a group of slowly progressive disorders characterized by their distinctive inheritance type and natural history, by the population of neurons involved, and by the type of pathologic lesion present. Predominant involvement of sensory neurons is referred to as inherited sensory neuropathy, of which there are four types: sensory neuropathy with foot ulcers and dissociated sensory loss (Type 1); acrodystrophic neuropathy (Type 2); dysautonomia or Riley-Day syndrome (Type 3); and recessively inherited insensitivity to pain (Type 4). Fabry's disease also involves peripheral sensory neurons.

Those disorders characterized by motor and sensory involvement are called hereditary motor and sensory neuropathies. There are eight such types. Most important are dominantly inherited hypertrophic neuropathy of peroneal muscular atrophy (Type 1); neuronal type of peroneal muscular atrophy, or Charcot-Marie-Tooth disease (Type 2); recessively inherited hypertrophic neuropathy, or Dejerine-Sottas disease, with ceramide hexoses and sulfate abnormality (Type 3); and recessively inherited hypertrophic neuropathy with excess of phytanic acid or Refsum's disease (Type 4). Several other genetically determined neuropathies with associated metabolic disturbances are recognized in addition to Refsum's disease, and recessively inherited hypertrophic neuropathy (Type 3). These include abetalipoproteinemia, metachromatic leukodystrophy, Tangier disease, and familial amyloidosis.

The diagnosis of the inherited neuropathies usually is based upon a positive family history, the detection of formes frustes among the relatives of a patient with a negative family history, physical clues such as bony abnormalities in the form of high arches, hammer toes, and curvature or kyphosis of the spine, "stork legs," and thickened peripheral nerves. Additional manifestations of diagnostic value include retinitis pigmentosa, ichthyosis, acanthocytosis of red blood cells, severe anesthesia to pain and temperature over the scalp, face, and limbs with sparing of distal parts, and progressive cerebral deterioration accompanying a neuropathy. Laboratory studies are important in the neuropathies caused by metabolic abnormalities. When necessary, nerve conduction determinations, needle electromyographic studies, and analysis of biopsied nerve tissue can be of considerable value in the diagnosis and classification of the inherited neuropathies.

Toxic Neuropathies

A large number of industrial agents and an increasing number of drugs have been associated with manifestations of peripheral neuropathy. Hundreds of new chemicals are being introduced each year into American industry, including many volatile solvents. New toxic euphoriant drugs and chemicals have been synthesized during the last two decades. The development of chemotherapeutic agents and other drugs has added to the increasing number of neuropathic toxins.

Diagnosis of intoxication from a specific drug or industrial agent is usually difficult because different agents frequently produce similar clinical manifestations. A high index of suspicion and a detailed occupational, hobby, and drug history are essential in the diagnosis of the toxic neuropathies. The search for a toxic cause relies more often on epidemiologic evidence than on laboratory investigation, since most organic compounds and drugs are inaccessible to chemical laboratory detection. However, as indicated in Tables 1 and 2, a number of industrial toxins, such as acrylamide, *n*-hexane, and dimethylaminopropionitrile produce highly distinctive symptoms and signs, which can serve as valuable clues to the diagnosis. The encephalopathy with delirium and visual loss seen in the methylmercury toxic neuropathy can be helpful in suggesting the diagnosis. A number of other drugs listed in Table 2 produce distinctive signs, such as optic neuritis (ethambutol); pure sensory neuropathy with an affinity for trigeminal nerves (stilbamidine); cranial neuropathy, particularly involving the trigeminal nerve (trichlorethylene); ascending paralysis and occasionally a pure motor neuropathy (nitrofurantoin); and ascending numbness, sensory neuropathy, visual signs, and myelopathy (clioquinol). These can be useful to the clinician in making a diagnosis. A markedly symmetric distal sensorimotor neuropathy of acute or subacute onset with predominantly sensory symptoms and signs is highly characteristic of most neuropathies caused by industrial and household toxins.

Clinical and laboratory differential diagnosis may be assisted by morphologic studies on specimens from sural nerve and muscle biopsy in addition to electrodiagnostic techniques. Electron microscopy can be of assistance in confirming axonal neuropathy or myelin degeneration. Electrodiagnostic studies can help to classify biologic types according to whether the toxic agents are acting on the neuronal perikarya, the distal axon, or the myelin (segmental demyelination). Classification of toxic neuropathies in relationship to the type of occupational exposure (occupation, life situation, medical problem) together with the biologic classifications may be of value in the diagnosis of unknown toxins.

AUTONOMIC NEUROPATHY

Autonomic symptoms and signs may occur as part of the more common acute and chronic polyneuropathies, such as acute idiopathic polyneuritis and diabetic, amyloid, and porphyric neuropathies. In amyloid neuropathy involvement of sympathetic neurons occurs so that pupillary paralysis and other glandular and smooth muscle functions are disturbed. Similar symptoms and signs are seen in Jewish children with the Riley-Day syndrome (familial dysautonomia), an autonomic and sensory polyneuropathy. Subacute combined degeneration, Tangier disease, paraneoplastic dysautonomia, and uremic and alcoholic neuropathies are additional causes of autonomic abnormality. Signs of autonomic dysfunction may consist of orthostatic hypotension, panhidrosis, pupillary paralysis, lacrimation and salivation deficits, impotence, impaired bladder and bowel function, reduced gastric acidity, and loss of pilomotor and vasomotor skin responses.

Table 1. Drugs Causing Distinctive Signs of Neuropathy

Drug	Signs
Vinca alkaloids	Early reflex loss with sensory neuropathy and painful paresthesias (feet)
Disulfiram	Peripheral sensory neuropathy
Chloramphenicol	Sensory neuropathy, optic neuritis
Isoniazid	Sensorimotor neuropathy, paresthesias (toes and feet)
Nitrofurantoin	Sensorimotor neuropathy, purely motor neuropathy, ascending paralysis, paresthesias
Gold	Asymmetric weakness, cranial nerves involved, sensory deficit
Sodium cyanate	Painful polyneuropathy
Ethambutol	Optic neuritis, peripheral neuropathy
Clioquinol	Visual loss, ascending numbness, myelopathy, predominantly sensory neuropathy
Stilbamidine	Purely sensory neuropathy, affinity for trigeminal nerves
Trichlorethylene	Cranial neuropathy: trigeminal, facial, and optic nerves

Table 2. Industrial and Household Toxins Causing Distinctive Signs of Neuropathy

Acrylamide	Prominent sweating and desquamation of palms, with severe ataxia
Dimethylaminoproprionitrile	Onset with bladder symptoms, impaired emptying, chronic distention, loss of bladder sensation; impotence; sensorimotor neuropathy with particular affinity for sacral segments
Hexacarbons (*n*-hexane)	Continued progression of symptoms and signs of peripheral neuropathy for 3 months following cessation of exposure
Organophosphates (triorthocresyl phosphate)	Sensorimotor neuropathy, calf pain and paresthesias, central nervous system dysfunction
Methylmercury	Delirious encephalopathy, loss of vision, peripheral neuropathy
Lead	Abdominal colic, anemia, wrist drop, increased urine and blood lead levels, increased urinary coproporphyrins and delta aminolevulinic acid
Arsenic	Hyperalgesic distal sensorimotor lower extremity neuropathy; gastrointestinal symptoms; elevated arsenic levels in blood, urine, nail clippings, and hair
Thallium	Sensory neuropathy, ataxia, retrobulbar neuritis, alopecia
Mercury	Peripheral neuropathy, fasciculations, atrophy, tremor

The neurologic history should include questions concerning postural dizziness, diarrhea, urinary or bowel incontinence, sweating, cold extremities, difficulty in focusing the eyes, dryness of the mouth and eyes, and impotence. Pulse and blood pressure should be determined to look for evidence of orthostatic hypotension.

Laboratory studies should include tests necessary to detect the most common causes of autonomic neuropathy.

If additional detailed evaluation is necessary, the combination of the intradermal histamine, acetylcholine, or methacholine tests with the cold pressor, thermal sweat, and denervation hypersensitivity tests may be of value in determining whether the autonomic abnormality is one involving postganglionic or preganglionic neurons.

CHRONIC INFLAMMATORY DEMYELINATING POLYRADICULONEUROPATHY

This chronic disorder consists of a sensorimotor polyradiculoneuropathy that has no association with carcinoma, multiple myeloma, diabetes or other systemic diseases and which is accompanied by normal erythrocyte sedimentation rate. It may follow a recurrent course, show a continuous or stepwise worsening over months or years, or have a prolonged monophasic course with worsening over months and years. The cerebrospinal fluid shows increased protein with little or no increase in mononuclear cells. Sural nerve biopsy reveals varying degrees of edema, mononuclear cells, and segmental demyelination, with or without onion-bulb formation. Nerve conduction velocities are diffusely low. The condition is associated with prolonged morbidity.

LABORATORY PROCEDURES

Laboratory procedures and biochemical determinations helpful in evaluating patients with peripheral neuropathies are listed in Table 3.

Lumbar Puncture

Elevated protein values above 100 mg/dl are found in many cases of acute idiopathic polyneuritis; chronic relapsing polyneuritis; amyloid, diabetic, and diphtheritic neuropathies; Dejerine-Sottas disease; Refsum's syndrome; and neuropathies associated with malignant tumors on a nonmetastatic basis.

Lymphocyctic pleocytosis (modest elevations) does occur in some cases of acute idiopathic polyneuritis. Acute herpes zoster with cranial nerve involvement is usually associated with elevated numbers of mononuclear cells.

Numbers of cells and protein level may be increased in brachial neuritis.

Low glucose values may occur in meningeal sarcoidosis and carcinomatosis.

Nerve Conduction and Electromyography

There are three types of involvement of alpha motor neurons: (1) degeneration of the entire neuron (neuronal degeneration), (2) axonal degeneration of the distal axon (dying-back) with or without secondary segmental demyelination, and (3) primary segmental demyelination. Nerve conduction velocity remains normal in the neuronal degeneration type until most of the nerve is damaged. Needle electromyography in this type of degeneration is characterized by denervation and increased motor unit potential size. In axonal degeneration, low conduction velocity is present only when axonal atrophy and secondary segmental demyelination have occurred. The electromyogram resembles that seen in anterior horn cell diseases. In primary segmental demyelination, nerve conduction velocity is reduced and muscle potentials are reduced in size. A decrease in amplitude and an increase in latency of the ulnar, median, and sural nerve action potential indicates an abnormality of the alpha primary afferent neuron.

Nerve conduction velocities are useful in distinguishing purely motor neuropathies from certain myopathies and anterior horn cell diseases. Values below 40 m/second are considered abnormal. Velocities are slowest in acute idiopathic polyneuritis, chronic relapsing polyneuritis, and some genetic neuropathies (Charcot-Marie-Tooth, Dejerine-Sottas, and Refsum's diseases). Normal or slightly reduced conduction velocities are present in most of the other major neuropathies.

Nerve Biopsy (Sural Nerve)

Nerve biopsy is of value in establishing the diagnosis in polyneuropathies such as leprosy, primary amyloidosis, metachromatic leukodystrophy, Fabry's disease, and the vasculitides. A presumptive diagnosis may be feasible in inflammatory neuropathies, lymphoproliferative disorders, and myxedema. Nerve biopsy may result in disagreeable side effects, such as painful numbness, and should be used with caution and only when indicated.

DIFFERENTIAL DIAGNOSIS

In the differential diagnosis of peripheral neuropathy, such entities as lesions of the cauda equina, cervical spondylosis with cervical myelopathy, primary diseases of muscle, spinal muscular atrophies, tabes dorsalis, and hysteria should be considered.

Lesions of the cauda equina nerve roots can produce distal motor and sensory deficits in the lower extremities, which may simulate a polyneuropathy. Prominent bladder or bowel manifestations should suggest a cauda equina lesion, and myelography may be necessary.

Cervical spondylosis with cervical myelopathy can result in a combination of motor and sensory manifestations, including glove-like sensory syndromes that may mimic polyneuropathies. Long tract signs in the form of pyramidal tract or posterior column signs, or both, may be helpful in suggesting a spinal cord problem. However, the combination of spinal cord syndromes and peripheral neuropathy may be seen in a number of conditions, particularly vitamin B_{12} deficiency and diabetes mellitus.

Primary diseases of muscle occasionally give rise to difficulties in diagnosis. Acute polymyositis can be mistaken for acute idiopathic polyneuritis when proximal muscles are involved. In rare cases a polymyositis may implicate the distal musculature and imitate a chronic polyneuropathy. Within the group of muscular dystrophies, uncommon cases of distal myopathy can be confusing. The onset with upper extremity involvement is helpful in suggesting this form of myopathy. Myotonica atrophica affects the distal muscles and seldom is a problem when the myotonic response, sternocleidomastoid and temporal muscle weakness, and the other characteristic features of this disorder are present. It is uncommon for myasthenia gravis to be confused with peripheral neuropathy with the exception of occasional childhood cases in which there is an acute onset with proximal limb weakness that may resemble acute idiopathic polyneuritis. The Eaton-Lambert syndrome with limb weakness and diminished tendon reflexes may be a more difficult problem, and electrophysiologic studies may be helpful in deciding whether a neurogenic or myopathic process is present.

Spinal muscular atrophies (motor neuron disease) may simulate predominantly motor neuropathies. Tendon reflexes may be diminished or absent. Fasciculations may or may not be present. The problem usually occurs in cases of motor neuron disease that begin with lower extremity involvement with loss of the Achilles tendon reflexes.

Tabes dorsalis may be confused with diabetes mellitus in that diminished tendon reflexes and a sensory ataxia may be present in both conditions, together with trophic changes in the form of perforating ulcers of the feet and neuropathic arthropathy. Electrophysiologic studies and serologic tests for syphilis can indicate the correct diagnosis.

Hysterical symptoms in the form of "glove and stocking" distribution of sensory patterns together with extremity paresthesias may simulate a peripheral neuropathy. However, inconsistent patterns, the fluctuating character of the physical findings, and the normal electrophysiologic studies usually suggest the proper diagnosis.

Table 3. Laboratory Tests for Evaluating Patients with Peripheral Neuropathy

Lumbar puncture (cells, glucose, protein)
Urinalysis (porphyrins and metachromatic material)
Tests for heavy metals (urine, hair, nails)
Vitamin B_{12}, free gastric acid, Schilling's test
Stool guaiac determinations
Gastrointestinal procedures
Chest x-ray
Hematologic studies
Bone marrow biopsy
Serum electrophoresis, Bence Jones protein
Liver function tests
Blood urea nitrogen determinations
Viral antibodies, test for infectious mononucleosis
Rheumatoid factor
Glucose tolerance test
Growth hormone determinations
Thyroid function tests
Erythrocyte sedimentation rate
Antinuclear antibodies
Phytanic acid levels
Uroporphyrinogen-1-synthetase in erthyrocytes (porphyric neuropathy)
Biopsy (rectal mucosa, gingiva, nerve, liver, or kidney) for amyloidosis

APPROACH TO PATIENTS WITH SUSPECTED PERIPHERAL NEUROPATHY

The approach to a patient with a likely diagnosis of peripheral neuropathy is two-pronged: (1) establish the presence of a peripheral neuropathy, and (2) determine its cause so that treatment possibilities and prognosis can be ascertained. To determine the etiologic background, it is important to consider the main categories or causes of peripheral neuropathy as outlined in Table 4 in addition to the course of the illness and the findings on the neurologic examination.

The combination of the clinical course of the illness and the neurologic findings may play an important role in suggesting certain categories of neuropathy.

Table 4. Causes of Peripheral Neuropathy

Toxins

Metals

- Arsenic
- Lead
- Mercury
- Antimony
- Thallium

Drugs

- Vincristine
- Maytansine
- 5-Flurouracil
- Hexamethylmelamine
- Procarbazine
- Doxorubicin
- Metronidazole
- Misonidazole
- Nitrofurantoin and related nitrofurazones
- Isoniazid
- Thalidomide
- Stilbamidine
- Phenytoin
- Chloramphenicol
- Tetra-ethylthiuram disulfide
- Clioquinols
- Procainamide
- Perhexiline
- Hydralazine
- Sodium cyanate
- Disulfiram
- Carbon disulfide
- Dapsone
- Trichlorethylene
- Ethambutol
- Methaqualone
- Amphetamines
- Glutethimide
- Gold

Organic Substances

- Organophosphates, including triorthocresyl phosphate
- DDT
- Dichlorophenoxy-acetic acid (2,4-D)
- Polychlorinated biphenyls (PCBs)
- *n*-Hexane
- Methyl-*n*-butyl ketone
- Toluene
- Methylethyl ketone
- Nitrous oxide
- Carbon monoxide
- Acrylamide
- Aromatic mercury fungicides
- Ethylene oxide
- Dimethylaminopropionitrile

Inflammatory States and Infections

- Acute idiopathic polyneuritis
- Polyneuropathy complicating acute or chronic infection, diphtheria, infectious mononucleosis, sarcoidosis
- Brachial neuritis
- Local nerve infection: Leprosy, herpes zoster

Metabolic Disorders and Deficiency States

- Diabetes mellitus
- Hypoglycemia
- Uremia
- Porphyria
- Amyloidosis
- Multiple myeloma
- Macroglobulinemia
- Lupus erythematosus
- Lung carcinoma
- Hypothyroidism
- Acromegaly
- Liver disease
- Polycythemia
- Lymphomas
- Leukemia
- Alcoholism
- Beriberi
- Pellagra
- Pregnancy
- Subacute combined degeneration
- Chronic gastrointestinal disease
- Pyridoxine deficiency

Vascular Abnormalities

- Rheumatoid arthritis
- Polyarteritis nodosa
- Systemic lupus erythematosus
- Scleroderma
- Sjögren's syndrome
- Cranial arteritis
- Wegener's granulomatosis

Hereditary Disorders

- Progressive hypertrophic polyneuropathy
- Charcot-Marie-Tooth disease
- Refsum's disease
- Leukodystrophies
- Fabry's disease
- Tangier disease
- Abetalipoproteinemia (Bassen-Kornzweig syndrome)
- Amyloidosis (primary and secondary)

Polyneuropathy of Obscure Origin

- Chronic progressive or recurrent polyneuropathy

An abrupt onset with pain may be representative of certain mononeuropathies and multiple mononeuropathies of ischemic origin, such as polyarteritis nodosa, rheumatoid arthritis, and the cranial nerve palsies or femoral neuropathy of diabetes mellitus. An abrupt onset with ascending motor or sensorimotor involvement is frequently characteristic of such neuropathies as acute idiopathic polyneuritis (Landry-Guillain-Barré syndrome), the neuropathies seen with infectious mononucleosis, hepatitis, diphtheria, porphyria, certain toxins (triorthocresyl phosphate), and the paraneoplastic and postvaccinal neuropathies. The combination of a subacute course and symmetric sensorimotor involvement should suggest (1) deficiency states, including alcoholism, pellagra, and vitamin B_{12} deficiency, (2) toxins, particularly heavy metals and industrial solvents, (3) drug intoxications, and (4) uremic polyneuropathy. A subacute course together with asymmetric sensorimotor neuropathy is characteristic of neuropathies secondary to diabetes, polyarteritis nodosa, sarcoidosis, and subacute idiopathic polyneuritis. A more chronic course associated with sensorimotor manifestations should alert the clinician to the possible presence of diabetes, connective tissue diseases, carcinoma and other malignancies, uremia, paraproteinemias, hypothyroidism, and amyloidosis. When the course of the illness is relapsing and chronic in character, idiopathic polyneuritis, porphyria, Refsum's disease, beriberi, or intoxications are the main considerations.

A positive family history for peripheral neuropathy, or the presence of formes frustes or peripheral nerve findings on the neurologic examination of relatives of a patient with a negative family history, suggests the presence of a genetically determined neuropathy. Within this group of genetic neuropathies, the presence of predominantly sensory findings on the neurologic examination is characteristic of a small group of sensory neuropathies. Mixed sensorimotor involvement is seen in the more common inherited neuropathies, such as dominant peroneal muscular atrophy (Charcot-Marie-Tooth disease) and dominant hypertrophic neuropathy of Dejerine-Sottas, and in those neuropathies with a known metabolic disorder, such as Refsum's disease and metachromatic leukodystrophy.

Establishing the presence of a peripheral neuropathy is easy when the patient presents with symmetric muscle weakness, with or without atrophy, diminished or absent reflexes, and distal sensory impairment. However, the absence of sensory symptoms or signs may present problems with the differential diagnosis of diseases involving the lower motor neuron. In such cases it is necessary to decide whether the weakness and reflex disturbance are due to a myelopathic, neuropathic, neuromuscular, or myopathic disorder. Pyramidal tract signs and a sensory level indicate the presence of a myelopathy. Muscle weakness, sensory abnormality, diminished reflexes, fasciculations, and distal involvement suggest a neuropathy. If the signs, symptoms, and diagnostic studies implicate a neurogenic disorder, it is then necessary to differentiate whether roots, plexus, or nerve trunks are involved and whether there is focal or diffuse pathology. Proximal limb involvement, radicular symptoms, radicular sensory impairment, and paraspinal denervation on the electromyographic study would favor root involvement. At times, there are insufficient symptoms and signs to differentiate disorders of the lower motor neuron. It is then necessary to utilize various laboratory procedures including measurement of nerve conduction velocity, electromyography (which distinguishes disorders of muscle, denervation, and neuromuscular block), cerebrospinal fluid studies (elevated protein level and cell counts with radicular and meningeal diseases), nerve (usually sural) and muscle biopsy, and biochemical determinations. Reduction or absence of sensory nerve fiber action potentials, low motor nerve conduction, and fibrillation potentials indicates a neuropathy. Low-amplitude polyphasic potentials would favor a myopathy. Myasthenia gravis, a disorder of the myoneural junction, is characterized by a fall in muscle action potential amplitude following supramaximal nerve stimulation (3 per second).

MOTOR NEURON DISEASES (ANTERIOR HORN CELL DISEASES)

By Linton C. Hopkins, M.D.
Atlanta, Georgia

DEFINITION

Motor neuron diseases are degenerative disorders of unknown cause in which skeletal muscle weakness and wasting are the dominant abnormality. Since the anterior horn cell in the spinal cord is affected, these are not "myopathies" or primary muscle diseases but are disorders of muscle innervation. However, the term "neuropathy" is usually not applied to these diseases but is reserved for disorders of the peripheral motor or sensory axons or peripheral nerve myelin. The most common anterior horn cell disease, adult-onset amyotrophic lateral sclerosis (ALS), is marked by the combination of upper and lower motor neuron findings. All types of degenerative anterior horn cell disease are marked by progressive deterioration in muscle strength.

INFANTILE SPINAL MUSCULAR ATROPHY (WERDNIG-HOFFMANN DISEASE)

Infantile spinal muscular atrophy (ISMA) should be considered in any infant under the age of 2 years who fails to meet motor milestones at expected times or shows deterioration in muscle performance. The most common and most severe form of this disease presents in the first year of life with poor head control, hypotonia, absence of tendon reflexes, and fasciculations of the tongue. Muscles of facial expression and extraocular muscles are usually spared. Because of early respiratory weakness the strength of the cry is reduced, and feeding problems commonly occur because of bulbar weakness. Muscle atrophy is not apparent initially because of the normal amount of adipose tissue in young infants, and fasciculations are usually not appreciated in peripheral muscles for the same reason. Tremor of the fingers is common and is most likely due to spontaneous motor unit discharges—contraction fasciculations. As in any progressive disorder that occurs when normal development is producing advancement in muscle power and in activity, the patient may still seem to be acquiring motor skills early in the course. Eventually new skills will not be acquired. Later, acquired skills will be lost. Death from respiratory infection or hypoventilation usually occurs by the age of 3 years.

A much less common, slowly progressive form of ISMA with onset in the first year also occurs, but although walking is acquired the patient does not survive for many years. Both types of ISMA are inherited as autosomal recessive traits.

Laboratory Tests

Laboratory procedures are of great importance in the diagnosis of this disease. Serum sarcoplasmic enzyme levels are usually normal but may be slightly elevated. Electromyography (EMG) is important and shows changes of denervation and reinnervation. There are fibrillation potentials and changes in the voluntary motor unit potentials—a reduction in number and an increase in size. In addition, fasciculations may be present. Muscle biopsy is also helpful. Most muscle fibers are atrophic but, oddly, large groups of hypertrophied type I (slow twitch) muscle fibers are usually present.

Differential Diagnosis

The major diagnostic dilemma or pitfall is in the differentiation of this very severe and invariably progressive infantile disease from more benign disorders and from disorders that can be treated. Congenital myopathies are rare and frequently nonprogressive but resemble ISMA. However, tongue fasciculations are not present in congenital myopathies, and the muscle biopsy shows specific alterations in the muscle cell that allows the identification of all morphologically specific congenital myopathies. The EMG does not show changes of denervation and reinnervation but does reveal changes indicative of mild myopathy. Also, ISMA must be differentiated from any cause of decreased muscle tone and decreased muscle activity in infants. A brief discussion of these disorders is present in the section on congenital myopathies.

Congenital and infantile myasthenia gravis does not produce tongue fasciculations, usually involves extraocular muscles, and can be distinguished from ISMA by a positive edrophonium chloride (Tensilon) test and by the usual absence of EMG changes indicating denervation and reinnervation. Biopsy does not show the changes noted in ISMA.

JUVENILE SPINAL MUSCULAR ATROPHY (KUGELBERG-WELANDER DISEASE)

Patients with juvenile spinal muscular atrophy (JSMA) present with proximal muscle weakness and atrophy, so clinically they may be suspected of having a myopathy. The first symptoms of weakness are usually noted between ages 5 and 15 years, but adults may also present with this syndrome. Unlike most patients with denervating diseases, these patients clinically appear to have a myopathy as their weakness, atrophy is proximal, and their complaints are due to proximal weakness. They have difficulty rising from chairs or ascending or descending stairs as well as difficulty with activities that involve reaching over their heads. Also, as with the myopathies, tendon reflexes may be preserved; however, usually with significant quadriceps weakness, the knee jerk is lost.

As with the infantile disease, JSMA follows an autosomal recessive pattern of inheritance.

Laboratory Tests

As in ISMA, laboratory studies are of importance. Serum sarcoplasmic enzymes (creatine kinase, aldolase) are usually normal or slightly increased, in sharp contrast to Duchenne type muscular dystrophy and other myopathies that clinically are similar. The EMG shows signs of denervation with fibrillations and fasciculations, enlargement of voluntary motor unit potentials, and reduction in their number. Muscle biopsy also is useful and usually provides diagnostic information. Muscle atrophy is the hallmark and, as in ISMA, groups of markedly hypertrophied fibers are present. Typical changes of myopathy — fiber necrosis and increased endomysial connective tissue — which are so prominent in dystrophy are usually absent or mild in JSMA.

Prognosis

The usual course is slow progression. These patients may have a normal life span, although one that is associated with significant muscle weakness and disability. More rapidly progressive forms are encountered, however, and severe respiratory weakness and the medical problems of the bedridden patient may appear after 10 or 15 years.

ADULT MOTOR NEURON DISEASE

Although rarely adults may present with genetically determined forms of motor neuron disease, the great majority are not familial. Acquired motor neuron disease in the adult may take several forms. The most common and most severe form, *amyotrophic lateral sclerosis,* is marked by the combination of upper motor neuron and lower motor neuron signs. As in the other anterior horn cell diseases already mentioned, the syndrome may be one of pure lower motor neuron disease with muscle wasting and weakness without upper motor neuron signs. This variety is called *progressive muscular atrophy.* Other varieties are *progressive bulbar palsy,* in which speech and swallowing muscles are primarily affected, and *primary lateral sclerosis,* a rare syndrome in which spastic paraparesis appears without evidence of lower motor neuron disease.

Amyotrophic Lateral Sclerosis

The most common form of adult motor neuron disease, ALS, is marked by the asymmetric onset of muscle wasting, prominence of fasciculations, muscle cramps, generalized distribution, and rapidly progressive course. It progresses more quickly than the other forms of adult motor neuron disease. Death usually occurs within 3 to 5 years after diagnosis. The disease usually begins with weakness and atrophy of one hand, or less commonly one foot, and then over months produces weakness and wasting in the other extremities and bulbar muscles. Extraocular muscle weakness and ptosis do not occur. As the disease is a pure motor syndrome, there are no sensory findings. In ALS, in which upper and lower motor neuron signs coexist, it is common to have an atrophied weak extremity with fasciculations yet an increase in tendon reflexes. Extensor plantar responses are usually present when the disease is well established.

Laboratory Tests. Laboratory studies are important. Serum sarcoplasmic enzymes (creatine kinase, etc.) are usually normal or slightly increased. Electromyography shows signs of denervation and reinnervation, with fibrillations and fasciculations, as well as enlargement and decreased number of voluntary potentials. Muscle biopsy shows changes of denervation. Fiber hypertrophy is not usually present. Single fiber atrophy of both types is the usual finding. As the disease advances, group atrophy and fiber type grouping appear. The latter is a histochemical change indicative of reinnervation.

Differential Diagnosis. Adult amyotrophic lateral sclerosis has an extensive differential diagnosis. In a patient who presents with atrophy of a single extremity, focal disorders must be considered. Tumors of plexus, nerve roots, or spinal cord will disturb innervation to the extremity.

The most common disorder that resembles motor neuron disease however, is cervical spondylosis, or degenerative arthritis of the cervical spine, which may compress nerve roots to the upper extremities and may produce a progressive spinal cord syndrome, spondylotic myelopathy. This differential diagnosis is occasionally difficult and requires extensive consultation and evaluation. Some clinical differences do exist, however. Most patients with compressive myelopathy due to spondylosis have disturbance of bladder function owing to compression and damage to the cervical spinal cord. Patients with motor neuron disease do not have disturbance of bladder function. In addition, cervical spondylosis produces changes seen with plain cervical spine films and cervical myelography that allow differentiation of this disorder from ALS. Occasionally, however, it is difficult to be certain whether the spondylosis is severe enough to produce spinal cord dysfunction. Cervical spondylosis and cervical spinal cord tumor may have lower motor neuron findings in the upper extremities, but not in the lower extremities, which will only show upper motor neuron signs from the cervical lesion. In contrast, patients with ALS usually have a combination of lower motor neuron and upper motor neuron signs in all four extremities. Occasionally, however, a patient with ALS has minimal lower motor neuron findings in the lower extremities, and these patients present the most difficult diagnostic dilemma. Cervical spondylosis does not produce involvement of bulbar muscles or muscles of swallowing and speech, whereas patients with well-established ALS usually have involvement of these muscles. When cervical spondylosis causes pressure on cervical nerve roots, it may be a painful process and produce sensory symptoms, numbness and tingling, in the extremity. Motor neuron disease produces cramps, but pain and sensory symptoms are not expected. However, cervical spondylosis may involve predominantly ventral roots, and atrophy may appear without pain and without numbness. When it is considered that patients over the age of 50 years commonly have mild disturbance of bladder function from other causes and that normal patients over 50 years old may have mild changes indicating denervation and reinnervation in intrinsic foot muscles on EMG, the diagnostic challenge posed by an individual patient becomes evident.

Spinal cord tumor, especially in the upper cervical-foramen magnum area, may resemble ALS. A well-planned myelogram with the assistance of computed tomography is commonly needed to adequately exclude foramen magnum tumor. A routine cervical myelogram will miss disease at the highest levels of the cervical cord.

Progressive Muscular Atrophy

Progressive muscular atrophy produces progressive generalized muscle atrophy without sensory symptoms and without upper motor neuron signs. Patients may have a positive family history, recessive or dominant, although most patients have an acquired disorder.

Initially distal weakness predominates although generalized weakness eventually appears. Patients complain of difficulty with fine finger manipulations and have weakness of finger abduction and difficulty in walking on heels and toes. Fasciculations may be present. Bulbar symptoms are either absent or mild, or occur late in the course, which is usually slowly progressive.

Laboratory Tests. Laboratory studies show normal or slight increase in creatine kinase (CK). EMG shows denervation and reinnervation. Nerve conduction studies show normal or slight reduction in motor conduction velocity, although evoked muscle potentials are usually small. Sensory potentials are normal.

Differential Diagnosis. Differentiation of motor neuron disease from other disorders of the peripheral nervous system may also pose real diagnostic difficulty. Occasionally peripheral neuropathies involve motor fibers with minimal or no involvement of the peripheral sensory system. Lead neuropathy is such a disorder and may produce a syndrome closely resembling adult motor neuron disease, although usually without the upper motor neuron findings. It resembles the progressive muscular atrophy form of adult-onset anterior horn cell disease. Patients with weakness who have had exposure to lead should be carefully studied with measurements of urine and serum lead, urine porphobilinogen, and urine delta-aminolevulinic acid, and they should be given chelation therapy if doubt exists, taking care to measure 24-hour urine lead for 48 hours after chelation. In addition, some patients with chronic idiopathic polyneuropathy, an immune disorder of the peripheral nervous system, have predominance of motor symptoms and such minor sensory systems that differentiation from progressive muscular atrophy is difficult. The differential diagnosis centers upon the nerve conduction velocity measurements, which are slowed in this demyelinating peripheral neuropathy but usually are normal or just slightly reduced in motor neuron disease. In addition, spinal fluid protein levels are usually increased in immune peripheral motor neuropathy and are normal in motor neuron disease.

Certain myopathies may resemble the progressive muscular atrophy form of motor neuron disease. Occasionally a patient with myasthenia gravis, particularly an elderly individual, poses diagnostic difficulty. These patients also have bulbar weakness, weakness of swallowing and speech, and extremity weakness, and in addition may have accompanying muscle atrophy. However, fasciculations do not occur in myasthenia gravis, and variability of weakness is expected, a feature not seen in motor neuron disease. Extensor plantar responses do not occur in myasthenia. In addition, extraocular muscle weakness with ptosis is expected in myasthenia gravis, although it is not invariably present. The diagnosis usually rests upon the response of patients with myasthenia to injected endrophonium chloride (Tensilon), response to repetitive stimulation of peripheral nerves, and the muscle biopsy, which shows change of denervation in ALS. Difficulties may still occur, however, as patients with myasthenia may have minor changes of denervation on muscle biopsy and 15 to 20 per cent of patients with motor neuron disease will have positive repetitive stimulation tests. Also, the Tensilon test may be difficult to interpret. Finally, motor neuron disease does not produce elevation of serum levels of antiacetylcholine receptor antibody, which is present in 80 to 90 per cent of myasthenic patients.

Inclusion body myositis, a variety of inflammatory myopathy, commonly presents with progressive weakness that is distal as well as proximal and can be confused with motor neuron disease. Levels of serum CK are usually increased to a greater extent than in motor neuron disease and the EMG shows myopathic changes instead of denervation and reinnervation. Muscle biopsy shows inflammation, fiber inclusions, and fiber necrosis rather than fiber atrophy alone, which is so typical of motor neuron disease.

A form of dominantly inherited motor neuropathy, *Charcot-Marie-Tooth disease,* affects axons rather than peripheral myelin and therefore has minimal slowing of nerve conduction velocities. It may be distinguished from motor neuron disease as patients with Charcot-Marie-Tooth disease usually have mild sensory findings, foot and toe deformities are common, tendon reflexes are diminished early, fasciculations are rare, and weakness is symmetric. Also, in dominantly inherited Charcot-Marie-Tooth disease, the physical examination and EMG of parents of patients will usually be abnormal.

The syndrome of benign fasciculations must be differentiated from motor neuron disease. For the most part, this condition is seen in young men with athletic build who have calf fasciculations. There is no weakness or atrophy and, except for the fasciculations, the EMG is normal. The cause is unknown. Rarely, patients will have fasciculations in a more generalized distribution in association with cramps and muscle aching and may even have evidence of axonal damage on EMG but do not develop weakness and disability. The cause of this syndrome is unknown, although it appears to be a benign axonal neuropathy.

Progressive Bulbar Palsy

Occasionally a patient who has motor neuron disease first shows weakness of swallowing and speech muscles and may continue to have major clinical weakness limited to these muscles. These patients are usually elderly. Their speech has a tight, spastic, dysphonic quality. Fasciculations and atrophy of the tongue are prominent. Laboratory studies show EMG evidence of denervation and reinnervation in the bulbar muscles, and there are usually mild changes in extremity muscles as well. Muscle biopsy of an extremity muscle may or may not show that the denervation is generalized.

The major pitfall in diagnosis is the distinction from bulbar myasthenia gravis, which usually has fluctuating symptoms, involvement of extraocular muscles, and fatigable ptosis. Antiacetylcholine antibody is present in 80 to 90 per cent of myasthenic patients but is not present in motor neuron disease.

Neoplastic involvement of lower cranial nerves by carcinomatous meningitis may cause bulbar palsy, but signs of systemic cancer are usually present and spinal fluid examination will demonstrate the abnormal cells, an elevated protein level, and commonly a reduced glucose level.

Benign and malignant tumors in the foramen magnum can also produce bulbar palsy but usually show signs of medullary or spinal cord compression with long-tract motor signs and bladder and bowel dysfunction, and these usually involve one, then the other, hypoglossal nerves, not both equally and simultaneously.

Progressive bulbar palsy usually shows the combination of upper and lower neuron disease expected in ALS, as the patient with an atrophic fasciculating tongue may have a preserved or increased gag reflex and jaw jerk.

Primary Lateral Sclerosis

This is a disease in which upper motor neuron signs are present without the lower motor neuron findings (fasciculations and wasting) of the more common ALS. Its existence as an acquired disorder is questionable, as extensive pathologic verification is lacking, but rarely a patient does have progressive spastic paraparesis in which no other disease can be found. A familial syndrome, *hereditary spastic paraparesis,* does exist and has been pathologically verified. It is usually dominantly inherited and very slowly progressive, with onset from the first to the fifth decades.

Primary lateral sclerosis is very rare, and the other causes of spastic paraparesis are numerous. Patients who have leg weakness with brisk reflexes and extensor plantar responses should undergo an extensive battery of diagnostic tests. The most common cause of spastic paraparesis in an adult over 40 years old is cervical spondylosis, which may not produce obvious upper extremity symptoms and signs and may be painless. Spinal cord tumor should also be considered; therefore, a complete myelogram is an essential part of the evaluation of spastic paraparesis. Attention should be directed to the thoracic area (a region difficult to study), to the cervical area, and particularly to the craniocervical junction, where tumors in the region of the foramen magnum may produce spastic paraparesis with minimal evidence of segmental bulbar muscle weakness. Pain is a common accompaniment of spinal cord tumor, and disturbance of bladder function usually occurs in cord compression by tumor or spondylosis. Bladder function is not affected in motor neuron disease. In addition, sensory symptoms and sensory signs are usual in patients with spinal cord tumor but are not expected in motor neuron disease.

Combined systems disease, caused by vitamin B_{12} deficiency, is an important and treatable metabolic spinal cord disorder that should be considered in any patient with spastic lower extremities. However, sensory symptoms and signs predominate in combined systems disease. Tingling and numbness in the hands and feet, reduction of joint position sense in hands and feet, and abnormal two-point discrimination in the fingertips are all present. Such major sensory signs are absent in the motor neuron diseases.

A form of chronic multiple sclerosis can be confused with primary lateral sclerosis. Most patients with multiple sclerosis have sensory and visual symptoms as well as ophthalmoplegia, nystagmus, or ataxia and can be easily distinguished from patients with motor neuron disease. Occasionally, however, multiple sclerosis produces a purely motor progressive paraparesis similar to primary lateral sclerosis. Patients with this disorder must be identified by diagnostic tests, such as visual and brain stem evoked responses and measurement of IgG in spinal fluid.

MYASTHENIA GRAVIS

By Donald B. Sanders, M.D.
Durham, North Carolina

DEFINITION

Myasthenia gravis (MG) is a disease in which abnormal neuromuscular transmission produces muscle weakness. The acquired form of MG is an autoimmune disease that results from an immunologic attack against the neuromuscular junction, with a subsequent reduction in the concentration of acetylcholine receptor molecules on the muscle endplate. This form of MG affects approximately 5 persons in 100,000. It can begin at any age in either sex but has peaks of incidence among young women and older men. In addition there are several congenital forms that do not have an immune basis and are much more rare.

SIGNS AND SYMPTOMS

Ocular and bulbar muscles are most frequently affected in acquired MG, although any voluntary muscles may be involved. Fluctuations in strength from time to time are highly characteristic, with weakness typically being greater after muscle activity. The most common presenting symptoms are ptosis and double vision, which are most marked after prolonged use of the eyes. Most patients will have these symptoms at some point in their illness. Early symptoms of bulbar weakness include nasal speech or hoarseness, especially after prolonged talking, intermittent choking, and nasal regurgitation of liquids. Involvement of jaw muscles may appear as weakness on chewing, especially of tough foods.

Bulbar and respiratory muscle weakness may be life-threatening. Abnormal swallowing may lead to aspiration of food or saliva, a weak cough will predispose to infection, and weakness of respiratory muscles produces hypoxia. Pneumonia may follow and contribute to these problems.

Weakness of extremity or respiratory muscles may be perceived by the patient as decreased "energy," stamina, or exercise tolerance. Many patients learn to pace themselves to avoid frank weakness, and questioning reveals a reduction in participation in activities that stress the neuromuscular system. With more severe involvement there may be dyspnea on exertion, inability to use the extremity muscles normally, and falling episodes.

Initially, symptoms may be mild and intermittent and are frequently recognized only in retrospect. In a small proportion of patients, the disease remains restricted to the ocular muscles. More often there is progression in the distribution and severity of weakness over a period of months to years. Onset or worsening of symptoms may follow emotional or physical stress, especially infections. Patients with MG have a heightened sensitivity to neuromuscular blocking agents, and the first manifestation of the disease may be prolonged paralysis after a surgical procedure during which one of these agents is used. Occasionally the onset may be acute, with rapid progression to severe weakness. After many years, chronically weak muscles become atrophic and no longer demonstrate the fluctuations in strength.

PHYSICAL EXAMINATION

The physical examination is normal except for the neuromuscular system. Weakness may be subtle when the disease is mild or between exacerbations. All muscle tests should include prolonged activity to demonstrate a fatigable component. When weakness is detected in this manner, the examination should be repeated after a period of rest to demonstrate any recovery.

Particular attention should be paid to the eyelids and ocular muscles. Ptosis of one or both lids may be present initially and become more marked with sustained upward gaze or may become apparent only during this maneuver. The most typical ocular pattern is asymmetric weakness of one or more muscles, especially the medial and superior rectus. Isolated weakness of the lateral rectus is not common in MG and should raise the question of a sixth nerve palsy. Very mild medial rectus weakness can be demonstrated when horizontal divergence develops on upward gaze ("V-phoria") or when the adducting eye is covered during lateral gaze. The use of a small focused light source as the target while testing eye movements can increase the yield by allowing the examiner to detect deviations from fixation when the corneal reflection moves from the center of the pupil.

The most sensitive evidence of facial muscle involvement is weak eye closure. The patient may not be able to bury his eyelashes, to resist forcible eye opening, or to maintain the sclerae covered. Weakness of lower facial muscles may be seen as loss of facial expression, inability to purse the lips or whistle, or inability to hold the jaw closed. A classic posture is that in which the patient props up the chin with the thumb and long finger of one hand, the index finger being extended up the side of the cheek.

Nasal speech indicates weakness of the palate. Slurred speech betrays weakness of the tongue or lips, the latter producing difficulty enunciating plosive sounds. Poor glottal closure produces a characteristic weak cough even when adequate air can be moved. Diaphragmatic weakness limits the ability to sniff sharply. Respiratory function can be assessed more quantitatively by measuring vital capacity, maximum midexpiratory flow rate or maximum expiratory force.

Muscle Testing

Observations of muscle function during the following maneuvers may reveal weakness that is otherwise unsuspected, even by the patient:

1. Rising on heels and toes.
2. Arising from a squat.
3. Stepping up onto a 12-inch stool.
4. Sit-ups from a supine position.
5. Holding each leg extended from a supine position.
6. Holding the arms outstretched for 2 minutes.
7. Reaching up toward the ceiling.
8. Holding the head off the bed for 2 minutes while supine.

Manual muscle testing can be used to quantitate the weakness in individual muscles. Neck flexors typically will be weak even when other extremity muscles are normal. It should be reiterated that weakness may become apparent on any of these tests only after sustained exertion.

Muscle tenderness, sensory abnormalities, changes in tone, or abnormal tendon reflexes are *not* produced by MG. Muscle atrophy may be seen in chronic untreated MG, accompanied by fixed weakness.

Change in muscle strength after administration of *cholinesterase inhibitors* is highly characteristic of MG. This can be demonstrated by assessing several muscle groups before and after administration of edrophonium chloride (Tensilon), a short-acting cholinesterase inhibitor. Ocular muscles are ideal for this purpose. Initially, 2 mg Tensilon is given intravenously in a 10 mg/ml solution. If there is no definite change and no adverse effects occur, another 8 mg can be given. Improvement occurs within 30 to 120 seconds and usually persists less than 10 minutes, although occasionally effects may be more long-lasting. Side effects of this drug include abdominal cramps, nausea, excessive salivation, sweating, fasciculations, and, rarely, bradycardia and hypotension. These can be suppressed by giving atropine, 0.5 mg, intramuscularly several minutes beforehand. To minimize observer bias and placebo effect, this test can be performed in a blinded fashion, although patients can frequently identify the drug by its side effects even when atropine has been given in advance.

In patients who are receiving cholinesterase inhibitors and in others with borderline neuromuscular compensation, Tensilon may produce worsening of strength. This response is also diagnostic but may be dangerous and must be anticipated.

Electromyographic tests can confirm the neuromuscular abnormality. Repetitive nerve stimulation at low frequencies produces a decrementing muscle response that can be reversed by Tensilon. This is the most commonly used electrodiagnostic test and can be performed in muscles of the hand, arm, shoulder, face, and leg. Results are more likely to be abnormal in proximal or face muscles, and they are less likely to be abnormal in patients with mild or purely ocular disease.

Single-fiber electromyography (*EMG*) is more sensitive but requires specialized equipment and extensive experience, and this method is not commonly available. Abnormalities of neuromuscular transmission can be demonstrated by single-fiber EMG in almost all patients with MG, including those with disease that is restricted to the ocular muscles clinically. Abnormal neuromuscular transmission can also be detected by this technique in neuropathies and myopathies, however, and these must be excluded by routine EMG studies when the single-fiber EMG is abnormal.

Other Tests

Antibodies to the human muscle acetylcholine receptor can be found in the serum of over 75 per cent of patients with MG, including over 60 per cent of those with ocular disease. When present, they are virtually diagnostic of MG, but their absence does not exclude the diagnosis. The assay for these antibodies is not universally available and should be regarded as complementing the EMG studies in confirming the diagnosis of MG.

Abnormalities of the thymus occur in 80 per cent of patients with MG. The majority of patients have hyperplasia, but 10 to 15 per cent of patients, most often in the older age group, will have a thymoma. Computed tomographic (CT) scan of the mediastinum is the most sensitive test for thymomas and should be performed, especially in the older patients.

All patients should be tested for thyroid disease, rheumatoid arthritis, and other autoimmune diseases, all of which occur more frequently with MG.

In some patients with mild disease that cannot be diagnosed conclusively by other means, a therapeutic trial of oral cholinesterase inhibitors, such as pyridostiomine (Mestinon), may help clarify the diagnosis.

Since the initial symptoms of MG are frequently vague and fluctuating, it is common for psychiatric disease to be suspected early on. When ocular muscle weakness is a prominent initial manifestation, intracranial pathology may be suspected.

Weakness that responds to Tensilon may also be seen in myopathies and denervating disease, especially amyotrophic lateral sclerosis (ALS). Appropriate electrodiagnostic tests will detect these.

DIAGNOSIS IN DISORDERS OF NEUROMUSCULAR TRANSMISSION

By Michael H. Rivner, M.D.
and Thomas R. Swift, M.D.
Augusta, Georgia

At the neuromuscular junction, information is transferred from the motor neuron to the muscle. Acetylcholine, the neurotransmitter, crosses a small gap at the neuromuscular junction and contacts receptors on the muscle cell membrane, generating an electrical potential that will ultimately lead to a muscle contraction. In normal muscle a nerve action potential in the axon will always result in a muscle contraction because no failures of transmission occur.

Normal transmission across the neuromuscular junction can be interfered with in many ways. In this article we will discuss various clinical conditions that can interfere with this process. The most common disease in this category, myasthenia gravis, will not be discussed in this section (see article on this topic). Factors interfering with neuromuscular transmission include congenital abnormalities, autoimmune diseases, and toxin, drug, and electrolyte effects. In almost all of these conditions a high index of suspicion on the part of the physician and access to an experienced physician electromyographer are essential for correct diagnosis.

MYASTHENIC SYNDROME (LAMBERT-EATON SYNDROME)

Myasthenic syndrome is a disorder of neuromuscular transmission characterized by generalized muscle weakness and fatigability. This disease usually occurs in patients older than 40 years of age and is five times more common in males than in females. Patients complain of symptoms related to proximal muscle weakness. Early difficulties are seen in climbing stairs or rising out of a chair. The strength of the patient typically improves temporarily following voluntary contraction. Extraocular, facial, and bulbar musculature usually is normal. Patients may also complain of dry mouth, dysuria, impotence, and constipation, indicating autonomic dysfunction. Muscle stretch reflexes are usually depressed but may improve temporarily following voluntary contraction. Despite peculiar leg sensations in many, the sensory examination is normal, as is the remainder of the neurologic examination. The weakness usually worsens unless therapy is given.

Myasthenic syndrome is frequently associated with carcinoma (70 per cent of men and 20 per cent of women with the symptoms), oat cell carcinoma of the lung being most likely. In many cases it is the first sign of a neoplasm. On physical examination additional symptoms may be found that are due to other remote effects of cancer, such as a polyneuropathy. In a few patients both myasthenic syndrome and myasthenia gravis have been reported simultaneously.

There are no specific blood or radiographic abnormalities associated with this syndrome. Electromyographic studies are the most useful laboratory tests in diagnosing this condition. The amplitude of the compound muscle action potential is abnormally low. The latency of the motor response is normal. Following either a tetanic nerve stimulation or voluntary contraction, the amplitude of the response will increase. With repetitive stimulation at low frequencies (2 Hz), the amplitude of the compound muscle action potential decreases further. At higher frequencies of stimulation, such as 20 Hz, the amplitude of the response increases. Conventional needle electromyography may show variability of motor unit potentials. Single fiber electromyography shows increased jitter and occasional blocking. Sensory nerve conduction studies are normal, unless a sensory neuropathy coexists.

Anticholinesterase drugs improve transmission in these patients, but the response is reduced compared to that in myasthenia gravis.

Muscle biopsy is of only limited value in this disorder. On light microscopy, atrophy of Type II fibers with Type I predominance may be seen. Electron microscopy demonstrates the postjunctional membranes either to be normal or to show an increase in the postsynaptic area. In these cases the postsynaptic endplate region has highly complex secondary clefts and folds.

Since myasthenic syndrome is frequently associated with an occult malignancy, all patients with these symptoms should be fully evaluated for this possibility. Myasthenic syndrome most commonly is associated with oat cell carcinoma of the lung, making chest X-ray mandatory in these patients. If evaluation of the chest fails to show a malignancy, the gastrointestinal tract should be evaluated fully.

Differential Diagnosis

The most common problem in diagnosing this condition is failure to suspect its presence. It is, therefore, necessary to have a high degree of suspicion when examining a patient who complains of proximal weakness. If a muscle response of low amplitude is noted on motor nerve conduction studies, it is important to test the patient to see if this response can be augmented following exercise or with high-frequency repetitive stimulation.

Distinguishing myasthenic syndrome from myasthenia gravis usually is not difficult. Myasthenia gravis presents with predominantly extraocular and bulbar muscle weakness that fatigues with exercise. Myasthenic syndrome presents with proximal limb weakness that frequently improves transiently following voluntary contraction. In myasthenic syndrome the extraocular and bulbar musculature usually is normal. In addition, the response to repetitive stimulation in these conditions differs.

Polymyositis may also present with proximal muscle weakness; however, in this condition the serum level of creatine kinase is usually elevated, and there may be muscle tenderness. In addition, no improvement is noted following voluntary contraction, and no electrophysiologic abnormalities are seen following repetitive stimulation. Also, the needle examination is usually abnormal, showing diffuse fibrillations and small-amplitude polyphasic units.

Inflammatory polyradiculopathy (Guillain-Barré syndrome) may present with proximal weakness. The onset of this condition is more rapid than that of myasthenic syndrome. In addition, this disorder usually follows a prodromal viral illness and frequently involves the bulbar musculature. Muscle stretch reflexes usually are reduced or absent, but a muscle contraction to direct percussion is seen. Spinal fluid protein level is elevated in most cases. The electromyographic findings in Guillain-Barré syndrome differ considerably from those of mysthenic syndrome. In Guillain-Barré syndrome, nerve conduction velocity may be slowed and distal latency prolonged. The muscle action potential in response to nerve stimulation is dispersed. In addition, the F-wave latency is prolonged. With high-frequency repetitive stimulation or exercise the amplitude of the muscle response does not increase in Guillain-Barré syndrome.

BOTULISM

Botulism is a disorder of neuromuscular transmission caused by the ingestion of a toxin produced by the bacterium *Clostridium botulinum,* most often following ingestion of improperly canned foods. A typical case begins 18 to 36 hours after the ingestion of the toxin; however, cases have occurred as early as 6 hours to as late as 8 days following ingestion of the toxin. Most patients suffer from gastrointestinal effects before the onset of neurologic symptoms. The symptoms include nausea, vomiting, constipation, and abdominal cramps. This may be followed by autonomic symptoms, such as dry mouth, dysuria, blurred vision, and xerophthalmia. Neurologic symptoms most commonly involve the cranial nerves first. Patients develop diplopia, dysphagia, dysphonia, and ptosis. Depending on the severity of the disease, the paresis progresses ultimately to involve the extremities and respiratory musculature. The pupils usually are dilated and poorly responsive to light. Mental status despite severe motor involvement is normal. Reflexes are decreased or absent in affected muscles. The course may vary from a mild weakness with only cranial nerve findings to a prolonged course with ventilatory insufficiency for several months. In addition to the typical case that is due to ingestion of the toxin, a similar syndrome may develop following a wound infected with *Clostridium botulinum.* The symptoms usually develop in these cases 4 to 12 days following the injury. The major complications of this condition are respiratory insufficiency and pneumonia.

The diagnosis of botulism is made by having a high index of suspicion and obtaining a history of ingestion of canned foods. Additional cases may present simultaneously if several people ate the same contaminated food item. The presence of a recent wound in an extremity with the development of neurologic symptoms should raise the possibility of wound botulism.

Serum, stool, and food specimens should be collected. These specimens should be tested for the presence of toxin and the stool cultured for the organism. Electromyographic studies are useful in making the diagnosis of botulism. The sensory and motor conductions and latencies are normal. Initially the amplitude of the motor potential is reduced. With high-frequency repetitive stimulation or following a tetanus, facilitation is usually but not invariably seen. Single-fiber electromyography shows increased jitter and blocking, which improves at high firing rates. Fibrillations may be seen in conventional needle electromyography (see separate article on botulism).

Differential Diagnosis

Guillain-Barré syndrome may present a picture similar to that of botulism. Usually the paralysis is of the ascending rather than the descending type seen in botulism. The spinal fluid protein level is elevated in Guillain-Barré syndrome but not in botulism. Guillain-Barré syndrome usually is associated with pain, and pupillary abnormalities are rare. Muscle stretch reflexes are reduced. The electromyographic findings of the two disorders differ as well.

Diphtheritic neuropathy can present with weakness of bulbar musculature and loss of accommodation. This may be followed in several weeks by a severe sensorimotor polyneuropathy. In this disease, in contrast to botulism, extraocular muscles are rarely affected. Sensory abnormalities are found in addition to the paralysis. In diphtheritic neuropathy elevated protein levels are found in the spinal fluid. There is slowing of both sensory and motor nerve conduction velocities. Culture of the throat may demonstrate *Corynebacterium diphtheriae* (see article on diphtheria).

Periodic paralysis may present with sudden profound weakness. Unlike the case with botulism, bulbar and extraocular muscles are usually not involved. Alterations of serum potassium level are usually associated with periodic paralysis. During a severe attack, muscles studied electromyographically are silent. (See article on the periodic paralyses).

Acute poliomyelitis may present as an acute paresis involving bulbar as well as spinal musculature. In addition, poliomyelitis may be associated with gastrointestinal tract abnormalities. Poliomyelitis usually follows a septic illness and is associated with a meningitis. Electromyography reveals evidence of denervation. (See article on poliomyelitis).

Myasthenia gravis also presents with ptosis and extraocular muscle weakness but without pupillary abnormalities. In addition, fatigue is noted in patients with myasthenia, and gastrointestinal symptoms are not seen. The onset of the weakness is not as rapid in patients with myasthenia gravis. The findings on electromyography and the response to edrophonium chloride (Tensilon) is also useful in distinguishing myasthenia gravis from botulism. (See article on myasthenia gravis.)

Tick paralysis may likewise be confused with botulism. The pattern of paralysis in this illness is of the ascending rather than the descending type noted in botulism. In addition, in cases of tick paralysis a tick should be found on the patient, usually in the scalp. The electromyographic findings in these conditions differ as well.

INFANT BOTULISM

Infant botulism is a condition characterized by weakness during the first 4 months of life caused by the toxin *Clostridium botulinum* that has colonized in the gastrointestinal tract of the infant. The infant is usually normal until the development of constipation between 5 and 20 weeks of age, after which cranial nerve signs and hypotonia occur. This weakness may progress to respiratory insufficiency. Infants with this disorder are hypotonic; show weak sucking, swallowing, and crying; and have pooling of oral secretions and diminished gag reflex. Because the infants are hypotonic they appear inactive but are usually alert. Reflexes are diminished in weak limbs. Because of generalized weakness, the infants have poor head control and diminished withdrawal response. Chest x-ray may reveal hypoinflated lung fields.

Serum specimens should be checked for the presence of botulinum toxin, but this has rarely been positive in cases of infant botulism. Fecal specimens should be investigated for the presence of both botulinum toxin and the microorganism. *Clostridium botulinum* has been isolated from the stool as long as 100 days after the patient's recovery.

Electromyographic examination shows similar results to those in adult botulism.

Differential Diagnosis

The diagnosis of botulism is one that must be thought of in any hypotonic infant. The initial diagnosis made in infants suffering from this disorder has ranged from meningitis to metabolic disorders. To make the diagnosis the clinician must ascertain that true hypotonia is present. In meningitis, sepsis, or encephalitis the infant is lethargic as a result of involvement of the central nervous system. In infant botulism the child is alert but weak. The spinal fluid in infant botulism is normal. To distinguish botulism from other causes of true hypotonia the history of progressive weakness, the association of constipation, and the absence of metabolic abnormalities in the serum and urine must be considered.

CONGENITAL MYASTHENIA GRAVIS

Congenital myasthenia gravis refers to a group of disorders in which the symptoms are similar to those found in acquired autoimmune myasthenia gravis, but all of them probably result from various congenital defects of the neuromuscular junction. Several of these disorders are caused by defects in the presynaptic synthesis, packaging, or release of acetylcholine. Acetylcholinesterase may be deficient in one of these syndromes. The other varieties of congenital myasthenia gravis result from postsynaptic defects. In one variety there is a defect in the acetylcholine receptor ion channel open time, and in another there is a deficiency of acetylcholine receptors.

These disorders all present as decreased muscle strength, usually starting in infancy. As in myasthenia gravis the extraocular and bulbar musculature is affected more than the distal musculature. Fatigue is seen following exercise. Muscle bulk of affected musculature is reduced and reflexes usually are diminished. The syndrome due to the abnormal ion channel open time may present initially in adolescence and may progress to severe muscle atrophy, whereas the other syndromes show little progression.

No antibodies to either striated muscle or acetylcholine receptors are found in these disorders. Edrophonium chloride (Tensilon) is effective in improving strength only in the presynaptic syndromes. In the other forms described it is ineffective. Sensory and motor nerve conductions are normal. With low-frequency repetitive stimulation a decrement is seen in all of these syndromes. In the two postsynaptic disorders, a repetitive motor response may occur following a single stimulus. Single-fiber electromyography reveals increased jitter and blocking.

Special biochemical, ultrastructural, and physiologic studies are needed to distinguish these disorders. In the case of a deficiency of acetylcholinesterase, no histochemical staining for this enzyme is seen. In vitro intracellular microelectrode studies are needed to further characterize these disorders. In the disorder of the postsynaptic receptors, there is a prolonged duration of the miniature endplate potential, whereas in presynaptic disorder the miniature endplate size is reduced, but the receptors appear normal.

Differential Diagnosis

These disorders will not be diagnosed correctly unless they are considered in pediatric patients who present with symptoms compatible with myasthenia gravis. Characteristics that differentiate this group of disorders from acquired myasthenia gravis are its onset at a young age, the absence of acetylcholine receptor antibodies, and familial occurrence. In addition, most patients with congenital myasthenia gravis do not respond to cholinesterase inhibitors, such as edrophonium.

DISORDERS DUE TO SNAKE ENVENOMATION

Certain poisonous snakes produce toxins that have potent effects on neuromuscular transmission. Most snakes that produce these toxins belong to two families, the *Elapidae* (cobras, coral snakes, mambas, and kraits) and the *Hydrophiidae* (sea snakes). In addition to these snakes, the South American rattlesnake (*Crotalus dirissus terrificus*) also produces a venom that has potent neuromuscular toxicity.

The symptoms following envenomation from an elapid snake begin with a preparalytic stage occurring from 30 minutes to 12 hours after the bite. During this stage, the victim's symptoms are headache, vomiting, visual disturbances, paresthesias, drowsiness, and hypotension. Only a small percentage of patients will develop the second or paralytic stage, which occurs from 30 minutes to 23 hours following the bite. Bilateral ptosis, ophthalmoplegia, and extraocular muscle weakness are followed by weakness of the tongue, larynx, and pharynx. The paralysis may continue to spread for up to 60 hours. In some cases ventilatory support is necessary. The paralysis gradually disappears over 3 to 10 days. Complications are due to pneumonia and respiratory compromise. Examination reveals a flaccid paralysis, normal sensation, absent stretch reflexes, and normal pupils. Because of enzymes contained in the venom, the area around the bite may become necrotic.

Electromyography reveals a compound muscle action potential of diminished size, which shows a decrement with low-frequency repetitive stimulation that improves following tetanic stimulation. As the patient's symptoms improve, the amplitude of the evoked muscle action potential increases. Cholinesterase inhibitors, such as edrophonium, improve strength.

Envenomation by a sea snake produces a slightly different clinical picture. The first symptoms appear several minutes to hours after the bite. The patient develops myalgias, muscle stiffness with increased passive resistance, and trismus, progressing to widespread rhabdomyolysis with myoglobinuria. Patients also develop parotid gland swelling, diaphoresis, nausea, and vomiting. Complications are due to respiratory paralysis, hyperkalemia, and renal failure due to rhabdomyolysis. Laboratory tests in this disorder show an elevated serum creatine kinase level and hyperkalemia. Myoglobinuria is seen as well. The electromyographic findings are probably similar to those seen in elapid snake envenomation, but few clinical studies have been reported.

Differential Diagnosis

Although the symptoms may superficially resemble myasthenia gravis, the temporal relationship to a snake bite and the rapid onset of symptoms would aid the clinician in making this diagnosis. In addition, effects of the venom on the cardiovascular system and skin will help differentiate this disorder from myasthenia gravis.

SPIDER BITES

Profound neuromuscular effects may be caused by the venom of the black and brown widow spiders. Symptoms begin from 10 to 60 minutes following the bite. The patient develops generalized piloerection, hypertension, vasoconstriction, and autonomic hyperactivity. The abdomen may develop board-like rigidity and extreme pain. Jaw and laryngeal spasm make intubation difficult. The symptoms usually subside in about an hour and are followed by a period of apnea and hypotension. These profound effects are due to the sudden release of transmitter at neuromuscular junctions as well as at sympathetic and parasympathetic ganglia.

DRUGS AFFECTING NEUROMUSCULAR TRANSMISSION

Many drugs have been associated with disorders of neuromuscular transmission. Most often the effects of these agents are seen in patients with subclinical myasthenia gravis, patients given muscle relaxants postoperatively, or patients with prexisting renal disease, or as part of a drug-induced immunologic disorder. Early symptoms are similar to those seen in myasthenia gravis, with extraocular paresis and ptosis. This may be followed by facial, bulbar, and proximal extremity weakness. Occasionally respiratory insufficiency may occur.

One major group of drugs that may block neuromuscular transmission is antibiotics. Neuromuscular transmission disturbances from these drugs usually occur when they are given coincidentally with a surgical procedure. Antibiotics producing this picture include the aminoglycoside antibiotics gentamicin, streptomycin, amikacin, kanamycin, and tobramycin. Other antibiotics producing disorders of neuromuscular transmission are polymyxin, lincomycin, clindamycin, tetracycline, rolitetracycline, colistin, and oxytetracycline. The anticonvulsants phenytoin, mephenytoin, trimethadione, and phenobarbital may interfere with neuromuscular transmission. Other drugs that are associated with neuromuscular transmission defects are quinidine, procainamide, propranolol, practolol, lithium, chlorpromazine, amantadine, trimethaphan camsylate, timolol, methoxyflurane, corticosteroids, and azathioprine. An autoimmune disturbance similar to acquired myasthenia gravis may be produced by either penicillamine or trimethadione. In most cases the easiest way to test for the effects of these drugs is to discontinue administration. Since the drugs may unmask subclinical cases of myasthenia gravis or myasthenic syndrome, patients presenting with drug-induced syndromes should be evaluated for these conditions as outlined earlier.

MAGNESIUM INTOXICATION

Neuromuscular transmission is blocked by elevated levels of magnesium. Toxicity may occur in eclamptic patients treated with parenteral magnesium or in their infants, patients with renal failure, or patients taking excess antacid and magnesium cathartics. The symptoms of magnesium intoxication include sedation, dry mouth, generalized weakness, and decreased muscle stretch reflexes. Serum magnesium level is generally greater than 4.0 mEq/liter in these patients. The electromyographic finding in this condition is a muscle action potential of decreased amplitude, which shows a decremental response with low-frequency repetitive stimulation. Following tetanus or at higher rates of stimulation, facilitation is seen.

MUSCULAR DYSTROPHIES

By Linton C. Hopkins, M.D.
Atlanta, Georgia

DEFINITION

Muscular dystrophies are defined by the following characterictics:

1. They are myopathies that have a genetic basis.
2. They have a progressive course.
3. They are disorders in which the pathologic diagnosis depends not on a single specific morphologic change in muscle fibers but instead on a combination of findings, each of which is nonspecific.
4. They are disorders of muscle in which a specific biochemical defect has not been identified.

This article focuses on the diagnosis of the four most common types of muscular dystrophy: X-linked recessive Duchenne's pseudohypertrophic muscular dystrophy, autosomal recessive limb-girdle muscular dystrophy, autosomal dominant facioscapulohumeral muscular dystrophy, and autosomal dominant myotonic muscular dystrophy. The diagnosis of any disease of muscle rests upon a triad of (1) clinical history and neurologic examination, (2) electromyography (EMG) and nerve conduction studies, and (3) muscle histopathologic studies. Each type of muscular dystrophy will be discussed with these in mind.

DUCHENNE'S PSEUDOHYPERTROPHIC MUSCULAR DYSTROPHY

The Duchenne variety of muscular dystrophy (DMD) is the most severe and most common muscular dystrophy. Only boys are affected, as it is an X-linked recessive disorder. Patients usually present for evaluation between the ages of 2 and 5 years with a history of toe-walking and difficulty in climbing stairs and in running. Parents frequently note calf enlargement. Examination reveals proximal muscle weakness and wasting as well as Achilles tendon contractures, which make it difficult for the patient to walk on his heels. When asked to rise from the floor, the child is noted to place his hands on his knees and push himself up (Gower's maneuver) rather than rising quickly under the power of his legs alone. The gait is waddling and unstable. Distal muscle strength is normal early. Facial weakness is usually not present, and eye movements remain normal throughout the course. The distribution of the weakness is symmetric and predominantly proximal. Muscles are not tender, and tendon reflexes are normal until severe weakness appears. Typically, posterior calf muscles are enlarged and firm. There are no sensory findings.

The course is one of progressive deterioration. Patients become confined to a wheelchair by the age of 12 to 15 years and death occurs by age 18 to 21 years.

The complications of DMD reflect the severity and extent of the muscle weakness and are predominantly respiratory. Early in the course, some involvement of respiratory muscles may be noted as the patient may have a weak cough and difficulty in clearing secretions. This complication becomes particularly severe when the patient is immobile in a wheelchair and develops scoliosis. Stasis pneumonia is a common fatal complication.

Laboratory Tests

Laboratory procedures that are of particular importance in the diagnosis of DMD are serum muscle enzymes studies, EMG and muscle biopsy.

Serum levels of sarcoplasmic enzymes (creatine kinase [CK], aspartate aminotransferase [AST, SGOT], lactate dehydrogenase [LDH], and aldolase) are always markedly elevated in DMD and are particularly high early in the course of the disease. Repeatedly normal serum CK levels are incompatible with the diagnosis. Values are usually over 5,000 milliunits/ml and values of 10000 or 15000 milliunits/ml are not unusual. EMG is always abnormal and shows a typical myopathic pattern with numerous short, small voluntary action potentials. However, EMG findings are in no way specific for this disease and merely show the effects of any severe chronic myopathy. Nerve conduction velocities are normal.

Muscle biopsy is useful in the diagnosis of DMD. The muscle to be biopsied should be a proximal muscle, preferably biceps or quadriceps, as artifacts from previous injections are less common than when deltoid and gluteus are used. The gastrocnemius should not be biopsied, since it is less affected than more proximal muscles when patients are walking and are undergoing initial diagnostic evaluation.

The pathologic changes in DMD are those of a chronic myopathy with increased connective tissue and fiber necrosis, hypertrophy, and atrophy. A typical pathologic change in DMD that is unusual in other disorders is the occurrence of necrotic and regenerating fibers in small groups.

Pitfalls in Diagnosis

Certain potential errors and pitfalls in diagnosis should be mentioned. When the first patient in a family with DMD comes to medical attention and the clinical findings indicate a myopathy, there might be some confusion with the childhood form of inflammatory myopathy, childhood dermatomyositis. This disease, in contrast to DMD, appears and progresses rapidly, and the history usually indicates perfectly normal development until several weeks or months before the patient presents with weakness. Also, a skin rash commonly is seen, which does not occur in DMD. The rash appears over the face and extensor surfaces of the joints, particularly the hands. In addition, CK level is usually elevated (200 to 1000 milliunits/ml but not as high as early in the course of DMD. The muscle biopsy also should help differentiate the two disorders; in inflammatory myopathy single-fiber necrosis is usual and inflammation is more common and more severe than in the occasional patient with DMD who has some inflammation. Perifascicular muscle atrophy found on biopsy, which is so common in childhood dermatomyositis, does not occur in muscular dystrophy.

Occasionally in a patient with DMD, pseudohypertrophy is mild and can best be appreciated by palpation, which will show abnormal firmness of the calf muscles. There may be superficial resemblance to any of the myopathies of childhood. Patients with congenital myopathies are commonly misdiagnosed as having muscular dystrophy. These myopathies are discussed elsewhere (see article on this topic) but are characterized by slowness or absence of progression, normal CK levels, and absence of contractures. Muscle biopsy will differentiate congenital myopathies from muscular dystrophy.

Early-onset juvenile spinal muscular atrophy (Kugelberg-Welander disease) may superficially resemble DMD as both conditions produce proximal weakness. This is an anterior horn cell disease, so EMG shows denervation and reinnervation, which is very different from the findings in DMD. CK level is normal or slightly increased. The biopsy results also are quite different in these two disorders.

In DMD and in the other muscular dystrophies a proper family history will give useful information. Only boys are affected in X-linked recessive dystrophies, of which DMD is the most common. Mothers and sisters may be carriers however. Spontaneous mutations occur, so that the mother is not necessarily a definite carrier if only one son has DMD. Carriers commonly have elevation of CK level in the serum and may even have abnormal EMG and biopsy results. The family history should include direct questioning about the patient's brothers and maternal uncles, as these are the members of the family likely to be affected. If other members of the family have had muscle disease, specific information on the clinical characteristics and muscle biopsies of the affected members should be obtained.

LIMB-GIRDLE MUSCULAR DYSTROPHY

This variety of muscular dystrophy is usually autosomal recessive, so that patients may have a negative family history. Differentiation from acquired myopathies may be difficult. The patients present with painless, slowly progressive proximal muscle weakness. Usually the weakness is mild when first noted and simply interferes with running, climbing, and rising from a low chair. Initial symptoms commonly appear in the third or fourth decade but the disease may begin at age 10 to 20 years or after the age of 40. A course of 20 to 30 years or even 40 years is not unusual, with patients becoming disabled after many years of muscle weakness. The disease is usually compatible with a normal life span but in more severe cases does limit life span, owing to involvement of respiratory muscles, which predisposes to pulmonary infection. The physical examination simply shows proximal muscle weakness and wasting. Contractures are rare and, as in DMD, tendon reflexes are usually spared. Pseudohypertrophy and facial weakness are not usually present. Laboratory procedures of specific help are determinations of serum sarcoplasmic enzyme levels (CK, LDH, and so forth), which are usually elevated but not as high as in DMD—CK is commonly 500 to 2000 milliunits/ml. EMG is also helpful in identifying the disorder as a myopathy, but no specific changes are noted. Also, muscle biopsy is always abnormal, but there are no specific pathologic changes in the muscle that allow a definitive diagnosis of limb-girdle dystrophy. The muscle is involved with a chronic myopathy. There is fiber hypertrophy, atrophy, necrosis, sarcolemmal nuclear proliferation, and, commonly, many bizarre necrotic forms. A potential error and pitfall in diagnosis lies in the differentiation of this form of muscular dystrophy (in which family history may be negative) from acquired myopathies, such as polymyositis or lipid and glycogen storage myopathies. Muscle biopsy may show diagnostic changes in the acquired myopathies, but limb-girdle dystrophy is a diagnosis of exclusion.

FACIOSCAPULOHUMERAL MUSCULAR DYSTROPHY

Facioscapulohumeral muscular dystrophy is an autosomal dominant disorder with a typical clinical presentation that is the most important feature in its recognition. All other aspects of this disease are nonspecific. The disorder involves both males and females equally, as it is dominantly inherited and, like other dominantly inherited neuromuscular diseases, it has a wide range of severity so that mildly affected patients may have offspring who are severely disabled. The facial muscles are involved, and patients have difficulty with whistling and usually weakness of eye closure and mouth retraction. Muscles that move and stabilize the shoulders are weak. Of all the muscular dystrophies, this is the most likely to have asymmetric muscle weakness and wasting. Unlike other myopathies, in the lower extremities the muscle first involved is the tibialis anterior, so some difficulty with heel walking is prominent when the disease is well established, and a neuropathic steppage-type gait may appear in advanced cases. The disease is generalized, although muscle weakness in the wrist and hand is unusual and proximal leg weakness is usually mild, so that ambulation is preserved except when the disease is severe or in late stages. The age of onset is highly variable, as it may present below the age of 10 years or as late as the fourth or fifth decade. In most cases the disorder is slowly progressive, but occasionally a patient is bedridden after a course of 10 or 15 years.

CK level is usually elevated to a degree similar to limb-girdle dystrophy, not as high as in DMD. EMG usually shows nonspecific myopathy. Inflammatory change may be prominent in muscle biopsy specimens so there may be confusion with a rare type of acquired inflammatory myopathy that has a facioscapulohumeral distribution.

The family history and examination of family members is most important, as mildly affected patients may be found who have inability to whistle, mild weakness of eye closure, or winging of one scapula. Mildly affected family members are usually unaware that they have any problem, and the family history may appear negative unless relatives are examined.

MYOTONIC MUSCULAR DYSTROPHY

Myotonic muscular dystrophy is also an autosomal dominant condition and, like facioscapulohumeral dystrophy, is marked by variation in severity. Patients usually present between the ages of 15 and 35 years complaining of trouble with their hands, which is due to the myotonic phenomenon of poor muscle relaxation after forceful contraction. When a tight fist is made, the patient experiences difficulty for several seconds in opening the fingers. Percussion of the thenar eminence will produce a sustained thumb contraction, but patients with far advanced weakness and wasting may not show this phenomenon. Usually the weakness is more severe distally in the hands and feet, but as the disease progresses all muscles become involved. Like facioscapulohumeral dystrophy, myotonic dystrophy usually has bifacial weakness as a prominent sign. Ptosis and ophthalmoplegia may occur. Fifteen per cent of babies born to women with myotonic dystrophy will have a congenital form of the disease and will have significiant muscle weakness, facial weakness, jaw deformity, and congenital hypotonia.

More than any other dystrophy, myotonic dystrophy involves nonmuscular tissues. The incidence of mental retardation is high, and other systemic abnormalities are common in both the congenital form and the form that appears during adult life. Low serum IgG values occur. Glucose intolerance is usual and is due to abnormal insulin production in response to a glucose load. Cataracts are common. Cardiac conduction abnormalities are also common complications and occasionally progress to complete heart block, which may cause sudden death. As in all severe chronic myopathies, involvement of respiratory muscles may occur and result in pneumonia. Unlike most dystrophies, tendon reflexes are usually depressed early in the course and absent when the disease is well established. Also quite different from the other common dystrophies, serum sarcoplasmic enzyme levels are either normal or only slightly increased.

Myotonic dystrophy, unlike other dystrophies, shows specific clinical features (percussion and grip myotonia) as well as specific findings on EMG, where the membrane abnormality of myotonia can be recorded, and on muscle biopsy, which shows characteristic changes. Muscle atrophy is the hallmark. Many fibers are so atrophic that only the nuclei remain. Long chains of nuclei may appear in longitudinal sections. Fiber necrosis is usually not prominent; this is reflected by the fact that the serum sarcoplasmic enzyme levels are either normal or only slightly elevated. Connective tissue is increased but not as much as in other dystrophies.

Pitfalls in Diagnosis

Pitfalls in diagnosis center on the fact that the phenomenon of myotonia is not specific for myotonic muscular dystrophy, although this is the most common disease in which myotonia occurs. A rare condition, Thomsen's disease, myotonia congenita, has prominent myotonia, of a more severe degree in proximal muscles rather than in the hands, but it is not associated with muscle weakness or wasting. In addition, the muscle biopsy does not show the abnormal changes noted earlier. Clinical myotonia may be seen in hyperkalemic periodic paralysis, and myotonia (by EMG only) can be seen in acid maltase deficiency, a glycogen storage myopathy that may appear in adult life. The myopathy of acid maltase deficiency is differentiated from myotonic muscular dystrophy by its proximal distribution of weakness, absence of clinical myotonia, and muscle biopsy findings that show numerous large vacuoles in fibers and reduction in acid maltase level when biochemical analysis of muscle tissue is performed. Since distal muscle weakness and wasting are prominent in myotonic dystrophy and tendon reflexes are reduced, there may be confusion with the most common dominantly inherited motor peripheral neuropathy, Charcot-Marie-Tooth (CMT) disease. Helpful distinctions are that in CMT facial weakness is rare, and ptosis and ophthalmoplegia are even rarer. Some sensory loss can usually be found in CMT and, most importantly, nerve conductions and EMG results differ. In CMT sensory nerve action potentials are absent or reduced in amplitude and motor nerve conduction velocities are usually reduced. However, a form of CMT exists in which nerve axons are affected rather than myelin so that the nerve conduction velocity may be normal. EMG provides the clearest difference—myotonia is not a feature of CMT and is present in hand muscles in myotonic dystrophy.

The congenital form of myotonic dystrophy, which appears in 10 to 15 per cent of children born to mothers with the disease, is difficult to diagnose by studying the patient. The mother must be examined and undergo EMG. Her disease may be so mild that a history alone may not reveal its presence. The congenital form presents as floppiness in the newborn, with a weak cry, poor sucking, and characteristic pursed lips. Clinical and EMG evidence of myotonia are not usually apparent in the infant in the first year, but they are present in the mother.

OTHER FORMS OF MUSCULAR DYSTROPHY

A more benign form of X-linked recessive dystrophy than the Duchenne type is *Becker's dystrophy.* It resembles DMD clinically in that there is hypertrophy of calves, marked elevation of enzyme levels, and progression; however, it appears later than DMD, at age 10 or 15 years, and progresses more slowly. *Oculopharyngeal muscular dystrophy* is a rare, usually dominantly inherited, late-life dystrophy presenting with difficulty in swallowing, ptosis, facial weakness, and ophthalmoplegia. It may be confused with myasthenia gravis. *Emery-Dreifuss humeroperoneal muscular dystrophy* is a rare X-linked recessive disease with contractures of posterior cervical muscles and elbow and Achilles tendons, as well as an atrial conduction abnormality that leads to complete heart block. Cardiac pacemaker insertion is necessary and ensures a normal or near-normal life span. *Scapuloperoneal dystrophy* is a disorder with prominent involvement of the upper arms and lower legs and may be autosomal dominant in inheritance. *Congenital muscular dystrophy* produces severe weakness, which appears at birth. It is differentiated from the more benign congenital myopathies by muscle biopsy and by clinical course.

DERMATOMYOSITIS AND POLYMYOSITIS

By Marcelo R. Olarte, M.D.
New York, New York

DEFINITION

Dermatomyositis is a clearly recognizable disease that is characterized by a typical skin rash and muscle weakness. The diagnosis is determined by the presence of the skin rash and acquired proximal myopathy with myopathic abnormalities of serum enzymes, muscle biopsy, and electrodiagnostic findings. Polymyositis is a syndrome with clinical and laboratory findings similar to those of dermatomyositis, but the rash is missing. The major of patients with dermatomyositis fall into two age groups: 5 to 15 years, and 45 to 60 years. Dermatomyositis is twice as frequent in females as in males.

Dermatomyositis at times (in 10 per cent of cases) is impossible to differentiate from scleroderma because of the presence of acrosclerosis and Raynaud's phenomenon. The pathogenesis of dermatomyositis and polymyositis is not known. It has been associated with malignancies, autoimmune diseases, viral illnesses, drugs, and toxic reactions.

SIGNS AND SYMPTOMS

The most important clinical signs are (1) symmetric weakness of limb-girdle muscles and neck flexors, developing in weeks or months, and limb weakness with or without respiratory muscle involvement, and (2) a skin rash that includes discoloration (described as "heliotrope" or violaceous) of the upper eyelids as well as erythema and edema of the face, anterior neck, torso, hands, knees, and elbows. There is also development of telangiectasia and Gottron's sign, consisting of erythema, scaling dermal atrophy, and dusky red patches or linear streaks over the knuckles. At times pruritus is a major problem, and bullous or ulcerative lesions may develop.

After a chronic course, skin lesions may be hyperpigmented or depigmented, and the affected skin becomes atrophic. In approximately one third of children and in a smaller percentage of adults subcutaneous calcifications occur in fingers, extensor joint surfaces, and buttocks. It might also involve fascial planes or erode through the skin. Calcinosis universalis (i.e., widespread) is common in dermatomyositis and is different from the calcinosis circumscripta (localized to the fingertips) of scleroderma.

There is proximal muscle involvement early in the course of the disease, characterized symptomatically by difficulty in climbing stairs, setting down in and rising from chairs, walking, running, and rising from a squatting position. Involvement of cranial nerves is rare and effects are usually restricted to swallowing; dysphagia occurs in 30 per cent of patients. There is usually no respiratory muscle involvement, and mechanical ventilation is usually not necessary.

At times there are also signs of systemic disease, with malaise, fever, muscle tenderness, weight loss, arthralgia, and hair loss. In children, gastrointestinal bleeding has been reported.

LABORATORY FINDINGS

An abnormal elevation of sarcoplasmic serum enzyme levels, especially creatine kinase (CK), serum glutamic-oxaloacetic transaminase (SGOT or aspartate aminotransferase, AST), serum glutamic-pyruvic transaminase (SGPT or alanine aminotransferase, ALT), aldolase, and lactate dehydrogenase (LD), occur, and enzyme measurements are helpful in making the diagnosis. CK is probably the most sensitive indicator of muscle inflammation, destruction, or abnormality of membrane permeability, but values may be normal in dermatomyositis or polymyositis, especially in the chronic stages. Abnormal muscle enzyme levels are not specific and elevations may also occur in denervating diseases (such as amyotrophic lateral sclerosis and peripheral neuropathy), muscular dystrophies, infections, hypothyroidism, sarcoidosis, and metabolic diseases of muscle (McArdle's disease, acid maltase deficiency).

The electrodiagnostic studies should be complete and should include motor and sensory nerve conduction velocities to exclude diseases of peripheral nerve or of anterior horn cells. Also, repetitive stimulation should be performed to exclude abnormalities of neuromuscular transmission (myasthenia gravis or Eaton-Lambert syndrome). Needle electromyography (EMG) should be performed on appropriate muscle groups, including paravertebral muscles. EMG changes during the acute stages of the disease include the classic triad of (1) polyphasic, short-duration, small motor units potentials, (2) fibrillations, positive sharp waves, and increased insertional activity, and (3) bizarre, high-frequency, repetitive discharges. The EMG may also be helpful in selecting the best site for biopsy. However, the site of needle penetration should not be chosen for biopsy because the needle tract may exhibit histologic changes similar to those of inflammatory myopathy.

Muscle biopsy is another important tool in the diagnosis of inflammatory myopathy. The abnormalities are varied and include necrosis of fibers, phagocytosis, and presence of regenerating fibers that are characterized by basophilia of the cytoplasm and large vesicular nuclei with prominent nucleoli. Also, there is an inflammatory cellular exudate, which may be restricted or widespread and is predominantly mononuclear. The process usually affects both Type I and Type II fibers, especially in a perifascicular distribution. If the disease is chronic, there is an increase in the endomysial or perimysial connective tissue, or of both, and replacement of muscle fibers by fat without inflammation. These changes may vary from patient to patient and also from one muscle to another. Some authors have even described changes ranging from normal findings to severe inflammation in the same specimen at different levels of section. At times calcifications occur, especially in the chronic stages.

A necrotizing vasculitis has been found in the childhood form of dermatomyositis and polymyositis, producing muscle infarction. It has been said that the myositis accompanying tumors is characterized by massive necrosis and minimal inflammation. Electron microscopy has sometimes shown intranuclear and intracytoplasmic inclusions resembling viral particles (myxovirus, picornavirus, and coxsackievirus). However, immunofluorescence, as well as animal and culture studies, have not added support to the theory of a viral basis for dermatomyositis. Polymyositis may result from infection with influenza virus or Toxoplasma.

Skin biopsies in dermatomyositis have shown nonspecific changes, at times similar to those found in systemic lupus erythematosus: poikiloderma, epidermal atrophy, basal cell layer degeneration, and vascular dilatation with perivascular lymphocytic or mononuclear infiltrates of the dermis. Mucin deposits resembling mucopolysaccharides have been found in involved and uninvolved skin. Other laboratory abnormalities include an elevated erythrocyte sedimentation rate and a diffuse increase in gamma globulin levels. Antinuclear antibodies, lupus erythematosus preparation and anti-DNA antibodies are usually negative except when the myopathy is part of the picture of mixed collagen-vascular disease.

ETIOLOGY AND PATHOGENESIS

Both dermatomyositis and polymyositis have been considered in the collagen-vascular category, and humoral or cellular mechanisms could be involved. There are reports of deposition in blood vessel walls of IgG, IgM, and the C3 portion of complement in patients with polymyositis and also in some with dermatomyositis.

Lymphocytes of patients with active polymyositis have been found to be cytotoxic to human muscle growth in culture.

In summary, it appears that cellular, humoral, or even viral factors could be involved in the pathogenesis of both diseases.

ASSOCIATED DISEASE

Dermatomyositis is associated with malignant neoplasia in about 10 per cent of cases, especially in patients older than 40 years of age. Virtually every tumor has been encountered, but especially cancer of the lung, stomach, prostate, breasts, and uterus. Some cases have improved after the removal of the tumor or appropriate chemotherapy. Polymyositis is commonly associated with collagen-vascular diseases, such as systemic lupus erythematosus, systemic sclerosis, rheumatoid arthritis, and Sjögren's syndrome.

COURSE AND PROGNOSIS

The myopathy of dermatomyositis is usually more severe and more likely to be fatal than that of polymyositis, especially if there is an associated malignancy, but if there is no tumor the course may be quite variable. It may be acute and fulminating, periodic with exacerbations and remission, or chronic and progressive, causing severe disability. In earlier trials one third of patients with dermatomyositis recovered, one third died, and one third were left with some disability. The mortality rate has not been clearly affected by the use of steroids, by antimicrobial therapy, or by caring for the patient in intensive care units. Death is usually due to respiratory failure, aspiration, and infection. Children have a better prognosis, but if the disease is associated with angiopathy the course may be severe.

COMPLICATIONS

Dermatomyositis and polymyositis may cause severe wasting, contractures, pain, disability, dysphagia, and respiratory insufficiency. In addition, dermatomyositis may be associated with painful calcinosis, abnormal gastrointestinal motility, and vascular lesions in skin, lungs, heart, liver, and kidneys. Therapeutic interventions with corticosteroids, immunosuppressants, or plasmapheresis may produce further complications, such as hypoglycemia, hypotension, sepsis, aseptic bone necrosis, hemorrhagic cystitis, and hypovolemia.

CRITERIA FOR THE DIAGNOSIS OF DERMATOMYOSITIS AND POLYMYOSITIS

To diagnose dermatomyositis a characteristic skin rash should be present. If this is lacking, the diagnosis of polymyositis should be made. The following points are common to the clinical diagnosis of both diseases:

1. The weakness develops in weeks or months (not years).
2. There should be proximal weakness and often dysphagia.
3. Muscle pain and tenderness occur in many but not all cases.
4. Laboratory findings should include "myopathic" EMG, "myopathic" findings on muscle biopsy, and increased serum enzyme levels.

CRITERIA SUGGESTIVE OF DIAGNOSES OTHER THAN DERMATOMYOSITIS AND POLYMYOSITIS

Patients showing the following features may have other conditions and should be investigated further:

1. Positive family history.
2. Cranial muscle abnormalities, especially involving the ocular muscles, and a response to anticholinesterase medication (edrophonium).
3. Overt endocrine disorders (thyroid, adrenal, parathyroid).
4. Specific biochemical disorders (of acid maltase, phosphorylase, or phosphofructokinase deficiency).

DIFFERENTIAL DIAGNOSIS

Dermatomyositis usually does not present diagnostic problems because of the characteristic rash and proximal muscle weakness. However, drug reactions, trichinosis, systemic lupus erythematosus, toxoplasmosis, mixed connective tissue disease, and pellagra may mimic dermatomyositis. Muscle biopsy and careful evaluation usually clarify the diagnosis.

The differential diagnosis of polymyositis is more complex because numerous illnesses cause proximal muscle weakness in association with other signs and symptoms. Among these are the following:

1. Infections: trichinosis, toxoplasmosis, schistosomiasis, cysticercosis, and influenza.
2. Toxins and drugs: alcohol, steroids, chloroquine, emetine, penicillamine, and azathioprine.
3. Endocrine disorders: hyper- or hypothyroidism, Cushing's disease, hyper-and hypoparathyroidism.
4. Collagen-vascular disease, in which the muscle weakness is part of the clinical picture (systemic lupus erythematosus, scleroderma, and mixed collagen-vascular disease).
5. Muscular dystrophy, especially the limb-girdle or the facioscapulohumeral type, in which the biopsy specimen sometimes shows inflammatory changes and the onset of symptoms is between the ages of 15 and 30 years.
6. Myopathy associated with thymoma, sarcoidosis, amyloidosis, plasma cell dyscrasia, malabsorption, and chronic renal disease.

ENDOCRINE MYOPATHIES

By Linton C. Hopkins, M.D.
Atlanta, Georgia

DEFINITION

Endocrine myopathies are syndromes of skeletal muscle weakness that are associated with endocrine diseases. They require no treatment other than correction of the underlying medical disorder.

The disorders that will be discussed in this article are the myopathies of hyperthyroidism, hypothyroidism, hyperparathyroidism, Addison's disease, and corticosteroid excess, both naturally occurring (in Cushing's disease) and due to the administration of corticosteroids.

SIGNS AND SYMPTOMS

Although the clinical manifestations of the underlying endocrine diseases are quite different, the signs and symptoms of skeletal muscle involvement are similar. They all produce painless proximal muscle weakness. With the exception of hypothyroidism, in which the serum creatine kinase (CK) level and that of other serum sarcoplasmic enzymes are usually elevated, enzyme levels are normal. Moreover, the most useful diagnostic procedures in muscle disease, electromyography (EMG) and muscle biopsy, do not show specific changes. The diagnosis of these disorders depends on the recognition by the physican that significant muscle weakness may be a major manifestation of commonly encountered endocrine disease. These treatable disorders should, therefore, be considered whenever proximal muscle weakness is encountered.

This brief discussion in no way reflects the importance of these disorders. When mild muscle weakness is considered, the endocrine neuropathies are among the most common of all neuromuscular diseases and are gratifying to diagnose and treat.

THE MYOPATHY OF HYPERTHYROIDISM

When mild weakness, fatigue, and performance of stressful physical tasks are considered, thyrotoxic myopathy is found to occur in most patients with hyperthyroidism. The clinical manifestations are simply those of proximal muscle weakness that is painless. Tendon reflexes are preserved or brisk, and proximal muscle wasting also occurs as a manifestation of the weight loss that usually accompanies this condition. Occasionally the skeletal muscle weakness and wasting may be severe and limit ability to walk. In elderly patients with apathetic hyperthyroidism, the myopathy dominates the clinical picture. As in any myopathy, patients experience difficulty rising from a low chair and climbing or descending stairs.

Enlargement and weakness of extraocular muscles occur in patients who have thyrotoxic exophthalmos. Upward gaze is more affected, though lateral and downward gaze may also be reduced. Facial weakness is unusual.

There is an association between myasthenia gravis and thyrotoxicosis. Only 0.5 to 1 per cent of patients with hyperthyroidism will also have myasthenia gravis, but of patients with myasthenia gravis, approximately 5 per cent will have hyperthyroidism. If the two diseases coexist, their symptoms and signs are additive. A patient with known hyperthyroidism who develops fluctuating ophthalmoparesis, fluctuating skeletal muscle weakness, weakness of swallowing, and weakness of muscles that control speech should have appropriate diagnostic studies to exclude myasthenia gravis. These include an edrophonium chloride (Tensilon) test, repetitive nerve stimulation, conventional EMG, and possibly single-fiber EMG.

Patients with thyrotoxicosis may have episodes of flaccid, areflectic muscle paralysis with either normal or reduced serum potassium level. Any patient being evaluated for periodic paralysis should have thyroid function tests performed.

Laboratory Tests

Laboratory procedures directed at analysis of skeletal muscle function usually yield nonspecific results. Levels of serum sarcoplasmic enzymes (CK, serum glutamic-oxaloacetic transaminase, lactate dehydrogenase, and aldolase) are normal. EMG is usually normal or mildly abnormal and is nonspecific. There may be reduction in the mean duration of voluntary motor unit potentials. Muscle biopsy is also abnormal but likewise is nonspecific. Atrophy of both types of muscle fibers is usually all that is present.

HYPOTHYROID MYOPATHY

As in hyperthyroidism, most patients with hypothyrodism have some abnormality of skeletal muscle. When their strength is compared to post-treatment levels, some skeletal muscle weakness can be appreciated in retrospect. Usually signs and symptoms of myxedema, such as lassitude and weight gain, predominate. Occasionally severe proximal myopathy with inability to walk occurs as a manifestation of hypothyroidism. Tendon reflexes are depressed and have a slow relaxation phase. The myopathy is usually painless, but occasionally patients have painful muscle spasms (Hoffmann's syndrome). Facial muscles and extraocular muscles are not weak in hypothyroid myopathy.

Laboratory Tests

Serum levels of sarcoplasmic enzymes (CK and others) are usually elevated in hypothyroidism even when there is no weakness and may be quite high in patients with significant myopathy. CK values may rise to several thousand milliunits per milliliter. Electromyography is usually very abnormal in hypothyroidism but shows nonspecific myopathy. Voluntary motor unit potentials are decreased in mean duration, as in any severe myopathy. Muscle biopsy is a useful but also nonspecific study in patients with hypothyroid myopathy. Fiber necrosis is common, and increase in endomysial connective tissue is usually seen. Inflammatory change is usually not present.

Differential Diagnosis

The most difficult differential diagnostic problem in patients with hypothyroid myopathy is distinguishing it from other acquired myopathies. As EMG and biopsy are nonspecific in hypothyroid myopathy, the differential diagnosis rests on the physician's being alert to the possibility of systemic hypothyroidism so that specific thyroid function tests will be performed whenever myopathy appears. Occasionally a patient with mild abnormalities of thyroid function will have significant myopathy, and differentiation from acquired inflammatory myopathy (polymyositis and other conditions) may be particularly difficult, especially when it is recognized that 25 per cent of patients with polymyositis and other inflammatory myopathies will not have evidence of inflammation on a muscle biopsy. Occasionally in these patients the diagnosis rests on the response of the patient to either replacement therapy with thyroid hormone or a trial of corticosteriods, which will not improve thyroid myopathy but may result in improvement in patients with inflammatory myopathy.

THE MYOPATHY OF HYPERPARATHYROIDISM

Both patients with primary hyperparathyroidism who have parathyroid adenomas and patients with secondary hyperparathyroidism may develop a similar muscle weakness syndrome, which is very nonspecific and marked simply by painless proximal muscle weakness and wasting. Reflexes are usually preserved. Facial and extraocular muscles are not involved.

Laboratory studies reveal normal sarcoplasmic enzymes levels, a normal or mildly myopathic EMG and atrophy of Type II muscle fibers on muscle biopsy. The diagnosis rests on the finding of an elevated serum calcium, reduced serum phosphorus, and elevated alkaline phosphatase, which should lead to specific parathyroid function tests and the proper diagnosis.

ADDISON'S DISEASE

Addison's disease, or hypoadrenalism, invariably produces muscle weakness and fatigue. Occasionally these symptoms predominate. The muscle syndrome is entirely nonspecific, however, and consists simply of mild proximal muscle weakness. The patients usually complain of difficulty in rising from a low chair and in climbing or descending stairs. Reflexes are usually preserved.

Laboratory studies are nonspecific in this disorder as well. Serum levels of sarcoplasmic enzymes are usually normal, and EMG and muscle biopsy findings are nonspecific. EMG is normal or shows mild myopathic change and muscle biopsy, when abnormal, usually shows nonspecific muscle atrophy The findings of an active myopathy, muscle cell necrosis, and connective tissue proliferation are not usually present in the myopathy of Addison's disease.

The diagnosis rests upon the physician's recognition of other symptoms and signs of Addison's disease.

THE MYOPATHY OF CUSHING'S SYNDROME AND STEROID MYOPATHY

As in other endocrine disorders, most patients with Cushing's syndrome have some muscle weakness and wasting when efforts are made to compare their premorbid strength to their muscle power at the time of presentation. Occasionally a patient may complain of weakness as the primary complaint. The syndrome is entirely nonspecific and consists of difficulty in rising from chairs or in descending or ascending stairs. Reflexes are preserved and, as in any other myopathy, there are no sensory findings. Facial and extraocular muscles are not clinically involved.

Laboratory studies show normal serum levels of sarcoplasmic enzymes, and EMG and muscle biopsy are both nonspecific. EMG is normal or shows mild myopathy, and the muscle biopsy change is that of type II muscle fiber atrophy.

In iatrogenic steroid myopathy, painless proximal muscle weakness and wasting are the only clinical abnormalities. The exact dose required to produce muscle weakness has not been determined, but the higher the dose the more likely the myopathy. The elderly are particularly sensitive to the effects of steroid hormones. Gluteus and quadriceps muscles become involved and weak after several weeks of high-dose prednisone therapy in many elderly patients. This limits ambulation and leads to instability ascending or descending stairs and to a tendency to fall, which is a distressing complication, particularly in elderly patients. The diagnosis should be suspected in any patient on steroids who develops proximal muscle weakness. Deep tendon reflexes are usually preserved. Facial and extraocular muscles are not involved.

Laboratory studies show normal levels of sarcoplasmic enzymes, and EMG is normal or mildly abnormal and shows mild reduction in duration of voluntary potentials, as in any other myopathy. Increased insertional activity, or fibrillation potentials, usually are not present or are present only rarely. Muscle biopsy findings are usually abnormal but nonspecific and show atrophy of Type II or fast-twitch muscle fibers.

Pitfalls in Diagnosis

The major pitfall in diagnosis is differentiating muscle weakness resulting from steroid therapy from muscle weakness caused by the underlying disorder for which steroids are being taken. The diagnosis is not difficult if the disorder being treated does not cause weakness, but it is a problem if a myopathy or chronic neuropathy is the underlying disease. This differential diagnosis is usually made by correlation of the clinical course of the weakness and CK level with the level of the steroid dose. The underlying clinical condition may initially improve on steroid therapy, but if with continuation of the drug muscle weakness returns, steroid myopathy is a major consideration. The diagnosis is less difficult if the disorder being treated is characterized by elevated levels of CK and other sarcoplasmic enzymes in the serum. As steroid myopathy does not produce elevation in the level of these enzymes, a patient whose strength is deteriorating while the muscle enzyme levels are falling is likely to have steroid myopathy. EMG and muscle biopsy do not help in this differential diagnosis if the underlying disorder being treated with steroids produces myopathic EMG changes and Type II muscle fiber atrophy. In muscle disease the most common disorder to be differentiated is inflammatory myopathy or polymyositis. Repeat muscle biopsy has been advocated as a way of telling the difference but, as the sample of muscle tissue taken is small and Type II muscle fiber atrophy occurs in both disorders, an accurate distinction cannot usually be made in this way. It is best to simply consider the clinical course of the weakness, the serum sarcoplasmic enzyme levels, and the steroid dose over time; make a decision; and either increase or decrease the steroid dose. The clinical response of the muscle strength will then allow differentiation between steroid myopathy and progression of the underlying disease.

THE PERIODIC PARALYSES

By Robert C. Griggs, M.D.
Rochester, New York

SUBGROUPS AND SYNONYMS

Hypokalemic periodic paralysis, hyperkalemic periodic paralysis (myotonic periodic paralysis), paramyotonia congenita.

DEFINITION

The periodic paralyses are a group of disorders, often inherited in an autosomal dominant fashion, in which attacks of episodic weakness occur. The term periodic paralysis is usually reserved for those conditions without a demonstrable definable underlying, metabolic disorder.

Table 1 lists a tentative classification of the periodic paralyses. Periodic paralysis is often divided into two broad categories: hypokalemic and hyperkalemic. However, it is only for hypokalemic periodic paralysis that a clear temporal relationship of attacks to alteration in potassium levels is demonstrable. Potassium level almost invariably falls during an attack. Such is not the case for hyperkalemic periodic paralysis, since potassium is not always elevated during attacks but may be normal or even low and may be high at times when no attack occurred. So-called normokalemic periodic paralysis is in most instances so similar to hyperkalemic periodic paralysis that it is not advisable to make a distinction between the disorders.

Attacks of thyrotoxic periodic paralysis are associated with hypokalemia and are similar in most respects to the attacks of hypokalemic periodic paralysis. Thyrotoxic periodic paralysis differs from hypokalemic periodic paralysis in that it typically occurs sporadically. The liability to develop thyrotoxic periodic paralysis, however, may be transmitted in an autosomal dominant fashion.

Thyrotoxic periodic paralysis is typically said to occur more frequently in Orientals, although there are many reports of thyrotoxic periodic paralysis occurring in members of other races. The age of onset of initial attacks of periodic paralysis in thyrotoxic periodic paralysis is higher than in hypokalemic periodic paralysis, since the majority of patients with thyrotoxic periodic paralysis experience their first attack between the ages of 20 and 30 years (versus the time of puberty for the hypokalamic variety). There is a marked male predominance in thyrotoxic periodic paralysis (20:1).

Paramyotonia congenita is characterized by paradoxical myotonia (i.e., myotonia that worsens with repeated activity), which is markedly exacerbated by cold; flaccid paresis of muscle on prolonged exposure to cold; and occasional attacks of generalized weakness unassociated with exposure to cold. Two subgroups of paramyotonia have been recognized (Table 1), and patients must be challenged with potassium and glucose-insulin (see later discussion) to adequately classify the disease. Treatment of these two subgroups is distinctly different.

Table 1. Classification of Periodic Paralysis

Hypokalemic
Familial and sporadic
Thyrotoxic
Hyperkalemic (potassium-sensitive): Includes myotonic periodic paralysis
Familial and sporadic
Paramyotonia with periodic paralysis
Paramyotonia congenita
Paralysis periodica paramyotonia

PRESENTING SIGNS AND SYMPTOMS

All types of periodic paralyses have some similar features, even though the terms hypokalemic and hyperkalemic suggest that the two disorders ought to be markedly different. It is largely the response to agents affecting potassium levels that clearly distinguishes the two disorders. Thus, all types of periodic paralysis usually present within the first three decades, are more severe in males, and are associated with myotonic phenomena. Attacks often occur on awakening and tend to take place following the rest period after exercise. When a family history can be established, an autosomal dominant inheritance pattern is usual. Hypokalemic periodic paralysis is frequently sporadic, with hyperkalemic periodic paralysis only rarely so.

Distinguishing clinical features of the periodic paralyses include the earlier age of onset of hyperkalemic periodic paralysis, in which diagnosis is often evident in the first year of life. The age of onset of hypokalemic periodic paralysis is characteristically near the time of puberty. Myotonic phenomena are often severe in hyperkalemic periodic paralysis and paramyotonia congenita. In hypokalemic periodic paralysis myotonic lid lag may be prominent, but other clinical evidence of myotonia is rare; electromyographically demonstrated myotonia is not evident.

The severity and duration of an attack are usually greater in hypokalemic periodic paralysis than in other forms of periodic paralysis. Total quadriplegia and respiratory involvement may occur, and attacks can last as long as 24 hours, occasionally even longer. Attacks of hyperkalemic periodic paralysis tend to be brief (usually 1 to 4 hours) and less severe. Attacks of hyperkalemic periodic paralysis are often associated with paresthesias, and Chvostek's sign is frequently present during the attack. Eye movements are spared in all forms of periodic paralysis. Attacks of hypokalemic periodic paralysis are often provoked by high-carbohydrate diets or sodium-containing foods, whereas hyperkalemic periodic paralysis is often triggered by fasting.

COURSE

In all forms of periodic paralysis, frequency of attacks tends to diminish with age. All forms have in common, however, the occurrence of progressive muscle weakness after a decade or more of attacks. The treatment and prevention of attacks has diminished this disabling problem.

COMPLICATIONS

Substantial cardiac involvement is uncommon in all forms of periodic paralysis, but significant arrhythmias can occur in either hypokalemic or hyperkalemic periodic paralysis. Thyrotoxicosis is associated with arrhythmias, and there may be a slightly greater risk of arrhythmia in thyrotoxic periodic paralysis. Respiratory failure is rare in all forms, even in severe attacks. Respiratory paralysis has occurred only in the hypokalemic form of periodic paralysis, and at least in some instances may have been the result of injudicious treatment with intravenous fluids.

PHYSICAL EXAMINATION

During attack-free intervals, examination of patients often gives normal results. The only finding to be anticipated in hypokalemic periodic paralysis is lid myotonia. Patients with hyperkalemic periodic paralysis may have more widespread myotonia, including grip, wrist percussion, and thenar percussion myotonia. Patients who have had frequent untreated attacks for more than 5 years may have persistent weakness *between* attacks. This weakness is particularly prominent in neck flexor and hip flexor muscles. After many years, a picture simulating limb-girdle muscular dystrophy can develop.

LABORATORY PROCEDURES AND DIAGNOSTIC EVALUATION

Most patients presenting with a history of episodic weakness do not have a primary periodic paralysis. When patients are first examined it is important to exclude secondary causes of paralysis, the most common of which are listed in Table 2. A good general rule is that patients presenting with episodic weakness after the age of 30 years probably have a secondary rather than primary periodic paralysis.

The importance of adequately studying the patient during an episode cannot be overemphasized. Serial electrolyte levels, electrocardiography, and glucose levels, as well as repeated examination of strength by both formal and functional testing, should be performed or determined. Muscle stretch reflexes and the presence or absence of myotonia should be determined.

Table 2. Some Disorders Secondarily Causing Episodic Paralysis

Hypokalemic Disorders
Primary hyperaldosteronism (Conn's syndrome)
Renal tubular acidosis—primary
Renal tubular acidosis—secondary to amphotericin B, toluene abuse
Juxtaglomerular apparatus hyperplasia (Bartter's syndrome)
Villous adenoma
Alcoholism
Diuretics, licorice, corticosteroids
Hyperkalemic Disorders
Addison's disease
Chronic renal failure
Hyporeninemic hypoaldosteronism
Recurrent rhabdomyolysis (e.g., McArdle's syndrome)
Disorders Without Change in Potassium Level
Sleep paralysis associated with narcolepsy
Myasthenia gravis
Eaton-Lambert syndrome
Multiple sclerosis
Transient ischemic attacks
Hypocalcemic tetany

Unfortunately, most patients with complaints of periodic weakness are not encountered during an attack, and provocative testing is necessary unless the patient is having frequent attacks or an attack can be precipitated with diet or activity change. The patient having provocative maneuvers should not be taking prophylactic medication and should not have significant coincident illness, such as cardiac or renal disease or diabetes. Small children require modifications of the procedures to be described. The order in which provocative testing is done depends on the index of suspicion for each disorder. Each test must be done on a separate day, and during loading tests the *electrocardiogram, muscle strength,* and *electrolytes* should be evaluated sequentially. The examiner must be prepared to terminate the test immediately if weakness or arrhythmia appears.

Hypokalemic Periodic Paralysis. Hypokalemic attacks may be precipitated by the administration of oral glucose, 1.5 gm/kg body weight (up to 100 gm). If no weakness is produced, on a subsequent day 1.5 to 3.0 gm/kg glucose may be administered intravenously over 60 minutes. Giving intravenous insulin (maximum 0.1 U/kg body weight at 30 and 60 minutes) during the infusion may aid in precipitating attacks. Maximum lowering of potassium level is seen 90 to 150 minutes after initiation of the test. Hypoglycemia often occurs 15 to 60 minutes following completion of glucose and insulin administration and must be anticipated. The administration of this amount of glucose can cause marked alteration in blood volume and osmolality, and *the test must be performed with caution.*

Hyperkalemic Periodic Paralysis. Oral potassium loading with 0.05 to 0.15 gm/kg body weight potassium chloride may precipitate weakness in patients with hyperkalemic periodic paralysis and in certain patients with paramyotonia. Myotonia may also be worsened. Oral loading should begin with the minimum amount before proceeding to larger doses. The maximum rise in circulating level of potassium following administration of potassium chloride occurs at 90 to 180 minutes. Diabetes and renal disease are contraindications to large potassium loads.

Since weakness may occasionally occur with glucose and insulin challenge in hyperkalemic periodic paralysis as well as in paramyotonia congenita, the majority of patients require both hypokalemic and hyperkalemic challenges.

Paramyotonia Congenita. Cold provocation (see later description) is usually adequate to confirm this diagnosis, but subclassification usually requires provocative tests with glucose and insulin, and with potassium. Glucose (and insulin) loading will produce weakness in true paramyotonia congenita, whereas potassium loading will produce weakness in paralysis periodica paramyotonia.

OTHER DIAGNOSTIC PROCEDURES

Careful evaluation for secondary causes of weakness and periodic paralysis, such as thyrotoxicosis (see

Table 2), is essential. Electromyography is often helpful in distinguishing hyperkalemic periodic paralysis or paramyotonia congenita from hypokalemic periodic paralysis. Myotonic discharges are seen only in hyperkalemic periodic paralysis and paramyotonia congenita, not in hypokalemic periodic paralysis.

Muscle biopsy is often indicated in the evaluation of patients with periodic paralysis when the diagnosis remains unclear, particularly in mild cases. In all types of periodic paralyses, vacuoles may be present in muscle fibers both during attacks and during attack-free intervals.

Cold provocation of weakness may be indicated for patients suspected of having paramyotonia congenita. Such patients will develop localized weakness after immersion of the hand in water at 10°C for 5 minutes. It should be stressed that myotonia will be worsened by cold and that it is the development of weakness, not stiffness, that distinguishes the patient with paramyotonia congenita.

THERAPEUTIC TESTS

Although it is essential to establish a diagnosis prior to initiating long-term treatment,the therapeutic response of patients with documented hypokalemia or hyperkalemia during an attack of paralysis may be of confirmatory value. The attacks of hypokalemic periodic paralysis are usually shortened by administration of oral KCl. Subsequent attacks often are not prevented, however, by even large prophylactic doses of potassium regardless of the schedule of such treatment. Treatment of presumed potassium-sensitive attacks with oral carbohydrate may be of confirmatory value.

POTENTIAL ERRORS AND PITFALLS IN DIAGNOSIS

Many patients whose symptoms suggest a periodic paralysis prove to have a negative evaluation for the disorders and for secondary causes of paralysis. Rarely a patient may have an undefined disorder that could be considered a "normokalemic" form of periodic paralysis. (Most such patients in the past have actually been shown to have a potassium-sensitive form of periodic paralysis.) A much larger subset of patients with negative evaluations give a history of episodic weakness but in fact do not have true *weakness,* but instead have *fatigue.* Such patients frequently defy specific categorization. Long-term follow-up in such cases usually does not disclose a cause for the symptoms. I have not known patients whose diagnostic and provocative tests were negative to subsequently be proved to have a periodic paralysis.

MYOGLOBINURIA AND MYOPATHY OF STORAGE DISEASE

By Salvatore DiMauro, M.D.
New York, New York

Disorders of glycogen or lipid metabolism of muscle cause two main syndromes (Fig. 1):

1. Acute, recurrent, reversible muscle dysfunction with myoglobinuria (with or without cramps) is characteristic of phosphorylase, phosphofructokinase (PFK), phosphoglycerate kinase (PGK), phosphoglycerate mutase (PGAM), and lactate dehydrogenase (LDH) deficiencies among the glycogenoses, and of carnitine palmitoyltransferase (CPT) deficiency among the disorders of lipid metabolism.

2. Progressive weakness is associated with acid maltase, debrancher, and brancher deficiencies among the glycogenoses, and with carnitine deficiency and other biochemically undefined lipid storage myopathies among the disorders of lipid metabolism.

METABOLIC DISORDERS CAUSING RECURRENT MYOGLOBINURIA

Myoglobinuria

Myoglobinuria, the presence of the muscle pigment myoglobin in the urine, is a symptom common to several disorders of different cause and is the consequence of acute muscle necrosis. During severe attacks, there is a characteristic discoloration of the urine, most often described by the patients as cola-colored. This is usually preceded (by 30 minutes to a few hours) by the onset of a variably severe but always rather dramatic clinical picture characterized by pain, tenderness, swelling, and weakness, either confined to certain muscle groups or generalized, but usually sparing facial and extraocular muscles. Involvement of respiratory muscles may require assisted ventilation. Acute tubular necrosis and renal insufficiency may occur; if not, complete spontaneous recovery of muscle function takes place in a matter of days or weeks. Although the association of acute muscle symptoms and pigment in the urine is characteristic, the diagnosis of myoglobinuria is often missed when the presentation is less dramatic. In some cases, muscle symptoms may be very mild and pigment may not be overtly present in the urine. Besides documentation of myoglobin in the urine and demonstration of greatly increased myoglobin concentration in serum, measurement of muscle enzymes in serum, particularly creatine kinase (CK), is a simple and important laboratory test. Serum levels of CK above 10,000 IU/liter in a patient with acute muscle symptoms is virtually diagnostic of myoglobinuria, even when a gross degree of pigment in the urine has not been noticed. Electrophoretic demonstration that the serum CK is represented predominantly or exclusively by the isoenzyme MM (typical of striated muscle), and the lack of clinical or ECG signs of heart involvement, help differentiate myoglobinuria from myocardial infarction.

Myoglobinuria is distinguished from hemoglobinuria by the sensitive and highly specific demonstration of myoglobin in urine and serum by radioimmunoassay as well as by the finding of a normal serum concentration of haptoglobin.

The most important *complication* of myoglobinuria is acute tubular necrosis, often leading to renal insufficiency. Dehydration and acidosis may contribute to cause renal failure. Urinary output should be carefully monitored in patients with myoglobinuria, adequate diuresis should be promoted, and, if necessary, hemodialysis should be provided.

Although *recurrent familial myoglobinuria* strongly suggests an underlying hereditary defect of muscle metabolism, it is important to remember that there are many causes of myoglobinuria besides metabolic myopathies. These include *strenuous exercise* in untrained individuals, particularly in hot weather, such as occurs in boot camp; *chronic alcoholism,* in which repeated episodes may follow weekend drinking binges; other *toxic agents,* including drugs (such as licorice or clofibrate) or animal poisons (for example, the exquisitely myotoxic poison of the Malayan sea snake); *infectious agents,* particularly influenza A virus; *trauma,* such as crush syndromes, sometimes caused by the weight of the patient's own body during states of deep coma; *other genetic diseases* of unknown cause, such as the autosomal dominant malignant hyperthermia (MH) syndrome.

When the cause of recurrent myoglobinuria is suspected to be one of the metabolic myopathies listed in Figure 1, several clues to the differential diagnosis may be derived from the clinical picture and from routine and provocative laboratory tests (Table 1).

Precipitating Factors. In patients with glycogenoses, myoglobinuria is always preceded by *exercise.* Although the type and amount of exertion needed to precipitate myoglobinuria may vary from patient to patient and even in the same patient from day to day, two forms of exercise are more commonly involved: (1) brief exercise of high intensity, such as carrying a heavy load, or (2) less intense but sustained activity, such as walking uphill. In CPT deficiency, exercise is a common but not obligatory cause of myoglobinuria. Also, in contrast to patients with glycogenoses, brief intense exercise is well tolerated by patients with CPT deficiency, whereas myoglobinuria is precipitated by prolonged although not necessarily intense exercise, such as long hikes. *Fasting* alone or in association with exercise is a very common precipitating factor in CPT deficiency, but it is never implicated in the glycogenoses. *Cramps* (that is, painful involuntary muscle shortening often manifested by "knotting" or swelling of affected muscles) are very common and often the sole complaint of patients with glycogenoses. Cramps are induced by exercise and precede myoglobinuria, thus representing a useful warning signal. In contrast, cramps are not a feature of CPT deficiency; patients do complain of muscle tightness and pain after prolonged exercise and during episodes of myglobinuria, but they do not describe real cramps. *Fixed weakness,* usually of moderate severity, may be

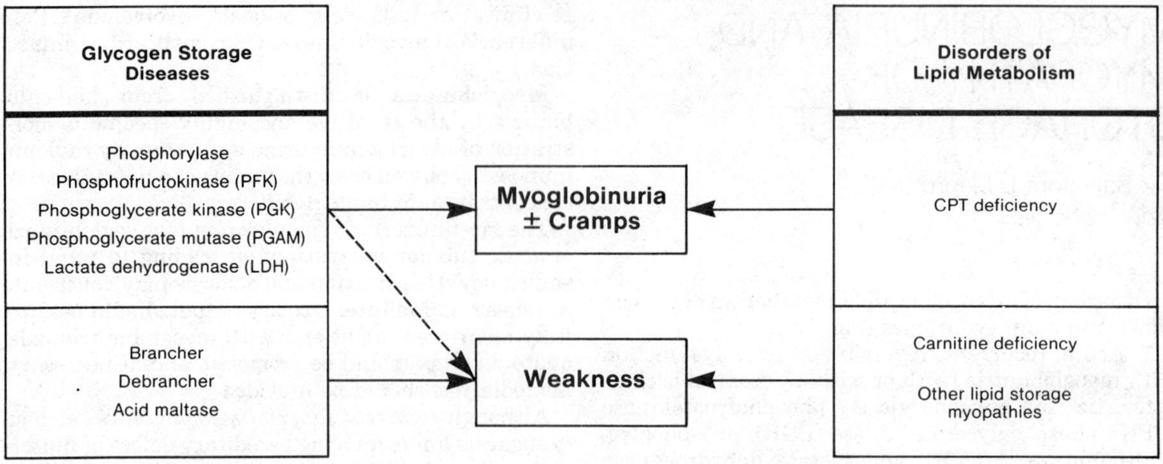

Figure 1. The main syndromes caused by disorders of glycogen or lipid metabolism of muscle. CPT=Carnitine palmitoyltransferase.

present outside episodes of myoglobinuria in patients with glycogen storage disease, especially with phosphorylase deficiency (McArdle's disease), whereas it is not seen in patients with CPT deficiency.

Routine Laboratory Tests. *Serum CK* level is often increased interictally in patients with glycogenoses, but not in those with CPT deficiency.

Electromyography (EMG) often shows mild myopathic features in patients with glycogenoses; results are usually normal in CPT-deficient patients. EMG of shortened muscles during cramps in patients with glycogenoses shows electrical silence (i.e., the cramps are contractures in a physiologic sense).

Provocative Tests. The *forearm ischemic exercise* is a simple and useful diagnostic tool in the identification of blocks of glycogen breakdown or glycolysis, which include not only all the glycogenoses causing cramps and recurrent myoglobinuria but also debrancher deficiency (Fig. 1). Thus, the test is *not* specific for any single enzyme defect.

I use the following protocol: an indwelling needle is placed in an superficial antecubital vein and a basal sample of blood is taken. A sphygmomanometer cuff is placed above the elbow and inflated above arterial pressure. The patient is asked to squeeze another rolled-up sphygmomanometer cuff repeatedly and vigorously enough to push the mercury column to the top of the scale. After 1 minute of exercise, the cuff around the arm is deflated and blood samples are drawn 1, 3, 6, and 10 minutes thereafter. In normal individuals, threefold to fivefold increase in lactate is seen in the first two samples, but levels gradually return to baseline values in the following specimens. In patients with phosphorylase or PFK deficiency, there is virtually no rise in lactate level; in patients with PGK, PGAM, and LDH deficiencies there may be a small increase of lactate level (1.5 or 2 times). An important limitation of this test is that the rise of venous lactate level depends on the ability and willingness of the patient to exercise vigorously; false-positive results may be obtained in weak or uncooperative patients. If a flat lactate response is obtained in an individual who does not seem weak, it is prudent to repeat the test, encouraging the patient to exercise to the best of his

Table 1. Metabolic Myopathies with Myoglobinuria: Differential Clinical and Laboratory Features

	Enzyme Defect	
	PPL, PFK, PGK, PGAM, LDH	*CPT*
Factors precipitating myoglobinuria	Intense exercise	Prolonged exercise Fasting No apparent cause
Cramps ("contractures")	+	−
Fixed weakness	±	−
Increased serum CK level at rest	±	−
Abnormal forearm ischemic exercise	+	−
Prolonged fasting:		
Increase of serum CK level	−	+
Decreased production of ketone bodies	−	+

Abbreviations: PPL = Phosphorylase; PFK = phosphofructokinase; PGK = phosphoglycerate kinase; PGAM = phosphoglycerate mutase; LDH = lactate dehydrogenase; CPT = carnitine palmitoyltransferase; CK = creatine kinase.

or her ability. The forearm ischemic exercise gives normal results in patients with CPT deficiency.

Fasting at rest (with the patient resting in bed in a clinical research center) for up to 72 hours may cause two types of abnormalities in patients with CPT deficiency: (1) absent or deficient rise of ketone bodies in the blood (reflecting involvement of the liver by the enzyme defect), and (2) increase of serum CK level (reflecting abnormal dependence of muscle on carbohydrate metabolism). Each abnormal result, however, is seen only in about one half of patients. Because prolonged fasting may cause severe myoglobinuria in patients with CPT deficiency, the fast should be conducted in a hospital and serum CK level should be monitored at frequent intervals.

Phosphorylase Deficiency (McArdle's Disease; Glycogenosis Type V)

Phosphorylase deficiency is an autosomal recessive myopathy caused by a genetic defect of the muscle isoenzyme of glycogen phosphorylase. There is a 2:1 predominance of males over females. Intolerance of strenuous exercise is present from childhood, but presentation is usually in adolescence with cramps after exercise. Myoglobinuria occurs in about one half of patients. If they avoid intense exercise, most patients can live normal lives; however, about one third of them develop some degree of fixed weakness, usually as a late-onset manifestation of the disease. In a few patients, weakness instead of exercise-related cramps and myoglobinuria characterizes the clinical picture.

In patients with myoglobinuria, renal insufficiency is a possible life-threatening complication. Physical examination between episodes of myoglobinuria may be completely normal or show some degree of weakness and, occasionally, wasting of some muscle groups.

Laboratory Procedures. Even outside episodes of myoglobinuria, most patients have increased serum CK levels. The forearm ischemic exercise (see earlier description) causes no rise of venous lactate level, and this is a useful but not specific test in McArdle's disease. EMG at rest shows nonspecific myopathic features in about one half of patients.

Muscle biopsy demonstrates subsarcolemmal "blebs" that contain periodic acid-Schiff (PAS)-positive material (glycogen). The histochemical stain for phosphorylase is negative, except in regenerating fibers. Biochemical documentation of the enzyme defect requires muscle biopsy because the defect is not expressed in more easily accessible tissues (leukocytes, erythrocytes, cultured fibroblasts).

Potential Diagnostic Errors. It is virtually impossible to distinguish McArdle's disease from the glycolytic defects (PFK, PGK, PGAM, and LDH deficiencies) on purely clinical grounds. Specific diagnosis requires muscle biopsy.

Phosphofructokinase Deficiency (Tarui Disease, Glycogenosis Type VII)

PFK deficiency is an autosomal recessive myopathy caused by a genetic defect of the muscle (M) subunit of the rate-limiting enzyme of glycolysis, PFK. There is a 2.4:1 predominance of males over females. Presenting symptoms are cramps after intense exercise, followed by myoglobinuria in about one half of patients. A few patients may have mild jaundice, reflecting excessive hemolysis, or typical symptoms and signs of gout. In patients with "typical" presentation, fixed weakness appears to be less common than in phosphorylase deficiency. On the other hand, in PFK deficiency, as in phosphorylase deficiency, a few patients have only weakness, without cramps or myoglobinuria. In addition to renal insufficiency due to myoglobinuria, other possible complications include renal colic due to urate stones and gouty arthritis.

Physical examination may show slight jaundice. Neurologic examination is normal. Serum CK level is variably increased in most patients. Forearm ischemic exercise causes no rise of venous lactate level. Serum bilirubin level is elevated in most patients, and the number of reticulocytes is increased. Serum uric acid level is also increased in most patients. EMG is usually normal. Muscle biopsy shows focal, mostly subsarcolemmal, accumulation of glycogen. In some patients, a small portion of the glycogen is abnormal by histochemistry (diastase-resistant) and by electron microscopy (finely granular and filamentous structure). The enzyme defect can be demonstrated by a specific histochemical reaction for PFK. Although a partial defect of PFK activity is manifested in erythrocytes from patients, firm diagnosis usually requires biochemical studies of muscle.

Phosphoglycerate Kinase (PGK) Deficiency

PGK deficiency is an X-linked recessive disease due to a genetic defect of PGK. The more common clinical presentation includes hemolytic anemia with or without central nervous system involvement (seizures, mental retardation). So far, only one patient, a 15-year-old boy, has been described with a purely myopathic syndrome, characterized by exercise-induced cramps and myoglobinuria. Between episodes of myoglobinuria, physical and neurologic examinations were normal. Forearm ischemic exercise caused contracture and no rise of venous lactate level.

Because the enzyme defect is expressed in almost all tissues, the diagnosis can be made by biochemical studies not only of muscle but also of erythrocytes, leukocytes, or cultured fibroblasts.

Phosphoglycerate Mutase Deficiency

This is an autosomal recessive myopathy caused by a genetic defect of the muscle (M) subunit of the enzyme PGAM. Three patients with this newly discovered enzyme deficiency have been identified so far.

The clinical picture includes cramps and recurrent myoglobinuria following intense exercise. Outside episodes of myoglobinuria, none of the patients was weak. Forearm ischemic exercise caused an increase of 1.5 to 2.0 times in venous lactate level, an abnormally low but not absent response. Muscle biopsy showed normal or only moderately increased glycogen concentration.

Because other accessible tissues, such as erythrocytes, leukocytes, and cultured fibroblasts, express a different isoenzyme, the diagnosis of PGAM-M subunit deficiency must be established by biochemical studies of muscle.

Lactate Dehydrogenase Deficiency

LDH deficiency is an autosomal recessive myopathy caused by a genetic defect of the muscle (M) subunit of the enzyme LDH. So far, one patient with this newly identified disease has been described. The clinical picture is characterized by cramps and myoglobinuria after intense exercise.

Forearm ischemic exercise showed a subnormal rise of lactate level, contrasting with an increased rise of pyruvate level. The diagnosis can be established by electrophoretic studies of LDH in serum, erythrocytes, and leukocytes, showing lack of subunit M–containing isoenzymes, but it should be confirmed by biochemical studies of muscle.

Carnitine Palmitoyltransferase Deficiency

This is an autosomal recessive myopathy caused by a genetic defect of the mitochondrial enzyme CPT. The disease has been identified in about 40 patients, with a marked prevalence of affected males (male: female ratio, 5.5:1).

The clinical manifestations are limited to attacks of myoglobinuria, not preceded by contractures and usually precipitated by prolonged exercise (of several hours' duration), prolonged fasting, or a combination of the two conditions. Less common precipitating factors include intercurrent infection, emotional stress, and cold exposure, but some episodes of myoglobinuria occur without any apparent cause. Most patients have two or more attacks, probably because the lack of muscle cramps deprives them of a warning signal of impending myoglobinuria.

For unknown reasons, some women seem to have milder symptoms, such as myalgia after prolonged exercise without pigment in the urine. This has been observed in sisters of men with recurrent myoglobinuria.

The only serious complication is renal failure following myoglobinuria.

Physical and neurologic examinations are completely normal. As described earlier, prolonged fasting at rest (to be conducted under close medical observation) causes a sharp rise of serum CK level in about one half of patients. Also in about half of patients, ketone bodies fail to increase normally after prolonged fasting. Forearm ischemic exercise causes a normal increase of venous lactate level. Outside episodes of myoglobinuria, serum CK level and EMG are normal. Muscle biopsy may appear completely normal or show variable, but usually moderate, accumulation of lipid droplets. Most patients with CPT deficiency benefit from a high-carbohydrate, low-fat diet, and the therapeutic response that takes place may serve as an indirect diagnostic clue. Because the enzyme defect appears to be generalized, tissues other than muscle (e.g., mixed leukocytes or isolated lymphocytes or platelets) can be used to demonstrate CPT deficiency, but the diagnosis should be confirmed in muscle.

METABOLIC MYOPATHIES CAUSING WEAKNESS

Acid Maltase Deficiency (AMD, Glycogenosis Type II

AMD is an autosomal recessive disease due to a genetic defect of the lysosomal enzyme acid maltase, an alpha-1,4- and alpha-1,6-glucosidase capable of digesting glycogen completely to glucose. Two major clinical syndromes are caused by AMD: a severe, generalized, and invariably fatal disease of infancy (Pompe's disease), and a less severe neuromuscular disorder beginning in childhood or in adult life.

Infantile, Generalized, Cardiomegalic AMD (Pompe's Disease). Pompe's disease usually becomes manifest in the first weeks or months of life, with failure to thrive, poor suck, and generalized hypotonia and weakness ("floppy infant" syndrome). Macroglossia is common, as is hepatomegaly, which, however, is rarely severe. There is massive cardiomegaly with congestive heart failure. Weakness of respiratory muscles makes these infants susceptible to pulmonary infection, and death occurs invariably before 2 years (usually before 1 year) of age.

Childhood- and Adult-Onset AMD. These forms of AMD cause symptoms and signs that are limited to the musculature, with progressive weakness of truncal muscles and of proximal more than distal limb muscles usually sparing facial and extraocular muscles. In the childhood form, onset is in infancy or childhood, and progression tends to be rapid. In the adult form, onset is usually in the third or fourth decade but occasionally even later, and the course is slower.

The clinical picture in male children can closely resemble the Duchenne type of muscular dystrophy, and in adults it mimics limb-girdle dystrophy or polymyositis. The early and severe involvement of respiratory muscles in most patients with AMD is a useful clinical clue to the correct diagnosis. Respiratory failure and pulmonary infection are the most common causes of death.

Physical Examination. Babies with Pompe's disease show massive cardiomegaly, hepatomegaly, and, in some cases, macroglossia. There are usually normal findings in the later-onset forms of AMD.

Neurologic Examination. In Pompe's disease severe generalized hypotonia, weakness, and hyporeflexia are seen. In childhood and adult AMD, there is proximal weakness with waddling gait and hyperlordosis, wasting of some muscle groups, and hyporeflexia.

Laboratory Procedures. Serum CK level is variably but consistently increased in all forms of AMD. Forearm ischemic exercise causes normal rise of venous lactate level in patients with childhood or adult AMD. The electrocardiogram is altered in Pompe's disease (short P-R interval, giant QRS complexes, and signs of left ventricular or biventricular hypertrophy) but is usually normal in the later-onset forms.

EMG shows myopathic features but also fibrillation potentials; bizarre, high-frequency discharges; and myotonic discharges.

Muscle biopsy shows vacuolar myopathy of very severe degree and affecting all fibers in Pompe's disease, but of varying degree and distribution in childhood and adult AMD.

In adult AMD, biopsy specimens from unaffected muscles may appear normal by light microscopy. The vacuoles contain PAS-positive material (glycogen). Electron microscopy shows the presence of abundant glycogen both within membranous sacs (lysosomes) and free in the cytoplasm.

The enzyme defect is expressed in all tissues, and the diagnosis can be made by biochemical analysis of urine, lymphocytes (mixed leukocytes do *not* give reliable results), or cultured skin fibroblasts. Fibroblasts cultured from amniotic fluid can be used for prenatal diagnosis of Pompe's disease.

Debrancher Deficiency (Glycogenosis Type III, Cori's Disease, Forbes' Disease)

Debrancher deficiency is an autosomal recessive disease caused by a genetic defect of the debranching enzyme. In its more common presentation, debrancher deficiency causes liver dysfunction in childhood, with hepatomegaly, growth retardation, fasting hypoglycemia, and seizures. Myopathy has been described in about 20 patients. In most of them, onset of weakness was in the third or fourth decade. Wasting of distal leg muscles and intrinsic hand muscles is common, and the association of late-onset weakness and distal wasting often suggests the diagnosis of motor neuron disease or peripheral neuropathy. The course is slowly progressive.

In a smaller number of patients, onset of weakness is in childhood, with diffuse weakness and wasting. The association of hepatomegaly and growth retardation facilitates the diagnosis.

Laboratory Investigations. Administration of glucagon or epinephrine produces no increase in blood glucose level, whereas a galactose load causes a normal increase.

After forearm ischemic exercise there is abnormally low rise or no increase in venous lactate level.

Serum CK level is variably and often markedly increased.

ECG shows left ventricular or biventricular hypertrophy in most patients.

EMG may show myopathic features alone or, more often, a pattern associated with fibrillations, positive sharp waves, and myotonic discharges. This "mixed" EMG pattern in patients with weakness and distal wasting often reinforces the erroneous diagnosis of motor neuron disease. Motor nerve conduction velocities were moderately decreased in one fourth of patients, suggesting the diagnosis of Charcot-Marie-Tooth disease or other neuropathies.

Muscle biopsy shows severe vacuolar myopathy with glycogen storage. On electron microscopy, the vacuoles correspond to pools of glycogen free in the cytoplasm.

The enzyme defect is generalized, and it has been demonstrated in erythrocytes, leukocytes, and cultured fibroblasts. In patients with myopathy, the diagnosis is securely established by measurement of debrancher activity in muscle biopsy specimens or by studies of iodine spectra of glycogen isolated from muscle; there is a shift in the spectrum toward lower wavelengths, indicating that the polysaccharide has abnormally short peripheral branches.

Branching Enzyme Deficiency (Glycogenosis Type IV, Andersen's Disease)

Branching enzyme deficiency is an autosomal recessive disease of infancy or early childhood typically causing liver dysfunction with hepatosplenomegaly, progressive cirrhosis, and chronic hepatic failure. Death usually occurs in childhood. Although muscle wasting and hypotonia are mentioned in several reports, only three patients had severe hypotonia, wasting, contractures, and hyporeflexia, suggesting the diagnosis of spinal muscular atrophy.

There are no diagnostic laboratory tests. Muscle biopsy may be normal or show focal accumulations of abnormal glycogen, which is intensely PAS-positive and partially resistant to diastase digestion. With the electron microscope, the abnormal glycogen is found to have a finely granular and filamentous structure.

Carnitine Deficiency

Primary carnitine deficiency is a clinically heterogeneous disorder of uncertain cause resulting in decreased concentration of carnitine (β-hydroxy-γ-trimethylaminobutyric acid) in skeletal muscle (myopathic form) or in muscle, liver, blood, and various other tissues (systemic form). Both myopathic and systemic forms of carnitine deficiency appear to be transmitted as autosomal recessive traits.

Clinically, *myopathic carnitine deficiency* is characterized by generalized weakness, starting in childhood in most patients and affecting mainly proximal limb and trunk muscles but sometimes also facial and pharyngeal muscles. The course is usually slowly progressive, but weakness may fluctuate in severity.

Laboratory investigations show normal or near-normal serum carnitine levels (an important differential feature from systemic carnitine deficiency) and variably increased serum CK levels. EMG shows myopathic features with or without spontaneous activity at rest. Muscle biopsy reveals severe triglyceride storage, best seen with the oil red O stain in frozen sections.

Systemic carnitine deficiency usually presents in early childhood with recurrent episodes of hepatic encephalopathy closely resembling Reye's syndrome; in fact, in all cases of "recurrent Reye's syndrome" the diagnosis of systemic carnitine deficiency should be considered and serum carnitine level measured.

The episodes are often triggered by mild intercurrent illnesses and are accompanied by nausea, vomiting, confusion, or coma. A progressive neuromuscular disorder similar to that of the myopathic form is also known. The prognosis for systemic carnitine deficiency is not as good as that for the myopathic form, and several patients have died of cardiorespiratory failure before the age of 20 years.

A special clinical presentation of systemic carnitine deficiency reported in two unrelated kindreds is dominated by cardiomyopathy rather than liver dysfunction; cardiomegaly and congestive heart failure occur in childhood.

Laboratory investigations in this form show decreased levels of serum carnitine, variably increased serum CK levels, and, during attacks of hepatic encephalopathy, hypoglycemia, ketoacidosis, lactic acidosis, increased activities of serum glutamic-oxaloacetic and glutamic-pyruvic transaminases (SGOT and SGPT), and increased urinary excretion of dicarboxylic acids. EMG shows nonspecific myopathic features.

Muscle and liver biopsy specimens show triglyceride storage and markedly decreased concentration of carnitine.

Oral administration of L-carnitine has proved to be beneficial in about one half of patients with hepatic symptoms, and it has been particularly effective in the patients with cardiomyopathy.

Secondary carnitine deficiency may occur as a consequence of several different disorders, such as severe malnutrition (usually associated with liver cirrhosis), Fanconi's syndrome, and intermittent hemodialysis. Carnitine replacement therapy should be instituted in these patients.

CONGENITAL MYOPATHIES AND MITOCHONDRIAL MYOPATHIES

By Linton C. Hopkins, M.D.
Atlanta, Georgia

Congenital myopathies are rare syndromes that cause muscle weakness, are present at birth, and have specific alterations in muscle fiber structure. Among the disorders discussed in this article are central core disease, centronuclear myopathies, nemaline myopathy (rod disease), congenital fiber type disproportion, myopathies with abnormality of other subcellular organelles, and mitochondrial myopathies.

It is most important that all disorders to be discussed in this article be differentiated from other causes of neonatal hypotonia and muscle weakness at birth. Fracture-dislocation of the cervical spine at birth, cerebral hypoxia, congenital or neonatal central nervous system infection, hypoglycemia, and hypocalcemia all may superficially resemble the rare muscle disorders discussed in this article.

In addition, two other neuromuscular diseases are known that are present at birth or in infancy but are not included with the congenital myopathies. They are infantile spinal muscular atrophy (Werdnig-Hoffmann disease) and congenital myotonic muscular dystrophy. These disorders are discussed elsewhere in this book (see articles on Motor Neuron Diseases and Muscular Dystrophies) but will be compared briefly to the congenital myopathies at the end of this article.

Although severe, even fatal, examples are known, the majority of patients with congenital myopathies do not have a progressively deteriorating course. This nonprogressive or static clinical course allows differentiation from progressive muscular dystrophy.

CONGENITAL MYOPATHIES

Congenital myopathies usually come to attention at birth, when the infant's muscle tone is found to be reduced, tendon reflexes are absent, and there is poor sucking and feeding, a weak cry, and a poor Moro reflex. Affected patients are floppy infants who have poor head control when lifted and tend to slip through the hands of the examiner when held under the arms. Motor milestones (turning over, crawling, walking, running) may be delayed.

If the condition is not severe, the patient may not present for evaluation until childhood or young adulthood, at which time complaints are of decreased endurance and poor muscle development, or the patient may appear for evaluation of scoliosis. Mild to moderate generalized muscle wasting and weakness is the expected physical finding in these diseases. As in all myopathies, sensory complaints and findings are absent. Serum levels of sarcoplasmic enzymes (creatine kinase, serum glutamic-oxaloacetic transaminase, lactate dehydrogenase, and adolase) are usually normal.

Central Core Disease

Patients with central core disease usually have hypotonia at birth and delayed motor milestones, but the disorder may be very mild, and affected children may have normal milestones and simply have mild, nonprogressive muscle weakness. Facial weakness is not present and extraocular muscles are not involved. The course is usually nonprogressive, in contrast to the dystrophies. Normal life span is expected. Scoliosis may appear when the child begins walking. In addition, central core disease appears to predispose to a serious complication of general anesthesia, malignant hyperthermia. Inheritance is usually autosomal dominant, and in these cases cores will be found in the muscle biopsy of a parent. However, sporadic cases have been described.

Laboratory examination is nondiagnostic and nonspecific with the exception of the muscle biopsy. Serum sarcoplasmic enzyme levels are usually normal and electromyography (EMG) shows a nonspecific myopathic pattern. The muscle biopsy, however, shows specific morphologic changes that can be seen when a histochemical stain is used that specifically stains mitochondria. The nicotinamide adenine dinucleotide (NADH) stain shows clear areas called cores, which contain no mitochondria, in the Type I or slow-twitch muscle fibers. Electron microscopy shows that the core regions are devoid of mitochondria and may demonstrate other significant structural alterations as well.

Centronuclear (Myotubular) Myopathy

This disorder varies from a mild type with difficulty in running and poor muscle development as the only complaints, to a more severe type with scoliosis but with preservation of ambulation, to a very severe myopathy involving respiratory muscles, which may be fatal in infancy. It is the morphologically specific congenital myopathy most likely to be associated with weakness of facial and extraocular muscles. As in the other congenital myopathies, poor muscle development, generalized muscle weakness, and hyporeflexia are expected. There are no sensory findings.

In addition, like the other congenital myopathies, the only helpful laboratory study is the muscle biopsy. Centronuclear myopathy always shows characteristic muscle fibers that have a single central nucleus and resemble fetal muscle fibers or myotubes. The biopsy may reveal fiber necrosis, increased connective tissue, and marked variation in fiber size as well. Sarcolemmal enzymes in the serum are usually normal. EMG is abnormal but nonspecific and shows myopathy.

A diagnostic pitfall is differentiating infants with centronuclear myopathy from infants with congenital or neonatal myasthenia gravis, who also have difficulty with eye movements and facial and respiratory weakness. This distinction rests upon the response of the weakness to injected edrophonium chloride (Tensilon) in myasthenia gravis and upon the typical pathologic features in muscle in centronuclear myopathy. Inheritance is either dominant with variable penetrance or X-linked recessive (one family).

Nemaline Myopathy (Rod Disease)

Patients with this congenital myopathy have rod-like structures in muscle fibers that stain red with Gomori trichrome stain. Patients present with generalized muscle weakness and wasting, which occasionally is severe, but which usually is nonprogressive. Dominant inheritance has been documented in some families, but other families have been described without an affected parent. Like patients with the other congenital myopathies, these children usually present in infancy with hypotonia, delayed motor milestones, and poor muscle development; they develop scoliosis when walking. Patients with nemaline myopathy are more likely to have bifacial weakness than are those with central core disease, and they usually have long, hatchet-shaped facies. The diagnosis rests upon the properly handled muscle biopsy, in which specimens demonstrate the typical diagnostic rod-like structure on light and electron microscopy. Serum sarcoplasmic enzyme levels are usually normal. The EMG is usually abnormal but shows only nonspecific myopathy.

The most common error in the evaluation of these patients occurs when the biopsy is stained only with hematoxylin and eosin, because the nemaline bodies may then be overlooked. Differentiation from progressive muscular dystrophy is another potential difficulty, but the more benign course of this illness, the typical muscle pathologic features, and the normal CK levels usually allow the distinction to be made.

Other Congenital Myopathies

Certain other congenital myopathies–congenital fiber type disproportion; myopathies with abnormality of other subcellular organelle, such as fingerprint myopathy; sarcotubular myopathy; and reducing body myopathy–are characterized by specific pathologic lesions of muscle but share the nonspecific muscle weakness of early onset that is typical of all congenital myopathies.

MITOCHONDRIAL MYOPATHIES

Mitochondrial myopathies are disorders of muscle in which the dominant morphologic abnormality is a disturbance in the structure and number of muscle mitochondria. This is a heterogeneous group of disorders, and a wide range of different clinical manifestations is possible. Clinically, patients with mitochondrial myopathies can be divided into (1) those who present with ophthalmoplegia; (2) those who have skeletal muscle weakness as their major complaint; and (3) those who have central nervous system dysfunction as the major feature.

Mitochondrial Myopathies With Progressive External Ophthalmoplegia

Progressive inability to move the eyes may be associated with the presence of abnormal muscle mitochondria, as seen in a muscle biopsy specimen of an arm or leg muscle. The terms *ocular muscular dystrophy, Kearns-Sayer syndrome,* and *ophthalmoplegia plus* refer to variants of the syndrome of progressive external ophthalmoplegia that may be associated with mitochondrial myopathy. The course is slowly progressive or nonprogressive. Physical examination shows inability to move the eyes. Ptosis is common. Bifacial weakness may occur, but skeletal muscle weakness is usually mild. Short stature and cardiac conduction abnormalities have been described in some varieties. The only specific diagnostic test is skeletal muscle biopsy, which shows abnormal collections of mitochondria as "ragged red fibers" on Gomori trichrome stain. When studied with electron microscopy, these fibers are found to contain abnormal mitochondria. Serum levels of sarcoplasmic enzymes are normal. The EMG may be abnormal but shows only nonspecific myopathy.

The major differential diagnosis is myasthenia gravis. Distinction may be difficult without a muscle biopsy, but can usually be made by the response of myasthenia to injected Tensilon, by repetitive nerve stimulation tests, and by conventional concentric needle EMG and single-fiber EMG.

Mitochondrial Myopathy With Progressive Proximal Muscle Weakness

This syndrome may demonstrate abnormal mitochondria on muscle biopsy but may have totally nonspecific clinical features. A muscle biopsy is required to differentiate myopathy associated with abnormality of mitochondrial structure from the other rare congenital myopathies noted in this article, and from muscular dystrophy and other childhood myopathies noted in other articles.

Mitochondrial myopathy with muscle weakness may show associated metabolic abnormalities that may suggest the diagnosis. One form is characterized by episodic weakness with salt craving and must be differentiated from periodic paralysis. Another type is associated with lactic acidosis and a third with nonthyroidal hypermetabolism (Luft's disease, Vera's disease.)

Mitochondrial Myopathy and Brain Disease

Recently reported rare syndromes with progressive intellectual deterioration, ataxia, and proximal weakness with extensor plantar responses and brisk reflexes have in some instances been found to be associated with abnormal mitochondria in skeletal muscle. Many patients with this disorder have myoclonic jerks and other types of seizures as well as hypoventilation. Some have been found to have specific deficiency of mitochondrial enzymes such as cytochrome B and cytochrome C oxidase.

A diagnostic pitfall is that when central nervous system signs predominate, peripheral skeletal muscle disease may not be considered. The mitochondrial disorders should be considered if the more usual causes of brain dysfunction in infants and children have been excluded.

OTHER DISORDERS TO BE DISTINGUISHED FROM CONGENITAL MYOPATHIES

Infantile spinal muscular atrophy (ISMA, Werdnig-Hoffmann disease) should be considered in the differential diagnosis in infants in the first year of life who show poor muscle movements and have hypotonia. It should be contrasted with the congenital myopathies. Eye movements are not affected, and tongue fasciculations are usually present. EMG and biopsy together will distinguish this autosomal recessive anterior horn cell disease, as definite evidence of denervation and reinnervation will be found. The EMG will show fibrillation potentials and voluntary motor unit potentials to be reduced in number and increased in size, in contrast to the normal or myopathic findings in the congenital myopathies. Biopsy results also differ and show small atrophic muscle fibers and groups of markedly hypertrophied Type I fibers. ISMA is always progressive, and death usually occurs by the age of 2 or 3 years.

Congenital myotonic muscular dystrophy also should be considered when a newborn is floppy and feeds poorly. The most important diagnostic test is the clinical examination and EMG of the mother, who will have grip and percussion myotonia and the other clinical stigmata of myotonic dystrophy. Importantly, she may be so mildly affected that she is unaware of her disorder and may deny having any medical or neuromuscular problem. Children with congenital myotonic dystrophy have generalized and bifacial weakness. Unfortunately, although the EMG is abnormal, it does not show the familiar myotonic discharges that are so diagnostic in the older child or adult with myotonic dystrophy. There is usually a diffuse increase in insertional activity, and voluntary potentials are small. Biopsy findings are usually abnormal but nonspecific.

Section Eleven

PSYCHIATRY

ANXIETY DISORDERS

By Jack M. Gorman, M.D.
New York, New York

Although anxiety disorders afflict approximately 5 per cent of the American population, this group of psychiatric illnesses has been relatively ignored by clinicians and researchers until recently. Part of the reason for this rests with the traditional concept that anxiety is at the core of all emotional disturbance and therefore does not represent a distinct entity. Indeed, the experience of anxiety is a ubiquitous human phenomenon as well as a feature of almost all psychiatric diseases. Nevertheless, it is now well recognized that there is a distinct group of psychiatric patients who suffer primarily from one of a group of forms of pathologic anxiety. As in all psychiatric illnesses, diagnosis of the anxiety disorders should follow the guidelines of the recently published *Diagnostic and Statistical Manual,* third edition (DSM III) of the American Psychiatric Association. Under this sophisticated system of diagnoses, the following anxiety disorders are included: panic disorder, agoraphobia with panic attacks, agoraphobia without panic attacks, simple phobia, social phobia, generalized anxiety disorder, obsessive-compulsive disorder, and post-traumatic stress disorder.

DEFINITION

In general terms, anxiety is the experience of fear, tension, worry, and autonomic nervous system hyperactivity out of proportion to the actual circumstances. It is not "anxiety" to experience fear during truly life-threatening situations. In the case of patients with panic disorder, generalized anxiety disorder, or post-traumatic stress disorder, some form of anxiety will be experienced without regard to environmental stimuli, even though certain events may make the symptoms worse. Patients with phobias will experience anxiety whenever they confront their particular phobic stimulus, always an irrational dread of some specific activity or object. Patients with obsessive-compulsive disorder will experience anxiety while contemplating their usual obsessive ruminations or if they try to avoid performing their compulsive ritual.

SYNONYMS

Anxiety neurosis; neurasthenia; neurocirculatory asthenia; globus hystericus; borderline; phobic anxiety depersonalization state; separation anxiety; soldier's heart; DaCosta syndrome; effort syndrome; irritable heart syndrome; hyperdynamic beta-adrenergic circulatory state; vasoregulatory asthenia.

SIGNS AND SYMPTOMS

In discussing the typical presenting signs and symptoms of patients with anxiety disorders, it is mandatory to take each specific anxiety disorder category in turn. Failure to make the correct distinctions among the various anxiety disorders can have as grave therapeutic consequences as failure to differentiate a primary anxiety disorder from an altogether different illness.

Panic Disorder

Patients with panic disorder often present to the physician or emergency room convinced they are in the midst of a dread physical illness. During the panic attack itself they complain of a cluster of symptoms that include the following: dyspnea; palpitations; chest pain or discomfort; choking or smothering sensations; dizziness or unsteady feelings; feeling that things appear unreal; paresthesias; hot and cold flashes; sweating; faintness; trembling or shaking; and the fear of dying, going crazy, or doing something uncontrolled.

In the beginning of the illness these attacks are spontaneous and not precipitated by known events. A typical attack lasts from 5 to 20 minutes, leaving the victim shaken and alarmed. After the initial few attacks the patient can generally be reassured that no dread physical event has occurred, but after a series of attacks reassurance often becomes impossible and the patient develops constant levels of anxiety, called *anticipatory anxiety,* as he or she awaits the next panic attack.

Panic disorder usually begins in late adolescence or early adulthood, appears to be inherited, and affects women over men by a ratio of about 4:1. About 50 per cent of these patients give a history of pathologic separation anxiety, usually manifested as school phobia, during their childhoods.

Agoraphobia

The term agoraphobia is misleading as a description of a clinical syndrome. While literally meaning "fear of open spaces," a more accurate description of an agoraphobic patient would concern someone afraid to be alone or in a place where he or she cannot get help immediately. In its most severe form, the patient with agoraphobia is afraid to leave home, experiencing severe panic attacks whenever venturing out the door. Some patients are able to go out if accompanied by a familiar person and if the place they go to is not physically confining. It is not uncommon for such patients to come to clinical attention only after many years of being housebound.

In almost all cases the patient will be able to give a history of having had a series of severe and spontaneous panic attacks preceding the onset of agoraphobic symptoms. Becoming afraid to experience one of these attacks in some situation in which help might not be immediately available, the patient gradually avoids many situations, such as travel in airplanes or automobiles, and eventually refuses to leave home. Such patients often still experience spontaneous panic attacks in addition to chronic levels of high anxiety. This is the most common and most severe form of phobia.

The condition usually begins in young adult life with 75 per cent of the patients being female. As is the case with panic disorder, half of the patients recall experiencing pathologic separation anxiety as children.

Simple Phobias

Simple phobias are persistent, irrational fears of certain specific objects or situations that the patient feels compelled to avoid. Under this rubric are included such phobias as claustrophobia (fear of closed-in spaces), astrophobia (fear of heights), and zoophobia (fear of animals). The most common phobia in the United States is small animal phobia. Such patients rarely come to clinical attention because the impact of the phobia on day-to-day life is not great. Therefore, estimates of the number of people who suffer from simple phobia are lacking.

Simple phobias are a normal part of childhood development, and the clinician is not alarmed by young children who are phobic of such things as the dark. When simple phobias do come to clinical attention, the patient is usually female, in her thirties, and apparently free of chronic anxiety. Only when presented, either in imagination or fact, with the actual phobic stimulus do these patients develop anxiety, respiratory difficulty, sweating, and tachycardia. Spontaneous panic attacks are not part of the syndrome. The patient will often tell a story of elaborate rearrangement of daily activity in order to avoid the phobic stimulus.

Social Phobia

Patients with social phobia are afraid of specific social situations in which they may be exposed to scrutiny by others. The patient complains that in this social situation, such as public speaking or parties, he fears that he will be embarrassed or humiliated. Like the simple phobic, the social phobic will not appear anxious during the clinical interview. Rather, this patient routinely experiences overwhelming physical sensations—notably blushing, trembling, sweating, and palpitations—only during whatever social confrontation is feared. Social phobia generally begins in the late teen-age years and seems to affect men and women equally. It is believed to be a relatively rare illness in its pure form, but can be extremely disabling, leading to severe restriction of lifestyle.

Generalized Anxiety Disorder

This is a category of pathologic anxiety developed to describe patients who suffer chronic feelings of nervousness, tension, autonomic hyperactivity, hyperattentiveness, and worry. These patients do not experience discrete panic attacks, but feel anxious all the time. The patients complain that they always feel jittery, restless, tense, fearful, and irritable. They have difficulty relaxing, feel cold and clammy, and experience rapid heart beat, sweating, frequent urination, stomach pain, and difficulty falling asleep. This is the patient who appears visibly anxious during the interview. If the condition persists for any length of time, patients often become secondarily demoralized, wondering whether the anxiety symptoms will ever subside or whether they will be plagued with apprehension for life. Epidemiologic data about this condition are being developed.

Obsessive-Compulsive Disorder

Obsessive-compulsive disorder is the rarest psychiatric illness, affecting 0.05 per cent of the population. It is characterized by one or both of two specific symptoms:

1. Recurrent and intrusive ruminative thoughts that the patient realizes are senseless but that he cannot stop thinking. The most common of these are thoughts of violence, contamination, doubt, or personal illness. It is important in making the diagnosis to note that the patient does not believe these thoughts are true reflections of reality. Patients who become convinced that their obsessive ruminations are true are suffering from psychotic delusions.
2. Repetitive, ritualistic behaviors that the patient recognizes are needless but that he cannot keep himself from performing. The most common compulsive rituals are handwashing, counting, checking rituals, and touching rituals. Each time the patient completes the ritual there is usually a temporary decrease in anxiety level that begins to increase again just before the next indulgence in the ritual. If the patient is prevented from completing a ritual, there will be intense feelings of panic and anxiety.

Obsessive-compulsive patients often appear quite depressed, but a careful history will reveal that obsessions and compulsions preceded the onset of dysphoric mood states and that depressed feelings are mainly related to the impact the obsessive-compulsive pathology has on life. In the most severe form of the illness, the patient will be completely incapacitated, having little time left for normal activities because of the distraction of constant obsessive ruminations or the demand to complete endless compulsive rituals. The condition can start in childhood, but usually has its onset in adolescence or early adulthood. Sex incidence is even between men and women.

Post-traumatic Stress Disorder

The patient in this category of anxiety disorder has undergone a real and recognizable life stress that would evoke symptoms in anyone. The patient presents to the clinician with a history of flashbacks to the traumatic event, nightmares about the event, and sudden feelings that the original traumatic event is reoccurring. For example, the war veteran who witnessed his best friend killed in action will relive the experience every time he hears loud noises reminiscent of gunfire. These patients experience a symptom called *emotional anesthesia*—loss of interest in significant activities, constricted affect, and feeling estranged from others. They may have insomnia, guilt about surviving the traumatic event, an exaggerated startle response, and difficulty concentrating. The condition can affect people of any age and either sex.

COURSE

Except for post-traumatic stress disorder, anxiety disorders do not seem related to obvious life stresses. The course of each condition is variable, but in general the anxiety disorders tend to wax and wane. Periods of symptomatic remission may last for months or even years, followed by a renewal of symptoms.

Patients with panic disorder may continue to have discrete panic attacks several times a week for years, with only a subgroup going on to develop phobic avoidance and frank agoraphobia. Once agoraphobia occurs, patients may have brief periods when they can be alone, but they usually remain severely restricted for years unless treatment is initiated.

Curiously, simple phobias often abate around the fifth decade of life.

Social phobia can be life-long, although some patients will muster the courage to confront the phobic situation at times and derive some relief.

Generalized anxiety disorder tends to be a recurring condition, characterized by varying levels of severity.

Obsessive-compulsive disorder is probably the most malignant of all the anxiety disorders; although there may again be symptom-free periods, the condition rarely remits spontaneously and often causes devastating disruption to life.

Post-traumatic stress disorders are considered *acute* if the symptoms last for only 6 months after the trauma and *chronic* if symptoms last beyond this point or begin more than 6 months after the traumatic event occurred. The more horrible the traumatic event causing the disorder, the longer and more severe the course of the illness.

COMPLICATIONS

Depression, substance abuse, and disarranged lives are the common complications of the anxiety disorders. After experiencing panic attacks, restricting phobias, compulsive behavior, and high anxiety for prolonged periods of time, many patients will become secondarily demoralized and despondent. They become convinced that their fears and anxiety will never remit and that normal life will not resume. Frank major depressive disorder with persistent dysphoria, anhedonia, and vegetative signs occurs in about one sixth of patients with panic disorder and in probably the same number of patients with the other anxiety disorders. However, the depressed mood experienced by patients with anxiety disorder is usually not persistent, and such individuals maintain the capacity for pleasure under the proper circumstances. Such typical depressive symptoms as early morning awakening, diurnal mood variation, weight loss, and psychomotor retardation are not common in anxiety disorder.

Unfortunately, many patients with anxiety disorder treat their condition themselves with alcohol or street drugs, a practice often leading to addiction. The astute clinician must be able to detect cases of alcoholism in which drinking began in response to panic attacks, chronic anxiety, or severe social phobia. Such patients can often be detoxified and successfully treated for the underlying anxiety condition. Because the anxiety disorders often have a severe impact on the ability to conduct normal daily activities, perhaps the most common complication of these illnesses is in terms of restricted capacity to engage in relationships and work. Patients with agoraphobia may be unable to travel to their jobs, while social phobics avoid parties and meetings. As they become accommodated to such disordered lifestyles, patients with anxiety disorder may appear as isolated and even eccentric people.

PHYSICAL EXAMINATION

Physical examination is performed to rule out the many physical conditions that can present as anxiety. Patients with panic disorder and agoraphobia have a higher incidence of mitral valve prolapse than is found in the normal population and may therefore have the classic mid- to late-systolic ejection click on cardiac auscultation. The patient may have labile hypertension related to anxiety symptoms, making it crucial to take blood pressure on more than one occasion and at different times of the day. A complete neurologic examination is mandatory because central nervous system lesions often present as anxiety before any other symptoms are apparent.

LABORATORY PROCEDURES

Like the case with the physical examination, laboratory procedures are performed to rule out medical conditions associated with anxiety. Probably the most important of these tests is a determination of thyroid hormone levels; both hyperthyroidism and hypothyroidism are associated with anxiety. Calcium levels should be obtained to rule out hyperparathyroidism. If anxiety attacks are associated with prominent flushing and warmth, a 24-hour urine screen for vanillylmandelic acid and total metanephrines may be deemed necessary to rule out pheochromocytoma.

Glucose tolerance tests are often performed on anxious patients in the mistaken belief that hypoglycemia is a common etiology of anxiety disorder. Actually, only the demonstration of low blood sugar at the exact time symptoms are actually occurring can link hypoglycemia to anxiety. To date, researchers have failed to implicate hypoglycemia as a reliable cause of any anxiety condition.

OTHER DIAGNOSTIC PROCEDURES

An electrocardiogram should be performed on patients with anxiety to be sure that dysrhythmias such as paroxysmal atrial tachycardia are not present. Usually, sinus tachycardia is the only finding. When there is suspicion that the patient who complains of constant palpitations or chest pain may indeed have a cardiac abnormality, 24-hour cardiac ambulatory monitoring and stress testing may be indicated. Echocardiography to look for mitral valve prolapse is indicated for patients with panic attacks. The dexamethasone suppression test appears to be positive in patients with obsessive-compulsive disorder. Sodium lactate infusions provoke panic attacks in patients with a history of spontaneous panic attacks, but never in normal patients. Therefore, intravenous infusion of half molar (0.5 M) sodium lactate in doses of 10 ml/kg over 20 minutes is now used at some centers to confirm the diagnosis of panic disorder.

PITFALLS IN DIAGNOSIS

It is altogether too common that patients suffering from anxiety disorder are dismissed from a physician's office or the emergency room with the advice, "Just relax, there is nothing really wrong with you." Clinicians often make the mistake of attributing anxiety symptoms to some obvious life stress and assume the condition is merely a reaction to personal problems. Panic attacks, compulsions, and phobias rarely respond to simple reassurance. Therefore, the clinician must be careful not to overlook formal symptoms of an anxiety disorder.

As discussed earlier, the diagnosis of an underlying anxiety disorder is often missed in patients presenting with drug or alcohol abuse. Affective disorder, notably depression, is often confused with anxiety disorder. Although patients with anxiety may become demoralized, they usually do not exhibit pervasively depressed mood or complete inability to experience pleasure.

Finally, because patients with anxiety disorder learn to accommodate their lifestyles to a variety of debilitating symptoms, they often lead isolated and even eccentric lives. For this reason, such patients are often called "neurotic" or labeled as having "character disorders." A careful search for the actual symptoms and their course of development will usually reveal that anxiety, panic, compulsions, or phobias preceded the onset of aberrant lifestyles.

In considering a diagnosis of anxiety disorder it is crucial that the clinician carefully elicit the patient's symptoms and attempt to fit them to one of the categories discussed. Even though anxiety is a routine accompaniment of 20th-century life, there are some people for whom pathologic anxiety becomes the dominant theme of life.

AFFECTIVE DISORDERS

By Madelaine M. Wohlreich, M.D.
and Layton McCurdy, M.D.
Philadelphia, Pennsylvania

Affective disorders are the most prevalent form of psychiatric illness and account for much suffering in affected individuals and their families. The prevalence of these illnesses, especially in primary care and nonpsychiatric practice, is impressive. As many as 30 per cent of the ambulatory medical patients seen by the primary physician may have a diagnosable affective disorder. Affective disorders may predispose the patient to other illnesses, such as alcoholism with all of its complications, as well as complicating compliance or pursuit of medical care for other ailments. The course of medical treatment may founder and fail because of the underrecognition of an affective disorder. Despite the best medical care, a patient may be lost to suicide if an affective disorder is not adequately recognized and treated by the physician.

DEFINITION

Affective disorders are, in essence, disorders of *mood.* While variations in mood or feeling are an essential part of human existence, when exaggerated, mood can incapacitate and cause the patient to become nonfunctional. Basically, mood disorders manifest as depression or mania.

Recognition of an affective or mood disorder is not an easy task for the physician. Few patients report an abnormal mood as a complaint to their physician. As with other medical illness, the patient presents with certain physical and behavioral signs and symptoms that the physician must put together as evidence of possible disease. Making the diagnosis of an affective illness can be rewarding to the physician and the patient, since these illnesses are among the most treatable psychiatric disorders.

Over the years, the classification of affective disorders has been subject to many changes—with resultant confusion. Recent attempts at classification have focused on differentiating this group of disorders into categories based on specified observable phenomena. This classification, published as the third edition of the *Diagnostic and Statistical Manual* (DSM III) of the American Psychiatric Association, will be used in this article whenever possible. Older terminology is still prevalent and reflects previous attempts to categorize the illnesses by etiology (e.g., endogenous vs.

reactive depression); by demography (e.g., involutional melancholia); or by other means.

The DSM III classification of affective disorders divides the illnesses into categories based on severity, duration, and degree of dysfunction caused by the illness (Table 1). The *major affective disorders* include the most severe forms of affective illness. *Dysthymic disorder* (or neurotic depression) is defined as a milder or less persistent form of affective illness; *cyclothymic disorder* describes a mild variation in mood that may shade into the normal ups and downs of feeling seen in most persons. It is the recognition of the major affective disorders that should most concern physicians and may most challenge their diagnostic skills, since complaints of mood per se are often not presented by the patient.

Major affective disorders are subdivided into the categories of *unipolar and bipolar disorders*. The unipolar disorders refer to those patients who show a history or presentation of major depression only, as will be described. Bipolar disorder implies that the patient exhibits evidence of manic illness *and* depression, or manic episodes alone, without episodes of depression. The manifestations of depression and the manifestations of mania, or manic illness, will be described separately.

Unipolar Disorders: Depression

Presenting Signs and Symptoms

One of the major difficulties in diagnosing depression is that the majority of patients do not present with complaints of disturbed mood or depression and often will not have any idea that their difficulties reflect a mood disturbance. This is particularly true for patients who seek help from a non-psychiatrist. The most frequent chief complaints in depressive disorders are vague, e.g., nonphysiologic patterns of fatigue. Headaches and gastrointestinal complaints are common. Even less specific problems may be the only presentation to the physician in the depressed patient; such as a feeling that "something is not right," or not feeling "up to par." The desire for a "check-up" in a patient who has not previously presented for routine care or who returns for medical care more frequently than recommended by the treating physician should alert the practitioner that depression may be the underlying problem prompting the request for treatment.

Table 1. Classification of Affective Disorders (DSM III Terminology)

Major Affective Disorders	Other (Milder) Affective Disorders
Major depression (major depressive episode)	Dysthymic disorder (neurotic depression)
Bipolar disorder	Cyclothymic disorder (neurotic depression alternating with hypomania)
Major depression alternating with manic episodes	
Manic episode(s) only	

The patient may note difficulty in concentrating or in performing routine tasks, but if the patient does not volunteer this information, the clinician should ask about these difficulties if depression is considered a possibility. Patients with a classic presentation of depression, if asked, will report a disturbance of sleep patterns, notably a change from a previously established pattern. Spontaneous awakening in the early morning hours with persistent fatigue is most common. Other patients may report hypersomnia with unrelieved exhaustion. In addition, disturbance and change of eating patterns, most commonly a loss of appetite, disinterest of food, and the sense that "food has lost its taste," is usually found. Weight loss corresponding to this complaint may be noticed by the patient or observed by the physician by the fit of clothing or comparison to a previously measured weight. Increased appetite and weight gain is less common.

Loss of sexual interest or libido is often present in depression, and depression should be considered when a change occurs in a previously established pattern of sexual function. Change in pattern is, again, more helpful than chronic difficulties in suggesting the diagnosis of depression.

Most depressed patients report a loss of interest in things that were previously interesting or important to them. Another consistent and reliable finding in depression is an inability to derive pleasure from previously enjoyable activities. For example, a housewife who usually takes great pride in maintaining a neat and orderly household may note she is disinterested in completing her chores and no longer cares about her home. An avid tennis player, when depressed, may find the game no longer fun or rewarding.

Recognition of depressed patients may be aided by their appearance and behavior in the physician's office. The patient may appear sad or tearful, withdrawn or apathetic, and may give evidence of lowered self-esteem by statements of self-reproach, guilt, or worry, the content of which may center on physical difficulties. Speech and thinking may be slowed considerably, and the patient may move as if made of lead. While some depressed patients manifest reduced movements, others will appear restless or agitated in their physical movements. The patient may seem unable to sit at rest and may rhythmically shake a foot or tap fingers as he or she is being interviewed or examined. Ruminations, or endlessly repeated painful thoughts or memories, may become apparent in the course of taking a history. In most severe cases, evidence of loss of contact with reality may be present in addition to the signs and symptoms. Delusions or hallucinations, if present, will also be of a depressive nature: for example, somatic delusions of cancer or hallucinations of the voice of God condemning the patient for past sins. Previously termed "psychotic depression," this is currently diagnosed as *major depression with psychotic features.*

Diagnosis of depression in the elderly patient can be particularly challenging. Geriatric patients with depressive illness may appear demented because of severe withdrawal from the world. In appearance they may seem distant, remote, and impassive. They may not answer questions, and their behavior could be mistakenly thought to result from organic brain change.

However, a medical work-up may fail to show evidence of an organic basis for the behavior. Careful questioning may prove that the patient is oriented, with recent memory more intact than would be expected for the degree of impairment if the clinical picture were due to dementia. A lack of neurologic findings for organicity and a normal CT scan in a patient who seems demented and withdrawn should alert the physician to consider depression in an elderly patient.

Pertinent History

Episodes of past difficulties similar to the current presentation, with or without diagnosis or treatment, are helpful in establishing a diagnosis of depression. Although many patients will experience recurrent depression, a past history of depression is not essential, since the current illness may be the first episode. The history may reveal a recent loss of a valued person, a goal, prestige, or some aspect of the person's preferred self-image. However, it is important to keep in mind that the degree of depression may not correspond to the severity of the loss. Any medical illness could be the trigger of a depression episode. A full-scale clinical depression may follow a minor loss, or the loss may not even be detectable by routine questioning. Again if present, this history is supportive of, but not essential to, the diagnosis of a depressive disorder.

Also important is a family history of depression, suicide, or substance abuse. If such a history is present, it may support the suspected diagnosis of depression.

Laboratory Examination

One of the most promising recent advances in the diagnosis of depression is the use of the dexamethasone suppression test (DST). The clinical finding of an abnormal lack of adrenal suppression after a dose of dexamethasone has been shown to correlate with clinical depression. While variations in administration of the DST have been reported, a simplified method of testing dexamethasone response is to draw a baseline 8 A.M. blood for cortisol measurement on day 1 of the test. One milligram of dexamethasone is administered orally to the patient at 11 P.M. On the following day, blood is drawn for cortisol measurement at 4 P.M. The finding of a cortisol level greater than or equal to 5 μg/dl on the day following dexamethasone administration (indicating an abnormal absence of adrenal suppression in response to dexamethasone) has been shown to correlate with the clinical type of depression described. This finding also appears to predict favorable response to antidepressant medication in the depressed patient.

Currently, the dexamethasone suppression test seems promising as a useful adjunct in supporting the diagnosis of major depression when the clinical picture is otherwise suggestive. It may also be useful in following the course of depression and predicting the outcome of treatment. However, limitations of the test include abnormalities of dexamethasone-induced adrenal suppression found in other medical conditions as well as with certain medications such as oral contraceptives. Additionally, recent studies suggest that the specificity of this test for depression, compared with other psychiatric illnesses, may not be as clear as originally believed.

Not all patients with clinical evidence of depression show the abnormal dexamethasone response. While a positive (abnormal) DST strongly suggests confirmation of the diagnosis of depression, less than 50 per cent of clinically depressed patients demonstrate this response to the test. Patients with less classic patterns of depression (also termed *atypical depression*) show even less clear correlation between results of the DST and diagnosis or response to treatment. Currently, the clinical usefulness of the dexamethasone suppression test appears to be changing so rapidly that it may be advisable to discuss its present status with a psychiatric consultant in order to be updated on this promising clinical tool in the diagnosis of depression.

Other laboratory test results may also be abnormal in depression. Investigators have found a correlation between depression and abnormal results of the thyrotropin-releasing hormone (TRH) test. Following administration of thyrotropin-releasing hormone, some depressed patients show a less than expected rise in thyroid-stimulating hormone (TSH) levels compared with nondepressed controls. Also being explored are other abnormal hormonal responses in depression, such as growth hormone response to insulin-induced hypoglycemia. At present, these laboratory abnormalities in depression are promising for the future, but their clinical usefulness in the confirmation and differential diagnosis of depression is not clearly established.

The use of a questionnaire-type depression inventory to be completed by the patient may be a useful clinical tool. The Hamilton and the Beck Depression indices have proved clinically valuable in the diagnosis of depression, but should not substitute for history taking, observation, and physical examination of the patient.

The question of which medical laboratory tests should be ordered to differentiate between depression and other organic medical pathology is best left to the assessment and knowledge of the treating physician, taking into account the differential diagnosis of the patient's presenting complaints and the physician's level of comfort in having ruled out other etiologies for the symptoms. However, it should be emphasized that thyroid function studies should always be included in the initial assessment of patients with suspected depression. Either hyperthyroidism or hypothyroidism can present with the clinical picture of depression, even in the absence of other data suggesting diagnosis of thyroid disease.

Bipolar Disorders: Manic Illness and Depression

Presenting Signs and Symptoms

While the frequency of bipolar disorders is less than that of unipolar affective illness in the general population, these disturbances are often extremely disruptive and destructive to patients and their families. As in unipolar disorders, diagnosis of bipolar affective illness is based on the clinical picture and history. Most patients with bipolar affective disorders suffer from episodes of depression and episodes of mania, but the diagnosis is also given to those rare patients who exhibit manic illness alone, without apparent history of depression. The most frequent form of bipolar illness consists of episodes of abnormal elation, euphoria, or irritability (mania) alternating with depressive episodes similar to those described previously. Also possible in patients with bipolar disorders are disturbances of mood with features of both depression and mania or hypomania simultaneously.

During the depressed phase of the illness, the patient's presentation is similar to the unipolar depressed patient, although subtle features of mania (to be described) may be noticeable even in depression. Between episodes of illness, some patients may function quite well with no trace of difficulty, while others may be incapacitated by rapidly cycling shifts of moods or by the social after-effects of extremely irrational behavior during the acute phases of the illness.

The bipolar patient in the midst of a full-blown manic episode may be brought to the attention of the physician by concerned family or community members. The patient is less likely to feel that there is something wrong with him. Frequently, in fact, the patient will feel euphoric and elated. These individuals may claim never to have felt better and may be extremely resistant to any medical attention. When manic, the patient may be unable to give a coherent history. It is often necessary to obtain information from family members of the patient.

Most bipolar patients demonstrate increased energy, with less need for sleep during their manic episodes. Increased productivity or creativity may be noted just prior to, or even during, the manic phase of illness. The mood of manic patients may be euphoric and elated, with exaggerated assessment of their capabilities, or the mood may be one of irritability, anger, and belligerence. The patient is often quick to anger and may be violent in the manic state. Also common in mania are rapid shifts between euphoria and rage, which may alternate on a moment-to-moment basis.

Speech is often non-stop and reflects a jumble of rapidly changing ideas or topics. It may appear that patients are unable to control the flood of thoughts they are expressing, and they may be unable to pause to answer questions appropriately. These features are referred to as "pressured speech" and "flight of ideas."

Loss of contact with reality is common, and judgment in manic illness is noticeably poor. This may lead to serious jeopardy of the patient's or others' personal property, or even life. Patients may go on wild buying sprees, make totally irrational and unrealistic business decisions, or gamble away life savings under the conviction that they can do no wrong. Even when faced with such consequences as loss of a job, bankruptcy, or legal arrest, these patients will remain grandiose and elated, with little or no understanding of the destructiveness of their behavior during the course of the manic episode.

Consistent with the loss of contact with reality in mania are the frequent findings of delusions in these patients. If present, the delusions reflect the grandiose ideas and wildly exaggerated sense of capabilities of the patient. For example, a patient may believe that he is a member of royalty or that he is more intelligent than anyone in the world.

Pertinent History

In the acutely manic patient, it is often necessary to obtain the history from a family member or friend of the patient, since true mania often renders the patient unable to cooperate with the demands of an organized interview. The clinical picture alone will often suffice to diagnose a bipolar disorder if the patient's behavior closely matches the description given for a manic episode.

Additional information of special value is a history of similar episodes in the patient's past, especially if there is evidence of some periodicity of depression and manic behavior. A relative or friend may give a description of a past depression in the patient, sometimes occurring just prior to the onset of the manic episode.

A family history of bipolar illness is often present, either by confirmed diagnosis or description of behavior.

Diagnosis of bipolar affective disorders is currently based on both the clinical picture and history of the patient and may be substantiated and supported by family history.

Laboratory Examination

At present, there is no pathognomonic test for bipolar affective disorder. The dexamethasone suppression test has not been found to be abnormal during manic episodes, although in the depressed phase bipolar patients may have results similar to those of the unipolar depressed patient. However, laboratory tests are extremely important to rule out other medical pathology that may coexist. In addition to the routine laboratory studies of general medical use, thyroid functions should always be checked in the work-up of suspected bipolar affective disorders. Either hyper- or hypothyroidism can present an affective illness, although presentation mimicking mania is less common than depression. In addition, thyroid function studies are also necessary as a baseline if the patient is to be treated with or begun on a therapeutic trial of lithium, which may be useful in determining the differential diagnosis between bipolar affective disorder and other psychiatric illnesses.

Blood and urine tests for toxic substances may also be important in differentiating an acute manic episode from a toxic psychosis and these should be ordered when the patient presents with an undiagnosed illness suggesting mania.

COURSE

The natural course of untreated major affective disorders is variable, but most patients who have experienced one episode of depression or mania will have future episodes of the same illness. Without treatment, a first episode of major depression usually remits spontaneously within an average of about 6 months. Recurrences are likely, especially at times of increased stress.

Patients who have had one manic episode are likely to experience future episodes of mania as well as depressive episodes, although there are some patients who will never manifest depressions. The patient may show regular cyclic alternation between periods of mania, depression and normal mood, with a periodicity of months to years. Others have less predictable episodes of affective illness or show more rapid cycling between mania and depression.

COMMON COMPLICATIONS

Affective disorders commonly result in a wide range of complications including job loss, marital and family discord, reduced work productivity, and personal suffering.

Sometimes these illnesses are recognized only when some medical complication has resulted. A suicide attempt, the most serious complication of affective disorder, may clearly suggest major depression. A less obvious complication which may also be a clue to diagnosis is the abuse of alcohol or drugs. A percentage of patients treated for substance abuse may have an affective disorder which they sought to relieve through the use of drugs or alcohol.

Another potentially serious complication of affective illness may be noncompliance with therapy for medical illnesses. Unrecognized affective illness, especially depression, may render the patient apathetic to personal hygiene or health care, even when the result is life-threatening.

POTENTIAL ERRORS AND PITFALLS IN DIAGNOSIS

Affective disorders have a close relationship to several nonpsychiatric medical illnesses. Often a patient will have a coexisting physical illness and will be depressed as well. This can be a source of confusion in diagnosis. A useful approach is to consider the diagnosis of an affective illness separately from other diagnoses under consideration, keeping in mind the high frequency of affective disorders in all patients.

Patients with medical illnesses have a higher incidence of depression than does the general population. Often patients respond with depression to the stress of a physical illness. Some medical illnesses, such as cancer or thyroid disease, may present as affective disorders. Drugs commonly used in medical treatment, such as reserpine, methyldopa, or propranolol, can cause depression.

Making the diagnosis is important because the treatment of a depressive disorder in the medically ill patient can greatly reduce suffering.

The medical work-up necessary to determine whether affective illness alone can account for the patient's presentation depends on the clinical judgment of the treating physician in ruling out other medical pathology. At times, only careful follow-up will answer the question. Of central importance is that affective disorders can *simulate* medical illnesses, can *complicate* medical illnesses, can be a *manifestation* of a medical illness, or can be a *reaction* to medical illness.

SOMATOFORM AND DISSOCIATIVE DISORDERS

By Donald E. Manning, M.D.
Atlanta, Georgia

SOMATOFORM DISORDERS

Definition

The chief feature of the somatoform disorders is the presence of or concern with physical symptoms suggesting a physical disorder for which there are no demonstrable organic findings to explain the symptoms. That is, the symptoms are assumed to result from psychological conflicts, not from a physical disorder.

The etiology of the disorders can be explained by utilizing the psychoanalytic theory of the neuroses. According to this theory, a current situation or life stress can make conscious or rekindle the affect attached to an old conflict. This old conflict, which can be conceptualized as a psychological trauma from the patient's developmental years, has been repressed utilizing mental or defense mechanisms. The new environmental stress renders the mental or defensive mechanism inadequate, and the old conflict becomes conscious and is felt as anxiety. In order to deal with this anxiety, the individual develops new and abnormal mental or defense mechanisms.

These abnormal or neurotic mechanisms that arise vary with different syndromes.

1. If the anxiety is changed into multiple somatic complaints, the mental or defense mechanism is called *somatization* and the resultant disorder is called the *somatization disorder.*
2. If the psychic symptom is changed into a discrete physical symptom isolated to a specific function of the voluntary nervous system or special neurosensory system, the mental or defense mechanism is called *conversion,* and the resulting disorder is called a *conversion disorder.*
3. If the anxiety is bound by focusing on a single pain, the resultant disorder is called *psychogenic pain disorder.*
4. If the anxiety is bound by focusing on multiple somatic concerns, the disorder is known as *hypo-chondriasis.*

There are four somatoform disorders. These disorders and their synonyms are as follows:

1. Somatization disorder (Briquet's syndrome).
2. Conversion disorder (conversion hysteria).
3. Psychogenic pain disorder (psychalgia).
4. Hypochondriasis (atypical somatiform disorder).

Presenting Signs and Symptoms

Somatization Disorder

This is the most common of the somatoform disorders. There are three essential elements:

1. There must be the onset of vague, dramatic, or complicated medical history prior to the age of 30.

2. There must be significant symptoms in many organ systems.

3. The individual usually consults many physicians without finding any apparent physical illness.

There are myriad physical complaints associated with this condition, including paralysis, blindness, difficulty swallowing, loss of voice, blurred vision, muscle weakness, urinary problems, convulsions, deafness, amnesia, syncopal episodes, abdominal pain, vomiting spells, bloating, diarrhea, chronic sexual difficulties, dyspareunia, musculoskeletal pain, and frequent headaches. The individual usually believes that he has been sickly most of his life. In addition to the physical symptoms, a further complicating symptom of the somatization disorder is depression. It is not uncommon for the depression to be associated with suicidal thoughts and gestures. Other associated disorders include personality disorders and substance abuse.

Conversion Disorder

The conversion disorder was classically described as having presenting symptoms that looked like neurologic diseases, including paralysis, anesthesia, blindness, or seizures. Other possible symptoms are vomiting and pseudocyesis (false pregnancy). In contrast to the somatization disorder, which is chronic and involves multiple organ systems, conversion disorder is usually of sudden onset in the face of marked stress, is short-lived, and remits completely. It is customary to recognize a primary and a secondary gain that the individual obtains as a result of a conversion symptom. The primary gain is generally seen as the alleviation of anxiety. The secondary gain is either support the individual receives from others or avoidance of something unpleasant because of the symptoms. The presence of these two gains allows the individual to maintain a quiet air of unconcern about the physical symptoms, referred to by its original French term, "la belle indifference."

Psychogenic Pain Disorder

The psychogenic pain disorder is defined as the presence of nonorganic pain instead of specific physical symptoms. This psychogenic pain is usually chronic, unrelenting, and unresponsive to treatment. At its onset, the pain may be viewed as a response to environmental stress or stimuli. It is generally felt that avoiding reinforcement of the pain and reducing the secondary gains at the onset will be helpful in preventing its chronicity.

Hypochondriasis

Hypochondriasis is a disorder wherein the individual is preoccupied with bodily function and fears various diseases. There are no physical symptoms and no complaints such as is seen in the somatization disorder, nor are there specific physical symptoms such as is seen in the conversion disorder. These individuals have the behavioral hallmark of repeated excessive medical consultation with subsequent excessive laboratory and diagnostic procedures that are ordered solely for the purpose of reassuring the patient with external data. Because of the hypochondriacal concerns, these laboratory and diagnostic procedures do nothing to alter the course of the patient's illness.

Course

The courses of somatization disorder and hypochondriasis are usually chronic and unrelenting. Psychologically, it is probable that the presence of the illness is reinforced by repeated medical intervention, whether it be frequent excessive diagnostic procedures or even frequent surgeries, usually of an exploratory nature. In addition, in the case of the somatization disorder, the potential for analgesic abuse and addiction is high and the use of analgesics should be avoided. The treatment of choice for both of these conditions is psychotherapy, and when secondary depressive episodes occur, antidepressant medication can be utilized.

The course of conversion disorders, in contrast to the other three somatoform disorders, is usually abrupt in onset, is time-limited, and responds favorably to treatment. Treatment measures that may be successfully employed include psychotherapy, amytal interview, and hypnosis. In some cases in which depressive or anxiety symptoms are prominent, psychotropic medication may be indicated.

DISSOCIATIVE DISORDERS

Definition

Dissociative disorders include a group of four conditions, each of which has dissociation as the predominant mental or defense mechanism producing a pathologic condition. In dissociation, a part of consciousness, a part of the identity, or a part of motor behavior is separated from the remainder of the conscious ego. This separation leads to symptoms of the different disorders in this class. As in conversion disorder, the primary gain of the dissociative mechanism is a repression and alleviation of anxiety produced from an unconscious conflict; there may also be a secondary gain of avoiding unpleasantness in the environment. Because of these primary and secondary gains, there may be "la belle indifference."

The dissociation may involve one of four separations of a part of the conscious ego.

1. If the separation is of a part of consciousness, the resultant disorder is *psychogenic amnesia.*

2. If the separation is of a part of motor behavior, the wanderings of the *psychogenic fugue* result.

3. If the separation is of a part of identity, the result may be the *multiple personality,* wherein the individual's customary identity is forgotten and a new identity takes over the individual's behavior.

4. It may be a *depersonalization disorder,* wherein the individual loses the sense of his own reality.

The dissociative disorders have also been called *hysterical neuroses, dissociative type.*

Presenting Signs and Symptoms

The dissociative disorders all present with dissociation of a part of the conscious ego.

Psychogenic Amnesia

This is the most common dissociative disorder. It is the sudden onset of an inability to recall important personal information registered and stored in memory. The amnesia begins suddenly, usually following severe psychological stress. During the episode, the patient is typically disoriented, perplexed, and indifferent. The episode is usually self-limiting and ends abruptly. There are four types of amnesia that may be seen in this condition:

1. In *localized* amnesia, there is an absence of memory for all events related to a fixed time.
2. In *selective* amnesia, there is an absence of memory for some events during a fixed time.
3. In *generalized* amnesia, there is a loss of memory for all events in one's life.
4. In *continuous* amnesia, there is a loss of memory for all events from a specific point in time to the present.

Psychogenic Fugue

Psychogenic fugue is extremely rare and is characterized by the sudden onset of travel away from home with loss of memory for one's identity, and following recovery there is memory loss for the fugue. Fugues may develop in the presence of alcohol or psychological stresses. The travel may be extensive and may include assumption of a new identity. The episode may extend from hours to months.

Multiple Personality

Multiple personality is a disorder that is exceedingly rare in which the individual has two or more complex, distinct, frequently opposite personalities. At any given time, one of the personalities will usually dominate the others. Transitions between the personalities may be abrupt and may be triggered by psychological stress.

Depersonalization Disorder

Depersonalization disorder is defined as the sudden onset of a sense of loss of one's own reality. It may be perceived as a feeling of unreality, of viewing oneself from a distance, of perceiving a distortion in one's extremities, or of a dream-like state. The depersonalization episodes are usually prolonged and last minutes to hours. Associated complaints include distortions of perception of the environment, dizziness, loss of a sense of time, and a feeling of derealization. There are usually recurrences at a weekly or monthly basis, but the individual is usually asymptomatic between episodes.

Course

All of the dissociative disorders are abrupt in onset, are predominantly a disease of adolescents and young adults, and become symptomatic during periods of psychological stress. Psychogenic amnesia and psychogenic fugue usually run a quite brief course, and patients rarely present for treatment for this condition alone. If the amnesia or fugue becomes recurrent or protracted, psychotherapy is indicated and produces good results. In contrast to psychogenic amnesia and psychogenic fugue, multiple personality and depersonalization disorder tend to be more protracted and recurrent. Both have a less favorable response to psychotherapy, but it remains the treatment of choice. In all four conditions, psychotropic medication should be avoided.

PSYCHOSEXUAL DISORDERS

By David B. Marcotte, M.D.
Fayetteville, North Carolina

Until the work of Masters and Johnson and others who applied the principles of learning theory to the treatment of sexual dysfunction, the vast majority of patients suffering from psychosexual disorders were literally an untreated population. Most medical colleges and residency training programs did not prepare physicians either to be knowledgeable about sexuality or to skillfully intervene to help patients suffering from sexual disorders, and patients with simple sexual problems that could be treated by the physician on the front line of medicine were referred for in-depth psychiatric treatment.

Beginning in the 1960s and continuing in the subsequent decade, practically all medical colleges and most residency programs, particularly those in psychiatry and obstetrics and gynecology, began to address physicians' lack of knowledge and skills in treating psychosexual disorders. Today a wide variety of health care specialists have been trained to deal with common as well as more complex psychosexual problems.

DEFINITION

Psychosexual disorders refer to two broad categories of problems. Both categories have a common origin, in that psychological developments and social influences have effected a change in sexual function. Psychosexual disorders do not include organic (physiologic, neurologic) causes of sexual dysfunction; however, every physician knows that physical problems such as coronary occlusion, stroke, alcoholism, breast amputation, or congenital deformities may indeed cause psychological changes that impair sexual functioning. Remarks in this article will be confined to those disorders that have their principal origins in psychological conflict.

Table 1. Psychosexual Disorders Affecting Relations between Sexes

Males	Females
Absence of self-stimulation	Vaginismus
Primary impotence	Primary nonorgasmia
Secondary impotence	Secondary nonorgasmia
Retarded ejaculation	—
Inhibited sexual desire	Inhibited sexual desire

The first category is sexual variations, more pejoratively termed by the lay individual "deviations" or "perversions." The vast majority of sexual variations that can be classified as disorders are prevalent in men. Rarely can the counterpart for sexual variations be found in women or, as in the case of same-sex orientation, with the same degree of frequency.

The second category refers to the psychosexual disorders that affect relationships between persons and are analogous between males and females (Table 1).

SEXUAL VARIATIONS

Disorders of sexual variation can be broken down into two categories of variation: (1) disorder of object (inanimate or person), related to a sexual object, and (2) disorders of aim, in which special conditions are required for sexual function to occur.

Disorders of Object

Age Differences. The choice of "appropriate" object varies from culture to culture and from social group to social group, and may change with age. An example of cultural sanction or disapproval for age-different choice of sexual partners can be easily seen, with older males being far more apt to choose much younger females as sexual partners whereas older women choosing younger male partners, i.e., a 70-year-old woman choosing a 30-year-old male, will call to question many more concerns regarding their relationship.

In our culture, the age of maturity influences when a person, male or female, chooses to be sexually active and give consent. Even though most states have laws that were formulated decades ago to protect minors under 18 years of age, the average age of puberty has dropped from 17 (in 1900) to 12, enabling younger males and females to experience increased interest and sexual ability at an earlier age than is permitted by law.

Disorder of age-inappropriate sexual variations occurs, therefore, in persons who seek out immature persons of the same or opposite sex for sexual activity, as in the case of the "child molester." The choice of a more mature child, i.e., age 16 to 17, by an adult differs significantly from the selection of prepubescent males or females. The greater the age difference between young child and older adult, the more potential damage to the child of engaging in sexual activity.

As with most sexual variations, the person does not usually seek out treatment for his or her "problem," but is referred by a legal or social agency or relative. The physician would do well to gather a complete sexual history and include sexual behavior, sexual education, sexual preferences, current sexual function, and use of fantasy. The majority of people who seek out immature sexual partners require special care that is beyond the scope of this article and are best referred to a specialist in the treatment of sexual disorders. Males who choose immature members of either sex tend to *repeat the behavior* and usually have inadequate adult-to-adult sexual relationships.

Animal/Human Sexual Contact. Although the physician who encounters a family member who has been referred because of animal sexual contact may become quite alarmed, the vast majority of animal sexual contact occurs in adolescent males as a substitute for self-stimulation. Such contact occurs especially with household pets and is usually *not* of great significance, but mainly requires reassurance on the physician's part that such activities occur with frequency of about 10 per cent in rural settings and 4 to 6 per cent in urban settings.

Same-Sex Behavior. The third disorder of object, same-sex attraction and/or bisexuality, which is a combination of both male and female partners, is beyond the scope of this article, as are more rare disorders such as transsexualism. The physician who interviews a person engaging in same-sex behavior, in addition to determining whether this pattern is a fixed pattern of adulthood (as differentiated from the same-sex play of adolescence that is common to both males and females), must assess whether the patient is dysphoric or has *strong emotional reaction to his or her own behavior.* The assessment of the patient's *discomfort with the behavior* is the most critical information to be obtained to assist in decisions regarding referral for treatment. The patient's use of erotic imagery will also help to distinguish whether an adolescent is struggling with same-sex orientation or same-sex activity because of social prohibition about sexual activity with the opposite sex. This is extremely common (75 per cent in young male adolescents and approximately 30 per cent in female adolescents).

Disorders of Aim

This second category of sexual variations refers to special circumstances that are *required* for sexual functioning. Again, each disorder of aim is almost exclusively a male disorder and usually the patient is not self-referred but may come to the attention of the physician after an arrest or a crisis.

The physician must assess whether the patient *requires or has to engage in* specific behavior in order to function sexually or whether the individual is expressing a preference that is truly volitional. The majority of males and females may experience erotic fantasies that include sadomasochistic or special conditions such as cross-dressing (wearing clothes of the opposite sex), but *rarely* do they put such behavior into practice. If they do, it is usually with a partner's consent and is not disconcerting to their sexual activity and indeed may enhance sexual pleasure and activity.

The first three subclassifications of disorders of aim are voyeurism, obscene phone calls, and exhibitionism. Persons with these disorders are similar in personality to sexual molesters of children. Their behavior is driven (repetitive), and they have usually very poor adult sexual activity with their usual sexual partners. An absence of sexual information and of permission to engage in sexual activity is commonly found in the patient's developmental background.

The other disorders of aim usually involve a sex partner of the appropriate age and gender, but sexual function can occur only when special ritualistic behavior or a special object is present (fetish). Disorder of aim involves an obligatory attraction to a person with special body parts, such as:

1. Partialism—long hair, the foot, or an amputee.
2. Fetishism—an article of clothing.
3. Cross-dressing and transvestitism.
4. Sadomasochism.
5. Bondage.

Partialism. Partialism refers to a specific body part or absence of body part as an object preference for function. The most common clinical problems are an unusual attraction for long hair, amputees, or obese partners. Here the importance of a physical characteristic may be *more* important to the patient than to the person who possesses the disorder or attribute.

Although body parts may hold special attraction such as large or well-shaped breasts (popular with males in our culture), if a male could sexually function only with large-breasted women, he would qualify for the definition of suffering from partialism or a body part fetish.

Fetishism. This refers to an object or article of clothing such as shoes, girdle, stocking, or other inanimate object that has overdetermined meaning for the patient. Common preferences are for filmy black nightgowns or stockings or other articles of clothing, well-known gifts to a sexual partner. Clinically, the *necessity* of such objects must be assessed before any treatment is conducted.

Transvestitism. Dressing in female clothing while engaging in sexual activity must be differentiated clinically from disorders of gender disturbance. Males who engage in cross-dressing *value* their genitalia and have no desire to change their sexual orientation or themselves as transsexuals do.

Sadomasochism. The incorporation of punishment or receipt of punishment simultaneously with sexual pleasure is very close to *bondage* (being forced or controlled by another while experiencing sexual pleasure). The majority of males who carry out such behavior prefer the role of being punished and dominated. The origin of the behavior can be traced to earlier traumatic developmental wounds that relate to guilt and shame over sexual desire and activity.

Course

Each of these disorders, if left untreated, remains as a part of the sexual repertoire of the patient. The reward (sexual pleasure) is considerable reinforcement for carrying out the behavior; lack of guilt, discomfort, and dysphoria over the behavior are poor prognostic indicators for motivation to remain in treatment.

All the sexual variations can be best treated with a combination of behavior therapy to control the behavior and substitution of more socially sanctioned activities, combined with intensive psychotherapy designed to uncover the origins of direct or indirect expression of hostility that have been fused with sexual expression.

If a partner is available, treatment of the *couple* (as in cross-dressing) offers the most favorable prognosis to alter the couple's sexual activity.

Physical Findings

The variations mentioned involve no physical or detectable endocrine abnormalities. Discovery of the presence of a variation may be accidental when the physician elicits a routine sexual history or offers the opportunity to a patient to discuss concerns relative to sexual fantasies or behavior.*

Once information and a detailed developmental psychosexual history are obtained, the physician can wisely refer patients who require specialized care or effectively reassure patients who frequently are concerned about being unique, "abnormal," or perverse, and who are experiencing common sexual preferences.

Complications

The chief complication of treatment of sexual variations is motivation to remain in treatment and to alter one's usual sexual expression. If the behavior is interfering with others (e.g., exhibitionism), legal coercion into treatment may assist the patient to remain in control of the behavior and, in spite of negative expectations of the motivation for treatment under these circumstances, may facilitate motivation to change behavior.

Pitfalls in Diagnosis

The most common clinical error in assessing a patient's psychosexual variation is to assume that behavior different from the physician's clearly is grounds for intensive treatment. The knowledge that the physician possesses may assist in recognizing common sexual fantasy or behavior and to discover the meaning of the behavior to the patient.

PSYCHOSEXUAL DYSFUNCTION

The second category of psychosexual disorders, in contrast to variations, is usually accompanied by distress and discomfort. Patients, if given the opportu-

*In order to learn how to take a review of systems of sexual behavior or a complete sexual history, the reader is referred to *Treatment Interventions in Human Sexuality* by Nadelson and Marcotte, New York, Plenum Press, 1983.

nity, will readily disclose to the physician their own or their partner's dysfunction.

Sexual dysfunctions can have their origin in:

1. Educational misinformation or lack of information.
2. Early attitudinal influences of the social-familial group, which inculcate unrealistic standards of thought and behavior.
3. Behavioral experiences, such as fear of failure after an episode of dysfunction, i.e., after stress or change in behavior.
4. Interpersonal conflicts with a specific partner.
5. Intrapsychic conflicts regarding sexual behavior, depression, or anxiety fear.

Finally, organic factors may initiate a sexual dysfunction that persists beyond the initial sexual dysfunction because of secondary stress such as fear of failure with erectile dysfunction or secondary nonorgasmia.

Female Sexual Dysfunctions

Vaginismus. Vaginismus, or spasm of the musculature of the vaginal area, can be caused by organic conditions that cause dyspareunia. When no organic features are present, vaginismus is usually seen in women who have fear of losing control, are frightened of sexual activity, and have been inculturated to believe that their own bodies are shameful and dirty. The physician can elicit the diagnosis upon pelvic examination if the patient will not or cannot submit to the examination.

Untreated, the patient and partner experience considerable humiliation and frustrations that may lead to severe marital problems and divorce. The treatment of choice is behavioral intervention designed to increase the female's comfort with an exploration of her own body. Vaginal dilators may be purchased and used *by the woman* to increase her comfort with penetration of the vagina.

Vaginismus may develop secondary to primary or secondary nonorgasmia, in which the patient does not become lubricated, which is the female analogue to erection in the male. Without lubrication the woman may engage in intercourse that is painful, resulting in increased avoidance of sexual activities and spasm of the vaginal barrel.

Primary and Secondary Nonorgasmia. These two categories refer to women who become aroused and lubricated, but do not experience orgasm in any circumstance (primary) or with their partner (secondary). The origin of primary nonorgasmia is usually a combination of lack of information about one's body and attitudinal or values conflicts associated with being a sexual person.

Secondary nonorgasmia more frequently is a communication problem between the couple in which lack of a sexual education, combined with misinformation of male and female sexual responsivity, collude to produce difficulty in achieving orgasm with one's usual partner.

Treatment. Treatment of primary nonorgasmia is best accomplished by behavior therapy in which permission-giving and encouragement of self-exploration and self-stimulation proceed to the ability to achieve orgasm solitarily. In essence, development of greater comfort with one's body and being sexual followed by recognition that the female is both capable of and responsible for her own sexual pleasure enables her to communicate those preferences to her partner.

Treatment of secondary nonorgasmia involves the classic model of behavioral treatment described by Masters and Johnson and elaborated by Kaplan. Such treatment consists of a paradox, which is forbidding sexual intercourse, accompanied by the gradual relearning of preferences of one's partner with reinforcement of specific verbal communication. The inclusion of more overtly genital sexual activity is gradually recommended as the couple is able to incorporate verbal communication into their sexual activity. Commonly, premature ejaculation in the male is linked to secondary nonorgasmia and/or other female sexual dysfunctions.

Pitfalls in Diagnosis. The greatest frequency of error in diagnosis results from the physician's inability to take a complete sexual history, the early use of laboratory testing to rule out organic causes such as diabetes, or the quick reliance on hormonal therapy.

Central to the understanding of primary nonorgasmia is the complete history of *self*-stimulation and sexual experiences with any partner, male or female. The physician must also inquire about vaginal lubrication. If vaginal lubrication is present, sexual arousal is occurring. With anxiety fear, the sexual response cycle is blocked and arousal is precluded. The same phenomenon exists with males who are unable to achieve erection secondary to fear, which precludes necessary parasympathetic stimulation.

Secondary nonorgasmia can be differentiated from primary if a complete sexual history is taken. Since the treatment of choice for secondary nonorgasmia is couple therapy and the treatment of choice for primary nonorgasmia is individual therapy, the importance of determining this point is significant.

Male Sexual Dysfunctions

Premature Ejaculation. The most frequent sexual complaint of males is premature ejaculation. Although many males ejaculate in the first 2 minutes of intromission, the patient with premature ejaculation has the impression that his ejaculation literally is "out of control" and that he has no way to prolong sexual activity.

The definition of "premature" ejaculation refers more to the "need" of the female, since if the female partner is orgasmic in 30 seconds, the male would not be considered premature. The definition is therefore quite flexible and has ranged from defining the number of pelvic thrusts, to timing intromission, to stating that if a male cannot "satisfy" his partner 50 per cent of the time he is premature. One readily sees that a female partner who is nonorgasmic, no matter how long her male partner thrusted, would therefore qualify him for a diagnosis of premature ejaculation using this definition.

The physician can be helpful by reassuring patients that:

1. Most males ejaculate within 1 to 2 minutes.

2. Intercourse is certainly the least likely sexual behavior to result in female orgasm.

3. The myth of simultaneous orgasm that many couples attempt to achieve is a rarity.

4. Many males can be paralyzed or unable to achieve erection and still lead active sexual lives with their partners.

Treatment. Beyond reassurance, methods are available both solitarily and with the couple for treatment of premature ejaculation. If the male is single without a regular partner, he can be taught to employ a Valsalva maneuver before ejaculatory inevitability occurs, which causes the pubococcygeus muscle to relax and diminishes the urge to ejaculate. The patient can practice this during self-stimulation to gain control over his own sexual response cycle. The male is also taught to recognize the situation *before* he reaches the point at which control of ejaculation is impossible (ejaculation inevitability, which occurs 10 seconds before ejaculation).

Two other methods are used for couple treatment of prematurity: the *Seaman's squeeze technique* and the *stop-and-start method.* Both encourage relearning touch techniques as described before. The male is encouraged to remain passive and supine. The male or female can be taught to squeeze the penis very firmly between thumb and two fingers; this results in diminished need to ejaculation and loss of some erection. The squeeze is applied over and over again to teach the couple that his orgasm can be under their control. The stop-and-start method follows the same principle, but has the advantage of not stopping intromission if the partners are engaged in intercourse. The male signals a halt to all pelvic thrusting until the urge to ejaculate has passed. This is again repeated in order to gain a mastery over the rapid ejaculation of previous sexual activities.

Primary Impotence. This condition is exceedingly rare and is defined as complete inability dating from adolescence to achieve erection with ejaculation. Most patients with primary impotence have severe interpersonal conflicts, very disordered psychosexual development, and harsh rigid ideas about sexuality. The differentiation from organic factors that cause lack of sexual desire can sometimes be determined simply if the physician inquires about nocturnal ejaculation, in which conscious control of sexual impulses is suspended. If a male has had nocturnal orgasm in dreams, there is no need to perform laboratory studies to determine endocrine function.

Secondary Impotence. This condition is extremely common and is defined as the inability to sustain erection once obtained so that intromission is not possible. Classically, the initial episode of loss of erection follows stress, fatigue, alcohol excess, or some other event. Subsequently, fear of failure or worry that an erection will be lost compounds the problem, leading to repetitive secondary impotence. Males may also pass from a stage of premature ejaculation to ejaculation without erection to secondary impotence. Theoretically, fear interferes with the male sex response cycle, preventing parasympathetic stimulation which is necessary for erection.

The treatment of secondary impotence is identical to that for secondary nonorgasmia and is the gradual relearning of non–goal-oriented sexual communication between partners.

Retarded Ejaculation. This is the inability to ejaculate or the delay of ejaculation for so long a period that hours may pass. This rare disorder can be differentiated by inquiring about self-stimulation. Usually the patient has little difficulty achieving orgasm when self-stimulating. Theoretically, males frequently have unresolved hostile or angry feelings toward their partner, or women in general, and referral for extensive evaluation is indicated.

Physical Findings

After adequate information is obtained about the dysfunction, including a sexual history, organic causes must be ruled out. Failure to obtain complete information, especially about self-stimulation and sexual experience outside of the committed partner relationship, and failure to inquire about male and female sleep orgasms are the most common errors.

Physical causes of sexual dysfunctions can be:

1. Biochemical/physiologic.
2. Infection or metastatic disease.
3. Mechanical or anatomic problems, e.g., rheumatoid arthritis.
4. Neurologic or vascular disease, e.g., diabetic peripheral neuritis, multiple sclerosis.
5. Endocrine disorders.
6. Genetic disorders, e.g., Turner's or Klinefelter's syndrome
7. Drugs, licit or illicit, especially hormones and antihypertensive medications.

Usually, physical illness influences all sexual expression and does not produce problems in one specific sexual area, i.e., erectile difficulty with intercourse without difficulty in self-stimulation.

Laboratory Findings

Only after a thorough sexual history, review of systems, and physical examination should laboratory assistance in diagnosis of the dysfunction be used. Laboratory studies can never be a substitute for adequate history taking.

Equipped with the skills necessary to gather information from patients about a highly emotionally charged area of life such as sexual behavior, the physician can intervene to provide information and reassure many patients who previously never discussed their sexual concerns with a physician.

SCHIZOPHRENIA

By Patricia M. Randels, M.D.
and Luis A. Marco, M.D.
Coatesville, Pennsylvania

DEFINITIONS

Schizophrenia is not a single syndrome but a congeries of chronic psychotic disorders characterized by deterioration of a previous level of functioning and by distinctive symptoms involving multiple psychological processes. The term "psychotic" has been defined variously in the past so that its meaning has become diffuse and imprecise. In the DSM III (*Diagnostic and Statistical Manual of Mental Disorders,* 3rd ed., American Psychiatric Association, 1980), on which this article is based, psychotic is redefined to denote impaired reality testing as manifested by any of the following symptoms:

1. Delusions.
2. Hallucinations.
3. Incoherence.
4. Looseness of associations.
5. Marked poverty of content of thought.
6. Marked illogicality.
7. Behavior that is grossly disorganized or catatonic.

Psychotic symptoms, however, are not pathognomonic of schizophrenia, because they also occur in other psychotic conditions such as affective disorders, organic brain syndrome, and drug abuse disorders. Therefore, in diagnosing schizophrenia, it is important to exclude other disorders with psychotic manifestations.

In the past, much emphasis was placed on a deteriorating course of schizophrenia; today the concept of schizophrenia is not limited to a progressively deteriorating course. It implies chronicity (symptoms present for a minimum of 6 months and a tendency toward recurrence) and a deterioration of a previous level of functioning concomitant with the presence of symptoms. The concept of onset in adolescence or early adult life has withstood the test of time. The term schizophrenia (schizo = split, phrenia = mind) implies a disruption of the functions of the mind, i.e., an idea and the corresponding mood do not occur at the same time. This split contrasts with the lay term "split or multiple personality," a dissociative disorder in which separate but intact personalities may occur at different times with amnesia during one state for the other.

In schizophrenia several mental functions such as orientation, memory, and consciousness are not disturbed, which makes the earlier synonym, dementia praecox, inappropriate. But other mental functions are impaired at some time during the course of the illness in all patients with schizophrenia. Disordered *associations;* loss of contact with reality, or *autism;* disordered *affect;* and *ambivalence* are fundamental. These symptoms are known as the "four A's." *Looseness of association* denotes that ideas are not connected in a logical sequence. Break with reality, or autism, indicates the schizophrenic's withdrawal from reality and preference for fantasy, delusions, or hallucinations. Abnormal emotional reactions and feeling tone are the hallmarks of a disordered affect. Everyone has ambivalences, and pathologic ambivalence exists in other psychiatric disorders; however, the schizophrenic feels torn in two opposite directions about almost everything. In other conditions, one attitude is often conscious and the opposing attitude unconscious although indirectly expressed. In schizophrenia both attitudes, though contradictory, may be conscious at the same time. According to some, hallucinations and delusions are secondary or derived from the four fundamental symptoms, but DSM III has reversed this position by establishing delusions and hallucinations as characteristic features of schizophrenia and relegating the "four A's" to a class of accessory symptoms. This approach is strongly influenced by the observation that certain types of delusions and hallucinations are, if not pathognomonic, characteristically found in schizophrenia. These are the "Schneiderian First Rank Symptoms" which are described in the section below.

CHARACTERISTIC PSYCHOLOGICAL SIGNS

Some of these can be objectively demonstrated and can provide distinctive evidence of schizophrenia. Others are considered "soft" signs because they are somewhat obscure, and examiners may have difficulty in agreeing on their presence or absence. Current nosology insists on the demonstration of the more objective signs at some time during the course of the illness. This group of manifestations is relatively homogeneous with regard to response to treatment, presence of a familial pattern, onset in early adult life, tendency toward recurrence, and level of impairment of functioning. These objective signs are described below.

Thought

Disorders are revealed in language and its thought content. Language disorders result from failure to follow grammatical rules, from deviations in rate or flow of associations, or from an illogical association of ideas. Although very characteristic of schizophrenia, language and communication disorders alone are not sufficient to establish a diagnosis.

Looseness of associations is one of the interesting and common disorders seen in schizophrenia. This is also called *derailment,* as in a classical description, ". . . the associations (i.e., a sudden switch from low whispering to loud screaming) lose their continuity .. . thinking operates with ideas and concepts which have no, or a completely insufficient, connection with the main idea and should therefore be excluded from the thought-process. The result is that thinking becomes confused, bizarre, incorrect, abrupt."

Neologisms are invented words with only autistic or private meaning.

Poverty of content of speech commonly occurs in schizophrenia, but is not limited to this condition. Little information is conveyed. This may be related to other characteristics of schizophrenic speech such as vagueness, tangentiality, too much concreteness, and stereotypy.

Vagueness means obscure or unclear responses. In *tangentiality,* responses veer off to a subject that appears unrelated to the topic of discussion. *Concrete responses* are too literal for the situation. *Stereotypy* is perseveration of ideas or the inclination to cling to a single thought which returns again and again. Generally, there is a marked dearth of ideas to the point of monoideaism.

"Blocking" indicates that the chain of thoughts is interrupted and sometimes becomes totally irretrievable. After such blocking, ideas may emerge which have no recognizable connection with preceding ones.

Delusions are a type of thought disorder consisting of false beliefs or ideas which are not culturally determined (not normative) and which are not readily amenable to change by logical proof. Superstitiousness, belief in clairvoyance or telepathy, or other peculiar ideas are borderline examples that could represent prodromal or residual symptoms of schizophrenia. Belief in astrology is currently widespread and therefore should probably be considered culturally determined. Overvalued ideas such as preoccupation with the special significance of particular dietary habits, prejudices, or extreme political beliefs may also be prodromal or residual symptoms, but are not generally considered to be delusions. Delusions of being controlled or influenced betray that the individual believes that his feelings, impulses, or actions are not his own but are imposed on him by some external force. Delusion of passivity is a synonym.

Thought withdrawal reflects the belief that thoughts have been removed from one's head. *Thought insertion* is a variant and represents the belief that thoughts are not one's own but have been planted by someone else. *Thought broadcasting* is the belief that an individual's thoughts are broadcast, as they occur, from his mind to the external world so that others can hear them. The delusions of being controlled, of thought withdrawal or insertion, and of thought broadcasting are all Schneider's First Rank Symptoms.

Somatic and *nihilistic delusions* occur in schizophrenia and other psychotic disorders, principally depression. The patient with somatic delusions believes that some bodily part is abnormal or decaying, that there is a growth in the stomach, or that the bones have turned to liquid or the heart to stone. Bizarreness distinguishes these delusions from mere *hypochondriasis,* in which beliefs about bodily problems are more realistic and do not border on the absurd. Nihilistic delusions are beliefs that the individual is doomed or that the world is coming to an end. They also occur in psychotic depression as well as in schizophrenia. Somatic delusions may also be nihilistic if the belief involves the nonexistence of the body or a body part.

Grandiose, persecutory, and religious delusions are typical in schizophrenia, but grandiose delusions are also often seen in mania. They take the form of exalted self-opinions, feeling the wealthiest, the most famous individuals, the most accomplished musicians or artists, the best fighters, and so on. Rarely seen any longer is a delusion in which the patient believes that he is some important individual such as Napoleon. Grandiose delusions occur especially in the paranoid subtype of schizophrenia and are often combined with delusions of persecution.

The individual obsessed with *persecutory delusions* believes that he is being chased, harassed, or conspired against. Often the agents of persecution cannot be identified from the patient's verbalizations.

Religious delusions also occur in the paranoid subtype of schizophrenia and occasionally in mania. Religious delusions may be closely akin to grandiose delusions, for example, the belief that one is Jesus or the Virgin Mary. It is sometimes necessary to be familiar with the patient's cultural background in order to differentiate religious beliefs from delusions. For false beliefs to be conceptualized as delusions, the idea must not be harbored, not even accepted, by other members of the patient's culture.

Perception

Hallucinations, or perceptions without an external stimulus, are the most important example. They are usually described in terms of the sensory modality affected which in schizophrenia is usually auditory. Other kinds of hallucinations should make one first think of an organic disorder rather than schizophrenia, although all types of hallucinations can occur in schizophrenia. A voice that keeps up a running commentary about the patient's actions or two voices conversing are said to occur only in schizophrenia. These two varieties of auditory hallucinations are also among Schneider's First Rank Symptoms.

Affect

The term "affect" is generally equivalent to emotions, although in psychiatry affect is usually restricted to the subjective aspects and emotion to the objectively determinable constellations (biochemical, physiologic, or behavioral). In schizophrenia, a disturbance in affective expression may be noted in that there is a deficiency in the capacity to modulate or adapt affect to changing thought content. There appears to be inadequate depth of affect. These abnormalities are referred to as blunted, flattened, or inappropriate affect. The patient with *blunted affect* may appear to be indifferent to all situations; the intensity of affective expression is severely limited. *Flatness of affect* is more extreme, there being virtually no evidence of affective expression. *Inappropriate affect* means that the feeling tone is not congruent with what the patient is talking about, and thus he may laugh as he describes something sad or painful. Lability of affect may also occur and implies sudden changes in affect for which no environmental provocation is apparent.

Sense of Self

Patients sometimes betray disturbances in this sphere as the experience of being unable to determine where they leave off and the world begins. This experience is also termed "loss of ego boundaries" or "oceanic feelings," and commonly leads to problems of identity. Altered states of consciousness due to multiple personality disturbance or to toxic states due to psychedelic drugs may cause similar disturbances and present a problem of differential diagnosis with schizophrenia.

Volition

Schizophrenia is a disorder in which there is a deterioration of a previous level of functioning. Disturbance in ability to function is an objective finding required for the diagnosis of schizophrenia. There is impairment in ability to work or to care for oneself. This may in part be related to a disturbance in self-initiated goal-directed activity, interest, will, or motivation. In part, this may be due to ambivalence, to autism, or to anhedonia. *Anhedonia* means the inability to experience pleasure from activities that would ordinarily generate it and is often thought to be a central problem in schizophrenia.

Relationship to the External World

In schizophrenia there is a tendency to withdraw from the external world and to become preoccupied with an inward and idiosyncratic world view or fantasies (autism) rather than dealing with the external world, which is more or less ignored or distorted.

Motor Behavior

Disorders are prominent in catatonic schizophrenia and in other subtypes. They may take various forms:

1. In *catatonic stupor* there is marked decrease in reactivity to the environment, with a reduction in spontaneous movements and activity, and the individual may appear unaware of his surroundings.
2. In *catatonic rigidity* the individual may maintain a rigid posture.
3. In *catatonic excitement,* apparently purposeless, stereotyped, and excited motor activity is exhibited to the point of exhaustion or heart failure.
4. In *catatonic posturing* the individual may assume inappropriate or bizarre postures.
5. In *flexibilitas cerea* (waxy flexibility) even uncomfortable postures are maintained when forced by an observer. Waxy flexibility, however, is not seen much nowadays. Weird mannerisms and grimacing are also prominent disturbances of motor behavior. Less extreme forms (i.e., pacing and rocking) are also seen in other types of schizophrenia. Apathy may lead to decreased movement. Tardive dyskinesia is a movement disorder linked to chronic antipsychotic medication. It is sometimes difficult to disentangle from the usual abnormalities of the motor sphere of schizophrenia proper. The history and pharmacologic manipulations are the best clues to establish a differential diagnosis.

COURSE

One must differentiate "true," "process," or "chronic" schizophrenia, which is thought to have a poor prognosis, from "reactive" (acute) schizophreniform disorder (see later), which has a better prognosis and is not, according to DSM III, any longer considered to be one of the schizophrenias. Evidence suggesting hereditability of schizophrenia applies to the true or chronic form but not to the schizophreniform (acute) type. Therefore, there are good empirical reasons for not linking these two disorders. But symptomatology does not always appear to reliably predict chronicity or recovery. Patients with Schneider's First Rank Symptoms have been found to have the same outcome as the less stringently diagnosed patients with no First Rank Symptoms, and no difference in outcome can sometimes be found between true schizophrenic and schizophreniform patients. Schizophrenic patients who manifest symptoms of depression, anxiety, mania, or confusion tend to have good prognosis, while patients with flatness of affect have poor prognosis. Indeed, flatness of affect may be the only sign that predicts poor outcome. Unfortunately, unless this feature is severe, it is not reliably assessed by psychiatrists or other trained observers. DSM III resolves the dilemma of schizophrenia versus schizophreniform disorder by length of time that symptoms last. If schizophrenic symptoms last less than 6 months, the illness is called schizophreniform. The problem with this is that the cut-off time period is somewhat arbitrary.

The onset of schizophrenia is usually insidious, even though relatives generally insist that it started acutely. Prodromal signs of disease take the form of nervous symptoms, character changes, or even direct overt schizophrenic manifestations. The illness begins most often during adolescence or early adulthood. The later the onset the better the prognosis. The patient's prepsychotic personality and adjustment will also affect the prognosis, such that being married or employed are adjustments that improve the outlook for recovery. Cultural background may also affect the outcome of schizophrenia. The risk of chronicity is greatest in those cultures in which insanity is viewed as a permanent disability. Recovery appears as a more likely outcome when the society views insanity as curable or, alternatively, as caused by some external agent. Schizophrenics in developing countries have been shown to have better course and outcome. These outcomes are independent of the views of the staff treating the patient. There are few long-term follow-up studies of schizophrenia to determine what is the natural course of the disease. However, retrospective assessment of a large collection of records reveals that about 25 per cent achieve full remission, 50 per cent reach at least a partial social remission, and 25 per cent remain social invalids whether or not they are hospitalized.

European psychiatrists have in recent years developed a different approach to classification of schizophrenic disorders, Type I and Type II syndromes. Type I syndrome, consisting of positive symptoms and often called the florid state (delusions, hallucinations, looseness of associations), and Type II syndrome or defect state, consisting of negative symptoms (flatness of affect, poverty of speech and loss of volition), may reflect two different underlying processes. The importance of this distinction is that the two syndromes predict different outcomes. The Type I syndrome allows the inference of a therapeutic response to antipsychotic drugs; the Type II syndrome augurs poor outcome regardless of drug treatment. In some chronic schizophrenic patients (Type II), there is computed tomographic (CT) scan evidence of increased ventricular size which is correlated with intellectual impairment and the presence of negative symptoms.

There are no specific physiologic or biochemical laboratory tests for the diagnosis of schizophrenia. However, all the neurodiagnostic, endocrine, and body fluid toxicologic studies can be vital, along with appropriate physical and neurologic examinations, to rule out conditions masquerading as schizophrenia. If Type I and Type II syndromes represent different dimensions of psychopathology, they nevertheless do not constitute separate diseases because they are often combined such that episodes of Type I syndrome not uncommonly progress into Type II syndrome, with or without the persistence of positive symptoms. This evidence suggests that chronic schizophrenia may sometimes evolve into an organic mental disorder with dementia. The proportion of schizophrenics with some brain damage remains to be determined, but it may be quite high. Although no specific damage has been associated with schizophrenia, a frontal lobe disorder would be compatible with findings from cerebral blood flow, positron emission tomography (PET) scanning, evoked potential, neuropsychological, and dopamine studies in schizophrenia. But the search for biologic "markers" of schizophrenia, so far, has been characterized by repeated failures and false starts, probably due to inherent nonspecificity, wide variability, and presence of different etiologies in a heterogeneous group of disorders.

DSM III DIAGNOSTIC CRITERIA FOR SCHIZOPHRENIA

The first three criteria that follow must be present and the fourth and fifth criteria must be absent to make a diagnosis of schizophrenia:

Characteristic Psychotic Symptoms. One or more of the following symptoms must be present during an active phase of the illness:

1. Bizarre delusions, such as being controlled; broadcasting, insertion, or withdrawal of thoughts.

2. Somatic, grandiose, religious, nihilistic, or other delusions with or without persecutory or jealous content, which may be accompanied by hallucinations of any type.

3. Auditory hallucinations in which either a voice keeps up a running commentary on the individual's behavior or thoughts as they occur or in which two or more voices converse with each other.

4. Auditory hallucinations on several occasions without affective content and not limited to one or two words.

5. Looseness of associations, marked illogicality, or marked poverty of speech, if accompanied by flat or inappropriate affect, delusions, or hallucinations, or behavior that is grossly disorganized or catatonic.

Deterioration of a Previous Level of Functioning. During the active phase of the illness, the characteristic symptoms are associated with significant impairment in two or more areas of daily functioning such as work, social relations, and self-care.

Chronicity. The diagnosis of schizophrenia cannot be made on the basis of a cross-sectional evaluation of a patient. Rather, symptoms must have persisted for at least 6 months at some time during the person's life. Thus, a longitudinal assessment is required.

Manic or Depressive Symptoms. These are not present or developed after the schizophrenic symptoms.

Origin. Not due to any organic mental disorder.

Thus the diagnosis of schizophrenia requires that continuous signs of the illness be present for at least 6 months during the person's life, and this time period must include an active episode of psychotic symptoms as described. The 6-month requirement may be met by the persistence of the active phase for 6 months or by any combination of active, prodromal, or residual symptoms as long as the total duration of symptoms was at least 6 months. Prodromal and residual symptoms are similar and include social isolation or withdrawal; marked impairment in role functioning or self-care; markedly eccentric or peculiar behavior; blunted, flat or inappropriate affect; tangential, vague, circumstantial, overelaborate, or metaphorical speech; odd or bizarre ideas or perceptual experiences.

DSM III PHENOMENOLOGIC SUBTYPES

Disorganized (Hebephrenic). This is characterized by frequently disorganized and incoherent thinking; shallow and inappropriate affect; silly or unpredictable and regressive behavior; weird mannerisms; frequent hypochondriacal complaints; absence of systematized delusions; and silly, incongruous, labile, or flat affect. The onset is usually early and insidious. The course is usually chronic, unremitting, and deteriorating. The prognosis is poor, but this subtype is rarely seen nowadays.

Catatonic. The patient often exhibits muscular rigidity, stupor, mutism, negativism, excitement, or posturing. Four types are distinguished: withdrawn, excited, rigid, and posturing. A given patient generally manifests only one type, but sometimes swift transitions from the withdrawn to the excited phases are observed. Both of these phases require careful monitoring. In the excited phase, the patient may be dangerous to himself or others, perhaps being driven to obey self-destructive or violent hallucinatory commands. In the severely withdrawn phase, the nutritional status requires careful attention because the patient might otherwise starve to death. Catatonic schizophrenia was once reported to be common, but now is relatively rare. The prognosis with treatment is fair, perhaps because many catatonic patients may in fact suffer from an affective disorder.

Paranoid. It is characterized by the presence of persecutory or grandiose delusions often associated with hallucinations. Delusions of jealousy and excessive religiosity are sometimes observed. Paranoid schizophrenic behavior is frequently hostile and aggressive and tends to be consistent with the content of the delusions. Although the prognosis is poor for recovery, most patients on neuroleptic medication are able to function outside the hospital.

Undifferentiated. This diagnosis is made when the episode of illness is manifested by psychotic symptoms that do not fit the preceding categories or when the symptoms are mixed and the patient could be classified in more than one category.

Residual. Reserved for patients who at some previous time had an episode involving florid psychotic symptoms of the disorganized type and who now have defect-state signs of schizophrenia such as blunted affect, eccentric behavior, communication disorder, or impairment in social relations, self-care, and work adjustments. Type II syndrome fits best here.

PERSONALITY DISORDERS

By Donald E. Manning, M.D.
Atlanta, Georgia

DEFINITION

Personality disorders are chronic, rigid, dysfunctional ways of behaving in relationship to the environment. These patterns of dealing with the environment must appear in the patient by the time he reaches late adolescence. From the onset of these fixed behavioral patterns, the severity of the dysfunction and the degree of subjective distress that the individual feels may vary from time to time or from situation to situation through most of adult life.

Personality disorders must be separated from *personality traits.* Personality traits are the predictable or usual style the individual has for dealing with his environment. Personality traits may have elements that closely resemble personality disorders. The key, however, for differentiating one from the other is that disorders are maladaptive and dysfunctional, whereas traits may be quite adaptive to the individual's lifestyle or the specific situation.

The concept of personality disorders presents three diagnostic problems:

1. These conditions do not fit the definition of illness as it is conceptualized by most physicians. Rather, there is rarely a clearly defined onset to the disorder, there is no predictable clinical course, and there is no termination to the disorder.
2. Our society in general as well as the legal structure does not generally consider personality disorders illnesses but instead "character flaws."
3. The degree of maladaption or dysfunction runs on a continuum from quite mild to quite severe. In the mild or moderate end of the spectrum, the individuals may be considered merely "eccentric" or "normal variants."

SYNONYMS

Personality disorders are also called *character disorders.* Contemporary psychiatry divides personality disorders into eleven syndromes:

1. Paranoid personality disorder—paranoiac personality.
2. Schizoid personality disorder—introverted personality disorder.
3. Schizotypal personality disorder—latent schizophrenia.
4. Histrionic personality disorder—hysterical personality disorder.
5. Narcissistic personality disorder—sociopath, psychopath, sociopathic character disorder.
6. Antisocial personality disorder—sociopath, psychopath, sociopathic character disorder.
7. Borderline personality disorder—unstable personality disorder.
8. Avoidant personality disorder—passive-dependent personality disorder.
9. Dependent personality disorder—passive personality disorder, inadequate personality disorder.
10. Compulsive personality disorder—obsessive-compulsive personality disorder.
11. Passive-aggressive personality disorder.

PRESENTING SIGNS AND SYMPTOMS

The eleven disorders are divided into three separate clusters because of distinctive features common to the disorders in each of the clusters: the *eccentric, erratic,* and *fearful.*

Eccentric Cluster

Individuals with personality disorders in the "eccentric" cluster rarely present for treatment for their disorder, but the disorder may complicate management of medical problems. The reason individuals rarely present for treatment of these personality disorders is twofold: they are not subjectively distressed by their disorders, or, if these individuals perceive a dysfunction at all, they are more likely to attribute it to a problem with the environment or society rather than to their own way of coping with the environment or society. There are three characteristics common to the three eccentric personality disorders:

1. The person appears "odd" or "eccentric,"
2. The person avoids intimate relationships and appear "cold," and
3. These disorders are related to more severe psychiatric conditions, particularly schizophrenia and paranoid schizophrenia.

There are three personality disorders in the eccentric cluster:

Paranoid Personality Disorder. Individuals with this disorder have a long-standing and pervasive suspiciousness and mistrust of people. These individuals tend to be overly sensitive and hypervigilant and are unwilling to relinquish suspicious ideas, even in the face of irrefutable data. Although the prevalence is unknown, the disorder may be overrepresented in mystical and esoteric religions, pseudoscientific groups, and quasipolitical groups.

Schizoid Personality Disorder. This disorder is characterized by the lack of capacity to form social relationships with a bland or constricted affect. These people are the true loners, hermits, hobos, and skid row bums.

Schizotypal Personality Disorder. In this disorder there are peculiarities of thinking, perception, communication, and behavior. In addition, individuals with this disorder have the characteristics of the schizoid personality disorder in that they are socially isolated with a bland or constricted affect.

Erratic Cluster

There are several characteristics common to the personality disorders in the "erratic" cluster. The individuals appear dramatic, are emotionally labile, have an often erratic behavior and maintain interpersonal relationships that are characteristically intense, superficial, manipulative, or unstable. In contrast to the eccentric cluster of personality disorders, individuals who have one of these disorders tend to have intermittent extreme subjective distress, but in common with the eccentric cluster personality disorders they tend to view the etiology of the problem as environmental or societal in nature and fail to recognize any personal or psychological reason for their distress.

There are four personality disorders considered to be a part of the erratic cluster:

Histrionic Personality Disorder. This includes those individuals who are superficially charming, appealing, and gregarious, but who on closer involvement become demanding, vain, and egocentric. Sexual adjustment tends to be poor with naïveté, coquettishness, promiscuity, and social inadequacy. Individuals with this disorder are prone to physical symptoms, depression, substance abuse, and suicide attempts.

Narcissistic Personality Disorder. This is characterized by a grandiose sense of the individual's self-importance and uniqueness, a preoccupation with fantasies of unlimited success, exhibitionism, and inability to handle criticism, with extreme responses of either cool indifference or overwhelming feelings of shame, inferiority, and emptiness. Individuals with a narcissistic personality disorder tend to have interpersonal relationships that include the expectation of special favors without reciprocal responsibility and lack of appreciation of how others feel.

Antisocial Personality Disorder. This category is reserved for those individuals who chronically violate the rights of others. The individual is unable to perceive the need for rules in society and cannot anticipate the consequences of breaking the rules. This personality disorder frequently appears before the age of 12 and invariably appears before the age of 15. Common symptoms are lying, stealing, fighting, truancy, early or aggressive sexual behavior, and alcohol and drug abuse. In adulthood, prevalent behaviors include sexual promiscuity, fighting, criminality, and vagrancy.

Borderline Personality Disorder. This disorder has as its hallmark instability. These individuals have intense relationships and can be impulsive and unpredictable. There are dysfunctions of mood, including feelings of loneliness, anger, emptiness, and boredom.

Fearful Cluster

Individuals who have disorders in the "fearful" cluster tend to have extreme subjective distress, similar to that of individuals in the erratic cluster. In contrast to the other two clusters of personality disorders, individuals with disorders in the fearful cluster tend to view the cause of their subjective distress as an intrapsychic or personal problem and not as a problem of the society or the environment.

There are four disorders in the fearful cluster:

Avoidant Personality Disorder. This category is applied to those individuals who are hypersensitive to rejection, and, although socially withdrawn, desire affection and acceptance. It is felt in most cases that they maintain their social withdrawal because of low self-esteem.

Dependent Personality Disorder. An individual with this disorder is characterized by the relinquishing of all responsibility for one's life to another. These individuals lack self-confidence, are painfully uncomfortable when alone, and frequently have anxiety and depression.

Compulsive Personality Disorder. This individual is characterized by an inability to express warmth and tender emotions. Individuals with this disorder are preoccupied with rules and details, and they are extremely dedicated to their work to the exclusion of pleasure. Because of a need to avoid the appearance of imperfection, they postpone or avoid making decisions.

Passive-Aggressive Personality Disorder. Individuals with this disorder are characterized by procrastination, stubbornness, and inefficiency. They express their hostility covertly and are resistant to demands for acceptable behavior either at work or socially.

COURSE

The usual course of all personality disorders includes an early onset of dysfunctional symptoms, usually during adolescence or young adulthood. The dysfunctional behavior continues in varying severity throughout adulthood, but the pathologic style of dealing with the environment usually remains throughout life. Treatment of all the personality disorders is difficult and protracted.

Individuals with diagnoses in the eccentric cluster usually present for treatment only when forced by an agency or legal process or when they have developed a psychotic disorder. Individuals with a diagnosis in the erratic cluster usually present for treatment during periods of extreme stress or after suffering a loss.

When the patient with a personality disorder presents for treatment, psychotherapy, either behavioral or psychodynamic, is generally the treatment of choice. Because of significant problems with addiction and substance abuse, medication should be avoided except for the treatment of transient psychotic episodes or depressive episodes.

SUBSTANCE USE DISORDERS

by Philip T. Ninan, M.D.
Atlanta, Georgia

DEFINITION

Considerable semantic confusion exists around the nonmedical use of drugs and other substances to modify mood and behavior. There are broad medical, legal, social, and moral issues involved that result in differing approaches to the problem. Thus, moderate use of alcohol, nicotine, and caffeine is widely accepted and practiced by society. A medical definition that liberally subsumes all use of substances to modify mood or behavior outside the sociocultural context is of limited value. Thus, according to the third edition of the *Diagnostic and Statistical Manual* (DSMIII) of the American Psychiatric Association (1980), *substance use disorders* encompass the pathologic use of a substance that results in a pattern of maladaptive behaviors causing impaired social or occupation functioning. This diagnostic category does not include the direct (acute or chronic) pharmacologic effects of the substance consumed (e.g., intoxication, idiosyncratic reactions, withdrawal effects), which are classified under *organic mental disorders.* Substance use disorders are further classified into those of (1) substance abuse and those of (2) substance dependence. Whether use of the substance will result in abuse or dependence is affected by a number of variables, including personality, sex and age characteristics, sociocultural factors, and pharmacology of the durg. Substance use can be continuous, episodic, or in remission.

SYNONYMS

Drug addiction as originally defined required the development of physical dependence, i.e., the development of a set of physiologic effects on partial or complete withdrawal of the drug. *Drug habituation* required only a psychological desire for the drug without the development of physical dependence. However, with the intense emotions surrounding the issue in the 1960s and 1970s and the broad political and moral overtones involved, the terms drug addiction and habituation were often used interchangeably with the resultant semantic confusion.

PRESENTING SIGNS AND SYMPTOMS

In *substance abuse* there is a pattern of pathologic use for a minimum period of a month, causing impairment of social or occupational functioning. Thus, frequent and chronic intoxication, with resulting deterioration in physical and psychological functioning, is necessary for this diagnosis. Moderate alcohol consumption without the complications of alcoholism would not be considered substance abuse. *Substance dependence* is a more severe form of substance abuse with the development of tolerance or of withdrawal symptoms. *Tolerance* is the development of diminishing effects with the same dose of the substance or an increasing dose being required to achieve the same effects. *Withdrawal* symptoms are a set of symptoms specific to the substance being used that occur on stopping or reducing its consumption.

Alcohol

Alcohol abuse is diagnosed when consumption of alcohol is frequent, excessive, and felt to be necessary for adequate functioning. Binges, black-outs, violence while intoxicated, medical complications (e.g., liver disease), and deterioration of work habits or social and family relations are indicative of alcohol abuse. Tolerance and a history of withdrawal symptoms (tremors, seizures, delirium tremens) would make the diagnosis *alcohol dependence.*

The organic mental disorders associated with alcohol abuse and dependence are

1. Alcohol intoxication,
2. Alcohol idiosyncratic intoxication,
3. Alcohol withdrawal,
4. Alcohol withdrawal delirium,
5. Alcohol hallucinosis,
6. Alcohol amnestic disorder, and
7. Dementia associated with alcoholism.

Barbiturates or Similarly Acting Sedative or Hypnotic Drugs

This group includes the benzodiazepines (e.g., diazepam, flurazepam), methaqualone, paraldehyde, chloral hydrate, and glutethimide. Though pharmacologic differences exist among the drugs in this group, each has the capacity to produce symptoms of intoxication and withdrawal that are similar to those caused by barbiturates. Like alcohol, barbiturates can cause abuse or dependence.

The organic mental disorders associated with the use of this class of compounds are (1) intoxication, (2) withdrawal, (3) withdrawal delirium, and (4) amnestic disorder.

Opioids

Opioids form the strongest analgesics known to man. They occur naturally (e.g., heroin and morphine) or are synthetically derived (e.g., meperidine and methadone). They can be taken orally, intranasally, subcutaneously, or intravenously. Opioid dependence is differentiated from opioid abuse with the development of tolerance or withdrawal symptoms. Roughly half of opioid abusers subsequently become dependent on opioids.

The organic mental disorders associated with opioid use are (1) intoxication and (2) withdrawal.

Cocaine

Cocaine can be taken intranasally, by smoking, or intravenously. Since a well-defined withdrawal syndrome does not develop with cocaine abuse, there is no diagnostic category of cocaine dependence.

The organic mental disorder associated with cocaine is intoxication.

Amphetamines and Similarly Acting Sympathomimetic Drugs

Amphetamines include dextroamphetamine and methamphetamines. Other substances in this category include methylphenidate and appetite suppressants. Both tolerance and withdrawal symptoms develop with chronic use of this group of drugs, and hence both abuse and dependence can develop for this category.

The organic mental disorders in this group are (1) intoxication, (2) delirium, (3) delusional disorders, and (4) withdrawal.

Phencyclidine (PCP) or Similarly Acting Arylcyclohexylamines

No clear tolerance or withdrawal symptoms are known to develop with the abuse of drugs in this group. Hence, only abuse without dependence exists in this category.

The organic mental disorders associated with this group of drugs are (1) intoxication, (2) delirium, and (3) a mixed organic mental disorder wherein there is progression from one organic brain syndrome to another.

Hallucinogens

This group includes lysergic acid diethylamide (LSD), dimethyltryptamine (DMT), and mescaline. Their common characteristic is the capacity to induce hallucinations. No dependence exists for this category of drugs.

The organic mental disorders associated with hallucinogens are (1) hallucinosis, (2) delusional disorder, and (3) affective disorder.

Cannabis

Cannabis abuse becomes cannabis dependence with the development of tolerance, although the existence of tolerance is debated. No withdrawal syndrome has been unequivocally demonstrated for cannabis.

The organic mental disorders for cannabis are (1) intoxication and (2) delusional disorder.

Tobacco

Tobacco dependence is seen in a person who has continuously used tobacco for at least a month; has made unsuccessful attempts to stop its use; or when such an attempt was made, had withdrawal symptoms; or continues to use tobacco despite the presence of medical conditions which are exacerbated by tobacco.

The organic mental disorder for tobacco is tobacco withdrawal.

COURSE AND COMPLICATIONS

Patients with substance use disorders often have underlying personality disorders. Mood disturbances are also frequently associated with substance abuse and dependence. Most substance use begins in the late teens and twenties, although alcohol use disorders usually appear in the third to the fifth decade.

Abuse and dependence in the barbiturate group of substances can develop from illegal use by young adults for recreational purposes or from use initially under medical supervision which, because of the effectiveness of these agents in reducing anxiety, proceeded to abuse. The course of substance use disorders is affected by life situations, personality make-up, life events, sociocultural contexts, and the development of complications. Frequent complications include the development of organic mental disorders, infection from unhygienic needles in intravenous drug use, allergic reactions, development of depressive symptoms, and legal difficulties.

BEHAVIORAL PROBLEMS IN CHILDREN AND ADOLESCENTS

By Gregory Prazar, M.D.
Exeter, New Hampshire
and Stanford B. Friedman, M.D.
Baltimore, Maryland

As the incidence and complications of major childhood diseases have decreased, emotional and adjustment problems have surfaced as more critical concerns for families. These concerns have been reinforced and amplified by expanding research in childhood and adolescent development. Moreover, there has been a proliferation of nonprofessional literature dealing with emotional health and child-parent relationships. Parents are encouraged to become actively involved in the maintenance and promotion of their child's emotional health, beginning in the delivery room or hospital birthing room. Self-help parenting courses (Systematic Training for Effective Parenting and Parent Effectiveness Training) encourage parents to improve their interactional skills. In fact, parents seek help from a variety of mental health advisors of widely divergent training and philosophy. No one group of therapists holds the exclusive "contract" for psychological therapy in our society. However, a large majority continue to look to their physicians for counseling and guidance.

Primary practitioners represent a logical choice for parents when a behavior problem arises. The practitioner has the unique opportunity to follow children through rapidly changing developmental and growth stages (e.g., weaning, toilet training, separation from parents, introduction and progression through formal learning processes, coping with sexual changes of adolescence). Therefore, parental reaction to the child's illnesses, physical and emotional growth, and emotional strengths and weaknesses can all be observed over time. Continuity of care allows the practitioner to develop comfortable rapport with parents and children. No other professional follows the family for such an extended period.

A discussion of all behavior problems exhibited by children and adolescents is beyond the scope of this article. The emphasis here will be on identifying problems during routine visits, helping families understand normal versus abnormal behavior, and evaluating and diagnosing a behavior concern once that concern has surfaced. Suggestions for the practitioner in the management of behavioral problems also will be given, as well as indications for referral.

ANTICIPATORY GUIDANCE

Longitudinal delivery of care to families does not ensure that behavioral concerns will be brought to the physician. Rather, the physician's approach to behavioral material often determines whether parents will verbalize their concerns. It is the responsibility of the physician to provide anticipatory guidance with respect to behavior problems during routine visits. Helping parents to *understand* what is normal behavior during specific childhood ages may forestall behavior problems or may at least allow discussion of problems before they reach crisis proportions.

Infancy

Beginning with infancy, well-child visits allow the physician opportunities to provide anticipatory guidance. Discussions concerning temperament during the child's first 3 months of life are important, since parents often misinterpret infant crying. Temperament can be again discussed during the second year of life, when temper tantrums and breath-holding spells begin. Parents often fail to appreciate that negativistic behavior represents an aspect of the normal developing toddler personality. Although *tantrums* and *negativistic behavior* herald the beginning of a child's necessary desire for separation and independence, parents need guidelines with respect to structuring daily activities and with respect to coping with the provocative conflicts of toddlerhood (e.g., sleep disorders, resistance to eating, toilet training). *Self-stimulating behaviors* (thumbsucking, masturbation, head banging) emerge during the first 3 years of life and usually are indicative of normal transitional behavior as the child separates from parents.

Preschool Years

Since separation and independence are crucial tasks of the normally developing preschool child, the physician should discuss with parents during well-child visits the importance of time away from the child. Parents who occasionally leave their infants and toddlers with responsible sitters provide their children with the security that adults can leave and *will* come back and can provide themselves with important "mental health holidays" from the rigors of parenting. Inability of parents to separate from the preschool child for even brief periods may indicate a problem that can be discussed before the child *must* separate to begin school.

School Years

Beginning school can be associated with the emergence of other emotional problems. Symptoms of the *attention deficit disorder* (formerly referred to as hyperactivity or "minimal brain dysfunction") may surface. Parents may not have noticed attention problems in the preschool years because the child was not previously required to concentrate in a room with other children. Impulsive behavior also is common among children with the attention deficit disorder.

Specific *learning problems* also are noted during school years. Evaluation of attention problems and learning disorders definitely requires cooperation and communication with the child's school. Behaviors of concern to the school may not be appreciated in the physician's office when a one-on-one situation, free of distractions, exists for the child. Since evaluation of children with attention deficit disorders or specific learning disabilities requires a multidisciplinary focus (school officials to provide background behavioral information and psychologists to administer and interpret specific tests), the practitioner may be of greatest benefit as a case coordinator and act as a communication-liaison professional among the different professions evaluating the child.

Other behavior problems frequently materialize during school years. Separation difficulties between parent and child may result in *school phobia.* School phobia rarely presents with the parent lamenting to the physician, "I can't get Johnny to attend school." Rather, since the problem involves separation conflicts, the presentation of the problem is usually masked by a somatic complaint. Long-standing abdominal pain or headaches are common presenting symptoms of school phobia. When information obtained at a visit suggests a long-standing symptom, the practitioner must ask how much school has been missed because of the illness. School phobia is a psychiatric emergency and requires communication between the school administration, the school nurse, and parents to adequately cope with the problem. The longer the child remains home from school, the more difficult school re-entry becomes. Interestingly, school phobia usually occurs in children who perform academically well when they are in school.

When the child reaches school age, behaviors that the family had previously tolerated as immature often are presented as problems, since school entry implies an increased level of maturity. *Enuresis* represents a neuromaturational problem which parents may not mention to the physician until the child starts school. Routine inquiries about enuresis at well-child visits provide the practitioner an opportunity to discuss this problem before families necessarily become upset. *Encopresis* (fecal soiling) represents a much more complex behavior problem that parents sometimes tolerate during preschool years, but obviously find disturbing once the child becomes involved in the "public sector." Evaluation of this problem usually requires the expertise of a physician with some psychological training.

Symptoms of *lying and stealing* often are brought to the attention of the practitioner by parents of the school age child. Lying and stealing may be tolerated at home in the preschool child. However, attendance in school places the child in the context of societal mores, which dictate truthfulness and respect for property. Too frequently parents overreact to symptoms of lying and stealing before analyzing all of the relevant information. As with many other behavior problems, lying and stealing can represent a spectrum of psychopathology, from a common transient developmental phenomenon to an ominous indication of severe psychiatric disturbance. It is the practitioner's responsibility to help the family evaluate the seriousness of the child's symptoms.

Adolescence

Adolescence represents a particularly difficult time for both parents and teen-agers. Parents frequently have never resolved feelings about their own adolescence when suddenly they begin to confront rebelliousness, anger, and mood swings in their child. Since teen-agers themselves unconsciously vacillate between wanting to be treated as an adult and as a child, parent-teenager communication becomes extremely difficult. Adolescents struggling to achieve autonomy frequently exhibit "out-of-control" behavior. Many parents and some practitioners fail to appreciate that out-of-control behavior is a spectrum. Such behavior may represent a transient loss of control (indicative of normal teen-age rebellion) or may intensify to a total lack of control (suggesting significant psychopathology). Therefore, conflicts regarding independence may be manifested by arguments about curfews or may terminate in runaway behavior. Anger toward parents may be displayed by habitually ignoring family rules (e.g., "forgetting" chores), or it may escalate to overt antisocial behavior (e.g., shoplifting).

If the family fails to resolve conflicts concerning adolescent struggles for independence, the adolescent may become depressed. Adolescent depression may be exhibited by delinquent behavior (an angry expression of helplessness), by substance abuse (an effort to control the depression), or by self-destructive acts (risk-taking behavior or suicide attempts as a final resignation to hopelessness).

Adolescence is not synonymous with years of tumultuous parent–teen-age conflict. Anticipatory guidance to families with respect to adolescent negativism and rebellion may forestall some behavior problems and attenuate others.

DIAGNOSTIC EVALUATION

Meeting with the Parent

When specific behavior concerns are mentioned by parents at routine visits, a special 30-minute appointment should be suggested to obtain more information. Parents should be advised that the fee will be greater for the consultation visit because more than the usual time will be spent and that a subsequent 20- to 30-minute appointment will be needed for the child or adolescent. Parents also should be told that on the basis of information obtained, referral to a mental health professional may be indicated. *Both* parents should be strongly encouraged to attend the appointment. The appointment should take place in an unhurried setting, free of interruptions.

The evaluation visit should provide the parents an opportunity to air their concerns. To this end, the practitioner will need to shift gears at this visit from directive, closed questions ("Does Joe steal?") to nondirective, open questions ("What worries you most about Joe's behavior?"). Although the interview should allow parents to ventilate their worries, some structure is necessary. Four crucial areas need to be assessed by the practitioner when any behavior problem is presented:

1. The child or adolescent's attributes as viewed by the family.
2. The child's functioning at home.
3. The child's functioning at school.
4. Peer relationships.

Attributes. Parents usually have no difficulty in enumerating the child's or adolescent's problems. Listing strengths may be much more difficult. In fact, inability to cite any strengths of the child or adolescent may indicate a parent-child relationship severely lacking in warmth and affection. A list of strengths may not only help the family feel less hopeless or pessimistic about the identified problem but also can provide the practitioner with a better understanding of the child's or adolescent's emotional resources and ability to cope.

Home. Evaluation of home functioning involves obtaining information about:

1. Parent-child separation problems.
2. Recurrent symptoms of physical or mental illness in the child or in family members.
3. How parents manage discipline problems.

Separation problems include situations in which parent or child has difficulty separating from the other and circumstances in which separation has been intense or severe, such as parental divorce, recent death in the family, or job or social commitments that keep parents away from their children. *Recurrent symptoms* of physical or mental illness in the family provide the practitioner information about family stresses and how the family copes with them. How parents handle *discipline issues* serves as a barometer of parent-child communication; e.g., are parents autocratic with discipline? Are expectations for the child's behavior inappropriate?

School. Information about school functioning helps the practitioner understand how the child or adolescent copes in a structured setting outside the home. Several issues should be explored:

1. What kind of grades does the child or adolescent receive and are parents satisfied with these grades?
2. Has there been a recent or progressive decline in academic performance?
3. Has the child ever repeated a grade?
4. Has the school defined any specific learning problems?
5. Does the school have specific concerns about the child's behavior?
6. How many school days has the child missed in the past year and for what reasons?

If significant concerns with respect to school functioning surface, school officials should be contacted to elicit their perspective about the child. A parental release form for this information must be obtained. The physician should contact the school principal first, since this is the person who administers the school, even if he or she may not be the most knowledgeable source about the patient.

Peers. Parental information regarding the child's peer relationships needs to be obtained:

1. Does the child have a best friend or does he prefer to be alone?
2. Are friends and activities age-appropriate?
3. Are most friends the same sex as the child?
4. How do the parents feel about the child's friends?
5. Has the child been involved in out-of-control behavior with friends (shoplifting, vandalism) and how did the parents react?

Meeting with the Child

Most of the preceding information can be obtained in a 30-minute appointment with the parents. A subsequent appointment will be necessary for the child or teen-ager to be seen alone by the practitioner. (Most children over 5 years of age can separate from parents for such an interview.) It should be emphasized to the parents during their interview that information provided to the physician by their child or teen-ager is confidential. It will not be shared with them unless such information involves possible danger to the child (e.g., suicide) or to others. This issue of confidentiality must be reiterated to the child or adolescent. Children and adolescents frequently distrust adults and envision their physician in collaboration with parents.

The evaluation session with the child or adolescent should be nondirective, candid, and nonthreatening. Specifically, effective physician-patient rapport is more readily established if at the beginning of the interview the physician honestly shares with the patient the nature of parental concerns. As with the parent interview, the physician should ask the child questions about:

1. *Family life.* Who hassles you most at home? Who is the easiest person to talk with at home?
2. *School.* What do you like most about school? What do you dislike most? What do you want to do when you graduate from school?
3. *Their peers.* Would you rather have friends or be alone? What do you like to do most with friends? Do you have a girlfriend or boyfriend?

Completing the Interview

At the completion of the two evaluation interviews, the physician should outline to the patient and parents his or her future approach to the defined problem. If the physician feels that more information is needed another appointment should be made. Clinicians often mistakenly assume that they should be able to clearly identify all pertinent issues in a single visit; in fact, a longer evaluation time may be more realistic. Similarly, families often erroneously assume that long-standing behavior problems can be diagnosed as quickly as an earache or sore throat.

REFERRAL

Although the practitioner is often best qualified to treat common behavior problems presented by a patient, there are definite indications for referral to mental health professionals:

1. If the diagnostic interviews reveal that there is dysfunction in more than one of the three critical areas (home, school, peers).
2. If parents request referral after the diagnostic interview. Parents' wishes should be respected even if the practitioner believes he or she could adequately treat the problem.
3. When the patient's problem creates uncomfortable feelings in the physician. Situations involving homosexual issues, seductive adolescent behavior, or adolescent acting-out problems may create feelings in the physician which can prevent an objective evaluation. It is as unrealistic to assume that a physician can adequately treat all psychological problems as it is to assume that he or she can treat all medical ones. Cognizance of one's own limitations is an important professional attribute.
4. When the patient or family member is a close social associate or a relative of the physician. Dealing with the emotional problems of a friend's child or of a relative's child is seldom appropriate. Obtaining personal details of family and sexual functioning is often indicated in the evaluation and may jeopardize the social relationship. Conversely, failure or hesitancy to obtain appropriate data may jeopardize subsequent effective problem resolution.

In all instances in which referral is suggested, parental and patient compliance with the referral is improved if that possibility has been mentioned as a contingency *early* in the evaluation process. The physician should always help families understand that seeing a psychiatrically trained professional *does not* connote "craziness." After the referral is made, continued physician contact with the family concerning the emotional problem helps assure compliance with the therapy appointments.

SUGGESTIONS TO THE PRACTITIONER

Certain caveats should be observed when behavior problems are presented to the practitioner. As previously stated, effective diagnostic evaluation of a behavior problem often may require more than two visits. The practitioner should avoid capitulating to parental pressure for quick advice after the first interview. Similarly, early reassurance by the practitioner with respect to problem behavior should be avoided until all facets of the problem have been explored. Practitioners are so well indoctrinated to a directive, advice-giving technique that a more nondirective, listening, and reflective approach may initially feel uncomfortable.

Responding to emotional problems may appear to have a more empirical framework than does diagnosing a physical problem. However, this is not the case and certainly does not justify an intuitive and personalized approach to behavior problems. Providing personal anecdotes regarding behavior of one's children as a form of reassurance to families or as an example of how to cope with problem behavior is inappropriate.

It is important to respect parental value systems when diagnosing and managing behavior problems and to observe child behavior in a relativistic way. For example, behaviors exhibited in the physician's office that upset the physician may not represent behaviors that upset parents. An inquisitive, explorative, and active 4-year-old may make the practitioner uneasy. To suggest to the parents that the child is overly active, if the parents have no problem with the child's behavior, imposes the practitioner's subjective opinion upon the family. The child may indeed display manifestations of the attention deficit disorder. However, if neither parents nor school officials have difficulty coping with the child, suggesting a problem is usually ill-advised.

SUMMARY

There is no dearth of child and adolescent patients with behavior problems and no scarcity of parents with concerns about their children. Helping parents understand the difference between normal and abnormal behaviors at routine well-child visits provides invaluable anticipatory guidance for optimal emotional growth and development. When a behavior problem surfaces, one or more extended visits will be needed to diagnose the problem adequately. Crucial areas to explore include emotional strengths and limitations, family functioning, school performance, and peer interactions. Referral to a mental health professional should be made if more than one of these critical areas appear significantly dysfunctional. The diagnosis and management of children and adolescents with emotional problems in practice can be rewarding, especially if the practitioner appreciates the importance of anticipatory guidance and the necessity of approaching behavior problems in an empathic, nondirective fashion.

Section Twelve

SKELETAL SYSTEM

RHEUMATOID ARTHRITIS

By Nancy L. Meryhew, M.D.
and Ronald P. Messner, M.D.
Minneapolis, Minnesota

DEFINITION

Rheumatoid arthritis (RA) is a chronic, systemic disease of unknown cause, whose major manifestation is symmetric polyarthritis and progressive joint destruction.

EPIDEMIOLOGY

Rheumatoid arthritis is a relatively common disease. It has an incidence of 0.1 to 1.0 per cent per year and a prevalence of 0.2 to 2.5 per cent per year. It is estimated that approximately 10 million people in the United States have this disease. The disease can occur at any age, although there is a peak distribution in the 40- to 60-year age group. Women are affected three times more often than men. There are no racial or geographic determinants; the disease has been reported in a worldwide distribution. A genetic determinant, HLA-DR4, has recently been described as occurring with increased frequency among RA patients; 20 per cent of a normal control population is DR4-positive, whereas 70 per cent of patients with RA have the DR4 haplotype. HLA-DR4 not only is a disease marker, but it also is associated with disease severity. RA patients with the DR4 haplotype are at greater risk for developing erosive arthritis as well as systemic complications of the disease.

ARTICULAR MANIFESTATIONS

The clinical hallmark of RA is symmetric polyarticular joint disease. The onset of arthritis is extremely variable and may be insidious, episodic, or explosive. Sixty to 70 per cent of RA patients have a slow onset over weeks to months, 15 to 20 per cent of patients have an intermediate onset with symptoms developing over days or weeks, and 8 to 15 per cent of patients have an acute onset with symptoms developing over hours to days. Symptoms of articular inflammation include joint pain, swelling, morning stiffness, and stiffness associated with prolonged rest. Joint symptoms may also be associated with prodromal symptoms of low-grade fever, malaise, fatigue, and weight loss.

Physical examination reveals a symmetric polyarthritis characterized by synovial proliferation and tenderness, warmth, effusion, and decreased range of motion. Synovial proliferation can be identified by the soft or spongy feel of the enlarged joint compared with the hard feel of hypertrophic bony spurring seen in osteoarthritis. The most commonly involved joints in RA are the metacarpal phalangeal (MCP, 87 per cent), wrist (82 per cent), and proximal interphalangeal (PIP, 63 per cent) joints. Characteristically, the second and third MCP and PIP joints are often involved early in RA. Temporomandibular, sternoclavicular, cervical spine, glenohumeral, acromioclavicular, elbow, hip, knee, ankle, and metatarsal phalangeal (MTP) joints are also frequently involved. The disease tends to spare the sacroiliac and lumbar spine joints as well as the interphalangeal joints of the toes. Progressive disease is associated with deforming arthritis and functional loss, including flexion contractures and muscle atrophy. Common deformities include ulnar deviation at the MCP joints; hyperextension of the PIP joints with flexion of the distal interphalangeal joints (DIP) (swan-neck deformity) or the reverse (boutonnière deformity), as well as "cock-up" and "hammer" toes. Bony ankylosis rarely occurs.

RADIOLOGIC FINDINGS

The radiographic features of RA include soft-tissue swelling secondary to synovial effusion, juxta-articular osteoporosis, uniform joint space narrowing secondary to destruction of articular cartilage, and bony erosions. The earliest sites of cortical surface erosion or marginal erosion correspond to the parts of the bone within the joint that are not covered by articular cartilage, the so-called "bare areas." More extensive erosions of the subchondral bone subsequently appear as the cartilage is destroyed and are associated with progressive, deforming RA. Osteophyte or new bone formation is not a radiologic feature of RA.

PATHOLOGY

Rheumatoid synovium is characterized histologically by chronic cellular infiltration and hypertrophy, resulting in pannus formation. The pannus is composed of a heterogeneous mixture of hyperplastic mesenchymal cells, new small blood vessels, lymphocytes, plasma cells, and macrophages. Lymphocytic infiltrates in RA synovium consists of 70 to 80 per cent T lymphocytes and 15 to 20 per cent B lymphocytes; monoclonal antibodies directed against T lymphocyte surface antigens have demonstrated increased suppressor lymphocytes in synovial fluid. Recent studies have also demonstrated an increased number of Ia (DR)-positive T lymphocytes in rheumatoid synovium. Ia or DR antigens are usually present on monocytes and B lymphocytes but also appear on T lymphocytes when they are activated. The pannus acts as a locally invasive tissue, destroying adjacent cartilage, bone, and capsular structures.

COURSE

The prognosis and natural course of rheumatoid joint disease is variable. Approximately 25 to 35 per cent of patients with RA will have an apparent self-limited disease course characterized by monocyclic involvement of less than 2 years' duration. A polycyclic disease course characterized by multiple exacerbations and remissions is more common, occurring in 50 per cent of patients. Unfortunately, 15 per cent of RA patients will have a progressive disease course characterized by relentless destruction of joints.

EXTRA-ARTICULAR MANIFESTATIONS

Although the clinical hallmark of RA is joint disease, it is important to recognize that systemic involvement may also occur. Joint disease per se is rarely fatal, but the systemic manifestations of RA can be. In general the number and severity of extra-articular features vary with the duration and severity of the joint disease. Arthritis usually precedes the extra-articular manifestations. Rheumatoid nodules, Felty's syndrome, and vasculitis are all extra-articular manifestations of RA. Systemic disease also includes pulmonary, cardiac, ocular, and neurologic involvement.

Subcutaneous rheumatoid nodules occur in 20 to 25 per cent of RA patients. They are usually found on extensor surfaces of the extremities, such as the olecranon process or the proximal ulna. The nodules may be firm or mobile and tender or nontender. They can occasionally suppurate. Rheumatoid nodules are associated with the presence of rheumatoid factor in the serum.

Felty's syndrome, the triad of RA, splenomegaly, and granulocytopenia (less than 2000 cells per cu mm), occurs in fewer than 1 per cent of patients. Splenomegaly without leukopenia is more common, occuring in 6.5 per cent of patients with RA. Patients with Felty's syndrome frequently have recurrent leg ulcers and are more prone to infection.

Rheumatoid lung disease includes pleural effusion, nodular lung disease, and interstitial fibrosis. Pleural fluid is characterized as an exudate with very low glucose and complement levels; rheumatoid factor may be present. Pulmonary nodules may be single or multiple and can occasionally cavitate. They cannot be distinguished radiographically from metastatic pulmonary disease. In *Caplan's syndrome,* a rare disorder, RA and pneumoconiosis occur synergistically.

Cardiac manifestations of RA include pericarditis, myocarditis, endocardial valve inflammation, conduction defects, coronary arteritis, and granulomatous aortitis. Pericarditis is the most common cardiac manifestation of RA, occurring in 30 to 50 per cent of patients as determined by echocardiography and autopsy studies; clinical pericardial disease, however, is less common. Cardiac tamponade and constrictive pericarditis can occur. Myocardial, endocardial, coronary arterial, and aortic disease occur in fewer than 1 per cent of all patients.

The most common *ocular manifestation* in RA is keratoconjunctivitis sicca (KCS) or "dry eyes" associated with Sjögren's syndrome. (See article on this topic.) Forty per cent of RA patients have Sjögren's syndrome, which is characterized by KCS and xerostomia or or dryness of the mouth. Other ocular manifestations include episcleritis, scleritis, and scleromalacia perforans.

Neurologic involvement includes entrapment neuropathy, peripheral neuropathy and cervical cord compression secondary to C1-C2 subluxation or basilar invagination. Entrapment neuropathies, such as carpal tunnel and tarsal tunnel syndromes, are compressive neuropathies secondary to rheumatoid synovial proliferation. Peripheral neuropathy may be either a benign sensory neuropathy or a combined motor-sensory neuropathy associated with mononeuritis multiplex. Mononeuritis multiplex, with an acute foot or wrist drop secondary to vasculitis of the vasa nervorum, may be the presenting sign of *rheumatoid vasculitis.* Rheumatoid vasculitis is also associated with cutaneous ulceration, infarction, and digital gangrene. Other visceral organ involvement, including bowel infarction, may occur, but nephritis is rare.

LABORATORY FEATURES

Anemia is the most common laboratory abnormality in RA, occurring in virtually all patients some time during their disease course. The anemia is usually a mild, normocytic hypochromic anemia of chronic disease with characteristic low serum iron levels, low total iron binding capacity, and normal reticuloendothelial iron stores. This form of anemia may coexist with iron deficiency secondary to gastrointestinal blood loss related to gastric irritation from aspirin or nonsteroidal anti-inflammatory drugs. In general, the anemia correlates with the erythrocyte sedimentation rate (ESR) and disease activity.

Rheumatoid factor (RF) occurs in 80 per cent of patients with RA and usually consists of IgM antibodies directed against antibodies of the IgG class. A rough correlation exists between the titer of RF and the severity of disease. In general, high titers are found in patients with extra-articular disease, particularly rheumatoid vasculitis. RF is not, however, diagnostic of RA; it is present in other connective tissue diseases as well as chronic infections, such as subacute bacterial endocarditis, tuberculosis, hepatitis, and others. In addition, RF has been reported in 10 to 40 per cent of apparently normal individuals over age 65 years, although usually in low titers.

Acute phase reactants, such as C-reactive protein, alpha$_2$-macroglobulin, haptoglobulin, fibrinogen, and ceruloplasmin, are usually elevated in RA. The ESR in particular is usually elevated and tends to parallel the activity of the disease. Increased values are found in 85 per cent of patients with mild severity, and in 95 per cent of patients with moderate or severe involvement.

Antinuclear antibodies (ANA) occur in 50 to 60 per cent of patients with RA and are associated with extra-articular manifestations of disease. ANAs are directed against histone or basic nuclear proteins and also cross react with rheumatoid factor in 50 per cent of patients.

Complement levels are usually normal or elevated in the serum and decreased in synovial fluid. Patients with rheumatoid vasculitis, however, may have hypocomplementemia. Sera from patients with rheumatoid vasculitis are also characterized by circulating immune complexes, cryoglobulins, eosinophilia, and thrombocytosis.

Synovial fluid is usually inflammatory, noninfectious type II fluid. The leukocyte count ranges from 2000 to 20,000 cells/cu mm. Immune complexes containing RF have been demonstrated in rheumatoid synovial fluid.

Differential Diagnosis

Perhaps the most important aspect in the differential diagnosis of any arthritis is establishing that joint tenderness is actually secondary to an inflammation of the synovial tissue. This is particularly important in the large shoulder and knee joints, in which inflammation of the surrounding bursa and tendons is associated with pain on motion. Localized tenderness over an area where bursa and tendon insertions are known to exist suggests inflammation of the periarticular tissue, not synovitis per se.

Once synovitis is confirmed, the differential diagnosis for RA includes other diseases that can present as a symmetric, inflammatory polyarthropathy. Certainly systemic lupus erythematosus (SLE), gout, and the axial arthropathies should be considered in the differential diagnosis. Although patients with SLE can have symmetric polyarticular disease, erosive or deforming arthritis rarely occurs. In addition, other systemic manifestations of SLE, such as cerebritis and nephritis, should help distinguish this disease from RA. Gout usually presents as an acute, monoarticular, or asymmetric oligoarticular arthritis, associated with hyperuricemia and uric acid crystals in the synovial fluid. Patients with polyarticular tophaceous gout, however, can have a symmetric arthritis that resembles RA with rheumatoid nodules. Demonstrating uric acid crystals within an involved joint, or performing a biopsy on the nodule to reveal its true nature as a tophus, should distinguish the two diseases. Rarely do gout and RA coexist.

Sacroiliac and lumbar spine involvement should identify a patient with an axial arthropathy. Patients with Reiter's syndrome or psoriatic arthritis, however, can present with polyarticular disease involving the small joints of the hands and feet. Characteristic involvement of the skin and mucosal membranes, involvement of the interphalangeal joints of the feet, heel tenderness, and absence of the serologic features of RA should distinguish these two diseases.

Osteoarthritis is the most common form of arthritis. It can easily be distinguished from RA by its clinical and radiographic features (Table 1). Osteoarthritis is usually not associated with clinical signs of joint inflammation, nor are erosive changes usually observed radiologically. A small subgroup of patients, usually middle-aged women, may have a variant form of osteoarthritis in which inflammation and bony erosion are prominent. Such erosive osteoarthritis primarily involves the DIP and PIP but spares the MCP joints of the hand; hence, it can be distinguished from RA on the basis of joint distribution.

Table 1. Differential Diagnosis of Rheumatoid Arthritis and Osteoarthritis

	Rheumatoid Arthritis	Osteoarthritis
History		
Age	20–60 years	Over 50 years
Sex	M:F ratio, 1:3	Probably equal
Pattern of onset	Symmetric polyarticular	Asymmetric with few joints involved
Stiffness	Hours	Usually less than 0.5 hour
Constitutional symptoms	Yes	No
Physical Examination		
Joints involved	MCP, wrist, PIP; symmetric peripheral joint involvement	DIP, knee, hip, first carpometacarpal joint; asymmetric involvement
Subcutaneous nodules	Yes	No
Heberden's nodes	No	Yes
Radiology		
Soft-tissue swelling	Yes	No
Bone density	Osteoporotic	Normal
Erosions	Yes	No
Osteophytes	No	Yes
Joint space narrowing	Uniform	Nonuniform

Abbreviations: MCP = Metacarpal phalangeal; PIP = proximal interphalangeal; DIP = distal interphalangeal.

JUVENILE RHEUMATOID ARTHRITIS

By Charles H. Spencer, M.D.
New Orleans, Louisiana

Juvenile rheumatoid arthritis (JRA) is a systemic inflammatory condition, or group of conditions, of unknown cause in which immunologic factors appear to contribute to the disease pathogenesis. The inflammation often causes widespread connective tissue injury, especially in diarthrodial joints. JRA affects as many as 250,000 children in the United States. The clinical features of JRA vary according to several subtypes (Table 1), which can be identified in the first 6 months of the illness by their relative systemic and joint involvement and associated laboratory abnormalities. The presence of these different subtypes suggests that JRA may actually represent several different diseases, yet until the causes of JRA and its varied subtypes are known, it is practical to consider JRA to be one disease with several subtypes. The diagnosis of the JRA subtype allows a more reliable prediction of the disease course to be expected in any individual child and facilitates selection of the appropriate anti-inflammatory treatment.

The diagnosis of JRA requires the presence for a minimum of 6 weeks of continuous arthritis in a child 16 years of age or less. The disease subtype (systemic, polyarticular, or pauciarticular) may be apparent at onset but often is not definitely established for several months. The diagnosis of JRA also requires a thorough consideration and exclusion of other rheumatic and nonrheumatic causes of arthritis and similar conditions in children (Table 2). This discussion will describe first the characteristic clinical and laboratory features of JRA and then the distinguishing features of the diseases that are commonly confused with JRA.

SUBTYPES OF JUVENILE RHEUMATOID ARTHRITIS

Systemic Juvenile Rheumatoid Arthritis

Systemic JRA is a clinically striking subtype characterized by fever and other extra-articular features. This subtype occurs in 20 per cent of JRA children and has an equal female-male incidence. If the principal clinical features are present, it is the easiest subtype to recognize. The cardinal feature is high fever (up to 41°C), which is usually present at disease onset. The fever is intermittent and brief, usually occurring in the afternoon and evening and returning to normal or subnormal levels. Severe constitutional symptoms, such as irritability, myalgias, chills, arthralgias, anorexia, and vomiting, often accompany the fever. Because of the myalgias, arthralgias, and general malaise, these children are utterly miserable at the time of high fever; once afebrile their disposition and personality are completely different and they often appear well. A typical rash usually accompanies the fever at disease onset. The rash consists of pale red macules, less than 1 cm in diameter, that frequently coalesce into large patches. The rash is evanescent and usually not pruritic. The presence of the characteristic fever and rash is strong evidence for the diagnosis of systemic JRA. Other extra-articular involvement in systemic JRA include lymphadenopathy and hepatosplenomegaly, which occasionally can be so severe that a malignancy is considered. Clinically mild pericarditis and pleuritis occur in over half

Table 1. The Subtypes of Juvenile Rheumatoid Arthritis

Number of Subgroups	Number of Joints Involved	Frequency	Sex Ratio (Male:Female)	Onset Characteristics	Joint Prognosis
Polyarticular					
I. Positive RF, nodules II. Negative RF	> 4	40%	1:4	Small-joint arthritis Mild constitutional signs	Poor Fair
Systemic (no subgroups)	Variable	20%	1:1	High fever Rash Organomegaly Lymphadenopathy Arthritis within 6 months Negative ANA, negative RF	Fair
Pauciarticular					
I. Young girls Positive ANA 25% iridocyclitis	≤ 4	40%	1:4	Usually knees, ankles, elbows, or wrists affected Mild or no constitutional signs	Good
II. Older boys Positive HLA-B27 Lower extremity arthritis					Fair to good
III. F > M, any age Negative ANA, negative HLA-B27					Good

of patients with systemic JRA at some time in their disease. Iridocyclitis is rare in this subtype.

The arthritis is usually present at the time of diagnosis, but it also may develop anytime in the next 6 months. The arthritis is usually chronic, but it may be episodic. Polyarticular involvement is the rule, affecting large and small joints. One to 2 years after diagnosis, the extra-articular involvement often decreases and the joint disease predominates.

Polyarticular Juvenile Rheumatoid Arthritis

The polyarticular subtype is characterized by a chronic synovitis in five or more joints detected in the first 6 months after disease onset. This subtype constitutes 40 per cent of all JRA patients. Girls outnumber boys by a 4:1 ratio. Constitutional symptoms, such as fever, anorexia, general malaise, arthralgias, and myalgias, are mild and occur less frequently than in children with systemic JRA. Rheumatoid rash and organomegaly are rare. Occasionally, lymph node enlargement can be severe. It is useful to divide this subtype into two subgroups.

The polyarticular subgroup I occurs throughout childhood and is characterized by the absence of the classic IgM rheumatoid factor. The polyarticular involvement affects both large and small joints. In contrast, subgroup II disease is characterized by a high incidence in adolescent girls, high-titer rheumatoid factor, and a symmetric, mostly small-joint arthritis. Subcutaneous nodules frequently develop during the course of disease. This JRA subgroup appears to be very similar to classic rheumatoid arthritis in adults and also has a poor joint prognosis. Iridocyclitis in this subgroup is unusual, but it does occur.

Table 2. Differential Diagnosis of Juvenile Arthritis

Rheumatic Diseases
- Juvenile rheumatoid arthritis
- Rheumatoid variants
  - Ankylosing spondylitis
  - Reiter's syndrome
  - Psoriatic arthritis
  - Inflammatory bowel disease
- Rheumatic fever
- Systemic lupus erythematosus
- Dermatomyositis
- Scleroderma
- Vasculitic diseases
  - Henoch-Schönlein purpura
  - Kawasaki syndrome
- Sarcoidosis

Nonrheumatic Diseases
- Infectious diseases
  - Pyogenic joint
  - Osteomyelitis
  - Viral arthritis
  - Tuberculous arthritis
  - Lyme arthritis
- Orthopedic syndromes
  - Traumatic joint
  - Legg-Perthes disease
  - Chondrolysis of the hip
  - Slipped femoral epiphysis
  - Osteochondritis dissecans
  - Chondromalacia patellae
  - Discitis
  - Transient synovitis
  - "Growing pains"
  - Reflex neurovascular dystrophy
- Malignancy
  - Acute lymphocytic leukemia
  - Lymphoma
  - Neuroblastoma

Pauciarticular Juvenile Rheumatoid Arthritis

Pauciarticular JRA may be diagnosed in a child if the arthritis affects four joints or fewer during the first 6 months after the disease onset and if no systemic manifestations are present. This subtype occurs in 40 per cent of all children with JRA and affects four girls for every boy. The arthritis usually affects large lower-extremity joints, particularly the knees and ankles. Initial monoarticular arthritis is very common and requires a careful evaluation for other diseases, particularly infections. Serious disability due to joint damage is uncommon in this subtype, and more than 75 per cent of the children recover without sequelae. There are three pauciarticular subgroups.

The pauciarticular subgroup I JRA occurs usually in young girls from 2 to 4 years of age. These children have a positive antinuclear antibody (ANA) titer and have a 25 per cent risk of developing chronic iridocyclitis at some point in the disease course. The iridocyclitis is insidious and often may be present for months without obvious symptoms or signs. In this early stage of this eye disease, routine ophthalmoscopy may not detect the eye abnormalities, and only a slit-lamp examination on a regular basis ensures early detection. The risks of the iridocyclitis include posterior synechiae, band keratopathy, cataracts, glaucoma, and blindness. The arthritis and iridocyclitis are often dissociated in disease activity. Occasionally, the eye disease precedes the arthritis.

These young patients have a mild arthritis that usually responds well to anti-inflammatory drugs. The arthritis occurs in the children's knees, ankles, wrists, and elbows in some combination. The arthritis usually causes mild to moderate pain and stiffness, but occasionally only a painless swelling is present.

Pauciarticular subgroup II JRA affects primarily boys from 8 to 16 years of age and is associated with the presence of the HLA-B27 antigen. Involvement of lower-extremity joints is common early in the disease. Sacroiliitis and spondylitis may develop late in the disease course. Acute iridocyclitis may occur in these children.

The pauciarticular subgroup II JRA condition may eventually evolve into a seronegative spondyloarthropathy, such as psoriatic arthritis, ankylosing spondylitis, or Reiter's syndrome. Early in the disease, though, it may be difficult to diagnose these seronegative spondyloarthropathy conditions owing to a lack of the necessary diagnostic criteria. Until these diseases can be diagnosed definitely, it is useful to include this condition under the umbrella of JRA.

The pauciarticular subgroup III JRA affects children of all ages and girls more frequently than boys. These children do not have positive ANA, lack HLA-B27, and usually do not develop iridocyclitis. This subgroup shares the lower-extremity joint involvement and good joint prognosis of the other two subgroups.

LABORATORY FINDINGS

No single laboratory test is available at this time that allows rapid and reliable laboratory diagnosis of JRA. In particular, conventional IgM rheumatoid factor is positive in only 15 per cent of definite JRA cases. Each JRA subtype has characteristic laboratory abnormalities that do support the diagnosis of JRA and exclude other diseases.

Systemic JRA. *Children with systemic JRA* have the most striking laboratory abnormalities. The white blood cell (WBC) count is often elevated during active disease, usually in the range of 20,000 to 40,000 cells per cu mm. Occasionally, a severe leukemoid reaction is seen and the WBC may exceed 100,000 cells per cu mm. The WBC differential count usually shows a shift to the left as well. A shift to the right should suggest acute lymphocytic leukemia. Children with systemic JRA often have thrombocytosis, in contrast to the leukemic child, who often has thrombocytopenia.

Anemia is common in systemic JRA patients, and the hemoglobin may be as low as 8 to 9 gm/dl at diagnosis. The red blood cell morphology is usually normocytic and normochromic. Occasionally the anemia is microcytic and hypochromic owing to poor iron absorption or mild gastrointestinal bleeding associated with drug therapy, particularly with aspirin. If bone marrow aspiration is done, a hyperplastic marrow with increased cellular elements is usually observed.

The erythrocyte sedimentation rate (ESR) is reliably elevated in children with systemic JRA at diagnosis, owing to increased production of acute phase reactants such as fibrinogen. A normal ESR in an untreated child with active arthritis is strong evidence against the diagnosis of systemic JRA. ANA titers and the IgM rheumatoid factor are negative in this subtype.

Other laboratory abnormalities commonly observed in these patients include elevated levels of liver enzymes, hypergammaglobulinemia, and mildly elevated antistreptococcal antibodies.

Polyarticular JRA. Patients with polyarticular JRA may have mild anemia, leukocytosis, and a left shift in the differential count. The ESR is usually elevated, occasionally very greatly, as when many joints are affected by the arthritis. The ANA is often positive, particularly in the subgroup II. By definition, the classic IgM rheumatoid factor is positive in subgroup II.

The "hidden rheumatoid factor" has been reported to be present in most JRA subtypes. This hidden factor appears to be bound to autologous IgG and is found to be positive only if the serum is treated chemically. This test may eventually be useful in the routine diagnosis of JRA but at present remains a research test, unavailable commercially. IgG rheumatoid factors have been found in JRA patients but appear to be present in other rheumatic diseases as well and thus have limited diagnostic usefulness.

HLA typing may eventually have a role in the diagnosis of JRA. Certain disease associations have been demonstrated, particularly linking HLA-B27 with pauciarticular subgroup II, HLA-DR4 with polyarticular subgroup II, and HLA-DR5 with pauciarticular subgroup I. HLA typing is expensive and DR typing is often not routinely available outside large metropolitan medical centers. For the present, HLA typing for the diagnostic work-up of JRA is usually limited to ordering an assay for HLA-B27 on an older boy (8 to 16 years of age) with arthritis.

Pauciarticular JRA. Children with pauciarticular JRA have the fewest laboratory abnormalities, reflecting the localized disease. There is usually no anemia, leukocytosis, or change in the differential count. The ESR is usually mildly elevated, but it may be normal. Because infection must be considered in monoarticular arthritis, synovial fluid from these patients is often examined, revealing an inflammatory picture. The synovial WBC count is elevated, often between 20,000 and 50,000 cells per cu mm. Occasionally this count can be extremely high, even over 150,000 cells per cu mm, suggesting a pyogenic joint. The synovial fluid glucose level is usually normal (greater than half the blood glucose), and the synovial fluid protein is usually two to three times normal.

Antinuclear antibodies are positive in patients with the polyarticular and especially the pauciarticular forms of JRA. By definition, children in the pauciarticular subgroup I have a positive ANA and a high risk of iridocyclitis. Also, children with pauciarticular subgroup III may be ANA-negative for a period of time and then convert to ANA-positive status and have a significant risk for developing the eye disease soon thereafter.

DIAGNOSTIC PITFALLS

JRA is the major chronic synovitis disease of childhood but to some extent it remains a diagnosis of exclusion. Several forms of JRA are clinically distinct and easily recognized, but others are easily confused with rheumatic and nonrheumatic conditions. To diagnose JRA properly, a physician must understand the criteria for JRA diagnosis, the JRA subtypes, and the varied diseases that can resemble JRA (Table 2).

As noted earlier, the diagnosis of JRA can be made only in a person 16 years of age or less who has had synovitis in one or more joints for a minimum of 6 weeks. More importantly, other infections, autoimmune diseases, and malignant causes of arthritis must be considered and ruled out. Frequently, the diagnosis must be tentative early in the illness, and close observation over the next year is necessary for diagnosis confirmation. Rheumatologists by necessity are cautious diagnosticians owing to these clinical overlaps and uncertainties.

Systemic JRA is the easiest JRA subtype to recognize. The high fever that returns to normal or subnormal levels, the distinct evanescent macular rash, the severe abnormalities found in laboratory values, the arthritis, and the severe myalgias and arthralgias together produce a remarkable clinical picture that is rarely imitated to a great extent by other diseases.

Both the pauciarticular subgroup I disease in young girls who have a positive ANA and the polyarticular seropositive disease (polyarticular subgroup II) are also distinct clinical syndromes. The remaining subtypes, polyarticular subgroup I and pauciarticular subgroups II and III, have features that are often found in other rheumatic and nonrheumatic disorders and often require tentative diagnoses.

Infections

Infectious causes of arthritis are the most important diseases to exclude. Pyogenic arthritis and osteomyelitis often cause high fevers, and joint or periarticular swelling; anemia, leukocytosis, a shift to the left in the differential count, and an elevated ESR are common. Prompt diagnosis is crucial because local tissue destruction and further spread of the bacterial infection occur quickly. Important clues lie in the general condition of the child and the results of the joint and bone examination. Children with bacterial infection usually appear more sick and "toxic" than those with JRA, even systemic JRA. Findings in the joint and bone examinations are more abnormal in patients with osteomyelitis and septic joints. These children have more pain, tenderness, and limitation of motion. The definitive diagnosis of these bacterial diseases requires isolation of the organism from the blood, synovial fluid, or bone aspirate; a positive Gram stain; or, in the case of a septic joint, at the least synovial fluid that is compatible with a septic joint with a high synovial fluid WBC count, elevated protein levels, and decreased glucose levels. When laboratory results are equivocal, serial physical examinations may be crucial in differentiating JRA from these infections. When the diagnosis is in doubt, the child should be treated for the infection and then observed carefully over the next few weeks for signs of JRA.

Gonococcal disease commonly causes fever and arthritis in adolescent girls. Joint involvement is usually polyarticular. The joints are quite painful, swollen, and red. The septicemic skin rash begins as a macule and may become vesicular and then pustular. Patients should be questioned for recent sexual contact, blood cultures should be done, cervical cultures should be obtained from females, and males should be examined for the urethral discharge. (See article on Gonococcal Infection.)

Viral arthritis should also be considered. Numerous viruses, including enteroviruses and rubella, mumps, mononucleosis, and hepatitis viruses, may produce a transient arthritis. This arthritis is usually mild and limited to a few large joints. Hepatitis in adolescent patients may produce severe joint pain, stiffness, and swelling in the anicteric phase. Liver enzymes and hepatitis-associated antigens and antibodies aid in this differentiation.

Tuberculous arthritis is an ever-present concern in the 1980s after a decade of increased immigration to the United States from areas of the world in which tuberculosis is endemic. Culture of synovial fluid for mycobacteria or synovial fluid biopsy is imperative in children with a pauciarticular arthritis, particularly if the purified protein derivative (PPD) of tuberculin is positive or equivocal or if there is a family history of tuberculosis.

Lyme arthritis should be considered in children with large joint arthritis in tick-infested areas of the United States (infestive tick, *Ixodes dammini*). The erythema chronicum migrans rash is helpful in the diagnosis. In addition, specific spirochete serology tests are available.

Orthopedic Syndromes

Numerous orthopedic syndromes may mimic JRA. Acute trauma to the joint may product a picture that resembles monoarticular onset of JRA. Bloody synovial fluid and resolution of the swelling with rest are characteristic. Legg-Perthes disease, chondrolysis of the hip, slipped femoral epiphysis, and osteochondritis dissecans may produce hip or knee pain in the older child or adolescent. Appropriate x-rays usually allow prompt diagnosis of these bone diseases. Chondromalacia patellae often causes knee pain in female adolescents and may be suspected by the characteristic tenderness on palpation on the medial patella and the association with recurrent lateral subluxation of the patella. Arthroscopy often is necessary for definitive diagnosis.

Discitis often presents a diagnostic problem. This nonspecific disc space inflammation is typically seen in infants and children aged 1 to 3 years. The child is irritable and refuses to walk or sit up. The joint examination of the lower extremity is normal. Tenderness over the lumbar spine is often present. The child may be febrile, may have mild leukocytosis, and may have an elevated ESR. The lumbar spine x-rays show disc space narrowing, usually L4-L5 or L5-S1, 1 to 2 weeks after onset. The technetium bone scan may show increased uptake in the involved disc space in the first week.

Transient synovitis syndromes are characterized by mild synovitis of a joint, particularly the hip, that is noninflammatory and brief in duration. Nonspecific muscle or joint pains ("growing pains") are very common in children and may at times resemble chronic synovitis. These pains are usually brief, mild, and unassociated with fever, swelling, rash, and other inflammatory features. The child appears well between bouts of these pains. Physical examination reveals no abnormalities. Findings on laboratory tests are normal or negative. Psychosocial factors may be prominent. Reflex neurovascular dystrophy, also associated with psychosocial problems, has more severe signs and symptoms. Exquisite sensitivity of an extremity to light touch is the cardinal feature, and pain, swelling, and color and temperature changes also occur. Disuse of the extremity is common. The severity of the pain, tenderness, and disuse easily distinguish this problem from chronic synovitis.

Malignancy

The most worrisome diagnosis to exclude is malignancy, particularly acute lymphocytic leukemia (ALL). Several clinical features of the musculoskeletal presentation of leukemia are helpful clues. The pain is much more severe in leukemic arthritis than in JRA and other rheumatoid diseases. The children will often cry spontaneously without any weight-bearing or movement of the involved joint. Rapidly developing anemia, leukocytosis or leukopenia, and thrombocytopenia are suggestive of malignancy as well. ALL is also suggested by the presence of a relative lymphocytosis despite severe inflammatory changes, a finding quite unusual in rheumatic diseases. Metaphyseal lucent lines are often present in long bone x-rays in leukemia. The average duration from onset to diagnosis in this presentation of ALL is 4 months. This delay has prompted some oncologists to suggest that all JRA patients undergo bone marrow aspiration at diagnosis. This radical approach is unnecessary if these clinical differences are appreciated.

Rheumatic Diseases

JRA often may resemble other rheumatic diseases. JRA subtypes, particularly pauciarticular subgroup II, may resemble the "rheumatoid variant" diseases, especially ankylosing spondylitis, Reiter's syndrome, and psoriatic arthritis. Ankylosing spondylitis frequently begins in adolescent boys who initially have lower extremity arthritis and the HLA-B27 antigen. The typical sacroiliitis is evident on radiographs after an average of 9 years. Reiter's syndrome also affects older boys; produces lower extremity arthritis, conjunctivitis, and urethritis; and is associated with the HLA-B27 antigen. Psoriatic arthritis is seen in adolescent girls, and occasionally the arthritis may occur before the rash. Pitting of the fingernails is a diagnostic sign. The first manifestation of inflammatory bowel disease may occasionally be arthritis. These children often have had substantial weight loss and appear more ill than JRA children. Children who have polyarticular subgroup I or pauciarticular subgroup II or III disease may eventually prove to have one of these rheumatoid variant diseases.

Rheumatic fever (RF) is uncommon in the 1980s in developed countries, but it must not be disregarded. The painful migratory arthritis that rapidly responds to aspirin, the presence of pancarditis, antistreptolysin O (ASO) or streptozyme titers two to three times normal, and a positive throat culture for Group A beta-hemolytic streptococci strongly favor RF over JRA. Other major Jones criteria for RF, such as chorea, erythema marginatum, and subcutaneous nodules, are now unusual but if present are very suggestive of RF. Solitary pericarditis is more characteristic of JRA rather than RF. The systemic JRA rash is an evanescent macular rash, whereas the erythema marginatum rash is usually raised and serpiginous, and it remains essentially unchanged for 1 to 2 weeks. (See article on Rheumatic Fever.)

Systemic lupus erythematosus (SLE) in children may initially present with a polyarthritic involvement that is indistinguishable from JRA. Laboratory tests are essential because the presence of high-titer ANA, anti-DNA antibodies, and depressed C3 and C4 complement levels supports the diagnosis of SLE. Another factor in favor of SLE is multisystem involvement (e.g., kidney, central nervous system). (See article on Systemic Lupus Erythematosus.)

Polyarthritis may occasionally develop in children who have juvenile dermatomyositis (JDMS). The proximal muscle weakness, typical violaceous eyelid rash, pink scaly rash over the knuckles, elbows, and knees, and elevated serum levels of muscle enzymes easily separate JDMS from JRA.

Scleroderma patients may have arthritis early in the disease course, rarely before the characteristic rash appears. The presence of this hard, indurated rash eliminates the possibility of JRA.

Two vasculitic disorders may be confused with JRA. Arthritis occurs in 50 per cent of patients with Kawasaki syndrome (KS), usually in the second to third week of the illness. The arthritis is brief in duration, but occasionally it may last for several months. KS is easy to distinguish from JRA by its multisystem involvement, particularly the conjunctivitis, variable rash, mucous membrane changes, and desquamation. The arthritis of Henoch-Schönlein purpura (HSP) is a painful polyarticular involvement. The typical purpuric rash of HSP of the lower extremity is not seen in JRA.

Sarcoidosis should be considered in young children with fever, rash, arthritis, and iridocyclitis. The sarcoid rash is papular and is not evanescent. Eye examination may detect typical sarcoid granulomas. Affected joints often have large, boggy synovial thickening and effusions with minimal limitation of motion. The sedimentation rate is often normal. The diagnosis of sarcoid should be further supported either by finding elevated levels of angiotensin-converting enzyme or by biopsy evidence of noncaseating granulomas. (See article on Sarcoidosis.)

ANKYLOSING SPONDYLITIS

By Jack M. Lockhart, M.D.
La Crosse, Wisconsin

SYNONYMS

Rheumatoid spondylitis, Marie-Strumpell disease, von Bechterew's disease, spondylitis deformans, pelvospondylitis ossificans, spondylitis ankylopoietica, spondylitis ossificans ligamentosa, atrophic spondylitis, and Pierre Marie's syndrome. The preferred name and the one currently favored by the American Rheumatism Association is ankylosing spondylitis.

DEFINITION

Ankylosing spondylitis is a chronic, usually progressive, form of inflammatory arthritis of unknown cause affecting primarily the axial skeleton. The sacroiliac joints are characteristically almost always involved, but the spinal apophyseal joints as well as the peripheral joints may be involved. There is a genetic predisposition for ankylosing spondylitis, with greater than 90 per cent of the patients being positive for the HLA-B27 antigen. In addition, there is a strong sexual preponderance, with approximately 75 to 90 per cent of the clinically obvious cases involving men.

PRESENTING SIGNS AND SYMPTOMS

The onset of ankylosing spondylitis is typically between the ages of 15 and 50 years, with the majority being between the ages of 20 and 40 years. The presenting symptom is most often low back pain and stiffness. The discomfort characteristically is worse at night and in the morning upon arising; the pain usually improves with activity. The discomfort can radiate in the sciatic nerve distribution, mimicking radiculopathy and, on occasion, can affect alternate sides ("alternating sciatica"). Neurologic findings are generally absent.

In approximately 20 per cent of patients, the initial manifestation may be peripheral arthritis. This is generally an asymmetric pauciarticular (five or fewer joints) or polyarticular arthritis affecting primarily large joints, usually in the lower extremities. Occasionally the peripheral arthritis can present as monoarticular arthritis. Peripheral arthritis is a common presenting feature of ankylosing spondylitis in children, and in young boys especially, pauciarticular juvenile rheumatoid arthritis (JRA) is commonly associated with the positive HLA-B27 antigen.

Less common presenting features include iritis, heel pain, acute back pain with fever, and systemic features (weight loss, fever, anorexia).

COURSE

Ankylosing spondylitis follows a variable course from patient to patient. At one end of the spectrum is essentially asymptomatic sacroiliitis discovered serendipitously, and at the other end is disease of explosive onset that leads rapidly (within a few months) to advanced immobility of the back. The great majority of patients with ankylosing spondylitis follow a course of exacerbations and remissions or have low-grade, steady low back pain with occasional exacerbations. The pain is typically worse at night and improves with exercise and activity during the day. There is characteristically stiffness, particularly in the morning. The pain of the typical case of ankylosing spondylitis begins in the sacroiliac area and slowly progresses cephalad. Virtually any level of the spine can be involved. With costovertebral involvement, chest expansion is diminished, and this can lead to progressive premature dyspnea, particularly if the patient has a smoking habit. With progressive involvement of the spine, a position of increasing kyphosis with concomitant hip contractures occurs and the classic end-stage appearance of a person fixed in a stooped position, walking with a slow, shuffling gait, with eyes fixed to the ground, develops.

The peripheral arthritis of ankylosing spondylitis rarely leads to the progressive erosive synovitis seen in other forms of inflammatory arthritis (e.g., rheumatoid arthritis). When it does, however, a peripheral erosive, destructive polysynovitis, difficult to distinguish from rheumatoid arthritis clinically, is seen.

Most patients with this condition do very well over the long run and lead essentially normal lives when treated appropriately with a program of a nonsteroidal anti-inflammatory drug plus exercise to maintain proper posture.

PHYSICAL EXAMINATION

The physical examination of the spine early in the course of ankylosing spondylitis will often elicit only tenderness to palpation over the sacroiliac joints and "flattening" of the normal lumbosacral lordosis with forward flexion. With progressive involvement of other levels of the spine, further loss of spinal motion occurs and pain on palpation of the vertebral processes (indicating ligamentous and periosteal inflammation) and on percussion of the vertebral processes (from apophyseal or synovial joint involvement) is often elicited. Inability to touch the head to the wall with the heels against the wall (occiput to wall test) suggests cervical involvement, whereas inability to touch the toes with the knees straight suggests early lumbosacral involvement. The Schober test, another test of early lumbosacral involvement, is performed by marking the patient's back at the level of L5 and then placing a second mark 10 cm above this. The patient then bends as far forward as possible and the distance between the two marks is measured. An increase of less than 5 cm is considered abnormal and indicative of lumbosacral involvement. Thoracic spine involvement is usually present when there is less than 5 cm of maximum chest expansion when measured at the nipple line.

The peripheral joints may show evidence of synovitis. Loss of motion of the hips and shoulders is the most common manifestation of articular involvement other than that involving the spine. The other peripheral joints are rarely deformed. Subcutaneous nodules are characteristically absent.

COMMON COMPLICATIONS

The most common complications of ankylosing spondylitis are iritis, pulmonary fibrosis, cardiac abnormalities, spinal fractures, and spondylodiscitis.

Iritis occurs in approximately 20 per cent of patients and occasionally is the presenting feature. It usually is unilateral. Cardiac complications include aortic regurgitation (2 per cent of patients with ankylosing spondylitis), first degree atrioventricular (AV) block (10 per cent of patients with ankylosing spondylitis), and rarely complete AV block. Pulmonary symptoms may be related to costovertebral and costosternal joint involvement, with diminished chest expansion, or to pulmonary fibrotic changes that occur in the upper lobes bilaterally. Spinal fractures often occur after even trivial trauma in patients with long-standing ankylosing spondylitis. The cervical region is most commonly involved, and unless neurologic damage occurs, the diagnosis may be overlooked.

Spondylodiscitis is a lesion seen in ankylosing spondylitis that mimics septic discitis or a fracture. The x-ray appearance characteristically shows erosions of vertebral bodies adjacent to a disc and marked sclerosis of the surrounding bone.

LABORATORY FEATURES

Ankylosing spondylitis has a strong genetic predisposition. Approximately 90 to 95 per cent of patients with ankylosing spondylitis are shown to have the HLA-B27 antigen. The HLA histocompatibility system consists of genes that code for cell surface antigens, the HLA antigens. Although the B27 antigen is present in over 90 per cent of patients with ankylosing spondylitis, the antigen is present in less than 8 per cent of the general Caucasian population.

Results of other laboratory studies are either normal or nonspecific. The erythrocyte sedimentation rate is elevated in up to 70 to 80 per cent of patients, but it may be normal and is not a useful test to rule out active inflammation with certainty. Serum is characteristically negative for rheumatoid factor, although it may be found in 5 to 10 per cent of patients.

RADIOGRAPHIC EVALUATION

The radiologic findings of ankylosing spondylitis are pathognomonic when present. These changes may take years to develop, however, and prior to the discovery of the association with HLA-B27, the diagnosis could be elusive in the early stages of the disease. The diagnosis is made by the radiographic finding of bilateral sacroiliitis. Often a routine pelvis film is adequate to demonstrate this, but early in the course, special views of the sacroiliac joints themselves may be necessary. The changes in the sacroiliac joints are initially apparent as erosions, often more apparent on the iliac side. These changes appear as erosions along the sacroiliac space, giving rise to so-called "pseudo-widening" of the joint space. Along with these changes, progressive sclerosis of the adjacent bone occurs. Ultimately, the sacroiliac joints are obliterated and radiographically bony ankylosis occurs. With vertebral column involvement, other changes may occur. Characteristic changes include: (1) squaring of the vertebral bodies, (2) calcification of the paraspinous ligaments and anulus fibrosus of the intervertebral discs, producing syndesmophytes and leading eventually to the classic "bamboo spine," with continuous intervertebral calcification, and (3) progressive fusion of the apophyseal joints. In those patients with peripheral involvement, erosion and cartilage loss of the hips and shoulders can be seen as well as periostitis of the ischial bones, calcaneus, and symphysis pubis.

DIFFERENTIAL DIAGNOSIS

The diagnosis of ankylosing spondylitis is confirmed in a patient with chronic low back pain who shows the radiographic changes characteristic of spondylitis. Before the typical x-ray changes become evident, the diagnosis can be suspected strongly in the setting of chronic low back pain that started slowly at a young age, is worse in the early morning, improves with exercise, and is found in an HLA-B27–positive patient. One controlled study of the evaluation of low back pain showed with 95 per cent sensitivity and 85 per cent specificity that the clinical history alone could differentiate between ankylosing spondylitis and other causes of low back pain. With four of the following five historical criteria, the diagnosis of ankylosing spondylitis was strongly likely: (1) insidious onset of low back pain, (2) onset of pain before age 40 years, (3) low back pain present for at least 3 months, (4) pain with morning stiffness, and (5) low back pain improving with exercise.

Other conditions that must be differentiated from ankylosing spondylitis include low back strain, degenerative joint disease of the spine, mechanical abnormalities (e.g., spondylolithiasis, spina bifida, scoliosis, and so forth), and degenerative disc disease with radiculopathy. These conditions can usually be differentiated from ankylosing spondylitis by the radiographic findings, the physical findings, or the history itself. Low back pain from musculoskeletal strain, which is often difficult to distinguish from early ankylosing spondylitis, can often be suspected and differentiated by using the five historical factors listed earlier. More difficult to differentiate historically and radiographically are psoriatic spondylitis, the spondylitis associated with inflammatory bowel disease, Reiter's syndrome with spondylitis, osteitis condensans ilii, and septic arthritis of the sacroiliac joint. Psoriatic arthritis, Reiter's syndrome, and inflammatory bowel disease can usually be differentiated on the basis of physical examination (conjunctivitis, typical psoriatic skin lesions, urethral discharge, perirectal fistulas, and other findings) or the history (recurrent diarrhea, bloody stools, dysuria). Osteitis condensans ilii is a condition seen primarily in young mothers that causes low back pain and appears radiographically as sclerosis limited to the ilium at the margins of the sacroiliac joint. Septic sacroiliitis is characteristically unilateral, and since ankylosing spondylitis causes bilateral sacroiliitis, it should not be confused with septic sacroiliitis. In the early stages, however, ankylosing spondylitis may involve only one of the sacroiliac joints, and an infectious cause would have to be ruled out. Tuberculous as well as fungal and pyogenic infections must be excluded in this setting.

Other diffuse connective tissue diseases, such as rheumatoid arthritis, systemic lupus erythematosus, rheumatic fever, polymyositis, and scleroderma are easily distinguished from ankylosing spondylitis by their typical clinical and serologic features, as well as by their general lack of lower back involvement.

OSTEOARTHRITIS

By George E. Ehrlich, M.D.
Summit, New Jersey

DEFINITION

Osteoarthritis should be thought of as an impairment of joints rather than as a disease. It afflicts diarthrodial joints and is characterized by degeneration of the hyaline articular cartilage, subchondral bone fractures, and remodeling of subchondral bone with the development of osteophytes. Cartilage is lost progressively, and exposed, denuded bone is worn as smooth as ivory in the process of "eburnation." However, these are late features, which permit diagnosis, and they are accompanied by characteristic roentgenographic evidence, namely narrowing of the joint, reshaping, marginal spurs (osteophytes), and sclerosis of juxta-articular bone. All of these changes are late to develop, and the process had been going on for some time before they are recognizable. Therefore, osteoarthritis may have a clinical definition that emphasizes the pathogenesis, and which recognizes that diagnosis is usually only suspected but can be verified on occasion through arthroscopy; the diagnosis is reached from observation of the clinical course long before x-rays confirm it.

In many parts of the world, the term "osteoarthrosis" is preferred. After all, to physicians and patients, "arthritis" implies inflammation and destruction and therefore implies a poorer prognosis than is seen in most instances; frequently the course avoids inflammation and even disability. Because trauma and inflammation are present at the inception of osteoarthritis at a point remote in time from the first clinical signs, and as secondary inflammation complicates the clinical course and probably accounts for the very painful symptoms that draw attention to this joint involvement, "osteoarthritis" is a better term to apply to the acutely symptomatic process, and "osteoarthrosis" to the underlying changes that often but not always result in clinical symptoms. Another term, "degenerative joint disease," advocated by the American Rheumatism Association, has little to recommend it. Osteoarthritis is a balance between destructive changes and repair, and so calling the disorder degenerative is not entirely apt and often implies an inevitable progression that is not warranted. As has been mentioned previously, the term "disease" rarely is an appropriate description and is applied logically to the syndrome of interphalangeal osteoarthritis, but probably not at all to isolated involvement of various major joints and the spine. Whether the labels primary and secondary when used in conjunction with the term osteoarthritis, have value remains controversial. These terms imply that primary osteoarthritis has no known antecedents, whereas secondary osteoarthritis results from identifiable causes. However, since the initial insult that results in osteoarthritis is quite remote in time, may be of seemingly minor import at the time, or may be repetitive but not identified as a source of the problem, it is unlikely that in most instances the cause will be remembered. Failure to associate the cause with the effect does not make the effect primary. Structural, metabolic, endocrine, and congenital factors all play a role in causation in some instances, and inflammation of joints by other identifiable diseases or trauma quite usually results in osteoarthritis.

Finally, the site of the primary lesion is still controversial. Some claim that changes in cartilage antedate all other changes, whereas some researchers have blamed subchondral bone fractures that occur from undue stresses as initiators of the process. Significantly, such fractures, breakage of collagen fibrils, swelling of cartilage proteoglycans, and alterations in joint fluid viscosity probably all figure in the pathogenesis. On the diagnostic level, specific joint involvement can usually be related to some vocational, avocational, or other use, disuse, or abuse of the afflicted joints, again with exception of the polyarticular syndrome, known as interphalangeal osteoarthritis.

PHYSICAL FINDINGS

Hands

The distal interphalangeal joints of the fingers are common sites for development of osteoarthritis. Heberden's nodes are bony enlargements at these joints, but their early development is often characterized by soft tissue swelling over the distal interphalangeal joints. The development of interphalangeal osteoarthritis is usually insidious and noticeable chiefly because of a certain clumsiness that the afflicted finger develops and because of sharp pains produced in the involved joint when it is mildly traumatized. Similar swellings, usually named Bouchard's nodes, may occur in the proximal interphalangeal joints. The interphalangeal joint of the thumb is also at risk. When these nodes become large, they tend to flex the joint slightly. Associated Dupuytren's contractures in the palm and trigger fingers, and rarely tenosynovitis near the metacarpophalangeal joint in the palm, are frequent accompaniments.

Occasionally, presentation of Heberden's nodes is dramatic, with marked redness, soft swelling, heat, tenderness, and considerable impairment of function. This syndrome is most common in women of middle life, with peak onset between the ages of 45 and 55 years; it may develop earlier if artificial menopause has been induced or there is a strong family history, or later if estrogen replacement therapy has been administered. Osteoarthritis is polyarticular, afflicting almost all of the distal and proximal interphalangeal joints in a symmetric fashion. Occasionally it involves even some metacarpophalangeal joints, chiefly those of the thumb and index finger, but including the first carpometacarpal joints as well. A remarkable symmetry characterizes this syndrome. The obvious signs of inflammation bring it to the patient's and the physician's attention, but they may be a secondary feature, with undetected nodose deformities perhaps having preceded the more severe inflammatory process. If the inflammatory process continues, it sometimes leads to dramatic phalangeal deformity and deviation, side-to-side instability, and, on x-ray, erosive changes. The term erosi ve osteoarthritis has been applied to this phase. Generally, treatment with nonsteroidal anti-inflammatory drugs and local measures to provide heat or stimulation effectively cause this syndrome to subside. Residual deformities are characteristic, but they do not usually preclude continued active use of the hands and rarely are prodromal for systemic disease. In some instances, rheumatoid arthritis supervenes some years later, but this occurs chiefly in those patients in whom ankylosis had previously been part of the osteoarthritic process. In erosive osteoarthritis, joints remote from the hands are not involved.

The syndrome termed primary generalized osteoarthritis probably included patients from all these groupings. It implied an osteoarthritic disease afflicting joints of the hands, neck, hips, and knees, and perhaps other joints as well. However, there is no statistical proof that this syndrome is more than a conjunction of symptoms and signs at various joints in the same person, rather than a causally related process.

Laboratory Tests. Laboratory investigations provide little help. The erythrocyte sedimentation rate (ESR) may be modestly elevated, but certainly not to the levels that usually accompany rheumatoid arthritis. There should be no influence upon the complete blood count or any other systemic laboratory tests, especially those of a serologic nature. Rheumatoid factor and other antibodies do not develop, although in patients in older age groups there often is a marginal titer of rheumatoid factor that will give positive results on the screening slide tests, even though it appears to be of no significance.

Pitfalls in Diagnosis. The most important feature of interphalangeal osteoarthritis is that it is not rheumatoid arthritis. Errors in diagnosis and confusion with rheumatoid arthritis frequently occur, leading to inappropriate treatment and prognosis. As a possible precursor to rheumatoid arthritis, interphalangeal osteoarthritis should be watched, but neither overtreatment nor unfavorable prognostic inferences are warranted.

One of the most interesting involvements in the hand is at the first carpometacarpal joint (trapeziometacarpal joint). This incongruous joint helps make it possible to appose the thumb to the other fingers, to rotate the thumb, and to use it for the firm grasp that distinguishes humans from the mammals. With osteoarthritic involvement of this joint, free use of the hands is limited, making it difficult or impossible for the patient to turn doorknobs, open jars, or participate in certain sports, notably bowling. Yet this joint most commonly is affected in the inflammmatory interphalangeal osteoarthritic syndrome, or it may be afflicted independently. Infrequently, the adjacent trapezioscaphoid joint is also involved, complicating the problem.

DeQuervain's disease, a stenosing tenosynovitis of the abductor muscle of the thumb, produces pain in the anatomic snuffbox area of the hand, and this can be confused with osteoarthritic joint involvement, which produces pain in much the same area. A differential point is that placing the thumb in the hand and forcibly abducting the hand aggravates the pain of DeQuervain's disease, whereas local palpation of the thickened and tender carpometacarpal area characterizes the osteoarthritic lesion. By fixing the wrist, the examiner can reproduce the painful symptom by rotating the first metacarpal distally while fixing it proximally. The first carpometacarpal joint area is squared, and this finding, together with an atrophic thenar eminence (similar to that seen in carpal tunnel syndrome, which often accompanies osteoarthritis of the hand), produces a characteristic appearance to this radial portion of the hand. This radial involvement also distinguishes osteoarthritis from rheumatoid arthritis in the hands, as the latter usually involves the wrist joint on the ulnar aspect. Swelling produced by rheumatoid arthritis tends to be diffuse; that produced by osteoarthritis is discrete. Although small nodules often form over joints and tendons in the hand in rheumatoid arthritis, mucous cysts will occasionally form over the joints in osteoarthritis.

Large Joints

Hips and knees, in particular, are involved by osteoarthritis, with shoulders, elbows, wrists, and ankles theoretically at risk but rarely involved, at least symptomatically. A diffusion of forces through the small bones of the carpus may help spare the wrist; a similar mechanism may be at work in the ankle. Because direct transmission of force from one bone to the next may play a role in pathogenesis, it is obvious that the knees and hips, which are the major weight-bearing joints, will most frequently show the characteristic changes. Shoulder involvement, often present but rarely symptomatic, becomes symptomatic chiefly in people who use the shoulders in a weight-bearing capacity, either at work or by leaning on assistive devices.

Hip

Except after unusual trauma, osteoarthritis of the hips and knees begins later in life, not necessarily because it is a process that occurs in the elderly but rather because it is a process that takes considerable time to develop into a clinically appreciable disorder. Osteoarthritis afflicts the hips more commonly in men, the knees more commonly in women. The hip on the longer side tends to be involved first, the knee on the shorter side. Dynamically speaking, this is a logical sequence: The femoral head on the longer side is driven into the acetabulum with each step more forcefully than that on the shorter side, and the forces are transmitted across the knee more forcefully on the shorter side than on the longer side. Although the symptoms are commonly unilateral, careful study will reveal osteoarthritis to be bilateral, at least in the later stages.

Osteoarthritis of the hip provokes dull, aching pain in the groin initially. This pain is worse and is accompanied by transient stiffness upon first arising and after any period of rest. However, unlike the stiffness of rheumatoid arthritis, this stiffness can be overcome by the simple expedient of moving about briefly or by the application of moist heat, as in a bath or shower. Pain and stiffness are aggravated by excessive use, so that the usual pattern is one of a brief period of discomfort in the morning and a more prolonged period of discomfort later in the day. In between, patients tend to feel reasonably well, and the pain can be relieved by rest. Thus, the patients are not awakened from sleep by the pain, although coincident leg and thigh cramps may occur during the night. Most patients state that they would be quite comfortable if they never had to get up. Clearly, this differentiates them from patients who have rheumatoid arthritis and similar inflammatory diseases, in which night symptoms are more intense and rest ultimately aggravates symptoms. Only in the last stages of osteoarthritis of the hip is night pain more severe, and then it is probably because of the superimposition of inflammation. Pain radiates from the groin to the inner aspect of the thigh, and often to the knee. In fact, many patients who have osteoarthritis of the hip present first with painful knees. Because some minor osteoarthritic changes can be found on the knee by x-ray, osteoarthritis of the hip may well be missed for some time.

Physical Examination. Osteoarthritis of the hip is best detected on examination by use of the FABERE maneuver. This is an acronym referring to flexion, abduction, external rotation, and extension, sequentially examined. Compromises in these motions will become apparent even early in the process. Adduction of the hip is also somewhat restricted. Patients will classically tell of being unable to tie their shoes, squat, or sit cross-legged. In women, sexual intercourse is difficult because of restrictive hip motion. However, osteoarthritis of the hip is much more common in men than in women. It is still referred to in international medical writings as morbus coxae senilis, erroneously suggesting that advanced age is causative; on the other hand, this term does abstract the problem so as not to imply that it is part of a generalized or systemic disease.

Radiographic Examination. On x-ray, loss of cartilage is demonstrated by diminution in the space between adjacent bones. At the hip, this narrowing takes place superiorly in almost all instances, rarely being axial or medial. Consequent to the narrowing is sclerosis, followed by eburnation, formation of osteophytes at the margins, and buttressing of the femoral neck. Bone cysts, also known as geodes, form, and ultimately there may be flattening of the femoral head superiorly with marked reshaping on the femoral and acetabular side of the hip.

Hip involvement is frequent in primary generalized osteoarthritis, but probably more often fortuitously, occurring in the patient at the same time as involvement of other joints but not as the result of the same disease process. Pain of similar nature and some restriction of motion of the hip can occur because of supratrochanteric bursitis or subischial bursitis, and these two common conditions must be sought for. They may be present despite x-ray changes in the hip that confirm early osteoarthritis, or they may be the source of pain when there are no x-ray changes, although the initial phases of osteoarthritis, as has already been said, need not be readily detectable radiographically. Paget's disease commonly involves this area as well, and aseptic necrosis of the femoral head consequent to connective tissue disorders, corticosteroid therapy, air embolism, and vascular disease will ultimately lead to secondary osteoarthritic change. Other metabolic diseases, such as ochronosis and hemochromatosis, will result in osteoarthritis of the hip. Gout rarely occurs here, although it may afflict the knee; in addition, chronic tophaceous gout and chondrocalcinosis, because of calcium pyrophosphate dihydrate deposition, can also provoke destructive changes of cartilage that will ultimately result in secondary osteoarthritis in the joint.

Laboratory Findings. There are no specific laboratory changes noted in osteoarthritis. Erythrocyte sedimentation rate is marginally elevated in some patients, but no other abnormalities are consistently demonstrable.

Knee

Knee involvement is more common in women. The narrowing tends first to be medial and only later becomes lateral, and there is sharpening of the tibial spines on x-ray. Mediolateral instability will be noted, in contrast to the fore-and-aft instability of rheumatoid arthritis. Large effusions may develop, and although these are hard to detect when they occur at the hip, they are readily detected at the knee. Initially, there will be a bulge sign: When fluid is massaged out of the knee on the medial aspect, massaging the lateral aspect of the knee to bring the fluid back will produce a fluid wave that is readily seen on the medial aspect. Just as in rheumatoid arthritis the knees tend to adopt a valgus position (knock-kneed), in osteoarthritis they commonly take a varus position (bow-legged). Again, stiffness and aching are worse after rest and are relieved by moving about, but dull pain is often the consequence of weight-bearing. The mechanical disadvantage of the reshaping at the knee, the malalignment, and the instability make patients with osteoarthritis become invalids quite readily.

A common additional problem is pain and exquisite tenderness at the medial aspect of the knee. In this area are found the anserine bursa and the medial fat pad, the latter occurring almost exclusively in women. These structures can become inflamed without the knee itself becoming inflamed. Usually, on x-ray, a small medial osteophyte will be seen deep to the area of pain, and it is assumed that this irritates the superficial fatty layer and the anserine bursa, thus accounting for a recalcitrant syndrome sometimes termed rather inelegantly fat lady's knee, or adiposa dolorosa juxta-articularis.

When effusions become quite large, they tend to bulge posteriorly, and, like the bubbles that form on inner tube tires under pressure, they will extend into the popliteal space as so-called popliteal (or Baker's) cysts. These outpouchings can dissect down the leg posteriorly to simulate thrombophlebitis, with calf tenderness, positive Homan's sign, and peripheral edema. Treatment is quite different than for thrombophlebitis, however, and this frequent complication of large knee effusions needs to be borne in mind.

Frequently, loss of cartilage takes place on the posterior aspect of the patella, so that patellofemoral osteoarthritis develops. This is sometimes confused with chondromalacia of the patella, and it restricts the excursion of the patella sufficiently to compromise knee motion. Knee flexion contractures often develop as a result of osteoarthritis, just as flexion contractures at the hips will develop in osteoarthritis of the hip. Naturally, whichever of these large joints is involved, the other will then reciprocate by also going into flexion contracture.

Pitfalls in Diagnosis. Osteoarthritis is often misdiagnosed as torn meniscus, but if the clinician recalls that torn menisci are relatively uncommon in elderly patients, whereas osteoarthritis of the knee is common, misdiagnosis is less likely.

Laboratory Findings. As at other joints, osteoarthritis of the knee develops after repeated trauma or in the presence of some predisposing disease. There are no specific laboratory findings. Fluid removed from the affected knee tends to be very viscous, resembling normal fluid, although it may be darker in color because of frequent bleeding into the joint. There should be few cells, although sometimes, especially during secondary inflammation, up to 5000 leukocytes/cu mm will be seen. Most of the cells will be lymphocytes, but occasionally some polymorphonuclear leukocytes will also be discovered. Tests for mucin clots tend to be normal. Inflammation will be seen in synovium on biopsy, and fluorescent staining of biopsy material from cartilage or synovium sometimes reveals deposits of immune complexes. Arthroscopy will confirm areas of denuding of cartilage, eburnation, and bone reshaping. Removed synovial material often contains a plethora of new blood vessels and aggregates of inflammatory cells, but the palisading and fibrinoid features of rheumatoid synovial membrane will not be found.

Other Tests. Arthrography can help differentiate between internal derangements and osteoarthritis at the knee. This is a relatively innocuous and simple procedure, and it should be used more often when diagnosis is in doubt.

Spine

Technically, osteoarthritis of the spine occurs only at the apophyseal articulations. Degenerative changes in the intervertebral discs and the associated osteophytic changes do not constitute osteoarthritis, although they are sometimes misread as this on x-ray. As a consequence, most backaches that are blamed on osteoarthritis are due to other causes. Ankylosing hyperostosis—or diffuse idiopathic skeletal hyperostosis, as it is now called—in which exuberant proliferation of bone anterior to the anterior ligament will be found, likewise is not osteoarthritis.

Midcervical and lower lumbar areas are the most commonly involved with osteoarthritis, although almost any mobile portion of the spine is at risk. Oblique x-rays are necessary to best demonstrate the lesions in the apophyseal joints. Encroachment from these joints into the neural foramina is common and is said to produce radicular pain. This will be associated with paresthesias, reflex changes, and motor and sensory deprivation. Acquired spondylolisthesis and spondylolysis can develop in both the lower lumbar and the lower cervical spines as a result of osteoarthritic changes.

Although pain ranges from localized dull aching to radicular shooting pains, the pain from osteoarthritic involvement of apophyseal joints is most common at C3-C4, C4-C5, and C6-C7 interspaces. In the lumbar spine, L4-L5 and L5-S1 are the sites most likely to be afflicted. There is slight restriction of forward bending because of osteoarthritis, which tends to differentiate this disorder from ankylosing spondylitis, in which the back flattens and little motion between adjacent segments is possible.

When there is considerable disc degeneration, leading to osteophyte formation, the syndrome of *spondylosis* is said to be present. Again, this is not osteoarthritis, as no diarthrodial joints are involved. Instead, the space between the vertebrae diminishes and the osteophytes can encroach on nerves and other structures. The symptoms produced depend upon the area involved; they may range from occipital neuralgia to lumbar stenosis, the latter a syndrome in which osteophytes encroach upon the spinal canal in its lower aspects. Neurologic changes occur at various levels, and include a syndrome that resembles intermittent claudication on a vascular basis. The patients have pain in the buttocks, thighs, and legs when they stand or attempt to walk, and this pain can be relieved by brief periods of rest.

Differential Diagnosis. In the age group in which spinal osteoarthritis and spondylosis are both common, other causes of back pain include polymyalgia rheumatica, in which the ESR is immoderately elevated and which is often associated with giant cell arteritis. A good differential diagnosis can help make the distinctions. Disc degeneration occurs uncommonly in this age group, so that herniated nucleus pulposus need not enter most differential diagnoses.

CONCLUSIONS

Osteoarthritis appears to be the consequence of work and play. To a lesser or greater extent, it involves almost all the joints, and almost all individuals will be affected in time. Although it causes some stiffness and perhaps even some sensitivity to weather changes, osteoarthritis rarely should be thought of as a disease. Often the precipitating factors can be deduced by careful history, but sometimes they remain elusive. They must be sought in the remote past for most individuals, unless some major trauma attended the development of osteoarthritis over a shorter period of time, as in the major joints of professional athletes.

Osteoarthritis seems to represent a balance between destruction and repair, so that the impediments to motion are seemingly part of the reason for the disorder, with diminished motion resulting in more rapid healing and less secondary inflammation. On occasion, osteoarthritic reshaping and joint narrowing have been seen to improve, giving some hope that other explanations and treatments can be found. It is most important to remember that all symptoms and signs need to be evaluated carefully, to avoid placing blame on changes that are radiographically demonstrable but not necessarily responsible for the symptoms and signs.

OSTEOPOROSIS

By Robert R. Recker, M.D.
Omaha, Nebraska

SYNONYMS

Postmenopausal osteoporosis, senile osteoporosis, idiopathic osteoporosis.

DEFINITION

Osteoporosis is a clinical syndrome characterized by reduction in bone mass to the extent that risk of fracture is high. The remaining bony material is normal. The disease most likely is due to a defect in bone remodeling.

SIGNS AND SYMPTOMS

The only important consequence of bone loss is fracture. Indeed, the presence of fracture is the hallmark of this disease, the morbid event. Fractures occur most commonly in the spine and femoral neck, although the entire skeleton may be involved. Spine fractures may occur gradually with very little pain. Many patients lose height and develop "dowager's hump" without ever seeking medical attention. Others suffer chronic back pain with or without episodes of acute pain.

Acute collapse of a vertebra is associated with severe localized pain and minimal lateral radiation. The pain increases with movement and with upright or weight-bearing posture. The acute pain gradually resolves and may be replaced by a more chronic muscular pain, or it may disappear altogether. Neurologic signs are very rare and their presence should suggest an alternative diagnosis. After several vertebrae have collapsed, chronic postural back pain is the rule. Acute episodes of back pain and vertebral collapse can result from mild trauma, such as picking up a cooking utensil, lifting a plant or window sash, or picking up a newspaper.

Hip fractures occur with trauma such as falling to the floor from a standing position. Some patients may fall *as a result of* a spontaneous femoral neck fracture, but this is difficult to document. A few patients will suffer spontaneous femoral neck fracture without a fall.

Although hip and spine fractures may occur in the same individual, most patients tend to suffer one or the other; in addition, a hip fracture does increase the chances that fracture will occur in the opposite hip.

NATURAL HISTORY

Spine fractures tend to occur in a series over 3 to 6 years, then stop. Eight inches or more of height can be lost. Many patients do not realize how much height they have lost until their height is measured. The natural course of spine fractures can be unpredictable, with some patients suffering no more than two or three collapsed vertebrae and others having all lumbar vertebrae and most of the thoracic vertebrae collapsed as well. The occurrence of hip fractures is influenced by the presence of unsafe conditions in the living environment, such as loose or wrinkled rugs.

Men suffer from spine and hip fractures, but they tend to have a lower incidence and the fractures occur later in life. This is a reflection of the fact that bone loss begins later in life in men and proceeds at a lower rate. Bone loss in women begins in the fourth decade and accelerates at menopause.

PHYSICAL EXAMINATION

The "dowager's hump" and increasing dorsal kyphosis are characteristic, but may not always be obvious until later in the course. With accumulation of fractures, the lower rib cage may descend onto the pelvic brim and the upper abdominal transverse skin fold may become quite prominent. Because of crowding of the upper abdominal cavity and loss of muscle tone, the lower abdomen may bulge outward. With acute vertebral compression there may be localized tenderness in the area of the fracture and considerable muscle spasm. Often, the entire paraspinous muscle system may be tender and rigid.

The characteristic physical findings of hip fracture are shortening and external rotation of the leg, along with severe pain and loss of motion.

LABORATORY FINDINGS

Serum calcium, phosphorus, and alkaline phosphatase levels and protein electrophoresis should be normal, and urine calcium excretion should not be excessive (less than 300 mg/24 hours). Occasionally the alkaline phosphatase level may be modestly elevated briefly following a fracture, and some patients show persistent alkaline phosphatase elevations for long periods without apparent cause. The clinician should be alert to the possibility of associated morbid conditions in the presence of an elevation in alkaline phosphatase level.

X-ray examination will show fractures or vertebral deformity such as wedging, compression, or ballooning of the intervertebral disc. Vertebrae that are not deformed may show accentuation of the end-plates and vertical striations. Prior to the development of fracture and in the unaffected vertebrae, demineralization may be noticed. Spinal x-ray films are notoriously inadequate for determination of mineral loss; however, 30 per cent of mineral content must be lost before there is any detectable amount of demineralization. A number of newer methods are available for measurement of skeletal mineral content, including single photon absorptiometry of the forearm, dual photon absorptiometry of the spine, and whole body neutron activation analysis. All of these methods can accurately determine bone mineral content, but they cannot predict the risk of fracture with precision; considerable overlap is found between fracture patients and age-matched, healthy controls. As a result, these methods are very useful in monitoring change in bone mass but are less helpful in making a diagnosis.

DIFFERENTIAL DIAGNOSIS

Since there is no specific biologic marker for the diagnosis of postmenopausal osteoporosis, the presence or absence of a cluster of clinical features must be relied on to distinguish the disease. As indicated earlier, the fundamental problem is bone loss with fracture. However, there are a number of diseases or conditions that result in bone loss as part of a separate cluster of features that form a distinct primary disease entity. For example, Cushing's disease with endogenous overproduction of adrenal corticosteroids or exogenous administration of corticosteroids will result in bone loss and increased risk of fracture. This may be superimposed on "naturally occurring" bone loss and greatly exaggerate the risk. Thus, a woman with plentiful bone mass and minor risk of fracture may be at high risk if exposed to excess steroids. She may even suffer extensive fractures and disability, which would not have occurred in the absence of exposure to steroids. The same can be said for other situations, such as hyperparathyroidism and hyperthyroidism. The classic radiologic findings of subperiosteal bone resorption and cyst formation may be absent in hyperparathyroidism, whereas bone loss may be prominent. Of course, the hallmark of this disease is elevation of serum calcium level.

Two diagnoses are often confused with osteoporosis: malignancy with metastases to the spine and multiple myeloma. Either may cause multiple vertebral compression fractures, but especially multiple myeloma. Further, diagnostic problems can occur when the cause of demineralization is the secretion by a malignant lesion of a peptide resembling parathyroid hormone. Usually, bone metastases can be recognized by the presence of several clinical clues:

1. A primary tumor is discovered by history or physical examination.
2. The pattern of vertebral collapse departs from that seen in osteoporosis, in which the T12 vertebra is most commonly the first to fracture, with decreasing frequency above and below this level; an isolated collapse of a lower lumbar or midthoracic vertebrae is suggestive of malignancy.
3. Elevation of serum alkaline phosphatase level.
4. Elevation of urinary calcium and sometimes serum calcium level.

Bone scanning may be helpful if "hot" spots are found outside the vertebral column, but this technology is not useful enough to be routinely performed.

Multiple myeloma should be detected in over 95 per cent of cases by serum protein electrophoresis. (See article on Multiple Myeloma and Other Plasma Cell Dyscrasias.) Bone biopsy may be necessary occasionally to rule out malignancy or multiple myeloma.

Osteomalacia should also be considered in patients with presenting features of osteoporosis; however, it is usually a co-morbid condition in these patients, contributing to skeletal fragility. Osteomalacia, defined as vitamin D deficiency, is not necessarily associated with bone loss, and it can occur without the classic features of lowered serum calcium and phosphorus levels and elevated serum alkaline phosphatase level. Measurement of serum 25-hydroxyvitamin D levels may give some information about the state of vitamin D nutrition, but it is still not clear how low these levels must be in order to affect the skeleton. Ultimately, bone biopsy after tetracycline labeling must be performed with undecalcified processing of the specimen in order to be certain about the vitamin D status of the skeleton. (See article on Rickets and Osteomalacia.)

In the United States, osteomalacia is rare, being found primarily in patients with renal tubular acidosis or malabsorption. However, in Great Britain it is much more common, especially among immigrants from the Middle East, and it may account for some of the increased incidence of fractures among the elderly.

Patients with a history of partial gastrectomy or other types of upper gastrointestinal tract surgery represent a special case. Many of them will have extensive bone loss, appearing with a typical syndrome of osteoporosis one or two decades later. These patients may have vitamin D deficiency because of occult malabsorption and should be investigated by measurement of serum 25-hydroxyvitamin D levels or bone biopsy if possible. Their problem is confounded by the presence of calcium malabsorption. These factors combine to result in severe osteoporosis developing at a younger than usual age.

Chronic renal, liver, and lung diseases seem to be associated with bone loss and a greater than expected incidence of osteoporosis. Chronic renal disease is a special case, in which the associated bone disease acquires distinctive features. However, patients with chronic liver and lung disease appear to acquire bone disease that resembles osteoporosis. Indeed, these conditions may simply cause acceleration of the usual age-related bone loss, resulting in fractures at an earlier age. Bone biopsy is particularly useful in the case of liver disease to rule out vitamin D deficiency resulting from insufficient hepatic production of 25-hydroxyvitamin D.

SEPTIC ARTHRITIS

By James Roberson, M.D.
Atlanta, Georgia

SYNONYMS

Infectious arthritis, bacterial arthritis, septic joint, pyogenic arthritis.

DEFINITION

Septic arthritis denotes an intra-articular infection by bacterial, mycoplasmal, or fungal organisms.

PRESENTING SIGNS AND SYMPTOMS

Findings at presentation are quite variable, depending upon the infecting organism and ability of the host to respond. Acute pyogenic arthritis usually causes obvious systemic evidence of infection, with chills and fever. Swelling, redness, and pain, especially with motion, tend to localize the involved joint. Significant guarding and spasm are usually present, and patients maintain a slightly flexed joint position as the capsule becomes distended with purulent fluid.

Chronic joint infections, such as tuberculous or fungal arthritis, usually have an insidious onset. Severe pain is often not an early finding, in contrast to acute pyogenic arthritis. There may be low-grade or even no fever, but often significant weight loss and malaise are present.

Important historical findings include recent surgery, contusion, or penetrating trauma to the area of the joint. Another recent site of infection is usually apparent when hematogenous seeding occurs. Immunosuppression, malnutrition, collagen vascular disease, renal disease, rheumatoid arthritis, and drug abuse predispose to septic arthritis.

CLINICAL COURSE

Untreated septic arthritis progresses rapidly to destruction of articular cartilage, and early superimposed osteoarthritis occurs with occasional spontaneous fusion. Bacteremia and even septic shock are possible. If treated aggressively early in the course, in the majority of cases sepsis can be controlled before marked joint destruction occurs, and a good result can be expected.

COMMON COMPLICATIONS

The most common adverse sequela of a septic joint is osteoarthritis. The primary determining factors are the time between onset and treatment, patient susceptibility, and virulence of the organism. Osteomyelitis can occur with inadequate or delayed treatment, and if a sequestrum develops, the condition becomes chronic, with intermittent or continuous drainage. Septicemia and hematogenous infection of other joints also occur.

PHYSICAL EXAMINATION

Physical findings are quite variable and are primarily determined by the virulence of the infecting organism and the patient's ability to respond. The most common and classic finding with acute pyogenic arthritis is pain, especially with motion of the involved joint. The patient assumes a position with the least amount of tension on the joint capsule. This is usually mild flexion, and passive or active motion is resisted by the patient. There may be considerable muscle spasm and guarding, and an effusion is essentially always present. The soft tissues around the joint are usually swollen, red, and warm. Elevated temperature is usually present. The skin around the joint should be examined for evidence of old abrasion, laceration, or puncture wound as the source of infection. Urethral discharge or a characteristic rash on the palms may be evidence of gonococcal infection.

Since septic arthritis occurs commonly in immunosuppressed hosts, the classic clinical presentation may not occur. Very little physical evidence may be present in the patient with severe rheumatoid arthritis or in the patient on chronic immunosuppressive therapy. These individuals are also vulnerable to organisms that are normally of low virulence and may present with a less fulminant course.

LABORATORY VALUES

As with most infections, leukocytosis and an elevated erythrocyte sedimentation rate are usually present, but by far the most valuable laboratory test is analysis of joint fluid. Blood cultures should be obtained, and aspiration of the joint should be performed at the earliest opportunity whenever a septic arthritis is suspected. It is extremely important that antibiotics not be started before adequate material for Gram staining and culture is obtained, and delay in obtaining this material causes needless damage of articular cartilage. Identification of a microorganism on culture and sensitivity tests confirms the diagnosis of infectious arthritis and determines the selection of the appropriate antibiotic and dose. Other factors, such as turbidity, viscosity, color, cell count, presence of crystals, volume, and glucose content of synovial fluid are helpful, but must be interpreted with the entire clinical picture, as considerable overlap exists with other causes of arthritis (Table 1).

Arthrocentesis technique varies with different joints. A large-gauge (No. 18) needle makes aspiration of purulent fluid easier, but in smaller joints it may be necessary to use smaller needles. Strict asepsis must be observed during both the aspiration and the handling of the fluid, as contamination may lead to misdiagnosis or selection of an inappropriate antibiotic. When fluid is obtained, it should be applied immediately to appropriate media or transported to the laboratory in a sealed syringe with air expressed, since anaerobic organisms may not remain viable for long periods if air is present. Fluid should then be placed in a tube containing heparin or ethylenediaminetetraacetic acid (EDTA) for cell count. Stains and cultures should be done for acid-fast and fungal organisms if there is reason to suspect the infection is caused by these organisms.

Aspiration of the hip is facilitated by fluoroscopic monitoring. If there seems to be adequate needle placement but no joint fluid is aspirated, nonbacteriostatic saline should be injected and aspirated for culture. Water-soluble contrast medium should then be injected to confirm needle placement by fluoroscopy.

Synovial fluid from an infected joint has a turbid appearance because of the numerous polymorphonuclear leukocytes present. Release of lysosomal enzymes gives the fluid a low viscosity, with a string sign of less than 2 cm, as opposed to approximately 5 cm for normal fluid. A white blood cell count greater than 50,000 cells per cu mm is suggestive and a count approaching 100,000 cells per cu mm is almost diagnostic for septic arthritis; lower cell counts are often seen, however.

Seventy-five per cent or more of the white blood cells are polymorphonuclear leukocytes in acute septic arthritis, and glucose levels in joint fluid are less than 50 per cent of serum levels. Examination of fluid for uric acid crystals or calcium pyrophosphate under polarized microscopy is necessary to exclude the possibility of gout or pseudogout.

RADIOLOGIC EXAMINATION

Radiographs of the involved joint should be examined for fracture or osteomyelitis. Effusion is often seen on x-ray, even though this is better determined clinically. Nuclear scans using technetium, gallium, or indium are often extremely helpful if the diagnosis is in doubt, but aspiration of the joint should not be delayed unnecessarily in order to obtain the scan. Late in the course, radiographs show chondrolysis with loss of joint space.

JOINT INFECTION FOLLOWING PROSTHETIC REPLACEMENT

A special category of septic arthritis with increasing frequency is infection involving joint prostheses. Assuming an infection rate of 1 to 2 per cent, 1500 of the 100,000 total hip replacements done each year in the United States will become infected. Infected prostheses may be classified as either acute, subacute, or late. The findings in the acute situation are very similar to those of any early postoperative infection. Within a few days or weeks of surgery the patient develops fever, chills, pain, and swelling or drainage at the wound site. The diagnosis is secured by Gram stain and culture results to confirm the clinical findings, and, if reasonable suspicion of infection exists, the wound should be aspirated or explored surgically.

With the advent of prophylactic antibiotics in joint replacement surgery, the incidence of early acute infections has decreased drastically, and subacute infections are now more common. The subacute infection is caused by organisms in the wound at the time of surgery. These are organisms that are not ordinarily pathogens, with those constituting the skin flora being most frequent. The presenting symptom is pain of gradually progressive severity. Systemic signs of infection are usually absent, and the incision appears well healed. The pain is present both at rest and with activity. A lucent line of progressing width is usually seen around the prosthetic components, and loss of bone substance is often seen as a result of lysis. The white blood cell count may be normal, but the erythrocyte sedimentation rate is usually increased. Many reports have found nuclear scans helpful in the diagnosis of the infected prosthesis, but in my experience they are very frequently equivocal. A gallium scan showing increased uptake, in conjunction with a technetium scan that does not, may be of more diagnostic significance. Indium specifically labels leukocytes and is currently being investigated as a radioactive label to diagnose infected prostheses. Although these procedures are helpful, the diagnosis is seldom made without positive culture results from aspiration or tissue at surgery.

Acute and subacute infections occur from contamination at the time of surgery, whereas late infections are generally hematogenous in origin. The most common sources include urinary tract infections, abscesses at any site, pneumonia, and oral or urologic surgery. The late hematogenous infection presents with the same findings as an acute postoperative infection, but with a healed incision and a history of satisfactory surgical result for several months. The diagnostic work-up is similar to that for acute infection.

DIAGNOSTIC PITFALLS

Most causes of acute arthritis can masquerade as infection. The majority of these are treated nonoperatively, but the treatment of septic arthritis is commonly incision and drainage and a course of antibiotics. Therefore, the failure to diagnose septic arthritis leads to inappropriate early treatment, with potentially disastrous results.

It is not uncommon to be faced with an initial work-up suggestive, but not diagnostic, of infection. The Gram stain may not reveal organisms and the joint fluid analysis may be equivocal. In this situation, a 24-hour waiting period for culture results is justified. Antibiotics appropriate for the most likely infecting organisms (Table 2) should be started after fluid for culture is sent. If this course is selected, reaspiration should be done within 24 hours to evaluate any reaccumulation of fluid. Indomethacin may also be used as a therapeutic trial if gout is suspected, as the clinical response is quite rapid.

Table 1. Examination of Synovial Fluid

	Normal	Noninflammatory	Inflammatory (Noninfectious)	Inflammatory (Infectious)
Color	Clear	Yellow	Yellow	Yellow
Clarity	Transparent	Transparent	Translucent	Opaque
WBC (cells/cu mm)	200	200–2,000	2,000–100,000	20,000–100,000
Viscosity	High	High	Low	Low
Mucin clot	Firm	Firm	Friable	Friable
Synovial glucose/ serum glucose	Equal	Equal	50%	50%

Table 2. Most Common Infecting Organisms in Septic Arthritis

Under 2 Years of Age
Hemophilus influenzae
Streptococcus pneumoniae
Staphylococcus aureus
Streptococcus spp.
2–15 Years of Age
Staphylococcus aureus
Streptococcus spp.
Neisseria gonorrheae
Pseudomonas
Over 15 Years of Age
Staphylococcus aureus
Neisseria gonorrheae
Streptococcus
Enterobacter

BURSITIS AND TENDINITIS

By Lewis Cogen, M.D.
Portland, Maine

Bursitis and tendinitis are common musculoskeletal disorders encountered by most physicians. The subdeltoid, olecranon, trochanteric, prepatellar, and anserine are the bursae most frequently involved; the tendons most often affected are in the regions of the shoulder, elbow, hand, and wrist. Achilles tendinitis and bursitis and plantar fasciitis are less commonly seen.

Bursae are thin-walled, flattened sacs lined by a synovial membrane and lubricated by a film of synovial fluid, which form where skin, bone, muscles, tendons, and ligaments are in close contact. Tendons are the strong cords composed of collagen by which muscles attach to bone. Where tendons insert into bone or are in close apposition to ligaments and retinaculae they are enclosed in a tube-like tendon sheath that has a synovial lining and contains synovial fluid. Bursae and tendon sheaths facilitate normal, painless motion by separating moving surfaces and decreasing the friction between them.

Inflammation in a bursa, tendon, or tendon sheath may result in thickening of the synovial lining and increase in fluid, which may cause pain and impaired function. Inflammation may occur as a consequence of repetitive activity, most commonly from work or sports, or from trauma, but for many patients there is no apparent precipitating event. Bursitis and tendinitis may have an abrupt onset with intense pain, or may begin gradually, with variable discomfort over long periods. Pain is usually made worse with activity and relieved by rest. Night pain and disability vary. In idiopathic or purely local tendinitis and bursitis, patients do not have constitutional sympotoms, such as malaise or fever, and the results of the erythrocyte sedimentation rate and other laboratory studies are normal.

Bursitis and tendinitis may be the initial manifestation of any of the rheumatic diseases that involve the synovium. Rheumatoid arthritis and polymyalgia rheumatica, for example, may be indistinguishable from one another early in their course, and either may present with shoulder bursitis or tendinitis or hip bursitis. Tenosynovitis at the wrist or involving the hand flexor tendons may be the first symptom of rheumatoid arthritis, psoriatic arthritis or other inflammatory joint disease. Achilles tendinitis and bursitis and heel pain are hallmarks of spondylitis and other HLA-B27 positive spondyloarthropathies. A careful history may disclose significant morning stiffness, fatigue, weight loss, and other symptoms of systemic rheumatic disease.

Gouty bursitis is most common in the olecranon and prepatellar bursae. Pseudogout more commonly affects joints rather than tendons and bursae. Hydroxyapatite crystal deposition disease is probably a relatively frequent cause of tendinitis at the shoulder, hand, and wrist. Fever may sometimes occur in crystal induced tendinitis and bursitis.

Although infrequent, infection should always be considered in patients with acute tendinitis and bursitis. Septic bursitis, usually a consequence of local trauma, is most common in the olecranon and prepatellar bursae, and it is most often caused by staphylococci. Gonococcemia may cause a migratory tenosynovitis. Tuberculosis and fungal infections are rare causes of tendinitis and bursitis.

When swelling is detected in a bursa, fluid should be aspirated and sent for culture, white blood cell, and differential counts; it should also be examined carefully for bacteria by Gram stain and for crystals by polarizing light microscopy. In traumatic bursitis the fluid may be either hemorrhagic or straw-colored, with a low white cell count, usually less than a few thousand cells per cubic millimeter. In infection, microcrystalline disease, or inflammatory arthritis the white cell counts are usually considerably higher. Aspiration of a tendon sheath is indicated if infection or crystal deposition disease is suspected; obtaining fluid from a tendon sheath, however, is sometimes very difficult.

SUBDELTOID BURSITIS

The subdeltoid bursa lies between the deltoid muscle and the rotator cuff of the shoulder (Fig. 1). The tendon of the supraspinatus muscle is the major tendon of the rotator cuff, and it inserts into the greater tuberosity of the humerus (Fig. 1). Subdeltoid and subacromial bursitis, calcific tendinitis and bursitis, and supraspinatus tendinitis and bursitis are sometimes described as separate processes, but they are considered together here as subdeltoid bursitis. Because the supraspinatus tendon and subdeltoid bursa are so anatomically close, inflammation of one involves the other and they cannot be distinguished by palpation.

Pain in subdeltoid bursitis may be poorly localized, but usually there is discomfort in the upper, lateral shoulder that radiates into the deltoid region of the arm. Sometimes pain is felt in the arm and not in the

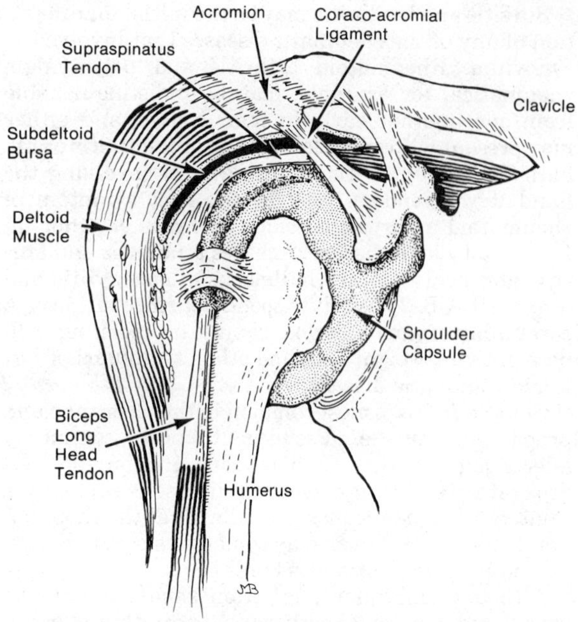

Figure 1. Subdeltoid bursa and bicipital tendon.

shoulder. Abduction and internal rotation aggravate the pain. Pain may be reproduced by forced abduction of the arm against resistance applied by the examiner. Night pain is common.

Shoulder motion may be limited by pain or adhesive capsulitis (fixed loss of passive shoulder motion). Pain can usually be reproduced by firm palpation of the subacromial space (Fig. 1). Clinically detectable swelling of the subdeltoid bursa is infrequent. Calcification in the supraspinatus tendon is a common finding and is best seen in the anteroposterior external rotation radiograph of the shoulder, but calcification is not required for diagnosis.

BICIPITAL TENDINITIS

The tendon of the long head of the biceps muscle arises from the superior rim of the glenoid and passes the shoulder anteriorly in the bicipital groove between the greater and lesser tuberosities of the humerus (Fig. 1). Pain in the anterior shoulder region usually indicates bicipital tendinitis. Pain is made worse with shoulder flexion and abduction and may be reproduced supination of the forearm against resistance (Yergason's sign). Loss of shoulder motion may be noted. Tenderness of the biceps tendon when it is palpated and rolled under the examining finger establishes the diagnosis. X-rays are seldom abnormal.

When subdeltoid bursitis and bicipital tendinitis fail to improve with treatment or recur frequently, there may be an *impingement syndrome,* in which the supraspinatus or the biceps tendon, or both, are compressed during shoulder motion between the head of the humerus and the anterior acromion or the coracoacromial ligament, or both (Fig. 1). An x-ray may show sclerosis of the inferior acromion. Suspected impingement syndrome requires an orthopedic evaluation.

Adhesive capsulitis, shoulder osteoarthritis, metastatic malignancy, and referred pain from the neck or viscera may simulate shoulder bursitis or tendinitis; when pain is referred, there is little or no local tenderness.

OLECRANON BURSITIS

The olecranon bursa lies between the skin and the tip of the olecranon process (Fig. 2). Bursitis in this location often follows trauma. Swelling is invariably present and may be considerable, but often patients have little or no pain. There is full motion of the elbow and no tenderness over the joint space. Nodules or tophi may be palpable within the bursa. X-rays usually show only soft-tissue swelling, but gouty tophi may calcify. Fluid is easily aspirated from the bursa and should be sent for complete synovial analysis, examination for crystals, Gram stain, and culture. Recurrent or bilateral olecranon bursitis suggests rheumatoid arthritis or gout.

EPICONDYLITIS

Most of the extensor tendons of the hand and wrist have their origin at the lateral condyle of the humerus (Fig. 2). Lateral epicondylitis (tennis elbow) commonly follows repetitive activity and racket sports, although few patients with this disorder actually play tennis. Symptoms are usually unilateral. Patients complain of pain at the lateral aspect of the elbow, which may radiate into the proximal forearm. Swelling rarely occurs. Elbow motion is usually normal. Considerable tenderness to palpation at the lateral condyle of the humerus confirms the diagnosis. Forced extension of the wrist, with the fingers flared and the elbow extended, against resistance applied by the examiner usually reproduces the pain. Inflammation of the medial condyle of the humerus, where most of the flexor

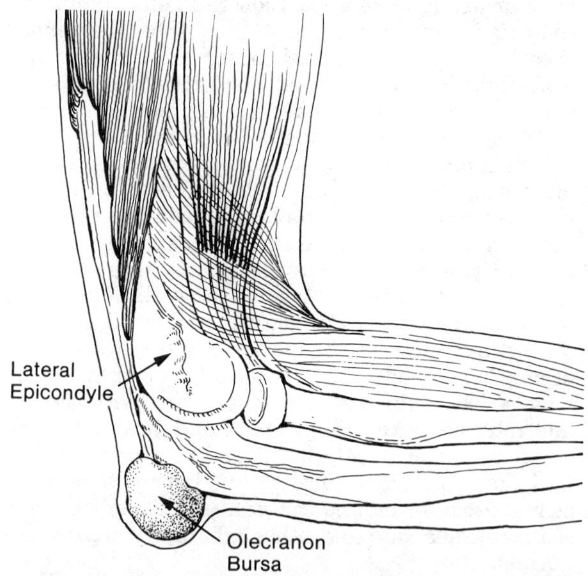

Figure 2. Olecranon bursa and site of "tennis" elbow.

tendons arise, is much less common. Elbow x-rays are usually normal.

DEQUERVAIN'S DISEASE

Tenosynovitis of the abductor pollicis longus and extensor pollicus brevis tendons of the thumb at the distal radius is called DeQuervain's tenosynovitis (Fig. 3). Local tenderness is present, and crepitance may be noted on palpation. Swelling of the tendons may occur and at times may be nodular and very firm. Ulnar deviation of the wrist when the thumb is flexed into the palm and compressed by the fingers reproduces the pain (Finkelstein's test).

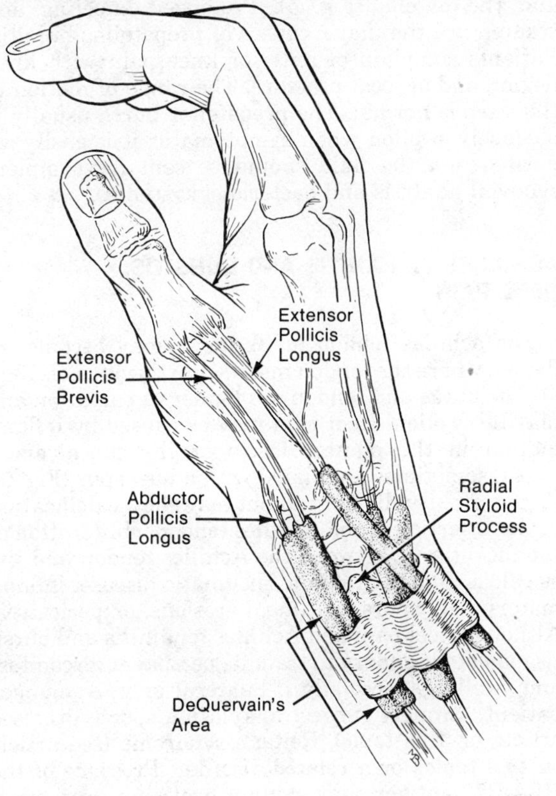

Figure 3. Site of DeQuervain's disease.

Flexor tenosynovitis (stenosing tenosynovitis) of the hands may result in painful motion and locking of the finger and thumb (trigger finger). Locking is commonly present when patients awaken in the morning. Tender crepitance and inflammatory nodules are usually palpable and are best appreciated when the examiner's finger pads are placed over the flexor tendons while the patient gently flexes and extends the involved finger. X-rays are usually normal in flexor tenosynovitis but may show soft-tissue swelling in DeQuervain's disease.

DeQuervain's disease and flexor tenosynovitis may occur in rheumatoid arthritis and other inflammatory joint diseases.

TROCHANTERIC BURSITIS

The trochanteric bursa forms at the insertion of the gluteus maximus muscle at the posterior and lateral portions of the greater trochanter (Fig. 4). Typically, patients complain of pain at the upper lateral thigh, often radiating down the side of the thigh to the knee. Pain may be poorly localized and diffuse, even when intense, and may mimic sciatica. Night pain is common, especially when patients sleep on the affected side. Trochanteric bursitis may be bilateral. Overweight women are particularly susceptible; leg length discrepancy and osteoarthritis of the hip predispose to this bursitis. Firm palpation over the greater trochanter, best accomplished with the patient lying on the opposite side (Fig. 4), establishes the diagnosis. Groin pain is absent unless there is also arthritis of the hip. Alleviation of pain after a local injection of lidocaine may be of diagnostic value. X-rays are usually normal, but may show calcification next to the greater trochanter or osteoarthritis of the hip.

ANSERINE BURSITIS

The anserine bursa is formed at the common insertion of the sartorius, gracilis, and semitendinosus muscles (pes anserinus) on the anteromedial tibia in

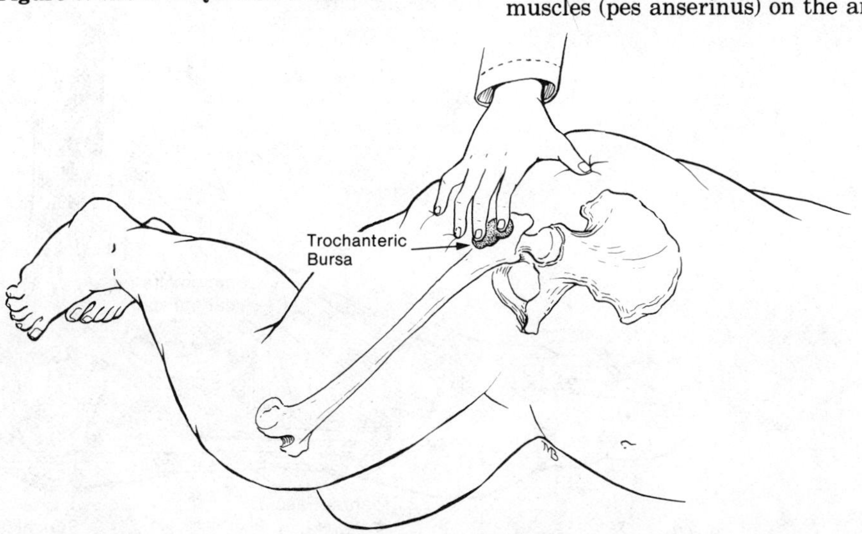

Figure 4. Trochanteric bursa.

an area below the joint line, anterior to the medial collateral ligament, and extending to as far as the level of the tibial tuberosity (Fig. 5). Patients complain of medial knee pain, worse when going up and down steps. Night pain is common and both knees may be involved. Firm palpation in the area of the anserine bursa usually elicits considerable tenderness when it is inflamed.

Anserine bursitis is more common in overweight women; pes planus deformity of the feet and osteoarthritis of the medial compartment of the knee are predisposing conditions. Swelling of the anserine bursa is seldom clinically apparent.

X-rays of the knee are usually normal but may show degenerative arthritis of the medial compartment of the knee. Anserine bursitis may be overlooked when medial knee pain is attributed to osteoarthritis: Since the bursa and knee do not communicate, injection of procaine hydrochloride into the knee joint does not alleviate the pain. A tear of the medial meniscus or the medial collateral ligament causes medial knee pain and may suggest anserine bursitis.

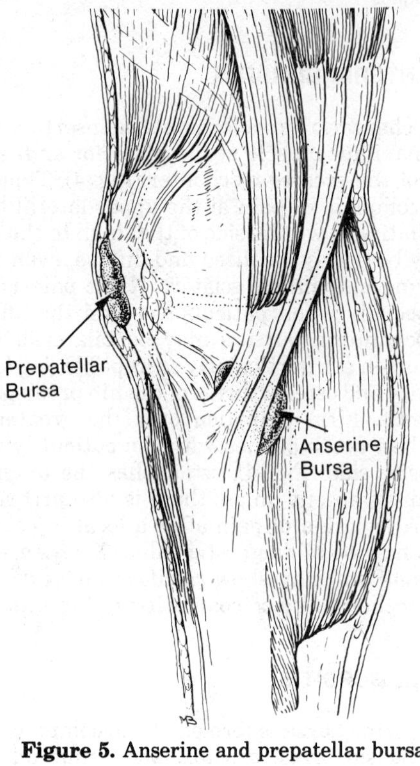

Figure 5. Anserine and prepatellar bursae.

PREPATELLAR BURSITIS (HOUSEMAID'S KNEE)

The prepatellar bursa is located between the skin and the patella (Fig. 5). Prolonged kneeling and trauma are the major causes of prepatellar bursitis. Patients complain of anterior knee pain with knee flexion and of local pressure. The range of motion of the knee is normal. The prepatellar bursa usually is obviously swollen when symptomatic; it is easily aspirated and the fluid should be sent for complete synovial analysis and bacteriologic studies.

ACHILLES TENDINITIS AND BURSITIS; HEEL PAIN

The achilles tendon or its bursa may become inflamed where the tendon inserts into the os calcis (Fig. 6). The bursa and tendon are tender to palpation and may be swollen. Heel pain may be caused by inflammation in the plantar fascia or the subcalcaneal bursa, sometimes associated with a heel spur (Fig. 6). X-rays are usually normal but may show calcification at the insertion of the Achilles tendon, obliteration of the lucent area between the Achilles tendon and the os calcis, and, in systemic rheumatic disease, inflammatory heel spurs, calcaneal erosions, or periostitis. Although heel pain and Achilles tendinitis and bursitis may be secondary to trauma, persistent discomfort and swelling, especially if bilateral or in a younger patient, strongly suggest ankylosing spondylitis (see article on this topic), Reiter's syndrome (see article on this topic), or a related disorder. Presence of the HLA-B27 antigen may explain heel pain even when other symptoms of a seronegative spondyloarthropathy are absent.

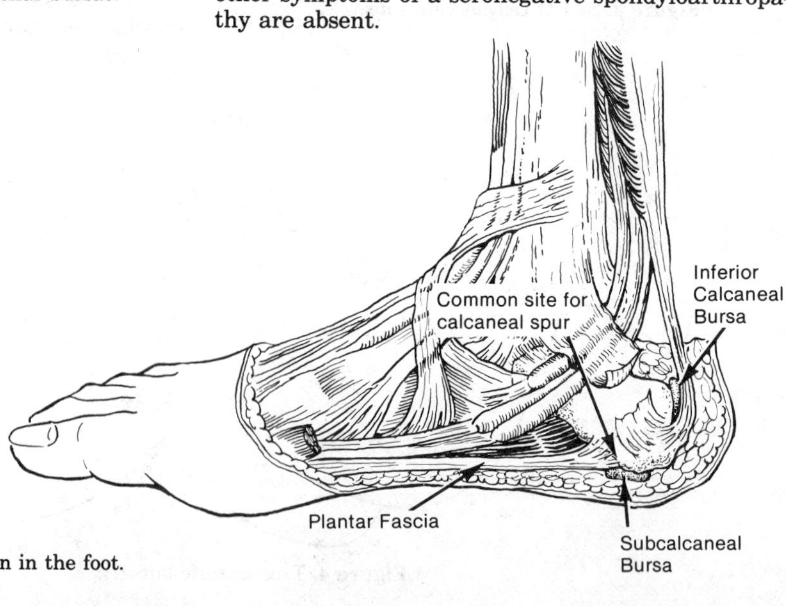

Figure 6. Common sites of inflammation in the foot.

Section Thirteen

GENITOURINARY SYSTEM

INFECTIONS OF THE URINARY TRACT

By S. Grant Mulholland, M.D.
and Louis L. Keeler, M.D.
Philadelphia, Pennsylvania

Urinary tract infection is second in incidence to respiratory and is the most prevalent nosocomial infection, accounting for nearly half, and in many institutions more than half, of these infections. Uncomplicated acute bacterial cystitis in the female has very little medical significance, but it is a significant problem to the patient, casuing considerable discomfort and financial burden. The progression of an acute urinary tract infection beyond the bladder is quite unusual. This progression is often accomplanied by some abnormality in the urinary tract that encourages the infection to invade the kidneys or the blood.

TERMINOLOGY

In order to thoroughly understand, diagnose, and treat urinary tract infections, the clinician should be familiar with common terminology. In so doing, the physician can classify the infection, thereby being able to communicate with other physicians as to the type of infection that a patient may have had and also to predict with reasonable accuracy the infecting organisms, proper treatment, and probability of cure.

Urinary tract infection refers to the invasion of the normally sterile urinary tract by pathogenic bacteria and the establishment of an infectious process. Urinary tract infections are classified according to (1) anatomic location (upper or lower urinary tract), (2) presence or absence of associated urinary tract abnormalities (complicated or uncomplicated), and (3) historical characteristics (acute or chronic, reinfection or relapse). The patient with an upper urinary tract infection may have the classic signs and symptoms of pyelonephritis, whereas a lower urinary tract infection will produce predominantly the symptoms of cystitis.

An *acute infection* is one occurring in a patient who has been free of infection for several months; a *chronic infection* is one that has been present continuously for a period of months. A *relapse* of infection is a recurrence with the same organism (identical serotype) previously cultured, which theoretically has persisted during and after therapy; a *reinfection* is a recurrence of infection with a different organism during or at any time after treatment.

Bacteriuria denotes the presence of bacteria in the urine in vivo. The method used to procure the urine specimen for this determination is crucial. Urine obtained by suprapubic needle aspiration of the bladder is normally sterile, but a specimen obtained by voiding (even a midstream specimen) or by urethral catheterization may become contaminated by the endogenous urethral flora. Therefore, the urine culture must include not only a qualitative evaluation but also a quantitative evaluation to rule out contamination. Significant bacteriuria ($> 10^5$/ml) is the bacterial count that indicates true colonization of the urinary tract rather than contamination of the specimen. Bacteriuria may be asymptomatic or symptomatic. A patient with *asymptomatic bacteriuria* has no symptoms suggestive of urinary tract infection and may have no past history of infection. This condition may be chronic, or it may alternate with intermittent episodes. In the latter case, patients should be treated as though they have a chronic rather than an acute infection.

EPIDEMIOLOGY

During the *neonatal period,* the incidence of bacteriuria in the male exceeds that in the female. Many urinary tract infections in neonates appear to be related to blood-borne infection, whereas in later life retrograde urethral ascent of organisms is more likely. The incidence of urinary tract infection in the neonate is similar to the incidence of neonatal septicemia (0.7 per cent in full-term and 2.9 per cent in premature infants). Vesicoureteral reflux is common in these patients, but usually resolves. Renal scarring is uncommon, but it can occur at this very early period in life.

The prevalence of bacteriuria in *preschool children* varies widely because of different methods of urine collection. There is a 2 per cent incidence of symptomatic urinary tract infection in female preschool children, while the incidence drops to near zero in males. The preschool child who presents with a urinary tract infection will have a high likelihood of significant radiologic abnormalities.

In *school-age girls,* the incidence of bacteriuria is approximately 1.7 per cent, which is 60 times higher than the rate for boys (0.03 per cent). The finding of radiologic abnormalities decreases as the age of the female child increases. Male urinary tract infections are rare, but when they occur they are often associated with significant structural abnormalities.

In the early years of sexual activity, bacteriuria affects 4 per cent of *young women.*

The incidence during *pregnancy* can be as high as 6 per cent.

Infection rate rises in *mature women* by 1 per cent per decade until the age of 60, at which time there is a rapid increase.

Males are affected in the two extremes of life; after the age of 60, incidence increases sharply to 10 per cent. This may be due to instrumentation, but is probably most directly related to lower urinary tract obstructive factors or associated medical diseases.

Interestingly, *chronic bacterial pyelonephritis* accounts for 11 per cent of the causes of renal insufficiency in transplant patients. However, a low percentage, possibly as few as 1 per cent, of all patients who have had urinary tract infections develop chronic bacterial pyelonephritis.

Urinary tract infections do not cause a high incidence of renal insufficiency; however, treatment involves a high annual cost, estimated at $20 billion, including hospitalization, investigative studies, surgical procedures, cultures, antibiotics, treatment of antibiotic reactions, time lost from work, dialysis, and transplantation.

CLINICAL MANIFESTATIONS

Cystitis

Signs and Symptoms. In true bacterial cystitis the signs and symptoms are due to irritation of the bladder mucosa and musculature by bacteria or their products. The patient usually complains of burning on urination or pain in the area of the urethra. Extreme urgency of urination with occasional incontinence may be reported. Most patients with cystitis have marked urinary frequency, voiding in small amounts as often as every 15 minutes. At times the patient may have the desire to void without being able to do so. It is extremely important to verify that the symptoms are present at night as well as during the day; nocturia is common and represents the continuation of daytime symptoms.

Hematuria is a sign of cystitis; although rare in males, it is not uncommon in females. When present, it is usually evident at the termination of voiding, but females may have total gross hematuria and may even pass clots.

In general, the patient may feel as though she has the "flu" with malaise and possibly a low-grade fever, sometimes accompanied by suprapubic discomfort or low back pain.

Diagnosis. Diagnosis may be difficult in the female, as some of these symptoms are also typical of the so-called urethral syndrome, which is due not to infection but to a low-grade inflammation of the urethra and trigone. This inflammation may be secondary to a vaginal inflammation, to the trauma of intercourse, or to a virus or atypical bacteria, or it may be psychosomatic.

Physical Examination. The abdomen is usually found to be normal. Although there may be some suprapubic discomfort, there is no flank tenderness. Examination of the male genitalia may reveal associated diseases such as epididymitis or urethritis. On rectal examination of the male, one may palpate an enlarged, boggy, tender prostate, indicating prostatitis. Pelvic examination in the female may reveal disorders commonly associated with cystitis, such as vaginitis, urethritis, cystocele, urethrocele, and urethral diverticulum.

Pyelonephritis

Signs and Symptoms. Typically, patients with acute pyelonephritis appear quite ill. They have marked weakness, malaise, anorexia, nausea, vomiting, fever, and possibly chills. The temperature may rise to 104°F (40°C). Unilateral or bilateral flank pain, which is usually a continuous ache of moderate intensity, is often present. Although predominantly in the lumbar area, pain sometimes radiates down the flank or into the midabdominal area. The latter characteristic may confuse the clinician with its implication of an intra-abdominal inflammatory process. Roentgenograms may reveal signs of a paralytic ileus. With acute pyelonephritis there is a 10 to 15 per cent incidence of gross or marked microscopic hematuria. Oliguria or anuria may occur, especially if acute pyelonephritis is superimposed upon chronic pyelonephritis. There may be abdominal distention, hypotonic bowel sounds, and tenderness in the lumbar area. The skin is cold and damp or, if the patient is dehydrated, warm and dry. If the patient is bacteremic, signs of septic shock may be evident. Symptoms of cystitis may precede those of pyelonephritis, but lower urinary tract infection is not necessarily concomitant.

In *neonates,* the signs and symptoms of pyelonephritis deviate significantly from the classic ones. Primary and secondary weight loss or failure to gain weight becuase of vomiting, diarrhea, and decreased food intake are usually the first signs of pyelonephritis. Fever is a common finding, although not as prominent in the first 10 days of life. Jaundice, cyanosis, paralytic ileus, increased blood urea nitrogen, and various neurologic symptoms may appear. These atypical signs in the neonate may be attributable to endotoxemia, since urinary tract infections in neonates are often hematogenous in origin. In general, fever, abdominal pain, frequency of urination, and neurologic symptoms are the main symptoms in the neonate with pyelonephritis.

In *young children* with pyelonephritis, gastrointestinal symptoms may be marked. The child may have loss of appetite, vomiting, diarrhea, abdominal pain, and distention.

After 5 years of age, the usual symptoms of the disease—fever, flank pain, urinary frequency, and dysuria—are more commonly found.

In the *elderly,* pyelonephritis may not be accompanied by fever. The patient is likely to be lethargic, weak, and anorexic, but may have no symptoms referable to the kidney.

Diagnosis. The diagnosis of pyelonephritis can be difficult, especially in children and elderly patients. Eighty-five per cent of cases of pyelonephritis are undiagnosed and are found at autopsy, partly because 35 to 50 per cent of all patients with pyelonephritis are asymptomatic or lack the common symptoms.

Course. Chronic pyelonephritis is a serious, progressive disease. Some patients with chronic pyelonephritis have had a long history of chronic cystitis. Presumably, they suffer transient bouts of pyelonephritis, which perhaps vary in presentation and may even be asymptomatic. Predisposing factors such as urinary obstruction, calculi, or reflux may be found. As the pyelonephritis progresses, the patient develops manifestations of end-stage renal disease. In addition, headache, weakness, malaise, anorexia, and nausea often appear with continuing intrarenal infection.

Alterations in Bacterial Flora

Although many different organisms cause urinary tract infections, patterns of infection are fairly predictable. Gram-negative organisms cause all but a very small percentage of urinary tract infections, both acute and chronic. The few infections caused by gram-positive organisms most commonly involve enterococci. Staphylococcus may be seen in the urine as a contaminant or in an infection combined with other organisms, and it is frequently associated with bacteremia.

In acute urinary tract infections, usually only one organism is found on culture—a specific serotype of *Escherichia coli.* As the patient develops additional urinary tract infections and is exposed to numerous antimicrobials, the flora changes. Not only does the incidence of *E. coli* as a causative organism decrease; more resistant *E. coli* infection and the other gram-negative bacteria appear. The percentages of infections caused by *E. coli* are greater in women than in men. Autoinfection with *E. coli* occurs less frequently in men; instrumentation is more often involved, and the organisms isolated are those commonly associated with nosocomial infections. Infections that are initiated within the hospital often are due to more resistant *E. coli* and the other pathogenic gram-negative organisms (e.g., Pseudomonas, Klebsiella, Proteus, Enterobacter).

LABORATORY DIAGNOSIS

Hospital Procedures

In the hospital setting, the physician who is suspicious of a urinary infection will want to make a bacteriologic diagnosis. This is commonly done by obtaining a voided, clean-catch, midstream specimen in the female and a two-glass specimen in the male. The physician should be sure that the staff is practicing proper collection procedures at all times, including nights and weekends. It may be necessary at times to obtain a catherized specimen in the adult female. Suprapubic needle aspiration of the urinary bladder is an accepted method of obtaining urine from children under 5 or 6 years of age, in whom the urinary bladder is an abdominal organ. An external collection device can also be used for young children and infants, although specimens obtained in this way will give less accurate results than clean-voided or aspirated urine.

Since urine at room temperature is an excellent culture medium, not only for urinary tract pathogens but also for contaminating organisms, the specimen should be examined or cultured without delay. If a delay is unavoidable, the urine must be refrigerated. The hospital bacteriology laboratory will then assume responsibility for accurate organism identification and appropriate sensitivity testing.

A culture report will be issued based on quantitative bacterial colony counts. With voided urines a bacterial count of greater than 10^5/ml indicates a true infection with that particular organism. If the bacterial count is less than 10^4/ml and the patient is not being treated, the urine should be considered sterile and the organism cultured is a contaminant. A bacterial colony of 10^4/ml with a classic urinary pathogen is suggestive of an infection in the female and usually represents a definite infection in the male.

Office Procedures

In the office setting, the physician can use the same methods of urine collection and then send the urine to the hospital or local laboratory for culture and sensitivity tests. However, this is very expensive and often not necessary. To be more cost-effective and to render proper treatment to the out-patient population more quickly, microscopic examination and possibly Gram stain of the spun urinary sediment in the office are as effective as the costly culturing method. This requires that the physician or the laboratory assistant become expert in microscopic examination of the spun urinary sediment.

Examination of the urine in the office should become as routine as examination of the heart with a stethoscope. An out-patient with a first acute urinary infection requires only microscopic examination of the spun urinary sediment for white blood cells and bacteria. Bacteria seen under high dry magnification represent a count of higher than 10^5/ml if the urine is cultured. Microscopic examination of the urine is 80 to 90 per cent accurate with experienced observers. In a patient with an acute uncomplicated infection, the bacterial species will be *E. coli* sensitive to all urinary antimicrobials. If there is any question as to the presence of organisms, practically always rods, then Gram stain of the spun urinary sediment may be done. A large number of these patients will have no bacteriuria at all. Those that do will respond to empirical antibiotic therapy. Of the total population who present to the physician's office with the first episode of cystitis, only about 3 per cent will fail a course of empirical antibiotic therapy and require subsequent culture of the urine and sensitivity tests.

Acute urinary infections, as demonstrated by a positive microscopic examination, that require immediate culture and sensitivity tests are those that:

1. Occur during or after hospitalization.
2. Are associated with a catheter or instrumentation.
3. Are recurrent or relapsing.
4. Have a history of stone disease.
5. Have signs of upper tract infection as previously described.
6. Occur with diabetes mellitus or other complicating medical diseases.

A patient with negative urine sample, either at the initial examination or following an appropriate course of therapy, generally needs no culture. If the clinician is very suspicious, a culture may be necessary on occasion.

Patients with significant pyuria, i.e., more than 10 white blood cells per high-power field on *uncentrifuged* urine, but without bacteriuria, should be evaluated for tuberculosis. Three first morning-voided specimens marked "for acid-fast smear and culture" are sufficient for diagnosis. The smear will be available in several days. The culture takes about 6 weeks.

Simplified Culture Techniques. Several commercially available culture techniques allow the physician to perform urine cultures in the office at extremely low cost. In most of these procedures, an accurately measured urine specimen is placed on an agar surface. After approximately 24 hours, the bacteria can be counted and in some instances partially identified. The literature supplied by the companies is accurate and should be thoroughly reviewed by the practitioner as to sensitivity and specificity before a decision is made regarding which to use in the office.

Various chemical tests are also available, including the tetrazolium reduction test, the nitrate reduction (Greis) test, the glucose oxidase test, and the catalase test. However, none of these accurately fulfills all the criteria for the determination of bacteriuria.

Evaluation. A common question asked by the clinician is: "When should evaluation of a urinary tract infection be undertaken?" It is accepted that at least an intravenous urogram should be ordered for all males and prepubertal females with one urinary tract infection and postpubertal females after the second or third documented urinary infection. In the following situations, evaluation of a urinary tract infection is wise:

1. In upper urinary tract signs and symptoms of pyelonephritis.
2. In urinary tract infection associated with medical diseases (e.g., diabetes mellitus, sickle cell anemia, lymphoma, neurologic diseases).
3. In infections associated with stone disease.
4. In patients who have hematuria with infection.
5. Infections caused by organisms other than *E. coli.*

ACUTE RENAL FAILURE

By T. K. Sreepada Rao, M.D.
Brooklyn, New York

Acute renal failure (ARF) is a clinical syndrome that can be defined as an abrupt reduction in glomerular and renal tubular function resulting in azotemia. Oliguria (urine output < 500 ml per day) or anuria with retention of urea, creatinine, uric acid, phosphorus and other nitrogenous products in the blood is a characteristic feature of this syndrome. However, a non-oliguric form (urine output > 1 liter per day) is frequently encountered in clinical practice. Other abnormalities such as metabolic acidosis, hyperkalemia, and hypocalcemia also occur with varying severity and frequency in ARF and depend largely on the duration of azotemia, associated tissue destruction or catabolism, and the nature of treatment undertaken.

DIAGNOSTIC APPROACH TO ARF

Acute renal failure has many causes (see Tables 1 to 3). A rational approach to patients with acute onset of renal failure involves a differentiation between pre-renal, intrinsic renal, and post-renal causes of azotemia.

Pre-renal Azotemia

The basic underlying mechanism of azotemia from pre-renal causes (Table 1) is a decrease in the effective arterial volume, resulting in renal hypoperfusion. A complete medical history and a thorough physical examination may uncover the underlying predisposing factor(s) such as dehydration or cardiac disease in most patients with pre-renal azotemia. Volume deficit may be indicated by the presence of shock, orthostatic hypotension, or a fast and feeble pulse rate. The skin

Table 1. Causes of Pre-renal Azotemia

Hypovolemia
Hemorrhage
Burns with plasma loss
Gastrointestinal (vomiting, diarrhea, nasogastric suction, colostomy)
Renal (diuretics, renal salt wasting, diabetes insipidus)
Excessive sweating
Increase in Vascular Capacity
Sepsis
Anaphylactic shock
Ganglionic blockade
Shift of Fluids into Extravascular Space
Ascites
Pancreatitis
Peritonitis
Cardiovascular Failure
Congestive heart failure
Myocardial infarction with shock
Cardiac tamponade

and mucous membranes may be dry, and signs of cardiac failure may be evident. In this entity, oliguria is usually associated with a benign urine sediment, a concentrated urine (high urinary specific gravity, a urine to plasma osmolality ratio of > 1.4), and a low urinary sodium concentration (< 20 mEq/liter or < 1 per cent fractional excretion of filtered sodium). The blood urea nitrogen (BUN)/creatinine ratio is disproportionately increased because urea clearance is reduced much more than creatinine clearance when there is a low urine flow rate (Table 2).

Another important diagnostic and therapeutic step in patients with pre-renal azotemia is the response following expansion of plasma volume with saline, albumin, plasma, blood, or other colloids, depending upon the clinical situation. In the presence of oliguria, fluids should be administered cautiously, and the patient's cardiovascular and hemodynamic status should be carefully monitored by central venous and/or pulmonary wedge pressure measurements. This will generally result in an improvement in the urine output with diminution in azotemia. If oliguria persists in spite of adequate volume expansion, 25 gm of mannitol should be administered intravenously as a bolus dose. If there is still no response, administration of 200 to 500 mg of furosemide* intravenously (despite absence of controlled studies) may produce diuresis in some patients. If all of these measures fail, a diagnosis of *acute tubular necrosis* (ATN) should be entertained (Table 2).

Acute Renal Azotemia

A complete medical history, physical examination, and routine blood chemistries are essential first steps that may identify some of the causes of azotemia listed in Table 3. It is important to be aware of the clinical context in which ATN is most likely to develop. This condition usually occurs secondary to renal ischemia following prolonged hypotension associated with trauma, surgery, or an obstetric event. In a medical setting, there may be history of ingestion of toxic chemicals or administration of nephrotoxic drugs or radiographic contrast agents, or mismatched blood transfusion. Patients may manifest external evidence of muscle injury with resultant rhabdomyolysis and myoglobinuria. This can be confirmed by demonstration of myoglobin in the blood or urine and indirectly

*This use of furosemide (Lasix) is not recommended by the manufacturer; directions for use state that furosemide is contraindicated in anuria.

Table 3. Causes of Acute Renal Azotemia

Acute Tubular Necrosis (Vasomotor Nephropathy)
- Ischemic injury (hypotension, shock)
- Post-traumatic, postsurgical
- Obstetric (septic abortions, placental abruption, uterine hemorrhage)

Nephrotoxins
- Ethylene glycol, mercury, carbon tetrachloride
- Aminoglycoside antibiotics, anesthetic agents (methoxyflurane)
- Radiographic contrast material
- Myoglobinuria—traumatic and nontraumatic rhabdomyolysis
- Intravascular hemolysis, mismatched blood transfusions
- Prostaglandin inhibitors—nonsteroidal anti-inflammatory agents

Vasculitides
- Polyarteritis nodosa
- Wegener's granulomatosis

Glomerular and Tubular
- Post-streptococcal, anti-GBM* antibody–induced, and other forms of glomerulonephritis
- Systemic lupus erythematosus
- Hemolytic-uremic syndrome
- Malignant hypertension, systemic sclerosis
- Allergic interstitial nephritis (antibiotics, anticonvulsants)
- Hypercalcemic and hyperuricemic nephropathy
- Hepatorenal syndrome
- Bilateral renal cortical necrosis

Vascular Obstruction
- Renal artery thrombosis, embolism, dissecting aortic aneurysm
- Renal venous thrombosis, vena caval occlusion

*GBM = Glomerular basement membrane.

Table 2. Differential Characteristics of Pre-renal Azotemia and Acute Tubular Necrosis

	Pre-renal Azotemia	Acute Tubular Necrosis
BUN/serum creatinine concentration*	> 10:1	≤ 10:1
Urine/plasma osmolality	> 1:4	1.0
Urinary sodium concentration	< 20 mEq/liter	> 20 mEq/liter
Fractional excretion of sodium†	< 1%	> 4%
Urine output	500–600 ml/day	< 400 ml/day
Urine sediment	Benign	Renal failure (broad granular) casts

*BUN = Blood urea nitrogen.

†Fractional excretion of sodium = $\frac{(\text{Urine Na}^+) \times (\text{Plasma Creatinine})}{(\text{Urine Creatinine}) \times (\text{Plasma Na}^+)} \times 100.$

by findings of elevated serum levels of muscle enzymes (creatine phosphokinase and aldolase). In ATN, urinalysis typically reveals broad, granular, pigmented casts; the urine is iso-osmolar to plasma, and the urinary sodium concentration is greater than 20 mEq/liter (Table 2). Clinically, ATN manifests an oliguric phase which lasts for 7 to 14 days (at times shorter or longer) and then a diuretic phase with a gradual recovery of renal function. The renal size is normal, and there is no evidence of urinary tract obstruction (discussed later).

In patients with glomerular and tubular disease, the urine may reveal red blood cell casts and massive proteinuria. Biochemical and serologic studies might confirm the diagnosis of *post-streptococcal infection, systemic lupus erythematosus* or other multisystem disease. Detection of circulating glomerular basement membrane (GBM) antibodies by radioimmunoassay may establish the diagnosis in patients suspected to have *Goodpasture's syndrome.* In *hemolytic uremic syndrome,* which usually affects infants and children, patients manifest severe renal failure, thrombocytopenia, and microangiopathic hemolytic anemia. *Allergic interstitial nephritis* is associated generally with a history of drug ingestion, eosinophilia, and eosinophiluria, which can be demonstrated by staining the urinary sediment. In *hepatorenal syndrome,* there is evidence of advanced liver disease such as ascites, jaundice, and abnormal liver functions. Urine shows a high specific gravity (osmolality) with a sodium concentration of less than 10 mEq/liter.

Search for Urinary Tract Obstruction: Post-renal Azotemia

The extent of diagnostic evaluation depends on the clinical situation (Table 4). A rectal examination in men to evaluate prostatic hypertrophy or pelvic examination in women to detect any masses is indicated in all patients. One of the simplest initial steps in the evaluation of an acutely azotemic patient is a single urinary bladder catheterization, which will effectively rule out urethral and bladder neck obstruction. A flat plate radiologic examination of the abdomen may reveal radiopaque stone(s). Intravenous urography for patients with azotemia not only is of little clinical value, but is contraindicated in most patients because of the nephrotoxicity of the dye. Renal ultrasonic examination is a most reliable and noninvasive way of determining the size of the kidneys and dilation of the collecting system. Renal sonography is associated with an absence of adverse side effects, and we employ it quite extensively in the evaluation of an azotemic patient. A normal kidney size on an ultrasound examination points generally to an acute intrinsic renal cause; the findings of a dilated calyceal system or renal pelvis indicate that the likely cause of azotemia is an obstruction to the urinary passage. Sonography is also a valuable tool in identifying cysts and other space-occupying lesions in the kidney. With ultrasound monitoring, antegrade pyelography can be performed to localize the site and determine the nature of urinary obstruction. In selected patients, retrograde ureteral catheterization and computed tomographic (CT) scans of the abdomen may be necessary to identify intrinsic and extrinsic causes of ureteral obstruction.

Table 4. Causes of Post-renal Azotemia

Ureteral obstruction bilateral, or in a solitary kidney by stones, blood clot, sloughed calyx, or extrinsic and intrinsic tumor
Retroperitoneal fibrosis
Surgical ligation of ureter(s)
Bladder neck obstruction—prostatic hypertrophy and cancer
Atonic bladder—autonomic neuropathy, spinal cord lesions
Urethral obstruction—stricture, stone

Direct assessment of renal perfusion by renal angiography is not necessary in most patients with ARF. However, in patients with abrupt anuria or following aortic surgery or renal angioplasty, the presence or absence of renal blood flow can be established by a radionuclide renal scan.

VALUE OF RENAL BIOPSY

In most patients with ATN and obstruction to the urinary tract, a renal biopsy is not indicated. When glomerular, interstitial, or tubular disease is suspected and the kidneys are not contracted or shrunken in size, biopsy may be the only way of determining the cause of renal diesase. In patients with anti-GBM antibody glomerulonephritis or Wegener's granulomatosis, renal biopsy is absolutely essential to establish the diagnosis and to institute a specific therapeutic program.

SUMMARY

Acute renal failure encompasses multiple etiologic factors. A comprehensive diagnostic approach, involving awareness, clinical examination of the patient, careful attention to urinary findings, and a few noninvasive radiologic techniques, should establish the cause of azotemia in most patients.

CHRONIC RENAL FAILURE

By W. Dallas Hall, M.D.
Atlanta, Georgia

DEFINITION

Azotemia refers to an excess of nitrogen (French *azote,* nitrogen) in the blood. This disorder can be diagnosed whenever the concentration of blood urea nitrogen (BUN) is increased above the upper limit of normal. Azotemia may be present with or without renal failure. For example, dehydration or an inadequate cardiac output can cause azotemia in the presence of normal kidneys. These settings, known as *prerenal azotemia*, are characterized by a ratio of BUN to serum creatinine (BUN:Cr) of 15:1 or more.

Uremia refers literally to the presence of urine (Greek *ouron,* urine) in the blood, although the term is used clinically to denote the occurrence of signs and symptoms of renal failure in azotemic patients.

Renal failure and *renal insufficiency* are terms that require the presence of intrinsic disease of the kidney or lower urinary tract that is severe enough to cause a reduction in the glomerular filtration rate and an increase in the level of serum creatinine that is above the upper limits of normal for the sex and age of the patient. Renal failure may be *acute* or *chronic.* It is usually deemed chronic when it is present or has been suspected for a period of 6 to 12 weeks or more. Chronic renal failure may be mild, moderate, or severe, defined broadly by ranges of serum creatinine between 1.6 to 2.9, 3.0 to 4.9, and 5.0 to 9.9 mg/dl, respectively.

End-stage renal disease connotes that chronic renal failure is severe enough to require replacement therapy in the form of chronic hemodialysis, chronic peritoneal dialysis, or kidney transplantation. In adults, laboratory criteria for end-stage renal disease usually require a serum creatinine level of 10 mg/dl or higher or a creatinine clearance of 7 ml/minute or less.

PRESENTING SYMPTOMS

Mild degrees of chronic renal failure are usually asymptomatic except for those complaints (i.e., dysuria, flank pain, and so forth) that are attributable to the underlying disease of the kidney or lower urinary tract. Hence, a diagnosis of mild chronic renal failure is made primarily from measurement of blood chemistries, specifically the serum creatinine.

Moderate degrees of chronic renal failure are generally symptomatic, although the symptoms may be so insidious that they are often overlooked by the patient as well as the physician. In the early stages, these subtle symptoms are primarily neurobehavioral and include lethargy, intermittent agitation, and disturbances in the usual pattern of sleep. Anorexia with weight loss, early morning nausea, a bitter taste in the mouth, and disagreeable breath are other early symptoms. All of these are often more apparent to a family member than to the patient.

In contrast, severe chronic renal failure is typically symptomatic. Anorexia, nausea, vomiting, weight loss, fatigue, lethargy, agitation, insomnia, memory loss, muscular twitching, pruritus, dry skin, and sexual disturbances produce an imposing constellation of complaints most often described by the patient as "just sick and not feeling well for the past few months." Severe chronic renal failure can, of course, progress to overt encephalopathy, seizures, and coma.

PRESENTING SIGNS AND PHYSICAL FINDINGS

The general appearance of the patient may provide the first clue to chronic renal failure. A pale and sallow complexion derives from the combination of anemia and retention of urochrome pigments. Visible concavity of the temporalis muscles and wasting of the interosseus muscles near the thumb are signs of weight loss and protein malnutrition. The skin may be dry and scaly. The fingernails may demonstrate transverse white bands (Muehrcke's lines) or discoloration of their distal half (Lindsay's half-and-half nails).

Elevation of the blood pressure is an important sign of chronic renal failure because it occurs in the early stages of most patients with primary glomerular or vascular diseases of the kidney, such as glomerulonephritis or diabetic nephropathy; it usually occurs later in the course of primary tubular or interstitial diseases of the kidney, such as pyelonephritis or hereditary nephritis. All patients with hypertension should have a urinalysis and measurement of serum creatinine to help exclude primary renoparenchymal disease and renal failure as a cause of their hypertension.

The cardiac apex impulse is often prominent and displaced because of hypertrophy and dilatation of the left ventricle. Auscultation usually reveals a prominent systolic ejection murmur located along the left sternal border and related to anemia. An S_4 gallop sound is usually present, and an S_3 gallop sound may be heard in the presence of circulatory overload or congestive heart failure. In advanced cases, a one-, two-, or three-component pericardial friction rub may be detected as well as a pleural friction rub or pleural effusion associated with uremic pleuritis.

Examination of the extremities may reveal edema related to hypoalbuminemia, circulatory overload, or both. Neurologic findings often include an altered level of consciousness as well as involuntary movements such as *asterixis* (flapping of the hands when the arms are outstretched and the wrists dorsiflexed) or *myoclonus* (sudden brief jerks or twitches of groups of muscles or a single muscle). Absent deep tendon reflexes and impaired joint position or vibratory sensation point to peripheral neuropathy.

LABORATORY FINDINGS

The most frequently used clinical tests of renal function are the (1) urinalysis, (2) BUN, (3) serum creatinine, (4) creatinine clearance, and (5) the 24-hour urinary excretion of protein.

Urinalysis

Most patients with chronic renal failure have defects in the normal concentrating and diluting mechanisms of the kidney. Hence, urine specific gravity usually approaches that of a protein-free ultrafiltrate of plasma, that is, about 1.010. Levels below 1.005 are unusual, as are levels above 1.020 unless there is glycosuria, heavy proteinuria, or recent administration of contrast media.

As estimated by dipstick techniques, a value of 1+ (about 30 mg/dl) or 2+ (about 100 mg/dl) proteinuria may be detected in any type of chronic renal failure, but a 24-hour excretion of more than 1 gm of protein suggests the presence of a primary glomerular disease. Glomerular disease is also likely when hematuria occurs in conjunction with significant proteinuria, whereas diseases of the lower urinary tract or a neoplasm of the kidney is more likely when hematuria occurs in the absence of significant proteinuria. Sickle cell trait (hemoglobinopathy AS), however, is a common cause of gross hematuria in black patients.

Pyuria of five or more white blood cells per (centrifuged) high-power field implies that there is inflammatory disease of the lower urinary tract or kidney parenchyma, provided that the specimen has been collected in a manner to avoid contamination from vaginitis in women.

White blood cell casts convey that the inflammation derives from the parenchyma of the kidney. They are usually associated with bacterial inflammation of the kidney, but they can also occur with nonbacterial inflammatory diseases, such as exudative glomerulonephritis, periarteritis nodosa, or renal infarction.

Hyaline and fine granular casts can occur in dehydrated or exercising patients with normal kidneys, whereas red blood cell casts usually imply active glomerular disease. Many of the casts seen in patients with chronic renal failure are unusually broad or convoluted, reflecting the classic dilatation and distortion of residual functioning tubules seen on histologic examination.

Blood Urea Nitrogen

The concentration of BUN reflects the physiology of urea reabsorption more than it reflects the functional status of the kidney. The level of BUN, representing 28/60 of the blood urea concentration, is an index of renal reabsorption of filtered urea. The normal kidney excretes over 10,000 mg of urea daily, and 40 to 60 per cent is reabsorbed. Excessive reabsorption of urea and increased levels of BUN occur during conditions of slow urine flow, dehydration, and decreased renal blood flow, whereas decreased reabsorption of urea and low levels of BUN occur during conditions of high urine flow, volume expansion, and increased renal blood flow. Hence, the BUN level may be considered only as a "poor man's index" of renal function.

Serum Creatinine

The level of serum creatinine is the best indicator of the degree of renal failure. The normal range for serum creatinine is often given as 0.6 to 1.5 mg/dl in adults, but this varies widely with the muscle mass of the individual. For example, a serum creatinine concentration of 1.5 mg/dl might be normal for a muscular young man, whereas a level of 1.3 mg/dl might be abnormal for an elderly or pregnant woman.

Creatinine Clearance

When specimens are properly collected, the creatinine clearance is the best practical test of nephron function and gives a better estimate of glomerular filtration rate than does the serum creatinine level. Normal values range from 80 to 130 ml/minute/1.73 square meters of body surface area. Precise collections of 24-hour urine samples, however, are fraught with difficulty. Invalid collections are often indicated by a creatinine coefficient (total mg creatinine excreted/kg of body weight/24 hours) below 10. Hence, the level of serum creatinine, or an index thereof, provides a valuable substitute under steady-state circumstances. One formula for the estimation of creatinine clearance (Ccr) from serum creatinine (Cr) is:

Table 1. Levels of Serum Creatinine and Creatinine Clearance Indicative of the Severity of Chronic Renal Failure

Severity	Serum Creatinine (mg/dl)	Creatinine Clearance (ml/minute)
Mild	1.6–2.9	40–60
Moderate	3.0–4.9	16–39
Severe	5.0–9.9	8–15
End-stage	⩾ 10	0–7

$$Ccr/70\ kg = \frac{(145 - Age)}{Serum\ Cr} - 3$$

For example, the estimated creatinine clearance of a 70-kg, 45-year-old man with a serum creatinine of 2.0 mg/dl would be 47 ml/min/70 kg. Another formula

$$\frac{(140 - Age) \times (Weight\ in\ kg)}{72 \times Serum\ Creatinine}$$

would give an estimated creatinine clearance of 46 ml/minute. Table 1 indicates the severity of chronic renal failure according to the level of serum creatinine and creatinine clearance.

24-Hour Urinary Excretion of Protein

The normal adult excretes less than 150 mg of protein per day. Delivered into a urine volume of 1000 to 2000 ml, this results in a urine protein concentration of 5 to 15 mg/dl, undetected by most dipstick methods.

Persistent proteinuria of 1+ or greater should be quantitated by chemical measurement of the 24-hour urine protein excretion. The severity of proteinuria is best considered by calculation of the permeability index (PI), the ratio of protein clearance to creatinine clearance according to the equation

$$PI = \frac{Urinary\ Protein\ (gm/liter)}{Serum\ Albumin\ (gm/dl)} \times \frac{Serum\ Creatinine\ (mg/dl)}{Urine\ Creatinine\ (mg/dl)} \times 10$$

The normal PI is less than 0.01. Values between 0.01 and 0.05 represent low-grade proteinuria, as from mild glomerular disease, nephrosclerosis, interstitial nephritis, pyelonephritis, vigorous exercise, congestive heart failure, febrile proteinuria, or benign orthostatic proteinuria.

Values of 0.05 or more represent high-grade proteinuria and usually indicate clinically significant glomerular disease, as from diabetic nephropathy, lupus nephritis, any type of glomerulonephritis, or any cause of nephrotic syndrome. Many patients with serious glomerular disease have a PI value of 0.05 or higher when the quantitative 24-hour protein excretion is below 3 gm/day. This is because impairment of renal function limits the filtration and excretion of protein. The permeability index will remain abnormally high under these circumstances; it can be determined from spot urine samples as well as from timed urine collections.

DIFFERENTIAL DIAGNOSIS

The reader is referred to the articles on the diagnosis of glomerulonephritis, diabetic nephropathy, and cystic disease of the kidney in this volume. Chronic renal failure may also be associated with chronic pyelonephritis, although there is no convincing evidence that recurrent urinary tract infections result in chronic pyelonephritis with progression to chronic renal failure unless there is an underlying anatomic abnormality (e.g., urinary tract obstruction, renal stones) or concomitant systemic disease of the kidney (e.g., diabetes, gout).

Significant pyuria, white blood cell casts and significant bacteriuria (more than 100,000 colonies/ml) are usually present intermittently in the course of chronic pyelonephritis. Intravenous pyelography can outline the contour of the kidney in most patients with levels of BUN or creatinine below 50 or 5 mg/dl respectively; at higher levels, drip infusion pyelography may provide enough detail to reveal or exclude hydroureter or hydronephrosis as signs of urinary tract obstruction. If renal failure is severe, renal ultrasonography is the preferred procedure for evaluation of kidney size and detection of obstruction.

The classic radiographic findings of chronic pyelonephritis include small and asymmetric kidneys. This contrasts with the small but symmetric kidneys that are typical of chronic glomerulonephritis or advanced nephrosclerosis. The renal cortex is usually irregular and thin, and there is blunting or dilatation of the calyceal structures.

In general, glomerular diseases of the kidney are characterized clinically by hypertension, hematuria, and high-grade proteinuria. Tubular and interstitial diseases of the kidney are characterized by a defect in the ability of the kidney to concentrate the urine, manifest clinically by the symptom of nocturia and in the laboratory by an inability to produce urine with an osmolality of 800 to 900 mOs/kg or more following a 12- to 14-hour overnight fast. Another early laboratory clue to interstitial diseases of the kidney is the presence of a hyperchloremic acidosis at a time when renal function may be only mildly impaired, as gauged by the level of creatinine or creatinine clearance.

COURSE AND COMPLICATIONS

Death, usually associated with hyperkalemia, congestive heart failure, gastrointestinal bleeding, pneumonia, or septicemia, is the major complication of chronic renal failure. Severe anemia, pericarditis, hyperparathyroidism, and nephrogenic bone disease may also occur during the natural course of progression from mild to end-stage disease. The rate of progression from one stage to another varies according to the underlying cause of the renal failure as well as the frequency of supervening acute complications. For example, most tubular and interstitial diseases tend to progress less rapidly than do glomerular diseases such as diabetic nephropathy. Recent evidence has shown, however, that even the rate of progression of diabetic nephropathy may be retarded by reduction of elevated blood pressure to levels of 140/95 mm Hg or less.

Death from chronic renal failure can be prevented by renal replacement therapy (chronic hemodialysis, chronic peritoneal dialysis, or transplantation) in patients who are appropriate candidates for these procedures. More importantly, however, the progression from mild to moderate or severe renal failure may be prevented or retarded by appropriate early management.

In general, diagnostic evaluation should begin as soon as even mild degrees of renal failure are detected. Procedures include determination of kidney size and contour by intravenous pyelography or renal ultrasonography as well as urine cultures, with referral to a urologist for cystoscopy and voiding cystourethrography when indicated by symptoms of inflammatory urinary tract disease. Additional metabolic or serologic tests in patients with suspected glomerular disease might include a glucose tolerance test, streptococcal antibody titers, serum protein electrophoresis, a screen for antinuclear antibodies, and measurement of the C3 and C4 components of complement. Early referral to a nephrologist should be considered for additional evaluation, possible renal biopsy, and follow-up consultations.

POTENTIAL ERRORS AND PITFALLS IN DIAGNOSIS

The most frequent diagnostic error is the failure to investigate thoroughly the possibility of reversible urinary tract obstruction. Urethral stricture, bladder neck contracture, prostatic hypertrophy, obstructive stone disease, and retroperitoneal fibrosis are but a few of the reversible conditions. The suspicion and pursuit of obstructive disease of the urinary tract are made even more difficult in patients who already have an established cause of chronic renal failure such as diabetes or primary hypertension.

A second common pitfall occurs during routine follow-up of patients with chronic renal failure. The outlook may not seem as dismal when the serum creatinine level is 2 mg/dl, although this can represent as much as a 50 per cent reduction in renal function. Successive 50 per cent reductions in renal function, however, will be associated with creatinine levels of 4, 8, and 16 mg/dl. Hence, patients frequently appear to deteriorate rapidly once the serum creatinine has reached levels between 4 and 8 mg/dl. This deterioration, however, can often be predicted by a logarithmic plot of the slope of deterioration of renal function over time.

NEPHROTIC SYNDROME

By Alan M. Robson, M.D.
and Linda C. Loney, M.D.
St. Louis, Missouri

DEFINITION

The nephrotic syndrome represents a clinical entity characterized by proteinuria, hypoproteinemia (predominantly hypoalbuminemia), edema, and hyperlipidemia. It is not appropriate to incorporate any arbitrary level of abnormality into this definition. For example, proteinuria in nephrotic syndrome typically exceeds 3 grams per day per 1.73 square meters of body surface area but may be less than one third of this level in children in relapse from *minimal change nephrotic syndrome,* especially if severe hypoalbuminemia is present. The existence of a nephrotic syndrome, however, in these children cannot be denied.

Once the presence of a nephrotic syndrome has been established, it is essential to define the underlying cause. Some of the more common ones are listed in Table 1. A glomerulopathy is responsible in approximately 95 per cent of patients; if the history, physical examination, or laboratory tests indicate that such a lesion is the cause, a complete histologic diagnosis should be established in the majority of patients by means of a renal biopsy (Table 2). The resulting information is helpful in determining the prognosis and in managing the patient. This approach is preferable to that sometimes advocated—of labeling all nephrotic patients with glomerulopathies as having *idiopathic nephrotic syndrome.* This term is misleading. In these disease states, the cause of the immune complex deposition in the kidneys may be unknown or idiopathic but the cause of the nephrotic syndrome is not.

Table 1. Diseases Associated with the Nephrotic Syndrome

1. Glomerulopathies not associated with known systemic disease (see Table 2 for more detail)
2. Malignancies: Hodgkin's disease, leukemia, carcinomas, multiple myeloma
3. Diabetes mellitus
4. Infectious diseases: syphilis, malaria, subacute bacterial endocarditis, cytomegalic inclusion disease, toxoplasmosis, schistosomiasis, pyelonephritis
5. Collagen vascular diseases: systemic lupus erythematosus, periarteritis, dermatomyositis
6. Cardiovascular diseases: renal vein thrombosis, inferior vena caval thrombosis, constrictive pericarditis, congestive heart failure
7. Nephrotoxins: organic and inorganic mercury, gold, bismuth
8. Allergens and drugs: bee stings, poison oak and ivy, milk allergy, snake bites; trimethadione, paramethadione, penicillamine, probenecid, heroin use
9. Congenital (Finnish and other types) nephrotic syndrome, hereditary nephritis
10. Miscellaneous conditions: amyloidosis, renal transplantation, pregnancy, obesity, sickle cell anemia

Table 2. Approximate Incidences of Diseases Found in Pediatric and Adult Patients with Nephrotic Syndrome*

Disease Entity	Relative Incidence (%) Children	Adults
Minimal change (nil) lesion	66	15
Focal glomerular sclerosis	9	10
Glomerulonephritis		
Membranous	3	22
Membranoproliferative	8	7
Other†	9	23
Other diseases‡	5	23
Total	100	100

* Figures averaged from selected, published series. Figures meant only as a guide. Comparable values in individual centers will vary depending on patterns of patient referral.

† Includes all other proliferative glomerulonephritides.

‡ For example, diabetes mellitus, systemic lupus erythematosus, amyloid, anaphylactoid purpura.

PRESENTING SIGNS AND SYMPTOMS

The reported prevalence of nephrotic syndrome is 1.2 to 2.3 new cases per year per 100,000 population, or 3.0 to 4.0 new cases per year per 100,000 children younger than 16 years old. The diseases that cause the nephrotic syndrome have varying incidences at different ages (Table 2). Thus, *minimal change disease* has a much higher incidence in children than in adults. In contrast, membranous glomerulonephritis and diseases such as diabetes mellitus are much more common causes in adult patients. Since the underlying cause modifies the patient's mode of presentation, signs and symptoms of the syndrome often differ in the child and in the adult.

Minimal change nephrotic syndrome may present at any age. It is rarely seen in the first year of life and has a peak age of onset in the third year of life. In childhood, the incidence in males is approximately 2.5 times that in females; in the adult age group, equal numbers of males and females are affected. There may be a positive family history for nephrotic syndrome. It has been reported that the incidence of the disease in a relative of an affected patient is approximately one hundred times the incidence in the general population.

Typically, patients present with edema. Not infrequently, an upper respiratory tract infection or other viral infection precedes by 2 or 3 days the appearance of the edema. Alternately, an allergic response to pollen, to bee stings, or to poison oak or ivy may appear to be the precipitating factor. Indeed, 40 per cent or more of children with minimal change nephrotic syndrome may have atopy. It is not unusual for the significance of the edema to be misinterpreted initially. Frequently, it is thought to be an integral part of the allergic illness. The patient or family may not recognize that some other problem has arisen until dependent edema develops in increasing amounts. The edema typically is more marked in the lower extremities after a period of exercise or standing, but it is predominantly in the periorbital or lumbosacral areas on awakening. Although variable in amount, periorbital edema may be sufficiently severe to interfere with vision, pedal edema may prevent patients from wearing their normal size of shoe, ascites may cause clothes to be too tight or result in respiratory difficulty, and either scrotal or labial edema may be incapacitating. After diagnosis, a patient frequently realizes that dependent or periorbital edema had been variably present for several weeks or months previously.

Sometimes the existence of the nephrotic syndrome may first be suspected from the finding of *proteinuria* on a routine urinalysis, or patients may mention excessive foaming of the urine, a consequence of massive proteinuria. Such patients may have had mild degrees of *edema* that are difficult to identify clinically even at the time the patient consults a physician. Typically, a patient must accumulate 2 or more liters of additional extracellular fluid per 1.73 square meters of body surface area before it can be detected as pitting edema. Nonspecific, vague symptoms of the nephrotic syndrome include malaise, fatigability, irascibility, depression, and loss of the feeling of well-being. These symptoms rarely dominate the clinical picture and are not the usual presenting ones. The pallor resulting from edema may be misinterpreted as indicating the presence of anemia. Rarely, the development of cellulitis, peritonitis, or pneumonia may be the first sign that eventually results in the diagnosis of an underlying nephrotic syndrome.

In patients with a nephrotic syndrome resulting from one of the *glomerulonephritides,* hematuria, hypertension, or the symptoms of renal insufficiency in addition to edema may prompt the patient to seek medical advice. Alternatively, the extrarenal signs of a systemic disease, such as systemic lupus erythematosus, or of the precipitating cause of the nephrotic syndrome, such as diabetes mellitus, may be the initial and dominant features of the patient's disease.

PHYSICAL FINDINGS

The presence of dependent edema is usually the most notable abnormal physical finding, irrespective of the cause of the nephrotic syndrome. When fluid retention is severe, anasarca is obvious. Ascites and pleural effusions should be looked for and may be sufficiently marked to embarrass respiration. The retina has a characteristic "wet" appearance. The normally white lunulae of the fingernails may be pink, in contrast to the remainder of the nail bed, which may be white secondary to subungual edema. Paired white lines (Mee's lines) may be seen on both the fingernails and toenails. Inguinal or umbilical hernias may be found, especially with severe or prolonged ascites. The elasticity of the auricular cartilage appears decreased.

Blood pressure in patients with *minimal change nephrotic syndrome* is usually normal, but mild hypertension may be found in up to 20 per cent of children and in up to 45 per cent of adults. Growth failure in children may be significant, especially in those who have had multiple relapses of the syndrome requiring long courses of steroids in high dosages. The presence of cellulitis may be readily apparent; less obvious infections such as peritonitis or pneumonia should be sought, especially in patients with fever or leukocytosis and who are taking steroids, since these drugs may mask the usual symptoms. Pallor consequent upon the edema and the clinical features of apparent hypothyroidism may also be noted on occasion, although characteristically patients are euthyroid. Patients often are irritable or may have depressive symptoms, especially when they have anasarca.

If *glomerulonephritis* is the underlying cause for the nephrotic syndrome, severe hypertension is found more frequently and may be associated with secondary changes such as a hypertensive retinopathy. Patients with glomerulonephritis may manifest the physical findings of azotemia, such as the characteristic earthen skin color or even asterixis. If a systemic disease is the underlying cause of the nephrotic syndrome, the clinical features of this disease may be readily apparent.

LABORATORY FINDINGS

Urine

Many urinary abnormalities are common to nephrotic patients, irrespective of the underlying cause. Proteinuria, usually 3 to 4+ by dipstick, varies from less than 1 to more than 25 grams per 1.73 square meters of body surface area per day. The values for adult patients usually exceed 3 grams per day. Pediatric patients frequently spill less protein even when corrections are made for the differences in body size. In part as a consequence of this proteinuria, the urine specific gravity is characteristically high. In minimal change nephrotic syndrome, values may be as high as 1.035; in diseases associated with renal failure, lower values are more typical.

The urine sediment often contains oval fat bodies. Lipiduria, however, is better diagnosed by examination of the urine sediment under polarized light when doubly refractile fat bodies ("Maltese crosses") may be seen, either in degenerative fatty vacuoles in the cytoplasm of desquamated renal epithelial cells or free in the urine as neutral fat droplets. Characteristically, urine samples with heavy proteinuria also contain hyaline casts.

Other urinary findings vary, depending upon the cause of the disease. In *minimal change nephrotic syndrome,* macroscopic hematuria is unusual, although microscopic hematuria of ten or fewer red blood cells per high-power field in a centrifuged urine sample may be found in up to one third of patients. In contrast, in patients with the nephrotic syndrome secondary to *glomerulonephritis,* the urine sediment tends to contain more cellular elements and casts including granular, cellular, and mixed hyaline casts. Unfortunately, patients with a minimal change lesion cannot always be differentiated from those with glomerulonephritis on the basis of urine sediment abnormalities alone. One exception to this general rule is the presence of a "telescoped" urine sediment, which indicates the presence of systemic lupus erythematosus or, less frequently, some other progressive glomerulonephritis.

Peripheral Blood

Proteins

Hypoalbuminemia is common to all nephrotic patients, and marked hyperlipidemia occurs in most. Total *serum protein* is characteristically reduced to between 4.5 and 5.5 gm/dl; *serum albumin* concentrations usually fall below 2 gm/dl and not infrequently to below 1 gm/dl. However, in some patients the concentrations of these proteins are remarkably well preserved despite massive proteinuria.

Serum *alpha$_1$-globulin* concentrations are usually normal or slightly decreased, whereas levels of serum alpha$_2$- and beta-globulins are characteristically increased. Although the concentration of *gamma globulin* determined by electrophoresis is normal or reduced, the levels of individual components vary. Serum IgG levels average approximately 20 per cent of normal; IgA levels are less severely reduced; IgM and IgE levels are increased, particularly in minimal change nephrotic syndrome.

Lipids

Serum total cholesterol concentration is almost always elevated. The average level is increased to approximately 400 mg/dl; values in excess of 1000 mg/dl have been reported.

Phospholipid may be increased, but the cholesterol-to-phospholipid ratio is almost invariably elevated, as are *serum triglyceride* levels. Despite these changes, the plasma of patients with nephrotic syndrome usually does not become lactescent until triglyceride levels exceed 400 mg/dl, or four times their normal level.

The lipoprotein profiles characteristic of the nephrotic syndrome are Types II and V in contrast to the Type IV profiles that are seen in uremic patients. Low-density and very low density lipoprotein levels are elevated early in the course of the disease; high-density lipoprotein levels may be moderately elevated, but tend to fall to subnormal levels with severe hypoalbuminemia.

Electrolytes

Despite massive amounts of edema, the *serum electrolytes* are usually within the normal range. If measured by flame photometry, the *serum sodium* may be low (e.g., to 130 mEq/liter) in the presence of marked hyperlipidemia. This artifact results from the high concentrations of blood lipid that contains no sodium; plasma water sodium concentration (and thus plasma osmolality) remains normal. Such pseudohyponatremia requires no treatment, in contrast to true hyponatremia, in which both plasma sodium and osmolality are reduced. More modern methods for measuring sodium concentration use ion-selective electrodes and avoid this artifact.

Serum total calcium may be reduced. Typically, this is due to hypoalbuminemia and a reduction in protein-bound calcium. On occasions, the hypocalcemia may be out of proportion to the hypoalbuminemia and ionized calcium levels may be reduced by 15 to 20 per cent as well, although symptoms of hypocalcemia rarely occur. Total and ionized serum calcium levels return to normal with remission of the nephrotic syndrome.

Serum phosphorus is normal unless the nephrotic syndrome is associated with renal insufficiency.

Blood Urea Nitrogen and Creatinine

In *minimal change nephrotic syndrome,* blood urea nitrogen (BUN) and serum creatinine values are characteristically normal, even though glomerular filtration rates, when measured by inulin clearance, average only 80 per cent of normal. In up to 20 per cent of patients with this syndrome, the glomerular filtration rate may be reduced to as low as 20 to 30 per cent of normal and both BUN and serum creatinine levels are increased accordingly. Such acute renal failure may be secondary to severe hypovolemia, and it reverses when the patient enters into remission from the nephrotic syndrome.

More often, *azotemia* results when the nephrotic syndrome is secondary to a *glomerulonephritis* or a systemic disease that is associated with nephron damage and loss. Thus, the presence or absence of azotemia cannot be used as a reliable indicator in the differential diagnosis of the nephrotic syndrome.

Hematologic Factors

Hemoglobin levels and hematocrit may be normal or even increased if there is hemoconcentration consequent upon hypoproteinemia. This may help to differentiate patients with *minimal change disease* from those with *renal insufficiency,* who most often have anemia. *Thrombocytosis* is not an uncommon finding in nephrotic syndrome.

Other Compounds, Enzymes, and Factors

Serum complement, and its components are normal in *minimal change nephrotic syndrome.* Reduced levels of the third component of complement (beta-1-C globulin) indicate that a *glomerulonephritis* underlies the nephrotic syndrome, but do not occur invariably with glomerulonephritis.

Plasma renin activity and urine excretion of *catechols* are increased in the nephrotic patient.

Abnormal plasma levels of *binding proteins* for hormones and metals may be accounted for by urinary loss. This is the proposed explanation for the decreased plasma 25-hydroxyvitamin D_3 and ionized calcium concentrations found in nephrotic patients. Similarly, losses of *thyroid-binding globulin* and *prealbumin* may result in the decreased half-life of thyroxine, which makes interpretation of the studies of thyroid function difficult in the nephrotic patient. These patients often appear hypothyroid, but they usually are euthyroid, despite low values for *serum protein-bound iodine* and increased uptake of iodine by the thyroid gland.

If an iron deficiency anemia develops in the nephrotic syndrome, it may well be due to urinary loss of *transferrin.* Copper or zinc deficiency can occur also in patients who have long-standing nephrotic syndrome.

Urinary losses of Factor B and serum hemolytic Factor D may result in decreased opsonization of *Escherichia coli* and may contribute to the susceptibility of nephrotic patients to infections. Decreased serum protein levels result in loss of drug-binding sites. This may alter drug metabolism and enhance toxicity.

Special Studies

Renal Biopsy

Virtually every patient presenting with the nephrotic syndrome after the age of 6 years warrants a renal biopsy to diagnose the underlying renal pathology, to help in selecting the appropriate therapeutic approach, and to determine prognosis. Patients 6 years or younger who have the typical clinical features of minimal change nephrotic syndrome may be given a therapeutic trial of steroids as described later. They require a biopsy only if there is no response to this therapy or if multiple relapses occur.

Renal biopsies should be performed only in centers familiar with the technique and where adequate facilities for examination using light microscopy, immunofluorescent microscopy, and electron microscopy are available.

The more common pathologic entities include:

1. *Minimal change lesion.* This is characterized by no remarkable glomerular findings on light or immunofluorescent microscopy. Electron microscopy demonstrates fusion of the podocytes (epithelial cell foot processes) in the glomeruli. This is now thought to be the consequence rather than the cause of the proteinuria. Apparent vacuolization in the cells of the proximal convoluted tubules is characteristic.

A similar picture complicated by mildly increased cellularity in the mesangial regions and by moderate deposition of IgM in the glomeruli has been described. It remains to be determined whether this represents a variant of the minimal change lesion or is a separate clinical entity.

2. *Focal glomerulosclerosis.* Light microscopic examination of renal tissue from patients with focal glomerulosclerosis demonstrates portions of glomeruli that are sclerotic. Characteristically, superficial nephrons obtained on renal biopsy are less severely involved, and the lesion may be missed by sampling error. Immunofluorescent microscopy may demonstrate no abnormality or nonspecific glomerular deposition of several plasma proteins, including albumin, fibrinogen, immunoglobulins, and complement in the sclerotic lesions. Electron microscopy shows foot process fusion, but has not helped elucidate the nature of the sclerotic lesions.

3. *Glomerulonephritis.* Common to all forms of glomerulonephritis is the glomerular localization of immunoglobulin or complement as demonstrated by immunofluorescent microscopy. Discussion of proposed pathologic classifications is presented in the article on glomerulonephritis. However, two diagnoses should be mentioned:

Membranous Glomerulonephritis. This disorder is characterized by glomerular capillary basement membrane thickening, usually without a remarkable increase in the number of cells in the glomerulus. Electron microscopy demonstrates abnormal electron-dense deposits on the epithelial side of the basement membrane. In more advanced disease, projections of basement membrane–like material are seen between the enlarging deposits and correspond to the silver-positive spikes seen on light microscopy. Eventually the basement membrane–like material appears to enclose the deposits, which become less electron-dense. Such changes may be classified according to Stages I through IV and tend to correlate with the duration of the disease. Basement membrane deposits do not resolve even if the patient enters a clinical remission. Glomerular foot process are greatly distorted, especially during periods of heavy proteinuria.

Membranoproliferative Glomerulonephritis. By light microscopy these patients have glomerular basement membrane thickening and glomerular hypercellularity. An increased number of mesangial deposits of immunoglobulin, complement, or both are seen on immunofluorescent microscopy. Two types are discernible by electron microscopy. Type 1 has predominantly subendothelial and mesangial immune complex deposits; Type 2 ("dense deposit disease") has unusually electron-dense deposits within the basement membrane. These two pathologic entities present with a similar clinical picture and can be separated only by biopsy.

Other Diseases. There remain a group of patients whose renal biopsies are diagnosed as glomerulonephritis but who do not fit into the aforementioned categories. The glomeruli in the biopsies of these patients are usually characterized by increased numbers of mesangial cells, leukocytic infiltration, or increased numbers of other glomerular cells (proliferation). Sometimes this is associated with glomerular crescents, glomerular necrosis, or mesangial expansion. In general, it may be stated that the presentation of necrosis in glomerular tufts or of crescents about the capillary tuft is an unfavorable pathologic feature.

Selectivity of Proteinuria

Proteinuria is selective in *minimal change nephrotic syndrome* so that the urinary clearance of albumin or transferrin is much greater than that of larger proteins such as IgG. In contrast, patients with *membranous* or *proliferative glomerular changes* typically have nonselective proteinuria characterized by disproportionately greater clearances of the larger proteins. Measurements of protein selectivity will separate groups of patients with different disease entities, but these determinations do not provide a reliable basis for diagnosis in the individual patient. In addition, a variety of technical problems have limited the usefulness of measuring selectivity of proteinuria as a clinical tool.

Coagulation Changes

Patients with the nephrotic syndrome have been shown to have significant elevations of Factors V and VIII, fibrinogen, plasminogen, and alpha-macroglobulin, with reduction in levels of fibrinolytic activity, antiplasmin activity, antithrombin III, and alpha$_1$-antitrypsin. These changes, along with hemoconcentration, may well account for the increased tendency to thrombosis observed in the nephrotic syndrome. Urinary loss of the smaller-molecular-weight coagulation Factors II, VII, IX, X, and possibly XI and XII may explain the hypocoagulable state that has been described in occasional nephrotic patients.

Other Studies

Circulating soluble immune complexes have been found in significantly higher titers in patients in relapse from steroid-responsive minimal change nephrotic syndrome than in control populations. The meaning of this observation is not known.

There is a significantly higher incidence of minimal change nephrotic syndrome in patients with the human leukocyte antigens (HLA) B12 or DR7. The presence of congenital nephrotic syndrome of the Finnish type can be diagnosed in utero by the finding of elevated concentrations of alpha-fetoprotein in the amniotic fluid, although neural tube defects are also associated with elevated amniotic concentrations of this protein.

Abnormalities of T cell function have been found in patients with nephrotic syndrome and have been proposed to represent the primary pathogenetic factor. Thus children in relapse may show negative skin tests to which they respond when in remission.

A *lymphokine,* referred to as vascular permeability factor, has also been reported in nephrotic patients.

Finally, it should be remembered that 10 per cent of adult patients with a nephrotic syndrome have an underlying malignancy.

THERAPEUTIC TESTS

Under certain circumstances, it is acceptable to determine the patient's responsiveness to steroids rather than performing a renal biopsy before treatment is started (see under Renal Biopsy). For such a therapeutic test, we recommend prednisone in a dose of at least 60 mg/day per 1.73 square meters of body surface area given as a single morning dose. A diuresis with loss of edema and disappearance of proteinuria is considered confirmatory evidence for a *minimal change renal lesion* in young children. However, a patient should not be considered unresponsive unless treatment has been given for 28 days without remission. In adults and in most children who present with nephrotic syndrome after the age of 6 years, we do not recommend steroid treatment until a pathologic diagnosis has been established.

COMPLICATIONS

A patient with nephrotic syndrome is particularly susceptible to acquiring infections. Pneumococcal peritonitis occurs less frequently than it did previously, but it still is a potential hazard and should be recognized early before treatment with steroids is begun. The use of pneumococcal vaccine (Pneumovax) will not necessarily prevent future pneumococcal infections in the nephrotic patient. The administration of other immunizations may precipitate a relapse of minimal change disease. Indeed, most nephrologists advise against immunizations in children with this disease until they have been in remission for 2 or more years or unless an epidemic of the disease to be protected against is present.

Gram-negative septicemia, periorbital cellulitis, cellulitis in the legs, erysipeloid eruptions, pneumonia, and septicemia are other infections that may be seen.

There is a significantly higher incidence of both arterial and venous thrombosis in patients with the nephrotic syndrome. This may involve the leg and axillary and subclavian veins as well as the pulmonary, femoral, coronary, and mesenteric arteries. Thrombosis of the renal veins may be a complication of the nephrotic syndrome and is associated with *membranous glomerulonephritis* and *amyloidosis.*

An occasional nephrotic patient may develop hypovolemia, shock, and even acute renal failure, especially at the time of a steroid-induced diuresis. Because this potential complication can be fatal, we prefer to keep nephrotic patients hospitalized under close observation until diuresis has been completed, urine output has returned to normal, and body weight has stabilized.

Patients with prolonged, massive proteinuria may develop negative nitrogen balance, and malnutrition has been described. We have never seen this complication in a pediatric patient with a minimal change lesion, but we advocate a high-protein diet in an attempt to replace urinary protein losses.

Progressive azotemia is not expected in a patient with minimal change lesion, although it is common in patients with nephrotic syndrome secondary to focal glomerulosclerosis or glomerulonephritis. Despite the lipidemia, only an occasional patient has been shown to develop atherosclerosis as a complication solely of the nephrotic syndrome. The side effects of steroid therapy include hypokalemia, weakness, obesity, osteopenia, personality changes, and depression. These may be striking in patients treated with steroids for prolonged periods.

In addition, the illness can have major psychological effects, especially in children, stemming from severe dietary restrictions, frequent visits to the physician, fear of relapse, and lost school days if relapses are frequent.

DIFFERENTIAL DIAGNOSIS

The diagnosis of nephrotic syndrome usually is not difficult, but other causes of hypoalbuminemia and generalized edema must be included in the differential diagnosis. These include heart failure, liver disease, malabsorption, and malnutrition, protein-losing enteropathy, or cystic fibrosis in infants, as well as local causes of edema such as lymphatic occlusion. Absence of significant proteinuria is helpful in separating most of these entities from the nephrotic syndrome.

COURSE

The course of the disease depends on the underlying etiology for the nephrotic syndrome. In general, patients with *minimal change disease* have a better prognosis than do those with *glomerulonephritis.* However, within any disease entity, prognosis cannot be reliably determined from severity of either proteinuria or symptomatology at the time of the patient's presentation. Criteria indicating that the patient should respond to treatment with steroids and have a good prognosis include age of onset of nephrotic syndrome between ages 1 to 6 years, normal renal function, normal C3 level, selective proteinuria, and absence of both hematuria and hypertension. Collectively, the predictive accuracy of these criteria is 95 per cent.

Minimal Change Nephrotic Syndrome

In the pre-antibiotic, pre-steroid era two thirds of patients with nephrotic syndrome died. The introduction of sulfonamides as antibacterial agents reduced this figure drastically to approximately 20 per cent, and the prognosis has improved even further by the introduction of newer antibiotics. The use of steroids has decreased morbidity dramatically, although it has had little effect on mortality.

An occasional patient with this syndrome will show a spontaneous remission. The majority, however, require treatment with steroids. Up to 90 per cent of patients respond to steroids with loss of edema and proteinuria. The onset of response in these "steroid-responsive" patients is usually heralded by a diuresis and progressive loss of edema that may begin within 6 days of commencing prednisone, but more often is seen after 2 weeks of treatment. Some patients do not respond for up to 28 days and occasionally for even longer, although such protracted therapy is recommended only in exceptional circumstances. Once started, the diuresis usually persists for 3 or 4 days with daily urine volumes of up to 2 liters or more. Urine protein concentration falls as urine volume increases, but proteinuria usually persists for several days after the diuresis has begun. The hypoproteinemia and hypercholesterolemia persist for several weeks or months, but values do return to normal.

Approximately 50 per cent of patients will relapse, the majority responding once again to a further course of steroids. A significant number will have multiple relapses, and if there are more than three relapses per year, such patients are referred to as "frequent relapsers." Patients who relapse as steroid therapy is being withdrawn are labeled "steroid-dependent."

Response to steroids within 4 weeks is a favorable indicator in minimal change nephrotic syndrome, and most patients with such a response have a good long-term outcome. Up to 15 per cent, however, may become steroid-resistant during later relapses. There is no way, at present, to identify such patients prospectively. A recent study showed that the number of relapses that occur during the first 6 months of the patient's course will predict the subsequent relapse rate. Twenty per cent or more of children will continue to have relapses 5 years after onset of disease.

Despite the frustrating course taken by many of the patients with frequent relapses, the long-term prognosis remains good. In one large series of pediatric patients, almost 70 per cent entered adult life in prolonged and presumed permanent remission with no evidence of any residual renal disease. Quite often, relapses stopped when the patient entered puberty. In this same series, an additional 20 per cent of the children were alive and well at the end of the follow-up period but spilled protein in their urine; 9 per cent of the patients died. In light of the fact that not all of these patients had the diagnosis of minimal change disease confirmed by histology, the prognosis for this disease may be shown subsequently to be even better. However, persistence of the nephrotic syndrome for 5 or more years has been associated with a death rate of 7 to 12 per cent even in patients with a proven minimal change lesion. More than 80 per cent of these deaths are nonrenal and are complications of infection or steroid therapy.

It has been recognized only recently that adult patients with minimal change disease entity have courses similar to those taken by children with the same pathologic diagnosis. In a series of 49 adult patients with proven minimal change glomerular lesions, follow-up extended for up to 19 years. Of the nine patients who died, only one was uremic; three deaths were probably related to complications of treatment. Eleven of the patients were still in relapse at the time follow-up was complete, but 29 patients were well and required no treatment.

Other Causes of Nephrotic Syndrome

The long-term prognosis for patients with nephrotic syndrome secondary to *glomerulonephritis* varies and depends on the nature of the renal disease, as well as on the stage in the disease course at which diagnosis is made. Many of the patients develop progressing azotemia and eventually require chronic hemodialysis. If renal transplantation is performed in these patients, the underlying disease may recur in the transplanted kidney. However, it is important to emphasize that with appropriate therapy edema can be controlled in the majority of patients and that this combined with other symptomatic treatment will often improve the patient's well-being, permitting a return to a more normal life.

Prognosis in the adult with *focal glomerulosclerosis* is not favorable; progressive renal failure not responsive to steroid therapy is to be expected. In children the prognosis is not always as bleak; 40 per cent of patients will show partial or complete remission of the nephrotic syndrome when treated with steroids.

The clinical course of *membranous glomerulonephritis* is highly variable. Twenty-five per cent of all patients have a spontaneous remission; an equal number develop progressive renal failure in addition to the nephrotic syndrome; the remaining 50 per cent of patients have persistent proteinuria but relatively stable, although reduced, renal function for many years.

Patients with *membranoproliferative glomerulonephritis* also have a variable course. The 10-year survival of those with the Type I lesion and persistent nephrotic syndrome is only 40 per cent. Patients with the same pathologic lesion but non-nephrotic proteinuria have an 85 per cent survival. The prognosis for Type II disease is worse than that for Type I, especially if the renal biopsy shows crescentic glomerular lesions. The outlook for children with this form of glomerulonephritis is not dissimilar from that for adults.

GLOMERULONEPHRITIS

By Yvonne E. Cummings, M.D.
and Dana L. Shires, Jr., M.D.
Tampa, Florida

Glomerulonephritis encompasses a large number of diseases whose common denominator is glomerular injury. The pathogenesis of this injury involves at least two immunologic mechanisms: *immune complex disease* and *antiglomerular basement membrane antibody disease.* These mechanisms produce many patterns of damage that can be characterized by clinical features, laboratory evaluation, and examination of renal biopsy specimens. Although clinical and laboratory presentations vary, the response of the kidney to glomerular injury is stereotyped to the extent that biopsy confirmation is mandatory for accurate diagnosis.

Analysis of renal biopsies and laboratory findings requires understanding of normal renal histology and function. The *nephron* is the functioning unit of the kidney, and the *glomerulus* is the filtering component of the nephron. The glomerulus has two basic areas (the capillary loop and the mesangium), and three basic cell types (endothelial, epithelial, and mesangial cells). The actual filtering process occurs in the *capillary loop.* The loop is lined on its inner aspect by an endothelial cell. A *basement membrane* surrounds most of the *endothelial cell,* and *epithelial cells* form an outer lining about the basement membrane. Discrete foot processes from the epithelial cells are in contact with the basement membrane. The *mesangial area* can be thought of as the inner support structure of the glomerulus. It is composed of mesangial cells and mesangial matrix. The mesangial cells also have significant reticuloendothelial cell functions.

MICROSCOPY

Adequate renal biopsy analysis should include examinations by three methods:

1. *Light microscopy,* the classic method, gives information about cellularity and can be used to make a gross estimate of glomerular basement membrane thickness.
2. Immunofluorescent microscopy is performed by staining glomeruli with fluorescent antisera to various factors involved in glomerular injury, such as the immunoglobulins and components of the complement system. If any of these components are present, a fluorescent pattern will be seen when the appropriate antiserum is used.
3. *Electron microscopy,* by means of its tremendous magnifying ability, gives a close view of the glomerular basement membrane and the epithelial foot processes, and will generally demonstrate, if they are present in the glomerulus, electron-dense deposits thought to be immune complexes.

PATTERNS OF GLOMERULAR INJURY

In *immune complex disease,* the kidney appears to be an "innocent bystander," inundated by circulating antigen-antibody complexes. The classic prototype of this is *serum sickness.* In serum sickness, a foreign protein, unrelated to the kidney, is administered. The antibodies made against the protein couple with it, forming complexes. When complexes of the appropriate size are formed at the stage of moderate antigen excess, deposition occurs in the glomeruli. Complement is fixed and activates a variety of noxious agents, producing glomerular damage. If the antigen is given in a single large injection, the process is self-limited; if it is given in small daily doses over a period of weeks, chronic, progressive disease occurs.

Recently, a second mechanism for immune complex deposition has been demonstrated. Antigens foreign to the glomerulus, if deposited there from the circulation, can attract circulating specific antibody to form complexes by a process of in situ combination. These "planted" antigens, in general, form immune complexes that localize to the subepithelial site. Indeed, it appears that the predominant mechanism in the formation of subepithelial deposits is in situ combination of antigen and specific antibody and represents one pattern of immune complex injury.

Multiple patterns of immune complex injury can be seen on microscopy. Immunofluorescent studies show deposition of complement and immunoglobulins. In some cases, the deposits are irregularly distributed and discrete, appearing under immunofluorescence in what has been described as a "lumpy, bumpy" distribution in poststrephococcal glomerulonephritis. Electron microscopy demonstrates the presence and distribution of immune complexes and any abnormalities of cell proliferation.

In contrast, in *antiglomerular basement membrane antibody disease,* antibodies to glomerular basement membrane are produced. The antibodies fix complement and set off the same mediators of membrane damage as in immune complex disease. Light microscopy reveals a variety of nonspecific types of glomerular damage, often with associated epithelial crescent formation. Immunofluorescence shows a linear, ribbon-like staining for immunoglobulins. Electron microscopy fails to show any electron-dense deposits.

LABORATORY EVALUATION

Laboratory investigation of glomerular injury begins with urinalysis. A dipstick evaluation gives gross estimates of proteinuria and hematuria. Microscopic examination of fresh urine allows for better quantification of hematuria. Two or three red blood cells per high-power field is accepted as normal. The presence of red cell casts implicates the kidney as the source of hematuria. These casts, however, do not persist in alkaline or hypotonic urine, and repeated examinations may be necessary to rule out their presence when a glomerular lesion is being sought. Blood urea nitrogen (BUN) and serum creatinine are used as rough measures of renal function. Creatinine is the normal end product of muscle metabolism and is produced at a relatively constant rate. It is primarily filtered and not reabsorbed. The production rate of urea, however, may vary significantly, depending upon the patient's rate of catabolism. Substantial amounts are reabsorbed in the renal tubules in patients with a diminished effective intravascular volume. Of the two, serum creatinine is the more reliable indicator of renal function. Unfortunately, a substantial decrease in renal function is necessary before clear-cut abnormalities of BUN or serum creatinine are seen.

A timed urine collection for calculation of the creatinine clearance is necessary for a more precise quantification of the glomerular filtration rate. A timed urine collection is also necessary to quantitate urinary protein losses. The clearance ratio of a relatively small and a relatively large protein molecule, e.g., transferrin and IgG, is used in estimating the degree of selectivity of proteinuria, which aids in defining the leakiness of the glomerular basement membrane. A high degree of selectivity—that is, excretion of primarily small protein molecules—is interpreted as reflecting a less porous glomerular basement membrane.

More sophisticated laboratory studies include the *fluorescent antinuclear antibody test* for collagen vascular disease, various screening tests for the presence of recent streptococcal infection, and a test to determine the profile of the complement system. Complement is composed of a series of factors found in normal serum that are activated in a sequential fashion. Activation of complement can lead to cellular injury. Complement is activated by either the classic or alternate pathways, each producing different serum complement profiles. Classic pathway activation, generally initiated by immune complexes, goes through C1, C4, and C2 to activate C3 and then through the remainder of the complement cascade. This tends to produce low serum levels of C1q, C4, and C3: Alternate pathway activation bypasses C1, C4 and C2, directly cleaving C3, and is caused by such agents as immunoglobulin aggregates, polysaccarides (inulin and zymosan), endotoxins, and properdin. This results in a normal serum C1q and C4 with a lower serum C3. Thus, precise complement profiles vary with different glomerular diseases.

Table 1 presents a convenient classification of glomerulonephritis based on immunologic mechanisms and subdivided according to biopsy characteristics. Following the outline of Table 1, the immune complex diseases are discussed first, followed by antiglomerular antibody disease and then several miscellaneous diseases. It needs to be emphasized that, although generalizations can and will be made about specific diseases, there may be wide individual variations in laboratory findings, chemical presentations, course, and outcome.

Table 1. Classification of Glomerulonephritis

I. Immune complex disease
   A. Proliferative
   B. Membranous
   C. Membranoproliferative
      1. Type I
      2. Type II (dense-deposit disease)
      3. Type III
   D. Focal glomerulonephritis
II. Antiglomerular basement membrane antibody disease with or without pulmonary hemorrhage
III. Miscellaneous
   A. Rapidly progressive glomerulonephritis
   B. Minimal change disease
   C. Focal glomerulosclerosis

IMMUNE COMPLEX DISEASES

Proliferative Glomerulonephritis

The prototype of proliferative glomerulonephritis is acute poststreptococcal glomerulonephritis (PSGN), a sequela of infection with a nephritogenic strain of streptococcus. Acute glomerulonephritis has also been reported in such diverse entities as viral infections, subacute bacterial endocarditis, and the Guillain-Barré syndrome.

Clinical Findings

Cellular proliferation is evident on light microscopy. Immunofluorescence demonstrates deposition of immunoglobulins and complement in a large granular pattern. Electron microscopy confirms immune complex deposition in a subepithelial distribution, very much as in acute serum sickness.

Acute PSGN has a classic presentation. Typically, acute manifestations of renal disease occur 7 to 21 days after the clinical manifestations of the streptococcal infection have subsided. A latent period less than 5 days suggests an exacerbation of pre-existing disease. PSGN may follow an episode of either pharyngitis or impetigo. Epidemic PSGN has been associated most commonly with skin infection, whereas the sporadic cases are most often seen following pharyngitis. Patients present with periorbital and ankle edema and frequently dyspnea. Urine volume is usually decreased, and the urine has the typical appearance of tea or is cola-colored because of hematuria. Abdominal pain, anorexia, nausea, and vomiting may be present. Hypertension is frequent and may present with signs of encephalopathy, including headache, lethargy, and convulsions. In most cases, the oliguria or anuria lasts only a few days.

Hematuria and red cell casts are the classic finding

on urinalysis. Proteinuria is characteristically present, but uncommonly exceeds 3.5 gm/day. The antistreptolysin-O titer (ASO titer), an indicator of previous streptococcal infection, becomes elevated in 1 to 3 weeks, peaks in 3 to 5 weeks, and returns to normal within 6 months in 50 per cent of patients. However, only 70 to 80 per cent of patients have an elevated ASO titer, and if the patient has been treated with antibiotics the percentage decreases to 10 to 15 per cent. Streptococcal skin infections may not be associated with substantial rises in the ASO titer. In this setting, measurement of anti-DNase B titers can confirm a recent streptococcal infection in more than 90 per cent of patients. Although complement levels vary, a common profile demonstrates a marked depression of C3 accompanied by depression of C1q or C4 or both. Serum C3 usually returns to normal in 3 to 6 weeks.

Course and Prognosis

Microscopic hematuria may persist for several years. Proteinuria has been reported to persist for more than 12 months in 61 per cent of these patients and for more than 24 months in 36 per cent. Urinalysis can remain abnormal long after the patient is asymptomatic. A poor prognostic indicator is an initial presentation with severe renal dysfunction and the presence of numerous epithelial crescents on biopsy. Adults fare substantially worse than children, and preschool children fare the best.

The incidence and overall outcome of acute PSGN are still matters of substantial controversy. Studies have demonstrated that many, if not most, people with acute PSGN are asymptomatic, their condition being discovered only when large groups are systematically screened by urinalysis and serum complement levels. These findings cast into doubt our past ideas on the incidence of the disease and suggest that past data on the natural history were based on inadequate samples. Some long-term studies indicate that acute PSGN may cause more residual damage than previously supposed.

Membranous Glomerulonephritis

Synonyms

Extramembranous glomerulonephritis, epimembranous nephropathy.

Clinical Picture

Membranous glomerulonephritis (MGN) is the most common cause of the idiopathic nephrotic syndrome in adults. Seventy-five to 80 per cent of patients with idiopathic MGN present with the nephrotic syndrome. It is associated with a variety of underlying diseases, including carcinomas, lymphomas, heavy metal intoxication, systemic diseases, numerous chronic infections, and drugs. There is a wide age range for the onset of this disease process, but the majority of patients present after the fourth decade; there is male predominance. In 85 to 90 per cent of patients, proteinuria is nonselective. Other findings that may be present at the time of diagnosis include microscopic hematuria, hypertension, and normal serum complement levels.

More recently, human leukocyte antigen (HLA) studies have shown that MGN is strongly associated with HLA DR3. On biopsy, subepithelial immune complexes are seen without evidence of significant cellular proliferation. The complexes are gradually incorporated into the glomerular basement membrane, ultimately resulting in a thickened irregular basement membrane. A characteristic appearance of "spikes" of glomerular basement membrane between deposits is seen with a silver stain on light microscopy. Immunofluorescence shows diffuse granular deposition of IgG and C3 in the capillary loops. Approximately 30 per cent of patients have deposits of IgM or IgA or both, and 20 per cent have deposition of early complement components. Electron microscopy confirms the findings of subepithelial (epimembranous) immune complex deposition.

Course and Outcome

The course of MGN is extremely variable, making evaluation of any therapy difficult. Under most circumstances, it should be regarded as an indolent and slowly progressive disease. Estimates are that approximately 25 per cent of patients will undergo a spontaneous remission, whereas 40 per cent will show sustained proteinuria and progression to some degree of chronic renal insufficiency.

Patients without nephrotic syndrome have a more benign course and rarely progress to end-stage renal disease. Children appear to do somewhat better than adults, with a higher remission rate and slower progression of the disease. Additionally, some authors have found that the natural history of MGN is more benign in women. Recurrence of the disease in renal allografts is rare.

Both chronic and acute unilateral or bilateral *renal vein thrombosis* may complicate the course of MGN. Renal vein thrombosis occurs more commonly in MGN than in other forms of the nephrotic syndrome. Clinical findings suggestive of renal vein thrombosis include acute flank pain, worsening of proteinuria, and decline in the glomerular filtration rate.

Except for its beneficial effect on thromboembolic phenomena, chronic anticoagulation has no proven efficacy in this situation.

Membranoproliferative Glomerulonephritis

Synonyms

Mesangiocapillary glomerulonephritis, hypocomplementemic glomerulonephritis.

Incidence

The majority of patients with membranoproliferative glomerulonephritis (MPGN) are between the ages of 5 and 15 years old.

Classification

Pathologically, there are two major subtypes of MPGN.

Type I. In Type I MPGN, there are subendothelial and mesangial immune complex deposits, an increase in mesangial matrix, and mesangial cell proliferation with intrusion of the mesangial cell matrix between the glomerular basement membrane and the endothelial cells. Duplication of the glomerular basement membrane or "splitting" with deposition of immunoglobulins and C3, is often present. Deposition of early-acting complement components C1q and C4 also occurs.

Type II. Type II MPGN is referred to as *dense-deposit disease.* It has a striking biopsy picture with the glomerular basement membrane greatly thickened and partially or totally replaced by an amorphous, homogeneous, highly electron-dense material. It has been suggested that this density may represent an intrinsic alteration of the glomerular basement membrane structure. All glomeruli are involved to a variable extent. Intramembranous deposition occurs in the tubular basement membranes in a segmental fashion. There is usually an associated mesangial cell proliferation and occasional crescent formation. Immunofluorescence shows granular or pseudolinear staining for C3 in a distribution identical to that of the intramembranous deposits and mesangial staining. Immunoglobulins, C1q, and C4 are either scanty or absent.

Comparison of Types I and II. Complement profiles are abnormal, but vary considerably. C3 is depressed initially in approximately 70 per cent of patients, but may fluctuate greatly during the course of illness. Type I MPGN is most often associated with classic pathway activation of complement with low C3, C4, and C1q. Type II is associated with alternate pathway activation of complement, low levels of C3, normal C4, and normal C1q. In addition, C3NeF, a heat-stable nonimmunoglobulin gamma globulin capable of activating complement at the C3 level, is often found in the plasma of patients with MPGN. C3NeF is more commonly found in Type II than in Type I.

Type III. More recently, Type III histologic changes have been described. Electron microscopy shows massive accumulation of electron-dense material on both sides of the basement membrane, associated with basement membrane disruption and duplication of lamina densa–like material. The clinical features and prognosis of patients with Type III MPGN appear to parallel those of other patients with Types I and II.

Clinical Course and Outcome

MPGN has been associated with a variety of underlying disorders such as partial lipodystrophy, hepatitis B virus infection, heroin abuse, and complete C2 or C6 deficiency. Despite these associations, the clinical presentation and clinical course, as well as the outcome, are similar for all three disease types.

MPGN is the cause of 5 to 10 per cent of the idiopathic nephrotic syndrome of childhood. The presentation varies; according to one estimate, approximately 50 per cent of the patients present with the nephrotic syndrome, 30 per cent present with asymptomatic proteinuria and recurrent hematuria, and 20 per cent present with an acute nephritic syndrome. Mild hypertension occurs in approximately one third of patients, and depressed renal function is common.

The prognosis is poor. In one large study, 5-year survival rates were 87 per cent, with 44 per cent of patients developing chronic renal insufficiency within 5 years. An actuarial analysis of patients with Type II MPGN suggests that 50 per cent develop end-stage renal disease by the tenth year. MPGN may recur in renal allografts, and current evidence suggests that Type II disease will recur in virtually all grafts.

Focal Glomerulonephritis

Pathologic Findings

The pathologic picture of focal glomerulonephritis is found in many diseases, including systemic lupus erythematosus, Henoch-Schönlein purpura, and idiopathic benign essential hematuria. The distinction between these diseases is made on clinical and laboratory grounds.

One form of idiopathic benign essential hematuria is called *IgA nephropathy,* or *Berger's disease.* It commonly presents in children or young adults as persistent microscopic or intermittent gross hematuria. The hematuria is often exacerbated by strenuous exercise or upper respiratory tract infections. Renal function is usually normal at time of diagnosis, and proteinuria mild, if present at all. Hypertension is not common until late in the disease. Serum complement levels are normal. An elevated serum IgA is usually present.

Renal biopsy reveals focal mesangial matrix increase, some mesangial cell proliferation, and mesangial immune complex deposits. The predominant immunofluorescent staining is for IgA in a mesangial distribution. There may be varying intensities of staining for IgG, IgM, and C3. C1q and C4 are usually not present.

Clinical Course and Outcome

This disease generally follows an indolent course, but up to 50 per cent of patients have been reported to develop end-stage renal disease over a 15- to 20-year period following diagnosis. Poor prognostic indicators are the presence of hypertension, proteinuria above 2 gm/24 hours, and decreased glomerular filtration rate at the time of biopsy. Recurrent disease is a risk in renal allografts.

ANTIGLOMERULAR BASEMENT MEMBRANE ANTIBODY DISEASE

This is an uncommon disease, with an estimated incidence of approximately 5 per cent of all cases of glomerulonephritis. Its hallmark is the presence of circulating glomerular basement membrane antibodies, in contrast to their absence in immune complex disease. In lieu of the demonstration of circulating antibodies, the presence of a linear immunofluorescent pattern for IgG is extremely strong evidence. A weak linear pattern may be seen in patients with diabetes mellitus; an extremely densely packed granular pattern can be mistaken for a linear pattern. Ten per cent of normal biopsies have been reported to have a linear "accentuation" of the glomerular basement membrane when stained for IgG; occasionally with quite advanced disease, no glomeruli with typical linear deposits are observed. Therefore, the immunofluorescent study alone at times can be misleading. The presence of linear tubular basement membrane antibody staining occurs in approximately 70 per cent of patients and supports the diagnosis. Electron microscopic findings are helpful in that they fail to reveal evidence of immune complexes. There are no light microscopy findings that are pathognomonic for glomerular injury induced by antiglomerular basement membrane antibody.

When associated with pulmonary hemorrhage, this disease is called *Goodpasture's syndrome.* Pulmonary disease precedes or is coincident with the onset of renal dysfunction in more than 70 per cent of patients with an average delay of approximately 3 months between the onset of the two symptoms. There is a striking preponderance of young adult males. Serum complement levels are normal. The renal disease is generally quite severe, but milder cases with remissions are now being reported. The diagnosis is strongly suggested by the combination of renal failure and pulmonary hemorrhage, but a similar picture may also occur with the vasculitides and immune complex forms of glomerular injury.

Current data suggest that the antiglomerular basement membrane antibody production is self-limited, with titers falling to undetectable levels over an average period of 7 to 8 months. If therapy can prevent irreversible renal damage during the period of antibody production, the prognosis should be substantially altered for the better. The disease may recur in renal transplants, but if the recipient has no detectable circulating antibodies before grafting, the recurrence is generally mild. Present policy is to defer transplantation until the disappearance of circulating antiglomerular basement membrane antibodies.

MISCELLANEOUS GLOMERULAR CONDITIONS

Rapidly Progressive Glomerulonephritis

Synonyms

Extracapillary proliferative glomerulonephritis, crescentic glomerulonephritis, subacute glomerulonephritis, malignant glomerulonephritis.

Etiology

Rapidly progressive glomerulonephritis (RPGN) appears to have a wide variety of causes, cutting across the immunologic classification given in Table 1. Therefore, it has been classified under the Miscellaneous heading in the table. Causes include streptococcal infections, the vasculitides, systemic lupus erythematosus, antiglomerular basement membrane antibody disease, and idiopathic disease.

Findings

There are extracapillary epithelial crescents in the majority of glomeruli. These crescents are formed by the cells lining Bowman's capsule that become hyperplastic and literally crush the glomerular capillaries.

Findings typical of immune complexes are seen in those cases associated with immune complex disease, and linear staining for IgG is seen in those cases associated with antiglomerular basement membrane antibody disease. An additional subdivision of patients with RPGN without immune complexes or only sparse deposits and no evidence of antiglomerular basement membrane antibody disease has recently been described. Substantial incidence figures have not been recorded to date; however, those available suggest that 20 to 30 per cent of patients may fall into this category, with the remainder being divided between antiglomerular basement membrane antibody disease and immune complex disease.

Clinical Features and Outcome

The clinical features and prognosis appear to be similar for all three types of RPGN. There is a slight male preponderance and an insidious onset with nonspecific signs and symptoms. The overall patient survival is 30 to 50 per cent without dialysis or transplantation. Serum complement levels are usually normal. The chances for recovery are slim if more than 70 per cent of glomeruli are extensively involved with crescents.

Course

RPGN is distinguished by its rapid downhill course and a striking biopsy picture. The clinical course is that of progressive loss of renal function occurring over weeks to months.

Minimal Change Disease

Synonyms

Lipoid nephrosis, nil disease, no-change-by-light-microscopy disease.

Clinical Features

Minimal change disease (MCD) is by far the most common cause of the idiopathic nephrotic syndrome of childhood and accounts for 10 to 30 per cent of the nephrotic syndrome in adults. The patients generally present with highly selective proteinuria, normal or near-normal renal function, an unremarkable urinary sediment, normal blood pressure, and normal serum complement levels. Occasional patients may have microscopic hematuria, and in adults poorly selective proteinuria is more often found. The glomeruli show little or no changes on light microscopy, and immunofluorescence is negative. Electron microscopy reveals fusion of the epithelial cell foot processes, but is otherwise negative. (See article on Nephrotic Syndrome.)

Etiology

There is no clear-cut evidence for either an antiglomerular basement membrane antibody or an immune complex etiology. It has been suggested that MCD results from an abnormality of T cell function, but this is still speculative. An association exists between MCD and Hodgkin's disease, and there are reports of patients developing MCD in association with exposure to allergens.

Course and Prognosis

This is a rather indolent disease in children, lasting for many years with periods of remission and relapse. An occasional patient may have progression to chronic renal failure. In adults, the prognosis does not appear to be nearly as good and a considerable number show progression to chronic renal failure.

Because up to 90 per cent of children respond promptly to steroid therapy, a therapeutic and diagnostic trial with steroids is often attempted in lieu of a renal biopsy. This is less frequently done in adults because of the much lower incidence of MCD. Initial steroid response rates for adults are fairly close to the rates for children. Approximately two thirds of patients responding to steroids will undergo relapse and require additional treatment, and 5 to 10 per cent of patients will have primary steroid resistance. Cyclophosphamide therapy has been shown to be beneficial in patients failing to respond to or having frequent relapses following steroid therapy, markedly reducing the frequency of subsequent relapses. Chlorambucil may even be more effective than cyclophosphamide in this setting, but an increased incidence of side effects has limited the use of this drug.

Minimal change disease has been reported to recur in renal allografts.

Focal Glomerulosclerosis

Focal glomerulosclerosis occurs in 5 to 15 per cent of children with the nephrotic syndrome and has been reported to occur in a similar or slightly higher percentage of adults.

Clinical Presentation

Differentiation between this syndrome and MCD is necessary because long-term prognosis may be quite different. Distinguishing features of focal glomerulosclerosis include:

1. A higher incidence of microscopic hematuria.
2. A higher degree of nonselective proteinuria.
3. A greater incidence of renal dysfunction at the time of initial diagnosis.
4. Hypertension.
5. A much lower incidence (less than 15 per cent) of steroid responsiveness.

In spite of these differences, a report of the International Study of Kidney Disease in Children, in which a multivariate analysis of clinical and laboratory evaluation of children with the idiopathic nephrotic syndrome was used, failed to demonstrate a good discrimination between these two diseases. Thus, biopsy is mandatory for a firm diagnosis.

Focal segmental areas of sclerosis without evidence of inflammation are seen in the glomeruli. There are no proliferative or membranous changes. Positive immunofluorescence for IgM and C3 in the affected lobules has been consistently reported. Occasional electron-dense deposits are seen in the same areas by electron microscopy. These changes are thought to first occur in the juxtamedullary glomeruli, and it is possible, if the biopsy specimen does not include this area, to miss the diagnosis. Focal segmental scarring is not specific for a single disease entity and may be simulated by glomerular scarring following proliferative glomerulonephritis. Similar changes have also been seen with chronic atrophic pyelonephritis, nephrosclerosis, and transplant rejection. To complicate the picture further, this histologic picture may also occur in patients with relapsing steroid-responsive MCD after the disease has been present for some 2 to 15 years. This overlap between the two entities complicates both our ability to diagnose and to prognosticate.

Prognosis

Although occasional remissions occur, focal glomerulosclerosis has a much poorer prognosis than MCD. The actuarial survival in one large series was 75 per cent at 5 years, 60 per cent at 10 years, and 38 per cent at 15 years. The recurrence rate of this disease in renal allografts may exceed 60 per cent.

OBSTRUCTIVE NEPHROPATHY

By Jonathan C. Boyd, M.D.
and William H. Boyce, M.D.
Winston-Salem, North Carolina

Obstructive nephropathy is obstruction of the flow of urine resulting in damage to the kidney. It can occur anywhere from the calyceal infundibulum to the urethral meatus and can be considered a type of, or end result of, *obstructive uropathy*, which is obstruction of the urinary flow resulting in damage to the urinary tract. Initially, obstructive uropathy results in hypertrophy, dilatation, and decompensation of the urinary tract. Scarring and inefficient transport of urine are the eventual results, and if uncorrected, they will lead to obstructive nephropathy. Obstructive nephropathy, in turn, causes renal failure by direct pressure of urine on the tubules and by pressure on the arteries, which causes ischemic atrophy.

Hydronephrosis (distention of the pelvis and calyces with urine) frequently, but not invariably, accompanies obstructive nephropathy. Acute onset of obstruction will cause symptoms before dilatation of the pelvis has occurred. The general term *hydronephrosis*

Table 1. Causes of Obstructive Nephropathy

Renal
Congenital anomalies
Infundibular stenosis
Calculus disease
Chronic infection
Neoplasm
Papillitis
Ureteral
Ureteropelvic junction obstruction
Strictures
Kinks
Chronic infection
Congenital valves
Retrocaval ureter
Calculus disease
External compression
Ureteritis cystica
Ovarian vein syndrome
Periureteral inflammation
Trauma
Pregnancy
Retroperitoneal fibrosis
Atony
Aperistalsis
Neoplasm
Bladder
Ureterovesicular junction obstruction
Ureterovesicular reflux
Neoplasm
Diverticulum
Calculus
Prolapsing ureterocele
Foreign bodies
Scarring
Neurogenic bladder
Cystitis
Prostatic
Benign prostatic hypertrophy
Prostatitis
Posterior urethral valves
Neoplasm
Urethral
Neoplasm
Stricture
Calculus
Genital anomalies
Strangulation (external compression of penis)
Meatal stenosis
Phimosis

should probably be replaced by the more specific terms *caliectasis, pelviectasis,* and *ureterectasis.*

The most common underlying causes of obstructive nephropathy are shown in Table 1.

PRESENTING SIGNS AND SYMPTOMS

Presentation of obstructive nephropathy varies from silent lesions compromising renal function without the patient's suspicion to incapacitating renal colic, which demands immediate diagnosis and treatment. Generally, the lower the degree of obstruction, the fewer the symptoms it will produce and the greater the renal failure that will occur before the diagnosis is made. Conversely, patients with a high degree of obstruction will have pronounced symptoms that will lead to early diagnosis and treatment before renal failure develops.

The symptoms and signs of obstructive nephropathy vary with the underlying cause, and symptoms from the underlying cause often will be noted before symptoms of obstructive nephropathy. Sometimes the symptoms from each are difficult to distinguish.

Pain. Pain is the most common presenting complaint of acute obstructive nephropathy of high degree. Renal colic classically begins at the costovertebral angle on the affected side and radiates down the flank to the loin, occasionally to the external genitalia. The pain is described as sharp; it eases and recurs, and no position assumed gives any relief.

Mass. Particularly in the newborn, chronic obstruction will cause parenchymal destruction and massive dilatation. These changes can occur before birth; if the obstruction is of low degree, changes may occur silently over a period of years. The result is a large sac of water instead of a kidney. Among the differential diagnoses of flank mass, particularly in the newborn, obstructive nephropathy should be high on the list. A lower abdominal mass may be the presenting sign of silent prostatism and obstructive nephropathy in psychiatric patients or in other patients unable to convey pain. Severe reversible azotemia is periodically encountered. Evaluation of a lower abdominal mass, even if nontender, always requires bladder catheterization or bladder irrigation if a catheter is indwelling.

Nausea and Malaise. A massive obstructive kidney, by its very size, can compress the digestive tract, causing nausea and malaise.

Symptoms of Urinary Tract Infection. Obstructed urinary systems are prone to stasis of urine and subsequent infection. Once infection occurs, symptoms range from cystitis to urosepsis.

Symptoms of Renal Failure. If the condition causing obstructive uropathy affects all renal units silently, renal failure and its stigmata may be the first signs of obstructive nephropathy. The presence of infection in the obstructed system accelerates the deterioration of renal function and may cause urosepsis.

COURSE

Without intervention, the course of obstructive nephropathy will be progressive renal atrophy leading to renal failure. If the condition affects one side, that unit will be destroyed. In bilateral disease, the result is progressive renal failure, uremia, and death. Fortunately, in many patients, renal function will improve or at least stabilize with release of obstruction. The prognosis depends on the duration of obstruction, the degree of obstruction, the presence of infection, and the degree of renal damage suffered. While relief of total obstruction after 6 months yields only limited recovery, the results after relief of partial obstruction are better, and renal function occasionally will continue to improve for several weeks after the release of obstruction. Generally, the earlier the diagnosis, the better the final renal function. Renal failure from obstruction can almost always be prevented by proximal diversion.

The nature of the underlying condition causing the obstructive nephropathy will frequently dictate the patient's ultimate course. Not uncommonly, metastasis to the retroperitoneum or compression of the ureter from tumor can be the cause of obstructive nephropathy, and in those instances, a patient's prognosis is clearly related to the type, extent, and growth pattern of the malignancy.

COMMON COMPLICATIONS

Clearly, renal failure is the major complication of obstructive nephropathy. Sepsis may intervene if the system becomes infected, and shock may follow if sepsis is not treated. Whenever renal failure is diagnosed, any degree of obstructive nephropathy must be determined. Even in patients in whom obstructive nephropathy causes only minimal or moderate renal impairment, proximal dilatation is common. This dilatation of the urinary tract causes urinary stasis, which promotes stone growth and infection, and some believe that it may lead to cancer.

DIAGNOSIS

Since such a wide variety of lesions are capable of causing obstructive nephropathy, making the diagnosis requires consideration of the entire urinary tract from the collecting tubules to the urethral meatus. The history may or may not lead to the point of obstruction. Ordinary physical examination may detect flank or abdominal masses involving the urinary tract. Examination of the external genitalia is essential to rule out a cause of obstruction there. Laboratory tests of urine and blood may suggest obstruction, but do not specify the level of obstruction. Generally, after the history has been obtained and the physical examination completed, the next step is radiologic evaluation.

Intravenous pyelography is the best single test to determine obstructive nephropathy wherever renal function is adequate for that test. Scout films of the abdomen may show a possibly obstructing mass or calculus, but contrast agents are necessary for diagnosis. Improvements in contrast agents, use of higher doses, and use of tomography when indicated have increased the diagnostic capabilities of intravenous pyelography. Dilatation of the collecting system to the point of obstruction is frequently apparent. Since there usually is a high degree of symmetry between renal units, enlargement on one side would suggest obstruction. When previous films are available, comparison with current films is useful in determining borderline changes. Often, in patients with normally large pelves, examination of the calyces for fine cupping or papillary atrophy will help make the diagnosis of obstructive nephropathy.

Intravenous pyelography is not free of complications. Renal failure, allergic reactions, and death have followed administration of contrast agents; fortunately, these complications are rare.

When visualization by excretory urography is inadequate because of renal failure, *sonography* is often helpful and is a noninvasive procedure. Although this test may yield false results, it can aid in diagnosis if its limitations are kept in mind when its results are interpreted.

On occasion, *retrograde pyelograms* are needed to determine whether or not obstructive nephropathy exists; frequently, they are necessary to determine the extent of the obstructing lesion before surgical correction is attempted.

Lesions of the bladder and urethra require *endoscopy* for exact delineation. *Cystograms* and *urethrograms* may be helpful in determining lower urinary tract lesions and are helpful in caring for the patients on a long-term basis.

Occasionally, a patient will present with renal failure suggestive of an obstructive nephropathy, but none of the diagnostic tests is conclusive. Placement of a ureteral or urethral *catheter* should bypass an obstruction if one exists. If repeat renal function studies show an improvement in renal function, it is safe to assume that this patient has obstruction and would benefit from its removal.

POTENTIAL ERRORS AND PITFALLS IN DIAGNOSIS

The patient with renal failure is particularly prone to infection, and the urinary tract is high on the list of potential sources. Despite routine precautions, endoscopy carries a significant risk of infection, and that complication should be anticipated when evaluating the patient with renal failure. When a renal unit is presumed to be entirely obstructed, the placement of a nephrostomy tube or ureteral catheter will drain the system; however, it will also introduce infection into the system. If this tube is removed, obstruction will recur, this time with bacteria in the kidney. Urosepsis may likely follow. The potential function of a kidney should be anticipated before a tube is placed. If good judgment is not used, a nonfunctioning kidney may be replaced by a pyonephrotic kidney.

The worst sin is that of omission, that is, not to suspect obstructive nephropathy. Since obstructive nephropathy is frequently reversible, it behooves the physician to rule out any degree of obstruction in any case of renal failure, recurrent urinary tract infection, or flank mass or pain. Suspicion is essential for early diagnosis and preservation of renal function.

LOWER URINARY TRACT OBSTRUCTION IN CHILDREN

By Robert L. Lebowitz, M.D.
Boston, Massachusetts

Congenital obstruction of the lower urinary tract in children occurs much more commonly in boys than in girls. It can be discovered in the fetus during maternal ultrasonography; or it can present at any age, either with nonspecific signs and symptoms, such as failure to thrive, vomiting, or urinary tract infection, or with quite specific symptoms, such as an abnormality in the force of the stream of urine (increased or decreased), dysuria, straining to void, or hematuria. The voiding cystourethrogram is the primary diagnostic tool, followed in patients in whom it is positive by endoscopy for both confirmation and often definitive therapy. Endoscopes are now available that can be used in all but the smallest premature boys. In most patients, endoscopy should *not* be performed without a voiding cystourethrogram for guidance.

Acquired obstructions are of two types, *strictures* and *voiding dysfunctional states,* and the former occur virtually always in boys.

CONGENITAL LESIONS

Posterior Urethral Valves

Posterior urethral valves are a congenital abnormality and consist of folds of tissue that extend distally from the verumontanum. They are well named, since they cause one-way obstruction to the flow of urine. They are present with all degrees of severity, and their effects on the urinary tract and patient vary widely, ranging from a newborn infant who presents with severe obstructive uropathy, including destroyed and/or dysplastic kidneys, urinary ascites, and pulmonary hypoplasia, to a healthy older child who presents with a minor micturition disturbance and who has normal kidneys and collecting systems. The diagnosis can be suspected in severe cases when bilateral hydroureteronephrosis and a thick-walled bladder are detected on maternal ultrasonography, ultrasonography of the child, or excretory urography. The definitive diagnosis is made only by voiding cystourethrography. In mild or moderate cases, there may be micturition signs or symptoms, but many times straining to void is *not* a prominent symptom. Before the overworked bladder tires, the stream may even be more forceful than usual because of increased voiding pressures that are forcing the urine through a lumen of decreased diameter. A boy with this condition will occasionally present with urinary retention. Voiding cystourethrography is best done under fluoroscopic guidance in the awake child. The retrograde urethrogram, because of the one-way nature of the obstruction, does not show the valves.

Posterior urethral valves do not actually "cause" vesicoureteric reflux, but when reflux coexists—because there is an independent abnormality at the ureterovesical junction—the degree of reflux is magnified and has very serious implications. The kidney affected by the combination of reflux and obstruction is usually more severely damaged or dysplastic than the kidney that faces obstruction alone.

On the voiding cystourethrogram, the narrowed stream, as it passes through the valvar obstruction, is eccentric and is located near the floor or ventral surface of the posterior urethra, just below the end of the verumontanum and below the beginning of the urethral sphincter (Fig. 1). This is why valves are not visible on the urethrogram when the bladder neck is open but the urethral sphincter has not yet relaxed.

Anterior Urethral Diverticulum

Sometimes mistakenly called *anterior urethral valves,* this congenital anomaly consists of a saccular diverticulum that extends beneath the floor of the anterior urethra. As a boy with such a condition urinates, the diverticulum fills and its anterior lip elevates, obstructing the urethral channel. The urinary stream is narrowed, or occasionally it may cease altogether. Thus, a story of intermittent obstruction during voiding is characteristic. In addition, at the end of voiding, the urine-filled diverticulum is often palpable on the undersurface of the penis; urine either dribbles out as the diverticulum empties or can be manually expressed.

The effects on the urinary tract vary, depending on the severity and duration of the obstruction. These effects range from a fetus or newborn with severe obstructive uropathy to an older boy with mild micturition symptoms.

A urethral catheter may be easily passed if it stays in the main channel, or it may be difficult to insert if it should coil in the diverticulum. The findings on voiding cystourethrography, done under fluoroscopic guidance, are pathognomonic (Fig. 2). Endoscopic examination is often mistakenly thought to be normal because the mouth of the diverticulum on the floor of the urethra can be easily overlooked.

Urethral Polyp

Fibroepithelial polyps are attached to the floor of the urethra at the verumontanum and prolapse downward during voiding to produce intermittent obstruction. The effects on the upper urinary tract vary, but are usually not as severe as in the previously described entities.

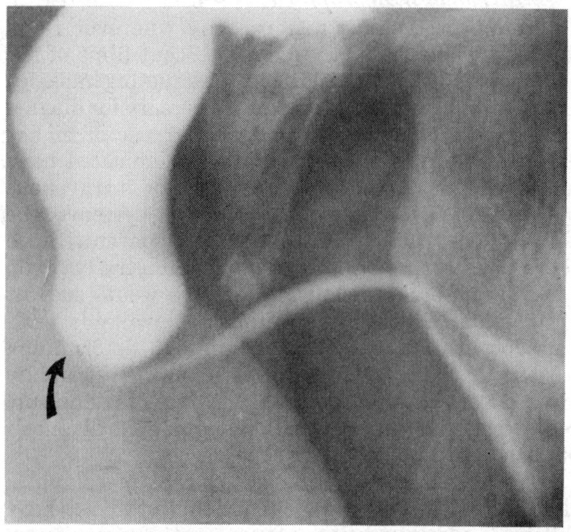

Figure 1. Posterior urethral valves (voiding cystourethrogram). There is marked dilatation of the posterior urethra above the obstructing valves. The tiny channel through which the urine must pass is characteristically eccentric and is located on the ventral aspect of the urethral lumen (i.e., along the "floor" of the urethra) (arrow).

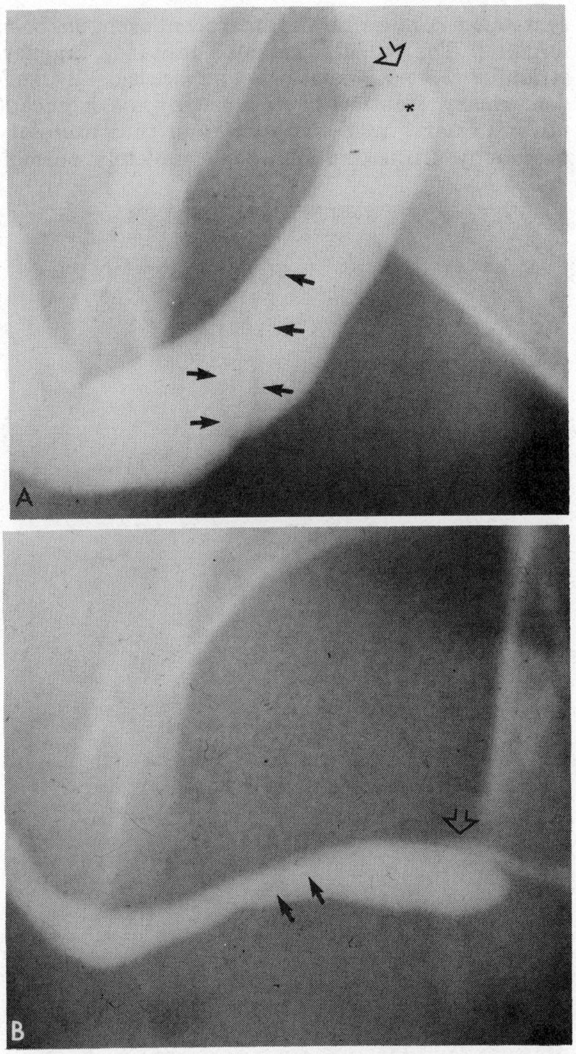

Figure 2. Anterior urethral diverticulum (voiding cystourethrogram). (A) A large contrast-containing diverticulum emanates from the floor of the proximal bulbous urethra. As the diverticulum fills during voiding, its anterior lip obstructs the lumen of the urethra (open arrow) and there is a sudden decrease in the caliber of the stream. Small arrows point to the floor of the urethra and the posterior lip of the diverticulum and an * marks the non-opaque stone caught in its blind distal end. (B) A smaller diverticulum. The anterior lip is beginning to obstruct the urethra distally (open arrow) and the posterior lip is faintly visible (closed arrows).

The findings on voiding cystourethrography under fluoroscopic control are pathognomonic when a polyp on a stalk is seen as a filling defect in the urine-contrast stream (Fig. 3). On retrograde urethrography the polyp can prolapse into the bladder and be missed. It may easily be overlooked at endoscopy, since the polyp is covered with the same epithelium as the surrounding urethra, and since the stream of water flowing into the urethra during the endoscopic procedure may cause the polyp to prolapse through the bladder neck and into the bladder.

Bladder Diverticulum

This is a rare cause of lower urinary tract obstruction in young boys. It causes symptoms that mimic those due to posterior urethral valves. The infant or boy presents with intermittent urethral obstruction or frank urinary retention. The voiding cystourethrographic findings (done under fluoroscopic guidance) are pathognomic. The diverticulum emanates from the posteroinferior aspect of the bladder and may cause ipsilateral vesicoureteric reflux. When the patient begins to void, the urinary stream divides, with some of the urine passing through the urethra and some passing into the diverticulum. As the diverticulum enlarges, it insinuates itself between the sacrum and the bladder neck and obstructs the posterior urethra (Fig. 4). It may extend well below the base of the bladder and displace the bladder up out of the pelvis. The contralateral (nonrefluxing) kidney is usually normal except for secondary dilatation because of urinary retention. Contralateral hydronephrosis is usually completely reversible when the bladder is emptied by a catheter or after the diverticulum is removed.

Prolapsed Ectopic Ureterocele

This entity is a rare cause of lower urinary tract obstruction in children of either sex. The ureterocele is associated with the upper moiety of a duplex collecting system approximately ten times more often than it is part of a single collecting system. The obstruction occurs when the child voids. The ureterocele prolapses into the bladder neck and then into the urethra. In boys it never extends beyond the posterior portion of the urethra, but in girls it can prolapse through the urethral meatus and present as a mucosal mass that occupies the region between the labia (Fig. 5). The obstruction is usually intermittent, except in the lat-

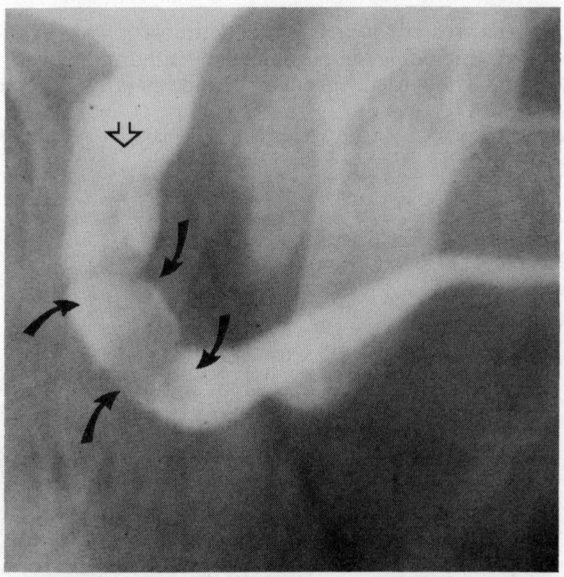

Figure 3. Urethral polyp (voiding cystourethrogram). Filling defect in the posterior urethra (curved arrows). This is a pedunculated polyp whose stalk arises from the verumontanum (open arrow). It prolapses down the lumen of the urethra as the boy voids.

ter instance when the prolapse may not be able to reduce spontaneously. The diagnosis is usually suggested from the typical findings on excretory urography or ultrasonography for ectopic ureterocele, but the definitive diagnosis is made by voiding cystography under fluoroscopic guidance when the ureterocele can actually be seen to prolapse with voiding.

Neurogenic Disturbances

Babies of either sex with myelomeningocele are occasionally born with urinary retention or develop it gradually as the months and years pass. The cause is a combination of bladder (detrussor) and urethral (sphincter) dysfunction, and it must be carefully searched for indefinitely in patients with this affliction. This is best done by means of periodic ultrasonographic examination of the kidneys. This can easily show not only the state of the upper collecting systems but also how well the bladder empties. Excretory urography can also be used if ultrasound is not available.

Urodynamic studies can accurately quantitate the degree of bladder and urethral dysfunction and can often predict which babies are at great risk for developing urinary retention.

This problem may be occult if, instead of myelomeningocele, the child's neurogenic dysfunction is secondary to sacral agenesis. This is seen most often in children whose mothers have diabetes, and the child may first be seen for problems with toilet training.

Bladder Neck Obstruction

Primary bladder neck obstruction, for practical purposes, does not exist in the child.

ACQUIRED CONDITIONS

Urethral Stricture

Strictures of the urethra are almost always traumatic (including iatrogenic) or inflammatory in origin. They occur gradually and usually become symptomatic long after the antecedent event has been forgotten. The symptoms include hesitancy, urgency, straining to void, hematuria, and, occasionally, sudden urinary retention. There is usually *not* significant upper urinary tract dilatation, and thus excretory urography/ultrasound may be completely normal.

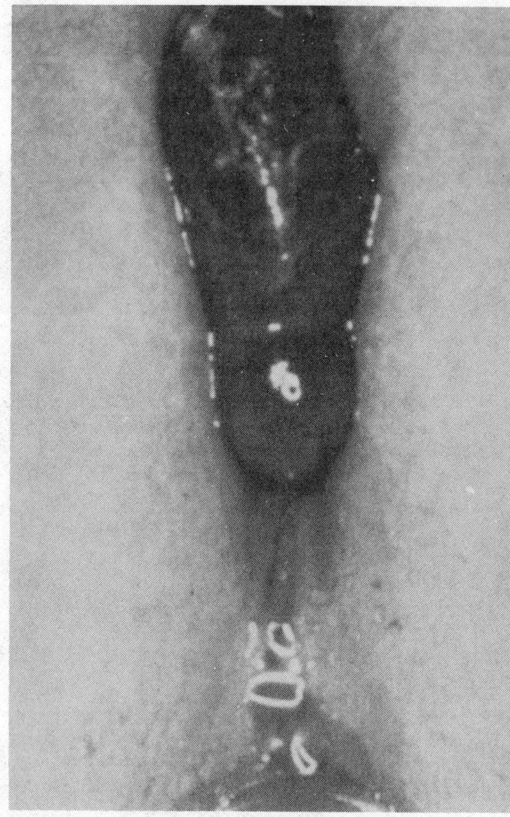

Figure 5. Prolapsed ectopic ureterocele. A glistening mucosal mass filling the interlabial region. This is the ureterocele that has prolapsed through the urethral meatus. It has a characteristic appearance and should not be mistaken for a vaginal tumor, an imperforate hymen, a periurethral cyst, or a prolapsed urethra.

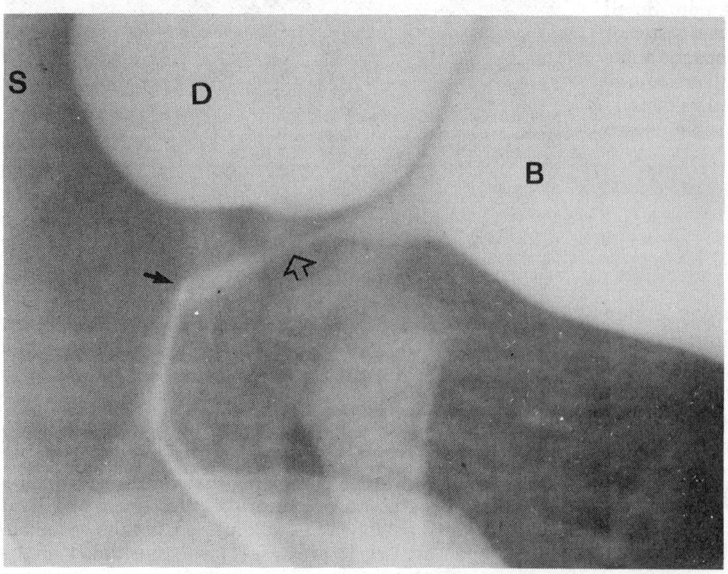

Figure 4. Posterior bladder Diverticulum (voiding cystourethrogram). As the boy begins to void, some of the urine leaves the bladder (B) via the urethra but some also exits aberrantly into the diverticulum (D). As the latter enlarges, it insinuates itself between the base of the bladder/posterior urethra and the sacrum (S) and obstructs the urethra (open arrow). As the flow through the urethra becomes impeded, the path of least resistance is into the diverticulum and a vicious cycle begins. The urethral catheter is just being withdrawn (small arrow).

The bladder may empty, albeit at slower rates of flow. The stricture characteristically occurs in the proximal portion of the bulbous urethra, and the diagnosis is made either by antegrade urethrography during an excretory urogram, by voiding cystourethrography, or by retrograde urethrography. When the stricture is first seen on the voiding cystourethrogram (Fig. 6*A*), a retrograde urethrogram is usually necessary to determine the length of the nondistensible segment (Fig 6*B*).

The degree of obstruction can be quantitated and then followed by formal determination of the urinary flow rate.

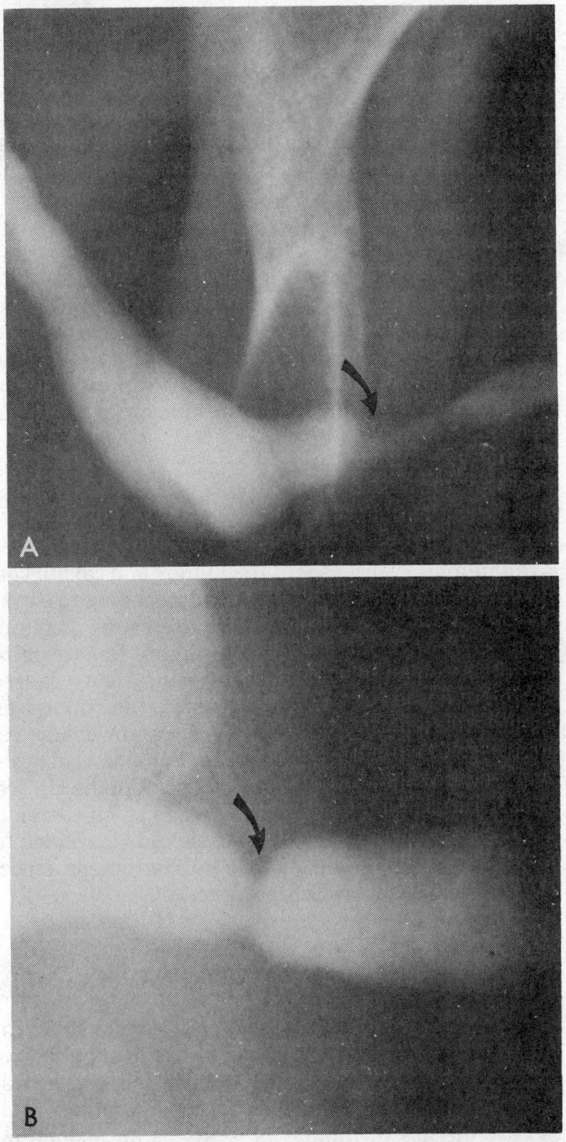

Figure 6. Acquired stricture of the urethra. (*A*) Voiding cystourethrogram. There is a sudden change in the caliber of the urethra in the proximal bulbous region (arrow). This is a characteristic location for an acquired stricture. The true length of the non-distensible segment cannot be determined because the rate of flow through the narrowed portion is not sufficient to distend the normal urethra beyond. (*B*) Retrograde urethrogram in the same boy shows a discrete area of narrowing (arrow). The urethra distal to the short stricture is normally distensible.

Meatal Stenosis

This entity is an acquired condition that occurs in circumcised boys (it is congenital only in those boys with minor degrees of hypospadias). The diagnosis is made by inspection of the meatus, which instead of being an oval slit becomes round as it becomes smaller. The stenosis begins inferiorly, and the urinary stream is thus not only narrowed but is also usually deflected upward.

The stenosis virtually never causes dilatation of the upper urinary tract, and uroradiologic examinations are usually not necessary.

Detrusor-Sphincter Dysfunction

The severest variety of this type of voiding dysfunction in children is also called *non-neurogenic neurogenic bladder* or *occult neuropathic bladder* because these boys and girls have urodynamic findings identical to those seen in some children with neurogenic bladder dysfunction from myelomeningocele, for example. Yet children with this acquired problem (they have learned abnormal patterns of control of urination) are neurologically intact.

Symptoms include chronic wetting day and night. Psychosocial problems are often present. Excretory urography shows hydronephrosis of varying degrees, while voiding cystography may reveal a spectrum of coexisting reflux (made worse by the dysfunction) and a trabeculated bladder that empties poorly, but no structural abnormalities of the urethra, for example, to obstruct the flow of urine. Urodynamic findings are those of incoordination of the detrusor and the sphincter.

A real hazard of not recognizing this condition is that if anti-reflux surgery is attempted without first treating the voiding disorder, it is doomed to fail.

CYSTIC DISORDERS OF THE KIDNEY

By Karl R. Herwig, M.D.
La Jolla, California

Cystic disorders of the kidney constitute the most common abnormality of this organ. Cysts occur in all ages, arise from numerous causes, and have varying significance in treatment.

NONHEREDITARY CYSTS

Simple Cysts

The most common cystic lesion of the kidney is the simple renal cyst. It arises at any age, but becomes more common with advancing age. It is estimated that as many as 50 per cent of people over 70 years of age have simple renal cysts. Simple cysts do not communicate with the renal collecting system, giving rise to the possibility that they represent acquired obstruction of a renal tubule or collecting duct. More than one cyst may be present in the same kidney, and both kidneys can be affected. Cysts vary in size from minute structures to large masses the size of a grapefruit.

Clinical Features

Simple renal cysts usually cause no symptoms and are usually found at the time of an intravenous urogram or abdominal computed tomographic (CT) scan performed for other reasons. On physical examination they may be large enough to palpate; however, this is uncommon. Unless a cyst becomes infected or ruptures—a rare occurrence—signs and symptoms of urinary tract disease such as pain or hematuria should not be attributed to a simple cyst and other causes of urinary tract disease should be sought.

Radiographic Features

The primary dilemma concerning simple renal cysts is their differentiation from renal tumors, since they can appear radiographically as "tumor deformities." Recent advances in radiologic diagnosis can make this differentiation accurately without resorting to operative renal exploration. Nephrotomography performed at the time of intravenous urography is valuable in delineating a simple cyst. Cysts do not tend to distort the renal collecting system, especially the calices, but rather displace them. Additionally, a cyst in the periphery of the kidney will often show a "rim" or "lip" of parenchyma along the border that sharply demarcates it from the surrounding renal parenchyma. *Tumors,* on the other hand, do not show the sharp demarcation and tend to distort and destroy the renal collecting system. Ultrasonography should be performed in all patients with renal tumor deformity. It can accurately differentiate a simple cyst from tumor, making further studies unnecessary, and is very cost effective. With ultrasonography, cysts have good sound transmission; have smooth, oval, or round outlines; do not have any internal echoes; and possess a clear demarcation of the far wall. Tumors have internal echoes and irregular outlines, and are thick-walled.

If any doubt exists after ultrasonography, which should be rare, CT scans, cyst puncture, and even arteriography should be used before operative renal exploration. CT scans are done without and with intravenous contrast to differentiate a cyst from a tumor. Cysts have homogeneous, low-attenuation values; indiscernible walls; and sharp delineation from the surrounding renal parenchyma, and they lack enhancement with contrast. Tumors, on the other hand, have attenuation coefficients close to those of the renal parenchyma, are contrast-enhanced, have an unsharp interface with the renal parenchyma, and may show spread outside the kidney.

Cyst puncture is unnecessary in simple renal cysts except in the rare instance in which previously described examinations remain equivocal. Cyst puncture can be performed with ultrasound or CT guidance. The fluid removed is studied for clarity and for cytologic properties, and contrast medium is injected into the cyst cavity. A simple cyst has clear fluid, negative cytologic findings, and a smooth wall. The fluid also contains no fat, cholesterol, or lactate dehydrogenase. Tumors have an abnormality in one of these parameters. If the fluid is bloody, tumor should be suspected. Calcification of a cyst wall also suggests tumor.

Simple cysts require no therapy, but periodically ultrasonography should be done to assess any changes in size or shape.

Parapelvic Renal Cysts

These are simple renal cysts in close proximity to the renal pelvis. They displace the renal pelvis, and evaluation of these cysts is the same as for simple renal cysts.

Cystic Renal Neoplasms

Many renal neoplasms, especially adenocarcinoma, present radiographically as renal cysts. By following the evaluation outlined previously, differentiation from benign cysts should be done efficiently and accurately.

Inflammatory Cysts

Inflammatory diseases of the kidney and calculi can cause obstruction of a collecting duct leading to a cyst or a caliceal diverticulum. These are usually asymptomatic. *Taenia echinococcus,* a minute tapeworm of sheep and cattle, infests humans and causes echinococcosis, which may occur in the kidney as echinococcal cyst. This disease occurs worldwide, especially in sheep-raising countries. Echinococcal cysts may cause pain, fever, or hematuria, but in the United States they are usually discovered as calcified renal masses. Aspiration of these cysts should be avoided to prevent spreading the disease to contiguous structures. (See article on Echinococcosis.)

Multicystic Disease of Childhood

An abnormality of ureteral bud development in utero can lead to artresia of the ureter or renal pelvis and will cause the renal blastema to develop as a multicystic structure similar to a "bunch of grapes." Multicystic disease of infants presents as an abdominal mass at birth and represents the most common abdominal mass of neonates. This condition usually involves only one kidney, and excretory urography will show absence of the kidney even with total body opacification. The involved kidney will transilluminate as multiple cysts in a dark room.

Another form of congenital cyst is found in infants with congenital obstruction of lower urinary tract such as urethral valves or vesical neck obstruction. (See article on Lower Urinary Tract Obstruction in

Children.) Infants with these problems may show failure to thrive and uremia. Oligohydramnios usually exists and can be diagnosed in utero with ultrasound. Recently, successful attempts have been made to relieve the bladder obstruction in utero utilizing ultrasound guidance.

HEREDITARY CYSTIC DISORDERS

Adult Polycystic Kidney Disease

The most common hereditary renal cystic disease is adult polycystic kidney disease (APCD). It is estimated to occur in 1 of 500 people. It is the third most common reason for renal transplantation. APCD affects males and females equally, usually presenting during the fifth or sixth decade. Most often it is discovered during evaluation of a patient for hematuria, hypertension, or renal failure. APCD is transmitted as an autosomal dominant trait, and patients affected often have a family history of renal failure in an ancestor. When found, genetic counseling of the patient and other family members becomes important in addition to searching for the disease in other family members.

Clinical Features

APCD can present as a symptomatic abdominal mass, hematuria, hypertension, or calculus disease. Hepatic cysts and berry aneurysms of the circle of Willis are often associated with APCD, and problems with these conditions may be the mode of presentation.

Radiologic Features

Intravenous urography characteristically shows large kidneys with displaced calices. Although both kidneys are involved, one kidney may show more involvement than the other. Multiple calcifications are often seen in both kidneys. Ultrasonography and CT scans may be used to confirm the diagnosis.

Polycystic Disease of Infants

Infantile polycystic disease is transmitted as an autosomal recessive trait and presents at various ages of infancy or childhood, depending upon the severity of the disease. It is usually associated with hepatic fibrosis and portal hypertension. Other names applied to this disease include *medullary cystic disease* and *juvenile nephronophthisis*. Clinically, the disease may present as renal failure or hepatosplenomegaly. Radiographically the kidneys have a mottled uptake of contrast that is very characteristic for the disease. There is no specific therapy, but genetic counseling of the parents is warranted.

Medullary Sponge Kidney

A benign condition with genetic transmission, medullary sponge kidney is often an incidental finding at the time of intravenous urography. Cystic dilatation of the collecting ducts appears as a blush or "fan" proximal to the renal pyramid during excretory urography. With retrograde pyelography, flow of contrast does not occur into the ducts and the pyelocaliceal system appears normal. Unless complications occur, these patients are entirely asymptomatic. Because of the dilatation of the collecting duct, however, stasis of urine can occur within the collecting ducts, thus leading to calculus formation. These calculi present in a fan shape proximal to the renal pyramid. Although both kidneys may be involved, it is not unusual to see only one area of a single kidney involved. Whether these patients have an increased risk of calculus formation or infection remains controversial; generally, the clinical presentation relates either to infection or to calcification if the condition is not noted incidentally.

Other Hereditary Renal Cysts

Renal cysts occur in the inherited diseases *tuberous sclerosis* and *von Hippel-Lindau disease,* in which they are associated with renal hamartomas. Patients with either of these conditions have increased risk of renal adenocarcinoma. Renal cysts have been reported in Meckel's syndrome, Jeune's asphyxiating thoracic dystrophy, Zellweg's cerebrohepatorenal syndrome, and trisomies D and E.

CARCINOMA OF THE KIDNEY

By Sam D. Graham, Jr., M.D.
and Samuel S. Ambrose, M.D.
Atlanta, Georgia

Carcinoma of the kidney is usually one of three pathologic types. In pediatric patients, the most common carcinoma is *Wilms' tumor;* in adults, the most common is *adenocarcinoma* of the kidney followed by *transitional cell carcinoma* of the collecting system. Adenocarcinoma of the kidney is the third most common genitourinary malignancy of adults. In 1982, there were estimated to be 18,100 new cases of renal adenocarcinoma, of whom approximately 8500 will die from their disease. The preponderance of this tumor is in men over the age of 50. Since surgery is the only treatment modality in renal adenocarcinoma that may be therapeutically successful, it is imperative that the diagnosis be made early so that treatment may be begun expeditiously. This article is devoted to the diagnosis of renal adenocarcinoma.

DIAGNOSIS

The diagnosis of renal adenocarcinoma is rapidly evolving from the traditional modalities of history and physical examination to high-technology radiographic techniques. Patients presenting with physical signs and symptoms frequently have advanced disease and are not curable. On the other hand, with the increased use of techniques such as intravenous pyelograms as diagnostic aids in the evaluation of hypertension and other diseases, a higher number of renal carcinomas are being identified as asymptomatic mass lesions. The incidence of carcinomas among all asymptomatic mass lesions of the kidney is only 2 to 4 per cent, but earlier diagnosis has begun to be reflected in the overall survival statistics for this disease. The pathway toward the diagnosis of renal carcinoma should be systematic and thorough, avoiding studies that offer little additional information or add unnecessary morbidity. However, a systematic approach should yield enough information for both the diagnosis and preoperative staging of each patient and thus should allow for individual flexibility. A suggested sequence of diagnostic procedures is shown in Figure 1.

HISTORY

By taking a careful history, the clinician may be able to delineate certain signs and symptoms that may be associated with renal cell carcinoma.

Gross painless hematuria is seen in approximately 50 per cent of patients and is usually characterized by dark blood, persisting throughout the entire voiding (i.e., not initial or terminal hematuria). The significance of this in renal cell carcinoma usually denotes invasion of the collecting system, a relatively poor prognostic sign of advanced disease.

Pain associated with renal cell carcinoma may be due to:

1. Clot obstruction of the ureter (colicky pain, with or without radiation to the groin).
2. Hemorrhage into the tumor with distention of the capsule, which may cause acute persistent sharp flank pain.
3. Invasion of perirenal nerves, which may present as radicular pain.
4. Metastases, which may present as bone pain and other symptoms. Associated with the pain may be nausea and vomiting as a secondary vagal response.

Flank mass is the third most common symptom of renal carcinoma, with an approximate incidence of 6 to 45 per cent. This presenting symptom is rarely noted by the patient, however, and again is associated with a poor prognosis, since it is usually indicative of massive disease.

The "classic triad" of a mass, gross hematuria, and pain is seldom seen and reflects advanced disease. Other signs and symptoms that may accompany renal carcinoma include fever, sweats, hypertension, weight loss, weakness, and other associated constitutional symptoms. With the wider use of the newer radiologic diagnostic modalities, however, a larger percentage of these tumors are being diagnosed prior to the advent of symptoms.

PHYSICAL EXAMINATION

On physical examination, the clinician should look for abdominal masses, which are usually firm and in the flank. Any mass should be assessed for mobility. The presence of a varicocele, especially if it is of sudden onset or right-sided, may indicate a renal carcinoma, but this is an uncommon sign. Jaundice may be seen in patients with renal cell carcinoma and is associated either with liver metastases or with a reversible hepatorenal dysfunction (*Stauffer's syndrome*). The latter is seen in 10 per cent of patients and is detailed in the discussion of paraneoplastic syndromes later in this article. Other significant findings on physical examination include signs referrable to metastases in the lung, liver, bone, lymph nodes, or central nervous system. Cutaneous nodules that represent metastatic deposits have also been described. Cardiac enlargement may be seen in association with arteriovenous (A-V) shunting within the tumor with a resulting high-output cardiac failure. Lower-extremity edema may accompany vena caval occlusion.

LABORATORY FINDINGS

Hematologic abnormalities include erythrocytosis (discussed under paraneoplastic syndromes), which is relatively uncommon ($<$10 per cent), and anemia, which is common (20 to 30 per cent). Anemia accompanying renal carcinoma is not necessarily associated with blood loss and is normochromic, normocytic. Advanced renal carcinoma may be associated with pancytopenia.

Chemical abnormalities found in renal carcinoma are usually due to the paraneoplastic syndromes found with renal carcinoma. These include elevation of hepatic enzymes and hypercalcemia. Adrenal metastases and replacement may demonstrate the electrolytic pattern of hypoaldosteronism as well as hypoadrenal corticalism. Elevated $alpha_2$ globulins have likewise been reported. At present, there are no reliable serum markers available for renal carcinoma. Examination of the urine may reveal microscopic hematuria or malignant cells. Rarely are there positive cytologic findings with renal cell carcinoma, although this is rather common with transitional cell carcinoma.

IMAGING PROCEDURES

Radiologic Diagnosis

The most important diagnostic tools for the preoperative identification of renal carcinoma are radiologic. These techniques are presented in Figures 2 through 7. The first study that should be done in a patient suspected of having a renal carcinoma is an intravenous pyelogram with nephrotomograms. With this one study, 90 to 95 per cent of renal masses can be detected. The plain scout film will show possible neoplastic calcification. Rapid tomography immediately following intravenous bolus injection of contrast will demonstrate the renal contours, delineate masses, and give some indication of the relative vascularity. Approximately 80 per cent of all renal cell carcinomas will be hypervascular, and 20 per cent will be hypovascular. The absence of a thin rim, the presence of abnormal calcification, and the absence of a "beak" at the junction of the mass with the kidney are highly suspicious for carcinoma, in contrast to simple cysts in patients demonstrating an avascular mass by this method. Intravenous pyelography without tomograms demonstrates the mass in only 70 to 80 per cent of cases.

The typical appearance on intravenous urography is a mass that protrudes from the normal contour of the kidney. There may also be splaying of the calices, distortion of the renal axis, or ureteral displacement. Other collecting system abnormalities may include "scalloping" of the ureter from nodal involvement or collateral vessels. Filling defects secondary to clots may also be seen. There may be a delay in visualization of the kidney due to the renal vein thrombosis. Pitfalls in the diagnosis of renal masses are primarily in tumors which are directly anterior or posterior, so as to be obscured by the renal shadow on the standard anteroposterior projection.

Computed Tomography

The most important advance in the diagnosis of renal carcinoma has been the computed tomography (CT) scan. With the newer generation of scanners, the

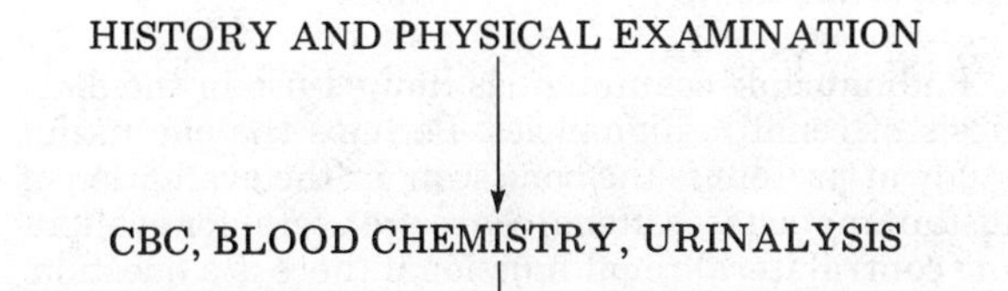

Figure 1. Suggested sequence of diagnostic procedures in patients with suspected renal tumors. Abbreviations: CBC = complete blood count; IVP = intravenous pyelogram; CT scan = computed tomography; DVI = digital venous imaging.

clarity of the image and resulting diagnostic accuracy have been spectacular. The relative density of an area of interest can be measured to identify fat (–30 to –50 Hounsfield Units [H]), water (0 to +20 H), and tissue (>+25 H). In using this mode, care must be taken that the measured units are true density measurements and not computer-averaged densities from adjacent structures. The measurements should be in multiple areas of the lesion in question and of a relatively small area to negate any such averaging errors. Contrast enhancement by intravenous injection of contrast material may be used during the CT scanning of vascular masses. CT scanning has other applications in the staging of renal neoplasms. For example, periaortic and pericaval lymphadenopathy may be seen, as well as extension outside the renal capsule, invasion of contiguous structures, liver or other visceral metastases, and vascular invasion, either vena caval or renal vein. If pulmonary metastases are suspected, CT scanning of the chest may help delineate the extent of the disease.

The typical CT appearance of a benign renal cyst is a homogeneous, well-circumscribed mass that shows no contrast enhancement and has a relative density of water. Renal tumors, on the other hand, usually are heterogeneous masses (showing contrast enhancement unless they are avascular), and are of tissue density. "Spidery tentacles," which may be seen extending into the perinephric fat, are usually due to either collateral vessels or tumor extension. Other masses that may radiographically resemble renal tumors include angiomyolipomas and renal abscesses. Angiomyolipomas typically have areas of fat density, thus making the CT scan the definitive preoperative study. Abscesses may show contrast enhancement and gas within the mass, yet it is at times very difficult to distinguish an abscess from a necrotic tumor.

Ultrasound

Ultrasonography has been replaced by CT scanning in the current management and diagnosis of renal carcinoma. Its limitations include poorer visualization of the mass and the interference of extraneous shadows cast by structures such as the ribs and spleen. The characteristic ultrasonographic picture of a renal carcinoma would show internal echoes and an irregularly defined posterior wall. Simple cysts, on the other hand, typically are sonolucent with a sharply defined posterior wall and an acoustical shadow. The primary use of ultrasonography at present is to confirm the diagnosis of simple cysts in patients with avascular lesions.

Angiography

Formal transfemoral transcutaneous angiography may be used as an adjunctive or therapeutic modality. *Arteriography* is typically used for (1) vascular mapping of the arteries, especially if partial nephrectomy is being considered, and (2) diagnosis. Renal tumors that are hypervascular will show abnormal neovascularity with corkscrew vessels, A-V shunting, vascu-

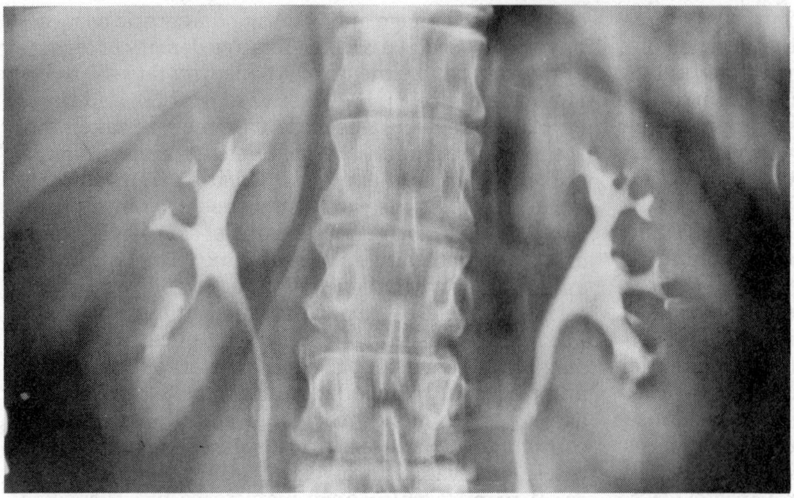

Figure 2. Case No. 1. Right renal cell carcinoma (arrows); routine intravenous pyelography. Film fails to demonstrate right renal mass but shows splaying of lower pole infundibulum and adjacent calyceal distortion.

lar puddling, and abnormal capsular vessels. Avascular tumors by arteriography require other diagnostic modalities. Selective arteriograms with and without epinephrine injection are used to identify questionable lesions. The neovascular vessels do not contain the medial layer within the vessel wall and are unable to constrict with epinephrine, thus showing a tumor "blush" with contrast injection. Currently, especially in right renal carcinomas in which caval extension is more common, a venogram or vena cavogram may be necessary to delineate the level of vena caval extension. Any patient who demonstrates renal vein or vena caval extension on CT scanning needs a venacavogram so that vascular control during surgery may be planned. Transcatheter embolization with autologous clot, Gianturcco coils, Gelfoam, or alcohol may also be done during the arteriogram. Liver metastases may be seen with a celiac axis injection during the aortogram.

Complications of these invasive procedures are significant. High doses of contrast are associated with acute tubular necrosis, especially in patients with partially compromised renal function. It is usually prudent to allow at least one day between arteriogram and surgery to watch the serum creatinine level. Diabetics and patients with elevated serum creatinine levels should be hydrated intravenously. Other complications include thrombosis of femoral vessels and renal arteries. Embolization adds the risk that the embolizing agent may migrate, especially if there is a large AV shunt, resulting in pulmonary emboli or arterial occlusion of other end arteries (renal, inferior mesenteric, femoral). Metal coils may make the cross-clamping of the renal artery during surgery difficult.

Digital venous imaging (DVI) may eventually replace the Seldinger technique. This technique involves an intravenous bolus of contrast material; the vascular pattern is produced by computed subtraction. These studies are quite useful in demonstrating the renal vessels and may be combined with a venogram to demonstrate the arterial and venous information previously obtainable only with more invasive techniques. As the quality of these venous imaging studies improves as a result of its relatively low incidence of complications and simplicity, it may be rare that formal angiography is used in the diagnosis of renal carcinomas.

Bipedal lymphangiography is another study that is rapidly being replaced by newer diagnostic modalities. Since CT scanning now allows detailed evaluation of periaortic and pericaval lymphadenopathy and since lymphangiography only has a 70 per cent accuracy rate, the lymphangiogram is no longer considered a necessary study in renal carcinoma.

Nuclear Medicine

Radionuclide scanning has limited use in the diagnosis of renal malignancies. Perhaps the one useful study at present is the bone scan for the evaluation of distant metastases. Renal scans are useful for evaluating contralateral renal function if there is a question, but they are of limited use in the diagnosis of a renal mass because the same information is available with CT scanning. Liver/spleen scans and brain scans likewise are of little use because there are more advanced technologic methods.

Chest X-rays and Tomography

Chest x-rays are of great benefit in the evaluation and staging of renal carcinoma. Since over 50 per cent of patients present with metastases and 44 per cent of the metastases are pulmonary, it is very important that this study be done as an adjuvant to the physical examination. Some centers are adding chest tomography or CT scans of the chest as a further diagnostic study because a significant number of pulmonary metastases may be missed on routine chest x-rays. Occasionally, fluoroscopy may be necessary for delineation of suspicious pulmonary nodules.

Nuclear Magnetic Resonance

This latest technique may revolutionize the diagnostic modalities for renal tumors. In nuclear magnetic resonance (NMR), the atomic orbital spin is measured while a strong external magnetic field is applied. When the field is stopped, the spins revert to their normal state. The image produced can distin-

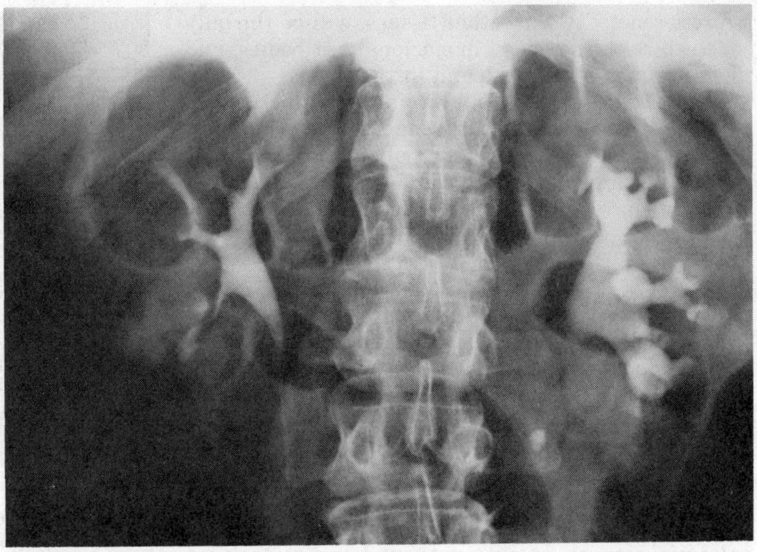

Figure 3. Case No. 1. Tumor extends off the lateral border of the right kidney (arrows). This nephrotomogram demonstrates the value of nephrotomography in the diagnosis of renal tumors.

guish molecular structure, and thus the metabolic activity, of tissues. How this modality will fit in the work-up will depend on further improvements in the resolution of the image and wider use of the instrument.

INVASIVE DIAGNOSTIC TECHNIQUES

Cyst Puncture. Cyst puncture and *cystography* (injection of contrast into the cyst cavity) are of limited usefulness. This technique is designed to distinguish cysts from cystic carcinomas by evaluation of cyst fluid for blood and cytologic findings as well as anatomic definition. Since CT scanning shows such clear anatomic detail and density of the fluid, it is rarely necessary to perform cyst punctures unless there is a massive cyst requiring drainage due to pain or significant compression.

Percutaneous Needle Biopsy. The use of percutaneous needle biopsy likewise has little practical use. Since the only effective treatment of renal carcinoma is surgical, any mass that is solid on CT scan or questionably carcinoma should be explored. The major possible impact of percutaneous needle biopsy will be most likely in the evaluation of suspicious pulmonary nodules, and that to only a limited extent.

Cystoscopy. Routine cystoscopy should be performed in patients with hematuria to rule out the chance of a concurrent urothelial bladder lesion. Occasionally retrograde pyelograms may be indicated if there is nonvisualization of a kidney, filling defects in the ureter, or questionable ureteral pathology.

FUTURE TRENDS

Monoclonal antibodies are being used in the identification of renal carcinomas in vitro. The potential in vivo applications include attachment of radionuclides for imaging and possibly therapeutic uses. Such technical considerations as the specificity toward renal carcinoma versus normal renal parenchyma, as well

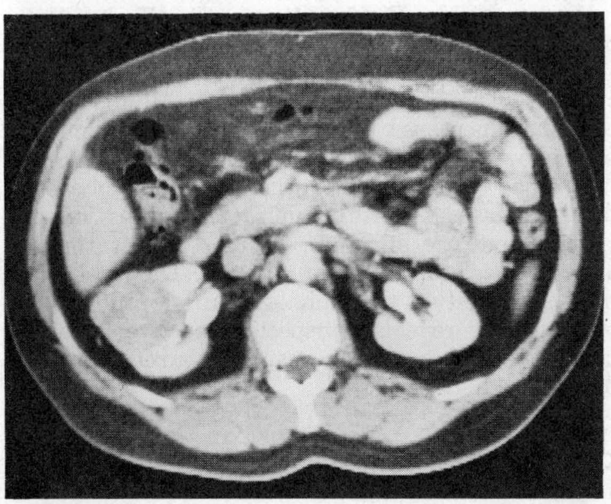

Figure 4. CT scan of tumor in Case No. 1 demonstrating the variable density of the renal mass.

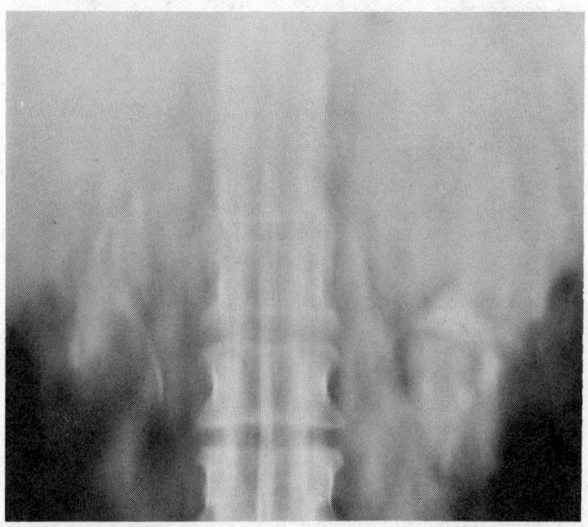

Figure 5. Case No. 2. Nephrotomogram shows a large left upper pole renal mass (arrows).

as cross-reactivity with other tissues, will be the only constraints on the use of monoclonal antibodies, and their use may rapidly expand in the future.

Other studies such as cellular immune function, circulating antibodies, enzyme markers (e.g., gamma glutamyl transferase, urinary polyamine levels, and viral DNA) are being used primarily as investigative tools and have very limited practical application at present.

PARANEOPLASTIC SYNDROMES

Renal cell carcinoma has been associated with various paraneoplastic syndromes that are not necessarily due to metastatic spread. These include hypercalcemia, erythrocytosis, and hepatic dysfunction.

Hypercalcemia. Hypercalcemia is not an uncommon finding in renal adenocarcinoma and is usually due to bony involvement with metastatic carcinoma. In a significant number of patients, however, hypercalcemia may be present without bony metastases. The presence of hypercalcemia in these patients appears to be due to the production of a parathormone-like substance by the tumor. Symptoms in these patients include polydypsia, polyuria, dysphagia, constipation, muscle weakness, and mental depression. In this subset of patients, nephrectomy may produce normocalcemic levels. Occasionally, the hypercalcemia may be rapidly progressive and fatal. Although hyperparathyroidism has been reported to be associated with renal cell carcinoma, usually the tumor-induced hypercalcemia is associated with hypokalemia, which tends to differentiate it from true hyperparathyroidism.

A second functional aspect of renal cell carcinomas that may also be responsible for hypercalcemia is prostaglandin (PG) production by the tumor. Both prostaglandin E(PGE) and prostaglandin F(PGF) have been reported as significantly elevated in metastases of renal cell carcinoma and clinical responses to indomethacin (prostaglandin synthetase inhibitor) have been reported. In tissue cultures of renal cell carcinomas, bone resorption mediated by PGE has been reported.

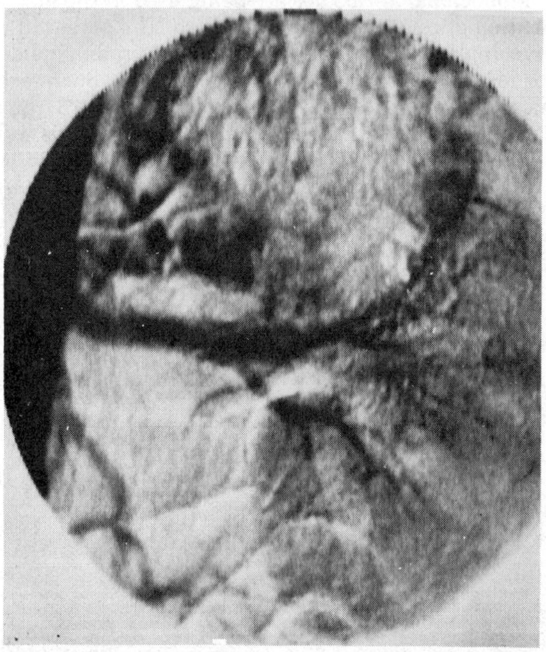

Figure 6. Digital venous angiogram of tumor in Case No. 2 showing the hypervascular mottled mass, which is the tumor. Image is distorted by the overlying stomach.

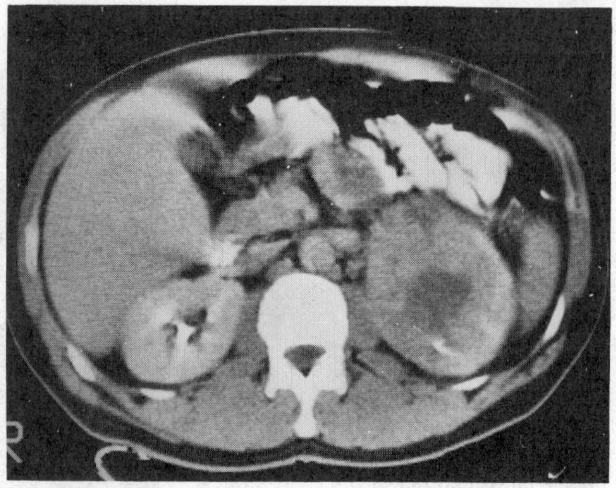

Figure 7. CT scan of left renal mass in Case No. 2 showing the solid and low-density nature of the tumor; the central low-density area represents tumor necrosis.

Erythrocytosis. Approximately 1.8 to 6 per cent of patients with renal cell carcinoma will present with erythrocytosis that is presumably due to elevated erythropoietin levels. Excessive erythropoietin levels have been shown to be common in patients with renal cell carcinomas, with one series reporting an incidence of 63 per cent. Usually these patients have an erythremia, not thrombocytosis or leukocytosis. The cause of the elevated erythropoietin levels is not completely understood, and may be due either to exogenous tumor production of erythropoietin (or possibly an erythropoietin activator) or to stimulation of erythropoietin production in the surrounding renal parenchyma either directly or by local ischemia. It is far more common for a patient with renal cell carcinoma to present with anemia, however, than with erythrocytosis.

Hepatorenal Dysfunction (Stauffer's Syndrome). Stauffer first described abnormal liver functions associated with nonmetastatic renal carcinomas. The reported incidence is 10 to 15 per cent, but increased awareness of the phenomenon may show the incidence to be significantly higher. Abnormalities include elevation of alkaline phosphatase, increased bromsulphalein (BSP) retention, increased indirect bilirubin, decreased prothrombin, and increased alpha$_2$-globulin levels. The most striking abnormality is the alpha$_2$-globulin level. Liver biopsy usually reveals nonspecific reactive hepatitis, and nephrectomy usually results in a return to normal of the abnormalities.

CONCLUSION

Successful therapy in renal cell carcinoma at present requires early and accurate diagnosis. Clinical awareness, coupled with improved diagnostic radiologic methods, especially renal tomography and the CT scan, have increased the overall survival by detecting lesions in earlier stages, when they are curable surgically. The advent of newer diagnostic methods such as NMR and monoclonal antibodies may further serve the clinician in the care and treatment of this disease.

TUMORS OF THE URETER AND URINARY BLADDER

By Randall G. Rowland, M.D., Ph.D.
and Robert A. Garrett, M.D.
Indianapolis, Indiana

The genesis of urothelial cancer is that of multifocal changes beginning with cellular atypia and hyperplasia, progressing to dysplasia and subsequently to carcinoma. The lesions may remain sessile or may become papillary in form. They may coexist in the bladder, renal pelvis, and ureter. Some become invasive in adjacent tissue and metastasize to local and regional lymph nodes, bones, and other viscera. The rate of progression along this spectrum is dependent on the biologic potential of each lesion. At any given time, individual tumors in a patient may be at variable stages of the natural history. The clinical evaluation of bladder and ureteral tumors attempts to determine the stage of the natural history that exists when the patient is first seen and is an effort to gather information that will assist in judging the future behavior of the tumor and in planning a therapeutic approach.

It is interesting to note that the relative incidence of transitional cell carcinoma (TCC) seems related to the pooling effect of urinary contact (50:3:1 = bladder:renal pelvis:ureter). The renal pelvis pools urine to a limited degree; the bladder, acting as a reservoir, markedly so; but the ureter, functioning as a conduit, minimally so. Recurrence of TCC in any one, two, or all three of the urothelium-lined segments is rather common, speaking for the urinary carcinogenic role and emphasizing the need for careful periodic urinary tract survey. In the bladder and ureter, TCC accounts for at least 90 per cent of the lesions, whereas squamous cell carcinoma and adenocarcinoma comprise almost all of the remainder. Melanosarcoma, leiomyosarcoma, endometriosis, and angiomas are exceedingly rare.

Some of the specifics of presentation, diagnosis, and staging of ureteral and urinary bladder tumors are described in the following sections.

URETER

Presenting Symptoms and Signs

Gross, often painless, hematuria is the initial symptom in the majority of patients with ureteral tumors. Frequency and discomfort on urination may occasionally be experienced. Mild to severe flank pain may indicate obstruction of the narrow ureteral channel by tumor or blood clots formed by bleeding from a ureteral tumor. Profound ureteral obstruction may develop, however, over a protracted period with no symptoms. Abdominal mass may be detected by careful bimanual ballottement in those few in whom obstruction has led to significant hydronephrotic dilatation.

Diagnosis

Radiography

The excretory urogram (IVP) is a useful preliminary screening examination that may in itself be strongly suggestive of the diagnosis. Unfortunately, the ureterogram in such studies is often incomplete or fragmentary, hence the need for retrograde ureterography in patients with gross hematuria and incomplete excretory ureterography. Poor visualization or nonvisualization of the upper urinary tract owing to obstruction demands retrograde studies. The excretory urogram as a periodic screening device in patients with TCC of the bladder may sporadically reveal otherwise unsuspected ureteral filling defects that prove to be tumor. Typically, ureteral tumors at ureterography display an intrinsic exophytic lesion above and below which the ureter is dilated. Retrograde ureterograms often show a characteristic "wine glass" or "meniscus" deformity distal to the lesion. Some few ureteral tumors, morphologically sessile, show irregular ureteral narrowing indistinguishable from inflammatory strictures.

Retrograde ureterography may not visualize the ureter above the obstructive neoplasm. Percutaneous antegrade pyeloureterography under ultrasonographic guidance may supplement retrograde studies not only to define the ureteral tumor but to visualize the renal pelvis for other urothelial tumors and evaluate renal function by radionuclide studies when the percutaneous nephrostomy tube is in place. Bilateral pyeloureteral TCC may necessitate renal parenchymal salvage in subsequent surgical management. Angiography of the ureteral vasculature is not regularly useful, but in rare instances may point out direct extension of tumor tissue to adjacent structures. Differential diagnosis of ureteral defects includes nonopaque stone, blood clot, sloughed renal papilla, ureteral stricture, periureteral fibrosis, ureteritis cystica, and disseminated pelvic endometriosis.

Cytology

Cytologic studies of voided urine sediments have a low yield and of themselves have no localizing potential. Urine aspirates from the suspected ureter and pelvis are more reliable. Accuracy can be enhanced by the "ureteral brushing" technique. This maneuver consists of passage of a ureteral catheter to the suspected tumor level. Through this catheter is passed a tiny bristle or wire brush that is twisted in contact with the suspected tumor. Clumps of cells enmeshed in the brush are available for cytologic evaluation. The success of all cytologic maneuvers is dependent upon an experienced cytopathologist.

URINARY BLADDER

Presenting Symptoms and Signs

Although gross hematuria is a common presenting complaint, recognition of the importance of accompanying or independent symptoms of vesical irritation, such as frequency, urgency, and dysuria, is essential to prompt recognition of patients with bladder tumors. Occasionally, a tumor mass in a strategic location may result in bladder outlet obstruction with its attendant symptoms of hesitancy or obstruction. The possibility that irritative bladder symptoms in the aging male may be due to neoplastic changes such as carcinoma in situ should not be dismissed despite the prevalence of symptoms caused by bladder neck obstruction from benign prostatic hyperplasia.

Occasionally, patients with bladder tumor will have no clinical symptoms. In these patients, the diagnosis of bladder tumors is made by evaluation of abnormal laboratory findings, such as microscopic hematuria, or incidental abnormalities noted on radiologic studies. In the majority of patients, symptomatic or epidemiologic history will prompt consideration of the diagnosis of bladder tumor. Physical findings, such as lower abdominal or rectal masses or renal enlargement, are found only in patients with far-advanced lesions. Bimanual examination is the most helpful maneuver of the physical examination; however, it is best performed under anesthesia at the time of bladder biopsy. If a mass is palpable, the size, consistency, location (including apparent involvement of other organs), and mobility should be noted.

Diagnosis

Laboratory Findings

Routine urinalysis (including microscopic evaluation of freshly voided, centrifuged urine) is essential in the evaluation of patients with symptoms suggestive of bladder tumor. Eighty to 90 per cent of all patients with bladder tumor will have gross or microscopic hematuria. The findings of pyuria and bacteriuria can help identify those patients whose symptoms are most likely due to infection; however, caution must be exercised in these patients, since bladder tumors can be secondarily infected. The findings on urinalysis are not specific for bladder tumors, with the exception of the rare instance in which tumor fragments may be recognized in the urinary sediment. Investigation of the causes of abnormalities on routine urinalysis, particularly microscopic hematuria, can lead to the diagnosis of an asymptomatic bladder tumor.

Urinary cytology is a sensitive, specific technique for making the initial diagnosis and for following patients with the history of bladder tumors. The reliability of cytology depends upon the adequacy of collection of specimens as well as the skill of the individual cytopathologist evaluating the smears. In the best of hands, the false-negative rate may exceed that of direct cystoscopic examination for the diagnosis of bladder tumors.

Hematologic findings are not specific for bladder cancer; however, anemia may be present in patients with far-advanced bladder tumor. Also, an elevation of blood urea nitrogen (BUN) and serum creatinine levels will be noted if there is significant obstruction of the upper urinary tracts by bladder tumors.

Cystoscopy

Cystoscopy is essential to evaluate the bladder and urethra accurately when a bladder tumor is suspected. In addition to looking for overt papillary and sessile lesions, the examiner should regard with suspicion any mucosal abnormalities, particularly encrusted or apparently inflammatory areas.

If a tumor or a suspicious area is seen, transurethral biopsies are made to establish the diagnosis and provide information about the grade, extent, depth, and biologic potential of bladder tumors. Biopsied sites should be carefully recorded for future reference with regard to treatment and recurrences.

A bimanual examination should be performed both before and after tumors are resected or biopsies are done. If a mass is noted, the size, location, extent of involvement, and fixation of surrounding tissue should be performed. Particular attention should be paid to the persistence of a mass or residual induration and fixation after removal of the bladder tumor.

Biopsy specimens can be taken by aspirating tissue samples with an open-end, blunt-tipped urethral catheter; with a cold cup biopsy forceps; or with a standard resectoscope. Each of these instruments has specific advantages and limitations. Biopsy specimen collection by either aspiration or cold cup can be performed without anesthesia and is particularly valuable for use in outpatients. The resectoscope is required for doing biopsies when muscle sections are needed to assess the extent of tumor invasion.

Both papillary and sessile lesions should be removed to the level of the bladder wall. The base of the tumor should be resected into the muscle and submitted separately for histologic study. If the size or location of the tumor(s) makes complete resection inadvisable, the tumor margin and base should be biopsied for accurate assessment of the extent of the tumor.

Studies have shown a high incidence of carcinoma in situ or severe atypia of the epithelium, both adjacent to overt bladder tumors and in apparently uninvolved areas distant from overt tumors. The most frequent sites of unapparent mucosal change are the left lateral, right lateral, and posterior walls, while the dome and trigone are relatively spared. In addition to biopsies of obvious and questionable lesions, random biopsies are performed to assess the status of the epithelium in the other frequently involved areas. Attempts are being made to identify areas of abnormal mucosa for biopsy by using ultraviolet light or lasers after certain marking chemicals have been instilled in the bladder.

Histologic Studies

Careful histologic examination of step-sections of the tissue biopsies is essential. From these studies, the cell type is identified and the grade of tumor or degree of differentiation is assigned (Table 1). The depth of invasion is used to assign an initial clinical stage using the terminology of Jewett or the International Union Against Cancer (UICC) (Table 2).

A close correlation between tumor grade and the likelihood of invasion has been observed. Of low-grade lesions (Grade I), approximately 6 per cent are invasive; of high-grade lesions (Grade III), 82 per cent are invasive. If multiple lesions are noted at a given time or if frequent recurrences are observed, the lesions are more likely to become invasive. Chromosomal analysis and the deletion of normally present ABO-isoantigens are currently being investigated as means of measuring the biologic potential of bladder tumors. In patients whose superficial bladder tumors show ABO antigen deletion, there is a 65 to 70 per cent likelihood that they will develop invasive bladder tumors within the next 5 years. If the antigens are still present on a bladder tumor, there is less than a 5 per cent probability that the patient will develop subsequent bladder tumors.

Additional Techniques for Staging

Cystoscopic examination and transurethral biopsies, even with information provided on bimanual examination, have definite limitations in distinguishing Stage B from Stage C lesions. Also, these techniques cannot identify Stage D disease unequivocally.

Information regarding higher stages of a bladder tumor can be obtained from intravenous pyelograms. Distal ureteral obstruction in the presence of a bladder tumor indicates an invasive lesion in approximately 98 per cent of patients. Also, maintenance of a fixed shape of the bladder wall at different bladder volumes seen during an intravenous pyelogram is indicative of an invasive lesion.

Double- and triple-contrast cystography and angiography, together or separately, have been developed to improve the accuracy of staging. Lymphangiography has been used to attempt to identify nodal metastases. The computed tomographic (CT) scan has virtually replaced the staging techniques mentioned earlier. The improved CT scans permit identification of extension of a tumor beyond the bladder wall in most cases. Often regional lymph nodes that have been enlarged by tumor can be identified. Also visceral, principally liver, metastases are usually visualized. In a particularily thin patient, the lack of perivesical fat can make it difficult to evaluate the degree of tumor extension because of loss of tissue planes. Whole lung tomograms, bone surveys, and bone scans are commonly used, but have infrequently provided useful information in our experience.

The development of transurethral and transrectal ultrasound probes has improved the usefulness of ultrasound in staging bladder cancer. Recent reports have noted accuracy in staging in the 90 to 95 per cent range. These studies are not as useful as a CT scan in demonstrating nodal involvement.

Table 1. Grading of Bladder Tumors

Grade	Cell Property
I	Well differentiated
II	Moderately well differentiated
III	Poorly differentiated
IV	Anaplastic

Table 2. Staging of Bladder Tumors

Depth of Invasion	Jewett Stage	UICC* Stage
Mucosa	O	TIS
Submucosa	A	T1
Superficial muscle	B_1	T2
Deep muscle	B_2	T3
Perivesical fat	C	T3
Metastases	D	T4

*UICC = International Union Against Cancer.

Pitfalls in Diagnosis

One of the most common errors in diagnosing bladder tumors is overlooking the incidental finding of microscopic hematuria on urinalysis. Another error is not considering bladder tumor as a diagnosis when treating irritative bladder symptoms. Cystoscopically the greatest errors in diagnosing and staging bladder tumors come from taking biopsy material that is inadequate for judging the depth of the tumor and for detecting random involvement of the bladder epithelium. Until recently, the significance of severe dysplasia or carcinoma in situ was not recognized.

The early and correct diagnosis of bladder cancer requires suspicion of bladder tumor in patients with hematuria or voiding symptoms, as well as in the patient who is asymptomatic but has microscopic hematuria. Accurate staging, coupled with information regarding grade, extent, and biologic potential, is critical to the rational management and assessment of results. Although the laboratory and x-ray examinations and the cystoscopic findings and biopsies provide valuable presumptive information, open surgical staging (including lymph node resection) is frequently required to obtain the desirable degree of accuracy in staging bladder tumors.

PROSTATITIS AND URETHRITIS

By Joseph N. Corriere, Jr., M.D.
Houston, Texas

PROSTATITIS

Many physicians apply the diagnosis of prostatitis to any man who complains of lower urinary tract symptoms; pelvic, low back, or perineal pain; or ejaculatory or erectile dysfunction. Frequently there are few or no abnormalities found on physical examination or on examination of the patient's urine or ejaculate. Except for true bacterial prostatitis, which is invariably associated with a positive urine culture, the diagnosis is based on such flimsy evidence as to be easily refuted. Unfortunately, the psychosocial stigma of having a diseased sexual organ is so great in our society that the damage to the patient by applying such a label in a frivolous fashion may be irreparable.

The best classification of this disorder is as follows: *bacterial prostatitis,* acute and chronic; *nonbacterial prostatitis;* and *prostatodynia.* Each of these entities will now be considered with regard to the signs and symptoms, and diagnostic procedures necessary to separate and treat these disorders of the prostate gland will be presented.

Bacterial Prostatitis

Acute Form. These patients are usually acutely ill with malaise, fever, and chills suggestive of systemic toxicity. The local prostatic inflammation will produce symptoms of urinary frequency, urgency, dysuria, and difficulty in voiding. Rectal examination will usually, but not always, reveal an enlarged, often hard and irregular-feeling, prostate gland. After examination, a purulent discharge frequently will be seen at the urethral meatus. The rectal examination must be done gently (mainly to rule out a prostatic abscess, which is a complication of acute prostatitis) to prevent bacteremia.

A microscopic examination of the urethral discharge shows evidence of inflammation. Sheets of white blood cells per high-power field as well as gram-negative rods are present. A midstream urine culture reveals over 100,000 colonies per ml of a gram-negative rod, usually *Escherichia coli,* Klebsiella, Pseudomonas, or enterococci.

No further diagnostic procedures should be done at this time, and the patient should be immediately treated with antibiotics appropriate for the organism that is present. Rest and hot sitz baths are also worthwhile therapeutic measures in these patients. Urethral manipulation should be avoided. If the patient develops urinary retention, catheterization, of course, will be necessary; if an abscess develops, it will have to be surgically drained, usually transurethrally. Post-therapy urine cultures should be done to prove that the patient's urine has been sterilized.

Chronic Form. In this condition, the patient's symptoms are entirely due to bacteriuria, namely frequency, urgency, nocturia, and dysuria. The prostate feels normal to examination. If prostatic secretions can be expressed by rectal palpation, a microscopic examination of this fluid will reveal greater than ten white blood cells per high-power field and possibly gram-negative rods. Urine cultures will be positive intermittently and should be treated by appropriate antibiotics, but up to half of the time the bacteriuria will recur. The organisms are most commonly *E. coli,* Klebsiella, Proteus, Pseudomonas, enterococci, and possibly *Staphylococcus epidermidis,* alpha streptococci, and diphtheroids.

Between episodes of infection, these patients will become asymptomatic. If the voided urine is segmented when it is collected, however, small numbers of bacteria may be shown to be present in the prostate even during these times. Segmented urine collections are performed by having the patient begin to void and by collecting the first part of the stream (urethral contaminants) separate from the true midstream portion (bladder urine), and then collecting a third aliquot of urine after prostatic massage (prostatic organisms). With this technique, colony counts of bacteria in the third specimen should be higher than colony counts in the first specimen and the bladder urine should be sterile to localize the infection to the prostate. Seminal fluid cultures are probably more confusing than helpful.

The hallmark of this disorder is relapsing bacterial urinary tract infections due to the same bacterial pathogen. Despite the fact that prostatic fluid is inherently antibacterial and the urine easily sterilized with appropriate antibiotics, recurrent symptomatic episodes occur. As the disease progresses, prostatic calculi may develop and may help perpetuate the problem. Transurethral resection of the prostate occasionally may remove infected prostatic foci, but chronic medical therapy is generally preferred.

Unfortunately, most antibiotics do not diffuse from plasma to prostatic fluid or enter the prostate gland. A drug must possess certain criteria to penetrate the prostate:

1. It must be lipid-soluble with basic properties.
2. It must have a pKa of 8.6 or higher.
3. It must have optimal activity against gram-negative bacteria at a pH of 6.6.
4. There should be as few protein-bound properties as possible.

It appears that trimethoprim, doxycycline, and possibly erythromycin come closest to satisfying these criteria.

Periodic emptying of the prostate glands and ducts by frequent ejaculation, either by sexual intercourse or masturbation, may help decrease the inoculum.

Nonbacterial Prostatitis

This disorder, sometimes called "prostatosis," is characterized by a variety of pelvic symptoms, usually suprapubic, perineal, scrotal or low back pain; by dysuria, frequency, or urgency; or by ejaculatory discomfort. Physical examination of these patients, particularly of the prostate, is entirely normal. However, examination of expressed prostatic secretions will reveal greater than ten white blood cells per high-power field, while the urine cultures are always sterile.

The cause of the inflammatory reaction in these patients is unknown. The presence of oval fat macrophages in the prostatic secretions, which sometimes appear dark brown, is said to be characteristic of this problem. Attempts to implicate Chlamydia, Ureaplasma, viruses, parasites, or anaerobes as definitive etiologic agents have all failed.

Since the cause of this common condition is unknown, curative therapy is not possible. Long-term antibacterial therapy is not warranted, is expensive, and may be psychologically harmful by supporting the belief that a mysterious incurable infection is present in the patient's genitals. Symptomatic therapy should be given as needed.

Prostatodynia

Patients who seek medical aid because of a perception of "pain" or "discomfort" in the prostate, with or without mild voiding symptoms, but who have no abnormalities on physical examination or analysis of urine or prostatic fluid are placed in this category by exclusion. They are identical to the patients with nonbacterial prostatitis except for the finding of white blood cells in the expressed prostatic secretions in the latter group. These patients do not have prostatic disease and are thought by many observers to have, on psychiatric testing, evidence of personality disorders. They may be helped by psychiatric counseling.

URETHRITIS

Urethritis in the male can be divided broadly into two categories: gonococcal urethritis and nongonococcal urethritis. This section will deal with the nongonococcal varieties, commonly called *nonspecific urethritis.* (See also the article on Gonococcal Infection).

Symptomatic patients with nongonococcal urethritis usually present with mild dysuria, frequency, occasionally nocturia, and a scanty white or clear mucoid urethral discharge. The discharge is commonly present first thing in the morning, and the patient may also complain that his urethral meatus is almost sealed shut when he first attempts to urinate. He will also state he has spots of pus in his undershorts and may say that his urethral meatus or urethra itches or burns between voids. Since the disease is venereal, the patient will have had sexual intercourse in the recent past. The incubation period may be as long as 3 weeks, and most of the time the contact will have been with a new sexual partner.

On physical examination, the urethral meatus may be hyperemic and pouting. Tenderness may be found along the pendulous urethra. Look at the man's underpants for telltale spots of dried discharge. Rectal examination of the prostate should be normal, but it may help elicit a discharge if the urethra is stripped toward the meatus after prostatic palpation.

A urethral discharge can almost always be discovered and should be placed on a glass slide for microscopic examination. A Gram stain will help rule out gonorrhea. If gonorrhea is strongly suspected, a urethral swab culture should be done at this time.

A voided urine specimen (not a midstream specimen) should now be taken—not prior to the physical examination. In fact, the longest possible interval after voiding is the best time to examine the patient, as urine will wash away any discharge present and, as mentioned, the prostatic and urethral stripping may enhance the "find" of discharge and white blood cells in the specimen.

Chlamydia trachomatis is responsible for 30 to 50 per cent of nongonococcal urethritis, *Ureaplasma urealyticum* 20 to 50 per cent, and Corynebacteria 20 to 30 per cent. *Trichomonas vaginalis, Candida albicans,* and various viruses and anaerobes have been implicated. Other than the appearance of Trichomonas parasites on the smear or microscopic examination of the urine, the only finding will be at least four polymorphonuclear leukocytes per high-power field on the urethral smear and urine sediment examination. Culturing these common pathogens is strictly a research technique and not clinically applicable.

Since the diagnosis is made on clinical grounds without the aid of definitive cultures, treatment is somewhat empirical, but at the same time can be looked upon as a therapeutic test. Chlamydia can be eradicated by 2 gm of tetracycline, the drug of choice, daily for 2 to 3 weeks. It is probably also effective against Ureaplasma, since more than 85 per cent of patients with nongonococcal urethritis are cured by this regimen. Because of the empirical nature of the therapy, failures are usually treated with erythromycin or a trimethoprim-sulfonamide combination. If the patient claims he was cured but quickly relapsed and has only one sexual partner, consider treating the partner at the same time. Chlamydia urethritis may go on to cause epididymitis and possibly Reiter's syndrome. Discussion of these entities may be found elsewhere in this book. (See the articles on Intrascrotal Masses and Tumors and on Reiter's Syndrome.)

Finally, the patient who returns after what appears to be successful treatment but continues to complain of some dysuria and minimal discharge must be mentioned. Many men become obsessed with their former problem and will spend time milking their urethra in search of a discharge. Invariably, some normal urethral secretion can be produced but will be found to be clear of white blood cells, as will the urinalysis on these patients. These men must be reassured that they do not have a disease and should be instructed not to strip their urethra, and their symptoms will abate.

BENIGN PROSTATIC HYPERTROPHY

By Paul C. Peters, M.D.
Dallas, Texas

Benign prostatic hypertrophy (BPH) is a common disease of the male of the human species. It begins shortly after puberty as a periurethral hyperplasia. The role of hormonal influences in prostatic growth, particularly testicular androgens and estrogens, has been the source of considerable research. The growth of the prostatic tissue secondary to the influence of androgen has been alluded to by research workers from Huggins through Wilson and Jacobi. More recent studies by Wilson, Walsh, and others have suggested that prostatic growth may be influenced greatly by the estrogen: androgen ratios, some of the largest prostates in experimental animals having been produced by a combination of 3-alpha-androstanediol and estradiol.

The process begins as a stromal proliferation in the periurethral tissue, usually just superior to the verumontanum, and later a glandular invasion of this hypertrophied stromal tissue occurs. The small nodules that subsequently develop along the course of the urethra from the apex of the prostate at the verumontanum to the base of the bladder may enlarge sufficiently to outweigh the original prostate by many times. The size of the prostate, however, does not directly correlate with the symptomatology. It is an axiom that a large prostate may not be the obstructing prostate; the small one may be.

As growth of the prostate proceeds, the patient may be completely asymptomatic. In studies of a series of patients presenting for surgery for prostate obstruction at many large medical centers, incidences of acute urinary retention range from 14 to 50 per cent, even in recent times. On the contrary, a small prostate associated with considerable fibrous tissue proliferation at the vesical neck may result in complete urinary retention and marked secondary changes in the urinary tract even though a small gland is palpable by rectal examination.

SYMPTOMS

The diagnosis of prostatic hypertrophy is suspected from the patient's history of progressive lower urinary tract obstructive symptoms. The history of diminishing size and force of the urinary stream, dribbling on urination, nocturnal frequency in micturition increasing in severity, hesitancy and dribbling, and the use of accessory aids to promote micturition (such as turning on the water faucet, flushing the toilet, or straining) serves to confirm the suspicion of the examiner that an obstructive process is present. At times the symptoms are telescoped by an associated prostate infarction; other patients are asymptomatic to the point of acute retention. The examiner occasionally sees the patient with urgency, frequency, and bladder irritability whose bladder has not yet decompensated and who has no residual urine.

Although urethral stricture must be ruled out by history and by passage of a catheter, it is common practice to defer such examinations until the initial examination of the prostate under anesthesia, at which time instrumentation of the urethra is also carried out, and the possibility of stricture may be confirmed or excluded. When the patient presents in acute retention, of course, catheterization is commonly done at the time to relieve this condition and to allow a preoperative period of catheter drainage to diminish back pressure on the urinary tract.

The presence of prostatic hypertrophy may be suspected from the history and confirmed by physical examination in the physician's office. Rectal examination will usually reveal enlargement of the prostate. A normal prostate is about 8 to 20 gm in weight, is shaped like a valentine heart, and is approximately 2.5 × 3 cm. in vertical and transverse diameters. The urinary bladder is easily palpated superior to the normal prostate. Physical examination of the prostate is best accomplished in the office by having the patient bend over an examining table about 3 or 4 feet in height and rest his elbows on it with the knees slightly bent and the toes pointed inward. Adequate lubrication of the perianal area is very important to allow the examiner to insert the examining index finger without causing undue discomfort.

Since the prostate is shaped much like a valentine heart, one can easily appreciate the lateral lobes, the apex of the prostate, the base of the prostate, and the median sulcus in the normal or slightly enlarged prostate. With a slight enlargement of the prostate (Grade 1), the examiner may notice that it is difficult, but still possible, to reach the superior surface of the prostate. This is the size of the majority of the prostates encountered clinically in patients who are candidates for transurethral resection. As the prostate enlarges still further in size (Grade 2), the examiner finds that with difficulty, the superior surface of the prostate can be reached. One would expect a prostate gland in the range of 40 to 60 gm in weight with this physical finding. With still further enlargement of the prostate, it is no longer possible for the examiner to place the index finger superior to the prostate and compress the urinary bladder. The lateral lobes will often be found to be quite enlarged, but they are still outlined by the examining finger. These prostates range from 60 to 80 gm in weight and are usually called Grade 3 enlargements. When the boundaries of the prostate can no longer be outlined by rectal palpation, the possibility of malignancy must be considered; in the case of prostatic hypertrophy, however, one would anticipate finding a quite large prostate, often greater than 100 to 200 gm in weight. In today's society, with many men obtaining medical attention quite early or even appearing for regular physical examinations by a physician, such prostates are infrequently encountered.

The apparent size of the prostate on rectal examination is usually a reliable index to the true size, though it is not infallible. Certainly, the size of the prostate by rectal examination does not always correlate with the degree of urinary tract obstruction. Median lobe enlargement, having arisen from the suburethral glands that have hypertrophied in response to changes in hormonal milieu or local tissue factors—both of which may have been incriminated—may account for obstruction of a greater degree than can be suspected by the size of the prostate on rectal palpation. The prostatic secretion obtained by gentle massage may be examined and usually is translucent, slightly sticky, and turgid. On microscopic examination, an occasional white blood cell can be found. The presence of more than ten white blood cells per high-power field and/or bacteria in the prostatic secretion should lead one to suspect the possibility of a complicating infection. Examination and culture of the expressed prostatic secretion (EPS) are indicated.

LABORATORY AND RADIOGRAPHY AIDS IN DIAGNOSIS

Microscopic examination of a freshly voided urine sample as well as EPS is a part of the work-up of the patient who is suspected of having prostatic hypertrophy. In the absence of infection, the normal, slightly yellow (straw-colored) urine with a specific gravity of 1.008 to 1.022 on a random specimen with an osmolality of 700 mM/kg (if such facilities are available) is confirmatory of renal function within a normal range. A blood sample for serum creatinine and for serum acid phosphatase should be drawn. The acid phosphatase sample is particularly important if suspicious areas of induration are felt in the prostate and should be drawn as a baseline study in patients with obstructive symptoms, even if surgery is not a prime consideration at the time of the examination because of the possibility of carcinoma of the prostate. Biopsy may be indicated in the presence of severe obstructive symptoms if urethral stricture has been ruled out and an indurated area is felt in the prostate.

Excretory urography is commonly performed in the preoperative evaluation of a patient with prostatic hypertrophy. The examination serves as a useful means of comparing, in a crude way, the function of the two kidneys and allows evaluation of anatomic changes in the urinary tract which may be secondary to prostatic obstruction and which may not be appreciated on physical examination (e.g., the presence of bilateral hydronephrosis or hydroureteronephrosis, thickening of the bladder, and the presence or absence of bladder diverticula). A crude estimate of the size of the prostate can be made by the appearance of displacement of the bladder silhouette superior to the symphysis pubis by a considerable distance, and an intravesical filling defect in the urinary bladder created by the prostate. Although one cannot accurately estimate the weight of the prostate by the magnitude of the intravesical filling defect, the bladder silhouette is often displaced superiorly from the symphysis pubis by marked lateral lobe enlargement of the prostate. Residual urine may be crudely estimated by noting the amount of residual contrast material remaining on the postvoiding film after the patient has been instructed carefully to empty the bladder completely, and thus catheterization may be avoided. Ultrasonography can help to estimate size and also detect nonpalpable malignancy.

There is no substitute for watching the patient void. One can detect certain mannerisms and certain reinforcing measures (such as the use of the water faucet, which the patient may have developed to aid in micturition), and the size and force of the urinary stream can be judged quite well by the experienced observer. The use of sophisticated urodynamics equipment, instrumentation flow rates, and anal sphincter electromyography is not part of the usual office examination in patients suspected of benign prostatic hypertrophy and cannot be considered cost-effective in the routine work-up of the individual with early obstructive complaints.

If neurogenic disease is suspected by the finding of a lax anal sphincter, the absence of ankle jerks, or the appearance of a pathologic reflex (such as the Babinski sign, a tremor, or evidence of previous neurologic disease as may be manifest by hemiparesis, hemiplegia, cranial nerve disturbances, or unilateral weakness in the arm or leg), further investigation of neurogenic dysfunction may be indicated.

Patients with diabetes present a particularly difficult problem because of the combination of neurologic changes and bladder hypotonia with obstruction from a hypertrophied prostate. Certainly, many patients with diabetes present with urinary frequency and may be mistaken for individuals with frequency and urgency secondary to lower urinary tract obstruction. The complicating neuropathic changes in the urinary bladder in unsuspected diabetic patients may mimic those of an individual with a large overdistended bladder from simple mechanical obstruction of the prostate (i.e., paradoxical or overflow incontinence).

As mentioned earlier, observing the patient void to note the size and force of urinary stream is an important practice in the office examination of the patient with prostatic hypertrophy. One must remember that the force of the urinary stream and the quantity of urine voided in a given period of time vary with the amount of urine in the patient's bladder at the time he is asked to void. A normal patient may empty the urinary bladder of 300 ml in 10 to 15 seconds with a flow rate greater than 15 ml/second (13.2 $\pm$ 2.0 ml/second). Individuals with quantities of less than 100 ml in the urinary bladder at the time they are asked to void may perform more poorly, and this must be taken into account. Reliance on a single observation is often faulty. Normal men experience a decline in flow rate of about 0.2 ml/second/year after age 40.

DIFFERENTIAL DIAGNOSIS

The differential diagnosis of prostatic hypertrophy, of course, includes carcinoma of the prostate, which may be suspected because of obstructive symptoms, or, more commonly, palpation of an area of induration in the prostate, and confirmed by biopsy and serum acid phosphatase measurement in suspicious cases. Acute bacterial prostatitis may present with high fever and symptoms of urinary tract obstruction. In extreme cases, acute urinary retention may result. Rectal examination must be performed cautiously in these acutely ill people. An enlarged, very tender prostate is palpated, and often a purulent urethral discharge may be easily expressed. Antibiotic therapy using broad-spectrum antibiotic treatment is indicated initially. Re-examination after completion of therapy in the asymptomatic patient may reveal striking reduction in the size of the prostate from the moment of presentation. Asymmetric enlargement of the prostate with fever, chills, and extreme tenderness, often with pain referred to the perineum, should cause one to suspect abscess of the prostate. This may be confirmed by sonographic studies, if available, or by simple needle aspiration of the prostate through a transperineal approach. Urologic consultation is indicated in such cases, as one may be dealing with a potentially serious situation with bacteremia and septicemia.

Congestive prostatovesiculitis, or *prostatosis,* often enters into the differential diagnosis. In this condition, the prostate is described as feeling "boggy" or "mushy" to palpation. Considerable quantities of fluid may be expressed. The patient often gets considerable symptomatic relief from massage of the prostate in such cases. Anxiety or guilt related to extramarital affairs is often elicited in these patients. Involvement or induration of the seminal vesicles should lead one to suspect the possibility of a granulomatous inflammation. This may be secondary to escape of seminal fluid or, rarely, to diseases such as tuberculosis. Lues is seldom seen today in the advanced stage, but the presence of a flaccid anal sphincter and infrequent voiding should call to mind the possibility of a tabetic state. Absence of ankle jerks, poor anal sphincter tone, a broad-based gait, a large-capacity bladder that nonetheless empties well, and the history of lightning-like upper abdominal pain of marked severity (the gastric crisis) may be sought in the history. Confirmation requires testing of the serum and cerebrospinal fluid using Fluorescent Treponema Antibody (FTA), *Treponema pallidum* immobilization (TPI), and Venereal Disease Research Laboratories (VDRL) methods.

The possibility of urethral stricture must be borne in mind with patients presenting with dribbling on urination, even when there is some associated prostatic enlargement. Instrumentation is usually not recommended prior to examination of the prostate under anesthesia. At times, however, it may be cost-effective and convenient to ask the urologist to perform cystoscopic examination in the office, and under such circumstances the stricture is usually easily identified. The urethra should not be calibrated in acutely infected patients or in febrile patients except in cases of acute retention when it may be necessary to leave in an indwelling urethral or suprapubic catheter for preoperative decompression of the chronically or acutely obstructed urinary tract.

When cystoscopic examination is performed in the evaluation of a patient with prostatic hypertrophy, the observer looks for objective evidence of obstruction. One anticipates seeing hypertrophy of the interureteric ridge and thickening of the muscle bundles of the urinary bladder, commonly called trabeculation. In addition, small outpouchings of the mucosa between the hypertrophied muscle bundles, called *cellules,* may be seen. In some cases associated with prostatic enlargement, large outpouchings of the vesical mucosa between hypertrophied muscle bundles may be seen, called *diverticula.* Rarely these are palpable by rectal examination. The presence of a stone in the urinary bladder above a hypertrophied prostate is not an uncommon finding and may account for the history of a sudden cessation of micturition during midstream, alleviated by a change of position of the patient, who may then resume micturition. In addition, diverticula should always be inspected carefully as a source of stone or tumor. One should not be misled by the relatively small appearance of a diverticulum on an excretory urogram, as it may be seen on voiding cystourethrography or on a postvoiding film after excretory urography to be quite large, sometimes larger than the bladder itself, and to contain residual contrast material. Stone in a diverticulum may be palpable by rectum; stone in a prostate may give the sensation of crepitus to palpation.

One cannot overemphasize the importance of the obstructive symptoms and the secondary changes in the urinary tract, including hypertrophy of the bladder muscle, dilatation of the upper urinary tracts, and diminution of glomerular filtration rate and fluid retention, that sometimes occur in a gradual and insidious manner in prostatic enlargement. Decompression of the chronically obstructed urinary tract must be contemplated with some caution and preparations made to handle a large water, sodium, or urea diuresis that sometimes ensues following decompression of the chronically obstructed urinary tract.

Lytton found that BPH occurred with an incidence of 0.6 per cent in males aged 10 to 14 and with an incidence of 42 per cent in men aged 70 to 74. The peak age for onset of symptoms is age 50 to 55, but growth of the prostate seems to be continuous throughout old age.

CARCINOMA OF THE PROSTATE

By Theodore V. Benderev, M.D.
and John T. Grayhack, M.D.
Chicago, Illinois

Carcinoma of the prostate has the second highest incidence of any malignancy found in males in the United States; only lung cancer surpasses this disease. Seventy-five thousand new cases of carcinoma of the prostate were expected in 1983 with 24,000 resulting deaths. The true prevalence of the disease is much higher than is apparent. Autopsy studies show that 30 per cent of all men over age 50 have clinically unrecognized carcinoma of the prostate, a figure that increases with age to nearly 100 per cent at age 90.

Adenocarcinoma accounts for 95 per cent of all cancers of the prostate, with transitional cell carcinoma, squamous carcinoma, and sarcoma making up most of the remainder.

SYMPTOMS

The appearance of symptoms of carcinoma of the prostate is dictated by the natural history of the disease. Carcinoma of the prostate usually begins in the periphery of the gland. As a consequence, early or localized carcinoma of the prostate is characteristically asymptomatic. The presence of symptoms implies an advanced form of the disease. As the tumor grows, it replaces the nonmalignant glandular tissue; and symptoms of bladder neck obstruction—namely, nocturia, frequency, hesitancy, and intermittency—develop. Asymptomatic or symptomatic dissemination of the tumor has frequently occurred before the onset of obstructive symptoms, since they require an appreciable local growth.

Carcinoma of the prostate disseminates over two major routes: the lymphatic system and the bloodstream. Metastases to the pelvic lymphatics rarely cause symptoms. However, the blood-borne metastases that commonly involve the skeletal system often produce back or leg pain, which may be the patient's initial complaint. This pain is often mistakenly diagnosed as arthritis. The pelvis, lumbar spine, femurs, thoracic spine, and ribs are involved in decreasing order of frequency. Paralysis can result at times from compression of the spinal cord by subdural metastasis. Hematogenous metastases to visceral organs such as the lung, liver, and brain may produce symptoms, but these instances are rare.

DIAGNOSIS

Diagnosis of carcinoma of the prostate depends, first, on recognition of patients with a high risk of the disease and, second, on histologic or cytologic confirmation. Various procedures, including rectal examination and chemical analysis of blood, urine, and prostatic fluid, have been and are being used to identify patients with high risk. Use of these techniques as screening or routine procedures is essential if the asymptomatic patient is to be identified early. Presently, only rectal examination and, possibly, prostatic fluid analysis seem likely to identify the patient with localized disease, and only the former is readily available and easily accomplished.

Recognition of Risk

Digital rectal examination remains the standard procedure to identify patients with a high risk of localized carcinoma of the prostate. The prostate is normally a compressible heart-shaped gland with a 4-cm broad base at the bladder neck. A prominent midline furrow and distinct lateral borders or sulci characteristically identify a normal gland. Alterations in the prostate varying from a slight change in consistency, through a discrete firm nodule, to a diffuse stony hard gland indicate a significant risk of carcinoma. Further evaluation is necessary in all such glands, since 50 per cent are histologically discovered to contain carcinoma. Other causes of such changes in the prostate are prostatic calculi, granulomatous prostatitis, focal benign prostatic hyperplasia, tuberculosis, and postoperative changes.

Several compounds in body fluids have been studied in an attempt to identify patients with a high risk of disease. In expressed prostatic fluid, the proteins transferrin and complement component C_3 are elevated in 70 and 80 per cent, respectively, of cases of cancer of the prostate. The ratio of isoenzymes LDH-5/1 in prostatic fluid has been found to be greater than 2:1 in 70 per cent of patients with prostate cancer. All of the biochemical changes observed in the prostatic fluid to date are nonspecific; however, the opportunity to evaluate these indicators over time increases their usefulness in identifying an increased risk of malignancy.

Confirmation of Cancer

Histologic verification by prostate biopsy is always necessary to establish the *diagnosis* of carcinoma of the prostate. Prostatic tissue may be obtained in a number of ways. Transurethral biopsy is usually unsatisfactory in early cancer of the prostate because of the peripheral location of the lesion. Cytologic examination of prostatic fluid also has limited usefulness in establishing the diagnosis.

The most frequently employed means of establishing the diagnosis of carcinoma of the prostate is transperineal or transrectal needle biopsy. It has a 70 to 90 per cent chance of sampling the diseased tissue, depending on the extent of the carcinoma and the skill of the operator. Since a negative test does not rule out malignancy, a repeat biopsy is performed if suspicion of carcinoma persists. Needle biopsy has a low morbidity, and tumor cell implantation has rarely occurred. A technique using a 22-gauge needle to aspirate a cytologic sample to confirm the presence of carcinoma has become popular. Its accuracy is similar to and its complications fewer than standard needle biopsy. No anesthesia is required. However, an experienced cytopathologist is vital for the accurate interpretation of the specimen.

Histologic examination of the biopsy specimen not only confirms the diagnosis but also provides evidence of its biologic activity. As with many other tumors, the grade of tumor correlates with the presence or development of metastasis. In carcinoma of the prostate, the chance of lymph node metastasis increases considerably in patients with clinically localized disease when the tumor is poorly rather than well differentiated.

STAGING

Classification

Proper staging of the tumor is essential in evaluating the appropriate therapeutic alternatives. Extraprostatic spread of the carcinoma, which is present in 75 per cent of newly diagnosed cases, markedly diminishes the likelihood of cure with available therapy. There are four clinical stages that reflect the natural history of prostate carcinoma. Stage A and B tumors are clinically localized, while stage C and D tumors show evidence of dissemination.

Stage A. Stage A disease is defined as a localized

cancer that is unsuspected clinically. It is discovered in 5 to 25 per cent of prostates examined histologically after removal to relieve bladder neck obstruction. This stage accounts for 10 per cent of cases of carcinoma of the prostate and is divided into substages A_1 and A_2. Patients with substage A_1 disease have limited focal microscopic disease and, unless they have a poorly differentiated lesion, can be expected to have a life span unlikely to be affected by their cancer. On the other hand, patients with substage A_2 disease have multifocal disease or an intragland mass that is more aggressive, with an approximate 35 per cent incidence of nodal metastasis (pathologic stage D).

Stage B. Stage B tumors are also confined to the prostate, but are recognizable on rectal examination. They are found in 10 to 15 per cent of cases of carcinoma of the prostate. This stage also has two subdivisions. Substage B_1 disease is characterized by induration limited to and occupying less than one lobe of the prostate. The incidence of lymph node metastasis is approximately 15 per cent. Induration involving all of one prostatic lobe or parts of both is classified as substage B_2 and has an approximate 35 per cent incidence of lymph node metastasis.

Stage C. Stage C tumors are recognized on rectal examination by evidence of extension locally through the prostatic capsule into the pelvic wall or perivesical areas. This stage includes 30 to 45 per cent of patients with carcinoma of the prostate. These patients have an approximately 55 per cent incidence of lymph node metastasis.

Stage D. Patients with clinical stage D tumors give evidence of metastasis by the clinical techniques to be described in the later sections of this article. Identification of pathologic stage D tumors depends on histologic demonstration of disseminated disease. These tumors account for 30 to 40 per cent of diagnosed cases of carcinoma of the prostate.

Assessment of Stage

The stage of prostate cancer is assessed in a standard manner using rectal examination, blood markers, bone x-rays, radionuclide studies, and, when indicated, surgery.

Rectal Examination

The rectal examination can enable the physician to distinguish between a clinical stage B and a stage C tumor. Whereas a clinical stage B tumor on rectal examination will have induration limited to the gland, a stage C tumor will have evidence of extension into the perivesical areas or into the pelvic wall, thus obscuring the lateral sulci. The examiner must be aware that the rectal examination will frequently understage the clinically localized tumor, since 50 per cent of clinical B_2 lesions have histologic evidence of extraprostatic extension (stage C).

Blood Markers

Serum acid phosphatase is an important marker in staging carcinoma of the prostate. In patients with diagnosed prostate carcinoma, an elevated serum acid phosphatase level implies disseminated disease. Of patients with disseminated prostate carcinoma, 70 per cent have elevations of this enzyme; patients with localized carcinoma rarely, if ever, show elevations.

Acid phosphatase can be found in a wide variety of tissues such as liver, platelets, and bone. As a consequence, although elevated serum levels of acid phosphatase in men over the age of 50 should suggest the likelihood of disseminated carcinoma of the prostate, these levels are also seen with such diverse disease states as cirrhosis, thrombocytopenia, Paget's disease of bone, multiple myeloma, rheumatoid arthritis, and cancers with osseous involvement, for example, osteosarcoma and cancer of the breast. Specific prostatic isoenzymes have been identified and can be measured by enzymatic and, more recently, immunologic methods. Unfortunately, while these techniques increase sensitivity, they decrease specificity. For example, in a recent general screening study 67 per cent of patients with elevated serum prostatic acid phosphatase as determined by radioimmunoassay had benign prostatic hyperplasia rather than cancer.

Transient elevations of serum acid phosphatase can result from manipulation of the prostate by rectal examination or urethral instrumentation. It is generally recommended that a serum acid phosphatase sample should not be drawn until 24 hours after a rectal examination.

Examination of bone marrow aspirates for acid phosphatase has been explored in an effort to document osseous metastasis, but this technique is not sufficiently accurate to be clinically useful.

The most frequently used marker after acid phosphatase is alkaline phosphatase. Serum alkaline phosphatase is elevated in 90 per cent of patients with bony metastasis, reflecting an increase in osteoblastic activity. Liver diseases such as hepatitis or cirrhosis can also increase total alkaline phosphatase. Measurement of the bone isoenzyme of alkaline phosphatase can be helpful in identifying bone involvement when liver disease is present.

Skeletal Evaluation

Examination of the skeleton for osseous metastasis by x-ray and radionuclide scanning is mandatory in staging carcinoma of the prostate. X-rays are more specific and bone scans more sensitive in the search for metastatic lesions. Osteoblastic lesions characterize bone involvement by cancer of the prostate and are present alone or with osteolytic changes in about 90 per cent of the patients with demonstrable bone metastases. Bone scans using technetium 99m polyphosphate have been found to indicate a high probability of bone metastases in up to 35 per cent of patients with negative skeletal surveys. The delayed recognition of metastasis on routine radiography is accounted for by the necessary 30 to 50 per cent replacement of bone by tumor before detection is possible by this technique.

In addition to the skeletal metastases due to prostate carcinoma, a variety of other metabolically active bone lesions such as arthritis, healing fractures, Paget's disease of bone, and osteomyelitis result in locally increased concentration of radionuclide. Therefore, despite the delay necessary to effect a recognizable change on x-ray, skeletal radiography has a significant role in specifically identifying stage D carcinoma of the prostate.

Lymphatic Evaluation

In patients without evidence of dissemination by the previously discussed staging modalities, accurate evaluation of the pelvic lymphatic drainage of the prostate is essential to rule out nodal metastasis. Bipedal lymphangiography and computed tomography (CT) provide inexact information but may allow the discovery of carcinoma when it is combined with thin needle aspiration. Presently, only pelvic lymphadenectomy provides unequivocal information regarding pelvic nodal metastases. This procedure can be combined with radical prostatectomy or radiation implants and has limited risks.

Other Imaging Studies

The intravenous pyelogram may demonstrate ureteral or bladder neck obstruction in carcinoma of the prostate. Deviation of the ureters by lymph node metastasis may also be apparent.

Ultrasound and CT scanning have limited usefulness in evaluating the extent of the local prostatic mass. The findings provided by these studies are nonspecific and are often difficult to interpret.

CONCLUSION

Diagnosing carcinoma of the prostate while it is still localized and potentially curable is the key to improving survival. While the search continues for better tests to be used in the clinician's practice to identify patients at high risk for having this disease, the digital rectal examination remains a satisfactory means of screening for prostate carcinoma. Proper employment of staging studies will allow identification of the stage of the natural history present in patients with a confirmed diagnosis of carcinoma of the prostate and will allow consideration and selection of the most appropriate treatment.

INTRASCROTAL MASSES AND TUMORS

By Rod Cherrie, M.D.
and Jean B. deKernion, M.D.
Los Angeles, California

The diagnosis of intrascrotal masses rests primarily on patient history; physical examination; various diagnostic maneuvers, such as transillumination; urinalysis and complete blood count (CBC); and occasionally intravenous urography and other standard laboratory tests. From these, one may either arrive at a final diagnosis or conclude that surgical exploration is required for diagnosis and appropriate treatment.

The timing of surgery is a matter of judgment. Vascular impairment secondary to strangulated hernia or torsion of the spermatic cord requires emergent intervention and must be treated in a timely manner. Other conditions may be dealt with electively.

We will discuss lesions of the testes, epididymis, appendages, tunics, and spermatic cord separately. Where appropriate, we will emphasize important differential diagnoses in disorders such as epididymitis, torsion of the spermatic cord, and testis tumors.

LESIONS OF THE TESTES

In this section we will consider lesions producing a testicular mass or swelling as well as traumatic rupture of the testes.

Traumatic Lesions

Rupture of the testis is a surgical emergency. Prompt diagnosis and intervention are required to avoid testicular loss and secondary infection and to diminish the morbidity of this injury.

Violent blunt trauma to the scrotum, crushing the testis against the pubic bone, is followed by painful swelling secondary to hemorrhage into the tunica vaginalis (hematocele). Scrotal ecchymosis and hematoma from ruptured vessels in the scrotal wall are common. The mass is tender, boggy, and purple and does not transilluminate. The intrascrotal contents cannot be delineated by palpation.

This presentation demands immediate scrotal exploration to evacuate the hematoma and to repair or remove the testis if it is indeed ruptured. When the diagnosis is in question, or when the suspected rupture seems to be minimal, producing only slight swelling and pain, close observation with bed rest, analgesics, and ice packs is acceptable. In general, however, the risks of surgery are less than the risk of loss of the testis by nonintervention.

Inflammatory Lesions

Acute Orchitis

The most common agent responsible for orchitis in the absence of epididymitis is the mumps virus. The testis may also be involved in epididymo-orchitis caused by Chlamydia or pyogenic bacteria, which will be discussed later. Either is attended by pain of somewhat gradual onset, swelling of the testis and scrotum, fever, and constitutional symptoms. On physical examination the testis is swollen and tender and usually can be distinguished from the epididymis, which is in the posterolateral position.

Chronic Orchitis

Luetic orchitis is vanishingly rare. It has been said a gumma of tertiary lues in the testis feels like a golfball in the scrotum and is about as common. Testicular swelling is painless and gradual. On examination, the testis is enlarged, indurated, and nontender. The diagnosis is mainly presumptive. Other stigmas of tertiary lues are present. The serologic test for syphilis (STS) is markedly elevated, and the manifestations resolve with antiluetic therapy.

Tuberculous orchitis is a consequence of tuberculous infection of the urine involving the prostate and extending down the vas deferens into the epididymis followed by invasion of the rete testis. Diagnosis rests on positive skin tests, positive urine culture for tuberculosis, and microscopic examination of excised portions of the testes and epididymis.

Vascular Lesions

Vascular compromise of the testis can occur after operations on the spermatic cord such as herniorrhaphy or ligation of the spermatic veins in which the gonadal artery may be divided or compressed. It is seen most often with intravaginal torsion of the spermatic cord on its axis, leading to twisting and occlusion of the vessels with subsequent ischemia of the testis and the epididymis.

Symptoms and Signs. The onset of pain is sudden, as is typical of vascular occlusion. A previous history of sudden testicular pain followed by sudden relief, either spontaneous or with manipulation, is virtually diagnostic, as is a history of prior contralateral "epididymitis" resulting in testicular atrophy.

If the patient is seen early, both the testis and epididymis are high in the scrotum and tender, and the epididymis is not in its usual posterolateral position. Soon after onset, edema and hyperemia of the scrotum and tunic occur, and it is impossible to delineate the testis and epididymis by palpation. One must then rely on history and laboratory tests.

Laboratory Findings. The urinalysis and CBC are usually unremarkable. We have found that the Doppler ultrasonic probe is useless and misleading in this condition. In patients in whom there is reasonable doubt as to diagnosis, the 99m technetium-pertechnate flow-scan may be useful in confirming or excluding torsion. In inflammatory conditions, the flow is increased (hot testicle); in torsion of the spermatic cord, the flow is absent (cold testicle); and in torsion of the appendages, the scan is normal. In testicular infarction (missed torsion), there is a central cold area with a surrounding hyperemic ring. Although this technique can be very accurate, it is not always readily available.

Deferring needed exploration of a clinically suspected torsion for a technetium scan wastes valuable time and is only to be condemned. The morbidity of exploration is negligible, whereas the morbidity of testicular infarction is quite substantial.

Differential Diagnosis. Torsion of the spermatic cord is most frequently confused with acute epididymo-orchitis. The pain of torsion is of sudden onset, often arousing the patient from a sound sleep, while that of epididymitis is more gradual. Initially, the pain of testicular ischemia is worse than the pain of epididymitis. High fever and chills are unusual in torsion, but are common in epididymitis. Most (but not all) patients with epididymitis have pyuria, bacteriuria, and leukocytosis. In epididymitis, one can usually distinguish the testes from the epididymis. If a reactive hydrocele is present, transillumination and aspiration of the hydrocele may assist the diagnosis. Extreme tenderness may make adequate palpation difficult, and infiltration of the cord just above the testes with 10 ml of 0.5 per cent lidocaine and 0.25 per cent Marcaine relieves the pain entirely and facilitates examination. Elevation of the scrotum is said to diminish the pain of epididymitis but not of torsion (Prehn's sign). However, this is often very unreliable.

Other entities that may present in similar fashion are strangulated hernia and testis tumor with sudden hemorrhage or necrosis. When torsion of the spermatic cord is suspected, expeditious exploration should be performed to confirm or exclude a torsion and to initiate appropriate treatment.

Testis Tumors

Testis tumors are usually found in young men, but can occur at any age. The majority are *germinal* tumors: embryonal carcinoma, teratoma, teratocarcinoma, choriocarcinoma, yolk sac tumor, and seminoma either alone or in combination with other germinal elements. *Nongerminal* tumors comprise 3 to 5 per cent of all testis tumors and include interstitial cell tumors, gonadoblastoma, and soft-tissue sarcomas. Metastatic tumors of the testis are rare and are usually incidental autopsy findings. They include leukemia, the lymphomas, hypernephroma, prostatic carcinoma, lung carcinoma, gastrointestinal carcinoma, and melanoma.

Symptoms and Signs. Certain aspects of the history are particularly pertinent. The incidence of malignancy in a cryptorchid testis is 20 to 40 times the norm unless orchiopexy was performed before the age of 6 years. Contrary to popular belief, testis tumors can be painful. A history of scrotal trauma can often be obtained that serves to call the patient's attention to his testicular abnormality. Hemorrhage into the tumor may occur following trauma, causing further swelling and pain. Gynecomastia may also be a common complaint.

Testis tumors are usually easily diagnosed by palpation, in the form of a discrete nodule or diffuse enlargement of the testis that is usually but not always nontender. The abdomen and supraclavicular nodes should be palpated for metastases. Gynecomastia may also be detected.

Laboratory Findings. Routine CBC, chemistry, and urinalysis are usually normal, but serum beta chain hCG or alpha-fetoprotein may be elevated and should be obtained whenever tumor is suspected. Chest x-ray or computed tomography (CT) scan of the lungs is essential to detect pulmonary metastases. Intravenous urography and CT scanning of the abdomen can be useful in detecting retroperitoneal disease, but a significant false-negative error accompanies CT scanning. When extensive retroperitoneal disease is suspected, however, CT is valuable in determining the gross extent of the disease which may require vigorous chemotherapy prior to surgery. Lymphangiography is utilized extensively in some institutions, often combined with CT scanning. We have not found this useful except in clinical staging of seminomas.

Differential Diagnosis. Testis tumor may cause acute pain and swelling and may be confused with epididymidis. A protracted mistaken diagnosis of epididymitis can have particularly tragic consequences in these patients. In doubtful cases, it may be appropriate to treat with antibiotics for 1 or 2 weeks. If clinical resolution of the pain and swelling is not prompt, exploration is imperative. In particularly difficult diagnostic problems, ultrasound of the testes may assist in determining the presence of a mass. Carefully performed, this can be a very sensitive and reliable test, capable of differentiating hydrocele from enlarged testes and identifying a solid mass in a suspiciously enlarged or painful testis. The ultimate diagnosis of testis tumor depends on inguinal exploration of the testis and histologic section.

LESIONS OF THE EPIDIDYMIS

Inflammatory Lesions

Acute Epididymitis

Acute epididymitis is usually caused by Chlamydia or pyogenic bacteria, and gonococcus is now a rare pathogen in the epididymis. Epididymitis may also follow scrotal trauma; untreated, it may progress to frank scrotal abscess. This is especially a threat in the severe diabetic.

Symptoms and Signs. A gradual onset of discomfort in the scrotum is typical. The pain rapidly becomes severe and may radiate up to the cord, to the ipsilateral lower quadrant or flank, or to the rectum if accompanying prostatitis is prominent. The pain is aggravated by motion, and the patient's gait is unmistakable. Fever, chills, malaise, and nausea are common. A recent history of dysuria, urethral discharge, or urethral instrumentation is usual but not invariable.

On examination, the epididymis is swollen, indurated, and tender and is in its normal anatomic position. Later, the scrotum becomes edematous and a reactive hydrocele may form. The role of local anesthesia, transillumination, and aspiration of the reactive hydrocele has been discussed earlier.

The spermatic cord is usually tender, and the prostate may also be boggy and tender.

Laboratory Findings. The white blood cell count is elevated with a shift toward immature granulocytes. Urinalysis often shows pyuria, though this finding is sometimes surprisingly absent. Bacteriuria is less common, since most cases in younger men are usually caused by Chlamydia. Gonococci may be seen on the Gram stain in cases of concomitant gonococcal and chlamydial infections. In postvasectomy epididymitis, or in postprostatectomy epididymitis secondary to reflux of sterile urine into the vas deferens, the urinalysis may be entirely normal.

If epididymitis is accompanied by infection of the urinary tract, the patient should have a cystoscopy and intravenous urogram after the acute process subsides in order to identify urinary tract abnormalities predisposing to infection.

Chronic Epididymitis

Old recurrent chronic epididymitis may present with variable symptoms of scrotal pain and a nodule. The epididymis is nodular, cystic, and mildly to moderately tender to palpation. The urinalysis and CBC are usually unremarkable. Sterile, chronic inflammation is usually found in the specimen if an epididymectomy is performed.

Tuberculous epididymitis does not occur in the absence of renal, prostatic, and seminal vesicular tuberculosis, since the bacilli travel down the vas deferens to the epididymis. The most frequent lesion is a nontender, cold abscess in the globus minor, but the entire epididymis may become filled with palpable abscesses and may become quite tender. A beaded, thickened vas deferens is suggestive of tuberculosis. Skin tests and urine cultures for tuberculosis are positive, and granulomas containing acid-fast bacilli will be found in the epididymectomy specimen.

Luetic epididymitis is quite rare and occurs in secondary or tertiary syphilis. The course is indolent and asymptomatic, with diffuse, nontender thickening of the globus major and sometimes a palpable rubbery nodule. Gummatous epididymitis is as rare as gummatous orchitis, and the diagnosis is usually presumptive. Other evidence of lues is present in the absence of other infection, and the manifestations resolve with antiluetic therapy.

Almost every other known organism has infected the epididymis at one time or another, but a detailed discussion of these varieties is beyond the scope of this article.

Sperm Granuloma

Sperm granulomas occur as a result of extravasation of sperm from the proximal vas deferens or from the epididymis after vasectomy. They can be painful and present as small, tender nodules that do not transilluminate. The final diagnosis is made by excision and microscopic examination.

Tumors of the Epididymis

Malignant tumors of the epididymis are quite rare and are almost always soft-tissue sarcomas: rhabdosarcoma, fibrosarcoma, liposarcoma, and undifferentiated mesenchymal tumors in descending order of frequency.

The most common *benign* tumor of the epididymis is the *adenomatoid tumor,* which is of obscure origin. It presents as a small, solid, painless mass in the lower pole of the epididymis.

Leiomyomata are the second most common benign tumors. Patients present with dull scrotal pain and a hydrocele. The epididymis is slightly enlarged, tender, and firm.

Cystadenomas are benign, cystic, epithelial tumors of the epididymis that are asymptomatic and are frequently found in patients with von Hippel-Lindau disease. The final diagnosis of all these is made by exploration and histologic section, and laboratory studies are of little value.

Other Lesions of the Epididymis

Spermatocele

Spermatoceles arise from the tubules connecting the rete testis to the globus major. They are cystic masses lying just above and posterior to the upper pole of the testis and are entirely separate from it. They are usually small and painless, but may become painful or achieve sufficient size to come to the patient's attention. Examination reveals a mobile cystic transilluminating mass posterosuperior to the testis. Aspirated fluid is cloudy and contains sperm.

Cyst

Epididymal cysts may accompany a spermatocele, or they may be a result of epididymitis. If large enough, they transilluminate and the postinflammatory variety usually are tender.

LESIONS OF THE APPENDAGES

The appendix testis is of müllerian origin and is located on the anterior aspect of the upper pole of the testis. The appendix epididymis is of wolffian origin and is located on the globus major of the epididymis. Small, soft, and somewhat polypoid, they are usually only incidental findings on physical examination. They can occasionally undergo torsion and infarction, but this is rare in the adult.

Symptoms and Signs. The patient with torsion of an appendix presents with pain of sudden onset in the involved hemiscrotum. The mass and tenderness can be usually localized to the given appendix, but inflammatory reaction may be severe enough to mimic torsion.

Laboratory Findings. Urinalysis and a CBC are usually unremarkable. In doubtful cases, the exact diagnosis is made by expeditious exploration of the testis.

LESIONS OF THE TUNICA ALBUGINEA

Various benign lesions of the tunica albuginea can present as testicular masses, and this diagnosis should be suspected when the lesion is small and painless and when it projects above the tunica albuginea. These include:

1. Fibromas.
2. Inclusion cysts, which may be single or multiloculated.
3. Chronically inflamed fibrous nodules.

Barring absolute certainty of the diagnosis, inguinal exploration of the testis should be performed and the lesion excised. However, small tunica albuginea cysts are very common and simply require reexamination and reassurance.

LESIONS OF THE TUNICA VAGINALIS

Tumors

The tunica vaginalis is an isolated portion of the coelomic cavity and can therefore give rise to a variety of mesothelial proliferative lesions, reactive or neoplastic. These occur in all age groups and present a similar picture to that of testis tumor—a firm, nontender, painless scrotal mass that does not transilluminate. Since it is impossible to separate paratesticular mesotheliomas into benign and malignant groups and since they probably are all capable of local invasion, the final diagnosis should be established by radical orchiectomy and histologic section.

Traumatic Lesions

Hematocele has been discussed previously along with traumatic rupture of the testis.

Hydrocele

Hydrocele is an accumulation of serous fluid between the parietal and vasceral layers of the tunica vaginalis that invests the testes. It may be secondary to inadequate fluid resorption (simple hydrocele) or to local inflammation (reactive hydrocele). Communicating hydrocele is actually a hernia; the patent processus vaginalis allows peritoneal fluid to enter the tunica vaginalis. This is usually seen only in children.

Signs and Symptoms. Hydroceles are usually painless, unless the cause of a reactive hydrocele produces discomfort. The mass is globular, feels cystic, and readily transilluminates. The cord and external ring are normal unless a hernia is present.

Differential Diagnosis. Indirect hernias do not transilluminate and are usually reducible, and the cord and ring are abnormal. An impulse is felt in the mass when the patient coughs and strains. All other scrotal masses should be readily differentiated from hydrocele by simple transillumination. When a mass is suspected in addition, ultrasound will usually delineate the testis clearly inside the hydrocele.

LESIONS OF THE SPERMATIC CORD

Vascular Lesions

Varicocele

A varicocele consists of elongated, dilated, tortuous veins of the pampiniform plexus in the spermatic cord, which are commonly on the left side (90 per cent). Right-sided varicoceles are usually found in cases of bilateral varicoceles secondary to incompetence of the valves of only the left spermatic vein with cross-circulation in the scrotum leading to bilateral varices. Varicocele is a relatively frequent cause of male infertility.

Patients may present either with infertility or with a dragging sensation and variable scrotal mass. In obvious cases the mass feels like a "bag of worms" and increases in size with an upright position and a Valsalva maneuver. Lifting and compressing the scrotum with the patient in the supine position cause the varicoceles to empty. In cases of infertility, the varicocele may be small but nonetheless significant. The Valsalva maneuver in the standing position can be helpful, and mild exercise or prolonged standing can be used to bring out a latent varicocele.

An acute onset of left varicocele or presence of a right unilateral varicocele, especially those that do not empty in the supine position, requires prompt evaluation for renal or other retroperitoneal tumor causing obstruction of the left renal vein or the vena cava.

Tumors

Benign and malignant tumors of the spermatic cord are rare. All are mesenchymal tumors, lipoma and liposarcoma being the most common. They appear as discrete, nontender masses in the cord and are entirely separate from the testis. Exploration and excisional biopsy establish the diagnosis. A rare but well-differentiated cause of spermatic cord masses is seeding of the cord from upper gastrointestinal (especially stomach) malignancies by "drop" metastases.

Hydrocele

Hydrocele of the spermatic cord itself is a fluid accumulation in a pinched-off portion of the processus vaginalis. It presents as a firm, nontender mass in the cord and may increase in size over time. Transillumination is not often helpful. The diagnosis is established at exploration.

Section Fourteen

GYNECOLOGIC MEDICINE

EVALUATION OF BREAST MASSES AND SYMPTOMS

By Blake Cady, M.D.
Boston, Massachusetts

Breast cancer is so common and has received so much attention in the public media that women's anxiety about breast symptoms creates a significant flow of patients to practitioners' offices. A logical scheme to cope with these patients while minimizing the ever-present danger of missing an occult or difficult to palpate carcinoma is much needed. Several techniques, practices, and understandings that were developed and became widely appreciated in recent years help the physician deal with these frequent problems.

First, it is important to realize that breast cancer is very common, occurring in the United States in about one of every 12 women (8 per cent) during her lifetime. The vast majority of cases, over 80 per cent, occur after the age of 45 years, but because of the infrequency of other fatal illnesses in younger adult women, breast cancer is the leading cause of all deaths in women between the ages of 35 and 50. In some diseases and some cancers, a high-risk group can be defined, and thus screening for early detection can focus on a small segment of the population. The risk of breast cancer, however, is distributed over the entire population, such that the patients in the Breast Cancer Detection and Demonstration Project (BCDDP) high-risk group had only twice the incidence of breast cancer as the remaining patients, a ratio that indicates the general ineffectiveness of selecting groups of women for screening programs and a need to consider the entire female population over the age of 45 years as at high risk. Consequently, the American Cancer Society recommends yearly mammograms for all women over the age of 40. One small but well-defined high-risk group, however, is premenopausal women with a first-degree relative (daughter, sister, or mother) who had premenopausal breast cancer, since there is a far higher genetic relationship in premenopausal breast cancer than in postmenopausal disease.

Another well-defined risk group is those women with biopsy-proven ductal or lobular abnormalities, such as florid atypical intraductal hyperplasia and lobular neoplasia (so-called lobular carcinoma in situ), of which the latter may have a risk of eventual invasive carcinoma of up to 30 per cent after 20 years or more. In half the cases the risk involves the contralateral breast. Thus, such women, whether subjected to mastectomy or not, need follow-up for the remainder of their lives. Of course, the highest risk group of all is women with a previous breast cancer, because contralateral cancer develops at a rate of about 1 or 2 per cent of the surviving population each year. Clearly this risk varies with the age of the patient and the prognosis of the first breast cancer, since the patients must live long enough to manifest the risk.

Techniques currently available to patients and physicians to separate common, benign lesions of the breast in young women from breast cancer, the only serious disease that occurs particularly in menopausal and postmenopausal women, are

1. Breast self-examination.
2. Physical examination.
3. Mammography.
4. Needle aspiration of masses.
5. Biopsy.

BREAST EXAMINATION

Self-Examination

Breast self-examination should be taught to all women in the early adult years so that by the age of 35 they are thoroughly conversant with their own anatomy and can report significant variations. Patient education pamphlets and movies can be obtained from the American Cancer Society and the National Cancer Institute and should be made available. Hospitals should consider displaying educational exhibits and showing teaching films for patients, visitors, and employees, stressing self-examination.

Cancers detected by women who practice breast self-examination are significantly smaller and have fewer lymph node metastases, as evidence of the benefits of this practice. It should be appreciated, however, that many women are reluctant or fearful about performing self-examination and need encouragement and support from physicians and nurses, as well as repeated exposure to educational material.

Physical Examination

Physical examination of the breast should be a part of the routine examination for women over the age of 30 and ideally should be performed at the middle of the menstrual cycle to minimize distortions caused by stimulation associated with the maximum estrogen level that occurs just premenstrually. A routine of both recumbent and erect examinations should be followed, with careful attention to the axillary contents and any nipple erosions or distortions, which should raise suspicion of Paget's disease, an early manifestation of breast cancer. Such an examination offers opportunities for instruction in self-examination as well as description of the concept of functional changes occurring in the premenopausal breast that may cause soreness, pain, and discomfort episodically and cyclically. These functional changes should always be described as such, and scrupulous avoidance of the term "fibrocystic disease" should be encouraged. Women who have sore or painful breasts and are told they have a "disease" will be anxious about it and make assumptions regarding the connection to breast cancer; such an association has not been proven to exist. Indeed, the very definition of "fibrocystic disease" is nebulous, since such pathologic changes are seen in the vast majority of women in routine autopsy studies. These changes are not related to illness or death, and they are manifested only by irregular and fluctuating episodes of discomfort and breast irregularities. By avoidance of the label "disease" and strict adherence to such terms as "lumpy breasts," "cystic breast," "functional changes," and "fibrocystic changes," much patient anxiety is successfully avoided. Almost all women who have episodes of even severe pain and discomfort will, with reassurance that they do not have a disease or a higher than average risk of developing cancer, wish to avoid active intervention with either drugs or surgery. Hormonal therapy is rarely, if ever, indicated, but occasionally women may benefit from diuretics.

Of course, any unilateral discrete mass should be viewed with suspicion, and a tissue diagnosis of persistent masses should be made within a short period of time to alleviate physician and patient anxiety. Any discrete mass in a menopausal or postmenopausal woman is considered to be cancer until proved otherwise. Almost all discrete masses in women 20 to 30 years old are benign; however, they are always viewed with alarm by patients and should be removed, with few exceptions, for determination of the nature and for peace of mind of both patient and physician.

Two symptoms need special comment. Unilateral nipple discharge of serous or blood-tinged serous fluid is usually the symptom of intraductal papilloma; however, intraductal cancer sometimes presents in this way, and therefore biopsies should be performed. At physical examination, it is important to confirm the patient's description of nipple discharge and note its location; this will offer clues for the appropriate siting of biopsy incisions. Greenish, blackish, or white nipple discharge in small quantities, which may be bilateral, is not of clinical significance and is not galactorrhea; determinations of prolactin concentrations to detect pituitary adenomas should be done only when there is copious bilateral secretion of a thin, nonserous fluid.

The most worrisome presentation of breast cancer occurs when no discrete mass is present but there is a diffuse thickening of the breast tissue, sometimes more apparent to the patient than to the physician. Women with such a finding know something is wrong with the breast but may not be able to describe an exact change, and the physician may not be able to document presence of a mass, distortion, or secondary signs of carcinoma, such as skin retraction. In some difficult-to-evaluate breasts, the patient may be convinced that something abnormal is occurring, and a mammogram, random needle aspiration cytology, or even open biopsy should be performed if there is clinical suspicion of any abnormality whatsoever or if the patient is convinced of an abnormality.

It should be kept in mind that a serious problem almost never occurs as a result of a biopsy, but numerous tragedies occur because of the failure to perform a biopsy on breasts that contain an abnormality.

Mammography

Mammography was designed as a screening technique for asymptomatic women and has been shown to be useful in detecting impalpable early breast cancer. It must be kept in mind, however, that it is *not* useful for confirmation of the nature of palpable masses and should *never* be used for this purpose. Mammography is negative in at least 15 to 25 per cent of known palpable carcinomas; this rate of false-negative reports prohibits its use for delineation of the nature of any palpable lesions. The purpose of mammography in women with palpable masses is to inspect the remainder of the breast tissue bilaterally, not to examine the palpable abnormality.

Breast cancer is rare in women under the age of 30, mammography is far less accurate in young women with active breast tissue, and the only evidence of breast cancer induction by radiation has been reported in women under the age of 30. Therefore, mammography should not be used in women below that age. Mammography should be used in women under the age of 35 only in high-risk circumstances, such as a strong family history of premenopausal breast cancer, a previous breast cancer in the patient herself, or high-risk pathology on previous biopsy. Between the ages of 35 and 40, there should be restrictive indications for the use of mammography and it should be utilized in women with some evidence of increased risk by physical examination or history. However, the current guidelines for mammography by the American Cancer Society suggest a single baseline mammogram sometime during this period for most American women.

After the age of 40, the use of mammography should become a routine. Although at present no clear data suggesting the ideal frequency of its use have been accepted, yearly intervals seem appropriate. In one prospective study, the routine use of mammography with yearly physical examinations was associated with a decreased death rate from breast cancer after both 5- and 10-year follow-up in postmenopausal women compared with similar patients not undergoing mammography routinely. Whether such reduction in death rate represents true avoidance of death or lead time bias is not completely defined at the present. Some abnormalities, such as lobular neoplasia (lobular carcinoma in situ) are detected that do not invariably lead to cancer if untreated, and thus some of the recent increased incidence of breast cancer and improvement in survival result from recording such benign-behaving lesions as cancer in registries of disease. Nevertheless, current practice suggests that the routine yearly use of mammography may reduce the death rate from breast cancer and its use should be encouraged at appropriate ages. Since no clear advantage of any particular type of mammography has been shown, either xeromammography or film mammograms are equally acceptable.

Thermography and Ultrasound

Neither thermography nor ultrasound has proved to be useful in breast cancer when applied routinely, and use of these techniques is not justified at present except for research purposes. Computed tomography is currently being evaluated but should not be used routinely.

Needle Aspiration

Needle aspiration of breast masses is to be encouraged, as it provides immediate definition and treatment of gross cysts and an opportunity to aspirate material from solid masses for cytologic studies which may permit a diagnosis of cancer to be made when slides are analyzed by experienced cytopathologists. Such aspiration cytology diagnoses may considerably simplify the management of breast cancer patients. The principal usefulness, however, remains the prompt resolution of breast cysts. When a cyst has been aspirated of nonbloody fluid and the mass has completely disappeared and has not recurred repeatedly, the clinical situation is resolved, since breast cancer rarely presents as a cystic lesion. Cyst fluid cytology is not useful and involves unnecessary expense if performed.

Cytologic studies of nipple discharges have not been found to be useful, generally because breast cancer does not commonly present in this fashion and because of the low yield of positive results when it does.

Biopsy

Breast biopsy should be performed whenever the definition of a breast mass is not clearly apparent by the procedures previously described and in any patient with a persistent discrete mass regardless of age. An unfortunate number of patients are still seen who have persistent mass that a physician has dismissed because of young age or a negative mammogram. Whether biopsies are excisional or incisional is less important. Generally, small cancers are removed by total excision, but large cancers may be handled best by small incisional biopsy to prove disease, after which appropriate surgery follows the necessary preoperative work-up. With the wide acceptance of outpatient biopsy of breast masses under local anesthesia, breast biopsy for any discrete palpable masses should be encouraged. A common ratio of benign to malignant biopsies in major centers and competently staffed general hospitals is about 3:1, indicating the necessity of liberal indications for biopsy. Very few patients require hospital admission or general anesthesia for breast biopsy, and I advise this only for patients with large breasts and impalpable, mammographically detected and localized microcalcification. When such lesions are biopsied, considerable time may be required to find the tiny clusters of microcalcification by x-ray directed frozen section of repeated tissue specimens.

The use of core needle biopsy under local anesthesia in the office is equivalent to formal open biopsy if the results demonstrate carcinoma. However, neither needle aspiration cytology nor core needle biopsy, when negative, can be considered definitive and must always be followed by open biopsy to ensure that adequate tissue was obtained and that a small cancer was not missed.

The greatest recent advance in management of patients with breast cancer has been to separate in time the definitive diagnosis by biopsy and the definitive treatment by either mastectomy or local excision and axillary dissection prior to radical radiotherapy. This time delay enables women to discuss therapeutic alternatives, seek opinions about management, and enter the primary surgery with a calmer state of mind. Since delays of up to 3 weeks do not detract from good results of definitive therapy, the sense of rush and panic that patients feel when subjected to general anesthesia, biopsy, and immediate mastectomy is avoided. Calmer, reasoned discussion concerning the definitive diagnosis and treatment ensues.

Estrogen Receptor Protein

Estrogen receptor protein (ERP) determination is obtained on all primary breast cancers because of its usefulness in directing therapy if metastatic disease ever occurs. The usefulness of this test in primary breast cancer management is uncertain at the present time, but it has become standard to obtain ERP determinations at the time of breast cancer removal either by biopsy or by mastectomy.

FUNCTIONAL MENSTRUAL DISORDERS

By Esther Eisenberg, M.D.
Philadelphia, Pennsylvania

Uterine bleeding when it occurs acyclically may be of great concern to the patient and present a diagnostic dilemma for the physician. This common clinical problem has been variously referred to as dysfunctional uterine bleeding, functional uterine bleeding, and anovulatory bleeding. Several descriptive terms serve to categorize the bleeding but do not indicate the cause. These include oligomenorrhea (menstrual bleeding which occurs less frequently than normal), polymenorrhea (bleeding which occurs more frequently than normal), menorrhagia or hypermenorrhea (increased amount or duration of bleeding or both). Prolonged intervals of amenorrhea (absence of bleeding) may occur in conjunction with the abnormal bleeding. Regardless of the pattern of bleeding, the diagnostic evaluation is similar.

Normal menstrual bleeding is the result of cyclic endometrial shedding, which occurs in response to the hormonal changes associated with ovulation. Generally, such cycles vary between 22 and 35 days and are characteristic for an individual. Menstrual flow normally lasts 3 to 8 days, with a range of 30 to 80 ml of blood loss per cycle. An average of three to four tampons or pads are used on the heaviest day of the cycle.

Dysfunctional uterine bleeding (DUB) may be irregular, excessive, scant, or prolonged. Of endometrial origin, it occurs in the absence of detectable organic lesions of the uterus and systemic conditions. By definition, DUB is a diagnosis of exclusion. No bleeding should be treated as DUB unless all other causes have been evaluated and corrected.

Aberrations of the hypothalamic-pituitary-ovarian axis that result in anovulation most frequently are manifested as abnormal uterine bleeding. Although this bleeding has no typical pattern and is usually not associated with other symptoms, it is uncharacteristic of the normal cycles experienced by an individual woman. Dysfunctional uterine bleeding most often occurs postpubertally and in the perimenopause. In fact, 75 per cent of DUB is found in the over-35-year age group. In the perimenarchal female, DUB often resolves spontaneously with time as the hypothalamic-pituitary-ovarian axis matures. In the older age group, DUB may be corrected through the diagnostic dilatation and curettage (D&C) performed (see later discussion) as part of the evaluation. Dysfunctional uterine bleeding may respond to medical therapy with progestational agents or may remit with the arrival of menopause. Approximately one third of women will have recurrence of DUB requiring further surgical therapy, either a repeat D&C or a hysterectomy.

The diagnostic process is directed toward excluding organic lesions of the reproductive tract, systemic disease, blood dyscrasias and trauma, as well as evaluating factors that may be responsible for anovulation (Table 1).

Table 1. Differential Diagnosis of Abnormal Uterine Bleeding

Reproductive Tract Pathology
Endometritis
Endometrial polyps
Uterine leiomyoma
Pregnancy
Threatened abortion
Ectopic pregnancy
Hydatidiform mole
Endometrial hyperplasia
Endometrial carcinoma
Cervical neoplasia
Endocrine Gland Dysfunction
Hypothyroidism
Hyperthyroidism
Pituitary adenoma
Systemic Disease
Hematologic disorder
von Willebrand's disease
Thrombocytopenia
Cirrhosis
Medications
Estrogen administration
Estrogen-containing vaginal creams
Combination oral contraceptives
Aspirin
Trauma
Foreign body: intrauterine contraceptive device
Ovulatory Dysfunction
Anovulation
Luteal phase deficiency

HISTORY

A careful history will elicit information about an alteration in menstrual pattern. Bleeding with clotting indicates brisk bleeding that has overcome the fibrinolytic system of the uterus. Inquiry should be made about each of the last menstrual periods in detail, whether there have been associated episodes of amenorrhea, and whether any other systemic symptoms, unusual bleeding from other organs, fever, frequency of urination, or bowel irregularity exists. These may direct further investigation. Specific inquiry about medications used is important. Aspirin in sustained use may cause a platelet dysfunction. Hormonal preparations, estrogens, or combinations of synthetic estrogen and progestin may cause abnormal uterine bleeding.

PHYSICAL FINDINGS

Physical examination will exclude signs of endocrine gland dysfunction or systemic illness. Breast examination should include milking of the breast with firm pressure toward the areola to search for the presence of galactorrhea. Pelvic examination is generally normal in women with functional menstrual disorders.

Uterine or adnexal enlargement or irregularity indicates the likelihood of a diagnosis other than DUB. Enlargement of the uterus may suggest pregnancy, uterine leiomyomas, or possible reproductive tract malignancy. Tenderness suggests the possibility of pelvic infection or intra-abdominal process. Gross lesions of the cervix and vagina are visible to inspection. Trauma related to a foreign body, if one is present, may be found.

LABORATORY INVESTIGATION

Hemoglobin and hematocrit determinations are obtained to establish the extent of anemia and to provide a baseline of hematologic status. Anemia, if found, should be corrected with iron replacement. A platelet count should be obtained. Persistent bleeding unresponsive to hormonal manipulation in the absence of organic pathology indicates the possibility of systemic blood dyscrasia. Bleeding time and tests of platelet function (ristocetin aggregation) may uncover von Willebrand's disease (see article on Hemophilia and other Hereditary Defects of Coagulation).

In the reproductive age group, any unusual bleeding is cause for suspecting a complication related to pregnancy. A serum pregnancy test should be obtained in this age group to exclude the possibility of intrauterine pregnancy, threatened abortion, ectopic pregnancy, or hydatidiform mole. Radioimmunoassay (RIA) of the beta subunit of human chorionic gonadotropin (β-hCG) is a highly sensitive and specific test of pregnancy. The RIA for β-hCG can detect as little as 0.0003 IU/ml in 4 hours. Radioreceptor assays are not as specific as the RIA for β-hCG but are faster to perform.

In the event of an ectopic pregnancy or threatened abortion, measured hCG is usually less than that expected from the date of the last normal menstrual period. The normal range of values for pregnancy should be available from the laboratory that performs the assay. If the hCG test is positive, a pelvic ultrasound examination in conjunction with the serum β-hCG level is helpful in establishing the diagnosis. When the level of β-hCG exceeds 5000 mIU/ml, a gestational sac or fetus should be visualized. Absence of a gestational sac suggests the possibility of ectopic pregnancy or missed abortion. With hydatidiform mole, the level of hCG will be markedly elevated above the expected range.

A reason for anovulation should be sought, with particular attention to tests of thyroid function (triiodothyronine, thyroxine, and thyroid-stimulating hormone) and serum prolactin determination. Hypothyroidism may be associated with menorrhagia. Hyperthyroidism is often associated with episodes of amenorrhea. Hyperprolactinemia may be associated with polymenorrhea or episodes of amenorrhea related to anovulation even in the absence of galactorrhea. Normal serum prolactin levels range from 5 to 25 ng/ml in the female. Evidence of hyperprolactinemia necessitates further investigation for pituitary micro- or macroadenoma by computed tomography (CT scan), using third- or fourth-generation CT scanners. These devices permit detection of microadenomas of the pituitary gland and have virtually made polytomography an outmoded radiographic technique for this problem.

Serum androgen levels (dehydroepiandrosterone sulfate and testosterone) may be helpful if there is physical evidence of hirsutism or virilization or suspicion of polycystic ovarian disease.

Diagnostic Procedures

Abnormal uterine bleeding in women under 35 years of age is most frequently due to anovulation. Charting of the basal body temperature (BBT) may be helpful in identifying this condition. In ovulatory cycles, the BBT recording generally reveals a thermal shift of approximately 0.6 °F lasting 12 to 14 days, characteristically found in the postovulatory phase of the cycle. A thermal shift is not present in anovulatory cycles. Another less frequent finding may be a thermal shift interval that is shorter than the expected 12 days. This finding suggests the possibility of luteal phase deficiency, which is due to inadequate progesterone production by the corpus luteum. Although these conditions are not life-threatening, fertility may be impaired.

Excessive or prolonged bleeding may be treated empirically in women under 35 years of age. The endometrium should also be shed periodically in women whose bleeding occurs less frequently than every 2 months. This is accomplished with a short course of progestin administration, referred to as a "medical curettage." Sometimes, cycles will resume and abnormal bleeding will remit. If the abnormal bleeding persists or recurs, a histologic evaluation of the endometrium is obligatory.

In women over 35 years of age and in those younger women who have failed medical therapy, endometrial sampling is crucial for the diagnosis of DUB. In most patients with DUB, the endometrium appears morphologically normal. Sampling of the endometrium permits detection of other more serious intrauterine pathology. Endometrial biopsy, although perhaps not representative of the entire endometrium, may be performed during an office visit. Endometrial aspiration (Vabra, Vacutage) is also an office procedure and provides a wider sampling of the endometrium. These sampling methods generally suffice for women less than 35 years of age. In women over 35 years who experience dysfunctional bleeding, and especially in the perimenopausal age group, a dilatation and fractional curettage is mandatory to exclude malignancy or endometrial hyperplasia.

Pathologic conditions of the endometrium, such as chronic endometritis, retained products of conception, endometrial polyps, hyperplasia, or carcinoma, may be discovered and will direct further therapy. Similarly, a submucosal leiomyoma may be suggested at the time of D&C by the contour of the uterine cavity. In this case, and in cases of persistent uterine bleeding unresponsive to hormonal manipulation, hysteroscopy may aid in determining an etiologic source. Hysteroscopy involves use of a fiberoptic endoscopic device that is placed within the endocervical canal as the uterine cavity is distended with medium, either CO_2, dextran, or 5 per cent dextrose in water. This technique enables the endometrium to be visualized directly, including submucosal myomas, endometrial polyps, lost intrauterine contraceptive devices, and intrauterine synechiae.

In the absence of the conditions cited earlier, the histologic appearance of the endometrium is either proliferative or secretory. When evaluated in relation to the onset of the next bleeding episode, knowledge of the histology is helpful in confirming either anovulation or luteal phase deficiency as a cause for the dysfunctional bleeding. Further therapy may be recommended with the assurance that potential life-threatening conditions have been excluded.

PREGNANCY

By J.T. Parer, M.D., Ph.D.
San Francisco, California

Pregnancy is the commonest cause of amenorrhea in the childbearing years. It is characterized by many physiologic and hormonal changes that affect almost every organ system. In some patients these normal changes simulate certain diseases. In addition, there are a number of abnormalities associated with gestation that can be deleterious to the pregnancy and may threaten the life and health of the mother.

DIAGNOSIS OF PREGNANCY

The missed menstrual period is the most frequent means by which a woman diagnoses pregnancy. In addition a substantial percentage of women have symptoms (nausea, breast tenderness, tiredness) that subjectively confirm pregnancy to them.

The most accurate means of confirming pregnancy is analysis of blood for human chorionic gonadotropin (hCG), or, more accurately, its beta subunit (β-hCG). This may be positive as early as 4 weeks after the last menses. Commercially available kits enable the woman to test her own urine for hCG, and these are quite reliable.

The next most common means of detecting pregnancy is by enlargement of the uterus and its softened consistency. This becomes fairly reliable at about 8 weeks of gestation. Detection of the fetal heart confirms the presence of a pregnancy. This can be heard by Doppler devices as early as 10 weeks in some patients, and almost always by 14 weeks. With the fetoscope (stethoscope), the heart beat is usually heard at 20 weeks.

Ultrasound imaging is more commonly being used to determine the integrity of an intrauterine pregnancy. A "gestational sac" can be seen by approximately 5 weeks after the missed menses, and if a fetus with heart motion is also seen, this will rule out certain abnormalities. Fetal heart movement is consistently seen by 8 weeks.

DIFFERENTIAL DIAGNOSIS

Ectopic Pregnancy

An ectopic pregnancy involves the implantation of the fertilized ovum in a region other than the endometrial cavity. The vast majority (about 98 per cent) implant in the tube, most commonly in the middle or distal third of the tube. The incidence of ectopic gestation varies widely in different populations and socioeconomic groups, but it approximates 1 per cent. The prime etiologic component is salpingitis. Ectopic pregnancy recurs with an incidence of approximately 10 per cent. Nontubal ectopic pregnancies occur in the following order of decreasing incidence: fimbrial, abdominal, cornual, ovarian, and cervical.

The signs and symptoms of ectopic pregnancy include amenorrhea, abnormal vaginal bleeding, pain, and, when internal or external bleeding is severe, shock. At times the diagnosis is missed because not all of the classic signs are present, and a chronic ectopic pregnancy may result. It is not uncommon for such patients to have had one or two courses of antibiotics in the belief that their pain was due to salpingitis.

Diagnosis is much more reliable now with the ready availability of radioimmunoassays for β-hCG in maternal serum. Virtually all patients will have detectable β-hCG levels, though often below the levels detected by routine urine pregnancy tests. Hence a sensitive and quantitative measurement in serum should be obtained. Ultrasound has proved useful in diagnosis if it reveals an intrauterine pregnancy when an ectopic gestation is suspected. It is less accurate for actually visualizing the ectopic site. Because of these advances, culdocentesis is now less important for diagnosis. Culdocentesis may be misleading if it is positive when there is retrograde tubal bleeding from a threatened abortion or spontaneous abortion. In adition, a culdocentesis negative for blood does not rule out an unruptured ectopic pregnancy.

When ectopic pregnancy is suspected but not certain, laparoscopy is often used to visualize the pregnancy. This has saved many women the added seriousness of a laparotomy when the findings are negative.

Threatened Abortion

Threatened abortion refers to any intrauterine pregnancy in which bleeding occurs in the first trimester. The prognosis can be optimistic if the uterus is appropriately enlarged, the bleeding is mild and self-limited, and cramping is absent. Should the symptoms and signs be severe, and the cervical os dilates, abortion is inevitable.

In cases of persistent threatened abortion, ultrasound imaging may assist if a moving fetus is visualized. However, nonvisualization of a fetus is not unequivocally associated with a blighted ovum, particularly at early gestational ages—e.g., less than 8 weeks or when the gestational sac size is 2.5 cm or less in diameter. Such findings require further confirmation.

Incomplete Abortion

Incomplete abortion is characterized by bleeding, cramps, and the passage of tissue, generally in the first trimester. Approximately 20 per cent of pregnancies result in spontaneous abortions, and 50 per cent of first trimester abortuses have chromosomal abnormalities. The diagnosis is made by determining that the cervical os is open (e.g., sufficiently to admit a ring forceps), and that there is passage of tissue (the products of conception) through the cervix. In some patients all of the products of conception are passed spontaneously; this is termed "complete abortion." This situation is characterized by a smaller uterus, virtual cessation of bleeding, and a closed cervical os. Unlike the incomplete abortion, the complete abortion does not require curettage.

Missed Abortion

Missed abortion is the death and partial resorption of the products of conception, usually the disappearance of the symptoms of pregnancy, continued amenorrhea, and no passage of the products of conception. The placental tissue may degenerate to such an extent that insufficient hCG is produced to give a positive pregnancy test (though hCG could be detected by more sensitive means).

Missed abortion is diagnosed by noting inadequate growth of the uterus, absence of fetal heart tones, and ultrasound imaging. It may be associated with coagulation disorders, although rarely until after 20 weeks of gestation. The coagulation disorder is usually characterized by decreasing fibrinogen levels beginning about 6 weeks after fetal death.

Trophoblastic Disease

Trophoblastic disease may be either hydatidiform mole or choriocarcinoma and always develops initially from a fertilized ovum. It may be suspected from inappropriate enlargement of the uterus, absence of fetal movement, or very early (e.g., 22 weeks) onset of preeclampsia (hypertension and proteinuria). Very high levels of hCG are present. Diagnosis in the office is aided by noting absent fetal heart tones, and a definitive diagnosis can be made by ultrasound imaging which shows characteristic diffuse vesicles without a fetus or placenta.

DATING OF PREGNANCY

Apart from the desire of the patients to know when their baby is due, there are a number of obstetrical reasons to determine when a pregnancy began. Such reasons are to determine premature labor, appropriateness of size for age, or postdatism of a pregnancy. The normal duration of a pregnancy is 280 days (40 weeks) after the beginning of the last menses, with a normal range of 38 to 42 weeks. Unless there are other fetal illnesses, outcome for the newborn is optimal if the baby is born within this period.

Methods of confirming duration of pregnancy are as follows:

1. *Last menstrual period.* This is accurate only if the patient's periods are regular and occur approximately every 28 days. If intervals are prolonged, pregnancy duration will be overestimated because conception occurs approximately 14 days *before* the next expected period. This method is inaccurate after the use of birth control pills, as the patient will have a withdrawal period after cessation of the pills, and may have some months of post-pill amenorrhea.

2. *Early pregnancy test.* A urine or blood pregnancy test at or about 6 weeks of gestation is a particularly valuable objective confirmation of the duration of pregnancy, especially in combination with several of the other clinical correlates. Because a minimum period of pregnancy can be determined from such information, it can often unequivocally confirm postdatism where it is suspected.

3. *Early uterine examination.* This can date a pregnancy to within about 2 weeks if the examination is done between 8 and 12 weeks of gestation. However, after this time it becomes progressively inaccurate.

4. *Quickening.* The first sensation of fetal movement is apparent at about 17 weeks, although there are quite large variations in individual patients.

5. *Auscultation of fetal heart tones.* Hearing fetal heart tones with the fetoscope is generally possible by 20 weeks, but once again there are quite large discrepancies; for example, it may be later if there is an anterior placenta.

6. *Top of fundus at umbilicus at 20 weeks of gestation.* This is the most reliable time to determine uterine size after the first trimester.

7. *McDonald's measurement.* After 20 weeks, the curved fundal height from the top of the uterine fundus to the pubic symphysis in centimeters approximates weeks of gestation. This is more important for determining rapidity or slowing of fetal growth than actual dating.

8. *Ultrasound imaging.* This is now the most popular means of dating pregnancy when duration is in doubt, but its accuracy in clinical usage is in fact often not much better than the methods already described. In the late first trimester, gestational age can be estimated by measuring crown-rump length and reading off the gestational age on a curve. Later, measurements are usually made of the fetal biparietal diameter, relating this to gestational age on a mean curve. The variance of this increases with gestational age, and its accuracy at any stage of gestation is rarely better than ± 2 weeks. It is particularly prone to error in the later third trimester, when the head may be deep in the pelvis, and the measurements may be distorted by molding.

THE MENOPAUSE

By John Studd, M.D.
London, England

In the latter part of the twentieth century women will live approximately one third of their lives after the cessation of reproductive potential. Far from being a welcome relief from fertility, these years are considered by doctors and patients alike as something more than a manifestation of the natural aging process. Current medical opinion clearly accepts that the postmenopausal woman is suffering a chronic endocrinopathy associated with varied symptomatic and degenerative changes that may be greatly affected by her sociocultural background. The symptoms in 25 per cent of women are severe enough to warrant specific replacement therapy. Fifty per cent of women have minimal symptoms that last a few months, and the remainder seem to be untouched by any characteristic climacteric problems.

The menopause occurs on average at age 50 and simply refers to the cessation of menstruation. This well-defined point in life may occur abruptly or after cycles of increasing length with decreasing menstrual flow. Heavy, frequent, or irregular periods at this time are not part of the normal approach to the menopause and should be investigated. Ovarian failure begins many years, perhaps as many as 10, before periods cease as the number of oocytes in the ovary diminishes in number by a progressive process of atresia. This prolonged time of failure of ovulation with the decreasing output of ovarian hormones is known as the climacteric. This may last for as long as 20 years, taking the woman through decreasing fertility, the menopause, and the atrophies of prolonged estrogen lack. The long-term effect of the climacteric may be particularly severe after oophorectomy in younger women or in those women who suffer a premature menopause.

PATHOLOGIC CHANGES

Pelvic tissues are the principal target organs for the sex steroids, and the changes are most readily observable in the vagina. The vaginal skin atrophies and loses its glycogen and protective acidic environment, allowing infection with commensal organisms. Vaginal cytology will show a preponderance of basal and parabasal cells with few mature, superficial cornified cells. Atrophic vaginitis may be obvious on examination. The uterus and fallopian tubes also involute, and the tiny cervix becomes flush with a narrowed vaginal vault. The labia and clitoris atrophy and become less sexually responsive. The bladder mucosa may show atrophic trigonitis, and the urethral tone decreases with resultant loss of urinary control. Estrogen deprivation leads to a negative nitrogen balance with a reduction in muscular strength as muscles become invaded with fibroblasts. The epidermis becomes thinner, and the subcutaneous fat atrophies with loss of elasticity and turgor. Similar changes occur in the breasts, causing them to lose contour. The ligaments surrounding joints lose their tone, giving rise to joint pain.

There are two important metabolic effects of estrogen deficiency, namely coronary thrombosis and postmenopausal osteoporosis. After ovarian failure the plasma levels of cholesterol, triglyceride, and β-lipoproteins rise. These are factors in the complex pathogenesis of coronary thrombosis, because before the menopause nonsmoking women have some immunity from coronary heart disease, but subsequently the incidence of myocardial infarction approaches that of men. The age at which the menopause occurs is significant, as epidemiologic studies in women who have suffered an early myocardial infarction demonstrate that an early menopause is a considerable risk factor, occurring in 18 per cent of the study population, compared with 3 per cent of controls.

Similarly, menopausal bone disease in the form of osteoporosis, with an increased incidence of fracture of the lower radius or the neck of the femur and crush fractures of the vertebrae, is now recognized as a hazard of estrogen deprivation. Estrogens act as an antiparathormone, being anticatabolic to bone formation. With ovarian failure, demineralization of the bone occurs to the extent of 1 to 3 per cent of body calcium per year, with a demonstrable increase in plasma calcium and alkaline phosphatase and an increased urinary calcium loss.

HORMONAL CHANGES

In the premenopausal woman the source of most estrone and estradiol is from direct ovarian secretion. The remainder is an insignificant amount from peripheral conversion of androstenedione and testosterone. Estrone and estradiol are interconvertible. On the other hand, there is virtually no ovarian production of steroids after menopause; estrone is produced by the peripheral conversion of adrenal androstenedione, and estradiol results from the conversion of estrone, testosterone, and androstenedione. Estrone and estradiol values fall to 20 and 30 per cent, respectively, of normal proliferative phase values. Testosterone levels remain essentially unchanged in the 30 years after the menopause, but androstenedione values fall to 40 per cent of normal values. The pituitary gonadotropins—follicle-stimulating hormone (FSH) and luteinizing hormone (LH)—are secreted in increased amounts in a vain attempt to stimulate ovulation even before the periods cease. The peak climacteric values are found 2 to 3 years after the menopause, with FSH being 13 times the levels of the proliferative phase and LH being three times the proliferative phase levels. However, the climacteric levels of LH never reach those of the periovulatory surge found in the reproductive phase of life. Consequently, an LH assay cannot be used as a simple diagnostic test of ovarian failure.

SYMPTOMS

The symptomatic response to the menopause will depend on the amount and rate of estrogen depletion, the inherited and acquired ability of the woman to succumb to or withstand the natural aging process, and, above all, the individual psychologic impact of the emotional implications of the change of life. The classic symptoms of the climacteric are those of vasomotor instability and vaginal atrophy. The hot flushes (or flashes) and sweats, particularly at night, tension or migrainous headaches, and palpitations are distressing symptoms that may antedate the menopause by several years. Disturbed sleep may lead to fatigue and loss of concentration. Dyspareunia, lack of lubrication, itching, and bleeding may follow the vaginal changes. Loss of libido, sometimes resulting from these local changes, may also be a manifestation of systemic decreases in estradiol and androgen levels in women who do not complain of a dry, uncomfortable vagina during intercourse.

Depression associated with low levels of free tryptophan is an integral part of the protean symptomatology, as is bone, joint, and muscle pain. Certainly these symptoms have a multifactorial cause, and the stressful social environment of the middle-aged woman should not be underestimated; but if these problems occur for the first time during middle age, it is likely that they are a direct result of loss of ovarian hormones. The bladder, urethra, and genital tract have a common embryologic origin, and the atrophy of the trigone and the periurethral vascular tissues is a cause of many cases of urinary frequency, urgency, and urge incontinence that are commonplace in women of this age group.

In 1969 the International Health Foundation undertook a survey by questionnaire of 2000 women between the ages of 46 and 55 in several European countries. It emerged that the symptoms most commonly experienced were flushes (55 per cent), tiredness (43 per cent), nervousness (41 per cent), sweating (39 per cent), headaches (38 per cent), insomnia (32 per cent), depression (30 per cent), irritability (29 per cent), joint and muscle pain (25 per cent), dizziness (24 per cent), palpitations (24 per cent), and pins and needles (22 per cent). However, *the order of symptoms complained of* was very different, the patients being worried most by depression, sexual difficulties, and faulty memory.

DIAGNOSIS

The diagnosis in a woman whose periods have ceased for a year or more should be straightforward. She is postmenopausal and will be estrogen deficient, although in some patients, particularly the obese, extraovarian conversion of adrenal androstenedione in the body fat and muscle may be responsible for considerable amounts of estrone. The symptoms outlined, if occurring close to the menopause, should be adequate for diagnosis without the need of any hormone assays. Cytologic studies of the cornification of vaginal cells may show an estrogen-deficient smear but, unless read by an expert cytologist, are useful only in those patients in whom the diagnosis is obvious without laboratory tests.

The difficulty in diagnosis occurs in the premenopausal woman and those who have previously had a hysterectomy with ovarian conservation. In the former the cycles may be anovulatory; in the other group progressive ovarian failure may occur unnoticed. The diagnosis, if suspected, can usually be made by a careful history eliciting mood change, dry vagina during intercourse, and recent loss of libido. It is important to establish that these are new symptoms, as psychologic problems abound at this age and one must be cautious of the chronic hypochondriacal psychoneurotic patient attempting to cure her long-term ills with estrogen therapy. The appearance of hot flashes and sweats should virtually clinch the diagnosis. If diagnostic proof is required, a single elevated plasma FSH result, a simpler assay than estradiol, or simply a trial of estrogen therapy should be sufficient.

DIFFERENTIAL DIAGNOSIS

It is possible in a state of therapeutic enthusiasm to ascribe spurious symptoms to the climacteric syndrome. Long-standing foibles of behavior or mood, reactive depression, and the domestic frustrations of middle age are not part of a deficiency state. Similarly, arthritis, backache, and headache may have other causes and require careful investigation. Hyperthyroidism may produce disorders of temperature response identical to those of vasomotor instability of the climacteric. Nevertheless, "common things occur commonly," and many debilitating symptoms occurring in women for the first time at about the time of the menopause are directly the result of the local and metabolic effects of estrogen loss.

INFECTION AND INFLAMMATION OF THE FEMALE GENITAL TRACT

By William E. Josey, M.D.
Atlanta, Georgia

A wide variety of infectious and inflammatory disorders may involve the vulva, vagina, and cervix uteri. This review excludes the classic venereal diseases (gonorrhea, syphilis, chancroid, granuloma inguinale, and lymphogranuloma venereum), which are discussed in other articles on these topics.

DIAGNOSTIC PRINCIPLES AND METHODS

The possible symptoms of genital tract infection and inflammation include itching or irritation (pruritus vulvae), local discomfort, and dyspareunia. Itching is experienced only on the vulvar skin but may be indicative of either primary disease of the vulva or, most commonly, primary vaginal disease with secondary vulvar irritation.

Abnormal vaginal discharge, with or without pruritus, may be related to either vaginitis or cervicitis. The term leukorrhea is used to signify vaginal discharge as an objective physical sign, although many discharges are not pure white in color, as this designation implies. It should be remembered that there are individual differences as well as cyclic variations in the quantity of the normal physiologic secretions. Moreover, increased volume of vaginal discharge may be caused by oral contraceptive drugs (due to hormone-induced secretions from the cervical glands) and by intrauterine contraceptive devices (due to their irritant effect on the endometrium and endocervix).

Diagnostic clues may emerge from careful history-taking, including the social, obstetric-gynecologic, and general medical histories. It is especially important to obtain information regarding sexual activity, contraceptive practices, and drug therapy for the current complaint or for other conditions. Often it is necessary to assist the patient in describing the exact nature of the problem; for example, a patient may say "I have an infection," meaning "I have a vaginal discharge."

It is important to bear in mind that most infectious diseases of the female genital tract are transmitted sexually. Also, some infections, such as candidiasis, although not ordinarily transmitted sexually, are acquired in this manner in some instances. Hence, coexistent infections are commonly observed, necessitating careful evaluation of the patient in all cases.

Appropriate treatment of genital tract infection and inflammation depends upon specificity of the diagnosis. The most important laboratory methods are the saline wet mount preparation, cytologic techniques, cultures for certain suspected microbial agents, and tissue biopsy. Each method has its pitfalls and limitations, and these should be taken into account in arriving at a diagnosis. Oftentimes the diagnosis can be made with confidence on the basis of the clinical appearance of the lesions, as in florid candidiasis. However, many vulvar lesions and most cases of leukorrhea require laboratory investigation.

VULVITIS

The vulva is subject to involvement with most of the infectious and inflammatory processes affecting the integument elsewhere. Among these are pyodermas, irritant and allergic reactions, and various other dermatoses, such as Behçet's syndrome, psoriasis, and lichen planus. Contact vulvitis or vulvovaginitis may result from hypersensitivity to topically applied medications, contraceptive chemicals, or hygienic preparations; true allergic reactions are relatively rare.

Seborrheic dermatitis is characterized by greasy and scaly eruptions arising from sebaceous gland overactivity. When present in the vulvar and pubic region, it is most often preceded by typical dandruff of the scalp.

Hidradenitis suppurativa, an infection of the apocrine glands, affects chiefly the vulva and axillae. The lesions are usually multiple and nodular, with eventual abscess formation.

Bartholinitis is usually recognized clinically by cystic enlargement of the gland and tenderness. Abscess formation is commonly noted.

Fungal Infections

The important fungal infections of the vulva are the tineas and candidiasis. Other mycoses involve the vulva very rarely. Laboratory diagnosis is made by microscopic examination of skin scrapings or by culture. Diabetic vulvitis is a special type of candidiasis presenting a characteristic appearance of intense erythema and edema with associated pustules and thrush patches. A similar but less erythematous picture is occasionally seen in the absence of diabetes.

Viral Infections

Viruses known to infect the vulva are herpes simplex viruses types 1 and 2, wart viruses, the virus of molluscum contagiosum, varicella-zoster virus, and vaccinia virus. Herpes zoster (shingles) represents an endogenous reactivation of varicella-zoster virus, initially acquired from an attack of varicella (chickenpox); rarely, herpes zoster may affect the vulva, chiefly in association with immunosuppressive drug therapy. Aberrant vaccinia of the vulva, which may be contracted by an unvaccinated child or adult through intimate exposure to a recently vaccinated person, is also rare.

Condyloma acuminatum (genital wart) is a sexually transmitted disease caused by a human papovavirus. The incubation period may be as long as several months. The disease commonly involves the vulva or perianal region, or both, but may also affect the cervix and vagina. Characteristically, the papillomatous lesions are multiple and have a tendency to spread and coalesce. Proliferation is influenced by immune factors, pregnancy, and oral contraceptive drugs. An uncommon but significant malignant potential is recognized. The diagnosis is confirmed by biopsy.

Genital herpes simplex infections are usually acquired through sexual contact, the majority of infections being due to herpes simplex virus type 2. Compared with cervical infection, a higher percentage of vulvar lesions are caused by herpes simplex virus type 1, but a differentiation of the two viral types of infection requires laboratory testing and at the present time is not of importance from a therapeutic viewpoint. Herpes simplex lesions of the vulva first appear as single or multiple vesicles on the outer labial skin, but the lesions are usually observed as shallow ulcers on the inner mucosal surfaces. In primary disease, in which there has been no exposure by the patient to either viral type prior to the current attack, the clinical course is likely to be more severe, with very painful ulcers, fever, and inguinal lymphadenopathy. In such patients the lesions may persist for 2 weeks or longer. On the other hand, recurrent lesions on the vulva cause only mild discomfort and are short-lived in patients with an intact immune system. Laboratory methods of diagnosis are discussed in the article on Herpes simplex virus infections.

Molluscum contagiosum is an innocuous epidermal disease of viral etiology. Sexually acquired infection may involve the mons pubis, inner aspect of the thighs, and vulva. The lesions are usually multiple and appear as tiny papules, 1 to 2 mm in diameter, umbilicated, and containing a caseous material. In questionable cases the diagnosis may be confirmed by microscopic demonstration of the large cytoplasmic inclusions (molluscum bodies).

Infections Caused by Insects

The principal parasitic disease of the vulva is pediculosis pubis, caused by the crab louse, *Phthirus pubis*. Examination with a magnifying lens may reveal the nits and parasites in the pubic hair.

Other insects, such as chiggers and the itch mite, *Sarcoptes scabei*, affect the vulva mainly as a part of a more generalized infestation.

Other Vulvar Lesions

Chronic white lesions of the vulva associated with pruritus are classified as the vulvar dystrophies. Hyperplastic dystrophy, lichen sclerosus, and mixed dystrophy are differentiated histologically in biopsy material. Some gynecologic pathologists consider hyperplastic dystrophy to be identical to lichen simplex chronicus (neurodermatitis). Progressive cellular atypical change, possibly indicating a malignant potential, is rare.

Finally, in the differential diagnosis of chronic pruritus vulvae one must include the burning vulva syndrome, in which there is no demonstrable disease. In the author's experience, most patients with this syndrome are overtly depressed or hostile, suggesting a psychosomatic disorder.

VAGINITIS

Candidiasis is the most frequently occurring infection of the vagina. The prevalence of vaginal candidiasis is influenced by a number of factors, including immune and metabolic factors, pregnancy, and therapeutic drugs, such as antibiotics, oral contraceptive drugs, and corticosteroids. Environmental factors, including increased genital moisture, also seem to play a role. The major symptoms are itching due to secondary vulvar involvement and vaginal discharge. The most characteristic sign is erythema of the vestibule. Thrush patches are seen on the vaginal mucosa in some cases. The discharge is variable in amount and must be differentiated from that of normal cellular dissolution. The diagnosis is made by wet mount examination or by culture on Sabouraud's medium.

Second in frequency of occurrence is *Gardnerella vaginalis* vaginitis, formerly known as *Haemophilus vaginalis* vaginitis or *Corynebacterium vaginale* vaginitis, and sometimes erroneously referred to as "nonspecific vaginitis." *Gardnerella vaginalis* vaginitis is a specific sexually transmitted infection in which there is colonization of desquamated vaginal epithelial cells by the bacterium, with practically no inflammatory reaction in the mucosa. The associated leukorrhea is typically homogeneous, grayish-white in color, and malodorous. When vaginal secretions are mixed with 10 per cent potassium hydroxide, a "fishy" odor is given off due to release of amines from superinfecting anaerobic organisms. The diagnosis is confirmed by wet mount examination or by culture.

Trichomoniasis is a sexually transmitted disease caused by the unicellular protozoan organism *Trichomonas vaginalis.* The discharge varies, but it is commonly purulent and malodorous. Identification of trichomonads in the wet mount preparation establishes the diagnosis. The organisms may also be demonstrated by culture techniques. Cytologic detection in routine Papanicolaou smears may be the first indication of infection in asymptomatic women.

Other parasitic infections of the vagina are rare in adults, but pinworm infestation (*Enterobius*) is a major cause of pediatric vaginitis. Amebiasis and schistosomiasis of the vagina occur mainly in underdeveloped areas of the world.

Extensive involvement of the vagina is uncommon as a manifestation of genital herpes simplex and wart virus infections, but may be seen in immunocompromised patients. Recently, attention has been called to occult flat warts of the vagina, best revealed by colposcopy.

The vaginal mucosa is highly resistant to bacterial infection; hence, primary vaginitis due to normal bacterial flora of the vagina rarely occurs. However, mention should be made of the recently identified *toxic shock syndrome* associated with toxins of *Staphylococcus aureus.* There is evidence pointing to tampon-produced mucosal ulcers as a possible portal of entry.

Atrophic vaginitis is related to loss of estrogen support as a consequence of menopause, castration, or ovarian failure from other causes. The mucosa appears thin and inflamed. The diagnosis is made by the finding of pus cells and a preponderance of intermediate and parabasal cells in the wet mount preparation.

Desquamative inflammatory vaginitis is the name given to a relatively rare condition of unknown etiology in which there is mucosal inflammation, mainly in the upper half of the vagina, in the presence of normal ovarian function.

CERVICITIS

The cervical squamous portio vaginalis is often involved in the vaginitides listed. Infections having their origin in the cervix affect chiefly the endocervical glandular epithelium and junctional zone. Herpes simplex cervicitis, which may occur with or without external lesions, usually gives the appearance of acute inflammation rather than discrete ulcers as seen on the vulva; the diagnosis can be made virologically or cytopathologically (see article on Herpes simplex virus infections). A large body of evidence implicates herpes simplex virus type 2 in cervical carcinogenesis. Herpetic cervicitis is also a major source of virus in intrapartum transfer of the infection from mother to the neonate. Cervicitis due to *Chlamydia trachomatis* is largely a subclinical infection, but it may have clinical significance in some patients as a source of tubal infection; cultures are not yet widely available. Cervical condyloma acuminatum probably is related to some cases of cervical neoplasia.

Almost all parous women and many who have not borne children show histologic evidence of chronic cervicitis. Clinically significant chronic cervicitis causes a malodorous discharge from the endocervical glandular epithelium. The cervix may appear inflamed, and nabothian cysts are commonly present. Dysplasia and carcinoma should be ruled out by biopsy prior to treatment.

ENDOMETRIOSIS

By D. Erskine Carmichael, M.D.
Birmingham, Alabama

Endometriosis describes the pathologic finding of ectopically located endometrial tissue.

When the endometrium locally invades the uterine musculature, the term *endometriosis interna* or *adenomyosis* is given. Endometrial tissue that becomes viably attached to structures outside the uterus is designated *endometriosis externa.* The latter is by far the more commonly noted form of endometriosis and is the type usually indicated when the term endometriosis is used.

The traditional division of endometriosis into internal and external types is still useful, since the manifestations of the pathologic processes and the implications for management of the two forms differ.

ENDOMETRIOSIS INTERNA (ADENOMYOSIS)

Endometriosis interna (adenomyosis) is characterized by the late onset of dysmenorrhea, menorrhagia, and dyspareunia. Lower midline abdominal discomfort may occur for several days before, during and after the menses. The condition occurs primarily in multiparous women, toward the end of their reproductive years. There seems to be a decline in fertility and frequency of ovulation after the diagnosis has been made.

The extent to which the basal layer of endometrium invades the uterine wall along the connective tissue channels between the muscle bundles determines the degree of uterine tenderness and anterior-posterior enlargement present. These aberrant endometrial cells, being derived from the basal layer of the endometrium, do not respond cyclically to the ovarian hormones to the same extent as the more superficial endometrium. Focal areas of bleeding sometimes may be seen. However, the tenderness and firmness of the uterus, especially near the menses, probably results primarily from the edema of the adenomyosis interposed among the irritated rigid muscle bundles.

The quantity and duration of menstrual bleeding is increased. This abnormality persists despite curettage and hormonal therapy. Estrogens and progestins may actually augment the symptoms.

Although the uterine enlargement generally is of no more than moderate degree and symmetric, localized concentrations of adenomyosis may produce an irregular surface indistinguishable from that encountered with leiomyomas. Interestingly, adenomyosis and leiomyomas of the uterus are frequently present in the same patient. Adenomyosis produces chiefly posterior uterine wall enlargement.

Endometriosis interna (adenomyosis) can be confirmed only by pathologic examination of the uterus. The diagnosis is strongly indicated and may warrant hysterectomy when persistent or increasing dysmenorrhea, menorrhagia, and dyspareunia are associated with an enlarged, tender, and firm uterus.

ENDOMETRIOSIS EXTERNA (ENDOMETRIOSIS)

Endometriosis externa consists of nests of endometrial-type cells that respond cyclically to the ovarian hormones, producing small amounts of blood. The accumulated blood accounts for the dark powder-burn or berry-like lesions that stimulate surrounding fibrosis as the body attempts to wall off the foreign tissue.

The diagnosis of endometriosis externa at this time still depends upon palpable or visual evidence leading to pathologic confirmation. How many patients experience pain or infertility from the presence of undetectable endometriosis is unknown, but it has become evident that patients exhibiting no endometriosis on surgical exploration may demonstrate, several months later, visual (on laparoscopy) or palpable evidence of the disease. Attempts are under way to find newer diagnostic methods, which may provide a means whereby endometriosis can be detected before it becomes observable and treated before the ravages of pain, infertility, and other sequelae are encountered.

At present, gynecologists are often required either to perform patch-up surgery for fertility enhancement in advanced cases of endometriosis or to remove the reproductive organs altogether, with the attendant surgical risks, in those who have completed their families or no longer wish to pursue fertility therapeusis. Earlier diagnosis leading to prevention of its disabling consequences is the ultimate goal of those interested in conquering this disease.

Estimates based on widely varying incidence reports place the prevalence of endometriosis externa as affecting about 20 per cent of all menstruating women, making it one of the more common gynecologic disorders. The disease is associated with infertility in about 30 per cent and with pain in about 45 per cent of patients. These observations, combined with the unknown additional number of undetectable cases of endometriosis, indicate the magnitude of the problem.

Endometriosis externa has been observed in women from the ages of 9 to 83 years. Most patients, however, present with signs or symptoms during their early to middle reproductive years, and activity generally ceases with menopause. A definite familial tendency exists, with the disease often affecting sisters or grandmother, mother, and daughter. Patients with a family history of endometriosis seem to have more severe and recurrent manifestations of the disease. The degree of pain associated with endometriosis is not necessarily correlated with the extent of disease, and infertility occurs in women with minimal disease.

History

The classic historical findings of patients with endometriosis externa are dysmenorrhea, dyspareunia, and occasionally diarrhea or painful defecation associated with menses. The miscarriage rate is increased in women with endometriosis. There is a suggestion that miscarriage may be the initial reproductive failure noted with endometriosis, with infertility being a later development. Menstrual irregularities may also be present, apparently due to corpus luteum dysfunction. Pelvic pain sometimes becomes a more constant feature, occurring intermittently throughout the menstrual cycle.

Physical Findings

On physical examination, the typical fine, sand-like irregularities or, in more advanced cases, larger indurated, roughened masses may be palpated along or between the uterine insertions of the uterosacral ligaments. It is not unusual to detect bowel adherent to the posterior aspect of the uterus at and above the level of the attachments of these ligaments, and frequently the uterus is held in retroversion by these adhesions. Decreased mobility or fixation of the ovaries may occur. Uterine leiomyomas are present with increased frequency in patients with endometriosis. Fortunately, the three most common sites of endometriosis (the ovaries, cul-de-sac, and sigmoid colon) can be evaluated by palpation. The rectovaginal examination is most useful for this purpose.

In some instances, endometriosis is more obvious if it occurs on the cervix or in a scar such as that of a vaginal vault, episiotomy, or abdominal incision. These lesions typically enlarge and become tender cyclically at or near the time of menses and may become visibly distended with blood. Cyclic vaginal bleeding has been noted following hysterectomy in patients with endometriosis of the vaginal vault. The diagnostic potential of the physical examination is enhanced if it is performed at the time of menses. Congenital anomalies causing obstruction of menstrual flow are often associated with endometriosis.

Diagnostic Procedures

Rarely, cyclic rectal bleeding, hematuria, or hemoptysis coinciding with menses may occur and should alert the clinician to the possibility of endometriosis of the respective organs. Radiologic or endoscopic examination of these areas will aid in making a diagnosis. Marked constriction of bowel or ureter may be found radiologically. The typical colonic constriction is localized and not annular as in the case of carcinoma. Endoscopically, the mucosa of bladder or bowel is usually intact even though bleeding may occur. These procedures should ideally be performed at the time of menstruation.

Laparoscopy has greatly facilitated the early diagnosis of endometriosis, especially when physical findings have been minimal or absent. Chronic pelvic pain or infertility has usually prompted such procedures. Biopsy confirmation may be obtained at the time of laparoscopy. Early diagnosis is most important in the prevention of serious sequelae, since treatment—surgical or medical—may be instituted while the disease process is minimal. Unfortunately, there are no radiologic, sonographic, or chemical studies by which general pelvic endometriosis can be diagnosed. A high degree of suspicion derived from a patient's history leading to a careful search via vaginal and rectovaginal examination will often establish the clinical diagnosis. Biopsy confirmation should be made whenever possible prior to initiating therapy.

Emergency Aspects

Although endometriosis usually produces symptoms of gradually increasing intensity, sometimes crises may arise requiring immediate attention. Should an endometrioma of the ovary rupture, the patient may present with an acute abdomen due to the expulsion of the bloody contents, which cause marked peritoneal irritation. Pain is severe, and laparotomy should be performed to relieve pain and to prevent adhesions and possible peritoneal implants. This sudden event most often occurs before or during a menstrual period. The findings may simulate those of a ruptured tubal pregnancy, but absence of pregnancy symptoms, intermenstrual bleeding, or delayed menses together with a negative radioimmunoassay pregnancy test make this diagnosis unlikely.

Several cases of hemoperitoneum with hypotension have followed erosion of a blood vessel from a tiny endometrial implant. Should the source of bleeding at exploratory laparotomy for abdominal hemorrhage be difficult to locate, this possibility should be considered.

Differential Diagnosis

The two diagnoses most often confused with endometriosis are pelvic inflammatory disease and ovarian carcinoma. The importance of differentiating these disease entities is obvious and demands a definitive diagnosis as early as possible.

Both endometriosis and pelvic inflammatory disease may be associated with recurrent pelvic pain, enlarged adnexa, and infertility. However, with endometriosis the pain more often occurs near a menstrual period and the adnexa are usually more firm, irregular, fixed, and perhaps less tender. Although mild leukocytosis and fever have been noted with endometriosis, these findings more often are associated with pelvic inflammatory disease. Nodularity in the cul-de-sac and dense adherence of bowel to the posterior uterus suggest endometriosis rather than an infectious process. When findings are minimal and a patient presents frequently with pelvic pain in the absence of a known infectious agent, laparoscopy should be performed to establish a diagnosis and institute an appropriate therapeutic plan.

Ovarian carcinoma, like endometriosis, frequently presents with nodularity in the pelvis and fixation of one or both adnexa. It may be impossible to differentiate these two entities by pelvic examination, and a definitive diagnosis should be reached surgically. When endometriosis is early and minimal findings are located in typical areas, the pathologic diagnosis may be reasonably delayed. However, ovarian carcinoma has been treated medically as endometriosis, causing serious postponement of treatment of the malignancy.

CLASSIFICATION OF ENDOMETRIOSIS

The American Fertility Society has introduced a classification of endometriosis. It is hoped that all physicians will utilize this format in describing the extent of disease in patients with endometriosis undergoing surgery.

Employment of a standard classification will allow physicians to communicate better descriptions of the location and extent of disease and will permit more accurate comparisons in research studies. Forms outlining the classification system are available free of charge from The American Fertility Society.*

---

*The American Fertility Society, 924 South 18th Street, Birmingham, Alabama 35205.

Recent research has revealed increased levels of prostaglandins in peritoneal fluid of patients with endometriosis, and an immune mechanism has been postulated as a possible cause for the infertility. Should a specific diagnostic factor be identified whereby serum analysis could be used to detect early, nonvisible and nonpalpable endometriosis, a giant step will have been made toward conquering this common and often disabling disease.

BENIGN AND MALIGNANT UTERINE CORPUS TUMORS

By Herbert J. Buchsbaum, M.D.
Pittsburgh, Pennsylvania
and Samuel Lifshitz, M.D.
Dallas, Texas

The uterine corpus, like the cervix, can be the seat of epithelial and mesenchymal tumors, but unlike the cervix, the corpus is not accessible to direct visual examination. The uterine corpus is the site of the most common benign pelvic neoplasm, leiomyomata uteri (fibroids), as well as the most common female genital malignancy, endometrial adenocarcinoma.

We will first outline techniques applicable in the diagnosis of benign and malignant tumors of the uterine corpus, then describe their use in specific pathologic entities.

DIAGNOSTIC TECHNIQUES

Abdominal and Pelvic Examination

A complete history and physical examination must be done in the assessment of any uterine neoplasm. Since the uterus is confined on two sides by the bony pelvis, enlargement can often be appreciated on abdominal examination. The symphysis pubis should be used as a reference point, and lesions should be described in centimeters above this point. Symmetry and mobility of the pelvic or abdominal tumor should also be recorded. Bimanual and rectovaginal pelvic examination can generally separate uterine from adnexal lesions. On bimanual examination, an attempt should be made to identify the relationship of the uterine corpus to the tumor mass—e.g., does it move when the uterus is moved, or does it appear to arise laterally, as from an ovary? Rectovaginal examination will help identify cul-de-sac lesions, which generally do not arise from the uterine corpus, as well as determine the integrity of the rectal mucosa.

Papanicolaou Smear

Cervical Papanicolaou smears are unreliable in detecting adenocarcinoma of the endometrium, missing the diagnosis in as many as 50 per cent of patients. Factors responsible for this poor yield are the acid pH of the vagina and the presence of lytic enzymes. The diagnostic accuracy of cytologic detection of endometrial cancer can be improved by the aspiration of material from the endocervical canal with a small pipette and a 25-ml rubber bulb. The improved accuracy (75 per cent) is due to better cellular preservation in the endocervical canal.

Endometrial Biopsy Techniques

A wide variety of instruments are available for the sampling of the endometrium. Some depend on cytologic, others on histologic, sampling. Most are used in office procedures requiring no anesthesia, since the instruments are small-diameter cannulas that can be passed through the cervical os without dilation. The accuracy of these techniques is noted in Table 1.

It must be remembered that an "inadequate" or "suspicious" biopsy report requires a fractional curettage (see later description) under anesthesia.

Dilatation and Curettage

Dilatation and curettage is ideally done under general anesthesia in an operating room, preceded by a thorough bimanual and rectovaginal pelvic examination. The cervix should be carefully examined before the fractional curettage is performed. The cervix is grasped with a tenaculum; the endocervical canal (2 to 5 cm in length) is curetted with a small, sharp curette; and the specimen is submitted in a container labeled "endocervical curettings." The uterus is then sounded with a calibrated uterine sound and the size recorded. The internal os is then progressively dilated with Hanks or Hegar dilators. The Goodell mechanical dilator should not be used. The endometrial cavity should be scraped with a large curette in either a clockwise or a counterclockwise manner to assure sampling of the entire cavity, and the specimen is submitted to the pathologist in a separate container. The surgeon must then explore the cavity with a Stone-Randall type polyp forceps so that any broad-based polyps that escaped the curette are identified. If any are grasped with the instrument, they are twisted free, removed, and submitted for histopathologic examination. Finally, any visible lesions on the cervix are biopsied.

Table 1. Reported Accuracy of Outpatient Methods of Detecting Endometrial Adenocarcinoma

Method	Accuracy (%)
Cervicovaginal smear	42.8
Endocervical aspiration	72.8
Endometrial lavage	81.6
Gravlee Jet Washer	81.7
Endometrial brush	87.4
Endometrial aspiration	88.7
Endometrial biopsy	90.0
Vabra curettage	98.0
Vacutage	100.0

Hysteroscopy

In hysteroscopy, an endoscope utilizing a lens system and a fiberoptic light source is introduced into the endometrial cavity and a seal created by occluding the cervix. The cavity is then distended by a liquid or gas medium, allowing examination of the endometrial cavity and its lining. This technique has found only limited application.

Contact Hysteroscopy

Contact hysteroscopy makes use of a newly introduced, small, and lightweight unit that operates on ambient light. No distention of the endometrial cavity is required. The limiting feature of this instrument is that the tip must be in intimate contact with the surface being examined, thus denying the operator a broad view of the endometrial cavity. Furthermore, the irregular shape of the uterus precludes complete examination and limits examination of the lower uterine segment.

Hysterosalpingography

Hysterosalpingography, a radiographic technique, allows assessment of the shape and contour of the endometrial cavity. Utilizing a special cannula and acorn, a radiopaque material is injected into the uterus and x-rays are obtained. Anteroposterior as well as oblique and lateral films help in evaluating the cavity. While used most commonly to assess tubal patency and uterine anomalies, submucosal myomas and endometrial polyps can also be identified.

Ultrasound

Pelvic ultrasonography is now widely available for evaluation of pelvic tumors. No risks to its use have yet been identified, so that it is suitable in distinguishing an early pregnancy from a uterine tumor if other studies are equivocal. The technique discriminates between solid and cystic tumors, and most often between uterine and adnexal lesions.

Computed Tomography (CT Scan)

Computed tomography is the most sensitive x-ray technique available. When used with contrast material in the gastrointestinal or genitourinary tracts, CT can give a three-dimensional image of any pelvic lesion. Newer machines have the ability to distinguish density of pelvic structures, thereby giving a clue to the type of tissue of which the tumor is composed.

Laparoscopy

Laparoscopy, an operative technique that can be done in day-surgery, offers direct visualization of the pelvic viscera and the uterine serosal surface. Performed under general anesthesia, a needle is introduced into the abdomen and a pneumoperitoneum created. Through a separate incision, a trocar and later an endoscope are inserted and the examination carried out.

Intravenous Pyelogram and Barium Enema

Intravenous pyelography and barium enema studies are radiographic contrast studies that occasionally are indicated in the assessment of pelvic tumors. The barium enema is helpful in distinguishing primary bowel disease (e.g., bowel cancer, ruptured appendix, or diverticulum) from genital pelvic tumors. The pyelogram is important in inflammatory and neoplastic lesions.

As noted earlier, an adequate history and abdominal and bimanual pelvic examinations are all important in the evaluation of uterine corpus tumors. There are *no* laboratory studies of value in diagnosing these tumors. Application of the techniques described will next be discussed in the diagnosis of the more common uterine tumors.

DIAGNOSIS OF UTERINE TUMORS

Leiomyomata Uteri

Uterine leiomyomas are smooth muscle tumors present in the uteri of nearly one third of women during reproductive years. Myomas are generally asymptomatic when small but may cause pressure on adjoining pelvic structures when large, i.e., producing the urge to defecate and/or urinate.

On bimanual examination the uterus is enlarged and smooth and may be multinodular. When tumors reach the size of a 14 to 16 weeks' gestation they become palpable on abdominal examination. Unless there is concomitant pelvic inflammatory disease or severe endometriosis, the uterus is generally mobile. If low-lying or intraligamentous myomas are suspected on pelvic examination, intravenous pyelography should be performed. Cervical and intraligamentous myomas may displace or obstruct one or both ureters, information important to the surgeon. If there is abnormal uterine bleeding, heavier than normal or prolonged periods, or intermenstrual bleeding, a fractional curettage should be performed. The myomas can be submucosal or intramural in location. Submucosal tumors can be appreciated during curettage as irregularity of the cavity and identified on hysterosalpingography; intramural lesions are identified by ultrasonography or CT scan.

Uterine Sarcoma

Uterine sarcomas are rare mesenchymal tumors, accounting for approximately 5 per cent of uterine neoplasms. They can occur at any age; the average for all histologic types is in the mid-50s. Thus, any uterine tumor increasing in size in a postmenopausal patient requires evaluation. Interestingly, nearly one third of mixed mesodermal tumors (sarcoma plus carcinoma) present with a lesion prolapsing through the external cervical os. Tissue prolapsing through the os in a younger woman probably represents products of conception; in the postmenopausal individual, the diagnosis of sarcoma must be seriously entertained. Dilatation and curettage will generally identify the mixed müllerian sarcomas.

Endometrial Carcinoma

Approximately 36,000 new adenocarcinomas of the endometrium are diagnosed annually in this country. Because bleeding, generally postmenopausal but rarely intermenstrual, occurs early in nearly 90 per cent of the patients, a fractional curettage will establish the diagnosis early. Early diagnosis and effective treatment generally result in an excellent prognosis. We do not believe that hysteroscopy and hysterosalpingography should be used in the diagnosis of endometrial adenocarcinoma. The information gained does not justify the potential risks of dissemination of the cancer via the fallopian tubes. The diagnosis of adenocarcinoma of the endometrium requires endometrial and endocervical curettings, as well as uterine sounding. The current International Federation of Gynecology and Obstetrics (FIGO) classification takes these important prognostic factors into account in the substaging of stage I. After histopathologic diagnosis is established, a thorough evaluation is required to appropriately stage the disease.

Adenomyosis

This condition is characterized by the presence of endometrial glands and stroma within the myometrium. Adenomyosis is present in over 50 per cent of uteri examined histopathologically. This ectopic endometrium may occupy a small area in the uterine wall and not be grossly evident, or it may occupy larger portions, causing a thickening and giving rise to symptoms of irregular vaginal bleeding and dysmenorrhea. The diagnosis is most frequently made on surgical specimens, although a diffuse thickening of the posterior wall can occasionally be appreciated on pelvic examination. CT scanning can establish the diagnosis preoperatively. Symptoms occur only in women of reproductive years or in postmenopausal women on estrogen replacement therapy. (See article on Endometriosis).

Endometrial Polyps

Endometrial polyps are pedunculated or sessile growths covered on three sides by endometrium and projecting into the endometrial cavity. They are most commonly found in women over 40 years old, in whom they give rise to intermenstrual bleeding or heavier than normal periods, or to bleeding in postmenopausal women. They can be single or multiple and of varying size; some have grown to fill the endometrial cavity. Not infrequently they prolapse through the external cervical os. The tip of the polyp may degenerate, giving those that prolapse into the vagina a disquieting appearance. There is only a remote danger that the surface endometrium will undergo malignant change, although hyperplasia is a common finding.

The diagnosis is generally established by endometrial curettage and probing of the endometrial cavity with a polyp forceps. Hysterography or hysteroscopy, or both, is indicated if bleeding persists after curettage.

OVARIAN TUMORS

By Samuel Lifshitz, M.D.
Dallas, Texas

Ovarian tumors constitute one of the most important conditions in gynecology. Such tumors can be functional or neoplastic, cystic or solid, endocrine active or inactive, benign or malignant. The physician's principal responsibility is to determine the precise nature of the ovarian tumor and the threat it presents to the patient's life and reproductive function. Of paramount importance is the differentiation between benign and malignant ovarian tumors. The prognosis of ovarian cancer relates to the stage of disease at the time of diagnosis. Over 60 per cent of patients with ovarian cancer have widespread intraperitoneal disease when the diagnosis is first established.

FUNCTIONAL TUMORS

Follicle and corpus luteum cysts are the most frequent cause of ovarian enlargement in women of reproductive age. They are pathologic variants of the normal physiologic events that affect the cyclic ovarian function and are characteristically unilateral, unilocular, and less than 10 cm in diameter. Theca lutein cysts result from overstimulation of the ovary by human chorionic gonadotropin (hCG), are uncommon in normal pregnancy, and more commonly are associated with hydatidiform mole and choriocarcinoma. These cysts are typically bilateral. They can reach enormous dimensions and regress spontaneously with decline in hCG stimulation. Anovulatory and hirsute women (Stein-Leventhal disease) may have bilateral ovarian enlargement characteristic of polycystic ovaries. Germinal inclusion cysts occur in postmenopausal women, are usually unilateral, and rarely exceed 3 to 4 cm in diameter.

Follicle and corpus luteum cysts are self-limiting. Clinical experience has taught that these cysts usually persist for only a few days or weeks. Serious problems develop only when these functional tumors undergo torsion of their pedicle with infarction or when they rupture.

NEOPLASTIC TUMORS

Neoplastic tumors of the ovary constitute a diverse group of lesions that can arise from the coelomic epi-

Table 1. Histologic Classification of Ovarian Tumors

Epithelial Tumors
Serous
Mucinous
Endometrioid
Clear cell
Brenner
Sex Cord–Stromal Tumors
Granulosa cell
Thecoma
Fibroma
Androblastomas (Sertoli-Leydig tumors)
Gynandroblastoma
Germ Cell Tumors
Dysgerminoma
Endodermal sinus tumor
Embryonal carcinoma
Polyembryoma
Choriocarcinoma
Teratomas
Immature
Mature
Monodermal (e.g., struma ovarii)
Mixed forms

thelium, the ovarian stroma, or the germ cells (Table 1). Tumors arising from the coelomic epithelium are by far the most common, accounting for 85 to 90 per cent of all ovarian neoplasms, and occur most commonly in perimenopausal and postmenopausal women. Germ cell tumors are found most frequently in children and adolescents. Gonadal stromal tumors can be hormone producing and occur in any age group.

Neoplastic ovarian tumors may be benign or malignant. The malignant tumors arise in their benign counterparts—i.e., serous and mucinous cystadenocarcinomas arise in serous and mucinous cystadenomas. The borderline tumors or tumors of low malignant potential are histologically intermediate forms that have been recently identified. These tumors may metastasize, but they have a very good long-term prognosis.

Ovarian neoplasms are the cause of more deaths than any other female genital cancer. There are about 20,000 new cases diagnosed each year, with about 11,000 deaths annually. One in 70 females born in the United States will develop ovarian carcinoma during her lifetime, and one in 100 will die of ovarian cancer. The ovary can also be the site of metastatic tumors, usually arising from a primary malignancy in the endometrium, breast, or bowel.

PRESENTING SIGNS AND SYMPTOMS

The symptoms of ovarian tumors are a reflection of tumor size and are generally related to pressure on the bladder, rectum, or other abdominal organs. Occasionally a rapidly growing ovarian tumor lying posterior to the uterus will displace the bladder anteriorly, producing some degree of urinary retention from urethral obstruction due to impingement of the vesical neck against the symphysis pubis. Impingement of an ovarian tumor against the rectosigmoid colon can produce signs and symptoms of large bowel obstruction. Torsion of the infundibulopelvic ligament with infarction or rupture of an ovarian tumor causes sharp abdominal pain and signs of peritoneal irritation.

Estrogen-producing ovarian tumors (granulosa-theca cell) cause postmenopausal bleeding in elderly women or premature sexual development in youngsters. Amenorrhea, virilization, and hirsutism with deepening of the voice accompany androgen-secreting tumors.

Ovarian cancer has an insidious onset. Symptoms often include vague abdominal discomfort, dyspepsia, nausea, and other mild gastrointestinal disturbances simulating primary gastrointestinal disorders. Abdominal distention resulting from ascites and shortness of breath are common presenting symptoms signaling extension of the neoplastic process to the abdominal cavity.

PHYSICAL EXAMINATION

The evaluation of an ovarian tumor requires a complete physical examination, with particular attention directed to the abdominal and pelvic organs. An adequate pelvic examination constitutes the most reliable means of detecting an early ovarian tumor.

Ovarian tumors are often palpable abdominally; the finding of a distended abdomen with ascites suggests a malignant ovarian neoplasm. Differentiation of ascites from a large ovarian cyst may be difficult. A fluid wave can be elicited in either condition. With the patient in the supine position, the tympanism of the small intestine should be central in a patient with ascites and lateral with a large ovarian cyst. On pelvic examination, mobile, unilateral cystic tumors are generally benign, whereas solid, fixed, and bilateral tumors are suggestive of malignant neoplasm (Table 2). An essential component of the pelvic examination is rectovaginal bimanual palpation of the pelvic structures. Small ovarian tumors, cul-de-sac nodules, and disease in the rectovaginal septum may be detected in this manner. The size of an ovarian tumor gives no clue as to its histologic nature. The largest ovarian tumors are usually mucinous cystadenomas.

LABORATORY STUDIES

Laboratory studies are of little value in the diagnosis of ovarian tumors. In early ovarian carcinoma there are no demonstrable hematologic, chemical, or enzymatic abnormalities; in advanced disease, anemia, hypoalbuminemia, hypercalcemia, and elevation of lactate dehydrogenase may be present.

With gonadal stromal hormone-producing tumors, there is elevation in serum estradiol or testosterone. Virilized women with a normal 24-hour 17-ketosteroid determination (<15 mg/24 hr) but an elevated serum testosterone (>1 ng/ml) are assumed to have an ovarian stromal tumor until proven otherwise.

Radioimmunoassay for hCG in ovarian choriocarcinoma and for alpha-fetoprotein in endodermal sinus tumor is of utility in the diagnosis and follow-up of

Table 2. Clinical Features of Benign and Malignant Ovarian Tumors

Clinical Findings	Benign	Malignant
Unilateral	+++	+
Bilateral	+	+++
Cystic	+++	+
Solid	+	+++
Mobile	+++	++
Fixed	+	+++
Irregular	+	+++
Smooth	+++	+
Ascites	+	+++
Cul-de-sac nodule	−	+++

patients with these rare germ cell tumors of the ovary. Radioimmunoassay for specific tumor markers to the more common epithelial tumors of the ovary is at present not sensitive or specific enough for clinical use.

RADIOLOGIC EVALUATION

A plain film of the abdomen frequently provides clues to the presence and nature of an ovarian tumor. Nearly half of ovarian dermoid cysts can be identified by the presence of calcification due to tooth or bone formation or by a radiolucent shadow cast by the lipid fluid filling the cyst. Papillary serous tumors, benign and malignant, may contain sufficient calcification to be visible radiographically. Metastases from malignant serous tumors may contain sufficient psammoma bodies to be visualized. A mottled pattern of calcification also may be seen with gonadoblastoma. Most ovarian tumors will produce nonspecific soft tissue densities on scout films of the abdomen.

An intravenous pyelogram is of great importance in evaluating the patient with an ovarian tumor, since it will identify the presence of ureteral obstruction and urinary tract anomalies, especially a pelvic kidney. Gastrointestinal contrast studies are helpful in excluding the presence of primary gastrointestinal malignancies and may also define intrinsic inflammatory lesions that may be confused with ovarian tumors.

A chest x-ray should be performed to exclude pulmonary metastases or pleural effusion. Lymphangiography, venography, and arteriography have no proven value in the evaluation of ovarian tumors.

OTHER DIAGNOSTIC PROCEDURES

Ultrasound imaging of the pelvic organs has been used extensively in the evaluation of ovarian tumors. Ultrasonography has the capability of localizing pelvic and intra-abdominal masses, can distinguish cystic from solid tumors, and allows for accurate assessment of dimension and consistency. Ultrasound may discriminate between uterine and adnexal masses and can also differentiate clinically occult ascitic fluid from intracystic fluid.

Isotope scans have no value in the diagnosis of ovarian tumors. Computed tomography (CT) has had limited application in the diagnosis of benign and malignant tumors. In advanced ovarian carcinoma CT permits estimation of tumor extent and response to therapy.

CYTOLOGY

Cervical cytologic examination (Papanicolaou smear) is of no value in the detection of early ovarian cancer. Generally, the Papanicolaou smear is positive only when ovarian carcinoma has metastasized to the uterine cavity or vagina. In these patients, endometrial sampling or vaginal biopsies are more rewarding. Endometrial hyperplasia and carcinoma may be found in women with estrogen-producing tumors of stromal origin. Very rarely, cells exfoliated from an ovarian cancer may be transported via the fallopian tube and uterine cavity to be detected by the Papanicolaou smear.

Abdominal distention resulting from ascites is a common presenting symptom of advanced ovarian carcinoma. Diagnostic paracentesis to detect malignant cells in the fluid is rarely indicated and should only be performed after a large fluid-filled cyst has been ruled out by ultrasonography.

LAPAROSCOPY

Laparoscopy has not been found to be of value in the evaluation of patients with suspected ovarian malignancy. Although laparoscopy may verify the presence of an ovarian tumor, visual examination alone is unreliable in determining whether an ovarian tumor is benign or malignant. Aspiration of fluid from an ovarian cyst at laparoscopy must be condemned because of the risk of spilling malignant cells into the peritoneal cavity. Similarly, the laparoscopic biopsy of ovarian tumors, cystic or otherwise, is contraindicated. In addition, it is impossible to estimate resectability of a tumor by laparoscopic examination alone, exploration of the abdominal contents is limited, and the retroperitoneal space cannot be assessed.

EXPLORATORY CELIOTOMY

Exploratory celiotomy (laparotomy) constitutes the definitive diagnostic procedure in assessing ovarian tumors. The decision as to which patient needs surgical exploration can best be determined by the patient's age and characteristics of the adnexal mass. Any ovarian mass that is greater than 10 cm, regardless of the patient's age, should be subjected to surgical exploration without delay.

During the reproductive years, ovarian tumors that are cystic and less than 10 cm in diameter can be presumed to be functional rather than neoplastic. The transitory nature of functional cysts is of prime importance in distinguishing them from true neoplasms. Oral contraceptives can be prescribed to these patients to accelerate the involution of the functional cyst on the presumption that these cysts are gonadotropin-dependent. Failure of the ovarian cyst to re-

Table 3. Differential Diagnosis of Adnexal Mass

Neoplastic
Ovarian neoplasm
Uterine myoma
Tubal carcinoma
Carcinoma of sigmoid, cecum, appendix
Retroperitoneal neoplasm
Non-neoplastic
Functional ovarian cyst
Para-ovarian cyst
Tubo-ovarian abscess
Diverticulitis
Pelvic kidney
Appendiceal abscess
Peritoneal cyst
Stool in sigmoid
Full bladder
Urachal cyst
Anterior sacral meningocele
Pregnancy (tubal, abdominal)
Abdominal wall hematoma or abscess

gress during a 4- to 6-week period of observation mandates surgical evaluation. In the premenarchal and postmenopausal women an ovarian tumor must be evaluated surgically without delay. During the postmenopausal years, the ovary becomes reduced in size and quiescent. The presence of a palpable ovary in these patients must alert the physician to the possibility of an underlying malignancy, and exploratory celiotomy is indicated.

Exploratory celiotomy in benign tumors and early ovarian cancer permits complete extirpation. In advanced ovarian carcinoma it allows the surgeon to assess the extent of the malignancy, perform reductive surgery, and obtain biopsy specimens for histologic examination in order to stage the disease. Ovarian carcinoma typically spreads by topical implantation to involve the parietal and visceral peritoneal surfaces of the abdominal organs. Malignant cells can also implant in the omentum and on the inferior surface of the diaphragm. For this reason, an adequate staging celiotomy for ovarian carcinoma should include visual and digital examination of the undersurface of the diaphragm, surface of the liver, small and large bowel serosa and their mesentery, paracolonic gutters, and the para-aortic lymph nodes. The pelvic organs and parietal peritoneum should be examined carefully and any suspicious lesions biopsied. All peritoneal fluid should be aspirated for cytologic examination. If no fluid is present in the peritoneal cavity, washings should be obtained from the pelvic and paracolonic gutters and from the undersurfaces of the diaphragm.

PITFALLS IN DIAGNOSIS

The greatest pitfall in diagnosis is the failure to differentiate an ovarian tumor from other causes of adnexal mass (Table 3), leading to an inordinate delay in surgical exploration because of unnecessary diagnostic procedures or prolonged observation.

TUMORS OF THE VULVA, VAGINA, AND CERVIX

By Edward W. Savage, M.D.
Los Angeles, California

The vulva, vagina, and cervix are parts of one organ system. Each is lined primarily by squamous epithelium and responds generally to the same stimuli, environmental and hormonal. Most of the tumors of this system are squamous. The small number of adenocarcinomas are derived primarily from appendages or glands that lubricate these structures. The remainder come from the columnar epithelium that lines the endocervix, and, in a high percentage of women, extends out onto the portio vaginalis.

VULVA

Benign Tumors of the Vulva

For the purpose of description, benign tumors of the vulva are divided into cystic and solid (Table 1).

Cystic Tumors

Bartholin Gland Cyst. Cystic dilatation of the duct of the vulvovaginal gland generally presents as a tender mass distorting the posterior labia and bulging frequently into the introitus. Such cysts usually occur in women during the reproductive years. Commonly, there is a history of prior infection. When the mass feels solid or nodular or occurs in older women, it should be totally excised for histologic examination.

Inclusion Cyst. Epidermal inclusion cysts generally occur secondary to surgery or trauma when there is disruption of the epithelium with inversion of the lining into the dermis. Frequently seen at the sites of previous scars and healed episiotomies, these cysts are usually localized, are painless, and are sometimes confused with sebaceous cysts. Diagnosis is made by simple excision and microscopic examination. Squamous cells line the cystic cavity.

Table 1. Benign Tumors of the Vulva

Cystic
Bartholin gland cyst
Inclusion cyst
Sebaceous cyst
Wolffian duct cyst
Hydrocele
Endometriosis
Solid
Fibroma
Lipoma
Condyloma
Angioma
Hydradenoma
Nevus
Granular cell myoblastoma

Sebaceous Cysts. Sebaceous cysts usually result from inflammatory blockage of the ducts of the sebaceous glands. They are usually small in size and are commonly seen on the inner surface of the labia majora and minora. The contents are cheesy or sebaceous. Ulceration and suppuration sometimes occur with the formation of small furuncles. In the absence of these phenomena, sebaceous cysts are generally asymptomatic. Definitive diagnosis is made by excision. When infection is present, the lining is not easily distinguishable and the cavity is filled with polymorphonuclear and foreign body giant cells. In the chronic stage, the cavity is lined by stratified squamous epithelium and is indistinguishable from the inclusion cyst. These cysts may occur at any age. Most are asymptomatic unless infection or trauma is present. The size varies from several millimeters to 3 to 4 cm. Sebaceous cysts are painless and well defined.

Wolffian Duct Cyst. Mesonephric or wolffian duct remnants are rare on the vulva. When large, they may project at the introitus. Diagnosis is by local excision and histologic examination.

Hydrocele. Hydrocele, a cyst of the canal of Nuck, forms where the round ligament inserts into the labium majus, carrying an investment of the peritoneum; where it becomes separated from the ligament, fluid may accumulate, forming a cyst. This cyst may present in the labium. The diagnosis is made by careful incision with dissection and exposure.

Endometriosis. In rare instances, implants of the endometrium into the vulva are seen. These are present most commonly in the region of the Bartholin gland, which suggests possible implantation at the time of surgery or drainage of a Bartholin cyst or abscess. The diagnosis is suggested by the cyclic recurrence of a painful nodule around the time of the menses.

Solid Tumors

Fibroma. Fibromas are of mesodermal origin and present as solid, round tumors in the labium majus. They are usually painless and small to moderate in size. They tend to become pedunculated if large. They may produce ulceration of the overlying skin. The microscopic picture is that of fibrous tissue with edema, and there may be an admixture of smooth and striated muscle elements. Special stains may be necessary to differentiate these growths from leiomyoma.

Lipoma. Lipomas are uncommon despite the presence of adipose tissue in the vulva, especially the labia majora. They are usually less than 4 cm in size, but large growths have been reported. They have the same clinical characteristics as those of fibromas, and the distinction is made by microscopic examination. The yellowish-appearing tumors are composed of groups of fat cells in a connective tissue stroma.

Condyloma. Condylomata acuminata, or vulvar warts, are usually seen in women during the reproductive years. They represent the most common form of the vulvar verruca and should be distinguished from the syphilitic lesion known as condyloma latum. Clinically they appear as individual or coalesced verrucous structures of the vulva and may involve the vagina or cervix. They usually begin as small papillae but may progress to the point that they form cauliflower-like masses. They appear in various sizes, are usually multiple, and may be scattered over the vulva, the adjacent perineum, buttocks, and inner thighs. They sometimes undergo pronounced enlargement during pregnancy, which may interfere with normal vaginal delivery. Some regress spontaneously post partum if not removed. Rarely malignancy may develop. Electron microscopic and other studies have confirmed a viral etiology. Microscopically the condyloma acuminatum has a tree-like structure with a central core of connective tissue covered with a hyperplastic, sometimes vacuolated epithelium characterized by acanthosis and parakeratosis. The stroma may be edematous and infiltrated with chronic inflammatory cells.

Angioma. Clinically and histologically, angiomas of the vulva have the same appearance as those of other areas of the body. Presence on the vulva, however, is rare and when the tumor is congenital it may be subjected to the irritation of diapers, urine, or feces. Most of the congenital types regress as the child grows.

Hydradenoma. Hydradenoma is also a rare lesion. It is painless, elevated, circumscribed, and usually found on the labium majus or perineum. It arises from the vulvar sweet gland and is almost always benign. Occasionally the overlying skin may be reddened or ulcerated. When ulcerated, slight bleeding may occur. The lesion has some significance because occasionally it may be mistaken microscopically for an adenocarcinoma. Histologically the tumor consists of slender papillary structures covered by a layer of columnar epithelial cells with slightly eosinophilic cytoplasm and distinct nuclei. Since it arises from the apocrine sweat glands, it is really an apocrine adenoma.

Nevus. Nevi are pigmented lesions composed of clusters of nevus cells. They range in color from black to tan and vary widely in size. They may be rough or smooth and occur with or without hair. They may be flat, raised, or pedunculated. Their importance lies in the fact that a disproportionate number of malignant melanomas in the female arise from the external genitalia. Of particular importance is the flat expanding pigmented lesion, of which three types are recognizable histologically.

1. Intradermal, in which the nevus cells are entirely located in the dermal layer and are separated from the overlying epidermis.
2. Compound, in which the nevus cells are located in both the dermal and the epidermal layers.
3. Junctional, in which the cells arise from the junction of the dermis and the epidermis.

These lesions should be excised with a wide margin if there is a change in color, an increase in size, ulceration, or bleeding. They should also be removed when located in areas that are chronically irritated by clothing, coitus, or other means. Since vulvar nevi are frequently junctional, they probably should be excised in most instances.

Granular Cell Myoblastoma. The name of this tumor is a misnomer since it arises from the myelin sheath of the nerve. It is composed of large, pale-staining cells with eosinophilic cytoplasmic granules. There are pseudoepitheliomatous changes that suggest, and occasionally are mistaken for, a squamous carcinoma. Clinically these tumors are solid neoplasms, which may be single or multiple and are generally well circumscribed. They are usually small and asymptomatic. Local excision provides tissue for diagnosis and should certainly be done if there is a change in size or consistency, or whenever the diagnosis is unclear.

White Lesions of the Vulva

Although many of the white lesions of the vulva are not truly neoplastic, they are grouped together for purposes of discussion (Table 2). White appearance of the vulvar skin may be due to two general types of change: absence or loss of pigment, or increased keratinization. Absence of pigment may be congenital, or loss may occur secondary to infection or trauma. Increased keratinization may be due to chronic infection or may be demonstrated in some benign tumors.

Dystrophies. The hyperkeratotic white lesions or leukoplakias may be productive of fairly severe symptoms, especially itching. The major significance, however, is the debilitation produced by these lesions and the fact that some of them are premalignant.

Lichen Sclerosus. Lichen sclerosus may present as a bluish-white papule and when many are present they may coalesce to produce a diffuse whitish change over the entire vulva and perineal area. In the later stages there is a loss of the subcutaneous tissue with flattening of the labial folds and constriction of the vaginal outlet. Lichen sclerosus frequently appears in the early post-menopausal years. The lesions initially are asymptomatic and tend to remain so unless collagenization becomes extensive. Although the appearance of these lesions is atrophic, metabolic activity has been demonstrated and correlated with anaplasia. Therefore, they must be followed carefully, for carcinoma may develop. Biopsies of suspicious areas are essential to diagnosis and follow-up. Vulvectomy may be necessary if anaplastic changes are noted in the tissue study. Toluidine blue, a vital dye, is useful in determining the area for biopsy; the more active anaplastic areas tend to retain the nuclear stain.

Table 2. Classification of White Lesions of the Vulva

I. Depigmentation—leukoderma or vitiligo
II. Hyperkeratosis
  A. Dystrophies
    1. Lichen sclerosus
    2. Hyperplasia
      a. Typical
      b. Atypical
    3. Mixed (combination of 1 and 2)
  B. Carcinoma in situ
  C. Invasive cancer

Hyperplasia. Hyperplasia denotes an increase in the normal cellular elements and more specifically is designated typical or atypical to denote the degree of proliferation and its malignant potential. Again, biopsy is essential and may be accomplished easily by using the Keyes punch under local anesthesia. The malignant potential of hyperplastic lesions depends on the degree of cellular aberrations. Particularly significant is abnormal maturation of epithelial cells in the basal layer.

Malignant Neoplasms of the Vulva

Carcinoma of the Vulva. Carcinoma of the vulva is the fourth most common genital cancer. It is exceeded in frequency by carcinoma of the uterine corpus, cervix uteri, and ovary. It accounts for approximately 3 to 4 per cent of primary malignancies of the female genitalia. Almost all of the lesions are squamous cell in origin, although adenocarcinoma of the Bartholin gland, basal cell carcinoma, malignant melanomas, and malignant sweat gland tumors also occur. Carcinoma is primarily a disease of the seventh decade, and delays on the part of both patient and physician frequently lead to unsuccessful treatment because of late diagnosis. The most common symptom of vulvar cancer is long-standing pruritus. Frequently an ulcer is noted. Treatment should always be preceded by biopsies for definitive diagnosis. This applies particularly to the white lesions, some of which may be treated medically to prevent development of malignant disease. Both hypertrophic and atrophic dystrophies respond to medical therapy.

Carcinoma in Situ. Carcinoma in situ represents 35 per cent of the vulvar cancers. There are no characteristic symptoms or lesions. A high index of suspicion is necessary to diagnose these lesions. Histologically most lesions are squamous, with surface keratinization. Carcinoma in situ is frequently multifocal, and multiple biopsies should be taken. Again, toluidine blue is helpful in directing attention to the site for biopsy. Unfortunately, the hyperkeratotic lesions tend not to take the stain. By definition, intraepithelial cancer of the vulva connotes full-thickness replacement of the lining epithelium by undifferentiated abnormal cells, characteristically spinal in type. Some degree of differentiation of the component cells is often found despite undeniable anaplasia. Terms such as Bowen's disease, erythroplasia of Queyrat, and others have been used to describe types of carcinoma in situ, but for all practical purposes these lesions all represent intraepithelial disease biologically and should be managed in the same fashion. Clinically the lesions may appear reddened, pigmented, whitish, flat, or slightly elevated, and commonly they are multicentric in origin. Paget's disease of the vulva, however, is a specific form of in situ cancer characterized grossly by a reddish lesion interspersed with white epithelial islands and microscopically by large pale "Paget cells." Rarely this lesion may be associated with an underlying adenocarcinoma.

Invasive Carcinoma. Basal cell carcinomas of the vulva are rare but when present have the same clinical and histologic pictures as basal cell carcinomas occurring in other areas of the body. In the usual form of vulvar carcinoma, the initial lesion becomes steadily larger, with induration, ulceration, and surrounding edema. As it progresses, it obviously involves the adjacent structures and the inguinal and femoral lymph nodes. From the superficial nodes, it spreads to the deep pelvic nodes. Careful evaluation is necessary for staging (Table 3). Treatment and prognosis correlate with the stage of the disease.

Other Vulvar Malignancies. Sarcoma of the vulva is exceptionally rare, as is malignant melanoma; however, malignant melanoma is the second most common malignancy of the vulva. Its origin is usually in pigmented moles. As with other vulvar lesions, diagnosis is established by biopsy and histologic examination.

VAGINA

Benign Lesions of the Vagina

Benign lesions of the vagina are divided into two categories, cystic and solid (Table 4).

Cystic Tumors

Cystic lesions, except those derived from müllerian duct remnants, arise in one of two ways, as follows.

Inclusion Cyst. These usually are seen at the lower portion of the vagina, most often on the posterior wall. They are caused by inclusion of the mucosa beneath the surface as a result of trauma or surgical repair. These cysts are lined by stratified squamous epithelium and the contents are usually mucoid.

Gartner Duct Cyst. Cysts of Gartner's duct arise from the remnants of the wolffian system. Embryologically these ducts course along the outer, anterior aspect of the vaginal canal. They are usually fairly small but may be large enough to bulge from the vaginal outlet. Microscopically, they are lined with varying types of epithelium: cuboidal, columnar, ciliated, nonciliated, and sometimes stratified squamous. When these cysts are small, asymptomatic, multiple, and arranged in a characteristic fashion, the diagnosis is fairly evident. Vaginal adenosis and adenocarcinoma of the vagina related to exposure to synthetic hormones should be considered. Exclusion

Table 3. FIGO* Classification of Carcinoma of the Vulva

T—Primary Tumor	
T1	Tumor confined to the vulva; 2 cm or less in larger diameter
T2	Tumor confined to the vulva; more than 2 cm in diameter
T3	Tumor of any size with adjacent spread to the urethra and/or perineum and/or the anus
T4	Tumor of any size infiltrating the bladder mucosa and/or the rectal mucosa, including the upper part of the urethral mucosa, and/or fixed to the bone
N—Regional Lymph Nodes	
N0	No nodes palpable
N1	Nodes palpable in either groin, not enlarged, mobile (not clinically suspicious of neoplasms)
N2	Nodes palpable in either one or both groins, enlarged, firm, and mobile (clinically suspicious of neoplasm)
N3	Fixed or ulcerated nodes
M—Distant Metastases	
M0	No clinical metastases
M1a	Palpable deep pelvic lymph nodes
M1b	Other distant metastases

Clinical Stage Groups

Stage I			Stage II		
T1	N0	M0	T2	N0	M0
T1	N1	M0	T2	N1	M0
Stage III			**Stage IV**		
T3	N0	M0	T1	N3	M0
T3	N1	M0	T2	N3	M0
T3	N2	M0	T3	N3	M0
T1	N2	M0	T4	N1	M0
T2	N2	M0	T4	N2	M0
			T4	N3	M0

All other conditions containing M1a or M1b.

*International Federation of Gynecology and Obstetrics.

Table 4. Benign Tumors of the Vagina

Cystic
Inclusion cyst
Gartner duct cyst
Solid
Condyloma
Endometriosis
Leiomyomas and fibromyomas
Vaginal adenosis

of these conditions is made by the presence of normal iodine staining of the vagina and the absence of a history of antenatal exposure to synthetic estrogens. The diagnosis can be confirmed by biopsy. Larger cysts may be removed by excisional biopsy for histologic diagnosis.

Solid Tumors

Condyloma. The most common solid tumor of the vagina is the wart. It is frequently seen in association with condylomas of the vulva and cervix. These tumors may proliferate markedly during pregnancy and produce bleeding during delivery if involvement is extensive; this may necessitate cesarean section. When these lesions occur in older patients, when there is a broad base, or when the clinical picture is atypical, biopsies are necessary to establish a definitive diagnosis.

Endometriosis. Endometriosis in the vagina may develop at the site of a previous operation or as a primary implant. From the posterior cul de sac, it may extend into the vagina. Frequently there are nodules containing chocolate-colored material with scarring around them. The endometrial glands and stroma may be identified histologically. Considerable inflammation and hemosiderin-laden macrophages may be present. On rare occasion endometriosis may occur as a diffuse process and simulate adenosis. Biopsy is usually necessary for diagnosis unless the endometriosis is a part of a generalized pelvic process.

Leiomyomas and Fibromyomas. These tumors are rare solid neoplasms. Clinically they present as firm, rubbery, solid masses that are spherical and shell out easily except for a relatively vascular stalk. Histologically they resemble the same tumor at other sites, with well-circumscribed margins and whorls of smooth muscle or fibrous tissue, or both.

Vaginal Adenosis. In 1970 several cases of adenocarcinoma of the vagina in young girls were reported. Later, evidence of the relationship between maternal diethylstilbestrol therapy and the appearance of this tumor was presented. Prior to that time, adenocarcinoma had been diagnosed primarily, and then only rarely, in older women. A high incidence of vaginal adenosis was also noted in female offspring of women treated with synthetic estrogen prior to the 18th week of gestation. Adenosis of the vagina was known before the advent of diethylstilbestrol, but the incidence was markedly increased in those who had been exposed to the drug.

This lesion is associated with leukorrhea and occasionally vaginal spotting, or the patient may be asymptomatic. Other associated abnormalities are a cervical hood, transverse ridges, and columnar epithelium covering most of the ectocervix. Histologically, there frequently is extensive metaplasia of the vaginal epithelium overlying areas of vaginal adenosis. Columnar epithelium may lie on the surface or may underlie the squamous epithelium. The columnar epithelium may be of the endocervical, endometrial, or fallopian tube glandular type. These cells may secrete mucus, as in their normal positions. Sometimes there is surrounding inflammation. The adenosis most frequently is found in the anterior upper third of the vagina; however, it may occur anywhere. The lesion is thought to result from the incomplete replacement of the müllerian epithelium by epithelium from the urogenital sinus during fetal development, i.e., from interference with normal development.

Since 1970 over 300 cases of adenocarcinoma of the vagina have been reported in young girls between the ages of 13 and 25 years. A majority of them had a history of antenatal exposure to synthetic estrogens. There have been no cases in which benign vaginal adenosis was documented and adenocarcinoma developed during subsequent observation. When there is a history of exposure, the girl should be examined carefully. This should include palpation of all aspects of the vagina, routine cytology on the full length of the vagina in quadrants, and, when necessary, Schiller staining and colposcopy. Biopsies of the nonstaining or colposcopically identified areas of adenosis should be undertaken initially to document the presence of the benign adenosis. These patients are generally followed from the time the history is obtained, and, in the absence of symptoms, full examination may be delayed until after menarche. With symptoms, however, the patient should be examined fully under anesthesia and biopsies obtained as needed. If the biopsies do not reveal any atypical changes, routine follow-up and examination appear to be sufficient without excision or other treatment. Over a period of time, metaplastic squamous epithelium normally replaces the surface adenosis.

Malignant Tumors of the Vagina

Primary vaginal neoplasia is rare and accounts for about 0.5 per cent of primary genital malignancies.

Carcinoma in Situ. Carcinoma in situ is also rare and is often found with, or subsequent to, the discovery of cervical or vulvar neoplasia. Thus, in the follow-up of any malignancy of the adjacent areas, the vagina should be inspected and thoroughly scraped for cytologic studies for evidence of malignancy. Schiller iodine staining and colposcopy are helpful for identifying the areas for biopsy.

Invasive Carcinoma. Squamous cell carcinoma constitutes approximately 92 to 95 per cent of all primary vaginal neoplastic lesions. The remainder of the lesions are adenocarcinoma, sarcoma, and melanoma, but all are extremely rare. When the cases of adenocarcinoma associated with diethylstilbestrol are excluded, carcinoma is usually found in the sixth decade of life.

The primary symptoms are bleeding and discharge. Later in the course of the disease a mass or pain may be present. The lesion is present most often on the anterior or posterior wall. Grossly it may be exfoliative or ulcerative. Early invasion of the bladder, rectum, or ectocervix may occur.

Sarcomas and melanomas are rare. The sarcoma may occur at any age. One rare type is the grape-like sarcoma botryoides, which is a highly malignant lesion. It arises from the proliferating stroma and is closely related to the uterine mixed mesodermal tumors. This type of sarcoma occurs almost exclusively in infants, although its presence in a few young adults has been reported. The grape-like mass is a pinkish, edematous, polypoid lesion protruding from the vagina. In advanced stages, the vagina may be completely filled, with extension to the cervix uteri, uterus, parametrium, and abdominal cavity. Sarcoma botryoides is almost uniformly fatal. The microscopic pattern is fairly innocuous. Squamous epithelium may be lifted up into multiple, edematous, papillary subepithelial accumulations of fusiform tumor cells. Sometimes they are rather sparse. Clinically the appearance is fairly typical, and the diagnosis is confirmed by biopsy and histologic evaluation.

Melanoma. This rare lesion may arise from the vagina. Its clinical manifestations are similar to those of other tumors of the vagina, depending upon the stage of the disease. Its behavior is simular to that of melanomas occurring in other areas of the body, and therefore the prognosis is poor.

CERVIX UTERI

Benign Neoplasms of the Cervix

Cervical Polyps. Cervical polyps are common and usually arise from the endocervical mucosa. They are almost always benign. Usually they are small, but they may become large enough to almost reach the vaginal introitus. They are usually single, but may be multiple, and are bright red in color with a thin pedicle. There is frequently an associated inflammation, edema, or ulceration. Clinically, the polyp may be seen protruding from the cervical os and is found on routine speculum examination. Polyps are usually asymptomatic but may produce postcoital spotting or intermittent bleeding. Histologically the polyp is covered with columnar or squamous epithelium, depending upon which mucosa it derives from. Commonly, the covering is columnar epithelium with some squamous metaplasia at the tip. The typical tall, cylindrical cells are found, with a light connective tissue stroma containing edema and round cell infiltration. Less commonly, the polyp may arise from the squamous epithelium.

Diagnosis may be made by palpation or inspection. Frequently the polyps may simply be twisted off, but larger ones may require excision, and when multiple an endocervical curettage should be performed. Curettage should also be performed when there is bleeding, especially if it cannot be ascertained whether the polyp is causal or if its origin is endometrial. Histologic examination should always be performed for confirmation of the diagnosis and to rule out the few cases of malignancy.

Nabothian Cysts. Nabothian cysts of the cervix are extremely common and result from metaplastic squamous epithelium growing across secreting columnar mucosa. When no opening is left for the escape of mucus, a cystic structure is formed. These cypts are easily recognized as benign structures because of a glistening, smooth surface and normally branching capillaries.

Condyloma Acuminatum. This wart was discussed earlier in this article (see *Vulva* and *Vagina*). The warts were thought to be relatively uncommon on the cervix until widespread use of the colposcope permitted closer scrutiny. They seem to be more common in pregnancy and may grow rapidly during that time. They are difficult to distinguish from papillomas except with special stains and other means of viral identification. Recently their association with intraepithelial neoplasia has been strongly suggested. Some forms may be difficult to distinguish colposcopically from intraepithelial neoplasia; therefore, they should be biopsied for accurate histologic assessment.

Endometriosis. Endometriosis may occur on the cervix, as in other areas of the genitalia. It may result from primary implantation or be secondary to surgical procedures performed around the time of the menses. This relatively rare lesion may be asymptomatic or may result in dysmenorrhea or dyspareunia. When dyspareunia is present, however, it is difficult to attribute it to the cervical lesion rather than to other implants in the pelvis. These implants range in color from dark purplish to brown or even black. The diagnosis is established by excision and microscopic evaluation.

Leiomyomas. Leiomyomas rarely occur on the ectocervix. They vary significantly in size and are usually associated with myomas of other parts of the uterine cervix or corpus. Depending upon size or symptoms, they should be excised for a definitive diagnosis. Other rare tumors consist of fibromas, lipomas, and hemangiomas. Diagnosis is made by biopsy.

Premalignant and Malignant Lesions of the Cervix

Cervical cancer remains one of the primary causes of death from cancer in women. Although it no longer occupies a preeminent position, there is still an incidence of approximately 16,000 new cases per year with about 7000 deaths. Cancer of the cervix is now the third most common genital malignancy, following carcinoma of the corpus uteri and ovary. Great strides have been made in conquering this disease because of its relatively easy detection in the early invasive or preinvasive stage, but it should be virtually nonexistent for the same reason. Regular Papanicolaou smear screening for all women should lead to disappearance of invasive disease. Diagnosis following an abnormal Papanicolaou smear is facilitated by the use of the colposcope, which permits accurate siting of the proper area for biopsy.

Much is known about the natural history of squamous carcinoma of the cervix. From the time of the earliest premalignant change in the cervix to invasive cancer, 15 years or more may elapse. It is now certain that cervical cancer is related to sexual activity, with the most important factor being the age of first sexual contact. Other factors may be multiple partners and frequent childbearing. Etiologic agents appear to be the herpesvirus and, as recent information suggests, the human papillomavirus. Although there has also been some evidence that the sperm itself may be causally related, this information has not been confirmed. Herpes antibodies have been found in up to 73 per cent of women with cervical cancer, compared with 33 per cent of controls.

Ninety-five per cent of cervical cancers are squamous. These lesions may easily be identified by cytologic screening. The peak incidence is between ages 40 and 50 years, with the peak incidence of in situ lesions approximately 10 years earlier. There is a continuing shift of both invasive and preinvasive lesions toward a younger age group. Whether this shift is due to changing sexual patterns is unknown. Fortunately, at the present time more lesions are diagnosed in the premalignant stage than in the malignant stage. This again is due to the widespread use of the Papanicolaou smear and the increasing acceptance of the use of the colposcope over the past decade.

Cytology

The Papanicolaou smear provides an accurate cytologic method for assessing asymptomatic women with a completely normal appearing cervix. This has led to the diagnosis of many cases of intraepithelial disease and early invasive cancer long before symptoms or early visible abnormalities become apparent.

A cervical smear should be obtained from every sexually active female on a yearly basis. The frequency should be increased or decreased depending on the patient's risk for developing the disease. This varies, depending upon age at the time of first sexual intercourse and the number of sexual partners. It has become apparent that the patient who has sexual activity with one person and began having sexual intercourse past the age of 20 years probably does not need a yearly Papanicolaou smear after she has had two or three successive normal smears. On the other hand, a patient who began sexual activity early and changes sexual partners frequently probably needs a smear more frequently. Other factors, such as number of children, venereal disease, and socioeconomic status, may also be used to determine the frequency with which smears should be obtained.

Smears should be reported from the laboratory according to the degree of abnormality, with an attempt to describe the findings in terms of benignity, infection, degree of dysplasia (mild, moderate, severe), carcinoma in situ, or invasive cancer. The term cervical intraepithelial neoplasia (CIN), grades 1, 2, and 3, which correlates with dysplasia and carcinoma in situ, may be used. The numbering system of classes 1 through 5 should be abandoned except in laboratories where lay personnel are used to separate the smears into categories for purposes of follow-up. The terms used should correlate closely with the suspected pathologic process.

The technique for obtaining the smear is important. A nonlubricated speculum should be used. A sample should be obtained from the endocervical canal and from the ectocervix. In older women a third sample from the vaginal pool may be of value. This specimen should be spread evenly and thinly over a clean glass slide and fixed immediately. In the presence of a cervical lesion, a biopsy should always be obtained after the smear is taken. Frequently, gross lesions may not be productive of an abnormal Papanicolaou smear because of the surface inflammation, necrosis, and ulceration. It must be remembered that a cytologic smear cannot be depended on for a definitive diagnosis. Whenever any degree of atypia is suggested, further evaluation and examination of tissue obtained by biopsy is necessary to establish the diagnosis. This process has been made easier and more accurate with the widespread acceptance of colposcopy over the last decade or more.

Colposcopy

The cervix is a site of junction between stratified squamous epithelium, which lines the vagina, and single layered columnar epithelium, which lines the endocervix. This junction may occur within the cervical canal, at the anatomic os, or on the portio vaginalis of the cervix. In some situations it may occur in the vagina. When the squamocolumnar junction is on the portio, the area surrounding the os appears red, designating the columnar epithelium. This condition is present in the majority of young women during the reproductive years.

Squamous and columnar epithelia of the cervix of early life are designated the original squamous and columnar epithelia, respectively. Later, the positions of these epithelial types change. The movement of the junction on the portio vanginalis toward the cervical canal is a result of metaplasia. It is believed that neoplasia usually begins at this site. Neoplastic change once developed may regress, remain the same, or progress to become invasive carcinoma.

The colposcope is a stereoscopic binocular microscope with a usual focal length of approximately 20 cm and a magnification of 10 to 40 times. When the cervix is viewed through this instrument, its topographic anatomy becomes visible. Normal findings consist of columnar epithelium, which has a grapelike appearance; a homogeneous smooth, pink epithelium, which is squamous; and an intervening area of metaplastic squamous epithelium called the transformation zone. This zone appears slightly different in color, with vestiges of columnar epithelium, such as nabothian cysts or gland openings. More importantly, the epithelial alterations with their vascular adaptations can be identified when abnormal. Using the Papanicolaou smear and the colposcope, a scheme for evaluation has been developed (Figure 1).

After being cleaned with dilute acetic acid, the squamous epithelium of the cervix seen through the colposcope appears smooth, pink, and semitranslucent. The squamocolumnar junction can be easily identified and studied. The columnar epithelium appears grapelike as a result of the accentuation of the villi and

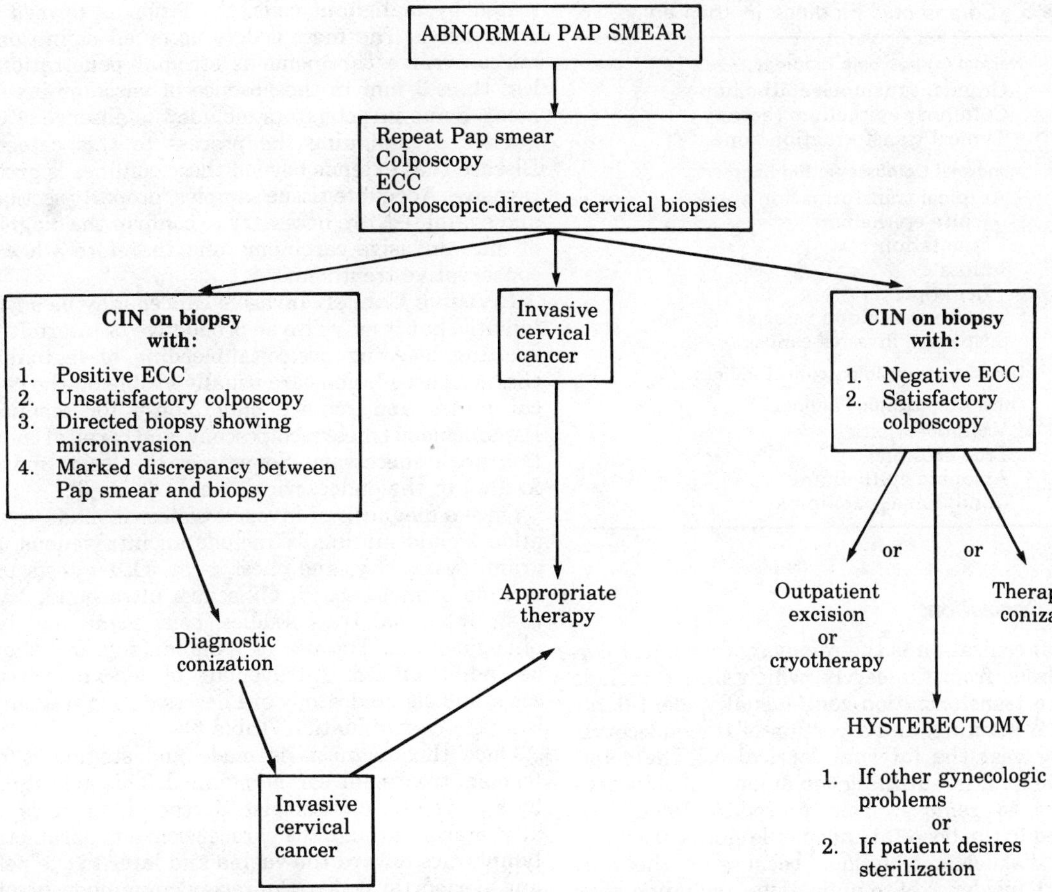

Figure 1. Diagnosis and management of the abnormal Papanicolaou smear. CIN = Cervical intraepithelial neoplasia; ECC = endocervical curettage.

clefts that extend into the connective tissue. The area of columnar epithelium usually does not stain with iodine. Areas covered by mature squamous epithelium are usually iodine-positive except in patients with hypoestrogenism, in whom the epithelium often stains poorly. The demarcation between squamous and columnar epithelium as seen through the colposcope may appear smooth and sharp or serrated, either before or after application of iodine.

In a majority of women, another type of epithelium in various stages of maturation lies between an original squamous epithelium and the area covered only by columnar epithelium. This transformation (transition) zone appears to originate from the squamocolumnar junction as gray tongues of tissue that project into the area covered by columnar epithelium. This process indicates growth of squamous epithelium from the periphery over the columnar epithelium toward the cervical os. However, islands of metaplastic tissue not connected directly to any peripheral squamous source occasionally occur within areas of the cervix covered only by columnar epithelium. In the early stages, metaplastic tissues are iodine-negative, but as the epithelium matures and produces glycogen it becomes histologically and topographically indistinguishable from the original stratified squamous epithelium of the cervix. Nevertheless, remnants of columnar epithelium may be present as nabothian cysts and gland openings.

In the majority of women, metaplasia proceeds in an orderly fashion to form a normal transformation zone but occasionally the normal process is disturbed. The changes may be recognized by variations in color and contour and abnormalities of the vascular patterns. The intercapillary distance may be increased, and there is a clarity of demarcation between the lesion and the surrounding normal epithelium. The terminology used to describe colposcopic findings is given in Table 5. These changes are easily recognized by the experienced colposcopist. Once the entire squamocolumnar junction is seen (satisfactory examination), it is possible to establish a definitive diagnosis with biopsies from the abnormal areas. An endocervical curettage may also be performed to assure the examiner that no lesions lie beyond the immediate area of visibility. The examination may be performed in the office and takes only a few minutes longer than the usual pelvic examination. If the examination is unsatisfactory, however, cervical conization must be done for a definitive diagnosis. This is necessary in only about 15 to 20 per cent of women within the child-bearing age group. Conization is also necessary when the diagnosis obtained by colposcopically directed punch biopsy is microinvasive carcinoma.

Table 5. Colposcopic Findings in the Cervix

Normal Colposcopic Findings
- Original squamous epithelium
- Columnar epithelium (ectopy)
- Typical transformation zone

Abnormal Colposcopic Findings
- Atypical transformation zone
  - White epithelium
  - Punctation
  - Mosaic
  - Leukoplakia
  - Abnormal blood vessels
- Suspected invasive cancer

Unsatisfactory Colposcopic Findings

Other Colposcopic Findings
- Vaginocervicitis
- True erosion
- Atrophic epithelium
- Condyloma, papilloma

Cervical Conization

Cervical conization is the removal of a conical portion of tissue from the cervix, which should include the entire transformation zone (usually identifiable by Schiller staining) and a portion of the endocervix extending near the internal cervical os. The colposcope is helpful in outlining the amount of ectocervical tissue to remove. This procedure should be performed in the hospital and should not be used as a primary diagnostic technique because of the relatively high incidence of complications, including hemorrhage, infection, cervical stenosis, and impaired fertility. On the other hand, the clinician should not hesitate to perform this procedure in the presence of an abnormal Papanicolaou smear when a definitive diagnosis cannot be established using colposcopically directed biopsy.

Cervical Neoplasia

Cervical Intraepithelial Neoplasia. This term was coined more than 20 years ago, and lesions can be divided into grades 1, 2, and 3. CIN grade 1 corresponds generally to mild dysplasia, grade 2 to moderate dysplasia, and grade 3 to severe dysplasia and carcinoma in situ. The term was used to promote the idea that dysplasia and carcinoma in situ represented a spectrum of increasing severity of the same disease. Intraepithelial neoplasia manifests itself by areas of abnormal cell growth characterized by the usual criteria of malignancy, i.e., loss of polarity, increase in mitosis, increased nucleocytoplasmic ratio signifying abnormalities in chromatin structure and content within the nucleus, and a decrease in some cellular elements. Histologically, the degree of severity is characterized by the extent to which the neoplastic process involves the thickness of epithelium. Carcinoma in situ thus represents full-thickness involvement, and other stages of neoplasia represent differing degrees of partial involvement.

Microinvasive Carcinoma. Once the lamina propria or basement membrane of the cervix is penetrated by malignant cells, the lesion is termed microinvasive. The most widely accepted definition of microinvasive carcinoma is stromal penetration of less than 3 mm in the absence of vascular involvement. Some investigators include the absence of confluence in assigning the process to this category. Disease that extends beyond those confines is grossly invasive. Adequate tissue samples, properly sectioned and evaluated, are necessary to confirm the diagnosis of microinvasive carcinoma and therefore allow for conservative treatment.

Invasive Cancer. Invasive cancer may be asymptomatic, but it may also be productive of intermittent spotting, bleeding, postcoital bleeding, or vaginal discharge. These lesions are usually visible on the cervical portio and require only biopsy for diagnosis. Papanicolaou smears, colposcopy, and cervical conization are unnecessary. Sometimes the lesion may be located in the endocervical canal (Table 6).

Once a diagnosis of invasive cancer is made, evaluation should minimally include an intravenous urogram, cystoscopy, and chest x-ray. Other tests used include sigmoidoscopy, CT scans, ultrasound, lower gastrointestinal tract studies, bone scans, and lymphangiograms. The use of lymphangiograms should be individualized. Intravenous pyelograms, cystoscopy, and sigmoidoscopy are necessary for staging, as is a pelvic examination (Table 6).

Once the diagnosis is made and staging is performed, treatment can be planned. This is best done by a gynecologic oncologist. Spread of cancer is usually lateral, through the paracervical and parametrial lymphatics toward the vagina and later to the pelvic and periaortic nodes. Supraclavicular node involvement is sometimes present when the disease is

Table 6. FIGO* Classification of Cancer of the Cervix

Stage 0:	Carcinoma in situ
Stage I:	Carcinoma confined to the cervix
IA:	Microinvasion (early stromal invasion)
IB:	(Occult cancer): Frank invasion recognized histologically but not clinically
IB:	All other cancers limited to the uterus
Stage II:	Involvement of the vagina but not the lower third on infiltration of the parametria but not out to the side wall
IIA:	Involvement of the vagina but no evidence of parametrial involvement
IIB:	Infiltration of the parametria but not out to the side wall
Stage III:	Involvement of the lower third of the vagina or extension to the pelvic side wall
IIIA:	Involvement of the lower third of the vagina but not out to the pelvic side wall if the parametria are involved
IIIB:	Involvement of one or both parametria out to the side wall
III	(Urinary): Obstruction of one or both ureters on intravenous pyelogram without the other criteria for stage III disease
Stage IV:	Extension outside the reproductive tract
IVA:	Involvement of the mucosa of the bladder or rectum
IVB:	Distant metastasis or disease outside the true pelvis

*International Federation of Gynecology and Obstetrics.

thought to be limited to the pelvis. After the initial spread laterally, the cancer may spread anteriorly to involve the bladder or posteriorly to involve the rectum. Ureteral compression is common in advanced disease. Metastasis may occur to other parts of the body. More commonly noted are metastases to the lung, liver, and bone. These all occur late in the course of the disease.

Adenocarcinoma. As mentioned previously, adenocarcinoma of the cervix is relatively uncommon, occurring in approximately 5 per cent of patients with cervical cancer. It usually begins within the cervical canal but may be seen first at or near the external os. Microscopically it is characterized by atypical gland patterns that are like the orderly distribution and appearance of normal cervical glands. There are marked variations in the degree of cellular and glandular pattern changes. Diagnosis and staging is the same as for squamous carcinoma.

Section Fifteen

IMMUNE SYSTEM

IMMUNODEFICIENCY

By Thomas F. Smith, M.D.
and David S. Gordon, M.D.
Atlanta, Georgia

Immunodeficiency diseases are a diverse group of disorders in which there is an increased susceptibility to infection as a result of one or more abnormalities of the immune system. The primary immunodeficiencies in general are congenital and hereditary, and their symptoms frequently present either in infancy or in early childhood. Primary immunodeficiencies occur relatively rarely. The incidence of hypogammaglobulinemia has been estimated at 1 case per 100,000 population; selective IgA deficiency may occur in 1 in 600 to 1 in 800. Secondary immunodeficiencies occur much more commonly and may result either from disease states such as malnutrition or neoplasia or from immunosuppressive drugs. It has been estimated that as many as 5 per cent of all hospitalized patients express secondary immunodeficiency. Although the possibility of immunodeficiency should be kept in mind in any patient with recurrent infections, it should be remembered that there are many nonimmunologic causes of recurrent infections as well (Table 1).

CLASSIFICATION

The primary immunodeficiencies may be classified according to the part of the immune system in which the defect occurs. Exclusive of selective IgA deficiency, antibody (B cell) immunodeficiencies are the most common and constitute approximately half of the primary immunodeficiencies. Cellular (T cell) immunodeficiencies constitute approximately 40 per cent of the total primary immunodeficiencies. Of these, three quarters have associated antibody deficiencies and, therefore, are combined immunodeficiencies. Phagocytic immunodeficiencies, which include either defects in the polymorphonuclear phagocytic or mononuclear phagocytic systems, make up about 6 per cent of the total primary immunodeficiencies. The remaining 4 per cent of the total are complement deficiency diseases.

Secondary immunodeficiencies frequently affect many components of the immunologic response and may result in deficiencies in any or all of the same four systems.

CLINICAL FINDINGS

The major feature of immunodeficiency is increased susceptibility to infection. This consists of an in-

Table 1. Disorders with Increased Susceptibility to Infection*

Type of Disorders	Conditions
Circulatory disorders	Sickle cell disease, diabetes, nephrosis, varicose veins, congenital cardiac defects
Obstructive disorders	Ureteral or urethral stenosis, bronchial asthma, allergic rhinitis, blocked eustachian tubes, cystic fibrosis
Integument defects	Eczema, burns, skull fractures, midline sinus tracts, immotile cilia
Unusual microbiologic factors	Antibiotic-induced overgrowth, chronic infection with resistant organism, continuous reinfection (water supply, infectious contact, contaminated inhalation therapy equipment)
Foreign bodies	Ventricular shunts, central venous catheter, artificial heart valves, urinary catheter, aspirated foreign bodies
Secondary immunodeficiencies	Malnutrition, prematurity, lymphoma, splenectomy, uremia, immunosuppressive therapy, protein-losing enteropathy
Primary immunodeficiencies	B cell immunodeficiencies, T cell immunodeficiencies, phagocytic immunodeficiencies, complement immunodeficiencies

*From Stiehm, E.R.: Immunodeficiency – general considerations. In Stiehm, E.R., and Fulginiti, V.A. (eds.): *Immunologic Disorders in Infants and Children.* Philadelphia, W.B. Saunders Company, 1980.

creased number of infections, increased severity of infection, prolonged infections, and infection with unusual or "opportunistic" organisms (organisms of low pathogenicity).

Recurrent respiratory infections commonly occur in immunodeficiency. These infections include rhinitis, acute otitis media, tonsillitis, bronchitis, sinusitis, and pneumonia. Patients who have these infections repeatedly frequently develop complications such as chronically draining ears or bronchiectasis. It should be kept in mind that many normal children have six to eight upper respiratory infections each year. Repeated respiratory infections are uncommon in adults and should indicate to the clinician the need to evaluate the patient for immunodeficiency. Repeated infections in the same lobe of the lung may indicate an anatomic defect, such as bronchiectasis; repeated infections in multiple lobes strongly suggest immunodeficiency.

Recurrent respiratory symptoms also occur in patients who have allergies or other atopic diseases. For example, a patient with eosinophilic nonallergic rhinitis may have recurrent episodes of acute otitis media on the basis of anatomic dysfunction. Likewise, a patient with untreated asthma may present with chronic cough and have x-ray changes during acute exacerbations of the disease which frequently are confused with pneumonia.

Severe bacterial infections, such as pneumonia, sepsis, and meningitis, frequently occur in patients with immunodeficiencies. Patients who have antibody deficiencies usually experience infections with gram-positive organisms, whereas those who have cellular immunodeficiencies experience infections with gram-negative bacteria, fungi, protozoa, mycobacteria, and viruses. Gastrointestinal symptoms, including chronic diarrhea, may also occur in immunodeficiency syndromes.

Past medical history may be as important in ruling out immunodeficiency as it is in ruling it in. For example, children who have responded normally to live-virus vaccine probably have intact cell-mediated immunity. The rash that occurs with viral exanthems and contact dermatitis also suggests intact cell-mediated immunity.

Family history is important in evaluating suspected immunodeficiencies. Severe infections in family members or early deaths of relatives should be investigated. A history of arthritis, collagen vascular disease, and allergy also should be explored. It should be kept in mind that several primary immunodeficiencies have an X-linked or autosomal recessive mode of inheritance (Table 2). Similarly, a variety of pharmacologic agents inhibit the effective immune response. Therefore, a drug history is important as well.

Table 2. Inheritance Patterns of the Primary Immunodeficiencies*

I. X-linked Inheritance
   A. Infantile agammaglobulinemia (Bruton type)
   B. Immunodeficiency with hyper-IgM
   C. Severe combined immunodeficiency (some)
   D. Wiskott-Aldrich syndrome
   E. Chronic granulomatous disease (most)
   F. X-linked lymphoproliferative disorder
   G. C1q deficiency (some)

II. Autosomal Recessive Inheritance
   A. Severe combined immunodeficiency (some)
   B. Immunodeficiency with enzyme deficiency
   C. Ataxia-telangiectasia
   D. Chronic mucocutaneous candidiasis (some)
   E. Chronic granulomatous disease (some)
   F. Chediak-Higashi syndrome
   G. C2 deficiency
   H. C3 deficiency
   I. C4 deficiency (one family)

III. Autosomal Co-dominant Inheritance
   A. C1r deficiency
   B. C4 deficiency (one family)
   C. C5 deficiency
   D. C6 deficiency
   E. C7 deficiency
   F. C8 deficiency

IV. Often Familial—Inheritance Pattern(s) Uncertain
   A. Selective IgA deficiency
   B. Immunodeficiency with normal immunoglobulin or hyperimmunoglobulinemia
   C. Chronic mucocutaneous candidiasis
   D. Short-limbed dwarfism
   E. Cellular immunodeficiency with abnormal immunoglobulin synthesis

*Adapted from Stiehm, E.R.: Immunodeficiency—general considerations. In Stiehm, E.R., and Fulginiti, V.A. (eds.): *Immunologic Disorders in Infants and Children.* Philadelphia, W.B. Saunders Company, 1980.

LABORATORY DIAGNOSIS OF IMMUNODEFICIENCY

The initial screening tests for immunodeficiency include a complete blood count, quantitative immunoglobulin determinations, a measurement of functional antibodies, and an evaluation for infection (Table 3). Other laboratory tests should be considered according to the past and present illness of the particular patient.

The complete blood count should include a white blood cell count, differential count, platelet count, and examination of the blood smear. Total absolute neutrophil and lymphocyte counts should be calculated. Absolute levels of IgG, IgM, and IgA immunoglobulins are measured either by single radial diffusion or by nephelometry. Levels of immunoglobulins probably should not be estimated from immunoelectrophoresis

Table 3. Initial Screening Tests for Immunodeficiency*

1. Complete blood count with differential: Granulocyte count, lymphocyte count, cell morphology, platelet count, hemoglobin
2. Protein electrophoresis: Gamma globulins, paraproteins
3. Quantitative immunoglobulins: IgG, IgA, IgM
4. Isohemagglutinins (IgM function): Anti-A, anti-B
5. Specific antibody titers (IgG function): Tetanus, diphtheria, rubella
6. Infection evaluation: Erythrocyte sedimentation rate, appropriate radiographs, appropriate cultures

*Adapted from Stiehm, E.R.: Immunodeficiency—general considerations. In Stiehm, E.R., and Fulginiti, V.A. (eds.): *Immunologic Disorders in Infants and Children.* Philadelphia, W.B. Saunders Company, 1980.

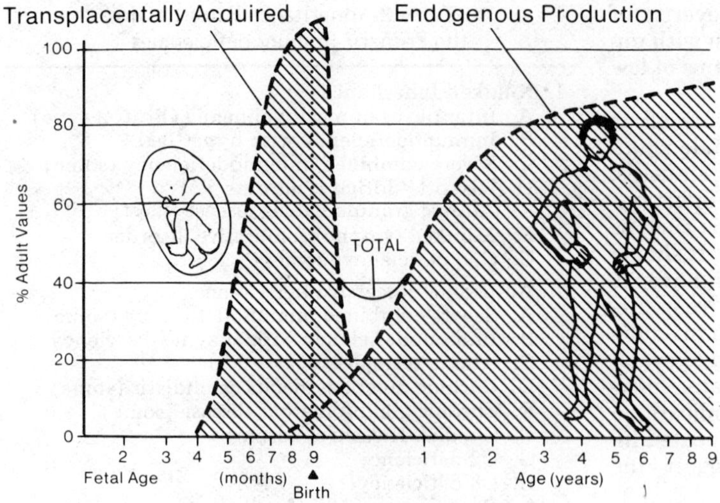

Figure 1. Temporal relationships between the placental transfer of IgG, the catabolism of maternal IgG, and the synthesis of IgG in the pre- and post-gestational periods. (Adapted from Goldman, A.S., and Goldblum, R.M.: Primary deficiencies in humoral immunity. Pediatr. Clin. North Am., 24:280, 1977.)

patterns. Levels of immunoglobulins vary according to age, and results measured from an individual patient should be interpreted accordingly (Figs. 1 and 2, Tables 4 and 5). Borderline low immunoglobulin levels must be correlated with functional antibody tests. It is also possible to have normal amounts of an antibody without functional activity. Functional antibody can be measured in several ways. Isohemagglutinin (anti-A, anti-B, or both) titers measure IgM function. Titers of at least 1:8 are present in most immunologically normal children over age 6 months and occur because of exposure to cross-reactive antigens. Isohemagglutinins are measured in hospital blood banks. Functional IgG usually is assessed by measuring titers against an immunizing agent. For example, diphtheria, tetanus, poliomyelitis, rubella, and rubeola titers frequently can be obtained in State Health Laboratories. An evaluation for infection should include erythrocyte sedimentation rate and appropriate radiographs and cultures. If these screening tests are positive or if the history is unusually suspicious for immunodeficiency, further testing is indicated (Table 6).

There are several ways of assessing B cell function in addition to quantitating immunoglobulin levels and measuring functional antibody titers. B cells can be enumerated in peripheral blood samples by immunofluorescence using polyvalent antiserum to human immunoglobulins. If a specific antibody titer is low, the antibody response to an immunizing agent can be measured. Diphtheria and tetanus toxoid commonly are used for this purpose, as is the pneumococcal vaccine.

The possibility of T cell immunodeficiency can be investigated by several tests in addition to simple estimation of total lymphocyte count and lymphocyte morphology. Delayed hypersensitivity skin tests can evaluate pre-existing cellular immunity to microbial agents or vaccine antigens. A battery of skin test antigens is now available on a multiple application device (Multitest CMI); this provides tetanus, diphtheria, streptococcus, candida, trichophyton, proteus, and tuberculin antigens as well as glycerin control. Over 90 per cent of a normal population will respond to one or more of these skin test antigens; total absence of reactivity indicates anergy and an underlying problem

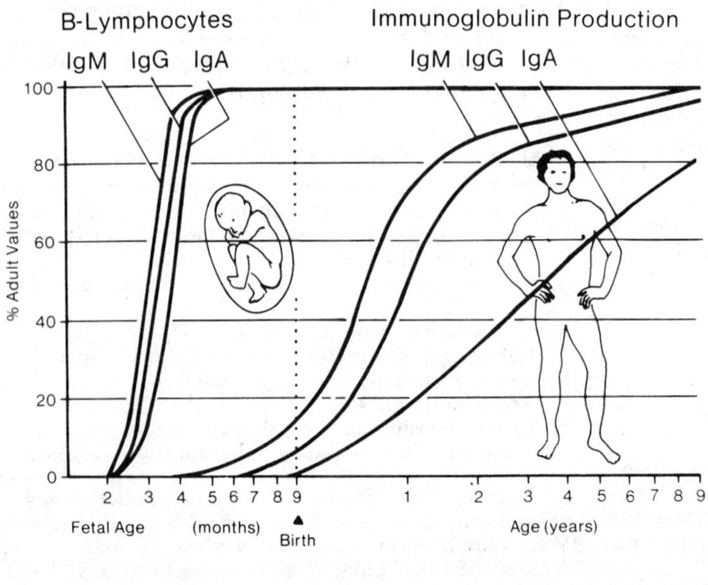

Figure 2. The development of B-lymphocytes and serum immunoglobulins in the pre- and postgestational periods. The serum concentrations of immunoglobulins are age-dependent. (Adapted from Goldman, A.S., and Goldblum, R.M.: Primary deficiencies in humoral immunity. Pediatr. Clin. North Am., 24:281, 1977.)

Table 4. Levels of Immunoglobulins in Sera of Normal Subjects, by Age*†

Age	IgG		IgM		IgA		Total Immunoglobulin	
	mg/dl	Per Cent of Adult Level	mg/dl	Per Cent of Adult Level	mg/dl	Per Cent of Adult Level	mg/dl	Per Cent of Adult Level
Newborn	1031 ± 200‡	89 ± 17	11 ± 5	11 ± 5	2 ± 3	1 ± 2	1044 ± 201	67 ± 13
1–3 mo.	430 ± 119	37 ± 10	30 ± 11	30 ± 11	21 ± 13	11 ± 7	481 ± 127	31 ± 9
4–6 mo.	427 ± 186	37 ± 16	43 ± 17	43 ± 17	28 ± 18	14 ± 9	498 ± 204	32 ± 13
7–12 mo.	661 ± 219	58 ± 19	54 ± 23	55 ± 23	37 ± 18	19 ± 9	752 ± 242	48 ± 15
13–24 mo.	762 ± 209	66 ± 18	58 ± 23	59 ± 23	50 ± 24	25 ± 12	870 ± 258	56 ± 16
25–36 mo.	892 ± 183	77 ± 16	61 ± 19	62 ± 19	71 ± 37	36 ± 19	1024 ± 205	65 ± 14
3–5 yr.	929 ± 228	80 ± 20	56 ± 18	57 ± 18	93 ± 27	47 ± 14	1078 ± 245	69 ± 17
6–8 yr.	923 ± 256	80 ± 22	65 ± 25	66 ± 25	124 ± 45	62 ± 23	1112 ± 293	71 ± 20
9–11 yr	1124 ± 235	97 ± 20	79 ± 33	80 ± 33	131 ± 30	66 ± 30	1334 ± 254	85 ± 17
12–16 yr.	946 ± 124	82 ± 11	59 ± 20	60 ± 20	148 ± 63	74 ± 32	1153 ± 169	74 ± 12
Adults	1158 ± 305	100 ± 26	99 ± 27	100 ± 27	200 ± 61	100 ± 31	1457 ± 353	100 ± 24

* From Stiehm, E.R.: Immunodeficiency—general considerations. In Stiehm, E.R., and Fulginiti, V.A. (eds.): *Immunologic Disorders in Infants and Children.* Philadelphia, W.B. Saunders Company, 1980.

† The values were derived from measurements made in 296 normal children and 30 adults. Levels were determined by the radial diffusion technique, using specific rabbit antisera to human immunoglobulins. (From Stiehm, E.R., and Fudenberg, H.H.: Serum levels of immune globulins in health and disease: A survey. Pediatrics, *37*:715, 1966, with permission.)

‡ One standard deviation.

with cell-mediated immunity. T cells may be quantitated by their ability to form rosettes with fresh sheep cells (E rosette). T cells also can be identified by immunofluorescence using monoclonal antibodies derived through hybridoma technology. T cell subsets can be quantitated using monoclonal antibodies of appropriate specificity with immunofluorescent or immunoperoxidase methodology. Cellular immunity is evaluated further by determining the ability of the patient's lymphocytes to proliferate under the influence of mitotic agents, such as phytohemagglutinin (PHA), pokeweed mitogen (PWM), or other antigens.

There are several ways to investigate the possibility of a phagocytic or complement deficiency. The nitroblue tetrazolium (NBT) dye test for chronic granulomatous disease measures the ability of stimulated leukocytes to reduce colorless nitroblue tetrazolium to a purple color after the dye has been ingested. It is a simple test that theoretically could be done in any physician's office. Chemotaxis is more difficult to assess and currently is measured only in research laboratories. Abnormal neutrophil chemotaxis frequently is found in children who have markedly elevated levels of IgE. Some research laboratories can also measure the ability of granulocytes and monocytes to ingest and kill microorganisms. Initial tests

Table 5. Levels of Serum IgE Immunoglobulin of Normal Subjects at Different Ages *†

Age	Number of Subjects	Range (IU/ml)	Geometric Mean (IU/ml)	Geometric Mean – 2 SD (IU/ml)	Geometric Mean + 2 SD (IU/ml)
0 days	24	< 0.1–1.5	0.22	0.04	1.28
6 weeks	17	< 0.1–2.8	0.69	0.08	6.12
3 months	15	0.3–3.1	0.82	0.18	3.76
6 months	15	0.9–28.0	2.68	0.44	16.26
9 months	16	0.7–8.1	2.36	0.76	7.31
1 year	12	1.1–10.2	3.49	0.80	15.22
2 years	18	1.1–49.0	3.03	0.31	29.48
3 years	6	0.5–7.7	1.80	0.19	16.86
4 years	7	2.4–34.8	8.58	1.07	68.86
7 years	18	1.6–60.0	12.89	1.03	161.32
10 years	17	0.3–215	23.66	0.98	570.61
14 years	19	1.9–159	20.07	2.06	195.18
18 to 83 years	96	1–178	21.20	Modal values 10–20 IU/ml)‡	

*From Stiehm, E.R.: Immunodeficiency—general considerations. In Stiehm, E.R., and Fulginiti, V.A. (eds.): *Immunologic Disorders in Infants and Children.* Philadelphia, W.B. Saunders Company, 1980.

†Ages 0 to 14 years from Kjellman, N.I.M., Johansson, S.G.O., and Roth, A.: Serum IgE levels in healthy children quantified by a sandwich technique (PRIST), Clin. Allergy, *6:* 51, 1976; ages 18 to 83 years from Nye, L., Merrett, T.G., Landon, J., and White, R.J.: A detailed investigation of circulating IgE levels in a normal population. Clin. Allergy, *1*:13, 1975. The method used was a double antibody assay.

‡Modal values—the most common values observed.

Table 6. Laboratory Tests for Immunodeficiency*

Antibody (B Cell) Immunodeficiency

Initial Tests

1. IgG, IgA, IgM levels
2. Isohemagglutinins (anti-A, anti-B titers)
3. Specific antibody titers (pre-existing levels)

Advanced Tests

1. B cell quantitation by surface immunoglobulin staining (sIg)
2. IgE level
3. Specific antibody response
4. IgG subclass levels
5. Secretory antibody levels
6. Lymph node biopsy
7. Immunoglobulin survival

Cellular (T Cell) Immunodeficiency

Initial Tests

1. Lymphocyte count, morphology
2. Delayed hypersensitivity skin tests (Multitest CMI)
3. Thymus x-ray

Advanced Tests

1. T cell quantitation (E rosettes)
2. T subsets (OKT antigens)
3. Lymphocyte proliferation to mitogens, antigens
4. Lymph node biopsy
5. Lymphokine assays (MIF, LT, etc.)
6. Enzyme assays (ADA, NP)
7. Thymic hormone assays

Phagocytic Immunodeficiency

Initial Tests

1. Granulocyte count, morphology
2. Nitroblue tetrazolium test
3. IgE level

Advanced Tests

1. White blood cell response (epinephrine, steroids)
2. Phagocytic and bactericidal assays
3. Random mobility
4. Chemotaxis
5. Metabolic assays (chemiluminescence)
6. Enzyme assays (myeloperoxidase, glucose-6-phosphate dehydrogenase)

Complement Immunodeficiency

Initial Tests

1. C3 level
2. C4 level
3. CH_{50} assay

Advanced Tests

1. Component assays—immunochemical or functional
2. Alternative pathway activity assay

*Adapted from Stiehm, E.R.: Immunodeficiency—general considerations. In Stiehm, E.R., and Fulginiti, V.A. (eds.): *Immunologic Disorders in Infants and Children.* Philadelphia, W.B. Saunders Company, 1980.

for complement abnormalities are measurement of serum total hemolytic complement (CH_{50}) and quantitation of serum C3 and C4 levels. Measurement of other complement components, both structurally and functionally, can be performed in a research setting.

PROGNOSIS

Long-term prognosis for patients with immunodeficiency is poor. Although acute infectious episodes frequently are controlled with antibiotics, chronic tissue damage may not be prevented and may contribute to both morbidity and mortality in these patients. It is true that occasionally an adult may recover the ability to synthesize antibodies spontaneously; in general, however, the primary immunodeficiencies are lifelong and incurable.

SPECIFIC IMMUNODEFICIENCY DISORDERS

This section briefly decribes selected immunodeficiency syndromes. The syndromes should be considered an illustrative but by no means a comprehensive listing.

X-Linked Hypogammaglobulinemia

This disorder is a syndrome (or group of syndromes) in boys that presents with recurrent pyogenic infections during infancy or early childhood. Patients with this disorder have low or absent serum immunoglobulins of all classes. Most of these patients lack B cells altogether, but some may have B cell precursors present in bone marrow. Peripheral blood lymphocytes from some patients with X-linked hypogammaglobulinemia can be shown to suppress differentiation of normal peripheral blood lymphocytes in vitro, but not all patients with this syndrome show this in vitro suppressor effect. Patients frequently present with recurrent bacterial infections beginning between 6 and 9 months of age. In addition to infections caused by pneumococci, *Haemophilis influenzae,* streptococci, and Pseudomonas, these children also may experience chronic infection with enteroviruses. Resistance to other infections, presumed to be dependent upon cell-mediated immunity, is intact. These patients experience problems with chronic otitis media, chronic sinusitis, and chronic pulmonary disease, including bronchiectasis.

Transient Hypogammaglobulinemia of Infancy

Transient hypogammaglobulinemia results from a delay in onset of normal immunoglobulin synthesis by the infant. Premature infants are especially prone to this disorder because of their lower levels of transplacental IgG at birth. There is no evidence of permanent abnormality of the immune function. Clinical manifestations are the same as those that occur in X-linked hypogammaglobulinemia. It has been suggested that the acquisition of allergy is connected to this syndrome in some patients.

Selective IgA Deficiency

Selective deficiency of IgA is the most common primary immunodeficiency. The clinical presentation is variable. Some patients are completely asymptomatic. The majority of patients with selective IgA deficiency have significant associated diseases. Many have autoimmune diseases, including systemic lupus erythematosus, dermatomyositis, and rheumatoid arthritis. Selective IgA deficiency is also associated with allergy and gastrointestinal tract disorders. Serum

IgA levels in these patients are less than 5 mg/dl. The levels of other immunoglobulins usually are normal but may be elevated on occasion. Patients with pulmonary symptions may have IgG subclass abnormalities. There is an increased incidence of autoantibodies in these patients.

Hyper-IgE Syndrome

This disorder is characterized by markedly elevated levels of serum IgE and recurrent staphylococcal abscesses involving the skin, lungs, joints, and other sites. Other clinical features of this syndrome include autosomal recessive inheritance, coarse facial features, and a pruritic dermatitis that differs from atopic eczema. Patients with this condition frequently have eosinophilia and strongly positive immediate hypersensitivity skin test responses to a variety of antigens. They frequently can be shown to have a chemotactic defect of monocytes or polymorphonuclear leukocytes. It should be noted that other patients with elevated IgE levels without the complete syndrome may from time to time have a neutrophil chemotactic defect. Elevated serum IgE concentrations have been reported in other immunodeficiency syndromes.

DiGeorge Syndrome (Thymic Hypoplasia)

DiGeorge syndrome is a congenital immunodeficiency disorder. It is characterized clinically by hypocalcemic tetany, congenital heart disease, facial dysmorphisms, and increased susceptibility to infections. The disorder results from a disturbance of the normal embryologic development of the third and fourth pharyngeal pouches; this results pathologically in the absence or hypoplasia of the thymus and parathyroid glands. There are abnormalities of structures derived from the first, second, and sixth pharyngeal pouches as well. These patients have partial or complete T cell immunodeficiency and normal or near normal B cell immune function.

Severe Combined Immunodeficiency Disease (SCID)

This is one of the several combined immunodeficiency diseases. Patients with SCID have significant deficiency of both T and B cell systems. Clinical findings, however, usually are associated with abnormal T cell function. Patients frequently develop pneumonia secondary to *Pneumocystis carinii* or various viruses. They also develop chronic oral candidiasis and may have chronic fungal skin infection. Often chronic diarrhea is present. The most discriminating laboratory test for SCID is the in vitro response of T cells to specific antigens.

Wiskott-Aldrich Syndrome

The Wiskott-Aldrich syndrome is an autosomal recessive immunodeficiency syndrome that is characterized clinically by thrombocytopenia, eczema, and recurrent infection. Characteristically, patients have markedly elevated serum levels of IgA and IgE and low levels of IgM. They consistently are unable to form antibodies to polysaccharide antigens. This may be seen as an inability to form isohemagglutinins (anti-A, anti-B). Abnormal T cell function has also been reported to occur in patients with Wiskott-Aldrich syndrome. The initial clinical manifestation frequently is bruising or bleeding occurring in the first 6 months of life. Eczema often occurs within this period as well. Older children with Wiskott-Aldrich syndrome frequently develop malignancies, including systemic reticuloendotheliosis and lymphomas. The average age at death of patients with Wiskott-Aldrich syndrome is 3½ years. Early death results from bleeding; children of older ages die from overwhelming infection or malignancy.

Ataxia-Telangiectasia

This is an autosomal recessive disorder. It is characterized clinically by telangiectasia and progressive ataxia. Children with ataxia-telangiectasia experience frequent pulmonary infections, which often result in bronchiectasis. They have a combined immunodeficiency disease, which usually includes selective IgA deficiency, cutaneous anergy, and depressed in vitro lymphocyte responses. In addition to recurrent infections, these children may develop lymphosarcoma and other malignancies.

Chronic Mucocutaneous Candidiasis

This disorder is a cellular immune deficiency syndrome characterized by persistent Candida infections. The primary defect is in the T cell response to Candida antigens; no other consistent immunologic abnormality has been described. Clinically patients present with Candida infection, most commonly on the oral mucous membranes. Fingernails and toenails often are involved, and infection of the skin of the face, hands, and feet also occurs. Up to 50 per cent of patients with chronic mucocutaneous candidiasis also have an endocrinopathy, usually hypothyroidism. In adults, this syndrome is occasionally seen in association with thymoma and various hematopoietic aplastic states, particularly red cell aplasia.

Chronic Granulomatous Disease of Childhood

This disease is an inherited disorder of leukocyte function wherein the patient's cells can ingest bacteria normally but are unable to kill them. Although most patients are males, females also inherit this disorder. Clinically, patients present with granulomatous lesions of the skin, lungs, and lymph nodes; hypergammaglobulinemia; anemia; and leukocytosis. Assessment of reduction of NBT by polymorphonuclear leukocytes is a simple and useful screening test for chronic granulomatous disease. In normal persons approximately 80 to 90 per cent of leukocytes reduce NBT during phagocytosis, but only 10 per cent of leukocytes in patients with chronic granulomatous disease will do so. Intermediate values are found in carriers.

Acquired Hypogammaglobulinemia

Patients with common variable immunodeficiency (acquired hypogammaglobulinemia) usually present with recurrent pyogenic infections, although these frequently are more chronic than the acute, overwhelming infections that occur in X-linked hypogammaglobulinemias. Patients also may present with autoimmune diseases. Their serum IgG level usually is less than 250 mg/dl; absence of IgA or IgM may or may not occur. Many individuals with this syndrome have cutaneous anergy. Most patients have normal numbers of circulating B cells; many have increased numbers of suppressor T cells or decreased numbers of helper T cells as well as abnormal proliferative responses. Patients often survive to the seventh or eighth decade. Many develop chronic lung disease in spite of adequate gamma globulin replacement. They are at increased risk of developing malignancy as well.

Complement Deficiencies

Deficiencies of complement are uncommon, but this in no way negates the importance of appropriate diagnosis. The best screening test is for total hemolytic (functional) complement. If a deficiency of hemolytic complement is found, specific component deficiencies should be sought. Deficiency of C1 esterase inhibitor leads to hereditary angioedema. Severe infections, similar to those seen in gamma globulin deficiencies, occur with C3 and C3 inactivator deficiencies. Deficiencies of the terminal components (C6, C7, C8) are associated with recurrent meningococcemia and gonococcemia.

Secondary Immunodeficiencies

Secondary immunodeficiencies may occur in a variety of situations (Table 7). The premature and the newborn infant may have depressed function of T and B lymphocytes, phagocytes, and complement system. Immunodeficiency appears in the context of chromosomal abnormalities such as Down's syndrome, malnutrition, sickle cell disease, immunosuppressive therapy, many viral infections, malignancy, and burns. It is beyond the scope of this discussion to describe these in detail. It is important to recognize that an increased susceptibility to infection occurs in a variety of clinical situations. In these situations, treatment includes prevention of exposure to infectious agents, careful surveillance for evidence of developing infection, and prompt institution of specific antimicrobial therapy.

Table 7. Secondary Immunodeficiencies*

I. The premature and the newborn
II. Hereditary and metabolic diseases
  A. Chromosome abnormalities
  B. Diabetes mellitus
  C. Exudative enteropathy
  D. Iron deficiency
  E. Malnutrition
  F. Myotonic dystrophy
  G. Nephrotic syndrome
  H. Sickle cell disease
  I. Uremia
III. Immunosuppressive agents
  A. Radiation
  B. Antilymphocyte globulin
  C. Corticosteroids
  D. Antimetabolites
IV. Infectious diseases
  A. Bacterial infections
  B. Viral infections
V. Infiltrative and hematologic diseases
  A. Histiocytosis
  B. Sarcoidosis
  C. Hodgkin's disease and lymphoma
  D. Leukemia
  E. Agranulocytosis and aplastic anemia
VI. Surgery and trauma
  A. Burns
  B. Splenectomy

*From Gotoff, S.P.: The secondary immunodeficiencies. In Stiehm, E.R., and Fulginiti, V.A. (eds.): *Immunologic Disorders in Infants and Children.* Philadelphia, W.B. Saunders Company, 1980.

DIAGNOSTIC PROBLEMS IN IMMUNOSUPPRESSED PATIENTS

By Bruce S. Rabin, M.D., Ph.D.
Pittsburgh, Pennsylvania

Children born with defective lymphocytic stem cell maturation have *severe combined immunodeficiency disease* (SCID). Without some type of intervention to restore the function of the immune system, children with SCID die from infectious disease. Other congenital immune deficiency diseases in which either the cellular immune component or the antibody-producing component of the immune system is deficient have provided evidence that different infectious diseases are prevented by various components of the immune system. Thus, we are reminded that the primary purpose of the immune system is prevention of invasion of the body by foreign pathogens.

Recently it has been learned that serum antibodies may induce physiologic changes in various tissues. For example, hyperthyroidism may be produced by an antibody to the thyroid-stimulating hormone receptor. Defects in muscle contraction may be induced by an antibody to the acetylcholine receptor at the motor endplate. These observations represent abnormal functions of the immune system that are associated with specific diseases (Graves' disease and myasthenia gravis). However, such abnormal immune responses are often of diagnostic significance and aid in determining the presence of a disease process. Thus, in addition to its protective role, the immune system can provide a diagnostic aid to the clinician.

Before considering the consequences of immunologic suppression, which most commonly is induced to prevent the rejection of transplanted tissue, some characteristics of immunosuppressive drugs will be reviewed.

ASPECTS OF IMMUNOSUPPRESSIVE THERAPY

1. Corticosteroids and irradiation are most effective when administered before the immune system encounters antigen.

2. Azathioprine, 6-mercaptopurine, and probably cyclosporine are most effective when used just after the immune system is exposed to antigen.

3. Cyclophosphamide is equally effective when administered prior to or after exposure of the immune system to antigen.

4. Some immunosuppressive drugs exert their primary effect on either the T or B lymphocyte populations. Thus, such drugs may be more effective in suppressing humoral or cellular immunity. An example of this type of immunosuppressive effect is demonstrated by cyclophosphamide, which has a greater effect upon B lymphocytes than on T lymphocytes.

5. It has been noted that certain types of immune responses are augmented following either low-dose irradiation or low-dose cyclophosphamide treatment in animals. Both cellular and humoral immune responses may be augmented by these procedures. Thus, it is possible that some types of immunosuppressive therapy may selectively deplete the suppressor lymphocyte population and allow more vigorous immune responsiveness.

6. Lymphocytes are highly radiosensitive, often being reduced to 25 per cent of baseline levels by 1000 rads of irradiation. The lymphocytes do not have to be undergoing cell division to be killed by irradiation. Generally, B lymphocytes are more radiosensitive than T lymphocytes, although different T lymphocyte populations have different sensitivities (for example, the suppressor lymphocyte is more radiosensitive than the helper lymphocyte).

7. In transplant immunology, cyclosporine is receiving a great deal of attention and increased use. The major reason for this is that the drug is highly specific for T lymphocytes and leaves other nucleated cells relatively intact. Thus, it does not affect the development of the erythroid and myeloid bone marrow elements. The exact means by which the drug is immunosuppressive is not certain, but it appears to prevent early activation processes of T lymphocytes. Examples of this are interference with the development of receptors for interleukin 1 and 2. The major problem in the use of cyclosporine is the development of B cell lymphomas while the drug is being taken. Most of these lymphomas appear to be due to Epstein-Barr virus infection and proliferation of a single lymphocyte into a malignant clone.

8. Injection of lymphocytes into a heterologous species can lead to the development of an antilymphocyte serum. Such sera are immunosuppressive. In humans, antilymphocyte serum can inhibit delayed hypersensitivity skin reactions to many different antigens. Skin graft survival may be prolonged by antilymphocyte serum, and rejection of transplanted tissue, such as heart allografts, can be reversed by injection of antilymphocyte serum. The use of monoclonal antibodies to specific lymphocyte populations permits the depletion of those populations. For example, monoclonal antibody specific for T helper or T suppressor cells has the theoretical capability of producing immunologic alteration by shifting the balance of the immune system. The clinical effectiveness of such antibodies is just beginning to be explored.

9. Total body lymph node irradiation has been found to reverse the ratio of helper to suppressor lymphocytes. Such treatment has been used in patients with rheumatoid arthritis and others receiving renal allografts. Immunosuppression results in the patients after lymph node irradiation. Interestingly, the reversal of the helper-suppressor ratio, which occurs in these patients, is not associated with infectious disease problems.

10. Glucocorticosteroids exert their effect on both immunologic and inflammatory responses. The exact mechanism by which these effects are obtained, however, is not well understood. It is important to remember that experimental animals, the mouse and rat, are highly sensitive to the effect of steroids, while normal lymphocytes of humans are steroid-resistant. Thus, it is important to note the species and doses of steroids used in experimental systems. In humans, the circulating mononuclear cells leave the intravascular space following exposure to corticosteroids and redistribute themselves. Decreases in lymphocyte counts in patients receiving corticosteroids are probably due to this phenomenon. Activated lymphocytes—those engaged in an immune response—may be sensitive to lysis by corticosteroids, however, and under certain circumstances the elimination of activated lymphocytes may be an important mechanism in immunoregulation. With regard to B lymphocytes and immunoglobulin levels, corticosteroids tend to reduce the levels of the immunoglobulins. IgG and IgA seem to be more sensitive to the suppressive effects of corticosteroids than is IgM.

IMMUNOSUPPRESSION AND INFECTIONS

The most common problem in patients who are immunologically suppressed relates to the development of infectious disease. Indeed, patients who are immunologically suppressed for organ transplantation or the treatment of an autoimmune or malignant disease may succumb not to the consequences of the original disease but to infection.

Fungal, bacterial, parasitic, and viral infections can occur in immunosuppressed patients. Examples of microbiologic agents causing central nervous system infections are *Listeria monocytogenes, Cryptococcus neo-*

formans, Toxoplasma gondii, and *Varicella zoster.* With central nervous system involvement, determination of the presence of infection may be difficult, as the inflammatory response is often impaired by the immunosuppressive treatment. Thus, more attention must be paid to the presence of headache or localizing neurologic signs in these patients. Subtle neurologic signs become extremely important and may indicate the necessity for performing a lumbar puncture. However, focal signs such as papilledema or decreased consciousness, which may indicate increased cerebrospinal fluid pressure, would be a contraindication to lumbar puncture. For these cases, computed tomography may be performed.

Fungal Infections

Fungal infections are a very frequent cause of death in immunosuppressed patients. In patients who are immunosuppressed, some of the fungal agents do not elicit antibody responses. An example of this is *Histoplasma capsulatum.*

The treatment used for many patients with fungal infection is amphotericin B, a drug with a high level of toxicity. This medication is best avoided unless a specific fungal infection is known to be present. Thus, isolation of the organism rather than serologic testing in immunosuppressed patients becomes extremely important. The usual fungal infections occurring in patients who are immunosuppressed are candidiasis, cryptococcosis, coccidioidomyocosis, histoplasmosis, and blastomycosis.

Bacterial Infections

Mycobacterial infections present an unusual complication in immunosuppressed patients. Normally, following infection with *Mycobacterium,* the cellular immune system reacts against the foreign pathogen. Tubercle bacilli are engulfed by macrophages and killed. However, a few of the bacilli remain in a dormant condition within the macrophages. If there is a decrease in cellular immune mechanisms, clinical reactivation of the mycobacterial infection can occur. Thus, a decrease in cell-mediated immunity increases the risk of dissemination of primary mycobacterial infection.

Parasitic Infections

A similar condition occurs with toxoplasmosis. *Toxoplasma gondii* is an obligate intracellular protozoan which is a common cause of latent infection in humans and is capable of persisting in tissue throughout the life of its host. In this regard, it is similar to mycobacteria. When an individual is immunosuppressed, the infection can become activated. Reactivation seems to involve primarily suppression of cell-mediated immunity. Some immunosuppressed patients are able to manifest a rising antibody titer to Toxoplasma infection; however, not all patients are capable of showing such a rise in titer.

Pneumocystis carinii infection occurs most commonly in patients who have T lymphocyte immunologic suppression, but it may also occur in patients with humoral immune suppression. Probably the most reliable means of diagnosing this infection is by open lung biopsy; on occasion, however, the organism may be demonstrated in sputum.

It may be useful to obtain serum from all patients being placed on immunosuppressive therapy prior to the initiation of such therapy. When a possible infection occurs for which a serologic assay is available, the original serum can be tested simultaneously with a serum obtained at the time of clinical symptomatology. Thus, changes in antibody levels may become apparent.

Viral Infections

Viral hepatitis provides a good disease model for the study of the role of cellular immune mechanisms in a disease pathogenesis. Patients with viral hepatitis have disease courses ranging from asymptomatic anicteric disease to fulminant hepatitis. Patients who have a congenital cellular immune deficiency (thymic alymphoplasia) rarely show any clinical evidence of liver damage following infection with a hepatitis-inducing virus. However, patients with a pure humoral immune deficiency develop fulminant hepatitis following infection. Thus, an immunocompromised patient will have an altered clinical course that depends upon the nature of the suppression.

Because of the paucity of clinical signs in an immunosuppressed patient with viral hepatitis, the diagnosis is extremely difficult. The diseases associated with susceptibility to hepatitis (chronic renal failure requiring hemodialysis, heroin addiction, Down's syndrome, Hodgkin's disease, lymphoproliferative disorders) should be kept in mind whenever there is a high degree of susceptibility to hepatitis.

IMMUNOSUPPRESSION AND MALIGNANCY

The incidence of malignancy in patients who are immunosuppressed, whether the immunosuppression is by a naturally occurring congenital or acquired immune deficiency disease or secondary to immunosuppression for tissue transplantation, strongly suggests that a normal functioning immune system is capable of protecting against the development of some types of tumors. In immunosuppressed patients, there is a marked increase in the incidence of lymphomas, with only a moderate increase in the incidence of epithelial tumors. As in patients with an intact immune system, the diagnosis of malignancy is based on a tissue diagnosis.

IMMUNOSUPPRESSION AND AUTOIMMUNITY

Autoimmune disease can occur in patients with hypogammaglobulinemia. For example, a syndrome resembling pernicious anemia occurs in such patients in association with gastric atrophy, megaloblastic anemia, and a quantitative deficiency of intrinsic factor. However, the patients lack parietal cell antibodies and intrinsic factor antibodies as well as a plasma cell infiltration in the gastric mucosa. Whether this pernicious anemia–like disease is due to T lymphocyte reactivity or, possibly, has a nonimmunologic basis has not been determined. Other diseases thought to be associated with autoimmune responses are vitiligo and alopecia, both of which occur with increased frequency in patients with hypogammaglobulinemia.

Role of Suppressor Cells

In considering autoimmune diseases, it is important to recognize that part of the immune system may be depressed, with a resultant susceptibility to the development of autoimmunity. There are various experimental indications that the immune system is held in check by a population of lymphocytes commonly referred to as suppressor cells. Immunization of an animal with pneumococcal polysaccharide leads to antibody production. If the thymus gland of the animal is removed prior to immunization, there is a marked increase in the amount of antibody produced. This would indicate that a loss of suppressor lymphocytes leads to increased amounts of antibody. In humans with common variable immunodeficiency diseases excessive numbers of suppressor lymphocytes are found, which inhibit the synthesis of antibody. Depletion of suppressor lymphocytes from human peripheral blood leads to the generation of autoreactive B lymphocytes. These observations suggest that as long as the balance between suppression and responsiveness is maintained, normal immunologic function exists. Once an imbalance occurs, however, either an immune deficiency disease or an autoimmune disease results.

Experimental evidence supporting this concept has been derived from New Zealand mice, which are prone to develop autoimmune diseases. These animals show a basic defect in their capacity to generate certain immune responses. The defect is present prior to the onset of autoimmunity. It has been suggested that, as one manifestation of this defect, these animals are unable to recognize and suppress the activity of autoreactive lymphocytes. In contrast, the immune system of normal animals is capable of suppressing the generation of self-reactive cells. Thus, this implicates defective suppressor activity as a fundamental abnormality in autoimmune diseases.

Role of Thymus in Defective Immune States

Suppressor activities have been attributed to a population of thymus-dependent lymphocytes. Therefore, abnormal thymic function may be a primary cause of defective regulatory mechanisms. This activity appears to be separable from the other activities of T lymphocytes, i.e., mediators of cellular immunity, "killer" function, and "helper" activity.

Autoimmune Disease in Immunosuppressed Patients

Consideration should be given to whether an immunologically suppressed individual is capable of manifesting immunologic disease. Examples of this are obtained by studying patients receiving tissue transplants who are immunosuppressed to prevent rejection of the transplant. Recurrence of the original immunologic disease or another immunologic disease would suggest that whereas immunosuppression may allow the survival of transplanted tissue, immunologic responses leading to disease can still occur.

Patients with systemic lupus erythematosus (SLE) have received renal allografts and have been immunologically suppressed to the point that the transplants were not rejected. In such patients SLE-associated damage to the transplanted tissue occurs. Indeed, such patients have the clinical and serologic manifestations of SLE. This includes dermatitis, pleuritis, and polyarthritis along with renal allograft lupus erythematosus. The type of serologic activity found in lupus patients (serum antinuclear antibodies, low serum complement) occurs in transplant individuals despite intensive immunosuppression.

Patients have been reported who have had biliary cirrhosis as a primary disease necessitating liver transplantation. Initially, following transplantation, the titer of antimitochondrial antibody dropped in the patients; however, all showed a rise in titer after the initial fall. Two years after transplantation, the antimitochondrial antibody titers are similar to or higher than those prior to transplantation. Thus, even though the patients were immunosuppressed, autoantibody formation occurred. Of course, it must be remembered that these antibodies did not develop in an antibody-negative individual, but recurred in an individual who had previously been positive.

The cited examples indicate that autoimmune disease can occur in immunosuppressed patients. There is little information regarding the development of autoimmune disease in patients who previously were normal. If the hypothesis that all normal individuals have low levels of autoantibody to autoantigens is correct, and disease is associated with the development of a high titer of antibody to an autoantigen, it may be assumed that autoantibodies can occur in patients who are immunosuppressed.

The development of autoantibodies in immunosuppressed patients would indicate that B lymphocyte function can proceed in the face of immunosuppression. If the assumption is made that immunosuppressive therapy primarily alters T lymphocyte function, the regulatory control of B lymphocytes would be expected to be decreased. This would suggest that B lymphocytes, which potentially are capable of manifesting autoantibody production but normally are impeded by suppressor T lymphocytes, could now become functional. Thus, it would be expected that many immunosuppressed patients would be prone to develop autoimmunity. That this does not occur may indicate that immunosuppressive agents interfere with B lymphocyte function or that autoimmune diseases do not always result from lack of regulation of B lymphocyte function. Certainly patients treated with drugs whose primary effect is on the suppressor lymphocyte population would be those in whom autoimmunity would most likely occur.

Examples of diagnostic information provided by the immune system in determining the presence of immunologically induced disease are given in Table 1.

Table 1. Diagnosis of Immune Disorders by Antibody Tests

Type of Antibody	Disease (Percentage of Patients with Antibody)
Antinuclear	Systemic lupus erythematosus (90–98%)
	Scleroderma (60%)
	Sjögren's syndrome (88%)
	Dermatomyositis (45%)
	Chronic active hepatitis (75%)
	Primary biliary cirrhosis (46%)
	Cryptogenic cirrhosis (38%)
	Rheumatoid arthritis (25%)
Antimitochondrial	Primary biliary cirrhosis (94%)
	Chronic active hepatitis (28%)
	Sjögren's syndrome (occasionally)
	Viral hepatitis (67%)
Anti–smooth muscle	Lupoid hepatitis (75%)
	Primary biliary cirrhosis (50%)
	Alcoholic cirrhosis (50%)
	Infectious mononucleosis (5%)
	Malignant tumors (5%)
Antithyroid	Pernicious anemia (55%)
	Myasthenia gravis (35%)
	Thyroid autoimmunity states (85%)
Anti-glomerular basement membrane	Glomerulonephritis—Goodpasture's syndrome (80%)
	Chronic active hepatitis (10%)
Anti-adrenal	Addison's disease (50%)
Anti–parietal cell	Pernicious anemia (90%)
	Atrophic gastritis, often in conjunction with iron deficiency anemia (60% in women)
Anti–striated muscle	Myasthenia gravis (50%)
	Thymus tumors (some)
Anti–islet cell	Newly diagnosed insulin-dependent diabetics (80%)
Anti-skin	Intercellular: *Pemphigus vulgaris* (85%)
	Pemphigus foliaceus (85%)
	Linear at basement membrane:
	Bullous pemphigoid (80%)
Antimyocardial	Dressler's syndrome (50%)
Antisperm	Infertile couples (10%)

In addition to immunosuppression produced by chemotherapy, naturally occurring immunosuppression does occur. For example, patients with congenital immune deficiency diseases (T lymphocyte, B lymphocyte, or combined T and B lymphocyte deficiencies) frequently will have life-threatening infections unless some type of immunologic reconstitution is initiated. Similarly, malignancy frequently will lead to immunologic suppression. Even patients undergoing surgery may have immunologic suppression following the surgical procedure. Sometimes this is associated with malnutrition, chronic stress, or chronic illness.

In summary, patients who are immunologically suppressed are prone to develop infectious and malignant diseases. Because a rise in antibody titer may not be a reliable indication for the diagnosis of infectious disease, it becomes increasingly important to isolate infectious agents. The diagnosis of malignancy in immunologically intact or immunologically suppressed individuals requires a tissue diagnosis. Autoimmune disease may recur in patients immunologically suppressed for tissue transplantation, but the initial development of autoimmunity in immunologically suppressed individuals is not clearly defined.

ACQUIRED IMMUNODEFICIENCY SYNDROME (AIDS)

By Thomas J. Spira, M.D.
and Russell K. Brynes, M.D.
Atlanta, Georgia

DEFINITION

The acquired immunodeficiency syndrome (AIDS) is a newly discovered disease manifested in its most severe form by a profound deficiency in cell-mediated immunity. Secondary to this immunodeficiency, opportunistic infections and certain malignancies may develop, most commonly Kaposi's sarcoma. The disease affects predominantly males, especially those in four high-risk groups. These are homosexual males, intravenous drug abusers, Haitians (both in Haiti and recent immigrants in other countries) and hemophiliacs. In addition, heterosexual partners and infants of members of risk groups have developed the disease, and cases have occurred in some individuals receiving blood transfusions. The peak incidence occurs between the third and fifth decades of life. Geographically about half the cases have occurred in New York state (the majority in New York City) and about one fifth in California (predominantly San Francisco and Los Angeles).

The disease is currently thought to be due to infection with a newly discovered human retrovirus known as lymphadenopathy-associated virus (LAV) or human T-cell lymphotropic virus III (HTLV III). This agent is specifically cytotoxic for T helper cells, thereby leading to immunodeficiency. It appears to be transmissible venereally as well as by blood or blood products.

The Centers for Disease Control (CDC) employ a definition for disease surveillance purposes that encompasses a majority of the severe cases of AIDS. This consists of Kaposi's sarcoma or an opportunistic infection (i.e., an infection that is moderately to highly predictive of a defect in cell-mediated immunity) occurring in a person without a known predisposing condition or known cause of cell-mediated immune deficiency, such as malignancy or immunosuppressive therapy. Patients need to be over 15 years and under 60 years of age. In addition to patients with severe involvement, there are other presentations, which are probably part of the full spectrum of AIDS. These include the occurrence of non-Hodgkin's lymphoma, autoimmune thrombocytopenic purpura, or chronic unexplained generalized lymphadenopathy in members of high-risk groups. The inclusion of these other conditions in the spectrum of AIDS is based on a variety of epidemiologic and laboratory data, and is being confirmed by the finding of antibodies to the presumed etiologic agent.

PRESENTING SIGNS AND SYMPTOMS

The onset of severe AIDS can be insidious—with a variety of vague constitutional symptoms, such as fever, night sweats, fatigue, malaise, weight loss, or diarrhea—or acute, with the rapid onset of an opportunistic infection, most commonly *Pneumocystis carinii* pneumonia. Since symptoms vary with the different manifestations, it is best to review them individually.

About one quarter of patients with severe cases have presented with Kaposi's sarcoma. This is a rare neoplasm that prior to the epidemic of AIDS was seen primarily in elderly males of Eastern European Jewish or Italian ancestry. It is characterized by multiple reddish-brown to violet macules or nodules of the skin, often on the extremities. Lesions are usually painless and can appear without any other signs or symptoms. In AIDS, Kaposi's sarcoma is also seen predominantly in males of similar ancestry but at a much younger age. In addition, it is commonly found at locations in the gastrointestinal tract from the oral cavity to the rectum as well as in lymph nodes. Kaposi's sarcoma is endemic in Central Africa, where AIDS patients have also been found.

Over one half of patients with severe AIDS have presented with *Pneumocystis carinii* pneumonia. This is heralded by several days of fever, dyspnea, and dry cough. In addition, there is often a history of weight loss, diarrhea, or oral thrush preceding the onset of pneumonia.

A variety of other opportunistic infections that may occur in individuals with severe AIDS are listed in Table 1. Their presentation is similar to that in other clinical situations in which immunosuppressive disease or therapy is encountered. Among these is infection caused by Cryptosporidium, which has only recently been found to be pathogenic to humans. This coccidian parasite causes a self-limited diarrhea in the normal host, which lasts about 1 week. In the immunodeficient AIDS patient it causes a chronic, profuse, watery diarrhea with weight loss, which may last several months or until the patient's death.

Individuals with chronic, generalized, unexplained lymphadenopathy may have an early or milder manifestation of AIDS. The sites of lymph node enlargement often include bilateral posterior and anterior cervical chains as well as axillary and inguinal nodes. Less frequently enlarged are occipital, supraclavicular, or epitrochlear nodes. Occasionally there is accompanying hepatomegaly or splenomegaly. Lymph nodes may vary in size over time but enlargement usually persists over a course of months to several years. They are usually asymptomatic, but occasionally patients have episodic or persistent tenderness. A variety of constitutional symptoms similar to those seen in the prodrome of severe AIDS are also found in these individuals, most commonly fatigue or malaise.

LABORATORY FINDINGS

The most prominent abnormalities in patients with severe AIDS are found in the immune system. Lymphopenia (less than 1500 cells/cu mm) is often present, and the absolute number of cells in the T helper/inducer subset is markedly depressed. T suppressor/cytotoxic cells are usually present in normal numbers unless there is extreme lymphopenia, in

Table 1. Severe Opportunistic Infections Seen in Patients with the Acquired Immunodeficiency Syndrome

Viral
- Disseminated cytomegalovirus infection
- Progressive or persistent herpes simplex virus infection
- Disseminated varicella-zoster virus infection
- Papovavirus infection (progressive multifocal leukoencephalopathy)

Fungal
- Oroesophageal candidiasis
- Cryptococcal meningitis or disseminated infection

Bacterial
- Disseminated *Mycobacterium avium-intracellulare* infection
- Disseminated *Mycobacterium tuberculosis* infection

Protozoal
- *Pneumocystis carinii* pneumonia
- *Toxoplasma gondii* encephalitis or disseminated infection
- *Cryptosporidium* enteritis

which case their numbers may also be depressed. The ratio of T helper/inducer cells to T suppressor/cytotoxic cells is often quite low (less than 1.0). Functionally the cells are hyporesponsive or unresponsive to lymphocyte mitogens and to specific recall antigens as measured by the in vitro lymphocyte blastogenesis test. In vivo there is usually cutaneous anergy to recall antigens as well. Humoral immunity, in contrast, is relatively intact, with the presence of normal numbers of B lymphocytes. Frequently a polyclonal hypergammaglobulinemia, usually of the IgG or IgA class, is present. High levels of circulating immune complexes are also commonly found.

Among other laboratory abnormalities identified in AIDS are the presence of a variety of autoantibodies. An increased incidence of antisperm antibodies has been found in homosexual AIDs patients. Antibodies to T lymphocytes, platelets (in patients with idiopathic thrombocytopenic purpura), neutrophils, and red cells have been reported. Elevations in the levels of an acid-labile alpha-interferon similar to that seen in systemic lupus erythematosus have also been identified in many patients. Antibodies to the human retrovirus(es) LAV/HTLV III have been found in AIDS patients and those with generalized lymphadenopathy, whereas others with immunosuppression of other origin lack antibodies. Antibodies are also found at increased prevalence in groups at high risk for AIDS. This is consistent with this virus being the etiologic agent for the disease, although the presence of antibodies does not indicate prognosis for those infected.

OTHER DIAGNOSTIC PROCEDURES

Biopsy is warranted in those individuals with chronic generalized unexplained lymphadenopathy. Frequently a histopathologic picture of reactive follicular and paracortical hyperplasia is seen. This may reflect an early or mild form of AIDS. However, lymphoid depletion with burned-out germinal centers often precedes development of opportunistic infections. Clinically unsuspected infections (tuberculosis, toxoplasmosis) or malignancies (non-Hodgkin's lymphoma) may also be diagnosed on occasion.

Kaposi's sarcoma manifested by the appearance of red-brown to violet cutaneous patches, macules, or nodules requires histopathologic confirmation. It may also present as primary lymph node or gastrointestinal disease.

CLINICAL COURSE

Patients with severe AIDS (meeting the CDC surveillance definition) have a poor prognosis. Those that present with Kaposi's sarcoma have a more prolonged course than those presenting with opportunistic infections, although in time the former also develop opportunistic infections. Mortality and morbidity are most often due to these infections rather than the Kaposi's sarcoma. The overall case-fatality rate is about 45 per cent, but 80 to 90 per cent of the patients diagnosed as having AIDS in 1979 and 1980 have already died. To date there is no evidence for the reversal of the immune deficiency in these patients. Lacking such a reversal, there is a sequence of opportunistic infections leading to death.

In patients with other manifestations of the spectrum of AIDS the situation is less clear. Patients with generalized lymphadenopathy are currently being followed to determine if this is a milder manifestation of the disease or part of the prodrome of the severe AIDS. To date, in only a small percentage of these patients has the condition progressed to the severe disease.

THERAPY

Therapy of severe AIDS has been symptomatic for the most part, treating the Kaposi's sarcoma or the infections rather than the underlying immune deficiency. Currently there is still no specific therapy for this disease.

SAFETY PRECAUTIONS

Information on the transmission of AIDS indicates that it is most often transmitted venereally or by blood and blood products. There is no evidence to date of AIDS transmission to hospital personnel from contact with patients or clinical specimens in the absence of another risk factor. The same precautions used in caring for patients with hepatitis B should be employed in managing AIDS or handling patients' clinical specimens.

Blood donations from AIDS patients and members of risk groups or their sexual contacts are currently being discouraged.

SJÖGREN'S SYNDROME

By Stuart S. Kassan, M.D.
Denver, Colorado
and Haralampos M. Moutsopoulos, M.D.
Ioannina, Greece

SYNONYMS

Other names given to this disorder have been primary Sjögren's syndrome (sicca complex), secondary Sjögren's syndrome, autoimmune exocrinopathy, and sicca syndrome.

DEFINITION

Sjögren's syndrome (SS) is a chronic, autoimmune disorder characterized by a lymphocyte-mediated destruction of exocrine glands that leads to diminished or absent glandular secretion and mucosal dryness. The disease affects primarily females. Women constitute at least 90 per cent of the patients in most studies, and the presence of the disease is highest in persons over 40 years of age. Sjögren's syndrome can occur alone or in association with other autoimmune diseases (most commonly rheumatoid arthritis and systemic lupus erythematosus).

The diagnosis of SS is most often made when objective evidence for two of the following three conditions is present: (1) xerophthalmia (with keratoconjunctivitis sicca); (2) xerostomia; and (3) another connective tissue disease.

Several studies have shown serologic, immunogenetic, and clinical differences between patients with SS alone and those with SS and rheumatoid arthritis. Because of these differences (see later description), SS alone is termed primary SS, and SS associated with rheumatoid arthritis or another connective tissue disease is termed secondary SS.

PRESENTING SIGNS AND SYMPTOMS

The main clinical manifestations of primary SS are xerophthalmia with keratoconjunctivitis sicca, xerostomia, and recurrent episodes of painful parotid or major salivary gland enlargement. The exocrine glands of the upper and lower respiratory tracts, gastrointestinal tract, genitalia, and skin are also often affected. Signs and symptoms of xerophthalmia (dry eyes) include injected conjunctivae often associated with a sensation of grittiness and an accumulation of thickened mucus, photosensitivity, blurred vision, burning, and decreased visual acuity. Xerostomia (dry mouth) may present with symptoms of "bad breath," altered taste, mouth soreness, and accelerated development of dental caries. Excessive ingestion of fluids is often noted both with and between meals as a result of the decrease in salivary gland secretions. Respiratory tract involvement may present with hoarseness, chronic cough (nonproductive), and increased incidence of upper and lower respiratory tract infections. Gastrointestinal tract involvement may result in mucosal atrophy of the esophagus, dysphagia, or atrophic gastritis. Dryness of the vagina may result in dyspareunia and pruritus. The skin may become excessively dry, and alopecia may occur when exocrine glands of the skin are involved. Extraglandular involvement in SS may present with significant lymphadenopathy, splenomegaly, or hepatomegaly. In addition nonthrombocytopenic purpura in the lower extremities with hypergammaglobulinemia (hypergammaglobulinemic purpura), Raynaud's phenomenon, interstitial pneumonitis (with dyspnea), peripheral neuropathy, and cryoglobulinemia may be present early in this disease process. In general, the extraglandular manifestations are most often found in primary SS.

CLINICAL COURSE

The clinical manifestations of SS represent an extremely wide spectrum of disease severity and organ involvement. Similarly, the clinical course in patients with SS remains quite variable. Patients with primary SS have a greater incidence of parotid gland enlargement, interstitial nephritis, myositis, pneumonitis, Raynaud's phenomenon, and purpura. The activity of disease in this group appears more indolent; however, a spontaneous waxing and waning of symptoms may be noted. In patients with secondary SS, the clinical course may mirror the course of the other associated connective tissue disease.

COMMON COMPLICATIONS

Progression of disease activity in SS results in glandular and extraglandular complications. Glandular involvement, as a result of lymphocytic infiltration, may predispose to parotid infection (parotitis) resulting from glandular obstruction. The most common offending organisms are the staphylococcus and streptococcus. Dry mouth may result in inflammation of the tongue and buccal cavity. Dryness of the nasal mucosa may cause epistaxis, and upper airway respiratory tract involvement may predispose to recurrent bronchitis.

Extraglandular complications may involve dependent hypergammaglobulinemic purpura, in which peripheral neuropathy may also be present as a result of vasculitic involvement of the vasa nervorum. Renal complications include latent or overt distal renal tubular acidosis and hyposthenuria. Glomerulonephritis may be seen in association with immune complex deposition.

Lymphocytic infiltration of the reticuloendothelial organs may be benign or malignant. Pseudolymphoma describes lesions that show tumor-like clusters of lymphoid cells but do not meet the criteria for malignancy. Lymphoma occurs in patients with primary and secondary SS with a relative risk 40 times that of controls. Waldenström's macroglobulinemia may be seen in SS, but the relative risk is unknown.

PHYSICAL EXAMINATION

Salient features of a careful physical examination include conjunctival erythema, a visibly dry conjunctival sac, and often enlarged lacrimal glands. A Schirmer's test, performed at the bedside, with filter paper wetting of less than 5 mm/5 minutes suggests clinically significant xerophthalmia but is associated with a high frequency of false-positive and false-negative results.

Evidence of oral mucosal dryness may include fissuring and cracking of the tongue and absence of secretions sublingually and at the orifice of Stensen's ducts (from the parotid glands), especially when parotid enlargement is present.

Evidence of extraglandular lymphoproliferation should be sought by examining for peripheral lymphadenopathy, splenomegaly, and hepatomegaly.

Vasculitic involvement may be detected by the presence of palpable purpura and altered peripheral sensory perception to touch or pain (suggesting a peripheral neuropathy).

In patients with secondary SS, evidence of another

associated connective tissue disease should be suggested by such findings as symmetric polyarthritis (in rheumatoid arthritis), sclerodermatous skin changes (in scleroderma), discoid lupus rash, or malar rash (in systemic lupus erythematosus).

LABORATORY PROCEDURES

Autoantibodies are common in SS. Tests for antinuclear antibodies (ANA) are positive in 50 to 80 per cent of patients. Rheumatoid factor is present in 75 to 90 per cent of SS patients. Fifty per cent have polyclonal hypergammaglobulinemia. In some patients hyperviscosity of the serum may be found as well as the presence of cryoglobulinemia. Circulating immune complexes have been detected by specialized laboratory procedures, but these have rarely been of clinical significance. Serum complement levels are infrequently depressed. Other, nonspecific laboratory abnormalities are commonly noted in SS. These include elevated erthyrocyte sedimentation rates; mild normochromic, normocytic anemia; and hypoalbuminemia.

Precipitating antinuclear antibodies in SS, specifically anti-SSB (La) antibody, are found in 54 to 73 per cent of patients with primary SS and in fewer than 10 per cent of patients with secondary S.

Histocompatibility antigens HLA-B8 and HLA-Dw-3/DRw3 have been found more frequently in patients with primary SS (75 per cent and 55 per cent respectively compared with normals (less than 15 per cent). In addition, HLA-Dw3 was found in a statistically greater percentage of those with primary SS than those with secondary SS.

DIAGNOSTIC PROCEDURES

Table 1 lists the tests commonly used in patients suspected of having SS. The Schirmer test (previously described) has been most commonly used, but the redictive value is extremely limited owing to the high percentage of false-positive and false-negative results found. The use of slit-lamp verification of keratitis with rose bengal corneal staining has been more specific in the appropriate clinical setting.

Techniques for examining the functional state of the salivary glands include parotid flow measurement and scintigraphy, the latter capitalizing on the selective ability of the salivary glands to concentrate radionuclides and to secrete them into saliva. Sialography, the introduction of radiopaque dye into the parotid ductal system, examines both anatomic and functional parotid gland abnormalities. In general, there is a fair correlation with the severity of xerostomia and the degree of abnormalities on sialogram in SS. These changes may include acinar and ductal atrophy with puddling, main duct enlargement, and retention of contrast material. These changes, however, are not specific and may be seen in chronic inflammation from other causes.

Table 1. Diagnostic Tests and Procedures in Sjögren's Syndrome

Tests of Functional Abnormalities
Schirmer's test
Parotid salivary flow rate
Radionuclide scan of parotid gland
Tests of Anatomic Abnormalities
Rose bengal staining of cornea
Parotid gland sialography
Biopsy
Minor salivary glands of lip and palate
Lacrimal gland
Parotid gland

Biopsy of the minor salivary glands located in the lip or soft palate is among the most specific of the diagnostic procedures available. Histologic changes are often similar to those found in the parotid, submaxillary, and lacrimal glands. The degree of focal lymphocytic infiltration detected in these biopsy specimens is a good index of severity and appears to be highly specific for SS.

POTENTIAL ERRORS AND PITFALLS IN DIAGNOSIS

The parotitis seen in SS may be confused with a bacterial or viral sialadenitis. In addition, coexistence of an infectious parotitis with the inflammatory parotitis of SS may also be seen, leading to further confusion over the true nature of this problem. Infiltrative processes such as sarcoidosis may also cause parotid gland enlargement and must be distinguished from SS by histologic means. Lymphoma or other malignancies that may cause parotid gland infiltration and enlargement and lymphadenopathy may also predispose to symptoms similar to those of SS. Sjögren's syndrome patients may also develop significant lymphadenopathy and splenomegaly, and in some cases the disease may progress to pseudolymphoma or frank lymphoma. In these patients, periodic histologic examination of affected lymph nodes may be indicated, as there is an increased relative risk for the development of non-Hodgkin's lymphoma in all SS patients compared with age- and sex-matched controls.

Medications with anticholinergic effects may mimic some of the clinical features of SS. The use of such medication may also enhance the symptoms of xerostomia and xerophthalmia in patients with pre-existent SS.

Finally, lipoproteinemia as well as amyloidosis can mimic the clinical features of SS.

Section Sixteen

ALLERGY

HAY FEVER

By Lawrence Zaslow, M.D.
New Orleans, Louisiana

DEFINITION

Hay fever, rose fever, and pollinosis are terms to describe seasonal allergic rhinitis. This is a form of immediate hypersensitivity that occurs in atopic individuals and is characterized by seasonal symptoms of nasal congestion, rhinorrhea, sneezing, lacrimation, and itching of the eyes, nose, and throat. Symptoms are recurrent and occur during the pollination season of the allergen to which the patient is sensitive.

Atopic individuals produce IgE that binds to the mast cells in the skin, nasal mucosa, and respiratory mucosa and causes generalized sensitization of the skin and mucosa. When the specific allergens in a sensitized individual contact the IgE–mast cell complex, chemical mediators such as histamine, kinins, and prostaglandins are liberated, producing the pharmacologic effect on blood vessels and glands to produce the symptoms of seasonal allergic rhinitis.

Hay fever, a seasonal form of allergic rhinitis, is caused by sensitivity to pollens and molds. It must be differentiated from perennial allergic rhinitis, which also occurs in atopic individuals sensitized to additional allergens such as dust, animal danders, and tobacco smoke, as well as pollen and molds. Perennial allergic rhinitis is characterized by continuous symptoms without seasonal variation. These patients have sneezing, rhinorrhea, and itching that are less severe than in seasonal rhinitis, and their main complaint is chronic nasal obstruction.

Seasonal allergic rhinitis is caused by pollen and mold allergy. Patients' symptoms recur yearly, and the symptoms are related to the time and duration of the pollinating season of the causative allergen. These airborne allergens depend upon the wind and atmospheric distribution for cross pollination. The pollinating season varies with the specific allergen and the geographic location. The pollinating season in a given location is fairly constant. Ragweed pollen is the most important allergen and causes the most severe form of seasonal rhinitis. Ragweed is found in the eastern as well as the midwestern portion of the United States. In general, ragweed pollinates in the late summer and early fall and pollen is present in the air until the first frost. Tree pollen occurs in the very early spring, and grass pollen predominates in late spring and early summer. Molds are found throughout the year but have a tendency to peak in the spring and late summer, especially during warm and humid months. There is usually a decrease in the spore count of molds with winter.

The more sensitive the patient, the more intense and prolonged are the symptoms. With increasing sensitization to additional allergens, the pollinosis has a tendency to worsen, with increased duration and severity. It is not common for spontaneous remission of symptoms to occur. Allergenic management, including avoidance of allergens when possible, medication, and immunotherapy, is very effective in rendering the patient symptom-free.

CLINICAL SIGNS AND SYMPTOMS

Typical symptoms of season allergic rhinitis are sneezing; thin watery rhinorrhea; itching of the nose, soft palate, and pharynx; and nasal obstruction. The nasal obstruction may be responsible for mouth breathing, snoring, and headaches, as well as "blocked-up ears." Postnasal secretions may cause coughing, hoarseness, and sore throat. Other associated symptoms are itching and watering of the eyes and loss of smell, as well as irritability and fatigue. These symptoms appear seasonally and recur, depending on the patient's sensitivity to the prevailing allergen. These patients also have symptoms of associated atopy, i.e., seasonal asthma, urticaria, and eczema.

PHYSICAL EXAMINATION

Many children demonstrate the "allergic salute." This is a rubbing of the nose in an upward and outward manner with the palm of the hand to relieve the itching. This maneuver may cause a transverse crease across the lower third of the nose. "Allergic shiners" are dark circles under the eyes and are probably due to venous stasis. The conjunctivae may be injected, and there may be edema of the eyelids. The lower eyelids may have a wrinkle or an accentuated line—the line of Denne. Examination of the nose may reveal clear secretions covering the boggy, edematous turbinates. These mucous membranes have a characteristic pale bluish color. Hyperplasia of the posterior pharyngeal lymphoid tissue may occasionally be found. With severe rhinitis, there may be increased swelling of the turbinates, leading to complete nasal obstruction. One third of children with severe seasonal rhinitis may have serous otitis media.

LABORATORY STUDIES

Many patients demonstrate mild or moderate peripheral eosinophilia of 4 to 8 per cent. However, nasal allergy may be present with normal values. Total eosinophil counts over 600/cu mm strongly suggest allergy. Hansel's stain of the nasal secretions usually reveals an eosinophilic predominance with the presence of more than 3 to 10 per cent eosinophils. Absence of eosinophils does not rule out seasonal rhinitis since upper respiratory tract infection may cause a predominance of neutrophils and lymphocytes. Serum IgE levels are increased in approximately 35 per cent of the patients. This level increases further during exposure and pollination, and it may fall after the season as well as with immunotherapy. IgE levels of normal and atopic individuals frequently overlap; therefore, an IgE level is seldom helpful in establishing a diagnosis of allergy. The radioallergosorbent test (RAST) is an in vitro method for measuring specific IgE antibodies to various allergens. Most studies show good correlation between positive skin tests and positive RAST, so that new information is not usually obtained from the RAST when skin tests can be done. The RAST is less sensitive and more expensive than conventional allergy skin tests. One major advantage the RAST has is in patients with extensive atopic eczema; skin tests may be difficult to perform and may aggravate the dermatitis of these patients.

Paranasal sinus x-rays may vary from normal studies in mild cases to those showing increased density over the maxillary and ethmoid sinuses in the most severe cases (see article on Disorders of the Paranasal Sinuses).

DIAGNOSIS

Skin testing is very important in confirming the initial impression in the patient with an atopic background having characteristic symptoms and physical findings. Skin testing should be performed by an allergist with the inhalant allergens found in the geographic area by scratch as well as the intracutaneous technique. Positive skin tests differentiate the allergic from the nonallergic patient, as demonstrated by the characteristic wheal and flare reactions that occur within 15 to 20 minutes after applying the allergen to the skin. Two common sources of inaccuracy of skin testing are prior administration of antihistamine, which would lead to false-negative responses, and dermographic skin, causing false-positive reactions. To prevent false-negative results, the patient should avoid antihistamines for 48 hours prior to testing. Corticosteroids, theophylline, and adrenergic agents do not alter skin reactivity and need not be discontinued before testing.

DIFFERENTIAL DIAGNOSIS

The early symptoms of the common cold may simulate seasonal allergic rhinitis; however, with time purulent secretions occur and may be associated with fever. Nasal obstruction due to a deviated septum or nasal polyps is easily detected by physical examination. Nasal polyps are rarely seen in allergic rhinitis. Vasomotor rhinitis is a condition with symptoms similar to those of allergic rhinitis; however, symptoms are caused by nonspecific stimuli, such as changes in temperature, humidity, and emotion, as well as fatigue and strong oder. Nonallergic rhinitis is frequently associated with nasal infection and nasal polyps, as well as with aspirin sensitivity and perennial asthma. Drugs such as rauwolfia, oral contraceptives, and the beta-adrenergic blockers can cause symptoms of nasal allergy. Prolonged use of topical vasoconstrictors in the form of nose drops or sprays can produce a chemical rhinitis (rhinitis medicamentosa).

COMPLICATIONS

Seasonal allergic rhinitis is usually associated with few complications. There is a tendency, however, for recurrent respiratory infections, sinusitis, and serous otitis media to occur.

ASTHMA IN CHILDHOOD

By Susan G. Marshall, M.D.
and C. Warren Bierman, M.D.
Seattle, Washington

DEFINITION

Asthma is a disorder of the tracheobronchial tree characterized by largely reversible mild to severe obstruction of airflow. In a given patient, the obstruction may improve spontaneously or may require intensive therapy. Symptoms are usually episodic and paroxysmal; they may last from hours to days or persist for months to years.

The clinical hallmark of asthma is wheezing, a squeaky expiratory sound made through partially obstructed airways. Cough is also a predominant characteristic.

Asthma is sometimes divided into two categories:

1. Intrinsic asthma, which is not mediated by IgE.
2. Extrinsic asthma, which is precipitated by allergens external to the body and is IgE-mediated.

In the vast majority of asthmatic children, specific IgE antibody can be demonstrated to a variety of allergens.

A common feature of asthma is the hyperreactivity of the tracheobronchial tree to various chemical mediators of inflammation. Alterations of mucosal permeability and abnormality of mechanisms associated with calcium flux may also be involved.

Precipitating factors in asthma include allergens, infectious agents, irritants, weather and climate changes, exercise, emotional factors, animals, drugs and chemicals, and upper respiratory tract inflammation.

Numerous physiologic mediators are activated or liberated in the inflammatory process, and many are probably important in asthma. These substances may act directly on target cells and induce bronchospasm, mucosal edema, or mucus secretion, or they may act indirectly through activation of other mediators or through recruitment of other mediator cells.

The tissue mast cell and the circulating basophil leukocyte are thought to be primary sources of inflammatory mediators, including preformed histamine and the mediators derived from arachidonic acid (such as the leukotrienes C, D, E, which previously were termed SRS-A or slow-reacting substance of anaphylaxis). These cells also liberate or activate various other substances that induce eosinophil or neutrophil chemotaxis, act on platelets, or activate kinins.

SYNONYMS

Asthma is also known as reversible obstructive airways disease, asthmatic bronchitis, allergic bronchiolitis, and WARI (wheezing associated with respiratory illness).

PRESENTING SIGNS AND SYMPTOMS

Asthma is characterized by episodes of respiratory obstruction, with expiratory obstruction predominating over inspiratory block. This obstruction is usually manifested by wheezing, a musical, high-pitched sound produced by airflow turbulence in the large airways. However, asthma can occur without wheezing if the obstruction involves primarily small airways—a form known as occult asthma. Wheezing also may disappear completely as obstruction becomes more severe and airflow becomes more limited.

Wheezing is generally accompanied by coughing, and occasionally cough may be the only symptom. Generally, symptoms are more severe at night and in the early morning.

Symptoms vary with age. The infant or young child may have a history of recurrent bronchitis, bronchiolitis, or pneumonia; persistent coughing with colds; recurrent croup; or a chronic chest rattle. Older children often develop a tight chest with colds, recurrent chest congestion, or persistent coughing or wheezing. Symptoms may be precipitated or aggravated by irritants, animal dander, molds, dusty areas, pollens, tobacco smoke, cold air, or exercise. Often the precipitating factor is unknown.

COURSE

A typical asthma attack may last 3 to 7 days. However, lung function, particularly airflow obstruction of small airways (beyond the 23rd generation of bronchi) may not return to normal for several weeks.

Initially asthma attacks may be episodic, with symptom-free intervals in between. As the disease becomes more chronic, the intervals between attacks may diminish.

In general, asthma is more severe in the younger child and tends to become less severe with anatomic development of the lungs. By age 6 years, adult configuration of the lungs is reached and severity of the disease tends to decrease, as measured by the number of hospital admissions. In adolescence, asthma may become more severe and require more intense pharmacologic therapy. By late adolescence most patients tend to improve, only to have recurrences of asthma in adulthood.

The course of asthma may be modified by several therapeutic factors. Long-term treatment involves:

1. Identification of exacerbating factors.
2. Elimination of specific exacerbating allergens or irritants.
3. Appropriate use of bronchodilator and antiasthmatic drugs, with corticosteroids reserved for acute exacerbations or when other medications are insufficient.
4. Immunotherapy against specific precipitating factors that cannot be avoided.

COMMON COMPLICATIONS

Complications of asthma include growth retardation, exercise-induced bronchospasm, school absenteeism, somatopsychic manifestations, and acute exacerbations which may require hospitalization (status asthmaticus). A rare complication of chronic asthma in North America is allergic bronchopulmonary aspergillosis (see article on Opportunistic Mycoses). An increasing number of patients with severe childhood asthma are recognized as having chronic, nonreversible obstructive disease as adults.

Complications of status asthmaticus include pulmonary and extrapulmonary factors. *Pulmonary* complications include acute respiratory failure, atelectasis, pneumothorax, and pneumomediastinum. *Extrapulmonary* complications include vasopressin (antidiuretic hormone) excess, flaccid paralysis of an arm or leg, sudden alteration in theophylline metabolism, and cardiac arrythmias. These factors may combine to cause acute respiratory failure, resulting in cardiorespiratory arrest, brain damage, and death.

CLINICAL EVALUATION OF PATIENTS WITH ASTHMA

History

Patients with asthma may present in a variety of ways, but most share certain common historical features and asthma often can be diagnosed by history alone. On history taking, it is essential that the patient or parent, or both, understand the meaning of the word wheezing. As previously mentioned, wheezing usually is accompanied by cough, although cough may be the only symptom. A history of symptomatic improvement after an epinephrine injection, inhaled or oral adrenergic drugs, or oral theopylline is important to note.

Physical Examination

The physical examination should focus on growth and development and on the eyes, ears, nose, paranasal sinuses, pharynx, chest, and skin.

Both asthma and the agents used to treat it can affect growth, and therefore weight and height should be recorded and plotted on a growth grid.

The physician should observe respiratory rate, color of lips and nail beds, dyspnea, prolongation of expiration, chest wall retractions, and use of accessory muscles in breathing. Evidence of clubbing of the fingers should be noted (this is not a concomitant of asthma). Round-shouldered posture with an increased anterior-posterior chest diameter may be appreciated. In children who develop asthma early, a pseudo-rachitic chest deformity from long-standing airway obstruction may be seen.

Blood pressure, along with cardiac rate and rhythm, should be noted because of the effects that several of the commonly used pharmacologic agents as well as the disease itself may have on these parameters.

The conjunctivae should be examined for edema, inflammation, and tearing. A slit-lamp examination for cataracts is indicated yearly in the chronic steroid-dependent asthmatic patient. Ear drums should be examined with a pneumatic otoscope for evidence of eustachian tube dysfunction and effusion, which can lead to conductive hearing loss or recurrent suppurative otitis. Examination of the nose classically reveals pale or bluish mucous membranes. However, the mucosa is frequently erythematous from chronic irritation. Rhinorrhea is typically clear unless there is superimposed infection. Allergy is an unusual cause of nasal polyposis, the presence of which suggests cystic fibrosis in the young child or paranasal sinusitis with aspirin sensitivity in the adolescent.

Examination of the lungs frequently reveals rhonchi or unequal breath sounds, which may clear upon changing position or coughing. Although wheezing is frequently elicited with a forced expiratory maneuver, occasionally only prolongation of the expiratory phase without wheezing may be appreciated. It is important to note air exchange, as some patients with severe asthma do not wheeze because too little air is exchanged to generate a wheezing sound. Wheezing from the lower respiratory tract should be differentiated from similar sounds that may emanate from the laryngeal area.

The texture of skin and subcutaneous tissue should be noted, as it relates to nutrition and fluid balance. Flexor creases and other areas of skin should be examined for active or healed atopic dermatitis.

LABORATORY DIAGNOSIS

Blood Counts

Often the complete blood count is normal. The stress of acute asthma and an injection of epinephrine may both induce a leukocytosis. Although eosinophilia is frequently thought to correlate with atopic tendencies, eosinophil counts may vary with adrenal function and severity of asthma or may reflect other disease states, including parasitic infestation.

Nasal Cytologic Examination

Nasal secretions may be obtained readily in children. Predominance of eosinophils suggests accompanying nasal allergy in children, although adolescents and adults can have nasal eosinophilia in the absence of allergy. A predominance of polymorphonuclear leukocytes (PMNs) and lymphocytes occurs with viral infections; PMNs and ingested bacteria are seen frequently in patients with sinusitis.

Serum Tests

Quantitative levels of serum immunoglobulins (IgG, IgM, and IgA) are useful to rule out immunodeficiency syndromes in children with recurrent or chronic bacterial infections. The finding of an elevated serum IgE level may be useful in the young child with recurrent bronchitis in whom there is a question of the role of allergy. A normal IgE level does not rule out allergy, nor does an elevated level mean the patient is allergic. In the child with shifting pulmonary infiltrates, a marked elevation in IgE should cause the physician to suspect bronchopulmonary aspergillosis.

Sweat Test

A sweat test should be performed on infants and children with chronic respiratory symptoms to rule out cystic fibrosis. However, cystic fibrosis and asthma are not mutually exclusive. The incidence of cystic fibrosis is the same in patients with asthma as in the general population, and cystic fibrosis patients may have a significant reactive airway component which should be treated (see article on Cystic Fibrosis).

Radiologic Evaluation

All children with asthma should have a chest x-ray early in their course to rule out parenchymal disease, congenital anomaly, or foreign body. A chest x-ray should be considered for children requiring hospitalization for asthma. Chest x-rays in patients with asthma may be normal, but with acute exacerbations hyperinflation, interstitial infiltrates, atelectasis, pneumothorax, and pneumomediastinum may be present.

Paranasal sinus films should be considered in children with persistent nocturnal coughing and headache.

OTHER DIAGNOSTIC PROCEDURES

Pulmonary Function Tests

Pulmonary function tests are objective, noninvasive, and extremely helpful in the diagnosis and follow-up of patients with asthma. Improvement following injected or inhaled beta-adrenergic agents, documented by pulmonary function tests performed prior to and after drug administration, may be helpful in ascertaining the presence of reversible airway disease.

Bronchial provocation or challenge tests using methacholine or histamine are helpful in diagnosing abnormal bronchial lability. The asthmatic attack can be characterized by decreased forced expiratory volume measured at 1 second, decreased vital capacity, and increased residual volume. The characteristic features, as well as the typical symptoms of asthma, can be induced in normal subjects and in asthmatic subjects by inhalation of aerosols containing histamine or cholinergic agonists. Patients with asthma are hyperresponsive to these bronchoconstrictors in that they respond to them at 1:100 to 1:300 of the concentration required to constrict normal airways. These tests may be useful in characterizing the patient with extreme airway sensitivity, and they are safe if performed in a well-equipped laboratory by an experienced physician.

Another challenge test involves the inhalation of specific allergens. Often this test induces a biphasic reaction, marked by an initial fall in lung function followed in 6 to 8 hours by more severe, protracted bronchospasm.

Bronchial provocation is not necessary in patients with obstruction, for whom bronchodilators or a short course of steroids is a better test.

Exercise Tests

An exercise test, which can employ a treadmill, a cycloergometer, or free running, can provide useful information regarding an individual's exercise tolerance. In exercise-induced bronchospasm, pulmonary functions begin to diminish after exercise, reaching a nadir 3 to 20 minutes after completion of exercise. Pulmonary function tests are generally measured before exercise and at 1, 5, 10, 15, and 20 minutes after. The response is usually expressed as a percentage of change from baseline. In general, a decrease of 15 per cent in either forced expiratory volume in one second (FEV_1) or peak expiratory flow rate (PEFR) is considered abnormal. A change of 30 to 40 per cent is considered moderately severe, and more than 45 per cent a severe response.

Allergy Tests

Skin testing or radioallergosorbent testing (RAST) is indicated in patients in whom specific allergic factors are believed to be important. Allergy testing is particularly important in children with severe asthma to rule out allergic factors that might contribute to exacerbations.

A variety of types of skin tests have been used in the specific diagnosis of reaginic (IgE-mediated) allergic disorders. These tests involve a small quantity of allergenic extract introduced below the epidermis. Within 15 to 20 minutes, a characteristic wheal and flare is observed in patients who have IgE antibodies that recognize one or more of the test allergens. This test is highly sensitive, cost-effective, and safe when used by experienced personnel.

The radioallergosorbent test is capable of detecting minute quantities of allergen-specific IgE antibodies that circulate in the serum of allergic patients. This test is now widely available.

Both tests have merits. Optionally performed, both skin tests and RAST detect IgE antibody accurately and reproducibly. The RAST is thought to be less sensitive than skin tests. Results of both tests usually correlate well with allergic symptoms and signs produced by exposure to the specific allergen tested. Results from either test can be used in deciding to institute immunotherapy. However, when RAST results are used as the basis for immunotherapy, a skin test with the planned initial dilution solution should be done to be certain that the patient tolerates in vivo administration of the allergenic extract. Skin tests are thought to be superior to currently available RASTs in the diagnosis of certain life-threatening anaphylactic states, particularly penicillin and hymenopteral allergy. Also, the results of skin tests are more immediately available. RAST is preferable in the child with generalized dermatitis, in the very young child, in the patient who is too ill for direct testing, and in the patient who must continually be on antihistamine therapy.

ERRORS AND PITFALLS IN DIAGNOSIS

There are a number of common conditions that should be differentiated from asthma at various stages of childhood. It is important to note that almost all can coexist with asthma. These include laryngotracheobronchomalacia, cystic fibrosis, chronic diseases due to respiratory viral infections, foreign body, croup, acute epiglottitis, hyperventilation syndrome, and mitral valve prolapse.

Just as not all wheezing indicates asthma, not all patients with asthma wheeze. In the absence of overt wheezing, the diagnosis may be missed, especially in children. For this reason an objective measurement of lung function is indicated. As already noted, pulmonary function tests are objective, noninvasive, and cost-effective. A simple mechanical spirometer from which an FEV_1 and forced vital capacity (FVC) can be calculated or a Wright Pediatric Flow Meter for younger children is useful in office practice. Children as young as 2 years of age can be taught to perform pulmonary function maneuvers with the aid of a birthday party favor.

Asthma is a greatly undertreated disorder in children, and its physical, psychological, and socioeconomic morbidity is unnecessarily high, especially in light of the diagnostic procedures and wide variety of beneficial pharmacologic agents available to our pediatric population.

ASTHMA IN ADULTS

By John M. O'Loughlin, M.D.
and John A. Saryan, M.D.
Burlington, Massachusetts

SYNONYMS

Other names for asthma in adults include hyperreactive airway disease, reversible obstructive airway disease, and asthmatic bronchitis.

DEFINITION

Asthma may be defined as intermittent reversible obstructive airway disease. It is a widespread disorder that affects between 9 and 10 million Americans and has been estimated to be fatal in 2000 to 3000 persons each year. Because of its chronicity, it can be a crippling and debilitating disease. Some patients have large airway obstruction; in others, small airway disease predominates as evidenced by a poor maximum midexpiratory flow rate. Still others have a combination of large and small airway obstruction. The bronchi narrow in response to stimuli by constriction of the peribronchial musculature, increased secretion of bronchial mucus, and edema of the mucous membranes.

In the past, asthma was (and still is by many) classified into two main forms:

1. Extrinsic or allergic, in which an allergen can be identified.

2. An intrinsic or idiopathic form, in which no offending allergen can be identified.

The extrinsic variety usually affects children and young adults and is characterized by paroxysms of bronchospasm, wheezing, shortness of breath, and other symptoms of respiratory distress following exposure to the offending allergen. Episodes are sudden in onset and usually brief, and the patient is relatively symptom-free between attacks. Patients often have other allergic manifestations, such as hay fever or eczema, or both. Dermal reactivity to allergens can usually be demonstrated in the form of IgE skin sensitizing antibody. Chronic wheezing may also be related to IgE mechanisms.

In contrast, intrinsic or nonallergic asthma usually begins in adults in the fourth decade, and allergic factors do not seem to play a role, nor can skin sensitizing antibody be demonstrated. The asthma attack is usually more severe and the prognosis less favorable. There are probably very few cases of pure extrinsic or intrinsic asthma. The majority of patients with this disease have a mixed type. An increased frequency of haplotypes HLA-1, HLA-8, and HLA-2 BB in white children with severe asthma is evidence of genetic predisposition to this disease.

The recurrent nature of asthma can restrict the patient severely and result in great economic loss. A decade ago, the average number of restricted activity days per person with asthma was 15 and the figure for bed disability days was 5.8. The natural course of asthma is extremely variable.

There is a slight male preponderance in adult asthmatics. About one third of patients have symptoms before the age of 16 years. A peak occurs during the third decade, and 1 in 10 cases begins after the age of 65.

Allergic rhinitis is not usually an antecedent disease, as was previously thought. Eczema is frequently found in allergic asthmatics. Asthma may be provoked by many stimuli in addition to identifiable allergens. After allergic causes, infections are the most commonly identifiable precipitating factor. Respiratory syncytial virus, parainfluenza virus, and influenza virus are the organisms most commonly involved.

The mechanisms involved in exercise-induced asthma have not been identified. Generally, there is a bronchodilation in the first 7 to 8 minutes of activity, followed by a bronchoconstriction. Some patients experience symptoms during exercise, and others note symptoms at the end of the exercise.

Irritability of the autonomic nervous system with predominance of the cholinergic system is found in many asthma patients. Cholinergic mechanisms are believed to be the cause when cold weather, emotional upsets, or irritants appear to precede the wheezing.

PRESENTING SIGNS AND SYMPTOMS

As in any specialty of medicine, carefully taken histories form a most important tool. Information obtained from many patients helps define and classify the major types of asthma. Responses to specific allergenic stimuli can occur with seasonal rhythmicity or on a year-round basis. The acute and initial episode may present with a variety of symptoms, including cough, shortness of breath, wheezing, or a feeling of tightness in the chest. These can occur at rest, or with exercise, or they may awaken the patient at night. Chest tightness is often the first of these symptoms, usually followed by dyspnea. With small airway obstruction, the patient and often the physician may not hear wheezes, and cough may be the only symptom. Cough may at first be dry and nonproductive. As the attack progresses, the patient will often begin to expectorate thick, colorless mucoid sputum. If infection complicates the picture, yellow- or green-colored phlegm may be produced. Usually as the patient begins to bring up the sputum, there is some relief of the symptoms. The wheezing may vary from high-pitched and musical to low-intensity, sonorous sounds. As breathlessness increases the patient may hyperventilate, using accessory muscles of respiration, and have sternal retractions. Occasionally cyanosis of the nail beds is seen. The periodicity of asthma is important in making the diagnosis as well as in pinpointing the probable etiologic agent. It is possible the patient may be seen at a symptom-free time and none of the usual signs will be present.

The following points should be emphasized in taking the patient's history. An individual who has symptoms in successive years at the same time of year usually has an allergic basis for symptoms. Pollens from trees and grasses are the airborne agents responsible for spring asthma, and ragweed is responsible for wheezing that begins in mid-August and lasts until the first frost. Symptoms that worsen in winter months could be due to animal dander and house dust exposure, since concentration and exposure to these allergens are greater in a closed environment. Mold spores are a problem during warm summer months and also into the fall until the temperature falls below freezing or a period of snow diminishes the production of the mold spores. Different parts of the country will have varying seasons when certain antigens are prevalent, and these should be recognized by the physician.

ENVIRONMENTAL FACTORS

Recurring symptoms during the week with freedom from wheezing at night suggests a precipitating factor at work. Symptoms occurring indoors with improvement outdoors suggests animal dander, dust, or mold from humidifiers and air conditioning units. Horsehair mattresses are uncommon but occasionally are found as causes of asthma. Feather pillows and down comforters may be aggravators during the night and early morning hours. Cold, dry air has been shown to precipitate wheezing, whereas cool humidified air can be helpful.

NONSPECIFIC STIMULI

Stimuli such as odors of perfumes or aftershave lotions can cause airway obstruction. Smoke, inorganic dusts, and temperature and barometric pressure changes have been believed to cause symptoms as well. An immunologic mechanism is probably not at work with these stimuli.

INFECTION

When infection precipitates wheezing, usually it is a viral infection, not a bacterial infection, that is responsible. Parainfluenza virus, respiratory syncytial virus, and influenza virus are the most frequent offending viral agents. Some authors have postulated that these agents cause damage to the lining of the respiratory system and result in post-infection wheezing of many month's duration and, in some patients, permanent symptoms of asthma.

CIRCADIAN FACTOR

Nocturnal asthma is frequent. Possible physiologic explanations include:

1. Pooled bronchial secretions with impairment in the mechanism of respiration resulting from the supine position,
2. Exposure to bedroom allergens,
3. Decrease in endogenous catecholamines and cortisol secretions with possible increased histamine levels in some,
4. Reflex changes of the parasympathetic nervous system,
5. Gastroesophageal reflux.

Many patients are free of symptoms during the day.

GENETIC FACTORS

Family or pre-existing personal history of allergy is found in most patients with allergic asthma. A history suggestive of wheezing with infection, frequent bronchitis, or croup is often elicited. Occasionally the family history will reveal alpha$_1$-antitrypsin deficiency, cystic fibrosis, or bronchiectasis.

FOODS AND DRUGS

Often the patient will volunteer the information that wheezing occurs with the ingestion of certain foods. High on the list of culprits are shellfish, other seafoods, nuts, and peanuts. Usually these are causes of acute explosive asthma attacks without sequelae. Certain drugs, dyes, and additives can cause wheezing. Aspirin, as well as other nonsteroidal antiinflammatory drugs, can cause acute wheezing in patients with adult-onset asthma, especially those with nasal polyps. Tartrazine dye (FD&C Yellow No. 5) which is found in many beverages, candies, and medicines, can precipitate acute wheezing. Metabisulfite, used as a preservative and antioxidant in alcoholic beverages (especially wines), salads, seafood, and fruits to prevent brownish discoloration, can cause severe acute dyspnea.

DIFFERENTIAL DIAGNOSIS

Bronchial asthma is frequently confused with emphysema and chronic bronchitis. Emphysema is nonreversible obstructive airway disease usually found in patients with a long history of cigarette smoking or occupational dust exposure. Chest x-rays show flattened diaphragms and hyperlucency. Smoking and air pollution are the most common precipitating factors in chronic bronchitis. Patients with this disorder have a long history of mucopurulent cough without remission.

Occasionally it is difficult to distinguish wheezing of cardiac origin from primary asthma. Acute wheezing can occur in paroxysmal nocturnal dyspnea of arteriosclerotic heart disease. Usually the signs of left heart failure, such as peripheral edema, liver congestion, and neck vein distention, help distinguish this form of asthma.

Pulmonary embolism may mimic acute asthma in patients without previous history of obstructive pulmonary disease. Radioisotope scanning is the most reliable screening procedure, although pulmonary angiography may be necessary.

Bronchial adenoma, bronchiectasis, cystic fibrosis, croup, and foreign bodies may also mimic asthma and should be ruled out, especially when conventional treatment is unsuccessful.

CLINICAL COURSE

Bronchial asthma is characterized by episodes of exacerbation and remission. Children suffering from asthma often become free of symptoms spontaneously in adolescence. Symptoms occurring in pregnancy are unpredictable, with both exacerbations and remissions being possible. Hyperreactivity of the airways remains during remission. This is demonstrated by exacerbation of symptoms upon contact with occupational allergens, irritant fumes, exercise, and cold weather. Allergic asthma may occur during well-defined allergic seasons. Patients who are better after moving to a new environment often develop symptoms after several years of sensitization to the antigens in that area.

Remissions are shorter and less likely to occur in nonallergic asthma. Nasal polyps and aspirin sensitivity often are present in adult-onset nonallergic asthma. Sinusitis frequently complicates the clinical course of asthma in these patients. Infections are often precipitating factors and cause prolonged periods of wheezing. Nonallergic asthma in adults frequently is unresponsive to conventional forms of therapy and may be fatal. Most deaths are sudden and unexpected and occur between 4 and 6 A.M. An increase in asthma deaths in Great Britain in the 1960s has been related (but not without controversy) to excessive use of Freon propellant inhalers. The abuse of certain beta-adrenergic agent aerosols can cause death by overperfusion of underventilated lungs, paradoxical bronchoconstriction caused by metabolic breakdown products of isoproterenol, or cardiac arrhythmia.

Rapport between patient and physician is critical. Communication should always be available to evaluate daily symptom changes and possible drug overuse. Prompt use of corticosteroids may be necessary when theophylline and beta-adrenergic medications are unsuccessful in controlling symptoms.

A patient who develops one or more of several critical criteria should be hospitalized for intensive care and possible intubation. These include pulsus paradoxus, tachycardia greater than 110 beats/minute, forced expiratory volume in one second (FEV_1) less than 1 liter, predicted expiratory flow rate (PEFR) less than 100 liters/minute, $Paco_2$ greater than 45 mm Hg or Pao_2 less than 50 mm Hg.

COMPLICATIONS

Complications that may occur in asthma include severe cough resulting in rib fractures or hemoptysis. Atelectasis with or without subsequent pneumonia may aggravate the clinical course. Mucus plugs can cause recurrent and peribronchial infections in the right middle lobe and lingula. Severe explosive attacks can be accompanied by pneumothorax or pneumomediastinum, or both. Both of these can also be precipitated by intermittent positive pressure breathing therapy. Obesity complicates asthma by forcing chronic hypoventilation. Medication can cause hypokalemia, hyperglycemia, cardiac arrhythmias, peptic ulcerations, weight gain, and osteoporosis. Acute adrenal insufficiency may occur from stress or infections in the steroid-dependent patient not given increased amounts of exogenous corticosteroid therapy.

Hypersensitivity to *Aspergillus fumigatus* may lead to a complication of asthma known as allergic bronchopulmonary aspergillosis (ABPA). Patients may have recurrent pneumonia, increased IgE levels, eosinophilia, brown plugs of mucus, and immediate and delayed skin test reactions to *Aspergillus fumigatus*.

PHYSICAL EXAMINATION

Although the traditional hallmark of asthma is wheezing, some patients may present with entirely normal physical findings and demonstrate abnormalities only with pulmonary function testing. This is frequently the case in cough-variant asthma. Asthma may be overlooked in individuals with mild disease unless a forced expiratory maneuver after complete inspiration is performed. Latent rhonchi and wheezes can be elicited by this technique as well as by a trial of exertion. In general, most symptomatic patients with chronic asthma will demonstrate prolonged expiration and wheezing or rhonchi on auscultation. The physical examination should also include an assessment of upper respiratory disease. The presence of nasal obstruction and discharge, nasal polyposis, and sinus tenderness may have an important bearing on lower airway disease. Clubbing of the extremities is not seen in uncomplicated asthma, and its presence suggests a complication or another disease. A barrel chest deformity secondary to chronic hyperinflation is occasionally seen.

In patients with acute asthma, emphasis is placed on determining the degree of aeration. The presence of diminished breath sounds and the use of accessory muscles of respiration are more important signs than the intensity of wheezing. The absence of wheezing (silent chest) is an ominous sign indicating poor air exchange. Hyperinflation, prolonged expiration, nasal flaring, and cyanosis may also be present in severe asthma. Elevation of the pulse and blood pressure may be seen as a result of an asthma attack or, more importantly, may be due to prior abuse of adrenergic drugs. A pulsus paradoxus greater than 10 to 20 mm Hg has been shown to be a reliable sign of airway obstruction. Anxiety and restlessness may occur as the attack progresses.

LABORATORY TESTS

The diagnosis of asthma is generally suspected on the basis of the history and physical examination. Laboratory tests are useful in distinguishing asthma from other diseases, in ascertaining the severity of an acute attack, and in determining whether an allergic basis exists.

Blood Counts

The presence of eosinophilia in the blood is helpful in distinguishing asthma from other disorders, such as chronic bronchitis. However, the presence of eosinophilia does not necessarily imply an allergic basis for asthma. Eosinophilia greater than 15 to 20 per cent may be seen in asthma but should raise suspicion of other disorders, such as parasitic diseases, allergic bronchopulmonary aspergillosis, drug reactions, malignancies, and periarteritis nodosa. Total eosinophil counts are more accurate than estimates of the eosinophil count from the white blood cell count and differential count. Values greater than 400 cells per cu mm represent elevated levels in adults. Infections and use of corticosteroids and epinephrine will decrease the number of circulating eosinophils. The erythrocyte sedimentation rate is normal in uncomplicated asthma. An elevated white blood cell count obtained prior to administration of epinephrine is supportive evidence for an intercurrent infection.

Sputum Examination

The sputum of asthmatic patients will vary considerably depending on the degree of inflammation, presence or absence of infection, and the patient's state of hydration. The presence of yellow or greenish sputum does not always signal infection; it may instead be due to eosinophils or cellular debris. Sputum eosinophilia greater than 5 to 10 per cent supports a diagnosis of asthma. Eosinophils may disappear during acute infections or with corticosteroid therapy. The presence of eosinophils, brown plugs, and fungal hyphae in the sputum suggests the diagnosis of ABPA. As was already mentioned, this is a complication of asthma.

In acute exacerbations of asthma, wet preparations of the sputum may be analyzed for the presence of eosinophils, which have large refractile granules. Sputum neutrophilia in the absence of eosinophilia would suggest an intercurrent infection.

Electrocardiography

Electrocardiography shows normal results in uncomplicated asthma but should be performed in acute attacks to look for the presence of arrythmias and signs of right heart strain. In asthma complicated by chronic bronchitis, signs of right heart strain such as right axis deviation, right bundle branch block, and cor pulmonale may be seen.

Skin Tests

Allergy skin testing for immediate or IgE-mediated hypersensitivity to airborne allergens is a valuable procedure in the assessment of patients with symptoms suggestive of chronic asthma. This procedure is the most important in distinguishing extrinsic from intrinsic asthma. The clinical significance of an immediate positive wheal and flare reaction depends on the ability to correlate the skin test reaction with a worsening of asthma symptoms on exposure to the particular allergen. A positive skin test, in the absence of immediate symptoms after exposure, does not necessarily exclude the possibility of clinical sensitivity, since delayed reactions do occur. Delayed or late-phase IgE-mediated reactions are gaining increased recognition. This can be demonstrated by bronchial (inhalation) challenge with an allergen. The late-phase reaction begins 2 to 8 hours after challenge and may last from 3 to 24 hours. This late-phase reaction is believed to be involved in the pathogenesis of chronic extrinsic asthma. Skin testing is performed with extracts of inhalants to which a patient is likely to be exposed. These include pollens, mold spores, animal danders, house dust, mites, feathers, kapok, and similar substances. A careful environmental history and knowledge of locally important pollens guides the selection of appropriate antigens for testing. Epicutaneous testing (prick or scratch test) is performed first. A more sensitive technique, intradermal testing, is then used for antigens that elicited a negative or borderline reaction. Routine skin testing for foods is not recommended, since positive reactions may or may not correlate with symptoms. Prick testing for foods may be done in selected instances in which a given food is suspected of causing symptoms. Testing should be done by experienced personnel trained in proper administration and scoring of test reactions. Current limitations of testing include improper techniques, loss of potency in extracts used for testing, and the lack of standardization of extracts by their content of active allergen. The only exception is ragweed pollen, which the Food and Drug Administration now requires to be labeled according to the amount of antigen E present.

Serum IgE Levels

Total serum IgE levels may be helpful in deciding whether a patient has extrinsic or intrinsic asthma, but considerable overlap between normal individuals and asthmatic patients exists. The presence of an IgE level greater than 300 IU/ml in patients with asthma is suggestive of atopy. A low or normal IgE level does not exclude the possibility of IgE-mediated hypersensitivity. The serum IgE level is most useful as an aid in the diagnosis and management of patients with allergic bronchopulmonary aspergillosis, since IgE levels fluctuate with exacerbations and remissions. The radioallergosorbent test (RAST) measures allergen-specific IgE in the serum. The significance of a positive RAST depends on its correlation with a patient's symptoms on exposure to the allergen. RASTs are currently available for a wide variety of foods and inhalants. Routine screening with RAST is not recommended, since it is more expensive than skin testing and less sensitive than the intradermal test. It may be useful in certain situations, such as widespread atopic dermatitis, dermatographism, and poor skin test reactivity, and as a research tool.

Pulmonary Function Tests

Carefully performed measurements of pulmonary function are indispensable in the office assessment and management of patients with chronic or acute asthma. Airway obstruction can easily be measured during performance of the forced expiratory maneuver with a spirometer. Spirometry measures the volume of air expelled from the lungs versus time. The most useful parameters are FVC (forced vital capacity), FEV_1 (forced expiratory volume in the first second), PFR (peak flow rate), and FEF $_{25-75\%}$ (forced expiratory flow during the middle 50 per cent of the vital capacity). Some newer spirometers are equipped with small computers capable of providing predicted values and percentages based on age, height, sex, and race. Values less than 75 to 80 per cent of predicted results are considered abnormal.

Baseline pulmonary function testing demonstrates the presence of airway obstruction and its severity. Improvement of greater than 20 per cent in a given parameter after inhalation of a bronchodilator establishes the presence of reversible airway obstruction or asthma. Failure to respond, however, does not rule out asthma. In some patients, a 2- to 4-week course of corticosteroids may be necessary to reverse long-standing obstruction secondary to chronic inflammation. Serial measurements of pulmonary function are useful in the management of patients hospitalized with acute asthma and in long-term office management of patients on bronchodilators or corticosteroids. The $FEF_{25-75\%}$ especially important since it is less dependent on effort and reflects small peripheral airway function, whereas the PFR, FVC, and FEV_1 are effort-dependent and represent large airway function. The $FEF_{25-75\%}$ is a particularly sensitive measure, since it may be decreased in ambulatory patients with no audible wheezing. In acute severe asthma, the FEV_1 is less than 15 to 30 per cent of predicted value and the FVC is less than 30 to 50 per cent of predicted level. Failure to show prompt, substantial improvement in the PFR or FEV_1 after the administration of epinephrine indicates a high likelihood that the patient will need hospitalization. A small hand-held peak flow meter may be quite useful for determining improvement.

More extensive pulmonary function testing in a well-equipped modern pulmonary laboratory, including determination of lung volumes, flow volume loops, and diffusion capacity, is indicated in patients with irreversible obstruction or in those with atypical features. Bronchial reactivity can be induced by methacholine or cold air challenge in patients with normal baseline spirometry who have symptoms suggestive of asthma. Bronchial challenge with allergens to look for immediate or delayed reactions may be useful in selected circumstances but is generally employed only as a research tool. Aspirin or tartrazine challenge may be useful in certain patients but should be done by experienced personnel in a laboratory setting.

Arterial Blood Gases

Arterial blood gas determinations are important in the assessment and management of acute severe asthma but are of little use for patients who have chronic asthma and are ambulatory. Hypoxemia may be seen in chronic asthma as a result of ventilation and perfusion mismatch. Poor ventilation of alveolar units results in underoxygenation and hypercapnia. During acute severe asthma, this defect is magnified, resulting in a fall of the Pa_{O_2} to less than 60 mm Hg. Signs of impending respiratory failure are a Pa_{O_2} less than 50 mm Hg and a Pa_{CO_2} greater than 45 mm Hg. In acute asthma, hyperventilation will result in a lowering of the Pa_{CO_2} but will not improve oxygenation. Unless airway obstruction is severe, the Pa_{CO_2} is generally low or normal. Arterial blood gas determinations should be obtained on all patients with respiratory distress who do not respond promptly to therapy. Serial measurements are especially important, since a rising Pa_{CO_2} indicates a worsening status and the need for intensive monitoring and treatment. Arterial pH is generally increased in less severe attacks as a result of the fall in the Pa_{CO_2}. In more severe episodes, the pH may be decreased as a consequence of respiratory or metabolic acidosis.

Other Tests

Other tests which may be helpful include tuberculin skin testing, particularly in patients who may need corticosteroids. Quantitative immunoglobulin levels to rule out an immune deficiency are indicated in patients who have recurrent sinopulmonary infections or evidence of bronchiectasis. Mild cystic fibrosis may not present until late adolescence or early adulthood. Symptoms of bronchiectasis and the presence of clubbing should warrant a sweat chloride determination (see article on Cystic Fibrosis).

RADIOGRAPHIC PROCEDURES

An initial chest x-ray should be obtained on all patients with a suspected diagnosis of asthma in order to rule out other disorders. The radiographic findings are usually normal, although hyperlucency of the lungs, increased peribronchial markings, and atelectasis secondary to mucous plugging may be seen. A routine chest x-ray is not necessary during every acute attack unless there is a poor response to treatment, evidence of infection, or signs and symptoms of pneumothorax or pneumomediastinum. X-rays of the paranasal sinuses are indicated in patients with unexplained exacerbations of asthma who have symptoms of nasal obstruction, postnasal discharge, purulent rhinorrhea, or sinus tenderness. A single Waters view is usually adequate to assess disease in the maxillary antra and frontal sinuses. Markedly thickened mucosal membranes, opacification, and air-fluid levels suggest the presence of acute or chronic sinusitis.

A barium esophagram may help identify some patients who have gastroesophageal reflux complicating their asthma; however, esophageal manometry, overnight pH recording in the distal esophagus, and esophageal biopsy may be necessary to identify other individuals with this problem.

POTENTIAL ERRORS IN DIAGNOSIS

Before making a diagnosis of bronchial asthma, the possibility of other diseases that may mimic asthma must be kept in mind. The differential diagnosis includes all diseases that may affect the lungs and tracheobronchial tree. The coexistence of asthma with another disease process should be considered a possibility. In patients in whom the diagnosis is not straightforward, demonstrating the reversibility of airway obstruction is mandatory before assuming that the patient has asthma.

Many patients with recurrent episodes of mild or moderate wheezing are often incorrectly diagnosed as having bronchitis and subjected to multiple courses of antibiotic therapy. Proper diagnosis may lead to early elimination of an offending agent(s) and institution of appropriate treatment of asthma. Another common error is the assumption that eosinophilia or positive allergy skin tests indicate an allergic basis. Eosinophilia is also seen in intrinsic asthma. The correlation of symptoms with skin test reactivity must be established before a patient is diagnosed as having allergic asthma.

DRUG REACTIONS

By Jeremy H. Thompson, M.D.
Los Angeles, California

Drugs are powerful chemicals that unfortunately may produce effects other than those sought by the prescriber. Such unsolicited effects are commonly called *adverse drug reactions;* they are usually inconvenient or trivial and only rarely fatal. A tremendous amount of attention has been given to their incidence and cost, but the precise role of such reactions in hospital admissions, office visits, duration of hospital stay, morbidity, and mortality is not known. Adverse drug reactions are obviously one facet of *iatrogenic disease,* and they may affect every body system.

The use of any drug inevitably entails some risk. No drug is so specific that it produces only desired effects in all patients. No clinically useful drug (not even a placebo) is entirely devoid of adverse effects. Both the patient and physician should recognize and accept these facts. The physician should neither become a therapeutic nihilist for fear of adverse drug reactions nor prescribe indiscriminantly. Before administering a drug, he or she should carefully consider its possible adverse effects and weigh these against the potential therapeutic benefits. In general, risks of unwanted reactions are acceptable if a serious disease is being treated. Potential adverse drug reactions are not acceptable in therapy of trivial illness. Most drugs are relatively safe, but some have so low a therapeutic ratio that there is little difference between the effective dose and the toxic dose. Knowledge of basic and clinical pharmacology, including the desired and adverse effects of drugs, permits rational use in respect to risk-benefit assessment.

Regrettably, every drug may cause adverse effects even when used according to recommended schedules of therapy. If a drug is used incorrectly, however, not only may it be less effective, but in addition adverse reactions are usually more likely. Furthermore, a drug response specifically sought in one patient may become an adverse effect in another when the same drug is used with a different indication. Serious adverse drug reactions usually occur in severely ill patients. Epidemiologically, important drugs producing adverse reactions include aspirin, digitalis, thiazide diuretics, antimicrobial agents, tranquilizers, antihypertensive drugs, anticoagulants, sulfonylureas, and glucocorticocosteroids—drugs with generally acceptable risk-benefit ratios.

DEFINITIONS OF ADVERSE DRUG REACTIONS

To minimize confusion, I use the term *adverse drug reaction* to cover any unsolicited effect produced by the drug in question. Numerous attempts have been made to classify adverse drug reactions, usually on the basis of pathogenesis, but such efforts are not too practical since many reactions are impossible to categorize. Commonly utilized operational definitions have included the following:

Side Effects. These are undesirable extensions of the drug's pharmacologic actions. Drowsiness following the use of H_1-antihistamines is a good example. Adverse drug reactions appearing as undesirable extensions of the drug's basic pharmacological actions are usually more readily recognizable than effects attributed to allergy or other mechanisms.

Toxic Effects. These are usually dose-dependent adverse drug reactions. An example is digitalis-induced toxicity.

Idiosyncratic Reactions. These are either normal responses to a subtherapeutic drug dose—for example, succinylcholine sensitivity (Table 1)—or unusual resistance to a drug, with very high doses being required to produce an effect—for example, sodium warfarin resistance (Table 1).

Allergic Reactions. Allergic reactions are mediated by specific antibodies or sensitized lymphocytes and can be classified into Coombs' and Gell's Types I, II, III, or IV (see later description). Many reactions presumed to be based on hypersensitivity phenomena are not readily classifiable, however.

Anaphylactoid Reactions. These reactions are dependent upon nonallergic release of mast cell mediators (Table 2).

Pseudoallergic Reactions. These refer to symptoms of cardiorespiratory collapse resulting from inadvertent intravascular administration of drugs such as procaine penicillin, which should be given intramuscularly.

Paradoxic Reactions. This term is self-explanatory; an example is cerebral excitement in children or in elderly individuals from the use of sedatives.

Drug Interactions. A drug interaction occurs whenever the prophylactic, therapeutic, or diagnostic action of a drug is altered in or on the body by a second chemical administered previously, concurrently, or in close sequence. The second substance (interactant) may be another drug, an excipient, ethanol, a component of tobacco smoke, a food, or a dietary or environmental chemical or contaminant. The frequency of significant deleterious drug interactions is not known, and their importance has probably been exaggerated. Drug interactions may result in therapeutic failure, an adverse drug reaction, or an additive or potentiated response.

Table 1. Some Important Genetically Determined Adverse Drug Reactions

Clinical Condition	Proposed Pathogenesis	Drug Involved
Favism and drug-induced hemolysis	Hemolysis secondary to a deficiency of erythrocytic glucose-6-phosphate dehydrogenase	Fava beans and various drugs (Table 4)
Suxamethonium sensitivity	Abnormal plasma pseudocholinesterase with reduced affinity for suxamethonium, thus prolonging muscle paralysis	Suxamethonium
Rapid and slow acetylation	Drug metabolism by acetylation is either rapid or slow depending upon enzyme characteristics	Isoniazid, hydralazine, procainamide, dapsone, phenelzine, some sulfonamides, (sulfasalazine, sulfapyridine)
Malignant hyperthermia	Uncontrolled rise in core body temperature possibly due to excessive muscle contraction.	Suxamethonium, halothane
Slow drug oxidation	Dose-dependent side effects due to less rapid drug breakdown (oxidation)	Carbamazepine, desipramine, diazepam, indomethacin, metoprolol, nortriptyline, phenylbutazone, phenytoin, primidone, warfarin
Porphyria	Symptoms of porphyria secondary to abnormal induction of δ-aminolevulinic acid synthetase	Barbiturates, griseofulvin
Warfarin resistance	Resistance of warfarin-induced anticoagulation secondary to increased sensitivity of the liver to vitamin K	Warfarin
Glaucoma	Unknown	Glucocorticosteroids

EPIDEMIOLOGY OF ADVERSE DRUG REACTIONS

The frequency of adverse drug reactions is not known, and precise figures are difficult to determine. Study has been hampered by numerous factors, especially lack of diagnostic criteria and availability of suitable controls. Symptoms usually ascribed to drug use are common in the absence of drug administration (adverse nondrug reactions) (Table 3), and specific drug reactions may be difficult to distinguish from symptoms of the disease being treated, since drugs may exacerbate or induce disease.

Allowing for imperfect diagnostic criteria, however, adverse drug reactions have accounted for 1 to 4 per cent of hospital admissions to general medical wards and for 0.3 to 1.0 per cent of all general hospital admissions. Furthermore, 5 to 40 per cent of patients in hospitals experience an adverse drug reaction; in addition 30 per cent of patients admitted for a drug

Table 2. Chemical Agents Releasing Histamine

Antihistamines (H_1-blockers)	Polymyxin B
Chymotrypsin	Polyvinylpyrrolidine
Compound 48/80	Propamidine
Desferoxamine	Reserpine
Detergents	Surface active agents
Dextran	Stilbamidine
DMSO (dimethylsulfoxide)	Toxins
Morphine	Tubocurarine
Pentamidine	Venoms
	X-ray contrast media

Table 3. Percentage of Subjects Reporting Each Symptom*

Symptom	Medical Subjects	Nonmedical Subjects
Skin rash	8	3
Urticaria	5	1
Bad dreams	8	3
Excessive sleepiness	23	23
Fatigue	41	37
Inability to concentrate	25	27
Irritability	20	17
Insomnia	7	10
Loss of appetite	3	6
Dry mouth	5	3
Nausea	3	2
Vomiting	0	0
Diarrhea	5	2
Constipation	4	3
Palpitations	3	3
Giddiness or weakness	2	3
Faintness or dizziness on first standing up	5	5
Headaches	15	13
Fever	3	1
Pain in joints	9	5
Pain in muscles	10	11
Nasal congestion	31	13
Bleeding or bruising	3	3
Bleeding from gums after brushing teeth	21	20
Excessive bleeding from gums after brushing teeth	1	1

*From Reidenberg, M.M., and Lowenthal, D.T.: Adverse, non-drug reactions. Reprinted by permission, from The New England Journal of Medicine, 279:678, 1968.

reaction have a further reaction while in the hospital, and the average length of hospital stay has been reported doubled for patients who experience a reaction.

The "incidence" of adverse drug reactions has increased in recent years. This increase may be due to a greater awareness of the problem; may be a result of more people taking more drugs, often for longer periods; may be due to more drugs being used concomitantly without a parallel increase in knowledge of their pharmacokinetics and the diseases for which they are being given; may be due to a changing pattern of diseases being treated, with a greater percentage being given to older patients or to those receiving chronic immunosuppressive therapy; or may be a result of a greater exposure to environmental agents that may alter the response to drugs.

In spite of their shortcomings, epidemiologic studies are of some use in evaluating the magnitude of the problem, in assessing cost factors, in calculating the relative rate of adverse drug reactions to individual agents, and in identifying some of the important predisposing factors.

The majority (70 per cent) of reported adverse drug reactions are minor functional gastrointestinal upsets, various skin disorders (rash, pruritus), fever, drowsiness, insomnia, headache, weakness, tremulousness, and muscle twitching. Many fatalities allegedly attributed to adverse drug reactions occur in patients who are seriously ill with an ultimately fatal underlying disease. Most adverse drug reactions are difficult to categorize definitely with respect to cause, owing to the characteristics of the reaction, the concomitant use of more than one drug, and the absence of specific diagnostic tests.

Not much is known concerning the epidemiology of drug-induced fetal abnormalities or drug-induced behavioral toxicity.

Many drugs are employed to influence disorders of behavior, mood, and psychomotor functioning. Thus, suppression of normal anxiety, impairment of memory, distortion of judgment, reduction in motivation, stimulation of inappropriate behavior, and interference with normal motor coordination are all potential adverse effects of drugs that are often difficult to recognize and even more difficult to quantitate.

Little is known concerning the epidemiology of adverse drug reactions in settings such as general office practice, since most of the published studies have analyzed university hospital data, usually from acute general medical inpatient services.

VARIABLES IN ASSESSING THE INCIDENCE OF ADVERSE DRUG REACTIONS

Many variables have been shown to influence the reported frequency of drug reactions. For example, diagnosis may be difficult or debatable, as with histamine H_1-antagonist–induced sedation, the response being either beneficial or adverse, depending upon the situation. Similarly, reaction rates differ widely, depending upon whether they were obtained prospectively or retrospectively, or on how the reactions were defined. Usually the number of prescriptions written or the extent of prescription and over-the-counter drug use is not known. If such figures are not available, no true incidence rates for adverse reactions can be calculated, and thus assessing the benefit-risk ratio of any agent for any patient is virtually impossible. This latter problem is compounded by errors in prescription filling and in drug administration, whether by nursing error or patient noncompliance. It is essential to establish whether the patient suspected of suffering an adverse drug reaction has in fact received the drug in question. Time factors are also important. Thus, adverse reactions to some agents (for example, x-irradiation, teratogens, gold salts) may not appear for months or years after the patient has been placed at risk, and with other drugs (for example, chloroquine), damage such as retinopathy may be seen only after chronic administration if cumulative effects occur.

Physicians may fail to recognize that a new "symptom" developing under therapy is in fact a drug reaction rather than some manifestation of the underlying disease. This is particularly likely if the reaction is either very common or highly unusual.

The patient who receives only a single drug is rare, with studies in hospital populations indicating that the "average" patient may receive between 10 and 15 different drugs. Thus, if a reaction develops during multiple drug administration, it may be impossible to decide which agent, if any, was responsible. Moreover, in this lawsuit-conscious age, many physicians fail to report adverse reactions for fear of legal complications.

Symptoms often listed as being typically caused by drugs are extremely common in the absence of drug administration. Failure to allow for these with an appropriate control group unduly biases the data (Table 3).

TIME OF ONSET OF DRUG REACTIONS

Depending on its pathogenesis, a reaction may appear within seconds (e.g., anaphylactic shock) to years (e.g., chloroquine-induced retinopathy) after drug administration. Most reactions, however, develop within 7 to 10 days of the start of therapy.

Some reactions may persist after the interacting drug has been excreted, such as catecholamine sensitivity occurring after administration of monoamine oxidase (MAO) inhibitors, in which situation the enzyme has been irreversibly inactivated. In such cases patients may remain sensitive to catecholamines for up to 3 weeks, during which time new MAO is being synthesized.

FACTORS PREDISPOSING TO ADVERSE DRUG REACTIONS

Although precise figures on the incidence of adverse drug reactions are unknown, many of the variables that influence their development have been identified. A review of these predisposing factors will facilitate diagnostic considerations at the bedside and aid in the prevention of adverse effects through more appropriate selection of drugs. In the discussion that follows, considerable overlap between individual categories will be evident.

Predisposing Factors Relating to Drugs

Chemical Characteristics

Highly polar or water soluble drugs (for example, aminoglycoside antibiotics and thiazide diuretics) are excreted primarily by the kidney unchanged and are thus likely to accumulate in patients with renal insufficiency. Conversely, nonpolar or fat-soluble drugs (for example, phenothiazines and barbiturates) require metabolic conversion to polar metabolites for their excretion. They also tend to be highly bound to plasma proteins and to cause enzyme induction or inhibition. Thus, knowledge of the chemical characteristics that determine a drug's polarity may facilitate prediction of adverse drug reactions in patients with disease of excretory organs as well as prediction of drug interactions at the level of plasma protein binding and hepatic metabolism. Similarly, appreciation of a drug's pK_a will facilitate prediction of certain drug interactions, since the pharmacokinetics of weak electrolytes are dramatically modified by altering the pH of the bowel lumen and the urine.

Chemical Similarities

Certain chemical groupings predictably yield adverse reactions, although they may occur in drugs with totally different pharmacologic properties. For example, hepatic damage induced by one hydrazine will almost invariably develop with another agent containing the grouping, and aniline-like drugs may produce hemolysis in subjects with glucose-6-phosphate dehydrogenase deficiency (Table 4).

Similarly, in persons hypersensitive to certain chemical groups, related drugs usually produce symptoms of allergy. A patient hypersensitive to a specific sulfonamide will usually show a similar response to all other antimicrobial sulfonamides and sulfones and to the chemically related but nonantibacterial sulfonylureas, thiazide diuretics, and acetazolamide.

Bioavailability

A drug is formulated (manufactured, compounded) with a variety of additional agents (excipients), such as buffers and flavoring agents (Table 5). Since the specific drug salt, the formulation process, and the number, type, and concentration of excipients are patentable, it is not surprising that the bioavailability of the active ingredient may vary in similar drugs from different manufacturers. Although the degree of bioavailability is important for most therapeutic agents, it is of critical importance with antiepileptic drugs, anticoagulants, digitalis, and endocrine agents. For example, switching from one generic antiepileptic agent to another supplied by a different manufacturer may lead to redevelopment of seizure activity if the bioavailability of the new formulation does not equal that of the initial preparation. In contrast, if the bioavailability of the second agent is greater than that of the initial preparation, an exaggerated therapeutic response or toxicity may ensue.

Table 4. Compounds That May Produce Hemolysis of Glucose-6-Phosphate Dehydrogenase–Deficient Red Cells*

Analgesics	**Nonsulfonamide Antibacterial Agents**
Acetanilid	Chloramphenicol‡
Acetophenetidin (phenacetin)	Furazolidone
Acetylsalicylic acid†	Furamethanol
Antipyrine	Neoarsphenamine
Pyramidone	Nitrofurantoin
Sulfonamides and Sulfones	Nitrofurazone
Dapsone	Para-aminosalicylic acid
N_2-Acetylsulfanilamide	**Miscellaneous**
Salicylazosulfapyridine	α-Methyldopa
Sulfacetamide	Dimercaprol†
Sulfamethoxypyridazine	Hydralazine
Sulfanilamide	Mestranol
Sulfapyridine	Methylene blue†
Sulfisoxazole†	Nalidixic acid
Sulfoxone†	Naphthalene
Thiazosulfone	Niridazole
Antimalarials	Phenylhydrazine
Chloroquine	Probenecid
Pamaquine	Pyridium
Pentaquine	Quinine§
Primaquine	Trinitrotoluene
Quinacrine	Vitamin K (water soluble)
Quinocide	

* Taken in part from Beutler E.: Glucose-6-phosphate dehydrogenase deficiency. In Stanbury, J.B., Wyngaarden, J.B., and Frederickson, D.S. (eds): *The Metabolic Basis of Inherited Disease*, 3rd ed. Copyright © 1974 by McGraw-Hill, Inc. Used by permission of McGraw-Hill Book Company, New York.

† Slightly hemolytic in blacks or hemolytic only in very large doses.

‡ Possibly hemolytic in whites but not in blacks or Orientals.

§ Hemolytic in whites but not in blacks.

Drug Degradation

Potentially unstable drugs are formulated with various excipient buffers and stabilizers and are supplied with an expiration date indicating the time period for which the manufacturer guarantees the product against decomposition under normal storage conditions. Owing to improper storage conditions, particularly extremes of temperature and humidity, some drugs may become degraded prematurely in spite of being buffered; out-of-date drugs are not necessarily degraded, but they should not be used. If a degraded drug is used, the patient is deprived of the active ingredient, and the degraded product may produce toxicity—for example, the Fanconi-like syndrome with degraded tetracyclines.

Drug Purity

Major advances in drug development and new drug regulations ensure in most instances a uniformity of response and relative safety with drug products. Thus it is rare that the active (drug) ingredient of any preparation is not what the manufacturer states it is, but mistakes do occur. In the United States, for example, some early preparations of digitalis glycosides were accidentally contaminated by estrogens that caused puzzling gynecomastia in several patients. Impure drugs rarely reach the market in the United States today. A tourist or alien, however, may bring in a drug

Table 5. Some of the Factors That May Alter Drug Bioavailability*

	Formulation and Manufacturing Factors	
Additives (adjuncts)	Excipients	Preservatives
Adjuvants	Flavors	Pressure of tablet punches
Binders	Formulation	Purity
Buffers	Friability	Solubility (of adjuncts)
Chelators	Granulators	Solubility (of drug)
Coating composition	Hardness	Solvation
Coating thickness	Hydration, degree of	Stereoisomeric stability
Coloring agents	Impurities	Stereoisomerism
Compactness of fill	Incompatibilities	Surface activity
Complexation	Lubricants	Surface area
Crystal structure	Packaging materials	Surfactants
Deaggregation rate	Particle size	Suspending agents
Diluents	pH	Uniformity of composition
Disintegrators	Porosity	Vehicles
Dissolution rate	Potency	Wettability
Emulsifying agents		
	Distribution Factors	
Age of drug product	Moisture, atmospheric	Stability of ingredients
Deterioration	Oxidation	Stereoisomeric shifts
Epimerization	Packaging	Storage conditions
Humidity	Radiation	Temperature of environment
Inertness of atmosphere	Reduction	Transportation stress

*Modified from Martin, E.W.: *Hazards of Medication*, 2nd ed. Philadelphia, J.B. Lippincott, 1978.

purchased abroad that, because of less stringent controls in its country of manufacture, contains contaminants. Similarly, with the increasing use of herbal teas and "natural" products, trace contaminants may be ingested, giving rise to puzzling hypersensitivity skin reactions or dose-dependent toxicity, such as occurs with plant glycosides.

More commonly, questions arise on the safety or dangers of contaminants or excipients. For example, the sodium content of antacids may pose a significant hazard to patients with compromised cardiovascular function, and drug solutions may become contaminated by bacteria. In recent years considerable publicity has been directed toward the potential dangers of particulate matter (fibers) in large-volume parenteral solutions for intravenous administration. Specific excipients may cause toxicity—for example, yellow dye–induced photodermatitis or allergy to procaine in intramuscular procaine penicillin G.

Because of the necessarily small number of patients evaluated in premarketing studies, practicing physicians have a great responsibility for early identification of suspected adverse drug reactions through various national reporting systems, such as those sponsored by the Food and Drug Administration (FDA).

Route of Drug Administration

Serious adverse reactions are usually more common after parenteral administration, particularly by the intravenous route, than after oral or topical administration. The topical application of some drugs, however—for example, the penicillins—is followed more frequently by sensitivity reactions than is parenteral administration. "Nonabsorbable" drugs given for an effect in the bowel lumen, such as sulfasalazine or magnesium and aluminum antacids, and neomycin are absorbed to a slight degree. Under normal circumstances such absorption is harmless, but with hypersensitivity to the compound or compromised excretory organ function, an allergic reaction or toxicity, respectively, may develop. Localized toxicity is also common when specific routes of drug administration are used; for example, thrombophlebitis may occur when too concentrated a drug solution is infused intravenously, or chemical meningitis and neuropathies may develop after poorly controlled intrathecal drug administration.

Too large a volume should not be injected intramuscularly since necrosis may result. Similarly, drugs intended for subcutaneous or intramuscular injection may be dangerous when accidentally administered intravascularly, and drugs formulated for intravenous injection may cause intense spasm of local arterioles if given intra-arterially.

Number of Drugs Administered

The number of adverse drug reactions increases exponentially with the number of drugs given. Considerable sophistication is required to evaluate the greatly increased potential for drug reactions when many drugs are given together. The benefit-risk ratio for each drug usually decreases when multiple drugs are given.

Drug Dosage and Duration of Treatment

In general, the longer the duration of treatment and the higher the dosage, the greater is the chance of development of adverse drug reactions. Interrupted short courses of some drugs, however, can be just as dangerous; with antibiotics for example, bacterial resistance may be more likely to develop under these circumstances.

Most responses to drugs are dose-dependent, but drugs may have more than one effect, each with a different dose response, such as sedation, antihistaminic actions, and anticholinergic effects with the H_1-blockers. Nevertheless, only minute quantities of a drug are needed to generate severe anaphylactic shock in subjects hypersensitive to that agent. Drug dosage must be individually tailored so that the optimally effective dose yielding the fewest side effects is given.

The rate at which some drugs are given may influence the development of reactions, especially when injected intravenously. Excessive plasma drug levels may result from differences in pharmacokinetic handling, altered bioavailability, or medication error. Suddenly stopping some drugs may be especially dangerous, as with the β-blockers clonidine and methyldopa, where with up-regulation of receptors the patient becomes supersensitive to otherwise tolerable stimuli when the drug is discontinued.

Addition or Antagonism of Pharmacologic Effects

If the pharmacologic effects of two drugs are additive, adverse drug reactions may develop. A patient taking para-aminosalicylic acid (PAS), for example, may develop salicylism on taking small doses of aspirin, or an individual taking apsirin may develop adverse effects on ingesting PAS. Similarly, atropinism may readily develop if an H_1-blocker and a phenothiazine are combined, since both drugs possess some parasympatholytic activity. Various additive and antagonistic drug effects may be observed with mixtures of antibiotics. Alcohol and H_1-blockers are the most common potentiators of central nervous system depressants, such as the benzodiazepines and barbiturates.

Combination of Drugs and Adjuvants

Excipients used as repository vehicles for drugs given parenterally may increase their sensitizing potential. Examples are the inclusion of procaine or benzathine in penicillin preparations or the use of heparin in oil.

Drug Cost

The high cost of some drugs may increase the rate of patient noncompliance or encourage the patient to "shop around" in an attempt to buy a generically available drug (with possibly altered bioavailability characteristics) more cheaply.

Effects After Use of Placebos

The basic emotional pattern of a patient may influence his or her response to drugs (see later discussion). This is particularly true of drugs affecting the central nervous system and of placebos. Many physicians have observed mild adverse reactions to placebos, such as depression, sleepiness, sleeplessness, anorexia, nausea, tremulousness, dizziness, palpitations, and lassitude. Some puzzling severe reactions to placebos have been reported, such as fixed drug eruptions, anaphylactic shock, and even death. Many "reactions" to placebos are in reality an expression of "adverse nondrug reactions" (Table 3).

A placebo is by definition innocuous. No substance should be used as a placebo if there is even remote danger of a harmful effect. Thus, aspirin should not be used, especially in children. Similarly, the ever-present danger of serum hepatitis and other transmissible disorders makes it impossible to guarantee the harmlessness of parenteral injections of normal saline, a common placebo. On the other hand, failing to recognize the need for precise treatment and substituting a placebo for necessary drug (or psychiatric) therapy is also dangerous. Megadoses of many vitamins frequently used (inappropriately) as placebos are potentially toxic.

Drug Interactions

As already noted, adverse drug reactions may develop through drug interactions (Table 6).

Intrinsic Predisposing Patient (Host) Factors

Patient variables may alter the pharmacodynamics or pharmacokinetics of drugs, producing adverse effects. Only a brief summary of these important variables will be given.

History of Drug Reaction

Patients with previous drug reactions are at greater risk of experiencing a second reaction (Table 7).

Age

At the extremes of life, the functions of absorption, metabolism, and excretion may be imperfectly developed (as in the newborn, particularly the premature infant) or diminished (as in the elderly subject). Furthermore, the responsiveness of certain tissues and homeostatic mechanisms may differ from those in the healthy adult and the ability of the body to oppose drug effects may be altered. Thus, therapy based on pharmacokinetic data derived from adults may lead to unexpected toxicity or failure of therapy. The developing fetus is particularly susceptible to drug effects (see later discussion).

Pediatric Age Group. Compared with adults, children have a more rapid gastrointestinal transit time, a higher body water content (70 to 75 per cent, compared with 60 per cent for adults), a relatively smaller body surface area, differences in tissue distribution of drugs (e.g., the relative permeability of the blood-brain barrier), a relatively low glomerular filtration rate and renal plasma flow, plasma proteins that do not bind drugs well, and difficulty (and therefore unreliability) with oral therapy.

Geriatric Age Group. In 60- to 70-year-old persons the risk of an adverse drug reaction is about double that in a young adult. This risk results predominantly from a diminution in the function of the organs of metabolism and excretion due to age or associated disease. For example, symptom-free patients of 65 years of age may have lost as much as 50 per cent of their renal glomerular and tubular functions. Dimin-

Table 6. Some Important Drug Interactions Causing Significant Drug Reactions

Agent	Interaction
Pharmaceutic Interactions	
Numerous examples are known; consult textbooks on this topic for details	
Gentamicin	Inactivates carbenicillin when both drugs are mixed in infusion bottles or syringes
Pharmacokinetic Interaction	
Metoclopramide	Accelerates the intestinal absorption of levodopa and many other agents by the small bowel
Anticholinergic agents	Reduce the intestinal absorption of many drugs (e.g., levodopa and sustained-release lithium)
Aluminum hydroxide	Slows intestinal absorption of many drugs, including digoxin, INAH, and chlorpromazine
Tetracycline antibiotics	Form poorly absorbable chelates with heavy metals in bowel lumen
Warfarin	Potentiated by phenylbutazone, clofibrate, and some sulfonamides through displacement from plasma proteins
Enzyme-inducing agents (see Table 15)	Accelerate the metabolism with subsequent reduced pharmacodynamic effects for a variety of agents, including oral anticoagulants, phenytoin, digitoxin, phenylbutazone, and oral contraceptive steroids
Phenylbutazone	Reduces renal clearance of chlorpropamide, salicylates, and probenecid, and some sulfonamides inhibit the renal excretion of methotrexate
Pharmacodynamic Interactions	
Aspirin and nonsteroidal anti-inflammatory agents	Potentiate the activity of oral anticoagulants
Cephaloridine	Nephrotoxic effect is potentiated by other nephrotoxic agents, including furosemide and ethacrynic acid
Central nervous system (CNS) depressants (sedatives, tranquilizers, antidepressants, narcotics, hypnotics, narcotic analgesic, alcohol, H_1-receptor antagonists)	Potentiate one another and produce excessive central nervous system depression
Diuretics	Induce hypokalemia, which increases digitalis myocardial toxicity
	Induce sodium loss, which potentiates lithium toxicity
Broad-spectrum antibiotics	Potentiate the action of warfarin
Nondepolarizing muscle relaxants	Potentiated by neomycin and other aminoglycosides, quinidine, colistin, and some local anesthetics
Aminoglycosides	Induce eighth cranial nerve toxicity, which is potentiated by furosemide and ethacrynic acid
Tricyclic antidepressants	Antagonize the antihypertensive effect of guanethidine

ished renal function is accentuated by such states as dehydration, congestive heart failure, urinary retention, and electrolyte abnormalities. Thus, drugs excreted by the kidney may rapidly achieve high plasma levels in geriatric patients if the dosage is not adjusted downward.

Geriatric patients may have reduced sensitivity (responsiveness) to some drugs compared with adults of younger ages. For example, a gradual loss in sensitivity of autonomic reflexes in the cardiovascular system may influence the response of patients to drugs such as guanethidine. Similarly, phenothiazines are more prone to produce Parkinson's disease in the elderly. Adverse drug reactions in elderly individuals are further compounded by impaired homeostatic mechanisms, which may result in inadequate compensation for excessive drug effects. Finally, emotional problems and cerebral arteriosclerosis can contribute to unintentional drug abuse, imperfect compliance, or an irrational attitude toward a drug reaction.

Race and Heredity

Genetic polymorphisms of drug metabolism can be responsible for the production of adverse drug reactions. This is a complex area with interaction of environmental factors often confusing the clinical picture. A summary is given in Table 1 of some of the important genetically determined adverse drug reactions.

Table 7. Incidence of Adverse Drug Reactions in Relation to History of Drug Reaction and to Drug Allergy

History	Reaction Rate	
	*United States** *(%)*	*United Kingdom†* *(%)*
No previous reaction	9	9
Previous reaction	14	28
No history of allergy	11	9
Previous allergies	13	28

*From Smith, J.W., Seidl, L.G., and Cluff, L.E.: Studies on the epidemiology of adverse drug reactions. Ann. Intern. Med., 65:629, 1966.

†Hurwitz, N.: Predisposing factors in adverse reactions to drugs. Br. Med. J., 1:536, 1969.

Physiologic Status

Effects on Reproduction. Parasympatholytic drugs, cimetidine, and many antihypertensive agents may produce impotence. Thorazine and related psychopharmacologic agents have been shown to interfere with ejaculation without affecting orgasm.

Pregnancy. Major alterations in body functions develop during pregnancy. It has been suggested, for example, that the increased demand for protein anabolism makes the liver more susceptible to drugs such as tetracyclines, which depress this function and which may produce fatal hepatic necrosis when given in doses greater than 2.0 gm/day. Moreover, during pregnancy the metabolism of some drugs (for example, succinylcholine) is delayed, and transport processes that clear drugs such as sulfobromophthalein through the liver cell are depressed. Changes in hemodynamics and renal function may alter drug clearance and response.

Effects During Intrauterine Development. Adverse drug effects are nowhere more dramatically evident than in the fetus and neonate. Most drugs with molecular weight of 1000 or less can easily cross the placental barrier (Table 8). The effects of some nonpharmacologic agents that cross the placenta, such as rubella virus (German measles), during the first trimester of pregnancy are well known. Of more importance but not as generally recognized is that many drugs can cause similar effects. A drug given in pregnancy may cause fetal death. During organogenesis, in the first trimester, malformations may be produced. Later in pregnancy or during labor, drugs may cause fetal morbidity or death. Morbidity in the perinatal period is more common in premature infants.

Drug exposure during pregnancy is unfortunately commonplace. Studies have reported that 82 to 92 per cent of women were given at least one drug during pregnancy, with four drugs being the average number prescribed; 4 per cent of patients were given 10 drugs or more during pregnancy.

Teratogenesis. The thalidomide disaster focused attention on the potential danger of administering drugs during pregnancy. The critical time during organogenesis for an individual tissue to be affected by teratogenic agents is usually considered to be the time that coincides with the greatest mitotic activity in that organ. For example, the limb buds exhibit maximal susceptibility between 18 and 28 days of gestation, or, in other words, 38 to 48 days after the first day of the last menstrual period. This indicates the importance of not exposing women of childbearing age to unnecessary medication, as teratogenic effects may be produced before pregnancy is diagnosed or even suspected.

Several potent pharmacologic agents, including anticancer drugs, sulfonylureas, and corticocosteroids, are suspected of being teratogenic.

Masculinization of the Female Fetus. Before embryonic sexual structures differentiate they are susceptible to the influence of exogenous endocrine agents. Female pseudohermaphroditism, for example, has been produced by testosterone (given for hyperemesis gravidarum) and by a variety of synthetic progestational agents commonly used in the treatment of habitual or threatened abortion.

Perinatal Effects. Drugs given to the mother before or during labor may cross the placenta, and the baby may be born still under their influence. Many drugs are excreted in breast milk (Table 9) and thus can produce adverse effects in breast-fed infants.

Neonatal Effects. The neonate is not just a miniature young adult. This point was discussed earlier under *Age.*

Circadian and Other Physiologic Variations. Many physiologic variations occur in the body during the day, and these functions may be altered if a patient is placed on a regimen of complete bed rest. For example, circadian fluctuations in urinary pH occur, particularly in relation to meals, and this may alter the excretion of weak electrolytes.

The normal human organism is populated by a variety of microorganisms, particularly in the gastrointestinal and genital tracts. That this microflora is important in drug metabolism is just beginning to be realized. For example, patients whose conditions have been stabilized on anticoagulants usually need to have the dose adjusted downward if broad-spectrum antibiotics are added to the drug regimen.

Concomitant Disease

Specific disease states may predispose to adverse drug reactions in several ways. For example, multiple drug therapy is often required (for example in infections, edema, heart failure, hypertension), a situation predisposing to adverse drug reactions (see earlier discussion).

Disease of the organs of drug absorption, metabolism, and excretion; congenital anomalies; or other drugs may significantly alter drug pharmacodynamics and pharmacokinetics, and drugs may exaggerate overt disease, promote latent disease, or precipitate disease (Table 10).

Little is known about the way disease states may alter drug handling or tissue sensitivity. Many diseases are associated with hypoproteinemia or hyperproteinemia, but whether plasma protein binding of drugs is significantly altered in these situations is not

Table 8. Drugs That Cross the Human Placental Barrier and That May Endanger the Fetus during Pregnancy or in the Prenatal Period

Drug	Adverse Effect
Acetophenetidin	Methemoglobinemia
Alphaprodine	Fetal respiratory depression
Aminopterin	Abortion, anomalies, cleft palate
Ammonium chloride	Acidosis
Androgens	Advanced bone age, clitoral enlargement, labial fusion, masculinization
Anesthetics (volatile)	Depressed fetal respiration
Barbiturates	Anomalies, depressed respiration
Bishydroxycoumarin	Fetal death and intrauterine hemorrhage
Bromides	Neonatal skin eruptions (bromoderma)
Busulfan	Cleft palate
Chloral hydrate (large doses)	Fetal death
Chlorambucil	Abortion, anomalies
Chloroquine	Thrombocytopenia
Chlorpromazine	Neonatal jaundice, prolonged extrapyramidal signs, neonatal goiter
Chlorpropamide	Prolonged neonatal hypoglycemia, neonatal goiter?
Cholinesterase inhibitors	Muscular weakness (transient)
Cortisone	Cleft palate
Cyclophosphamide	Defects of extremities, stunting, fetal death
Cyclopropane	Neonatal respiratory depression
D-Amphetamine sulfate	Transposition of vessels?
Estrogens	Advanced bone age, clitoral enlargement, labial fusion, masculinization, vaginal cancer (20 years later)
Ether	Neonatal apnea
Ethyl biscoumacetate	Fetal death, neonatal hemorrhage
Ganglionic blocking agents	Neonatal ileus
Heroin	Initial neonatal addiction, neonatal death, respiratory depression
Hexamethonium bromide	Neonatal ileus, death
Iodides	Goiter
Iophenoxic acid	Hypothyroidism, retardation
Iothiouracil	Neonatal goiter
Isoniazid	Retarded psychomotor activity
Levorphanol	Fetal respiratory depression
Lithium carbonate	Neonatal goiter
Lysergic acid diethylamide	Chromosomal damage, stunted offspring
Mecamylamine	Fetal neonatal ileus
Mepivacaine	Fetal bradycardia, neonatal depression
Methadone	Fetal respiratory depression
Methimazole	Neonatal goiter, hypothyroidism, mental retardation
Methotrexate	Abortion, anomalies, cleft palate
Morphine	Initial neonatal addiction, respiratory depression, neonatal death
Nicotine (smoking)	"Small for dates" neonates
Nitrofurantoin	Fetal hemolysis
Nitrous oxide	Respiratory depression
Oral progestogens	Clitoral enlargement, labial fusion, masculinization
Paraldehyde	Respiratory depression
Phenmetrazine	Multiple skeletal and visceral anomalies
Phenobarbital	Respiratory depression, death
Phenylbutazone	Neonatal goiter
Phenytoin	Anomalies
Podophyllum	Fetal resorption, deformities
Potassium iodide	Cyanosis, goiter, mental retardation, respiratory distress
Propylthiouracil	Neonatal goiter, hypothyroidism, mental retardation
Quinine	Deafness, thrombocytopenia
Radioactive iodine	Congenital goiter, mental retardation, hypothyroidism
Reserpine	Nasal block, respiratory obstruction
Salicylates	Anomalies, neonatal bleeding
Smallpox vaccination	Fetal vaccina
Sodium warfarin	Intrauterine hemorrhage, fetal death
Streptomycin	Hearing loss, eighth cranial nerve damage, micromelia, multiple skeletal anomalies
Sulfonamides (long-acting)	Kernicterus, hyperbilirubinemia, acute liver atrophy, anemia, neonatal goiter
Sulfonylureas	Neonatal goiter, prolonged neonatal hypoglycemia
Tetracyclines	Discolored teeth, inhibition of long bone growth, micromelia, syndactyly
Thalidomide	Phocomelia, hearing defects, fetal death
Thiazides	Neonatal death, thrombocytopenia
Thiouracil	Hypothyroidism, neonatal goiter, mental retardation
Tolbutamide	Congenital anomalies and prolonged neonatal hypoglycemia

Table continued on following page

Table 8. Drugs That Cross the Human Placental Barrier and That May Endanger the Fetus during Pregnancy or in the Prenatal Period (Continued)

Drug	Adverse Effect
Tribromoethanol	Depressed fetal respiration
Vitamin A (large doses)	Cleft palate, congenital anomalies, eye damage, syndactyly
Vitamin D (large doses)	Hypercalcemia, mental retardation
Vitamin K analogues (large doses)	Hyperbilirubinemia, kernicterus

clear. Certainly, low serum albumin levels have been associated with increased phenytoin, diazepam, chlordiazepoxide, and prednisone toxicity; reduced protein binding of many drugs (for example, the sulfonamides, phenytoin, clofibrate, chlorpropamide, and thyroxine) occurs in uremia. This results in a therapeutic level of unbound drug at lower plasma concentrations mandating reduction of drug dose to avoid toxicity. Such is especially true with drugs that are highly protein-bound and those with narrow therapeutic ratios, such as chlorpropamide.

Drug reactions are more likely to develop in patients with infections. The reason is unclear, but experimentally the toxicity of some drugs to the central nervous system is increased in the presence of fever.

The measurement of blood urea nitrogen (BUN), serum creatinine, or creatinine clearance may facilitate the selection of proper dosage of specific drugs during renal failure. Certain agents (aminoglycoside antibiotics, polymyxin B, colistin, amphotericin B, cephaloridine, and lithium) are liable to produce renal tubular damage.

Allergic Diathesis

Hypersensitivity (allergic) reactions represent the largest single group of adverse drug reactions. Approximately 200,000 hospitalized patients suffer allergic drug reactions each year, and approximately 50,000 patients are hospitalized for allergic drug reactions on an annual basis. Drug allergy may be more likely to develop in patients with an "allergic diathesis" (history of eczema, hay fever, asthma, hives, urticaria, angioedema) than in nonhypersensitive per-

Table 9. Some Drugs Excreted in Human Milk

- Acetaminophen
- Alcohol
- Allergens (e.g., peanuts, others)
- Ambenonium chloride
- Aminophylline
- Amphetamines
- Anthraquinone cathartics
- Antihistamines (H_1-blockers)
- Arsenical salts
- Aspirin
- Atropine
- Barbiturates
- Bishydroxycoumarin
- Bromides
- Brompheniramine
- Caffeine
- Calomel
- Cascara
- Chloral hydrate
- Chloramphenicol
- Chloroform
- Chlorpromazine
- Codeine
- Copper
- Cortisone
- Cyclophosphamide
- Cyclopropane
- Cycloserine
- D-Amphetamine
- Danthron
- DDT
- Diazepam
- Diphenhydramine
- Ephedrine
- Ergot alkaloids

- Erythromycin
- Estrogens
- Ether
- Ethinamate
- Ethyl biscoumacetate
- Folic acid
- Heroin
- Hexachlorobenzene
- Hydroxyzine
- Imipramine
- Iodine-131
- Iopanoic acid
- Isoniazid
- L-Propoxyphene
- Mandelic acid
- Mefenamic acid
- Meperidine
- Methadone HCl
- Methdilazine
- Methimazole
- Methocarbamol
- Metronidazole
- Morphine
- Narcotics
- Neomycin sulfate
- Niacin
- Nicotine
- Nitrofurantoin
- Oral contraceptives
- Oxacillin
- Oxyphenbutazone
- Pantothenic acid
- Papaverine
- Para-aminosalicylic acid
- Penethamate hydriodide
- Penicillin G

- Pentazocine
- Phenacetin
- Phenaglycodol
- Phenolphthalein
- Phenylbutazone
- Phenytoin
- Potassium iodide
- Prochlorperazine
- Propoxyphene
- Propylthiouracil
- Pseudoephedrine
- Pyrimethamine
- Quinidine
- Quinine sulfate
- Reserpine
- Rhubarb
- Riboflavin
- Salicylates
- Scopolamine
- Senna
- Sodium salicylate
- Streptomycin
- Sulfadimethoxine
- Sulfamethoxazole
- Sulfanilamide
- Sulfapyridine
- Sulfathiazole
- Tetracyclines
- Thiamine
- Thiazide diuretics
- Thiopental
- Thiouracil
- Thyroid hormones
- Tolbutamide
- Trifluoperazine
- Vitamins A, B, B_{12}, C, D, E, K

Table 10. Some Important Drug-Induced Metabolic Diseases

Condition	Drug
Hyperkalemia	Potassium salt (e.g., KCl), potassium salt of drug (e.g., potassium penicillin), aldosterone antagonists, lithium
Hypokalemia	Diuretics, cathartics (chronic), corticosteroids, insulin, carbenoxolone, any drug producing chronic diarrhea, amphotericin B
Hypernatremia	Sodium salts of drugs (e.g., methicillin), sodium in drugs (e.g., antacids), corticosteroids
Hyponatremia	Diuretics, laxatives
Hypercalcemia	Vitamin D, thiazide diuretics, corticosteroids
Hyperuricemia	Thiazide diuretics, chlorthalidone, ethacrynic acid, furosemide, aspirin, ethionamide, pyrazinamide, methotrexate
Hyperglycemia	Thiazide diuretics, corticosteroids, oral contraceptive steroids, chlorthalidone, ethacrynic acid, furosemide, growth hormone, diazoxide
Porphyria, acute	Aminopyrine, androgens, barbiturates, chlordiazepoxide, phenytoin, estrogens, griseofulvin, meprobamate, oral contraceptives, sulfonamides, sulfonylureas, glutethimide, rifampin
Porphyria, cutaneous	Androgens, barbiturates, chloroquine, estrogens, ethyl alcohol, hexachlorobenzene, oral contraceptives, sulfonylureas

sons. In patients with ulcerative gastrointestinal disease, allergy to orally administered drugs may be more likely to develop than in other persons. A patient known to have suffered an allergic drug reaction should not be exposed again to the offending agent or to related chemicals without full consideration of the risk of inducing fatal anaphylaxis. In one study, the penicillins, streptomycin, barbiturates, meprobamate, codeine, quinidine, sulfonamides, and thiazide diuretics were responsible for 70 per cent of the allergic reactions encountered. Penicillin allergy is covered more fully later; little is known about allergies to other drugs.

Reactions Associated with Allergy

To give rise to an allergic reaction, the drug, drug metabolite(s), or drug contaminant must initiate antibody production. However, our understanding of how antibodies are produced is far from clear. Antibodies against the offending drug or its metabolites cannot be demonstrated in every case of suspected drug allergy, and re-exposure of the patient to the original drug may not elicit an allergic reaction. Additionally, the development of specific diagnostic tests is difficult since in most instances not all the drug metabolites are known (either because of interlocking complex pathways of biodegradation or because of interindividual variations in metabolism), and only a trace quantity of a potential allergen is in fact necessary to initiate antibody production.

According to the Coombs and Gell classification, there are four main categories of allergic (drug) reactions: Type I (anaphylaxis), Type II (cytotoxic), Type III (hypersensitivity), and Type IV (delayed hypersensitivity). These reactions as they relate to penicillin are indicated in Table 11.

Type I Reactions. Type I reactions depend upon an antigen binding and bridging two specific membrane-bound antibodies (IgE) on the surface of mast cells or basophils. Binding is followed by a series of intracellular metabolic steps, which results in the extrusion of various potent vasoactive substances, including histamine, slow-reacting substance of anaphylaxis (leukotrienes C and D), and numerous others. Clinical symptoms will depend upon the route of antigen exposure and the magnitude of mediator release; they include hives, urticaria, bronchospasm, hypotension, angioedema, and, in severe cases, anaphylactic shock.

Type II Reactions. Type II reactions are mediated by IgG or IgM antibody directed against a cell surface antigen. In the presence of complement, the cell is damaged, causing lysis or rendering the cell susceptible to phagocytosis. Several mechanisms are known whereby drugs can initiate Type II responses; the specific antibody may attack the drug affixed to a cell by covalent linkage, thereby destroying the cell directly or indirectly. A good example is seen in penicillin-induced hemolytic anemia (Table 11). Specific drugs may initiate antibodies against tissue-specific antigens. For example, methyldopa induces specific antibodies that cross-react with human red cells, producing hemolytic anemia. Drugs or their reactive metabolites may alter host tissue, rendering it antigenic. Procainamide and other agents (Table 12) may alter nuclear material, stimulating the formation of antinuclear antibodies, which in certain circumstances results in a lupus erythematosus-like state.

Type III Reactions. Type III reactions are caused by circulating soluble complexes of antigen and IgG or IgM antibody. In the presence of complement, these complexes become deposited on endothelial surfaces and with activation of complement chemotactic factors are generated locally, initiating an inflammatory response. Serum sickness following the administration of foreign protein is a good example. Penicillin is the most common drug cause of a serum sickness today (Table 11).

Antigen-antibody complexes may be passively absorbed by an "innocent bystander" cell, which is then destroyed through the mediation of complement. A good example is apronalide-induced thrombocytopenia. Some consider that this "innocent bystander" type III reaction is in reality a Type II reaction in

Table 11. Some Important Sensitivity Reactions to Penicillin

Type of Allergy	Antigen	Antibody	Clinical Response	Comment
Type I	PCN, PC, and PI; occasionally PO	IgE	Anaphylaxis, laryngeal edema, early onset (< 72 h) of urticaria	Symptoms of anaphylaxis usually develop within 0 to 20 minutes of exposure
Type II	PO	IgG	Coombs' positive hemolytic anemia	Specific IgG binds to the PO/red blood cell complex and activates complement. Hemolysis subsequently occurs in the reticuloendothelial system
Type III	PO (probably soluble)	IgG and IgM	Serum sickness	Site of injury is nonspecific, reflecting the intravascular lodgment of antigen-antibody-immune complexes. Complement is activated.
Type IV		T cell	Contact dermatitis	Rarely seen today because topical penicillin therapy is no longer used. May be seen in those persons exposed accidentally to topical penicillin (pharmaceutical employees, pharmacists, nurses, patients in whom back leakage of the antibiotic occurs after an intramuscular injection)
Unknown but strongly suspected to be present	(?)	(?)	Drug fever, maculopapular (excluding "ampicillin rash") and other skin rashes, including erythema nodosa, erythema multiforme, Stevens-Johnson syndrome, late onset of urticaria, eosinophilia, hepatitis/nephritis, neutropenia	Negative prospective testing for IgE or other parameters of "allergy" does not provide evidence for or against the development of these reactions

Abbreviations: PCN = Penicillin G; PC = penicilloate; PI = penilloate; PO = penicilloyl.

which the antigen-antibody complex stays only transiently on the red cell membrane (as an example). Before the complex dissociates, complement is activated and remains bound to the red cell membrane, rendering it susceptible to destruction. Under these circumstances the Coombs test is positive only if antibody to complement is used instead of anti-immunoglobulins.

Type IV Reactions. Type IV reactions involve specifically sensitized lymphocytes. On contact with antigen, these cells undergo mitotic division and produce soluble factors called lymphokines, which are responsible for mediating an inflammatory response. Type IV reactions develop slowly, and those induced by drugs are classic examples of contact dermatitis.

Table 12. Drugs That May Produce Lupus Erythematosus–like Illness

Aminosalicylic acid	Paramethadione
Barbiturates (long-term?)	Penicillamine
Chlorpromazine	Penicillins
Chlortetracycline	Phenothiazines
Digitalis (long-term)	Phenylbutazone
Ethosuximide	Phenytoin
Gold compounds (long-term)	Primaclone
Griseofulvin	Procainamide
Hydralazine	Propranolol
Isoniazid	Propylthiouracil
Mephenytoin	Quinidine
Methsuximide	Reserpine (long-term)
Methyldopa	Streptomycin
Methylthiouracil	Sulfadimethoxine
Oral contraceptives (mestranol?)	Sulfamethoxypyridazine
	Tetracycline (degraded)
Oxyphenisatin	Thiazides (long-term)
Para-aminosalicylic acid	Trimethadione

It should be stressed that many adverse reactions to drugs of a presumed allergic nature do not fall into the categories of clinical Types I to IV as typified by those described for penicillin (Table 11).

Penicillin Allergy. It is now clear that the important antigens mediating penicillin allergy are penicilloyl (the major antigenic determinant) and penicillin, penicilloate, and penilloate (the minor antigenic determinants) (Table 11). Penicilloyl coupled with polylysine has been available commercially for some time. The minor antigenic determinants have recently been field tested by the National Institute of Allergic and Infectious Diseases (NIAID) and should soon be licensed for distribution and available for general use.

A history of penicillin allergy is unreliable in predicting allergic responses to penicillin, and such patients should not be denied penicillin without the benefit of skin testing. Patients with a positive history who do not respond to penicilloyl or the minor antigenic determinants can receive penicillin if it is indicated clinically; many physicians would still, however, use an initial test dose under these circumstances.

Patients with a positive skin test to penicilloyl polylysine have a greater than 50 per cent chance of an accelerated or urticarial reaction if given penicillin, and patients with a positive reaction to minor antigenic determinants have an almost 100 per cent chance of developing anaphylaxis if given penicillin.

Patients with a positive history but with negative skin tests, and who have been given penicillin without problem, should be skin tested before receiving their next course of penicillin, since they remain potentially allergic and may form sufficient IgE from accidental or environmental exposure.

Whereas a few possible cases of cross allergy of a Type I nature have been reported between penicillins and cephalosporins, this reaction, if it occurs, must be very, very rare. If cross allergy does occur between cephalosporins and the penicillins, it probably involves cross reactivity with non–IgE antibodies, producing Type II or Type III reactions. Detailed analysis of cephalosporin allergy is hampered by the fact that the probable antigens are not known. The stability of the cephalosporoyl group in vivo is not too strong and, unlike the penicillins, this configuration probably does not act as an antigen. Furthermore, cephalosporin allergy is probably dependent on side-chain substitutions not present in the penicillins.

Skin Color

Cutaneous melanin protects against injury by external agents, such as radiant energy (of ultraviolet or near ultraviolet wavelengths). Thus, photodermatitis, either phototoxic or photoallergic, is very rare in black subjects, is not uncommon in white persons, and is frequent in albinos of any race.

In addition, drug photosensitivity has been documented in at least three diseases: porphyria, lupus erythematosus, and pellagra. Phototoxic reactions (Table 13) occur when a nontoxic substance is converted into a toxic one in the patient's skin by the absorption of photoenergy. Photoallergic reactions, on the other hand, occur when the absorption of photoenergy by a chemical converts it into a metabolite that may then sensitize the patient. Photosensitization may also arise after topical exposure of various compounds, particularly antiseptics and antibiotics in soaps, hair rinses, shampoos, perfumes, and antiseptic creams. Photoallergic rashes may persist for long periods after termination of drug exposure. The patient may remain permanently sensitized to the offending drug, even in the absence of sunlight.

Weight and Body Composition

Body weight and composition (especially fat content) may be important in drug metabolism and excretion. For example, phenobarbital (a nonpolar drug) rapidly accumulates in adipose tissue, from where it is released slowly to act on the central nervous system. Thus, the pattern and deviation of pharmacologic effects of this agent will vary with the amount of body fat. In general, drugs should be given in doses based on ideal rather than actual body weight.

Sex

Although various sex differences in drug distribution, response, and metabolism have been described in animals, these are not of major importance in hu-

Table 13. Characteristics of Drug-Induced Photosensitivity*

Reaction	Phototoxic	Photoallergic
Reaction possible on first exposure	Yes	No
Incubation period necessary after first exposure	No	Yes
Chemical alteration of photosensitizer	No	Yes
Covalent binding with carrier	No	Yes
Clinical changes	Usually like sunburn	Varied morphology
"Flares" at distant previously involved sites possible	No	Yes
Persistent light reaction possible	No	Yes
Cross reactions to structurally related agents	Infrequent	Frequent
Broadening of cross reactions following repeated photo-patch testing	No	Possible
Concentration of drug necessary for reaction	High	Low
Incidence	Usually relatively high (theoretically 100%)	Usually very low (but theoretically could reach 100%)
Action spectrum	Usually similar to absorption spectrum	Usually higher wavelength than absorption spectrum
Passive transfer	No	Possible
Lymphocyte stimulation test	No	Possible
Macrophage migration inhibition test	No	Possible

*From Baer, R.L., and Harber L.C.: Reactions to light, heat, and trauma. In Swater, M. (ed.): *Immunologic Diseases.* Volume II. Boston, Little, Brown & Co., 1971.

mans, with the exception of those associated with pregnancy and lactation (see earlier discussion). Epidemiologic studies have shown that drug reactions are two to three times more common in women than in men. For example, blood dyscrasias associated with use of phenylbutazone, aminopyrine, and chloramphenicol have an unexplained 3:1 preponderance in women. The reason for this preponderance is not known, but women may have a greater tendency to seek care or report reactions. Furthermore, many reactions may be due specifically to treatment of obstetric or gynecologic conditions. For example, oral contraceptive steroids retard drug metabolism, whereas androgens are enzyme inducers, and the half-lives of some drugs vary with the menstrual cycle.

Sex differences influence the severity of some diseases in humans—for example, essential hypertension. Since hypertension is usually associated with greater end-organ damage in men than in women, more potent drugs tend to be used by men. Finally, sex-linked genetic factors may be important, such as glucose-6-phosphate dehydrogenase deficiency (Table 1).

Temperament and Social Awareness

Emotional, sensitive, frail, asthenic, high-strung, and hypochondriacal subjects report more adverse drug reactions and tend to be greater responders to placebos than more stable and more stoic persons. Geriatric patients may have wide swings of mood owing to cerebral arteriosclerosis and other factors and thus may suffer more "subjective" drug reactions.

A patient's expectations and perspectives about drug reactions and effects often vary depending on societal values and personal traits. Thus, for example, American women complained more of the adverse effects of oral contraceptives than did women of a non-American social environment, even though the groups experienced similar drug effects.

Patient Noncompliance and Errors of Drug Administration

Patients may interfere with therapy either by not following directions or by self-medication. The patient who does not comply with drug therapy is usually poorly compliant with other aspects of management, such as dietary restrictions, termination of tobacco smoking, and exercise regimens. Patients may take either more or less than the prescribed dose; both usually result in suboptimal therapy. The common (and fallacious) reasoning behind taking more than the prescribed dose is "if three of these pills a day are making me better, six of them a day will make me better twice as quickly." However, taking drugs irregularly is far more common than overmedication.

Noncompliance rates of 20 to 80 per cent have been reported in studies involving antibiotics, antacids, antidepressants, and antimalarials. Noncompliance may be serious; for example, in a study of patients with congestive heart failure, 92 per cent continued to take digitalis as prescribed, whereas 83 per cent took thiazide diuretic and only 60 per cent continued to take potassium supplements, thus encouraging digitalis toxicity.

Noncompliance is more difficult to predict than to detect, since the causes are poorly understood; however, correlations between noncompliance and various factors have been determined (Table 14). Two important points are clear: Noncompliance increases with the increasing number of tablets and the number of different drugs prescribed, and in many instances, failure to comply results from failure of the physician to fully inform the patient about the drug, its purpose, its dosage schedule, and what is meant by expressions such as "three times a day," or "take with (before, during, or after?) meals."

Consequences of Noncompliance. The consequences of noncompliance are either adverse drug reactions or apparent therapeutic failure. For example, failure to take an antibiotic regularly often leads to relapse of the original infection, emergence of resistant organisms, or suprainfections.

The best remedy for noncompliance is prevention. The physician should explain drug therapy to the patient thoroughly, giving the drug name, describing its purpose, and explaining how it should be taken. In addition, any prescription drugs, over-the-counter drugs, or foods that might interfere with the agent's action should be identified.

Self-Medication. Self-medication with drugs remaining from previous prescriptions or with over-the-counter preparations (tonics, vitamins, aspirin, antacids, iron tablets, cold remedies, laxatives, dimethylsulfoxide) is not unusual and may lead to drug interactions. Similarly, care must be taken with regard to drugs the patient may be taking concomitantly that were prescribed by another physician. In addition, the hospitalized patient may surreptitiously be brought drugs by visitors, which may interfere significantly with therapy or produce specific drug interactions.

One of the most important parts of history taking is a thorough inquiry into the nature and dosage of all drugs taken in the immediate past. It is common for patients to be cared for by several physicians simultaneously and thus duplicative, additive, counteractive, or synergistic drugs may be given inadvertently unless care is taken.

Table 14. Patients Likely to Be Noncompliant or Factors Contributing to, or Associated with, Patient Noncompliance

Children, particularly when poorly supervised
Geriatric subjects
Disadvantaged subjects
Patients living alone
Single or divorced patients
Low socioeconomic status
Psychiatric disease or other personality disorder
Occurrence of an adverse drug reaction
Unfamiliar or uncommunicative physician
Unhelpful or uncommunicative pharmacist
Drug administration more frequent than once per day
Chronic illness with chronic therapy
Increasing number of drugs

Table 15. Some Drug-Metabolizing Enzyme Inducers and Inhibitors

Inducers			
Alcohol (ethanol)	Chlorcyclizine	Hexobarbital*	Phenacetin
Aldrin	Chlorobutanol	Imipramine*	Phenaglycodol
Aminopyrine*	Chlordane	Insecticides, halogenated	Phenobarbital*
Amobarbital*	Chlordiazepoxide	Lindane	Phenylbutazone*
Androstenedione	Chlorinated hydrocarbons	Meprobamate*	Phenytoin*
Antihistamines	Chlorinated insecticides	Methoxyflurane*	Prednisolone
Barbiturates*	Chlorpromazine*	Methylphenylethylhydantoin	Prednisone*
Bemegride	Cortisone	Methyprylon	Probenecid*
Benzene*	Cotinine	Nicotine (tobacco smoking)	Promazine
3,4-Benzpyrene (charcoal broiled meats, cigarette smoke)*	o,p-DDD	Nikethamide	Pyridione
Butabarbital	Dieldrin	Nitrous oxide	Secobarbital*
Carbromal	Diphenhydramine	Norethynodrel	Stilbestrol*
Carbutamide	Ethchlorvynol	Orphenadrine*	Testosterone and its derivates
Carcinogens (polycyclic aromatic hydrocarbons)	Glutethimide*	Paramethadione	Tolbutamide*
Chloral betaine	Griseofulvin	Pentobarbital*	Trifluperidol
Chloral hydrate	Haloperidol	Pesticides	Triflupromazine
	Heptabarbital		Urethane
	Heptachlorepoxide		
	Hexachlorocyclohexane		
Inhibitors			
Acetohexamide	Chlorpropamide	Methylphenidate	Procarbazine
Allopurinol	Clofibrate	Metronidazole	Prochlorperazine
p-Aminosalicylic acid	Coumarins	Mushrooms (*Coprinus atramentarius*)	Quinacrine
Anabolic steroids	Disulfiram	Nialamide	SKF-525A
Androgens	Estrogens	Nitrofurantoin	Sulfonylureas
Anticholinesterases	Furazolidone	Norethandrolone	Sulfaphenazole
Bishydroxycoumarin	Insecticides	Oral contraceptives	D-Thyroxine
Calcium carbimide	Iproniazid	Pargyline	Tolbutamide
Carbon disulfide	Isocarboxazid	Phenelzine	Tranylcypromine
Chloramphenicol	Isoniazid	Phenyramidol	Triparanol
Chlordiazepoxide	MAO inhibitors	Prednisolone	Warfarin
Chlorpromazine	Methandrostenolone		

*These drugs stimulate their own metabolism either in test animals or in humans during chronic administration.

Extrinsic Predisposing Patient (Host) Factors

Foods may alter the rate or degree of drug absorption, and tobacco smoking and ethanol are potent enzyme inducers. For example, tobacco smoking increases the activity of hepatic oxidases, and heavy cigarette smokers are less likely than nonsmokers to suffer excessive sedation from benzodiazepines. Similarly, tobacco smoking interferes significantly with theophylline pharmacokinetics, posing a threat to the proper management of asthma.

Exposure to DDT and other insecticides is unavoidable for almost everybody in the United States, and some foodstuffs contain up to 5 ppm of DDT, a concentration that causes enzyme induction in animals. Many other common substances produce enzyme induction (Table 15), and some industrial solvents can produce hepatic or renal damage. Extreme heat or cold is associated with hypovolemia or hypervolemia, respectively; concomitantly there are changes in pH and electrolytes in tissue fluids. Hypoxia (such as occurs with living at high altitude) is a stimulus to enzyme induction. Picas, such as clay or starch eating, can be associated with drug interactions, through chelation of the components in the bowel lumen. Undoubtedly, numerous other environmental and dietary factors are yet unknown. Many common substances are potent enzyme inhibitors (Table 15).

DIAGNOSTIC APPROACH TO THE PATIENT WITH A SKIN REACTION

What should be done when a patient develops a cutaneous reaction that may be drug-induced? The obvious answer is to stop all medications, but this may not be possible. Whereas some drugs may be stopped with impunity, others may need to be continued. A practical approach to the problem of diagnosis is to ask the following questions:

1. Can a coincident specific skin disease be excluded?
2. Are the observed changes compatible with a drug-induced condition?
3. If a drug is suspected, which is the most likely candidate?

Table 16. Drugs That May Produce an Acneiform Eruption

Adrenocorticotropic hormone	Iodides
Anabolic steroids	Isoniazid
Androgenic steroids	Methandrostenolone
Barbiturates	Oral contraceptives
Bromides	Phenytoin
Glucocorticosteroids	Troxidone
	Vitamin B_{12}

Table 17. Drugs That May Cause Lichenoid and Lichen Planus–like Reactions

Amiphenazole	Phenothiazines
Chloroquine	Propylthiouracil
Chlorpropamide	Quinacrine
Gold salts	Quinidine
Methyldopa	Thiazide diuretics
Organic arsenicals	
Para-aminosalicylic acid	

4. Can any specific investigations be performed to confirm the clinical impression?

Can a Coincident Specific Skin Disease Be Excluded?

In many instances the skin lesion may resemble a specific dermatologic disorder. On the other hand, some specific skin disorders may be exacerbated by drugs; for example, acne (Table 16) and lichen planus (Table 17). In addition, drugs such as chloroquine, quinacrine, and lithium may exacerbate psoriasis.

Are the Observed Changes Compatible with a Drug-Induced Condition?

Drugs are notorious for causing completely different eruptions in different patients. Similarly, pharmacologically unrelated agents may cause similar eruptions. There are a few classic reaction patterns that are often drug-induced. Some of the more common ones are listed below. Whereas few drugs have escaped the stigma of causing disease, a direct cause-and-effect relationship is rarely apparent.

Allergic vasculitis: This is a Type III allergic disorder (see earlier description) in which antigen-antibody complexes are deposited on the endothelium of small blood vessels, leading to inflammatory changes. Clinically, a range of lesions from urticaria through necrotic ulceration may appear. Drugs occasionally associated with this reaction are the sulfonamides, phenytoin, the nonsteroidal anti-inflammatory agents, and the penicillins.

Table 18. Drugs That May Cause Bullous Eruptions

Acetophenitidin	Gold salts
Aminoglycosides	Griseofulvin
Aminopyrine	Insulin
Antipyrine	Iodides
Arsenicals	Mercurial diuretics
Atropine	Penicillins
Barbiturates	Phenolphthalein
Bismuth	Phenothiazines
Bromides	Phenytoin
Chloral hydrate	Quinine
Cinchophen	Salicylates
Digitalis	Streptomycin
Diuretics	Sulfonamides
Ergot	

Table 19. Drugs That May Produce Contact Dermatitis

Acriflavin	Menthol
Amethocaine	Meprobamate
Aminoglycosides	Mepyramine
Antazoline	Mercurials
Antihistamines (H_1-blockers)	Neomycin
Arsphenamine	Nitrofurazone
Bacitracin	Para-aminosalicylic acid
Benzocaine	Parabens
Benzoyl peroxide	Penicillins
Cetrimide	Peru balsam
Chloramphenicol	Phenindamine
Chlorcyclizine	Phenol
Chlorhexidine	Potassium hydroxyquinoline sulfate
Chlorhydroxyquinoline	Procaine
Chloroxylenol	Promethazine
Chlorphenesin	Propamidine
Chlorpromazine	Pyribenzamine
Crotamiton	Quinacrine
Cyclomethycaine	Quinine
Domiphen bromide	Resorcin
Ephedrine	Salicylates
Formaldehyde	Selenium sulfide
Gold salts	Sulfonamides
Halogenated phenolic compounds	Sulfur and salicylic acid ointment
Iodine and iodides	Tetracyclines
Iodochlorhydroxyquinoline	Thiamine
Isoniazid	Thimerosal
Lanolin	

Bullous eruptions (see Table 18).

Contact dermatitis (see Table 19).

Erythema nodosum (see Table 20).

Erythema multiforme, Stevens-Johnson syndrome: In these conditions the target-like lesions are confined to the limbs (erythema multiforme), and when the mucous membranes are effected, the condition merges with the Stevens-Johnson syndrome (see Table 21).

Eczema: This is usually a response in patients previously sensitized systemically (see Table 22.)

Exfoliative dermatitis (see Table 23).

Fixed drug eruptions: These consist of well-demarcated erythematous plaques that characteristically reappear each time the drug is given. Excessive pigmentation may remain after clearing. Common drugs causing fixed eruptions are listed in Table 24.

Hair loss (see Table 25).

Hirsutism (see Table 26). Hirsutism is a logical consequence to the use of sex hormones. It may also be seen in some people taking glucocorticosteroids and minoxidil.

Table 20. Drugs That May Cause Erythema Nodosum–like Lesions

- Bromides
- Iodides
- Oral contraceptive steroids
- Para-aminosalicylic acid
- Penicillins
- Salicylates
- Sulfonamides

Table 21. Drugs That May Cause Erythema Multiforme–like Lesions or Stevens-Johnson Syndrome

Acetophenetidin	Paramethadione
Aminoglycosides	Penicillins
Aminopyrine	Phenolphthalein
Antihistamines (H_1-blockers)	Phenothiazines
Antipyrine	Phensuximide
Arsenicals	Phenylbutazone
Barbiturates	Phenytoin
Belladonna	Quinine
Bismuth	Salicylates
Bromides	Smallpox vaccine
Carbamazepine	Streptomycin
Chloramphenicol	Sulfadimethoxine
Chlorpropamide	Sulfamethoxpyridazine
Cinchophen	Sulfisomidine
Codeine	Sulfonamides
Erythromycin	Sulfonylureas
Ethasoximide	Tetracyclines
Gold salts	Thiacetazone
Hydralazine	Thiazide diuretics
Iodides	Thiouracil
Measles vaccine	Trimethadione
Meprobamate	Triple sulfonamides (sulfadiazine, sulfamethazine, sulfamerazine)
Mercurial diuretics	
Methylhydantoin	
Para-aminosalicylic acid	

Table 22. Drugs That May Cause Eczematous Dermatitis

Antibiotics	Lanolin
Antihistamines (H_1-blockers)	Mercurials
Arsenicals	Neomycin
Bromides	Para-aminosalicylic acid
Chloral hydrate	Penicillins
Cosmetics (various)	Phenothiazines
Iodides	Quinacrine
Local anesthetics (topical)	Streptomycin
	Sulfonamides

Table 23. Drugs That May Cause Exfoliative Dermatitis

Acetazolamide	Mesantoin
Allopurinol	Methotrimeprazine
Aminoglycosides	Nitroglycerin
Antimony compounds	Para-aminosalicylic acid
Arsenicals	Penicillins
Barbiturates	Phenacetamide
Bismuth	Phenindione
Carbamazepine	Phenothiazines
Chloroquine	Phenylbutazone
Demeclocycline	Phenytoin
Furosemide	Quinacrine
Gold salts	Quinidine
Griseofulvin	Streptomycin
Hydroflumethiazide	Sulfonamides
Iodides	Sulfonylureas
Isorbide	Tetracyclines
Isoniazid	Thiazide diuretics
Measles virus vaccine	Vitamin A
Mercurials	

Table 24. Drugs That May Cause a Fixed Drug Eruption

Acetanilid	Meprobamate
Acetarsone	Mercury salts
Acetophenetidin	Methenamine
Acetylsalicylic acid	Neoarsphenamine
Acriflavine	Opium alkaloids
Aminoglycosides	Oxophenarsine
Aminopyrine	Oxytetracycline
Amobarbital	Para-aminosalicylic acid
Amodiaquine	Penicillins
Amphetamine sulfate	Phenacetin
Anthralin	Phenobarbital
Antimony potassium tartrate	Phenolphthalein
Antipyrine	Phenylbutazone
Arsphenamine	Phenytoin
Barbital	Potassium chlorate
Barbital sodium	Pyrimidine derivatives
Belladonna	Quinacrine
Bismuth salts	Quinidine
Bromides	Quinine
Chloral hydrate	Reserpine
Chloroguanide	Saccharin
Chloroquine	Salicylates
Chlorothiazide	Santonin
Chlorpromazine	Scopolamine
Chlortetracycline	Sodium salicylate
Cinchophen	Streptomycin
D-Amphetamine	Strychnine
Diallylbarbituric acid	Sulfadiazine
Diethylstilbestrol	Sulfaguanidine
Digilanid	Sulfamerazine
Digitalis	Sulfamethazine
Dimenhydrinate	Sulfamethoxypyridazine
Diphenhydramine	Sulfapyridine
Disulfiram	Sulfarsphenamine
Ephedrine	Sulfathiazole
Epinephrine	Sulfisoxazole
Ergot alkaloids	Sulfobromophthalein sodium
Erythrosine	Tetracyclines
Eucalyptus oil	Thiambutosine
Formalin	Thonzylamine hydrochloride
Frangula	Tripelennamine
Gold salts	Trisodium arsphenamine sulfate
Griseofulvin	Tryparsamide
Iodine	Vaccines and immunizing agents
Ipecac	
Karaya gum (Sterculia gum)	
Magnesium hydroxide	

Table 25. Drugs That May Cause Alopecia

Allopurinol	Methotrexate
α-Methyldopa	Norethindrone acetate
Amphetamine	Oral contraceptives
Anticoagulants	Phenytoin
Arsenic	Propylthiouracil
Aspirin	Quinacrine
Clofibrate	Selenium sulfide
Cyclophosphamide	Sodium warfarin
Ethionamide	Thallium
5-Fluorouracil	Trimethadione
Gentamicin	Triparanol
Gold salts	Uracil mustard
Heparin	Vinblastine
Iodine	Vincristine
Mepesulfate	Vitamin A
Mephenytoin	
Methimazole	

Table 26. Drugs That May Cause Hirsutism

Sex hormones
Glucocorticosteroids
Minoxidil

Lichenoid eruptions (see Table 17). Characteristically, the mouth is not affected.

Lupus erythematosus-like skin lesions: These may be present with or without fever and with systemic manifestations, such as myalgia, polyarthritis, and polyserositis. Many drugs have been incriminated in producing this disorder (see Table 12).

Photosensitivity (see Table 27): this was discussed earlier.

Pigmentation (see Table 28). A variety of pigmentary changes may occur following drug administration. For example, phenothiazines may yield a bluish-gray or brownish-yellow pigmentation. Quinacrine may produce yellowish discoloration and chloroquine a bluish-black to slate gray pigmentation of the nails and palate, with depigmentation of hair. Various pigmentary disturbances can be seen following heavy metal use, and oral contraceptives can produce the changes of chloasma. Argyria is extremely uncommon today. Pigmentary changes resulting from dietary idiosyncrasies, cyanosis jaundice, severe anemia, or methemoglobinemia are not considered.

Pruritus: Pruritus may be a manifestation of hypersensitivity reactions, as discussed earlier. However, generalized pruritus may arise secondary to biliary stasis and obstructive jaundice. Pruritus ani and

Table 28. Drugs That May Produce an Alteration in Skin Pigmentation

Adrenocorticotropic hormone	Gold salts
Arsenic	Lucanthone
Bismuth	Nitrofurantoin
Bleomycin	Phenothiazines
Bromides	Phenolphthalein
Busulfan	Phenytoin
Catecholamines	Potassium iodide
Chloroquine	Quinidine
Chlorpromazine	Quinacrine
Cyclophosphamide	Silver salts
Cytotoxic agents	Sulfonamides
Estrogen-containing oral contraceptives (stimulate melanocytes)	Vitamin A
	Zinc oxide

pruritus vulvi are commonly produced by candidal suprainfections.

Purpura: Drug-induced purpuric lesions may arise either from thrombocytopenia, from disorders of blood coagulation, or from a vasculitis (see Table 29). Common drug causes of purpura are sulfonamides, quinine, the barbiturates, the thiazide diuretics, sulfonylureas, and the nonsteroidal anti-inflammatory agents (see Table 30).

Serum sickness (see Table 31).

Toxic epidermal necrolysis: When seen in infants, this disorder is due to a staphyloccocal suprainfection, but in adults it may follow treatment with several drugs (see Table 32).

Table 27. Drugs and Chemicals That May Cause Photodermititis

Acetohexamide	Demeclocycline	8-Methoxypsoralen	Quinine
Acridine dyes	Desipramine	Monoglycerol para-aminobenzoate	Reserpine
Agave lechuguilla (amaryllis)	Dibenzopyran derivatives	Mustards	Rose bengal perfume
Agrimony	Dicyanine-A	Nalidixic acid	Rue
9-Aminoacridine	Diethylstilbestrol	Naphthalene	Salicylanilides
Aminobenzoic acid	Digalloyl trioleate	Nortriptyline	Salicylates
Angelica	Dill	Oral contraceptives	Sandalwood oil (perfume)
Anthracene	Diphenhydramine hydrochloride	Oxytetracycline	Silver salts
Arsenicals	Doxycycline	Para-dimethylaminoazobenzene	Stilbamidine isethionate
Barbiturates	Estrone	Paraphenylenediamine	Substituted benzoic acids (sunscreens)
Bavachi (corylifolia)	Fennel oil	Perloline	Sulfonamides
Benzene	Fentichlor	Perphenazine	Sulfonylureas
Benzopyrine	Fluorescein dyes	Phenanthrene	Tetrachlorsalicylanilide
Bergamot (perfume)	5-Fluorouracil	Phenazine dyes	Tetracyclines
Bithionol	Furosemide	Phenolic compounds	Thiazide diuretics
Blankophores (sulfa derivatives)	Glyceryl para-aminobenzoate	Phenothiazine	Thiophenes
Bromchlorsalicylanilid	Gold salts	Phenoxazines	Thiopropazate dihydrochloride
Bulosemide (Jadit)	Griseofulvin	Phenylbutazone	Tribromosalicylanilide
4-Butyl-4-chlorosalicylanilide	Hexachlorophene	Phenytoin	Trichloromethiazide
Carbamazepine	Imipramine	Prochlorperazine	Triethylene melamine
Carbinoxamine	Isothipendyl	Promazine hydrochloride	Triflupromazine hydrochloride
Carbutamide	Lantinin	Promethazine hydrochloride	Trimeprazine tartrate
Cedar oil	Lavender oil	Protriptyline	Trimethadione
Chlordiazepoxide	Lime oil	Psoralens	Trypaflavine
Chlorpromazine	Meclothiazide	Pyrathiazine hydrochloride	Trypan blue
Chlorpropamide	Mepazine	Pyridine	Vanillin oils
Chlortetracycline	9-Mercaptopurine	Quinethazone	Water ash
Citron oil	Methotrimeprazine	Quinidine	Xylene
Coal tar	Methoxsalen		Yarrow
Cyclamates	5-Methoxypsoralen		

Table 29. Drugs That May Cause Blood Dyscrasias

Drug	Agranulocytosis (Leukopenia)	Aplastic Anemia	Hemolytic Anemia	Megaloblastic Anemia	Pancytopenia	Thrombocytopenia
Acetanilid			•			
Acetazolamide	•	•			•	•
Acetophenitidin		•	•		•	•
Acetylphenylhydrazine			•			
Acetylsalicylic acid	•	•	•		•	•
Allyl-isopropyl-aceticarbamide						•
Aminopyrine	•	•	•			
Antihistamines (H_1-blockers)	•					
Antineoplastics	•	•			•	
Antipyrine			•			
Arsenicals	•					
Arsenobenzenes						•
Barbiturates		•		•	•	•
Busulfan		•		•	•	•
Carbamazepine	•	•				•
Cephalothin sodium			•			•
Chloramphenicol	•	•	•		•	•
Chloroquine	•		•			
Chlorothiazide	•	•			•	•
Chlorpromazine	•		•			
Chlorpropamide		•			•	•
Cinchophen	•					
Clofibrate	•					
Colchicine		•		•		
Corticotropin	•					
Cycloserine				•		
Cytarabine	•		•	•		•
Diaminodiphenylsulfone			•			
Digitalis glycosides	•	•			•	•
Dimercaprol			•			
Dipyrone	•					
5-Fluorouracil				•		
Furazolidone			•			
Gamma benzene hexachloride	•					
Glutethimide				•		
Gold compounds	•	•			•	•
Hydralazine	•					
Hydrochlorothiazide						•
Imipramine	•					
Indomethacin		•				
Iothiouracil	•					
Irradiation (radioactive drugs)		•				
Isoniazid			•			
Mepazine	•	•			•	
Meprobamate	•	•			•	
6-Mercaptopurine	•	•		•	•	•
Metformin				•		
Methiamazole	•	•			•	•
Methophenobarbital				•		
Methotrexate	•	•		•	•	•
Methyldopa	•	•	•		•	•
Methylene blue			•			
Neomycin				•		
Nitrofurantoin			•	•		
Nitrofurazone			•			
Oral contraceptives				•		
Oxyphenbutazone	•					
Pamaquine			•	•		
Para-aminosalicylic acid			•	•		
Penicillin	•	•	•		•	
Penindione	•					
Pentamidine isethionate				•		
Pentaquine			•			
Phenacetin	•					

Table continued on following page

Table 29. Drugs That May Cause Blood Dyscrasias (Continued)

Drug	Agranulocytosis (Leukopenia)	Aplastic Anemia	Hemolytic Anemia	Megaloblastic Anemia	Pancytopenia	Thrombocytopenia
Phenantoin		•	•		•	
Phenothiazines	•					
Phenylbutazone	•	•			•	•
Phenylhydrazine			•			
Phenytoin	•	•		•		
Primaquine			•			
Primaclone				•		
Probenecid			•			
Procainamide	•					
Prochlorperazine	•					
Promazine	•					
Propylthiouracil	•					
Pyrimethamine				•		
Quinacrine	•	•	•			•
Quinidine	•	•	•		•	•
Quinine			•			•
Rifampin						•
Salicylates	•					
Stibophen			•			
Streptomycin	•	•		•		
Sulfonamides	•	•	•		•	•
Sulfoxone			•			
Tetracyclines	•		•		•	•
Thiazides	•					
Thiazolsulfone			•			
Thioridazine	•					
Thiouracil	•					•
Tolbutamide	•	•			•	•
Triamterene				•		
Trimethadione	•	•			•	
Trimethoprim				•		
Tripelennamine	•					
Vitamin K water-soluble analogues			•			

Table 30. Drugs That May Produce Purpura

Acetophenetidin	Ergot
Adrenocorticotropic hormone	Fluoxymesterone
Allopurinol	Gold salts
Anticoagulants	Griseofulvin
Antihistamines (H_1-blockers)	Heparin
Antipyrine	Insulin
Arsenicals	Iodides
Arsenobenzols	Isoniazid
Barbiturates	Mepesulfate
Bismuth	Meprobamate
Bromides	Nirvanol
Carbamides	Para-aminosalicylic acid
Cephalosporins	Penicillins
Chloral hydrate	Phenothiazines
Chloramphenicol	Phenylbutazone
Chlorothiazide	Phenytoin
Chlorpromazine	Quinidine
Chlorpropamide	Quinine
Cinchophen	Salicylates
Corticosteroids	Sulfonamides
Digitalis	Thiazide diuretics
Digitoxin	Thiouracils
	Trifluoperazine

Toxic erythema: This is probably the most common skin reaction to drugs. The reaction is usually accompanied by systemic symptoms of malaise and fever. Common drugs producing this reactions are listed (see Table 33).

Uticaria: Urticaria (see Table 34) is seen as a component of allergic reaction. It was discussed earlier. Urticaria may also arise in pseudoallergic reactions owing to nonspecific histamine release (see Table 2).

Which Drug Is Most Likely to Be Responsible?

Regrettably, very few drugs are so specific as to cause a characteristic eruption, and most drugs at one time or another have been associated with every conceivable dermatologic rash. A complete listing of the behavior of individual drugs is beyond the scope of this article, and in the tables supplied, only commonly associated agents have been listed. Appropriate reference sources should be consulted for more detailed information.

Once a statistically based guess has been advanced

Table 31. Drugs and Other Agents That May Produce Serum Sickness

Antihistamines	Penicillins
Arsenicals	Phenylbutazone
Barbiturates	Phenytoin
Bismuth	Procainamide
Digitalis	Quinidine
Heparin	Salicylates
Hydralazine	Sera
Insulin	Streptomycin
Iodides	Sulfonamides
Mercurial diuretics	Thiouracils
	Vaccines

and the appropriate drug discontinued (when possible), the lesion will usually start to improve within several days. Some drug reactions, however, may persist for days or weeks and clear more slowly. Continued exposure to the sensitizing substance in an unusual form—for example, penicillin in milk or iodine or digitalis glycosides in herb teas—may confuse diagnostic considerations.

Discontinuance of the suspected drug followed by disappearance of the reaction provides presumptive evidence of drug-induced illness. In addition, reappearance of the reaction with cautious readministration of the drug suspected of causing the symptoms may provide confirmation of the association, if such confirmation will add useful information to the continuing management of that patient without entailing undue risk.

Can Any Specific Investigations Be Performed to Confirm the Clinical Impressions?

The diagnosis of most drug-induced cutaneous allergy is presumptive, based on clinical appearance and a temporal association between drug administration and clinical response. In most cases this is sufficient because the drug in question can be discontinued or substituted. Occasionally a diagnosis is confirmed, or even excluded, when the drug in question is administered a second time, often inadvertently. It is extremely hazardous to continue to administer drugs suspected of causing an allergic reaction, since the potential for fatal anaphylactic shock is always present.

Patch Tests. Patch tests are of limited value since they are useful only in diagnosing Type IV allergic reactions. The possible allergen is placed on the skin and covered with tape for 24 to 48 hours; suitable control tape is also used. It should be remembered that the test may be positive on the plaque of a fixed drug eruption but negative on uninvolved skin.

Prick and Scratch Tests. These tests are used to detect IgE-mediated Type I reactions, and they are always of potential danger since they may be followed by a severe allergic response. The object is to introduce a trace quantity of the possible allergen into the dermis. Most drugs are, unfortunately, simple chemical compounds that require complexing with an endogenous or exogenous macromolecule in order to become antigenic. In most instances of allergic reaction the allergen is not known, which hampers the

Table 33. Drugs and Other Agents That May Produce Toxic Erythema

Aminoglycosides	Methaminodiazepoxide
Anticonvulsants	Nitrofurantoin
Anticholinergics	Organic extracts
Antihistamines (H_1-blockers)	Para-aminosalicylic acid
Atropine	Penicillins
Barbiturates	Phenothiazines
Bromides	Phenylbutazone
Chloral hydrate	Phenytoin
Chlordiazepoxide	Primaclone
Chloroquine	Quinacrine
Chlorothiazide	Quinine
Chlorpromazine	Reserpine
Diethylstilbestrol	Salicylates
Erythromycin	Sera
Gold salts	Sulfonamides
Griseofulvin	Sulfones
Insulin	Tetracyclines
Meprobamate	Thiouracil
Mercurials	

Table 32. Drugs That May Cause Toxic Epidermal Necrolysis

Acetazolamide	Nalidixic acid
Allopurinol	Neomycin sulfate
Aminopyrine	Nitrofurantoin
Antihistamines (H_1-blockers)	Nonsteroidal anti-inflammatory agents
Antipyrine	Opium powder
Barbiturates	Penicillins
Bromides	Phenolphthalein
Brompheniramine	Phenylbutazone
Chenopodium oil	Phenytoin
Ethylmorphine HCl	Polio vaccine
Gold salts	Sulfonamides
Iodides	Sulfones
Ipecac	Tetanus antitoxin
Isoniazid	Tetracyclines
Methyl salicylate	Tolbutamide

Table 34. Drugs and Other Agents That May Cause Urticaria

Adrenocorticotropic hormone	Meprobamate
Aminoglycosides	Mercurials
Barbiturates	Nitrofurantoin
Bromides	Opiates
Chloramphenicol	Penicillinase
Dextran	Penicillins
Enzymes	Phenolphthalein
Erythromycin	Phenothiazines
Glutethimide	Phenytoin
Griseofulvin	Propoxyphene
Insulin	Salicylates
Iodides	Sera
Iodopyracet	Streptomycin
Liver extracts	Sulfonamides
Meperidine	Tetracyclines
	Thiouracil

development of an appropriate testing material. In the case of penicillin, skin testing with penicilloyl polylysine (PPL) is of some use in predicting a Type II or Type III reaction, and the use of the minor determinants of penicillin (pencillin, penicilloate, and penilloate) can be used to predict anaphylaxis (see earlier discussion).

Various in vitro tests, such as the basophil degranulation test, the lymphocyte transformation test, and the leukocyte migration test, are still experimental.

The Skin Window Technique. In this test a drop of the possible allergen is applied onto an abraded area of skin and covered with a glass cover slip for a period of time. The cover glass is subsequently removed and stained for the presence of cells. The technique has not achieved widespread use.

Detection of Antibodies. The detection of antibodies—for example, hemagglutinating antibodies of the IgG type—is of limited diagnostic value since a positive result indicates only that the patient has developed an antibody to the appropriate drug; it does not necessarily mean that the drug is responsible for the symptoms produced. Most patients receiving a given drug will develop hemagglutinating antibodies to that agent without any relationship to an adverse effect. Both the direct and indirect Coombs test, various complement fixation tests, and mixed antiglobulin reactions have been used to diagnose Type II reactions. Measurement of circulating immune complexes (C1q precipitation) and the identification of antigen-antibody-complement complexes by immunofluorescence may be valuable in Type III reactions.

The Radioallergosorbent Test (RAST). In RAST the possible antigen is coupled to an insoluble carrier, such as a paper disc. The fluid containing the suspected antibody (for example, serum) is then added to the disc and rinsed off. If antibody is present in the serum, it binds to the paperbound antigen, and then can be detected with the subsequent addition of a radioactive antibody to the bound antibody. The RAST is widely used to detect allergens such as pollens, but so far has not proved successful in the identification of IgE to minor antigenic determinants of penicillin or other drugs.

Section Seventeen

COLLAGEN DISEASES

SYSTEMIC LUPUS ERYTHEMATOSUS

By John Seaman, M.D.
Wright Patterson AFB, Ohio
and James C. Steigerwald, M.D.
Denver, Colorado

SYNONYMS

SLE, lupus erythematosus.

DEFINITION

Systemic lupus erythematosus (SLE) is a multisystem disease characterized by the presence of serum autoantibodies that participate in immunologically mediated tissue injury. Of the connective tissue diseases (CTD), it is second in occurrence only to rheumatoid arthritis with an incidence of SLE in the United States of 7.6 cases per 100,000 population per year. SLE occurs more commonly in females (9:1 female to male preponderance), but this marked difference occurs only after puberty. It is more prevalent in black females aged 15 to 64 years in the United States, in whom there is 1 case per 245 women; in comparison, the rate in all females aged 15 to 64 years is 1 case per 700.

Estrogens appear to play a role in this increased prevalence in females, for (1) there are reported cases in which monozygotic twins were discordant for SLE, with the non-affected twin having undergone castration at an early age; (2) oral contraceptive therapy increases the risk of a flare in SLE patients; and (3) SLE is associated with Klinefelter's syndrome, in which there is evidence for persistent estrogenic stimulation.

There also appears to be some genetic predisposition to the disease. In one report of 16 pairs of monozygotic twins, 11 of the pairs were concordant for clinical SLE and only five pairs were discordant. Additionally there appears to be an increased percentage of two of the histocompatibility locus antigens (HLA-DR2 and HLA-DR3) in patients with SLE.

In 1982, the American Rheumatism Association modified the preliminary criteria for the classification of SLE. The new classification is based on 11 criteria (Table 1). The diagnosis of SLE can be made if at least four of the 11 criteria are present serially or simultaneously during the period of observation. Of interest is that two of the earlier criteria, Raynaud's phenomenon and alopecia, were dropped because of lack of specificity, while others were modified (i.e., the amount of proteinuria was reduced from greater than 3.5 gm/24 hr to greater than 0.5 gm/24 hr).

PRESENTING SIGNS AND SYMPTOMS

The onset of SLE may mimic many other diseases, especially when only one organ system is initially involved. Thus, thrombocytopenia may be present for months to years and diagnosed as idiopathic thrombocytopenic purpura (ITP) until involvement of other organ systems occurs and the correct diagnosis is made. Because of this and the fact that any organ system may be involved at the onset of the disease, we find it useful to consider each organ system individually.

Cutaneous Manifestations

Up to 80 per cent of patients will have skin involvement sometime in the course of their disease, with approximately 25 per cent having cutaneous involvement as a presenting feature of the disease.

Skin lesions related to SLE may be classified into three groups: chronic, subacute, and acute. Discoid lesions constitute the most common chronic form, characterized by atrophic scarring lesions surrounded by erythematous and hyperkeratotic scaling, which, if unroofed, frequently show follicular plugs of keratin. These lesions occur most frequently on the head, neck, and scalp but may also be more widespread, occurring over the extensor surfaces of the arms, hands, back, and chest. A hypertrophic or verrucous form has also been described. Approximately 10 per cent of patients presenting with only discoid lesions eventually develop SLE, whereas the others continue to suffer from discoid lupus erythematosus (DLE).

A less common chronic skin lesion in SLE is *lupus profundus,* a panniculitis that is initially painful, later forming depressed, firm nodules and occurring on the head, chest, back, thighs, and arms. These lesions frequently occur in association with DLE. The subacute variety of skin disease, termed *subacute cutaneous lupus erythematosus* (SCLE), occurs as a much more widespread erythematous, superficial, nonscarring, pleomorphic skin rash with a significant tendency for hyper- or hypopigmentation. In contrast to the more persistent and permanent scar-forming

Table 1. The 1982 Revised Criteria for Classification of Systemic Lupus Erythematosus*

Criterion	Definition
Butterfly rash	Fixed erythema, flat or raised, over the malar eminences, tending to spare the nasolabial folds
Discoid lupus	Erythematous raised patches with adherent keratotic scaling and follicular plugging; atrophic scarring may occur in older lesions
Photosensitivity	Skin rash as a result of unusual reaction to sunlight, diagnosed by patient history or physician observation
Oral ulcers	Painless oral or nasopharyngeal ulceration observed by a physician
Arthritis	Nonerosive arthritis involving two or more peripheral joints, characterized by tenderness, swelling, or effusion
Serositis	Pleuritis—convincing history of pleuritic pain or rub heard by a physician or evidence of pleural effusion, *or* Pericarditis—documented by ECG or rub or evidence of pericardial effusion
Renal disorder	Persistent proteinuria greater than 0.5 gm/d or greater than 3+ if quantitation not performed, *or* Cellular casts—may be red cell, hemoglobin, granular, tubular, or mixed
Neurologic disorder	Seizures—in the absence of offending drugs or known metabolic derangements (e.g., uremia, ketoacidosis, or electrolyte imbalance), *or* Coma—in the absence of offending drugs or known metabolic derangements (e.g., uremia, ketoacidosis, or electrolyte imbalance)
Hematologic disorder	Hemolytic anemia with reticulocytosis, *or* Leukopenia—less than 4000/cu mm total on two or more occasions, *or* Lymphopenia—less than 1500/cu mm on two or more occasions, *or* Thrombocytopenia—less than 100,000/cu mm in the absence of offending drugs
Immunologic disorder	Positive LE cell preparation, *or* Antibody to native DNA (n-DNA) in abnormal titer, *or* Antibody to Sm nuclear antigen, *or* False-positive STS for patients known to be positive for at least 6 months and confirmed by TPI or FTA tests
Antinuclear antibody	An abnormal titer of ANA by immunofluorescence or an equivalent assay at any point in time and in the absence of drugs known to be associated with drug-induced lupus erythematosus syndrome

*For the purpose of identifying patients in clinical studies, a person shall be said to have systemic lupus erythematosus if any four or more of the 11 criteria are present, serially or simultaneously, during any interval of observation.
Abbreviations: TPI = *Treponema pallidum* immobilization; FTA = fluorescent treponema antibody.

lesion of DLE, this variety usually follows an episodic course and has the potential for complete healing.

Acute forms of cutaneous SLE such as malar (butterfly) erythema or a more diffuse, macular erythema occur in 30 to 40 per cent of the patients. These disorders frequently are seen in conjunction with a flare of systemic disease, may appear abruptly after sun exposure, and may be associated with significant swelling. The widespread eruption may mimic a drug eruption, erythema multiforme, or bullous disease but, in contrast to the latter two, does not involve the cornea and only rarely involves the mucosal membranes.

A number of other nonspecific but frequently associated cutaneous findings in SLE deserve mention, including a wide spectrum of cutaneous necrotizing vasculitis; urticaria; livido reticularis; indolent ulcers, particularly of the legs; superficial thrombophlebitis; and Raynaud's phenomenon. Purpura may be seen either as a manifestation of leukocytoclastic vasculitis (palpable purpura) or related to thrombocytopenia.

Musculoskeletal Manifestations

Polyarticular joint pain is the most common feature of SLE, occurring in 80 to 95 per cent of patients. Characteristically it involves the distal joints of the extremities and may be associated with swelling, tenderness, and limited range of motion. Typical swan-neck and boutonnière deformities may develop. Volar subluxation of the metacarpophalangeal joints resembling rheumatoid arthritis in SLE is termed *Jaccoud's deformity*. These anatomic derangements occur because of tendon laxity and intrinsic muscle tightness. Cartilage destruction, subchondral cysts, and erosions are not usual features of SLE.

Muscle weakness may result from a primary myopathy, but more frequently it is caused by disuse or medications used to treat other features of SLE, such as corticosteroids or hydroxychloroquine.

Lung Involvement

Parenchymal and pleural involvement in SLE is common. Pleuritic chest pain, occasionally severe, may occur in as many as 80 per cent of patients. Pleural effusions, usually small in size, occur in 15 to 40 per cent. Analysis of pleural fluid is essential not only for confirming the diagnosis but also for distinguishing this effusion from a septic process, which is always a consideration in this immunosuppressed population.

Parenchymal lung involvement in SLE may take either an acute or a chronic form. A majority of patients, even those who are asymptomatic, have a mild to moderate restrictive pattern and low diffusion capacity by pulmonary function testing. Interstitial fibrosis may be seen on chest x-rays and on occasion may lead to disabling dyspnea and death. The more subacute picture of fibrosing alveolitis with patchy bilateral basilar pulmonary infiltrates and severe dyspnea may be more steroid-responsive than is chronic interstitial fibrosis. *Acute lupus pneumonitis* frequently presents a dramatic clinical picture. The patient typically appears toxic, with fever, dyspnea, and hypoxemia. A dry cough is usually present, and despite the fact that there may be widespread diffuse alveolar infiltrates physical findings in the lung may be minimal. Even with aggressive therapy, the mortality rate is high.

Massive pulmonary hemorrhage is also an acute complication of SLE, but fortunately it is rare. The true cause of this hemorrhagic disorder is unknown, as patients may have a normal bleeding time and normal platelet counts. Circulating and fixed immune complexes in lung tissue are thought to play a role. A sudden drop in hematocrit at the onset of respiratory distress may provide a valuable differential clue.

Two other pulmonary conditions relating to SLE deserve mention. *Pulmonary hypertension* may progress relentlessly despite control of other manifestations of SLE (see article on Pulmonary Hypertension). *Diaphragmatic dysfunction,* suggested by loss of lung volume on chest x-ray or pulmonary function tests ("the shrinking lung"), can be confirmed by the inability of the patient to produce negative intrathoracic inspiratory pressure. Patients with this syndrome may complain of dyspnea when supine, but they tend to show improvement on long-term follow-ups.

Cardiac Manifestations

Cardiac disease also occurs frequently in SLE. *Pericarditis* is by far the most common manifestation, occurring in up to one third of the patients, and it is often seen in conjunction with pleuritis. Recumbent or pleuritic chest pain, pericardial friction rubs, and ST and T wave abnormalities on electrocardiography (ECG) suggest pericarditis, but asymptomatic pericardial effusions can be detected by echocardiography in as many as two thirds of patients. Pericardial tamponade and constrictive pericarditis may occur.

Clinical *myocarditis* may be detected in up to 10 per cent of patients. Contributing factors to its development include small vessel arteritis, inflammatory myositis, hypertension, and renal failure. Noninfective verrucous endocarditis (Libman-Sacks disease) is a well-established complication of SLE but is only rarely associated with secondary infection, peripheral embolization, or valvular insufficiency. The most commonly involved valve is the mitral, but the aortic and tricuspid valves can be involved as well.

Ischemic coronary artery disease may occur as a result of small vessel vasculitis but much more commonly is related to accelerated coronary atherosclerosis. Hyperlipidemia is a common risk factor, as are corticosteroid use, hypertension, and the nephrotic syndrome, all of which may be seen in SLE.

Conduction system disease is only occasionally seen in adults with SLE, but newborn infants of mothers with SLE having anti-SS-A (anticytoplasmic) antibodies are at risk for congenital heart block.

Gastrointestinal Manifestations

Gastrointestinal symptoms occur in over half of SLE patients. Most are nonspecific, and frequently they are related to drugs used in treatment. Episodes may be severe or life-threatening in as many as 15 per cent of cases. Abdominal pain is often attributed to serositis of the peritoneum and may be associated with ascites. *Spontaneous bacterial peritonitis,* often due to gram-positive organisms, and *mesenteric vasculitis* with subsequent visceral perforations of large or small bowel must also be considered in the differential diagnosis. Visceral vasculitis usually occurs in the setting of cutaneous vasculitis and active SLE. Bloody diarrhea due to mucosal infarction may mimic acute inflammatory bowel disease.

Pancreatitis has also been reported in patients with SLE. Its pathogenesis is unknown but in some cases may be related to the use of corticosteroids for treatment.

Clinically significant liver disease is unusual in SLE, but hepatomegaly can be found in as many as one third of the patients. Low-grade elevations of transaminase, alkaline phosphatase, and bilirubin occur, but histologic findings are nonspecific. *Lupoid hepatitis* is really a subset of chronic active hepatitis, but its association with antinuclear antibodies and symptoms of SLE frequently make this a difficult clinical differentiation. For unknown reasons, some patients with SLE are predisposed to hepatotoxicity from aspirin. These changes resolve if the drug is discontinued or if the dose is lowered.

Neuropsychiatric Manifestations

Nervous system disorders appear as the initial symptom of SLE in roughly 10 per cent of patients, most frequently in the form of generalized motor seizures or psychiatric illness. Significant neuropsychiatric dysfunction occurs sometime during the course of disease in 50 per cent of patients and overall is the second most common organ-related cause of death. These disorders may take a multitude of forms: seizures, psychosis, organic brain syndrome, demyelinating lesions, cerebral infarcts, and peripheral neuropathies. Other, less common events are also implicated in SLE, including choreiform movements, tremor, aseptic meningitis, cranial nerve palsies, and visual disturbances. When coma occurs, it is a particularly ominous sign, even with prompt and aggressive therapy. Meningitis, especially in view of the immunosuppressed nature of the patient, may be caused by a number of opportunistic organisms. Psychiatric disease frequently takes the form of mood disturbances or schizophrenia. Since many of these patients are taking corticosteroids or have recently increased their dosage, the differentiation from medication-induced psychosis may be difficult. Organic features of brain disease, such as intellectual impairment and memory deficits, are present in the majority of patients with SLE-induced psychosis, and these signs are generally not thought to be due to steroids. There are very few diagnostic procedures that aid in the differential diagnosis of lupus cerebritis. An abnormal cerebrospinal fluid occurs at most in one half of patients and may consist only of slightly elevated protein levels.

Renal Manifestations

Nephritis is the initial manifestation in SLE in roughly 5 per cent of patients, although 50 to 75 per cent will ultimately have clinical renal involvement. Despite this high frequency, death from renal failure occurs in fewer than 10 per cent of patients. Clinical signs of significant renal disease include hypertension, nephrotic syndrome (or lesser degrees of proteinuria), hematuria, pyuria, active urinary sediment, and renal failure, which may present in an acute or chronic form. It should also be pointed out that even in patients without clinical features of renal involvement, a majority will show some changes in renal biopsy.

A widely accepted histologic classification of lupus nephritis subdivides this disease into four categories: focal proliferative, mesangial, diffuse proliferative, and membranous glomerulonephritis. Patients with focal proliferative and mesangial glomerulonephritis may have active sediment or significant proteinuria, but they very rarely develop renal failure. Diffuse proliferative glomerulonephritis connotes widespread glomerular sclerosis and proliferative change frequently with accompanying interstitial tubular atrophy. If untreated, the majority of these patients develop some degree of azotemia and consequently have a poorer prognosis. Membranous glomerulonephritis resembles idiopathic membranous nephritis without cellular infiltration or necrosis by light microscopy. Although hypertension and frank azotemia are less common, profuse proteinuria is characteristic. This subgroup also carries a less favorable prognosis for long-term survival.

COURSE

The course of SLE is unpredictable, with multiple flares and remissions being common. Certain clinical manifestations, however, carry a more ominous prognosis. Thus, patients with diffuse proliferative glomerulonephritis, active central nervous system disease, acute lupus pneumonitis, or pulmonary hemorrhage tend to do poorly. Overall, however, more than 90 per cent of patients are alive 10 years after the onset of the disease.

PHYSICAL EXAMINATION

The findings on physical examination depend on the organ system involved; thus, even with significant disease (e.g., renal disease) signs may be few or lacking completely.

When present, the most characteristic findings on physical examination are the cutaneous lesions. A malar rash and discoid lesions are found in no other condition, with the possible exception of mixed connective tissue disease. Other findings on physical examination that suggest a diagnosis of SLE include recurrent fevers in the absence of infection, oral or nasal ulceration, alopecia, and a persistent inflammatory arthritis, which either is nondeforming or causes easily reducible swan-neck or boutonnière deformities of the hands. The presence of multiple fluffy white exudates (cytoid bodies) in the retina should also alert the physician to the diagnosis of SLE. Other findings, such as pleural or pericardial friction rubs, reflect an underlying pleuritis and pericarditis but are not specific for SLE.

COMMON COMPLICATIONS

Complications seen in SLE are primarily related to the immune status of the patient or are secondary to the treatment of disease. In some series of patients, infection has now become the leading cause of death in those with active disease. The presence of multiple autoantibodies, some of them directed against white blood cells, in itself predisposes patients to more frequent infection. When corticosteroids or other immunosuppressive agents are added to the treatment plan the patient is even more immunosuppressed and at great risk for the development of bacterial, mycobacterial, fungal, or viral infections. Organisms that usually are not considered pathogenic in humans may frequently cause disseminated disease in SLE patients. Thus, the onset of fever in SLE can never be assumed to be related to a flare of the disease until an extensive search has been made for an infectious cause for the fever.

Specific complications from drugs used to treat SLE can include an increase in liver enzymes or a decline in renal function related to the use of salicylates or other nonsteroidal anti-inflammatory drugs. The antimalarials can cause proximal muscle weakness or retinal toxicity. Corticosteroids, although life-saving, in many instances cause multiple problems, especially when they need to be used on a long-term basis. Posterior subcapsular cataracts and severe osteopenia with compression fractures are particularly bothersome problems. Premature atherosclerosis may also be related to prolonged corticosteroid therapy. Another complication, aseptic necrosis or avascular necrosis of bone, may either be related to the disease itself or result from the prolonged use of corticosteroids. In some patients who are otherwise doing well, joint problems related to aseptic necrosis, particularly of lower extremity joints, have prevented the patients from returning to an active lifestyle.

Immunosuppressive therapy, when needed, is also associated with definite risks. Besides the previously mentioned increased problems with infections, cyclophosphamide can cause hemorrhagic cystitis, alopecia, and sterility. There also appears to be an increased risk of malignancy in patients with SLE.

This may in part be related to their altered immune system, but the addition of immunosuppressive drugs would seem to increase this risk even further.

LABORATORY FINDINGS

The hallmark of SLE is the wide variety of autoantibodies produced by virtually all patients. These antibodies are directed not only against nuclear and cytoplasmic components but also against circulating proteins and cell membranes (Table 2). The LE cell phenomenon is an example of an autoantibody (antinucleoprotein antibody) interaction with antigen (nuclear debris), which in turn is engulfed by a phagocytic cell (the polymorphonuclear cell, or PMN).

Detection of Antibodies

The detection of these antibodies requires a number of special techniques. The fluorescent antinuclear antibody (ANA) test is the most commonly used screening method. This gives a number of fluorescent patterns, commonly classified as diffuse (homogeneous), rim (peripheral), speckled, or nucleolar. These patterns may appear mixed, reflecting the detection of more than one type of antibody. The rim pattern is the most specific for SLE, but the speckled and diffuse patterns are seen more commonly. ANAs detected by this technique are by no means diagnostic for SLE, but are also seen in high titers in mixed connective tissue disease and in low titers in many other rheumatic and nonrheumatic diseases. Subtyping the ANAs requires other techniques available at specialized laboratories. Detecting these antibodies is useful for a number of reasons. Antibodies to the Sm antigen are considered to be markers for SLE, while high-titer antibody to native DNA (n-DNA) is seen almost exclusively in SLE. Antibodies to n-DNA can be further subdivided according to immunoglobulin subclasses and also according to whether or not they fix complement. This appears to be clinically useful, since most patients with active lupus nephritis have IgG complement-fixing antibody to n-DNA. Furthermore, many patients with lupus nephritis demonstrate increased levels of anti-n-DNA antibody during an exacerbation of their renal disease. This is frequently accompanied by a decrease in levels of either total hemolytic serum complement or complement components, such as C3 or C4. There have also been suggestions that those patients with low titers of antibodies to n-DNA and specificities limited to Sm or ribonucleoprotein (RNP) have less renal involvement. Clinicians are certainly more comfortable with the diagnosis of SLE if antinuclear antibodies are detected, but approximately 5 per cent of patients remain repeatedly negative. In many of these, anticytoplasmic antibody (SS-A) is detected.

In addition to their role in diagnosing SLE, antinuclear antibodies have been shown to play a significant role in producing organ damage, particularly in renal, skin, and vascular tissues. Complexes of anti-DNA antibody and DNA have been detected in the dermoepidermal junction of the skin, in the glomerulus, and as free circulating immune complexes. The activation of complement by these complexes induces an inflammatory response that results in tissue damage. Furthermore, antibodies bound to circulating proteins or cell membranes have been shown to produce functional defects in the respective protein or cells (for example, antibodies to white blood cells may be related to the leukopenia frequently seen in SLE).

Table 2. Classification of Antinuclear Antibodies

Type of Antibody	Relevance to SLE
Antibodies to DNA	
Single stranded (ss) DNA	Present in many diseases
Double stranded (ds) DNA	High titers in 70% of patients with SLE, lower titers in other rheumatic diseases
Antinucleoprotein	
Requires DNA, protein complex	LE cell in SLE and other rheumatic diseases
Antibodies to histones	Drug-induced LE and idiopathic SLE (30% of patients)
Antibodies to nonhistone proteins	
RNP	High titer in MCTD, other rheumatic diseases
Sm	Probably specific for SLE (25% of patients)
SS-A (Ro)	"ANA-negative" SLE, other rheumatic diseases
SS-B (La)	Sjögren's syndrome, other rheumatic diseases
Scl-70	High specificity for PSS
PCNA	SLE (7% of patients)
Anticentromere antibodies	PSS, CREST syndrome
Antinucleolar antibodies	PSS, other rheumatic diseases, especially in association with Raynaud's phenomenon

Abbreviations: ANA = Antinuclear antibodies; MCTD = mixed connective tissue disease; PSS = progressive systemic sclerosis; SLE = systemic lupus erythematosus; RNP = ribonucleoprotein; CREST = calcinosis, Raynaud's phenomenon, esophageal hypomotility, sclerodactyly, and telangiectasia; PCNA = proliferating cell nuclear antigen; Sm = Smith antigen, named after the first patient in whom the antibody was described SS-A, SS-B = Sjögren's syndrome antibodies A, B.

Detection of Complement Components

Activation of the complement cascade is found in 60 to 75 per cent of patients with SLE. This is best determined by measuring total hemolytic complement activity in the serum, since it reflects the function of the entire cascade. Unfortunately, either this determination must be done immediately or the serum must be frozen at –70°C to prevent spontaneous consumption of the complement components. Detection of the complement components C3 and C4 by immunodiffusion, although less sensitive, is a more practical method of following complement activation and one that is available in most laboratories. Complement levels may be useful not only in the diagnosis of SLE, but also in following disease activity, since they often drop with any flare in the disease.

Detection of Immune Complexes

Detection of the presence of immune complexes could also be very helpful in monitoring the activity of SLE. Multiple assays are available, but except for searching for cryoglobulins, which are present in approximately 50 per cent of SLE patients, none of the other assays is sufficiently standardized; even then they would be available only in research laboratories. Thus, at present they do not appear to be a useful laboratory method for following disease activity.

Blood Cell Disorders

Disorders of both quantity and function of blood elements and coagulation occur frequently in patients with SLE. Anemia occurs in 60 to 80 per cent of patients. The most frequent finding is a hypoproliferative normocytic, normochromic anemia with either normal or increased erythroid elements and normal stainable iron on bone marrow examination. Hematocrit values less than 28 per cent are unusual unless blood loss, hemolysis, or uremia supervenes. Although approximately 30 per cent of SLE patients have a positive Coombs' test result, fewer than 10 per cent have significant hemolytic anemia. This type of hemolysis is due to IgG and IgM antibodies directed against red cell surface antigens. These surface-bound immunoglobulins activate complement and are cleared by the spleen (IgG-mediated) or liver (IgM-mediated). Autoimmune hemolytic anemia alone or combined with thrombocytopenia (Evans' syndrome) may precede the full expression of SLE.

Thrombocytopenia in SLE similarly is mediated by IgG bound to the platelet surface, resulting in clearance by the spleen. As in autoimmune hemolytic anemia, antibody-dependent thrombocytopenia presenting as typical ITP may antedate the clinical expression of SLE. In some cases, differences in splenic histology may help differentiate the two causes. Platelet dysfunction occurs frequently in patients with SLE, manifested by an increased bleeding time. This in part is due to a circulating serum factor that interferes with platelet aggregation. Even though platelet quantity appears sufficient, it is thus advisable to obtain bleeding time before invasive procedures are contemplated. Severe thrombocytopenia may be treated with corticosteroids.

Autoimmune granulocytopenia with peripheral white counts of 2000 to 4500 per cu mm likewise is not uncommon. There may be an increased number of band forms on peripheral smear. Surface-bound IgG appears to be responsible for the shortened survival of the circulating granulocytes. In addition, defects in granulocyte phagocytosis have been demonstrated, as well as circulating factors that can suppress production of any individual myeloid element.

T cell function appears to play a major role in the altered immune state. Most patients with active SLE demonstrate a defect in the ability to form T suppressor cells. There is also a polyclonal activation of B cells, which results in the production of numerous autoantibodies and the hypergammaglobulinemia seen in the disease.

Blood Clotting Disorders

Hemostatic disorders in SLE relate not only to the platelet system but also the coagulation cascade. Circulating anticoagulants occur in as many as 10 per cent of patients, but unless there is associated prothrombin deficiency or other isolated factor deficiencies or thrombocytopenia, they rarely cause bleeding. The most common anticoagulation activity in SLE is an interference with a platelet phospholipid complex manifested as a prolonged partial thromboplastin time (PTT), but with a normal or slightly prolonged prothrombin time (PT). These circulating anticoagulants are not specific for SLE but occur in a wide variety of disease states as well as in normal individuals. If the situation dictates, reversal of anticoagulant activity can be achieved with corticosteroids.

Urinary Disorders

Urinary abnormalities occur sometime during the course of disease in approximately 75 per cent of patients with SLE. Proteinuria is the most common finding and if present should be quantitated, since nephrotic range proteinuria most often indicates either membranous or diffuse proliferative glomerulonephritis. Urinary sediment should be examined on a regular basis, since the presence of white blood cells, red blood cells, and especially red blood cell casts indicates active renal disease. Twenty-four hour urine collection for creatinine clearance is also very helpful in assessing renal function. Adequate collections, however, are sometimes difficult to obtain, especially on an outpatient basis, so we follow the serum creatinine level routinely and tend to repeat 24-hour urine collections only if there is a rise in the serum creatinine level.

Synovial Fluid Changes

Synovial fluid findings in SLE may be helpful in establishing a diagnosis when there is a white blood cell count ranging from 2000 to 5000 cells per cu mm. In contrast, rheumatoid arthritis, the articular disease that may resemble SLE, has a more inflammatory picture, with white blood counts most often in the range of 10,000 to 20,000 cells per cu mm. Although occasionally a patient with SLE may have a white blood cell count in this range, a septic arthritis should definitely be suspected, especially if the differential count demonstrates a predominance of polymorphonuclear white blood cells.

Effusions

Pleural, pericardial, or peritoneal effusions can also be seen in patients with SLE. The while blood cell count in these effusions rarely exceeds 3000 cells per cu mm and there is a predominance of PMNs. Protein content usually ranges from 3.0 to 4.5 gm/dl, and glucose content is usually within 80 per cent or more of the serum glucose level. The pH typically is greater than 7.35, opposed to the more acidic effusions of tuberculosis, rheumatoid disease, and empyema. Lactate dehydrogenase concentration in SLE effusions is lower than 500 IU/liter. Complement levels (either C4, C3, or CH_{50}) when corrected for total protein are generally depressed, reflecting either the low value in serum or a local complement consumption. Levels of immunoglobulin and antinuclear antibodies also parallel those in serum and therefore have limited value as a differential test.

BIOPSY FINDINGS

Histopathology and direct immunofluorescence of skin biopsy specimens can be very helpful in diagnosis. Histologically, discoid lesions are characterized by hyperkeratosis, epidermal atrophy, follicular plugging, and a mononuclear cell infiltrate around appendicular structures such as sebacious glands and hair follicles. These changes are less prominent in subacute and acute lesions. Direct immunofluorescence demonstrates granular deposition of IgG, IgM, or IgA with frequently associated complement components C3 and C4 at the dermoepidermal junction and in the blood vessels. Immunofluorescent staining is seen in 75 per cent of biopsy specimens from nonlesional skin of patients with systemic lupus erythematosus, but this finding is unusual in nonlesional skin of patients with DLE. Interestingly, subepidermal immunoglobulin is present in only about 50 per cent of biopsy specimens of lesion in subacute cases, perhaps reflecting a different immunopathogenic potential of the SSA antibody found in SCLE.

Although the value of renal biopsy in the overall management and prognosis of lupus nephritis remains controversial, the biopsy may in certain instances provide information on the activity of the immune complex deposition and extent of irreversible damage. In addition, we find a biopsy particularly useful in patients who demonstrate significant serologic abnormalities (high levels of antibody to n-DNA and depressed serum complement values) but have normal or minimal urinary findings. If a biopsy is done, the specimen should be submitted for routine histologic, immunofluorescent, and electron microscopic examination. Typical immunofluorescent studies of renal biopsy specimens from the majority of SLE patients stain for IgG, and occasionally for IgM and IgA, with variable association with complement components and fibrin. Electron microscopic examination may reveal subendothelial or mesangial and subepithelial electron-dense deposits, which presumably represent immune complexes.

PITFALLS IN DIAGNOSIS

Features of SLE may occur in combination with features of other CTD. This syndrome is referred to as mixed connective tissue disease (MCTD) if certain serologic findings are present (high titers of antibody to RNP) or "overlap" syndrome if anti-RNP antibodies are absent. The major overlap in MCTD occurs with progressive systemic sclerosis (PSS) or polymyositis/dermatomyositis, although occasionally patients will have some features of rheumatoid arthritis. Because of this overlap, severe Raynaud's phenomenon, sclerodermatous skin changes, esophageal dysmotility, and a significant myositis, along with findings of SLE, should alert you to this diagnosis. These patients rarely develop severe renal or central nervous system disease but may develop progressive pulmonary fibrosis. The diagnosis may be further confirmed by the findings of high-titer antibody to RNP.

A lupus erythematosus-like syndrome has also been well described in association with certain drugs, most notably procainamide, hydralazine, and phenytoin. It is also seen but much less frequently with the phenothiazines, isoniazid, and penicillamine. Clinically, patients with this syndrome have prominent skin lesions, arthralgias or arthritis, pericarditis, and pleuritic lung involvement. Renal and central nervous system diseases are very rare in drug-induced LE and would suggest that the patient has SLE instead. Serologic studies are also quite helpful in differentiating drug-induced LE from SLE. Although essentially all patients with drug-induced LE do demonstrate antinuclear antibodies in their serum, they rarely have antibodies directed against n-DNA. In procainamide- and hydralazine-induced LE the antinuclear antibody found is directed against histones.

Finally, since SLE can begin with involvement of any organ system, a high degree of suspicion should be maintained in any unusual or difficult-to-diagnose systemic disease. Indeed it has been said that SLE is the "syphilis of the 1980s" in that its clinical presentation may mimic almost any type of disease.

PERIARTERITIS NODOSA

By Austin J. Corbett, M.D.
and Daniel E. Furst, M.D.
Iowa City, Iowa

In 1755 Michaelis and Matanni published a paper describing the lesions of diffuse vasculitis. In 1866 Kussmaul and Maier described what is now considered to be classic periarteritis nodosa (PAN). Since then many attempts have been made to classify systemic vasculitis in a consistent and understandable way.

CLASSIFICATION

Frequently, classification has been based on a histologic picture, with syndromes being defined by the size of vessels involved, the presence or absence of vascular necrosis, the type of inflammatory infiltrate in the vessel walls, the location and distribution of the vascular lesions, or other histologic features. The classic definition of PAN is that of a segmental, necrotizing vasculitis involving small- and medium-sized muscular arteries, with distal spread to involve arterioles and even, occasionally, adjacent veins. Vascular lesions in all stages of development are found with (1) acute polymorphonuclear infiltrates throughout all layers of the vascular walls in earlier lesions, followed later by mononuclear infiltrates, and (2) vascular wall degeneration, fibrinoid necrosis, thrombosis, and intimal proliferation. Histologic findings vary, depending on the age and severity of the lesion.

In general, pulmonary and splenic effects are not considered characteristic of PAN, but they *are* sometimes seen, often in association with peripheral eosinophilia. When pulmonary involvement occurs in conjunction with a granulomatous component in the vessels on biopsy and the patient has a history of extrinsic asthma or allergy, the diagnosis of *Churg-Strauss syndrome* or *allergic granulomatosis* may be used. Eosinophilia is a marker for the *overlap syndrome* or *systemic necrotizing vasculitis* type of PAN, and usually occurs in several "PAN-like" syndromes, which are also characterized by smaller vessel involvement, such as: vasculitis as a consequence of trichinosis; vasculitis in association with the hypereosinophilic syndrome; and vasculitis after hyposensitization therapy for atopic respiratory disease. Thus, eosinophilia and small vessel involvement are features common to several distinct clinical syndromes whose essential "overlapping" characteristic is vasculitis. Smaller vessel involvement is also noted in *hypersensitivity angiitis,* first described by Rich in 1942, in association with serum sickness and sulfonamide hypersensitivity. McCombs and others have hypothesized that exposure to an antigenic or infectious agent (such as hepatitis B virus) must be involved in most cases of vasculitis, regardless of the size of the vessels involved, but this formulation remains only an hypothesis.

In adults, then, PAN might be classified into three general categories: (1) classic PAN; (2) allergic granulomatosis (Churg-Strauss syndrome); and (3) overlap syndrome or systemic necrotizing vasculitis. The term *hypersensitivity angiitis* is used to designate a histologic picture dominated by small vessel inflammation, with the histologic lesions all of the same age. These findings are characteristic of several clinical syndromes, either idiopathic or associated with a known toxic exposure. Not surprisingly, this histologic picture can and often does present the clinical features of classic PAN.

Febrile mucocutaneous lymph node syndrome (also called *infantile periarteritis nodosa* or *Kawasaki's disease*) is histologically quite similar to adult PAN. It occurs in children, has a predilection for coronary arteries, and in most cases exhibits less vascular necrosis than classic PAN. Clinically, the disease has a better prognosis.

These two exceptions to our categorization of PAN (hypersensitivity angiitis and Kawasaki's disease) point out that the classification of PAN is not yet completely satisfactory.

PATHOGENESIS

The pathogenesis of PAN, as for most vasculitic syndromes, is believed to be closely associated with immune complex deposition. Antigen combines with antibody either intravascularly or after deposition of antigen in vessel walls, and the resulting immune complexes fix complement and activate the complement cascade. The resulting chemotaxis of polymorphonuclear cells and lymphocytes produces endothelial injury and eventual activation of the clotting cascade and platelet aggregation. This, in turn, results in vascular necrosis, thrombosis, and eventual fibrosis. In support of this theory is the finding that concentrations of immune complexes rise and fall concomitantly with disease activity; further, immune complexes are sometimes found in high percentages of patients during time of disease activity (93 per cent in one study). Hepatitis B surface antigen–associated PAN is thought to result from just such a mechanism.

An alternative hypothesis postulates the deposition of antigen (e.g., virus) in blood vessel walls and tissues. The secondary formation of immune complexes results in damage to the vessels as innocent bystanders.

The eosinophil may play a role in some patients with PAN. This statement stems from the observation in the hypereosinophilic syndrome (HES) that substances released from the eosinophil (and found in high concentrations in sera of HES patients) can be toxic to vascular endothelium and are thrombogenic. Thus, the eosinophil could possibly be involved in pathogenesis of that subset of PAN associated with hypereosinophilia and small vessel vasculitis—i.e., systemic necrotizing vasculitis.

CLINICAL FEATURES

As would be expected from the histopathology and pathogenesis just outlined, periarteritis can present in any one of a large variety of ways. Indeed, multisystem involvement is typical of PAN and should suggest the diagnosis when typical features are pres-

In memoriam to Carl M. Pearson, M.D.

Table 1. Clinical Signs and Symptoms Plus Selected Laboratory Findings in Periarteritis Nodosa

	Overall Incidence (%)*	Initial Findings (%)†
Constitutional		71
Fever	75	
Weight loss, malaise	67	
Skin		58
Purpura	33	
Rash	28	
Subcutaneous nodules	16	
Urticaria	3	
Neurologic		55
Peripheral neuropathy (including mononeuritis multiplex)	50	
Central nervous system (including confusion, visual loss, aphasia subarachnoid hemorrhage)	11	
Cardiovascular		28
Edema or ascites	33	
Congestive heart failure	12	
Myocarditis	3	
Phlebitis	6	
ECG abnormalities or cardiomegaly on x-ray	50	
Gastrointestinal		40
Abdominal pain and diarrhea	65	
Bleeding or abdominal catastrophe	12	
Hepatomegaly	50	
Renal		8
Proteinuria, hematuria	66	
Azotemia (⩾ 40 BUN)	24	
Hypertension	36	
Musculoskeletal		55
Arthralgias or arthritis	66	
Muscular pain and weakness	26	
Laboratory		
Anemia	67	
Elevated ESR	89	
Leukocytosis	54	
HBsAg	20–50	
Lung		38
Asthma	13	
Pneumonia or pleurisy	33	
Eosinophilia	31	

* From 377 cases in four literature series.
†From a study of 130 patients.
Abbreviations: BUN = Blood urea nitrogen; ESR = erythrocyte sedimentation rate; HBsAg = hepatitis B surface antigen.

ent. Table 1 gives a general view of the incidence and type of organ involvement. The first column details overall involvement in four series of patients, while the second column presents the frequency of organ involvement at initial presentation from a study of 130 patients. It is clear from the table that nearly any organ may be involved at any point in the course of PAN.

Without obtaining tissue or angiographic evidence of the typical vascular abnormalities, the unequivocal diagnosis of PAN is extremely difficult. Nonetheless, there are some features which, although infrequent, are very helpful diagnostically when they do occur. Thus, the presence of mononeuritis multiplex (without diabetes or other conditions) is highly suggestive. Tender subcutaneous nodules suggest PAN and in addition offer accessible lesions for biopsy. Myocardial infarction in a young man or sudden renal failure and progressive hypertension in a middle-aged man should also suggest the possibility of PAN.

Systemic Manifestations

Constitutional symptoms are a frequent clue to diagnosis. The fever found in PAN has no characteristic pattern, although fever is commonly present at some point in the disease. Weight loss and malaise are among the most common presenting symptoms and may be out of proportion to the rest of the clinical picture.

Skin Lesions

Nonspecific skin lesions are present more frequently than the classic nodules of PAN and include petechiae, purpura, skin ulcers, urticaria, and nonspecific maculopapular eruptions. In aggregate they occur in up to 58 per cent of patients.

Neurologic Manifestations

Neurologic involvement produces both central and peripheral nervous system signs and symptoms. Involvement of the central nervous system may be nonspecific, ranging from confusion, disorientation, and delirium to blurred vision, transient blindness, hemiplegia, convulsions, and subarachnoid bleeding. Distal sensory or sensorimotor neuropathy is more frequent, although less distinctive, than mononeuritis multiplex, and occurs about 50 per cent of the time.

Cardiovascular Manifestations

Cardiovascular signs and symptoms (excluding hypertension, which will be mentioned under renal disease) are also frequent (up to 50 per cent), although they may be as nonspecific as disproportionate tachycardia. Symptoms include those associated with congestive heart failure, myocarditis, or even myocardial infarction. Cardiomegaly may be seen on chest x-ray, while electrocardiographic signs can include nonspecific ST-T wave changes, arrhythmias, or heart block.

Gastrointestinal Manifestations

Gastrointestinal manifestations range from nonspecific abdominal pain and diarrhea to massive gastrointestinal or hepatic infarction. Occasionally, PAN may present with localized involvement of one visceral organ, such as the gallbladder or appendix, without major systemic manifestations. Usually, however, gastrointestinal involvement is ominous and may be catastrophic. Bowel infarction, gastrointestinal ulceration, and hemorrhagic infarction of the pancreas are characteristic, although unusual (12 per cent of patients). Abnormal liver function tests range in frequency from 5 to 40 per cent in different series and may be associated with hepatomegaly and jaundice, but they are no more frequent when hepatitis B surface antigen is present than when it is absent. Approximately half of reported massive liver infarctions are due to PAN. Rheumatoid factor and cryoglobulinemia are more frequent in patients with mesenteric arteritis, and rheumatoid factor seroconversion may occur with the onset of the abdominal vasculitis.

Urinary Manifestations

Abnormal urinary findings are extremely common. Proteinuria and hematuria are present at some time in the disease course in 60 to 70 per cent of patients. Glomerulonephritis is the most frequent pathologic finding (in up to 30 per cent of patients), and renal arteritis is occasionally seen on biopsy. Azotemia is usually a late finding and implies a poor prognosis. Hypertension was the initial finding in 25 per cent of patients in one series and in young males should alert the physician to possible PAN. Although hypertension does not correlate with urinary sediment abnormalities, it frequently correlates with renal ischemia, hyperreninemia, and secondary hyperaldosteronism. Metabolic abnormalities associated with hyperaldosteronism should be expected and have been described. These patients typically respond dramatically to small doses of captopril. Recently treatment, particularly with cytotoxic drugs, has been shown to reverse both accelerated hypertension and renal dysfunction.

Musculoskeletal Manifestations

Musculoskeletal symptoms, most commonly arthralgias and myalgias, are present in about 60 per cent of patients. They tend to be transient and migratory, but may be very severe. Frank arthritis, with objective swelling and tenderness, has been reported in 8 to 27 per cent of patients and may affect any joints in a symmetric or asymmetric pattern. Most commonly the arthritis is of short duration and affects large joints such as the knees and wrists. Muscular atrophy, tenderness, or weakness on physical examination occurs in 20 to 30 per cent of patients.

Pulmonary Manifestations

As mentioned earlier, pulmonary involvement is not characteristic of classic PAN, but it may be present in the subtype with peripheral eosinophilia. This subtype includes patients with asthma (13 per cent), pneumonia, pleurisy, hemoptysis, and dyspnea. X-rays are nonspecific, and pulmonary function tests can show either obstructive or restrictive disease.

The great variety of clinical signs and symptoms associated with PAN emphasizes the need to consider the diagnosis in any patient with an unexplained multisystem disorder, particularly when associated with fever, malaise, or weight loss; with mononeuritis multiplex; or with unexpected or unexplained hypertension or renal failure.

LABORATORY FINDINGS

The erythrocyte sedimentation rate (ESR) is elevated in approximately 90 per cent of patients; for one series of 124 patients the average ESR was 75 mm/hour. Leukocytosis (greater than 10,000 per cu mm) occurs in over 50 per cent of patients and anemia is common. The significance of eosinophilia, occurring in up to 30 per cent of patients with pulmonary involvement, has been mentioned.

Serologic abnormalities may be seen but cannot be considered characteristic of PAN per se. Positive rheumatoid factor (RF) or antinuclear antibodies (ANA) are most often seen in patients who also have rheumatoid arthritis, systemic lupus erythematosus, or liver disease. The significance of rheumatoid factor seroconversion was already mentioned with respect to abdominal vasculitis. The hepatitis B surface antigen (HBsAg) has been detected in 20 to 50 per cent of patients with PAN, although its presence does not correlate with active vasculitis. The actual risk of developing PAN in the presence of the hepatitis B surface antigen is not known. In a recent study in a population of dialysis patients, 3 of 266 HBsAg carriers had PAN, whereas none of 384 HBsAg-negative patients had the disease. Most of the 266 HBsAg-positive carriers had immune complexes but no vasculitis, suggesting an individual susceptibility in those patients who do develop PAN. Immune complex concentrations tend to correlate with disease activity, although their clinical usefulness is *not* well established. The incidence of immune complexes is high (in up to 93 per cent of patients) when determined using polyethylene glycol precipitation, but usually a negative result is obtained with C1q or Raji cell assays. Thus, the physical characteristics of the immune complexes may determine their pathogenicity.

The frequency of abnormal findings in the renal sediment has been noted, but it should be added that red and white cell casts, indicative of glomerulonephritis, can be seen in one third of patients.

DIAGNOSIS

As already noted, given the protean clinical manifestations of PAN and the generally nonspecific nature of the laboratory findings, the diagnosis may be extremely difficult to make.

Definitive diagnosis of PAN usually relies on biopsy of the involved tissues or organs. Occasionally, multiple biopsies of various tissues are negative and patients with negative biopsies but characteristic findings of PAN by angiography have been included in recent series.

Angiography

The angiographic features of polyarteritis have been known for many years. Recently the use of abdominal arteriography (usually including the renal, hepatic, and mesenteric circulations) yielded evidence of definite, multiple aneurysm formation in 60 per cent of biopsy-proven cases. The presence of these abnormalities did not correlate with evidence of clinical involvement of a particular organ system. Nor are the angiographic findings absolutely specific for PAN, since they may be seen in Wegener's granulomatosis, systemic lupus erythematosus (SLE), thrombotic thrombocytopenic purpura (TTP), atrial myxoma, and hypernephroma. Finally, regression or persistence of arteriographic lesions need not correlate with clinical course, so that the prognostic significance of a positive test is not known.

Biopsy

It is important, when searching for histopathologic evidence of PAN, to biopsy clinically involved tissues and organs. In general, only 20 to 30 per cent of antemortem biopsies, unless taken from clinically involved tissue, will be diagnostic. Only 13 to 32 per cent of blind muscle biopsies are positive in the absence of localized symptoms, and only 22 per cent of blind testicular needle biopsies can be expected to be positive. If biopsies of nonspecific rashes are performed, they must be at least deep enough (deep dermis and panniculus) to obtain specimens of muscular arteries or arterioles. Many organs (e.g., kidneys, sural nerve, or superficial skin) often reveal only nonspecific nondiagnostic changes when biopsy is done without localizing signs or symptoms.

Biopsy of skin lesions may yield typical findings of PAN. However, PAN may be limited to the skin in some patients, in whom the longterm prognosis is excellent (see below). The finding of typical vascular immune deposits in the skin (in the absence of characteristic changes by light microscopy) may suggest the diagnosis of PAN, but the *exact* diagnostic predictive value of this finding is not known.

Although the usual considerations relating to ruling out infection, malignancies, allergic reactions, and other connective tissue diseases must be heeded, particular attention with respect to PAN should be paid to patients with (1) unexplained prominent fever, weight loss, and myalgias with elevated ESR, particularly those who are in their 40s and 50s and are male; (2) unexplained multisystem disease, particularly involving the central nervous system, peripheral nerves, or kidneys, or associated with abdominal catastrophes; (3) myocardial infarction or disease in the young; or (4) unexplained sudden onset of hypertension and renal failure, particularly in middle-aged males.

Kawasaki's Disease

Kawasaki's disease, or febrile mucocutaneous lymph node syndrome, was first described in 1967 and is now thought to be identical with infantile periarteritis nodosa. The disease seems to be much more prevalent in Japan than in the United States. Characteristic symptoms include fever (95 per cent); bilateral conjunctival congestion (90 per cent); peripheral edema (75 per cent) followed by erythema of the palms and soles (90 per cent); desquamation of the finger tips (95 per cent); red, dry, fissured lips (90 per cent) associated with stawberry-like swelling of the tongue papillae (80 per cent); diffuse reddening of the oral and periungual mucosa (90 per cent); a vesicular or crusting truncal rash (90 per cent); and cervical adenopathy of 1.5 cm or more in diameter (75 per cent). Nonspecific ECG abnormalities are found in the majority of patients, and coronary angiography reveals aneurysms in 20 per cent. High resolution echocardiography is an acceptable way of screening for cardiac involvement if it is performed sequentially (during the acute attack and in later stages of the illness). The usual cause of death in this disease is coronary thrombosis, but the mortality rate is less than 2 per cent. Histologically, the coronary arteries are involved segmentally with a panarteritis, associated with fibrinoid necrosis in some cases.

COURSE AND PROGNOSIS

In adults the prognosis of PAN has changed over the years. In 1938, the 1-year survival rate in a study of 152 patients was 13 per cent, most patients dying of renal failure. By 1967, with the use of corticosteroids alone, the 5-year survival was 50 to 60 per cent in most series. Several recent series, which have included patients treated with combined steroids and immunosuppressive agents, have reported a similar 5-year survival rate. There are data to suggest, however, that aggressive early treatment of severe disease with steroids and immunosuppressive drugs, cyclophosphamide in particular, may result in a significantly improved rate of survival (up to 80 per cent survival at 5 years). The highest mortality rate occurs in the first 3 to 6 months, with the presence of significant renal disease being the poorest prognostic sign. The presence of hypertension has not been shown to correlate with a poorer prognosis in several series, unless it was associated with clinical renal involvement. After 6 months, death from infection, unrelated disease, or drug-related disease is more frequent than death from vasculitis.

A unique subset of patients with PAN are those who initially present with only skin involvement, often associated with arthritis and occasionally with peripheral neuropathy. The prognosis is often excellent, despite evidence of medium-sized muscular artery involvement on skin biopsy. The use of high doses of steroids and immunosuppressive agents should not be automatic in these patients, and their treatment should be individualized based on the clinical course.

SCLERODERMA

By M. Bashar Kahaleh, M.D.
and E. Carwile LeRoy, M.D.
Charleston, South Carolina

SYNONYMS AND SUBSETS

Systemic sclerosis (progressive systemic sclerosis, PSS):

1. Diffuse, generalized.
2. CREST syndrome (calcinosis, Raynaud's phenomenon, esophageal hypomotility, sclerodactyly, telangiectasis).
3. Overlap syndromes, including sclerodermatomyositis, undifferentiated connective tissue syndromes, and scleroderma features associated with classic lupus erythematosus or rheumatoid arthritis.

Localized or cutaneous forms:

1. Morphea, including plaque-like, guttate, nodular, symmetric, and generalized.
2. Linear scleroderma, including scleroderma en coup de sabre with or without facial hemiatrophy.

DEFINITION

Scleroderma is a multisystem disease of unknown cause characterized by inflammatory, vascular, and fibrotic changes in the skin and certain internal organs, notably the gastrointestinal tract, lungs, heart, and kidneys. In its advanced form, scleroderma is one of the most easily recognized of rheumatic syndromes. However, early in its course scleroderma is most difficult to diagnose. The difficulty lies in the fact that the disorder evolves in unpredictable, multiple stages, and the clinical expression of each stage varies in a spectrum of severity from mild and slowly progressing to severe and rapidly evolving disease.

Early stages consist of vascular instability (Raynaud's phenomenon) followed after months to years by a puffy, edematous stage, which in turn evolves into a fibrotic stage. This cycle recurs in various sites at different intervals; thus, a patient may have hidebound skin on the hands and puffy skin on the forearms. As a result, a number of fundamental problems arise in terms of early diagnosis, differential diagnosis, assessment of disease activity and prognosis, evaluation of therapy, and validity of interseries comparisons. It is crucial to consider each stage of scleroderma separately with regard to the particular system suspected of being involved. Taut skin proximal to the metacarpophalangeal joints has been identified by an American Rheumatism Association (ARA) cooperative study to be the major diagnostic criterion for scleroderma. The same study identified sclerodactyly, digital pitting scars, and bilateral basilar pulmonary fibrosis on chest roentgenograms as minor criteria. Presence of the major criterion or of two or more minor criteria documents the diagnosis of scleroderma. In actual practice, many features precede the appearance of fibrosis, which, if recognized, offer the promise of earlier detection and possible therapeutic control. Attempts at defining subgroups of patients with scleroderma (e.g., those with CREST syndrome and acrosclerosis) for purposes of prognosis have not been entirely satisfactory. Also, the belief that the disorder is progressive (i.e., progressive systemic sclerosis) does not take into account those patients whose cutaneous involvement remains stable or improves spontaneously. Localized forms of scleroderma (morphea, linear scleroderma, en coup de sabre, and so forth) should be considered separately, since almost without exception they are not associated with visceral disease.

EARLY SIGNS AND SYMPTOMS

In the majority of patients, the disease starts with Raynaud's phenomenon months to years before hidebound skin changes or visceral involvement make the diagnosis of scleroderma obvious.

Raynaud's phenomenon defines an episodic constriction of the small arteries and arterioles of the fingers, toes, and occasionally the face in response to cold or emotional stimuli. The episodes are characterized by triphasic segmental color changes consisting of pallor, cyanosis, and rubor. One or more of these color changes may be observed in individual patients. Numbness and stiffness are usually present during the phases of pallor and cyanosis; pain and tingling are often experienced during the phase of rubor. On examination, the fingers may be abnormally cool (if the process has been particularly severe or prolonged) and there may be ulceration at the tips of digits or scars of healed ulcerations. At times, this may be manifested as flattening or concavity of the distal finger pulp. There may also be loss of hair over the proximal phalanx or tautness of the skin over the distal fingers dorsally (sclerodactyly). The toes and occasionally the nose or ears may be similarly involved.

The major challenge to each physician who cares for patients with Raynaud's phenomenon is to select those destined to develop scleroderma, systemic lupus erythematosus, or other connective tissue disorder. This must be done with minimum risk, cost, and alarm to the patient. By using the earliest and most sensitive detectors available, at times it is possible to detect organ damage and support function before the patient's life or quality of life is threatened.

Detection of the earliest stages of scleroderma in patients begins with the recognition of Raynaud's phenomenon and puffy hands; patients may also note fatigue and a lack of energy. The puffy hand syndrome can be seen as an early feature not only of scleroderma but also of systemic lupus erythematosus, dermatopolymyositis, and rheumatoid arthritis. All patients with puffy hands should be designated as having undifferentiated disease until such time as their condition evolves into a classic rheumatic syndrome. The presence of antibodies to double-stranded DNA or to Sm antigens favors systemic lupus erythematosus, whereas erosive arthritis favors rheumatoid arthritis. At present, the most promising pre-scleroderma features in the early setting are morphologic and flow abnormalities of the cutaneous microvascular bed and the presence of anticentromere antibodies (see Table 2 in the article on SLE).

Morphologic studies of nailfold capillaries with wide-field capillary microscopy led to the recognition of scleroderma-specific capillary changes, consisting of enlargement of capillary loops, loss of capillaries, and disruption of the orderly appearance of normal capillary beds. In a prospective study of Raynaud's phenomenon, capillary changes, as well as serum antinuclear antibodies, were found to be associated with future development of connective tissue disease, particularly scleroderma.

CLINICAL FEATURES

Commonly seen features of scleroderma include flexion contractures of hands; loss of normal skin wrinkles; development of immobile, expressionless facies with decrease in the maximal oral aperture; skin hyperpigmentation, often stippled, with spotty or patchy depigmentation giving rise to a salt-and-pepper appearance; telangiectasia chiefly on fingers, palms, lips, and face; painful skin ulcerations, particularly over bony eminences, often secondarily infected chiefly by staphylococci; subcutaneous calcifications on finger tips, extensor surface of forearms, olecranon bursa, and prepatellar area.

Systemic involvement is critical to prognosis, but it can be subtle in its presentation. Esophageal hypomotility is the most common visceral manifestation. It is often asymptomatic, but can be suspected if the patient has a feeling of tightness under the sternum after eating or, occasionally, if a person chokes on a pill, a piece of meat, or cold liquid. The documentation of esophageal hypomotility by barium swallow, or more sensitively by esophageal manometrics, supports the early diagnosis of scleroderma. If esophageal involvement is found, the small and large bowel should be evaluated for dilatation, sacculations, and malabsorption.

Cardiopulmonary involvement may be subtle and relatively far advanced before it is recognized clinically. Mild pitting edema of the legs, slight loss of stamina, and mild degrees of shortness of breath should be evaluated by careful physical examination to detect dry rales at the lung bases and signs of pulmonary hypertension (increased P_2 and a fixed A_2–P_2 interval) (see article on Pulmonary Hypertension). Pulmonary function tests of diffusion capacity should be carried out on all patients, even those who are asymptomatic and whose chest-x-rays are unremarkable. Electrocardiography and echocardiography are helpful for cardiac evaluation. The echocardiogram is particularly useful in detecting pericardial effusion and possibly pulmonary hypertension, two of the most common cardiopulmonary abnormalities of scleroderma. Pulmonary hypertension can be missed even by experienced echocardiographers.

Renal involvement is the most common cause of death in scleroderma; unfortunately, it may be sudden in onset, with the occurrence of headache, blurred vision, hypertension with retinopathy and papilledema, oliguria, and sudden death. In actuality, the arterial proliferative lesion probably progresses in the kidney, as in the other affected organs, at a more or less constant pace throughout the course of the disease. The sudden shutdown of renal cortical blood flow, precipitated by a complex interaction of structural vascular disease, intravascular coagulation, and vasoconstriction with vessel damage via the renin-angiotensin pathway, ushers in the final events of renal scleroderma. It is important to identify patients with scleroderma who are suspected of developing renal involvement. At present, the best method for this identification is to monitor all patients with scleroderma for proteinuria, azotemia, a change in baseline blood pressure levels, microangiopathic hemolytic anemia, para-aminohippurate (PAH) clearance, and hyperreninemia. The appearance of any of these features should lead to more intensive evaluation of renal blood flow by isotopic clearance, angiography, or renal biopsy. Patients should be shown how to take their own blood pressure measurements and take them daily. The stakes are high, because patients who would have died are alive and functional through renal support and aggressive antihypertensive therapy.

DIFFERENTIAL DIAGNOSIS

The differential diagnosis of scleroderma includes scleredema; eosinophilic fasciitis; scleromyxedema; carcinoid syndrome; reflex dystrophy, such as shoulder-hand syndrome; porphyria cutanea tarda; amyloidosis; and vinyl chloride-, pentazocine-, and bleomycin-induced fibrosis. These rare conditions may mimic sclerodermal skin disease but are distinguished by the lack of the classic sclerodermal visceral involvement and by characteristic clinical features of their own. Because of their rare occurrence, they will not be discussed in detail.

COURSE AND PROGNOSIS

Individual patients with scleroderma show a wide variety of organ involvement and variable rate of progression. Prognosis depends on the degree of renal, lung, heart, and bowel involvement. It is important to emphasize to patients the fact that prior to specific visceral involvement, skin and musculoskeletal scleroderma of themselves do not affect life expectancy. In patients with long-standing cutaneous scleroderma, the dense hidebound skin changes have been noted to improve spontaneously. On the other hand, patients with Raynaud's syndrome and limited skin involvement have been observed to develop oliguric renal failure. The proper role for physicians treating patients with scleroderma is to encourage patients, detect organ involvement, treat symptoms as they occur, and reassure patients that the disease may stop at any stage.

Section Eighteen

DISORDERS OF GROWTH AND DEVELOPMENT

FAILURE TO THRIVE

By Pasquale Accardo, M.D.
St. Louis, Missouri

SYNONYMS

Failure to thrive, organic failure to thrive, nonorganic failure to thrive, reactive attachment disorder of infancy, maternal deprivation, psychosocial dwarfism of early childhood, reversible hyposomatotropic dwarfism, severe malnutrition, marasmus, marasmic kwashiorkor, and kwashiorkor.

DEFINITION

There are three essential components to the syndrome of failure to thrive: (1) growth failure, (2) perception of illness, and (3) absence of obvious cause.

Growth Failure

With regard to growth failure, there are no universally recognized criteria. A weight (in younger infants) or a height (in older children) persistently below the third percentile (2 standard deviations [SD] below the mean) for age, a weight less than 80 per cent of the ideal weight for age, and failure to maintain a previously established growth pattern are several possible criteria for growth failure. The crossing of percentile curves by 2 SD is probably the only absolute indicator of growth failure; the child who is small but gaining steadily, following his own growth curve, and developing normally should not be considered as failing to thrive. If weight for height, skinfold thickness, and other growth indicators are taken into account, constitutional short stature and slow growth secondary to intrauterine growth retardation will not be found in the list of final diagnoses for failure to thrive. From a diagnostic perspective, the onset of weight gain in the hospital is an unreliable point by which to discriminate organic from nonorganic failure to thrive, but when a child presents with height, weight, and head circumference all below the third percentile, there is an increased probability of an organic cause. Finally, for the growth failure to be compatible with failure to thrive, it must be persistent rather than acute; in infants up to 5 months old, a duration of 56 days has been suggested, and in infants over 5 months, a duration of 90 days has been suggested.

Perception of Illness

An incidence of almost 10 per cent of growth failure to some degree in a primary care setting has been used to suggest that much growth delay follows a generally benign course. A "perception of illness" criterion (to a degree subjective) is needed to distinguish failure to thrive from this type of benign growth delay: failure to thrive is growth failure about which the physician is concerned. The suspicion of illness that a particular case of growth failure raises for the experienced clinician is not necessarily one relating exclusively to organic disorders. The concern is that if this growth failure continues untreated, the child's general health and well-being will be compromised.

Absence of Obvious Cause

The single criterion contributing most to the vagueness of the syndrome is the fact that the reason for the growth failure is not immediately apparent to the attending physician after a careful history and physical examination. Some of the rarest causes of growth failure will be immediately apparent to a specific physician, whereas a less esoteric cause will lead another practitioner to seek hospitalization and consultation. Indeed, many of the retrospective studies from tertiary care centers obviously relied on the least experienced physician (house staff in training) to make the initial classification. Inexact terminology contributes further to the confusion: even after an evident factor has been documented to cause the growth failure, the final diagnosis not infrequently reads "failure to thrive secondary to . . . " rather than "growth failure associated with/secondary to. . . . " This distinction applies equally well to obvious nonorganic causes; the infant or young child exhibiting growth failure on a deprivational basis can sometimes be classified immediately as having "reactive attachment disorder of infancy" or "psychosocial dwarfism" without first being considered as "failing to thrive." It must be remembered that failure to thrive is not a diagnosis but a presenting symptom, an initial impression. Although some degree of growth failure is a sine qua non of the syndrome, both a perception of illness on the part of the examining physician and the absence of an obvious cause are also required. Epidemiologic data are not available, but failure to thrive represents approximately 5 per cent of admissions to pediatric in-patient hospital ward services.

Failure to thrive is usually divided into two major etiologic categories: organic and nonorganic.

Organic Type

In the organic type the growth failure results from some occult underlying pathologic process involving a particular organ system in the child. In the nonorganic type the growth failure is secondary to emotional factors and reflects a disorder of bonding between the infant and the mother. Although this distinction is an important first step, it is not always rewarding to force each child having failure to thrive into a particular diagnostic category. Many cases of failure to thrive have multiple precipitating factors. For example, prior to the development of gastroenteritis, infants with low body weights are more susceptible to a disaccharide intolerance. Again, since malnutrition impairs the body's ability to respond to infection, marginal undernutrition with a supervening infection may progress to overt malnutrition. This interaction between causal factors need not be restricted to disorders with organic causes. The identification of an organic disease causing growth failure does not rule out a nonorganic component to the failure to thrive. The potential contribution of maternal intelligence, social stresses, prematurity, early separation of infant and mother, and physical deformity to a mother's reaction to a baby with an organic condition causing growth failure needs to be assessed. Similarly, multiple psychosocial factors might combine to produce nonorganic failure to thrive. The evaluation of such complex, multifaceted interactions can benefit from a team approach.

Nonorganic Type

In the third edition of its Diagnostic and Statistical Manual (DSM-III), the American Psychiatric Association describes what pediatricians would categorize as nonorganic failure to thrive under the diagnosis "reactive attachment disorder of infancy" (Table 1). This nosology stresses the fact that this type of failure to thrive often is less the child's problem than the parent's. In this perspective, failure to thrive is viewed as a disorder of parenting, a failure of bonding. The older term maternal deprivation lacks precision and is best discarded. Psychosocial dwarfism is synonymous with reversible hyposomatotropinism. It is a condition of growth failure that occurs in children above the DSM-III age cut-off for reactive attachment disorder (8 months) and is marked by bizarre behavior, measurable endocrine changes that have been caused by prolonged emotional deprivation, and a striking lack of growth in height. When weight for age is below 80 per cent of the expected value the child is undernourished; when weight drops below 60 per cent of the expected value a state of marasmus exists.

Table 1. Diagnostic Criteria for Reactive Attachment Disorder of Infancy*

A. Age at onset less than 8 months.

B. Lack of the type of care that ordinarily leads to the development of affectional bonds to others, e.g., gross emotional neglect, imposed social isolation in an institution.

C. Lack of developmentally appropriate signs of social responsivity, as indicated by at least several of the following (the total number of behaviors looked for will depend on the chronological age of the child, corrected for prematurity):
   1. Lack of visual tracking of eyes and faces by an infant more than 2 months of age.
   2. Lack of smiling in response to faces by an infant more than 2 months of age.
   3. Lack of visual reciprocity in an infant of more than 2 months; lack of vocal reciprocity with caregiver in an infant of more than 5 months.
   4. Lack of alerting to and turning toward caregiver's voice by an infant of more than 4 months.
   5. Lack of spontaneous reaching for the mother by an infant of more than 4 months.
   6. Lack of anticipatory reaching when approached to be picked up by an infant more than 5 months of age.
   7. Lack of participation in playful games with caregiver by an infant of more than 5 months.

D. At least three of the following
   1. Weak cry.
   2. Excessive sleep.
   3. Lack of interest in the environment.
   4. Hypomotility.
   5. Poor muscle tone.
   6. Weak rooting and grasping in response to feeding attempts.

E. Weight loss or failure to gain appropriate amount of weight for age unexplainable by any physical disorder. In these cases usually the failure to gain weight (falling weight percentile) is disproportionately greater than failure to gain length; head circumference is normal.

F. Absence of physical disorder, mental retardation, or infantile autism.

G. The diagnosis is confirmed if the clinical picture is reversed shortly after institution of adequate caregiving, which frequently includes short-term hospitalization.

*Modified from the *Diagnostic and Statistical Manual*, 3rd ed. (DSM-III), 313.89, American Psychiatric Association, 1980.

Kwashiorkor (weight below 80 per cent of expected) and marasmic kwashiorkor (weight below 60 per cent of expected) result from a disproportional deficiency of protein reflected in the clinical finding of edema. Marasmus, marasmic kwashiorkor, and kwashiorkor are rarely encountered in developed countries.

CLINICAL MANIFESTATIONS AND COURSE

Clinical findings in failure to thrive relate to three distinct areas:

1. Signs of malnutrition.
2. Markers for specific etiologic diagnoses.
3. Secondary behavioral manifestations.

Malnutrition

In infancy, if malnutrition persists over time, weight is affected first, length next, and head circumference last. Height will be affected more than weight in endocrine disorders and constitutional short stature, but there is a proportional reduction of both height and weight in growth disturbances secondary to primordial dwarfism or severe central nervous system lesions. Signs of malnutrition are presented in Table 2. The possibility of recovery of weight, height, and head circumference depends on the underlying cause as well as the duration of the untreated state.

Diagnostic Indicators

Failure to thrive in infancy and early childhood can be caused by a variety of developmental anomalies, organic disease, and environmental disorders. An exhaustive differential diagnosis would include almost every item indexed in a standard encyclopedic pediatric text. Since, by definition, the cause of the growth failure is not immediately apparent even to the experienced clinician and may require an in-patient diagnostic evaluation and feeding trial, the signs indicating specific etiologic factors will be fairly subtle (also as implied by the definition) and open only to a careful and methodic probing of each more general clue, such as feeding history, vomiting, diarrhea, or constipation.

Behavioral Manifestations

Although a number of behavioral signs are directly attributable to malnutrition or to the malaise that accompanies an underlying organic illness, a more extensive behavioral profile exists that characterizes the child with failure to thrive on a nonorganic basis. Psychopathology of this sort does not arise de novo in infants; it needs to be understood as a reaction of the child to a complementary psychological profile that can be observed in the mother (Table 3). Psychosocial dwarfism presents after infancy, usually between the second and sixth year of life, and is best interpreted as nonorganic failure to thrive in the older child although with more severe underlying psychopathology in both the child and the caregiver (Table 4). Whatever the age of onset, the factors that influence the strength of maternal attachment (Table 5) need to be carefully assessed. With the more protracted course of psychosocial dwarfism, the normalization of the behavioral constellation, the reinstitution of growth, and the reversal of the endocrine abnormalities—all of which are required to confirm the diagnosis—may take as many months as the deprivation has persisted in years.

The high prevalence of either mental retardation or other significant neurodevelopmental disabilities, either during the initial failure to thrive evaluation or in the long-term follow-up period, raises the question

Table 2. Signs of Malnutrition

Signs
Physical Signs
Decreased lean body mass/adiposity, decreased skinfold thickness, prominent ribs, "skin and bones"
Hair sparse, thin, dry, lifeless, easily pulled out, dull brown or reddish yellow (kwashiorkor)
Pallor (anemia)—"pastel children"
Excessive perspiration, especially about the head
Face: lined, aged, pinched appearance with sharp features and sunken cheeks (loss of Bichat suctorial fat pads), "fish-mouth face of misery"
Skin: an "old look"—wrinkled, poor turgor, folds hanging on inner thighs and buttocks
Heart murmur (from anemia)
Protuberant abdomen, hepatomegaly, edema ("sugar baby" type)
Disturbed sleep cycle
Abnormal stool pattern (constipation or diarrhea)
Decreased pulse, blood pressure, temperature
Decreased physical activity, mental apathy, hypotonia, tonic immobility
Intercurrent infections with higher morbidity or mortality rate
Laboratory Signs
Low fasting blood sugar
Diabetic-type glucose tolerance test (GTT) curve
Hypoproteinemia: low transferrin and albumin
Low urea nitrogen and creatinine excretion, decreased creatinine to height index
Decreased urinary hydroxyproline and branched-chain amino acids

Table 3. Behavioral Characteristics in Nonorganic Failure to Thrive

Child	Mother
Developmental delay	Poor self-esteem
Apathy, lethargy, withdrawal	Depression
Floppiness or (plastic) rigidity	Anger
Wide-eyed gaze	Anxiety
Difficulty with change in routine	Poor eye contact
Decreased vocalization	Holds child clumsily or facing away from herself
Sad or apprehensive facies	Poor perception of child's needs
Decreased stranger anxiety or indiscriminate affection	Views child as overly demanding
Tactile defensiveness	Demonstrates little affection
Abnormal sleep pattern	Negative perception of mothering or child-rearing role
Irritability and antisocial behavior	
Self-stimulatory behavior	

of whether it is possible to distinguish between brain damage existing prior to (and contributing via multiple pathways to) malnutrition from the various degrees of brain dysfunction resulting from severe malnutrition. Although there are no true "critical periods" in human development, the impact of severe, prolonged malnutrition on the developing infant brain probably reflects a "sensitive period" of increased vulnerability. Early malnutrition does affect brain cell size, number, neurotransmitter production, and myelin deposition. Long-term follow-up studies of individuals with severe malnutrition in developing countries nevertheless support a considerable plasticity and ability of the infant brain to recover from or compensate for the central nervous system effects of prolonged undernutrition.

In addition to the one fifth of cases of organically based failure to thrive with a neurologic cause, a large number of infants malnourished for other reasons also exhibit neurodevelopmental abnormalities that may confuse the diagnosis. On the one hand, transient neurologic findings such as hypotonia ("floppy baby") or hypertonia (in a pattern suggestive of spastic diplegia) are common in infants who are severely malnourished on a nonorganic basis. On the other hand, cerebral palsy with or without oral motor involvement is both difficult to diagnose before the age of 18 months and quite commonly associated with poor physical growth. Similarly for cognition, the child with failure to thrive tends to exhibit psychomotor retardation that responds to refeeding and environmental stimulation, whereas the child with undiagnosed retardation may feed poorly, interact poorly with the mother, and contribute significantly to his own growth failure. When objective measurements are lacking, clinical impressions of developmental progress during realimentation in hospital need to be viewed with skepticism; qualitative improvements in affect and behavior are quite probable during careful refeeding of a retarded infant although there may be little or no change in the developmental quotient. Fully recognizing the limitations under which it must be interpreted, a comprehensive neurodevelopmental assessment should be both performed and repeated after an appropriate interval for all children with failure to thrive.

Table 4. Symptoms of Psychosocial Dwarfism (Reversible Hyposomatotropinism)

Disorders of eating and drinking: polydipsia, polyphagia alternating with meal refusal, drinking from toilet bowls, eating from garbage cans, roaming and foraging
Eccentric sleep patterns
Enuresis and encopresis
Social distancing
Pain agnosia and self-injurious behavior
Delayed puberty
Mental retardation and language delay
Pathogenic family relationships
Neuroendocrine changes: low levels of growth hormone
Behavior and symptom reversal with change in domicile

LABORATORY AND OTHER DIAGNOSTIC TESTS

Approximately 75 per cent of diagnoses are ascertained from the history and 25 per cent from the physical examination, with laboratory tests being used as

Table 5. Factors Associated with a Weak Bond of Maternal Attachment

Previous Experience of the Mother (Caregiver)
Early parental life deprivations
Loss of parent figures early in life of parent
Illness during childhood
Death or illness in prior children
Pregnancy
Emotional or physical illness
Death or major illness of key family figures
Other loss of significant relationships
Perinatal Events
Complications of delivery causing prolonged separation of mother and child
Acute illness in mother or infant
Prematurity
Congenital defects
Other diseases and disturbances
Current Life Events
Marital stress
Mental or medical illness causing caregiver to be unavailable
Drugs and alcohol
Financial crisis

needed to confirm these diagnoses or monitor treatment. Despite an average of more than a dozen laboratory tests per patient, when the history and physical examination do not furnish a lead, the test results are consistently unhelpful. Suppose test X diagnoses disease Y, and the history and physical examination do not suggest disease Y. In such a case a 0 per cent incidence of X positives in a given number of cases says very little about the usefulness of test X unless the atypical presentation of disease Y has an occurrence rate of at least the same magnitude. For example, some series of failure to thrive cases may have a 0 per cent incidence of cystic fibrosis or hypothyroidism; the absence of these diagnoses from a biased sample of 100 to 200 cases of growth failure does not exclude them from clinical consideration. Although uncommon presentations of common diseases are more frequent than common presentations of uncommon diseases as causes, to a certain extent all failure to thrive cases are uncommon.

There is no "routine work-up" for failure to thrive, and it is not the purpose of this section to propose one. History, physical findings, and neurologic and developmental assessments should take precedence over laboratory tests. Noninvasive procedures should be completed before pursuing more invasive tests (Table 6). The detailed pediatric history needs to stress feeding, development, and previous and familial growth patterns, as well as a careful review of systems for signs of rare syndromes or unusual presentations. Although the importance of a detailed history cannot be overemphasized, it is also true that many parents of children with failure to thrive tend to be poor historians. A lack of health care continuity frequently makes the obtaining of old medical records difficult and unrewarding. An adequate history should prevent patients with simple feeding problems and constitutional short stature from being admitted to hospital for evaluation. A small percentage of infants, whether breast-fed or bottle-fed, will not cry as an indication that they are being underfed. Height, weight, and head circumference need to be plotted and compared with one another with regard to both percentiles and mean age (the age for which a particular measurement is at the fiftieth percentile). The pattern generated by these plots when they correlate past, present, and follow-up growth data with life history events, onset of clinical signs, and response to different therapeutic interventions will be the single most important contribution to achieving a diagnosis. Low birth weight (with the baby being small for gestational age [SGA]) should make the physician suspect an intrauterine cause for growth failure, such as congenital infection or genetic defect; major organ system involvement and minor malformations consistent with suspected syndromes should be diligently sought. It must be remembered that biochemical variations may reflect the state of malnutrition rather than an underlying organic disorder; if not diagnostically helpful, these laboratory values can supplement anthropometrics in monitoring realimentation. While some cases of failure to thrive may be diagnosed and treated on an outpatient basis, short-term hospitalization is frequently utilized for both diagnostic and therapeutic purposes (Table 7). Increased weight gain in a hospital environment is a classic diagnostic finding in nonorganic failure to thrive.

Table 6. Evaluation of Failure to Thrive

History
Physical examination
Neurologic assessment
Developmental evaluation
Calorie count (plus intake and output, frequent weight measurements)
Complete blood count (hemoglobin, hematocrit, differential count, and indices)
Blood chemistries (Na, K, Cl, CO_2 content, blood urea nitrogen, creatinine, Ca, P, alkaline phosphatase, serum glutamic-oxaloacetic transaminase, bilirubin, blood sugar, glucose tolerance test)
Urinalysis (pH, specific gravity, reducing substances, ketones, protein, blood, microscopic examination, culture, creatinine, amino acids)
Stool examination (pH, reducing substances, fat balance)
Radiologic examination (chest, intravenous pyelography, upper and lower gastrointestinal series, trauma survey, bone age)
Endocrine tests (especially thyroid function tests)
Sweat test
Serology (VDRL test, immunoglobulins)
Electrocardiography
Chromosome studies

PITFALLS IN DIAGNOSIS

Since growth represents a final common pathway for the interaction between organic and environmental variables, the diagnostic evaluation of failure to thrive needs to assess the contribution of both organic and nonorganic factors simultaneously; the diagnostician does not rule out every possible rare organic disease and then begin to investigate potential emotional causes. Many cases of failure to thrive have multiple causes; organic factors may be found to interact with social stresses and psychological variables, with both infant and mother contributing to the pathogenesis. The overwhelming majority of organic causes for failure to thrive are identified by the history and physical examination. Any routine labora-

Table 7. Indications for Hospitalization in Failure to Thrive

Strong suspicion of organic cause
Signs of physical abuse
Suspected neglect
- Poor infant hygiene (e.g., severe cradle cap, diaper rash, long dirty fingernails)
- Parental unconcern
- No previous medical attention

History of frequent vomiting or diarrhea
Infant over 2 months of age and still near birth weight
Infant between 3 and 6 months of age with minimal weight gain over previous 2 months
Potentially life-threatening malnutrition
Mother overtly depressed or rejecting baby
History of bizarre diet
Insignificant weight gain after 1 month of outpatient management

tory protocol that is followed independently of guidelines received from a meticulous physical examination and history is almost certainly doomed to failure and represents, at the least, a disservice to the patient. Some laboratory abnormalities may reflect the general state of malnutrition rather than an underlying organic cause. Celiac disease and diencephalic syndrome tend to be missed because of their rarity; cystic fibrosis and hypothyroidism represent more common and more frequently correctly diagnosed conditions that will cause the clinician difficulty only when they present atypically. Unusual etiologic factors not often considered include excessive crying and the improper use of elimination diets. The identification of organic pathology is not the same as the identification of the cause of the failure to thrive; some conditions such as heart murmurs and developmental delay may be coincidental or contributory without being the primary cause of the growth failure. Although nonorganic failure to thrive can be part of a continuum of child neglect and abuse, such a cause should not be entertained or acted upon without positive evidence; environmental influences need to be carefully investigated and not assumed on the basis of race, social class, or identified risk factors.

DELAYED DEVELOPMENT

By Katerina Haka-Ikse, M.D., F.R.C.P.(C)., F.A.A.P.
Toronto, Ontario

SYNONYMS

Developmental delay, slow development, developmental retardation, developmental disability, developmental subnormality, and developmental deficit.

DEFINITION

The abilities of infants and children are measurable and can be compared to established norms. Such norms vary according to racial, cultural, and socioeconomic factors. Delayed development is defined as the failure of a child to demonstrate skills according to an expected timetable for its particular sociocultural and racial cohort.

Developmental processes in children are induced by neurologic maturation, which in turn is affected by genetic, constitutional, and environmental (experiential or socioemotional) factors or combinations of these. Regarding the environmental factors, it is of paramount importance to consider that the child's relationship with the human and physical environment is transactional; the child's actions affect the environment and are in turn modified by the changes elicited. This premise may explain why certain children cope successfully with the same developmental deficits that may seriously limit the functioning of others.

Developmental abilities are divided into distinct areas as follows:

1. Gross motor, or body movements.
2. Fine motor, or hand-digital movements.
3. Cognitive-adaptive, or nonverbal intelligence.
4. Visuoperceptual, or capacity for proper mental representation of visual stimuli.
5. Expressive language, or ability to express verbally needs, wants, and thoughts.
6. Receptive language, or ability to comprehend what others say.
7. Social-emotional, or the ability to develop and experience feelings, acquire controls over feelings and drives, and relate meaningfully and appropriately with others.

PRESENTING SIGNS AND SYMPTOMS

The delay in achieving milestones may be (1) global, affecting all areas of developmental abilities although often each one of them to a different degree, or (2) partial, affecting one or more developmental areas.

Global Delayed Development

Early signs of delay include sucking and feeding difficulties, lack of regular sleeping patterns, somnolence or irritability, and unresponsiveness to soothing practices. These children smile, vocalize, and become alert visually, auditorially, and socially later and less frequently than their normal counterparts. Parents may not notice or consider significant such early signs and become concerned only in the second half of the first year of the child's life, when the child fails to present concrete evidence of progress, such as ability to sit independently, creep, and walk.

In the second year, when parents expect the child to be able to communicate, they become aware of the lack of meaningful speech sounds, and lack of gestures, facial expressions, or body language signs of communication. The child likewise fails to respond to spoken language and may show lack of interest in people speaking. At this stage, a common parental concern is that the child may be hearing impaired. In the preschool age group, prolonged negativism, temper tantrums, and difficulty in acquiring toilet training, selffeeding, and dressing skills or in relating to peers become major areas of concern, together with the slow progress in acquiring other milestones. If the disorder remains undetected and the child joins a regular nursery school or kindergarten group, he or she cannot participate in group activities, follow routines, play and communicate with the other children, or respond to teacher's directions.

Global developmental delay can be mild, moderate, or severe; thus, the degree of these symptoms varies.

Partial Delayed Development

Language delay is the most common isolated developmental deficit, with the child progressing normally in other areas. More often, both expressive and receptive language is affected, although not uncommonly the child may comprehend the language of others without being able to produce it. At times language delay is so severe that even the gestural system is involved and cannot be used as an alternative form of communication. As language is an important tool in relating to others and acquiring social skills, as well as in developing controls over one's own impulses, children with serious language deficits experience difficulties in these areas as well.

Speech impediment—i.e., inability to articulate clearly—is quite frequent, either alone or in combination with language delay. Other related difficulties are delayed acquisition of correct syntax; limited vocabulary of single words; dysnomia, i.e., use of a word that is close to but not exactly what is meant (for example, saying "rain" or "rainthing" instead of umbrella); repetitions; or tangential verbalizations out of context with the situation.

Gross motor delay is quite common as well, although more often than not it is combined with language delay.

Fine motor or visuoperceptual delay may exist alone or in various combinations with language or gross motor deficits. These deficits, although isolated, may influence adversely the child's social-emotional development as they delay acquisition of feeding and manipulatory skills necessary for activities of daily living, impede competitiveness with peers, and increase the child's frustration level.

Cognitive deficits usually occur in combination with delayed language, fine motor, or visuoperceptual delay. The same is true about social-emotional deficits. The latter are, however, quite common in all permutations of developmental deficits and may present under the form of difficult temperament, low frustration tolerance, attention deficit disorder, and impulsivity. It is possible that in most cases temperamental difficulties and easy frustration may not be primary deficits but rather the consequences of having to deal with one's own limitations and the social consequences of being different. Indeed, adults tend to consider that children who do not perform according to expectations are "bad" and "unwilling," instead of being unable to perform in certain area(s).

In terms of what may cause the signs and symptoms of delayed development the following provides a useful framework:

1. Uniformly and significantly low skills usually indicate mental retardation, such as syndromic condition.
2. Scattering and unevenness of developmental skills may be indicative of brain dysfunction of prenatal or perinatal causation.
3. Mildly delayed language, motor, and visuoperceptual skills are often due to familial-constitutional low endowment, with one or both parents or other members of the family having a history of slow development and limited school achievements.
4. Isolated speech or language, visuoperceptual, or motor delay may be familial-constitutional or the result of localized brain dysfunction.
5. Attention deficits, impulsivity, low frustration tolerance, and a difficult temperament can be constitutional, secondary to brain damage, the result of adverse family and sociocultural environment, or a combination of some or all of these.
6. Deprivation of care and an adverse sociocultural and family environment, often coupled with familial-constitutional low endowment, may be manifested by verbal, cognitive, and motor deficits apart from the previously described behavioral manifestations.
7. Behavior problems, difficulties in acquiring independence and socialization skills, and later school problems are seen in children whose families are dysfunctional owing to parental discord, parental psychopathology, and family disorganization.
8. Chronic illnesses and neuromuscular disorders affect variously the psychomotor development of children as a result of physical debility, experiential deprivation, hospitalization, and psychological invalidism.
9. Children of various cultural and subcultural groups may appear slow or atypical in their development if compared with mid–North American standards, whereas they may conform well to the accepted norms of their own cultural group.
10. Stressful events may provoke temporary developmental regression in many children.

COURSE

Despite developmental limitations, children continue to progress although their rate of development usually remains below that of their age counterparts. The majority of children with motor and language delay ambulate and acquire useful language for communication purposes. Cognitive, visuoperceptual, fine motor, and attentional deficits or behavioral manifestations also improve with time, particularly if proper and timely remedial intervention is instituted. Early delayed development, however, is more often than not associated with school learning difficulties, particularly when early language, visuoperceptual, and attention deficits coexist. Ultimately, the majority of children with delayed development are capable of leading useful, productive and satisfying lives provided that they are given early remedial intervention and later proper vocational training.

Moderate and severe degrees of mental retardation, severe forms of cerebral palsy, aphasia (central language disorder), and communicative-emotional disorders (autism) have a considerably more limited prognosis for acquisition of skills for independent and productive existence. Nevertheless, there are increasingly more medical, social, and nursing services to assist families in the care of such individuals.

PHYSICAL EXAMINATION

Particular emphasis should be given to looking for dysmorphic signs that may indicate a specific syndrome associated with delayed development. Clusters of minor dysmorphic signs may not be diagnostic of a particular syndrome, yet they are found more frequently in children with delayed development than in the general population. The head circumference should be noted, as small head size is prevalent in children with delayed development; conversely, hydrocephalus, subdural hematoma, or megaencephaly should be ruled out. The physical growth and nutritional state of the child, among other data, provide

THE HOSPITAL FOR SICK CHILDREN
DEVELOPMENTAL CLINIC
PSYCHOMOTOR DEVELOPMENT SCREENING TEST

Patient Name: ______

Birth Date: ______ Sex: ______ History No: ______

Address: ______

Phone: ______

Date: ______ Tested By: ______

INSTRUCTIONS:

1. This is a simple test to help you evaluate the Developmental Age of a child. The purpose is to determine whether Development is in the broad range of normal and if not whether the child should be referred for a more precise assessment.
2. Start with scoring (+) or (−) at one level below the child's age. Go as high as the child may have successes.
3. Supplement your own observations by questioning the mother. Score as (+) successes reported by the mother even if these are not observed by you.
4. Under "Remarks":
   a) Note problem areas in development and behaviour reported by the mother.
   b) Note activity level, alertness, mood, attention span, unusual behaviour.
   c) State your own impressions of, and predictions about, the child.
5. Items indicate performance in one of the following areas: (M) Motor, (A) Adaptive, (L) Language, (PS) Personal-Social
6. Materials needed; Red Wool yarn, one inch wooden blocks, crayons and paper, a rubber ball, a picture vocabulary.

AGE	SCORE		PSYCHOMOTOR DEVELOPMENT SCREENING TEST
4 Weeks		M	Rotates head when placed in prone position
		A	Responds to sound by changing activity
		A	Focuses eyes on bright object (red wool yarn—stethoscope) and follows it for a short distance
		PS	Interest in examiner (focuses eyes for a while on examiner's face – activity deminishes)
	Remarks:		
8 Weeks		M	Holds head erect briefly in pull-to-sit (pull by the hands until the child is in sitting position)
		M	Holds head 45° up in prone position (child raises head and shoulders off crib level)
		A	Follows object with his eyes past midline
		L	Vocalizes single vowels –"AH" "EH" "UH"
		PS	Social smile (smiles at the approach of mother or examiner)
	Remarks:		
16 Weeks		M	Raises self up on hands in prone position
		M	Reaches for toys – grasps toy actively if it is near his hand
		A	Follows object with eyes through 180° horizontally and vertically
		L	Coos and laughs
		PS	Recognizes mother (responds promptly and more to her than to other persons)
	Remarks:		
24 Weeks		M	Raises legs in extension in supine position and touches feet with hands
		M	Rolls over both ways
		A	Approaches and grasps objects in the midline, brings other hand to the object
		L	Babbles
		PS	Aware and/or apprehensive of strangers
	Remarks		
36 Weeks		M	Sits unsupported 5–10'
		M	Crawls on abdomen
		A	Plays with two toys simultaneously
		L	Vocalizes "mama" – "dada", non-meaningfully
		PS	Responds to pick up gesture
	Remarks:		

Figure 1. Example of a developmental screening test.

Figure continued on opposite page.

Age		Item
44 Weeks	M	Creeps on hands and knees and pulls self up to stand
	M	Grasps small objects (piece of paper – bread crumbs) with thumb and index finger
	A	Imitates behaviour: speech sounds, clapping hands, waving bye-bye
	A	Matches two toys together – places one object into another
	L	Vocalizes "mama" – "dada" and another word, meaningfully
Remarks:		
12 Months	M	Walks if one hand is held
	A	Attempts to pile two blocks after is shown how
	L·	Imitates words–has two words plus "mama" and "dada"–baby word count if used consistently for a certain object
	L	Responds to simple orders accompanied by gestures: "give me", "no-no" etc.
	PS	Attempts to feed himself with his fingers
Remarks:		
18 Months	M	Walks well, begins to run
	M	Climbs on furniture
	A	Piles 3 – 4 Blocks
	L	Follows simple directions – no gestures "give me", "give to", "come here"
	L	Vocabulary of ten words
	PS	Attempts to feed himself with spoon
Remarks:		
2 Years	M	Walks up and down stairs alone (one step at a time–does not need to hold on to the rail)
	M	Kicks ball without being shown how
	A	Imitates vertical and circular strokes
	L	Combines 2–3 words together
	PS	Names and identifies objects and parts (at least 4) of own body
	PS	Imitates domestic activities, (sweeping, dusting, washing)
Remarks:		
3 Years	M	Jumps down from a small chair
	M	Balances on one foot briefly
	A	Copies circle and imitates cross with crayon
	L	Asks "what" questions
	L	Knows name, sex and age
	PS	Puts on shoes, and simple pieces of clothing
	PS	Co-operates in play with peers
Remarks:		
4 Years	M	Stands on one foot for 6–10 seconds
	M	Walks heel to toe
	A	Copies cross
	A	Draws a two-part man
	L	Names fourteen or more of the Stanford-Binet picture vocabulary
	L	Recognizes and names three or more colors
	PS	Separates from mother easily – plays specific role in games
Remarks:		

Figure 1. Example of a developmental screening test. *(Continued)*

useful information in the diagnosis of deprivation failure to thrive, malnutrition, and so forth. Neurologic findings, including functional assessment of the child's neuromotor apparatus; presence or absence of primary reflexes in the case of young infants; abnormalities of tonus or protective reactions; presence of associated movements; finger agnosia; delayed acquisition of, or mixed, hand dominance; and disturbances of movement should all be carefully recorded, as they are often found in slow developing children. Examination of hearing and visual acuity is particularly important, as sensory deficits may present under the guise of developmental delay; also, sensory deficits are common among developmentally slow children and, if present, may further hamper the children's developmental progress.

DEVELOPMENTAL SCREENING

To ascertain the child's developmental level, the physician should not rely only on parental reports or on his or her own impression. A standardized, reliable, and valid developmental screening test should be administered routinely during well baby and child visits to detect as early as possible signs of slow or atypical development. The use of such a test not only organizes observations and provides reminders of normal milestones and the need to measure all areas of development but also is an excellent, concise way to record findings and follow the child's developmental progression. Such records are very useful in medicolegal situations as well.

The Denver Developmental Screening Test (DDST) and its more recent abbreviated form (DDST–R) are recommended as they are widely used and easy to administer.

Figure 1 is an example of another abbreviated developmental screening test.

Unstructured observations of the child's spontaneous behavior and the parent-child interaction during the examination are necessary. They should be complemented by a thorough history from the parents, including family history of delayed development, birth and health data of the child, developmental milestones, and daily functioning and behavior, as all these form integral parts of developmental screening.

LABORATORY, RADIOLOGIC, AND OTHER PROCEDURES

Judicious use of some of the following procedures may help in establishing the cause of delayed development: amino acid and organic acid or specific enzyme determinations; metabolic screening; chromosome studies, including banding techniques and search for fragile X-chromosome; skull x-rays and computed tomography; electroencephalography; auditory and visual evoked potentials in case of inconclusive conventional sensory examination; electromyography and nerve conduction time.

A different but most important source of information should be to utilize social agencies and the services of visiting nurses to obtain information about the sociocultural environment within which the child is growing up, the type of care and rearing practices the child is receiving, and the opportunities the child has for experiential, social, and emotional learning. Referral to a developmental pediatrician, child psychologist, or speech pathologist is necessary if the physician is in doubt about the presence, degree, or nature of the developmental delay.

POTENTIAL ERRORS AND PITFALLS IN DIAGNOSIS

A common error in diagnosis of delayed development is not to search for it, either because the child is considered too young or because the physician does not include developmental screening in routine examination of the child. Careful assessment may uncover signs of developmental delay as early as the newborn period.

Another common error is to dismiss parental concerns about the child's development with reassurance that the child will outgrow the problem or that little or nothing can be done about it. Children may continue to develop at their own slow pace, but unless their condition is diagnosed early they are denied the advantage of the various and effective early remedial programs that are available. Also, unless the developmental deficit is recognized early and its implications are explained clearly, the parents meet considerable difficulties in offering proper support, learning experiences, and behavioral management to their developmentally delayed child.

Gross motor development is as a rule an unreliable predictor of future development; physicians should not assess a child's development on the basis of this parameter alone. The assessment should cover all areas of development and include pertinent knowledge of the family and circumstances within which the child grows.

Conversely, caution should be exercised and the physician should recognize that delayed development may at times be transient and not indicative of a permanent developmental deficit. The younger the child, the more cautious the physician should be in prognosticating about the degree of disability and its permanence, nature, and significance for the developmental future of the child. In case of doubt, the physician should not hesitate to consult specialists in child development at the earliest suspicion of developmental delay. Finally, the diagnosis of delayed development should not be considered as an end in itself but as the beginning of a remedial process on behalf of the child and the family. Serial developmental diagnostic procedures will be necessary to monitor and set ongoing goals for remedial therapy as the child grows.

SHORT STATURE

By S. Douglas Frasier, M.D.
Los Angeles, California

One of the more common problems seen by any physicians who care for children and adolescents is short stature. Most short patients have no significant underlying pathology, and some are short only in the eyes of their parents. However, a variety of disorders may become manifest as short stature or poor growth. Table 1 presents a classification of the more common disorders and conditions that may present in this way.

Chronic nonendocrine disorders (category I) and endocrine abnormalities (category II) are characterized by both short stature and a subnormal growth velocity, whereas the common nonendocrine conditions (category III) listed in the table are characterized by short stature and a growth velocity that is normal for the patient's age. Thus, the initial differential diagnosis of short stature, after a complete history and physical examination has been obtained, depends on comparison of the patient's height with normal standards and calculations of the patient's growth rate.

GROWTH STANDARDS

Accurate serial measurements of height and weight and an accurate record of growth are essential components of the clinical evaluation of all children. Maintenance of a growth chart allows comparison of an individual child with a large population in terms of both percentile ranking and the determination of "height age": the chronological age at which the patient's height falls on the 50th percentile. The growth chart also facilitates observations of the pattern of growth and provides the basis for calculation of growth velocity.

Until recently, growth standards used in the United States were based on data accumulated over 30 years ago. Newer standards have been set by the National Center of Health Statistics (NCHS) of the United States Public Health Service, and growth charts based on these data are now generally available. Table 2 summarizes the NCHS standards for length between birth and 3 years of age; Table 3 summarizes these standards for height between 2 and 18 years of age.

The growth rate can be calculated from serial measurements plotted on the growth curve. The definition of normal growth velocity varies with age and sex. For practical purposes, a growth rate below 5.0 cm per year in both boys and girls between 5 years of age and the beginning of rapid adolescent growth is subnormal. Because younger children normally grow more rapidly, the lower limit of normal for height velocity must be raised with decreasing age. A growth rate between birth and 6 months of age below 16.0 cm in girls and 17.0 cm in boys should be evaluated. Between 6 and 12 months, both boys and girls should grow at least 8.0 cm. A growth rate between 1 and 2 years of age below 11.0 cm in girls and 10.0 cm in boys is less than that expected for age. Between 2 and 5 years of age both boys and girls should grow 6.0 cm per year.

The pattern of growth is of great help in the assignment of a patient to a general diagnostic category. As shown in Figure 1, children with a congenital condition interfering with growth show persistent deviation from the normal curve from a very early age. At times this occurs before 3 to 6 months of age, and it is almost always apparent within the first 12 to 18 months of life. Children with an acquired abnormality affecting growth follow a normal curve for a variable period of time and then begin to deviate from the norm. In contrast, the child with one of the common nonendocrine conditions leading to short stature, such as constitutional delay in growth and adolescence, will grow at a normal rate.

The determination of body proportions provides additional useful differential clinical information. The proportions that have been most widely used are the

Table 1. Causes of Short Stature

Chronic Disease of a Nonendocrine Organ System
- Cardiac
- Pulmonary
- Renal
- Gastrointestinal
- Liver
- Central nervous system
- Bone and cartilage

Endocrine Disorders
- Hypothyroidism
- Abnormalities of the X chromosome
- Growth hormone deficiency
- Deprivation (psychosocial) dwarfism
- Cortisol excess

Common Nonendocrine Conditions
- Constitutional delay in growth and adolescence
- Familial (genetic) short stature
- Intrauterine growth retardation

Table 2. National Center for Health Statistics Percentiles for Length, Boys and Girls, Birth to 36 Months

Age (Months)	Males (Percentiles) 5th	50th	95th		Females (Percentiles) 5th	50th	95th
Birth	46.4	50.5	54.4	cm	45.4	49.9	52.9
	18¼	20	21½	inches	17¾	19¾	20¾
3	56.7	61.1	65.4	cm	55.4	59.5	63.4
	22¼	24	25¾	inches	21¾	23½	25
6	63.4	67.8	72.3	cm	61.8	65.9	70.2
	25	26¾	28½	inches	24¼	26	27¾
12	71.7	76.1	81.2	cm	69.8	74.3	79.1
	28¼	30	32	inches	27½	29¼	31¼
18	77.5	82.4	88.1	cm	76.0	80.9	86.1
	30½	32½	34¾	inches	30	31¾	34
24	82.3	87.6	93.8	cm	81.3	86.5	92.0
	32½	34½	37	inches	32	34	36¼
30	87.0	92.3	98.7	cm	86.0	91.3	96.9
	34¼	36¼	38¾	inches	33¾	36	38¼
36	91.2	96.5	103.1	cm	90.0	95.6	101.5
	36	38	40½	inches	35½	37¾	40

Table 3. National Center for Health Statistics Percentiles for Height, Boys and Girls, Age 2 to 18 Years

Age (Years)	Males (Percentiles) 5th	50th	95th		Females (Percentiles) 5th	50th	95th
2	82.5	86.8	94.4	cm	81.6	86.8	93.6
	32½	34¼	37¼	inches	32¼	34¼	36¾
2½	85.4	90.4	97.8	cm	84.6	90.0	96.6
	33½	35½	38½	inches	33¼	35½	38
3	89.0	94.9	102.0	cm	88.3	94.1	100.6
	35	37¼	40¼	inches	34¾	37	39½
4	95.8	102.9	109.9	cm	95.0	101.6	108.3
	37¾	40½	43¼	inches	37½	40	42¾
5	102.0	109.9	117.0	cm	101.1	108.4	115.6
	40¼	43¼	46	inches	39¾	42¾	45½
6	107.7	116.1	123.5	cm	106.6	114.6	122.7
	42½	45¾	48½	inches	42	45	48¼
7	113.0	121.7	129.7	cm	111.8	120.6	129.5
	44½	48	51	inches	44	47½	51
8	118.1	127.0	135.7	cm	116.9	126.4	136.2
	46½	50	53½	inches	46	49¾	53½
9	122.9	132.2	141.8	cm	122.1	132.2	142.9
	48½	52	55¾	inches	48	52	56¼
10	127.7	137.7	148.1	cm	127.5	138.3	149.5
	50¼	54¼	58¼	inches	50¼	54½	58¾
11	132.6	143.3	154.9	cm	133.5	144.8	156.2
	52¼	56½	61	inches	52½	57	61½
12	137.6	149.7	163.3	cm	139.8	151.5	162.7
	54¼	59	64	inches	55	59¾	64
13	142.9	156.5	169.8	cm	145.2	157.1	168.1
	56¼	61½	66¾	inches	57¼	61¾	66¼
14	148.8	163.1	176.7	cm	148.7	160.4	171.3
	58½	64¼	69½	inches	58½	63¼	67½
15	155.2	169.0	181.9	cm	150.5	161.8	172.8
	61	66½	71½	inches	59¼	63¾	68
16	161.1	173.5	185.4	cm	151.6	162.4	173.3
	63½	68¼	73	inches	59¾	64	68¼
17	164.9	176.2	187.3	cm	152.7	163.1	173.5
	65	69¼	73¾	inches	60	64¼	68¼
18	165.7	176.8	187.6	cm	153.6	163.7	173.6
	65¼	69½	73¾	inches	60½	64½	68¼

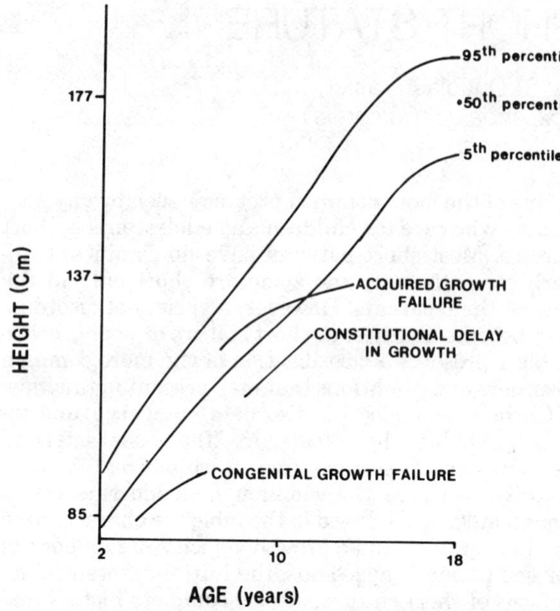

Figure 1. Characteristic growth patterns plotted against a growth curve based on National Center for Health Statistics standards. (From Frasier, S.D.: *Abnormalities of Growth in Pediatric Endocrinology.* New York, Grune & Stratton, 1980.)

ratio of upper body segment to lower body segment and the relationship between arm span and height. The average measurements for these two proportions as a function of age and sex are shown in Table 4. The lower segment is the distance from the top of the symphysis pubis to the heel, with the ankle at 90 degrees. In practice, the upper segment measurement is obtained by subtracting the lower segment from the total height. Arm span is measured with the arms fully extended. Short patients with primary disorders of bone and cartilage, or with long-standing hypothyroidism, have relatively short extremities. Their arm span is shorter than their height, and their upper/lower segment ratio is greater than expected. Other short children are normally proportioned.

CHRONIC DISEASE OF A NONENDOCRINE ORGAN SYSTEM

As shown in Table 1, chronic disease of any major organ system may interfere with growth and lead to short stature. Disorders in this group are far more common than are endocrine abnormalities and they should be considered first. The history, physical examination, and routine laboratory evaluation will uncover the clues that allow the diagnostic search to be narrowed to a particular system and eventually to a specific disorder. The growth pattern in children with nonendocrine based chronic illness is that of acquired growth failure. Body proportions are normal except in disorders primarily affecting bone and cartilage, in which the limbs are shorter than expected.

Table 4. Body Proportions: 50th Percentile Standards for Upper: Lower Segment Ratio and Arm Span Compared to Height

Age	Upper:Lower Segment Ratio Female	Male	Arm Span Minus Height (cm) Female	Male
Birth	1.70	1.70	−2.5	−2.5
6 months	1.60	1.62	−3.0	−2.5
12 months	1.52	1.54	−3.3	−2.5
18 months	1.46	1.50	−3.3	−2.7
24 months	1.41	1.42	−3.5	−3.0
3 years	1.30	1.35	−4.0	−2.7
4 years	1.22	1.24	−3.8	−3.0
5 years	1.15	1.19	−3.5	−3.3
6 years	1.10	1.12	−3.3	−2.5
7 years	1.06	1.07	−2.0	−2.5
8 years	1.02	1.03	−1.8	−1.2
9 years	1.01	1.02	−1.2	0
10 years	1.00	0.99	−1.0	0
11 years	0.99	0.98	0	0
12 years	0.99	0.98	0	+2.0
13 years	1.00	0.97	0	+3.3
14 years	1.01	0.97	0	+3.3
15 years	1.01	0.98	+1.2	+4.3

Short patients growing at a subnormal rate for their age should have a screening hematologic evaluation and routine urinalysis with particular attention to the presence of reducing substances and protein, as well as urine specific gravity and pH. A screening chemistry panel should be performed to evaluate electrolyte and acid-base status, as well as kidney and liver function. The further evaluation of children with disorders in this category will depend on the results of these screening procedures.

ENDOCRINE DISORDERS

After chronic nonendocrine disease has been eliminated in the short child who is growing slowly, endocrine disorders become diagnostic possibilities. The major endocrine disorders that must be considered in the differential diagnosis of short stature are also listed in Table 1.

Hypothyroidism

Children with acquired primary hypothyroidism (see article on Hypothyroidism) often present with the complaint of growth failure. If short stature is due to hypothyroidism, associated symptoms can usually be elicited. These include cold intolerance, increased need for sleep, constipation, muscle aches and weakness, decreased activity, and mental dullness. Hypothyroid children are both short and growing at a subnormal rate. Their growth curve is that of acquired growth failure. If growth is impaired from an early age, body proportions may be relatively infantile with a greater than expected upper:lower segment ratio and short arm span in relation to height.

When hypothyroidism has been present for more than 6 to 12 months, patients may appear pale and puffy. Speech may be slow, with the voice hoarse and lowpitched. The skin is usually thickened, dry, coarse, and cool. Scalp hair may be dry and brittle. Some patients show an unusual type of hirsutism in which there is an increase in fine, dark lanugo-like hair over the back, shoulders, and upper arms. Dental development is frequently delayed. There may be bradycardia and an elevation in diastolic blood pressure. Although muscle weakness is present, the muscles of the extremities may be hypertrophied. There is characteristic delay in the relaxation phase of the deep tendon reflexes, most easily demonstrated at the ankle. Goiter is frequently present, and the thyroid is two or three times normal in size. The surface is generally irregular but not nodular, and the consistency of the gland is firm and rubbery.

The diagnosis of acquired primary hypothyroidism is confirmed by the demonstration of a decreased serum concentration of thyroxine and an elevated serum concentration of thyroid-stimulating hormone (TSH). After chronic disease of a nonendocrine organ system has been eliminated from consideration, these two tests of thyroid function should be performed in all short children who are growing at a subnormal rate. Antibodies to thyroglobulin and thyroid microsomes should be sought in all hypothyroid patients.

Epiphyseal maturation is usually significantly delayed in acquired hypothyroidism. At times, characteristic epiphyseal stippling (epiphyseal dysgenesis) is seen. This abnormality may not become evident until therapy is begun, and it is frequently present during the resolving phase of hypothyroidism.

Abnormalities of the X Chromosome

The unifying expressions of a wide variety of X-chromosome abnormalities are short stature and gonadal dysgenesis. Abnormalities of the X chromosome (see article on Chromosomal Disorders) must be considered in the evaluation of any short girl whether or not associated abnormalities or sexual immaturity is present. Short stature has been present from birth in up to half of the patients. In almost all patients height is below that expected by age 4 or 5 years. The growth rate is subnormal and there is no pubertal acceleration of growth

Patients with gonadal failure usually show no estrogen effect at the time of expected puberty. However, the increase in adrenal androgen production that is part of normal pubertal development does occur, and girls with gonadal failure develop pubic and axillary hair. In a few patients in whom sufficient gonadal tissue is present, pubertal development may advance and menarche may occur.

If no chronic illness is present, all euthyroid girls being evaluated for short stature should have chromosome analysis of peripheral lymphocytes. Since no more than half of the patients with abnormalities of the X chromosome are chromatin-negative, the buccal smear is not a satisfactory method of diagnosis and a karyotype is necessary. The presence of primary gonadal failure can be confirmed by demonstrating elevated concentrations of follicle-stimulating hormone (FSH) and luteinizing hormone (LH). Because of the association between abnormalities of the X chromosome and autoimmune thyroiditis, thyroid function should be evaluated and antithyroid antibodies should be measured at regular intervals. Epiphyseal development is delayed in most patients with short stature owing to an abnormality of the X chromosome.

Growth Hormone Deficiency

Although growth hormone (GH) deficiency is a relatively rare cause of short stature, it should be looked for after chronic nonendocrine disease, hypothyroidism, and abnormalities of the X chromosome have been eliminated as diagnostic possibilities.

If growth hormone deficiency is congenital, growth failure is usually noted by 12 to 18 months of age. Children with acquired GH deficiency have the growth curve of acquired growth failure. Children deficient in growth hormone are normally proportioned, and their upper:lower segment ratio and the relationship between arm span and height are normal. Many patients share a number of physical features regardless of the underlying cause which, when taken together, produce a common appearance (Fig. 2). Patients tend to be overweight, and their height age is less than their weight age. Although the excess fat deposition does not spare the extremities, it is frequently concentrated over the chest and abdomen. Head size may also be more consistent with chrono-

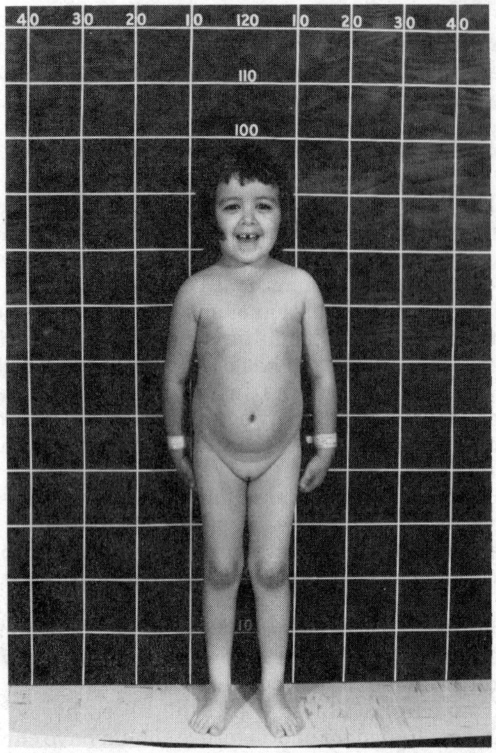

Figure 2. Growth hormone deficiency in an 8-year-old girl. Height age is 3 years, 5 months; weight age is 3 years, 9 months. Note the normal body proportions and the missing deciduous single central incisor. (From Frasier, S.D.: Growth disorders in children. Pediatr. Clin. North Am., 26:1, 1979.)

logical age than height. This overall appearance has been described as "doll-like" or "cherubic." The voice may be high-pitched and squeaky owing to immaturity of the facial bones. Congenital growth hormone deficiency may first become manifest in early infancy as hypoglycemia with convulsions, cyanosis, and shock. In the male, associated congenital gonadotropin deficiency may lead to micropenis, and the combination of microgenitalia and hypoglycemia is due to multiple pituitary hormone deficiencies, which include growth hormone.

Since growth hormone is often undetectable in the serum of normal persons, a random determination of the concentration of growth hormone is of no value. Children in whom the diagnosis of growth hormone deficiency is suspected on clinical grounds should be screened for GH deficiency by performing an exercise test. Patients are instructed to have nothing by mouth for 3 or 4 hours and to rest quietly for 30 minutes after coming to the office or are studied between 8:00 A.M. and 9:00 A.M., after an overnight fast, without a rest period. A control blood sample is drawn and the patient either walks on a level surface for 15 minutes and then runs up and down one flight of stairs for 5 minutes or performs 20 minutes of parent-supervised vigorous exercise consisting of jumping jacks, running, or whatever is preferable for the patient. A post-exercise blood sample is then obtained. Between 80 and 90 per cent of normal children will respond to exercise with a rise in the serum concentration of growth hormone to 6 ng/ml or more. Pretreatment with propranolol (20 mg in children weighing less than 30 kg, and 40 mg in heavier children) enhances the response. A propranolol-primed test should be performed in children who fail to respond to exercise alone prior to proceeding to definitive testing. Children who are too young to perform standardized exercise should be given levodopa, as described for definitive testing, with samples obtained at 0, 60, and 90 minutes.

Tests for Growth Hormone Deficiency

Children who fail to respond to a screening test need definitive testing. The tests that have been standardized for this purpose are insulin-induced hypoglycemia, intravenous arginine, oral levodopa, and intramuscular or subcutaneous glucagon. Confirmation of the diagnosis of growth hormone deficiency requires failure to respond to two of these stimuli.

Hypoglycemia is induced by the intravenous injection of regular insulin in a dose of 0.05 to 0.1 unit/kg of body weight. Blood samples are obtained for the determination of both blood glucose and growth hormone concentrations at 10- or 15-minute intervals over an initial hour, and at 20- or 30-minute intervals over a second hour. A 50 per cent fall in the concentration of blood glucose results in a rise in the concentration of growth hormone in serum to 8 ng/ml or more in over 85 to 90 per cent of normal children. The peak serum concentration of growth hormone is usually observed at 30 to 60 minutes after the administration of insulin. Symptoms of hypoglycemia may be seen between 15 and 45 minutes after administration. The person performing the test must be prepared to administer 50 per cent glucose intravenously or 1 mg of glucagon intramuscularly, or both, if termination of the test is indicated.

Arginine hydrochloride, which is available as a 10 per cent solution for use as a diagnostic reagent, is administered as an intravenous infusion over 30 minutes. The dose is 0.5 gm/kg of body weight up to a maximum of 30 gm. Blood samples are obtained every 15 minutes for the first hour and at 30-minute intervals over a second hour. Between 80 and 85 per cent of healthy children will respond with a peak serum growth hormone level of 8 ng/ml or more, usually at 30 to 60 minutes. Girls are somewhat more likely to respond than are boys. The intravenous infusion of arginine is essentially without side effects.

When levodopa is administered by mouth, there is a prompt release of GH from the pituitary. The dose of levodopa is 125 mg for children weighing less than 15 kg, 250 mg for children weighing 15 to 30 kg, and 500 mg for children weighing more than 30 kg. Blood samples are obtained every 30 minutes over 2 hours. A peak serum growth hormone concentration of 8 ng/ml or more is seen in 85 to 90 per cent of normal children in the 30- or 60-minute sample. Unpleasant side effects, particularly nausea or vomiting, are induced by levodopa in a significant number of children.

The intramuscular or subcutaneous administration of glucagon in a dose of 0.03 mg/kg up to 1.0 mg results in a significant rise in the serum concentration of GH as a relatively late response. Blood samples are obtained at 30-minute intervals over 3 hours following glucagon injection, and a maximum GH concentration of 8 ng/ml or more is observed between 120 and 150 minutes in 75 to 80 per cent of normal children. No significant side effects have been reported following glucagon administration.

Propranolol may be given 30 minutes prior to testing with either levodopa or glucagon, as described for exercise testing. Administration of this agent increases the likelihood of a good response in a normal child.

Abnormalities in the growth hormone system have been described in which patients appear to have the clinical characteristics of growth hormone deficiency, but have a normal growth hormone response to standard definitive stimuli. Patients who fall into this category may have an inability to generate somatomedin. The serum concentration of somatomedin-C should be measured, and if it is subnormal, evaluation of the somatomedin-C response to exogenous growth hormone may be useful. Human growth hormone (hGH), 0.2 International Units (IU)/kg, is given intramuscularly daily for 5 days. The somatomedin-C concentration is measured before the first hGH injection and 24 hours after the fifth injection. If the serum concentration of somatomedin-C fails to increase, the diagnosis is probably Laron dwarfism. If the somatomedin-C concentration increases significantly, the patient may have biologically inactive endogenous hGH and may benefit from exogenous hGH therapy.

Deprivation (Psychosocial) Dwarfism

The syndrome of deprivation dwarfism, or psychosocial dwarfism, is characterized by emotional disturbances and abnormalities in behavior that are associated with reversible growth failure and transient impairment of pituitary function.

The age of onset of growth failure is highly variable. At the time of initial evaluation, patients are well below average height for their age and are growing at a subnormal rate. Their growth curve cannot be distinguished from that seen in acquired growth hormone deficiency. The growth retardation is proportional. The relationship between span and height is normal and the upper:lower segment ratio is appropriate for the patient's height. While there is a tendency for the patients to be underweight for height, this is a variable finding and some patients are mildly or even moderately obese. There may be a protuberant abdomen and thin extremities, which suggest the possibility of intestinal malabsorption.

In most patients, the characteristic behavioral abnormalities begin before the age of 2 years. Disturbed behavior is centered on drinking, eating, and sleeping. Almost all patients show bizarre polydipsia. It is usual for them to drink from toilet bowls, sprinkler heads, gutters, or fish tanks. Water is frequently requested throughout the night. Most affected children have voracious appetites. They frequently eat from garbage cans, and beg or steal food from friends, neighbors, or food stores. Rumination and cyclic vomiting are sometimes seen. Insomnia and roving nighttime behavior are common. Many patients have difficulty with bladder and bowel training. Apparent retardation of intellectual development and speech is frequent.

The family is usually disrupted. The incidence of divorce and separation is higher than expected, and the father is frequently out of the home. One or both parents are often alcoholic. There may be clear evidence of estrangement between the parents and child, particularly the mother and the patient. A past history or current physical evidence of child abuse is often found. The child with psychosocial dwarfism tends to be isolated and does not participate in family activities.

The diagnosis depends primarily on past history and subsequent clinical course. When tests of pituitary function are performed during the time that growth is impaired, there is usually evidence of growth hormone deficiency. Many patients also have adrenocorticotropic hormone (ACTH) deficiency. Thyroid function is normal. If pituitary function is studied during the recovery phase when growth is accelerated, growth hormone and ACTH secretion are found to be normal. The bone age is markedly retarded during the period of growth failure, and epiphyseal maturation normalizes during the phase of catch-up growth.

Figure 3 shows a patient with deprivation dwarfism before and after her environment was changed.

Glucocorticoid Excess

Glucocorticoid excess in infancy and childhood almost always leads to a subnormal growth rate, short stature, and delayed epiphyseal maturation. Occa-

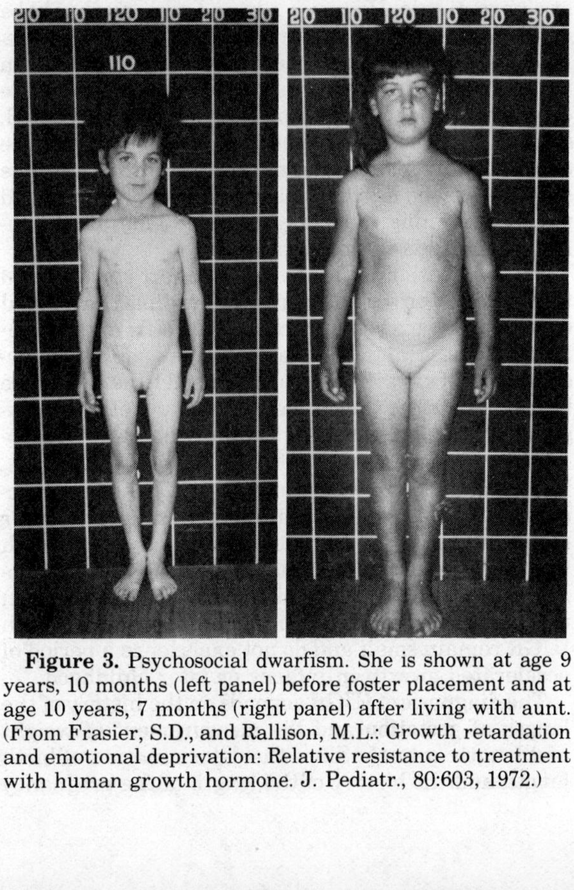

Figure 3. Psychosocial dwarfism. She is shown at age 9 years, 10 months (left panel) before foster placement and at age 10 years, 7 months (right panel) after living with aunt. (From Frasier, S.D., and Rallison, M.L.: Growth retardation and emotional deprivation: Relative resistance to treatment with human growth hormone. J. Pediatr., 80:603, 1972.)

sionally growth failure is the primary or only clinical manifestation. This diagnosis should be considered, and appropriate tests for cortisol excess should be performed whenever the cause of growth failure is obscure, as well as when there are more classic symptoms and signs of increased glucocorticoid secretion.

COMMON NONENDOCRINE CONDITIONS

Table 1 lists several nonendocrine conditions that require consideration in the differential diagnosis of short stature. These are not really disorders, but rather are variations of normal that show more or less characteristic clinical pictures and patterns of growth.

Children with constitutional delay in growth and adolescence are normal in height and length at birth. They grow normally for several months or longer and usually deviate from a normal growth pattern for some period of time between 6 and 36 months of age. After that time, the growth rate is normal and their growth pattern parallels the normal growth curve. When seen for evaluation, these children are usually growing at a normal rate for age. Puberty is delayed, and there is a later than average adolescent acceleration of growth. However, normal adult height is attained and normal sexual development occurs. There is usually a family history of a similar pattern of childhood and adolescent growth in one parent or other first degree relative. The great majority of children who fall into this category are short boys who are otherwise normal.

The general screening studies previously described are not necessary in short children who are growing at a normal rate. However, a bone age x-ray should be obtained for prognostic purposes. The bone age is delayed and is more consistent with height age than with chronological age. Tests of thyroid function are often performed but are only sometimes indicated, since the diagnosis of hypothyroidism can usually be eliminated by history and physical examination. The short child who is active, alert, and clearly euthyroid in the examining room does not need laboratory confirmation of his or her normality.

Patients with familial or genetic short stature tend to be short at birth. Their growth parallels the normal curve but is below the fifth percentile from early infancy. Adolescent development and the adolescent acceleration of growth occur at the usual time. Ultimate height is short for the patient's racial and ethnic background but is consistent with family height. All laboratory results are normal, including bone age.

Intrauterine growth retardation (IUGR), which occurs both as an isolated abnormality and in a number of conditions in which short stature is associated with multiple congenital malformations, is usually sporadic. There is no family history of a similar pattern of growth. A significant number of children with IUGR remain small and do not experience a period of accelerated growth in infancy or later childhood.

The diagnosis of IUGR depends on the history of the length of gestation and the measurement of weight and length at birth. Since the determination of birth length and the history of the length of the pregnancy are notoriously inaccurate, the diagnosis is frequently based on birth weight and the best estimate of the length of pregnancy.

All laboratory studies of endocrine function show normal results. The bone age of patients with IUGR is variable when compared with both height age and chronological age. In general, patients who remain short generally have delayed epiphyseal maturation.

SUMMARY

Short stature in childhood has many possible causes, only a minority of which are endocrine disorders. In addition to a complete history and physical examination, the most important information that can be brought to bear on the differential diagnosis of short stature is accurate serial measurements of length or height or both. When these data are used to calculate growth velocity and are plotted on a standard growth curve, short children can quickly be classified into those growing at a subnormal rate and likely to have a significant underlying problem and those whose growth rate is normal and who are very unlikely to have an underlying problem. In general, diagnostic studies may be limited to short children who are growing at a subnormal rate. Endocrine disease should be considered only after chronic illness of a nonendocrine organ system has been eliminated from consideration. The possibilities of hypothyroidism, an abnormality of the X chromosome in short girls, and growth hormone deficiency should be evaluated sequentially. The unusual diagnoses of deprivation dwarfism and glucocorticoid excess must be kept in mind. The vast majority of short children seen in practice are growing at a normal rate and are boys with constitutional delay in growth and adolescence. A bone age x-ray is extremely helpful in arriving at a prediction of their mature height, which is almost always within the range expected from their family pattern. The reassurance provided by this procedure usually makes any further diagnostic studies unnecessary.

MENTAL RETARDATION

By Herbert J. Cohen, M.D.
and Ruth K. Kaminer, M.D.
Bronx, New York

SYNONYMS

Mental subnormality and mental deficiency.

DEFINITION

Mental retardation refers to significantly subaverage intellectual functioning existing concurrently with deficits in adaptive behavior and manifested during the developmental period. This is a condition based on a level of functioning which should be determined by individual psychological testing using a standard instrument. It is not a disease in the usual sense.

Mental retardation is a disorder of considerable importance to physicians, educators, and other professionals because of its common occurrence, the multiplicity of etiologic factors, and the enormous worldwide economic consequences of the problem. Those affected have significant medical needs and requirements for special education, habilitation, vocational training, and other services. The impact of the problems of the mentally retarded on families is another serious issue of concern to all service providers.

Although physicians do not usually have the primary responsibility in the treatment of most patients with mental retardation, they have a vital role in early diagnosis, initial medical and surgical management of some infants and young children, provision of more comprehensive early intervention services, supervision of physical rehabilitation programs, and provision of general medical care; they also are instrumental in the important area of prevention.

CLASSIFICATION

In the past few decades, the classification and terminology used to describe the degree of mental retardation present in an individual have changed. Two approaches are now used: intelligence testing and level of adaptive functioning. The level of performance on types of intelligence testing and the corresponding categorization of degree of retardation are summarized in Table 1. The functional levels of affected individuals from those classified as "borderline" to those testing as definitely mentally retarded (from the mild to the profound range) are outlined in Table 2, which incorporates information on general guidelines about the academic potential, expected accomplishments in activities of daily living (ADL), travel capability, and vocational potential of affected individuals. It should be noted that borderline intelligence is a category in which the individual functions above the retarded level but below the average range.

Table 1. Level of Retardation Indicated by IQ Range Obtained on Measure of General Intellectual Functioning*†

Term	IQ Range for Level	Code
Mild mental retardation	50–55 to approx. 70	(317.0)
Moderate mental retardation	35–40 to 50–55	(318.0)
Severe mental retardation	20–25 to 35–40	(318.1)
Profound mental retardation	Below 20 or 25	(318.2)
Unspecified		(319.0)

*From Grossman, H.J.: Classification in Mental Retardation. Washington, D.C., American Association on Mental Deficiency, 1983.

†Note. Levels of retardation are identified with the same terms as those used in previous AAMD manuals. The IQ ranges for levels are generally consistent with those suggested by the American Psychiatric Association in their *Diagnostic and Statistical Manual III*, but a narrow band at each end of each level was used to indicate that clinical judgment about all information, including the IQs, and more than one test, the information about intellectual functioning obtained from other sources, etc., is necessary in determining level. Thus, someone whose Full Scale Wechsler IQ is 53 might be diagnosed as having either mild or moderate retardation, depending on other factors, such as the relative difference in Performance and Verbal IQ or results of other tests.

ETIOLOGY

The causes of mental retardation are numerous, and defining specific factors is a complex task. Satisfactory anatomic and etiologic classifications do not exist to assist the practitioner. In cases of mild mental retardation, social class and environmental factors appear to play an important role, since numerous studies have verified the higher incidence of mental subnormality among individuals whose families have the lowest socioeconomic status (SES) in their locales. Many clinicians support the view that lower SES predisposes individuals to higher risks of neurologic dysfunction owing to a greater exposure to adverse prenatal, perinatal, or postnatal conditions—e.g., from higher rates of infection, poorer nutrition, greater dangers of exposure to toxic substances, and less adequate prenatal and perinatal care. The interaction of biologic, sociocultural, and psychological factors in producing maladaptive social adaptation and sub-par intellectual functioning is portrayed in Figure 1. A listing of biologic factors involved in the causation of mental retardation is presented in Table 3. It must be noted, however, that even this comprehensive list of factors is identifiable in fewer than half of patients with mental retardation, though the incidence is higher among children with an intelligence quotient (IQ) of less than 50.

EPIDEMIOLOGIC ISSUES

Mental retardation is reported to be present in 3 per cent of the population based on the number of individuals scoring more than 2 standard deviations (SD) below the mean on formal IQ tests (see Table 1). However, recent reports from Scandinavian countries suggest that only about 0.5 per cent of the population is affected. The figure is considered to be higher in the United States. The incidence of IQs below 50 has been more clearly shown, in both the United States and Great Britain, to be between 3 to 4 per 1000. About 75 per cent of mental retardation is classified as mild, 20 per cent as moderate, and 5 per cent as severe and profound.

PRESENTING SIGNS AND SYMPTOMS

Mental retardation presents with different findings at different ages. More severely impaired individuals are identified at a younger age. The common theme

Table 2. Prognosis and Expected Functional Level Based on Degree of Retardation*

Level	Academic Potential	Activities of Daily Living (ADL)†	Travel Capability	Vocational Ability
Borderline	Educable, with potential up to about 6th grade level	Fully independent	Independent	Employable without special help though may need vocational training for competitive employment
Mild	Educable to 4th or 5th grade level (or less). Capable of reading and writing	Relatively independent in all areas; some training might be required	May require travel training to use public transportation	Employable, but often needs some special training if competitive employment is feasible.
Moderate	May read or write but very limited (1st or 2nd grade level)	Trainable for all ADL. Can dress, be toilet trained, prepare food	Travels only with special training. Usually requires special transport	No real competitive employment except in restricted setting; sheltered employment likely with specialized training
Severe	Very unlikely to read or write	Partially trainable. Should acquire most ADL skills. Is toilet trainable, can dress, but may require assistance	Very limited independent travel potential	Sheltered employment only, special training required
Profound	None	May sometimes be toilet trained and dress with assistance. Generally very dependent	May or may not be ambulatory. Requires special transport	Very limited trainability for vocational functions

*From Cohen, H.J.: *Introduction to Mental Retardation.* Pediatric Annuals, vol. 11, No. 5, 1982, Charles Slack and Co., Thorofare, N.J.

†Dressing, feeding, bathing, routine self care, toileting.

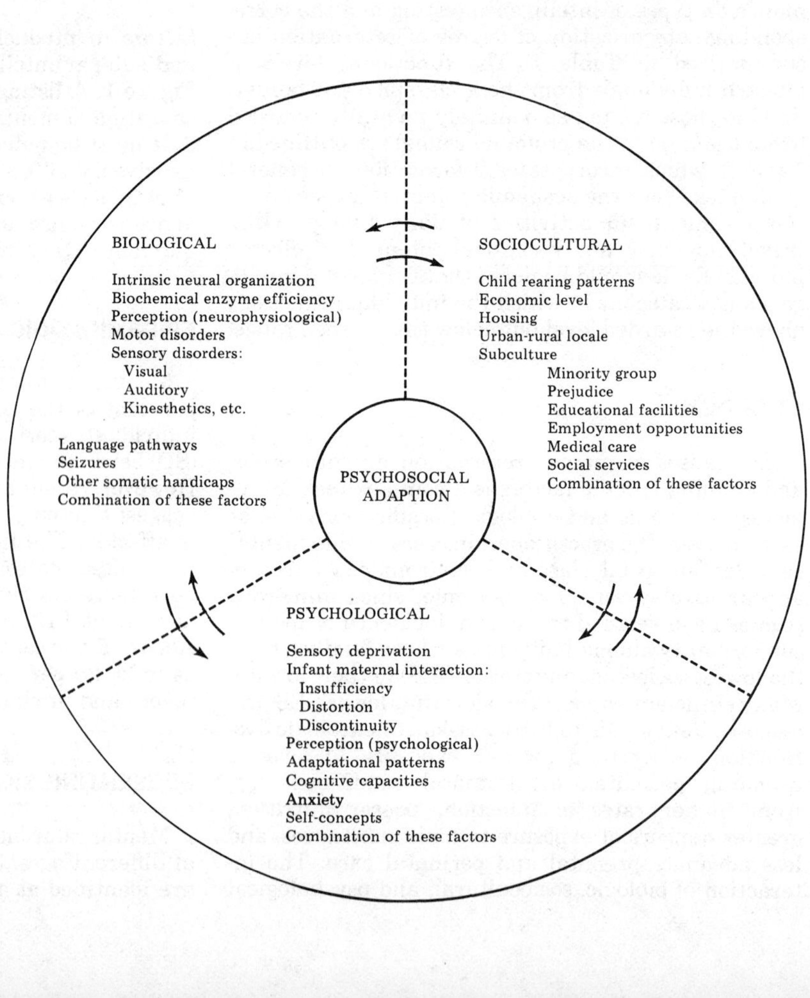

Figure 1. Interacting factors in abnormal mental development. (Adapted from Garrard, S.D., and Richmond, J.B. In H. Lief, V. Lief and N. Lief, eds.: *The Psychological Basis of Medical Practice.* New York, Harper and Row, 1963. Originally from Richmond, J.B., and Lustman, L.L.: J. Med. Educ., 29:23, 1954).

Table 3. Biologic Factors in Causation of Mental Retardation

Prenatal Factors

Chromosomal anomalies:

- Autosomes: nondisjunction (trisomies), translocation, deletion or partial deletion of chromosome material, mosaicism
- Sex chromosome anomalies

Effects of abnormal genes:

- Homozygous genes: produce identifiable recessive disorders of metabolism of amino acids (PKU, nonketotic glycinemia), lipids (leukodystrophies, lipidoses), carbohydrates (galactosemia, mucopolysaccharidoses), purines (hyperuricemia)
- Heterozygous genes: carrier states (maple syrup urine disease, Tay-Sachs disease), dominant disorders (some anencephalies, osteogenesis imperfecta)
- X-linked recessive disorders
- Unknown causation: identifiable syndromes of unknown etiology

Deleterious intrauterine influences

- Maternal illness, infection, nutritional deficiency, hormonal imbalance
- Teratogens: maternal drug ingestion, including alcohol, phenytoin, antimetabolities, nicotine, quinine; environmental toxins (lead, cadmium), radiation
- Uterine disease, malformations, dysfunction
- Multiple pregnancy
- Placental dysfunction, malimplantation
- Isoimmunization
- Trauma: foreign body in uterus; direct blow or accident
- Prematurity (resulting from intrauterine problems but also associated with perinatal difficulties)

Perinatal Factors (Including Those Associated with Trauma or Hypoxia)

- Prolonged labor due to malpresentation of fetus, cephalopelvic disproportion, uterine inertia, placental abnormalities, placenta previa, abruptio placentae
- Umbilical cord prolapse, torsion, looping around neck
- Maternal hypotension: hemorrhage, anesthesia
- Neonatal sepsis or meningitis
- Asphyxia neonatorum and respiratory distress
- Kernicterus

Postnatal Factors

- Anoxia (drowning, plastic bag over head)
- Cerebrovascular accidents: hemorrhage, thrombosis, embolism
- Degenerative diseases: leukodystrophies, Tay-Sachs disease
- Encephalopathies: postimmunization, associated with common childhood infections, secondary to toxins; metabolic (e.g., hypoglycemia)
- Endocrine disorders (e.g., hypothyroidism)
- Head trauma: falls, auto accidents, child abuse
- Central nervous system infections: meningitis, encephalitis
- Severe nutritional deficiencies
- Poisons and environmental toxins: lead or mercury ingestion, carbon monoxide, other contaminants of food, water, or air
- Space-occupying lesions: neoplasms, abscesses, subdural hematomas
- Anatomic factors: premature synostosis, hydrocephalus

Modified from Taft, L., and Cohen, H.J.: In Barnett, H. (ed.): *Pediatrics*. 16th Ed. New York, Appleton-Century-Crofts, 1977.

throughout all age groups is a delay in acquiring skills at expected milestones of development compared with normal children of the same age. The quality of interest in materials and in the environment may be less among retarded children. The most common findings in various age groups are as follows:

Birth to 1 Year. Delayed motor milestones are the most common presenting sign, including delays in gaining head control, rolling over, sitting, crawling, or standing. Other findings include abnormalities of muscle tone, abnormal patterns of primitive reflexes, especially their failure to disappear at the appropriate ages, and delay in appearance of adaptive reflexes. In addition, there may be a limited response to spoken language and no attempt at expressive language, especially mimicry, failure to recognize familiar people, or failure to display stranger anxiety.

1 to 3 Years. Delay in development of expressive language is the most common chief complaint in mildly to moderately retarded children, with delays in all developmental areas (motor, personal-social, and adaptive) common in the moderate, severe, and profound groups.

3 to 5 Years. Common findings include continued delayed language development and failure to acquire skills in activities of daily living, including toileting, dressing, and feeding. Motor clumsiness may also be evident. Social skills vary with the degree of social stimulation. Moderately retarded children are usually identified in the preschool years. Mildly retarded children who tend to be unstigmatized and have normal motor skills may be considered normal at this age unless developmental screening is performed. Behavior problems are common, often due to the child's inability to meet parental expectations based on his chronological, not mental, age.

5 to 7 Years. Findings include failure to acquire academic skills on a par with peers, with the degree of difficulty proportional to the degree of retardation; fine and gross motor coordination may be deficient. Mildly retarded children are often identified at this age level.

7 to 16 Years. If the retardation was undetected previously, then school failure and difficulty in acquiring self-care skills, particularly the latter in the more severely involved population, are common problems. Speech and language problems consist of poor articulation and difficulties in understanding or using more complex language.

16 Years and Older. Mental retardation other than mild degrees in individuals not attending school is rarely undetected at these ages. Functional deficits will vary with the degree of retardation (see Table 2).

COURSE

The level of accomplishment and functioning of the mentally retarded individual depends on two key factors: (1) the intrinsic intellectual potential and (2) the type, amount, and effectiveness of intervention. Reasonable expectations for mentally retarded adults in different categories of retardation are outlined in Table 2. However, early intervention and effective education and training with care in a normalizing home-like environment are more likely to promote normal social behavior, and these help the patient in achieving the highest levels of academic and vocational potential. In vocational areas, even severely retarded individuals have been trained to complete assembly tasks of a complex nature using behavior modification and reinforced sequencing techniques. Behavior modification has also been effective in achieving successful toilet training in severely and profoundly retarded children and adults.

COMMON COMPLICATIONS

The most common complications are associated with inadequate management. These include failure to recognize and treat associated sensory deficits and medical problems or to promote normal psychological and social development.

When mental retardation is associated with a genetic or chromosomal abnormality, such as Down's syndrome, or an early perinatal insult, the frequency of associated congenital deficits is higher. Recognition and treatment of hydrocephalus and cardiac, renal, or infectious complications is essential. In cases of associated neuromuscular disturbance with pseudobulbar difficulties, prevention or early treatment of respiratory infections is important. When mental retardation is associated with significant brain damage, early recognition and treatment of seizures is required. In infants who were born prematurely, those with anoxia, and/or those with an infectious disorder such as meningitis, concerns about visual and auditory functioning are appropriate. Among profoundly retarded patients, particularly the institutionalized or understimulated population, as well as those with Lesch-Nyhan syndrome, self-abusive behavior must be prevented. In the psychosocial area, when the social and psychological needs of the patient are improperly met, acting out or aggressive or antisocial behavior can become a problem requiring use of medication or special behavioral interventions. Finally, sorrow and guilt related to having a retarded child and fear of its potential disruptive effects on families may require considerable psychological support, counseling, and assistance to parents and siblings of the affected individual.

PHYSICAL EXAMINATION

Since mental retardation has diverse causes, the physical findings vary. Children with chromosomal abnormalities or with brain damage associated with first trimester prenatal insults are more likely to have some of the following physical stigmata or other congenital defects:

Head: Abnormalities of head shape or size, including microcephaly or hydrocephalus

Eyes: Abnormal slants (mongoloid or antimongoloid), colobomas, cataracts, strabismus, microphthalmias

Ears: Abnormal shape of the pinnae, low-set ears

Nose: Flat bridge, unusual shapes

Philtrum: Too short or too long

Mouth: Small orifice, cleft lip or palate, high-arched palate, scrotal tongue or abnormally shaped or sized tongue

Hair: Hirsutism, low hairline, abnormal quality of hair, eyebrow hair meeting in midline

Neck: Short, webbed neck (Turner's and Noonan's syndrome)

Chest: Broad, shield-like, small nipples (Turner's and Noonan's syndromes)

Genitalia: Small, undescended testes, hypospadias

Heart and Kidney: Congenital defects

Extremities: Abnormal number or shape of digits, incurved fifth digit, webbing of fingers and toes, abnormal dermatoglyphics, simian creases

Skin: Café au lait spots or vitiligo (tuberous sclerosis or neurofibromatosis), unusual rashes in some metabolic disturbances

When there is brain damage, the neurologic examination indicates abnormalities of tone, reflexes, balance, and gross and fine motor coordination, as well as the presence of pathologic reflexes.

LABORATORY PROCEDURES

Laboratory procedures are generally of limited value in cases of mental retardation, except, in a few instances, as aids in determining the cause and associated complications or abnormalities. Useful tests include the following:

Metabolic Screening. Urine or blood samples are useful in newborn infants and some children not screened or diagnosed as retarded in infancy to rule out common inborn errors of metabolism, such as phenylketonuria (PKU) or hypothyroidism.

Antibody Titers. These tests may detect congenital infectious causes, such as rubella, syphilis, herpes simplex, cytomegalic inclusion disease, or toxoplasmosis.

Electroencephalography (EEG). Electroencephalograms are generally of limited value except for the identification of associated seizure disorders.

Cytogenetic Studies. These are indicated when a chromosomal disorder is suspected, including the more obvious abnormalities associated with trisomy or deletion syndromes or more subtle findings, such as occur with Klinefelter's or fragile X syndromes (see article on Chromosomal Disorders).

Toxicologic Studies. These may be used to detect elevated lead or mercury levels or presence of other heavy metals known to produce brain damage, when a history of significant exposure exists.

RADIOLOGIC STUDIES

Routine x-rays usually are not indicated. However, skull x-rays may confirm premature closure of sutures or occasional cases of toxoplasmosis or cytomegalic inclusion disease in which periventricular calcification may be present. Tuberous sclerosis may be associated with calcifications, as may Sturge-Weber syndrome, both associated with difficult-to-control seizure disorders. Sophisticated techniques such as computed tomography (CT) or, more recently, nuclear magnetic resonance (NMR) scans or positron emission tomography (PET) can locate smaller areas of brain damage or structural defects to a greater extent, and without the need for invasive procedures, than was possible in the past.

OTHER DIAGNOSTIC PROCEDURES

Important diagnostic procedures in children suspected of mental retardation include the following:

1. Psychological testing by an experienced professional; this is a precondition to making the diagnosis.
2. Audiologic testing to rule out hearing impairment as a cause of delay in language, social, and adaptive functioning, or as an associated finding in patients in whom brain or nerve damage is present.
3. Vision testing, since satisfactory vision is required to promote normal learning unless special assistance is provided.
4. Speech and language evaluation to assess the need for specialized training, including a feeding program, if necessary.
5. Social evaluation to assess the family's need for special assistance or counseling.
6. Psychiatric evaluation to rule out a primary psychiatric problem that may be confused with mental retardation, or to assess the extent that secondary psychological problems are present.
7. Physiatric, orthopedic, occupational therapy, or physical therapy examination, if associated physical disabilities or neuromuscular problems are evident.
8. Educational or vocational evaluations to assess the educational or vocational needs and to prescribe required treatment.

POTENTIAL ERRORS AND PITFALLS IN DIAGNOSIS

There are many potential pitfalls in establishing the correct diagnosis. Conditions that may either be confused with or make patients appear mentally retarded include the following:

Child Abuse and Neglect. Fearful, anxious, inhibited, or deprived children may test poorly on standardized testing, particularly soon after the period of trauma. Retesting after a period of stability in the child's life, by a nonthreatening examiner, is essential (see article on Child Abuse).

Hearing Impairment. Children with a hearing loss should have their intellectual functioning tested with nonverbal approaches using instruments such as the Leiter scale. Similar concerns and approaches also apply to aphasic children.

Cerebral Palsy and Related Neuromuscular Disorders. The presence of physical disability or a movement disorder that impairs gross and fine motor coordination may adversely affect the child's ability to complete test procedures at an appropriate age. Special caution must be exercised in predicting future intellectual functioning of young physically handicapped children because of the inhibiting effects of the physical disability and the possibility of limited social exposure or stimulation.

Emotional Disturbance. Children who are withdrawn and who do not relate well to others may test more poorly than their ultimate potential may, in fact, be. However, most autistic children do eventually test in the mentally retarded range.

Other Possible Pitfalls. Other pitfalls and concerns about which clinicians must be aware include the following:

1. Psychological testing must be conducted by experienced testers.
2. Screening tools such as the Denver Developmental Screening Test are not complete psychometric tests and are not intended as reliable predictors of future IQ or adaptive functioning.
3. Some formal tests do have a cultural bias and, in addition, if not administered in the individual's native language, can produce spuriously low test results.
4. Another factor influencing test results may be the health of the child. The presence of an acute illness makes testing difficult, and with chronic illness the child's energy level, motivation, and attention span can adversely affect test results.
5. Hyperactive children may also be difficult to test.
6. Hospitalized children may respond adversely to a new and often anxiety-producing setting. Optimally, testing should occur when a child is healthy and should be performed by an experienced examiner in a non-threatening outpatient or home-like setting.

PREVENTION

Insufficient attention is often paid to the issue of prevention, an area in which the medical role is quite significant.

Primary prevention involves directly preventing the condition from occurring. Relevant examples include:

1. Use of genetic counseling, which is of particular importance when a previous hereditary or genetic disorder is known or suspected.
2. Amniocentesis for antenatal diagnosis.
3. Satisfactory prenatal and perinatal care, especially in high-risk situations.
4. Early treatment of hyperbilirubinemia and metabolic disorders.
5. Avoidance of asphyxia, anoxia, and serious infections in both the prenatal and postnatal periods.
6. Prevention of accidents, poisonings, and abuse or neglect.

Secondary prevention involves ameliorating a condition or mitigating its adverse effects. The physician's role is significant in the secondary area in early detection of developmental delay and referral for intervention for the child, and counseling, support, or assistance for the family.

SUMMARY AND CONCLUSION

Mental retardation is a serious problem with lifelong implications for the child and family. The causes are numerous, with social, medical, environmental, and psychological factors all relevant, alone and in combination. More mentally retarded individuals are now remaining in the community, and they require either specialized or general health care and treatment. Although the major required interventions are educational, the other important factors affecting prognosis are the types of social environment and stimulation the affected individual experiences, and the type and quality of health care offered. The physician must be attuned to early diagnosis and to treatment of associated medical problems, and should be well informed about resources available to help the patient. The physician is an important advocate for the patient's or client's needs, a counselor for the family, and a key contributor to prevention activities, the area with potentially the greatest long-range benefits.

DELAYED SEXUAL MATURATION AND SEXUAL PRECOCITY

By Frank B. Diamond, Jr., M.D.
and Allen W. Root, M.D.
St. Petersburg, Florida

NORMAL SEXUAL MATURATION

Puberty or adolescence is the period of transition between the sexually immature and adult states of growth and reproductive capability. Marked changes in linear growth, body weight and composition, primary and secondary sexual characteristics, and function of the reproductive endocrine system occur during this phase of life. The physical changes of the secondary sexual characteristics as defined in the Tanner classification are shown in Table 1.

A number of hormonal changes precede and accompany the physical alterations of puberty (Tables 2 to 5). These may be listed as follows:

1. Serum concentrations of the adrenal androgens, dehydroepiandrosterone (DHEA) and its sulfate (DHAS), and androstenedione begin to increase between 6 and 8 years of age and increase steadily thereafter to adult values (the adrenarche).
2. Serum concentrations of luteinizing (LH) and follicle-stimulating hormones (FSH) begin to increase at 8 to 10 years. In girls the rise in FSH levels precedes the increase in LH values.
3. There is enhanced sleep-associated secretion of LH beginning in the late prepubertal period and continuing until late puberty in both sexes. In pubertal boys, serum testosterone concentrations also increase during sleep.
4. The secretion of LH becomes demonstrably episodic—i.e., LH is released irregularly and serum concentrations fluctuate rapidly. Episodic LH secretion may also be observed in prepubertal subjects when highly sensitive assays are utilized. In girls the secretion of LH and FSH becomes cyclic.
5. The biologic activity of circulating LH increases.
6. Administration of gonadotropin-releasing hormone (GnRH) results in increased LH secretory responsivity. GnRH-induced secretion of FSH in the female declines with advancing puberty. Infusion of GnRH demonstrates two pools of LH in the pubertal subject—an immediately releasable LH pool and a more slowly releasable pool.
7. There is decreasing inhibitory ("negative feedback") sensitivity to the gonadotropin-suppressing effects of gonadal sex steroids.
8. By midpuberty in girls a "positive feedback" effect of estrogens is demonstrable—i.e. administration of estrogen provokes LH release.
9. There are increasing serum concentrations of testosterone and estradiol.
10. In boys the testosterone secretory response to human chorionic gonadotropin (hCG) increases.
11. Serum concentrations of prolactin increase in girls during puberty as estrogen values rise.

DELAYED SEXUAL MATURATION

Puberty is considered delayed if sexual development has not begun by age 13 years in girls or 14 years in boys.

In 2.5 per cent of normal males, the onset of sexual development will be delayed more than 2 years after the usual age, and in 0.1 per cent the delay will be more than 3 years. In the male, the initial manifestation of puberty is enlargement of the testes to a length greater than 2 cm, which occurs on the average at approximately 11 years of age. If male genital development has not begun by 14 years, if it is incomplete more than 4.7 years after onset of puberty, or if Tanner genital stage V has not been reached by 17.1 years of age, evaluation is indicated (Table 1).

In the female, breast budding is the first physical sign of puberty and occurs on the average at 10.5

Table 1. Tanner Classification of Sexual Development

	Age at Onset (Years)	
A. Stages of Male Genital Development	*Mean*	*Range*
I Prepubertal: testicular length less than 2 cm	—	—
II Testicular length more than 2 cm, less than 3.2 cm; enlargement and reddening of scrotal skin	11.6	9.5–13.8
III Testicular length more than 3.3 cm, less than 4.0 cm; further enlargement and thinning of scrotum, lengthening of penis	12.9	10.8–14.9
IV Testicular length more than 4.1 cm, less than 4.9 cm; darkening and enlargement of scrotum, increase in penile width, length, and glans size	13.8	11.7–15.8
V Adult: testicular length more than 5 cm; scrotum pigmented and thickened; penis of adult size and configuration	14.9	12.7–17.1

	Age at Onset (Years)	
B. Stages of Female Breast Development	*Mean*	*Range*
I Prepubertal	—	—
II Areolar widening, pigmentation, and subareolar breast tissue present	11.2	8.0–13.3
III Further breast enlargement	12.2	10.0–14.3
IV Further breast enlargement with mounding of areola above plane of breast in most	13.1	10.8–15.3
V Adult (variable size)	15.3	11.9–18.8

	Age at Onset (Years)			
	Boys		Girls	
C. Stages of Pubic Hair Growth	*Mean*	*Range*	*Mean*	*Range*
I Prepubertal (hair absent)	—	—	—	—
II Sparse, long, slightly curly and pigmented hair at the base of phallus or scrotum (boys) or on labia majora or mons veneris (girls)	13.4	11.2–15.6	11.7	9.3–14.1
III Increased quantity of coarsely pigmented, curled hair on mons veneris	13.9	11.9–15.0	12.4	10.2–14.6
IV Curled, coarse hair covering mons veneris	14.4	12.2–16.5	13.0	10.8–15.1
V Hair of adult quality and quantity covering entire mons veneris and medial aspect of thighs	15.2	13.0–17.3	14.4	12.2–16.7
VI Extension of hair growth up linea alba (boys)	—	—	—	—

Table 2. Gonadotropin Concentrations During Growth and Sexual Maturation*

	Serum iLH (mIU/ml)†		Serum iFSH (mIU/ml)†	
	Male	*Female*	*Male*	*Female*
Prepubertal Stage				
Birth–1 year	<1–60	<1–40	<1–12	<1–20
1–8 years	<1–6	<1–6	<1–6	<1–4
9–10 years	<1–10	<1–4	<1–10	2–8
11–12 years	<1–12	<1–9	2–12	3–11
13–14 years	3–15	3–10	3–15	3–15
15–20 years	5–25	4–25	5–20	4–20
Pubertal Stage				
I	<1–5	<1–6	<1–5	2–4
II	<1–8	<1–9	<1–10	2–10
III	3–15	3–15	3–15	3–15
IV	3–20	3–20	3–20	3–20
V	5–25	4–25	5–20	4–20
Adult	5–25	4–25	5–20	4–20

*Modified from Reiter, E., and Root, A.: *Children Are Different*. Columbus, Ohio Ross Laboratories, 1978, p. 73.
†Range.
Abbreviations: iLH= Immunoreactive luteinizing hormone; iFSH= immunoreactive follicle-stimulating hormone.

Table 3. Gonadotropin Secretion Following Intravenous Bolus Injection of Gonadotropin-Releasing Hormone*

Developmental Stage	Serum iLH (mIU/ml)		Serum iFSH (mIU/ml)	
	Basal	*Peak*	*Basal*	*Peak*
Prepubertal				
Male	1.8 ± 0.2†	4.0 ± 0.3	2.1 ± 0.3	5.1 ± 0.6
Female	1.9 ± 0.4	4.2 ± 0.7	2.5 ± 0.4	9.3 ± 3.2
Pubertal				
Male	3.1 ± 0.3	12.5 ± 0.8	3.0 ± 0.2	4.6 ± 0.3
Female	4.0 ± 0.6	10.9 ± 2.0	4.9 ± 0.6	10.6 ± 2.1
Adult				
Male	12 ± 1.5	96 ± 7.5	9.0 ± 1.2	19 ± 1.8
Female				
Midfollicular	5–15	30–90	8–12	15–20
Midluteal	10–50	140–220	6–10	15–20

*Modified from Reiter, E., and Root, A.: *Children Are Different*. Columbus, Ohio, Ross Laboratories, 1978, p. 73.
†Mean ± SE.
‡Range.
Abbreviations: iLH= Immunoreactive luteinizing hormone; iFSH= immunoreactive follicle-stimulating hormone.

Table 4. Serum Sex Steroid Concentrations During Growth and Sexual Maturation in the Male*

	Testosterone (ng/dl)	Androstene-dione (ng/dl)	Estrone (pg/ml)	Estradiol (pg/ml)	Dehydroepi-androsterone (ng/dl)	Dehydroepiandro-sterone Sulfate (μg/dl)
Age (Years)						
2–3	< 20				< 60	< 40
4–5		< 50				
6–7	10–30		< 20	< 10	20–132	10–60
8–9	< 20–30	60–70			20–316	10–150
10–11	< 20–60	30–80			40–480	25–200
12–13	< 20–250	60–90	15–50	< 30	60–620	50–250
14–15	40–620	85–140		5–40	135–775	75–250
Genital Stage					*Pubic Hair Stage*	
I	< 20		< 20		25–290	20–260
II	< 20–85	60	15–40	< 10	50–260	40–475
III	50–330		20–50		120–600	40–470
IV	135–530	40		10–20		
V	290–560	80	30–50	15–30	175–650	60–390
Adult	300–800	100–180	15–50		200–700	100–600

* Adapted from Reiter, E., and Root, A.: Med. Clin. North Am., 59:1289, 1975.

years. Breast growth is usually complete 4.0 years after initiation, but as many as 9 years may elapse. Pubic hair growth is usually complete within 2.5 years after onset, but 3.1 years may elapse. Sixteen per cent of girls develop pubic hair before breast growth begins. Menarche occurs after the time of peak height velocity has passed and corresponds with breast stage IV in 60 per cent of girls. In 99 per cent of females, menarche occurs within 5 years after onset of breast development. The hormonal changes of puberty are listed in Tables 2 to 5.

Causes of Delayed Sexual Development

Constitutional delay in growth and development (Table 6) is a variant of the normal growth pattern and is by far the most common form of delayed adolescence encountered by the clinician. It occurs in both males and females, although physicians tend to see more boys than girls with this growth and maturational pattern. This is probably due to social factors and pressures, which seem to bear more heavily on the male. Hypogonadism may be due to decreased synthesis or secretion of hypothalamic GnRH or pituitary gonadotropins (secondary hypogonadism or hypogonadotropic hypogonadism), or to gonadal dysfunction (primary hypogonadism or hypergonadotropic hypogonadism).

Constitutional Delay in Growth and Development

Individuals with constitutional delay in growth and development are those whose timing of pubertal events is shifted to later years. This pattern of growth is often familial, with similar growth and developmental histories being elicited from parents or other family members. The clinical presentation is characterized by short stature, normal growth velocity, absent or very early sexual development, bone age retarded within 75 per cent of chronological age, and absence of symptoms of systemic or endocrine disease. The diagnosis of constitutional delay in growth and development is a diagnosis of exclusion, and it is necessary to follow these patients to be certain that the

Table 5. Serum Sex Steroid Concentrations During Growth and Sexual Maturation in the Female*

	Estrone (pg/ml)	Estradiol (pg/ml)	Testosterone (ng/dl)	Androstenedione (ng/dl)	Dehydroepi-androsterone (ng/dl)	Dehydroepiandro-sterone Sulfate (μg/dl)
Age (Years)						
1–7	< 20	< 10	< 20	< 80	< 100	< 50
8–10	< 30	< 10	< 30	40–120	180–300	10–100
10–12	20–67	10–200	10–65		150–600	25–150
12–14	20–177	10–270	20–80	40–150	150–700	50–150
14–16	20–100	15–400	20–85		200–700	125–225
Breast Stage					*Pubic Hair Stage*	
I	< 20	< 10	< 20		< 100	10–250
II	10–53	5–60	< 20–65	< 100	< 400	30–180
III	15–90	10–125	20–80			30–370
IV	15–180	10–270	20–85	40–150	800	50–340
V	30–80	15–400				
Adult	20–180	15–400	< 20–85	40–180	200–700	60–390

* Adapted from Reiter, E., and Root, A.: Med. Clin. North Am., 59:1289, 1975.

Table 6. Causes of Delayed Adolescence

I. Constitutional delay in growth and development
II. Hypogonadotropic hypogonadism
  A. Hypothalamic pituitary disorders
    1. Isolated deficiency of GnRH
    2. Isolated deficiency of growth hormone
    3. With multiple anterior pituitary hormone deficiencies
    4. With congenital anomalies—anosmia, midline defects, cryptorchidism, Prader-Willi syndrome, Laurence-Moon-Biedl syndrome, Friedreich's ataxia, congenital adrenal hypoplasia
    5. Trauma
    6. Post-encephalitis/meningitis
    7. Infiltrative disease (histiocytosis X)
    8. Tumor—hypothalamic, pituitary
      a. Craniopharyngioma
      b. Optic glioma
      c. Prolactinoma
      d. Chromophobe adenoma
    9. Radiation
    10. Aplasia, hypoplasia of pituitary
    11. Isolated deficiency of LH and/or FSH
    12. Biologically inactive LH
    13. Hypophysitis
    14. Repetitive transfusions, hemochromatosis
    15. Idiopathic
  B. Functional gonadotropin deficiency
    1. Chronic systemic or endocrinologic disease
      a. Cardiovascular—congenital, acquired heart disease
      b. Respiratory—asthma, cystic fibrosis
      c. Gastrointestinal—inflammatory bowel disease
      d. Renal—renal failure, renal tubular acidosis
      e. Endocrine—hypothyroidism, glucocorticoid excess, uncontrolled diabetes mellitus
      f. Collagen-vascular—lupus erythematosus, rheumatoid arthritis
    2. Emotional disorders
    3. Drugs
      a. Cannabis
      b. Cimetidine
III. Hypergonadotropic hypogonadism
  A. Gonadal abnormalities
    1. Congenital
      a. Gonadal dysgenesis (Turner's syndrome)
      b. Seminiferous tubule dysgenesis (Klinefelter's syndrome)
      c. Anorchia
      d. 17-α-hydroxylase deficiency (female)
      e. Galactosemia
      f. Myotonia dystrophica
      g. Pseudo-Turner's syndrome
      h. Prader-Willi syndrome
      i. Marinesco-Sjögren's syndrome (ataxia, cataract, mental retardation)
      j. Primary resistance to gonadotropins
    2. Acquired
      a. Oophoritis—isolated or with other autoimmune disease
      b. Orchitis
      c. Trauma, torsion, surgical excision, or vascular insult
      d. Antimetabolites
      e. Radiation
      f. Neoplasms
IV. Hyperprolactinemia
V. Hyperandrogenism (female), PCOS
VI. Uterine and vaginal disorders
  A. Absence of uterus, vagina, or both
  B. Imperforate hymen
  C. End-organ insensitivity to androgens (testicular feminization)

Abbreviations: PCOS = Polycystic ovarian syndrome; GnRH = gonadotropin-releasing hormone; LH = luteinizing hormone; FSH = follicle-stimulating hormone.

anticipated pattern of growth and development occurs. If the patient fails to grow and mature as the bone age reaches 12 to 13 years, further evaluation is indicated.

Hypogonadotropic Hypogonadism

Decreased secretion of LH and FSH (hypogonadotropic hypogonadism) may result from isolated absence of GnRH. Congenital central nervous system anomalies, such as septo-optic dysplasia, agenesis of the olfactory bulb (Kallmann's syndrome), and other midline craniofacial deformities, may be associated with sexual infantilism. In Kallmann's syndrome, end-organ resistance to the action of gonadotropins or a primary Leydig cell defect, or both, may also be present. Hypoxic or traumatic perinatal events may result in hypogonadism presenting in later life. A variety of insults to the hypothalamus or pituitary such as trauma, radiation, infections (in utero or postnatally acquired) or infiltrative disease may impair gonadotropin secretion. Tumors of the hypothalamus, such as optic gliomas, craniopharyngiomas, pinealomas, or germinomas and astrocytomas, interfere with GnRH release. Pituitary tumors may destroy the gonadotropin-producing cells. Hyperprolactinemia presents with hypogonadism or galactorrhea, or both, in both sexes. Decreased secretion of LH and FSH may occur as isolated defects or in association with other anterior pituitary hormone deficiencies, most commonly growth hormone deficiency. In patients with isolated deficiency of growth hormone, puberty is delayed; puberty occurs spontaneously at an appropriate bone age (11 to 12 years). Isolated deficiency of either LH or FSH probably reflects a defect in synthesis of the specific beta-gonadotropin subunit. A male patient with normal immunoreactive but biologically inactive LH has also been reported.

Inherited disorders associated with deficiencies of gonadotropin secretion of probable hypothalamic origin include familial hypogonadism with ataxia (X-linked and autosomal dominant), Friedreich's ataxia (X-linked), and cytomegalic congenital adrenal hypoplasia (X-linked). Three syndromes with obesity and hypomentia have associated hypogonadotropic hypogonadism. These are the Prader-Willi syndrome (hypotonia, carbohydrate intolerance, growth retardation, small hands and feet, autosomal recessive inheritance), the Laurence-Moon-Biedl syndrome (retinitis pigmentosa, polydactyly, X-linked recessive inheritance), and the male-limited X-linked recessive syndrome of gynecomastia and short stature. Occasionally a patient with Prader-Willi syndrome will manifest hypergonadotropic hypogonadism.

Poor nutritional states may also affect hypothalamic function and impair release of LH and FSH. This may be due to anorexia nervosa or simple weight loss or to underlying systemic illness, such as cystic fibrosis, severe congenital heart disease, or chronic inflammatory bowel disease. Decline in body weight greater than 20 per cent below ideal weight depresses LH and FSH secretion. Delayed menarche and amenorrhea also occur in women who have normal body weight but decreased fat content relative to lean body mass, such as ballet dancers, marathon runners, and dedicated joggers. There is reported to be a 5-month delay in menarche for each year of athletic training before menarche. Gonadotropin secretion and cyclic functioning may also be inhibited by emotional factors, even without weight loss. The emotional stress of leaving home to attend summer camp or school is often associated with amenorrhea ("boarding school amenorrhea") and may result from altered cerebral-hypothalamic neurotransmitter synthesis or function. Severe zinc deficiency will also delay pubertal development.

In young adult males, reduced testosterone levels and impaired spermatogenesis may result from cannabis abuse. Long-term ingestion of cimetidine also has been reported to depress LH levels while increasing prolactin values. Insulin-dependent diabetes or primary hypothyroidism developing in early adolescence may delay the onset of adolescence. Amenorrhea associated with hyperthyroidism is probably the result of accelerated catabolism of gonadotropins. Hematologic causes of delayed puberty include sickle cell anemia, which is associated with hyperzincuria and low body zinc stores, and hemosiderosis due to repetitive transfusion for thalassemia major or other chronic form of anemia.

Hypergonadotropic Hypogonadism

In patients with hypergonadotropic hypogonadism, a primary gonadal defect is present, and greatly increased serum and urinary levels of LH and FSH reflect loss of the suppressive mechanisms controlling gonadotropin secretion. Klinefelter's syndrome in males and gonadal dysgenesis and its variants (Turner's syndrome) in females result from chromosomal abnormalities. Other gonadal insults include infection (mumps orchitis), surgery, exposure to drugs or toxins (cyclophosphamide), radiation, or autoimmune disease. Anorchia is present in males with the "vanishing testes syndrome." Primary gonadal dysfunction occurs in patients with myotonica dystrophica and galactosemia. In females, deficiency of the adrenal enzyme 17-α-hydroxylase results in sexual infantilism because of inability to synthesize the sex steroids and in hypertension, presumably due to excessive mineralocorticoid synthesis. The polycystic ovarian syndrome (PCOS), previously thought to occur in the third and fourth decades, is now being recognized in adolescent and occasionally in preadolescent females, who present with signs of androgen excess—precocious sexual hair growth, acne, and hirsutism (hair appearing on the face, chest, abdomen, thighs, upper arms, and back)—or arrested pubertal development. In one study, virtually all patients with primary amenorrhea and Tanner stage V breast development had PCOS. LH concentrations are modestly elevated while FSH values are normal in such girls. Circulating LH levels may also be elevated in patients with isolated FSH deficiency.

End-organ insensitivity to testosterone (the syndrome of testicular feminization and its variants) often presents with primary amenorrhea in phenotypic females (genotypic males), and may be present in subtle form in some phenotypic males with desultory sexual development and gynecomastia.

Clinical and Laboratory Manifestations

Genitalia and Growth

In the newborn male, prenatal gonadotropin deficiency is often manifested by small external genitalia, micropenis, and cryptorchidism. When associated with hypoglycemia these findings may indicate deficiencies of growth hormone and corticotropin, which may be life-threatening if not recognized and treated.

During childhood, gonadotropin deficiency is not generally apparent. Penile size may be below norms for age; linear growth rate is usually normal, but bone age may be delayed. In the hypogonadotropic girl, the genitalia remain infantile and there is no breast development, uterine growth, or menses. When growth hormone as well as gonadotropins is affected, there is usually decreased growth velocity, with consequent extreme short stature. Patients with isolated deficiency of gonadotropins often are of normal height for chronological age, whereas patients with constitutional delay in growth and development are short, with height age approximately equal to bone age. In both conditions, growth rate does not increase at the time of expected puberty owing to the lack of the adolescent growth spurt. However, the child with constitutional delay in growth and development eventually begins sexual maturation and attains a pubertal growth spurt and peak height velocity at the appropriate bone age of 14 years.

Central Nervous System Tumors or Other Lesions

Clinically, central nervous system mass lesions present with headaches, visual disturbances, weakness, incoordination, symptoms of diabetes insipidus, or growth retardation. Visual field defects, optic atrophy, or papilledema may be found on physical examination. Craniopharyngioma, a common neoplasm associated with sexual infantilism, is usually suprasellar but may be completely within the sella. Extrasellar tumors that arise in or impinge upon the hypothalamus may produce diabetes insipidus and either sexual infantilism or precocious puberty. Prolactin-secreting adenomas occur most commonly in the later teen-age years and present with primary or secondary amenorrhea. In patients with Hand-Schüller-Christian disease (histiocytosis X) there is often diabetes insipidus, loose or absent teeth, and cystic areas in flat bones and mandible. Infiltration of the orbit may lead to exophthalmos; mastoiditis and temporal bone involvement may produce chronic otitis media with drainage. In septo-optic dysplasia, searching eye movements suggest blindness, while the optic nerve itself is small, pale, and dysplastic. Associated hypothalamic defects may result in growth hormone deficiency, diabetes insipidus, and deficient production of corticotropin, thyrotropin, and gonadotropins. Other congenital midline defects associated with hypothalamic dysfunction form a continuum from complete dysraphism and holoprosencephaly to cleft lip and cleft palate.

Kallmann's Syndrome

In Kallmann's syndrome, anosmia or hyposmia results from abnormality of olfactory lobe function associated with hypothalamic deformities and GnRH deficiency. Affected individuals often do not notice the impaired sense of smell, and testing with graded dilutions of pure scents may be necessary. Associated findings include cleft lip or cleft palate, shortened metacarpals, and cryptorchidism. The syndrome may be transmitted as an X-linked dominant characteristic with variable penetrance and occurs in both males and females. Males with cerebellar ataxia and deficient gonadotropin production have been reported in kindreds with X-linked inheritance, and an X-linked form of congenital adrenal hypoplasia with sexual infantilism has been described. Isolated LH deficiency causes deficient testosterone production in the presence of spermatogenesis (the fertile eunuch syndrome). In the presence of isolated absence of LH secretion in the female, estradiol levels are low and there is primary amenorrhea and minimal breast development.

Isolated Growth Hormone Deficiency

In patients with idiopathic isolated growth hormone deficiency there is often delayed puberty; such patients ultimately exhibit spontaneous pubertal developmental without exogenous sex steroid therapy when skeletal maturation approaches that characteristic of 12 years. Patients with associated gonadotropin deficiency do not undergo puberty even when their bone age advances to the pubertal stage as a result of treatment.

Effects of Malnutrition

The child in whom nutritional deprivation may be an important factor in a delayed pattern of growth and development is one whose body weight is more than 10 per cent below that weight approximate for height. Anorexia nervosa is a disorder occurring primarily in adolescent girls, characterized by severe weight loss (the patient usually is more than 25 per cent underweight for height), distorted body image, food avoidance (or induced vomiting), and primary or secondary amenorrhea. Cessation of menses may precede the onset of weight loss and may persist for months after renewed weight gain, indicating the role of factors other than weight loss in this process. Other findings include hyperactivity, cold intolerance, constipation, hypotension, hypertrichosis (manifestations of hypotriiodothyroninemia), and occasionally peripheral edema when the patient is severely hypoproteinemic.

In other chronic systemic diseases it is necessary to distinguish the effects of malnutrition that can produce functional hypogonadotropic hypogonadism from the primary effect of the disease. If adequate nutrition and body weight are restored in patients with chronic infections or chronic lung or renal disease, gonadotropin secretion usually resumes.

Signs of Hypergonadotropic Hypogonadism

The clinical manifestations and course of patients with hypergonadotropic hypogonadism depend on the underlying cause. The diagnosis of Klinefelter's syndrome is commonly made at the age of expected puberty, although the testes are abnormally small even prior to adolescence. Body proportions are eunuchoid with inappropriately low upper to lower and height to span ratios for age. Patients tend to be tall because of continued linear growth in the presence of delayed epiphyseal closure. Testes are characteristically small and firm, but the penis may be of normal size. Pubic hair may be normal or reduced in quantity and distribution. Although these patients are commonly slim, truncal obesity may develop, and gynecomastia is present in 50 per cent of cases. Behavioral problems are seen with increased frequency; in addition, mental retardation occurs in about 5 per cent of patients with this syndrome. There may be reduced libido and impotence, but many patients mature normally and present in early adulthood for evaluation of infertility (see article on Chromosomal Abnormalities).

Females with gonadal dysgenesis (Turner's syndrome, 45X) are small, with a characteristic phenotype consisting of typical facies (micrognathia, epicanthal folds, fish mouth), highly arched palate, webbed neck, low-set hairline, shield chest with hypoplastic areolae, increased carrying angle, shortened metacarpals and metatarsals, excessive nevi, and left-sided cardiac lesions (see article on Chromosomal Abnormalities). In the newborn, the diagnosis may be suggested by the presence of prominent webbing of the neck or peripheral lymphedema (Bonnevie-Ullrich syndrome). As a child, the patient is short and the pubertal height spurt does not occur. Bone age is usually normal until the age of adolescence and then fails to progress. Because of the absence of functional ovaries, primary amenorrhea and sexual infantilism occur. However, girls with variants of the syndrome may have no clinical stigmata, normal height, pubertal feminization, menses, and even fertility. Females with sex chromosome mosaicism (45X/46XX and others) often have fewer clinical manifestations. Similarly, patients with structural abnormalities of the X chromosome (deletion, isochromosome) may have variable clinical findings of Turner's syndrome. Lack of genetic material from either the long or the short arm of the X chromosome causes decreased gonadal function, whereas loss of all or part of the short arm leads to the physical stigmata of Turner's syndrome. The 45X/46XY pattern of sex chromosome mosaicism (mixed gonadal dysgenesis) varies in its clinical presentation from the classic Turner's syndrome to ambiguous genitalia to phenotypic male, and gonadal tissue may range from streak gonads to mixed gonadal tissue to functioning testes. Patients with an abnormality of sexual development associated with a Y chromosome are at increased risk for neoplastic degeneration of dysgenetic gonads into gonadoblastomas, which may secrete either testosterone or estrogen. The development of sexual characteristics in a previously sexually infantile teen-ager with this variant of gonadal dysgenesis may indicate the occurrence of a gonadoblastoma and should be evaluated.

Pure gonadal dysgenesis refers to a condition in

which the patient is phenotypically female, with sexual infantilism, eunuchoid habitus, streak gonads, and 46XX or 46XY sex chromosome composition. Incomplete forms of 46XX pure gonadal dysgenesis with desultory menses followed by secondary amenorrhea may occur. Some familial cases have been associated with sensorineural deafness. In some patients with 46XY gonadal dysgenesis, the dysgenetic gonad may produce testosterone, which causes slight clitoromegaly at birth and later virilization at puberty. Incomplete forms may present with ambiguous genitalia.

The "pseudo-Turner syndrome" occurs in both boys and girls. These patients have a phenotype typical of Turner's syndrome, variable gonadal function, right-sided heart lesions, and often normal sex chromosome composition.

Gonadal Disorders

Autoimmune oophoritis may lead to pubertal failure and secondary amenorrhea in early adolescence. Signs of autoimmune disease, such as vitiligo, alopecia, and candidiasis, may be present. The condition may be associated with clinical findings suggesting Addison's disease, Hashimoto's thyroiditis, or pernicious anemia. Radiation of the ovaries or testes may result in gonadal dysfunction in patients with abdominal or pelvic neoplasms or leukemia. Cyclophosphamide treatment of the nephrotic syndrome in prepubertal males has caused Sertoli and germ cell damage. Ovarian failure has been associated with galactosemia (galactose is toxic to the developing ovary), ataxia-telangiectasia, DiGeorge syndrome, and cerebellar ataxia. In germinal cell aplasia (the Sertoli-cell-only syndrome) puberty is not delayed, but FSH values are elevated and oligospermia is present. A defect in ovarian function has been reported to result from end organ insensitivity to gonadotropins. This defect is now recognized, along with thyroid insensitivity to thyroid-stimulating hormone as part of the syndrome of pseudohypoparathyroidism. Gonadotropin levels are elevated and an exaggerated LH secretory response to GnRH is present. Histologically, no growing follicles are present in the ovary.

Bioactive and immunoreactive LH levels are moderately elevated in about half of adolescent women with PCOS. This is a heterogeneous group of disorders presenting with oligomenorrhea or amenorrhea, obesity, acne, and male pattern hirsutism. This may progress to frank virilization with clitoromegaly, deepening of the voice, and male pattern muscular development. In contrast to findings in adults, palpable ovaries are rarely present on pelvic examination in teen-agers.

Phenotypic Abnormalities

Sexual infantilism occurs in girls with 17-α-hydroxylase deficiency because of their inability to synthesize estrogens. A eunuchoid habitus is present. A genotypic male with 17-α-hydroxylase deficiency will present with a female phenotype or ambiguous genitalia and sexual infantilism. Associated cortisol deficiency and increased mineralocorticoid secretion in this condition lead to hypertension, decreased potassium concentrations, and metabolic alkalosis.

The phenotypic male with XY karyotype and without palpable testes may have intra-abdominal testes or, alternatively, the vanishing testes syndrome, in which no testes are found at laparotomy. The presence of male phenotype and internal duct structure suggests that functional testes were present during fetal life but then degenerated. Cryptorchidism may be due to a primary testicular defect or to decreased gonadotropin secretion. Cryptorchid testes, even if replaced in the scrotum, have the same small but definite risk of malignant change as do abdominal testes.

Diagnostic Evaluation

History and Physical Examination

Evaluation of the patient with delayed adolescence begins with a thorough historical review and physical examination (Fig. 1). In the history the patterns of growth and sexual maturation are determined, and evidence for a perinatal, postnatal, or later insult or a systemic or familial disease is sought. The physical examination may disclose findings characteristic of a disorder such as gonadal dysgenesis, Klinefelter's syndrome, or hypothyroidism. The stages of sexual development (breast, genitalia, pubic hair) are identified. The degree of skeletal maturation is then assessed. In the patient with an unremarkable history, with normal growth velocity, and with bone age approximately equal to height age and not less than 75 per cent of chronological age, the most likely diagnosis is constitutional delay in growth and development, particularly if there are physical signs consistent with early puberty (breast budding, testicular enlargement). The diagnosis is confirmed by continued growth and sexual maturation while the patient is seen at follow-up visits.

Laboratory Tests

Additional laboratory and roentgenographic studies are indicated in the prepubertal patient (1) who is 14 to 15 years of age, (2) whose bone age is greater than 12 years, (3) whose height is more than 3 standard deviations (SD) below the mean for age, (4) where sexual development, once initiated, has not progressed normally or has arrested, or (5) who is suspected of having a systemic or endocrinologic disorder. Screening tests for underlying systemic disease include blood count, urinalysis, sedimentation rate, and determinations of thyroxine, creatinine, albumin, and electrolyte levels. Patients with inflammatory bowel disease, for example, often present with delayed growth and development prior to the onset of gastrointestinal symptoms; these children have increased sedimentation rates and decreased levels of serum albumin.

Tests for Hypogonadotropic Hypogonadism

In patients of pubertal bone age, elevated basal levels of LH and FSH differentiate patients with primary gonadal disorders from those with hypogonadotropic hypogonadism due to dysfunction of the central ner-

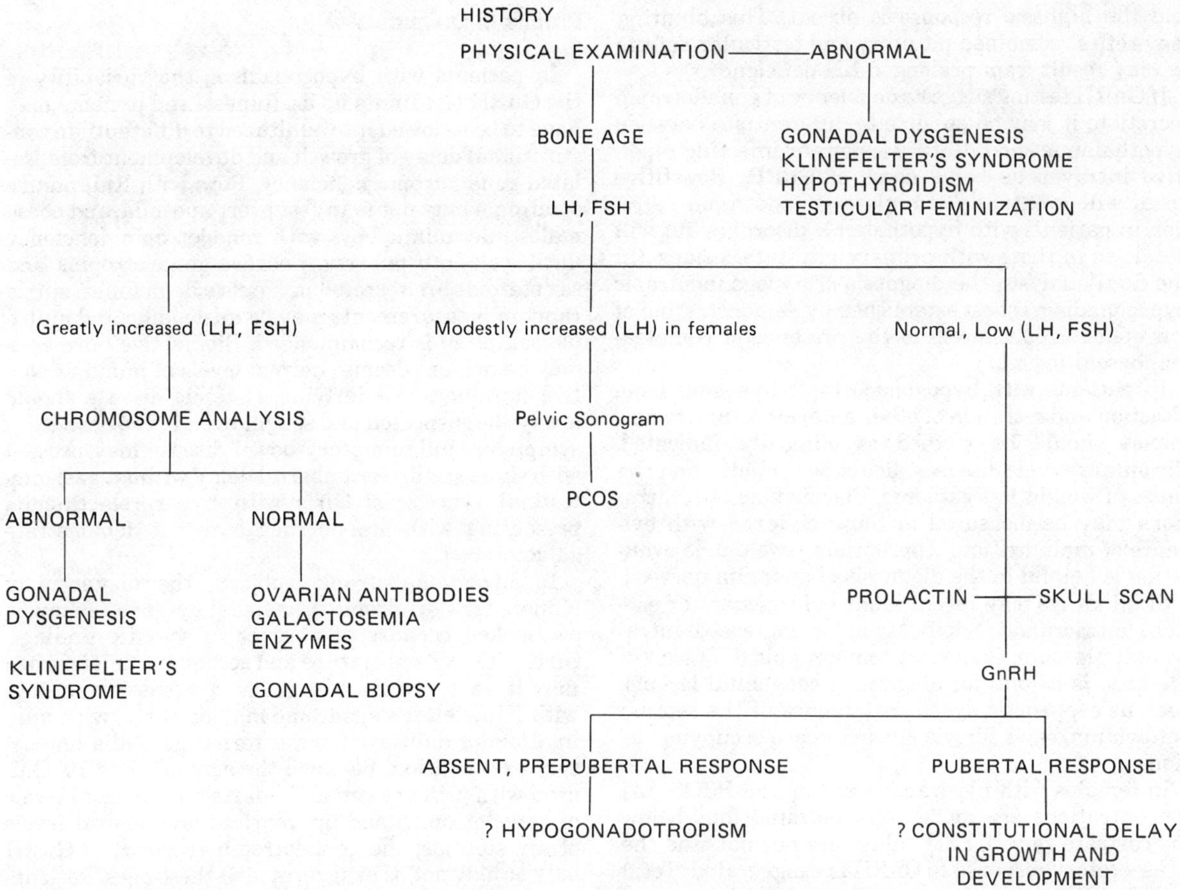

Figure 1. Evaluation of the patient with delayed adolescence. LH = Luteinizing hormone; FSH = follicle-stimulating hormone; PCOS = polycystic ovarian syndrome; GnRH = gonadotropin-releasing hormone.

vous system, hypothalamus, or pituitary. The patient with hypogonadotropic hypogonadism has persistently low basal LH and FSH values in serum and urine as well as decreased gonadal sex steroid levels. Patients with constitutional delay in growth and development also have low gonadotropin values for chronological age. Differentiation between the latter two conditions may be difficult, requiring prolonged observation and repeated study. Because of the pulsatile secretory pattern of gonadotropins and sex steroids, frequent sampling over several hours may be helpful in determining basal gonadotropin and sex steroid levels. The pubertal sleep-associated surge of gonadotropins, which occurs in early and midpubertal subjects, is absent in hypogonadotropic children. Serum levels of the adrenal androgens dehydroepiandrosterone (DHEA) and its sulfated conjugate (DHAS) are appropriate for chronological age in hypogonadotropic children; they are low for chronological age but appropriate for bone age in patients with constitutional delay in growth and development, and they are very low in patients with hypopituitarism associated with corticotropin deficiency.

The LH and FSH secretory responses to GnRH administration (Table 3) are blunted or absent in hypogonadotropic individuals. In the child with constitutional delay of growth and development, GnRH-evoked LH and particularly FSH secretion either is appropriate for the normal prepubertal subject if there is no clinical sign of sexual development or approximates the early pubertal response even if only minimal pubertal changes are present. However, considerable variability exists in the normal prepubertal GnRH response. In addition, as many as 30 per cent of patients with isolated gonadotropin deficiency may have normal gonadotropin response to a single, acutely administered GnRH bolus. Thus, neither absent nor normal gonadotropin responses to GnRH provide absolute certainty of subsequent normal or abnormal gonadotropin secretion in adulthood. In obese, sexually immature males, an absent or blunted gonadotropin secretory response to GnRH is not diagnostic of gonadotropin deficiency even with skeletal age of 12 years or greater. In such patients, prolonged observation often reveals progressive sexual maturation in the absence of any significant weight loss. The testosterone secretory response to GnRH infusion may be helpful diagnostically. In patients with constitutional delay in growth and development, testosterone levels increase several-fold after GnRH administration; in hypogonadotropic subjects, testosterone concentrations do not change. The testosterone secretory response to human chorionic gonadotropin may also be blunted in patients with hypogonadotropism, and the biphasic response is absent. This blunting may reflect combined pituitary and testicular defects or may result from prolonged LH deficiency.

If GnRH testing suggests deficiency of gonadotropin secretion, it may be possible to differentiate between hypothalamic and pituitary lesions by injecting repetitive intravenous bolus doses of GnRH. Repetitive doses will eventually stimulate gonadotropin secretion in patients with hypothalamic disorders but will not do so in those with primary pituitary lesions. (In the final analysis, the diagnosis of hypogonadotropic hypogonadism is best established by demonstration of low gonadotropin levels in the presence of complete epiphyseal fusion.)

In patients with hypogonadotropic hypogonadism, olfaction and secretion of other anterior pituitary hormones should be studied as clinically indicated. Chronic systemic diseases should be excluded and the cause of weight loss explored. Plasma zinc concentrations may be measured in those children with evidence of malnutrition. Appropriate psychiatric evaulation is helpful in the diagnosis of anorexia nervosa.

Skull x-rays may reveal sellar enlargement or erosion, intracranial calcification, or increased intracranial pressure. Computed tomographic (CT) scan of the head is helpful for diagnosing congenital lesions, such as septo-optic dysplasia (absence of the septum pellucidum), and for visualizing space-occupying lesions.

In females with hyperandrogenism and PCOS, LH concentrations are moderately elevated (but below the castrate range), FSH values are normal, and the LH secretory response to GnRH is exaggerated. Total and free testosterone concentrations and levels of other androgens are often elevated while the level of sex hormone–binding globulin (testosterone/estradiol–binding globulin) is low. Pelvic sonography often, but not always, reveals an echogenic pattern consistent with PCOS.

Basal concentrations of prolactin are increased in patients with prolactin-secreting adenomas (see article on Hyperprolactinemia). Roentgenographic studies (CT and tomograms) of the sella turcica may reveal an adenoma, but often differentiation of adenoma from functional hyperprolactinemia may be difficult. Secondary or drug-induced causes of increased prolactin secretion must be sought in the history.

Tests for Hypergonadotropic Hypogonadism

The diagnosis of Turner's and Klinefelter's syndromes may be suspected clinically and confirmed by abnormal sex chromatin patterns on buccal smears (negative in phenotypic females, positive in phenotypic males) and by karyotype analysis. Serum LH and FSH concentrations are in the castrate range in patients over 12 years of age. In other sexually immature patients without obvious somatic abnormalities, serum LH and FSH levels may be high. Often sex chromosome mosaicism will be found in these patients. In other patients, pelvic sonogram, laparoscopy, and biopsy of gonadal tissue may be required for final diagnosis. Antiovarian antibodies should be measured in the girl with suspected autoimmune disease.

Pitfalls in Diagnosis

In patients with hypogonadism, the variability of the GnRH test limits its usefulness, and patients may have to be followed into adulthood to differentiate constitutional delay of growth and development from isolated gonadotropin deficiency. Boys with Kallmann's syndrome may not manifest overt anosmia, and obese males may mimic boys with gonadotropin deficiency until well into puberty. Because gonadotropins and sex steroids are secreted in a pulsatile manner, single random measurements may be misleading and multiple sampling is recommended. Bioinactive hormones may be present despite normal levels of immunoreactive hormones. Underlying systemic disease should always be suspected and sought even in the absence of symptoms. Inflammatory bowel disease may present with short stature or pubertal delay without gastrointestinal symptoms. Girls with hyperprolactinemia presenting with amenorrhea may not demonstrate galactorrhea.

In hypergonadotropic subjects the diagnosis of Klinefelter's syndrome or gonadal dysgenesis may be overlooked because of absence of somatic findings. Girls with normal stature and secondary amenorrhea may have a variant of gonadal dysgenesis and boys with Klinefelter's syndrome may be obese, with minimal abnormalities of the external genitalia on cursory examination. Between the ages of 4 and 10, children with primary gonadal failure have normal levels of gonadotropins and appropriate prepubertal levels of sex steroids; the gonadotropin response to GnRH may or may not be exaggerated at these ages. Patients with PCOS often present with normal testosterone levels, but owing to decreased levels of sex hormone-binding globulin free testosterone levels are usually elevated. Although such patients may be hirsute, no obvious physical findings may be present initially. PCOS is a more common cause of aberrations of adolescent development in the female than is generally recognized.

SEXUAL PRECOCITY

Sexual precocity is present when any sign of sexual development occurs before 8 years in the girl or 9 years in the boy (more than 2.5 SD below the mean). *Isosexual precocity* is abnormally early sexual development consistent with the child's phenotype, whereas *heterosexual precocity* is sexual development at variance with phenotype. *True and complete isosexual precocity* implies premature maturation of the hypothalamic-pituitary-gonadal axis and may be idiopathic or due to congenital or acquired lesions of the central nervous system (Table 7.) *Pseudoprecocious puberty* is sexual development occurring independently of the normal mechanisms regulating the hypothalamic-pituitary-gonadal axis. It is associated with excessive gonadotropin, androgen, or estrogen secretion by gonads, adrenals, or neoplasms. *Incomplete isosexual precocity* refers to isolated pubertal changes such as breast development (premature thelarche) or pubic hair growth (premature pubarche). *Premature thelarche* with evidence of mild intermittent estrogenization is sometimes termed premature gonadarche.

Table 7. Causes of Isosexual Precocity

I. True and complete isosexual precocity
  A. Idiopathic
  B. Familial: Male-limited
  C. Congenital anomalies
    1. Septo-optic dysplasia
    2. Hydrocephalus
  D. Tumors of the central nervous system
    1. Glioma of optic nerve or hypothalamus (neurofibromatosis)
    2. Astrocytoma
    3. Ependymoma
    4. Germinoma
    5. Teratoma (hCG-producing)
    6. Hamartoma
    7. Craniopharyngioma
    8. Suprasellar cysts
    9. Sarcoid granuloma
    10. Pinealoma
  E. Post-inflammatory: Meningitis, encephalitis, brain abscess
  F. Post-traumatic
  G. Other
    1. Polyostotic fibrous dysplasia (McCune-Albright syndrome)
    2. Tuberous sclerosis
    3. Silver syndrome
    4. Primary hypothyroidism
    5. Following late treatment of congenital adrenal hyperplasia
    6. Isolated LH secretion (?)

II. Pseudoprecocious puberty
  A. hCG-secreting tumors
    1. Hepatoma
    2. Chorioepithelioma (gonadal, extragonadal)
    3. Teratoma
  B. Gonadal
    1. Ovarian
      a. Granulosa or theca cell tumor
      b. Follicular luteal cysts
    2. Testicular
      a. Leydig cell tumor or hyperplasia
      b. Adrenal rest tumor
  C. Adrenal
    1. Congenital adrenal hyperplasia
    2. Adrenal neoplasm—virilizing or feminizing
  D. Iatrogenic, surreptitious, or drug-contaminated sex hormone or hCG administration

III. Incomplete isosexual precocity
  A. Premature thelarche
  B. Premature adrenarche

IV. Other
  A. Adolescent male gynecomastia
  B. Vaginitis, foreign body
  C. Vaginal or uterine neoplasm

Abbreviations: hCG = Human chorionic gonadotropin; LH = luteinizing hormone.

Premature pubarche with laboratory evidence of elevated adrenal androgen levels is referred to as premature adrenarche.

Etiology and Manifestations (Table 7)

True and Complete Isosexual Precocity

In true and complete isosexual precocity the secretory pattern of gonadotropins and sex steroids is within the pubertal range and a pubertal GnRH response is found. There is an associated adolescent growth spurt with advancement of bone age. In many girls with this aberration, no organic lesion of the central nervous system can be identified but nonspecific electroencephalographic abnormalities are common. However, in 50 per cent of boys with true and complete isosexual precocity, a central nervous system lesion or insult can be identified. This condition appears to represent premature decline in the sensitivity of the hypothalamus to the negative feedback or inhibitory effects of sex steroids upon the secretion of gonadotropins. Testicular enlargement under gonadotropin stimulation precedes other signs of puberty in boys, whereas breast development and enlargement of labia minora are the presenting signs in girls. The progression of puberty follows the normal pattern. Rarely, true precocious puberty may be familial.

True and complete isosexual precocity may also be due to disorders of the central nervous system that interrupt inhibitory input to the hypothalamus. These include lesions such as hydrocephalus, septo-optic dysplasia, head trauma, meningitis, brain abscess, encephalitis, suprasellar cysts, sarcoid or tuberculous granulomas, and various neoplasms. Sexual precocity as the presenting sign of tumors of the central nervous system is more common in boys than in girls. These tumors include optic and hypothalamic gliomas (some associated with neurofibromatosis), astrocytomas, ependymomas, craniopharyngiomas, cysts, and possibly GnRH-producing hypothalamic hamartomas. Hypothalamic teratomas may cause precocious puberty through mass effects or by the secretion of hCG. Pineal tumors may also cause sexual precocity. The incidence of sexual precocity is about three times greater in nonparenchymatous tumors than in parenchymous tumors of the pineal, suggesting that in such tumors sexual precocity may be due to the absence of a normal pineal inhibitory factor rather than to destructive effects upon inhibitory tracts. In fact, solid tumors of the pineal are often associated with delayed sexual maturation, particularly in boys. Pineal tumors (germinomas) may also secrete hCG. Central nervous system tumors may present with signs of increased intracranial pressure, headaches, visual disturbances, optic atrophy, or hydrocephalus. However, midline lesions may be asymptomatic, and sexual precocity may be the only clinical manifestation of such tumors.

Sexual precocity may occur as a primary abnormality of hypothalamic function, perhaps associated with hypersecretion of hypothalamic releasing factors in diseases such as the McCune-Albright syndrome, which consists of the triad of irregularly edged café au lait spots, polyostotic fibrous dysplasia, and isosexual precocity. There is also a high incidence of Cushing's syndrome, acromegaly, and hyperthyroidism in affected patients. The Silver syndrome is characterized by intrauterine growth retardation, short stature, hemihypertrophy, and sexual precocity. Precocious puberty may occur in patients with neurofibromatosis, perhaps because of the frequent association of this disease with lesions of the central nervous system. An autosomal dominant disorder with variable penetrance, neurofibromatosis is characterized by multiple smooth-edged café au lait spots, freckling of the axilla, cutaneous and deep neurofibromas, bone cysts, hemihypertrophy, and scoliosis. In patients with congenital adrenal hyperplasia, when diagnosis is delayed and the bone age is advanced at initiation of treatment, suppression of adrenal androgen production with glucocorticoids may be followed by activation of the hypothalamic-pituitary-gonadal axis and result in true and complete isosexual precocity in both sexes. Isolated increase in LH secretion associated with heterosexual precocity in the female and isosexual precocity in the male has been described.

Pseudoprecocious Puberty

Pseudoprecocious puberty is sexual development occurring independently of the normal mechanisms regulating the hypothalamic-pituitary-gonadal axis and may be isosexual or heterosexual.

Female Children. In asymptomatic prepubertal girls, small follicular cysts are common and may be related to intermittent elevation of FSH secretion. In some instances cysts may enlarge and elaborate sufficient estrogen to cause breast and nipple development and dulling of the vaginal mucosa. With cyst regression, withdrawal vaginal bleeding may occur and a pattern of involution and recurrence may rarely mimic normal menses. Larger cysts may be associated with plasma estrogen levels similar to those found with ovarian neoplasms. Granulosa or theca cell tumors of the ovary are rare causes of pseudoprecocious puberty. In many instances, these neoplasms are palpable on bimanual examination. Less commonly, tumors such as hepatomas, hepatoblastomas, teratomas, or teratocarcinomas secrete an hCG-like material that directly stimulates gonadal sex hormone release. In addition to secreting hCG, choriocarcinomas increase estrogen levels by converting adrenal androgens such as DHEA and DHAS to estrogens. Gonadoblastomas associated with streak gonads, lipoid ovarian tumors, cystadenomas, ovarian carcinomas, hilus cell tumors, and adrenal rests are all capable of secreting estrogens or androgens. Primary hypothyroidism is frequently associated with sexual precocity in both sexes. In these patients, LH and prolactin levels may be elevated and regress after treatment with thyroxine. This syndrome is characterized by breast development and galactorrhea in girls, testicular enlargement in boys, growth arrest, and scant growth of sexual hair. In hypothyroid females, luteal cysts may occur as a result of prolonged ovarian exposure to LH, while galactorrhea has been attributed to hyperprolactinemia, a consequence of unopposed secretion of hypothalamic thyrotropin-releasing hormone (TRH). In experimental models of hypothyroidism, prolactin increases ovarian estrogen responsiveness to hCG, presumably by induction of ovarian LH receptors, suggesting a primary role of prolactin in the sexual prococity of hypothyroidism. Prolonged biologic activity of the gonadotropins in hypothyroidism may also be attributed to decreased catabolism of LH and FSH due to the hypometabolic state.

In females with heterosexual pseudoprecocious puberty, virilization may result from ovarian tumors such as arrhenoblastomas, lipoid tumors, cystadenomas, carcinomas, and gonadoblastomas. Adrenal carcinomas and teratomas often secrete significant amounts of DHEA and DHAS and cause rapid virilization. Several forms of congenital adrenal hyperplasia (CAH) virilize the female fetus (deficiency of 21-hydroxylase, 11-hydroxylase, and 3β-hydroxysteroid dehydrogenase enzymes). In Cushing's syndrome, increased adrenal secretion of androgens may cause premature growth of pubic hair.

Male Children. Male isosexual pseudoprecocious puberty may be caused by virilizing adrenal tumors or congenital adrenal hyperplasia (21-hydroxylase and 11-hydroxylase deficiencies). In such patients testicular size is disproportionately small in relation to phallic size and sexual hair growth. Leydig cell tumors may present with testicular asymmetry or masses. Leydig cell hyperplasia is a state of gonadotropin-independent hyperfunctioning of the interstitial cells of the testes. Adrenal rests (heterotopic adrenal tissue in the testes) may enlarge under endogenous corticotropin stimulation in boys with untreated or inadequately treated CAH and may mimic unilateral or bilateral interstitial cell tumors. Boys with gonadotropin-secreting neoplasms have slightly enlarged testes, and may be difficult to differentiate from boys with true precocious puberty on physical examination. The liver is enlarged, firm, and irregular in patients with hepatomas and hepatoblastomas. Some teratomas or chorioepitheliomas in the hypothalamic and pineal regions, the mediastinum, the gonads, or the retroperitoneum may cause isosexual precocity in boys by secreting large amounts of hCG.

Male heterosexual pseudoprecocious puberty manifested primarily by gynecomastia may be due to feminizing adrenal adenomas or carcinomas, estrogen-producing teratomas, choriocarcinomas, or neurofibromatosis. Adolescent gynecomastia occurs in approximately 70 per cent of normal early pubertal males and is due to increased estrogen secretion by the normal pubertal testes. Breast enlargement may be unilateral or bilateral and of varying degree. This condition usually resolves spontaneously within 2 years of onset. Gynecomastia also occurs in males with Klinefelter's syndrome, enzymatic disorders of testosterone synthesis, and end-organ resistance to testosterone, such as Reifenstein's syndrome or partial testicular feminization.

Incomplete Isosexual Precocity

Incomplete forms of sexual precocity are by definition not due to an underlying disease process. Unilateral or bilateral breast enlargement occurring as an isolated nonprogressive finding (premature thelarche) is common in girls before the age of 4 years. Breast development may be arrested or regress after several months and normal puberty commence at an appropriate age. Linear growth is not accelerated and skeletal maturation is normal for chronological age. Other signs of estrogen effect, such as nipple development and dulling of the vaginal mucosa, are absent. Vaginal cytologic findings and serum estrogen levels are usually prepubertal. A prepubertal GnRH test helps to distinguish premature thelarche from true and complete isosexual precocity. In some patients with a clinical picture of benign premature thelarche, evidence of mild intermittent estrogenization is obtained, which is referred to as premature gonadarche. Such findings may represent the activity of small ovarian cysts.

Other Conditions

The appearance of pubic or axillary hair without other pubertal changes is termed premature pubarche. This condition is perhaps more common in females than males and usually occurs after 6 years of age. This is a nonprogressive disorder; further secondary sexual development occurs at the normal age of puberty. Bone and height ages may be slightly advanced for chronological age. Some patients have normal levels of measured circulating androgens. However, in many instances, early pubertal levels of serum DHEA and DHAS and urinary 17-ketosteroids are present. Premature pubic hair growth may be the only manifestation of mild 21-hydroxylase–deficient congenital adrenal hyperplasia. In such patients serum 17-hydroxyprogesterone levels will be elevated. Development of the PCOS has been observed in some girls who were initially found to have premature adrenarche.

Vaginal bleeding may also reflect local trauma, foreign body, infection, or neoplasm. Exogenous androgens or estrogens are a very significant cause of sexual precocity and such sources should be carefully sought in each patient being evaluated. Foodstuffs, cosmetics, or vitamins may be contaminated with estrogens. Estrogen dust may be inhaled and absorbed. In addition to breast development, pigmentation of the areola and linea alba may occur in children exposed to estrogen. In males, extended use of hCG may stimulate secretion of testosterone sufficient to cause isosexual precocity.

Diagnostic Evaluation

History and Physical Examination

Evaluation of the patient with sexual precocity begins with the historical review and physical examination (Fig. 2). Historical data that should be obtained include type of sexual development; age at initiation and rate of progression; possible exposure to exogenous steroids or gonadotropins; perinatal abnormalities or head injuries; previous infections of the central nervous system, intercurrent illnesses, or head trauma; neurologic symptoms, such as headaches, visual disturbances, or motor incoordination; symptoms of hypothyroidism; family history of sexual precocity, congenital adrenal hyperplasia, neurofibromatosis, or thyroid disease.

Physical examination should define the stage of sexual development according to the Tanner classifications. Previous height and weight measurements are plotted to determine growth pattern and velocity. In males the correlation between testicular and phallic size is assessed; penile enlargement in the presence of testes of prepubertal size suggests an exogenous or extratesticular source of androgens. If the testes or scrotum is asymmetrical in configuration or a palpable mass is found, the possibility of a Leydig cell tumor or of adrenal rest tissue should be considered. Breasts should be palpated for the presence of gynecomastia and galactorrhea. In girls, the external genitalia are inspected for signs of estrogenization, labial fusion, or clitoromegaly. Rectal examination is performed to seek ovarian masses or vaginal foreign bodies. If a vaginal foreign body or neoplasm is suspected, vaginal examination under anesthesia is indicated. Examina-

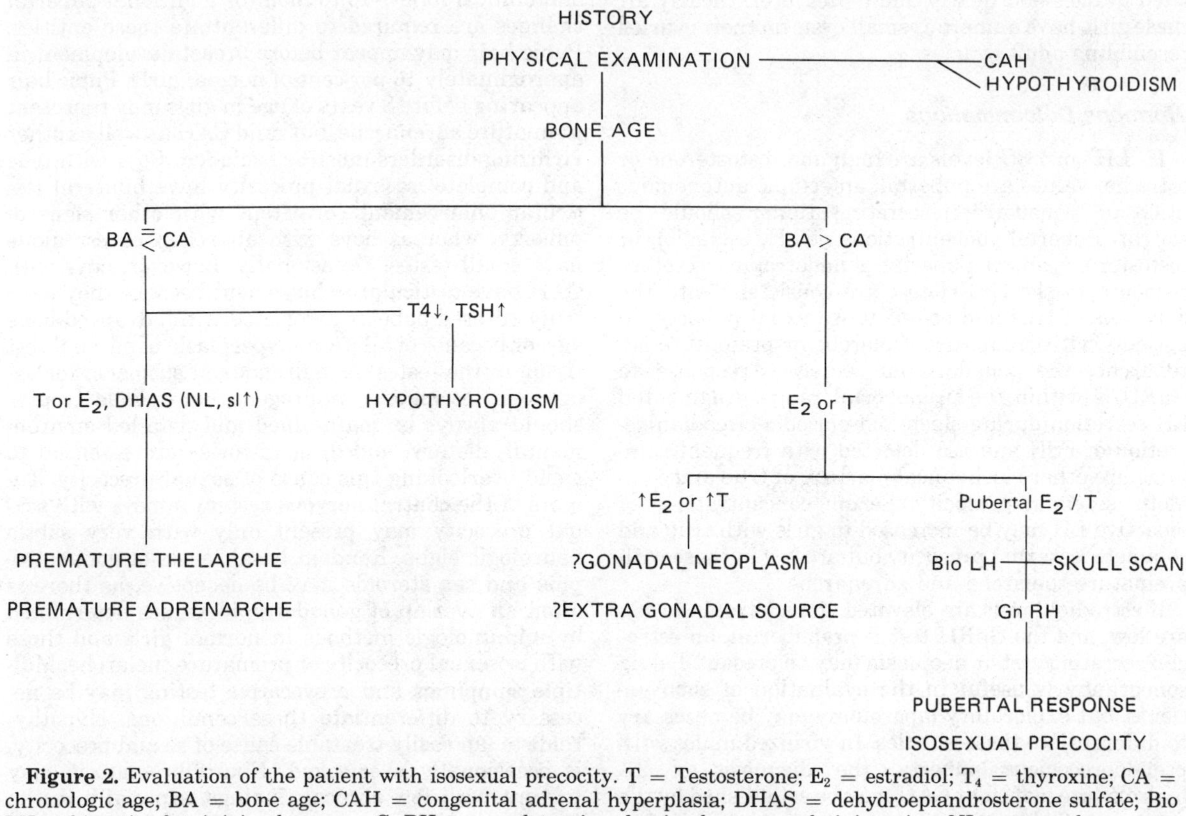

Figure 2. Evaluation of the patient with isosexual precocity. T = Testosterone; E_2 = estradiol; T_4 = thyroxine; CA = chronologic age; BA = bone age; CAH = congenital adrenal hyperplasia; DHAS = dehydroepiandrosterone sulfate; Bio LH = bioactive luteinizing hormone; GnRH = gonadotropin-releasing hormone administration; NL = normal.

tion for acne, facial and body hair distribution, muscular development, and axillary odor is performed in both sexes. The skin is inspected for neurofibromas or café au lait spots, carotenemia, dryness, coolness, and sebaceous gland activity. Careful ophthalmologic examination with attention to the assessment of visual fields and careful neurologic examination are important.

Radiologic Examination

A valuable radiologic procedure is determination of bone age. Significant advancement of skeletal maturation in relation to chronological age suggests excessive and prolonged exposure to sex steroids, while delayed bone age might be associated with hypothyroidism or Cushing's syndrome. In children with premature adrenarche or thelarche, bone age is reasonably similar to chronological age. Skull x-rays may reveal intracranial or perisellar abnormalities but may be negative in the presence of significant pathologic features. Detailed views of the optic foramina should be obtained in patients with visual defects or neurofibromatosis. Cranial CT is essential in any girl or boy with true and complete isosexual precocity or in whom neurologic findings are present. Pneumoencephalography may be indicated if skull x-rays and CT scans are negative but tumor is strongly suspected because of neurologic signs on physical examination. Polyostotic fibrous dysplasia may be diagnosed by a bone survey, ordered if clinically indicated. Computed tomography of the suprarenal or pelvic areas and pelvic sonography may be informative in specific patients. In children with true and complete isosexual precocity, pelvic ultrasonography demonstrates adult-sized ovaries and nearly adult-sized uteri; nearly all these girls have numerous small cysts on their ovaries resembling adult ovaries.

Hormone Determinations

If "LH" or hCG levels are high and testosterone or estradiol values are pubertal, an ectopic autonomous hCG- or gonadotropin-secreting tumor should be sought. Pubertal concentrations of LH, estradiol, or testosterone and a pubertal gonadotropin secretory response in the GnRH test are consistent with the diagnosis of true and complete isosexual puberty. In patients with premature thelarche or premature adrenarche, the gonadotropin secretory response to GnRH is within the prepubertal range. Augmented LH secretion during sleep and episodic circadian secretion of FSH and LH detected with frequent sampling are other biochemical markers of true and complete isosexual precocity. Serum concentrations of bioactive LH may be increased in girls with true and complete isosexual precocity but are low in those with premature thelarche and adrenarche.

If estradiol levels are elevated, gonadotropin levels are low, and the GnRH test is prepubertal, an estrogen-secreting cyst or neoplasm may be present. Pelvic sonography is useful in the evaluation of such patients, but exploratory laparotomy may be necessary to differentiate these entities. In virilized males with pseudoprecocious puberty, the diagnosis of 21-hydroxylase–deficient CAH may be established by the presence of elevated serum concentrations of 17-α-hydroxyprogesterone and increased urinary excretion of 17-ketosteroids and pregnanetriol, all of which may be suppressed by administration of hydrocortisone. The diagnosis of Leydig cell hyperplasia often requires testicular biopsy after demonstrating increased testosterone independent of gonadotropin control. In newborn females with virilized external genitalia, a similar diagnosis must be considered. In an occasional girl with premature sexual hair growth, elevated 17α-hydroxyprogesterone values may be found, consistent with a mild (attenuated, late onset) form of CAH. In patients with 11-hydroxylase deficiency CAH, hypertension may be present and there are increased serum concentrations of 11-deoxycortisol (Compound S) and urinary excretion of tetrahydro-Compound S. Patients with deficiency of 3β-hydroxysteroid dehydrogenase activity have elevated values of DHAS and Δ5-pregnenelone in serum and increased levels of pregnenetriol and 17-ketosteroids in the urine. In patients with adrenal adenoma or carcinoma, urinary 17-ketosteroid values are markedly elevated and DHAS levels are high and are not suppressible with glucocorticoids, as they are in CAH. Leydig cell tumors in males are associated with high testosterone levels, whereas adrenal feminizing tumors cause elevated estrogen values. In patients with primary hypothyroidism presenting as precocious puberty, the thyroxine concentration is low while levels of thyrotropin are elevated.

Pitfalls in Diagnosis

True and complete isosexual precocity presenting as breast enlargement in girls may be misdiagnosed as premature thelarche. Appropriate diagnostic testing and clinical follow-up to monitor additional pubertal changes are required to differentiate these entities. Pubic hair may appear before breast development in approximately 16 per cent of normal girls. Pubic hair appearing before 8 years of age in girls may represent premature adrenarche, but mild CAH as well as other virilizing disorders must be excluded. Boys with true and complete isosexual precocity have bilateral testicular enlargement consistent with other signs of puberty, whereas boys with androgen excess alone have small testes. Occasionally, however, boys with CAH have testicular enlargement because they have truly entered puberty associated with advanced bone age, or because of bilateral hyperplasia of adrenal rest tissue in the testes. A high index of suspicion for exogenous estrogens, androgens, or gonadotropins should always be maintained and detailed environmental, dietary, and drug histories are essential to avoid overlooking this cause of sexual precocity. Tumors of the central nervous system in boys with sexual precocity may present only with very subtle neurologic signs. Random basal levels of gonadotropins and sex steroids may be deceptive, as there is often an overlap of gonadotropin values determined by immunologic methods in normal girls and those with isosexual precocity or premature thelarche. Multiple samplings and provocative testing may be necessary to differentiate these conditions. Hypothyroidism, an easily treatable cause of sexual precocity, is occasionally overlooked. Neurofibromatosis may present with few clinical findings, especially in the first year of life.

Section Nineteen

RECOGNIZABLE CONGENITAL SYNDROMES

CHROMOSOMAL DISORDERS

By Jean H. Priest, M.D.
Atlanta, Georgia

Defects involving whole or parts of chromosomes detectable at the resolution of the light microscope generally cause defects in multiple organ systems. Frequently the diagnosis is made in the neonatal period, although detection may be delayed until puberty in the case of sex chromosome defects. Prenatal diagnosis is also available by means of amniocentesis and chromosome studies on cells cultured from amniotic fluid.

The frequency of genetic disorders generally, including those with chromosomal bases, is discussed in Dr. Dumars' article, Approach to Genetic Disease. Briefly, chromosome aberrations are a significant cause of birth defects and fetal loss, being present in an estimated 0.5 per cent of live births (about equally distributed between sex chromosomal and autosomal abnormalities) and in up to half of all spontaneous abortions. A format for normal human chromosomes is shown in Figure 1. An excellent reference describing all types of congenital defect syndromes, including those of chromosomal origin, is the book by David W. Smith, *Recognizable Patterns of Malformation* (Philadelphia, W. B. Saunders, 3rd edition, 1982).

INDICATIONS FOR CHROMOSOME ANALYSIS

1. Multiple congenital anomalies involving different organ systems.
2. Mental retardation, mild to profound, of unknown origin, associated with major or minor congenital anomalies.
3. Confirmation of a clinically diagnosed chromosomal disorder, particularly Down's syndrome.
4. Multiple (two or more) unexplained spontaneous abortions or infertility.
5. Family history of Down's syndrome or other autosomal trisomy or translocation.
6. Ambiguous genitalia.
7. Short stature and primary amenorrhea.

INTERPRETING A CHROMOSOME REPORT

Most cytogenetic reports give both the standard chromosome nomenclature symbols and a narrative diagnosis using clinical terminology, but in some cases both terminologies are the same. For instance, +21 is now common in medical terminology and frequently is used instead of Down's syndrome or trisomy 21. When the plus sign comes before the chromosome number it means that an extra chromosome is present. A plus sign after the chromosome number means something entirely different—the presence of extra material on a chromosome. Some of the more common cytogenetic symbols are listed in Table 1.

Table 1. Symbols and Nomenclature Used in Describing Chromosomal Abnormalities*

Symbol	Definition
A to G	Chromosome groups
1 to 22	Autosome numbers
X and Y	Sex chromosomes
/	Separates cell lines in describing mosaicism
+ or −	*Before* a symbol means an additional or missing chromosome; *after* a symbol means increase or decrease in the length of part of a chromosome
del	Deletion
dic	Dicentric
h	Secondary constriction or negatively staining region
i	Isochromosome
inv	Inversion
mar	Marker chromosome
mat	Maternal origin
p	Short arm of chromosome (for petit)
pat	Paternal origin
q	Long arm of chromosome
r	Ring chromosome
s	Satellite
t	Translocation

*Chromosome shorthand is used as follows: The first item to be recorded is the total number of chromosomes, followed by a comma, then the sex chromosome constitution. The autosomes are specified only when an abnormality is present. Examples:

45, X	45 chromosomes, including one X
47,XX,+21	47 chromosomes, including 2 X chromosomes; a chromosome 21 is extra

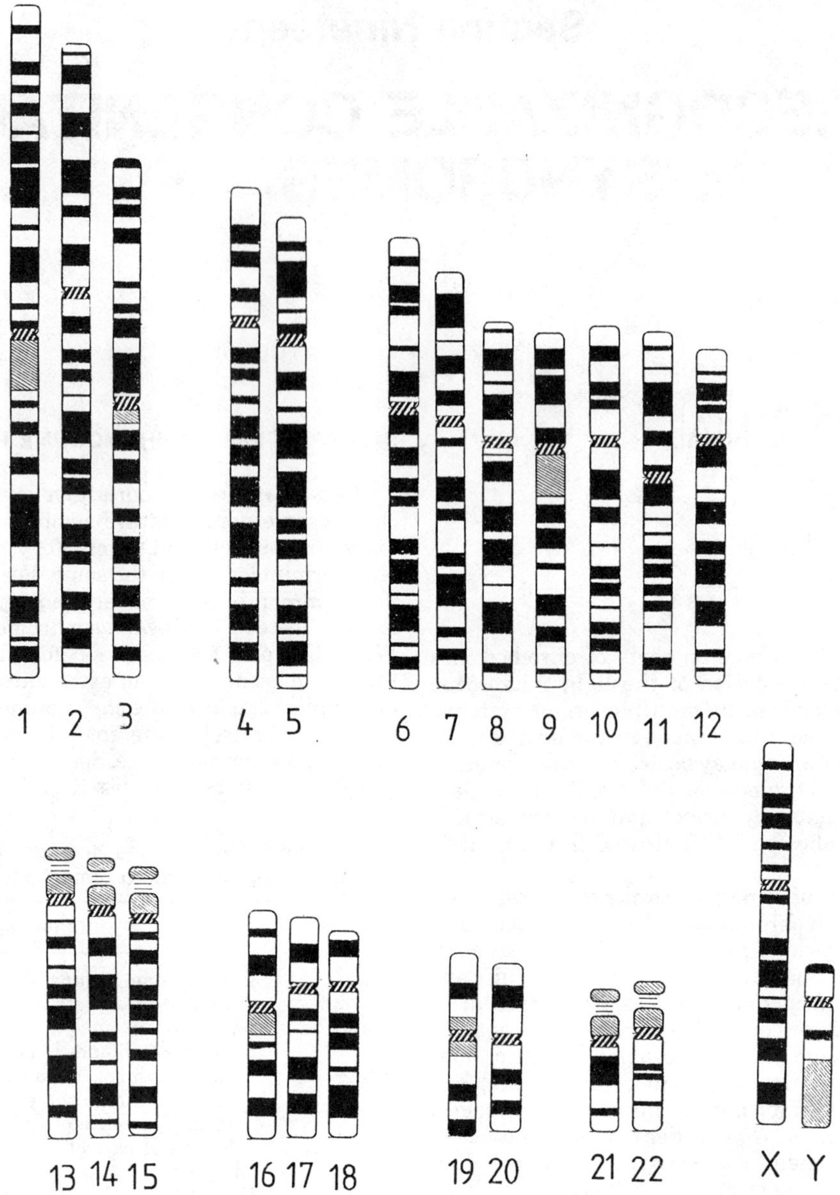

Figure 1. Normal human banded chromosomes. Sex chromosomes X and Y are shown as well as one member of each identical autosomal pair. The total number of bands shown (including the cross-hatched areas, which stain variably) is approximately 550. This number is considered to represent good resolution for detection of morphologic abnormalities in chromosomes.

ARRANGING FOR CHROMOSOME STUDIES

The usual approach for chromosome analysis is to obtain a heparinized peripheral blood specimen. Sodium heparin, not lithium heparin, is required. Transport to the laboratory as soon as possible is recommended. The blood specimen is placed in culture medium along with an agent, phytohemagglutinin, which induces the lymphocytes (T cells) to divide. The usual culture time is 3 days before slides can be prepared for chromosome analysis, and usually several more days are needed to have the slides in proper condition for banded analysis. Microscopy and photography take an average of another 2 weeks. Therefore, results of chromosome studies should not be expected in less than about 3 weeks. When the type of therapy depends on a chromosomal diagnosis, or in the case of ambiguous sex in a newborn before sex can be assigned, a "chromosomal emergency" may exist. The laboratory can speed up a diagnosis and may be willing to provide a preliminary report before all definitive stains and photographic records are complete.

Remember that a chromosome analysis is an expensive test because it requires special light microscopes with high resolution optics and cameras. Expertise that is not at present part of usual medical technology training is required. It is helpful for the laboratory to know what to look for, as judged from clinical findings. A simple request for chromosome analysis with no indication of why the test is needed is likely to provide less than the optimal answer. As an example, longer chromosomes giving greater band resolution are now obtained by pretreatment of the cultures prior to analysis. The laboratory needs to know ahead of time if small morphologic changes are to be detected by an "extended banding" approach. Wilms' tumor–aniridia is now known to be associated with a small deletion in the short arm of chromosome 11; retinoblastoma with a deletion in the long arm of chromosome 13; and Prader-Willi syndrome with a deletion in the long arm of 15. Frequently these more subtle abnormalities will remain undetected without extended banding. On the other hand, do not waste money or time to look at fine chromosome details when evaluation of total chromosome number is more important. For instance, if chromosomal mosaicism or numerical abnormality is a possibility, more cells need to be counted.

USING SEX CHROMATIN AS A DIAGNOSTIC TEST

A buccal smear is easier to obtain and is a less expensive test to examine than a chromosomal analysis, but it is only a screening test for genetic sex. Buccal smear analysis alone may be appropriate in the case of hypospadias or undescended testes, when further abnormality of sex differentiation is not in question. Delayed onset of puberty in an otherwise normal girl of below average height may be an indication for buccal smear sex chromatin analyses, as well as for follow-up visits to decide if further testing is indicated. In suspected sex chromosome defects, both sex chromatin and chromosome analyses are advisable because they sample different tissues and can give an indication of tissue mosaicism, more frequent in sex chromosomal than in autosomal defects. Remember that a satisfactory examination for sex chromatin includes analysis for both female sex chromatin (X-bodies, X-chromatin, Barr bodies) and male sex chromatin (Y-bodies, Y-chromatin). Female sex chromatin is examined after a nuclear DNA stain; male sex chromatin after fluorescent stain and microscopy. Rules are as follows: $n + 1 =$ number of X chromosomes where n is the number of Barr bodies; $n =$ number of Y chromosomes where n is the number of Y-bodies.

ANALYSIS OF DERMAL RIDGING

Analysis of the fine ridging pattern on palms and feet is a precise form of inspection during physical diagnosis and can be done without the aid of printing. Printing, however, gives a permanent record and is advisable for documentation of abnormality or quantitative analysis. Magnification with a good lens is helpful either for direct inspection or for analysis of prints. A distal axial triradius on the palm is frequently mentioned as a minor sign accompanying more major features of congenital defect syndromes, such as Down's syndrome. Distal refers to a position approaching half-way up the palm from the wrist crease. Triradius refers to a joining point of three major ridging pattern areas to form a triangular pattern. Four variations are shown:

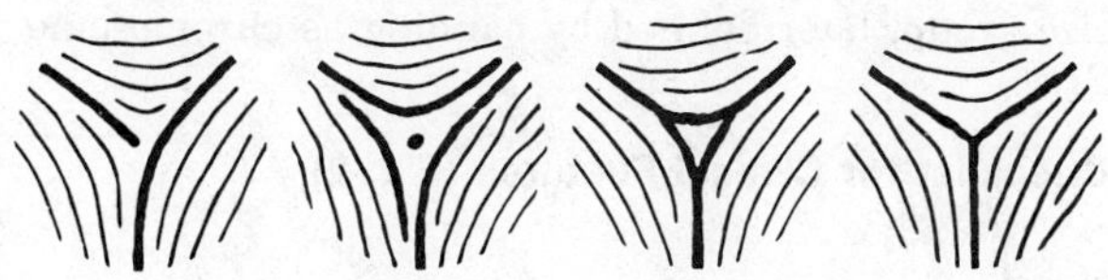

Several other dermal ridging patterns are characteristic of particular chromosomal syndromes. The flat arch on most or all fingertips is seen in trisomy 18:

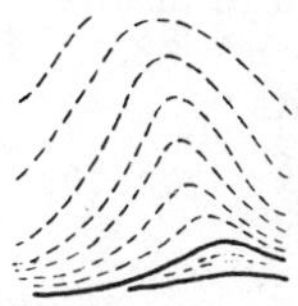

An arch opening to the tibial side of the foot is seen in the plantar hallucal area (base of the great toe) in Down's syndrome:

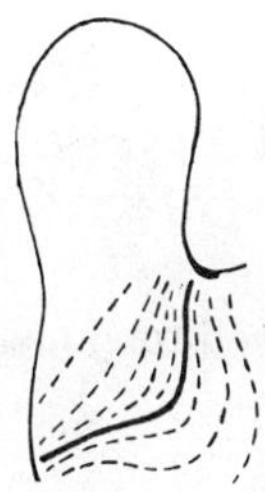

An arch opening to the fibular side of the foot, sometimes with an S shape, is seen in trisomy 13:

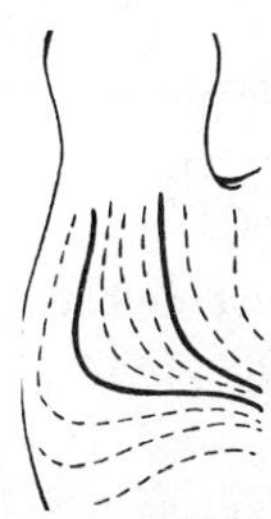

Abnormal flexion creases, not strictly speaking a part of dermal ridging, are nevertheless useful clues in congenital defect syndromes. Good examples are the single, deep, transverse palmar crease; the single flexion crease of the fifth finger; and the deep crease between the first and second toes—all seen frequently in Down's syndrome.

TRISOMY 21 (DOWN'S SYNDROME)

Langdon Down in 1866 provided the first clinical report of this syndrome in the medical literature. The chromosomal basis was established by Lejeune (1959), who described an extra chromosome in the smallest size group, later defined by banding as chromosome 21.

Checklist for Clinical Features (Fig. 2)

Head

1. Persistent open fontanel
2. Small
3. Flat occiput

Eyes

4. Upslanting palpebral fissures
5. Epicanthal folds
6. Chronic blepharitis
7. Strabismus
8. Speckling of iris
9. Refractive errors
10. Lens opacities

Ears

11. Malformed
12. Low-set

Nose

13. Flat nasal bridge

Mouth

14. Large and furrowed tongue
15. High palate
16. Malformed teeth
17. Open mouth
18. Low voice

Neck

19. Broad
20. Short
21. Loose folds in posterior neck (infancy)

Chest

22. Congenital heart defects, especially atrioventricularis communis

Abdomen

23. Umbilical hernia
24. Diastasis recti

Genitalia

25. Underdeveloped external genitalia (M and F)
26. Cryptorchidism (M)
27. Irregular or absent menstruation (F)
28. Absent breast development (F)

Skeleton

29. Short stature
30. Pelvis—shallow acetabular angle
31. Hyperextensible joints

Hands

32. Short
33. Broad
34. Palmar horizontal lines
35. Short fingers
36. Incurved fifth fingers
37. Single flexion crease, fifth finger
38. Distal palmar axial triradius
39. Dermal ridge pattern: loop in third interdigital area

Feet

40. Gap between toes 1 and 2
41. Plantar furrow
42. Dermal ridge pattern: arch opening to tibial side in plantar hallucal area

General

43. Hypotonia
44. Marmoration of skin
45. IQ less than 70
46. Retarded development
47. Frequent infections
48. Maternal age may be over 35 years
49. Other congenital malformations are frequent

Laboratory

50. Extra chromosome 21 material

Natural History

Incidence is estimated at about 1 in 1000 births. If cardiac abnormalities are absent, life span may be nearly normal. Infections are frequent, especially in early life. Muscle tone tends to improve with age. Early developmental enrichment programs and rearing within families rather than in institutions improves the rate of progress and development of social skills in young children. Intellectual capacity remains limited, and guardianship is required throughout life. Down's syndrome children are usually easy to manage, tend toward mimicry, have happy moods, and are friendly, but mischievousness and obstinacy may be problems. In later life societal pressures may remove some of the positive behavioral qualities of infancy.

Etiology

At least 90 per cent of cases result from an extra chromosome 21, either of maternal age–dependent or maternal age–independent types. When maternal age is not a factor, paternal age, environmental exposures (especially to ionizing irradiation), parental mosaicism, and other factors yet to be understood may be involved. Relative contributions of these causes other than maternal age are not established. Approximately 3 per cent of cases are caused by translocation (see article on Approach to Genetic Disease), and about one half of these are familial. Another 2 to 3 per cent of cases are caused by trisomy and normal mosaicism, and, depending on the percentage of normal cells, clinical features are less apparent.

Special Comments

Genetic evaluation, as described in the article on Approach to Genetic Disease, is an essential part of the diagnosis. In the case of +21 Down's syndrome, parents should be advised of the availability of prenatal chromosomal diagnosis for subsequent pregnancies. Similar advice is given in the case of translocation Down's syndrome. Chromosome analysis of peripheral blood is also recommended to evaluate carrier status in a parent or other family members. Reproducing women over 35 years of age without a positive history should also be offered prenatal chromosomal diagnosis.

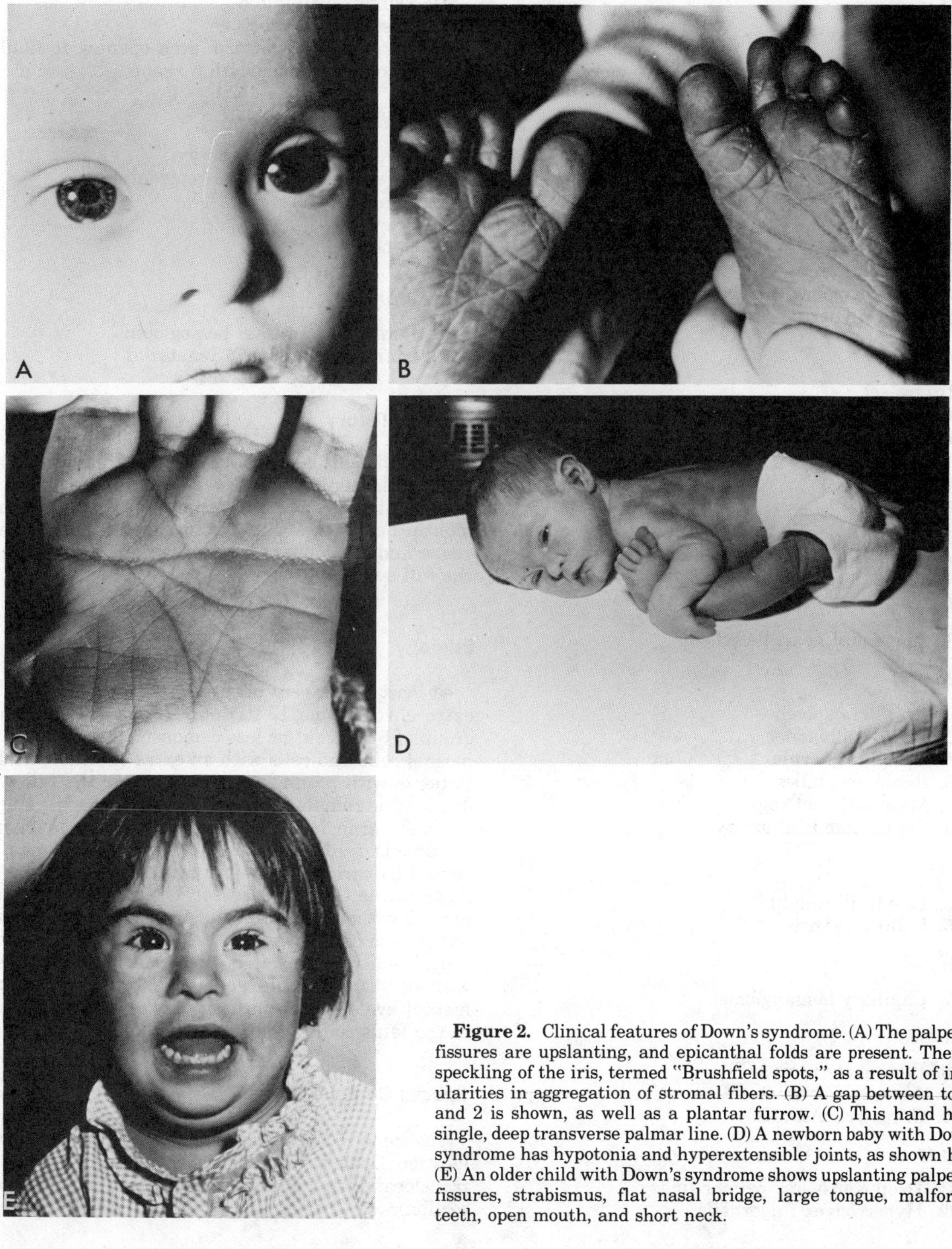

Figure 2. Clinical features of Down's syndrome. (A) The palpebral fissures are upslanting, and epicanthal folds are present. There is speckling of the iris, termed "Brushfield spots," as a result of irregularities in aggregation of stromal fibers. (B) A gap between toes 1 and 2 is shown, as well as a plantar furrow. (C) This hand has a single, deep transverse palmar line. (D) A newborn baby with Down's syndrome has hypotonia and hyperextensible joints, as shown here. (E) An older child with Down's syndrome shows upslanting palpebral fissures, strabismus, flat nasal bridge, large tongue, malformed teeth, open mouth, and short neck.

TRISOMY 13 (PATAU SYNDROME)

In 1960, 1 year after an extra G group chromosome was described in Down's syndrome, Patau and coworkers found an extra D chromosome in a baby with many birth defects. The extra chromosome was later shown to be chromosome 13.

Checklist for Clinical Features (Fig. 3)

Head

1. Sloping forehead
2. Microcephaly
3. Wide sagittal sutures
4. Wide fontanel
5. Arhinencephaly
6. Localized scalp defects

Eyes

7. Iris coloboma
8. Anophthalmia
9. Microphthalmia
10. Small palpebral fissures
11. Ocular hypertelorism

Ears

12. Low-set
13. Malformed
14. Deafness

Nose and Mouth

15. Cleft lip
16. Cleft palate
17. Flat nasal bridge

Chest

18. Congenital heart defects

Abdomen

19. Accessory spleen
20. Large gallbladder
21. Umbilical hernia
22. Renal anomalies
23. Malrotation of colon
24. Single umbilical artery

Trunk

25. Low birth weight
26. Failure to thrive

Skin

27. Capillary hemangiomas

Genitalia

28. Bicornuate uterus (F)
29. Abnormal scrotum (M)
30. Cryptorchidism (M)

Hands

31. Deep transverse palmar lines
32. Hyperconvex fingernails
33. Narrow fingernails
34. Retroflexible thumbs
35. Overlapping of flexed fingers
36. Deviation of hands
37. Postaxial polydactyly
38. Distal palmar axial triradius

Feet

39. Posterior prominence of heels
40. Rockerbottom
41. Dorsiflexed big toe
42. Postaxial polydactyly
43. Dermal ridge pattern: arch opening to fibular side of foot; sometimes with S shape

Central Nervous System

44. Severe mental retardation
45. Severe developmental retardation
46. Apneic spells
47. Seizures
48. Hypertonia

Laboratory

49. Persistence of fetal hemoglobin
50. Extra chromosome 13 material

Natural History

The incidence is not more frequent than about 1 in 7000 births. Trisomy 13 is a severe disorder, fatal in about half of affected liveborn infants within the first month. Fewer than 5 per cent survive more than 5 years, and this longer survival is related to absence of the full syndrome.

Etiology

At least 80 per cent of cases are associated with an extra chromosome 13 (trisomy 13 or +13). Another group of 5 per cent or less demonstrate mosaicism of normal cells and cells with an extra chromosome 13. Patients with mosaicism may not have the full syndrome. The remainder of cases with chromosomal basis have translocation trisomy, usually involving another D group chromosome. Translocation can be caused by carrier state in one parent (see article on Approach to Genetic Disease). The syndrome may be present without chromosomal abnormality. In this situation, the clinical features would be called "phenocopy," which means that the phenotype is present without demonstrable genetic defect. An environmental event disrupting critical organ development in the fetus could produce a phenocopy.

Special Comments

The same recommendations for trisomic and translocation Down's syndrome also apply if trisomy or translocation involves chromosome 13 (see previous section).

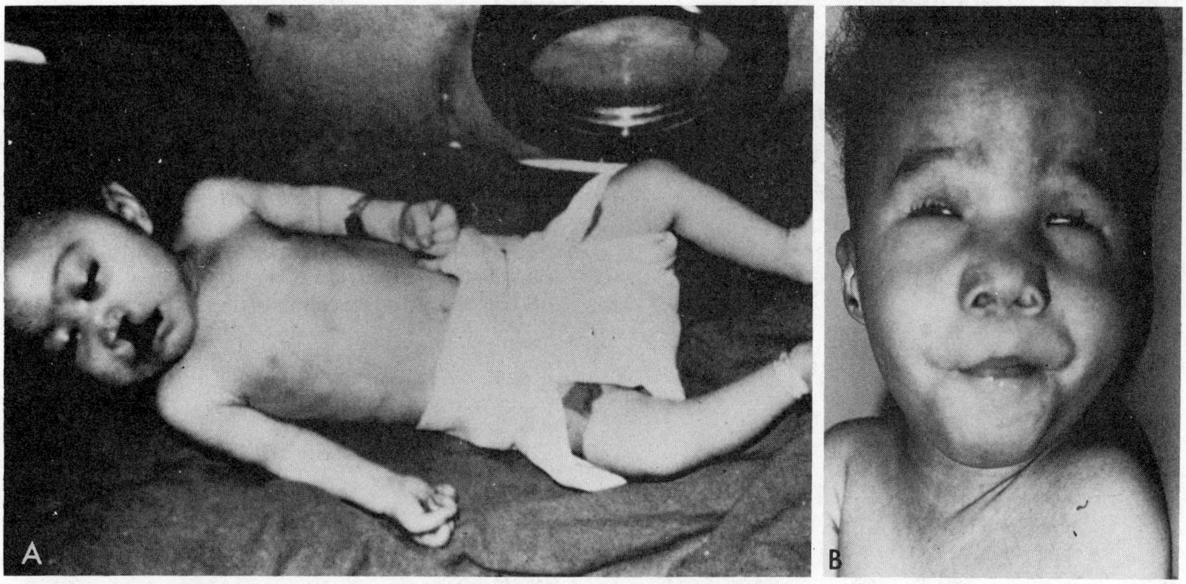

Figure 3. Clinical features of trisomy 13. (*A*) Positive findings include microcephaly, low-set and malformed ears, cleft lip, polydactyly, overlapping and flexed fingers, posterior prominence of heels, and severe developmental retardation. (*B*) Arhinencephaly and associated sloping forehead, as well as anophthalmia or microphthalmia, are cardinal features.

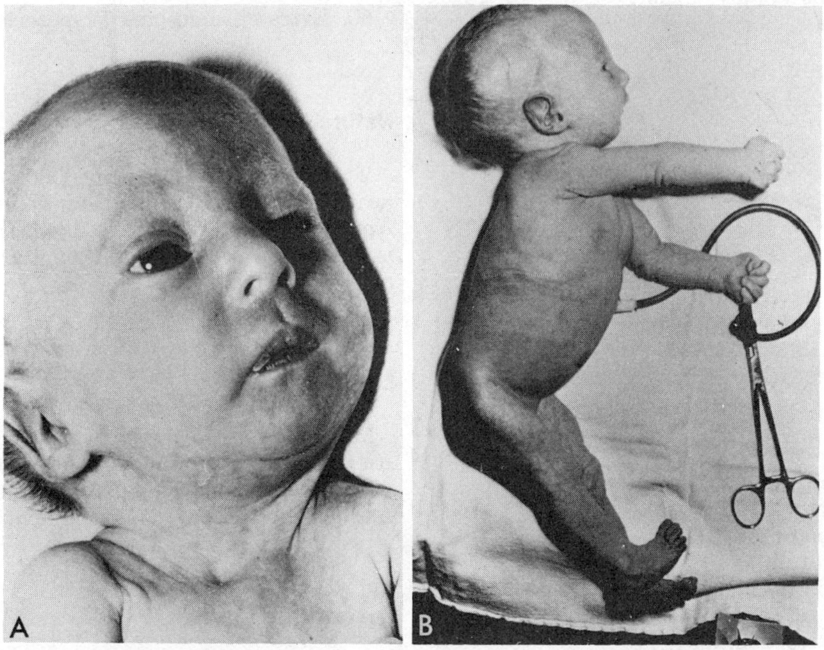

Figure 4. Clinical features of trisomy 18. (A) Ptosis of eyelids, small palpebral fissures, low-set and malformed ears, short upper lip, small and receding mandible, short neck with loose skin folds, and hypermobility of shoulders. (B) Prominent occiput, malformed ears, small and receding mandible, flexed and overlapping fingers, dorsiflexed big toes, hypertonia, and decreased muscle mass.

TRISOMY 18 (EDWARDS' SYNDROME)

In 1960 Edwards and co-workers described an extra E group chromosome in a baby with multiple defects. The extra chromosome was later shown to be chromosome 18.

Checklist for Clinical Features (Fig. 4)

Head

1. Prominent occiput
2. Large fontanel
3. Small

Eyes

4. Epicanthal folds
5. Ptosis of lids
6. Small palpebral fissures
7. Corneal opacity

Ears

8. Low-set
9. Malformed

Nose

10. Flat nasal bridge
11. Short upper lip
12. Posterior choanal atresia

Mouth

13. Small mandible, receding
14. Narrow palate, may be cleft
15. Bifid uvula
16. Small

Neck

17. Loose skin folds
18. Short

Chest

19. Shield chest, wide-spaced nipples
20. Small circumference
21. Short sternum
22. Cardiac anomaly

Abdomen

23. Inguinal or umbilical hernias
24. Small pelvis
25. Eventration of diaphragm
26. Renal abnormality
27. Malrotation of colon
28. Accessory spleen
29. Meckel's diverticulum
30. Single umbilical artery

Genitalia

31. Small or absent labia (F)
32. Cryptorchidism (M)

Trunk

33. Low birth weight
34. Failure to thrive
35. Scoliosis

Hands

36. Flexed and overlapping fingers
37. Partial syndactyly (also of feet)
38. Small hypothenar muscles
39. Distal palmar axial triradius
40. Simple arch dermal ridge pattern on fingers

Feet

41. Equinovarus
42. Hypoplastic dorsiflexed big toes

Central Nervous System

43. Hypertonic
44. Retarded development and mental retardation
45. Weak

General

46. Feeble cry, poor feeding
47. Retarded bone age
48. Decreased muscle mass
49. Hypermobility of shoulders

Laboratory

50. Extra chromosome 18 material

Natural History

The incidence is about 1 in 8000 newborns. The majority of trisomy 18 fetuses abort spontaneously. Among infants who are live-born, the mean survival is only several months, although a few may live to older childhood.

Etiology

Most patients have an extra chromosome 18. A few are mosaics for trisomic and normal cells, and these are ones who survive longer. Translocation involving another chromosome is uncommon.

Special Comments

As is true for trisomy 21, increasing maternal age is a risk factor and therefore reproducing women over the age of 35 years should be offered prenatal chromosomal diagnosis. This test is also recommended for younger women who have already had a trisomic child.

5p PARTIAL MONOSOMY (5p– or CRI DU CHAT SYNDROME)

Lejeune and co-workers first described this syndrome in 1963. The name of cri du chat comes from the resemblance of the cry of an affected child to the mewing of a cat. The chromosome abnormality first reported was a partial short arm deletion of a B group chromosome, later shown to be chromosome 5. The total chromosome number is the correct count of 46. Therefore, discovery of the chromosomal basis for this syndrome represented development of cytogenetic skills to the point of detecting changes in morphology as well as in number of human chromosomes.

Checklist for Clinical Features (Fig. 5)

Head

1. Small
2. Round facies (infancy)
3. Long, thin face (older individuals)
4. Facial asymmetry
5. Large frontal sinuses
6. Mild premature graying of hair

Eyes

7. Strabismus
8. Antimongoloid slant
9. Epicanthal folds
10. Hypertelorism
11. Optic atrophy

Ears

12. Low-set
13. Narrow ear canals

Nose

14. Broad base
15. Flat nasal bridge

Mouth

16. Micrognathia (infancy)
17. High palate
18. Dental malocclusion

Chest

19. Congenital heart disease
20. Respiratory stridor
21. Laryngomalacia

Abdomen

22. Inguinal hernia

Genitalia

23. Cryptorchidism (M)

Musculoskeletal System

24. Low birth weight
25. Failure to thrive
26. Small wings of ilia
27. Poor muscle development

Hands

28. Deep transverse palmar creases
29. Small
30. Short metacarpals
31. Distal palmar axial triradius

Feet

32. Short metatarsals
33. Small
34. Pes planus

Natural History

Incidence estimates vary, but the average is about 1 in 50,000 among live births. Growth retardation persists through adult life, as may the hypotonia. This disorder is estimated to account for about 1 per cent of institutionalized retardates with lowest intelligence.

Etiology

Most cases are sporadic, but about 10 per cent of patients are the offspring of translocation carriers. For this reason, parental chromosome studies are recommended when the diagnosis is first established. If the carrier state is detected, these individuals should be advised of increased risk for subsequent pregnancies and of the availability of prenatal diagnosis.

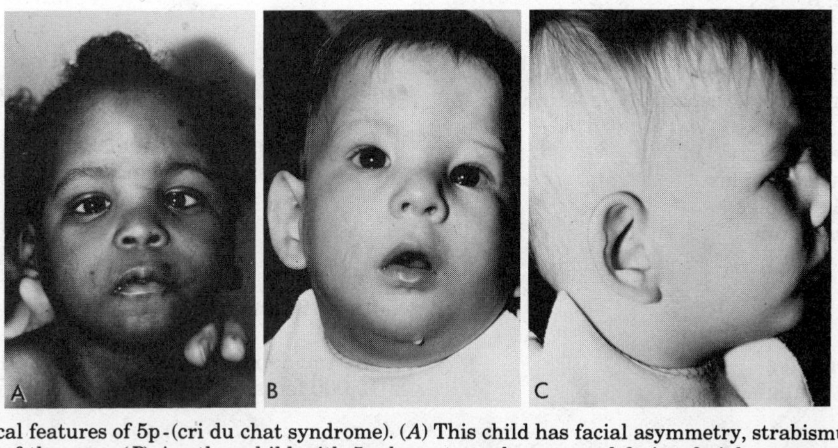

Figure 5. Clinical features of 5p-(cri du chat syndrome). (*A*) This child has facial asymmetry, strabismus, hypertelorism, and a broad base of the nose. (*B*) Another child with 5p-karyotype shows round facies, facial asymmetry, antimongoloid slant of the eyes, epicanthal folds, hypertelorism, low-set ears, and a broad nasal bridge. (*C*) A lateral view of the child shown in B illustrates micrognathia.

TURNER'S SYNDROME

In 1938 Turner first described a syndrome of sexual infantilism in females, congenital webbed neck, and cubitus valgus in female children. Later, in 1954, Polani and co-workers noted that some individuals with Turner's syndrome were missing a Barr body and thus did not have female sex chromatin. By 1959 Ford and co-workers had found the chromosomal basis for some cases of Turner's syndrome when they reported an X chromosome to be missing.

Checklist for Clinical Features (Fig. 6)

Head

1. Abnormal sella
2. Unusual facies

Eyes

3. Strabismus
4. Ptosis
5. Refractive error
6. Epicanthal folds
7. Blue sclera

Ears

8. Anomalous and prominent
9. Low-set
10. Deafness

Mouth

11. Narrow, high palate
12. Small mandible
13. Dental malocclusion

Neck

14. Low posterior hairline
15. Short
16. Webbed

Chest

17. Idiopathic hypertension
18. Cardiac anomalies, especially coarctation of aorta
19. Broad, shield-like
20. Widely spaced nipples
21. Hypoplastic nipples
22. Pectus excavatum

Abdomen

23. Renal anomalies
24. Intestinal telangiectases

Genitalia

25. Primary amenorrhea
26. Sterility
27. Streak gonads
28. Failure of development of secondary sex characteristics

Musculoskeletal System

29. Short stature
30. Varying skeletal anomalies
31. Delayed bone age
32. Metaphyseal dysplasia or osteoporosis
33. Lax joints

Hands (Arms)

34. Lymphedema (infancy)
35. Short fourth metacarpal
36. Single deep transverse palmar line
37. Narrow, hyperconvex nails
38. Increased carrying angle of the elbow
39. Clinodactyly
40. Distal palmar axial triradius

Feet (Legs)

41. Lymphedema (infancy)
42. Medial tibial exostosis

Central Nervous System

43. Defective space-form perception

Skin

44. Excessive pigmented nevi
45. Cutis laxa
46. Keloid formation

Laboratory

47. Increased pituitary gonadotropins
48. Decreased estrogen
49. Abnormal sex chromatin
50. Abnormal X chromosome

Natural History

The incidence of XO Turner's syndrome is about 1 in 10,000 female births. There is a high rate in spontaneous abortions, estimated to constitute about 20 per cent of all chromosomally abnormal abortuses. Affected patients usually have normal intelligence, often with spatial-perceptual deficit, and can live a normal although nonreproductive life.

Etiology

Only about 60 per cent of Turner's syndrome patients are missing an X chromosome. The remainder have other types of X chromosome defects, including most commonly mosaicism for XO and XX cells or cells containing one normal X and one X isochromosome. This isochromosome is composed of two X chromosome long arms and is the result of abnormal separation at the centromere during cell division. Patients with these latter "Turner variant" genotypes may not have all or even most of the clinical features, although short stature and gonadal dysgenesis are common denominators. Absence of one X chromosome does not appear to be related to maternal age and most cases are sporadic. Mosaicism for X chromosome defects with clinical features of Turner's syndrome is reported in multiple generations within a family, usually associated with subfertility. A Turner's syndrome phenotype can be present in males or females without chromosome abnormality, most such cases fitting the diagnosis of Noonan's syndrome. Distinction between the two syndromes can be made by absence of the full Turner's syndrome phenotype and different cardiac lesions, usually pulmonic valvular or infundibular stenosis, in Noonan's syndrome. Chromosomal studies are definitive in the differential diagnosis.

Special Comments

Most individuals with mosaicism for XO and XY cells have female phenotype and some features of Turner's syndrome. Embryonic gonadal tumors (gonadoblastomas) occur in these patients, often early in life. Chromosomal diagnosis is helpful for calling attention to the risk of tumor.

The chromosomal diagnosis of trisomy X (triple X female) strictly speaking does not automatically classify a case as a variant in the Turner's syndrome group. Triple X females may be infertile and show a few features of Turner's syndrome, but most patients do not have a particular constellation of clinical features. Their condition is likely to remain undiagnosed unless it is detected during newborn screening. Through such studies the incidence of XXX is judged to be about 1 in 1000 females. A few patients are identified in infertility clinics or institutions for the mentally retarded, although this type of ascertainment is more likely in individuals with XXXX or XXXXX. All of these multiple X patients may have mosaicism for at least two distinct cell lines.

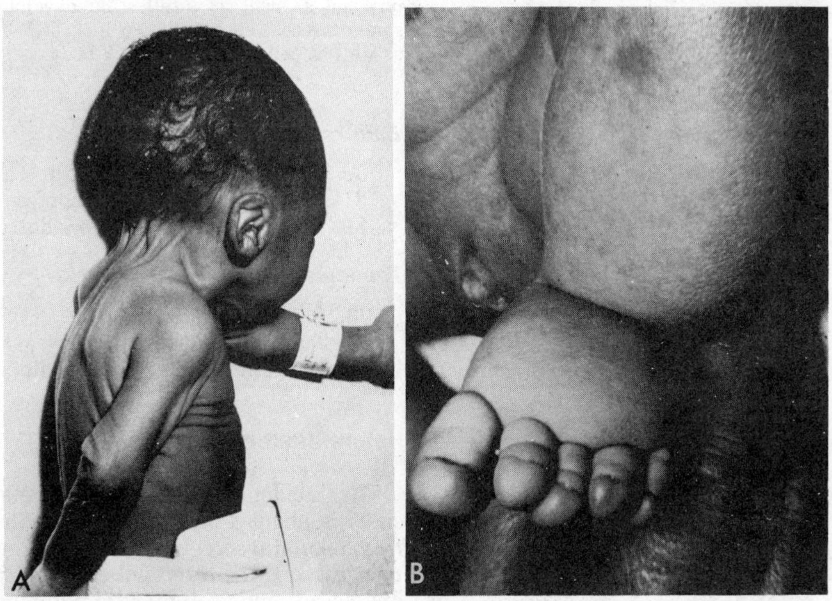

Figure 6. Clinical features of Turner's syndrome. *(A)* In a baby the webbed neck may appear as abundant and loose skin folds. *(B)* Lymphedema in a newborn is illustrated.

KLINEFELTER'S SYNDROME

In 1942 Klinefelter and co-workers described a syndrome involving males who were usually tall and sterile, with small or undescended testes and some feminization. When the technique for Barr body analysis became available in 1957, some of these patients were found to have female sex chromatin. Then, in 1959, Jacobs and Strong demonstrated an extra X chromosome.

Checklist for Clinical Features (Fig. 7)

Head

*1. Brachycephaly
*2. Low hairline

Face

3. Little hair after puberty

Eyes

*4. Refractive error
*5. Strabismus

Ears

*6. Congenital deafness
*7. Minor defects of auricles

Chest

8. Gynecomastia after puberty
*9. Chronic pulmonary disease

Genitalia

10. Small, firm testes after puberty
*11. Undescended testes
*12. Small penis
13. Sterility
14. Impotence

Trunk

15. Tall
16. Decreased upper:lower segment ratio
17. Obesity
18. Feminine habitus
19. Scanty body hair after puberty

Skeleton

*20. Scoliosis, lordosis, kyphosis
*21. Sacralization of lumbar vertebrae
*22. Osteoporosis
*23. Radioulnar synostosis
24. Long arms and legs
*25. Pes planus
*26. Clinodactyly of fifth fingers
*27. Single transverse palmar line

Central Nervous System

28. Behavioral and mental disturbance
29. Mild mental retardation

*Less regularly occurring features.

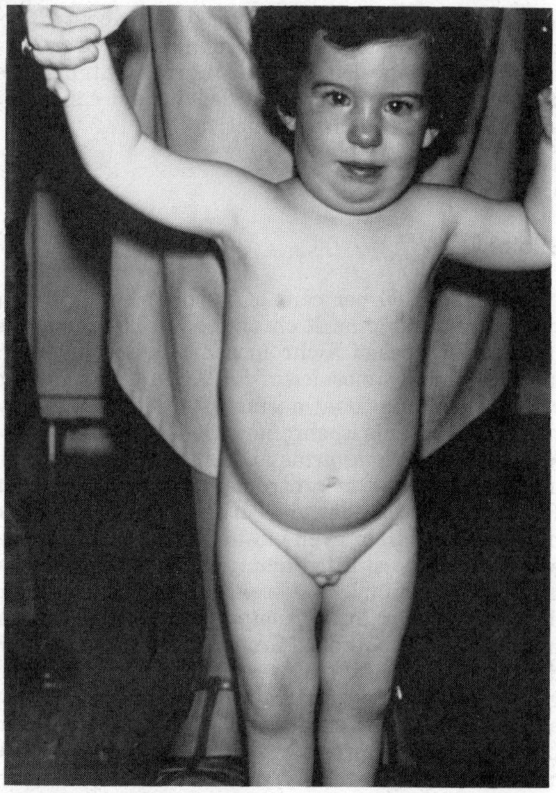

Figure 7. Clinical features of Klinefelter syndrome in a 3-year-old boy with mosaicism for multiple additional X chromosomes. This boy has mosaicism for 48,XXXY and 49,XXXXY metaphases. This type of variant Klinefelter syndrome is associated with more severe defects in sexual and mental development. Illustrated in this photograph are truncal obesity, micropenis, and underdeveloped scrotum with undescended testes. The child is delayed in physical as well as intellectual development. The buccal smear has cells each with two or three X-bodies (Barr bodies) as well as cells with a single Y-body.

Laboratory

30. Abnormal sex chromatin
31. Abnormal sex chromosomes
32. Increased pituitary gonadotropin

Testicular Biopsy

33. Aspermatogenesis
34. Tubular hyalinization
35. Interstitial cell hyperplasia

Natural History

The incidence of 47,XXY Klinefelter's syndrome cases is about 1 in 1000 male births as determined from neonatal screening. The syndrome is usually not recognized until after puberty and may remain undiagnosed among nonfertile adult males in the general population.

Etiology

An extra X chromosome is the prototype chromosome abnormality in Klinefelter's syndrome. However, less commonly XXXY and XXXXY also occur and as a general rule the additional X chromosomes cause more severe dysmorphisms and defects in sexual and mental development. It is estimated that about 15 per cent of individuals with Klinefelter's syndrome have mosaicism of two or more distinct cell lines. One mosaic form is XY/XXY, and because some normal male cells are present, the clinical features are less severe. Other types of mosaicism involve different numbers of X and Y chromosomes. The term "Klinefelter variant" is used to describe these cases with chromosome abnormalities other than 47,XXY. Some patients with features of the syndrome have normal male chromosomes, but the typical histologic pattern in testicular biopsy is absent. Maternal age is advanced in XXY patients. It is estimated that about 60 per cent of cases result from divisional error of maternally derived X chromosomes, but the remainder involve divisional error of paternally derived chromosomes. Risk of recurrence in a subsequent pregnancy is not significantly increased. However, women over 35 years old with negative family history should be made aware of the availability of prenatal chromosomal diagnosis if a pregnancy is anticipated.

Special Comments

The chromosomal diagnosis of XYY (males with an extra Y chromosome) strictly speaking does not automatically classify a case as a variant in the Klinefelter's syndrome group. Double Y males are tall but may not have other features of Klinefelter's syndrome and in fact may not have a particular constellation of clinical features. Most with this condition remain undiagnosed unless detected during neonatal screening. Through such studies the incidence of XYY is estimated to be about 1 in 1000 males. The association of XXY and XYY with aggressive, psychopathic, or criminal behavior is suggested by the increased incidence of these cytogenetic defects in tall adult males in prisons and mental institutions. It is probable that a predisposition to behavioral problems is present in some individuals with XXY or XYY chromosome constitution, but complex environmental influences are important in formation of their adult behavioral patterns.

RECOGNIZABLE CONGENITAL SYNDROMES DUE TO SINGLE-GENE ABNORMALITIES

By Kenneth W. Dumars, M.D.
Irvine, California

It is not feasible to describe all recognizable genetic disorders. This article describes representative single-gene disorders presenting with aberrations of linear growth, facial configuration, extremities, and cognitive development; late-onset diseases; and one type of male pseudohermaphroditism.

SMALL STATURE

Seckel's Syndrome

Synonyms. Bird-headed dwarfism, dwarfism.

Mode of Inheritance. Autosomal recessive.

Incidence. Seckel's syndrome occurs in approximately 1 in 10,000 live births. Microcephaly, a cardinal manifestation of Seckel's syndrome, occurs commonly. It is estimated that approximately 20 per cent of the cases of microcephaly are genetic in origin and Seckel's syndrome is but one example of genetic microcephaly.

Clinical Manifestations. This disorder is apparent at birth and the characteristic findings include proportionate short stature (below 3rd percentile), small for gestational age (SGA), microcephaly, and unusual facial features that include large eyes, prominent beaklike nose, and narrow facies with micrognathia (Fig. 1). Associated abnormalities can occur, such as hypoplastic thumbs, congenitally dislocated hips, scoliosis, strabismus, and anomalies of the genitourinary tract. The children are slow to develop and when tested at the appropriate age, function at a retarded level. They are ambulatory, social children who learn to speak, but usually they are unable to function and live independently. The level of retardation varies from moderate to severe, the latter often due to the

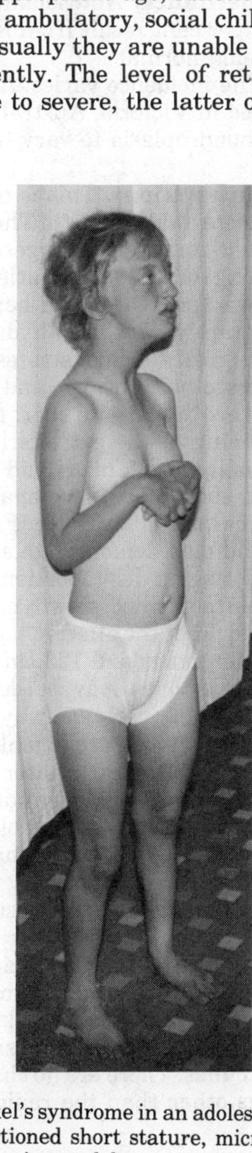

Figure 1. Seckel's syndrome in an adolescent female. Note normally proportioned short stature, microcephaly, psittacorhina, and prominent globes.

absence of social stimulation as a result of placement in large, impersonal institutions. Children with Seckel's syndrome have a normal life expectancy.

Confirmatory Tests. There are no specific laboratory markers for this disorder. The diagnosis rests with the small stature, microcephaly, and characteristic facial features.

Recurrence Risks and Prenatal Diagnosis. Seckel's syndrome is an autosomal recessive characteristic; thus, for the patient's biologic parents there is a one in four (25 per cent) risk of recurrence with each pregnancy. Normal sibs, if they are carriers, are at risk of having affected children only if the other partner is a carrier, and as yet there is no test available to detect the heterozygous state. The patient's children are at risk, again, only if the other parent is a carrier or also has the syndrome. As yet, prenatal diagnosis has not been described.

Achondroplasia

Synonyms. Chondrodystrophia fetalis, chondrodystrophy.

Mode of Inheritance. Autosomal dominant. Approximately 80 per cent result from fresh mutations, both parents being normal.

Incidence. The incidence varies. A recent 10-year survey conducted in Victoria, Australia, revealed the incidence of achondroplasia to vary from 1 in 19,670 to 1 in 38,000.

Clinical Manifestations. This is one of the chondrodystrophies detectable at birth. The infant's linear growth is less than anticipated for gestational age owing to shortening of the extremities, resulting in short-limbed dwarfism. Often the head is disproportionately large, rarely a result of hydrocephalus. The face characteristically demonstrates a prominent forehead, depressed nasal bridge, and a small, button nose. The hands are broad, with short fingers ("trident hands"). Shortening of the extremities is more pronounced proximally; the humeri and femora are disproportionately shortened in comparison with the bones of the forearm and lower leg (Fig. 2*A*). Even in infancy, the child may demonstrate a relatively long trunk with lordosis and disproportionately large buttocks. Rimoin has published growth curves for achondroplasia; the height of the affected individual seldom exceeds 132 cm in males and 123 cm in females. Although motor milestones may be delayed in childhood, normal mentality can generally be anticipated.

Complications rarely can occur and include spinal cord compression in infancy. In later life, nerve root irritation or cauda equina claudication can occur as a result of a gibbus (usually thoracolumbar), a herniated disc, or osteophytes. Individuals with achondroplasia are frequently employed in a theatrical setting, or more specifically, the circus. Historically, individuals with achondroplasia were often depicted as court jesters, a role imposed by society. Life span is normal in the absence of serious complications.

Confirmatory Tests. Achondroplasia can be detected early in life, and the diagnosis can be made upon clinical grounds. There are no characteristic laboratory findings other than the radiographic abnormalities. These may ultimately be supplemented by ultrasonographic changes, thus avoiding the theoretic risks of ionizing radiation. The characteristic x-ray findings vary with age and include disproportionate shortening of the humeri and femora in infancy, "square ilia," small sacrosciatic notches, decreased anterior-posterior diameter of the ossified proximal femora, characteristic broad and short proximal and middle phalanges, and a small foramen magnum (Fig. 2*B–E*). Additionally, in childhood, there is a narrow sacrum, narrowing of the interpeduncular space, and short lumbar vertebral pedicles. In adulthood there is an absence of the normal ilial flare and a narrow and horizontal positioning of the sacrum. As in infancy, the head appears large. A conductive or sensorineural hearing loss may be present.

Recurrence Risks and Prenatal Diagnosis. The risk of occurrence to children of an affected mother or father is 1 in 2 or 50 per cent. The risk of recurrence to subsequent children of nonaffected parents who have had an affected child is no greater than that for the general population. If both parents are affected, which is not uncommon, the risk for a heterozygous affected child is 1 in 2 or 50 per cent for achondroplasia and 1 in 4 or 25 per cent for the fatal homozygous state.

To date, ultrasound during the second trimester has been successful in detecting short-limbed dwarfism, but it cannot specifically identify achondroplasia.

FACIAL ABNORMALITIES

KBG Syndrome

Synonyms. Syndrome of short stature, characteristic facies, mental retardation, macrodontia, and skeletal anomalies.

Mode of Inheritance. Autosomal dominant.

Incidence. The incidence of this syndrome is unknown. "Mental retardation" is not a diagnosis. The population of individuals functioning at a retarded level is composed of individuals suffering from a number of entities due to specific causes. Understanding the cause or mode of inheritance is the first step to specific treatment or prevention. The KBG syndrome (an acronym suggested by Hermann and colleagues, using the first initial of the last name of the first three families described) is one of these entities, attributable to an autosomal dominant mutant gene.

Clinical Manifestations. Unless the disorder has occurred previously in a parent or a sibling, the KBG syndrome in a child may not be recognized early. Usually the affected individual presents with short stature, at or below the third percentile, with a normal-sized brachycephalic head, rounded facies with telecanthus, and wide eyebrows extending onto the upper lid (Fig. 3). The individual has a broad mouth with a thin upper vermilion border, a full lower vermilion border giving a (hunter's) bow-shaped mouth. Micrognathia is often present, with poorly aligned large teeth. The external ears are often prominent and the nares are anteverted. The children so far identified are developmentally delayed and when old enough for formal intelligence tests fall below the norm.

Table 1. Incidence of Craniosynostosis in 50,282 Newborn Infants

Ethnic Group	Number	Rate
White (22,811)	15	0.66
Black (24,030)	6	0.25
Puerto Rican (3441)	5	1.45
Total (50,282)	26	0.52

Skeletal x-rays may reveal cervical ribs, segmentation defects of the cervical vertebra, hands with short tubular bones, and irregular upper and lower plates of the thoracic vertebra with tonguing or notching of the anterior vertebral outline. Dental films often reveal fusion of teeth, producing macrodontia.

Confirmatory Tests. The diagnosis is determined by clinical evaluation and the already cited x-ray changes.

Recurrence Risk and Prenatal Diagnosis. The syndrome can vary in its expressivity. In all cases so far described, a parent has been affected. Thus, the risk to each subsequent child is 50 per cent. In the event that conclusive evidence is lacking on whether a parent is affected, the propositus presumably had suffered a mutation. In that event, there is no increased risk in subsequent generations. However, too few cases have been described to determine penetrance, and if the syndrome is nonpenetrant, this would influence risk assessment upon ascertainment of the first case in a family.

There is no prenatal test available.

Crouzon's Craniofacial Dysostosis

Synonyms. Crouzon's syndrome, facial and cranial dysostosis.

Mode of Transmission. Autosomal dominant with variable expression.

Prevalence or Incidence. In the Perinatal Collaborative Study which included 50,282 newborn infants, craniosynostosis was found in 26 of the 50,282 infants, with a slightly greater incidence in the Puerto Rican infants (Table 1).

Over 40 syndromes have been described that include craniosynostosis as part of the entity. Crouzon's

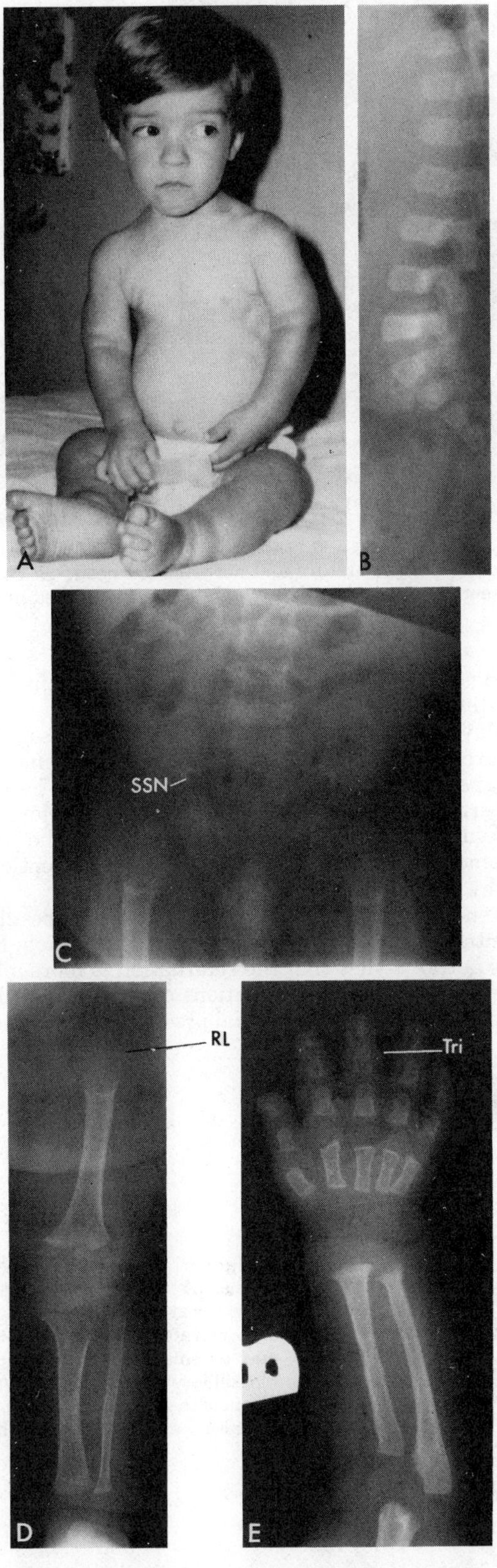

←

Figure 2. Achondroplasia. (*A*) A 32-month-old male. Note the relatively large head, proximal segment shortening of the upper extremities (rhizomelic), and normal-sized trunk. (*B*) X-rays of lumbar vertebrae reveal progressive shortening of the pedicles and the spines in both anteroposterior and lateral projections (*C*). The pelvis shows hypoplasia of the inferior portion of both ilia and small sacro-sciatic notches (SSN). There is rhizomelic shortening of the extremities, with flaring of the long bone metaphyses. (*D*) The lower extremity reveals a typical rounded lucency (RL) of the proximal femur. (*E*) The metacarpals are short, the distal phalanges are peg-shaped, and there is a V-shaped separation between the third and fourth digits, producing the trident deformity (Tri).

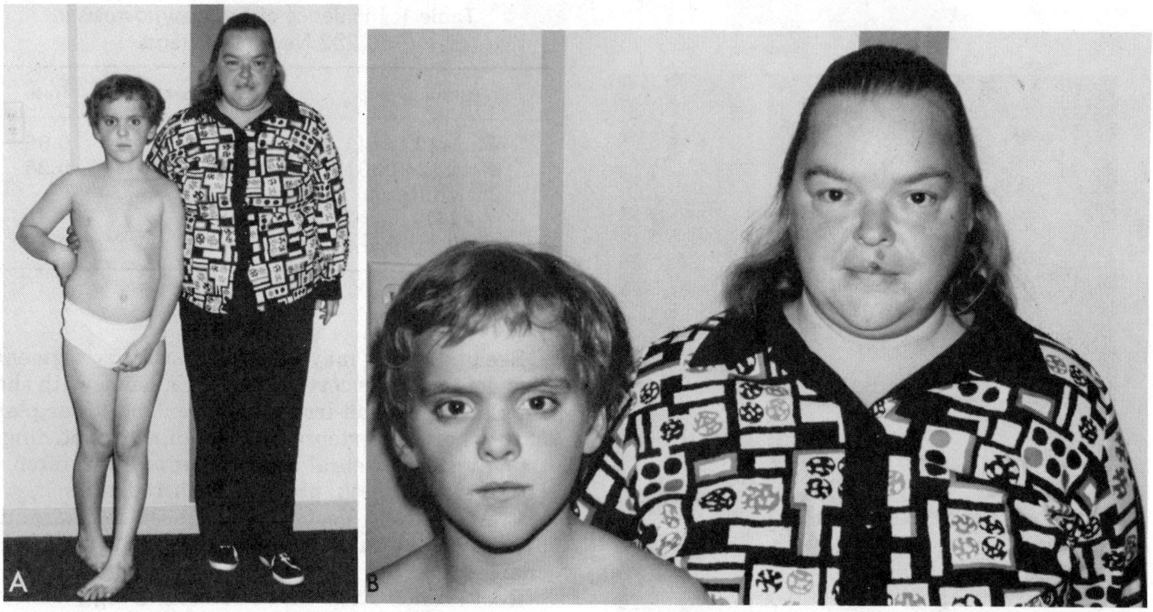

Figure 3. KBG syndrome. (*A*) Mother and son are both affected. Note short stature and normal-sized head. (*B*) Facial view. Both mother and son have generous eyebrows, bow-shaped mouth, and telecanthus, the latter more marked in the mother.

craniofacial dysostosis is one of those 40 entities and was one of the earliest recognized as genetic in etiology. Approximately 25 per cent of the patients with Crouzon's syndrome are a result of a new mutation.

Clinical Manifestations. Although Crouzon's craniofacial dysostosis may vary in expression, the anomaly is usually detectable at or very shortly after birth. Classically the head is brachycephalic, the nose is beaked (psittacorhina), and the mandible quite prominent. Within 6 to 12 months the child's brachycephaly becomes more pronounced. Decreased growth of the maxilla produces midface hypoplasia. The brachycephaly is due to a short anterior fossa and maxillary hypoplasia. These changes produce shortening of the roof and floor of the orbit, resulting in a small orbit and exophthalmos (Fig. 4).

Movement at the coronal, and often the sagittal, sutures cannot be detected. The psittacorhina and prognathism become more marked, the eyes become hyperteloric, and strabismus frequently develops. As a result of abnormal bony changes about the optic foramen or increased intracranial pressure, optic atrophy can develop.

A number of children may demonstrate developmental delay and ultimately mental retardation. It is this author's view that the retardation is more often due to associated malformations of the brain rather than to increased intracranial pressure. This does not

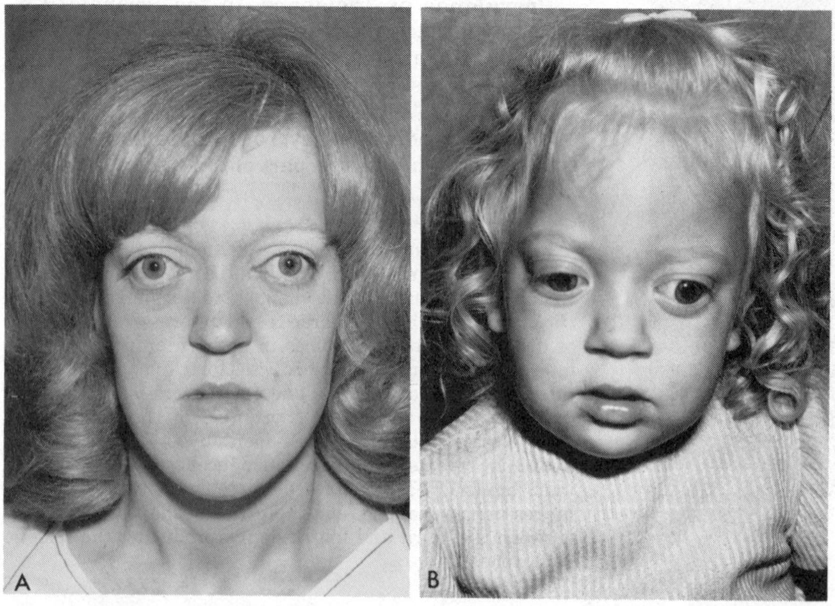

Figure 4. Crouzon's syndrome. (*A* and *B*) Mother and daughter are both affected. Both demonstrate prominent globes due to small orbit prominent mandible with a relative hypoplasia of the midface. The daughter also has a marked strabismus.

mean surgical correction of the synostosed sutures is unnecessary, for in those children who develop optic nerve compression or severe exophthalmos, neurosurgical intervention may be useful. Surgical treatment for cosmetic reasons may also be desirable.

Rarely additional anomalies can occur, such as cleft palate, atresia of the auditory meatus, and anterior subluxation of the head of the radius.

Since expressivity is highly variable, in some individuals the condition may be clinically inapparent. Skull films taken by 10 years of age should detect those patients with minimal involvement.

Confirmatory Tests. Clinical suspicions can be confirmed with skull films, which demonstrate the brachycephaly, shallow orbits, and premature synostosis of the coronal sutures. Computed tomographic (CT) scan is useful if hydrocephalus is suspected.

Recurrence Risk and Prenatal Diagnosis. If a parent is affected there is a 50 per cent risk with each pregnancy. If a parent clearly is not affected, only the affected child has a risk for occurrence in offspring.

To the present time, prenatal detection has not been successful; however, with the rapid improvements in ultrasonography, prenatal diagnosis will soon be possible.

LIMB ABNORMALITIES

Congenital Contractural Arachnodactyly (CCA)

Synonyms. Hereditary dysplasia of bone with kyphoscoliosis, contractures, and abnormally shaped ears; Beals-Hecht syndrome.

Mode of Inheritance. Autosomal dominant with variable expression.

Incidence. The incidence of this disorder is unknown. Beals and co-workers proposed that the patients originally described by Marfan suffered from CCA rather than the entity that now bears Marfan's name.

Clinical Manifestations. The etiology of contractures is varied and can be associated with different clinical entities. The evaluation of a patient with contractures, usually a child, must include a family pedigree, pregnancy history, and a description of the child's appearance at birth. Evaluation of the patient should document which joints are involved (i.e., proximal or distal); the extent of limitation of movement; and whether it is fixed and in what position it occurs at rest. Are there associated malformations? What is the neurologic status? Is the muscle mass normal? Is the overlying skin thickened and atrophic? And lastly, is there bony or soft-tissue fusion of the joint(s)?

Contractures can result from intrauterine constraints. Limitation of motion can result from primary muscle or neurologic disease; for example, the child with myelomeningocele can and does develop increasingly severe contracture of the joints in the area below the level of the neurologic lesion. Contracture occurs in metabolic diseases characterized by abnormal storage of mucolipids or mucopolysaccharides. Contracture also commonly occurs in diseases affecting the connective tissue, such as dermatomyositis and, obviously, the arthritides. CCA can be confused with arthrogryposis multiplex congenita; in the latter, however, the contractures are more severe and seldom improve spontaneously.

Individuals with CCA are often taller than expected in view of parental heights. CCA is characterized by contractures of the hips, knees, ankles, shoulders, elbows, wrists, and digits. The digits are long (arachnodactyly), and often contracture is in a flexed position, with the thumb in a flexed and adducted position (Fig. 5). The contractures may improve spontaneously. Kyphoscoliosis can occur, and the patient walks in an anteflexed position (Fig. 6).

Associated abnormalities are often seen, such as pectus excavatum and pectus carinatum. The external ears present a crumpled appearance, with a small, folded superior helix. Unlike the finding in Marfan's syndrome, the eyes are normal. There may be an associated congenital heart disease. Intelligience is normal.

With aging, the contractures may become more severe and kyphoscoliosis also increases in severity.

Confirmatory Tests. Diagnosis is based upon the family history and the clinical appearance. There are no diagnostic laboratory tests available.

Recurrence Risk and Prenatal Diagnosis. CCA is a dominant disorder, and thus an affected parent faces a 50 per cent chance of having an affected child. Because of the rarity of the disorder, the mutation rate as well as the penetrance is unknown.

Ectrodactyly

Synonyms. Split-hand deformity, lobster-claw deformity.

Mode of Inheritance. Autosomal dominant.

Incidence. Ectrodactyly, commonly called split-hand or lobster-claw deformity, is readily detectable at birth and occurs in 1.5 to 8 of 100,000 live-born infants.

Clinical Manifestations. Like many genetic disorders, ectrodactyly presents with a high degree of cosmetic and functional variability as well as genetic heterogeneity. The typical split-hand anomaly is characterized by two main anatomic variations. Type I

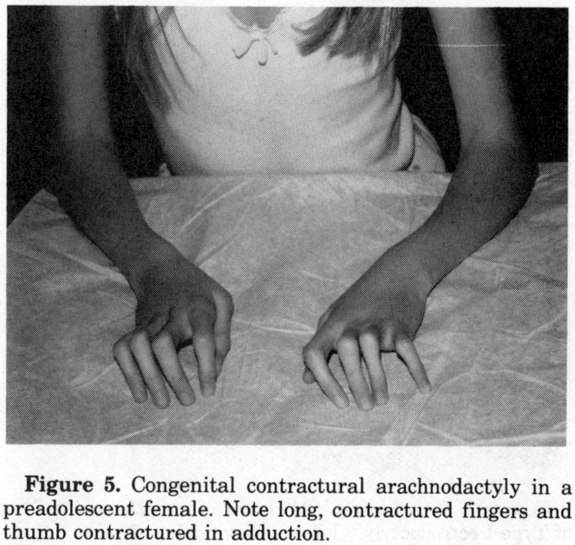

Figure 5. Congenital contractural arachnodactyly in a preadolescent female. Note long, contractured fingers and thumb contractured in adduction.

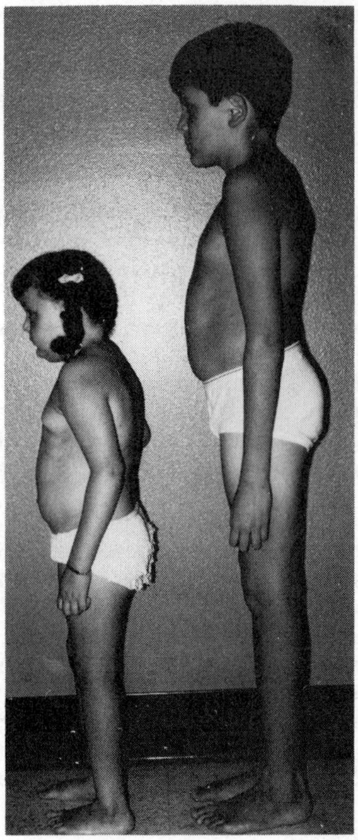

Figure 6. Siblings with congenital contractural arachnodactyly (CCA), lateral view. Both children are large, and even at this early age the girl, especially, stands in anteflexed position.

lobster-claw deformity results from an absence of central rays, with the hand thus being divided into two parts by a deep groove at the site of the absent third digit. The digits lateral to the groove may be syndactylous, as there may be only a first and fifth digit separated by this deep groove (Fig. 7). Characteristically, this affects both upper and lower extremities. Type II or monodactyly presents with absence of the radial rays, no cleft formation, but preservation of the fifth digit (monodactyly). The split-hand deformity can also be associated with unilateral or bilateral absence of the long bones, especially the femur, tibia, and fibula, less often the radius and ulna. Even within the typical split-hand deformity there appears to be a degree of genetic heterogeneity.

Atypical cases of split-hand deformity have also been reported that are unilateral, in contradistinction to the typical bilateral variety. The atypical split-hand syndrome occurs sporadically and thus is not genetic.

Ectrodactyly can also occur as part of a syndrome associated with other anomalies, such as perceptive deafness, congenital nystagmus, or orofacial malformation, the EEC (ectrodactyly, ectodermal dysplasia, and cleft lip/cleft palate) syndrome. The individual with the typical split-hand deformity functions very well. With the Type I deformity apposition of the thumb is present and these individuals may become very adept at fine motor activities. Even the monodactylous individual learns to function quite well. Individuals with Type I and Type II ectrodactyly do not have delayed development and function at a normal level.

Confirmatory Tests. There is no associated chromosomal or biochemical abnormality. X-rays of the hands and feet reflect changes seen clinically.

Recurrence Risks and Prenatal Diagnosis. The recurrence risk is high. In the typical variety of split-hand deformity, many families demonstrate the expected risk of 50 per cent; however, in other families the risk may be appreciably lower, to about 15 per cent.

Prenatal diagnosis with the use of ultrasound is possible, but this author questions its necessity in view of the normal function of these patients.

MENTAL RETARDATION

X-linked Mental Retardation with Fragile X

Synonyms. Congenital normofunctional testicular hyperplasia and mental deficiency; X-linked mental retardation and an X-chromosome marker; marker X

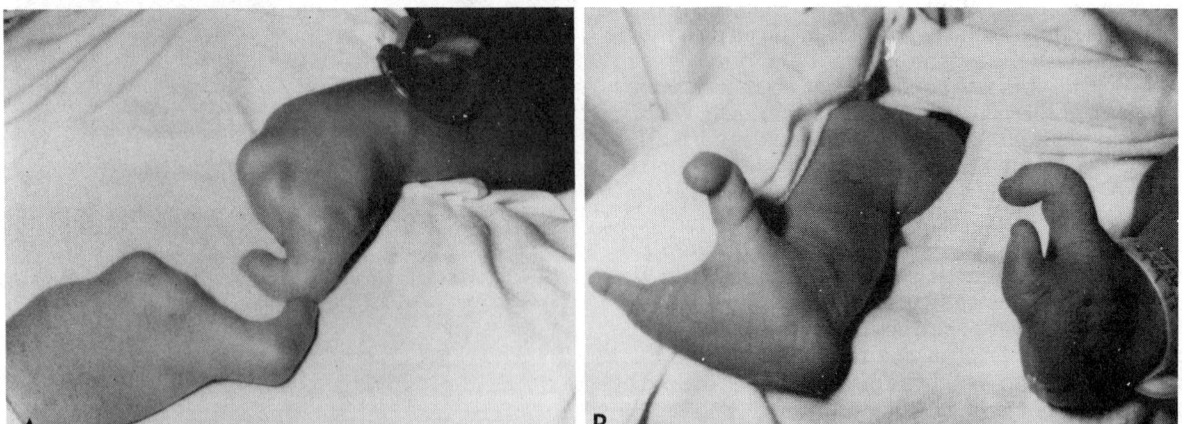

Figure 7. Ectrodactyly. (*A*) Hands of a mother with Type II monodactylous ectrodactyly. (*B*) Child's feet, characteristic of Type I ectrodactyly ("lobster claw" deformity).

chromosome, mental retardation, and macro-orchidism; X-linked mental deficiency and megalotestis syndrome.

Mode of Inheritance. Autosomal recessive.

Incidence. Penrose in 1938 noted a 25 per cent excess of males in a selected population of retarded individuals. Many surveys conducted since that time, including 1980 United States Census figures, reveal a significant excess of males. A significant proportion of the excess retardation in the male population is due to X-linked mental retardation (XLMR), and a subset of those with XLMR have associated megalotestis and a chromosome marker on the long arm of the X chromosome (Xq27) (Fig. 8). The absolute incidence of the fragile X (fra X) chromosome marker in males and females is not known, but Turner estimates that the prevalence of fra X in males to be 0.92 in 1,000 and in females 2.5 in 10,000.

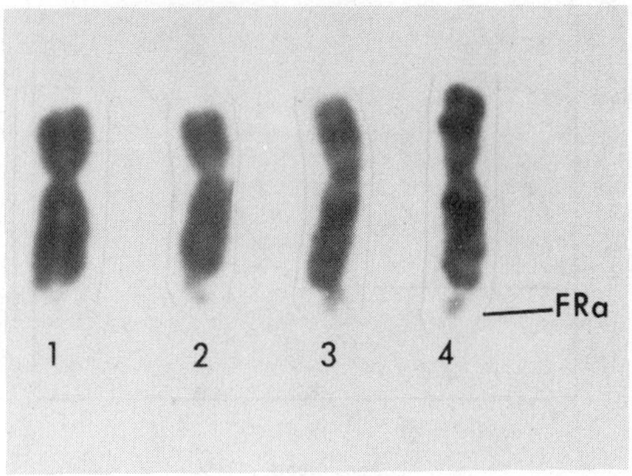

Figure 8. Four unbanded X chromosomes, each demonstrating characteristic fragile site (FRa) at the distal end, long arm of the X chromosome.

Clinical Manifestations. Not all males with XLMR manifest a fragile site on the X chromosome and megalotestis; however, for purposes of this description, only those males with XLMR and fra X with and without megalotestis are included.

Upon clinical examination of the affected male patient, few phenotypic abnormalities are found. The boys often are blue-eyed and tend to have prominent external ears, which upon measurement are longer than the norm (Fig. 9A, 9B). The testicular enlargement, when present can be subtle, but by actual measurement is characterized by a testicular volume greater than the norm. The testicular volume can be calculated by the formula $\pi/6 \times$ length $\times$ width squared. Alternatively, testicular models of varying sizes can be matched with the patient's testis (Fig. 10).

As the child progresses there is a delay in development; however, the children walk, talk, and can function in society. Measurement of their intelligence reveals a slight to moderate degree of mental retardation. The children have no neurologic abnormalities.

XLMR with fra X can produce mental retardation in girls. Lyonization can result in inactivation of the normal X; thus, gene expression by the mutant X results in mild to moderate degrees of mental retardation.

The male patients produce normal numbers of sperm, and reproduction has been reported, which means all of the sons are normal and all of the daughters will be hemizygous for the mutant X chromosome. The female hemizygote produces equal numbers of ova containing normal and mutant X chromosomes, so there is a 50 per cent chance a male fetus will receive the mutant X and a priori be retarded, and a 50 percent chance that a female fetus will receive a mutant X and, dependent upon lyonization, be retarded.

Confirmatory Tests. In early childhood, the presence of megalotestis may be the first clue to XLMR. The definitive test is the chromosome karyotype. In order to demonstrate fra X, the culture medium must be deficient in folic acid. If the medium is not deficient in folic acid, the fra X marker will not be visible. Folic acid treatment of patients with XLMR and fra X is currently under investigation; however, preliminary data are not encouraging

Risk of Occurrence and Prenatal Diagnosis. XLMR is believed to be second only to Down's syndrome as a cause of moderately severe mental retardation in the male, and any male presenting with mental retardation should be investigated for the fragile site on the X chromosome. Detection of the carrier mother is not always easy, for the presence of fra X seems to decrease with age. However, in any

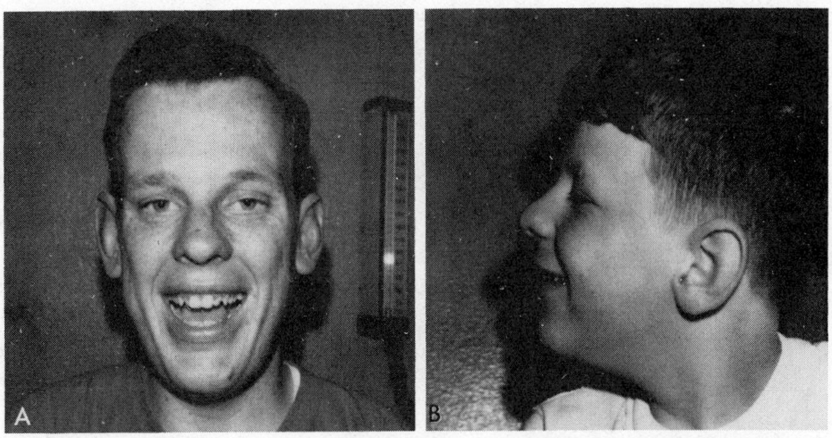

Figure 9. (*A* and *B*) X-linked mental retardation in siblings; the fragile site is at the distal end, long arm of X chromosome (Xq27). Both have normal-appearing facies with prominent external ears. Both also had megalotestis.

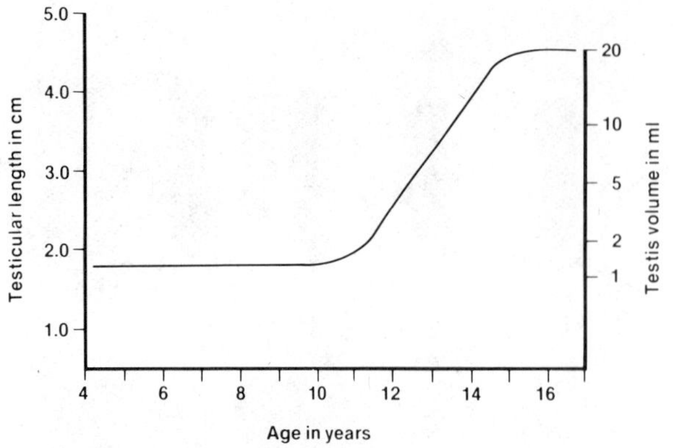

Figure 10. Normal values for testicular length and volume by age. Volume can be determined by measuring length and width or by use of testicular models (manufactured by Prader Company, Germany).

family with mental retardation associated with fra X, there is a 50 per cent chance that any male offspring will be affected and a 50 per cent chance that any female offspring will be a carrier. Amniocentesis during the second trimester has been successful in demonstrating the fragile X in the fetal karyotype, thus identifying a conceptus at risk for mental retardation.

Incontinentia Pigmenti (IP)

Synonym. Bloch-Sulzberger syndrome.

Mode of Inheritance. Probably X-linked dominant, with lethality in the male.

Incidence. IP is a rare disorder that is manifested by marked pleiotrophy and variable expression and is probably lethal in males. According to Lenz, 355 cases have been reported in females and 6 in males.

Clinical Manifestations. Incontinentia pigmenti is characterized by pigmentary disturbances of the skin variably associated with alopecia and dental, ocular, osseous, and neurologic abnormalities. The name IP is based upon the mistaken notion that melanin "leaks" from the basal layer of the epidermis, producing tattooing of the skin. The lesions at birth are located primarily on the trunk and typically present a swirling pattern of melanin resembling "marble cake" (Fig. 11). This characteristic appearance may be preceded by an inflammatory stage with redness, bullae, and scarring. The inflammatory stage is replaced by the "marble cake" melanin pigment patterns, which may come and go and often disappear by the third decade.

The skin lesions are usually associated with abnormal dentition and alopecia. These may be the only manifestations, and affected individuals, primarily females, can live normal lives, including reproductive capacity.

However, there is a subset of females affected with IP who can have more severe manifestations, including minor cosmetic abnormalities, supernumerary tragi, and extra ribs, but more importantly loss of vision due to retrolental fibroplasia; varying degrees of neurologic disturbance, including seizures; spastic quadriparesis; and mental retardation of varying degrees.

Confirmatory Tests. There are no specific tests available. Skin biopsy can be supportive of the diagnosis; however, the diagnosis is based upon clinical findings. Minimal criteria for the diagnosis include the pigment abnormalities, impaired dentition, and usually alopecia.

Recurrence Risk and Prenatal Diagnosis. If the mother is affected, there is a 50 per cent risk to each conceptus. Since the disorder is usually lethal to males, it is uncommon for a father to be affected, but if so, his sons are not at risk, but all of his daughters will be affected.

There is no prenatal diagnostic test available for IP.

LATE ONSET DISORDERS

Huntington's Disease

Synonyms. Progressive chorea, Huntington's chorea.

Mode of Inheritance. Autosomal dominant.

Incidence. Incidence within the United States and Western Europe varies between 1 in 15,000 to 1 in 20,000. New mutations seldom occur. It is of interest that a child manifesting Huntington's disease more

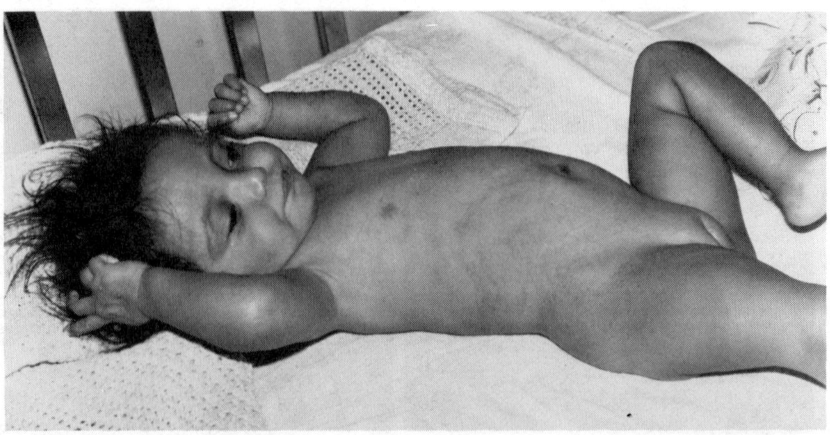

Figure 11. Female infant demonstrating developmental delay due to neurologic manifestations occasionally found in incontinentia pigmenti. The "marble cake" pattern of pigment distribution is seen over the lower right side of the abdomen onto the right upper thigh.

frequently inherits the disorder from the father than from the mother.

Clinical Manifestations. Features characteristic of Huntington's disease include a movement disorder most often choreiform in nature. The disease can begin at any age (Fig. 12), but commonly initial symptoms appear by 40 years of age. The onset is insidious, preceded oftentimes by years of anxiety and often depression. The latter, particularly, can be part of the disease process; however, the extreme anxiety and fear of the disease process can affect virtually all at-risk individuals. Suicide is not uncommon in those at risk, often before they have even developed the disease. Early in the course, the patient stumbles, drops objects, and generally seems clumsy. Accidents occur in the conduct of everyday tasks, for example, in cooking or using the stairs. Cigarettes are often left burning or dropped, resulting in injury to the patient as well as to others. Memory lapses occur and the individual may exhibit a labile disposition. Repetitive movements and restlessness, with constant shifting of position, occur. The purposeless repetitive movements become more frequent and progress to choreiform movements involving the extremities, trunk, and face. The gait assumes a shuffling nature and is accompanied by writhing motions of the trunk (Fig. 13). Speech becomes slurred and indistinct. Behavior, as well as body movements, becomes unpredictable, but with time the movement disorder becomes constant during waking hours.

Children often present with what appears to be mental retardation, delayed and difficult speech, and occasionally convulsions. The juvenile form often presents with rigidity similar to that seen in Parkinson's disease and progresses to the choreiform stage.

Physical examinations in the early stage may be

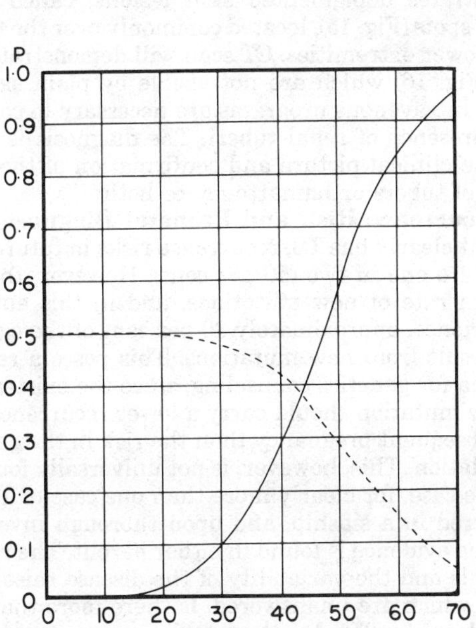

Figure 12. Profile of Huntington's disease. Age of onset is depicted on horizontal axis, and probability of development is shown (solid line) on the vertical axis. Note decreasing probability with increasing age (dashed line).

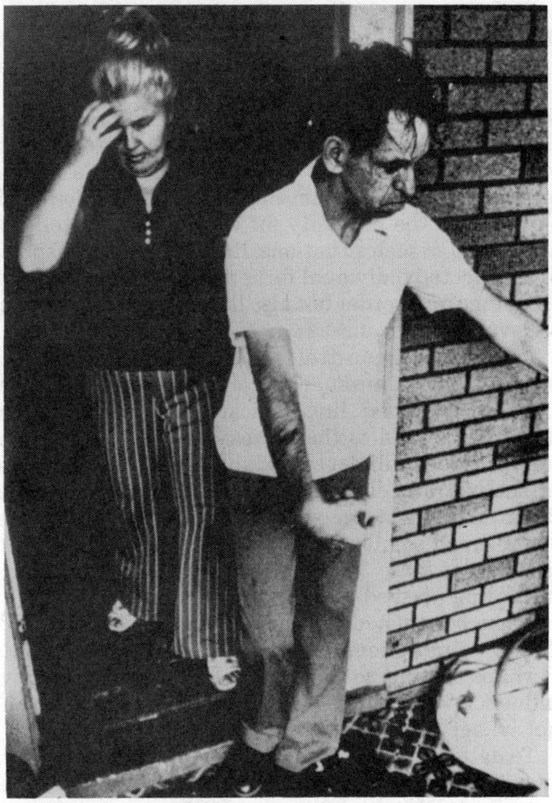

Figure 13. The man is affected with Huntington's disease. The photo poignantly depicts the movement disorder and the sadness of the patient's spouse.

unremarkable other than the reported clumsiness and dropping of objects; however, the patient soon develops upper motor neuron signs with increased tendon reflexes, positive great toe signs, and clonus. The patient's facies become mask-like, interspersed with grimacing. Sadly, within 10 to 20 years the patients cannot care for themselves and become bedfast and totally dependent. Debilitation resulting in pneumonia or aspiration is oftentimes the terminal event. It is this writer's view that the progress of the disease is enhanced *without* a sympathetic support system, and yet support of a patient with Huntington's disease becomes trying because of the unpredictable and labile mood swings, the seeming irresponsibility, and, occasionally, violence.

Confirmatory Tests. There is no satisfactory confirmatory test. A documented, accurate family history is essential. Prior to the symptomatic period, individuals may be given dopa, which temporarily produces signs of the disease, thus presaging the ultimate onset of Huntington's disease. However, the absence of such a response *does not* guarantee that the patient *will not* develop Huntington's disease. Psychological testing reflects the disease process. The CT scan demonstrates a characteristic atrophy in the region of the putamen, which may be earlier and more accurately reflected by positron emission tomography.

Treatment is symptomatic, and recent studies indicate vigorous attempts to control the movement disorder pharmacologically may enhance progression of the dementia.

Recurrence Risks and Prenatal Diagnosis. This is a disease of truly tragic proportions, for even though an at-risk person may have seemed healthy throughout life and may die of some unrelated disease or accident at 60 years of age, Huntington's disease may ultimately have developed in that person. This emphasizes the necessity for expert postmortem examination in such situations. In general, any offspring of an affected individual faces a 50 per cent chance of escaping the disorder but also has a 50 per cent chance of developing the disease.

Figure 12 demonstrates the relationship between age and time of onset. This can be used to refine risk figures. The solid line indicates age of onset, the dashed line reflects the decreasing probabilities that an individual will develop Huntington's disease as he or she becomes older. An at-risk person who reaches 50 or 60 years of age without developing the disease has a much smaller risk of developing it than an individual at 20 to 30 years. Also note that the probability line (dashed line) never reaches zero.

It has been noted that juvenile onset Huntington's disease is more commonly transmitted by the father. Perhaps there is some maternally derived protective influence when the disease occurs in the mother and not in her children.

To date, there is no prenatal test available for identification of the at-risk conceptus. With the use of the promising DNA probes, an accurate presymptomatic test for Huntington's disease may become available prior to satisfactory available specific therapy. This raises the ethical dilemma of telling an individual who seems well that he or she may develop a devastating disease.

Tuberous Sclerosis

Synonyms. Bourneville syndrome; Adenoma sebaceum, seizures, and mental retardation.

Mode of Inheritance. Autosomal dominant with a high frequency of new mutations.

Incidence. Because of the pleiotropic nature of the disease, the true incidence is not clear, but it is believed to be 1 in 15,000 to 1 in 20,000.

Clinical Course. There are no universally accepted criteria for tuberous sclerosis (TS); however, Berberich and Hall have suggested the following as minimal criteria for diagnosis: presence of multiple depigmented macules, angiofibromas, shagreen patches, or retinal hamartomas, alone or in combination with seizures or mental retardation. Alternatively, any three less commonly found features, such as subependymal nodules, renal hamartomas, gingival or subungual fibromas, astrocytomas, or lung cysts, also constitute adequate criteria for diagnosis.

The natural history of TS varies widely. In the florid state, TS presents during infancy with seizures, skin lesions, and a high risk for severe mental handicap (Fig. 14). The seizures are generalized, can be quite frequent, and are difficult to control. The mental handicap can be severe, rendering a patient quite dependent. The angiofibromas can be disfiguring. Control of the seizures and coping with the behavioral aberrations and cognitive deficits tries the endurance of even the most tolerant parent and physician. With this degree of severity, life expectancy is limited, for patients often do not survive into their mid-20's.

Another group of patients with TS may present with seizures, skin lesions, and less severe cognitive deficits. This author has cared for patients who have social skills and are capable of independent living, but who are troubled primarily by the recurring seizures and the persisting and unattractive angiofibromas. Their life expectancy is little different from the norm.

A third group of patients is made up of adults whose disorder is undetected until they have a child with the florid disease. Only then, as a result of laboratory investigation, is an isolated intracranial or renal tuber found in the parent.

TS is a multisystem disease. In addition to the involvement of the skin and central nervous system, hamartomas can occur within the eye and in the kidney, as can cysts within bone and lung.

Infrequently, the cerebral glial nodules undergo malignant transformation. More commonly the nodules may, by their position or growth, cause obstruction of the cerebrospinal fluid pathway and an increase in intracranial pressure. Optic atrophy may be the end result. The rupture of a cyst within the lung parenchyma may produce a pneumothorax. More commonly, progressive dyspnea, hemoptysis, and pulmonary hypertension occur if the lung is involved. Tumors located within the kidney can cause obstruction, leading to pyelonephritis and uremia. Rhabdomyoma of the heart is almost pathognomonic of TS, and the tumor can cause congestive heart failure.

Confirmatory Tests. A useful technique is examination of the skin with a Wood's light. This often demonstrates depigmented skin lesions, called "ash-leaf" spots (Fig. 15), located commonly over the flanks and lower extremities. CT scan will demonstrate tubers (Fig. 16) which are not visible by plain skull x-rays. Intravenous urograms are necessary to confirm the presence of renal tuberi. The diagnosis is made by the clinical picture and confirmation of the presence of tubers or hamartoma, or both.

Recurrence Risk and Prenatal Diagnosis. If a parent clearly has TS, recurrence risks in future children are one in two (50 per cent). However, there is a high rate of new mutations, and in this author's experience, approximately 80 per cent of the cases of TS result from new mutations. This poses a real dilemma for genetics counseling, since the existence of a new mutation should carry a lower recurrence risk in subsequent pregnancy than the risk in the general population. This, however, is not universally found to be the case, for clearly more than one case of TS has occurred in a sibship, and upon thorough investigation no evidence is found in either parent. The reason for this and the variability of the disease raise questions which are unanswered. Is there more than one gene locus for TS? Are there truly nonpenetrant cases of TS? Does germinal mosaicism occur? And, finally, are there modifying genes that prevent the expression of the mutant gene or conversely enhance the mutant gene's expression? To date, there has been no case of TS identified in a conceptus by prenatal diagnosis.

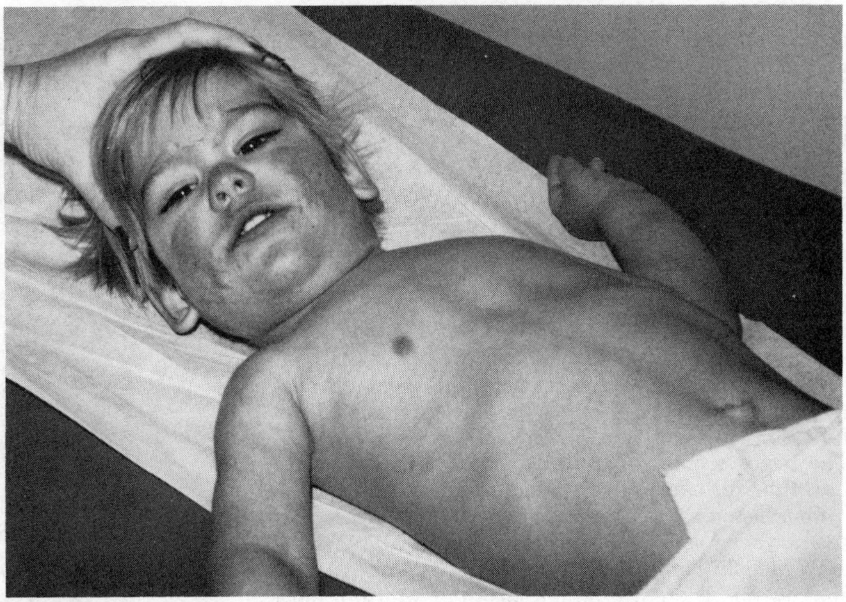

Figure 14. Tuberous sclerosis in a 16-month-old child. The child presented with major motor seizures, developmental delay, and "adenoma sebaceum" (facial angiofibromas), the latter an erythematous papular rash becoming confluent over the malar area.

However, the advent of improved ultrasound or more particularly gene linkage or gene probe studies makes the prenatal diagnosis of TS imminent.

MALE PSEUDOHERMAPHRODITISM

Androgen Resistance Syndrome

Synonyms. *Complete type*: Androgen insensitivity syndrome; testicular feminization syndrome. *Incomplete type*: Incomplete male pseudohermaphroditism, Type I (Wilson and Goldstein); feminizing male pseudohermaphroditism (Jones); incomplete testicular feminization syndrome; incomplete feminizing testes syndrome; Lubs' syndrome; Gilbert-Dreyfus syndrome.

Mode of Inheritance. X-linked recessive.

Incidence. It is estimated that complete androgen resistance occurs in approximately 1 in 60,000 to 1 in 65,000 live-born males. Due to the evolving clinical picture of incomplete androgen resistance, the actual incidence is unknown. Whether the two disorders are allelic has not been proved; however, it seems probable.

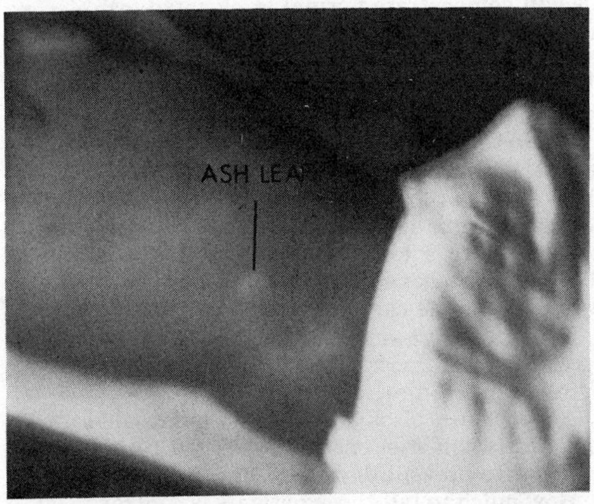

Figure 15. Ash leaf spot, seen only with ultraviolet light and a Woods filter.

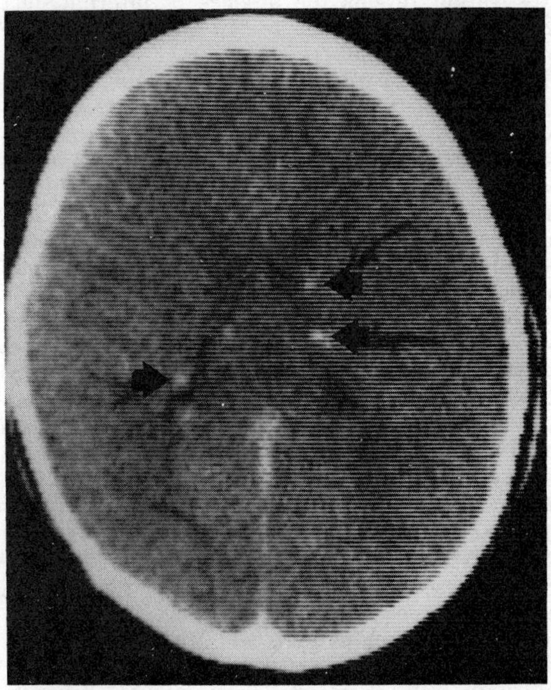

Figure 16. CT scan demonstrating calcified tubers in the brain (arrows).

Clinical Manifestations. Androgen resistance syndromes are the most common form of male pseudohermaphroditism. Wilson ranks androgen resistance syndromes as the third most common cause of primary amenorrhea in the phenotypic female, ranking behind gonadal dysgenesis and congenital absence of the vagina. Individuals with the androgen resistance syndromes have an XY male genotype. The fetal gonad at 40 days' gestation differentiates into a testis and produces testosterone; however, the target organs are insensitive to the testosterone. Owing to a defect in a specific cytosol-binding protein, there is no response to the testosterone produced by the fetal testis and therefore no wolffian duct structures develop. The müllerian suppressive factor in the male remains normally active and so inhibits the development of the fallopian tubes, uterus, cervix, and proximal vagina. The testosterone resistance can be complete or partial, thus influencing the phenotype.

Complete androgen resistance is seldom detected in the newborn period, as the external genitalia are unambiguously feminine. However, the vagina is quite shallow and there are no müllerian or wolffian duct structures. There is an absence of uterus, cervix, fallopian tube, and proximal portion of the vagina. The gonads are testes and remain either in the pelvis or in the labia. Simpson estimates that 50 per cent of patients with the complete variety develop a gonad-containing inguinal hernia; thus, in any phenotypic female who presents with an indirect inguinal hernia, appropriate cytogenetic procedures should be completed. The affected patient undergoes normal secondary sexual development; however, there is scant axillary and pubic hair (Fig. 17). Usually the diagnosis is not suspected until the patient fails to menstruate. At that time, a chromosome karyotype will reveal 46,XY or, less commonly, 47,XYY or 47,XXY. Further investigation reveals the absence of internal duct structures and the gonads to be testes. Reproductive ability is improbable.

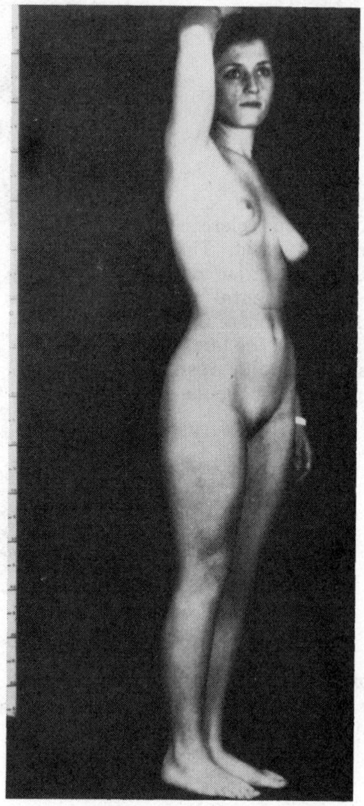

Figure 17. A paucity of body hair is demonstrated in a phenotypic woman with complete androgen resistance.

An infant with *incomplete testosterone resistance* can be identified at birth, for the genitalia are ambiguous, presenting with clitoromegaly and varying degrees of labioscrotal fusion. Further investigation reveals intra-abdominal testes, absence of müllerian duct structures, and absent or vestigal wolffian duct structures. Pubertal breast development, amenorrhea, and infertility occur, as may varying degrees of virilization.

In both types of androgen insensitivity syndromes, the risk of testicular cancer is increased. The tumors generally do not occur until the third decade. It seems advisable to allow patients to reach adolescence normally and then remove the testes. If the testes are removed prior to adolescence, substitution hormonal therapy will be necessary for the development of normal secondary sex characteristics.

The androgen resistance syndromes must be differentiated from other types of male pseudohermaphroditism presenting with a female phenotype. Other disorders include pure gonadal dysgenesis with an XY karyotype, in which patients will not become feminized at adolescence, have bilateral streak gonads, and are usually taller than individuals with XO Turner's syndrome; disorders due to deficiency of enzymes necessary for normal testosterone formation; agenesis of Leydig cells; and, rarely, the autosomal recessive disorder agonadism.

Confirmatory Tests. A chromosome karyotype should be completed for any phenotypic female born to a family known to have a child with the androgen resistance syndrome. A karyotype is also recommended in the evaluation of the phenotypic female with an inguinal hernia, a phenotypic female who fails to menstruate at adolescence, or individuals with ambiguous genitalia. Measurement of hormonal levels will demonstrate normal or elevated testosterone and elevated plasma luteinizing hormones. As a diagnostic test, fibroblasts obtained from a skin biopsy in the genital area should be examined for presence of cytosol androgen receptors.

Recurrence Risk and Prenatal Diagnosis. The androgen resistance syndromes are believed to result from either an X-linked recessive or a sex-limited autosomal dominant mutation, so that any genetic male born to a carrier female has a 50 per cent risk for this disorder. Any genetic female offspring has a 50 per cent risk for the carrier state.

Prenatal diagnosis may be possible upon demonstration of XY karyotype plus a defect in androgen cytosol binding protein.

A word must be said about treatment and counseling. Castration after onset of puberty is recommended in order to prevent development of testicular tumor.

How much to tell these patients is controversial. It is this author's belief that the patient and parents should be informed of all aspects. In light of the availability of medical records, including information on insurance forms, the patient and family will at some time discover the facts. It is preferable to provide this information to the patient and family gradually, dependent upon the patient's and family's assessed ability to deal with this threatening information. The alternative too often is for the patient or family to accidentally or inappropriately discover the facts.

TERATOGENIC AGENTS

By James W. Hanson, M.D.
and James A. Bartley, Ph.D., M.D.
Iowa City, Iowa

Teratogens are agents that can cause birth defects when present in the environment of the developing fetus. It is increasingly clear that such factors singly or in combination with other genetic or environmental agents account for a substantial proportion of all congenital defects. As these are often avoidable hazards, it is important for physicians who care for children and pregnant, or potentially pregnant, women to be familiar with these disorders. This will not only facilitate diagnosis leading to improved care, but also may allow primary preventive steps to be taken.

INDICATORS OF POTENTIAL TERATOGENICITY

As a group, teratogens characteristically produce prenatal-onset growth deficiency, reproductive loss, and alterations of nervous system performance in addition to defects of morphogenesis. As a result, the clinician may deal with teratogenic concerns prior to pregnancy, during pregnancy, or after pregnancy. In addition, some teratogens are also associated with a mutagenic or carcinogenic potential.

Defects of morphogenesis especially raise concerns about prenatal exposure to a teratogen. However, as genetic factors (see article on Approach to Genetic Diseases) can also contribute to such anomalies, it is important for the clinician to recognize specific patterns of defects associated with particular agents. In addition, the clinician should be aware of the substantial variability in effects manifested among any group of affected children. This variability can be attributed to four sources:

1. *Variations in exposure dosage.* The higher the dose, the greater is the likelihood of an effect and the likelihood that the effect will be severe.
2. *Variations in exposure timing.* There are susceptible periods, especially during organogenesis, when teratogens may act. At other times, the fetus may not be damaged by an exposure.
3. *Variations in host susceptibility.* Inborn genetic differences, such as in drug metabolism, may predispose some fetuses to the teratogenic effects of an agent.
4. *Interactions with other environmental factors.* Pregnant women may be exposed to a variety of potentially hazardous agents. Combinations of these agents may have additive or other types of interactions in the fetus.

CATEGORIES OF TERATOGENS

Teratogenic agents can be grouped into four broad categories: infectious agents, physical agents, drugs and chemicals, and maternal metabolic and genetic factors. An exhaustive discussion of each agent is beyond the scope of this article. However, a summary of agents about which concerns are frequently expressed is presented in Tables 1 through 4. More detailed information can be obtained from standard reference resources.

DIAGNOSTIC AIDS

Vital to the diagnosis of a teratogenic disorder is the identification and documentation of a hazardous exposure. In the case of infectious disorders, microbiologic cultures and serologic investigations may provide objective evidence of fetal infection. Likewise, appropriate laboratory investigation of possible maternal health problems, such as diabetes mellitus, myotonic dystrophy, or phenylketonuria, can help to confirm the teratogenic etiology of fetal abnormalities. However, a carefully taken prenatal history, buttressed by the observations of independent individuals, may be the only source of information about exposure to many other agents, such as drugs of abuse and alcohol.

In all instances a careful search for the specific defects associated with a particular teratogen is crucial to such a diagnosis. Teratogens do not produce defects at random. The search may include radiographic, ophthalmologic, and psychologic studies.

PITFALLS IN DIAGNOSIS

Because most teratogenic exposures are associated with wide variation in outcomes, substantial overlapping of effects among these agents may be expected. Likewise, some genetic disorders may produce similar patterns of abnormalities. This can lead to substantial diagnostic confusion, especially in the absence of a positive family history.

SPECIFIC TERATOGENIC DISORDERS

A few relatively common teratogenic disorders deserve special comment because of their frequency or medical therapeutic implications.

Fetal Alcohol Syndrome

Synonym

Fetal alcohol effects.

Table 1. Infectious Teratogenic Agents

Agent	Effects			
	Fetal Death	Growth Deficiency	Mental Deficiency	Congenital Abnormalities
Viruses				
Rubella	+	+	+	Ocular and cardiovascular anomalies, deafness, microcephaly, immune and endocrine disturbances, delayed skeletal development
Cytomegalovirus	+	?	+	Ocular and cardiovascular anomalies, deafness, microcephaly, hydrocephaly, ? gastrointestinal tract anomalies
Herpes simplex	+	?	+	Ocular anomalies, microcephaly, patent ductus arteriosus, hypoplastic distal phalanges
Varicella zoster	?	+	+	Ocular anomalies, microcephaly, hypoplastic limbs, neurogenic muscular atrophy, cutaneous defects
Bacteria				
Treponema pallidum	+	+	+	Ocular, dental and skeletal anomalies, hydrocephaly, microcephaly, cutaneous lesions, nerve palsies, nephrosis
Mycoplasmas	+	?	?	?Neural tube defects, ?aneuploidy
Parasites				
Toxoplasma	+	+	+	Ocular anomalies, microcephaly, hydrocephaly, deafness
Possibly Hazardous Agents				
Influenzavirus	+	?	?	?Neural tube defects, ?hydrocephaly
Measles virus	+	?	?	?
Mumps virus	+	?	?	?Endocardial fibroelastosis, diabetes mellitus
Lymphocytic choriomeningitis virus	?	?	?	?Hydrocephaly
Polioviruses	?	?	?	?Paralysis
Coxsackie B viruses	?	?	?	?Heart defects
Condyloma acuminatum virus	?	?	?	?Laryngeal papillomata

? = Proposed association; magnitude of risk uncertain; more information needed.

Definition

The fetal alcohol syndrome is a pattern of altered growth and development near the extreme end of a spectrum of fetal effects resulting from prenatal exposure to ethanol. Although previous descriptions of the effects of ethanol on the fetus had been published, the disorder was most clearly described and investigated by Jones and Smith in the early 1970s. Subsequent studies by others using both human data and experimental animals confirm the hazards of prenatal ethanol exposure.

It is now clear that use of ethanol by pregnant women can result in a wide spectrum of fetal abnormalities. The frequency and severity of these anomalies appear to be dose-related, and range from apparently clinically unaffected children to severely affected children with the so-called fetal alcohol syn-

Table 2. Physical Hazards to the Fetus

Agent	Effects
Radiation	
High levels	Microcephaly, ?ocular defects, mutations, malignancy
Low levels	?Mutations, ?malignancy, no clear association with birth defects
Heat or fever	Neural tube defects, ?other CNS anomalies, ?mental retardation
Mechanical factors	
Oligohydramnios, multiple gestation, uterine malformation	Positional deformities, ?limb reduction defects, ?mandibular hypoplasia
Amniotic bands	Syndactyly, prenatal limb amputations, atypical facial clefts, exencephaly, encephalocele, thoracogastroschisis, ocular defects

? = Proposed association; magnitude of risk uncertain; more information needed.

Table 3. Drug and Chemical Hazards to the Fetus

Agent	Congenital Abnormalities
Environmental Chemicals	
Organic mercurials	Microcephaly, cerebral palsy, mental retardation
Polychlorinated biphenyls (PCBs)	"Cola-colored" babies, growth deficiency, natal teeth, exophthalmos
Xylene*	?Caudal regression syndrome
"Agent Orange" and dioxin*	No clear evidence of association with malformations, dioxin may be mutagenic, risk to exposed fetuses probably low
Pesticides*	?Little information available
Heavy metals*	?Little information available
Nonprescription drugs	
Thalidomide	Limb reduction malformations; cardiac, renal, gastrointestinal, ocular, and aural anomalies
Ethyl alcohol	Fetal alcohol syndrome; mental and growth deficiency; fetal death; cardiac, ocular, central nervous system, and skeletal malformations; cleft palate; characteristic facies
Tobacco	Growth deficiency; fetal death; no clear association with human malformations
Salicylates*	?Growth deficiency, ?patent ductus arteriosus
Opiates*	Growth deficiency; no clear association with human malformations
Caffeine*	No clear link to human malformations
Other "street drugs" (e.g., amphetamines, LSD, hallucinogens, marijuana)*	No clear link to human malformations
Prescription drugs	
Anticancer agents	
Folic acid antagonists (e.g., methotrexate)	Fetal death; growth and mental deficiency; characteristic facies; central nervous system, ocular, and skeletal malformations; cleft palate
Alkylating agents (e.g., chlorambucil, nitrogen mustards)	Fetal death; growth and mental deficiency; ocular, genitourinary, and limb malformations; cleft palate
Other agents	Insufficient information, probably hazardous
Anticoagulant agents	
Coumarin derivatives	Fetal death; growth and mental deficiency; characteristic facies; central nervous system and skeletal anomalies; choanal atresia
Heparin*	?Fetal death
Antibiotics	
Tetracyclines	Dental abnormalities
Streptomycin	Hearing loss
Kanamycin	?Hearing loss
Aminoglycosides (e.g., gentamicin)	?Hearing loss
Chloroquine	?Ocular defects, ?hearing loss
Pyrimethamine	No consistent association with human malformations
Penicillins*	No consistent association with human malformations
Sulfonamides*	No consistent association with human malformations
Anticonvulsants	
Oxazolidines (e.g., trimethadione)	Trimethadione syndrome; fetal death; growth and mental deficiency; characteristic facies; cardiac, central nervous system, gastrointestinal, genitourinary, and limb malformations; cleft palate
Hydantoins (e.g., phenytoin)	Hydantoin syndrome; growth and mental deficiency; characteristic facies; cardiac, skeletal, and limb malformations; cleft palate; possible association with neuroblastoma
Barbiturates (and primidone)	?Possible syndrome; present evidence inconclusive
Valproic acid	?Possible syndrome; meningomyelocele; cardiac malformations
Diazepam	?Low risk for facial clefts
Others	Insufficient information
Endocrine agents	
Female sex hormones	
Diethylstilbestrol	Vaginal anomalies, vaginal adenocarcinoma, ?uterine malformation, testicular abnormalities, ?testicular malignancy
Progestins	Masculinization of females

Table continued on following page

Table 3. Drug and Chemical Hazards to the Fetus (Continued)

Agent	Congenital Abnormalities
Prescription drugs (continued)	
Endocrine agents (continued)	
Female sex hormones (continued)	
Estrogen/progestin combinations (e.g., birth control pills)	?Possible very low risk for cardiac and other anomalies
Clomiphene*	?Neural tube defects, ?Down's syndrome, ?positional deformities
Adrenal corticosteroids*	No consistent association with human malformations
Antithyroid agents (e.g., methimazole, propylthiouracil)	Possible hypothyroidism and mental deficiency, ?limb and scalp defects
Psychotropic agents	
Lithium	?Cardiac anomalies
Amphetamines*	?Cardiac anomalies
Phenothiazines*	?Limb and cardiac anomalies
Tricyclic antidepressants*	?Limb anomalies
Meprobamate*	?Brain, heart, palate, and limb defects
Benzodiazepines*	?Cleft palate
Butyrophenones*	?Limb reduction malformations
Barbiturates	?Cardiac and brain defects
Other agents	
Antihistamines*	No consistent association with human malformations
Diuretics*	No consistent association with human malformations
Anesthetic gases	?Fetal wastage; no consistent association with human malformations
Spermicides*	?Limb malformations
Penicillamine	Abnormal connective tissue syndrome
Retinoic acid (isoretinoin)	?Brain and craniofacial malformations

*These drugs have not been clearly associated with congenital defects, and available information is insufficient to ascribe specific risk estimates. In each case, if the risk is increased at all, it is estimated to be very low.
? = Proposed association; magnitude of risk uncertain; more information needed.

drome, often born to women with severe chronic alcoholism. Current evidence suggests that the average daily consumption of as little as two drinks per day in the early parts of pregnancy or periodic binge drinking in early pregnancy may be associated with recognizable (although milder) abnormalities in a significant percentage of exposed newborns. At the more severe end of the spectrum, there would appear to be a 50 per cent or greater risk of severe abnormalities of growth and performance in the offspring of chronic alcoholics. Recent data suggest that in both humans and animals, alcohol consumption during pregnancy is associated with an increased risk of fetal death that is dose-related.

Epidemiologic studies suggest that prenatal damage from maternal abuse of alcohol may be one of the most frequent recognizable causes of mental deficiency in the United States. This is particularly tragic, since virtually all such exposures are unnecessary and avoidable. Increased levels of ethanol abuse by children and adolescents suggest that this problem may well become more prevalent in the near future. At

Table 4. Hazardous Maternal Metabolic and Genetic Factors for the Fetus

Factor	Effects
Diabetes mellitus (insulin-dependent)	Cardiovascular, renal, and neural tube defects; facial clefts; holoprosencephaly; caudal regression syndrome
Phenylketonuria	Mental retardation, growth deficiency, microcephaly, ?heart defects, ?vertebral defects, ?fetal death
Myotonic dystrophy	Severe early-onset myotonic dystrophy, arthrogryposis, ?heart defects, ?hernia, ?hydrocephaly, ?hydronephrosis, ?facial clefts
Malnutrition	Growth deficiency; no clear link with human malformations

? = Proposed association; magnitude of risk uncertain; more information needed.

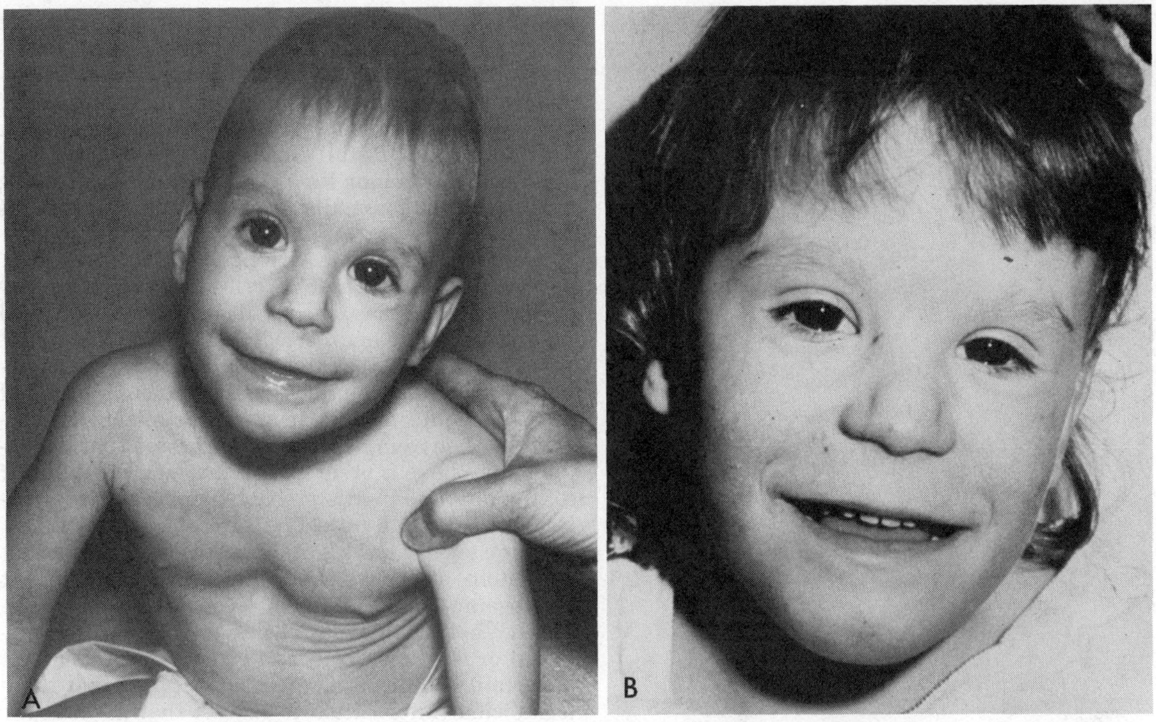

Figure 1. Facial features of the fetal alcohol syndrome at 4 months (*A*) and 2 years (*B*) of age.

the present time, it would seem prudent to suggest that pregnant women or women who might become pregnant avoid ethanol as much as possible, with the safest amount being none at all.

Clinical Manifestations and Course

The fetal alcohol syndrome is characterized by a distinctive facial appearance, prenatal-onset growth deficiency, an increased frequency of developmental and mental retardation, and an increased frequency of major congenital anomalies. Children with this syndrome display a rather flat midface with narrow palpebral fissures; a low nasal bridge; short, upturned nose; and rather long, convex philtrum, with narrow vermilion border of the upper lip (Fig. 1). Presenting as small-for-gestational-age babies in the newborn period, they continue to grow poorly and often are admitted to the hospital for evaluation of so-called failure to thrive. In the newborn period, the babies may be described as jittery or tremulous, a feature that often results in confusion with drug withdrawal symptoms. However, these neurologic abnormalities persist, and in addition to showing developmental delay and frank mental retardation such children often show poor coordination, tremulousness, and sometimes "hyperactivity" in later life. A wide variety of congenital anomalies has been associated with this syndrome, including cleft palate, cardiac malformations (especially atrial and ventricular septal defects), microphthalmia, joint anomalies, and a variety of dermal and skeletal abnormalities. Neuropathologic examination has often revealed significant abnormalities of neuronal migration, occasionally associated with microcephaly, hydrocephaly, absence of the corpus callosum, and cerebellar abnormalities.

Pitfalls in Diagnosis

The fetal alcohol syndrome has been confused with a wide variety of other conditions, including Noonan's syndrome, Williams' syndrome, trisomy 18 syndrome, Aarskog's syndrome, fetal hydantoin syndrome, and neurofibromatosis. Particular attention should be directed at the exclusion of these and other, similar disorders, especially in more mildly or atypically affected individuals from whom a clear history of ethanol abuse cannot be elicited.

Fetal Hydantoin Syndrome

Synonyms

Fetal hydantoin effects, fetal Dilantin syndrome.

Definition

The fetal hydantoin syndrome is a pattern of altered growth and development attributable to prenatal exposure to phenytoin and other hydantoin anticonvulsants. Although concern regarding the possible role of hydantoin anticonvulsants, specifically phenytoin, in the production of birth defects was voiced as early as 1972, there is still widespread disagreement about the frequency and severity of defects in infants exposed prenatally to this agent. In 1975 a distinct syndrome, the fetal hydantoin syndrome, was described. Subsequent investigations suggest that approximately 10 per cent of exposed infants may be sufficiently affected to be diagnosed in infancy, whereas an additional 30 per cent may show lesser degrees of alteration. In addition, familial occurrence of this pattern of altered growth and development has

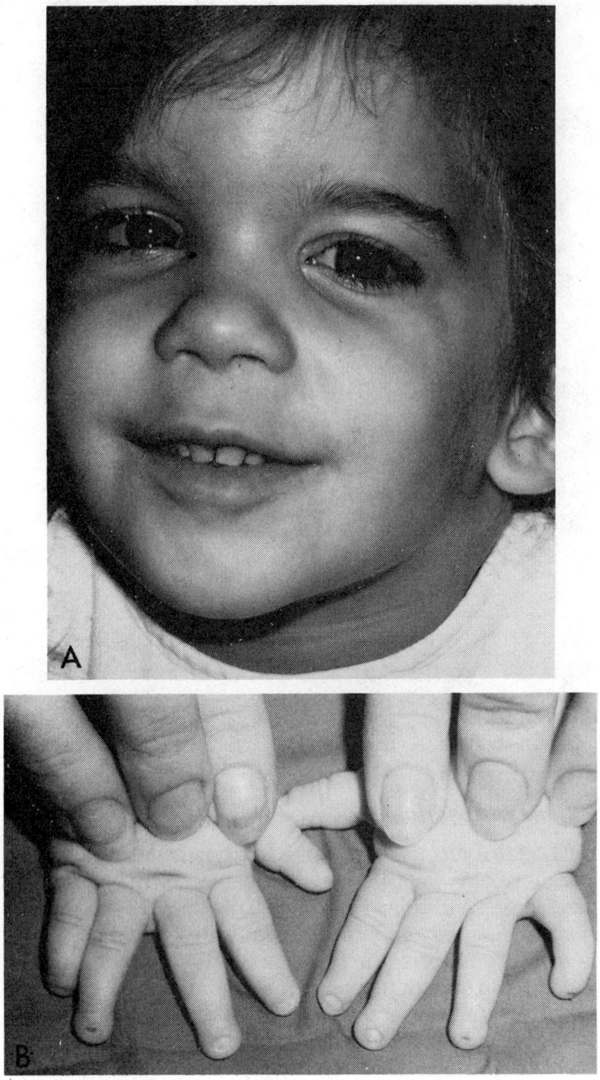

Figure 2. Facial features (*A*) and distal phalangeal hypoplasia (*B*) in a child with fetal hydantoin syndrome.

been seen in several families, whereas other families have been described in which no child seems to be affected. This has raised the possibility that individual differences in drug metabolism may contribute in some fashion to this pattern of altered growth and development. An animal model of the fetal hydantoin syndrome has been developed that supports the conclusion that this pattern of altered growth and development is attributable to drug therapy.

Clinical Manifestations and Course

The abnormalities found in children exposed prenatally to hydantoin anticonvulsants include a characteristic facial appearance, with hypoplasia of the midface, low nasal bridge, ocular hypertelorism, and an accentuated cupid's bow of the upper lip (Fig. 2). Prenatal-onset growth deficiency, including poor growth for weight, length, and head circumference, is occasionally seen. However, no information linking the use of phenytoin to early miscarriage has yet been presented. Children with this characteristic pattern of altered growth and development often show alterations of central nervous system performance, including mental deficiency. In addition, an increased risk of developing major malformation—particularly cleft lip and palate, distal phalangeal hypoplasia, and other, usually minor limb reduction malformations, cardiovascular anomalies, and skeletal defects, has been noted.

Recently four infants with signs of the fetal hydantoin syndrome have been described who subsequently developed neuroblastomas; a fifth child was identified with a melanotic neuroectodermal tumor of infancy. In view of the association of hydantoins with lymphomatous changes in adults and the observation of an epoxide intermediate in one of the metabolic pathways of phenytoin, it has been suggested that hydantoins may have a prenatal carcinogenic potential. If so, the absolute risk is probably very low. Nevertheless, this possibility deserves further evaluation.

Taken together, these findings strongly suggest that hydantoin anticonvulsants may have a significant teratogenic potential for at least some exposed infants. Whether this may be due to differences in maternal or fetal metabolism of genetic origin is as yet uncertain. However, it would now appear that there is sufficient information to suggest that all epileptic women, especially those receiving phenytoin, should be cautioned, prior to beginning pregnancy, of the potential adverse outcomes for their offspring. In some instances a trial off drug therapy prior to pregnancy may be warranted. In other cases, when it is deemed unsafe to remove the mother from such drug therapy, she should be placed on the least number of anticonvulsant agents and the lowest dosages compatible with adequate seizure control, and the potential hazards of anticonvulsant therapy to the offspring should be discussed in detail.

Fetal Warfarin Syndrome

Synonyms

Synonyms include fetal warfarin effects and fetal coumarin syndrome.

Definitions

The fetal warfarin syndrome is a pattern of altered growth and development attributable to prenatal exposure to coumarin anticoagulants characterized by Hall during the past decade. Published case reports and review of pregnancies in which coumarin derivatives were used reveal that there is an increase in abortion, stillbirth, and prenatal growth deficiency in exposed infants.

Clinical Manifestations and Course

Overall, approximately one third of exposed fetuses or infants die prenatally or suffer serious teratogenic consequences. At most, two thirds of exposed infants appear to be normal at the time of birth. The period of greatest concern for the production of fetal anomalies extends from approximately 6 to 9 weeks after conception. During this time period a characteristic syndrome of craniofacial anomalies (Fig. 3) and other defects is often produced. Affected infants characteristically demonstrate prenatal-onset growth deficiency with subsequent failure to thrive, developmental delay, mental deficiency, and other neurologic abnormalities, including hypotonia and seizures. Facial features are strikingly abnormal in many cases, with a severe degree of hypoplasia that may also affect the ethmoid complex, resulting in choanal atresia.

Microcephaly is common, and optic atrophy has repeatedly been observed. Radiographic studies often reveal a lag in skeletal maturation with stippling of epiphyseal growth centers. Other serious malformations occur less frequently.

Beyond 9 weeks of age, ocular defects and midline central nervous system malformations may be produced. Children with these abnormalities often have a poor prognosis. Survivors not suffering from mental retardation, however, usually do relatively well except for the various craniofacial cosmetic abnormalities.

PATERNAL EXPOSURES

Concern is often voiced regarding the potential role of paternal exposures to teratogenic agents in the pathogenesis of birth defects. It is important to emphasize that it seems unlikely that such paternal exposures could produce a birth defect in a particular infant other than by means of the mechanism of mutation. Although the possibility of mutation certainly exists for many agents to which fathers might potentially be exposed, the overall risk for mutation would presumably apply to many different genetic loci, each at a relatively low frequency. Thus, there would not be expected to be any consistent pattern of fetal abnormalities among the offspring of an exposed male. Rather, a low-frequency increase in a variety of categories, particularly related to new autosomal dominant mutations, would be anticipated. Such reports have not occurred at the present time, although it is possible that such exposures contribute to the increased paternal age effect seen with a number of autosomal dominant and X-linked recessive single-gene disorders. Thus, it would appear likely that preconceptional paternal exposures to most potentially teratogenic agents in general present minimal absolute risks to the fetus and certainly none at all if the exposure occurred subsequent to conception.

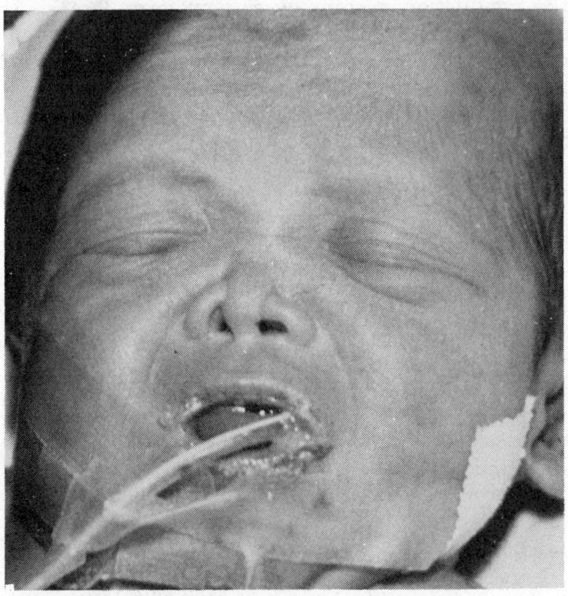

Figure 3. Facial features of the fetal warfarin syndrome. Note severely hypoplastic midface and nose.

COUNSELING FOR TERATOGENIC EXPOSURE

The essence of prevention of birth defects from teratogenic exposures is the exclusion of the teratogen from the prenatal environment. Although this is not always possible at the present time, increased attention should be paid by physicians to patient education in this respect. It is incumbent upon both patients and treating physicians to be aware of the teratogenic potential of many agents and to avoid unnecessary drug exposure or exposures to other potentially teratogenic agents during pregnancy, particularly during the first trimester, whenever possible. In situations in which there is a clear need for drug therapy, the potential risks and benefits should be discussed with the patient in advance of drug therapy, and preferably in advance of pregnancy. In the final analysis, decisions regarding the use of potentially dangerous agents during pregnancy are best left to an informed couple armed with knowledge provided by a sensitive and supportive physician. Failure to inform a pregnant or potentially pregnant patient of hazards relating to medical treatment or procedures may place the physician in legal jeopardy.

Concern is often voiced that informing couples of the adverse effects of a drug, chemical agent, or other potential teratogen on a child with birth defects may create serious psychologic problems, particularly in situations that may involve maternal drug abuse, such as excessive consumption of ethanol. It must be stressed that only through such a frank approach will it be possible to prevent teratogenic effects in other children. It is clear, however, that the sharing of such information may indeed produce psychologic problems. Under these circumstances it is extremely important to provide long-term support to affected families through existing agencies and health care mechanisms.

The evaluation of children suspected to have been damaged by a teratogen or in whom a teratogenic exposure has occurred prenatally begins with a high index of suspicion. A careful search of the prenatal history for such exposures should be made and the child examined for abnormalities known to be associated with such exposures. In many instances, a firm diagnosis can only be made through long-term follow-up and the exclusion of alternative explanations for any abnormalities identified.

Section Twenty

DISEASES OF UNKNOWN CAUSE

SARCOIDOSIS

By Robert L. Hackney, Jr., M.D.
Roscoe C. Young, Jr., M.D.
and Willie McDaniel, M.D.
Washington, D.C.

Sarcoidosis is a condition in which there are noncaseating granulomas in many organs of the body, resulting in dysfunction of varying degrees depending on the intensity of granuloma formation. Clinically, the lungs and lymph nodes are by far the most frequently affected, but the skin, eyes, heart, liver, spleen, and many other organs may be involved. The disease most often is mild in its presentation and clinical course; however, a small number of patients die, most often from respiratory failure.

Over a century has passed since Hutchinson's initial description of this condition, and although a greater understanding of the pathogenesis of the disorder as an immunologic disease has emerged, no additional light has been shed on the initiating factor(s). Diagnosis cannot be based on etiology but depends upon the clinical features, roentgenographic and nuclear imaging changes in the lungs and other organs, certain blood studies, and the pathologic picture of excised tissues.

EPIDEMIOLOGY

Sarcoidosis has been reported throughout the world, and a mass chest x-ray film survey suggested a prevalence of 20 per 100,000 population. Most series show that women are more likely to have sarcoidosis than men by a ratio of 2:1 or 3:1. The majority of patients are between 20 and 40 years of age. In the United States, the disease affects blacks 10 to 12 times as often as whites. In South Africa, the predominance of sarcoidosis in blacks over whites is similar to that found in the United States.

CLINICAL FEATURES

Most individuals found to have sarcoidosis come to medical attention because of an abnormal routine chest x-ray film rather than because of symptoms. These symptoms are usually relatively mild, but most patients will admit to some complaints when the history is taken after the chest roentgenogram is found to show lesions suggestive of the disorder. Symptoms are related to the sites of granulomatous infiltration. Table 1 demonstrates this fact, revealing that the most common symptoms are pulmonary, since over 90 per cent of the patients have lung lesions.

The symptoms listed in the table are seldom definitive enough to diagnose sarcoidosis, since many disorders may cause the same problems. Respiratory symptoms are significant because of their frequency, and suspicion should be raised when dyspnea is moderate in the presence of a chronic, nonproductive cough in a young black woman. Cervical lymphadenopathy should raise the suspicion that sarcoidosis is present when the nodes are not fluctuant or hard. Skin lesions of the face and extremities are fairly common in sarcoidosis, especially if they are nodular and not pruritic. When facial paralysis occurs in a young black person who has not had trauma to the facial nerve, sarcoidosis is a very good possibility. If this is combined with parotid enlargement and blurred vision, sarcoidosis is almost certain to be present.

Dizziness in a young individual may represent the effects of cardiac arrhythmia owing to infiltration of the conduction system by sarcoid granulomas. Abdominal discomfort in either upper quadrant may be due to hepatic or splenic enlargement, both of which are fairly common in these patients.

Table 2 shows the spectrum of organ system involvement in sarcoidosis.

Pulmonary Sarcoidosis

Lung lesions occur in more than nine of ten patients with sarcoidosis. These lesions are so common that the physician should be very careful about making a diag-

Table 1. Presenting Symptoms in Sarcoidosis

Most Common	Rare
Dyspnea	Cardiac arrhythmias
Nonproductive cough	Hepatosplenomegaly
Easy fatigue	Destruction of the nasal cartilage
Less Common	Subcutaneous nodules
Cervical lymphadenopathy	Facial paralysis
Blurred vision	
Cutaneous lesions	
Nonpleuritic chest pain	

Table 2. Organ System Involvement in Sarcoidosis by Relative Frequency

Most Common	Less Common (cont'd)
Lungs	Nervous system
Hilar and mediastinal lymph nodes	Bones
Skin	**Rare**
Less Common	Kidney
Cervical lymphadenopathy	Genitourinary tract
Eye	Gastrointestinal tract
Heart	Parotid glands
Liver and spleen	Lacrimal glands
	Endocrine glands

nosis of sarcoidosis if bilateral infiltrative disease is not present in the chest film except, of course, when bilateral hilar lymphadenopathy is seen.

These patients may have a nonproductive cough initially, but it may become productive of whitish sputum as the disease progresses, or of purulent material if infection complicates the disease. Hemoptysis may occur if the cough is hard and frequent; in this instance the amount of blood is small. When there is a cavity with a fungus ball, bleeding may be profuse and life-threatening. Obviously, tuberculosis should be considered if a patient presents with hemoptysis, but sarcoidosis should be suspected if sputum is consistently negative for *Mycobacterium tuberculosis* by both smears and cultures.

Dyspnea is frequent when there are diffuse bilateral lesions, as is usual in sarcoidosis. Often, however, the dyspnea may be slight or even absent when the lesions are granulomatous, but as the process progresses to fibrosis, dyspnea worsens. When fibrosis and destruction of the lungs occur, shortness of breath becomes the main symptom of the disease and it is usually associated with progressively worse hypoxemia (leading to the need for continuous oxygen administration), and death.

Lymphadenopathy

Enlargement of the hilar and mediastinal lymph nodes is characteristic of sarcoidosis and may occur with or without pulmonary infiltrations. Lymph node enlargement is practically always bilateral and occurs in about 80 per cent of patients with sarcoidosis. The nodes produce no symptoms and can only be discovered by chest x-rays. Cervical nodes are easily palpable and sometimes visible. They are not tender, red, or fluctuant, and in the scalene area nonpalpable nodes commonly show noncaseating granulomas. Lymphadenopathy is an important sign because it is so characteristic of sarcoidosis, and an enlarged node is such a convenient and productive source of biopsy material. The nodes usually decrease in size over a period of months with or without treatment. No evidence of enlarged nodes is left on the chest x-ray film as they diminish; however, in rare cases calcification of hilar nodes has been described. Rarely, also, hilar nodes may remain enlarged for a period of years.

Other organ system involvement is considerably less common than pulmonary disease and lymphadenopathy. It is usually very difficult to associate nonpulmonary involvement with sarcoidosis when lung lesions are absent. In most instances, extrapulmonary sarcoidosis can be diagnosed only when this disorder has also been recognized in the lungs or peripheral or hilar lymph nodes.

Cutaneous Lesions

Cutaneous lesions occur in about 9 per cent of cases and often are associated with sarcoid granulomas in many other areas of the body. For this reason, they may represent a marker of multisystem disease. The lesions may be maculopapular or nodular, and they may also be subcutaneous. They are most often found on the face and the extremities. Erythema nodosum is seen in almost 20 per cent of cases worldwide, but it is uncommon in black persons. The skin lesions respond to steroid therapy quite well, but atrophic depigmented lesions may be left in the affected areas. Cutaneous disease recurs often, and it provides a good clinical sign of activity of the disease.

Ocular Involvement

About 25 per cent of patients have eye lesions. The most common finding is granulomatous uveitis. When it is acute, watering, redness, and photophobia are the principal symptoms and signs. Conjunctival lesions, scleral plaques, and papilledema are present in a few cases, and the disease may progress to glaucoma which, if untreated, may leave the patient blind. When uveitis is associated with parotid gland enlargement and fever, it is called Heerfordt's syndrome. This is often accompanied by unilateral facial paralysis. The syndrome is virtually pathognomonic of sarcoidosis. Response to therapy is good.

Cardiac Sarcoidosis

The heart is involved in just under 5 per cent of cases. Arrhythmias, either supraventricular or ventricular, are the most likely evidence of the presence of cardiac infiltration by the granulomas. The patient may be asymptomatic or have episodes of dizziness when arrhythmia occurs, and death may result. Arrhythmias in young females may occur in mitral valve prolapse and cause confusion when sarcoidosis is also present; the differentiation is important because the conduction defect is benign in valve prolapse and dangerous in sarcoidosis. It usually responds to steroids when it is sarcoidosis-related. A patient with this combination of problems was seen at this institution in 1983, and a negative thallium scan made it clear that sarcoidosis was not responsible for the arrhythmia.

Cor pulmonale occurs in patients with advanced pulmonary disease.

Bone, Muscle, and Joint Manifestations

Lesions of the bones produce no symptoms and are discovered on x-ray films of the extremities. The lesions are cystic in the terminal phalanges and may be present in any patient with the disease; rarely they occur with hilar and mediastinal lymphadenopathy without pulmonary disease, but much more commonly they are found with advanced lung lesions. Joint disease may present as pain without roentgenographic abnormalities or as acute inflammation with x-ray films suggestive of rheumatoid arthritis.

A small number of patients may have significant weakness of the muscles of the extremities, suggesting muscular dystrophy. Muscle biopsy may be of value in establishing the diagnosis of sarcoidosis.

Liver and Spleen Disease

About one of every seven sarcoidosis patients has an enlarged liver, but most will be asymptomatic for evidence of hepatic disease, although fever is present in more than 33 per cent of cases. In almost all instances, the liver will return to a normal size in a matter of several months even without treatment. A few patients will develop hepatic failure, and deaths do occur. Within the past 2½ years, two patients at our institution have died because of hepatic failure due to sarcoidosis.

The diagnosis of hepatic sarcoidosis may present a problem despite the finding of granulomas in the liver since similar lesions may be relatively common in the livers of patients without sarcoidosis. In this instance, the diagnosis should be made only if other markers of this condition are present—e.g., typical chest x-ray film abnormalities and granulomas in other areas, such as the lung or lymph nodes.

The spleen is enlarged less than half as frequently as the liver; occasionally both are enlarged in the same patient. The spleen is usually only moderately larger than normal, but it may reach a huge size and cause a full sensation in the left upper abdominal quadrant as well as hypersplenism. This may cause a diagnostic dilemma if other features of sarcoidosis are absent, and splenectomy may become necessary for diagnosis. The spleen will return to normal with steroid treatment within several months, but in some patients the spleen has not become normal in size until after more than a year of therapy.

Nervous System Involvement

The most common sign of nervous system sarcoidosis is unilateral facial paralysis. This may often occur in association with uveoparotid fever (Heerfordt's syndrome) and represents early sarcoidosis. Facial paralysis and other peripheral neuropathies disappear rapidly, and uveoparotid fever with or without unilateral facial paralysis can be considered pathognomonic of sarcoidosis.

Other signs of nervous system sarcoidosis are more widespread and may present as meningitis due to granulomas in the meninges or as diffuse intracerebral lesions suggesting multiple sclerosis. On rare occasions, a mass of sarcoid lesions may simulate a brain tumor. When evidence of meningitis is present, a careful search for microorganisms must be made, particularly in patients receiving steroid therapy. In these patients, there is a strong possibility that tuberculosis or an opportunistic infection is responsible, not sarcoidosis.

Organ Systems Rarely Involved in Sarcoidosis

Parotid and Lacrimal Glands. It is generally said that these structures are rarely involved in sarcoidosis; however, if the parotid glands are examined carefully they frequently appear enlarged, perhaps in up to one in five or ten patients with early sarcoidosis. Gallium scans confirm involvement of the parotid and lacrimal glands far more often than is generally stated, particularly in disease of recent onset. When involved, both parotid and lacrimal glands are almost always enlarged bilaterally, and enlargement may be associated with fever and acute uveitis (Heerfordt's syndrome), a finding that is considered pathognomonic of sarcoidosis.

Except for the Heerfordt's syndrome, parotid and lacrimal gland involvement is usually asymptomatic.

Kidney. Renal sarcoidosis is extremely uncommon and may present with (1) granulomatous infiltration of the kidneys, (2) nephrocalcinosis and stone formation, or (3) glomerulonephritis.

Granulomatous disease of the kidney is rare and causes proteinuria and sterile pyuria. Response to corticosteroids is good initially, but long-term therapeutic results have not been adequately studied as yet. Nephrocalcinosis and renal stones result from hypercalcemia and hypercalciuria and may lead to pyelonephritis and renal failure. Glomerulonephritis is extremely rare in sarcoidosis, and it has not been established whether this condition is due to sarcoidosis or if it represents a chance occurrence of two unrelated diseases. The course is that of glomerulonephritis progressing to end-stage renal disease.

Genitourinary and Gastrointestinal Tracts. Involvement of these systems is extremely rare. There have been reported cases of lesions in the intestines, esophagus, and peritoneum, but stomach lesions are more common. We have seen several cases of sarcoidosis of the stomach, one of which had an ulcer surrounded by granulomatous tissue that proved to be noncaseating on biopsy. Patients are usually asymptomatic. Genitourinary involvement with sarcoidosis is extremely rare.

LABORATORY FINDINGS

In general, most laboratory studies are nonspecific and are only diagnostically supportive. They assume greater significance when other evidence of sarcoidosis is present, particularly a characteristic chest x-ray film and biopsy findings of noncaseating granulomas. On the other hand, laboratory findings vary in importance, with some being considerably more specific as sarcoidosis indicators than others. Table 3 categorizes laboratory studies according to their value in the diagnosis of this disorder.

Hematologic Findings

Leukopenia and lymphopenia occur commonly in sarcoidosis patients and are unrelated to splenomegaly or lymphadenopathy. The disease is likely active

Table 3. Laboratory Abnormalities in Sarcoidosis

Low Specifity
Leukopenia, lymphopenia
Eosinophilia
Elevation of IgA, IgG, IgM, IgE
Elevation of alkaline phosphatase
Hypercalcemia
Moderate Specifity
Elevation of angiotensin-converting enzyme
Elevation of serum lysozyme activity
Elevation of transcobalamin II
Chest x-ray film
Kveim-Siltzbach test
Hydroxyprolinuria
Negative tuberculin test
High Specifity
Gallium scan
Noncaseating granuloma on biopsy
Bronchoalveolar lavage

when the white blood cells are decreased, but normal numbers of these cells do not place the diagnosis in doubt. No clinical syndrome is associated with lymphopenia and the attendant leukopenia. The eosinophilia is slight and is not related to an allergic phenomenon.

Blood Chemistry

Elevation of serum alkaline phosphatase occurs in sarcoidosis and is related to hepatic involvement; thus it is a sign of disease activity but is of little diagnostic value. Serum immunoglobulins IgA, IgG, IgM, and IgE have been elevated in sarcoidosis patients, particularly those who are black. There does not appear to be any correlation between serum immunoglobulin increases, chest x-ray changes, or other laboratory or clinical parameters.

Hypercalcemia and Hypercalciuria

Elevation of the serum calcium level occurs in about 12 per cent of sarcoidosis patients. It is more common in males and occurs mainly in long-term disease. It appears without good reason and disappears within weeks with therapy, but it also may revert to normal spontaneously. Hypercalcemia is not related to bone lesions because there is no correlation between a high serum calcium level and bone changes. Hypercalciuria may be present along with hypercalcemia, but increases in urinary calcium are much more frequent than high serum calcium levels.

Renal stones are rare despite the relatively great frequency of hypercalcemia and hypercalciuria. When calcium is elevated in the urine or serum, or in both, confusion with other problems may exist. If a patient is given 5 to 10 mg of prednisone every 8 hours by mouth for 10 to 12 days, calcium levels will return to normal when hypercalcemia is caused by sarcoidosis, adrenal insufficiency, or Vitamin D intoxication, but serum calcium levels will not be changed in hyperparathyroidism.

Serum Enzymes and Other Serum Abnormalities

In 1976, Lieberman reported that more than 80 per cent of sarcoidosis patients had increased levels of serum angiotensin-converting enzyme (ACE). As more investigators began to measure ACE in these patients, it became obvious that this test was not as valuable as first reported; some studies showed ACE elevations in as few as 35 per cent of known sarcoidosis patients. Of interest is that patients with bilateral hilar lymphadenopathy and lung lesions have elevated ACE levels about 67 per cent of the time, whereas only 33 per cent of those without pulmonary infiltration have ACE elevations. Finally, ACE may be elevated in many conditions other than sarcoidosis: leprosy, Gaucher's disease, silicosis, miliary tuberculosis, primary biliary cirrhosis, lymphoma, talc granulomatosis, asbestosis, berylliosis, and several other disorders. This fact diminishes the specifity of ACE as a diagnostic aid, but the test may have value as a parameter to follow the course of the disease, since ACE elevation drops rapidly during corticosteroid therapy and when the disease is inactive.

Serum lysozyme (SL) levels were found to be increased in just over one half of 73 sarcoidosis patients in one study. Another study found only 37 per cent had elevated SL levels. Thus, SL levels are of limited value as diagnostic aids in sarcoidosis.

Transcobalamin II, a fraction of Vitamin B_{12} binding capacity, was found to be elevated in the serum of 54 per cent of a group of sarcoidosis patients. Gaucher's disease, lymphoproliferative conditions. Waldenström's macroglobulinemia, multiple myeloma, and liver disease are all characterized by elevations of transcobalamin II. Thus, this measurement cannot be considered important in the diagnosis of sarcoidosis at this time.

Chest X-Ray Film

Despite the clinical features noted earlier, the overwhelming majority of sarcoidosis patients are discovered because of an abnormal chest roentgenogram. Because of the high prevalence of pulmonary lesions, the most commonly used classification of this disease is based on the chest x-ray film findings: Stage 0—normal chest; Stage I—bilateral hilar lymphadenopathy (BHL) alone; Stage II—BHL with pulmonary infiltrations; Stage III—pulmonary infiltrations without BHL. Pulmonary lesions may be: (1) fine nodular early in the course; (2) large nodular; (3) fluffy, resembling pulmonary edema; (4) interstitial fibrosis; and (5) interstitial or massive fibrosis with cavities, most often in the upper lobes and occasionally containing fungus balls.

When pulmonary lesions are fine granulomas, large nodular lesions, or fluffy lesions they frequently disappear spontaneously within a few months even when no treatment is given. If the lesions persist, fibrosis will follow and they will not disappear even if therapy is administered. Many physicians will use steroids in these patients since the presence of some granulomas cannot be ruled out when fibrosis is the main feature in the film. Hilar and mediastinal nodes will generally disappear within a few months without therapy, although a small number of patients will have lymphadenopathy persisting over a period of years. Calcification of the nodes has been reported.

The chest x-ray film is not pathognomonic of sarcoidosis, but bilateral hilar lymphadenopathy with or without pulmonary infiltration in a young black individual almost always represents sarcoidosis. Tuberculosis and Hodgkin's disease may simulate sarcoidosis in this situation; therefore biopsy proof should always be obtained. When large nodular lesions are present, metastatic carcinoma should be considered. Interstitial granulomas or fibrosis suggests many disorders, making the need for biopsy unquestioned. Finally, cavitary sarcoidosis resembles old tuberculosis, which cannot be ruled out until it can be established that acid-fast bacilli are not present.

Gallium Scan

^{67}Gallium is used to identify active sarcoidosis lesions. The test is performed by the intravenous injection of 3 to 8 mCi of ^{67}Gal citrate, and at 48 hours multiple anterior and posterior scans of the head, thorax, abdomen and pelvis, and upper and lower extremities are performed.

The granulomatous infiltration of sarcoidosis may involve any organ system; however, the most frequent sites detected on scans include the spleen, salivary and lacrimal glands, hilar and paratracheal lymph nodes, and pulmonary parenchyma. Although gallium scans are in wide use for the evaluation of sarcoidosis, they are by no means completely reliable for the demonstration of active progression. It was found that the accuracy of normal gallium scans for the prediction of clinical inactivity was 87 per cent, whereas abnormal scans were an accurate predictor of clinical activity in only 63 per cent of the patients studied. Gallium is taken up in many lung diseases—e.g., carcinoma, hypersensitivity pneumonitis, pneumoconiosis, and lymphoma. It is not specific for sarcoidosis, but it has its greatest use in providing a parameter of activity of the disease.

Tissue Biopsy

Sarcoidosis cannot be diagnosed without tissue that shows noncaseating granulomas with no evidence of acid-fast organisms on the smear or of *Mycobacterium tuberculosis* on culture. The granulomas are usually similar in age, but it should be kept in mind that a number of other conditions may produce lesions that are indistinguishable from sarcoidosis. Thus, noncaseating granulomas may be seen in tuberculosis, histoplasmosis, allergy to metals such as beryllium, hypersensitivity pneumonitis, lymphomas, other malignancies, syphilis, regional ileitis, primary biliary cirrhosis, leprosy, and infestation with helminths. This emphasizes the fact that sarcoidosis should be diagnosed only when the compatible clinical complex accompanies the finding of noncaseating granulomas.

Important here is the biopsy site employed. The diagnostic yield, the ease of the procedure, and the safety of the procedure must all be taken into consideration. Disfiguring surgical scars should be avoided where possible. This is especially true for blacks, some of whom tend to form keloids. Unfortunately, this is the group with the highest prevalence of sarcoidosis.

Biopsy Sites. It is apparent from Table 4 that a number of biopsy methods and sites are available; however, there are obvious disadvantages to most of the procedures.

Biopsies of skin lesions and cervical nodes have the advantages of being easy to perform, of being safe, and of having a 100 per cent success rate in obtaining diagnostic tissue. Some individuals, however, may reject these procedures because unattractive scars often form.

Open lung biopsy in the presence of pulmonary infiltration is almost perfect from a point of view of yield; however, it carries a small but significant morbidity rate and may be dangerous in patients with advanced lung disease, especially when respiratory failure is present.

Scalene node biopsy was once popular because diagnostic material could be obtained even when cervical nodes were not palpable. It lost favor because the yield was relatively small compared with *mediastinoscopy.* In the latter procedure nearly 100 per cent of biopsies are positive when hilar or mediastinal lymph nodes, or both, are visible on the chest x-ray film. With greater use of the CT scan of the chest, nodes may be seen when the chest film fails to show them; thus, mediastinoscopy will become even more valuable. The same comment may be made about *mediastinotomy.* The disadvantages here are the formation of a surgical scar and possible of keloids in normally exposed parts of the body.

Percutaneous biopsy of the liver will result in the finding of granulomas in 70 per cent of sarcoidosis patients; however, the lesions cannot be differentiated from those of a number of other diseases—e.g., tuberculosis, primary biliary cirrhosis, and lymphoma, to name a few. Percutaneous lung biopsy has the disadvantages of producing a very small, often inadequate, piece of tissue; the danger of a pneumothorax in a patient with marginal pulmonary function; and pulmonary hemorrhage of varying degrees. Conjunctival biopsy has too low a yield to be of significant value.

Transbronchial biopsies through the fiberoptic bronchoscope may yield positive results in over 60 per cent of patients with pulmonary sarcoidosis. Some authors have reported finding granulomas in more than 90 per cent of patients who have had multiple bronchoscopies. Fiberoptic bronchoscopy with biopsy has

Table 4. Biopsy Sites or Methods

With External Lesions
Skin
Cervical or other lymph nodes
Without External Lesions
Bronchus and lung (transbronchial)
Mediastinoscopy
Mediastinostomy
Scalene node
Conjunctival
Percutaneous liver
Percutaneous lung
Open lung

become the most popular diagnostic procedure used because it is easy to perform and can be done safely in extremely ill patients. Patient acceptance of repeat examinations is good, and when done under local anesthesia it can be carried out in almost any individual, including those with respiratory failure. Complications are infrequent and easily treatable. Pneumothorax may occur rarely during biopsy, but it is usually small and the lung will re-expand if the patient is kept at rest for a day or two. Hemorrhage is expected after biopsy but rarely amounts to more than a few milliliters and seldom lasts more than a few hours. The transbronchial biopsy through the fiberscope is now the preferred method of diagnosing sarcoidosis.

Bronchoalveolar Lavage

This is performed through the fiberscope. Normal saline is instilled into a distal airway and the fluid is collected by suction. In normal nonsmokers, more than 90 per cent of the cells in the lavage fluid are pulmonary alveolar macrophages, fewer than 10 per cent are lymphocytes, and fewer than 1 per cent are polymorphonuclear leukocytes. Patients with alveolitis due to pulmonary sarcoidosis have predominantly activated T lymphocytes, and the ratio of immunoglobulin G (IgG) to albumin is less than 1. The intensity of the alveolitis can be measured by the increased number of T lymphocytes. For this reason, bronchoalveolar lavage provides a good indicator of activity in patients with sarcoidosis and, when diffuse interstitial lung disease is present, may suggest this diagnosis if T cell predominance exists.

On the basis of these factors, then, the specific diagnosis of sarcoidosis is best accomplished by obtaining lung tissue by biopsy through the fiberoptic bronchoscope. Bronchoalveolar lavage can also be done through the fiberscope, providing a measure of activity, and if it is repeated it can define the course of disease and the response to therapy.

OTHER STUDIES

Pulmonary Function

Studies of respiratory physiologic parameters are not diagnostic but simply define how the lung function is disturbed by sarcoidosis. Patients with Stages 0 and I disease may show little or no change in pulmonary function. Even when diffuse pulmonary granulomas are present, it is surprising that function remains relatively good. As fibrosis develops, the lung becomes stiff and the restrictive pattern is seen, although the pattern can be mixed restrictive and obstructive as bronchial anatomy becomes distorted by the lung scarring. Diffusing capacity may be reduced.

Microbiologic Studies

A careful search for *M. tuberculosis* should be made in every case of sarcoidosis. This has been recognized for many years, since the pathology and epidemiology of tuberculosis and sarcoidosis are similar. Stage II pulmonary lesions may be fine and nodular, resembling hematogenous tuberculosis, and Stage III lesions may suggest chronic tuberculous infection, especially when cavitation is present. Most physicians who see large numbers of sarcoidosis patients can cite instances in which acid-fast bacilli were found in "typical" sarcoidosis. On rare occasions, noncaseating granulomas have revealed acid-fast bacilli on smear and *M. tuberculosis* on culture. It is important to rule out tuberculosis before steroid therapy is started for sarcoidosis. A number of patients with tuberculosis who were given corticosteroids have had massive intrapulmonary or hematogenous dissemination of the disease, leading to death.

Skin Tests

Tuberculin Test. For many years it has been known that most patients with sarcoidosis have negative tuberculin tests. Despite this, other skin tests may be positive and circulating antibody formation is not diminished in these patients. If tuberculosis complicates sarcoidosis, the tuberculin test will convert from negative to positive. It is difficult to determine whether the decreased cell-mediated immunity has any practical significance in this disorder.

Kveim-Siltzbach Test. This test is performed by injecting a saline suspension of sarcoidal spleen or lymph node intracutaneously. A nodule is formed at the injection site within 2 to 6 weeks when active sarcoidosis is present. The nodule is biopsied and is considered positive when noncaseating granulomas are seen. Two problems decrease the worth of the Kveim-Siltzbach test: (1) a potent validated antigen is not widely available, and (2) the test is positive most often when very large lymph nodes or erythema nodosum is present—i.e., when sarcoidosis is easiest to diagnose. False-positive reactions have occurred in patients with regional enteritis, infectious mononucleosis, chronic lymphocytic leukemia, and nonspecific lymphadenitis. For these reasons, the Kveim-Siltzbach test is not commonly used as a diagnostic aid in sarcoidosis.

THE DILEMMA OF DIAGNOSTIC SARCOIDOSIS

This disorder may simulate many other conditions, primarily because it has no characteristics that are peculiar to it which are rare in other diseases. Even its pathologic features are shared by tuberculosis, histoplasmosis, berylliosis, lymphomas and other malignancies, and several other conditions. The chest roentgenogram can be easily confused with the picture for tuberculosis. Relatively recent diagnostic tools thought to be helpful in diagnosing sarcoidosis are being found to produce positive results in other diseases; this compounds the diagnostic dilemma. The serum angiotensin-converting enzyme may be elevated in Gaucher's disease, primary biliary cirrhosis, asbestosis, talc granulomatosis, and chronic lymphocytic pneumonitis; in the conditions already noted; and in sarcoidosis. The same comment can be made about serum transcobalamin II. The gallium scan findings in sarcoidosis may be confused with those in many other diseases.

What best makes the diagnosis of sarcoidosis? The five most important findings are (1) typical clinical picture; (2) Stage I, II, and III chest x-ray findings; (3) positive gallium scan; (4) pathologic picture; and (5) negative studies for *M. tuberculosis.*

REITER'S SYNDROME

By Andrei Calin, M.D., M.R.C.P.
Bath, England

SYNONYMS

Reiter's syndrome may be referred to as Reiter's disease, post–nonspecific urethritis Reiter's disease (endemic Reiter's disease), postdysenteric Reiter's disease (epidemic Reiter's disease), the Fiessinger-Leroy-Reiter syndrome, or sexually acquired reactive arthritis.

DEFINITION

"Reiter's syndrome" was originally applied to the triad of conjunctivitis, urethritis, and arthritis. It is now well recognized that many patients also have circinate balanitis, keratoderma blennorrhagicum, mouth ulcers, dactylitis, sacroiliitis, and other features. A subcommittee of the American Rheumatism Association has recently suggested that Reiter's disease should be defined as a period of arthropathy occurring within 1 month of nonspecific urethritis or cervicitis. Alternatively, others have thought of Reiter's syndrome as an oligoarthropathy occurring predominantly in large lower limb joints, sometimes in association with the various stigmata already mentioned. The connotation "sexually acquired" reactive arthritis is unfortunate, since many patients have the postdysenteric form of disease or features that are unrelated to obvious sexual or dysenteric events. Some authors have favored the term "incomplete" Reiter's syndrome for those individuals not demonstrating the full triad. However, since the term "overcomplete" is not used for patients with more than three features, I consider it better to use the name Reiter's syndrome to include the entire spectrum of disease.

PRESENTING SIGNS AND SYMPTOMS

Patients can present with an acute arthropathy and fever, arthropathy alone, the classic triad of features, or seven or more problems, including mucocutaneous changes, lymphadenopathy, diarrhea, ruptured popliteal cyst, tendinitis, dactylitis, nail changes, and other features.

In certain parts of the world, postdysenteric Reiter's disease is most commonly seen, whereas in other regions post–nonspecific urethritis Reiter's disease is seen more frequently. In my experience, the most common form of Reiter's disease has had no obvious precipitating factor.

COURSE

The course is variable. Some patients have self-limited disease that lasts for 2 or 3 weeks, whereas others develop progressive destructive multisystem disease that affects virtually every system in the body. In my experience of more than 200 patients with Reiter's syndrome, roughly 20 per cent had a self-limited episode, in 20 per cent the disease progressed with multisystem involvement and the patients often needed continuous medication that resulted in loss of work, and the remaining 60 per cent of patients had various degrees of severity between these two ends of the spectrum. In some 20 per cent of cases, ankylosing spondylitis complicated the initial Reiter's syndrome, and these patients frequently had a course that mimicked that of typical spondylitis.

COMMON COMPLICATIONS

Patients may go blind with chronic iridocyclitis. Ankylosing spondylitis occurs in a minority of patients. Persistent arthropathy may complicate the course. Progressive skin lesions may be a major event. Ruptured popliteal cysts can occur early in the syndrome and aortic regurgitation much later.

PHYSICAL EXAMINATION

The patient may look unwell, with fever, lymphadenopathy, anemia, and other nonspecific findings. Neuropsychiatric symptoms occasionally occur.

Conjunctivitis or uveitis, or both, occurs in two thirds of patients at the outset or during the course of the disease. The changes may be unilateral or bilateral.

Urethritis may be present in the history with no findings on examination, or may be absent in the history with evidence of a discharge found on examination of the underwear or urethral orifice.

Arthritis and dactylitis are the main features, with a polyarthropathy occurring in the majority of patients. Dactylitis is found at some stage of the course in about 25 to 50 per cent of patients. The arthritis may be acute or chronic and typically involves the feet, ankles, and knees, as well as the upper limb joints to a lesser extent. Sacroiliac joint involvement occurs in about 25 per cent of patients and may be associated with ascending spinal disease and resulting decreased mobility of the back in all directions.

The important clinically silent and almost diagnostic features of shallow mouth ulcers and other mucocutaneous lesions typified by balanitis must be searched for. Keratoderma blennorrhagicum usually occurs on the palms and soles of feet but may involve the shaft of the penis and other sites.

Tendinitis can occur at any site, but typically the insertion of the Achilles tendon is affected, with or without plantar fasciitis. Nail involvement with hyperkeratotic nail changes and occasionally a subungual discharge of toothpaste-like material may be seen.

A ruptured popliteal cyst may mimic a deep vein thrombosis.

A striking feature of the clinical findings is the dissociation between the degree of joint or extraarticular swelling and the degree of pain; some patients with dramatic swelling have little pain, and vice versa.

LABORATORY PROCEDURES

The sedimentation rate (Westergren) varies from 1 to 2 mm/hour to over 100 mm/hour. There seems to be little correlation between rate and disease activity.

The patient may be anemic, with a mild leukocytosis. HLA-B27 is present in some 75 per cent of patients but should not be used as a diagnostic indicator.

RADIOLOGIC EVALUATION

X-ray changes occur frequently at the site of ligament insertion into bone. Thus, there may be fluffy spurs at the site of the insertion of the Achilles tendon or plantar fascia. Sacroiliac disease occurs in a quarter of patients and, in contrast to sacroiliitis or ankylosing spondylitis, the inflammatory disease may be unilateral.

POTENTIAL ERRORS AND PITFALLS IN DIAGNOSIS

Without doubt, the most common error in management is the failure to recognize the disease. The silent but important mucocutaneous disease, when missed, may prevent the correct diagnosis from being reached. That not all patients have obvious urethritis or diarrhea must be remembered. The difficulty in recognizing urethritis and cervicitis in women results in the diagnosis frequently being missed in this sex. Gonococcal septicemia typically occurs in women, not men; thus, in any male with a diagnosis of gonococcal septicemia, Reiter's syndrome should be considered sooner rather than later.

Section Twenty-One

LABORATORY REFERENCE VALUES OF CLINICAL IMPORTANCE

By Rex B. Conn, M.D.
Atlanta, Georgia

INTRODUCTION

The quantitative procedures carried out in a clinical laboratory represent measurements of substances normally present within rather narrow ranges of concentration. In order to use such data, we must know the values to be expected in a normal individual and what is considered a significant deviation from normal. Actually, there can be no sharp dividing line between abnormal and normal values, since there is a gradual transition during any pathological process from what is clearly normal to what is clearly a pathological condition.

In medicine, it is a logical impossibility to define normality, and the term "reference values" has replaced the earlier term "normal values." Reference values are derived from statistical studies on subjects believed to have no condition that might affect the measurements under consideration. The traditional and most widely used statistical approach is to carry out the measurement on a large group of subjects and to set the reference limits at the mean value plus or minus two standard deviations. Since values obtained for many measurements are not Gaussian in distribution, additional steps are frequently used in calculation of the reference ranges. The important consideration is that the reference ranges derived by these statistical methods contain only 95 per cent of the reference population. Thus, a value slightly outside the reference range might be due either to chance distribution or to an underlying pathological process.

A single reference range for all individuals may be inadequate for some clinical measurements. Values obtained on presumably normal persons may vary because of age, sex, body build, race, environment, and state of gastrointestinal absorption. The use of reference ranges obtained on a mixed population of adults is particularly misleading when applied to interpretation of studies done on infants.

A universal caveat in the use of published tables of reference values is that for many procedures the reference range will vary with the method used. This is particularly true for enzyme measurements and measurements based upon immunochemical principles.

THE INTERNATIONAL SYSTEM OF UNITS FOR LABORATORY MEASUREMENTS (LE SYSTÈME INTERNATIONAL D'UNITÉS)

An extensive modification of the metric system has been adopted by clinical laboratories in many countries. This adaptation is the International System of Units (Le Système International d'Unités), usually abbreviated S.I. Units. Whereas the metric system utilizes the centimeter, the gram, and the second as basic units, the International System uses the meter, the kilogram, and the second as well as four other basic units.

The International System is a coherent approach to all types of measurement that utilizes seven dimensionally independent basic quantities: mass, length, time, thermodynamic temperature, electric current, luminous intensity, and amount of substance. Each of these quantities is expressed in a clearly defined *basic unit* (Table 1).

Two or more basic units may be combined to provide *derived units* (Table 2) for expressing other measure-

Table 1. BASIC UNITS

Property	Basic Unit	Symbol
Length	metre	m
Mass	kilogram	kg
Amount of substance	mole	mol
Time	second	s
Thermodynamic temperature	kelvin	K
Electric current	ampere	A
Luminous intensity	candela	cd

Table 2. DERIVED UNITS

Derived Property	Derived Unit	Symbol
Area	square metre	m^2
Volume	cubic metre	m^3
	litre	l
Mass concentration	kilogram/cubic metre	kg/m^3
	gram/litre	g/l
Substance concentration	mole/cubic metre	mol/m^3
	mole/litre	mol/l
Temperature	degree Celsius	C = K − 273.15

ments such as mass concentration (kilograms per cubic meter) and velocity (meters per second). Standardized prefixes (Table 3) for basic and derived units are used to express fractions or multiples of the basic units so that any measurement can be expressed in a value between 0.001 and 1000.

Medical Applications

The most profound change in laboratory reports will result from expressing concentration as amount per volume (moles per liter) rather than mass per volume (milligrams per 100 milliliters). The advantages of the former expression can be seen in the following:

Conventional Units

1.0 gram of hemoglobin
Combines with 1.37 ml. of oxygen
Contains 3.4 mg. of iron
Forms 34.9 mg. of bilirubin

S.I. Units

1.0 mmol of hemoglobin
Combines with 4.0 mmol of oxygen
Contains 4.0 mmol of iron
Forms 4.0 mmol of bilirubin

Chemical relationships between lactic acid and pyruvic acid and the glucose from which both are derived, as well as the relationship between bilirubin and the binding capacity of albumin, are other examples of chemical relationships that will be clarified by using the new system.

There are a number of laboratory and other medical measurements for which the S.I. Units appear to offer little advantage, and some that are disadvantageous

Table 3. STANDARD PREFIXES

Prefix	Multiplication Factor	Symbol
atto	10^{-18}	a
femto	10^{-15}	f
pico	10^{-12}	p
nano	10^{-9}	n
micro	10^{-6}	μ
milli	10^{-3}	m
centi	10^{-2}	c
deci	10^{-1}	d
deca	10^{1}	da
hecto	10^{2}	h
kilo	10^{3}	k
mega	10^{6}	M
giga	10^{9}	G
tera	10^{12}	T

because the change would require replacement or revision of instruments such as the sphygmomanometer. The cubic meter is the derived unit for volume; however, it is inappropriately large for medical measurements, and the liter has been retained. Thermodynamic temperature expressed in kelvins is not more informative for medical measurements. Since the Celsius degree is the same as the Kelvin degree, the Celsius scale is used. Celsius rather than centigrade is the preferred term.

Selection of units for expressing enzyme activity presents certain difficulties. Literally dozens of different units have been used in expressing enzyme activity, and interlaboratory comparison of enzyme results is impossible unless the assay system is precisely defined. In 1964, the International Union of Biochemistry attempted to remedy the situation by proposing the International Unit for enzymes. This unit was defined as the amount of enzyme that will catalyze the conversion of 1 micromole of substrate per minute under standard conditions. Difficulties remain, however, as enzyme activity is affected by the temperature, pH, the type and amount of substrate, the presence of inhibitors, and other factors. Enzyme activity can be expressed in S.I. Units, and the katal has been proposed to express activities of all catalysts, including enzymes. The katal is that amount of enzyme that catalyzes a reaction rate of 1 mole per second. Thus, adoption of the katal as the unit of enzyme activity would provide no more information than is obtained when results are expressed in International Units.

Hydrogen ion concentration in blood is customarily expressed as pH, but in S.I. Units it would be expressed in nanomoles per liter. It appears unlikely that the very useful pH scale will be discarded.

Pressure measures, such as blood pressure and partial pressures of blood gases, would be expressed in S.I. Units using the Pascal, a unit that can be derived from the basic units for mass, length, and time. This change probably will not be adopted in the early phases of the conversion to S.I. Units. Similarly, a proposed change in expressing osmolality in terms of the depression of freezing point is inappropriate, because osmolality may be calculated from vapor pressure as well as freezing point measurement.

Conventions

A number of conventions have been adopted to standardize usage of S.I. Units:

1. No periods are used after the symbol for a unit (kg not kg.), and it remains unchanged when used in the plural (70 kg not 70 kgs).

2. A half space rather than a comma is used to divide large numbers into groups of three (5 400 000 not 5,400,000).

3. Compound prefixes should be avoided (nanometer not millimicrometer).

4. Multiples and submultiples are used in steps of 10^3 or 10^{-3}.

5. The degree sign for the temperature scales is omitted (38 C not 38°C).

6. The preferred spelling is metre not meter, litre not liter.

7. Report of a measurement should include infor-

mation on the system, the component, the kind of quantity, the numerical value, and the unit. For example: *System,* serum. *Component,* glucose. *Kind of quantity,* substance concentration. *Value,* 5.10. *Unit,* mmol/l.

8. The name of the component should be unambiguous; for example, "serum bilirubin" might refer to unconjugated bilirubin or to total bilirubin. For acids and bases, the maximally ionized form is used in naming the component; for example, lactate or urate rather than lactic acid or uric acid.

Tables of Reference Values

Tables accompanying this article indicate "normal values" for most of the commonly performed laboratory tests. The title of the tables has been changed from the "normal values" of previous years to "reference values" to conform to current usage. The reference value is given in conventional units, and the value in S.I. Units is calculated from these figures. Notes (page 1322) provide additional information.

REFERENCE VALUES IN HEMATOLOGY

	Conventional Units		S.I. Units		Notes
Acid hemolysis test (Ham)	No hemolysis		No hemolysis		
Alkaline phosphatase, leukocyte	Total score 14–100		Total score 14–100		
Carboxyhemoglobin	Up to 5% of total		0.05 of total		a
Cell counts					
Erythrocytes					
Males	4.6–6.2 million/cu. mm.		4.6–6.2 × 10^{12}/l		
Females	4.2–5.4 million/cu. mm.		4.2–5.4 × 10^{12}/l		
Children (varies with age)	4.5–5.1 million/cu. mm.		4.5–5.1 × 10^{12}/l		
Leukocytes					
Total	4500–11,000/cu. mm.		4.5–11.0 × 10^{9}/l		
Differential	*Percentage*	*Absolute*			
Myelocytes	0	0/cu. mm.	0/1		b
Band neutrophils	3–5	150–400/cu. mm.	150–400 × 10^{6}/l		
Segmented neutrophils	54–62	3000–5800/cu. mm.	3000–5800 × 10^{6}/l		
Lymphocytes	25–33	1500–3000/cu. mm.	1500–3000 × 10^{6}/l		
Monocytes	3–7	300–500/cu. mm.	300–500 × 10^{6}/l		
Eosinophils	1–3	50–250/cu. mm.	50–250 × 10^{6}/l		
Basophils	0–0.75	15–50/cu. mm.	15–50 × 10^{6}/l		
Platelets	150,000–350,000/cu. mm.		150–350 × 10^{9}/l		
Reticulocytes	25,000–75,000/cu. mm. 0.5–1.5% of erythrocytes		25–75 × 10^{9}/l		b
Bone marrow, differential cell count	*Range*	*Average*	*Range*	*Average*	
Myeloblasts	0.3–5.0%	2.0%	0.003–0.05	0.02	a
Promyelocytes	1.0–8.0%	5.0%	0.01–0.08	0.05	
Myelocytes: Neutrophilic	5.0–19.0%	12.0%	0.05–0.19	0.12	
Eosinophilic	0.5–3.0%	1.5%	0.005–0.03	0.015	
Basophilic	0.0–0.5%	0.3%	0.00–0.005	0.003	
Metamyelocytes	13.0–32.0%	22.0%	0.13–0.32	0.22	
Polymorphonuclear neutrophils	7.0–30.0%	20.0%	0.07–0.30	0.20	
Polymorphonuclear eosinophils	0.5–4.0%	2.0%	0.005–0.04	0.02	
Polymorphonuclear basophilis	0.0–0.7%	0.2%	0.00–0.007	0.002	
Lymphocytes	3.0–17.0%	10.0%	0.03–0.17	0.10	
Plasma cells	0.0–2.0%	0.4%	0.00–0.02	0.004	
Monocytes	0.5–5.0%	2.0%	0.005–0.05	0.02	
Reticulum cells	0.1–2.0%	0.2%	0.001–0.02	0.002	
Megakaryocytes	0.3–3.0%	0.4%	0.003–0.03	0.004	
Pronormoblasts	1.0–8.0%	4.0%	0.01–0.08	0.04	
Normoblasts	7.0–32.0%	18.0%	0.07–0.32	0.18	
Coagulation tests					
Antithrombin III (synthetic substrate)	80–120% of normal		0.8–1.2 of normal		
Bleeding time (Duke)	1–5 min.		1–5 min		
Bleeding time (Ivy)	Less than 5 min.		Less than 5 min		
Bleeding time (Template)	2.5–9.5 min.		2.5–9.5 min		
Clot retraction, qualitative	Begins in 30–60 min. Complete in 24 hrs.		Begins in 30–60 min Complete in 24 h		

Table continued on following page

REFERENCE VALUES IN HEMATOLOGY (*continued*)

	Conventional Units	S.I. Units	Notes
Coagulation time (Lee-White)	5–15 min. (glass tubes)	5–15 min (glass tubes)	
	19–60 min. (siliconized tubes)	19–60 min (siliconized tubes)	
Euglobulin lysis time	2–6 hr. at 37°	2–6 h at 37 C	
Factor VIII and other coagulation factors	50–150% of normal	0.50–1.5 of normal	a
Fibrin split products (Thrombo-Wellco test)	Less than 10 mcg./ml.	Less than 10 mg/l	
Fibrinogen	200–400 mg./dl.	5.9–11.7 μmol/l	c
Fibrinolysins	0	0	
Partial thromboplastin time, activated (APTT)	20–35 sec.	20–35 sec.	
Prothrombin consumption	Over 80% consumed in 1 hr.	Over 0.80 consumed in 1 h	a
Prothrombin content	100% (calculated from prothrombin time)	1.0 (calculated from prothrombin time)	a
Prothrombin time (one stage)	12.0–14.0 sec.	12.0–14.0 s	
Tourniquet test	Ten or fewer petechiae in a 2.5 cm. circle after 5 min.	Ten or fewer petechiae in a 2.5 cm circle after 5 min	
Cold hemolysin test (Donath-Landsteiner)	No hemolysis	No hemolysis	
Coombs' test			
Direct	Negative	Negative	
Indirect	Negative	Negative	
Corpuscular values of erythrocytes (values are for adults; in children, values vary with age)			
M.C.H. (mean corpuscular hemoglobin)	27–31 picogm.	0.42–0.48 fmol	d
M.C.V. (mean corpuscular volume)	80–96 cu. micra	80–96 fl	
M.C.H.C. (mean corpuscular hemoglobin concentration)	32–36%	0.32–0.36	a
Haptoglobin (as hemoglobin binding capacity)	100–200 mg./dl.	16–31 μmol/l	d
Hematocrit			
Males	40–54 ml./dl.	0.40–0.54	a
Females	37–47 ml./dl.	0.37–0.47	
Newborn	49–54 ml.dl.	0.49–0.54	
Children (varies with age)	35–49 ml./dl.	0.35–0.49	
Hemoglobin			
Males	14.0–18.0 grams/dl.	2.17–2.79 mmol/l	d
Females	12.0–16.0 grams/dl.	1.86–2.48 mmol/l	
Newborn	16.5–19.5 grams/dl.	2.56–3.02 mmol/l	
Children (varies with age)	11.2–16.5 grams/dl.	1.74–2.56 mmol/l	
Hemoglobin, fetal	Less than 1% of total	Less than 0.01 of total	a
Hemoglobin A_{1c}	3–5% of total	0.03–0.05 of total	a
Hemoglobin A_2	1.5–3.0% of total	0.015–0.03 of total	a
Hemoglobin, plasma	0–5.0 mg./dl.	0–0.8 μmol/l	d
Methemoglobin	0–130 mg./dl.	4.7–20 μmol/l	e
Osmotic fragility of erythrocytes	Begins in 0.45–0.39% NaCl	Begins in 77–67 mmol/l NaCl	
	Complete in 0.33–0.30% NaCl	Complete in 56–51 mmol/l NaCl	
Sedimentation rate			
Wintrobe: Males	0–5 mm. in 1 hr.	0–5 mm/h	
Females	0–15 mm. in 1 hr.	0–15 mm/h	
Westergren: Male	0–15 mm. in 1 hr.	0–15 mm/h	
Females	0–20 mm. in 1 hr.	0–20 mm/h	
(May be slightly higher in children and during pregnancy)			

REFERENCE VALUES FOR BLOOD, PLASMA AND SERUM

(For some procedures the reference values may vary depending upon the method used)

	Conventional Units	S.I. Units	Notes
Acetoacetate plus acetone, serum			
Qualitative	Negative	Negative	
Quantitative	0.3–2.0 mg./dl.	3–20 mg/l	
Adrenocorticotropin (ACTH), plasma			
6 A.M.	10–80 picogm./ml.	10–80 ng/l	
6 P.M.	Less than 50 picogm./ml.	Less than 50 ng/l	
Alanine aminotransferase *see* Transaminase			
Aldolase, serum	0–11 milliunits/ml. (30°)	0–11 units/l (30 C)	f
Aldosterone			
Adult, supine	3–10 ng./dl.	0.08–0.3 nmol/l	
standing			
male	6–22 ng./dl.	0.17–0.61 nmol/l	
female	5–30 ng./dl.	0.14–0.8 nmol/l	
Alpha amino nitrogen, serum	3.0–5.5 mg./dl.	2.1–3.9 mmol/l	
Ammonia (nitrogen), plasma	15–49 mcg./dl.	11–35 μmol/l	
Amylase, serum	25–125 milliunits/ml.	25–125 units/l	
Anion gap	8–16 mEq./l.	8–16 mmol/l	
Ascorbic acid, blood	0.4–1.5 mg./dl.	23–85 μmol/l	
Aspartate aminotransferase *see* Transaminase			
Base excess, blood	0 ± 2 mEq./liter	0 ± 2 mmol/l	
Bicarbonate, serum	23–29 mEq./liter	23–29 mmol/l	
Bile acids, serum	0.3–3.0 mg./dl.	3.0–30.0 mg/l	
Bilirubin, serum			
Direct	0.1–0.4 mg./dl.	1.7–6.8 μmol/l	
Indirect	0.2–0.7 mg./dl. (Total minus direct)	3.4–12 μmol/l (Total minus direct)	
Total	0.3–1.1 mg./dl.	5.1–19 μmol/l	
Calcium, serum	4.5–5.5 mEq./liter 9.0–11.0 mg./dl. (Slightly higher in children) (Varies with protein concentration)	2.25–2.75 mmol/l (Slightly higher in children) (Varies with protein concentration)	a
Calcium, ionized, serum	2.1–2.6 mEq./liter 4.25–5.25 mg./dl.	1.05–1.30 mmol/l	
Carbon dioxide content, serum			
Adults	24–30 mEq./liter	24–30 mmol/l	
Infants	20–28 mEq./liter	20–28 mmol/l	
Carbon dioxide tension (P_{CO_2}), blood	35–45 mm. Hg	35–45 mm Hg	g
Carotene, serum	40–200 mcg./dl.	0.74–3.72 μmol/l	
Ceruloplasmin, serum	23–44 mg./dl.	230–440 mg./l	h
Chloride, serum	96–106 mEq./liter	96–106 mmol/l	
Cholesterol, serum			
Total	150–250 mg./dl.	3.9–6.5 mmol/l	
Esters	68–76% of total cholesterol	0.68–0.76 of total cholesterol	a

Table continued on following page.

REFERENCE VALUES FOR BLOOD, PLASMA AND SERUM (*Continued*)

(For some procedures the reference values may vary depending upon the method used)

	Conventional Units	S.I. Units	Notes
Cholinesterase			
Serum	0.5–1.3 pH units	0.5–1.3 pH units	f
Erythrocytes	0.5–1.0 pH unit	0.5–1.0 pH unit	f
Copper, serum			
Males	70–140 mcg./dl.	11–22 μmol/l	
Females	85–155 mcg./dl.	13–24 μmol/l	
Cortisol, plasma			
(8 A.M.)	6–23 mcg./dl.	170–635 nmol/l	
(4 P.M.)	3–15 mcg./dl.	82–413 nmol/l	
(10 P.M.)	Less than 50% of 8 A.M. value	Less than 0.5 of 8 A.M. value	
Creatine, serum	0.2–0.8 mg./dl.	15–61 μmol/l	
Creatine kinase, serum (CK, CPK)			
Males	12–80 milliunits/ml. (30°)	12–80 units/l (30 C)	f
	55–170 milliunits/ml. (37°)	55–170 units/l (37 C)	f
Females	10–55 milliunits/ml. (30°)	10–55 units/l (30 C)	f
	30–135 milliunits/ml. (37°)	30–135 units/l (37 C)	f
Creatine kinase isoenzymes, serum			
CK-MM	Present	Present	
CK-MB	Absent	Absent	
CK-BB	Absent	Absent	
Creatinine, serum	0.6–1.2 mg./dl.	53–106 μmol/l	
Cryoglobulins, serum	0	0	
Fatty acids, total, serum	190–420 mg./dl.	7–15 mmol/l	i
nonesterified, serum	8–25 mg./dl.	0.30–0.90 mmol/l	
Ferritin, serum	20–200 nanogm./ml.	20–200 μg/l	
Fibrinogen, plasma	200–400 mg./100 ml.	5.9–11.7 μmol/l	c
Folate, serum	1.8–9.0 nanogm./ml.	4.1–20.4 nmol/l	
Erythrocytes	150–450 nanogm./ml.	340–1020 nmol/l	
Follicle-stimulating hormone (FSH), plasma			
Males	4–25 milliunits/ml. (I.U.)	4–25 IU/l	
Females	4–30 milliunits/ml. (I.U.)	4–30 IU/l	
Postmenopausal	40–250 milliunits/ml. (I.U.)	40–250 IU/l	
Gamma glutamyltransferase			
Males	6–32 milliunits/ml. (30°)	6–32 units/l (30 C)	f
Females	4–18 milliunits/ml. (30°)	4–18 units/l (30 C)	f
Gastrin, serum	0–200 picogm./ml.	0–200 ng/l	
Glucose (fasting)			
Blood	60–100 mg./dl.	3.33–5.55 mmol/l	
Plasma or serum	70–115 mg./dl.	3.89–6.38 mmol/l	
Growth hormone, serum	0–10 nanogm./ml.	0–10 μg/l	
Haptoglobin, serum	100–200 mg./dl. (As hemoglobin binding capacity)	16–31 μmol/l (As hemoglobin binding capacity)	d
Hydroxybutyric dehydrogenase, serum (HBD)	0–180 milliunits/ml. (30°)	0–180 units/l (30 C)	f
17-Hydroxycorticosteroids, plasma	8–18 mcg./dl.	0.22–0.50 μmol/l	j
Immunoglobins, serum			
IgG	550–1900 mg./dl.	5.5–19.0 g/l	
IgA	60–333 mg./dl.	0.60–3.3 g/l	
IgM	45–145 mg./dl.	0.45–1.5 g/l	
IgD	0.5–3.0 mg./dl.	5–30 mg/l	
IgE	<500 nanogm./ml. (Varies with age in children)	<500 μg/l (Varies with age in children)	

Insulin, plasma (fasting)	5–25 microunits/ml.	5–25 milliunits/l	
Iodine, protein bound, serum	3.5–8.0 mcg./dl.	0.28–0.63 μmol/l	k
Iron, serum	75–175 mcg./dl.	13–31 μmol/l	
Iron binding capacity, serum			
Total	250–410 mcg./dl.	45–73 μmol/l	
Saturation	20–55%	0.20–0.55	a
Lactate, blood, venous	4.5–19.8 mg./dl.	0.5–2.2 mmol/l	
arterial	4.5–14.4 mg./dl.	0.5–1.6 mmol/l	
Lactate dehydrogenase, serum (LD, LDH)	45–90 milliunits/ml. (I.U.) (30°)	45–90 units/l (30 C)	f
	100–190 milliunits/ml. (37°)	100–190 milliunits/ml (37 C)	
LDH_1	22–37% of total	0.22–0.37 of total	a
LDH_2	30–46% of total	0.30–0.46 of total	
LDH_3	14–29% of total	0.14–0.29 of total	
LDH_4	5–11% of total	0.05–0.11 of total	
LDH_5	2–11% of total	0.02–0.11 of total	
Leucine aminopeptidase, serum	14–40 milliunits/ml. (30°)	14–40 units/l (30 C)	f
Lipase, serum	0–1.5 units (Cherry-Crandall)	0–1.5 units (Cherry-Crandall)	f
Lipids, total, serum	450–850 mg./dl.	4.5–8.5 g/l	m
Lipoprotein cholesterol, serum			
LDL cholesterol	60–180 mg./dl.	600–1800 mg/l	
HDL cholesterol	30–80 mg./dl.	300–800 mg/l	
Luteinizing hormone (LH), serum			
Males	6–18 milliunits/ml. (I.U.)	6–18 IU/l	
Females, premenopausal	5–22 milliunits/ml. (I.U.)	5–22 IU/l	
midcycle	3 times baseline	3 times baseline	
postmenopausal	Greater than 30 milliunits/ml. (I.U.)	Greater than 30 IU/l	
Magnesium, serum	1.5–2.5 mEq./liter	0.75–1.25 mmol/l	
	1.8–3.0 mg./dl.		
5′-Nucleotidase, serum	3.5–12.7 milliunits/ml. (37°)	3.5–12.5 units/l (37 C)	f
Nitrogen, nonprotein, serum	15–35 mg./dl.	10.7–25.0 mmol/l	
Osmolality, serum	285–295 mOsm./kg. serum water	285–295 mmol/kg serum water	n
Oxygen, blood			
Capacity	16–24 vol. % (varies with hemoglobin)	7.14–10.7 mmol/l (varies with hemoglobin)	o
Content Arterial	15–23 vol. %	6.69–10.3 mmol/l	o
Venous	10–16 vol. %	4.46–7.14 mmol/l	o
Saturation Arterial	94–100% of capacity	0.94–1.00 of capacity	a
Venous	60–85% of capacity	0.60–0.85 of capacity	a
Tension, pO_2 Arterial	75–100 mm. Hg	75–100 mm Hg	g
P_{50}, blood	26–27 mm. Hg	26–27 mm. Hg	g
pH, arterial, blood	7.35–7.45	7.35–7.45	p
Phenylalanine, serum	Less than 3 mg./dl.	Less than 0.18 mmol/l	
Phosphatase, acid, serum	0.11–0.60 milliunits/ml. (37°)	0.11–0.60 units/l	f
	(Roy, Brower, Hayden)		
Phosphatase, alkaline, serum (ALP)	20–90 milliunits/ml. (30°)	20–90 units/l (30 C)	f
	(Values are higher in children)	(Values are higher in children)	
Phosphate, inorganic, serum			
Adults	3.0–4.5 mg./dl.	1.0–1.5 mmol/l	
Children	4.0–7.0 mg./dl.	1.3–2.3 mmol/l	

Table continued on following page

REFERENCE VALUES FOR BLOOD, PLASMA AND SERUM (*continued*)

(For some procedures the reference values may vary depending upon the method used)

	Conventional Units	S.I. Units	Notes
Phospholipids, serum	6–12 mg./dl.	1.9–3.9 mmol/l	
	(As lipid phosphorus)	(As lipid phosphorus)	
Potassium, serum	3.5–5.0 mEq./liter	3.5–5.0 mmol/l	
Prolactin, serum			
Males	1–20 nanogm./ml.	1–20 μg/l	
Females	1–25 nanogm./ml.	1–25 μg/l	
Protein, serum			
Total	6.0–8.0 grams/dl.	60–80 g/l	m
Albumin	3.5–5.5 grams/dl.	35–55 g/l	q
	52–68% of total	0.52–0.68 of total	a
Globulin			
$Alpha_1$	0.2–0.4 gram/dl.	2–4 g/l	m
	2–5% of total	0.02–0.05 of total	a
$Alpha_2$	0.5–0.9 gram/dl.	5–9 g/l	m
	7–14% of total	0.07–0.14 of total	a
Beta	0.6–1.1 grams/dl.	6–11 g/l	m
	9–15% of total	0.09–0.15 of total	a
Gamma	0.7–1.7 grams/dl.	7–17 g/l	m
	11–21% of total	0.11–0.21 of total	a
Protoporphyrin, erythrocyte	27–61 mcg./dl. packed RBC	0.48–1.09 μmol/l packed RBC	
Pyruvate, blood	0.3–0.9 mg./dl.	0.03–0.10 mmol/l	
Sodium, serum	136–145 mEq./liter	136–145 mmol/l	
Sulfates, inorganic, serum	0.8–1.2 mg./dl.	83–125 μmol/l	
Testosterone, plasma			
Males	275–875 nanogm./dl.	9.5–30 nmol/l	
Females	23–75 nanogm./dl.	0.8–2.6 nmol/l	
Pregnant	38–190 nanogm./dl.	1.3–6.6 nmol/l	
Thyroid-stimulating hormone (TSH), serum	0–7 microunits/ml.	0–7 milliunits/l	
Thyroxine, free, serum	1.0–2.1 nanogm./dl.	13–27 pmol/l	
Thyroxine (T_4), serum	4.4–9.9 mcg./dl.	57–128 nmol/l	
Thyroxine binding globulin (TBG), serum (as thyroxine)	10–26 mcg./dl.	129–335 nmol/l	
Thyroxine iodine, serum	2.9–6.4 mcg./dl.	229–504 nmol/l	k
Tri-iodothyronine (T_3), serum	150–250 nanogm./dl.	2.3–3.9 nmol/l	
Tri-iodothyronine (T_3) uptake, resin (T_3RU)	25–38%	0.25–0.38 uptake	a
Transaminase, serum			
SGOT (aspartate aminotransferase, AST)	8–20 milliunits/ml. (30°)	8–20 units/l (30 C)	
	7–40 milliunits/ml. (37°)	7–40 units/l (37 C)	
SGPT (alanine aminotransferase, ALT)	8–20 milliunits/ml. (30°)	8–20 units/l (30 C)	f
	5–35 milliunits/ml. (37°)	5–35 units/l (37 C)	f
Triglycerides, serum	40–150 mg./dl.	0.4–1.5 g/l	r
		0.45–1.71 mmol/l	
Urate, serum			
Males	2.5–8.0 mg/dl.	0.15–0.48 mmol/l	
Females	1.5–7.0 mg./dl.	0.09–0.42 mmol/l	
Urea			
Blood	21–43 mg./dl.	3.5–7.2 mmol/l	
Plasma or serum	24–49 mg./dl.	4.0–8.2 mmol/l	
Urea nitrogen			
Blood	10–20 mg./dl.	7.1–14.3 mmol/l	k
Plasma or serum	11–23 mg./dl.	7.9–16.4 mmol/l	
Viscosity, serum	1.4–1.8 times water	1.4–1.8 times water	
Vitamin A, serum	20–80 mcg./dl.	0.70–2.8 μmol/l	
Vitamin B_{12}, serum	180–900 picogm./ml.	133–664 pmol/l	

REFERENCE VALUES FOR URINE

(For some procedures the reference values may vary depending upon the method used)

	Conventional Units	S.I. Units	Notes
Acetone and acetoacetate, qualitative	Negative	Negative	
Albumin			
Qualitative	Negative	Negative	
Quantitative	10–100 mg./24 hrs.	10–100 mg/24 h	q
		0.15–1.5 μmol/24 h	
Aldosterone	3–20 mcg./24 hrs.	8.3–55 nmol/24 h	
Alpha amino nitrogen	50–200 mg./24 hrs.	3.6–14.3 mmol/24 h	
Ammonia nitrogen	20–70 mEq./24 hrs.	20–70 mmol/24 h	
Amylase	1–17 units/hr.	1–17 units/h	f
Amylase/creatinine clearance ratio	1–4%	0.01–0.04	
Bilirubin, qualitative	Negative	Negative	
Calcium			
Low Ca diet	Less than 150 mg./24 hrs.	Less than 3.8 mmol/24 h	
Usual diet	Less than 250 mg./24 hrs.	Less than 6.3 mmol/24 h	
Catecholamines			
Epinephrine	Less than 10 mcg./24 hrs.	Less than 55 nmol/24 h	
Norepinephrine	Less than 100 mcg./24 hrs.	Less than 590 nmol/24 h	
Total free catecholamines	4–126 mcg./24 hrs.	24–745 nmol/24 h	s
Total metanephrines	0.1–1.6 mg./24 hrs.	0.5–8.1 μmol/24 h	t
Chloride	110–250 mEq./24 hrs.	110–250 mmol/24 h	
	(Varies with intake)	(Varies with intake)	
Chorionic gonadotropin	0	0	
Copper	0–50 mcg./24 hrs.	0–0.80 μmol/24 h	
Cortisol, free	10–100 mcg./24 hrs.	27.6–276 mmol/24 h	
Creatine			
Males	0–40 mg./24 hrs.	0–0.30 mmol/24 h	
Females	0–100 mg./24 hrs.	0–0.76 mmol/24 h	
	(Higher in children and during pregnancy)	(Higher in children and during pregnancy)	
Creatinine	15–25 mg./kg. body weight/24 hrs.	0.13–0.22 mmol · kg^{-1} body weight/24 h	
Creatinine clearance			
Males	110–150 ml./min.	110–150 ml/min	
Females	105–132 ml./min.	105–132 ml/min	
	(1.73 sq. meter surface area)	(1.73 m^2 surface area)	
Cystine or cysteine, qualitative	Negative	Negative	
Dehydroepiandrosterone	Less than 15% of total 17-ketosteroids	Less than 0.15 of total 17-ketosteroids	a
Males	0.2–2.0 mg./24 hr.	0.7–6.9 μm/24 h	
Females	0.2–1.8 mg./24 hr.	0.7–6.2 μm/24 h	
Delta aminolevulinic acid	1.3–7.0 mg./24 hrs.	10–53 μmol/24 h	
Estrogens			
Males			
Estrone	3–8 μg./24 hrs.	11–30 nmol/24 h	
Estradiol	0–6 μg./24 hrs.	0–22 nmol/24 h	
Estriol	1–11 μg./24 hrs.	3–38 nmol/24 h	
Total	4–25 μg./24 hrs.	14–90 nmol/24 h	u
Females			
Estrone	4–31 μg./24 hrs.	15–115 nmol/24 h	
Estradiol	0–14 μg./24 hrs.	0–51 nmol/24 h	
Estriol	0–72 μg./24 hrs.	0–250 nmol/24 h	
Total	5–100 μg./24 hrs.	18–360 nmol/24 h	u
	(Markedly increased during pregnancy)	(Markedly increased during pregnancy)	

Table continued on following page.

REFERENCE VALUES FOR URINE (*continued*)

	Conventional Units	S.I. Units	Notes
Glucose (as reducing substance)	Less than 250 mg./24 hrs.	Less than 250 mg/24 h	
Hemoglobin and myoglobin, qualitative	Negative	Negative	
Homogentisic acid, qualitative	Negative	Negative	
17-Hydroxycorticosteroids			
Males	3–9 mg./24 hrs.	8.3–25 μmol/24 h	j
Females	2–8 mg./24 hrs.	5.5–22 μmol/24 h	
5-Hydroxyindoleacetic acid			
Qualitative	Negative	Negative	
Quantitative	Less than 9 mg./24 hrs.	Less than 47 μmol/24 h	
17-Ketosteroids			
Males	6–18 mg./24 hrs.	21–62 μmol/24 h	l
Females	4–13 mg./24 hrs.	14–45 μmol/24 h	
	(Varies with age)	(Varies with age)	
Magnesium	6.0–8.5 mEq./24 hrs.	3.0–4.3 mmol/24 h	
Metanephrines (see Catecholamines)			
Osmolality	38–1400 mOsm./kg. water	38–1400 mmol/kg water	n
pH	4.6–8.0, average 6.0	4.6–8.0, average 6.0	p
	(Depends on diet)	(Depends on diet)	
Phenolsulfonphthalein excretion (PSP)	25% or more in 15 min.	0.25 or more in 15 min	a
	40% or more in 30 min.	0.40 or more in 30 min	
	55% or more in 2 hrs.	0.55 or more in 2 h	
	(After injection of 1 ml PSP intravenously)	(After injection of 1 ml PSP intravenously)	
Phenylpyruvic acid, qualitative	Negative	Negative	
Phosphorus	0.9–1.3 gm./24 hrs.	29–42 mmol/24 h	
Porphobilinogen			
Qualitative	Negative	Negative	
Quantitative	0–0.2 mg./dl.	0–0.9 μmol/l	
	Less than 2.0 mg./24 hrs.	Less than 9 μmol/24 h	
Porphyrins			
Coproporphyrin	50–250 mcg./24 hrs.	77–380 nmol/24 h	
Uroporphyrin	10–30 mcg./24 hrs.	12–36 nmol/24 h	
Potassium	25–100 mEq./24 hrs.	25–100 mmol/24 h	
	(Varies with intake)	(Varies with intake)	
Pregnanediol			
Males	0.4–1.4 mg./24 hrs.	1.2–4.4 μmol/24 h	
Females			
Proliferative phase	0.5–1.5 mg./24 hrs.	1.6–4.7 μmol/24 h	
Luteal phase	2.0–7.0 mg./24 hrs.	6.2–22 μmol/24 h	
Postmenopausal phase	0.2–1.0 mg./24 hrs.	0.6–3.1 μmol/24 h	
Pregnanetriol	Less than 2.5 mg./24 hrs. in adults	Less than 7.4 μmol/24 h in adults	
Protein			
Qualitative	Negative	Negative	
Quantitative	10–150 mg./24 hrs.	10–150 mg/24 h	m
Sodium	130–260 mEq./24 hrs.	130–260 mmol/24 h	
	(Varies with intake)	(Varies with intake)	
Specific gravity	1.003–1.030	1.003–1.030	
Titratable acidity	20–40 mEq./24 hrs.	20–40 mmol/24 h	
Urate	200–500 mg./24 hrs.	1.2–3.0 mmol/24 h	
	(With normal diet)	(With normal diet)	
Urobilinogen	Up to 1.0 Ehrlich unit/2 hrs. (1–3 P.M.)	Up to 1.0 Ehrlich unit/2 h (1–3 P.M.)	
	0–4.0 mg./24 hrs.	0–4.0 mg/24 h	
Vanillylmandelic acid (VMA) (4-hydroxy-3-methoxymandelic acid)	1–8 mg./24 hrs.	5–40 μmol/24 h	

REFERENCE VALUES FOR THERAPEUTIC DRUG MONITORING

Drug	Therapeutic Range	Toxic Levels	Proprietary Names
Antibiotics			
Amikacin, serum	15–25 mcg./ml.	Peak: >35 mcg./ml. Trough: >5–8 mcg./ml.	Amikin
Chloramphenicol, serum	10–20 mcg./ml.	>25 mcg./ml.	Chloromycetin
Gentamicin, serum	5–10 mcg./ml.	Peak: >12 mcg./ml. Trough: >2 mcg./ml.	Garamycin
Tobramycin, serum	5–10 mcg./ml.	Peak: >12 mcg./ml. Trough: >2 mcg./ml.	Nebcin
Anticonvulsants			
Carbamazepine, serum	5–12 mcg./ml.	> 12 mcg./ml.	Tegretol
Ethosuximide, serum	40–100 mcg./ml.	> 100 mcg./ml.	Zarontin
Phenobarbital, serum	10–30 mcg./ml.	Vary widely because of developed tolerance	
Phenytoin, serum (diphenylhydantoin)	10–20 mcg./ml.	>20 mcg./ml.	Dilantin
Primidone, serum	5–12 mcg./ml.	>15 mcg./ml.	Mysoline
Valproic acid, serum	50–100 mcg./ml.	> 100 mcg./ml.	Depakene
Analgesics			
Acetaminophen, serum	10–20 mcg./mlds.	>250 mcg./ml.	Tylenol Datril
Salicylate, serum	100–250 mcg./ml.	>300 mcg./ml.	
Bronchodilator			
Theophylline (aminophylline)	10–20 mcg./ml.	>20 mcg./ml.	
Cardiovascular drugs			
Digitoxin, serum	15–25 nanogm./ml. (Specimen obtained 12–24 hrs. after last dose)	>25 nanogm./ml.	Crystodigin
Digoxin, serum	0.8–2 nanogm./ml. (Specimen obtained 12–24 hrs. after last dose)	>2.4 nanogm./ml.	Lanoxin

Table continued on following page.

REFERENCE VALUES FOR THERAPEUTIC DRUG MONITORING (*continued*)

Drug	Therapeutic Range	Toxic Levels	Proprietary Names
Disopyramide, serum	2–5 mcg./ml.	>5 mcg./ml.	Norpace
Lidocaine, serum	1.5–5 mcg./ml.	>5 nanogm./ml.	Anestacon Xylocaine
Procainamide, serum	4–10 mcg./ml. *10–30 mcg./ml. (*Procainamide + N-Acetyl Procainamide)	>16 mcg./ml. *>30 mcg./ml.	Pronestyl
Propranolol, serum	50–100 nanogm./ml.	Variable	Inderal
Quinidine, serum	2–5 mcg./ml.	>10 mcg./ml.	Cardioquin Quinaglute Quinidex Quinora
Psychopharmacologic drugs			
Amitriptyline, serum	*120–150 nanogm./ml. (*Amitriptyline + Nortriptyline)	*>500 nanogm./ml.	Amitril Elavil Endep Etralon Limbitrol Triavil
Desipramine, serum	*150–300 nanogm./ml. (*Desipramine + Imipramine)	*>500 nanogm./ml.	Norpramin Pertofrane
Imipramine, serum	*150–300 nanogm./ml. (*Imipramine + Desipramine)	*>500 nanogm./ml.	Antipress Imavate Janimine Presamine Trofranil
Lithium, serum	0.8–1.2 mEq./liter (Specimen obtained 12 hrs. after last dose)	>2.0 mEq./liter	Lithobid Lithotabs
Nortriptyline, serum	50–150 nanogm./ml.	>500 nanogm./ml.	Aventyl Pamelor

REFERENCE VALUES IN TOXICOLOGY

	Conventional Units	S.I. Units	Notes
Arsenic, blood	3.5–7.2 mcg./dl.	0.47–0.96 μmol/l	
Arsenic, urine	Less than 100 mcg./24 hrs.	Less than 1.3 μmol/24 h	
Bromides, serum	0	0	
	Toxic levels: Above 17 mmol/l	Toxic levels: Above 17 mmol/l	
Carbon monoxide, blood	Up to 5% saturation	Up to 0.05 saturation	
	Symptoms occur with 20% saturation	Symptoms occur with 0.20 saturation	
Ethanol, blood	Less than 0.005%	Less than 1 mmol/l	
Marked intoxication	0.3–0.4%	65–87 mmol/l	
Alcoholic stupor	0.4–0.5% mcg./dl.	87–109 mmol/l	
Coma	Above 0.5%	Above 109 mmol/l	
Lead, blood	0–40 mcg./dl.	0–2 μmol/l	
Lead, urine	Less than 100 mcg./24 hrs.	Less than 0.48 μmol/24 h	
Mercury, urine	Less than 10 mcg./24 hrs.	Less than 50 nmol/24 h	

REFERENCE VALUES FOR CEREBROSPINAL FLUID

	Conventional Units	S.I. Units	Notes
Cells	Fewer than 5/cu. mm.; all mononuclear	Fewer than 5/μl; all mononuclear	
Chloride	120–130 mEq./liter	120–130 mmol/l	
	(20 mEq./liter higher than serum)	(20 mmol/l higher than serum)	
Electrophoresis	Predominantly albumin	Predominantly albumin	
Glucose	50–75 mg./dl.	2.8–4.2 mmol/l	
	(20 mg./dl. less than serum)	(1.1 mmol/l less than serum)	
IgG			
Children under 14	Less than 8% of total protein	Less than 0.08 of total protein	a,m
Adults	Less than 14% of total protein	Less than 0.14 of total protein	
Pressure	70–180 mm. water	70–180 mm water	g
Protein, total	15–45 mg./dl.	0.150–0.450 g/l	m
	(Higher, up to 70 mg./dl., in elderly adults and children)	(Higher, up to 0.70 g/l, in elderly adults and children)	

REFERENCE VALUES FOR GASTRIC ANALYSIS

	Conventional Units	S.I. Units	Notes
Basal gastric secretion (1 hour)			
Concentration	(Mean ± 1 S.D.)	(Mean ± 1 S.D.)	
Males	25.8 ± 1.8 mEq./liter	25.8 ± 1.8 mmol/l	
Females	20.3 ± 3.0 mEq./liter	20.3 ± 3.0 mmol/l	
Output	(Mean ± 1 S.D.)	(Mean ± 1 S.D.)	
Males	2.57 ± 0.16 mEq./hr.	2.57 ± 0.16 mmol/h	
Females	1.61 ± 0.18 mEq./hr.	1.61 ± 0.18 mmol/h	
After histamine stimulation			
Normal	Mean output 11.8 mEq./hr.	Mean output 11.8 mmol/h	
Duodenal ulcer	Mean output 15.2 mEq./hr.	Mean output 15.2 mmol/h	
After maximal histamine stimulation			
Normal	Mean output 22.6 mEq./hr.	Mean output 22.6 mmol/h	
Duodenal ulcer	Mean output 44.6 mEq./hr.	Mean output 44.6 mmol/h	
Diagnex blue (Squibb): Anacidity	0–0.3 mg. in 2 hrs.	0–0.03 mg in 2 h	
Doubtful	0.3–0.6 mg. in 2 hrs.	0.3–0.6 mg in 2 h	
Normal	Greater than 0.6 mg. in 2 hrs.	Greater than 0.6 mg in 2 h	
Volume, fasting stomach content	50–100 ml.	0.05–0.11	
Emptying time	3–6 hrs.	3–6 h	
Color	Opalescent or colorless	Opalescent or colorless	
Specific gravity	1.006–1.009	1.006–1.009	
pH (adults)	0.9–1.5	0.9–1.5	p

GASTROINTESTINAL ABSORPTION TESTS

	Conventional Units	S.I. Units	Notes
d/Xylose absorption test	After an 8 hour fast, 10 ml./kg. body weight of a 0.05 solution of d-xylose is given by mouth. Nothing further by mouth is given until the test has been completed. All urine voided during the following 5 hours is pooled, and blood samples are taken at 0, 60, and 120 minutes. Normally 0.26 (range 0.16–0.33) of ingested xylose is excreted within 5 hours, and the serum xylose reaches a level between 25 and 40 mg./100 ml. after 1 hour and is maintained at this level for another 60 minutes.	No change	
Vitamin A absorption	A fasting blood specimen is obtained and 200,000 units of vitamin A in oil is given by mouth. Serum vitamin A level should rise to twice fasting level in 3 to 5 hours.	No change	

REFERENCE VALUES FOR FECES

	Conventional Units	S.I. Units	Notes
Bulk	100–200 grams/24 hrs.	100–200 g/24 h	
Dry matter	23–32 grams/24 hrs.	23–32 g/24 h	
Fat, total	Less than 6.0 grams/24 hrs.	Less than 6.0 g/24 h	
Nitrogen, total	Less than 2.0 grams/24 hrs.	Less than 2.0 g/24 h	
Urobilinogen	40–280 mg./24 hrs.	40–280 mg/24 h	
Water	Approximately 65%	Approximately 0.65	a

REFERENCE VALUES FOR IMMUNOLOGIC PROCEDURES

	Conventional Units
Lymphocyte Subsets	
T cells	60–85%
B cells	1–20%
Helper cells	35–60%
Suppressor cells	15–30%
H/S ratio	1.5–2.5
Complement	
C3	85–175 mg./dl.
C4	15–45 mg./dl.
CH_{50}	25–55 H_{50} units/ml.
Tumor Markers	
Carcinoembryonic Antigen (CEA)	
(Roche)	Less than 5 nanog./ml.
(Abbott)	Less than 4.1 nanog./ml.
Alpha-fetoprotein (AFP)	Less than 10–30 nanog./ml. (depends on method)

REFERENCE VALUES FOR SEMEN ANALYSIS

	Conventional Units	S.I. Units	Notes
Volume	2–5 ml.; usually 3–4 ml.	2–5 ml; usually 3–4 ml	
Liquefaction	Complete in 15 min.	Complete in 15 min	
pH	7.2–8.0; average 7.8	7.2–8.0; average 7.8	p
Leukocytes	Occasional or absent	Occasional or absent	
Count	60–150 million/ml. Below 60 million/ml. is abnormal	60–150 million/ml Below 60 million/ml is abnormal	
Motility	80% or more motile	0.80 or more motile	a
Morphology	80–90% normal forms	0.80–0.90 normal forms	a

ORAL GLUCOSE TOLERANCE TEST

The oral glucose tolerance test (OGTT) may be unnecessary if the fasting plasma glucose concentration is elevated (venous plasma ≥140 mg/dl or 7.8 mmol/l) on two occasions. The OGTT should be carried out only on patients who are ambulatory and otherwise healthy and who are known not to be taking agents that elevate the plasma glucose (see reference 10). The test should be conducted in the morning after at least 3 days of unrestricted diet (≥150 grams of carbohydrate) and physical activity. The subject should have fasted for at least 10 hours but no more than 16 hours. Water is permitted during the test period; however, the subject should remain seated and should not smoke throughout the test.

The dose of glucose administered should be 75 grams (1.75 grams per kg of ideal body weight, up to a maximum of 75 grams for children). Commercial preparations containing a suitable carbohydrate load are acceptable. If criteria for gestational diabetes are used, a dose of 100 grams of glucose is required.

A fasting blood sample should be collected, after which the glucose dose is taken within 5 minutes. Blood samples should be collected at 30 minute intervals for 2 hours (for gestational diabetes fasting 1, 2 and 3 hours). The following diagnostic criteria have been recommended by the National Diabetes Data Group:

Normal OGTT in Nonpregnant Adults	Fasting venous plasma glucose <115 mg/dl (6.4 mmol/l) ½ h, 1 h, or 1½ h OGTT venous plasma glucose <200 mg/dl (11.1 mmol/l) 2 h OGTT venous plasma glucose <140 mg/dl (7.8 mmol/l)
Diabetes Mellitus in Nonpregnant Adults	Both the 2 hour sample *and* some other sample taken between administration of the 75 gram glucose dose and 2 hours later must show a venous plasma glucose ≥200 mg/dl (11.1 mmol/l)
Impaired Glucose Tolerance in Nonpregnant Adults	Three criteria must be met: Fasting venous plasma glucose <140 mg/dl (7.8 mmol/l) ½ h, 1 h, or 1½ h OGTT value ≥200 mg/dl (11.1 mmol/l) 2 h OGTT venous plasma glucose between 140 and 200 mg/dl (7.8 and 11.1 mmol/l)
Gestational Diabetes	Two or more of the following values after a 100 gram oral glucose challenge must be met or exceeded: (values are for venous plasma glucose)

Fasting	105 mg/dl	5.8 mmol/l
1 h	190 mg/dl	10.6 mmol/l
2 h	165 mg/dl	9.2 mmol/l
3 h	145 mg/dl	8.1 mmol/l

NOTES

a. Percentage is expressed as a decimal fraction.
b. Percentage may be expressed as a decimal fraction; however, when the result expressed is itself a variable fraction of another variable, the absolute value is more meaningful. There is no reason, other than custom, for expressing reticulocyte counts and differential leukocyte counts in percentages or decimal fractions rather than in absolute numbers.
c. Molecular weight of fibrinogen = 341,000 daltons.
d. Molecular weight of hemoglobin = 64,500 daltons. Because of disagreement as to whether the monomer or tetramer of hemoglobin should be used in the conversion, it has been recommended that the conventional grams per deciliter be retained. The tetramer is used in the table; values given should be multiplied by 4 to obtain concentration of the monomer.
e. Molecular weight of methemoglobin = 64,500 daltons. See note d above.
f. Enzyme units have not been changed in these tables because the proposed enzyme unit, the katal, has not been universally adopted (1 International Unit = 16.7 nkat).
g. It has been proposjed that pressure be expressed in the Pascal (1 mm Hg = 0.133 kPa); however, this convention has not been universally accepted.
h. Molecular weight of ceruloplasmin = 151,000.
i. "Fatty acids" includes a mixture of different aliphatic acids of varying molecular weight. A mean molecular weight of 284 has been assumed in calculating the conversion factor.
j. Based upon molecular weight of cortisol 362.47.
k. The practice of expressing concentration of an organic molecule in terms of one of its constituent elements originated when measurements included a heterogeneous class of compounds (nonprotein nitrogenous compounds, iodine-containing compounds bound to serum proteins). It was carried over to expressing measurements of specific substances (urea, thyroxine), but the practice should be discarded. For iodine and nitrogen 1 mole is taken as the monoatomic form, although they occur as diatomic molecules.
l. Based upon molecular weight of dehydroepiandrosterone 288.41.
m. Weight per volume is retained as the unit because of the heterogeneous nature of the material measured.
n. The proposal that osmolality be reported as freezing point depression using the millikelvin as the unit has not been received with universal enthusiasm. The milliosmole is not an S.I. unit, and the unit used here is the millimole.
o. Volumes per cent might be converted to a decimal fraction; however, this would not permit direct correlation with hemoglobin content, which is possible when oxygen content and capacity are expressed in molar quantities. One millimole of hemoglobin combines with 4 millimoles of oxygen.
p. Hydrogen ion concentration in S.I. units would be expressed in nanomoles per liter; however, this change has not received general approval. Conversion can be calculated as antilog (−pH).
q. Albumin is expressed in grams per liter to be consistent with units used for other proteins. Concentration of albumin may be expressed in mmol/l also, an expression that permits assessment of binding capacity of albumin for substances such as bilirubin. Molecular weight of albumin is 65,000.
r. Most techniques for quantitating triglycerides measure the glycerol moiety, and the total mass is calculated using an average molecular weight. The factor given assumes a mean molecular weight of 875 for triglycerides.
s. Calculated as norepinephrine, molecular weight 169.18.
t. Calculated as metanephrine, molecular weight 197.23.
u. Conversion factor calculated from molecular weights of estrone, estradiol, and estriol in proportions of 2:1:2.

REFERENCES

1. AMA Drug Evaluations, 4th ed. Chicago, American Medical Association, 1980.
2. Baron, D. N., Broughton, P. M. G., Cohen, M., Lansley, T. S., Lewis, S. M., and Shinton, N. K.: J. Clin. Path. 27:590, 1974.
3. Dybkaer, R.: Am. J. Clin. Path. *52*:637, 1969.
4. Gilman, A. G., Goodman, L. S., and Gilman, A.: Pharmacologic Basis of Therapeutics, 6th ed. New York, Macmillan, 1980.
5. Henry, J. B.: Clinical Diagnosis and Management by Laboratory Methods, 17th ed. Philadelphia, W. B. Saunders Company, 1984.
6. Henry, R. J., Cannon, D. C., and Winkleman, J. W.: Clinical Chemistry—Principles and Techniques, 2nd ed. New York, Harper & Row, 1974.
7. International Committee for Standardization in Hematology, International Federation of Clinical Chemistry and World Association of Pathology Societies: Clin. Chem. *19*:135, 1973.
8. Lehmann, H. P.: Am. J. Clin. Path. *65*:2, 1976.
9. Miale, J. B.: Laboratory Medicine—Hematology, 6th ed. St. Louis, C. V. Mosby, 1982.
10. National Diabetes Data Group: Diabetes *28*:1039, 1979.
11. Page, C. H., and Vigourex, P.: The International System of Units (S.I.). U.S. Department of Commerce, National Bureau of Standards, Special Publication 330, 1974.
12. Physicians' Desk Reference. 38th ed. Oradell, N.J., Medical Economics Company, 1984.
13. Scully, R. E., McNeely, B. U., and Galdabini, J. J.: N. Engl. J. Med. *302*:37, 1980.
14. Tietz, N. W.: Clinical Guide to Laboratory Tests. Philadelphia, W. B. Saunders Company, 1983.
15. Tietz, N. W.: Reference ranges and laboratory values of clinical importance. *In* Wyngaarden, J. B., and Smith, L. H. Jr.: Cecil Textbook of Medicine, 16th ed. Philadelphia, W. B. Saunders Company, 1982.
16. Williams, W. J., Beutler, E., Erslev, A. J., and Lichtman, M. A., Hematology, 3rd ed. New York, McGraw-Hill Book Company, 1983.
17. Young, D. S.: N. Engl. J. Med. *292*:795, 1975.

Some of the values have been established by the Clinical Pathology Laboratories, Emory University Hospital, Atlanta, Georgia, and have not been published elsewhere.

Index

Note: Page numbers in *italics* indicate illustrations; page numbers followed by (t) refer to tables. The expression "vs." has been used to denote "differential diagnosis." For example, "Tetanus, vs. rabies" would be the equivalent of "Tetanus, differential diagnosis from rabies."